Brain's Diseases of the Nervous System

ELEVENTH EDITION

Edited by

Michael Donaghy

Reader in Clinical Neurology, University of Oxford;
Honorary Consultant Neurologist, the Radcliffe Infirmary;
Honorary Civilian Consultant in Neurology to the Army.

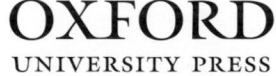

OXFORD
UNIVERSITY PRESS

OXFORD

UNIVERSITY PRESS

Great Clarendon Street, Oxford OX2 6DP

Oxford University Press is a department of the University of Oxford.
It furthers the University's objective of excellence in research, scholarship,
and education by publishing worldwide in

Oxford New York

Auckland Bangkok Buenos Aires Cape Town Chennai Dar es Salaam
Delhi Hong Kong Istanbul Karachi Kolkata Kuala Lumpur Madrid
Melbourne Mexico City Mumbai Nairobi São Paulo Shanghai Taipei
Tokyo Toronto

Published in the United States
by Oxford University Press Inc., New York

First published 1933
Sixth edition published 1962
Seventh edition published 1969
Eighth edition published 1977
Ninth edition published 1985
Tenth edition published 1993
Eleventh edition published 2001

A catalogue record for this title is available from the British Library

Library of Congress Cataloguing in Publication Data
(Data available)

ISBN 0 19 262618 3

10 9 8 7 6 5 4 3

Typeset by EXPO Holdings, Malaysia
Printed in Italy
on acid-free paper by Legoprint S.p.A.

Preface to the eleventh edition

Dr Russell Brain originally published Brain's Diseases of the Nervous System in 1933 having perceived the need to digest those 20 years of advance which marked the start of neurology as we know it now. Professor John Walton joined Lord Brain in revising the 7th edition, a task which coincided with the founding author's death in 1966. Walton carried Brain's Diseases forward as sole author for its 8th and 9th editions, an increasingly immense and daunting task. In 1989, after a dinner at Green College, Sir John asked if I would consider joining him as the co-author for the 10th edition of Brain's Diseases. Armed with post-prandial courage, I declined this tempting invitation. It seemed that clinical neurology had become simply too vast in scope, and too sub-specialized, for two authors alone to provide the depth and authority required of a large reference book. So the 10th edition of Brain's Diseases, published in 1993, was the product of a team of 13 authors, revising 24 chapters under the editorship of Lord Walton. Roughly half of the chapters from the previous edition were substantially or completely reorganized and rewritten. Lord Walton decided to step down after the 10th Edition. Neurologists throughout the world owe a debt of gratitude to him for guiding Brain's Diseases into the modern era.

The chapter headings of this, the 11th Edition of Brain's Diseases, have been completely reorganized. Now there are 35 chapters contained within seven sections, and contributed by 14 authors. The text has been completely rewritten with a great increase in the number of illustrations and tables. Most of the chapters represent monographs addressing the clinical problem areas so readily identifiable in neurological practice, such as stroke, epilepsy, polyneuropathy, meningitis, headache, brain tumour, spinal cord disorder, or long-term disability. Such clinical topics will be easily recognized by every doctor possessing a basic knowledge of clinical neurology. Thus readers can consult a single chapter knowing that the entirety of the relevant clinical problem area will be covered by only one author. This avoids the unevenness, lack of perspective, and omissions so often evident when vast and diverse authorships contribute to a medical reference text.

We hope Brain's Diseases will serve two functions. First to continue to be a textbook, thereby providing a programme of advanced instruction in the subject. To this quest, each chapter includes sections outlining a clinical approach to the topic in question. Secondly, to provide a reference book of the depth and completeness required by the busy specialist of today. Some of the chapters address matters of background importance to contemporary clinical practice in neurology. The main neurological investigations are discussed from the perspective of neurologists who use and interpret these tests. Knowledge of the biology of degeneration and regeneration is crucial for understanding the long term consequences of neurological diseases, and their prospects for repair and recovery. Our introductory chapter describes a practical approach to evaluating clinical problems, the differential diagnosis of ubiquitous symptoms such as muscular weakness, the importance of psychological factors in generating neurological complaints, and the historical development of clinical neurology.

The present authors are cognisant of the disparate forces which have shaped their practice and inspired their understanding of clinical neurology. All of us are deeply grateful for the influence of our mentors, junior colleagues, students, research collaborators, and patients for provoking and moulding our thinking. Our secretaries have played an immense role in bringing this book to fruition; in particular Mrs Joanna Wilkinson has been responsible for rendering our piecemeal contributions into a form digestible by Oxford University Press. Warm thanks must go to Dr Robert Surtees of the Institute of Child Health for his extensive work in preparing Tables 4.1 and 4.2 summarizing paediatric neurometabolic disorders. Many of our colleagues have been generous enough to advise upon, or comment on chapters. The following deserve especial thanks for their expert advice on individual topics: Professor Peter Goadsby, Professor Neva Haites, Dr Robin Kennett, Mr Michael Powell and Dr Kevin Talbot. Also we are immensely grateful to Dr Philip Anslow, Professor Dian Donnai, Dr Darren Forward, Dr Waney Squier, Dr John Stevens, Mr Nick White, and the technical graphics staff of Oxford University Press for their help with the book's many illustrations. Effective teamwork is crucial in producing a book demanding such huge contributions from each individual author. I must add warm and personal thanks to each of my fellow authors for underpinning their skill and scholarship with forbearance and industry, and to the editorial and production staff of Oxford University Press for their unstinting work in bringing this volume to fruition.

Michael Donaghy
Oxford
April 2001

Preface to the first edition

The last twenty years have witnessed a remarkable development in neurology. Investigation of the effects of war injuries of the spinal cord has greatly increased our knowledge of reflex action in man. The appearance of encephalitis lethargica and the multiplication of forms of acute disseminated encephalitis have added a new field to clinical neurology and brought it into relationship with the new branch of bacteriology which studies the filterable viruses. The discovery of important metabolic centres in the hypothalamus has enhanced the importance of neurology to general medicine. Advances in the technique of neurological surgery have aroused fresh interest in the symptoms and in the pathology of intracranial tumours. Other developments, scarcely less important, have occurred.

Much of this new knowledge is physiological, and in one respect I have departed from the traditional arrangement of a textbook of nervous diseases. Neurology is more dependent than many other branches of medicine upon anatomy and physiology. These subjects, the essential basis of neurological diagnosis, are usually dismissed in a few introductory pages, with the result that much clinical neurology is apt to be both unintelligible and uninteresting to the student. In the first part of this book, as an introduction to the subject, I have discussed—at greater length than usual—the application of anatomy and physiology to the interpretation of the physical signs of nervous disease. Elsewhere will be found sections dealing with anatomy and physiology as introductions to clinical sections. In planning the clinical sections I have used what seemed the most practical, if not always the most logical, arrangement, for there is no entirely satisfactory way of arranging subjects, many of which might be placed in more than one group.

Limitations of space restrict the number of references which it is possible to quote. I have, therefore, chosen only those of special interest and those which form the best introduction to a subject, or are themselves useful sources of references. To the many other writers upon whose work I have freely drawn I express my indebtedness. I am indebted also to a number of my colleagues for the loan of illustrations.

Finally, I welcome this opportunity of expressing my gratitude to my colleagues at the London Hospital for their teaching, encouragement, and help, especially to Dr Charles Miller, Professor Arthur Ellis, and Dr George Riddoch, under whom I had the privilege of working on the Medical Unit, and to Mr Hugh Cairns, Dr Dorothy Russell, and Dr S. Phillips Bedson.

London
June 1933

W. Russell Brain

Contents

Contributors

Milne Anderson, FRCP(Ed), FRCP
Consultant Neurologist, Queen Elizabeth
Neuroscience Centre, Edgbaston,
Birmingham, B15 2TH, UK

David Chadwick, DM, FRCP
Professor of Neurology in the University of Liverpool,
Walton Centre for Neurology and Neurosurgery,
Lower Lane, Liverpool L9 7LJ,
UK

Alastair Compston, PhD, FRCP
Professor of Neurology in the University of
Cambridge, Department of Neurology,
Addenbrooke's Hospital, Hills Road, Cambridge CB2
2QQ, UK

Michael Donaghy, DPhil, FRCP
Reader in Clinical Neurology in the University of
Oxford, Department of Clinical Neurology,
Radcliffe Infirmary, Woodstock Road, Oxford
OX2 6HE, UK

Nicholas Fletcher, MD, FRCP
Consultant Neurologist, Walton Centre for Neurology
and Neurosurgery, Lower Lane, Liverpool L9 7LJ,
UK

Robert Grant, MD, FRCP(Glasg)
Consultant Neurologist, Department of Clinical
Neurosciences, Western General Hospital, Crewe
Road, Edinburgh EH4 2XU, UK

David Hilton-Jones, MD, FRCP, FRCP(Ed)
Consultant Neurologist, Department of
Clinical Neurology, Radcliffe Infirmary,
Woodstock Road, Oxford OX2 6HE,
UK

Christopher Kennard, PhD, FRCP
Professor of Clinical Neurology at Imperial College of
Science, Technology, and Medicine, Division of
Neuroscience and Psychological Medicine, Charing
Cross Hospital, Fulham Palace Road, London W6
8RF, UK

David Mendelow, PhD, FRCS(Ed)
Professor of Neurosurgery in the University of
Newcastle upon Tyne, Department of Neurosurgery,
Newcastle General Hospital, Westgate Road,
Newcastle upon Tyne NE4 6BE, UK

David Miller, MD, FRCP
Professor of Clinical Neurology at University College
London, Institute of Neurology, National Hospital for
Neurology and Neurosurgery, Queen Square, London
WC1N 3BG, UK

Brian Neville, FRCP
Professor of Paediatric Neurology at University
College London, Neuroscience Unit, Institute of Child
Health, 30 Guilford Street, London WC1N 1EH, UK

Martin Rossor, MD, FRCP
Professor of Clinical Neurology at University College
London, Dementia Research Group, National
Hospital for Neurology and Neurosurgery, Queen
Square, London WC1N 3BG, UK

Derick Wade, MD, FRCP
Professor of Neurological Disability in the University
of Oxford, Rivermead Rehabilitation Centre,
Abingdon Road, Oxford OX1 4XD, UK

Charles Warlow, MD, FRCP
Professor of Medical Neurology in the University of
Edinburgh, Department of Clinical Neurosciences,
Western General Hospital, Crewe Road, Edinburgh
EH4 2XU, UK

Plates

Abbreviations

ACA	anterior cerebral artery	AZOOR	acute zonule occult outer retinopathy
ACE	angiotensin-converting enzyme	BAEP	brainstem auditory evoked potential
ACh	acetylcholine	BBB	blood-brain barrier
AChR	acetylcholine receptor	BCNU	carmustine
ACoA	anterior communicating artery	BDNF	brain-derived nerve growth factor
ACTH	adrenocorticotrophic hormone	BIH	benign intracranial hypertension
ADC	apparent diffusion coefficient OR	BMD	Becker muscular dystrophy
	activated diffusion coefficient	BOAA	β-N-oxalylamino-L-alanine
ADH	antidiuretic hormone	BPPV	benign paroxysmal positional vertigo
ADHD	attention deficit/hyperactivity disorder	BrdU	bromodeoxyuridine
ADL	activities of daily living	CAA	cerebral amyloid angiopathy
A & E	accident and emergency	CADASIL	cerebral autosomal dominant
AED	antiepileptic drug		arteriopathy with subcortical infarcts
AEP	auditory evoked potential		and leucoencephalopathy
AF	atrial fibrillation	CAR	cancer-associated retinopathy
AFP	α-fetoprotein	CAT	computer-assisted tomography
AIDP	acute idiopathic demyelinating	CBF	cerebral blood flow
	polyradiculoneuropathy	CBV	cerebral blood volume
AIDS	acquired immune deficiency syndrome	CCA	common carotid artery
AION	anterior ischaemic optic neuropathy	CCD	central-core disease
ALS	amyotrophic lateral sclerosis	CCF	carotid-cavernous fistula
AMAN	acute motor axonal neuropathy	CCM	chemical cleavage of mismatched DNA
AMP	adenosine monophosphate	CCNU	lomustine
AMPA	α-amino-3-hydroxy-	CD	cluster-defined
	5-methylisoxazo1e-4-propionate	cDNA	complementary DNA
ANCA	antineutrophil cytoplasmic antibodies	CGRP	calcitonin-gene related peptide
4-AP	4-aminopyridine	Cho	choline-containing compounds
APP	amyloid precursor protein	CHOP	cyclophosphamide, doxorubicin,
APS	antiphospholipid syndrome		vincristine, prednisolone
A-R	Argyll Robertson (pupils)	CIDP	chronic inflammatory demyelinating
ARMS	amplification-resistant mutation		polyneuropathy
	system	CIE	polysaccharide countercurrent
ASO	allele-specific oligonucleotide		electrophoresis
AST	aspartate transaminase	CJD	Creutzfeldt-Jakob disease
ATLS	advanced trauma life support	CK	creatine kinase
AV	arteriovenous	CKBB	creatine kinase BB isoenzyme
AVM	arteriovenous malformation	CMAP	compound muscle action potential

CMD	congenital muscular dystrophy
$CMRo_2$	cerebral metabolic rate of oxygen
CMR_{glu}	cerebral metabolic rate of glucose
CMT	Charcot-Marie-Tooth disease
CN	cranial nerve
CNPase	$2',3'$-cyclic nucleotide $3'$-phosphohydrolase
CNS	central nervous system
CNTF	ciliary neurotrophic factor
COMA	congenital ocular motor apraxia
CPAP	continuous positive airway pressure
CPEO	chronic progressive external ophthalmoplegia
CPP	cerebral perfusion pressure
CPSE	complex partial status epilepticus
Cr	creatine/phosphocreatine
CRAO	central retinal artery occlusion
CRP	C-reactive protein
CRPS	complex regional pain syndrome
CSF	cerebrospinal fluid
CSI	craniospinal irradiation
CT	computed tomography
CTA	CT angiography
CVS	continuing vegetative state
2,4-D	2,4-dichlorophenoxyacetic acid
DAI	diffuse axonal injury
DHPR	dihydropyridine receptor
DM	dermatomyositis
DMD	Duchenne muscular dystrophy
DGGE	denaturing gradient gel electrophoresis
DIDMOAD	diabetes insipidus, diabetes mellitus, optic atrophy, and deafness
DLPFC	dorsolateral prefrontal cortex
DMD	Duchenne muscular dystrophy
DML	distal motor latencies
DNET	dysembryoplastic neuroepithelial tumours
DRPLA	dentatorubropallidoluysian atrophy
DTPA	diethylenetriaminepentaacetic acid
DVT	deep-vein thrombosis
DWI	diffusion-weighted imaging
EBV	Epstein-Barr virus
ECA	external carotid artery
ECG	electrocardiogram
ECoG	electrocochleography
EDSS	expanded disability status scale
EEG	electroencephalogram
EGF	epidermal growth factor
EGFR	epidermal growth factor receptor
EMA	eyelid myoclonia with absences
EMG	electromyogram
ERG	electroretinogram
ESR	erythrocyte sedimentation rate
FASE	fast asymmetric spin-echo
FEF	frontal eye field
FGF	fibroblast growth factor
FISH	fluorescent *in situ* hybridization
FLAIR	fluid-attenuated inversion recovery

FMD	fibromuscular dysplasia
fMRI	functional MRI
FSH	facioscapulohumeral
FTT	Fibrinolytic Therapy Trialists
FV	flow velocity
GABA	γ-aminobutyric acid
GalC	galactocerebroside
GAD	glutamic acid decarboxylase
GAP	GTPase activating protein
GBM	glioblastoma multiforme
GBS	Guillain-Barré syndrome
GCA	giant cell arteritis
GCSE	generalized convulsive status epilepticus
G-CSF	granulocyte-colony stimulating factor
GDNF	glial cell-line-derived nerve growth factor
GEFS+	generalized epilepsy with febrile seizures plus
GFAP	glial fibrillary acidic protein
GGF	glial growth factor
GMP	guanosine monophosphate
β-hCG	β-human chorionic gonadotrophin
HIV	human immunodeficiency virus
HMSN	hereditary motor and sensory neuropathy
HNPP	hereditary neuropathy with liability to pressure palsies
HSAN	hereditary sensory and autonomic neuropathies
5-HT	5-hydroxytryptamine
HTLV-I	human T-cell leukaemia virus-I
IBM	inclusion-body myositis
ICA	internal carotid artery
ICAM	intercellular adhesion molecule
ICH	intracerebral haematoma or haemorrhage
ICP	intracranial pressure
IFN	interferon
IGF	insulin-like growth factor
IHS	International Headache Society
IL	interleukin
INC	interstitial nucleus of Cajal
INO	internuclear ophthalmoplegia
i.v.	intravenous
IvIg	intravenous immunoglobulin
IVM	intracranial vascular malformations
J_vo_2	jugular vein oxygen
KSS	Kearns-Sayre syndrome
LGMD	limb-girdle muscular dystrophy
LHON	Leber's hereditary optic neuropathy
LIF	leukaemia inhibitory factor
LP	lumbar puncture
MAG	myelin-associated glycoprotein
MBP	myelin basic protein
MCA	middle cerebral artery
MCAD	medium-chain acyl-CoA dehydrogenase
MCI	mild cognitive impairment
MEB	muscle–eye–brain disease
MEK	methylethylketone
MELAS	mitochondrial encephalomyopathy, lactic

	acidosis and stroke-like episodes
MERRF	myoclonic epilepsy with ragged red fibres
MEUDS	multiple evanescent white dot syndrome
MH	malignant hyperthermia
MHC	major histocompatibility complex
mI	myoinositol
MLF	medial longitudinal fasciculus
MLP	mitral leaflet prolapse
MNBK	methyl n-butyl ketone
MOG	myelin oligodendrocyte glycoprotein
MPTP	1-methyl-4-phenyl-1,2,3,6-tetrahydropyridine
MRA	magnetic resonance angiography
MRI	magnetic resonance imaging
mRNA	messenger RNA
MRS	magnetic resonance spectroscopy
MRV	magnetic resonance venography
MS	multiple sclerosis
MSRV	multiple sclerosis-associated retrovirus
MST	medial superior temporal (visual area)
MT	middle temporal (visual area)
mtDNA	mitochondrial DNA
MTLE	mesial temporal-lobe epilepsy
MUAP	motor unit action potential
NAA	N-acetyl aspartate
NARP	neurogenic atrophy, ataxia and retinitis pigmentosa
NART	National Adult Reading Test
NEA	non-epileptic attack
NF	neurofibromatosis
NGF	nerve growth factor
NGPSE	National General Practice Survey of Epilepsy
NIRS	near infrared spectroscopy
NMDA	N-methyl-D-aspartate
NMJ	neuromuscular junction
NMR	nuclear magnetic resonance
NREM	non-rapid eye movement (sleep)
NSE	neuronal specific enolase
NT	neurotrophin
OCD	obsessive–compulsive disorder
OEF	oxygen extraction fraction
OKN	optokinetic nystagmus
ON	optic neuritis
ONTT	optic neuritis treatment trial
OSA	obstructive sleep apnoea
OTR	ocular tilt reaction
PAN	periodic alternating nystagmus
PCR	polymerase chain reaction
PCV	packed cell volume
PDGF	platelet-derived growth factor
PDS	paroxysmal depolarization shift
PEF	posterior eye field
PET	positron emission tomography
PGFE	pulsed-field gel electrophoresis
PICH	primary intracerebral haemorrhage
PLEDs	periodic lateralized epileptiform discharges
PLP	proteolipid protein
PM	polymyositis
PMA	perioral myoclonia with absence
PMP	peripheral myelin protein
PMR	polymyalgia rheumatica
PNET	primitive neuro-ectodermal tumour
PoCA	posterior communicating artery
POEMS	peripheral neuropathy, organomegaly, endocrine disorders, M protein, and skin disease
PROMM	proximal myotonic myopathy
PPRF	paramedial pontine reticular formation
PSP	progressive supranuclear palsy
PVS	persistent vegetative state
RAPD	relative afferent pupillary defect
RCT	randomized controlled trial
REM	rapid eye movement (sleep)
RFLP	restriction fragment length polymorphism
riMLF	rostral interstitial nucleus of the medial longitudinal fasciculus
ROM	rifampicin, ofloxacin, and minocycline
RT	radiotherapy
SABP	systemic arterial blood pressure
SAH	subarachnoid haemorrhage
SC	superior colliculus
SCA	spinocerebellar ataxia
SCARMD	severe childhood autosomal recessive muscular dystrophy
SEF	supplementary eye field
SEP	somatosensory evoked potentials
SLE	systemic lupus erythematosus
SMA	spinal muscular atrophy OR supplementary motor area
SMON	subacute myelo-optic neuropathy
SNAP	sensory nerve action potential
SNpr	substantia nigra, pars reticular
snRNA	small nuclear RNA
SPECT	single-photon emission computed tomography
SPSE	simple partial status epilepticus
SR	sarcoplasmic reticulum
SRS	stereotactic radiosurgery
SRT	stereotactic radiotherapy
SSCP	single-stranded conformational polymorphism
SSPE	subacute sclerosing panencephalitis
SSRI	selective serotonin re-uptake inhibitor
SUDEP	sudden unexpected death in people with epilepsy
SUNCT	short-lasting unilateral neuralgiform headache attacks with conjunctival injection and tearing syndrome
SWJ	square wave jerks
T_3	tri-iodothyronine
T_4	thyroxine
TACS	total anterior circulation syndrome
TAP	peptide transporter gene products
TCD	transcranial Doppler

TCDB	Traumatic Coma Data Bank	UPSIT	University of Pennsylvania Smell Identification Test
TCR	T-cell receptor		
TDM	therapeutic drug monitoring	VDRL	Venereal Disease Research Laboratory
TDS	transcranial Doppler sonography	VEGF	vascular endothelial growth factor
TE	echo time	VEP	visual evoked potentials
TEA	tetraethylammonium 4-aminopyridine (4-AP)	VER	visual evoked response
TENS	transcutaneous electrical nerve stimulation	VGCC	voltage-gated calcium channels
TGA	transient global amnesia	VGKC	voltage-gated potassium channels
TGF	transforming growth factor	VGNC	voltage-gated sodium channels
TIA	transient ischaemic attack	VIP	vasoactive intestinal polypeptide
TNF	tumour necrosis factor	VNTR	variable number of tandem repeats
tPA	tissue plasminogen activator	VOR	vestibulo-ocular system
TR	repetition time	VP	ventriculo-peritoneal
TSH	thyroid-stimulating hormone	WAIS	Wechsler Adult Intelligence Scale
TTP	thrombolic thrombocytopenic purpura	WEBINO	wall-eyed bilateral internuclear ophthalmoplegia

Introduction

CHAPTER 1

Clinical diagnosis

Michael Donaghy, Alastair Compston, Martin Rossor, and Charles Warlow

1.1 A short history of the approach to clinical diagnosis

1.1.1 Introduction

More than any other branch of medicine, the practice of neurology uses the classical method of intuitive conversation, structured examination, and selective investigation. We teach the importance of eliciting an accurate neurological history. The key symptoms are identified and their course defined. For the experienced clinician, this process becomes routine, efficient, and quick. The competent neurologist is one who instinctively senses relevant components of the history, appreciates the most likely underlying mechanism, reliably elicits the physical signs, knows which investigations are necessary and assesses their relevance, provides a sensible clinical formulation, and communicates the situation accurately and sensitively. One piece of information directs the subsequent logic and steers questions down anatomical, physiological, and pathological lines of enquiry.

This system evolved over several centuries, during which knowledge accumulated on structure and function, localization in health and disease, the reliability of physical signs and laboratory investigations, and the nosology of disease. The brief account that follows is unashamedly Anglocentric. It focuses, but not exclusively, on the major contributions to clinical neuroscience from Great Britain—Thomas Willis, Robert Whytt, John Hughlings Jackson, William Gowers, Charles Sherrington, and Gordon Holmes. Several distinguished names do not appear and the references are highly selective. Many better balanced and more detailed histories of neurology are available: *Garrison's History of Neurology* by Lawrence McHenry (1969) is comprehensive but often inaccurate; J. D. Spillane's *The Doctrine of the Nerves* (1981) is detailed and engaging but selective, with significant omissions; *Morton's Medical Bibliography* by J. M. Norman (1991) lists all significant publications, books, and articles in the history of medicine, including discoveries relating to the nervous system; Haymaker and Schiller's *The Founders of Neurology* (1970) contains biographies, and portraits or photographs where available, of all significant neuroscientists arranged by discipline.

1.1.2 The structure of the nervous system

It was the need for Renaissance artists better to depict the external form of the human body through an improved knowledge of its inner arrangements that first provided an accurate anatomical account of structure in the nervous system. That process started with Leonardo da Vinci [1452–1519] but soon reached full maturity through the work of Andreas Vesalius [1514–1564]. His first detailed depiction of human anatomy (1543), including the brain, dislodged the medieval cell doctrine, developed in classical times, which had remained largely unchallenged for almost 11 centuries. Vesalius's work epitomizes the role of the printing press in moving science and

culture from the medieval to the modern. Still largely untranslated from the original Renaissance Latin, *De fabrica* is famous for its woodcuts, last reprinted from the original pearwood blocks in 1934. These were destroyed soon after during the Allied bombing of Munich.

Others quickly borrowed, refined, and extended Vesalius's neuroanatomy, with major schools developing in The Netherlands, Germany, and Italy. In Great Britain, anatomy improved through the work of Thomas Willis [1621–1675], John Browne [1642–1702], William Cowper [1666–1709], who serially stripped away the muscles, leaving his flayed exemplars otherwise represented intact in rural landscapes, and Humphrey Ridley [1653–1708]. Willis improved on primitive depictions of the arterial anastomosis at the base of the brain and explained its physiology. In *Cerebri Anatome* (1664: translated 1681), he described a patient (dying from carcinoma of the stomach) in whom the left carotid artery was occluded yet the brain had not suffered since the right carotid was increased to three times its normal size. Willis concluded that a connection must exist between the circulation on the two sides. The famous illustration is by Christopher Wren [1632–1723]. Vesalius and Willis were concerned with gross anatomy of the normal brain, nerves, and muscles, but an understanding of how the brain works ultimately required knowledge of its cellular structure and organization.

Microscopes were developed in the 1640s and a range of histological stains, suitable for distinguishing cell types within intact tissue, became available during the nineteenth century. It was Camillo Golgi's [1843–1926] silver stain and the use to which this was put by Santiago Ramon y Cajal [1852–1934] that culminated in definitive studies of the cellular architecture of the central nervous system. From this work emerged the neuron theory for which Cajal and Golgi were jointly awarded the 1906 Nobel prize for medicine. Cajal's work is relatively

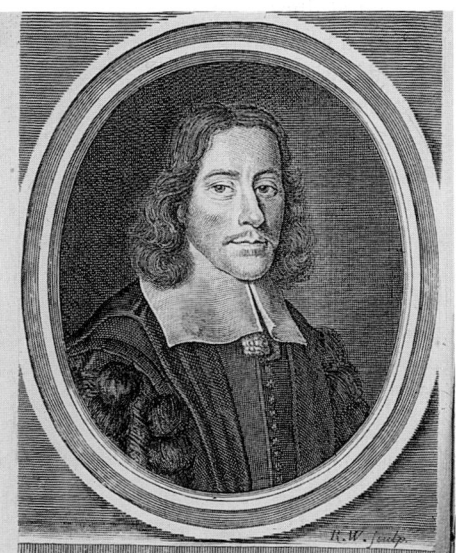

Fig. 1.1. Thomas Willis [1621–1675].

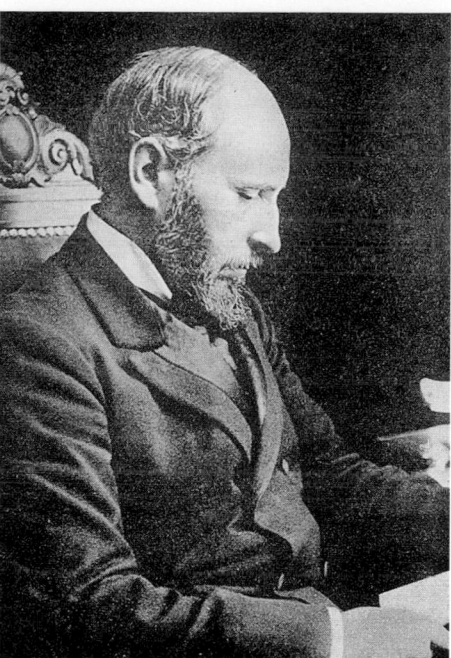

Fig. 1.2. Santiago Ramon y Cajal [1852–1934].

unread, but translations have appeared in recent years and his treatise on *Textura del Sistema Nervioso del Hombre y de los Vertebrados*, first published between 1897 and 1904, updated and translated into French (1909–1911), is now undergoing its second English version (first from the French and now from the Spanish text) since 1995. Arguably, Cajal will be seen as the most significant neuroscientist of the twentieth century. He described accurately the distinguishing features of neurons and glia within discrete regions of the brain and spinal cord; he characterized their local organization, supplementing the descriptions with beautiful drawings based on Golgi's silver stains; and he consolidated the neuron doctrine. Preceded in this work by Jan Purkinje [1787–1869], Wilhelm His [1831–1904], and Fridtjof Nansen [1861–1930: neuroscientist, arctic explorer, and humanist], Cajal perfected Golgi's method and advanced his discoveries through the study of developing nervous systems in order to overcome the limitation of poor silver staining of myelinated fibres. He overturned the reticular theory of neural organization, showing histologically the variability of dendritic arborizations and axon terminations, establishing that axon cylinders end freely but form contacts, and conceiving that the nerve impulse is conducted between axons, dendrites, and the cell body of neighbouring neurons. Everything we know about structure, function, and physiology in the nervous system at the cellular level, in health and disease, evolves from the concept that organization is through the connectivity of functionally independent neurons and their processes. His most detailed studies were of the cerebellum but, in time, no part of the brain or spinal cord went unexplored. Paradoxically, Cajal and Golgi disagreed publicly on the neuron doctrine when they gave their 1906 Nobel lectures in Stockholm.

1.1.3 The function of the nervous system

Some of those who first described the structure of the nervous system in the sixteenth and seventeenth centuries also formulated primitive concepts of reflex activity—that is, function. Historical guides to knowledge on reflex function are to be found in Franklin Fearing's *Reflex Action: a Study in the History of Physiological Psychology* (1930) and E. G. T. Liddell's *The Discovery of Reflexes* (1960), a tribute to his teacher Sir Charles Sherrington [1857–1952].

Thomas Willis likened muscle contraction to an explosion of gunpowder, with new spirits being supplied to muscle by the blood (1670, translated 1681), extending the ideas of William Croone [1633–1684] who (in *De Ratione Motus Musculorum*, 1664: often wrongly attributed to Thomas Willis) postulated an interaction of spirituous juice from the nerves and blood agitating the space between muscle fibres and transmitting to them a force which expanded their width and shortened their length. Willis later elaborated these ideas (1667, translated 1681): 'the first designation of motion is in the Brain or Cerebel: its transmission … is performed by the spirits within the nerves … implant[ing] a contracture or elastick force'.

Robert Whytt [1714–1766] of Edinburgh consolidated the reflex theory of function in the nervous system, settling a debate polarized by Rene Descartes [1596–1650] and Willis on the dependence of intact reflexes on integrity of peripheral nerve plexuses. His experiments on the frog (1751) established that reflex activity depends on segmental integrity of the spinal cord. He also described the reflex pupillary response to light.

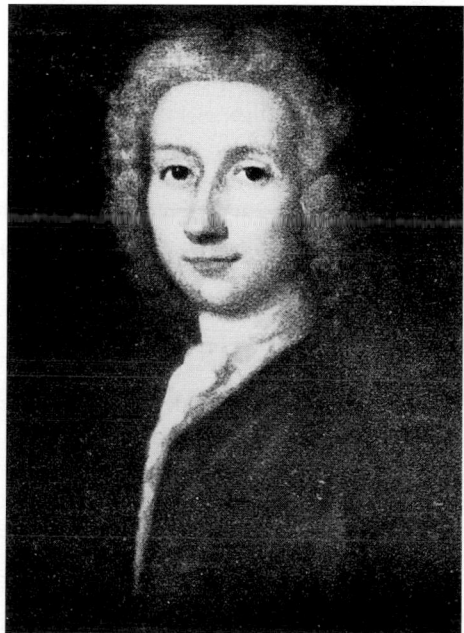

Fig. 1.3. Robert Whytt [1714–1766].

Against this background, the themes that underpin the modern concept of facilitation and inhibition of (spinal) reflexes as the basis for organization of neural systems and behaviour were: recognition that the nervous system consists of nerve cells connected through synapses to their neighbours (see above); evidence for (animal) electricity as the basis for passage of the nerve impulse (work associated especially with Luigi Galvani [1737–1798]); and the accurate designation of afferent and efferent components of the reflex arc.

Charles Bell [1774–1842] comes out second best in the Bell–Magendie wrangle. Bell was much excited by his deliberations on the workings of the brain. He had grasped the principles of afferent connections, central processing, and efferent output, but attributed both motor and sensory functions to the anterior roots and oversimplified the central functions of the cerebellum and cerebrum. It is difficult to guess whether François Magendie [1783–1855] saw a copy of Bell's *Idea of a New Anatomy of the Brain* (1811) before correctly assigning anterior and posterior nerve root functions in 1822. Whatever the truth of Magendie's position, Bell was soon putting around modified views which neatly corrected, but did not formally retract, his earlier error.

Marshall Hall [1790–1857] coined the term reflex arc and documented methodically the range and variety of reflex responses of isolated portions of the animal nervous system (1837). Later, he extended these principles to the interpretation of clinical observations, including spinal shock—rather unsatisfactorily in the opinion of Spillane (1981).

John Hughlings Jackson [1835–1911] sought to understand the organizational principles that determine how the brain works. He was not an experimentalist but used clinical observation to inform his analyses. He learned much from colleagues at the West Riding Lunatic Asylum and the philosopher Herbert Spencer [1820–1903]. Jackson's concept of functional localization passed to Sigmund Freud [1856–1939] and Sir Henry Head [1861–1940], who concluded that function is not normally localized but depends on complex orchestration, even though disorder at specific sites yields precise and predictable clusters of clinical deficits. Beyond this rather pragmatic view of cerebral localization lay a more sophisticated philosophy which postulated three layers of organization determining function in the central nervous system. In disease, subservient systems in this hierarchy are released, creating syndromes consisting of negative (loss of function) and positive (release) symptoms. The lowest level is concerned with vegetative function and operates through reflex activity at the spinal level. The next tier (cortex, striatum, and long tracts) determines movement and sensation. The most elevated system is the pre-frontal region, providing higher functions and co-ordination of the more elementary components. Jackson is revered but largely unread. He left no major synthesis of his views and his papers (1932: edited by James Taylor [1859–1946]) are somewhat impenetrable.

Sir David Ferrier [1843–1928] set out to confirm experimentally, what Jackson had proposed theoretically on destructive and discharging lesions of the nervous system, and to deal

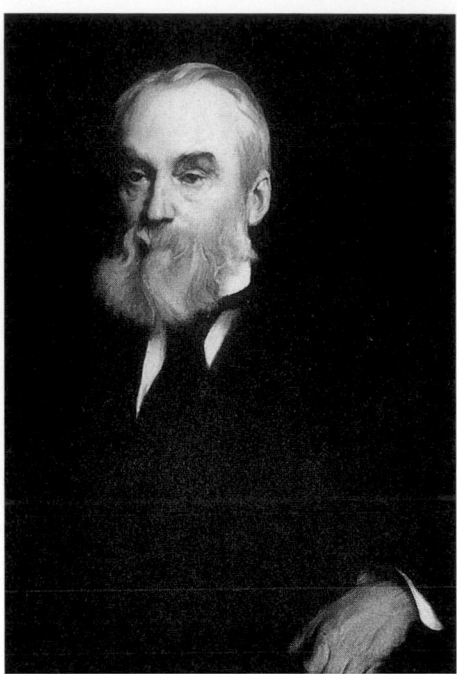

Fig. 1.4. John Hughlings Jackson [1835–1911].

with the issue of cerebral localization. Using electrical stimulation and local excision of the monkey and canine cortex, together with clinical analyses, Ferrier (1876) concluded that certain areas of the cortex do possess defined functions and that lesions at different sites will generate predictable syndromes. Inevitably his work was scientifically and socially controversial—famously at the medical Congress of 1881 when he demonstrated the lesioned dog that so impressed Jean-Martin Charcot [1825–1893] and argued openly with Friedrich Goltz [1834–1902]—but Ferrier pioneered neurosurgery and his work culminated in the first human operative intracranial procedure in December 1884.

Only four people attended the last of Sherrington's celebrated Silliman Lectures in 1904. The published version (1906) offered a summary of functional organization in nervous systems which ranks, in its overall synthesis and stature, with the greatest works in medicine. Sherrington's book is probably the single most significant publication in clinical neuroscience of the twentieth century, and the author has been dubbed the Harvey of the Nervous System—although several others have staked this claim, for themselves or on behalf of third parties. Sherrington begins with a restatement of the neuron doctrine: 'nowhere in physiology does the cell theory reveal its presence more frequently in the very framework of the argument than in the study of nervous reactions'. Against this background, and the certain knowledge of animal electricity and reflex function of the isolated spinal cord, he formulated ideas on propagation of the nerve impulse through synapses, mainly using observations on the scratch reflex of dogs. He defined the efferent and afferent properties of nerve and muscle, and characterized the physiology of the tendon stretch reflex. Sherrington argued that

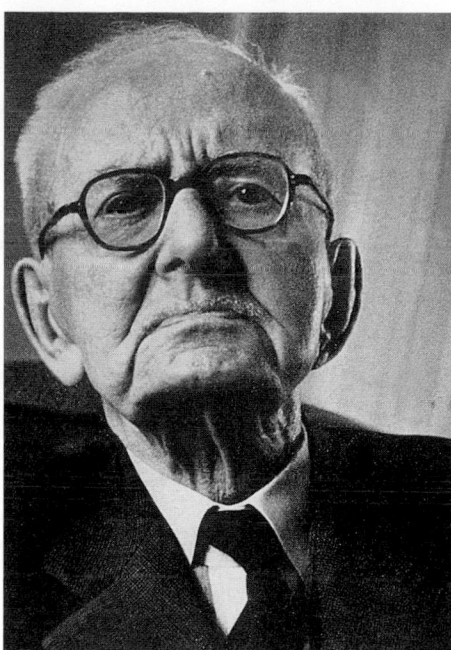

Fig. 1.5. Charles Sherrington [1857–1952].

trate his dissections of the cranial and peripheral nerves. He acknowledged the propensity of the brain to manifest striking disturbances of function on the basis of apparently trivial disorders of structure. Swan published three monographs on the normal anatomy of the cranial, spinal, and peripheral nerves between 1825 and 1830. Bright (1827–1831) introduced a classification based on inflammation, pressure, irritation, and inanition, but no details were provided of his patients' physical signs in life. Carswell (1838) also showed consummate artistry in use of the colour spectrum as organs affected by inflammation (pink), analogous tissues (crimson), atrophy, (yellow and ochre: with the first illustrations of multiple sclerosis), hypertrophy (brown), pus (yellow and green), mortification (blue-black), haemorrhage (purple), softening (yellow), melanoma (jet black), carcinoma (orange and green), and tubercle (back to red) are pictured and described. The first separate work on neuropathology, by Robert Hooper (1826), anticipated Carswell in attempting a classification (inflammation, tumour, diseased structure and unnatural appearance without tumefaction, and fluid collected around the hemispheres or extravasated), with descriptions of diseases as they affect the meninges, brain, nerves, blood vessels, and sinuses.

activities such as walking depend on temporal and spatial regulation of reflex activity; orchestration of the separate segments, dependent on integrity of the spinal cord, requires interaction of neighbouring segments and reciprocal inhibition and facilitation of agonists and antagonists, as the basis for tonic and phasic contraction of muscles concerned with posture and stepping.

1.1.4 The pathological anatomy of the nervous system

Giovanni Morgagni [1682–1771] first suggested classifications of pathological anatomy (1761) but not until the early nineteenth century were anatomical and clinical descriptions of neurological disease systematically correlated and illustrated.

Many attended the Parisian clinical demonstrations and dissections in which Philippe Pinel [1745–1826] and Xavier Bichat [1771 1802] consolidated the discipline of pathological anatomy in the first half of the nineteenth century. This school reached its continental zenith with the *livraisons* published by Jean Cruveilhier [1791–1874] between 1828 and 1842. Pathological anatomy also flourished in the British Isles during the first few decades of the nineteenth century because a few clinician scientists with artistic temperaments met in a culture which was becoming liberated with respect to anatomical examination of the sick. The principal activists in this school were Matthew Baillie [1761–1823], Robert Hooper [1773–1835], (Sir) Charles Bell (see above), Richard Bright [1789 1858], Joseph Swan [1791–1874], and (Sir) Robert Carswell [1793–1857].

Baillie (1793, 1798–1803) established organ-based pathology as a separate science in the United Kingdom. Bell (1802) produced exquisitely artistic images of normal structure to illus-

1.1.5 Examination of the nervous system

Willis described symptoms and made observations; James Parkinson [1755–1824] noted the tremor, posture, and slowness of movement of those who shuffled through Hoxton Square. But physical examination did not feature in these early descriptions of neurological disease. The first systematic textbooks of the nineteenth century started to combine accounts of symptomatology with objective evidence for impairments; and these methods were fully in place by the time the great treatises, manuals, textbooks, and systems of Moritz Romberg [1795–1873], William Gowers [1845–1915] (see below), Carl Wernicke [1848–1905], Hermann Oppenheim [1858–1919] (who wrote in a style reminiscent of Kinnier Wilson (see below): 'I may be permitted to add that my textbook contains all that is essential'), and Jules Dejerine [1849–1917] duly appeared.

On the clinical art of eliciting (tendon) reflexes, the catalogue of methods collated by Robert Wartenberg (1945 [1887–1956]) carried a warning from Foster Kennedy [1884–1952] in its forward: 'the open season for the hunting of the reflex was the thirty years around the turn of the century ... the present generation has inherited these impedimenta of variety without variance ... shrill claims to be the Prometheus of the pyramidal tracts'.

The evolution of the method for physical examination peaked with Joseph Babinski's [1857–1932] presentation to the Biological Society of Paris (1896). Parallel themes based on experimental and clinical work provided the basis for Babinski's discovery. These included the demonstration of cutaneous and tendon reflexes, and the contributions of Charcot and Alfred Vulpian [1826–1882] in observing other aspects of the upper motor neuron lesion. Charles Edouard Brown-Sequard

[1817–1894] knew of a paraplegic American whose valet would relieve spasticity and clonus (Charcot's spinal epilepsy) by forcible flexion of toes; and others undoubtedly stroked the plantar surface in order to induce reflex flexion of the leg.

Monographs dedicated to examination of the nervous system first appeared in the 1920s. The Norwegian G. H. Monrad Krohn offered no short cuts (1921). After a history supplemented with leading questions, he advocated a thorough collection of the signs without speculation on the diagnosis, ordered tabulation of the findings, focal diagnosis by applying the rules of functional anatomy, and pathological interpretation. His book introduced many components of the examination which survive: there is the recall of prime ministers, recitation of serial digits forwards and in reverse, interpretation of proverbs, mental arithmetic on mythical shopping trips, tongue twisters such as 'West Register Street' and the 'British Constitution', and sensory examination—preferably spread over 2 days. Tips on how to test the main muscles and assign their nerve and root supply anticipate the monograph (1943) published by the Medical Research Council (War Memorandum number 7) under the chairmanship of Brigadier (Dr) George Riddoch [1888–1947]. The model is Dr M. J. (Sean) McArdle [1909–1989], who succeeded Dr William Ritchie Russell [1903–1980]—foundation professor of neurology in the University of Oxford—as neurologist to Scottish Command in 1942; the photographs were taken at Gogarburn with assistance from the department of medical illustration of the University of Edinburgh.

Sir Gordon Holmes [1876–1965] published a system for clinical examination of the nervous system (1946) orientated around motor and sensory systems, vision and eye movements, aphasia and related disorders, mental state, and autonomic function—all based on physiological and anatomical principles of organization—which is still in routine use. The three-page practical summary is minimalist but complete. Written at the age of 70, after a professional career in which (like Hughlings Jackson) Holmes had mainly depended for his insights on opportunities made available through clinical neurology (especially gunshot injuries sustained in the First World War, following the example of Silas Weir Mitchell [1829–1914]), Holmes's manual synthesizes his many insights into structure and function of the cerebellum, visual system, and spinal cord.

J. D. Spillane's photographic summary of clinical neurology (1968) takes in a few names not mentioned here but (happily) prioritizes the same key figures. Not inhibited by present-day restrictions on identification of individuals and other discretions, the subjects tell not only the story of neurological anatomy, nosology, and pathology, but also provide a medico-social account of conditions common in mid-twentieth-century international and provincial neurological practice. Many of the photographs are by (Professor) Ralph Marshall. The power of black and white, use of shadow, and creative construction of images (scotoma, hemianopia, and trigeminal neuralgia; and stills from movie sequences used to great effect in explaining the subjective experience of movement disorders) are organized

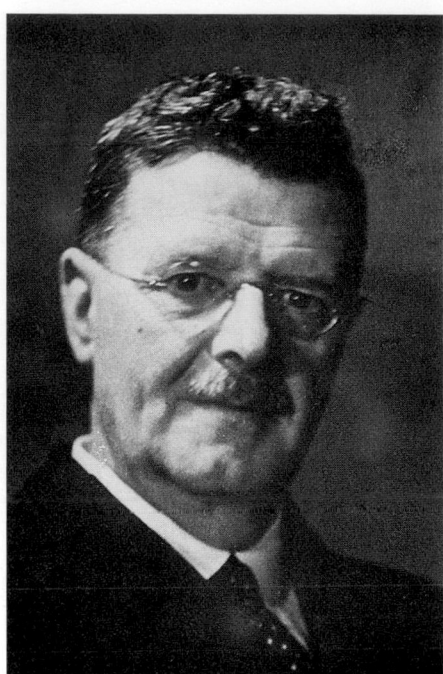

Fig. 1.6. Gordon Holmes [1876–1965].

around head and neck, cranial nerves, acute and chronic polyneuritis, peripheral nerve lesions, muscle and neuromuscular disease, and neurodegeneration. Spillane rightly pays tribute to the two outstanding non-photographic medical artists of the twentieth century—Max Brodel [1870–1941] and Frank Netter [1906-1991].

1.1.6 The origins of clinical neurology

Thomas Willis is the most significant figure in British neurology. He coined the term: 'we shall institute the whole neurology or the doctrine of the nerves'. In addition to the anatomical contributions, Willis described accurately an astonishing number of general medical and neurological disorders, based on experience gathered in his medical practices in Oxford and London. Willis's casebook reveals the origin of the clinical methodology on which modern medicine is based—symptoms as the patient describes them, social aspects of the illness, examination, formulation of the problem, a list of pathophysiological alternatives, an approach to treatment, an assessment of prognosis, and communication with patients and their families.

Willis (1667, translated 1681) proposed that seizures are not an affection of the part that moves but a remote consequence of activity in the brain, albeit in response to a peripheral stimulus, or of the blood entering the brain: 'to wit that the spirits inhabiting it being disposed to explosions, and there being exploded, bring on or cause every Falling Evil'. He distinguished what would now be classified as complex partial seizures, symptomatic epilepsy, and pseudo-seizures, and described several movement disorders. On hysteria, Willis rejected the concept of uterine displacement and the theory of pulmonary congestion, and preferred to consider this as a disorder of the brain. This is what he means by 'convulsion', using the term 'epilepsie' for all types of the falling sickness. Willis wrote on the soul of *brutes* (1672, translated 1683) as a device for deflecting criticism from the Church on the physical basis for reason and human behaviour—man having both a brutal and rational soul—allowing Willis to get on with his analysis of structure, function, and disease in the nervous system. In addition to further accounts of epilepsy, he describes headache, apoplexy, neurosyphilis, narcolepsy, mental retardation, paracusis, head and spinal-cord trauma and a range of psychiatric syndromes; 'there is another kind depending on the scarcity of the spirits in which the motion is performed weakly … those being troubled are able to move their arms in the morning … but before noon … they are scarce able to move hand or foot … [and] after long speaking become mute … and [do] not recover the use still after an hour or two' is taken as the first description of myasthenia gravis.

Robert Whytt's textbook of neurology (1765) is psychiatrically flavoured—the distinction between nervous, hypochondriac, and hysteric disorders being only the frequency and duration with which his patients experienced somatic manifestations of emotional states. Not until the nineteenth century did physicians systematically correlate knowledge gathered from pathological anatomy into systems of neurological disease. John Cooke [1756–1838] wrote a thorough history of contributions to clinical neurology from ancient times to modern (1820–1823), with sections on apoplexy, palsy, and epilepsy, and in which he first drew attention to James Parkinson's description of the shaking palsy. The contributions to an astonishing range of topics in clinical neurology attributa-

ble to Charcot were faithfully recorded and published by his students (1872–1887, translated 1877–1889). The clinical demonstrations, although selectively translated, are still only available in the original edition (1887, revised and reprinted 1892). Many of his school at the Salpetrière themselves later wrote definitive accounts of clinical and experimental neurology—notably Pierre Marie [1853–1940] and Gilles de la Tourette [1857–1904]. They (and others, including Charcot's son—the Antarctic explorer) are gathered in the famous painting by Pierre Brouillet of Charcot demonstrating hysteria at the Salpetrière during one of his Tuesday lectures; Babinski is catching the swooning Blanche Wittmann, one of the many hysterics accommodated long-term at the hospital in return for serial examinations of themselves and, eventually, their tissues.

In the United Kingdom, books summarizing contemporary knowledge on clinical neurology emerged mainly from the National Hospital. Its early history is recorded by Sir Gordon Holmes (1954). Multi-author systems were edited, for example, by John Russell Reynolds [1828–1896] with contributions from many of the foundation staff. Sir William Gowers (1886–1888) wrote the bible of nineteenth-century neurology; of him it could reasonably be said that, neurologically, what he knew not was not knowledge. The book is decorated with his own line drawings of patients and pathological features of disease. Its production was timely, coinciding with the dawn of descriptive clinical neurology. Few of his accounts can be improved upon and many remain accurate to this day. Gowers' authority was usually his own experience, without much delving into the published literature. Organized by anatomical region, the table of contents would do well as a nomenclature of contemporary

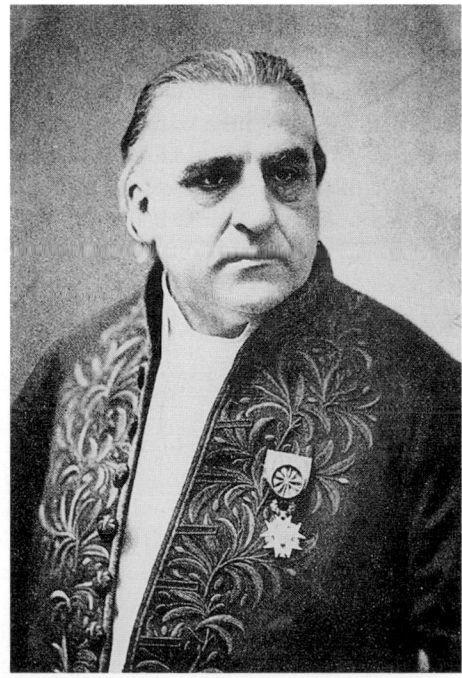

Fig. 1.7. Jean-Martin Charcot [1825–1893].

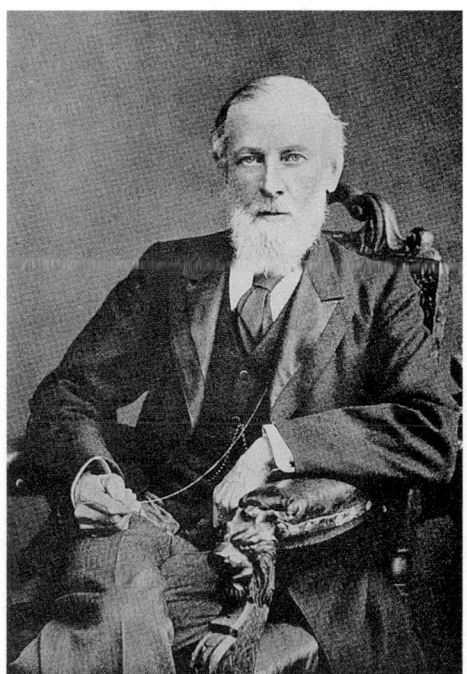

Fig. 1.8. William Gowers [1845–1915].

neurology. The manual summarizes knowledge gathered by the greatest clinical observer in the history of neurology. It appeared at the peak of Gowers' career (according to Foster Kennedy, later he declined)—after his writings on pseudo-hypertrophic (Duchenne) muscular dystrophy, medical ophthalmoscopy (Gowers was not the first to use systematically the ophthalmoscope introduced by Hermann von Helmholz [1821–1894], but he made it popular; it was also used by Hughlings Jackson and Sir Clifford Allbutt [1836–1925]), epilepsy, and the published lectures delivered at University College; only the essay on the borderland of epilepsy, lectures given at the National Hospital, and a speculative work on the dynamics of life lay ahead.

Russell Brain [1895–1966] wrote the textbook which has most influenced neurology in the English-speaking world (1933). Brain wrote six editions up to 1962; John Walton [born 1922] completed the seventh, published in 1969, and this volume (the first to lack his guiding editorial hand) is the eleventh. Lords Brain and Walton reviewed developments in clinical neurology over a period in which more was learned about the nervous system in health and disease than at any other time in history. In 1933, the symptoms of Parkinson's disease could best be alleviated by riding in a motor car; in 2001, this requires striatal transplantation of embryonic stem cells. The 900-odd pages of the 1933 edition are remarkable for having first been written by a 38-year-old who sustained this effort single handed until his death at 71. Is there any neurologist trained since the 1930s who has not repeatedly used a copy of whichever edition was then current? But the book had its critics. John Walton relates how he was advised waspishly by F. M. R. Walshe [1885–1973] to 'put some red cells' into the 1967 revision. Walshe himself wrote a book on disease of the nervous system for practitioners and students (1940) which was popular but not on the same scale. As a neurologist, Brain's lasting discoveries were the syndromes of

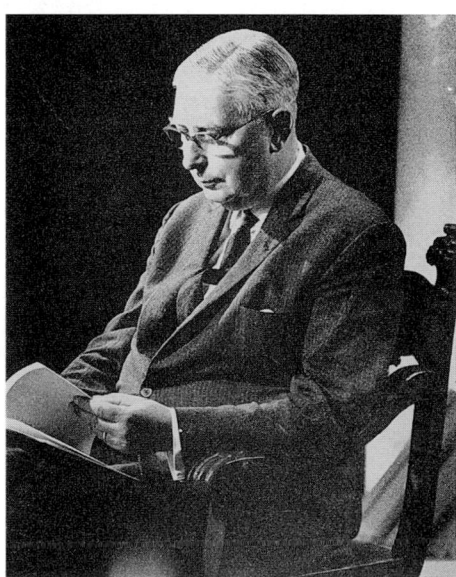

Fig. 1.9. Russell Brain [1895–1966].

median nerve compression in the carpal tunnel, disc prolapse as a cause of cervical myelopathy, and paraneoplasia.

In some respects, Brain's prestige was short lived, for in 1940 appeared the last of the great single-author textbooks, largely written by Samuel Alexander Kinnier Wilson [1878–1937] but seen through the press by Alexander Ninian Bruce [1882–1968], to whose father the book is jointly dedicated. Wilson was one for the subtleties of symptomatology and signs in early diagnosis—an abdominal reflex that can be tired, a few kicks of nystagmus—and lightened his text with clinical anecdotes, such as the patient who convulsed the ward with a Rabelaisian peal of laughter through reference to the condition of his trousers in answer to a question on bladder control (Wilson's penchant for music-hall humour was well known to his colleagues). Unlike Gowers or Brain, Wilson's opinions are supported extensively by citations from the (often non-anglophone) literature of the 1920s and 1930s. Each chapter has a brief but well-researched historical synopsis. Written in an era when infections usually ran their natural course, and substances of abuse were becoming associated with recognizable clinical complications, the emphasis is on toxi-infective disease of the nervous system. Wilson insisted on hepato-lenticular degeneration being known as Kinnier-Wilson's disease—and the eponym stuck. In 1940, diseases of uncertain nature included the epilepsies, narcolepsies, headache, and myasthenia gravis. With the exception of Parkinson's disease and the choreas, all movement disorders were considered by Kinnier Wilson to be entirely functional. Out of print since 1954 (in an edition revised by Russell Brain and including his own monograph on aphasia), the discerning neurologist wanting to confirm a clinical fact, not only in the context of diseases which are now less prevalent in everyday neurology, can turn to 'Kinnier Wilson' and invariably come away better informed.

An apocryphal story summarizes the tradition at the National Hospital, Queen Square when clinical neurology was at its zenith: the ideal team to handle a case was Sir Charles Symonds [1890–1978] to take the history, Sir Gordon Holmes to examine the patient, and W. D. Adie [1886–1935] to explain matters to the family—it seems that, then as now, clinical wisdom and a good pastoral approach were not always set on the same pair of magisterial shoulders.

1.1.7 The investigation of the nervous system

It was not until 1875 that Richard Caton [1842–1926], working in Liverpool, extended knowledge on the electrical basis for nerve action, discovered by Luigi Galvani [1737–1798] in 1791 and developed by Emil du Bois Raymond [1818–1896] in 1848, to the brain. Hans Berger [1873–1941] recorded this activity through the intact skull and the technique was perfected by E. D. (Edgar) Adrian [1889–1977], who also developed methods for recording electrical activity from peripheral nerves. Intracellular recordings eventually led to elucidation of the conduction of the nerve impulse by Sir Andrew Huxley [born

1917] and Sir Alan Hodgkin [1914–1998]. The exploration of human brain function by evoked potential methods originates from the observations of George Dawson [1912–1983]. Subsequently the group of Martin Halliday [born 1928] and Ian McDonald [born 1933] moved electrical exploration of conduction in the central nervous system into clinical practice.

The most direct method of examining body fluids which reflect brain activity was the introduction of lumbar puncture in life (Domenico Cotugno [1736–1822] removed fluid from cadavers). First used at the Middlesex Hospital in London to treat children with tuberculous meningitis (described by Robert Whytt in 1768) by Walter Essex Wynter [1860–1945], the procedure was applied routinely in neurology by Henirich Iraneaeus Quincke [1842–1922] from 1891. He measured the pressure and examined the chemical constituents of spinal fluid; qualitative features of the protein content were described by CGR Lange [1883–nk] in 1912 and by Elvin Kabat [1914–2000] in 1942.

Definitive textbooks on neuroradiology began to appear within a few years of Wilhelm Roentgen's [1845–1923] X-ray demonstration of the bone in his wife Bertha's hand. It was an imaginative next step to adapt this technique using substances, including radiopaque dies, injected in and around the brain and spinal cord to define their structure. In 1918, Walter Edward Dandy [1886–1946] outlined the outer and inner contours of the brain using air introduced directly into the ventricles or lumbar sac. Jean Athanase Sicard [1872–1929] replaced air with iodinized oil and produced images of the spinal canal by myelography in 1921. The most colourful of these early pioneers was Antoni Caetano de Abreu Egas Moniz [1875–1955] who, after signing the Versailles treaty for Portugal in 1918, returned to neurology and introduced arteriography (1927). He was best known for pioneering frontal leucotomy and other forms of psychosurgery (receiving the Nobel prize in 1949 but nearly losing his life at the hands of a gun-crazed schizophrenic patient in his office).

It is fitting to end this patchy history of neurology and its methods with reference to brain imaging. Neurologists trained since 1973 must find it hard to imagine the confidence needed to localize structural lesions accurately, as the sufficient basis for surgical exploration, using nothing more than clinical analysis. Even when neuroradiology was introduced, the procedures offered limited information, showing only the grossest abnormalities, and failing to depict most processes that affect tissue integrity. And even those who witnessed this transition would not have imagined the possibilities (revisiting the glorious age of eighteenth- to nineteenth-century phrenology) for demonstrating focal brain activity during a host of behavioural activations, real and imagined.

No procedure has so revolutionized the everyday practice of medicine and opened up methods for studying normal and disordered function as the introduction of computerized axial tomography (Hounsfield 1973), from which evolved techniques for depicting structure and function of the brain using magnetic resonance imaging and positron emission tomography. If award of the Nobel prize (for medicine) is about ingenuity,

step-changes in knowledge, promotion of human health, and opening up unimagined opportunities for illuminating medicine—motives which inspired Vesalius and Willis—the recognition of Sir Godfrey Hounsfield [born 1919] as the unrivalled contributor of the latter half of the twentieth century is surely not contested.

1.2 The frequency of neurological diseases

Some neurological disorders (e.g. stroke) are so common and serious that reducing their burden features in the public health goals of many countries. Others are about as common, and treatable, but—rightly or wrongly—are regarded as having less public health importance (e.g. epilepsy, migraine). Yet more are common, but as yet untreatable (e.g. Alzheimer's disease). Multiple sclerosis is, thankfully, not all that common, but it is still the most frequent cause of disability in young adults. And then there are a myriad of less common disorders, many of which are hopelessly incurable (e.g. motor neuron disease), but a few very rare diseases are extremely treatable (e.g. Wilson's disease, tetanus). Perhaps the rarest of all, variant Creutzfeldt–Jakob disease, is of most political, economic, and public-health concern, at least in the UK. So, neurologists have to deal with a huge range of disorders and the challenge of handling a large number of patients with common disorders while, at the same time, keeping alert to the once-in-a-professional-lifetime patient with a treatable disease who slips in to the end of a busy clinic (MacDonald *et al.* 2000). It makes sense for neurologists to subspecialize, at least to the extent of taking on the management of rare disorders such as myasthenia gravis and inflammatory muscle disease, and the difficult end of the spectrum of more common disorders such as Parkinson's disease with intractable on/off periods. In this way patients are treated by physicians who have as much experience as possible of their disorder.

1.2.1 Measuring disease frequency

The three traditional measures of disease frequency are mortality, incidence, and prevalence. Which measure to use depends on the frequency of the disease in question, whether it is likely to be fatal, and whether it is an acute one-off event or chronic, and also on logistic and methodological issues to do with recording and coding the disease itself. Furthermore, because the frequency of almost every disease varies by age, and sometimes also by sex, any rates must be in given in strata of age and by sex (i.e. age- and sex-specific rates). Of course, frequencies of disease based on hospital data are hopelessly flawed because one has no idea of the size of the population from which the patients came, nor why some patients were referred to hospital and others not.

Mortality data (the number of deaths from a particular disease per annum in a population of known size) are routinely collected in developed countries from death certificates. However, there are many problems of erratic classification of disease and poor coding practice. Even more problematic is that some diseases are not fatal (e.g. migraine); the disease may be fatal but lingers in such a chronic fashion that the patient's death is due to, and is coded as, something quite different (e.g. multiple sclerosis patients may die of cancer); and some diseases have mild forms which are seldom fatal (e.g. lacunar stroke). On the other hand, mortality data are usually based on large numbers and are likely to be precise as a result. None the less, mortality is a very crude approximation of disease frequency and unhelpful when asking rather specific questions, such as how often patients with epilepsy die suddenly, and what the deaths are due to.

1.2.2 Incidence of neurological disorders

Incidence is the number of new cases of a disease appearing in a defined population of known size per annum. To measure it one must therefore have good census data to define the population denominator, multiple and overlapping case-finding methods to identify all the patients, a clear idea of when the disease actually starts (which is easy for stroke but more difficult for gradually progressive disorders such as motor neuron disease), and a large-enough number of patients with the disease to calculate precise estimates of frequency over a defined time period. All this is hardly possible outside prospective community-based studies, although if all the community is getting healthcare in one place and the records system is seriously well organized and funded (such as in Rochester, Minnesota, USA), then retrospective estimates of incidence are reasonably accurate, and probably the only sensible method to use for rare diseases. However, any method relying on the examination of patient records would be threatened if society insists that researchers, or others, must first obtain the explicit consent of every patient.

Table 1.1 provides some estimates of the incidence of various neurological disorders in the conventional way (number of new cases per 100 000 population per annum, but not divided by sex). In addition, it emphasizes that even the common neurological disorders, such as multiple sclerosis, are not all that common in primary care, where physicians have to be extraordinarily alert to recognize and diagnose disorders that they may not have seen since medical school. Perhaps, therefore, in medical education we should concentrate on the common diseases and on the general principles of recognizing that a patient has a neurological disorder, so they can be referred to neurologists for diagnosis, and not on the details of rare diseases, however interesting.

1.2.3 Prevalence of neurological disorders

The prevalence of a disease is the number of patients with that disease at a particular point in time, usually expressed per 100 000 population. Again this requires good census data or some other method of measuring the population denominator (e.g. a UK family practice computerized age–sex register), and

then finding all the patients with the disease of interest in that population and confirming they actually have the disease. This is surprisingly difficult to do, and tedious, particularly when the disease is rare. Of course, prevalence will tell one nothing about fatalities. Furthermore, for episodic diseases (such as transient ischaemic attacks), an episode many years before may well have been forgotten and, even if not, it may be difficult to diagnose in retrospect. None the less, for some chronic and persisting disorders estimates of prevalence can be illuminating (Table 1.2). This table again shows just how rare many neurological disorders are, even in a family practice of five doctors looking after 10 000 people. If one knows the incidence and the proportion of patients who die, then prevalence can be calculated and does not have to be measured directly.

1.3 Principles of clinical diagnosis

Just under 10 per cent of the population consult their general practitioner about a neurological symptom each year in the United Kingdom. About 10 per cent of these are referred for a specialist opinion, usually to a neurologist. The most common diseases or clinical problems encountered in a general neurological outpatient clinic are shown in Table 1.3. Together these nine conditions account for roughly 75 per cent of general neurological referrals and are diagnosed initially on purely clinical grounds and frequently managed purely in an outpatient setting (Stevens 1989; Perkin 1989). The remaining 25 per cent of neurological consultations concern the huge range of other neurological disorders, many rare. Such disorders are particularly likely to require highly specialist investigation and treatment, to need in-patient care, and continuing follow-up care. Naturally these broad statistics will vary in different healthcare settings which may not be based upon general practice, and as the demand for, and availability of, neurological services changes.

This section is concerned with a practical, everyday approach to diagnosing neurological disorders. It does not aim for the exhaustive completeness familiar in traditional accounts of the neurological examination. However, there are times at which a more detailed approach to clinical assessment is necessary, for instance in elucidating the neuroanatomical site of the lesion responsible for muscle weakness (Section 1.5) or a somatosensory disturbance (Section 1.6). Also it is important to document the different reflexes that can be elicited, giving some indication of their usefulness (Section 1.4). These more traditional clinical approaches to such problems are presented separately, later in this chapter.

1.3.1 History taking

History taking is fundamental to neurological diagnosis. For instance, epilepsy or migraine are diagnosed solely on the basis of the history, with the examination merely ensuring there is no evidence of associated underlying structural disorders of the brain. The history is usually much more informative than

Table 1.1. The approximate incidence of various neurological disorders and how often a new case will be seen in primary care by a general practitioner (family doctor) with a list size of 2000 people

	Incidence/100 000/annum	Number of years between consecutive new cases seen by a general practitioner with a list size of 2000 people
Stroke	200	0.25
Carpal tunnel syndrome	100	0.5
First epileptic (non-febrile) seizure	50	1.0
Transient ischaemic attack	50	1.0
Bell's palsy	25	2.0
Essential tremor	24	2.1
Parkinson's disease	20	2.5
Primary brain tumour	15	3.3
Secondary brain tumour	14	3.6
Multiple sclerosis (Scotland)	12	4.2
Subarachnoid haemorrhage	10	5.0
Essential tremor	8	6.3
Giant-cell arteritis	6	8.3
Migrainous neuralgia	6	8.3
Unexplained motor symptoms	5	10
Trigeminal neuralgia	4	13
Meningococcal meningitis (UK)	3	17
Transient global amnesia	3	17
Guillain–Barré syndrome	2	25
Intracranial vascular malformation	2	25
Motor neuron disease	2	25
Neuralgic amyotrophy	2	25
Progressive supranuclear palsy	1	50
Diabetic amyotrophy	1	50
Benign intracranial hypertension	1	50
Focal dystonia	1	50
Myasthenia gravis	1	50
Polymyositis/dermatomyositis	1	50
Hemifacial spasm	0.8	63
Multiple system atrophy	0.6	83
Gilles de la Tourette syndrome	0.5	100
Pneumococcal meningitis (UK)	0.5	100
Herpes simplex encephalitis	0.3	250
Creutzfeldt–Jakob disease (sporadic)	0.1	500
Tetanus	0.1	500
Subacute sclerosing panencephalitis	0.03	1667
New variant Creutzfeldt–Jakob disease (UK)	0.02	2500

These figures are all very approximate. They have been taken from various, more-or-less sound, community-based epidemiological studies in Europe or North America and a large survey of general practice in the UK (MacDonald *et al.* 2000). When more than one study is available, an approximate average rate has been used. The exact rates will generally depend on the age and sex structure of the population (which varies between communities), the size of the population (which will influence the precision of any estimate), and on the precise diagnostic criteria (which also vary). However, the rates give a general idea of incidence and how common, or rare, some neurological disorders are.

examination, which generally is either reassuringly normal or merely confirms features anticipated from the history. However, sometimes examination is crucially helpful. For instance, in localizing the cause of muscle weakness, specific physical signs will reveal whether the lesion affects the upper motor neuron, the lower motor neuron, or the muscle. An unanticipated physical sign, such as an extensor plantar response, signifying pyramidal-tract damage, or papilloedema, signifying raised

Table 1.2. The approximate prevalence of various neurological disorders and how frequently they are present in an average general practice (family practice) of 10 000 people looked after by five doctors

	Prevalence/100 000	Number of cases in a general practice with 10 000 people
Migraine	10 000	1 000
Chronic tension headache	3 000	300
Stroke	800	80
Alzheimer's disease	800	80
Active epilepsy	500	50
Essential tremor	300	30
Multiple sclerosis (Scotland)	200	20
Chronic fatigue syndrome	200	20
Parkinson's disease	160	16
Migrainous neuralgia	40	4
Unexplained motor symptoms	38	4
Neurofibromatosis (type 1)	13	1
Myasthenia gravis	10	1
Hemifacial spasm	10	1
Narcolepsy syndrome	10	1
Huntington's disease	8	<1
Myotonic dystrophy	7	<1
Syringomyelia	7	<1
Progressive supranuclear palsy	5	<1
Motor neuron disease	5	<1
Duchenne muscular dystrophy	4	<1
Fascioscapulohumoral dystrophy	3	<1
Mitochondrial cytopathy	2	<1
Multiple system atrophy	2	<1
Chronic inflammatory demyelinating neuropathy	1	<1
Tuberous sclerosis	1	<1
Wilson's disease	0.4	<1

These figures are all very approximate. They have been taken from various, more-or-less sound, community-based epidemiological studies in Europe or North America and a large survey of general practice in the UK (MacDonald *et al.* 2000). When more than one study is available, an approximate average rate has been used. The exact rates will generally depend on the age and sex structure of the population (which varies between communities), the size of the population (which will influence the precision of any estimate), and on the precise diagnostic criteria (which also vary). However, the rates give a general idea of prevalence and how common, or rare, some neurological disorders are.

intracranial pressure, will alter one's diagnostic view fundamentally if the history has pointed to diagnoses such as psychologically determined weakness or benign tension headache.

With experience one recognizes that patients often describe the symptoms of certain disorders in a very distinctive way. Intuitive recognition of a characteristic history plays a large part in diagnosis. There is no particular list of questions to ask. It is best to invite the patient to describe their symptoms in the order in which they occurred, with approximate dates. Important detail can be clarified by specific questioning during or after the patient's account. It is helpful to determine whether the patient's symptoms are so 'disabling' as to prevent crucial everyday activities or work, or whether they merely constitute a 'nuisance'. This will guide the decision as to whether a symptom such as headache needs treatment.

Some features of the history provide important clues to the neurological diagnosis. Questions about them should be phrased in open terms which do not influence the patient's response:

Time course

Symptoms of abrupt or instantaneous onset usually indicate epilepsy (sudden loss of consciousness) or cerebrovascular disease (instantaneous headache of subarachnoid haemorrhage, or sudden hemiparesis due to middle cerebral artery embolus). Symptoms that deteriorate subacutely, over hours, days, or even a few weeks are generally caused by inflammatory or demyelinating disorders. Slowly deteriorating symptoms over some weeks, months, or years point to the growth of a tumour, or a neurodegenerative process. Relapsing and remitting symptoms,

Table 1.3. Most common conditions seen by neurologists (from Donaghy 1997)

Headache and face pain
Blackouts and epilepsy
Peripheral nerve and root disorders
Cerebrovascular disease
Multiple sclerosis
Parkinsonism and movement disorders
Dementia
Giddiness and vertigo
Psychologically determined symptoms

which come and go over weeks, are typical of multiple sclerosis, whereas recurrent headaches, each lasting 3 hours to 3 days, are typical of migraine.

Negative symptoms

Negative symptoms are those in which normal neurological functions are lost, and are the most common symptoms of damage to the nervous system. Examples include the hemiparesis due to cerebral-hemisphere infarction, memory loss due to Alzheimer's disease, muscle weakness due to motor neuron degeneration, or the loss of micturition control due to a cauda equina tumour.

Positive symptoms

Positive symptoms are novel phenomena which often suggest specific diagnoses. A 'pill-rolling' tremor of the fingers and thumb at rest is characteristic of Parkinson's disease. Flashing lights (photopsia) or zigzag lines (fortification spectra) preceding a headache are diagnostic of classical migraine. Repetitive twitching of the fingers or the corner of the mouth occurs in focal motor seizures. A hallucination of an odd smell, often like burning rubber, is typical of an epileptic discharge in the temporal lobe. Tingling in the toes and fingers is typical of acquired, rather than inherited, peripheral neuropathy.

Neuroanatomical localization

Sometimes enquiry about other specific symptoms is necessary to localize the disease process anatomically. For example, a patient with suspected motor neuron disease should be asked whether there are sensory or sphincter symptoms which might point to the alternative diagnoses of generalized peripheral neuropathy or to spinal cord compression. A patient with sensory symptoms in the legs should be asked whether their hands are also affected; this would be a pointer to a polyneuropathy or cervical myelopathy rather than a focal lesion of the cauda equina or thoracic spinal cord. Determine whether a patient with dysphasia also has impaired spatial abilities, such as a dressing apraxia or getting lost in familiar places; this would point to a generalized dementing process involving both cerebral hemispheres rather than a focal lesion of the left hemi-

sphere causing isolated dysphasia. Question a patient with gait unsteadiness about vertigo or double vision, which would imply damage to the brainstem rather than to the cerebellum or somatosensory pathways.

Eye witness description

Patients with blackouts are unaware of what they did while unconscious and may not recollect the onset of the blackout. Thus, an eye witness description of a convulsion or automatic behaviour is diagnostic of epilepsy. In a patient with early dementia, it is often the spouse who provides the evidence for loss of intellectual function: forgetting the grandchildren's names, inability to do the usual crossword, or personality change. Patients with motor neuron diseases are often unaware of their limb muscle fasciculations, yet their spouse may have noticed their occurrence while in bed.

Previous neurological history

This is vital for establishing the diagnosis of multiple sclerosis, a neurological disorder which is disseminated in space and time. Thus, a history of temporary unilateral visual loss due to optic neuritis a decade previously suggests multiple sclerosis in a 30-year-old woman with unsteady gait and urgency of micturition due to an incomplete spinal cord lesion.

Familial disorders

Many neurological disorders are genetic, although each of these is usually rare. Examination of the relatives of a patient with longstanding muscle wasting and weakness below the knees, and with high foot arches (pes cavus), may reveal autosomal dominant inheritance of a similar disorder, so allowing diagnosis of hereditary motor and sensory neuropathy, otherwise known as Charcot–Marie–Tooth disease. First-cousin marriage between the parents may be a clue to autosomal recessive disorders in offspring with neurological disease. Sex-linked recessive disorders, transmitted on the X chromosome and occurring in males, will not manifest in the mother, but may be present in the males of earlier or parallel generations.

Contributory general medical disorders

Progressively deteriorating neurological symptoms should prompt questions about a possible underlying cancer affecting the nervous system: smoking, weight loss, haemoptysis, bowel symptoms, and recent breast and gynaecological check-ups. In a patient with stroke, a previous history of ischaemic or valvar heart disease, hypertension, diabetes, oral contraceptive usage, migraine, or cocaine abuse may be relevant. Unusual neurological disorders, such as opportunistic infections or lymphoma of the central nervous system, are particularly likely in the increasing numbers of immunosuppressed patients who are HIV infected, or have received organ transplants. Typical neurological side-effects of medicines are headache, giddiness, tremulousness tinglings, and peripheral neuropathy; a patient's drugs should be checked in a pharmacopoeia for side-effects, and the onset of the symptoms related to the introduction of the drug. The travel history may increase the likelihood that a patient's symptoms are due to an underlying infection such as leprosy, schistosomiasis, malaria, diphtheria, or borreliosis. Patients addicted to alcohol or recreational drugs are notorious for underestimating or denying consumption, which may be directly relevant to disorders such as ataxia and stroke, respectively.

1.3.2 General neurological examination

Present-day neurology has acquired a reputation for being both complicated and arcane because of the huge diversity of examination techniques that have been described. This has led, in turn, to the notion that there is an excessively lengthy entity called 'a full neurological examination' which utilizes this vast panoply of examination manoeuvres. Also, there is a commonly held belief that if one religiously executes all those manoeuvres, a diagnosis will miraculously appear. In reality, the diagnostic process is one of intuition, which involves devising a selective examination to answer diagnostic hypotheses posed by the symptoms of the particular patient in question. For instance, it is usually pointless to undertake cognitive testing in a patient who has given a cogent history of paraesthesiae in an arm, or to undertake detailed muscle power examination in a patient presenting with cognitive decline.

Many of the described examination manoeuvres are simply alternative methods of detecting the same pathological signature. Therefore to use more than one of them introduces unnecessary redundancy and repetition to the examination. For instance, a cerebellar lesion affecting the arm can be detected by the finger–nose test, by dysdiadochokinesis, by demonstrating 'cerebellar hypotonia' (Section 1.5.2), or by showing 'underdamping' when the outstretched arm is displaced with the eyes closed. Experienced neurologists develop sensitive and critical, yet economical, examination skills. They may recognize that a properly conducted finger–nose test is the only test that need be performed to demonstrate a cerebellar disorder of the

Table 1.4. A general neurological examination (after Donaghy 1997)

1. During history-taking note:		Speech and cognition
		Facial expression
		Involuntary movements
2. With patient standing note:		Normal gait
		Heel–toe gait
		Romberg's test
3. With patient sitting note:	Cranial nerves:	Fundoscopy (IInd cranial nerve)
		Visual fields (II)
		Horizontal eye movements (III, VI)
		Pupil–light responses (afferent II; efferent III)
		Facial sensation (V)
		Facial movements (VII)
		Hearing (VIII)
		Palatal movement (X)
		Tongue movement (XIII)
	The arms:	Inspection
		Tone
		Power (shoulder abduction and finger spreading)
		Finger–nose co-ordination
4. With the patient lying, note:	The arms (cont.):	Tendon reflexes (biceps and triceps)
	The legs:	Inspection
		Ankle clonus
		Power (hip flexion and ankle dorsiflexion)
		Tendon reflexes (knee and ankle)
		Plantar responses
5. Then carry out additional examination tests as required by history or by abnormalities on the examination thus far		

arm. A valuable physical sign offers proof that an abnormality is present. Less valuable signs merely suggest one. The worth of trying to elicit different signs varies accordingly.

Many tests are of limited usefulness because they do not provide objective evidence of abnormality. Examples include the patient's subjective responses to visual or somatosensory testing, or the influence of psychological factors on exertion of muscle power. Consequently a useful neurological examination will be rich in manoeuvres which can provide unequivocal evidence of pathology. These include inspection for papilloedema, testing pupil–light reflexes and eye movements, examining for cogwheel rigidity, noting muscle wasting and detecting absent tendon reflexes, extensor plantar responses, or sustained ankle clonus. For this reason it is recommended that physicians develop a brief basic neurological examination for routine use which is rich in testing for such unequivocal physical signs (Donaghy 1997).

Such basic neurological examinations need take only a few minutes. The ensuing example of a quick screening examination includes practical advice, such as how to phrase instructions, where to place the hands for best effect, and how to interpret fundamentals such as abnormal reflexes. This basic examination is quite adequate for examining a patient with uncomplicated headache or epilepsy, or as part of a general medical examination for a patient without neurological symptoms. Other tests should be added on to this examination if the patient's symptoms suggest a particular disease, or if abnormalities requiring further assessment are encountered during the basic examination.

It is practical to perform this basic examination in four stages: first, during history-taking; secondly, while the patient is walking; thirdly, while the patient is sitting facing you; and, fourthly, while the patient is lying down (Table 1.4) (Donaghy 1997).

During history taking

Speech and cognition

Abnormalities of speech, thought, or memory raise questions of dysphasia or generalized dementia. Dysarthic speech is slurred. Dysphonic speech is quiet.

Facial expression

An impassive face suggests Parkinson's disease, or occasionally a bilateral facial palsy. A melancholy facial expression occurs in depression. Dementia reduces the use of facial expression and gesture for non-verbal communication.

Involuntary movements

Pill-rolling tremor of the fingers at rest is characteristic of Parkinson's disease. Sudden choreiform movements of the hands, which may look like fidgets, occur in Huntingdon's disease and are often disguised as mannerisms. Spasms of closure of one eye occur in hemifacial spasm. Fixed or spasmodic head rotation to the side occurs in torticollis.

With the patient standing

Gait

In the wide-based gait of ataxia the feet cross more than the usual 5 cm apart, and the stride length is irregular. Uniformly small strides occur in the gait apraxia of frontal-lobe disease. Difficulty in starting, shuffling, and then progressively lengthening strides occur in parkinsonism. Arm swing is lost in Parkinson's disease, usually unilaterally early on. Floppy foot drops occur in peripheral nerve or nerve root disease. Stiff foot drops occur in spastic upper motor neuron lesions, or occasionally in dystonia. A waddling gait, with drop of the pelvis on the striding side, occurs in proximal muscle weakness due to myopathy.

Heel-to-toe walking

This is a sensitive screen for cerebellar disease, or sensorimotor abnormalities affecting the limbs. It is best tested by instructing 'Please walk heel-to-toe, like this' while the examiner demonstrates two or three such steps. Patients will stumble to the side if they have ataxia due to cerebellar disease, or loss of leg proprioception due to peripheral neuropathy or dorsal column disease.

Romberg's test

This is an excellent test for loss of proprioceptive feedback from the legs in peripheral neuropathy or dorsal column disease. In patients with abnormal heel-toe walking, it differentiates those with ataxia due to loss of proprioceptive feedback from those with ataxia due to cerebellar disease. It is best tested by the examiner instructing 'stand with your feet together like this (while demonstrating), get your bearings, and now close your eyes—I won't let you fall', while preparing to steady the patient's shoulders with his hands if the patient begins to topple. Romberg's test is positive if the patient falls, or is unable to maintain balance without corrective movements of the feet. It is important to realize that a correctly performed Romberg's test does not merely test balance with the eyes closed, but compares stability with and without vision. A truly positive Romberg's test takes some moments to develop, with an increasing amplitude of slow swaying until a critical degree of lean occurs, beyond which the patient can no longer remain upright. Not uncommonly one encounters patients who promptly fall in one direction immediately upon closing their eyes; this usually results from lack of confidence or is otherwise psychologically determined, and rarely indicates structural disease of the nervous system.

With the patient sitting

Ophthalmoscopy

Inspect the optic nerve head, also called the optic disc. It is most important to understand the location of the optic nerve head (which corresponds to the blind spot) within the visual field and its corresponding position in the eye. This enables the patient's direction of gaze to be aligned so that the examiner can look into their eye confident of looking directly at, or very near to, the optic disc. The blind spot, which represents the optic disc, lies about 20° of visual angle lateral to the point of fixation in each eye. It also lies just below the horizontal. This determines the 'line of attack'. Therefore the patient should be asked to fixate on a point behind the examiner chosen for height so that he is able to look into the eye comfortably from just below its horizontal meridian. The particular fixation point chosen will depend upon the relative heights of the examiner's and the patient's heads. The ophthalmoscope should be used with one's right eye to examine the patient's right eye, and vice versa for the left, looking into the eye from about 20° lateral to the line of fixation, and from just below the line of sight.

Examine whether the edge of the optic disc is sharply defined as is normal, or has blurred edges, suggesting disc swelling due to papilloedema resulting from raised intracranial pressure. A pale or white disc is due to optic atrophy. Having inspected the optic disc, the vessels and more peripheral parts of the retina can be scrutinized, for instance if diabetic retinopathy is suspected. The foveal pit, or macula, can be inspected while the patient stares directly at an ophthalmoscope beam adjusted to the small spot.

Visual fields

It is time-consuming and rarely rewarding to carry out detailed examination of the peripheral and central portions of the visual fields of each eye separately unless the patient has symptoms of visual or pituitary disease. The following quick manoeuvre is a simple screen for homonymous heminanopia (an identical visual field deficit in both eyes due to cerebral-hemisphere disease), and for sensory inattention (due to parietal lobe lesions). The patient is asked to 'keep looking at my nose and point to whichever of my index fingers moves'. The examiner's arms are raised so as to position the index fingers at about 80° peripheral in each visual field. After a moment the tips of both index fingers should be moved once while keeping the rest of the arm still; the patient should point immediately to both sides. If the patient has sensory inattention or a homonymous hemianopia, they will only see movement on one side despite simultaneous movement of the fingers on both sides, and further analysis of the deficit can be undertaken. A red pinhead, or perimetry techniques, are often required for accurate detection and delineation of more subtle visual field defects. These

include red desaturation monocularly in the temporal field in optic chiasm lesions, or the monocular partial central scotoma so common in optic neuritis.

Eye movements

Inspection of the patient's face when gazing straight ahead will show the drooping eyelid of ptosis. This is easier to detect when unilateral. In a definite ptosis, the eyelid will overlap the edge of the pupil.

To test eye movements, ask the patient 'to hold your chin with one hand (in order to prevent head movements) and then follow my finger with your eyes'. A finger or a stick is held vertically and moved laterally to about 50 or 60°. After holding it still for a moment, ask the patient whether he sees it as single or double. Simultaneously inspect the eyes carefully to detect nystagmus or any paralysis of ocular movement. Vertical eye movements can be tested similarly by holding a finger horizontally and moving it up and then down by about 45°. Many elderly patients develop clinically insignificant loss of upgaze.

Pupils

To test the pupil–light reflex, the patient should be asked to fixate the examiner's nose while he notes the size of the pupils before light stimulation. If it is very difficult to see the pupil because of dim illumination, or a darkly pigmented iris, it helps to shine the torch beam at the bridge of the nose so that light scatter is enough to make the pupil visible, without stimulating the pupil–light response by shining the light directly into the eye. Secondly, shine the torch directly into the left eye and observe that both pupils constrict equally; this elicits the direct pupil–light response on the left and the indirect (or consensual) response on the right. Thirdly, swing the torch beam quickly across to the right eye and check that there is no further dilatation or constriction of either pupil. This swinging torch test compares the amplitude of the direct and consensual pupil responses of each eye. If there were an optic nerve lesion on the right, both pupils would dilate slightly when the torch was shone in the right eye, compared to their normal constriction following left eye stimulation. This way of comparing the pupil responses has the sensitivity to detect relative, rather than absolute, afferent pupillary defects due to partial optic nerve lesions, as may occur in optic neuritis.

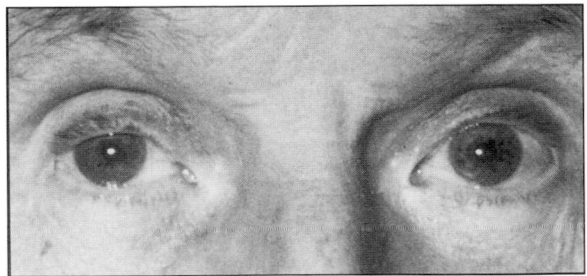 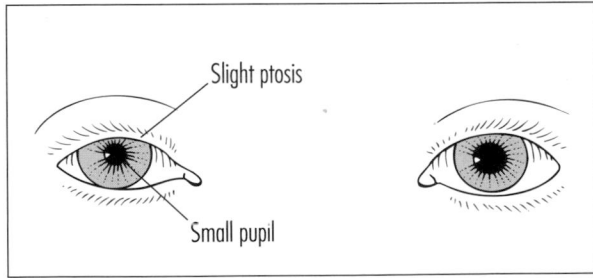

Fig. 1.10. Right-sided Horner's syndrome showing a slight degree of ptosis and a small pupil (from Donaghy 1997).

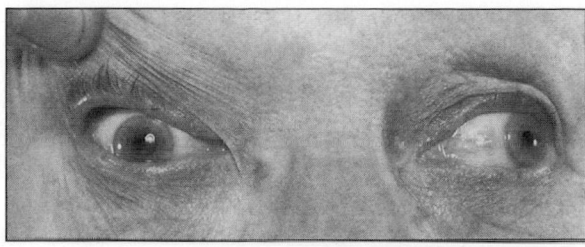 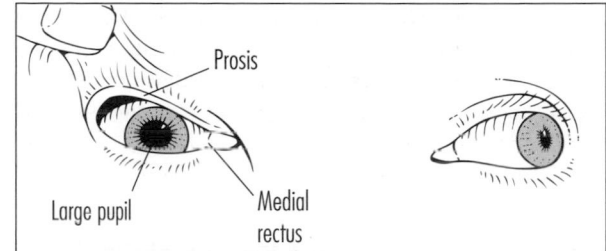

Fig. 1.11. Right-sided third nerve palsy showing marked ptosis, a dilated pupil, and medial rectus weakness (from Donaghy 1997).

A unilaterally small pupil is most usually due to a cervical sympathetic pathway lesion (Horner's syndrome) which will be associated with no more than a slight degree of eyelid drooping (ptosis) (Fig. 1.10).

A unilaterally, fixedly dilated pupil is typical of an oculomotor nerve lesion (cranial nerve III) (Fig. 1.11), in which there will also be impairment of adduction and vertical eye movement, and the ptosis will be usually much more marked than in Horner's syndrome.

Facial sensation

The fingertips of both the examiner's hands are lightly drawn on both sides simultaneously across the patient's forehead, to the cheek and nose, and then onto the chin. While covering all three territories of the trigeminal nerve, frontal (V_1), maxillary (V_2) and mandibular (V_3), he should ask 'Do my fingers feel normal and the same on each side?'. Any area of altered sensation can be tested in more detail and mapped out using a pin or a wisp of cotton wool. Testing the corneal reflex with a wisp of cotton wool is not necessary as a routine.

Facial movements

Subtle degrees of facial weakness, such as unilateral slowing of movement, are best seen if the examiner steps back a couple of paces so as to see both sides of the patient's mouth simultaneously within his central vision. Movement of the mouth can be produced by saying 'show me your teeth like this' or 'give me a smile'; if smiled at while hearing this instruction, patients often respond with an involuntary grin which demonstrates facial movements perfectly. Observe whether both sides of the mouth move equally quickly, and produce similar elevation and deepening of the nasolabial skin creases. If the mouth movement is asymmetrical, indicating unilateral weakness, ask the patient to 'raise your eyebrows' to see whether both sides of the frontalis muscle in the forehead contract equally. Lower motor neuron lesions of the seventh nerve will affect movements of both the forehead and the mouth. Unilateral upper motor neuron facial paralysis affects only the mouth and lower face, but not the forehead.

Hearing

The patient is instructed 'Could you repeat this number?' while the examiner lightly rubs the tip of his finger in the left ear to create a masking noise and whispers a number from about 2 feet (60 cm) away so as to test hearing in the right ear, and vice versa to test the left ear. Unilateral or bilateral deafness should be assessed further by Weber's and Rinne's tests (Section 1.3.3) to distinguish between conductive and sensorineural deafness, and by otoscopic examination of the eardrum.

Palatal movements

These are best tested by asking the patient to open his or her mouth and say 'ah' while illuminating the throat with a torch. If the elevation of the palate and uvula is normal and symmetrical, and there is no swallowing difficulty or dysphonia, there is no need for the discomfort of eliciting the gag reflex as a routine. When necessary, the gag reflex is elicited by stimulating one side of the soft palate with a stick and watching the resultant rise of both sides of the palate.

Tongue movement

It is best to inspect the tongue for wasting or fasciculations while it is relaxed on the floor of the mouth during examination of the palatal movements. It is misleading to look for fasciculations while the tongue is being actively protruded since most normal tongues show ripples and flickers under such circumstances. Tongue movements can be tested by asking the patient to 'stick out your tongue and move it from side to side like this' and demonstrate this movement. A lower motor neuron lesion affecting a hypoglossal nerve causes the tongue to be wasted on, and deviate towards, the same side as the lesion (Figs. 11.11 and 11.12). If an upper motor neuron lesion is bilateral, the tongue becomes spastic and square in profile and its movements limited and slow. In a cerebellar lesion, alternating tongue movements will be slowed and irregular.

The arms

Inspection

The profile of the upper arms should be inspected for muscle wasting or fasciculations, with the patient sitting facing towards the examiner. Then the hands should be inspected for muscle wasting, by looking particularly at the first dorsal interosseous muscles on the dorsum of the hand between the thumb and forefinger (innervated by the ulnar nerve), and the abductor pollicis brevis in the lateral part of the thenar eminence (innervated by the median nerve).

Tone

Either the extrapyramidal rigidity of Parkinson's disease, or the spasticity of an upper motor neuron lesion can be detected reliably in the arms. Different techniques are used to test for these tone changes. Which one is chosen should be determined by which of these conditions is suspected. Spasticity should be sought by holding the patient's hand with the elbow flexed, and abruptly supinating the forearm to detect a sudden jerk of spastic resistance known as a 'pronator catch'. The 'cogwheel rigidity' of Parkinson's disease is best detected by holding the patient's wrist with one hand, and repeatedly flexing and extending the fingers and wrist by gripping the tips of the fingers with the other hand. The term 'cogwheel rigidity' merely describes lead-pipe rigidity with superimposed tremor.

Power

For general screening purposes, it is sufficient to test one proximal and one distal muscle in each arm. The best proximal muscle to test is shoulder abduction to 90° by deltoid (C5 root, axillary nerve). A good distal muscle to test is the first dorsal interosseous (T1 root, ulnar nerve), which spreads the fingers apart. Its power can be compared with the examiner's own first dorsal interosseous muscle. Additional muscles should be tested if a lesion of a particular peripheral nerve or root is suspected.

Coordination

The finger–nose test is the most reliable but is only sensitive if the patient is required to stretch their arm out fully from the shoulder to touch the examiner's target finger. The examiner should stand well behind his own outstretched target finger so as to detect the randomly distributed inaccuracies in the patient's pointing known as ataxia or dysmetria. Dysmetria on this test usually indicates cerebellar disease (cerebellar ataxia), or loss of proprioceptive feedback (sensory ataxia), but can occur in proximal muscle weakness. If ataxia is detected, pseudoathetosis indicative of loss of sensory feedback can be sought by asking the patient to hold out the arms horizontally with the eyes closed, with the fingers extended and spread apart; if pseudoathetosis is present, the fingers wander and fail to remain in position (Fig. 12.16).

With the patient lying down

Arm tendon reflexes

The biceps reflexes (musculocutaneous nerve; fifth and sixth cervical roots) should be tested from the patient's right side. The examiner's thumb should be used to transmit a firm blow from the tendon hammer to the biceps tendon within the cramped space of the antecubital fossa so as to elicit a visible or palpable contraction of the biceps muscle. When testing the triceps reflex (radial nerve; seventh and eighth cervical roots), the hammerhead should hit the tendon at right angles just above the elbow, because the triceps muscle has an extremely short tendon. The brachioradialis reflex (radial nerve; sixth cervical root) is difficult to elicit reliably and rarely adds extra information unless a C6 root lesion is suspected, or the examiner is trying to localize or detect a radial nerve lesion. Tendon reflexes are brisk in upper motor neuron lesions. An absent tendon reflex will be due to a peripheral nerve or nerve root lesion. Before concluding that a reflex is absent, reinforcement should be undertaken by asking the patient to 'bite your teeth together when I say "bite"' while you try simultaneously to elicit the reflex.

The legs

Inspection

The bulk of the vastus medialis component of quadriceps just above and medial to the kneecap can be observed by asking the patient to 'tighten your kneecaps'. The bulk of more distal muscles can be demonstrated by asking the patient to 'cock your toes up towards you' while checking that the tibialis anterior muscle bulges in front of the anterior border of the tibial bone. The leg muscles should be inspected for fasciculations, which are visible flickering contractions within the muscle belly, insufficient to produce movement around the joint. They signify disease of the lower motor neuron, for instance in motor neuron disease. Sometimes fasciculations are visible in other-

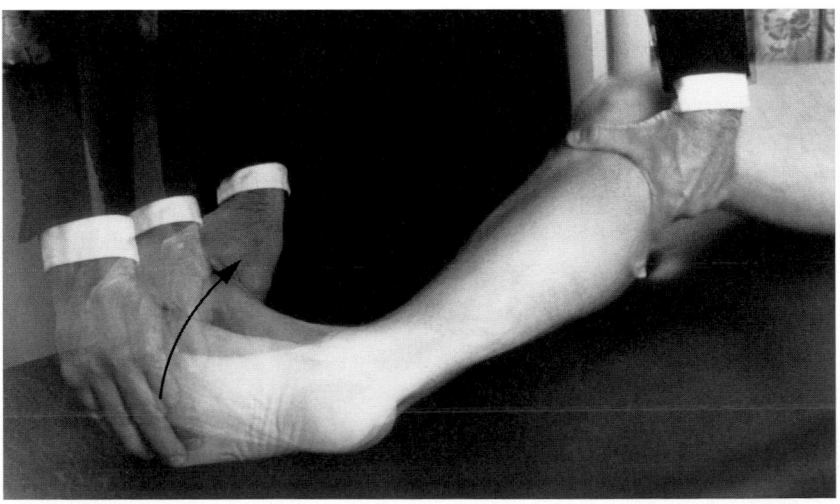

Fig. 1.12. Eliciting ankle clonus (from Donaghy 1997).

wise normal calf muscles of healthy individuals, particularly after exercise. Skin ulcers, burns, or disrupted joints (Charcot joints) may be trophic changes resulting from loss of protective pain sensation.

Tone

The spasticity of an upper motor neuron lesion, observed as clonus, is the most reliably objective tone change detectable in the legs. Ankle clonus is elicited by externally rotating the foot and holding the knee slightly flexed with one hand, while sharply jerking the sole of the foot upwards with the other hand (Fig. 1.12). For a few seconds the foot should be held firmly in sustained dorsiflexion since the rhythmic downward beatings of clonus may take a moment or two to become evident. Sustained clonus, or unsustained clonus of more than six beats, is generally regarded as definite evidence of an upper motor neuron lesion.

Power

Testing of one proximal and one distal muscle in each leg is sufficient to screen for the weakness of unexpected myopathies (proximal), peripheral neuropathy (distal) or upper motor neuron lesions (both proximal and distal). Proximal leg power is reflected by hip flexion (iliopsoas muscle, first and second lumbar roots), best tested by instructing the patient to 'push your leg up to 45 degrees' and then for the examiner to press downwards just above the knee. A distal muscle, the tibialis anterior (peroneal nerve, fifth lumbar root), is tested by asking the patient to 'cock your foot up towards you' while the examiner tries to overcome this dorsiflexion at the ankle. The tibialis anterior is a particularly valuable muscle to test, since it will be weakened by upper motor neuron lesions, polyneuropathy, common peroneal nerve lesions, and in L5/S1 root lesions due to prolapsed intervertebral disc. Some leg muscles are so naturally powerful that milder degrees of weakness cannot be detected reliably by bedside testing. For instance, mild weakness of knee extension by quadriceps (femoral nerve; third and fourth lumbar roots) may be revealed best by asking a patient to stand up from a chair without using his or her arms. Ankle plantar flexion by gastrocnemius (posterior tibial nerve; first

and second sacral roots) is best tested by asking a patient to stand on tiptoe or even to hop.

Tendon reflexes

The knee jerk or quadriceps tendon reflex (femoral nerve; L3/4) is elicited by lifting and flexing both knees over the examiner's left arm by 60–90°, and then striking the two patellar tendons in turn to compare the reflex on both sides. The ankle jerk or gastrocnemius or Achilles tendon reflex (posterior tibial nerve; S1/S2) is best tested by externally rotating the foot with the knee slightly bent, gently dorsiflexing the knee, and then striking the Achilles tendon firmly with the hammer (Fig. 1.13). Poor technique is often responsible for apparent absence of the ankle jerks; the examiner may not have struck the Achilles tendon sufficiently firmly, or the patient may be 'helping' by holding the foot rigidly in dorsiflexion. Brisk tendon reflexes point to an upper motor neuron lesion, in which case sustained ankle clonus or an extensor plantar response would also be expected. Slightly brisk reflexes may occur in anxious, tense patients. The reflexes are absent in peripheral nerve or root lesions. The ankle jerks are absent in many people over the age of 70. As with the arm reflexes, reinforcement should be undertaken before finally declaring a reflex absent.

Plantar responses

An extensor plantar, or Babinski, response (Fig. 1.14) is a definite sign of an upper motor neuron lesion. It is present from the moment of the upper motor neuron lesion, well before sufficient spasticity has developed to allow clonus or hyperreflexia.

Technique is all-important for eliciting the plantar response reliably (Fig. 1.15). The patient should be lying down, unable to see his or her toes. The examiner should passively move the great toe up and down beforehand, both to ensure relaxation, and also to detect hallux rigidis, which would mask the toe movement. Then, lightly holding the leg just above the ankle with the left hand, a thin stick or a key is held in the right hand and slowly but firmly drawn up the outer aspect of the sole and across the ball of the foot. During this the examiner should watch the great toe from the side so as to detect whether its first

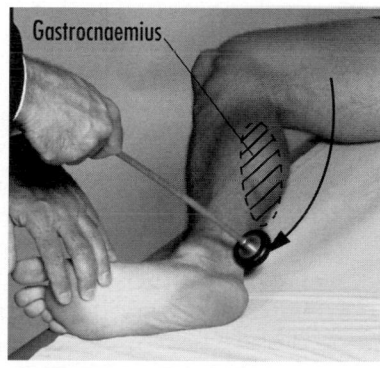

Gastrocnaemius

Fig. 1.13. Eliciting the ankle tendon jerks (from Donaghy 1997).

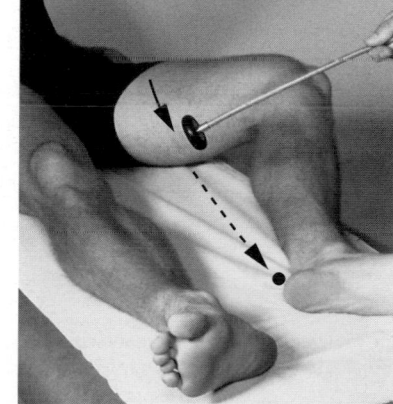

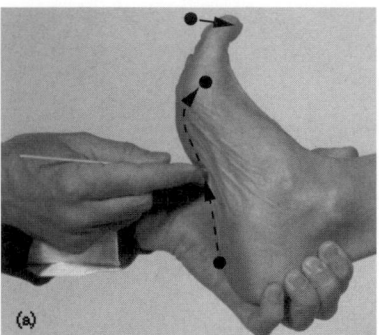
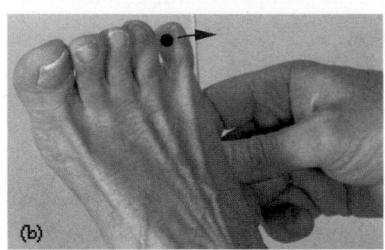

Fig. 1.14. An extensor plantar response, or Babinski's sign, showing (a) dorsiflexion of the great toe and (b) fanning of the little toe (from Donaghy 1997).

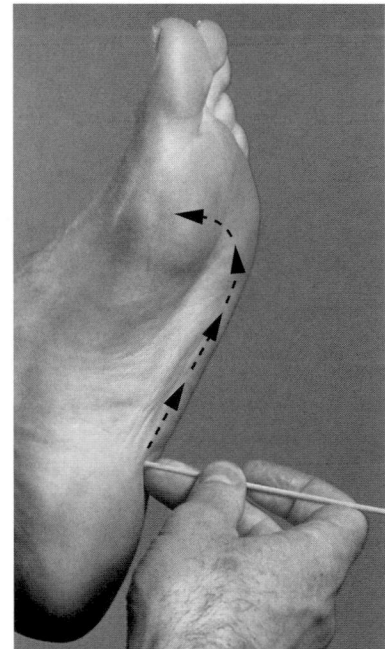

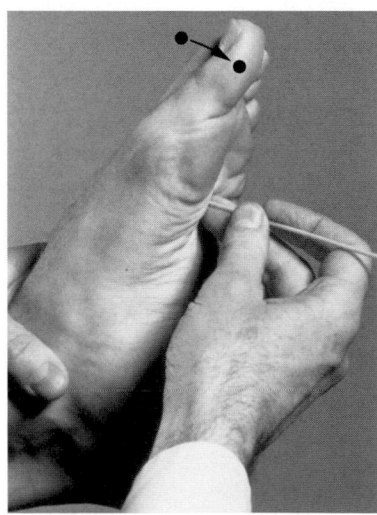

Fig. 1.15. Technique for eliciting the plantar response (a) showing a normal (flexor) response (b) (from Donaghy 1997).

movement is downwards (flexor and normal) or upwards (extensor and abnormal).

Sensory examination

In a patient without sensory symptoms, such as deadness or tingling, and whose Romberg test is normal, sensory examination is rarely abnormal. Generally it is not worth performing as a routine if disease of the sensory pathways is not suspected.

1.3.3 Specific clinical circumstances

The following examples show how other examination manoeuvres can be added to the general neurological examination (Section 1.3.2) if the patient's symptoms suggest a specific disorder, or if the basic examination has revealed abnormalities requiring further evaluation. More details concerning these examination findings and their interpretation are given in relevant chapters later in this volume.

Individual cranial nerves

The general neurological examination outlined in Section 1.3.2 does not test every cranial nerve in detail. The following main functions of each cranial nerve are easily testable, should the clinical situation require it:

I Olfactory. Test the ability to detect a smell in each nostril, while the other nostril is blocked, with the eyes closed. It is not necessary that the patient identify a particular smell. Easily available odours such as coffee, soap, or orange peel are quite adequate for testing.

II Optic. Fundoscopy; visual acuity using a Snellen chart held at 6 m; pupil–light response (afferent); visual fields can be tested either by confrontation, to detect movement of a finger, or by comparing the field within which a hatpin becomes seen as red (usually out to about 40°) when it is moved slowly in from the periphery exactly midway between examiner and patient. Visual fields can be tested with both eyes open when a homonymous field defect due to a lesion of the pathway after the optic chiasm is suspected. The visual field of each eye must be tested separately if a lesion of the retina, optic nerve, or optic chiasm is suspected.

III **Oculomotor**. Eye movements (horizontal adduction, up, down); eyelid elevation; pupil–light response (efferent).

IV **Trochlear**. Eye movement (down and in) is easily tested by asking the patient to 'look towards the tip of your nose'.

V **Trigeminal**. Jaw closure (masseter and temporalis); jaw opening (pterygoids); facial sensation; corneal reflex (afferent) using a wisp of cotton wool.

VI **Abducens**. Eye movement (horizontal abduction).

VII **Facial**. Facial muscles (test eyebrow elevation and smiling movements of the corners of the mouth); corneal reflex (efferent).

VIII **Auditory**. Hearing a whisper in each ear; Weber's and Rinne's tests with 512 Hz tuning fork to distinguish between conductive and sensorineural deafness. Weber's test involves putting the vibrating tuning fork on the middle of the forehead and asking 'is it louder on one side or in the middle?' Normally it is loudest in the middle, in sensorineural deafness it is louder on the opposite side, and in conductive deafness it is louder on the same side. Rinne's test compares the loudness of bone conduction at the mastoid process with air conduction in front of the pinna for each ear. Normally air conduction is louder, whereas bone conduction will be louder in conductive deafness. Otoscopic examination of the eardrum should be carried out if conductive deafness is detected.

IX **Glossopharyngeal**. An orange stick is used to test palatal sensation and to stimulate the gag reflex (afferent).

X **Vagus**. Palatal elevation; gag reflex (efferent); vocal cord movement (speaking, sharp cough).

XI **(Spinal) Accessory**. Shoulder shrugging and scapular rotation to abduct the arm beyond 90° (trapezius); head rotation laterally (sternomastoid).

XII **Hypoglossal**. Tongue protrusion.

A weak, areflexic, or numb limb

Commonly patients complain of neurological symptoms affecting a single limb. In such cases, or if abnormalities are found on general neurological examination, a wide range of muscles and sensory territories must be examined using a strategy to distinguish between polyneuropathy, root lesions, mononeuropathy, and myopathy. For example, if a patient has weakness of the first dorsal interosseous muscle (ulnar nerve, T1 root), but the abductor policis brevis (median nerve, T1) is normally strong, it is clear that there is an ulnar nerve lesion rather than a polyneuropathy or a T1 root lesion. Muscle strength can be assessed particularly sensitively in the arms by testing the strength of individual muscles, such as biceps or finger flexors and extensors, using the identical muscle in the examiner (Fig. 1.16). Full details of muscles innervated by individual peripheral nerves are given in Chapter 13.

Frequently tested muscles in the arm are:

◆ Shoulder abduction (0–15° supraspinatus, suprascapular nerve, C5 root; 15–90° deltoid, axillary nerve, C5 root).

◆ Biceps: elbow flexion (musculocutaneous nerve, C5/6 root). The patient's power of elbow flexion is compared with that of the examiner.

◆ Triceps: elbow extension (radial nerve, C7/8). The patient's power of elbow extension is compared with that of the examiner.

◆ Finger extensors: (radial/posterior interosseous nerve, C7). The examiner can use his own extended fingers to try and overcome the patient's extended fingers.

◆ Flexor digitorum profundus: terminal interphalangeal joint flexion (anterior interosseous branch of median nerve (index finger) or ulnar nerve (little finger), C7/8). The power of flexion of the terminal phalanx of the finger can be directly compared with the examiner's (Fig. 1.16).

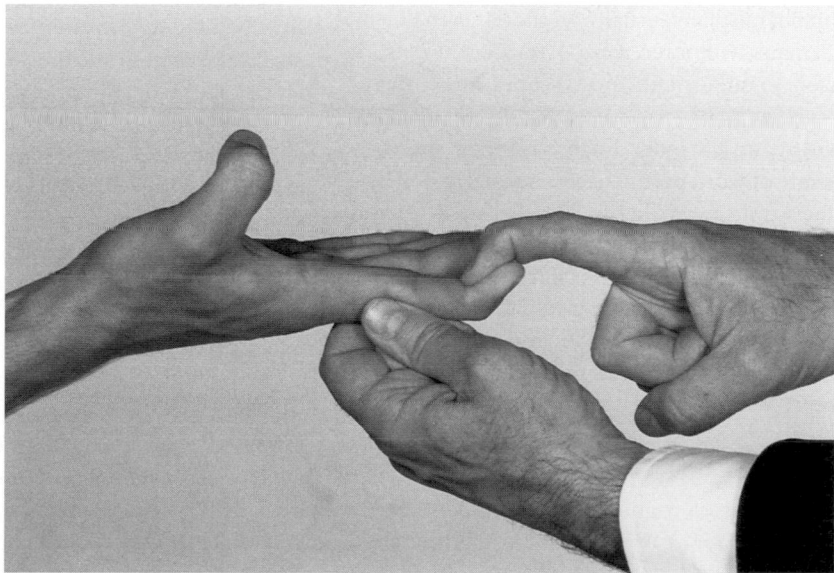

Fig. 1.16. Testing flexor digitorum profundus power. Compare the power of flexion at the distal interphalangeal joint by pulling against the patient's finger (from Donaghy 1997).

◆ Dorsal interosseous: finger abduction (ulnar nerve, T1).

◆ Abductor pollicis brevis: abduction of thumb at right angles to the palm (median nerve, T1).

Useful muscles to test in the leg include:

◆ Iliopsoas: hip flexion (innervated by lumbar plexus, L1/2 roots).

◆ Gluteus maximus: hip extension (inferior gluteal nerve, L5/S1). If hip extension is of normal power, the examiner can raise the patient's buttocks off the bed by lifting upwards at the ankle.

◆ Quadriceps: knee extension (femoral nerve, L3/4). This very powerful muscle must be tested with the knee starting flexed by at least 45°.

◆ Tibialis anterior: ankle dorsiflexion (peroneal nerve, L5).

◆ Gastrocnemius: ankle plantar flexion (tibial nerve, S1/2).

Speech disorders

Dysphonia is an inability to create noise properly from the larynx. The voice is quiet and somewhat featureless because the larynx produces sound inefficiently; patients are unable to shout. Attempts at producing a sharp, explosive cough are 'bovine' because the larynx cannot be tightly closed then suddenly opened. Dysarthria is an inability to shape that noise accurately into recognizable words. The tongue, pharynx, and lips are uncoordinated on trying to pronounce consonants. This becomes particularly obvious on repeating words rich in consonants, such as 'uNiVeRSiTy' or 'WeST ReGiSTeR STReeT' or 'BRiTiSH CoNSTiTuTioN'. Cerebellar incoordination makes these consonants slurred and slow, with 'scanning speech'. A pseudobulbar palsy produces a spastic immobile tongue with 'hot potato speech' or total anarthria (inability to speak at all).

Dysphasias are abnormalities of the understanding of, or the generation of, language. They result from damage to the speech areas of the cerebral hemisphere, usually on the left even in left-handed people. Patients with a receptive, Wernicke, or sensory dysphasia are unable to understand and execute a simple three-stage command such as 'When I clap my hands, please touch your right ear with your left index finger'. Yet their speech is fluent, in that the rate of word production is normal, but meaningless because the words are wrong or jumbled up. It should be noted that some patients are unable to execute commands because of dyspraxia, which is common in left cerebral-hemisphere lesions. A motor or Broca's dysphasia causes non-fluent speech, with a slowed rate of word production. Also there are obvious difficulties in finding the correct word and gestures are often used to compensate for the lack of verbal meaning.

Dementia

Dementia is a diffuse loss of cognitive function, particularly involving memory, due to generalized disease of both cerebral hemispheres. Diagnosing early dementia can be difficult and the spouse's observations are all-important. Initially minor symptoms may have been attributed to absent-mindedness. Then patients are noted to develop uncharacteristic errors of judgement, inability to perform their customary intellectual tasks, such as puzzles or games, loss of interest in hobbies and recreations, and inability to remember the names of friends and family. As the disease becomes more advanced, the personality is lost and patients may become disinhibited about the usual social codes of excretion or sexuality. Ultimately the patient becomes mute and unresponsive, wanders aimlessly, is incontinent, and dependent on feeding. Demented patients are vague or rambling during history taking, although this is sometimes masked by preserved social skills. Simple bedside clues to dementia involve checking the orientation for date and place; orientation for person usually being preserved except in psychiatric disease or simulated dementia. Calculation ability is usefully tested by serial subtraction of 7 from 100. General knowledge of everyday and historical events should be assessed, to judge whether it is consistent with the patient's educational and social background. Memory loss may be indicated by impaired immediate and 5-minute recall of a simple three-line address or of three objects. Cognitive estimates such as 'Roughly how long is a man's spine?' or 'How many camels are there in Holland?' may be abnormal in frontal lobe disease. If the patient's demeanour is flat or gloomy, it suggests depression, which may be a clue to potentially treatable pseudo-dementia. Self-neglect may be evident, as may be failure to use facial expression and gesture for non-verbal communication. Right parietal lobe spatial functions can be tested by asking the patient to draw or copy a three-dimensional cube. If a dysphasic component prevents understanding of such instructions, impaired spatial functioning may be revealed by dressing apraxia, in which the patient is unable to put on a dressing gown or shirt correctly when one of the sleeves has been pulled through the wrong way.

Impaired sphincter control

In a patient with hesitancy of micturition, or retention or incontinence of urine, the following aspects of examination are crucial. Extensor plantar responses point to a spinal-cord lesion affecting the upper motor neurones. Absent ankle jerks point to cauda equina compression or peripheral neuropathy. Blunted perianal pinprick sensation occurs in cauda equina lesions. The anal reflex can be tested by stroking the anal verge firmly with an orange stick, and looking for a reflex contraction which crinkles the anal skin. This reflex is lost in cauda equina lesions but is difficult to elicit reliably, with the response being particularly uncertain in older patients or those with a patulous anus.

Stroke

Cardiovascular examination is usually more informative than neurological examination to elucidate the underlying cause of stroke or transient ischaemic attacks. Cardiac arrhythmia, particularly atrial fibrillation, or hypertension may be significant. Possible sources of cerebral emboli may be revealed by ausculatation for cardiac murmurs indicative of valvar disease, and to the carotid arteries just below the angle of the jaw for the bruit of an internal carotid artery stenosis. When listening for carotid bruits, it is important to ask the patient to hold his breath so that breath sounds are not confused with a bruit. Cranial bruits, for instance due to a vascular malformation, are best heard by applying the stethoscope bell over the closed eyelid, and listening when the patient has opened the other eye and is fixating. This avoids distracting eye movement noises. Atrial septal defects, potentially allowing paradoxical emboli from the venous circulation, are suggested by the subtle finding of fixed splitting of the second heart sound during respiration.

Systemic malignancy

Progressive focal neurological abnormalities of the brain, spinal cord, or nerve roots raise the question of compression or infiltration by tumour. In such cases, the search for a primary systemic tumour should include examination of all lymph node groups, the breasts, testicles, chest (including chest radiograph), abdomen, rectum, and prostate or vagina.

Sciatica

Straight leg raising will be limited by pain to less than the normal 80–90° on the side of a prolapsed intervertebral disc affecting the L5 or S1 nerve roots. Muscles innervated by the different nerve roots under suspicion should be tested, particularly ankle dorsiflexion (L5). The briskness of the ankle jerks should be compared carefully on the two sides, if necessary from behind, with the patient kneeling on a chair. Pinprick sensation in the L5 dermatome on the dorsum of the foot and lateral leg below the knee, and in the S1 dermatome on the sole of the foot and back of the calf, should be compared on the two sides. The lumbar spine should be examined for focal tenderness or deformity, which might indicate a tumour deposit or infection in a vertebra.

Parkinsonism

During history-taking the patient may exhibit a paucity of facial expression or a characteristic pill-rolling tremor of the finger and thumb at rest. Observe walking for a slow and shuffling start, or loss of arm swing. Unilateral loss of arm swing whilst walking may be the earliest sign of Parkinson's disease. Cogwheel rigidity of the arms is a valuable objective

January 1995:   Before Treatment

July 1997:   After L–Dopa

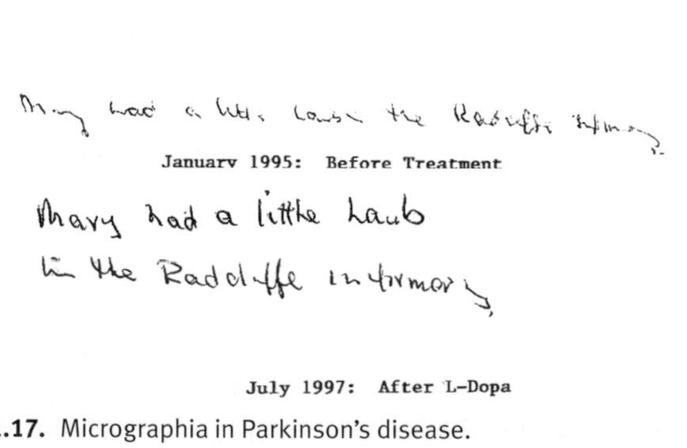

Fig. 1.17. Micrographia in Parkinson's disease.

test and is often more pronounced when the patient waves the other arm in the air. Test writing for micrographia (Fig. 1.17) in which the letters get smaller during the writing of a word, but note that some patients have learned to compensate for this by writing long words in batches of a few letters at a time, momentarily stopping or lifting the pen from the paper between these groups of letters.

Coma

A completely different strategy is required to examine unconscious patients, because of their inability to carry out instructions. The general medical examination may reveal cardiovascular shock, arrhythmia, respiratory failure, pyrexia, alcohol intoxication, pinpoint pupils of opiate overdose, or head trauma. Blood sugar testing with Dextrostix® will reveal hypo- or hyperglycaemia, and blood should be sent for toxicological analysis and creatinine measurement. Neck stiffness due to meningism is usually found in subarachnoid haemorrhage or meningitis, careful technique will detect mild neck rigidity (Fig 1.18). Regular or spontaneous breathing may be disrupted by damage to brainstem respiratory nuclei; Cheyne–Stokes respiration (irregular waxing and waning of respiration) is typical of cerebral-hemisphere lesions. The depth of unconsciousness is reflected by the extent of any withdrawal response to painful squeezing of the fingernails or toenails. If withdrawal is particularly reduced on one side, it points to a contralateral cerebral lesion. The plantar responses are usually bilaterally extensor in unconscious patients and have little specific diagnostic or localizing value. Decerebrate posturing, in which the limbs become stiffly extended, usually indicates a brainstem lesion. Generalized or focal seizures may be evident in status epilepticus or encephalitis, and can particularly affect the corner of the mouth, with repetitive twitching. Brainstem function can be tested by eliciting the vesibulo-ocular reflex of compensatory eye movement induced by head rotation, or by irrigation of the ears with cold water, the so-called caloric response. Brainstem integrity is also reflected by the corneal reflex of bilateral eye closure when one cornea is stimulated with a wisp of cotton wool, and by the cough and gag responses to laryngeal or pharyngeal stimulation with a sucker or stick.

1.3.4 Children

When parents bring their child to a neurologist they bring their most precious aspirations and very often their gravest concerns. This is the emotional setting to paediatric neurology. Clinical neurological evaluation of children requires a child-friendly environment with lack of medical equipment and white coats that could worry the child. A great deal of the child's ability to relax and perform is dependent upon the parent's confidence in the environment and in the person that they are speaking to. Toys for different aged children are required. Many children with neurological disease have a degree of cognitive delay and their ability to help with history and comply with examination is dependent upon developmental age, communicative intent,

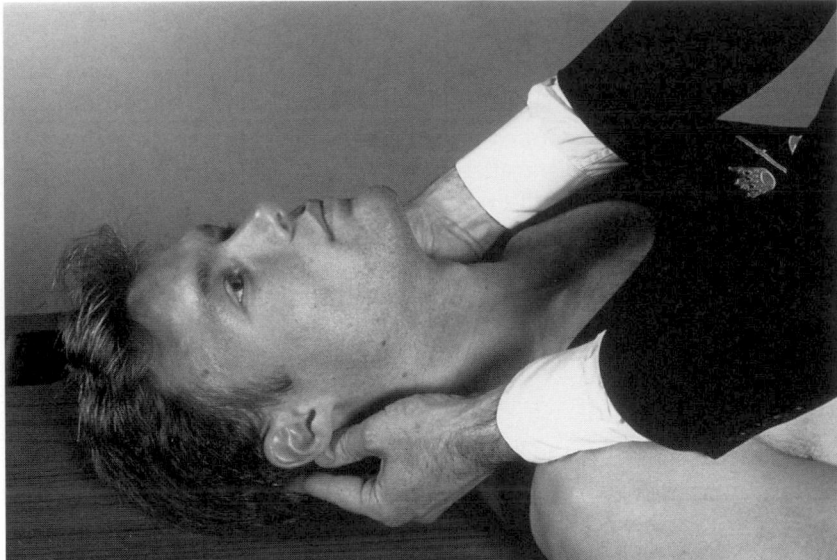

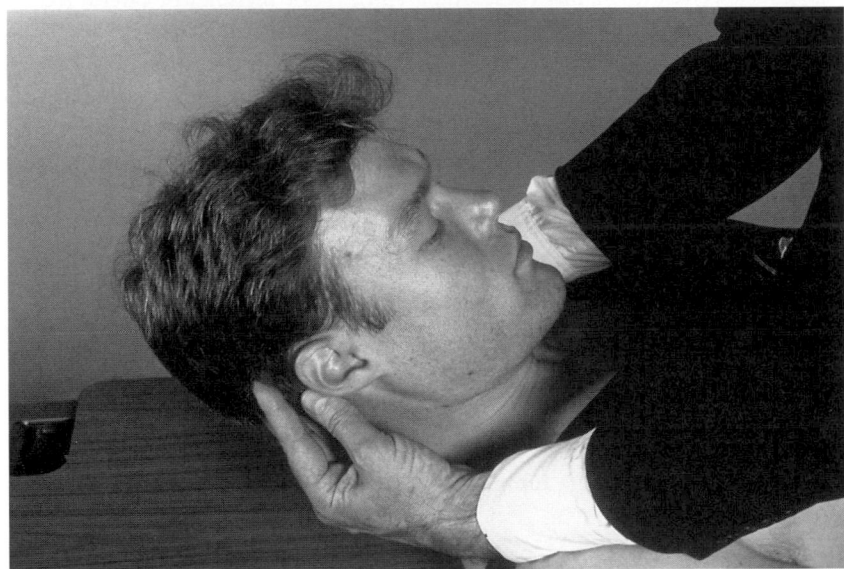

Fig. 1.18. A sensitive method to examine for neck stiffness in suspected meningitis or subarachnoid haemorrhage. The pillow should be removed to extend the neck, the extensor aspect of the examiner's wrists should be rested on the patient's shoulders, while inserting the fingers behind the mastoid processes to assess the degree of resistance while flexing the neck. (From Donaghy 1997.)

bulbar function, and attention control. Children are much more upset by intercurrent illness, such as otitis media which may temporarily but seriously impair a child's performance. Neurological assessment of children and infants follows the same principles as for adults, but that of neonates lies beyond the scope of this text.

History

Younger children cannot respond as specifically as adults to detailed questions about symptoms, particularly their time course. Children find it hard to give meaningful accounts of sensory symptoms or pain. Young children are often surprisingly undisturbed by serious negative symptoms involving loss of functions such as vision.

The parent or guardian's presence is important to reassure the child, to summarize the history and its chronology, to give their own observations of their child's condition, to provide consent, and to chaperone the physical examination. However, one should always try to obtain the child's own version, however rudimentary. Not only is history taking the most powerful diagnostic tool but it is also the situation in which we have most chance to provide the early phase of support for the family. It should not be highly detailed clinically at the expense of the family feeling dangerously exposed. When history taking is difficult, it is the duty of the doctor to discover the reason for this or acknowledge that the problem is unsolved. There can be various reasons for difficulty in obtaining a history: overwhelming anxiety about serious illness may have arisen from information gleaned from texts, support groups, the internet, other doctors, or from first-hand exposure to a similar illness in a relative or friend. If the disease is familial, this can alter the clinical transaction to include consideration of the whole family, examples being fragile-X syndrome, dystrophia myotonica, attention deficit hyperactivity disorder, Asperger's syndrome, or Tourette syndrome. Parents aim to see the best in their children and may compensate for their difficulties, for example, overestimating language comprehension because they are familiar with their child's non-verbal communication. Exceptionally, a parent will fabricate part or all of the child's illness, or sometimes invent a plausible explanation to divert attention from abuse or violence as causes of symptoms.

Apart from hearing a verbatim account of the child's symptoms, often best presented chronologically, a number of specific enquiries need to be considered, many of which relate to pre-natal factors. Prior to birth, a maternal history of alcoholism or of infections such as rubella, cytomegalovirus, syphilis, HIV, or toxoplasmosis can each cause brain damage, although such infections may have been subclinical in the mother. Drugs consumed during pregnancy, both medicinal and recreational, should be checked in a formulary for their potential to cause congenital damage. Abnormalities of pregnancy, its duration, or of the delivery may have caused ischaemic brain damage. Low birth weight, especially if associated with pre-term delivery, predisposes to neurological disorders, a particular example being the increased risk of cerebral palsy if the birth weight was less than 1000 g.

Developmental milestones

Paediatric developmental history enquires about milestones for attainment of visual and social responses, walking, and speech. Often the quality of these activities matter rather more than their exact timing. Early lively social and visual responsiveness, walking steadily with progression to running, and using sentences to communicate spontaneously are more important than the exact age at which they first occur. The attention devoted to the developmental history should depend on the diagnostic question. It is unlikely to be very discriminating in an older child with headache who is making satisfactory progress at school. However, the early history and comparison with any previous assessments will be crucial in deciding if a long-standing gait or cognition disorder is progressive or static.

Brain disorders in infants and young children often become suspected only when the parents sense that behaviour, or specific skills, are failing to develop as anticipated. Parents will detect such developmental abnormalities at an earlier age if they have previous experience of bringing up children. Where there has been an early abnormality or insult to brain development, the affected skills show slow but steady progress but with a lower trajectory. Less often, the rate of development will have decelerated due to the onset of a new brain disorder, such as hydrocephalus or a genetically determined storage disorder.

Cerebral palsy is a condition of delayed motor development due to damage to the developing brain. It is non-progressive, and with normal or near-normal underlying intellect. In contrast, children with cognitive impairments are backward in all aspects of development, with varying involvement of motor function. Initially they may be thought to have impaired vision

or hearing responses, and some fail to develop close emotional bonds with their mother. Children with severe cognitive impairments are at high risk of epilepsy and additional behaviour disturbances. These include attention deficit hyperactivity disorder (Section 4.4.4), autistic spectrum features (Section 4.4.1), persisting immaturities of behaviour, and the development of stereotypies such as repetitive rocking and vocalization.

Because of the high rate of cognitive and special-sense impairments in paediatric neurological disease, it is important that the developmental history contains a statement about gross motor, fine motor, speech and communication, and social development. Assessment using simple play materials like wooden cubes allow observation of co-ordination, developmental level, and attention. The use of such methods, including vision and hearing assessment, is well described (Egan 1990). Multidisciplinary assessment is usually required for children with complex impairments.

The mother should be asked when the child mastered certain skills. The following milestones are easy to remember:

◆ Were fetal movements normal?

◆ 1–2 months: social smiling.

◆ 4 months: head control while sitting supported.

◆ 6 months: starts sitting unaided.

◆ 10–16 months: walks.

◆ 15 months: a few words in addition to 'mum' and 'dad'.

◆ 2 years: simple sentences.

◆ 3–4 years: uses lavatory.

◆ 5 years: dresses independently.

Neurological examination

For children developmentally at a 5-year level or more, this should follow the same outline as for adults. Younger children will be unable or unwilling to co-operate with complicated or protracted physical examination and are best examined on a parent's lap. Often the examination is better conducted more informally than in adults, with an emphasis on natural activities that the child understands, such as running and rising from the floor to test balance and leg power, or reaching to pluck objects as a test of vision and co-ordination and so as to observe eye movements. In uncooperative children, the main information may come from observing how they play with bricks and beads, and run about. Neurological examination of neonates lies beyond the scope of this book.

General examination should include any specific features pertinent to the diagnosis in question. Head circumference should be measured in children under 2 years, usually towards the end of the examination. Any question of hydrocephalus in older children should prompt measurement of head circumference to be plotted against standard values. The posterior fontanelle normally closes by 6 weeks of age and the anterior by 10–20 months. Foot deformity, particularly when combined with urinary incontinence, should provide a search for caudal spinal canal disorders, such as spina bifida. Children with epilepsy may have tuberous sclerosis and examination may reveal amelanotic patches, epiloia on the face, or periungual fibromas of the nails; Wood's light should be used to reveal shagreen patches on the trunk. In children with foot deformity, examination may show that one parent also has hereditary motor and sensory neuropathy.

Motor examination cannot be conducted by the usual formal commands if the child is too young to understand, or if the child is too apprehensive to co-operate. It is informative simply to observe the use of the limbs and eyes during play, walking, and in response to visuomotor stimulation with balls or dolls. Delayed motor milestones, asymmetry of limb usage, failure of visual following, incoordination, or involuntary movements will be obvious. By 3 months of age an infant should follow with his eyes, by 7 months can transfer objects from hand to hand, and by 10 months can pick up small objects using finger–thumb opposition. By 3–4 months head control is good when sitting or lying and no longer does the head lag when the infant is pulled from lying to sitting.

Examination of the reflexes is often unrewarding in the very young because of inability to stay still or a tendency to stiffen and withdraw at the prospective tendon hammer blow. A child may be reassured by the charade of seeing the reflexes elicited in their parent, or on a doll. It helps to use a finger of your left hand to transmit the tendon hammer's blow to the tendon, both to prevent pain and to stabilize the limb in the necessary position. The plantar responses are extensor until about 1 year of age. Infants below 20 weeks of age show the Moro reflex (Section 1.4.5) which is elicited by holding the infant supine and dropping the head into extension by a few centimetres. The normal response is symmetrical extension and adduction of the arms and extension of the legs.

Sensory testing is difficult in children below the age of 8 years and it is impossible to carry out more than rudimentary testing of pain and touch appreciation in infants.

Language and cognitive function require specialist testing if they are important for diagnostic purposes or to plan education. Cerebral dominance for hand and foot can be deduced from observing behaviours such as writing, throwing, and kicking. Handedness is rarely apparent before 2 years, and mild hemiparesis should be suspected if clear hand preference is displayed at an earlier age. Analysis of drawings and application of age-related intelligence quotient (IQ) tests give an accurate measure of overall intelligence. An informal view of intelligence can be derived from talking to a child about a picture or a story and by testing numerical tasks suitable for the age. Developmental dyspraxia represents a difficulty with voluntary movements despite an intact motor apparatus and is often associated with attention deficits or perceptual difficulties. It may be evident while the child is dressing or using writing implements, and can be tested by asking the child to imitate gestures. Conversation will reveal the extent of a child's vocabulary, their ability to understand instructions and questions, whether sentence construction has progressed beyond the single-word stage which predominates in children younger than 3 years, and whether the grammatical use of pronouns has developed correctly.

1.3.5 The elderly

A large proportion of those presenting with neurological disorders are elderly. Stroke, Parkinson's disease, dementia, and cervical spondylotic myelopathy are common disabling neurological conditions in this age group. Furthermore, troublesome neurological symptoms which evade formal diagnosis are common in patients in their seventh decade and beyond. Examples include mild degrees of memory difficulty, dizziness and dysequilibrium, falls (Section 1.7.5), or unwitnessed blackouts. High-level gait disorders (Section 1.7.4), without a demonstrable frontal lobe abnormality on scanning, are a common problem for the very old. These may be difficult to distinguish from the mild gait deterioration which is almost universal by the age of 80. Elderly patients with neurological disorders are just as deserving as younger patients of expert neurological evaluation and investigation. A particular effort should be made to pursue diagnoses which may lead to improvement or stabilization of the disorder during the patient's natural life span. Examples include detection and treatment of subdural haematoma, meningioma, Parkinson's disease, herpes encephalitis, hydrocephalus, idiopathic demyelinating polyneuropathy, lumbar canal stenosis, and myasthenia gravis.

The neurological examination becomes less discriminating in elderly patients. Absent ankle tendon jerks, loss of vibration sense from the feet, mild weakness of ankle dorsiflexion, and general loss of muscle bulk are frequent age-related findings. These only assume clear pathogenic significance if unilateral, or if they emerge at an unexpectedly rapid rate during sequential examinations. Steadily diminishing pupil size, and loss of upgaze or convergence are frequent asymptomatic ocular signs in the elderly. Hearing, smell, and taste all deteriorate with ageing. Gait in the elderly often shows small strides, uncertainty, a widened base, use of a stick, and a tendency to walk carefully around corners. Romberg's test is frequently positive. Heel–toe walking is often impossible for elderly patients without being clearly related to an identifiable and deteriorating disease process.

1.4 The reflexes

1.4.1 Reflex arcs

A reflex is the simplest form of involuntary response to a stimulus. The anatomical basis of a reflex arc consists of: (1) a receptor organ; (2) an afferent path running from the periphery to the brainstem or spinal cord; (3) one or more intercalated neurons in the central nervous system linking the afferent path to the efferent path (4), which leaves the neuraxis by the lower motor neuron axons to reach (5), the effector organ. Reflexes are elicited by afferent sensory stimuli such as touch, pain, sudden muscle stretch, light, or noise. The efferent response consists of muscular contraction, a modification in muscle tone, or glandular secretion. Important though visceral reflexes are, the neurologist investigating the state of the nervous system is mainly concerned with reflexes that excite responses in the somatic musculature.

Reflexes play an important role in diagnostic neurology because they reflect the integrity of, or alterations in, the neural structures responsible for their arc. Loss of a reflex may be due to interruption of the afferent path by a lesion involving the first sensory neuron in the peripheral nerves, plexuses, spinal nerves, or dorsal roots, by damage to the central paths of the arc in the brainstem or spinal cord, by lesions of the lower motor neuron at any point between the anterior horn cells and the

muscles, of the muscles themselves, or by the neural depression produced by neural shock. In clinical practice, the most useful and oft-elicited reflexes are the tendon reflexes of the limbs, the jaw jerk, the plantar response, the superficial abdominal reflexes in adults and the Moro reflex in infants. The place of these particular reflexes in the routine neurological examination is outlined in Section 1.3.2. This section describes the elicitation and significance of these reflexes and of a wide variety of others which are used occasionally.

1.4.2 Tendon reflexes

Physiological basis

The physiological basis of the tendon reflex is the myotatic reflex, which is the reflex contraction of a muscle or part of a muscle in response to stretch. It is monosynaptic; mediated by a

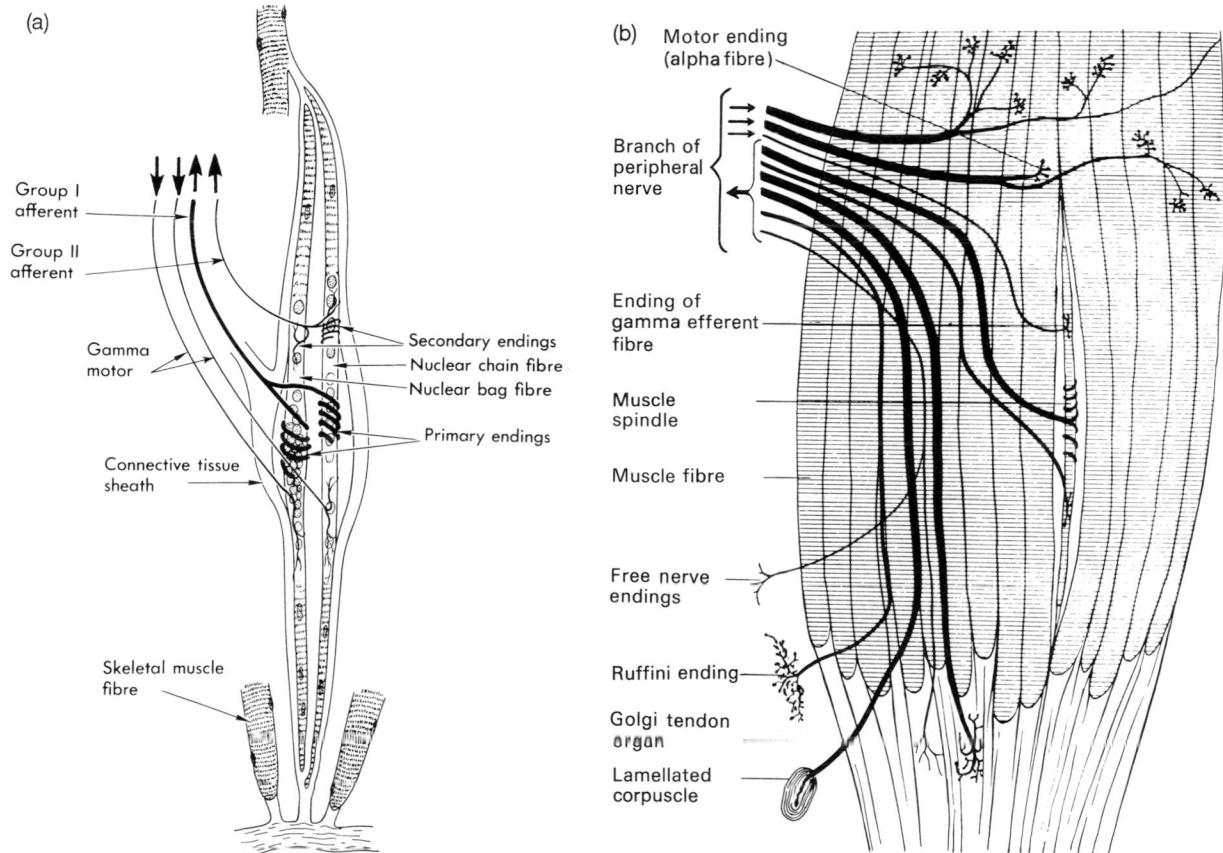

Fig. 1.19. (a) Schematic representation of a muscle spindle. The end parts of three skeletal muscle fibres are shown (cross-striated, nuclei at edge). Inside the connective-tissue sheath of the spindle are two muscle fibres (thinner than extrafusal skeletal muscle fibres, with central nuclei, and striations minimal or absent in the region of the sensory endings). Sensory nerve fibres form primary (annulospiral) and secondary (flower-spray) endings, the primary endings arising from the large fibres. Small nerve fibres (gamma efferents) form motor endings at each end of the spindle muscle fibres. Motor discharges over gamma efferents cause the muscle spindle fibres to contract at each end, thus stretching the intervening, non-contractile sensory region and activating the sensory endings. Arrows indicate direction of impulse conduction. (Courtesy of Gardner (1975).) (b) Schematic representation of a muscle and its nerve supply. Arrows indicate direction of impulse conduction. Each extrafusal muscle fibre has a motor ending from a large myelinated (alpha) fibre. The intrafusal muscle fibres within a muscle spindle have motor endings from small myelinated (gamma) fibres. Muscle nerves contain many sensory fibres. Some are large myelinated fibres from primary (annulospiral) endings in spindles, from neurotendinous spindles (Golgi tendon organs), and from Pacinian corpuscles in the connective tissue within and external to the muscle. Smaller myelinated and non-myelinated fibres arise from Ruffini endings in the connective tissue in and around muscle, and in joints. Finally there are small myelinated and non-myelinated fibres that form free endings in the connective tissue in and around muscle. (Courtesy of Gardner (1975).)

reflex arc consisting of two neurons with one synapse between them. The afferent input of the tendon reflex is transmitted by large myelinated sensory peripheral nerve fibres which innervate the muscle spindles. These, in turn, are connected in parallel with the main contractile extrafusal muscle fibres. Their nuclear chain fibres signal the actual length of the spindle, while the nuclear bag fibres detect the velocity of change of length (Fig. 1.19). The overall sensitivity of the muscle spindle is determined by its efferent supply from gamma-motor neurons, which control contraction of its intrafusal muscle fibres (Fig. 1.19). Tendon reflexes must be distinguished from the tonic stretch reflex, which results from slow or prolonged stretch of a muscle and which is a polysynaptic response, probably involving cortical pathways (Marsden *et al.* 1973). The activity of many bulbar and spinal reflexes is profoundly influenced by the state of the muscle spindles and of the gamma efferent system of motor nerve fibres. In conditions causing hypotonia (e.g. cerebellar lesions) the tendon reflexes are depressed. By contrast, the hypertonia associated with increased gamma efferent discharge exaggerates reflexes; such enhancement is greater in spasticity than in extrapyramidal rigidity. Anxiety, tensing, and painful conditions may also cause some increase in the deep tendon reflexes. Paradoxically, in severe long-standing spinal cord lesions or spastic diplegia, the spasticity is so severe that sometimes the tendon reflexes in the lower limbs may be difficult to elicit. Perhaps this is due to fibrotic muscular shortening resulting from chronic spasticity, or else the flexor withdrawal reflex may be so dominant as to inhibit the tendon jerks.

Tendon reflexes

A tendon reflex or jerk is a sharp muscular contraction evoked by suddenly stretching the muscle. The sudden stretch may be brought about by tapping the tendon, or by suddenly displacing the segment of a limb into which the muscle is inserted (Fig. 1.20). The response, a muscular contraction is most evident in the muscle stretched, but may not be confined to this muscle. A tendon reflex is diminished or abolished by a lesion interrupting either the afferent, central, or efferent paths of the reflex arc, or by a disorder which makes the muscle incapable of responding to the nervous impulse.

If initially absent, reinforcement of tendon jerks may be achieved by simultaneous voluntary muscle contraction elsewhere in the body such as biting the teeth together, clenching a fist, or by pulling the flexed fingers of the two hands against each other (Jendrassik's manoeuvre). This increases activity in the gamma efferent system. Reflex activity in the legs may be recorded electrophysiologically as 'H' reflex, a contraction in the calf muscles which is elicited by stimulating afferents in the medial popliteal nerve. The H response, which is a monosynaptic reflex evoked by stimulation of Group I afferent fibres in the nerve, follows the so-called M response evoked in the muscle by the direct effect of the nerve stimulus upon alpha efferent fibres. In early polyneuropathy the tendon reflexes may be lost before sensory loss is detectable clinically, although abnormalities of conduction usually are detectable electrically. Rarely, the tendon reflexes are congenitally absent. Some or all of the tendon reflexes may be well-nigh impossible to elicit, despite reinforcement, in well-muscled young men who are completely healthy. Table 1.5 gives the principal tendon reflexes, the mode of elicitation, and their innervation.

Clonus

Clonus is a rhythmical series of contractions evoked by maintaining stretch and tension in a muscle. It is associated with increased gamma efferent discharge, and is often elicitable

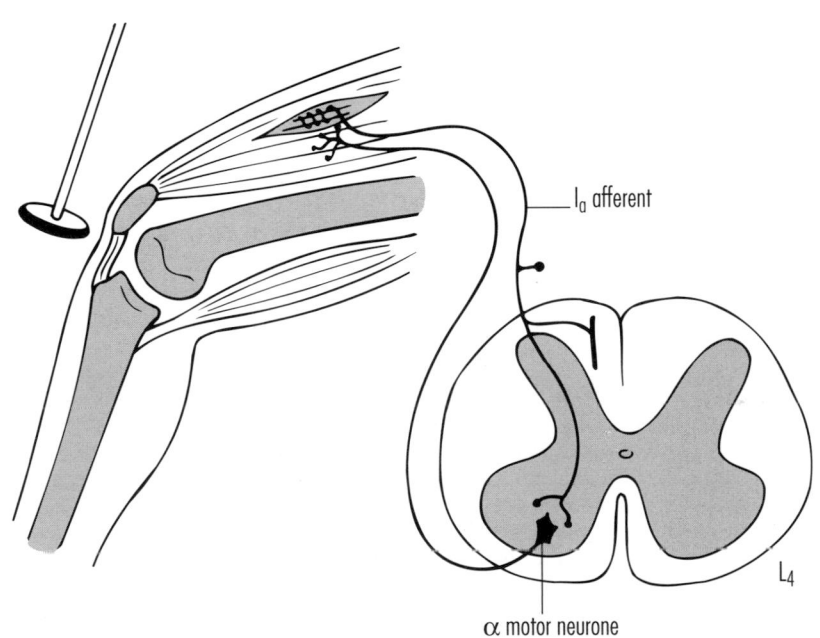

Fig. 1.20. The components of the monosynaptic stretch reflex elicited by percussing the patellar tendon of the quadriceps muscle (from Donaghy 1997).

Table 1.5. The tendon reflexes

Reflex	Mode of elicitation	Response	Segment	Peripheral nerve
Jaw-jerk	A downwards blow on the chin	Closure of the mouth	Trigeminal	Trigeminal
Biceps-jerk	A blow upon the biceps tendon	Flexion of the elbow	Cervical 5–6	Musculocutaneous
Triceps-jerk	A blow upon the triceps tendon	Extension of the elbow	Cervical 6–7	Radial
Brachioradialis-jerk	A blow at the distal end of the radius stretching brachioradialis	Visible contraction of brachioradialis	Cervical 6	Radial
Flexor finger-jerk	A blow upon the palmar surface of the semiflexed fingers	Flexion of the fingers and thumb	Cervical 7–8	Median and ulnar
Knee-jerk	A blow upon the patellar tendon	Extension of the knee	Lumbar 3–4	Femoral
Ankle-jerk	A blow upon the Achilles tendon	Plantar flexion at the ankle	Sacral 1–2	Sciatic/posterior tibial

when the tendon reflexes are exaggerated after a corticospinal lesion. Clonus of the quadriceps, patellar clonus, is best elicited by a sudden sharp downward displacement of the patella. Ankle clonus is obtained by sharply dorsiflexing the ankle (Fig. 1.12). Clonus in the finger flexors can sometimes be elicited by suddenly extending the fingers.

Hoffmann's reflex

The patient's hand is pronated and the observer grasps the terminal phalanx of the middle finger between his forefinger and thumb. With a sharp flick the phalanx is passively flexed and suddenly released. A positive response consists of a sharp twitch of adduction and flexion of the thumb and flexion of the fingers. This reflex is physiologically identical with the *flexor finger-jerk*, which is elicited by tapping the palmar surface of the slightly flexed fingers. It is an index of muscular hypertonia rather than proof of a corticospinal lesion as such. It is not always positive in the presence of such a lesion, and may be elicitable in a nervous individual with no organic disease; if present only unilaterally it is likely to be significant.

Reflex spread

In states of muscular hypertonia, a reflex response may spread beyond the muscles stretched, as when a tap on the styloid process of the radius elicits a contraction not only of the brachioradialis, but also of the long flexors of the fingers.

Inverted reflexes

In the upper limbs, so-called 'inverted reflexes' may be a useful sign of lesions of the cervical spinal cord. For instance, a lesion at C5–6 may both interrupt the arc for reflexes innervated by that segment, and also compress the corticospinal tracts to give exaggeration of reflexes subserved by lower segments. Thus tapping the biceps tendon may fail to elicit the biceps jerk but gives contraction of triceps (the inverted biceps jerk). Similarly, the radial jerk may be absent but the attempts to elicit it cause finger flexion (the inverted radial jerk). An inverted knee jerk (contraction of the hamstrings with knee flexion when the quadriceps tendon is tapped) may also be a sign of a spinal-cord lesion at L2–4 (Boyle *et al.* 1979) but is much less common.

1.4.3 Superficial reflexes

The palmomental reflex

To elicit this reflex, an orange stick is firmly scratched across the base of the thenar eminence. A positive response consists of contraction of the ipsilateral mentalis muscle, giving a dimpling of the chin. The reflex may be present bilaterally in normal individuals or in states of reflex hyperexcitability. But when present on one side only, it may be indicative of a corticospinal-tract lesion (Wartenberg 1945).

The superficial abdominal reflexes

These are cutaneous reflexes consisting of a brisk unilateral contraction of a part of the abdominal wall in response to a cutaneous stimulus, such as a light stroke with an orange stick. It is convenient to elicit them at three levels on each side—just below the costal margin (T8), at the level of the umbilicus (T10), and just above the inguinal ligament (T12)—using stimuli oriented to run along the respective thoracic dermatomes. The abdominal and erector spinae reflexes are polysynaptic, and are reactions of the trunk to potential injury. They are plurisegmental, and lead to a local withdrawal from the stimulus. They are normally dependent upon the integrity of the corticospinal tract, for reasons not fully understood. Hence a corticospinal lesion is usually associated with diminution or loss of the superficial abdominal reflexes upon the same side. Loss of the abdominal reflexes is not always proportional to the severity of the lesion. In multiple sclerosis, for example, they may be lost early, at a stage of the disease when other signs of corticospinal-tract dysfunction are slight. In spastic diplegia and motor neuron disease, on the other hand, they are often retained, despite frank spasticity of the legs.

The reflex arcs of the superficial abdominal reflexes are localized in the spinal cord from the seventh to the twelfth dorsal segments. Lesions involving the arcs themselves may produce diminution or loss of the reflexes, for instance a structural lesion of the spinal cord at those segmental levels. One such lesion is damage to the lower motor neuron by poliomyelitis. These reflexes may be absent in in the aged, the obese, those with abdominal scars, and the fecund (Madonick 1957).

The cremasteric reflex

The cremasteric reflex is a cutaneous reflex closely related to the abdominal reflexes. The stimulus is a light scratch along the inner aspect of the upper part of one thigh. The response is a contraction of the cremaster muscle, with elevation of the testicle on that side. This reflex, mediated by the first lumbar spinal segment, is diminished or abolished by a corticospinal-tract lesion or a lesion of the reflex arc. It is usually extremely brisk in children, in whom it may sometimes be elicited by a stimulus applied to any part of the lower limb. It is often diminished or absent on the affected side in a patient with a varicocele.

The gluteal reflex

The gluteal reflex is physiologically akin to the abdominal reflexes. A scratch on the buttock evokes contraction of the glutei. The spinal segments concerned are L4 and 5.

The plantar reflex

The plantar reflex is one of the most important of all reflexes to the neurologist, because, if extensor, it provides unequivocal evidence of an upper motor neuron lesion. The plantar reflex normally becomes flexor after the first year of life. The stimulus which evokes it is a longitudinal scratch upon the lateral aspect of the sole of the foot from the heel towards the toes (Fig. 1.15). The normal response is plantar flexion of the toes, sometimes associated with dorsiflexion of the foot at the ankle, contraction of the tensor fasciae latae muscle, and other variable muscular contractions. It is a spinal segmental reflex mediated by the first sacral segment of the cord and akin to the abdominal reflexes.

The extensor plantar response, or Babinski response, occurs in the presence of a corticospinal-tract lesion. The normal reflex response is replaced by an upward, extensor movement of the great toe (Fig. 1.14). Extension of the great toe is not an isolated phenomenon of the abnormal plantar reflex, but is part of a general reflex flexion of the whole lower limb. This relates to the primitive flexor withdrawal reflex in response to a nociceptive stimulus to the lower limb seen in animals after division of the spinal cord. Clinical and physiological studies in humans show that the distinction between the flexor and extensor plantar reflexes is not absolute (Brain and Wilkinson 1959). Both are nociceptive reflexes, but 'the unique feature of the pathological extensor response is the recruitment of extensor hallucis longus into contraction with tibialis anterior and extensor digitorum longus' (Kugelberg and Hagbarth 1958). The afferent focus, or region from which it is easiest to elicit this reflex, is the outer border of the sole and the transverse arch of the foot (Dohrmann and Nowack 1973). The motor focus, or minimal response, is a contraction of the inner ham-string muscles which may be present even when the great toe fails to move. When fully developed, the extensor plantar reflex consists of flexion at all joints of the lower limb with dorsiflexion of the great toe and abduction or fanning of the other toes.

There are several points of practical importance in eliciting the plantar reflex, some of which are discussed in Section 1.3.2. The stimulus should always be applied first along the outer border of the sole; an extensor response may sometimes be obtained here when the inner border of the sole yields a flexor response. The response is more consistently obtained if the stimulus is then continued medially across the anterior arch of the sole of the foot. Oppenheim's reflex, dorsiflexion of the great toe, evoked by firm, moving pressure on the skin over the tibia, is physiologically the same as Babinski's reflex, differing only in the site of the stimulus. The same is true of Chaddock's and Gordon's reflexes. Chaddock's (also called the external malleolar sign) is an extensor plantar response elicited by scratching the skin in the region of the external malleolus. In Gordon's reflex (also called the paradoxical flexor reflex) the stimulus consists of squeezing the calf muscles. The extensor plantar reflex is not an all-or-none reaction: minor degrees of corticospinal-tract damage lead to an incomplete flexor response or a failure of the great toe to move up or down (an 'equivocal' response). In experienced hands such equivocal responses carry reasonably reliable diagnostic implication if clearly unilateral.

Bilateral extensor plantar reflexes are often observed during sleep and deep coma from any cause, and for a short time after an epileptic convulsion. They are usually extensor in the first year of life, when the corticospinal fibres are incompletely developed. An extensor plantar response has been noted sometimes in patients in whom no anatomical lesion of the corticospinal tract was subsequently discovered. Occasionally the plantar response remains clearly flexor despite the presence of such a lesion (van Gijn 1978). It may occur transiently as a result of physical fatigue. In the presence of a corticospinal-tract lesion, the Babinski response may be lost if an associated lower motor neuron lesion paralyses the extensor hallucis muscle. This is a common problem in amyotrophic lateral sclerosis, where denervation of the distal leg musculature obscures the presence of the associated upper motor neuron lesion.

The bulbocavernosus reflex

The bulbocavernosus reflex consists of contraction of the bulbocavernosus muscle, which can be detected by palpation, in response to squeezing the glans penis. The spinal segments concerned are sacral 2, 3, and 4. This reflex is abolished in lesions of the cauda equina.

The anal reflex

The anal reflex consists of contraction of the external sphincter ani in response to a firm scratch on the skin of the anal verge. It is hard to illicit in the elderly and those with a patulous anus. The spinal segments concerned are sacral 4 and 5.

1.4.4 Cranial reflexes

The pupil–light reflex

The pupil–light reflex is discussed in Section 8.9.1.

The corneal reflex

The stimulus that evokes the corneal reflex is a light touch upon one cornea with a wisp of cotton wool. The normal response is bilateral blinking. The afferent path is through the first division of the fifth cranial nerve. The central path consists of fibres uniting the spinal nucleus of the fifth nerve with both facial nuclei. The efferent path passes through the facial nerves to both orbiculares oculi muscles. A lesion involving the fifth nerve or its spinal nucleus, since it interrupts the afferent path, causes bilateral loss of blinking in response to stimulation of the cornea on the side of the lesion. A lesion involving the nucleus or fibres of one seventh nerve interrupts the efferent path and hence causes loss of the reflex on the side of the lesion only, while the blink response remains on the other side. Loss of the corneal reflex is often an early sign of a lesion of the fifth nerve and may occur before any cutaneous anaesthesia can be detected. Apart from lesions involving the reflex arc, the corneal reflex is lost in states of deep coma.

The glabellar tap

A brisk tap on the glabella above the bridge of the nose causes bilateral blinking. In the normal individual, on repeated tapping the blinking ceases after two or three taps, but in patients with parkinsonism it may continue in time with the taps (the 'glabellar tap' sign). Electrophysiological recordings from the orbicularis oculi have shown that there is an initial monosynaptic reflex response of low amplitude, followed by a larger response of longer latency which is clearly polysynaptic (Gandiglio and Fra 1967). This habituates in normal individuals but not usually in parkinsonism.

The vestibulo-ocular reflex

This is also known as the oculocephalic reflex. The term 'doll's head phenomenon' is misleading because the eyes of some dolls are fixed, whereas those of others counter-rotate. When the eyelids are held open and the head is rotated sharply from side to side, the eyes show conjugate deviation away from the side to which the head is moved. On flexion of the neck they move upwards; after each such movement they return slowly to the mid position, even if the head remains rotated or flexed. The reflex persists in blind individuals and after occipital lobectomy (Plum and Posner 1980). It is impaired when there are lesions of the oculomotor nerves. Its absence usually indicates a brainstem lesion.

The caloric or oculovestibular reflex

This has much in common with the vestibulo-ocular reflex. Irrigation of an external auditory meatus with warm or cold water causes nystagmus in normal individuals. As this reflex depends upon the integrity of the vestibular nuclei, its absence

may be a valuable sign of pontine damage if there is no reason to suspect a labyrinthine or eighth-nerve lesion. Repeated absence of the caloric reflex is an important criterion in diagnosing brainstem death (Section 25.14.2).

The jaw jerk

In response to a tap upon the chin, depressing the lower jaw, there is a bilateral contraction of the elevators of the jaw. The jaw jerk is best elicited with the mouth half open, with the examiner resting a finger on the centre of the mandible to cushion the blow of the tendon hammer. Both afferent and efferent paths pass through the trigeminal nerve. This reflex is a stretch reflex, and, like other such reflexes, becomes exaggerated as a result of bilateral corticospinal-tract lesions. It is often weakly present in normal individuals, and is only clearly enhanced if notably brisk and of large amplitude, or if it provokes jaw clonus.

The sucking reflex

In the infant the contact of an object with the lips evokes sucking movement of the lips, tongue, and jaw. This sucking reflex is lost after infancy but may reappear in states of severe cerebral degeneration, such as senile dementia (Paulson and Gottlieb 1968). It may be unilateral, and associated with a grasp reflex on the same side.

The 'snout' and 'pout' reflex

Although the two terms are often used interchangeably, it is more accurate to consider the 'snout' and 'pout' reflexes as separate entities. The pout reflex is evoked by a brisk tap upon the closed lips, and, if positive, produces an immediate pouting response. This represents an enhanced myotatic reflex of the orbicularis oris muscle which appears in bilateral corticospinal tract lesions at or above the upper brainstem. The term 'snout' reflex is better reserved for the slower 'rooting' reflex in which the lips follow and seek out a gentle tactile stimulus on the lips or adjacent face. This snout reflex is normal in infants, and re-emerges in frontal lobe lesions.

The palatal reflex

The palatal ('gag') reflex consists of bilateral elevation of the soft palate in response to a touch on one side. The afferent path is by the glossopharyngeal nerve; the efferent by the vagus. The palatal reflex is variable in intensity in normal individuals. It is abolished by glossopharyngeal nerve lesions causing anaesthesia of the palate, and by lesions of the vagus nuclei. In lesions of a single vagus nerve, the response is unilateral, irrespective of the side of the stimulus, and the uvula is displaced towards the normal side.

The pharyngeal reflex

The pharyngeal reflex consists of constriction of the pharynx in response to a touch upon the posterior pharyngeal wall. Its afferent path runs in the glossopharyngeal nerve, its efferent path in the vagus. It is abolished by lesions causing pharyngeal anaesthesia and by lesions of the vagus nuclei. In cases of unilateral paralysis of the vagus musculature, the response is confined to the opposite half of the pharynx.

1.4.5 Postural and grasping reflexes

These are reflexes in which the response consists not of a brief muscular contraction but of a sustained modification in the posture of one or more sections of the body.

Tonic neck reflexes

In the decerebrate animal, changes in the position of the head relative to the body cause reflex modifications of limb tone and posture. These reflexes, which are excited from the proprioceptors of the cervical spine, are known as tonic neck reflexes, and may sometimes be observed in severe cerebral diplegia. Passive turning of the head to one side evokes extension of the arm and leg on the side to which the head is turned; the contralateral limbs flex.

Associated reactions

Associated reactions, or associated movements, are automatic modifications of the posture of parts of the body when vigorous voluntary or reflex movement of some other part occurs. They are best observed in the paralysed upper limb in hemiplegia, following a vigorous grasping movement with the sound hand. Other patterns of associated movement occur. Such semivoluntary activities as yawning, stretching, and coughing often evoke associated movements in the paralysed limbs in hemiplegia, and may arouse false hopes of recovery.

Grasp reflex of the hand

In some patients the contact of an object with the palmar surface of the fingers, especially the region between the thumb and the index finger, causes reflex flexion of the fingers and thumb so that the hand involuntarily grasps the object. The patient is unable to relax his grasp voluntarily, and efforts to pull the object away only cause it to be held more firmly. The patient may even notice that when he is holding an object he is unable to relinquish hold of it. This phenomenon is known as the grasp reflex. In some cases, when the patient's eyes are closed, if the palmar surface of the hand or fingers is lightly touched, the fingers close upon the object and the hand and arm move towards the stimulus, and in this way may be drawn in any direction—forced groping or the instinctive grasp reaction. Even an object presented to vision may be groped for (Seyffarth and Denny-Brown 1948). Forced grasping and groping, which have been considered a regression to the infantile stage of the function of grasping, usually indicate a lesion involving the upper part of the opposite frontal lobe. A unilateral grasp reflex in a fully conscious patient is of localizing value. Its value is much less when the reflex is bilateral or the patient semicomatose. If the causative lesion produces a progressive hemiplegia, the grasp reflex disappears when paralysis becomes complete; this indicates that it utilizes the corticospinal tract as part of its motor path.

The grasp reflex of the foot

A similar grasp reflex is sometimes seen in the foot. Light pressure or a stroking movement applied to the distal half of the sole and plantar surface of the toes evokes tonic flexion and adduction of the toes without other associated movements. Like the fingers, the toes may grasp and hold an object. This reflex is present in the normal infant up to the end of the first year, and in 50 per cent of children with Down's syndrome. It may occur either with or without the hand-grasp reflex, and results from similar lesions.

The avoiding and grab reflexes

The avoiding reflex, which is in many respects the converse of the grasp reflex, is seen in animals with lesions of the parietal lobe. When an object is brought close to the hand on the affected side, the limb is drawn away instead of grasping the object. Although phenomena similar to avoiding are sometimes seen in human subjects with parietal-lobe lesions, this reflex is rarely seen in clinical practice and is thus of little value. The so-called 'grab reflex' which causes flexion of the terminal phalanx of the thumb when the hand is passively displaced radially at the wrist is also unlikely to be of diagnostic value (Traub *et al.* 1980).

The Moro reflex

The Moro reflex is normally present at birth and disappears by 20 weeks of age; persistence suggests a diffuse central nervous system disorder. It is elicited by holding the infant supine with the head slightly flexed, and then dropping the head through about 30°. The normal response is of symmetrical abduction, extension, and rotation of the arms. An asymmetrical Moro response occurs in brachial plexus injury or hemiparesis.

The Landau reflex

The Landau reflex should be present by 10 months of age and will be absent in diplegia or tetraplegia. The infant is held prone, supported by the examiner's hand. The normal response is extension of the neck, trunk, and legs. If abnormal, the infant tends to collapse into flexion around the examiner's hand.

1.5 Diagnosing muscle weakness

Anatomical localization of the lesion responsible for muscle weakness is a common purpose of neurological examination.

1.5.1 Symptoms

Surprisingly often patients do not complain of weakness itself, but rather of difficulty in using a limb for certain manoeuvres, or to walk. Particularly for the hand, an integrated motor–sensory organ, the early symptoms of difficulty in manipulating buttons or pens, or dropping things, can be remarkably similar in pure motor and pure sensory disorders. Furthermore, a patient who proffers the complaint of weakness may be suffering in reality from numbness, disinclination to use a painful limb, incoordination, or even the aesthenic effects of cardiorespiratory disease. Patients may use the term 'weakness' when referring to other motor disorders which do not involve loss of raw muscle power, such as the bradykinesia of an extrapyramidal disorder (Chapter 32), or apraxia (Section 26.4.3), which is an inability to formulate and execute a complex movement despite normal upper and lower motor neuron and muscular function. Weakness accompanied by exhaustion may be a complaint of patients with chronic fatigue syndrome. However, such patients are usually capable of exerting normal muscle strength, at least momentarily, if encouraged adequately.

Weakness of certain muscles often produces distinctive complaints. Proximal arm muscle weakness usually causes difficulty in doing the hair, hanging out washing, or lifting objects from high shelves. Patients rarely notice isolated weakness of small hand muscles, but sometimes complain of loss of grip, for instance in trying to unscrew bottle tops. Weakness of individual arm muscles can be distinctively symptomatic, such as difficulty in sliding the hand into a pocket with weakness of finger extension due to posterior interosseous nerve lesions, or difficulty in pushing the car gear lever forward with focal triceps weakness. Proximal leg muscle weakness, particularly if it affects quadriceps, leads to difficulty in climbing or descending stairs, standing out of the bath, or arising from sitting without using the arms. Distal leg muscle weakness shows as ankle instability or foot drop, inability to scrunch up the toes into plantar flexion so as to keep loose shoes on, or to grip the edge of a swimming bath so as to dive.

The pattern of the weakness and the presence of other symptoms have considerable implications for localizing the lesion and determining the pathology. Predominantly proximal muscle weakness points to myopathy or myasthenia. Increasing weakness of muscles on usage, and during the course of the day, suggests myasthenia gravis. Hemiparesis, affecting both the arm and the leg on one side only, is typical of a cerebral-hemisphere lesion. Weakness of both legs, or paraparesis, points to thoracic spinal cord or cauda equina disease. Weakness of all four limbs, known as quadriplegia or tetraplegia, suggests cervical spinal cord or brainstem disease, or diffuse neuromuscular disease. Difficulty in swallowing is typical of motor neuron diseases, myasthenia, inclusion-body myositis and some muscular dystrophies, and acute polyneuropathies such as Guillain–Barré syndrome or diphtheria. Although patients usually notice wasting of their proximal muscles, such as biceps or quadriceps, often they are oblivious of advanced atrophy of distal muscles, such as the dorsal interossei.

Concurrent alteration of sphincter control should provoke prompt attempts to diagnose and treat the cause of associated limb weakness. Urgency of micturition with frequent voiding of small quantities, and sometimes incontinence, reflects the small, spastic, irritable bladder typical of bilateral upper motor neuron lesions, particularly those affecting the spinal cord. Retention of urine, or sometimes dribbling incontinence, occurs in cauda equina disease. Erectile impotence is an early feature of either spinal cord or cauda equina disease. It is rare for anal sphincter control to be impaired in a manner that is characteristically diagnostic before obvious abnormalities of micturition or potency. Rapidly developing impairment of sphincter control implies compression of the spinal cord or cauda equina and requires emergency investigation.

1.5.2 Differentiating upper and lower motor neuron lesions

If examination reveals muscle weakness, it is necessary to differentiate between lesions of the upper or lower motor neurons, the neuromuscular junction, or primary muscle disease. Also, one should recognize that distinctive patterns of fluctuating weakness may be due to psychological factors, loss of kinaesthetic feedback, or pain. The key features to this differential diagnosis are the presence of wasting or fasciculations, the pattern of muscle power loss, changes in tone, tendon reflex

Table 1.6. Physical signs used to differentiate between muscle weakness due to diseases affecting the upper motor neuron, lower motor neuron, and muscle and psychogenic weakness (from Donaghy 1997)

Sign	Upper motor neuron damage		Lower motor neuron damage	Primary muscle disease	Psychogenic disorder
	Cerebral hemisphere	Spinal cord			
Wasting			Present	Present	
Fasciculations			Present		
Reflexes	Brisk	Brisk	Absent	Normal	Normal
Tone	Spastic	Spastic	Flaccid	Normal	Normal
Plantars*	↑↓	↑↑	↓↓	↓↓	↓↓
Sensory loss	Sometimes	Usually	Usually	No	Often
Distribution of weakness	Hemiplegic	Paraplegic or quadriplegic	Individual peripheral nerve or root; distal in polyneuropathy	Proximal	Variable

* ↑, Extensor plantar response; ↓, flexor plantar response.

abnormalities, plantar responses, and the topography of any associated sensory loss (Table 1.6).

Wasting

Wasting is typical of a denervated muscle, or one affected by primary muscle disease. Other causes are much rarer (Section 13.1.4). In polyneuropathy the wasting will be predominantly distal, in myopathy it is predominantly proximal. The wasting follows the distribution dictated by the innervation in individual peripheral nerve lesions (Sections 13.10, 13.11) or spinal root lesions (Section 21.2). Wasting develops in any muscle that has been significantly denervated for 4–6 weeks. Muscle atrophy is not a feature of myasthenia.

Disuse atrophy of muscles occurs in patients who have been recumbent for general medical reasons. It may affect muscles acting at a diseased joint, such as quadriceps with knee arthritis. Disuse atrophy can be distinguished from the wasting due to lower motor neuron or muscle diseases because the reflexes and tone are normal, and no fasciculations occur. But, most importantly, strength is relatively well preserved in a disuse-atrophied muscle, whereas a pathologically wasted muscle will be profoundly weakened.

Pseudohypertrophy is an unusual physical sign in which a pathologically weakened muscle is hypertrophied. It is a particular sign in the calves in Duchenne muscular dystrophy (Section 15.2.1) and is a rare feature of polyneuropathies such as hereditary motor and sensory neuropathy (Section 12.4) and multifocal motor neuropathy (Fig. 12.18) (Section 12.11.3).

Fasciculations

Fasciculations occur during subacute partial denervation of muscles, and are a particularly common feature of motor neuron disease. A fasciculation is a flickering contraction, visible for a moment within the belly of a muscle. It represents simultaneous contraction of all the muscle fibres in the motor unit innervated by a single motor neuron (Fig. 1.21). Fasciculations are most easily visualized in those muscles with large motor units containing hundreds of muscle fibres, such as powerful proximal limb muscles, rather than in those muscles with small motor units that are used for fine motor control,

such as the small hand muscles. However, electromyography will detect fasciculation discharges in such muscles even though they may be invisible to the naked eye. Fasciculations are only definitely pathological if associated with wasting or weakness of the muscle (Section 14.1.2).

Tone

The tone of a muscle is the response it shows to passive stretching. A completely relaxed and resting muscle is not in a state of continuous partial contraction and is electrically silent; it has elasticity, but no tone. Therefore tone can be assessed only when the muscle is stretched or when it is maintaining posture against an applied force, such as gravity. Postural tone is the state of partial contraction of certain muscles needed to maintain the posture of body parts.

In neurological practice, tone is usually assessed by moving a limb and observing the reaction which occurs in the muscles that are being stretched. The moment stretch begins, the muscle spindles give out afferent stimuli and reflex partial contraction results. The responses to momentary and to more prolonged stretching are different—the former being responsible for the tendon jerks, the latter eliciting more complex responses, often in the form of tonic contraction. Variations in the sensitivity of these reflexes account for the alterations in tone which occur as a result of nervous disease. Forceful continued contraction of a group of muscles (e.g. biting or clenching one fist or pulling firmly with the flexed fingers of both hands) temporarily causes an increased flow of afferent impulses in the sensory fibres from the spindles. In turn, this increases the rate of discharge in gamma-motor neurons throughout the body, thus causing a generalized slight increase in sensitivity of the spindles to stretch. The tendon reflexes become brisker as the state of contraction of its intrafusal fibres is increased. This phenomenon, also known as reinforcement, or Jendrassik's manoeuvre, is often used to elicit tendon reflexes which at first seem absent. In spasticity and in extrapyramidal rigidity, the 'set' of the spindles is continuously increased.

On stretching, the tone of a muscle may be increased (spasticity, rigidity, or hypertonia) or reduced (flaccidity or hypotonia); these alterations are of great value in neurological

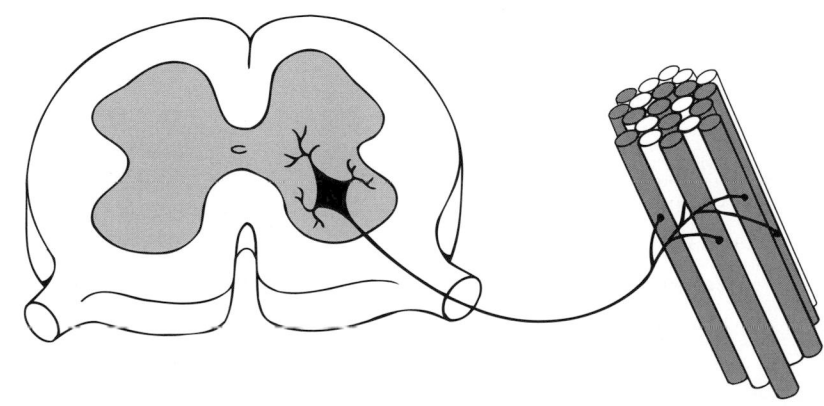

Fig. 1.21. Schematic illustration of a motor unit, consisting of a group of muscle fibres innervated by a single motor neuron. Note that the muscle fibres of a motor unit may be widely scattered throughout the belly of the muscle. (From Donaghy 1997.)

diagnosis. Muscle tone is normally regulated by reticulospinal fibres, which accompany the pyramidal tract and exert an inhibitory effect upon the stretch reflex. This inhibition balances the background facilitatory impulses conveyed by the pontine reticulospinal and lateral vestibulospinal pathways. In turn, these are influenced by multisynaptic reflex arcs traversing the cerebellum, basal ganglia, and brainstem. Dorsal reticulospinal fibres appear specifically to inhibit flexor lower-limb reflexes. When lesions of the pyramidal and reticulospinal tracts release stretch reflexes from inhibition, the resultant increase in tone is initially associated with hyperactivity of dynamic fusimotor neurons. If such increased tone persists (spasticity), increased alpha-neuron discharge develops, so that spasticity may be associated with increases in both gamma- (dynamic fusimotor) and alpha-motor neuron activity.

Spasticity

Spasticity results from lesions of the pyramidal and often of the reticulospinal pathways. The stretch reflexes become hyperactive because of increased excitability of dynamic fusimotor neurons and alpha-neurons, which have been released from descending inhibitory influences. If the dorsal reticulospinal system is also damaged, there is disinhibition of afferent flexor reflex pathways. Release of such flexor reflexes may give flexor spasms in the lower limbs in response to stimulation of the legs, bladder, bowels, or skin. The 'extensor' plantar or Babinski reflex (Section 1.4.3) is one component of the primitive flexor withdrawal reflex. Usually in spasticity the affected limb shows increased resistance to passive stretching. This is particularly severe initially, but then 'gives' suddenly as the movement is continued. This sign is seen particularly well in the legs of a patient with a spastic paraplegia due to bilateral pyramidal-tract disease, and is known as 'clasp-knife' rigidity. Hyperactivity of tendon reflexes is often accompanied by clonus (Section 1.3.2) in which sustained stretch of muscle evokes repetitive contraction and relaxation due to reverberating activity in the hyperexcitable fusimotor system. Spasticity, in the form of sustained ankle clonus, or a pronator catch in the forearm (Section 1.3.2) is an incontrovertible sign of pyramidal-tract disease.

Extrapyramidal rigidity

Extrapyramidal rigidity differs from spasticity. It occurs in patients with disease of the basal ganglia such as parkinsonism. The rigidity is uniform in degree throughout the entire range of passive movement, known as 'plastic' or 'lead-pipe' rigidity. If a tremor is superimposed, it is referred to as 'cogwheel' rigidity. In dystonia there is simultaneous contraction of agonists and antagonists so that the reciprocal inhibition of antagonists is impaired and there is increased alpha-neuron discharge. As a consequence, parts of the body become virtually fixed in an abnormal posture.

Decerebrate rigidity

Decerebrate rigidity occurs in animals when a transverse lesion across the midbrain at about the level of the superior colliculus or red nucleus releases the brainstem, cerebellum, and spinal cord from cerebral control. Strong continuous contraction in extensor groups of muscles occurs, so that an animal placed upright with support will remain standing, but if pushed over cannot rise. This contraction may occur intermittently, leading to episodes of decerebrate posturing. This predominance of extensor activity is mediated by the reticulospinal and vestibulospinal pathways, and is aroused by a further lesion induced at the level of the vestibular nuclei. In humans, a similar state may accompany severe midbrain lesions, which usually also cause loss of consciousness. In such a case, all four limbs are rigidly extended, the back is arched, and there may be neck retraction. Thus the patient, if lying supine, is virtually supported by the back of the head and the heels, a posture known as opisthotonos. The arching of the back can be increased by any sensory stimulus and there is striking resistance to any attempt at flexing the limbs passively. Tonic neck reflexes (Section 1.4.5) can usually be elicited; turning the head to one side gives extension of the limbs on that side and flexion on the other.

Decorticate rigidity

Decorticate rigidity usually occurs with lesions of the cerebral white matter, or thalamus and internal capsule. The arm is flexed and adducted while the leg is stiffly extended, the familiar posture of a chronic spastic hemiplegia.

Flaccidity

Flaccidity, or hypotonia, is a reduction in tone. It may be due to cerebral or spinal shock, resulting from acute and extensive brain or spinal-cord lesions which transiently suppress all motor reflex activity. It is a common manifestation of cerebellar disease, associated with diminished gamma efferent activity. It also occurs whenever a lesion of the afferent or efferent pathway interrupts the spinal reflex arc. In severe hypotonia, as in patients with total flaccid paralysis, all resistance to passive stretch is lost and the limbs are limp and flail-like. Lesser degrees of hypotonia in the upper limbs can be elicited by asking the patient to hold out his arms horizontally. The forearms are then tapped briskly. When one limb is hypotonic, the recoil is slowed and the arm swings through a wider range as though 'underdamped'. If a hypotonic patient is asked to raise his arms above his head with the palms facing forwards, the palm of a hypotonic limb is seen to be externally rotated. In practice, hypotonia has limited diagnostic usefulness, being overshadowed by more prominent features of cerebellar disease, such as dysmetria, or of spinal reflex arc disease, such as areflexia.

Pattern of weakness

Severe upper motor neuron lesions cause complete paralysis of the limb. Less severe upper motor neuron lesions cause distinctive patterns of weakness. In the arm, extensor muscles are most markedly affected: deltoid, triceps, finger and wrist extensors, and the dorsal interossei. In the leg, hip flexion due to iliopsoas is usually affected earliest, and hamstring and ankle dorsiflexion weakness is often pronounced. As a general rule, weakness is symmetrically distributed distally in polyneuropathy and proximally in myopathies. The pattern of weakness follows the innervation pattern in mononeuropathy or spinal-nerve root lesions.

Tendon reflexes

Tendon reflexes (Section 1.4.2) are crucial to differentiating between upper and lower motor neuron disorders, being brisk in the former, and often absent or hypoactive in the latter. Although areflexia is common in lower motor neuron lesions, this is mainly due to coexisting involvement of the muscle spindle sensory afferent fibres within peripheral nerves or roots. For example, the tendon reflexes are preserved even with quite advanced muscle denervation in motor neuron disease, because the sensory afferent pathways are not affected. Tendon reflexes are preserved in primary muscle disease, except when chronic fibrosis of the muscle or damage to the muscle spindle have occurred. Areflexia occurs in the rare disorder of Eaton–Lambert myasthenic syndrome.

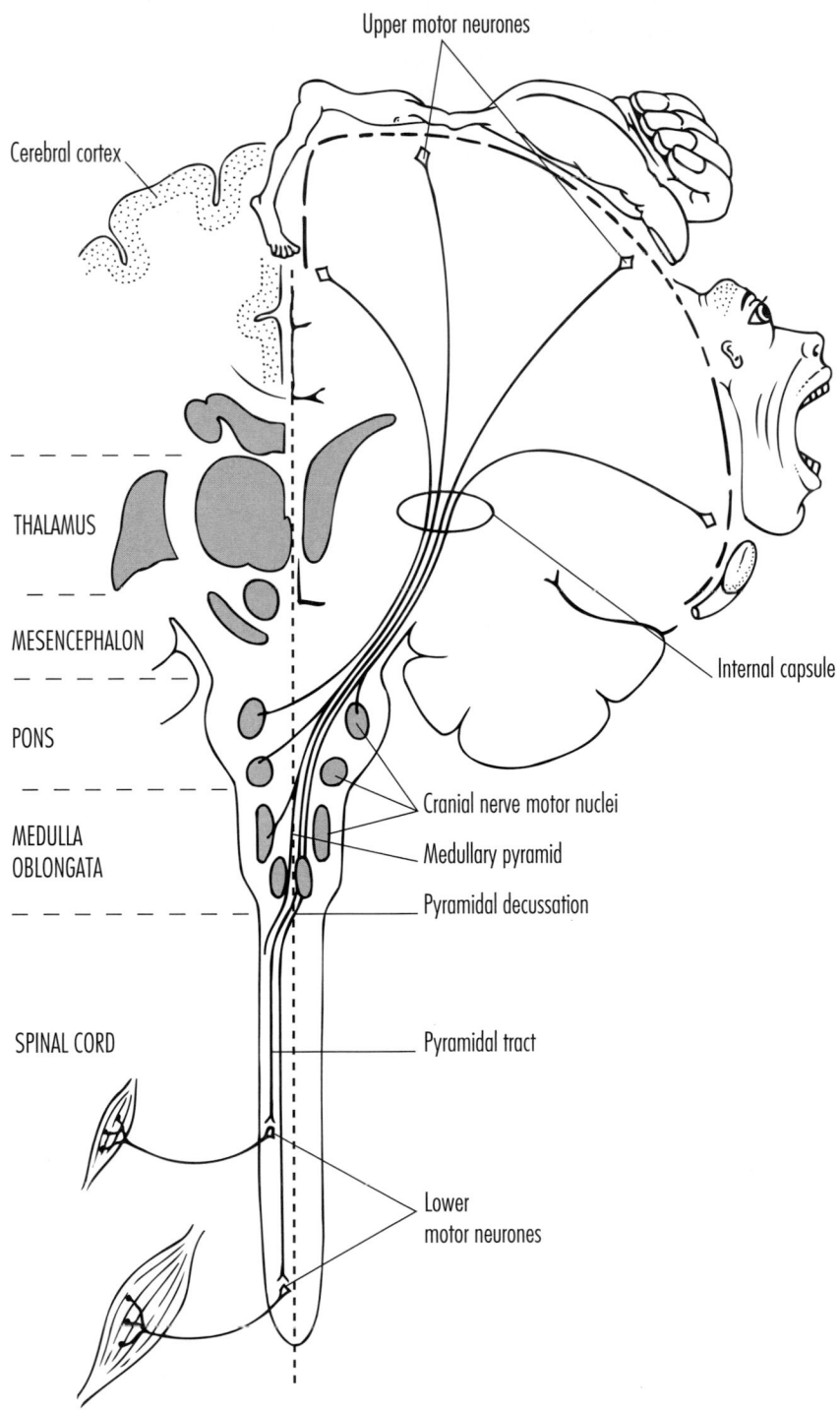

Fig. 1.22. Schematic representation showing the course of the pyramidal tract, the homuncular organization of the motor cortex in the precentral gyrus, the concentration of the motor output within the internal capsule, and the decussation of the pyramidal tract in the medulla oblongata (from Donaghy 1997).

There are only three objective conclusions with clear pathological implications that can be made about any individual tendon reflex viewed alone. Either it is normal, or it is absent despite reinforcement, or it is pathologically brisk in that one or more clonic beats occur during elicitation. A normal reflex may vary from being only obtainable with reinforcement, to being quite brisk in anxious individuals. It is often valuable to compare the briskness of reflexes in different regions of the body. For instance, upper motor neuron lesions will produce brisker tendon reflexes on the side of a hemiplegia, or in the legs compared to the arms in thoracic spinal-cord lesions. A focally hypoactive reflex occurs in the territory of a diseased spinal-nerve root or peripheral nerve. The ankle jerks may be markedly hypoactive compared to the knee and arm reflexes in polyneuropathy.

An extensor plantar reflex (Section 1.4.3) represents incontrovertible evidence of an upper motor neuron lesion. Circumstantial evidence of an upper motor neuron lesion may be provided by absent superficial abdominal reflexes (Section 1.4.3).

1.5.3 Cerebral-hemisphere lesions

Unilateral cerebral-hemisphere lesions cause contralateral hemiparesis, often including the lower facial musculature. The

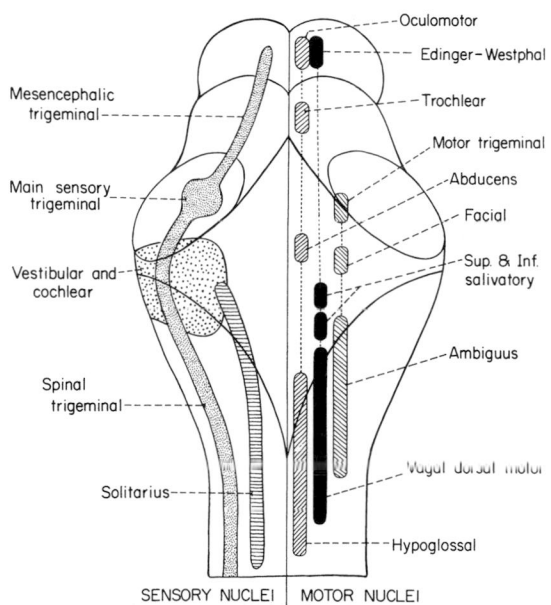

Fig. 1.23. Cranial-nerve nuclei in surface projection on a schematic posterior view of the brainstem. The cerebellum has been removed by a cut through the cerebellar peduncles, so that the floor of the fourth ventricle is revealed. Caudally, the medulla is severed at about the transition to the spinal cord. Rostrally, the superior and inferior colliculi of the midbrain are indicated. The cranial-nerve sensory nuclei are shown on the left side and the motor nuclei on the right. These motor and sensory nuclei are grouped according to the functional categories of the efferent and afferent fibres and associated brainstem nuclei. (Reproduced from Patton, Sundsten, Crill, and Swanson (1976), *Introduction to basic neurology*, Saunders Philadelphia, by kind permission of the authors and publisher.)

forehead, tongue, and bulbar musculature will be spared unless an upper motor neuron lesion is bilateral. Focal lesions affecting only a portion of the motor cortex produce paralysis of the body part represented by that point of the homunculus (Fig 1.22). An example is the 'cortical hand' in which weakness affects all movement of the hand, including finger extension, flexion, and abduction. Complete hemiplegia is a common result of even small lesions in the internal capsule, where the corticospinal-tract fibres are crowded together. Focal motor, or Jacksonian, epileptic attacks, often picking out only one side of the mouth, the finger and thumb, or the great toe, are typical of irritative lesions of the motor cortex. Predominantly proximal or limb-girdle patterns of hemiparesis result from high motor cortex lesions and often result from ischaemia in the watershed between middle and anterior cerebral artery territories. Cortical or subcortical lesions often cause associated cognitive deficit.

By contrast, a lesion deep in the white matter, particularly one affecting the internal capsule, usually produces dense hemiplegia without cognitive loss. Milder hemiparesis with prominent dysarthria or ataxia points to lacunar infarction in the posterior limb of the internal capsule. If a hemiparesis is associated with a cranial nerve lesion on the opposite side, this socalled 'alternating hemiplegia' signifies a brainstem location of the lesion.

1.5.4 Brainstem lesions

The clue to a brainstem lesion causing weakness is an associated disorder of a cranial nerve (Fig. 1.23), or of the intrinsic pathways of the brainstem, such as the cerebellar or vestibular connections. The majority of lesions of the brainstem are due to demyelination, ischaemia, or tumour deposits, and are often patchy and unstereotyped in their location and effects. Pyramidal-tract damage in the brainstem can be either unilateral or bilateral, depending upon the topography of the lesion; asymmetrical bilateral lesions are the most common. Because the pyramidal tract decussates in the lower medulla, all brainstem lesions above this level will produce contralateral weakness. Lesions of the cerebellum or its peduncles are often associated with damage to the adjacent brainstem itself. Cerebellar hemisphere damage causes ipsilateral dysmetria or ataxia, and hypotonicity. Midline damage to the cerebellar vermis causes gait ataxia, truncal ataxia, dysarthria, and slowed, irregular side-to-side tongue movements. Lesions of the flocculonodular lobe, or vestibulocerebellum, produce various eye-movement abnormalities, including skew deviation and head tilt, inaccurate saccades, square-wave jerks, loss of smooth pursuit, and opsoclonus.

Midbrain lesions

Midbrain lesions cause various syndromes which can be associated with weakness if the cerebral peduncles are involved. A lesion of one cerebral peduncle produces an ipsilateral third nerve lesion and contralateral hemiparesis (Weber's syndrome) (Fig. 1.24). Lesions affecting the red nucleus cause ipsilateral third nerve lesions and contralateral tremor (Benedikt

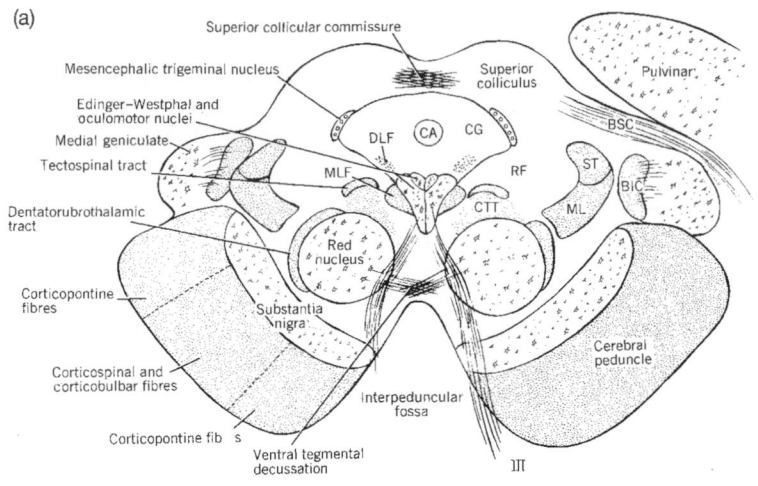

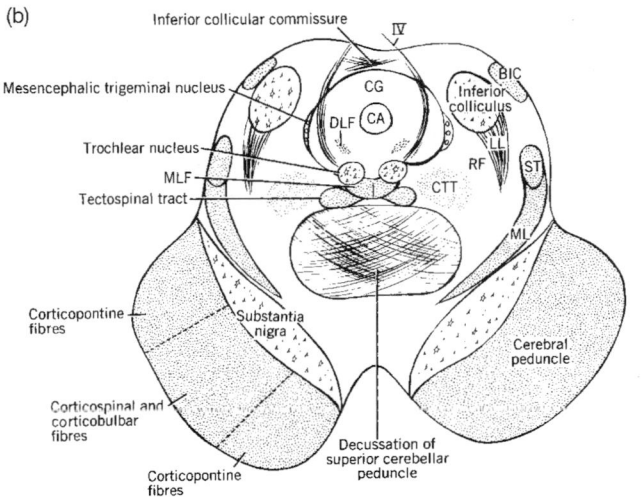

BIC, brachium of the inferior colliculus;
CA, cerebral aqueduct;
CG, central grey matter;
CTT, central tegmental tract;
DLF, dorsal londitudinal tract;
MLF, medial longitudinal fasciculus;
RF, reticular formation;
ST, spinothalamic tract.

Fig. 1.24. Cross-section of the midbrain at rostral (a), caudal (b) levels.
(a) The midbrain at the level of the superior colliculus and oculomotor nerve (III). Fibres of the oculomotor nerve are leaving to enter the interpeduncular fossa. The medial lemniscus (ML) is in the lateral part of the tegmental field. The brachium of the inferior colliculus (BIC) is entering the medial geniculate, and the brachium of the superior colliculus (BSC) is entering the superior colliculus. Fibres from the decussation of the superior cerebellar peduncle have formed at the lateral margin of the red nucleus as the dentatorubrothalamic tract; it sends fibres to the red nucleus and to the ventralis lateralis nucleus of the thalamus. Rubrospinal fibres from the red nucleus cross at the ventral tegmental decussation, and at a more caudal level will join the fibres in the central tegmental tract (CTT), finally ending in the spinal cord.
(b) The midbrain at the level of the inferior colliculus and the trochlear nerve (IV). Fibres of the trochlear nerve are leaving dorsally. The medial lemniscus (ML) is rotating into a dorsoventral position in the lateral tegmental field. The lateral lemniscus (LL) is entering the nucleus of the inferior colliculus. Fibres from the cerebellum are crossing though the tegmentum as the decussation of the superior cerebellar peduncle. (Reproduced from Patton, Sundsten, Crill, and Swanson (1976), by kind permission of the authors and publisher.)

syndrome). Lesions of the central and posterior midbrain produce various eye movement abnormalities, especially affecting vertical eye movements, pupil reactions, and altered eyelid movements. The Parinaud syndrome is an example involving loss of upgaze, eyelid retraction, dissociation of near-light pupil responses and convergence–retraction nystagmus.

Pontine lesions

Pontine lesions (Fig. 1.25) are notably variable in their effects. These include dysarthria, contralateral ataxia, trigeminal (V), abducens (VI), facial (VII), or auditory (VIII) nerve lesions

(Fig. 1.25). Complex eye-movement disorders are common too: ipsilateral gaze palsy, internuclear ophthalmoplegia, one-and-a-half syndrome, and skew deviation. Owing to the higher level of the corticofacial fibres, a unilateral corticospinal lesion in the pons does not cause weakness of the opposite side of the face, but only of the opposite limbs. But the lesion may also involve the facial nucleus or the intrapontine fibres of the facial nerve on the same side, thus causing one form of 'crossed hemiplegia'. Different forms of this have been described. The Millard–Gubler syndrome consists of paralysis of one lateral rectus, due to involvement of the sixth-nerve

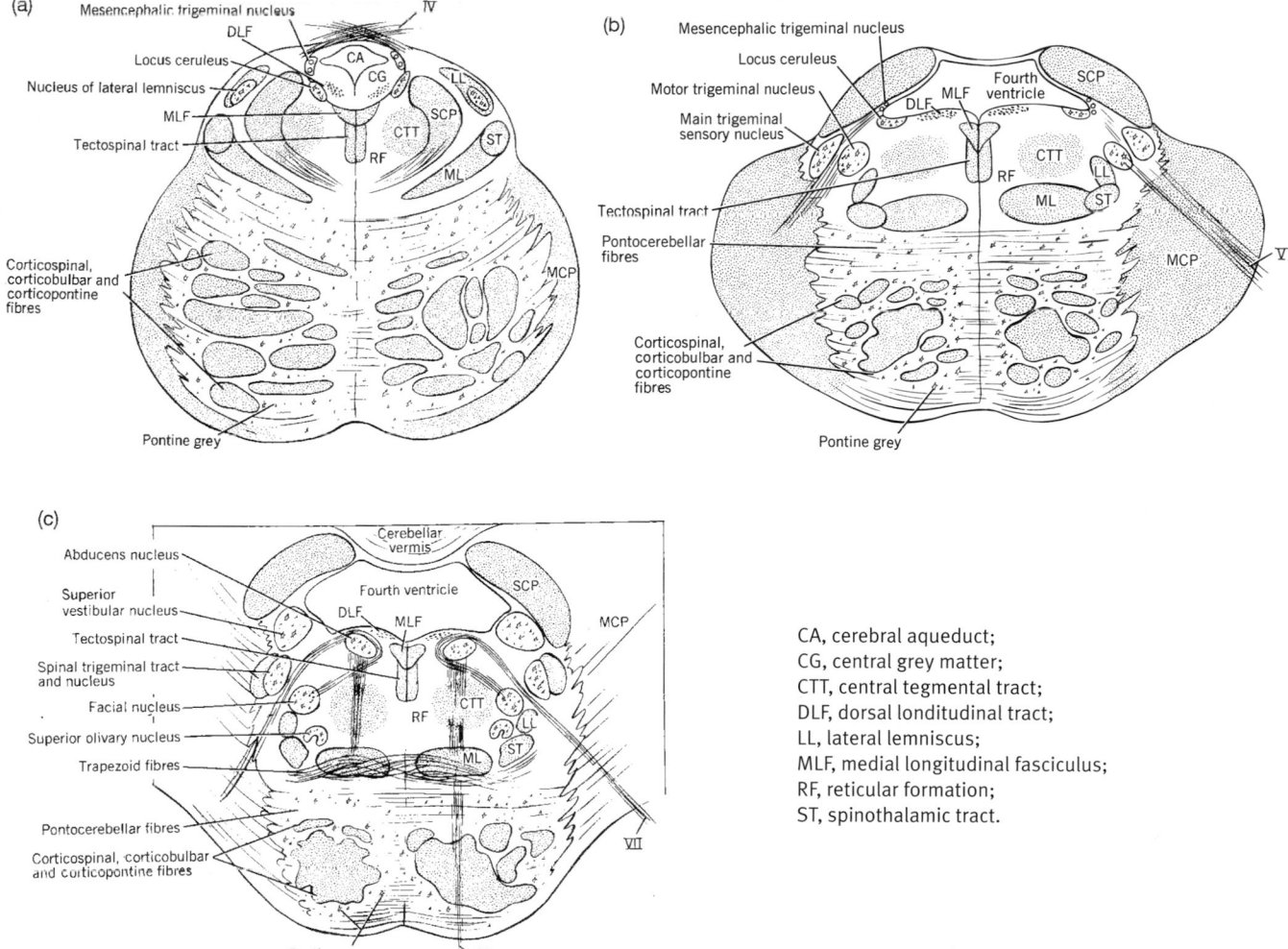

CA, cerebral aqueduct;
CG, central grey matter;
CTT, central tegmental tract;
DLF, dorsal londitudinal tract;
LL, lateral lemniscus;
MLF, medial longitudinal fasciculus;
RF, reticular formation;
ST, spinothalamic tract.

Fig. 1.25. Cross-sections of the pons at rostral (a), mid (b) and caudal (c) levels.

(a) The rostral pons at the isthmus. Fibres of the trochlear nerve (IV) are crossing as they leave dorsally. The medial lemniscus (ML) is moving laterally and beginning to rotate to a dorsoventral position. The superior cerebellar peduncle (SCP) is moving towards the midline. The rostral-most edge of the middle cerebellar peduncle (MCP) is present. The corticospinal, corticobulbar, and corticopontine fibres, which constitute the cerebellar peduncle, are separating as they plunge into the basilar pontine grey matter.

(b) The midpons at the level of the trigeminal nerve (V). Fibres of the trigeminal nerve separate the main sensory trigeminal and motor trigeminal nuclei. The cell bodies of proprioceptive trigeminal afferents constitute the mesencephalic nucleus. The trigeminal nerve leaves through the middle cerebellar peduncle (MCP). The medial lemniscus (ML) has begun to move laterally towards the spinothalamic tract (ST). The superior cerebellar peduncle (SCP) forms the lateral wall of the fourth ventricle as it descends from the cerebellum towards to midbrain tegmentum. Pontocerebellar fibres (receiving input from the corticopontine fibres) are streaming across the midline to form the middle cerebellar peduncle. The corticospinal, corticobulbar, and corticopontine fibres are scattered throughout the basilar pontine grey matter.

(c) The caudal pons at the level of the abducens (VI) and facial (VII) nerves. The abducens nerve leaves ventrally through the basal pons near the midline; the facial nerve loops medially around the abducens nucleus and then courses laterally to emerge at the caudal edge of the middle cerebellar peduncle (MCP). The pontine grey matter is sending pontocerebellar fibres across the midline to form the middle cerebellar peduncle. The superior cerebellar peduncle (SCP) is projecting towards the midbrain. The medial lemniscus (ML) has rotated to a mediolateral position and is obscured by trapezoid fibres of the auditory system that cross the midline; the trapezoid fibres will turn rostrally to ascend in the lateral lemniscus. Primary afferents from the trigeminal nerve have formed the spinal trigeminal tract. (Reproduced from Patton, Sundsten, Crill, and Swanson (1976), by kind permission of the authors and publisher.)

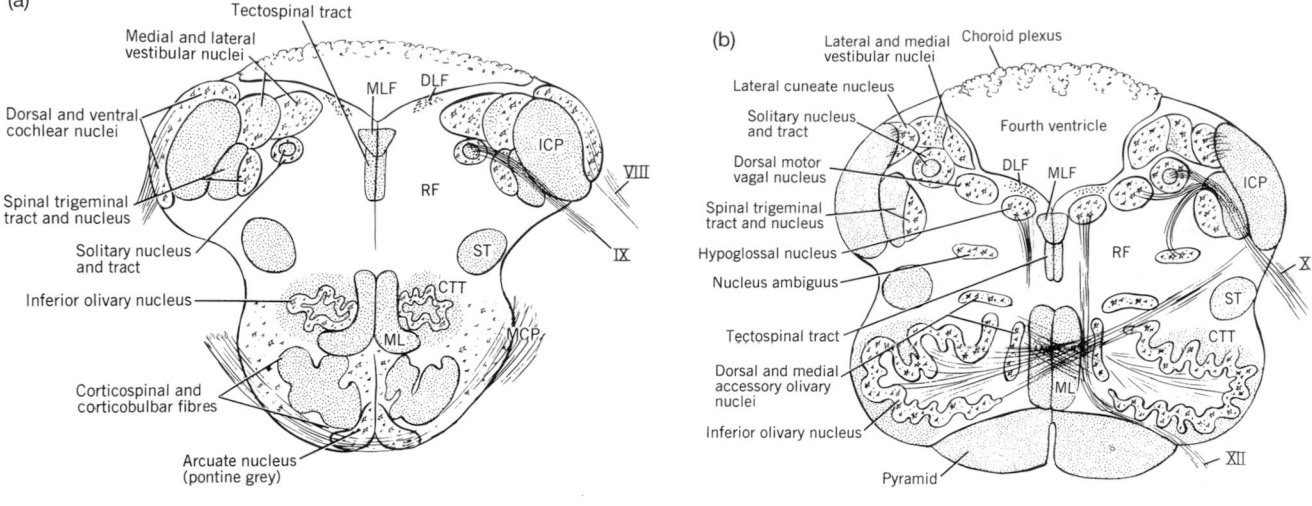

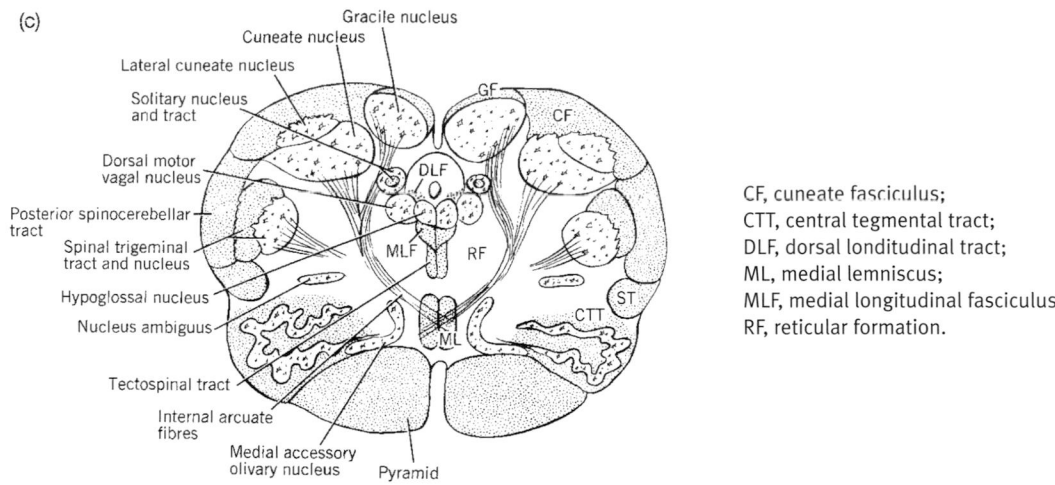

CF, cuneate fasciculus;
CTT, central tegmental tract;
DLF, dorsal londitudinal tract;
ML, medial lemniscus;
MLF, medial longitudinal fasciculus;
RF, reticular formation.

Fig. 1.26. Cross-sections of the medulla oblongata at rostral (a) mid (b) and caudal (c) levels.
(a) The rostral medulla at the level of the vestibulocochlear (VIII) and glossopharyngeal (IX) nerves. The cochlear nuclei cap the lateral surface of the inferior cerebellar peduncle (ICP). The medial lemniscus (ML) is still situated medially along the midline. Its trigeminolemniscal components (not shown) would be in its most dorsal part; the laterally placed spinothalamic tract (ST) would also contain trigeminothalamic components. The rostral pole of the inferior olivary nucleus appears in the course of the descending central tegmental tract (CTT), some of whose fibres terminate there; another component of the central tegmental tract will continue its descent to the spinal cord (rubrospinal tract). The corticospinal and corticobulbar fibres are closely grouped as the pontine grey matter thins out; just cordal to this section they will form the medullary pyramids. The caudalmost edge of the middle cerebellar peduncle (MCP) is present.
(b) The midmedulla at the level of the vagus (X) and hypoglossal (XII) nerves. The vagus nerve leaves lateral to the inferior olivary nucleus, whereas the hypoglossal nerve does so between it and the pyramid. Motor components of the vagus are shown coming from the dorsal motor vagal nucleus and nucleus ambiguus; visceral afferents are forming the tractus solitarius. The medial lemniscus is orientated dorsoventrally along the midline above the pyramid; the spinothalamic tract (ST) is in the lateral part of the tegmental field. Olivocerebellar fibres are crossing and will enter the inferior cerebellar peduncle (ICP). The lateral cuneate nucleus is also sending fibres into the inferior cerebellar peduncle. The descending corticospinal and corticobulbar fibres have grouped together to form the pyramids.
(c) The caudal medulla at the level of the sensory decussation. Most of the fibres of the gracile fasciculus (GF) have already synapsed in the gracile nucleus. Internal arcuate fibres from the cuneate and gracile nucleus are crossing to form the medial lemniscus (ML). Second-order fibres from the spinal trigeminal nucleus are extending towards the midline. They will cross, some forming a component of the medial lemniscus and others mixing with the spinothalamic fibres. The spinothalamic tract (ST) is in the lateral tegmental field. The posterior spinocerebellar tract is lateral to the spinal trigeminal tract and will enter the inferior cerebellar peduncle rostral to this level. (Reproduced from Patton, Sundsten, Crill, and Swanson (1976), by kind permission of the authors and publisher.)

nucleus, with or without lower motor neuron facial paralysis on the same side and supranuclear paralysis of the limbs on the opposite side. Foville's syndrome is similar to the Millard–Gubler syndrome, except that paralysis of the conjugate ocular deviation to the side of the lesion takes the place of lateral rectus paralysis.

Medulla oblongata lesions

Medulla oblongata lesions are more likely to cause weakness if medially situated. The lower the medullary lesion, the more likely is involvement of the pyramidal decussation. A medial medullary lesion produces an ipsilateral hypoglossal (XII) nerve deficit and contralateral sensory loss, affecting vibration sense and joint position in addition to the contralateral hemiparesis (Fig 1.26). More lateral medullary lesions cause the Wallenberg syndrome of ipsilateral trigeminal (V) territory sensory loss, Horner's syndrome, nystagmus, loss of gag reflex (IX and X cranial nerves) and contralateral spinothalamic tract damage with pain and temperature loss below the face.

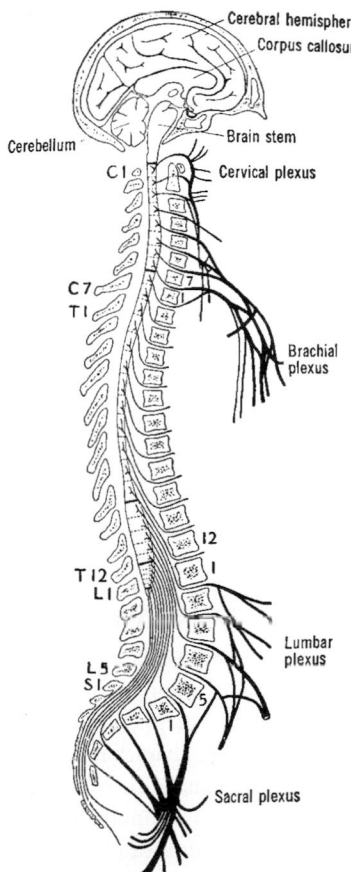

Fig. 1.27. Drawing of the brain and spinal cord *in situ*. The brain is shown sectioned in the median plane. Although not illustrated, the first cervical vertebra articulates with the base of the skull. The letters along the vertebral column indicate cervical, thoracic, lumbar, and sacral. Note that the cord ends at the upper border of the second lumbar vertebra. (Reproduced from Gardner (1975) by kind permission of the author and publisher.)

1.5.5 Spinal cord lesions

The distinctive clinical features of a spinal cord lesion are paralysis below the level of the lesion with signs of upper motor neuron damage, impaired sphincter control, and a sensory level. It should be noted that the spinal cord is shorter than the vertebral column and thus the segmental localization of a lesion will correspond to a higher vertebral level (Fig. 1.27). If the dorsal columns are substantially affected, there will be gait ataxia, Rombergism and altered joint position and vibration sensations in the feet. The tendon reflex arc may be interrupted at the level of the lesion, and associated muscle wasting and weakness may reflect anterior horn cell destruction at that segment.

1.5.6 Neuromuscular disease

Lower motor neuron lesions produce patterns of weakness which reflect pathology localized to the anterior horn cells, a spinal-nerve root, or an individual peripheral nerve.

Spinal roots

The myotomal pattern of weakness occurring with spinal-nerve root lesion is usually accompanied by dermatomally distributed sensory disturbance and loss of the tendon reflex subserved by that segment. In reality, most muscles receive spinal root innervation from at least two segments, and single nerve-root lesions usually produce relatively mild degrees of weakness (Table 1.7). Furthermore there is some variation in the exact spinal segment that makes the major contribution to a muscle, depending upon whether the brachial or lumbosacral plexus is pre-fixed or post-fixed (Section 13.6.1).

Peripheral neuropathy

A detailed account of the muscles innervated by individual peripheral nerves of the arm and leg is given elsewhere (Sections 13.10 and 13.11, respectively). Polyneuropathy produces weakness which is symmetrical, and predominantly distally located; additional weakness of proximal muscles may occur in acquired demyelinating polyneuropathies affecting proximal nerve

Table 1.7. Myotomes of use in localizing spinal nerve root lesions

Spinal segment	Muscle
C5	Deltoid, Spinati
C6	Brachioradialis
C7	Triceps, Extensor digitorum
C8	Flexor digitorum profundus
T1	Dorsal interossei
L1, L2	Iliopsoas
L3	Thigh adductors
L3, L4	Quadriceps
L4, L5	Tibialis anterior
L5	Extensor hallucis longus
S1, S2	Gastrocnemius, Soleus

segments and roots. Lesions of the brachial or lumbosacral plexus produce patterns of weakness, and sensory and reflex loss, which cannot be accounted for by lesions either of an individual spinal nerve root or an individual peripheral nerve (Section 13.1.2).

Primary muscle disease

Primary muscle disease characteristically affects the proximal limb muscles symmetrically. Various forms of muscular dystrophy (Section 15.2) pick out specific muscle groups, facio-scapulohumeral and oculopharyngeal dystrophies being examples. Myasthenia gravis (Section 15.10.1) may present with proximal limb muscle weakness, with pharyngeal and palatal weakness, or with ptosis and eye-movement abnormalities; characteristically muscle bulk will be preserved, reflexes are normal, and fatiguability is demonstrable. Proximal muscle weakness also occurs in the Lambert–Eaton myasthenic syndrome (Section 15.10.2), but there are associated autonomic features such as dry mouth. Furthermore, the tendon reflexes, although initially absent, show post-tetanic potentiation in which the reflex appears when retested after sustained maximal contraction of its muscle. Neck extensor muscle weakness is uncommon and occurs in myasthenia, motor neuron diseases, myotonic dystrophy, and some myopathies. Muscle and neuro-muscular junction diseases do not produce sensory disturbance.

1.5.7 Fluctuating weakness

Not uncommonly, patients demonstrate momentarily fluctuating, inconsistent, or collapsing patterns of weakness. There are three possible causes of this: loss of sensory feedback, pain or, most usually, psychological factors. Fluctuating weakness due to loss of kinaesthetic feedback usually affects the hand, and is often associated with pseudoathetosis. Normality of underlying muscle power can be demonstrated by asking the patient to look at his or her hand while making a simple elemental movement, such as abducting the index finger. This will reverse weakness that had been apparent during a more complex movement, such as spreading all the fingers apart. Collapsing weakness due to pain in a joint may be accompanied by complaints of discomfort; the raw power of the muscles can be assessed by instructing the patient to 'push as hard as you can just for a moment when I count to three'. Psychologically determined weakness (Section 1.9.3) fluctuates, is inconsistent, may be improved temporarily by firm encouragement, and is discordant with obviously better use of the limb during natural activities such as dressing. It may be associated with theatrical grunting and sighing in a charade of effort, and the collapsing element may occur more from the trunk than from the limb itself.

1.6 Somatosensory abnormalities

1.6.1 Sensory symptoms

Patients express their symptoms of sensory dysfunction in a multitude of ways, and only careful enquiry by the neurologist will determine their likely pathophysiological relevance.

Numbness

Numbness is a term that is used confusingly. Most doctors mean by it 'a loss of sensation', but many patients really mean weakness or clumsiness. It is less ambiguous to ask about 'deadness of skin sensation'. Polyneuropathy produces numbness in a glove-and-stocking distribution. When patients describe numbness or 'pins and needles' extending on to the trunk, it is most commonly due to myelitis, an inflammation of the spinal cord, which may occur as part of multiple sclerosis. Some patients with numb feet describe a feeling of walking on cotton wool. Those with numb hands may feel as though they are touching things through a plastic bag.

Paraesthesiae

Paraesthesiae are spontaneous abnormal sensations, most usually described as 'pins and needles'. They may be physiological, especially during hyperventilation, but in such cases they are generalized, especially perioral, and only intermittent. Continuous paraesthesiae are an important indicator of acquired, rather than congenital disease of the nervous system. They are particularly likely in idiopathic demyelinating polyneuropathy, and less commonly in lesions of central sensory pathways. Attacks of focal paraesthesiae can occur in focal epilepsy of the sensory cortex. Focal paraesthesiae, occurring intermittently, are common in compressive mononeuropathy, a common example being the finger paraesthesiae at night and after hand usage in carpal tunnel syndrome.

Dysaesthesiae

Dysaesthesiae are unpleasant distorted sensations resulting from actual sensory stimuli. Usually they occur in focal peripheral nerve damage or polyneuropathies that involve axonal degeneration.

Spontaneous pain

Spontaneous pain can occur in association with paraesthesiae in peripheral nerve disorders. It is a particular and early feature in the sensory territory of a nerve affected by vasculitis. Lancinating pain radiating in a dermatomal distribution down a limb, like an electric shock, suggests spinal-nerve root compression by prolapsed intervertebral disc. Painful disorders of an internal viscus, joint, or muscle may be referred to an area of skin either overlying or remote to the abnormality. Spontaneous pain in the limbs, trunk, or face can arise from posterior thalamic lesions and has a particularly unpleasant burning character, often with 'tearing' or 'grinding' qualities. Similar sensations of continuous burning, warmth, or cold may result from a spinothalamic-tract lesion, but are clearly localized to within an area of altered skin sensation. Spontaneous pain occurs in causalgia and reflex sympathetic dystrophy (Section 13.4).

Analgesia and thermoanaesthesia

Reduced ability to feel pain and temperature sensations occurs in peripheral neuropathies affecting unmyelinated and small myelinated fibres and in lesions of the spinothalamic tract, including syringomyelia and posterior thalamus. Painless burns, or unfelt wounds, may occur in the analgesic area.

Lhermitte's symptom

Lhermitte's symptom consists of an electric shock or strong paraesthesiae radiating down the trunk, and often into the limbs, on sudden flexion of the neck. It is particularly common in myelitis due to multiple sclerosis, and also occurs in cervical spondylitic myelopathy, vitamin B_{12} deficiency, and some sensory neuropathies involving both the central and peripheral axons of the dorsal root ganglia.

Tight bands and size distortions

Tight bands and size distortions, such as feeling that the toes are swollen, are abnormal sensations occurring in the fingers and feet of patients with acquired demyelinating polyneuropathy and lesions of the dorsal columns in the spinal cord.

Clumsiness and Rombergism

Clumsiness and Rombergism are due to loss of kinaesthetic feedback via large myelinated peripheral nerve sensory fibres or the dorsal column–medial lemniscus system. Hand clumsiness particularly affects the complex motor–sensory integration involved in activities such as doing up buttons or underwear clips, particularly when the eyes cannot monitor the action. 'Dropping things' may be an associated complaint; although this symptom in isolation rarely denotes disease. Loss of joint position sense from the legs causes gait unsteadiness. This is particularly noticeable when the patient tries to walk in the dark or close their eyes in the shower, and is known as Rombergism.

Astereognosis

Astereognosis occurs in patients with parietal lobe lesions. Such patients may complain of being unable to identify coins manually in their pockets or with their eyes closed.

1.6.2 Sensory examination

Many complex and time-consuming methods have been described for semiquantitative assessment of different sensory modalities. In most clinical situations these make little or no extra contribution to diagnosis over and above what can be achieved by simple testing of superficial skin sensation using the fingertips or a pin, routine testing of vibration and joint position sense, and Romberg's test. What is important is to examine each patient with a clear strategy for resolving the diagnostic hypotheses. The neurologist must instruct the patient clearly in how to respond to stimuli, and must present these stimuli unambiguously. In general, superficial sensation is assessed by taking the patients' view as to whether the stimulus 'feels normal'. By contrast, joint position and vibration sensations can be assessed more objectively by using the principles of blinding (in which the patients' eyes are closed), coupled with forced-choice (in which the patient has to respond 'up' or 'down'), or time-locked response (in which the patient has to say 'now' immediately the tuning fork stops vibrating).

Superficial skin sensation

The boundary of an area of sensory loss is mapped best by starting within the numb area and working outwards until the normal area is reached. Traditionally, an unused pin or a wisp of cotton wool are recommended. However, neither patients nor doctors are familiar with the thresholds for such sensations on different parts of the body. This can make it difficult for the patient to report whether the quality of sensation is altered, unless there is a clear boundary; it is rare for skin sensation to be lost completely. However, everyone is familiar with the feeling of fingertips on every part of their body skin and patients can tell you instantly whether the finger 'feels normal' when you lightly stroke any patch of skin. Furthermore, the examiner can use both forefingers to present simultaneously comparable stimuli to the two sides of the patient's body. Thus the use of fingertip stroking is recommended for routine testing of superficial sensation and will reveal abnormalities of spinothalamic (tickle) or dorsal column (pressure) pathways. Only rarely is it necessary to test temperature sensation; if so, the cold metal of a tuning fork generally provides a sufficient stimulus. A tube of warm water can be used to test warm sensation in those rare occasions when it is necessary to test the unmyelinated thermal fibres in isolation. Occasionally superficial sensory testing produces hyperpathia, in which any background loss of sensation is overshadowed by an abnormal, and sometimes unpleasant, additional quality to the sensory experience. In such situations it can be difficult to determine which is the abnormal side, because of this apparent heightening of sensation.

Vibration sensation

Vibration sensation should be tested using a 128 Hz tuning fork struck in such a way that it does not produce audible high-frequency harmonics that can be heard, rather than felt, by the patient. Place it on the patient's sternum and ask 'Can you feel it

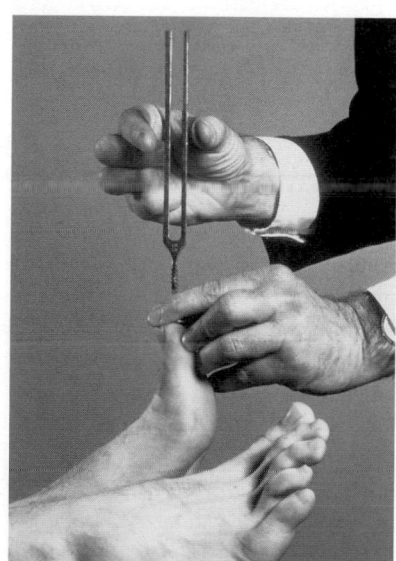

Fig. 1.28. Testing vibration sense. The fingers of one hand are positioned ready to stop the tuning fork vibrating. (From Donaghy 1997.)

buzzing?' Then move it to the tip of the great toe, or a finger, and ask the patient to 'Close your eyes, and tell me as soon as it stops buzzing'. The patient should respond promptly when the examiner stops the buzzing prongs with the fingers of his other hand (Fig. 1.28).

If vibration sense is absent from the toes, testing should be repeated more proximally on the ankle malleolus, tibial bone, knee, anterior superior iliac crest, and finally the rib cage. Vibration sense abnormalities usually mean that there is a polyneuropathy affecting large myelinated sensory fibres, or a spinal-cord lesion. Vibration sense is not affected by a lesion restricted to the somatosensory cerebral cortex. Vibration sense is lost from the lower legs of many elderly people as a natural phenomenon of ageing.

Joint position sensation

With the patient's eyes open, move the great toe up and then down, showing to the patient 'this is up and this is down'. Then ask the patient to close his or her eyes and identify small movements (Fig. 1.29). The distal interphalangeal joints of the fingers can be tested similarly. Usually joint position sensation is lost in similar conditions to loss of vibration sensation. It is particularly likely to be abnormal in patients with sensory ataxia or Rombergism. But, unlike vibration sensation, joint position perception is also lost in lesions of the somatosensory cortex.

Romberg's test and pseudoathetosis

Romberg's test and pseudoathetosis provide evidence of loss of kinaesthetic sensory feedback from the legs and hands, respectively. They are abnormal in disorders of large myelinated sensory peripheral nerve fibres and of the dorsal column–

medial lemniscus system. Romberg's test has been described previously (Section 1.3.2). Pseudoathetosis is demonstrated by asking patients to close their eyes and extend their hands and fingers in front of them. The fingers and wrist 'wander' slowly in random directions, of which the patient is unaware (Fig. 12.16).

Sensory inattention

Sensory inattention occurs with lesions of the parietal lobe insufficient to cause gross cortical sensory loss, but sufficient to cause perceptual rivalry between the two sides of the body. The patient is able to appreciate stimuli when applied separately to either side of the body. However, when two similar stimuli are applied simultaneously to the same skin area on each side, one side will be ignored. This finding implies a disturbance in function of the sensory area of the contralateral cerebral cortex. The phenomenon does not occur if the interval between the two contacts is more than 3 seconds (Critchley 1953).

Astereognosis

Astereognosis is another sign which may occur in patients with lesions of the arm representation of the opposite sensory cortex. They are unable to appreciate the form and texture of objects placed in the hand with the eyes closed. Correctly this should be called *stereoanaesthesia*, but the term *astereognosis* is more often used. Strictly speaking, the latter term should be reserved for failure to recognize objects, such as coins, when the primary sensory modalities are intact. This is an agnosic defect,

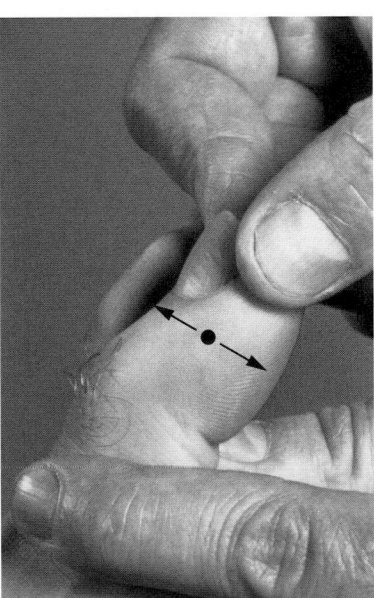

Fig. 1.29. Testing joint position sense at the great toe. The proximal phalanx is steadied with one hand while the toe is moved up and down. (From Donaghy 1997.)

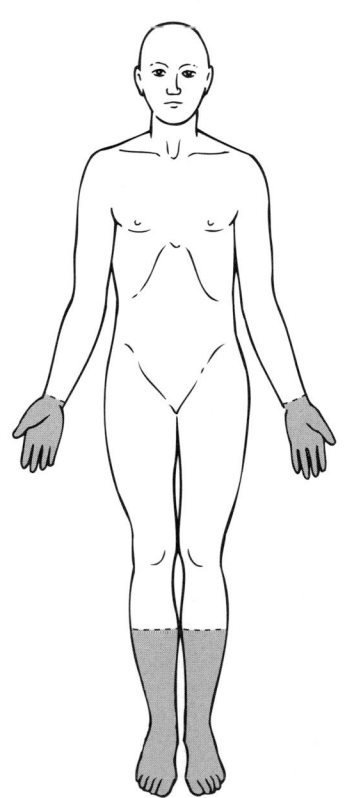

Fig. 1.30. Glove and stocking sensory loss in polyneuropathy (from Donaghy 1997).

due to a disorder of sensory association and akin to the other more complex disorders of parietal-lobe function.

Two-point discrimination abnormalities and graphaesthesia

Two-point discrimination abnormalities and graphaesthesia occur in patients with a lesion of the sensory cortex. The threshold for two-point discrimination is much greater on the abnormal than on the normal side, and there may be inability to recognize figures or letters drawn on the skin. Sensory stimuli are also incorrectly localized on the affected side.

1.6.3 Patterns of sensory loss

Polyneuropathy

A distal stocking, and later glove, distribution of diminished skin sensation is typical of polyneuropathy (Fig. 1.30). Usually the border between normal and reduced sensation gradually changes over some centimetres, rather than being abrupt.

Focal neuropathy

The pattern of superficial sensory loss corresponds to the territory of innervation of the affected peripheral nerve (Fig. 1.31). The border between normal and reduced sensation is reasonably well-defined, although not abrupt. Usually the area of sensory loss for touch is larger than that for pain or temperature.

Spinal root lesions

Spinal root lesions cause loss of superficial sensation in the corresponding dermatome (Fig. 1.32). In the earlier stages of a single root lesion, tingling or pain in the dermatome may occur without demonstrable superficial sensory loss, because there is same overlap of innervation from adjacent roots.

Spinal cord lesions

Spinal cord lesions produce patterns and modalities of sensory loss which depend upon the level of the lesion, the degree of damage to the spinothalamic tracts in the arterolateral cord, which carry pain and temperature sensations from the oppo-

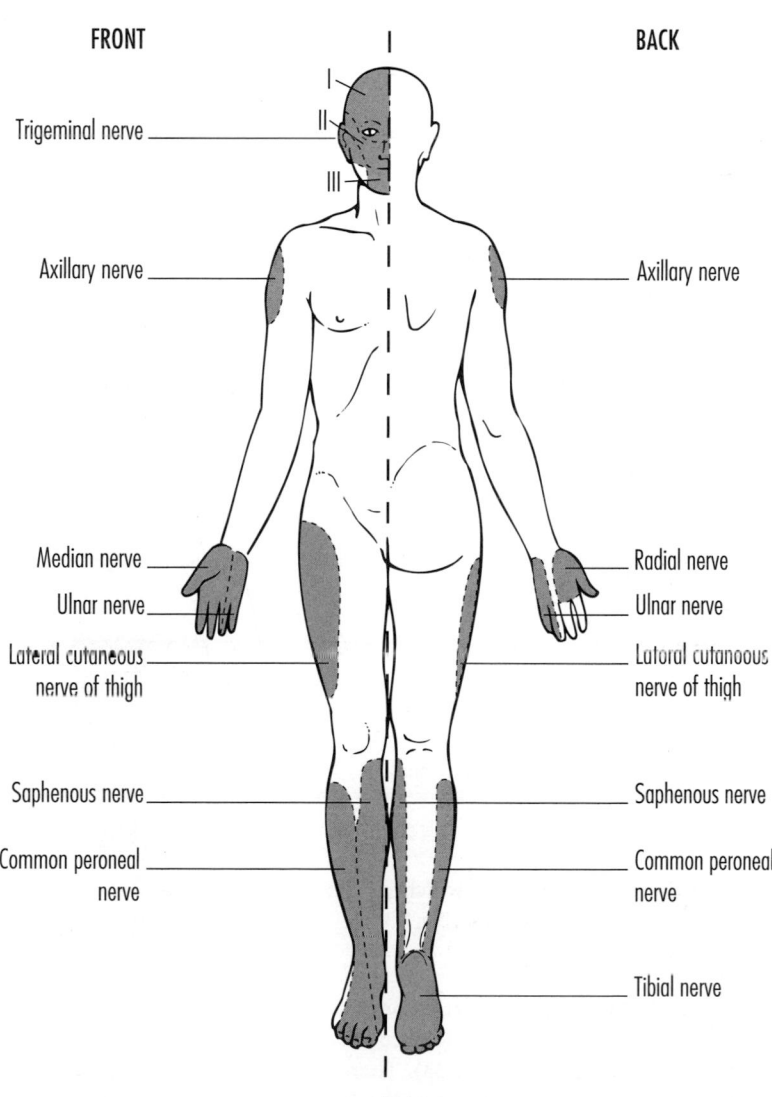

FRONT   BACK

Trigeminal nerve

Axillary nerve   Axillary nerve

Median nerve   Radial nerve

Ulnar nerve   Ulnar nerve

Lateral cutaneous nerve of thigh   Lateral cutaneous nerve of thigh

Saphenous nerve   Saphenous nerve

Common peroneal nerve   Common peroneal nerve

Tibial nerve

Fig. 1.31. Skin territories of some commonly damaged peripheral nerves. Skin territories of all named cutaneous nerves are shown in Fig. 13.1. (From Donaghy 1997.)

FRONT   BACK

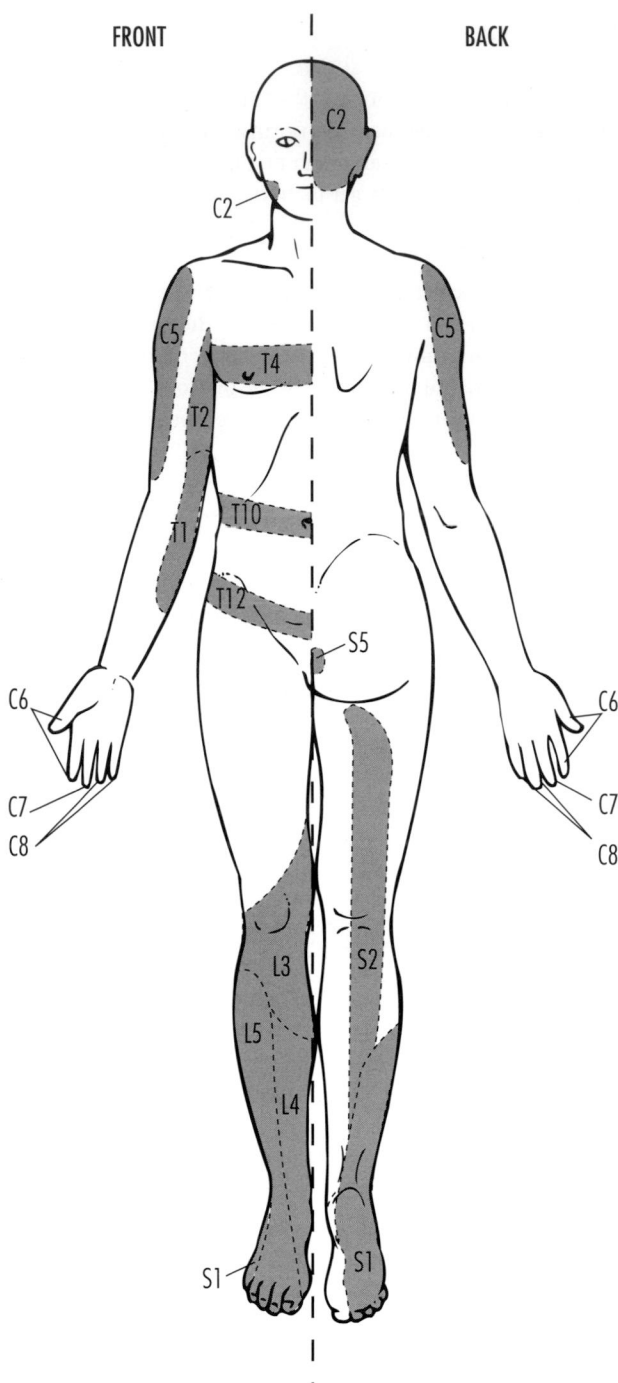

Fig. 1.32. Some memorizable dermatomal landmarks (from Donaghy 1997).

above the lesion. External compression of the spinal cord often produces early loss of pain and temperature sensation in the sacral dermatomes, because the fibres subserving these lowest segments travel most superficially within the spinothalamic tracts.

Intramedullary spinal cord lesions

Intramedullary spinal cord lesions initially affect the decussating spinothalamic tracts within the spinal cord at the level of the lesion (Fig. 1.35a). This produces a 'cape-like' pattern of suspended sensory loss affecting pain and temperature sensations, but not touch or kinaesthesia (Fig. 1.35b); a pattern typical of syringomyelia (Section 20.6.2). Expanding intramedullary lesions within the spinal cord usually spare pain sensation from the sacral dermatomes, because these fibres travel the most superficially in the spinothalamic tracts.

Brown–Séquard syndrome

The Brown–Séquard syndrome follows damage to one half of the spinal cord (Fig. 1.36). Below the level of the lesion there is ipsilateral weakness and loss of vibration and joint position sensations and contralateral loss of pain and temperature sensations. Elements of light touch sensation may be preserved bilaterally since it is a composite sensation involving both spinothalamic and dorsal column pathways.

Myelitis

Myelitis can produce relatively restricted patterns of sensory loss which characteristically extend onto the trunk, may spare

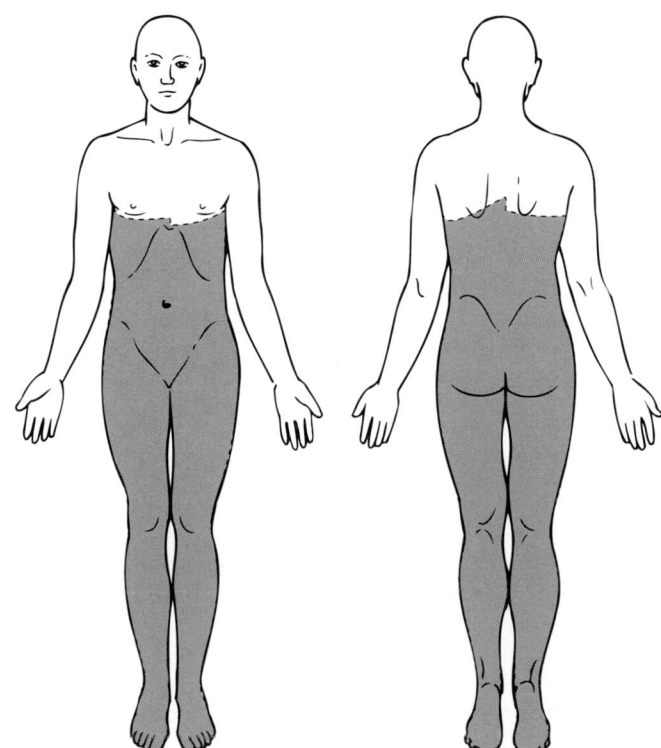

Fig. 1.33. A 'sensory level' in compression of the spinal cord at the T5 level (from Donaghy 1997).

site side (Fig. 1.34a), and to the dorsal columns, which carry vibration and joint position sensations ipsilaterally (Fig.1.34b).

Spinal cord compression

Spinal cord compression or transection causes reduction or loss of all modalities of sensation below the dermatomal level corresponding to the segment of the transection (Fig. 1.33). There may be a zone of hyperaesthesia in the dermatome immediately

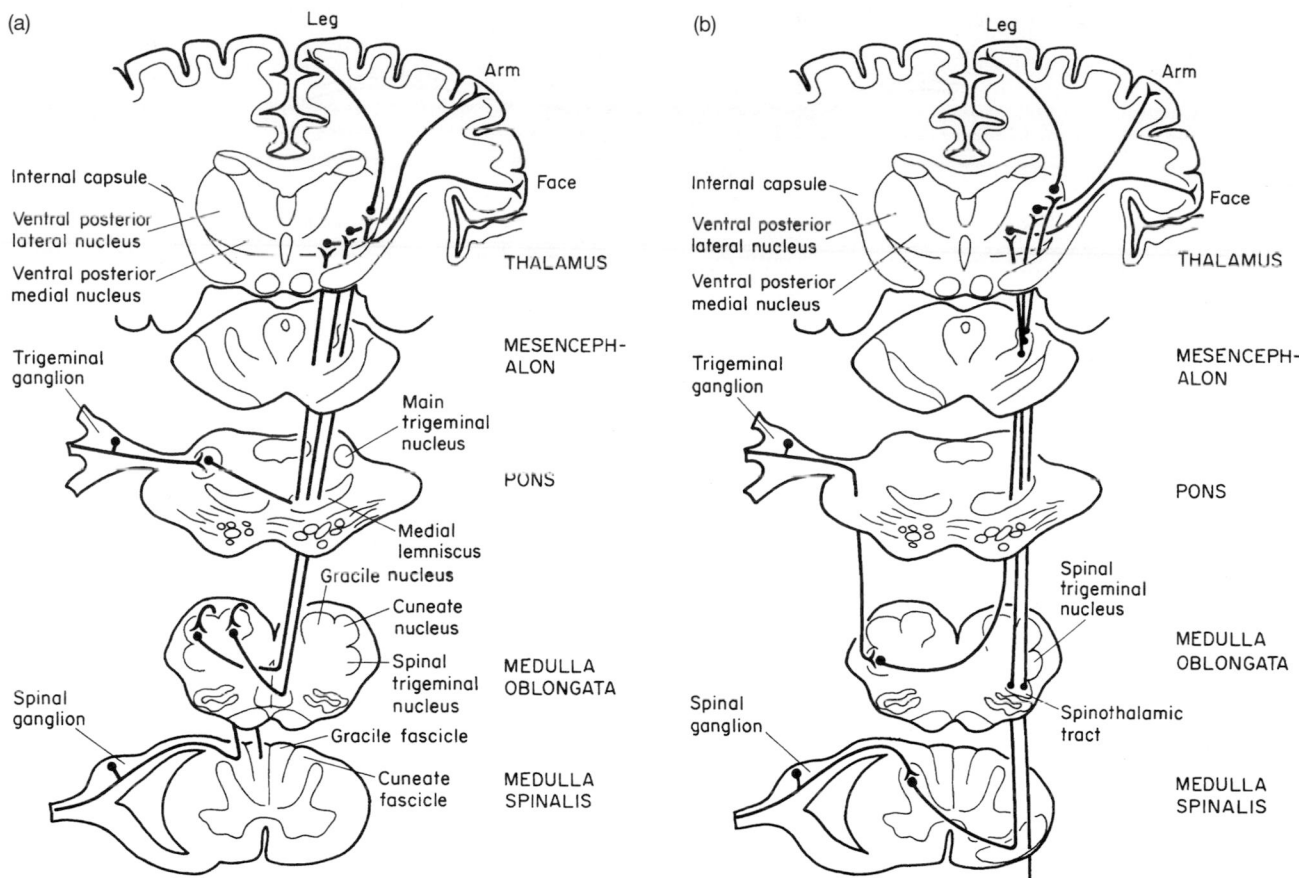

Fig. 1.34. Spinal-cord sensory pathways. (a) The spinothalamic tract. This is the main pathway for transmission of signals from nociceptors and thermoreceptors. (b) The dorsal column–medial lemniscus pathway. This is the main pathway for transmission of signals from low-threshold mechanoreceptors. Fibres transmitting impulses from mechanoreceptors in the face join the medial lemniscus in the brainstem. (From P. Brodal (1992), *The central nervous system*, Oxford University Press.)

the hand or foot, and may be strictly unilateral (Fig. 1.37). Depending upon the location of the myelitis within the spinal cord, spinothalamic and dorsal column sensations may be differentially affected. Sometimes a Brown–Séquard syndrome is encountered if only one half of the spinal cord is involved. Severe forms of myelitis produce impairment of all modalities of sensation below the level of the lesion.

Foramen magnum lesions

Foramen magnum and high cervical spinal cord compressive lesions can cause loss of vibration sense limited to the arms and upper ribcage if the lesion affects the decussation of the medial lemniscus. External compressive lesions at the foramen magnum may produce symptoms of 'rotating sensory loss' in which sensory symptoms start in one limb, for instance a foot, and later rotate to the other foot and the hand on the same side, before eventually reaching the remaining hand.

Brainstem lesions

Brainstem lesions produce sensory abnormalities interpretable on an anatomical basis. Dissociated sensory loss in the face can result from syringobulbia, due to involvement of the descend-

ing fibres from the trigeminal nerve. Lesions of the pons and medulla can give facial sensory impairment on one side, due to a lesion of the trigeminal nucleus, with hemianaesthesia or hemianalgesia of the trunk and limbs on the opposite side due to involvement of ascending sensory tracts. A lesion of the upper pons or midbrain can give complete contralateral sensory loss. An infarct in the midbrain involving the third-nerve nucleus, red nucleus, and medial lemniscus may give a unilateral third-nerve palsy with contralateral static tremor, hemianaesthesia (Benedikt's syndrome), and hemianalgesia. More often, such unilateral sensory loss is dissociated, involving only pain and temperature sensation, owing to selective involvement of ascending fibres of the spinothalamic tract, as in the lateral-medullary (Wallenberg's) syndrome due to vertebral or posterior inferior cerebellar artery thrombosis. Occasionally in such cases there is a sensory level on the trunk on the affected side (Matsumoto *et al.* 1988).

Thalamic lesions

Thalamic lesions can produce patchy contralateral hemianaesthesia and hemianalgesia. Often there is also spontaneous pain of a peculiar, unpleasant, and disturbing nature on the partially

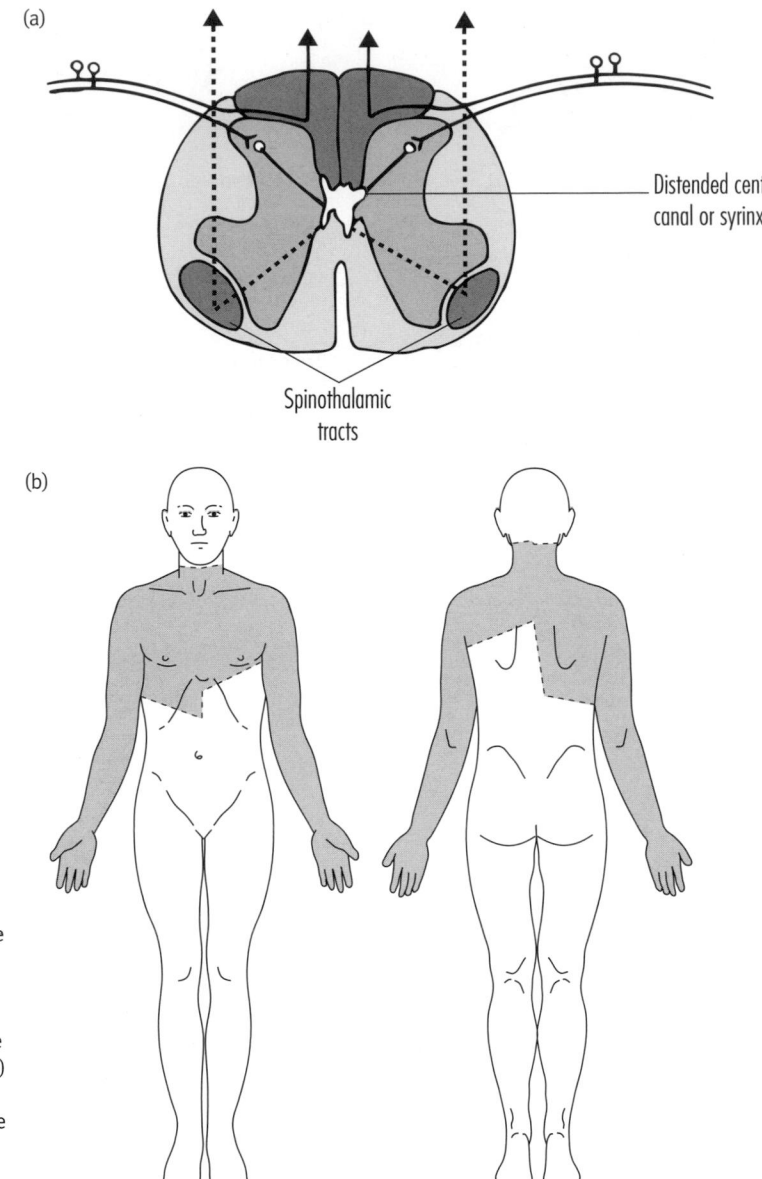

Fig. 1.35. Sensory loss in intramedullary spinal cord lesions, such as syringomyelia. (a) Diagram showing how the decussating spinothalamic tract fibres (pain and temperature) are interrupted by the enlarged central canal or syrinx. The dorsal column fibres (joint position and vibration sense) are unaffected. (From Donaghy 1997) (b) A 'cape-like' pattern of suspended pain and temperature loss in syringomyelia affecting the cervical and upper thoracic segments of the spinal cord.

anaesthetic side. Fortunately, this thalamic pain syndrome, usually resulting from infarction, is rare. The discomfort most often affects the face, arm, and foot. Surprisingly, extensive thalamic lesions such as neoplasms often produce comparatively little sensory loss. Sometimes more anterior thalamic infarcts impair appreciation of posture, passive movement, light touch, and tactile discrimination with little effect upon pain and thermal sensibility. Sharply defined hemisensory loss is an unusual phenomenon, occurring only in lesions of the thalamus or immediately adjacent internal capsule.

Cortical sensory loss

Lesions restricted to the somatosensory cortex characteristically impair joint position sensation and two-point discrimination, while vibration sense is preserved. Graphaesthesia is common

in cortical lesions and best tested by asking patients, with closed eyes, to identify numbers outlined with a stick on the palm of their hand.

Psychologically determined sensory loss

Psychologically determined sensory loss (Section 1.9.3) often has implausibly sharply defined boundaries, which may shift in position, and which do not obey anatomical distributions.

1.6.4 Pain

When a patient complains of pain, the neurologist must determine whether it is a neuropathic pain, due to disease directly affecting the nervous system, rather than a musculoskeletal pain.

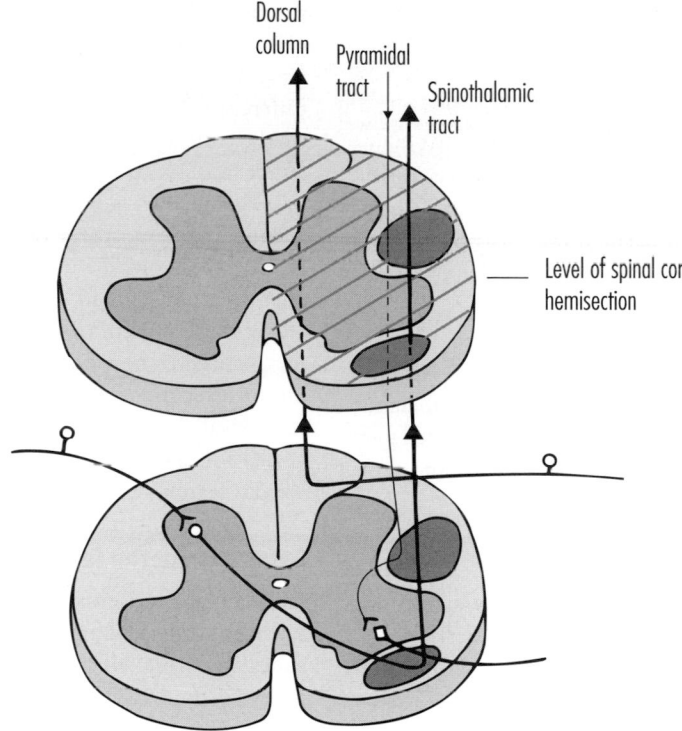

Fig. 1.36. A Brown–Séquard syndrome due to hemisection of the spinal cord. There is ipsilateral weakness due to pyramidal tract damage, ipsilateral loss of joint position and vibration sensations due to dorsal column damage, and contralateral loss of pain and temperature sensation due to spinothalamic tract damage. (From Donaghy 1997.)

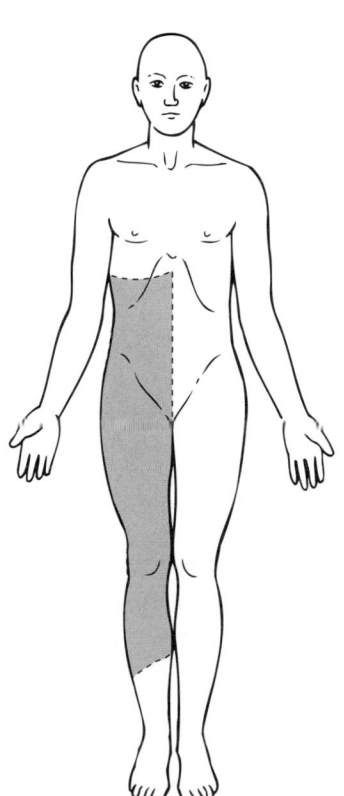

Fig. 1.37. A characteristic pattern of sensory loss in mild myelitis. The exact distribution depends upon the segmental level and pathways of the spinal cord that are affected. (From Donaghy 1997.)

Local tenderness, or discomfort on passively moving a joint, are signs suggestive of disease or strain injuries affecting bones, joints, tendon, muscles or other organs. Localization of the painful area is diagnostically helpful in spinal-root, and cranial or peripheral nerve lesions. However, pain may be localized imprecisely in reflex sympathetic dystrophy or cerebral lesions.

Referred pain

Painful lesions of the muscles or viscera sometimes give pain perceived to be in the overlying skin, or in a remote cutaneous area. Such painful sensations seem not to be coming from the viscus involved but from the body surface. But this apparent error in localization, giving what is alternatively called *pseudo-visceral pain,* is systematically related to the dermatomes innervated by those dorsal roots that supply the diseased viscus. Thus afferent pain fibres from the myocardium enter the T1–5 dorsal root ganglia and myocardial pain is referred to the anterior chest wall and down the inner aspect of the left or of both arms. Similarly, pain fibres from the diaphragm travel in the phrenic nerve (C3–4) so that diaphragmatic pain is often referred to the C3 and 4 dermatomes in the neck and shoulder.

Cutaneous nerve lesions

Cutaneous nerve lesions produce pain which is prickly, associated with paraesthesiae and often dysaesthetic to the extent that patients avoid contact or tight clothing. Despite this apparent increase in sensitivity, background thresholds for sensation will be impaired if, for instance, a wisp of cotton is used to compare the two sides.

Spinal nerve root pain

Spinal nerve root pain is worsened by stretching movements such as the straight leg-raising test in sciatica, by other movements, or by sneezing, all of which increase the degree of compression. The pain radiates in a dermatomal distribution and may be out of all proportion to the degree of demonstrable sensory or motor loss.

Spinal cord and brainstem lesions

Spinal cord and brainstem lesions affecting the spinothalamic tracts occasionally produce a burning and poorly localized pain associated with demonstrable impairment of pain and temperature sensations.

Thalamic pain

Thalamic pain, known as the Dejerine–Roussy syndrome, results from lesions within, or just behind, the posterior thalamus. Appreciation of sensory stimuli is impaired on the contralateral body, but stimuli such as pain, cold, and touch induce marked pain (Section 1.6.3).

Cortical lesions

Cortical lesions produce pain only rarely. A pseudothalamic burning pain syndrome can result from damage to the deep part of the Sylvian cortex and may be associated with hemiplegia.

1.7 Gait disorders

Walking is a complex motor performance which can be affected by a wide variety of different diseases, and which undergoes natural change with ageing. Everybody's gait differs in a characteristic way—one can normally recognize an acquaintance by her walk even when too far away to see her face. Non-neurological disorders, such as hip-joint disease are important in the differential diagnoses of gait abnormalities. Particularly in the elderly, gait disorders may be multifactorial, for instance involving a neurological disease such as parkinsonism, the mild gait apraxia of natural senescence, and degenerative arthritis of the hip joints. Gait disorders are conveniently classified hierarchically into low-, middle-, and high-level gait disorders, reflecting the level of the nervous system lesion (Nutt *et al.* 1993).

1.7.1 Normal gait

Normal walking requires equilibrium, so as to maintain a balanced upright posture, coupled with locomotion (Nutt *et al.* 1993). Equilibrium involves various righting reflexes for assumption of the upright posture, antigravity supporting reactions to maintain that posture, postural reflexes to maintain balance during weight transfers, rescue reactions to avoid falling if postural reflexes prove inadequate, and protective reactions if all else fails and falling starts. Locomotion involves gait ignition mechanisms followed by rhythmic stepping. Unsurprisingly, this complex motor task is controlled by many different brain regions. The brainstem appears to have a particular role in righting reflexes, synergizing proximal and trunk muscles to maintain balance, and in gait ignition. The basal ganglia are not involved in the rhythm of walking, but lesions impair postural responses and gait ignition. Chronic cerebellar lesions do not eliminate equilibrium reactions or alter their pattern, but do alter the scaling of responses, generally rendering them too large. The frontal cortex is important for postural responses, and cortical mechanisms are responsible for executive control of whether, when, where, and how fast to walk.

Bedside diagnosis of disordered gait requires analysis of how various features of the patient's walking differ from normal.

Separation of the feet

Normally the feet cross within a few centimetres of each other during a stride, leading to occasional scuffs on the inner heel of shoes. In normal efficient gait, the feet loop slightly round each other so that the footprints of the two feet lie almost in a straight line (Fig. 1.38a). A wide-based gait occurs in cerebellar and sensory ataxias (Fig. 1.38b), probably as a compensation to preserve balance and so the feet don't catch on one another when crossing on dysmetric strides. A slightly wide-based gait can also occur in apraxia (Fig. 1.38d) or Parkinson's disease (Fig. 1.38c), but the stride length is short in these conditions. The feet cross in wide arcs in spastic gaits, because the stiffly extended leg and foot cannot be flexed slightly in the normal manner so as to clear the ground during a stride (Fig. 1.38e,f).

Stride length

People normally hit their standard stride length with their first step and it varies little thereafter (Fig. 1.38a). In ataxia the stride length varies, elongated strides may lead to overbalancing behind a foot which has landed too far ahead, or sometimes shortening causes a stumble over a foot which has gone down too soon (Fig. 1.38b). Shortened, shuffling strides occur in Parkinson's disease. The gait ignition failure of more advanced Parkinson's disease leads to a hesitant start to a walk, and acceleration associated with increasing stride length (Fig. 1.38c). Gait apraxias, or frontal gait disorders, cause short striding of constant length from the start, a marche à petits pas (Fig. 1.38d). Such patients have particular difficulty in turning corners, being unable to spin round at a single step, and sometimes getting their feet hopelessly tangled up, or having to walk around corners (Fig. 1.38d).

Foot drop

Foot drop interferes with normal gait because it prevents the patient from swinging their striding leg through underneath their body without it catching on the ground. Stiffly held foot drops usually result from spasticity, less often from dystonia. Walking with a spastic leg requires laborious circumduction of

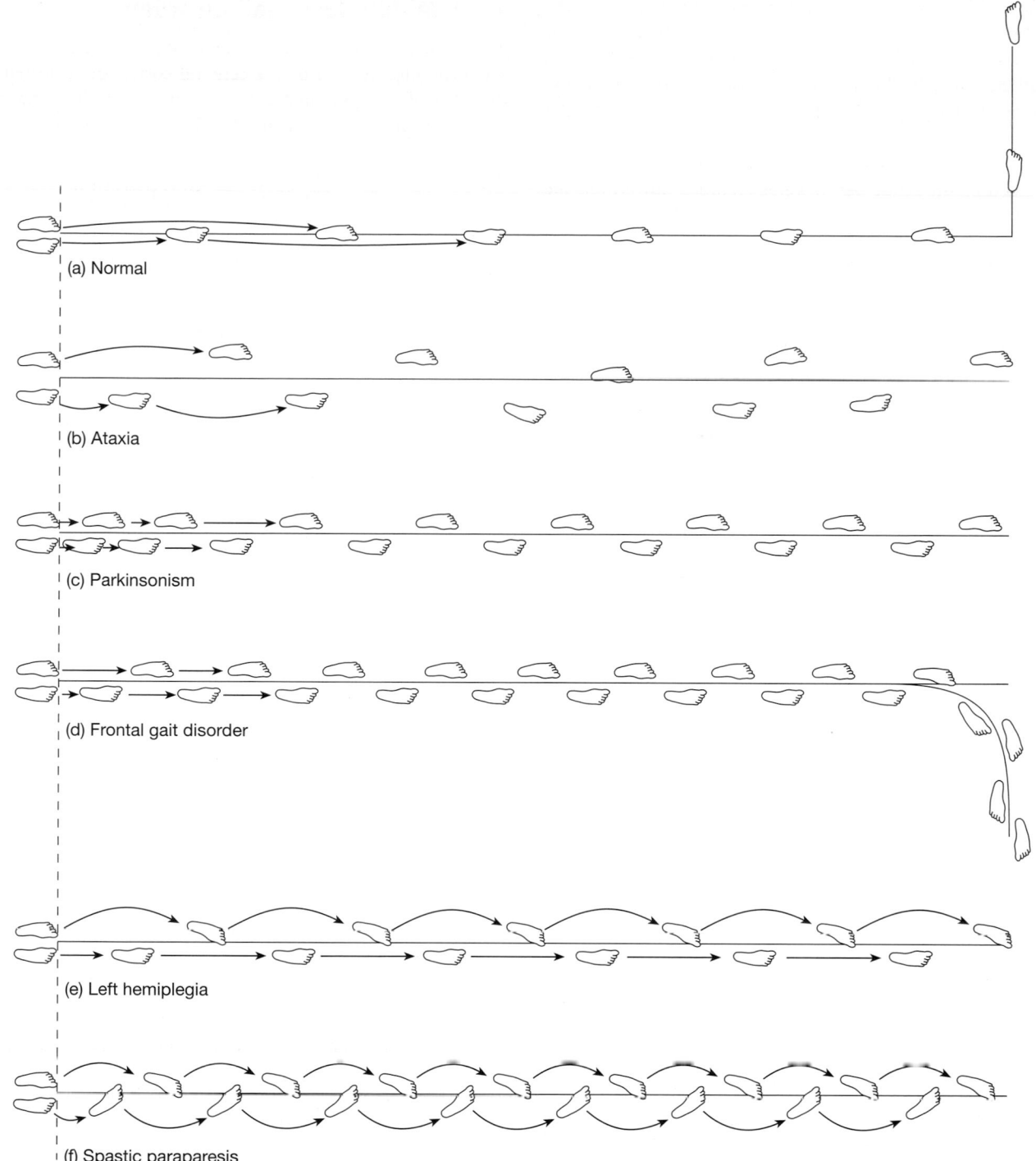

Fig. 1.38. Stride patterns in various gait disorders. (a) The stride pattern in normal gait, showing how a fixed stride length is hit immediately, and varies little thereafter, how the feet cross close to one another, and how a corner is taken in a single step by body rotation through a right angle. (b) Ataxia, showing wide separation of the feet and an irregular stride length. (c) Parkinsonism, showing short strides, with a shuffling start. (d) Frontal gait disorder, gait apraxia, or marche à petits pas, showing the short steps and the walking round corners, rather than spinning round them. (e) and (f) Showing a left hemiplegia and spastic paraparesis respectively, with circumduction of the spastic leg(s). (Based on Donaghy 1997.)

the stiffly extended leg and foot in a wide lateral arc so as to avoid catching the toe (Fig. 1.38e), a compensatory manoeuvre required bilaterally in spastic paraparesis (Fig. 1.38f). This scissors gait is exhaustingly inefficient and throws unnatural stresses upon the low back and pelvic girdle, which can result in further gait deterioration due to secondary degenerative arthritis. Circumduction of the striding leg is not so marked in dystonic foot drop because usually the patient retains the ability to lift the foot by flexing the leg at the hip and knee and raise the pelvis while striding. Floppy foot drops occur with lower motor neuron weakness of tibialis anterior due to motor neuron, spinal root, or peripheral nerve diseases. In order to swing the dangling foot through during a stride without catching it on the ground, and the hip and knee are flexed exaggeratedly, with lifting of the pelvis, and the leg is kicked out in front at the end of the stride before being stamped down onto the ground.

Pelvic tilt

Normally the pelvis remains horizontal, or even elevates slightly, when the weight is taken by only one leg during a stride. This stabilization of pelvic height is achieved principally by gluteus medius contraction on the weight-bearing side. Gluteal muscle weakness will cause the pelvis to flop downwards towards the side on which the leg has been lifted to stride out, giving the gait a waddling appearance. This is the typical gait of proximal myopathy.

Arm swing

Normally balance is assisted by swinging the arm opposite to the striding leg, familiar in its most exaggerated form in military marching. Loss of arm swing is characteristic of Parkinson's disease, occurring unilaterally in early disease. The physician should not make the patient aware that it is his arm swing which is of particular interest. However, later in the examination it should be ensured that the shoulder is not immobile simply due to joint disease. Arm swing of irregular amplitude, sometimes of a slightly wild nature, may occur in ataxia, in part as a balance compensatory mechanism.

Rising and standing

Rising and standing depend upon righting reflexes and supporting responses, respectively. Withstanding pushed displacements demonstrates reactive postural responses. The response to larger displacement pushes, or spontaneous imbalances, demonstrates the integrity of rescue and protective reactions, but should be tested with care to avoid injury.

1.7.2 Low-level gait disorders

Central nervous system equilibrium reactions and locomotor generation are well able to compensate for the gait disorder resulting from disorders of the musculoskeletal or peripheral motor and sensory systems. The musculoskeletal gait disorders of limping due to arthritis or prosthetic limbs, waddling due to proximal muscle weakness, and foot drop due to lower motor neuron disorders are easy to recognize. Ataxia due to loss of proprioceptive, visual, or vestibular feedback usually leads to cautious locomotion, and compensatory maintenance of equilibrium is efficient. Such conditions produce a major threat to independent walking when associated with other middle- or high-level disorders of gait which impair these compensatory mechanisms.

1.7.3 Middle-level gait disorders

The mechanisms for maintaining equilibrium and implementing locomotor control by the cerebral cortex are distorted by disorders of the pyramidal tract, cerebellum, and basal ganglia, and superimposed movement disorders such as chorea or dystonia. For instance, cerebellar ataxia causes dysmetria of striding and postural adjustment mechanisms. Early Parkinson's disease and pyramidal-tract lesions impair postural responses. It is only when very severe, or conjoined with another gait disorder, that walking ability is completely abolished by middle-level disorders.

1.7.4 High-level gait disorders

These are the least well understood gait disorders and have attracted varying and confusing descriptive labels. They are defined as disorders of those high-level processes, presumably cortical and subcortical in the frontal lobes, responsible for selecting postural responses and locomotor behaviour suitable for the particular circumstance of the patient at that time. By definition, they cannot be explained by middle-level gait disorders. In general neurological practice they are often called gait apraxias, marches à petits pas, and sometimes atherosclerotic parkinsonism, but the precise manifestations and disabilities clearly vary widely between patients. These disorders usually occur in the elderly, or in those with acquired bilateral disease of the frontal lobes, due to ischaemia or demyelination. Five component entities have been described (Nutt et al. 1993), although some overlap of features is evident:

1. *Cautious gaits* are common the elderly, who are often conscious of disequilibrium and a real risk of falling; they walk slowly with small steps, a slightly wide base, and walk carefully round corners.

2. *Subcortical dysequilibrium* is associated with poor or aberrant postural responses, such as neck extension and backwards falling, and are often associated with oculomotor abnormalities, dysarthria, or extrapyramidal signs.

3. *Frontal dysequilibrium* impairs a patient's ability to stand up, to remain standing or sitting independently, to organize their leg and trunk movements so as to bring their feet under their centre of gravity, or to avoid tangling their feet when attempting to corner.

4. *Gait ignition failure* is familiar as part of parkinsonism. It can be an isolated phenomenon with freezing attacks provoked by diversion of attention or narrow spaces, such as an open doorway. Walking is often easier if the patient concentrates on a rhythmically recurring feature, such as paving stone cracks, the tip of their walking stick, or simply by counting.

5. *Frontal gait disorders* result from multiple forebrain lesions and involve varying combinations of a wide-based gait, short steps, shuffling, initiation hesitations, and dysequilibrium.

1.7.5 **Falls in the elderly**

Thirty per cent of people aged over 65 fall each year, a quarter of whom are seriously injured; 1 in 20 fracture bones, particularly the hip (Tinetti *et al.* 1988). These injuries are an important cause of either temporary or permanent disability and sometimes death.

Gait disorders are a leading cause of such falls, particularly the high-level disorders which are particularly common in the elderly (Section 1.7.4) (Sudarsky 1990). Many such gait disorders are slowly progressive, often presumably due to non-specific neurodegenerative disease which merges with normal age-related changes in gait. Stepwise progression of a gait disorder points to cerebrovascular disease (Sections 27.4 and 32.3.11) and interventions which may prevent further events should be considered. The gait disorder associated with Parkinson's disease may improve with dopaminergic treatment (Section 32.3), although the associated impairment of postural adjustment mechanisms often responds poorly. Patients with signs of spinal cord disease should be investigated for potentially operable compressive lesions (Section 20.5). Rapidly evolving high-level gait disorders should be investigated for potentially operable structural cerebral disease, such as frontal tumours, subdural haematoma (Section 16.8.3), obstructive hydrocephalus (Section 17.3), or normal-pressure hydrocephalus (Section 17.3.8).

Drop attacks, postural hypotension, inadequate vision, poor illumination, and trips over environmental hazards are the other important cause of falls in the elderly (Sheldon 1960). Drop attacks are momentary losses of postural tone while standing, without loss of awareness or consciousness, and usually the patient is aware of the fall before hitting the ground. More than 80 per cent of such patients have become free of drop attacks at a mean follow-up of 6.5 years, whether or not there is an associated medical condition (Meissner *et al.* 1986). The average number of attacks experienced is 11 and they are not a predictor of stroke, suggesting that their pathogenesis is not vascular. Postural hypotension is another important cause of falls in the elderly, often being precipitated by antihypertensive and vasodilator drugs, and occasionally being due to peripheral or central autonomic failure.

1.8 **Autonomic disorders**

1.8.1 **Clinical features**

Generally, symptoms of autonomic nervous system disease develop insidiously and reflect loss of function or failure of autonomic regulation. Occasionally paroxysms of autonomic hyperactivity occur in diseases such as Guillain–Barré syndrome (Section 12.10.1), causing wide fluctuations in blood pressure and heart rate which predispose to cardiac arrhythmias, episodic skin flushing, sweating disturbances, paralytic ileus, pupil abnormalities, and micturition disturbances. Autonomic dysreflexia occurs in high spinal-cord lesions

(Section 6.3.5). Stimuli originating in the skin, muscles, or internal organs below the level of the lesion lead to hypertension, bradycardia, and sweating. Bladder distension is a noteworthy precipitant of autonomic dysreflexia.

The early symptoms of autonomic failure can be relatively unnoticed for years because of compensatory mechanisms. Persistent postural hypotension when standing leads to recurrent faintness, dizziness, episodes of vision draining away and blacking out, feelings of weakness, aching across the shoulders and posterior neck, or attacks of abrupt unconsciousness with falling. Food, alcohol, drugs, hot baths, or exercise can provoke these symptoms. These symptoms are reversed by lying down. Gastrointestinal autonomic dysfunction causes either nocturnal diarrhoeal attacks or pseudo-obstruction. Such obstruction may be generalized, or localized as in achalasia of the cardia or Hirschprung's disease; commonly laparotomy has been performed to exclude mechanical bowel obstruction. Autonomic denervation of the bladder and genitalia impairs voiding, causes erectile impotence, and can allow retrograde ejaculation. Patients are usually unaware that they have lost sweating, but direct questioning can reveal that the palms no longer sweat and the finger skin has lost that moist adhesive quality required for effective gripping of paper. An autonomically denervated foot becomes warm and red due to loss of cutaneous vasoconstriction, and dry due to loss of sweating; the resultant lack of skin lubrication may contribute to cracking, fissuring, and ulcer formation.

Some autonomic disorders are focal, examples being Horner's syndrome (Section 8.9.5), Adie's pupil (Section 8.9.4), gustatory sweating, idiopathic palmar or axillary hyperhidrosis, or surgical sympathectomy.

1.8.2 **Autonomic function testing**

A wide variety of possible investigations of autonomic function have been described (Mathias and Bannister 1999). Most of these are too complex for routine clinical use. They include thermoregulatory and sweat testing, gastrointestinal function testing, sympathetic skin responses, measurement of noradrenaline and renin responses to head-up tilt, urodynamic studies and sphincter electrophysiology, and penile plethysmography. Simple clinical tests for autonomic failure include the following.

Sweating

Lack of moistness may be noted on the palms and soles of patients with peripheral neuropathies involving autonomic fibres. Sweating can be provoked by putting a hand in a plastic bag to prevent evaporation and warming it under a light for a few minutes. Indicator dyes, such as Ponzo red, which turn red on becoming wet, can be dusted onto the skin, or placed under pieces of transparent tape stuck to the skin.

Lying and standing blood pressure

Normally on standing the blood pressure is unchanged or rises slightly and the pulse rate increases slightly. In autonomic

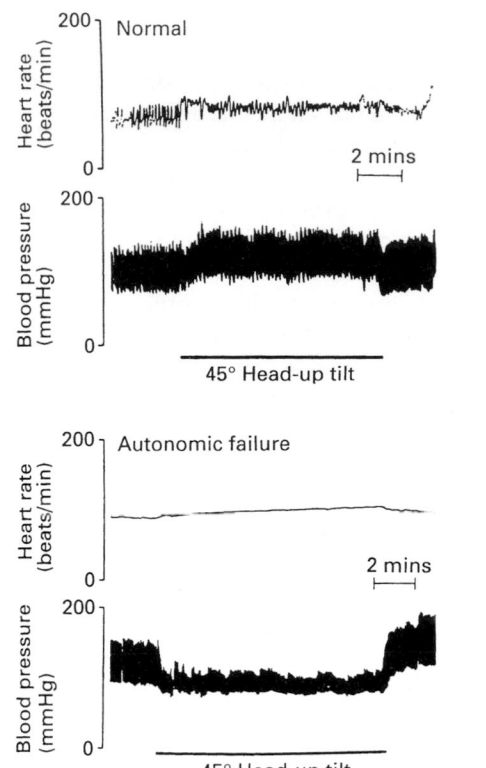

Fig. 1.39. Blood pressure and pulse rate recordings before, during, and after head-up tilt in a normal subject (top) and a patient with pure autonomic failure (bottom). Whereas blood pressure does not fall with upright posture in the normal subject, a marked fall without compensatory tachycardia occurs in autonomic failure (After Mathias and Bannister 1999, with permission.)

failure the blood pressure falls and there may be no compensatory tachycardia (Fig. 1.39). Baseline blood pressure normally tends to fall slightly on repeated testing so it is advisable to measure blood pressure in the sequence lying–standing–lying and to compare the second pair of readings.

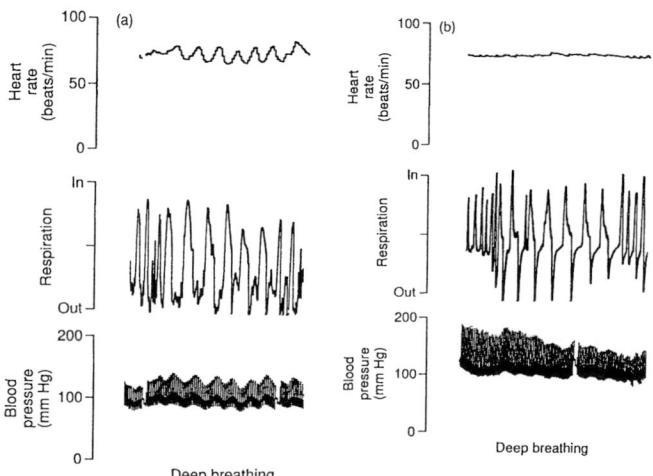

Fig. 1.40. Sinus arrhythmia of the cardiac rate during deep breathing in a normal subject (a). This variation in cardiac rate during respiration is lost in autonomic failure (b). (Courtesy of Mathias and Bannister 1999).

Sinus arrhythmia

Normally the heart rate rises during inspiration and falls during expiration. This sinus arrhythmia is mediated by the cardiac vagus nerves. Loss of variation in the R–R interval when the electrocardiogram is recorded during deep breathing occurs in autonomic neuropathy (Fig. 1.40).

Valsalva manoeuvre

When a normal subject attempts to exhale forcibly against a voluntarily closed glottis, the blood pressure drops, with loss of venous return to the heart, and the heart rate rises. When this intrathoracic pressure increase is released, the blood pressure overshoots because of continued sympathetic drive, and the heart rate drops below the basal level due to baroreflex activation (Fig. 1.41). Autonomic neuropathies abolish this second blood pressure overshoot and the associated reflex bradycardia (Fig. 1.41). If the baroreflex arc remains intact, as may be the case in high spinal-cord lesions and some forms of central autonomic failure, the cardiac rate rises during the initial phase of falling blood pressure. In formal quantitative testing the subject is asked to exhale against a standard resistance of 40 mmHg.

1.8.3 Causes of autonomic failure

A wide variety of disorders cause autonomic dysfunction, usually associated with other neurological or general medical disorders (Table 1.8). In everyday clinical practice the most

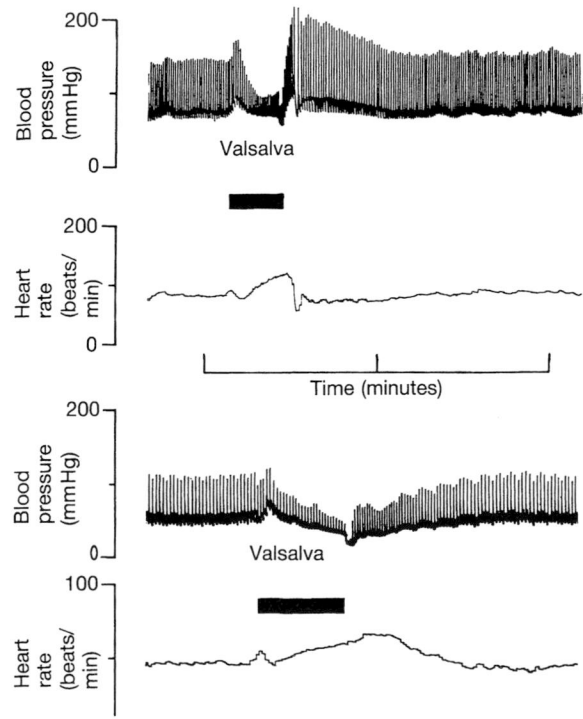

Fig. 1.41. Valsalva manoeuvre. The blood pressure and heart rate responses to exhaling against a resistance of 40 mmHg are shown for a normal subject (top) and a patient with autonomic failure (bottom). (Courtesy of Mathias and Bannister 1999).

Table 1.8. Classification of disorders resulting in autonomic dysfunction (after Mathias and Bannister 1999, with modifications)

Primary (aetiology unknown)

Acute/subacute dysautonomias (section 12.10.4)

    Pure cholinergic dysautonomia

    Pure pandysautonomia

    Pandysautonomia with neurological features

Chronic autonomic failure syndromes

    Pure autonomic failure (section 32.3.8)

    Multiple system atrophy (Shy–Drager syndrome) (section 32.3.8)

    Autonomic failure with Parkinson's disease (section 32.3.1)

Secondary

Congenital

    Nerve growth factor deficiency

Hereditary

    Familial amyloid neuropathy (section 12.9.1)

    Porphyria (section 12.8.6)

    Hereditary sensory and autonomic neuropathies (section 12.6)

    Familial dysautonomia—Riley–Day syndrome (section 12.6.4)

    Dopamine β-hydroxylase deficiency

    Aromatic L-amino acid decarboxylase deficiency

    Anderson–Fabry disease (section 12.8.5)

Metabolic diseases

    Diabetes mellitus (section 12.17.1)

    Chronic renal failure (section 12.17.2)

    Chronic liver disease

    Vitamin B_{12} deficiency (section 12.21.3)

    Alcohol-induced (section 12.18.1)

Inflammatory

    Guillain–Barré syndrome (section 12.10.1)

    Transverse myelitis (section 20.4.5)

Infections

    Bacterial—tetanus (section 35.7)

    Viral—human immunodeficiency virus infection (section 12.14.2)

    Parasitic—trypanosomiasis cruzi; Chagas disease

    Prion—fatal familial insomnia (section 24.2.6)

Neoplasia

    Brain tumours—especially of third ventricle or posterior fossa

    Paraneoplastic, to include Lambert–Eaton syndrome (section 15.10.2)

    Primary amyloidosis (section 12.9.2)

Connective tissue disorders

    Rheumatoid arthritis

    Systemic lupus erythematosus

    Mixed connective tissue disease

Surgery

    Regional sympathectomy—upper limb, splanchnic

    Vagotomy and drainage procedures—'dumping syndrome'

    Organ transplantation—heart, kidney

Table 1.8. *Continued*

Trauma

    Spinal cord transection (section 6.3.5)

Neurally mediated syncope (section 23.1.2)

    Vasovagal syncope

    Carotid sinus hypersensitivity

    Micturition syncope

    Cough syncope

    Swallow syncope

    Associated with glossopharyngeal neuralgia

Drugs, chemicals, poisons, and toxins

common neurological diseases causing autonomic failure are diabetic polyneuropathy and Parkinson's disease, it is usually relatively asymptomatic in both cases.

1.9 Psychologically determined abnormalities

1.9.1 Occurrence

Neurologists frequently see patients with symptoms or inconsistent signs that are not explicable in terms of any recognized neurological disease process. Often it is clear that such symptoms and signs are being manufactured psychologically, either by a conscious or, more often, an unconscious process. Such patients are often polysymptomatic, and may have a long history of consulting other specialists, particularly abdominal and gynaecological surgeons. They run the risk of developing secondary abnormalities induced by surgical and other invasive procedures.

Individuals vary considerably in their response to illness and in what being ill means to them and to their families. For some, significant disease is shrugged off whereas for others, trivial symptoms may be dramatized and elaborated. Both ends of the spectrum can be challenging to the physician but it is those who elaborate their symptoms that run the risk either of a missed diagnosis or of being overinvestigated. Moreover, somatization of symptoms relating to psychological disorders is common. Indeed, the term abnormal illness behaviour (Pilowsky, 1969) reflects more society's view of what is normal and what is abnormal in terms of a patient's response to illness. Considered separately (Section 26.10) are patients who are frankly malingering or those with a conversion disorder. Clearly, patients whose symptoms and signs are greater than one might anticipate from the underlying neurological disease, overlap with patients who develop somatic symptoms in association with psychological and psychiatric disorder (Section 26.10). Because of the range of symptoms associated with neurological disease and the anxiety which such disorders can generate, it is not surprising that many patients present with apparent abnormal illness behaviour.

Somatization is very common (Smith *et al.* 1986; Carson *et al.* 2000) and in the UK 25 per cent of patients present without a clear neurological illness that could explain all their symptoms (Perkin 1989). The danger is always that the doctor is mistaken in believing that underlying neurological disease is either absent or insufficient to explain the symptoms. The influential study by Slater (1965) found that up to 50 per cent of patients followed with a diagnosis of hysteria turned out to have significant neurological or psychiatric disease. More recent series with the benefit of improved investigation, find a much lower misdiagnosis rate (Crimlisk *et al.* 1998). Nevertheless, it is a sobering thought that many of the diseases previously thought to be non-neurological, such as spastic dysphonia and writer's cramp, are now understood in neurological terms. It is likely that some patients currently considered to have 'non-organic' disorders, will subsequently prove to be explicable in neurobiological terms. In the case of sensory symptoms, for example, the body is constantly receiving a barrage of afferent information, even when no discrete external stimulus is present. Normal perception involves developing a threshold level below which such stimuli are considered normal and remain unnoticed. Abnormal interpretation of body state may involve erroneous positioning of this boundary between interpreting afferent information as normal or abnormal.

1.9.2 Symptoms

The manner in which patients with psychologically generated disorders describe their symptoms may be discordant with the actual symptoms themselves. Relatively trivial symptoms such as tingling may be described in a vivid, florid, and exaggerated manner. Or a totally paralysed limb may be described in a smiling and unconcerned manner. This is a difficult diagnostic area which sometimes misleads the most skilful diagnostician. Often the symptoms need full investigation before you can come to a definite conclusion that they originate psychologically. It is particularly difficult when psychologically determined symptoms occur in someone also suffering from a definite disease. Common examples include an exaggerated gait disorder in multiple sclerosis, pseudo-seizures in an epileptic, or exaggerated disability in an injured person seeking compensation.

Common psychologically determined symptoms include headache, facial pain, spinal pain, tinglings, patches of sensory loss, sensory disturbance and dropping things on the non-dominant side, tremor, blackouts, clumsiness, paralyses, memory blocks, dementia, and gait disorders.

Depression underlies many instances of tension headache, facial pain, and apparent dementia. Anxiety states may be responsible for tinglings, tremors, blackouts, or memory blocks, and sometimes these symptoms are due to hyperventilation. Typically, anxiety-provoked symptoms fluctuate markedly and may resolve for part of the day. For instance, the tingling of a true polyneuropathy does not disappear for half of the day.

Malingering takes a number of forms, not all necessarily fully conscious; self-delusion can be prominent. Many patients are seeking compensation for alleged personal injury in road traffic accidents or at the hands of doctors. These usually feign a disabling symptom such as pain, which is difficult to disprove, or paralysis. Drug-addicted malingerers may feign intractable pain so as to obtain opiates. Mildly incapacitating symptoms which create a state of dependency can occur in domestic situations, for example in the 'empty-nest syndrome' in middle-aged women whose children are leaving home. True conversion hysteria is uncommon. Such patients seem to accept quite placidly that their paralysis or gait disorder is an incurable condition. Almost all are female and frequently have a long history of gynaecological and sexual symptoms, and surgical operations. Such patients can be permanently wheelchair-bound, and no treatment seems to help.

1.9.3 Interpreting physical signs

Muscle power

The most characteristic feature of psychologically determined weakness is the fluctuating production of power by the muscles (Section 1.5.7). None the less the muscle can exert full power momentarily after encouragement. Muscular contraction may collapse after being normal for a moment. Co-contraction of antagonist and agonist muscles may be evident. Inconsistencies in muscle power may be demonstrated. For instance, the patient may be unable to flex the hip against gravity on the couch, but will be observed to stand and flex the hip normally to put on trousers or tights. The patient may have weakness of plantar flexion when tested on the couch, but be able to stand on tiptoe. Patients with psychologically determined weakness sometimes accompany their unimpressive efforts with copious and theatrical grunting and sighing.

Sensation

Psychologically determined patches of sensory loss are often implausibly sharply defined with instantaneous transition from complete anaesthesia to normal sensation. It may be possible to demonstrate that these apparently sharp boundaries shift in position when the stimulus is presented at different speeds or from different directions, particularly if the patient's eyes are shut. Sometimes it can be demonstrated that the numb limb changes sides when the patient is rolled over and retested. The sensory findings may vary greatly on retesting a few days later. Generally, psychologically determined patches of numbness do not obey the anatomical territories of peripheral nerves or nerve roots. For instance, a sensory boundary may occur at the lower border of the mandible with facial sensory disturbance extending into the middle of C2 territory. One may observe apparent loss to vibration sensation when tested with a tuning fork on just one side of the sternum. Or patients may be observed to have apparent gross loss of proprioception in the fingers and yet are able to manipulate an object in their hand successfully when tested for astereognosis. Sharply demarcated hemisensory loss is commonly determined psychologically, but always raises the question of a thalamic lesion (Section 1.6.3). In all of these situations, however, care must be taken not to enter into a battle of wits between the clinician and the patient but merely to observe the phenomena.

Visual disturbances

Visual disturbances which are determined psychologically are commonly associated with spiralling of the visual fields and tunnel vision. Inconsistencies can be brought out on examination in patients who complain of unilateral blindness by the use of prisms in which movement of the ocular axis can be observed in order to achieve binocular vision. Similarly, one eye may be covered with a red, and the other with a green glass, the patient being then asked to read a word-test of alternate red and green letters. Since one colour is invisible to each eye, if all the letters are read the patient must be using both eyes. The development of optokinetic nystagmus with a rotating drum can also be useful with complaints of total loss of vision. Abnormalities of eye movement due to convergence spasm may be suggested by the observance of pupillary constriction. Care must be taken, though, in patients with visual disorientation in whom there may be little to find on examination and even at times normal visual acuity, but in whom there may be gross everyday visual dysfunction.

Gait disorders

Psychologically determined gait disorders are often extremely athletic or even balletic. For instance, patients may momentarily balance on one foot in midstride, which indicates extremely good motor control. Psychologically determined gaits may improve when the patients think they are not being observed. Patients with psychologically determined gait disorders are often able to transverse an open space only to fall theatrically once they are able to grasp nearby furniture or an observer. However, bizarre gaits may also be observed in patients with dystonia, hereditary spastic paraparesis, or gait apraxia. Similarly, gross truncal ataxia due to midline cerebellar lesions may be misinterpreted because of the normal examination on the couch.

References

Babinski, J. (1922). Reflexes de defense. *Brain*, **45**, 149–84.

Baillie, M. (1793). *The morbid anatomy of some of the most important parts of the human body*, p. 314. Johnson and Nicol, London.

Baillie, M. (1798–1803). *A series of engravings accompanied with explanations which are intended to illustrate the morbid anatomy of some of the most important parts of the human body*, p. 288. Bulmer and Co., London.

Bell, C. (1803). *The anatomy of the brain explained in a series of engravings*. Longman and Rees, London.

Bell, C. (1811). *Idea of a new anatomy of the brain*, p. 36. Strahan and Preston, London.

Boyle, R. S., Shakir, R. A., Weir, A. I. *et al.* (1979). Inverted knee jerk: a neglected localizing sign in spinal cord disease. *J. Neurol. Neurosurg. Psychiat.*, **42**, 1005–7.

Brain, W. R. (1933). *Diseases of the nervous system*, p. 899. Oxford University Press, London.

Brain, W. R. and Wilkinson, M. (1959). Observations on the extensor plantar reflex and its relationship to the functions of the pyramidal tract. *Brain*, **82**, 297–320.

Bright, R. (1827–1831). *Reports of medical cases, selected with a view of illustrating the symptoms and cure of diseases by a reference to morbid anatomy*, pp. 231, 724. Longmans, London.

Cajal, S. R. (1897–1904). *Textura del sistema nervioso del hombre y de los vertebrados*, 3 volumes. Madrid 1897; 1899; 1904. Translation by L. Azoulay (1909–1911) *Histologie du systeme nerveux de l'homme et des vertebres*, 2 volumes. Paris. [Translated into English by N. Swanson and L. W. Swanson (1995) *Histology of the nervous system of man and vertebrates*, 2 volumes, pp. 805; 806. Oxford University Press, New York. Also translated by P. Pasik and T. Pasik (1999) *Texture of the nervous system of man and the vertebrates*, Vol. 1 (all published), p. 631. Springer, Wien.]

Carson, A. J., Ringbauer, B., Stone, J. *et al.* (2000). Do medically unexplained symptoms matter? A prospective cohort study of 300 new referrals to neurology outpatient clinics. *J. Neurol. Neurosurg. Psychiat.*, **68**, 207–10.

Carswell, R. (1838). *Pathological anatomy; illustrations of the elementary forms of disease*. Longman, Orme, Brown, Green and Longman, London.

Caton, R. (1875). The electric currents of the brain. *BMJ*, **2**, 278.

Charcot, J. M. (1872–1887). *Leçons sur les Maladies du Systeme Nerveux faites a la Salpetrière*, A. Delahaye and E. Lecrosnier. Progrès Medicale, Paris. Translated into English by G. Sigerson (1877–1889) as *Lectures on the diseases of the nervous system delivered at the Salpetrière*, pp. 325, 399, 438. The New Sydenham Society, London.

Charcot, J. M. (1887). *Leçons du Mardi a la Salpetrière*, p. 638. A. Delahaye et Progrès Medicale, Paris.

Cooke, J. (1820–1823). *A treatise on nervous diseases*, pp. 469, 215, 235. Longman, Hurst, Rees, Orme and Brown, London.

Crimlisk, H. L., Bmatia, K., Cope, H. *et al.* (1998). Slater revisited: 6 year follow up study of patients with medically unexplained motor symptoms. *BMJ*, **316**, 582–586.

Critchley, M. (1953). *The parietal lobes*. Arnold, London.

Cruveilhier, J. (1835–1842). *Anatomie pathologique du corps humain; descriptions avec figures lithographiées et coloriées; des diverses alterations morbides dont le corps humain est susceptible*. J. B. Baillière, Paris.

Dandy, W. E. (1918). Ventriculography following the injection of air into the cerebral ventricles. *Ann. Surg.*, **68**, 5–11.

Dohrmann, G. J. and Nowack, W. J. (1973). The upgoing great toe: optimal method of elicitation. *Lancet*, **i**, 339.

Donaghy, M. (1997). *Neurology*. Oxford University Press, Oxford.

Egan, D. F. (1990). Developmental examination of infants and pre-school children. *Clin. Develop. Med.*, **112**, 1–84.

Egas Moniz, A. C. de (1927). L'encephalographie arterielle, son importance dans la localisation des tumeurs cerebrales. *Rev. Neurologique*, **34**, 72–90.

Fearing, F. (1930). *Reflex action*. Williams and Wilkins, Baltimore.

Ferrier, D. (1876). *The functions of the brain*, p. 323. Smith Elder, London.

Gandiglio, G. and Fra, L. (1967). Further observations on facial reflexes. *J. Neurol. Sci.*, **5**, 273–85.

Gardner, E. (1975). *Fundamentals of neurology*, 6th edn. Saunders, Philadelphia.

Gowers, W. R. (1886–1888). *A manual of disease of the nervous system*, 2 vols, pp. 463, 975. J. and A. Churchill, London.

Hall, M. (1837). *Memoirs on the nervous system*, p. 113. Sherwood, Gilbert and Piper, London.

Haymaker, W. and Schiller, F. (1970). *The founders of neurology*, 2nd edn, p. 616. C. C. Thomas, Illinois.

Holmes, G. (1946). *An introduction to clinical neurology*, p. 183. E. and S. Livingstone, Edinburgh.

Holmes, G. (1954). *The National Hospital Queen Square 1860–1948*, p. 98. E. and S. Livingstone, Edinburgh.

Hooper, R. (1826). *The morbid anatomy of the human brain being illustrations of the most frequent and important organic diseases to which that viscus is subject*, p. 36. Longman, Rees, Orme, Brown, and Green, London.

Hounsfield, G. N. (1973). Computerised transverse axial scanning (tomography). *Br. J. Radiol.*, **46**, 1016–22.

Hughlings Jackson, J. (1932). *Selected writings*, (ed. J. Taylor), pp. 500, 510. Hodder and Stoughton, London.

Kugelberg, E. and Hagbarth, K. E. (1958). Spinal mechanism of the abdominal and erector spinae skin reflexes. *Brain*, **81**, 290–304.

Liddell, E. G. T. (1960). *The discovery of reflexes*, p. 174. Oxford at the Clarendon Press.

MacDonald, B. K., Cockerell, O. C., Sander, J. W. A. *et al.* (2000). The incidence and lifetime prevalence of neurological disorders in a prospective community-based study in the UK. *Brain*, **123**, 665–76.

Madonick, M. J. (1957). Statistical control studies in neurology: 8. The cutaneous abdominal reflex. *Neurology*, **7**, 459–65.

Marsden, C. D., Merton, P. A., and Morton, H. B. (1973). Is the human stretch reflex cortical rather than spinal? *Lancet*, **I**, 759.

Mathias, C. J. and Bannister, R. (1999). *Autonomic failure. A textbook of clinical disorders of the autonomic nervous system*, 4th edn. Oxford University Press.

Matsumoto, S., Okuda, B., Imai, T. *et al.* (1988). A sensory level on the trunk in lower lateral brainstem lesions. *Neurology*, **38**, 1515–19.

McHenry, L. (1969). *Garrison's history of neurology*, p. 552. C. C. Thomas, Illinois.

Meissner, I., Wiebers, D. O., Swanson, J. W. *et al.* (1986). The natural history of drop attacks. *Neurology*, **36**, 1029–34.

Monrad-Khrohn, G. H. (1921). *The clinical examination of the nervous system*, p. 135. H. K. Lewis, London.

Morgagni (1761). *De Sedibus, et Causis Morborum per Anatomem Indigatis Libri Quinque*, pp. 298, 452.

Norman, J. M. (1991). *Morton's medical biography*, p. 1243. Scholar Press, Aldershot.

Nutt, J. G., Marsden, C. D., and Thompson, P. D. (1993). Human walking and higher-level gait disorders, particularly in the elderly. *Neurology*, **43**, 268–79.

Paulson, G. and Gottlieb, G. (1968). Developmental reflexes; the reappearance of foetal and neonatal reflexes in aged patients. *Brain*, **91**, 37–52.

Perkin, G. D. (1989). An analysis of 7836 successive new outpatient referrals. *J. Neurol. Neurosurg. Psychiat.*, **52**, 447–8.

Pilowsky, I. (1969). Abnormal illness behaviour. *Br. J. Med. Psychol.*, **42**, 347–51.

Plum, F. and Posner, J. B. (1980). *The diagnosis of stupor and coma*, 3rd edn. Blackwell, Oxford.

Quincke, H. I. (1891). Die Lumbarpunction des Hydrocephalus. *Berlin klinisches Weschrift*, **33**, 965–8.

Riddoch, G., Rowley Bristow, W., Cairns, H. W. B. *et al.* (1943). Aids to investigation of peripheral nerve injuries, p. 54. Medical Research Council, London.

Seyffarth, H. and Denny-Brown, D. (1948). The grasp reflex and the instinctive grasp reaction. *Brain*, **71**, 109–83.

Sheldon, J. H. (1960). On the natural history of falls in old age. *BMJ*, **2**, 1685–90.

Sherrington, C. S. (1906). *The integrative action of the nervous system*, p. 411. Constable, London.

Sicard, J. A. (1921). Methode radiographique d'exploration de la cavité epidurale par la lipodol. *Rev. Neurologique*, **28**, 1264–6.

Slater, E. (1965). Diagnosis of hysteria. *BMJ*, **1**, 1395–9.

Smith, G. R., Monson, R. A., and Ray, D. C. (1986). Psychiatric consultation in somatisation disorder. A randomised controlled study. *N. Engl. J. Med.*, **314**, 1407–13.

Spillane, J. D. (1968). *An atlas of clinical neurology*, p. 376. Oxford University Press, Oxford.

Spillane, J. D. (1981). *The doctrine of the nerves: chapters in the history of neurology*, p. 467. Oxford University Press, Oxford.

Stevens, D. L. (1989). Neurology in Gloucestershire: the clinical workload of an English neurologist. *J. Neurol. Neurosurg. Psychiat.*, **52**, 439–46.

Sudarsky, L. (1990). Geriatrics: gait disorders in the elderly. *N. Engl. J. Med.*, **322**, 1441–6.

Tinetti, M. E., Speechley, M., and Ginter, S. F. (1988). Risk factors for falls among elderly persons living in the community. *N. Engl. J. Med.*, **319**, 1701–7.

Traub, M. M., Rothwell, J. C., and Marsden, C. D. (1980). A grab reflex in the human hand. *Brain*, **103**, 869–84.

van Gijn, J. (1978). The Babinski sign and the pyramidal syndrome. *J. Neurol. Neurosurg. Psychiat.* **41**, 865–73.

Vesalius, A. (1543). *De humani corporis fabrica libri septum.* p. 663. Oporini, Basel.

Walshe, F. M. R. (1940). *Disease of the nervous system*, p. 288. E. and S. Livingstone, Edinburgh.

Wartenberg, R. (1945). *The examination of reflexes*, p. 222. Year Book Publishers, Chicago.

Whytt, R. (1751). *An essay on the vital and involuntary motions of animals*, p. 392. Hamilton, Balfour and Neill, Edinburgh.

Whytt, R. (1765). *Observations on the nature causes and cure of those disorders which have been commonly called nervous hypochondriac or hysteric etc.*, p. 520. Becket, Edinburgh.

Willis, T. (1681). *The remaining medical works etc*, pp. 178, 192, 106, (30). Dring, Harper, Leigh and Martyn, London.

Willis, T. (1683). *Two discourses concerning the soul of brutes*, p. 234 (8). Dring, Harper and Leigh, London.

Wilson, S. A. K. (1940). *Neurology. Disseminated sclerosis*, 2 vols, p. 1838. E. Arnold and Co., London.

CHAPTER 2

Investigation

David Chadwick, Alastair Compston, Michael Donaghy,
Nicholas Fletcher, David Hilton-Jones, David Miller, Martin
Rossor, and Charles Warlow

2.1 Imaging of the nervous system

Advances in non-invasive methods of neuroimaging have been enormous in the past 25 years, and have revolutionized the diagnostic work-up of patients with suspected disease of the central nervous system in particular. Computer-assisted tomography (CAT) X-ray scanning was the first major advance when it was introduced in the mid 1970s. It was followed about 10 years later by magnetic resonance imaging (MRI), which has made an even greater impact. While a place still remains for more invasive investigations, such as conventional arteriography (Section 2.2) and, to a much more limited extent, myelography, some previously disagreeable investigations (e.g. air encephalography) have been rendered obsolete. Because it has become the tool par excellence for imaging the central nervous system, most of this section will concern the principles and applications of MRI. The role of CT scanning, magnetic resonance spectroscopy, and positron emission tomography will also be discussed.

2.1.1 Computed tomography scanning

Computed tomography (CT) scanning applies many small X-ray beams at different angles within single planes in order to build up a set of multi-slice tomographic images of the tissue structure. Tissues are distinguished by their electron density. Highly electron dense tissues, such as cortical bone, calcification, or acute haematomas, are seen as bright areas (high attenuation); cerebrospinal fluid is dark (low attenuation). Grey matter has a higher attenuation than white matter (Fig. 2.1). Iodine-based contrast agents produce areas of high attenuation where they become concentrated (e.g. in vascular malformations, highly vascular tumours, or areas of blood–brain barrier leakage due to a variety of pathologies). CT scanners are widely available, and are extremely valuable in neurological practice. However, as MRI has become widely available in the past decade, it has replaced CT as the investigation of choice in many situations.

2.1.2 Magnetic resonance imaging

To produce a nuclear magnetic resonance (NMR) signal, an atomic nucleus must be mobile and contain an odd number of protons or neutrons. Magnetic resonance (MR) images are constituted from the NMR signal derived from such nuclei. Conventional MR images are obtained from hydrogen (^{1}H) nuclei because of their great abundance in the water and fat of living organisms, in comparison to alternatives such as ^{31}P or ^{23}Na. Different tissues, normal or pathological, are discriminated by differences in the density and macromolecular environment of their mobile protons—in the brain and spinal cord, these are almost all water protons since the lipid protons in myelin are immobile and thus do not produce an NMR signal.

The production of satisfactory images from humans required the development of large-bore magnets with very homogeneous

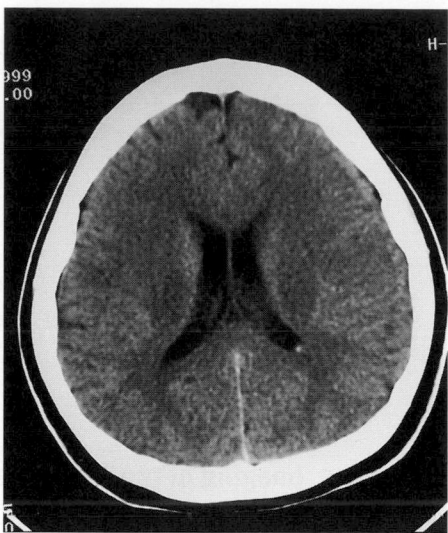

Fig. 2.1. CT scan of a normal individual. Axial slice through the level of the lateral ventricles. (Courtesy of Dr T Cox.)

magnetic fields, together with an efficient method of spatial localization of the acquired NMR signals. These requirements were met in the early 1980s when the first whole-body MR scanners were built and two-dimensional Fourier transformation was used to constitute the images. MR images can be reconstructed in various planes, with coronal images frequently used to image the temporal lobes and sagittal images to visualize the brainstem and craniocervical junction (Fig. 2.2).

MRI scanners are in essence large magnets; their use is therefore contraindicated in patients with cardiac pacemakers or berry aneurysm clips. Most scanners in clinical use have field strengths ranging from 0.5 to 1.5 tesla. Within this range satisfactory images can be obtained in a reasonable period of time with 3–5 mm-thick slices and an in plane resolution of 1 mm^2. However, as signal-to-noise ratio is proportional to the square root of field strength, 1.5 tesla systems allow more accurate imaging of smaller structures (e.g. auditory canal, spinal cord and nerve roots, cranial nerves, pituitary fossa). The resolution of MR angiography is significantly better at 1.5 tesla (Section 2.2.4) and this field strength or higher is necessary if a MR spectroscopy examination is being performed.

The MR image intensity of any given tissue is influenced mainly by three parameters: its mobile proton density, T1 and T2 relaxation times. Although the three parameters all contribute to some extent when using conventional sequences, strategies are employed to allow one or other to dominate the image. Thus in practice, three sequences are commonly employed: proton density-weighted (long repetition time [TR], short echo time [TE]), T1-weighted (short TR, short TE) and T2-weighted (long TR, long TE) (Fig. 2.3). Intravenous MRI contrast agents containing gadolinium chelates (e.g. gadolinium-diethyltriaminepentacetic acid) produce enhancement by reducing proton mobility in areas in which they accumulate (e.g. regions with an abnormal blood–brain barrier) and this appears as an area of high signal on T1-weighted sequences. It

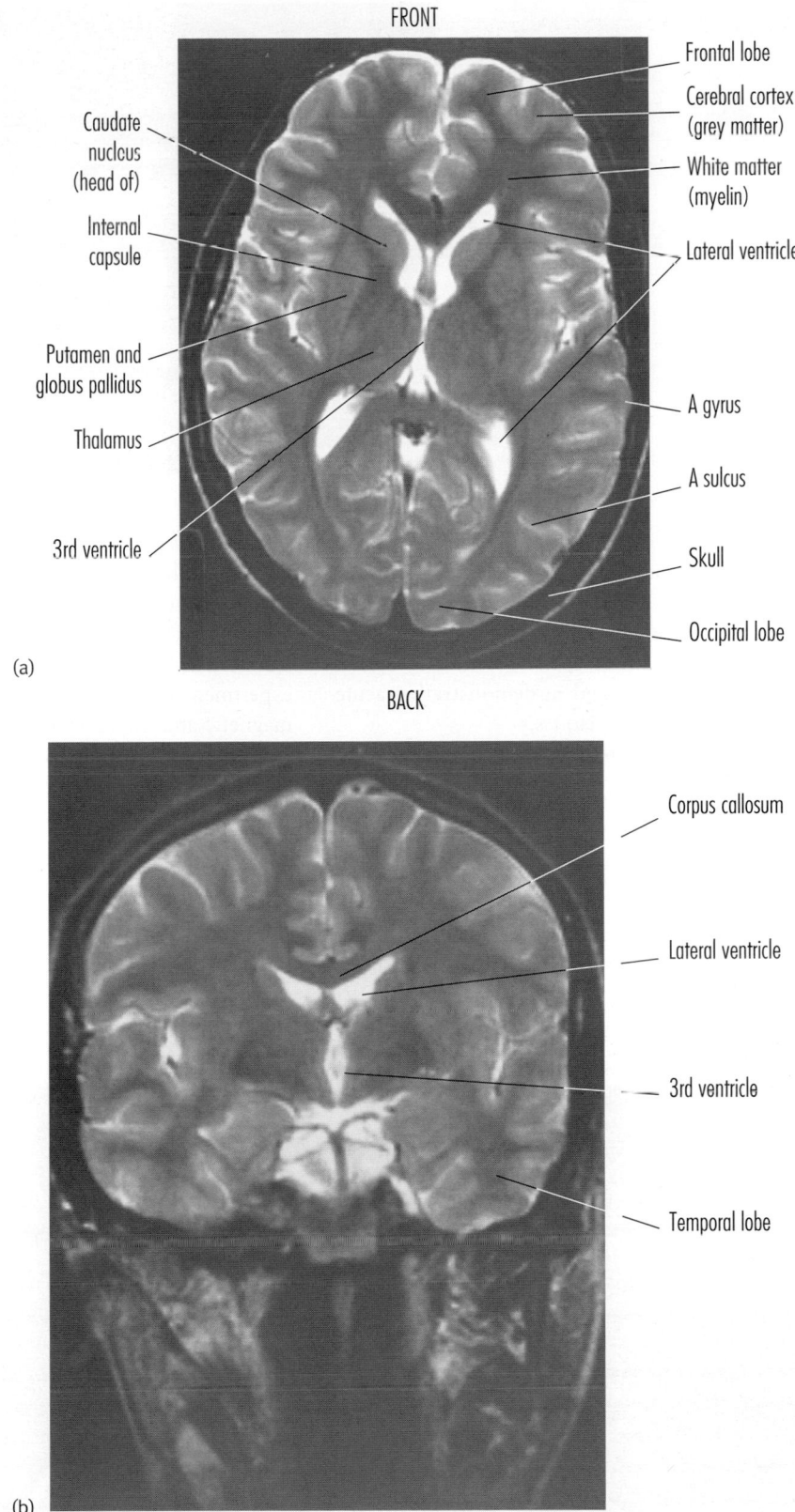

FRONT

Caudate nucleus (head of)

Internal capsule

Putamen and globus pallidus

Thalamus

3rd ventricle

Frontal lobe

Cerebral cortex (grey matter)

White matter (myelin)

Lateral ventricle

A gyrus

A sulcus

Skull

Occipital lobe

(a)

BACK

Corpus callosum

Lateral ventricle

3rd ventricle

Temporal lobe

Fig. 2.2. Normal MRI brain scans in the horizontal (a), coronal (b), and sagittal (c) planes, with labelling of common anatomical structures (from Donaghy 1997).

(b)

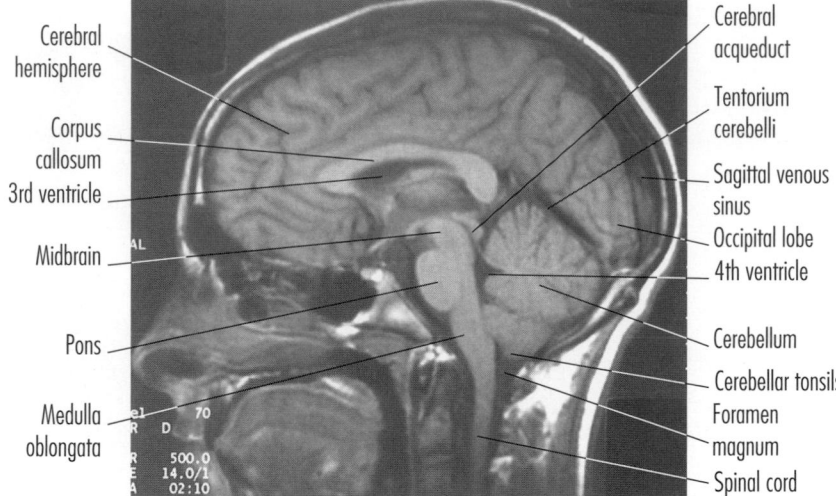

Labels (left, top to bottom): Cerebral hemisphere, Corpus callosum, 3rd ventricle, Midbrain, Pons, Medulla oblongata

Labels (right, top to bottom): Cerebral acqueduct, Tentorium cerebelli, Sagittal venous sinus, Occipital lobe, 4th ventricle, Cerebellum, Cerebellar tonsils, Foramen magnum, Spinal cord

Fig. 2.2. Cont (c)

is useful in a wide range of clinical situations; for example, imaging the optic chiasm; small intracanalicular acoustic neuromas; detection of meningiomas which are sometimes iso-intense with normal central nervous system tissue on T2- and T1-weighted unenhanced sequences; intramedullary spinal tumours; leptomeningeal disease; and in demonstrating acute inflammation in multiple sclerosis plaques.

Less often, special sequences are used which highlight other physical properties of the tissue protons: thus one may obtain images that are diffusion weighted, perfusion weighted, or sensitive to flow (MR angiography) and changes in blood oxygenation (functional MRI). Diffusion, perfusion, and functional MRI sequences are best performed using echo planar hardware and high field systems. Diffusion and perfusion MR sequences are being used increasingly in the early evaluation of acute cerebral infarction, in which context changes on diffusion MRI precede those seen on conventional T2-weighted sequences.

Functional MRI (fMRI), in examining focal changes in cerebral blood flow and oxygen utilization in response to a variety of activation paradigms, is providing enormous insights into the anatomical basis of brain functioning, both in health and disease. The basis of the MRI signal changes seen during a fMRI experiment is due to the fact that deoxyhaemoglobin is paramagnetic and therefore an alteration in its amount (as occurs with focal changes in neuronal metabolism and blood flow) is detected using appropriate rapid-acquisition MR sequences. The role of fMRI as a diagnostic or prognostic tool in everyday clinical practice is currently very limited.

2.1.3 Clinical applications of MRI and CT

The value of MRI and CT are well established in diagnosis of many central nervous system (CNS) disorders. Their use in peripheral nerve and muscle disease are much more limited. In

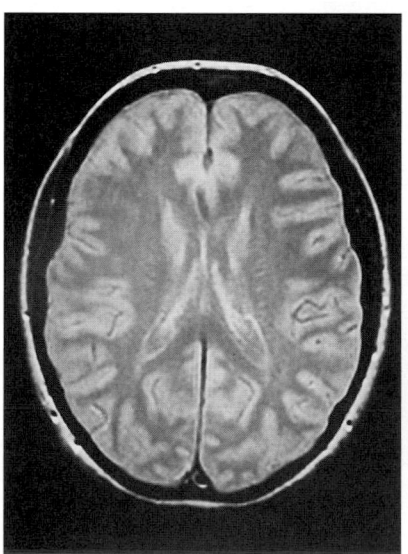
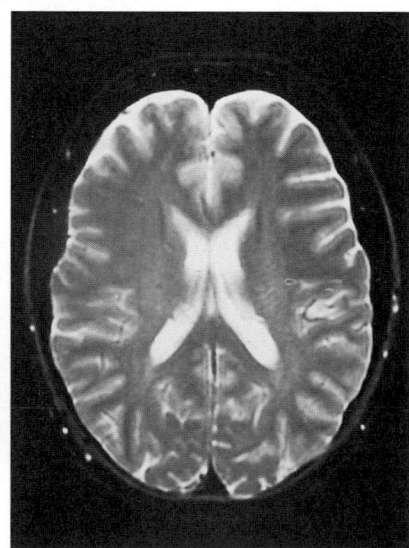
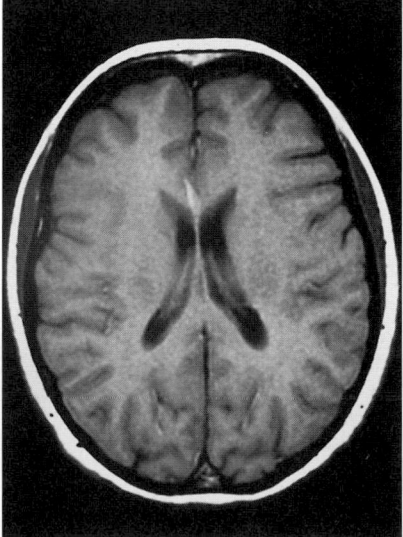

Fig. 2.3. MRI scan of a normal individual: (a) proton-density, (b) T2-weighted, and (c) T1-weighted axial slices at the level of the lateral ventricles (courtesy of Mr D. G. MacManus).

the CNS, because of immunity to bone-hardening artefacts (which are a problem with CT scanning), a capacity for multiplanar imaging, and exquisite sensitivity to white matter disease, MRI is of particular value in the investigation of spinal cord, brainstem, and cerebellar syndromes, and in the work-up of patients with suspected demyelinating disease. It is therefore appropriate to consider both the site and pathological nature of the problem when considering the investigation of choice. The relative values of both modalities are now discussed in such a context.

Cerebral hemisphere mass lesions

Gliomas, metastases, and abscesses are better defined on MRI than CT in terms of their nature, extent, and number (Brandt-Zawadski 1988). However, above the tentorium, CT scanning is also often adequate for diagnostic purposes. In acquired immunodeficiency syndrome, MRI sometimes reveals multiple lesions where CT showed only one, the former being of practical management importance in favouring a diagnosis of toxoplasmosis rather than cerebral lymphoma.

Occasionally tumours (especially low-grade astrocytomas) are poorly defined on CT and display little mass effect leading to diagnostic uncertainty—MRI can sometimes more clearly define the tumour and distinguish it from surrounding oedema. Non-enhanced MRI is less sensitive than contrast-enhanced CT in detecting meningiomas, especially if they are small and calcified. Calcium is poorly visualized on MRI and about 20% of meningiomas are isointense with normal brain on standard MRI sequences. However, gadolinium-enhanced MRI has an excellent sensitivity in showing meningiomas and is in fact slightly more sensitive than enhanced CT, especially in the skull base where bone-hardening artefacts are troublesome when using CT.

Vascular disease

Once established, large cerebral infarcts are readily seen with either CT or MRI. However, CT abnormalities may not appear for a day or two, whereas conventional T2-weighted MRI becomes abnormal within a few hours of the arterial occlusion. Diffusion-weighted images become abnormal even sooner—in experimental studies, areas of reduced diffusion, thought to be due to cell swelling, are seen within minutes of arterial occlusion. Perfusion-weighted images also reveal abnormalities very early after occlusion, and the mismatch of diffusion and perfusion abnormalities may identify the location and size of the potentially salvageable ischaemic penumbra. Such information is now being acquired as a prelude to trials of acute interventional therapies within the first few hours of ischaemic stroke (e.g. thrombolytic therapy), and in the future may have a role in assigning prognosis and selecting those most suitable for aggressive early therapeutic interventions.

MRI also demonstrates haemorrhagic changes in a cerebral infarct with a greater sensitivity than CT. Haematomas, be they parenchymal, subdural, or extradural, are detected better with MRI than CT. Because of the magnetic properties of deoxy-haemoglobin, methaemoglobin, and haemosiderin, characteristic serial MRI changes are seen which identify the age of the haematoma. MRI provides evidence of old haemorrhages at a time when CT has returned to normal. However, in acute subarachnoid haemorrhage (within the first few days of bleeding), CT scanning is better than MRI in demonstrating subarachnoid blood.

Arteriovenous malformations are seen with either enhanced MRI or CT. Cavernous angiomas, which are small (2–20 mm) vascular malformations, are a frequent incidental finding on MRI. They occasionally produce symptoms due to bleeding. The MRI appearances are highly characteristic, with a reticulated central core of mixed signal intensity surrounded by an area of decreased signal on T2-weighted sequences. With recent bleeding there may be a slight mass effect as well as methaemoglobin-induced paramagnetic effects. Cavernous angiomas are often not visible or produce only non-specific changes on CT or angiography. Their detection on MRI may obviate the need for invasive investigations such as angiography or even brain biopsy.

White-matter disease

MRI is far superior to CT in detecting white-matter pathology, and is the investigation of choice in the work-up of a patient with suspected multiple sclerosis (MS). Nevertheless, the differential diagnosis of MRI white-matter lesions is large (Table 2.1). The most common difficulty is distinguishing the white-matter lesions of MS from those due to arteriosclerotic small-vessel disease. The latter become increasingly frequent with ageing, being present in about 30 per cent of the population over the age of 50 years; they are more common in those with a history of hypertension or symptoms of cerebrovascular disease. Pathologically, they are associated with arteriosclerosis,

Table 2.1. Causes of white-matter abnormalities on MRI

Common	
Cerebrovascular disease	
'Normal' ageing	
Multiple sclerosis	

Other	
Acute disseminated encephalomyelitis	Migraine
Behçet's disease	Mitochondrial encephalopathy
Decompression sickness	Motor neuron disease
Fat embolism	Neurosarcoidosis
HIV encephalitis	Phenylketonuria
HTLV-1 associated myelopathy	Progressive multifocal leucoencephalopathy
Hydrocephalus	Subacute sclerosing panencephalitis
Irradiation	Systemic lupus erythematosus
Leucodystrophies (many)	Trauma

dilated perivascular spaces, vascular ectasia, and, occasionally, lacunar infarction.

Although no feature is absolute, there are patterns more characteristic of vascular disease or of multiple sclerosis. In vascular disease, smooth periventricular changes are seen, along with lesions in the centrum semiovale discrete from the ventricles. Basal ganglia lesions are frequent, but infratentorial lesions are less common and, when they occur, tend to be located centrally in the pons. In subcortical arteriosclerotic encephalopathy, the subcortical U fibres are usually spared. In multiple sclerosis, periventricular changes usually predominate and are asymmetrical and irregular. Other common and characteristic findings include ovoid-shaped lesions, involvement of the corpus callosum and corticomedullary junction white matter, and infratentorial lesions. Lesions are often seen around the floor of the fourth ventricle, or extending to the surface of the brainstem.

Leucodystrophies characteristically cause a symmetrical pattern of abnormality. Predominant involvement of posterior parietal and occipital white matter is a feature of adreno-leucodystrophy, whereas frontal predominance is a feature of Alexander's disease. In metachromatic leucodystrophy, the white-matter changes are generalized. About 70 per cent of patients with motor neuron disease have high signal involving the corticospinal tract in the centrum semiovale, posterior limb of internal capsule, and cerebral peduncles. Inflammatory, multifocal disorders, such as acute disseminated encephalomyelitis, systemic lupus erythematosus, Behçet's disease, and sarcoidosis may sometimes be difficult to distinguish radiologically from multiple sclerosis. Useful points of distinction are that subcortical white-matter lesions often predominate in systemic lupus, neuro-Behçet's disease characteristically involves the brainstem and diencephalon, and gadolinium enhancement of meninges and cortical structures may be seen in sarcoidosis. Acute disseminated encephalomyelitis may be indistinguishable from multiple sclerosis on a single scan, but with follow-up, partial lesion resolution and an absence of new lesions is a feature of the former condition, whereas new lesion formation is often seen in the latter.

Temporal lobes

MRI has considerable advantages over CT in this region, being able to demonstrate normal and pathological anatomy in the absence of bone-hardening artefacts from adjacent skull (cortical bone produces a signal void on MRI). Multiplanar imaging also improves the detection of pathology using MRI. In herpes simplex encephalitis, the focal inferior frontal and temporal lesions, which are a characteristic finding, are better defined on MRI.

In patients with intractable complex partial seizures or secondary generalized epilepsy, MRI occasionally detects temporal-lobe tumours and hamartomas not seen on CT. Mesial temporal sclerosis is the most common abnormality in patients with intractable seizures of temporal-lobe origin. The two pathological features of this condition are focal loss of neurons in the hippocampus along with focal gliosis in the same region. Rarely, a unilaterally dilated temporal horn on CT will give a clue to this pathology. However, high-field MRI using coronal sections perpendicular to their long axis reveals abnormalities in the majority of hippocampi that are thought to be the epileptic focus from clinical and EEG investigations. Three-dimensional T1-weighted sequences allow the construction of 1 mm thick slices through these structures and precise quantitation of hippocampal volumes, which are characteristically reduced in mesial temporal sclerosis. FLAIR or T2-weighted imaging may also reveal high signal in the hippocampus. Three-dimensional sequences also allow the detection of extratemporal epileptiform foci in some patients with intractable epilepsy, e.g. cortical dysgenesis, small hamartomas, or vascular malformations. High-resolution MRI thus has an indispensable role in the management of patients with epilepsy (Duncan 1997).

Posterior fossa/foramen magnum

The posterior fossa is a difficult area to study with CT because of bone-hardening artefacts. Brainstem tumours, arteriovenous malformations, infarcts, and plaques are readily identified with MRI but may be poorly visualized or missed altogether on CT. Cerebellopontine angle tumours are better seen with MRI, and gadolinium-enhanced imaging with thin slices (down to 1.5 mm) is the most sensitive method for detecting small intracanalicular acoustic neuromas. As a result, it is a key investigation in patients with unexplained sensorineural deafness. A variety of spinocerebellar degenerations show characteristic abnormalities in the cerebellum or brainstem, including both atrophy and intrinsic parenchymal signal changes.

Congenital craniocervical junction abnormalities can present with a mixture of spinal cord, cerebellar, and brainstem signs simulating multiple sclerosis. The foramen magnum is difficult to visualize with either CT or myelography. MRI clearly and unequivocally demonstrates such abnormalities.

Spinal cord/cauda equina

MR imaging of the spinal cord is technically more demanding than that of the brain, because of the small size of the cord and motion artefact from the adjacent pulsating cerebrospinal fluid (CSF). However, technical developments in the past few years have greatly improved the quality of spinal MRI. These include the use of phased array surface coils, which allow the whole cord to be included in a single sagittal image. High-field scanners (1.5 tesla), which improve resolution and signal-to-noise ratio, are preferable to lower-field systems for the investigation of spinal pathology. The fast spin echo sequence has also allowed good-quality T2-weighted images to be obtained in a clinically acceptable time frame.

Spinal-cord compression due to extradural tumours, cysts, and intervertebral disc prolapses are readily identified by MRI, with a sensitivity equal or superior to that of combined CT/myelography and, except when contraindicated, the former has replaced the latter as the imaging investigation of choice in virtually all cases of myelopathy. Gadolinium-enhanced imaging is needed to investigate meningeal pathology, including infective, inflammatory, and malignant processes.

MRI clearly demonstrates intradural extramedullary tumours such as neurofibroma and meningioma. Enhancement improves the detection of meningiomas. MRI is much superior to CT and myelography in displaying intramedullary spinal-cord lesions, such as syringomyelia and tumours, and distinguishes cystic from solid swellings. The appearances of lipomas are distinctive because of the characteristically high signal of fat on unenhanced T1-weighted sequences. Plaques of multiple sclerosis are seen in the spinal cord in about 75 per cent of those with a clinically definite diagnosis, and this can be of considerable diagnostic value, especially when brain imaging is normal or in older subjects where brain white-matter abnormalities have a lower specificity. High-resolution MRI also detects the majority of spinal angiomas—features on T2-weighted images include serpiginous voids over the surface of the cord due to dilated veins, and swelling with increased signal in the adjacent cord; enhancement may be seen on gadolinium-enhanced T1-weighted images. Spinal angiography is less often needed for diagnosis of spinal arteriovenous malformations, although this is frequently used to identify the level of the fistula and for therapeutic embolization procedures.

Lumbosacral intervertebral disc disease, or cauda equina tumour, is usually detectable with MRI. Both CT and MRI are better than myelography in demonstrating lateral disc prolapses. CT is superior to MRI in detecting calcified discs. However, MRI has the advantage that all levels of the cauda equina and the conus medullaris are imaged in sagittal slices and that multiplanar imaging can assist in more fully characterizing abnormalities. Gadolinium-enhanced MRI can help to distinguish postoperative fibrosis from recurrent disc prolapse in the patient with recurrent symptoms following lumbar laminectomy.

Orbits/optic chiasm

Standard MR sequences result in chemical shift artefact at the nerve–fat interface which makes for rather poor-quality images of the orbit. Furthermore, the fat has a rather high signal which makes the detection of pathology more difficult. However, fat suppression techniques are available which improve the quality of orbital imaging and make MRI competitive with CT for the investigation of orbital pathology. Intrinsic signal change in the optic nerve is seen in optic neuritis with a sensitivity approaching that of visual evoked potentials—the latter, however, will usually suffice as a diagnostic tool.

MRI, especially with gadolinium enhancement, is better able than CT to demonstrate intracranial extension of orbital pathology, such as optic nerve glioma or meningioma. Enhanced MRI is also more accurate in showing the relationship of pituitary and other tumours in the chiasmal region to the chiasm itself, such information being particularly useful to the neurosurgeon.

Basal ganglia

A decrease in signal intensity of T2-weighted sequences in the putamen has been reported in some Parkinsonian syndromes,

especially in multiple system atrophy. High signal on T2-weighted images in the basal ganglia can have many causes, including hypoxia, prion disease, and numerous metabolic disorders, including Wilson's disease and mitochondrial disease.

Meningeal disease

Gadolinium enhancement is required to demonstrate meningeal pathology, although CSF examination is also necessary and overall is more sensitive and specific as a diagnostic tool. Nevertheless, meningeal enhancement is a feature of many meningeal disorders, e.g. infective (including tuberculosis and borrelia), inflammatory (e.g. sarcoidosis), and malignant infiltration.

2.1.4 MRI as a tool to monitor treatment

MRI is being used as a surrogate tool to evaluate treatment efficacy in a number of neurological disorders, perhaps most notably in multiple sclerosis (Miller *et al.* 1996). Serial scanning in relapsing remitting and secondary progressive multiple sclerosis has revealed 5–10 new or gadolinium-enhancing lesions for every clinical relapse; this marked increase in sensitivity has enabled therapeutic effects to be demonstrated within a matter of months in small numbers of patients. A number of drugs substantially reduce new lesion activity, most notably β-interferons which reduce activity by about 70 per cent. The main limitation of conventional T2-weighted and gadolinium-enhanced MRI as a surrogate is that the findings correlate only weakly with clinical evolution, both in treated and untreated patients. Newer MR methods which directly study tissue and axonal damage (MR spectroscopy or progressive brain and spinal cord atrophy) appear to correlate more closely with clinical progression and should enhance the value of MRI as a surrogate tool in future clinical trials.

In Alzheimer's disease, serial three-dimensional T1-weighted sequences can be co-registered and subtracted, with an ability to display small but significant reductions in brain volume over a year or so (Fox *et al.* 1996). Such a surrogate tool holds promise in evaluating potential new therapies for this disease. There is future potential to use MRI and spectroscopy to evaluate the course and treatment of other progressive degenerative disorders that result in atrophy and neuronal loss.

In acute stroke, the very early changes seen on diffusion- and perfusion-weighted MRI offers both a surrogate tool with which to evaluate the efficacy of acute treatment interventions, and also a potential tool for selecting those most suitable for therapeutic intervention. Further studies will be required to define the role of MRI in these areas.

2.1.5 MR spectroscopy

MR spectroscopy (MRS) allows the study of individual compounds that contain a specified atomic nucleus capable of producing an NMR signal. Such nuclei include ^{1}H, ^{31}P, ^{23}Na, and ^{13}C. A high-field system is required to obtain useful spectroscopic data (at least 1.5 tesla). The single NMR peak consists of a series of smaller peaks separated by a few hertz. They arise from chemically different compounds containing the same atomic nucleus; this chemical shift occurs because the magnetic field experienced by the atomic nucleus is slightly modified by its immediate chemical environment. MR spectroscopy demonstrates this frequency shift in parts per million. An example is the protons of water which resonate about 3–5 parts per million distinct from the protons in the methyl group of fat.

The nuclei most studied to date are ^{1}H and ^{31}P. The height and sharpness of the spectral peaks depend on the concentration and mobility of nuclei within each compound. NMR-visible metabolites are generally present in small (millimolar) concentrations, thus implying limits to spatial resolution. This is especially so for ^{31}P spectroscopy, where approximately 30 ml of tissue needs to be sampled to get adequate signal-to-noise at 1.5 tesla. Resolution is better using water-suppressed ^{1}H spectroscopy; good-quality spectra may be obtained from voxels as small as 1 ml at a field strength of 1.5 tesla. Furthermore, chemical-shift imaging techniques are available which allow a single slice of data to be collected in which there are multiple voxels containing spectra—thus it is feasible to survey a relatively large region of the brain. Methods for automated calculation of absolute concentrations of metabolites have been developed (Provencher 1993), and these provide a more reliable estimate of metabolite abnormalities than the measurement of ratios which have used the creatine/phosphocreatine (Cr) peak as an internal standard (alterations in the concentration of Cr have been described in a number of pathological conditions).

In ^{1}H spectroscopy, the major peaks are due to N-acetyl aspartate (NAA), choline-containing compounds (Cho), Cr, and myoinositol (mI). NAA is contained almost exclusively within neurons in adult brain and therefore provides an indication of neuronal/axonal dysfunction, damage, or loss. Cho are prominent in membranes. Myoinositol may act as an osmolyte. Smaller peaks from glutamate, glutamine, and γ-aminobutyric acid (GABA) may be detectable when short echo times and spectral editing techniques are used. Lactate may appear when anaerobic metabolism is occurring, and peaks due to mobile lipids, which are small in normal brain on short echo studies, may become prominent in acute demyelinating lesions, probably as a result of myelin breakdown.

A variety of spectral abnormalities have been reported in numerous CNS diseases (e.g. reduced NAA in tumours, infarcts, multiple sclerosis plaques, and a variety of neurodegenerative disorders; increased NAA in Canavan's disease; increased Cho in some tumours and acute multiple sclerosis plaques; reduced Cho in spinocerebellar degeneration; increased glutamate/glutamine peaks in hepatic encephalopathy; increased mI in Alzheimer's disease and multiple sclerosis plaques; and increased lactate in infarctions, some tumours, mitochondrial disease, and Huntingdon's disease). However, the role of MRS as a diagnostic tool has to date been limited for two reasons. First, it is technically difficult to acquire and to obtain reproducible quantitative measurements. Secondly, many of the abnormalities reported are non-specific, i.e. are common to several diseases. A greater role in the future cannot be excluded as techniques for resolving and quantitating metabolite abnormalities improve.

2.1.6 Positron emission tomography

This imaging technique employs radioactive isotopes and can study a variety of functional or chemical features in normal and pathological brain which are inaccessible to other imaging modalities. A positron is a positively charged electron, and in positron emission tomography (PET) imaging, a biological tracer is labelled with a positron-emitting radionuclide. The tracer is given by intravenous injection or gaseous inhalation, and its distribution in the brain can be demonstrated on tomographic images. Despite the existence of PET for over 20 years, its role in everyday clinical practice of neurology remains small. It is an expensive tool, requires immediate access to a cyclotron and the opportunity for serial examinations is limited by the constraints of radiation exposure.

PET studies have, however, provided considerable insights into aspects of normal brain function and as well disease pathogenesis and pathophysiology. Using radio-isotopes such as $[^{15}O]$- or $[^{18}F]$deoxyglucose, it has been possible to quantify cerebral blood flow and metabolism in vivo. Valuable insights have been obtained into the varying anatomical patterns of altered metabolism and flow in a wide range of neurodegenerative diseases, and the patterns of flow and oxygen utilization in infarcts and their surrounding ischaemic penumbra. Functional MRI has, in many instances, superseded PET as a tool to study blood flow and oxygenation changes in normal and abnormal states, because of superior anatomical resolution and the ability to perform serial studies safely. Radio-isotope labels are also used in PET studies to evaluate receptor binding, e.g. the study of dopaminergic receptors in extrapyramidal disease.

Single-photon emission computed tomography (SPECT) is technically less sophisticated and demanding when compared with PET, but provides lower-resolution images. It can be used to evaluate regional variations in blood flow, but its role in everyday clinical practice is, like that of PET, a small one.

2.2 Imaging the cerebral circulation

2.2.1 Introduction

Cerebral angiography, introduced by Egas Moniz in Portugal in the 1930s, was the first method to display the cerebral circulation during life (Moniz 1934). Originally it required the direct intracarotid, and sometimes even intracardiac, injection of material which was opaque to X-rays. Over the years, the basic principal has remained the same but nowadays the femoral artery route is easier, less traumatic catheters are used, the catheters can be controlled and advanced into any intracranial vessel as small as cortical branches of the middle cerebral artery, X-ray contrast material has become far less toxic, and better imaging equipment exploits the ease and speed of computerized digitization rather than photographic images based on silver-based chemical methods. But the indications have radically shrunk. Before the introduction of axial imaging of the brain in the early 1970s, first by CT and then by MRI, catheter angiography was used to show not just abnormalities of the vessels, but also to outline and display, albeit indirectly, intracranial mass lesions, hydrocephalus, and other structural abnormalities. Nowadays, catheter angiography is more or less confined to displaying arterial stenosis and occlusion due to vascular disease (atheroma, vasculitis, dissection, etc.), intracranial venous thrombosis, intracranial aneurysms, and intracranial vascular malformations. But even the small risks of modern catheter angiography have become unacceptable, and non-invasive—and so safer—vascular imaging is reducing its role still further: first ultrasound imaging, then MR angiography, and now CT angiography (Sellar 1995). However, catheter angiography is certainly not redundant, although it is far less used than even 5 years ago. Furthermore, it remains the 'gold standard' against which all other vessel imaging methods must be compared, both for the extracranial and intracranial arteries and veins. Catheter angiography also provides the underpinning access and imaging for the interventional neuroradiological treatment of aneurysms and vascular malformations, and possibly of stenoses using angioplasty, all of which are eroding the role of surgeons.

2.2.2 Catheter X-ray angiography

Even these days, catheter angiography is still inconvenient, invasive, uncomfortable, costly, carries a risk, and normally requires hospital admission for at least a day if the patient is not already in hospital. During and immediately after angiography of patients with atherothrombotic arterial disease, about 4 per cent have a transient ischaemic attack (TIA) or stroke, one-quarter of them permanent. Indeed, the risk is probably higher if the patient has severe carotid disease who, with prior duplex sonography screening, is precisely the sort of patient now selected for angiography with a view to carotid surgery (Hankey et al. 1990a,b; Davies and Humphrey 1993; Heiserman et al. 1994). TIAs and strokes occur because the catheter dislodges atheromatous plaque or dissects the arterial wall during insertion, injection, or flushing; thrombus may form at the catheter tip or in blood contaminating the contrast-containing syringe; and exceptionally as a result of the almost inevitable injection of at least some air (Gerraty et al. 1996). In addition, there are systemic and allergic adverse effects of the contrast material, particularly during intravenous digital subtraction angiography, where very large quantities are used: bradycardia, hypotension, angina, shortness of breath, nausea, vomiting, headache, epileptic seizures, transient bilateral blindness, periorbital oedema, urticaria, bronchospasm, and renal failure. Some patients develop a haematoma, aneurysm, or nerve injury at the site of arterial puncture (which is usually into the femoral artery in the groin), and the occasional patient develops de novo, or has worsened symptoms of, peripheral vascular disease in the leg distal to the puncture site, sometimes even

leading to amputation. The cholesterol embolization syndrome is very rare, but it can be fatal (Section 27.4.2). The neurological risks involved in investigating patients for ruptured or unruptured aneurysms and intracranial vascular malformations are much less, partly perhaps because the patients are generally younger and partly because their arteries do not contain so much friable and easily dislodged material (Cloft et al. 1999).

Compared with cut-film selective intra-arterial catheter angiography recorded directly onto X-ray film, intra-arterial digital subtraction angiography is quicker, less contrast is used, and the images are easier to manipulate and store, contrast resolution is better although the spatial resolution is less, but there is no evidence that it is much safer (Warnock et al. 1993). Neither intravenous digital subtraction nor arch aortography are satisfactory alternatives to selective intra-arterial cut-film or digital angiography, because so often the images are poor and stenoses impossible to measure (particularly with the former method), vessels may overlap, there is no accurate information about intracranial vessels and so aneurysms, and the techniques are not necessarily safer (Pelz et al. 1985; Rothwell et al. 1998).

2.2.3 Ultrasound of the extra- and intracranial vessels

Duplex sonography

This technique combines real-time ultrasound imaging to demonstrate the anatomy of the neck arteries, along with pulsed Doppler analysis of blood flow at any point of interest in the vessel lumen. Its accuracy is enhanced, and it is technically easier to do, if the Doppler signals are colour-coded to show the direction of blood flow and its velocity, and also with power Doppler which is extremely sensitive to moving blood in any direction (Furst et al. 1992; Griewing et al. 1996). The amount of luminal stenosis is calculated not just from the real-time ultrasound image, which can be difficult to see when the stenotic lesion is echolucent or calcification scatters the ultrasound beam, but also from the blood-flow velocities derived from the Doppler signal.

Although duplex sonography is non-invasive, widely available, and hospital admission is not required, there are some difficulties which any ultrasound service must acknowledge and deal with: it is very operator dependent and so requires skill, training, and considerable experience to be sure of accurate measurements of stenosis and the avoidance of pitfalls, such as confusing the external with the internal carotid artery; it may be difficult to interpret, particularly if there is plaque or periarterial calcification; it is not completely reliable in distinguishing very severe (>90 per cent) stenosis (which is operable) from occlusion (which is not), unless used and interpreted with very great care (Furst et al. 1999); it is not completely sensitive and specific for severe (70–99 per cent) carotid bifurcation stenosis; different machines vary in their accuracy in measuring carotid stenosis (Howard et al. 1996); and it provides little information about the arterial anatomy proximal to the carotid bifurcation which, as it happens, is seldom affected by severe disease, and

Table 2.2. Methodological criteria for comparing a non-invasive vessel imaging method against the 'gold standard' of intra-arterial catheter angiography

Prospective study design

Rigorously consecutive series of patients, or random sample

Adequate description of the study population, the inclusion and exclusion criteria

A spectrum of vessel disease severity over the clinically relevant range

No exclusion of patients with poor images

Adequate detail of *both* imaging techniques

Adequate detail of exactly how *both* imaging techniques are used, and stenotic or other lesions are interpreted and measured

Reproducibility of measurements reported

Images assessed by one technique 'blind' to the images of the other technique

All relevant data presented

Proper statistical methodology for comparing continuous and discontinuous variables in a clinically relevant manner

Analysis based on individual patients, not just on arteries

Appropriate sample size for adequate power

none at all about distal anatomy (e.g. the position of the upper limit of a high stenotic lesion, intracranial arterial stenosis, and intracranial aneurysms) (Griffiths *et al.* 1996).

As staff change and machines are updated, constant audit of the results against any subsequent catheter angiography is essential, but this is becoming more and more problematic as fewer catheter angiograms are being done (Elgersma *et al.* 1998). Another problem is that the ultrasound techniques are changing so fast, and hopefully improving, that any conclusions about their accuracy in measuring the severity and character of carotid lesions are constantly out of date, and must anyway be applied in the context of one's own institution (Ringelstein 1995; Carpenter *et al.* 1996). Unfortunately, the literature comparing the accuracy of ultrasound, and other non-invasive imaging methods, versus the 'gold standard' of catheter angiography is bedevilled by poor epidemiological and statistical methodology and publication bias, and seldom conforms to very standard guidelines for evaluating this kind of diagnostic test (Blakeley *et al.* 1995; Rothwell 2000; Rothwell *et al.* 2000; Table 2.2). None the less, with stringent quality control, and confirmation of any stenosis by an independent observer, duplex sonography is now the most common way that carotid stenosis severe enough to warrant surgery is diagnosed.

There are no standard and commonly used definitions for the ultrasound appearance of plaques (soft, hard, calcified, etc.) and there is also considerable variation in reporting between, and even within, the same observers at different times (Arnold *et al.* 1999). Therefore, although unstable and ulcerated plaques are more likely to be symptomatic than stable plaques with fibrous caps, the ultrasound inaccuracy obviously compromises any study of the relationship between plaque characteristics on duplex and the risk of later stroke (Gronholdt 1999). But,

bearing all these limitations in mind, duplex is a remarkably quick and simple investigation in experienced hands and it is neither unpleasant nor risky. Very rarely, the pressure of the ultrasound Doppler probe on the carotid bifurcation can dislodge thrombus or cause enough carotid sinus stimulation to lead to bradycardia or hypotension (Rosario *et al.* 1987; Friedman, 1990).

Transcranial Doppler sonography

Essentially, transcranial Doppler sonography (TCD) provides information on blood-flow velocity, and its direction in relation to the ultrasound probe, in the major intracranial arteries at the base of the brain (Fig. 2.4). It can display occlusion of the middle cerebral artery trunk if not its branches, of the anterior cerebral artery, and, less easily, of the basilar and posterior cerebral arteries. However, stenosis can be difficult to distinguish from hyperaemia because velocity flow is increased in both situations. It is non-invasive, repeatable on demand, can be done at the bedside in sick patients, or in outpatients, is not expensive and not too difficult to perform accurately. Furthermore, it is very safe, although during tests involving compression of the carotid artery it is conceivable that emboli could be released from an underlying atheromatous plaque (Khaffaf *et al.* 1994; Karnik *et al.* 1995). However, the patient has to keep reasonably still; the examination can take as long as an hour; the skull is impervious to ultrasound in 5–10 per cent of cases, more with increasing age and in females, but less if intravenous echo contrast is used; exact vessel identification may be difficult, but colour-flow real-time imaging makes this easier; diagnostic criteria vary; and the technique is not always accurate in comparison with catheter angiography, although not all that many patients have been properly compared (Ley-Pozo and Ringelstein 1990; Bornstein and Norris 1994; Baumgartner *et al.* 1997; Gerriets *et al.* 1999).

Despite the fact that TCD, like positron emission tomography (PET), has increased our knowledge of the cerebral circulation in health and disease, and even though it is inexpensive and quite widely available (very unlike PET), it still has rather a minor role in routine clinical management: monitoring carotid endarterectomy under general anaesthesia (Section 27.10.3); the diagnosis of patent foramen ovale (Section 27.4.5); detecting 'vasospasm' in patients with subarachnoid haemorrhage (Section 27.7.4); and detecting major arterial occlusion before using thrombolytic treatment in acute ischaemic stroke (Section 27.8.4); perhaps in the future in helping define long-term stroke risk (Babikian *et al.* 1997; Molloy and Markus 1999); and it may have a role in displaying intracranial aneurysms (Wardlaw and White 2000).

2.2.4 **MR angiography**

Magnetic resonance angiography (MRA) provides images of blood vessels which are open, by displaying the flow voids of moving blood within them (Graves 1997). Like any other MR technique, the pictures can be in any plane, and it is applicable

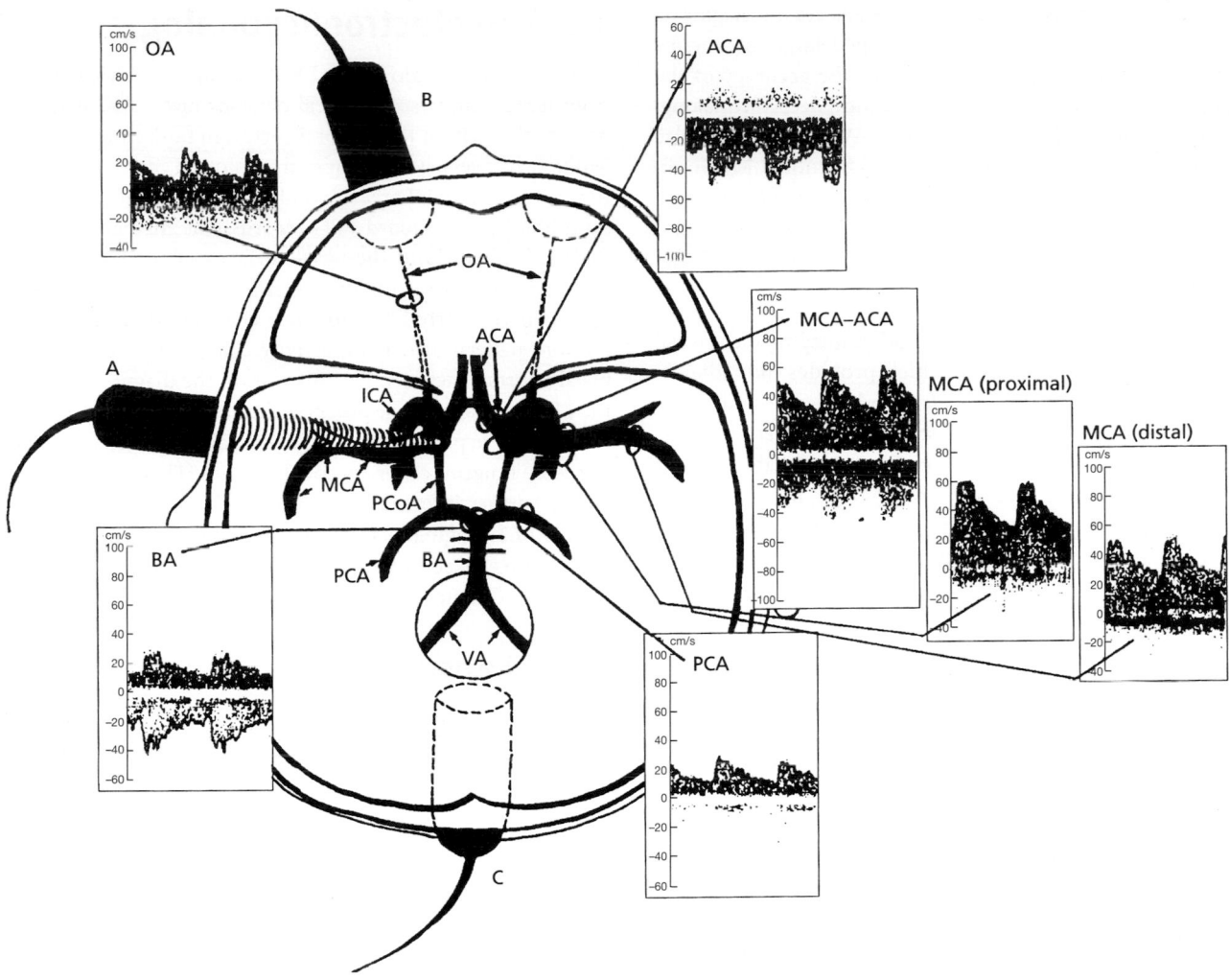

Fig. 2.4. Technique of transcranial Doppler sonography. Diagram of the head looked at from above (eyes at the top of the diagram) to illustrate the cranial sonographic windows (A, temporal; B, orbital; C, foramen magnum) and typical waveforms obtained from the major intracranial arteries. Note that the power output of the transducer must be reduced to 10 per cent of the maximum for the transorbital approach to avoid damage to the eyes. ACA, anterior cerebral artery; ICA, internal carotid artery; MCA, middle cerebral artery; BA, basilar artery; OA, ophthalmic artery; PCA, posterior cerebral artery; PCoA, posterior communicating artery; VA, vertebral artery. (From Warlow, C. P., Dennis, M. S., van Gijn, J. *et al.* (1996). *Stroke: a practical guide to management*. Blackwell Science Ltd, Oxford.)

as much to the intracranial as the extracranial circulation, and to the intracranial venous sinuses as well as the cerebral arteries.

Although non-invasive and safe, and it is certainly an outpatient procedure, MRA alone is unlikely to be sufficiently accurate in estimating carotid bifurcation stenosis, at least at the present stage of development. The pictures are not always adequate to allow measurement of the stenosis (movement and swallowing artefacts are particular problems); the severity of the stenosis tends to be overestimated; there may be a flow gap distal to a stenosis of only 60 per cent, probably due to loss of laminar flow and increased residence times of the blood, making precise measurement impossible; irregularity/ulceration is not well seen; and severe stenosis can be confused with occlusion (Siewert *et al.* 1995; Levi *et al.* 1996). So far, there have not been enough methodologically sound comparisons of MRA with intra-arterial catheter angiography to assess bias and

imprecision over the whole range of stenosis in appropriate patient groups; and the comparative studies that have been done have frequently been overtaken by changes, if not improvements, in MR technology. Anyway, at present, MRA is expensive, not readily available, claustrophobic for some people, requires the patient to lie still for several minutes, and may be contraindicated if there is any metal in the body. It is certainly not sensitive or specific enough to image cerebral arterial beading and stenosis of the sort that can be found in vasculitis and other conditions (Table 28.2).

In acute ischaemic stroke it would, of course, be interesting to image the intracranial circulation, but it is difficult to look after acutely ill patients in the MR scanner, and in confused patients who move around the images are corrupted by artefact. The same problems arise in imaging aneurysms in acute subarachnoid haemorrhage. Although MRA is more tolerable in well patients when unruptured aneurysms are the diagnostic issue, particularly the more easily imaged large aneurysms causing a third nerve palsy for example, the accuracy of the technique may well be insufficient for clinical decision-making, compared with catheter angiography (Wardlaw and White 2000). MR venography, along with cross-sectional MR brain imaging, is now the first and often the best method to diagnose definitively intracranial venous thrombosis (Section 27.11.2).

2.2.5 CT angiography

This still-evolving non-invasive method of imaging the arterial system uses helical (spiral) CT which provides immediately adjacent and overlapping images from which two- and three-dimensional images can be reconstructed (Brink et al. 1997). But, to image blood vessels, the patients must be able to hold their breath for several seconds; unlike MRA, a large dose of intravenous contrast is required to outline the lumen and this has complications of its own (Section 2.2.2); the contrast bolus must not become too dispersed, which is problematic with cardiac failure; there is radiation exposure, which is a problem if repeated imaging is required; the images obtained depend on the proficiency of the operator in their selection; and so far CT angiography (CTA) has not been well evaluated against the gold standard of selective intra-arterial catheter angiography. However, it does provide multiple viewing angles, three-dimensional reconstruction, and imaging of calcium deposits separately from the vessel lumen outlined by the contrast (Heiken et al. 1993; Leclerc et al. 1995). Moreover, compared with MRA, it is quicker, much less claustrophobic, and sick patients can be better looked after in the scanner. Therefore, it has an emerging role in imaging both extracranial arterial stenosis and intracranial aneurysms (Fig. 2.5).

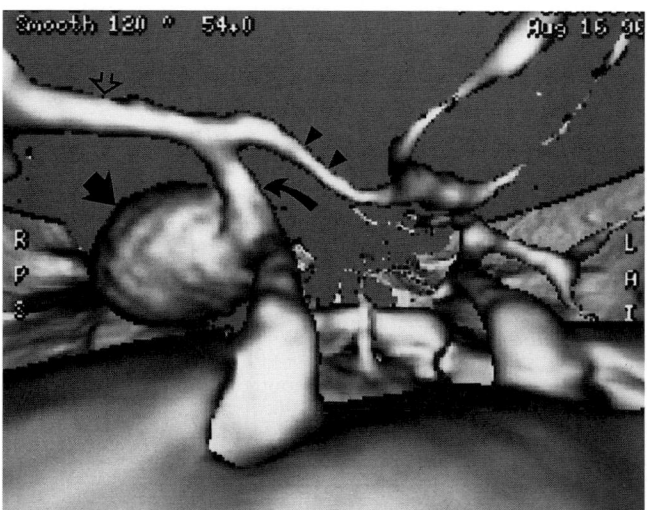

Fig. 2.5. CT angiogram showing a large aneurysm (black arrow) arising from the terminal internal carotid artery (curved arrow) before it divides into the middle (open arrow) and anterior (arrowheads) cerebral arteries.

2.3 The electroencephalogram

The electroencephalogram (EEG) averages electrical activity from large numbers of cortical neurons orientated parallel to one another within the cerebral cortex, in both time and space. While it has very good temporal resolution, its spatial resolution is very limited. Large areas of the cortex are too remote for sampling from standard EEG records (the medial surfaces of the hemispheres and the basal surfaces of the frontal lobe). Because of the averaging that takes place during recording, the EEG is particularly likely to show changes when the normal, random pattern of cortical activity changes to more synchronized neuronal activity. For this reason, the diagnostic value of the EEG is greatest in disorders such as epilepsy (which is essentially one of hypersynchrony of neuronal hyperexcitability) and in a wide range of other encephalopathies (Ebersole and Pedley 1990). Further information can be extracted from the EEG by the use of averaging techniques time-locked to sensory stimuli to produce evoked potentials (Section 2.4). The EEG in sleep is covered in Chapter 24.

2.3.1 The normal EEG

Alpha rhythm is the most striking component of the normal EEG. It is of regular and moderate amplitude with a frequency of between 8 and 13 Hz. It occurs during wakefulness with the eyes closed, is attenuated by eye opening, and disappears during sleep, and is most clearly demonstrated in posterior leads (Fig. 2.6).

Beta activity is defined as any rhythmic activity with a frequency of more than 13 Hz. It is usually generalized and may be seen in normal subjects who are tense or anxious about the procedure, and also as a drug-induced effect in patients receiving sedative or tranquillizing drugs.

Theta activity has a frequency of 4–7 Hz. It is a normal component of the EEG of children and adolescents, particularly over the temporal regions, but becomes more sparse with maturation. The finding of temporal theta activity represents a non-specific abnormality in adult patients with a variety of neurological disorders.

Artefactual changes

Numerous physiological and technical artefacts may be seen during EEG recording. These include large-amplitude frontal potentials due to eye movements, activity of very short duration due to muscle activity, ECG, and electrode artefacts. The elimination of these problems demands a high level of technical expertise.

2.3.2 Abnormal EEG activity

Delta activity is defined as activity with a frequency of less than 4 Hz. Although delta activity may occur in normal individuals during sleep, and in children, its presence in the waking state in adults is abnormal. Generalized delta activity is seen postictally in patients with metabolic or drug-induced encephalopathy,

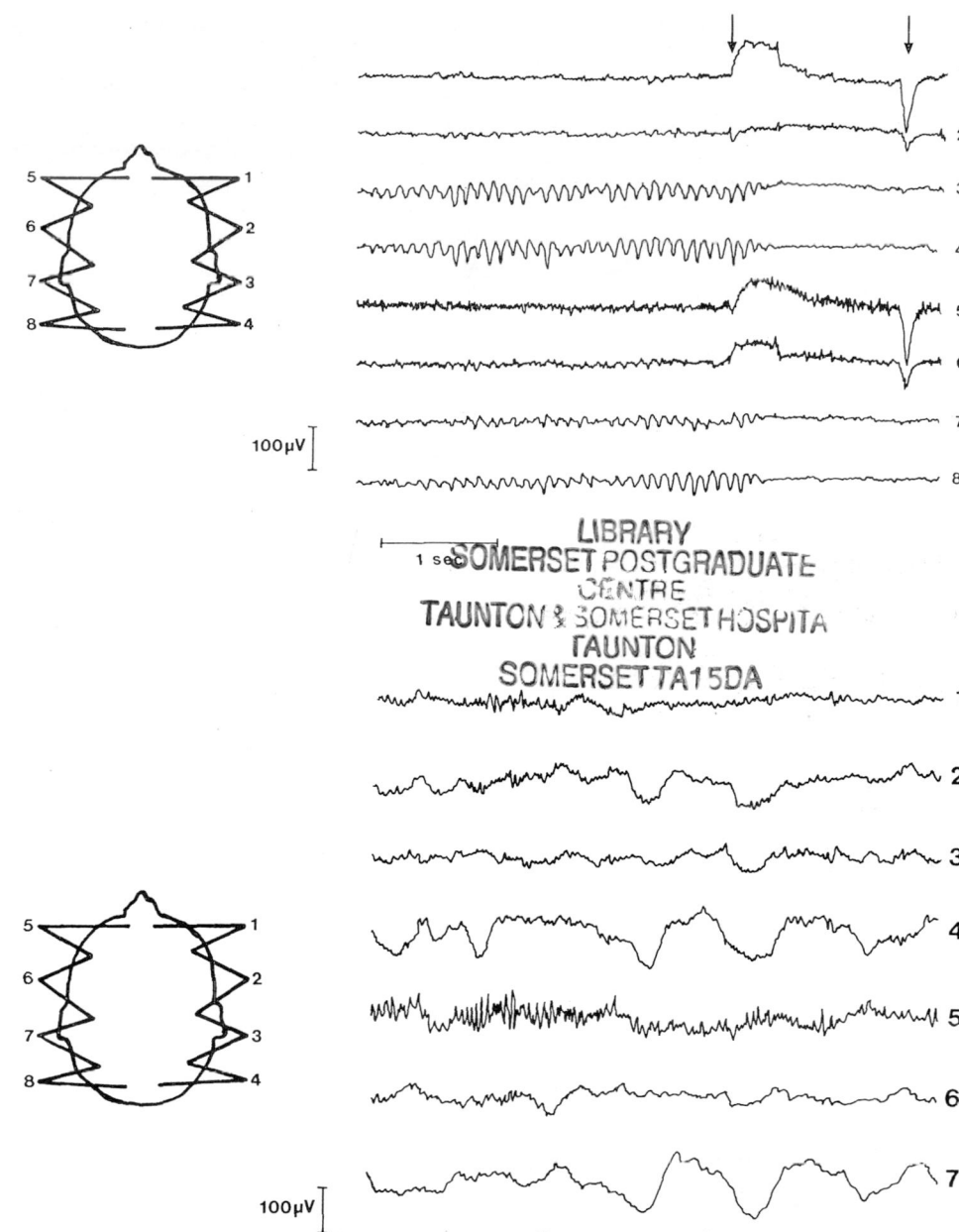

Fig. 2.6. A normal EEG with eye-movement artefact marked by arrows.

100μV

1 sec

Fig. 2.7. Generalized slow (delta) activity of high amplitude, maximal in posterior leads, in a patient in coma due to a viral encephalitis.

100μV

and in patients with a diffuse encephalitis (Fig. 2.7). When it is localized to one area of the hemisphere it is usually indicative of some form of structural pathology (Fig. 2.8). However, it is impossible to differentiate between tumour and infarction on the basis of localized delta activity.

Spike discharges or sharp waves with a duration of up to 200 ms are the characteristic interictal abnormality found in epileptic patients. When they are generalized, interictal spikes are most commonly associated with following slow waves. When they are localized, although spikes and sharp waves may be associated with slow activity, they may occur independently. Sharp waves may be induced by drugs and alcohol withdrawal.

Paroxysmal activity may be defined as activity of very sudden onset and termination. This obviously includes spike wave activity, but also describes bursts of faster theta activity, seen as part of an epileptic process, other more non-specific activity and periodic complexes (see below).

2.3.3 EEG responses to activation

Hyperventilation leads to a general slowing of activity, often with the development of paroxysmal high-voltage delta activity. These changes are most evident in younger patients and diminish with increasing age. Hyperventilation may provoke spike

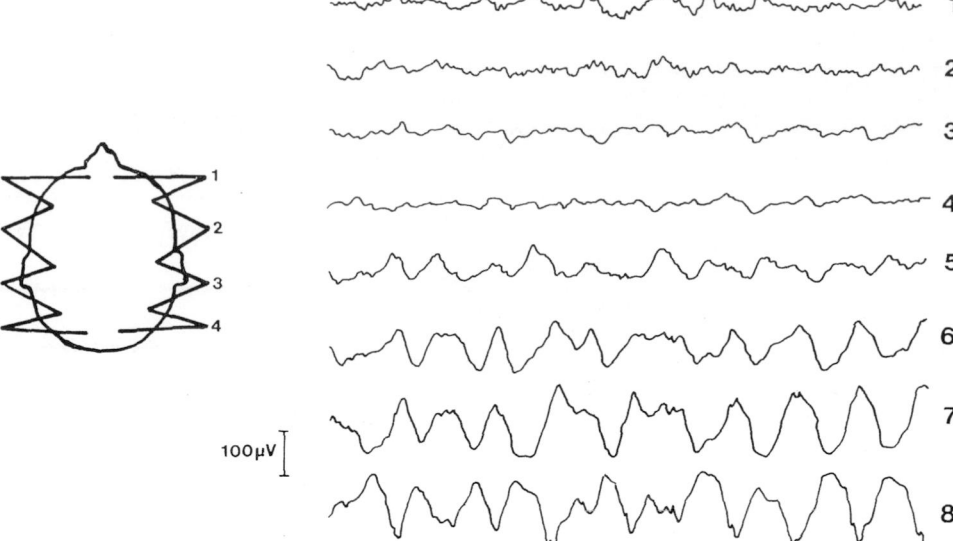

Fig. 2.8. Slow (delta) activity of high amplitude arising from the left hemisphere in a patient with a massive hemisphere infarction.

100μV

wave discharges in patients with absence and other forms of idiopathic generalized epilepsy. Occasionally hyperventilation may enhance local abnormalities in the EEG.

Photic stimulation is performed with a stroboscopic stimulus, usually with the eyes closed and open. This generates some posterior rhythmic activity that is time-locked to the rate of stroboscopic stimulation. In some instances photo-myoclonic responses may be generated, with muscle activity most commonly localized around the eyelids, occurring at the rate of stimulation. However, in patients with photosensitive epilepsy, a photo-convulsive response occurs, consisting of bursts of spike–slow wave activity which are usually bilateral and synchronous, and which persist briefly after the termination of the stroboscopic stimulus. This abnormality is seen in patients with idiopathic and symptomatic generalized epilepsies.

Historically, drugs have been used to 'activate' the EEG. This is now rarely performed, though sodium methohexitone may be used in the specialized investigation of patients being assessed for temporal lobectomy.

Recordings during natural sleep show a significant modification of EEG activity. There tends to be a generalized slowing of activity with loss of alpha rhythm, and quite dramatic activity with K complexes and bursts of sleep spindles may occur; however, a full description of these is beyond the scope of this chapter. The main value of sleep recording is in the detection of abnormalities in patients with suspected partial seizures, and in the investigation of sleep apnoea.

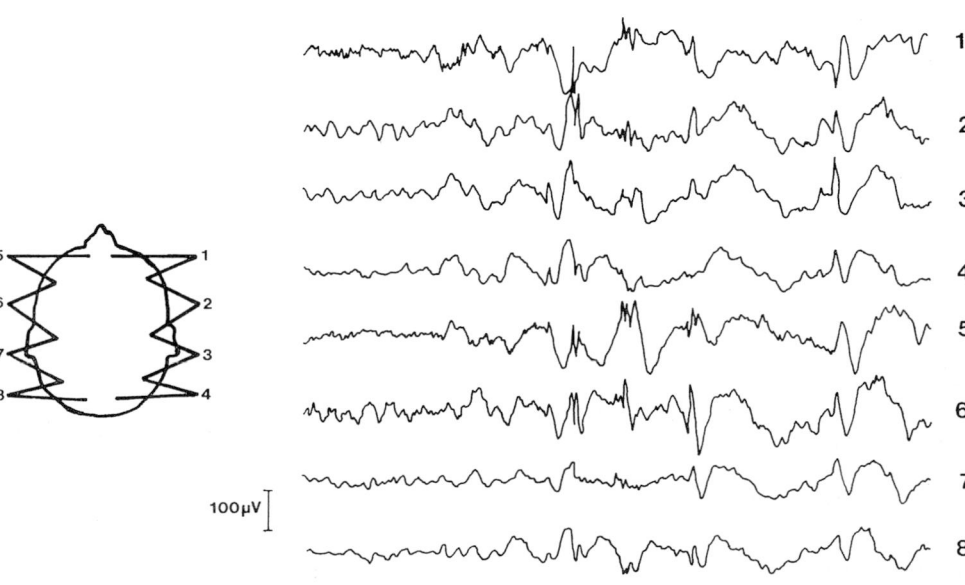

Fig. 2.9. Irregular, generalized slow spike wave activity in a child with Lennox–Gastaut syndrome.

100μV

2.3.4 **The EEG in epilepsy**

Synchronous postsynaptic potentials and paroxysmal depolarization shifts will be detected in the scalp EEG when they occur synchronously in large enough populations of neurons. They will produce spikes or sharp waves that are usually electronegative over the cortex. These are commonly followed by slow waves associated with hyperpolarization of pools of neurons and reduced firing patterns. This is the basic electroencephalographic signature of the epilepsies, and may be seen in focal distributions in the partial epilepsies and more generalized distributions in the generalized epilepsies (Sections 23.2, 23.4).

The patterns of EEG activity occurring during seizures vary considerably with the type of seizure. It is a general rule that diagnostic interictal and ictal EEG abnormalities will be found much more frequently in the generalized than in partial epilepsies. For childhood absence epilepsy, an EEG that shows no 3/second spike wave activity during a period of hyper-

ventilation will, for practical purposes, exclude the diagnosis, hyperventilation being strongly provocative of spike wave activity in this and other generalized epilepsies. Atypical absences are more commonly associated with slower, more irregular spike wave activity associated with a more abnormal EEG background (Fig. 2.9).

In patients with myoclonic seizures, both ictal and interictal discharges consist of spike and polyspike and wave slow activity (Fig. 2.10), and a high proportion will exhibit a photoconvulsive response with photic stimulation.

Tonic–clonic seizures will usually obscure the EEG during the tonic phase, but during the clonic phase rhythmic spike wave activity is seen, proceeding to a generally flat postictal EEG. In contrast, tonic and atonic seizures are often associated with low-voltage fast activity or electrodecremental events at the onset of seizures.

Well-localized spike wave activity is most commonly seen in the temporal-lobe epilepsies (Fig. 2.11). Frontal-lobe epilepsies can sometimes be associated with relatively normal EEG

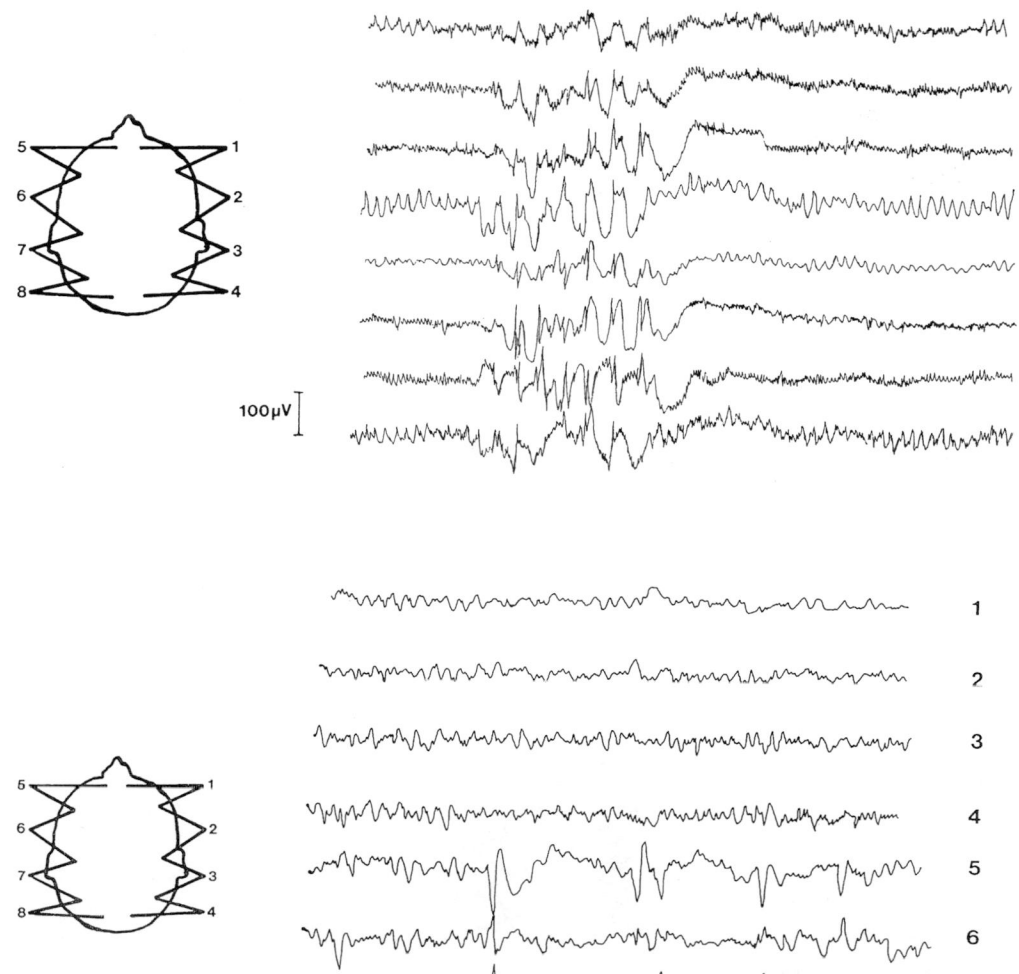

Fig. 2.10. A short burst of 4–6 Hz spike and polyspike and wave activity in a patient with juvenile myoclonic epilepsy.

100 µV

Fig. 2.11. Focal spike activity showing phase reversal in the left frontotemporal region (between leads 5 and 6) in a patient with complex partial epilepsy.

00 µV

recordings, both ictally and interictally. On other occasions, frontal-lobe epilepsies may produce somewhat atypical bi-frontal spike wave activity that may be difficult to differentiate from discharges of a generalized epilepsy. Ictal recordings of partial epilepsies usually begin with localized fast activity which builds in amplitude and become more rhythmic, eventually transforming to spike wave activity. Seizure activity commonly spreads rapidly to the homotopic area of the contralateral hemisphere, and to other parts of the ipsilateral hemisphere.

Issues concerning the sensitivity and specificity of the EEG for the diagnosis of epilepsy are dealt with elsewhere (Section 23.9.1).

2.3.5 Specialized recording techniques in epilepsy

The usefulness and yield of the EEG in epilepsy can be increased in some patients by the use of specialized techniques, either to prolong recording or to increase the spatial sampling. Ambulatory recording is usually undertaken using a slowly running electromagnetic tape, but may alternatively be recorded on other mass storage devices such as flash cards and miniature hard discs. While it is increasingly possible to combine this with synchronized video-recording, more commonly ambulatory records are undertaken without such benefit. The main use of ambulatory recording is in differentiating convulsive pseudoseizures from true tonic–clonic seizures, and also potentially for studying the links between different states of responsiveness and subtle seizures in individuals with severe epilepsy.

Video-telemetry has, in the past, allowed more extensive recording, with up to 128 channels and, in addition, synchronized video-recording to document behavioural correlates of seizure activity. This greatly enhances the diagnostic capabilities for non-convulsive events and allows the use of the EEG for

lateralization and localization of seizure onsets in patients being evaluated for surgery.

Intracranial recording may further support the localization of seizure onsets. A number of different techniques are available. Foramen ovale recording is relatively non-invasive and is very sensitive in identifying seizures starting in the medial temporal structures. For extratemporal epilepsies, subdural mats, with or without stereotactically implanted depth electrodes, may be used.

Many systems are available which allow the production of isopotential maps. The production of these maps eliminates the temporal element of EEG recording, which is in fact the EEG's greatest strength. It is doubtful whether these maps provide any additional information that cannot be derived from a conventional EEG by a reasonably experienced observer.

2.3.6 The EEG and non-epileptic disorders

The EEG will exhibit gross changes of slowing of background activities, with ultimately burst suppression types of periodic activity, in a number of metabolic, drug-induced, neurodegenerative, infective, and post-hypoxic states. In a few instances, the findings of generalized slow activity or periodic activity may be diagnostically useful within a well-defined clinical setting.

The EEG may be particularly useful in the differentiation of psychogenic coma-like states from true coma. The presence of typical occipital alpha rhythms in an unresponsive subject is, for practical purposes, diagnostic of pseudocoma. Periodic complexes (Fig. 2.12), when they occur on the background of subacute dementing illness, are reasonably specific for subacute sclerosing panencephalitis (SSPE) in children and young adults, and for classical Creutzfeldt–Jakob disease in older subjects. Localized periodic activity in one or other frontotemporal regions is a relatively late feature of herpes simplex encephalitis.

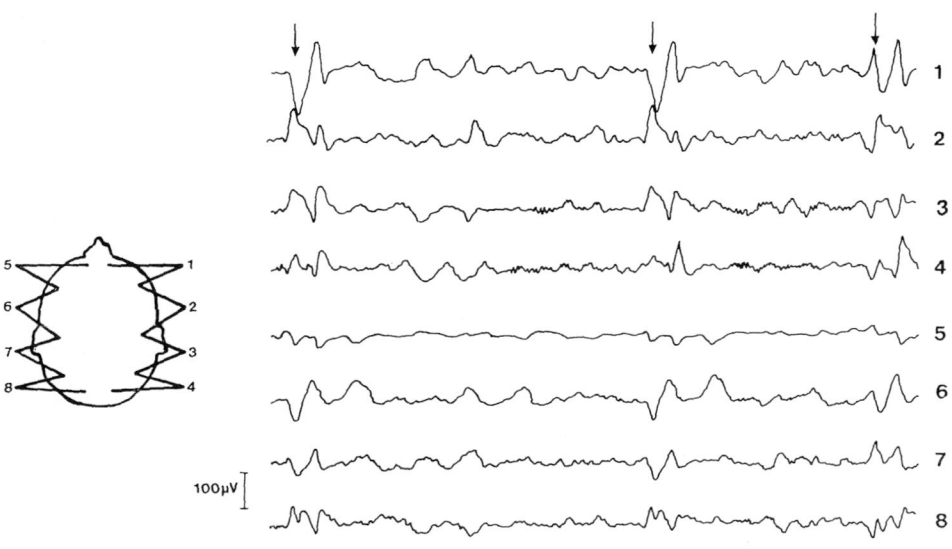

Fig. 2.12. Periodic activity (marked by arrows) separated by periods of relatively featureless EEG in a patient with subacute sclerosing panencephalitis.

100μV

2.4 Evoked potentials

2.4.1 General principles

Evoked potentials were first used in clinical practice to explore the integrity of myelinated pathways in the central nervous system when it became clear that averaging techniques could be used to distinguish the slowing of conduction in focal demyelination from the near normal physiological properties of surviving fibres in pathways with partial axonal degeneration (Fig 2.13). These principles of clinical neurophysiology had been pioneered in the peripheral nervous system.

The systematic use of evoked potentials began with the introduction of pattern-reversed stimulation of the visual system (Halliday *et al.* 1972). This was soon extended to the exploration of other central afferent pathways (sensory (Small *et al.* 1978) and auditory (Robinson and Rudge 1977)), descending motor tracts using electrical (Merton and Morton 1980) and magnetic (Barker *et al.* 1985) stimulation of the cortex, and cognition through event-related potentials (see Heinze *et al.* 1999). Because slowing of conduction characterizes both the anatomical site and pathophysiological properties of demyelination, evoked potentials were soon used routinely to provide laboratory support for the diagnosis of demyelinating disease and related disorders (Halliday *et al.* 1973; Cowan *et al.* 1984). Abnormalities of the latency and amplitude of the evoked response are seen in a variety of conditions affecting the central nervous system, including compression and neurodegeneration. Specific methods, such as imaging and molecular analysis, are increasingly available and preferred for detecting these conditions. Evoked potentials are used in peroperative assessment of spinal surgery which potentially threatens the cord, such as correction of scoliosis, but for practical purposes the main clinical application remains the detection of demyelinated pathways.

2.4.2 Visual evoked potentials

Using a chequerboard pattern of black and white squares subtending approximately 50 min of arc at the retina and reversing at 2 Hz, the visual evoked response is transiently decreased in amplitude (or absent if acuity is less than 6/24) in acute optic neuritis (Fig. 2.14). Typically it stabilizes at a prolonged latency (by about 35 ms) with normal amplitude in the postacute phase. The latency routinely returns to normal in the majority of affected children (Kriss *et al.* 1988). There is also evidence for progressive shortening of the latency of the evoked response for up to 3 years after an episode of acute optic neuritis in adults, consistent with remyelination, but this is not associated with sustained improvement in vision, perhaps through the establishment of irreversible axonal changes in the previously demyelinated nerve (Brusa *et al.* 1999).

Where the absolute latency is not prolonged, demyelination may be marked by an asymmetry in response between the two eyes. Half-field stimulation can demonstrate demyelinating lesions of the chiasm and posterior visual pathway. Evoked potentials are particularly useful in supporting the diagnosis of non-organic visual loss. Normal amplitude, waveform, and latency with a visual acuity of 6/24 or less, not due to refractive error, suggests a functional disturbance of vision. Conversely, delayed latency may guide the interpretation of dubious visual symptoms.

The visual evoked potential (VEP) is delayed in approximately 70 per cent of patients suspected of having widespread demyelination and in the majority of those with clinically definite multiple sclerosis (McDonald 1998). Asymptomatic delay in a patient with isolated demyelination affecting the other optic nerve or another part of the central nervous system increases the probability of subsequent clinical conversion to multiple sclerosis.

Compression of the optic nerve usually produces a visual evoked potential of irregular form without a convincing

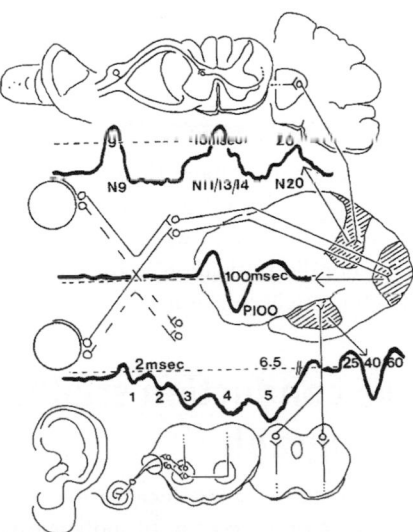

Fig. 2.13. Cartoon to illustrate the principal wave forms obtained by visual, somatosensory, and auditory evoked potentials.

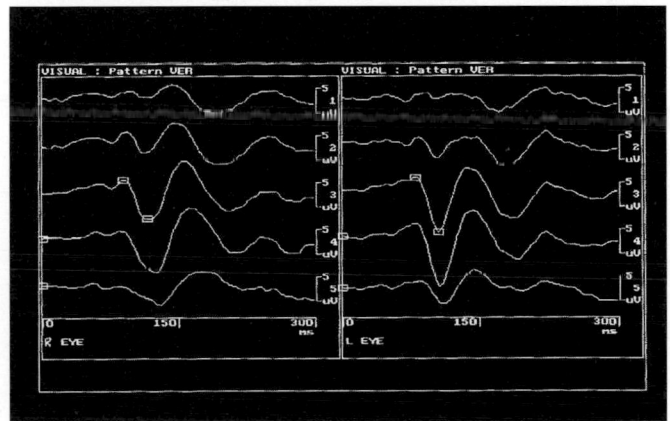

Fig. 2.14. Visual evoked response (VER) to full field pattern reversal stimulation, in a patient with multiple sclerosis, showing a delayed latency (115 ms) and a normal latency (105 ms) from the left and right eyes, respectively, and a larger amplitude from the right of the occiput (lower channels).

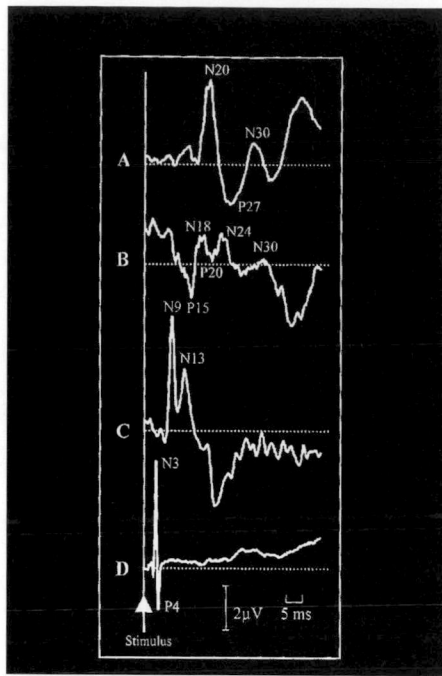

Fig. 2.15. Somatosensory evoked potential (SEP) from stimulation of the median nerve at the wrist, showing normal responses at the elbow (D), Erb's point (C), the neck (B), and scalp (A).

increase in latency of the main response (Halliday *et al.* 1976), although compression can produce focal conduction block with slowing of conduction in the visual system and spinal cord.

2.4.3 Somatosensory evoked potentials

The standard method for evoking somatosensory potentials is by suprathreshold electrical stimulation of the median or posterior tibial nerves recording over the spinal cord and sensory cortex at 20 ms and 40 ms (Fig 2.15). The somatosensory evoked potential (SEP) is reduced or absent in the acute phase of demyelinating myelopathy involving the dorsal part of the cord, and this abnormality often persists after clinical recovery. The frequency of abnormality is around 80 per cent for clinically definite multiple sclerosis but lower in less definite diagnostic categories (Small *et al.* 1978).

2.4.4 Brainstem auditory evoked potentials

Potentials of short latency (within 10 ms) can be obtained from scalp electrodes after auditory stimulation (Fig. 2.16). Of the five normal waves, I and II originate from the eighth nerve external to the brainstem, III from the cochlear nucleus, and IV and V from the region of the superior olivary complex (McPherson and Starr 1993). Demyelinating disease is characterized by an increase in latency between the first two and later waves (Robinson and Rudge 1977). The sensitivity in detecting involvement of brainstem pathways is marginally less than for visual or somatosensory systems in clinically definite (*c.* 50–75 per cent) and suspected (*c.* 25 per cent) multiple sclerosis (McPherson and Starr 1993) and end-organ failure is a more

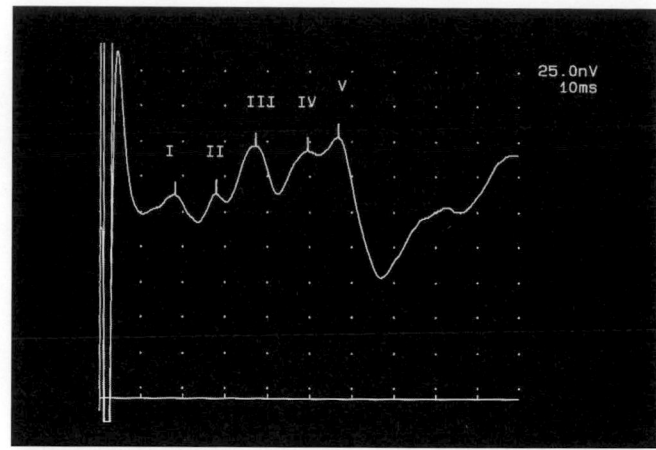

Fig. 2.16. Brainstem auditory evoked potential (BAEP) to stimulation of one ear, showing normal responses from the auditory nerve (I), the cochlear nucleus (II), the superior olive (III), lateral lemniscus (IV), and inferior colliculus (V).

common cause of alteration in the auditory evoked potential than in other afferent systems.

2.4.5 Central motor conduction

Motor evoked responses, following either electrical or magnetic stimulation, are somewhat variable, reflecting their passage through multiple synapses between cortex and peripheral limb muscle. Long delays (*c.* 20 ms) are more likely to result from demyelination than degeneration (Thompson *et al.* 1987)—although either may be present in patients with multiple sclerosis—and they have rather a low prevalence of asymptomatic abnormality.

2.4.6 Event-related potentials

Event-related potentials reflect the summation of cognitive processes, including attention, memory, language, and responses (see Heinze *et al.* 1999). Being complex, they do not easily define precise cognitive functions and so have a limited role in clinical neurology. The most accessible measurement is the p300, based on auditory stimulation; its latency extends to 700 ms when the visual system is stimulated. The p300 is considered to reflect evaluation more than response time and to depend on activity in several parts of the cerebrum. It is typically delayed in dementia, with a specificity of around 70 per cent but poor discrimination across the range of clinical conditions affecting intellectual function.

2.5 Nerve conduction studies and electromyography

Nerve conduction studies allow localization of compressive focal neuropathy and detection of polyneuropathy, with distinction between demyelinating, axonal degeneration and conduction block neuropathies. Electromyography detects denervation of muscle, helps to distinguish between myopathic and neuropathic weakness, and is diagnostic of myotonias and neuromyotonias (Section 15.1.3). Single-fibre electromyography and neuromuscular transmission studies are particularly important for diagnosing myasthenia gravis and the Lambert–Eaton myasthenic syndrome (Section 15.10).

2.5.1 Motor conduction studies

Maximal motor conduction velocity is measured by applying a supramaximal stimulus to a motor nerve at two or more different points along its course through bipolar electrodes applied to the skin over the trunk of the nerve (Fig. 2.17). The evoked compound muscle action potential from a muscle supplied by this nerve is recorded. Measurement of the latency from the stimulus to the initial rise of the compound muscle action potential, and of the distance between the pairs of stimulating electrodes, allows calculation of the conduction velocity in m/s along various segments of the nerve. In the case of the median nerve (Fig. 2.17) the interval between the stimulus applied at the wrist and the initial rise of the muscle action potential in the abductor pollicis brevis is known as the distal motor latency. Motor conduction velocities generally exceed 48 m/s in the arms and 40 m/s in the leg nerves. Distal motor latencies (DMLs) vary depending upon the particular nerve, the site of stimulation, and the technique employed; for the median nerve following stimulation at the wrist, the normal DML is less than 4.2 m/s but will be prolonged in carpal tunnel syndrome or demyelinating neuropathy. F-wave latencies, which reflect the time taken for the antidromic volley to depolarize the motor neuron cell bodies within the spinal cord, and then for the passage of the resultant action potential to travel orthodromically to the muscle, reflect conduction over proximal segments of the nerve and root, and the normal values are dependent upon height. Well-established methods are now available for studying motor conduction in the median, ulnar, and radial nerves in the arm, and in the common peroneal and posterior tibial

nerves in the leg, and the normal ranges for motor conduction parameters have been extensively documented (Liveson and Ma 1992; Binnie *et al.* 1995). Temperature has a profound effect upon nerve conduction, so the skin temperature of the limb should be maintained at 25–30 °C, if necessary by prior immersion in warm water or by a radiant heat lamp.

Blockage of impulse conduction is recognized increasingly as an important cause of weakness due to peripheral nerve disease. This conduction block usually reflects failure of action potential propagation through axons at sites of severe compression or through segments that are demyelinated. It is especially seen in acutely demyelinated nerves within the first few weeks before sodium channel redistribution to the denuded internodal segments of the axon allows resumption of conduction, albeit at slowed velocity. Recently it has been recognized

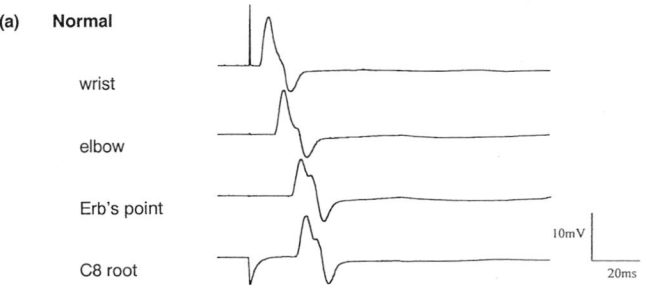

(a)   Normal

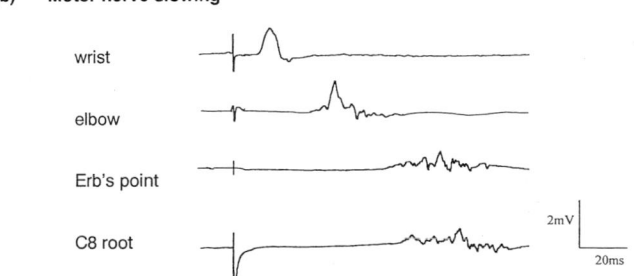

(b)   Motor nerve slowing

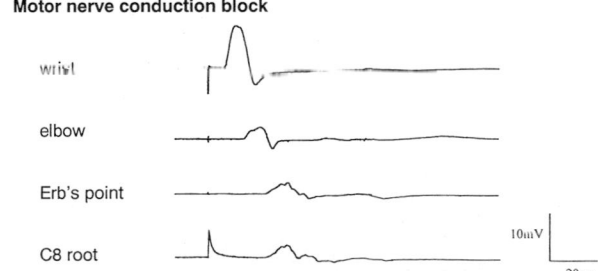

(c)   Motor nerve conduction block

Fig. 2.18. Abnormalities in motor conduction along the median nerve recorded with surface electrodes over abductor pollicis brevis. (a) Normal, showing constant amplitude compound muscle action potentials (CMAP) with normal latency. (b) Demyelinating neuropathy, showing slowing and dispersion of CMAPs. (c) Multifocal motor neuropathy with conduction block in the forearm segment, causing reduced CMAP amplitudes following stimulation at the elbow and above, but with preserved conduction velocity (courtesy of Dr M. Busby).

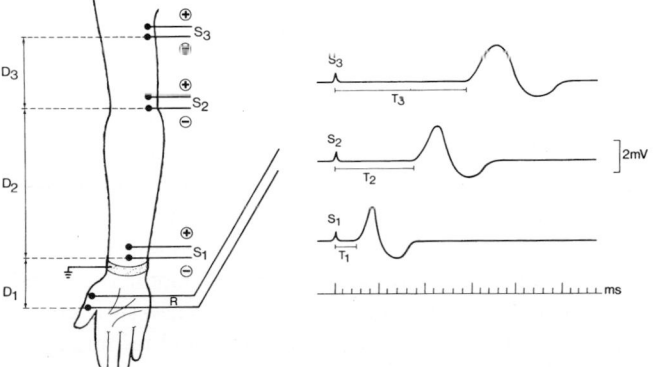

Fig. 2.17. Measuring motor conduction velocity along the median nerve: diagrammatic representation with stimulating electrodes (S_1, S_2, S_3) at various points along the course of the nerve and measurement of the compound muscle action potential using surface electrodes (R) over abductor pollicis brevis (reproduced from Bradley 1974).

that there are neuropathies in which conduction block appears to be the primary pathophysiological process. In such neuropathies, the block often occurs without sufficient associated conduction slowing to point to underlying demyelination; multifocal neuropathy with conduction block (Section 12.11.13) is an important example. Most frequently, conduction block is partial rather than total and it may be diffusely distributed along a length of nerve, rather than being tightly localized to a particular site. This has led to difficulty and dispute about the quantificative definition of conduction block. Partial conduction block leads to three electrophysiological abnormalities:

1. Reduced amplitude and area of the compound muscle action potential evoked by nerve stimulation at proximal sites compared to distal (Fig. 2.18); different authors quote degrees of reduction ranging from 20 to 60 per cent (Lewis and Sumner 1982; Cornblath *et al.* 1991).

2. Dispersion of the compound muscle action potential waveform; however, this abnormal temporal dispersion can lead to phase cancellation, resulting in the misleading appearance of amplitude reduction of the compound muscle action potential.

3. Absent or sparse F-wave responses if the conduction block affects proximal nerve segments or the nerve roots.

2.5.2 Sensory nerve action potentials

Sensory conduction in the median, ulnar, and radial nerves can be measured by applying stimuli through ring electrodes upon a finger (Fig. 2.19) and then recording the sensory nerve action potential through cutaneous electrodes applied over the trunk of the nerve (orthodromic conduction). For other nerves, such as the sural, the nerve trunk is stimulated and sensory nerve action potentials recorded from surface electrodes (antidromic or orthodromic conduction). The sensory nerve action potential (SNAP) is so small that averaging techniques are required

following multiple stimuli, and occasionally needle recording electrodes inserted close to the nerve are required (Kimura 1983; Liveson and Ma 1992; Binnie *et al.* 1995).

Sensory nerve action potential amplitudes generally range from 5 to 50 μV, depending upon the particular nerve being studied, and drop in amplitude, or absence of the potential, occurs in axonal degenerative, demyelinating, or compressive neuropathies. Thus a diminished SNAP cannot in itself distinguish between these types of neuropathy. Sensory nerve action potentials reflect the integrity of the distal axonal branch of the dorsal root ganglion sensory neurons. They remain normal in disease such as spondylitic radiculopathy affecting the spinal nerve roots containing the proximal axonal branches because the dorsal root ganglia cell bodies lie outside the intervertebral foramina (Aminoff *et al.* 1985). The only exception to this can occur in the lower lumbar and sacral nerve roots, in which the dorsal root ganglia can lie within the intervertebral foramina, and loss of sensory nerve action potentials may occur with spinal disease as well as with peripheral nerve disease. Radiculopathy may be confirmed by the finding of denervation within limb and paraspinal muscles innervated by the same segment. Sensory nerve conduction latencies and velocities can be measured but generally find little usefulness in diagnostic clinical practice. Routine techniques for measuring possible conduction block in sensory nerves have not been established.

2.5.3 Uses of nerve conduction studies

Nerve conduction studies are principally used to diagnose focal mononeuropathies, usually due to nerve compression, and to detect polyneuropathy and determine whether it is due to demyelination or axonal degeneration. The additional uses of detecting conduction block neuropathies (Section 2.5.1) and in discriminating nerve root disease from polyneuropathy (Section 2.5.2) are dealt with above.

Focal compressive neuropathy

Focal compressive neuropathy can be diagnosed electrophysiologically for most limb nerves and some truncal nerves. This is particularly useful for median nerve compression in the carpal tunnel and the ulnar nerve at the elbow. Conduction distal to a neurapraxial lesion of a peripheral nerve may remain normal at a time when its function is severely impaired. When a nerve is compressed, as in entrapment neuropathies, motor and sensory conduction across the site of the lesion may be either lost or greatly reduced in speed. This leads to reduction or loss of the sensory action potential in that nerve, and prolongation of the distal motor latency. Localized slowing of motor conduction can be demonstrated at some entrapment sites, such as compression of the ulnar nerve at the elbow, and techniques are now available for measuring conduction over short segments of nerve in presumed entrapment neuropathies (Liveson and Ma 1992). Electromyographic sampling of muscles supplied by a trapped nerve will show to what extent axonal degeneration has caused denervation. This generally implies a poorer prospect

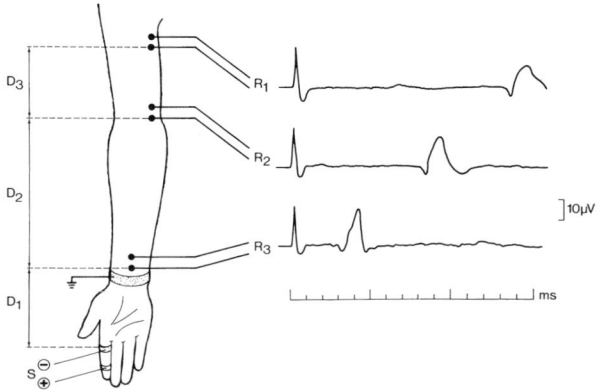

Fig. 2.19. Diagrammatic representation of the technique of measuring the sensory nerve action potential (SNAP) in the median nerve (at points R₁, R₂, R₃) after orthodromic stimulation of the finger(s) (reproduced from Bradley 1974).

for recovery of nerve function following surgical release of the compression.

Changes in the electromyogram (EMG), tactile sensibility, and nerve conduction after suture or compression of peripheral nerves in human subjects have been studied longitudinally (Buchthal and Kühl 1979). Enlargement of re-innervated motor units and marked dispersion of motor unit action potentials persisted long after suture. The sensory nerve action potential recovered five times as quickly, and tactile sensibility 10 times, after correction of a compressive lesion as after releasing a suture. After relief of compressive lesions, the maximum motor and sensory conduction velocity recovered to 80–90 per cent of normal within 1 year, but after nerve suture it had only reached 65–75 per cent of normal after 40 months.

Demyelinating polyneuropathies

Demyelinating polyneuropathies markedly slow conduction along affected nerve trunks. Sometimes difficulty can arise because reduced velocities are seen in profound axonal loss when there are no surviving fast-conducting fibres remaining to a grossly denervated muscle. If demyelination chiefly affects the proximal segments of motor fibres, it will be associated with normal conduction velocity measurements along distal segments. In this case, prolonged F-wave responses are a clue to proximal conduction slowing. Criteria have been proposed for defining a neuropathy as demyelinating in nature (Ad Hoc Subcommittee of American Academy of Neurology AIDS Task Force 1991). In outline these require three out of four of the following abnormalities, affecting two or more nerves:

(1) reduction of motor velocity to less than 80 per cent of the lower limit of normal (which represents <39 m/s for arm nerves and <34 m/s for leg nerves);

(2) partial conduction block of greater than 20 per cent, or abnormal temporal dispersion causing greater than 15 per cent change in duration not attributable to an entrapment neuropathy;

(3) prolonged distal motor latencies exceeding more than 125 per cent of the upper limit of normal;

(4) prolonged F-wave latencies greater than 125 per cent of the upper limit of normal.

Such stringent criteria, while useful in established disease, are not met early in the course of mild forms of chronic idiopathic demyelinating polyneuropathy. Furthermore, sometimes these criteria can only be satisfied by exhaustive electrophysiological study of numerous individual peripheral nerves. Most demyelinating neuropathies also involve sensory fibres, with reduced amplitude or absent sensory nerve action potentials.

Axonal degeneration polyneuropathies

Axonal degeneration polyneuropathies usually involve a dying back process which mainly affects the longest axons. The earliest evidence of axonal polyneuropathy is electromyographic evidence of denervation of foot and hand muscles, coupled with reduced amplitude or absence of sensory nerve action potentials in the feet and hands. The muscle denervation is evident on surface electromyography by reduction in the amplitude of compound muscle action potentials, which normally range from 10 to 25 mV in hand muscles. Concentric needle electrodes inserted into denervated muscle will reveal fibrillation potentials and positive sharp waves (Section 2.5.5). Early on, the motor conduction velocity in surviving axons will be normal, or only marginally reduced. However, as severe denervation sets in and the large-diameter axons are lost, the motor conduction velocity can fall markedly but rarely to less than 80 per cent of the lower limit of normal, and the distal motor latency can rise, but rarely above 125 per cent of the upper limit of normal (Cornblath et al. 1992). This means that primarily demyelinating polyneuropathies can be distinguished electrophysiologically from axonal degeneration. However, in practice, a number of polyneuropathies involve mixed elements of demyelination and axonal degeneration and sometimes evade confident clinical or electrophysiological classification into either category.

2.5.4 Age and nerve conduction

Infants and children

Infants and children show reduced nerve conduction velocity compared to adults. Motor conduction velocity in the newborn is approximately half of the adult speed and only reaches the adult range at 3–5 years of age (Ouvrier et al. 1990). Compound muscle action potential amplitudes also increase with age. Sensory nerve action potential amplitudes are normally less than half of adult values, which are attained by 3 years of age.

The elderly

The elderly show variable reduction in nerve conduction velocity and in median and sural sensory nerve action potential amplitudes during their seventh and eighth decades (Bouche et al. 1993). By 80 years of age, all patients will show reduction in these parameters and reduced compound muscle action potential amplitudes.

2.5.5 Electromyography

Routine electromyography (EMG) records the electrical activity of a muscle at rest, during minimal voluntary contraction, and during full contraction. Two techniques may be used. Surface electrodes may identify which muscle or muscle groups are participating in voluntary movement and allow quantification of the compound muscle action potential during motor conduction studies. But for diagnostic work it is necessary to insert a concentric needle electrode into the muscle so as to detect changes of acute and chronic denervation or myopathy (Binnie et al. 1995). The needle electrode records the activity of about 10 muscle fibres in a vicinity. The particular use of EMG to diagnose primary muscle disease is discussed in Section 15.1.5.

Modern electromyographic recording techniques allow easy quantification of parameters relating to motor unit wave form and duration. The amplitude and duration of motor unit potentials increases with age.

Normal muscle

Normal muscle at rest shows no electrical activity. On slight voluntary contraction motor unit potentials of 300–2000 μV in amplitude and 6–10 m/s in duration are recorded. These are usually monophasic, biphasic, or triphasic in shape, but 10–25 per cent of potentials recorded from normal muscle may be polyphasic. On vigorous voluntary muscular contraction an interference pattern develops. Since the patient recruits as many motor units as possible, and they fire asynchronously, each one interferes with the waveforms of ones that precede and follow it (Fig. 2.20

Denervated muscle

About 2 weeks after complete transection of a nerve, fibrillation potentials can be recorded from the resting muscle (Fig. 2.21).

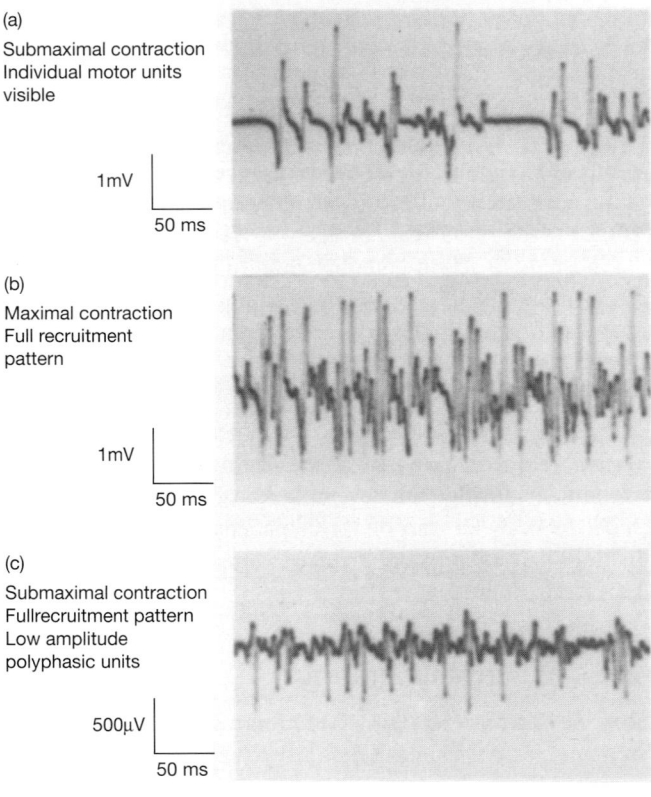

(a)
Submaximal contraction
Individual motor units visible

1mV

50 ms

(b)
Maximal contraction
Full recruitment pattern

1mV

50 ms

(c)
Submaximal contraction
Fullrecruitment pattern
Low amplitude
polyphasic units

500µV

50 ms

Fig. 2.20. The electromyogram (EMG) in normal muscle and in myopathy. (a) The normal electromyogram on submaximal contraction. Note that the individual motor units here vary between 1.5 and 3 mV in amplitude and are of approximately 6–7 ms duration. (b) During maximal contraction in the normal muscle there is a full interference pattern. The spikes of greater amplitude represent action potentials derived from motor units lying relatively close to the recording electrode, while those of lower amplitude are derived from motor units lying some distance away. (c) The electromyogram in myopathy. The constituent motor units are greatly reduced in amplitude and duration and many are polyphasic. (Courtesy of Dr R. Weiser.)

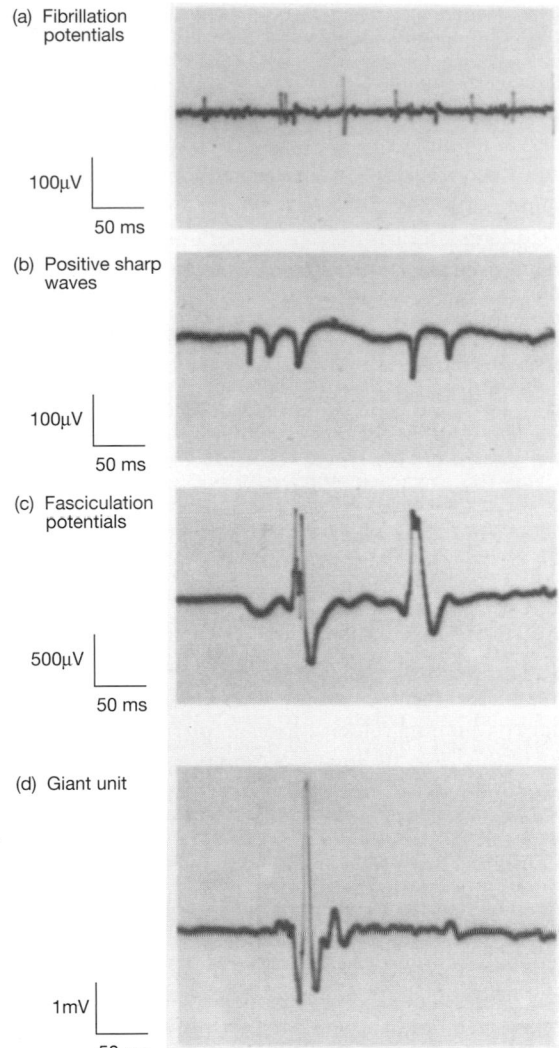

(a) Fibrillation
potentials

100µV

50 ms

(b) Positive sharp
waves

100µV

50 ms

(c) Fasciculation
potentials

500µV

50 ms

(d) Giant unit

1mV

50 ms

Fig. 2.21. The electromyogram in denervation. (a) Spontaneous fibrillation recorded from resting muscle; the individual potentials measure 100 μV or less in amplitude and about 1 ms duration. (b) Positive sharp waves (saw-tooth potentials) recorded from resting denervated muscle. (c) Fasciculation potentials firing spontaneously recorded from resting muscle in motor neuron disease; these potentials are morphologically indistinguishable from motor unit action potentials. (d) A giant motor unit action potential of approximately 5 mV in amplitude, occurring during volitional activity in a patient with motor neuron disease. (Courtesy of Dr R. Weiser.)

A fibrillation potential results from spontaneous contraction of a single muscle fibre, and is usually 50–100 μV in amplitude, 1–2 ms in duration, and monophasic or biphasic in shape. Total absence of motor unit potentials is evident on attempted voluntary contraction, whether the lesion is neurapraxial or due to neurotmesis or axonotmesis (Sections 13.2.4 and 13.2.5). However, in neurapraxia, fibrillation does not occur; hence if no fibrillation potentials appear 2 or 3 weeks after total paralysis of a muscle, the lesion is probably compressive without axonal transection. On the other hand, if fibrillation potentials are recorded, it does not necessarily mean that every motor axon has been severed. Another type of spontaneous activity sometimes recorded from resting denervated muscle is that of so-called positive sharp waves or 'saw-tooth' potentials. The EMG recorded from partially denervated muscle shows a mixture of positive sharp waves and fibrillation potentials, along with an interference pattern of reduced density. The EMG differs in acute and chronic denervation. If the denervating process is acute and active, fibrillations and positive sharp waves are prominent, but such activity may be absent or sparse if the denervation is very chronic or has become arrested. However, in cases of chronic denervation, fasciculation potentials may be recorded, occurring spontaneously and repetitively when the muscle is at rest. Fasciculation potentials are morphologically indistinguishable from motor unit action potentials. They often point to a lesion within the anterior horn cell. Fasciculation may also be a benign phenomenon (Section 14.1.3). In chronic denervating processes, surviving axons often produce collateral sprouts which re-innervate denervated muscle fibres. As a consequence, some surviving motor units become much larger than normal in both amplitude and duration. These 'giant motor units' are particularly common in muscles previously affected by acute poliomyelitis (Section 14.5.3).

Myopathic muscle

Spontaneous fibrillation and fasciculations are less commonly seen in primary muscle diseases, but fasciculations can be seen in thyrotoxic and hypoparathyroid myopathies. In some cases of myopathy, especially polymyositis, fibrillation potentials do occur because the disease process may affect intramuscular nerve endings, or focal necrosis of part of a muscle fibre may separate the remainder of the fibre from its motor end-plate. On slight voluntary contraction the duration and amplitude of the motor unit potentials is diminished, and many are broken up or polyphasic because the content of normal muscle fibres within a motor unit is reduced (Fig. 2.20). On maximal contraction, the same number fire: complex polyphasic motor unit action potentials (MUAPs) of prolonged duration can fill the oscilloscope interference pattern at very low forces, but usually maximum voluntary contraction produces a complete interference pattern but low tension.

Myotonias

Myotonias cause high-frequency discharges of single muscle fibres. These are provoked by movement of the exploring needle within the muscle and produce a typical recurring 'dive-bomber' sound in the loudspeaker. Myotonic discharges start at a crescendo, and then fade gradually. They must be distinguished from other bizarre 'pseudomyotonic' high-frequency discharges which begin and end abruptly and give a more constant sound; these occur in disorders as diverse as motor neuron disease, polyneuropathy, muscular dystrophy, and many metabolic myopathies, and they lack diagnostic specificity, unlike true myotonic discharges. Neuromyotonia causes motor units to fire spontaneously and irregularly as doublets, triplets, or multiplets with high intraburst frequencies of up to 120 Hz (Section 14.9).

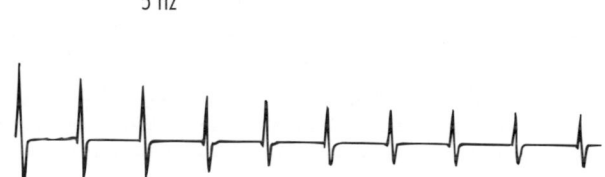

5 Hz

Fig. 2.22. Progressive decline in size of the compound muscle action potential amplitude with repetitive stimulation in myasthenia gravis (from Donaghy 1997).

Repetitive stimulation

Normally the amplitude of the compound muscle action potential evoked by nerve stimulation remains relatively constant on repetitive stimulation. In myasthenia gravis the initially normal muscle potential steadily diminishes for the first four or five stimuli delivered to the nerve at 3–5/second (Fig. 2.22). In Lambert–Eaton myasthenic syndrome the muscle potential is initially small, but progressively enlarges at tetanic rates of nerve stimulation between 20 and 50/second.

2.5.6 Single-fibre electromyography

The technique of single-fibre electromyography employs a specially constructed electrode for simultaneously recording from a number of individual muscle fibres within the motor unit supplied by a single motor neuron. Normally these adjacent muscle fibres will fire in a close temporal relationship to one another; if this interval varies it is known as jitter. Blocking is the phenomenon when one of the muscle fibre potentials fails to fire during muscular contraction. Jitter and blocking generally indicate a failure of neuromuscular transmission at the motor end-plate and occur particularly in myasthenia gravis, but also, to a lesser extent, in neuropathies and motor neuron disease.

2.6 Cerebrospinal fluid

2.6.1 Introduction

Quinke introduced the technique of diagnostic spinal puncture in 1891 and by the turn of the century it was in widespread clinical usage. For many decades it was one of the few investigative techniques available to neurologists and few patients escaped in-patient admission without encountering its ritual. Later, the development of myelography gave another reason for spinal puncture, and until the advent of MRI many patients (e.g. with a paraparesis and a differential diagnosis of multiple sclerosis or a structural lesion affecting the spinal cord) underwent the process of lumbar puncture with cerebrospinal fluid (CSF) removal, followed by instillation of contrast medium. Arguably, MRI has removed the need for CSF examination in certain instances, including multiple sclerosis.

CSF is most frequently obtained by lumbar puncture, because that is the easiest and safest site for dural puncture, and that is the only technique that will be discussed in any detail in this section. Alternative techniques exist and may be required in a few rare specific circumstances. CSF can be obtained from the cisterna magna (cisternal puncture) or cervical spine (lateral cervical puncture), but it needs little imagination to appreciate the potential hazards, particularly in inexperienced hands. A previous indication was the need to introduce contrast medium for myelography to determine the upper level of a spinal block, but MRI has removed that need. Occasionally CSF examination may be required in a patient in whom the lumbar approach is impossible or contraindicated (e.g. local sepsis, previous spinal surgery, obesity, arachnoiditis, severe spinal disease).

2.6.2 Cerebrospinal fluid

The CSF is secreted by the choroids plexuses of the ventricles. Flow is caudal, through the fourth ventricle, and out through the foramina of Luschka and Magendie into the subarachnoid space, which covers the entire surface of the brain and spinal cord. The subarachnoid space is contained by the pia mater over the brain and spinal cord and, externally, by the arachnoid membrane. The subarachnoid space is bridged by numerous trabeculae and by blood vessels and nerves, and the surfaces of all of these structures are covered by mesothelial cells. The blood vessels entering the brain and cord carry an extension of the arachnoid and pia mater, forming the Virchow–Robin spaces.

The brain and spinal cord are bathed in CSF. The fluid flows upwards, over the hemispheres, to be absorbed into the venous sinuses through the arachnoid villi. The total CSF volume is about 120 ml. CSF is produced at the rate of about 0.35 ml/minute, indicating a turnover of the total volume several times a day.

A major function of the CSF is to provide physical support for the brain. A clinical indication of this function is provided by the headache that develops, due to stretching of pain-sensitive structures by the sagging brain, when the CSF volume is reduced, for example following lumbar puncture. The CSF also acts as a dumping ground for cerebral metabolites, although overall their clearance under normal circumstances is probably mainly through the transcapillary route and the venous outflow from the brain. There is also some evidence that CSF may act as an intracerebral transporter, carrying neuro-active substances, such as hormones and releasing factors, from one part of the brain to another.

Although lists are often published of the numerous constituents of the CSF, and their normal concentrations, only very few are assayed in routine clinical practice. These are discussed below.

2.6.3 Indications for spinal puncture

Broadly speaking, spinal (usually lumbar, as noted above) puncture is performed for either diagnostic or therapeutic purposes (Table 2.3).

Air encephalography is now redundant, and myelography has largely been replaced by MRI. Spinal anaesthesia is not important in the present discussion. Thus, the main indications for dural puncture are either related to pressure measuring or manipulation, or to the need to obtain CSF for diagnostic purposes.

Although the CSF pressure is raised in numerous pathologies, the only indications to perform dural puncture specifically in order to measure the pressure are suspected benign intracranial hypertension and some cases of communicating hydrocephalus. Indeed, in most other causes of raised pressure, such as tumour or haemorrhage, lumbar puncture is contraindicated. Dural puncture, with removal of a relatively large quantity of CSF, is an important therapeutic manoeuvre in benign intracranial hypertension.

By far and away the most frequent indication for lumbar puncture (LP) is the need to obtain CSF for diagnostic purposes. Broadly speaking, LP may be performed in the emergency or (relatively) non-emergency situation (Table 2.4).

2.6.4 Contraindications to spinal puncture

There are several contraindications to lumbar puncture, some absolute, some relative (Table 2.5). By far and away the most

Table 2.3. General indications for spinal puncture

Diagnostic
CSF examination
CSF pressure measurement
Instillation of radiological contrast media
Therapeutic
Reduction of CSF pressure
Instillation of drugs and contrast media
Spinal anaesthesia

Table 2.4. Diagnostic indications for lumbar puncture

Emergency
Suspected infection
Meningitis (viral, bacterial, fungal)
Encephalitis
Suspected subarachnoid haemorrhage
Unexplained confusional state
Non-emergency
Multiple sclerosis
Malignancy
Carcinomatous meningitis
Lymphoma
Sarcoidosis
Demyelinating polyneuropathy
Infection (syphilis, chronic fungal)
CNS vasculitis
Benign intracranial hypertension

Table 2.5. Contraindications to lumbar puncture

Raised CSF pressure due to an intracranial mass lesion

Local lumbar skin sepsis

Warfarin or heparin therapy

Coagulation defect

Spinal block

dangerous situation is the presence of raised intracranial pressure due to a mass lesion. There is considerable risk of tentorial or cerebellar herniation, which may be fatal. Broadly speaking, the presence of lateralizing abnormal physical signs is a contraindication to LP, at least until CT or MRI has excluded a mass lesion causing shift or distortion. The symptoms and signs associated with a spinal canal block may also be exacerbated by the shift caused by removal of CSF from below the block. Local skin sepsis is a contraindication, although in practice it is vanishingly rare for LP to give rise to secondary CSF infection, even in the presence of septicaemia. Any disorder of coagulation increases the risk of local haemorrhage.

2.6.5 **Lumbar puncture**

To learn how to perform a lumbar puncture well, watch an expert (not once but several times) and then practise the procedure under expert supervision. There are two types of 'traumatic tap'. The presence of blood in the CSF is discussed below. The other describes emotional and physical trauma to the patient who goes off and tells her friends of the 'lumbar punch' and vows never to let a doctor with a needle near her again! With appropriate clinical skills, this situation should never arise.

Method

One can only learn properly by watching, not by reading a detailed, turgid, account of the method—no surgeon should embark on his first operation of a type having only read about it! The following points note some of the more common questions, errors, and problems.

Position

The standard position is the left lateral decubitus—because it is the best position. It is sometimes suggested that if difficulties are encountered, then puncture is easier with the patient sitting-up. If that were truly the case, then why are not most LPs done in this position? If a tyro has failed in the lateral position, that he has at least attempted a few times before, then the chance of success in a position he has never previously attempted is probably even less.

Posture

The patient lies with his or her left shoulder, trunk, and hip lying along the near-edge of the bed/couch. The spine, hips, and knees should be flexed as much as is comfortable for the patient—having an assistant forcibly flexing the patient is unnecessary and will only contribute to the patient's trauma. The spine should be horizontal and not twisted—twisting is avoided by placing a pillow between the patient's knees and making certain that the upper, right shoulder remains directly above the lower, left shoulder. Failure to get the patient in the correct position is the major reason for failure of the procedure.

Level

A line drawn between the anterior superior iliac spines runs through the level of the L3 vertebra. In adults, the LP should be performed between either L2 and L3, or L3 and L4. In children, the spinal cord terminates lower, and LP should be performed at L3/4 or L4/5.

Local anaesthesia

It is arguable whether local anaesthesia is necessary. Only the skin and immediate subcutaneous tissues appear to contribute significant discomfort—it may well be that the discomfort of local anaesthetic infiltration is as great as would be experience by simply inserting the spinal needle (which is of similar or smaller calibre). If local anaesthesia is used, then only the superficial tissues should be infiltrated, and the volume required is no more than 0.5 ml (lignocaine, 1 or 2 per cent). Using larger volumes causes such swelling that it becomes impossible to feel the essential landmarks (the tips of the spinous processes).

Needle size

As noted below, there is a clear correlation between needle size and the incidence of post-LP headache. A 26G needle gives rise to a very low incidence of headache, but its very narrow calibre and lack of rigidity lead to several problems:

(1) insertion, without using a larger-diameter short needle to act as a guide, is difficult, particularly for the inexperienced operator;

(2) removal of reasonable quantities of CSF may take a considerable time; and

(3) pressure measurements, particularly 'dynamic' measurements, are difficult because of the slow flow.

In practice, a 26G needle is used by anaesthetists and radiologists for instilling drugs and contrast media, but for diagnostic purposes a 21- or 22G needle is used. The needle should be inserted with the bevel horizontal, as there is evidence that this reduces the incidence of post-LP headache (the theory being that this parts rather than severs the longitudinally running fibres of the dura mater).

The 'careful' LP

It is sometimes suggested that LP may be safer if only a small quantity of CSF is removed, for example in situations of raised intracranial pressure. Nonsense! Probably in most cases much more CSF leaks out from the dural hole after the procedure than is ever removed by the operator.

Pressure measurement

As noted above, there are only a few specific indications for pressure measurement, which is achieved using a simple manometer. Indeed, in many situations (such as obtaining CSF for protein studies in suspected multiple sclerosis), measuring the pressure is not only unnecessary but the fiddling around with the needle and apparatus increase the chance of getting blood and other contaminants (e.g. talc from the gloves) into the CSF, invalidating further studies.

CSF collection

The requisite amount of fluid should be collected in the appropriate tubes. Err on the side of generosity, particularly for cytological studies. If the initial sample is bloodstained, collect three or more subsequent specimens in separate tubes (see below).

Bedrest

There is no evidence that bedrest (whether with the patient lying prone or supine, or with one end of the bed elevated) reduces the incidence of post-LP headache. Bedrest for 24 hours simply delays the onset of headache by the same period. Therefore, unless there are other indications, there is no reason to confine the patient to bed.

Traumatic tap

This term, in its medical sense (see above), means that blood was introduced into the CSF during the procedure, and its major implication is the confusion that it causes in identifying pre-existing subarachnoid haemorrhage. It also interferes with protein electrophoresis studies. Contrary to popular belief, a traumatic tap is not primarily due to technical difficulties or clumsiness on the part of the operator, although these might slightly increase its occurrence, but rather to penetration of one of the numerous veins in the region. It occurs in about 1 in 10 punctures and is not necessarily anything to be ashamed about.

The traditional method of distinguishing traumatic tap, which although not foolproof is still reasonably reliable, is to collect three sequential samples of about 3 ml each and to note by visual inspection, backed up by laboratory red cell counts, that the blood clears. In pre-existing subarachnoid haemorrhage the red cell count in each sample will be the same. Equally important, on obtaining bloodstained CSF, is to centrifuge the sample and observe the supernatant—with a traumatic tap it will be clear, with previous subarachnoid haemorrhage, as long as a reasonable time interval has elapsed (e.g. 8 hours), it will be xanthochromic. Further confirmation, and detection of blood breakdown products of insufficient concentration to render the sample visibly xanthochromic, can be obtained by spectrophotometric analysis.

Complications

The most serious complication, which should generally be avoided by not performing LP on inappropriate patients in the first place, is cerebral or cerebellar herniation. Otherwise, serious complications of LP are very rare.

Following diagnostic LP, somewhere between one-quarter and one-third of patients develop headache, but in only a small proportion of these is it severe. There are several risk factors to the development of haemorrhage, but needle size is the most important (see above). The cause of headache is CSF hypotension consequent upon continued CSF leakage through the hole left by the needle. If the headache does not settle with rest and simple analgesics, then almost immediate relief can be obtained by injecting 10 ml of the patient's blood into the epidural space at the level of the previous puncture ('blood patch'). Complications of this procedure include back and radicular (i.e. like sciatica) pain (which occur in up to one-third) and, because of these, blood patching cannot be recommended as a routine, prophylactic procedure.

Post-LP headache has a number of very specific characteristics that allow it to be distinguished from other non-specific headaches, and these should generally be present before considering blood patching. The most important feature is its postural dependence—it is exacerbated by sitting-up and standing, and typically resolves rapidly on lying. It is often throbbing in character, and may be associated with neck pain and stiffness.

Another complication of persistent low pressure is the formation of subdural fluid collections, typically below the tentorium cerebelli. This may occur following diagnostic LP but is also seen in cases of spontaneous CSF hypotension due to dural tears and fistulae.

Rarely, and usually accompanied by significant post-LP headache, there may be symptoms and signs of cranial nerve dysfunction, including dizziness, tinnitus, deafness, and diplopia (due to a VIth nerve lesion).

Local haemorrhage at the site of puncture is really only seen in patients with disordered clotting. If severe it can lead to paraplegia.

2.6.6 CSF pressure

The opening CSF pressure is measured with a simple manometer. In the conventional position, with the patient in the left lateral decubitus position, the normal CSF pressure is in the range 70–180 mm of CSF. As noted, the pressure needs to be measured in only a few clinical situations. One of these is suspected benign intracranial hypertension. This is most common in obese females, and, importantly, obesity is a major cause of a 'false-positive' result. In an otherwise normal obese person, the act of flexing the spine and lower limbs creates pressure on the abdomen, which in turn increases the CSF pressure, up to as much as 300–400 mm CSF. This may be taken to confirm a diagnosis of benign intracranial hypertension in a patient with the not uncommon combination of obesity and tension-type headache. In this situation, asking the patient to relax by slightly extending their hips and taking the pressure off their abdomen leads to an immediate fall of the CSF pressure.

Measurement of the closing pressure, after CSF sampling and just before removal of the needle, is often performed in patients with benign intracranial hypertension, to determine the effect of CSF extraction. It is of dubious validity, given that CSF will continue to leak through the dural hole for some time after the procedure.

2.6.7 CSF analysis

The specific findings in individual disorders are discussed throughout the text. In routine clinical practice assessment is generally limited to following areas listed below and summarized in Table 2.6

Appearance

Normal CSF is often described as being 'gin-clear'—vodka or clean water would be equally descriptive, as would 'crystal-clear'! Purulent CSF in bacterial meningitis is cloudy or turbid, and green-tinged if gross. Following subarachnoid haemorrhage the supernatant following centrifugation of the blood-stained CSF is xanthochromic (yellow) due to haemoglobin breakdown products, although this may not be evident to the naked eye until up to 12 hours after the initial haemorrhage. The value of spectrophotometry is discussed above and elsewhere. After several days the CSF will remain xanthochromic, but the red cells will have disappeared. A high protein level also causes xanthochromia. A markedly xanthochromic CSF with a protein content of less than 1.5 g/l is almost always secondary to

Table 2.6. Common CSF analyses

Appearance
  Naked eye
  Spectrophotometric
Proteins
  Total protein content
  Albumin and globulin
  Immunoglobulin assay
  Isoelectric focusing
Cells
  Lymphocyte and polymorphonuclear cell count
  Identification of other cell types, including malignant cells
  Cell-typing in certain malignancies
Microbiology
  Stains (Gram, Ziehl–Neelsen, Indian ink, etc.)
  Polysaccharide countercurrent electrophoresis (CIE)
  Polymerase chain reaction (PCR)
  Fungal antigens
Biochemistry
  Glucose
  Lactate and pyruvate assay
  Angiotensin-converting enzyme (ACE)

previous haemorrhage. The CSF may also appear discoloured in severe jaundice, with dietary hypercarotenaemia, and in the presence of certain drugs (e.g. rifampicin).

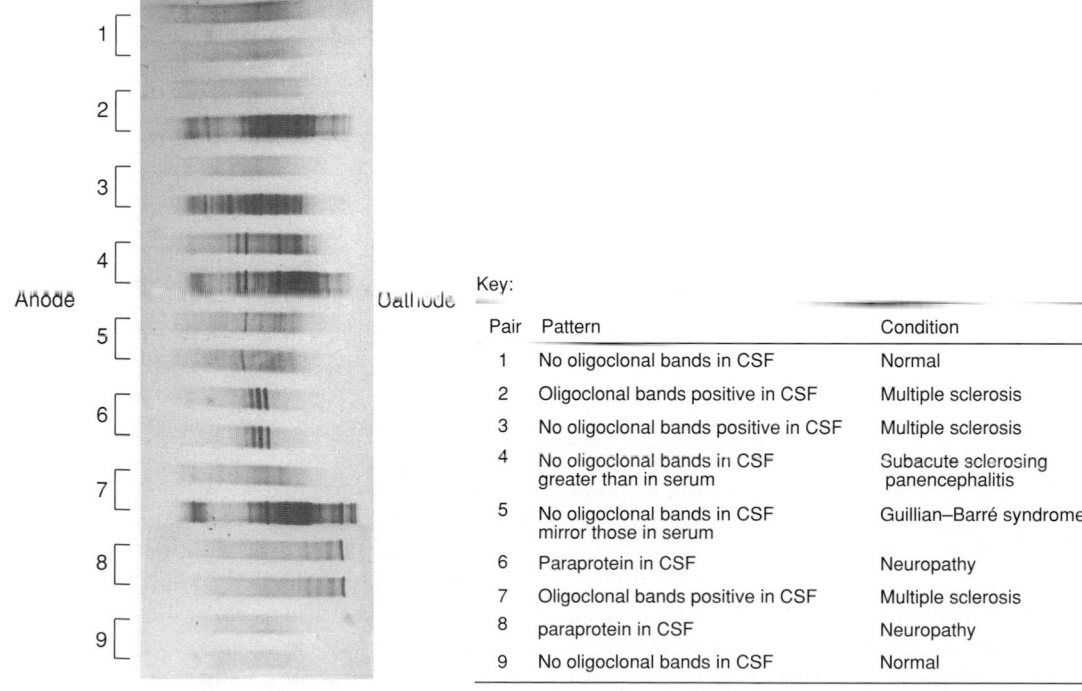

Key:

Pair	Pattern	Condition
1	No oligoclonal bands in CSF	Normal
2	Oligoclonal bands positive in CSF	Multiple sclerosis
3	No oligoclonal bands positive in CSF	Multiple sclerosis
4	No oligoclonal bands in CSF greater than in serum	Subacute sclerosing panencephalitis
5	No oligoclonal bands in CSF mirror those in serum	Guillian–Barré syndrome
6	Paraprotein in CSF	Neuropathy
7	Oligoclonal bands positive in CSF	Multiple sclerosis
8	paraprotein in CSF	Neuropathy
9	No oligoclonal bands in CSF	Normal

Fig. 2.23. CSF isoelectric focusing. The figure shows nine pairs (upper, serum; lower, CSF) illustrating typical banding patterns on isoelectric focusing (courtesy of Professor E. J. Thompson).

Proteins

The normal total protein content of lumbar CSF is in the range 0.1–0.5 g/l. The quoted range varies slightly between laboratories and it is impossible to state an absolute upper limit of normal. Protein levels are lower in ventricular and cisternal CSF.

The total CSF protein is elevated in many disorders and therefore changes lack specificity. The highest levels, sometimes exceeding 10 g/l, are seen in purulent meningitis, tuberculous meningitis, tumour (particularly causing spinal block), and arachnoiditis. When the protein level is very high, clots may form.

Quantitative and qualitative assessments of CSF immunoglobulins have achieved importance in providing laboratory support for the diagnosis of multiple sclerosis, and are discussed in detail in the relevant section. Paramount has been the technique of CSF isoelectric focusing (Fig. 2.23).

Cells

Normal CSF contains fewer than 5 lymphocytes/mm³, and no other cell type. The cell count is elevated in many conditions. In multiple sclerosis the count rarely exceeds 100, and contains predominantly lymphocytes. Moderately elevated counts (several hundred) are seen in viral meningitis—typically lymphocytes predominate, but polymorphonuclear cells may be the dominant cell type in early stages. Very high counts (thousands) are seen in bacterial meningitis, with polymorphonuclear cells predominating, except that in the earliest stages the cell count may be low and lymphocytes predominate—misdiagnosis of a viral process may be made. In tuberculous meningitis polymorphonuclear cells may predominate in the early stages, but later lymphocytes gain the ascendancy and typically number up to 500/mm³. The findings in fungal meningitis are similar to those of tuberculous meningitis.

In the search for malignant cells, CSF sampling may have to be repeated several times before a positive result is obtained. Yield is also increased by taking larger quantities of CSF.

Microbiology

The importance of cell type and count in differentiating different causes of infection is noted above. Specific diagnosis is achieved through one or more of the microbiological methods listed in Table 2.6. In partially treated meningitis (i.e. patient already given an antibiotic), immunoelectrophoretic methods may be valuable. Antigen studies are also particularly useful in fungal meningitides. Polymerase chain reaction studies remain an ancillary rather than first-line diagnostic test, and are most useful in viral encephalitides.

Biochemistry

The only frequent biochemical estimation, apart from protein, is glucose. It should be measured in cases of suspected infection or of carcinomatous meningitis. This has to be compared with a simultaneous blood glucose level. The CSF : blood glucose ratio is typically about 2 : 3. The ratio falls in the presence of hyperglycaemia (e.g. diabetes mellitus). Ratios between 1 : 3 and 2 : 3 may be normal, values below 1 : 3 are invariably abnormal. CSF glucose levels are usually very low in cases of purulent meningitis.

CSF, and indeed serum, lactate estimation is an ancillary investigation in cases of suspected mitochondrial cytopathy. Levels are elevated, as is the lactate : pyruvate ratio, but in general other, more specific, investigations are more likely to lead to the correct diagnosis.

2.7 Neuropsychology

2.7.1 General principles

Cognitive assessment is an important component of the neurological examination; it is essential for accurate assessment of disorders of the cerebral cortex (Hodges 1994). Classically, identification of the pattern of cognitive impairment has led to a topographical diagnosis, identifying which areas of cerebral cortex are involved. Although the recognition of specific topographical syndromes remains important (Section 26.2), the advent of non-invasive imaging has shifted the emphasis towards diagnosis of the underlying disease process, understanding of the cognitive deficits in functional terms, and measurement of change in cognitive performance.

Neuropsychological tests have become increasingly sophisticated as our understanding of brain function in modular terms has advanced (McCarthy and Warrington 1990). Any test of clinical value will need to be valid. Thus it should measure what is intended, and needs to produce similar results reliably in comparable circumstances. Any test should be of graded difficulty to avoid ceiling effects, particularly important in subtle disease. Ideally, tests should be of comparative difficulty across different domains. It is important to ensure that a pattern of deficit reflects the underlying disease process and not the pattern of difficulty of the tests used. It follows that interpretation of performance on a neuropsychological test requires knowledge of how a control population of comparable age, education, and gender to the patient (normative data) would perform. The neuropsychological tests used in clinical practice vary in the extent to which they meet these requirements.

With an appropriate battery of tests it is possible to identify patterns of deficit which can be diagnostically useful. For example, in the diagnosis of frontotemporal degeneration or Alzheimer's disease, it is possible to tell whether impairment, for example in memory, is outside normal limits and thus indicative of Alzheimer's disease as opposed to normal ageing or depression. Identification of an inconsistent pattern of performance may distinguish the patient with a psychologically generated abnormal illness behaviour (Section 26.10). Measurement of change is also essential for identifying deterioration, which may trigger an intervention, or for measuring the success of such an intervention. Finally, an understanding of the nature of the deficit, for example visual disorientation or dynamic aphasia, may assist in the management of the deficit and an explanation of the deficit for the patient and family (Cipolotti and Warrington 1995).

An adequate neuropsychological assessment should include an assessment of:

(1) general intelligence and pre-morbid ability;

(2) memory;

(3) language and calculation;

(4) visuoperceptual and visuospatial function;

(5) problem solving and executive functions;

(6) speed and attention.

Although a number of tests may be administered by neurologists or psychiatrists with appropriate training, a comprehensive assessment will be carried out by a qualified clinical psychologist. Routine administration of tests and uncritical acceptance of the resulting numerical data may lead to erroneous conclusions. The choice and interpretation of tests must be made within the overall clinical context, and therein lies the contribution of a skilled clinical psychologist. An adequate assessment is unlikely to take less than an hour, and may take much longer, depending upon which additional tests are chosen to explore particular deficits, and on the stamina of the patient. Some patients find assessments stressful and, indeed, may have a catastrophic reaction to failure. This is important to recognize and thus avoid overinterpretation of poor performance; reassessment the following day may be necessary.

In summary, neuropsychological assessment is now a major part of the neurological investigative armamentarium. It has taken the qualitative pattern recognition of classical behavioural neurology to the quantitative assessment of rigorous science. However, like all investigations, the information derived must be interpreted in the light of the clinical picture.

2.7.2 General intelligence and pre-morbid ability

The Wechsler Adult Intelligence Scale (WAIS) is a cornerstone of the neuropsychological assessment and involves six verbal and five non-verbal subtests exploring various skills. The revised test (WAIS-R) is now the standard test, with normative data available for the elderly (Ryan *et al.* 1990). Other widely used tests of intelligence are the Raven's tests of coloured progressive matrices, the standard progressive matrices, and advanced progressive matrices.

In order to assess deterioration in a patient at first presentation, some impression of pre-morbid intelligence needs to be formed. Pre-morbid test results would be available only rarely, although some indication may be given by educational attainment and occupation. An additional approach derives from the observation that patients with a variety of disorders, but particularly degenerative diseases such as Alzheimer's disease, have relative preservation of verbal skills and, in particular, reading. Moreover, such skills have an overall association with intelligence in the normal population. Thus, the National Adult Reading Test (NART) assesses ability to read and pronounce correctly 50 irregular words (Nelson and O'Connell 1978). Clearly, such a test is of limited use if lexical skills are selectively involved in a focal degenerative condition.

2.7.3 Memory

Impairment of memory is widely used to refer to failure to remember day-to-day events, or to remember to do something in the future. Although this is a salient feature in clinical practice, memory is now seen to be multidimensional, with discrete components which may be selectively involved in a disease process. A distinction is made between short-term memory, i.e. limited capacity with a short duration of about 30 seconds, and long-term memory. Both short- and long-term memory may also be divided on the basis of whether visual or verbal information is being retained. Short-term verbal memory is routinely tested with the digit span.

Long-term memory may be divided into episodic memory and semantic memory. Episodic memory deals with day-to-day events and provides the basis of our autobiographical memory. By contrast, semantic memory deals with our lifetime acquisition of knowledge. Semantic memory is usually explored in language tests. Episodic memory is assessed with either recall or recognition test paradigms. Examples of the former would be a story recall or the Rey–Osterreith figure for the verbal and visual domains respectively. An example of recognition memory tests would be the recognition tests for words and faces (Warrington 1984), which provide tests of comparable difficulty, such that patterns of deficit can reflect the left–right hemisphere asymmetry in verbal and visual processing of information.

2.7.4 Language, literacy skills, and calculation

A variety of tests have been developed to explore the main linguistic components for spoken language, namely phonology, syntax, and semantics. A number of aphasia batteries have been developed, such as the Boston Diagnostic Aphasia Examination, and are widely used. However, none of these batteries necessarily explores in depth all the domains of language that recent cognitive psychology has delineated. Written, as opposed to spoken language, can be explored by tests such as the NART (see above) and the Schonell Graded Reading Test. There are similar graded tests for spelling and for calculation.

2.7.5 Visuoperceptual and visuospatial function

Bedside cognitive tests by clinicians will often identify major patterns of memory, language, and frontal dysexecutive failure. Visuoperceptual and visuospatial failure are less easily identified and need to be specifically explored. A variety of tests have been developed which explore visuoperceptual function from early visual processing, such as shape detection, point localization and colour discrimination, through to the ability to form a complex visual percept. Such patients have difficulty with degraded visual stimuli or unusual as opposed to canonical views of common objects.

2.7.6 Frontal executive skills

Frontal-lobe deficits have proved difficult to measure reliably. Frontal-lobe behaviour may be only too apparent to the clinician but when tested formally, the patient may perform surprisingly well on a whole range of tests. Even tests that are sensitive to frontal-lobe function may provide variable scores over time, and patients may fail on one particular test but pass well on others. Tests believed to be sensitive to frontal-lobe function include cognitive estimates, verbal fluency, Stroop tests, and the Hayling sentence completion test. Quantitative tests of frontal-lobe function have proved difficult in the same way that the reliable measurement of praxis has been elusive. Bedside qualitative, as opposed to quantitative, assessments of dyspraxia and frontal-lobe function remain an important contribution of the clinical neurologist.

2.8 Neurogenetics

2.8.1 Patterns of inheritance

Although the impact of molecular genetics in neurology has been considerable, both in terms of clarifying mechanisms of disease and the development of diagnostic tests, it remains vital that the clinician knows about the main patterns of inheritance at a clinical level. When considering autosomal inheritance, it is the observed phenotypic expression of a gene that is dominant or recessive rather than the gene itself. In other words, pathological phenotypes are dominant or recessive characteristics of mutant genes and produce corresponding patterns of inheritance within families. The recognition of patterns of inheritance can be difficult when environmental factors are important or when the family history is incomplete. A common problem is the conclusion that a patient's family history is 'negative' when it is in fact unreliable and limited. For example, there may be little or no information about the state of health of relatives who died prematurely or lost contact with the patient years previously. This is common, for example, in families with Huntington's disease.

Terminology in genetics can be confusing; when describing individuals within families, the *proband* (or *index case*) is the individual by which the family was detected (ascertained) and affected relatives are referred to as *secondary cases*. Nearly all somatic cells contain two copies of autosomal genes and the two versions of a given gene are referred to as *alleles*; thus an individual may be a *homozygote* with two mutant alleles or a *heterozygote* with one mutant and one normal allele; individuals with two different mutant alleles are termed *compound*

heterozygotes. The *segregation ratio* of a hereditary disorder is the proportion of clinically affected individuals within a generation. This is difficult to observe in single families due to the effects of chance and small numbers of children. Segregation ratios usually need to be calculated from observations of many families.

Autosomal dominant inheritance

In autosomal dominant inheritance, the effect of the mutant gene is evident in heterozygotes. Homozygotes are only occasionally encountered, due to the rarity of the abnormal gene, but they may be either more severely affected than heterozygotes or clinically indistinguishable (as in Huntington's disease). The pattern of transmission of an autosomal dominant condition within a family is vertical (generation to generation) and the risk of the disorder appearing in a child born to an affected individual is 1 in 2. Overall, the segregation ratio among siblings, children, and parents of those affected is 0.5 (50 per cent). Both sexes are affected and either sex can transmit the condition to children. This classical pattern of autosomal dominant inheritance is not always obvious. *Sporadic cases* may arise due to new *mutation* within a family; the proportion of cases of an autosomal dominant disorder arising by fresh mutation is higher if it reduces the ability of affected individuals to reproduce. Therefore, an autosomal dominant disease which is lethal before reproductive age or confers a reproductive disadvantage for any reason is unlikely to be transmitted to children and most, if not all cases, will therefore arise sporadically because of the constant background rate of mutation of the relevant gene within the population. Conversely, a condition which is associated with normal reproductive ability will usually appear in the children of affected people and only a small proportion of cases are accounted for by new mutation. Other cases may appear to be sporadic if the family history is inaccurate. In some autosomal dominant conditions, only some gene carriers are affected and the segregation ratio in children or siblings will be lower than 0.5; the proportion of heterozygotes who have the clinical phenotype is the *penetrance* of the gene. In addition, the clinical phenotype itself may be variable in nature or severity; this is referred to as variable *expressivity* of the gene.

Autosomal recessive inheritance

In autosomal recessive inheritance, the condition is only seen in those homozygous for the disease-related allele, as for example in Friedreich's ataxia. Sometimes an autosomal recessive disorder appears in individuals who carry two different disease-related alleles, so-called compound heterozygotes. In autosomal recessive inheritance, there is horizontal transmission of the disorder with normal parents and one or more affected children; both sexes are affected. Both parents, although clinically normal, are heterozygous carriers of the mutation; consequently the chances of a child being homozygous for the mutant allele (and therefore affected), a heterozygous carrier or being homozygous for the normal allele are

1 in 4, 1 in 2, and 1 in 4 respectively. Therefore, with small families, many cases will appear sporadically, but among the siblings of affected patients overall, the segregation ratio will be 0.25. Children of affected patients must be heterozygotes (an affected person cannot transmit a normal allele) but are clinically normal. Very rarely, a person with an autosomal recessive condition may transmit the condition to a child if the other parent is a heterozygous carrier (pseudo-dominance) but the chance of this occurring is small, due to the low frequency of any one mutation in the population. An autosomal recessive disorder is more likely to appear if there is parental consanguinity, due to the increased likelihood of both parents carrying the same mutant allele.

X-linked recessive inheritance

In X-linked recessive inheritance, a condition is seen almost exclusively in males (in whom the allele on the single X chromosome may be normal or a mutation) but not usually in heterozygous females because of the corresponding normal allele. An example is Duchenne muscular dystrophy. The affected males have normal parents and children; sons cannot be affected (they must inherit their X chromosomes from their mothers) and all daughters are carriers. The disease is transmitted only by carrier females, with a 50 per cent risk to sons of being affected and 50 per cent risk to daughters of being cariers. Sometimes daughters of affected males are affected if the mother is by chance a carrier, but this is unusual. Females may also be affected because of the normal process of X-chromosome inactivation (lyonization). Usually X-chromosome inactivation is random, so that equal numbers of normal and mutant alleles are inactivated. If, by chance, X inactivation is non-random and mostly normal alleles are inactivated, a female will be affected, but not normally as severely as an affected male; such females are referred to as *manifesting carriers*, as seen in adrenoleucodystrophy.

X-linked dominant inheritance

X-linked dominant inheritance is much less common and resembles autosomal dominant transmission, except that affected males cannot transmit the disorder to sons and always do so to daughters.

Multifactorial inheritance

In multifactorial inheritance, a disease phenotype is the result of the interaction of many different genes and environmental factors. Such disorders are common and, although many affected individuals appear to be sporadic cases, the incidence of affected relatives is higher than would be expected by chance. At a clinical level, there may be clues to this type of inheritance. The risks to parents, children, and sibs are low, but should be similar (approximately $1/\sqrt{q}$, where q = the population prevalence of the disorder), while the risks to second- and third-degree relatives are minimal. The risk to relatives of the less commonly affected sex is higher than that to those related to index cases of the more commonly affected sex. Parental consanguinity will be slightly increased, but not as high as that seen with autosomal recessive inheritance. In addition, there will be a greater concordance in monozygotic twins compared with dizygotic pairs; the degree of the concordance increase is a guide to the relative importance of genetic and environmental factors.

Maternal inheritance

In maternal inheritance, a phenotype is transmitted only through the female line; although affected individuals may be male or female, only females may pass on the gene or the phenotype. This is seen with mitochondrial disorders; spermatozoa do not contain mitochondria, which are exclusively transmitted in ova.

2.8.2 Chromosomes and genes

The human genome consists of DNA approximately 3×10^9 base pairs (bp) in length. *Chromosomes* are huge molecules of genomic DNA in highly compact form, associated with structural proteins of two types, either basic histones or acidic non-histone proteins. The DNA–protein complex is termed *chromatin*. Human chromosomes are composed of 22 pairs of homologous autosomes and the two sex chromosomes (XX or XY). If metaphase chromosomes are stained with a basic dye (usually Giemsa stain after exposure to trypsin) they are seen to have characteristic *bands* (G-bands) which vary such that the individual chromosomes can be distinguished and identified (Fig. 2.24). The dark-stained bands consist of histone-rich *heterochromatin* and contain mostly structural DNA. The polypeptide-encoding genes are mainly located within the unstained bands of non-histone *euchromatin*. The *map positions* of genes refer to the number of the chromosome, the part of the chromosome (long arm q, short arm p, centromere, or telomere), and the band number within which the gene is situated. These positions are approximate, as each band contains approximately 5–10 megabases (Mb) and may contain several genes.

The genes themselves have a complex structure (Fig 2.25) and are split into *exons* (coding sequences) and intervening non-coding *introns*. The *transcription* process reads the DNA in the 5′ to 3′ direction and a primary messenger RNA (mRNA) transcript is synthesized by RNA polymerase. Subsequently the primary mRNA is processed by the addition of a 7-methyl guanosine cap at the 5′ end, a polyadenylate tail at the 3′ terminal and the removal of the intron sequences by a *splicing* procedure regulated by small nuclear RNA molecules (snRNAs). The much smaller polypeptide-encoding mature mRNA transcript is then transported to the cytoplasm.

The level of transcription of a gene is regulated by sequences upstream of the 5′ end which influence the activity of RNA polymerase; these are referred to as *promoters* (such as TATA sequences) and *enhancer elements* (e.g. CCAAT sequences) (Fig. 2.25). Transcription is also affected by chromatin structure and the level of *methylation* of the cytosine bases within

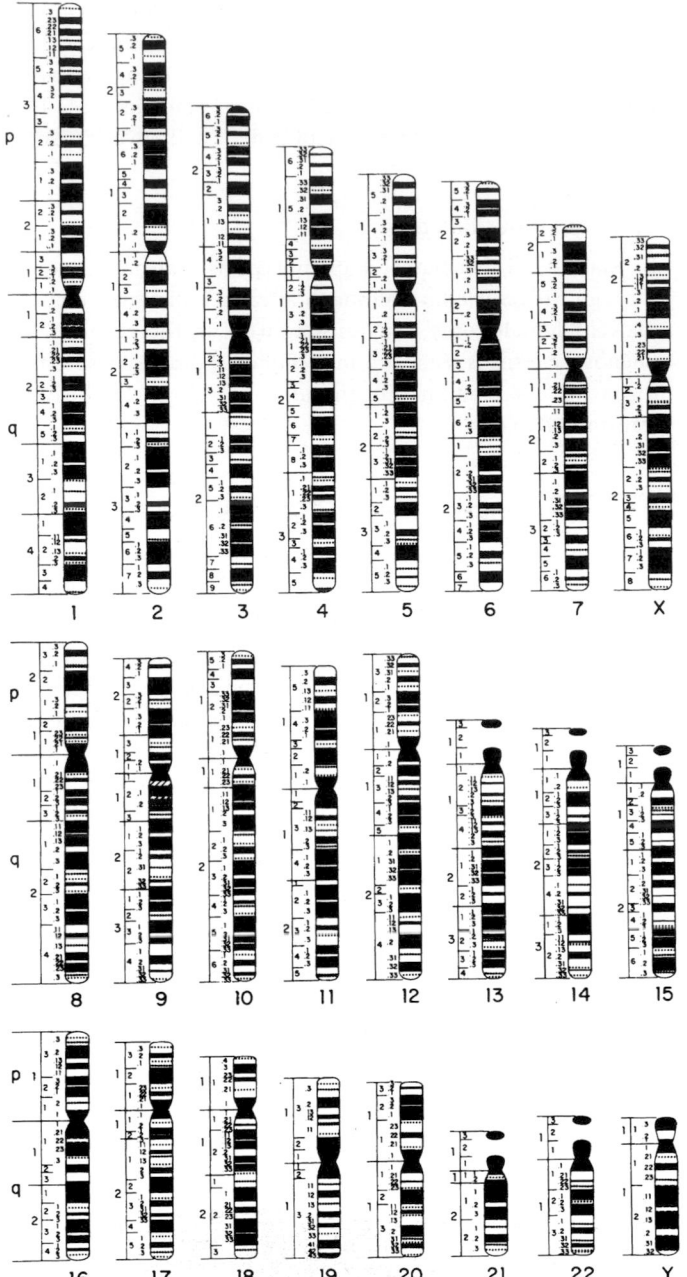

Fig. 2.24. Banding patterns of human chromosomes. Black G-bands are those seen at the prometaphase 850-band stage; dashed bands are those seen only in late prophase (1300-band stage) and mid prophase (1700-band stage). (From Fig 2.16 in Vogel, F. and Motulsky, A. G. (eds) (1986). *Human genetics*, (2nd edn). Springer Verlag, Berlin. This figure was originally published in Yunis (1980). *Human Genetics*, **56**, 296.)

the DNA. Transcription is less likely to occur in histone-rich heterochromatin regions and in regions where there is a high degree of DNA methylation.

In addition to protein-coding genes, the great majority of the genome contains non-coding DNA. This consists of structural DNA, inactive pseudogenes and *repetitive sequences*. A common example of the latter is the numerous Alu sequences, 300 bp in length and containing restriction sites for the enzyme *Alu*I; the function of these repetitive sequences is unclear.

An important feature of genomic DNA is that it contains frequent variations (*polymorphisms*). These variations take several forms, are stable, and can be inherited in a Mendelian manner. Polymorphisms may be *single base changes* or variations in the number of consecutive repeats of sequences of DNA (*variable number of tandem repeats*; VNTRs). Such VNTR polymorphisms may be based on repeats of a sequence of about a dozen base pairs, so that the different polymorphisms differ by thousands of base pairs (minisatellites). Other VNTRs are based on repeats of only a few base pairs, so that there are polymorphisms differing by only tens of base pairs (microsatellites) or repeats of only a single base.

2.8.3 Mitochondria and genes

Mitochondria are intracellular organelles whose main function is to synthesize ATP utilizing the mitochondrial respiratory chain and oxidative phosphorylation system. Each mitochondrion contains 2–10 circular DNA molecules (mtDNA) of about 16 kb. The mtDNA forms about 1 per cent of the total cellular DNA and has a slightly different genetic code, no introns and very little non-coding DNA. mtDNA replicates with each cell division and both strands contain coding sequences. Mitochondrial genes include 13 protein-encoding (*mit*) genes for seven subunits of respiratory complex I, three subunits of cytochrome oxidase (COX, complex IV), two subunits of ATP synthetase (complex V), and apocytochrome *b* (complex III). There are also 24 (*syn*) genes encoding RNAs required for mitochondrial protein synthesis, two ribosomal rRNAs, and 22 transfer tRNAs. All other proteins needed for mitochondrial replication and function are encoded by nuclear genes. In most cells there are thousands of copies of mtDNA, which can be variable (*heteroplasmy*). Mitochondria are not transmitted by spermatozoa, so inheritance of mtDNA is exclusively maternal.

Mutations of mtDNA are the basis of several mitochondrial diseases (Zeviani and Taroni 1994; Leonard and Schapira 2000). These tend to affect tissues with low cell turnover, such as the nervous system, muscle, and heart, in which mutant mtDNAs are able to persist, rather than be gradually depleted during repeated mitotic cell division. Mutations of mtDNA are either point mutations or deletions; duplications are unusual. Point mutations are specified by the mtDNA nucleotide position at which they have occurred. A summary of the important mutations and their associated mitochondrial diseases is given in Table 2.7. The clinical features associated with mitochondrial diseases are discussed in Section 8.5.2 (Leber's disease), Section 15.6.3 (myopathy), Chapter 32 (movement disorders), and Section 31.7.8 (ataxia) which also contains a summary in Table 31.8.

Genetic counselling in mitochondrial diseases is difficult, but in general, risks are low to the offspring of women carrying mtDNA deletions, which are usually sporadic. For those with point mutations the risks to offspring are low unless the proportion of mutant mtDNA in their cells is very large (Chinnery and Turnbull 1997). Males cannot transmit mtDNA mutations.

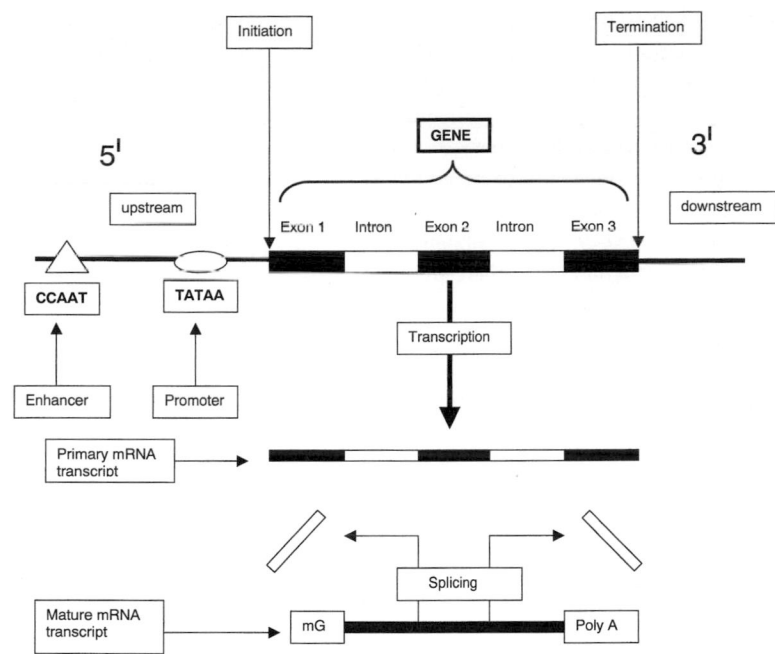

Fig. 2.25. A simplified diagram of a human gene, transcription, and RNA processing. mG, Methyl guanosine cap; poly A, polyadenylated tail. Sites of initiation and termination of transcription are indicated.

Table 2.7. Mutations of mitochondrial DNA and associated disorders (adapted from Zeviani and Taroni 1994)

Inheritance	Disease	RRF in muscle	Mutation	Gene involved
Maternal	LHON	No	11778	Complex
			3460	Complex
			Other point mutations	Various
	NARP	No	8993	ATP synthetase (complex V)
	MELAS	Yes	3243	tRNA
			3271	tRNA
	MERRF	Yes	8344	tRNA
			8356	tRNA
			3243 MELAS	tRNA
	CPEO	Yes	Various point mutations including 3243 MELAS and others	tRNA
	Myopathy	Yes		tRNA
	Cardiomyopathy	No		tRNA
	Deafness	No		rRNA
Sporadic	CPEO	Yes	Deletion	Various
	KSS	Yes	Deletion	Various
	Pearson syndrome	Yes	Deletion	Various
Autosomal dominant	CPEO plus	Yes	Multiple deletions	Various

LHON, Leber's hereditary optic neuropathy; NARP, neurogenic atrophy, ataxia and retinitis pigmentosa; MERRF, myoclonic epilepsy with ragged red fibres; MELAS, mitochondrial encephalomyopathy, lactic acidosis, and stroke-like episodes; CPEO, chronic progressive external ophthalmoplegia; KSS, Kearns–Sayre syndrome.

The situation is different in rare families in which multiple mtDNA deletions occur as a result of mutations of nuclear genes; in this situation the mitochondrial disorder (Table 2.7) is transmitted by either sex as an autosomal dominant trait.

2.8.4 DNA analysis

A comprehensive review of laboratory molecular genetic methods is beyond the scope of this chapter and only a very brief summary of techniques likely to be of interest to clinicians will be attempted here. More detail is available in other texts (Davies and Read 1992; Conneally 1993). DNA is extracted from blood, or sometimes other tissues (e.g. muscle), and may then be stored at low temperatures for long periods (*DNA banking*). For different regions of the DNA to be analysed, genomic DNA must be cut into manageable fragments. This is achieved with *restriction endonucleases*. These enzymes cut DNA at certain sequences only (*restriction sites*); there are many restriction endonucleases, each recognizing a particular DNA cleavage sequence. The resulting DNA pieces are referred to as restriction fragments, within an overall restriction digest. These must then be analysed by other methods; some important techniques are as follows.

Agarose gel electrophoresis allows the physical separation of DNA fragments based on their size. Small fragments migrate further through the gel in the direction of the current than larger fragments; several different DNA samples can be analysed simultaneously in different lanes within the gel. Only fragments up to 20–30 kb can be separated in this way. The DNA can be visualized in the gel by chemical staining, but individual fragments cannot be distinguished. The two techniques for identifying a selected fragment within a restriction digest are *PCR amplification* of the fragment of interest prior to electrophoresis so that it is present in much greater quantities on the gel than any other fragment (see below) or, alternatively, *Southern blotting* onto a membrane after electrophoresis and hybridization with a labelled probe specific for the fragment (see below).

Pulsed-field gel electrophoresis (PFGE) uses an alternating-direction electrophoretic current to separate large DNA fragments up to 10 000 kb in length. Such large fragments are produced initially with restriction endonucleases which recognize infrequent, widely separated restriction sites.

Fragments may be rendered single stranded and then hybridized to DNA or RNA *probes* labelled with a radionucleotide or chemical. A probe is a fragment of DNA or RNA with a complementary sequence to that of the DNA fragment of interest and so will hybridize with this fragment and not other fragments with different DNA sequences. In this way the fragment of interest may be detected visually or by autoradiography. Probes may be fragments of DNA with the same sequence as a known gene (complementary or cDNA probes), RNA transcripts from a given gene, or simply DNA sequences whose chromosomal localization is known. cDNA is synthesized from a mature RNA transcript by the enzyme reverse transcriptase; accordingly it contains only the exon DNA sequences of the gene in question.

Cloning of a DNA sequence involves introducing the fragment into the genome of a bacterial or viral *vector* which then replicates *in vitro* to yield many copies of the amplified sequence for further analysis.

The *polymerase chain reaction* (PCR) allows *in vitro* DNA replication of many copies of a selected DNA region or restriction fragment, therefore hugely amplifying a selected fragment

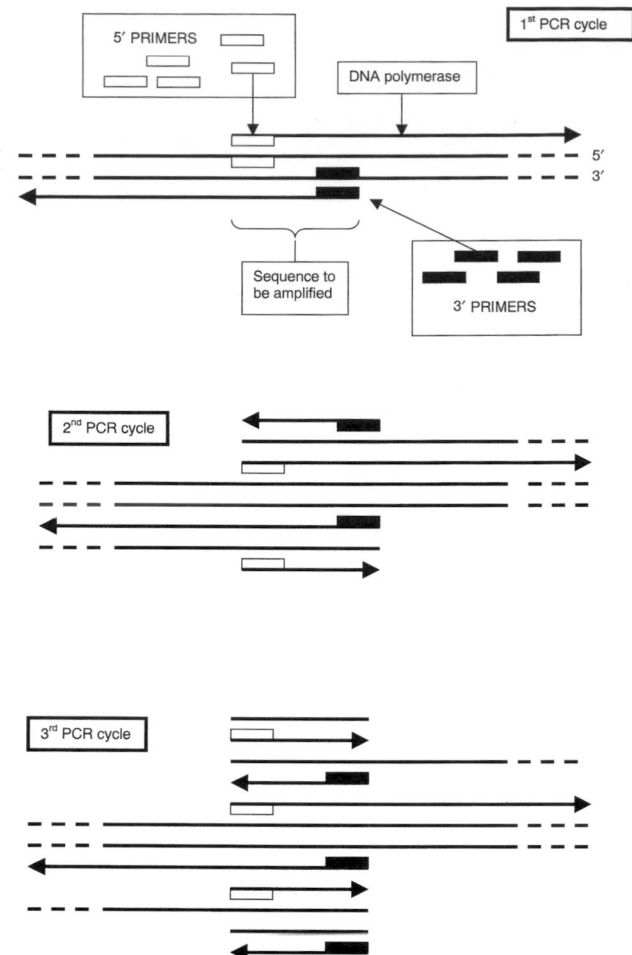

Fig. 2.26. The polymerase chain reaction. The sense strand of the DNA to be copied runs in a 5′ to 3′ direction, the antisense strand runs 5′ to 3′ in the opposite direction due to the antiparallel arrangement of the DNA double helix. DNA polymerase always proceeds in a 5′ to 3′ direction. The 5′ end of the target sequence on the sense strand is therefore defined by a 5′ primer complementary to the 3′ end of the sequence on the antisense strand (open rectangle). The 3′ end of the target sequence on the sense strand (filled rectangle) is defined by a directly complementary primer (3′ primer). Note that both long and short fragments of DNA are synthesized but that as more cycles are completed, the proportion of short fragments complementary to the target sequence increases.

within a DNA sample. The DNA to be amplified is designated by the use of *primers* which are complementary to sequences at its 5′ and 3′ boundaries. The 5′ primer hybridizes at the 5′ end of the sense strand of the designated fragment while the 3′ primer hybridizes to the 5′ end of its complementary antisense strand (Fig. 2.26). There are three steps: DNA denaturation at high temperature renders the DNA single stranded and therefore able to hybridize with primers; hybridization then occurs between the complementary sequences of the primers and the DNA fragment to be amplified; DNA synthesis (which can only proceed in a 5′ to 3′ direction) then occurs using a heat-stable DNA polymerase. Synthesis has to start from the primer sequences only, therefore yielding many copies of the

DNA within the primer hybridization sites. The resulting amplified fragment is then available for gel electrophoresis (the amplified DNA can be visualized directly in the gel after chemical staining), DNA sequencing, cloning into vectors, or detection of polymorphisms and mutations in the amplified sequence.

Southern blotting is the process of transferring electrophoresed DNA fragments from an agarose gel to a membrane. The DNA binds to the membrane and may then be transferred to a solution containing a probe which has a sequence complementary to the fragment to be identified. The choice of probe therefore determines the fragment to be detected. The radioactive or chemically labelled probe hybridizes to the selected DNA fragment whose position on the membrane is detectable by autoradiography. To increase sensitivity, Southern blotting can be carried out after gel electrophoresis of a restriction digest of PCR-amplified DNA.

PCR, Southern blotting, or both may be used to identify *polymorphisms* which alter the length of a restriction fragment created by a particular restriction endonuclease at a particular genetic locus. The locus can be specified by the use of a probe known to hybridize to a particular chromosomal locus or PCR primers complementary to the known DNA sequence at a particular locus. Single-base-change polymorphisms throughout the genome will cause some restriction sites to be lost and new ones to be created, therefore producing *restriction fragment length polymorphisms* (RFLPs). VNTR polymorphisms also lead to variable lengths of restriction fragments at particular loci near to a VNTR sequence. The size of a RFLP or VNTR polymorphism is given by the distance travelled by the relevant restriction fragment during gel electrophoresis; this is visualized by direct staining if prior PCR amplification has been used or by Southern blotting and probe detection.

Other *single-base-change polymorphisms* do not alter restriction sites and cannot be detected by RFLP analysis. These may be detected by several methods:

1. *Allele-specific oligonucleotide* (ASO) probes will only hybridize to an exactly complementary sequence of PCR-amplified DNA and not if there is a single base change.

2. *Amplification-resistant mutation system* (ARMS) is a PCR reaction which will only work if the DNA sequence of the 3′ primer exactly matches the target sequence but not if a single base change is present.

3. Single-stranded DNA shows different electrophoretic mobility with even a single base change, which can be detected by gel electrophoresis after PCR and denaturing of the DNA to render it single stranded. The base change therefore creates a *single-stranded conformational polymorphism* (SSCP).

4. *Chemical cleavage of mismatched DNA* (CCM) relies on the imperfect hybridization of PCR-amplified DNA containing a base change to another DNA strand or RNA probe of the correct complementary sequence (*heteroduplex formation*); there is slight separation of the heteroduplex at the site of the base mismatch, allowing, under the correct conditions, enzymatic cleavage of the altered fragment at the site of the polymorphism. This produces two bands instead of one after gel electrophoresis of the fragments.

5. Heteroduplexes in which there is a single base mismatch caused by a base change polymorphism also show altered electrophoretic mobility through a special type of gel (*denaturing gradient gel electrophoresis*; DGGE).

DNA fragments may also be analysed by DNA sequencing of the PCR-amplified or cloned DNA sequence or fragment. Usually this will involve analysis of all or part of a gene. Many normal (wild-type) genes have now been amplified or cloned and sequenced to determine their normal DNA structure as well as the nature of any pathogenic mutations (see below).

2.8.5 Gene mapping and linkage analysis

Genes (or any other unique DNA sequences) may be localized to particular chromosomal locations to produce a genetic map of the chromosome or ultimately of the entire genome (the basis of the ongoing human genome project). Many genes have now been localized (mapped) to particular chromosomal loci. There are two approaches, either *physical mapping* or *genetic mapping*.

Physical mapping

Physical mapping involves the direct assignment of a DNA sequence (either a gene or a random restriction fragment) to a particular chromosomal locus.

1. *Fluorescent in situ hybridization* (FISH) uses chemical labelling of the DNA sequence and hybridization to a metaphase chromosome preparation to detect the chromosome and subregion to which the sequence has hybridized.

2. *Somatic cell hybrids*, created by fusing mouse and human cells, yield cell lines containing different mixtures of human and mouse chromosomes, either as whole chromosomes or parts of them. By determining which cell lines hybridize with the human sequence to be mapped and which do not, its chromosomal location can be determined.

3. *Chromosomal abnormalities* detectable by cytogenetic methods such as visible deletions, inversions, or translocations (particularly of the X chromosome) can reveal the location of a gene if they are associated with a disease phenotype. This is because the function of a gene is likely to be disrupted if it is located at the site of a deletion or chromosomal break point.

Genetic mapping

Genetic mapping or *linkage analysis* reveals the chromosomal location of a DNA fragment by establishing close physical proximity to another fragment (a genetic *marker*), the map position of which is known already. The two fragments (the one to be mapped and the genetic marker) are tracked together through several generations of several human families. If they are very close, they will tend to be inherited together because of the low probability of a genetic crossover between them during meiotic recombination. If they are widely separated, they will be inherited together only at chance level 50 per cent of the time. The recombination fraction, θ, is calculated from the frequency of crossovers between the loci and is an indicator of genetic distance. Thus if recombinations (crossovers) are seen in 10 per cent of meioses, $\theta = 0.1$. Genetic distance is measured in centi-Morgans (cM), 1 cM being equivalent to a 1 per cent recombination frequency ($\theta = 0.01$). As a rough guide, 1 cM = 1 Mb (10^6 bp), but this is not a reliable calculation because of unequal recombination frequency at different parts of the genome. It should be noted that there is a prior probability of establishing 50 per cent co-segregation of two markers by chance alone. It is therefore necessary to calculate the likelihood of linkage of two loci; this is expressed as the logarithm of the odds in favour of linkage at a given value of θ (*lod score*). A lod score of 3.0 is equivalent to a 95 per cent probability of linkage at a given genetic distance. These calculations are usually based on data from numerous families and are complex, so that specialized computer programs are used to determine lod scores for different values of θ. The method can be refined by testing for linkage between the DNA fragment to be mapped and multiple other markers, the chromosomal map positions of which are known (*multi-locus linkage*), therefore searching for linkage over a wider area of a chromosome. In practice, linkage analysis is limited by the need for multiple highly polymorphic markers, limited human family sizes in which there are only a few informative meioses, and the often limited family histories and available DNA samples from human families.

It is very important to realize that linkage analysis can be used in exactly the same way to map a disease gene by using the phenotype as a marker for the *disease gene*. The gene can therefore be mapped to a chromosomal locus by linkage analysis without knowing anything about its DNA sequence. Many genes have been mapped in this way, leading to subsequent analysis of the relevant part of the chromosome in order to detect and sequence the gene itself. There are other less accurate methods of linkage analysis using the disease phenotype and genetic markers.

1. *Sib pair analysis* involves searching for allelic markers shared by affected sibs more often than would be expected by chance (25 per cent). This is useful in autosomal recessive inheritance where affected siblings share the same mutant allele at a given locus and are therefore more likely to have the same alleles at loci very close to the disease gene.

2. *Linkage disequilibrium* refers to the existence of a particular allele at a locus linked to the disease gene more often than would be expected by chance. In the normal population, the particular alleles seen at two linked loci will be determined by the frequency of those alleles in the overall population. If a new pathogenic mutation occurs at one of the loci and causes a disease phenotype which is then transmitted to future generations, it will usually occur in association with the particular alleles that were present at closely linked loci at the time of the

mutation. Only after many generations, when there have been frequent recombinations between the linked loci, will this linkage disequilibrium disappear. Therefore, alleles which occur in association with a disease phenotype more often than would be expected from their population frequency may lie close to the disease locus, in linkage disequilibrium with it.

2.8.6 Mechanisms of mutation

Point mutations involve the change of a single DNA base; a transition involves a change of one purine (A or G) or one pyrimidine (T or C) to the other while a transversion involves a change of a purine to a pyrimidine. The effects of such subtle mutations can be severe. Pathogenic point mutations alter gene function by damaging the action of 5′ upstream promoter or enhancer elements (transcriptional mutants), by altering a base triplet (codon) so that transcription is prematurely terminated (nonsense mutation), by changing the codon specifying one amino acid to that for another (missense mutation), or by disrupting RNA processing by altering spicing sites. If a single base is deleted from within an exon, the whole sequence of base triplets is changed, leading to a completely different amino-acid sequence (frameshift mutation).

Other mutations involve the deletion of segments of DNA removing part or even all of one or more genes (e.g. Duchenne muscular dystrophy). In other situations, part of a chromosome is duplicated, disrupting genes involved in the duplicated region (e.g. the 17p11.2 duplication in hereditary motor and sensory neuropathy type Ia). Some genes contain unstable trinucleotide repeats; these are similar to microsatellite VNTR polymorphisms but the trinucleotide repeat sequences have expanded into an abnormally large mutation with a repeat number beyond the normal range and consequent disruption of gene function and a deficiency or functional abnormality of the protein product. These mutations are associated with a tendency to undergo greater expansion during meiosis in one sex than in the other; for example the fragile X and myotonic dystrophy mutations tend to undergo greater expansion during maternal transmission, while the expansions causing Huntington's disease or the autosomal dominant (SCA) cerebellar ataxias are more unstable during paternal meiosis. There is also a tendency for these expansions to become longer during successive meioses. As greater repeat length tends to be associated with earlier age of disease onset, the phenomenon of anticipation (earlier onset in succeeding generations) is a characteristic clinical feature of trinucleotide repeat disorders. Several diseases are now known to be associated with this recently discovered mechanism of mutation (Table 2.8).

2.8.7 Detection of mutations

DNA testing in neurology is carried out for one of two reasons and it is vital that the neurologist is quite clear about which reason applies when a test is requested. In diagnostic testing, a clinically affected patient is investigated to test a diagnostic hypothesis; for example frataxin gene testing in a teenager with

Table 2.8. Trinucleotide repeat disorders

Disease	Inheritance	Gene locus	Gene	Trinucleotide	Normal size range (repeats)[a]	Mutation size range (repeats)[a]
X-linked bulbospinal neuronopathy (Kennedy syndrome)	XL	Xq13–21	Androgen receptor	CAG	7–34	38–68
Huntington's disease	AD	4p16.3	Huntingtin	CAG	11–34	36–121
Myotonic dystrophy	AD	19q13.2–3	Protein kinase MT-PK (3′)	CTG	5–37	41–4000+
Fragile X syndrome	XL	Xq27.3	FMR1 (5′)	CGG	5–50	>200
Friedreich's ataxia	AR	9q13	Frataxin	GAA	7–29	66–1700
SCA1	AD	6p23	Ataxin 1	CAG	7–34	38–68
SCA2	AD	12q24	Ataxin 2	CAG	14–31	35–59
SCA3	AD	14q32	Ataxin 3	CAG	13–44	65–84
SCA6	AD	19p13	α-1A calcium channel	CAG	4–16	21–27
SCA7	AD	3p12	Ataxin 7	CAG	7–17	38–160
DRPLA	AD	12p13	Atrophin 1	CAG	5–35	49–85

SCA, spinocerebellar ataxia; DRPLA, dentatorubropallidoluysian atrophy; AD, autosomal dominant; AR, autosomal recessive; XL, X linked.
3′ indicates expansion located in 3′ flanking region of the myotonic dystrophy gene; 5′ indicates expansion located in 5′ flanking region of FMR1 gene.
[a] Repeat sizes vary among different reports and approximate repeat numbers in normal and affected individuals are quoted.

ataxia and areflexia. In presymptomatic or predictive testing, the test is carried out to determine the genetic status of an asymptomatic individual in order to predict whether or not a genetic disease will develop in future; the usual example of this is predictive testing in Huntington's disease. Prenatal testing is a special form of predictive testing usually undertaken by clinical geneticists.

The methods used for detection of mutations in individuals are varied and depend on the type of mutation and whether the gene sequence or only its chromosomal locus is known. If the gene has been sequenced and the type of mutation is known, *direct mutation detection* is possible. Direct methods include:

1. PCR amplification and gel electrophoresis to detect small deletions or expansions (especially trinucleotide repeat mutations) which alter the specified DNA fragment size. Southern blotting and probe hybridization may also be used to reveal abnormally sized restriction fragments.

2. Large deletions (as in Duchenne muscular dystrophy; DMD) require PGFE to reveal abnormally sized restriction fragments from the large DMD gene.

3. Deletions may be detected by failure of a probe to hybridize to the deleted sequence, but this is only reliable in males with X-linked deletions, due to the presence of the DNA from the normal allele; densitometric methods can be used to get around this problem (e.g. in detection of DMD female carriers) but are not reliable enough for clinical use.

4. Known specified point mutations may be detected by allele-specific oligonucleotide (ASO) probes or ARMS (see above).

5. Unknown point mutations (which are often variable within the same gene in different families) can be detected by SSCP, heteroduplex cleavage by CCM, or DGGE (see above), but often require sequencing of the gene for their detection.

If the sequence of the disease gene and the type of mutation is unknown, as is the case in many disorders in which the gene is mapped but not cloned or sequenced, *indirect* gene tracking is used to detect affected individuals. This uses markers known to be tightly linked to the disease gene, such as RFLP or VNTR polymorphisms. The marker can be analysed in DNA samples from as many family members as possible to determine its transmission through the family. This may reveal whether an individual is likely to have inherited the mutant or normal allele at the disease locus. There are considerable difficulties with this approach: DNA from several individuals in three generations is usually required and may not be available; some individuals in the family may not be heterozygous for the linked marker and are therefore uninformative; an inaccurate family history, non-paternity, and reduced gene penetrance may all confound the interpretation of gene marker studies; and finally, the possibility of recombination between the disease gene locus and the linked marker introduces some uncertainty into the results. The accuracy of indirect mutation testing can be increased by the use of multiple linked markers or RFLPs known to lie within the gene to be tracked (intragenic RFLPs). The indirect approach has been used mainly for the detection of mutations in unaffected individuals who wish to know whether they carry a mutation which is segregating within the family; a previous example of this was presymptomatic diagnosis of Huntington's disease. As more genes are sequenced and their mutations characterized, direct mutation screening is increasingly used for this purpose, as well as for the detection of specific mutations for diagnosis of affected persons.

2.8.8 Ethical aspects

One of the most important aspects of DNA testing is consent. The patient must understand the nature of the test, the reasons for it, and the potential consequences (for their family as well as themselves) of a positive result. This enables the patient to make an informed decision about the investigation. In diagnostic testing, there are unlikely to be problems if the patient has given informed consent, but there should be follow-up information about the implications of the result and the prognosis, so that sensible informed decisions about the future can be made. As with all aspects of patient care, confidentiality is essential, but special care is needed with genetic testing because of interest in the results from relatives (who sometimes request test results via their own doctors) and sometimes employers and insurance companies. Consent and avoidance of adverse psychological and social consequences are much more difficult in predictive testing. Careful counselling is needed before this is done, and in some patients psychiatric evaluation may be appropriate if problems such as suicide following a positive test are a possibility. The first instinct of many relatives of patients with autosomal dominant disorders is to request a DNA test, but it is surprising how many reconsider this once the possible consequences of a positive predictive test in terms of employment, insurance, and personal relationships are thought through. In general, predictive testing should not be undertaken in the neurological outpatient clinic but only in the context of a predictive testing programme conforming to nationally agreed guidelines (World Federation Research Group on Huntington's disease 1990); such programmes are available in departments of clinical genetics. It is inappropriate to request genetic testing for conditions such as Huntington's disease or autosomal dominant cerebellar ataxia in a patient with vague neurological symptoms, unless there is a genuine clinical suspicion of such a disorder. Otherwise a predictive test may inadvertently be carried out with potentially unfortunate consequences. Problems may also arise with predictive testing when a person at 25 per cent risk of an autosomal dominant condition because of an affected grandparent wishes to be tested, but the intervening parent, at 50 per cent risk, does not. It may be difficult to resolve this situation but caution is required when considering such tests. Children pose another difficulty; it is not uncommon for patients with hereditary neurological disorders to request that their children are tested for the disorder. However, the child is unable to make an informed decision and, in most situations, an adverse result is unlikely to be helpful to the child. For adult-onset conditions for which there is no treatment, predictive testing of minors is not advisable.

2.8.9 Identified neurological disease genes

The number of identified neurological disease genes continues to increase rapidly. Up-to-date information can be obtained from online genetic databases such as Online Mendelian Inheritance in Man (OMIM) at http://www.ncbi.nlm.nih.gov/Omim/. The morbid map at this site is a particularly helpful summary of disease genes. Table 2.9 summarizes of some of the more important neurological genes and their chromosomal loci.

Table 2.9. Neurological disease genes

Disorder	Locus
Adrenoleucodystrophy/adrenomyeloneuropathy	Xq28
Aicardi syndrome	Xp22
Alzheimer's disease 1 (APP related)	21q21.3–q22.05
Alzheimer's disease 2 (late onset)	19cen–q13.2
Alzheimer's disease 3 (presenilin related)	14q24.3
Alzheimer's disease 4 (presenilin related)	1q31–q42
Alzheimer's disease 5	12p11–q13
Amyloid neuropathy	18q11.2–12.1
Aneurysm (familial)	2q31
Ataxia telangiectasia	11q22.3
Ataxia with vitamin E deficiency (AVED)	8q13
Benign familial infantile convulsions	19q
Benign heredity chorea	14q
CADASIL	19p13
Canavan disease	17pter–p13
Cavernous haemangiomas (familial)	7q11.2–q21
Cavernous haemangiomas (familial)	7p15–p13
Cerebellar ataxia (autosomal dominant) (SCA 1)	6p23
Cerebellar ataxia (autosomal dominant) (SCA 2)	12q24
Cerebellar ataxia (autosomal dominant) (SCA 3)	14q32
Cerebellar ataxia (autosomal dominant) (SCA 4)	16q22
Cerebellar ataxia (autosomal dominant) (SCA 5)	11cen
Cerebellar ataxia (autosomal dominant) (SCA 6)	19p13
Cerebellar ataxia (autosomal dominant) (SCA 7)	3p12
Cerebellar ataxia (X linked)	Xp11.21–q21.3
Cerebral amyloid angiopathy	20p11.2
Cerebral amyloid angiopathy (Dutch type)	21q21
Cerebral amyloid angiopathy (Finnish type)	9q34
Cerebrotendinous xanthomatosis	2q33–qter
Ceroid lipofuscinosis 1 (infantile)	1p32
Ceroid lipofuscinosis 2 (classic late infantile)	11p15.5
Ceroid lipofuscinosis 3 (juvenile)	16p12.1
Ceroid lipofuscinosis 4 (variant late infantile)	13q21–q32
Ceroid lipofuscinosis 5 (variant late infantile)	15q21–q23
Ceroid lipofuscinosis (variant juvenile type)	1p32
Charcot–Marie–Tooth disease (CMT) 1A	17p11.2

Table 2.9. *Continued*

Disorder	Locus
Charcot–Marie–Tooth disease (CMT) 1B	1q22
Charcot–Marie–Tooth disease (CMT) 2A	1p36–p35
Charcot–Marie–Tooth disease (CMT) 2B	3q13–q22
Charcot–Marie–Tooth disease (CMT) 2D	7p14
Charcot–Marie–Tooth disease (CMT) 4A	8q13–q21.1
Charcot–Marie–Tooth disease (CMT) 4B	11q23
Charcot–Marie–Tooth disease (CMT) X1 (Connexin 32)	Xq13.1
Charcot–Marie–Tooth disease (CMT) X2	Xp22.2
Choreoathetosis, paroxysmal dystonic	2q33–35
Cockayne syndrome 1	5
Cockayne syndrome 2 (ERCC6)	10q11
Creutzfeldt–Jacob disease (PRNP gene)	20pter–p12
DRPLA	12p13.31
Dysautonomia, familial	9q31–q33
Dystonia (DYT6) (Mennonite)	8p21–q22
Dystonia (DYT7) (segmental)	18p
Dystonia, dopa responsive (DYT5)	14q22
Dystonia, dopa responsive, tyrosine hydroxylase deficiency	11p15.5
Dystonia, primary torsion (DYT1)	9q34
Dystonia, X linked (DYT3)	Xq13.1
Dystonia, myoclonic (DYT11)	7q21
Dystonia, rapid onset dystonia-parkinsonism	19q13
Epilepsy, benign neonatal type 1	20q13
Epilepsy, benign neonatal type 2	8q24
Epilepsy, idiopathic generalized	8q24
Epilepsy, idiopathic generalized	2q22–23
Epilepsy, juvenile myoclonic	15q14
Epilepsy, juvenile myoclonic	6p
Epilepsy, juvenile myoclonic	2q22–23
Epilepsy, adult myoclonic	8q23–24
Epilepsy, nocturnal frontal lobe	20q13
Epilepsy, nocturnal frontal lobe	1p21
Epilepsy, nocturnal frontal lobe	15q24
Epilepsy, partial	10q23–q24
Epilepsy, progressive myoclonic (Unverricht Lundborg)	21q22.3
Episodic ataxia type 1 (with myokymia)	12p13
Episodic ataxia type 2	19p13
Essential tremor (ETM1)	3q13
Essential tremor (ETM2)	2p22–25
Fabry disease	Xq22
Familial amyloid polyneuropathy (several alleles)	18q11
Febrile convulsions, familial type 1	8q13–q21
Febrile convulsions, familial type 2	19p13.3
Fragile X syndrome	Xq27.3
Friedreich's ataxia	9q13–q21.1
Geniospasm	9q13–q21
Giant axonal neuropathy	16q24.1

Table 2.9. *Continued*

Disorder	Locus
GM2 gangliosidosis (AB variant)	5q31–q33
GM2 gangliosidosis (Tay–Sachs)	15q23–q24
Hemiplegic migraine, familial	19p13
Hereditary spastic paraplegia 1, X linked (L1CAM)	Xq28
Hereditary spastic paraplegia 2, X linked (PMD gene)	Xq22
Hereditary spastic paraplegia 3a	14q11.2–q24.3
Hereditary spastic paraplegia 4	2p21–24
Hereditary spastic paraplegia 5a	8p12–q13
Hereditary spastic paraplegia 6	15q11.1
Hereditary spastic paraplegia 7 (paraplegin gene)	16q24.3
Hereditary spastic paraplegia 8	8q23–24
Hereditary spastic paraplegia 9	10q23.3–q24.1
Hereditary spastic paraplegia 10	12q13
Hereditary spastic paraplegia 11	15q13–15
Hereditary spastic paraplegia 12	19q13
Hereditary spastic paraplegia 13	2q24
Hereditary spastic paraplegia 14	3q27–28
Hereditary spastic paraplegia 16	Xq11.2
Hereditary spastic paraplegia, recessive (Sjögren–Larsson)	17p11.2
Huntington's disease	4p16.3
Huntington's disease (non 4p16 linked)	4p15.3
Huntington's disease (non 4p16 linked)	20p
Hydrocephalus, aqueduct stenosis (L1CAM)	Xq28
Hyperekplexia, dominant	5q32
Hyperekplexia, recessive	5q32
Hyperkalaemic periodic paralysis	17q23–q25
Hypokalaemic periodic paralysis	1q32
Joulbert syndrome	9q34.3
Klippel–Feil syndrome	5q11.2
Krabbe's disease	14q31
Lafora body disease	6q24
Lesch–Nyhan syndrome	Xq26–q27
McArdle's disease	11q13
McLeod phenotype	Xp21.1–p21.2
Meningiomatosis (autosomal dominant)	22q12–qter
Metachromatic leucodystrophy	22q24–q32
Moebius syndrome type 1	13q12–q13
Moebius syndrome type 2	3q21–q22
Motor neurone disease (SOD related)	21q22.1
Motor neurone disease (with frontal dementia)	9q21–22
Muscular dystrophy (Becker)	Xp21.2
Muscular dystrophy (Duchenne)	Xp21.2
Muscular dystrophy (Emery–Dreifuss)	Xq28
Muscular dystrophy, congenital (Fukuyama)	9q31–q33
Muscular dystrophy, fascioscapulohumeral	4q35
Muscular dystrophy, limb girdle, type 1a	5q22–q31
Muscular dystrophy, limb girdle, type 1b	1q11–q21

Table 2.9. *Continued*

Disorder	Locus
Muscular dystrophy, limb girdle, type 1c	3p25
Muscular dystrophy, limb girdle, type 2a	15q15–q21
Muscular dystrophy, limb girdle, type 2b	2p13.3–p13.1
Muscular dystrophy, limb girdle, type 2c	13q12
Muscular dystrophy, limb girdle, type 2d	17q12–q21
Muscular dystrophy, limb girdle, type 2e	4q12
Muscular dystrophy, limb girdle, type 2f	5q33
Muscular dystrophy, limb girdle, type 2g	17q11–q12
Muscular dystrophy, limb girdle, type 2h	9q31–34.1
Muscular dystrophy, merosin deficient	6q22–q23
Muscular dystrophy, desmin deficient	11q22.3–23.1
Muscular dystrophy, with spinal rigidity	1p36–p35
Myasthenia gravis, familial infantile	17p13
Myasthenia gravis, transient neonatal	2q33–q34
Myasthenic syndrome, slow channel syndrome	2q24–q32
Myasthenic syndrome, slow channel syndrome	17p11–p12
Myopathy, carnitine palmitoyl transferase II deficiency	1p32
Myopathy, congenital	12q13
Myopathy, desmin type	2q35
Myopathy, distal	14q
Myopathy, nemaline type 1	1q22–q23
Myopathy, nemaline type 2	2q21–q22
Myopathy, phosphoglycerate mutase deficiency	7p12–p13
Myopathy, scapuloperoneal	12q13–q15
Myopathy, succinate dehydrogenase deficiency	1p35–p36
Myotonia congenita (acetazolamide responsive)	17q23–q25
Myotonia congenita (Becker type, reccessive)	7q35
Myotonia congenita (Thomsen type, dominant)	7q35
Myotonic dystrophy	19q13.2–q13.3
Myotonic dystrophy type 2	3q
Neimann–Pick disease type C1 (autosomal recessive)	18q11–q12
Neimann–Pick disease type C2 (autosomal recessive)	14q24.3
Neurocanthocytosis	9q21
Neurofibromatosis type 1	17q11.2
Neurofibromatosis type 2	22q12.2
Neuropathy, hereditary sensory and autonomic	9q22
Optic atrophy, dominant, type 1	3q28–q29
Optic atrophy, X linked	Xp11.4–p11.21
Ornithine transcarbamylase deficiency	Xp21.1
Paramyotonia congenita	17q23–q25
Parkinson's disease, atypical (Parkin)	6q25.2
Parkinson's disease, autosomal dominant	2p13
Parkinson's disease, autosomal dominant	4p15
Parkinson's disease, autosomal dominant (alpha synuclein)	4q21–q22
Pelizaeus–Merzbacher disease (PMD)	Xq22
Phenylketonuria	12q24.1

Table 2.9. *Continued*

Disorder	Locus
Phenylketonuria, DHPR deficiency	4p15.31
Phenylketonuria, PTS deficiency	11q22–q23
Porphyria, acute intermittent	11q23.3
Progressive external ophthalmoplegia (autosomal dominant)	10q23–q24
Progressive external ophthalmoplegia (autosomal dominant)	3p14–p21
Progressive subcortical gliosis	17q21–q22
Ptosis, hereditary congenital	1p32–p34
Refsum's disease	10pter–p11.2
Rett's syndrome	Xq28
Sandhoff disease	5q13
Schindler's disease	22q11
Sialidosis type 2	6p21.3
Spinal muscular atrophy, congenital non-progressive of legs	12q23–q24
Spinal muscular atrophy, distal	7p
Spinal muscular atrophy, scapuloperoneal	12q24
Spinal muscular atrophy, type IV	12q24
Spinal muscular atrophy, types I, II, III	5q12.2–q13.3
Spinal muscular atrophy, X linked (Kennedy syndrome)	Xq11–q12
Spinal muscular atrophy, X linked lethal	Xp
Tourette syndrome	11q23
Tuberose sclerosis 1	9q34
Tuberose sclerosis 2	16p13.3
Von Hippel–Lindau disease	3p26–p25
Wilson's disease	13q14.3–q21.1

References

Ad Hoc Subcommittee of American Academy of Neurology AIDS Task Force (1991). Research criteria for diagnosis of chronic inflammatory demyelinating polyneuropathy (CIDP). *Neurology*, **41**, 617–18.

Aminoff, M. J., Goodin, D. S., Parry, G. J., *et al.* (1985). Electrophysiologic evaluation of lumbosacral radiculopathies: electromyography, late responses, and somatosensory evoked potentials. *Neurology*, **35**, 1514–18.

Andersson, M., Alvarez-Cermeño, J., Bernardi, G., *et al.* (1994). Cerebrospinal fluid in the diagnosis of multiple sclerosis: a consensus report. *J. Neurol. Neurosurg. Psychiat.*, **57**, 897–902.

Arnold, J. A., Modaresi, K. B., Thomas, N. *et al.* (1999). Carotid plaque characterization by duplex scanning: observer error may undermine current clinical trials. *Stroke*, **30**, 61–5.

Babikian, V. L., Wijman, C. A. C., Hyde, C. *et al.* (1997) Cerebral microembolism and early recurrent cerebral or retinal ischaemic events. *Stroke*, **28**, 1314–18.

Barker, A. T., Freeston, I. L., Jalinous, R. *et al.* (1985). Magnetic stimulation of the human brain. J. Physiol. (London), **369**, 3P.

Baumgartner, R. W., Mattle, H. P., Aaslid, R. *et al.* (1997). Transcranial colour-coded Duplex sonography in arterial cerebrovascular disease. *Cerebrovasc. Dis.*, **7**, 57–63.

Binnie, C. D., Cooper, R., and Fowler, C. J. (1995). *Clinical neurophysiology. EMG, nerve conduction and evoked potentials*. Butterworth-Heinemann Ltd, Oxford.

Blakeley, D. D., Oddone, E. Z., Hasselblad, V. *et al.* (1995). Noninvasive carotid artery testing. A meta-analytic review. *Ann. Intern. Med.*, **122**, 360–7.

Bornstein, N. M. and Norris, J. W. (1994) Transcranial Doppler sonography is at present of limited clinical value. *Arch. Neurol.*, **51**, 1057–9.

Bouche, P., Cattelin, F., Saint-Jean, O. *et al.* (1993). Clinical and electrophysiological study of the peripheral nervous system in the elderly. *J. Neurol.*, **240**, 263–8.

Bradley, W. G. (1974). *Disorders of peripheral nerves*. Blackwell, Oxford.

Brandt-Zawadski, M. (1988). MR imaging of the brain. *Radiology*, **166**, 1–10.

Brink, J. A., McFarland, E. G., and Heiken, J. P. (1997). Helical/spiral computed body tomography. *Clin. Radiol.*, **52**, 489–503.

Brusa, A., Jones, S. J., Kapoor, R. *et al.* (1999). Long-term recovery and fellow eye deterioration after optic neuritis, determined by serial visual evoked potentials. *J. Neurol.*, **246**, 776–82.

Buchthal, F. and Kühl, V. (1979). Nerve conduction, tactile sensibility and the electromyogram after suture or compression of peripheral nerve: a longitudinal study in man. *J. Neurol. Neurosurg. Psychiat.*, **42**, 436–51.

Carpenter, J. P., Lexa, F. J, and Davis, J. T. (1996). Determination of duplex Doppler ultrasound criteria appropriate to the North American Symptomatic Carotid Endarterectomy Trial. *Stroke*, **27**, 695–9.

Chinnery, P. and Turnbull, D. (1997). Clinical features, investigation and management of patients with defects of mitochondrial DNA. *J. Neurol. Neurosurg. Psychiat.*, **63**, 559–63.

Cipolotti, L. and Warrington, E. K. (1995). Neuropsychological assessment. *J. Neurol. Neurosurg. Psychiat.*, **58**, 655–64.

Cloft, H. J., Joseph, G. J, and Dion, J. E. (1999). Risk of cerebral angiography in patients with subarachnoid hemorrhage, cerebral aneurysm, and arteriovenous malformation: a meta-analysis. *Stroke*, **30**, 317–20.

Conneally, M. (1993). *Molecular basis of neuorology*. Blackwell Scientific Publications, Boston.

Cornblath, D. R., Sumner, A. J., Daube, J. *et al.* (1991). Conduction block in clinical practice. *Muscle and Nerve*, **14**, 869–71.

Cornblath, D. R., Kuncl, R. W., Mellits, E. D. *et al.* (1992). Nerve conduction studies in amyotrophic lateral sclerosis. *Muscle and Nerve*, **15**, 1111–15.

Cowan, J. M. A., Dick, J. P. R., Day, B. L. *et al.* (1984). Abnormalities in central motor pathway conduction in multiple sclerosis. *Lancet*, **2**, 304–7.

Davies, K. N. and Humphrey, P. R. (1993). Complications of cerebral angiography in patients with symptomatic carotid territory ischaemia screened by carotid ultrasound. *J. Neurol. Neurosurg. Psychiat.*, **56**, 967–72.

Davies, K. and Read, A. (1992). *Molecular basis of inherited disease*. Oxford University Press, Oxford.

Donaghy, M. (1997). *Neurology*. Oxford University Press, Oxford.

Duncan, J. S. (1997). Imaging and epilepsy. *Brain*, **120**, 339–77.

Ebersole, J. F. and Pedley, T. A. (2001). *Current Practice of Clinical Electroencephalography*, (3rd edn.), p. 72, Lippincott, Williams, and Wilkins.

Elgersma, O. E. H., Van Leersum, M., Buijs, P. C. *et al.* (1998). Changes over time in optimal duplex threshold for the identification of patients eligible for carotid endarterectomy. *Stroke*, **29**, 2352–6.

Fishman, R. A. (1992). *Cerebrospinal fluid in diseases of the nervous system*, (2nd edn). W. B. Saunders, Philadelphia.

Fox, N. C., Freeborough, P. A., and Rossor, M. N. (1996). Visualisation and quantification of rates of atrophy in Alzheimer's disease. *Lancet*, **348**, 94–7.

Friedman, S. G. (1990). Transient ischaemic attacks resulting from carotid duplex imaging. *Surgery*, **107**, 153–5.

Furst, G., Saleh, A., Wenserski, F. *et al.* (1999). Reliability and validity of noninvasive imaging of internal carotid artery pseudo-occlusion. *Stroke*, **30**, 1444–9.

Furst, H., Hartl, W. H., Jansen, I. *et al.* (1992). Color-flow Doppler sonography in the identification of ulcerative plaques in patients with high-grade carotid artery stenosis. *Am. J. Neuroradiol.*, **13**, 1581–7.

Gerraty, R. P., Bowser, D. N., Infeld, B. *et al.* (1996). Microemboli during carotid angiography. Association with stroke risk factors or subsequent magnetic resonance imaging changes? *Stroke*, **27**, 1543–7.

Gerriets, T., Seidel, G., Fiss, I. *et al.* (1999). Contrast-enhanced transcranial color-coded duplex sonography: efficiency and validity. *Neurology*, **52**, 1133–7.

Graves, M. J. (1997). Magnetic resonance angiography. *Br. J. Radiol.*, **70**, 6–28.

Griewing, B., Morgenstern, C., Driesner, F. *et al.* (1996). Cerebrovascular disease assessed by color-flow and power Doppler ultrasonography: Comparison with digital subtraction angiography in internal carotid artery stenosis. *Stroke*, **27**, 95–100.

Griffiths, P. D., Worthy, S., and Gholkar, A. (1996). Incidental intracranial vascular pathology in patients investigated for carotid stenosis. *Neuroradiology*, **38**, 25–30.

Gronholdt, M. L. (1999.) Ultrasound and lipoproteins as predictors of lipid-rich, rupture-prone plaques in the carotid artery. *Arterioscl. Thromb. Vasc. Biol.*, **19**, 2–13.

Halliday, A. M., McDonald, W. I., and Mushin, J. (1972). Delayed visual evoked response in optic neuritis. *Lancet*, **i**, 982–985.

Halliday, A. M., McDonald, W. I., and Mushin, J. (1973). Visual evoked response in diagnosis of multiple sclerosis. *BMJ*, **4**, 661–4.

Halliday, A. M., Halliday, E., and Kriss, A. *et al.* (1976). The pattern-evoked potential in compression of the anterior visual pathways. *Brain*, **99**, 357–374.

Hankey, G. J., Warlow, C. P. and Molyneux, A. (1990a). Complications of cerebral angiography for patients with mild carotid territory ischaemia being considered for carotid endarterectomy. *J. Neurol. Neurosurg. Psychiat.*, **53**, 542–8.

Hankey, G. J., Warlow, C. P., and Sellar, R. J. (1990b). Cerebral angiographic risk in mild cerebrovascular disease. *Stroke*, **21**, 209–22.

Heiken, J. P., Brink, J. A., and Vannier, M. W. (1993). Spiral (Helical) CT. *Radiology*, **189**, 647–56.

Heinze, H. J., Munte, T. F., Kutas, M. *et al.* (1999). Cognitive event-related potentials. In *Recommendations for the practice of clinical neurophysiology. Guidelines of the International Federation of Clinical Neurophysiology*, (EEG Suppl. 52), (ed. G. Deuschl and A. Eisen), pp. 91–5. Elsevier Science BV, Amsterdam.

Heiserman, J. E., Dean, B. L., Hodak, J. A. *et al.* (1994). Neurologic complications of cerebral angiography. *Am. J. Neuroradiol.*, **15**, 1401–7.

Hilton-Jones, D. (1984). What is postlumbar puncture headache and is it avoidable? In *Dilemmas in the management of the neurological patient*, (ed. C. Warlow and J. Garfield). Churchill Livingstone, Edinburgh.

Hodges, J. R. (1994). *Cognitive assessment for clinicians.* Oxford University Press, Oxford.

Howard, G., Baker, W. H., Chambless, L. E, *et al.* (1996). An approach for the use of Doppler ultrasound as a screening tool for hemodynamically significant stenosis (despite heterogeneity of Doppler performance). A multicenter experience. Asymptomatic Carotid Atherosclerosis Study Investigators. *Stroke*, **27**, 1951–7.

Karnik, R., Winkler, W. B., Valentin, A. *et al.* (1995). Carotid sinus massage and the risk of cerebral embolization. *Stroke*, **26**, 1124–5.

Kennett, R. P. (1996). Electromyography. In Handbook of muscle disease, (ed. R. J. M. Lane). Dekker, New York.

Khaffaf, N., Karnik, R., Winkler, W. B. *et al.* (1994). Embolic stroke by compression maneuver during transcranial Doppler sonography. *Stroke*, **25**, 1056–7.

Kimura, J. (1983). *Electrodiagnosis in diseases of nerve and muscle.* Davis, Philadelphia.

Kriss, A., Francis, D. A., Cuendet, F. *et al.* (1988). Recovery after optic neuritis in childhood. *J. Neurol. Neurosurg. Psychiat.*, **51**, 1253–8.

Leclerc, X., Godefroy, O., Pruvo, J. P. *et al.* (1995). Computed tomographic angiography for the evaluation of carotid artery stenosis. *Stroke*, **26**, 1577–81.

Leonard, J. V. and Schapira, A. H. V. (2000). Mitochondrial respiratory chanin disorders 1: mitochondrial DNA defects. *Lancet*, **355**, 299–304.

Levi, C. R., Mitchell, A., Fitt, G., *et al.* (1996). The accuracy of magnetic resonance angiography in the assessment of extracranial carotid artery occlusive disease. *Cerebrovasc. Dis.*, **6**, 231–6.

Lewis, R. A. and Sumner, A. J. (1982). The electrodiagnostic distinctions between chronic familial and acquired demyelinative neuropathies. *Neurology*, **32**, 592–6.

Ley-Pozo, J. and Ringelstein, E. B. (1990). Noninvasive detection of occlusive disease of the carotid siphon and middle cerebral artery. *Ann. Neurol.*, **28**, 640–7.

Liveson, J. A. and Ma, D. M. (1992). *Laboratory reference for clinical neurophysiology.* F. A. Davis, Philadelphia.

McCarthy, R. A. and Warrington, E. K. (1990). *Cognitive neuropsychology. A clinical introduction.* Academic Press, London.

McDonald, W. I. (1998). In *McAlpine's multiple sclerosis*, (ed. D. A. S. Compston, G. C. Ebers, H. Lassmann, *et al.*), pp. 251–79. Churchill Livingstone, London.

McPherson, D. and Starr, A. (1993). Auditory evoked potentials in the clinic. In *Evoked potentials in clinical testing*, (ed. A. M. Halliday), pp. 359–81. Churchill Livingstone, Edinburgh.

Merton, P. A. and Morton, H. B. (1980). Stimulation of the cerebral cortex in the intact human subject. *Nature*, **285**, 227.

Miller, D. H., Albert, P. S., Barkhof, F. *et al.* (1996). Guidelines for using magnetic resonance techniques in monitoring the treatment of multiple sclerosis. *Ann. Neurol.*, **39**, 6–16.

Molloy, J. and Markus, H. S. (1999). Asymptomatic embolization predicts stroke and TIA risk in patients with carotid artery stenosis. *Stroke*, **30**, 1440–3.

Moniz, E. (1934). *L'angiographie cerebrale*. Masson and Cie, Paris.

Nelson, H. E. and O'Connell, A. (1978). Dementia: the estimation of premorbid intelligence levels using the New Adult Reading Test. *Cortex*, **14**, 234–44.

Ouvrier, R. A., McLeod, J. G., and Pollard, J. D. (1990). *Peripheral neuropathy in childhood*. Raven, New York.

Pelz, D. M., Fox, A. J., and Vinuela, F. (1985). Digital subtraction angiography: Current clinical applications. *Stroke*, **16**, 528–36.

Provencher, S. L. (1993). Estimation of metabolite concentrations from localised *in vivo* proton NMR spectra. *Magnet. Reson. Med.*, **30**, 672–9.

Ringelstein, E. B. (1995). Skepticism toward carotid ultrasonography: A virtue, an attitude, or fanaticism? *Stroke*, **26**, 1743–6.

Robinson, K. and Rudge, P. (1977). Abnormalities of the auditory evoked potentials in patients with multiple sclerosis. *Brain*, **100**, 19–40.

Rosario, J. A., Hachinski, V. A., Lee, D. H. *et al.* (1987). Adverse reactions to Duplex scanning. *Lancet*, **2**, 1023.

Rothwell, P. M. (2000). Analysis and presentation of data in studies of imaging and measurement of carotid stenosis: lessons for the validation of continuous measurements in cerebrovascular disease. *J. Neurol.*, in press.

Rothwell, P. M., Gibson, R. J., Villagra, R. *et al.* (1998). The effect of angiographic technique and image quality on the reproducibility of measurement of carotid stenosis and assessment of plaque surface morphology. *Clin. Radiol.*, **53**, 439–43.

Rothwell, P. M., Pendlebury, S. T., Wardlaw, J. *et al.* (2000). A critical appraisal of the design and reporting of studies of imaging and measurements of carotid stenosis. *Stroke*, **31**, 1444–50.

Ryan, J. J., Paolo, A. M., and Brungardt, T. M. (1990). Standardization of the Wechsler adult intelligence scale-revised for persons 75 years and older. *Psychol Assess. J. Consult. Clin. Psychol.*, **2**, 408–11.

Sellar, R. J. (1995). Imaging blood vessels of the head and neck. *J. Neurol. Neurosurg. Psychiat.*, **59**, 225–37.

Siewert, B., Patel, M. R., and Warach, S. (1995). Magnetic resonance angiography. *The Neurologist*, **1**, 167–84.

Small, D. G., Matthews, W. B., and Small, M. (1978). The cervical somatosensory evoked potential in the diagnosis of multiple sclerosis. *J. Neurol. Sci.*, **35**, 211–24.

Thompson, P. D., Day, B. L., Rothwell, J. C. *et al.* (1987). The interpretation of electromyographic responses to electrical stimulation of the motor cortex in diseases of the upper motor neurone. *J. Neurol. Sci.*, **80**, 91–110.

Wardlaw, J. M. and White, P. M. (2000). The detection and management of unruptured intracranial aneurysms. *Brain*, **123**, 205–21.

Warnock, N. G., Gandhi, M. R., Bergvall, U. *et al.* (1993). Complications of intraarterial digital subtraction angiography in patients investigated for cerebral vascular disease. *Br. J. Radiol.*, **66**, 855–8.

Warrington, E. K. (1984). *Recognition Memory Test*. NFER-Nelson, Windsor, UK.

World Federation research group on Huntington's disease (1990). Ethical issues policy statement of Huntington's disease molecular genetics predictive test. *J. Med. Genet.*, **27**, 34–8.

Zeviani, M. and Taroni, F. (1994). *Mitochondrial diseases*. *Baillières Clin. Neurol.*, **3**, 315–34.

Headache

Martin Rossor

3.1 Introduction

3.1.1 Prevalence and economic burden

It is a rarity never to have suffered a headache. Indeed, so common is it that a headache at sometime can be viewed as a normal phenomenon. A lifetime prevalence study revealed that as many as 93 per cent of men experienced a headache at some time; the most common cause being tension-type headache (69 per cent). For women, the lifetime prevalence was 99 per cent, again tension-type headache being the most common (88 per cent) (Rasmussen *et al.* 1991). Although such a high prevalence suggests a commonplace, almost trivial, symptom, it can nevertheless be a symptom of grave significance. It is thus a major cause for attendance in neurological outpatient clinics, representing approximately 15 per cent of routine neurological attendance (Murray 1977; Perkin 1989) and reflecting the anxiety amongst both patients and doctors that headache may be due to a sinister cause. Thus every patient with headache requires careful consideration and sometimes thorough investigation (reviewed by Silberstein *et al.* 1998). Headache in children is considered in Section 4.3.

Although most patients with headache will not contact their doctor, those with frequent headache, and those with migraine constitute a significant public health and economic problem. A pharmoco-economic study of migraine in the USA calculated that the annual loss of productivity due to migraine cost more than $1 billion per year (Stang *et al.* 1996) and some studies have suggested that the cost might be as much as $17 billion per year (Osterhaus *et al.* 1992).

3.1.2 Classification

In 1985, the International Headache Society (IHS) established a classification committee which published the first international headache classification in 1988, including operational diagnostic criteria (Headache Classification Committee of the International Headache Society 1988) (Table 3.1). This has been adopted by the World Federation of Neurology and the World Health Organization, which has incorporated the main features in the international classification of diseases (ICD-10). The classification provides 13 broad categories which are then subdivided to allow for coding up to a four-digit level. The extent of the subclassification thus depends upon the degree of sophistication required. The classification has been an important advance, primarily for research but increasingly for clinical management. It is gradually replacing the previous variable terminology which included classic migraine, classical migraine, combined headache, psychogenic headache, and essential headache.

Revisions of the IHS classification have been proposed. For example, refocusing on the old problem of patients with very frequent headache, often referred to as chronic daily headache (Silberstein *et al.* 1994, 1995), or addition of new entities, such as the short-lasting unilateral neuralgiform headache attacks with conjunctival injection and tearing (SUNCT) syndrome (Goadsby and Lipton 1997).

Table 3.1. Classification of headache (data from Headache Classification Committee of the International Headache Society 1988)

Migraine
Tension-type headache
Cluster headache and chronic paroxysmal hemicrania
Headache associated with head trauma
Headache associated with vascular disorders
Headache associated with non-vascular intracranial disorders
Headache associated with substances and their withdrawal
Headache associated with non-cephalic infection
Headache associated with metabolic abnormality
Headache or facial pain associated with disorders of cranium, neck, eyes, ears, nose sinuses, teeth, mouth, or other facial or cranial structures
Cranial neuralgias, nerve trunk pain, and deafferentation pain
Other types of headache or facial pain
Headache not classifiable

3.1.3 Anatomy and physiology of headache

All the tissues covering the cranium are sensitive to pain, especially the arteries but also the muscles and pericranium. The skull bone itself is insensitive. Within the cranium, the venous sinuses and their tributaries, the dura mater and the cerebral arteries, and the fifth, ninth, and tenth cranial nerves are the chief pain-sensitive structures. The main factors causing headache (Lance 1981) have been considered to be:

(1) inflammation involving pain-sensitive structures of the head;

(2) referred pain;

(3) meningeal irritation;

(4) traction on or dilatation of blood vessels;

(5) pressure upon or distortion of pain-sensitive structures caused by tumours or other lesions; and

(6) psychological causes, when the pain is considered in some instances to be due to tension in the muscles of the scalp and neck.

However, such a classical view of headache production does not readily explain the mechanisms of headache in migraine and tension-type headache. A more precise understanding is now emerging which implicates all levels of the innervation of cranial structures (reviewed by Goadsby and Silberstain, 1997). The somatosensory innervation to the head is primarily the trigeminal nerve and upper cervical spinal-cord segments. The original studies by Penfield and colleagues on awake patients during surgery identified that traction of the pain-sensitive meninges and meningeal vessels could give rise to severe headache, but by contrast, the brain parenchyma was not pain sensitive. The trigeminal innervation of the meninges and meningovascular structures is via small, unmyelinated C fibres

**PAIN PROCESSING AND MECHANISMS
AND BRAINSTEM CONTROL**

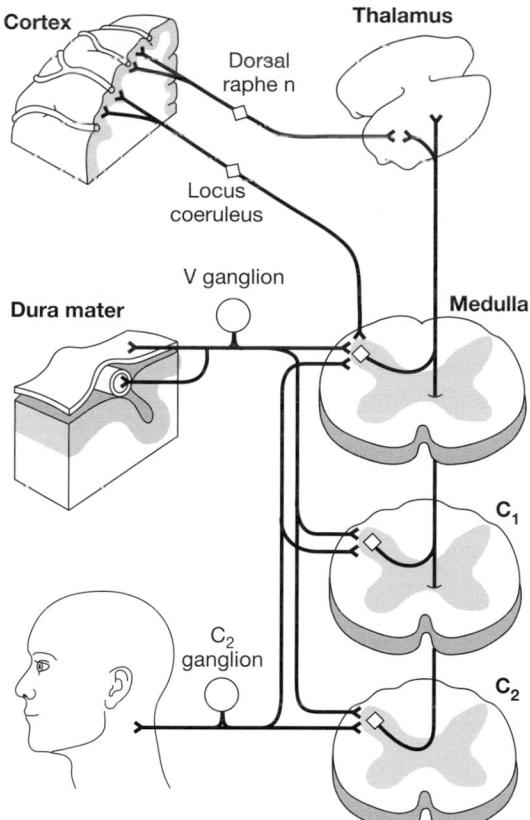

Fig. 3.1. Diagram of the main connections of the trigeminovascular system. (Reproduced with permission from Silberstein, Lipton, and Goadsby (1998) *Headache in clinical practice*, Figure 5.12. Isis Medical Media, Oxford.)

to the caudal trigeminal nucleus, which extends into the upper spinal cord; the spinal nucleus relating to afferents from the posterior fossa (Arbab *et al.* 1986). Activation of the caudal trigeminal nucleus and the dorsal horn at the C1/2 level can be demonstrated by c-*fos* immunocytochemistry, a method for showing activation of cells following stimulation of both vessels and meninges in animals (Strassman and Vos 1993). Activation of trigeminovascular fibres is also accompanied by release of the neuropeptides, substance P, and calcitonin-gene-related peptide (CGRP) (Goadsby *et al.* 1988). The second-order pathway from the caudal trigeminal nucleus is via the quintothalamic tract primarily to the ventroposteromedial nucleus of the thalamus (Zagami and Lambert 1990) (Fig. 3.1).

Sensitization of the trigeminal pathway may be important in the generation of some headaches, for example that associated with migraine which can be exacerbated by coughing and sudden head movement. Exacerbation by movement is a classic feature of the headache associated with intracranial pathology, when it is thought to be due to the mechanical stimulation of meningeal vessels. In animals, recording of primary afferent neurons in the trigeminal ganglion has shown that chemical

stimulation of the dural receptive field with inflammatory mediators directly excites the neurons, but in addition, enhances their mechanical sensitivity. Thus neurons may be strongly activated by mechanical stimuli that normally excite little or no response (Strassman *et al.* 1996).

In addition to mapping the early components of pain processing, cognitive factors are increasingly recognized as being important in the central modulation of headache pain. Attentional mechanisms are important, particularly the anticipation of pain. For example, in the study by Bayer *et al.* (1991), normal volunteers who had dummy electrodes placed on their heads, experienced headache if they were told that they would be electrically stimulated. Moreover, patients with frequent and severe tension-type headaches have been found to show high scores on questionnaires that measure fear of pain (Hursey and Jacks 1992).

3.1.4 **Differential diagnosis and clinical approach**

In taking the history, attention must be paid to the following points. How long has the patient suffered from headache? Is it increasing in severity? Is it constant or paroxysmal and, if paroxysmal, what is the duration of the attacks and do they occur at any special time of day? Are the headaches precipitated by any circumstance or activity, and how, if at all, can they be relieved? What is the character of the headache and its situation? Is there associated tenderness of the scalp or skull, with visual disturbances, vomiting, or vertigo? Has there been a head injury? Are there symptoms of nasal obstruction or discharge, either from the nose or into the pharynx? Is the patient anxious, tense, or depressed? Physical examination should include a general assessment which must include the blood pressure.

Investigations will be dictated by the history and the findings; ranging from the ESR and temporal artery biopsy in patients whose history is indicative of cranial arteritis, through to neuroimaging. The decision of when to undertake neuroimaging can be difficult. Many features may influence the decision, including the anxiety of the patient and referring physician. However, patients with long-standing symptoms of tension-type headache are rarely found to have an underlying structural lesion. Similarly, patients with a typical history of migraine need not undergo neuroimaging. Thus, in a study of 547 patients with a typical history and normal examinations, only four had an abnormality on CT scan (Alter *et al.* 1994). Clearly the presence of a neurological deficit demands imaging, as does recent onset in the elderly or headache, without the features of migraine, that awaken the patient early in the morning or is becoming relentlessly more severe.

3.2 **Tension headache and depression**

Headache is an extremely common phenomenon, experienced by most people, particularly in settings of stress and fatigue.

Tension headache in children is considered in Section 4.3.3. One of the most common is a sense of pressure over the vertex or the sense of a tight band that is present most of the day, but is usually worse in the evening. It is quite often felt in association with anxiety and in some patients with depression, although it may be difficult to know which is cause and effect. The IHS classification uses the term 'tension-type headache', to imply in some patients an abnormality of pericranial muscle. It is classified either as episodic or chronic. It is likely that the underlying pathophysiology is heterogeneous. Although there may be sensitive trigger points in pericranial muscles, it has been difficult to demonstrate abnormalities consistently with electromyogram (EMG) studies. Patients with other headaches, such as migraine, often suffer from coexistent tension-type headache. The headache does not usually interfere with daily activity and is less often exacerbated by physical activity than migraine. Similarly, photophobia, phonophobia, and nausea are much less prominent than with migraine and typically the headache is bilateral rather than unilateral.

Tension headache can be difficult to treat. Simple analgesics may provide relief, and ibuprofen is generally the first choice before aspirin (Nebe *et al.* 1995). The use of a tricyclic antidepressant as a prophylactic, starting at a low dose (for example 10–25 mg of amitriptyline), can be beneficial (Lance and Curran 1964). A danger in the treatment of tension-type headache, however, is a vicious circle of increasing medication, with the emergence of drug-induced headache which can change the pattern of episodic tension type headache into a chronic one. Drug-induced headache is most commonly recognized in headache clinics, where patients present with a long history which has often started with migraine or, less commonly, tension-type headache (Olesen 1995). The withdrawal of analgesics in regular users can result in a rebound headache, thus leading to sustained high levels of analgesic consumption. Withdrawal of caffeine, which is used in a number of migraine medications, can also result in rebound headache (Silverman *et al.* 1992). A careful analgesic drug history is important, and although withdrawal of analgesics and/or caffeine may initially exacerbate symptoms, it can often change chronic tension headache into a more manageable episodic pattern.

Patients with established depressive illness will often have coexistent headache, which can assume a delusional quality. Sometimes these patients will present with night-time headache or early morning headache due to the disturbance of sleep pattern with early morning wakening. Fitzpatrick and Hopkins (1981) found that, in a follow-up study of patients with headache not due to defined structural disease, many feared organic disease but few had overt psychiatric symptoms.

3.3 Migraine

3.3.1 Introduction

Migraine has been known to medical science for nearly 2000 years. In the first century of the Christian era, Aretaeus of

Table 3.2. Classification of migraine (data from Headache Classification Committee of the International Headache Society 1988)

Migraine without aura
Migraine with aura
Migraine with typical aura
Migraine with prolonged aura
Familial hemiplegic migraine
Basilar migraine
Migraine aura without headache
Migraine with acute-onset aura
Ophthalmoplegic migraine
Retinal migraine
Childhood periodic syndromes that may be precursors to or be associated with migraine
Benign paroxysmal vertigo of childhood
Alternating hemiplegia of childhood
Complications of migraine
Status migrainosus
Migrainous infarction
Unclassifiable migraine-like disorder

Cappadocia referred to it as heterocrania, and the term hemicrania (from which the word migraine was derived) was introduced by Galen (AD 131–201). A key feature of migraine headache is that it is periodic, with attacks lasting usually between 4 and 72 hours. Typical features, although not exclusive, are that it is unilateral and pulsatile. Operational diagnostic criteria (International Headache Classification) require that the headache is accompanied by nausea or vomiting and/or photophobia or phonophobia. The headache itself may or may not be associated with an aura of preceding neurological symptoms. During the latter, characteristic changes in cerebral blood flow may be demonstrated.

The International Headache Classification (Headache Classification Committee of the International Headache Society 1988) distinguishes between migraine with aura and migraine without aura (Table 3.2). The former subsumes a number of migraine subtypes or variants. This classification replaces the earlier terms of classic/classical migraine, referring to those with aura, and common or simple migraine, referring to those without. The new classification is quite explicit and avoids confusion. Migraine with and without aura can, of course, both occur in an individual patient.

Migraine is extremely common. Recent epidemiological studies, using the IHS criteria, suggest a prevalence in women of between 15 and 20% and in men between 5 and 10% (Stewart *et al.* 1992) and in some studies even higher in women (Rasmussen *et al.* 1991). Migraine in children is considered in Section 4.3.2. There is a strong family history reported in migraine sufferers, particularly in those suffering from migraine with aura (Russell and Olesen 1995).

3.3.2 **Pathophysiology**

The traditional view of the pathophysiology of migraine has been that of arterial spasm within the internal carotid territory resulting in the aura, followed by dilatation in the distribution of the external carotid artery, resulting in the headache. The original evidence in support of this included the observation that amyl nitrite could temporarily abolish the visual scotoma and that cerebral infarction or occlusion of retinal arteries could both occur during the aura phase. Schumacher and Wolff (1941) showed that the headache is due to arterial dilatation, mainly of the extracerebral arteries of the dura and scalp, and other branches of the external carotid, with the clinical concomitants of congestion of the conjunctiva and nasal mucosa in some patients and pulsation of the superficial temporal artery on the same side that the headache is experienced. The specific therapeutic effect of ergotamine is thus interpreted as being due to the constriction of the branches of the external carotid artery. This simple interpretation, particularly with respect to vasoconstriction, has been challenged following the seminal observations by Olesen *et al.* (1981) of focal hyperaemia followed by a slow spread of reduced blood flow which outlasts the aura. This slow spread of oligemia which transcends specific arterial territories has been compared to the spreading depression of Leao (Leao 1944). Spreading depression occurs as an experimental phenomenon in the rodent following direct stimulation of the brain. Neuronal depolarization is followed by suppression of neuronal activity, which spreads at a rate of approximately 3–4 mm/min, independently of the vascular territory. This is similar to the rate of spread of reduced blood flow and the calculated rate of spread of neuronal dysfunction in the occipital cortex to account for the slow progression of the visual scotomata. The opportunistic study of a patient undergoing a positron emission tomography study who developed a migraine,

has confirmed bilateral hypoperfusion starting in the occipital lobes and spreading anteriorly at a constant rate, independent of cerebral artery territory. The maximal decreases in flow were in the order of 40 per cent (Woods *et al.* 1994) (Fig. 3.2). Similar studies with functional magnetic resonance imaging demonstrate significant reductions in perfusion during the aura phase (Cutrer *et al.* 1998). Additional evidence relating these changes directly to alterations in neuronal excitability have been provided by magnetoencephalography with suppression of neuronal signal during the migraine aura (Barkley *et al.* 1990). These imaging studies during migraine headache with aura, increasingly support the view that perfusion changes are secondary to a primary neuronal dysfunction.

A number of biochemical correlates of the migraine attack have been observed. The most consistent and extensively explored has been that relating to serotonin (5-hydroxytryptamine; 5-HT) (Raskin 1991). Serotonin constricts large arteries and dilates arterioles and capillaries, and there is a widespread subcortico-cortical projection system from the midbrain raphe nucleus which utilizes serotonin as its neurotransmitter. The urinary excretion of the serotonin metabolite 5-hydroxyindolacetic acid is increased in severe attacks, indicating release of serotonin into the circulation (Sicuteri *et al.* 1961). Injection of reserpine, which causes release of serotonin, can also precipitate attacks in vulnerable subjects. Platelets release serotonin, and platelet aggregation is abnormal in migraineurs. Platelets have also been demonstrated to have decreased monoamine oxidase activity (Glover *et al.* 1977). These observations of platelet abnormality and the fact that they release serotonin has given rise to the theory that peripheral platelet function is a principal factor in the pathogenesis of migraine (Hanington 1986). It now seems unlikely that an impairment of peripheral function is directly responsible,

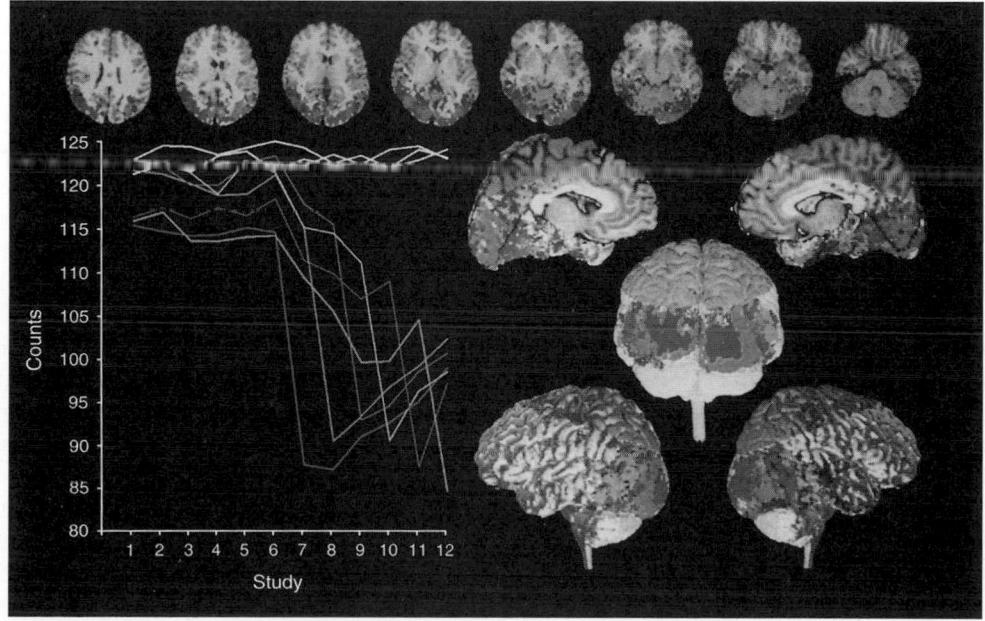

Fig. 3.2. Spreading oligaemia in a young woman during a spontaneous migraine attack demonstrated by positron emission tomography. (Reproduced with permission from Woods, R. P. *et al.* (1994). Bilateral spread cerebral hypoperfusion during spontaneous migraine headache. *N. Engl. J. Med.*, **331**, 1689–1692, Figure 1.) Also shown in colour in Plate 1.

although it might reflect a more general abnormality of serotonin function. Alternatively, these peripheral events may be neurally mediated since trigeminal stimulation leads to platelet aggregation and mast-cell degranulation (Dimitriadou *et al.* 1992). Importantly, sumatriptan and other newer drugs of the same class are potent 5-HT$_1$ agonists. Recent cloning of the 5-HT receptor subtypes has resulted in more precise classification and, specifically, sumatriptan and its analogues are 5-HT$_{1B}$ (vascular) and 5-HT$_{1D}$ (presynaptic neuronal) agonists (Hartig *et al.* 1996).

There is no generally accepted theory that encompasses all of the observed vascular changes and the central and biochemical correlates of migraine. However, considerable advance has been made from the animal model of head pain developed by Moskowitz (1984). In this model, electrical stimulation of the trigeminal ganglion results in local vasodilatation and plasma extravasation (neurogenic inflammation) via an axon reflex. A refinement of this trigeminovascular model involves a stretching stimulus to the sagittal sinus (Goadsby and Zagami 1991). A variety of vasoactive peptides, including calcitonin-gene-related peptide, are shown to be released using this model (Goadsby *et al.* 1988). The release of peptides and the plasma extravasation can be blocked by sumatriptan.

Stimulation of the superior sagittal sinus or meningeal irritation also causes activation of the caudal trigeminal nucleus and its extension into the upper cervical cord. This can be demonstrated by c-*fos* immunocytochemistry which indirectly demonstrates cellular activation. Activation can also be blocked by antimigraine drugs such as dihydroergotamine (Hoskin *et al.* 1996). Since the sinus and trigeminal nerve supply are stimulated directly, the pharmacological antagonism must be central. Importantly, neocortical spreading depression will also provoke c-*fos* immunoreactivity within the trigeminal nucleus (Moskowitz *et al.* 1993). Recently, a PET study during an acute migraine headache attack demonstrated an increase in cerebral blood flow within medial brainstem structures which persisted for a time after symptom relief with sumatriptan. The precise location of the increased blood flow was beyond the resolution of the imaging system, but might have related to the locus coeruleus and dorsal raphe nuclei (Weiller *et al.* 1995).

No adequate theory yet exists to encompass all of these observations and, no doubt, many further molecular candidates will be proposed. The discovery of the importance of nitric oxide as a transmitter, both centrally and peripherally, has also directed attention to a possible role in migraine (Olesen *et al.* 1994).

Finally, important advances can be anticipated arising from the impact of molecular genetics on our understanding of migraine. A major clue has come from studies of families with cerebral autosomal dominant arteriopathy with subcortical infarcts and leucoencephalopathy (CADASIL). The clinical phenotype in some pedigrees has included migraine (Chabriat *et al.* 1995); in some this has had the features of familial hemiplegic migraine and in others a predisposition to arteriographic complications. Following demonstration of linkage to chromosome 19 in CADASIL families, similar linkage was observed in patients with familial hemiplegic migraine. The gene for CADASIL has recently been cloned, and shown to be the *Notch 3* gene (Joutel *et al.* 1996), a gene with some functional similarities to the presenilins (see Chapter 26). The potential relationship of mutations in this gene to those families with coincidental migraine is unclear. By contrast, the linkage to chromosome 19 in families with hemiplegic migraine has been established as being due to mutations in a brain-specific P/Q-type calcium channel α1-subunit gene, *CACNL1A4* (Ophoff *et al.* 1996). The role of this channel in migraine pathophysiology is not yet clear, but progress can be anticipated from transgenic mouse models.

3.3.3 Clinical features

The age of onset is often at, or shortly after, puberty and less frequently in middle or later life (Stewart *et al.* 1992), although in women onset around the menopause does occur, sometimes without the accompanying headache, which can lead to diagnostic difficulties. Migraine is less common before puberty, but cyclical vomiting and travel sickness are common in children who subsequently develop migraine. The frequency of attacks varies enormously; in an unlucky few, they may occur two or three times a week, whereas others may have only one or two attacks in a lifetime. One or two attacks per month is a common pattern. They may be more frequent at the time of menstruation and commonly diminish in frequency during pregnancy. The general pattern is towards reduction in frequency with age, and sometimes the headache disappears leaving only an aura (Fisher 1980).

It is often said that migraine sufferers have a perfectionist or obsessional character, but in a disease that is so common this is difficult to establish. Certainly migraine can occur after a period of excitement or excessive work. Sometimes this is due to extra sleep at a time of relaxation, so-called weekend migraine. Minor trauma can also precipitate migraine (Matthews 1972), as can bright lights and, in some patients, strong smells, such as wet paint. Dietary precipitants are often sought, but rarely found. Those thought to be responsible include dairy products, particularly cheese, chocolate, fruit, and most commonly caffeine and alcohol. Missing meals may also precipitate an attack.

Headache is the most characteristic symptom of migraine and the one from which it derives its name. It may be the only manifestation, where it is referred to as migraine without aura (common migraine); indeed this is probably four times as common as migraine with aura (classical migraine). The headache may be preceded by premonitory symptoms—the most common of which are lassitude, hunger, and slight looseness of the bowels. On occasions the patient may feel exceptionally well and energetic before an attack. The onset may occur during the day, but can awake the patient in the morning, particularly from a heavy, deep sleep. Rarely, the attack may awaken the patient during the night. Typically the pain is localized to one side, often in the temple, and starts as a boring pain, which then gradually spreads until the whole side of the head is affected. As it increases in intensity it tends to acquire a throbbing character, which is intensified by stooping and by all forms of exertion. Although usually unilateral, a significant number of cases become bilateral and often, late in an attack, the pain moves posteriorly to an occipital distribution. The headache builds up to a maximum over about 30 min and lasts from hours to 1 or 2 days. It is usually relieved by sleep, although patients may be left feeling fatigued and with a mild headache on awaking the next day. In the majority of cases nausea occurs, but only in about 50 per cent is there vomiting. There is occasional diarrhoea. Photophobia and phonophobia occur during the attacks and patients usually prefer to lie quietly in the dark, in contrast to cluster headache, when the patient will move around.

Vasomotor changes are often conspicuous. The face is often pale and the extremities cold, until improvement begins, but congestion of the face, conjunctiva, and nasal mucosa may occur, often confined to the side of the headaches. There may even be subconjunctival haemorrhage or bruising around the eyes. The superficial temporal artery on the affected side is often seen to be congested and pulsating vigorously, and some patients can obtain temporary relief by pressing over the temporal artery or the carotid, although release of compression often results in worsening of the headache after a minute or so. There is quite often polyuria following recovery from the attack.

When the headache is accompanied by an aura (migraine with aura) this usually precedes, but may accompany, the headache. The headache is indistinguishable from that which occurs with migraine without aura, although it may be more commonly unilateral. Patients often have a combination of headache attacks, both with and without auras.

Visual disturbances are the commonest auras. These are usually homonymous, involving the corresponding halves of both visual fields, although patients often experience them as being worse in one eye than the other. The visual disturbance is commonly characterized by positive phenomena at the outset, with a bright spot appearing near the centre, or in the periphery, which gradually expands, the advancing edge exhibiting scintillating figures (teichopsia) which may be coloured and angular. The zigzag patterns are characteristic and referred to as fortification spectra. The spreading scintillation leaves behind it an area of blindness, so that when it reaches the periphery or the centre of the half-fields the patient is hemianopic, although this is often more difficult to demonstrate on examination. The progression of the visual disturbance lasts from 15 to 20 min and the hemianopia then gradually fades away, the whole disturbance lasting about half an hour, although objects in the affected fields may appear less bright than normal for several hours. The disturbance may have a homonymous quadrantic distribution, or much less commonly, all peripheral vision is lost in both fields, leaving only a 'telescopic' field of vision. Exceptionally, the hemianopia is bilateral, giving temporary blindness. Patients may also experience macropsia or micropsia.

Auras of paraesthesiae and numbness occur next in frequency. These symptoms occur in a 'cortical' distribution, involving the periphery of the limbs and the circumoral region. The upper limb is more often affected, paraesthesiae beginning in the fingers and gradually spreading up the limb, taking 5–20 min to do so. The proximal part of the arm is often relatively spared. The lips, face, and tongue may be subsequently affected on one or both sides, or can be involved without the upper limb. Frequently, patients give a history of only half of the tongue being affected. The lower limb is only rarely affected. Paraesthesiae usually develop shortly after the onset of the visual disturbances, but may occur without the latter as the first symptom, or after the headache has been present for several hours. Olfactory and auditory hallucinations have been reported, but are rare. Mild weakness of the limb, usually the upper, may develop following the paraesthesiae, and in rare instances transient hemiparesis occurs with each attack ('hemiplegic migraine', see below). Aphasia is usually of the expressive type and is accompanied by dysgraphia. In right-handed people it is usually associated with visual disturbance in the right hemifield and paraesthesiae in the right hand and face. Patients often complain of difficulties with concentration, and may feel disorientated in space and time.

The characteristic feature of migraine attacks is the slow speed of the developing neurological disturbance. This has been attributed to spreading cortical depression which travels over the cortex at a rate of about 3 mm/min (Section 3.3.2), by contrast to the rapid neural excitatory spread of focal seizures. Similarly, transient ischaemic attacks have a much more rapid progression. The characteristic history is of great importance when one encounters patients who have the migrainous aura without headache. Attacks often become less frequent with age, with lessening of the headache and vomiting, and patients may ultimately only experience the aura (Fisher 1980).

3.3.4 Treatment

Education with explanation of the nature of migraine is important. If there are identified trigger factors, such as loss of sleep, excessive sleep, change in diet, and caffeine withdrawal, then these can be avoided. Extensive changes in diet are usually unrewarding. Concomitant drugs should be reviewed, such as vasodilator drugs and the oral contraceptive.

Drug treatment can be divided into two categories, namely treatment of the attack and prophylaxis. Many attacks can be controlled by aspirin, paracetamol, or other simple analgesics, in combination with an antiemetic such as domperidone. The key is to take the drug early in the treatment. Narcotic analgesics should be avoided. The mainstay of symptomatic treatment has, in the past, been ergotamine or dihydroergotamine. This still has a role, although one has to be aware of the dangers of exceeding a weekly dose of 2–4 mg, the problems of frequent, even small doses, and the fact that ergotamine in itself can cause headache in overdose. Recently, the introduction of the 5-HT$_{1B/1D}$ agonist, sumatriptan, and similar drugs such as naratriptan, rizatriptan, and zolmitriptan, are rapidly becoming first-line treatment for the acute attack (Tfelt-Hansen et al. 2000). Sumatriptan is effective in migraine with or without aura, both as an oral and a subcutaneous preparation. Subcutaneous administration of 6 mg of sumatriptan improves nearly 90 per cent of migraine attacks (Goadsby and Olesen 1996). The headache, in responders, settles in 30 min or so, and only a few patients require further doses.

The decision of when to use prophylactic medication is difficult and depends on both the frequency and severity of attacks, but, in general, patients who suffer weekly attacks are likely to benefit from such medication. Migraine attacks in relation to the menstrual cycle can be treated prophylactically on a more circumscribed basis. Aspirin, twice daily, may be effective (O'Neill and Mann 1978), but the three mainline drugs are the 5-HT antagonist pizotifen, the β-adrenoreceptor antagonist propanolol, and sodium valproate. These all have a broadly similar efficacy. However, each has side-effects, and propanolol is contraindicated in patients with asthma, and sodium valproate should be used with caution in women of childbearing age who may become pregnant.

Methysergide is highly effective, but in view of the side-effect of retroperitoneal fibrosis, is only reserved for treatment-resistant cases. Some patients, particularly those with more frequent attacks, respond well to tricyclic antidepressants, often in low dosage, such as amitriptyline (Goadsby and Olesen 1996).

Patients with status migrainosus are best admitted to hospital for fluid replacement, correction of electrolyte imbalance, and management of the nausea and vomiting. Some patients may benefit from treatment with steroids.

3.3.5 Migraine variants

Ophthalmoplegic migraine

This term has been applied to recurrent attacks of headache, usually orbital or retro-orbital, associated with paralysis of one or more oculomotor nerves. Although transient diplopia may occur with migraine, the isolated oculomotor palsies of ophthalmoplegic migraine can rarely persist for days or weeks after the attack, and sometimes become permanent (Cruciger and Mazow 1978). The third nerve is most commonly involved, but rarely the fourth, and the first division of the fifth may be implicated. The diagnosis should be accepted with care when used to account for ocular palsies lasting more than an hour or two, as many such cases hitherto described may have had intracranial aneurysms. However, in a review of the ophthalmological complications of migraine, Pearce (1968) found that the ophthalmoplegia, either isolated or recurrent, occurring in migrainous attacks, often remained unexplained despite full investigation.

Ophthalmoplegic migraine appears to be extremely rare. Many of the earlier descriptions and reports of series of cases did not have the detailed neuroimaging now available. Many structural lesions can give rise to a similar feature, and in particular, Tolosa–Hunt syndrome, which is responsive to steroids, can mimic ophthalmoplegic migraine. The diagnosis should not be accepted without scrupulous investigation and neuroimaging.

Hemiplegic migraine

Heaviness and mild weakness of a limb, usually the arm, is not uncommon, but occasionally recurrent attacks are each accompanied by transient hemiparesis. Hemiplegic migraine can be sporadic or familial; the EEG in attacks may show slow waves over the hemisphere contralateral to the hemiplegia, but neuroimaging is usually normal (Gastaut et al. 1981). Respiratory arrest in an attack, leading to death, has been described (Neligan et al. 1977). Occasionally a mild CSF pleocytosis occurs. In sporadic hemiplegic migraine, the weakness can affect alternate sides. In the familial form, it is usually on the same side. A mutation in a brain-specific calcium channel α1-subunit gene has been linked to familial hemiplegic migraine (Ophoff et al. 1996).

Basilar artery migraine

In 1961, Bickerstaff described attacks of migraine, starting most commonly during adolescence, in which the symptoms of the aura suggested ischaemia in the distribution of the posterior circulation (Bickerstaff 1961a). The attacks commonly begin with classical visual disturbances of migraine which are usually bilateral, followed by paraesthesiae of the lips, hands, and feet. Dysarthria and diplopia in association with severe occipital headache may then follow. Impairment of consciousness with stupor has been attributed to involvement of the brainstem reticular formation (Bickerstaff 1961b; Swanson and Vick 1978).

Retinal migraine

Unilateral photopsia, monocular altitudinal defects, and transient monocular blindness all indicate involvement of the retinal circulation and, when occurring in isolation with migraine headache, suggest a diagnosis of retinal migraine. Thrombosis of the central retinal artery and of single branches may occur (Graveson 1949), and recurrent attack of retinal ischaemia may lead to bilateral optic atrophy due to ischaemic papillopathy (McDonald and Sanders 1971). Some cases of the typical retinal migraine history are found to have associated aortic valve abnormalities on echocardiography (O'Sullivan et al. 1992).

Lower-half migraine

Some patients experience episodic pain which is predominantly in the nose, ear, and neck, referred to as lower-half headache or facial migraine. Recurrent attacks of cervical pain with tenderness over the carotid (carotidynia) may occur in association with migrainous headaches, and in such cases the symptoms usually respond to antimigraine preparations (Raskin and Prusiner 1977).

3.3.6 Complications of migraine

Occasionally patients develop very frequent attacks, and ultimately the migraine, with a recurring or persistent aura, may last for many days with little or no relief (status migrainosus). Dehydration and fatigue may be secondary contributing factors.

Rarely, a permanent hemiparesis may develop or persist in cases of hemiplegic migraine; similarly, a hemianopia may persist and, less commonly, may be associated with prolonged positive visual phenomena. In these instances neuroimaging evidence of ischaemic infarction is found (Rothrock *et al.* 1988). Some patients with the antiphospholipid antibody syndrome develop increasing attacks of migraine and are at risk of migraine-associated cerebral infarction. The presence of antiphospholipid antibodies is an independent risk factor for cerebral infarction and such patients with a combination of migraine and antibodies should be anticoagulated. It is often assumed that in patients with a permanent visual field defect, hemiparesis, aphasia, or opthalmoplegia, an intracranial vascular anomaly (e.g. aneurysm or angioma) will be present, but a review of cases of 'complicated migraine' showed that investigations designed to demonstrate such lesions are usually negative (Pearce and Foster 1965).

An association between migraine and epilepsy has been found in some studies (Basser 1969), and occasionally an epileptic attack may occur at the height of a severe attack of migraine.

3.4 Cluster headache

3.4.1 Migrainous neuralgia

The term cluster headache was introduced by Kunkle (Kunkle *et al.* 1952) referring to the characteristic pattern of attacks occurring in clusters. This has superseded the earlier term of 'periodic migrainous neuralgia' applied by Harris (Harris 1926) and histamine headache (Horton 1941). Syndromes referred to by earlier neurologists as ciliary neuralgia, vidian neuralgia, and sphenopalatine neuralgia are almost certainly the same condition (Sjaastad 1993), the terminology reflecting various theories of pathogenesis in vogue at the time.

The headache is highly distinctive and involves chiefly the eye and frontal region on one side and is characterized by its periodicity. Attacks may occur once or several times in 24 hours and last from 10 minutes to, rarely, several hours. The pain is intense, even leading to attempted suicide; it is continuous and of 'boring' or 'burning' character. Typically the attacks may awaken the patient from sleep in the early morning, coincident with the first REM (rapid eye movement) state. During the attack, the patient paces up and down, in contrast to the behaviour in migraine attacks. A bout tends to last for several weeks, after which the patient is free from symptoms for months or even 1–2 years before the headache recurs. Lacrimation and nasal congestion on the affected side occur during the attack; some patients have a sense of facial and palatal swelling ipsilaterally, which can occasionally be observed. There are no abnormal physical signs, although a Horner's syndrome, either transient or permanent, sometimes develops on the affected side and has been attributed to damage to the sympathetic fibres in the wall of the carotid artery. Cluster headache is most common in males and usually begins in the third or fourth decade.

Cluster headache is far less common than migraine. In headache clinics, the ratio of migraine to cluster headache

patients has been reported to be as high as 10 : 50 (Sjaastad 1993). However, patients with cluster headache are far more likely to be referred to a specialist clinic and this overestimates the prevalence. Population-based studies in the USA suggest a prevalence for men of 0.4 per cent and for women of 0.08 per cent (Kudrow 1980). A detailed review of the medical records of the population of the Republic of San Marino (27 792) gave a prevalence of 0.07 per cent (D'Alessandro *et al.* 1986). Overall prevalence is unlikely to be more than 0.1 per cent. The fact that it can be precipitated by vasodilator drugs such as nitroglycerine and histamine or by alcohol, and that acute attacks are relieved by oxygen, has suggested that vasodilation might be involved. However, this is difficult to demonstrate. The autonomic features are those of parasympathetic activation. During an attack, an increase in neuropeptides, namely calcitonin gene related peptide (CGRP) and vasoactive intestinal polypeptide (VIP), the latter a marker for parasympathetic activity, have been found in ipsilateral jugular blood (Goadsby and Edvinsson 1994).

In view of the clustering, prophylactic treatment during the period of attacks is the mainstay of treatment for those with very regular attacks. Education and explanation is important, including the avoidance of triggering factors, such as alcohol, during a cluster. Altitude may also precipitate attacks. Verapamil (80 mg four times a day) is an effective prophylactic, followed by lithium with appropriate monitoring of levels. Combination with a late-night ergotamine preparation, either orally or as a suppository, may help those patients whose attacks are typically triggered during early sleep. Prednisolone (40 mg daily in a reducing period over 3 weeks) can be valuable but should only be given in a short course. Other drugs that may have benefit include propranolol, methysergide, and pizotifen.

For acute attacks, ergotamine preparations are efficacious, and subcutaneous sumatriptan (6 mg) is effective in the majority of patients (The Sumatriptan Cluster Headache Study Group 1991). Oxygen inhalation in effective but the equipment can be cumbersome (Kudrow 1981).

The typical history provides the diagnosis and extensive investigation is not required. The non-specialist may misinterpret the history as being trigeminal neuralgia, and in some instances, an overlap syndrome can occur, the so-called 'cluster–tick syndrome', often related to vascular compression (Solomon *et al.* 1985). Glaucoma should rarely cause confusion but is an important diagnosis not to miss. Occasionally, cluster headache can be symptomatic of lesions in the cavernous sinus, and atypical histories or those occurring for the first time in the young or old should prompt investigation.

In some patients, the periodicity does not occur. The Headache Classification Committee criteria for chronic cluster headache is that the attacks of pain occur for more than a year on a daily basis without a remission lasting longer than 2 weeks. This chronic cluster headache may develop *de novo* or follow episodic cluster headache with increasing periods of attack and reducing remission time. Patients with chronic cluster headache often require lithium (Pearce 1980).

3.4.2 **Paroxysmal hemicranias**

Paroxysmal hemicrania shares with cluster headache the uni-lateral severe ocular or periorbital and frontal pain with associated autonomic disturbance of lacrimation, rhinorrhoea, and conjunctival injection. The attacks are very frequent, ranging from 2 to as many as 40 times a day, and tend to be shorter than those of cluster headache, ranging from a couple of minutes to half an hour (Antonaci and Sjaastad 1989). The key feature of chronic paroxysmal hemicrania is the response to indo-metacin in a dose of 150 mg a day or less. This is an absolute criterion for the diagnosis.

More recently, episodic paroxysmal hemicrania has been described with a periodicity similar to that of cluster headache, but otherwise the same features as chronic paroxysmal hemi-crania. Hemicrania continua can also be episodic or chronic and is characterized by a constant hemicranial headache with exacerbations that can be associated with ipsilateral auto-nomic features (Sjaastad *et al.* 1984). The *sine qua non* of the diagnosis of the hemicranias is the absolute responsiveness to indometacin.

Short-lasting, unilateral neuralgiform headache attacks with conjunctival injection and tearing (SUNCT) syndrome (Sjaastad *et al.* 1989; Goadsby and Lipton 1997) is character-ized by very brief attacks of unilateral headache with auto-nomic phenomena. The attacks only last from 30 seconds to 2 minutes and may occur many times in an hour. These paroxysmal headaches are all very rare.

3.5 **Trauma**

In severe head injury, headache is apt to be masked by impaired consciousness and, on recovery, may be overshadowed by the other symptoms of cerebral trauma. It is, however, a prominent symptom of the post-traumatic syndrome and it normally occurs in association with symptoms of poor concentration, dizziness, and irritability (Section 16.8.6). The occurrence of headache in the post-traumatic syndrome appears not to bear a direct relationship to the severity of injury and can occur without loss of consciousness. It is also frequently seen with whiplash injuries, in association with neck pain. The headache itself can resemble tension headache or can be hemicranial, and is often exacerbated by noise, excitement and exertion, or head movement. The IHS classification of post-traumatic headache stipulates that headaches should occur within 2 weeks of injury, but headache is often observed to come on later than this. Headache persisting after 2 months is referred to as chronic post-traumatic headache, and certainly, those persisting after 6 months tend to have a less good prognosis (Packard and Ham 1993). The headache symptoms have been considered by some to be neurotic and to relate to impending litigation in relation to the trauma, although the headache does not necessarily resolve with satisfactory resolution of the litigation (Packard 1992). Moreover, with the advent of MRI scanning, minor changes, such as small haemorrhages and features indicative of

diffuse axonal injury, are increasingly demonstrated, even with relatively modest trauma.

The headache of subdural haematoma can be severe and is the most common symptom, except in the elderly, in whom a change in behaviour and drowsiness often predominate. The headache may be generalized or unilateral, and characteristi-cally increases with time. Following blunt trauma to the neck, throbbing, unilateral headache with ipsilateral mydriasis and facial sweating may develop—post-traumatic dysautonomic cephalalgia. This is believed to result from cervical sympathetic overactivity related to carotid damage, and the symptoms may respond to propranolol (Vijayan and Dreyfus 1975). Minor head trauma can also result in migraine-type headache, even in those not normally suffering from migraine (Matthews 1972). In some patients the post-injury headache can have the features of orthostatic headache, in which case a CSF leak needs to be considered.

3.6 **The headache of intracranial lesions and changes in intracranial pressure**

3.6.1 **Brain tumours and other space-occupying lesions**

The headache resulting from mass lesions is predominantly due to distortion of the dura mater, the pain-sensitive intracranial vessels, and the cranial nerves carrying pain sensation (V, VII, IX, X). The pain is often paroxysmal at first and may last from a few minutes to more than an hour, and as the mass increases the pain becomes more frequent and will ultimately be contin-uous; this suggests that there is an accompanying disturbance of CSF dynamics. The pain is characteristically worsened by changes in posture, particularly bending down, and is improved by rest. It may be worse on waking. It is accentuated by exer-tion, coughing, sneezing, vomiting, and straining at stool. However, these features overlap with migraine headache. The headache is often generalized, but if unilateral, is more likely to be on the side of the lesion. Posterior fossa tumours are pa-ticularly liable to give rise to headache due to early disturbance of CSF dynamics, and can give rise to orbital pain due to the innervation of the superior aspect of the tentorium cerebelli by the first division of the trigeminal nerve; more commonly, they give rise to occipital and neck pain.

Headache is said to be a classical feature of cerebral tumours and, certainly, in early neurology textbooks would be described as a consistent feature, usually with an early morning pattern. However, with the earlier diagnosis of neoplasms by neuro-imaging, headache is now found in only about a half of patients with cerebral tumour (Forsyth and Posner 1993), and in less than 10 per cent is it the presenting feature (Vazquezbarquero *et al.* 1994). Headache in patients presenting to a neurology clinic is thus rarely due to a tumour.

Sudden exacerbation of headache may represent haemorrhage into the tumour; this may occur in pituitary tumours, causing a poorly localized central headache (pituitary apoplexy). Of particular note is the headache that arises with colloid cysts of the third ventricle, but can also occur with other intraventricular tumours. Sudden obstruction of CSF flow, which may accompany changes in posture, can result in a rapid crescendo headache and subsequent loss of consciousness. Rarely, brain tumours can be associated with headache and migrainous features (Schlake *et al.* 1991). The overlap between the headache found with brain tumours and tension-type headache or migraine can create diagnostic difficulties (Silberstein and Marcelis 1992); an important feature in guiding investigation is a recent change in pattern, particularly in the older age group.

3.6.2 Meningeal irritation

The headache of meningeal irritation is one of the most severe. When it is due to irritation of the meninges by blood, as in subarachnoid haemorrhage, it is of very sudden onset. With infective meningitis, however, it is of subacute onset, and in both instances the pain is severe, generalized, constant, and associated with neck stiffness and pain in the back, with a positive Kernig's sign. Photophobia, phonophobia, and irritability are characteristic. The headache of malignant meningitis due to neoplastic infiltration is of slow onset, but gives rise to an unremitting, severe headache, which may have less of a throbbing nature and remains unaltered by posture or by coughing. It is very difficult to treat and usually requires opiates.

3.6.3 Raised CSF pressure headache

Intermittent or chronic increases in CSF pressure, as with congenital hydrocephalus or normal pressure hydrocephalus, are rarely associated with headaches. Rapid changes and, in particular, falls of pressure are more likely to result in headache. Indeed the classic studies by Kunkle *et al.* (1943) suggest that raised pressure *per se* may not lead to headache. They studied the effect of experimentally induced rise and falls in CSF pressure by injection of isotonic saline intrathecally They found that a fall from an artificially raised pressure resulted in headache, as did artificial lowering; headache could be resolved by restoring the pressure to normal. Raised pressure of itself, even up to 500 mm of water, did not necessarily result in head pain. This can be most readily interpreted in terms of the distortion of pain-sensitive structures because of pressure and volume changes between intracranial compartments.

Benign intracranial hypertension

Benign intracranial hypertension (BIH), or pseudotumour cerebri (Section 17.1.4), is associated with headache which can be severe, particularly in the morning. It is the presenting feature in over 90 per cent of cases seen by neurologists. Visual obscurations, tinnitus, and diplopia are common and, rarely,

other cranial nerve palsies can be seen (Wall 1991; Ramadan 1996). The cause is not clear, but most theories implicate increased CSF outflow resistance and there is some evidence for elevated cerebral venous pressure (Karahalios *et al.* 1996). There is a clear association with obesity and hormonal change in women. A number of medications have been implicated, most consistently hypervitaminosis A, tetracycline, and, occasionally, steroid withdrawal.

Investigation requires neuroimaging to rule out any structural lesion, ideally with an MRI. An MR venogram will also exclude cerebral venous thrombosis, which is increasingly recognized in association with the clinical picture of BIH (Cremer *et al.* 1996). A lumbar puncture is also mandatory; the CSF pressure is usually above 250 mm of CSF and sometimes up to 600 mm, and the CSF constituents are normal. Treatment is aimed at preventing visual loss and relieving the headache. The diagnostic lumbar puncture itself can relieve symptoms and can be repeated on two or three occasions, but repeated lumbar puncture is not a long-term management solution and itself can transform the headache into that of a low CSF pressure headache. Acetazolamide and a short course of prednisolone may also relieve symptoms. In patients who do not respond to medical treatment, the main surgical options are optic nerve sheath fenestration and lumbar peritoneal shunting (Burgett *et al.* 1997). The former appears to be associated with fewer side-effects but there has been no formal comparison.

3.6.4 Low CSF pressure headache

Low CSF pressure is more consistently associated with headache than raised CSF pressure. The pain is attributed to traction on meninges and cranial nerves, particularly V, IX, X, and the upper cervical nerves together with the bridging veins. It is exemplified by post-lumbar puncture headache; a characteristic feature is the occipital and frontal pain that occurs on standing and which is relieved by lying down. The IHS criteria dictate that the headache occurs or worsens less than 15 minutes after assuming the upright position and disappears or improves less than 30 minutes after resuming the recumbent position (Headache Classification Committee of the International Headache Society 1988). The headache can be associated with vomiting, photophobia, neck stiffness, tinnitus, and occasionally sixth nerve palsies (Berlit *et al.* 1994).

Low CSF pressure headache is most commonly encountered after lumbar puncture, when it occurs in up to 30 per cent of cases. It may last from hours to up to 2 weeks, and resolution coincides with cessation of leakage of CSF from the lumbar theca. Anecdotally, steroids may be helpful, as may a period of recumbancy following puncture, but neither are proven. The only precaution of established efficacy is the use of a small-bore needle (Kuntz *et al.* 1992), although this is not always feasible.

Low CSF headache may also occur following shunt procedures and increasingly has been recognized as a spontaneous syndrome or associated with precipitating events such as minor trauma, e.g. falling on the buttocks, sneezing or coughing, vigorous exercise including marathon running, and sexual intercourse. These are most commonly related to rupture of spinal epidural cysts or tears in the dural nerve sheath. Leakage of CSF can also occur through the cribriform plate or into the petrous or ethmoidal regions, giving rise to CSF rhinorrhoea or otorrhoea. Diagnostically, lumbar puncture may be required to show a low pressure but is often technically difficult. Radio-isotope cisternography or CT myelography may demonstrate a leak, and recently MRI scanning has shown diffuse meningeal enhancement in cases of spontaneous low CSF pressure (Mokri et al. 1993).

The majority of cases of low-pressure headache will resolve with conservative management. Although steroids have been used, their efficacy is not clearly demonstrated. Epidural blood patching involving the infusion of 10–20 ml of autologous blood into the epidural space is widely practised (Gaukroger and Brownridge 1987), although its mode of action is not clearly understood as the siting of the patch need not necessarily correspond with the demonstration of leakage (Raskin 1990).

3.7 Headaches of vascular origin

A paroxysmal throbbing headache which on occasions has a bursting quality and is exacerbated by head movement is common in a number of clinical situations and believed to reflect changes in the calibre, and possibly in the permeability, of cranial vessels. These throbbing headaches are seen in a number of systemic disorders, such as fever, acute anaemia, high altitude, hyperthyroidism, and hypoglycaemia. Carbon dioxide retention (hypercapnia) due to chronic pulmonary disease or sleep apnoea can give rise to headache which may be nocturnal, present on waking, and chronic. Untreated hypercapnia can lead to raised intracranial pressure with papilloedema. The headache that follows generalized seizures may also result from hypercapnia and/or oxygen desaturation.

Hypertension has often been cited as a cause of headache, and although in some reports it occurs more commonly than in normal subjects, there is no clear relationship between the severity of hypertension and the presence of headache. Rapid and major increases in blood pressure may be associated with headache, as is seen in phaeochromocytoma when, characteristically, the headache can develop dramatically. Similarly, headache may occur in pregnancy complicated by pre-eclampsia, with exacerbation of headache at the time of delivery.

A number of drugs are associated with headache which may also have a vascular origin, e.g. amyl nitrate, calcium-channel blockers, and less commonly now, the headache that can occur in patients who are taking monoamine-oxidase inhibitors and are exposed to dietary tyramine. The oral contraceptive, withdrawal of steroid drugs, excessive coffee and tea drinking, caffeine withdrawal, and alcohol are all associated with headaches. Hangover headache is probably further exacerbated by dehydration. Headache associated with substances and their withdrawal, and headaches associated with metabolic abnormalities, have their own designation under the IHS classification.

By contrast with the vascular headache that is believed to relate to arterial dilatation, headache following a cold stimulus is believed to be due to reflex vasoconstriction. This is familiar to many people as 'ice-cream headache' with mid-frontal or supra-orbital unilateral pain occurring within 5 seconds and peaking in about 20–40 seconds after an intense cold stimulus to the palate or incisor teeth. The pain subsides over the same period of time and is more common in migraineurs. The hypothesis that it is due to reflex vasoconstriction is supported by an observed fall in skin temperature over the forehead when the pain develops (Mumford 1979).

3.7.1 Subarachnoid haemorrhage

The rupture of an intracranial aneurysm or arterial–venous malformation is explosive, and the headache of such a sudden onset that the patient may believe that they have been hit over the head. It is often accompanied by an additional pain in the neck which may radiate down the back and into the legs. There may be loss of consciousness shortly afterward. There is usually photophobia, phonophobia, and often drowsiness. Patients who present with subarachnoid haemorrhage from cerebral aneurysm or arterial venous malformations may give a history of earlier, less severe 'sentinel' headaches, presumed to relate to small warning leaks. The significance is often missed but clearly important to recognize when possible (Gorelick et al. 1986). More controversial is the question whether arteriovenous malformations or unruptured intracranial aneurysms can give rise to headaches per se. This is unlikely unless an arterial venous malformation is very large, when throbbing pain may occur, or if an aneurysm is large enough to press on pain-sensitive structures such as the trigeminal nerve, as in the case of internal carotid and posterior communicating artery aneurysms. However, Day and Raskin (1986) described a woman who suffered three severe headaches of instantaneous onset referred to as 'thunderclap headaches'. At surgery there was no evidence that the aneurysm had leaked and it was considered that this might represent haemorrhage into the wall of the aneurysm or vasospasm of the adjacent vessels, causing pain.

3.7.2 Parenchymal haemorrhage and subdural haematomas

Parenchymal haemorrhage may give rise to headache by tissue distortion, obstruction of CSF flow, or rupture into the subarachnoid space. The headache is of acute or subacute onset, but not as dramatic as a primary subarachnoid haemorrhage. Cerebellar haemorrhage may give rise to a more rapid onset of occipital and neck pain, with subsequent loss of consciousness due to brainstem compression. Classical teaching suggested that the association of a hemiparesis with headache indicated a haemorrhage, whereas infarctions were more commonly painless. Modern imaging has disproved this, with many small haemorrhages being painless and cerebral infarction often being associated with a pulsatile headache ipsilateral to the side of the lesion (Section 3.7.4).

Bleeding into the subdural space to cause subdural haemotomata is usually due to damage to the bridging veins. They normally occur over the convexity of the cerebral hemispheres, but can occur within the posterior fossa. Not all patients will give a history of head trauma. Headache is the most common symptom, but this can be fluctuating and intermittent and come on insidiously before additional neurological features emerge. Subdural haematoma should be considered together with cranial arteritis in the emergence of headache in the elderly. The headache usually disappears or improves on resolution of the haematoma.

3.7.3 Cranial arteritis

The headache of cranial arteritis in the elderly is of particular importance since prompt treatment not only resolves the headache, but prevents the potential complication of loss of vision. It is a disease of the elderly, never occurring below the age of 50 years and rarely below 60 years. The headache may be severe and throbbing, and is associated with scalp tenderness. It is often worse at night and the scalp tenderness may be exacerbated by contact with the pillow. The headache is almost invariably accompanied by systemic symptoms of malaise, weight loss, anorexia, low-grade fever, and occasionally night sweats. Indeed, these may be the only symptoms, with the headache not mentioned by the patient. The indurated, tender temporal artery is pathognomonic (Fig. 3.3), but is only seen in a minority of cases.

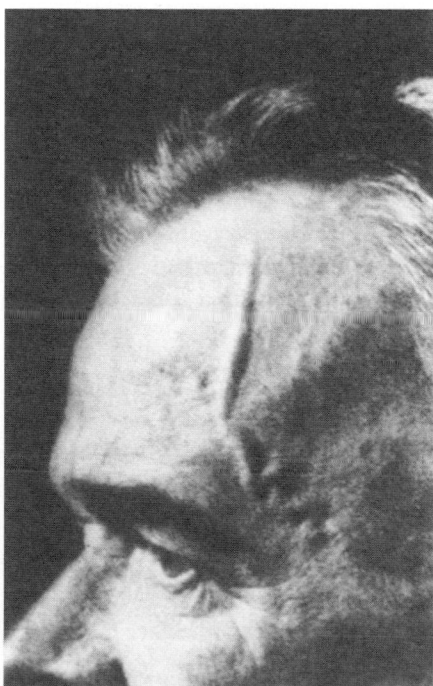

Fig. 3.3. Indurated, tender temporal artery in cranial arteritis (from Brain and Bannister (1992), *Clinical neurology*, Fig. 3.3. Oxford University Press, Oxford).

The involvement of other medium or large vessels is common; inflammation of branches of the external carotid artery also gives rise to facial pain and jaw claudication (Caselli *et al.* 1988). Involvement of the ophthalmic, posterior ciliary, or central retinal arteries can lead to severe visual loss or blindness, most commonly due to ischaemic optic neuropathy and less commonly to retinal infarction. It is the feared complication of this disease and the reason for considering cranial arteritis as a medical emergency. Visual impairment is reported in 15–50 per cent of cases, importantly, in the majority of those with visual loss, there have been promonitory transient symptoms (Font *et al.* 1997). Rarely, involvement of vertebral arteries and, much less commonly, carotid arteries can lead to transient ischaemic attacks and strokes.

The pathology is a granulomatus vasculitis with fragmentation of the internal elastic lamina (Fig. 3.4). Pathological studies have shown a much wider distribution involving all branches of the aorta, although there are some suggestions that cranial arteritis, with selective involvement of the extracranial external carotid, represents a distinct biological subgroup (Brack *et al.* 1999). The inflammation is confined to the extracranial arteries and where they penetrate the dura, also where the internal elastic lamina ceases, the inflammation terminates (Wilkinson and Russell 1972). Biopsy of the temporal artery is the mainstay of diagnosis with a good yield if the artery itself is tender. At least 2 cm of the artery biopsy needs to be biopsied because of the patchy distribution of the inflammation. Other investigations will reveal in most cases a high ESR and cranial arteritis is one of the few diseases where this can exceed 100 mm/h. It is not however, an invariable finding. A raised C-reactive protein, mild normochromic normocytic anaemia, raised platelet count, and mildly abnormal liver function tests complete the typical profile.

Treatment is with steroids, starting with a dose of prednisolone (60 mg or 80 mg daily), maintained for between 2 and 4 weeks and then gradually reduced using the ESR and recurrence of symptoms as a guide. Steroids can be started while awaiting the biopsy, as long as this is completed within 1–2 days. The biopsy-proven clinical diagnosis makes subsequent management much easier. Characteristically there is very rapid resolution of headache and systemic features within 24–48 hours of starting steroid therapy. Treatment needs to be continued for at least a year with a high relapse rate if steroids are withdrawn early and, on average, 2–4 years is required before the disease becomes inactive (Kyle and Hazleman 1993).

3.7.4 Cerebral thrombosis and arterial dissection

Prior to non-invasive neuroimaging, headache was used as a distinguishing clinical feature between haemorrhage and cerebral ischaemia. However, cerebral infarction, whether embolic or occlusive, is frequently associated with headache. It is usually of a throbbing nature but can occasionally be sudden and severe. In general, infarction within the carotid territory leads to frontotemporal pain, and to occipital pain in relation to the

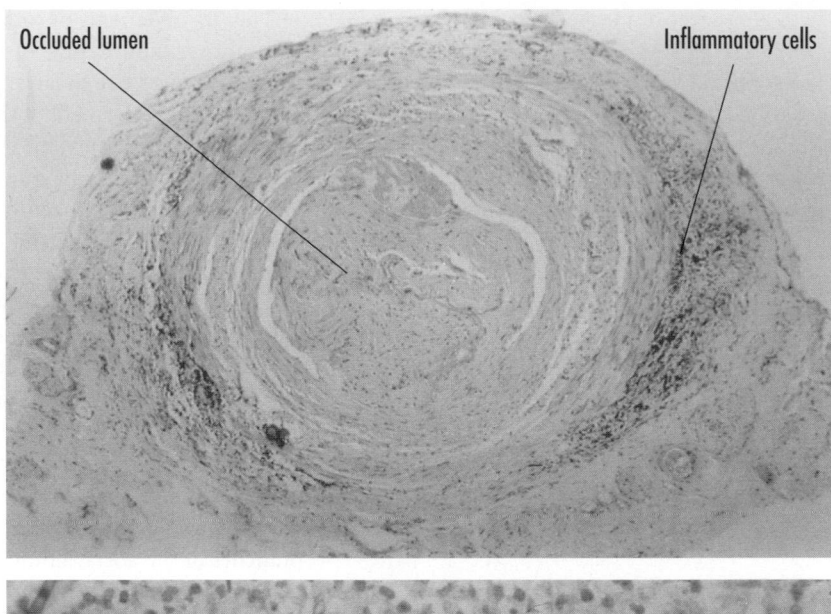

Occluded lumen   Inflammatory cells

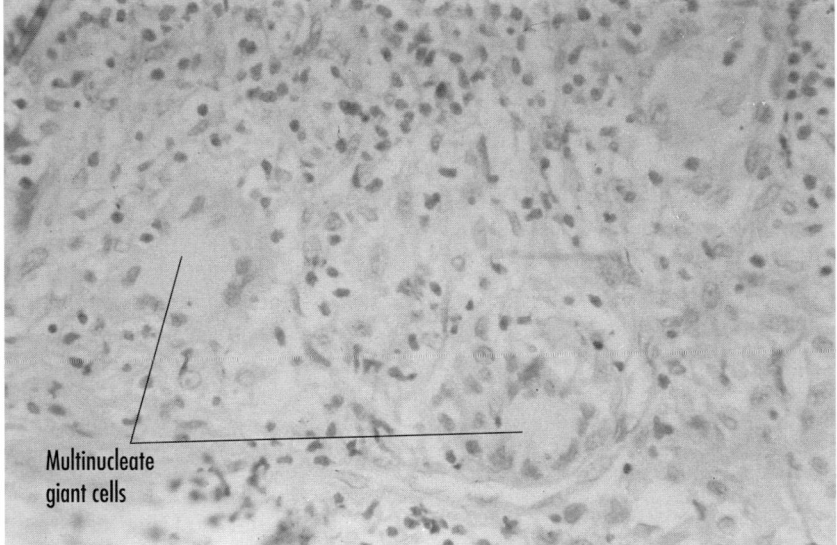

Multinucleate
giant cells

Fig. 3.4. Temporal (giant cell) arteritis. (a) Transverse section of temporal artery showing disruption of the vessel wall, infiltration with cells, and obliteration of the lumen; (b) multinucleate giant cells. (Reprinted from Donaghy 1997).

vertebrobasilar territory (Mitsias and Ramadan 1992). Cerebellar infarcts may give severe headache with rapid worsening due to significant mass effect and subsequent obstructive hydrocephalus. Haemorrhage into an established infarct can be associated with an exacerbation of headache. Carotid occlusion is often associated with orbital pain, probably due to dilatation in anastomotic vessels. Tight carotid stenosis can also produce an ipsilateral headache, presumably by the same mechanism. Cerebral venous sinus thrombosis may also present with a thunderclap headache mimicking subarachnoid haemorrhage (Debruijn *et al.* 1996).

Headache is an important clinical feature of both internal carotid and vertebral artery dissection. It is the initial manifestation of carotid dissection in about 80 per cent of cases. The headache is normally unilateral to the side of the dissection. Orbital and facial pain commonly occurs with carotid dissection and neck pain more commonly with vertebral dissection (Silbert *et al.* 1995). The headache precedes the neurological

features or may coincide; it rarely follows. In up to 20 per cent of patients, the onset may be severe and sudden, with the features of 'thunderclap headache'.

3.8 Diseases of the skull and extracranial structures

3.8.1 Sinus disease

Acute sinusitis is an important cause of headache, which is usually clinically obvious. Chronic sinusitis has been traditionally implicated as a cause of headache, but is rarely so in adults; it can be a cause of persisting headache in children. The distribution of pain depends partly on the sinus involved, although can be poorly localized. Frontal sinus disease tends to be associated with frontal headache and maxillary sinus with pain over the face and cheeks. The pain in sphenoidal and ethmoidal sinusitis can be more difficult to locate, is often behind the eyes or referred to the vertex, and clinically is a more difficult diagnosis in the absence of imaging. It can be worse on standing. In general however, change in posture with symptoms worsening on bending and lying down is the characteristic feature of sinusitis. Severe frontal sinusitis can progress to an epidural and intracerebral abscess, although this is rarely seen. Nasopharyngeal carcinoma is an important diagnosis to be considered in the elderly; it may give unremitting head pain before the development of the characteristic cranial nerve palsies.

3.8.2 Dental and temporomandibular joint disorders

Pain arising from dental disease with a root abscess is usually fairly readily localized, but incomplete tooth fracture can be more diffuse; temperature sensitivity is a frequent accompaniment. Arthritic change in the temporomandibular joint or malocclusion and subluxation can all give rise to facial and head pain (Costen's syndrome). The pain is characteristically worsened with jaw movement, which may also be limited or asymmetric. Clicking is frequently reported (Reik and Hale 1981). Temporomandibular joint dysfunction is frequently diagnosed, and indeed, some of the symptoms and signs of temporomandibular joint dysfunction are frequently found in control populations (Dworkin *et al.* 1990). Management should be conservative in the first instance and further treatment undertaken with the assistance of a maxillofacial surgeon, only with a secure diagnosis.

3.8.3 Ocular causes of headache

Frontal and periorbital headache may arise from opthalmological disease. Refractive errors, particularly hypermetropia or latent strabismus, are often implicated, although care should be taken in attributing headache to this cause (Waters 1970). Of greater diagnostic importance is the orbital head pain that can arise with glaucoma and which represents a medical emergency. The patient may have severe pain with vomiting, but usually the ocular nature is obvious, with injected sclera. In established glaucoma, patients may develop eye and frontal pain due to ciliary muscle spasm following the installation of pilocarpine eyedrops.

3.8.4 Diseases of the skull

Osteitis of the cranial bones secondary to suppuration in the middle ear or paranasal sinuses is now rare, as is syphilitic osteitis, but Paget's disease is relatively common. Headache due to these causes is of a burning, boring character and may be accompanied by tenderness of the skull, which often feels warmer than normal. Local or general thickening of the cranium is often present, and the radiological changes are characteristic. Metastases in skull bones, whether osteolytic (for example in bronchial or breast carcinoma) or osteosclerotic (as in carcinoma of the prostate), and multiple myelomatosis may also give a similar headache.

3.8.5 Headache and the neck

Pain referred to the head from disease in the neck is an important cause of headache but probably overdiagnosed. Cervical spondylosis is often cited as being the cause of headache, but there are no reliable epidemiological data. Cervical spondylosis is most common in the mid and lower cervical spine, whereas referred pain to the head relates to pathology in the upper cervical spine. The convergence and overlap of the first three cervical roots and the trigeminal nerve (especially nociceptive fibres from the first division) provides the anatomical basis for referred pain. Moreover, stimulation of the C1 dorsal root can give pain in the forehead and periorbitally (Bogduk 1997). A number of specific cervical headache syndromes have been described, not all of which have been readily accepted. Sjaastad *et al.* (1990) described a unilateral headache precipitated by neck movement with pain radiating from the neck forward to the front of the head, accompanied by nausea and vomiting and occasionally difficulty in swallowing. C2 neuralgia arises from disorders of the lateral atlantoaxial joint and results in a lancinating pain in the occipital region, usually associated with lacrimation. Complete relief is provided by local anaesthetic blockade of the C2 spinal root (Jansen *et al.* 1989). Irritation of the C3 root subsequent to osteoarthritis of the C2/3 hypophyseal joint or 'third occipital headache' (Bogduk and Marsland 1986) is common among whiplash injury patients (Lord *et al.* 1994). The 'neck–tongue' syndrome describes a sharp pain in the occiput or upper cervical area with accompanying numbness of the ipsilateral tongue occurring on head movement. This has been interpreted as being due to irritation of the ventral ramus of C2 which carries proprioceptor fibres from the tongue via the hypoglossal nerve (Lance and Anthony 1980). Paroxysmal and intense pain radiating from the occiput to the vertex may occur with entrapment of the greater or lesser occipital nerves. In between the paroxysms, there is often a persisting occipital discomfort, and pressure over the occipital nerves will reproduce the symptoms. Injection of local anaesthetic and steroid can provide both diagnostic confirmation and treatment.

3.9 Miscellaneous causes of headache

3.9.1 Exertional or cough headache

This is a distinctive, brief, but often severe 'bursting' kind of pain experienced after coughing, or with exertion involving a Valsalva manoeuvre, most commonly seen in middle-aged men. The patient may clasp his head when he coughs in an attempt to relieve it. The pain usually lasts only seconds or a few minutes, but can be longer. In many cases it is benign and disappears spontaneously (Symonds 1956), but with the availability of MRI scanning, an increasing number of such patients are found to have cerebellar ectopia.

3.9.2 **Coital headache**

Cervical and occipital headache may build up during intercourse and is believed to be due to sustained contraction of the cervical and scalp musculature. In addition, however, an explosive headache may occur at the time of orgasm and persist for several minutes or even hours. Both types of headache are more common in males (Lance 1976). The headache is sufficiently severe to suggest the diagnosis of subarachnoid haemorrhage, which may need to be excluded; typically, however, recurrent attacks become less severe. Some patients respond to propanolol prophylaxis (Porter and Jankovic 1981). Sudden severe headache can also occur at other times, so called 'thunderclap headache', mimicking a subarachnoid haemorrhage, but with normal investigations and a good prognosis (Wijdicks *et al.* 1988).

3.9.3 **Ice-pick headache**

This graphic term refers to patients who experience extremely brief but very sharp jabs of pain which can be felt anywhere in the head, including the orbits. The latter has sometimes been referred to as ophthalmodynia fugax. Treatment is rarely required but some patients with very frequent attacks respond to indomethacin, suggesting some overlap with paroxysmal hemicrania.

References

Alter, M., Daube, J. R., and Franklin, G. (1994). Practice parameter: The utility of neuroimaging in the evaluation of patients with normal neurological examinations. *Neurology*, **44**, 1353–4.

Antonaci, F. and Sjaastad, O. (1989). Chronic paroxysmal hemicrania (CPH): a review of the clinical manifestations. *Headache*, **29**, 648–56.

Arbab, M. A. R., Wiklund, L., and Svendgaard, N. A. (1986). Origin and distribution of cerebral vascular innervation from superior cervical, trigeminal and spinal ganglia investigated with retrograde and anterograde wga-hrp tracing in the rat. *Neuroscience*, **19**, 695–708.

Barkley, G. L., Tepley, N., Nagelleiby, S. *et al.* (1990). Magnetoencephalographic studies of migraine. *Headache*, **30**, 428–34.

Basser, L. (1969). The relation of migraine and epilepsy. *Brain*, **92**, 285.

Bayer, T. L., Baer, P. E., and Early, C. (1991). Situational and psychophysiological factors in psychologically induced pain. *Pain*, **44**, 45–50.

Berlit, P., Bergdammer, E., and Kuehne, D. (1994). Abducens nerve palsy in spontaneous intracranial hypotension. *Neurology*, **44**, 1552.

Bickerstaff, E. R. (1961*a*). Basilar artery migraine. *Lancet*, **i**, 15.

Bickerstaff, E. R. (1961*b*). Impairment of consciousness in migraine. *Lancet*, **ii**, 1057.

Bogduk, N. (1997) Headache and the Neck. In *Headache*, (ed. P. J. Goadsby and S. D. Silberstein), pp. 369–81. Butterworth-Heinemann, Boston.

Bogduk, N. and Marsland, A. (1986). On the concept of third occipital headache. *J. Neurol. Neurosurg. Psychiat.*, **49**, 775–80.

Brack, A., Martinez, T. V., Stanson, A. *et al.* (1999). Disease pattern in cranial and large-vessel giant cell arteritis. *Arthritis Rheum.*, **42**, 311–17.

Burgett, R. A., Purvin, V. A., and Kawasaki, A. (1997). Lumboperitoneal shunting for pseudotumor cerebri [see comments]. *Neurology*, **49**, 734–9.

Caselli, R. J., Hunder, G. G., and Whisnant, J. P. (1988). Neurologic disease in biopsy-proven giant-cell (temporal) arteritis. *Neurology*, **38**, 352–9.

Chabriat, H., Vahedi, K., Iba Zizen, M. T. *et al.* (1995). Clinical spectrum of CADASIL: a study of 7 families. Cerebral autosomal dominant arteriopathy with subcortical infarcts and leukoencephalopathy. *Lancet*, **346**, 934–9.

Cremer, P. D., Thompson, E. O., Johnston, I. H. *et al.* (1996). Pseudotumor cerebri and cerebral venous hypertension. *Neurology*, **47**, 1602–3.

Cruciger, M. P. and Mazow, M. L. (1978). An unusual case of ophthalmoplegic migraine. *Am. J. Ophthalmol.*, **86**, 414–17.

Cutrer, F. M., Sorensen, A. G., Weisskoff, R. M. *et al.* (1998). Perfusion-weighted imaging deficits during spontaneous migrainous aura. *Ann. Neurol.*, **43**, 25–31.

D'Alessandro, R., Gamberini, G., Benassi, G. *et al.* (1986). Cluster headache in the Republic of San Marino. *Cephalalgia*, **6**, 159–62.

Day, J. W. and Raskin, N. H. (1986). Thunderclap headache—symptom of unruptured cerebral aneurysm. *Lancet*, **2**, 1247–8.

Debruijn, S. F. T. M., Stam, J., and Kappelle, L. J. (1996). Thunderclap headache as first symptom of cerebral venous sinus thrombosis. *Lancet*, **348**, 1623–5.

Dimitriadou, V., Buzzi, M. G., Theoharides, T. C. *et al.* (1992). Ultrastructural evidence for neurogenically mediated changes in blood vessels of the rat dura mater and tongue following antidromic trigeminal stimulation. *Neuroscience*, **48**, 187–203.

Donaghy, M. (1997). *Neurology*. Oxford University Press, Oxford.

Dworkin, S. F., Huggins, K. H., LeResche, L. *et al.* (1990). Epidemiology of signs and symptoms in temporomandibular disorders: clinical signs in cases and controls. *J. Am. Dental Assoc.*, **120**, 273–81.

Fisher, C. M. (1980). Late-life migraine accompaniments as a cause of unexplained transient ischemic attacks. *Can. J. Neurol. Sci.*, 7, 9–17.

Fitzpatrick, R. and Hopkins, A. (1981). Referrals to neurologists for headaches not due to structural disease. *J. Neurol. Neurosurg. Psychiat.*, 44, 1061–7.

Font, C., Cid, M. C., Coll, V. B. *et al.* (1997). Clinical features in patients with permanent visual loss due to biopsy-proven giant cell arteritis. *Br. J. Rheumatol.*, 36, 251–4.

Forsyth, P. A. and Posner, J. B. (1993). Headaches in patients with brain-tumors—a study of 111 patients. *Neurology*, 43, 1678–83.

Gastaut, J. L., Yermenos, E., Bonnefoy, M. *et al.* (1981). Familial hemiplegic migraine: EEG and CT scan study of two cases. *Ann. Neurol.*, 10, 392–5.

Gaukroger, P. B. and Brownridge, P. (1987). Epidural blood patch in the treatment of spontaneous low csf pressure headache. *Pain*, 29, 119–22.

Glover, V., Sandler, M., Grant, E. *et al.* (1977). Transitory decrease in platelet monoamine-oxidase activity during migraine attacks. *Lancet*, 1, 391–3.

Goadsby, P. J. and Edvinsson, L. (1994). Human *in vivo* evidence for trigeminovascular activation in cluster headache. Neuropeptide changes and effects of acute attacks therapies. *Brain*, 117, 427–34.

Goadsby, P. J. and Lipton, R. B. (1997). A review of paroxysmal hemicranias, SUNCT syndrome and other short-lasting headaches with autonomic feature, including new cases. *Brain*, 120, 193–209.

Goadsby, P. J. and Olesen, J. (1996). Diagnosis and management of migraine. *BMJ*, 312, 1279–83.

Goadsby, P. J. and Silberstein, S. D. (1997). *Headache*. Butterworth-Heinemann, New York.

Goadsby, P. J. and Zagami, A. S. (1991). Stimulation of the superior sagittal sinus increases metabolic activity and blood-flow in certain regions of the brain-stem and upper cervical spinal-cord of the cat. *Brain*, 114, 1001–11.

Goadsby, P. J., Edvinsson, L., and Ekman, R. (1988). Release of vasoactive peptides in the extracerebral circulation of humans and the cat during activation of the trigeminovascular system. *Annals of Neurology*, 23, 193–6.

Gorelick, P. B., Hier, D. B., Caplan, L. R. *et al.* (1986). Headache in acute cerebrovascular-disease. *Neurology*, 36, 1445–50.

Graveson, G. S. (1949). Retinal arterial occlusin in migraine. *BMJ*, 2, 838.

Hanington, E. (1986). The platelet and migraine. *Headache*, 26, 411–15.

Harris, W. (1926). *Neuritis and neuralgia*, Oxford University Press, London.

Hartig, P. R., Hoyer, D., Humphrey, P. P. A. *et al.* (1996). Alignment of receptor nomenclature with the human genome—classification of 5-ht1b and 5-ht1d receptor subtypes. *Trends Pharmacol. Sci.*, 17, 103–5.

Headache Classification Committee of the International Headache Society (1988). Classification and diagnostic criteria for headache disorders, cranial neuralgias and facial pain. *Cephalalgia*, 8 (Suppl. 7), 1–96.

Horton, B. T. (1941). Histamine cephalalgia. *J. Am. Med. Assoc.*, 116, 377.

Hoskin, K. L., Kaube, H., and Goadsby, P. J. (1996). Central activation of the trigeminovascular pathway in the cat is inhibited by dihydroergotamine—a c-fos and electrophysiological study. *Brain*, 119, 249–56.

Hursey, K. G. and Jacks, S. D. (1992). Fear of pain in recurrent headache sufferers. *Headache*, 32, 283–6.

Jansen, J., Bardosi, A., Hildebrandt, J. *et al.* (1989). Cervicogenic, hemicranial attacks associated with vascular irritation or compression of the cervical nerve root C2. Clinical manifestations and morphological findings. *Pain*, 39, 203–12.

Joutel, A., Corpechot, C., Ducros, A. *et al.* (1996). Notch3 mutations in cadasil, a hereditary adult-onset condition causing stroke and dementia. *Nature*, 383, 707–10.

Karahalios, D. G., Rekate, H. L., Khayata, M. H. *et al.* (1996). Elevated intracranial venous pressure as a universal mechanism in pseudotumor cerebri of varying etiologies. *Neurology*, 46, 198–202.

Kudrow, L. (1980). *Cluster headache: mechanisms and management*. Oxford University Press, Oxford.

Kudrow, L. (1981). Response of cluster headache attacks to oxygen inhalation. *Headache*, 21, 1–4.

Kunkle, E. C., Ray, B. S., and Wolff, H. G. (1943). Experimental studies on headache: Analysis of the headache associated with changes in intracranial pressure. *Arch. Neurol. Psychiat.*, 49, 323.

Kunkle, E. C., Pfeiffer, J. B., and Wilhoit, W. M. E. A. (1952). Recurrent brief headache in 'cluster' pattern. *Trans. Am. Neurol. Assoc.*, 77, 240.

Kuntz, K. M., Kokmen, E., Stevens, J. C. *et al.* (1992). Postlumbar puncture headaches—experience in 501 consecutive procedures. *Neurology*, 42, 1884–7.

Kyle, V. and Hazleman, B. L. (1993). The clinical and laboratory course of polymyalgia rheumatica/giant cell arteritis after the first two months of treatment. *Ann. Rheum. Dis.*, 52, 847–50.

Lance, J. W. (1976). Headaches related to sexual activity. *J. Neurol. Neurosurg. Psychiat.*, 39, 1226–30.

Lance, J. W. (1981). Headache. *Ann. Neurol.*, 10, 1–10.

Lance, J. W. and Anthony, M. (1980). Neck–tongue syndrome on sudden turning of the head. *J. Neurol. Neurosurg. Psychiat.*, **43**, 97–101.

Lance, J. W. and Curran, G. A. (1964). Treatment of chronic tension headache. *Lancet*, **i**, 1236.

Leao, A. P. P. (1944). Spreading depression of activity in the cerebral cortex. *J. Neurophysiol.*, **7**, 359.

Lord, S. M., Barnsley, L., Wallis, B. J. *et al.* (1994). Third occipital nerve headache: a prevalence study. *J. Neurol. Neurosurg. Psychiat.*, **57**, 1187–90.

Matthews, W. B. (1972). Footballer's migraine. *BMJ*, **2**, 326–7.

McDonald, W. I. and Sanders, M. D. (1971). Migraine complicated by ischaemic papillopathy. *Lancet*, **2**, 521–3.

Mitsias, P. and Ramadan, N. M. (1992). Headache in ischemic cerebrovascular-disease. 1. Clinical features. *Cephalalgia*, **12**, 269–74.

Mokri, B., Krueger, B. R., Miller, G. M. *et al.* (1993). Meningeal gadolinium enhancement in low-pressure headaches. *J. Neuroimaging*, **3**, 11.

Moskowitz, M. A. (1984). The neurobiology of vascular head pain. *Ann. Neurol.*, **16**, 157–68.

Moskowitz, M. A., Nozaki, K., and Kraig, R. P. (1993). Neocortical spreading depression provokes the expression of c- fos protein-like immunoreactivity within trigeminal nucleus caudalis via trigeminovascular mechanisms. *J. Neurosci.*, **13**, 1167–77.

Mumford, J. M. (1979). Thermography and ice cream headache. *Acta Thermograph.*, **4**, 33.

Murray, T. J. (1977). Concepts in undergraduate neurological teaching. *Clin. Neurol. Neurosurg.*, **79**, 273–84.

Nebe, J., Heier, M., and Diener, H. C. (1995). Low-dose ibuprofen in self-medication of mild-to-moderate headache—a comparison with acetylsalicylic-acid and placebo. *Cephalalgia*, **15**, 531–5.

Neligan, P., Harriman, D. G., and Pearce, J. (1977). Respiratory arrest in familial hemiplegic migraine: a clinical and neuropathological study. *BMJ*, **2**, 732–4.

Olesen, J. (1995). Analgesic headache [editorial]. *BMJ*, **310**, 479–80.

Olesen, J., Larsen, B., and Lauritzen, M. (1981). Focal hyperemia followed by spreading oligemia and impaired activation of rcbf in classic migraine. *Ann. Neurol.*, **9**, 344–52.

Olesen, J., Thomsen, L. L., and Iversen, H. (1994). Nitric-oxide is a key molecule in migraine and other vascular headaches. *Trends Pharmacol. Sci.*, **15**, 149–53.

O'Neill, B. P. and Mann, J. D. (1978). Aspirin prophylaxis in migraine. *Lancet*, **2**, 1179–81.

Ophoff, R. A., Terwindt, G. M., Vergouwe, M. N. *et al.* (1996). Familial hemiplegic migraine and episodic ataxia type-2 are caused by mutations in the Ca^{2+} channel gene cacnl1a4. *Cell*, **87**, 543–52.

Osterhaus, J. T., Gutterman, D. L., and Plachetka, J. R. (1992). Health care resources and lost labor costs of migraine headaches in the United States. *Pharmacoeconomics*, **2**, 67.

O'Sullivan, F., Rossor, M., and Elston, J. S. (1992). Amaurosis fugax in young people [see comments]. *Br. J. Opthalmol.*, **76**, 660–2.

Packard, R. C. (1992). Posttraumatic headache—permanency and relationship to legal settlement. *Headache*, **32**, 496–500.

Packard, R. C. and Ham, L. P. (1993). Posttraumatic headache—determining chronicity. *Headache*, **33**, 133–4.

Pearce, J. (1968). The ophthalmological complications of migraine. *J. Neurol. Sci.*, **6**, 73–81.

Pearce, J. and Foster, J. B. (1965). The opthamological complications of migraine. *J. Neurol. Sci.*, **6**, 73.

Pearce, J. M. (1980). Chronic migrainous neuralgia: a variant of cluster headache. *Brain*, **103**, 149–59.

Perkin, G. D. (1989). An analysis of 7836 successive new outpatient referrals. *J. Neurol. Neurosurg. Psychiat.*, **52**, 447–8.

Porter, M. and Jankovic, J. (1981). Benign coital cephalalgia. Differential diagnosis and treatment. *Arch. Neurol.*, **38**, 710–12.

Ramadan, N. M. (1996). Headache caused by raised intracranial pressure and intracranial hypotension. *Curr. Opin. Neurol.*, **9**, 214–18.

Raskin, N. H. (1990). Lumbar puncture headache—a review. *Headache*, **30**, 197–200.

Raskin, N. H. (1991). Serotonin receptors and headache. *N. Engl. J. Med.*, **325**, 353–4.

Raskin, N. H. and Prusiner, S. (1977) Carotidynia. *Neurology* **27**, 43–46.

Rasmussen, B. K., Jensen, R., Schroll, M. *et al.* (1991). Epidemiology of headache in a general-population—a prevalence study. *J. Clin. Epidemiol.*, **44**, 1147–57.

Reik, L. and Hale, M. (1981). The temporomandibular joint pain-dysfunction syndrome: a frequent cause of headache. *Headache*, **21**, 151–6.

Rothrock, J. F., Walicke, P., Swenson, M. R. *et al.* (1988). Migrainous stoke. *Arch. Neurol.*, **45**, 63–7.

Russell, M. B. and Olesen, J. (1995). Increased familial risk and evidence of genetic-factor in migraine. *BMJ*, **311**, 541–4.

Schlake, H. P., Grotemeyer, K. H., Husstedt, I. W. *et al.* (1991). 'Symptomatic migraine': intracranial lesions mimicking migrainous headache—a report of three cases. *Headache*, **31**, 661–5.

Schumacher, G. A. and Wolff, H. G. (1941). Experimental studies in headache. *Arch. Neurol. Psychiat., Chicago*, **45**, 199.

Sicuteri, F., Testi, A., and Anselmi, B. (1961). Biochemical investigations in headache; increase in the hydroxyindolacetic acid excretion during migraine attacks. *Internat. Arch. Allergy*, **19**, 55.

Silberstein, S. D. and Marcelis, J. (1992). Headache associated with changes in intracranial-pressure. *Headache*, **32**, 84–94.

Silberstein, S. D., Lipton, R. B., Solomon, S. *et al.* (1994). Classification of daily and near-daily headaches—proposed revisions to the IHS criteria. *Headache*, **34**, 1–7.

Silberstein, S. D., Lipton, R. B., and Sliwinski, M. (1995). Assessment for revised criteria of chronic daily headache. *Neurology*, **45**, A 394–A 394.

Silberstein, S. D., Lipton, R. B., and Goadsby, P. J. (1998). *Headache in clinical practice*, (1st edn). ISIS Medical Media, Oxford.

Silbert, P. L., Mokri, B., and Schievink, W. I. (1995). Headache and neck pain in spontaneous internal carotid and vertebral artery dissections. *Neurology*, **45**, 1517–22.

Silverman, K., Evans, S. M., Strain, E. C. *et al.* (1992). Withdrawal syndrome after the double-blind cessation of caffeine consumption. *N. Engl. J. Med.*, **327**, 1109–14.

Sjaastad, O. (1993). Cluster headache syndrome. In *Major problems in neurology*, Anonymous. Saunders, London.

Sjaastad, O., Spierings, E. L., Saunte, C. *et al.* (1984). 'Hemicrania continua'. An indomethacin responsive headache. II. Autonomic function studies. *Cephalalgia*, **4**, 265–73.

Sjaastad, O., Saunte, C., Salvesen, R. *et al.* (1989). Shortlasting unilateral neuralgiform headache attacks with conjunctival injection, tearing, sweating, and rhinorrhea. *Cephalalgia*, **9**, 147–56.

Sjaastad, O., Fredriksen, T. A., and Pfaffenrath, V. (1990). Cervicogenic headache: diagnostic criteria. *Headache*, **30**, 725–6.

Solomon, S., Apfelbaum, R. I., and Guglielmo, K. M. (1985). The cluster-tic syndrome and its surgical therapy. *Cephalalgia*, **5**, 83–9.

Stang, P., Sternfeld, B., and Sidney, S. (1996). Migraine headache in a prepaid health plan—ascertainment, demographics, physiological, and behavioral-factors. *Headache*, **36**, 69–76.

Stewart, W. F., Lipton, R. B., Celentano, D. D. *et al.* (1992). Prevalence of migraine headache in the United States—relation to age, income, race, and other sociodemographic factors. *J. Am. Med. Assoc.*, **267**, 64–9.

Strassman, A. M. and Vos, B. P. (1993). Somatotopic and laminar organization of fos-like immunoreactivity in the medullary and upper cervical dorsal horn induced by noxious facial stimulation in the rat. *J. Comp. Neurol.*, **331**, 495–516.

Strassman, A. M., Raymond, S. A., and Burstein, R. (1996). Sensitization of meningeal sensory neurons and the origin of headaches. *Nature*, **384**, 560–4.

Swanson, J. W. and Vick, N. A. (1978). Basilar artery migraine 12 patients, with an attack recorded electroencephalographically. *Neurology*, **28**, 782–6.

Symonds, C. (1956). Cough headache. *Brain*, **79**, 557.

Tfelt-Hansen, P., Saxena, P. R., Dahlof, C. *et al.* (2000). Ergotamine in the acute treatment of migraine: a review and European consensus. *Brain*, **123**(1), 9–18.

The Sumatriptan Cluster Headache Study Group (1991). Treatment of acute cluster headache with sumatriptan. *N. Engl. J. Med.*, **325**, 322–6.

Vazquezbarquero, A., Ibanez, F. J., Herrera, S. *et al.* (1994). Isolated headache as the presenting clinical manifestation of intracranial tumors—a prospective-study. *Cephalalgia*, **14**, 270–2.

Vijayan, N. and Dreyfus, P. M. (1975). Posttraumatic dysautonomic cephalalgia. Clinical observations and treatment. *Arch. Neurol.*, **32**, 649–52.

Wall, M. (1991). Idiopathic intracranial hypertension. *Neurol. Clin.*, **9**, 73–95.

Waters, W. E. (1970). Headache and the eye. A community study. *Lancet*, **2**, 1–4.

Weiller, C., May, A., Limmroth, V. *et al.* (1995). Brain-stem activation in spontaneous human migraine attacks. *Nature Medicine*, **1**, 658–60.

Wijdicks, E. F., Kerkhoff, H., and van, G. J. (1988). Long-term follow-up of 71 patients with thunderclap headache mimicking subarachnoid haemorrhage. *Lancet*, **2**, 68–70.

Wilkinson, I. M. and Russell, R. W. (1972). Arteries of the head and neck in giant cell arteritis. A pathological study to show the pattern of arterial involvement. *Arch. Neurol.*, **27**, 378–91.

Woods, R. P., Iacoboni, M., and Mazziotta, J. C. (1994). Brief report—bilateral spreading cerebral hypoperfusion during spontaneous migraine headache. *N Engl J Med.*, **331**, 1689–92.

Zagami, A. S. and Lambert, G. A. (1990). Stimulation of cranial vessels excites nociceptive neurons in several thalamic nuclei of the cat. *Exp. Brain Res.*, **81**, 552–66.

CHAPTER 4

Paediatric neurology

Brian Neville

4.1 Introduction

Paediatric neurology has a number of distinctive features. Pathological changes occur in a developing nervous system and this has the following consequences:

1. Methods of examining and investigating the nervous system have to be age appropriate and are intrinsically more difficult.

2. Acquisition of skills may be expected from the undamaged part of the nervous system in a static encephalopathy and in the early phases some degenerative encephalopathies.

3. Some conditions are entirely confined to the early years of life, either because they happened to be age-locked, for example the syndrome of infantile spasms, or because of short life expectancy.

4. The very large number of conditions, particularly those that are genetically determined, occurring in the developing nervous system is daunting.

5. The extent and severity of a static encephalopathy may only be revealed as the child develops.

6. Progressive metabolic disease that starts *in utero* may present a picture of dysmorphic features plus an extra-uterine progressive syndrome. There is therefore now considerable emphasis on intrauterine and perinatal medicine in paediatric neurology.

7. Disability and acute neurology are in the main different perspectives on similar diseases. Children and their families require comprehensive acute and disability-orientated medical services, which include therapy and specialist medical inputs.

8. The social and emotional aspects of paediatric neurology are crucial. Families have a major role in both the recognition of abnormality and in providing therapy and care. On occasions they may even contribute to the severity of the disability. Medical and educational management are closely interrelated.

9. Cognitive function is very important in describing both individual children and in delineating syndromes. Involvement of special senses is very common and very high rates of psychiatric illness are found in chronic disability of cerebral origin in childhood.

10. Traditional lesion-based neurology has not been very effective in describing the consequences of global damage to the developing nervous system. This has mainly been because of the lack of working hypotheses about the interrelationships between, for example, motor and intellectual disabilities and epilepsy. A functional description of what the child can do is essential and often of more use than a neurological examination based on the model of acquired damage to the adult brain.

11. As intensive care and specialist treatments improve, the need for sophisticated monitoring of cerebral and spinal-cord function increases, specifically looking for early warning of impaired perfusion, oxygenation, and energy supply. This is a rapidly expanding area of paediatric neurology which is revealing the selective vulnerability of the developing nervous system to different insults.

12. Research into the efficacy of therapy in a developmental setting is difficult. The conditions themselves often show wide variation and age-dependent norms are required. Long-term follow-up into adult life is essential if we are to understand the natural history of, for example, the cerebral palsies or epilepsies. Thus medical practice in paediatric neurology has developed ahead of a sound scientific basis.

13. It has become clear that although clinical phenomenology has been the foundation of clinical practice, research into mechanisms and prevention requires *in vivo* assessment of pathological change, which modern imaging is now providing.

14. In young children illness often has much more general manifestations which may render the child neurologically inaccessible. For example, the degree of motor delay and general developmental delay which can coexist with chronic gastrointestinal illness or severe infection that does not directly involve the nervous system, requires considerable paediatric experience to make a sensible neurological assessment.

15. In a general account of neurological disease, therefore, it is useful to discuss the areas of paediatric neurology which provide an insight into adult practice: for example, many children suffering from the epilepsies and metabolic diseases and from conditions such as the cerebral palsies survive to adult life and require continued medical advice.

4.2 The cerebral palsies

The cerebral palsies are a group of conditions and not a single clinical or pathological entity; thus their definition is arbitrary. Different definitions may therefore be required for specific purposes. They comprise motor disorders with neurological signs resulting from 'brain damage' which is static and has occurred in early life. In order to give an adequate picture of the manifestations of damage to the developing nervous system, it is necessary to include statements about motor, cognitive, sensory, and behavioural aspects of the patients, and the presence or absence of epilepsy. By convention, a number of situations are excluded from the cerebral palsies: motor delay without specific neurological signs, including hypotonia in association with mental retardation, spinal-cord damage; hydrocephalus; brain tumours; metabolic disease; well-documented syndromes with a motor component; motor problems of cerebral origin in spina bifida; and disorders of fine motor control. The underlying purpose of the definition is an attempt to include conditions with static cerebral pathology, but the generally accepted exclusions clearly indicate the arbitrary nature of some of these decisions. Several detailed clinical studies have been well documented in monographs and texts (Crothers and Paine 1959; Ingram 1964; Brett 1997). This account is of a group of syndromes which have proved to be of use in clinical practice; these include spastic diplegia, spastic tetraplegia, spastic hemiplegia, dyskinetic cerebral palsy, ataxic cerebral palsy, and the Worster-Drought syndrome or bulbar variant.

Approaches to a pathological classification through magnetic resonance imaging (MRI) are developing quickly (Krägeloh-Mann et al. 1993a,b). It is customary to include a mixed group for those who truly fall between the definitions of the syndromes listed above. This should not be confused with the fact that mixed signs are present in many of the above. What we are aiming for diagnostically is the best fit and the identification of treatable pathology. Since detailed investigation by imaging and metabolic investigation is not feasible on all patients with static cerebral pathology, the following guidelines should be used to determine which patients with an apparently static motor disorder should be investigated:

(1) the lack of an obvious cause;

(2) any hint of progressive loss of skills, or even a plateauing of skills in the first 2 or 3 years of life;

(3) familial occurrence;

(4) episodes of encephalopathy;

(5) the presence of an aspect of a neurological syndrome which is not recognized as a regular part of the cerebral palsies, e.g. ocular nystagmus, pure chorea, dystonia, or cerebellar ataxia.

Clearly neurological signs that could implicate either a spinal-cord or lower motor neuron lesion will also require further investigation. In all but congenital hemiplegia, unexplained cerebral palsy carries an increased genetic risk, particularly if investigations fail to reveal a non-genetic cause.

4.2.1 Incidence and prevalence

The prevalence of cerebral palsies in developed countries fell in between 1950 and 1970 to 1.3/1000 but then rose to above 2/1000 live births (Hagberg et al. 1975a and b, 1976, 1984, 1989, 1993; Stanley and Alberman 1984). These global figures hide a rise in cases that follow preterm birth because of increased survival and a fall in those associated with full-term perinatal problems. There are many underlying pathologies, including variably timed embryological defects, some of which may be genetic, pre- and postnatal infections, focal and global ischaemia, hypoxia, and injury, and these all contribute to each of the cerebral palsy syndromes, although with varying relative importance. In this complex situation causation is best expressed as risk factors which often appear to act together but sometimes may be part of the primary mechanism (Nelson and Ellenberg 1986).

Where there is sufficient intrapartum compromise of cerebral perfusion/oxygenation to be associated with the development of a neurological defect, a neonatal encephalopathy is usually seen (Volpe 1987). The manifestations of this are reduced tone, poor feeding, and, quite commonly, epileptic seizures of obvious or subtle type which usually begin in the first 2 days of life. There is often clinical and imaging evidence of cerebral oedema and this condition has a significant mortality and a high morbidity. There is virtually always a motor component to any subsequent neurological syndrome (Nelson 1988). It is important to emphasize that statements about the cause of a chronic neurological disorder should not be made unless full information has been obtained about all aspects of the pregnancy and perinatal period. There is no doubt that there are significant discrepancies between the legal analysis of preventable cause and the scientific evidence about risk factors. The most common problem is that a neurologically abnormal fetus will often show abnormal behaviour during the birth process.

The motor disability in spastic cerebral palsy is caused mainly by lack of fine motor control and weakness or slowness in producing selective movements. It is rare that the spastic phenomenon of itself causes major disability. Thus, treatments aimed at reducing spasticity usually are only dealing with a small part of the problem.

A number of important 'schools' of therapy have developed in this difficult area (Scrutton 1984). The work of the Gothenburg group led by Professor Bengt Hagberg, has, over the past 40 years, been crucial to our understanding the epidemiology, risk factors, and clinical manifestations of the cerebral palsies.

4.2.2 Spastic diplegia

This condition accounts for 33 per cent of most series of patients with cerebral palsy, and prematurity is a risk factor in 55 per cent. Even in the premature group, only 50 per cent have purely perinatal risk factors. The clinical picture is of bilateral, but not necessarily symmetrical, pyramidal involvement of the legs more than the arms. There is a range of severity from a mild condition in which only the legs appear to be involved and walking is only moderately delayed, to a severe condition with no prospect of eventual walking and quite disabling upper-limb involvement. Typically there is little bulbar involvement, and intellectual function is relatively preserved, particularly in those with only mild upper-limb involvement. Epilepsy is uncommon and, as for all forms of cerebral palsy except hemiplegia, its incidence is closely related to the degree of mental retardation. The pathology in the premature is usually cystic periventricular leucomalacia, which is regarded as ischaemic in origin, and this pathology can also occur in some full-term infants (Wiklund and Uvebrant 1990).

The presentation is of an infant with primary motor delay, typically not affecting feeding or social functioning. Sitting, standing, and walking are delayed, and there is a variable effect on early hand function. Pyramidal signs are usually apparent early, i.e. towards the end of the first year, but outcome is not specifically dependant on their presence and severity, but upon the rate of motor progress. It is possible to find pyramidal signs in some premature babies with little or no motor delay. The presence of dystonia either in the form of global rigidity or focal involvement of one leg is often a poor prognostic sign. Extrapyramidal involvement appears to limit severely the potential for improvement using physiotherapy or orthopaedic treatment. The dystonic element may not become obvious until the second or third year of life. The usual approach is to introduce physical management early and not to attempt too precise a prediction of outcome until the child has been managed for at least a year. The physical management consists of advice on handling and postural development, passive stretching, and the use of light splints, particularly ankle–foot orthoses where dynamic equinus is a problem. Surgical treatment is reserved for two quite specific situations. First, it is used in those who are ambulant and have significant and potentially treatable fixed or mobile deformity, commonly internal rotation and adduction of the hip, flexion at the knees, and equinus. Although practices vary, the common modern management is to leave surgery until relatively late, that is, after the age of 5, and to perform a balanced, multiple procedure, perhaps even at hip, knee, and ankle levels (Bleck 1987). Isolated lengthening of the tendo achilles is now performed much less commonly because of the hazards of a worsened crouch posture. Surgery has to cope with secondary bony abnormalities, particularly torsion forces on both the femora and tibiae. It is in this situation that sophisticated gait analysis is being used increasingly (Gage 1991). Gait is often at its best in the latter part of the first decade. The important factors limiting further motor progress are weakness or relative slowness in the production of selective movements, particularly at hip level. A plateauing of motor skills and even deterioration is common in people with moderately severe cerebral palsy, but its pathogenesis is little researched. Factors believed to be involved in this process are: the mechanical disadvantage of increased linear growth, realistic decisions on the part of the adolescent about the value of therapeutic walking, and psychiatric illness. However, some adolescents and young adults appear to suffer a true neurological deterioration, e.g. of bulbar function in the presence of a presumably stable post-birth asphyxia dyskinetic motor disorder. Degenerative joint changes may also be important. Orthopaedic surgery is also used where progressive dislocation of one or both hips occurs.

A variant of diplegia is mixed ataxic/spastic diplegia, in which ataxia and disequilibrium occur with pyramidal signs. It should not be assumed that this disorder specifically involves the cerebellum, and, interestingly, the outcome for motor function tends to depend more on intellectual function than upon the physical signs.

An important differential diagnosis of diplegia is hydrocephalus. The motor disorder that occurs with hydrocephalus, either aqueduct stenosis or communicating hydrocephalus, is of a mixed spastic/ataxic diplegia with a slow but clearly postnatal onset and usually accompanied by loss of intellectual function,

visual failure and symptoms of raised intracranial pressure, and the presence of a large head (Kirkpatrick et al. 1989). However, the neuropathology of extreme prematurity commonly includes post-haemorrhagic ventriculomegaly or frank hydrocephalus (Hagberg and Hagberg 1989) and thus pressure monitoring may be required if there is any doubt about the static nature of the pathology.

Metabolic disease, particularly the very rare arginase deficiency, may produce a clinical picture very similar to that of spastic diplegia but in which the disorder tends to come on as a concomitant of acute encephalopathy (Antonizzi and Leuzzi 1987). The cerebral illness may, however, be subacute, and if it occurs in the first year of life the initial progression may be missed. The recurrence risk for unexplained symmetrical spasticity, including diplegia, of about 1 in 9 (Bundey and Griffiths 1977) indicates the need for investigation of unexplained diplegia by MRI and metabolic encephalopathy investigations. These latter investigations will include blood and urine amino acids and organic acids, at least a blood lactate or, ideally, a cerebrospinal fluid (CSF) lactate and a blood ammonia level. This series of investigations is designed to look for both treatable diseases and clues to genetic counselling. An uncommon, recessively inherited ataxic/disequilibrium syndrome associated with severe learning disorder emerged from the Gothenburg epidemiological studies (Hagberg et al. 1972). In a number of centres the word 'quadriplegia' is used for the severe end of diplegia, in which there is considerable upper-limb involvement and some bulbar involvement, but the overall picture of more severe lower-limb involvement is maintained. Such patients are included under the diagnosis of diplegia in this chapter.

4.2.3 Spastic tetraplegia

This disorder has a prevalence in childhood of approximately 8/100 000 (Edebol-Tysk et al. 1989). It is therefore uncommon. Children with this disorder are amongst the most disabled members of society and there is, as a consequence, a very high burden of care. By definition they have total body (four limbs and bulbar) involvement and the clinical syndrome includes severe learning problems, usually with microcephaly (in approximately 80 per cent of all cases). In the Gothenburg study of 96 children, all were severely mentally retarded and lacked speech; 94 per cent had epilepsy, 47 per cent had severe visual disability, and 80 per cent a bulbar palsy. Hip subluxation was present in 75 per cent, usually combined with multiple contractures, and scoliosis was present in 72 per cent (Edebol-Tysk 1989).

The early presenting features include: feeding difficulty, poor motor and visual behaviour, and epilepsy. The feeding problems are often extreme, and carers may spend many hours per week in this activity. Nevertheless, secondary nutritional growth failure is common. This has prompted a range of assessment and management techniques. Early nasogastric-tube feeding is commonly used and long-term gastrostomy feeding is now in increasing use in this situation (Morton et al. 1993). Congenital upper motor neuron bulbar palsies are commonly associated with problems of fore-gut control, which manifests with inhalation, gastro-oesophageal reflux, and vomiting. Motor examination in a young child usually shows marked hypotonia, but episodes of axial stiffening in extension are often seen. Tone rises with age and in a distal to proximal progression from the latter part of the first year, and the final picture combines rigidity with pyramidal signs. There is a high rate of intercurrent illness, particularly upper and lower respiratory infection. All of these factors cause a mortality of at least 10 per cent in childhood, which, though significant, still means that there is a need to plan for survival into adult life, particularly by strategies for minimizing secondary disability.

The medical management of children with spastic tetraplegia involves a multidisciplinary team with agreed specific aims. One problem of non-ambulant children with four-limb cerebral palsy, which also occurs in children with very severe mental retardation and gross motor delay, is the development of the windswept hip deformity (Scrutton 1978). This begins with asymmetry, which is initially postural, with both hips habitually deviating to the same side in a semi-flexed position. The adducting hip is at high risk of progressive posterior subluxation and eventual dislocation. The natural history of hips in four-limb cerebral palsy now allows clearer definition of hips at risk (Scrutton 1997). This is commonly associated with scoliosis and can, by adolescence, leave the person unable to be sat in any position of comfort or function, and is commonly associated with pain in the hip. Therefore one aim of management is to support symmetrical postures by seating and to intervene surgically early if deformity is developing.

Any cause of bilateral severe cerebral cortical damage can form the pathological basis for tetraplegia, including malformations, hypoxic–ischaemic damage, and severe intrauterine infection. The full clinical picture can also be caused by postnatal damage in the first year of life. If the cause of spastic tetraplegia is unexplained, there is a similar recurrence risk to that of unexplained spastic diplegia. In the Gothenburg series only 12 per cent of cases were of unknown cause, and many of the adverse factors were multiple.

4.2.4 Dyskinetic cerebral palsies

This group of disorders, also known as athetoid palsy or dystonic cerebral palsy, with whole-body involvement, has a very high rate of identifiable perinatal risk factors, which are thought to cause damage, particularly but not exclusively in the basal ganglia (Kyllerman 1983). Hyperbilirubinaemia causing the syndrome of kernicterus is now very uncommon and the most common identifiable cause is perinatal asphyxia in full-term babies. However, interestingly, in this group, a proportion of cases are of relatively low weight for length at birth, indicating that multiple risk factors have been involved.

The typical history is of a neonatal hypoxic–ischaemic encephalopathy with seizures, reduced conscious level, and lack of feeding, followed by severe motor delay with hypotonia. The mobile stereotyped movements of the limbs and variable hypertonus appear later, at any time from 6 months to 2 years, or on rare occasions much later. The eventual motor disorder is of mobile dystonic spasms, usually with a degree of pyramidal involvement as well. The distribution can range from diplegic with quite early walking to severe four-limb and bulbar involvement, precluding anything but the most primitive motor output. Cognitive function is commonly in the normal or mild/moderate learning impairment range. Early clues to preserved intellectual functioning are a normal rate of head growth, parental accounts of a child's understanding, and perhaps a relatively pure extrapyramidal motor disorder itself. Pure chorea is not seen in this setting. There is a need for detailed investigations of cause of unexplained extrapyramidal disorders. This should include a trial treatment with L-dopa. Within this unexplained group are some genetic disorders, some with progressive symptoms (Fletcher and Marsden 1996). Therapy is specifically aimed at postural control, seating, communication, and environmental control, and is a lifelong task. Contractures are uncommon (Kyllerman 1977).

4.2.5 Hemiplegic cerebral palsy

This condition, which comprises approximately 36 per cent of the cerebral palsies, is defined as a unilateral motor disorder of early onset caused by static brain pathology (Neville and Goodman 2000). A degree of minor dysfunction on the opposite side is usually accepted within this definition. In a detailed computed tomography (CT) study from Sweden of 111 children, 17 per cent showed defective organogenesis or histogenesis (schizencephaly, pachygyria, and heterotopic grey matter), 42 per cent showed central or periventricular atrophy of varying distribution, 12 per cent showed cortical and subcortical atrophy, 3 per cent miscellaneous lesions, and 26 per cent were reported as normal (Wiklund et al. 1990). Interestingly, this study was able to document appropriately timed potential aetiological factors in the majority. The incidence of epilepsy and learning impairments was related to the degree of cortical involvement. The proportion of cases with mental retardation has varied in reported series because of the methods of ascertainment and assessment techniques used. At least 25 per cent have significant learning problems. It is clear that speech is relatively well preserved despite early left-hemisphere damage and that the coexistence of epilepsy is an adverse factor for selective and global cognitive outcome (Vargha-Khadem et al. 1992). Important studies based upon the London Hemiplegia Register have shown psychiatric disorder in at least one-third of the cases, though again without any effect of hemispheric lateralization (Goodman and Graham 1996). This tends to indicate that problems of learning, and emotional and social adjustment, are often the major disability in people with congenital hemiplegia. The first evidence of congenital hemiplegia, if partial motor seizures do not occur early, is of strongly developed hand preference, which would not normally be expected in the first year of life. Despite asymmetry of gait, independent walking is at most only mildly delayed, and most children with hemiplegia walk by 18 months of age. If walking is not achieved by the age of 2 years, it is likely that there is additional pathology and/or impairments.

The neurological signs may be purely pyramidal or a varying degree of dystonia may be present. Usually the upper limb is more severely involved, with major problems in hand function, but an interesting subgroup was found in the Gothenburg series, with predominant involvement in the leg, which correlated with periventricular lesions of CT scanning, thus being, in effect, half of a diplegia (Wiklund and Uvebrant 1990). The severity of the hemiplegia varies from severe to a condition so mild that it can go unrecognized into adult life. From the point of view of gait disturbance, this has been classified into four grades of severity: from the mildest, with a purely dynamic equinus; through fixed equinus, limited knee motion; and, in the severest, a disturbance of hip movement. Orthotic and orthopaedic intervention is prescribed on the basis of these findings (Winters *et al.* 1987).

4.2.6 Ataxic cerebral palsy

This group of disorders includes mixed ataxic/spastic diplegia, and the disequilibrium syndrome associated with severe learning problems which are referred to under diplegia. Any child with a predominantly cerebellar ataxic disorder should be investigated on the suspicion that the disorder is not due to static pathology and may also be genetically determined.

4.2.7 The Worster-Drought syndrome or bulbar variant of cerebral palsy

This disorder comprises a predominantly bulbar disorder with minor limb involvement but usually a significant degree of cognitive delay problems. It may be regarded as a mild tetraplegia. The diagnosis is often made quite late (Worster-Drought 1956).

There are usually no obvious causative factors. The presentation is with primary feeding problems in the severest cases, with sucking difficulty of sufficient severity to necessitate several months of nasogastric feeding. In less severe cases the major problems are encountered on introducing solid food. These difficulties include problems with lip closure and tongue mobility so that food is not propelled posteriorly or cleared efficiently from the buccal cavity or hard palate. Chewing is often impaired and disordered, and swallowing may lead to inhalation. These problems may persist for many years or remit gradually over the first 2–3 years. The second major clinical problem is usually severe speech delay, which may amount to anarthria. Mild degrees of limb incoordination are common and gradually the degree of learning difficulty emerges over the first few years of development.

The typical signs are of lack of voluntary lip, tongue, and sometimes palatal movement, with brisk facial and jaw jerks. The limb signs may be merely a lack of fine movement control but usually signs of mild spasticity and incoordination can be elicited. There is evidence to link this disorder with the bilateral perisylvian syndrome (Clark *et al.* 2000).

Management of the feeding and communication difficulties is symptomatic and often very long term (Neville 1997).

4.2.8 Kernicterus

This term has been applied to a disorder of infancy in which pathological examination of affected brains reveals yellow staining of the meninges, choroid plexus, basal ganglia (especially the globus pallidus), the dentate nuclei, vermis, hippocampus, and medullary nuclei. In the affected areas there is widespread neuronal degeneration and secondary astrocytosis.

The condition is associated with an elevated blood level of unconjugated bilirubin to 20 mg/100 ml or more in the neonatal period. Many reported cases were due to erythroblastosis fetalis (haemolytic disease of the newborn) due to Rh or other blood-group incompatibility (Gerrard 1952). However, with exchange transfusion and, more recently, other methods of treatment and prevention, especially the use of anti-D immunoglobulin (*British Medical Journal* 1981), kernicterus due to this cause has virtually disappeared. The mechanism of damage to the nervous system is complex and appears to involve several factors. In addition to hyperbilirubinaemia in preterm infants (Arnato *et al.* 1987) it may also be that lower levels of bilirubin are a risk factor for cerebral palsies in general (Newman and Maisels 1989). The classical syndrome is of a neonatal encephalopathy, starting with irritability and a high-pitched cry, usually on the second to fourth day, followed by continuous and paroxysmal extensor spasms. The later clinical picture is of a severe extrapyramidal motor disorder, a supranuclear defect of vertical more than horizontal gaze, and nerve deafness, with relative preservation of intellect (Evans and Polani 1950). Isolated deafness may occur in mildly affected children (De Vries *et al.* 1985).

4.2.9 Management of hypertonia

Spasticity has appeared an attractive therapeutic target in the cerebral palsies (Neville and Albright 2000). However, such treatment can have no effect upon lack of selective motor control or weakness that may dominate the picture. Selective posterior rhizotomy has been widely used in spastic diplegia in North America (Peacock and Staudt 1990) but with concerns about long-term outcome. Recent randomized studies cast doubt upon the long-term benefits of this procedure (McLaughlin *et al.* 1997).

Botulinum toxin A has been used in diplegia and hemiplegia, with reports of useful benefits. The scientific basis of this work has been criticized (Forssberg and Tedroff 1997). The use of intrathecal baclofen in spastic cerebral palsy has been reported by Albright, but its general applicability is still uncertain. However, one of the most surprising benefits has been seen in some children with severe dyskinetic cerebral palsy with marked reductions in dystonic movements (Albright *et al.* 1995; Albright 1996).

4.3 Headache, migraine, and hydrocephalus in childhood

4.3.1 General considerations

Headache occurs at some time in at least 60 per cent of children. Population studies have shown that approximately 7 per cent of children have non-migrainous headaches and 4 per cent have migraine as a significant problem (Barlow 1984). Although the headache of raised intracranial pressure tends to occur in sleep or on waking and to be exaggerated by coughing and straining, these characteristics are not reliably diagnostic in many children. Over 90 per cent of children with raised intracranial pressure, however, have neurological signs or skull X-ray abnormalities at an early stage (Honig and Charney 1982). The indications for proceeding to CT or MRI scanning include the presence of neurological signs, sleep-related headaches, a large head, persistent vomiting or anorexia, major problems in school progress, behaviour change, epilepsy, persistently focal head pains, complex 'migraine' with hemiplegia, and failure to relieve headaches which are presumed to be migrainous or psychogenic.

4.3.2 Migraine

Migrainous headaches in childhood may not be of a throbbing character and only a minority of children reports a hemicranial distribution, in contrast to adults (Section 3.3). A feeling of dizziness or light-headedness not amounting to vertigo is reported in about 20 per cent of children in whom migraine is the eventual diagnosis. Provoking factors include upper respiratory infection, family stress, hypoglycaemia, specific foods, minor head trauma, menarche, flickering lights, and sleep deprivation. The 'periodic syndrome' in younger children is regarded as an early manifestation of migraine. It consists of cyclical bouts of illness lasting for up to 3 days with vomiting, abdominal pain, headache, and fever. The alternative diagnosis of recurrent metabolic encephalopathy is excluded by the absence of a reduced conscious level and neurological signs and the occurrence of full recovery between episodes. If there is doubt, specific metabolic conditions need to be excluded by investigation.

4.3.3 Tension headache

Headaches are a common feature of older children who are unhappy or suffering stress, and represent the counterpart of tension headache in adults (Section 3.2). They are typically continuous over several days or weeks and do not have any specific characteristics. Although the history may reveal evidence of depression, with loss of interest in friends and activities, sleep disturbance, and spontaneous crying, it is important to realize that the cause may be hidden in family psychopathology, including sexual abuse.

4.3.4 Hydrocephalus

Simple hydrocephalus secondary to aqueduct stenosis or basal cistern block may present with an excessive rate of head growth and global regression in the first year of life (Section 17.3.6), or at a later age with dementia, visual failure, and a mixed ataxic and spastic motor disorder in a diplegic distribution. A remarkable degree of neurological recovery can occur following surgical treatment. Headache in this situation may be surprisingly intermittent or absent, despite clear evidence of raised intracranial pressure. In one study of children presenting with hydrocephalus at a later age, the clinical features were: a large head in 60 per cent, pyramidal signs in 40 per cent, cognitive delay and visual loss in 37 per cent, gait disturbance in 35 per cent, epilepsy in 22 per cent, nausea and vomiting in 20 per cent, and headaches in 15 per cent (Kirkpatrick et al. 1989). MRI is required to exclude slow-growing tumours as a cause of aqueduct stenosis.

A much more difficult diagnostic problem occurs in the child with an apparently fixed neurological deficit who has recurrent vomiting or is severely anorexic and has communicating hydrocephalus. Monitoring of intracranial pressure is often required to make the diagnosis and decide on the need for treatment.

The most difficult clinical problem within the general rubric of hydrocephalus is in premature babies who have a combination of intraventricular haemorrhage, ventriculomegaly, the ischaemic brain lesion of periventricular leucomalacia, and high susceptibility to infection, particularly if foreign bodies are introduced into the ventricles. A high mortality and very high morbidity of cerebral palsy and developmental delay is the rule. In one study, only 15 per cent were normal at 1 year and that figure will undoubtedly be reduced at an older age when the final toll of psychological and psychiatric disorder is revealed. This phenomenon is the product of increased survival of very premature babies (de Vries et al. 1988).

When hydrocephalus occurs with open spina bifida, the underlying pathology is the Chiari malformation, in which the medulla is more caudally placed. The possibility of hydrocephalus is therefore raised at birth and ventricular size can be monitored using real-time ultrasound. In the presence of a Chiari malformation, the clinical presentation of hydrocephalus, either initially or as a recurrence, often includes cranial nerve palsies, particularly causing stridor and sometimes facial palsy. Unless the cause of hydrocephalus is definitely acquired, a genetic issue arises.

4.4 Neuropsychiatric disorders

4.4.1 The autistic spectrum of disorders

The currently used definition of autism includes:

(1) a disturbance of reciprocal social integration;

(2) a disturbance of communication, including language;

(3) a marked limitation of behavioural repertoire, including imaginitive play; and

(4) the onset is usually under the age of 3 years.

Because of the range of clinical manifestations, the term 'autistic spectrum' is in common usage for children with the above features.

Although cognitive impairment coexists in the majority, the early feature of discrepant lack of social awareness and interaction is noticed in the first 2 years of life by 80 per cent of parents, and as the child grows older a lack of empathy is apparent. A need for apparently idiosyncratic 'order' in the child's life and curious sensitivity to sensory stimuli may cause severe problems in early management. These children change over years, however, and should not be labelled for life. A prevalence of about 1 per 1000 for the full syndrome but with around 5/1000 for Asperger's syndrome (Gillberg 1995) is now the agreed figure. Using the above broad definition, autistic-spectrum disorders are now increasingly recognized. The prevalence is higher in boys.

The organic nature of the disorder is strongly supported by the coexistent impairments—about 75 per cent with global cognitive impairment; 30–40 per cent with epilepsy, problems of motor control, and hyperactivity. Investigation for causes of developmental delay and deviance are appropriate, particularly if there is a period of developmental deterioration or arrest, which is quite often reported in the second year of life (see also atypical presentations of Landau–Kleffner syndrome).

4.4.2 Asperger's syndrome

Asperger's syndrome is often regarded as high-functioning autism, i.e. without global cognitive impairment, and there are genetic studies that link these two syndromes. In Asperger's syndrome the social impairments predominate, with poor peer group interactions and inappropriate behaviour, based upon their great difficulty in understanding other people's perspective. Narrow interests are prominent and rigidity of behaviour imposed upon self and others can make life very difficult. A lack of appropriate social skills is often quite striking. These children and adults are not deliberately isolating themselves, and recognition of their predicament can be very helpful. A prevalence of 3–7/1000 has emerged from various studies, particularly those of Gillberg in Sweden, with a 3 : 1 male : female ratio.

A very clear genetic predisposition is seen (Gillberg and Gillberg 1989) with an affected close relative quite often making the recognition of the problem more difficult. A number of causes of non-progressive early brain damage may be associated with the development of Asperger's syndrome, but making such a diagnosis often doesn't influence management.

4.4.3 Tourette syndrome

This neuropsychiatric disorder (Section 6.6.3) is becoming increasingly recognized as a troublesome and misunderstood condition, beginning usually between the ages of 5 and 21 years. It is commonly familial. The diagnostic criteria include multiple motor, including vocal, tics which are frequent and wax and wane in severity and site. In many children attention deficits, a general fidgetiness and irritability, and repetitive behaviours, sometimes amounting to obsessive–compulsive disorder (OCD), are common and may predominate. Much of the management is to provide children, families, and teachers with insight into the organic nature of the disorders. Drug treatment for tics with dopamine blockers, e.g. haloperidol and pimozide, which carry a small risk of tardive dyskinesia is reserved for those with disabling tics when other measures have failed. Drug treatment for OCD can be very effective, but methylphenidate, used for attention deficit, is difficult to use because it tends to worsen the tics. Recent work indicates an association between streptococcal infection and OED and other features of Tourette syndrome with cross-reacting antibodies to basal ganglia (Heyman 1997).

4.4.4 Attention deficit/hyperactivity disorder

Although problems of definition exist, it is clear that there are a lot of children whose main neurological problem is one of attention, i.e. distractability and of having a high activity level and impulsivity, and that many can be helped by a combination of drug (particularly methylphenidate) and behavioural treatment. It is therefore a useful diagnosis, which may help the child and family to function better. The prevalence in school-aged children is between 3 and 9 per cent (Landgren *et al.* 1996). Features of this condition are common in association with intractable epilepsy, learning disability, and in children with organic brain disease in which, however, drug treatment is often effective. It is also seen in Tourette syndrome and autism, in which the usual drugs are rarely used because of lack of response and side-effects. Phenobarbitone quite commonly causes attention deficit/hyperactivity disorder (ADHD), for which the remedy is obvious.

The diagnosis is only usefully made for children who are failing despite reasonable measures to help them in nursery or school. Bright young children are often very active but do not fail, except perhaps to please. Treatment with methylphenidate is very well studied, with a much higher response rate than, for example, dietary manipulation, which helps a much smaller proportion of children.

The terminology in this area has been confusing, with such terms as 'minimal brain dysfunction or damage' being used, but one cannot easily defend these. The implication that a number of mild cognitive, behavioural, and motor problems coexist is, however, common experience. Gillberg has suggested the term 'DAMP' (for deficits in attention motor control and perception) for this group and has drawn attention to the significant risks of additional psychiatric disorder.

4.5 Neural tube defects

4.5.1 Terminology and aetiology

Neural tube defects include anencephaly (Section 4.6.2). Various terminologies have been used, causing confusion. Congenital defects of spinal-cord closure (spinal dysraphism) may be usefully divided into those with a skin covering (closed spina bifida) and those without (open spina bifida). The term spina bifida occulta is reserved for the presence of a narrow bony cleft of L5/S1 which is present in at least 5 per cent of normal people and is usually regarded as of no clinical significance.

In the early embryo the nervous system is represented by the neural groove, the lateral folds of which unite dorsally to form the neural tube. Arrest of this developmental process leads to defective closure of the neural tube, associated with a similar defective closure of the bony vertebral canal—spina bifida. Several varieties of spina bifida are described, differing in respect to the nature and severity of the spinal defect. In the severe form, a sac protrudes through the vertebral opening, yields an impulse on crying and coughing, and the compression of the sac in the infant increases the tension of the fontanel. The sac may contain meninges only—menigocele; in more severe cases it contains both meninges and the flattened, opened, or bifid spinal chord—myelocele or meningomyelocele. When the cutaneous covering is incomplete, there may be leakage of CSF. The central canal of the chord may be closed but dilated—syringomyelocele. Talwalker and Dastur (1970) distinguish six anatomical varieties of meningocele, depending upon the association of such additional defects as fistulae, aberrant neural tissue, and tethering of the chord or roots; and three varieties of meningomyelocele, which they prefer to call 'ectopic spinal chord'. In the least severe cases there is no protrusion, but a defect in the laminae may be palpable as a depression, which is sometimes covered by a dimple or a tuft of hair (Fig. 4.1). Often, however, there is no visible or palpable abnormality and the laminal defect is only then detected by imaging.

4.5.2 **Closed spina bifida**

The Newcastle group reported on an operated series of 200 patients with this defect (which they called spina bifida occulta) (James and Lassman 1981). The pathology represented in this series included a low conus, a split cord, lipomas, meningoceles, dermoid cysts and sinuses, and pure bony defects. Seventy six per cent had skin lesions, which included lumbosacral lipoma (30 per cent) hypertrichosis (19 per cent), a sinus or dimple above the sacrum (10 per cent), scarring and the presence of a naevus in a small number.

Neither the level of the bony abnormality nor the type of lesion determines the clinical manifestations. These included asymmetric shortening of one leg and foot, which may be unilateral. Equinovarus and calcaneovalgus feet occur according to the level of motor root deficiency, and a general deficiency of muscle below the knee is often seen. L5 and/or S1 sensory loss is common and is a hazard for pressure and infection because these children are ambulant.

A neuropathic bladder commonly coexists and may be diagnosed at a late stage if not specifically looked for. Some of the most severe bladder problems, high pressure with bladder sphincter dyssynergia and upper-tract damage, occur in children with the mildest of lower limb deficits and, interestingly, often in the absence of any evidence of pyramidal disease (Borzyskowski and Neville 1981). Major neuropathic bladder problems may coexist in a child with intact anal reflexes and normal buttock sensation. It this situation the bladder requires early video-urodynamic studies and careful lifelong management by a multidisciplinary team (Borzyskowski and Mundy 1990).

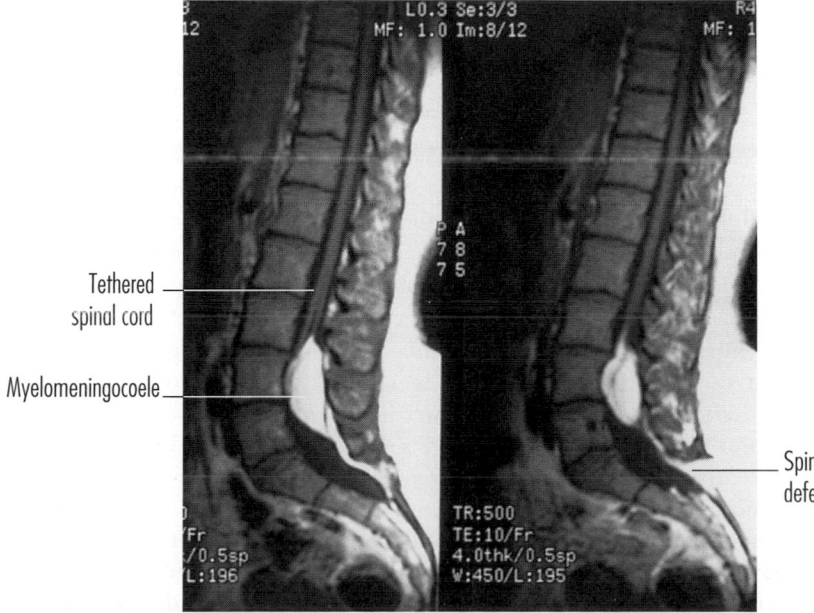

Fig. 4.1. Spina bifida showing the myelomeningocele, tethered spinal cord, and the vertebral bone defect (MRI) (courtesy Dr G. Quaghebeur).

Tethered spinal cord

Myelomeningocoele

Spinal defect

The bony changes on X-ray include defects of laminar fusion of the vertebral body, narrow disc spaces, a wide canal, bony spurs, pedicle erosion, sacral dysgenesis, and scoliosis.

The issue of progressive neurological deficits in the setting of closed spina bifida is contentious. Much of the deficit is prenatally fixed, and to some degree progressive deformity may be merely a result of growth and postural effects. However, the progression of deformity, and sometimes the late presentation of bladder dysfunction, strongly suggests that in some cases the neurological deficit has progressed. In these clinical situations surgery is usually recommended, provided, of course, that there is a surgically treatable lesion. The issue of prophylactical 'untethering' of a low attached conus is not settled.

Sacral dysgenesis (see below) is a part of this embryological sequence and has a very high rate of severe bladder problems. It has a specific association with maternal diabetes.

4.5.3 Open spina bifida

Pathology

The most common site of spina bifida is the lumbosacral region. Occasionally it is found in the thoracic region, very rarely in the cervical. In lumbosacral spina bifida the spinal chord often retains its fetal length and extends down to the sacrum. Spina bifida may be associated with other congenital abnormalities, such as hydrocephalus due to atresia of the aqueduct or the Chiari type I (ectopia of the cerebellar tonsils) (Fig. 4.2a) or type II (lengthened posterior vermis and brainstem displaced into the spinal canal) malformation (Fig. 4.2b); the latter is often called the Arnold–Chiari malformation (see below) (Spillane and Rogers 1959; Emery and MacKenzie 1973).

The most common lesion is a myelomeningocele in which uncovered flat or bulging neural tissue is present, most commonly at the lumbar or thoracolumbar levels. All of the lesions present in closed spina bifida may coexist and, in addition, hydromyelia is commonly present. After surgical treatment, the appearances of tethering are almost universal (McEnery et al. 1992). Although hydromyelia may be associated with scoliosis, the clinical significance of both narrow clefts in the cord and tethering are uncertain.

Symptoms, signs, and management

At birth careful assessment will give both a motor and sensory level for the neurological deficit. Specific syndromes of deformity and disability are associated with different levels of neurological lesion (Brocklehurst 1976). In general, quadriceps activity is required for useful future walking. The issue of surgical closure of the lesion in babies with total lower limb paralysis or other major malformations, including severe hydrocephalus, requires discussion with parents, often on a number of occasions. Increasingly, these lesions are found prenatally and there has also been an unexplained reduction in the incidence, so that this difficult neonatal problem arises much less commonly than 10–20 years ago. Nevertheless, even if an

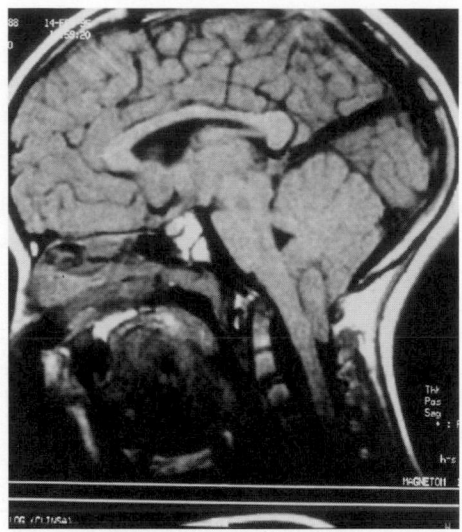

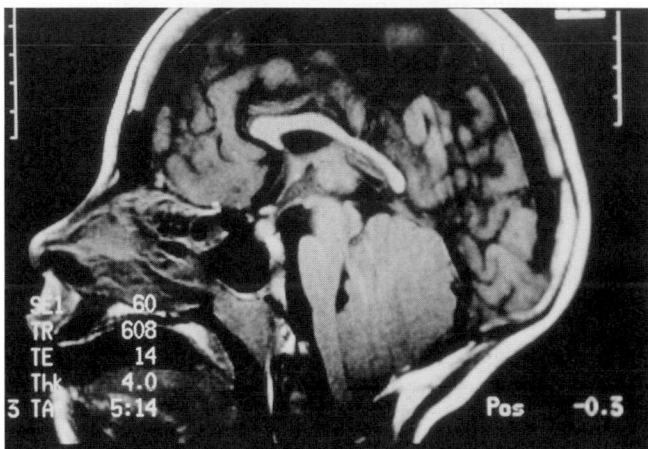

Fig. 4.2. (a) Chiari I malformation, showing ectopia of the cerebellar tonsils (sagittal MRI; courtesy of Dr Kling Chong). (b) Chiari II malformation, showing slit-like fourth ventricle and lengthened posterior vermis and brainstem into the spinal canal (sagittal MRI; courtesy of Dr Kling Chong).

initial decision is made not to operate, the baby may survive and later surgery may be required. The family should also understand that no operation will cure any of the neurological deficits.

Since hydrocephalus is very common, the use of ultrasound to follow ventricular size is routine. It is clear, however, that learning problems can occur even with effective early management of hydrocephalus or untreated mild ventriculomegaly (Section 17.3).

A neuropathic bladder is almost universally present. Ultrasound of the bladder before and after micturition and of the upper tract are important screening procedures. Reference is made in the section on closed spina bifida to use of video-urodynamic studies, particularly looking for bladder–sphincter dyssynergia, which is associated with a high risk of upper-tract damage. Modern management of neuropathic bladder includes clean intermittent catheterization, infection prophylaxis, and the use of drugs and selective surgery to the bladder and urethra. With such measures, most children can be rendered continent and their renal function preserved (Borzyskowski and Mundy 1990). Surgical diversions are very uncommon now and thus the attendant physical and psychological problems are usually avoided.

The management of a neuropathic bowel is often neglected but constipation and soiling are very important disabling problems and are amenable to simple measures (McCarthy 1990).

The necessary physiotherapy and the orthotic and orthopaedic management of the lower limbs is dealt with by a number of authors (Bleck 1987; McCarthy 1992). The pattern of contractures of the lower limbs follows that expected for the level of the motor deficit. It is clear that despite the best endeavours of methods of rehabilitation the results of multiple orthopaedic procedures have been disappointing. The conviction that there is a progressive element to the lower-limb problems of children with spina bifida has developed from this evidence, and it has suggested that untethering of the cord may prevent this process. As yet, no convincing evidence of this has been published.

Spina bifida and its management offer a good test of specialist medical and community services. Many children in this situation require co-ordinated care of hydrocephalus, learning problems, a neuropathic bladder and bowel, paralysed and anaesthetic lower limbs, scoliosis, and mobility, as well as the effective psychosocial support that takes them smoothly through childhood into independent adult life. Achieving medical efficiency in this area is very difficult. The predicament of these families and children can be assisted by the involvement of professional psychological help and lay support groups. It is important to understand the process whereby parents with expectations of a normal child deal with the disaster with which they have been presented (Taylor 1992).

Genetics

Studies of neural-tube defects—open and closed spina bifida and anencephaly—show that these conditions carry a recurrent risk of around 1 in 25 for a further child with a neural-tube defect, not necessarily the one that the first child suffered. There is also an increased risk of isolated hydrocephalus. If two children in a sibship have been born with neural-tube defect, the risk rises to 10 per cent. The risk of a recurrence in the offspring of an adult with spina bifida is approximately 3 per cent. The teratogenic factors known to increase the risk of neural-tube defects include sodium valproate in pregnancy (Stanley and Chambers 1982) and the specific relationship between maternal diabetes and sacral agenesis (Baraitser 1982). Antenatal diagnosis of neural-tube defects is discussed with anencephaly (Section 13.6.1).

4.5.4 Caudal dysplasia (sacral agenesis)

This rare developmental anomaly, also called the caudal regression syndrome, is characterized by clinical and radiographic evidence of agenesis of the sacrococcygeal segments of the vertebral column and spinal cord; there is associated severe atrophy

of the related spinal roots and nerves with grossly impaired innervation of the lower limb musculature (Price et al. 1970; Sarnat et al. 1976). Patients so affected have neurological abnormalities ranging in severity from mild impairment of bladder control to total motor and sensory paralysis below the level of the lesion. Other developmental anomalies (often of the cervical spine, such as Klippel–Feil deformity or multiple hemivertebrae, and of the abdominal viscera) are often found in such cases.

4.5.5 The Arnold–Chiari malformation

Arnold–Chiari malformations are commonly associated with hydrocephalus (Section 17.3.1) and the Chiari type I anomaly with syringomyelia (Section 20.6.2). It is of interest to note that Arnold–Chiari malformation, and sometimes an encephalocele, may be produced in animals by excess vitamins A, arsenate, or clofibrate (Marin-Padilla 1980; Marin-Padilla and Marin-Padilla 1981). In humans, headache, ataxia, and dysphagia are sometimes the presenting symptoms, but in some cases oscillopsia, diplopia, and blurred vision with vertical nystagmus (Spooner and Baloh 1981) or progressive upper-limb paralysis with sensory loss (Gol and Hellbusch 1978) also occur. The Chiari type I (Fig. 4.2a) and Type II (Fig. 4.2b) malformations are clearly defined by MRI. In the former case suboccipital surgical decompression, in the latter rerouting of cervical nerve roots achieved by removal of part of the floor of the neural canal or facetectomy, may relieve the symptoms.

4.6 Cerebral malformations

4.6.1 Normal development of the central nervous system

- *2 weeks*: the three primary layers of ectoderm, mesoderm, and endoderm form, and the notocord, a dorsal column of mesoderm, induces a plate of ectoderm above it to develop into the dorsal neural plate.

- *2–4 weeks*: the neural plate forms a groove which develops into the neural tube which closes anteriorly at day 24 and posteriorly at day 29. Defects at this stage cause the dysraphic states, which range from anencephaly to spina bifida. Anteriorly the forebrain (prosencephalon) midbrain (mesencephalon), and hindbrain (rhombencephalon) develop from the second week with the rest of the neural plate forming the spinal cord. A secondary group of cells forms lateral to the neural tube, the neural crest, which provides a stream of elements of the peripheral nervous system and non-neural elements, e.g. melanocytes and parts of the face.

- *5–6 weeks*: the main division of the forebrain into the primary elements of the cerebrum, basal ganglia, and diencephalon. The holoprosencephaly sequences occur at this stage.

- *8–16 weeks*: cellular proliferation and the beginnings of differentiation of neuroblasts and glioblasts from the ventricular surface. Neuroblasts migrate radially along a glial fibrillary framework. This is followed by the formation of a primordial plexiform layer, or preplate, which forms a framework for the migration of nerves to the final six layers of the mature cerebral cortex. The superficial layers migrate late and the deep layers, e.g. pyramidal cells of layers V and VI, early. This process is largely completed by 20 weeks, although some migration in the cerebellum and hippocampus continues well beyond this time, albeit at a slow rate. During this phase up to half of the cells formed die in an apparently programmed fashion known as apoptosis. During this phase microcephaly and the migrational disorders of the cortex and agenesis of the corpus callosum occur, with more minor cortical dysplasias occurring after 24 weeks, when gyri, and secondary and tertiary sulci appear.

The processes of dendritic development and synaptogenesis continue until 3–4 years, with particularly fast growth and pathway selection in the first year of extrauterine life. Myelination starts at 30 weeks *in utero* but is mainly extrauterine.

Infantile hydrocephalus (Sections 4.3.4 and 17.3.6), syringomyelia, and associated conditions (Section 20.6.2) are considered elsewhere, and developmental anomalies of the skull and skeleton, such as the craniosynostoses (4.7), may also affect the central nervous system. Mentioned below are some of the more common congenital malformations of the brain.

The genetic factors influencing normal and deviant central nervous system development have been the subject of a great deal of research, with a number of mouse models providing close analogies to human diseases. The identification of chromosome and single-gene defects with predominant effects upon the CNS has increased, and approximately one-third of the human genome has effects upon the nervous system, particularly timed developmental effects. Environmental influences, which include maternal illness and a large number of teratogens, have also been explored so that genetic risks and preventive measures can be defined more precisely (Harding and Copp 1997).

One group of disorders arises from abnormal morphogenesis, i.e. the major primary structural process of neuroblast migration and neurepithelial elaboration, including neural-tube defects and neuronal migration defects. A second group of disorders arises from defects in the regional specification of neurepithelium by organizing genes, particularly the *HOX* genes. A third area of great interest in developmental neurobiology is the phenomena of programmed cell death, whereby large numbers of neuroblasts and neurons fail to survive development through a process of cell death quite distinct from necrosis, i.e. apoptosis. There is a great deal of interest in the interaction of environmental and genetic effects in the developing cortex. The classic model of lack of development of the visual cortex and amblyopia with congenital cataracts has prompted the search for other 'amblyopias' secondary to lack of stimulus and experience.

4.6.2 Anencephaly

This is the most common major malformation of the CNS seen in the West, varying in incidence from 0.65 per 1000 live births in Japan to 3 per 1000 in the British Isles (Gabriel 1980). There has been a remarkable decline in its incidence in the Netherlands and Australia (Danks and Halliday 1983; Romijn and Treffers 1983). No cause for this reduction in neural tube defects of all types is evident. Evidence of the value of multivitamins, particularly folic acid, in a preventative role is conflicting (Smithells *et al.* 1981; Mills *et al.* 1989). In anencepholy it is clear that genetic factors are important in all neural-tube defects (Carter 1976) and that sodium valproate (Robert and Guibaud 1982) and a number of other maternal drugs and illnesses are possible factors in causation (Lindhout and Schmidt 1986). In anencephaly, the cephalic neural folds fail to fuse into a neural tube, with consequential degeneration of all forebrain germinal cells. The spinal cord, brainstem, and cerebellum are small, but the cord shows no descending tracts; above this level there are only a few glial and vascular tangles and remnants of midbrain. The eyes are normal but the optic nerves are absent and the calvarium is rudimentary. Fifty per cent of anencephalic fetuses are aborted spontaneously, but if pregnancy goes to term the infants quickly succumb, showing only slow, stereotyped movements and frequent decerebrate posturing. Like spina bifida, anencephaly can be detected early in pregnancy by measuring α-fetoprotein (AFP) in the maternal serum or amniotic fluid (Brock and Sutcliffe 1972; Seller *et al.* 1973). After AFP estimation, the presence of anencephaly can be confirmed confidently by ultrasonic examination (Cuckle 1994).

4.6.3 Holoprosencephaly

This defect, which varies in severity (Gabriel 1980) is one of failure of the primary cerebral vesicle (telencephalon) to divide and expand bilaterally. In its most severe form there is a single large cerebral ventricular cavity within an undivided prosencephalic vesicle (alobar holoprosencephaly) and there is a single median eye (cyclopia). Less severe forms are associated (semilobar and lobar) with hypoplastic olfactory bulbs and tracts (arhinencephaly) and various midline facial malformations, including hypertelorism and/or cleft lip and palate (Fig. 4.3). The most common associated intracerebral abnormality is hydrocephalus. The less severely affected infants show severe mental retardation, rigidity, seizures, and attacks of apnoea. Facial abnormality is not invariable. Prenatal diagnosis is often possible (Nyberg *et al.* 1987).

4.6.4 Septo-optic dysplasia

This generally sporadic anomaly comprises optic nerve hypoplasia and variable absence of the septum pellucidim (Fig. 4.4). It is commonly associated with pituitary and hypothalamic endocrine disturbances. The degree of visual and cognitive impairment varies (Williams *et al.* 1993).

4.6.5 Schizencephaly

The schizencephalies (Yakovlev and Wadsworth 1946*a,b*; Gabriel 1980) comprise a number of developmental defects in

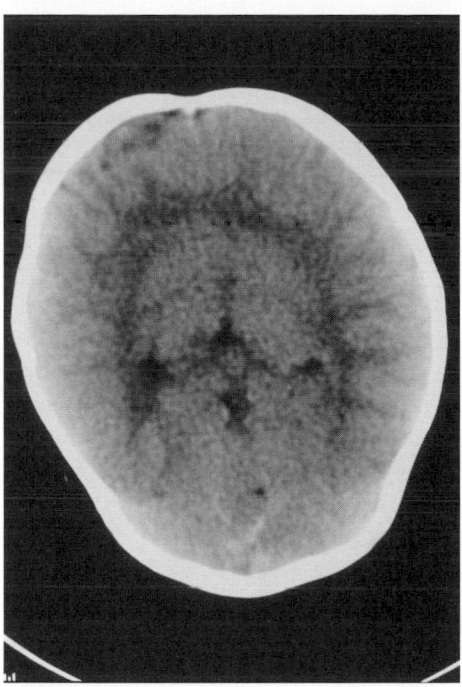

Fig. 4.3. Holoprosencephaly, showing fusion of the frontal lobe (CT scan; courtesy of Dr Kling Chong).

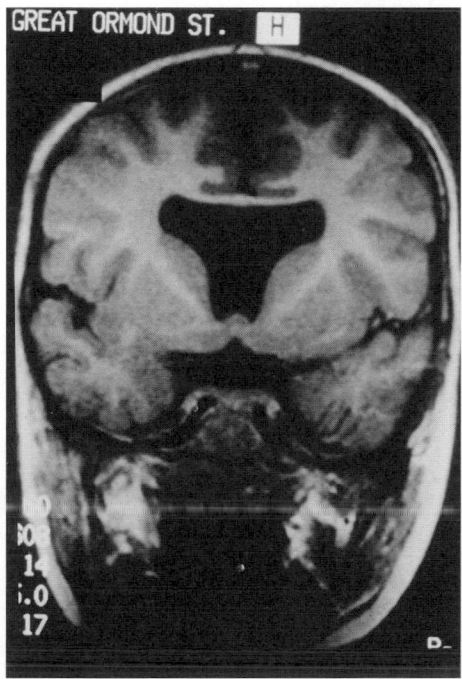

Fig. 4.4. Septo-optic dysplasia, showing agenesis of the septum pellucidum and hypoplasia of the optic nerves and chiasm (coronal MRI; courtesy of Dr Kling Chong).

which there are unilateral or bilateral congenital clefts in the cerebral mantle, which extend from the cortical surface to the underlying ventricular cavities; the brain proximal to or below its clefts may be relatively normal, while that above is hypo-

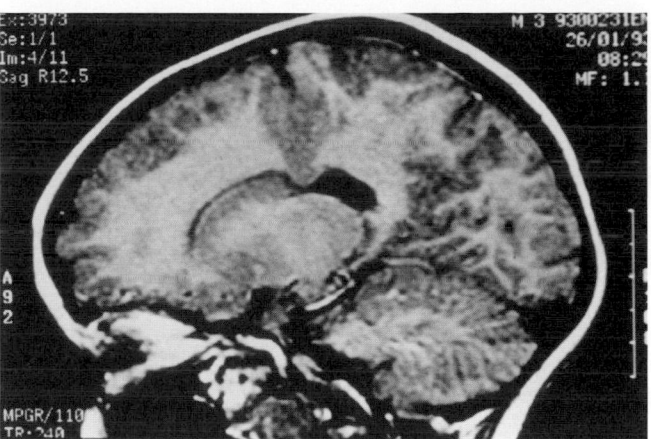

Fig. 4.5. Closed-lips schizencephaly, showing a narrow and mostly virtual cleft lined by heterotopic grey matter (MRI; courtesy of Dr Kling Chong).

plastic or rudimentary, so that the upper part of the cerebrum on both sides may be represented by a cyst covered with a paper-thin layer of nervous parenchyma. The differential diagnosis from *acquired porencephaly* (which is usually unilateral and due to focal infarction or other injury in fetal life or early infancy) may then arise, but that from *congenital porencephaly* (with absence of the corpus collosum and septum pellucidum and large ventricles) may be much more difficult. MRI will show the extent of clefting and associated heterotopic grey matter, and other abnormalities in which the lips of the cleft may be open or closed (Fig. 4.5). Severely affected individuals show spastic tetraplegia, severe mental retardation, and seizures. Modern imaging has demonstrated that there are more mildly affected children with limited, and sometimes unilateral, deficits, with partial seizures, milder learning problems, and focal motor deficits. Eighty per cent have epilepsy (Granata *et al.* 1996).

4.6.6 The agyria-pachygyria disorders

This group of disorders of cortical neuronal migration may arise from primary agenesis and also from secondary destruction of the cortex at an early stage of formation (Evrard *et al.* 1989). The most extreme manifestation is a smooth brain (lissencephaly) but usually there is some evidence of gyri and sulci. Pachygyria implies some evidence of primary and secondary gyration (Fig. 4.6). Polymicrogyria (see below) may also coexist.

Type I lissencephaly is the severest end of the range, with a thick, four-layered cortex and maximal developmental arrest. Although often sporadic, a dysmorphic syndrome, the Miller–Dieker syndrome, which is associated with a deletion on chromosome 17p13 (Van Tuinen *et al.* 1988; Ledbetter *et al.* 1992), is the best described example of type I lissencephaly. The deletion may be small and the dysmorphology absent. Type II lissencephaly has a thin, disorganized cortex and is a feature of the Walker–Warburg syndrome (Pagon *et al.* 1983).

There are more than 15 syndromes associated with this group of disorders, some clearly genetic and others of uncertain

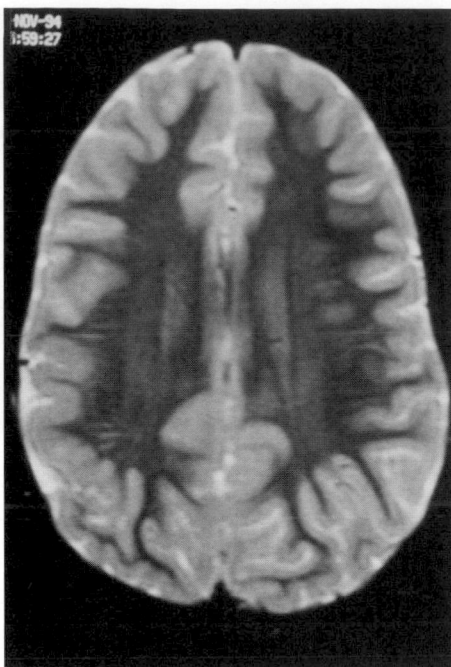

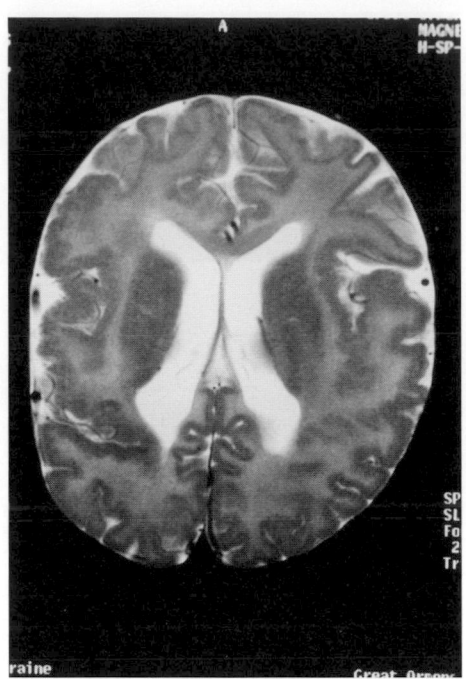

Fig. 4.6. Pachygyria, showing right parietal thickness and poor cortical gyration (MRI; courtesy of Dr Kling Chong).

Fig. 4.7. Polymicrogyria, showing widespread excess of small abnormal gyri, perisylvian and parietal (MRI; courtesy of Dr Kling Chong).

cause (Winter and Baraitser 1991). They are discovered by CT or MRI. The range of clinical manifestations varies widely, with focal unilateral pachygyria presenting as focal epilepsy at the milder end of the spectrum (Andermann *et al.* 1987). The classification of this group of disorders is developing rapidly (Dobyns and Truwit 1995).

4.6.7 Colpocephaly

In this uncommon condition a fetal configuration of the cerebral ventricles persists into postnatal life and the occipital horns are disproportionately large and dilated (Garb 1982). Agenesis of the corpus collosum and optic nerve may coexist (Coupland and Sarnat 1990).

(a)

(b)

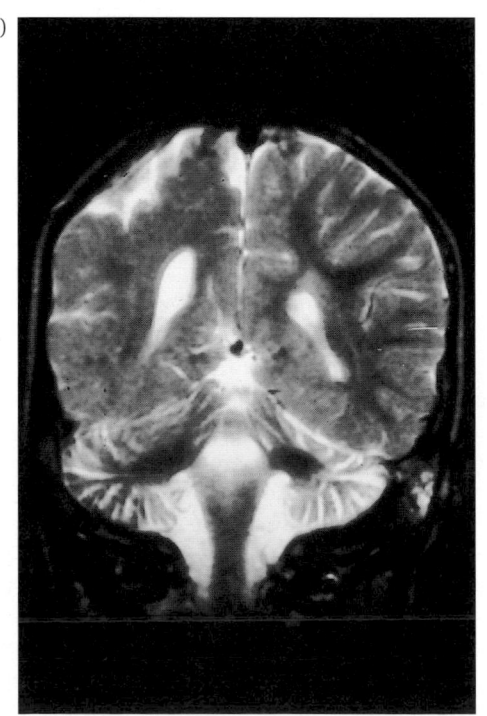

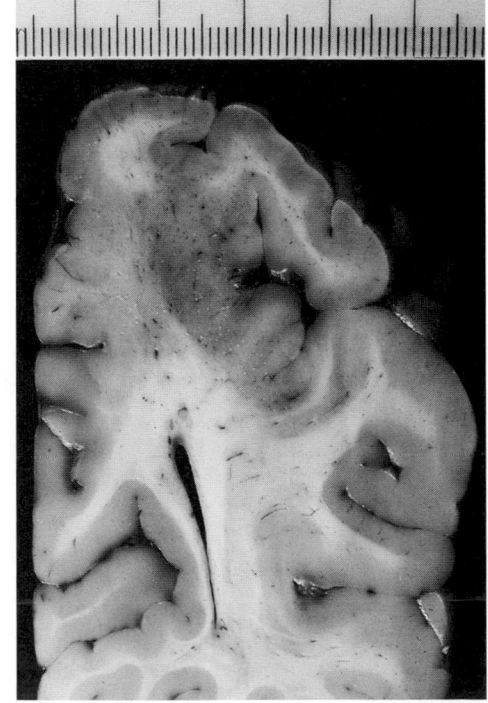

Fig. 4.8. Focal cortical dysplasia.
(a) Coronal MRI, showing an area of focal cortical thickening with additional changes in the underlying white matter.
(b) Coronal fixed brain slice from the same patient, showing the area of thickened cortex. Note the associated poor definition of the cortical margin with groups of nerve cells which have not migrated normally. (Courtesy of Dr W. Squier.)

4.6.8 Polymicrogyria

This pathological description is of a cortex with many narrow gyrae in an abnormal pattern and it is often combined with other underlying malformations (Friede 1989) (Fig. 4.7). Since this abnormality may be associated with a variety of biochemical, genetic, and ischaemic lesions that can cause damage *in utero*, it should not be regarded as a distinct entity.

4.6.9 Cortical dysplasia

Focal cortical dysplasia is a localized disturbance of the cerebral cortex, with giant neurons and astrocytes and chaotic organization (Fig. 4.8). This was recognized as an important cause of partial epilepsy (Taylor *et al.* 1971) and can now sometimes be recognized by MRI (Kuzniecky *et al.* 1988).

The cortical dysplasias comprise microdysgenesis (a purely microscopic abnormality), focal cortical dysplasia (as described above), macrogyria, polymicrogyria, pachygyria, and hemimegalencephaly.

4.6.10 Microcephaly

This term, literally meaning small brain, is used to identify certain primary developmental anomalies (primary microcephaly) as well as secondary microcephaly, which results from shrinkage of the brain (in neonatal hypoxia or encephalomalacia) or physical restriction of its development (as in craniostenosis, Section 4.7). Primary microcephaly can be inherited as an autosomal recessive trait, in which case the brain at birth may weigh as little as 500 g, and may also show agyria, macrogyria, micropolygyria, corpus callosum agenesis, and neuronal heterotopias (Sugimoto *et al.* 1993). Genetically determined microcephaly may show a trajectory of head growth, which drops from being in the normal range at birth to being below the third centile by the end of the first year. Many such individuals demonstrate long survival, but with moderate mental retardation, epilepsy and hyperkinetic behaviour, and variable spastic weakness of the limbs (Gabriel 1980). Microcephaly is also seen in some chromosomal disorders associated with mental retardation, and as a result of maternal irradiation or intrauterine infection with *Toxoplasma*, cytomegalovirus, or rubella.

4.6.11 Rett syndrome

This disorder (Hagberg *et al.* 1983) is confined to girls and is due to an X-linked lethal mutation. It has a prevalence of approximately 1 : 12 500 (Hagberg 1985). Typically, the clinical features are of normal or near-normal development for the first 6 months to up to 3 years of age, when purposive hand movements are lost, with the appearance of stereotyped wringing movements or sucking of the hands. Dementia, usually profound and with autistic features, develops rapidly with, at a later stage, development of pyramidal and extrapyramidal signs, often with kyphoscoliosis. Secondary microcephaly occurs in those whose onset is early. Epilepsy with a characteristic EEG may be useful in diagnosis (Robb *et al.* 1989). Abnormal breathing patterns are commonly seen. The management is of all the multiple problems of these very disabled children who usually survive to adult life.

Since the classic disease was recognized an increasing number of variants have been recognized, some with severe epilepsy and others with milder features and later onset. Until a diagnostic test is widely used, the extent of the clinical phenotype will not be clear (Hagberg 1993; Hagberg and Skjeldal 1994). The causative X-chromosome gene mutations in 80% of cases involve the methyl-CpG-binding protein 2 locus (Amir *et al.* 1999).

4.6.12 Hemimegalencephaly

Hemimegalencephaly involves a major dysgenetic process in one cerebral hemisphere and sometimes of the cerebellum, in which the volume of the abnormal brain is increased (Friede 1989) (Fig. 4.9). This group of conditions presents with developmental delay and usually intractable hemiseizures and hemiparesis. Where the epilepsy is not controlled by drugs, early hemispherectomy is usually indicated, but with concern about bilateral involvement (Chugani 1996). A number of conditions are associated with hemimegalencephaly, including the linear sebaceous naevus syndrome (Levin *et al.* 1984), neurofibromatosis (Ross *et al.* 1989), and Proteus syndrome (Cohen 1988).

4.6.13 Macrocephaly

A large head is a feature of a large number of neurological conditions of childhood. These include:

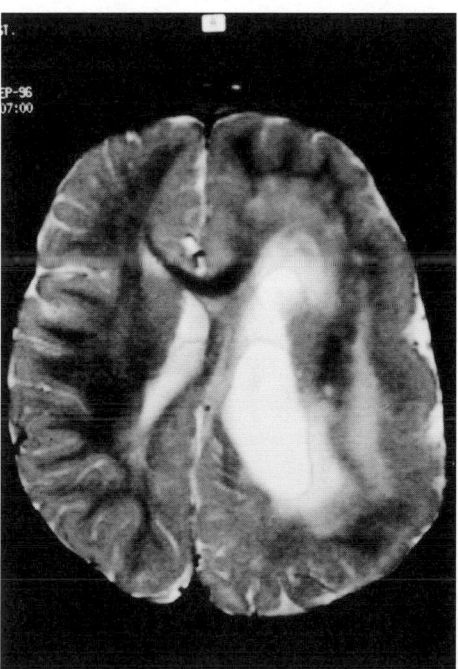

Fig. 4.9. Hemimegalencephaly, showing an enlarged and markedly disorganized left hemisphere (MRI; courtesy of Dr Kling Chong).

(1) hydrocephalus and subdural effusions;

(2) abnormalities of venous drainage;

(3) skeletal dysplasias;

(4) brain malformations; for example, agenesis of the corpus callosum and hemimegaloencephaly;

(5) early onset tumours;

(6) neurocutaneous syndromes, including neurofibromatosis, tuberous sclerosis and haemangiomatosis, and Proteus syndrome;

(7) dysmorphic syndromes, particularly Sotos and Beckwith–Widemann;

(8) metabolic diseases, particularly GM_2 gangliosidosis, mucopolysaccharidosis and Canavan's and Alexander's leucodystrophy.

It may be an isolated primary abnormality, with or without cerebral impairments.

Since head circumference measurements are part of the physical examination of young children, it may be the presenting feature, despite its non-specific nature.

4.6.14 Agenesis of the corpus callosum

This relatively common malformation may be partial or complete, and isolated or combined with a variety of other malformations (Barkovitch and Norman 1988). It is found

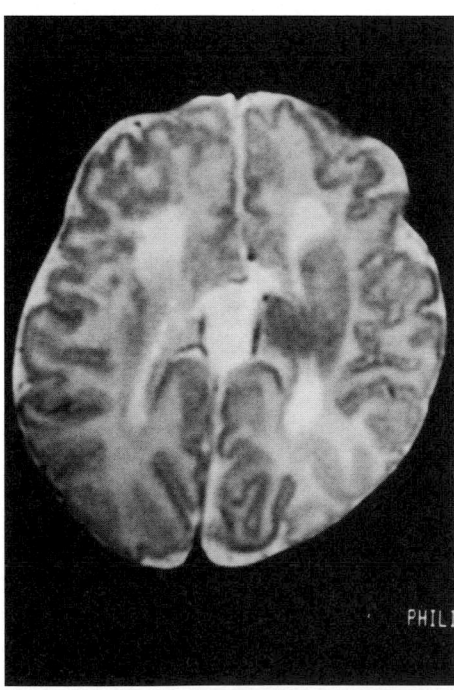

Fig. 4.10. Aicardi syndrome, showing widely spaced lateral ventricles with a high third ventricle, typical of agenesis of the corpus callosum, and a large mass of heterotopic grey matter in the left hemisphere (MRI; courtesy of Dr Kling Chong).

increasingly now that non-invasive imaging is used widely, and may be associated with very little neurological deficit. It is a feature of at least 12 syndromes (Aicardi 1998). Of particular interest is the Aicardi syndrome, which is associated with periventricular heterotopias, choroido-retinal lacunae, and vertebral anomalies (Fig. 4.10). This condition, which is confined to girls, presents with severe mental retardation and early onset infantile spasms. In Shapiro's syndrome there are features of hypothalamic dysfunction, particularly hypothermia (Shapiro *et al.* 1969). Agenesis of the corpus callosum may also occur in a number of metabolic diseases of the nervous system (Section 4.10).

4.7 Craniosynostosis

Craniosynostosis (or craniostenosis) is the early fusion of skull sutures (Fig. 4.11). Sutures allow growth of the skull bone at right angles to their axis. Skull X-rays show narrow, straight, or obliterated sutures and thickened bone, with increased convolutional markings close to the suture (Fig. 4.12). The metopic suture closes antenatally and the rest have fibrous union by 6 months and bony union by 8 years.

Early union of the metopic suture causes a narrow, pointed frontal region with a ridge in the line of the suture and is of little clinical significance. Early closure of the sagittal suture is the most common type of craniosynostosis (Hunter and Rudd 1976). It is more common in boys. It causes a long, narrow head which is recognizable at birth. Although not associated with symptomatic raised intracranial pressure, it is usually treated surgically for cosmetic reasons.

Early closure of the coronal suture is more common in girls (Hunter and Rudd 1977). Unilateral closure causes an asymmetric skull deformity, which should be treated surgically for cosmetic reasons but is not usually associated with raised intracranial pressure. Bilateral synostosis may cause raised intracranial pressure and primary or secondary optic atrophy. Although cognitive impairment may occur, this is not purely related to raised pressure. The skull is short and wide. There may be mainly a skull-vault abnormality (Fig. 4.13) or this may be combined with basal suture synostosis in the coronal plane,

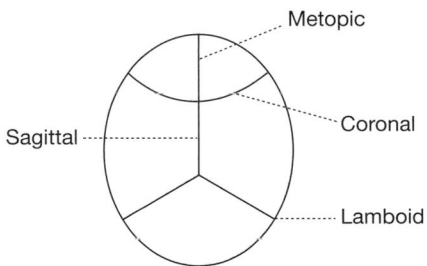

Fig. 4.11. Diagrammatic illustration of the various skull sutures, premature fusion of any of which may lead to craniosynostosis.

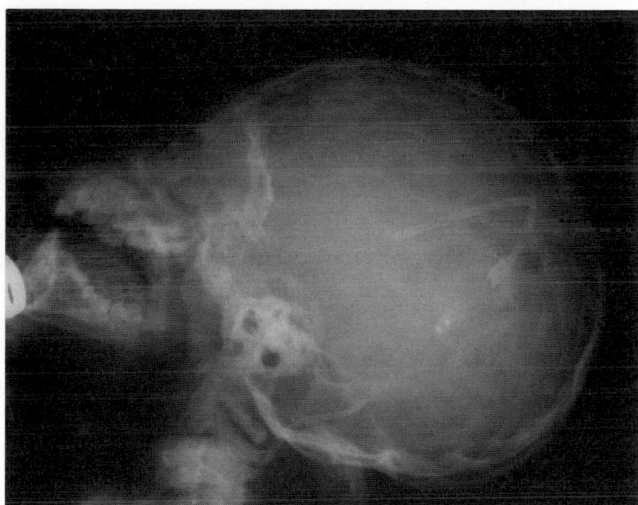

Fig. 4.12. Craniostenosis. Lateral skull x-ray showing copper-beating reflecting the identation of growing gyri within the skull. A ventriculoperitoneal shunt is in situ. (Courtesy of Dr P. Anslow.)

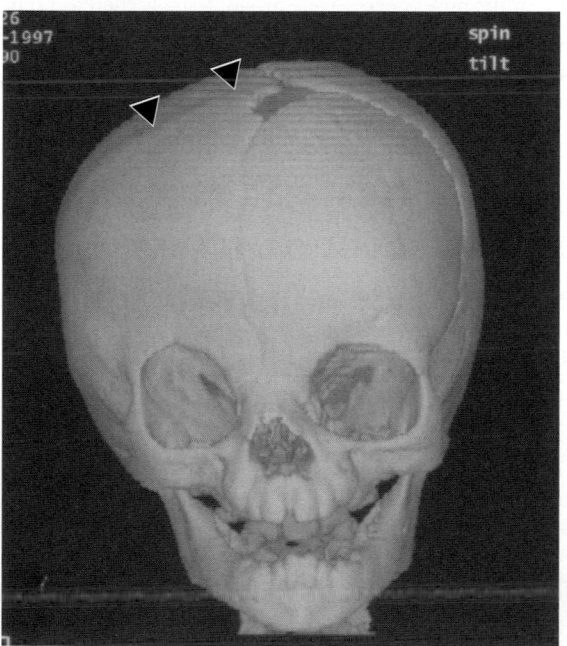

Fig. 4.13. Craniostenosis. CT reconstruction of a skull showing right unicoronal synostosis with a ridge (arrowheads) indicating premature fusion of the right coronal suture, and the early development of a Harlequin eye (courtesy of Dr P. Anslow).

in which case a characteristic facial deformity occurs, with widely spaced eyes, shallow orbits with proptosis, and hypoplasia of the maxillae. This is the appearance seen in Crouzon syndrome, one of the many syndromes that include craniosynostosis. Early surgical treatment of the skull vault is used, but for the facial deformities much more extensive reconstruction procedures are now used.

Unilateral lambdoid synostosis is very uncommon and produces a characteristic deformity if not surgically treated. It is important that the very uncommon unilateral coronal and lambdoid synotosis are separated from the common problem of postural plagiocephaly. In this situation the baby has a right or left head turn preference, probably from intrauterine life, and this is associated with flattening of the skull, eg. left posterior and right anterior flattening for a left preferred head turner, so that the head has developed a predictable postural deformity (Jones *et al.* 1997). In unilateral coronal or lambdoid synostosis, the skull flattening would be on the same side anteriorly and posteriorly. Postural plagiocephaly is more common in relatively inactive babies, in whom a similar deformity of the chest may also occur. Postural plagiocephaly does not require surgical treatment. Total craniosynostosis is rare and causes a small head with very marked convolutional markings on skull X-ray, which distinguish it from primary microcephaly secondary to lack of brain growth in which convolutional markings are diminished or absent. Total craniostenosis requires early surgery. Surgical details of all such procedures are available in specialist texts (Sun and Persing 1999). There is a strong genetic background to craniosynotosis and several discrete syndromes in which multiple additional impairments occur. It is important to recognize that such neurological impairments are not usually caused by raised intracranial pressure but appear to be primary. The gene locations of several of these are known (Aicardi 1998).

4.8 Other craniovertebral anomalies

4.8.1 Basilar impression

Basilar impression is an abnormality of the skull base in which the angle between the basisphenoid and the basilar portion of the occipital bone—normally between 110° and 140°—is widened. In the congenital form, the foramen magnum is deformed and the medulla is unusually low, so that it and the upper part of the cervical spinal cord may be compressed by the odontoid process of the axis. In a lateral radiograph, the line drawn from the posterior end of the hard palate to the posterior lip of the foramen magnum normally lies above the cervical spine, but in basilar impression it crosses the odontoid process at some point (Chamberlain 1939); Bull *et al.* (1955) pointed out that the plane of the axis relative to that of the hard palate is a more reliable guide. The condition is often identified, particularly in American literature, by the term 'platybasia', but the latter term, which simply means a flat base of skull, can equally be applied to the changes that occur, for instance, in Paget's disease. Basilar impression may be present without platybasia (Spillane *et al.* 1957). Basilar impression is the name best reserved for the congenital abnormality of the occipital bone, the posterior part of the atlas vertebra being partially invaginated into the cranial cavity.

Basilar impression may lead to hydrocephalus and perhaps to the Arnold–Chiari syndrome (Gustafson and Oldberg 1940), but the latter is more probably an associated congenital abnormality. It may occur secondarily to osteogenesis imperfecta or be part of a wider craniocervical anomaly, e.g. Klippel–Feil syndrome (Hurwitz and McSwiney 1960). The spinal cord may show hydromyelia, but there is also a clear association with syringomyelia (Foster *et al.* 1969; Barnett *et al.* 1974). In adults the clinical picture may resemble multiple sclerosis, syringomyelia, or a high cervical tumour. The most common clinical features are those of a spastic tetraparesis with marked impairment of position and joint sense in both hands, and to a lesser extent in the legs, but in some cases there are also signs of involvement of lower cranial nerves, cerebellar ataxia, and/or hydrocephalus due to obstruction to the outflow of CSF from the fourth ventricle (O'Connell and Aldren Turner 1950; Michie and Clarke 1968). Symptoms suggesting dysfunction of the C8–T1 segments of the spinal cord in some such cases have been attributed to venous obstruction and stagnant hypoxia in the cervical cord (Taylor and Byrnes 1974). The head is sometimes mushroom-shaped and the neck abnormally short, but the diagnosis can only be made by X-ray examination. If symptoms occur, the treatment of choice is surgical decompression (Gordon 1969; Harkey *et al.* 1990).

In children, basilar impression may be asymptomatic until the second decade. Vertigo, ataxia, and occipital pain may precede the long-term symptoms and signs outlined above. Hydromyelia is often associated with localized scoliosis at the site of the cord lesion.

4.8.2 Klippel–Feil syndrome

The Klippel–Feil syndrome consists of fusion of the bodies of some cervical vertebrae. It may, however, occur without associated craniovertebral malformation and is often an incidental finding on X-ray (Fig. 4.14); some such patients show 'mirror movements' in the upper extremities, so that a voluntary movement carried out with one hand is mimicked spontaneously by the other (Gunderson and Solitare 1968).

4.8.3 Achondroplasia

Achondroplasia may cause not only spinal-cord compression but also internal hydrocephalus without platybasia or basilar impression, possibly due to shortening of the skull base (Spillane 1952). Symptoms of high cervical-cord compression may result from atlantoaxial subluxation with separation of the odontoid process of the axis; this may be a congenital maformation or the result of trauma, but also occurs spontaneously in rheumatoid arthritis (Stevens *et al.* 1971). It is also an important complication of Down's syndrome (Pueschel 1983). The radiology of the craniovertebral anomalies was reviewed in detail by Wackenheim (1974). Transoral decompressive surgery has vastly improved the outlook for many of these patients (Crockard *et al.* 1990).

4.9 Hypertelorism

In this developmental disorder the distance between the eyes is increased; there may be a vertical ridge on the forehead and the bridge of the nose is excessively broad. Usually there is no neurological defect, but in occasional rare and severe cases associated maldevelopment of the forebrain causes cognitive impairment (Currarino and Silverman 1960).

4.10 The investigation of possible neurometabolic disorders of the nervous system in infancy and childhood

Although individually rare, collectively neurometabolic disorders are quite common. Suspicion of a neurometabolic dis-

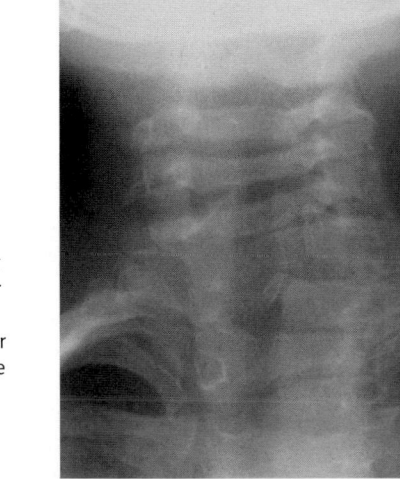
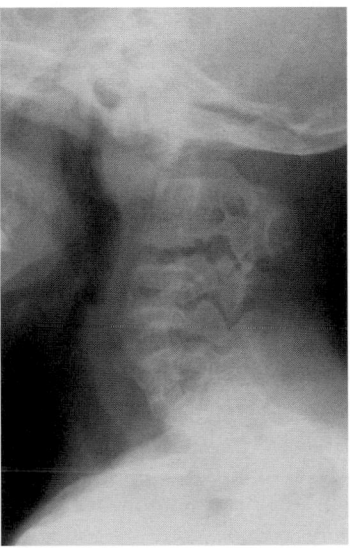

Fig. 4.14. Klippel–Feil syndrome. Plain X-rays showing failure of segmentation of lower cervical vertebrae. This is frequently associated with other vertebral anomalies, in this case of the cervico-cranial junction and thoracic hemivertebrae. (Courtesy of Dr P. Anslow and Mr J. Wilson-MacDonald.)

order depends upon the recognition of progressive neurological disease occurring after a free interval. This may not be easy. The recognition of progressive disease may be very difficult in the young child (under 3–4 years) where the developmental process may obscure the progressive pathology, resulting in developmental slowing rather than loss of acquired skills. Some progressive disorders can evolve over many years, sometimes decades, before clear loss of skills can be demonstrated. Alternatively, progressive deformity complicating a static motor disorder, the increasing discrepancy in cognitive abilities with time in severe static learning difficulty, and the natural evolution of some static encephalopathies may be misinterpreted as progressive disease. A period of normal development may be impossible to demonstrate in very early onset neurometabolic disease.

Additional clues may point to a neurometabolic disease. There may be a family history of unexplained illness or sudden infant death. Often there are earlier unexplained symptoms in the child that may be gastrointestinal (anorexia, vomiting, failure to thrive) or neurological (developmental delay, seizures). The symptoms may be accompanied or preceded by an acute event, or associated with a mild metabolic disturbance. The presence of these should heighten suspicion of a neurometabolic disease.

Not all progressive neurological disease is neurometabolic. Infection, especially in the immunocompromised host, cerebrovascular disease, hydrocephalus, and poorly controlled epilepsy may all produce progressive symptoms that may be reversible on treatment of the underlying condition.

When a neurometabolic disease is suspected, the problem requires careful thought and focused investigation. There is no simple 'metabolic screen'. For the purpose of planning investigation, it is convenient to segregate progressive neurometabolic disorders of infancy and childhood into those occurring *without* acute encephalopathy (Table 4.1) and those with episodes of acute encephalopathy (Table 4.2).

Table 4.1. Progressive neurological diseases without acute metabolic encephalopathy (kindly prepared by Dr Robert Surtees)

I. **AMINO-ACID DISORDERS**

1. **Hyperphenylalaninaemia syndromes:**

   a. **Phenylketonuria (phenylalanine hydroxylase deficiency).** Identified by neonatal screening, dietary treatment prevents classical phenotype of severe dementia, behaviour disorder and epilepsy. Nevertheless a significantly lowered IQ, behaviour difficulties and abnormalities of myelin on MRI are present in treated young adults. Some adults develop a severe neurological disease if diet is stopped in late childhood. Severe teratogenic effects of untreated maternal PKU

   Screening tests: plasma amino acids (raised phenylalanine, reduced tyrosine); phenylalanine and tetrahydrobiopterin loads

   Diagnosis: liver phenylalanine hydroxylase activity, DNA

   b. **Tetrahydrobiopterin (BH$_4$)** deficiencies. BH$_4$ is the cofactor for phenylalanine hydroxylase, tyrosine and tryptophan mono-oxygenases, and nitric oxide synthase. Severe forms (usually recessive) present in infancy with hyperphenylalaninaemia and parkinsonism–dystonia (due to dopamine deficiency). Less severe forms (may be dominant) may present later in life with symptoms of dopamine deficiency alone (dopa-responsive dystonia)

      i. Dihydropteridine reductase and pterin-4 α-carbinolamine dehydratase deficiencies prevent recycling of BH$_4$

      ii. GTP-cyclohydrolase, 6-pyruvoyltetrahydropterin synthase and, in theory, sepiapterin reductase are defects of tetrahydrobiopterin synthesis

   Screening tests: plasma amino acids, CSF or urine pterin analysis

   Diagnosis: red cell dihydropteridine reductase activity, white cell GTP-cyclohydrolase or 6-pyruvoyltetrahydropterin synthase activity

2. **Glutathione metabolism defects:**

   a. **Oxoprolinuria (pyroglutamic aciduria).** Learning difficulties, spasticity; haemolysis and severe metabolic acidosis in newborn period

   Screening tests: urine amino acids

   Diagnosis: red cell glutathione synthetase activity

   b. **Glutamylcysteine synthetase deficiency.** Adult spinocerebellar degeneration, haemolysis, peripheral neuropathy, generalized aminoaciduria

   Screening tests: urine amino acids

   Diagnosis: red cell glutamylcysteine synthetase

3. **Hyperornithinaemia.** Progressive choroidoretinitis (gyrate atrophy) and subcapsular cataract: night blindness in first 10 years, complete blindness in 5th decade. Mild proximal muscular weakness, late white matter degeneration

   Screening tests: plasma amino acids (raised ornithine, modest decrease in glutamate, glutamine, lysine, and creatinine)

   Diagnosis: fibroblast ornithine aminotransferase; DNA

4. **Homocystinuria:**

   a. **Cystathionine β-synthase** deficiency. Learning difficulties, psychiatric illness, osteoporosis, lens dislocation, marfanoid features, vascular disease

   Screening tests: plasma amino acids (raised methionine; homocystine and mixed disulphides present), plasma total homocysteine, urine amino acids, methionine load

   Diagnosis: fibroblast cystathionine β-synthase activity

Table 4.1. *Continued*

    b. **Inborn errors of folate metabolism**. The range of severity of these is great, from severely affected infants to asymptomatic adults. Dementia, motor disorders, seizures, and psychiatric

    c. **Some inborn errors of cobalamin metabolism**. The range of severity of these is great, from severely affected infants to adults with a disorder mistaken for multiple sclerosis. Dementia, motor disorders, seizures, and psychiatric

5. **Tyrosinaemia**

    a. **Type I (fumarylacetoacetase deficiency)**. Liver and renal tubular disease, peripheral neuropathy and porphyric crises

    b. **Type II (tyrosine aminotransferase deficiency)**. Palmar–plantar keratosis, corneal erosions, mental retardation in 50 per cent (Richner–Hanharts syndrome)

    c. **Type III (4-hydroxyphenylpyruvate bisoxygenase deficiency)**. Delayed maturation can cause benign transient neonatal tyrosinaemia

      Screening tests: plasma amino acids (raised tyrosine), urinary succinylacetone (Type 1)

      Diagnosis: white cell or fibroblast FAA activity; liver TAT and PHPPD activities; DNA

6. **Arginase deficiency**. Progressive spastic paraparesis, seizures, learning difficulties, metabolic stroke. May have episodes of encephalopathy

    Screening tests: plasma ammonia, amino acids (raised arginine)

    Diagnosis: red cell arginase activity

II. ORGANIC ACID DISORDERS

1. **Canavan's disease**. Macrocephaly, dementia, optic atrophy, demyelination, death in early childhood. Milder variants (juvenile) exist

    Screening tests: urine *N*-acetylaspartate

    Diagnosis: fibroblast aspartoacylase activity; DNA

2. **L2-hydroxyglutaric aciduria**. Early onset ataxia and mild learning difficulties, later myoclonus, extrapyramidal movement disorder, dementia in teens, characteristic demyelination

    Screening tests: urine L2-hydroxyglutaric acid, CSF lysine

2a. **D2-hydroxyglutaric aciduria**. Early onset intractable epilepsy, severe learning difficulties, cardiomyopathy. Later onset of a variety of neurological problems (ascertainment bias?)

    Screening tests: urine D2-hydroxyglutaric acid

3. **4-hydroxybutyric aciduria**. Non-progressive ataxia, hypotonia with depressed reflexes, less commonly hyperkinesis, seizures and supranuclear ophthalmoplegia

    Screening tests: urine 4-hydroxybutyric acid

    Diagnosis: fibroblast succinate semialdehyde dehydrogenase activity; DNA

4. **3-methylglutaconic aciduria**. Some evidence to suspect that, excepting hydratase deficiency, these syndromes may be secondary to mitochondrial oxidative phosphorylation defects

    a. **Type I**. Delayed speech and macrocephaly

      Screening tests: urine 3-methylglutaconic, 3-methylglutaric and 3-hydroxyisovaleric acids

      Diagnosis: fibroblast 3-methylglutaconylCoA hydratase activity

    b. **Type II (Barth's X-linked cardiomyopathy and neutropaenia syndrome)**

    c. **Type III (Costeff's optic atrophy)**. Early onset optic atrophy, later chorea, paraparesis, ataxia and nystagmus

      Screening tests: urine 3-methylglutaconic and 3-methylglutaric acids

    d. **Type IV (unclassified)**

5. **Glutaric aciduria type 1**. One of the more common metabolic diseases causing neurological disease, often misdiagnosed as cerebral palsy. One-third have gradual onset dystonia in infancy, less commonly seizures and learning difficulties

    Screening tests: urine glutaric, 3-hydroxyglutaric and glutaconic acids, glutarylcarnitine and glutarylglycine; reduced plasma free carnitine, increased plasma acylcarnitine or glutarylcarnitine

    Diagnosis: fibroblast or white cell glutarylCoA dehydrogenase activity; DNA

6. **Mevalonic aciduria**. Progressive multisystem disorder. Learning difficulties, progressive ataxia, progressive myopathy and cardiomyopathy, failure to thrive, dysmorphism punctuated by recurrent crises of fever, rash, arthralgia and diarrhoea and vomiting

    Screening tests: urine mevalonic acid, plasma mevalonic acid, creatine kinase (raised) and ubiquinone-10 (reduced)

    Diagnosis: fibroblast or white cell mevalonate kinase activity

III. MITOCHONDRIAL DISORDERS

1. **Pyruvate carboxylase deficiency**. Type A learning difficulties and lactic acidosis. Type B lactic acidosis, seizures, hypotonia, stridor, dystonia, dementia, liver failure and early death (less than 3 months)

    Screening tests: CSF and plasma lactate, plasma alanine. Plasma ammonia, citrulline and lysine increased in type B

    Diagnosis: fibroblast pyruvate carboxylase activity

Table 4.1. *Continued*

2. **Pyruvate dehydrogenase deficiency.** Variable clinical features. Brain malformation syndromes, through lethal neonatal lactic acidosis, Leigh's disease to carbohydrate-induced episodic ataxia in males

Screening tests: CSF and plasma lactate, plasma alanine

Diagnosis: fibroblast pyruvate dehydrogenase activity

3. **Respiratory chain defects.** A complex group of disorders with both nuclear and mitochondrial inheritance. May have any, and combinations, of: dementia, seizures, spasticity, ataxia, dystonia, retinopathy, optic atrophy, ophthalmoplegia, deafness, peripheral neuropathy, extraneural symptoms. 'Any symptom, any organ, at any age'. Recognizable syndromes include Pearson's marrow–pancreas syndrome, Leigh's disease, Leber's hereditary optic neuritis, Kearns–Sayre, MERRF, MELAS, NARP and MNGIE syndromes; considerable overlap occurs in childhood

Screening tests: CSF and plasma lactate and alanine, muscle histology and histochemistry

Diagnosis: muscle respiratory chain complex assays; mitochondrial and nuclear DNA

a. **Pearson's syndrome.** Sideroblastic anaemia and exocrine or endocrine pancreatic failure. Variable CNS involvement. Survivors may develop Kearns–Sayre syndrome later. Normally large deletion mitochondrial DNA

b. **Leigh's disease.** A post-mortem diagnosis where necrosis, gliosis and neovascularization are seen in, predominantly, the basal ganglia and brainstem. In life, the disease may be suspected when there is the stuttering onset of brainstem or extrapyramidal symptoms, raised CSF lactate and neuroimaging findings of symmetrical basal ganglia or periaqueductal lesions. Usually nuclear DNA mutations, although some families have private mitochondrial DNA mutations

c. **Leber's hereditary optic neuritis.** Subacute onset optic neuritis in early adulthood with permanent visual impairment. Multiple or large-scale deletions mitochondrial DNA

d. **Kearns–Sayre syndrome.** Chronic progressive external ophthalmoplegia, cardiac conduction defects, short stature, myopathy, and a variety of CNS defects. Most due to a large deletion or duplication of mitochondrial DNA

e. **MERRF.** *My*oclonic *e*pilepsy with *r*agged *r*ed *f*ibres on muscle biopsy. Most due to a deletion of mitochondrial DNA

f. **MELAS.** *M*itochondrial myopathy, *e*ncephalopathy, *l*actic *a*cidosis and *s*troke-like episodes. Most due to a deletion of mitochondrial DNA

g. **MNGIE.** *My*oneural, *g*astro*i*ntestinal *e*ncephalopathy. Early-onset intestinal pseudo-obstruction followed by myopathy and encephalopathy in adulthood

IV. PEROXISOMAL DISORDERS

A group of diseases with either absence of peroxisomes (at least 13 different types) or deficiencies of the oxidative or synthetic enzymes contained within

1. **Peroxisomal biogenesis disorders**

a. **Zellweger's syndrome.** Craniofacial abnormalities (high forehead, upslanting palpebral fissures, hypoplastic supraorbital ridges, and epicanthic folds), severe weakness and hypotonia, deafness, neonatal seizures, absent development, retinal pigmentation, optic nerve hypoplasia, cataract, corneal clouding, hepatomegaly, renal cysts. Neuroimaging may show polymicrogyria, pachygyria, neuronal migration defects and abnormal myelination

Screening tests: plasma very long chain fatty acids, red cell plasmalogens, plasma and urinary bile acids, X-ray patella/acetabulum (for stippling)

Diagnosis: liver biopsy, DNA

b. **Neonatal adrenoleucodystrophy.** Less severe Zellweger's syndrome with mild adrenal hypofunction

Screening tests: as for Zellweger; no calcific stippling/renal cysts

2. **Disordered peroxisome enzyme import**

a. **Rhizomelic chondrodysplasia punctata.** Disturbed endochondral bone formation and short proximal limbs, learning difficulties, ichthyosis, cataract. Both phenotypic and genotypic variability

Screening tests: X-ray patella or acetabulum (calcific stippling), plasma phytanate, red cell plasmalogens, plasma and urinary bile acids

Diagnosis: red cell dihydroxyacetonephosphate acyltransferase

3. **Defects single peroxisomal enzymes**

a. **Pseudo-Zellweger syndrome.** Clinical features similar to classical form in 15%

Screening tests: plasma very long chain fatty acids, pipecolic acid and bile acid intermediates increased but peroxisomes present on liver biopsy; plasmalogens normal

Diagnosis: liver peroxisomal 3-oxoacylCoA thiolase, acylCoA oxidase, and bifunctional enzyme activity

b. **X-linked adrenoleucodystrophy.** Severe childhood cerebral form dementia, seizures, motor disorder, adrenal dysfunction; neuroimaging shows a leucodystrophy. Adrenomyeloneuropathy form progressive paraparesis with sphincter involvement, adrenal dysfunction in 60%

Screening tests: plasma very long chain fatty acids, synacthen test, urine glycerol (glycerol kinase deficiency causes neurological disease with adrenal insufficiency)

Diagnosis: DNA

Table 4.1. *Continued*

---

c. Refsum's disease. Tetrad of retinitis pigmentosa, peripheral neuropathy, cerebellar ataxia and increased CSF protein, may have neural deafness, anosmia, and ichthyosis

Screening tests: plasma phytanic acid

Diagnosis: fibroblast phytanate α-oxidase

V. LYSOSOMAL ENZYMES

1. Mucopolysaccharidoses

All develop some features of Hurler syndrome, excrete glycosaminoglycans in urine, and have white cell inclusions. The clinical features of Hurler's disease include hepatosplenomegaly, characteristic bony features of brachymetacarpal dwarfism, stiff joints, coarse facies, mental deterioration, and corneal cloudiness. Behaviour problems are frequent and early

Screening tests: skeletal survey, vacuolated lymphocytes, urine glycosaminoglycans

Diagnosis: white cell enzyme (below); DNA

   a. MPS I H: Hurler disease (α-L-iduronidase deficiency)

   b. MPS I S: Scheie disease (α-L-iduronidase deficiency). Normal CNS. Carpal tunnel syndrome

   c. MPS I H/S (α-L-iduronidase deficiency)

   d. MPS II XR: Severe Hunter disease (iduronate sulphatase deficiency)

   e. MPS II XR: Mild Hunter disease (iduronate sulphatase deficiency). Normal IQ

   f. MPS III A: Sanfilippo disease (Heparan N-sulphatase deficiency). Progressive dementia with only mild MPS features

   g. MPS III B (N-acetyl-A-D-glucosaminidase deficiency)

   h. MPS III C (acetyl-CoA:α-glucosaminide N-acetyl-transferase deficiency)

   i. MPS III D (Acetyl-CoA:α-glucosaminide 6-sulphatase deficiency)

   j. MPS IV A: Morquio disease (galactosamine 6-sulphate sulphatase deficiency). Skeletal and corneal involvement, normal IQ but atlantoaxial dislocation. Some CNS, including meningeal, involvement

   k. MPS IV B (β-galactosidase deficiency). No CNS involvement

   l. MPS VI: Severe Maroteaux–Lamy disease (arylsulphatase B deficiency). Mainly skeletal with risk of cervical cord compression

   m. MPS VI: Intermediate Maroteaux–Lamy disease (arylsulphatase B deficiency)

   n. MPS VI: Mild Maroteaux Lamy disease (arylsulphatase B deficiency)

   o. MPS VII: Sly disease (β-glucuronidase deficiency). Very variable phenotype

2. Pompé disease. Infantile progressive proximal muscle weakness, anterior horn cell disease, cardiomyopathy and early death. Later onset progressive proximal muscular weakness

Screening tests: vacuolated white cells, muscle histology

Diagnosis: white cell or muscle acid α-glucosidase; DNA

3. Abnormal lysosomal enzyme phosphorylation. Prevents normal trafficking of enzymes to lysosomes. Hurler-like features with variable time of onset

Screening tests: vacuolated white cells, plasma lysosomal enzymes (10–20 fold increase in β-hexosaminidase, arylsulphatase A, and iduronate sulphatase), urine glycosaminoglycans (normal)

Diagnosis: fibroblast UDP-GlcNAc: lysosomal enzyme precursor GlcNAc1-phosphotransferase activity

   a. I-cell disease (mucolipidosis II)

   b. Pseudo-Hurler (ML III)

4. Schindler disease. Severe: onset in second year, hypotonia, dementia, upper and lower motor neuropathy, brainstem disease. Mild: mild learning difficulties, angiokeratoma

Screening tests: skin nerve electron microscopy (axonal spheroids)

Diagnosis: white cell α-N-acetylgalactosaminidase; DNA

5. Abnormal glycoprotein degradation and structure

   a. α-Mannosidosis. Hurler features, dementia, angiokeratoma

   Screening tests: vacuolated white cells, urinary oligosaccharides

   Diagnosis: white cell α-mannosidase A & B

   b. β-Mannosidosis. Hurler features, variable neurological phenotype

   Screening tests: vacuolated white cells, urine oligosaccharides

   Diagnosis: white cell β-mannosidase

Table 4.1. *Continued*

c. Fucosidosis. Mild Hurler features, dementia and seizures, retinopathy

Screening tests: vacuolated white cells, urine oligosaccharides

Diagnosis: white cell fucosidase activity

d. Sialic acid storage disorders (Salla disease, sialic acid lysosomal transport deficiency). Dementia, extrapyramidal and cerebellar signs. Infantile and later onset

Screening tests: vacuolated white cells, urine sialic acid

Diagnosis: white cell sialic acid

e. Sialidosis (ML I). Infantile onset and juvenile onset

i. Normosomic. Cherry-red spot, action myoclonus, seizures, ataxia, normal facies and bones; burning feet; often no vacuolated lymphocytes

ii. Dysmorphic (may be associated with partial β-galactosidase deficiency). Cherry-red spot, myoclonus, mild MR, coarse Hurler-like facies, bony changes, ataxia

Screening tests: vacuolated white cells and foam cells, urine oligosaccharides

Diagnosis: white cell neuraminidase activity

f. Aspartylglucosaminuria. Mild Hurler features, learning difficulties

Screening tests: urine aspartylglucosamine, vacuolated white cells

Diagnosis: white cell aspartylglucosaminidase activity

g. Carbohydrate-deficient glycoprotein syndromes. Syndromes defined by the isoelectric focusing pattern of transferrin

i. Type 1a. Infantile onset: learning difficulties, squint and supranuclear ophthalmoplegia, hypotonia; abnormal fat distribution, inverted nipples; hepatomegaly, cardiomyopathy, pericardial effusions; cerebellar hypoplasia. Later onset: learning difficulties, ataxia, peripheral neuropathy, strokes, epilepsy; thoracic deformity, hypogonadism; cerebellar hypoplasia

ii. Type 2. Severe learning difficulties and hypotonia

iii. Type 1x. Severe learning difficulties, optic atrophy, epilepsy

iv. Type 2x. Intractable seizures, movement disorder, microcephaly, optic atrophy, tetraparesis

Screening tests: plasma albumin, thyroid binding globulin, haptoglobin, coagulation factors, lysosomal enzymes (increased)

Diagnosis: transferrin isoelectric focusing, fibroblast phosphomannomutase activity (type 1a), phosphomannose isomerase activity (type 1b), fibroblast *N*-acetylglucosaminyltransferase activity (type 2). Types x have transferrin pattern of 1 or 2 but no enzyme defect

6. Wolman's disease. Hepatosplenomegaly; severe gastrointestinal illness; neurological deterioration; calcification of adrenals

Screening tests: vacuolated lymphocytes and lipid inclusions in bone marrow cells

Diagnosis: white cell acid lipase activity

7. Farber's disease. Infantile onset swollen, very painful joints, joint and tendon nodules; laryngeal involvement; anterior horn cell disease, myopathy foveal grey spot

Diagnosis: white cell ceramidase activity

8. Niemann–Pick disease A & B. A: hepatosplenomegaly, hypotonia, dementia, foveal grey or cherry red spot. B: hepatosplenomegaly with no CNS involvement or mild ataxia alone

Screening tests: vacuolated white cells, bone marrow foamy histiocytes

Diagnosis: white cell acid sphingomyelinase; DNA

9. Niemann–Pick disease C. Progressive vertical supranuclear ophthalmoplegia, ataxia, dystonia and dementia. Variable early hepatosplenomegaly and failure to thrive. Neonatal hepatitis in 60%

Screening tests: foam cells in marrow, white cell sphingomyelinase activity (normal)

Diagnosis: fibroblast lysosomal cholesterol accumulation; DNA

10. Gaucher's disease

a. Type 1. Chronic non-neuronopathic form. Can present from infancy to adult life; early splenomegaly; hypersplenism and bone pain; late neurological problems in some

b. Type 2. Acute neuronopathic form. First year; hepatosplenomegaly; trismus, strabismus, retroflexion of head, progressive spasticity and dementia

c. Type 3. Subacute neuronopathic form. Half have onset in first 10 years dementia, spasticity, ataxia, movement disorder, supranuclear horizontal ophthalmoplegia; splenomegaly

Screening tests: raised non-tartrate inhibitable acid phosphatase (types 1 and 2), bone marrow for Gaucher cells

Diagnosis: white cell glucocerebrosidase activity

Table 4.1. *Continued*

11. **Krabbe's disease (globoid cell leucodystrophy)**
    a. Infantile. Early irritability, opisthotonus, dementia, peripheral neuropathy, optic atrophy, pyramidal signs, raised CSF protein
    b. Juvenile. Cortical blindness; spasticity, or extrapyramidal signs
    Screening tests: neuroimaging
    Diagnosis: white cell galactocerebrosidase activity

12. **Metachromatic leucodystrophy (sulphatide lipidosis)**. Variable time of onset and features; 5 subtypes recognized although only 3 given for simplicity. Occasional rare case of MLD without ASA deficiency. Pseudodeficiency gene is common
    a. Infantile. Ataxia, dementia, pyramidal tract signs and demyelinating peripheral neuropathy
    b. Juvenile. 3–20 years; psychosis, dementia, pyramidal tract signs, and dystonia
    c. Adult. Like juvenile, or pure dystonia
    Screening tests: neuroimaging, urinary sulphatide excretion, metachromatic inclusions in fresh urinary sediment
    Diagnosis: white cell arylsulphatase A activity, pseudodeficiency gene, fibroblast sulphatide load, sphingolipid activating protein

13. **Fabry's disease**. X-linked recessive. Angiokeratoma corporis diffusum; limb pains; retinopathy, variable neurology, stroke; severe renal disease
    Diagnosis: white cell α-galactosidase A activity

14. **GM$_1$ gangliosidosis**
    a. GM$_1$ type I. Hepatosplenomegaly, Hurler features, dementia, cherry red spot
      Screening tests: vacuolated white cells; Bone marrow foam cells
      Diagnosis: white cell β-galactosidase activity
    b. GM$_1$ type II – Morquio B. Later onset; mild bony involvement, ataxia, dementia; spasticity
      Screening tests: vacuolated white cells; bone marrow foam cells
      Diagnosis: white cell β-galactosidase activity

15. **GM$_2$ gangliosidosis**
    a. GM$_2$ type I – Tay–Sachs disease
      i. Early onset. Hyperacusis; visual failure, cherry red spot; dementia; hypotonia and pyramidal tract signs
      ii. Juvenile. Dystonic stammer, ataxia, extrapyramidal disease, anterior horn cell disease, dementia
      Diagnosis: white cell hexosaminidase A activity
    b. Sandhoff disease. Clinically like Tay–Sachs disease
      Diagnosis: white cell hexosaminidase A & B activity

16. **Batten's disease (ceroid lipofuscinosis)**
    a. Infantile (Santavuori). Early onset (8–12 months); knitting hyperkinesia, extrapyramidal and pyramidal signs, dementia, epilepsy, retinal degeneration, progressive reduction in EEG activity
      Screening tests: EEG and ERG/VEP may be suggestive
      Diagnosis: white cell electron microscopy, neural histopathology on rectal (full thickness) or skin biopsy; fibroblast or white cell palmitoyl-protein thioesterase activity; DNA
    b. Late infantile (Jansky–Bielschowsky). Myoclonic epilepsy and other seizures; ataxia; dementia; visual failure is a late feature
      Screening tests: loss of ERG with large VER to slow rates of flicker
      Diagnosis: neural histopathology on rectal (full thickness) biopsy; white cell tripeptidyl peptidase I activity (not the variant forms); DNA (not the variant forms)
    c. Juvenile (Spielmeyer–Vogt). Rapidly progressive retinitis pigmentosa, then disintegrative psychosis and dementia; seizures; late pyramidal and extrapyramidal movement disorder
      Screening tests: vacuolated white cells; ERG/VER
      Diagnosis: neural histopathology on rectal (full thickness) biopsy; DNA
    d. Adult (Kufs). May exhibit seizures, psychiatric and extrapyramidal features
      Diagnosis: neural histopathology on rectal (full thickness) biopsy

VI. PURINE AND PYRIMIDINES

1. **Purine defects**
    a. Lesch–Nyhan syndrome. X-linked. Learning difficulties, hypotonia and chorea in the first year, self-mutilation, dystonia, and spasticity at some stage in childhood
      Screening tests: plasma urate, urine urate to creatinine ratio (both increased; urine test more sensitive because of high renal urate clearance)
      Diagnosis: red cell hypoxanthine–guanine phosphoribosyl-transferase activity; DNA

Table 4.1. *Continued*

b. **Phosphoribosylpyrophosphate synthetase superactivity**. X-linked. Variable neurology. Learning difficulties, deafness

Screening tests: plasma urate, urine urate to creatinine ratio (both increased; urine test more sensitive because of high renal urate clearance)

Diagnosis: red cell phosphoribosylpyrophosphate synthetase activity

c. **Adenylosuccinase deficiency**. Severe learning difficulties with autism, later epilepsy. Milder variants occur related to degree enzyme deficiency

Screening tests: plasma succinyladenosine and succinylaminoimidazole carboxamide riboside

Diagnosis: red cell adenylosuccinase activity; DNA

d. **Adenosine deaminase deficiency**. Combined immunodeficiency; spasticity and ataxia

Screening tests: white cell count, serum immunoglobulins. Plasma adenosine and deoxyadenosine (both increased), red cell deoxyadenosine triphosphate (increased) and *S*-adenosylhomocysteine hydrolase activity (decreased)

Diagnosis: red cell ADA activity; DNA

e. **Purine nucleoside phosphorylase deficiency**. Combined (mostly cellular) immunodeficiency; spasticity (diplegia), learning difficulties, ataxia and tremor

Screening tests: white cell count, serum immunoglobulins. Plasma urate and urine urate to creatinine ratio (both decreased)

Diagnosis: red cell PNP activity; DNA

2. **Pyrimidine defects**

a. **Dihydropyrimidine dehydrogenase deficiency**. No consistent neurological consequences. Epilepsy, learning difficulties and microcephaly

Screening tests: urine thymine, 5-hydroxymethyluracil and uracil (increased)

Diagnosis: fibroblast or white cell dihydropyrimidine dehydrogenase activity

b. **Dihydropyrimidinase deficiency**. No consistent neurological consequences. Epilepsy, learning difficulties and microcephaly

Screening tests: urine dihydrothymine, dihydrouracil (increased) and 5-hydroxymethyluracil (not detected)

Diagnosis: liver dihydropyrimidinase activity

c. **Ureidopropionase (β-alanine synthase) deficiency**. Learning difficulties, hypotonia and dystonia

Screening tests: urine dihydrothymine, dihydrouracil, ureidopropionate, ureidoisobutyrate (increased) and 5-hydroxymethyluracil (not detected)

Diagnosis: liver ureidopropionase activity; DNA

d. **Hyper-β-alaninaemia**. Seizures and dementia

Screening tests: plasma and urine amino acids

Diagnosis: liver β-alanine-α-ketoglutarate aminotransferase

VII. METALS

1. **Copper metabolism**

a. **Wilson's disease**. Liver disease; progressive dystonia and other involuntary movements, Kayser Fleischer rings

Screening tests: plasma copper (total) and caeruloplasmin (reduced), urine copper (increased), penicillamine load

Diagnosis: liver copper (increased); DNA

b. **Menke's syndrome**. X-linked. Steely or kinky hair; hypothermia; osteoporosis with flared epiphyses, fractures; haemorrhages; seizures, dementia, early death

Screening tests: plasma copper and caeruloplasmin (reduced)

Diagnosis: fibroblast copper uptake; DNA

2. **Iron metabolism**

a. **Atransferrinaemia**. Dystonia and dementia

Diagnosis: serum transferrin

b. **Hallervorden–Spatz disease**. Progressive dystonia, retinopathy and dementia in some

Screening tests: neuroimaging, ERG, acanthocytes, lipoprotein electrophoresis

3. **Molybdenum cofactor deficiency**. Combined sulphite oxidase and xanthine oxidase deficiency, symptoms caused by sulphite oxidase deficiency which may exist as an isolated defect. Neonatal-onset feeding difficulties and seizures, dementia, lens dislocation, pyramidal tract signs

Screening tests: plasma urate (reduced), urine sulphite

Diagnosis: fibroblast sulphite oxidase activity

4. **Primary hypomagnesaemia**. Onset before 4 months, irritability, feeding difficulties, tetany, seizures

Screening tests: plasma magnesium and calcium (reduced), urine magnesium (reduced)

Table 4.1. *Continued*

VIII. VITAMINS

1. Tetrahydrofolate metabolism

a. Congenital folate malabsorption. Infantile onset severe megaloblastic anaemia, learning difficulties, later dementia, pyramidal and extrapyramidal motor disorder, intracranial calcification, demyelination

Screening tests: plasma total homocysteine. Serum, red cell and CSF 5-methyltetrahydrofolate, oral folate load

Diagnosis: small bowel folate transporter activity; DNA

b. 5,10-methylenetetrahydrofolate reductase deficiency. Variable severity of symptoms from severely affected infants to asymptomatic adults. Dementia, motor disorders, demyelination, seizures and psychiatric; vascular; no megaloblastic anaemia

Screening tests: plasma total homocysteine. Serum, red cell and CSF 5-methyltetrahydrofolate

Diagnosis: fibroblast 5,10-methylenetetrahydrofolate reductase activity; DNA

c. Forminoglutamic aciduria. Variable neurological picture and uncertain whether causes disease. **Type 1**: learning difficulties and hypotonia. **Type 2**: mild speech delay

Screening tests: serum and red cell folate (raised), histidine load

2. Cobalamin (vitamin B$_{12}$) metabolism. Very variable symptoms depending upon site and severity of the metabolic block

a. Defects in absorption and transport

i. Intrinsic factor deficiency. Onset second to fifth year of life, failure to thrive, irritability, muscular weakness, drowsiness, megaloblastic anaemia

ii. Immerslund–Gräsbeck syndrome. Onset after second year, gastrointestinal symptoms and developmental delay, proteinuria

iii. Transcobalamin 2 deficiency. Onset first year, failure to thrive, weakness, megaloblastic anaemia, developmental stagnation

iv. R-binder deficiency. Of uncertain disease-causing status, demyelination in adulthood

Screening tests: blood count, serum cobalamin, plasma total homocysteine, urinary methylmalonate, double isotope Schilling test

Diagnosis: serum transcobalamin 2 activity, fibroblast TC2 production

b. Defects in intracellular processing

i. MethylmalonylCoA mutase defects alone (cblA, *cblB* and cblH). Neonatal or late onset forms. Failure to thrive, developmental delay, acute encephalopathy

ii. Methionine synthase defects alone (cblE and cblG). Onset usually in first year, failure to thrive, megaloblastic anaemia, learning difficulties, seizures

iii. Combined defects (cblC, cblD and *cblF*). Infantile and late-onset forms. **Infantile**: microcephaly, failure to thrive, megaloblastic anaemia, learning difficulties, seizures, retinopathy, demyelination, severe systemic vasculitis. **Late onset**: anorexia, irritability, dementia, myelopathy, psychiatric

Screening tests: blood count, serum cobalamin, plasma total homocysteine, urinary methylmalonate

Diagnosis: fibroblast complementation studies

3. Biotin metabolism

a. Biotinidase deficiency. Seizures, ataxia, hyperventilation or stridor, dementia, deafness, optic atrophy, rash and alopecia

Screening tests: urine lactate, methylcitrate, propionylglycine, 3-hydroxypropionate, 3-methylcrotonylglycine, 3-hydroxyisovalerate may only be apparent late in the course of the disorder. Plasma lactate and alanine. CSF lactate

Diagnosis: plasma biotinidase activity

b. Holocarboxylase synthetase deficiency. Neonatal onset, apnoea, hypotonia, seizures, coma

Screening tests: blood acidosis and hyperammonaemia, urine lactate, methylcitrate, propionylglycine, 3-hydroxypropionate, 3-methylcrotonyl-glycine, 3-hydroxyisovalerate and tiglylglycine

Diagnosis: fibroblast carboxylase activities

4. Pyridoxine metabolism

a. Pyridoxine dependency. Intractable neonatal seizures, CNS malformations. Milder variants with later onset of tractable seizures may be more common

Screening tests: CSF 4-aminobutyric acid

Diagnosis: trial of pyridoxine

5. Nicotinamide metabolism. No enzymatic diagnoses made, but patients present with a photosensitive rash (pellagra-like), learning difficulties and ataxia

Screening tests: urine kynurenine pathway metabolites

Table 4.1. *Continued*

IX. LIPOPROTEINS

1. **Abetalipoproteinaemia**. Malabsorption; retinopathy; peripheral neuropathy; ataxia

   Screening tests: acanthocytes on wet blood film, decreased serum cholesterol, triglycerides and vitamin E

   Diagnosis: absent apolipoprotein B; DNA

2. **Tangier disease**. Tonsil abnormality; corneal opacification; hepatosplenomegaly; mononeuritis multiplex in adults

   Screening tests: decreased serum cholesterol, normal or raised triglycerides

   Diagnosis: absent apolipoprotein A-I

X. TRANSPORT DEFECTS

1. Lysosomal transport

   a. Sialic acid storage disorders

      i. **Infantile free sialic acid storage disease**. Severe Hurler-like phenotype

      ii. **Salla disease**. Infantile-onset learning difficulties and ataxia

   Screening tests: vacuolated white cells, urine sialic acid

   Diagnosis: white cell sialic acid

   b. **Cystinosis**. Renal failure mid-childhood. Surviving adults may develop myopathy, anterior horn cell disease and central demyelination

      Screening tests: corneal crystals on slit-lamp examination

      Diagnosis: increased fibroblast or polymorphonucleocyte cystine; DNA

2. **Lowe's syndrome**. X-linked. Prenatal cataract and other ocular abnormalities, hypotonia with absent tendon reflexes, learning difficulties

   Screening tests: renal Fanconi syndrome (bicarbonaturia, renal tubular acidosis, aminoaciduria, phosphaturia, tubular proteinuria, impaired urine concentration)

   Diagnosis: DNA

3. **Lysinuric protein intolerance**. Can have encephalopathic episodes (*vide infra*) but protein avoidance more usual; hepatosplenomegaly; sparse hair; hypotonia, psychiatric disturbance

   Screening tests: decreased plasma lysine, ornithine and arginine; increased plasma ammonia, glutamate, alanine, serine, proline, citrulline and glycine. Massive urine lysine excretion

   Diagnosis: fibroblast cationic amino acid transporter activity; DNA

4. **Hartnup disease**. Around 10% develop intermittent symptoms of pellagra (photosensitive rash, ataxia)

   Screening tests: neutral aminoaciduria, but not proline, cystine, lysine, and ornithine

XI. RED CELL GLYCOLYTIC DEFECTS

1. **Triose phosphate isomerase deficiency**. Haemolytic anaemia; cardiomyopathy and early death; jerky dystonia, pyramidal tract, anterior horn cell disease

   Diagnosis: red cell TPI activity

2. **Phosphoglycerate kinase deficiency**. X-linked. Haemolytic anaemia; variable neurology – learning difficulties, dystonia, psychiatric

   Diagnosis: red cell PGK activity

XII. DNA REPAIR DEFECTS

1. **DNA excision repair defects**

   Screening tests: fibroblast chromosome ultraviolet sensitivity

   Diagnosis: DNA (in some)

   a. **Cockayne syndrome**. Sun sensitivity, short stature, dysmorphism; microcephaly, demyelination, intracerebral calcification, retinitis pigmentosa, dementia, neuropathy. Milder variant recognized, three complementation groups

   b. **Xeroderma pigmentosa**. Sun sensitivity and neoplasia; dementia, deafness, ataxia, neuropathy. Seven complementation groups

   c. **Trichothiodystrophy**. Sulphur-deficient, brittle hair, short stature, learning difficulties, late movement disorder

2. **Ataxia telangiectasia**. Ataxia, dystonia, supranuclear ophthalmoplegia; immunodeficiency; neoplasia

   Screening tests: serum α-fetoprotein, immunoglobulins and IgG subclasses

   Diagnosis: white cell chromosome radiation sensitivity; DNA

Table 4.1. *Continued*

XIII. CLASSICAL WHITE MATTER DISORDERS

Diagnosis requires expert neuroradiology and magnetic resonance imaging in addition to biochemical and other investigations

1. Leukodystrophies

 a. **Metachromatic leucodystrophy.** *See above*

 b. **Krabbe leucodystrophy.** *See above*

 c. **Adrenoleucodystrophy.** *See above*

 d. **Canavan's disease.** *See above*

 e. **Alexander's disease.** Failure to thrive; dementia, leucodystrophy, megalencephaly

 f. **Aicardi–Goutiere syndrome.** Microcephaly, intracranial calcification, demyelination, CSF pleocytosis, raised CSF α-interferon

 g. **Cockayne syndrome.** *See above.*

 h. **Megalencephalic cystic leucoencephalopathy (van der Knaap leucodystrophy).** Macrocephaly in first year, motor disorder by fifth year, seizures and dementia in teens

 i. **Cerebellar ataxia central hypomyelination/vanishing white matter disease.** Encephalopathy followed by spastic/ataxic motor disorder, late bulbar involvement and optic atrophy

2. Brain dysmyelinating disorders

 a. **Pelizaeus–Merzbacher disease.** X-linked. Onset in first year nystagmus, spastic paraparesis, movement disorder

 b. **Merosin-deficient congenital muscular dystrophy.** Weakness and contractures at birth. No CNS symptoms

 c. **3-phosphoglycerate dehydrogenase deficiency (serine biosynthesis deficiency).** Microcephaly, intractable seizures, developmental stagnation

XIV. OTHERS

1. **Rett syndrome.** Females. From 6 months to 2 years; hand stereotypies and loss of hand function, dementia, acquired microcephaly, seizures; later pyramidal tract signs and neuropathy. DNA diagnosis (MECP2 gene).

2. **Progressive neuronal degeneration of childhood (Alpers' disease).** Early onset dementia, myoclonus and seizures; rapid deterioration, late liver involvement. Brain or liver biopsy may show characteristic changes. Some cases due to mitochondrial respiratory chain defects (*see above*)

3. **Infantile neuroaxonal dystrophy (Seitelberger's disease).** Onset at end of first year; profound hypotonia, dementia, pyramidal signs, anterior horn cell disease, optic atrophy and squint. Atypical cases include a juvenile variant with progressive myoclonic epilepsy and sometimes retinopathy. Axonal spheroids found on electron microscopy of brain, nerve, conjunctival or skin biopsy. Schindler's disease is a variant (*see above*).

4. **Unvericht–Lundborg disease.** Onset 8–13 years; progressive myoclonic epilepsy, action myoclonus, dementia

5. **Lafora-body disease.** Onset 11–18 years; myoclonic seizures, focal occipital seizures, dementia. Lafora bodies in apocrine sweat glands

6. **Idiopathic torsion dystonias.** Childhood onset progressive dystonia, usually sparing orobulbar musculature. DYT 1 gene accounts for some dominantly inherited forms, recessive inheritance also occurs

7. **Hereditary spastic paraplegias.** Childhood onset progressive spastic paraparesis. Usually dominantly inherited with variable penetrance

8. **Friedreich's ataxia.** Late childhood onset ataxia, axonal neuropathy and cardiomyopathy. DNA diagnosis

9. **Sjögren–Larssen syndrome.** Ichthyosis at birth; spastic diplegia and mental retardation developing before 3 years; macular changes. Skin alcohol dehydrogenase activity

10. **Chediak–Higashi syndrome.** Partial albinism, hepatosplenomegaly, lymphadenopathy; learning difficulties, cerebellar degeneration, nystagmus, peripheral neuropathy

11. **Guanidinoacetate methyltransferase deficiency (creatine biosynthesis defect).** Developmental stagnation, intractable seizures, dystonia. Low plasma creatinine, increased urine guanidinoacetate, absent creatine plus creatine phosphate peak on proton magnetic resonance spectroscopy. White cell guanidinoacetate methyltransferase activity and DNA

Table 4.2. Progressive neurometabolic disorders with episodes of acute metabolic encephalopathy (kindly prepared by Dr Robert Surtees)

I. CARBOHYDRATE DISORDERS

1. **Galactosaemia.** Liver failure with hepatosplenomegaly; cerebral oedema; cataracts. Later dyspraxia, variable learning difficulties, later still dystonia

 Screening tests: urine galactose, red cell galactose-1-phosphate

 Diagnosis: red cell galactose-1-phosphate-uridyl transferase or UDP-glucose epimerase activity

2. **Hereditary fructose intolerance.** Drowsiness, apathy; liver disease

 Diagnosis: liver fructose-1-phosphate-aldolase deficiency

Table 4.2. *Continued*

II. AMINO ACID DISORDERS

1. **Maple syrup urine disease.** Accumulating keto-acids have an aroma of maple syrup or fenugreek seeds

   a. **Classical.** Acute newborn presentation with severe ketoacidosis

   b. **Intermittent.** Ketoacidosis; ataxia, lethargy, slurred speech during attack; neurological handicap varies

   c. **Intermediate.** Learning difficulties without ketoacidosis

   d. **Thiamine responsive.** Learning difficulties

   e. **E_3 deficient form.** Progressive encephalopathy in first year

   Screening tests: raised plasma and urine leucine and 2-oxo-isocaproic acid

   Diagnosis: fibroblast branched chain keto-acid carboxylase activity

2. **Non-ketotic hyperglycinaemia.** Neonatal encephalopathy with apnoea and myoclonus. Later intractable seizures, pyramidal and extrapyramidal movement disorder; developmental stagnation

   Screening tests: raised plasma, urine, CSF and CSF/plasma (>0.09) glycine

   Diagnosis: fibroblast glycine cleavage enzyme activity; DNA

3. **Urea cycle disorders.** Ataxia, lethargy and coma, especially during decompensation, seizures. May present as Reye-like illness, stroke and intermittent ataxia

   Screening tests: plasma ammonia and amino acids, urine orotic acid

   Diagnosis: liver enzyme activity; DNA (for OCT deficiency)

   a. **N-acetylglutamate synthetase deficiency.** Very severe

   b. **Carbamoylphosphate synthetase deficiency.** Suspected by normal citrulline, arginosuccinic acid and arginine. No orotic acid in urine

   c. **Ornithine carbamoyl transferase deficiency.** X-linked, with manifesting carriers; liver disease. Orotic aciduria, low plasma arginine

   d. **Arginosuccinate synthetase deficiency (citrullinaemia).** Can be mild. Orotic aciduria, no arginosuccinic acid, citrulline high

   e. **Arginosuccinate lyase (argininosuccinic aciduria).** Metabolic acidosis, hepatomegaly; trichorrhexis nodosa and ataxia. Orotic acidaemia

   f. **Arginase deficiency (arginaemia).** See Table 4.1

   g. **Hyperornithinaemia, hyperammonaemia, homocitrullinaemia.** Ataxia, growth failure, learning difficulties

III. ORGANIC ACID DISORDERS

1. **Propionic acidaemia.** Severe acidosis, osteoporosis, neutropaenia, thrombocytopaenia, hyperglycinaemia. Neurological deficits acquired in acute attacks, and as late onset chorea

   Screening tests: blood count and gases, raised plasma glycine, raised urine methylcitrate, propionylglycine

   Diagnosis: white cell propionylCoA carboxylase activity

2. **Methylmalonic aciduria.** Severe acidosis, neutropaenia, thrombocytopaenia, hyperglycinaemia. Severe extrapyramidal disorder with low attenuation in globus pallidus following acute decompensation. Cobalamin responsive forms (cblA and cblB, see Table 4.1) do better

   Screening tests: blood count and gases, raised plasma glycine and methylmalonate, raised urine methylmalonate

   Diagnosis: fibroblast methylmalonylCoA mutase activity

3. **Isovaleric acidaemia.** Acquired neurological deficits; sweaty feet smell

   Screening tests: urine *N*-isovalerylglycine and 3-hydroxyisovaleric acid

   Diagnosis: white cell or fibroblast isovalerylCoA dehydrogenase

4. **Glutaric aciduria type I.** See Table 4.1. Approximately two-thirds present with an encephalopathic crisis and on recovery have dystonia and chorea; macrocephaly

   Screening tests: urine glutaric, 3-hydroxyglutaric and glutaconic acids, glutarylcarnitine and glutarylglycine. Reduced plasma free carnitine, increased plasma acylcarnitine or glutarylcarnitine

   Diagnosis: fibroblast or white cell glutarylCoA dehydrogenase activity; DNA

5. **Glutaric aciduria type II (multiple acylCoA dehydrogenase deficiency).** Dysmorphic features, coma, hypoglycaemia (acidosis, hyperammonaemia); renal cysts; sweaty feet smell. Classically with early death, but milder variants

   Screening tests: urine lactate, ethylmalonic, glutaric, adipic, 2-hydroxyglutaric, suberic and sebacic acids

   Diagnosis: fibroblast electron transfer flavoprotein or ETF-ubiquinone oxidoreductase activity

V. MITOCHONDRIAL FAT OXIDATION DEFECTS

1. **Carnitine transporter defect.** Early onset: hypoglycaemia (hypoketotic, hyperammonaemia), myopathy and cardiomyopathy. Late onset: progressive myopathy and cardiomyopathy

   Screening tests: decreased plasma carnitine

   Diagnosis: white cell or fibroblast carnitine transporter activity

Table 4.2.   *Continued*

2. **Carnitine palmitoyltransferase I deficiency**. Encephalopathy, seizures; hepatomegaly; hypoglycaemia

    Screening tests: normal or raised plasma carnitine, no abnormal urinary metabolites

    Diagnosis: white cell or fibroblast CPT I activity

3. **Carnitine palmitoyltransferase II deficiency**. Early onset: myopathy and cardiomyopathy. Adult: episodic myoglobinuria

    Screening tests: normal or raised plasma carnitine

    Diagnosis: muscle, white cell or fibroblast CPT II activity

4. **Carnitine/acylcarnitine translocase deficiency**. Hypoglycaemia (hyperammonaemia); myopathy and cardiomyopathy

    Screening tests: plasma carnitine normal

    Diagnosis: fibroblast CAT activity

5. **Medium chain acylCoA dehydrogenase deficiency**. Fasting induced encephalopathy, Reye's-like illness, no myopathy; hypoglycaemia (hyperammonaemia)

    Screening tests: plasma 4-**cis**-decenoic acid and low free carnitine, urine C_{6-12} dicarboxylic acids

    Diagnosis: fibroblast MCAD activity; DNA

6. **Very long-chain acylCoA dehydrogenase deficiency**. Fasting induced encephalopathy, hypoglycaemia, lethargy, muscle weakness, cardiomyopathy

    Screening tests: raised plasma urate, low plasma free carnitine, urine; C_{6-10} dicarboxylic acids

    Diagnosis: fibroblast LCAD activity; DNA

7. **Short chain acylCoA dehydrogenase deficiency**. Variable failure to thrive, myopathy

    Screening tests: urine ethylmalonate and methylsuccinate

    Diagnosis: fibroblast SCAD activity

8. **Long chain 3-hydroxyacylCoA dehydrogenase deficiency**. Fasting encephalopathy, myopathy, cardiomyopathy, retinitis pigmentosa, neuropathy

    Screening tests: plasma free carnitine reduced, urine C_{6-14} hydroxydicarboxylic acids

    Diagnosis: fibroblast LCHAD activity; DNA

9. **Short chain 3-hydroxyacylCoA dehydrogenase deficiency**. Fasting encephalopathy, myopathy, cardiomyopathy

    Diagnosis: muscle SCHAD activity

V. OTHERS

1. **Glycerol kinase deficiency**. X-linked

    Screening tests: urine glycerol

    Diagnosis: white cell or fibroblast GK activity

    a. **Juvenile onset**. Encephalopathy, vomiting, acidosis

    b. **Adult**. Benign (artefactual hypertriglyceridaemia)

    c. **Complex**. Contiguous gene defect possibly involving Xpter–*adrenal hyperplasia congenita–glycerol kinase–Duchenne muscular dystrophy–ornithine carbamoyl transferase*–cen

2. **The porphyrias**. Intermittent neuropathic symptoms in 10%, triggered by drug, hormonal, nutritional or unknown factors. Abdominal pain and vomiting; neuropathic pain and neuropathy (motor, sensory, cranial or autonomic), psychiatric

    a. **δ-aminolevulinic acid dehydratase porphyria**. Recessive

    Screening tests: increased urine δ-aminolevulinic acid, normal porphobilinogen

    Diagnosis: red cell δ-aminolevulinic acid dehydratase activity

    b. **Acute intermittent porphyria**. Dominant

    Screening tests: increased urine δ-aminolevulinic acid and porphobilinogen

    Diagnosis: red cell porphobilinogen deaminase activity

    c. **Hereditary coproporphyria**. Dominant, photosensitivity in 30%

    Screening tests: increased urine and faecal coproporphyrinogen III

    Diagnosis: hepatic coproporphyrinogen oxidase activity

    d. **Variegate porphyria**. Dominant, photosensitivity

    Screening tests: faecal protoporphyrinogen IX and coproporphyrinogen III

    Diagnosis: hepatic protoporphyrinogen oxidase activity

References

Aicardi, J, (1998). *Diseases of the nervous system in childhood.* MacKeith Press, Oxford.

Albright, A. L. (1996). Baclofen in the treatment of cerebral palsy. *J. Child Neurol.*, **11** (2), 77–83.

Albright, A. L., Barry, M. J., Fasick, M. P. *et al.* (1995). Effects of continuous intrathecal baclofen infusion and selective posterior rhizotomy on upper extremity spasticity. *Paediatr. Neurosurg.*, **23** (2), 82–5.

Amir, R. E., Van den Vyver, I. B., Wan, M. *et al.* (1999). Rett syndrome is caused by mutations in X-linked MECP2, encoding methyl-CpG-binding protein 2. *Nature Genetics*, **23**, 185–8.

Andermann, F., Olivier, A., Melanson, D. *et al.* (1987). Epilepsy due to focal cortical dyplasia with macrogyra and the form fruste of tuberous sclerosis: a study of 15 patients. In *Advances in epileptology*, (ed. P. Wolf, M. Darn, D. Janiz, and F. E. Dreifuss), p. 35. Raven Press, New York.

Antonizzi, I. and Leuzzi, V. (1987). Hyperargininaemia: case report. *J. Inher. Metab. Dis.*, **10**, 200.

Arnato, M., Fauchere, J. C., and Von Muralt, G. (1987). Relationship between periventricular–intraventricular hemorrhage and neonatal hyperbilirubinemia in very low birth weight infants. *J. Perinatology*, **4**, 275.

Baraitser, M. (1979). *The genetics of neurological disorders*, (3rd edn). Oxford University Press, Oxford.

Barkovitch, A. J. and Norman, D. (1988). Anomalies of the corpus callosium: correlation with further anomalies of the brain. *Am. J. Neuroradiol.*, **11**, 523–31.

Barlow, C. F. (1984) Headaches and migraine in childhood. *Clin. Develop. Med.*, **91**. Spastics International Medical Publications with Blackwell Scientific, London; J. B. Lippincott, Philadelphia.

Barnett, H. J. M., Foster, J. B., and Hudgson, P. (1974). *Syringomyelia.* Saunders, London.

Bleck, E. E. (1987). Orthopaedic management in cerebral palsy. *Clin. Develop. Med.*, **99/100**. MacKeith Press with Blackwell Scientific, London; J. B. Lippincott, Philadelphia.

Borzyskowski, M. and Mundy, A. R. (1990). Neuropathic bladder in childhood. *Clin. Develop. Med.*, **111**. MacKeith Press with Blackwell Scientific, Oxford.

Borzyskowski, M. and Neville B. G. R. (1981). Neuropathic bladder and spinal dysraphism. *Arch. Dis. Child.*, **56**, 176.

Brett, E. M. (1997). *Paediatric neurology*, (3rd edn). Churchill Livingstone, London.

British Medical Journal (1981). Prevention of haemolytic disease of the newborn due to due anti-D. *BMJ.*, **282**, 676.

Brock, D. J. H. and Sutcliffe, R. G. (1972). Alpha-fetoproteinin the antenatal diagnosis of anencephaly and spina bifida. *Lancet*, **ii**, 197.

Brocklehurst, G. (ed.) (1976). Spina bifida for the clinician. *Clin. Develop. Med.*, **57**. Spastics International Medical Publications and Heinemann, London.

Bull, J., Nixon, W. L. B., and Pratt, R. T. C. (1955). The radiological criteria and familial occurrence of primary basilar impression. *Brain*, **78**, 229.

Bundey, S. and Griffiths, M. I. (1977). Recurrence risks in families of children with symmetrical spasticity. *Devel. Med. Child Neurol.* **19**, 179–91.

Carter, C. O. (1976). Genetics of common single malformations. *Br. Med. Bull.*, **32**, 21–6.

Chamberlain, W. E. (1939). Basilar impression (platybasia). *Yale J. Biol. Med.*, **11**, 487.

Clarke, M., Carr, L., Reilly, S., Nerille, B. G. R. (2000). Worster-Drought syndrome, a mild Ectraplegic perisylvian cerebral palsy: A review of 47 cases. *Braik*, **123**, 2160–70.

Cohen, M. M. (1988). Understanding Proteus syndrome, unmasking the Elephant Man, and stemming elephant fever. *Neurofibromatosis*, **1**, 260–80.

Coupland, S. G. and Sarnat, H. B. (1990). Visual and auditory evoked potential correlates of cerebral malformations. *Brain Develop.*, **12**, 466–72.

Crockard, H. A., Clader, I., and Ransford, A. O. (1990). One-stage transoral decompression and posterior fixation in rheumatoid atlanto-axial subluxation. *J. Bone Joint Surg.*, **72**, 682–5.

Crothers, B. and Paine, R. S. (1959). *The natural history of cerebral palsy.* Harvard University Press, Cambridge, MA. (Reprinted 1988: MacKeith Press with Blackwell Scientific, London; J. B. Lippincott, Philadelphia.)

Cuckle, H. S. (1994). Screening for neural tube defects. In *Neural tube defects*, (ed. G. Bock and J. Marsh), Cubi Foundation Symposium 181, pp. 253–66. John Wiley, Chichester.

Currarino, G. and Silverman, F. N. (1960). Orbital hypertelorism, arhinenvephaly and trigonocephaly. *Radiology*, **74**, 206.

Danks, D. M. and Halliday, J. L. (1983). Incidence of neural tube defects in Victoria, Australia. *Lancet*, **i**, 65.

De Vries, L. S., Lary, S., and Dubowitz, L. M. S. (1985). Relationship of serum bilirubin levels to oxotoxicity and deafness in high risk low birth weight infants. *Pediatrics*, **76**, 351.

De Vries, L. S., Larroche, J. C., and Levine, M. (1988). Intracranial sequelae. In *Fetal and neonatal neurology and neurosurgery*, (ed. M. I. Levine, M. J. Bennett, and J. Pant). Churchill Livingstone, Edinburgh.

Dobyns, W. B. and Truwit, C. L. (1995). Lissencephaly and other malformations of cortical development, 1995 update. *Neuropaediatrics*, **26**(3), 132–47.

Edebol-Tysk, K. (1989). Epidemiology of spastic tetraplegic cerebral palsy in Sweden. I: Impairments and disabilities. *Neuropediatrics*, **20**, 41–45.

Edebol-Tysk, K., Hagberg, B., and Hagberg, G. (1989). Epidemiology of spastic tetraplegic cerebral palsy in Sweden. II: Prevalence, birth data and origin. *Neuropediatrics*, **20**, 46–52.

Emery, J. L. and MacKenzie N. (1973). Medullo-cervical dislocation deformity (Chiari II deformity) related to neurospinal dysraphism (meningomyelocele). *Brain*, **96**,155.

Evans, P. R. and Polani, P. E. (1950). The neurological sequelae of Rh sensitisation. *Quart. J. Med.*, **19**, 129.

Evrard, P., de Saint-Georges, P., Kadhim, H., and Gadisseux, J. F. (1989). Pathology of prenatal encephalopathies: In *Child neurology and developmental disabilities*, (ed. J. H. French, S. Harel, and P. Caesar), pp. 153–76. P. H. Brookes.

Fletcher, N. A. and Marsden, C. D. (1996). Dyskinetic cerebral palsy: a clinical and genetic study. *Develop. Med. Child Neurol.*, **38**, 873–80.

Forssberg, H. and Tedroff, K. B. (1997). Botulinum Toxin treatment in cerebral palsy: intervention with poor evaluation? *Develop. Med. Child Neurol.*, **39**, 635–40.

Foster, J. B., Hudgson, P., and Pearce, G. W. (1969). The association of syringomyelia and congenital cervico-medullary anomalies: pathological evidence. *Brain*, **92**, 25.

Friede, R. L. (1989). *Developmental neuropathology*, (2nd edn). Springer, Berlin.

Gabriel, R. S. (1980). Malformations of the central nervous system. In *Textbook of child neurology*, (ed. J. H. Menkes), (2nd edn), p. 161. Lea and Febiger, Philadelphia.

Gage, J. R. (1991). Gait analysis in cerebral palsy. *Clin. Develop. Med.*, **121**. MacKeith Press with Blackwell Scientific, London; Cambridge University Press, New York.

Garb, B. P. (1982). Colpocephaly: en error of morphogenesis. *Arch. Neurol.*, **39**, 243.

Gerrard, J. (1952). Kernicterus. *Brain*, **75**, 526.

Gillberg, C. (1995). *Clinical neuropsychiatry*. Cambridge University Press, Cambridge.

Gillberg, I. C. and Gillberg, C. (1989). Asperger syndrome—some epidemiological considerations: a research note. *J. Child Psychol. Psychiat.*, **30**, 631–8.

Gol, A. and Hellbusch, L. C. (1978). Surgical relief of progressive upper limb paralysis in Arnold–Chiari malformation. *J. Neurol. Neurosurg. Psychiat.*, **41**, 433.

Goodman, R. and Graham, P. (1996). Psychiatric problems in children with hemiplegia: cross sectional epidemiological survey. *BMJ*, **312**, 1065–9.

Gordon, D. S. (1969). Neurological syndromes associated with cranio-vertebral anomalies. *Proc. R. Soc. Med.*, **62**, 725.

Granata, T., Battaglia, G., D'Incerti, L. *et al.* (1996). Schizencephaly: neurologic and epileptologic findings. *Epilepsia*, **37**, 1185–93.

Gunderson, C. H. and Solitare, G. B. (1968). Mirror movements in patients with the Klippel–Feil syndrome. *Arch. Neurol.*, **18**, 675.

Gustafson, W. A. and Oldberg, E. (1940). Neurologic significance of platybasia. *Arch. Neurol. Psychiat.*, **44**, 84.

Hagberg, B. (1985). Rett's syndrome: prevalence and impact on progressive severe mental retardation in girls. *Acta Paediat. Scand.*, **74**, 405–8.

Hagberg, B. (1993). Rett syndrome—clinical and biological aspects. *Clin. Develop. Med.*, **127**. MacKeith Press, London.

Hagberg, B. and Hagberg, G. (1989). Epidemiology of spastic tetraplegic cerebral palsy in Sweden. II: Prevalence, birth data, and origin. *Neuroped.*, **20**, 46.

Hagberg, B. and Skjeldal, O. H. (1994). Rett variants: a suggested model for inclusion criteria. *Paediat. Neurol.* **11**, 5–11.

Hagberg, B., Hagberg, G., and Olow, I. (1975a). (i) The changing panorama of cerebral palsy in Sweden 1954–1970. I. Analysis of the general changes. *Acta Paediat. Scand.*, **64**, 187–92.

Hagberg, B., Hagberg, G., and Olow, I. (1975b). The changing panorama of cerebral palsy in Sweden 1965–1970. II. Analysis of the various syndromes. *Acta Paediat. Scand.*, **64**, 193–200.

Hagberg, B., Hagberg, G., Olow, I. (1976). The changing panorama of cerebral palsy in Sweden. III: The importance of foetal deprivation of supply. *Acta Paediat. Scand.*, **64**, 403–8.

Hagberg, B., Aicardi, J., Dias, K., and Ramos, O. (1983). A progressive syndrome of autism, dementia, ataxia and loss of purposeful hand use in girls: Rett syndrome: report of 35 cases. *Ann. Neurol.*, **14**, 471–9.

Hagberg, B., Hagberg, G., and Olow, I. (1984). The changing panorama of cerebral palsy in Sweden. IV. Epidemiological trends 1959–1978. *Acta Paediat. Scand.*, **73**, 433–40.

Hagberg, B., Hagberg, G., Olow, I. *et al.* (1989). The changing panorama of cerebral palsy in Sweden. V. The birth year period 1979–1982. *Acta Paediat. Scand.*, **78**, 283–90.

Hagberg B., Hagberg, G., and Olow, I. (1993). The changing panorama of cerebral palsy in Sweden. VI. Prevalence and origin during the birth year period 1983–1986. *Acta Paediat. Scand.*, **82**, 387–93.

Hagberg, G., Sanner, G., and Steen, M. (1972). The dysequilibrium syndrome in cerebral palsy. *Acta Paediat. Scand.*, Suppl. 226.

Harding, B. and Copp, A. J. (1997). Malformations. Chapter 8 in *Greenfield's neuropathology*, (ed. D. Graham and P. L. Lantos), Vol. 1. Arnold, London.

Harkey, H. L., Crockard, H. A., Stevens, J. M. *et al.* (1990). The operative management of basilar impression in osteogenesis imperfecta. *Neurosurg.*, 27, 782.

Heyman, I. (1997). Children with obsessive compulsive disorder. *BMJ*, 315, 444.

Honig, P. T. and Charney, E. B. (1982). Children with brain tumour headaches. *Am. J. Dis. Child.*, 136, 121–4.

Hunter, A. G. W. and Rudd, N. L. (1976). Craniosynotosis. I. Sagittal synostosis: its genetics and associated clinical findings in 214 patients who lacked involvement of the coronal suture(s). *Teratology*, 14, 185–93.

Hunter, A. G. W. and Rudd, N. L. (1977). Craniosynostosis. II. Coronal synostosis: its familial characteristics and associated clinical findings in 109 patients lacking bilateral polysyndactyly or synbdactyly. *Tyeratology*, 15, 301–10.

Hurwitz, L. J. and McSwiney, R. R. (1960). Basilar impression and osteogenesis impertecta in a family. *Brain*, 83, 138.

Ingram, T. T. S. (1964). *Paediatric aspects of Cerebral Palsy*. Churchill-Livingstone, Edinburgh.

James, C. C. M. and Lassman, L. P. (1981). *Spina bifida occulta: orthopaediatric, radiological and neurosurgical aspects*. Academic Press, London.

Jones, B. M., Hayward, R., Evans, R., and Britto, J. (1997). Occipital plagiocephaly: an epidemic of craniosynotosis? *BMJ*, 315, 693–4.

Kirkpatrick, M., Engleman, H., and Minns, R. A. (1989). Symptoms and signs of progressive hydrocephalus. *Arch. Dis. Child.*, 64, 124–8.

Klemmer, R. N., Snoke, P. O., and Cooper, H. K. (1931). Cleidocranial dysostosis. *Am. J. Roetgen.*, 25, 710.

Krägeloh-Mann I., Hagberg G., Meisner C., *et al.* (1993a). Bilateral spastic cerebral palsy—a comparative study between South West Germany and Western Sweden I clinical patterns and disabilities. *Develop. Med. Child Neurol.*, 35, 1037–47.

Krägeloh-Mann, I., Hagberg, G., Meisner, C. *et al.* (1993b). Bilateral spastic cerebral palsy- a comparative study between South West Germany and Western Sweden II Epidemiology. *Develop. Med. Child Neurol.*, 36, 473–83.

Kuzniecky, R., Berkovic, S., Andermann, F. *et al.* (1988). Focal cortical myoclonus and rolandic cortical dysplasia: clarification by magnetic resonance imaging. *Ann. Neurol.*, 23, 317–25.

Kyllerman, M. (1977). Dyskinetic cerebral palsy. An analysis of 115 Swedish cases. *Neuropadiatrie*, 8 (Suppl.), S28–S32.

Kyllerman, M. (1983). Reduced optimality in pre- and perinatal conditions in dyskinetic cerebral palsy. Distribution and comparison to controls. *Neuropediatrics*, 14, 29–36.

Landgren, M., Pettersson, R., Kjellman, B., and Gillberg, C. (1996). *DAMP/MBD hos 6–7 åringar, metodik för BVC och preliminära resultat*. Läkarstämman, Stockholm. [In Swedish.]

Ledbetter S. A., Kuwano A., Dobyns W. B., and Ledbetter D. H. (1992). Microdeletions of chromosome 17p13 as a cause of isolated lissencephaly. *Am. J. Hum. Genet.*, 50, 182–9.

Levin, S., Robinson, R. O., Aicardi, J., and Hoare, R. D. (1984). Computed tomographic appearance in the linear sebaceous nevus syndrome. *Neuroradiology*, 26, 469–72.

Lindhout, D. and Schmidt, D. (1986). In-utero exposure to valproate and neural tube defects. *Lancet*, 1, 1392.

Marin-Padilla, M. (1980). Morphogenesis of experimental encephalocele (cranioschisis occulta). *J. Neurol. Sci.*, 46, 83.

Marin-Padilla, M. and Marin-Padilla, T. M. (1981). Morogenesis of experimentally induced Arnold–Chiari malforamtion. *J. Neurol. Sci.* 50, 29.

McCarthy, G. T. (1990). Management of the neuropathic bowel. In *Neuropathic bladder in childhood*, (ed. M. Borzyskowski and A. R. Mundy), pp. 72–80. *Clin. Develop. Med.*, 111. MacKeith Press with Blackwell Scientific, Oxford.

McCarthy, G. T. (1992). *Physical disability in childhood*. Churchill Livingstone, Edinburgh.

McEnery, G., Borzyskowski, M., Cox, T. C. S., and Neville, B. G. R. (1992). The spinal chord in neurologically stable spina bifida: a clinical and MRI study. *Develop. Med. Child Neurol.*, 34, 342.

McLaughlin, J. F., Bjornson, K. F., Astley, S. *et al.* (1997). Efficacy of selective dorsal rhizotomy in spastic diplegia: changes in spasticity and mobility after 24 months. *Devel. Med. child Neurol.*, 39, 15.

Michie, I. and Clarke, M. (1968). Neurological syndromes associated with cervical and craniocervical anomalies. *Arch. Neurol., Chicago*, 18, 241.

Mills, J. L., Rhoads, C. G., Simpson, J. L., *et al.* (1989). The absence of a relation between the periconceptional use of vitamins and neural-tube defects. *N. Engl. J. Med.*, 321, 430–5.

Morton, R. E., Bonas R., Fourie, B., and Minford, J. (1993). Videofluoroscopy in the assessment of feeding disorders of children with neurological problems. *Develop. Med. child Neurol.*, 35, 388–95.

Nelson, K. B. (1988). What proportion of cerebral palsy is related to birth asphyxia? *J Pediat.*, 112, 572–4.

Nelson, K. B. and Ellenberg, J. (1986). Antecedents of cerebral palsy. Multivariate analysis of risk. *N. Engl. J. Med.*, **315**, 81–6.

Neville, B. G. R. (1997). The Worster-Drought syndrome: a severe test of paediatric neurodisability services. *Develop. Med. Child Neurol.*, **39**, 782–4.

Neville, B. G. R. and Albright, A. L. (2000). *The management of spasticity in children and adolescents*, Churchill Livingstone, London.

Neville, B. G. R. and Goodman, R. (2000). *Congenital hemiplegia*. MacKeith Press, Cambridge.

Newman, T. B. and Maisels, M. J. (1989). Bilirubin and brain damage: what do we do now? *Pediatrics*, **83**, 1062.

Nyberg, D. A., Mack, L. A., Bronstein, A., *et al.* (1987). Holoprosencephaly: prenatal sonographic diagnosis. *Am. J. Radiol.*, **149**, 1051–8.

O'Connell, J. E. A. and Aldren Turner, J. W. (1950). Basilar impression of the skull. *Brain*, **73**, 405.

Pagon, R. A., Clarren, S. K., Millam, D. F., and Hendrickson, A. E. (1983). Autosomal recessive eye and brain anomalies: Warburg syndrome. *J. Paediat.*, **102**, 542–6.

Peacock W. J. and Staudt, L. A. (1990). 'Spasticity in cerebral palsy and the selective posterior rhizotomy procedure. *J. Child Neurol.*, **5**, 179–85.

Price, D. L., Dooling, E. C., and Richardson, E. P. (1970). Caudal dyplasia (caudal regression syndrome). *Arch. Neurol.*, **23**, 212.

Pueschel, S. M. (1983). Atlanto-axial subluxation in Down syndrome. *Lancet*, **i**, 980.

Robb, S. A., Harden, A., and Boyd, S. G. (1989). Rett syndrome: an EEG study in 52 girls. *Neuropaediatrics*, **20**, 192–5.

Robert, E. and Guibaud, P. (1982). Maternal valproic acid and congenital tube defects. *Lancet*, **2**, 937.

Romijn, J. A. and Treffen, P. E. (1983). Anencophaly in the Netherlands: a remarkable decline. *Lancet*, **i**, 64.

Ross, G. W., Miller, J. Q., Persing, J. A. *et al.* (1989). Hemimegalencephaly, hemifacial hypertrophy and intracranial lipoma: a variant of neurofibromatosis. *Neurofibromatosis*, **2**, 69–77.

Sarnat, M. B., Case, M. E., and Graviss, R. (1976). Sacral agenesis: neurologic and neuropathologic features. *Neurology*, **26**, 1124.

Scrutton, D. (1978). Developmental deformity and the profoundly retarded child. In *Care of the handicapped children*. Spastics International Medical Publications, London; William Heineman Medical Books.

Scrutton, D. (ed.) (1984). Management of the motor disorders of children with cerebral palsy. *Clin. Develop. Med.*, **90**. Spastics International Medical Publications with Blackwell Scientific, London; J. B. Lippincott, Philadelphia.

Scrutton, D. (ed.) (1997). Telling is not always answering. *Develop. Med. Child Neurol.*, **39**, 71.

Seller, M. J., Campbell, S., Coltart, T. M., and Singer, J. D. (1973). Early termination of of anencephalic pregnancy after detection by raised alpha-fetoprotein levels. *Lancet*, **ii**, 73.

Shapiro, W. R., Williams, G. H., and Plum, F. (1969). Spontaneous recurrent hypothermia accompanying agenesis of the corpus callosum. *Brain*, **92**, 423–36.

Smithells, R. W., Sheppard, S., Schorah, C. J., *et al.* (1981). Apparent prevention of neural tube defects by periconceptional vitamin supplementation. *Arch. Dis. Child.*, **56**, 911–18.

Spillane, J. D. (1952). Three cases of achondroplasia with neurological complications. *J. Neurol. Neurosurg. Psychiat.*, **15**, 246.

Spillane, J. D. and Rogers, L. (1959). Lumbrosacral spina bifida cystica with craniovertebral anomalies: report of two cases presenting with neurological disorder in adult life. *J. Neurol. Neurosur. Psychiat.*, **22**, 144.

Spillane, J. D., Pallis, C., and Jones, A. M. (1957). Developmental abnormalities in the region of the foramen magnum. *Brain*, **80**, 11.

Spooner J. W. and Baloh, R. W. (1981). Arnold–Chiari malformation: improvements in eye movements after surgical treatment. *Brain*, **104**, 51.

Stanley, F. J. and Alberman, E. (1984). The epidemiology of the cerebral palsies. *Clin. Develop. Med.*, **87**. Spastics International Medical Publications with Blackwell Scientific, London; J. B. Lippincott, Philadelphia.

Stanley, O. H. and Chembers, T. L. (1982). Sodium valproate and neural tube defects. *Lancet*, **ii**, 1282.

Stevens, J. C., Cartlidge, N. E., Saunders, M. *et al.* (1971). Atlanto-axial subluxation and cervical myelopathy in rheumatoid arthritis. *Quart. J. Med.*, **40**, 391.

Sugimoto T., Yasuhara, A., Nishida, N., *et al.* (1993). MRI of the head in the evaluation of microcephaly. *Neuropediatrics*, **24**, 4–7.

Sun, P. P. and Persing, J. A. (1999). Craniosynotosis. In *Principles and practice of pediatric neurosurgery*, (ed. A. L. Albright, I. F. Pollack, and P. D. Adelson), pp. 219–42. Thième, New York.

Talwalker, V. C. and Dasur, D. K. (1970). 'Meningoceles' and 'meningomyelocles' (ectopic spinal chord). Clinicopathological basis of a new classification. *J. Neurol. Neurosurg. Psychiat.*, **33**, 251.

Taylor, A. R. and Byrnes, D. P. (1974). Foramen magnum and high cervical cord compression. *Brain*, **97**, 473.

Taylor, D. C. (1992). Mechanisms of coping with handicap. In *Physical disablity in childhood*, (ed. G. T. McCarthy), pp. 53–64. Churchill Livingstone, London.

Taylor, D. C., Falconer, M. A., Briton, C. J., and Corsellis, J. A. N. (1971). Focal dysplasia of the cerebral cortex in epilepsy: *J. Neurol. Neurosurg. Psychiat.*, **34**, 369–87.

Van Tuinen, P., Dobyns, W. B., Rich, D. C., *et al.* (1988). Molecular detection of microscopic and submicroscopic deletions associated with Miller–Dieker syndrome. *Am. J. Hum. Genet.*, **43**, 587–96.

Vargha-Khadem, F., Isaacs, E. B., Van der Werf, S., Robb, S., and Wilson, J. (1992). Development of memory in children with hemiplegia cerebral palsy: the deleterious consequences of seizures. *Brain*, **115**, 315–29.

Volpe, J. J. (1987). *Neurology of the newborn*, (2nd edn). W. B. Saunders, Philadelphia.

Wackenheim, A. (1974). *Roentgen diagnosis of the cranio vertebral region*. Springer-Verlag, Berlin.

Wiklund, L. M. and Uvebrant, P. (1990). *Periventricular leukomalacia at full-term birth—a lesion of prenatal origin*. University of Gothenburg.

Wiklund, L. M., Uvebrant, P., and Flodmark, O. (1990). Morphology of cerebral lesions in children with congenital hemiplegia: a study with computed tomography. *Neuroradiology*, **32**, 179–86.

Williams, J., Brodsky, M. C., Griebel, M., *et al.* (1993). Septo-optic dysplasia: the clinical insignificance of an absent septum pellucidum. *Devel. Med. Child Neurol.*, **35**, 490–501.

Winter, R. M. and Baraister, M. (1991). *Multiple congenital anomalies*. Chapman & Hall, London.

Winters, T. F. Jr, Gage, J. R., and Hicks, R. (1987). Gait patterns in spastic hemiplegia in children and young adults. *J. Bone Joint Surg.*, **69A**, 437–41.

Worster-Drought, C. (1956). Congenital suprabulbar paresis. *J. Laryngol. Otol.*, **70** 453–63.

Yakovlev, P. I. and Wadsworth, R. C. (1946a). Schizencephalies: a study of the congenital clefts in the cerebral mantle. I. Clefts with fused lips. *J. Neuropath. Exp. Neurol.* **5**, 116.

Yakovlev, P. I. and Wadsworth, R. C. (1946b). Schizencephalies: a study of the congenital clefts in the cerebral mantle. II. Clefts with hydrocephalus and lips separated. *J. Neuropath. Exp. Neurol.* **5**, 169.

CHAPTER 5

Toxic and environmental disorders

Michael Donaghy

5.1 Introduction

This chapter addresses those toxins and environmental insults which predominantly affect the nervous system, or which produce noteworthy long-term neurological consequences. The peripheral nervous system is particularly vulnerable to the toxic effects of drugs, metals, and industrial and agricultural poisons; these manifestations are covered in Chapter 12. Overdosage with an enormous range of drugs and chemicals causes acute poisoning syndromes which affect multiple organ systems, including the nervous system. Such systemic poisonings are not covered below and the reader is referred to comprehensive toxicology reference texts such as Ellenhorn *et al.* (1997).

5.2 Alcohol toxicity

Acute alcohol intoxication adversely affects judgement, restraint, and co-ordination. In high dosage it starts to have general anaesthetic effects, but at lower dosage it affects neurotransmitter systems including γ-aminobutyric acid (GABA)-mediated inhibition, increasing opioid effects, and inhibiting glutamate neurotransmission. The behavioural effects contribute to the neurological injury caused by motor vehicle accidents and violent behaviour. Alcohol intoxication predisposes to casual sexual contacts, thereby promoting the acquisition of sexually transmitted infections. In this regard the nervous system may be affected by the human immunodeficiency virus, herpes simplex virus type II, or syphilis. Pre-existing cerebral conditions, such as subdural haematoma or infection, dispose the sufferer to apparent intoxication after ingestion of lesser amounts of alcohol than usual. This phenomenon is known as pathological drunkenness.

Habitual heavy drinkers may become physically dependent upon ethanol: alcoholism. There is an inherited predisposition to alcoholism. This leads to a variety of neurological disorders, described below. These result from the direct toxic effects of alcohol and its metabolites, or from secondary malnutrition, particularly of thiamine. Many alcoholic patients exhibit combinations of various alcohol-related neurological disorders. The biological effects of alcohol upon the nervous system are reviewed in detail by Charness *et al.* (1989).

5.2.1 Ethanol withdrawal and delirium tremens

Withdrawal symptoms develop in established alcoholics who are starved of alcohol for more than a few hours. They are particularly likely in those deprived of their usual access to alcohol by prostration due to acute infection, accidents, or surgical operations. The 'shakes', a generalized course tremor of the face, tongue, and hands, appears earliest and may be the only symptom in mild cases. Frank delirium tremens develops in more serious cases. These patients experience nausea and vomiting, terrifying visual hallucinations often of animals, acute confusion, agitation, tachycardia, sweating, and hyperpyrexia.

Generalized tonic–clonic convulsions may occur. These symptoms are maximal about 36 hours after alcohol withdrawal. The mortality of delirium tremens is considerable, and is paticularly caused by uncontrolled convulsions and by cardiac arrhythmias due to autonomic nervous system dysfunction. On recognizing these symptoms, alcoholics usually resume drinking to suppress them. Medical treatment of delirium tremens consists of the administration of sedative drugs such as chlordiazepoxide (50 mg orally 6 hourly for 3 days), benzodiazepines, or chlomethiazole to control agitation and reduce the incidence of seizures (Thompson *et al.* 1975; Saitz and O'Malley 1997); β-blockers (such as atenolol) to control autonomic manifestations (Kraus *et al.* 1985); and thiamine parenterally. Neuroleptic drugs are useful adjunctive therapy for troublesome hallucinations and agitation, but may provoke seizures. In addition, any associated infection, dehydration, or hypoglycaemia should be treated. Although delirium tremens is a self-limited disorder, which resolves spontaneously, the majority of patients resume their habit and are vulnerable to further attacks.

5.2.2 Seizures and alcohol

Alcoholics usually develop seizures, either as a result of cerebral trauma or due to ethanol withdrawal. Occasionally acute alcohol intoxication provokes seizures within a few hours (Brennan and Lyttle 1987). Seizures due to cerebral trauma sustained during alcoholic binges constitute a diagnosis of epilepsy and should be treated with long-term anticonvulsant therapy. Alcohol withdrawal seizures are generally accompanied by other features of delirium tremens and should be investigated only if the seizures are focal, more than six in number, occur over a period exceeding 6 hours, or are associated with protracted post-ictal confusion, evidence of cranial trauma, or focal neurological signs (Charness *et al.* 1989). Anticonvulsant drug therapy is not usually recommended for alcohol withdrawal seizures, either over the short or the long term (Simon 1988). Other associated features of alcohol withdrawal should be treated as outlined above. Benzodiazapine or chlomethiazole infusions are usually effective for recurrent withdrawal seizures or status epilepticus.

The role of prior alcohol consumption has been studied in an unselected population of patients presenting with their first-ever seizure. Large daily levels of alcohol consumption correlate with an increased risk of seizure. Seizures are most frequent within 48 hours of last drinking alcohol. However, only half of all seizures occur within the conventional period for alcohol withdrawal symptoms, 6–48 hours after the cessation of drinking (Ng *et al.* 1988).

5.2.3 Wernicke–Korsakoff syndrome

Wernicke's encephalopathy is a reversible cerebral disorder due to thiamine deficiency. In most patients with Wernicke's encephalopathy, there is an underlying permanent disorder of memory known as Korsakoff's psychosis. Because of the usual concurrence of these two disorders, they are often referred to jointly as the Wernicke–Korsakoff syndrome (Victor *et al.* 1989) (Section 26.5).

Wernicke's encephalopathy is a reversible complication of thiamine deficiency in alcoholics, particularly those who are malnourished. Other causes of thiamine deficiency, such as starvation or gastrointestinal disease, and protracted hyperemesis gravidarum, may also lead to Wernicke's encephalopathy (Reuler *et al.* 1985). Neurological symptoms develop over hours or days and may be precipitated by a high carbohydrate intake. The typical clinical triad consists of encephalopathy, ataxia, and ophthalmoplegia. The encephalopathy produces somnolence and disorientation and eventually progresses to coma. Ataxia results from the combination of polyneuropathy and cerebellar dysfunction. Abnormal eye movements are crucial to the diagnosis of Wernicke's encephalopathy in life. There may be bilateral lateral rectus palsies, nystagmus, or complex ophthalmoplegias, and occasionally the pupils become small and unreactive. Patients may be hypothermic or hypotensive. Atypical presentations are common and post-mortem studies suggest that only 20 per cent of those reaching autopsy had been diagnosed in life (Harper 1983). On suspicion of the diagnosis at least 100 mg of thiamine should be given intravenously and continued regularly thereafter: without treatment mortality approaches 20 per cent. The response to thiamine replacement is dramatically fast. Within 1–6 hours, the ocular palsies begin to resolve and conscious level improves.

Underlying Korsakoff's psychosis of variable severity is evident in most patients following thiamine treatment of their associated Wernicke's encephalopathy. Patients exhibit retrograde amnesia (in which they are unable to recall information) and anterograde amnesia (in which they cannot register novel information). Confabulation may also be present. Useful recovery from Korsakoff's psychosis occurs in less than a quarter of these patients, despite adequate treatment of their associated Wernicke's disease with thiamine. Mammillary body atrophy and neuronal loss from the dorsal medial thalamus, periaqueductal grey matter of the midbrain, vagal nuclei, and cerebellar vermis are characteristic neuropathological features of Wernicke–Korsakoff disease (Victor *et al.* 1989). Mammillary body atrophy is particularly characteristic and may be demonstrated in life by magnetic resonance scanning (Charness and de la Paz 1987).

Red cell transketolase enzyme activity is reduced in thiamine deficiency. However, the delay in obtaining results of this enzyme assay precludes its use in diagnosing Wernicke–Korsakoff syndrome; treatment with thiamine should be started immediately once the disorder is suspected on clinical grounds. Some patients with Wernicke–Korsakoff disease have an inherited anomaly of the transketolase enzyme, affecting the binding of thiamine pyrophosphate (Blass and Gibson 1977).

5.2.4 Alcoholic cerebellar degeneration

Long-standing alcoholics may develop gait ataxia due to degeneration of cerebellar cortex Purkinje cells (Section 31.1.8). Although generally of gradual onset, alcoholic cerebellar ataxia may evolve relatively acutely, sometimes in the context of Wernicke's encephalopathy. Early on, demonstrable ataxia may be limited to the gait alone, but severely affected patients show ataxia if the legs or arms are tested individually. Dysarthria or nystagmus are unusual (Victor *et al.* 1959). In many patients, an alcoholic or thiamine deficiency peripheral neuropathy contributes to the ataxia. The incidence of cerebellar ataxia does not correlate with the extent of lifetime alcohol consumption (Estrin 1987) or with the occurrence of cerebellar atrophy on computed tomography of the brain (Hillbom *et al.* 1986). Quantitative histological studies show Purkinje cell loss from the cerebellum in alcoholics, which is particularly severe in those with additional Wernicke–Korsakoff syndrome (Phillips *et al.* 1987). These observations make it likely that cerebellar degeneration does not only result from the direct toxic effects of alcohol or its metabolites, but may also reflect some other factor, such as thiamine deficiency. Thiamine replacement and prolonged abstinence from alcohol should be recommended in all patients. Prolonged abstinence decreases the amplitude of body sway associated with alcoholic ataxia, suggesting some capacity for the ataxia to improve (Diener *et al.* 1984).

5.2.5 Alcoholic dementia

Cognitive impairment is common in alcoholics. It usually reflects varying combinations of acute intoxication, Wernicke– Korsakoff syndrome, mild delirium tremens, depressive pseudo-dementia, pre-morbid cognitive impairments, previous cerebral trauma, and the diffuse alcoholic brain damage otherwise known as alcoholic dementia. Less frequently, the cognitive impairment is due to sub-dural haematoma, metabolic encephalopathy, nicotinic acid deficiency, or Marchiafava– Bignami disease.

Whether diffuse alcoholic brain damage is an important and frequent cause of dementia in alcoholics (Lishman 1981) is questioned on the grounds that autopsy studies usually show evidence of inactive and chronic Wernicke–Korsakoff disease (Victor 1994). Generally it is assumed that alcoholic dementia involves generalized cognitive abnormalities, which distinguishes it from the selective amnesia of the Wernicke–Korsakoff syndrome. Neuropsychological studies show that alcoholic dementia predominantly affects problem-solving abilities, whereas memory is selectively impaired in the Wernicke–Korsakoff syndrome (Carlen *et al.* 1981). Alcoholic patients with dementia display cortical shrinkage and ventricular dilatation on computed tomography of the brain (Carlen *et al.* 1981; Ron *et al.* 1982). This cerebral shrinkage is only partially reversible following a period of abstinence in chronic alcoholics. Quantitative neuropathological studies show reduced numbers of neurons within the superior frontal cortex in such patients, despite preserved neuronal populations in the motor cortex (Harper *et al.* 1987).

5.2.6 Central pontine myelinolysis

Alcoholics are particularly prone to central pontine myelinolysis, particularly if they are chronically hyponatraemic (Slager 1986) (see also Section 29.5). This can also occur in alcoholics with a normal serum sodium (McKee *et al.* 1988). The clinical picture often develops an average of 6 days after correction of chronic hyponatraemia with intravenous fluids at rates exceeding 12 mmol/l of sodium per day. Accordingly, if intravenous therapy is deemed necessary, it is recommended that the serum sodium concentration should be increased by less than 8 mmol/l/day (Sterns *et al.* 1986).

Central pontine myelinolysis affects primarily the corticospinal tracts in the central brainstem. It produces a symmetrical paraparesis or quadriparesis with extensor plantar responses. In some patients the bulbar and facial musculature is also paralysed. Gaze palsies occasionally occur. The full-blown state produces a locked-in syndrome in which the patient is incapable of any voluntary movements except vertical eye movements, yet consciousness is preserved. Many patients die, and the remainder suffer substantial chronic disability; worthwhile recovery is rare. Autopsy studies show a characteristic large area of demyelination within the central pons; axons are spared (Wright *et al.* 1979). Computed tomography is relatively insensitive in detecting the large area of pontine demyelination, but magnetic resonance scanning demonstrates such lesions (Miller *et al.* 1988). It is not yet known how frequently mild degrees of clinically inapparent central pontine myelinolysis occur.

5.2.7 Marchiafava–Bignami disease

In this distinctive disorder, usually associated with underlying cirrhosis, demyelinating lesions develop in the corpus callosum. These are similar histologically to those in the brainstem in central pontine myelinolysis. Patients develop gait apraxia, dementia, spasticity, and dysarthria. Most patients die, or survive for many years with severe dementia; recovery is rare. The demyelinating lesion in the corpus callosum and adjacent cerebral white matter is demonstrable by magnetic resonance imaging or high-resolution CT scanning (Kawamura *et al.* 1985). The disorder was originally noted in malnourished Italian red wine drinkers but is now known to occur also in other groups of alcoholics.

5.2.8 Alcohol and stroke

Some have noted heavy alcohol intake to be a risk factor for ischaemic stroke, particularly in young males during or immediately following a bout of acute intoxication (Hillbom and Kaste 1983; Gill *et al.* 1986). A case control study has shown both ischaemic and haemorrhagic strokes to be less frequent in moderate consumers of alcohol, whereas the incidence of both types of stroke was increased in heavy drinkers (Gill *et al.* 1991).

5.2.9 Alcoholic peripheral neuropathy

The peripheral neuropathies due to alcohol or disulfiram (Antabuse®) are discussed in Section 12.18 and that due to thiamine deficiency associated with alcoholism (dry beriberi) in Section 12.21.1.

5.2.10 Alcoholic myopathy

Alcoholic myopathy may develop chronically or acutely (Section 15.9.1). Episodes of acute deterioration frequently punctuate an insidious background myopathy. Chronic alcoholic myopathy is a relatively painless affliction predominately affecting proximal muscles. In many alcoholics mild myopathy is an incidental asymptomatic finding on examination. Established myopathy occurs in those chronic alcoholics with a cumulative lifetime consumption exceeding 13 kg ethanol per kg body weight (a standard measure of spirits, wine, or a half-pint of beer contains approximately 10 g of alcohol). Malnutrition or electrolyte imbalance are not thought to be important contributing factors (Urbaro-Marquez *et al.* 1989). An associated cardiomyopathy is common. The serum creatine kinase levels are elevated in one-third of patients. Muscle biopsies show varying degrees of necrosis and atrophy, particularly affecting type II fibres. Electromyography shows non-specific myopathic features, fibrillations occur in the more acute myopathies. Episodes of acute alcoholic muscle weakness due to rhabdomyolysis often follow bouts of massive alcohol ingestion and are associated with dark urine containing myoglobin. Abstinence leads to some improvement. Downhill progression occurs in persistent drinkers (Martin *et al.* 1985).

5.2.11 Methanol poisoning

Consumption of doses of methylated spirits containing more than 30 g of methanol is often fatal. Methanol causes a toxic confusional state. Misty vision, central scotomata, or blindness are associated with optic disc oedema, and optic atrophy eventually develops (Sharpe *et al.* 1982). A Parkinsonian syndrome unresponsive to L-dopa has been described and involves bilateral infarction of the frontal white matter and putamen (McLean *et al.* 1980). These permanent neurological complications, and death when it occurs, are thought to be due to the accumulation of formic acid. This metabolite of methanol forms within 12 hours of ingestion and causes metabolic acidosis (*Lancet* 1983). Early treatment with haemodialysis is indicated for mental or visual changes, metabolic acidosis, if the blood methanol level exceeds 0.5 g/l, or following ingestion of more than 30 g of methanol (*Lancet* 1983).

5.3 Recreational drug abuse

This section addresses the neurological consequences of recreational drug abuse. It does not cover the associated social, epidemiological, or psychiatric aspects. It should be noted that multiple drug abuse is common and may include alcohol; that violent injuries are common in the drugs underworld; that pressure palsies of peripheral nerves may result from periods of stuporous immobility; and that intravenous drug abusers are prone to blood-borne infection, particularly with human immunodeficiency virus. Cerebrovascular disease in young adults should always provoke the question of drug abuse causing cerebral vasospasm (Sloan *et al.* 1998).

5.3.1 Cocaine

Cocaine is a currently fashionable central nervous system stimulant used to induce pleasurable euphoria and hypersexuality. It is usually absorbed through the mucous membranes by sniffing ('snorting') or by chewing. Highly purified free-base cocaine ('crack') may be inhaled. Cocaine is occasionally used intravenously, usually in polydrug abusers. Overdosage sometimes follows rupture of cocaine-loaded condoms within body cavities in smugglers. The common neurological consequences of cocaine are seizures and strokes. Cerebrospinal fluid rhinorrhoea has followed protracted cocaine sniffing and poses the risk of meningitis (Sawicka and Trosser 1983). Cocaine may induce choreo-athetoid movements, so-called 'crack dancing' (Daras *et al.* 1994).

Seizures may follow acute intoxication with cocaine, generally occurring within 90 minutes of abuse (Pascual-Leone *et al.* 1990). Most such seizures are generalized but focal attacks do occur. The seizures are generally single and are particularly likely following the use of 'crack'. Persistent neurological features and encephalographic or computed tomographic abnormalities are not subsequently evident. Cocaine-provoked seizures are the reason for coming to medical attention in approximately 10 per cent of those with cocaine-induced medical problems. There is an increased frequency of seizures in pre-existing epileptics who abuse cocaine.

Cocaine abuse is generally regarded as a risk factor for cerebrovascular disease in young adults. It is a potent vasoconstrictor and ischaemic and haemorrhagic strokes occur. Strokes may develop within minutes of 'crack' abuse and are frequently associated with headache. Intracerebral and subarachnoid haemorrhages may derive from pre-existing aneurysms or arteriovenous malformations, and may be provoked by hypertension during acute cocaine intoxication (Nolte *et al.* 1996). However, a case control study of young adults with stroke in a United States city failed to establish a clear association with episodes of crack cocaine usage (Qureshi *et al.* 1997). Cocaine associated cerebral infarction may affect any arterial territory of the brain (Levine *et al.* 1990) Stroke syndromes affecting the thalamomesencephalic regions are noteworthy since they are otherwise uncommon (Rowley *et al.* 1989). The pathogenesis of cocaine-related cerebral infarction is uncertain but probably relates to its powerful vasoconstrictive properties. Although cerebral angiography may reveal narrowed segments and beading of arteries, it is probable that this reflects focal vasospasm rather than a true vasculitis (Aggarwal *et al.* 1996). Habitual cocaine abusers develop computed tomographic evidence of diffuse cerebral atrophy, but it is not known whether there is associated dementia (Pascual-Leone *et al.* 1991).

5.3.2 Opiates

Acute overdosage with heroin and other opiates may cause coma associated with pinpoint pupils. Acute ischaemic stroke has been noted either immediately, or within hours of injecting heroin (Caplan *et al.* 1982a). Heroin 'mainlining' may also cause bacterial endocarditis, with the attendant risks of haemorrhage due to mycotic cerebral aneurysm and of blood-borne cerebral abscess. Seizures and choreiform movements have been noted soon after heroin administration but resolve spontaneously. Inhalation of poisoned heroin vapours (pyrolysate) has led to a spongiform leucoencephalopathy which initially causes apathy, bradyphrenia, motor restlessness, cerebellar ataxia, and pseudo-bulbar dysarthria; death may follow (Walters *et al.* 1982). Aspergillosis of the cerebral ventricles (Morrow *et al.* 1982) and cerebral mucormycosis (Masucci *et al.* 1982) have occurred in heroin abusers. Lumbosacral and brachial plexus neuropathies have occurred in those injecting adulterant heroin mixtures (Sections 13.6 and 13.7) (Challenor *et al.* 1973; De Gans *et al.* 1985). These plexus lesions are thought to represent hypersensitivity reactions and may respond to high-dose steroid therapy (Herdmann *et al.* 1988).

5.3.3 Lysergic acid diethylamide

Lysergic acid diethylamide (LSD) is usually taken orally. Acute panic attacks and psychotic reactions may lead to delusion-driven self-trauma. Seizures and ischaemic stroke occasionally occur (Lieberman *et al.* 1974).

5.3.4 Amphetamines

These central nervous system stimulants are generally consumed orally but can be inhaled or injected. Amphetamine psychosis with prominent paranoia usually occurs in chronic abusers. Acute neurological side-effects most commonly follow injection. Intracranial haemorrhage is signalled by sudden onset of headache within minutes of amphetamine administration. Both subarachnoid and intracerebral haemorrhage are well-recognized complications (Delaney and Estes 1980; Harrington *et al.* 1983). Seizures, ischaemic strokes due to vasospasm, and intracranial infection all occur in intravenous amphetamine abusers (Caplan *et al.* 1982b). Methylphenidate, an amphetamine analogue, has been associated with exacerbation or the onset of Gilles de la Tourette syndrome (Golden 1977).

Ecstasy (MDMA; 3,4-methylenedioxymethamphetamine) is an orally consumed amphetamine derivative, popularly used at 'rave' dance parties to induce euphoria and a sense of familiarity. Sweating, tachycardia, and jaw grinding may accompany its use, and hypertensive crises, paranoid psychosis, convulsions, stroke, and sudden death may occur (Henry 1992).

5.4 Toxic gases and asphyxia

5.4.1 Carbon monoxide

Carbon monoxide intoxication is a leading cause of death or brain damage due to poisoning. Accidental or suicidal exposure to vehicle exhaust fumes or coal-gas leaks, fires, or paint removers may all be responsible. Carbon monoxide replaces the oxygen in haemoglobin with the formation of carboxyhaemoglobin, thus causing hypoxic brain damage. In fatal cases of carbon monoxide poisoning there is multifocal neuronal loss, particularly affecting the cerebral cortex, basal ganglia, and limbic system, resembling that in anoxic encephalopathy. Prolonged or permanent neurological sequelae are usually seen only in patients rendered unconscious by the initial exposure. Such patients should be treated immediately with 100 per cent oxygen, and if promptly available, hyperbaric oxygen therapy. Hyperbaric oxygen therapy helps eliminate carboxyhaemoglobin and enhances the oxygen dissolved in plasma, but its practical role in treating carbon monoxide poisoning is uncertain. It should be considered when the carboxyhaemoglobin level exceeds 40 per cent in patients with significant neurological abnormalities within a few hours of the exposure (Ellenhorn *et al.* 1997). Those patients who regain consciousness go through variable periods of restlessness, confusion, disorientation, and amnesia. Multifocal neurological abnormalities may appear and fluctuate considerably: agnosias, dyspraxias, dysphasias, dysgraphias, akinesias, rigidity, a Parkinsonian syndrome, deafness, epilepsy, incontinence, and involuntary movements (Garland and Pearce 1967; Lacey 1981; Klawans *et al.* 1982;). Low-density lesions may be evident on brain computed tomography as early as 24 hours after exposure, usually bilaterally in the globus pallidus. The presence of such lesions signals a poorer prognosis (Saweda *et al.* 1980). Some neurological recovery occurs in most patients. However, permanent neurological sequelae are common, particularly residual disturbances of gait and memory. An encephalopathy starting some weeks after the initial carbon monoxide exposure has been noted occasionally. This is due to delayed onset of demyelination in the cerebral hemispheres (Plum *et al.* 1962; Sawa *et al.* 1981).

5.4.2 Hypoxic–ischaemic encephalopathy

Diffuse cerebral injury occurs in a variety of anoxic circumstances, including temporary cardiorespiratory arrest, anaesthetic accidents, cardiopulmonary bypass operations, near-miss drownings, and attempted strangulation or suffocation. The clinical manifestations closely resemble those of carbon monoxide poisoning (Section 5.4.1). Cessation of oxygenated blood flow to the brain for more than 3–5 minutes is likely to cause long-term cerebral injury. Diffuse cerebral anoxic injury is unlikely if the patient has not been rendered unconscious by the initial insult. During the first 24 hours following anoxia, a poor prognosis for independent daily functioning is signalled by absent pupillary light reflexes, disconjugate and disoriented eye movements, absent or extensor motor responses, and lack of response to commands (Levy *et al.* 1985). Gradual recovery occurs over weeks or months but is of variable extent. Severe anoxic–ischaemic insults may result in a permanent vegetative state in which there is no evidence of cognitive awareness despite recovery of brainstem responses (Dougherty *et al.* 1981). Focal cerebral lesions may occur in patients with pre-existing cerebral vascular disease. Persistent amnesia, parkinsonism, movement disorders, or action myoclonus can all follow anoxic brain injury. Up to a fifth of children satisfactorily resuscitated from near-miss drownings have minor visuomotor impairments or subtle disparities between verbal and performance intelligence quotients; but hard neurological signs are rare (Pearn 1977). Post-mortem studies of hypoxic–ischaemic brain damage show relatively symmetrical multifocal lesions affecting either the cerebral cortex or the cerebral white matter, and perhaps involving the caudate nucleus or cerebellum (Dougherty *et al.* 1981).

Occasionally a secondary neurological deterioration occurs days or a few weeks after the initial cerebral anoxic–ischaemic insult. After a good initial recovery, such patients abruptly become irritable, apathetic, and confused, and exhibit a shuffling gait with muscular rigidity (Plum *et al.* 1962). Autopsy studies show demyelination within the cerebral hemispheres.

5.4.3 Nitrous oxide

Chronic repeated recreational inhalation of nitrous oxide can lead to sensorimotor polyneuropathy and a myelopathy, with abnormalities of visual evoked responses and sensory nerve action potentials. Improvement occurs with abstinence (Heyer *et al.* 1986). The neurological abnormalities resemble those seen in vitamin B_{12} deficiency and it is of interest that normally nontoxic doses of nitrous oxide can produce neurological deterioration in patients with pre-existing vitamin B_{12} deficiency (Holloway and Alberico 1990).

5.4.4 Ethylene oxide

Ethylene oxide is used as an industrial chemical precursor and for sterilizing heat-sensitive medical equipment. An encephalopathy manifesting with fatiguability, poor concentration, and impaired co-ordination, or a polyneuropathy, may result from prolonged exposure (Gross *et al.* 1979).

5.4.5 Toluene

Paints and glues containing toluene have been popular with solvent abusers because of their euphoric effects. Two-thirds of a group of chronic abusers showed cognitive, pyramidal tract, cerebellar, brainstem, or cranial nerve abnormalities (Hormes *et al.* 1986). Accidental massive exposure to toluene diisocyanate leads to immediate euphoria, ataxia, and impaired consciousness, with persistent memory, mood, and personality changes (Le Quesne *et al.* 1976).

5.5 Therapeutic and diagnostic agent toxicity

This section addresses noteworthy or permanent neurological side-effects of some drugs and radiographic contrast agents. Many drugs produce mild temporary side-effects, such as giddiness, headache, or concentration difficulties; these are not covered in this section. Tardive dyskinesia (Section 32.9.2) and acute dystonic reactions (Section 32.4.13) due to neuroleptic drugs, and drug-induced peripheral neuropathy (Section 12.18) are covered elsewhere.

5.5.1 Oral contraceptives

Stroke is the most common serious neurological consequence of oral contraceptive use. A threefold increased incidence of ischaemic stroke is noted in women using oral contraceptives containing oestrogen (WHO 1996*a*), with a higher risk for pills containing ≥50 μg oestrogen. Hypertension, regular cigarette smoking and age over 35 years are important compounding risk factors for stroke in women using the pill. Haemorrhagic stroke is significantly increased in those pill-taking women aged over 35, with a history of hypertension, and who smoke (WHO 1996*b*). Migraine is also a risk factor for ischaemic, but not haemorrhagic, stroke and this risk is increased in oral contraceptive users, particularly with higher oestrogen dosages (≥50 μg) and in those who also smoke or have high blood pressure (Chang *et al.* 1998). Cerebral venous sinus thrombosis is also attributable to oral contraceptive use (Atkinson *et al.* 1970). Chorea may occur in patients taking oral contraceptives (Section 32.5.7). Carpal tunnel syndrome has been reported after oral contraceptive use (Sabour and Fadel 1970).

5.5.2 Neuroleptic malignant syndrome

This life-threatening drug reaction produces fever accompanied by autonomic and extrapyramidal abnormalities (Section 32.9.1). It is generally under-recognized and can produce permanent neurological abnormalities which may reflect a form of heatstroke. It usually occurs in patients receiving neuroleptic drugs, either acutely or chronically, either for psychiatric disorders, or as anti-emetics, or as premedication (Buckley and Hutchinson 1995). It has also been noted following cessation of dopaminergic therapy for Parkinson's disease. Neuroleptic malignant syndrome usually develops subacutely over 1–3 days, even in those patients who have been taking neuroleptic drugs for a long time. A review of the clinical manifestations of a large number of cases shows that muscular rigidity and hyperthermia (sometimes greater than 41 °C) are almost always present (Rosenberg and Green 1989). Other common features include mutism, tachycardia, tachypnoea, sweating, and hypertension. Tremor, mask-like facies, hyporeflexia, and obtundation are less common manifestations. The serum creatine phosphokinase level is elevated in approximately 70 per cent of patients, often to extreme levels. Pneumonia and respiratory failure are the most common life-threatening medical complications of the condition. Prompt recognition of the disorder and initiation of specific therapy greatly diminishes the chance of death, which occurs in up to 30 per cent of untreated patients. The offending causative drug should be stopped, and the patient rehydrated and treated with antipyretics. Bromocriptine (5 mg orally or nasogastrically 4 times daily) or dantroline (2–3 mg/kg/day intravenously) significantly improve the recovery time (Rosenberg and Green 1989). Cerebellar degeneration has been described in a patient with a particularly hyperpyrexic form of neuroleptic malignant syndrome and it is proposed that such permanent neurological features may reflect heat-related nervous system injury (Lee *et al.* 1989).

The differential diagnostic considerations in a typical case include heatstroke, idiopathic lethal catatonia, malignant hyperthermia associated with anaesthesia, drug interactions with monoamine-oxidase inhibitors, and a central anticholinergic syndrome which can be caused by the anticholinergic effects of several neuroleptic drugs.

5.5.3 Lithium

Lithium carbonate is commonly used to treat bipolar affective disorders. It produces tremor in more than 50 per cent, generally mild in degree. This tremor resolves with reduction or cessation of lithium therapy. Overdosage with lithium can produce peripheral neuropathy (Section 12.18.15). Seventeen patients have been reported with persisting neurological deficits after lithium therapy, commonly female, often associated with toxic blood levels (Donaldson and Cunningham 1983). These permanent deficits include Parkinsonian syndromes with akinetic hypertonicity or cogwheel rigidity, tremors, drooling, dysarthria, mask-like facies, and a positive glabella tap sign. Less frequent permanent features include choreo-athetosis, corticospinal tract damage, oculogyric crises, opisthotonic attacks, ataxia, impaired ocular conjugation, myoclonus and grand mal seizures. Downbeat nystagmus in the primary position can persist after cessation of lithium therapy (Williams *et al.* 1988). A subacute dementing syndrome associated with myoclonus has occasionally occurred and is associated with periodic complexes on EEG resembling Creutzfeldt–Jacob disease (Smith and Kocen 1988). Such patients recover after withdrawal of lithium.

5.5.4 Cancer chemotherapy

A number of therapeutic agents used to treat cancer may induce encephalopathies which should be distinguished from cerebral secondary deposits, malignant meningitis, opportunistic infections, metabolic disorders, and paraneoplastic neurological syndromes. Peripheral neuropathy may result from treatment with cisplatinum, misonidazol, taxol, or vincristine (Section 12.18).

Intrathecal or intravenous methotrexate may cause three distinct encephalopathies (Glass *et al.* 1986). First, a slowly progressive intellectual loss and personality change may occur, sometimes with seizures and ataxia. Secondly, acute encephalopathy may develop within 24 hours of cranial radiotherapy combined with intrathecal methotrexate; headache, papilloedema, coma, and seizures develop. These patients usually recover within 3 days but may exhibit residual neurological deficits. Thirdly, high-dose intravenous methotrexate therapy for osteogenic sarcoma may cause transient focal neurological abnormalities. These usually develop 7–14 days after the second or third administration of methotrexate (Glass *et al.* 1986). Such patients may abruptly develop gaze palsies, hemiparesis, focal seizures, sensory deficits, or behaviour abnormalities. These may worsen for up to 3 days before slowly resolving completely; computed tomographic scans are normal.

Cytosine arabinocide, used in high intravenous dosage to treat leukaemia, induces encephalopathy with seizures or cerebellar dysfunction in 12 per cent of recipients (Hwang *et al.* 1985). Permanent neurological deficits may occur in those receiving a total cumulative dose exceeding 24 g/m^2.

Adjuvant therapy for 15–19 weeks with 5-fluorouracil and levamisole for colonic adenocarcinoma has caused encephalopathy which progressively worsens over 2 or 3 weeks and is associated with MRI and biopsy evidence of central nervous system demyelination (Hook *et al.* 1992). Declining intellect, ataxia, or episodic loss of consciousness have occurred, with subsequent improvement, and the syndrome is most likely to represent 5-fluorouracil toxicity.

α-Interferon can induce cognitive dysfunction of mild to moderate severity, often associated with a Parkinsonian syndrome, which is not reversible on stopping the drug (Meyers *et al.* 1991).

5.5.5 Radiological contrast agents

Catheter-induced arterial embolization accounts for most cases of focal cerebral deficit or spinal-cord damage occurring during arteriography. The direct toxic effects of angiographic contrast media include seizures, which occur most commonly in patients with an underlying disorder of the blood–brain barrier. Spinal myoclonus may occur after selective spinal angiograms (Junck and Marshall 1983). Intravenous administration of contrast agents for computed tomography occasionally causes seizures, most commonly if the blood–brain barrier is impaired due to an underlying tumour.

Acute or chronic arachnoiditis has been associated with the use of oil-based myelographic contrast media such as iophendylate (Pantopaque®) or iophenylundecylate (Myodil®) (Keogh 1974; Jorgensen *et al.* 1975; Junck and Marshall 1983). The acute reactions usually involve meningismus associated with CSF pleocytosis, and settle in a few days. Chronic reactions produce an adhesive arachnoiditis after an interval of some months or more. Chronic back pain and lumbar or sacral root symptoms occur. Patients may be more vulnerable to chronic arachnoiditis if they received myelograms and operations in close succession, making this a possible cause for the 'failed back surgery syndrome' (Jørgensen *et al.* 1975). Magnetic resonance imaging of the lumbar spine defines the changes of lumbar arachnoiditis (Ross *et al.* 1987). The most typical changes are clumping of nerve roots into small groups, and adhesion of the nerve roots to the dural tube. The treatment of chronic arachnoiditis is primarily symptomatic. Some recommend attempts to remove any residual contrast medium which is still mobile (Junck and Marshall 1983). Pantopaque® and Myodil® were generally superseded as myelographic contrast agents during the early 1980s by the water-based compound metrizamide. Metrizamide can produce seizures or transient encephalopathy with confusion, hallucinations, asterixis, and myoclonus (Bertoni *et al.* 1981; Junck and Marshall 1983). Metrizamide has since been replaced by less toxic water-based myelographic contrast media, such as iohexol. In turn, myelography itself is generally being replaced by non-invasive magnetic resonance scanning.

5.5.6 Epidural and spinal anaesthesia

Neurological complications follow about 1 in 10 000 epidural, intrathecal, and caudal local anaesthetic blocking procedures (Puke *et al.* 1989). Often these neurological problems are not evident until persisting neurological symptoms or signs are noted 12 hours or more after the last injection of anaesthetic, by which time the nerve block should have worn off.

Direct needle trauma to a cauda equina roots, or to the conus medullaris of the spinal cord, usually causes immediate neuralgic pain, often in a radicular distribution, usually accompanied by sudden involuntary movements of a leg, and is sometimes followed by permanent neurological damage within the distribution of the affected nerve root. Spinal epidural haematoma is particularly likely in patients with pre-existing coagulation deficits and usually presents with low back pain associated with progressive leg paralysis over a few hours and loss of sphincter control; urgent scanning is required with a view to early neurosurgical decompression so as to try and prevent permanent neurological damage.

Accidental puncture of the dura mater occurs during intended epidural anaesthesia in about 2–5 per cent of patients, and the subsequent local anaesthetic infusion can lead to total intrathecal blockade with unconsciousness and cardiorespiratory failure; complete recovery is the rule with suitable intensive care. Presumed ischaemic lesions of the spinal cord or cauda equina occur, and may be particularly likely after accidental dural puncture and injection of local anaesthetic mixtures containing adrenaline. However, no pathogenetic mechanism is ever established in many cases of permanent neurological damage following epidural or spinal anaesthesia. Spinal epidural abscess or late adhesive arachnoiditis of the cauda equina are rare, but represent serious causes of neurological damage developing days, weeks, or months after the anaesthetic procedure (Parnass and Schmidt 1990). Headache in the upright position due to spinal fluid hypotension, and aseptic meningitis, are other recognized transient complications of dural puncture during local anaesthesia.

5.6 Complications of organ transplantation

Neurological disorders make a major contribution to the mortality and morbidity of organ transplantation, often developing many months or years later. The range of neurological disorders is large, but particularly common disorders include stroke, cerebral lymphoma, intracranial infections, polyneuropathy, and side-effects of immunosuppressant drugs.

The first diagnostic step requires the patient's neurological syndrome to be categorized (Table 5.1) (Donaghy 1998).

Table 5.1. Neurological syndromes in transplant recipients

1. Diffuse encephalopathy
Meningitis
Encephalitis
Electrolyte disturbances
Rejection encephalopathy
Hypertensive encephalopathy
Hypoxic, hypotensive encephalopathy
Remote effects of systemic sepsis
Multifocal cerebral lymphoma
Pulmonary, liver, or renal failure
Cyclosporin toxicity
FK506 toxicity
OKT3 antibody meningo-encephalopathy

2. Focal neurological abnormalities
Cerebral lymphoma
Ischaemic stroke
Intracerebral haematoma
Focal cerebral infection
Central pontine myelinolysis

3. Seizures
Cyclosporin toxicity
Hypomagnesaemia
Hyponatraemia
Rejection encephalopathy
Cerebral lymphoma
Meningitis/encephalitis

4. Neuromuscular disease
Perioperative focal nerve damage
Guillain–Barré syndrome
Chronic inflammatory demyelinating polyneuropathy
FK506 neuropathy
Critical illness polyneuropathy
Polymyositis
Myasthenia gravis
Rhabdomyolysis

5.6.1 **Diffuse encephalopathy**

This may range from mild confusion or ataxia to deep coma, sometimes with headache, seizures, or meningeal irritation, depending upon the underlying cause. Cyclosporin or FK506 toxicity usually appear within 3 months and may include tremors, seizures, or visual disturbances, such as hallucinations or cortical blindness. *Listeria* meningoencephalitis usually develops more than a month after transplantation and often includes prominent features of brainstem dysfunction, such as abnormal eye movements or dysarthria. Cryptococcal meningitis is usually delayed for at least 6 months after transplantation.

A syndrome of rejection encephalopathy in young transplant recipients, which includes papilloedema, may reflect cumulative physiological and metabolic insults, including hypertension and electrolyte disorders, rather than representing a direct consequence of rejection. Cardiac or pulmonary transplant recipients may develop hypoxic–hypotensive encephalopathy perioperatively. Encephalopathy regularly occurs in the weeks following bone marrow or liver transplantation, although the pathogenesis often remains unclear. Patients require brain imaging to detect multiple mass lesions, such as multifocal lymphoma, masquerading as diffuse encephalopathy. If the brain scan is normal, spinal fluid examination will detect infections. As well as being itself a cause of encephalopathy, it should be noted that hyponatraemia may be a secondary feature of other neurological disorders, such as meningitis.

5.6.2 **Focal cerebral abnormalities, lymphoma, and stroke**

Hemiparesis, dysphasia, or homonymous hemianopia are usually due to ischaemic or haemorrhagic stroke, or primary cerebral lymphoma. Focal cerebral infection with *Toxoplasma* or *Aspergillus* may become evident as early as 2 weeks post-transplant, whereas *Nocardia* brain abscess tends to present later than 3 months. Central pontine myelinolysis is particularly likely in hepatic transplant recipients, particularly in the presence of blood sodium disorders (Winnock *et al.* 1993).

The risk of cerebral lymphoma in transplant recipients is estimated at 2 per cent, between 30 and 350 times higher than normal (Patchell 1988). The median interval from transplantation to clinical detection of primary cerebral lymphoma in transplant recipients is 9 months, with a range of 5.5 to 46 months (Hochberg and Miller 1988). The cerebral lymphoma is multifocal in a third and generally affects the cerebral hemispheres. High-dose steroid therapy should be avoided prior to neurosurgical biopsy, since dramatic tumour shrinkage can occur within a few days and confuse the histological picture. The treatment of cerebral lymphoma in transplant recipients should follow the usual lines (Section 18.8.3), although the prognosis appears to be poorer than in immunocompetent patients with lymphoma.

Stroke is a major cause of morbidity and mortality, both early and late after transplantation. Cerebral ischaemic events occurred in nearly 10 per cent of 10-year survivors in the early days of renal transplantation, but the impression is that these are less frequent now high doses of steroids have been replaced by cyclosporin for the prevention of graft rejection. Perioperative stroke is a particular risk in cardiac transplantation, due to air or solid embolism, or cerebral hypoperfusion (Montero and Martinez 1986). Haemorrhagic stroke is a noteworthy problem in bone marrow and liver transplant recipients, and can reflect underlying septicaemia, endocarditis, thrombocytopenia, or sickle-cell disease (Patchell *et al.* 1985; Wijdicks *et al.* 1995).

5.6.3 **Convulsions**

A multiplicity of factors is generally responsible for convulsions in transplant recipients. Cyclosporin toxicity is a common cause, sometimes exacerbated by hypomagnesaemia, particularly early after liver transplants (Kahan *et al.* 1987). Focal cerebral lesions such as lymphoma, infarction, or infection should be sought by scanning if convulsions develop after the immediate post-transplant period. If seizures persist in cyclosporin recipients, despite reducing the dosage if the blood level is high, the choice of an anticonvulsant drug is difficult. Phenytoin, carbamazepine, and phenobarbital all induce hepatic enzymes, which poses difficulties for achieving adequately immunosuppressive blood levels of cyclosporin. Sodium valporate is the recommended anticonvulsant in patients simultaneously receiving cyclosporin (Hillebrand *et al.* 1987).

5.6.4 **Neuromuscular disorders**

Focal peripheral neuropathies may complicate transplant surgery (Donaghy 1998). Self-retaining retractors in the pelvis can cause femoral nerve palsies in renal transplant recipients. Diabetics undergoing renal transplantation are vulnerable to lumbosacral plexus lesions of presumed ischaemic cause. Phrenic nerve lesions can complicate lung transplantation and prolong ventilator dependence postoperatively. Various mononeuropathies complicate liver transplantation, especially brachial plexus injury due to arm malpositioning.

Acute polyneuropathies of Guillain–Barré type are usually seen in bone marrow or hepatic transplantation, and can follow renal transplantation from a cytomegalovirus-infected donor. Chronic inflammatory demyelinating neuropathy can occur in the months following liver transplantation, sometimes after immunosuppression with FK506, and shows the usual good response to steroids, plasma exchange, or intravenous immunoglobulin. Although cyclosporin often produces tinglings in the fingers and toes, this is a 'hyperexcitability' phenomenon which does not reflect underlying polyneuropathy.

Myopathies occur in bone marrow or liver transplant recipients. Chronic graft-versus-host disease can cause polymyositis or myasthenia gravis. A recoverable quadriplegia can occur in liver transplant recipients; its cause is generally unknown, although a few cases are due to rhabdomyolysis.

5.6.5 **Cyclosporin and FK506 toxicity**

Cyclosporin is used widely because of its effectiveness in preventing rejection of organ transplants. Up to a quarter of patients experience neurological side-effects (Kahan *et al.* 1987; Walker and Brochstein 1988). Tremors are most common, but seizures, dysaesthesia of the extremities, depression, sleepiness, ataxia, and visual hallucinations have all been reported (Kahan *et al.* 1987; Walker and Brochstein 1988; Steg and Garcia 1991). Occasionally patients with cyclosporin neurotoxicity are hypomagnesaemic (Thompson *et al.* 1984). Some others have toxic blood levels of cyclosporin or its metabolites. Symptoms generally resolve on reducing or stopping the drug, but this should only be undertaken by those supervising the organ transplant, for fear of precipitating graft rejection. Mild tremor or parasthesiae, the most common complications, are often tolerated without reduction in drug dosage. If anticonvulsant therapy is needed for seizures, sodium valproate is recommended because of the risk that enzyme induction by phenytoin, carbamezepine, or phenobarbital will produce low cyclosporin blood levels (Walker and Brochstein 1988).

An acute encephalopathy with cortical blindness and other focal deficits may occur, associated with cerebral white matter hypodensity on computed tomographic scan (Rubin and Kang 1987). This leucoencephalopathy recovers after drug withdrawal, but sometimes recurs on reintroduction of cyclosporin (Walker and Brochstein 1988).

FK506 provides an alternative immunosuppressant to cyclosporin, and is a useful alternative in cases of neurological or other side-effects. But FK506 itself produces neurological side-effects in up to 30 per cent; speech disturbance, seizures, tremor and ataxia, encephalopathy, nightmares, or agitation have been reported and usually resolve with dosage reduction (Wijdicks *et al.* 1994). A more serious leucoencephalopathy may occur, resembling that caused by cyclosporin, and presents with headache, vomiting, seizures, and visual disturbance (Small *et al.* 1996).

5.7 Metal toxicity

Please see also Section 12.18.13 for the peripheral neuropathies due to toxicity from gold, and Section 12.19 for neuropathies due to arsenic, lead, mercury, and thallium.

5.7.1 **Aluminium**

Aluminium has been implicated in the pathogenesis of Alzheimer's disease. X-ray spectrometry shows aluminium accumulation in neuronal fibrillary tangles (Perl and Brody 1980). A geographical correlation has been noted between drinking water aluminium concentration and the incidence of dementia, as judged by computed tomography scanning requests (Martyn *et al.* 1989). Despite these findings, any possible causative relationship between ingested aluminium and Alzheimer's disease is generally regarded as being conjectural.

Aluminium toxicity was responsible for the encephalopathy which used to occur in patients receiving long-term renal dialysis using aluminium-rich dialysis fluids. Such patients developed progressive dementia with noteworthy speech abnormalities, myoclonic jerkings, and epilepsy. They have increased aluminium levels in the cerebral cortex, bone, and blood (Alfrey *et al.* 1976). The incidence of dementia correlates closely both with the incidence of fracturing dialysis osteodystrophy and with the aluminium content of the water used in preparing the dialysis fluids (Parkinson *et al.* 1979). Over the past decade, reduction of the aluminium content in the diasylate has massively reduced the incidence of severe dialysis encephalopathy. However, subtle alterations in psychomotor function can still be detected in dialysis patients with only mildly elevated serum aluminium levels (Altman *et al.* 1989). This has led to the suspicion that dietary sources of aluminium, including gastrointestinal phosphate binders, may also lead to toxic aluminium accumulation in dialysis patients.

5.7.2 Bismuth

Encephalopathy has been noted in patients taking bismuth salts for chronic gastrointestinal disorders, particularly for the control of output from colostomies (Burns *et al.* 1974). Confusion, tremors, myoclonus, and a prominent gait abnormality develop. The blood bismuth level is raised. Recovery occurred when bismuth was withdrawn, sometimes with residual memory deficits.

5.7.3 Lead

Inorganic lead toxicity usually follows ingestion of lead-containing paints by children, or occupational exposure of adult metal workers. There are public health concerns about the degree to which lead from vehicle exhaust fumes and domestic water supply pipes can cause subtle developmental intellectual abnormalities. In adults, inorganic lead poisoning leads to a purely or predominantly motor peripheral neuropathy (Section 12.19.2). In children, inorganic lead poisoning causes a subacute encephalopathy with irritability or listlessness, sometimes associated with anaemia. This may be followed by clumsiness, seizures, and evidence of elevated intracranial pressure with vomiting, headache, and papilloedema. Childhood lead poisoning may be fatal, and autopsy studies of the brain show exudative oedema and widespread patchy cerebral necrosis (Smith *et al.* 1960). Lead lines may be evident in X-rays of the epiphyseal plates of long bones. Mildly impaired cognitive and psychomotor development in children has been correlated with chronic low-level lead exposure, as judged by blood and tooth lead contents (Fulton *et al.* 1987). These mild neurobehavioural abnormalities persist into young adulthood (Needleman *et al.* 1990).

Organic lead intoxication usually follows exposure to tetraethyl lead, the antiknock compound of petroleum. Neurological disease has been reported in industrial workers in the petroleum industry (Cassells and Dodds 1946) and in recreational petroleum inhalers (Kaelan *et al.* 1986). The first symptoms consist of altered sleep patterns, dreams, irritability, and anorexia. Confusion or psychosis subsequently develops. In severe toxicity, myoclonic jerks, ataxia, and hallucinations are evident. Death may occur and autopsies characteristically show loss of neurons from Ammon's horn in the hippocampus and of cerebellar Purkinje and granule cells. Late cognitive decline has been noted in former organolead manufacturing workers (Schwartz *el al.* 2000).

5.7.4 Manganese

Manganese neurotoxicity has been reported in ore miners, particularly in Chile, and in steel workers. Chronic manganese poisoning generally follows exposure for more than 1 year and

produces a clinical picture resembling Parkinson's or Wilson's diseases (Cook *et al.* 1974; Huang *et al.* 1989). The initial symptoms consist of psychomotor excitement, somnolence, gait unsteadiness, slurred speech, and manipulatory difficulties. More chronic toxicity produces typical features of parkinsonism, with notably prominent slurred speech of low volume, oral tremors, dystonias, and neuropsychiatric abnormalities, which may progress even 10 years after ceasing exposure (Huang *et al.* 1998). There is a characteristic gait abnormality in which patients walk on the metatarsophalangeal joints in the talipes equinus position, a so-called 'cock walk' (Cook *et al.* 1974). During exposure, blood and hair manganese levels are elevated (Huang *et al.* 1989). Levels of manganese in tissues other than the brain slowly revert to normal after patients are removed from the exposure, although the neurological syndrome does not improve. Although minor neurological improvements have been noted after metal chelation therapy with eidetic acid, significantly prolonged benefit does not generally result (Cook *et al.* 1974). Indeed, chronic asymptomatic manganese exposure in miners causes subtle movement disorders later in life, such as tremors (Hochberg *et al.* 1996). L-Dopa therapy may improve the motor abnormality in some patients (Huang *et al.* 1989).

5.7.5 Mercury

Two forms of mercury poisoning occur: exposure to inorganic or elemental forms occurs in the manufacture of mirrors and scientific instruments, whereas inorganic mercurial compounds may be consumed in foods such as fish (which have ingested them) or grain (which has been treated with mercurial fungicide). The peripheral nervous system bears the main brunt of inorganic mercury toxicity (Section 12.19.3). Depression, tremor, emotional outbursts, and insomnia may also occur, and chelation therapy may improve symptoms (Hargreaves *et al.* 1988). Methyl mercury poisoning produces paraesthesia in the limbs and mouth, gait ataxia, concentrically restricted visual fields or cortical visual loss, and intellectual loss, which may persist until death (Davis *et al.* 1994). Mercury levels are increased in affected cortical areas showing neuronal loss and gliosis.

5.7.6 Tin

Triethyl tin and trimethyl tin toxicity have been associated with different syndromes of neurological disease; elemental or inorganic tin compounds are not neurotoxic. Over 200 patients were poisoned when triethyl tin contaminated the antibacterial drug stalinon (Alajouanine *et al.* 1958). The main clinical features were raised intracranial pressure, generalized seizures, and muscle weakness; 50 per cent of patients died. Autopsies showed intramyelinic oedema in the brain. Trimethyl tin poisoning has been reported less frequently, recently in six patients exposed to the vapour (Besser *et al.* 1987). Symptoms generally developed 3–5 days after exposure and consisted of deafness, cognitive impairment, behavioural abnormalities, seizures, ataxia, limb sensory disturbances, and hyperphagia. Death may occur and recovery may be incomplete in the more severely affected patients. Urinary organo-tin levels are elevated for 15–20 days after exposure. Attempts to reduce body tin levels using penicillamine were not thought to be clinically beneficial. Autopsy showed evidence of neuronal damage in the cerebellar Purkinje layers and the amygdala.

5.8 Pesticide poisoning

Chronic peripheral neuropathies due to insecticides (organophosphates and carbamates, Section 12.20.8), organo-metal rodentocytes (arsenic, thallium, and organic mercury, Section 12.19), fumigants (methylbromide, Section 12.20.7), and herbicides (2,4-D, Section 12.20.5) are covered in Chapter 12.

5.8.1 Organo-phosphorous compounds

Organo-phosphorous insecticides are the leading cause of systemic poisoning due to agricultural chemicals. Human disease has been most frequently described following discrete episodes of intense exposure, such as tri-ortho-cresyl phosphate contamination of moonshine whisky in 1930s prohibition America (Jamaica ginger extract) or of Moroccan cooking oil in the 1950s. Nowadays suicidal consumption is common in India and Sri Lanka (Agarwal 1993) and accidental agricultural exposures are frequent, especially during crop spraying. The possible neurological effects of repeated low-dose exposure have not been defined.

Three distinct phases of neurological illness may follow organo-phosphorus poisoning. The most common manifestation, which occurs within hours of exposure, consists of an acute cholinergic crisis with weakness, and autonomic and cerebral dysfunction. Occasionally, an intermediate paralytic syndrome develops after 1–4 days. Finally, after a delay of 1 or 2 weeks, some patients develop a sensorimotor polyneuropathy which progresses over subsequent weeks (Section 12.20.8). It is uncommon for all three phases of organo-phosphate poisoning to occur in the same patient. There are more than 80 organophosphorous compounds in use, with varying degrees of toxicity (Ellenhorn et al. 1997).

Acute cholinergic phase

Organo-phosphates irreversibly phosphorylate acetylcholinesterase. This inactivates the enzyme, causing a build-up of acetylcholine at muscarinic, nicotinic, and central nervous system cholinergic synapses within 12 hours of exposure (Namba et al. 1971). Muscarinic autonomic symptoms invariably occur: miosis, copious bronchosecretions, salivation and lacrimation, bronchoconstriction, bowel and bladder hyperactivity, bradycardia, and arrhythmias. Roughly half of patients also develop weakness due to depolarization block of neuromuscular transmission. In such patients, fasciculations precede the areflexia and weakness, particularly of proximal muscles. Various central nervous system manifestations may occur: impaired consciousness, agitation, tremors, confusion, ataxia, and convulsions. Respiratory failure is the usual mode of death

in untreated patients and results from the combination of bronchoconstriction and bronchosecretions, respiratory muscle weakness, and impaired central respiratory drive. Because of the clinical urgency posed by organo-phosphorus poisoning, decisions concerning specific treatment should be based upon the clinical features and history of possible exposure. A test dose of 1 mg atropine intravenously should confirm the diagnosis within 10 minutes by producing pupil dilation, tachycardia, confusion, and an ileus (Ellenhorn et al. 1997). The diagnosis may be confirmed subsequently by measurement of the red blood cell cholinesterase activity, which remains depressed for up to 2 months after intense exposure (Coye et al. 1987).

The immediate aim of therapy is to prevent death due to respiratory failure. Endotracheal incubation with suction and assisted ventilation may be necessary. Repeated large doses of atropine should be given parenterally to reduce secretions and bradycardia. Pralidoxime or obidoxime specifically reverse cholinesterase inactivation by organo-phosphorous compounds if given within 24 hours of exposure (Namba et al. 1971). Diazepam should be used to treat seizures. Prompt and adequate treatment of the cholinergic phase allows complete recovery in less than 2 weeks.

Carbamate insecticides can produce an acute cholinergic syndrome similar to that caused by organo-phosphorous compounds (Ellenhorn et al. 1997). However, central nervous system effects are less, inactivation of cholinesterase is less complete and lasts for a shorter duration because the enzyme binding is reversible, and pralidoxime therapy may exacerbate the cholinergic excess.

Certain organo-phosphorous compounds have been designed as chemical warfare nerve agents to produce rapidly fatal cholinergic crises (Gunderson et al. 1992). Tabun, Sarin, and Soman can cause death by respiratory failure within 5 minutes of inhalation of aerosols created by explosions. Agent VX is oil-based and absorbed through the skin from surfaces which may have been contaminated weeks previously (Dunn and Sidell 1989). Armies preparing to face nerve-agent warfare should carry atropine and autoinjectors of an oxime, such as pralidoxime, for administration at the first symptoms of exposure. Pre-treatment with pyridostigmine, itself a carbamate inhibitor of cholinesterase, appears to protect cholinesterase from inactivation by organo-phosphorous nerve agents.

Subacute neurotoxicity

An intermediate syndrome of muscle paralysis has been described which begins 1–4 days after organo-phosphorus poisoning, and is separate from the preceding cholinergic crisis (Senanayake and Karalliede 1987). This delayed syndrome of muscle paralysis typically affects the neck, respiratory, cranial nerve, and proximal limb muscles, and may require assisted ventilation. It lasts for less than 20 days. It has been described in patients who have already received pralidoxime for the preceding cholinergic phase of the poisoning. The pathogenesis of this delayed paralytic syndrome is not understood.

Chronic neurotoxicity

There is considerable interest currently in whether permanent neurological sequelae follow organo-phosphate poisoning. A number of studies show relatively minor long-term impairment on neurobehavioural tests or altered sensory testing thresholds (Steenland *et al.* 1994). Whether chronic subclinical exposure can produce similar impairments has become a contested issue.

5.8.2 Carbon disulphide-based pesticides

Carbon disulphide and carbon tetrachloride mixtures are used extensively in the grain industry for controlling insects. Abnormal finger tremor at 5–7 Hz has been noted in chronically exposed grain workers, and some workers display Parkinsonian syndromes which also include rigidity and gait abnormalities (Chapman *et al.* 1991). Peripheral neuropathy due to carbon disulphide exposure is described in Section 12.20.2.

5.8.3 Strychnine

Strychnine is a plant extract present in some commercial rodenticides. It blocks inhibitory actions of the neurotransmitter glycine in the central nervous system. Symptoms usually occur within 1 hour of poisoning, with anxiety, extensor spasms, opisthotonos, and convulsions, usually with preservation of consciousness in the initial stages (O'Callaghan *et al.* 1982). In patients who survive, recovery occurs over a few days. In severely poisoned patients, therapy should include respiratory assistance using endotracheal incubation and neuromuscular blockade, and treatment of seizures with diazepam or barbiturates (Ellenhorn *et al.* 1997).

5.8.4 Vacor®

This rodenticide is related to streptozotocin, a diabetogenic toxin. The acute onset of diabetes mellitus and severe autonomic failure, and a glove-and-stocking disturbance of pinprick sensation have been recorded after suicidal consumption of Vacor® (Pont *et al.* 1979). The autonomic failure is permanent with prominent disturbance of blood pressure and bladder control.

5.8.5 Endrin®

Convulsions may occur as an early feature of poisoning by this chlorinated hydrocarbon pesticide of the cyclodiene group. Small epidemics of poisoning have been reported from Pakistan in which patients, usually children, became suddenly ill within a few hours of consuming food presumed to be contaminated with Endrin® (Rowley *et al.* 1987). Vomiting, headache, and muscle fasciculation were noted in some patients in addition to tonic–clonic convulsions. Seizures can be resistant to intravenous therapy with diazepam or phenobarbital, and death may occur. Blood Endrin® levels may be elevated.

5.9 Environmental and physical insults

5.9.1 Radiation damage

The occurrence of radiation-induced damage to the brain and spinal cord depends upon the radiation dosage, the scheduling of fractionation, technical aspects of beam focusing, and different individual susceptibilities (Henson and Urich 1982). Because of these variations, it has proved hard to define 'threshold dosages' for the development of radiation-induced neurological injury. Accepted 'safe' dosage regimens are now in general use, with the result that radiotherapy-induced injury to the nervous system is less common nowadays. Radiation injuries to the brachial and lumbosacral nerve plexuses are covered in Section 13.5.3.

The pathogenesis of nervous system injury involves prominent endothelial damage, and the resulting radiation-induced vasculopathy seems to be a common feature to the different syndromes discussed below. Of interest has been the preliminary report that some such patients improve with anticoagulation (Glantz *et al.* 1994).

Radiation myelopathy

Various clinical syndromes of radiation-induced spinal-cord damage occur. By analogy with animal studies, acute spinal-cord damage might be expected within hours or days of inadvertently high dosages of irradiation. An early and benign form of spinal-cord damage may develop within 6–18 weeks of treatment to fields that had included the cervical cord (Jones 1964). Paraesthesia may radiate through all four limbs, and this syndrome usually resolves within 6 months. Lhermitte's symptom of electric shock sensations in the limbs evoked by neck flexion is common in this benign myelopathy. Also, Lhermitte's sign occasionally occurs early on in the progressive form of radiation myelopathy described below (Godwin-Austen *et al.* 1975).

Delayed progressive radiation myelopathy may develop at any time from a few months to 6 years after radiotherapy (Godwin-Austen *et al.* 1975; Henson and Urich 1982). Patients experience progressive deterioration in the sensory, motor, and sphincteric functions of the spinal cord below the irradiated level. Sensory disturbance is the most common initial symptom. Early on the signs may be referable to unilateral damage of the spinal cord with monoparesis or a Brown-Séquard syndrome. Ultimately signs of bilateral spinal-cord damage develop. Progression over months or years leads to clinically complete loss of spinal-cord function. Stabilization with incomplete spinal-cord lesions can occur. The chief differential diagnosis is from spinal-cord compression due to recurrence or metastasis of the underlying cancer. Vertebral body deposits may be revealed by plain spine X-rays. More commonly, myelography or magnetic resonance imaging of the spinal canal may be required to exclude spinal-cord compression. Both these investigations may reveal diffuse spinal-cord swelling in post-irradiation myelopathy. Many patients die from the effects of radiation-induced spinal-cord disease. Pathological studies reveal necrosis of the spinal cord confined to the irradiated segments. White-matter tracts are affected preferentially and the lesions may be patchy. Fibrinoid necrosis or hyaline fibrosis of associated blood vessels suggests a vascular basis for the spinal-cord damage in some cases.

Post-irradiation lumbosacral radiculopathy

A lower motor neuron degeneration can affect the legs 3–25 years after radiotherapy to the lower thoracic or lumbar spine (Bowen *et al.* 1996) (Section 14.7). This rare syndrome has usually followed radiation treatment with more than 40 Gy for testicular tumours or Hodgkin's disease. Minor sensory and sphincter symptoms are common.

Radiation encephalopathy

Radiation-induced brain damage generally follows treatment of cerebral tumours, extracerebral head and neck tumours, or neuraxis irradiation in the treatment of leukaemia.

A transient encephalopathy may develop a few weeks after irradiation. This presents with drowsiness, clumsiness, and headache, which resolve over subsequent months (Henson and Urich 1982). Bilateral low-attenuation areas may be seen in the brain on computed tomographic scan. Death has resulted from a brainstem form of this early delayed encephalopathy in which demyelination was noted at autopsy. A variant of early transient post-irradiation encephalopathy occurs in leukaemics receiving combined treatment with radiotherapy and chemotherapy. This is known as treatment encephalopathy (Section 5.5.4).

The more usual type of post-irradiation encephalopathy develops months or years after radiotherapy and progressively deteriorates. The onset of symptoms is most common after an interval of 9 months to 2 years. It is particularly likely if standard brain tumour irradiation doses of 5000 to 7000 rad are administered in daily fractions exceeding 200 rad (Martins *et al.* 1977). The focal neurological deficit in post-irradiation encephalopathy often parallels that of the underlying brain tumour to which radiotherapy had been directed originally. Progressive dysphasia, hemianopia, cognitive dysfunction, or hemiparesis may be features of radiation encephalopathy of the cerebral hemisphere. Focal or secondarily generalized seizures and features of raised intracranial pressure may occur (Henson and Urich 1982).

The diagnosis of post-irradiation encephalopathy is easy if such a neurological syndrome develops in a patient without a pre-existing brain tumour, who had received radiotherapy for an extracerebral tumour of the head or neck. The diagnosis is usually difficult in patients who had received radiotherapy for an underlying brain tumour. Without further brain biopsy, the distinction from tumour regrowth often remains uncertain. Computed tomography in radiation necrosis usually shows a focal low-density cerebral lesion with mass effect, and often with enhancement, which may be impossible to differentiate from tumour (Martins *et al.* 1977; Rottenberg *et al.* 1977;

Henson and Urich 1982). Magnetic resonance imaging may show multifocal lesions which contrast enhance, sometimes in a ring pattern, within the field of previous radiotherapy, and the appearance of these waxes and wanes with time, unlike the steady growth of recurrent tumour (Peterson *et al.* 1995). Neuropathological studies show necrotic areas of brain which particularly involve white matter, and associated fibrinoid necrosis, hyaline thickening, or thrombosis of vessels (Martins *et al.* 1977). Without treatment, radiation necrosis of the brain tends to worsen progressively, causing death. Occasionally it stabilizes spontaneously. Dexamethasone therapy may control symptoms (Martins *et al.* 1977). Surgical excision of the swollen area of necrotic brain can lead to permanent improvement (Rottenberg *et al.* 1977). Such surgical treatment is best confined to patients with cerebral necrosis following radiotherapy for extracerebral malignancies, and who are not going to be intolerably disabled by extirpation of the affected brain area.

Cerebral and carotid arteries may be damaged by irradiation and occlusive stroke may occur many years later. Angiography in such cases shows arterial narrowings within the previously irradiated field (Murros and Toole 1989).

A follow-up of children irradiated for scalp ringworm shows an increased incidence of brain tumours 7–16 years later (Modan *et al.* 1974). Most of these radiation-induced tumours of the nervous system are not gliomas.

Radiation-induced cranial nerve palsies

Progressive visual failure from optic nerve and chiasm damage has followed external irradiation therapy for pituitary tumours and craniopharyngiomas (Atkinson *et al.* 1979). Such patients may also suffer radiation-induced hypothalamic damage. Any cranial nerve may be compromised as a delayed effect of radiotherapy. The hypoglossal nerve appears to be particularly susceptible following earlier radiotherapy for tonsular, pharyngeal, and supraglottic pharyngeal tumours and prominent bulbar palsy may develop (Shapiro *et al.* 1996).

5.9.2 Heatstroke

Heatstroke is defined as a state of acute onset in which the rectal temperature exceeds 40 °C, accompanied by hypotension, tachycardia, and hyperventilation, with hot and yet dry skin, and with an associated neurological disturbance (Yaqub *et al.* 1986; Simon 1993). It occurs in various circumstances, including protracted exertions such as marathon running, in unacclimatized visitors to hot climates, in alcoholics, and in those with cardiovascular disease, particularly if elderly and exposed to a heat wave. Various drugs predispose to heatstroke, including diuretics, phenothiazines, anti-Parkinsonian drugs, anticholinergics, β-blockers, tricyclic antidepressants, and amphetamines (Hart *et al.* 1982). Heat injury may cause some aspects of neurologic dysfunction in the neuroleptic malignant syndrome, particularly in those patients who develop residual neurological abnormalities (Sections 5.5.2 and 32.9.1).

Altered consciousness is the main presenting neurological sign of heatstroke. The pupils are characteristically tightly constricted. Skin temperature may be substantially less than the rectal core temperature, which should exceed 40 °C. Patients in deep coma may lose brainstem and tendon reflexes and have a poor prognosis even if they receive prompt assisted ventilation and cooling (Yaqub 1987). Convulsions may occur, especially during cooling. The creatine phosphokinase level is elevated and a wide range of metabolic and electrolyte disturbances have been recorded, most notably raised liver enzyme levels or frank hepatic failure (Hart *et al.* 1982; Yaqub 1987).

Heatstroke constitutes a medical emergency and body cooling should be started immediately. The entire body surface should be exposed and wrapped in a continually moistened sheet in a cool room while evaporation is promoted by multiple fans (Yaqub *et al.* 1986). Such evaporative cooling should be continued until the rectal temperature reaches 38.5 °C. A bad prognosis is signalled by an initial rectal temperature exceeding 42 °C and failure to achieve cooling within 1 hour. Death occurs in approximately 10 per cent of all patients with heatstroke (Yaqub *et al.* 1986). Permanent neurological abnormalities may persist after satisfactory cooling in a few patients. Cerebellar syndromes are most common (Yaqub 1987) and spinal-cord lesions with motor neuron loss also occur (Delgado *et al.* 1985).

5.9.3 Cold injury

Two forms of tissue injury result from extreme cold. Noteworthy peripheral nerve injury occurs in the trench and immersion foot syndromes, which represent non-freezing cold injury resulting from prolonged immersion of the limbs in cold liquid mud in warfare trenches, or in cold, waterlogged life rafts (Kennett and Gilliatt 1991). Freezing injury, or frostbite, produces a localized area of generalized tissue necrosis, and peripheral nerve injury remains more or less confined to this area.

The clinical features of the trench and immersion foot syndromes are similar, although not identical. An affected limb becomes numb and clumsy. Pain and tingling are uncommon but calf cramps may occur. The skin passes through a hyperaemic red and oedematous phase before becoming 'sickly yellow' or mottled (Ungley *et al.* 1945). On removing the tight boots encasing oedematous feet and rewarming, the limb goes through a hyperaemic phase lasting up to 10 weeks. During this, signs of a predominantly sensory and autonomic neuropathy are present. Pain and heat sensations are impaired in a glove-and-stocking distribution, and the limb is warm and dry. Over the long term, skin colour and temperature return to normal, sweating returns and may be excessive, and sensory and motor function returns towards normal. Chronic pain is reported by many patients, particularly a burning dysaesthesia in the region of the metatarsal heads exacerbated by walking (Blair *et al.* 1957). Hyperhidrosis or signs of distal sensorimotor neuropathy may persist. Histopathological studies show Wallerian degeneration in the early stages of cold immersion injury, particularly affecting interdigital nerves.

5.9.4 Altitude sickness

Acute mountain sickness afflicts climbers who ascend rapidly to heights of at least 3000 m without intermediate periods of acclimatization. Symptoms develop a few hours or days after ascent. Headache, ataxia, cognitive impairment, and vomiting due to cerebral oedema may be accompanied by dyspnoea due to pulmonary oedema (Johnson *et al.* 1984). Subtle aphasic errors and impaired verbal learning and memory may persist for at least a month after ascents to altitudes above 5000 m (Hornbein *et al.* 1989). Climbers with a history of repeated conquests of peaks exceeding 8500 m without using supplementary oxygen show long-term impairments of concentration and memory (Regard *et al.* 1989). Death may result from acute mountain sickness. Acetozolamide pretreatment reduces the incidence of altitude sickness (Birmingham Medical Research Expeditionary Society Mountain Sickness Study Group 1981). Rapid descent provides the definitive treatment for mountain sickness. However, patients may benefit from dexamethasone if descent proves impractical (Levine *et al.* 1989). Chronic mountain sickness can produce migranous headaches, cognitive and depressive disorders, and paraesthesiae due to mild sensory polyneuropathy (Thomas *et al.* 2000).

5.9.5 Diving

Decompression sickness, or the 'bends', occurs in deep-sea divers returning to the surface without adequate decompression. It has also occurred in aviators ascending in unpressurized aircraft. It is advised that at least 24 hours should elapse between diving and going to altitude. Compressed air sickness was originally called caisson disease when it was noted following the introduction of high-pressure chambers for underwater work. The neurological illness is generally believed to result from the formation of intravascular gas bubbles, causing arteriolar or venular blockage. The most common manifestation of acute decompression sickness is 'limb-bends' in which musculoskeletal pains flit from joint to joint. The 'chokes' refers to an acute respiratory decompression sickness which may occur after a latency of several hours. Neurological complications occur in roughly a quarter of patients, particularly if recompression has not been undertaken at the first sign of the 'bends'. Neurological symptoms follow the 'bends' by 1–36 hours. Spinal-cord damage or 'spinal bends' is the most common neurological manifestation (Kimbro *et al.* 1997). Minimal limb weakness or paraesthesia may progress to complete paraplegia or tetraplegia in less than 1 hour. Minor degrees of spinal-cord damage may be discovered at autopsy in medically fit divers dying for unrelated reasons, or in divers who have made a full functional recovery from 'spinal bends' as a result of prompt recompression (Palmer *et al.* 1987). Occasionally there is evidence of brain involvement with visual blurring, diplopia, dysarthria, deafness, or cognitive disturbances. Migraine-like symptoms have been described in aviators after descent. Treatment of decompression sickness consists of immediate inhalation of a high concentration of oxygen, and immediate transport to a hyperbaric oxygen chamber for recompression. The nitrogen may be eliminated more quickly if recompression uses a helium–oxygen mixture rather than oxygen alone (Melamed *et al.* 1992).

5.9.6 Electrical and lightening injuries

The site of the neurological injury is mainly determined by the part of the body receiving the electric shock or lightening strike. The immediate consequences of electrical injury include the electrical tinglings familiar to all of us and, for more severe strikes, there may be temporary unconsciousness with retrograde amnesia, temporary tinnitus and deafness, complex visual disturbances, and temporary or permanent cardiorespiratory arrest. A wide variety of longer-lasting or permanent neurological sequelae have been recorded following electrical injury. These may be present from the time of the shock, or develop after delays of days, weeks or even months. Immediate onset of transient paraplegia with sensory loss has followed lightening strikes, and may recover in less than 24 hours. Permanent spastic quadriplegia with small hand muscle wasting has followed electric shock to the arm. The onset of quadriplegia may be delayed for some days after the electric shock, and sometimes eventually recovers partially some months later (Farrell and Starr 1968). Electric shocks or lightening strikes to the head can produce an immediate or delayed onset of hemiparesis, aphasia, or unilateral extrapyramidal syndromes (Farrell and Starr 1968). Cerebral damage with delayed onset may reflect electrically induced damage to cerebral vessels. Persisting fatigue and concentration difficulties are reported in survivors of lightening strikes sufficient to render them unconscious (Van Zomeren *et al.* 1998). Seizures or myoclonic jerks may occur as an immediate sequel of electrical injury. Peripheral nerve damage is usually restricted to the shocked limb. Permanent peripheral nerve damage occurs within the area of generalized tissue burn, most generally affecting the median or ulnar nerves in the hand, but more extensive peripheral nerve damage may ensue (Hawkes and Thorpe 1992). Electrical muscle injury may produce substantial subfascial oedema, and early fasciotomy may be required to prevent secondary peripheral nerve damage or distal ischaemia (Di Vincenti *et al.* 1969).

5.10 Plant and fungus poisoning

A vast range of plants and fungi can produce systemic poisoning syndromes after ingestion, which may include autonomic, neurological, or psychiatric features. These are too numerous for comprehensive discussion here and the reader is referred to detailed reference texts for further details (Ellenhorn *et al.* 1997).

5.10.1 Buckthorn

Progressive ascending polyneuropathy resembling Guillain–Barré syndrome has followed consumption of the poisonous buckthorn shrub, *Karwinskia humboldtiana*, which grows in Mexico and Texas. Patients develop an areflexic quadriplegia,

and may have weakness of respiratory and bulbar muscles. Sensory loss is relatively mild. Patients who survive recover completely over a matter of months. The spinal-fluid protein content is typically normal, in contrast to Guillain–Barré syndrome. Sural nerve biopsy shows acute segmental demyelination (Calderon-Gonzalez and Rizzi-Hernandez 1967). Supportive treatment should follow the guidance outlined for Guillain–Barré syndrome (Section 12.10).

5.10.2 Cicutoxin

Water hemlock, or *Cicuta*, contains the poison cicutoxin. The plant is sometimes accidentally consumed after misidentification as wild parsnip, artichoke, or potato. The symptoms of poisoning reflect cholinergic excess at muscarinic and central nervous system synapses. Abdominal pain, sweating, bronchosecretion, brachycardia, hypotension, and pupillary abnormalities are common early features. Convulsions are frequent and may lead to status epilepticus. Non-convulsive involuntary movements may occur, causing trismus, opisthotonos, and hemiballismus. It is likely that cicutoxin has a direct toxic effect on muscles, causing tenderness and weakness of trunk and proximal limb muscles. Creatine phosphokinase levels are elevated and severe metabolic acidosis may occur. Infusions of thiopentone sodium control the abnormal muscle movements and seizures (Starreveld and Hope 1975).

5.10.3 *Gloriosa*

Acute ascending polyneuropathy has followed ingestion of *Gloriosa superba*, the glory lily, a tuber found in tropical Africa, Asia, and North America (Angunawela and Fernando 1971). *Gloriosa* contains colchicine, which is known to cause a neuromyopathy when given for therapeutic purposes (Section 12.18.7). In massive overdose, colchicine may cause confusion and signs of cerebral oedema, leading ultimately to brain death (Heaney *et al.* 1976).

5.10.4 Mushrooms

The wide range of poisoning syndromes that may follow ingestion of different species of mushrooms include hepatorenal failure, gastroenteritis, parasympathomimetic syndromes due to muscarinic effects, and disulfiram-like ethanol sensitivity (Ellenhorn *et al.* 1997). Primarily neurological and psychiatric syndromes follow poisoning with the hallucinogenic mushrooms, of which *Psilocybe* has been popular for recreational abuse. Patients may develop confusion, visual hallucinations, distorted perceptions, and ataxia, sometimes accompanied by signs of parasympathetic abnormalities. Symptoms usually develop within 90 minutes of ingestion and resolve within 4–12 hours. Seizures or hyperthermia occur occasionally (McCormick *et al.* 1979). Sedation with benzodiazepines may be necessary. Gut decontamination should be considered within the first few hours of large overdoses, particularly in children. Major tranquillizers should be used sparingly, if at all, to control psychotic features, because of their propensity to lower seizure thresholds. Self-injury may occur if the poisoning precipitates aggressive or suicidal behaviour. Disturbing psychiatric 'flash-back' symptoms may persist after the acute poisoning (Benjamin 1979).

5.10.5 Podophyllin

Podophyllin is an antimitotic drug derived from the May apple, of the genus *Podophyllum*, which has been used for topical treatment of warts. Human toxicity has followed excessive skin absorption or oral ingestion, including overdosage with herbal laxative tablets containing podophyllin (Filley *et al.* 1982; Dobb and Edis 1984). Confusion or impaired consciousness, hallucinations, and ataxia may all occur during the first week of toxicity. Evidence of an axonal degeneration sensorimotor peripheral neuropathy commences during the second week, although absent tendon reflexes may have been noted earlier. The neuropathy may worsen for up to 3 months before slowly improving (Filley *et al.* 1982; Dobb and Edis 1984).

5.10.6 Solanine

Green or sprouting potatoes may contain solanine, which causes illness 7–19 hours after ingestion. Solanine poisoning from potatoes is uncommon if the green skins are not eaten and if the potato has been boiled thoroughly; baking does not detoxify solanine. Outbreaks of poisoning have occurred in institutions such as schools (McMillan and Thompson 1979). Solanine depresses human pseudocholinesterase activity. Vomiting, diarrhoea, and fever are the most common symptoms. Some patients develop confusion, delirium, hallucinations, headaches, convulsions, paraesthesiae, and muscle spasms. Recovery occurs over a few days, but more persistent visual blurring or giddiness have been noted.

5.11 Animal poisons, bites, and stings

Poisons produced by organisms have survival benefit for those organisms either in terms of offence (e.g. the poison produced by snakes enables them to immobilize their prey) or defence (e.g. the toxins produced by sea algae discourage their consumption). Some biological toxins have highly specific effects upon nerve conduction or synaptic transmission and are of interest as molecular probes of excitable tissues. This section discusses human poisonings due to bungarotoxin and latrotoxin, both of which interfere with cholinergic neurotransmission, and tetrodotoxin, saxitoxin, brevitoxin, and ciguatoxin, all of which interfere with sodium-channel function in excitable membranes.

5.11.1 Ciguatera fish poisoning (ciguatoxin)

Ciguatoxin occurs in certain predatorial fish from tropical reefs in the Atlantic and Pacific: barracuda, red snapper, grouper, and amberjack. The toxin originates in dinoflagellate plankton of the *Gambierdiscus* genus which are ingested by small fish which, in turn, are themselves eaten by larger predators. Within 12 hours of a meal, patients develop vomiting, diarrhoea, cramps or myalgias of distal muscles, paraesthesiae, and gait ataxia (Chretien *et al.* 1981). Life-threatening respiratory muscle paralysis occurs in severe cases. Symptoms generally undergo gradual resolution over approximately 4 weeks. There is no specific antidote. Polymyositis has been reported in some patients who had suffered severe myalgias in the early weeks of their ciguatera fish poisoning (Stommel *et al.* 1991).

5.11.2 Puffer-fish poisoning (tetrodotoxin)

Tetrodotoxin reduces the excitability of nerve and muscle membranes by reducing their permeability to the inflow of sodium ions. Poisoning has usually followed ingestion of puffer fish, particularly in Japan and Australia, or occasionally after consuming porcupine fish. It has also followed envenomation from the bite of the blue-ringed octopus (Bower *et al.* 1981). Vomiting occurs within 1 hour of ingestion due to tetrodotoxin's direct action on the area postrema. Perioral tinglings occur, followed by limb sensory disturbances, muscle twitching and increasing paralysis, and severe hypotension. Respiratory muscle paralysis may cause death, with preservation of consciousness until the last (Bower *et al.* 1981). There is no specific antidote to tetrodotoxin poisoning and treatment is supportive. Recovery of muscle power may be accelerated by the use of anticholinesterase drugs (Chew *et al.* 1984).

5.11.3 Shellfish neurotoxicity

Paralytic shellfish poisoning (saxitoxin)

Outbreaks of paralytic shellfish poisoning have followed consumption of mussels and other shellfish obtained from waters where 'red tides' have been observed. These 'red tides' are due to toxic dinoflagellate sea algae of the genus *Protogonyaulax*. These algae contain saxitoxin and are ingested and concentrated by shellfish (Sakamoto *et al.* 1987). Outbreaks of poisoning have occurred in a wide variety of countries bordering on the Atlantic and Pacific oceans (Mills and Passmore 1988). Symptoms develop within less than an hour of the shellfish meal. Paraesthesiae are initially circumoral and later affect the limbs. In more severe cases there is progressive muscular paralysis leading to death by asphyxia. There are no specific antidotes to saxitoxin poisoning. Survivors generally recover within a week.

Neurotoxic shellfish poisoning (brevitoxin)

The dinoflagellate alga *Ptychodiscus brevis* produces brevitoxin and is another cause of 'red tides' around the southern USA. The alga is concentrated by shellfish, and human disease follows within 3 hours of their consumption (Sakamoto *et al.* 1987). Diarrhoea, abdominal pain, and circumoral paraesthesiae are the initial symptoms. Tingling later extends to the limbs and trunk. Vertigo, ataxia, and repeated seizures may all occur in severe poisonings. The poisoning is generally milder than paralytic shellfish poisoning due to saxitoxin, and no deaths have been notified.

Excitotoxic shellfish poisoning (domoic acid)

An outbreak of neurological illness has followed ingestion of mussels contaminated with domoic acid, which is related to the excitatory transmitter substance glutamate (Teitelbaum *et al.* 1990). Patients developed gastrointestinal symptoms within 12 hours of consumption. These were followed by various combinations of confusion, altered consciousness, seizures, myoclonus, unsteadiness, weakness, fasciculations, alternating hemiparesis, and ophthalmoplegia. Many months later survivors displayed anterograde amnesia and evidence of a predominantly motor axonal peripheral neuropathy. Autopsy studies showed hippocampal damage in a pattern resembling that caused by excitotoxins.

5.11.4 Snake envenomation (bungarotoxin)

Various polypeptide neurotoxins are present in the venoms of different snakes. Some of these block synaptic transmission, particularly at the neuromuscular junction. Some snake venoms also contain other toxins causing severe bleeding disorders, rhabdomyolysis, renal failure, and hypovolaemic shock and pulmonary oedema due to increased capillary permeability (see Ellenhorn *et al.* 1997).

Krait (genus *Bungarus*) venom contains bungarotoxins, principally α-bungarotoxin which binds powerfully to postsynaptic acetylcholine receptors, thereby blocking neuromuscular transmission. Kraits are found in South-East Asia, India, Indonesia, Taiwan, and China, and usually bite their sleeping victims at night (Warrell *et al.* 1983). Not all bites envenomate sufficiently to cause paralysis. After the bite, the preparalytic phase usually lasts 1–3 hours, but delays of up to 12 hours have been recorded. Ptosis is often the earliest sign of impending generalized muscular paralysis. Complete muscular paralysis may occur, with death from respiratory failure unless assisted ventilation is instituted promptly. Muscle fasciculations may be observed. Both antivenom and edrophonium may improve muscle strength, and adequate doses of neostigmine by infusion may be indicated. With prompt ventilation and adequate supportive care, full recovery occurs within a few days.

Post-synaptic neuromuscular blockade also occurs after cobra (*Naja*) envenomation, presenting a similar clinical picture to that of krait envenomation. A myasthenic decrement may be noted neurophysiologically after cobra envenomation, and positive Tensilon® (edrophonium) test responses may occur. Unassisted respiratory function may be maintained by infusion of adequate doses of neostigmine (Watt *et al.* 1986).

Russell's viper, common in Sri Lanka and India, produces a mixed clinical picture after envenomation. The venom's neurotoxicity produces external ophthalmoplegia, ptosis, and lower cranial nerve palsies, respiratory failure, and limb paralysis. There is no response to Tensilon® (edrophonium), suggesting that the neurotoxin inhibits presynaptic release of acetylcholine

at the neuromuscular junction, rather than causing postsynaptic blockade. Generalized muscle tenderness and myoglobinuria indicate that the venom also causes rhabdomyolysis (Phillips *et al.* 1988). Generalized rhabdomyolysis is the most serious consequence of bites from a wide variety of other snakes, including sea snakes, some Australian snakes (taipan, tiger snake, mulga snake, and small-eyed snake), and the tropical rattlesnake in Brazil (Phillips *et al.* 1988). It is likely that the phospholipase A group of neurotoxins are responsible for both the presynaptic blockade of neuromuscular transmission and the rhabdomyolysis.

The Papuan taipan's venom contains taipoxin, a phospholipase A_2, which acts on presynaptic nerve endings to abolish transmitter release, with a latency of around 9 hours before the clinical onset of paralysis. Paralysis predominates in the cranial, trunk, and proximal limb muscles, and artificial ventilation may be necessary. Compound muscle action potential amplitudes are low, but repetitive stimulation produces a distinctive brief potentiation in amplitude followed by an enhanced decrement unaffected by edrophonium (Connolly *et al.* 1995).

5.11.5 Spider venom (latrotoxin)

Envenomations by black- and brown-widow spiders (genus *Latrodectus*) include toxins such as α-latrotoxin, which destroys motor nerve terminals, causing failure of neuromuscular transmission (Okamoto *et al.* 1971). Spider bites are rare in humans. The unlucky victims experience pain at the site of the envenomation, abdominal pain, and leg weakness. Death is rare. Recently, it has been concluded that horse-serum antivenom does not promote recovery and should be considered only in potentially life-threatening poisonings. The antivenom has the disadvantage of causing allergic reactions (Moss and Binder 1987).

5.11.6 Tick paralysis

Prolonged attachment to the body in the early summer by various species of gravid female tick can cause ascending flaccid paralysis of the limbs, culminating in bulbar and respiratory muscle weakness. This mainly occurs in north-western USA, but can occur elsewhere in North America, Australia, South Africa, and southern Europe. Tick paralysis of animals, particularly sheep, was once an economic setback to farmers. Children are particularly likely to be affected, and tick envenomation enters the differential diagnosis of the acutely weak child. The presence of an attached tick should be sought, usually to be found in the scalp or ears. Ascending paralysis usually occurs after the tick has been attached for 5 days or more. Areflexia and ptosis are frequent. Although paraesthesiae may occur, sensory loss is uncommon. Bulbar paralysis can develop within 2 days of the onset of weakness. Neurophysiological studies show reduced amplitude of sensory nerve action potentials and muscle action potentials but only a moderate slowing of motor nerve conduction (Grattan-Smith *et al.* 1997). The spinal fluid is usually normal. Clinical and electrophysiological improvement occurs within a few days of removing the tick, and recovery can be complete in less than a week. This form of tick paralysis is due to a toxin and should not be confused with the polyradiculopathy caused by the *Borrelia* infection transmitted by tick bites, which is known as Lyme disease or Bannwarth's syndrome (see 12.14.3).

References

Agarwal, S. B. (1993). A clinical, biochemical, neurobehavioural, and sociopsychological study of 190 patients admitted to hospital as a result of acute organophosphorus poisoning. *Environ. Res.*, **62**, 63–70.

Aggarwal, S. K., Williams, V., Levine, S. R. *et al.* (1996). Cocaine-associated intracranial haemorrhage: absence of vasculitis in 14 cases. *Neurology*, **46**, 1741–3.

Alajouanine, T., Derobert, L., and Thieffry, S. (1958). Etude clinique d'ensemble de 210 cas d'intoxication par les sels organiques d'étain. *Rev. Neurol. (Paris)*, **98**, 85–96.

Alfrey, A. C., Le Gendre, G. R., and Kaehny, W. D. (1976). The dialysis encephalopathy syndrome. Possible aluminium intoxication. *N. Engl. J. Med.*, **294**, 184–8.

Altman, P., Dhanesha, V., Hamon, C. *et al.* (1989). Disturbance of cerebral function by aluminium in haemodialysis patients without overt aluminium toxicity. *Lancet*, **2**, 7–12.

Angunawela, R. M. and Fernando, H. A. (1971). Acute ascending polyneuropathy and dermatitis following poisoning by tubers of Gloriosa. *Ceylon Med. J.*, **16**, 233–5.

Atkinson, A. B., Allen, I. V., Gordon, D. S. *et al.* (1979). Progressive visual failure in acromegaly following external pituitary radiation. 4123 cases—two with pathology including one with frontal lobe necrosis. *Clin. Endocrinol.*, **10**, 469–79.

Atkinson, E. A., Fairburn, B., and Heathfield, K. W. J. (1970). Intracranial venous thrombosis as complication of oral contraceptives. *Lancet*, **1**, 914–18.

Benjamin, C. (1979). Persistent psychiatric symptoms after eating psilocybin mushrooms. *BMJ*, **i**, 1319–20.

Bertoni, J. M., Schwartzman, R. J., Van Horn, G. *et al.* (1981). Asterixis and encephalopathy following metrizamide myelography: investigations into possible mechanisms and review of the literature. *Ann. Neurol.*, **9**, 366–370.

Besser, R., Kramer, G., Thumler, R. *et al.* (1987). Acute trimethyltin limbic-cerebellar syndrome. *Neurology*, **37**, 945–50.

Birmingham Medical Research Expeditionary Society Mountain Sickness Study Group (1981). Acetozolamide in control of acute mountain sickness. *Lancet*, **1**, 180–3.

Blair, J. R., Schatzki, R., and Orr, K. D. (1957). Sequelae to cold injury in one hundred patients. *JAMA*, **163**, 1203–8.

Blass, J. P. and Gibson, G. E. (1977). Abnormality of a thiamine-requiring enzyme in patients with Wernicke–Korsakoff syndrome. *N. Engl. J. Med.*, **297**, 1367–70.

Bowen, J., Gregory, R. P., Squier, M. *et al.* (1996). The post-irradiation lower motor neurone syndrome. Neuronopathy or radiculopathy? *Brain*, **119**, 1429–39.

Bower, D. J., Hart, R. J., Matthew, P. A., *et al.* (1981). Nonprotein neurotoxins. *Clin. Toxicol.*, **18**, 813–63.

Brennan, F. N. and Lyttle, J. A. (1987). Alcohol and seizures: a review. *J. Roy. Soc. Med.*, **80**, 571–3.

Buckley, P. F. and Hutchinson, M. (1995). Neuroleptic malignant syndrome. *J. Neurol. Neurosurg. Psychiat.*, **58**, 271–3.

Burns, R., Thomas, D. W., and Barron, V. J. (1974). Reversible encephalopathy possibly associated with bismuth subgallate ingestion. *BMJ*, **1**, 220–3.

Calderon-Gonzalez, R. and Rizzi-Hernandez, H. (1967). Buckthorn polyneuropathy. *N. Engl. J. Med.*, **277**, 69–71.

Caplan, L., Hier, D., and Banks, G. (1982a). Current concepts of cerebrovascular disease-stroke: stroke and drug abuse. *Stroke*, **13**, 869–72.

Caplan, L., Thomas, C., and Banks, G. (1982b). Central nervous system complications of 'T's and blues' addiction. *Neurology*, **32**, 623–8.

Carlen, P. L., Wilkinson, D. A., and Wortzman, G. (1981). Cerebral atrophy and functional deficits in alcoholics without clinically apparent liver disease. *Neurology*, **31**, 377–85.

Cassells, D. A. K. and Dodds, E. C. (1946). Tetra-ethyl lead poisoning. *BMJ*, **2**, 681–5.

Challenor, Y. B., Richter, R. W., Bruun, B. *et al.* (1973). Nontraumatic plexitis and heroin addiction. *JAMA*, **225**, 958–61.

Chang, C. L., Donaghy, M., and Poulter, N. *et al.* (1999). Migraine and stroke in young women: a case control study. *BMJ*

Chapman, L. J., Sauter, S. L., Henning, R. A. *et al.* (1991). Finger tremor after carbon disulfide-based pesticide exposures. *Arch. Neurol.*, **48**, 866–70.

Charness, M. E. and de la Paz, R. L. (1987). Mammillary body atrophy in Wernicke's encephalopathy: antemortem identification using magnetic resonance imaging. *Ann. Neurol.*, **22**, 595–600.

Charness, M. E., Simon, R. P., and Greenberg, D. A. (1989). Ethanol and the nervous system. *N Engl J Med*, **321**, 442–54.

Chew, S. K., Chew, L. S., Wang, K. W., *et al.* (1984). Anticholinesterase drugs in the treatment of tetrodotoxin poisoning. *Lancet*, **2**, 108.

Chretien, J. H., Fermaglich, J., and Garagusi, V. F. (1981). Ciguartera poisoning. Presentation as a neurological disorder. *Arch. Neurol.*, **38**, 783.

Connolly, S., Trevett, A. J., Nwokolo, N. C. *et al.* (1995). Neuromuscular effects of Papuan Taipan snake venom. *Ann. Neurol.*, **38**, 916–20.

Cook, D. G., Fahn, S., and Brait, K. A. (1974). Chronic manganese intoxication. *Arch. Neurol.*, **30**, 59–64.

Coye, M. J., Barnett, P. G., Midtling, J. E. *et al.* (1987). Clinical confirmation of organophosphate poisoning by serial cholinesterase analysis. *Arch. Int. Med.*, **147**, 438–42.

Daras, M., Koppel, B. S., Atos-Radzion, E. (1994). Cocaine-induced charcoatheroid movements (Crack dancing). *Neurology*, **44**, 751–2.

Davis, L. E., Kornfeld, M., Mooney, H. S. *et al.* (1994). Methymercury poisoning: long-term clinical, radiological, toxicological, and pathological studies on an affected family. *Ann. Neurol.*, **35**, 680–8.

De Gans, J., Stam, J., van Wijngaarden, G. K. (1985). Rhabdomyolysis and concomitant neurological lesions after intravenous heroin abuse. *J. Neurol. Neurosurg. Psychiat.*, **48**, 1057–9.

Delaney, P. and Estes, M. (1980). Intracranial haemorrhage with amphetamine abuse. *Neurology*, **30**, 1125.

Delgado, G., Tunon, T., Gallego, J. *et al.* (1985). Spinal cord lesions in heat stroke. *J. Neurol. Neurosurg. Psychiat.*, **48**, 1065–7.

Diener, H. C., Dichgans, J., Bacher, M. *et al.* (1984). Improvement of ataxia in alcoholic cerebellar atrophy through alcohol abstinence. *J. Neurol.*, **231**, 258–62.

Di Vincenti, F. C., Moncrieff, J. A., and Pruitt, B. A. (1969). Electrical injuries: a review of 65 cases. *J. Trauma*, **9**, 497–507.

Dobb, G. J. and Edis, R. H. (1984). Coma and neuropathy after ingestion of herbal laxative containing podophyllin. *Med. J. Aust.*, **140**, 495–6.

Donaghy, M. (1998). Neurological considerations. In *Transplantation*, (ed. B. C. Ginns, A. B. Cosimi, and P. J. Morris), Chapter 25. Blackwell Scientific, Cambridge, Mass.

Donaldson, I. M. and Cunningham, J. (1983). Persisting neurologic sequelae of lithium carbonate therapy. *Arch. Neurol.*, **40**, 747–51.

Dougherty, J. H., Rawlinson, D. G., Levy, D. E. *et al.* (1981). Hypoxic–ischaemic brain injury and the vegetative state: clinical and neuropathologic correlation. *Neurology (Minneapolis)*, **31**, 991–7.

Dunn, M. A. and Sidell, F. R. (1989). Progress in medical defense against nerve agents. *JAMA*, **262**, 649–52.

Ellenhorn, M. J., Schonwald, S., Ordog, G. *et al.* (1997). *Ellenhorn's Medical Toxicology*, (2nd edn). Williams & Wilkins, Baltimore.

Estrin, W. J. (1987). Alcoholic cerebellar degeneration is not a dose-dependent phenomenon. *Alcoholism*, **11**, 372–5.

Farrell, D. F. and Starr, A. (1968). Delayed neurological sequelae of electrical injuries. *Neurology, Minneapolis*, **18**, 601–6.

Filley, C. M., Graff-Radford, N. R., Lacy, J. R. *et al.* (1982). Neurologic manifestations of podophyllin toxicity. *Neurology*, **32**, 308–11.

Fulton, M., Raab, G., Thompson, G. *et al.* (1987). Influence of blood lead on the ability and attainment of children in Edinburgh. *Lancet*, **i**, 1221–6.

Garland, H. and Pearce, J. (1967). Neurological complications of carbon monoxide poisoning. *Quart. J. Med.*, **36**, 445–55.

Gill, J. S., Zezulka, A. V., Shipley, M. J. *et al.* (1986). Stroke and alcohol consumption. *N. Engl. J. Med.*, **315**, 1041–6.

Gill, J. S., Shipley, M. J., Tsementzissa *et al.* (1991). Alcohol consumption—a risk factor for haemorrhagic and non-haemorrhagic stroke. *Am. J. Med.*, **90**, 489–97.

Glantz, M. J., Burger, P. C., Friedman, A. H. *et al.* (1994). Treatment of radiation-induced nervous system injury with heparin and warfarin. *Neurology*, **44**, 2020–7.

Glass, J. P., Lee, Y.-Y., Bruner, J. *et al.* (1986). Treatment-related leukoencephalopathy. A study of three cases and literature review. *Medicine Baltimore*, **65**, 154–62.

Godwin-Austen, R. B., Howell, D. A., and Worthington, B. (1975). Observations on radiation myelopathy. *Brain*, **98**, 557–68.

Golden, G. S. (1977). The effect of central nervous system stimulants on Tourette syndrome. *Ann. Neurol.*, **2**, 69–70.

Grattan-Smith, P. J., Morris, J. G., Johnston, H. M. *et al.* (1997). Clinical and neurophysiological features of tick paralysis. *Brain*, **120**, 1975–87.

Gross, J. A., Haas, M. L., and Swift, T. R. (1979). Ethylene oxide neurotoxicity. Report of four cases and review of the literature. *Neurology*, **29**, 978–83.

Gunderson, C. H., Lehmann, C. R., Sidell, F. R. *et al.* (1992). Nerve agents. A review. *Neurology*, **42**, 946–50.

Hargreaves, R. J., Evans, J. G., Janota, I. *et al.* (1988). Persistent mercury in nerve cells 16 years after metallic mercury poisoning. *Neuropath. Appl. Neurobiol.*, **14**, 443–52.

Harper, C. (1983). The incidence of Wernicke's encephalopathy in Australia—a neuropathological study of 131 cases. *J. Neurol. Neurosurg. Psychiat.*, **46**, 593–8.

Harper, C., Kril, J., and Daly, J. (1987). Are we drinking our neurones away? *BMJ*, **294**, 534–6.

Harrington, H., Heller, A., Dawson, D. *et al.* (1983). Intracerebral haemorrhage and oral amphetamines. *Arch. Neurol.*, **40**, 503–7.

Hart, G., Anderson, R., Crumpler, C. *et al.* (1982). Epidemic classical heat stroke: clinical characteristics and course of 28 patients. *Medicine*, **61**, 189–97.

Hawkes, C. H. and Thorpe, J. W. (1992). Acute polyneuropathy due to lightening injury. *J. Neurol. Neurosurg. Psychiat.*, **55**, 388–90.

Heaney, D., Derghazarian, C. B., Pines, G. F. *et al.* (1976). Massive colchicine overdose: a report on the toxicity. *Am. J. Med. Sci.*, **271**, 233–8.

Henry, J. A. (1992). Ecstasy and the dance of death: severe reactions are unpredictable. *BMJ*, **305**, 566.

Henson, R. A. and Urich, H. (1982). *Cancer and the nervous system*. Blackwell, Oxford.

Herdmann, J., Benecke, R., Meyer, B. U. *et al.* (1988). Successful corticoid treatment of lumbosacral plexus neuropathy in heroin abuse. Clinical aspects, electrophysiology, therapy and follow-up. *Nervenartzt*, **59**, 683–6.

Heyer, E. J., Simpson, D. M., Bodiswollner, I. *et al.* (1986). Nitrous oxide: clinical and electrophysiologic investigation of neurologic complications. *Neurology*, **36**, 1618–22.

Hillbom, M. and Kaste, M. (1983). Ethanol intoxication: a risk factor for ischaemic brain infarction. *Stroke*, **14**, 694–9.

Hillbom, M., Muuronen, A., Holm, L. *et al.* (1986). The clinical versus radiological diagnosis of alcoholic cerebellar degeneration. *J. Neurol. Sci.*, **73**, 45–53.

Hillebrand, G., Castro, L. A., van Scheidt, W. *et al.* (1987). Valproate for epilepsy in renal transplant recipients receiving cyclosporine. *Transplantation*, **43**, 915–16.

Hochberg, F. H. and Miller, D. C. (1988). Primary central nervous system lymphoma. *J. Neurosurg.*, **68**, 835–53.

Hochberg, F., Miller, G., Valenzuela, R. *et al.* (1996). Late motor deficits of Chilean manganese miners. *Neurology*, **47**, 788–95.

Holloway, K. L. and Alberico, A. M. (1990). Postoperative myeloneuropathy: a preventable complication in patients with B_{12} deficiency. *J. Neurosurg.*, **72**, 732–6.

Hook, C. C., Kimmel, D. W., Kvols, L. K. *et al.* (1992). Multifocal inflammatory leukoencephalopathy with 5-Fluorouracil and levimasole. *Ann. Neurol.*, **31**, 262–7.

Hormes, J. T., Filley, C. M., and Rosenberg, N. L. (1986). Neurologic sequelae of chronic solvent vapour abuse. *Neurology*, **36**, 698–702.

Hornbein, T. F., Townes, B. D., Schoene, R. B. *et al.* (1989). The cost to the central nervous system of climbing to extremely high altitude. *N. Engl. J. Med.*, **321**, 1714–19.

Huang, C.-C., Chu, N.-S., Lu, C.-S. *et al.* (1989). Chronic manganese intoxication. *Arch. Neurol.*, **46**, 1104–6.

Huang, C.-C., Chu, N.-S., Lu, C.-S. *et al.* (1998). Long-term progression in chronic manganism. Ten years of follow-up. *Neurology*, **50**, 698–700.

Hwang, T.-L., Yung, W. K. A., Estey, E. H. *et al.* (1985). Central nervous system (CNS) toxicity with high-dose Ara-C. *Neurology*, **35**, 1475–9.

Johnson, T. S., Rock, P. B., Fulco, C. S. *et al.* (1984). Prevention of acute mountain sickness by dexamethasone. *N. Engl. J. Med.*, **310**, 683–6.

Jones, A. (1964). Transient radiation myelopathy (with reference to Lhermitte's sign of electrical paraesthesiae). *Br. J. Radiol.*, **37**, 727–44.

Jørgensen, J., Hansen, P. H., Steenskov, V. *et al.* (1975). A clinical and radiological study of chronic lower spinal arachnoiditis. *Neuroradiology*, **9**, 139–44.

Junck, L. and Marshall, W. H. (1983). Neurotoxicity of radiological contrast agents. *Ann. Neurol.*, **13**, 469–84.

Kaelan, C., Harper, C., and Viera, B. I. (1986). Acute encephalopathy and death due to petrol sniffing: neuropathological findings. *Aust. NZ J. Med.*, **16**, 804–7.

Kahan, B. D., Flechner, S. M., Lorber, M. I. *et al.* (1987). Complications of cyclosporine–prednisone immunosuppression in 402 renal allograft recipients exclusively followed at a single centre for from one to five years. *Transplantation*, **43**, 197–204.

Kawamura, A., Shiota, J., Yagashita, T. *et al.* (1985). Marchiafava–Bignami disease: computed tomographic scan and magnetic resonance imaging. *Ann. Neurol.*, **18**, 103–4.

Kennett, R. P. and Gilliatt, R. W. (1991). Nerve conduction studies in experimental non-freezing cold injury: 1 local nerve cooling. *Muscle Nerve*, **14**, 553–62.

Keogh, A. J. (1974). Meningeal reactions seen with myodil myelography. *Clin. Radiol.*, **25**, 361–5.

Kimbro, T., Tom, T., and Neuman, T. (1997). A case of spinal cord decompression sickness presenting as partial Brown-Séquard syndrome. *Neurology*, **48**, 1454–5.

Klawans, H. L., Stein, R. W., Tanner, C. M. *et al.* (1982). A pure Parkinsonian syndrome following acute carbon monoxide intoxication. *Arch. Neurol.*, **39**, 302–4.

Kraus, M. L., Gottlieb, L. D., Horwitz, R. I. *et al.* (1985). Randomised clinical trial of atenolol in patients with alcohol withdrawal. *N. Engl. J. Med.*, **313**, 905–9.

Lacey, D. J. (1981). Neurologic sequelae of acute carbon monoxide intoxication. *Am. J. Dis. Child.*, **135**, 145–7.

Lancet (1983). Methanol poisoning. *Lancet*, **i**, 910–12.

Lee, S., Merriam, A., Kim, T.-S. *et al.* (1989). Cerebellar degeneration in neuroleptic malignant syndrome: neuropathologic findings and review of the literature concerning heat-related nervous system injury. *J. Neurol. Neurosurg. Psychiat.*, **52**, 387.

Le Quesne, P. M., Axford, A. T., McKerrow, C. B. (1976). Neurological complications after a single severe exposure to toluene diisocyanate. *Br. J. Indust. Med.*, **33**, 72–8.

Levine, B. D., Yoshimura, K., Kobayashi, T. *et al.* (1989). Dexamethasone in the treatment of acute mountain sickness. *N. Engl. J. Med.*, **321**, 1707–13.

Levine, S. R., Brust, J. C. M., Futrell, N. *et al.* (1990). Cerebrovascular complications of the use of the 'crack' form of alkaloidal cocaine. *N. Engl. J. Med.*, **323**, 699–704.

Levy, D. E., Caronna, J. J., Singer, B. H. *et al.* (1985). Predicting outcome from hypoxic-ischaemic coma. *JAMA*, **253**, 1420–6.

Lieberman, A. N., Bloom, W., Koshore, P. S. *et al.* (1974). Carotid artery occlusion following ingestion of LSD. *Stroke*, **5**, 213–15.

Lishman, W. A. (1981). Cerebral disorder in alcoholism: syndromes of impairment. *Brain*, **104**, 1–20.

Martin, F., Ward, K., Slavin, G. *et al.* (1985): Alcoholic skeletal myopathy, a clinical and pathological study. *Quart. J. Med.*, **55**, 233–51.

Martins, A. N., Johnson, J. S., Henry, J. M. *et al.* (1977). Delayed radiation necrosis of the brain. *J. Neurosurg.*, **47**, 336–45.

Martyn, C. N., Barker, D. J. P., Osmond, C. *et al.* (1989). Geographical relation between Alzheimer's Disease and aluminium in drinking water. *Lancet*, **1**, 59–62.

Masucci, E. F., Fabara, J. A., Saini, N. *et al.* (1982). Cerebral mucormycosis (phycomycosis) in a heroin addict. *Arch. Neurol.*, **39**, 304–6.

McCormick, D. J., Avbel, A. J., and Gibbons, R. B. (1979). Non-lethal mushroom poisoning. *Ann. Int. Med.*, **90**, 332–5.

McKee, A. C., Winkelman, M. D., and Banker, B. Q. (1988). Central pontine myelinolysis in severely burned patients: relationship to serum hyperosmolality. *Neurology*, **38**, 1211–17.

McLean, D. R., Jacobs, H., Mielke, B. W. (1980). Methanol poisoning: a clinical and pathological study. *Ann. Neurol.*, **8**, 161–7.

McMillan, M. and Thompson, J. C. (1979). An outbreak of suspected solanine poisoning in school boys: an examination of criteria of solanine poisoning. *Quart. J. Med.*, **48**, 227–43.

Melamed, Y., Shupak, A., and Bitterman, H. (1992). Medical problems associated with underwater diving. *N. Engl. J. Med.*, **326**, 30–5.

Meyers, C. A., Scheibel, R. S., and Forman, A. D. (1991). Persistent neurotoxicity of systemically administered interferon-alpha. *Neurology*, **41**, 672–6.

Miller, G. M., Baker, H. L., Okazaki, H. *et al.* (1988). Central pontine myelinolysis and its imitators. *Radiology*, **168**, 795–802.

Mills, A. R. and Passmore, R. (1988). Pelagic paralysis. *Lancet*, **I**, 161–4.

Modan, B., Baidatz, D., and Mart, H. (1974). Radiation-induced head and neck tumours. *Lancet*, **i**, 277–9.

Montero, C. G. and Martinez, A. J. (1986). Neuropathology of heart transplantation: 23 cases. *Neurology*, **36**, 1149–54.

Morrow, P., Wong, B., Finkelstein, W. E. *et al.* (1982). Aspergillosis of the cerebral ventricles in a heroin abuser. *Arch. Int. Med.*, **143**, 161–4.

Moss, H. S. and Binder, L. S. (1987). A retrospective review of Black Widow spider envenomations. *Ann. Emerg. Med.*, **16**, 188–92.

Murros, K. E. and Toole, J. F. (1989). The effect of radiation on carotid arteries. *Arch. Neurol.*, **46**, 449–55.

Namba, T., Nolte, C. T., Jarkrel, J. *et al.* (1971). Poisoning due to organophosphate insecticides. *Am. J. Med.*, **50**, 475–92.

Needleman, H. L., Schell, A., Bellinger, D. *et al.* (1990). The long-term effects of exposure to low doses of lead in childhood. *N. Engl. J. Med.*, **322**, 83–8.

Ng, S. K. C., Hauser, W. A., Brust, J. C. M. *et al.* (1988). Alcohol consumption and withdrawal in new-onset seizures. *N. Engl. J. Med.*, **319**, 666–73.

Nolte, K. B., Brass, L. M., and Fletterick, C. F. (1996). Intracranial haemorrhage associated with cocaine abuse: a prospective autopsy study. *Neurology*, **46**, 1291–6.

O'Callaghan, W. G., Joyce, N., Counihan, H. E. *et al.* (1982). Unusual strychnine poisoning and its treatment: report of eight cases. *BMJ*, **285**, 478.

Okamoto, M., Longenecker, H. E., Riker, W. F., *et al.* (1971). Destruction of mammalian motor nerve terminal by black widow spider venom. *Science*, **172**, 733–6.

Palmer, A. C., Calder, I. M., and Hughes, J. T. (1987). Spinal cord degeneration in divers. *Lancet*, **ii**, 1365–6.

Parkinson, I. S., Ward, M. D., Feest, T. G. *et al.* (1979). Fracturing dialysis osteodystrophy and dialysis encephalopathy. An epidemiological study. *Lancet*, **1**, 406–9.

Parnass, S. M. and Schmidt, K. J. (1990). Adverse effects of spinal and epidural anaesthesia. *Drug Safety*, **5**, 179–94.

Pascual-Leone, A., Dhuna, A., Altafullah, I. *et al.* (1990). Cocaine-induced seizures. *Neurology*, **40**, 404–7.

Pascual-Leone, A., Dhuna, A., and Anderson, D. C. (1991). Cerebral atrophy in habitual cocaine abusers: a planimetric CT study. *Neurology*, **41**, 34–8.

Patchell, R. A. (1988). Primary central nervous system lymphoma in the transplant patient. *Neurol. Clinics*, **6**, 297–303.

Patchell, R. A., White, C. L., Clark, A. W. *et al.* (1985). Neurologic complications of bone marrow transplantation. *Neurology*, **35**, 300–6.

Pearn, J. (1977). Neurological and psychometric studies in children surviving freshwater immersion accidents. *Lancet*, **i**, 7–9.

Perl, D. P. and Brody, A. R. (1980). X ray spectrometric evidence of aluminium accumulation in neurofibrillary tangle-bearing neurones. *Science*, **208**, 297–9.

Peterson, K., Clark, H. B., Hall, W. A. *et al.* (1995). Multifocal enhancing magnetic resonance imaging lesions following cranial irradiation. *Ann. Neurol.*, **38**, 237–44.

Phillips, R. E., Theakston, R. D. G., Warrell, D. A., *et al.* (1988). Paralysis, rhabdomyolysis and haemolysis caused by bites of Russell's viper (*Vipera russelli pulchella*) in Sri Lanka: Failure of Indian (Haffkine) antivenom. *Quart. J. Med.*, **68**, 691–716.

Phillips, S. C., Harper, C. G., and Kril, J. (1987). A quantitative histological study of the cerebellar vermis in alcoholic patients. *Brain*, **110**, 301–14.

Plum, F., Posner, J. B., and Hain, R. F. (1962). Delayed neurological deterioration after anoxia. *Arch. Int. Med.*, **110**, 56.

Pont, A., Rubino, J. M., Bisop, D. *et al.* (1979). Diabetes mellitus and neuropathy following Vacor ingestion in man. *Arch. Int. Med.*, **139**, 185–7.

Puke, M., Arnér, S., and Norlander, O. (1989). Complications of regional anaesthesia, with special reference to epidural, spinal and caudal anaesthesia. In *General anaesthesia*, (5th edn), (ed. J. F. Nunn, J. E. Utting, and B. R. Brown), Chapter 92. Butterworth, Oxford.

Qureshi, A. I., Akbar, M. S., Czander, E. *et al.* (1997). Crack cocaine use and stroke in young patients. *Neurology*, **48**, 341–5.

Regard, M., Oelz, O., Brugger, P. *et al.* (1989). Persistent cognitive impairment in climbers after repeated exposure to extreme altitude. *Neurology*, **39**, 210–13.

Reuler, J. B., Girard, D. E., and Cooney, T. G. (1985). Wernicke's encephalopathy. *N. Engl. J. Med.*, **312**, 1035–9.

Ron, M. A., Acker, W., Shaw, G. K. *et al.* (1982). Computerised tomography of the brain in chronic alcoholism: a survey and follow-up study. *Brain*, **105**, 497–514.

Rosenberg, M. R. and Green, M. (1989). Neuroleptic malignant syndrome. Review of response to therapy. *Arch. Int. Med.*, **149**, 1927.

Ross, J. S., Masaryk, T. J., Modic, M. T. *et al.* (1987). MR imaging of lumbar arachnoiditis. *Am. J. Neuroradiol.*, **8**, 885–92.

Rottenberg, D. A., Chernick, N. L., Deck, M. D. F. *et al.* (1977). Cerebral necrosis following radiotherapy of extracranial neoplasms. *Ann. Neurol.*, **1**, 339–57.

Rowley, D. L., Rab, M. A., Hardjotanojo, W. *et al.* (1987). Convulsions caused by Endrin poisoning in Pakistan. *Paediatrics*, **79**, 928–34.

Rowley, H. A., Lowenstein, D. H., and Rowbotham, M. C. (1989). Thrombo-mesencephalic strokes after cocaine abuse. *Neurology*, **39**, 428–30.

Rubin, A. M. and Kang, H. (1987). Cerebral blindness and encephalopathy with Cyclosporin-A toxicity. *Neurology*, **37**, 1072–6.

Sabour, M. S. and Fadel, H. E. (1970). The carpal tunnel syndrome—a new complication ascribed to the pill. *Am. J. Obstet. Gynaecol.*, **107**, 1265–7.

Saitz, R. and O'Malley, S. S. (1997). Pharmacotherapies for alcohol abuse. *Med. Clin. North Am.*, **81**, 881–907.

Sakamoto, Y., Lockey, R. F., and Krzanowski, J. J. (1987). Shellfish and fish poisoning related to the toxic dinoflagellates. *South. Med. J.*, **80**, 866–72.

Sawa, G. M., Watson, C. P., Terbrugge, K. *et al.* (1981). Delayed encephalopathy following co intoxication. *Can. J. Neurol. Sci.*, **8**, 77–9.

Saweda, Y., Takahashi, M., Ohashi, N. *et al.* (1980). Computerised tomography as an indication of long-term outcome after acute carbon monoxide poisoning. *Lancet*, **1**, 783–4.

Sawicka, E. H. and Trosser, A. (1983). Cerebrospinal fluid rhinorrhoea after cocaine sniffing. *BMJ*, **286**, 1476–7.

Schwartz, B. S., Stewart, W. F., Bolla, K. I. *et al.* (2000). Past adult lead exposure is associated with longitudinal decline in cognitive function. *Neurology*, **55**, 1144–50.

Senanayake, N. and Karalliede, L. (1987). Neurotoxic effects of organo-phosphorus insecticides. An intermediate syndrome. *N. Engl. J. Med.*, **316**, 761–3.

Shapiro, B. E., Rordorf, G., Schwamm, L. *et al.* (1996). Delayed radiation-induced bulbar palsy. *Neurology*, **46**, 1604–6.

Sharpe, J. A., Mostovsky, M., Bilbao, J. M. *et al.* (1982). Methanol optic neuropathy: a histopathological study. *Neurology*, **32**, 1093–100.

Simon, H. D. (1993). Hyperthermia. *N. Engl. J. Med.*, **329**, 483–7.

Simon, R. P. (1988). Alcohol and seizures. *N. Engl. J. Med.*, **319**, 715–16.

Slager, U. T. (1986). Central pontine myelinolysis and abnormalities in serum sodium. *Clin. Neuropathol.*, **5**, 252–6.

Sloan, M. A., Kittner, S. J., Feeser, B. R. *et al.* (1998). Illicit drug-associated ischaemic stroke in the Baltimore–Washington young stroke study. *Neurology*, **19**, 1688–93.

Small, S. L., Fukui, M. B., Bramblett, G. T. *et al.* (1996). Immunosuppression-induced leukoencephalopathy from Tacrolimus (FK506). *Ann. Neurol.*, **40**, 575–80.

Smith, J. F., McLaurin, R. L., Nichols, J. B. *et al.* (1960). Studies in cerebral oedema and cerebral swelling. 1. The changes in lead encephalopathy in children compared with those in alkyl tin poisoning in animals. *Brain*, **83**, 411–24.

Smith, S. J. M. and Kocen, R. S. (1988). A Creutzfeldt–Jacob like syndrome due to lithium toxicity. *J. Neurol. Neurosurg. Psychiat.*, **51**, 120–3.

Starreveld, E. and Hope, C. E. (1975). Cicutoxin poisoning (water hemlock). *Neurology*, **25**, 730–4.

Steenland, K., Jenkins, B., Ames, R. G. *et al.* (1994). Chronic neurological sequelae to organophosphate pesticide poisoning. *Am. J. Public Health*, **84**, 731–6.

Steg, R. E. and Garcia, E. G. (1991). Complex visual hallucinations and cyclosporine toxicity. *Neurology*, **41**, 1156.

Sterns, R. H., Riggs, J. E., and Schochet, S. S. (1986). Osmotic demyelination syndrome following correction of hyponatraemia. *N. Engl. J. Med.*, **314**, 1535–42.

Stommel, E. W., Parsonnet, J., and Jenkyn, L. R. (1991). Polymyositis after Ciguatera toxin exposure. *Arch. Neurol.*, **48**, 874–7.

Teitelbaum, J. S., Zatorre, R. J., and Carpenter, S. *et al.* (1990). Neurologic sequelae of Domoic acid intoxication due to the ingestion of contaminated mussels. *N. Engl. J. Med.*, **332**, 1781–7.

Thomas, P. K., King, R. H. M., Feng, S. F. *et al.* (2000). Neurological manifestations in chronic mountain sickness: the burning feet–burning hands syndrome. *J. Neurol. Neurosurg. Psychiat.*, **69**, 447–52.

Thompson, C. B., June, C. H., Sullivan, K. M. *et al.* (1984). Association between cyclosporin neurotoxicity and hypomagnesaemia. *Lancet*, **2**, 1116–20.

Thompson, W. L., Johnson, A. D., and Maddrey, W. L. (1975). Diazepam and paraldehyde for treatment of severe delirium tremens: a controlled trial. *Ann. Int. Med.*, **82**, 175–80.

Ungley, C. C., Channell, G. D., and Richards, R. L. (1945). The immersion foot syndrome. *Br. J. Surg.*, **33**, 17–31.

Urbaro-Marquez, A., Estruch, R., Navarro-Lopez, F. *et al.* (1989): The effects of alcohol on skeletal and cardiac muscle. *N. Engl. J. Med.*, **320**, 409–15.

van Zomeren, A. H., ten Duis, H.-J., Minderhoud, J. M. *et al.* (1998). Lightening stroke and neuropsychological impairment: cases and questions. *J. Neurol. Neurosurg. Psychiat.*, **64**, 763–9.

Victor, M. (1994). Alcoholic dementia. *Can. J. Neurol. Sci.*, **21**, 88–99.

Victor, M., Adams, R. D., and Mancall, E. L. (1959). A restricted form of cerebellar cortical degeneration occurring in alcoholic patients. *Arch. Neurol.*, **1**, 579–688.

Victor, M., Adams, R. D., and Collins, G. H. (1989). *The Wernicke–Korsakoff syndrome and related neurologic disorders due to alcoholism and malnutrition.* Contemporary Neurology Series. F. A. Davis, Philadelphia.

Walker, R. W. and Brochstein, J. A. (1988). Neurologic complications of immunosuppressive agents. *Neurol. Clin.*, **6**, 261–78.

Walters, E. C., van Wijgaarden, G. K., Stam, F. C. *et al.* (1982). Leucoencephalopathy after inhaling 'heroin' pyrolysate. *Lancet*, **2**, 1233–7.

Warrell, D. A., Looareesuwan, S., White, N. J. *et al.* (1983). Severe neurotoxic envenoming by the Malayan krait *Bungarus candidus* (Linnaeus): response to antivenom and anticholinesterase. *BMJ*, **286**, 678–80.

Watt, G., Theakston, R. D. G., Hayes, C. G. *et al.* (1986). Positive response to edrophonium in patients with neurotoxic envenomation by cobras (*Naja Naja philippinesis*). *N. Engl. J. Med.*, **35**, 1444–8.

WHO collaborative study of cardiovascular disease and steroid hormone contraception (1996*a*). Ischaemic stroke and combined oral contraceptives: results of an international, multicentre, case-control study. *Lancet*, **348**, 498–505.

WHO collaborative study of cardiovascular disease and steroid hormone contraception (1996*b*). Haemorrhagic stroke, overall stroke risk, and combined oral contraceptives: results of an international, multicentre, case-control study. *Lancet*, **348**, 505–10.

Wijdicks, E. F. M., Wiesner, R. H., Dahlke, L. J. *et al.* (1994). FK-506-induced neurotoxicity in liver transplantation. *Ann. Neurol.*, **35**, 498–501.

Wijdicks, E. F., de Groen, P. C., Wiesner, R. H. *et al.* (1995). Intracerebral haemorrhage in liver transplant recipients. *Mayo Clinic Proc.*, **70**, 443–6.

Williams, D. P., Troost, B. T., and Rogers, J. (1988). Lithium-induced downbeat nystagmus. *Arch. Neurol.*, **45**, 1022–3.

Winnock, S., Janvier, G., Parmentier, F. *et al.* (1993). Pontine myelinolysis following liver transplantation: a report of two cases. *Transpl. Int.*, **6**, 26–8.

Wright, D. G., Laureno, R., and Victor, M. (1979). Pontine and extrapontine myelinolysis. *Brain*, **102**, 361–85.

Yaqub, B. A. (1987). Neurologic manifestations of heat stroke at the Mecca pilgrimage. *Neurology*, **37**, 1004–6.

Yaqub, B., Al-Harthi, S., Al-Orainey, I. *et al.* (1986). Heat stroke at the Mekkah Pilgrimage: clinical characteristics and course of 30 patients. *Quart. J. Med.*, **59**, 523–30.

CHAPTER 6

Disability, rehabilitation, and spinal injury

Derick Wade

6.1 General principles

Diseases of the nervous system account for the majority of patients with severe disability living in the community. Although schizophrenic illness is the single most common cause, it is managed by psychiatrists. People with learning disability are also managed by a separate specialist service in most countries. Neurologists will be involved with patients suffering almost all the other diseases that leave people severely dependent. It is likely that many, if not most, patients with severe acquired disability will be seen by a neurologist at some stage of their illness. Consequently neurologists potentially have a pivotal role in ensuring that the disability is managed properly. In many cases the neurologist can be the lead physician. This chapter aims to enable the neurologist to ensure that their patient has effective rehabilitation.

Effective rehabilitation depends upon specific knowledge and skills, and both depend upon having a good understanding of the nature of disability. Consequently the neurologist must have a good working knowledge of a conceptual model of disability and the processes involved in rehabilitation. This chapter starts with a description of the most widely used illness framework, that put forward by the World Health Organization (WHO) in their International Classification of Impairments, Disabilities and Handicaps (ICIDH). Although a new version is due out in the year 2000 with some changes in terminology (discussed later), the model is still referred to as the WHO ICIDH model of illness.

After explaining the WHO ICIDH model of disability, and developing a more comprehensive model, the chapter moves on to explain rehabilitation, defining its aims, the processes involved, and the organizational requirements. The explanation will demonstrate the close parallels between normal 'medical neurology' and 'disability neurology' (i.e. neurological rehabilitation). It will also review briefly the wide range of rehabilitation interventions that may occur.

Rehabilitation, like normal medical processes, depends upon tools to diagnose and measure aspects of a patient's situation. The third part of this chapter concentrates upon assessment procedures and measures that may be useful to practising neurologists. It also emphasizes that assessment is a process which helps the neurologist understand the patient's clinical state and plan future management, whereas measurement is simply a tool that allows the clinician to quantify some observations.

With this important conceptual basis explained fully, the chapter then moves on to review selected areas of neurological rehabilitation. As far as possible, evidence will be provided to support any recommendations.

The evidence supporting well-organized specialist disability services is strong, and this is the starting point. Additional discussion of some specific processes, such as goal planning, will be incorporated into this section.

The chapter then discusses four types of disabling neurological illness: those with acute onset, initially severe disability; those with slowly progressive disability; those with unpredictable and fluctuant courses; and those where there is no underlying pathology. Specific coverage of the rehabilitation of all diseases and all problems lies beyond the scope of this chapter, but it does cover specifically spasticity and spinal-cord injury.

The main messages are as follows. The WHO ICIDH framework and associated definitions of rehabilitation do provide a very powerful analytic and management tool. Clinically useful measures and assessment procedures that can be used profitably by neurologists do exist (and some are illustrated here). Well-organized, multi-professional, co-ordinated specialist rehabilitation services are cost-effective in reducing disability. The evidence relating to many specific interventions is less strong, and clinical judgement is still important. The nature of the problems generated will be determined in part by the time course of the illness. The neurologist's roles are to recognize disability when present, to perform an initial assessment to determine whether further action is needed, and to refer on to other professions within his/her own team or refer on to a specialist disability service, according to the patient's needs and local service availability.

6.1.1 The WHO ICIDH model of illness

Illness is used in this context to encompass both the subjective experience and the external observations associated with ill health.

Models of illness are important (Brown and Hughson 1993; Ekdawi and Conning 1994). They form the implicit basis for all decisions, including political decisions, on the allocation of resources. They can help in the analysis and understanding of clinical cases; they can form a framework for research and for planning intervention; and they can help in developing and constructing services. Neurologists already routinely use one model of illness, which is based on neurophysiology, neuro-anatomy, and neuropathology, to make the diagnosis of the disease underlying their patient's presenting complaints. This model requires the doctor to (1) localize the site(s) of the lesion(s) and (2) characterize the nature of the pathological process(es) within the lesion. The neurologist can then usually make a diagnosis without much further investigation. A different model is needed when considering disability.

There are many models of disability and illness (Brown and Hughson 1993; Ekdawi and Conning 1994; Post *et al.* 1999). However, most are similar to the World Health Organization's

Table 6.1. Rehabilitation model—the WHO ICIDH-2 framework

Level of illness

Term	Synonym	Comment
Pathology	Disease/diagnosis	Refers to abnormalities or changes in the structure and/or function of an *organ or organ system*
Impairment	Symptoms/signs	Refers to abnormalities or changes in the structure and/or function of the *whole body* set in *personal context*
Activity (was *disability*)	Function/observed behaviour	Refers to abnormalities, changes, or restrictions in the interaction between a person and his/her environment or *physical context* (i.e. changes in the *quality or quantity of behaviour*)
Participation (was *handicap*)	Social positions/roles	Refers to changes, limitations, or 'abnormalities' in the *position* of the person in their *social context*

Contextual factors

Domain	Examples	Comment
Personal	Previous illness	Primarily refers to *attitudes, beliefs, and expectations*, often arising from previous experience of illness in self or others, but also to personal characteristics
Physical	House, local shops, carers	Primarily refers to local physical *structures* but also includes people as *carers* (not as social partners)
Social	Laws, friends, family	Primarily refers to *legal* and local *cultural* setting, including expectations of important others.

This model is usually prefaced with the words: 'In the context of illness, ...'

model of Impairment, Disability (now termed Activities) and Handicap (now termed Participation) (Badley 1993; WHO 1999). It is usually referred to as the WHO ICIDH model, and its development and acceptance has been the greatest single advance in the field of rehabilitation over the past 10 years (Wade and de Jong 2000).

The original model, published in 1980 (Wood 1980, Wade 1996) has been recognized as being incomplete, and it has recently been revised and expanded (WHO 1999) to draw attention to three aspects of the patient's context: the person's own personal past experiences, which may determine their attitudes, beliefs, and expectations (i.e. their 'internal environment'); the person's external environment, including other people as helpers; and the person's social or cultural environment. The terminology has also been revised.

An outline of the model is shown in Table 6.1. In essence it follows a systems analytic approach to illness, and suggests that illness can be considered as a hierarchy of interacting systems best considered to have four levels. The first level is that of the organ (the nervous system and muscles in this book); the second level is that of the whole person; the third level is the person's interaction with his/her environment; and the last level is the person's position or status within their own society. These systems or levels of illness are also influenced by three other 'environmental' systems: the person's given internal state;

the person's given physical environment; and the person's given social environment.

The model fails to recognize two important aspects of illness. The first is the person's experience or perception of the illness at each level. The second is the person's overall response to their situation, their perception of their 'quality of life'. More recent and complex models have incorporated these aspects (Post *et al.* 1999) and a model derived from the ICIDH-2 and Post *et al.* (1999) is shown in Table 6.2, incorporating both quality of life and the subjective aspects of illness.

This model of illness is of practical value in that certain consequences or lessons flow from it. Table 6.3 outlines briefly many of the aspects of health and illness that may be understood or analysed more easily using this model. Only two consequences are explored in detail here.

Neurologists are frequently confronted by patients with symptoms or signs for which there is no obvious underlying cause (Sections 1.9 and 26.10). Quite apart from headache, it is estimated that about 10–30 per cent of patients have no specific diagnosis (Carson *et al.* 2000). This phenomenon would be predicted by any systems model. For example, stress at the level of handicap (e.g. a failure to gain promotion at work, or other role conflicts) or stress at the level of disability (e.g. a patient functioning at the limits of his endurance) would be expected to cause changes at the level of impairment (i.e. symptoms or

Table 6.2. Expanded model of illness

System	Experience/location	
	Subjective/internal	Objective/external
Level of illness		
Person's organ: *pathology*	*Disease*: label attached by person, usually on basis of belief	*Diagnosis*: label attached by others, usually on the basis of investigation
Person's body: *impairment*	*Symptoms*: somatic sensation, experienced moods, thoughts, etc.	*Signs*: observable abnormalities (absence or change), explicit or implicit
Person in environment: *behaviour*	*Perceived ability*: what person feels they can do, and feeling about quality of performance	*Disability/activities*: what others note person does do, quantification of that performance
Person in society: *roles*	*Role satisfaction*: person's judgement (valuation) of their own role performance (what and how well)	*Handicap/participation*: judgement (valuation) of important others (local culture) on role performance (what and how well)
Context of illness		
Internal, personal context	'*Personality*': person's beliefs, attitudes, expectations, goals, etc.	'*Past history*': observed/recorded behaviour prior to and early on in this illness
External, physical context	*Salience*: person's attitudes towards specific people, locations, etc.	*Resources*: description of physical (buildings, equipment, etc.) and personal (carers, etc.) resources available
External, social context	*Local culture*: the people and organizations important to person, and their culture; especially family and people in same accommodation	*Society*: the society lived in and the laws, duties, and responsibilities expected from, and the rights of, members of that society
Totality of illness		
Quality of life: *summation of effects*	*Happiness*: person's assessment of and reaction to achievement or failure of important goals *and* sense of being a worthwhile person	*Status*: society's judgement on success in life; material possessions

Table 6.3. Lessons from the model

Implication	Comment
Time	
The time frames are different at each level	Change and management at levels of pathology and impairment are generally quick (hours/days), but change and management at levels of disability and handicap are generally slow (weeks/months/years)
Health services	
Hospitals and health services focus on pathology	Hospitals are environmentally unsupportive of disability; hospital systems are procedurally set in short time frames (hours/days); health-service data are usually predicated on a definite diagnosis which is often not available, certainly at presentation
Dependence at the level of disability determines main cost of long-term ill health	Supportive care provided is the main resource used in healthcare, even in the acute phase. The resources used are not related reliably to pathological diagnosis
Disability and context	
Disability refers not only to 'quantity' (e.g. dependence or otherwise) but also to quality	For some people it matters more how normally they act than whether they can undertake an activity; the social implications of altered behaviour may restrict that behaviour; measures rarely take account of the quality of task performance
Disability is strongly influenced by the goals of the patient (the personal context)	All behaviour is goal-directed, and so disability cannot be considered 'context free'; many factors, including financial considerations, may determine the activities undertaken by a patient
Observed disability also depends upon the physical and social context	How someone behaves is inevitably affected by environmental factors and may be significantly constrained by the environment. The 'environment' includes the capabilities, wishes and expectations of relevant others
Relationship between levels	
The nature and extent of the relationships between levels are weak	For example, patients may have 'silent' pathology (i.e. disease without symptoms or signs). This gives scope for rehabilitation. It also implies that measures of the extent of pathology are poorly related to the extent of disability in many cases
Causal relationships may extend in any direction, 'up' or 'down' the hierarchy	The relationships are not all one way from pathology through to handicap. Changes in behaviour may 'cause' pathology. For example, electively not moving a shoulder may lead to the pathology of adhesive capsulitis (frozen shoulder)
Not all illness need start from pathology	A systems analysis of the model would predict that illness may start at any level, and interact down the systems as well as up the systems. Abnormal beliefs (part of personal context) may cause as much disability as pathology (abnormal organ structure or function)
Prognosis depends upon pathology (if present)	The prognostic field for an individual patient is usually determined by the specific disease, but the specific prognosis within that field for a particular patient is usually related to impairments and other factors
Measurement and normality	
Measures should only encompass items from one level	It is invalid to add scores from items or measures covering domains from different levels
'Normal' becomes much less easy to define, and becomes increasingly personal	*The metric against which structure, function, behaviour, or performance is judged varies:*
Pathology:	Structure or function measured against any human, with some allowance for age and gender
Impairment:	Structure or function measured against humans matched for age, gender, and other demographic characteristics
Activities:	Behavioural performance and repertoire measured against: • Socially normative behaviour for some activities • Previous personal behaviour for some activities • Desired behaviour for some activities • Expected (e.g. by family) behaviour for some activities
Participation:	Social role performance and social position measured against: • Socially valued and expected roles for whole society • Culturally valued and expected roles for local, personal society • Personally valued and expected roles

Table 6.3. *Continued*

Implication	Comment
Miscellaneous	
The terminology used all assumes abnormality	There are currently no good words for the opposite of impairment, disability or handicap
Interventions may occur at many points	While removal of the prime cause of an illness is the ideal, and this prime cause will often be at the level of pathology, interventions at other points are often also effective, especially when there is no pathology or when pathology cannot be altered

signs). The nature of this phenomenon is being discussed more openly now. The most common single label applied within neurology to this phenomenon is probably 'conversion hysteria' or hysterical motor loss (although it could be argued that headache is the neurologist's equivalent of irritable bowel syndrome, another somatoform disorder.) The equivalence of many similar diagnoses across different specialities has recently been emphasized (Wessely *et al.* 1999). The causes of and mechanisms underlying conversion hysteria are still unknown, and treatment methods are still not researched (Halligan *et al.* 2000).

Second, the neurologist must always recognize that a patient's disability arises not simply from the observed impairments, but that it is strongly influenced by many other factors, both internal and external. Furthermore the neurologist will need to understand that there is no clear, direct and consistent relationship between pathology and impairment, or between impairment and disability, both within a patient over time and also between patients. For example, it is not uncommon to see patients with large areas of cerebral infarction but few symptoms, signs, or disabilities.

Thus when confronted by a patient whose disability is not easily explained the neurologist should ask two series of questions. The first series revolves around understanding the goals of the patient:

- Are there personal, contextual factors that are driving the patient? For example:
    - fear of worsening state, based on belief or experience?
- Are there factors in the patient's social context that are driving the patient? For example:
    - expectation that his or her financial state may be worsened if disability lessens?
    - expectation that he or she will lose a valued social role or social contacts if disability improves?
- Does some factor of the patient's physical context motivate the patient? For example:
    - expectation that she or he will get a better house if she or he remains disabled?

The second series of questions revolves around exploring factors that may be constraining behaviour that have not been recognized:

- Are there impairments that are not yet documented? For example:

- pain, incontinence, loss of initiation, apraxia, etc.?
- Is there a second pathology (or is the primary diagnosis itself in error)? For example:
    - development of hydrocephalus after head injury, or development of osteo-arthritis?
    - illness without pathology, rather than multiple sclerosis?

In difficult cases it may sometimes be helpful to admit a patient to a different environment (e.g. to a rehabilitation ward). First, this allows more prolonged observation of behaviour, thus identifying whether observed disability is consistent, and is consistent with the stated disability. Secondly, the new environment may precipitate change if the normal environment was in fact the major determinant of the disability. Another approach to understanding difficult cases is to imagine the situation from the point of view of the patient in his or her situation.

6.1.2 Rehabilitation

The development of, and discussion about, models of disability has fostered and clarified discussions about the nature of rehabilitation. While there is still no universally agreed definition of rehabilitation, it is now recognized that definitions of rehabilitation may refer to the:

- **structure** (i.e. the *operational characteristics* of a rehabilitation service);
- **process** (i.e. *how* rehabilitation services work); and
- **outcome** (i.e. the *aims* of rehabilitation services).

Definitions of all three aspects of rehabilitation are given in the Tables 6.4, 6.5, and 6.6.

It is worth noting that the processes involved in rehabilitation are identical to those involved in normal neurological practice. Medical diagnosis is the process of collecting and collating sufficient information to understand the patient's situation so as to influence the pathology; rehabilitation assessment is the process of collecting and collating sufficient information to understand the nature and genesis of the disability sufficiently to intervene. They both have the same purpose, but focus on different levels. Goal planning in rehabilitation involves identifying long-term goals and a set of actions needed to achieve those long-term goals. The main features differentiating goal planning from a medical plan of management are that the long-term goals are longer term and concern social

Table 6.4. Structure: the operational characteristics of rehabilitation services

The characteristics of a service that specializes in rehabilitation are that:

- It comprises a multidisciplinary group (team) of people who:
- Work together towards common goals for each patient;
- Involve and educate the patient and family in the process;
- Have relevant expertise and experience (knowledge and skills); and
- Can, between them, resolve most of the common problems faced by their patients

Table 6.5. Process: the stages of rehabilitation

Rehabilitation is a re-iterative active, educational, problem-solving process, focused on a patient's behaviour (disability), with the following components:

- Assessment, the identification of the nature and extent of the patient's problems and the factors relevant to their resolution
- Goal setting
- Intervention, which may include either or both of:

    Treatments, which affect the process of change

    Support (care), which maintains the patient's life and safety
- Evaluation, to check on the effects of any intervention

Table 6.6. Outcome: the aims of rehabilitation

The three aims of the rehabilitation process are to:

- Maximize the participation of the patient in his/her social setting
- Minimize the pain and distress experienced by the patient
- Minimize the distress of and stress on the patient's family and/or carers

functioning, and that the nature and number of further assessments or diagnostic tests and interventions are usually different and greater in range and number. Supportive care is essential in both medical and rehabilitation practice, and treatments (i.e. interventions to affect the process of change) are common to both. And in both circumstances evaluation after intervention is important.

Three *specific core skills* are particularly associated with rehabilitation:

(1) an ability to assess all relevant aspects of a patient's situation (and not simply their disease and its symptoms and signs), formulating the important interactions;

(2) an ability to set realistic but challenging goals in both the short and long term, a skill that depends upon an accurate evaluation of the likely prognosis and scope for effective intervention; and

(3) an ability to participate in teamwork, working co-operatively with a group of other experts towards agreed common goals.

Specialists in neurological disability (rehabilitation) will obviously be expert in all three areas, but most neurologists should be able to undertake these roles in relatively straightforward cases. They will also have an invaluable contribution to make to teams involved with more complex cases when there are no other medical rehabilitation experts available.

6.1.3 Assessment

Assessment is the collection and interpretation of the data needed to formulate sensible goals. In complex cases this will usually require input from several professions over several days or weeks, but in many cases it will require simple questioning and the use of appropriate measures, and it can be undertaken by a neurologist alone.

Most neurologists will be expert at assessing neurological impairments such as neglect, poor memory, aphasia, visual acuity, and severity of motor loss, although few will necessarily be familiar with detailed measures. However, the neurologist should also become familiar with a few of the more commonly used assessments of disability, such as those shown below. For more extensive information on various assessments, specialist texts should be consulted (Wade 1992; Herndon 1997).

Every neurologist should be able to document formally a patient's independence in personal activities of daily living (ADL), and the Barthel ADL index (Collin *et al.* 1988) (see Table 6.7) is strongly recommended because it is the most widely used, it is short and simple, and it probably gives as much information as any of the longer, more complex measures used in some places. It is important to note that this records the patient's observed (or reported or self-reported) performance—what he does do, not what he can do.

Most patients value mobility highly, and it is often affected, and so most neurologists should also record this routinely. Simple measures include the Rivermead Mobility Index (RMI; Table 6.8) (Forlander and Bohannon 1999) and the time taken to walk 10 metres (Collen *et al.* 1990). Both are short, simple, and reliable, and have demonstrated good utility and sensitivity in studies. Specifically the RMI is a better measure of disability in multiple sclerosis that the Kurtzke Expanded Disability Status Scale (EDSS) (Vaney *et al.* 1996), although there are other, more comprehensive, disease-specific measures. Finally, the number of falls experienced over some set time should also be recorded.

Measures of dexterity do exist, such as the nine-hole peg test (Heller *et al.* 1987). An alternative measure, in stroke at least, is grip strength. However, most neurologists will not have the equipment easily available in the clinic. Thus, in practice, asking a few specific questions can be very helpful; no set of questions has yet been studied to determine validity or reliability, but the questions shown in Table 6.9 should be sufficient in most cases.

Assessment is more than the simple documentation of the nature and extent of impairments and disabilities. The ultimate aim of assessment is to gain sufficient insight into a patient's situation to allow one to make plans for future management.

Table 6.7. The Barthel ADL index

	Day								
	Month								
	Year								

Bowels

0 = Incontinent of faeces (or is given enemas)

1 = Occasional accident (less than 1×/24 hours)

2 = Continent

Bladder

0 = Incontinent, or catheterized/convene drain and unable to manage it him/herself

1 = Occasional accident (maximum 1×/24 hours)

2 = Continent (for last 7 days)

Grooming

0 = Needs help (supervision, prompts, or practical help)

1 = Independent in washing face, doing teeth, shaving or putting on make-up, brushing hair

Toilet use

0 = Dependent, unable to wipe self

1 = Needs help, but can wipe self

2 = Independent in transfers and managing clothes off/on

Feeding

0 = Unable; is fed, has gastrostomy, or feeds self minimally

1 = Needs help cutting food, spreading butter, prompts/supervision, etc.

2 = Independent with food provided/selected

Transfer

0 = Unable; hoisted and/or unable to sit in wheelchair

1 = Major help; one or two people, much physical effort

2 = Minor help; one person, prompts/supervision or minor physical effort

3 = Independent bed-chair

Mobility

0 = Immobile; unable to get from bedroom to dining area

1 = Wheelchair independent (electric or self-propelled) at least bedroom to dining area

2 = Walks with help of one person (physical, or prompts/supervision) from bedroom to dining area

3 = Independent. May use stick, rollator, etc. if necessary

Dressing

0 = Dependent

1 = Needs help, but does about half (e.g. top or bottom independently, or minor prompts and/or physical help)

2 = Independent, including shoes, laces, buttons, etc.

Stairs

0 = Unable

1 = Needs help, physical or supervision/prompts or carrying equipment

2 = Independent up and down stairs (any means, including stair lift)

Bathing

0 = Dependent

1 = Independent (bath or shower) including getting in and out, washing, and drying and hair

TOTAL

Table 6.8. Rivermead Mobility Index

Ask the patient each question. Observe for question 5. Score 1 for 'yes', 0 for 'no'

Topic and question	Day						
	Month						
	Year						
Turning over in bed Do you turn over from your back to your side without help?							
Lying to sitting From lying in bed, do you get up to sit on the edge of the bed on your own?							
Sitting balance Do you sit on the edge of the bed without holding on for 10 seconds?							
Sitting to standing Do you stand up from any chair in less than 15 seconds and stand there for 15 seconds, using hands and/or an aid if necessary?							
Standing unsupported Observe standing for 10 seconds without any aid _Ask to stand_							
Transfer Do you manage to move from bed to chair and back without any help?							
Walking inside (with an aid if necessary) Do you walk 10 metres, with an aid if necessary, but with no standby help?							
Stairs Do you manage a flight of stairs without help?							
Walking outside (even ground) Do you walk around outside, on pavements, without help?							
Walking inside, with no aid Do you walk 10 metres inside, with no caliper, splint, or other aid (including furniture or walls) without help?							
Picking up off floor Do you manage to walk 5 metres, pick something up from the floor, and then walk back without help?							
Walking outside (uneven ground) Do you walk over uneven ground (grass, gravel, snow, ice, etc.) without help?							
Bathing Do you get into/out of a bath or shower and to wash yourself unsupervised and without help?							
Up and down four steps Do you manage to go up and down four steps with no rail, but using an aid if necessary?							
Running Do you run 10 metres without limping in 4 seconds (fast walk, not limping, is acceptable)?							
TOTAL							

Table 6.9. Some questions relating to dexterity

Question	Comment
Can you hold and use a knife/fork in your right/left hand?	
Can you do up buttons and zips?	
Can you hold a pen and write?	
Can you use a keyboard?	
Can you drink from a cup?	
Do you spill fluid from a cup?	
Can you clean your teeth (or shave)?	
Can you tie shoelaces?	
Can you pick up a saucepan safely?	

The starting point in rehabilitation is of course to determine the level of activities undertaken by the patient. However, sufficient information must also be identified: (1) to under-stand the genesis of the observed disability (i.e. the factors causing it); and (2) to predict, as far as possible, the prognosis and what interventions might improve matters.

Therefore it is vital to know the underlying pathology (if any) in order to judge prognosis and to specify what impairments are likely to be present. One very specific role for the neurologist is to inform the patient and the rehabilitation team of the prognosis for the disease and to suggest what impairments should specifically be sought. The impairments present are not only often the main influences upon disability, but they also often help determine prognosis.

It is also vital, when planning interventions, to know as much as possible about the patient's context, especially their beliefs and aspirations. Contextual information will often only be gathered over time by a variety of people. When a neurologist (or a rehabilitation team) is confronted by a patient whose disability is not readily explained by the known disease and associated impairments, it is particularly important to gather information about the patient's social and physical context, their attitudes and expectations, and the social position both in the past and now. It is often easiest to understand the patient's disability by simply trying to put oneself in the patient's situation.

In rehabilitation practice it is usual to have a structured way of assessing a patient, just as neurologists use structured methods to achieve diagnosis. The neurologist should have an abbreviated structured disability assessment for routine use, probably focused on the Barthel ADL index and Rivermead Mobility Index, and a single question about the nature of the patient's main way of occupying time during the day (work, leisure, or watching television?).

6.1.4 Goal planning and teamwork

In neurological medical practice there is usually only one treatment for any pathology, but in neurological rehabilitation there are almost always multiple simultaneous interventions—this is one great contrast between rehabilitation and traditional neurological practice. Furthermore, and again in contrast to neurological medical practice, many different professions and different people may be involved, and indeed many of the interventions may involve people outside the health services. In other words, rehabilitation is likely to involve a much bigger and more extensive team of people than is involved in medical management. Multiple interventions by several professions is, of course, now more the case in the management of malignant tumours, where specialist teams again provide a more effective service.

As discussed in more detail below, effective rehabilitation depends upon effective teamwork. Effective teamwork requires that all team members work towards common goals; this is a working definition of a team. Therefore one defining characteristic of rehabilitation is that it has a procedure for identifying, agreeing, and setting goals.

The process of goal setting in rehabilitation, and the evidence in support of this process, has been reviewed in detail elsewhere (Wade 1998a, 1999a) and it is not necessary to cover the detail here. It is important to recognize that good rehabilitation practice should:

- set meaningful, challenging, but achievable goals;

- involve the patient in goal setting, and the family if appropriate;

- set both short- and long-term goals;

- set goals both at the team level and at the level of an individual clinician; *but* should

- avoid using the progress of individual patients against goals set (goal attainment scaling) as the sole or major means of determining further rehabilitation in individual patients.

The neurologist may have several important roles in rehabilitation teamwork and goal setting. First, setting goals depends upon all interested parties meeting together to negotiate agreed achievable goals. Sometime the doctor may need to chair the meeting, either as the person with most experience of chairing meetings or as the person with least direct involvement, able to take a more dispassionate point of view. Secondly, the neurologist must ensure that goals set are realistic, given the patient's clinical state and prognosis. Thirdly, the neurologist may well be surprised at how much their own accumulated knowledge can contribute to the process of setting rehabilitation goals. The need for a systematic approach to goal planning, and details on what it is and how it may be undertaken, has been reviewed in detail (Wade 1999b,c,d).

6.1.5 Rehabilitation interventions

The major difference between rehabilitation interventions and most other medical (neurological) interventions is that they focus on disability (activities), not on pathology. While in most medical and surgical specialities great attention is paid to relieving symptoms and to the non-pathological aspects of a patient's illness, none the less the main focus is on diagnosing and then alleviating the underlying pathology. In contrast, the focus in rehabilitation is on alleviating the restriction on, or alteration in, activities, while still being concerned with knowing and, if possible, treating the underlying pathology.

This difference in focus has three major consequences. First, and discussed in more detail below, it might explain in part why traditional medical systems have so much difficulty in diagnosing, understanding, and managing patients with 'conversion hysteria', 'abnormal illness behaviour', or 'non-organic disability'. Secondly, it means that once all diagnostic and management processes focused on pathology have been completed, the medical system is no longer especially concerned with the patient's continuing disability; it is the system or organization that loses interest, not the individual clinicians. Thirdly, as illustrated in Fig. 6.1, the number of influences on a patient's activity is great, and consequently the range and number of potential interventions is usually greater than that normally met in medical practice.

Figure 6.1 illustrates the factors that might influence (cause, exacerbate, or reduce) disability in any one patient. It only shows the direct and a few indirect pathways, and in reality there will be many more links and cross-pathways. The figure does illustrate that observed activities (i.e. disability) may arise in very many ways, and that the link to and influence of the underlying disease process may be quite limited.

It is also important to remember that activities, the behaviours exhibited by the patient, are goal directed and will reflect the wishes, expectations, and beliefs of the patient. These internal factors will themselves be the result of past experience, cultural background, education, and many other, often unknown, factors. Two very important other factors, often forgotten, are the beliefs and expectations of the patient and the family and friends.

Interventions can, in principle at least, be classified into two main types. The first is support. This refers to any intervention needed or given to maintain the status quo without any specific

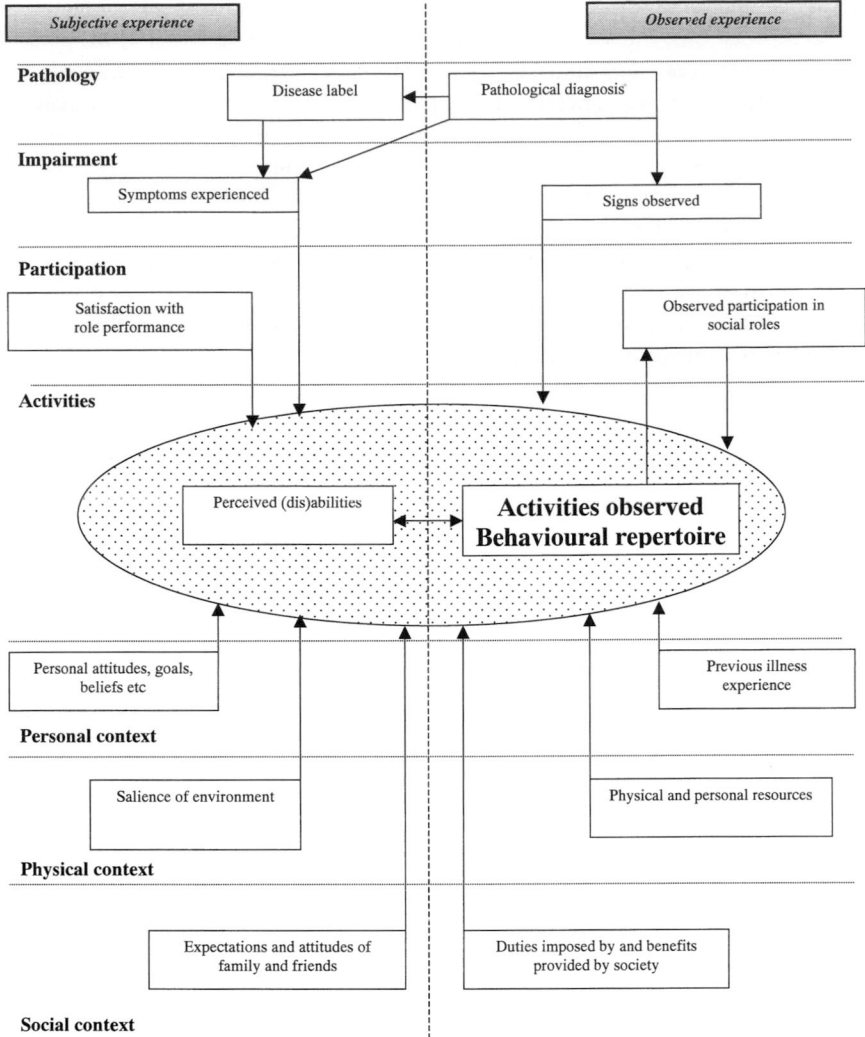

Fig. 6.1. Influences on a patient's activity (disability).

expectation of altering the natural history of the condition. Examples might include undertaking maintenance stretches of joints not being moved normally, helping someone with dressing, preparing food for someone, or providing gastrostomy feeding. The second class of intervention is any action that is expected to lead to a sustained change in the situation. Most 'therapy', provision of any equipment, and giving information are all examples of this class of intervention. This class of intervention may be referred to as treatment, but the interventions extend well outside the normal concept of treatment, which is often constrained to therapy alone.

In reality the distinction is not always easy to make, and in some instances treatment will inevitably include support, for example when dressing someone while teaching them how to dress themselves. The best way to distinguish treatment from support is to consider whether the intervention will be continued indefinitely; if so, it is probably support. This distinction is of some importance. First, long-term support is funded differently from treatment in most healthcare systems. At the same

time, however, the provision of support is often major resource attributable to a patient receiving treatment in the healthcare system. Secondly, support rarely requires general expertise (although the individual care worker may need specific training to manage a specific situation). Thirdly, the patient and family should not anticipate further progress from support, whereas they will correctly expect treatment to be associated with change, usually progress.

There has been little research into the provision of support: how can one assess how much is appropriate; how is it best delivered; who should give it; how should it be funded, etc. Indeed, providing support may not always be appropriate. For example, some patients ask for, or are offered, more support than they strictly need (i.e. they could manage the activity in its absence), and this might reinforce or prolong their dependence. Making this judgement is difficult and there are no easy ways of determining need.

Some specific areas of intervention will now be considered. The WHO ICIDH-2 framework from Table 6.1 is used, taking

Table 6.10. Rehabilitation interventions, some examples

Level (*term*)	Intervention	Comment
Level of illness		
Organ (*pathology*)	Prevent disease Reverse or remove pathology Replace lost physiological function (e.g. insulin) Give information and advice	Important to know pathology for prognosis and likely impairments. 'Cure' often not possible **Note** Pathology is not always present in an illness
Person (*impairment*)	Prevent occurrence or worsening of impairment Reverse or improve impaired skill Replace lost skill or part with external or internal 'aid'	May use therapy, drugs, orthoses, prostheses, surgery, etc. May learn technique to overcome loss **Note** Impairment may improve secondary to functional practice
Person in environment (*activities*)	Prevent patient learning abnormal behaviours Teach how to undertake activities in presence of immutable impairments Practise activities, advising on risks, techniques, etc.	Involves altering behaviour in one way or another. Will often also involve changing the environment. May involve changing patient's goals or goals of others **Note** Takes time and depends upon learning
Person in society (*participation*)	Prevent loss of social contacts and roles Help identify new roles, and how to develop them Ensure has opportunities to develop new or maintain old roles	Will almost always involve other people. May involve change in accommodation. For most people work is a central role **Note** Takes a long time
Context of illness		
Personal context	Prevent development of maladaptive beliefs and expectations Alter beliefs and expectations if necessary, usually through giving information and psychological therapy	Beliefs and expectations are major determinants of behaviour; but consequences of behaviour may also affect beliefs and expectations
Physical context	Avoid loss of familiar environment if possible Adjust environment physically, including through providing support from other people	Could include environmental control equipment, mobility aids, housing adaptations, etc.
Social context	Adjust or help patient find new social context; or help adapt to new social context	Usually strongly linked to accommodation and work
Totality of illness		
Quality of life	Full rehabilitation	

some of the additional aspects shown in Table 6.2. Table 6.10 lists some examples, and some aspects of intervention at each level and in each context will be discussed below.

It is always important to establish the pathological diagnosis (or the absence of any disease). The diagnosis determines the general prognosis (i.e. the prognostic field), and suggests the impairments likely to be present, and that should be sought specifically. However, it is also important to consider what disease the patient believes he has and, of more importance, what he believes the implications of that diagnosis to be. For example, some people recently diagnosed with multiple sclerosis believe they should rest excessively, or that they should not become pregnant, or that they will die within a few years; there is no evidence to support any of these beliefs.

Intervention at this level must concentrate first upon reversing, removing, or controlling any pathology. The rehabilitation focus should be on providing accurate and understandable relevant information to the patient and family (and others as needed), and should especially focus on dispelling inaccurate or unfounded fears and beliefs. A second, possible area that should interest both neurologists and rehabilitationists is that of increasing secondary neural change directly. It has been shown that amphetamine coupled with physical therapy may increase neurophysiological recovery after stroke (Walker-Batson *et al.* 1995). It has also been shown that some drugs probably impede neurophysiological recovery after stroke (Goldstein 1995). Serotoninergic drugs may increase functional recovery after stroke (Dam *et al.* 1996; Miyai and Reding, 1998), it has recently been shown that lofepramine and phenylalanine (with vitamin B_{12}) may reduce impairment seen with multiple sclerosis (unpublished observations). These two drugs increase central noradrenaline, which is similar to the effect of amphetamine, and future research may build on these observations.

Establishing what impairments are present, and what skills are preserved, is important in trying to understand the genesis of any observed disability and in trying to predict what treatments might help. It is particularly important to consider whether some impairments that are unusual or unusually severe are in fact due to another pathology, or whether they indicate significant emotional distress or unsubstantiated beliefs about the illness.

There are many interventions at this level, and most neurologists will be familiar with those that involve the use of drugs, such as the use of baclofen or botulinum toxin for spasticity, the use of botulinum toxin for cervical dystonia (Lew *et al.* 1997), and the various ways of controlling pain. Further, outside their normal expertise, there are many orthoses and prostheses for replacing or supporting lost skills or functions: ankle–foot orthoses for foot drop, diaries and notebooks for amnesia, artificial limbs, splints, etc. Surgery may be used to lengthen or transfer tendons, and to correct or ameliorate other impairments. There is little research into these treatments. Therapy, such as physiotherapy or cognitive therapy, is sometimes thought to act directly on impairments. However, there is little evidence in support of this contention, and it is probable that task-oriented therapy will itself reduce impairment (Lord *et al.* 1998).

Rehabilitation services will always pay much attention to the patient's physical context, exploring the current physical environment and ways that it can be made more appropriate for the individual. The range of interventions is huge, extending from simple peri-personal changes in clothing and the provision of a walking aid, through complex equipment such as computer-based environmental control systems and electric wheelchairs, on to major building changes in accommodation. At the same time the availability of people to provide direct physical help or supervision must be considered, and any people involved must be taught the necessary skills.

The patient's own social and cultural context must always be taken into account. First, it may determine where someone lives, and the patient's family, friends, and colleagues may all have particular views on the way that 'disabled people' should behave. In some cultures (and subcultures) people with a disease are expected to be dependent, and independence is not an all-important goal as it is in many Western cultures. In other cultures, people with disability are considered of no value, and in yet other cultures such people are thought to be been made disabled as a punishment for past misdemeanours in this life or in a previous existence. All these social beliefs must be known about and considered. Secondly, society may provide perverse incentives favouring certain behaviours. For example, for some people there is a financial disincentive to work or to be more independent unless complete normality can be achieved, because partial improvement from the present situation may lead to complete loss of financial support without gaining a full salary or income. Other people may remain dependent because it is the only way they can obtain any social contact through the day.

Intervention at the level of an individual's social and cultural context is difficult, if not impossible, but it is vital to take these factors into account when planning other interventions.

Next, one must always remember the person's own context, their beliefs, expectations, goals, and experiences. These are perhaps the most potent determinants of behaviour. If it can be achieved, changing erroneous or maladaptive beliefs and attitudes may be more effective as an intervention than any other single intervention.

Returning to the four levels of illness, it is possible to intervene at the level of participation. Social participation depends upon being able to meet and interact with other people in social settings and activities. Consequently, one may need to organize transport to allow someone to attend Church or some other wanted activity, or one may need to refer someone on to a social group appropriate to their interests and skills. Or one may sometimes need to suggest that the person would have a better 'quality of life' if they moved from living alone in the community to living in suitable residential accommodation where they could develop a fuller social life with more social roles. In other words, although one cannot force increased participation, one should always ensure that every person has the opportunities to participate in society as fully as they wish within their limitations.

The final level to consider is that of activity. Within rehabilitation there remains a continuing and unresolved debate between those who believe that treatments should aim at reversing the underlying impairments and those who believe that treatment should simply aim at improving task performance, regardless of how this is achieved. This can be characterized with two modern examples of unanswered questions: should stroke patients practise walking on a treadmill with harness support from the earliest possible opportunity (Visintin *et al.* 1998), or should they try to learn better control of movement and tone? And should patients with cognitive losses participate in 'cognitive retraining', or should they practise the activities they need to undertake (Kalra *et al.* 1997)?

The traditional approach, still the most widely practised, is to focus on reducing the impairment. However, there is now increasing evidence that a task-oriented approach is at least as effective, and probably more efficient (Lord and Hall 1986; Richards *et al.* 1993, Lin *et al.* 1997). At present it is certainly true that neither approach can be rejected on the evidence.

Finally, when faced with an individual patient, it is important to remember that the effective intervention may be unique to your patient. Evidence may guide you as to the best approach, and may suggest that certain traditional interventions will or will not help, but each patient's combination of circumstances is unique and the solution may be unique. The key is to spend time considering the most efficient and effective way to increase the patient's level of participation.

6.1.6 Effectiveness of rehabilitation

Rehabilitation undoubtedly 'works'. A meta-analysis of data from trials of stroke unit rehabilitation has shown that rehabilitation services are effective at reducing both mortality and morbidity, possibly without any extra resources (Stroke Unit

Trialists' Collaboration, 1997, 1998). Furthermore, there is evidence that these benefits can be achieved in actual practice in unselected hospitals (Rudd *et al.* 1999), and they may last for many years (Indredavik *et al.* 1998). The meta-analysis was especially important because it helped characterize the probable important ingredients of effective rehabilitation: co-ordination, expertise, and education. These three factors relate to the overall structure and process of rehabilitation, emphasizing the need for dedicated, multidisciplinary expert teams involved in rehabilitation of patients with neurological disability.

Evidence in support of specialist co-ordinated rehabilitation services is less strong in other fields, but trials have shown benefits for patients with multiple sclerosis (Di Fabio *et al.* 1998; Freeman *et al.* 1999), and mild or moderate head injury (Wade *et al.* 1998). Consequently, the presumption should now be that most patients with neurological disability will benefit from being seen by a specialist, co-ordinated, neurological rehabilitation service. It is no longer tenable to depict rehabilitation as an expensive placebo service. There are continuing debates about the advantages and disadvantages of yet more focused disease-specific services as against relatively generic neurological disability services.

The evidence concerning each part of the process of rehabilitation is much more difficult to identify and evaluate.

The evidence would suggest that a process of formal structured assessment of patients with a disability by a team of people specialized in rehabilitation does improve outcome, although (obviously) only when taken as a part of the whole process (Wade 1998*b*). Assessment in isolation is not helpful, and it is important that more than one profession is involved (Cunningham *et al.* 1996) because otherwise it is probable that important impairments or disabilities will not be identified and because different people do not agree on 'rehabilitation potential' (Cunningham *et al.* 2000).

The evidence relating to goal planning has been reviewed recently (Wade 1998*a*, 1999*a*) and, although it is not susceptible to meta-analysis and although it is difficult to review systematically, there is reasonable support for a systematic approach to setting goals for disabled patients participating in rehabilitation.

The evidence concerning specific interventions is very extensive, with more than 80 randomized studies of rehabilitation intervention for acute stroke alone (Inter-collegiate Working Party for Stroke 2000). Unfortunately, because rehabilitation covers a huge range of treatments, often not specifically tied to single diseases, it is difficult to construct an analytic framework (Wade 1998*c*), let alone access and review the large volume of information. However, recent research, mostly related to stroke, does support various hypotheses.

First, there is now evidence that even quite small levels of intervention can have quite powerful and specific effects (Kwakkel *et al.* 1999) and there is some evidence of a dose–response relationship between therapeutic input and outcome (Kwakkel *et al.* 1997). However, there is currently no evidence to identify a minimum or maximum effective level of direct therapeutic input.

Secondly, there is strong evidence that assessment for and provision of simple equipment is extremely cost-effective (Mann *et al.* 1999). This observation demonstrates that it is not correct simply to equate rehabilitation with the provision of face-to-face therapy. The therapist also needs expertise to know what equipment may be helpful, how to define the specific characteristics of the piece of equipment, and, most importantly of all, how to find and fund the equipment. This all takes time, a fact often not appreciated by patients or by funding agencies.

Thirdly, there is some evidence that even the simple provision of information may be effective in a variety of diseases (Mant *et al.* 1998; Wade *et al.* 1998). Again this demonstrates that effective interventions extend well beyond simply giving direct, face-to-face treatment, and that effective rehabilitation depends crucially upon the clinician's expertise and time. Giving information is simply one aspect of the therapeutic relationship between a patient and the doctor or other healthcare professional. There are no studies that investigate the benefits or disbenefits of a therapeutic relationship between a clinician and a patient. However, the benefits of service dogs for people with long-term mobility disability has been shown in relation to dogs (Allen and Blascovitch 1996) and it seems probable that this may, in part, be related to the existence of an animal–patient relationship. Thus it seems probable that acting on the patient's personal context (knowledge and beliefs) may well be an undervalued component of rehabilitation.

Fourthly, there is evidence that drugs can have both beneficial and harmful effects upon a patient's performance (Section 6.1.5). In many instances the neurologist will be helping the patient recover independence without specifically realizing that it is part of rehabilitation, for example through prescribing analgesics, giving antidepressant medication, etc. The neurologist does have two important roles in relation to drugs. The first is always to review whether the drugs being taken are still giving more benefit that harm. Too frequently drugs are started for sound reasons but are continued without further thought. Patients should be encouraged to seek review of medication at regular intervals, perhaps every 6 months. Drugs that may need the dose altering or may need withdrawing include: antispastic drugs, anticonvulsant drugs, antidepressant drugs, and minor and major tranquillizers. Most of these drugs have cognitive side-effects and some may effect adversely the process of recovery (Goldstein 1995). The second is to be aware of the use of drugs to treat specific impairments. This task requires both the initial identification of the impairment and knowledge of the intervention, which may be difficult because information is not easily collated. Examples include the use of gabapentin to improve visual acuity when nystagmus is present (Averbuch-Heller *et al.* 1997), identifying and treating neuropathic pain, identifying and treating urinary urgency and incontinence, the use of amantadine for fatigue in multiple sclerosis (Krupp *et al.* 1995), and the use of bromocriptine to ameliorate reduced initiation after frontal lobe damage (Powell *et al.* 1996).

There is virtually no useful evidence concerning the second aspect of intervention, the provision of support and care. However, this is often the major intervention provided to patients, and one should take a critical approach to this.

Finally, the process of rehabilitation includes the formal evaluation of any intervention. Again, there is little evidence to guide one on the nature or frequency of this evaluation, or on the best method. Some studies suggest that goal attainment scaling is one sensitive way of measuring change (Rockwood *et al.* 1997). This may be so for the individual patient. However, it is not clear whether it is better than any other method. More importantly, goal attainment scaling should not be used to determine whether a specific rehabilitation intervention should be reimbursed or continued; it is one method for the clinician to use, but, as with all information, the information obtained must be interpreted in the whole context of the patient. Using goal attainment scaling as the main measure of effectiveness is subject to major risks: unchallenging goals may be set, with lowering of the morale of both the patient and the clinician; and other unpredictable factors may intervene.

In summary, the evidence strongly supports the effectiveness of the process of specialist neurological rehabilitation, but the evidence is not able to give any detail about the process. The patchy nature of the evidence for specific interventions must not detract from the most important fact to remember about rehabilitation, namely that the evidence supports rehabilitation services which show the following characteristics:

◆ good organization, delivering a coordinated service; *from*

◆ a multi-professional team; *with*

◆ expertise and experience in the conditions they treat; and *also involving*

◆ continuing education of both staff, and patients and their families.

Such a service is likely to use:

◆ structured assessment procedures or protocols;

◆ goal-setting procedures that involve the patient and family as well as all relevant agencies;

◆ a wide range of interventions at many levels and in many contexts;

◆ some system of evaluating the effects of interventions in a re-iterative way.

6.2 Patterns of disability

6.2.1 Acute-onset disability

The paradigmatic disease for acute-onset disability is obviously stroke (Chapter 27). The evidence for the effectiveness of rehabilitation has been reviewed recently in the British National Clinical Guidelines for Stroke (Inter-collegiate Working Party for Stroke 2000). This section simply reviews some of the more general characteristics of acute-onset disability and how these might impact on management. This refers not only to acute onset in single-episode disease, such as herpes simplex encephalitis or head injury, but also to acute deterioration in diseases such as multiple sclerosis.

Common sense and methodological completeness requires that prevention should be a key component of managing this situation. There are two ways that acute-onset neurological disability could be prevented. First, the incidence of the pathological process itself might be reduced. Programmes to identify and control hypertension will reduce stroke incidence; accident prevention programmes (e.g. reducing alcohol abuse) will reduce accidents that cause head injury; wearing seat belts and bicycle helmets will reduce traumatic brain damage in those accidents that do happen; β-interferon may reduce relapse rate in multiple sclerosis; vaccination against meningitis or polio will reduce infections, and so on.

More importantly in the context of hospital-based neurological services, effective acute management may minimize the extent of permanent neurological loss in individual patients. Obvious examples include the timely use of antibiotics or antiviral agents to treat infections, the use of intravenous immunoglobulin (Ig) for Guillain–Barré syndrome, and surgical removal of extradural haematomas after head injury. The importance of rapid, accurate diagnosis of pathology followed by rapid intervention is obvious. In order to achieve reduction or prevention of brain damage in individual patients, it is vital that all patients with an acute neurological illness are seen within a setting that includes the relevant expertise and resources. This often does not occur. For example, secondary brain damage after acute head injury in an accident continues to be common, despite recognition of the problems and promotion of easy solutions for many years. In the UK only a minority of acute neurological illnesses are managed by appropriate experts (i.e. neurologists)—the cost of this 'policy' in terms of neurological disability has not been investigated. It is of note that well-organized expert stroke services reduce mortality, which presumably reflects prevention of pathological processes within the brain or elsewhere.

Neurologists have an important role to play in the prevention of disability, both directly, in minimizing neurological damage in their individual patients, and indirectly (and probably more effectively) through ensuring that the system of healthcare and public health locally is organized efficiently. In both instances the neurologist should concentrate on achieving a well-organized system that applies current evidence-based best practice in a consistent way.

Prevention of avoidable disabling secondary complications should also be a high priority. This, too, is most effectively carried out by well-organized expert services. Obvious examples include pressure sores and the development of joint contractures. Less obvious, and often overlooked or ignored, are the emotional consequences of acute-onset severe disability which can, in themselves, have a major impact on the long-term outcome.

Most acute illnesses are unexpected. Consequently, patients and their families may experience considerable secondary emotional trauma. This can take several forms. Many people search for the 'cause' or reason for the event, often with a degree of guilt and blame being attached either to the patient and family, or to external others. This can become an overwhelming process. Some people develop significant secondary anxiety or depression, with the extreme form being labelled post-traumatic stress syndrome. In some people the illness may precipitant a crisis in family relationships with separation or divorce; usually this is simply the end stage of a process that started before the onset, possibly due to pre-existing stresses. Whatever the aetiology, the emotional sequelae of an acute-onset disabling illness can be severe. Furthermore, the emotional consequences can themselves cause significant impairments such as poor memory and concentration, weight loss, and multiple symptomatology, and thus cause increased disabilities. In addition, the emotional consequences will almost always worsen the effects of any impairments caused directly by the pathology. The emotional sequelae may become the dominant cause of prolonged disability. Ideally, this complication should be prevented. Unfortunately there is no evidence to support any particular intervention, such as counselling. Evidence related to treatment is equally sparse, but, in general, the usual psychiatric approaches are used: cognitive behavioural therapy; giving information; reassurance; antidepressant medication; and minor and major tranquillizers.

The family and others may also experience significant emotional distress. This can have a direct effect on the patient's rehabilitation. It is important that the rehabilitation team always considers the emotional state of the family, especially if there are unexplained difficulties in the rehabilitation process.

Emotional problems may also arise later in the illness. Most acute-onset illnesses are followed by a period of recovery that may extend for weeks, months, or even years. While this naturally leads to optimism, it is rarely possible to give an accurate prognosis in an individual case, even in a condition such as stroke. The failure to fulfil expectations, or unrealistic hopes, can then lead to significant delayed-onset emotional consequences. For example, the patient and family may not realize that significant longer-term sequelae may exist, or may deny the possibility. When full recovery does not occur, anger may follow.

In summary, acute-onset disability is often considered the easiest to manage, because recovery occurs and may be complete. However, the stress of the unexplained and unexpected onset and the slowness of recovery, which is often incomplete and uncertain, both may cause significant emotional problems which can directly or indirectly impede rehabilitation.

6.2.2 Slowly progressive disability

The opposite extreme, in terms of time course, is any illness where the patient slowly but inexorably worsens over many months or years. This leads to a different set of problems which vary, depending upon whether or not the disease process affects cognition.

When the patient has a disease that does not affect cognition, the patient is often able to adapt their behaviour to the increasing level of impairment. Typical examples include most forms of muscular dystrophy (Chapter 15) and motor neuron disease (Chapter 14). Such patients rarely need the specialist skills of a rehabilitation service, but they will sometimes need access to the specialist knowledge about specialist equipment. The only skills they require are the assessment for equipment, and being taught how to use equipment. Such patients can usually teach even rehabilitation specialists something about the management of progressive impairment. Moreover, it is often difficult to understand how the patient can manage with such severe impairment.

In the situation where the patient has a disease that primarily affects cognition, it is often the family that slowly adapts, learning how to manage the situation. The patient, or more correctly the family, will normally need some help and advice from the specialist rehabilitation service. This will be to help them cope with the increasing amnesia and the practical problems that follow, especially the risk of harm.

In some circumstances, especially multiple sclerosis, the patient may have progressive impairment of both cognition and motor control. This is perhaps the most difficult situation to manage. In the early stages, when cognition is relatively intact and the other impairments relatively mild, the patient will usually benefit from active intervention. Ironically, however, the more dependent the patient becomes, the less likely she or he is to benefit from intervention. In an individual patient it is important to have an accurate knowledge of the level of cognitive function in relation to the cognitive demands of the proposed intervention.

Therefore in any slowly progressive illness it may well be worth referring the patient to a specialist disability service at an early stage. However, the main purpose of this referral will depend upon the nature of the underlying disease.

For patients with primary non-cognitive impairments or with almost exclusively cognitive impairments, the purposes will be to establish a baseline measure of the impairments and disabilities, and of the context, to establish medical contact, and to give the patient information about how to make contact again in future. The patient (or the family) should then be made responsible for contacting specialist services when help is needed. Guidance on likely circumstance may be helpful. In reality the neurological service may well undertake regular follow-up for some reason, in which case the neurologist should check that any problems arising have been resolved satisfactorily.

For patients with mixed impairments, the service will often need to become involved actively over the course of the illness. Initially this may focus on minimizing the patient's disability, and over time it is likely to focus increasingly on supporting the family and organizing appropriate care and support.

Whatever the nature of the disease process, it is always important to inform the patient about any local voluntary sector support services. Such organizations often provide invaluable aid. The support available usually includes good information, social support, and social networks of people facing similar difficulties. Sometimes voluntary sector organizations will also provide or identify financial support and other physical resources (e.g. specialist wheelchairs). However, it is wise to be aware of the nature of the specific support organization. Some are very political, campaigning but not helping individual patients; others are very exclusive, not necessarily welcoming all potential recruits; some are overoptimistic, suggesting unrealistic goals; others are unduly pessimistic, emphasizing the worst possible outcomes.

Therefore the neurologist has several important roles to play, whether working as part of a specialist rehabilitation service or working in isolation. In every case the patient and the family should be given as accurate information as possible about the future prognosis and how to make use of all available resources, both locally and further afield. In some cases it may be appropriate to refer the patient on to a specialist rehabilitation service for early assessment and advice. In other cases the neurologist may well remain the primary contact.

There is no evidence to guide routine follow-up arrangements. It could be argued that the rehabilitation service or neurology service should see every patient with a progressive disorder regularly, to monitor the situation. Quite apart from any resource considerations, it is worth realizing that this process may have adverse effects. The patient and family may retain unrealistic hopes of a cure. The patient and family become reinforced in a belief that they are 'medically ill', with the result that others, such as employers or friends, may similarly believe that cure is imminent. One solution might be to undertake a yearly review by post, telephone, or email.

In a relatively small minority of patients with slowly progressive disability the patient or the family may experience significant emotional distress. They should be referred to a clinical psychology service or to a psychiatry service.

In summary, slowly progressive disorders are usually associated with successful adaptation over time by the patient and family, because cognition is usually preserved in one or both parties. The role of specialist services is to provide expert advice on supportive adaptations, equipment, and services as the need arises. The role of the neurologist undertaking regular follow-up is to monitor the adaptation of the patient and to refer on if necessary.

6.2.3 Multiple sclerosis and other fluctuant diseases

The most common fluctuating disease is multiple sclerosis. Other diseases with longer-term fluctuation might include the neurological aspects of systemic lupus erythematosus and other autoimmune diseases. Such diseases pose some very specific problems.

First, the prognosis for an individual patient is usually quite unknown. The patient, and the patient's family, therefore have to live with constant uncertainty. For many patients this constant uncertainty is extremely demoralizing. The emotional stress can itself then worsen the effects of the disease. Unfortunately, the neurologist is not in a position to reduce the level of uncertainty. However, it is important that the doctor at least recognizes this emotional stress, and recognizes how it may exacerbate or exaggerate the consequences of the disease process itself. It is also important for the neurologist to emphasize that there is no evidence that the prognosis can be altered through most of the 'alternative' therapies offered, and to protect the patient against any suggested treatments that may pose significant risk or expense.

Secondly, in multiple sclerosis itself and in some other similar diseases, individual patients can suffer one of an extremely wide range of specific impairments. No two patients are the same. None the less patients and their families, and often professional staff too, will base their actions and expectations on their observation of other patients with the same disease. This can be extremely counter-productive. Patients and professional staff should be encouraged to consider the patient's specific range of impairments, not the disease label.

One major consequence of this uncertainty and variability is that it is very difficult to organize services. As has been stated, the key aspect of a successful rehabilitation service is organization. The problems of organizing services for patients with multiple sclerosis have been discussed elsewhere (Wade 1997). In essence patients present with problems that require the expertise of many different people, usually employed by different organizations and having different budgets. An audit of services for patients with multiple sclerosis in Oxfordshire revealed the complete chaos, and showed how patients suffered as a result of the disorganization. The audit also showed that most patients were in contact with their general practitioner (family doctor), and that the second most common contact was with a neurologist. This reinforces the need for doctors, including the neurologist, to be well aware of the disabling consequences of any disease.

Fluctuation on a much shorter time scale also occurs. The archetypal disease is Parkinson's disease and the neurologist has a major role to play in optimizing the drug regime (Section 32.3.1) to smooth out the fluctuations in motor performance. However, it is worth noting that short-term fluctuation may occur in almost any patient with chronic neurological disease. Sometimes there may be simple explanations, such as changes in temperature, but often there is no explanation. In most circumstances the patient simply needs to accept that fluctuation will occur, and adapt accordingly.

6.3 Spinal-cord injury

Spinal injury services give perhaps the best evidence of the benefits of well-organized, specialist rehabilitation services. Furthermore, these benefits have been accepted worldwide without a single randomized, controlled trial! None the less the evidence is dramatic: before 1930 almost all patients died within a few months, whereas now almost all patients will probably survive for the majority of their expected lifespan. This extraordinary reversal of prognosis has occurred in the absence of any specific medical intervention whatsoever, demonstrating that the process of specialist, well-organized rehabilitation is itself extremely effective, even when the underlying pathology and impairments cannot be changed.

The key to this success is the attention given to all aspects of prevention: prevention of pressure sores (decubitus ulcers); prevention of urinary tract damage; prevention of contractures, etc. And the method of achieving this success is to ensure that patients are managed by a specialist service as soon as possible. Although there are no randomized controlled data, observational evidence shows that a delay of even 1 day is associated with a poorer outcome (De Vivo *et al.*, 1990).

The other key principle underlying the success of spinal-cord rehabilitation is that the patient should be fully educated about, and responsible for, as much of his or her management as possible. Consequently, whenever the neurologist is asked to see a patient late after injury, she or he would be well advised to ask the patient or the family for their opinion about any specific problem relating to the injury being consulted about. This will immediately make a good relationship between neurologist and patient, particularly useful if the patient is incorrect in their assessment or suggested plan.

6.3.1 Epidemiology

The annual incidence of spinal-cord trauma varies in different countries, from 1.3 to 5.0 per 100 000 population (Kurtzke 1975; Kraus 1985). Road traffic accidents, especially motor cycle accidents, are responsible for over half such injuries; about a quarter occur at work or in the home by falling down stairs,

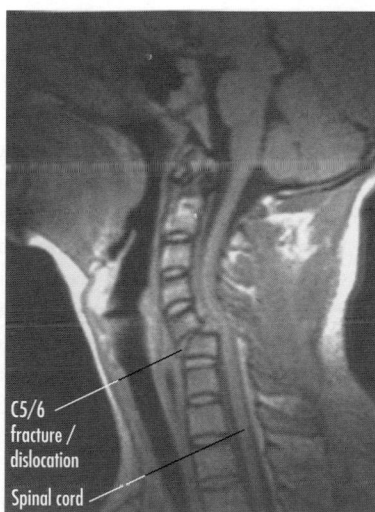

Fig. 6.2. Traumatic tetraplegia due to fracture–dislocation between the C5 and C6 vertebrae with spinal cord compression (MRI) (from Donaghy 1997).

scaffolding, or ladders; and approximately one-fifth result from sporting injuries, notably diving into shallow water, rugby, and horse-riding (Grundy *et al.* 1990). The most common sites of injury in civilian life are the lower cervical region and the thoracolumbar junction, followed by the upper cervical region. In a series of admissions to a spinal injuries unit in the UK, 55 per cent of cases had cervical injuries, 35 per cent thoracic injuries, and 10 per cent lumbosacral injuries.

The cord may be damaged directly, or secondarily by fractures, dislocations, or fracture—dislocations of the vertebral column (Fig. 6.2). Most cervical injuries are due to forcible flexion. A blow on the head causing flexion and compression of the neck may result in anterior displacement of the odontoid and anterior subluxation of C1 and C2. In the lower cervical spine, a dislocation or acute central herniation of an intervertebral disc may occur. A vertical compression force may cause a Jefferson fracture of the atlas, in which the occipital condyles of the skull are driven downwards, fracturing the atlas, pushing the lateral masses outwards and sometimes rupturing the transverse ligament. More commonly, extension–compression forces may fracture the posterior arch of the atlas. Hyperextension of the upper cervical spine can fracture the odontoid and displace it posteriorly, with posterior subluxation of C1 on C2. When extension of the neck is accompanied by distraction, the pedicles of the atlas may fracture, with an anterior slip of C2 on C3. Pre-existing cervical spondylosis, with or without congenital narrowing of the cervical canal (Kessler 1975), greatly increases the risk of damage to the spinal cord by injuries that cause forcible neck extension. Thus in older people, severe spinal-cord injuries may occur in the absence of fractures or dislocations, and in children a similar discrepancy may be seen because the spine is more supple and can accommodate distortions that damage the cord without causing a fracture.

The spinal cord may occasionally be injured in the infant during birth as a result of violent traction. Such injuries may arise in three ways. Traction on the head may cause dislocation of the upper cervical spine, which is usually immediately fatal. Traction separating the head and shoulders, by exerting tension on the brachial plexus and cervical spinal roots, may injure the spinal cord while also producing a brachial plexus palsy. And, in a breech presentation, violent traction may cause fracture dislocation in the thoracic or lumbar regions.

6.3.2 Pathology

The interpretation of the pathology of spinal-cord trauma is complicated by the fact that approximately 30 per cent of cases have significant additional injuries, some of which may contribute to hypoperfusion or hypoxia prior to the arrival of medical assistance. Even when no significant encroachment upon the spinal canal can be detected, the cord shows bruising without rupture of the pia mater. The contused cord is swollen and may show small haemorrhages. Microscopically, besides oedema and punctate haemorrhage there is swelling of axis cylinders and disintegration of their myelin sheaths. In severe cases both completely disappear and the cord may be markedly softened. Ascending and descending degeneration of the long tracts follows the focal lesion. The structural, vascular, physiological, and biochemical changes which follow experimental cord contusion were reviewed by Dohrmann (1972). In humans acute contusion is often followed by progressive haemorrhagic necrosis or softening, which is at a maximum in the centre of the cord. Cord damage due to acute ischaemia during aortic surgery is also most severe in the central grey matter (Kim *et al.* 1988) and the area of infarction often extends several segments or more below the level of the clinical lesion. Injuries to the thoracic spinal cord are particularly likely to give rise to central necrosis, presumably because there is less potential space within the thoracic spinal canal than at other levels and tissue pressures after injury may therefore be higher. Laceration implies an injury of greater severity than contusion, with rupture of the pia mater and partial or complete transection of the cord. When a wound penetrates the dura mater, meningitis is liable to occur as a complication of spinal injury. Rupture of the pia in such cases increases the risk of pyogenic myelitis. Injuries of the vertebral column may also damage spinal roots and nerves as they pass through the intervertebral foramina.

In addition to the acute pathological changes, patients may show delayed pathological changes: post-traumatic spinal cysts and syrinxes. Barnett *et al.* (1973) and Nurick *et al.* (1970) showed that a progressive myelopathy due to ascending cavitation of the cord above the level of the lesion may develop in some cases of traumatic paraplegia some years after the injury. Until the advent of magnetic resonance imaging (MRI) these complications were thought to affect up to 2 per cent per annum of survivors of acute spinal cord injury, the onset of symptoms being delayed by at least 2 months up to a maximum reported of 36 years, with a mean of 8–9 years. It is now clear that cysts and syrinxes can form without causing detectable new signs or symptoms and the incidence and prevalence of such cysts may thus be far higher in survivors than was previously thought, and their clinical implications correspondingly more benign. In patients who do show late deterioration in symptoms and signs, MRI may identify cysts, myelomalacia, or a syrinx in at least 50 per cent; approximately 10 per cent have additional pathology that had not previously been suspected and the others may show evidence of continuing compression associated with the original injury (Sett and Crockford 1991).

Syrinxes occur most commonly after mid-thoracic cord lesions. The mechanism of their formation is unclear, but MRI scanning has demonstrated that cysts developing in damaged central areas of the cord can progress to a syrinx, and that separate cystic areas (presumably due to ischaemic degeneration) can, over time, coalesce to form a large syrinx. Late extension of the syrinx cavity occurs also after many other forms of spinal-cord damage. It is thought to result from repeated pressure changes in the CSF and in the intraspinal veins, the effects of which are possibly accentuated by restriction of the normal mobility of the cord by adhesions or arachnoiditis.

6.3.3 Symptoms and signs

The neurological assessment of a patient with acute spinal-cord damage may be complicated by coexisting injuries to the head, thorax, abdomen, or limbs. Between 10 and 20 per cent of patients with a spinal injury, especially a cervical spine injury, also have a head injury. Conversely, patients with an injury to the forehead, which is often associated with hyperextension trauma to the cervical spine, must, if unconscious, be assumed also to have a cervical spine injury until X-rays of the entire cervical spine have excluded this. Evidence of local tenderness, bruising, or deformity of any part of the spine should be specifically sought.

Complete interruption of the spinal cord leads immediately to flaccid paralysis with loss of all sensation and most reflex activity below the site of the lesion, and paralysis of the bladder and rectum. Lesions above T7 cause paralytic ileus for approximately 48 hours and mask the classical signs of peritoneal irritation from intra-abdominal injury. Priapism indicates a high spinal-cord lesion.

Cervical lesions paralyse the intercostal muscles and the patient then has to rely for survival on diaphragmatic ventilation. Complete lesions of the cord above C4 usually cause death through paralysis of the diaphragm and hypoxia. In traumatic tetraplegia, the thoracolumbar sympathetic outflow is interrupted and hypotension and bradycardia may occur. The level of the lesion can be deduced from the distribution of impaired power, sensation, and altered reflexes. Within the first 24–48 h of injury the level of the lesion as assessed clinically may rise temporarily by 1–3 segments, probably due to oedema or ischaemia of the cord, or a combination of the two. A patient whose ventilation is initially satisfactory but then deteriorates is likely to regain independent ventilation after this complication resolves, normally within a few days.

Clinically, partial spinal-cord lesions may fall into one of four syndromes. The anterior-cord syndrome is usually caused by a flexion–rotation injury producing an anterior dislocation or compression fracture of the vertebral body and damage in the territory of the anterior spinal artery, affecting corticospinal and spinothalamic tract functions (weakness and loss of pain, temperature, and some touch sensation). The central-cord syndrome is seen in hyperextension of the cervical spine in the presence of anterior compression from cervical spondylosis and in thoracic-cord lesions. In the cervical spine, the corticospinal fibres to the arms are more severely affected than the more laterally placed fibres going to the legs, giving a characteristic pattern of flaccid weakness of the arms with a less pronounced spastic weakness of the legs. The posterior-cord syndrome involves damage principally to the posterior columns (touch and proprioception) and is most common in hyperextension injuries with fractures of the vertebral arch. The Brown-Séquard syndrome, or 'hemitransection', is associated with lateral mass fractures of the vertebrae or stab wounds, and impairs power, light touch, and proprioception on the same side as the lesion, and pinprick and temperature sensation on the opposite side.

Fracture–dislocation of the spine below the first lumbar vertebra damages only the nerves of the cauda equina. In civil life unilateral injuries here are rare, although the severity and extent of the nerve damage may differ on the two sides. Paralysis of the bladder, rectum, and sexual functions follow immediately. The motor, sensory, and reflex disturbances are similar to those produced more gradually by slow compression of the cauda equina.

The diagnosis is usually made on the basis of the above clinical findings supplemented by plain radiographs. These require considerable skill in their interpretation because of the crucial need to stabilize and control the position of the spine until structural instability has been totally excluded. Where possible, X-rays should be taken in the radiology department with a doctor in attendance, rather than by mobile equipment, which usually gives pictures of inferior quality on which lesions may be missed. For cervical injuries, both lateral and antero-posterior radiographs must be taken, including an open-mouth view of the odontoid process. Oblique views with the patient log-rolled from the horizontal help confirm the presence of subluxation or dislocation of the facet joints. For thoracolumbar injuries, antero-posterior and lateral views are taken and may need to be supplemented in the T1–4 region by lateral tomography. MRI scanning, when available without risk to the patient, is helpful in delineating the location and extent of compression and identifying ligamentous damage, root compression, or prolapsed disc material in the spinal canal (Fig. 6.2). Bony abnormalities and loose fragments are better delineated by CT scanning. The clinical efficacy of these two forms of imaging is continually being re-evaluated in the light of technical advances and accumulating clinical experience.

6.3.4 Early management

Specially trained acute recovery services increase survival. They can give appropriate treatment and prevent further cord damage at the scene of the accident by stabilizing the fractured spine and by minimizing hypoxia and arterial hypotension (without causing pulmonary oedema by overperfusing the patient). High-dose intravenous methyprednisolone given within 8 hours of injury (30 mg/kg bolus over 15 minutes, then 5.4 mg/kg/h for 23–48 hours) may reduce long-term losses (Bracken 2000).

Respiration

Respiration should be monitored and maintained. In high cervical-cord lesions, there is an immediate risk of respiratory failure. Respiratory insufficiency is also likely when ribs have been fractured, and can be compounded by abdominal distension secondary to paralytic ileus. In addition, the inability to cough allows secretions to accumulate, and there may be neurogenic ventilation–perfusion mismatch. A vital capacity of 500 ml or less often necessitates endotracheal intubation and ventilation, following the administration of atropine to prevent reflex cardiac arrest. If a muscle relaxant is needed, a non-depolarizing drug must be used, as suxamethonium in acute spinal injury has caused sudden hyperkalaemia leading to cardiac arrest(Grundy et al. 1990). Cardiac arrest may occur as a result of respiratory failure or after lesions above T1, through unopposed vagal stimulation induced by laryngeal suction or intubation.

Thromboembolism

Once the patient is medically and surgically stable, the most frequent cause of death in the next 3 weeks is pulmonary embolism (3–4 per cent), especially in patients over the age of 40 years, whose risk of death in one recent series of 1419 subjects was approximately 14 per cent, compared with a risk to younger patients of 0.4 per cent (Waring and Karunas 1991). Therefore, in the absence of contraindications, anticoagulation with heparin and then by oral anticoagulants should be initiated 24–36 hours after the injury, to prevent deep-vein thrombosis and pulmonary embolism. Graded-support stockings should be worn. Anticoagulation should be continued for 3–6 months unless there are reasons for continuing longer.

Vertebral damage

Patients with cervical fractures should be managed by skeletal traction using 1–2 kg for upper cervical injuries and 3–5 kg for lower cervical fractures without dislocation. Much higher forces may be needed to reduce dislocations. Unstable fractures associated with partial cord lesions may require operative fusion, notably C7–T1 facet dislocations which cannot be reduced by traction. If non-union and atlantoaxial instability persist after immobilization and traction for odontoid fractures, posterior atlantoaxial fusion is necessary. Penetrating injuries may require surgery for débridement or removal of foreign bodies. Most thoracolumbar injuries in most spinal injury units are treated conservatively for 8–12 weeks before mobilization. If the injury is unstable, especially in fractures of the upper cervical spine, which may be associated with a fracture of the sternum, or there is marked deformity, operative reduction with fusion may be performed, with the insertion of Harrington distraction rods and bone grafting. The threshold for deciding upon surgical stabilization is lower in patients with clinical partial cord lesions, because of the further loss of neurological function if instability persists. There continue to be differences of opinion about the indications for surgery in the acute or early phases of recovery, and controlled clinical trials will probably be needed to settle current areas of controversy.

Nutrition

Nutrition of the paraplegic patient is of the utmost importance. The average recommended calorific intake is 3500 kcal per 24 hours, including 125 g of protein and a high vitamin intake. A high calcium intake (for example, milk) should be avoided be cause of the risk of urinary calculi. Absorption from the gut may be impaired, as in other forms of trauma, and a dramatic loss of muscle bulk is unavoidable in complete flaccid paraplegia. There is experimental clinical evidence that extended periods of electrical stimulation of muscles can maintain a significant proportion of muscle bulk (Taylor *et al.* 1993).

Deformities

Deformities due to contractures of muscle and joint capsules must be prevented by careful passive mobilization and positioning, as part of the regular nursing care needed to prevent the development of pressure sores. The latter are always preventable by careful lifting of the patient (avoiding shearing of the skin by dragging it across bedding) and turning to a new position every 2–3 hours. If a red mark appears on the skin which does not fade after 30 minutes, all further pressure on that area must be avoided until all redness and induration disappears.

Bladder and bowels

Two alternative methods of bladder drainage are currently favoured in acute and early phases of recovery, when the bladder is mainly atonic. One is intermittent urethral catheterization with a 12 FG or 14 FG Nelaton catheter every 6 hours, restricting fluid intake to 1500 ml/24 hours. The other is suprapubic catheterization using a 10 or 15 FG catheter, which avoids the risks associated with urethral catheterization and allows a high fluid intake if necessary. As involuntary reflex detrusor activity appears, voiding may be achieved by a combination of suprapubic abdominal stimulation and compression ('tapping and expression') which usually results in a 'trained bladder' 6–12 weeks after the injury. This mechanism may not be necessary for patients with paraplegia who are able to perform intermittent catheterization on themselves. If infection becomes established in the bladder, continuous drainage using a small (12 or 14 FG) urethral catheter with a 5 ml balloon may be used, with weekly or twice-weekly bladder wash-outs, if necessary, to prevent the formation of calculi (Grundy *et al.* 1990). During the period of spinal shock, the bowel must be prevented from overdistension by gentle manual evacuation daily or every other day until, by careful attention to diet and the judicious use of aperients, a satisfactory routine can be established.

Psychological stresses

Psychological stresses and needs of patients recovering from acute spinal injury have been reviewed by Judd and Burrows (1986). Only 50 per cent of patients are initially aware or able to recognize that they are paralysed. Moreover the circumstances of such injuries are usually frightening and may also evoke considerable guilt or anger because of the perception that the injury could have been avoided. Patients experience acute anxiety in relation to their immediate prospects of survival, persisting pain, disorientation due to lack of sleep and an absence of time cues, and a perceived lack of information. The effects of sensory deprivation are accentuated by the enforced immobility of spinal traction and may induce a state of panic.

The patient's ability to cope may be further compromised by other injuries, especially by the effects of concurrent head injury. In a recent series, between 40 and 60 per cent of acutely injured patients showed altered cognitive function, notably a poor attention span, limited initial learning ability, poor concentration and problem-solving ability, and impaired memory (Roth *et al.* 1989). These formidable sources of suffering and obstacles to communication may be accentuated by difficulties in communication between members of the hospital team and the patient, reflecting a mismatch between their respective priorities and objectives (Glass *et al.* 1991). It is essential, therefore, that the psychological state of the patient is carefully assessed and monitored, and that those looking after the patient and liaising with relatives are trained to recognize and deal appropriately with their psychological needs. This is likely to require flexibility in relation to the patient's immediate environment and to ward routines.

The previous personality of the patient predicts to some extent their vulnerability to psychological stress. Those who are male, older, and lacking in formal education, who have passive personality traits, previous dependence on drugs or alcohol, low self-esteem, and little personal ambition are especially at risk from severe psychological stress and depression. That these factors are important to recognize from the outset is illustrated by a series of 423 consecutive patients studied in Los Angeles. During the first 4 years after leaving hospital, 43 per cent of all recorded deaths were due to suicide (Wilcox and Staffer 1972).

6.3.5 Later management

There are some specific long-term problems where the neurologist may be asked for help: the acute management of autonomic dysreflexia, the diagnosis of possible post-traumatic syringomyelia, the management of spasms and spasticity, and the management of chronic neuropathic pain. The neurologist is unlikely to be asked about the long-term management of the bladder, which is in the domain of the urologist, or the long-term management of the bowels, where nursing expertise is most relevant. Pressure sores also require the expertise of other specialists.

Autonomic dysreflexia

Autonomic dysreflexia is an uncontrolled sympathetic reflex response to normally noxious stimuli, such as distension of bladder or bowels, or pain from any lower-body trauma or urinary tract infection. The clinical effects are a rise in blood pressure, a pounding headache, and other symptoms or signs of sympathetic overactivity. The danger arises from the uncontrolled rise in blood pressure and fatalities do occur each year. Autonomic dysreflexia occurs after injury at the level of T6 or above, and most commonly occurs between 3 and 18 months after injury.

Prevention, through avoiding the precipitating causes, is obviously the most important factor, but is not always easy. Pharmacologically, terazosin or phenoxybenzamine may be used prophylactically if the patient is known to suffer the problem and is likely to experience a precipitating event.

The immediate management includes sitting the patient upright and removing or reversing the precipitating cause. However, care must be taken not to increase noxious stimulation in the process. For example, rectal examination to check for faecal impaction might cause or worsen the situation and it is wise to use local anaesthetic when examining the rectum. Control of the hypertension using nifedipine (5–10 mg sublingually) or phentolamine (5–10 mg intravenously) or other drugs such as prazosin or nitrates may be necessary at times. The incidence of autonomic dysreflexia is not known, but most patients are aware of the complication and how to avoid it and how to treat it.

Late deterioration

Patients who show late deterioration in symptoms and signs should be investigated, usually by MRI scan which may identify cysts, myelomalacia, or a syrinx in at least 50 per cent; approximately 10 per cent have additional pathology that had not previously been suspected; and the remainder may show evidence of continuing compression associated with the original injury (Sett and Crockford 1991).

6.3.6 Rehabilitation

Patients with spinal-cord injury should be managed by services with specialist experience and expertise, and the primary role of any neurologist is to ensure rapid transfer in the acute phase, and appropriate referral when patients present with later problems outside the expertise of the neurologist.

The principles are much as in all other areas of rehabilitation. Prevention of known avoidable complications carries the highest priority. Obvious examples include: prevention of pressure sores (decubitus ulcers) through good skin care and regular pressure relief; avoidance of urinary tract infections through good bladder routines; avoidance of constipation; prevention of contracture development though regular mobilization and stretching of joints; and maintaining good mental health and reducing the risk of suicide.

Although one cannot reverse any motor or sensory losses, it is important to maximize the use of residual motor function. This involves both maintenance of strength, where appropriate, and teaching the patient how to use residual motor skills most effectively. In addition, one may use surgical translocation of tendons to increase the function of an arm.

Environmental adaptation is central to spinal injury rehabilitation. This involves provision of a wide range of equipment (e.g. wheelchairs, adapted clothing, special cutlery, hoists, etc.) and ensuring that accommodation is adapted as necessary. The patients will need to be taught how to use all equipment. Furthermore it involves teaching all those involved in providing support and care how to do so.

Effective rehabilitation must also consider both how to minimize any emotional sequelae and how to maximize employment and other social role functions. Both are vital if the patient is to have a good quality of life in the long-term. A sys-

tematic review suggests that benefit does follow from psychosocial interventions (McAweeney *et al.* 1997) such as coping effectiveness training (King and Kennedy 1999). Among other roles that rehabilitation may help is that of becoming a father through providing advice on achieving ejaculation (Beckerman *et al.* 1993).

Finally, patients should learn how to manage their condition. Patients with spinal cord injury usually have well-preserved cognition. Consequently, perhaps the most important single skill they should be taught is that of managing their own illness. They should learn to recognize (diagnose) all likely complications, what investigations might be needed, and what management options there are. They should know how to organize and undertake all preventative care, and where to go for help. This degree of independence can be threatening to some doctors, but its presence is a sign of an effective rehabilitation programme.

6.4 Specific topics

There are many specific topics that may fall within the sphere of neurological rehabilitation: spasticity, behavioural disturbance associated with brain injury; hysterical conversion disorder, etc. Some of these are discussed below.

6.4.1 Spasticity

Spasticity is still 'a neurological demon' with an 'emperor's new therapy' (Landau 1974), although the therapy is now both more expensive and, possibly, more effective. The demonic aspects are getting agreement on, first, the nature or definition of spasticity and, secondly, whether it should be considered primarily an impairment worthy of treatment in its own right or simply a phenomenon associated with upper motor neuron weakness.

In practice one finds that the term 'spasticity' may be used to refer to one or more of:

- any presumed upper motor neuron weakness;
- a pattern of movement seen following central neurological damage;
- associated movements seen when the patient makes an effort;
- involuntary associated movements, for example arm stretching in association with yawning;
- overactive tendon jerks, with or without clonus;
- involuntary flexor or extensor muscle spasms;
- reduced range of passive movement at a joint; and
- stiffness in muscles.

Many neurologists will reject instantly many of these suggestions as being nothing to do with spasticity at all; unfortunately each reader will reject a different set! Therefore when considering spasticity it is important to be as clear as possible about the phenomenon or phenomena being treated. In this section spasticity will refer generally to such phenomena as an increased sensitivity of the stretch reflex, stiffness and slowness in movement, and spasms. At present there is no good evidence to support making direct attempts to control spasticity (or abnormal tone) in the expectation that improved function will follow.

Specific treatment of spasticity should only be undertaken in particular circumstances. The most common is when spasticity or spasms are sufficiently troublesome to cause distress, pain, or undue difficulty in providing care and maintaining range of passive movement at a joint. However, general spasticity in the arms is rarely present when there is also sufficient motor control to envision functional use, and so the use of more general treatment such as baclofen is unlikely ever to improve arm function. In the legs generalized spasticity is as often helpful, allowing the legs to take weight, as it is a hindrance.

There may be occasions when local spasticity is thought to be a significant specific cause of reduced functional ability, and local treatments may be tried. For example, botulinum toxin injection may improve function when spasticity follows focal spinal-cord damage (Richardson *et al.* 1997). Focal spasticity will usually be best treated with intramuscular botulinum toxin, and this may also be associated with functional benefit on mobility after stroke (Burbaud *et al.* 1996). There is no evidence to support routine use of EMG guidance when giving botulinum toxin. Other localized treatments include destruction of nerves using phenol or alcohol injection and cutting of nerves or tendons. There is no evidence to guide one on when, or whether, or how to use such techniques, but in the hands of those expert in their use they may undoubtedly help some patients.

A more recent treatment is intrathecal baclofen, delivered through an implanted pump. Although there is little doubt that this can be effective, the cost–benefit ratio and rates of success and complication have yet to be established (Creedon *et al.* 1997) and its use should be restricted to patients with severe intractable and very troublesome spasticity or spasms of the legs.

In clinical practice, antispastic drugs are most commonly helpful for spasms associated with spinal cord damage or disease, and sometimes for more general spasticity, making it difficult to maintain a range of movement. The useful drugs include baclofen, tizanidine, dantrolene, clonazepam, and diazepam. With all drugs it is vital to start with a low dose and to increase slowly (at weekly intervals) according to response. It may be useful to use two drugs together at times. Other methods of controlling spasticity, especially when more generalized, include reduction of any noxious stimulation and pain, regular (once or twice daily) stretching of joints, well-adjusted positioning in (wheel)chairs, and sometimes the use of ice, TENS machines, etc.

6.4.2 Abnormal illness behaviour; disability without disease

Neurologists will be referred many disabled patients bearing a neurological diagnosis attached to them but who, in fact, have abnormal illness behaviour or non-organic disability (Sections 1.9 and 26.10). In some cases this neurological diagnosis will be attributed to the patient by the referring doctor. In some cases it will be the patient, or the patient's family, who have attached the neurological label. In a significant proportion of cases the neurologist will discover that the patient either does not have any neurological disease at all, or that the patient has an alternative neurological disease, or that the disability is not accounted for by the known neurological disease.

This is a common problem. Experience of unselected patients referred to or attending a Young Disabled Unit suggests that 5–10 per cent of all patients referred have disability that has no basis in 'organic disease'. Misdiagnosis is common (Teasell and Shapiro 1997), but is important to recognize this situation as soon as possible in an attempt to manage it successfully. Some neurologists will wish to take on the management for themselves. In some areas referral is most appropriately made to an interested psychiatrist. In many areas it is appropriate to refer such patients on to the specialist neurological disability service, provided they have an interest and suitable expertise.

The management of patients presenting with disability that is not due to any known neurological disease, or that is grossly exaggerated in relation to the known neurological disease, is extremely difficult. The usual approach is to adopt a functional, behavioural treatment programme (Shapiro and Teasell 1997). In other words, one chooses to state that although there is no pathology, the impairments are like those seen with stroke, multiple sclerosis, or whatever, and that a similar therapeutic treatment will be used. This may work sometimes, but it may also fail.

One newly described approach uses a 'double-bind' that capitalizes on the patient's prejudice against psychological explanations (Shapiro and Teasell 1997). In essence the patient and family are told that a vigorous treatment programme should allow them to regain completely full normal function without any risk of later relapse or of developing other symptoms, and they are also told that failure of this programme proves that they need to see a psychiatrist as their illness must then have a psychological basis. This approach allows them to recover with good justification ('the treatment got me better') without challenging them about the cause. It should prevent them from simply manifesting with other impairments and disabilities. It utilizes the family in the same way. However, it does not address the issue of the putative mechanism (i.e. the psychological causes) and it may reinforce their stigmatizing view of psychological illness. None the less dramatic results have been reported in one uncontrolled but convincing study (Shapiro and Teasell 1997).

Other treatments may work. If one assumes that this form of illness is similar to many other types of non-organic illness (Wessely *et al.* 1999) then one may draw on the evidence relating to somatization disorder (Wade 2001). This evidence suggests that treatment with amitriptyline and other antidepressants often helps, and that cognitive behavioural therapy may help.

However, at present the most important aspects of managing these patients are, first, to recognize as soon as possible that there is no specific neurological pathology present and then to limit the inappropriate and potentially risky use of further investigative or treatment interventions, and, thirdly, to minimize the inappropriate use of scarce rehabilitation therapy resources and support resources. This must be done in a non-judgemental, non-punitive way, and must acknowledge that such patients may have needs for physical or other support that must be met.

References

Allen, K. and Blascovitch, J. (1996). The value of service dogs for people with severe ambulatory disabilities. A randomised controlled trial. *JAMA*, **275**, 1001–6.

Averbuch-Heller, L., Tusa, R. J., Fuhry, L. *et al.* (1997). A double-blind controlled study of gabapentin and baclofen as treatment for acquired nystagmus. Ann. Neurol., **41**, 818–25.

Badley, E. M. (1993). An introduction to the concepts and classifications of the International Classification of Impairments, Disabilities and Handicaps. *Disabil. Rehabil.*, **15**, 161–78.

Barnett, H. J. M., Foster, J. B., and Hudgson, P. (1973). In *Syringomyelia*, (ed. J. N. Walton). Major Problems in Neurology Series. Saunders, London.

Beckerman, H., Becher, J., and Lankhorst, G. J. (1993). The effectiveness of vibratory stimulation in anejaculatory men with spinal cord injury: review article. *Paraplegia*, **31**, 689–99.

Bracken, M. B. (2000). *Pharmacological interventions for acute spinal cord injury*. Cochrane Collaboration review; Update Publications, issue 1.

Brown, R. I. and Hughson, E. A. (1993). *Behavioural and social rehabilitation and training*, (2nd edn). Captus Press, Toronto; Chapman & Hall, London.

Burbaud, P., Wiart, L., Dubos, J. L. *et al.* (1996). A randomised, double-blind, placebo-controlled trial of botulinum toxin in the treatment of spastic foot in hemiparetic patients. *J. Neurol. Neurosurg. Psychiat.*, **61**, 265–9.

Cardol, M., Brandsma, J. W., de Groot, I. J. M. *et al.* (1999*a*). Handicap questionnaires: what do they assess? *Disabil. Rehabil.*, **21**, 97–105.

Cardol, M., de Haan, R. J., van den Bos, G. A. M. *et al.* (1999*b*). The development of a handicap assessment questionnaire: the Impact on Participation and Autonomy (IPA). *Clin. Rehabil.*, **13**, 411–19.

Carson, A. J., Ringbauer, B., Stone, J. *et al.* (2000). Do medically unexplained symptoms matter? A prospective cohort study of 300 new referrals to neurology outpatient clinics. *J. Neurol. Neurosurg. Psychiat.*, **68**, 207–10.

Collen, F. M., Wade, D. T., and Bradshaw, C. M. (1990). Mobility after stroke: reliability of measures of impairment and disability. *Internat. Disabil. Studies*, **12**, 6–9.

Collin, C., Wade, D. T., Davis, S. *et al.* (1988). The Barthel ADL Index: a reliability study. *Internat. Disabil. Studies*, **10**, 61–3.

Creedon, S. D., Dijkers, M. P., and Hinderer, S. R. (1997). Intra-thecal baclofen for severe spasticity: a meta-analysis. *Internat. J. Rehabil. Hlth*, **3**, 171–85.

Cunningham, C., Horgan, F., Keane, N. *et al.* (1996). Detection of disability by different members of an interdisciplinary team. *Clin. Rehabil.*, **10**, 247–54.

Cunningham, C., Horgan, F., and O'Neill, D. (2000). Clinical assessment of rehabilitation potential of the older patient: a pilot study. *Clin. Rehabil.*, **14**, 205–7.

Dam, M., Tonin, P., De Boni, A. *et al.* (1996). Effects of fluoxetine and maprotiline on functional recovery in post-stroke hemiplegic patients undergoing rehabilitation therapy. *Stroke*, **27**, 1211–14.

De Vivo, M. J., Kartus, P. L., Stover, S. L. *et al.* (1990). Benefits of early admission to an organized spinal cord injury care system. *Paraplegia*, **28**, 545–55.

Di Fabio, R. P., Soderberg, J., Choi, T. *et al.* (1998). Extended outpatient rehabilitation: its influence on symptom frequency, fatigue, and functional status for persons with progressive multiple sclerosis. *Arch. Phys. Med. Rehabil.*, **79**, 141–6.

Dohrmann, G. J. (1972). Experimental spinal cord trauma. *Arch. Neurol.*, **27**, 468–73.

Ekdawi, M. Y. and Conning, A. M. (1994). Guiding models and philosophies. In Psychiatric rehabilitation. a practical guide, (eds M. Y. Ekdawi and A. M. Conning), Ch. 2, pp. 16–35. Chapman & Hall, London.

Forlander, D. A. and Bohannon, R. W. (1999). Rivermead Mobility Index: a brief review of research to date. *Clin. Rehabil.*, **13**, 97–100.

Freeman, J. A., Langdon, D. W., Hobart, J. C. *et al.* (1999). The impact of inpatient rehabilitation on progressive multiple sclerosis. *Ann. Neurol.*, **42**, 236–44.

Glass, C. A., Krishnan, K. R., and Bingley, J. D. (1991). Spinal injury rehabilitation. Do staff and patients agree on what they are talking about? *Paraplegia*, **29**, 343–9.

Goldstein, L. B. (1995). Common drugs may influence motor recovery after stroke. The Sygen In Acute Stroke Study Investigators. *Neurology*, **45**, 865–71.

Grundy, D., Russell, J., and Swain, A. (1990). *ABC of spinal cord injury*. British Medical Journal, London

Halligan, P. W., Bass, C., and Wade, D. T. (2000). Conversion hysteria: an illness in search of a disease. *BMJ*, **320**, 1488–9.

Heller, A., Wade, D. T., Wood, V. A. *et al.* (1987). Arm function after stroke: measurement and recovery over the first three months. *J. Neurol. Neurosurg. Psychiat.*, **50**, 714–19.

Herndon, R. M. (1997). *Handbook of neurologic rating scales.* Demos Vermande, New York

Indredavik, B., Bakke, F., Slordahl, S. A. *et al.* (1998). Stroke unit treatment improves long-term quality of life. A randomised controlled trial. *Stroke,* **29**, 895–9.

Inter-collegiate Working Party for Stroke (2000). *National clinical guidelines for stroke.* Clinical Effectiveness and Evaluation Unit, Royal College of Physicians, London.

Judd, F. K. and Burrows, G. D. (1986). Liaison psychiatry in a spinal injuries unit. *Paraplegia,* **24**, 6–19.

Kalra, L. P. I., Gupta, S., and Wittink, M. (1997). The influence of visual neglect on stroke rehabilitation. *Stroke,* **28**, 1386–91.

Kessler, J. T. (1975). Congenital narrowing of the cervical spinal canal. *J. Neurol. Neurosurg. Psychiat.,* **38**, 1218–24.

Kim, S. W., Kim, R. C., Choi, B. H. *et al.* (1988). Non- traumatic ischaemia myelopathy: a review of 25 cases. *Paraplegia,* **26**, 262–72.

King, C. and Kennedy, P. (1999). Coping effectiveness training for people with spinal cord injury: preliminary results of a controlled trial. *Br. J. Clin. Psychol.,* **38**, 5–14.

Kraus, J. F. (1985). Epidemiological aspects of acute spinal cord injury: a review of incidence, prevalence, causes and outcome. In *Central nervous system trauma status report 1985,* (ed. D. P. Becker and J. T. Povlishcock), p. 313. National Institute of Health, Bethesda, Maryland.

Krupp, L. B., Coyle, P. K., Doscher, C. *et al.* (1995). Fatigue therapy in multiple sclerosis: results of a double-blind, randomised, parallel trial of amantadine, pemoline, and placebo. *Neurology,* **45**, 1956–63.

Kurtzke, J. F. (1975). Epidemiology of spinal cord injury. *Exp. Neurol.,* **48**, 163–236.

Kwakkel, G., Wagenaar, R. C., Koelman, T. W. *et al.* (1997). Effects of intensity of rehabilitation after stroke. A research synthesis. *Stroke,* **28**, 1550–6.

Kwakkel, G., Wagenaar, R. C., Twisk, J. W. R. *et al.* (1999). Intensity of leg and arm training after primary middle-cerebral-artery stroke: a randomised trial. *Lancet,* **354**, 191–6.

Landau, W. M. (1974). Spasticity: the fable of a neurological demon and the emperor's new therapy. *Ann. Neurol.,* **31**, 28–33.

Lew, M. F., Adornato, B. T., Duane, D. D. *et al.* (1997). Botulinum toxin type B: a double-blind, placebo-controlled, safety and efficacy study in cervical dystonia. *Neurology,* **49**, 701–7.

Lin, K., Wu, C., Tickle-Degnen, L., and Coster, W. (1997). Enhancing occupational performance through occupationally embedded exercise: a meta-analytic review. *Occupat. Ther. J. Res.,* **17**, 25–47.

Lord, J. P. and Hall, K. (1986). Neuromuscular re-education versus traditional programs for stroke rehabilitation. *Arch. Phys. Med. Rehabil.,* **67**, 88–91.

Lord, S. E., Wade, D. T., and Halligan, P. W. (1998). A comparison of two physiotherapy treatment approaches to improve walking in multiple sclerosis: a pilot randomised controlled trial. *Clin. Rehabil.,* **12**, 477–86.

Mann, W. C., Ottenbacher, K. J., Fraas, L. *et al.* (1999). Effectiveness of assistive technology and environmental interventions in maintaining independence and reducing home care costs for the elderly. *Arch. Family Med.,* **8**, 210–17.

Mant, J., Carter, J., Wade, D. T. *et al.* (1998). The impact of an information pack on patients with stroke and their carers: a randomised controlled trial. *Clin. Rehabil.,* **12**, 465–76.

McAweeney, M. J., Tate, D. G., and McAweeney, W. (1997). Psychosocial interventions in the rehabilitation of people with spinal cord injury: a comprehensive methodological inquiry. *Spinal Cord Injury Psychosoc. Process,* **10**, 58–66.

Miyai, I. and Reding, M. J. (1998). Effects of anti-depressants on functional recovery following stroke. A double-blind study. *J. Neurol. Rehabil.,* **12**, 5–13

Montgomery, E. B., Lieberman, A., Singh, G. *et al.* (1999). Patient education and health promotion can be effective in Parkinson's disease: a randomised controlled trial. PROPATH Advisory Board. *Am. J. Med.,* **97**, 429–35.

Nurick, S., Russell, J. A., and Deck, M. J. F. (1970). Cystic degeneration of the spinal cord following spinal cord injury. *Brain,* **93**, 211–22.

Post, M. W. M., de Witte, L. P., and Schrijvers, A. J. P. (1999). Quality of life and the ICIDH: towards an integrated conceptual model for rehabilitation outcomes research. *Clin. Rehabil.,* **13**, 5–15.

Powell, J. H., al-Adawi, S., Morgan, J. *et al.* (1996). Motivational deficits after brain injury: effects of bromocriptine in 11 patients. *J. Neurol. Neurosurg. Psychiat.,* **60**, 416–21.

Richards, C. L., Malouin, F., Wood-Dauphinee, S. *et al.* (1993). Task-specific physical therapy for optimisation of gait recovery in acute stroke patients. *Arch. Phys. Med. Rehabil.,* **74**, 612–20.

Richardson, D., Edwards, S., Sheean, G. L. *et al.* (1997). The effect of botulinum toxin on hand function after incomplete spinal cord injury at C5/6: a case report. *Clin. Rehabil.,* **11**, 288–92.

Rockwood, K., Joyce, B., and Stolee, P. (1997). Use of goal attainment scaling in measuring clinically important change in cognitive rehabilitation patients. *J. Clin. Epidemiol.,* **50**, 581–8.

Roth, E., Davidoff, G., Thomas, P. *et al.* (1989). A controlled study of neuropsychological deficits in acute spinal cord injury patients. *Paraplegia,* **27**, 480–9.

Rudd, A. G., Irwin, P., Rutledge, Z. *et al.* (1999). The national sentinel audit of stroke: a tool for raising standards of care. *J. Roy. Coll. Phys.*, **33**, 460–4.

Sett, M. S. and Crockford, H. A. (1991). The value of magnetic resonance imaging (MRI) in the follow-up management of spinal injury. *Paraplegia*, **29**, 396.

Shapiro, A. P. and Teasell, R. W. (1997). Strategic–behavioural intervention in the inpatient rehabilitation of non-organic (factitious/conversion) motor disorders. *Neuro Rehabilitation*, **8**, 183–92.

Stroke Unit Trialist's Collaboration (1997). Collaborative systematic review of the randomised trial of organised inpatient (stroke unit) care after stroke. *BMJ*, **314**, 1151–9.

Stroke Unit Trialists' Collaboration (1998). Organised inpatient (stroke unit) care for stroke (Cochrane Review). In *The Cochrane Library*, Issue 1.

Taylor, P. N., Ewins, D. J., Fox, B. *et al.* (1993). Limb blood flow, cardiac output and quadriceps muscle bulk following spinal cord injury and the effect of training for the Odstock Functional Electrical Stimulation Standing System. *Paraplegia*, **31**, 303–10.

Teasell, R. W. and Shapiro, A. P. (1997). Diagnosis of conversion disorders in a rehabilitation setting. *NeuroRehabilitation*, **8**, 163–74.

Umbach, I. and Heilporn, A. (1991). Post spinal cord injury syringomyelia. *Paraplegia*, **29**, 219–21.

Vaney, C., Blaurock, H., Gatter, B. *et al.* (1996). Assessing mobility in multiple sclerosis using the Rivermead Mobility Index and gait speed. *Clin. Rehabil.*, **10**, 216–26.

Visintin, M., Barbeau, H., Korner-Bitensky, N. *et al.* (1998). A new approach to retrain gait in stroke patients through body weight support and treadmill stimulation. *Stroke*, **29**, 1122–8.

Wade, D. T. (1992). *Measurement in neurological rehabilitation.* Oxford University Press, Oxford.

Wade, D. T. (1996). Epidemiology of disabling neurological disease: how and why does disability occur? *J. Neurol. Neurosurg. Psychiat.*, **61**, 242–9.

Wade, D. T. (1997). Services for patients with multiple sclerosis. *J. Neurol. Neurosurg. Psychiat.*, **63**, 275–8.

Wade, D. T. (1998*a*). Evidence relating to goal planning in rehabilitation. *Clin. Rehabil.*, **12**, 273–5.

Wade, D. T. (1998*b*). Evidence relating to assessment in rehabilitation. *Clin. Rehabil.*, **12**, 183–6.

Wade, D. T. (1998*c*). A framework for considering rehabilitation interventions. *Clin. Rehabil.*, **12**, 363–8.

Wade, D. T. (1999*a*). Goal planning in stroke rehabilitation: evidence. *Topics Stroke Rehabil.*, **6**(2), 37–42.

Wade, D. T. (1999*b*). Goal planning in stroke rehabilitation: why? *Topics Stroke Rehabil.*, **6**(2), 1–7.

Wade, D. T. (1999*c*). Goal planning in stroke rehabilitation: what? *Topics Stroke Rehabil.*, **6**(2), 8–15.

Wade, D. T. (1999*d*). Goal planning in stroke rehabilitation: how? *Topics Stroke Rehabil.*, **6**(2), 16–36.

Wade, D. T. (2001). Rehabilitation for hysterical conversion states: A critical review and conceptual reconstruction. In (ed. P. Halligan and C. Bass). Oxford University Press, Oxford.

Wade, D. T. and De Jong, B. A. (2000). Recent advances in rehabilitation. *BMJ*, **320**, 1385–8.

Wade, D. T., King, N. S., Wenden, F. J. *et al.* (1998). Routine follow-up after head injury: a second randomised controlled trial. *J. Neurol. Neurosurg. Psychiat.*, **65**, 177–83.

Walker-Batson, D., Smith, P., Curtis, S. *et al.* (1995). Amphetamine paired with physical therapy accelerates motor recovery after stroke. Further evidence. *Stroke*, **26**, 2254–9.

Waring, W. P. and Karunas, R. S. (1991). Acute spinal cord injuries and the incidence of clinically occurring thromboembolic disease. *Paraplegia*, **29**, 8–16.

Wessely, S., Nimnuan, C., and Sharpe, M. (1999). Functional somatic syndromes: one or many? *Lancet*, **354**, 936–9.

WHO (1999). *ICIDH-2: International Classification of Functioning and Disability.* Beta-2 draft. World Health Organisation, Geneva.

Wilcox, N. E. and Stauffer, E. S. (1972). Follow-up of 423 consecutive patients admitted to the spinal cord centre, Rancho Los Angeles Hospital, 1 January to 31 December 1967. *Paraplegia*, **10**, 115–22.

Wood, P. (1980). *International classification of impairments, disabilities and handicaps: a manual of classification relating to the consequences of disease.* World Health Organization, Geneva.

CHAPTER 7

Development, degeneration, and regeneration of the central nervous system: neuroimmunology

Alastair Compston

7.1 Development of the nervous system

The evolution of nervous systems allowed primitive organisms to respond to their environment. The need to sense external threat was met by the reflex withdrawal response. Then it became expedient to explore the external environment through the development of goal-directed activities. Nervous systems began to control some aspects of the internal environment, contributing to homeostasis. With time, protective and discriminative sensation, the special senses, movement and co-ordination underpinned the development of new motor and cognitive behaviours, which further enhanced interaction of the individual with its physical and social environment. At the organizational level, these abilities depend on neurons connected to their neighbours by axons and with dendritic arborizations extending the local range of connections. This is the cell doctrine formulated by Ramon y Cajal in the 1890s. Order is achieved by grouping neurons into defined structures or nuclei, and by arranging their axonal projections into bundles which reach a specific set of preferred targets through anatomically coherent pathways. These neuronal systems may subserve local circuits or constitute the major highways and byways of the central nervous system and spinal cord. In turn, several systems can interact in determining a particular function. For example, in order to achieve tasks such as reaching or walking, motor control requires the integration of frontal and prefrontal cortex, descending corticospinal pathways, the additional influence of closed loops constituting the extrapyramidal and cerebellar systems, vestibulospinal influences on muscle tone, and feedback from sensory circuits. Even now, some aspects of where the main planning and assessment of movement are regulated remain unclear.

Communication between interconnected axons and dendrites occurs across synapses, propagation of the nerve impulse releasing chemical transmitters which depolarize receptors on the postsynaptic membrane. Different chemicals are involved in the separate systems but with some sharing within the broad categories of facilitatory and inhibitory transmission. However, the strengthening of preferred anatomical connections and the selective deployment of individual neurotransmitters at their synapses create additional specificity and give rise to the major chemically defined systems. Thus, for example, we think of that system within the basal ganglia which facilitates the planning and regulation of movement as dopaminergic (although the nerve fibres using dopamine actually inhibit inhibitory interneurons); and the hippocampal circuits involved in memory are cholinergic.

This chemical activity occurs at synapses. It is adaptable and forms the basis for plasticity in the central nervous system. The presynaptic membrane has vesicles which contain the locally active neurotransmitter. This is released in response to the nerve impulse and controlled by calcium influx. It drifts across the synapse, binds to receptors on the postsynaptic membrane, causing direct or indirect opening or closure of ion channels, mediated through G proteins and second messengers systems, with effects on conductance of the postsynaptic membrane. Ion channels gate the entry, in either direction, of sodium, potassium, calcium, and chloride, producing local current. The main excitatory neurotransmitter is glutamate, whereas glycine and γ-aminobutyric acid (GABA) are inhibitory. Small molecular weight transmitters include acetylcholine, catecholamines, and many neuroactive peptides. The intracellular signals used in indirect activity of ion channels are cyclic adenosine monophosphate (cAMP), inositol phosphates, arachidonic acid metabolites, and protein kinases. It is the binding by neurotransmitters or peptides to postsynaptic receptors and their effect on ion channels which leads either to propagation of a facilitatory or inhibitory nerve impulse.

Not all synapses deploy chemical transmission. Some are entirely electric. In order to maintain close contact between the pre- and postsynaptic surfaces, there is a need to prevent the intrusion of glial processes into the electrically and chemically active gap junctions. This turns out to be one further contribution of inhibitory molecules (in this instance, laminin 11) expressed on cell surfaces and extracellular matrix (Patton *et al.* 1998).

Specificity within systems is therefore an integral of focal activation in nuclei or co-ordinated regions; simultaneous conduction of the nerve impulse down anatomical pathways; a transient shift in neurotransmission at nerve endings, leading to the activation of receptors; the opening of ion channels which propagate continuation of the facilitatory or inhibitory nerve impulse; and simultaneous orchestration of many interrelated circuits.

Additional structure and function are provided by glial cells (Fig. 7.1). In their different ways, macroglia (oligodendrocytes and astrocytes) and microglia contribute to the cellular archi-

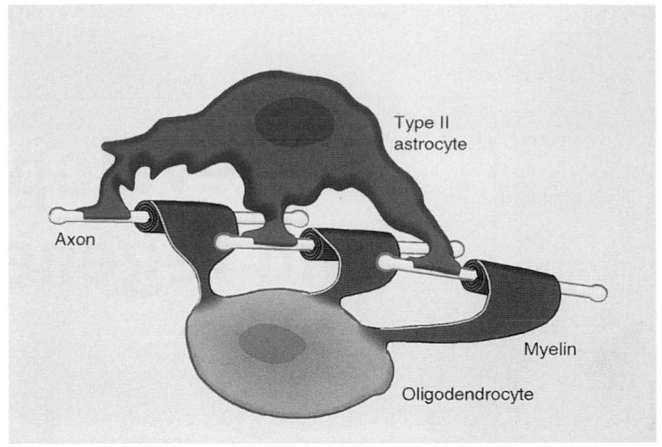

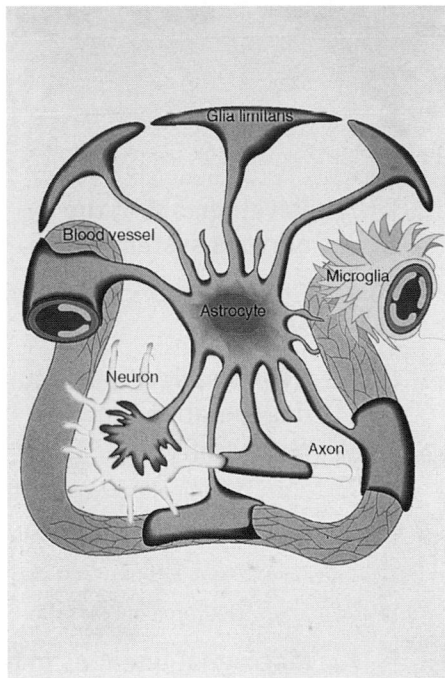

Fig. 7.1. (a) The cellular architecture of myelinated axons. (b) The functions of astrocytes in the central nervous system. (Reproduced with permission from Compston 1998.) Also shown in colour in Plate 2.

tecture of the central and peripheral nervous systems. Oligodendrocytes synthesize and maintain the myelin sheath which extensively coats nerve fibres in white matter and achieves saltatory conduction. These are terminally differentiated cells with a limited response to injury and they depend on the availability of precursors for renewal. Astrocytes provide an architecture for neurons and define anatomical boundaries; they act as a source of growth factors and cytokines, assume a physiological role in conduction of the nerve impulse, and participate in the response to injury. Microglia are bone-marrow-derived cells of the macrophage lineage, which provide the nervous system with a degree of immunological competence. Astrocytes and microglia are each highly reactive cells which orchestrate the response to injury but they play an ambiguous role in health and disease, contributing to tissue injury and scar formation, respectively.

Development in the central nervous system begins when embryonic mesoderm induces the overlying dorsal midline ectoderm to form neuroectodermal cells of the neural plate. This becomes invaginated along its length to form the neural groove, the lips of which eventually fuse so that neuroepithelial cells comprising the neuroectoderm form a neural tube surrounding what will become the ventricle. Neuroepithelial cells lining the ventricle rapidly proliferate and cells migrate along the neural tube from this layer to form a specialized subventricular zone where further division continues. These precursors lose their bipotentiality and develop into cells committed either to the neuronal or glial lineages. At first, most cells in the subventricular zone are neuronal and have a low rate of division, whereas the glial lineage has a greater capacity for mitosis and fewer cells are found in the germinal zones. In terms of lineage commitment, it is instructive that neuronal progenitors identified in one region of the developing nervous system acquire different phenotypes, which may not even be neuronal,

depending on the location in which they are allowed to mature (Suhonen *et al.* 1996). This emphasizes the role of growth factors and other environmental conditions in orchestrating the timing and specificity of maturation in the central nervous system (Fig. 7.2).

The long-held belief that the adult mammalian brain is incapable of neurogenesis is under revision. The source of adult neural stem cells is subventricular zone ependymal cells. These generate neurons and glia in response either to growth factors or tissue injury (Johansson *et al.* 1999). Others consider that subventricular zone cells of the astrocyte lineage are the source of neural stem cells (Doetsch *et al.* 1999).

An essential feature of stem cells is proliferation. In marmosets, proliferation is seen in the hippocampus under conditions which suggest that this is a local response of neurons (Gould *et al.* 1998) rather than just the export of cells from a pre-existing precursor depot to deprived areas of the damaged adult central nervous system. The imaginative use of brain tissue removed as part of surgical treatment for epilepsy has resolved the issue of whether stem cells are present in the adult human nervous system. Adult human subventricular zone cells and occasional cortical cells express precursor markers. These are committed to a neuronal fate and show proliferation, prolonged survival, and enhanced neurite outgrowth in response to FGF-2 (basic fibroblast growth factor) and brain-derived nerve growth factor (BDNF; Pincus *et al.* 1998). Patients given bromodeoxyuridine (BrdU) to assess mitotic activity in primary tumours outside the central nervous system, and studied at autopsy up to 2 years later, have proliferating neurons in the hippocampus (Eriksson *et al.* 1998). Most recently, embryonic stem cells which are totally unrestricted and can, in theory, be driven to any cell-specific fate have been described in the adult (Thompson *et al.* 1998).

The need to select survivors from cells overproduced in the developing nervous system involves apoptotic programmed cell death. Survival is probable for cells which receive adequate amounts of trophic factors. The lack of a positive signal provided by neighbouring cells is seen as the most likely mechanism of programmed cell death. Apoptosis differs from necrosis in that the cell contents are contained and do not elicit a local inflammatory response, the debris being removed by microglia. It is a feature both of development and pathological processes (for review, see Raff 1998). Programmed cell death makes it safe to retain a source of mitotic precursors in the mature nervous system, while avoiding uncontrolled growth. This is a more efficient way of allowing cellular plasticity than suppressing the ability to generate new cells. Work in invertebrates has characterized the *ced-3* and *ced-4* genes in *Caenorhabditis elegans* which programme for cell death, and *ced-9* which regulates these suicide genes. *Ced-3* encodes an interleukin-1-converting enzyme, closely related to several caspases present in humans. They cleave proteins supporting the nuclear membrane and cause apoptosis by activation of the endonuclease which digests DNA. Anti-apoptotic molecules which protect cells from programmed cell death include the mammalian mitochondrial

neocortex
Human CNS stem cells transplanted into the neonatal rat brain

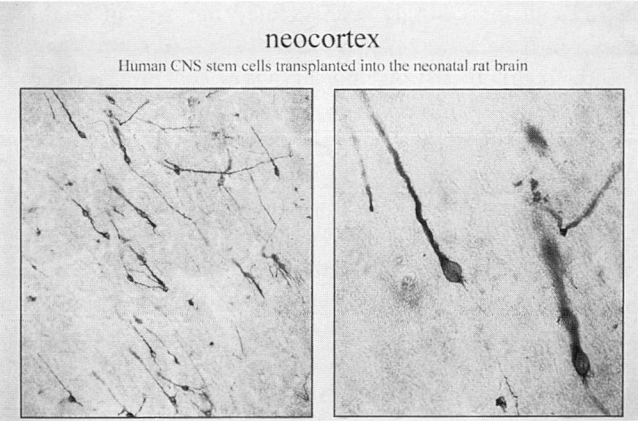

Striatum
Human CNS stem cells transplanted into the neonatal rat brain

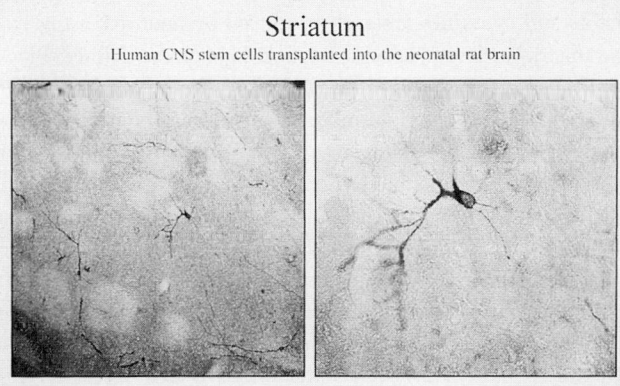

Fig. 7.2. (a) Morphological features of cortical neurons, shown by human neurosphere cells implanted into the neocortex. (b) Morphological features of striatal neurons, shown by identical human neurosphere cells implanted into the striatum. (Kindly provided by Dr Anne Rosser.) Also shown in colour in Plate 3.

product Bcl-2, whose homologue is encoded by *ced-9* in the worm. The Bcl-2 family includes several anti-apoptotic (Bcl-X) and pro-apoptotic molecules (Bax, Bad, and Bid).

7.2 Growth factors for neurons and glia

Acting together or in sequence, growth factors orchestrate development within the nervous system, influencing proliferation, migration, and differentiation. Many also support survival of fully differentiated cells. More is known concerning nerve than glial growth factors, but several have actions both on neurons and glia (Fig. 7.3). Some show autocrine or paracrine effects and cytokines also possess trophic activity.

Neural stem cells proliferate in response to epidermal growth factor (EGF) and when this is withdrawn they differentiate into neurons, astrocytes, and oligodendrocytes. A multipotent EGF-responsive neural stem cell can be isolated from the adult mammalian central nervous system (Reynolds and Weiss 1992). EGF and FGF-2 act sequentially in regulating neuronal development from stem cells. Glial cell-line-derived nerve growth factor (GDNF) induces a bias towards glial differentiation within cultured neural crest cells (Shah *et al.* 1994) but there may also be a role for FGF-2 in steering the development of stem cells in a glial direction (Qian *et al.* 1997). Some of these findings based

on mammalian neurobiology are now being validated in humans. Embryonic neurospheres can be expanded with EGF. Their default pathway for differentiation is GABA-ergic neurons, but they can be directed towards dopaminergic and non-neuronal fates (Rosser *et al.* 1997). Human neurospheres initially expanded with FGF-2 and then allowed to differentiate increase their yield of oligodendrocytes when stimulated with Tri-iodothyronine (Murray and Dubois Dalcq 1997).

Factors which regulate growth and survival of neurons include nerve growth factor (NGF), BDNF, neurotrophin (NT)-3, NT-4/5, GDNF, FGF-1 and FGF-2, and ciliary neurotrophic factor (CNTF). Each preferentially (but not exclusively) supports one (or more) functional or anatomical neuronal systems. Thus (for example), NGF, BDNF, and NT-3 are growth and survival factors for some sensory neurons; but NGF and BDNF also support cholinergic neurons. Conversely, GDNF has potent actions both on dopaminergic and motor neurons. In the visual system, NT-4 can rescue neurons in the lateral geniculate body, which do not otherwise survive experimental deprivation of vision in one eye; and BDNF increases the dendritic arborization of optic axons developing *in vivo* from retinal ganglion cells. This list of system-specific neuronal and growth factor dependence is not encyclopaedic and merely illustrates an increasingly sophisticated network of relationships.

Growth, differentiation, and survival of glial progenitors and their progeny are influenced by GDNF, FGF-2, platelet-derived growth factor (PDGF), insulin-like growth factors (IGF-1 and 2), NGF, NT-3, CNTF, retinoic acid, glial growth factors (GGFs), interleukin (IL)-6, and leukaemia inhibitory factor (LIF). GGF promotes the development of Schwann cells in the peripheral nervous system, as does a newly described mitogen, Reg-2, produced by axons and regulated by local production of LIF and CNTF; it is associated with enhanced regeneration, providing further evidence for the link between growth promotion and Schwann cells (Livesey *et al.* 1997).

Given the complex network of cell–cell interactions operating during development, it is logical that many of these growth factors and cytokines are each produced by neurons, astrocytes, and microglia. Several specific relationships can be defined. PDGF is mitogenic for oligodendrocyte progenitors but they differentiate after a defined number of divisions; however, FGF-2 indefinitely suspends their maturation and promotes migration. EGF, NT-3, thyroxine and Tri-iodothyronine, retinoic acid, and glucocorticoids each also stimulate oligodendrocyte progenitor differentiation and maturation *in vitro* (Barres *et al.* 1994). A neuronal factor which is mitogenic for oligodendrocyte progenitors but not cells that have acquired the early oligodendrocyte differentiation marker, O4, or those that are fully committed to astrocyte differentiation, has been characterized as GGF-2 (Canoll *et al.* 1996). Survival factors for the oligodendrocyte lineage include IGF-1 and -2, LIF, IL-6, and NT-3, as well as PDGF and CNTF (Barres *et al.* 1992). Several astrocyte-derived molecules which have yet to be characterized also exert proliferative and survival effects on cells of the oligodendrocyte lineage.

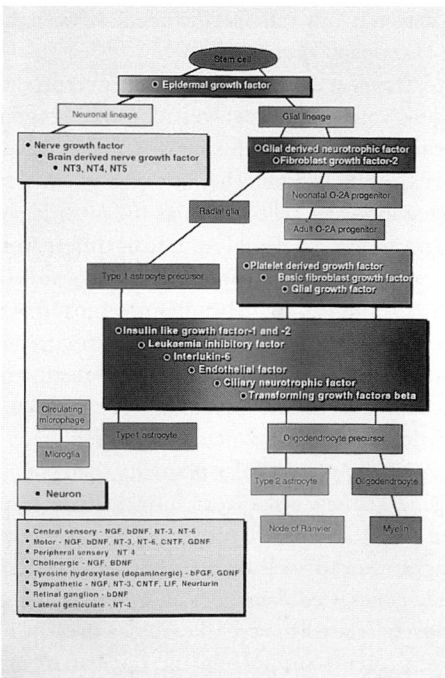

Fig. 7.3. Growth factors which influence proliferation, migration, differentiation, or survival of neurons and glia are shown; most have effects on more than one cell type. Also shown in colour in Plate 4.

7.3 Neuronal development, degeneration, and regeneration

7.3.1 Neuronal development

Neurons develop from the most anterior vesicle of the neural tube and cells destined for the cortex migrate along radial glia, forming columns. To some extent there is significant topographical and lineage scatter, reflecting developmental plasticity provided by local environmental factors, including afferent activity on neurons in the developing cortex. Elongation of axons occurs through the extension of growth cones which form connections with targets at remote sites in the developing brain. Pathfinding proceeds in fits and starts; growth cones stall and the developing axon retracts in association with calcium transients within the developing neurite (Gomez and Spitzer 1999). The awkward path which many axons take indicates that additional guidance is provided *en route*; subplate cells provide signposts for growing axons by switching their orientations, especially at points where bundles of axons are converging; thus developing commissural neurons of the spinal cord are attracted by netrin, receive a survival signal from as yet unidentified factors produced midway as they reach the floor plate, and are then guided home by neurotrophin (Wang and Tessier-Lavigne 1999). Axons appear to grow along pre-formed scaffolds formed by reciprocally innervating afferent and efferent pathways going to and from the same brain regions; and although many growth cones use guidance channels vacated by their predecessors, it remains uncertain how pioneer axons find their targets. Boundaries and orientations seem to be established by regional variation in the expression of genes which govern cell-surface adhesion and repulsion molecules (for example, the *Derailed* receptor tyrosine kinase; Bonkowsky *et al.* 1999), and by regulating molecules which determine cell differentiation schedules. Alterations in the local environment and contact-mediated inhibition induce stop signals, terminal differentiation and the development of dense dendritic arborizations; and cessation of growth occurs with calcium-dependent alterations in the actin cytoskeleton and tubulin polymerization of the advancing growth cone.

7.3.2 Neuronal degeneration

Physiologically active neurons respond to molecules which bind receptors, open ion channels, and transduce signals across the cell membrane. These trigger changes in intracellular calcium and protein kinases, induce immediate early genes, and enhance transcription of cell-specific products. Paradoxically, many forms of cell injury converge on this same final common pathway and threaten cell survival. An uncontrolled rise in calcium destabilizes the cell, committing it to irreversible injury. Calcium overload mediated by glutamate has been proposed as a common mediator of excitotoxicity. The entry of calcium and associated intracellular signals shows different temporal and spatial organization when physiological events switch to calcium overload and cell injury (reviewed by Berridge *et al.* 1998). The response to injury and recovery of cell homeostasis require rapid alterations in gene expression and protein synthesis. Immediate early genes are usually expressed at low or undetectable levels in quiescent cells but are rapidly induced by growth factors and other events occurring at the cell membrane. A sustained but transient rise in intracellular calcium, lasting several minutes, is sufficient to induce immediate early gene expression, but their transcription may be differentially sensitive to intracellular calcium. The best-characterized immediate early gene is the proto-oncogene *c-fos* (Sheng and Greenberg 1990). Immediate early gene expression is followed by increased expression of factors which secure cell survival and restore specialist or luxury properties of the threatened cell but may also precede programmed cell death *in vivo* (Smeyne *et al.* 1993).

Growth factors protect from injury neurons that they themselves support during development and maintain in the postmitotic state. For example, BDNF protects dopaminergic neurons from metabolites of 1-methyl-4-phenyl-1,2,3,6-tetrahydropyridrine (MPTP) (Hyman *et al.* 1991) and from axonal injury (Yan *et al.* 1992). Hippocampal neurons are saved from excitotoxic injury by FGF-2. This and other growth factors protect a range of hippocampal, septal, and cortical neurons from hypoglycaemic and hypoxic injury; and their tissue expression increases following ischaemic and other insults *in vivo*. NGF and bFGF released close to the striatum reduce the excitotoxic effects of glutamate receptor analogues in a model of Huntington's disease. Many of these effects are mediated by stabilizing the oscillating or sustained rise in intracellular calcium. CNTF may also be important as a survival factor in response to injury; it is transported in increased amounts to the cell body in axotomized nerve (Curtis *et al.* 1993) and influences the fate of nerve fibres threatened by injury, including motor neurons (Sendtner *et al.* 1992; Lindholm *et al.* 1993).

Other metabolic interactions are involved in excitotoxicity. Oxygen radicals and nitric oxide are generated in response to the rise in intracellular free calcium. Tissue damage resulting from excitotoxicity can be modified by antagonists of excitotoxins and inhibition of oxygen radical and nitric oxide formation. The demonstration of mutations in the gene for superoxide dismutase on chromosome 21 in familial motor neuron disease has suggested that selective motor neuron death results from oxidative stress (Rosen *et al.* 1993). In fact, this metabolic cascade has been proposed as the final common pathway of damage occurring in a variety of neurodegenerative situations, including ischaemia, Huntington's disease, Parkinson's disease, Alzheimer's disease, and motor neuron disease. Experimental studies show that mice transgenic for superoxide dismutase have selective susceptibility of spinal compared with cortical neurons. This correlates with the level of mutated gene expression and free radical production (Liu *et al.* 1998). Creatine acts to stabilize mitochondrial activity, participating in the cell buffer systems which orchestrate energy production and consumption; creatine protects motor neurons and the substantia nigra in animals with mutations of superoxide dismutase (Klivenyi *et al.* 1999). Free radicals cause local damage by capturing nearby electrons to fill their own unpaired electrons, leading to lipid peroxidation and other changes which precipitate cell death. In several neurodegenerative disorders, oxygen radicals may interact with tyrosine kinase receptors, resulting in growth factor deprivation, through the ability to react with conserved nitrate tyrosine residues. The glutamate and free-radical hypotheses for death of motor neurons are not necessarily incompatible. Embryonic rat motor neurons are directly injured by glutamate stimulation of *N*-methyl-D-aspartate (NMDA) and α-amino-3-hydroxy-5-methylisoxazole-4-proprionate (AMPA) receptors—an effect which is increased and independently mediated by nitric oxide. This is made *in vivo* by a variety of neurons which protect themselves by also producing a soluble cyclic guanosine monophosphate (cGMP) analogue. However, motor neurons which lack a protective mechanism are thereby exposed to the double hit of exposure to glutamate and nitric oxide (Urushitani *et al.* 1998). An histological study, in which increased modification of proteins by lipid peroxidation was reported in patients with motor neuron disease (Pedersen *et al.* 1998), linked free-radical production and impaired glutamate transport as the basis for excitotoxicity.

Protection from free radicals occurs physiologically through the action of superoxide dismutase and this can be increased by scavengers such as vitamins C and E. Certain molecules (including iron), donate electrons more readily than others and free-radical stress is enhanced if these are regionally concentrated. There are also rival, but not necessarily competing, theories for the mechanism of tissue injury in Parkinson's disease. These include local iron accumulation in affected tissue and the inherent capacity for dopaminergic neurons to generate oxygen radicals, exposure to toxic metabolites analogous to 6-hydroxy-dopamine or 1-methyl-4-phenyl-1,2,3,6-tetrahydropyridine (MPTP) and its MPP$^+$ metabolite, and a decrease in complex 1 of the mitochondrial respiratory chain.

Excitotoxicity caused by calcium overload and mediated by glutamate or its analogues operating through ligand-gated calcium channels has been suggested as an alternative mechanism of cell injury in motor neuron disease. Amongst the evidence is the observation that toxicity of motor neurons occurs following exposure to the cycad nut in the Guam dementia–motor neuron disease, with the further modification that a primary immunological insult first injures motor neurons, altering their threshold for excitotoxic injury. Others have shown that glutamate transport is defective in motor neurons from affected regions of the nervous system in patients with motor neuron disease and that this is disease and region specific, leading to glutamate accumulation and calcium overload (Rothstein *et al.* 1992). Zhang *et al.* (1998) report that pathogenic mutations in the presenilin-1 gene destabilize the β-catenin family of signalling proteins and thereby promote amyloid-β protein-induced apoptotic degradation of neurons. Hippocampal neurons from presenilin-1 mutant mice show increased vulnerability to glutamate excitotixity associated with calcium overload and oxidative stress (Guo *et al.* 1999).

A major advance in the taxonomy of neurodegenerative disease is provided by the recognition that many phenotypically distinct disorders share the presence of intranuclear inclusions as a defining neuropathological feature. They exist either as rare familial genetic forms or more common sporadic disease. The inclusions consist of abnormal filaments. The molecular component of the extracellular fibrils of Alzheimer's and Pick's diseases is identified as amyloid β peptide; the intraneuronal paired helical and straight filaments consist of hyper-phosphorylated tau. This is also deposited in dementias with parkinsonism (supranuclear palsy, corticobasal degeneration, and frontotemporal dementia). Three phenotypically distinct Parkinsonian disorders (Parkinson's disease, dementia with Lewy bodies, and multiple system atrophy) are characterized by inclusions which contain α-synuclein. Filaments containing expanded glutamine repeats are also present in Huntington's disease and other trinucleotide-repeat-associated disorders, especially the hereditary ataxias (reviewed by Goedert *et al.* 1998). Increasingly coherent ideas are now emerging on how the products of these gene mutations accumulate through failure of normal proteolytic processes to cause neuronal loss.

7.3.3 Axon regeneration

A marked difference exists in the extent to which axon regeneration occurs in the central and peripheral nervous systems. Characterizing and comparing biological properties of the response to axotomy of central and peripheral nerve fibres has provided many insights into axon regeneration, and led to several strategies for manipulating events so as to secure functional recovery in clinical practice. However, with the exception of some success with re-implantation of avulsed peripheral nerve roots into the spinal cord, most of this work remains experimental. Nevertheless, a dividend from the application of these advances in neurobiology, leading to improved outcome after spinal-cord injury, is anticipated.

Although the failure of central axons to regenerate following injury to the adult central nervous system can be explained in part by intrinsic growth-limiting properties, several inhibitory effects on axon growth mediated by components of the developing vertebrate nervous system have been identified. In one sense, the lack of axonal regeneration which characterizes adult mammalian nervous systems can be considered as the price paid for needing an inhibitory environment to guide axons during development, for stabilizing arrangements in the post-mature nervous system, and for inhibiting uncontrolled axonal exploration. *In vitro* studies indicate that astrocytes, mammalian oligodendrocytes, and central myelin each actively inhibit neurite growth (Fig. 7.4).

Astrocytes block axon regeneration through a mechanism which induces the normal stop signals on growth cones. Extracellular matrix molecules produced by astroglia which have growth-inhibitory properties include fibronectin, laminin, neural cell adhesion molecule, januscin, tenascin, and chondroitin sulphate proteoglycans (Fawcett and Asher 1999). The ability of embryonic growth cones to penetrate their surround-

(a)

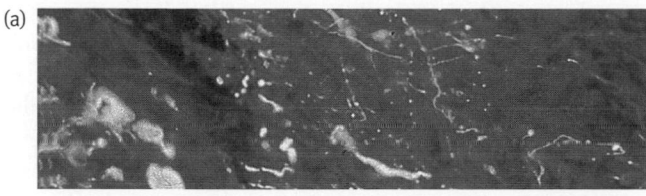

(b)

Fig. 7.4. (a) Axonal processes of neurons grow through a three-dimensional culture of Schwann cells (top); (b) failure of rat axons to penetrate oligodendrocytes in culture (bottom). (Kindly provided by Dr James Fawcett.) Also shown in colour in Plate 5.

ing astrocyte matrix depends on local secretion of proteases in response to bFGF, IL-1, and tumour necrosis factor α (TNF-α) (Fok-Seang *et al.* 1998). The failure of axon regeneration correlates with the amount of local reactive glial extracellular matrix (marked by proteoglycan expression) and, if axons can traverse that impediment, normal white matter is relatively permissive (Davies *et al.* 1997).

Axon growth inhibition is associated with myelin proteins, known as Nogo (formerly NI-35 and NI-250), produced by mature oligodendrocytes. Nogo, a member of the reticulin family, forms part of the endoplasmic reticulum of oligodendrocytes but not Schwann cells. Products of the *Nogo* gene are therefore intracellular but may act to contain axons within their nerve bundles in health; after fibre-tract injury, Nogo spills from the disrupted oligodendrocyte–myelin unit and acts, unhelpfully, to inhibit neurite outgrowth and axon regeneration (for review and citation of the primary literature, see Goldberg and Barres 2000). Bregman *et al.* (1995) showed that anti-NOGO antibodies placed in the parietal cortex of animals undergoing spinal hemisection partially restore motor function by enhancing recovery of brainstem, spinal or corticospinal fibres, and promoting plasticity of surviving serotonergic and adrenergic descending motor neurons. Another candidate moleule for mediating growth inhibition of specific axons (embryonic cerebellar and adult dorsal root ganglion cells) is myelin-associated glycoprotein (MAG), which is involved in the initial adhesion between the processes of myelinating cells and axons (McKerracher *et al.* 1994; Mukhopadhyay *et al.* 1994). Chen *et al.* (1997) showed that, in addition to improved cell survival through the inhibition of apoptosis, Bcl-2 enhances the regeneration of retinal ganglion cells towards the (murine) tectum. The mechanism may involve increasing the response of injured axons to growth-promoting factors by effects on their signal transduction pathways. In addition to these discrete manipulations of axon growth, it is clear that (experimentally), saturating spinal-cord lesions with stem cells having the potential to re-establish elemental neuronal and

glial populations enhances structural and functional recovery (McDonald *et al.* 1999).

Inflammation can be both neuroprotective and enhance axon regeneration. Macrophages release IL-2 which transiently removes the inhibitory constituents from oligodendrocytes and astrocytes. The poor regenerative response of the central (compared to the peripheral) nervous system) is associated with slower recruitment of macrophages in response to injury (Hirschberg and Schwartz 1995). Neuronal survival in the crushed optic nerve is enhanced if myelin-specific autoimmune T cells are injected locally, perhaps by a mechanism which involves transient reduction in energy requirements due to reduced nerve activity (Moalem *et al.* 1999). The functional advantage of allowing inflammation to enhance axon regeneration is shown by Rapalino *et al.* (1998), who observed enhanced motor recovery in rats, made paraplegic by complete spinal-cord transection, transplanted with macrophages first primed *in vitro* against peripheral nerve. Neuroprotection after spinal-cord injury is also provided experimentally by systemic immunization with myelin basic protein specific autoreactive T cells (Hauben *et al.* 2000). Functional recovery is associated with reconstitution of nerve fibres across the lesion and restoration of motor conduction. No additional repair is achieved by manipulating growth factors within the lesions.

7.3.4 Neuronal implantation

The possibility that reconstitution of neuronal depletion occurring as part of a disease process might be achieved by cell implantation has stimulated a new field of research which, although yet to deliver in terms of routine clinical interventions, has nevertheless driven an increase in knowledge concerning the development, plasticity, and potential for repair of focal or system-based neurological disorders. The biological events needed for restoration of structure and function include cell survival, axon growth (generally through a non-permissive environment), connectivity, and the production of neurotransmitters.

Implanted embryonic axons grow through white matter tracts which are not yet myelinated, and adult neurons regenerate best through unmyelinated pathways—observations which confirm that myelin-associated molecules are important in the inhibition of axon growth in the mature central nervous system. Paradoxically, neuroblasts transplanted from the embryonic human nervous system into rat brain and spinal cord have an enhanced growth potential compared with rodent cells; these results can be interpreted as reflecting the longer period of growth, and the greater distance which needs to be covered by the developing human nervous system. They also illustrate the relative growth potential of some neurons released from an inhibitory environment. Axon regeneration improves when central myelin and oligodendrocytes are replaced by the more permissive environment of peripheral glia. Schwann cells within intact peripheral nerves promote axon regeneration in the central nervous system, perhaps by making available neurotrophic factors (NGF, BDNF, and CNTF) and expressing

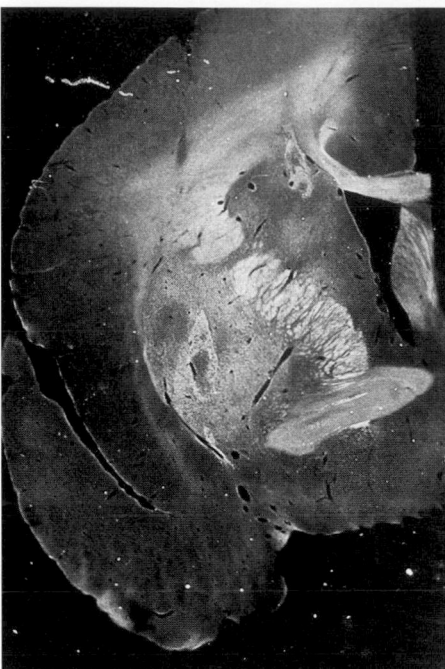

Fig. 7.5. Implantation of mesencephalic neurons into the marmoset striatum survive and connect locally, restoring selected motor functions. (Kindly provided by Professor Stephen Dunnett.) Also shown in colour in Plate 6.

adhesion molecules which support neurite outgrowth. Another candidate for creating a permissive growth-promoting environment for central axons is the olfactory bulb ensheathing cell.

Surveying the entire range of experimental situations in which neural grafting has been assessed, it is clear that a wide variety of systems can be reconstituted and these include visual, endocrine, cognitive, and motor pathways. The formation of local synapses may not be sufficient to restore complex behaviours if implanted cells fail to migrate from sites of engraftment (Fig. 7.5). Ectopic graft placement overcomes this limitation but restricts the extent to which implanted cells can explore their target area and connect extensively. Thus, the limitations on migration and axonal growth in the central nervous system represent a trade-off between restoration of orthodox anatomical arrangements and what can realistically be achieved.

Of particular interest is the demonstration that neural progenitors implanted into the cerebral ventricles of newborn mice are found distributed throughout the neuraxis at maturity (Fishell *et al.* 1993). This demonstrates the potential for rapid and widespread dissemination of implanted cells throughout the nervous system, at least during development. As expected, the viability of transplanted neurons is enhanced by factors that promote growth and survival of these same neurons *in vitro*; and, for example, graft protection by increasing the availability of free-radical scavengers improves the survival of implanted dopaminergic neurons into the striatum.

Assessment of the extent to which neural grafts restore connectivity and function has required the development of behavioural tasks which can reliably be reproduced in experimental animals and which (ideally) mimic the defects of neurodegenerative disease. In the prototypic models of Parkinson's disease, learned tasks of motor and cognitive performance in rodents and primates show that grafting restores akinesia, sensory neglect, and memory. Neural transplantation has been carried out systematically in patients with Parkinson's disease, but experimental studies indicate that there may also be opportunities for patients with Huntington's disease. Striatal grafts restore structure and (cognitive and motor) function after excitotoxic injury of the rat and primate putamen with quinolinic acid. In a model designed to show restoration of motor activity, connectivity was established histologically without uncontrolled or inappropriate growth, and synapses formed which had the neurotransmitter properties of medium spiny neurons, producing dopamine and staining for tyrosine hydroxylase (Kendall *et al.* 1998). Subsequently, Palfi *et al.* (1998) confirmed the restoration of motor activity and showed that grafting the caudate and putamen bilaterally also improves tests of cognition. Caspase inhibitors reduce apoptosis of implanted cells, enhancing their survival and improving functional recovery in models of parkinsonism (Schierle *et al.* 1999). Ideas are also developing on the possibility for repairing focal areas of cortical damage resulting from ischaemic injury. Fetal neocortex grafts have been assessed using sensory stimulation, monitored by deoxyglucose utilization in grafted areas of focal ischaemia with neuronal degeneration; thalamic projections capture and connect with the engrafted neurons but the extent to which these restore independent cortical activity remains uncertain (Grabowski *et al.* 1993).

Now that the concept of reconstructing defined regions of the brain and restoring function is established, research is moving towards the production of alternative cells for implantation so as to circumvent the logistic and ethical limitations of depending on human fetal tissue. Zawada *et al.* (1998) used cloned transgenic bovine cells to create fetuses which yielded viable mesencephalic tissue providing a source of cells, some of which survived transplantation despite an otherwise high immunological rejection rate, and restored features of parkinsonism (rotational behaviour) in rats.

7.4 Macroglial lineages in the rodent and human nervous system

7.4.1 Astrocytes

Most information concerning glial development derives from studies of rodent nervous systems, but there is now also a growing body of evidence from human studies. As stem cells start to differentiate, the first conspicuous morphological change in glia is the appearance of radial cells which stretch in parallel arrays from the subventricular zone to the subpial brain surface (Cameron and Rakic 1991). Initially, these are bipolar, with a short process connecting the cell body to the adjacent ventricular zone, and a longer process penetrating the developing cortical plate, reaching to the pial surface and terminating in the glial limiting membrane. Outward migration of the cell body then occurs, altering the relative length of the two processes; as movement occurs towards the cortex, the descending process is lost, the ascending one elaborates and the cell begins to resemble the mature astrocyte with randomly orientated processes. The radial network coincides with neuronal histogenesis, suggesting that this is a scaffold for nerve cells migrating from their germinal zones towards the developing cortex. This wave of neuronal growth is associated with inhibition of cell proliferation in the glial network. But as nerve cells switch from the phase of migration and distribution to the establishment of their synaptic connections, radial glia start to differentiate and develop into multipolar astrocytes.

Morphological studies have identified several astrocyte subtypes and specific functions have periodically been assigned to each. Type-1 astrocytes contribute to formation of the glia limitans, which defines the boundaries of the central nervous system and contributes to formation of the blood–brain barrier. The intimate anatomical relationship between astrocytes and axons at the node of Ranvier initially led to the suggestion that astrocytes act as a source of sodium channels and this property was assigned to the type-2 astrocyte, although this cell has an ambiguous status *in vivo*. In the original analysis, neonatal O-2A progenitors that encountered an altered environment were shown to differentiate into type-2 astrocytes. CNTF temporarily induced the astrocyte phenotype and, in association with an unidentified extracellular matrix molecule, promoted

O-2A differentiation. Oncostatin and LIF exert a similar influence. However, in long-term culture, the type-2 astrocyte has an unstable phenotype and begins to look rather like a type-1 astrocyte in terms of ion-channel profile, morphological appearance, and antigen expression. Furthermore, the use of marker dyes to reveal *in vivo* glial arrangements in the optic nerve show only astrocytes that contact nodes of Ranvier, blood vessels, and the pial surface, substantiating claims that the separate morphological arrangements proposed for type-1 and -2 astrocytes are *in vitro* artefacts (Butt and Ransom 1989). Taken together, one interpretation is that astrocytes develop from a progenitor which is distinct from the O-2A cell. This is committed either to oligodendrocyte development or self-renewal as an adult O-2A cell (Fig. 7.6).

Astrocyte reactivity, marked by increased expression of glial fibrillary acidic protein (GFAP), is aimed primarily at increasing the availability of growth and neuroprotective factors. The origin of reactive astrocytes is not resolved. *Some* are cells which have migrated into lesions. Others have proliferated locally. Most are resting cells which react and change their phenotype. Eventually, astrocyte reactivity leads to glial scar formation consisting of hypertrophied astrocytes, fibroblasts, and meningeal cells. Eddleston and Mucke (1993), reviewing the literature on *in vivo* and *in vitro* studies of astrocytes, list more than 100 molecules which are upregulated on astrocytes in response to more than 300 stimuli; these include adhesion, antigen-presenting, calcium-binding, cytokine, cytoskeletal, immediate-response, eicosanoid, enzyme, defined-epitope, receptor, transport, and various miscellaneous markers.

Most cytokines and growth factors produced by resting astrocytes *in vitro* are also released by reactive astrocytes *in vivo*. Several are simultaneously produced by microglia, but astrocytes are a major source of soluble mediators of inflammation synthesized locally as part of the response to injury. FGF-2 and EGF stimulate the division of astrocytes, as does GGF in addition to its effect on Schwann cells, whereas proliferation is inhibited by transforming growth factor α (TGF-α). Although normally expressed at low levels in the central nervous system, TGF-α1 expression is increased after penetrating wounds of the cerebral cortex; TGF-α1 can be detected for up to 14 days in neurons and glia which are either the targets for focal injury or orchestrate its response. TGF-α1 increases the availability of neurite growth-promoting molecules, limits the infiltration of macrophages and microglia, and acts to organize the formation of a glial limiting membrane made up of reactive astrocytes.

Clearly, the damaged brain needs to steer a course between promoting reactive changes in astrocytes, which usefully encapsulate the area of tissue injury and provide mediators for the promotion of recovery, while avoiding formation of a dense astrocytic scar which would then exclude beneficial cytokines, growth factors, and cells needed to repair neurons and glia. This conflict between protection and injury is no less delicately balanced for microglia (Section 7.6.4).

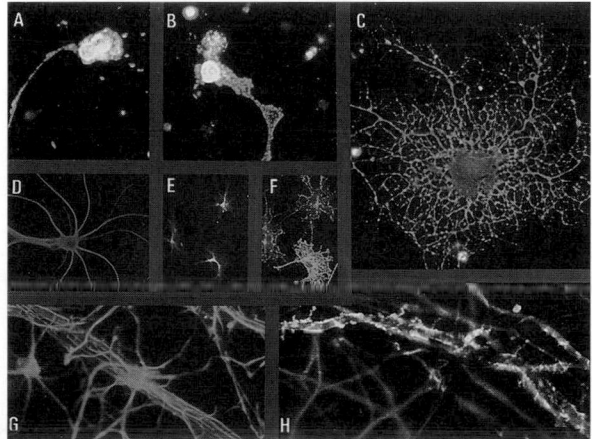

Fig. 7.6. The rodent glial lineage. (a) A bipolar A2B5 positive rat cortex neonatal progenitor undergoing division (bromdeoxyuridine uptake shown in yellow). (b) A unipolar (rat hindbrain) adult progenitor undergoing division. (c) A differentiated oligodendrocyte stained for galactocerebroside. Astrocyte subtypes: (d) the type-1 astrocyte stained for GFAP; (e) the type-2 astrocyte stained for GFAP; (f) the type-2 astrocyte stained for A2B5; (g) the type-2 astrocyte stained with GFAP seen contacting a bundle of axons. (h) Triple staining for axons (blue), asytocytes (red), and oligodendrocytes (green/yellow) to show the interactions of O-2A progenitor progeny and nerve fibres. (Originals kindly provided by Dr John Zajicek.) Also shown in colour in Plate 7.

7.4.2 **Oligodendrocytes**

The proliferative cells which give rise to mammalian oligo-dendroglia during embryogenesis are born around the lateral ventricles, the fourth ventricle, and in the ventral spinal cord. As cells which are committed *in vivo* to the oligodendrocyte lineage proliferate and migrate into white and grey matter, they start to express maturation markers. One much characterized step in the process of oligodendrocyte development features the O-2A progenitor, which can be recovered from the rodent optic nerve, cerebrum, and hindbrain; this bipolar, migratory, and proliferative cell is characterized by the development *in vitro* both of oligodendrocyte and astrocyte progeny, depending on local growth-factor conditions (Raff *et al.* 1983; see Fig. 7.6). Although certain features cannot be characterized *in vivo*, definition based on the detection of PDGF-receptor α-chain mRNA permits identification of O-2A progenitors in the spinal cord and ventricular zone during embryonic development. Glial progenitors which migrate away from germinal zones retain developmental plasticity, differentiating either into astro-cytes or oligodendrocytes (Levison and Goldman 1993). The next step in differentiation of the oligodendrocyte progenitor is marked by expression of O4. This pre-oligodendrocyte proliferates and is bipotential but no longer motile.

Cells having the properties of neonatal O-2A cells can also be recovered from the adult rodent nervous system (ffrench Constant and Raff 1986). Adult progenitors behave as stem cells, dividing asymmetrically (at least *in vitro*) to produce one daughter O-2A cell and one oligodendrocyte. In this way, they maintain a pool of cells in the adult nervous system capable of self-renewal and generating new oligodendrocytes through asymmetric division and differentiation (Wren *et al.* 1992). They can re-enter a more proliferative phase, perhaps by resuming the phenotype, growth factor responsiveness, and behaviour of their neonatal O-2A counterparts, increasing their rate of division prior to final differentiation and so maximizing the production of oligodendrocytes ultimately derived from the adult O-2A progenitor pool (Engel and Wolswijk 1996). Resting microglia and their supernatants increase the survival of mature oligodendrocytes *in vitro* through a mechanism which promotes both the survival and differentiation of oligodendro-cyte progenitors (Nicholas *et al.* 2001). The effect is mediated through PDGF. In contrast to the effect on oligodendrocytes, activated microglial stimulate astrocyte proliferation which, in turn, increases the availability of oligodendrocyte lineage growth factors.

Human oligodendrocyte precursors are born in many parts of the central nervous system, including the spinal cord (Weidenheim *et al.* 1994; Yu *et al.* 1994), by 7–9 weeks' gestation, and they can be identified 2–3 weeks before the onset of myelination. They increase progressively within the ventral and lateral portions of the cervical and then the lumbar cord, thereafter populating the lateral and dorsal regions by the time myelination starts, at embryonic day 83 (Hajihosseini *et al.* 1996). However, their constitutive proliferative response does not increase in response to PDGF or FGF-2 (Satoh and

Kim 1994). Rivkin *et al.* (1995) studied human cerebra from 15–18-week fetuses and generated cultures in which large numbers of O-2A cells differentiated both to pre-oligodendro-cytes and fully differentiated oligodendrocytes over the ensuing weeks.

Turning to the adult human central nervous system, the pre-oligodendrocyte, equivalent to the rodent pro-oligodendrocyte, which expresses O4 but not galactocerebroside (GalC) and is neither bipotential nor proliferative *in vitro* was first identified (Armstrong *et al.* 1992). Scolding *et al.* (1995), using normal-appearing temporal lobe white matter, removed during epilepsy surgery, then identified bipolar cells positive for A2B5 but nega-tive for O4 and markers of mature oligodendrocytes or astro-cytes. These proliferated and were bipotential *in vitro*, but although the adult human progenitor divides on a monolayer of human astrocytes, no proliferation is observed in response to PDGF, FGF-2, or NT-3 (alone or in combinations)—stimuli known to promote rat neonatal O-2A progenitor division (Fig. 7.7). The human pre-oligodendrocyte and its progenitor have each now been identified in the lesions of multiple sclero-sis (Scolding *et al.* 1998; Wolswijk 1998). The fact that pro-

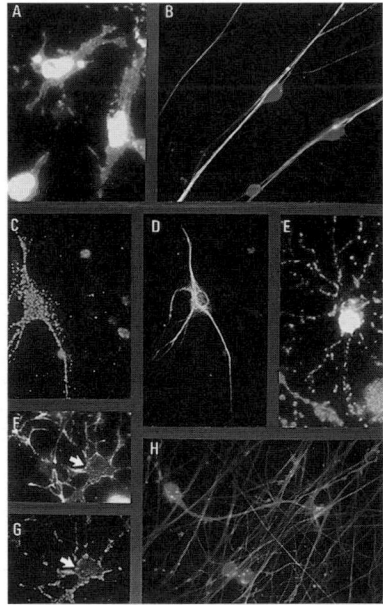

Fig. 7.7. The adult human oligodendrocyte lineage. (a) The oligodendrocyte progenitor stained red with A2B5 proliferates in response to astrocyte-derived factors. (b) The bipolar oligodendrocyte progenitor associates with (rat) dorsal root ganglion neurons stained blue for neurofilament. (c) The progenitor differentiates into an astrocyte stained red with A2B5. (d) The progenitor differentiates into an astrocyte stained green with GFAP. (e) The O4-positive pro-oligodendrocyte stained red with O4 and showing BrdU uptake is considered to have divided as a progenitor and then differentiated. (f) The progenitor differentiates into an oligodendrocyte stained green with antibody for galatocerebroside. (g) The differentiating progenitor stains red with A2B5. (h) Differentiated human glial oligodendrocytes (stained red with galactocerebroside) develop processes which associate with several (rat) dorsal root ganglion axons. (Originals kindly provided by Professor Neil Scolding and Dr Christopher Shaw.) Also shown in colour in Plate 8.

genitors are present within persistently demyelinated lesions suggests that these have not engaged naked axons. However, Capello *et al.* (1997) detected a developmental isoform of the myelin basic protein (MBP) gene which does correlate with remyelination, suggesting that either through the role of primitive cells or differentiated oligodendrocytes, the formation of new myelin involves recapitulation of ontogenic events.

7.5 Axon–glial interactions and myelination

The relationship between axons and glia is reciprocal and complex. Myelination occurs when the membranous processes of mature oligodendrocytes contact and ensheathe axons of diameter 1 μm or more, and compact to form the myelin lamellae needed for saltatory axonal conduction. Oligodendrocyte progenitors need to orientate their processes and maximize points of contact with the unmyelinated nerve fibre. Neurons are less sensitive than cells of the oligodendrocyte lineage to topographical information, and their progenitors use smaller topographical cues than neurites during pathfinding. The migration of oligodendrocyte progenitors occurs along established axonal tracts which provide a migration substratum consisting of parallel aligned axons (Colello *et al.* 1994). The movement of migrating cells is influenced by receptor–ligand adhesions with the extacellular matrix, and integrins are one of several molecules which determine cell–cell interactions in the developing and post-mature nervous system (Shaw *et al.* 1996). Stable myelination depends on cell-surface and extracellular matrix molecules which promote and maintain interactions between myelin and axons; these include janusin, tenascin, laminin, and fibronectin.

Although it is the oligodendrocyte which ultimately synthesizes and maintains myelin around short segments of neighbouring axons, there is some unresolved debate on which cells within the lineage possess or can re-acquire myelinating potential. The myelinating cell must divide and since the fully differentiated oligodendrocyte cannot, remyelination is mainly considered to be a property of its progenitor. But the relationship is reciprocal and oligodendrocyte progenitors are also influenced by their axonal environment. For example, neurons are mitogenic for cells of the oligodendrocyte lineage. The molecular basis involves both diffusible and membrane-associated signals which include PDGF (Zajicek and Compston 1994), also produced by astrocytes. Electrical activity in axons also influences oligodendrocyte progenitor proliferation (Barres and Raff 1993). Whatever the stimulus, the number of mature oligodendrocytes is matched to the local axon density, survival being orchestrated by the number of axons requiring myelination (Burne *et al.* 1996).

Although glia undoubtedly inhibit axon regeneration, a factor derived from oligodendrocytes promotes the survival, growth, and calibre of retinal ganglion cells in the developing optic nerve (Colello *et al.* 1995; Meyer-Franke *et al.* 1995;

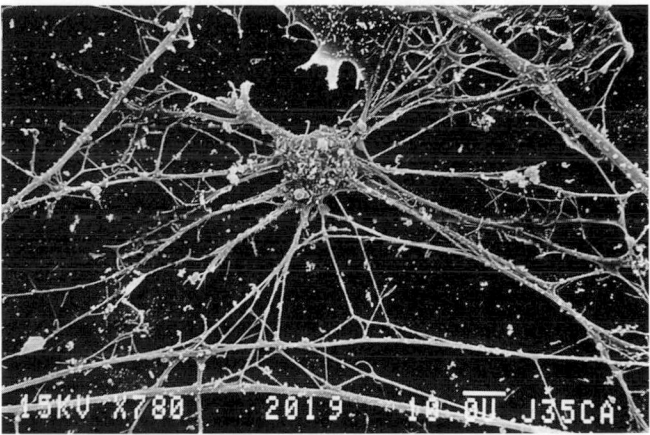

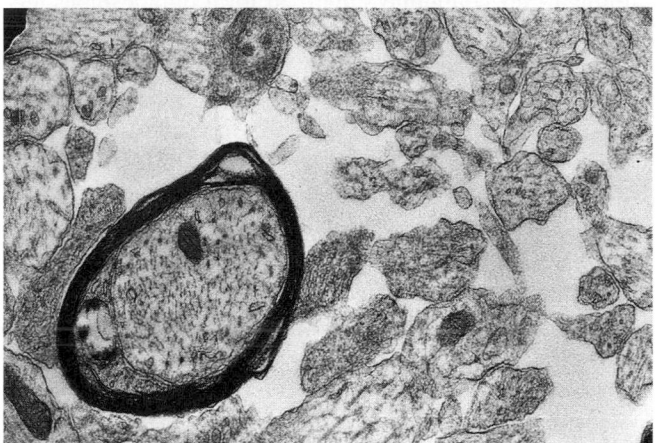

Fig. 7.8. (a) Rat O-2A progenitors associate *in vitro* with several bundles of dorsal rat ganglion axons shown by scanning electron microscopy. (b) The formation of compact myelin sheaths is shown by transmission electron microscopy. (Reproduced with permission from Zajicek and Compston 1994.)

Sanches *et al.* 1996). Oligodendrocytes, but not astrocytes, secrete a factor needed for the sodium channels to cluster at intervals appropriate for the diameter of developing axons in preparation for propagation of the nerve impulse (Kaplan *et al.* 1997). Unlike oligodendrocytes, myelinating Schwann cells are fully permissive for axon growth, both in the peripheral and central nervous system, due to the production of trophic factors, including NGF, BDNF, and CNTF, and expression of cell-adhesion molecules known to promote neurite growth. A further effect of axons is to bias differentiation of the oligodendrocyte precursor. Since astrocytes are involved in the formation of internodes, careful orchestration is needed to juxtapose progenitors alongside axons, and to ensure that differentiation does not proceed along one route to the exclusion of the other. The bipotential oligodendrocyte progenitor shows an increase in astrocyte differentiation on contact with axons (Zajicek and Compston 1994). One interpretation is that axonal signals alter the differentiation schedule of bipotential O-2A cells so as to make available each cell type needed to complete cellular architecture at the node of Ranvier (Fig. 7.8).

Once stable axon–glial contact is established, the elongated oligodendrocyte processes form a cup around the axon at the point of contact, extending lengthwise to form a trough, the two lips of which advance around the circumference of the axon until they meet. One then passes beneath the other to become the inner tongue of the future sheath which rotates many times around the axon to form the multiple membrane layers, or lamellae. During compaction, the cytoplasmic content of all except the innermost and outermost lamellae of the developing spiral sheath is gradually extruded, and the two inner leaflets of the surface membrane lipid bilayer thus become opposed. These fuse to form the major dense line visible in ultrastructural cross-section. The two outer leaflets of adjacent layers of the spiral process are also closely opposed, and although they commonly appear to form only a single, less-dense intraperiod line, electron microscopy confirms that they do not fuse and that the intraperiod line comprises two separate leaflets. Inner and outer tongues of cytoplasm remain where the corresponding central and outermost lamellae have not compacted. Radial components visible in ultrastructural cross-sections of myelin probably correspond to stacks of tight junctions arrayed in lines from outermost to innermost lamellae. These are thought to seal adjacent lamellae together and to anchor the outer cytoplasmic tongue.

The developing myelin sheath extends lengthwise in both directions along the axon to form an internodal segment, but at the advancing edge, each layer of the spiral retains a bead of cytoplasm where the two inner leaflets of the surface membrane remain separate. In three dimensions, this bead comprises a ring of cytoplasm around the axon and is termed the lateral loop. Transverse bands, regularly arranged sites of close membrane apposition spaced 10–15 nm apart, later develop between the end of each lateral loop and the underlying axolemma. There are as many lateral loops at the leading edge of the advancing sheath as there are lamellae, and these become stacked in a regular way, those of the outermost lamellae being distal to those of the innermost. The complement of lateral loops at one end of each developing internode abuts onto its adjacent counterpart, and together these form the paranodal region next to the node of Ranvier.

Compact myelin thereby consists of a condensed lipid-rich membrane wrapped spirally many times around axons to form a segmented sheath. This is interrupted periodically along the course of the axon at the (unmyelinated) nodes of Ranvier, areas where electrical resistance is low due to the high concentration of sodium channels, and where depolarization is thereby facilitated. In myelinated axons, the action potential induced by depolarization generates electrical currents which in turn trigger depolarization not at the immediately adjacent myelinated (and insulated) internode, but preferentially at the next node of Ranvier; this saltatory conduction is considerably more rapid than continuous propagation of the nerve impulse.

Central myelin is mainly composed of lipid (cholesterol, phospholipid, and galatolipid) with some protein. The glycoproteins are GalC, MAG, and myelin oligodendrocyte glyco-protein (MOG), the latter constituting less than 1% of myelin proteins. The two major proteins are proteolipid protein (PLP) and MBP. A further structural component is the myelin-specific enzyme 2′,3′-cyclic nucleotide 3′-phosphohydrolase (CNPase). Bronstein et al. (1996) described a novel oligodendrocyte-specific protein related to peripheral myelin protein-22 which is widely distributed and follows a developmental profile similar to PLP; its role in myelinogenesis and relevance for demyelinating disease remain to be determined. The separate roles of these structural components are not fully explained. MAG is believed to have an important role in stabilizing the initial glial–axon contact as the spiral process begins, in anticipation of compaction, but myelination proceeds normally in transgenic mice which are deficient in the gene for MAG (Montag et al. 1994). There are some differences in myelination between central nerve fibres and peripheral nerves. Unlike the oligodendrocyte which myelinates short segments of several neighbouring axons, Schwann cells contact only a single peripheral nerve fibre. Peripheral nerve myelin consists of MAG, Po, and MBP but no PLP.

Much of the preceding analysis is based on rodent studies. Whittemore et al. (1993) showed that, although human oligodendrocytes can be maintained on rat dorsal root ganglion cells and tend to associate with their axons, they do not form myelin sheaths. Neurons improve the survival of human oligodendroglia in vitro but there is no proliferation, even in the presence of bFGF, PDGF, IGF, BDNF, NT-3, NT-4/5 (alone or in combination), or rat astrocyte or neuroblastoma cell line (B-104)-conditioned medium (Scolding et al. 1999). Turning to what happens in vivo, Hunter et al. (1997) conclude, on the basis of spatial and temporal patterns of myelin formation in the retina, that some non-myelinating oligodendrocytes use phylogenetically older axons as a substrate for migration, whereas other more mature oligodendrocyte progenitors myelinate well into adult life but operate over a much shorter range.

The pioneering experimental studies of demyelination and remyelination showed that remyelination occurs endogenously both in young and adult nervous systems and that the capacity for repair by oligodendrocyte precursors is exhausted by repeated insult. This work involves mechanical and gliotoxin-induced methods for inducing demyelination, but with anti-galactocerebroside antibody mediated demyelination of the feline optic nerve, Carroll et al. (1998) identified small glial cells, derived from precursors located outside the demyelinating lesion, which differentiate into remyelinating oligodendrocytes and achieve extensive remyelination. They concentrate early at the margins of the lesions, suggesting an origin from residents of the optic nerve and not distant migrants. This remyelinating cell is beyond reasonable doubt the in vivo counterpart of the oligodendrocyte progenitor, characterized extensively in vitro. Komoly et al. (1992) and Yao et al. (1995) have provided evidence that reactive gliosis brings to the experimental demyelinating lesion cytokines or growth factors (IGF-1) which promote repair, and the same properties are associated with reactive astrocytes in the lesions of multiple sclerosis (Malik et al. 2000).

also upregulates the expression of an heterogeneous group of receptors on microglia involved in the phagocytosis of opsonized particles. These include the FcR1 (CD64), FcRII (CD32), and FcRIII (CD16) receptors, which increase after exposure to γ-IFN and β-IFN (Williams *et al.* 1992; Hall *et al.* 1997). Peritoneal macrophages and microglia have receptors for the complement components C1q and iCR3. Human microglia possess chemotactic receptors for C5a, IL-8, and the bacterial peptide fMet–Leu–Phe (Lacy *et al.* 1995). These and other receptor–ligand interactions allow the microglia to recognize and then deliver a lethal signal to target cells.

Perivascular macrophages express the low-affinity NGF receptor which binds neurotrophin but does not transduce signals unless the tyrosine kinase receptor is also present and activated. CNTF has been shown to induce expression of the low-affinity NGF receptor and the CD4 antigen, and to increase expression of CR3 *in vivo* and *in vitro*. There is now evidence that microglia contribute to the degenerative process in several disorders where inflammatory events are not traditionally considered to be involved. Interactions are described between β-amyloid and microglia. Chemokines are released by astrocytes and oligodendrocytes in response to β-amyloid, acting as chemoattractants for microglia (Johnstone *et al.* 1999). Meda *et al.* (1999) describe a synergistic effect between β-amyloid and γ-IFN in triggering the release of reactive oxygen metabolites, TNF-α and IL-1β but not IL-6 or IL-10, from (murine) microglia; these activated microglia are then able to injure neurons *in vitro*. There are similarities between the transcriptional change induced in response to aggregated β-amyloid and that seen during neuronal apoptosis in response to growth factor withdrawal. Barger and Harmon (1997) have narrowed the component of β-amyloid precursor protein which activates microglia (leading to the production of IL-1β and inducible nitric oxide) to the secreted derivative s-APP-α. This effect is inhibited by apolipoprotein-E3. Clearly, these findings have potential implications for the role of inflammatory mechanisms in the pathogenesis of neuronal degeneration in Alzheimer's disease.

The pro-inflammatory responses of microglia are limited by the production of IL-4, IL-10, prostaglandin-E$_2$ and TGF-β (Morgan *et al.* 1993), which suppress several behaviours (proliferation, activation, adhesion, migration, phagocytosis, co-stimulation, and mediator production), and by apoptosis of autoreactive T cells using perforin and the Fas/Fas-ligand pathway. Microglia are themselves killed by apoptotic mechanisms in response to TGF-β and are not protected by Bcl-2. The balance at any one time of these pro- and anti-inflammatory responses may influence the stability of axon–glial interactions. With some variations, the same checks and balances are provided by anti-inflammatory cytokines on the pro-inflammatory behaviour of astrocytes (Xiao and Link 1998).

The terms 'professional' and 'non-professional' usefully define antigen-presenting cells which can initiate antigen-specific primary or secondary immune responses respectively, reflecting differences in the quality of stimulation required for naive as opposed to memory T-cell activation. The issue of

whether antigen presentation occurs exclusively within the central nervous system or uses cells (of peripheral or brain origin) which encounter antigen in draining lymph nodes (Weller *et al.* 1996) and stimulate lymphocytes which migrate into the central nervous system, is not fully resolved. Theoretically, antigen presentation could also result from interactions between cells which straddle but do not pass the endothelial barrier and communicate with those resident on the abluminal surface.

The first candidate for the role of antigen-presenting cell in the central nervous system was the astrocyte, following claims that it can present antigen to T cells *in vitro* in a recall assay (Fontana *et al.* 1984). However, human astrocytes do not express the co-stimulatory molecule B7 spontaneously or following activation (Meinl *et al.* 1994). Microglia are better equipped for antigen presentation, secreting IL-1 and constitutively expressing class II MHC and B7 (De Simone *et al.* 1995) following activation. Co-stimulation is most effectively delivered through CD28 and B7, and/or CD40 and its ligand. These co-stimulatory molecules are upregulated by γ-IFN, activation of the system leading to TNF-α production; and downregulated by anti-inflammatory cytokines, especially the Th-2-associated products IL-4, IL-10, and TGF-β1. That microglia can act as non-professional antigen-presenting cells is generally accepted and less controversial than their putative role in activation of naive T cells (Williams *et al.* 1993).

The most recent evidence questions the role of microglia even as non-professional antigen-presenting cells, since if adult rodent microglia are separated by flow cytometry *in vitro*, it is the CD45^{high}CD11b/c$^+$ perivascular macrophage rather than the CD45^{low}CD11b/c$^+$ parenchymal microglia which activates T cells. Unlike perivascular macrophages, microglia fail to produce IL-2, resulting in limited T-cell proliferation and the promotion of apoptosis (Ford *et al.* 1996). These observations have led to the conclusion that the main antigen-presenting cell of the central nervous system is the perivascular macrophage, which, in this respect, is distinguished from the microglial cell despite their common origin as bone marrow monocytes.

Antigen presentation by microglia to memory T cells results in cytokine release, which reciprocally activates naive microglia, indicating that recall antigen presentation results in an environment which propagates the immune response (Hall *et al.* 1999). The effect is predominantly mediated by γ-IFN but amplified by TNF-α. Both are blocked by IFN-β through an effect on class II expression (Hall *et al.* 1997) and by inhibition of protein kinases (Hellendall and Ting 1997). Histocompatibility determinants are also induced after virus infections, tumour development, and in neurodegenerative disorders. Recent observations indicate that neurons have a crucial role in regulating histocompatibility antigen expression in the central nervous system. Electrically active neurons strongly downregulate histocompatibility antigen expression on their own membrane and surrounding glia cells. Paralysis of neuronal activity leads to the prompt induction of histocompatibility determinants, rendering neurons vulnerable to T-cell derived perforin but not Fas-ligand killing (Rensing-Ehl *et al.* 1996). It is not clear whether this negative signalling is mediated by diffusible neurotransmitters (glutamate, vasoactive intestinal peptide, catecholamines), or results directly from electrical activity (Neumann *et al.* 1995, 1997). IL-4 also induces microglial proliferation, having a synergistic effect when used with IL-3 and G-CSF. Expression of a novel brain-specific cytokine, designated neurotactin and produced by microglia, which attracts neutrophils, is enhanced in experimental brain inflammation (Pan *et al.* 1997). Horwitz *et al.* (1997) overexpressed γ-IFN on the oligodendrocytes of transgenic mice. Demyelination and clinical signs occurred without oligodendrocyte depletion; the main histological finding was removal of myelin by activated microglia with increased class II antigen expression and levels of pro-inflammatory cytokines (IL-12, TNF-α, lymphotoxin-B, and IL-1 but not IL-6, IL-10, β-IFN, and TGF-β).

Relative lack of co-stimulatory molecules may account for the limited antigen-presenting properties of microglia. One analysis is that the interaction of microglia with lymphocytes entering the nervous system is more likely to induce their apoptotic death, and so protect the brain parenchyma, rather than promote T-cell proliferation and amplification of the immune response (Perry 1998). However, others retain the option that this situation will differ if there is a recall response, in which case microglia may propagate the immune response. Although the best candidates for a brain-derived antigen-presenting cell are microglia or bone-marrow-derived macrophages, astrocytes, cerebral vascular endothelial cells, and pericytes are all capable of re-stimulating lymphocytes (Xiao and Link 1998)—and there is now experimental evidence that dendritic cells can migrate from the periphery and trigger the immune response (Perry 1998).

7.6.5 Oligodendrocyte injury

Ludwin (1997) and Raine (1997) have summarized the available evidence on factors likely to be present in the central nervous system during health or disease and which are known from *in vivo* and *in vitro* studies to be capable of injuring oligodendrocytes or disrupting axon–glial interactions.

Oligodendrocytes are almost as susceptible to anoxia and excitotoxic damage (kainate and glutamate) mediated by oxygen radicals as hippocampal neurons (Yoshioka *et al.* 1995). But they are especially sensitive to mediators of inflammation. Because they lack a factor (CD59) which normally protects cells from autologous complement injury by regulating assembly of the membrane-attack complex, rat oligodendrocytes activate complement *in vitro* but can be protected from complement attack by re-incorporating CD59 on the cell surface. Oligodendrocyte progenitors are also complement sensitive. Piddlesden and Morgan (1993) confirmed that mature rat oligodendrocytes are sensitive *in vitro* to complement activation because they lack sufficient CD59 to inhibit formation of membrane attack complexes. The sensitivity of oligodendrocytes differentiating from neonatal progenitors *in vitro* increases despite no change in expression of CD59, suggesting that, with differentiation, oligodendrocytes acquire the lethal combination of a molecule which activates complement and the lack of CD59 needed to protect from membrane-attack complex formation. Alternatively, Agoropoulou *et al.* (1998) showed that, although they lack CD59, oligodendrocytes which ensheathe axons are insensitive to complement attack because they have no cell-surface C3; hence it is the initial step of activation rather than formation of the membrane-attack complex which distinguishes the injury of oligodendrocytes in serum from those co-cultured with axons.

Cells exposed to sublytic concentrations of complement or perforin show a transient increase in intracellular calcium, during which pores forming in the membrane are gathered into vesicles and shed from the cell surface, thereby restoring membrane integrity and leaving the oligodendrocyte metabolically intact (Scolding *et al.* 1989). Oligodendrocytes exposed to T-cell-derived perforin show increased membrane permeability, identical to that seen following complement attack, and both cause an abrupt rise in cytosolic free calcium. The association of oligodendrocyte recovery with calcium oscillation suggests that the complex calcium signal following insertion of the membrane-attack complex stimulates protective mechanisms and repair at the cellular level (Wood *et al.* 1993). Recovery from membrane permeabilization mediated by any pore-forming agent occurs rapidly *in vitro*. Single-cell studies demonstrate heterogeneity in the response of individual oligodendrocytes, and allow certain conclusions to be reached concerning the dynamics and mechanisms of membrane repair. Even when successful recovery from a single cycle of injury has been achieved, oligodendrocytes remain unduly susceptible to repeated complement attack. Although this evidence draws attention to the reversible nature of oligodendrocyte injury, the direct relevance of these findings for the induction or amplification of immune-mediated damage *in vivo*, and in humans, is uncertain.

Preliminary evidence suggests that complement activation is not a property of human oligodendrocytes which, unlike rat cells, do appear to possess the complement regulatory protein CD59 (Zajicek and Compston 1995). Other receptor–ligand interactions may therefore be more important in mediating damage to human oligodendrocytes by microglia. Of particular relevance to multiple sclerosis is the demonstration that antibody in low concentration, coating the surface of the oligodendrocyte or its myelin sheath, opsonizes the target cell for lytic damage by microglia using their Fc receptors (Scolding and Compston 1991). Demyelinated axons are coated with anti-MOG antibody in the lesions of acute multiple sclerosis (Genain *et al.* 1999). The potential role of MOG is further suggested by the high prevalence of intrathecal anti-MOG and anti-MBP antibodies, persistent in multiple sclerosis from an early stage in the illness, unlike the evolving pattern of antibody responses to MBP, but transient in other inflammatory diseases of the central nervous system (Reindl *et al.* 1999).

The main relevance of complement activation in the context of inflammatory brain disease may therefore be the breakdown

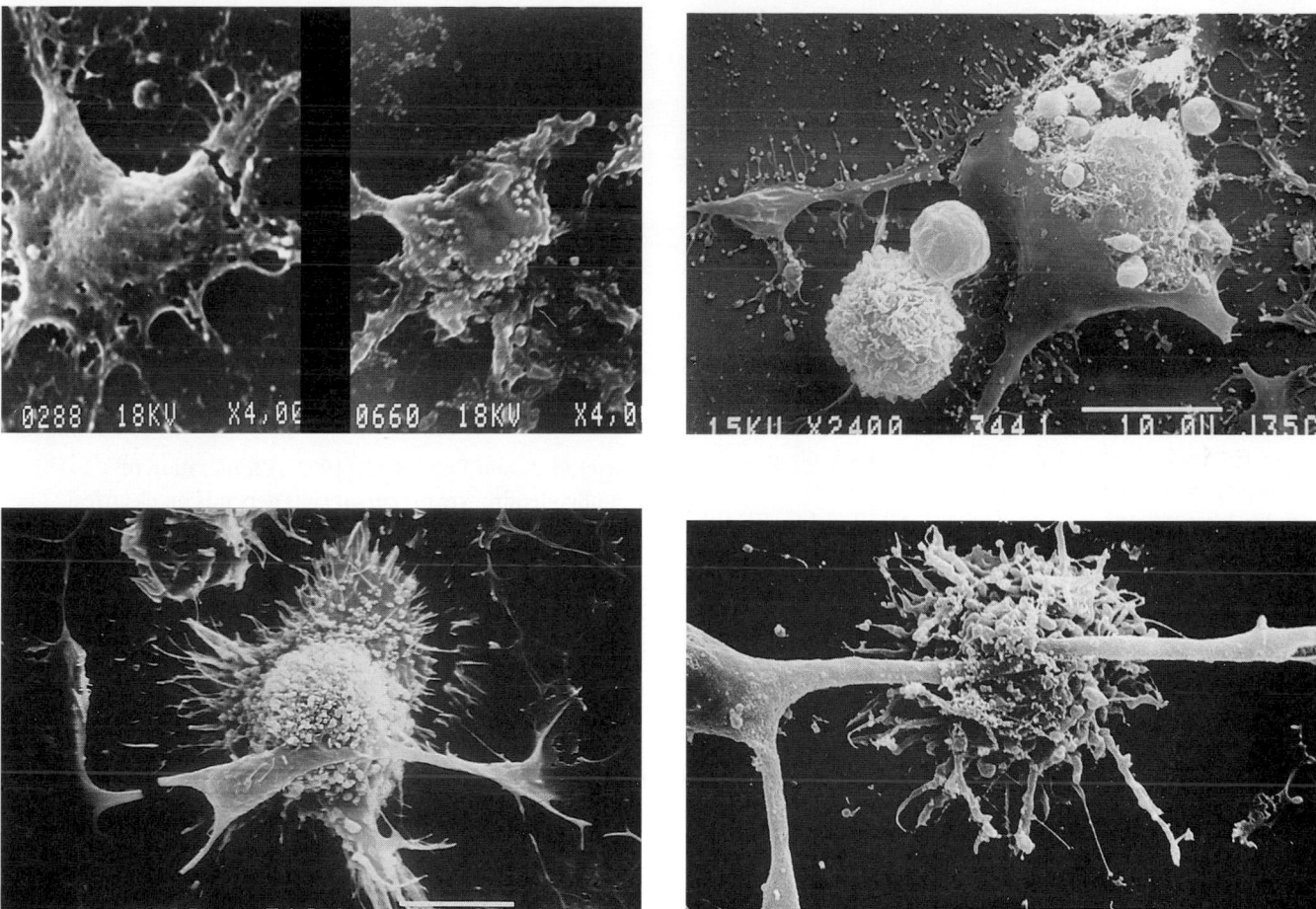

Fig. 7.11. Reversible injury of oligodendrocytes by membrane vesiculation. (a) Oligodendrocytes are shown before initiating non-lethal injury with complement. (b) After 3 minutes, numerous vesicular structures staining brightly with anti-C9 antibody and avidin gold appear on the cell and its processes. These vesicles have disappeared at 6 minutes. (Reproduced with permission from Scolding *et al.* 1989.) (c) Scanning electron microscopy to show that activated microglia adhere to oligodendrocytes but do not induce lethal injury. (d) Activated microglia adhere to and injure oligodendrocytes opsonized with sublethal concentrations of antigalactocerebroside antibody. (Reproduced with permission from Scolding and Compston 1991.) (e) Activated microglia adhere to and injure oligodendrocytes opsonized with sublethal concentrations of complement. (Reproduced with permission from Zajicek *et al.* 1992.)

of C3, releasing membrane-bound and fluid-phase products which determine interactions between oligodendrocytes and macrophages or microglia. Selmaj *et al.* (1991) report that soluble TNF-α directly injures and lyses oligodendrocytes *in vitro*. Others have been unable to reproduce this finding using physiological concentrations of TNF-α. Even though they are resistant to physiological concentrations of soluble TNF-α, oligodendrocytes are vulnerable to cell-surface TNF-α present on activated microglia (Zajicek *et al.* 1992: Fig. 7.11). van der Laan *et al.* (1996) confirm that uptake of myelin by macrophages is enhanced by opsonization with complement, involves the CR3 receptor, induces a rise in intracellular calcium, and is associated with the production of TNF-α and nitric oxide by these activated macrophages. Aside from the issue of whether the oligodendrocyte is more susceptible to cell bound than soluble TNF-α, the fact that it possesses receptors for TNF-α and the related molecule Fas, provides a basis for

signalling events which activate both apoptotic and necrotic death pathways (D'Souza *et al.* 1995, 1996). TNF-α may also inhibit the maturation of oligodendrocyte precursors (Cammer and Zhang 1999). Köller *et al.* (1996) showed that TNF-α induces a rise in intracellular calcium within astrocytes which has consequences for axon–glial interactions and saltatory conduction of the nerve impulse.

Intravitreal injection of TNF-α leads to demyelination of mouse optic nerve axons, and its injection into murine spinal cord causes an inflammatory response which reproduces many features of autoimmune encephalomyelitis. Butt and Jenkins (1994) injected optic nerve oligodendrocytes with lucifer yellow and showed swollen myelin processes which then unravelled, eventually losing continuity with the oligodendrocyte cell body in TNF-α injected nerves. Merrill *et al.* (1993) showed in co-cultures of rat amoeboid microglia and oligodendrocytes in serum-containing medium that antagonists of nitric oxide, as well as anti-TNF-α antibodies or the presence of TGF-β, each protect rat oligodendrocytes from necrotic cell death mediated by nitric oxide, γ-IFN and TNF-α, acting alone or in combination.

CNTF protects oligodendrocytes from injury by TNF-α but not complement attack (Louis *et al.* 1993). Scolding and Compston (1995) used a variety of growth factors to protect rat oligodendrocytes from complement attack, deploying this as a model of injury and repair in the nervous system at the single-cell level, but were unable to control the rise in calcium or to alter the threshold for vesicular recovery. Conversely, inhibiting the intracellular calcium-activated protein calmodulin, using W7, lowered the threshold for complement lysis by blocking vesiculation; under these circumstances, concentrations of serum from which oligodendrocytes were normally protected by vesicle formation proved lethal.

Fully differentiated oligodendrocytes stimulated to divide by exposure to bFGF or NGF, transduce the mitotic signal and enter the cell cycle but cannot divide and either enter a resting non-myelinating state or die by apoptosis (Muir and Compston 1996; Bansal and Pfeiffer 1997). Casaccia-Bonnefil *et al.* (1996) have also shown that mature post-natal rat cortical oligodendrocytes, but not their progenitors (or astrocytes), are selectively killed by exposure to NGF, through binding to the p75 receptor when trkA is not co-expressed, whereas no such effect is seen with brain-derived nerve growth factor (BDNF) or NT-3; p75 receptor may be upregulated on oligodendrocytes within the lesions of multiple sclerosis (Dowling *et al.* 1999). This apparent paradox is not so surprising since the trkA and p75 NGF receptors are part of the cell death pathway involving Fas and the TNF-α receptor. Thus, there may be diametrically opposite effects of growth factors on cells of the same lineage depending on the expression of receptors, the signals transduced, and their ability to enter the cell cycle.

From this and other evidence emerges the general principle that the signals transduced by cells during growth and physiological activity are the same as those which become overloaded during pathological events leading to cell injury and death. The extent to which a cell can survive injury is modulated by its growth-factor-dependent state of health; it follows that cell death may occur in response to a state of injury from which protection would be anticipated under more favourable growth-factor conditions; and conversely, optimal growth factor conditions may save cells from otherwise lethal events occurring at the cell membrane.

References

Agoropolou, C., Piddlesden, S. J., Lachmann, P. J., and Wing, M. G. (1998). Neuronal protection of oligodendrocytes from antibody-independent complement lysis. *Neuroreport*, 9, 927–32.

Archelos, J. J. and Hartung, H.-P. (1997). The role of adhesion molecules in multiple sclerosis: biology, pathogenesis and therapeutic implications. *Mol. Med. Today*, 3, 310–21.

Armstrong, R. C., Dorn, H. H., Kufta, C. V. *et al.* (1992). Pre-oligodendrocytes from adult human CNS. *J. Neurosci.*, 12, 1538–47.

Bansal, R. and Pfeiffer, S. E. (1997). FGF-2 converts mature oligodendrocytes to a novel phenotype. *J. Neurosci. Res.*, 50, 215–28.

Barger, S. W. and Harmon, A. D. (1997). Microglial activation by Alzheimer amyloid precursor protein and modulation by apolipoprotein E. *Nature*, 388, 878–81.

Barnett, S. C., Alexander, C. L., Iwashita, Y. *et al.* (2000). Identification of a human olfactory ensheathing cell that can effect transplant-remediated remyelination of demyelinated CNS axons. *Brain*, 123, 1581–8.

Barres, B. A. and Raff, M. C. (1993). Proliferation of oligodendrocyte precursor cells depends on electrical activity in axons. *Nature*, 361, 258–60.

Barres, B. A., Hart, I. K., Coles, H. S. R. *et al.* (1992). Cell death and control of cell survival in the oligodendrocyte lineage. *Cell*, 70, 31–46.

Barres, B. A., Raff, M. C., Gaese, F. *et al.* (1994). A crucial role for neurotrophin-3 in oligodendrocyte development. *Nature*, 367, 371–5.

Berridge, M. J., Bootman, M. D., and Lipp, P. (1998). Calcium—a life and death signal. *Nature*, 395, 645–8.

Bonkowsky, J. L., Yoshikawa, S., O'Keefe, D. O. *et al.* (1999). Axon routing across the midline controlled by *Drosophila* Derailed receptor. *Nature*, 402, 540–4.

Bregman, B. S., Kunkel-Bagden, E., Schnell, L. *et al.* (1995). Recovery from spinal cord injury mediated by antibodies to neurite growth inhibitors. *Nature*, 378, 498–501.

Bronstein, J. M., Popper, P., Micevych, P. E., and Farber, D. B. (1996). Isolation and characterisation of a novel oligodendrocyte-specific protein. *Neurology*, 47, 772–8.

Burne, J., Staple, J. K., and Raff, M. C. (1996). Glial cells are increased proportionally in transgenic optic nerves with increased numbers of axons. *J. Neurosci.*, 16, 2064–73.

Bush, T. B., Puvanachandra, N., Horner, C. H. *et al.* (1999). Leukocyte infiltration, neuronal degeneration, and neurite outgrowth after ablation of scar forming reactive astrocytes in adult transgenic mice. *Neuron*, 23, 297–308.

Butt, A. M. and Jenkins, H. G. (1994). Morphological changes in oligodendrocytes in the intact mouse optic nerve following intravitreal injection of tumour necrosis factor. *J. Neuroimmunol.*, 51, 27–33.

Butt, A. M. and Ransom, B. R. (1989). Visualisation of oligodendrocytes and astrocytes in the intact rat optic nerve by intracellular injection of lucifer yellow and horseradish peroxidase. *Glia*, 2, 470–5.

Cameron, R. S. and Rakic, P. (1991). Glial cell lineage in the cerebral cortex: a review and synthesis. *Glia*, 4, 124–37.

Cammer, W. and Zhang, H. (1999). Maturation of oligodendrocytes is more sensitive to TNF-α than is survival of precursors and immature oligodendrocytes. *J. Neuroimunol.*, **97**, 37–42.

Campbell, R. D. and Trowsdale, J. (1997). A map of the human major histocompatibility complex. *Immunol. Today*, **18** (inserted wall chart).

Canoll, P., Musacchio, J., Hardy, R. *et al.* (1996). GGF/neuregulin promotes the proliferation and survival and inhibits the differentiation of cells of the oligodendrocyte lineage. *Neuron*, **17**, 229–43.

Capello, E., Voskuhl, R. R., McFarland, H. F., and Raine, C. S. (1997). Multiple sclerosis: re-expression of a developmental gene in chronic lesions correlates with remyelination. *Ann. Neurol.*, **41**, 797–805.

Carroll, W. M., Jennings, A. R., and Ironside, L. J. (1998). Identification of the adult resting progenitor cell by autoradiographic tracking of oligodendrocyte precursors in experimental CNS demyelination. *Brain*, **121**, 293–302.

Casaccia-Bonnefil, P., Carter, B. D., Dobrowsky, R. T., and Chao, M. V. (1996). Death of oligodendrocytes mediated by the interaction of nerve growth factor with its receptor p75. *Nature*, **383**, 716–19.

Chao, C. C., Molitor, T. W., and Hu, S. (1993). Neuroprotective role of IL-4 against activated microglia. *J. Immunol.*, **151**, 1473–81.

Chen, D. F., Schneider, G. E., Martinou, J.-C., and Tonegawa, S. (1997). Bcl-2 promotes regeneration of severed axons in mammalian CNS. *Nature*, **385**, 434–9.

Colello, R. J., Pott, U., and Schwab, M. E. (1994). The role of oligodendrocytes and myelin on axon maturation in the developing rat retinofugal pathway. *J. Neurosci.*, **14**, 2594–605.

Colello, R. J., Devey, R. L., Imperato, E., and Pott, U. (1995). The chronology of oligodendrocyte differentiation in the rat optic nerve: evidence for a signalling step initiating myelination in the CNS. *J. Neurosci.*, **15**, 7665–72.

Compston, D. A. S. (1998). Neurobiology of multiple sclerosis. In *McAlpine's Multiple Sclerosis*, (ed. D. A. S. Compston, G. C. Ebers, H. Lassmann, *et al.*), pp. 283–321. Churchill Livingstone, London.

Curtis, R., Adryan, K. M., Zhu, Y. *et al.* (1993). Retrograde axonal transport of ciliary neurotrophic factor is increased by peripheral nerve injury. *Nature*, **365**, 253–5.

Davies, J. A., Fitch, M. T., Memberg, S. P. *et al.* (1997). Regeneration of adult axons in white matter tracts of the central nervous system. *Nature*, **390**, 680–3.

Davies, M. and Bjorkman, P. (1988). T cell antigen receptor genes and T cell recognition. *Nature*, **344**, 395–402.

De Simone, R. Giampaolo, A., Giometto, B. *et al.* (1995). The costimulatory molecule B7 is expressed on human microglia in cultured and in multiple sclerosis acute lesions. *J. Neuropath. Exp. Neurol.*, **54**, 175–87.

Doetsch, F., Caille, I., Lim, D. A. *et al.* (1999). Subventricular zone astrocytes are neural stem cells in the adult mammalian brain. *Cell*, **97**, 703–16.

Dowling, P., Ming, X., Raval, S. *et al.* (1999). Up-regulated p75[NTR] neurotrophin receptor on glial cells in MS plaques. *Neurology*, **53**, 1676–82.

D'Souza, S. D., Alinauskas, K. A., McCrea, E. *et al.* (1995). Differential susceptibility of human CNS-derived cell populations to TNF-dependent and independent immune mediated injury. *J. Neurosci.*, **15**, 7293–300.

D'Souza, S. D., Bonetti, B., Balasingam, V. *et al.* (1996). Multiple sclerosis: Fas signalling in oligodendrocyte cell death. *J. Exp. Med.*, **184**, 2361–70.

Eddleston, M. and Mucke, L. (1993). Molecular profile of reactive astrocytes—implications for their role in neurologic disease. *Neuroscience*, **54**, 15–36.

Engel, U. and Wolswijk, G. (1996). Oligodendrocyte-type-2 astrocyte (O–2a) progenitor cells derived from adult-rat spinal-cord—in-vitro characteristics and response to PDGF, bFGF and NT-3. *Glia*, **16**, 16–26.

Eriksson, P. S., Perfilieva, E., Bjork-Eriksson, T. *et al.* (1998). Neurogenesis in the adult human hippocampus. *Nature Medicine*, **4**, 1313–17.

Fawcett, J. W. and Asher, R. A. (1999). The glial scar and central nervous system repair. *Brain Res. Bull.*, **49**, 377–91.

ffrench Constant, C. and Raff, M. C. (1986). Proliferating bipotential glial progenitor cells in adult rat optic nerve. *Nature*, **319**, 499–502.

Fishell, G., Mason, C. A., and Hatten, M. E. (1993). Dispersion of neural progenitors within the germinal zones of the forebrain. *Nature*, **362**, 636–8.

Fok-Seang, J., DiProspero, N. A., Meiners, S. *et al.* (1998). Cytokine-induced changes in the ability of astrocytes to support migration of oligodendrocyte precursors and axon growth. *Europ. J. Neurosci.*, **7**, 2400–16.

Fontana, A., Wierz, W., and Wekerle, H. (1984). Astrocytes present myelin basic protein to encephalitogenic T-cell lines. *Nature*, **307**, 273–6.

Ford, A. L., Goodsall, A. L., Hickey, W. F., and Sedgwick, J. D. (1995). Normal adult microglia separated from other central nervous system macrophages by flow cytometry sorting. *J. Immunol.*, **154**, 4309–21.

Ford, A. L., Foulcher, E., Lemckert, F. A., and Sedgwick, J. D. (1996). Microglia induce CD4 T lymphocyte final effector function and death. *J. Exp. Med.*, **184**, 1737–45.

Franklin, R. J. M., Crang, A. J., and Blakemore, W. F. (1991). Transplanted type-1 astrocytes facilitate repair of demyelinating lesions by host oligodendrocytes in adult rat spinal cord. *J. Neurocytol.*, **20**, 420–30.

Franklin, R. J. M., Bayley, S. A., and Blakemore, W. F. (1996). Transplanted CG-4 cells (an oligodendrocyte progenitor cell line) survive, migrate and contribute to repair of areas of demyelination in X-irradiated and damaged spinal cord but not in normal spinal cord. *Exp. Neurol.*, **137**, 263–76.

Gay, D. and Esiri, M. M. (1991). Blood–brain barrier damage in acute multiple sclerosis plaques. An immunocytochemical study. *Brain*, **114**, 557–72.

Genain, C. P., Cannella, B., Hauser, S. L., and Raine, C. S. (1999). Identification of autoantibodies associated with myelin damage in multiple sclerosis. *Nature Medicine*, **5**, 170–5.

Goedert, M., Spillantini, M.-G., and Davies, S. W. (1998). Filamentous nerve cell inclusions in neurodegenerative diseases. *Curr. Opin. Neurobiol.*, **8**, 619–32.

Goldberg, J. L. and Barres, B. A. (2000). Nogo in nerve regeneration (news and views). *Nature*, **403**, 369–70.

Gomez, T. M. and Spitzer, N. C. (1999). In vivo regulation of axon extension and pathfinding by growth-cone calcium transients. *Nature*, **397**, 350–5.

Gould, E., Tanapat, P., McEwen, B. S. *et al.* (1998). Proliferation of granule cell precursors in the dentate gyrus of adult monkeys is diminished by stress. *Proc. Natl Acad. Sci., USA*, **95**, 3168–71.

Grabowski, M., Brundin, P., and Johansson, B. B. (1993). Functional integration of cortical grafts in brain infarcts of rats. *Ann. Neurol.*, **34**, 362–8.

Groves, A. K., Barnett, S. C., Franklin, R. J. M. *et al.* (1993). Repair of demyelinated lesions by transplantation of purified O-2A progenitor cells. *Nature*, **362**, 453–5.

Guo, Q., Fu, W., Sopher, B. L. *et al.* (1999). Increased vulnerability of hippocampal neurons to excitotoxic necrosis in presenilin-1 mutant knock-in mice. *Nature Medicine*, **5**, 101–6.

Hajihosseini, M., Tham, T. N., and Dubois-Dalcq, M. (1996). Origin of oligodendrocytes within the human spinal cord. *J. Neurosci.*, **16**, 7981–94.

Hall, G., Wing, M. G., Compston, D. A. S., and Scolding, N. J. (1997). Beta-interferon regulates the immunoregulatory activity of neonatal rodent microglia. *J. Neuroimmunol.*, **72**, 11–19.

Hall, G. L., Girdlestone, J., Compston, D. A. S., and Wing, M. G. (1999). Recall antigen presentation by gamma interferon activated microglia results in T cell proliferation, cytokine release and propagation of the immune response. *J. Neuroimmunol.*, **98**, 105–11.

Hauben, E., Nevo, U., Yoles, E. *et al.* (2000). Autoimmune T cells as potential neuroprotective therapy for spinal cord injury. *Lancet*, **354**, 286–7.

Hellendall, R. P. and Ting, J. P.-Y. (1997). Differential regulation of cytokine-induced major histocompatibility complex class II expression and nitric oxide release in rat microglia and astrocytes by effectors of tyrosine kinase, protein kinase C, and cAMP. *J. Neuroimmunol.*, **74**, 19–29.

Hirschberg, D. L. and Schwartz, M. (1995). Macrophage recruitment to acutely injured nervous system is inhibited by a resident factor: a basis for an immune-barrier. *J. Neuroimmunol.*, **61**, 89–96.

Horwitz, M. S., Evans, C. F., McGavern, D. B. *et al.* (1997). Primary demyelination in transgenic mice expressing interferon-γ. *Nature Medicine*, **3**, 1037–41.

Hunter, S. F., Leavitt, J. A., and Rodriguez, M. (1997). Direct observation of myelination *in vivo* in the mature human central nervous system. A model for the behaviour of oligodendrocyte progenitors and their progeny. *Brain*, **120**, 2071–82.

Hyman, C., Hofer, M., Barde, Y.-A. *et al.* (1991). BDNF is a neurotrophic factor for dopaminergic neurons of the substantia nigra. *Nature*, **350**, 230–2.

Jeffery, N. D. and Blakemore, W. F. (1997). Locomotor deficits induced by experimental spinal cord demyelination are abolished by spontaneous remyelination. *Brain*, **120**, 27–37.

Johansson, C. B., Momma, S., Clarke, D. L. *et al.* (1999). Identification of a neural stem cell in the adult mammalian central nervous system. *Cell*, **96**, 25–34.

Johnstone, M., Gearing, J. H., and Miller, K. M. (1999). A central role for astrocytes in the inflammatory response to β-amyloid; chemokines, cytokines and reactive oxygen species are produced. *J. Neuroimmunol.*, **93**, 182–93.

Kaplan, M. R., Meyer-Franke, A., Lambert, S. *et al.* (1997). Induction of sodium channel clustering by oligodendrocytes. *Nature*, **386**, 724–8.

Kendall, A. L., Rayment, F. D., Torres, E. M. *et al.* (1998). Functional integration of striatal allografts in a primate model of Huntington's disease. *Nature Medicine*, **4**, 727–9.

Kiersted, H. S. and Blakemore, W. F. (1997). Identification of post mitotic oligodendrocytes incapable of remyelination within the demyelinated adult spinal cord. *J. Neuropathol. Exp. Neurol.*, **56**, 1191–201.

Kiersted, H. S., Levine, J. M., and Blakemore, W. F. (1998). Response of the oligodendrocyte progenitor cell population (defined by NG2 labelling) to demyelination of the adult spinal cord. *Glia*, **22**, 161–70.

Klivenyi, P., Ferrante, R. J., Matthews, R. T. *et al.* (1999). Neuroprotective effects of creatine in a transgenic animal model of amyotrophic lateral sclerosis. *Nature Medicine*, **5**, 347–50.

Köller, H., Bucholz, J., and Siebler, M. (1996). Cerebrospinal fluid from multipole sclerosis patients inactivates neuronal Na⁺ current. *Brain*, **119**, 457–63.

Komoly, S., Hudson, L. D., deF Webster, H., and Bondy, C. A. (1992). Insulin-like growth factor 1 gene expression is induced in astrocytes during experimental demyelination. *Proc. Natl Acad. Sci., USA*, **89**, 1894–8.

Lacy, M., Jones, J., Whittemore, S. R. *et al.* (1995). Expression of the receptors for the C5a anaphylatoxin, interleukin-8 and FMLP by human astrocytes and microglia. *J. Neuroimmunol.*, **61**, 71–8.

Leppert, D., Waubant, E., Burk, M. R. *et al.* (1996). Interferon beta 1b inhibits gelatinase secretion and *in vitro* migration of human T cells: a possible mechanism for treatment efficacy in multiple sclerosis. *Ann. Neurol.*, **40**, 846–52.

Levison, S. W. and Goldman, J. E. (1993). Both oligodendrocytes and astrocytes develop from progenitors in the subventricular zone of postnatal rat forebrain. *Neuron*, **10**, 201–12.

Lindholm, D., Dechant, G., Heisenberg, C.-P., and Thoenen, H. (1993). Brain-derived neurotrophic factor is a survival factor for cultured rat cerebellar granule neurons and protects them against glutamate induced neurotoxicity. *Europ. J. Neurosci.*, **5**, 1455–64.

Liu, R., Althaus, J. S., Ellerbrock, B. R. *et al.* (1998). Enhanced oxygen radical production in a transgenic mouse model of familial amyotrophic lateral sclerosis. *Ann. Neurol.*, **44**, 763–70.

Livesey, F. J., O'Brien, J. A., Li, M. *et al.* (1997) A Schwann cell mitogen accompanying regeneration of motor neurons. *Nature*, **390**, 614–18.

Liwei, L., Hua, B. S., Liu, H. *et al.* (1998). Selective inhibition of human glial inducible nitric oxide synthase by interferon-B: implications for multiple sclerosis. *Ann. Neurol.*, **43**, 384–7.

Louis, J.-C., Magal, E., Takayama, S., and Varon, S. (1993). CNTF protection of oligodendrocytes against natural and tumor necrosis factor-induced death. *Science*, **259**, 689–92.

Ludwin, S. K. (1997). The pathobiology of the oligodendrocyte. *J. Neuropathol. Exp. Neurol.*, **56**, 111–24.

McDonald, J. W., Liu, X.-Z., Q Y *et al.* (1999). Transplanted embryonic stem cells survive, differentiate and promote recovery in injured rat spinal cord. *Nature Medicine*, **12**, 1410–12.

McKerracher, L., David, S., Jackson, D. L. *et al.* (1994). Identification of myelin associated glycoprotein as a major myelin-derived inhibitor of neurite growth. *Neuron*, **13**, 805–11.

Meda, L., Baron, P., Prat, E. *et al.* (1999). Proinflammatory profile of cytokine production by human monocytes and murine microglia stimulated with β amyloid[25–35]. *J. Neuroimmunol.*, **93**, 45–52.

Meinl, E., Aloisi, F., Erd, B. *et al.* (1994). Multiple sclerosis: immunomodulatory effects of human astrocytes on T-cells. *Brain*, **117**, 1323–32.

Merrill, J. E., Ignarro, L. J., Sherman, M. P. *et al.* (1993). Microglial cell cytotoxicity of oligodendrocytes is mediated through nitric oxide. *J. Immunol.*, **151**, 2132–41.

Meyer-Franke, A., Kaplan, M. R., Pfeiger, F. W., and Barres, B. A. (1995). Characterisation of the signalling interactions that promote the survival and growth of developing retinal ganglion cells in culture. *Neuron*, **15**, 805–19.

Moalem, G., Leibowitz-Amit, R., Yoles, E. *et al.* (1999). Autoimmune T cells protect neurons from secondary degeneration after central nervous system axotomy. *Nature Medicine*, **5**, 49–54.

Montag, D., Giese, K. P., Bartsch, V. *et al.* (1994). Mice deficient for the myelin associated glycoprotein show subtle changes 1abnormalities in myelin. *Neuron*, **13**, 229–46.

Morgan, T. E., Nichols, N. R., Pasinetti, G. M., and Finch, C. E. (1993). TGF-beta1 mRNA increases in macrophage/microglial cells of the hippocampus in response to deafferentation and kainic acid-induced neurodegeneration. *Exp. Neurol.*, **120**, 291–301.

Muir, D. and Compston, D. A. S. (1996). Growth factor stimulation triggers apoptic cell death in mature rat oligodendrocytes. *J. Neurosci. Res.*, **44**, 1–11.

Mukhopadhyay, G., Doherty, P., Walsh, F. S. *et al.* (1994). A novel role for myelin associated glycoprotein as an inhibitor of axonal regeneration. *Neuron*, **13**, 757–67.

Murray, K. and Dubois Dalcq, M. (1997). Emergence of oligodendrocytes from human neural spheres. *J. Neurosci. Res.*, **50**, 146–56.

Neumann, H., Cavalie, A., Jenne, D. E., and Wekerle, H. (1995). Induction of MHC class I genes in neurons. *Science*, **269**, 549–52.

Neumann, H., Schmidt, H., Cavalie, A. *et al.* (1997). MHC class I gene expression in single neurons of the central nervous system: Differential regulation by interferon-γ and tumor necrosis factor-α. *J. Exp. Med.*, **185**, 305–16.

Nicholas, R. St J., Compston, D. A. S., and Wing, M. G. (2001). Microglia regulate oligodendrocyte lineage survival and maturation through the PDGF pathway and then transcription factor NF-$_\kappa$B. *Eur. J. Neurosci.* (in press).

Palfi, S., Conde, F., Riche, D. *et al.* (1998). Fetal striatal allografts reverse cognitive deficits in a primate model of Huntington's disease. *Nature Medicine*, **4**, 963–6.

Pan, Y., Lloyd, C., Zhou, H. *et al.* (1997). Neurotactin, a membrane-anchored chemokine upregulated in brain inflammation. *Nature*, **387**, 611–17.

Patton, B. L., Chiu, A. Y., and Sanes, J. R. (1998). Synaptic laminin prevents glial entry into the synaptic cleft. *Nature*, **393**, 698–701.

Pedersen, W. A., Fu, W., Keller, J. N. *et al.* (1998). Protein modification by the lipid peroxidartion product 4-hydroxynonenal in the spinal cords of amyotrophic lateral sclerosis patients. *Ann. Neurol.*, **44**, 819–24.

Perry, V. H. (1998). A revised view of the central nervous system microenvironment and major histocompatibility complex class II antigen presentation. *J. Neuroimmunol.*, **90**, 113–21.

Piddlesden, S. J. and Morgan, B. P. (1993). Killing of rat glial cells by complement: Deficiency of the rat analogue of CD59 is the cause of oligodendrocyte susceptibility to lysis. *J. Neuroimmunol.*, **48**, 169–76.

Pincus, D. W., Keyoung, M., Harrison-Restelli, C. *et al.* (1998). Fibroblast growth factor-2/brain derived nerve growth factor-associated maturation of new neurons generated from adult human subependymal cells. *Ann. Neurol.*, **43**, 576–85.

Pryce, G., Male, D., Campbell, I., and Greenwood, J. (1997). Factors controlling T-cell migration across rat endothelium *in vitro. J. Neuroimmunol.*, **75**, 84–94.

Qian, X., Davis, A. A., Goderie, S. K., and Temple, S. (1997). FGF2 concentration regulates the generation of neurons and glia from multipotent cortical stem cells. *Neuron*, **18**, 81–93.

Raff, M. C. (1998). Cell suicide for beginners. *Nature*, **396**, 119–22.

Raff, M. C., Miller, R. H., and Noble, M. (1983). A glial progenitor that develops *in vitro* into an astrocyte or an oligodendrocyte depending on culture medium. *Nature*, **303**, 390–6.

Raine, C. S. (1997). The Norton Lecture: a review of the oligodendrocyte in the multiple sclerosis lesion. *J. Neuroimmunol.*, **77**, 135–52.

Rapalino, O., Lazarov-Spiegler, O., Agranov, E. *et al.* (1998). Implantation of stimulated homologous macrophages results in partial recovery of paraplegic rats. Nature Medicine, **4**, 814–21.

Reindl, M., Linington, C., Brehm, U. *et al.* (1999). Antibodies against the myelin oligodendrocyte glycoprotein and the myelin basic protein in multiple sclerosis and other neurological diseases: a comparative study. *Brain*, **122**, 2047–56.

Rensing-Ehl, A., Malpiero, U., Irmler, M. *et al.* (1996). Neurons induced to express major histocompatibility complex class I antigen are killed via the perforin and not the Fas (APO-1/CD95) pathway. *Europ. J. Immunol.*, **26**, 2771–4.

Reynolds, B. A. and Weiss, S. (1992). Generation of neurons and astrocytes from isolated cells of the adult mammalian central nervous system. *Science*, **255**, 1707–10.

Rieckmann, P., Michel, U., Albrecht, M. *et al.* (1995). Soluble forms of intercellular adhesion molecule-1 (ICAM-1) block lymphocyte attachment to cerebral endothelial cells. *J. Neuroimmunol.*, **60**, 9–15.

Rivkin, M. J., Flax, J., Mozell, R. *et al.* (1995). Oligodendroglial development in human fetal cerebrum. *Ann. Neurol.*, **38**, 92–101.

Rosen, D. R., Siddique, T., Patterson, D. *et al.* (1993). Mutations in Cu/Zn superoxide dismutase gene are associated with familial amyotrophic lateral sclerosis. *Nature*, **362**, 59–62.

Rosser, A. E., Tyres, P., ter Borg, M. *et al.* (1997). Co-expression of MAP-2 and GFAP in cells developing from rat EGF responsive precursor cells. *Develop. Brain Res.*, **98**, 291–5.

Rothstein, J. D., Martin, L. J., and Kuncl, R. W. (1992). Decreased glutamate transport by the brain and spinal cord in amyotrophic lateral sclerosis. *N. Engl. J. Med.*, **326**, 1464–8.

Sanches, T., Hassinger, L., Paskevich, P. A. *et al.* (1996). Oligodendroglia regulate the regional expansion of axon calibre and local accumulation of neurofilaments during development independent of myelin formation. *J. Neurosci.*, **16**, 5095–105.

Satoh, J. and Kim, S. U. (1994). Proliferation and differentiation of fetal human oligodendrocytes *in vitro. J. Neurosci. Res.*, **39**, 260–72.

Schierle, G., Hansson, O., Leist, M. *et al.* (1999). Caspase inhibition reduces apoptosis and increases survival of nigral transplants. *Nature Medicine*, **5**, 97–106.

Scolding, N. J. and Compston, D. A. S. (1991). Oligodendrocyte-macrophage interactions *in vitro* triggered by specific antibodies. *Immunology*, **72**, 127–32.

Scolding, N. J. and Compston, D. A. S. (1995). Growth factors fail to protect oligodendrocytes against humoral injury *in vitro. Neurosci. Lett.*, **183**, 75–8.

Scolding, N. J., Morgan, B. P., Houston, W. A. J. *et al.* (1989). Vesicular removal by oligodendrocytes of membrane attack complexes formed by complement. Nature, **339**, 620–2.

Scolding, N. J., Rayner, P. J., Sussman, J. *et al.* (1995). A proliferative adult human oligodendrocyte progenitor. *NeuroReport*, **6**, 441–5.

Scolding, N., Franklin, R., Stevens, S. *et al.* (1998). Oligodendrocyte progenitors are present in the normal adult human CNS and in the lesions of multiple sclerosis. *Brain*, **121**, 2221–8.

Scolding, N. J., Rayner, P. J., and Compston, D. A. S. (1999). Early oligodendrocyte progenitors and *type-2* astrocytes are present in adult human white matter. *Neuroscience*, **89**, 1–5.

Seilhean, D., Gansmuller, A., Baron-van Evercooren *et al.* (1996). Myelination by transplanted human and mouse central nervous system tissue after long-term cryopreservation. *Acta Neuropathol.*, **91**, 82–8.

Selmaj, K., Raine, C. S., Cannella, B., and Brosnan, C. F. (1991). Identification of lymphotoxin and tumor necrosis factor in multiple sclerosis lesions. *J. Clin. Invest.*, **87**, 949–54.

Sendtner, M., Holtmann, B., Kolbeck, R. *et al.* (1992). Brain-derived neurotrophic factor prevents the death of motoneurones in newborn rats after nerve section. *Nature*, **360**, 757–9.

Shah, N. M., Marchionni, M. A., Isaacs, I. *et al.* (1994). Glial growth factor restricts mammalian neural crest stem cells to a glial fate. *Cell*, **77**, 349–60.

Shaw, C. E., Milner, R. M., Compston, D. A. S., and ffrench Constant, C. (1996). Integrin expression during axo-glial interactions: a developmental comparison of oligodendrocytes and Schwann cells. *J. Neurosci.*, **16**, 1163–72.

Sheng, M. and Greenberg, M. E. (1990). The regulation and function of c-*fos* and other immediate early genes in the nervous system. *Neuron*, **4**, 477–85.

Smeyne, R. J., Vendrell, M., Hayward, M. *et al.* (1993). Continuous c-Fos expression precedes programmed cell death *in vivo*. *Nature*, **353**, 166–9.

Smith, K. J., Blakemore, W. F., and McDonald, W. I. (1981). The restoration of conduction by central remyelination. *Brain*, **104**, 383–404.

Stuve, O., Dooley, N. P., Uhm, J. H. *et al.* (1996). Interferon β-1b decreases the migration of T lymphocytes *in vitro*: effects on matrix metalloproteinase-9. *Ann. Neurol.*, **40**, 853–63.

Suhonen, J. A., Peterson, D. A., Ray, J., and Gage, F. H. (1996). Differentiation of adult hippocampus-derived progenitors into olfactory neurons *in vivo*. *Nature*, **383**, 624–7.

Sun, D., Coleclough, C., Cao, L. *et al.* (1998). Reciprocal stimulation between TNF-α and nitric oxide may exacerbate CNS inflammation in experimental autoimmune encephalomyelitis. *J. Neuroimmunol.*, **89**, 122–30.

Targett, M. P. *et al.* (1996). Failure to remyelinate rat axons following transplantation of glial cells obtained from the adult human brain. *Neuropath. Appl. Neurobiol.*, **22**, 199–206.

Thompson, J. A., Itskovitz-Eldor, J., Shapiro, S. S. *et al.* (1998). Embryonic stem cell lines derived from human blastocysts. *Science*, **282**, 1145–7.

Urushitani, M., Shimohama, S., Kihara, T. *et al.* (1998). Mechanism of selective motor neuronal death after exposure of spinal cord to glutamate: involvement of glutamate-induced nitric oxide in motor neuron toxicity and non-motor neuron protection. *Ann. Neurol.*, **44**, 796–807.

van der Laan, L. J. W., Ruuls, S. R., Weber, K. S. *et al.* (1996). Macrophage phagocytosis of myelin *in vitro* determined by flow cytometry: phagocytosis is mediated by CR3 and induces production of tumor necrosis factor-A and nitric oxide. *J. Neuroimmunol.*, **70**, 45–152.

Wang, H. and Tessier-Lavigne, M. (1999). *En passant* neurotrophic action of an intermediate axonal target in the developing mammalian CNS. *Nature*, **401**, 765–9.

Weidenheim, K. M., Epshteyn, I., Rashbaum, W. K., and Lyman, W. D. (1994). Patterns of glial development in the human foetal spinal cord during the late first and second trimester. *J. Neurocytol.*, **23**, 343–53.

Wekerle, H., Linington, C., Lassmann, H., and Meyerman, R. (1986). Cellular immune reactivity within the CNS. *Trends in Neurosci.*, **9**, 271–7.

Weller, R. O., Engelhardt, B., and Phillips, M. J. (1996). Lymphocyte targeting of the central nervous system: a review of afferent and efferent CNS-immune pathways. *Brain Pathol.*, **6**, 275–88.

Whittemore, S. R., Sanon, H. R., and Wood, P. M. (1993). Concurrent isolation and characterisation of oligodendrocytes, microglia and astrocytes from adult human spinal cord. *Internat. J. Develop. Neurosci.*, **11**, 755–64.

Williams, K., Bar-Or, A., Ulvestad, E. *et al.* (1992). Biology of adult human microglia in culture: comparison with peripheral blood monocytes and astrocytes. *J. Neuropathol. Exp. Neurol.*, **51**, 538–49.

Williams, K., Ulvestad, E., Cragg, L. *et al.* (1993). Induction of primary T cell responses by human glial cells. *J. Neurosci. Res.*, **36**, 382–90.

Wolswijk, G. (1998). Chronic stage multiple sclerosis lesions contain a relatively quiescent population of oligodendrocyte precursor cells. *J. Neurosci.*, **18**, 601–9.

Wood, A., Wing, M. G., Benham, C. D., and Compston, D. A. S. (1993). Specific induction of intracellular calcium oscillations by complement membrane attack on oligodendroglia. *J. Neurosci.*, **13**, 3319–32.

Wren, D., Wolswijk, G., and Noble, M. (1992). *In vitro* analysis of the origin and maintenance of O-2A^adult progenitor cells. *J. Cell Biol.*, **116**, 176–186.

Xiao, B. G. and Link, H. (1998). Immune regulation within the central nervous system. *J. Neuroimmunol.*, **157**, 1–12.

Yan, Q., Elliott, J., and Snider, W. D. (1992). Brain-derived neurotrophic factor rescues spinal motor neurons from axotomy-induced cell death. *Nature*, **360**, 753–5.

Yao, D.-L., Liu, X., Hudson, L. D., and Webster, H. deF. (1995). Insulin-like growth factor 1 treatment reduces demyelination and up-regulates gene expression of myelin related proteins in experimental autoimmune encephalomyelitis. *Proc. Natl Acad. Sci., USA*, **92**, 6190–4.

Yednock, T. A., Cannon, C., Fritz, L. C. *et al.* (1992). Prevention of experimental autoimmune encephalomyelitis by antibodies against α4β1 integrin. *Nature*, **356**, 63–6.

Yoshioka, A., Hardy, M., Younkin, D. P. *et al.* (1995). Alpha-amino-3-hydroxy-5-methyl-4-isoxazoleproprionate (AMPA) receptors mediate excitotoxicity in the oligodendroglial lineage. *J. Neurochem.*, **64**, 2442–8.

Yu, W. P., Collarini, E. J., Pringle, N. P., and Richardson, W. D. (1994). Embryonic expression of myelin genes: Evidence for a focal source of oligodendrocyte precursors in the ventricular zone of the neural tube. *Neuron*, **12**, 1353–62.

Zajicek, J. P. and Compston, D. A. S. (1994). Myelination *in vitro* of dorsal root ganglia by glial progenitor cells. *Brain*, **117**, 1333–50.

Zajicek, J. P. and Compston, D. A. S. (1995). Human oligodendrocytes are not sensitive to complement—a study of CD59 expression in the human central nervous system. *Lab. Invest.*, **73**, 128–38.

Zajicek, J. P., Wing, M., Scolding, N. J., and Compston, D. A. S. (1992). Interactions between oligodendrocytes and microglia, a major role for complement and tumour necrosis factor in oligodendrocyte adherence and killing. *Brain*, **115**, 1611–31.

Zawada, W. M., Cibelli, J. B., Choi, P. K. *et al.* (1998). Somatic cell cloned transgenic bovine neurons for transplantation in parkinsonian rats. *Nature Medicine*, **4**, 569–74.

Zhang, Z., Hartmann, H., Minh Do, V. *et al.* (1998). Destabilization of β-catenin by mutations in presenilin-1 potentiates neuronal apoptosis. *Nature*, **395**, 698–702.

Disorders of special senses

CHAPTER 8

Neuro-ophthalmology

Christopher Kennard

8.1 Introduction

Neuro-ophthalmology is a discipline comprising a wide variety of disorders that overlap the fields of neurology, ophthalmology, and general medicine. Diagnosis in this field requires a good knowledge of the anatomy and physiology of the visual pathways and ocular motor system, as well as the ability to carry out a thorough neuro-ophthalmological examination. It is this examination which should enable a full differential diagnosis to be reached, so that the appropriate investigative techniques, such as imaging or electrophysiology, can be appropriately performed and directed. Comprehensive coverage of all aspects of clinical neuro-opthalmology is to be found in the five volume compendium *Walsh and Hoyt's Clinical Neuro-opthalmology* (Miller and Newman 1998).

8.2 Assessment of visual sensory function

Vision is one of the major sensory inputs in humans, and defects at any point along the visual pathway, from eye to cortex, often rapidly become obvious to the patient as impaired visual acuity or localized defects in their field of vision. Therefore the first requirement when a patient presents with impaired vision is to determine the best corrected visual acuity and, by clinical evaluation, to attempt to localize the site of the lesion. This is vital if the sophisticated imaging and electro-physiological techniques currently available are to be directed at the appropriate site along the visual pathways.

8.2.1 Visual acuity

The visual acuity is determined for each eye using a Snellen chart, and refraction is used if there is any impairment. A simpler method for the bedside is to retest the acuity with the patient observing the chart through a pinhole (multiple pinholes with diameters 2.0–2.5 mm are best). This improves acuity in uncorrected refractive errors and with abnormalities of the cornea, its tear film, and the lens. It should be remembered that the cornea is the main refractory surface of the eye and damage to it or its tear film by local inflammatory adnexal disease, poor lid coverage, or diminished blinking may all result in complaints of impaired vision. Determining visual acuity can offer clues as to the presence of field defects, e.g. a patient with a hemianopia may only read one side of the chart, and one with a central scotoma searches the chart to try and see round the scotoma.

If the acuity is still reduced, the eye must be carefully assessed ophthalmologically to exclude any opacities in the ocular media or lesions of the fundus. This can only be adequately performed with a properly dilated pupil and the benefits derived from this simple procedure far outweigh the exceedingly small risk of precipitating glaucoma. If no obvious cause for the visual loss is found in the fundus, it is still possible that minimal changes in the retina or retinal pigment epithelium may be the cause. The *brightness test* may be used to differentiate between this and optic nerve disease. A bright light is simply shone into each eye in turn and the patient is asked if the light is of equal brightness. If a difference is noted, this can be roughly quantitated by asking the patient to give the normal stimulus a value of 100 per cent, and then give the degree of brightness in the other eye an appropriate value. If a diminution in brightness is found in one eye this is likely to be due to optic nerve disease rather than macular lesions or pigmentary abnormalities. The *photostress test*, in contrast, is abnormal when retinal lesions are present. In this test the best corrected acuity of the patient is assessed and a bright light is directed into one eye for 10 seconds. The recovery time taken for the patient to read the next larger line on the acuity chart is recorded and the test repeated on the other eye. A comparison of the recovery times for the two eyes is made, and if there is a marked prolongation in one this is likely to be due to macular receptor disease.

8.2.2 Pupil–light reflex

A further useful specific indicator of optic nerve disease is the finding of a relative afferent pupillary defect (Marcus Gunn pupil) using the *swinging flashlight test*. The technique for performing this test is described in Section 8.9.2. If an afferent pupillary defect is detected, further confirmation of optic nerve disease is obtained by tests of *colour perception*.

8.2.3 Colour perception

This can be performed quickly by asking the patient to compare the red colour, e.g. of the top of a mydriatic bottle, viewed separately by each eye. Even quite large choroido-retinal lesions fail to produce a gross impairment of colour recognition. However, optic nerve disease may result in the red colour appearing faded, grey, orange, or pink. A more formal examination of colour vision can be made using pseudo-isochromatic plates (Hardy–Rand–Rittler, Ishihara). Optic nerve lesions classically produce red–green defects of variable intensity.

8.2.4 Visual fields

If these tests show that there is visual loss due to a neuroretinal lesion, the next step is the examination of the *visual fields*. *Simple confrontation tests* can be used as a screening test at the bedside and, if carefully performed, will identify most neurologically produced visual field defects. These allow examination of two important regions: the central field (especially the fixational area) in the diagnosis of optic nerve disease, and the fields about the vertical meridian in the diagnosis of chiasmal and hemianopic defects. Hand or colour comparison is tested by asking the patient to monocularly fixate the examiner who places his two hands (or two equal red objects) in front of the patient on either side of the vertical meridian, first in the upper quadrants and then in the lower ones. The patient then compares them for colour, brightness, and clarity and reports any difference. If the hand or object is abnormally perceived, it is slowly moved towards the vertical meridian, the patient being asked to indicate when it appears normal compared with the stationary object. For example, in an early temporal field defect due to a chiasmic lesion, the target will demonstrably 'brighten' or its colour become normal when it passes through the vertical meridian into the nasal field.

The central visual field may be explored by moving a 5–10 mm red or white hatpin away from or towards the central point of fixation. The patient is asked if the target changes in colour or brightness or if it disappears indicating that it is a relative or absolute scotoma respectively.

Another useful method is the Amsler grid, which consists of a series of lined and patterned grids for testing the central 20° at reading distance. Although mainly used by ophthalmologists for patients with macular disease, these plates can quickly identify small central or paracentral scotomas that occur in optic nerve disease.

More detailed examination of the visual fields may be made using a tangent (Bjerrum) screen for the central 20–40° of the visual field. The central and paracentral regions, as well as the blind spot, can be examined. In addition, both horizontal and vertical 'steps' and the degree of congruity of binocular field defects can be sought. For accurate recording of a field defect and comparison of changes with time, a Goldmann perimeter is best used but its detailed description is beyond the scope of this chapter.

Examination of the visual fields in infants and children may be difficult. Visually elicited movements constitute a useful technique in which a bright or large stimulus, e.g. a picture of Donald Duck, is presented in the child's peripheral field. This normally initiates a reflex movement, bringing the target on to the fovea, and provides a test of gross function in the peripheral field. This technique is a valuable method for testing infants, but may also be used in partially sighted patients and for bitemporal or homonymous hemianopic field defects. The other method useful for children is the finger counting test, and one may ask them to mimic the number of fingers presented.

The localization of a lesion in the visual pathways producing visual loss can often be achieved by the visual field examination and, although details of specific field defects are described in subsequent sections, a brief summary will be given here (Fig. 8.1).

The first important distinction to be made is between those *field defects* that have a nerve fibre bundle configuration and those that have a clear hemianopic defect. The former, usually involving the central, caecal, or arcuate region, indicates a lesion either in the retinal nerve fibre layer or in the anterior part of the optic nerve, whereas the latter suggests a chiasmic or retrochiasmic lesion. If a monocular nerve fibre bundle type field defect is found, the chances that it is due to a compressive lesion are extremely small (approximately 3 per cent). If, however, a unilateral or bilateral hemianopic field defect is detected in association with impaired visual acuity, a compressive, chiasmal lesion is extremely probable.

The ganglion cell axons show a specific pattern which can give rise to specific visual field defects when they are damaged. A central scotoma results from a lesion of the fibres from ganglion cells passing directly from the foveal region to the optic disc (Fig. 8.2A), whereas a centrocaecal scotoma involves fibres from both the macula and the area between the macula and the optic disc. Nerve fibres from the temporal region course above and below the papillo-macular bundle, and a lesion here gives rise to an arcuate scotoma (C). Finally, if the nasal retina fibres are involved, a wedge-shaped scotoma results, with its apex at the blind spot (Fig. 8.2D).

The ganglion cell axons from the peripheral retina assume a position deeper within the nerve fibre layer than those arising from ganglion cells closer to the optic nerve. As a result, fibres from the posterior pole congregate in the centre of the optic

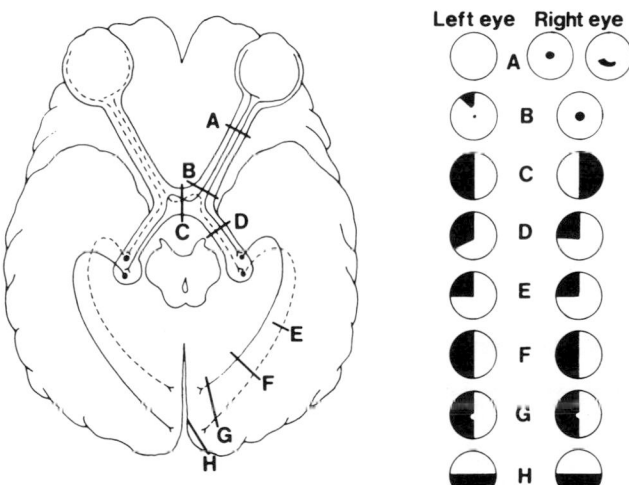

Fig. 8.1. Patterns of visual field loss: (A) Optic nerve lesions result in a central scotoma or arcuate defect. (B) Optic nerve lesions just prior to the chiasm produce junctional scotoma due to ipsilateral optic nerve involvement with the inferior contralateral crossing fibres (dotted line). (C) Chiasm lesions produce a bitemporal hemianopia. (D) Optic tract lesions result in incongruous hemianopic defects. (E, F) Lesions of the optic radiation result in either homonymous quadrantinopia or hemianopia, depending on the extent and location of the lesion (upper quadrant, temporal lobe; lower quadrant, parietal lobe). (G) Lesions of the striate cortex produce a homonymous hemianopia, sometimes with macular sparing, particularly with vascular disturbances. (H) Partial lesions of the superior or inferior bank of the striate cortex cause inferior or superior altitudinal field defects, respectively.

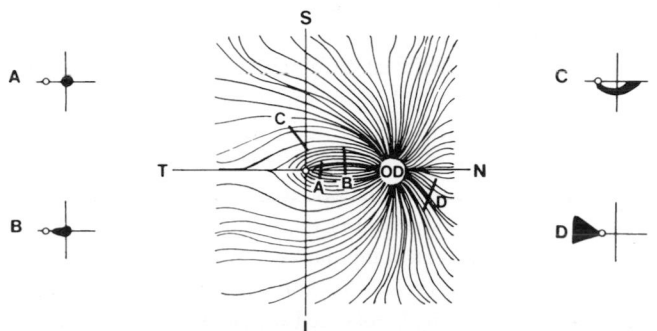

Fig. 8.2. Retinal nerve fibre layer defects (see text for description).

nerve, whereas those from the periphery are arrayed around the outer aspects of the nerve.

Hemianopic field defects indicate disease of the chiasmal or retrochiasmal visual pathways. These defects have a border aligned to the vertical meridian, but do not necessarily involve the whole hemifield. The classic bitemporal hemianopia of a lesion of the optic chiasm is rarely symmetrical. In such cases the optic nerve is also often involved, resulting in impaired acuity. Various characteristic field defect are found in chiasmic lesions. Lesions involving the retrochiasmic visual pathway mainly produce field defects which are congruent, except when the optic tract or lateral geniculate nucleus is involved. Depending on the extent of involvement of the optic radiation, a homonymous quadrantanopia or hemianopic field defect is produced. Homonymous altitudinal field defects normally result from lesions of the upper or lower calcarine (visual) cortex. The presence of macular sparing of vision indicates that the hemianopia is due to a lesion of the posterior occipital lobe; but it should be noted that lesions of the occipital pole can produce a small, central, homonymous hemianopic field defect, which may be missed if only the peripheral visual field is examined.

8.3 Retinal disorders

8.3.1 Anatomy

The retina is a multilaminated structure which extends from the ora serrata anteriorly to the optic nerve posteriorly. The retinal layers consist of a number of different cell types, which include photoreceptors (rods and cones), pigment epithelial cells, bipolar cells, horizontal cells, amacrine cells, ganglion cells, and Müller cells. The retina is strikingly laminated in cross-section. The outermost layer consists of the pigment epithelial cells which send out finger-like processes which interdigitate between the outer segments of the receptor cells. The outer nuclear layer of the retina consists of the inner segments of the receptors which contain many mitochondria and nuclei. Moving towards the inner surface of the retina, there is the outer plexiform layer, which consists of synaptic contacts between the photoreceptors and the dendrites of bipolar cells, the cell bodies of which constitute the *nuclear layer*. In addition this layer contains horizontal cells, which connect the photoreceptors and amacrine cells which form connections between terminals of the bipolar cells and the dendrites of ganglion cells. The inner plexiform layer consists of connections between bipolar terminals and dendrites of ganglion cells, the nuclei of which form the *innermost cell layer* of the retina. The inner surface of the retina contains the axons of the ganglion cells which course along the inner surface of the retina to enter the optic nerve at the optic disc. The pregenicular visual pathway can be reviewed simplistically as consisting of three cell types: the photoreceptor, bipolar cell, and ganglion cell. Only injury to the ganglion cell or its axon will result in optic atrophy, whereas damage to the bipolar cells or photoreceptors alone do not lead to disc pallor.

The distribution of the two types of photoreceptors across the retina is non-uniform. Whereas rods are widely dispersed, cones are mainly located in the central macula area. The fovea itself is rod free and consists of some 100 000 slender cones. The retinal ganglion cells also show a non-uniform distribution, being four or five cells thick in the parafoveal zone, thinning rapidly towards the retinal periphery to a single non-contiguous cell layer.

8.3.2 Retinal degenerations

Degenerative diseases which affect the photoreceptors and/or the retinal pigment epithelium of the outer retina often produce a variety of symptoms, for which terms such as retinitis pigmentosa, pigmentary retinopathy, tapeto-retinal degeneration, and retinal dystrophy are often used interchangeably (Newsome 1988). A number of other aetiologies such as inflammation, toxic causes, ischaemia, and trauma can lead to secondary retinal degeneration. The principal clinical features are poor night vision, diminished peripheral fields, narrowed retinal vessels, waxy pallor of the disc and abnormal pigment deposits called 'bone spicules' observed in the peripheral region of the fundus. This pigmentary retinopathy may be absent in early cases which typically demonstrate fine white spots scattered over the retina (retinitis punctata albescens), or may be restricted to one sector of the retina, often giving rise to superior temporal visual field defects, sometimes causing confusion with chiasmal compressive lesions. More typically a visual field defect starts as a ring scotoma which gradually enlarges out towards the periphery and in towards fixation.

The aetiology is usually genetic, with a variety of patterns of inheritance including autosomal dominant, autosomal recessive, X-linked, and mitochondrial.

Although the diagnosis of retinal photoreceptor degeneration can often be made clinically, several investigations may be helpful, including fluorescein angiography and the electroretinogram (ERG), which shows a marked diminution or extinction.

Cone dystrophy (cone–rod degeneration)

In this condition a cone dystrophy leads to diminished central acuity and reduced colour vision, and clinical examination reveals a central scotoma, generalized field constriction, ring scotoma, pseudo-altitudinal defects and centro-caecal scotoma, nystagmus, and a bull's-eye macula appearance (Krauss and Heckenlively 1982). Nyctalopia (night blindness) may not be present at the outset. The ERG shows a severely depressed photic response.

Leber's congenital amaurosis

In this congenital form of retinitis pigmentosa, infants are born blind or nearly so. Although the fundus may initially appear normal, the ERG is extinguished, and subsequently typical bone spicule changes and retinal vessel narrowing appear. This entity accounts for a large proportion of all blindness in children in some countries, but it is not thought to be associated with severe intellectual impairment or poor educability, as was once considered.

Retinal degeneration associated with mitochondrial DNA deletions

A 'salt and pepper' retinopathy is found in Kearns–Sayre syndrome which, in addition, is associated with progressive ophthalmoplegia and at least one of either cardiac conduction abnormalities, cerebellar dysfunction, or elevated spinal fluid (CSF) protein. In rare cases of mitochondrial myopathy, encephalopathy, lactic acidosis, and stroke-like episodes (MELAS) a pigmentary retinopathy has been observed (Holt *et al.* 1990).

Paraneoplastic retinal degenerations

The principal symptom reported by patients with cancer-associated retinopathy (CAR) is of bizarre entopic phenomena, which include intermittent shimmering or flashing lights and floaters (Chung and Selhorst 1992). There is usually a progressive decline in vision associated with a ring scotoma, and fundoscopy shows retinal arterial attenuation. An initial search for a metabolic or toxic cause is negative and some months later a remote cancer is discovered. It is likely that the cancer leads to the development of anti-photoreceptor antibodies.

Specific idiopathic retinal degenerations: acute zonule occult outer retinopathy; big blind spot syndrome; multiple evanescent white dot syndrome

In recent years a number of idiopathic syndromes have been described in which there is rapid visual loss of an area of outer retinal function which is associated with photopsia and minimal fundoscopic abnormalities (Gass 1993). The abnormalities usually affect one or both eyes, and the condition is found predominantly in young women. In one variety of acute zonule occult outer retinopathy (AZOOR), scotomas are centred around the normal blind spot, giving rise to the big blind spot syndrome. In a further variant, multiple evanescent white dot syndrome (MEUDS), acute white outer retinal lesions and vitreous haze are seen, which fade rapidly. With time, retinal pigment epithelium atrophy develops, but the field defects usually persist (Hamed *et al.* 1989). It is important to be aware of these conditions, which may be misdiagnosed as cases of optic neuritis, cancer associated retinopathy, or acute neuroretinitis.

8.3.3 Vascular occlusive disease

Temporary or partial occlusion of the retinal arteries and veins, either separately or jointly, may lead to transient monocular blindness (amaurosis fugax) or a permanent, complete, or partial monocular visual failure.

Central retinal artery occlusion

In central retinal artery occlusion the onset of painless blindness is usually sudden. A relative afferent pupillary defect is usually found and fundoscopy reveals, within the first few

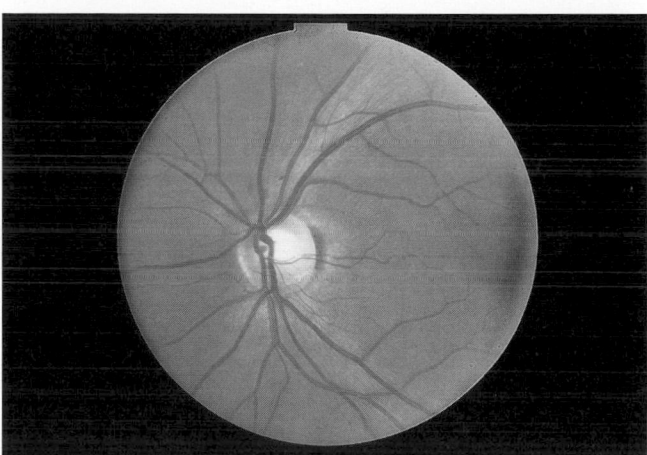

Fig. 8.3. A normal fundus and optic disc (see also colour Plate 10).

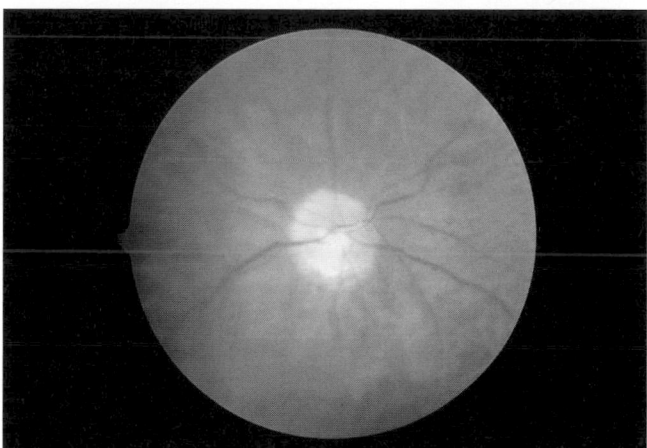

Fig. 8.4. Central retinal artery occlusion (see also colour Plate 11).

minutes of the onset, 'cattle truck' segmentation of the venous blood column, associated with arterial narrowing. After about an hour the affected retina becomes pale, and a cherry-red macular spot is observed at the fovea (Figs 8.3, 8.4). Such changes fade, usually to be replaced by optic atrophy and a markedly narrowed arterial tree. Several different causes of central retinal artery occlusion have been described, which include embolic obstruction from carotid atheroma or calcific cardiac valve disease, local artery atheroma, arteritis, drug abuse, and vasospasm associated with migraine.

In some cases temporary, complete or altitudinal visual loss (amaurosis fugax) may occur in an eye prior to the onset of central retinal artery occlusion (CRAO). Retinal emboli are usually composed of cholesterol, platelets, or calcium, but occasionally they can be due to fat emboli as a result of long-bone fractures or pancreatitis, and foreign bodies such as talc in intravenous drug abusers.

The acute treatment of CRAO is still controversial, since irreversible damage to the retina usually occurs within 2–4 hours. It is, however, worth attempting certain treatments within the first 12 hours. These include ocular massage, with the aim of lowering the intraocular pressure in an attempt to dislodge an embolus into the peripheral circulation, intravenous acetazolamide, and CO_2 rebreathing.

Lesser degrees of visual field loss, usually taking the form of an altitudinal hemianopia or ocular scotoma, are usually found with branch retinal artery occlusions. These are usually due to an embolus lodging at a first- or second-order bifurcation of the central retinal artery. Fundoscopy reveals a pallid retinal oedema in an area which corresponds to the visual field defect. Further details about the investigation and management of patients with amaurosis fugax are to be found in Chapter 27.

Chronic ocular ischaemia

In patients with occlusion of one carotid artery in association with severe stenosis of the remaining carotid and vertebral arteries, severe chronic ocular ischaemia may occur due to inadequate blood supply via the ophthalmic artery. Initially this presents with venous stasis retinopathy in the posterior pole, but with time leads to anterior segment abnormalities (Riordan-Eva *et al.* 1994).

In addition to carotid disease, other systemic diseases, such as hyperviscosity syndromes, blood dyscrasias, or severe anaemia, which lead to a reduced oxygen supply to the eye may give rise to a similar condition.

Patients with this condition may complain of blurring of vision, but may also experience a dazzling phenomenon when exposed to bright light, which is thought to be due to hypoxia of the photoreceptors. The initial venous stasis retinopathy has many features which are similar to those found in diabetic retinopathy and central vein occlusion. These include microaneurysms, dot-and-blot retinal haemorrhages, venous congestion, and irregular-calibre retinal veins. In addition, there may be macular oedema and mild disc swelling, but as the condition progresses retinal neovascularization develops, often with iris/angle neovascularization, corneal oedema, uveitis, episcleral vascular congestion, and sluggish pupillary light reactions. Light pressure on the eyeball while observing the retinal artery by ophthalmoscopy, will lead to induced pulsation due to the lowered central artery pressure.

Therapy for this condition depends on the ability to restore an adequate blood supply to the ophthalmic artery. It is essential to prevent the ischaemic oculopathy from developing, since visual prognosis by this stage is poor.

Carotid–cavernous fistulas

See Section 8.12.5.

8.3.4 Metabolic storage diseases

Although there are a wide variety of different metabolic storage diseases, the most frequent disorders affecting the retina are the sphingolipidoses and ceroid lipofuscinoses.

In the sphingolipidoses the metabolic by-product accumulates in retinal ganglion cells, thereby producing a characteristic cherry-red spot in the macula. The cherry-red spot may

clear as the disease progresses, leaving only optic atrophy (Kivlin *et al.* 1985). Many other storage diseases, in addition to the most well-known, Tay–Sachs disease, produce a similar fundus picture.

The lipofuscinoses characteristically show a retinal pigmentary retinopathy, in contrast to the ganglion cell deposition of the sphingolipidoses. Further details of these conditions are to be found in Chapter 4.

8.3.5 Phakomatoses

The phakomatoses are a group of disorders characterized by cutaneous lesions and hamartomatous growths elsewhere in the body. A hamartoma is a tumour composed of tissues normally present in the organ of origin with limited capacity for proliferation.

Tuberous sclerosis (Bourneville's disease)

This condition, which is inherited as an autosomal dominant trait, is usually associated with the triad of epilepsy, retinal tumours, and adenoma sebaceum (see Section 19.1). However, all tissues are involved. The main retinal abnormality is astrocytic hamartomas, which are typically smooth, dome-shaped semi-translucent greyish and white lesions located anywhere in the retina, but found preferentially in the pericapillary region (Zimmer Galler and Robertson 1995) (Fig. 8.5). They may be calcified and, when in the pericapillary area, may be mistaken for optic drusen.

Neurofibromatosis types 1 and 2 (von Recklinghausen's disease)

Although orbital and ocular adnexal involvement in neurofibromatosis (NF) are common, fundoscopic abnormalities are distinctly uncommon. Neurofibromatosis types 1 and 2 (NF1 and NF2) are now considered separate diseases, which map to separate chromosomes—17 for NF1 and 22 for NF2—and developmental hamartomas arise in both types (Ragge 1993)

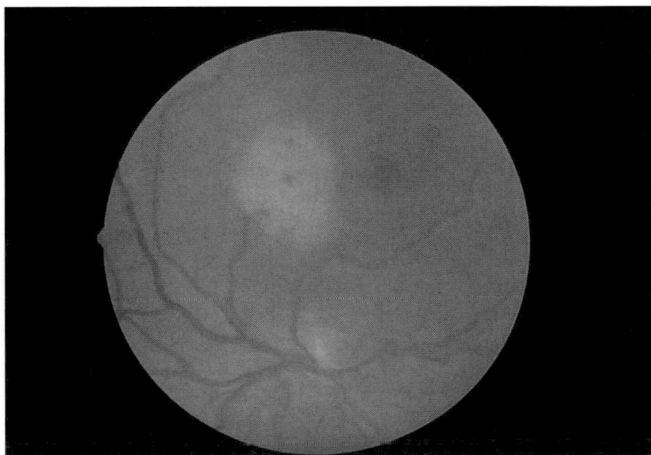

Fig. 8.5. Fundus, showing retinal haematoma associated with tuberous sclerosis (see also colour Plate 12).

(see Section 19.2). Retinal and choroidal hamartomas are occasionally seen in NF1, but they are more typical features of NF2. The ocular features of NF1 include iris hamartomas (Lisch nodules), congenital glaucoma, anterior subcapsular cataract, retinal vascular occlusions, and optic nerve gliomas (Mustonen *et al.* 1997).

The much rarer NF2 often have premature visual loss due to cataract and, in addition to the retinal hamartomas, may have epi-retinal membranes, optic disc gliomas, retinal haemangiomas, medullated nerve fibres, choroidal naevi, uveal melanomas, and choroidal hamartomas.

Encephalo-trigeminal angiomatosis (Sturge–Weber disease)

This condition is characterized by a facial 'port wine' stain, which is in fact a cavernous haemangioma, usually in the ophthalmic division of the trigeminal nerve (see Section 19.3). In addition, lepto-meningeal angiomatosis, seizures, cerebral calcification, unilateral glaucoma, and choroidal haemangioma may occur. Ipsilateral to the facial lesion may be found an intracranial calcifying occipitoparietal lepto-meningeal angiomata. Choroidal haemangiomas are diffuse, minimally elevated subretinal lesions of deep red colour, which may easily be overlooked. They may also occur in the conjunctiva and episclera. In some patients, asymptomatic retinal vascular tortuosity, serous retinal detachment, retinal degeneration, and iris heterochromia may also be noted (Sullivan *et al.* 1992).

Cerebello-retinal angiomatosis (von Hippel–Lindau disease)

This is a autosomal dominantly inherited disorder, characterized by a predisposition to develop haemangioblastomas of the CNS and retina, and in addition renal cell carcinoma, phaeochromocytoma, and renal, pancreatic, and ependymal cysts (see Section 19.4). As visual symptoms may antedate symptoms due to involvement of other organs, it is imperative that the retinal lesions be properly diagnosed, so that appropriate investigation for systemic involvement can be initiated in a timely manner (Maher *et al.* 1990).

The most frequent initial manifestation is retinal angiomatosis which, by the age of 60, has developed in more than 70 per cent of patients. These lesions may be incipient or fully developed, the former being frequently located at the equator or beyond, and therefore more effectively observed using indirect ophthalmoscopy (Welch 1970). The lesions are about the size of diabetic microaneurysms and consist of a tight network of small vascular channels, with an arterial feeding and venous draining vessel. When the lesion is fully developed, these feeding and draining vessels are dilated and tortuous, while the lesion itself is berry-like in configuration. Fluoroscein angiography is required for the detection of nascent preclinical lesions. Exudative retinopathy and retinal detachment usually account for visual morbidity.

In an affected individual, annual ophthalmological examination should be carried out, and when screening at-risk relatives their eyes should be examined from the age of five (with fluorescent angiography from age 10).

Racemose haemangiomas

Racemose haemangiomas of the retina may occur, in addition to those involving the thalamus and midbrain (Wyburn–Mason syndrome). These uncommon haemangiomas show a massive dilatation and tortuosity of retinal vessels without clear differentiation between arteries and veins. Visual function is often impaired to a point where the eye may be blind. Similar vascular malformations may occur along the visual pathway, including the optic nerve, chiasm, optic tract, and mesencephalon.

8.3.6 Acquired immune deficiency syndrome

Patients with acquired immune deficiency syndrome (AIDS) may often show fundoscopic abnormalities, which include cotton-wool spots, cytomegalovirus retinitis, conjunctival Kaposi's sarcoma, retinal periphlebitis, and acute retinal necrosis (Jabs 1995).

8.4 Abnormalities of the optic disc

8.4.1 Optic disc anomalies

Optic nerve hypoplasia

Hypoplasia of the optic nerve may be mild or severe, unilateral or bilateral, and may be associated with normal or impaired visual function. It may occur in isolation, or be associated with central nervous system anomalies.

When the condition is extreme, the disc is small, with a yellow and white depigmented halo surrounded by a pigmented rim. In less severe cases, it is important to identify the small amount of nerve tissue in relation to the surrounding, exposed, scleral ring. There is only a reasonable correlation between the extent of optic disc hypoplasia and impaired visual acuity. In some instances there may be a peripheral field loss associated with good central vision. In such cases the individual may be unaware of the field defect.

Optic nerve hypoplasia may be isolated, but if bilateral is often associated with a variety of facial and intracranial anomalies, for example aniridia, ocular colobomas, Duane's syndrome, and hemifacial spasm. A particular association with intracranial developmental abnormalities is the *De Morsier's syndrome (septo-optic dysplasia)* (Brodsky 1991). This syndrome is associated with bilateral optic nerve hypoplasia, nystagmus, and short stature. An important feature is the absence of the septum pellucidum. The condition is frequently associated with growth hormone deficiency and pituitary dysfunction. It is therefore essential for both imaging and endocrine assessment to be undertaken in all cases of bilateral optic nerve hypoplasia.

Although most cases of optic nerve hypoplasia are idiopathic and sporadic, the condition has been associated with maternal exposure to LSD, crack cocaine use, anticonvulsants, and quinine, and it may occur in association with the fetal alcohol syndrome.

Optic nerve dysplasia

Optic nerve dysplasia presents with a spectrum of abnormalities, including optic nerve colobomas, optic pits, and the morning glory syndrome, all considered to be associated with abnormal closure of the embryonic fetal optic stalk and cup fissure. They are important to recognize, since they are sometimes associated with basal encephalocoeles and other forebrain anomalies (Brodsky and Glaser 1993).

Optic disc colobomas

These are deeply evacuated nerve-head anomalies with blood vessels exiting from the margins, which are associated with defects in the retinal nerve fibre layer, leading to an appropriate visual field loss.

Optic pits

Optic pits are crater-like depressions in the optic disc with a dark grey hue, usually situated in the temporal disc margin with an accompanying nerve fibre layer defect. They may be associated with blind-spot enlargement or arcuate field defects. Optic pits may be associated with a serious detachment of the macula produced by vitreous fluid seeping into the subretinal space through the pit.

The morning glory syndrome

In this condition, an enlarged dysplastic disc is associated with an elevated centrally retained mass of glial and embryonic glial and vascular material, which radiates outwards in a sunburst pattern (Pollack 1987).

Tilted discs

An asymmetrically shaped, tilted disc is produced when the optic nerve leaves the globe at an extremely oblique angle. It is often associated with a crescentric zone of exposed sclera along one edge. The vessels may appear to be displaced in a superior division, or appear to originate from the temporal side of the disc, rather than the nasal in *situs inversus*. The disc may appear hypoplastic, and patients with this condition often have moderately high myopia and oblique astigmatism.

However, it is an important condition to recognize, since it results in elevation of the superior disc margin, which may be incorrectly diagnosed as pathological disc swelling. Because the infero-nasal margin of the disc is usually deficient, this may result in temporal field defects, which may cause confusion with chiasmal compressive processes (Apple *et al.* 1982).

Optic nerve drusen

Drusen of the optic disc can give rise to an elevation of the optic nerve head. Drusen are intrapapillary, prelaminar refractile concretions which are though to arise from degenerating nerve fibre damage due to compression as they leave the globe

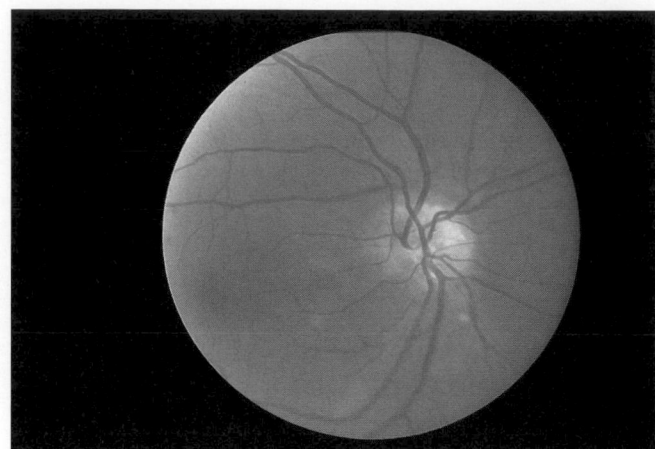

Fig. 8.6. Pseudopapilloedema showing optic nerve head drusen (see also colour Plate 13).

through a congenitally narrow scleral canal. Anomalous discs due to drusen are usually smaller than normal, have an absent central optic disc cup, and exhibit an aberrant branching pattern of the central retinal vessels. Initially the drusen are buried with simple elevation of the disc, but become more apparent in later years when they appear to give rise to a typical lumpy disc, with a scalloped margin (Rosenberg *et al.* 1979) (Fig. 8.6).

There is evidence that disc drusen are inherited as an autosomal irregular dominant trait. It is therefore worthwhile examining the fundi of parents and siblings, when trying to decide whether or not a patient has pseudo-papilloedema due to drusen. Other methods to determine the presence of drusen are to retro-illuminate the disc, which can be achieved by directing the ophthalmoscope beam at the margin rather than the centre of the disc itself, thereby causing the drusen to glow with an opalescent quality. Drusen also exhibit nodular autofluorescence when viewed with a cobalt blue light. Finally, CT scanning through the optic nerve head reveals drusen as calcific densities.

Drusen may sometimes be associated with visual field defects, usually arcuate scotomas or an infero-nasal depression, and with haemorrhagic complications (Savino *et al.* 1979).

It should be remembered that the presence of drusen does not prevent the patient from harbouring a brain tumour, that chronic papilloedema and optic nerve sheath meningiomas can produce intra-capillary refractile bodies resembling drusen, and finally that occasionally disc drusen can occur in patients with retinitis pigmentosa.

It should be remembered that along with optic disc drusen, other causes of anomalous disc swelling are tilted discs with asymmetric elevation and the physiologically elevated discs found in hypermetropic eyes.

8.4.2 Myelinated nerve fibres

In slightly less than 1 per cent of the population, some portion of retinal nerve fibres are myelinated, although normally optic nerve myelination stops at the lamina cribrosa. It appears on

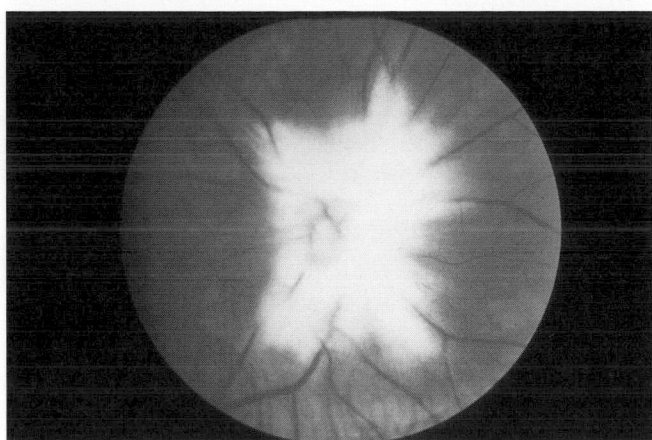

Fig. 8.7. Myelinated retinal nerve fibres (see also colour Plate 14).

fundoscopy a white area, usually adjacent to the disc, which has a centrifugal feathered edge (Fig. 8.7).

8.4.3 Optic disc swelling

Although optic disc swelling and papilloedema have been used synonymously, it is now usual to only refer to papilloedema as optic disc swelling when it is associated with a raised intracranial pressure. Other cases of optic disc swelling are either due to local abnormalities in the eye, nerve, or orbit, or due to congenital anomalies, as described above.

Local causes of optic disc swelling are usually associated with impaired visual acuity and colour vision, central, arcuate or altitudinal field defects, often an afferent pupillary defect, which contrasts with papilloedema when the acuity remains normal, except in the final stages, and is usually bilateral.

Papilloedema

The evolution of the disc changes in papilloedema due to raised intracranial pressure are usually classified into four stages: early, fully developed, chronic, and atrophic (Neetens and Smets 1989).

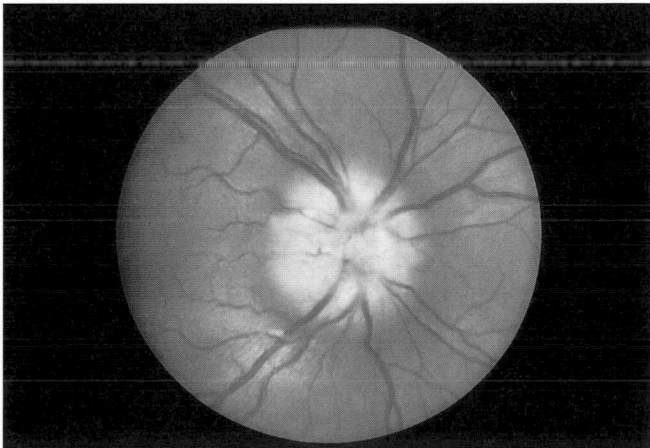

Fig. 8.8. Papilloedema due to raised intracranial pressure (see also colour Plate 15).

In *early* papilloedema there is disc hyperaemia, mild disc swelling with blurring of the fine peripapillary nerve fibre layer striations, dilatation of retinal veins with loss of spontaneous venous pulsations, and occasionally fine splinter haemorrhages at the disc margin (Fig. 8.8).

In fully developed papilloedema, disc elevation is moderate to marked, and there is increased venous distension or tortuosity, increasing number of peripapillary haemorrhages, cotton-wool spots, and dilated capillaries on the disc surface. The retinal blood vessels and disc margin become increasingly indistinct, due to the increasing opacification of the retinal nerve fibres. A hemimacular star figure may occur in the nasal macula.

In chronic papilloedema, there is resolution of the haemorrhages and exudates, leaving a dome-shaped ('champagne cork') disc swelling, which often contains hard exudates. White refractile bodies may appear on the disc surface, known as corpora amylacea. As time goes on there is increasing nerve fibre attrition, leading to progressive visual field loss.

Finally, the end result is post-papilloedema (consecutive) atrophy, in which the disc acquires a milky opalescence and the retinal vessels are sheathed.

Clinical features

Usually papilloedema is bilateral and there is an absence of visual symptoms. However, unilateral or bilateral transient obscurations may occur, which last a few seconds and are often associated with postural changes. Although it has been suggested that such obscurations herald permanent visual loss, there is no evidence to support this view. The longer the papilloedema persists, the more likely there is to be progressive visual field loss, which usually starts as a peripheral field constriction. Occasionally, sudden visual loss occurs in a patient with papilloedema due to ischaemic optic neuropathy (Orcutt *et al.* 1984).

Pathogenesis

Papilloedema is due to impairment of axonal transport in the retinal nerve fibres, leading to axonal distension, which is seen as disc swelling at the level of the pre-laminar optic nerve. The raised intracranial pressure compromises elements of retrograde axonal axoplasmic transport at the lamina cribrosa, leading to axonal distension. It is mainly the slow component of axonal transport which is primarily affected (Hayreh 1977).

Aetiology

There is a vast array of different causes leading to increased intracranial pressure (Table 8.1) (see also Chapter 17).

Management

Treatment depends primarily on the underlying cause of the raised intracranial pressure. If due to a mass lesion which cannot be completely removed, or due to a non-surgically remediable cause, then a shunting procedure or medical measures, such as osmotic agents or diuretics such as acetazolamide, may be used. Increasingly, optic nerve sheath fenestration is

Table 8.1. Causes of optic disc swelling due to raised intracranial pressure

1. Mass lesions: tumours, aneurysms, granulomas, parasitic cysts
2. Intracranial haemorrhage: subdural haematoma, epidural haematoma, subarachnoid haemorrhage
3. Arterio-venous malformations
4. Intracranial infections: brain abscess, meningitis, encephalitis
5. Obstructed cranial venous outflow: dural venous sinus thrombosis; dural venous sinus infiltration; jugular vein compression; dural venous sinus arteriovenous malformation
6. Obstructive hydrocephalus
7. Brain oedema following trauma
8. Spinal cord tumours
9. Benign intracranial hypertension
   (a) idiopathic
   (b) secondary to metabolic and endocrine disorders: Addison's disease, diabetic ketoacidosis; thyrotoxicosis; hypoparathyroidism; chronic uraemia
   (c) secondary to toxic causes: tetracycline; naladixic acid; steroid therapy; lithium; hypervitaminosis A
10. Guillain–Barré syndrome
11. Craniostenoses
12. Mucopolysaccharoidoses
13. Systemic illness: Behçet's syndrome; status epilepticus; Reye's syndrome; Whipple's disease; systemic lupus erythematosus; systemic hypertension; chronic respiratory insufficiency

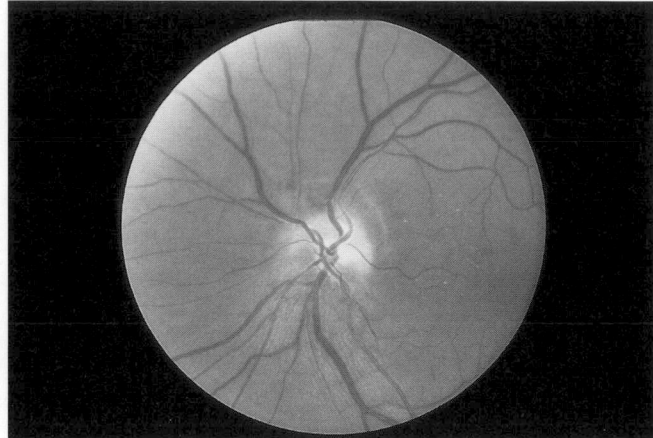

Fig. 8.9. Anterior ischaemic optic neuropathy (see also colour Plate 16).

being used for patients with intractable papilloedema who are developing early visual loss. A small window is made in the retro-laminar optic nerve sheath, which may lead to a reduction in the pressure around the optic nerve, thereby preventing axoplasmic stasis.

8.4.4 Ischaemic optic neuropathy

Ischaemic optic neuropathy is due to infarction of the optic nerve head, and can either be arteritic, as part of giant cell arteritis, or non-arteritic (idiopathic ischaemic neuropathy, anterior ischaemic optic neuropathy, AION), which is the more common form of the condition.

Non-arteritic ischaemic optic neuropathy

This tends to occur in patients aged between 45 and 80 years, and is characterized by abrupt and painless, and generally non-progressive, visual loss, associated with an arcuate or altitudinal visual field loss (Boghen and Glaser 1975). In nearly all cases, there is optic disc oedema, which may be diffuse or sectoral, often associated with one or more splinter haemorrhages at the disc margin (Fig. 8.9). Although previously considered irreversible, as many as 40 per cent of patients may show improvements by three or four lines at 6 months following the acute episode (Ischemic Optic Neuropathy Decompression Trial Research Group 1995).

A small proportion of patients with non-arteritic AION develop progressive stepwise visual loss for as long as 6 weeks. This is rare, although a significant proportion of cases do progress over a 48-hour period. Although subsequent involvement of the same eye is unusual, there is a 40 per cent chance of involvement of the fellow eye within 5 years. Optic atrophy rapidly ensues after the ischaemic event.

The cause of AION remains obscure, although it has been associated with haemodynamic shock, carotid artery occlusion, hyperviscosity states, and acquired defects of thrombosis and haemostasis regulation (Hayreh *et al.* 1994). Recently attention has been focused on its association with the absence of a cup at the optic nerve head, often associated with hypermetropic eyes (Burde 1993).

There is no treatment of proven benefit for patients with AION. However, if the patient is seen at a very early stage acetazolamide can be given to raise the optic nerve head perfusion pressure, in association with lying the patient flat. Although in the past few years there has been a vogue for using optic nerve sheath decompression, a recent control-led trial showed it to be of no value (Ischemic Optic Neuropathy Decompression Trial Research Group 1995). In view of their age, a number of these patients may be found to have hypertension, but vigorous lowering of the blood pressure can lead to worsening.

The most important aspect of management is to exclude the possibility of the arteritic form, since in such cases the fellow eye is vulnerable to similar involvement.

Arteritic ischaemic optic neuropathy

The arteritic form of ION usually occurs in giant cell (cranial, temporal) arteritis (GCA), but also occurs rarely in lupus and polyarteritis nodosa (see Section 3.7.3).

Anyone with AION over the age of 50 should be suspected of having GCA. This often occurs in the context of headache, malaise, weight loss, anorexia, anaemia, proximal muscle ache or stiffness, temporal artery tenderness, jaw claudication, and fever. These symptoms and signs usually precede the visual loss.

The disc infarction is similar to that seen in non-arteritic AION, except the degree of disc pallor tends to be more prominent. The infarction is believed to be due to occlusion of the short posterior ciliary vessels (Liu *et al.* 1994).

A high index of suspicion is required for GCA, and if suspected an urgent erythrocyte sedimentation rate (ESR) and temporal artery biopsy should be arranged. At the same time as the blood is taken for ESR, the patient should be started immediately on systemic steroids (prednisolone 80 mg daily, plus 200 mg i.v. hydrocortisone immediately). In most patients the ESR is markedly elevated, as is the C-reactive protein. Occasionally the ESR may be normal. A biopsy of the superficial temporal artery should be obtained as soon as possible after the diagnosis has been considered. The biopsy will not be affected by the use of corticosteroids for up to at least 48 hours. A positive temporary artery biopsy confirms the diagnosis of giant cell arteritis, but in 25 per cent of patients skip areas are found in biopsy specimens, and therefore a negative biopsy can sometimes occur in consequence.

Steroid treatment should not be tapered or withdrawn too early, since a relapse of symptoms is common. The dose of prednisolone can be gradually tapered after 2–3 weeks to maintain a normal ESR and the patient asymptomatic. Treatment should be continued for at least 6–12 months.

Papillo-phlebitis

Papillo-phlebitis, is also known as optic disc vasculitis or 'the big blind spot' syndrome, occurs in healthy young individuals, and is characterized by unilateral disc swelling with venous engorgement and peripapillary haemorrhages, without any significant visual symptoms. The blind spot may be enlarged, with only mild central visual blurring. In most cases this resolves within a few months, although some may progress to profound visual loss.

8.4.5 Optic atrophy

Optic atrophy is the final result of a variety of disturbances to the optic nerve or retina. The disc appears pale, and there is an absence of disc vasculature and retinal nerve fibres (Fig. 8.10). An ischaemic process is most likely to have occurred, when arteriolar narrowing and sheathing occur. A cupped atrophic disc usually denotes end-stage glaucoma. Retrograde atrophy from lesions of the optic tract result in band or 'bow tie' atrophy of the contralateral disc with generalized atrophy of the ipsilateral optic disc.

However, as a general maxim the ophthalmoscopic appearance of optic atrophy is usually non-specific and non-diagnostic. If the preceding pathological process is unknown, it is essential to conduct imaging to exclude a compressive lesion.

Optic atrophy results from any diseased process which results in death of the retinal ganglion cells with a dying back of their nerve fibres. This can, therefore, be due to diseases which directly involve the ganglion cells themselves or from damage to the axons in the pre-geniculate visual pathway, resulting in

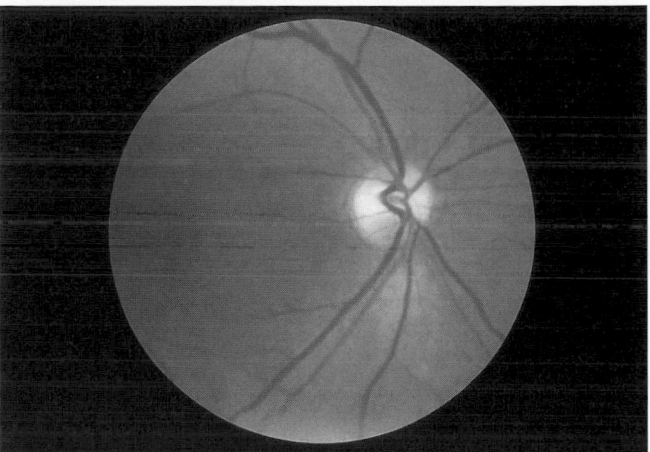

Fig. 8.10. Optic atrophy (see also colour Plate 17).

retrograde atrophy. The development of optic atrophy is usually slow, dependent on its cause, but takes some 6 weeks to first appear after optic nerve transection due to trauma. In most instances the optic atrophy is bilateral, the disc appearing chalky-white in colour with clearly defined margins. Although previously a distinction was made between 'primary' and 'secondary' or 'consecutive' optic atrophy due to subtle ophthalmoscopic differences, it has now been realized that the pathological process is the same in both instances so the distinction is

Table 8.2. Causes of optic atrophy

A Deficiency states
  1. Thiamine ('tobacco–alcohol amblyopia')
  2. B_{12} (pernicious anaemia; 'tobacco amblyopia'?)
B Drugs/toxins
  1. Ethambutol
  2. Chloromycetin
  3. Streptomycin
  4. Isoniazid (INH)
  5. Chlorpropamide
  6. Digitalis
  7. Chloroquine
  8. Placidyl
  9. Antabuse
  10. Heavy metals
C Hereditary optic atrophies
  1. Dominant (juvenile)
  2. Leber's
  3. Associated heredodegenerative neurological syndromes
  4. Recessive, associated with juvenile diabetes
D Demyelination
E Graves' disease
F Atypical glaucoma
G Macular dystrophies

no longer made. The differential diagnosis of optic atrophy is considered in Table 8.2.

The ophthalmoscopic appearance of the fundus usually fails to assist in making the diagnosis, although sometimes accompanying blood vessel changes and nerve fibre layer alterations may provide some useful clues. For example, central retinal artery occlusion and anterior ischaemic optic neuropathy produce optic atrophy that is accompanied by narrowing and sheathing of the retinal arterial tree. Retrograde atrophy from lesions of the optic tract may result in band or 'bow tie' atrophy of the contralateral disc and generalized atrophy of the ipsilateral nerve head. Although a cupped optic disc usually accompanies end-stage glaucoma, it can occasionally result from a compressive lesion.

8.4.6 Infiltrative papillopathy

Rarely the optic nerve head is infiltrated with cells from optic nerve glioma, metastatic carcinoma, leukaemia, and sarcoidosis, as well as other rarer conditions. The visual acuity is often reduced in these conditions.

8.5 Optic nerve lesions

8.5.1 Optic neuritis

Optic neuritis (ON) is a term used to describe an idiopathic optic neuropathy, or one resulting from inflammatory, infectious, or a demyelinating aetiology (see Section 29.3.2). In the majority of cases the optic disc is normal on ophthalmoscopy and the term retrobulbar neuritis is used. In those cases in which the optic disc is swollen then the terms papillitis or anterior ON are used.

Typical optic neuritis

Clinical features

It is important to distinguish between those features of typical optic neuritis of idiopathic or demyelinating causation from atypical optic neuritis. In typical ON there is usually acute unilateral loss of visual acuity and of visual field, which may progress over hours or a few days, reaching its maximal effect within 1 week. Ninety per cent of cases complain of ocular pain which is noted especially with eye movement, and which may precede the visual impairment by a few days (Lepore 1991). There may also be some mild tenderness of the globe at onset. The visual loss may range from contrast defects but maintained acuity to no light perception. The patient is usually aged under 40 years, although ON may occur at any age, and improvement takes place in most patients (90 per cent) to normal or near normal visual acuity over several weeks. There may be persistent subtle residual defects of colour vision, depth deception, and contrast sensitivity, which may continue for several months. Subsequent disc pallor may occur but does not correlate closely with the level of visual recovery (McDonald and Barnes 1992).

Less common features of the disorder include movement phosphates (light flashes provoked by eye movement) and an

Table 8.3. Causes of typical and atypical optic neuritis

Unknown aetiology
Multiple sclerosis
Viral infections of childhood (measles, mumps, chicken pox) with or without encephalitis
Viral encephalitides
Postviral, paraviral infections
Infectious mononucleosis
Herpes zoster
Contiguous inflammation of meninges, orbit, sinuses
Granulomatous inflammations (syphilis, tuberculosis, cryptococcosis, sarcoidosis)
Intraocular inflammations

afferent pupillary defect is present in over 90 per cent of patients with acute ON. Although ON is generally associated with a central scotoma, recent studies have shown that a wide variety of field defects may be found, ranging from a central scotoma to altitudinal and nerve fibre layer defects (Keltner et al. 1993).

Atypical ON may involve bilateral simultaneous onset of ON in an adult patient. There is often lack of pain and there may be other ocular findings suggestive of an inflammatory process, such as an anterior uveitis. Other features include a worsening of visual function beyond 14 days of onset, in a patient outside the 20- to 50-year age span. They may also have evidence of other systemic conditions, particularly inflammatory or infectious diseases.

A number of disorders may be associated with typical or atypical ON (Table 8.3).

The evaluation of patients with ON rather depends on whether or not it is a typical or atypical case. Typical ON probably does not necessitate any additional laboratory investigations, although an MRI brain scan gives some indication of the likely development of multiple sclerosis. This varies between the published series, but of patients presenting with optic neuritis and an abnormal brain MRI, from 36 per cent to as high as 82 per cent have been reported to have gone on to develop definite MS within 3–5 years. This compares with less than 10 per cent of those with a normal MRI (Morrisey et al. 1993).

Those patients with atypical ON should have a chest X-ray and laboratory tests, including a blood count, biochemistry, and tests for collagen and vascular disease and syphilis serology. Examination of the spinal fluid (CSF) is probably justified in this group of patients.

Management

The clinical management of patients with acute ON has been significantly enhanced by the multicentre prospective optic neuritis treatment trial (ONTT). It was concluded that patients receiving oral prednisolone would not recover any more quickly or achieve a better final acuity than those given oral placebo. Those given intravenous methylprednisolone did have a more rapid visual recovery, but at the end of 6 months their visual acuity was no better than that of those receiving placebo (Beck *et al.* 1992). Although there has been some suggestion that patients who receive methylprednisolone had a reduced risk of developing multiple sclerosis, this has not been accepted by many and awaits a further trial.

As a result of this trial and of others, steroid treatment of patients with typical ON is unnecessary, unless there is severe ocular pain which cannot be managed with analgesics, or if there is already poor vision in the fellow eye due to some other disease process.

Atypical optic neuritis

Atypical ON may occur in a variety of different circumstances. It occurs in the context of systemic lupus erythematosus (SLE), when it has been considered that although elements within the optic nerve may be susceptible to autoantibody-mediated attack (Kupersmith *et al.*, 1988*a*), it is likely that the ON may be due to small-vessel occlusive disease. In several other conditions, such as Sjögren's syndrome and vascular disease (for example, polyarteritis nodosa or Churg–Strauss syndrome), inflammation takes place in blood vessel walls, leading to an ischaemic rather than an inflammatory mechanism. Supposedly immunologically mediated ON has also been observed following bee stings and the use of interleukin-2 and α-interferon.

ON may also occur following several different viral illnesses, including chickenpox, rubella, infectious mononucleosis, and mumps (Selbst *et al.* 1983). Such cases may be bilateral, occur within 7–10 days of the onset of the illness, and there is usually a spontaneous and full recovery. It may also occur after vaccinations against both bacterial and viral infection.

Outside the context of acquired immunodeficiency syndrome (AIDS), primary infection of the optic nerve is rare (Nichols and Goodwin 1992). However, with AIDS the optic nerve can develop a granulomatosis perineuritis due to tuberculosis, aspergillosis, syphilis or cryptococcosis. Acute retinal necrosis due to herpes viruses is also sometimes encountered.

Difficulties may sometimes be encountered when atypical ON presents with visual loss and disc swelling due to infiltration of the intraorbital nerve sheath or the nerve itself. This may be due to tuberculosis, sarcoidosis, cryptococcosis, or idiopathic granulomatous meningeal disease. Acute and chronic presentations may sometimes occur. In such cases of atypical ON due to granulomatous inflammation it is necessary to carefully examine the optic media and retina in addition to the optic nerve. Frequently vitreous infiltrates, retinal vasculitis, and choroidal lesions may be observed, but in some cases these are absent. Some of these cases may be steroid dependent, a term used to indicate that following withdrawal of systemic steroid therapy vision usually drops again. This feature may also be observed in patients with infiltrations of the optic nerve head in meningeal involvement by non-Hodgkin's lymphoma or metastatic carcinoma of the breast or lung.

8.5.2 Heredo-familial optic neuropathies

The hereditary optic neuropathies can be divided into those which are autosomal dominant or recessive, and those which are due to point mutations in mitochondrial DNA.

Autosomal recessive optic atrophy

A rare condition, which may occur in very simple form in which visual impairment is noted before the age of 4 years, associated with disc pallor, and sometimes retinal arterial attenuation. A more complex form occurs when the optic atrophy is associated with spinocerebellar degenerations and cerebellar ataxia, known as Behr's syndrome. It also occurs in association with metabolic disturbances, such as diabetes mellitus and diabetes insipidus and hearing loss (DIDMOAD: diabetes insipidus, diabetes mellitus, optic atrophy, and deafness) (Barrett *et al.* 1995).

Autosomal dominant optic atrophy

This condition is characterized by moderately poor visual acuity (20/40–20/200), which begins between the ages of 4 and 8 years, and is associated with slow progression and temporal disc pallor (Kjer 1959). There is also a centro-caecal blind spot enlargement and blue–yellow dyschromatopsia. In some families there is associated nystagmus. Impairment in this disorder is considerably more mild than in either recessive optic atrophy or Leber's optic atrophy. The gene defect has now been isolated to chromosome 3 (Kjer *et al.* 1996).

Leber's hereditary optic neuropathy

Leber's hereditary optic neuropathy (LHON) develops primarily in males (approximately 14 per cent of women) in the second to third decade of life, characterized by an abrupt loss of central vision in one eye, usually followed by a loss of vision in the remaining eye weeks, months or sometimes years later. Occasionally visual loss may occur simultaneously in the two eyes. There is no associated pain on eye movement, in contrast to acute ON, and the visual loss is usually permanent with optic atrophy and large absolute central scotomas. However, the fundoscopic picture in the acute phase often shows the swelling of the papillary nerve fibre layer, circumpapillary telangiectatic microangiopathy, and tortuosity of the retinal vessels. Fluorescein angiography does not show disc leakage (Riordan-Eva *et al.* 1995).

Although the visual loss usually occurs in isolation, in some cases there may be associated cardiac dysrhythmias (pre-excitation syndromes). A maternal pattern of inheritance has been known for some time, and a number of point mutations in mitochondrial DNA, particularly at the 11778 location and less frequently at 3460 and 14484, have been identified (Mackey 1994). The significance of the point mutation at 14484 is that a much higher percentage (37 per cent as opposed to 4 per cent) of patients show some visual recovery when compared with patients who have a defect at the 11778 location. It is, therefore, appropriate to carry out genetic testing in those individuals presenting with atypical ON of the appropriate sex and age, even if a positive family history is not available. There is no effective treatment for this condition. It is of some interest that earlier suggestions of cyanide toxicity in predisposed individuals, which led to the use of hydroxycobalamin, may relate to recent observations that tobacco and alcohol may play a role in phenotypic expression of the mitochondrial mutations.

8.5.3 Nutritional and toxic optic neuropathies

Bilateral, slowly progressive central visual loss with centro-caecal scotomas, and usually normal or mild temporal atrophic optic discs, characterizes optic nerve failure due to either nutritional deficiency or a toxic cause. Once a family history of one of the hereditary familial diseases has been excluded, this condition should be considered, and is usually due to a combination of alcohol abuse, deficiencies within the B vitamin complex, and, frequently, high tobacco consumption. With treatment by abstinence of the likely toxic agents and vitamin supplementation, recovery of vision usually occurs, unless the condition is so long-standing that optic atrophy has intervened.

Recent epidemics of optic neuropathy in Cuba (Sadun *et al.* 1994) and in West Africa have probably been related to multiple dietary deficiencies.

A wide variety of substances have been cited as causing toxic optic neuropathy, which include ethambutol, chloramphenicol, halogenated hyroxyquinolones, lead, isoniazid, and vincristine. The toxic effects may be either dose dependent or idiosyncratic (Grant and Schuman 1993).

8.5.4 Tumours of the optic nerve

Optic nerve sheath meningiomas

Although optic nerve sheath meningiomas may arise directly from the optic nerve sheath, usually in the orbital regions of the nerve, they frequently arise from the tuberculum sellae, sphenoid wing, and olfactory groove, leading to secondary invasion or compression of the nerve. Primary optic nerve sheath meningiomas, most frequently found in middle-aged women, are usually unilateral but if bilateral raise the possibility of central neurofibromatosis (NF2). Although most patients will have mild (2–4 mm) proptosis at the time of their initial consultation, ocular prominence is not their presenting symptom. Rather, they complain of dimming of vision and decreased colour vision. Usually an afferent pupillary defect is observed, peripheral field constriction, or a centro-caecal scotoma. Transient visual obscurations are common and, in some cases, amaurosis has been reported. Visual loss progresses over years, with optic disc swelling gradually being supplanted by optic atrophy, with or without the evolution of optociliary venous (retino-choroidal anastamoses) shunt vessels (Dutton 1992) (Fig. 8.11).

Meningiomas may invade the orbit by trans-sheath extension, and intracranial spread through the optic canal is always a

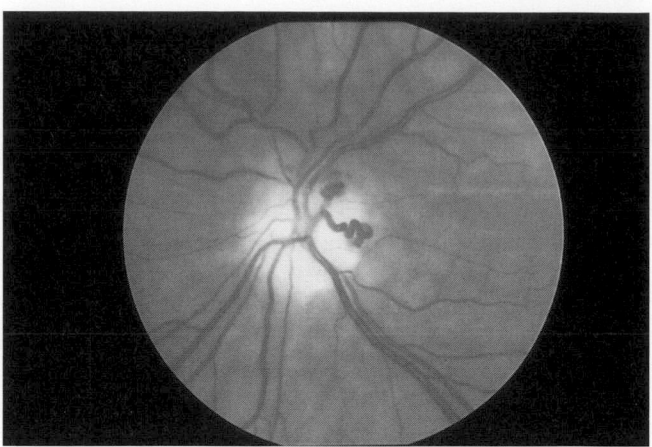

Fig. 8.11. Optociliary shunts due to an optic nerve sheath meningioma (see also colour Plate 18).

possible danger, particularly in children, when the tumour sometimes behaves in a more aggressive fashion.

The CT picture in patients with these tumours is most often one of diffuse narrow enlargement of the optic nerve, with bulbous swellings of the nerve in the region of the globe and orbital apex. 'Railroad-track' calcification of the optic nerve sheath in the orbit is a characteristic feature. Use of MRI has enabled optic nerve sheath meningiomas to be dis--tinguished from optic nerve gliomas, where both may cause a uniform enlargement in the orbital region. In meningiomas but not gliomas the nerve and optic nerve sheath are readily distinguished (Lindblom *et al.* 1992).

Management of patients with optic nerve sheath meningiomas is controversial (Kennerdell *et al.* 1988). While there is general agreement that nerve sheath tumours are most aggressive in children and become progressively more indolent with advancing age, there is no consensus as to the best way to treat these lesions. Clinical resection, particularly when there is intracranial spread, is usually incomplete. These patients rarely die from the meningioma and it is probably best to observe. In some instances radiotherapy has shown to result in some visual improvement, but there is no agreement as to its value. Endocrine treatments suitable for optic nerve meningiomas, such as progesterone antagonists, have not been reported as successful.

Optic nerve gliomas

Optic nerve gliomas, which may also involve the chiasm, are of two distinct types. By far the commonest is the benign glioma of childhood, and the other the malignant glioblastoma which occurs in adults (Dutton 1994). Approximately a quarter of cases occur in the setting of NF1.

Benign optic nerve gliomas usually present within the first two decades of life, with a peak incidence from 1 to 6 years of age. The usual presenting manifestations are proptosis and visual loss, which may be so mild as to be undetectable, although a profound reduction in acuity is more common. The fundus picture may be that of either papilloedema or optic atrophy, and further diagnostic confusion is sometimes caused by the finding of optociliary shunt vessels, more commonly associated with nerve sheath meningiomas.

The clinical course of childhood optic nerve gliomas is highly variable. In some, tumour enlargement proceeds slowly for a time but then reaches a plateau, while in others the enlargement proceeds unabated (Hoyt and Bagdassarian 1969). Necropsy material shows an absence of mitotic figures, and the fact that these gliomas grow with or without tumour cell division has suggested that they are in fact hamartomas rather than true neoplasms. Optic nerve gliomas are generally managed conservatively, although some favour radiation therapy for lesions with chiasmal involvement, and surgery for at least those tumours restricted to the orbit (Klug 1982).

Optic nerve gliomas of adulthood, on the other hand, are malignant gliomas which usually arise in males aged 40–60 years. These patients often present with a rapid onset of visual failure, which on some occasions may mimic acute ON. The tumour progresses rapidly, as occurs with glioblastoma multiforme tumours elsewhere in the brain, and the patient usually dies within a short period.

Other optic nerve tumours

Metastatic cancer may lead to optic nerve involvement, either as a result of infiltration of the meninges, as occurs with cancer of the breast and lung, or by direct tumour infiltration, as with lymphoproliferative disorders and certain types of leukaemia and non-Hodgkin's lymphoma. Paraneoplastic optic neuropathy has also been described in patients with small cell carcinoma of the lung (Malik *et al.* 1992).

8.6 Optic chiasm disorders

8.6.1 Clinical features

Approximately 25 per cent of all brain tumours occur in the chiasmal region, and since half of these cases present initially with visual loss, an appreciation of the various field abnormalities is important (Hollenhorst and Younge 1973). Although there are a number of other causes for the chiasmal syndrome, e.g. trauma and demyelination, these are rare and will be discussed later. The neuro-ophthalmological signs of a compressive optic chiasm lesion are primarily a field defect and deterioration of visual acuity, which depend on the relationship of the chiasm to the pituitary. In 79 per cent of cases it lies directly over the pituitary, in 17 per cent it is over the tuberculum sellae (pre-fixed), and in the remaining 4 per cent it is over the dorsum sellae (post-fixed). The classical field defect of a chiasmal lesion is a bitemporal hemianopia. This may be complete or incomplete and may or may not be symmetrical. Sometimes the defect is only paracentral and may, therefore, be missed if the central field is not explored during visual field testing. It is unusual to have a bitemporal hemianopia without some reduction in central visual acuity in at least one eye, due to the optic nerve being compromised in addition to the

chiasm. Whether a bitemporal hemianopia is more marked in the inferior or superior field is not helpful in deciding whether the compression is from above or below.

The anterior junction syndrome gives rise to another characteristic field defect due to an anterior chiasmic lesion. This is seen mainly with a post-fixed optic chiasm when the optic nerve close to the chiasm is mainly involved. This results in an ipsilateral central scotoma with reduced visual acuity, and a contralateral superior temporal visual field depression. The latter is due to involvement of contralateral inferior nasal optic fibres, which decussate and then pass a little way anteriorly into the ipsilateral optic nerve (von Willebrand's knee) before turning into the chiasm and contralateral optic tract. While prechiasmal compression only involves the intracranial portion of the optic nerve, a central scotoma is the only visual field defect. Since there are no differentiating features of such a scotoma resulting either from an inflammatory process (e.g. ON) or from compression, apart from temporal compression, the latter possibility must always be considered when this defect is found. However, if the optic tract is mainly involved, then an incongruous homonymous hemianopia, with reduced visual acuity in one eye, is found which is particularly suggestive of a pre-fixed chiasm, and is often found with craniopharyngiomas.

It is important to remember that not all cases of bitemporal field loss are due to chiasmal disease. Such field defects are also found in centro-caecal scotomas, tilted discs, dysplastic optic discs, refractive scotomas, massive papilloedema due to blind spot enlargement, and overhanging redundant upper eyelids. In a large series of patients with pituitary tumours the most common field defect was a bitemporal hemianopia (67 per cent), with less frequent junctional scotoma (29 per cent), homonymous hemianopia (7 per cent), and prechiasmal field loss (2 per cent) (Hollenhorst and Younge 1973). The mechanisms by which field defects occur in chiasmal compression are not certain, but direct pressure on the fibres, resulting in impaired axonal transport, and interference with the vascular supply, producing ischaemia, have both been considered. A rapid return of acuity and visual field loss, which sometimes occurs within 48 hours of decompression, supports the former hypothesis. Other signs found in chiasmal lesions include optic disc pallor, which was found in 50 per cent of eyes in one series. Its absence usually denotes a virtual complete return of visual function with successful decompression. Papilloedema is frequently associated with a suprachiasmal tumour but rarely with intrasellar tumours. Involvement of the extraocular nerves may occur in association with parachiasmal lesions such as pituitary tumours, and an unusual phenomenon, see-saw nystagmus, may occur in young patients with a tumour of the chiasm and diencephalic regions.

The main symptom resulting from the chiasmal syndrome is usually deterioration of vision, often with associated dimming of the visual field, particularly temporally. This is usually a progressive deterioration over a period of months or years, except when due to pituitary apoplexy, when the acuity loss usually precedes the field defect. However, a fairly frequent symptom in patients with the chiasmal syndrome is diplopia. This may be a vertical or horizontal separation of images, which usually occurs in the absence of a demonstrable ocular motor paresis. An explanation for this phenomenon is the absence of the temporal field in each eye, which normally acts as a physiological linkage for the two nasal fields and has been called the hemifield slide phenomenon. Minor ocular motor imbalance, which does not normally affect binocular fusion, now results in an inability to maintain the two fields in juxtaposition. Some patients will also complain of a disturbance of depth deception, experiencing problems with such tasks as sewing, threading needles, or using precision tools. This phenomenon, called chiasmic postfixation blindness, is due to the presence of a blind area beyond the fixation point. The image of objects located in this area falls on the nasal retina which is blind (Kirkham 1972).

8.6.2 Specific causes of the chiasmal syndrome

As has already been mentioned, the most common cause of chiasmal compression is pituitary adenomas (50–55 per cent) (see Section 18.7.1). Other tumours include craniopharyngiomas (20–25 per cent) (see Section 18.8.5), meningiomas (10 per cent) (see Section 18.7.2), and gliomas (7 per cent) (see Section 18.8.1), which are described elsewhere. Other rare non-tumorous causes of chiasmal compression include aneurysms of the circle of Willis, posterior ethmoid or sphenoid sinus mucocoeles, pituitary abscess, distension of the third ventricle, and suprasellar arachnoid cysts. There are numerous non-compressive causes of bitemporal hemianopia, some of which will be discussed below.

The empty sella syndrome

In this condition there is an extension of the subarachnoid space into the pituitary fossa, through a deficient diaphragma sellae. This may mimic pituitary disease and may occur either spontaneously or following surgery or radiotherapy to the sella region. It may rarely cause symptoms suggestive of a pituitary tumour, including a moderate hyperprolactinaemia, headaches, and, rarely, a progressive visual loss following transnasal hypophysectomy (Neelon et al. 1973).

Chiasmal arachnoiditis

This is due to meningitis, especially tuberculosis, syphilis, sarcoidosis, or carcinoma and occurs rarely. Head trauma may also produce a chiasmal syndrome, the result of a variable combination of contusion, haemorrhage, necrosis, or actual tear. Intrinsic lesions of the optic chiasm are best exemplified by plaques of demyelination found in multiple sclerosis, which, despite being an apparent common site of demyelination, rarely give rise to appropriate visual field defects. Vascular abnormalities, such as arteriovenous malformations, involving the chiasm may occur.

Radionecrosis

Following irradiation to the sella region for pituitary tumours, progressive visual impairment may occur due to radionecrosis of the chiasm, optic tract, and intracranial optic nerves (Morris et al. 1994). The onset of the visual loss is usually 6 months to 3 years after completion of therapy, with a peak incidence of 12–18 months. Pathological examination of radionecrosis indicates a microvasculopathy and occlusive endarteritis. Patients most at risk are those who have received in excess of 200 cGy per day or a total dose in excess of 6000 cGy. The management of this condition is uncertain, but it has been suggested that anticoagulation with intravenous heparin followed by warfarin treatment given early, may help to arrest further visual loss (Glantz et al. 1994). Others have claimed benefits from hyperbaric oxygen therapy.

8.7 Disorders of the optic tract, optic radiation, and occipital lobe

8.7.1 Optic tract lesions

Lesions of the optic tract, although rare (less than 3 per cent of visual field defects in a series of 100 homonymous hemianopias), often produce specific signs and visual field abnormalities which allow definitive diagnosis (Newman and Miller 1983). The optic tract is the first point in the visual pathways where the ipsilateral temporal and contralateral nasal retinal nerve fibres come together, and so the field defect is usually a partial or complete homonymous hemianopia. When partial, there is often gross incongruity between the visual field defects found in each eye, which may also be found with lesions of the lateral geniculate nucleus and, more rarely, the optic radiations.

Lesions of the optic tract without involvement of the chiasm or optic nerve result in normal visual acuity, but pupillary abnormalities have often been reported. A relative afferent defect may be found in the eye with the temporal field loss (contralateral to the side of the lesion) (Bell and Thompson 1978). In pupillary hemiakinesia described by Wernicke, there is a decreased or absent pupillary reaction when the 'non-seeing' portion of the retina is stimulated, compared to the 'seeing' portion. Because of light scatter, this phenomena has often been difficult to observe. A second pupillary sign, described by Behr, of the pupil ipsilateral to the homonymous field defect being larger than that contralateral to the field defect, has again not been consistently observed.

Ophthalmoscopically optic pallor due to retrograde degeneration may be observed. This takes a characteristic form with band or 'bow tie' atrophy in the eye opposite to the lesion, due to loss of nasal retinal fibres. Ipsilateral to the lesion, temporal pallor is found due to loss of arcuate fibres from the temporal hemiretina (Savino et al. 1978).

The most frequently encountered lesions causing the optic tract syndrome are aneurysms, craniopharyngiomas, and pituitary tumours.

8.7.2 Lateral geniculate nucleus

Lesions of the lateral geniculate nucleus have been found to produce incongruous wedge-shaped homonymous field defects, but when the aetiology is ischaemic the defect is usually congruous (Gunderson and Hoyt 1971). The lateral geniculate nucleus receives its blood supply from the distal anterior choroidal and lateral choroidal arteries, and occlusion of one or other artery may result in a specific syndrome. A loss of the upper and lower homonymous sectors in the visual field with corresponding sectoral optic disc pallor characterizes the distal anterior choroidal artery syndrome, whereas a horizontal sectoral defect with appropriate disc pallor is found in the lateral choroidal syndrome (Frisén et al. 1978). Other causes for lateral geniculate nucleus involvement include tumours and demyelination. Since the pupillomotor fibres leave the optic tract to ascend in the superior brachium, a geniculate lesion results in normal pupillary responses.

8.7.3 The optic radiations

As the geniculo-striate fibres leave the lateral geniculate nucleus, the ventral fibres (subserving the superior visual field) pass anteriorly around the temporal horn of the lateral ventricle to form Meyer's loop. Lesions in this region usually result in a congruous homonymous field defect, mainly affecting the superior quadrant. This is often wedge-shaped and may extend into the inferior quadrant. The visual acuity and pupillary responses are both normal. The cause of lesions involving the optic radiation are either vascular occlusion, tumours (intrinsic or metastatic), or abscesses. Temporal lobectomy for the treatment of epilepsy does not involve fibres of the optic radiation so long as the resection is confined to the anterior 4–5 cm only (Tecoma et al. 1993). Some degree of incongruity may be found in the resulting field defects.

Although lesions of the dorsal optic radiation in the parietal lobe may result in a homonymous hemianopia, primarily affecting the lower fields, large lesions usually result in a complete homonymous hemianopia with macular splitting. Damage to the parietal or occipitoparietal cortex may result in the phenomenon in the contralateral visual field called unilateral visual inattention or visual extinction (Bender and Furlow 1945). A test object presented in this field is perceived normally but, when an identical object is similarly presented equidistant from the fixation point in the ipsilateral visual field, the stimulus in the field contralateral to the parietal lobe lesion disappears. Visual inattention may be found during the recovery phase of a homonymous hemianopia, but it should be noted that it may also be found rarely in lesions of the frontal lobe, thalamus, and mesencephalon.

8.7.4 Occipital lobe

On reaching the occipital lobe there is a high degree of order in the fibres of the optic radiation, and lesions, which are usually due to infarction, trauma, or tumour, produce congruent field defects which are homonymous. The only features of the field defect which help localize the lesion to the occipital lobe, rather than the anterior optic radiation, is the presence of macula sparing or a temporal crescent in a homonymous hemianopia.

In macula sparing there is preservation of the visual field within a region of 1–2° up to 10° around the fixation point in the hemianopic field. In the more usual situation the hemianopic field is split along the vertical meridian through the fixation point (macula splitting). Although it has been argued that macula sparing is a result of poor fixation during visual field testing, this would only account for about 1–2° of sparing (Bishoff et al. 1995). Despite the continued controversy concerning the cause of macula sparing, there appear to be two main anatomical factors which may explain this phenomenon. First, there is evidence that there is a vertically orientated median strip centred on the fovea in which retinal ganglion cells project either ipsilaterally or contralaterally (Fukuda et al. 1989). The macula, therefore, is bilaterally represented, but since this strip is at most responsible for 2° of the central field this is insufficient to explain many cases of macula sparing. The second, more probable, explanation is the rich anastomotic network between terminal branches of the middle cerebral artery and the posterior cerebral artery, which supply the area of the striate cortex containing the macula representation in the occipital pole (Sugishita et al. 1993).

Lesions at the pole of the occipital lobe result in small homonymous central scotomas, which may lead the patient to present with reading difficulties and may be missed if only the peripheral field is examined to confrontation. The central 10° occupies approximately 60 per cent of the primary visual cortex (Horton and Hoyt 1991). More anterior lesions of the occipital lobe involving the more anterior part of the calcarine fissure, which contains the representation of the unpaired peripheral nasal retina, results in a monocular defect in the peripheral temporal field, called the 'temporal crescent', between 60 and 90° from the fixation point. However, it should be remembered that the most common cause for such peripheral visual field defects is a retinal lesion rather than a intracranial one. The converse of this defect may be found, in which there is sparing of the temporal crescent in a homonymous hemianopia. This usually occurs with a vascular lesion affecting the more posterior striate cortex (Benton et al. 1980).

Bilateral lesions of the occipital lobes may result in varying degrees of homonymous hemianopia, ranging from small bilateral central homonymous scotomas to complete blindness. The extent of the abnormality may vary between the two halves, being partial or complete, hemianopic or quadrantic. Sometimes restricted bilateral lesions of the occipital lobes may result in small bilateral homonymous central scotomas (or 'ring' scotomas, if there is some degree of macular sparing in addition). Altitudinal field defects usually occur as a result of trauma (rarely tumours or vascular events) involving both upper and lower occipital poles (Holmes 1918). Inferior altitudinal defects are mainly found, since patients with inferior occipital lobe injury (i.e. a superior altitudinal defect) often die as a result of haemorrhage from lacerated dural sinuses.

Cortical blindness

Cortical blindness usually indicates selective involvement of the occipital visual cortex, but may be difficult to distinguish from bilateral homonymous hemianopia due to bilateral lesions in

Table 8.4. Causes of cortical blindness

Trauma
Schilder's disease
Cerebral angiography
CO poisoning
Meningitis
Air embolism
Neoplasm
Tentorial herniation
Cardiac arrest
Systemic lupus erythematosis
Dialysis disequilibrium

the optic radiation. Marquis (1934) described the essential features as:

(1) complete loss of all visual sensation;

(2) loss of reflex lid closure to threat;

(3) normal pupillary light reactions;

(4) normal retina and full extraocular eye movements.

Although the most commonest aetiology is hypoxia of the striate cortex, cases have been reported in a number of different conditions (Table 8.4).

Patients with cortical blindness may sometimes be unaware of their visual defect (anosognosia) and vigorously deny it, known as Anton's syndrome. This may occur with lesions elsewhere causing total blindness. There is no satisfactory explanation for this syndrome and the various hypotheses are discussed by Lessell (1975). Various suggestions include an alteration in emotional reactivity, 'psychiatric' denial as an accentuation of a common response to illness, a memory disorder, for example in Korsokoff's syndrome, and associated lesions elsewhere in areas of the brain responsible for the recognition and interpretation of visual images.

Transient cortical blindness may occur in a number of different situations, e.g. after cardiac or respiratory arrest, head trauma, and meningitis. Greenblatt (1973) has detailed three clinical patterns:

(1) in children (up to 8 years) transient cortical blindness (1–6 hours) is associated with irritability, somnolence, and vomiting, and has a good prognosis;

(2) in the age range 8–20 years there may be delay before the onset of blindness, which recovers over hours with full return of function; and

(3) in adults transient cortical blindness, with onset often immediately following head trauma, may last many days and result in some degree of permanent visual loss.

Rare cases of transient cortical blindness have also been reported following seizures.

8.8 Disorders of higher visual processing

8.8.1 Residual visual function in hemianopias

In his classic work, Holmes (1918) showed that striate cortex damage results in a complete hemianopia. However, incomplete damage to the occipital lobe may result in retention of some aspects of visual perception, the most commonly observed being the ability to perceive small moving objects in the homonymous hemianopia (Riddoch 1917). Riddoch's phenomenon may be the first evidence of recovery of a homonymous hemianopia. This is then usually followed by perception of static targets and finally colour perception returns. Unfortunately the Riddoch phenomenon is not only found in occipital lesions, but has been reported in patients with lesions in the anterior visual pathways (Safran and Glaser 1980).

The retention of the ability to localize objects in space and limited pattern discrimination in monkeys in whom both striate cortices had been removed, led to interest in the possible visual functions in the hemianopic field of human patients (Weiskrantz 1986). Since these patients are unaware of any residual visual capacity and appear blind by standard clinical perimetric methods, this visual capacity has been termed 'blindsight' (Weiskrantz et al. 1974, Weiskrantz 1986). Using forced-choice discrimination methods such patients have revealed their ability to locate stimuli, both by saccadic eye movements and by pointing (Cowey and Stoerig 1991). The extent of the residual visual capacity is varied amongst the patients so far reported, and as yet there is poor correlation with the precise location of lesions in the occipital lobe.

8.8.2 Functional visual loss in prestriate lesions

There is increasing evidence from electrophysiological studies in primates that once initial processing of visual information has occurred in the striate cortex, segregation of different properties of the visual stimulus occurs in the prestriate cortex (Zeki and Shipp 1988; Zeki 1993). Here there are a number of individual representations of the contralateral hemifield, each containing neurons with a particular response characteristic. For example, some areas contain neurons which are selective for colour (V4), and another for motion (V5, middle temporal gyrus, MT). There appears, therefore, to be parallel processing of different aspects of visual information in these various cortical areas before an organized synthesis of the visual scene can be generated. Specific lesions in one or other of these areas might be expected to give rise to an appropriate specific loss of a visual modality. In this section such specific losses are described for colour (achromatopsia), movement (akinetopsia), and faces (prosopagnosia).

Colour

Acquired disorders of colour vision due to lesions of the central nervous system are of two types. In one the colour sense is normal but the naming and recognition of colour is impaired. This can occur as part of an aphasia, e.g. Wernicke's or anomic, in the syndrome of alexia without agraphia, or as one feature of visual agnosia (see below). In the second type there is an inability to see colours (dyschromatopsia or achromatopsia) (Zeki 1990).

Patients with lesions in the region of the lingual and fusiform gyri, which lies in the anterior inferior region of the occipital lobe and is considered to be the human homologue of the monkey visual area V4, complain that they cannot see colours and that everything looks grey or in varying shades of black and white (Meadows 1974a). They are unable to identify the figures on pseudo-isochromatic test plates, although they are able to name correctly the colours of brightly coloured objects. In addition, they are unable to perform normally on the Farnsworth–Munsell 100-hue test. Patients with cerebral dyschromatopsia may or may not realize that their colour sense is impaired. Other functions such as visual acuity, object recognition, and depth perception are all normal, but there is often an associated visual field defect, usually a bilateral superior homonymous quadrantanopia, sometimes also associated with prosopagnosia.

Movement

A case has been reported of a woman who exhibited a selective deficit of movement perception (Zihl et al. 1983). She had no impression of movement in depth and could only discriminate between a stationary and a moving target in the periphery of her otherwise intact visual fields. The patient had bilateral lesions involving the lateral occipito-parieto-temporal junction, which PET has revealed is specifically activated during motion perception and, therefore, appears to be the human homologue of the monkey visual area V5 (Zeki 1991).

8.8.3 Visual associated agnosia

The term visual agnosia refers to a rare condition in which there is an inability to recognize and name or demonstrate the use of an object presented visually, in the absence of a language deficit, general intellectual dysfunction, or attentional disturbances. The patient is, however, able to name the object when using other sensory modalities such as touch, sound, etc. Teuber (1965) described visual agnosia as a 'percept stripped of its meaning'.

Visual agnosia has been classified in a number of different ways. One classification depends on the specific category of visual material which cannot be recognized. This is a disturbance of recognition of objects (object agnosia), faces (prosopagnosia), and colour (colour agnosia), which may occur in isolation or in various combinations. Lissauer's (1890) classic dichotomous classification of visual agnosia is, however, still relevant today. When a patient is able to copy and match-to-sample objects that he fails to name or recognize visually, his agnosia is termed associative; but if he fails on all these tasks or demonstrates perceptual abnormalities his agnosia is termed apperceptive (Tranel and Damasio 1996).

Apperceptive visual agnosia

Well-documented cases of apperceptive visual agnosia are rare (Warrington and James 1988). They show an inability to copy or match-to-sample drawings which they cannot recognize, and recognition and matching of all other stimuli which demand shape or pattern perception is also affected. Most cases have been associated with cerebral damage due to cardiac arrest, carbon monoxide poisoning, or bilateral cerebrovascular infarction. Less severe apperceptive disorders are associated with unilateral and generally right cerebral damage.

Associative visual agnosia

Unlike apperceptive agnosia there is no doubting the existence of associative agnosia as a definite neuropsychological syndrome, since a number of well-documented cases have been reported (Humphreys and Riddoch 1993).

These cases exhibit the ability to copy and/or match-to-sample items which they fail to identify visually, without any evidence of primary sensory or sensory motor disturbance. The syndrome is commonly associated with colour agnosia, prosopagnosia, and alexia in various combinations. This may reflect task and processing similarities between recognition, e.g. faces and objects, resulting from defects of both. Alternatively, lesions giving rise to object agnosia may involve adjacent areas specific for colour or face processing.

Patients with associative visual agnosia show an increasing difficulty in identifying an object when presented as an object itself, or as a picture or a line drawing. Auditory and tactile recognition are usually intact. There is no uniformity about the field defects which are often present. A further commonly found feature is the strong tendency these patients have to perseverate, either previously viewed objects or, more commonly, the verbal response to them.

A number of hypotheses to explain visual agnosia have been proposed. Geschwind (1965) suggested that agnosia was not a defect of a unitary process of recognition, but rather a special form of a modality-specific naming defect. Using a disconnection explanation similar to that given for dyslexia without dysgraphia and colour agnosia, he suggested that the confabulatory verbal responses are due to a pathological disconnection of the intact speech area from the intact sensory area. Ratcliff and Newcombe (1982) have argued, however, that since object recognition, as opposed to naming, is mediated by the semantic system, disconnection must be a visual–semantic one and not merely visual–verbal. However, patients with surgically sectioned cerebral commissures are able to extract meaning from words and pictures when visual input is restricted to the right hemisphere, making it unlikely that this disconnection of an intact right hemisphere would be sufficient to cause agnosia.

A second hypothesis, proposed by Warrington (1975), suggests that the disorder is due to a disturbance of access to visual semantic information itself, since in her patient 'all links of associations were lost, not just verbal' and hence a visuo-verbal disconnection was not a sufficient explanation. She regarded preservation of the ability to make same/different judgements with respect to photographs of objects taken from different angles as evidence of preserved 'perceptual classification'. However, other authors have suggested a defect of visual categorization in their patients (Albert *et al.* 1975). It has to be concluded that both the anatomical basis and clinical criteria for associative visual agnosia are still uncertain, but there are excellent reviews by Farah (1990) and Tranel and Damasio (1996).

8.8.4 Prosopagnosia

Prosopagnosia is a specific inability to recognize familiar faces despite a normal ability to recognize everyday objects, and is therefore, different from visual agnosia (Meadows 1974*b*). Although facial recognition is a visual pattern discrimination of great complexity, patients with prosopagnosia have no difficulty in discriminating unfamiliar faces and matching faces correctly. Indeed there appears to be no disturbance of visual perception, patients being able to recognize accurately many stimuli which are visually more complex than human faces. It appears that the disorder is not specific to faces but to complex non-verbal visual stimuli that belong to a group where individual members are visually similar and yet individually different. For example, prosopagnosics cannot recognize their own car and do not recognize different makes of car; however, they can distinguish different classes of vehicle, e.g. ambulance or fire engine. Similarly, a case has been reported of a farmer suddenly becoming unable to distinguish individual animals within his herd and of a birdwatcher developing an inability to recognize different species of birds.

Prosopagnosics appear, therefore, to be unable to match a current visual stimulus within a class such as faces, with the memory traces of other members of this specific class which have been built up from past experience (De Renzi 1997). Pathophysiologically there is disorder of visually triggered contextual memory. Under normal circumstances after multiple exposures to a stimulus, a template of the stimulus is stored, perhaps at several levels, but in prosopagnosics there is a defect in activating this template. Recent brain-imaging studies have suggested that these processes involve the inferior temporal lobe and also the ventrolateral frontal cortex (Haxby *et al.* 1996). Certainly, in monkeys electrophysiological recordings from the superior temporal sulcus have identified neurons with a response specific for faces, which may well be involved in the facial recognition process (Perrett *et al.* 1984).

Most cases of prosopagnosia are due to infarction, head injury, or hypoxia resulting in bilateral lesions in the ventromedial aspects of the occipitotemporal region (Damasio *et al.* 1982).

8.8.5 Visual illusions

Visual illusions occur when the visually perceived target appears altered in size, shape, colour, position in space, and in number of images (Kölmel 1993). The illusory type of defects may occur in the entire field of vision, or may affect only the object or the background. The term 'dysmetropsia' indicates the apparent smallness (micropsia), largeness (macropsia), or irregularity of shape (metamorphopsia) of objects. Dysmetropsia usually occurs as a result of retinal disease, due to distortion of the relative distance between rods and cones. However, these distortions can also occur as a result of cortical dysfunction, for example in the aura of migraine or epilepsy, chiasmic compression, or focal cerebral lesions. Visual allesthesia is a transfer of visual images from one half field to the other (Jacobs 1980). There may also rarely be an inversion of the visual scene or tilting of the environment in patients with the lateral medullary syndrome (Wallenberg's syndrome) (Hornstein 1974). This relates to a disturbance of the vestibular inputs required for normal visual perception.

8.8.6 Visual hallucinations

Visual hallucinations occur under many circumstances, e.g. drug withdrawal, anoxia, migraine, infection, and schizophrenia, in addition to those related to focal neurological disease. Those in the latter category may be unformed, consisting of flashes of light (coloured or white), lines, or simple shapes, or they may be complex, highly organized hallucinations of people, objects, etc. (Kölmel 1993).

Although it is considered that simple visual hallucinations signify involvement of the occipital lobe, and complex ones involvement of the temporal lobe, this is not always the case; for example, complex hallucinations have been observed by patients with hemianopias due to occipital lobe lesions (Kölmel 1985).

It has long been considered that visual hallucinations could result from irritative foci analogous to epileptic discharges, and certainly electrical stimulation of the occipital and temporal lobes (Penfield and Perot 1963) support this suggestion. Another mechanism may be a release phenomenon to be found in the context of sensory deprivation (Charles Bonnet syndrome, in which visual cortical areas are deprived of normal visual impulses so releasing cortical activity which normal visual inputs keep suppressed). This is the explanation usually given to hallucinations occurring in elderly patients who have impaired vision (Teunisse *et al.* 1995). The term 'peduncular hallucinations' was first described by Lhermitte (1922) to describe visual hallucinations which appear animated, slow moving, cartoon-like, and are usually frightening for the patient. This type of hallucination is usually associated with inversion of the sleep–wake cycle, with diurnal somnolence and nocturnal insomnia, and occurs with lesions in the upper brainstem (McKee *et al.* 1990).

8.8.7 Palinopsia

Palinopsia is a rare disorder in which there is persistence (perseveration) or recurrence of visual images after the exciting stimulus has been removed (Bender *et al.* 1968). Although in the literature both perseveration and recurrence of visual images have been lumped together under the term palinopsia, it has been argued that they may be distinct (Blythe *et al.* 1986).

It most commonly occurs during the progressive evolution or resolution of a homonymous hemianopic field defect, usually resulting from a posterior cerebral hemisphere lesion due to neoplasia (Bender *et al.* 1968), vascular disease, or trauma.

Bender *et al.* (1968) suggested four possible mechanisms for this phenomenon: sensory seizures, psychogenic elaboration or fantasies, visual after-images, or hallucinations. Although some patients with palinopsia have had seizures, most have no evidence of seizure activity on the electroencephalogram, and the palinopsia does not respond to treatment with anticonvulsants. Patients with palinopsia show no signs of psychopathology and, therefore, it is unlikely that they are due to psychogenic elaborations. Similarly, there is no evidence that visual after-effects in patients with palinopsia are enhanced, and such an explanation would not explain the late recurrence of the image (by some several minutes) which occurs in some patients. However, palinopsia may be a type of release phenomenon as described for visual hallucinations. In favour of this possibility is the fact that formed release hallucinations can occur in patients with palinopsia and that in both conditions there is evidence of an interruption of cortical visual processing.

Specific types of palinoptic phenomena are illusory visual spread and polyopia. In illusory visual spread (Critchley 1951) there is an extension of visual perception over an area greater than that excited by the object presented to the observer. In the time domain, visual perseveration of moving objects has also been reported and one patient experienced accelerated movement of a perseverated image.

In instances of usually right-sided occipital lesions patients may experience monocular diplopia or more commonly polyopia (the seeing of multiple images) which persist whichever eye is closed. Rare cases of cerebral induced monocular diplopia emphasize the importance of ensuring that this phenomena is not present in patients complaining of diplopia. Other causes for monocular diplopia include ocular causes such as corneal irregularities, iris lesions, and retinal detachment.

Certain cases of polyopia may be due to epileptic phenomena (Bender and Sobein 1963), but Bender (1945), in a description of four cases, tried to explain the phenomenon as a result of impaired fixation.

8.9 Disorders of the pupil

A detailed account of the anatomy, physiology, and clinical applications of the pupil is to be found in the comprehensive monograph by Loewenfeld (1999).

8.9.1 The pupillary light reflex

The afferent pupillary light reflex pathway is a three-neuron reflex arc originating in the retinal ganglion cells, which project to the pretectal nucleus in the midbrain (Loewenfeld 1999) (Fig. 8.12). Interneurons from this area project to the Edinger–

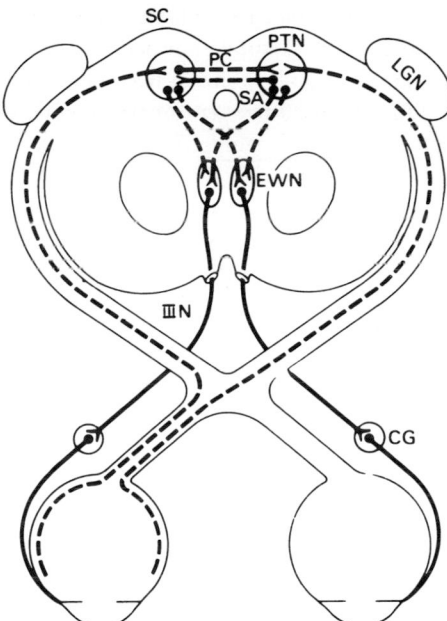

Fig. 8.12. Pupillary light reflex pathway. PC, posterior commissure; PTN, pretectal nucleus; SA, Sylvian aqueduct; LGN, lateral geniculate nucleus; EWN, Edinger–Westphal nucleus; SC, superior colliculus; CG, ciliary ganglion.

Westphal subnucleus of the oculomotor nucleus. Passing from the Edinger–Westphal nucleus preganglionic, parasympathetic efferent pupillary fibres lie in the periphery of the oculomotor nerve, where they are particularly susceptible to compression by aneurysms of the posterior communicating artery. They then pass via its inferior division to the ciliary ganglion lying in the floor of the orbit, and reach the iris sphincter muscle via the short ciliary nerves. Interruption of this pathway from the mesencephalon to the sphincter muscle causes pupillary dilatation and decreased speed and amplitude of constriction.

At the optic chiasm a slightly higher proportion of afferent fibres cross into the contralateral optic tract, with a ratio of crossed : uncrossed fibres which has been estimated at 53 : 47 (Kupfer *et al.* 1967). This may explain the afferent pupillary defect which is sometimes observed in patients with isolated retrochiasmal lesions. In the Edinger–Westphal nucleus there is a functional dissociation, with the rostral portion containing mainly efferent neurons relating to accommodation and the caudal neurons involved in pupil constriction.

The pupillary near response results from accommodative effort induced by retinal image blur or conscious near fixation. It is part of the 'near triad', which consists of pupillary constriction, lens accommodation, and convergence of the visual axes. It is possible for a number of neural lesions to give rise to a dissociation of components of the near triad, in which there is absent pupillary constriction with the other components remaining intact; but preservation of pupillary constriction with absence of convergence and lens accommodation does not occur.

The size of the pupil is in a constant state of flux, adjusting to a variety of external stimuli, such as ambient illumination and fixation distance, as well as psychosensory stimuli. Pupillary diameter tends to be smaller in infants and older adults compared to young adults. A subtle anisocoria is often observed, and a difference in pupillary size of 0.4 mm or more is easily identified clinically in 20 per cent of the normal population. This so-called simple (physiological) anisocoria is associated with a pupil inequality which is the same under all lighting conditions, and the pupillary light reactions are equally brisk.

8.9.2 Lesions of the afferent pupillary pathway

A unilateral lesion of the afferent pupillary pathway results in an impaired direct light reflex of the affected eye, sparing the consensual response elicited by stimulating the contralateral eye. If there is a complete lesion, either in the retina or optic nerve, there will be a complete failure of the direct light reflex. However, in most instances there is an impaired response, which is best identified clinically by using the swinging light test. It is performed by using a hand-held torch with a bright light beam, which is moved back and forth from one eye to the other, the light being held on each eye for approximately 1 second. When the light is shining in the normal eye the pupil is constricted and the contralateral consensual response is maximal. When the light is then shifted to the eye with the impaired vision the direct light reflex is now reduced in comparison with the former consensual response, resulting in further dilatation of the pupil (Thompson 1966). It is best to perform the test in a dimly lit room. The magnitude of the relative afferent pupillary defect (RAPD) (Marcus-Gunn pupil) may be estimated by placing neutral density filters over the normal eye until the responses from the two eyes are balanced (Thompson et al. 1981). A RAPD does not occur as a result of refractive errors, opaque optic media, amblyopia, or functional visual loss.

Retina

The degree to which an RAPD is identified due to retinal disease depends on the degree and location of the lesion. A small retinal detachment involving the macula may not result in an RAPD, whereas a complete detachment will certainly do so. A useful clinical guide is that if ophthalmoscopy reveals a normal macula, the presence of an RAPD is unlikely to be due to retinal disease. Suppression amblyopia does not result in an RAPD.

Optic nerve

Optic nerve disease is commonly associated with a RAPD, the magnitude of which correlates closely with the extent of the visual field defect and the visual acuity, particularly when due to optic neuritis (Ellis 1979). The absence of an RAPD in a patient with unilateral visual loss and an otherwise normal eye, should raise the possibility of bilateral optic nerve disease or non-organic visual loss. Bilateral optic nerve disease is suggested by a disassociation between the direct light reflex and the amplitude of the pupillary near response. Recovery of optic neuritis leads to a reduction in the RAPD but not usually to its absence.

Optic tract

A RAPD may be observed in some patients with optic tract disease in association with a homonymous hemianopia (Bell and Thompson 1978). The RAPD is in the eye with the temporal field loss, and is thought to be due to the asymmetric decussation of optic nerve fibres at the chiasm, as described above.

Pretectal nucleus and brachium of the superior colliculus

The pupillary fibres coming from the ipsilateral optic tract to the pretectal nucleus, via the brachium of the superior colliculus, may be involved by a unilateral lesion such as an arteriovenous malformation, infarction, or tumour (Wilhelm et al. 1996). This may produce a contralateral RAPD without any loss of visual acuity or colour vision, and without any visual field defect, although the RAPD may occasionally be associated with an ipsilateral or contralateral trochlear nerve paresis.

8.9.3 Lesions of the central pupillary pathway

Argyll Robertson pupils

For over a century, since the original description by Douglas Argyll Robertson in 1869 of the pupillary abnormalities subsequently shown to be associated with neurosyphilis, there has been controversy regarding the site of the lesion. The most widely held current view (Loewenfeld 1999) is that the classic Argyll Robertson pupil (A-R) is the result of neuronal damage in the region of the Sylvian aqueduct in the rostral midbrain. Diffuse damage around the sylvian aqueduct and the posterior portion of the third ventricle is a prominent finding in patients with Argyll Robertson pupils who have died from tabes or general paralysis. In this location the damage interferes with the light reflex fibres and the supranuclear inhibitory fibres as they approach the visceral oculomotor nuclei. The essential features of A-R pupils, which are usually bilateral and symmetric, are miosis with poor dilation in darkness, absence or marked impairment of the light reflex, and relative preservation of the near response (light–near dissociation). In addition, the pupil may be irregular due to iris damage, and shows impaired dilatation to mydriatic drugs.

As the incidence of tertiary syphilis has declined since the introduction of penicillin, the percentage of non-syphilitic patients with A-R pupils has increased. Typical A-R pupils have been observed in patients with diabetes mellitus (Smith and Smith 1983), chronic alcoholism, encephalitis, multiple sclerosis, age-related and degenerative diseases of the CNS, some rare midbrain tumours, and rarely in systemic inflammatory diseases, including sarcoidosis and neuroborreliosis. However, the main differential diagnosis is with bilateral tonic pupils, which after many years become small, unreactive to light, and show light–near dissociation. The major distinguishing feature is the presence of tonicity of the near response

Mesencephalic lesions

Pressure on the dorsal mesencephalon may produce Parinaud's syndrome, also known as the dorsal midbrain syndrome or the sylvian aqueduct syndrome. This syndrome, due to damage in the region of the posterior commissure, includes a supranuclear vertical gaze palsy, disturbances of pupillary function, accommodation difficulties, and, frequently, convergence retraction nystagmus. The pupils are usually dilated, fail to constrict to light or do so very poorly, and show relative preservation of the reaction to near vision (light–near dissociation). Dilated pupils due to an impaired light reflex may be the first sign of a pineal or other tumour that compresses or infiltrates the dorsal midbrain, or from hydrocephalus, particularly if caused by aqueductal stenosis or a blocked shunt.

Mesencephalic lesions in the region of the oculomotor nerve nucleus nearly always damage both the sympathetic and parasympathetic pathways to the eye, resulting in slightly unequal and irregular pupils. Rarely in midbrain lesions a phenomenon called correctopia occurs in which there is an upward, inward displacement of the pupil (Selhorst *et al.* 1976a).

8.9.4 Lesions of the efferent pupillary pathway

Involvement of the preganglionic parasympathetic fibres located in the periphery of the oculomotor nerve results in a dilated pupil which has an impaired or absent direct, consensual, and near response. Although such a finding suggests significant intracranial pathology, such as an unruptured posterior communicating artery aneurysm, there is usually in addition some degree of ptosis and ophthalmoplegia.

However, a dilated pupil which fails to respond either to light or to the near reflex raises the possibility of accidental or deliberate instillation of a pharmacologically active agent such as scopolamine, atropine, or some plant juices containing belladonna alkaloids. This can be reversed by instilling 1 per cent pilocarpine, in contrast to the pupillary dilatation which occurs due to an oculomotor nerve palsy or a tonic pupil. The possibility of acute-angle closure glaucoma must be considered in any patient presenting with pupillary inequality with reduced visual acuity or pain.

A rare condition of episodic unilateral transient pupillary dilatation with headache has been described in young women (Edelson and Levy 1974).

Tonic pupil

The most common cause of abnormal unilateral pupillary light reactions and a dilated pupil is the tonic pupil, due to a lesion involving the preganglionic parasympathetic neuron. The essential feature of a tonic pupil is a slow, steady near pupil response followed by the pupil holding its contraction for a few seconds when the patient is asked to look back into the distance. The tonic pupil is the result of damage to the ciliary ganglion or the short ciliary nerves, resulting in denervation and subsequent re-innervation of the iris sphincter and the ciliary muscle. Several different causes have been found, which have been classified by Thompson (1979):

(1) Holmes–Adie syndrome, associated with tendon areflexia;

(2) local tonic pupils, associated with orbital disease or following orbital surgery; and

(3) neuropathic tonic pupils, associated with peripheral or autonomic neuropathy.

Holmes–Adie syndrome

This is a relatively uncommon syndrome, which usually occurs between 20 and 50 years of age, has a clear predilection for women (women 70 per cent; men 30 per cent), and is unilateral in 80 per cent of cases. The onset is usually acute, with the patient often complaining of photophobia, particularly when going outdoors into bright sunlight, blurred near vision, an enlarged pupil and headaches. The essential features of the pupil abnormality are a delayed and reduced-amplitude light reaction. When the iris is viewed via a slit lamp, in about 90 per cent of cases it can be seen that there is segmental contraction of the sphincter muscle, with other segments appearing paralysed. This is in contradistinction to a tonic pupil due to pharmacological anticholinergic blockade, in which the entire sphincter is paralysed. The near response which is tonic, however, results in contraction of all the sphincter muscle. The pupillary dilatation is also tonic. As a result of denervation hypersensitivity the tonic pupil constricts with a low concentration of pilocarpine (0.125 per cent), but a normal pupil will not. However, the value of this pharmacological test has been questioned recently because of the false-positive results due to the variable corneal penetration of pilocarpine. Deep-tendon hyporeflexia or areflexia, particularly of the ankle and triceps jerks, can be demonstrated in a substantial number of patients with Holmes–Adie syndrome (Thompson *et al.* 1979a).

The pathology of the Holmes–Adie syndrome is considered to be degeneration of neurons in the ciliary ganglion, as has been observed in two post-mortem studies. The hyporeflexia or areflexia is probably due to a central lesion within the spinal cord. In one case degeneration was observed in the gracile and cuneate fascicles (Selhorst *et al.* 1984).

Two pathophysiological explanations have been proposed for the pupillary abnormalities. In the first Loewenfeld and Thompson (1967) proposed that some of the fibres originally destined for the ciliary muscle resprouted randomly, with some of the fibres reaching the iris sphincter and causing miosis every time the ciliary muscle was innervated. There is also a marked predominance of fibres arising from the ciliary ganglion passing to the ciliary muscle compared to those passing to the iris sphincter (97 per cent : 3 per cent), making such aberrant reinnervation a likely outcome of damage to the ganglion. This explanation was challenged by Wirtschafter and colleagues (1978), who proposed that the iris sphincter remains permanently denervated and that the pupillary near-vision constriction results from acetylcholine released by the accommodative nerve endings in the ciliary muscle. This then diffuses to the pupillary sphincter via the aqueous fluid. On the basis of several clinical observations this hypothesis is not widely supported (Thompson 1979).

Follow-up of patients with the Holmes–Adie syndrome have shown the following changes over time (Thompson *et al.* 1979*b*):

(1) recovery of the accommodation paresis;

(2) progressive impairment of the pupillary light reaction;

(3) increasing hypometria of the deep-tendon reflexes;

(4) the affected pupil gradually becomes smaller; and

(5) the other eye may become involved.

Local causes

An acute internal ophthalmoplegia followed by the development of a tonic pupil has been reported following a variety of infections, inflammations, and infiltrative processes which involve the ciliary ganglion. These include infections by herpes zoster, chickenpox, measles, diphtheria, syphilis, rheumatoid arthritis, sarcoidosis, primary and metastatic choroidal and orbital tumours, blunt injury to the orbit and penetrating injuries, as well as following various ocular and orbital surgical procedures (Lowenstein and Loewenfeld 1965).

Neuropathic tonic pupils

This category consists of tonic pupils which are a result of involvement of the ciliary ganglion or short ciliary nerves as part of a generalized peripheral or autonomic neuropathy. These include those with chronic alcoholism, diabetes mellitus, Guillain–Barré syndrome and the Miller Fisher variant and some hereditary neuropathies. Those autonomic neuropathies which can result in a tonic pupil include acute pandysautonomia, Shy–Drager syndrome, and Sjögren's syndrome, in which the pupil abnormality may be the presenting sign.

8.9.5 Lesions of the sympathetic pathway

A lesion anywhere along the long sympathetic pathway results in a typical Horner's syndrome with miosis and ptosis. The central, first-order, neuron lies in the ipsilateral hypothalamus, and its axon passes to the ciliospinal centre in the intermediolateral grey column via the dorsolateral medulla. Here it synapses with the preganglionic second-order neuron in the upper three dorsal segments of the spinal cord. The axon from the preganglionic neuron exits the spinal cord at this level, passes across the pulmonary apex to ascend to the superior cervical ganglion via the inferior and middle cervical ganglia. The postganglionic, third-order, neuron passes from the superior cervical ganglion up along the internal carotid artery, where it is termed the carotid plexus. It leaves the internal carotid artery in the cavernous sinus, to briefly join the abducens nerve before leaving it to join the ophthalmic division of the trigeminal nerve, entering the orbit with its nasociliary branch.

The ptosis in Horner's syndrome is usually slight, due to paralysis of the sympathetically innervated smooth muscle (Müller's muscle) in the upper eyelid. Similar smooth muscle fibres in the lower eyelid are denervated, leading to a slight elevation of the lower lid, producing an 'upside-down' ptosis. Combined, these result in a narrowed palpebral fissure and an apparent enophthalmos.

The miosis is due to complete or partial sympathetic denervation of the iris dilator muscle, leading to constriction of the iris sphincter, producing a small pupil. The weakness of the dilator muscle is greatest in the dark when the anisocoria is most apparent, and may be almost absent in the light. The extent of the anisocoria varies in extent, depending on a number of factors which include completeness of the lesion and the extent of re-innervation, the alertness of the patient, the degree of denervation supersensitivity, and the level of circulating adrenergic substances in the blood.

The paresis of the dilator muscle can be detected by observing a dilation lag of the affected pupil compared to the normal pupil when the lights are turned out. This is best performed by holding a torchlight on the eyes from below and turning the room lights out (Loewenfeld 1999). A simultaneous sudden noise accentuates the lag, due to enhanced sympathetic activation of the intact pupil.

Depigmentation of the affected iris is rarely observed in acquired Horner's disease, although hypochromia of the iris is a common finding in the congenital form.

Horner's syndrome is also associated with characteristic vasomotor and sudomotor changes on the affected side of the face, such as loss of sweating (anhidrosis) and occasionally facial flushing. These changes are most frequently observed following preganglionic lesions, since the fibres for sweating pass onto the external carotid artery from the superior cervical ganglion.

On some occasions the presence or absence of a Horner's syndrome may be in doubt, in which case pharmacologic testing can be applied. Cocaine blocks the reuptake of noradrenaline in the sympathetic nerve endings so, when applied to the eye, leads to a dilatation of the pupil (Thompson 1977). When two drops of a 2–10 per cent solution of cocaine are applied to each eye in turn, after 30–40 minutes the affected pupil is found to have dilated less than the normal pupil. This occurs because the sympathetic denervation leads to a reduced release of noradrenaline and a reduced amount accumulates at the receptors of effector cells. It is important to observe the diameter of the pupils in a dimmed room since the background ambient illumination may lead to pupillary constriction, thereby obscuring the pharmacologically induced anisocoria. The cocaine test will be positive for a Horner's syndrome associated with a lesion anywhere along the sympathetic pathway.

Localization of the site of damage giving rise to a Horner's syndrome usually depends on the associated clinical findings (Fig. 8.13). Lesions affecting the first-order and second-order neurons may be accompanied by signs of dysfunction of the brainstem and cervicothoracic spinal cord respectively. Lesions involving the third-order, postganglionic neuron are accompanied by signs of lesions affecting structures around the common and internal carotid arteries. The various aetiologies of Horner's syndrome at these different levels are listed in

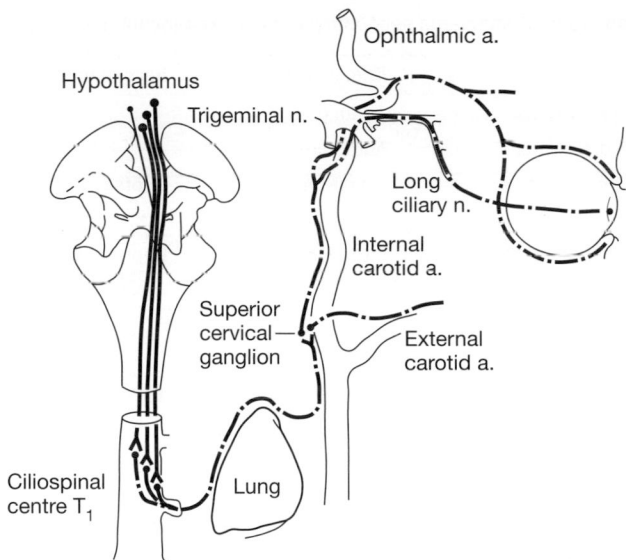

Fig. 8.13. The sympathetic pathway to the pupil. Note that the sympathetic fibres to the face pass on to the external carotid artery.

Table 8.5. When trying to determine the location of the sympathetic lesion further pharmacological can be of assistance. Hydroxyamphetamine (1 per cent) causes the release of noradrenaline from sympathetic nerve endings and, if applied to the normal eye, results in pupil dilation (Van der Wiel and van Gijn 1983). It can, therefore, be used to differentiate between a postganglionic and a preganglionic or central Horner's syndrome, since in the former the nerve endings are destroyed and there are no noradrenaline stores to release and there is therefore no mydriatic effect. If the lesion involves the preganglionic or central neuron, the pupil will dilate fully.

Table 8.5. Aetiology of Horner's syndrome

Central (first neuron)
    Lateral medullary infarction
    Other brainstem infarction
    Cerebral infarction
    Cerebral haemorrhage
    Intracranial tumour
    Trauma (including surgery)
    Multiple sclerosis
    Syrinx
    Transverse myelopathy
    Other/unknown

Preganglionic (second) neuron
    Thoracic and neck tumour
    Trauma
      surgical
      non-surgical
    Other/unknown

Postganglionic (third) neuron
    Intracranial tumour (cavernous sinus)
    Trauma (including surgical)
    Carotid artery dissection
    Vascular headache
    Other unknown
Unknown localization

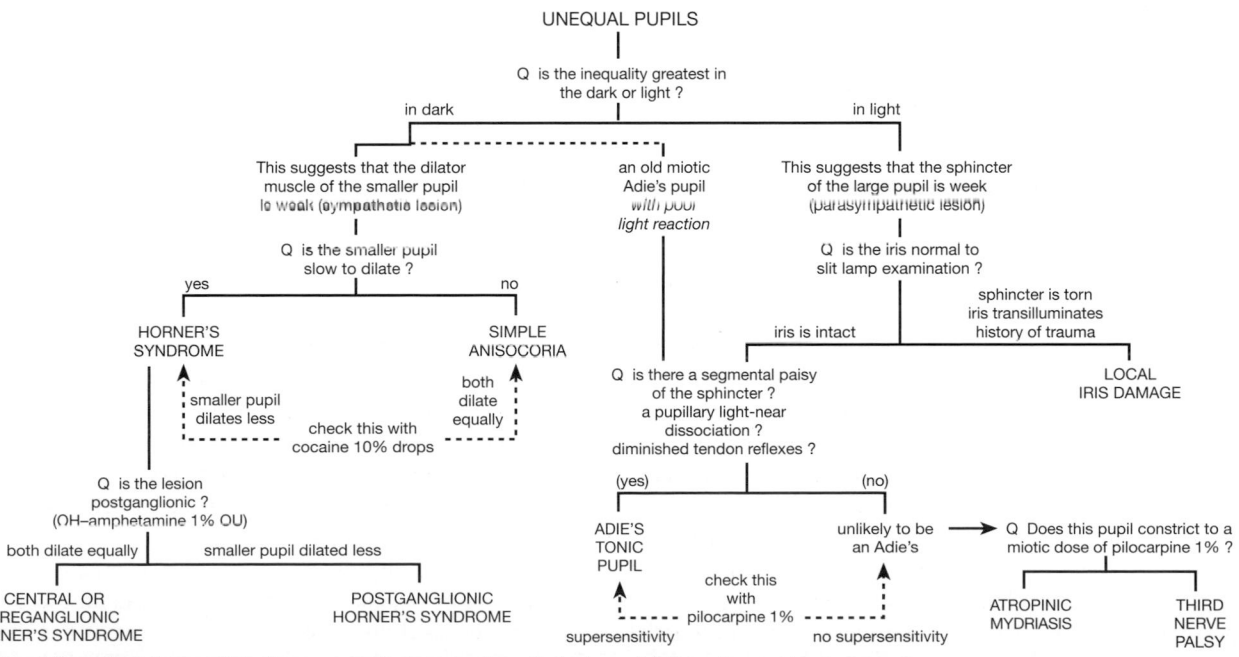

Fig. 8.14. A flow chart for the clinical assessment of unequal pupils (anisocoria) (from Czarnecki *et al.* 1979).

8.9.6 Differentiation of anisocoria

Using some straightforward principles Thompson and Pilley (1976) have described a straightforward approach to determine the cause for anisocoria. If the anisocoria is more apparent in light compared with darkness, this suggests that there is a defect in the parasympathetic system or the sphincter muscles, since this implies that both pupils dilate in the dark but one pupil does not respond to light stimulation. If the opposite is observed, that is the anisocoria is more evident in darkness than in light, this suggests that the parasympathetic pathway and the iris sphincter are intact, since both pupils constrict in the light yet one pupil dilates more in darkness than the other.

In a flow chart (Fig. 8.14) indicating the various steps to differentiate between the different causes of anisocoria, the first step is to check the light reaction. A normal light reaction in both eyes suggests that the anisocoria is due either to simple anisocoria or a Horner's syndrome. These two conditions can be differentiated using 10 per cent cocaine. A positive cocaine test may call for a hydroxyamphetamine test on another occasion to differentiate a postganglionic from a preganglionic and central sympathetic lesion.

If the light reaction in one or both eyes is impaired, the patient has a parasympathetic lesion or a damaged iris sphincter. The iris is then viewed with a slit lamp to identify any iris damage. At this point it is necessary to differentiate a pharmacologically blockaded pupil from a neurogenic cause: 0.1 per cent pilocarpine can be used to detect denervation supersensitivity of the parasympathetic system as occurs in a tonic pupil syndrome. If neither pupil constricts, then a 1 per cent solution of pilocarpine will identify a dilated pupil due to pharmacological blockade, since the pupil will fail to constrict.

8.10 Disorders of eye movements

A detailed description of the neural control of eye movements and their disorders can be found in the excellent monograph by Leigh and Zee (1999).

8.10.1 Examining eye movements

Actions of the extraocular muscles

Each eye is rotated by six muscles: four recti and two obliques. It should be noted that the actions of the muscles are dependent on the starting position of the eye. For example, the superior rectus, because of the anatomy of its insertion into the sclera, acts as a pure elevator only when the globe is abducted by 23°. With increasing adduction of the eye from this position, the superior rectus acts more as an intorter and less as an elevator. Similarly, the superior oblique acts purely as a depressor only when the eye is adducted, and more as an intorter with increasing abduction of the eye. The primary and secondary actions of the different extraocular muscles are shown in Table 8.6.

The other important feature is that the yoke pair of muscles from each eye (e.g. right medial rectus and left lateral rectus,

Table 8.6. Primary and secondary action of extraocular muscles

Muscle	Primary action	Secondary action
Lateral rectus	Abduction	–
Medial rectus	Adduction	–
Superior rectus	Elevation	Intorsion
Inferior rectus	Depression	Extorsion
Superior oblique	Intorsion	Depression
Inferior oblique	Extorsion	Elevation

left superior rectus and right inferior oblique) receive equal innervation (Hering's law of motor correspondence) so that eye movements are conjugate. It should be noted that the fixating eye determines the innervational input to both eyes. This is of importance in the assessment of the cover test, and in the interpretation of investigations such as the Hess screen test.

The assessment of diplopia

It is first essential (Shaunak *et al.* 1997) to decide whether the patient is complaining of diplopia due to a disparity in retinal stimulation between the two eyes (binocular diplopia), or, more rarely, when it is present in one eye only (monocular diplopia). Monocular diplopia occurs, with few exceptions, when there are abnormalities of the ocular refractive surfaces and media, producing multiple overlapping images on the retina. The most common cause is myopic astigmatism, but monocular diplopia may occur in early cataracts, especially under conditions of dim illumination. Other causes include abnormalities of the cornea and iris, foreign bodies in the aqueous or vitreous humour, retinal disease, occipital cortex pathology, and psychogenic causes.

If the diplopia is alleviated by covering one eye, a systematic approach to evaluation is required. As well as determining the nature of the separation of the two images and the direction of maximal separation, enquiries as to the presence of a family history of strabismus, or a childhood history of orthoptic treatment should be made. If the eyes are misaligned, it should be ascertained at an early stage if one is dealing with a non-comitant or comitant strabismus; the degree of misalignment varies with gaze position in the first, but does not vary with gaze position in the second. Non-comitance suggests a recent paretic or restrictive aetiology. Comitance is characteristic of childhood strabismus, and diplopia in such circumstances is usually due to decompensation of a long-standing phoria (a deviation of the visual axes when only one eye is viewing), normally kept in check by fusional mechanisms (a latent deviation). The term tropia, as used later, refers to a deviation of the visual axes when both eyes are viewing, which is not kept in check by fusion (a manifest deviation).

Patients with diplopia may adapt a compensatory head posture, and the position of the chin, head, and face should therefore be carefully observed. The purpose of the abnormal head posture is to turn the eyes as far as possible from the field of action of the weak muscle. Hence, if one of the muscles that mediates conjugate gaze to the right is underacting, the face will be turned to the right. Underaction of the superior and inferior recti, which act primarily to move the eyes in the vertical plane, is compensated by head flexion and extension respectively. Torsional diplopia usually arises from underaction of the superior and inferior oblique muscles, and patients with this symptom often tilt their head towards the shoulder opposite to that of the weak muscle.

Identification of the paretic muscle

In the cover/uncover test the patient, wearing appropriate refractive correction, is asked to fixate a distant target (e.g. a letter on the Snellen chart) with the eyes in the primary position, repeating the test in the nine cardinal positions of gaze and with near fixation (Fig. 8.15). For each position in turn each eye is covered and then uncovered and initially the movements of the uncovered eye are observed. Cover tests rely on the fact that foveation occurs in an eye that is forced to fixate. If the retinal image was not directed on to the fovea before the eye took up fixation, a movement of redress will be noted as the eye fixates, which gives an indication of the degree of misalignment of the visual axes. If the uncovered eye moves to take up fixation, it can be assumed that under binocular viewing conditions the eye was not aligned with fixation, and a manifest deviation was present (a tropia). Inward movement of the uncovered eye indicates an exotropia, and an outward movement an esotropia. A vertical deviation may be either a hypotropia or a hypertropia, depending on whether the eye moves up or down, respectively. The examiner should determine whether the tropia is comitant or non-comitant by seeing if the magnitude of the deviation varies with the position of the eye. If no tropia is present, and the uncovered eye is observed to assume fixation just after it is uncovered, a latent deviation (a heterophoria) is present. Depending on the direction of the deviation this may be classified as an exophoria, esophoria, hypophoria, or a hyperphoria. The test is then repeated, and the same observations made while covering the other eye. It should be noted that the convention is that if there is a vertical deviation of the eyes, the higher of the two is referred to as hypertropic/hyperphoric, regardless of which eye is at fault.

The alternate cover test is more dissociating that the cover/uncover test, and is used to fully dissociate the eyes and show the maximal deviation While the patient fixates a target the occluder is quickly switched from eye to eye to prevent binocular viewing, allowing sufficient time for the eyes to settle in their new position after each transfer. The test should be performed in the nine cardinal positions of gaze to determine the direction of gaze that elicits the maximal direction, and the eye in which fixation in that field of gaze causes the maximal devia-

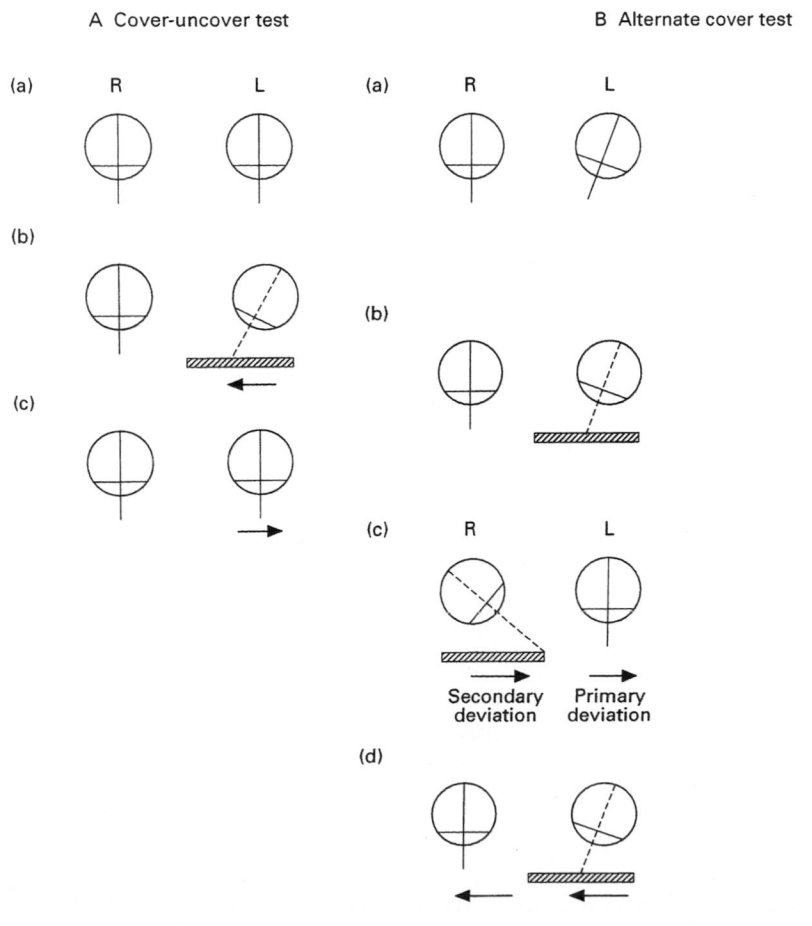

Fig. 8.15. A. Cover/uncover test, showing the presence of an esophoria. Dotted lines indicate the position of the eye when under cover. (a) At rest the visual axes are aligned correctly. (b) When the cover is placed before the left eye, the eye no longer fixates and moves inwards. (c) On removal of the cover the eye moves outwards to take up fixation, indicating an esophoria. B. The alternate cover test, showing the presence of an esotropia. (a) At rest, with both eyes viewing, there is a manifest inward deviation of the left eye. (b) A cover placed before the non-fixating left eye causes no movement. (c) When the right eye is occluded, the left eye is forced to fixate, and a movement of redress occurs (the primary deviation). The resulting additional innervation to the contralateral yoke muscle leads to deviation of the sound eye under the cover (the secondary deviation). Note that the secondary deviation is greater than the primary deviation. (d) When the cover is transferred to the left eye both eyes assume their original position.

tion. While ensuring that the patient is never allowed to regain fixation during transfer of the occluder, the examiner notes the movement of the uncovered eye as the occluder is transferred from one eye to the other. Movement of the uncovered eye may indicate either a heterotropia or a heterophoria, and the alternate cover test will not differentiate between the two. The cover/uncover test should therefore be performed first to determine if a tropia is present.

When there is a vertical deviation of the visual axes, the hypertropic (higher) eye always gives rise to the lower image. This may be due either to a paresis of the depressor muscles of the hypertropic eye or the elevators of the other eye. There are now four possible defective muscles, which can be further reduced to two by asking the patient to look to the left and the right and state in which direction the deviation is maximal. Finally, determining which of these two muscles is paretic is decided by finding whether the deviation is maximal in up or down gaze.

In some instances there may be no differential vertical deviation; this situation occurs with chronic palsies due to an adaptive phenomenon, termed 'spread of comitance'. To work out which vertical muscle is paretic the Bielschowsky head-tilt test is performed. In this test the vertical deviation is compared with the alternate cover test in right and left head-tilt positions. The degree of misalignment will increase when the head is tilted to the side of the paretic muscle if the ipsilateral intorters (superior oblique and superior rectus) are weak, and to the opposite side if the extorting muscles (inferior oblique and inferior rectus) are weak. In practice, an increased misalignment on head tilt is usually indicative of an ipsilateral superior oblique palsy. The test is less often positive with palsies of the vertical recti or inferior oblique muscles.

The explanation for the effect lies in the fact that a head tilt to either shoulder induces an ocular counter-rolling, which is mediated by the ipsilateral intorters (superior rectus and superior oblique) and the contralateral extorters (inferior rectus and inferior oblique). If, for example, the ipsilateral superior oblique is paretic, the superior rectus on the same side receives excessive innervation to intort the eye and, by virtue of its relatively unopposed primary action, elevates the eye.

8.10.2 Oculomotor nerve palsies

The oculomotor (third cranial nerve) nerve, in addition to innervating the superior, medial, and inferior rectus, and inferior oblique eye muscles, also supplies the levator palpebrae superioris muscle and carries the parasympathetic nerve fibres to the sphincter muscle of the pupil and the ciliary body. A complete oculomotor palsy is easily recognized by ptosis, a fixed dilated pupil, and an eye which is deviated 'down and out' due to the unopposed action of the lateral rectus and superior oblique, although partial palsies are more common (Fig. 8.16). The nerve may be damaged anywhere along its course from the nuclear complex to the muscles, and the combination of an oculomotor palsy with other cranial nerve deficits (cranial nerves II, IV, V, or VI) and the long-tract signs usually enables accurate localization of the site of the lesion. Numerous causes

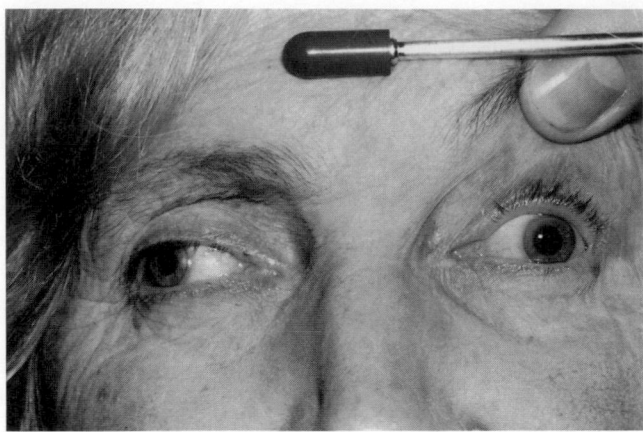

Fig. 8.16. Third cranial nerve palsy. A left oculomotor nerve palsy showing ptosis, pupillary dilation, and abduction of the eye due to the unopposed action of the lateral rectus muscle.

of oculomotor nerve palsies have been described (Table 8.7), and in adults the most common are either an aneurysm or presumed peripheral nerve vascular microinfarction, although evidence is growing that fascicular damage in the brainstem may be a more frequent cause than previously thought (Rush and Younge 1981). These infarcts are commonly associated with arteriosclerosis, hypertension, and diabetes mellitus. Infarcts and aneurysms each account for approximately 20 per cent of the total number of oculomotor palsies. The next most common are tumours or trauma, which each account for 10–15 per cent of cases (Richards *et al.* 1992).

The oculomotor nuclear complex is a paired structure lying beneath the aqueductal grey matter of the rostral midbrain at the level of the superior colliculus. The nuclear complex is divided into distinct motor pools subserving individual extraocular muscles. From the clinical point of view the following features should be noted: the caudal nucleus is a single midline structure supplying the levator palpebrae superioris muscles; the nuclei for each superior rectus muscle lie dorsally, close to the midline, and the axons cross the midline to innervate the contralateral muscle. Two patterns of ocular motility are characteristic of lesions of the oculomotor complex, either an isolated complete bilateral ptosis or a unilateral palsy of the medial rectus, inferior rectus, and inferior oblique together with a contralateral superior rectus palsy. Daroff (1970) has suggested the following clinical rules to decide whether or not a disorder of the oculomotor nerve is due to a nuclear lesion.

1. Conditions which cannot represent nuclear lesions:

   (a) unilateral external ophthalmoplegia (with or without pupil involvement) associated with normal contralateral superior rectus function;

   (b) unilateral internal ophthalmoplegia;

   (c) unilateral ptosis.

2. Conditions which may be nuclear:

   (a) bilateral total third nerve palsy;

   (b) bilateral ptosis;

Table 8.7. Causes of oculomotor nerve palsy

Nuclear
    Congenital hypoplasia
    Infarction
    Tumour (metastatic)

Fascicular
    Infarction
    Demyelination (rare)
    Tumour

Subarachnoid
    Aneurysm
    Meningitis
    Infarction
    Tumour
    Neurosurgical complication

At the tentorial edge
    Uncal herniation
    Pseudotumour cerebri
    Trauma

Cavernous sinus and superior orbital fissure
    Aneurysm
    Thombosis
    Carotid–cavernous fistula
    Tumour (pituitary adenoma, meningioma, nasopharyngeal, and other
        metastases)
    Pituitary apoplexy
    Tolosa–Hunt syndrome
    Sphenoidal sinusitis
    Mucormycosis and other fungal infections
    Herpes zoster
    Nerve infarction (associated with hypertension and diabetes)

Orbit
    Trauma
    Pseudotumour

Localization uncertain
    Viral infections and infectous mononucleosis
    Following immunization
    Migraine
    Arteritis
    Guillain–Barré and Miller Fisher syndromes

(c) bilateral internal ophthalmoplegia;

(d) bilateral medial rectus palsy;

(e) isolated single muscle involvement (except levator and superior rectus).

3   Obligatory nuclear lesions:

(a) unilateral third nerve palsy with contralateral superior rectus and bilateral partial ptosis;

(b) bilateral third nerve palsy (with or without internal ophthalmoplegia) associated with spared levator function.

Infarction of this region of the mid-brain often involves more rostral structures, resulting in supranuclear vertical gaze disorders. Isolated nuclear oculomotor nerve palsies of vascular origin usually occur as a result of selective embolic or thrombotic occlusion of small dorsal perforating branches of the mes-

encephalic portion of the basilar artery, or less often, from occlusion of the distal portion of the basilar artery itself ('top of the basilar syndrome'). Other aetiologies include haemorrhage, infiltration by tumour, inflammation, and brainstem compression (Bogousslevsky *et al.* 1994).

It has been proposed that both medial rectii subnuclei may be damaged in patients who show bilateral adduction failure with exotropia and loss of convergence. This has been called 'WEBINO' (wall-eyed bilateral internuclear ophthalmoplegia) (Daroff and Hoyt 1971).

The fascicles of the oculomotor nerve pass ventrally through the medial longitudinal fasiculus, red nucleus, substantia nigra, and the medial cerebral peduncle. Lesions of the nerve in this location are normally either due to infarction or tumours, and their precise anatomical location determines the associated neurological signs. Thus, a lesion in the red nucleus results in a contralateral cerebellar tremor (Nothnagel's syndrome), or is associated with contralateral involuntary movements (Benedikt's syndrome). If the lesion is in the cerebral peduncle, the oculomotor palsy is associated with a contralateral hemiparesis (Weber's syndrome). When the lesion is more extensive, involving the red nucleus and cerebral peduncle, all these signs are present (Claude's syndrome). Palsies of one extraocular muscle may occur due to a lesion within the oculomotor nerve fascicles due to their topographic organization. It is suggested that the most medial fibres are for the pupil, followed by fibres for the inferior rectus, levator, medial rectus, superior rectus and, most laterally, the inferior oblique (Castro *et al.* 1990).

The fascicles emerge from the midbrain as several rootlets in the interpeduncular space, where basal tumours and the rare basilar artery aneurysm may compress the nerve and the cerebral peduncle in an extrinsically produced Weber's syndrome. The nerve then passes below the uncus of the temporal lobe lying lateral to the posterior communicating artery. During cerebral herniation due to a unilateral mass lesion the nerve is compressed against the tentorial edge, petroclinoid ligament, or clivus by the uncus. Since the pupillary fibres travel superficially and superonasally in the nerve they are normally affected first during compression leading to mydriasis, to be followed by ptosis and then extraocular muscle weakness. Aneurysms of the posterior communicating artery damage the oculomotor nerve by haemorrhage into the nerve itself or into the aneurysm sac, which causes enlargement and stretching of the nerve to which it is adherent. These aneurysms are often associated with orbital or facial pain, which may precede the oculomotor paresis by up to 2 weeks. It is very unusual for an aneurysm to present with an oculomotor nerve with sparing of the pupil, i.e. normal pupillary function, and in such cases the pupil usually becomes involved within 10 days (Nadeau and Trobe 1983; Trobe 1988; Cullom *et al.* 1995).

An important cause for an oculomotor palsy is trauma, which usually has to be severe enough to lead to skull fractures and loss of consciousness. The nerve may be damaged at three different locations: as it emerges from the midbrain (rootlet avulsion), in the subarachnoid space where the nerve is fixed as it penetrates the dura, and finally in relation to fractures of the superior orbital fissure. Mild head injury resulting in an oculo-motor palsy should always raise the possibility of a tumour in the skull base (Eyster *et al.* 1972). As the nerve lies in the sub-arachnoid space it is vulnerable to damage from inflammatory processes, particularly infection such as tuberculosis, meningo-coccus, and syphilis.

Shortly after piercing the dura lateral to the posterior clinoid process, the oculomotor nerve enters the cavernous sinus where it lies above the trochlear nerve. In this location it is usual for the nerve to be involved with the other ocular motor nerves, and the first and second divisions of the trigeminal nerve. A partial involvement of the nerve, often with sparing of the pupilloconstrictor fibres, is common. Involvement of the nerve in this location may be due to local infection or inflammation, compression by aneurysms of the intracavernous portion of the internal carotid artery, in which case there is often accom-panying orbital or facial pain, or by meningiomas or lateral extensions of pituitary tumours.

In the rostral part of the cavernous sinus or in the superior orbital fissure the oculomotor nerve divides into a superior division, which supplies the superior rectus and levator pal-pebrae superioris muscles, and an inferior division, which sup-plies the medial and inferior rectii and the inferior oblique muscles as well as the parasympathetic pupilloconstrictor fibres. Isolated palsy of the superior branch has been described due to intracavernous internal carotid artery aneurysm, and of the inferior branch to trauma and tumour. Presumed post-infectious isolated branch palsies have also been reported. However, since the oculomotor nerve has a divisional topo-graphic arrangement beginning in the brainstem, a divisional oculomotor nerve palsy can arise from a lesion anywhere along its course.

One of the most common causes for an isolated oculomotor nerve palsy is microvascular infarction, which may be associ-ated with diabetes mellitus, hypertension, atherosclerosis, or collagen vascular disease. Under these circumstances there is usually partial or complete sparing of the pupil (Goldstein and Cogan 1960). Pathological studies have shown focal demyel-ination without axonal degeneration due to occlusion of intraneural arteries in the intracavernous or subarachnoid seg-ments, with relative sparing of the peripherally located para-sympathetic fibres which are supplied by the vasa nervorum (Asbury *et al.* 1970). Rarely, the pupil may be involved with vas-cular oculomotor nerve lesions. Clinically the palsy may be pre-ceded by orbital or facial pain which disappears with the onset of the paresis. In diabetes mellitus the palsy may be the present-ing symptom, but in an established diabetic, if associated with other ocular motor palsies, a paranasal sinus or orbital infection by mucormycosis must be considered.

Injury of the oculomotor nerve often results in subsequent *aberrant regeneration*. The most common clinical findings are lid elevation when the globe is adducted or depressed (pseudo-von Graefe phenomenon), with absence of, or only partial, ver-tical eye movement. In addition, lid depression on abduction and pupil constriction on adduction or depression despite

absent pupillary reflexes may occur (Forster *et al.* 1969). Aberrant regeneration may occur after trauma, aneurysm, con-genital third nerve palsy, and migraine, but not after micro-infarction due to hypertension or diabetes mellitus, presumably due to preservation of axonal continuity. In addition, it may occur without a history of preceding oculomotor palsy—primary aberrant regeneration. In this case an intracavernous meningioma or carotid aneurysm should be sought (Cox *et al.* 1979). The hypothesis which has been used traditionally to explain this oculomotor synkinesis is that at the site of nerve injury axons become misdirected and eventually innervate muscles for which they were not originally intended. Although there is good support for this hypothesis, both experimentally and clinically, other explanations have had to be considered to explain both primary aberrant regeneration, in which there is no acute nerve injury, and the transient nature of the phenome-non in some patients (Lepore and Glaser 1980). These have included ephaptic transmission, in which synkinetic move-ments may arise from interaxonal cross-activation (ephaptic) at the site of the injury, or, as a result of peripheral axonolysis, there may be reorganization of neuronal central connections which unmask previously encoded synkinetic movements. Currently there is no single explanation which explains ade-quately all the clinical features of oculomotor synkinesis.

Isolated oculomotor palsy in infancy and childhood is rare and most often congenital (Victor 1976; Kodsi and Younge 1992). They probably result from ischaemic or hypoxic insults to the brainstem *in utero*, which may lead to hypoplasia of the nucleus. Some probably result from traction to the subarach-noid portion of the nerve during labour. These palsies are often incomplete and show evidence of aberrant regeneration. The acquired causes include trauma, inflammatory disease, tumour, aneurysms, and ophthalmoplegic migraine (Miller 1977). Slowly progressive isolated palsies should undergo imaging every 2 years, with the expectation of eventually detecting a small tumour somewhere along the course of the nerve. An unusual phenomenon is *cyclic oculomotor paresis*, which usually occurs in early childhood, but may be noted at birth. In this condition oculomotor paresis alternates every 2 minutes, with the shorter spasms of oculomotor 'overactivity' lasting 10–30 seconds when the ptotic lid elevates, the globe begins to adduct, the pupil constricts, and accommodation increases. The condition usually persists unchanged throughout life (Loewenfeld and Thompson 1975).

Ophthalmoplegic migraine has its onset in childhood and occurs in the setting of headache, photophobia, cyclical vo-miting, or other migrainous symptoms. A family history of migraine is usually absent. The oculomotor palsy may persist for some time after the headache has resolved, and may in fact develop as the headache phase abates. The cause of the palsy is considered to be either compression of the oculomotor nerve by a swollen dilated carotid or basilar artery, or a delayed ischaemic neuropathy (Walsh and O'Doherty 1960). When such a condition occurs in a young child there is obviously concern about the possibility of an aneurysm. However, presentation of a Berry aneurysm under the age of 10 years is exceptionally rare, and if the palsy recovers along with the other symptoms, angiography is not indicated. In a teenager, MR angiography is advisable.

Patients with *ocular neuromyotonia* experience paroxysmal diplopia due to involuntary contraction of muscles supplied by the oculomotor nerve, although the abducens and trochlear nerves may also be involved. This condition usually, but not always, occurs in the context of a patient who has previously received radiotherapy for skull-base or thalamic tumours. The presumed cause is a radiation-induced cranial neuropathy manifesting as a spontaneous discharge from axons with unstable cell membranes. This produces a tonic contraction of one or more muscles, and the paroxysms occur 20–30 times daily. The paroxysms, which last several minutes, may be induced by sudden shifts of gaze into the field of action of the involved muscles. Most patients respond satisfactorily to carbamazepine (Ezra *et al.* 1996).

8.10.3 **Trochlear nerve palsies**

The trochlear nerve (fourth cranial nerve) passes from its nucleus to decussate with the contralateral nerve in the anterior medullary velum, which forms the anterior roof of the fourth ventricle just caudal to the inferior olive. It is unique amongst motor nerves since it emerges from the dorsal surface of the brain, and then passes round the midbrain tectum, crossing the inferior cerebellar artery to reach the free edge of the tentorium, where it enters the dura to run forward into the cavernous sinus. It finally enters the orbit through the superior orbital fissure to innervate the superior oblique muscle. It is the most slender of all the cranial nerves and has the longest intracranial course.

A trochlear nerve palsy is the most common cause for vertical extraocular muscle weakness, but is less common than palsies of the other ocular motor nerves (Richards *et al.* 1992; Tiffin *et al.* 1996). The aetiological causes of trochlear nerve palsies are listed in Table 8.8. However, as with an isolated lateral rectus muscle paresis, other orbital causes for an isolated paresis of the superior oblique muscle must be sought before it can be attributed to a trochlear nerve lesion. These include skew deviation, myasthenia gravis, dysthyroid myopathy and other restrictive ocular myopathies, childhood strabismus syndromes, and *Brown's superior oblique tendon sheath syndrome*. In the latter condition there is restricted elevation of the adducted eye, which may be congenital due to a shortened superior oblique tendon, or acquired when it is caused by a tenosynovitis or neoplastic infiltration of the tendon as it passes through the trochlear pulley (Brown 1973).

Clinically the patient with a trochlear nerve paresis usually complains of vertical and torsional diplopia accentuated by looking down. There is usually a compensatory head tilt to the side opposite the affected eye, with the chin down. In the majority of cases there is a hypertropia of the affected eye with an increased vertical deviation of the two images when the head

Table 8.8. Causes of trochlear nerve palsy

Nuclear and fascicular
   Infarction or haemorrhage
   Aplasia
   Demyelination
   Trauma
Subarachnoid
   Trauma
   Tumour
   Neurosurgical procedure
   Mastoiditis
   Meningitis
Cavernous sinus and superior orbital fissure
   Tumour
   Thrombosis
   Aneurysm
   Tolosa–Hunt syndrome
   Herpes zoster
Orbit
   Ethmoidectomy
   Ethmoiditis or maxillary sinusitis
   Trauma
Localization uncertain
   Infarction (associated with hypertension and diabetes)

is tilted to the side of the paretic muscle (Bielschowsky manoeuvre). A unilateral trochlear nerve paresis is usually associated with torsional diplopia on downgaze, with the false image tilted outwards. Torsion greater than 10° is usually indicative of a bilateral weakness of the superior obliques, as does a V-pattern esotropia.

It is impossible to differentiate clinically a lesion of the nucleus from a nerve lesion. The nucleus may be congenitally hypoplastic or damaged by haemorrhage or tumour. The only clue to a lesion of the nucleus or fascicle is the association of a trochlear nerve paresis with a unilateral Horner's syndrome and a relative afferent pupillary defect without evidence of an optic nerve or tract syndrome (Mansour and Reinecke 1986). More commonly the nerve is affected in its long subarachnoid course, especially from head trauma, both severe and minor. The nerve is particularly prone to damage due to its position in respect to the edge of the tentorium. Blunt injury to the forehead or skull leads to a contrecoup contusion of the midbrain tectum by the free tentorial edge. The resulting trochlear nerve palsy is often bilateral (Lepore 1995).

The second most common cause of an isolated trochlear nerve paresis is microinfarction, often associated with hypertension or diabetes mellitus (Keane 1993). This has a better prognosis than a traumatic nerve lesion, although unlike oculomotor nerve palsies there has been no clinicopathological correlation. The nerve may be affected in the cavernous sinus and the superior orbital fissure by other diseases, such as tumours and aneurysms, but it is usual for the other ocular motor and trigeminal nerves also to be involved. The sudden onset of vertical diplopia, without any predisposing cause, should always be considered clinically to be due to an underacting superior oblique muscle, which when occurring from late childhood up to 50 years of age is due to a decompensated congenital trochlear nerve palsy. Old photographs of the patient may show a head tilt in infancy. These patients tend to have large fusional amplitudes. In many patients with isolated trochlear nerve pareses no cause can be found (after tensilon testing, CT scanning, and a glucose tolerance test), and in this situation recovery usually occurs spontaneously.

A rare disorder is *superior oblique myokymia*, in which there are bursts of small amplitude, high frequency torsional oscillations of one eye (Hoyt and Keane 1970; Miller 1996). This results in symptoms of recurring vertical or torsional diplopia, monocular blurring of vision, and tremulous sensations in the eye. These episodes last less than 10 seconds and occur many times per day. The attacks may be induced by looking downward, tilting the head toward the side of the affected eye, or by blinking. The oscillations may be difficult to observe on gross examination but can be readily observed with the ophthalmoscope or slit lamp, asking to the patient to move the eyes in the direction known to induce the oscillations. Electromyographic studies have suggested that this condition is due to neuronal damage with subsequent regeneration leading to desynchronized contraction of muscle fibres (Komerell and Schaubele 1980). The condition is usually benign, although rare cases have been reported following trochlear nerve palsy, after mild head trauma, associated with MS, and after a brainstem infarction. Superior oblique myokymia spontaneously resolves in some patients, and in others the symptoms are not troublesome. In those patients whose symptoms are distressing a range of medical treatments are available, including membrane stabilizing drugs such as carbamazepine and phenytoin, baclofen, and systemically administered β-adrenergic blocking agents. If drug therapy fails, surgical procedures such as superior oblique tenectomy with myectomy of the ipsilateral inferior oblique muscle are available.

8.10.4 Abducens nerve palsies

An abducens (sixth cranial nerve) nerve palsy, which results in a lateral rectus muscle paresis is the most common type of ocular nerve palsy (Fig. 8.17) (Richards *et al.*, 1992), but it is import-

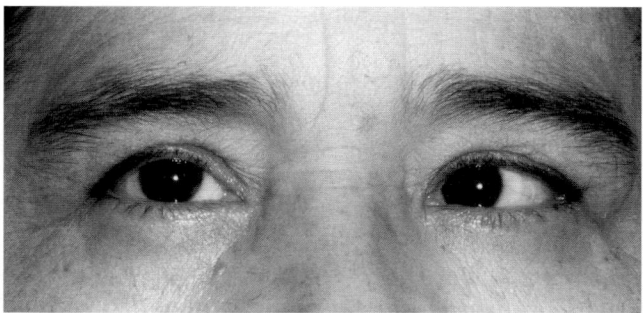

Fig. 8.17. Sixth cranial nerve palsy. A right abducens nerve palsy due to multiple sclerosis, causing failure of abduction.

Table 8.9. Causes of abducens nerve palsy

Nuclear
  Congenital, e.g. Möbius syndrome
  Tumour
  Infarction
  Wernicke–Korsakoff syndrome
Fascicular
  Demyelination
  Infarction, tumour
Subarachnoid
  Meningitis
  Subarachnoid haemorrhage
  Post-infectious
  Clivus tumour
  Trauma
  Compression by aneurysm or ectatic vessels
  Sarcoidosis
Petrous
  Mastoid or petrous bone tip infection
  Fracture of petrous bone
  Aneurysm
  Thombosis of inferior petrosal sinus
  Downward displacement of brainstem by supratentorial mass (raised intracranial pressure)
  Following lumbar puncture, epidural anaesthesia
  Trigeminal schwannoma
Cavernous sinus and superior orbital fissure
  Aneurysm
  Tumour (meningioma, nasopharyngeal carcinoma, pituitary adenoma)
  Carotid–cavernous fistula
  Thrombosis
  Dural arteriovenous malformation
  Tolosa–Hunt syndrome
  Herpes zoster
  Sinusitis
Orbital
  Tumour
Localization uncertain
  Infarction (often associated with hypertension or diabetes)
  Migraine

ant to differentiate it from disorders of the neuromuscular junction such as myasthenia gravis, and extraocular muscles, e.g. dysthyroid eye disease or orbital inflammation (pseudotumour). Other conditions which need to be excluded include orbital trauma (ethmoid blowout), convergence spasm, and congenital innervation abnormalities (Duane's and Möbius syndromes). The various causes of abducens nerve palsies at different locations along its course are listed in Table 8.9.

The abducens nucleus lies in the floor of the fourth ventricle and contains, in addition to motor neurons that supply the ipsilateral lateral rectus muscle, interneurons with axons that cross the midline to ascend in the medial longitudinal fasciculus to the contralateral oculomotor nucleus (medial rectus subnucleus). Therefore lesions of the nucleus never produce ipsilateral abduction weakness, but always result in an ipsilateral conjugate gaze palsy, often associated with an ipsilateral lower motor neuron palsy of the facial nerve, the fascicles of which course around the abducens nucleus (Henn and Büttner 1982). The abducens nucleus is susceptible to abnormalities of development, such as Duane's syndrome, and acquired lesions mainly due to metastatic tumours and vascular infarction. Patients with Wernicke–Korsakoff syndrome often develop horizontal paralysis of conjugate gaze, presumably from a metabolic insult to the abducens nuclei.

Involvement of the abducens nerve fascicles in the lateral tegmentum due to infarction in the territory of the anterior inferior cerebellar artery produces abduction paresis, ipsilateral lower motor neuron facial palsy, loss of taste from the anterior two-thirds of the tongue, ipsilateral Horner's syndrome, ipsilateral analgesia of the face and ipsilateral peripheral deafness (Foville's syndrome). As the abducens nerve fascicles pass ventrally through the pontine tegmentum they pass lateral to the pyramidal tract. An infarction at this site results in an ipsilateral abducens paresis, ipsilateral facial palsy, and contralateral hemiplegia (Millard–Gubler syndrome). Other causes for a fascicular abducens nerve palsy are brainstem glioma or metatasis, and demyelination which commonly results in bilateral palsies (Silverman *et al.* 1995).

The abducens nerve may leave the caudal border of the pons as a single or double trunk, the latter possibility explaining the partial palsies which may occur due to trauma or raised intracranial pressure. The nerve passes almost vertically in front of the clivus where it may be damaged by an enlarged ectatic basilar artery or by tumours such as a chordoma, meningioma, or nasopharyngeal carcinoma (Volpe and Lessell 1993). Minor head trauma resulting in an abducens paresis should raise the suspicion of a clivus or parasellar tumour. In the subarachnoid space the nerve is liable to damage from meningeal inflammation, especially due to secondary carcinoma and any infective organism, particularly tuberculosis. The nerve then enters the dura, medial to the trigeminal nerve, and passes under the petroclinoid ligament in Dorello's canal. It is fixed at this point and hence downward displacement of the brainstem due to a supratentorial lesion may result in unilateral or bilateral abducens palsies. Partial palsies have been reported after lumbar punctures, not necessarily associated with raised intracranial pressure (Bell *et al.* 1994).

Before the nerve passes into the cavernous sinus, it lies on the medial tip of the petrous temporal bone where it is susceptible to damage from trauma, particularly as a result of a longitudinal fracture of the temporal bone. The most common cause for abducens nerve involvement at this site is infection, usually in the middle ear or mastoid, leading to a petrositis with or without thrombosis of the inferior petrosal sinus. The trigeminal ganglion and facial nerve lie nearby, often resulting in associated pain in the face or eye, and a facial paresis may occur in addition to the abducens palsy (Gradenigo's syndrome).

On entering the cavernous sinus the nerve lies lateral to the internal carotid artery and medial to the ophthalmic division of the trigeminal nerve, in close proximity to the oculomotor and trochlear nerves. Despite this, lesions in the sinus often lead to an isolated abducens nerve palsy, probably because it is not tethered to the dural wall. For a short distance the pupillo-sympathetic fibres run with the abducens nerve as they pass from the internal carotid artery to the first division of the trigeminal nerve. Tumour, inflammation, dural arteriovenous malformation, or intracavernous aneurysm of the internal carotid artery may affect the abducens nerve in this location. An isolated palsy may also be the first indication of the contralateral spread of a cavernous sinus thrombosis. When the nerve passes through the superior orbital fissure to innervate the lateral rectus muscle it may be compressed by tumours of the skull base, such as nasopharyngeal carcinoma, often with involvement of the other ocular motor nerves, when facial pain and proptosis may also be a feature. Although isolated chronic abducens nerve palsies require investigation, many have benign causes (Savino *et al.* 1982). Bilateral abducens nerve palsies, in contrast to unilateral palsies, are more commonly due to demyelination, subarachnoid haemorrhage, meningitis, tumours, Wernicke's encephalopathy, and raised intracranial pressure. These palsies need to be differentiated carefully from convergence spasm and divergence paresis.

A transient abducens palsy is occasionally present in the newborn, which resolves within approximately 6 weeks (Knox *et al.* 1967). It is important to differentiate this from congenital abnormalities such as Duane's syndrome or congenital esotropia with cross-fixation. Full abduction can be achieved in the latter by the doll's head manoeuvre or by patching one eye for a week. Several diseases in children lead to isolated abducens palsies, which may be the first sign of a posterior fossa tumour (Robertson *et al.* 1970). When it is associated with a gaze palsy, a brainstem glioma is suggested, and if associated with cerebellar dysfunction, an astrocyoma, ependymoma, or medulloblastoma. An abducens nerve palsy sometimes follows an upper respiratory tract infection or measles immunization, or develops during a chickenpox infection, usually with full recovery. It should, however, always be remembered when a child develops a sudden ocular deviation that this may be due to a unilateral loss of vision resulting from a tumour of the retina or anterior visual pathways, or the battered child syndrome.

8.10.5 Combined ocular motor nerve palsies

It is important to distinguish multiple ocular motor palsies from orbital disease due to dysthyroid eye disease, myasthenia gravis, and progressive myopathy (chronic progressive external ophthalmoplegia). This can usually be achieved by careful consideration of the tempo of progression and associated signs, e.g. pupil involvement, response to edrophonium, and the forced duction test. Unilateral multiple ocular motor nerve palsies are usually associated with lesions involving the cavernous sinus or superior orbital fissure but, if bilateral, a wide range of possible diagnoses must be considered (Table 8.10). An isolated or multiple ocular motor nerve palsy associated with pain in or around the eye constitutes the syndrome of painful

Table 8.10. Causes of multiple ocular motor palsies

Brainstem
    Tumour
    Infarction
    Motor neuron disease
    Leigh's disease

Subarachnoid
    Meningitis (infective and neoplastic)
    Trauma
    Clivus tumour
    Aneurysm

Cavernous sinus and superior orbital fissure
    Aneurysm
    Tumour (meningioma, pituitary adenoma with apoplexy; metastases,
        especially nasopharyngeal carcinoma)
    Thrombosis
    Tolosa–Hunt syndrome
    Herpes zoster
    Neurosurgical complication
    Infarction
    Carotid–cavernous fistula
    Mucormycosis and other fungal infections
    Sphenoid sinus mucocoele

Orbital
    Trauma
    Tumour
    Sinusitis

Localization uncertain
    Toxins
    Postinflammatory neuropathy (Guillain–Barré and Fisher syndrome)
    Arteritis
    Behçet disease

Table 8.11. Painful ophthalmoplegia syndromes

Subarachnoid
    Aneurysm (posterior communicating artery or basilar)
    Carcinomatous meningitis

Cavernous sinus and superior orbital fissure
    Aneurysm
    Tumour (meningioma, chordoma, pituitary adenoma,
        nasopharyngeal carcinoma, lymphoma, metastases)
    Cavernous sinus thrombosis
    Tolosa–Hunt syndrome
    Herpes zoster
    Carotid–cavernous fistula
    Sphenoid sinus carcinoma
    Petrositis (Gradenigo's syndrome)

Orbital
    Metastatic tumour
    Lymphoma
    Inflammatory pseudotumour
    Contiguous sinusitis
    Mucormycosis or other fungus infections

Localization uncertain
    Migrainous ophthalmoplegia
    Diabetic ophthalmoplegia
    Cranial arteritis

ophthalmoplegia, which again has a wide differential diagnosis (Table 8.11).

When multiple ocular nerve palsies occur as a result of trauma the head injury is usually severe and associated with fractures of the sphenoid, petrous temporal, or orbital bones (Lepore 1995). They can be confused with blowout fractures of the orbit which lead to restricted eye movements, particularly of upward gaze, which is due to prolapse of the inferior rectus muscle through the bony defect in the orbital floor.

Many different disease processes may affect the ocular motor nerves in the cavernous sinus; differentiation between lesions at this site or at the orbital apex is suggested by sensory disturbance in the trigeminal distribution in the former, and by proptosis and visual loss in the latter. The most common causes for multiple ocular motor palsies in the cavernous sinus are aneurysms and tumours. In a large series of cases of cavernous sinus syndrome Thomas and Yoss (1970) found that differentiation was not possible clinically by analysis of the mode of onset, presence or absence of pain, the pattern of neurologic deficit, or the response to steroids. However, in a series of patients with meningiomas and aneurysms of the cavernous sinus Trobe *et al.* (1978) found that patients with meningiomas tended to be aged over 70 years, systemically healthy and pain free, with a subtle onset of symptoms and insidious progress. Aneurysms presented in patients (who were usually women over 70 years with hypertension or cardiovascular disease), with acute severe orbital pain or trigeminal (first and second divisions) dysaesthesiae at onset, early abduction defect, and with negligible or an explosive progression. Intracavernous aneurysms may expand rapidly but rarely rupture, in which case the dural envelope of the cavernous sinus usually contains the haemorrhage and a carotid–cavernous fistula is formed, with obvious physical signs. A fistula may be treated electively, but otherwise the only indication for surgery is severe intractable facial pain, when common carotid ligation with progressive clamping is undertaken.

In the *cavernous sinus syndrome* it is commonly found that when the oculomotor nerve is compressed there appears to be relative pupil sparing. It has been suggested that this is due to coincident sympathetic and parasympathetic paresis. It is often difficult to differentiate clinically between meningioma, intracavernous aneurysm, and nasopharyngeal carcinoma or other metastatic tumours, which are the most common cause (20 per cent) of a cavernous sinus syndrome. In the case of multiple ocular motor nerve palsies, with or without pain, in which CT and MRI scanning have failed to localize a lesion, a 'blind' nasopharyngeal biopsy may be positive even in the absence of visible tumour. Metastases from other sites may infiltrate the cavernous sinus, and progressive involvement of the ocular motor and other cranial nerves may be the presenting signs of carcinomatous meningitis.

Pituitary tumours may suddenly expand laterally into the cavernous sinus. This is usually due to infarction of the tumour, giving rise to what is called pituitary apoplexy. Patients with this condition usually present with a sudden onset of severe headache, multiple ocular motor palsies, which are often bilateral, variable degrees of visual loss, and signs of endocrine insufficiency.

Cavernous sinus thrombosis may occur as a complication of infectious and non-infectious processes. Septic thrombosis of the cavernous sinuses most commonly follows infections of the middle third of the face due to *Staphylococcus aureus*. Other antecedent sites of infection include paranasal (usually sphenoid) sinusitis, dental abscess and, less often, otitis media. Fever is a nearly constant feature, but headache may not be prominent. Periorbital oedema, chemosis, proptosis, and limitation of extraocular movements (especially lateral gaze) develop in almost all recognized cases. Involvement of the opposite eye frequently appears within 2 days following the onset of unilateral signs. Although CT scanning may be helpful, MRI is the diagnostic procedure of choice. Treatment includes appropriate antibiotics and often surgical drainage of the primary site of infection. Less than half the patients recover completely, and the mortality is approximately 30 per cent.

The development of an acute or subacute painful ophthalmoplegia demands extensive investigation of the patient to exclude an aneurysm, tumour, or one of the rarer causes. In diabetics the urgent exclusion of a mucormycosis infection by sinus mucosal biopsies is important, since favourable outcome with amphotericin B is only possible if treatment is instituted early.

Once these other causes have been excluded, then the diagnosis of a non-specific granulomatous inflammation in the region of the cavernous sinus resulting in the *Tolosa–Hunt syndrome* should be considered (Lakke 1962; Kline 1982). The criteria for the diagnosis of the syndrome (Hunt *et al.* 1961) are:

1. The pain may precede the ophthalmoplegia, is located behind the eye, and has a steady 'boring' or 'gnawing' quality.

2. Any combination of ocular motor nerves may be involved, with or without the ophthalmic branch of the trigeminal nerve and oculosympathetic nerves, and rarely the optic nerve or maxillary branch of the trigeminal nerve.

3. The symptoms are acute or subacute in onset, lasting for days or weeks, and spontaneous remissions may occur with partial or complete regression of deficits.

4. The symptoms often respond rapidly to large doses of corticosteroids.

5. Attacks may recur at intervals of months or years.

6. Exhaustive studies, including CT, MRI imaging, and angiography show no evidence of involvement of structures outside the cavernous sinus

It is clear that the so-called Tolosa–Hunt syndrome may be caused by a spectrum of inflammatory processes, both granulomatous and non-granulomatous inflammation. This condition cannot be distinguished clearly from the painful superior orbital fissure syndrome.

Orbital venography is a useful investigation in these cases, often showing obstruction of the cavernous sinus or superior ophthalmic vein. In addition, irregularities of the intracavernous portion of the internal ophthalmic artery may be found. MR imaging often shows an abnormal soft-tissue area in the cavernous sinus, with intermediate to high signal on T1-weighted images and enhancement of the abnormal area with gadolinium. These abnormalities reflect the low-grade inflammatory response in the cavernous sinus, which has been found pathologically and which has been shown to disappear with corticosteroids.

It is important to note that a similar systemic steroid responsiveness may be observed with other lesions in the superior orbital fissure and cavernous sinus, including tumours and aneurysms. It is therefore important that complete neuroradiological investigations are carried out in patients with the syndrome of painful ophthalmoplegia.

The aetiology of the Tolosa–Hunt syndrome is poorly understood. Mathew and Chandy (1970) identified a high prevalence of parasitic infections and tuberculosis in their patients, which suggested that the syndrome may be the result of an unusual immune reaction to endemic infections. Most cases of the condition have no evidence of systemic disease, although some cases have positive tests for LE cells and a raised ESR. The evidence for a generalized connective tissue disease or endemic infection as being the underlying cause is poorly substantiated. An excellent review of the painful ophthalmoplegia syndrome, and Tolosa–Hunt syndrome in particular, has been written by Kline (1982).

Involvement of the third, fourth, and sixth cranial nerves may occur in typical Guillain–Barré syndrome. In the variant of this condition, the *Miller Fisher syndrome*, an external, and often internal, ophthalmoplegia develops in association with ataxia and areflexia. Because the ophthalmoplegia is often incomplete and the resulting paresis symmetrical, suggesting a horizontal or vertical gaze palsy, some authors have suggested that some cases of the syndrome may be due to a central lesion, although the majority of cases are probably associated with a peripheral demyelinating neuropathy (Berlit and Rakicky 1992). As in Guillain–Barré syndrome, cases have been found to have evidence of *Campylobacter jejuni* infection, and to have autoantibodies against certain gangliosides in their serum, particularly anti-GQ1b IgG antibody (Chiba *et al.* 1992). Most patients with the Miller Fisher syndrome improve completely in 8–12 weeks without treatment.

8.10.6 Disorders of the neuromuscular junction and muscle

Disorders of the neuromuscular junction

A number of different diseases affecting transmission at the neuromuscular junction may produce ocular motor disorders. Contaminated food or infected wounds may lead to an elaboration of the toxin of *Clostridium botulinum* (Miller and Moses 1977). This neurotoxin blocks release of acetycholine from nerve terminals and may lead to varying degrees of internal and external ophthalmoplegia.

Myasthenia gravis

The most common disorder affecting the neuromuscular junction is myasthenia gravis, an autoimmune disorder affecting the postsynaptic acetylcholine receptor (Weinberg *et al.* 1994) (see Section 15.10.1). The presenting symptoms are ocular (levator palpebrae superioris or extraocular muscles) in about 70 per cent of cases, and during its course ocular involvement occurs in 90 per cent (Oosterhuis 1982). Approximately 20 per cent of all myasthenic patients remain with ocular involvement alone—ocular myasthenia. The risk of developing generalized involvement after presentation with ocular myasthenia reduces to about 15 per cent after 2 years (Bever *et al.* 1983). Since the disorder is one of muscle fatiguability and spontaneous remissions, it is not surprising that the ocular signs and symptoms fluctuate over hours or weeks. The most common sign is lid ptosis, which is usually asymmetrical and may be especially pronounced on sustained upgaze. The contralateral lid may be elevated due to the increased innervation required by the ptotic lid, which, when covered, results in the normal lid returning to normal. Rapid shifts of ptosis from one eye to the other are considered pathognomonic of the disorder (Osserman 1957), as is the lid 'twitch' sign described by Cogan (1965). In this, rapid refixations from downgaze to the primary position result in transient lid retraction followed by a slow droop to the ptotic position, or else the lid twitches several times before settling into a stable position. Forced eyelid closure may lead to fatigue of the orbicularis oculi muscle, resulting in the eye 'peeking' at the examiner. Patients with myasthenia gravis have an increased prevalence of thyroid eye disease, which may result in bilateral or unilateral eyelid retraction, the latter without contralateral ptosis.

Myasthenia gravis is the 'great mimicker' of ocular motor disorders and may produce pseudostrabismus; oculomotor (without pupil involvement), trochlear, and abducens palsies; and mimic conditions which are normally associated with central lesions, such as internuclear ophthalmoplegia (with abducting nystagmus) and conjugate gaze palsies. The medial rectus is the most commonly affected muscle, but muscle fatigue may be seen on sustained upward and lateral gaze. Apart from these ophthalmoplegias, myasthenia can result in a number of saccadic abnormalities, including slow saccades, slowing after repeated refixations, and saccadic dysmetria, as well as increasing nystagmus on sustained lateral gaze. It is still not clear why there is a predilection for the levator and extraocular muscles in myasthenia gravis, although several hypotheses have been proposed:

(1) extraocular muscles show several anatomical and physiological differences from limb muscles;

(2) these properties of extraocular muscles make them particularly sensitive to a loss of functional acetylcholine (ACh) receptors;

(3) the antigenic properties of extraocular muscles may differ from those of skeletal muscle;

(4) minimal weakness of extraocular muscles are likely to be symptomatic, in contrast to limb muscles (Kaminsky *et al.* 1990).

It is generally agreed that pupillary reflexes in patients with myasthenia gravis appear clinically normal.

Prolonged ocular involvement in myasthenia gravis may lead to a chronic or 'fixed' ophthalmoplegia, which fails to improve with anticholinesterase medication. The resulting symmetrical external ophthalmoplegia, ptosis, and facial weakness may make separation from chronic progressive external ophthalmoplegia difficult, but a slow symmetric progressive course without fluctuations or remissions favours the latter.

When there is a moderate or marked deficit of lid elevation or ocular motility, the diagnosis of myasthenia gravis is best confirmed by the edrophonium (Tensilon) test. To increase the objective sensitivity of the test, the response of the ophthalmoplegia can be assessed by the Hess chart, prisms, or the Lancaster red–green test performed before and 1–2 minutes after the injection of edrophonium. Ocular deviations may actually get worse if the muscles are differentially responsive to edrophonium, in which case the test is still considered positive. Seventy-five per cent of patients with pure ocular myasthenia were found to have antiacetylcholine receptor antibody, and abnormal jitter on single fibre electromyographic examination of skeletal muscle was found in 50 per cent of such cases (Kelly *et al.* 1982). Another simple test which has a high degree of sensitivity and specificity is the ice-test (Ertas *et al.* 1994), in which local cooling is used to eliminate ptosis in patients suspected of having myasthenia. A bag containing ice is placed over the ptotic lid for 2 minutes and, following removal, the size of the palpebral fissure is measured and compared with the size before cooling. Patients with myasthenia gravis usually show a difference of greater than 2 mm. Because a thymic tumour is found in about 10 per cent of patients with myasthenia gravis, part of the evaluation of a patient suspected of having the disease should include a CT scan of the mediastinum.

It is commonly found that the paresis of the extraocular muscles responds poorly to anticholinesterase drugs, although the ptosis may respond more favourably. For this reason steroid therapy has been used in ocular myasthenia and often results in considerable, and sometimes complete, resolution of ocular symptoms (Oosterhuis 1982). Patients with ocular myasthenia can be commenced on low doses of daily or alternate-day steroids (equivalent to 10 mg/day). The dose is gradually increased until the desired effect is achieved. A year later a gradual reduction should be attempted to see if the symptoms reappear (Weinberg *et al.* 1994).

When diplopia becomes troublesome, occlusion of one eye is the best initial measure; prisms are unhelpful because of the fluctuations in the angle of the optical axes. The ptosis may be relieved with a ptosis hook attached to spectacles but, if chronic, the patient may be helped by ptosis surgery.

In contrast to myasthenia gravis, ocular symptoms are rare in Lambert–Eaton myasthenic syndrome, but both clinical and subclinical ocular motor involvement does occur in some patients (see Section 15.10.2).

Ocular myopathies

A progressive limitation of ocular motility, accompanied by ptosis but usually without diplopia or pupillary abnormalities,

Table 8.12. Classification of progressive ophthalmoplegia

1. Site uncertain
   (a) Ophthalmoplegia and ptosis, congenital and late forms, sporadic and genetic
      (i) Ophthalmoplegia alone
      (ii) Ptosis alone
2. Ocular myopathies
   (a) Ocular and other cranial muscles
      (i) Oculopharyngeal muscular dystrophy (genetic)
      (ii) Oculopharyngeal myopathy (sporadic)
   (b) Ocular and proximal limb muscles
   (c) Ocular and distal limb muscles
   (d) Myotonic muscular dystrophy
   (e) Myotubular or centronuclear myopathy
   (f) Ophthalmoplegia, glycogen storage, and abnormal mitochondria
   (g) Ophthalmopathy of Graves disease (euthyroid, hypothyroid, hyperthyroid)
   (h) Ocular myositis (orbital pseudotumour)
   (i) Congenital myopathic ptosis or ophthalmoplegia
      (i) Limb weakness
      (ii) Anomalous insertion of ocular muscles
      (iii) Some cases of Möbius syndrome
3. Disorders of neuromusclar junction
   (a) Curare-sensitive ocular myopathy
   (b) Myasthenia gravis
4. Neural ophthalmoplegias
   (a) Nuclear and supranuclear abnormalities
      (i) Congenital: Möbius syndrome; isolated ophthalmoplegia
      (ii) Ophthalmoplegia with central myelopathy or encephalopathy of later onset: mental retardation, hereditary ataxias, hereditary spastic paraplegia, hereditary multisystem disease, dystonia musculorum deformans, abetalipoproteinaemia (Bassen–Kornzweig), progressive supranuclear bulbar palsy (Steele–Richardson–Olszewski)
      (iii) Ophthalmoplegia with motor neuron disease: infantile spinal muscular atrophy (Werdnig–Hoffman), juvenile spinal muscular atrophy simulating muscular dystrophy (Wohfart–Kugelbertg–Welander)
      (iv) Ophthalmoplegia, retinitis, cardiopathy, and neural disorder (Kearns–Sayre)
   (b) Peripheral neuropathies

occurs in many diseases (Table 8.12). There are several subgroups of myopathies predominantly affecting the extra-ocular muscle—*chronic progressive external ophthalmoplegia* (CPEO)—these are often accompanied by a variety of other findings and have been called 'ophthalmoplegia plus' (Drachman 1968; Petty *et al.* 1986).

Oculopharyngeal dystrophy

This is inherited as an autosomal dominant trait mapped to chromosome 14q11.2–q13 in the region of the gene for myosin (see Section 15.2.6). The marked ptosis with some restriction of ocular motility is associated with wasting of the temporalis muscle and weakness of the bulbar muscles. The onset is usually in the fifth and sixth decades and mild ptosis usually precedes the dysphagia by years (Murphy and Drachman 1968). Sporadic isolated cases have been reported but may represent poor case ascertainment or reduced penetrance. Myotonic dystrophy may give rise to slowed eye movements due to involvement of the extraocular muscles (Ter Bruggen *et al.* 1990).

Kearns–Sayre syndrome

Although CPEO may occur in association with a number of other defects, those found in the Kearns–Sayre syndrome are the most varied (Kearns and Sayre 1958). The onset of this condition is within the first or second decades, without any family history, and is associated with retinal pigmentary degeneration, cardiac conduction abnormalities, raised cerebrospinal fluid protein, excessive ragged red fibres in peripheral muscle with trichrome staining methods, and various other features (Table 8.13). The sequence of manifestations varies and the cardiomyopathy may be delayed for years. Pathologically there is a spongy degeneration of the brain. The disease is now characterized as a mitochondrial cytopathy in which a deletion from the circular strand of mitochondrial DNA may result in defects of the intracellular respiratory chain.

CPEO must be differentiated from a number of conditions. In progressive supranuclear palsy full ocular rotations to oculocephalic manoeuvres are maintained. Chronic ocular myasthenia may be confused with CPEO, especially since there may be a lack of response to edrophonium; but a progressive course lacking fluctuations or remissions favours CPEO. Dysthyroid restrictive myopathy usually has associated lid retraction, proptosis, or congestive conjunctival signs that are absent in CPEO.

Table 8.13. Features associated with chronic progressive external ophthalmoplegia

Cardinal manifestations
  CPEO onset <20 years
  Retinal pigmentary degeneration
  Heart block
  Elevated CSF protein
  Negative family history
  Myopathy affecting skeletal muscles (ragged red fibres)
  Spongiform encephalopathy
Association manifestations
  Short stature
  Hearing loss
  Cerebellar ataxia
  Corticospinal tract signs
  Subnormal intelligence
  Cranial muscle weakness (face, palate, neck)
  Peripheral neuropathy
  Corneal clouding
  Scrotal tongue
  Slowed EEG
  Hypogonadism
  Endocrine abnormalities (steroid, calcium, glucose metabolism)

8.10.7 **Congenital abnormalities**

A number of different congenital abnormalities have been described in which there is ocular motor paresis, often associated with synkinesis of movement of other eye and lid muscles. It is important that these congenital conditions should be distinguished from acquired ocular motor disorders so that unnecessary investigations are not undertaken.

Möbius syndrome

In this condition there is a variable degree of facial diplegia associated with a disturbance of horizontal eye movements. Other abnormalities include tongue atrophy, cleft palate, and various musculoskeletal dysplasias involving the head and neck, chest, and upper extremities. The diversity of pathological findings in patients with Möbius syndrome suggests that the syndrome is actually a heterogeneous group of congenital disorders which, in some cases, are due to developmental defects, and in others due to acquired hypoxic or other insults (Towfighti *et al.* 1979).

Duane's retraction syndrome

This syndrome is due to abnormal development of the abducens nucleus (Miller *et al.* 1982), and is so named because of the retraction of the globe and narrowing of the palpebral fissure, which occurs on attempted adduction, in association with limitation or absence of abduction. Duane's syndrome is usually unilateral, the left eye being more frequently affected than the right, and is bilateral in 15–20 per cent of cases. The condition may be familial and sometimes associated with other congenital abnormalities, such as Klippel–Fiel anomaly, deafness, urinary tract abnormalities, and cardiac defects.

The condition occurs in three forms (Huber 1974): type I, which is the most common, consists of limited or absent abduction with relatively normal adduction; in type II there is impaired adduction and full abduction; and in type III there is impairment of both adduction and abduction. A number of electromyographic and oculographic studies have indicated abnormal innervation patterns, compatible with the clinicopathological studies which have shown hypoplastic abducens nuclei, and partial or complete innervation of the lateral rectus from branches of the inferior division of the oculomotor nerve. Patients with Duane's syndrome usually have excellent visual adaptation, resulting in absence of diplopia, good stereopsis and fusion in directions of gaze where the visual axes are aligned.

Congenital elevator palsies

In the congenital 'double elevator palsy' there is paresis of both the superior rectus and inferior oblique muscles. Since the eyes are straight in the primary position and the Bell's phenomenon is preserved, it is considered to be a supranuclear paresis of monocular elevation. This condition may develop in later life, when it is usually due to a small, discrete vascular lesion in the pretectum.

Marcus Gunn jaw-winking phenomenon

This is an example of anomalous innervation in which a unilateral ptosis of variable extent is noted shortly after birth.

When the baby suckles the ptotic lid jerks rhythmically and is intermittently retracted, as it does later with chewing and jaw movements. Two major groups are described: the most common is external pterygoid-levator synkinesis with lid elevation when the jaw is moved to the opposite side, and the other is internal pterygoid-levator synkinesis with lid elevation on clenching the jaw closed (Sano 1959).

8.11 **Central disorders of eye movement**

Many different disease processes affecting the central nervous system from the brainstem to the cortex can lead to supranuclear disorders of eye movements. Examination of eye movements offers a number of advantages to the neurologist over skeletal movements. These include: eye movements are directly related to the activity of brainstem neurons, since the extraocular muscles lack a stretch reflex; eye movements have limited degrees of freedom, so that disordered movements lend themselves to analysis (clinical or quantitative) in three planes—horizontal, vertical, and torsional; finally there are several functional classes of eye movements, each with special physiological properties that suit a particular purpose and which have a separate and well-segregated neural substrate. This enables the clinician to examine these various types of eye movements and identify abnormalities, which can then provide information regarding anatomical, physiological, and pharmacological lesions (Leigh and Zee 1999).

8.11.1 **Types of eye movement**

Types of eye movement and their examination

The various types of functional classes of eye movements all subserve the same goal, the projection of an image of the object of interest on to the most sensitive part of the retina, the fovea. Rapid conjugate eye movements, saccades, enable the line of gaze to be redirected to bring the image of a new object of interest on to the fovea, and the dysjunctive or vergence eye movements ensure that these images are placed simultaneously on both foveae, regardless of their distance from the observer. There is also a need to stabilize the image of the object of interest on the fovea when the object itself moves, achieved by the smooth pursuit system, or when the subject's head or body moves, as occurs during locomotion, when the vestibular and optokinetic ocular motor reflexes are activated. These different functional types of eye movements can each be tested rapidly at the bedside (Shaunak *et al.* 1997).

Saccades

Voluntary saccade initiation should be assessed by instructing the patient to look from side to side and up and down. The patient is then asked to fixate two targets alternately—for example, a pen in one hand and a raised finger of the other—so that each time they are briefly moved and their distance from each other varied. This generates reflexive saccades, which are tested in the horizontal and vertical planes, and the examiner should observe saccadic variables such as speed of initiation (latency), accuracy, and velocity. Any slowing of saccades can be accentuated by using an optokinetic striped drum or tape, when the repositioning saccades will appear slowed. This is of particular help when showing slowed adducting saccades in a partial internuclear ophthalmoplegia. To accentuate this abnormality another method used involves oblique targets. Because the velocity is slowed in the horizontal and not the vertical plane, the resulting saccade is L-shaped. Predictive saccades can be tested by alternately raising a finger of one hand and then the other in a predictable regular pattern, and asking the patient to make saccades to the target. Finally, the patient should be observed for any head movements or blinks before making a saccade, as occurs in Huntington's disease and ocular motor apraxia.

Smooth pursuit

Smooth pursuit can be tested by asking the patient to track a small target at a distance of about 1 m while keeping his or her head still. Assessment of both horizontal and vertical smooth pursuit should be performed. The target should be moved initially at a slow, uniform speed and the pursuit eye movements observed to determine whether they are smooth, or broken up by catch-up saccades. This is a non-specific sign if present in both directions—for example, due to ageing or cerebellar disease—or it may indicate a focal posterior cortical lesion if only present in one direction, in which case the abnormal pursuit is in the direction of the lesion. The speed should be gradually increased, but at high velocities all smooth pursuit eye movements will be broken up by saccades, even in normal subjects. The optokinetic nystagmus (OKN) drum and tape is a useful method to elicit a series of pursuit movements, and does not elicit true optokinetic eye movements.

Optokinetic nystagmus (OKN)

The optokinetic system cannot be tested as part of the clinical examination, because the OKN drum and tape commonly used tests smooth pursuit and not the optokinetic system. A full-field revolving striped drum is required to elicit OKN.

Vestibular system

If the vestibulo-ocular system (VOR) is functioning normally, passive rotation of the patient's head should result in a slow eye movement so that the eyes deviate in the opposite direction to that of the head movement. This is known as the doll's head (oculocephalic) manoeuvre and should be performed both horizontally and vertically. This technique is not only valuable for assessing vestibular function, but also for differentiating between infranuclear and nuclear and supranuclear gaze palsies, and in the evaluation of brainstem function in comatose patients. It should be noted that the eye movements elicited in unconscious patients by this procedure largely reflect the integrity of the semicircular canals and their central connections, although in conscious patients the effects of visual input on eye movements may influence the response to head rotation.

A rough estimate of any deterioration of vestibular gain (head velocity divided by eye velocity) can be obtained by asking the patient to read a Snellen chart while their head is being passively rotated. If there is an abnormality, the visual acuity will show a deterioration compared with the acuity obtained when the head is stationary. Another bedside test of the horizontal VOR is for the examiner to observe the patient's optic disc with an ophthalmoscope while the patient tries to fixate a distant object and shake their head from side to side. If the gain of the VOR is normal (unity), the examiner will not see any movement of the optic disc; and if abnormal, the disc will repeatedly slip from view.

The VOR can be suppressed by activating the smooth pursuit system. This may be tested by asking the patient to fixate their thumbnail with their arms outstretched while rotating their head and trunk in harmony. Impaired cancellation of the VOR, and hence abnormal smooth pursuit, is shown by observing the eye repeatedly moving off fixation due to the VOR, followed by refixation saccades. This is a particularly useful technique for testing pursuit in patients with gaze-evoked nystagmus.

Further details of tests used to assess the vestibular system are to be found in Section 9.5.

8.11.2 Brainstem and cerebellar disorders

Anatomy and physiology of horizontal and vertical gaze

There are two main features of the brainstem neural control of horizontal and vertical gaze: an anatomic separation so that the neural substrate for horizontal gaze is located in the pons and that for vertical gaze in the midbrain, and the requirement to overcome viscous drag and resist elastic restoring forces in the orbit when making dynamic eye movements. An understanding of the neural mechanisms that generate a horizontal saccade will serve as an illustration of the principles involved. A rapid phasic contraction of the extraocular muscle, e.g. lateral rectus muscle, is required to overcome the orbital viscosity, and a rapid, high-frequency burst of nerve impulses, the pulse, is transmitted to the muscle via the ocular motor nerve. The premotor inputs to the motor neurons in the abducens nucleus arise from neurons in a region of the reticular formation which lies ventral and anterior to the nucleus, the paramedial pontine reticular formation (PPRF). The equivalent premotor region for vertical gaze is the rostral interstitial nucleus of the medial longitudinal fasciculus (riMLF) in the midbrain, rostral to the oculomotor nucleus at the level of the red nucleus. The pulse, a velocity signal, is generated by cells called burst neurons, and must be of an appropriate size to ensure that the eye is brought to the target. Once the saccade has been completed, it is necessary to maintain the new position of the eye against orbital elastic restoring forces. The muscle must, therefore, maintain a sustained tonic contraction, and this is achieved by the tonic innervation, the step, which is a position signal the motor neuron receives from so-called integrator neurons lying in the nucleus prepositus hypoglossi and the medial vestibular

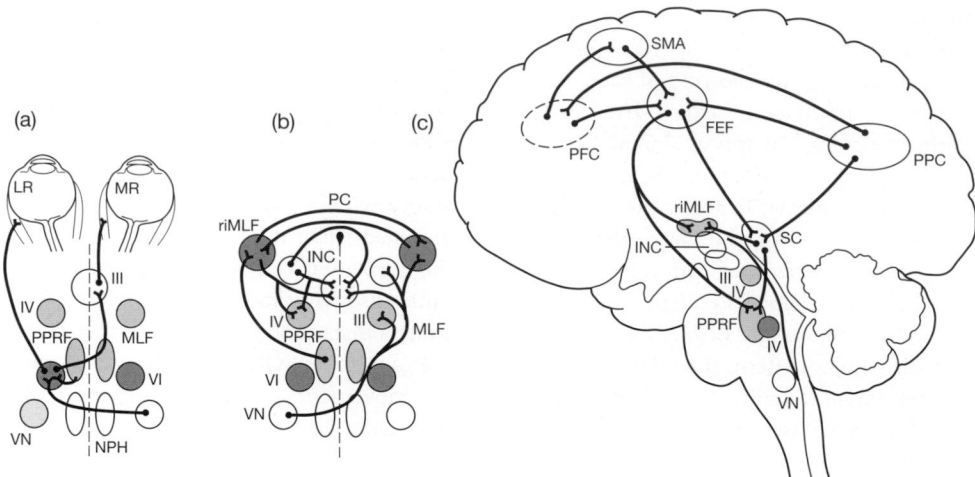

Fig. 8.18. Summary of eye movement control. (a) The brainstem pathways for horizontal gaze. Axons from the cell bodies located in the abducens nucleus travel to the ipsilateral lateral rectus muscle (LR), and the axons of abducens internuclear neurons cross the midline and travel in the medial longitudinal fasciculus (MLF) to the portion(s) of the oculomotor nucleus (III) concerned with the medial rectus (MR) function (in the contralateral eye). (b) The brainstem pathways for vertical gaze. Important structures include the rostral interstitial nucleus of the medial longitudinal fasciculus (riMLF), paramedial pontine reticular formation (PPRF), the interstitial nucleus of Cajal (INC), and the posterior commissure (PC). Note that axons from cell bodies located in the vestibular nuclei (VN) travel directly to the abducens nuclei and, mostly via the MLF, to the oculomotor nuclei. IV, trochlear nucleus. (c) The supranuclear connections from the frontal eye fields (FEF) and the posterior parietal cortea (PPC) to the superior colliculus (SC), riMLF, and the PPRF. The FEF, PPC, and SC are involved in the production of saccades.

nucleus. The pulse and step must be perfectly matched to prevent drift of the eye back to the primary position at the end of the saccade. Faulty neural integration leads to an inadequately maintained step, and after a saccade the eye drifts back in an exponential manner due to the unopposed orbital elastic restoring forces, followed by a saccade to refixate the target. This pattern leads to gaze-evoked nystagmus and is observed in cerebellar disease and anticonvulsant or sedative intoxication. An abnormal pulse may either be of reduced duration or of reduced firing frequency. If the step is appropriately matched, the former will result in a reduced amplitude (hypometric) saccade and the latter a saccade of reduced velocity but of normal amplitude.

Abnormalities of horizontal eye movements

The abducens nucleus contains two populations of neurons: motor neurons innervating the ipsilateral lateral rectus muscle and interneurons. The axons for the interneurons cross the midline and ascend in the medial longitudinal fasciculus (MLF) to the contralateral medial rectus subdivision of the oculomotor nerve nucleus (Fig. 8.18a). The final instructions for horizontal conjugate eye movements lie within the abducens nucleus itself, so that its activation results in an ipsilaterally directed horizontal conjugate gaze movement.

Unilateral horizontal gaze palsy

A lesion of the abducens nucleus will, therefore, result in an ipsilateral horizontal gaze palsy for all types of conjugate movements (saccades, pursuit, and vestibular). Vergence movements of the eyes are spared, however, so that adduction is possible

with a near stimulus (Müri *et al.* 1996). The palsy is usually associated with an ipsilateral lower motor neuron facial nerve palsy due to involvement of the genu of the facial nerve, which passes around the abducens nerve (Fig. 8.19). A selective horizontal gaze palsy involving only saccades, including the quick phases of vestibular and optokinetic nystagmus, occurs when the lesion involves the PPRF in isolation, since the vestibular and pursuit inputs pass directly to the abducens nucleus. The most common causes for horizontal gaze palsies are either vascular infarction and haemorrhage or demyelination.

Bilateral horizontal gaze palsy

A bilateral pontine lesion involving the PPRF can cause a bilateral selective saccadic palsy with preservation of vestibular and optokinetic eye movements (Hanson *et al.* 1986). Such a lesion may impair vertical eye movements, since signals for vertical vestibular and smooth pursuit eye movements ascend in the MLF and other pathways through the pons. The most common causes for a bilateral horizontal gaze palsy, with sparing of vertical gaze, are neurodegenerative diseases such as Huntington's disease or Gaucher's disease.

Internuclear ophthalmoplegia

A lesion of the MLF produces an internuclear ophthalmoplegia (INO), in which there is weakness of adduction ipsilateral to the side of the lesion (Zee 1992) (Fig. 8.20). In a partial INO, adduction will be slowed, but will be completely absent in a complete lesion. Since the fibres of the MLF carry the horizontal gaze commands subserving all types of conjugate eye movements, this adduction paresis involves not only saccades but

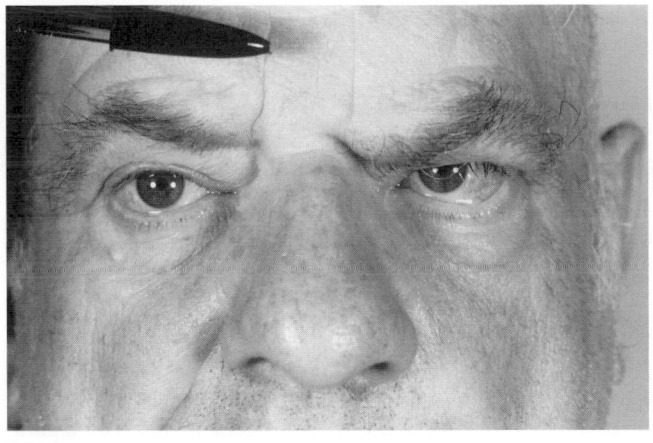
(a)

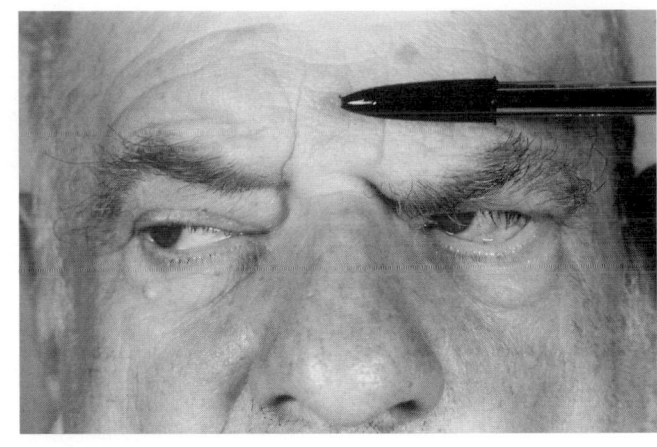
(b)

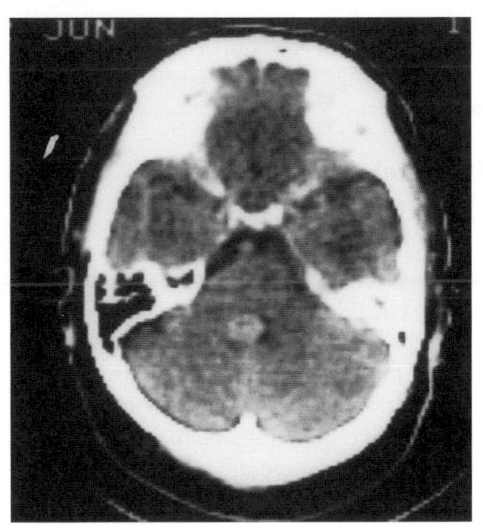
(c)

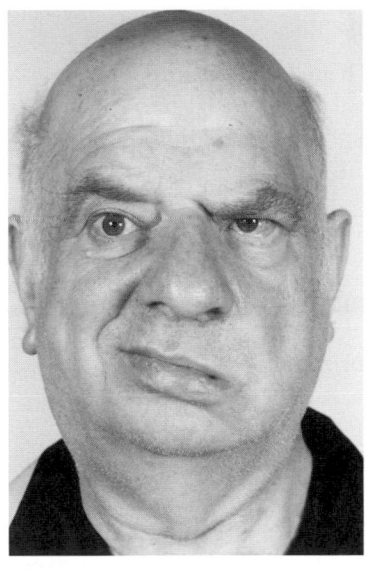
(d)

Fig. 8.19. A left conjugate gaze palsy (a, b) due to an arteriovenous malformation involving the left abducens nucleus (shown on CAT scan (c)). No eye movement, including vestibulo-ocular, could be made into the left field of gaze. This was associated with a left lower motor neuron facial nerve palsy (d).

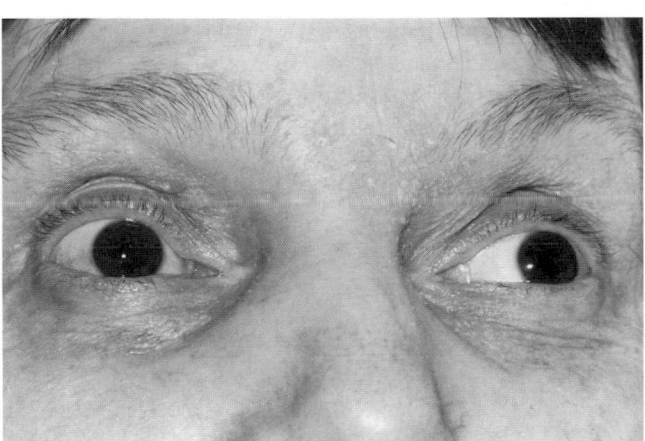

Fig. 8.20. Right unilateral internuclear ophthalmolplegia.

also pursuit and vestibular eye movements. The presence of intact convergence in the absence of voluntary adduction implies that the medial rectus subdivision of the oculomotor nerve is intact, and that the INO is due to a caudal lesion.

Cogan (1970) called this a posterior INO, in contrast to patients with an INO and absent convergence which he called 'anterior'. However, such patients do not necessarily have a lesion involving the medial rectus subdivision of the oculomotor nucleus.

The second major feature of an INO is the nystagmus on abduction in the contralateral eye. This consists of a centripetal (inward) drift, followed by a corrective saccade. Several different mechanisms have been proposed to explain the abducting nystagmus (Zee 1992). These include:

(1) a gaze-evoked nystagmus;

(2) impaired inhibition of the medial rectus contralateral to the lesion;

(3) an increase in convergence tone;

(4) adaptation to the contralateral medial rectus weakness.

The latter is generally considered the most appropriate explanation.

A skew deviation (a vertical misalignment of the visual axes due to a disturbance of prenuclear inputs) is often observed in

Table 8.14. Causes of internuclear ophthalmoplegia

Multiple sclerosis
Brainstem infarction
Brainstem and IV ventricular tumours
Arnold–Chiari malformation
Wernicke's encephalopathy
Infection
Metabolic disorders
Drug intoxications: phenothiazines, tricyclic antidepressants, lithium, barbituates
Syphilis
Trauma, subdural haematoma
Hydrocephalus
Progressive supranuclear palsy
Pseudo-internuclear ophthalmolplegia: myasthenia gravis, Miller Fisher syndrome

patients with a unilateral INO, with the higher eye usually on the side of the lesion. Patients with bilateral INOs have bilateral adduction weakness and abducting nystagmus. In addition, they also have impaired vertical pursuit and vestibular eye movements, and impaired vertical gaze-holding with gaze-evoked nystagmus on looking up or down (Ranalli and Sharpe 1988).

Patients with an INO are usually asymptomatic, although if there is a complete adduction failure they may complain of diplopia, especially during shifts of horizontal gaze. Occasionally they may complain of oscillopsia. A number of different aetiologies lead to an INO (Table 8.14), but if unilateral, the most common is ischaemia, and if bilateral, demyelination associated with multiple sclerosis.

A rarer, so-called posterior internuclear ophthalmoplegia of Lutz has been described in which there is an impairment of abduction (not adduction) of saccades and pursuit, but not vestibular eye movements. This is different to the posterior INO described by Cogan, in which convergence is intact. The pathogenesis of the posterior INO of Lutz is unclear (Thömke *et al.* 1992).

One-and-a-half syndrome

A combined lesion of the abducens nucleus or PPRF and the adjacent MLF on one side of the brainstem results in an ipsilateral horizontal gaze palsy and INO (Wall and Wray 1983). The only preserved horizontal eye movement is abduction of the contralateral eye, and the condition is therefore termed the 'one-and-a-half' syndrome. Although the majority of patients have no deviation or an esotropia in the primary position of gaze, some patients may habitually fixate with the horizontally immobile ipsilesional eye, which results in exotropia of the contralesional eye that has intact lateral rectus innervation. This condition is called paralytic pontine exotropia (Sharpe *et al.* 1974). Some MLF lesions cause an adduction palsy due to INO that is bilateral and exotropic in the primary position, termed a 'wall-eyed' bilateral INO (WEBINO).

The main causes of a one-and-a-half syndrome are brainstem ischaemia, haemorrhage, and tumour. The syndrome can

be mimicked by a bilateral INO with an ipsilateral abducens nerve palsy.

Lateropulsion

This is a feature of lateral medullary infarction (Wallenberg's syndrome), in which there is a compelling sensation of being pulled toward the side of the lesion, accompanied by appropriate eye movement signs. During voluntary eye closure and sometimes even during blinks, the eyes deviate toward the side of the lesion, and have to make corrective saccades on eye opening to refixate the target. All ipsiversive saccadic eye movements overshoot the target (hypermetric), and saccades directed away from the side of the lesion undershoot the target (hypometric) (Baloh *et al.*. 1981). Vertical saccades have a parabolic ipsiversive trajectory. This ipsipulsion is in contrast to the overshooting of contralateral saccades (saccadic contrapulsion) observed in patients with infarction in the territory of the superior cerebellar artery. The eye signs of lateropulsion are considered to be due to damage to olivo-cerebellar projections (Soloman *et al.* 1995).

Abnormalities of vertical eye movements

Disturbances of vertical gaze are usually associated with damage to one or more of three structures in the mesencephalon, the posterior commissure, the riMLF, and the interstitial nucleus of Cajal (Fig. 8.18b). The only exceptions are an apparent vertical gaze palsy due to mechanical restriction of extraocular muscles in orbital disorders such as thyroid eye disease; large acute pontine lesions involving the PPRF bilaterally producing a temporary vertical saccadic palsy, in addition to the permanent horizontal saccadic palsy; and certain degenerative disorders of the nervous system such as progressive supranuclear palsy or adult Niemann–Pick disease.

Dorsal midbrain syndrome (Parinaud's syndrome)

This syndrome is due to a lesion which involves the posterior commissure and is associated with a variety of aetiologies (Table 8.15) and clinical features, some of which may not be present in an individual patient (Baloh *et al.* 1985). The essential sign is a loss of upward gaze involving all types of eye movement, although the VOR and Bell's phenomenon may sometimes be spared. When acute, the eyes may be deviated downwards (the setting-sun sign), and may be observed in premature infants following intraventricular haemorrhage, and

Table 8.15. Causes of disorders of vertical gaze

Tumour: pineal germinoma or teratoma, pineocytoma glioma, metastasis
Hydrocephalus
Vascular: midbrain or thalamic haemorrhage or infarction
Metabolic: e.g. Niemann–Pick variants, Gaucher's disease
Degeneration: progressive supranuclear palsy, Huntington's disease, cortico-basal degeneration
Drug-induced: barbituates, carbamazepine, neuroleptics
Miscellaneous: MS, Whipple's disease, hypoxia, syphilis

when a ventricular shunt becomes acutely blocked. Downward saccades may be of reduced velocity.

The dorsal midbrain syndrome may also be associated with an impairment of convergence, which is usually paralysed but may rarely be excessive and cause convergence spasm, convergence-retraction nystagmus (see Section 8.11.5), eyelid retraction (Collier's sign), and a pupillary light-near dissociation.

Selective vertical gaze palsy due to riMLF lesion

A unilateral or bilateral lesion of the riMLF produces a down-gaze palsy, mainly affecting saccades, or more rarely a complete vertical gaze palsy (Büttner-Ennever *et al.* 1982). Patients with unilateral midbrain lesions can develop combined upgaze and downgaze palsies, isolated upgaze palsies, an uniocular upward ophthalmoplegia with no primary position hypotropia (monocular double elevator palsy), and a vertical one-and-a-half syndrome which describes the combination of a vertical gaze palsy in one direction and a monocular vertical ophthalmoplegia in the other direction, with no primary position heterotropia (Hommel and Bogousslavsky 1991).

The ocular tilt reaction and lesions of the INC

A lesion of the INC, which lies immediately caudal to the riMLF and rostral to the oculomotor nucleus, produces two distinct deficits: an ocular tilt reaction (OTR), and a deficit in vertical pursuit and vertical gaze holding (Halmagyi *et al.* 1990). The OTR is a head–eye postural synkinesis that consists of a skew deviation with a head tilt (towards the side of the hypometric eye), and torsion of the eyes (incyclotropia of the hypermetric eye and excyclotropia of the hypometric eye). Such patients also show a deviation of their subjective vertical. Although the OTR is produced by a lesion of the INC, it can be found whenever peripheral or central lesions cause an imbalance of otolithic inputs (Brandt and Dieterich 1993).

Thalamic lesions

Thalamic lesions can give rise to disorders of both horizontal and vertical eye movements (Clark and Albert 1995). Conjugate deviation of the eyes contralateral to the lesion (so-called wrong-way deviation) is associated with haemorrhage in the medial thalamus. Thalamic haemorrhage may also lead to forced downward deviation of the eyes, associated with convergence and miosis. Caudal lesions in the thalamus have been associated with esotropia, which although usually associated with a downward gaze deviation, may be present as an isolated finding. A paralysis of downgaze is associated with a caudal thalamic infarction, due to occlusion of the proximal portion of the posterior cerebral artery or its perforator branch, the thalamosubthalamic paramedian artery. However, the ocular motor deficit may well be due to damage to the riMLF or its immediate premotor inputs.

Cerebellar lesions

Although it is generally accepted that the cerebellum plays an important role in the control of eye movements in humans, pure lesions of the cerebellum without some brainstem involve-ment are unusual (Lewis and Zee 1993). This creates some difficulty in determining eye movement abnormalities specific for cerebellar dysfunction. It is appropriate to segregate lesions to three main regions of the cerebellum, each of which has a particular ocular motor syndrome: the dorsal vermis and underlying fastigial nucleus, the nodulus and ventral uvula, and the flocculus and paraflocculus. The dorsal vermis and underlying fastigial nucleus are involved in controlling saccadic accuracy and smooth pursuit. Lesions in this region lead to saccadic dysmetria and mild deficits of smooth pursuit. The nodulus and ventral uvula are involved in the control of the low-frequency response of the VOR, and disorders in this region give rise to periodic alternating nystagmus, positional nystagmus, and impaired habituation of the VOR, with increased duration of the vestibular responses. The flocculus and paraflocculus are concerned with retinal-image stabilization, e.g. smooth tracking with the head still, gaze-holding, control of the VOR and its suppression, and pulse-step matching. Lesions of this region, therefore, lead to impaired pursuit and VOR cancellation, with gaze-evoked, rebound, centripetal, and downbeat nystagmus; and inappropriate amplitude of the VOR. Other signs which have been associated with cerebellar lesions, although precise localization is not available, include torsional nystagmus during vertical pursuit (lesion in the middle cerebellar peduncle), square wave jerks, esotropia with alternating skew deviation, divergent nystagmus, primary position upbeating nystagmus, and centripetal nystagmus.

The cerebellum is also important in generating long-term adaptive responses which enable eye movements to be kept appropriate to the visual stimulus. For example, when wearing lens corrections there is a magnifying or minifying effect which requires adaptive changes in the gain of the VOR. These take a few hours to days to occur and explain why some individuals experience difficulties when prescribed new lenses.

8.11.3 Disorders of the voluntary control of gaze

Anatomy and physiology of voluntary gaze

The cerebral hemispheres are extremely important for the programming and co-ordination of both saccadic and pursuit conjugate eye movements (Fig. 8.18c). Since different areas are involved in these two types of eye movements, they will be dealt with separately, always realizing that for fully effective ocular motor control, co-ordination between these subtypes of eye movement is essential.

Saccadic system

There appear to be four main cortical areas in the cerebral hemispheres involved in the generation of saccades. In the frontal lobe in humans there is the frontal eye field (FEF) which lies laterally at the caudal end of the second frontal gyrus in the premotor cortex (Brodmann area 6), and the supplementary eye field (SEF) which lies mesially at the anterior region of the supplementary motor area in the first frontal gyrus (Brodmann area 6). The third area is in the dorsolateral prefrontal cortex (DLPFC), which lies anterior to the FEF in the second frontal gyrus (Brodmann area 46). Finally, a posterior eye field (PEF) lies in the parietal lobe, possibly in the superior part of the angular gyrus (Brodmann area 39) and the adjacent lateral intraparietal sulcus. Studies in monkeys reveal that these areas are all interconnected with each other, and they all appear to send projections to the superior colliculus (SC) and the premotor areas in the brainstem controlling saccades.

It appears that there are two parallel pathways involved in the cortical generation of saccades. First, an anterior system originating in the FEF projecting both directly, and via the SC, to the brainstem saccadic generators. This pathway also passes indirectly via the basal ganglia to the SC. The second, or posterior, pathway originates in the PEF, passing to the brainstem saccadic generators via the SC. Only after bilateral lesions to both the FEF and SC in monkeys is there a failure to trigger saccades.

Although the precise functions of these various cortical areas in saccade generation have not been determined, a number of general statements can be made. The FEF is involved in triggering volitional saccades which, for example, may be predictive (in anticipation of the appearance of a target), memory-guided (to a previously seen target), or scanning (searching for a particular target of interest). The PEF could be involved in triggering reflexive saccades to the sudden appearance of novel visual or auditory stimuli, and appears to be involved in visuo-spatial integration. The DLPFC may be responsible for maintaining a spatial map of the environment in short-term memory, providing spatial information for memory-guided saccades and other volitional saccades. There is also evidence that it contains circuits responsible for inhibiting unwanted misdirected reflexive saccades. The SEF appears to be involved in the generation of sequences of saccades.

A subsidiary neural circuit related to saccade generation is from the frontal lobe to the superior colliculus via the basal ganglia. Projections from the frontal cortex pass to the substantia nigra, pars reticular (SNpr), via a relay in the caudate nucleus. An inhibitory pathway from the SNpr projects directly to the SC. This appears to be a gating circuit related to volitional saccades, especially of the memory-guided type.

Smooth pursuit system

To maintain foveation of a moving target the smooth pursuit system has developed relatively independently of the saccadic oculomotor system, although there have to be interconnections between the two. It is first necessary to identify and code the velocity and direction of a moving target. This is carried out in the extrastriate visual area known as the middle temporal visual area (MT) (also called visual area V5), which contains neurons sensitive to visual target motion. In humans, this lies immediately posterior to the ascending limb of the inferior temporal sulcus at the occipitotemporal border (Brodmann area 19/37 junction). Area MT sends this motion signal to the medial superior temporal visual area (MST), which in monkeys is located on the anterior bank of the superior temporal sulcus, but in humans is considered to lie superior and a little anterior to area MT within the inferior parietal lobe. Damage to this area results in an impairment of smooth pursuit of targets moving towards the damaged hemisphere. Evidence of a possible contribution of the FEF to the generation of smooth pursuit has recently been obtained in the monkey.

Both area MST and the FEF send direct projections to a group of nuclei which lie in the basis pontis of the pons. In the monkey, the dorso-lateral and lateral groups of pontine nuclei receive direct cortical inputs related to smooth pursuit. Lesions of similarly located nuclei in humans result in abnormal pursuit. These nuclei transfer the pursuit signal bilaterally to the posterior vermis, contralateral flocculus and fastigial nuclei of the cerebellum. Finally, the pursuit signal passes from the cerebellum to the brainstem, specifically the medial vestibular nucleus and nucleus prepositus hypoglossi, and thence to the PPRF and possibly directly to the ocular motor nuclei. This circuitry therefore involves a double decussation, firstly at the level of the midpons (pontocerebellar neuron) and secondly in the lower pons (vestibulo-abducens neuron).

8.11.4 Specific disorders of eye movements

Disorders of saccadic eye movements

Disorders of saccades can be considered in terms of abnormalities of the saccadic pulse–step innervation pattern. A change in the amplitude (width × height) of the pulse, either too big or too small, leads to saccadic hypermetria (overshoot) or hypometria (undershoot), respectively. Such a saccadic pulse dysmetria is associated with a lesion of the dorsal vermis in the cerebellum. A decrease in the height of the pulse, which implies disturbed function of the burst neurons in the PPRF or riMLF, leads to slow saccades. Many causes of slow saccades, several of which involve these areas, have been described (Table 8.16). A mismatch between the size of the pulse and the step (pulse–step mismatch) results in post-saccadic drifts and glissades. They are observed in diseases involving the vestibulocerebellum. If the pulse is not followed by a step (a *saccadic pulse*) the eye drifts back to its previous position in a decreasing velocity, exponential, smooth eye movement. Both conjugate and monocular saccadic pulses occur in patients with multiple sclerosis.

Table 8.16. Causes of slow saccades

Olivopontocerebellar atrophy
Huntington's chorea
Wilson's disease
Parkinson's disease
Ataxia telangiectasia
Lipid storage disease
Progessive supranuclear palsy
Lesions of the paramedial pontine reticular formation
Internuclear ophthalmoplegia
Peripheral nerve palsy or muscle weakness
Drug intoxications

Disturbances in the initiation of saccades may lead to a prolonged latency, or the addition of a head movement or blink to initiate the saccade. This may be seen in congenital or acquired oculomotor apraxia, and various degenerative conditions, including Parkinson's disease (O'Sullivan and Kennard 1998), Huntington's disease (Lasker and Zee 1997), and Alzheimer's disease (Fletcher and Sharpe 1986).

Saccades may also occur inappropriately, particularly during attempted fixation. *Square wave jerks* (SWJ) are small-amplitude (up to 5°) saccades that take the eyes off fixation, followed some 200 ms later by a corrective saccade. Many normal subjects have low-frequency SWJ (<15/min), but elderly subjects often have a higher frequency. They are most prominent in cerebellar disease, progressive supranuclear palsy, and multiple system atrophy. *Macrosquare wave jerks* (5–40°) are encountered in multiple sclerosis and olivopontocerebellar degeneration. Patients with diffuse cerebral cortex damage often exhibit large-amplitude saccades away from the object of regard. After an interval of several hundred milliseconds the patient makes a saccade back to the target. These anticipatory saccades are observed particularly in Alzheimer's disease.

Ocular motor apraxia is a term used for failure to generate saccades to commands, and may be of a congenital (COMA) (Cogan 1952) or acquired type (Pierrot-Deseilligny *et al.* 1988). COMA may be recognized shortly after birth, when the child does not appear to be fixating upon objects normally. At around 4–6 months the child develops the characteristic thrusting horizontal head movements, sometimes with blinking, when the child wants to change fixation. This manoeuvre serves to use the intact VOR to drive the eyes into an extreme eccentric position in the orbit. As the head moves past the target, the eyes are dragged along in space until they align with the target. The head then rotates back and the VOR ensures that fixation is maintained until the eye is in the primary position (Harris *et al.* 1996). The cause of COMA is unknown. It is sometimes associated with developmental abnormalities such as delayed psychomotor development, infantile hypotonia, and with associated anomalies such as agenesis of the corpus callosum and cerebellar dysplasia and hypoplasia (for example, as part of Joubert's syndrome). Patients with COMA usually improve with age. In certain diseases affecting the brainstem a similar clinical syndrome to COMA may occur. These include ataxia-telangiectasia, cerebral Whipple's disease, Gaucher's disease, Niemann–Pick's disease, vitamin E deficiency, and many other storage diseases and aminoacidureas.

Disorders of smooth pursuit

A number of different disturbances of smooth pursuit are found (Morrow and Sharpe 1993). The most common abnormality is a low gain (gain = eye velocity/target velocity), which appears as deficient pursuit in which pursuit is broken by small catch-up saccades. Low-gain pursuit can occur as a result of tiredness and inattention, as a side-effect of medications such as sedatives and anticonvulsants, or due to lesions in the vestibulocerebellum. Generally, bilateral low-gain pursuit has no localiz-

ing value. This is not the case with asymmetrical low-gain pursuit, which usually occurs as a result of a lesion in the ipsilateral parietal lobe, thalamus, midbrain tegmentum, dorsolateral nucleus of the pons, and vestibulocerebellum (Heide *et al.* 1996). Occasionally a disturbance of pursuit 'tone' (balance) occurs due to cerebral hemisphere lesions, when the eyes drift towards the side of the lesion. Disturbances of direction can occur, for example, in congenital nystagmus in which there is an apparent 'inversion' of pursuit when the eyes move in an opposite direction to the motion of the target.

Disorders of vergence eye movements

The most common causes of disturbed vergence are congenital abnormalities. Various forms of convergence or divergence excess or insufficiency are usually accompanied by a concomitant strabismus. Although this may not give rise to diplopia in childhood, it can present as intermittent diplopia later in life. Acquired forms of vergence disorders commonly occur in association with disturbances of vertical gaze, as in the dorsal midbrain syndrome, and in Parkinson's disease and progressive supranuclear palsy. Spasm of the near triad (convergence spasm) is only rarely due to organic disease and is usually a voluntary convergence in patients with a conversion syndrome (Sarkies and Sanders 1985). The patients often complain of discomfort and the convergence, which only lasts for a brief period on each occasion, may be associated with visual blurring, diplopia, and 'eye strain'. An important clue to this diagnosis is the strong pupillary miosis which accompanies the convergence.

Disorders of vestibular eye movements

These will be covered in Section 9.2 in this volume.

8.11.5 Saccadic oscillations and nystagmus

There is an important distinction between saccadic oscillations, which are sustained oscillations that are initiated by fast saccadic eye movements, and nystagmus where the oscillations are initiated by smooth eye movements, i.e. the fast phase in jerk nystagmus is corrective and not primary.

Saccadic oscillations

Saccadic oscillations are bursts of saccades, which may be intermittent or continuous, causing a disruption of fixation. Two main types can be identified, those with intersaccadic intervals and those composed of back-to-back saccades.

The oscillations with intersaccadic intervals include *square wave oscillations* consisting of sequences of SWJs which can occur in Parkinson's disease and progressive supranuclear palsy. *Macrosaccadic oscillations* straddle the intended fixation position. The amplitudes (up to 40°) of sequential saccades increase in amplitude and then decrease in a crescendo–decrescendo pattern (Selhorst *et al.* 1976b). This type of oscillation is usually observed in acute damage to the dorsal cerebellum involving the deep cerebellar nuclei, as in demyelination, tumour, or haematoma.

Oscillations without any intersaccadic interval (back-to-back) include opsoclonus, ocular flutter, and convergence–retraction saccadic pulses. *Opsoclonus* consists of multidirectional (including oblique and torsional) back-to-back saccades of varying amplitude (Averbuch-Heller and Remler 1996). It has been suggested that the disorder arises due to disordered pause cell function in the PPRF. A variety of posterior fossa disorders can give rise to the condition, including infective agents such as coxsackie virus type B and *Haemophilus influenzae* meningitis. It can also occur in neonates associated with myoclonus—'dancing eye and dancing feet'. This appears to be a maturational deficit which resolves over approximately 6 weeks. Opsoclonus also occurs as a paraneoplastic (non-metastatic) disorder, which in children is associated with occult neuroblastoma and in adults with small cell carcinoma of the lung and carcinoma of the breast and uterus. *Ocular flutter* consists of bursts of back-to-back saccades in the horizontal plane only. It can therefore be observed in patients recovering from opsoclonus. Isolated ocular flutter is most often observed in patients with multiple sclerosis and signs of cerebellar disease. A voluntary form of flutter (voluntary flutter) can be induced by about 8 per cent of the population, usually by convergence. It consists of salvoes of horizontal back-to-back saccades. Lesions of the dorsal midbrain are often associated with upward-gaze palsies and *convergence–retraction nystagmus* (Ochs et al. 1979). This is incorrectly termed a nystagmus since it actually consists of adducting saccades and should be redesignated convergence–retraction saccadic pulses. Finally, a further type of saccadic oscillation is *ocular bobbing* (Susac et al. 1970). This consists of rhythmic, sudden, downward jerks of the eyes followed by slow return to the midposition, either immediately or after a short delay. The typical type, associated with pontine haemorrhage or infarction, is associated with paralysis of horizontal eye movements. Atypical bobbing is similar, except horizontal eye movements are intact, and occurs in metabolic encephalopathy, obstructive hydrocephalus, or cerebellar haematoma. When the fast movement is upward followed by a delayed slow return, the condition is known as reverse bobbing.

Nystagmus

Nystagmus is an oscillation which is initiated by a slow eye movement. When this slow movement is accompanied by a fast (saccadic) eye movement it is called jerk nystagmus. Although the direction of the nystagmus is conventionally determined by the direction of the quick phases, it is important to remember that it is the smooth eye movement imbalance which is responsible for the nystagmus. If both phases are smooth eye movements, pendular nystagmus is observed.

The most common form of jerk nystagmus is *vestibular nystagmus*, which most frequently results from labyrinth or vestibular nerve dysfunction (further details in Section 9.2). Several different types of central vestibular nystagmus are described, all of which show no change in intensity with the removal of fixation (by using Frenzel goggles). This is in contrast to peripheral vestibular nystagmus, in which removal of fixation leads to an increased intensity of the nystagmus.

Downbeat nystagmus may or may not be present in the primary position; if it is, it beats directly downwards and is often accentuated in lateral gaze (Halmagyi et al. 1983). When it is present in the primary position, a disturbance of the cerebellar flocculus is found, commonly due to a disturbance at the craniocervical junction, such as an Arnold–Chiari malformation. Other causes include cerebellar degenerations, anticonvulsant drugs, lithium intoxication, and intra-axial brainstem lesions. In about half of the patients with downbeat nystagmus, no cause can be found.

Upbeat nystagmus, when present in the primary position, is usually associated with focal brainstem lesions in the tegmental grey matter, either at the pontomesencephalic junction or at the pontomedullary junction, involving the nucleus prepositus hypoglossi or the ventral tegmental pathway of the upward vestibulo-ocular reflex (Fisher et al. 1983). Multiple sclerosis, tumour, infarction, and cerebellar degeneration are the most common causes.

Torsional nystagmus is a jerk nystagmus around the antero-posterior axis. It is commonly associated with other types of nystagmus. However, when it is pure it indicates a lesion of the lateral medulla involving the vestibular nuclei. Occasionally it may be due to a midbrain–thalamic lesion, involving the INC.

Periodic alternating nystagmus (PAN) is a primary position horizontal nystagmus that changes direction in a crescendo–decrescendo manner, characteristically approximately every 90 s (Fletcher 1993). Between each directional change there is a null period of 0–10 s. There is a congenital form, and acquired forms are due to Chiari malformations, multiple sclerosis, fourth ventricle tumours, spinocerebellar degenerations, and anticonvulsant intoxication. Baclofen has been shown to be an effective treatment (Halmagyi et al. 1980).

Gaze-evoked nystagmus is a common clinical observation with limited localizing value. It is a jerk nystagmus which is absent in the primary position and is only present on eccentric gaze. It usually signifies cerebellar parenchymal disease, particularly involving the flocculus or its projections to the brainstem. Bilateral horizontal, together with vertical, gaze-evoked nystagmus commonly occurs with structural brainstem and cerebellar lesions, diffuse metabolic disorders, and drug intoxication. A variant of gaze-evoked nystagmus is *rebound nystagmus*, in which there is a jerk nystagmus that beats away from the previous direction, present in eccentric gaze, lasting for 3–25 s after the eyes return to the primary position. It is also associated with parenchymal cerebellar disease.

Pendular nystagmus is either congenital or acquired due to cerebellar and brainstem disease, usually multiple sclerosis (Fletcher 1993). Acquired pendular nystagmus may have both horizontal and vertical components, and the amplitude and phase relationships of the two sine waves determine the trajectory of the eyes, e.g. oblique, circular, or elliptical. It can affect one eye or both, equally or unequally, and is often symptomatic, resulting in oscillopsia. It may be associated with oscillations of other structures, such as the palate, head, or limbs. When it is present in association with palatal myoclonus, *oculopalatal myoclonus*, the lesion is usually in Mollaret's triangle, which consists of the red nucleus, dentate nucleus, and inferior olivary nucleus (Nakada and Kwee 1986). The latter nucleus usually shows pseudohypertrophic degeneration. A combination of a convergence-induced pendular nystagmus and synchronous jaw contractions, called *oculomasticatory myorhythmia*, is characteristic of Whipple's disease (Schwartz *et al.* 1986). In *see-saw nystagmus* one eye intorts and rises while the other eye extorts and falls in a rapidly alternating sequence. In this pendular form there is often a bitemporal hemianopia, and the condition is associated with large parasellar masses which have expanded up into the third ventricle and are distorting structures in the mesencephalic–diencephalic region (Daroff 1965).

Congenital nystagmus is almost invariably a horizontal conjugate nystagmus which is unaltered by vertical position. It is generally of jerk type with accelerating slow phases, and has an eccentric null position. Fixation effort enhances congenital nystagmus. Less commonly, the nystagmus is of a pendular type. Reversed optokinetic nystagmus, beating in the direction of the target motion, is a feature of congenital nystagmus. Patients may show a head turn or occasionally a head oscillation (Dell'Osso and Daroff 1975).

Latent nystagmus is a type of congenital nystagmus that is only present on monocular viewing and which then beats toward the viewing eye (Gresty *et al.* 1992). It is absent on binocular viewing. If the patient has amblyopia in one eye, latent nystagmus is present with both eyes viewing, when it is called manifest latent nystagmus.

8.12 Orbital disease

8.12.1 Anatomy and examination

The orbit has a pear-like shape with the optic canal as the stem. The orbital walls, which are made up of seven bones (maxillary, frontal, zygomatic, ethmoid, sphenoid, palatine, and lacrimal), are of variable thickness and pierced by several fissures and foramina. The superior orbital fissure admits to the orbit the three ocular motor cranial nerves (CN III, IV, VI), the ophthalmic division of the trigeminal nerve, and some sympathetic fibres. In addition, the superior ophthalmic vein, which drains most of the orbit, passes through this fissure. The remainder of the venous drainage passes through the inferior orbital fissure to join the pterygoid plexus. Since there are no valves in the orbital venous drainage system, a carotid-cavernous fistula leads to reversed flow in the venous system, accounting for the marked venous congestion and orbital oedema.

The apex of the orbit is very crowded, with the optic nerve emerging through the canal of Zinn, to which are attached the rectus muscles. This explains why enlargement of the extra-ocular muscles, as in dysthyroid ophthalmopathy, may lead to optic nerve compression. Several sinuses (ethmoid, sphenoid,

maxillary, and frontal) surround the orbit, which allows spread of disease, especially infection and tumour, from these spaces to the orbit.

Clinical examination

Although several imaging modalities, including ultrasound, CT, and MRI scanning, are available to aid the localization and diagnosis of orbital disease, a systematic clinical examination enables one to use them appropriately.

First, the eyelids are examined for disturbance of position, such as ptosis or retraction, abnormalities of movement, in particular lid lag and fatiguability, and the presence of swelling or a mass. The conjunctivae are next examined for evidence of oedema (chemosis), dilated vessels, or neoplastic infiltration. The globe may show axial or non-axial proptosis. This is best judged by inspection alone and may be difficult to determine because of significant interindividual and racial variation. Viewing the position of each cornea relative to the other from a vantage point above and behind the patient can be helpful. Up to 2 mm of asymmetry is within normal limits, as measured by exophthalmometry. Looking at old photographs can be helpful in estimating the time of onset of protrusion of the eye. The degree of retrocessability of the globe can be estimated by gentle backward pressure through the closed lid. Retrobulbar mass lesions will reduce the ability to push the globe back into the orbit, whereas blood-filled spaces, such as varices, allow compression and repositioning of the exophthalmic globe. Pain to palpation may accompany orbital infection and inflammation, while being uncommon in dysthyroidism and orbital tumours. Auscultation over the globe with the lids closed may reveal vascular bruits. Finally, ophthalmoscopy may reveal disc oedema and optic atrophy with optociliary shunts, suggestive of an optic nerve sheath meningioma. Choroidal folds and acquired hyperopia usually imply a retrobulbar mass lesion deforming the globe from behind.

A wide range of disorders can give rise to orbital involvement and are listed in Table 8.17 (Wright 1988).

8.12.2 Dysthyroid eye disease

Dysthyroid eye disease (Graves' ophthalmopathy, dysthyroid ophthalmopathy, endocrine ophthalmopathy) is the most

Table 8.17. Causes of orbital disease

Cellulitis
Sequelae of trauma
Graves' disease
Pseudotumour of orbit
Lymphoma
Cavernous haemangioma
Lacrimal gland tumour
Peripheral nerve tumours
Meningioma
Mucocoele
Metastatic and secondary tumours

common systemic disorder, associated with diplopia, ophthalmoparesis, and infiltration of extraocular muscles (Sergott and Glaser 1981). It is usually accompanied by biochemical and immunological evidence of thyroid dysfunction, although this may not be apparent for months or years. Pathological examination of extraocular muscles in patients with dysthyroid eye disease reveal infiltration by lymphocytes and plasma cells. The nature of the orbital antigen recognized by the infiltrating T lymphocyte is unknown. Cytokines released by these lymphocytes appear to be responsible for the proliferation of orbital fibroblasts and increase their synthesis of glycosoaminoglycans. As the disease progresses, the infiltration and oedema of the extraocular muscles produce loss of muscle tissue, and the muscles become fibrotic (van der Gaag *et al.* 1996).

The early symptoms of this condition may take the form of ocular irritation or scratchiness, which is typically worse when the patient first awakes. This may be associated with a feeling of orbital fullness and intermittent vertical diplopia. Photophobia and tearing are usual and blurred vision may be due to corneal exposure due to the proptosis or a central scotoma associated with a compressive optic neuropathy.

In the acute phase there is usually unilateral or bilateral lid retraction, accompanied by lid lag on downgaze, and lid puffiness (Fig. 8.21). Conjunctival chemosis and injection overlying the insertions of the horizontal rectus muscles are routine. Periorbital oedema varies in degree and may be extreme. These signs usually precede the disturbed ocular motility which is frequently observed in this disease, and is usually due to a restrictive myopathy of the inferior rectus muscle, leading to impaired ocular elevation (Fells *et al.* 1994). In more advanced cases the affected eye becomes hypotropic, and if the medial rectus is similarly affected esotropia may result. If these ocular motility disturbances are found in the context of other typical signs of dysthyroid eye disease, diagnosis is assured. However, in others the florid stage is limited and subclinical and the patient presents with an ophthalmoparesis which has to be differentiated from an ocular motor nerve palsy. To differentiate this from the restrictive myopathy of thyroid eye disease, the forced duction

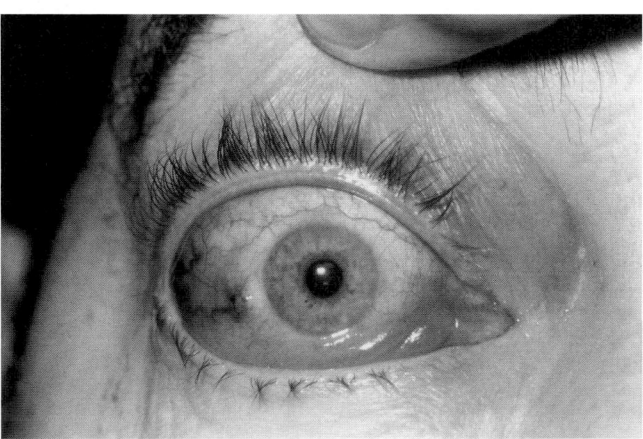

Fig. 8.21. Thyroid eye disease, causing proptosis, chemosis, and lid oedema.

test in used. In this test an attempt is made to move the globe, with a forceps under topical anaesthesia, into its appropriate field of gaze. CT or MRI of the orbit reveals characteristic enlargement of the rectus muscles, the most frequently affected being the medial and inferior rectii. Although the diagnosis is supported by the demonstration of thyroid-associated auto-antibodies and abnormal thyroid function, it is important to remember that these may be absent, and this should not dissuade the clinician from a diagnosis of dysthyroid eye disease if the clinical signs are compatible.

Since it is impossible to predict which patients will develop an orbitopathy, initial management of the condition is based on rendering the patient euthyroid and using symptomatic therapy such as topical drops and ointments, and elevation of the head of the bed at night for oedema. Worsening of the symptoms can be managed by immunosuppression using systemic corticosteroids in doses up to 120 mg daily (Wiersinga 1996). Benefit is usually apparent within 3 weeks. Lens sparing, low-dose (2000 cGy) orbital radiotherapy should be used if there is a failure to adequately respond to steroids, usually with good results. Failure to respond to either therapies, particularly if a compressive optic neuropathy or severe proptosis with corneal exposure keratitis are present, requires surgical orbital decompression. In the fibrotic phase of the disease restrictive myopathy may require extraocular muscle surgery to restore binocular single vision, and retracted lids may require plastic surgery.

8.12.3 Idiopathic orbital inflammation

Idiopathic inflammatory inflammation (orbital pseudotumour) is the term used for a syndrome consisting painful proptosis, orbital congestion, periorbital oedema, diplopia, and sometimes visual loss, for which a cause cannot be found after diseases such as syphilis, tuberculosis, sarcoidosis, Wegener's granulomatosis, or collagen vascular disease have been excluded (Lakke 1962; Kline 1982). It may be diffuse or selectively affect any orbital structure, resulting in only one specific symptom or sign. Some accounts of this condition divide it into different entities depending on the structure involved, e.g. sclera (posterior scleritis), lacrimal gland (dacryoadenitis), cavernous sinus/superior orbital fissure (Tolosa–Hunt syndrome), extraocular muscle (myositis), but they are probably all due to the same pathological process. Orbital lymphoma is particularly difficult to exclude, even with biopsy material.

The condition is usually unilateral, although occasionally it may be bilateral, and it affects both children and adults. Involvement of one or more extraocular muscles may lead to a painful ophthalmoplegia. Many patients experience a general malaise. The condition may run a chronic remitting course with gradual worsening, or spontaneous remissions may occur.

The CT appearance of orbital pseudotumour varies, depending on the orbital structures which are preferentially affected, and includes retrobulbar fatty infiltration, proptosis, extraocular muscle enlargement, apical fat oedema, optic nerve thickening, and uveoscleral thickening. It may also show muscle tendon sheath involvement, which is spared in dysthyroid eye disease. MRI studies show that on T2-weighted images the lesions are isointense or only mildly hyperintense to fat, in contradistinction to the hyperintense signal obtained from orbital metastasis, a not infrequent differential diagnosis.

Patients with this constellation of signs, in whom no other cause can be found, should be given a course of systemic corticosteroid treatment, failing which orbital radiotherapy can be of value.

8.12.4 Orbital tumours

A variety of tumours may involve structures within the orbit (Shields *et al.* 1984). The location of the mass in the orbit is often a clue to their nature. They may be intraconal (within the cone of the extraocular muscles), extraconal, and periorbital (outside the orbit, but impinging on its structures).

Intraconal tumours cause forward displacement of the globe. These include tumours which may be primary, such as optic nerve sheath meningiomas and optic nerve gliomas which have been discussed in Section 8.5.4, or secondary, due to metastases. One of the most common orbital tumours in adults, which has an affinity for the intraconal space, is the *cavernous haemangioma*. This usually presents as a painless proptosis and slowly enlarges over a period of many years. Its CT appearance is of a well-circumscribed homogeneous mass which shows marked enhancement with contrast. Complete surgical excision is the treatment of choice.

Proptosis may be due to venous anomalies (varices). These may exhibit increased proptosis on Valsava manoeuvre or on bending forward. Their CT appearance is characteristic, and non-intervention is appropriate.

The most common *metastatic tumours* to the orbit come from breast (42 per cent), lung (11 per cent), and prostate (8.3 per cent). Although patients may present with proptosis, scirrhous breast carcinoma may cause enophthalmos. Any proptotic patient who has a history of treatment of cancer must be suspected of having an orbital metastasis. Histological verification is mandatory before treatment.

Orbital tumours in the extraconal space cause downward or upward displacement of the globe, when located in the superior and inferior orbital spaces, respectively. They may arise in the extraconal space, extend into it from surrounding structures, or be metastatic from distant sources. A rapidly developing unilateral proptosis in a child is likely to be an orbital rhabdomyosarcoma. Tumours frequently located in the superior orbital space are dermoid tumours and mucocoeles, and less frequently lesions of the lacrimal gland and fibrous dysplasia.

8.12.5 Vascular disorders

The main types of neuro-ophthalmic vascular disorders are the high-flow *carotid–cavernous sinus fistulas* (CCF) and the low-flow spontaneous *dural–cavernous sinus shunts* which produce overlapping clinical syndromes (Keltner *et al.* 1987). This communication between the arterial and venous systems leads to a rise in the venous pressure in the globe, resulting in a fall in the arterial perfusion pressure, and a major drop in perfusion pressure.

Fistulas may be classified (Barrow *et al.* 1985) according to the velocity of blood flow through the shunt into low- and high-flow fistulas; the anatomic origin of the arteries supplying the fistula; and the aetiology, which may be spontaneous or traumatic.

◆ Type A: communication between internal carotid artery (ICA) and cavernous sinus (CS); high flow; direct tears.

◆ Type B: communication between meningeal branches of ICA and CS; slow flow; indirect dural artenovenous malformation (AVM).

◆ Type C; communication between external branches of external IC (EIC) and CS; slow flow; indirect dural AVM.

◆ Type D; communication between meningeal branches of ICA, external carotid artery (ECA), and CS; slow flow; indirect dural AVM.

Direct carotid–cavernous fistula; Type A

This may occur at any location along the length of the intracavernous portion of the INC and commonly occurs as a result of both penetrating or non-penetrating head trauma and from aneurysmal rupture. There may be a delay of days, or even weeks, for symptoms to develop following injury. The common signs are proptosis associated with chronic conjunctival injection and oedema, and an audible bruit. The conjunctival veins may be arterialized (Fig. 8.22a). Because of connections between the two CSs a unilateral fistula may give rise to bilateral ocular signs. Damage to cranial nerves and sympathetic and parasympathetic fibres in the CS may lead to diplopia and pupillary abnormalities. The most commonest cause for diplopia is an abducens nerve palsy. The definitive diagnosis of CCF is made by selective cerebral angiography (Fig. 8.22b).

There are several potential causes for the visual loss commonly seen in CS fistulas, including corneal damage due to exposure; retinal artery occlusion; glaucoma due to raised episcleral venous pressure or, rarely, to iris neovascularization; macula involvement due to ischaemia, haemorrhage, or cystoid oedema; anterior segment ischaemia. Ophthalmoscopy reveals features of a slow-flow retinopathy, which include blot haemorrhages, microaneurysms, mild disc swelling, and venous congestion and tortuosity. Occasionally a picture similar to a complete central vein occlusion may occur (Brosnaham *et al.* 1992).

Without treatment the ocular abnormalities will progress, leading to blindness. A variety of endovascular procedures have been developed for CS fistulas with the aim of closing the fistula and maintaining the patency of the distal ICA. These include electrometallic thrombosis using coils and detachable balloon occlusion.

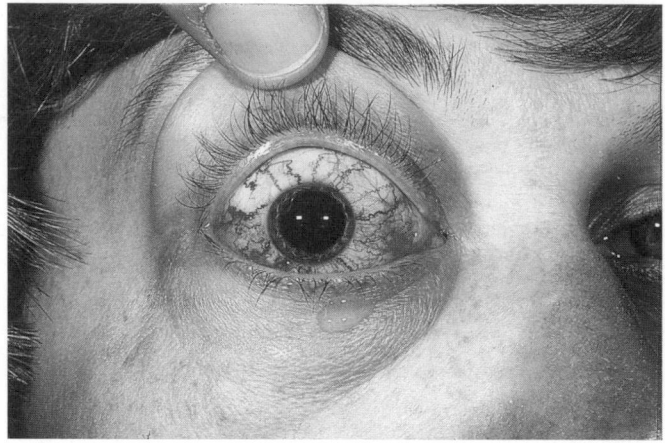

(a)

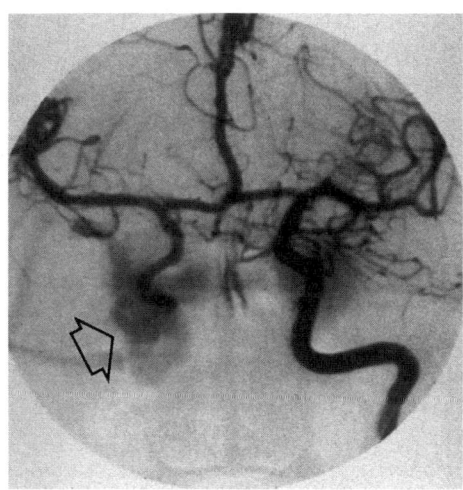

(b)

Fig. 8.22 Carotid-cavernous sinus fistula. (a) Chronic conjunctival injection and oedema with aterialisation of the conjunctival veins. (b) Left carotid arteriogram illustrating a right direct carotid-cavernous sinus fistula (arrow).

Spontaneous dural–cavernous sinus shunts; Types B–D

These slow-flow, indirect cavernous fistulas are thought to occur due to rupture of congenital arteriovenous anomalies, which usually occur in middle-aged women. The clinical manifestations depend on the direction of venous outflow from the fistula. If anterior, then the signs are similar, but less dramatic, to those which occur with direct CCF, including conjunctival venous arterialization, orbital congestion, and proptosis. Posterior drainage may cause cranial nerve palsies, most commonly of the abducens nerve. A bruit may not be present. Less commonly, choroidal detachment and angle-closure glaucoma develop as a result of altered venous outflow.

Treatment should be conservative, as between 20 and 50 per cent of spontaneous dural CCFs close spontaneously, not infrequently after carotid angiography. If vision is threatened,

then endovascular therapy is indicated (Kupersmith *et al.* 1988*b*).

8.12.6 Orbital infections

Proptosis, periorbital swelling, and ophthalmoplegia in a febrile patient suggest orbital cellulitis. Most patients will have contiguous sinus disease, commonly of the ethmoid sinus, with the frontal and maxillary sinuses being involved less frequently. If the cellulitis occurs in the context of trauma, scanning must be performed to locate any foreign body, which must then be removed.

The causative agent must be sought by culture of both the blood and any purulent wound drainage. The most likely organisms are *Haemophilus influenzae* (in children), *Staphylococcus aureus,* and *Streptococcus pneumoniae.* As soon as cultures have been obtained, the patient should be treated with broad-spectrum antibiotics to cover the possible causative organisms, until the specific organism has been identified.

Patients presenting with an orbital cellulitis who have diabetes mellitus or who are immunocompromised should be considered to have mucormycosis until proven otherwise. Early symptoms include sinusitis, orbital pain, and sudden visual loss (Gass 1961). The organism causes an obliterative arteritis which results in necrotic lesions appearing in the skin, orbit, nasal mucosa, or palate, although this is infrequently present at the onset of symptoms. If mucormycosis infection is suspected, a complete nasal examination should be undertaken to identify the typical black eschars of *Mucor*. Prompt treatment with amphotericin B and surgical débridement ensuring adequate sinus and orbital drainage is essential.

8.12.7 Proptosis

The clinical approach to diagnosing a patient presenting with proptosis depends on aspects of the history as well as a careful examination (see Section 8.12.1). The patient's past medical history may provide evidence of previous thyroid disease, suggesting thyroid eye disease; diabetes mellitus, raising the possibility of a mucormycosis infection; or of previous tumour surgery, suggesting possible metastatic infiltration. The family history may also provide clues; for example, if members of the family have a history of skin lesions, epilepsy, or brain tumours, this raises the possibility of an optic nerve glioma being the cause of the proptosis due to neurofibromatosis.

The tempo of development of the proptosis and the presence or absence of pain are also important features to ascertain. A rapidly developing proptosis in a child would immediately raise the suspicion of a malignant tumour, such as a rhabdomyosarcoma or metastatic neuroblastoma. Such a rapid painless onset in adults suggests a metastatic tumour, but if associated with pain the diagnosis includes orbital cellulitis and inflammatory orbital pseudotumour, all of which may be associated with diplopia. If there is a history of intermittent, painful proptosis, the likely aetiology are venous varices or lymphangiomas.

When the tempo of development of the proptosis is unclear, evidence for earlier proptosis than recognized by the patient can be derived from viewing antecedent photographs. If the history or photographs suggest a more slowly progressive painless course, thyroid eye disease or an orbital tumour should be considered. If the tumour is associated with visual impairment due to associated involvement of the optic nerve, which occurs some time after the onset of the proptosis, the mass is probably within the anterior or mid-third of the orbit. If, however, the visual loss precedes the proptosis, the mass is more likely to lie in the posterior third of the orbit. More anterior lesions tend to cause horizontal diplopia, whereas apical or posterior masses cause vertical diplopia due to impaired vertical gaze.

Other symptoms should be sought, such as swishing noises in the head, suggestive of a carotid–cavernous fistula; a history of chemosis and lid swelling upon rising in the morning associated with photophobia, lacrimation, and burning, suggestive of thyroid eye disease; and increasing proptosis with raised intra-abdominal pressure (Valsalva manoeuvre) or change in position, suggestive of an orbital varix or mucocoele.

Painful proptosis is relatively uncommon, and the differential diagnosis includes acute orbital inflammation, metastases, acute thrombosis of orbital varices and of the enlarged veins associated with an arteriovenous (AV) fistula. It should be remembered that there are other causes for orbital pain, including the superior orbital fissure/cavernous sinus syndrome or referred from the dura.

Once a satisfactory history has been obtained, an examination of the orbit and its contents, as described above, should be undertaken. This should help to refute or substantiate clues to the diagnosis obtained from the history, and enable the clinician to order the appropriate investigations necessary to confirm the diagnosis.

References

Albert, M. L., Reches, A., and Silverberg, R. (1975). Associative visual agnosia without alexia. *Neurology*, 25, 322–6.

Apple, D. J., Rabb, M. F., and Walsh, P. M. (1982). Congenital anomalies of the optic disc. *Surv. Ophthalmol.*, 27, 3–41.

Asbury, A. K., Aldredge, H., Hershberg, R. *et al.* (1970. Oculomotor palsy in diabetes mellitus: A clinico-pathological study. *Brain*, 93, 555–66.

Averbuch-Heller, L. and Remler, B. (1996). Opsoclonus. *Sem. Neurol.*, 16, 21–6.

Baloh, R. W., Yee, R. D., and Honrubia, V. (1981). Eye movements with Wallenberg's syndrome. *Ann. NY Acad. Sci.*, 374, 600–13.

Baloh, R. W., Furman, J. N., and Yee, R. D. (1985). Dorsal midbrain syndrome: clinical and oculographic finding. *Neurology*, 35, 54–60.

Barrett, T. G., Bundley, S. E., and Macleod, A. F. (1995). Neurodegeneration and diabetes: UK nationwide study of Wolfram (DIDMOAD) syndrome. *Lancet*, 346, 1458–62.

Barrow, D. L., Spector, R. H., Braun, I. F. *et al.* (1985). Classification and treatment of spontaneous carotid—cavernous sinus fistulas. *J. Neurosurg.*, 62, 248–56.

Beck, R. W. and ONTT Study Group (1992). A randomised, controlled trial of corticosteriods in the treatment of acute optic neuritis. *N. Engl. J. Med.*, 326, 581–8.

Bell, II. A., McIlllwain, G. G., and O'Neill, D. (1994). The iatrogenic lateral rectus nerve palsies: a series of post-myelographic cases. *J. Neuro-Ophthalmol.*, 14, 205–9.

Bell, R. A. and Thompson, H. S. (1978). Relative afferent pupillary defect in optic tract hemianopias. *Am. J. Ophthalmol.*, 85, 538–40.

Bender, M. B. (1945). Polyopsia and monocular diplopia of cerebral origin. *Arch. Neurol. Psych.*, 54, 323–38.

Bender, M. B. and Furlow, L. T. (1945). Phenomenon of visual extinction in homonymous fields and psychologic principles involved. *Arch. Neurol. Psychol.*, 53, 29–33.

Bender, M. B. and Sobein, A. J. (1963). Polyopia and palinopia in homonymous fields of vision. *Trans. Am. Neurol. Ass.*, 88, 56–7.

Bender, M. B., Feldman, M., and Sobein, A. J. (1968). Palinopsia. *Brain*, 91, 321–38.

Benton, S., Levy. I., and Swash, M. (1980). Vision in the temporal crescent in occipital infarction. *Brain*, 103, 83–95.

Berlit, P. and Rakicky, J. (1992). The Miller Fisher syndrome: review of the literature. *J. Clin. Neuro-Ophthalmol.*, 12, 57–63.

Bever, C. T., Aquino, A. V., Penn, A. S. *et al.* (1983). Prognosis in ocular myasthenia. *Ann. Neurol.*, 14, 516–19.

Bishoff, P., Lang, J., and Huber, A. (1995). Macular sparing as a perimetric artifact. *Am. J. Ophthalmol.*, 119, 72–80.

Blythe, I. M., Bromley, J. M., Kennard, C. *et al.* (1986). A study of systemic visual perseveration involving central mechanisms. *Brain*, 109, 661–75.

Boghen, D. R. and Glaser, J. S. (1975). Ischaemic optic neuropathy: the clinical profile and natural history. *Brain*, 98, 689–708.

Bogousslevsky, J., Maeder, P., Regli, F. *et al.* (1994). Pure mid-brain infarction: clinical syndromes, MRI and aetiologic patterns. *Neurology*, 44, 2032–40.

Brandt, T. and Dieterich, M. (1993). Skew deviation with ocular torsion: a vestibular brainstem sign of topographic diagnostic value. *Ann. Neurol.*, 33, 528–34.

Brodsky, M. C. (1991). Septo-optic dysplasia: a reappraisal. *Semin. Ophthalmol.*, 6, 227–32.

Brodsky, M. C. and Glaser, C. M. (1993). Optic nerve hypoplasia: clinical significance of asociated central nervous system abnormalities on magnetic resonance imaging. *Arch. Ophthalmol.*, 111, 66–74.

Brosnaham, D., McFadzean, R. M., and Teesdale, E. (1992). Neuro-ophthalmic features of carotid cavernous fistulas and their treatment by endoarterial balloon embolisation. *J. Neurol. Neurosurg. Psych.*, 55, 553–6.

Brown, H. W. (1973). True and simulated superior oblique tendon sheath syndromes. *Doc. Ophthalmol.*, 34, 123–36.

Burde, R. M. (1993). Optic disc risk factors for nonarteritic anterior ischaemic optic neuropathy. *Am. J. Ophthalmol.*, 115, 759–63.

Büttner-Ennever, J. A., Büttner, U., Cohen, B. *et al.* (1982). Vertical gaze paralysis and the rostral interstitial nucleus of the medial longitudinal fasiculus. *Brain*, 105, 125–49.

Castro, O., Johnson, L. N., and Mamourian, A. C. (1990). Isolated inferior oculomotor paresis from brainstem infarction. Prospective oculomotor fascicular organisation in the ventral mid-brain pigmentum. *Arch. Neurol.*, 47, 235–7.

Chiba, A., Kusunoki, S., Shimuzi, T. *et al.* (1992). Serum IgG antibody to ganglioside GQ1b is a possible marker of Miller Fisher syndrome. *Ann. Neurol.*, 31, 677–9.

Chun, S. M. and Selhorst, J. B. (1992). Cancer associated retinopathy. *Ophthalmol. Clin. North Am.*, 5 (3), 587–96.

Clark, J. M. and Albert, G. W. (1995). Vertical gaze palsies from medial thalamic infarctions without mid-brain involvement. *Stroke*, 26, 1467–70.

Cogan, C. G. (1952). A type of congenital ocular motor apraxia presenting with jerky head movements. *Trans. Am. Acad. Ophthalmol.*, 56, 853–62.

Cogan, D. G. (1965). Myasthenia gravis: a review of the disease and a description of lid twitch as a characteristic sign. *Arch. Ophthalmol.*, 74, 217–21.

Cogan, T. G. (1970). Internuclear ophthalmoplegia: typical and atypical. *Arch. Ophthalmol.*, 84, 583–9.

Cowey, A. and Stoerig, P. (1991). The neurobiology of blindsight. *Trends Neurosci.*, 14, 140–5.

Cox, T. A., Wurster, J. B., and Godfrey, W. A. (1979). Primary aberrant oculomotor degeneration due to intracranial aneurysm. *Arch. Neurol.*, 36, 570–1.

Critchley, M. (1951). Types of visual perseveration, palinopsia and illusory visual spread. *Brain*, 74, 267–99.

Cullom, M. E., Savino, P. J., Sergott, R. C. *et al.* (1995). Relative pupillary sparing 3rd nerve palsies; arteriogram or not? *J. Clin. Neuro-Ophthalmol.*, 15, 136–41 [also see commentary].

Czarnecki, J. S. C., Pilley, S. F. J., and Thompson, H. S. (1979). The analysis of anisocoria. *Can. J. Ophthalmol.*, 14, 297–302.

Damasio, A. R., Damasio, H., and Van Hoesen, G. W. (1982). Prosopagnosia: Anatomic basis and behavioural mechanisms. *Neurol.*, 32, 331–41.

Daroff, R. B. (1965). See-saw nystagmus. *Neurol.*, 15, 874–7.

Daroff, R. B. (1970). Ocular motor manifestations of brainstem and cerebellar dysfunction. In *Neuro-ophthalmology*, Vol. 5, (ed. J. L. Smith), pp. 104–18. Hoffmann, Florida.

Daroff, R. B. and Hoyt, W. F. (1971). Supranuclear disorders of ocular control systems in man. Clinical, anatomical and physiological correlations – 1969. In *The control of eye movements*, (ed. P. Bach-y-Rita, C. C. Collins, and J. E. Hyde). Academic Press, New York.

De Renzi, E. (1997). Prosopagnosia. In *Behavioural neurology and neuropsychology*, (ed. T. E. Finberg and M. J. Farah), pp. 245–55. McGraw-Hill, New York.

Dell'Osso, L. F. and Daroff, R. B. (1975). Congenitital nystagmus waveforms and foveation strategy. *Doc. Ophthalmol.*, 39, 155–82.

Drachman, D. A. (1968). Ophthalmolplegia plus: the neurodegenerative disorders associated with progressive external ophthalmolplegia. *Arch. Neurol.*, 18, 654–74.

Dutton, J. J. (1992). Optic nerve sheath meningiomas. *Surv. Ophthalmol.*, 37, 167–83.

Dutton, J. J. (1994). Gliomas of the anterior visual pathway. *Surv. Ophthalmol.*, 38, 427–52.

Edelson, R. N. and Levy, D. E. (1974). Transient benign unilateral pupillary dilation in young adults. *Arch. Neurol.*, 31, 12–14.

Ellis, C. J. K. (1979). The afferent pupillary defect in acute optic neuritis. *J. Neurol. Neurosurg. Psych.*, 42, 1008–17.

Ertas, M., Arac, N., Kumral, K. *et al.* (1994). Ice test as a simple diagnostic test for myasthenia gravis. *Acta Neurol. Scand.*, 89, 227–9.

Eyster, E. F., Hoyt, W. F., and Wilson, C. B. (1972). Oculomotor palsy from minor head trauma. *JAMA*, 220, 1083–6.

Ezra, E., Spalton, D., and Sanders, M. D. (1996). Ocular neuromyotonia. *Br. J. Ophthalmol.*, 80, 350–5.

Farah, M. J. (1990). *Visual agnosia: Disorders of optic recognition and what they tell us about normal vision.* MIT Press, Cambridge, Mass.

Fells, P., Kousoulides, L., Pappa, A. *et al.* (1994). Extraocular muscle problems in thyroid eye disease. *Eye*, 8, 497–505.

Fisher, A., Gresty, M., Chambers, B. *et al.* (1983). Primary position up-beating nystagmus. A variety of central positional nystagmus. *Brain*, 106, 949–64.

Fletcher, W. A. (1993). Nystagmus: an overview. In *The vestibular-ocular-reflex and vertigo*, (ed. J. A. Sharpe and H. O. Barber), pp. 195–215. Raven Press, New York.

Fletcher, W. A. and Sharpe, J. A. (1986). Saccadic eye movement dysfunction in Alzheimer's disease. *Ann. Neurol.*, **20**, 464–71.

Forster, R. K., Shatz, N. J., and Smith, J. L. (1969). A subtle eyelid sign in aberrant regeneration of the 3rd nerve. *Am. J. Ophthalmol.*, **67**, 696–8.

Frisén, L., Holmegaard, L., and Rosencrantz, M. (1978). Sectorial optic atrophy and homonymous horizontal sectoranopia: a lateral choroidal artery syndrome? *J. Neurol. Neurosurg. Psych.*, **41**, 374–80.

Fukuda, Y., Sawai, H., Watanbe, M. *et al.* (1989). Nasotemporal overlap of crossed and uncrossed retinal ganglion cell projection in the Japanese monkey (*Macaca fuscata*). *J. Neurosci.*, **9**, 2353–73.

Gass, J. D. M. (1961). Acute orbital mucormycosis. *Arch. Ophthalmol.*, **65**, 214–20.

Gass, J. D. M. (1993). Acute zonal occult outer retinopathy. *J. Clin. Neuro-Ophthalmol.*, **13**, 79–97.

Geschwind, N. (1965). Disconnection syndromes in animal and man. *Brain*, **88**, 237–94, 585–644.

Glantz, M. J., Burger, P. C., Friedman, A. H. *et al.* (1994). Treatment of radiation-induced injury with heparin and warfarin. *Neurol*, **44**, 2020–7.

Goldstein, J. E. and Cogan, D. G. (1960). Diabetic ophthalmoplegia with special reference to the pupil. *Arch. Ophthalmol.*, **64**, 592–600.

Grant, W. M. and Schuman, J. S. (1993). *Toxicology of the eye*, (4th edn). Charles C. Thomas, Springfield IL.

Greenblatt, S. H. (1973). Post traumatic transient cerebral blindness: association with migraine and seizure diatheses. *JAMA*, **225**, 1074–6.

Gresty, M. A., Metcalfe, T., Timms, C. *et al.* (1992). Neurology of latent nystagmus. *Brain*, **115**, 1303–21.

Gunderson, C. H. and Hoyt, W. F. (1971). Geniculate hemianopia: Incongruous homonymous field defects in two patients with partial lesions of the lateral geniculate nucleus. *J. Neurol. Neurosurg. Psych.*, **34**, 1–6.

Halmagyi, G. M., Rudge, P., Gresty, M. A. *et al.* (1980). Treatment of periodic alternating nystagmus. *Ann. Neurol.*, **8**, 609–11.

Halmagyi, G. M., Rudge, P., Gresty, M. A. *et al.* (1983). Down-beating nystagmus: a review of 62 cases. *Arch. Neurol.*, **40**, 777–84.

Halmagyi, G. M., Brandt, T., Dieterich, M. *et al.* (1990). Tonic controversive ocular tilt reaction due to unilateral mesodiencephalic lesions. *Neurology*, **40**, 1503–9.

Hamed, L., Glaser, G. S., Gass, J. D. M. *et al.* (1989). Protracted enlargement of the blind-spot in multiple evanescent white dot syndrome occurring in the same patients. *Arch. Ophthalmol.*, **107**, 194–8.

Hanson, M. R., Hamid, M. A., Thomsak, R. L. *et al.* (1986). Selective saccadic palsy caused by pontine lesions: clinical, physiological and pathological correlations. *Ann. Neurol.*, **20**, 209–17.

Harris, C., Shawkat, F., Russell-Eggitt, I. *et al.* (1996). Intermittent horizontal saccade failure, 'ocular motor apraxia', in children. *Br. J. Ophthalmol.*, **80**, 151–8.

Haxby, J. V., Ungerleider, L. G., Horwitz, B. *et al.* (1996). Face encoding and recognition in the human brain. *Proc. Natl Acad. Sci. USA*, **93**, 922–7.

Hayreh, S. S. (1977). Optic disc edema in raised intracranial pressure – V. Pathogenesis. *Arch. Ophthalmol.*, **95**, 1553–65.

Hayreh, S. S., Joos, K. M., Podhajsky, P. A. *et al.* (1994). Systemic diseases associated with nonarteritic anterior ischaemic optic neuropathy. *Am. J. Ophthalmol.*, **118**, 766–80.

Heide, W., Kurzidin, K., and Kompf, D. (1996). Deficits in smooth pursuit eye movements after frontal and parietal lesions. *Brain*, **119**, 1951–69.

Henn, V. and Büttner, U. (1982). *Disorders of horizontal gaze: functional basis of ocular motility disorders*, (ed. G. Lennerstrand, D. S. Zee, and E. L. Keller), pp. 239–45. Pergamon Press, Oxford.

Hollenhorst, R. W. and Younge, B. R. (1973). Ocular manifestations produced by adenomas of the pituitary gland: Analysis of 1000 cases. In *Diagnosis and treatment of pituitary tumours*, (ed. P. O. Kohler and G. T. Ross), pp. 53–64. Elsevier, New York.

Holmes, G. (1918). Disturbances of vision by cerebral lesions. *Br. J. Ophthalmol.*, **2**, 353–84.

Holt, I. J., Harding, A. E., Petty, R. K. H. *et al.* (1990). A new mitochondrial disease associated with mitochondrial DNA heteroplasmy. *Am. J. Hum. Genet.*, **46**, 428–33.

Hommel, B. and Bogousslavsky, J. (1991). The spectrum of vertical gaze palsy following unilateral brainstem stroke. *Neurology*, **41**, 1229–34.

Hornstein, G. (1974). Wallenberg's syndrome, Part I: General symptomatology, with special reference to visual disturbances and imbalance. *Acta Neurol. Scand.*, **50**, 434–46.

Horton, J. C. and Hoyt, W. F. (1991). The representation of the visual field in human striate cortex: a revision of the classic Holme's map. *Arch. Ophthalmol.*, **109**, 816–24.

Hoyt, W. F. and Bagdassarian, S. A. (1969). Optic glioma of childhood: natural history and rationale for conservative management. *Br. J. Ophthalmol.*, **53**, 793–8.

Hoyt, W. F. and Keane, J. R. (1970). Superior oblique myokymia. *Arch. Ophthalmol.*, **84**, 461–7.

Huber, A. (1974). Electrophysiology of the retraction syndromes. *Br. J. Ophthalmol.*, **58**, 293–300.

Humphreys, G. W. and Riddoch, M. J. (1993). Object agnosias. In *Visual perceptual visual defects*, (ed. C. Kennard), pp. 339–59. Baillière Tindell, London,

Hunt, W. E., Meagher, J. N., LeFever, H. E. *et al.* (1961). Painful ophthalmoplegia. *Neurology*, 11, 56–62.

Ischemic optic neuropathy decompression trial research group (1995). Optic nerve decompression sugery for nonarteritic anterior ischemic optic neuropathy (NAION) is not effective and may be harmful. *JAMA*, 273, 625–32.

Jabs, D. A. (1995). Ocular manifesations of HIV infection. *Trans. Am. Ophthalmol. Soc.*, 93, 623–83.

Jacobs, I. (1980). Visual allesthesia. *Neurology*, 30, 1059–63.

Kaminsky, H. J., Maas, E., Spiegel, P. *et al.* (1990). Why are eye muscles frequently involved in myasthenia gravis? *Neurology*, 40, 1663–9.

Keane, J. R. (1993). Forth nerve palsy: historical review and study of 215 inpatients. *Neurology*, 43, 2439–43.

Kearns, T. P. and Sayre, G. P. (1958). Retinitis pigmentosa, external ophthalmoplegia and complete heart block. *Arch. Ophthalmol.*, 60, 280–9.

Kelly, J. J., Daube, J. R., Lennon, V. A. *et al.* (1982). The laboratory diagnosis of mild myasthenia gravis. *Ann. Neurol.*, 12, 238–42.

Keltner, J. L., Satterfield, D., Dublin, A. B. *et al.* (1987). Dural and carotid cavernous sinus fistulas: diagnosis, management and complications. *Ophthalmology*, 94, 585–1600.

Keltner, J. L., Johnson, C. A., Spurr, J. O. *et al.* (1993). Baseline visual field profile of optic neuritis: the experience of the Optic Neuritis Treatment Trial. *Arch. Ophthalmol.*, 111, 231–4.

Kennerdell, J. S., Maroon, J. C., Malton, M. *et al.* (1988). The management of optic nerve sheath meningiomas. *Am. J. Ophthalmol.*, 106, 450–7.

Kirkham, T. H. (1972). The ocular symtomatology of pituitary tumours. *Proc. Roy. Soc. Med.*, 65, 517–18.

Kivlin, J. D., Sanborn, G. E., and Myers, G. G. (1985). The cherry-red spot in Tay–Sachs and other storage diseases. *Ann. Neurol.*, 17, 356–60.

Kjer, B. (1959). Infantile optic atrophy with dominant mode of inheritance. A clinical and genetic study of 19 Danish families. *Acta Ophthalmol.*, 37, (Suppl.54).

Kjer, B., Eibergh, H., Kjer, P. *et al.* (1996). Dominant optic atrophy mapped to chromosome 3Q region. II Clinical and epidemiological aspects. *Acta Ophthalmol. Scand.*, 74, 3–7.

Kline, L. B. (1982). The Tolosa–Hunt syndrome. *Surv. Ophthalmol.*, 27, 79–95.

Klug, G. L. (1982). Gliomas of the optic nerve and chiasm in children. *Neuro-Ophthalmol.*, 2, 217–23.

Knox, D., Clark, D., and Schuster, F. (1967). Benign VI nerve palsies in children. *Paediatrics*, 40, 560–4.

Kodsi, S. R. and Younge, B. R. (1992). Acquired oculomotor, trochlear and abducens cranial nerve palsies in pediatric patients. *Am. J. Ophthalmol.*, 114, 568–74.

Kölmel, H. W. (1985). Complex visual hallucinations in the hemianopic field. *J. Neurol. Neurosurg. Psych.*, 48, 29–38.

Kölmel, H. W. (1993). Visual illusions and hallucinations. In *Visual perceptual defects*, (ed. C. Kennard), pp. 243–64. Baillière Tindall, London.

Komerell, G. and Schaubele, G. (1980). Superior oblique myokymia. An electromyographic analysis. *Trans. Ophthalmol. Soc.*, 100, 504–6.

Krauss, H. R. and Heckenlively, J. R. (1982). Visual field changes in cone-rod degenerations. *Arch. Ophthalmol.*, 100, 1784–90.

Kupersmith, M. J., Burde, R. M., Warren, F. A. *et al.* (1988*a*). Auto-immune optic neuropathy: evaluation and treatment. *J. Neurol. Neurosurg. Psych.*, 51, 1381–6.

Kupersmith, M. J., Berenstein, A., Choi, I. S. *et al.* (1988*b*). Management of non-traumatic vascular shunts involving the cavernous sinus. *Ophthalmology*, 95, 121–30.

Kupfer, C., Chumbley, L., and Downer, J. (1967). Quantitative histology of optic nerve and optic tract nucleus of man. *J. Anat.*, 101, 393–402.

Lakke, J. P. W. F. (1962). Superior orbital fissure syndrome: report of a case caused by local pachymeningitis. *Arch. Neurol.*, 7, 289–300.

Lasker, A. G. and Zee, D. S. (1997). Ocular motor abnormalities in Huntington's disease. *Vis. Res.*, 37, 3639–45.

Leigh, R. J. and Zee, D. S. (1999). *The neurology of eye movements*, (3rd edn). Oxford University Press, Oxford.

Lepore, F. E. (1991). The origin of pain in optic neuritis. Determinants of pain in 101 eyes with optic neuritis. *Arch. Neurol.*, 48, 748–9.

Lepore, F. E. (1995). Disorders of ocularmotility following head trauma. *Arch. Neurol.*, 52, 924–6.

Lepore, F. E. and Glaser, J. S. (1980). Misdirection revisited: a critical appraisal of acquired ocularmotor nerve synkinesis. *Arch. Ophthalmol.*, 98, 2206–9.

Lessell, S. (1975). Higher disorders of visual function: negative phenomina. In *Neuro-ophthalmology*, Vol. 8, (ed. J. S. Glaser and J. L. Smith), pp. 1–26. CV Mosby, St. Louis.

Lewis, R. F. and Zee, D. S. (1993). Ocular motor disorders associated with cerebellar lesions: pathophysiology and topical diagnosis. *Rev. Neurol.*, 149, 665–77.

Lhermitte, J. (1922). Syndrome de la calotte du pedoncule cerebral: les troubles psychosensoriels dans les lesions du mesocephale. *Rev. Neurol. (Paris)*, 38, 359–65.

Lindblom, B., Truit, C. L., and Hoyt, W. F. (1992). Optic nerve sheath meningioma: definition of intraorbital, intracanlicular and intracranial components with magnetic resonance imaging. *Ophthalmology*, **99**, 560–6.

Lissauer, H. (1890). Ein fall von Seelenblindheit nebst einem Beitrage zur Theorie derselben. *Arch. Psychiatr. Nervenkr.*, **21**, 22–70.

Liu, G. T., Glaser, J. S., Shatz, N. J. *et al.* (1994). Visual morbidity in giant cell arteritis: Clinical characteristics and prognosis for vision. *Ophthalmology*, **101**, 1779–85.

Loewenfeld, I. E. (1999). *The pupil: anatomy, physiology and clinical applications*. Butterworth Heinemann, Boston.

Loewenfeld, I. E. and Thompson, H. S. (1967). The tonic pupil: a reevaluation. *Am. J. Ophthalmol.*, **63**, 46–87.

Loewenfeld, I. E. and Thompson, H. S. (1975). Ocular motor paresis with cyclic spasms. A critical review of the literature and a new case. *Surv. Ophthalmol.*, **20**, 81–124.

Lowenstein, O. and Loewenfeld, I. E. (1965). Pupillotonic pseudo-tabes. *Surv. Ophthalmol.*, **10**, 130–85.

Mackey, D. A. (1994). Three subgroups of patients from the United Kingdom with Leber's hereditary optic neuropathy. *Eye*, **8**, 431–6.

Maher, E. R., Yates, J. R., Harries, R. *et al.* (1990). Clinical features and natural history of von Hippel–Lindau disease. *Quart. J. Med.*, **77**, 1151–63.

Malik, A., Furlan, A. J., Sweeney, P. J. *et al.* (1992). Optic neuropathy: a rare paraneoplastic syndrome. *J. Clin. Neuro-Ophthalmol.*, **12**, 137–41.

Mansour, A. M. and Reinecke, R. D. (1986). Central trochlear palsy. *Surv. Ophthalmol.*, **30**, 279–97.

Marquis, D. G. (1934). Effects of removal of visual cortex in mammals with observations on the retention of light discrimination in dogs. In *Proceedings of the Association for Research in Nervous and Mental Disease*, Vol. 13, p. 558. William & Wilkins, Baltimore.

Mathew, N. T. and Chandy, J. (1970). Painful ophthalmoplegia. *J. Neurol. Sci.*, **11**, 243–56.

McDonald, W. I. and Barnes, D. (1992). The ocular manifestations of multiple sclerosis. I. Abnormalities of the afferent visual system. *J. Neurol. Neurosurg. Psych.*, **55**, 747–52.

McKee, A. C., Lavine, D. N., Kowll, N. W. *et al.* (1990). Peduncular hallucinosis associated with isolated infarction of the substantia nigra, pars reticulata. *Ann. Neurol.*, **27**, 500–4.

Meadows, J. C. (1974*a*). Disturbed perception of colours associated with localised cerebral lesions. *Brain*, **97**, 615–32.

Meadows, J. C. (1974*b*). The anatomical basis of prosopagnosia. *J. Neurol. Neurosurg. Psych.*, **37**, 489–501.

Miller, N. R. (1977). Solitary oculomotor nerve palsy in childhood. *Am. J. Ophthalmol.*, **83**, 106–11.

Miller, N. R. (1996). The clinical manifestations, natural history and results with treatment of superior oblique myokymia. *Am. Orthopt. J.*, **46**, 189–94.

Miller, N. R. and Moses, H. (1977). Ocular involvement in wound botulism. *Arch. Ophthalmol.*, **95**, 1788–9.

Miller, N. R. and Newman, N. J. (eds) (1988). Walsh and Hoyt's clinical neuro-opthalmology, 5th edn. Williams and Wilkins, Baltimore.

Miller, N. R., Kiel, S. M., Green, W. R. *et al.* (1982). Unilateral Duane's retraction syndrome (Type 1). *Arch. Ophthalmol.*, **100**, 1468–72.

Morris, J. G. L., Grattam-Smith, P., Panegyres, P. K. *et al.* (1994). Delayed cerebral radiation necrosis. *Quart. J. Med.*, **87**, 119–29.

Morrisey, S. P., Miller, D. H., Kendall, B. E. *et al.* (1993). The significance of brain magnetic resonance imaging abnormalities at presentation with clinically isolated syndromes suggestive of multiple sclerosis. *Brain*, **116**, 135–46.

Morrow, M. J. and Sharpe, J. A. (1993). Smooth pursuit eye movements. In *The vestibular-ocular reflex and vertigo*, (eds J. A. Sharpe and H. O. Barber), pp. 141–62. Raven Press, New York.

Müri, R. M., Chermann, J. F., Kohen, L. *et al.* (1996). Ocular motor consequences of damage to the abducens nucleus area in humans. *J. Neurol. Ophthalmol.*, **16**, 191–5.

Murphy, S. F. and Drachman, D. M. (1968). The oculopharyngeal syndrome. *J. Am. Med. Ass.*, **203**, 1003–8.

Mustonen, E., Poyhonen, M., and Leisti, E.-L. (1997). Neuro-ophthalmological findings in neurofibro matosis: Clinical and neuroradiological study of 125 patients. *Neuro-Ophthalmol.*, **17**, 117–26.

Nadeau, S. E. and Trobe, J. D. (1983). Pupil sparing in oculomotor palsy: a brief review. *Ann. Neurol.*, **13**, 143–8.

Nakada, T. and Kwee, I. L. (1986). Oculo-palato myoclonus. *Brain*, **109**, 431–41.

Neelon, F. A., Goree, J. A., and Lebovitz, H. E. (1973). A primary empty sella: clinical and radiographic characteristics and endocrine function. *Medicine*, **52**, 73–84.

Neetens, A. and Smets, R. M. (1989). Papilloedema. *Neuro-Ophthalmol.*, **9**, 81–101.

Newman, S. A. and Miller, N. R. (1983). Optic tract syndrome: Neuro-Ophthalmic considerations. *Arch. Ophthalmol.*, **101**, 1241–50.

Newsome, D. A. (ed.) (1988). *Retinal dystrophies and degenerations*. Raven Press, New York.

Nichols, J. W. and Goodwin, J. A. (1992). Neuro-ophthalmic complications of AIDs. *Semin. Ophthalmol.*, **7**, 24–9.

Ochs, A. L., Stark, L., Hoyt, W. F. *et al.* (1979). Opposed adducting saccades in convergence-retraction nystagmus. A patient with Sylvian aqueduct syndrome. *Brain*, **102**, 497–508.

Oosterhuis, H. J. G. H. (1982). The ocular signs and symptoms of myasthenia gravis. *Doc. Ophthalmol.*, **52**, 363–78.

Orcutt, J. C., Page, N. G. R., and Sanders, M. D. (1984). Factors affecting visual loss in benign intracranial hypertension. *Ophthalmology*, **91**, 1303–12.

Osserman, K. E. (1957). *Myasthenia gravis*. Grune and Stratton, New York.

O'Sullivan, E. P. and Kennard, C. (1998). Neuro-ophthalmology of movement disorders. In *Parkinson's disease and movement disorders*, (ed. J. Jankovic and E. Tolosa), pp. 869–86. Williams Wilkins, Baltimore.

Penfield, W. and Perot, P. (1963). The brain's record of auditory and visual experience. *Brain*, **86**, 596–696.

Perrett, D. I., Smith, P. A. J., and Potter, D. D. *et al.* (1984). Neurones responsive to faces in the temporal cortex: studies of functional organisation, sensitivity to identity and relation to perception. *Hum. Neurobiol.*, **3**, 197–208.

Petty, R. K., Harding, A. E., and Morgan-Hughes, J. A. (1986). The clinical features of mitochondrial myopathy. *Brain*, **109**, 915–38.

Pierrot-Deseilligny, C., Gautier, J. C., and Loron, P. (1988). Acquired ocular motor apraxia due to bilateral fronto-parietal infarcts. *Ann. Neurol.*, **23**, 199–202.

Pollack, S. (1987). The morning glory disc anomaly: contractile movement, classification and embryogenesis. *Doc. Ophthalmol.*, **65**, 439–60.

Ragge, N. K. (1993). Clinical and genetic patterns of neurofibromatosis 1 and 2. *Br. J. Ophthalmol.*, **77**, 662–72.

Ranalli, P. J. and Sharpe, J. A. (1988). Vertical vestibulo-ocular reflex smooth pursuit and eye head tracking dysfunction in internuclear ophthalmoplegia. *Brain*, **111**, 1299–317.

Ratcliff, G. and Newcombe, F. (1982). Object recognition: some deductions from the clinical evidence. In *Normality and pathology of cognitive function*, (ed. A. Ellis), pp. 147–71. Academic Press, New York.

Richards, B. W., Jones, F. R., and Younge, B. R. (1992). Causes and prognosis in 4,278 cases of the oculomotor, trochlear and abducens cranial nerve palsies. *Am. J. Ophthalmol.*, **113**, 489–96.

Riddoch, G. (1917). Dissociation in visual perceptions due to occipital injuries, with special reference to appreciation of movement. *Brain*, **40**, 15–57.

Riordan-Eva, P., Restori, M., Hamilton, A. M. P. *et al.* (1994). Orbital ultrasound in the ocular ischaemic syndrome. *Eye*, **8**, 93–6.

Riordan-Eva, P., Sanders, M. D., Govan, C. G. *et al.* (1995). The clinical features of Leber's hereditary optic neuropathy defined by the presence of a pathogenic mitochondrial DNA mutation. *Brain*, **118**, 319–37.

Robertson, D. N., Heinz, J. D., and Rucker, C. W. (1970). Acquired sixth nerve paresis in children. *Arch. Ophthalmol.*, **83**, 574–9.

Rosenberg, M. A., Savino, P. J., and Glaser, J. S. (1979). A clinical analysis of pseudo-papilloedema: I. population, laterality, acuity, refractive error, ophthalmoscopic characteristics, and coincident disease. *Arch. Ophthalmol.*, **97**, 65–70.

Rush, J. A. and Younge, B. R. (1981). Paralysis of cranial nerves III, IV and VI. Cause and prognosis in 1000 cases. *Arch. Ophthalmol.*, **99**, 76–9.

Sadun, A. A., Martone, J. F., Muci-Mendoza, R. *et al.* (1994). Epidemic optic neuropathy in Cuba: eye findings. *Arch. Ophthalmol.*, **112**, 691–9.

Safran, A. B. and Glaser, J. S. (1980). Statokinetic dissociation in lesions of the anterior visual pathways. *Arch. Ophthalmol.*, **98**, 291–5.

Sano, K. (1959). Trigemino-oculomotor synkineses. *Neurologia*, **1**, 29–51.

Sarkies, N. J. C. and Sanders, M. D. (1985). Convergence spasm. *Trans. Ophthalmol. Soc.*, **104**, 782–6.

Savino, P. J., Paris, M., Schatz, N. *et al.* (1978) Optic tract syndrome: A review of 21 patients. *Arch. Ophthalmol.*, **96**, 656–63.

Savino, P. J., Glaser, J. S., and Rosenberg, M. A. (1979). A clinical analysis of pseudopapilloedema: II. Visual field defects. *Arch. Ophthalmol.*, **97**, 71–5.

Savino, P. J., Hilliker, J. K., Cassell, G. H. *et al.* (1982). Chronic sixth nerve palsies: are they really harbingers of serious intracranial disease? *Arch. Ophthalmol.*, **100**, 1442–4.

Schwartz, M. A., Selhorst, J. B., Ochs, A. L. *et al.* (1986). Oculomasticatory myorhythmia: a unique movement disorder occurring in Whipple's disease. *Ann. Neurol.*, **20**, 677–83.

Selbst, R. G., Selhorst, J. B., Harbison, J. W. *et al.* (1983). Para-infectious optic neuritis. *Arch. Neurol.*, **40**, 347–50.

Selhorst, J. B., Hoyt, W. F., Feinsord, M. *et al.* (1976a). Midbrain correctopia. *Arch. Neurol.*, **33**, 193–5.

Selhorst, J. B., Stark, L., Ochs, A. L. *et al.* (1976b). Disorders in cerebellar ocular motor control. II Macrosaccadic oscillation and oculographic control system and clinicoatomical analysis. *Brain*, **99**, 509–22.

Selhorst, J. B., Madge, G., and Ghatack, N. (1984). The neuropathology of the Holmes–Adie syndrome. *Ann. Neurol.*, **16**, 138.

Sergott, R. C. and Glaser, J. S. (1981). Grave's ophthalmopathy. A clinical and immunologic review. *Surv. Ophthalmol.*, **26**, 1–21.

Sharpe, J. A., Rosenberg, M. A., Hoyt, W. F. *et al.* (1974). Paralytic pontine exotropia. A sign of acute unilateral gaze palsy and internuclear ophthalmoplegia. *Neurology*, **24**, 1076–81.

Shaunak, S., O'Sullivan, E., and Kennard, C. (1997). Eye movements. In Neurological investigations, (ed. J. A. C. Hughes), pp. 253–82. BMJ, London.

Shields, J. A., Bakewell, B., Augsberger, J. J. *et al.* (1984). Classification and incidence of space-occupying lesions of the orbit—a survey of 145 biopsies. *Arch. Ophthalmol.*, **102**, 1606–11.

Silverman, I. E., Liu, G. T., Volpe, N. J. *et al.* (1995). The crossed paralysis: the original brainstem syndromes of Millard–Gubler, Foville, Weber and Raymond–Cestan. *Arch. Neurol.*, **52**, 625–38.

Smith, S. A. and Smith, S. E. (1983). Evidence for a neuropathic aetiology in the small pupil of diabetes mellitus. *Arch. J. Ophthalmol.*, **67**, 89–93.

Solomon, D., Galetta, S. L., and Liu, G. T. (1995). Possible mechanisms for horizontal gaze deviation and lateropulsion in the lateral medullary syndrome. *J. Neuro-Ophthalmol.*, **15**, 26–30.

Sugishita, M., Hemmi, I., Sakuma, I. *et al.* (1993). The problem of macular sparing after unilateral occipital lesions. *J. Neurol.*, **241**, 1–9.

Sullivan, T. J., Clarke, M. P., and Morin, J. D. (1992). The ocular manifestations of Sturge–Weber syndrome. *J. Paed. Ophthalmol. Strabismus*, **29**, 349–56.

Susac, J. O., Hoyt, W. F., Daroff, R. D. *et al.* (1970). Clinical spectrum of ocular bobbing. *J. Neurol. Neurosurg. Psych.*, **33**, 771–5.

Tecoma, E. S., Laxer, K. D., Barbaro, N. M. *et al.* (1993). Frequency and characteristics of visual field defects after surgery for mesial temporal sclerosis. *Neurology*, **43**, 1235–8.

Ter Bruggen, J. P., Bastiaensen, A. K., Turssen, C. C. *et al.* (1990). Disorders of eye movement in myotonic dystrophy. *Brain*, **113**, 463–73.

Teuber, H. L. (1965). Somatosensory disorders due to cortical lesions. *Neuropsychologia*, **3**, 287–94.

Teunisse, R. J., Cruysberg, J. R. M., Verbeek, A. *et al.* (1995). The Charles Bonnet Syndrome. A large prospective study in The Netherlands. *Br. J. Psych.*, **166**, 254–7.

Thomas, J. E. and Yoss, R. E. (1970). The parasellar syndrome: Problems in determining etiology. *Mayo Clin. Proc.*, **45**, 617–23.

Thömke, F., Hopf, H. C., and Krämer, G. (1992). Internuclear ophthalmoplegia of abduction: clinical and electrophysiological data on the existence of abduction paresis of prenuclear origin. *J. Neurol. Neurosurg. Psych.*, **55**, 105–11.

Thompson, H. S. (1966). Afferent pupillary defects. *Am. J. Ophthalmol.*, **62**, 860–73.

Thompson, H. S. (1977). Diagnosing Horner's syndrome. *Trans. Am. Ophthalmol. Otolaryngol.*, **83**, 840–2.

Thompson, H. S. (1979). A classification of tonic 'tonic pupils'. In *Topics in neuro-ophthalmology*, (ed. H. S. Thompson, R. Daroff, L. Friesen *et al.*), pp. 95–6. Williams and Wilkins, Baltimore.

Thompson, H. S. and Pilley, S. F. J. (1976). Unequal pupils: a flow chart for sorting out the anisocorias. *Surv. Ophthalmol.*, **21**, 45–8.

Thompson, H. S., Bourgon, P., and van Allen, M. W. (1979*a*). The tendon reflex in Adie's syndrome. In *Topics in neuro-ophthalmology*, (ed. H. S. Thompson, R. Daroff, L. Frisen *et al.*), pp. 104–13. Williams and Wilkins, Baltimore.

Thompson, H. S., Bell, R. A., and Bourgon, P. (1979*b*). The natural history of Adies syndrome. In *Topics in neuro-ophthalmology*, (ed. H. S. Thompson, R. Daroff, L. Frisen *et al.*), pp. 96–9. Williams and Wilkins, Baltimore.

Thompson, J. S., Corbett, J. J., and Cox, T. A. (1981). How to measure the relative afferent pupillary defect. *Surv. Ophthalmol.*, **26**, 39–42.

Tiffin, P. A., MacEwen, C. J., Craig, E. A. *et al.* (1996). Acquired palsy of the oculomotor, trochlear and abducens nerves. *Eye*, **10**, 377–84.

Towfighti, J., Marks, K., Palmer, E. *et al.* (1979). Möbius syndrome: neuropathologic observations. *Acta Neuropathol.*, **48**, 11–17.

Tranel, D. and Damasio, A. R. (1996). Agnosias and apraxias. In *Neurology in clinical practice*, (ed. W. G. Bradley, T. C. B. Daroff, G. H. Fenichel *et al.*), pp. 119–29. Butterworth Heinemann, Boston.

Trobe, J. D. (1988). Third nerve palsy and the pupil. *Arch. Ophthalmol.*, **106**, 601–2.

Trobe, J. D., Glaser, J. S., and Post, J. D. (1978). Meningiomas and aneurysms of the cavernous sinus. *Arch. Ophthalmol.*, **96**, 457–67.

van der Gaag, R., Schmidt, E. D., Zonneveld, F. W. *et al.* (1996). Orbital pathology in thyroid-associated ophthalmopathy. *Orbit*, **15**, 109–17.

Van der Wiel, A. L. and van Gijn, J. (1983). Localisation of Horner's syndrome. Use and limitations of the hydroxyamphetamine test. *J. Neurol. Sci.*, **59**, 229–35.

Victor, D. I. (1976). The diagnosis of congenital unilateral third nerve palsy. *Brain*, **99**, 711–17.

Volpe, N. J. and Lessell, S. (1993). Remitting sixth nerve palsy in skull based tumours. *Arch. Ophthalmol.*, **111**, 1391–5.

[Published erratum appears in *Arch. Ophthalmol.*, **112**, 1118, 1994.]

Wall, M. and Wray, S. H. (1983). The one-and-a-half syndrome—a unilateral disorder of the pontine tegmentum: a study of 20 cases and review of the literature. *Neurology*, **33**, 971–80.

Walsh, F. B. and O'Doherty, D. S. (1960). A possible explanation of the mechanism of ophthalmoplegic migraine. *Neurology*, **10**, 1079–84.

Warrington, E. K. (1975). The selective impairment of semantic memory. *Quart. J. Expl Psychol.*, **27**, 635–58.

Warrington, E. K. and James, M. (1988). Visual aperceptive agnosia: a clinco-anatomical study of three cases. *Cortex*, **24**, 13–32.

Weinberg, D. A., Lesser, R. L., and Vollmer, T. L. (1994). Ocular myasthenia: A protean disorder. *Surv. Ophthalmol.*, **39**, 169–210.

Weiskrantz, L. (1986). *Blindsight: a case study and implications.* Clarendon Press, Oxford.

Weiskrantz, L., Warrington, E. K., Sanders, M. D. *et al.* (1974). Visual capacity in the hemianopic field following a restricted occipital ablation. *Brain*, **97**, 709–28.

Welch, R. B. (1970). Von Hippal–Lindau disease: the recognition and treatment of early angiomatosis retinae and the use of cryosurgery as an adjunct to therapy. *Trans. Am. Ophthalmol. Soc.*, **68**, 367–424.

Wiersinga, W. M. (1996). Advances in medical therapy of thyroid-associated ophthalmopathy. *Orbit*, **15**, 177–86.

Wilhelm, H., Wilhelm, B., Petersen, D. *et al.* (1996). Relative afferent pupillary defects in patients with retrogeniculate lesions. *Neuro-Ophthalmol.*, **16**, 219–24.

Wirtschafter, J. D., Volk, C., and Sawchuk, R. J. (1978). Transaqueous diffusion of acetylcholine to denervated iris sphincter muscle: a mechanism for the tonic pupil syndrome. *Ann. Neurol.*, **4**, 1–5.

Wright, J. E. (1988). Doyne Lecture: Current concepts in orbital disease. *Eye*, **2**, 1–11.

Zee, D. S. (1992). Internuclear ophthalmoplegia: clinical and pathophysiological consideration. In *Ocular motor disorders in the brainstem*, (ed. U. Büttner and T. Brandt), pp. 455–70. WB Saunders, London.

Zeki, S. (1990). A century of cerebral achromatopsia. *Brain*, **113**, 1727–77.

Zeki, S. (1991). Cerebral akinetopsia (visual motion blindness). A review. *Brain*, **114**, 811–24.

Zeki, S. (1993). *A vision of the brain.* Blackwell, London.

Zeki, S. and Shipp, S. (1988). The functional logic of cortical connections. *Nature*, **335**, 311–17.

Zihl, J., von Cramon, D., and Mai, N. (1983). Selective disturbance of movement vision after bilateral brain damage. *Brain*, **106**, 313–40.

Zimmer Galler, I. E. and Robertson, D. M. (1995). Tuberose sclerosis: long term observation of retinal lesions in tuberose sclerosis. *Am. J. Ophthalmol.*, **119**, 318–24.

CHAPTER 9

Deafness, vertigo, and imbalance

Christopher Kennard

Disturbances of the eighth or vestibulocochlear cranial nerve and its central connections lead to various combinations of deafness, vertigo, and imbalance. The cochlear division of the nerve supplies the cochlea and is concerned with hearing, whereas the vestibular division supplies the semicircular canals, the utricle, and saccule, and is concerned in postural and equilibratory functions.

9.1 Anatomy and physiology of hearing

9.1.1 Mechanical transduction

The outer, middle, and internal ear are illustrated in Fig. 9.1. Sound passing via the pinna or auricle into the external auditory canal impinges on the tympanic membrane which transmits vibrations into the middle ear. The chain of auditory ossicles (malleus, incus, and stapes) in turn transmit the sound vibrations across the middle ear cavity, which is air filled, to the oval window of the cochlear where they are conveyed to the cochlear endolymph. The cochlear contains the apparatus for transforming the physical motion of the oval window membrane into an auditory response. This process can be modified by two muscles, the tensor tympani (innervated by a branch from the motor division of the trigeminal nerve) and the stapedius (innervated by the facial nerve), attached to the ossicular chain, which can reduce energy transmission and subserve a reflex protective function by protecting the ear against sound of exceptional intensity. In Bell's palsy hyperacusis may be noted as a result of paralysis of the stapedius.

9.1.2 The cochlea

The structure and function of the inner ear is complex (Dallos *et al.* 1996). The bony labyrinth contains fluid (perilymph,

closely resembling CSF) within which is the membranous labyrinth filled with endolymph, which closely resembles intracellular fluid except that the anion content is extracellular in type. The three parts of the labyrinth are the semicircular canals (containing the semicircular ducts), the vestibule (containing the utricle and saccule), and the cochlea (containing the cochlear duct or scala media). Of these, the former two parts are concerned with balance and equilibrium (see below), the

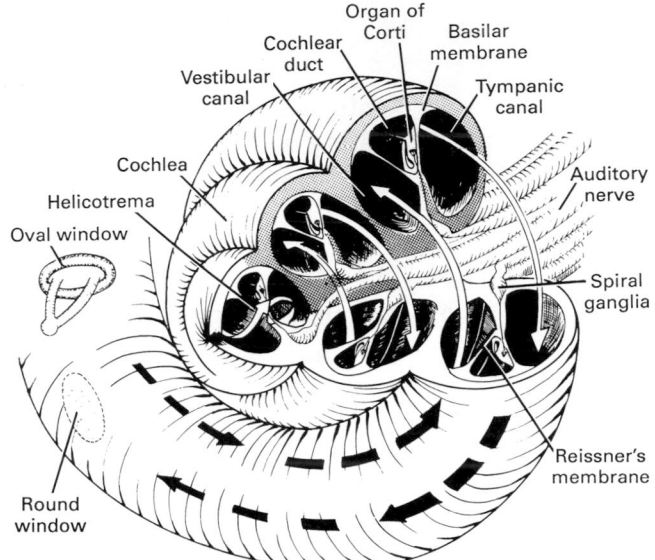

Fig. 9.2. The cochlea and the organ of Corti. Diagram of the cochlea cut through to show the partition of the cavity by the basilar membrane and cochlear duct (scala media). Arrows show the pathway of transmission of pressure waves originating at the oval window. (Reproduced from Patton, Sundsten, Crill, and Swanson (1976) and previously published in Curtis, Jacobson, and Marcus (1972), by kind permission of the authors and publishers.)

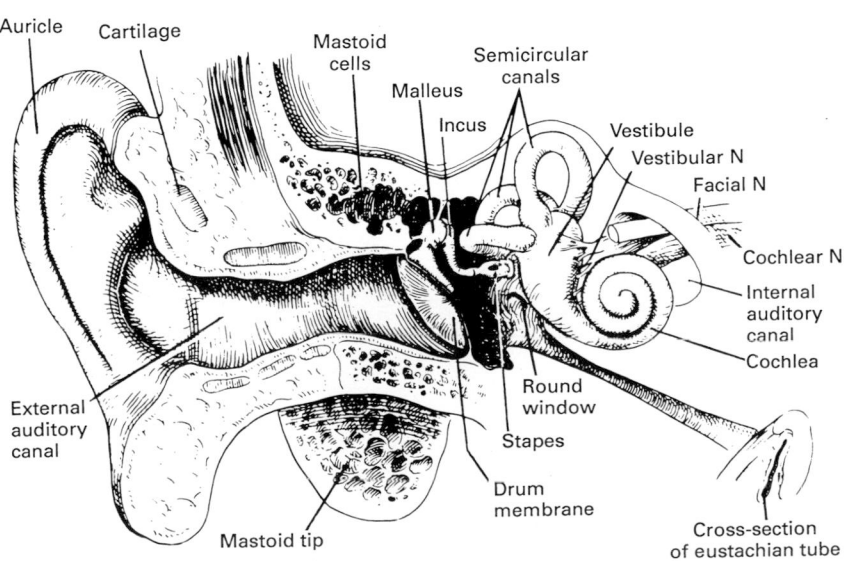

Fig. 9.1. The peripheral auditory apparatus. The cochlea is turned slightly to show its coils. The Eustachian tube runs forward as well as downward and inward. (Reproduced from Patton, Sundsten, Crill, and Swanson (1976) and previously published in Davis and Silverman (1970), by kind permission of the authors and publishers.)

cochlear portion solely with hearing. The cochlea makes two and a half turns around a central bony core, the modiolus, from which a bony ledge projects into the canal. Attached to the free edge of this shelf is the basilar membrane, which supports the sensory structures. It is bounded by Reissner's membrane, which separates the endolymph from the perilymph in the scala vestibuli which is continuous with that of the vestibule, and peripherally by the stria vascularis, which contains columnar cells responsible for controlling the composition of the endolymph. Below the basilar membrane is the scala tympani, filled with perilymph, above it the cochlear duct filled with endolymph (Fig. 9.2). At the apex of the cochlea, the scala tympani and the scala vestibuli communicate through a tiny opening, the helicotrema; the scala tympani ends below at the round window, closed by a membrane separating it from the middle ear.

The basilar membrane is wider and less stiff at its apical end than at the basal end so that it is broadly tuned (similar to a piano keyboard) with high frequencies vibrating the basal end and the lower frequencies vibrating progressively more apically. The response of the basilar membrane establishes a place code in which different locations of membrane are maximally deformed by different sound frequencies. The organ of Corti, the final cochlear sensory receptor organ, lies on the dorsal surface of the basilar membrane (Fig. 9.3). It contains a mixture of supporting cells, the rods of Corti, and transducing hair cells. The outer hair cells act as motors, finely tuning the vibration of the basilar membrane, and the inner hair cells are sensory, sending afferent nerve impulses to the brain, conveying hearing. Although there are approximately five times more outer hair cells compared with inner hair cells, some 95 per cent of the 35 000–50 000 neurons in the spiral ganglion communicate with the former. This means that most of the information leaving the cochlea comes from the responses of inner hair cells. The large number of outer hair cells, however, appear to have an important role in sound transduction. They contain motor proteins which can change the length of the outer hair cell, and it has been found that they respond to sound with both a receptor potential and a change in length. These cells, therefore, are able to alter the physical relationship between the cochlear membranes, whereby they are able to amplify the response of the basilar membrane to produce a greater response in the auditory nerve. The response of outer hair cells can also be affected by inputs from about 1000 efferent fibres which project from the brainstem toward the cochlea. They can cause alterations to the shape of these cells, thereby regulating auditory sensitivity.

9.1.3 Central projections

On entering the brainstem the auditory nerve projects to ipsilateral dorsal and ventral divisions of the cochlear nuclei. The tonotopic arrangement of fibres, first observed in the auditory nerve, is maintained in the central auditory pathways. From the cochlear nuclei fibres project to the superior olivary nucleus on both sides of the brainstem. Axons of the olivary neurons ascend in the lateral lemniscus to innervate the inferior colliculus in the midbrain. Collicular neurons project to the medial geniculate nucleus, which in turn projects to the auditory cortex.

Whereas neurons in the spiral ganglion each have a characteristic frequency response, a frequency tuning which is observed all the way along the central auditory pathways, the further along this pathway one progresses the more diverse and complex become the neuronal response properties.

9.2 Pathophysiology of hearing

The importance of the outer hair cells is indicated by the fact that most noxious stimuli lead to damage of these cells in advance of damage to the inner hair cells. These stimuli, which include excessive exposure to antibiotics such as streptomycin, mechanical trauma, noise trauma, and hypoxia, lead to a loss of auditory sensitivity and frequency resolution. Nerve deafness is deafness associated with the loss of neurons in either the auditory nerve or the hair cells of the cochlea, and it is often very difficult to determine in which the primary pathology occurs.

One of the more common problems presenting to the neurologist is whether a patient's hearing loss is due to a deficit in the conductive or sensorineural mechanism, and if the latter, whether the cochlea or retrocochlear structures involving the auditory nerve or central auditory pathways are involved. A large number of audiological tests have been designed to locate the site of the lesion. These can be divided into two groups: psychoacoustical tests, which study the relation between subjective awareness and acoustical stimuli; and neurophysiological tests, which study biophysical responses which can be recorded after auditory stimulation.

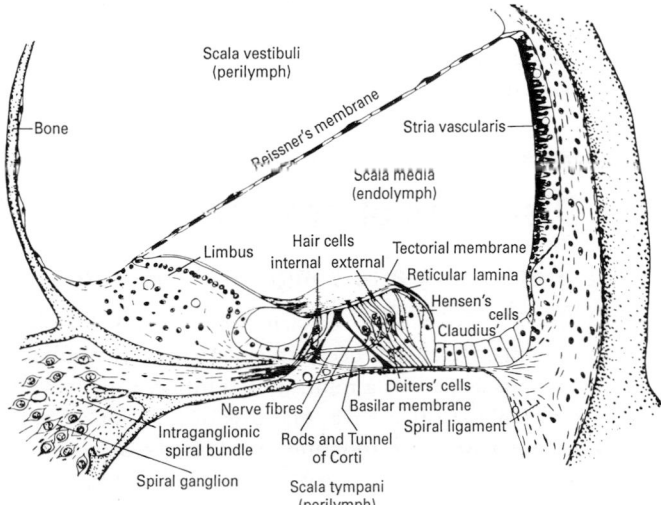

Fig. 9.3. The cochlear partition and the organ of Corti. (Reproduced from Patton, Sundsten, Crill, and Swanson (1976) and previously published in Davis and Silverman (1970), by kind permission of the authors and publishers.)

9.2.1 Bedside testing

As a bedside test a vibrating tuning fork (C = 256) is applied to the forehead or vertex in the midline and the patient is asked whether the sound is heard in the midline or is localized in one ear (Weber's test). In normal individuals the sound appears to be in the midline. In conductive deafness it is usually localized in the affected ear, in nerve deafness in the normal ear. This is because in sensorineural or nerve deafness bone-conduction is reduced as well as air-conduction, whereas in conductive deafness air-conduction is reduced but bone-conduction is relatively enhanced.

In *Rinne's test* a vibrating tuning fork is applied to the patient's mastoid process, the ear being occluded by the observer's finger. The patient is asked when the sound ceases, and the fork is then held at the acoustic meatus. In conductive deafness the sound cannot be heard by air-conduction after bone-conduction has ceased to transmit it. In sensorineural or nerve deafness, as in normal individuals, the reverse is the case. It is usual also to occlude the opposite ear during the test; even so, the results of Rinne's test may be misleading in unilateral nerve deafness when the sound of the tuning fork applied to the mastoid process of the deaf ear is heard in the opposite, normal ear.

9.2.2 Audiometry

A formal psychophysical detection test, *pure-tone audiometry*, applies similar principles to Rinne's test. The extent of a hearing loss and its distribution in the frequency range are mapped by measurements of auditory thresholds of pure-tone stimuli of frequencies between 125 and 8000 Hz. The test can distinguish between conductive and sensorimotor hearing loss by threshold measurements of air- and bone-conduction.

Loudness recruitment is a technique of particular value in detecting unilateral sensorineural deafness (due to cochlear end-organ disease, as in Menière's disease) (Dix *et al.* 1948). A pure tone of constant frequency is applied with increasing intensity (in decibels) to each ear alternately. In conductive deafness and in nerve deafness due to disease of the cochlear nerve central to the sensory end-organs, the ratio between the intensities required to produce sounds of equal loudness in both ears remains constant; in sensorineural deafness, however, with increasing intensity the sound can eventually seem equally loud in both ears.

Speech audiometry is a psychoacoustical identification test in which the patient is required to repeat a spoken, recorded message. Several variations on this basic test have been developed in attempts to increase the test's sensitivity. These include presenting the speech signal in background noise (speech in noise test), free-field speech audiometry, and dichotic speech audiometry in which the ability of the auditory system to use the signals from the two ears is studied (Pinheiro and Musiek 1985).

Impedance audiometry is a physiological method which utilizes the impedance the ear exerts to incoming sound. The mechanical properties of the tympanic membrane and the middle ear can be studied by tympanometry. Of particular value is the *acoustic reflex threshold (stapedius reflex test)* in which the minimum intensity of sound at a particular frequency that produces contraction of the stapedius muscle is measured. The stapedius muscle contraction alters the acoustic impedance of the middle ear, which is measured by using an impedance bridge. The test can be used to diagnose conductive hearing loss and to differentiate between cochlear, retrocochlear, and brainstem lesions (Hirsch and Anderson 1980*a,b*).

9.2.3 Electrophysiological tests

Evoked otoacoustical emissions are low-level acoustic signals of cochlear origin, which can be recorded in the external auditory canal, in response to cochlear stimulation by clicks or short tone bursts. They are considered to originate from biomechanical activity in the outer hair cells of the organ of Corti, and their presence therefore indicates that cochlear function is normal and the subject of normal peripheral hearing (Probst 1990).

Auditory evoked potentials (AEPs) are obtained by averaging the electrical activity in the auditory system in response to a series of repetitive sound stimuli. Receptor potentials in the cochlea and the whole nerve action potential generated in the cochlear nerve are recorded by *electrocochleography* (ECoG) (Eggermont and Odenthal 1977).

The more commonly used measurement is of the short-latency potentials recorded in response to repetitive click stimuli, known as the *brainstem auditory evoked potentials* (BAEP). There are five such potentials occurring in the first 8 ms after the stimulus, which are believed to originate in the auditory nerve and the brainstem nuclei (Møller *et al.* 1988). Measurements of their interwave intervals, amplitude ratios, and responses to changing stimuli rates are used to aid localization of brainstem lesions in adults and children. Intermediate latency components occurring 8–50 ms after the stimulus, and even less well-defined long-latency waves, probably reflect activity in the auditory cortex and associated areas, but have not proved to be of much diagnostic value.

9.3 Disorders of hearing

9.3.1 Hereditary and congenital disorders

Hereditary and congenital sensorineural hearing loss is a common entity, which can occur in isolation, with vestibular dysfunction, or as part of a multisite syndrome. Patients with inner ear dysplasia often have total loss of function of both cochlear and vestibular function. In *Michel's defect* there is a complete absence of the otic capsule and eighth cranial nerve. In *Mondini–Alexander dysplasia* there is incomplete development of both the bony and membranous labyrinth, whereas only the membranous labyrinth is affected in *Bing–Siebenmann dysplasia*. With *cochleo-saccular (Scheibe) dysplasia* the cochlea and the saccule are involved, but not the utricle or the semicircular canals.

A number of hereditary conditions which involve both the auditory and vestibular systems have been described. *Usher syndrome*, an autosomal recessive disorder, is characterized by sensorineural hearing loss and retinitis pigmentosa (Kimberling *et al.* 1989). Usher I patients, who account for about 90 per cent of cases, have profound congenital hearing loss and absent vestibular function, whereas Usher II patients typically present with congenital moderate to severe sloping sensorineural hearing loss with normal vestibular function. The Usher II gene (*USH2*) has been mapped to 1q31 region, and one form of the Usher I to chromosome 11q due to a mutation in the gene encoding myosin VIIa (Weil *et al.* 1995).

Alport's syndrome, usually inherited as a X-linked condition but which may occasionally be autosomal recessive, is characterized by a slowly progressive sensorineural hearing loss and haemorrhagic nephritis (Schuknecht 1993). The pattern of high-frequency hearing loss and milder vestibular dysfunction are suggestive of hair cell abnormality, and the abnormal gene leads to a defect in type IV collagen, an important component of basement membranes of the inner ear and kidney (Mochizuki *et al.* 1994).

Secondary degeneration of the auditory nerve has been reported in association with other defects in many syndromes. With *Waardenburg syndrome* profound deafness is common and vestibular hypofunction is a frequent finding. Some syndromes are associated with metabolic disturbances. *Pendred's syndrome* is characterized by congenital hypothyroidism, hearing loss, and vestibular dysfunction. Hearing loss and vestibular abnormalities are a frequent finding in a number of inherited spinal degenerations, ataxias, neuropathies, and myopathies.

9.3.2 Infection

The auditory nerve may be damaged by viral, bacterial, and mycotic organisms, due to direct invasion of the nerve and blood vessels of the internal auditory meatus, secondary to meningoencephalitis, and finally by blood-borne infection (Schuknecht 1993).

The best example of a *viral mononeuritis* affecting the auditory nerve is the *Ramsey Hunt syndrome*, or *herpes zoster oticus*. (Blackley *et al.* 1967) Initially there is a deep burning pain in the ear, which is followed some days later by a vesicular eruption in the external auditory canal. Hearing loss and vertigo then develop, and may be accompanied by a facial palsy. Viruses other than varicella zoster that can cause cochleovestibular destruction are Portbilli virus, cytomegalovirus, and Epstein–Barr virus. Mumps virus can cause unilateral deafness, and prenatal rubella may lead to bilateral deafness.

Bacterial infection of the inner ear produces dramatic symptoms of acute unilateral deafness and severe vertigo. When due to a bacterial meningitis, most commonly seen in neonates and young children, it may lead to profound hearing loss. The most common bacteria to involve the cochlea or nerve are *Neisseria meningitidis*, *Streptococcus pneumoniae*, and *Haemophilus influenzae*. Meningitis may lead to unilateral or bilateral deafness. More subacute sensorineural hearing loss may result from syphilis (Steckelberg and McDonald 1984) and borreliosis (*Lyme disease*). The eighth cranial nerve may be involved in the petrositis which affects the petrous temporal bone due to a chronic bacterial labyrinthine infection. *Gradenigo's syndrome*, associated with an abducens nerve palsy and pain behind the ipsilateral eye, occurs when the infection from an otitis media reaches the tip of the petrous temporal bone.

9.3.3 Vascular disease

The internal auditory artery, which is an end artery, provides the blood supply to the inner ear. Disturbance of this blood supply causes sudden unilateral hearing loss and vestibular loss, producing severe vertigo. This situation may occur as an isolated event or as part of an anterior inferior cerebellar artery occlusion (Oas *et al.* 1992). This artery may develop aneurysms and loops which compress the eighth cranial nerve and give rise to auditory and vestibular dysfunction.

9.3.4 Toxic disorders

Many drugs have ototoxic properties (Hawkins and Preston 1975). Aminoglycoside antibiotics, although predominantly involving the vestibular system, can damage the cochlea symmetrically, particularly involving the high frequencies. Other ototoxic drugs include thalidomide, which can lead to aplasia of the eighth cranial nerve, and vincristine. Lead and mercury poisoning may lead to both auditory and vestibular symptoms.

9.3.5 Trauma

Head injury may lead to hearing problems via a number of different mechanisms. Hearing loss may be conductive, indicating disruption of the ossicular chain. Cochlear hearing loss or total deafness may result from concussion of the inner ear with concomitant secondary neural degeneration, or a temporal bone fracture, particularly if transverse involving the vestibule of the inner ear (Schuknecht 1993). *Barotrauma*, increasingly seen in divers, may result in rupture of the round window membrane or the stapes footplate and can occur in association with a perilymph fistula (Shupak *et al.* 1991).

9.3.6 Neoplasia

The most common tumour involving the eighth cranial nerve is the vestibular schwannoma, also called incorrectly acoustic neurinoma, which accounts for 10 per cent of all intracranial tumours (Sections 18.7.3 and 19.2.4). Deafness and tinnitus are the most common presenting symptoms.

Schwannomas of other adjacent cranial nerves (V, VII, IX, or XI) may compress the eighth cranial nerve, as may other tumours in the cerebellopontine angle, such as meningiomas and epidermoid cysts. Leukaemia may invade the inner ear by leukaemic infiltration or haemorrhage. Involvement of the temporal bone can occur in association with metastatic neoplasms, particularly from breast, lung, stomach, and kidney, and multiple myeloma (Schuknecht *et al.* 1968). Deafness may occur as a result of carcinomatous and lymphomatous meningitis.

9.3.7 Metabolic

Various reports have indicated frequent damage of the cochlea and rarer involvement of the eighth cranial nerve and brainstem in patients with *diabetes mellitus* (Colletti *et al.* 1985). Hearing loss in severe *renal failure* may be due to abnormalities of the cochlear and the eighth cranial nerve.

9.3.8 Temporal bone abnormalities

In *otosclerosis* of the bony labyrinth the stapes usually becomes immobilized, leading to a conductive hearing loss, although in some cases there may also be compression of neural elements (Schuknecht 1993). *Paget's disease* may also give rise to auditory and vestibular symptoms. The hearing abnormality is usually a bilateral sensorineural hearing loss, although there may, in addition, be a conductive component.

9.3.9 Autoimmune disorders

A variety of autoimmune diseases can affect the inner ear (Stevens *et al.* 1982; Moscicki 1994). *Cogan's syndrome* is a systemic vasculitis in which interstitial keratitis and audio-vestibular symptoms are present. There is diffuse degeneration of all neural elements of the inner ear, resulting in a predominantly cochlear-type hearing loss. Similar abnormalities have been reported in *Vogt–Koyanagi–Harada syndrome*. Involvement of the cochlear nerve has been suggested in patients with various autoimmune disorders, including polyarteritis nodosa, Wegener's granulomatosis, and rheumatoid arthritis. *Autoimmune sensorineural hearing loss* is a clinical diagnosis ascribed to patients with hearing loss occurring over a period of weeks or months, and sometimes accompanied with vertiginous episodes. Women at middle age are most at risk, and about half of these patients go on to develop systemic autoimmune conditions.

9.3.10 Tinnitus

Tinnitus is a symptom in which the person hears noises in the ears or head in the absence of any sound stimulus. It is a common complaint, which is only significant when its intensity overrides the normal environmental sounds to reach consciousness. The subjective sensations can take many forms which include buzzing, humming, hissing, roaring, clicking, or some similar description. It is usually constant, but some patients describe it as intermittent, pulsating, or fluctuating. Tinnitus is usually a high-frequency tone, although if associated with a conductive rather than a sensorineural hearing loss, it may be lower in frequency. The onset of a loss of hearing, which is usually associated with the condition, may precede, follow, or occur simultaneously with the tinnitus.

Although several hypotheses have been proposed to explain the pathophysiology of tinnitus, it is still unclear (Møller 1984; Jastreboff and Hazell 1993). The hypotheses include an abnormality of spontaneous resting activity of primary auditory fibres, derangement of the temporal pattern of auditory nerve discharges, or derangement of the efferent fibres in the auditory nerve, leading to abnormal auditory behaviour.

Subjective tinnitus is an auditory sensation which is only heard by the patient, whereas objective tinnitus, which is much rarer, may be perceived by the examiner as well (Tyler 1997). The latter includes vascular causes, such as fistulae or arteriovenous malformations, or mechanical causes, as in palatal myoclonus due to abnormal contractions of the nasopharynx.

It is important to recognize that tinnitus is a symptom which, in addition to the common inner ear causes such as Menière's disease, may herald a number of disorders, such as a glomus tumour, tumours of the internal auditory meatus or cerebellopontine angle, or a vascular abnormality in the temporal bone or skull. Appropriate otological, audiological, and neurological examination and investigation should therefore be undertaken to exclude such causes. If the patient presents with persistent, isolated tinnitus which after investigation is unexplained, it is necessary to arrange regular follow-up.

Management of patients with tinnitus is difficult, and includes applying external masking sound into the affected ear, thereby eliminating the perception of the tinnitus, biofeedback, and counselling (Lenarz 1998). Pharmacological therapy is of limited value, although carbamazepine may occasionally be of value.

9.3.11 Assessment of deafness

A pure conductive hearing loss may be due to a variety of causes, including congenital abnormalities of the external ear, otitis media, impacted cerumen, perforated tympanic membrane, and otosclerosis. Patients with this type of hearing loss usually tend to have the same loss of sensitivity for sounds of all frequencies, speech discrimination is generally unimpaired, they often complain of low-frequency tinnitus, and generally speak at a reduced intensity level because they can hear themselves well by bone conduction.

Sensorineural hearing loss occurs as a result of disorders between the cochlea and the brainstem. Patients with this type of hearing loss tend to speak with excessive loudness, and have better hearing for the lower frequencies than for the high frequencies. This enables such patients to hear voices at normal intensity, due to intact low-frequency hearing, but they do experience difficulty understanding what is being said to them. They also have a disproportionate difficulty hearing against a noisy background. Tinnitus is also a frequent complaint in patients with sensorineural hearing loss. It tends to be a constant buzzing or ringing noise, of a higher pitch than occurs in conductive hearing impairments. Audiometry usually reveals normal hearing up to about 1000 Hz and then a rapid drop off at higher frequencies. Loudness recruitment is usually present in the most common type of sensorineural hearing loss, which is due to damage of the cochlea.

An important diagnostic problem for the neurologist in a patient with a sensorineural hearing loss is the differentiation of a cochlear lesion from a tumour in the cerebellopontine angle. Audiometric evaluation can provide some pointers but cannot determine the specific disease process. Pure-tone audiometry usually shows a unilateral loss of low frequencies in patients with a cochlea disturbance, due for example to Menière's disease, whereas a schwannoma leads to high-frequency deficits. Not infrequently, patients present with a mixed unilateral hearing loss, consisting of both a conductive and a sensorineural component.

9.4 Anatomy and physiology of the vestibular system

Excellent reviews of the aetiology, diagnosis, and management of patients with disturbances of the vestibular system are to be found in Baloh and Halmagyi (1996) and Brandt (1999).

The vestibular portion of the eighth cranial nerve conveys impulses from the receptors of the vestibular labyrinth concerned with the spatial orientation of the body into the central nervous system, where the information is correlated with visual and proprioceptive inputs, in order to control and modulate posture, balance, and other motor activity.

Each vestibular labyrinth includes the three semicircular canals and the utricle and saccule, each of which contains a sensory epithelium containing receptor hair cells and supporting structures (Figure 9.1). The semicircular canals on each side are mirror images, so that they normally function in pairs to provide information concerning linear acceleration. The lateral semicircular canal is largely in the horizontal plane and acts with the opposite lateral semicircular canal to give information in this plane. The superior and vertical semicircular canals lie in vertical planes with approximately 90° separation. The right anterior canal acts with the left posterior semicircular canal to give information in a vertical axis passing at a 45° angle passing from left to right; while the right anterior semicircular canal acts with the left posterior semicircular canal to give information in the vertical plane passing from right to left. At one end of each semicircular canal there is a dilatation or *ampoule* containing the receptor organ or *crista ampullaris*; a gelatinous *cupula* covers the hair cells of this organ, each of which has numerous short steriocilia and a single longer koniocilium. Movement of endolymph in the membranous labyrinth bends the cupula towards or away from the utricle; such a deflection bends the steriocilia towards the koniocilium and evokes increased discharge in the afferent vestibular nerve fibres, while a deflection in the opposite direction reduces such neuronal firing. It is the extent of the angular deflection of the cupula which determines the frequency of firing in the vestibular neurons.

In the utricle and saccule, the sensory epithelium is called the *macula*, which contains hair cells like those of the crista ampullaris but, in addition, crystals of calcium carbonate or *otoliths* lie in the gelatinous material overlying other hair cells. As these organs lie horizontally, movement of the upright head produces deflection of the hair-cell cilia; and tilting the head, with the effect of gravity upon the otoliths, also causes deflections. Hence, these organs, *static vestibular receptors,* are not affected, like the semicircular canals, by velocity of head movement, but by change of position of the head with respect to gravity.

The cell bodies of the vestibular neurons lie in *Scarpa's ganglion* in the internal auditory canal; most of the axons travel to the vestibular nuclei in the lateral pons and medulla, but a few pass through the nuclei without synapsing to enter the cerebellar flocculonodular lobe. There are medial, lateral (Dieter's), superior, and inferior vestibular nuclear groups, which are connected with the spinal cord via the vestibulospinal tracts; with the third, fourth, and sixth cranial nerve nuclei and proprioceptive pathways from the neck muscles via the medial longitudinal fasciculus; and with the cerebellum via the inferior cerebellar peduncle. Ocular deviation to the opposite side with nystagmus induced by stimulation of one horizontal semicircular canal is mediated via the medial longitudinal fasciculus, as in the oculocephalic or vestibulo-ocular reflexes.

Thus the function of the vestibular system is to assist the motor system in maintaining equilibrium by providing a continuing inflow of information into the nervous system relating to the effects of movement and the gravitational forces upon the body. If there is excessive output from the system, as in rapid rotation, or differing input from the two sides because of pathological processes, an illusion of movement or *vertigo* (see below) results. Such vertigo is nearly always accentuated by closing the eyes and lessened by opening them.

9.5 Tests of vestibular function

9.5.1 Nystagmus

Tonic vestibular input on one side causes deviation of the eyes to the opposite side which is, however, quickly overcome by cerebral cortical mechanisms concerned with saccadic eye movements so that there is a rapid recoil (saccade). Thus a vestibular lesion may cause a spontaneous nystagmus (Section 8.11.5) with a slow phase towards the side of the lesion and a saccade in the opposite direction. While the tonic vestibular component of the nystagmus is the slow phase, it is customary in clinical practice to describe the direction of nystagmus as being that of the quick phase, which is normally therefore away from the affected labyrinth. However, unlike the nystagmus which results from central brainstem lesions, that of labyrinthine origin is not affected by the direction of voluntary gaze and is inhibited by fixation.

In dysfunction of the semicircular canals or their peripheral neurons, the nystagmus is always accompanied by vertigo, which is of limited duration due to central compensation. If nystagmus persists for more than a few weeks, it is usually due to an abnormality in the central vestibular pathways. With central lesions, subjective symptoms are less severe, and nystagmus may be multidirectional, dissociated in the two eyes, and unchanged by eye closure (cessation of visual fixation). The electronystagmographic recording of spontaneous nystagmus in light conditions, in darkness, and after eye closure can be helpful for diagnostic purposes where nystagmus is not clinically obvious.

9.5.2 Induced manifestations

Induced manifestations of vestibular dysfunction are shown by various clinical tests for vestibular function. Caloric tests and tests for positional and optokinetic nystagmus are necessary for diagnosis. Electronystagmography makes it possible to record details of the nystagmus (Hood 1977).

Caloric test

The caloric test of Fitzgerald and Hallpike (1942) is a method of demonstrating dysfunction of the canal and tonic elements of the vestibular system, although it predominantly tests the lateral canal only.

A moderate but effective thermal stimulus is applied to each labyrinth separately. The stimulus is water at 7 °C below and 7 °C above body temperature. This produces equal and opposite horizontal nystagmus lasting approximately 2 minutes in the normal individual.

During the test the patient lies on a couch with the head raised 30° from the horizontal. In this position the lateral semicircular canals are vertical, the position of maximal thermal sensitivity. The patient is asked to fix his gaze on a suitable spot throughout. Water at 30 °C is run into one ear continuously for 40 s, not less than 24 ml being used. In the normal subject, second-degree nystagmus away from the stimulated labyrinth occurs. The time is recorded in seconds from the beginning of irrigation to the point when nystagmus can no longer be seen with a good light at a distance of 25 cm. Irrigation at 30 °C is

repeated in the other ear. Water at 44 °C is then used in each ear in turn, when the induced nystagmus is towards the irrigated side. Accuracy of temperature and duration of irrigation are essential. Experience in observing the end point and in interpreting the patterns is also necessary.

The caloric test (Fig. 9.4) is of great value in the diagnosis of organic lesions at all levels of the vestibular system. It may show suppression of activity on one side, canal paresis, as shown by a greater than 20 per cent asymmetry. After a canal paresis has occurred, central vestibular mechanisms attempt to rebalance the subject and this results in a directional preponderance to the opposite side to the lesion. The nystagmus in one direction, from whichever canal it is obtained, is stronger and lasts longer than in the other direction, according to whether the canal or tonic elements of the vestibular system are affected (Fig. 9.5). Combined responses showing directional preponderance and canal paresis frequently occur (Fig. 9.6).

In cerebral lesions involving the posterior temporal lobe, the cortical centre for the tonic pathway, marked directional preponderance of caloric nystagmus towards the side of the lesion is found.

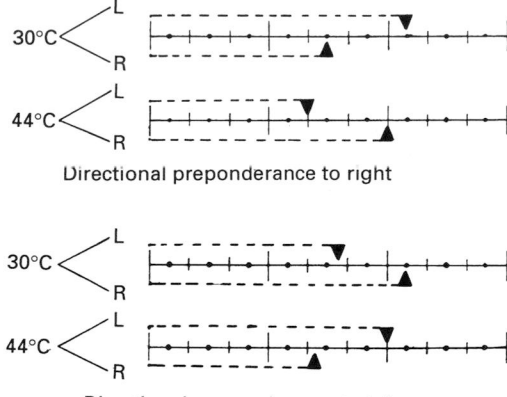

Fig. 9.5. Caloric responses: directional preponderance. (Reproduced from Fitzgerald and Hallpike (1942) by kind permission of the authors and editor.)

THE CRANIAL NERVES

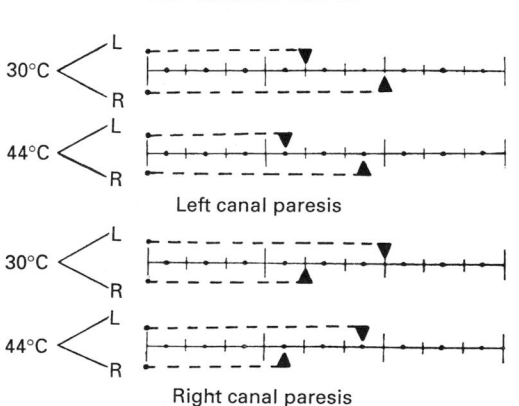

Fig. 9.4. Caloric responses: canal paresis. (Reproduced from Fitzgerald and Hallpike (1942) by kind permission of the authors and editor.)

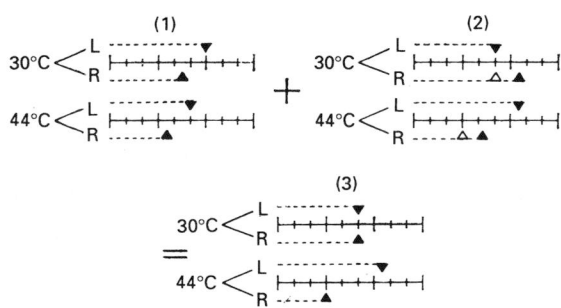

Fig. 9.6. Caloric responses: from a case of Menière's disease of the right labyrinth. Combination of right-canal paresis (1) and directional preponderance to the left (2). (Reproduced from Hallpike (1965) by kind permission of the author and editor.)

In brainstem lesions, directional preponderance away from the lesion is found more often than canal paresis, which occurs when the lesion is at or above the level of entry of the eighth cranial nerve. Combined responses sometimes occur. Simple stimulation of one ear with a small quantity of ice-cold water is a useful rapid test of the responsiveness of pontine vestibular nuclei in comatose patients; absence of nystagmus implies a severe disturbance of brainstem function (Section 25.14.2).

In peripheral lesions the most common abnormality is canal paresis, due to a lesion of the lateral semicircular canal or its peripheral neurons. Canal paresis is found in most patients with Menière's disease, vestibular neuronitis, and acoustic neuroma. Directional preponderance of caloric nystagmus alone is found less often in peripheral disease. Various quantitative vestibulo-ocular test batteries, involving the recording of eye-movement responses to precise vestibular and ocular stimuli such as caloric-induced nystagmus, smooth ocular pursuit, optokinetic nystagmus, and rotational tests (involving sinusoidal acceleration) with computer analysis, have been developed to improve diagnostic accuracy (Baloh and Honrubia 1990).

Positional and positioning tests

Positional tests, in which any nystagmus is recorded in response to slow changes of the patient's head position, are of limited value. However, the positioning test of Hallpike (1955) is of value, particularly in patients suspected of having benign paroxysmal positioning vertigo (BPPV). The patient is seated on a couch. His head is held and he is briskly laid back to bring his head 30° below the horizontal and rotated 30–40° toward the observer (Fig. 9.7). In the normal subject no nystagmus or vertigo occurs. In BPPV, after a short characteristic latent period, severe vertigo and rotary nystagmus towards the lowermost ear (the affected one) occur and lasts for several seconds. If the critical position is maintained, the nystagmus and vertigo gradually stop. On returning to a sitting position a similar, though less severe, episode occurs. If the test is then repeated, the phenomenon may not be seen as adaptation occurs rapidly.

Central lesions can produce nystagmus in this test, for example posterior fossa lesions, such as ependymomas or metastases in the fourth ventricle, or in brainstem demyelination due to multiple sclerosis. In contrast to those with a benign peripheral lesion, in these individuals nystagmus develops without a latent period, neither adapts nor fatigues, and is variable in direction depending upon how the head is moved; there is less severe subjective vertigo or even none at all.

Tests of stance and gait

Several tests of stance and gait have been used to detect vestibular disturbances, although none show a high sensitivity. The *Romberg test*, in which the patient is required to stand with eyes closed, feet together, and arms to the side, although originally devised to detect proprioceptive instability, does result in body sway towards the side of an uncompensated peripheral vestibular lesion. The *Unterberger test*, requires the patient with eyes closed to stretch his hands out in front and to step up and down in the same place, like a soldier marching on the spot. Normal subjects, after 15 seconds, usually do not rotate by more than 15° to either side, and a greater deviation is suggestive of a peripheral vestibular lesion. Several commercially developed *computerized body sway tests* are available, in which the patient stands on a special sensor plate and various visual and proprioceptive inputs are generated and the patient's response measured. There is still no agreement as to their superiority over other cheaper clinical tests already mentioned (Fetter and Dichgans 1996).

9.6 The nature of vertigo

Vertigo may be defined as an awareness of disordered orientation of the body in space. The derivation of the term implies a sense of rotation of the patient or of his surroundings, but this, though often present, is not invariable. As Brandt and Daroff (1980*a*) have suggested, vertigo occurs with either physiological stimulation or pathological dysfunction of any of the three stabilizing sensory systems: vestibular, visual, and somatosensory (Fig. 9.8). It has two principal forms:

1. The external world may appear to move, often in a rotatory manner, but other forms of movement, such as oscillation, may be experienced.

2. The body itself may be felt to be moving, either in rotation or as a sensation of falling, or the movement may be referred to within the body, e.g. within the head.

The motor accompaniments of vertigo consist of involuntary movements of the whole body, such as falling, and disordered orientation of its parts, manifested in the eyes as nystagmus or rarely diplopia, and in the limbs as pass pointing, while visceral disturbances, such as pallor, sweating, alterations in the pulse rate and blood pressure, nausea, vomiting, and diarrhoea may be present.

The maintenance of an appropriate position of the body in space depends, in humans, upon several groups of afferent inputs, of which the following are the most important:

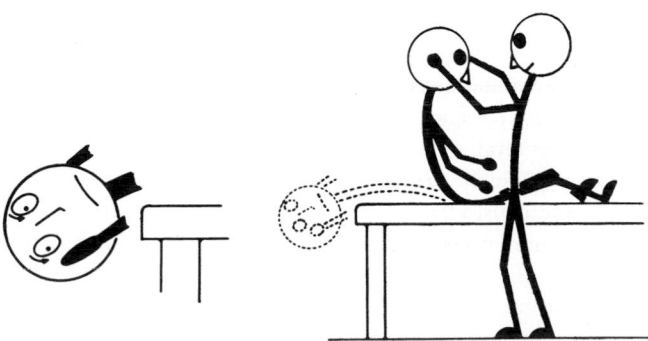

Fig. 9.7. The method of eliciting positional nystagmus. (Reproduced from Hallpike (1955) by kind permission of the author and editor.)

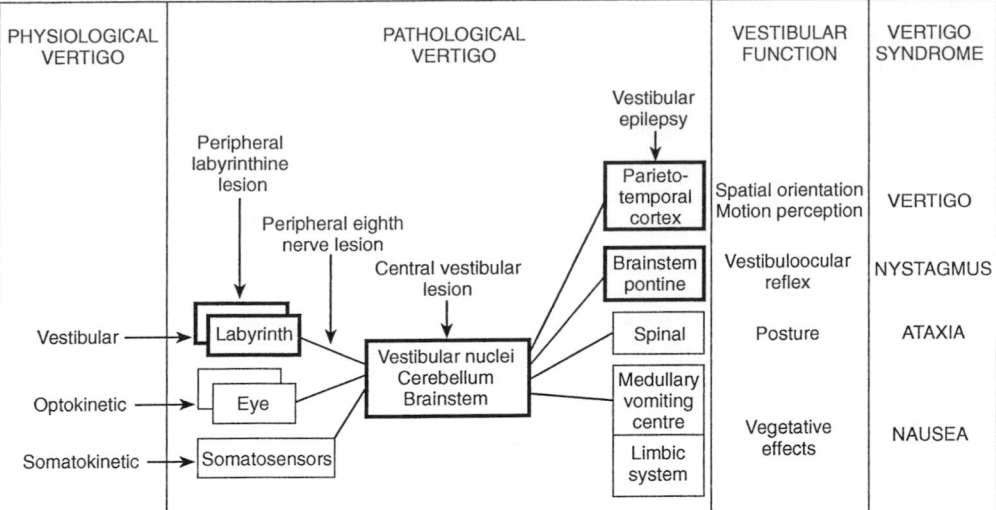

PHYSIOLOGICAL VERTIGO	PATHOLOGICAL VERTIGO	VESTIBULAR FUNCTION	VERTIGO SYNDROME

Fig. 9.8. Classification and origin of different types of vertigo. These are not clinical entities but different multisensory syndromes arising from unusual stimulation or lesional dysfunction. (Reproduced with permission from Brandt and Daroff 1980a.)

1. From the retina are derived inputs which, in contributing to our perception of visual space, are intimately concerned in spatial orientation.

2. The labyrinth is a highly specialized spatial proprioceptor. The otoliths are mainly concerned with the orientation of the organism with reference to gravity, while the semicircular canals respond to movement and angular momentum.

3. The proprioceptors of the joints and muscles of the neck are important in relating labyrinthine impulses, which convey information solely concerning the position of the head, to the attitude of the rest of the body.

4. The proprioceptors of the lower limbs and trunk are concerned with the position of the body in relation to such acts as sitting, standing, and walking.

The afferent inputs derived from these various sense organs are integrated by central mechanisms, of which the cerebellum, the vestibular nuclei, the medial longitudinal fasciculus, and the red nuclei are probably the most important, and which constitute reflex pathways by which the position of the body is normally appropriately orientated. From these lower centres, impulses reach the cerebral cortex mainly in the temporal and parietal lobes and so influence voluntary movement. Vertigo may result from disordered function of the sensory end-organ, of the afferent paths, or of the central mechanisms concerned, which lead to a mismatch of the various inputs.

9.7 Peripheral vestibular disorders

The most common peripheral vestibular nerve and labyrinthine vertigo disorders encountered in clinical practice, in order of frequency, are benign paroxysmal positioning vertigo, vestibular neuritis, and Menière's disease. The management of these disorders is well summarised by Brandt (2000).

9.7.1 Acute vestibulopathy (vestibular neuritis)

The chief symptoms associated with acute unilateral (idiopathic) vestibular paralysis, also known as vestibular neuritis, are acute rotational vertigo associated with spontaneous nystagmus, postural imbalance, and nausea without any auditory symptoms. Although the precise cause is still controversial, a viral aetiology is likely in view of the epidemic occurrence of the condition, the frequency of associated upper respiratory tract infection, and, in the few reported post-mortem examinations, evidence of cell degeneration in vestibular nerve trunks (Schuknecht and Kitamura 1981). The condition mainly affects individuals aged between 30 and 60, without a gender preference. The associated nystagmus is always horizontal–rotatory, with the fast phase directed away from the side of the lesion, reduced in frequency by optic fixation and enhanced by eye closure or Frenzel lenses, and increases in amplitude on eccentric gaze toward the fast phase (Alexander's law). Caloric testing shows a partial or complete canal paresis.

The condition is usually self-limiting, with recovery from symptoms taking place over a period of 1–6 weeks, although rapid head movements may continue to cause mild oscillopsia and impaired balance. Management of the patient in the acute phase consists of the use of vestibular sedatives such as the antihistamine dimenhydrilate (Dramamine®), or the anticholinergic scopolamine, which, if necessary, can be administered parenterally. However, it is important not to prolong the use of such drugs any longer than is necessary to relieve the nausea, since they are likely to inhibit the normal central compensatory mechanisms. Similarly, such compensation is enhanced by active eye and head movements as are promoted by the Cawthorne–Cooksey (Cawthorne 1944) or other vestibular exercises, which should be commenced as soon as possible once the acute symptoms are resolving.

9.7.2 **Benign paroxysmal positional vertigo**

Benign paroxysmal positional vertigo (BPPV), also called benign positioning vertigo, is a syndrome which can be the sequela of several inner ear diseases, and often follows mild to moderate head injuries. In about 50 per cent of cases no cause can be found.

The typical clinical presentation of BPPV is a patient experiencing repeated brief episodes of vertigo, with nystagmus lasting less than 30 seconds, usually precipitated by a positional change, such as turning in bed, getting in and out of bed, extending the neck to look up, and bending over and straightening up. The condition is diagnosed by obtaining a positive head positioning test, described above. Originally considered to be due to a lesion of the otolith organs by Bárány (1921), support for this came with the finding of basophilic deposits on the cupula of the posterior canals in two patients with BPPV ante-mortem (Schuknecht 1969). On the basis of this observation, Schuknecht proposed the cupulolithiasis theory, which states that the cupula of the posterior canal becomes heavier than the surrounding endolymph due to the degenerating utricular macula clot of calcium carbonate which settles on it. The cupula, normally of equal specific gravity to the endolymph and a transducer of only angular accelerations, now should become sensitive to changes in head position relative to the gravitational vector. The stereotyped torsional vertical nys-

tagmus in BPPV is consistent with the known excitatory connections of the posterior canal to the vertical oculomotor neurons. However, if the degenerate macula material is attached to the cupula, the nystagmus should persist as long as the head-hanging position is maintained. To deal with this objection the canalithiasis theory has been proposed (Epley 1992; Brandt and Steddin 1993), which better explains the characteristic features of the syndrome. It is proposed that a clot of calcium carbonate forms in the most dependent part of the posterior canal with the patient sitting upright. When the patient's head moves back and to the side in the plane of the posterior canal (as occurs in the head positioning test) the clot moves in an ampullofugal direction, and acting as a plunger in a narrow canal, causes an ampullofugal deflection of the cupula. The typical fatiguability is explained by dispersion of particles from the clot, reducing the effectiveness of the plunger. The latency before onset can be explained by delay in setting the clot in motion. The brief duration of the vertigo and nystagmus is explained by the slow return of the cupula to its primary position once the clot has reached its lowest point in the canal with respect to gravity. Finally, the most convincing argument is the impressive response of BPPV to positional manoeuvres designed to move the clot from the posterior canal into the utricle (Epley 1992) (Fig. 9.9).

Management of the condition includes repeated precipitation of head positions over a period of weeks, with the aim of

Fig. 9.9. Positional manoeuvre designed to remove debris from the posterior semicircular canal. (A) In the sitting position the clot of calcium carbonate crystals lies at the lowest position within the posterior canal. (B) Movement to the head-hanging position causes the clot to move away from the cupula, producing an excitatory burst of activity in the ampullary nerve from the posterior canal (ampullofugal displacement of the cupula). (C) Movement across to the other head-hanging position causes the clot to move further around the canal. (D) The patient then rolls onto the side facing the floor, causing the clot to enter the common crus of the posterior and anterior semicircular canals. (E) Finally, the patient sits up, and the clot disperses in the utricle. The manoeuvre is repeated until no nystagmus is induced, and the patient is then instructed not to lie flat for 48 hours (to prevent the debris from re-entering the canal). (Adapted from Epley 1992.)

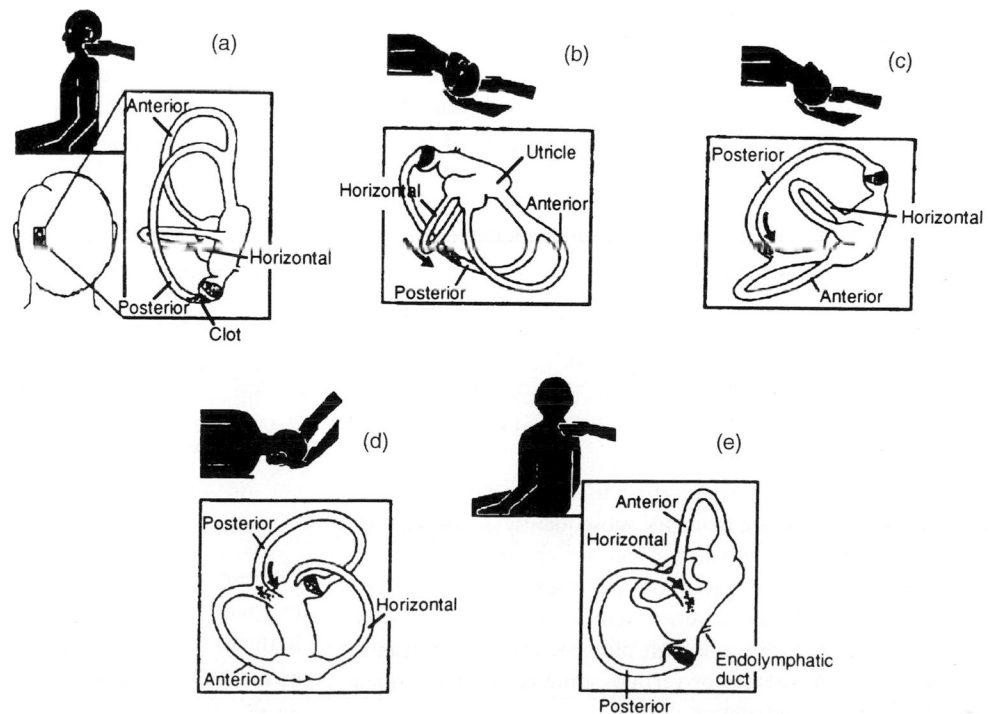

dispersing the clot (Brandt and Daroff 1980*b*), but now the positioning manoeuvres such as those described by Epley (1992) usually result in relief. In the few cases with intractable BPPV a surgical procedure such as singular neurectomy or a canal-plugging procedure may be considered. Drug therapy with antivertiginous medications have not proved particularly effective.

9.7.3 Menière's disease

Menière's disease is an inner ear disorder, first described by Menière in 1861, characterized by episodic symptoms of vertigo, hearing loss, tinnitus and aural fullness, which often, but not always, occur together. The condition can be severely debilitating, with attacks occurring without warning. The condition is thought to result from idiopathic distension of the endolymphatic system (endolymphatic hydrops) and periodic ruptures of the membranes separating endolymph from perilymph. There is a prevalence of between 218 and 370/100 000 of the population. It is slightly more common in men than in women, and usually develops in late or middle life, the mean age of onset being around 50 years of age (reviewed by Brandt 1999).

Clinical features

Based on the nature of the symptoms, the disease can be considered in two phases: early and late. In the early phase it is always unilateral and the symptoms are episodic. Some patients may initially present with only one set of symptoms, for example, attacks of vertigo or hearing loss, but usually within a year virtually all symptoms become manifest.

In the early phase most patients have disabling attacks of vertigo, described as a whirling sensation, associated with nausea and vomiting which often lasts for several hours. The vertigo builds up over minutes and towards the end slowly subsides, although the patient may experience milder symptoms of dizziness an unsteadiness for hours or days. The hearing loss is described as fluctuant due to its episodic nature. It tends to come on acutely within seconds, leading to distortion of sound in addition to loss of function. With repeated attacks full recovery of hearing is less complete. Often associated with the hearing loss, although occurring sometimes independently, is tinnitus. This is usually low in frequency and described as a 'roar' or 'similar to the ocean'. Even in the early stages, tinnitus may never resolve completely. Although not always present, many patients experience an aural fullness, similar to the sensation of pressure normally associated with Eustachian tube dysfunction.

Although in the early stages the patient is usually symptom free between attacks, the majority subsequently develop slowly progressive tinnitus and hearing loss, which show a degree of fluctuation unusual for other inner ear disorders. During these late phases patients have a severe sensorineural loss, constant tinnitus, which may become high pitched, and, in addition to the acute disabling attacks of vertigo, some patients describe a constant feeling of imbalance.

There is no pathognomonic test with which to diagnose Menière's disease, and in the early stages of the disease there may be diagnostic difficulties.

Management

Since the acute attack is self-limiting, it is usually only necessary to give vestibular sedatives, such as dimenhydrinate, promethazine, or perphenazine, which can be administered parenterally, for severe nausea or vomiting.

During remission the aim of treatment is to prevent further attacks. Although a wide variety of different dietary regimes and drugs have been advocated, most have not stood the test of time. Strict dietary sodium restriction, aiming for a urinary sodium less than 50 mmol/day is, however, worth instituting. The histamine derivative, betahistine, is probably the most useful drug (Brookes 1996).

Surgical procedures, including intratympanic gentamicin (Longridge and Mallinson 2000), for patients with Menière's disease experiencing severe repeated attacks of vertigo can often stop the attacks, but do not affect the hearing problems.

9.7.4 Perilymph fistula

The otic capsule surrounding the perilymphatic fluids of the inner ear have two comparatively vulnerable areas to trauma; the round window and the oval window. These windows are vulnerable to damage, particularly in ears with congenital deformations, after head injury (or physical exhaustion), barotrauma, and stapedectomy surgery. Perilymph fistulas may lead to episodic vertigo and sensorineural hearing loss of a high-frequency type, in combination or separately (Seltzer and McCabe 1986). Tinnitus is also common, and so may be a feeling of aural fullness. Some patients may find that the hearing loss or vertigo is worse after lying down on the affected side. The condition is therefore difficult to differentiate from both Menière's disease and BPPV, and an awareness of the clinical situations in which it may occur is valuable:

(1) hearing loss preceded by trauma (head trauma, barotrauma);

(2) new-onset sensorineural hearing loss in a child with craniofacial anomalies;

(3) fluctuating or progressive hearing loss;

(4) new-onset hearing loss in an only hearing ear;

(5) progressive hearing loss in patients with CT-documented inner ear anomalies;

(6) history of recurrent meningitis or labyrinthitis;

(7) unexplained vestibular or balance abnormalities with or without hearing loss (Shott and Pensak 1992).

Some fistulas appear as a solely otolithic vertigo, in which the patient experiences a distressing to-and-fro movement of both the body and the surroundings with sudden head movements, gait ataxia, and unpleasant tilt symptoms on tilting the head.

Unfortunately there is no satisfactory diagnostic test for peri-lymph fistulas. Audiometry reveals a progressive (usually step-wise) sensorineural hearing loss, and there may be significant deterioration after lying the patient on the affected side for 20 minutes or more. If the pressure in the external auditory canal is suddenly increased (produced by a Politzer balloon or pneu-matic otoscope) a fistula is indicated by the sudden onset of ocular deviation, nystagmus, oscillopsia, vertigo, or postural imbalance (Hennebert's sign). However, a positive result occurs in only about 25 per cent of cases.

Although 65 per cent of leaks are thought to heal sponta-neously, in patients in whom symptoms persist after head injury, or in whom the diagnosis is a strong possibility, it is necessary to carry out an exploratory tympanotomy, usually under local anaesthesia. Closing the leak often helps considerably. However, treatment of suspected perilymph fistula when the diagnosis is in doubt should consist of a trial of bedrest with head elevation and the avoidance of any Valsalva manoeuvre (e.g. bending, lifting, straining, or nose blowing) (Wall and Rauch 1996).

9.7.5 Acoustic neurinomas

Acoustic neurinomas (schwannomas) usually arise from the vestibular portion of the eighth cranial nerve in the internal audi-tory meatus, and usually present with hearing loss. If the tumour becomes particularly large, it may cause dizziness, although this may be due to compression of brainstem structures. Further details about these tumours are to be found in Section 19.2.

9.7.6 Post-traumatic vertigo

Post-traumatic vertigo is a common sequela to head and neck injury and barotrauma, yet the causation for it is often unclear and in some cases multifactorial (Luxon 1996). In some cases of severe head injury contusion or haemorrhage in the brainstem results in a central cause. In other cases, typical benign paroxys-mal positional vertigo, which occurs days or weeks after the injury, is recognized. Phobic postural vertigo is another common cause, particularly if there is no improvement in the vertigo after 4–6 weeks (Section 9.8.6). A third frequent cause is *traumatic otolith vertigo* without cupulolithiasis. In this condition patients describe a non-rotatory, to-and-fro vertigo, often associated with an unsteadiness of gait resembling walking on pillows. The otolith is a sensitive accelerometer, particularly vulnerable to head accel-eration, and the symptoms resemble those associated with otolith dysfunction (Brandt and Daroff 1980*a*). Presumably the calcare-ous material embedded in the gelatinous matrix may loosen, and even become free. Whether or not this disruption is associated with BPPV is determined by the position of any debris in the membranous labyrinth.

9.8 Central vestibular vertigo

9.8.1 Vestibular epilepsy

Vestibular epilepsy is a cortical vertigo syndrome secondary to focal discharge from either the temporal or parietal lobe, each of which receive bilateral vestibular projections from the thalamus. Vestibular seizures are either simple or complex partial with ver-tigo as the major component. Patients experience the sudden onset of dysequilibrium with rotational or linear vertigo, usually accompanied by contraversive body, head, and eye rotation. These symptoms usually last for several seconds only, and may be ac-companied by mild nausea, and occasionally tinnitus. *Vesti-bulogenic epilepsy*, a form of sensory-evoked epilepsy, occurs following a peripheral labyrinthine stimulation and results in simple, complex, or grand mal seizures. Finally, *paroxysmal dys-arthria, vertigo, and ataxia* is a well-recognized episodic symptom complex in multiple sclerosis, and is considered to be due to ephaptic activation of partially demyelinated axons in the brain-stem.

9.8.2 Vertebrobasilar insufficiency

Vertebrobasilar ischaemia is commonly associated with vertigo, as well as other symptoms of brainstem dysfunction (Section 27.5). When the other features occur, ischaemia of the brain-stem is clear, but in patients with recurrent episodes of vertigo alone, which are ascribed to vascular insufficiency, it is likely that these are due to transient ischaemia of the vestibular labyrinth, since the labyrinth is particularly susceptible because the labyrinthine circulation is an end circulation with minimal collaterals (Oas *et al.* 1992).

9.8.3 Basilar artery migraine

Basilar artery migraine is a form of migraine most commonly observed in adolescent girls (Bickerstaff 1961). It is associated with the sudden onset of symptoms of brainstem dysfunction which include vertigo, diplopia, dysarthria, drop attacks, visual phenomena and, in some cases, loss of consciousness. This aura usually develops over a few minutes to an hour, and it usually followed by a severe throbbing headache in the occipital region, associated with vomiting. There is a striking relationship with menstrual periods, and usually a family history of migraine. Basilar artery migraine may occur alone or in a patient already having typical attacks of classic migraine. It is important to differentiate this condition from hyperventilation. Migraine as a cause of episodic vertigo should also be considered (Dietrich and Brandt 1999).

9.8.4 Benign paroxysmal vertigo

This condition of childhood, first described by Basser (1964), is characterized by attacks of acute rotational vertigo, often causing the child to drop to the ground or cry out while clutching for support. The episodes, which are usually accompanied by nystag-mus and postural imbalance, last up to 5 minutes, and usually occur in the first 4 years of life and spontaneously resolve before 8 years. There is often a family history of migraine and many chil-dren subsequently develop classic migraine.

9.8.5 The ocular tilt reaction

The ocular tilt reaction (OTR), a vestibular disorder involv-ing the otolithic graviceptive pathways, is an oculocephalic synkinesis with a triad of ipsilateral lateral head tilt, a skew deviation (hypotropia of the undermost eye), and ocular torsion (few degrees up to 20°), which can only be determined by fundus photography. Despite this, patients do not complain about a perceptual tilt, although when their subjective vertical is measured it usually shows a significant deviation in the direction of the head tilt.

This triad was first observed by Westheimer and Blair (1975) with electrical stimulation of the midbrain in the region of the interstitial nucleus of Cajal (INC) in the monkey. However, in humans it is associated with lesions anywhere along the graviceptive pathways from the labyrinth (otoliths), via the vestibular nuclei, to the rostral midbrain tegmentum and the INC. The OTR is ipsiversive with medullary lesions and contraversive with mesodiencephalic (Dieterich and Brandt 1993; Brandt and Dieterich 1993) lesions. The most common aetiologies are brainstem infarction and tumours, although cases have been reported following brainstem haemorrhage, multiple sclerosis, and basilar artery migraine.

9.8.6 Psychogenic vertigo

Vertigo, a subjective symptom, occurs in a number of psychiatric disorders, including anxiety, depression, and personality disorders, although rarely in psychosis. In addition, vertigo as a symptom due to vestibular dysfunction can itself lead to the development of psychiatric disorders, including anxiety, panic attacks, and depression. This may, in turn, lead to the persistence of symptoms of persistent dizziness and postural imbalance after central compensation or remission of a peripheral vestibular disorder. This occurs particularly in individuals with an obsessive personality.

Several specific disturbances have a psychological basis, including *acrophobia*, in which there is a fear of heights, and *agoraphobia*, a fear of wide, open spaces. *Phobic postural vertigo* is a common disorder characterized by a combination of nonrotational vertigo with subjective postural imbalance and unsteadiness, mainly in patients with either an obsessive–compulsive or hysterical personality. The diagnosis is based on six characteristic features (Brandt *et al.* 1994):

1. Dizziness and subjective disturbance of balance in the upright posture and during gait, despite normal clinical balance tests.

2. Postural vertigo described as fluctuating unsteadiness, often taking the form of attacks, or sometimes the perception of illusory body perturbations for fractions of seconds.

3. Anxiety (57 per cent) and stressful vegetative symptoms accompanying and subsequent to the vertigo, elicited by direct questioning, although most patients experience vertigo attacks with and without excess anxiety.

4. Vertigo attacks that can occur spontaneously, but upon specific questioning are found to be almost invariably associated with particular constellations of perceptual stimuli from which the patients have difficulty withdrawing and that they recognize as provoking factors. There is a tendency for rapid conditioning, generalization, and avoidance behaviour to develop.

5. Typically an obsessive–compulsive type of personality in patients, who are often found to have affective lability and mild (reactive) depression.

6. Frequently, the onset of the condition follows periods of particular stress or after the patient has been through an illness, usually a vestibular disorder (21 per cent).

Brandt (1999) has proposed that this condition involves a transient uncoupling of efference and efference copy, leading to a mismatch between anticipated and actual movement. Management of this condition consists of giving a detailed explanation of the mechanism that causes, and the factors that provoke, vertigo attacks.

References

Baloh, R. M. and Halmagyi, G. M. (ed.) (1996). *Disorders of the vestibular system*. Oxford University Press, Oxford.

Baloh, R. W. and Honrubia, V. (1990). *Clinical neurophysiology of the vestibular system*, pp. 130–71. F. A. Davis, Philadelphia.

Bárány, R. (1921). Diagnose von Krankheitserschirnungen im Bereiche des otolithenapparates. *Acta Otolaryngol. (Stokh)*, **2**, 434–7.

Basser, L. S. (1964). Benign paroxysomal vertigo of childhood. *Brain*, **87**, 141–2.

Bickerstaff, E. R. (1961). Basilar artery migraine. *Lancet*, **1**, 15–17.

Blackley, B., Friedmann, I., and Wright, I. (1967). Herpes zoster auris associated with facial nerve palsy and auditory nerve symptoms: a case report with histopathological findings. *Acta Otolaryngol. (Stockh)*, **6**, 533–40.

Brandt, T. (1999). *Vertigo: Its multisensory syndromes*, (2nd edn). Springer-Verlag, London.

Brandt, T. (2000). Management of vestibular disorders. *J. Neurol.*, **247**, 491–9.

Brandt, T. and Daroff, R. B. (1980*a*). The multisensory physiological and pathological vertigo syndromes. *Ann. Neurol.*, **7**, 195–203.

Brandt, T. and Daroff, R. B. (1980*b*). Physical therapy for benign paroxysmal positional vertigo. *Arch. Oto-laryngol.*, **106**, 484–5.

Brandt, T. and Dieterich, M. (1993). Skew deviation with ocular torsion: a vestibular brainstem sign of topographic diagnostic value. *Ann. Neurol.*, **33**, 528–34.

Brandt, T. and Steddin, S. (1993). Current view of the mechanism of benign paroxysmal positional vertigo: Cupulolithiasis or canalithiasis? *J. Vest. Res.*, **3**, 373–82.

Brandt, T., Huppert, D., and Dieterich, M. (1994). Phobic postural vertigo: a first follow-up. *J. Neurol.*, **241**, 191–5.

Brookes, J. B. (1996). The pharmacological treatment of Ménières disease. *Clin. Oto-Laryngol.*, **21**, 33–7.

Cawthorne, T. (1944). The physiological basis for head exercises. *J. Chart. Soc. Physiother.*, **30**, 106–7.

Colletti, V., Fiorino, F. G., Sittoni, V. *et al.* (1985). Auditory evaluation in diabetes mellitus. *Adv. Audiol.*, **3**, 121–32.

Curtis, B. A., Jacobson, S., and Marcus, E. M. (1972). *An introduction to the neurosciences.* Saunders, Philadelphia.

Dallos, P., Popper, A. N., and Fay, R. R. (ed.) (1996). *The cochlea.* Springer-Verlag, New York.

Davis, H. and Silverman, S. R. (1970). *Hearing and deafness.* Holt, Rinehart, Winston, New York.

Dieterich, M. and Brandt, T. (1993). Ocular torsion and tilt of subjective visual vertical are sensitive brainstem signs. *Ann. Neurol.*, **33**, 292–9.

Dietrich, M. and Brandt, T. (1999). Episodic vertigo related to migraine (90 cases): vestibular migraine? *J. Neurol.*, **246**, 883–92.

Dix, M. R., Hallpike, C. S., and Hood, J. D. (1948). Observations upon the loudness recruitment phenomenon with special reference to the differential diagnosis of disorders of the internal ear and 8th nerve. *Proc. R. Soc. Med.*, **41**, 516–26.

Eggermont, J. J. and Odenthal, D. (1977). Potentialities of clinical electrocochleography. *Clin. Otolaryngol.*, **l2**, 275–86.

Epley, J. M. (1992). The canalith repositioning procedure for treatment of benign paroxysmal positional vertigo. *Otolaryngol. Head Neck Surg.*, **107**, 399–404.

Fetter, M. and Dichgans, J. (1996). Vestibular tests in evolution. II posturography. In *Disorders of the vestibular system*, (ed. R. W. Baloh and G. M. Halmagyi), pp. 256–73. Oxford University Press, Oxford.

Fitzgerald, G. and Hallpike, C. S. (1942). Studies in human vestibular function. *Brain*, **65**, 115–32.

Hallpike, C. S. (1955). Ménières disease. *Postgrad. Med. J.*, **31**, 330–6.

Hallpike, C. S. (1965). Clinical otoneurology and its contribution to theory and practise. *Proc. Roy. Soc. Med.*, **58**, 185–92.

Hawkins, J. E. and Preston, R. E. (1975). Vestibular ototoxicity. In *The vestibular system*, (ed. R. F. Naunton), pp. 321–49. Academic Press, Orlando, Florida.

Hirsch, A. and Anderson, H. (1980*a*). Elevated stapedius reflex thresholds and pathologic reflex decay: clinical occurrence and significance. *Acta Oto-Laryngol. Suppl.*, **368**, 1–28.

Hirsch, A. and Anderson, H. (1980*b*). Audiologic test results in 96 patients with tumors affecting the eighth nerve: a clinical study with emphasis on the early audiological diagnosis. *Acta Oto-Laryngol. Suppl.*, **369**, 1–26.

Hood, J. D. (1977). Whither vestibular tests? *Proc. Roy. Soc. Med.*, **70**, 675 82.

Jastreboff, P. J. and Hazell, J. W. P. (1993). A neurophysiological approach to tinnitus: clinical implications. *Br. J. Audiol.*, **27**, 7–17.

Kimberling, W. J., Møller, C. G., Davenport, S. L. H. *et al.* (1989). Usher syndrome: clinical findings and gene localisation studies. *Laryngoscope*, **99**, 66–72.

Lenarz, T. (1998). Diagnosis and management of tinnitus. *Laryngol. Rhino-Otology*, **77**, 54–60.

Longridge, N. S. and Mallinson, A. I. (2000). Low-dose intratympanic gentamycin treatment for dizziness in Ménière's disease. *J. Otolaryngol.*, **29**, 35–9.

Luxon, L. M. (1996). Posttraumatic vertigo. In *Disorders of the vestibular system*, (ed. R. W. Baloh and D. M. Halmagyi), pp. 381–95. Oxford University Press, Oxford.

Mochizuki, T., Lemmink, H. H., Mariyama, M. *et al.* (1994). Identification of mutations in the alpha 3(IV) and alpha (IV) collagen genes in autosomal recessive Alport syndrome. *Nature Genet.*, **8**, 77–81.

Møller, A. R. (1984). Pathophysiology of tinnitus. *Ann. Oto-Rhino-Laryngol.*, **93**, 39–44.

Moller, A. R., Jannetta, A. P. J., and Sekhar, L. N. (1988). Contributions from the auditory nerve to the brain stem auditory evoked potentials (BAEPs): results of intracranial recording in man. *Electroencephalog. Clin. Neurophysiol.*, **71**, 198–210.

Moscicki, R. A. (1994). Immune-mediated inner ear disorders. In *Neurotology*, (ed. R. W. Baloh), pp. 547–63. Baillière Tindall, London.

Oas, J. G., Baloh, R. W., Demer, J. L. *et al.* (1992). The effect of target distance and stimulus frequency on horizontal eye movements induced by linear acceleration on a parallel swing. *Ann. NY Acad. Sci.*, **656**, 874–6.

Patton, H. D., Sundsten, J. W., Crill, W. E. *et al.* (1976). *Introduction to basic neurology.* Saunders, Philadelphia.

Pinheiro, M. L. and Musiek, F. E. (ed.) (1985). *Assessment of central auditory dysfunction. Foundations and clinical correlates.* Williams & Wilkins, Baltimore.

Probst, R. (1990). Otoacoustic emissions: an overview. *Adv. Otolaryngol.*, **44**, 1–99.

Schuknecht, H. F. (1969). Cupulolithiasis. *Arch. Oto-laryngol.*, **90**, 765–78.

Schuknecht, H. F. (1993). *Pathology of the ear*, (2nd edn). Lea & Febiger, Philadelphia.

Schuknecht, H. F. and Kitamura, K. (1981). Vestibular neuritis. *Ann. Otol. Rhinol. Laryngol. (Suppl.)*, **78**, 1–19.

Schuknecht, H. F., Alluam, A. F., and Murakami, Y. (1968). Pathology of secondary malignant tumours of the temporal bone. *Ann. Oto-Laryngol.*, **77**, 5–22.

Seltzer, S. and McCabe, B. F. (1986). Perilymph fistula: the Iowa experience. *Laryngoscope*, **94**, 37–49.

Shott, S. R. and Pensak, M. L. (1992). Perilymphatic fistula. *Ear Nose Throat J.*, **71**, 568.

Shupak, A., Doweck, L., Greenberg, E. *et al.* (1991). Diving related inner ear injuries. *Laryngoscope*, **101**, 173–9.

Steckelberg, J. M. and McDonald, T. J. (1984). Otologic involvement in late syphilis. *Laryngoscope*, **94**, 753–7.

Stevens, S. D. G., Luxon, L. M., and Hinchcliffe, R. (1982). Immunological disorders and auditory lesions. *Audiol.*, **21**, 128–48.

Tyler, R. S. (1997). Perspectives on tinnitus. *Br. J. Audiol.*, **31**, 381–6.

Wall, C. and Rauch, S. D. (1996). Perilymph fistula. In *Disorders of the vestibular system*, (ed. R. W. Baloh and D. M. Halmagyi), pp. 396–406. Oxford University Press, Oxford.

Weil, D., Blanchard, S., Kaplan, J. *et al.* (1995). Defective myosin VIIa gene responsible for Usher syndrome type 1b. *Nature*, **374**, 60–1.

Westheimer, G. and Blair, S. M. (1975). The ocular tilt reaction—a brainstem oculomotor routine. *Invest. Ophthalmol.*, **14**, 833–9.

CHAPTER 10

Abnormalities of smell and taste

Christopher Kennard

Since both the sensation of smell (olfaction) and taste (gustation) rely on chemical stimuli to excite their receptors, they are known as the chemosensory system (Smith and Shepherd 1999). Both of these senses are interdependent, together providing the sensation of flavour of food and drink, but dysfunction of one may be misinterpreted as an abnormality of the other. Although loss of either sensation is rarely a major handicap, they are essential to detect noxious odours, such as smoke or gas, and to avoid spoiled food or potential poisons. Their loss could, therefore, have serious consequences. In addition, loss of smell or taste may indicate serious intracranial or systemic disease.

10.1 Olfaction

10.1.1 Anatomy and physiology of olfaction

Odours, which must be volatile and soluble in water, are detected by specialized olfactory receptor cells in the olfactory epithelium, located in the mucous membrane of the upper and posterior parts of the nasal cavity (superior turbinates and nasal septum), which measures 2–5 cm^2, and by the free nerve endings of the trigeminal nerve. The olfactory epithelium contains three cell types, the olfactory or receptor cells (approximately 6–10 million in each nasal cavity), sustentacular or supporting cells, which maintain the electrolyte concentration in the extracellular milieu (especially K$^+$), and basal cells, which are the source of new receptor and sustentacular cells, since the former have a life span of only 4–8 weeks.

The olfactory receptor cell is a bipolar sensory neuron with a thin, single, dendritic knob which extends into the mucus layer of the nasal cavity. The mucus layer contains immunoglobulins A and M, lactoferrin, lysoenzyme, and odorant-binding proteins. These molecules are thought to prevent the passage of noxious pathogens into the intracranial cavity via the olfactory nerve. From the knob protrude 10–30 non-motile cilia which bear the specific membrane receptor proteins, and where signal transduction is initiated. When an odour binds to a receptor there is activation of a membrane-bound GTP-dependent adenyl cyclase (G protein), which then activates a second messenger, leading to conformational changes in the transmembrane receptor and a series of intracellular events leading to the generation of axon potentials (Shepherd 1994; Smith and Shepherd 1999). Since the odour receptor cells respond to wide range of odorants, odour quality is presumably coded by some form of cross-fibre pattern. Very thin unmyelinated nerve axons leave the receptor cells and converge into small fascicles, enwrapped by Schwann cells, which pass through the cribriform plate of the ethmoid bone to the olfactory bulb. These axons collectively constitute the olfactory or first cranial nerve, and terminate within the olfactory glomeruli of the olfactory bulb. Here they form synaptic contacts with interneurons that have processes restricted to the bulb and with output neurons (mitral and internal tufted cells) that contribute axons to the lateral olfactory tract. From the olfactory tract axons project to terminate in primitive cortical areas, known as the primary olfactory cortex. In the human this probably includes small portions of the uncus, hippocampal gyrus, amygdaloid complex, and entorhinal cortex (Fig. 10.1).

10.1.2 Classification of olfactory disorders

Disturbances of olfaction can be grouped into four main subtypes:

1. Quantitative abnormalities: a total (general anosmia) or partial (partial anosmia) ability to detect olfactory sensations. There may also be a complete (general hyposmia) or incomplete (partial hyposmia) insensitivity to odorants, or heightened sensitivity (partial or total hyperosmia).

2. Qualitative abnormalities: distortions or illusions of smell (dysosmia or parosmia).

3. Olfactory delusions or hallucinations associated with disorders of the temporal lobe and psychiatric disease.

4. Olfactory agnosia in which there is an inability to recognize an odour sensation despite intact olfactory sensory processing, language, and general intellectual function.

10.1.3 Evaluation of olfactory function

In the clinical examination of olfactory function it is necessary to discriminate between deficits due to nasal obstruction, which prevent volatile substances from reaching the olfactory epithelium (transport olfactory loss), and neurogenic loss, which may be due to abnormalities of the receptors or their axons (sensory olfactory loss) or due to pathological processes affecting the central pathways. Transport olfactory loss can result from a variety of causes, including rhinitis, upper respiratory infection, polyps, sinusitis, and neoplasms. The symptoms of impaired olfactory detection, discrimination, or distortion of normal smells are no different to those accompanying sensory olfactory loss, which may be due to impaired receptor cell turnover resulting from radiation or chemotherapeutic drugs, or damage

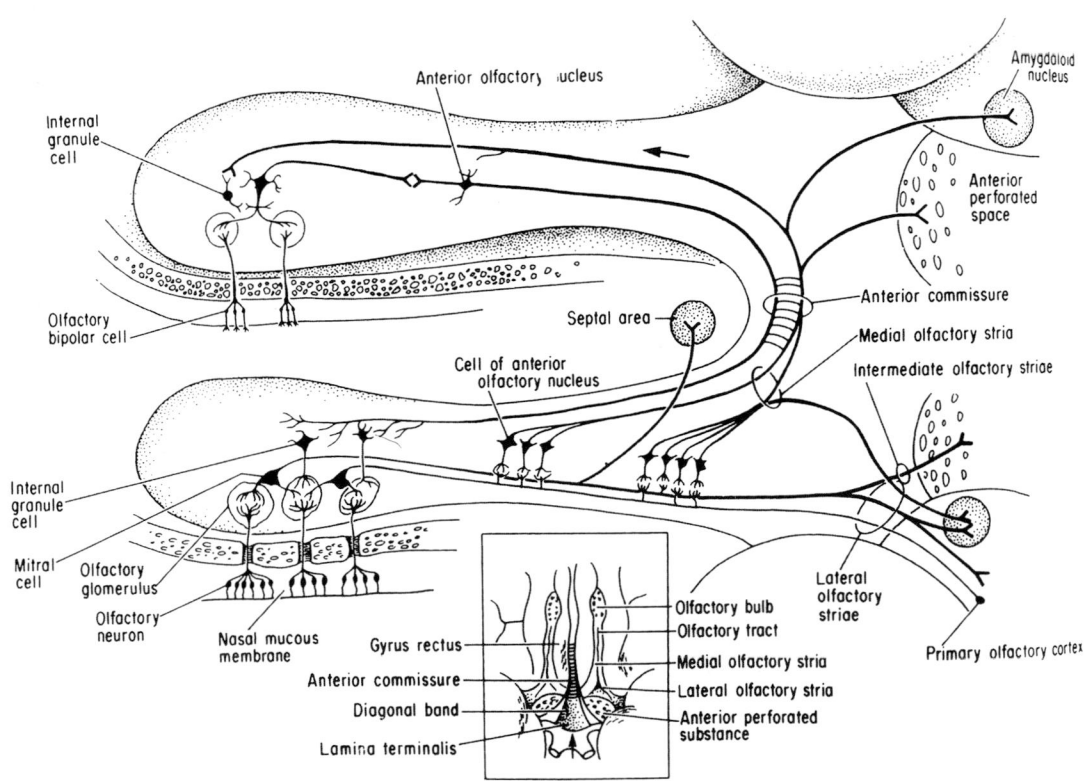

Fig. 10.1. Diagram illustrating the relationships between the olfactory receptors in the nasal mucosa and neurons in the olfactory bulb and tract. Cells of the anterior olfactory nucleus are found in scattered groups caudal to the olfactory bulb. Cells of the anterior olfactory nucleus make immediate connections with the olfactory structures via the anterior commissure. Inset: diagram of the olfactory structures on the inferior surface of the brain. (Reproduced from Adams *et al.* 1997, with permission.)

to the olfactory axons due to closed head injury, toxic substances, and viral infection.

It is therefore essential that, in addition to taking a full history and testing smell and taste, careful examination of the nose, mouth, and nasopharynx is undertaken. Examination of smell is usually carried out using a variety of familiar odiferous substances such as coffee, oil of peppermint, tobacco, oil of cloves, and vanilla. A bottle of each is held under one nostril with the other being occluded by a finger. The patient is asked whether or not he can detect an odour and, if so, whether or not he can identify it. If the odour can be detected even if it cannot be described, it may be assumed that the olfactory nerves are relatively intact. Malingering can be detected by using ammonia, which stimulates the trigeminal nerve. If the patient denies noticing the stimulus, the anosmia is likely to be bogus.

A more refined assessment of olfaction can be performed using the 40-item 'scratch 'n sniff' test developed and standardized by Doty and colleagues (1984) (the University of Pennsylvania Smell Identification Test, UPSIT). This test is highly reliable and allows the classification of patients into discrete categories of dysfunction.

10.1.4 Disorders of olfaction and their management

This subject is reviewed by Doty (1979). The most common causes of loss of smell are nasal and paranasal sinus disease, viral infection of the upper respiratory tract, and closed head injury. Hypertrophy and hyperaemia of the nasal passages, from whatever cause, leads to hyposmia or anosmia, due to odours being unable to reach the olfactory epithelium. Chronic rhinitis and sinusitis of allergic, infective, or vasomotor origin are frequent causes. Nutritional and endocrinological disorders, such as thiamine deficiency, adrenal insufficiency, vitamin A deficiency, cirrhosis, renal failure, hypothyroidism, Cushing syndrome, may also have similar effects, due to sensorineural dysfunction (Doty *et al.* 1992). A frequent cause of hyposmia is heavy smoking. Infections due to influenza, herpes simplex, and hepatitis viruses can lead to hyposmia or anosmia due to destruction of the receptor cells, and recovery may not occur if the basal cells are also destroyed. There are several congenital diseases in which the receptor cells are absent or hypoplastic. These include Kallmann's syndrome (anosmia and hypogonadotrophic hypogonadism), Turner's syndrome, and albinism.

Loss of smell in head trauma is usually due to the severing of the delicate axons of the receptor cells, as they pass through the cribriform plate, but may also occur due to damage of the olfactory bulb and possibly cerebral cortical injury. The incidence of smell dysfunction following head trauma is 5–10 per cent and is proportional to the severity of the injury. Anosmia or hyposmia may be unilateral or bilateral. Recovery of smell occurs in about a third of cases, but is unlikely to occur if the loss of smell has been present for more than 1 year after injury (Sumner 1967). The olfactory epithelium can be damaged by a variety of toxic agents, including organic solvents such as benzene, and drugs such as antimicrobial agents (ampicillin, griseofulvin, streptomycin, tetracyclines), anti-inflammatory agents (allopurinol, colchicine, gold, D-penicillamine, phenylbutazone), antiproliferative agents (methotrexate, vincristine, doxorubicin), and other drugs, including phenindione, amphetamines, cocaine, corticosteroids.

Impaired odour detection or discrimination has been described in Parkinson's disease and Alzheimer's disease (Devanand *et al.* 2000). Alcoholics with Korsakoff's psychosis have a defect of odour discrimination, as have some patients with temporal lobe epilepsy. A similar deficit is found in patients in whom anterior temporal lobe or orbitofrontal cortical excision has been performed. Anosmia may be the first symptom of an olfactory groove meningioma, which may involve the olfactory bulb and tract, and extend posteriorly to involve the optic nerve, leading to atrophy (Foster Kennedy syndrome).

There is no specific treatment for patients with hyposmia or anosmia, unless there is a local, remediable cause. However, these patients are at potential risk from inhaling noxious fumes and failing to detect burning, so it is important to advise them of the necessary precautions. These should include the use of domestic smoke and gas detectors, and the provision of adequate ventilation in enclosed areas in which toxic solvents are being used.

The most common cause of *parosmia*, the distortion of normal smell, is a local nasopharyngeal condition such as sinusitis. Other causes include temporal lobe seizure, partial injuries of the olfactory bulb, and depression. The majority of patients have associated hyposmia or anosmia.

Olfactory hallucinations are always of central origin, and are most often due to temporal lobe seizures (uncinate seizures). Other causes include Alzheimer's disease, endogenous depression, schizophrenia, and alcohol withdrawal (Pryse-Phillips 1975).

10.2 Gustation

Disturbances of taste are far less frequent than disorders of smell, and frequently patients with lack or loss of taste turn out to have impaired olfaction with normal taste sensation. Several disorders of taste are recognized: ageusia (loss of taste), hypogeusia (diminished sensitivity), dysgeusia or parageusia (distortions of normal taste) and, finally, gustatory hallucinations.

10.2.1 Anatomy and physiology of taste

The peripheral receptors for taste—the taste buds—are mainly located on the surface of the tongue and in smaller numbers over the soft palate, the pharynx, larynx, and oesophagus (Fig. 10.2). Each taste bud consists of about 200 vertically orientated receptor cells, such that the superficial portion of the bud is marked by an exacuation, the taste pit or pore, into which the microvilli of the receptor cells project. Receptor cells have a limited life span of about 10 days and undergo constant

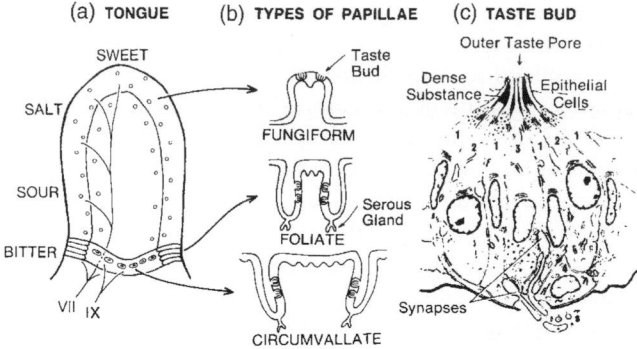

Fig. 10.2. (a) Distribution of taste buds, innervation pattern, and lowest threshold regions for different tastes in the human tongue. (b) Main types of taste papillae, containing taste buds. (c) Fine tructure of a taste bud. (Reproduced with permission from Murray 1973.)

replacement from adjacent basal epithelial cells. Fine, unmyelinated sensory fibres pass up through the base of the bud to innervate the receptor cells, which have no axons. Taste afferent fibres from the anterior two-thirds of the tongue course through the lingual nerve, a branch of the trigeminal nerve, which they leave via the corda tympani to join the facial nerves, the nervus intermedia portion, with their cell bodies in the geniculate ganglion. The posterior third of the tongue and the pharynx are supplied by the glossopharyngeal nerve, with cell bodies in the nodose ganglion. Afferents from taste buds on the palate travel with the superficial petrosal nerve, and from the larynx and oesophagus via the vagal afferents. Gustatory fibres from these nerves project to the ipsilateral solitary tract, from which they project via the gustatory lemniscus to the thalamus and then to the postrolandic sensory cortex.

The taste receptors respond to chemical substances in solution, the four primary taste sensations being salty, bitter, sweet, and sour. More complex taste sensations are derived from combinations of these four basic tastes and from olfaction (Smith and Shepherd 1999).

10.2.2 **Clinical assessment**

Patients presenting with a disturbance of taste should be asked about any associated disorder of smell, and any associated medical conditions or medications (Doty *et al.* 1992). In addition to testing smell and taste it is essential to examine the oral cavity carefully, noting any evidence of infection, masses, and atrophy and dryness of the tongue, gums, and dentition.

Taste can then be assessed using standard solutions of sugar, sodium chloride, acetic acid, and quinine. Electrical stimulation of the tongue (electrogustometry) can also be used as a sour stimulus by simply applying a low-voltage direct current. If the taste loss is bilateral, the solutions can be swished around the mouth and the patient asked to identify the taste. The solution is then spat out and the mouth rinsed with water before the next solution is tried. If the taste loss is unilateral or focal, the tongue is protruded and gently held with a piece of gauze.

Crystals of salt or sugar are then placed on the tongue and the patient asked to identify the taste.

10.2.3 **Disorders of gustation and their management**

Disturbances of taste are due either to local causes involving the tongue or taste buds, or damage to the peripheral or central neural pathways. The most common associated cause of hypogeusia is an upper respiratory tract infection and smoking (Henkin *et al.* 1975). Deficiency (as in Sjögren's syndrome) or hyperviscosity of saliva (as in cystic fibrosis, pandysautonomia, and after irradiation of the head and neck), resulting in dryness of the mouth (xerostomia), leads to disturbed taste, because taste stimuli are only effective in a fluid medium. There may also be an accompanying reduction in the number of papillae and taste buds, which may possibly be due either to the loss of the lubricating effect of saliva or of trophic factors contained with in it. Unfortunately, artificial saliva or regular water mouthwashes do not appear to restore normal taste in patients with xerostomia. Other causes of ageusia or hypogeusia include scleroderma, hypothyroidism, adrenocortical insufficiency, Cushing's syndrome, diabetes mellitus, chronic renal failure, liver cirrhosis, niacin (vitamin B_6) deficiency, zinc deficiency, and neoplasia of the oral cavity and base of skull. Disorders (reduced or distorted function) of taste not infrequently occur following influenza-like infections. A unilateral loss of taste is often found in cases of Bell's palsy.

Post-traumatic ageusia is far less common than post-traumatic anosmia, occurring in less than 1 per cent of serious head injuries (Sumner 1967). However, it always occurs in association with anosmia, and often the ageusia resolves within a few weeks. The cause for such ageusia is unclear. Although bilateral lesions near the frontal operculum and paralimbic areas would result in both ageusia and anosmia, this would not explain the frequent recovery of ageusia in advance of the anosmia. It is likely that many cases of ageusia are in fact mislabelled cases of anosmia.

Gustatory hallucinations occur much less frequently than olfactory ones in association with epileptic seizures. Such an aura, which may represent primary taste (e.g. sweet, bitter) or as peculiar and rotten, usually occurs in a seizure originating from the frontoparietal (suprasylvian) cortex or the uncal region (Hausser-Hauw and Bancaud, 1987),

Management of taste disorders includes the use of various salivary substitutes for xerostomia, the correction of any nutritional deficiency, and, in some cases, flavour enhancers.

References

Adams, R. D., Victor, R., and Ropper, A. H. (1977). *Principles of neurology*, (6th edn). McGraw-Hill, New York.

Devanand, D. P., Michaels-Marston, K. S., Liu, X. H. *et al.* (2000). Olfactory deficits in patients with mild cognitive impairment predict Alzheimer's disease at follow-up. *Am. J. Psychiat.*, **157**, 1399–1405.

Doty, R. L. (1979). A review of olfactory dysfunctions in man. *Am. J. Oto-Laryngol.*, **1**, 57–79.

Doty, R. L., Shaman, P., and Dann, M. (1984). Development of the University Pennsylvania Smell Identification Test: A standardised micro-encapsulated test of olfactory function. *Physiol. Behav. (Monograph)*, **32**, 489–502.

Doty, R. L., Kimmelman, C. P., and Lesser, R. (1992). Smell and taste and their disorders. In *Diseases of the nervous system*, (2nd edn), (ed. A. K. Asbury, G. M. McKhann, and W. I. MacDonald), pp. 390–403. Saunders, Philadelphia.

Hausser-Hauw, C. and Bancaud, J. (1987). Gustatory hallucinations in epileptic seizures. *Brain*, **110**, 339–60.

Henkin, R. I., Larson, A. L., and Powell, R. D. (1975). Hypogeusia, dysgeusia, hyposmia and dysosmia following influenza like infection. *Ann. Otol.*, **84**, 672–9.

Murray, R. G. (1973). The ultrastructure of taste buds. In *The ultrastructure of sensory organs*, (ed. I. Friedmann), pp. 1–81. Elsevier, New York.

Pryse-Phillips, W. (1975). Disturbances in the sense of smell in psychiatric patients. *Proc. R. Soc. Med.*, **68**, 26–32.

Shepherd, G. M. (1994). Discrimination of molecular signals by the olfactory receptor neurone. *Neurone*, **13**, 771–90.

Smith, D. V. and Shepherd, G. M. (1999). Chemical senses: taste and olfaction. In *Fundamental neuroscience*, (ed. M. J. Zigmond, F. E. Bloom, S. C. Landis *et al.*), pp. 719–59. Academic Press, Santiago.

Sumner, D. (1967). Post-traumatic ageusia. *Brain*, **90**, 187–97.

Nerve and muscle disease

CHAPTER 11

Lower cranial nerves and dysphagia

David Hilton-Jones

11.1 The fifth (trigeminal) nerve

11.1.1 Functional anatomy

The trigeminal nerve contains both sensory (afferent) and motor (efferent) fibres. Sensory information is conveyed from the skin of the face and forehead (Fig. 11.1), from the mucous membranes of the nasal sinuses and oral cavities, from the teeth, and from the dura of the anterior and middle cranial fossae. Efferent fibres innervate the masseter, temporalis, and pterygoid muscles (the muscles of mastication). Whereas the organization of the motor pathways is relatively straighforward, the sensory system is complex, with three major peripheral branches (each with several smaller branches), and two central pathways each subserving different sensory modalities. The peripheral distribution will be discussed first followed by a description of the central connections.

Peripheral sensory pathways

The cell bodies of the afferent fibres lie in the trigeminal ganglion (also known as the Gasserian or semilunar ganglion)

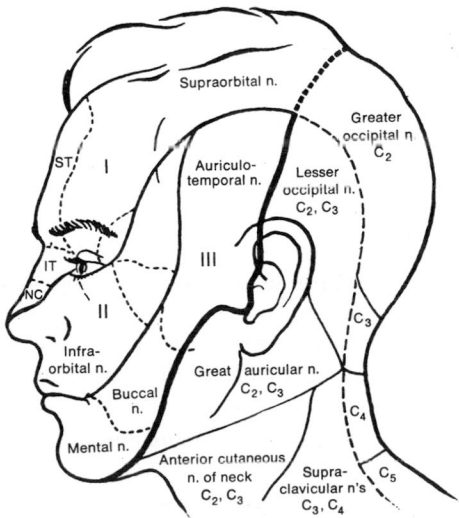

Fig. 11.1. The cutaneous distribution of the trigeminal nerve and its branches. ST, supratrochlear nerve; IT, intratrochlear nerve; NC, nasociliary nerve. (Reproduced from Brodal (1981) Neurological Anatomy, Oxford University Press.)

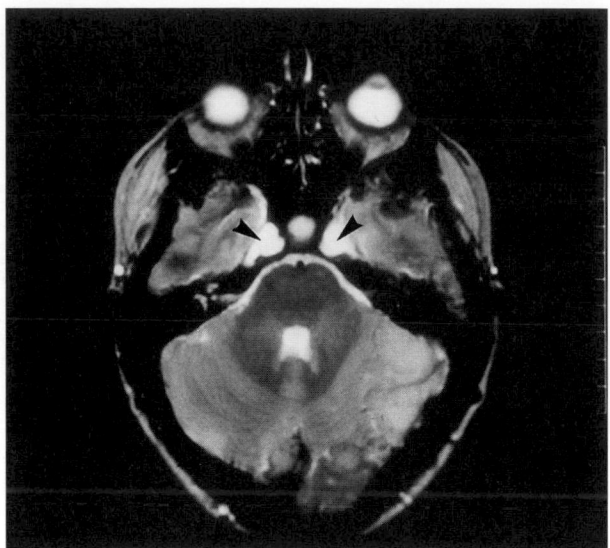

Fig. 11.2. MRI (axial T2 image) showing position of Meckel's cave (arrows) (courtesy of Dr P. Anslow).

which sits in a dural cavity (Meckel's cave) near the tip of the petrous apex bone (Fig. 11.2). The peripheral processes of these unipolar ganglion cells give rise to the three main divisions of the trigeminal nerve: the ophthalmic, maxillary, and mandibular branches, often conveniently referred to as V_1, V_2 and V_3. The central processes form the sensory root which enters the pons on its lateral aspect.

The ophthalmic nerve passes forwards in the lateral wall of the cavernous sinus, where it lies close to the third, fourth, and sixth cranial nerves, and enters the orbit through the superior orbital fissure. Branches of the nerve supply sensation to the scalp, forehead and nose, to the mucous membrane of the frontal sinus and upper part of the nasal cavity, and to the eye (conjunctiva and cornea), the latter providing the afferent limb of the corneal reflex. The area of cutaneous distribution is clearly defined (Fig. 11.1) but often misunderstood. Posteriorly, the nerve supplies the scalp as far back as the lambdoidal suture. Non-organic sensory loss over the face and forehead often extends only to the hairline, but care must be taken in interpretation because such apparently non-anatomical distribution of sensory loss may be seen in organic disease. The lateral extent of the cutaneous distribution and the boundaries with the areas of supply of the maxillary and mandibular divisions are shown in Fig. 11.1.

The maxillary nerve passes through the inferior part of the cavernous sinus and leaves the skull through the foramen rotundum. A major branch, the infraorbital nerve, enters the orbit through the inferior orbital fissure and exits through the infraorbital foramen. The area of cutaneous supply is shown in Fig. 11.1. The nerve also supplies the mucous membrane of the upper lip, hard palate, and anterior part of the soft palate, the mucous membrane of the maxillary sinus and of the lower nasal cavity, and the teeth of the upper jaw.

The mandibular nerve fuses with the motor root and leaves the skull through the foramen ovale. The cutaneous distribution is shown in Fig. 11.1. The angle of the jaw is not supplied by the mandibular nerve, but in non-organic facial sensory loss this area is often affected. As noted for ophthalmic sensory loss, caution must be taken in interpreting this sign. The area of sensory supply includes part of the pinna, external auditory meatus, and tympanic membrane. The nerve also supplies the mucous membrane of the cheek, floor of the mouth and anterior two-thirds of the tongue, and the teeth of the lower jaw. The lingual branch carries taste fibres from the anterior two-thirds of the tongue, which then join the facial nerve via the chorda tympani.

Peripheral motor pathways

The motor fibres emerging from the pons pass under the trigeminal ganglion and fuse with sensory fibres to form the mandibular nerve, which leaves the skull through the foramen ovale. They innervate the temporalis, masseter, and medial and lateral pterygoid muscles. Other muscles are supplied by the mandibular nerve, but they cannot be tested at the bedside and their involvement in isolation is not associated with specific clinical features.

Central connections

The sensory root, formed by the central processes of the trigeminal ganglion cells, enters the lateral pons and divides into short ascending and long descending branches. The short ascending fibres terminate in the principal sensory nucleus of the trigeminal nerve, which lies in the substantia gelatinosa of the lateral tegmentum of the upper pons. These fibres subserve tactile and pressure sensation (in clinical practice, lesions impair light-touch sensation and the corneal reflex). The long descending fibres form the spinal trigeminal tract, which reaches down as far as the upper cervical spinal cord (C2 level). As the tract descends, the fibres gradually terminate in the medially placed substantia gelatinosa, forming the spinal trigeminal nucleus which therefore can also be seen to extend from the pons down to the upper cervical cord. This pathway subserves pain and thermal sensation (in clinical practice, lesions impair pinprick and temperature sensation). There is a specific but complex topographical arrangement of fibres within the trigeminal tract; fibres from the ophthalmic division lie most ventrally, and those from the mandibular division most dorsally.

The secondary trigeminal pathways arise from the primary sensory nucleus and from the spinal trigeminal nucleus. Crossed and uncrossed fibres are important in various reflex pathways, discussed below, but the major sensory pathways involve crossed fibres. The secondary fibres arising from the principal sensory nucleus cross the midline in the pons and ascend as the quintothalamic tract, in close association with the medial lemniscus. Secondary fibres arising from the long spinal trigeminal nucleus cross the midline raphe and ascend in association with the medial lemniscus. Secondary trigeminal pathways, from both the principal sensory nucleus and the spinal trigeminal nucleus, terminate in the thalamus.

Trigeminal reflexes

Secondary crossed and uncrossed fibres from the two trigeminal nuclei are involved in several reflex pathways, including lacrimation, sneezing, and vomiting. In clinical practice the most important are the corneal reflex and the jaw jerk.

Stimulation of the cornea sends afferent impulses via the ophthalmic division to the trigeminal nucleus. Secondary fibres project bilaterally to the facial nuclei which, with the facial nerves, complete the reflex arc. Unilateral corneal sensation evokes bilateral blinking. In the presence of a facial-nerve palsy, ipsilateral corneal stimulation will cause contralateral blinking. Corneal stimulation on the side of an ophthalmic nerve lesion will produce no response, but contralateral corneal stimulation will produce bilateral blinking.

The jaw jerk is a monosynaptic reflex. Jaw tapping invokes bilateral contraction of the masseter and temporalis muscles. The reflex is not noticeably affected by a unilateral upper or lower motor neuron lesion of the trigeminal nerve, but is exaggerated in the presence of bilateral upper motor neuron lesions.

11.1.2 Lesions of the trigeminal nerve

Trigeminal nerve function may be affected by supranuclear (upper motor neuron), nuclear, or peripheral lesions.

Supranuclear lesions

The motor nuclei receive bilateral supranuclear (corticobulbar) innervation. A unilateral upper motor neuron lesion (e.g. a hemispheric stroke) causes no clinically discernible weakness of the trigeminal nerve-innervated muscles. Bilateral upper motor neuron lesions (e.g. bilateral hemispheric strokes, occurring simultaneously or consecutively, or an upper brainstem lesion affecting both corticobulbar pathways) result in a pseudobulbar palsy with dysarthria, dysphagia, and a brisk jaw jerk.

Nuclear lesions

Lesions involving the motor nucleus in the pons will cause ipsilateral weakness and wasting of the muscles of mastication. Masseter and temporalis can be seen and felt to be wasted, on jaw closure, and on jaw opening the jaw will deviate to the affected side because of weakness of the pterygoid muscles.

Isolated involvement of the pontine primary sensory nucleus would be expected to produce ipsilateral loss of facial light-touch sensation, with preservation of pinprick sensation, but in practice lesions invariably also involve descending fibres and both sensory modalities are impaired. Lesions in this area affecting trigeminal motor and sensory function also frequently cause contralateral hemiplegia and spinothalamic sensory loss. Common pathologies include vascular disease, demyelination, and tumour. Rarer causes are a variety of vascular malformations and (very rare) syringobulbia.

Lesions in the medulla and upper cervical cord may affect the spinal trigeminal tract and nucleus, causing ipsilateral loss of facial pain (pinprick) and temperature sensation, with preservation of light-touch and the corneal reflex. By far the most common cause is infarction of the lateral medulla secondary to occlusion of the vertebral artery or the posterior inferior cerebellar artery (the lateral medullary syndrome of Wallenberg). Further symptoms include hiccoughs, dizziness, dysarthria, and dysphagia. Ipsilateral signs, in addition to the facial sensory loss, include Horner's syndrome, palatal and vocal cord paresis, and cerebellar ataxia. Contralaterally there is limb and trunk spinothalamic (pinprick and temperature) sensory loss.

In syringomyelia a central cord lesion (a syrinx or cavity) gradually extends upwards from the cervical spinal cord into the medulla (when it is referred to as syringobulbia) and possibly as far as the pons. Spinal cord tumours may behave in the same fashion. In these situations there is bilateral involvement of the trigeminal tract and nuclei and, due to the topographic organization of nerve fibres, a particular pattern of facial sensory loss (to pinprick and temperature) evolves, which has been likened to an onion-skin or the wearing of a balaclava helmet. Thus, the sensory loss gradually progresses forwards and medially towards the nose.

Peripheral lesions

Numerous pathologies can affect the intracranial parts of the trigeminal nerve complex (the motor and sensory roots, trigeminal ganglion, and the three major nerve divisions). These include tumours (metastases, carcinomatous meningitis, acoustic neuromas, trigeminal neuromas, meningiomas, nasopharyngeal carcinoma), infections (viral, acute and chronic meningitis, abscesses, osteitis), Paget's disease, trauma, aneurysms, and granulomatous processes. Depending upon the site of the lesion, other cranial nerves may be involved and particular syndromes can be identified (Table 11.1).

A lesion affecting both the sympathetic nerve fibres around the internal carotid artery and the trigeminal ganglion may

Table 11.1. Cranial nerve syndromes involving the trigeminal nerve

Cranial nerves	Site of lesion	Common causes
III, IV, V_1, VI	Superior orbital fissure	Tumours Carotid aneurysm Granulomata
III, IV, V_1, VI; occasionally V_2	Cavernous sinus	Carotid aneurysm Sinus thrombosis Tumours Granulomata
V, VI	Apex of petrous bone	Tumour Osteitis (Gradenigo's syndrome)
V, VII, VIII; rarely IX	Cerebellopontine angle	Acoustic neuroma Meningioma Embryonic tumours

produce a Horner's syndrome (without anhydrosis as sudomotor fibres travel along the external carotid artery) and trigeminal nerve involvement (either with pain alone or with a demonstrable sensorimotor neuropathy). This combination is referred to as Raeder's paratrigeminal syndrome, and causes include carotid aneurysm, infection, tumours, and trauma. Such lesions may involve the optic nerve and cranial nerves III, IV, and VI in the parasellar region.

Peripheral branches of the three main nerves may be damaged by blunt or penetrating, or surgical, trauma, resulting in areas of sensory disturbance, sometimes accompanied by continuous or neuralgic pain. Those most commonly affected are the supraorbital, infraorbital, and inferior alveolar nerves. The rather specific numb cheek and chin syndromes are discussed below.

11.1.3 Trigeminal neuralgia

This is the most frequently encountered disorder of the trigeminal nerve. It may be symptomatic of an underlying structural disorder affecting the nerve, but in the majority of patients no specific cause is identified. It is more common in the second half of life, cases in younger people more often being symptomatic, is slightly more frequent in women, and has an overall prevalence of the order of 3–5 per 100 000 population.

Clinical features

These are highly characteristic, but despite this the diagnostic label is frequently applied erroneously to many other causes of facial pain, particularly atypical facial pain and dental disease. In trigeminal neuralgia, pain, typically very severe, occurs in paroxysms, each episode lasting only a few seconds. The frequency of attacks may vary from several in a minute to days between episodes, and in the early stages spontaneous remission for months or years may occur. Unfortunately, permanent remission is rare and with time the bouts of pain become more frequent. Patients often provide graphic descriptions which indicate the severity and quality of the pain—like a dagger, or red hot needle, or poker. Clinicians use the word lancinating. When attacks are frequent, secondary depression is common. Many patients identify one or more triggers to their attacks. These include touching a very specific part of the face, a cold draught, talking, swallowing, chewing, and brushing their teeth. Tactile triggers may prevent the patient washing their face or shaving.

The pain is strictly within the trigeminal distribution, most commonly in the maxillary and mandibular divisions. The ophthalmic division is involved in less than 10 per cent of cases. Typically, pain is felt in only part of the region supplied by the affected division, at least initially, but may then spread to the rest of the divisional area. In later stages both the mandibular and maxillary areas may become involved, but spread to the ophthalmic area is unusual.

Between the paroxysms, particularly if they are frequent, there may be a dull background ache that is not severe. Trigeminal neuralgia never causes continuous discomfort without the characteristic paroxysms. The stabs of pain may be accompanied by involuntary contraction of the facial muscles, giving rise to the synonymous term 'tic douloureux'. Occasional patients develop typical symptoms bilaterally but do not experience bilateral pain at the same time.

Physical examination is normal in idiopathic trigeminal neuralgia. Abnormal physical signs suggest symptomatic trigeminal neuralgia.

Aetiology

It has long been recognized that trigeminal neuralgia may be symptomatic of underlying disease. Thus, about 4 per cent of patients with multiple sclerosis experience it, although it is very rare as a presenting symptom. Primary tumours of the trigeminal nerve and compression of the nerve (e.g. by a tumour or aneurysm) very rarely produce symptoms identical to those of trigeminal neuralgia, but more commonly produce complaints of continuous pain or numbness, and on examination abnormal physical signs can be detected.

Excluding these rare causes of symptomatic trigeminal neuralgia one is left with a majority of patients in whom no physical cause is readily apparent, and thus the disorder might be considered to be one of altered function rather than structure. However, it has been suggested that in a significant number of these patients (over 90 per cent) the cause is a misdirected or ectatic blood vessel in the posterior fossa compressing the trigeminal sensory roots, and that symptomatic improvement can be gained by surgically separating the root from the aberrant blood vessels (Jannetta 1977; Haines et al. 1980). In another series, vascular compression was found in only 11 per cent of patients (Adams et al. 1982). Increasingly sensitive MRI techniques may shed further light on this issue—scans may show vessels apparently impinging on the trigeminal nerve (Fig. 11.3), but a cause–effect relationship remains to be proved.

Differential diagnosis

Rare symptomatic causes of trigeminal neuralgia have been discussed above and it was noted that they are often accompanied by abnormal physical signs. A substantial number of patients initially diagnosed as having trigeminal neuralgia prove to have other conditions. By far the most common confusion centres around the teeth. Dental disease, such as apical abscess, may cause paroxysmal as well as continuous pain, but the overall features and specific trigger factors should readily distinguish this from trigeminal neuralgia. Conversely, every specialist will have seen patients with trigeminal neuralgia who have had healthy teeth removed. Apart from dental disease, referred facial pain may be caused by sinus disease and eye disease (e.g. glaucoma). Angina may cause lower jaw pain.

Other causes of trigeminal nerve-related pain, which can be distinguished from trigeminal neuralgia on the basis of the history and physical signs, include brainstem lesions, postherpetic neuralgia, and tabes dorsalis. Local irritative lesions

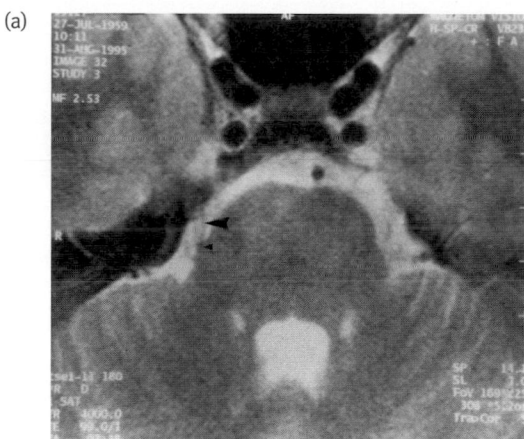

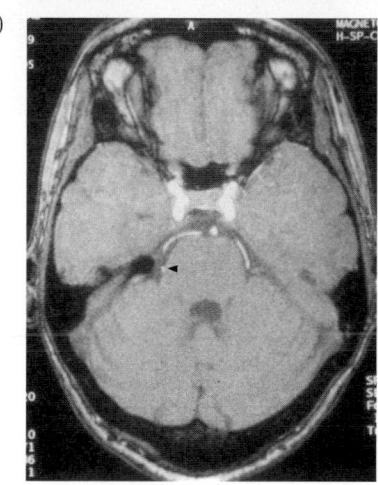

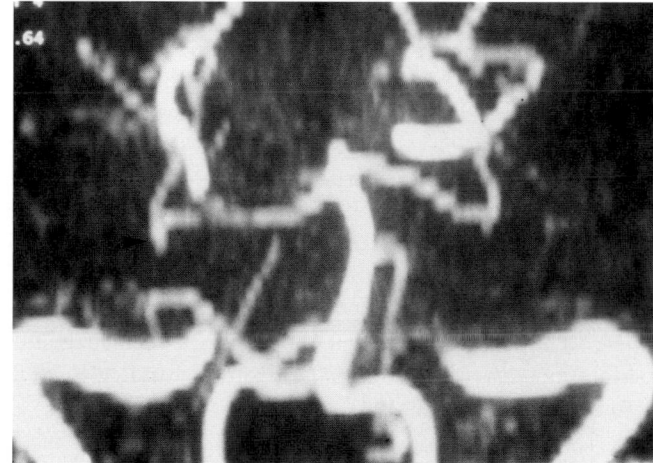

Fig. 11.3. MRI showing blood vessel 'impinging' on the trigeminal nerve. (a) High-resolution axial T2 sequence, showing the motor and sensory roots of the trigeminal nerve (large arrowhead). Immediately next to these is a blood vessel (small arrowhead), seen as a flow-void. That it is a blood vessel is confirmed on magnetic resonance angiography: (b) axial image from MR angiography sequence. The aberrant blood vessel appears white (arrowhead). (c) MR angiography (MIP projection). The looping blood vessel can be seen (arrowhead). These findings were confirmed at surgery. Separation of the vessel and nerve proved therapeutic. (Courtesy of Dr P. Anslow.)

and trauma in the regions of exit from the skull of the supraorbital and infraorbital nerves can cause localized neuralgic pain.

Facial pains attributed to temporomandibular joint dysfunction (Costen's syndrome) and maladjustment of the bite are possibly overdiagnosed.

Atypical facial pain, despite its name, is a characteristic disorder seen mainly in young and middle-aged women. They complain of a dull, constant ache in the upper jaw/cheek region which may extend to the whole of the side of the head and down into the neck. Often, but not always, there is clear evidence of an anxiety or depressive disorder. There may be a response to antidepressant drugs.

Cluster headache (migrainous neuralgia) is a highly characteristic condition that really should not be confused with trigeminal neuralgia, but sometimes is. The duration, distribution and characteristics of the pain, the different triggering factors, the accompanying symptoms, and the pattern of attacks distinguish the condition from trigeminal neuralgia.

Glossopharyngeal neuralgia (Section 11.3.3) causes attacks of identical character but in a different distribution.

Treatment

Carbamazepine gives good or excellent symptomatic relief in up to 70 per cent of patients. A reasonable starting dose is 100 mg twice daily increasing, as required, over a 1–2 week period to either the lowest effective dose or the maximal tolerable dose. This is a much more rapid increase than would be used for treating epilepsy (and is done because of the frequency and severity of the attacks) and consequently side-effects are more common, although patients may be happy to trade these off against the relief from pain. Common dose-related side-effects include nausea, unsteadiness, and visual disturbance. Up to 10 per cent of patients develop an idiosyncratic drug rash which usually necessitates stopping the drug.

If carbamazepine does not work or cannot be tolerated, other drugs that can be tried include sodium valproate, phenytoin, lamotrigine, clonazepam, and baclofen, but success rates are much lower than with carbamazepine.

Spontaneous remission may occur, especially in the early stages. Therefore, if drug treatment leads to resolution of symptoms, it is appropriate to attempt discontinuing treatment when the patient has been pain free for several weeks.

In some patients even very determined attempts with drug treatment prove unsuccessful, whereas in others there may be partial or complete relief but only at the cost of unacceptable side-effects. In such circumstances some form of surgical intervention should be considered.

If the pain is localized within the distribution of a single peripheral nerve (e.g. supraorbital or infraorbital), relief for up to 18 months may be obtained by sectioning the nerve or by injecting the nerve or trigeminal ganglion with alcohol or phenol (Loeser 1978). Such techniques have largely been superseded by radiofrequency thermal coagulation of the trigeminal ganglion, in which an electrode is inserted percutaneously, through the foramen ovale, into the ganglion (Sweet and

Wepsic 1974). Pain appreciation may be abolished, while pre-serving light-touch. Most patients have good initial relief of pain but late recurrence is not uncommon. The procedure can be repeated.

Posterior fossa exploration, looking for neurovascular abnormalities, has been discussed above. Success rates over 90 per cent have been reported (Jannetta 1977), but others have been less impressed (11 per cent by Adams *et al.* 1982) and recurrence rates may be high (Breeze and Ignelzi 1982). If a neurovascular abnormality is not identified, an alternative approach during posterior fossa surgery is partial trigeminal nerve root section, which will produce complete numbness in the relevant areas.

A recent review concluded that radio frequency rhizotomy is the treatment of choice for most patients undergoing a first operative procedure for V^2 and V^3 neuralgia, but that microvascular decompression is more appropriate for V^1 neuralgia because there is a lower risk of corneal anaesthesia (Taha and Tew 1996).

An area of numbness rather than pain might seem to be an acceptable exchange, but up to 10 per cent of patients develop extremely distressing dysaesthesiae in the anaesthetic area (Fig. 11.4) and this is very resistant to treatment. A further complication is that of keratitis, if the surgical treatment produces anaesthesia in the ophthalmic nerve territory. These complications are more likely to occur if there is extensive surgically induced sensory loss, but conversely the less sensory impairment there is, the higher the risk of recurrence of trigeminal neuralgia (Hardy 1991).

11.1.4 Herpes zoster ophthalmica

Shingles is due to reactivation of herpes zoster virus lying dormant in a sensory root ganglion. In youth it most frequently affects the trunk, less often the limbs, but with increasing age

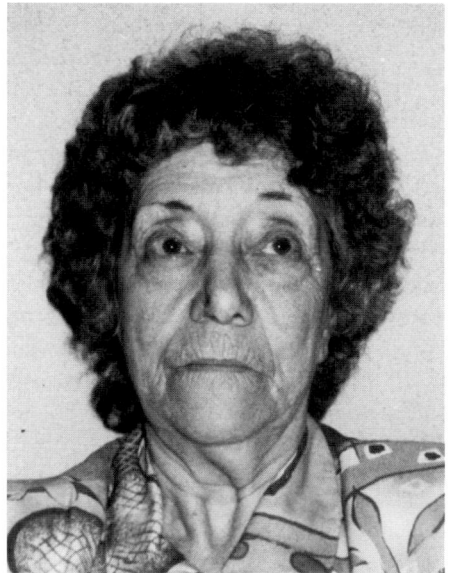

Fig. 11.4. Ulcerated area on right side of nose. Patient with trigeminal neuralgia secondary to multiple sclerosis, treated by RF thermocoagulation. The anaesthetic area was intensely itchy and repeated scratching caused ulceration.

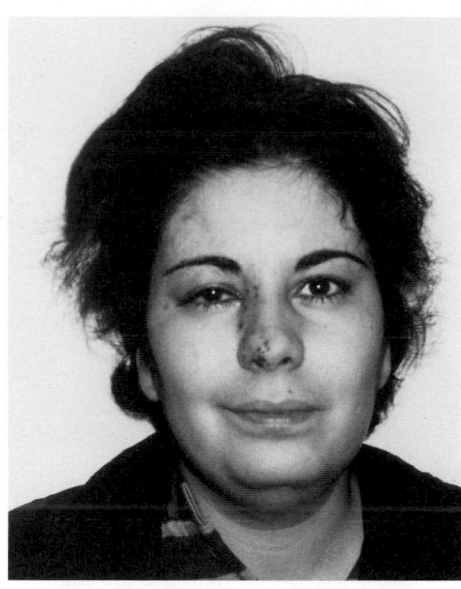

Fig. 11.5. Herpes zoster ophthalmica (patient with myasthenia gravis on immunosuppression).

facial involvement becomes more common. Reactivation of virus in the trigeminal ganglion usually affects only the ophthalmic division, producing herpes zoster ophthalmicus. Early ophthalmic complications and later neurological sequelae are common (Harding 1993, Marsh and Cooper 1993).

Most cases occur apparently spontaneously, but sometimes the trigger appears to be an intercurrent infection, or a state of drug- or disease-induced immunosuppression. Unilateral pain in the distribution of the ophthalmic nerve is followed within hours or days by a vesicular skin eruption (Fig. 11.5). The rash resolves spontaneously.

Treatment is based on oral aciclovir, with the addition of topical steroids if there is evidence of anterior segment involvement, such as iritis.

Important sequelae of herpes zoster ophthalmica include ocular complications, post-herpetic neuralgia, cranial nerve lesions, and cerebral involvement.

Ocular complications

These occur in up to 50 per cent of patients and include corneal perforation, uveitis, keratitis, entropion, and glaucoma (Womack and Liesegang 1983).

Post-herpetic neuralgia

This is the most common neurological complication of herpes zoster ophthalmica, occurring in over 10 per cent of cases, and much more frequently in the elderly. The initial acute pain and the rash resolve, leaving the patient complaining of a continuous severe pain, often burning in quality, in the affected area. The pain is notoriously resistant to treatment (Watson 1995). As noted above, measures in the acute phase may reduce the risk of its development. When established, the major approach to treatment is with tricyclic antidepressants such as amitriptyline, which may be combined with sodium valproate.

The role of topical capsaicin remains uncertain but it may have a modest effect.

Cranial neuropathy

Cranial nerve lesions may develop several weeks after the acute episode. The ocular motor nerves (III, IV, and VI) are most frequently affected, either alone or in combination, sometimes resulting in an orbital apex or superior orbital fissure syndrome (Womack and Liesegang 1983; Gupta and Vishwakarma 1987; Harding *et al.* 1987). The pathogenesis is unclear and the extent of recovery very variable.

Cerebral involvement

Rarely, at any time up to 1 month after the acute episode, patients develop contralateral hemiparesis, dysphasia, or hemianopia (Womack and Liesegang 1983). Angiography shows segmental arteritis of the carotid artery and its proximal branches ipsilateral to the shingles, and pathologically there is granulomatous arteritis with viral particles in the smooth muscle cells of the arterial wall (Linnemann and Alvira 1980).

11.1.5 Trigeminal sensory neuropathy

This term describes a syndrome with rather variable clinical features and several pathological causes. The only constant feature is sensory disturbance confined to the distribution of the trigeminal nerve. This is usually numbness, with or without pain, and may affect one or more divisions of the nerve, unilaterally or bilaterally, symmetrically or asymmetrically. The onset may be acute or insidious. Ipsilateral taste sensation may be affected. Motor involvement is rare. The corneal reflex may be impaired. Trophic ulceration/self-mutilation may be seen in anaesthetic areas (Lecky *et al.* 1987; Hagen *et al.* 1990).

There is a strong association with connective-tissue disorders (Hagen *et al.* 1990; Forster *et al.* 1996), particularly systemic sclerosis and mixed connective tissue disease, and with autoantibodies (Lecky *et al.* 1987).

11.1.6 Numb cheek and chin syndromes

The development of numbness or paraesthesiae affecting the chin, lips, or cheek (usually unilaterally) should immediately raise concern because of the strong association with tumours, particularly breast and lung metastases and lymphoproliferative disorders (Horton *et al.* 1973; Lossos and Siegal 1992). Several mechanisms may produce these symptoms. Meningeal involvement in the region of the trigeminal roots may not be associated initially with other features of carcinomatous meningitis. Basal skull deposits may affect the trigeminal ganglion and the major branches of the trigeminal nerve in their exit foramina (the mandibular division being the most frequently involved). Metastases in the mandible may damage the mental nerve, causing localized chin numbness (Horton *et al.* 1973).

Extensive investigation is required, but an underlying cause is not always found. In the elderly, simple bone atrophy leading to

mental foramen stenosis may produce chin paraesthesiae (Furukawa 1990).

11.2 The seventh (facial) nerve

11.2.1 Functional anatomy (Fig. 11.6)

The facial nerve has two roots. The larger contains the motor nerve fibres which supply the ipsilateral facial muscles. The smaller root, the intermediate nerve, contains fibres conveying taste sensation from the anterior two-thirds of the tongue, cutaneous sensory fibres from the posterior part of the ear, and preganglionic parasympathetic fibres that innervate the lacrimal and submandibular glands.

Motor pathways

The facial-nerve motor nucleus lies in the ventrolateral tegmentum of the pons. The efferent fibres arising from the nucleus

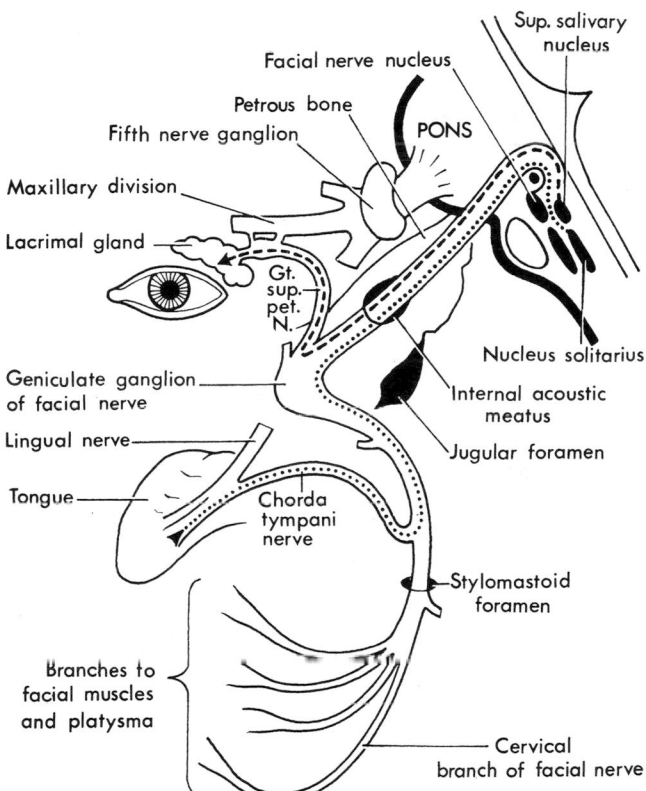

Fig 11.6. The facial nerve. Lesions involving the facial-nerve trunk above the geniculate ganglion will cause loss of lacrimation (greater petrosal nerve) and loss of taste in the anterior two-thirds of the tongue (chorda tympani nerve), as well as paralysis of both upper and lower facial muscles. Lesions between the geniculate ganglion and the point where the chorda tympani nerve leaves the facial nerve (6 mm above the stylomastoid foramen), will cause loss of taste sensation in the anterior two-thirds of the tongue, as well as paralysis of the facial muscles, but lacrimation will still be present. Lesions below the point where the chorda tympani nerve leaves the facial nerve will cause paralysis of the facial muscles, but both taste and lacrimation will be present. (Redrawn from an original drawing by Mr Charles Keogh.)

sweep dorsomedially, to the floor of the fourth ventricle, loop sharply around the sixth nerve nucleus, and then pass ventro-laterally to emerge from the lateral border of the caudal pons, at the cerebellopontine angle. The facial nerve is medial to the eighth nerve and between the two lies the intermediate nerve. These three nerves pass through the internal acoustic meatus and then the facial nerve and intermediate nerve enter the facial canal. In the facial canal, on the medial side of the middle ear, the facial nerve turns sharply (the genu of the facial nerve), moving posteriorly and inferiorly, gives off a branch to the stapedius muscle, and exits from the skull through the stylomastoid foramen.

After leaving the stylomastoid foramen the facial nerve sends branches to the stylohyoid muscle and to the posterior belly of the digastric, and then passes through the parotid gland, dividing into several branches which supply platysma and all of the muscles of facial expression, excluding levator palpebrae superioris (which is supplied by the oculomotor nerve—thus, facial-nerve lesions do not cause ptosis).

Corticobulbar pathways

The facial nucleus is composed of a number of distinct cell groups, each innervating specific facial muscles. Those supplying the upper facial muscles receive bilateral supranuclear (corticobulbar) innervation, whereas those supplying the lower facial muscles receive mainly crossed fibres from the contra-lateral hemisphere. In addition to direct corticobulbar fibres, there are several indirect pathways between the cortex and facial nuclei, involving the thalamus and reticular formation.

Sensory pathways

In the facial canal there is an expansion of the facial nerve as it makes its sharp backwards turn, at the genu. This expansion is the geniculate ganglion and is formed by the cell bodies of the nerves that give rise to the two sensory components of the facial nerve.

Special visceral afferent fibres convey taste sensation from the anterior two-thirds of the tongue. From the tongue these fibres travel first in the lingual nerve, and then in the chorda tympani which enters the skull, crosses the tympanic cavity, and joins the facial nerve in the facial canal. From the geniculate ganglion, the central connections pass via the intermediate nerve and terminate in the nucleus solitarius in the medulla.

Cutaneous nerve fibres arise from a small area, which includes the posterior part of the external auditory meatus and the skin behind the ear and in front of the mastoid. They enter the facial canal just proximal to the stylomastoid foramen. From the cell bodies in the geniculate ganglion the fibres pass centrally in the intermediate nerve and terminate in the spinal trigeminal tract. Sensory loss is not a clinically detectable feature of facial-nerve lesions, presumably because of overlap from adjacent cutaneous nerve territories, but the presence of this sensory pathway probably explains the symptom of pain in the mastoid region which is so common in patients with Bell's palsy (see below).

Autonomic pathways

Preganglionic parasympathetic fibres arise from the superior salivary nucleus, in the dorsolateral reticular formation. They travel in the intermediate nerve and at the genu of the facial nerve divide into two groups. One group passes with the greater superficial petrosal nerve to the pterygopalatine ganglion. Postganglionic fibres innervate the lacrimal gland and mucous membrane of the nose and mouth. The other group of fibres travels in the chorda tympani and terminates in the sub-mandibular ganglion. Postganglionic fibres innervate the submandibular and sublingual salivary glands.

Facial-nerve reflexes

In clinical practice the corneal reflex (see Section 11.1.1) and, to a lesser extent, the glabellar tap reflex, are of value. The glabellar tap reflex is polysynaptic and comprises tapping the forehead over the bridge of the nose and observing contraction of or-bicularis oculi (i.e. blinking) bilaterally. After several taps there is habituation and blinking stops. In early childhood and in Parkinsonian syndromes there is failure of habituation and blinking continues in time with the tapping.

Other reflexes include the naso-lacrimal reflex (lacrimation in response to stimulation of the nasal mucosa), naso-mental reflex (tapping the side of the nose causes elevation of the upper lip), and the stapedius reflex (contraction of stapedius in response to a loud noise). These and other similar reflexes are of little importance at the bedside but some, such as the stape-dial reflex, may be studied in the laboratory and can help with localization of facial nerve lesions.

11.2.2 Lesions of the facial nerve

Lesions of the facial nerve, its nucleus or supranuclear pathways, may produce facial muscle weakness; but only peripheral lesions, affecting the facial nerve itself, affect taste sensation and autonomic function. As noted above, numbness is not an expected finding in facial-nerve lesions, although symptomatic complaints of sensory disturbance are common in Bell's palsy (see below).

Supranuclear lesions

The upper facial muscles have almost equal bilateral cortical representation, whereas the lower facial muscles receive mainly crossed fibres from the contralateral hemisphere. Thus, a uni-lateral upper motor neuron lesion causes contralateral facial weakness, with the lower part of the face being more affected than the upper (NB it is relative rather than absolute sparing of the upper facial muscles). As noted above, there is more than one pathway of supranuclear innervation and, depending upon the site of the lesion, spontaneous emotional movements may be more affected than voluntary movements, and vice versa.

Nuclear and peripheral lesions

A lesion of the nucleus or facial nerve generally causes equal weakness of all ipsilateral facial muscles and the clinical features are exemplified by Bell's palsy, described below. Occasionally, partial lesions of the nucleus or nerve may selectively affect the lower facial muscles, thus mimicking the appearance seen with an upper motor neuron lesion.

Considering the origins and sites of union with the facial nerve of the greater superficial petrosal nerve, the nerve to stapedius and the chorda tympani (Fig. 11.6), the presence of impaired lacrimation, hyperacusis or an impaired stapedial reflex, or altered taste sensation can help in localizing the site of a facial-nerve lesion. The absence of such features is not of localizing value.

The facial nucleus may be affected by pontine lesions, and the nerve by lesions in the cerebellopontine angle, within the petrous temporal bone and outside the skull.

Pontine lesions

These rarely affect the facial nucleus or nerve fibres in isolation, and associated features include ipsilateral lateral rectus or conjugate gaze palsy, trigeminal motor and sensory involvement, and contralateral hemiparesis and hemisensory loss. Common pathologies include vascular lesions, multiple sclerosis, and tumours, less common disorders being brainstem encephalitis, syringobulbia, and poliomyelitis. Bilateral facial paralysis due to agenesis of the facial nuclei (Möbius' syndrome) is a rare disorder that may be associated with other cranial nerve lesions and dysmorphic features.

Cerebellopontine angle lesion

The most common lesions at this site, which affect the facial nerve, intermediate nerve, and eighth nerve, are acoustic neuromas and meningiomas. Less common lesions include secondary tumours, nasopharyngeal carcinoma, developmental tumours, cholesteatomas, and any basal meningitic process (e.g. sarcoid).

Petrous temporal bone lesions

In the facial canal the nerve may be affected by infection spreading from the middle ear or mastoid, or by surgical procedures in that area. Inflammation and swelling of the facial nerve in the facial canal and at the stylomastoid foramen is presumed to be present in Bell's palsy. In the Ramsay Hunt syndrome swelling of the geniculate ganglion due to reactivation of latent herpes zoster infection may compress the motor fibres, or there may be direct infection of the motor nerve. The resultant facial palsy is accompanied by a rash, typically seen in the external auditory meatus, although it is often more extensive than this and involves the trigeminal distribution (e.g. the anterior pillar of the fauces) and cervical dermatomes. There is often pain around the ear.

Lesions outside the skull

Benign and malignant lesions of the parotid gland may involve some or all of the branches of the facial nerve.

Bilateral facial palsy

Bilateral, as well as unilateral, lower motor neuron facial weakness may be seen in Guillain–Barré syndrome, sarcoidosis (due to basal meningeal or parotid involvement), Lyme disease (often accompanied by facial rash and induration), HIV infection (at seroconversion), and Melkersson's syndrome. In the latter disorder, recurrent episodes of unilateral or bilateral facial swelling and facial palsy are associated with a deeply furrowed tongue.

11.2.3 Bell's palsy

Bell's palsy is, by definition, an acute lower motor neuron facial palsy of unknown cause. It is generally accepted that there is inflammation and oedema of the nerve in the facial canal but, not surprisingly, there have been few pathological studies. A viral aetiology is suspected. There are conflicting reports of clustering of cases, suggesting an infective aetiology, and recurring reports implicating herpes viruses (Morgan et al. 1995; Bauer and Coker 1996).

The incidence of Bell's palsy is about 23/100 000/annum (Hauser et al. 1971). It affects both sexes equally and is less frequent in children than adults. It shows relatively weak associations with hypertension and diabetes, particularly in older patients (Hauser et al. 1971). Recurrence, on the same or opposite side, is relatively common.

The major causes of non-idiopathic acute facial palsy are head injury, multiple sclerosis, sarcoidosis, Guillain–Barré syndrome, and infection, including herpes zoster (Ramsay Hunt syndrome), Lyme disease, and HIV infection. Some of these may cause simultaneous bilateral facial palsies, whereas bilateral idiopathic (i.e. Bell's) palsy is very rare.

Clinical features

The entire course of Bell's palsy may be painless, but frequently patients complain of pain behind the ipsilateral ear, in the mastoid region, for a day or two before the onset of weakness, and this may continue for a week or more. Paralysis develops rapidly and may reach maximum severity within a few hours. Continuing progression for 24–48 hours is not uncommon and rarely may be over as long as 5 days.

All of the muscles on the affected side of the face are involved, but the degree of weakness may range in severity from mild to complete (about 70 per cent of patients). The appearance (Fig. 11.7) of even an incomplete palsy, is striking and it is not surprising that it causes the patient and sometimes their medical attendant considerable alarm. In elderly patients, presumably due to greater laxity of supporting tissues, the resultant facial deformity is more evident than in younger patients. The eyebrow droops and cannot be elevated, and the brow looses its furrows and becomes smooth. The lower eyelid everts (ectropion) causing impaired drainage of the tears, which overflow onto the cheek. The eye cannot close voluntarily or on blinking but there will be some lowering of the upper lid due to reflex inhibition of levator palpebrae superioris. The nasolabial fold becomes shallower, the angle of the mouth droops and cannot be retracted, the cheek billows on respiration, and food tends to accumulate between the cheek and teeth. There is mild

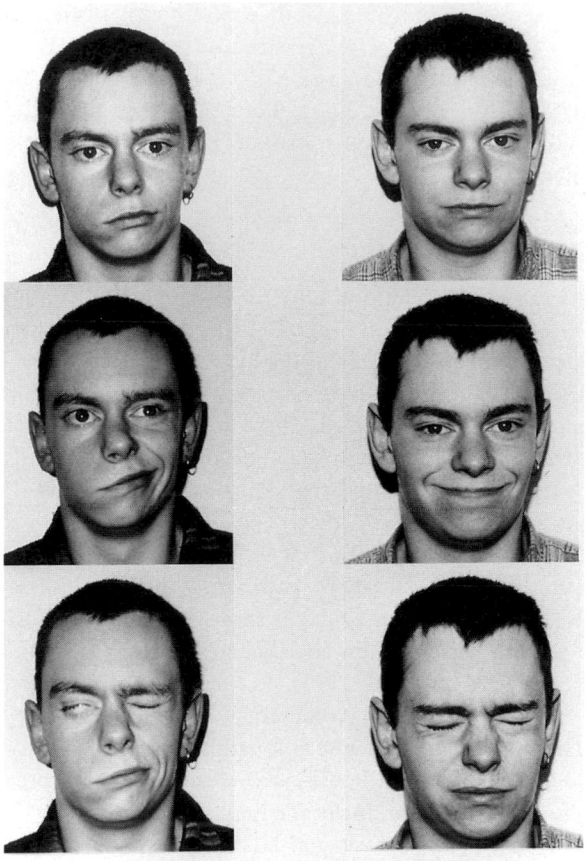

Fig. 11.7. Bell's palsy. Left panel: 5 days after onset; right panel: 3 months later. From above down: face at rest, smiling, forceful eye closure.

dysarthria. If the nerve is involved proximal to the point where it is joined by the chorda tympani, or higher still, affecting the nerve to stapedius (see above), then the patient may complain of impaired taste sensation or hyperacusis (an unpleasant quality to louder sounds).

Many patients complain of numbness over the affected side of the face and, sometimes, tongue. This may be objective, in the sense that the patient will say that light-touch and pinprick sensation are less on the affected side. The corneal reflex is always preserved. There is no obvious anatomical explanation for such sensory symptoms and they are usually attributed to distorted perception caused by the drooping musculature, skin, and associated tissues.

Prognosis

In about 80 per cent of patients improvement starts early and there is full recovery within a few weeks from the onset. Pathologically it is presumed that the weakness in these cases is due entirely to conduction block, from segmental demyelination, from which recovery is rapid. In the remaining 20 per cent of patients, in addition to conduction block, there is Wallerian degeneration of some or all of the axons, and full recovery will

not occur, although most patients have a satisfactory cosmetic outcome. Nerve regeneration starts from the point of interruption but re-innervation, and thus functional recovery, does not develop until at least 3 months after the onset of the palsy, and is never complete, leaving some residual weakness. Some of the regenerating axons become misdirected and innervate muscles that they did not originally supply. Thus, movement in one area may be accompanied by associated movement (synkinesis) elsewhere. This and other complications are discussed below.

An incomplete palsy is the most favourable prognostic sign. Adverse features may include advanced age, diabetes, hypertension, severe pain, loss of taste, and hyperacusis, but none is a reliable indicator of prognosis. Neurophysiological studies, particularly if performed more than 1 week after onset, may offer prognostic information. Whether the findings indicate a good or poor prognosis doesn't alter management, and so they are rarely performed in clinical practice.

Complications

Associated movements (synkinesis) are the result of aberrant re-innervation by regenerating axons (Fig. 11.8). Common patterns include eye closure on lip movement, or elevation of the angle of the mouth on blinking or when the eyebrow is raised. Occasionally the synkinetic movements may be very extensive.

There may also be aberrant parasympathetic nerve re-innervation, giving rise to the phenomenon of crocodile tears—profuse watering of the affected eye when eating. The simplest explanation is that regenerating fibres destined to innervate the submandibular salivary glands become misdirected and reach the lacrimal gland. An alternative explanation is that glossopharyngeal nerve fibres, destined for the parotid gland, in the lesser superficial petrosal nerve send branches to the greater superficial petrosal nerve, where they lie close together, and then innervate the lacrimal gland.

When recovery is incomplete there is often some contracture of the affected muscles. This may be evident as narrowing of the palpebral fissure or deepening of the nasolabial fold.

Treatment

It is likely that the outcome of Bell's palsy is determined within days of the onset. If the inflammation and oedema of the facial nerve causes only conduction block, then full recovery will occur independent of treatment. If the inflammatory process is more severe and results in axonal degeneration, then recovery will be incomplete. Thus, the aim of treatment must be to reduce the oedema and self-compression of the nerve within its bony canal before axonal degeneration occurs. It is impossible, on available evidence, to commend surgical decompression. To be effective it would have to be performed within days of the onset of the palsy. There are no clinical or neurophysiological pointers in those first few days to which patients are going to have a poor prognosis, and it would clearly be unjustified to operate on all patients given that the vast majority will, in any case, have a satisfactory outcome

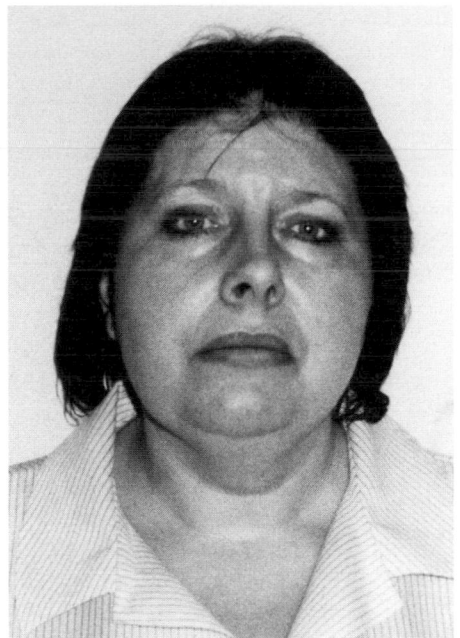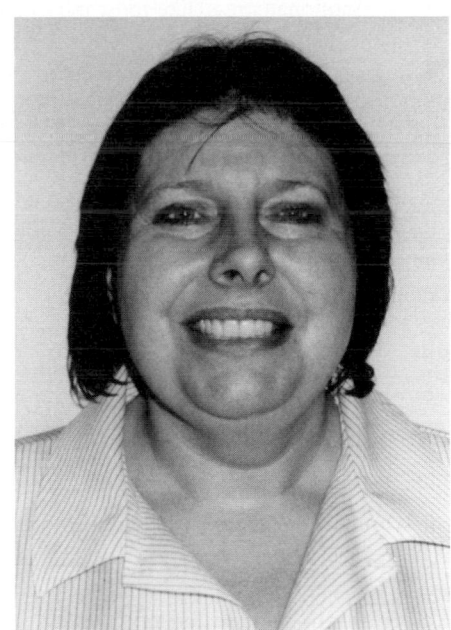

Fig. 11.8. Synkinetic movements (due to aberrant re-innervation) following previous left Bell's palsy. Smiling causes narrowing of the palpebral fissure.

Whether or not corticosteroids are helpful remains an unanswered question (Matthews 1982). In the absence of contraindications it is very common practice for patients seen within 1 week of onset of the palsy to be given a short course of oral steroids. A typical regimen might start with prednisolone 1 mg/kg body weight/day, with gradually diminishing doses over the next 10–14 days.

The normal tear film is disturbed in Bell's palsy. Despite anatomical considerations, a dry eye or underproduction of tears due to denervation of the lacrimal gland is very uncommon. Rather, tear drainage is affected due to the ectropion and this, together with reduced blinking, often causes mistiness of vision and associated patient anxiety. Corneal sensation is normal and corneal damage is rare in Bell's palsy. Tarsorrhaphy is rarely required but the patient may find it more comfortable to tape the eye closed in bed, and to use glasses to protect the eye from dust and wind. If tear production is impaired, methylcellulose eye drops should be used.

There is no effective treatment for synkinetic movements. In those few patients with severe residual weakness, various plastic surgery procedures can improve the cosmetic appearance. Because of the slow rate of nerve regeneration, no surgical intervention, except occasionally tarsorrhaphy, should be considered until at least 6, and probably 12, months after the onset of the palsy.

Crocodile tears may be treated by section of the tympanic nerve which carries the glossopharyngeal salivary fibres.

A major element in the management of Bell's palsy is reassurance of the patient and detailed explanation of what has happened and the generally favourable prognosis. There is no good evidence that physiotherapy or electrical stimulation are of specific value. However, some patients benefit from taking an active part in the management of their problem, for example by regularly massaging their face or exercising it in front of a mirror.

11.2.4 Hemifacial spasm

This painless but distressing condition develops in middle age or later, and is more common in women. It is characterized by unilateral repetitive involuntary contractions of the facial muscles.

Aetiology

The condition may be symptomatic of an irritative lesion of the facial nerve. Rarely, this may be a mass lesion such as a tumour or aneurysm. Considerable controversy still surrounds the suggestion that the irritative lesion is often an aberrantly placed artery compressing the nerve (Kaye and Adams 1981; Barker *et al.* 1995). In many patients even detailed investigation fails to find a structural abnormality, and so most frequently the conclusion is that hemifacial spasm is an idiopathic disorder, or that it is cryptogenic (i.e. there is an unidentified structural cause). Very rarely there is an antecedent history of Bell's palsy. There have been no detailed studies using modern imaging methods, but MRI would seem to be an appropriate investigation in most patients.

Electromyography shows rhythmical high-frequency discharges during an attack and evidence of synkinesis between episodes. The likely pathophysiological basis is ephaptic excitation of neighbouring nerve fibres.

Clinical features

The disorder evolves slowly over many years. In the early stages the involuntary contractions are confined to one area, such as the corner of the mouth or, most often, the lower followed by the upper eyelid, causing spasmodic eye closure. They are worsened by fatigue and emotional stress, like most movement disorders. The extent of the contraction slowly spreads until the whole of the side of the face and platysma are involved. Individual contractions, although sometimes very frequent, are usually brief, lasting a few seconds, although occasionally they may persist for several minutes.

As the condition advances it is clear, between attacks, that there is weakness of the facial muscles on the affected side and synkinetic movements are apparent. Spontaneous remission rarely occurs.

Treatment

Drug treatment is almost invariably disappointing and should not be tarried with long before trying more effective methods. Carbamazepine, sodium valproate, baclofen, and anticholinergic drugs have occasionally been reported to be of some benefit but adequate and sustained improvement is rarely achieved, or only at doses causing unacceptable side-effects.

At present, the main treatment choice is between injection of botulinum toxin into the affected muscles, or posterior fossa exploration. Botulinum injections are effective and have a relatively low incidence of side-effects (ptosis and diplopia), but have to be repeated indefinitely, every 3–6 months (Elston 1986). The rationale behind posterior fossa exploratory surgery is to decompress the nerve from aberrant blood vessels (Barker *et al.* 1995). Such compressive lesions are not always found, but it appears that simply moving and wrapping the nerve may be effective treatment (Kaye and Adams 1981). Surgery is clearly not without hazards and recurrence of hemifacial spasm may occur. Present evidence suggests that physicians prefer botulinum and surgeons surgery (Barker *et al.* 1995).

11.2.5 Other involuntary facial movements

Bilateral involuntary facial movements are seen in a number of dyskinetic syndromes (e.g. orofacial dyskinesia, Breughel's syndrome) discussed elsewhere in this text, and facial chorea may be striking in Huntington's disease. Focal epilepsy can give rise to unilateral facial contractions. Gross fasciculation of the facial muscles is seen in Kennedy's syndrome (X-linked bulbospinal neuronopathy).

In facial myokymia there is an irregular writhing movement of the facial muscles, typically of the cheek, sometimes rather graphically described as 'creeping flesh'. It is usually unilateral and most commonly due to multiple sclerosis (when it is transient) or to a brainstem glioma (when it progresses). Whether the cause is interruption of supranuclear pathways, or damage to the nucleus or intrapontine part of the facial nerve, is unclear. Bilateral myokymia may rarely be seen in Guillain– Barré syndrome.

11.3 The ninth (glossopharyngeal) nerve

Although the glossopharyngeal nerve contains sensory, motor, and parasympathetic fibres, only its sensory function is testable at the bedside and for all practical purposes its other functions can be ignored. Functionally and anatomically it is closely related to the vagus nerve and, together with the accessory nerve, all three nerves may be affected by lesions in the jugular foramen. Isolated glossopharyngeal nerve lesions are rare, but this nerve alone is affected in the rare syndrome of glossopharyngeal neuralgia.

11.3.1 Functional anatomy

Three components of the glossopharyngeal nerve are of little interest in everyday clinical neurology. Special visceral afferent fibres subserve taste sensation from the posterior one-third of the tongue. Symptomatic loss of taste sensation from lesions of the nerve is not seen and there are no practical tests of this function at the bedside. General visceral efferent fibres give rise to parasympathetic fibres which stimulate secretion from the parotid gland. Special visceral efferent fibres innervate the stylopharyngeus, but this muscle cannot be assessed clinically.

Peripheral course

The glossopharyngeal nerve is formed by a series of radicles which enter and leave the medulla, in the posterior lateral sulcus, rostral to the vagus nerve. The nerve crosses the posterior fossa and leaves the skull, together with the vagus and accessory nerves, through the jugular foramen. It crosses in front of the internal carotid artery to reach the lateral wall of the pharynx. The nerve contains two peripheral ganglia, the superior ganglion which lies in the jugular foramen and the inferior (petrosal) ganglion which is extracranial. The ganglia contain the cell bodies of primary sensory neurons that subserve general somatic and general visceral sensation.

Sensory pathways

General visceral afferent fibres convey sensory impulses (tactile, thermal, and pain) from the posterior one-third of the tongue, tonsil, posterior wall of the upper pharynx and Eustachian tube, via the inferior ganglion, to the solitary fasciculus and its nucleus. Clinically, this particular sensory pathway is the most important function of the nerve and the only function readily assessed at the bedside. General somatic afferent fibres carry sensation from the posterior part of the ear, via the superior ganglion, and terminate in the spinal trigeminal tract and nucleus.

11.3.2 Lesions of the glossopharyngeal nerve

As noted above, clinically the most important function of the glossopharyngeal nerve is its provision of sensory input from the upper pharynx. It thus provides the afferent limb of the gag or palatal reflex, the efferent limb of which is provided by the vagus. This reflex is too gross a test of glossopharyngeal function. If a lesion is suspected, the sensation on each side of the posterior pharyngeal wall should be tested using an orange stick or a firmly secured pin. Most patients will gag, and the palate will be seen to move, but what is more important is for the patient to state whether the sensation is the same on both sides.

Supranuclear and nuclear lesions

Supranuclear lesions have no specific discernible effect on glossopharyngeal nerve function, although involvement of stylopharyngeus may contribute to pseudobulbar palsy. Nuclear lesions in isolation are rarely, if ever, seen and other cranial nerve nuclei, particularly the vagus, are usually also involved. The most common cause is a vascular lesion, with other causes including primary and secondary neoplasia and syringobulbia.

Peripheral lesions

Between the medulla and jugular foramen the nerve may be affected by meningeal disease (e.g. inflammatory and neoplastic processes) and metastases. In the jugular foramen probably the most common lesion, which of course may also affect the vagus and accessory nerves, is a glomus tumour. Neuromas of any of these three nerves may arise in or near the jugular foramen and each nerve may be affected by basal skull fracture and basilar invagination. Metastatic disease may affect the nerve anywhere along its course, intracranially or extracranially.

11.3.3 Glossopharyngeal neuralgia

Although much rarer, glossopharyngeal neuralgia shares many similarities with trigeminal neuralgia with respect to aetiology, treatment, and the characteristics of the paroxysms of pain. Most cases are idiopathic but neuralgia may be symptomatic of lesions affecting the glossopharyngeal nerve, particularly neoplastic disorders, and there is evidence that new cases, like trigeminal neuralgia, may be caused by compression of the nerve by an aberrantly situated artery (Laha and Jannetta 1977).

Clinical features

The paroxysms of pain may occur in clusters, with long periods of remission, or may be chronic. The pain is experienced in the back of the throat, below the angle of the jaw, and within the ear. The stabbing or lancinating quality is similar to that occurring in trigeminal neuralgia. Precipitants include eating, swallowing, talking, head turning, coughing, sneezing, and touching the outer ear. Syncope may occur in association with pain and is due to sinus bradycardia or asystole (Jacobson and Ross-Russell 1979), reflecting the intimate associations between the glossopharyngeal and vagus nerves.

Treatment

The treatment of choice is carbamazepine, but if this does not work, or can not be tolerated, then the same drugs as used in trigeminal neuralgia (e.g. phenytoin, sodium valproate, baclofen, and lamotrigine) may be tried before resorting to surgical techniques, which include microvascular decompression, nerve section, and medullary tractotomy.

11.4 The tenth (vagus) nerve

11.4.1 Functional anatomy

The vagus nerve has the most extensive course of any of the cranial nerves and is anatomically complex, with different courses for the main nerve trunks and their branches on each side of the body. The nerve carries motor, sensory, and autonomic fibres, but with respect to structural lesions only the motor pathways are of great clinical importance. Disturbances of autonomic function are discussed elsewhere.

Sensory and autonomic pathways

General somatic afferent fibres subserve sensation from the skin over the back of the ear and the posterior wall of the external auditory meatus. The cell bodies are situated in the superior ganglion, which sits in or just below the jugular foramen, and centrally the fibres enter the spinal trigeminal tract in the medulla. General visceral afferent fibres, from the pharynx, larynx, trachea, oesophagus, and thoracic and abdominal viscera have their cell bodies in the inferior ganglion, and centrally the fibres enter the nucleus and tractus solitarius.

Preganglionic parasympathetic fibres (general visceral efferent) arise from the dorsal motor nucleus of the vagus nerve, situated in the floor of the fourth ventricle, and are destined to innervate the thoracic and abdominal viscera.

Motor pathways

Special visceral efferent fibres innervate the voluntary striated muscles of the pharynx and larynx. They originate in the nucleus ambiguus (which also gives rise to the special visceral efferent fibres of the glossopharyngeal nerve and cranial part of the spinal accessory nerve) which lies in the medullary reticular formation between the inferior olive and the spinal trigeminal nucleus.

Peripheral course

The trunk of the vagus nerve is formed by a series of rootlets which emerge from the medulla, anterior to the inferior cerebellar peduncle, in line with the radicles of the glossopharyngeal and accessory nerves (Fig. 11.9). The nerve leaves the skull through the jugular foramen, intimately associated with the accessory nerve and separated from the glossopharyngeal nerve only by a fibrous septum. In the neck it lies in the carotid sheath, initially between the internal carotid artery and internal jugular vein, and then between the common carotid artery and internal jugular vein. Below the root of the neck the course of the nerve is different on the two sides of the body.

On the right, the nerve crosses the subclavian artery and descends through the superior mediastinum posterior to the brachiocephalic vein and to the right of the trachea, to reach the posterior aspect of the lung root. On the left, the nerve passes between the common carotid and subclavian arteries to enter the thorax. It descends through the superior mediastinum, behind the phrenic nerve and brachiocephalic

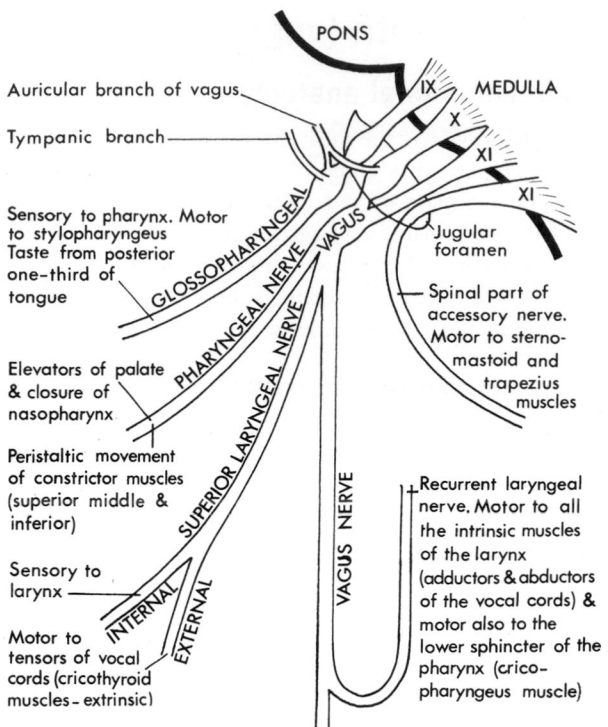

Fig. 11.9. The motor and sensory nerves supplying the pharynx and larynx, explaining the various patterns of paralysis commonly met with. (Redrawn from an original drawing by Mr Charles Keogh.)

vein and crosses the left side of the aortic arch, reaching the posterior surface of the lung root.

The nerves branch behind the lung roots, and these branches unite with fibres from thoracic sympathetic ganglia to form the right and left posterior pulmonary plexuses. Fibres from these form the posterior and anterior oesophageal plexuses, respectively. Trunks, containing fibres from both vagus nerves, are re-formed from these plexuses and pass into the abdomen, through the oesophageal opening, where they undergo complex further branching before supplying the abdominal viscera.

On each side, the vagus nerve has important branches arising in the jugular foramen, neck, and thorax. From the superior ganglion arises a *meningeal* branch, which innervates the dura in the posterior fossa, and an *auricular* branch which subserves sensation from the posterior auricle and external auditory meatus. The *pharyngeal* branch arises from the inferior ganglion and is the main motor nerve to the pharynx and soft palate. The *superior laryngeal* nerve also arises from the inferior ganglion. It has two branches: the internal, which is the main sensory nerve of the larynx, and the external, which is motor to the inferior pharyngeal constrictor and cricothyroid muscles. The *recurrent laryngeal* nerves have a different origin and course on each side of the body. On the right, this nerve arises from the vagus at the root of the neck, in front of the subclavian artery. It winds below and behind that vessel and ascends beside the trachea and behind the common carotid artery. At the level of the thyroid gland the nerve is closely related to the inferior thyroid artery. On the left, the nerve arises from the vagus at

the level of the aortic arch. It winds under the arch and then ascends along the side of the trachea. On both sides the recurrent laryngeal nerves ascend in a groove between the oesophagus and trachea, pass closely next to the medial surface of the thyroid gland, and enter the larynx to supply all of the laryngeal muscles except the cricothyroid.

11.4.2 Lesions of the vagus nerve and its branches

Supranuclear, nuclear, nerve trunk, and branch lesions may affect swallowing and phonation, the exact pattern of symptoms depending upon the site and chronicity of the lesion.

Supranuclear lesions

Because the nuclei receive both crossed and uncrossed corticobulbar fibres, unilateral supranuclear lesions do not usually cause persisting problems with phonation and swallowing, although dysphagia may be prominent following an acute hemispheric stroke. Bilateral lesions are associated with the syndrome of pseudobulbar palsy, in which dysphagia and dysarthria are due to disordered movements of the pharyngeal and laryngeal (and tongue) muscles rather than frank paralysis. Common causes include upper brainstem or bilateral hemispheric strokes, motor neuron disease, and demyelination.

Nuclear lesions

A unilateral nuclear lesion will cause ipsilateral palatal, pharyngeal, and laryngeal paralysis. On phonation the soft palate does not rise on the affected side and the uvula is drawn to the normal side. Dysphagia is variable but usually mild. Phonation is affected not only because of laryngeal muscle weakness but also by accumulation of frothy mucus which collects near the opening of the oesophagus and overflows into the larynx as a result of impaired pharyngeal emptying. The voice and cough are weak and there is difficulty clearing the voice. Bilateral lesions, in the syndrome of bulbar palsy, produce much more severe symptoms. The speech is nasal and on attempting to swallow fluids regurgitate through the nose due to palatal weakness. There may be snoring and inspiratory stridor. Coughing is paralysed, leading to a high risk of bronchial aspiration. Acute bulbar palsy is life threatening and tracheostomy is required.

Unilateral nuclear lesions rarely occur in isolation and are usually accompanied by involvement of other cranial nerve nuclei and long tracts. Causes include vascular lesions (e.g. lateral medullary syndrome) and tumour. Bilateral nuclear lesions, sometimes asymmetric, may be due to vascular lesions, motor neuron disease, tumour, syringobulbia, encephalitis, poliomyelitis, and rabies.

Nerve-trunk lesions

The clinical features of a lesion affecting the vagus nerve trunk between its origin and the jugular foramen are as described above for a unilateral nuclear lesion. Thus, there is unilateral paralysis of the soft palate, pharynx, and larynx. Causes include primary (glomus jugulare, meningioma) and secondary tumour, meningitic processes, and basal skull fracture. There is frequently involvement of other cranial nerves (IX, XI, and XII).

The inferior ganglion lies just below the jugular foramen and from it arise the pharyngeal and superior laryngeal nerves, which supply the muscles of the soft palate and pharynx, and the tensors of the cords (cricothyroids). A lesion of the vagus nerve trunk below the inferior ganglion thus spares these muscles and the pattern of laryngeal paralysis is the same as is seen with an isolated lesion of the recurrent laryngeal nerve.

Recurrent laryngeal nerve lesions

In practice, isolated vagus nerve trunk lesions are rare, but recurrent laryngeal nerve palsies are common. A unilateral lesion causes paralysis of the ipsilateral larynx and lower sphincter of the pharynx. The vocal cord is immobile and lies near the midline. Dysphagia is not a major feature, because the pharyngeal nerve is unaffected, although following an acute lesion there may be transient difficulties swallowing fluids. In the acute phase there may also be dysphonia but despite the paralysed vocal cord compensatory mechanisms are so efficient that the voice may remain or soon return to normal.

The left recurrent laryngeal nerve is more commonly involved than the right, as a result of mediastinal lesions, particularly neoplasia but less frequently aortic aneurysm and enlargement of the left atrium. In the neck the nerve may be affected unilaterally or bilaterally by trauma, surgery, cervical lymph gland enlargement (inflammatory or neoplastic), thyroid enlargement, and oesophageal carcinoma. Up to one-third of cases of recurrent laryngeal nerve palsy are idiopathic. They may be persistent or show partial or complete recovery (Blau and Kapadia 1972).

11.5 The eleventh (accessory) nerve

This is a purely motor nerve. It is formed from cranial and spinal roots which, as the accessory nerve, run together for only a very short distance. The cranial component is essentially part of the vagus nerve and is distributed mainly to the pharyngeal and recurrent laryngeal branches of that nerve, whereas the spinal component innervates sternomastoid and trapezius.

11.5.1 Functional anatomy

Spinal and cranial origins

The spinal nucleus of the accessory nerve lies in the lateral part of the anterior horn grey matter and extends from the pyramidal decussation to the fifth cervical segment. The fibres arising from it emerge from the lateral aspect of the cord, between the dorsal and ventral roots, and unite to form a trunk which ascends posterior to the denticulate ligament and enters the skull through the foramen magnum, dorsal to the vertebral

artery. The cranial root is formed by nerve fibres arising from the lower part of the nucleus ambiguus. Rootlets emerge from the lateral medulla, below the origin of the vagus.

Peripheral course

The cranial and spinal components unite for a short distance and leave the skull through the jugular foramen, in close relationship to the vagus nerve to which the cranial root fibres are distributed. The spinal part runs backwards and laterally between the internal jugular vein and internal carotid artery and crosses the transverse process of the atlas. It passes deep to the sternomastoid muscle, which it supplies, and emerges from its posterior border from where it crosses the posterior triangle, lying on levator scapulae. In this part of its course it is quite superficial, thus subject to trauma, and also related to cervical lymph nodes. The nerve then passes under the anterior border of the trapezius and unites with branches of the third and fourth cervical nerves (C3 and C4) to form a plexus which innervates the muscle. The pattern of innervation of the different parts of trapezius is probably quite variable but, in general, the accessory nerve appears to supply the upper part of the muscle, and fibres derived from C3 and C4 supply the lower part.

11.5.2 Lesions of the accessory nerve

Unilateral sternomastoid weakness is asymptomatic because it normally acts in concert with other cervical muscles which can compensate. Bilateral, but otherwise isolated, nerve lesions must be vanishingly rare. Bilateral sternomastoid weakness, with symptomatic weakness of neck flexion, is seen in myotonic dystrophy, inflammatory myopathies, various muscular dystrophies, myasthenia gravis, and motor neuron disease, but in all of these cases other cervical muscles are also involved.

Trapezius weakness is symptomatic (Fig. 11.10). The shoulder droops slightly and there is mild scapular winging at rest, with the scapular rotated outwards and downwards. The winging is exacerbated by abduction of the arm, whereas winging due to serratus anterior weakness is most evident on forward flexion of the arm. The patient notices difficulty in shrugging the shoulder, abducting the arm above 90° (Fig. 11.10) and carrying the extended arm backwards. Bilateral trapezius weakness causes the head to fall forwards. This is rarely the result of bilateral nerve-trunk involvement but is seen in myasthenia gravis, motor neuron disease, and various myopathies.

Supranuclear lesions

The cortical representation is mainly ipsilateral for sternomastoid and contralateral for trapezius. Thus, following a major hemisphere stroke, trapezius is weak on the paralysed side but sternomastoid is weak on the side of the hemispheric event.

Nuclear and nerve-trunk lesions

The spinal cord nucleus is rarely involved in isolation. The anterior horn cells may be affected by motor neuron disease and

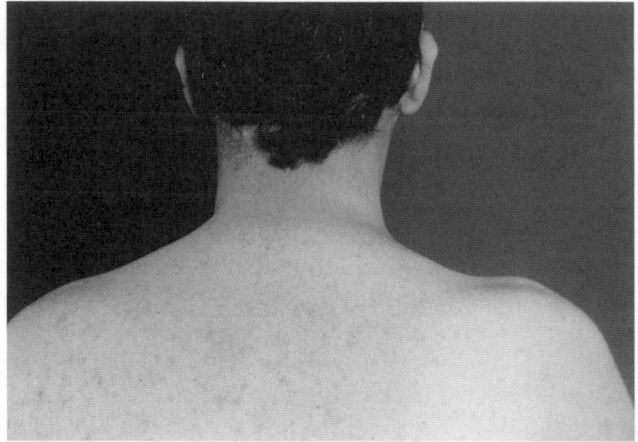

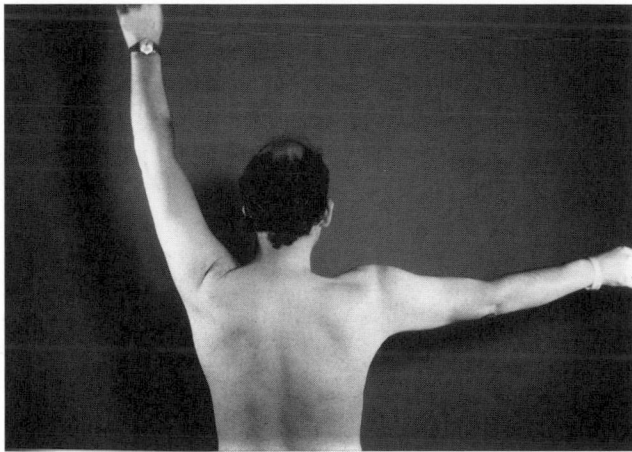

Fig. 11.10. Trapezius wasting and weakness (skull-base tumour affecting the accessory nerve). (From Donaghy M. *Neurology* 1997, Oxford University Press.)

poliomyelitis and the nuclei may be compressed by upper cervical cord tumours and syringomyelia.

In the posterior fossa, lesions affecting the accessory nerve often also involve cranial nerves IX, X, and XII. Common pathologies include primary and secondary tumours, meningitic processes, and basal skull fracture through the jugular foramen.

Outside the skull the most common site of damage is in the posterior triangle (giving rise to trapezius but not sternomastoid weakness). The nerve may be damaged by trauma or during surgical procedures (particularly removal of cervical lymph glands) including carotid endarterectomy (Sweeney and Wilbourn 1992).

Up to one-third of accessory nerve palsies are idiopathic, probably often as a forme fruste of neuralgic amyotrophy.

11.6 The twelfth (hypoglossal) nerve

This motor nerve innervates all of the muscles of the tongue through general somatic efferent fibres. Although it contains

some afferent fibres, their function is unclear and they are of no importance in clinical practice.

11.6.1 Functional anatomy

Nucleus

The nucleus, which is nearly 2 cm long, lies in the central grey matter of the medial eminence and extends from the stria medullaris to the most caudal part of the medulla. The axons arising from it pass ventro-laterally and emerge as a series of rootlets on the ventral aspect of the medulla between the inferior olivary complex and the pyramid.

Peripheral course

The rootlets pass behind the vertebral artery and unite as they exit the skull through the hypoglossal canal, which lies about 1 cm anterior, inferior, and medial to the jugular foramen. Immediately outside the skull the nerve is in close proximity to cranial nerves IX, X, and XI, the internal jugular vein, and the internal carotid artery. At the level of the angle of the mandible it sweeps antero-laterally, looping below the occipital artery and crossing the external carotid artery and then the loop of the lingual artery just above the hyoid bone. It then passes deep to the digastric muscle and terminates through multiple branches in the intrinsic and extrinsic tongue muscles.

11.6.2 Lesions of the hypoglossal nerve

A unilateral lesion of the nucleus or nerve trunk causes ipsilateral wasting and weakness of the tongue (Figs 11.11 and 11.12). Fasciculation may be prominent, especially in infantile spinal muscular atrophy and classical motor neuron disease. The epithelium is thrown into folds (Fig. 11.12), which accumulate fur. In the acute stage, articulation and swallowing may be slightly impaired but chronic lesions are typically asymptomatic. The tongue deviates to the affected side on protrusion. Bilateral lower motor neuron lesions cause weakness of both

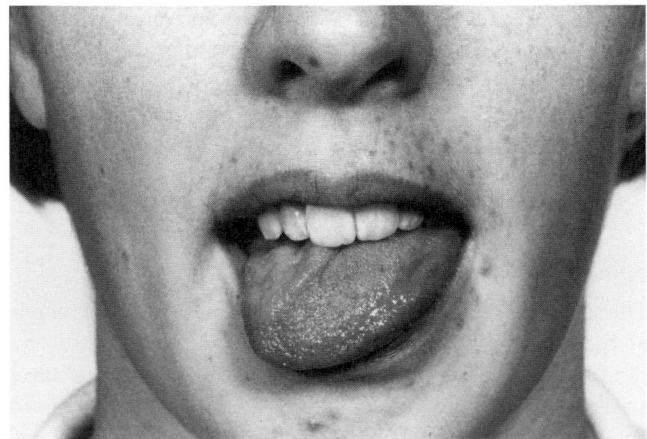

Fig. 11.11. Idiopathic right hypoglossal nerve palsy. Deviation of the protruded tongue to the affected side.

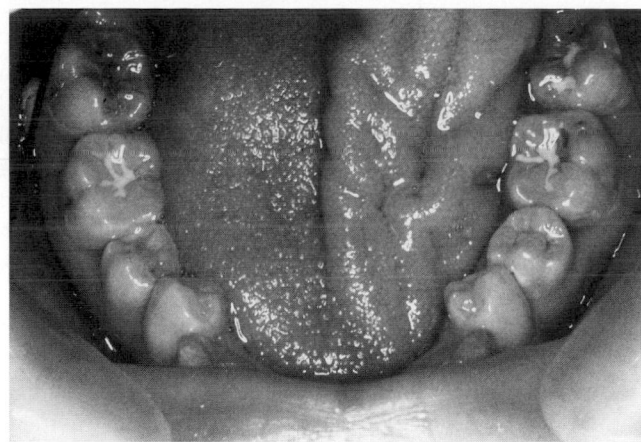

Fig. 11.12. Unilateral tongue wasting in a left hypoglossal nerve palsy. Fur tends to accumulate in the folds (courtesy of Dr M. Donaghy and Oxford University Press).

sides of the tongue with inability to protrude the tongue, marked dysarthria, and mild swallowing difficulties. Such bilateral lesions are rare in isolation and are usually part of the syndrome of bulbar palsy, in which other bulbar muscles are affected and in which there is significant dysphagia. In one large series of cases of hypoglossal nerve palsy, 49 of 100 cases were due to tumour (Keane 1996).

Supranuclear lesions

The nuclei have bilateral cortical representation so that a unilateral upper motor neuron lesion may have no observable effect, although occasionally the tongue may deviate to the contralateral side. Bilateral upper motor neuron involvement is seen as part of the syndrome of pseudobulbar palsy. The tongue is weak, clumsy, and contracted secondary to spasticity, but not wasted. Causes include bilateral hemispheric vascular disease, upper brainstem stroke and tumours, multiple sclerosis, and motor neuron disease.

Nuclear lesions

Unilateral nuclear damage may be caused by tumours or vascular lesions, in both of which cases other structures are usually involved. Thus, a vascular event in the lower medulla might cause a unilateral hypoglossal nerve palsy and contralateral hemiplegia due to corticospinal tract involvement. Bilateral, but sometimes asymmetric, hypoglossal nuclear lesions may result from vascular lesions, tumours, syringobulbia, spinal muscular atrophy, motor neuron disease, and poliomyelitis.

Nerve-trunk lesions

In the posterior fossa the hypoglossal nerve rootlets may be affected, often together with cranial nerves IX, X, and XI, by primary (e.g. glomus jugulare, meningioma) and secondary neoplasms and basal meningitic processes. Unilateral or bilateral palsies may arise as a result of congenital or acquired bony abnormalities around the foramen magnum (basilar impression, Paget's disease).

In the neck, the nerve may be damaged by external trauma, during surgery (including carotid endarterectomy), by tumours, and as a late consequence of radiotherapy to the region. Vascular causes include aberrantly placed arteries, carotid artery dissection, and as a complication of central venous catheterization. As with cranial nerves X and XI, idiopathic cases occur.

11.7 Dysphagia

Difficulty in swallowing (dysphagia) is a common neurological problem and the most important sequelae include aspiration and malnutrition (Wiles 1991). Often it is these complications, particularly aspiration, that first draw the clinician's attention to the possibility of a swallowing disorder. Dysphagia may be due to mechanical factors, upper and lower motor neuron disorders, myasthenic syndromes, and myopathy.

11.7.1 Swallowing mechanisms

A complex sequence of movements, some voluntary but most involuntary or reflex, ensure that food is safely transferred from the outside world to the stomach. Normal swallowing depends upon the integrity of sensory and motor pathways of several cranial nerves: V, VII, IX, X, and XII. These events can be broken down into separate stages. In the first stage food is contained within the mouth, chewed, formed into a bolus, positioned on the tongue, and pushed into the oropharynx. The swallowing reflex is initiated as the bolus passes between the pillars of the fauces. The individual elements of this reflex include elevation of the soft palate (thus preventing nasal regurgitation), elevation of the larynx and closure of the entry to the trachea, and peristaltic propulsion of the bolus through the cricopharyngeal sphincter into the oesophagus. Co-ordinated peristalsis carries the bolus through the lower oesophageal sphincter, into the stomach.

11.7.2 Causes of dysphagia

In neurological practice dysphagia is most often seen in association with other, obvious, neurological problems. Apart from in oculopharyngeal muscular dystrophy, it is relatively rare as a sole presenting symptom, although occasionally this is seen in motor neuron disease, myasthenia gravis, and inclusion-body myositis. Conversely, in general medical practice, there are many mechanical or structural disorders which may have dysphagia as the presenting feature. In some of the disorders listed in Table 11.2, notably motor neuron disease, both upper and lower motor neuron dysfunction may contribute to the dysphagia.

11.7.3 Symptoms

The patient's description of their swallowing problem may give a clear indication as to the level of the problem. Oropharyngeal

Table 11.2. Causes of dysphagia

Anatomical basis	Typical causes
Mechanical	Oropharyngeal or oesophageal tumour
	Goitre
	Anterior cervical osteophytes
	Scleroderma
	Strictures
	Post-surgical
	Hiatus hernia
	Diverticula
Pseudobulbar palsy	Cerebrovascular disease
	Upper brainstem tumours
	Amyotrophic lateral sclerosis (Section 14.2)
	Demyelination (Chapter 14)
Bulbar palsy	Motor neuron disease
	Lower brainstem tumour
	Bilateral medullary infarction
	Syringobulbia (Section 20.6.2)
	Polyneuropathy (Sections 12.10, 12.11, 12.14.4)
	Poliomyelitis (Section 14.5)
Neuromuscular junction disorders	Myasthenia gravis (Section 15.10.1)
Myopathies	Oculopharyngeal muscular dystrophy (Section 15.2.6)
	Inflammatory myopathies (Section 15.7)
	Inclusion-body myositis (Section 15.7.3)
	Myotonic dystrophy (Section 15.3)
Extrapyramidal, cerebellar, and autonomic disorders	Spinocerebellar degenerations (Section 31.2)
	Parkinson's disease (Section 32.3.1)
	Autonomic neuropathies

disorders cause symptoms on swallowing or immediately after—there may be nasal regurgitation, coughing, and choking due to aspiration, a sensation of blockage in the neck, and sometimes pain. With oesophageal problems, symptoms come on a little later and patients locate the site of blockage and discomfort to the lower throat or retrosternal region. As a generalization, obstructive causes of dysphagia, such as oesophageal carcinoma, initially give rise to greater problems with solids than fluids, whereas in neuromuscular disorders dysphagia for fluids may be a relatively early feature.

As noted above, when considering individual cranial nerves, unilateral upper or lower motor lesions generally do not cause major problems with dysphagia, particularly if of gradual onset. An important exception is the dysphagia, sometimes severe, seen transiently following hemispheric stroke. This is a major contributing factor to aspiration pneumonia.

It cannot be overemphasized that aspiration may be silent, without symptoms such as coughing and choking, and without abnormal physical signs on bedside examination. If a patient with a disorder that might cause swallowing problems develops a chest infection then, even in the absence of specific features pointing towards such a problem, further investigation, such as videofluoroscopy, should be performed.

11.7.4 Examination and investigation

More often than not, the history and findings on examination (particularly those related to the lower cranial nerves) will identify the neurological disorder causing the dysphagia, or will at least point to the likely nature of the problem (e.g. a myopathy, neurogenic problem, or upper motor neuron disorder) and thus the direction of further investigations. In patients with mechanical oesophageal problems, physical examination may, of course, be normal.

Endoscopy is of limited value in neurological practice, but of course invaluable when investigating structural disorders of the oesophagus. Videofluoroscopy (essentially a combination of a barium swallow with video-recording, allowing frame-by-frame playback and detailed analysis) is useful in establishing the anatomical level and nature of the dysphagia, but in the neurological setting it is very unlikely to point to a specific diagnosis. However, the results may be of great value in deciding therapeutic approaches and, as noted above, may point towards silent aspiration. Oesophageal manometry remains largely a research tool.

11.7.5 Management

Once dysphagia has been identified as a real or potential problem, the patient should undergo expert evaluation by a clinician and, perhaps particularly, by a speech therapist, prior to any attempt at feeding. Videofluoroscopy may be required. If there is any doubt, it is best to achieve adequate nutrition through the use of a fine-bore nasogastric tube and to reassess swallowing periodically.

If the degree of dysphagia is slight, then the patient may be able to achieve an adequate nutritional intake, safely, by eating food of appropriate consistency, perhaps with the addition of high-energy food supplements. They will require close supervision by a speech therapist and dietitian. With a slightly greater degree of dysphagia, some patients may cope with a combination of nasogastric feeding and limited oral intake. If it is clear that long-term tube feeding will be required, then many patients will prefer to opt for a gastrostomy (performed endoscopically).

Surgery, other than gastrostomy, has a limited role in the management of dysphagia. If it can be shown, by videofluoroscopy, that the dysphagia relates to failure of relaxation of the cricopharyngeal sphincter, then cricopharyngeal myotomy, which is a relatively minor procedure, may be helpful.

Limited studies have shown that the motility stimulant cisapride may benefit some patients but side-effects, particularly excessive bowel motility, are common. Cisapride has recently been withdrawn because of concern about cardiac side-effects. Pyridostigmine appears to help some patients, and there is anecdotal evidence for its use in motor neuron disease. Again, bowel symptoms can be a problem, although they can be counteracted by propantheline or atropine. Anticholinergic drugs may benefit patients with severe dysphagia by reducing saliva production (drooling and choking on their own saliva is common in patients with motor neuron disease). Scopolamine transdermally is convenient to use. It may be difficult to achieve a satisfactory balance, with an excessively dry mouth being an unacceptable outcome. Drooling may also be helped by postural manoeuvres and the use of portable suction apparatus.

Many of the neuromuscular diseases that can lead to severe dysphagia can also cause respiratory failure, so that some patients will also require tracheostomy. Although a cuffed tracheostomy tube offers protection against the consequences of aspiration, it may further impair swallowing because of the restrictive effect it has on laryngeal movement and because it impairs coughing.

References

Adams, C. B. T., Kaye, A. H., and Teddy, P. J. (1982). The treatment of trigeminal neuralgia by posterior fossa microsurgery. *J. Neurol. Neurosurg. Psych.*, **45**, 1020–6.

Barker, F. G., Jannetta, P. J., Bissonette, D. J., *et al.* (1995). Microvascular decompression for hemifacial spasm. *J. Neurosurg.*, **82**, 201–10.

Bauer, C. A. and Coker, N. J. (1996). Update on facial nerve disorders. *Otolaryngol. Clin. North Am.*, **29**, 445–54.

Blau, J. N. and Kapadia, R. (1972). Idiopathic palsy of the recurrent laryngeal nerve: a transient cranial mononeuropathy. *BMJ*, **4**, 259–61.

Breeze, R. and Ignelzi, R. J. (1982). Microvascular decompression for trigeminal neuralgia. *J. Neurosurg.*, **57**, 487–90.

Elston, J. S. (1986). Botulinum toxin treatment of hemifacial spasm. *J. Neurol. Neurosurg. Psych.*, **49**, 827–9.

Forster, C., Brandt, T., Hund, E., *et al.* (1996). Trigeminal sensory neuropathy in connective tissue disease. *Neurology*, **46**, 270–1.

Furukawa, T. (1990). Numb chin syndrome in the elderly. *J. Neurol. Neurosurg. Psych.*, **53**, 173.

Gupta, D. and Vishwakarma, S. K. (1987). Superior orbital fissure syndrome in trigemino-facial zoster. *J. Laryngol. Otol.*, **101**, 975–7.

Hagen, N. A., Stevens, J. C., and Michet, C. J. (1990). Trigeminal sensory neuropathy associated with connective tissue diseases. *Neurology*, **40**, 891–6.

Haines, S. J., Jannetta, P. J., and Zorub, D. S. (1980). Microvascular relations of the trigeminal nerve. *J. Neurosurg.* **52**, 381–6.

Harding, S. P. (1993). Management of ophthalmic zoster. *J. Med. Virol. Suppl.*, **1**, 97–101.

Harding, S. P., Lipton, R. J., and Wells, J. C. D. (1987). Natural history of herpes zoster ophthalmicus: predictors of post-herpetic neuralgia and ocular involvement. *Br. J. Ophthal.*, **71**, 353–8.

Hardy, D. G. (1991). Trigeminal neuralgia. In *Clinical neurology*, (ed. M. Swash and J. Oxbury), pp. 364–70. Churchill Livingstone, Edinburgh.

Hauser, W. A., Karnes, W. E., Annis, J., and Kurland, L. T. (1971). Incidence and prognosis of Bell's palsy in the population of Rochester, Minnesota. *Mayo Clin. Proc.*, **46**, 258–64.

Horton, J., Means, E. D., Cunningham, T. J., and Olson, K. B. (1973). The numb chin in breast cancer. *J. Neurol. Neurosurg. Psych.*, **36**, 211–16.

Jacobson, R. R. and Ross-Russell, R. W. (1979). Glossopharyngeal neuralgia with cardiac arrhythmia: a rare but treatable form of syncope. *BMJ*, **1**, 379–80.

Jannetta, P. J. (1977). Treatment of trigeminal neuralgia by suboccipital and transtentorial cranial operations. *Clin. Neurosurg.*, **24**, 538–49.

Kaye, A. H. and Adams, C. B. T. (1981). Hemifacial spasm: a long term follow-up of patients treated by posterior fossa surgery and facial nerve wrapping. *J. Neurol. Neurosurg. Psych.*, **44**, 1100–3.

Keane, J. R. (1996). Twelfth-nerve palsy. Analysis of 100 cases. *Arch. Neurol.*, **53**, 561–6.

Laha, R. K. and Jannetta, P. J. (1977). Glossopharyngeal neuralgia. *J. Neurosurg.*, **47**, 316–20.

Lecky, B. R. F., Hughes, R. A. C., and Murray, N. M. F. (1987). Trigeminal sensory neuropathy. *Brain*, **110**, 1463–85.

Linnemann, C. C. and Alvira, M. M. (1980). Pathogenesis of varicella-zoster angiitis in the CNS. *Arch. Neurol.*, **37**, 239–40.

Loeser, J. D. (1978). What to do about tic douloureux. *JAMA*, **239**, 1153–5.

Lossos, A. and Siegal, T. (1992). Numb chin syndrome in cancer patients. *Neurology*, **42**, 1181–4.

Marsh, R. J. and Cooper, M. (1993). Ophthalmic herpes zoster. *Eye*, **7**, 350–70.

Matthews, W. B. (1982). Treatment of Bell's palsy. In: Recent advances in clinical neurology, Vol. 3, (ed. W. B. Matthews and G. H. Glaser), pp. 239–48. Churchill Livingstone, Edinburgh.

Morgan, M., Moffat, M., Ritchie, L. *et al.* (1995). Is Bell's palsy a reactivation of varicella zoster virus? *J. Infect.*, **30**, 29–36.

Sweeney, P. J. and Wilbourn, A. J. (1992). Spinal accessory (11th) nerve palsy following carotid endarterectomy. *Neurology*, **42**, 674–5.

Sweet, W. H. and Wepsic, J. G. (1974). Controlled thermocoagulation of trigeminal ganglion and rootlets for differential destruction of pain fibres. *J. Neurosurg.*, **40**, 143–56.

Taha, J. M. and Tew, J. M. (1996). Comparison of surgical treatments for trigeminal neuralgia. *Neurosurgery*, **38**, 865–71.

Watson, C. P. (1995). The treatment of postherpetic neuralgia. *Neurology*, **45**, (Suppl. 8), S58–60.

Wiles, C. M. (1991). Neurogenic dysphagia. *J. Neurol. Neurosurg. Psych.*, **54**, 1037–9.

Womack, L. W. and Liesegang, T. J. (1983). Complication of herpes zoster ophthalmicus. *Arch. Ophthal.*, **101**, 42–5.

CHAPTER 12

Polyneuropathy

Michael Donaghy

12.1 **Diagnosis of polyneuropathy**

Peripheral neuropathy has a multitude of causes, many of which can be diagnosed simply by careful clinical and electro-physiological evaluation. A fundamental distinction should be made between polyneuropathy, which is a generalized neuropathy affecting all peripheral nerve fibres, and focal neuropathy, which affects individual peripheral nerves either singly or multiply. Recognized causes of (multi)focal peripheral neuropathy are listed in Table 13.1. In focal neuropathy the muscle wasting and weakness, reflex loss, and sensory disturbance are restricted to the territories of the affected peripheral nerve(s) or root(s). Occasionally widespread vasculitic involvement of the peripheral nervous system may produce a clinical picture resembling symmetrical polyneuropathy, rather than the multiple mononeuropathies more usually associated with vasculitis.

12.1.1 **Clinical features**

Typically polyneuropathy will cause the combination of distal limb muscle weakness, loss of tendon reflexes, and reduced distal limb sensation. There is variable loss of the autonomic innervation, causing a dry, vasodilated foot or hand. Loss of tendon reflexes is a cardinal sign of polyneuropathy, often restricted to the ankle jerks in axonal degeneration, but involving more proximal reflexes in demyelinating neuropathies affecting more proximal segments or the nerve roots. Clinical features suggestive of demyelinating or conduction block polyneuropathy include:

(1) a relative lack of muscle wasting in relation to the degree of weakness, because no denervation has occurred;

(2) weakness of proximal muscles as well as distal, because of nerve root involvement; and

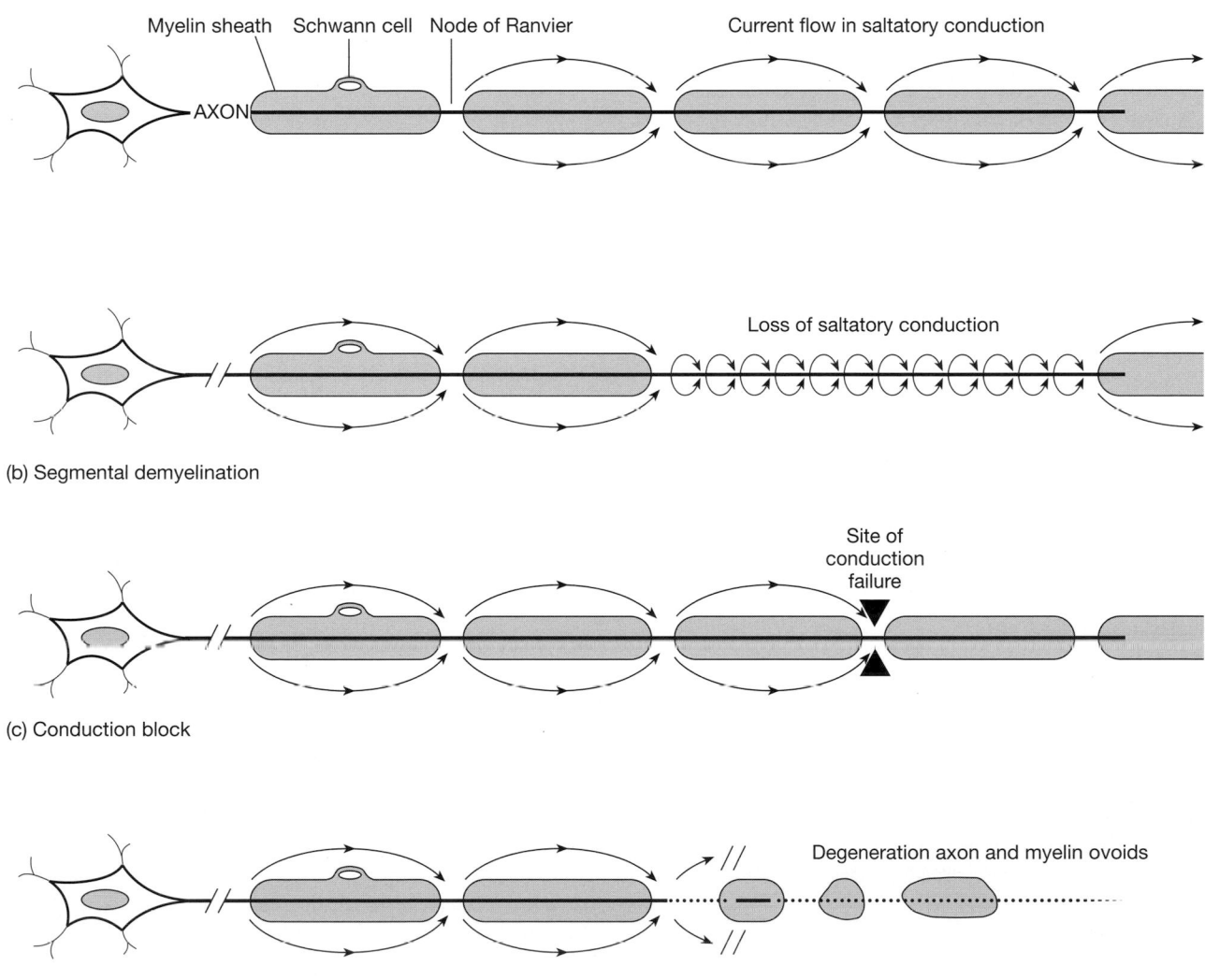

Fig. 12.1. Schematic illustration of axonal impulse conduction in (a) normal axon, (b) segmental demyelination after repopulation of the demyelinated segment of axon with sodium channels, (c) conduction block due to a local blocking factor or acute segmental demyelination, and (d) Wallerian axonal degeneration.

(3) disproportionate loss of joint position and vibration sensations compared to relative preservation of pain and temperature sensations which are carried by unmyelinated fibres.

Nerve-conduction velocity measurements and electromyography (Section 2.5) should be used to distinguish between primarily demyelinating, axonal degeneration, or conduction block polyneuropathies (Fig. 12.1). Nerve-conduction studies in demyelinating polyneuropathy show prolonged distal motor latencies, slowed motor conduction velocities, and prolonged F-wave latencies. Evidence of conduction block is particularly likely in acquired forms of demyelinating polyneuropathy. Demyelinating polyneuropathies generally hold a better prospect for recovery than axonal degeneration polyneuropathies. Causes of demyelinating polyneuropathy are shown in Table 12.1.

Inherited polyneuropathy usually holds a poor prospect for recovery and other family members may require genetic counselling. Inherited polyneuropathy must be considered if there is a family history of neuropathy or parental consanguinity. Compared to acquired polyneuropathy, it tends to evolve slowly, and even marked degrees of weakness may not excite complaint by the patient. Positive sensory symptoms, such as paraesthesiae, spontaneous pains, or thermal sensations, suggest an acquired neuropathy, although they do occur in the polyneuropathy of the inherited metabolic disorders metachromatic leucodystrophy and Fabry disease. Often the suspicion of an inherited basis for a patient's polyneuropathy can only be confirmed by clinical or electrophysiological examination of relatives or molecular genetic studies.

Table 12.1. Causes of demyelinating polyneuropathy

Inherited
  Hereditary motor and sensory neuropathy type I (12.4.2)
  Hereditary motor and sensory neuropathy type III (Dejerine–Sottas disease) (12.4.4)
  Hereditary neuropathy with liability to pressure palsies (12.5)
  Adrenoleucodystrophy (12.8.4)
  Krabbe's disease (12.8.3)
  Leigh's disease (12.8.10)
  Metachromatic leucodystrophy (12.8.2)
  Refsum disease (phytanic acid accumulation) (12.8.1)

Acquired
  Guillain–Barré syndrome (12.10.1)
  Chronic inflammatory demyelinating neuropathy (12.11.1)
  Multifocal motor neuropathy with conduction block (12.11.3)
  Pure motor demyelinating neuropathy (12.11.4)
  Neuropathies associated with lymphoproliferative disorders (12.12) or carcinoma (12.13)
  Diphtheria (12.14.4)

Toxic
  Amiodarone neuropathy (12.18.3)
  Perhexiline neuropathy (12.18.19)
  Hexacarbon neuropathy (12.20.6)

These are discussed in the sections indicated in parentheses.

Table 12.2. Causes of sensory peripheral neuropathy

Inherited
  Hereditary sensory and autonomic neuropathies (12.6)
  Anderson–Fabry disease (12.8.5)
  Tangier disease (12.8.7)
  Familial amyloidosis (12.9.1)

Acquired
  Acute sensory neuropathy (12.10.3)
  Chronic idiopathic sensory (ataxic) neuropathy (12.11.5)
  Sjögren's syndrome (12.13.1)
  Primary amyloidosis (12.9.2)
  Paraneoplastic sensory neuropathy (12.13.1)
  Acquired immune deficiency syndrome (late) (12.14.2)
  Leprosy (12.14.1)
  Lyme disease (*Borrelia* infection) (12.14.3)
  Sensory perineuritis (12.16.1)
  Migrant sensory neuritis of Wartenberg (12.16.2)
  Diabetes mellitus (12.17.1)
  Vitamin B_{12} deficiency (12.21.3)
  Vitamin E deficiency (12.21.4)

Toxic
  Almitrine (12.18.2)
  Cisplatin (12.18.5)
  Didanosine (12.18.9)
  Metronidazole (12.18.16)
  Misonidazole (12.18.17)

These are discussed in the sections indicated in parentheses.

Neuropathies purely or predominantly involving sensory fibres are shown in Table 12.2. Some purely *sensory neuropathies* spare large myelinated fibres, only affecting unmyelinated and small myelinated fibres. In such cases tendon reflexes are preserved and sensory nerve conduction is normal. However, there is usually associated dysfunction of unmyelinated autonomic fibres, with postural hypotension and dry, red feet.

Purely or predominantly *motor neuropathies* are detailed in Table 12.3.

Ageing: after the age of 65, an increasing proportion of asymptomatic people without neuropathic risk factors have unobtainable ankle jerks or loss of vibration sense from the feet, and a few have more extensive abnormalities, such as mild distal muscle weakness (Bouche *et al.* 1993). Such features cannot be taken as sole evidence for peripheral-nerve disease in the elderly and merely reflect the natural age-related loss of peripheral-nerve axons (Jacobs and Love 1985).

Table 12.3. Causes of motor peripheral neuropathy

Hereditary motor and sensory neuropathy (some patients) (12.4)
Porphyric neuropathy (12.8.6)
Guillain–Barré syndrome (12.10.1)
Acute motor axonal neuropathy (12.10.2)
Multifocal motor neuropathy with conduction block (12.11.3)
Pure motor demyelinating neuropathy (12.11.4)
Diphtheria (12.14.4)
Dapsone (12.18.8)
Lead poisoning (12.19.2)
Organophosphate poisoning (12.20.8)

These are discussed in the sections indicated in parentheses.

12.2 Nerve biopsy

Biopsy of peripheral nerves makes a major diagnostic impact only in a small selected group of patients with peripheral neuropathy (Gabriel *et al.* 2000). It is of particular use in those patients suspected of suffering from the treatable conditions of vasculitic or leprous neuropathy, or sensory perineuritis. It may establish the diagnosis in rare conditions such as giant axonal neuropathy or neuroaxonal dystrophy. Traditionally nerve biopsy has been used to demonstrate amyloidosis, but rectal biopsy is similarly sensitive and less invasive. Hereditary pressure-sensitive (tomaculous) neuropathy is diagnosable by nerve biopsy, but this is being replaced by molecular genetic tests. Views vary as to the role of nerve biopsy in establishing a diagnosis of acute or chronic

inflammatory demyelinating polyneuropathy. Occasionally in these conditions, examination of teased nerve fibres may show segmental demyelination in suspected cases where motor-nerve conduction velocities are insufficiently slow to be diagnostic.

The nerve most commonly chosen for biopsy is the sural nerve at the ankle, less commonly the radial nerve at the wrist or the superficial peroneal nerve in the calf. The biopsy is carried out under local anaesthesia. Some favour fascicular, rather than full-thickness nerve biopsy, on the grounds that it leaves less residual sensory deficit. However, comparison of the long-term outcome of fascicular and full-thickness nerve biopsies shows no differences in the degree of subsequent sensory loss or dysaesthetic pain (Pollock *et al.* 1983a). Full-thickness biopsy is advisable if vasculitis is suspected, so as to permit

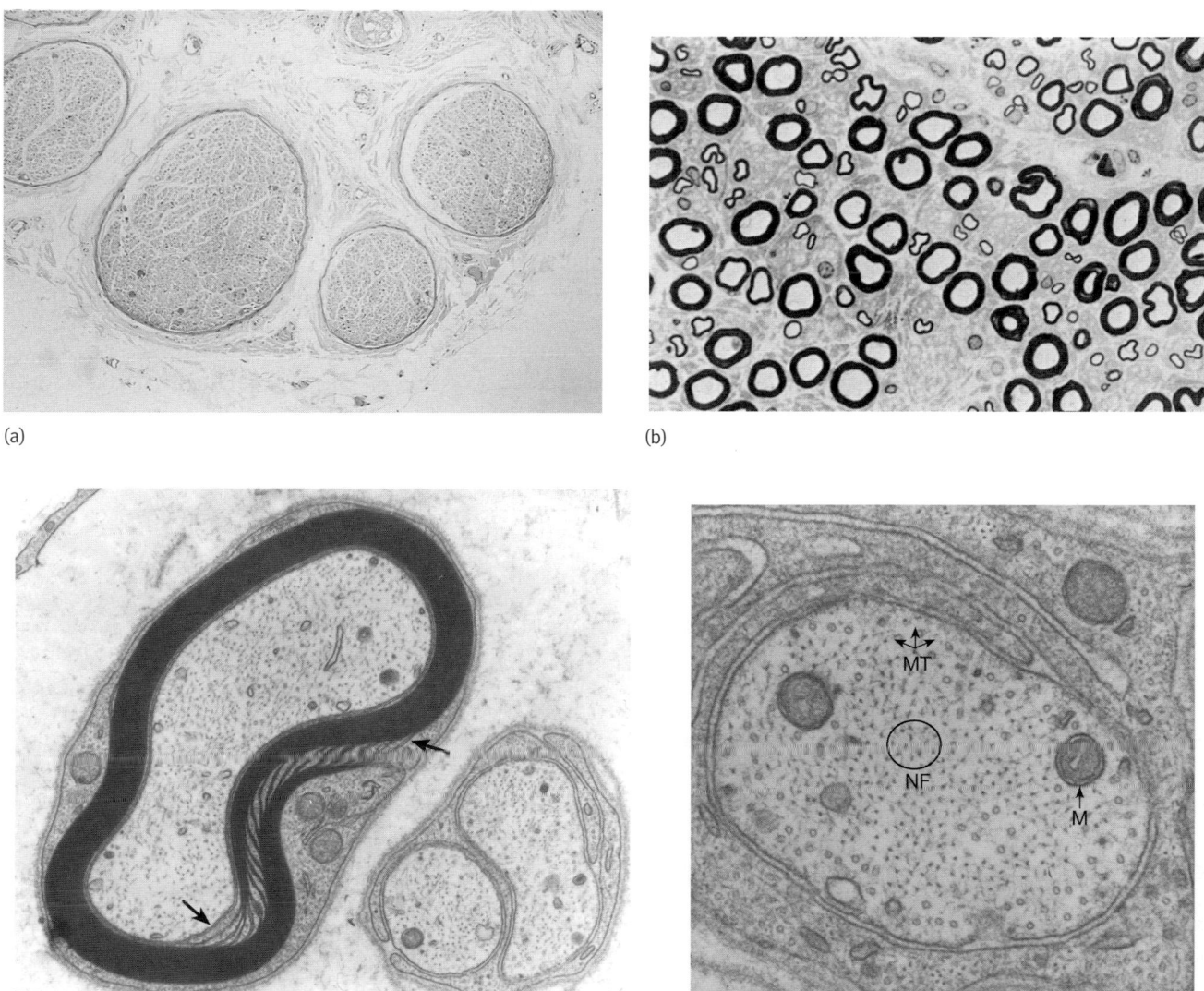

(a)

(b)

(c)

(d)

Fig. 12.2. Transverse sections of a peripheral nerve: (a) low-power section (light microscopy) of a complete nerve showing the fascicular organization and epineurial blood vessels; (b) higher power, showing the myelinated axons and endoneurial cells (light microscopy, semi-thin section, toluidine blue stain); (c) electron microscopy of a myelinated fibre from a 3 month old infant showing a Schmidt–Lanterman incisure in the myelin sheath (arrowed); (d) electron microscopy of an unmyelinated nerve fibre showing the intra-axonal microtubules (MT), neurofilaments (NF) and mitochondria (M). ((a) Courtesy of Professor M. Esiri; (b) from Jacobs and Love (1985), by permission of S. Love; (c) and (d) courtesy of Dr R. King.)

inspection of the maximum number of epineurial blood vessels. The most common complications of nerve biopsy are failure of wound healing, or infection, particularly in patients receiving steroid therapy. Significant pain or paraesthesiae attributable to the biopsy occur in less than 10 per cent of patients after 1 year.

The specimen should be processed immediately by a laboratory experienced in peripheral-nerve pathology. It should be divided to provide material for paraffin embedding, and for glutaraldehyde and osmium tetroxide fixation for single nerve fibre teasing, and for electron and light microscopy on 1 mm plastic-embedded sections; additional material may be frozen for immunofluorescent studies (Fig. 12.2). Morphometric analysis may be required to reveal subtle differences in the density of myelinated or unmyelinated fibres, or alterations in the fibre size distribution; this process is time-consuming and technically demanding. Control morphometric values have been established for a wide age range (Jacobs and Love 1985), and the characteristic pathological changes in a wide variety of diseases (Richardson and De Girolami 1995) will be referred to in the following sections.

Quantitative assessment of immunohistochemically stained epidermal nerve fibres in small punch biopsies of skin is a valuable development in assessing small unmyelinated fibre involvement in neuropathies. This technique seems more sensitive than morphometry of sural nerve biopsies, is less technically complex, and detects unmyelinated fibre involvement in a wide range of polyneuropathies involving sensory fibres (Herrmann *et al.* 1999). Skin biopsy provides a repeatable tool for assessing progression of neuropathy or the effects of treatments. It can demonstrate loss of nerve fibres in those oft-encountered patients with painful burning feet, in whom conventional clinical examination, nerve-conduction studies, and sural nerve biopsy fail to reveal abnormalities (Periquet *et al.* 1999).

12.3 Treatment of polyneuropathy

12.3.1 General principles

Accurate diagnosis of the cause is essential to ensure that correct therapy is provided for certain conditions, e.g. immunosuppression for vasculitic neuropathy and chronic inflammatory demyelinating neuropathy; intravenous immunoglobulin for multifocal motor neuropathy with conduction block; plasma exchange or intravenous immunoglobulin for the Guillain–Barré syndrome; cessation of toxic exposure to chemicals, drugs, or alcohol; vitamin replacement; diet modification in Refsum disease; and surgical release of peripheral-nerve compression. Hence, some general principles underlying treatment will be considered before detailed description of the different varieties of peripheral-nerve disease.

Physiotherapy is important to prevent muscle contractures and keep joints mobile, so that when regeneration of nerve fibres occurs, the limb may be in the best possible condition to profit by the return of nervous function. In the past, firm splinting was commonly employed in order to keep a paralysed muscle in a relaxed position and to preclude movement which

Table 12.4. Total neuropathy score (reproduced from Cornblath *et al.* 1999, with permission)

Parameter	Score				
	0	1	2	3	4
Sensory symptoms	None	Symptoms limited to fingers or toes	Symptoms extend to ankle or wrist	Symptoms extend to knee or elbow	Symptoms above knees or elbows, or functionally disabling
Motor symptoms	None	Slight difficulty	Moderate difficulty	Require help/assistance	Paralysis
Autonomic symptoms, *n*	0	1	2	3	4 or 5
Pin sensibility	Normal	Reduced in fingers/toes	Reduced up to wrist/ankle	Reduced up to elbow/knee	Reduced to above elbow/knee
Vibration sensibility	Normal	Reduced in fingers/toes	Reduced up to wrist/ankle	Reduced up to elbow/knee	Reduced to above elbow/knee
Strength	Normal	Mild weakness	Moderate weakness	Severe weakness	Paralysis
Tendon reflexes	Normal	Ankle reflex reduced	Ankle reflex absent	Ankle reflex absent, others reduced	All reflexes absent
Vibration sensation (QST vibration)	Normal to 125% ULN	126–150% ULN	151–200% ULN	201–300% ULN	>300% ULN
Sural amplitude	Normal/reduced to <5% LLN	76–95% of LLN	51–75% of LLN	26–50% of LLN	0–25% of LLN
Peroneal amplitude	Normal/reduced to <5% LLN	76–95% of LLN	51–75% of LLN	26–50% of LLN	0–25% of LLN

QST = quantitative sensory test; ULN = upper limit of normal; LLN = lower limit of normal.

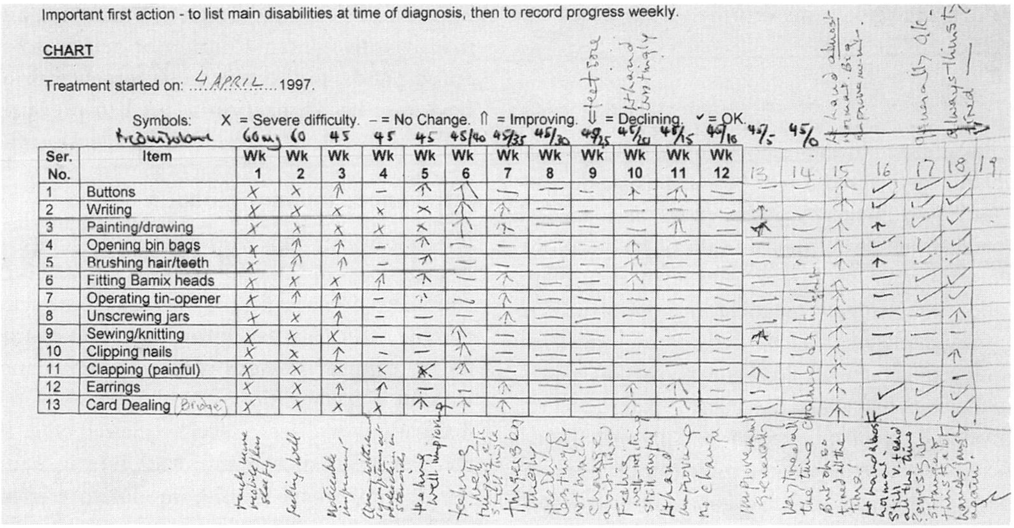
Important first action - to list main disabilities at time of diagnosis, then to record progress weekly.

CHART

Treatment started on: 4 APRIL 1997.

Symbols: X = Severe difficulty. – = No Change. ⇑ = Improving. ⇓ = Declining. ✓ = OK.

Ser. No.	Item	Wk 1	Wk 2	Wk 3	Wk 4	Wk 5	Wk 6	Wk 7	Wk 8	Wk 9	Wk 10	Wk 11	Wk 12
	Prednisolone	60mg	60	45	45	45	45/40	45/35	45/30	45/25	45/20	45/15	45/10
1	Buttons	X	X	↑	–	↑	↑	–	–	–	↑	↑	–
2	Writing	X	X	X	X	X	↑	↑	–	–	–	–	–
3	Painting/drawing	X	X	X	X	X	↑	↑	–	–	–	↑	–
4	Opening bin bags	X	↑	↑	–	↑	–	–	–	–	↑	–	–
5	Brushing hair/teeth	X	↑	↑	–	↑	–	–	–	–	↑	–	–
6	Fitting Bamix heads	X	X	X	↑	↑	–	↑	–	–	↑	–	–
7	Operating tin-opener	X	↑	↑	–	↑	–	↑	–	–	–	–	–
8	Unscrewing jars	X	X	↑	–	–	–	↑	–	–	–	–	–
9	Sewing/knitting	X	X	X	–	–	↑	–	–	–	–	–	–
10	Clipping nails	X	X	↑	–	–	↑	–	–	–	–	–	–
11	Clapping (painful)	X	X	X	X	X	↑	–	–	–	–	–	–
12	Earrings	X	X	↑	↑	–	–	↑	–	–	↑	↑	–
13	Card Dealing (Bridge)	X	X	X	X	↑	↑	↑	–	–	↑	↑	–

Fig. 12.3. The diary of a patient with chronic inflammatory demyelinating neuropathy, showing improving weekly performance on a variety of useful everyday tasks when treated with prednisolone.

was thought to promote contracture of antagonists. Seddon (1975) reviewed the objective evidence in detail and concluded that except in cases of Erb's paralysis, when the arm should be splinted at the shoulder in a position of abduction and external rotation, splinting generally has little to commend it, as immobilized muscles tend to atrophy and become fibrotic more quickly.

12.3.2 **Assessing recovery**

The advent of effective therapies for disabling neuropathies brings the need for reliable assessment of recovery. This is useful both for formal clinical trials of treatments and for assessing effectiveness of a trial of treatment in an individual patient. In general, the recent trend has been to regard estimates of functional ability, such as walking, as more reliable and useful than quantification of physical signs, such as strength of individual muscles. When assessing an individual's response to treatment, a set of measurements relevant to that patient's disability should be drawn up and measured pre- and post-treatment, paying particular attention to those which signify improvement of use in everyday life.

Various quantitative measures of the neurological examination can be undertaken. Muscle strength can be graded using the MRC scale: Grade 0 = no contraction, Grade 1 = flicker of contraction, Grade 2 = active movement with gravity eliminated, Grade 3 = active movement against gravity, Grade 4 = active movement against gravity and resistance, Grade 5 = normal power (Guarantors of Brain 1986). However, this MRC grading is relatively unreliable and unreproducible for the majority of neuropathies encountered in a civilian and non-surgical practice, in which most weakness is either grade 3 or 4. Nerve-conduction studies can be quantified, particularly the velocity of motor conduction, the degree of block of motor conduction, or the amplitude of sensory nerve action potentials. However, such neurophysiological measures often shown surprisingly little improvement, even with clear-cut clinical improvement in conditions such as demyelinating neuropathy. Quantitative sensory testing devices have been developed, particularly for vibration and thermal sensation. The most recent proposal to integrate various clinical and electrophysiological parameters is the total neuropathy score, shown in Table 12.4 (Cornblath *et al.* 1999).

In many circumstances a restricted set of measures can provide reliable evidence of improvement. For instance regaining the ability to heel–toe walk, stand on tiptoe, or perform Romberg's test provide clear-cut and reproducible evidence. Measurement of outstretched arm times, peg-sorting tasks, stair-climbing speed, or walking speed is also reliable unless you suspect that psychological factors may influence the patient's performance. It is useful for patients to monitor treatment against a variety of everyday tasks (Fig. 12.3). Overall motor function can be quantified in acute neuropathies such as Guillain–Barré syndrome using a simple scale, assessable by telephone if need be: disability grade 0 = healthy, no signs or symptoms, Grade 1 = minor symptoms or signs and able to run, Grade 2 = able to walk 5 m without assistance, Grade 3 = able to walk 5 m with assistance or sticks, Grade 4 = chair- or bed-bound, Grade 5 = requiring assisted ventilation (Plasma Exchange/Sandoglobulin Guillain–Barré syndrome Trial Group 1997). Similar criteria can be applied to other clinical situations.

12.3.3 **Immunomodulation**

Immunomodulatory treatments are used successfully in a range of acquired neurological diseases, including acute idiopathic polyneuritis (Section 12.10), chronic idiopathic polyneuropathies (Section 12.11), neuropathies associated with lymphoproliferative disorders (Section 12.12), vasculitic neuropathy (Section 12.15), central nervous system vasculitic and collagen vascular disorders (Chapter 28), multiple sclerosis (Section 29.4.7), inflammatory myopathy (Section 15.7), myasthenias (Section 15.10), and cranial arteritis (Section 3.7.3). Although detailed discussion of these immunomodulatory treatments and their side-effects lies outside the scope of this book, knowledge of important general principles is necessary for managing these diseases.

Steroids

Steroids are given as oral prednisolone for chronic maintenance treatment, intravenous methylprednisolone for acute disorders, or dexamethasone for raised intracranial pressure. Consideration should be given to alternate-day administration of prednisolone in neuromuscular disorders requiring long-term treatment. Increased susceptibility to infections, including opportunistic organisms, is a significant risk, particularly with long-term therapy. Steroid-induced diabetes mellitus, or exacerbation of previously controlled diabetes, may occur. Steroid myopathy (Section 15.8.1) may occur with long-term therapy, especially with fluorinated steroids such as dexamethasone. Steroids can produce, or exacerbate, psychiatric conditions such as paranoia or depression. To offset the osteoporosis induced by chronic steroid therapy, prophylactic therapy with a biphosphonate or a calcitriol should be given from the outset, and hormone replacement therapy considered in post-menopausal women.

Azathioprine

Azathioprine is often used as a steroid-sparing treatment when long-term immunosuppression is required. It, too, increases susceptibility to infection, mediated at least in part by leuco-penia related to dose-related bone-marrow suppression. Hypersensitivity reactions, often involving abdominal pain and abnormal liver function tests, are not uncommon and necessitate permanent withdrawal. Regular full blood count and liver function testing are required; weekly for the first 4–8 weeks of therapy, and 3-monthly thereafter. Although the question of azathioprine causing lymphoproliferative disorders has been raised, especially in the setting of renal transplantation, there is no evidence of this complication when it is used in neurological disorders (Amato et al. 1993). Some female patients may wish to continue azathioprine during pregnancy so as to avoid deterioration in their neurological disorder. If so, they should be advised that although there are occasional reports of chromosomal abnormalities and neonatal haematological disorders, the teratogenic risk is generally considered small to minimal, and that the vast majority of such pregnancies end happily.

Cyclophosphamide

Cyclophosphamide is used in vasculitis and may be given either orally or pulsed intravenously. Susceptibility to infection is the chief early side-effect and the full blood count should be monitored closely for dose-related bone-marrow suppression. Simultaneous administration of mesna helps avoid haemorrhagic cystitis, and it should be noted that cyclophosphamide greatly increases the risk of future bladder cancer.

Plasma exchange

Plasma exchange is generally carried out by centrifugal or filtration methods, generally for 5 days, exchanging 50 ml plasma/kg body weight at each exchange. The rationale is removal of pathogenic antibodies in the plasma fraction, and replacement is usually with human albumin or gelatin solutions. In experienced hands, the technique is largely free of complications. Low-dose heparinization is used to prevent thrombosis and embolization from the indwelling venous catheter.

Intravenous immunoglobulin

Intravenous immunoglobulin (IvIg) therapy is generally given in high doses of 0.4 g/kg body weight/day for 5 days. Repeated administration every 6–10 weeks is required in the treatment of chronic neuropathies. Domiciliary administration may use different regimes, provides effective maintenance administration without hospitalization, and avoids loss of time from work or fluctuations in disease severity (Sewell et al. 1997). The precise mechanism(s) of the action of IvIg in neurological disease remains unknown; immunomodulatory effects, anti-idiotypic antibodies, cytokine alterations, and direct effects on conduction block or remyelination are all possibilities (Stangel et al. 1999). Significant side-effects are unusual, although 5 per cent may experience mild, self-limited reactions of headache, myalgia, fever, rash, or vasomotor reactions, which are generally controllable by varying the infusion rate or by using antihistamines (van der Meché and van Doorn 1997). IgA-deficient patients may develop anaphylactic reactions. Rarely self-limited aseptic meningitis similar to that with OKT3 monoclonal antibodies (Section 5.6.1), viscosity-induced thromboembolic events, acute oligutic renal failure, or haemolytic anaemia have occurred. Naturally patients will be concerned about possible transmission of infections by IvIg; no case of HIV infection has been described, and the solvent detergent step currently employed in purification inactivates HIV and hepatitis viruses.

12.4 Hereditary motor and sensory neuropathy

Hereditary motor and sensory neuropathy (HMSN) is the most common cause of the peroneal muscular atrophy syndrome of distal leg muscle wasting and weakness, usually accompanied by pes cavus foot deformity (Figs 12.4 and 12.5). It is also known as peroneal muscular atrophy, Charcot–Marie–Tooth disease (CMT), hereditary hypertrophic neuropathy, Roussy–Lévy syndrome, and Dejerine–Sottas disease. HMSN comprises a range of demyelinating and axonal loss neuropathies with various patterns of inheritance. Patients generally present in childhood or adolescence, but symptoms may become evident at any age from birth to senescence. Asymptomatic, yet affected, elderly relatives may be identified. In the two most common forms of HMSN, types I and II, it is males who are more likely to be symptomatic and severely affected, whereas females are more often asymptomatic (Harding and Thomas 1980b). The presenting symptoms are usually difficulty in walking or foot deformity. Positive sensory symptoms, such as paraesthesiae, would make the diagnosis of HMSN unlikely and should suggest an acquired neuropathy. Occasionally HMSN is associ-

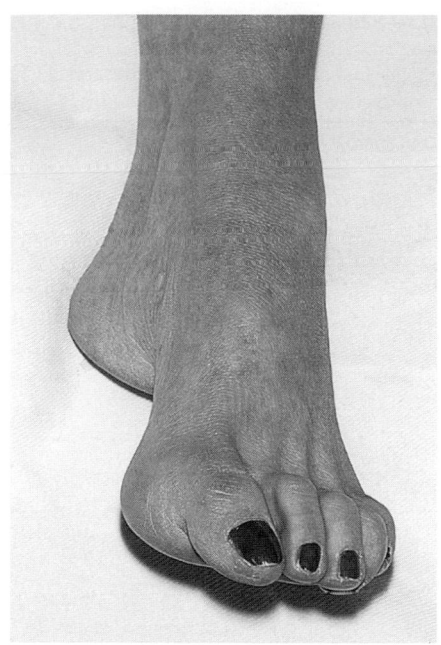

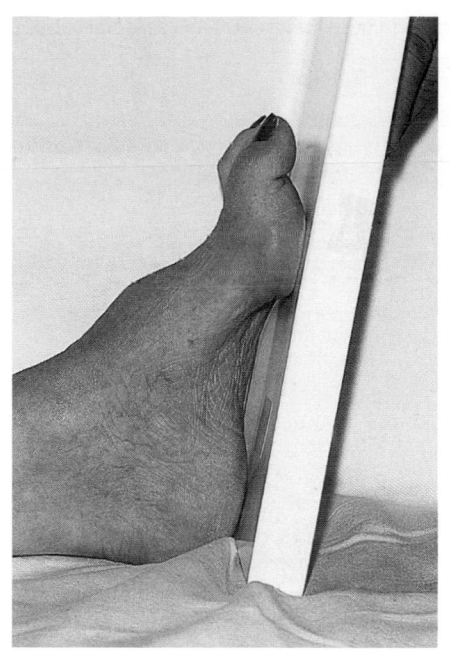

(a)   (b)

Fig. 12.4. Pes cavus in hereditary motor and sensory neuropathy. (a) The hammer toe deformity. (b) A defining feature of pes cavus is the ability to see daylight through the foot arch when the sole is placed against a flat surface.

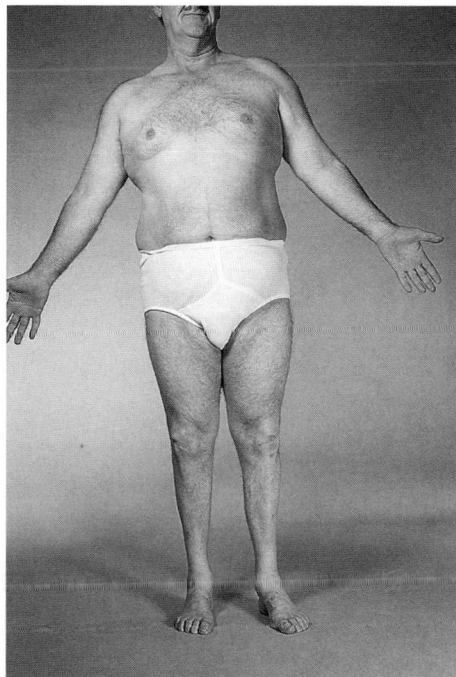

Fig. 12.5. Peroneal muscular atrophy in hereditary motor and sensory neuropathy, showing the typical 'inverted champagne bottle' appearance of the legs due to muscle wasting below the knees.

ated with other neurological features, such as spastic paraparesis, optic atrophy, pigmentary retinal degeneration, deafness, or mental retardation, or the dysmorphic Noonan syndrome (Frith *et al.* 1994; Silburn *et al.* 1998; Stojkovic *et al.* 1999).

HMSN can be classified either on a clinical and electrophysiological basis into types I–V, or on the basis of identified molecular genetic abnormalities. Correlation between these two classification systems is increasingly incomplete. In general, the most common form, autosomal dominantly inherited HMSN IA, is associated with 17p11.2 reduplications, and sex-linked recessive forms of HMSN I are associated with various mutations of connexin-32. The traditional clinical classification has consisted of types I (adult-onset demyelinating), type II (adult-onset axonal), type III (Dejerine–Sottas disease; infantile or childhood onset), type IV (Refsum disease; phytanic acid accumulation), type V (HMSN with other nervous system involvement) (Dyck *et al.* 1993*a*). Currently, this classification mainly finds practical utility in the electrophysiological differentiation of types I (demyelinating) and II (axonal) forms of the disorder. However, there are increasingly extensive subclassifications and overlaps of these two types, often correlating with newly described mutations or linkage loci.

HMSN should be distinguished from hereditary distal spinal muscular atrophy (Section 14.3.4), the other common cause of the peroneal muscular atrophy syndrome (Meadows and Marsden 1969). Patients with spinal muscular atrophy are less likely to have upper limb weakness, their tendon reflexes are relatively preserved, the sensory examination is normal, and the sensory-nerve action potentials are normal (Harding and Thomas 1980*a*). Symptoms of distal spinal muscular atrophy usually start in childhood, although onset as late as 60 years has been recorded. Both autosomal dominant and recessive forms occur, the former tending to present earlier in life. The condition rarely produces overwhelming disability.

12.4.1 **Molecular genetic abnormalities**

An ever-widening range of genetic abnormalities (Table 12.5) underlies the various forms of hereditary motor and sensory neuropathy (Nelis *et al.* 1999). Some are used for routine diag-

Table 12.5. Identified genetic abnormalities in hereditary motor and sensory neuropathy (HMSN) (see Nelis *et al.* 1999 and Section 12.4.1)

Gene	Locus	Mutation	Mode of inheritance	Usual clinical picture	Other described phenotypes
PMP22 (peripheral myelin protein 22)	17p11.2	Duplication	AD	HMSN IA	
		Deletion	AD	HNPP	
		Point mutations	AR, AD		HNPP DSS HMSNIA
MPZ (myelin protein Po)	1q 22–23	Point mutations/polymorphisms	AD	HMSN IB	HMSN II DSS CH CIDP
NDRG1 (*N-myc* downstream regulated gene 1)	8q24.3	?	AR	HMSN I+ deafness (LOM)	
Cx-32 (connexin-32)	Xq13.1	Point mutations Deletions	XR	HMSN I	HMSN II Deafness
EGR (early growth response 2)	10q21.1–22.1	Point mutations	AD AR	HMSN I	CH
?	5q23–33	?	AR	HMSN I	
?	1p35–36	?	AD	HMSN IIA	
?	3q13–22	?	AD	HMSN IIB	
?	?	?	AD	HMSN IIC	
?	7p14	?	AD	HMSN IID	
-NF-L (neurofilament light chain)	8p21	Point mutation	AD	HMSN IIE + hypekeratosis	–
?	X	?	XR	HMSN II	

AD, autosomal dominant; AR, autosomal recessive; CH, congenital hypomyelination; CIDP, chronic inflammatory demyelinating polyneuropathy; DSS, Dejerine–Sottas syndrome; HNPP, hereditary liability to pressure palsies; XR, X-linked recessive.

nostic testing: the 17p11.2 duplication, and mutations of the myelin protein P0 and connexin-32 genes. Distinctive clinical and electrophysiological syndromes generally characterize the most common mutations of particular genes. However, this is not always the case, which has led to some blurring of the distinction between HMSN I, HMSN II, and HMSN III as separate clinical and electrophysiological syndromes.

PMP 22

Seventy per cent of HMSN I (type IA) is associated with a duplication of the gene for peripheral myelin protein 22 (*PMP22*) on chromosome 17 due to unequal crossover during meiosis, particularly on the father's side. This same myelin protein gene is affected by a mutation in the hypomyelinating *Trembler* mouse mutant (Timmerman *et al.* 1992) and is deleted in hereditary liability to pressure palsies (Section 12.5), a condition of hypermyclination (Lenssen *et al.* 1998). Thus increased copies of the *PMP22* gene are associated with decreased growth of the myelin spiral. Unsurprisingly, the HMSN Ia phenotype occurs in Down syndrome trisomy 17 (Chance *et al.* 1992).

Po

The myelin protein P0 (MPZ) gene is an adhesive protein responsible for compaction of the myelin sheath. Abnormally wide spacing of the myelin lamellae results from some of its mutations (Gabreëls-Festen *et al.* 1996). More than 50 point mutations of the P0 gene occur (Nelis *et al.* 1999; Donaghy *et al.* 2000). These are variably associated with the phenotypes HMSN I, HMSN II, Dejerine–Sottas syndrome, and congenital hypomyelination. Also they can be associated with a syndrome resembling chronic inflammatory demyelinating polyneuropathy which also occurs in P0 knockout mice (Shy *et al.* 1997; Donaghy *et al.* 2000).

Connexin-32

X-linked forms of HMSN I are associated with more than 150 point mutations in the connexin-32 (*Cx-32*) gene, which encodes the gap junctions occurring at the Schmidt–Lanterman incisures (Fig 12.2c) and the paranodal regions of the myelin sheath. These *Cx-32* mutations may interfere with rapid transport of small molecules across adjacent myelin lamellae.

Mutations of the early growth response gene 2 (*EGR*) can lead to HMSN I or congenital hypomyelination in both mice and humans (Warner *et al.* 1998). None of the genes responsible for type II HMSN have been identified as yet. Novel forms of autosomal dominant HMSN unassociated with any of the above genes or loci are described (De Jonghe *et al.* 1999b). So far, three different types of autosomal recessive demyelinating HMSN have been identified:

(1) hemizygous mutations of the *PMP22* gene (Numakura *et al.* 2000);

(2) linkage to a novel locus on chromosome 5q23–q33 (Gabreëls-Festen *et al.* 1999);

(3) a form linked to chromosome 8q24 associated with deafness and occurring in Bulgarian gypsies (Kalaydjieva *et al.* 2000).

It is intriguing to discover that broadly similar HMSN phenotypes result from such an eclectic array of disturbances of cell biology.

12.4.2 **Type I hereditary motor and sensory neuropathy**

This demyelinating neuropathy is the most common form of HMSN. It is also known as Charcot–Marie–Tooth disease type 1 (CMT1). Motor-nerve conduction in the median nerve is substantially slowed and nerve biopsy shows segmental demyelination, usually accompanied by hypertrophic 'onion-bulb' changes (Fig. 12.6) (Harding and Thomas 1980b). These concentric layers of Schwann-cell proliferation around axons represent previous cycles of recurrent demyelination followed by attempted remyelination. The inheritance is usually autosomal dominant, with a high degree of intrafamilial concordance for the velocity of motor slowing in keeping with the under-lying genetic heterogeneity (Harding and Thomas 1980b). Seventy per cent of patients with the autosomal dominant form have reduplication of the *PMP22* gene (type IA) (Thomas *et al.* 1997) and many of the remainder have point mutations of myelin protein P0 (type IB) (De Jonghe *et al.* 1999a) (Section 12.4.1). Sex-linked recessive forms, sometimes mildly expressed in female carriers, are usually associated with connexin-32 mutations, and may progressively deteriorate involving permanent axonal degeneration (Birouk *et al.* 1998). Autosomal recessive forms occur occasionally and generally produce more severe disability with even lower motor conduction velocities (Harding and Thomas 1980c).

Clinical features

Distal leg muscle atrophy and weakness, or pes cavus foot deformity (Fig. 12.4) are usually evident in the first or second decades of life. Leg weakness can become severe. Distal wasting may be such that the legs resemble inverted champagne bottles (Fig. 12.5). The ankle-jerks are usually lost, but generalized areflexia occurs in only half the patients. Some hand weakness eventually occurs in most patients with HMSN type I. A few develop tremor or ataxia of the limbs, the so-called 'Roussy– Lévy syndrome' which is not genetically distinct from HMSN type I. All modalities of sensation may be impaired distally in the limbs. Occasional patients develop acrodystrophic changes secondary to severe sensory loss. Scoliosis, pupil abnormalities, or extensor plantar responses occasionally occur. Diaphragmatic weakness may cause dyspnoea or respiratory failure (Hardie *et al.* 1990). Palpable nerve thickening, best detected at the great auricular nerve (Fig. 12.7) is found in about a quarter and is specific to the demyelinating forms of HMSN, types I and III (Harding and

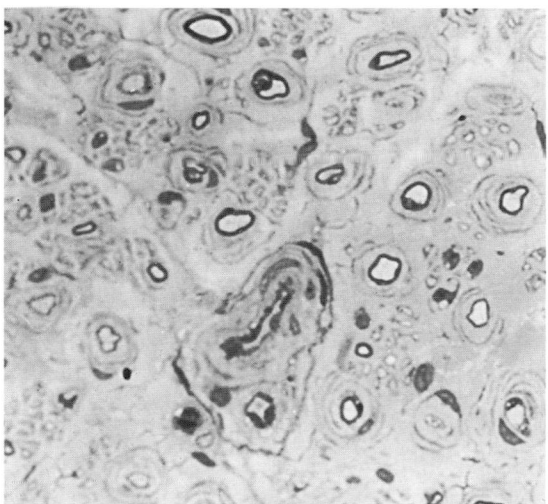

Fig. 12.6. Hereditary motor and sensory neuropathy type 1 (HMSNI). Transverse section of a 1 mm araldite section of peripheral nerve stained with toluidine blue, showing multiple 'onion-bulbs'; sural-nerve biopsy. (Courtesy of Dr R. Madrid.)

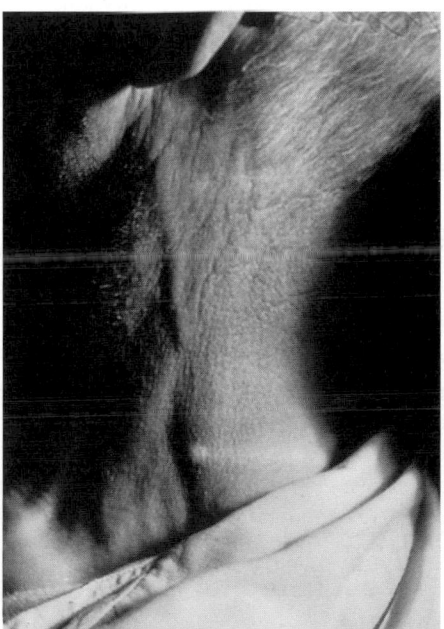

Fig. 12.7. Palpable enlargement of the greater auricular nerve in hereditary motor and sensory neuropathy type 1. (Courtesy of Professor W. B. Matthews.)

Thomas 1980*b*). Neurophysiological examination of the patient and first-degree relatives is crucial for diagnosis.

Nerve conduction

The median nerve motor conduction velocity is 38 m/s or less, which distinguishes the condition from the neuronal form of HMSN (type II). Generalized motor slowing is already evident in infancy and early childhood (Garcia *et al.* 1998). Sensory-nerve action potentials are absent or reduced in all patients, allowing distinction from distal spinal muscular atrophy (Harding and Thomas 1980*b*). Motor conduction velocities in HMSN type I rarely lie below 12 m/s, and if so, the diagnosis of HMSN type III should be considered (Ouvrier *et al.* 1987). Sural-nerve biopsy shows hypertrophic onion-bulb changes (Fig. 12.6) and reduced myelinated fibre density. The spinal-fluid protein is usually normal, but is occasionally elevated to 1 g/l or higher (Ouvrier *et al.* 1987).

Management

No treatment is known to reverse the neuropathy. Downhill progression is slow, noteworthy symptoms usually appear in the second decade of life and patients rarely become wheelchair-bound (Garcia *et al.* 1998). Weakness is generally restricted to the limbs and the disease does not significantly shorten life. Plastic moulded splints should be used to correct footdrop. Specialist orthopaedic advice should be sought if there is severe foot or spinal deformity.

Differential diagnosis

The most important differential diagnosis is from chronic inflammatory demyelinating polyneuropathy (CIDP), which is treatable (Section 12.11.1). CIDP, too, is associated with reduced motor conduction velocity and with segmental demyelination on nerve biopsy, occasionally with onion-bulb changes. Pointers in favour of HMSN type I are pes cavus, palpable nerve thickening, preserved proximal limb muscle power, a spinal fluid protein of less than 0.8 g/l, a slow rate of progression of symptoms, a lack of positive sensory symptoms such as tingling, and onion-bulb changes on nerve biopsy. The diagnosis of HMSN may be positively established by molecular genetic testing or by examining close relatives for signs of neuropathy, even if they are asymptomatic. Cases of HMSN with ataxia (the Roussy–Lévy syndrome) should be distinguished first from Refsum disease (Section 12.8.1) in which the serum phytanic acid is elevated, and secondly from Friedreich's ataxia, in which nystagmus and extensor plantars are usual, inheritance is autosomal recessive, the GAA trinucleotide expansion of intron 1 of the Frataxin gene is present, and motor-nerve conduction velocity is not markedly slowed.

12.4.3 Type II hereditary motor and sensory neuropathy

Otherwise known as the neuronal form of Charcot–Marie–Tooth disease, HMSN type II reflects a reduction in the number of primary motor and sensory neurons. HMSN type II is less common than type I. Motor-nerve conduction velocities are

normal or only slightly reduced and inheritance is usually autosomal dominant (Harding and Thomas 1980*b*).

Syndromes

Four clinical and genetically distinct syndromes of dominantly inherited HMSN II are recognized (Table 12.5). The most common form, type IIA, involves distal weakness and wasting, with lesser degrees of sensory loss and areflexia, starting in the second or third decade and linked to chromosome 1 (Othmane *et al.* 1993). Type IIB shows a younger age of onset, often with foot ulceration and preserved ankle tendon reflexes, and is linked to chromosome 3 (De Jonghe *et al.* 1997); an Austrian kinship without such genetic linkage is also described (Auer-Grumbach *et al.* 2000). Type IIC involves vocal cord or diaphragm paralysis in some members of the kinship (Dyck *et al.* 1994; Donaghy and Kennett 1999). Type IID characteristically produces more severe arm than leg muscle involvement and is linked to chromosome 7 (Ionasescu *et al.* 1996). A German kinship with HMSN type II has been described with sural-nerve axonal swellings filled with neurofilaments (Vogel *et al.* 1985), but the dominant pattern of inheritance and the normal hair distinguish this family from giant axonal neuropathy (Section 12.7.1). In Russia, an autosomal dominant form Type IIE coupled with hyperkeratosis is associated with point mutation of the neurofilament light chain (Mersiyanova *et al.* 2000). Autosomal recessive forms of HMSN II are encountered occasionally, with an earlier onset of symptoms than the dominant form (Harding and Thomas 1980*c*). Rare X-linked dominant forms with childhood onset have been linked to loci on the long arm of the X-chromosome (Hahn *et al.* 1990). In these X-linked kinships, males are severely affected and females may suffer subclinical or mild disease; no male-to-male transmission occurs. HMSN II, often associated with Adies Pupil deafness and elevated creative kinase levels, occurs with some myelin Po (MPZ) mutations (Misu *et al.* 2000).

Clinical features

Clinical features of HMSN type II resemble those of HMSN type I, but the onset of symptoms is generally later, usually in the second or third decade of life (Harding and Thomas 1980*b*). Onset can be delayed until old age. Patients most commonly present with difficulty in walking due to distal leg muscle weakness and wasting. Pes cavus foot deformity is less frequent than in HMSN type I. The ankle jerks are usually absent. Hand weakness, tremor or ataxia of the arms, marked sensory loss, or generalized loss of tendon reflexes are less frequently encountered in HMSN type II than in HMSN type I (Harding and Thomas 1980*b*). Palpable nerve thickening does not occur in HMSN type II. Many patients with HMSN type II show little or no deterioration, even when reassessed at intervals of many years, and serious disability is uncommon. The median-nerve motor conduction velocity is usually just within the normal range, and should not lie below 38–40 m/s. The median-nerve sensory action potential is absent or reduced in amplitude (Harding and Thomas 1980*b*). The spinal-fluid protein level is normal in HMSN type II. Nerve biopsies show axonal loss with little evidence of demyelination. Hypertrophic 'onion-bulb' changes are observed only rarely.

Differential diagnosis

Late-onset HMSN type II should be distinguished from chronic idiopathic axonal polyneuropathy (Section 12.11.6). Sensory features predominate and progression occurs in this latter condition (Teunissen *et al.* 1997). The dominant inheritance should distinguish ataxic forms of HMSN type II from inherited causes of vitamin E deficiency (Section 12.21.4) and from Friedreich's ataxia, which has a poorer prognosis. Abnormal sensory nerve conduction distinguishes patients with predominantly motor forms of HMSN type II from distal spinal muscular atrophy.

12.4.4 Type III hereditary motor and sensory neuropathy

This heterogeneous and relatively uncommon progressive sensorimotor demyelinating neuropathy starts in infancy or early childhood and is inherited either autosomally recessively or dominantly (Lynch *et al.* 1997). It is also known as Dejerine–Sottas syndrome or congenital hypomyelination neuropathy. It is caused by various point mutations of the PMP 22, MPZ, and EGR2 genes (Table 12.5) (Tyson *et al.* 1997). Affected children usually show delayed onset of walking and often develop ataxia and skeletal deformity. Palpable nerve thickening is common. One form of HMSN III, congenital hypomyelination neuropathy, presents at birth. It has a particularly poor prognosis; patients are unable to walk by their teens and may die at any age due to respiratory insufficiency. The prognosis is better if the onset is in childhood, but severe motor disability is usually evident by early adult life. Motor-nerve conduction is extremely slow, to less than 12 m/s. This is lower than that generally measured in HMSN type I (Ouvrier *et al.* 1987). Spinal-fluid protein is usually elevated to between 0.7 and 2.1 g/l. This can pose difficulties in distinction from the steroid-responsive chronic inflammatory demyelinating polyneuropathy of infancy and childhood (Section 12.11.1). In HMSN III, nerve biopsies show extensive onion-bulb formation and marked thinning of the myelin sheaths surrounding axons of all diameters (Ouvrier *et al.* 1987). Many axons are completely devoid of myelin sheaths in congenital hypomyelination neuropathy (Guzzetta *et al.* 1982). The ataxic forms may cause severe disability and can be distinguished from early onset Friedreich's ataxia by their slow motor conduction velocities, and from Refsum disease by measurement of the serum phytanic acid level.

12.5 Hereditary neuropathy with liability to pressure palsies

Some families exhibit autosomal dominant inheritance of a tendency to develop mononeuropathies due to the fact that their nerves are unusually vulnerable to pressure or traction (hereditary neuropathy with liability to pressure palsies, HNPP). This condition is also known as hereditary suscept-

ibility (or liability) to pressure palsies or tomaculous neuropathy. Exposed nerves, such as the radial or lateral popliteal, are especially vulnerable. Painless brachial plexus lesions may result from sleeping in awkward postures or from the shoulder straps of heavy backpacks. Patients present with motor and sensory features typical of the mononeuropathy in question, and recovery occurs over days or weeks. Typically patients experience deadness or tingling of the fingertips when using scissors. Permanent disability may develop after recurrent episodes of paralysis affecting the same nerve (Earl *et al.* 1964; Behse *et al.* 1972). In roughly half, nerve-conduction studies show generalized slowing of distal motor latencies or sensory nerve action potentials and minor slowing of motor conduction velocities (Andersson *et al.* 2000). This can be useful in detecting asymptomatic affected family members, or in raising suspicion of this hereditary neuropathy when investigating a seemingly uncomplicated peripheral-nerve palsy. In approximately 80 per cent there is a deletion of the *PMP22* gene at 17p11.2, and more pronounced evidence of background polyneuropathy (Lenssen *et al.* 1998). New mutations account for up to 5 per cent of all patients encountered with hereditary liability to pressure palsies.

Teased fibres from nerve biopsies show characteristic 'tomaculous' (Latin: sausage) swellings due to redundant myelin loops as a result of overgrowth of the myelin spiral (Fig. 12.8) (Behse *et al.* 1972; Madrid and Bradley 1975). Similar sausage-shaped swellings are found in peripheral-nerve fibres in hereditary brachial plexus neuropathy (Section 13.6.5). Less-pronounced tomaculous change can also occur in the Ehlers–Danlos syndrome (Schady and Ochoa 1984), in paraproteinaemic neuropathy (Vital *et al.* 1985), and in a syndrome of recurrent acute ascending polyneuropathy (Joy and Oh 1989). These more recent findings show that tomaculous change is not pathognomonic of hereditary pressure-sensitive neuropathy.

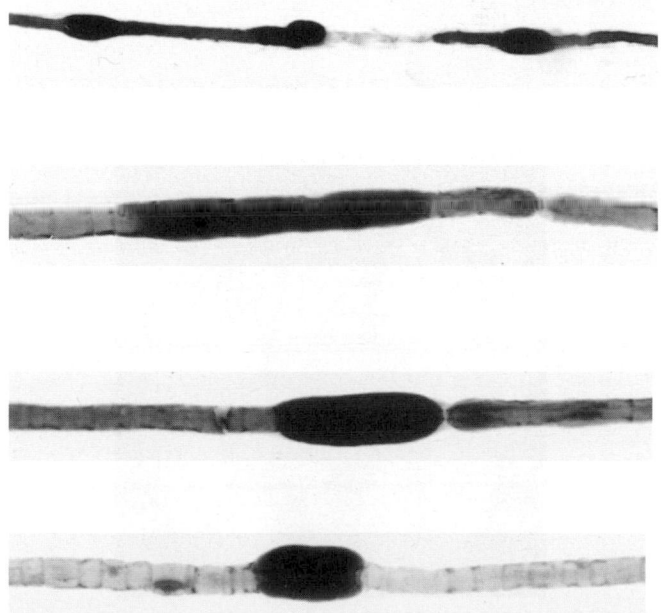

Fig. 12.8. Sausage-shaped myelin swellings on teased sural-nerve fibres from a patient with hereditary pressure-sensitive ('tomaculous') neuropathy. (Reproduced from *Greenfield's neuropathy*, (5th edn), by permission of Edward Arnold.)

12.6 Hereditary sensory and autonomic neuropathies

Hereditary sensory and autonomic neuropathies (HSAN) reflect failure of development, or degeneration, of sub-populations of peripheral sensory and autonomic neurons. Lack of self-protection due to impaired pain appreciation leads to the development of a mutilating acropathy (Fig. 12.9), with skin ulceration and fissuring, long-bone fractures, Charcot joints, and digit amputation. The precise symptoms and signs of each neuropathy, and whether accompanied by nerve-conduction abnormalities, is determined by which sub-population of sensory neurons is most affected. Prior to the recognition that peripheral neuropathy underlies these disorders, they were termed as lumbosacral syringomyelia, inherited perforating ulcers or whitlows, acrodystrophic neuropathy, and congenital insensitivity to pain. Also some such patients were considered to suffer from congenital indifference or asymbolia to pain, a term which should be reserved for the rare situation in which there is lack of concern to a painful stimulus which is well received and in which the peripheral nerves are normal. Patients with HSAN should be instructed to avoid situations likely to cause thermal burns and trauma to the limbs, to be assessed regularly by a chiropodist, and to ensure that their shoes are well fitting and do not contain stones or sharp objects. HSAN should be distinguished from familial amyloidotic polyneuropathy (Section 12.9.1), which often affects sphincter control and sexual functioning, both of which remain normal in HSAN.

There is no consensus for the classification of hereditary sensory and autonomic neuropathies. Here the descriptive classification of Donaghy *et al.* (1987) will be followed, indicating the corresponding classification of Dyck *et al.* (1983) into HSAN types I–V.

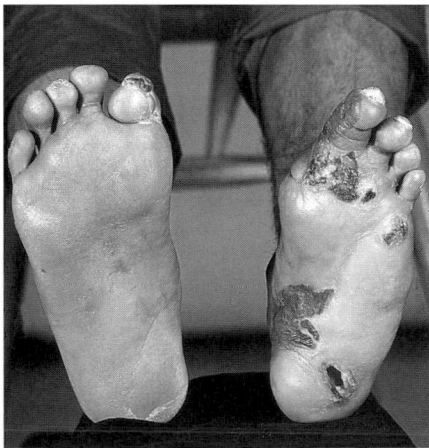

Fig. 12.9. Feet of a patient with herediatry sensory and autonomic neuropathy, showing chronic ulceration, loss of the left hallux, and shortening of the right hallux due to previous fracture. (Reproduced from Donaghy *et al.* (1987))

12.6.1 Autosomal dominant sensory neuropathy (HSAN type I)

Patients with this condition gradually lose all modalities of sensation from the distal part of their limbs, particularly pain and temperature sensations. Spontaneous shooting pains in the legs may occur early in the disease. Foot ulcers, calluses, and foot deformity develop in many patients (Denny-Brown 1951). Anhidrosis may occur in the regions of impaired sensation. The ankle jerks are usually absent. Some patients eventually develop mild distal muscle wasting and weakness, raising the question of overlap with more sensory forms of hereditary motor and sensory neuropathy. Sensory-nerve action potentials are reduced or absent and motor conduction velocity is just within the normal range. Autopsy studies show loss of dorsal root ganglion neurons, with replacement by nodules of Nageotte, indicating that sensory neurons have degenerated, rather than failing to develop. The condition is linked to chromosome 9q22 (Bejaoui *et al.* 1999). Dominantly inherited HSAN can be associated with deafness and intellectual impairment (Horoupain 1989).

12.6.2 Autosomal recessive sensory neuropathy (HSAN type II)

Otherwise known as congenital sensory neuropathy, this autosomal recessive condition presents in infancy or childhood with impairment of all modalities of sensation in the limbs and on the trunk. Marked distal-limb mutilation occurs, with whitlows, paronychia, plantar ulcers, painless long-bone fractures, and Charcot joints. Motor function is preserved. Tendon reflexes are usually lost. Anhidrosis of the hands and feet adversely affects skin texture and contributes to ulceration. Sensory-nerve action potentials are usually absent. The cutaneous sensory nerves are virtually devoid of myelinated fibres and depleted of unmyelinated fibres. The neuropathy seems to worsen progressively and patients progressively accumulate acrodystrophic changes (Nukada *et al.* 1982). The prognosis is uncertain, but since published reports usually relate to patients under the age of 20, a shortened life span is inferred (Ohta *et al.* 1973). The genetic locus is as yet unidentified. A similar form of HSAN may be inherited as an X-linked recessive trait (Jestico *et al.* 1985). Autosomal recessive HSAN may be associated with spastic paraplegia (Cavanagh *et al.* 1979).

12.6.3 Hereditary anhidrotic sensory neuropathy (HSAN type IV)

Patients with this autosomal recessive neuropathy suffer from congenital insensitivity to pain. They present in infancy with bouts of pyrexia, failure to thrive, retarded development, failure to respond to painful stimuli, anhidrosis, and mild mental retardation. The peripheral nerves are virtually devoid of unmyelinated axons and small neurons are absent from dorsal root ganglia (Swanson *et al.* 1965). The condition is rare and leads to premature death, often associated with a bout of unexplained fever. Mutations of a nerve growth factor receptor gene are associated with this neuropathy (Indo *et al.* 1996).

12.6.4 **Familial dysautonomia (HSAN type III)**

Otherwise known as the Riley–Day syndrome, this rare congenital disorder is autosomally recessively inherited, principally by Ashkenazi Jews. It is linked to chromosome 9q31–q33 (Blumenfeld *et al.* 1993). Affected infants vomit, have impaired body temperature control, sweat excessively, develop patchy skin blotching, have impaired tear formation, and are prone to pulmonary infection. Fungiform papillae are typically absent from the tongue. There is insensitivity to painful stimuli applied to the skin or eyes. The sensory deficit worsens with age, eventually involving kinaesthesia. There is areflexia and postural hypotension. Motor involvement eventually occurs. Nerve biopsy shows reduced numbers of unmyelinated fibres and a lack of large-diameter sensory myelinated fibres. Intradermal histamine injection fails to cause the erythematous flare of the triple response. A quarter of the patients die by the age of 20 (Axelrod and Abularrage 1982).

12.6.5 **Deficiency of small myelinated sensory fibres (HSAN type V)**

A large Kashmiri kinship has shown autosomal recessive inheritance of a mutilating acropathy associated with bilateral corneal opacification due to neurotrophic keratitis (Donaghy *et al.* 1987). Pain and temperature sensation are absent from the limbs and there is patchy anhidrosis. Motor function, the tendon reflexes, and kinaesthetic sensations are normal. Motor and sensory nerve fibre conduction, which reflect the fastest conducting fibres, are normal. Sural nerve biopsy shows selective reduction of the smaller myelinated fibre population. An identical neuropathy has also occurred sporadically, but associated with normal corneas (Dyck *et al.* 1983).

12.6.6 **Congenital indifference to pain**

True indifference to pain is rare. Most patients so described probably had hereditary sensory neuropathies with selective lack of small myelinated or unmyelinated sensory fibres. This was overlooked because there were no neuropathic abnormalities on examination and sensory nerve conduction was normal, given that large myelinated fibres were preserved in such neuropathies. One family has been described with dominantly inherited indifference to painful stimuli over the whole body and with normal morphometric examination of peripheral nerves (Landrieu *et al.* 1990).

12.7 **Other inherited polyneuropathies**

12.7.1 **Giant axonal neuropathy**

This rare progressive disorder of childhood involves both the peripheral and central nervous systems, causing peripheral neuropathy, ataxia, intellectual loss, and pyramidal tract dysfunction. It is characterized by accumulations of abnormally

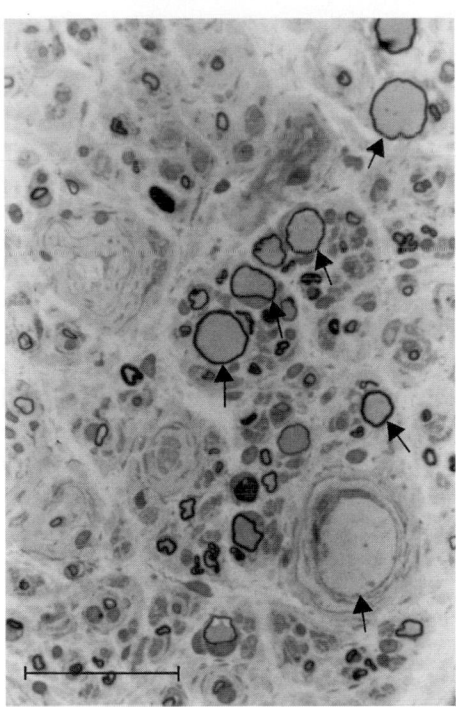

Fig. 12.10. Giant axonal neuropathy: semi-thin section of sural nerve showing numerous giant axonal swellings, some unmyelinated. Giant axonal profiles are shown by arrows; bar = 50 μm. (Reproduced with permission from Donaghy *et al.* (1988)).

closely packed neurofilaments within swollen peripheral-nerve axons (Fig. 12.10). The disorder is not restricted to neurofilaments and affects intermediate-filament organization in all cell types, including glial fibrillary acidic protein in Schwann cells (Donaghy *et al.* 1988). Most patients have characteristic tightly curled hair, reflecting an abnormality of keratin, another intermediate-filament protein. However, such hair is only variably present, even within affected kinships. The inheritance is autosomal recessive. Patients present in childhood, before dying from progressive disease in their second or third decade. A more benign autosomal recessive form with later onset, normal hair, and a better prognosis occurs in Tunisia (Ben Hamida *et al.* 1990). Toxic neuropathy due to hexacarbons causes a similar histological picture, but the hair is normal, there is a history of exposure to glues or other solvents, and the age of onset is generally later (Section 12.20.6).

12.7.2 **Neuropathy in Friedreich's ataxia**

Friedreich's ataxia (Section 31.4.1) affects the peripheral as well as the central nervous system. A stocking distribution of impaired light-touch sensation spreads proximally with age. The Achilles tendon reflexes are lost early, and vibration and joint-position sensations are impaired in the feet. Pes cavus may occur. The amplitude of sensory-nerve action potentials is markedly reduced and sural-nerve biopsy shows severe loss of the large myelinated fibres (Caruso *et al.* 1987). Despite the clinical evidence of progression, actively degenerating fibres are only relatively rarely encountered in biopsies, and the marked absence of large myelinated fibres is unlikely to be explicable by degeneration alone.

12.7.3 Chédiak–Higashi syndrome

This rare autosomal recessive disease usually presents in infancy or childhood with febrile episodes, pyogenic infections, and partial oculocutaneous albinism. Death within the first two decades usually follows an accelerated phase with lymphoma-like proliferation. Peripheral blood granulocytes contain pathognomonic giant peroxidase-positive lysosomal granules. Patients develop features of spinocerebellar degeneration, and peripheral neuropathy is particularly likely to occur during the accelerated phase. Prednisolone and vincristine may be effective in controlling the neurological manifestations (Pettit and Berdal 1984).

12.7.4 Multiple symmetric lipomatosis

Patients with this condition (also known as Madelung's disease) develop disfiguring multiple subcutaneous lipomata over the upper trunk and proximal arms (Fig. 12.11). The buttocks and legs are spared and are often relatively devoid of the usual sub-cutaneous fat. Up to 80 per cent of patients develop an axonal peripheral neuropathy, usually sensorimotor but occasionally with autonomic features. The neuropathy presents insidiously in middle age, is usually mild, and has a heterogeneous basis. Excessive alcohol consumption was observed in many Italian patients, suggesting that alcoholism caused the neuropathy

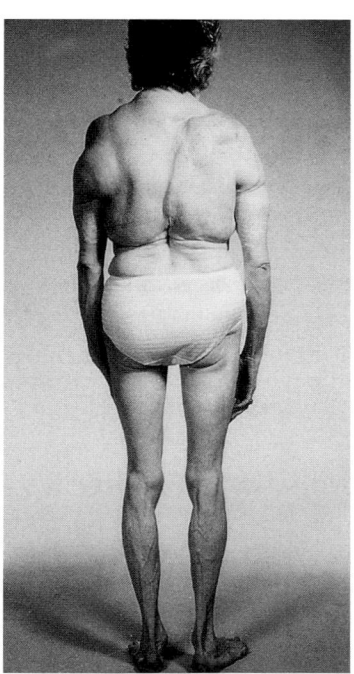

Fig. 12.11. Multiple symmetrical lipomatosis. Multiple lipomata are present on the neck, back, and upper arms, with scars from plastic surgery. Subcutaneous fat is sparse on the legs. (Reproduced with permission from Chalk et al. (1990)).

(Enzi et al. 1986). However, a large kinship has shown invariant association of peripheral neuropathy with multiple symmetrical lipomatosis, with possible autosomal recessive inheritance. Since no members of this kinship were alcoholic, the neuro-pathy of multiple symmetrical lipomatosis is likely to be deter-mined genetically (Chalk et al. 1990). Other patients have abnormalities in complex IV and multiple deletions of mito-chondrial DNA (Klopstock et al. 1994).

12.7.5 Chorea-acanthocytosis

Muscle wasting and areflexia may occur in patients with limb chorea and orofacial dyskinesias associated with acanthocytes in peripheral blood. Nerve-conduction studies show an axonal degeneration neuropathy. The condition is often familial (Sobue et al. 1986). It should be differentiated from the peri-pheral neuropathy and acanthocytosis which occurs in abeta-lipoproteinaemia (Bassen–Kornzweig disease), which is treatable with vitamin E (Section 12.8.8).

12.7.6 Mitochondrial cytopathy

A quarter of all patients with various forms of mitochondrial cytopathy (Section 15.6.3) have clinical features of mild senso-rimotor neuropathy. Asymptomatic electrophysiological evi-dence of peripheral neuropathy is somewhat more common (Yiannikas et al. 1986). Sural nerve biopsies show loss of large myelinated fibres, evidence of axonal degeneration, and the Schwann-cell cytoplasm may contain abnormal mitochondria with paracrystalline inclusions.

12.7.7 Thermosensitive neuropathy

A French family has shown autosomal dominant inheritance of reversible episodes of ascending muscle weakness, para-esthesiae, and areflexia which seemed to be triggered by pyrexia over 38.5 °C (Magy et al. 1997).

12.8 Inherited metabolic disorders causing polyneuropathy

This section addresses the peripheral nerve manifestations of a number of diseases, the central nervous system manifestations of which are discussed in Chapter 4. In addition to those disor-ders to be discussed in detail, mild polyneuropathy has been described in lysosomal-storage diseases (Niemann–Pick, Gaucher, or GM gangliosidosis), hyperoxaluria, defective DNA repair (xeroderma pigmentosum, ataxia telangiectasia), and Cockayne's syndrome. Focal entrapment neuropathies may occur in the mucopolysaccharidoses.

12.8.1 Refsum disease

Refsum disease is also known as phytanic acid oxidase defi-ciency, heredopathia atactica polyneuritiformis, hereditary motor and sensory neuropathy type IV, and phytanic acid accumulation. Demyelinating polyneuropathy is a central feature of Refsum disease, associated with retinitis pigmentosa, cerebellar ataxia, and a markedly raised spinal-fluid protein. Most patients also show hearing loss, anosmia, ichthyosis, skeletal abnormalities, and cardiomyopathy. The disease is rare, generally occurring in people of northern European racial stock (Refsum *et al.* 1984).

A deficiency of phytanic acid α-hydroxylation is inherited as an autosomal recessive trait. This results in a failure to oxidize exogenous phytol, with resultant conversion to phytanic acid, which accumulates. The diagnosis is confirmed by demonstrating a high serum phytanic acid level. Phytates are derived chiefly from dietary dairy products and other animal fats; the chlorophyll of green vegetables is a less well-absorbed source. Symptoms first develop at any time from childhood to the third decade, and may be provoked by infections. Recurrent attacks of polyneuropathy have been described. The neuropathy is usually predominantly distal and motor, and generally preceded by night blindness. Severe disability may develop. Peripheral nerves may be palpably hypertrophied. Motor-nerve conduction velocities are greatly slowed. Nerve biopsy confirms the demyelinating nature of the neuropathy, and may reveal hypertrophic changes and round paracrystalline inclusions within Schwann cells. The diagnosis of Refsum disease is of importance, since dietary restriction of phytate ingestion improves or stabilizes the neuropathy, with increased motor-nerve conduction velocities. Plasma exchange also helps to lower the phytanic acid level, and is particularly valuable soon after diagnosis before dietary restriction becomes effective (Harari *et al.* 1991).

12.8.2 **Metachromatic leucodystrophy**

In this rare group of autosomal recessive diseases, also known as sulphatide lipidosis and arylsulphatase deficiency, a severe demyelinating sensorimotor neuropathy accompanies psychomotor retardation and seizures due to disease of the cerebral white matter (Section 29.6.4). Motor-nerve conduction velocity is slowed substantially (McFaul *et al.* 1982) with elevated spinal-fluid protein. The different metachromatic leucodystrophies present variously in late infancy, childhood, or adulthood; presentation as late as the sixth decade is recorded (McFaul *et al.* 1982). Sulphatides accumulate in nervous tissue because of defects in the arylsulphatase A gene, accounting for the varying age of onset and diverse clinical picture (Draghia *et al.* 1997). The diagnosis is confirmed by measuring reduced activity of the lysosomal enzymes arylsulphatase A and B in peripheral blood leucocytes. Metachromatic granules may be demonstrated in an early morning urine deposit. Nerve biopsy shows evidence of demyelination and remyelination, and the presence of metachromatic granules in Schwann-cell cytoplasm after staining with aniline dyes. Electron microscopy shows zebra-like bodies, and tuffstone and prismatic inclusions (Martin *et al.* 1982). Identical histological features have been demonstrated in the sural nerve of a patient with typical clinical features of metachromatic leucodystrophy, but with normal activity levels of leucocyte arylsulphatase A and B and cerebroside sulphatase (Hahn *et al.* 1982). The prognosis is poor, with early death particularly likely in those with infantile onset. Optimistic progress occurred in a child with infantile onset treated by bone-marrow transplantation (Krivit *et al.* 1990).

12.8.3 **Krabbe's disease**

This rare autosomal recessive disease is also known as globoid cell leucodystrophy, galactosylceramide lipidosis, and galactosylceramide-β-galactosidase deficiency. It usually presents in infancy with psychomotor retardation. Demyelinating sensorimotor peripheral neuropathy generally develops later. Protruding ears may be a feature. A late-onset form has been described (Phelps *et al.* 1991). After an initial phase of hyperreflexia, which reflects central nervous system disease (Section 29.6.2), patients become areflexic as the peripheral neuropathy develops. Motor-nerve conduction velocity is substantially reduced. The diagnosis is confirmed by demonstrating reduced leucocyte galactosylceramide-β-galactosidase levels. A wide range of mutations in the galactosylceramide gene underlie the late-onset and classical forms, but observations such as late onset despite completely abolished enzyme activity suggest that other factors contribute to the phenotypic expression (De Gasperi *et al.* 1996).

12.8.4 **Adrenoleucodystrophy**

X-linked adrenoleucodystrophy (ALD) (Section 29.6.3) is also known as adrenomyeloneuropathy. It causes adrenal insufficiency and neurological dysfunction associated with raised plasma levels of very-long-chain saturated fatty acids, such as hexacosanoic, pentacosanoic, and tetracosanoic acids. Different phenotypes occur with different ages of onset, within the same kinship, and even between monozygotic twins (Sobue *et al.* 1994). Over a 100 mutations in the ALD gene are identified, with little genotype–phenotype correlation (Dodd *et al.* 1997). The peripheral neuropathy is generally mild and causes little disability compared to the associated spastic and ataxic paraparesis. Nerve conduction may be slowed, but a mixed axonal and demyelinating picture is usual; female carriers may show electrophysiological evidence of neuropathy (van Geel *et al.* 1996).

12.8.5 **Anderson–Fabry disease**

This X-linked disorder is also known as angiokeratoma corporis diffusum or α-galactosidase deficiency. It presents in childhood or early adult life with burning pain and paraesthesiae distally in the limbs. Discrete crises of pain may be provoked by exercise or heat. These can be sufficiently severe to prevent or impede walking. Anhidrosis may occur. Most patients have angiokeratoma corporis diffusum, a characteristic crimson maculopapillar rash in the 'bathing-trunks' area, which may be overlooked on cursory examination (Fig. 12.12).

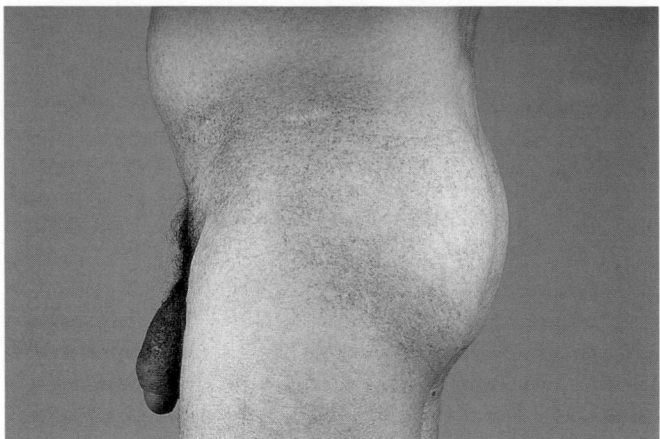

Fig. 12.12. Anderson–Fabry disease. The typical crimson angiokeratoma corporis diffusum rash in the 'bathing-trunks' area.

Strokes, hypertension, renal failure, and corneal opacification are common. Muscle strength, kinaesthetic sensation, and nerve-conduction studies are usually normal. Excess lysosomal storage of glycosphingolipids occurs in blood vessel walls, and selected populations of neurons, including ganglia (de Veber *et al.* 1992). The diagnosis is confirmed by measuring blood leucocyte lysosomal α-galactosidase. Numerous different mutations of the α-galactosidase A gene are responsible for the classical severe form of Fabry disease (Blanch *et al.* 1996).

12.8.6 Porphyric neuropathy

Neurological symptoms occur in all three autosomal dominantly inherited hepatic porphyrias: acute intermittent, hereditary coproporphyria, and variegate porphyria. All three exhibit similar neuropsychiatric features during acute porphyric attacks. Only hereditary coproporphyria and variegate porphyria produce photosensitive skin lesions. Acute attacks may be diagnosed by measuring elevated levels of δ-aminolevulinic acid in the plasma, of porphobilinogen in the urine, and of faecal porphyrins. The underlying enzyme defects can be identified in cultured fibroblasts.

Acute attacks are provoked by a wide variety of drugs, hormones, intercurrent infections, by reduced dietary carbohydrate intake, or by lead intoxication (Section 12.19.2). Lead-exposed workers whose blood and urine lead levels lie within accepted safety limits may, none the less, develop wrist drop due to plumboporphyria (Dyer *et al.* 1993). During an acute attack, the urine characteristically turns red on standing, due to oxidation of porphobilinogen. The first manifestation is usually abdominal pain. This is often associated with constipation, tachycardia, sweating, tremor, fever, and hypertension. These features reflect acute sympathetic outflow activity and may be associated with sudden death. They are followed by the neuropsychiatric features of insomnia, confusion, hallucinations, delusion, or depression (Ridley 1969). Seizures may occur. A dilutional hyponatraemia may contribute to the central nervous system dysfunction.

A wide variety of neuromuscular manifestations have been described (Ridley 1969; Suarez *et al.* 1997). Acute weakness may start symmetrically in proximal muscles, preceded by myalgias and cramps. The onset may be restricted to only one limb for the first few hours or days. Weakness can take weeks to develop fully, and eventually may be most marked distally. The resultant tetraplegia is often maximal in the arms. Dysphagia, facial paralysis, and diplopia may occur in severe cases. Assisted ventilation may be required for diaphragm weakness. Tendon reflexes are absent or diminished in nearly all patients; characteristically the ankle jerks are most likely to be preserved. Paraesthesiae, dysaesthesiae, or numbness of the limbs may be present from the outset. Distal glove and stocking diminution of superficial sensation, and vibration sense abnormalities can be evident. It is unusual for the sensory disturbance to precede motor weakness. Some patients develop truncal sensory deficits, either in band-like distributions or in a bathing-trunks distribution. Postural hypotension and urinary retention can occur, reflecting autonomic neuropathy. Nerve-conduction studies in established attacks are consistent with an axonal degeneration neuropathy. However, nerve conduction may be normal early in an attack, although mild myopathic features may be noted on electromyography of affected muscles (Samuels *et al.* 1984). We still lack a cogent pathogenic explanation for the early weakness. The early proximal muscle involvement and relatively prompt recovery suggest a reversible myopathic or conduction block element, rather than axonal degeneration.

The treatment should aim to control pain with opiate analgesics. Sedation with phenothiazines is helpful. Epilepsy should be treated with low-dose clonazepam or sodium valproate and by correcting the underlying dilutional hyponatraemia. Other major anticonvulsants such as phenytoin, carbamazepine, or barbiturates are likely to worsen the severity of the underlying porphyric attack. The porphyric attack itself should be terminated by withdrawing precipitating drugs, by treating any underlying infections, by rehydration, and by administration of a high carbohydrate load either parenterally or orally. If the attack is severe or unresponsive to the preceding measures, haematin infusion may be effective (Bosch *et al.* 1977). The neurological deficit recovers gradually over months. Permanent deficits may result.

Identical neurological crises may occur in children with autosomal recessive hereditary tyrosinaemia (Mitchell *et al.* 1990) and in patients with lead poisoning. δ-Aminolevulinic acid excretion is increased in both these conditions, as in porphyria.

12.8.7 Tangier disease

Plasma high-density lipoproteins are severely reduced in this rare autosomal recessive disorder which is also known as familial high-density lipoprotein deficiency or analphalipoproteinaemia. Cholesterol esters accumulate in body tissues, producing splenomegaly and visibly swollen, orange-coloured pharyngeal tonsils. Most patients eventually develop peripheral neuropathy, which can take either of two forms. Most commonly there is a relapsing and remitting multiple mononeuropathy. Less often there is a slowly progressive symmetrical sensory neuropathy in which the distribution of the sensory disturbance resembles syringomyelia, with dissociated sensory loss affecting the upper limbs and wasting of the arm and facial muscles. These two contrasting peripheral neuropathies reflect focal demyelination and axonal degeneration, respectively (Pollock *et al.* 1983*b*; Pietrini *et al.* 1985). There is no specific treatment.

12.8.8 **Abetalipoproteinaemia**

This rare autosomal recessive disorder is also known as Bassen–Kornzweig disease or acanthocytosis. Associated with the acanthocytes in peripheral blood, there is fat malabsorption, retinitis pigmentosa, and a spinocerebellar degeneration resembling early onset Friedreich's ataxia. The associated axonal degeneration peripheral neuropathy produces areflexia and impaired vibration and joint-position sensation (Brin *et al.* 1986). It is due to deficiency of the microsomal triglyceride transfer protein (Wetterau *et al.* 1992). High-dose vitamin E therapy may prevent progression of the neurological symptoms and can produce improvement (Muller *et al.* 1985).

12.8.9 **Cerebrotendinous xanthomatosis**

Cholestanol accumulates in the tissues in this rare autosomal recessive disorder, which is due to a block in hepatic bile acid synthesis. A sensorimotor peripheral neuropathy is associated with dementia, spastic paraparesis, cerebellar ataxia (see Section 31.7.1), and tendon xanthomas (Fig. 12.13). A high blood level of cholestanol confirms the diagnosis. Chenodeoxycholic acid therapy may produce some minor neurological improvement, including increased nerve-conduction velocities (Donaghy *et al.* 1990). Presymptomatic detection of the mutation in at-risk family members allows presymptomatic treatment to try and stave off clinical disease (Meiner *et al.* 1994).

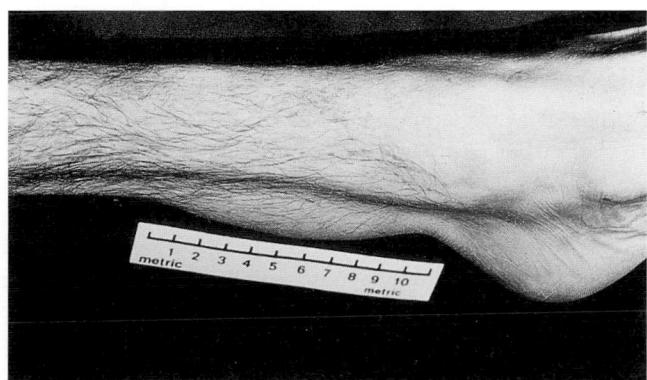

Fig. 12.13. Cerebrotendinous xanthomatosis. Achilles tendon xanthoma.

12.8.10 **Leigh's disease**

Demyelinating sensorimotor neuropathy occurs in infants and children with this disorder, which is also known as subacute necrotizing encephalomyelopathy (Goebel *et al.* 1986). Neuropathy is rarely, if ever, the presenting feature of the disorder and the associated nervous system dysfunction is generally the major cause of disability (Section 4.10).

12.9 **Amyloid neuropathy**

Amyloidotic polyneuropathy results from deposition within nerves of various non-branching, fibrillar proteins which all possess the crystallographic characteristic of forming a β-pleated sheet (Glenner and Murphy 1989). Histologically, amyloid material is recognized by its property of staining with Congo-red dye and exhibiting apple-green birefringence when viewed in polarizing light (Fig. 12.14).

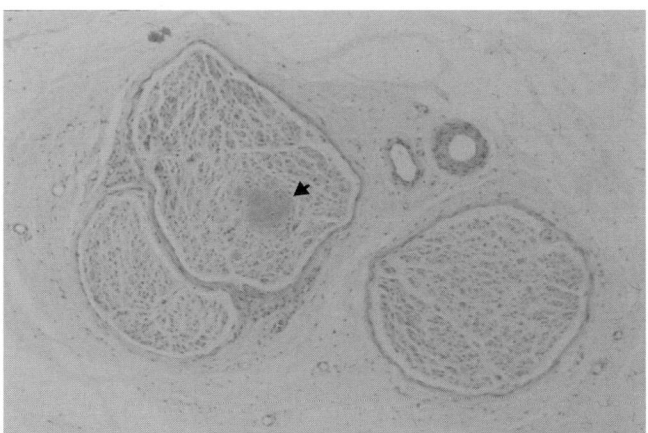

(a)

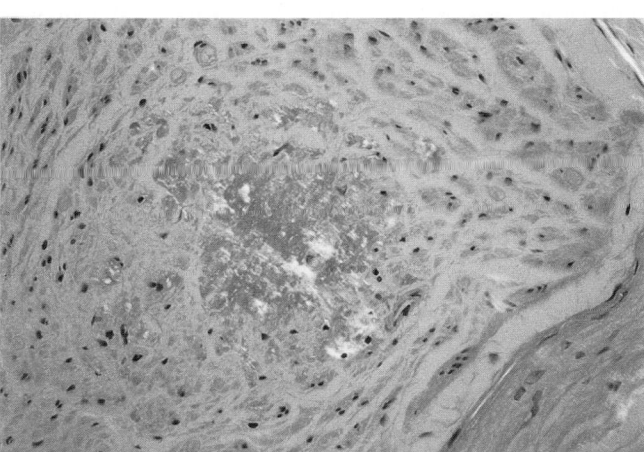

(b)

Fig. 12.14. Amyloid due to immunoglobulin light-chain deposition in peripheral nerve. (a) Eosinophilic deposit within a nerve fascicle (arrowed) (low power, haematoxylin and eosin); (b) apple-green birefringence of the amyloid deposit in polarized light (Congo red, higher power) (see also colour Plate 19).

Amyloidotic neuropathy occurs in two main groups of patients. The familial amyloidotic neuropathies reflect inherited substitutions of single amino acids in the proteins which are deposited: transthyretin (pre-albumin) or, less frequently, apolipoprotein A-I or gelsolin. Primary amyloidosis is due to tissue deposition of immunoglobulin light chains, usually derived from benign or malignant plasma cell tumours. It is rare for peripheral neuropathy, apart from carpal tunnel syndrome, to complicate the reactive or secondary amyloidoses, associated with circulating serum amyloid A protein, which result from chronic inflammatory conditions.

12.9.1 Familial amyloidosis

Genetics

These neuropathies are inherited as autosomal dominant traits. Onset of neuropathic symptoms is usually in the third to sixth decades. The original clinical classification into types I–IV is being replaced by classification based upon genetic mutations. Types I (Portuguese) and II (Indiana/Swiss) are due to the deposition of abnormal transthyretin within the body tissues, including the peripheral nerves. At least 32 different point mutations have been identified in the transthyretin gene on chromosome 18 (Reilly et al. 1995; Planté-Bordeneuve et al. 1998). Of these, the methionine 30 (Met30) mutation is by far the most common. Molecular genetic analysis can now be applied to affected families for diagnostic, presymptomatic, and prenatal testing. Type III (Iowa) familial amyloidosis is due to deposition of mutant apolipoprotein A-I, resulting from a single base-pair substitution in the gene (Nichols et al. 1988). Type IV (Finnish) is due to gelsolin gene mutations (Paunio et al. 1995).

Clinical features

The polyneuropathy is similar in all these different types of familial amyloidosis. Numbness is usually associated with impaired pain and temperature sensations in the hands and feet. This may eventually lead to trophic ulceration. Spontaneous pains occur in the limbs. Areflexia develops. Weakness generally follows the sensory disturbance and affects distal muscles, particularly the small hand muscles and ankle dorsiflexors (Andrade 1952). Autonomic involvement affects the pupillary reactions to light, impairs gastrointestinal motility, and produces impotence and postural hypotension. The spinal-fluid protein is often raised. Nerve-conduction studies show an axonal degeneration neuropathy. Proteinuria, renal failure, and cardiac involvement contribute to premature death.

There are some noteworthy variations in the presentation of these different forms of familial amyloidosis. In type II the earliest symptom is usually a carpal tunnel syndrome, due to deposition of amyloid in the flexor retinaculum at the wrist. Renal and sphincter involvement do not occur in type II amyloidosis. Type IV presents with lattice dystrophy of the cornea and patients may develop amyloid infiltration of the facial skin and involvement of the facial and auditory nerves.

Pathology

Nerve biopsies show amyloid deposition within nerve fascicles and around endoneurial blood vessels. At autopsy, widespread amyloid deposition is seen in the peripheral nervous system, affecting nerve plexuses, dorsal root and sympathetic ganglia. Multiple mechanisms probably contribute to the peripheral-nerve damage. Amyloid deposits in the dorsal root ganglia may cause a sensory neuronopathy. Ischaemic changes may result from amyloid deposition around endoneurial blood vessels. Multifocal interruption of axons by small amyloid deposits along the course of a nerve may summate distally to produce a picture of diffuse fibre loss (Hanyu et al. 1989).

Treatment

Liver transplantation has been introduced to treat transthyretin-related amyloid polyneuropathy on the grounds that the liver produces more than 90 per cent of this protein. Transplantation reduces mutated transthyretin in the blood and halts the progression of polyneuropathy, with additional benefits for general health and gastrointestinal symptoms. There is little objective evidence of significant improvement in the neuropathy but further loss of myelinated axons from peripheral nerves largely ceases (Adams et al. 2000). Transplantation carries a significant mortality in amyloidosis, with only 60 per cent survival at 5 years (Parrilla et al. 1997). Poor prognosis is predicted by an already heavy load of amyloid deposition prior to transplantation, as revealed by symptomatic postural hypotension, urinary incontinence, or cardiac involvement. In principle, liver transplantation should be considered early in the disease so as to forestall amyloid deposition in the nerves and other organs.

12.9.2 Primary amyloidosis

Systemic amyloidosis due to immunoglobulin light-chain deposition is unusual before middle age. The peripheral nervous system is affected in about one-third of all cases (Duston et al. 1989). Various underlying lymphoproliferative disorders may be responsible for the monoclonal immunoglobulin production, ranging from malignant myeloma to benign paraproteinaemia. Serum paraproteinaemia and/or free light chains in the urine (Bence Jones protein) may be detected. This form of amyloidosis is occasionally associated with hypernephroma.

Clinical features

Peripheral neuropathy is the presenting symptom in about 10 per cent of patients with primary amyloidosis and these patients tend to have the longest survival (Duston et al. 1989). The initial symptoms tend to be sensory or, less frequently, autonomic. Impaired pain and temperature sensations and numbness affect the limbs. Spontaneous lancinating or burning dysaesthetic pains occur and may respond to carbamazepine therapy. Sometimes these lancinating pains are focal, for instance picking out a particular finger for a few weeks. Muscle weakness and areflexia occur later in the course of the neuropathy. Autonomic symptoms include postural hypotension, impotence, constipation, anhidrosis, and hypoactive pupils (Kelly *et al.* 1979). Sensorimotor symptoms can be distributed asymmetrically, suggesting that individual peripheral nerves or dorsal root ganglia may be infiltrated to differing degrees by amyloid. Involvement of the ocular motor, trigeminal, or facial cranial nerves may be prominent (Traynor *et al.* 1991). Other features suggesting a diagnosis of primary amyloidosis include macroglossia, hepatosplenomegaly, proteinuria or nephrotic syndrome, and paraproteinaemia. Muscular stiffness, hypertrophy, and weakness occasionally complicate amyloid deposition in muscles (Yamada *et al.* 1988). Nerve-conduction studies show an axonal degeneration neuropathy. The spinal-fluid protein is usually elevated (Kelly *et al.* 1979). The diagnosis is confirmed by demonstrating amyloid deposition within biopsied peripheral nerves. However, it is simpler to establish the diagnosis of amyloidosis by rectal biopsy, which can be positive even when a nerve biopsy has not shown amyloid (Wokke *et al.* 1996). The neuropathological features at autopsy resemble those of familial amyloidotic polyneuropathy (Section 12.9.1).

Treatment

The neuropathy progresses relentlessly. Eighty per cent of patients die within 3 years, usually due to associated renal or cardiac disease. Attempts at drug therapy have been generally unsuccessful, although there are recent glimmers of hope. Chemotherapy with melphalan and prednisolone does not alter perceptibly the downhill course of the neuropathy (Kelly *et al.* 1979). However, trials have shown enhanced survival in amyloidosis patients treated with melphalan and prednisolone compared to colchicine, and retrospective analysis has shown that colchicine doubles the median survival compared to no treatment (Kyle *et al.* 1985; Cohen *et al.* 1987). There are recent reports of stabilization or improvement of primary amyloidosis following intravenous melphalan chemotherapy and peripheral blood stem-cell support (Comenzo *et al.* 1999). However, there has been no systematic study of how these more aggressive therapeutic approaches may benefit the polyneuropathy.

12.10 Acute idiopathic polyneuropathies and the Guillain–Barré syndrome

These conditions produce acute and diffuse demyelination or conduction block, or less frequently axonal degeneration affecting the spinal roots and peripheral nerves, and occasionally the cranial nerves. They are usually post-infective and recover spontaneously. The term Guillain–Barré syndrome includes two main entities only recently recognized as distinct: acute idiopathic demyelinating polyradiculoneuropathy (AIDP) (Section 12.10.1) and acute motor axonal neuropathy (AMAN) (Section 12.10.2).

12.10.1 Acute idiopathic demyelinating polyneuropathy

The term Guillain–Barré syndrome (GBS) tends to be used interchangeably with acute idiopathic demyelinating polyneuropathy. Other names used for the condition have included: acute post-infective polyradiculoneuropathy, acute infectious polyneuritis, Landry–Guillain–Barré–Strohl syndrome, and post-infective polyneuritis.

Epidemiology

The Guillain–Barré syndrome is one of the most common forms of polyneuropathy. Many cases were observed among troops during the First World War (Guillain *et al.* 1916). The condition may occur in either sex, with slight male preponderance, and at any age, occasionally including infancy. The mean age of onset is around 40 but many series have shown a binodal distribution with peaks in the third and sixth decades of life. There is no obvious seasonal clustering of cases. The crude average annual incidence rate varies in different countries from 0.6 to 1.9 per 100 000 people (Ropper *et al.* 1991).

Antecedent infections

Over half of Guillain–Barré syndrome patients experience symptoms of viral respiratory or gastrointestinal infections during the 1–3 weeks prior to the onset of neurological symptoms (Winer *et al.* 1988*b*). Serological studies have implicated a wide range of infective agents. Cytomegalovirus (13 per cent) and *Campylobacter jejuni* (in approximately 30 per cent) are the most common. Epstein–Barr virus (10 per cent), *Mycoplasma pneumoniae* (5 per cent), human immunodeficiency virus (HIV), and childhood exanthems are also reported (Cornblath *et al.* 1987; Winer *et al.* 1988*b*; Rees *et al.* 1995; Jacobs *et al.* 1998). The Guillain–Barré syndrome may accompany primary infection with HIV at a stage before viral antibodies are detectable in the serum; measurement of the p24 capsid antigen proving the underlying infection.

Cytomegalovirus and campylobacter infections precipitate differing forms of Guillain–Barré syndrome. That associated with cytomegalovirus tends to occur in younger patients, with a high occurrence of respiratory muscle weakness, cranial nerve involvement, and significant sensory involvement (Visser *et al.* 1996). By contrast, *Campylobacter jejuni* infection is associated with preceding diarrhoeal illness in 70 per cent, a pure motor disorder (AMAN) is common (Section 12.10.2), the electrophysiology often points to axonal dysfunction rather than demyelination, and recovery can be markedly slow (Rees *et al.* 1995). Forms of Guillain–Barré syndrome precipitated by both campylobacter and cytomegalovirus show delayed recovery compared to cases unassociated with these two infections (Visser *et al.* 1996).

When *Campylobacter jejuni* enteritis has precipitated Guillain–Barré syndrome, stool culture may be positive and serum IgM antibodies detected. Preceding *Campylobacter jejuni* infections can evoke Guillain–Barré syndrome even if there has been prompt treatment with antibiotics. Unusual forms of acute polyneuritis may occur following campylobacter infection, including variants with ophthalmoplegia.

After immunization in 1976 of more than 40 million adults in the United States with swine influenza virus vaccine (A/New Jersey/76) more than 500 cases of Guillain–Barré syndrome were reported in vaccinated individuals. It is estimated that this vaccine resulted in an excess incidence of one case of Guillain–Barré syndrome per 100 000 population, approximately doubling the normal incidence (Schonberger *et al.* 1981). No other causal relationship linking Guillain–Barré syndrome to vaccination with other strains of influenza virus has been shown. A prospective case-control study in England showed no significant excess of any form of vaccination during the 3 months preceding the Guillain–Barré syndrome (Winer *et al.* 1988*b*). Occasionally the Guillain–Barré syndrome may be associated with underlying lymphoma, usually Hodgkin's disease (Lisak *et al.* 1977). It can appear in patients already being treated with substantial doses of steroids (Steiner *et al.* 1986), and is occasionally seen after renal transplantation from a cytomegalovirus-positive donor, and after bone-marrow or hepatic engraftment (Section 5.6.4).

Immunopathogenesis

An autoimmune basis for the Guillain–Barré syndrome seems likely but remains unproven. Although antibodies to various gangliosides are described in Guillain–Barré syndrome, particularly following campylobacter infection (Section 12.10.2), it is unclear whether these antibodies are pathogenic (Hartung *et al.* 1995*a, b*; Ang *et al.* 1999). Certainly no single antibody is ubiquitous for Guillain–Barré syndrome. Guillain–Barré syndrome bears a strong histological resemblance to experimental allergic neuritis, an acute monophasic disorder induced by immunization of experimental animals with peripheral-nerve myelin proteins, particularly P2 and galactocerebroside (Hughes 1990). It is likely that diverse immunopathogenic mechanisms occur, including both antibody- and cell-mediated immune mechanisms (Hartung *et al.* 1995*a*). Prominent neural inflammatory infiltrates can occur in both Guillain–Barré syndrome and experimental allergic neuritis.

Circumstantial support for autoantibody mediation of the neuropathy comes from the finding that plasma exchange shortens the duration of the disease. However, unlike most organ-specific autoimmune diseases, the Guillain–Barré syndrome shows no clear association with other autoimmune diseases or with MHC (major histocompatibility complex) antigens. There is controversy as to whether demyelination or conduction block can be induced by injection of Guillain–Barré sera into animal nerves.

Pathology

The peripheral nerves in acute Guillain–Barré syndrome often show inflammatory cell infiltrate, with associated areas of demyelination, resembling experimental allergic neuritis (Asbury *et al.* 1969). This inflammatory infiltrate is mainly

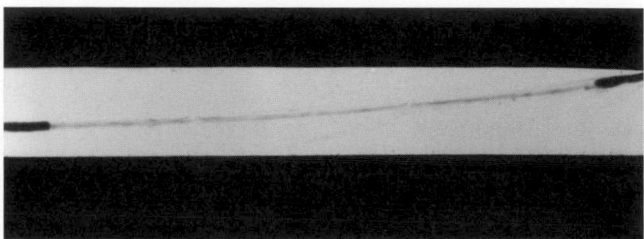

Fig. 12.15. Segmental demyelination: demyelinated internode of a teased sural-nerve fibre.

perivascular and comprised of lymphocytes and macrophages. Electron microscopy shows that macrophages cause the myelin damage, and penetrate the basement membrane around nerve fibres before stripping myelin sheaths off axons (Prineas 1981). Spinal nerve roots may be particularly affected, but changes are found at all levels of the peripheral nervous system. Teased peripheral sensory nerve fibre preparations may show marked segmental demyelination (Fig. 12.15). Some Wallerian degeneration may occur. Biopsy of the sural nerve may show surprisingly few abnormalities in comparison to the marked clinical severity of the neuropathy; this may reflect the distal and purely sensory nature of the sural nerve. Sensory nerve biopsy is generally unhelpful in establishing the diagnosis of Guillain–Barré syndrome; more typical demyelinative changes being present in motor nerves, which are not amenable to routine biopsy (Hall *et al.* 1992). Clinical criteria, spinal-fluid protein elevation, and nerve-conduction abnormalities remain the mainstay of diagnosis.

Occasional patients display motor–sensory axonal, rather than demyelinating, forms of Guillain–Barré syndrome. Opinion has been divided as to whether this represented secondary axonal degeneration induced by severe oedematous swelling of nerve roots, or whether it represented a primary attack on axonal antigens; evidence tends to support the latter (Lu *et al.* 2000). Characteristically, these patients have electrically inexcitable motor nerves early in their illness, electromyographic evidence of denervation within 2–5 weeks, marked muscle wasting, and protracted weakness with a generally poor recovery (Feasby *et al.* 1986).

Clinical features

The neurological illness is preceded by symptoms of respiratory tract infection in approximately 40 per cent and gastrointestinal infection in less than 20 per cent in an English series; 8 per cent had undergone an operation in the preceding 3 months (Winer *et al.* 1988*b*). Neurological symptoms first develop 1–4 weeks after this infection. The Guillain–Barré syndrome produces a relatively symmetrical areflexic tetraparesis; the essential diagnostic criteria consist of progressive motor weakness of more than one limb, coupled with areflexia (Asbury and Cornblath 1990). Although sensory symptoms usually occur first, it is profound muscle weakness which is the main clinical feature in most patients once the disease is established.

Sensory features

In three-quarters of patients, the first neurological symptom is of paraesthesiae in the toes, less often in the fingers. Simultaneously, or soon afterwards, patients develop progressive limb weakness, often first noted as difficulty in walking (Löffel et al. 1977). Despite the sensory nature of the initial symptoms, it is unusual for the eventual sensory loss to be particularly severe when compared to the profound motor loss. When sensory signs are present, they usually consist of impaired vibration and joint-position sensations (Winer et al. 1988a). Half the patients experience severe pain which may be present from the outset. It is generally maximal in the back and buttocks and may require short-term opiate analgesia. It usually resolves as recovery starts.

Motor features

Muscle weakness usually starts in the legs and ascends to the arms. Proximal muscle weakness may be prominent from the outset. The weakness is fairly symmetrical and usually involves the trunk musculature. It is unusual for the arms to be more severely weakened than the legs (Winer et al. 1988a). Maximal weakness generally develops within 12–14 days of the onset of neurological symptoms. Although cessation of symptom progression within 4 weeks is often regarded as a necessary criterion for the diagnosis of Guillain–Barré syndrome (Asbury and Cornblath 1990), it is clear that in a small proportion of patients symptoms and signs continue to increase for up to 6 weeks from the onset (Löffel et al. 1977; Winer et al. 1988a). At the height of the disease, the majority of the patients are bed-bound and many of these have complete paralysis of all four limbs. Only 12 per cent remain able to walk throughout the illness (Winer et al. 1988a). Those patients who become bed-bound and ventilator-dependent within 5 days tend to have the most prolonged disability and may develop severe permanent weakness (Ropper 1986). Significant sphincter dysfunction does not occur in Guillain–Barré syndrome, although urinary retention may result from abdominal wall weakness, particularly in patients with pre-existing urinary outflow tract obstruction.

Reflexes

Tendon reflexes are usually lost early in the disease. Total areflexia occurs in over 80 per cent of patients at some stage of the illness. The remainder usually lose their ankle jerks in isolation (Winer et al. 1988a).

Cranial nerves

Approximately half the patients develop cranial-nerve palsies, usually in the wake of severe ascending limb weakness (Löffel et al. 1977; Winer et al. 1988a). Isolated unilateral or bilateral facial palsy is the most common cranial-nerve lesion in Guillain–Barré syndrome. If weakness of the face is out of proportion to that of the limbs, Bannwarth syndrome or Lyme disease (Section 12.14.3) should be considered, especially if the spinal-fluid cell count is raised. Bulbar palsy and weakness of the muscles of mastication are the next most common cranial-

nerve abnormalities. With bulbar weakness there is a considerable risk of aspiration, leading to acute respiratory failure or pneumonia, and endotracheal intubation should be performed if this seems likely to occur. Ocular palsy only occurs in about 10 per cent of patients, usually following severe limb and respiratory muscle weakness.

Breathing

Respiratory failure of sufficient severity to require assisted ventilation occurs in one-quarter of patients, although milder degrees of respiratory muscle involvement are much more common. Patients with imminent respiratory failure may complain of orthopnoea and may be unable to complete more than a brief phrase of speech before pausing for breath. All patients with evolving Guillain–Barré syndrome need to have their vital capacity and diaphragmatic movements assessed regularly so as to predict their requirement for assisted ventilation before a respiratory crisis occurs. Usually ventilation needs to be considered when the vital capacity falls below 1 litre in adults with otherwise normal lungs.

Autonomic dysfunction

Autonomic dysfunction is common in the Guillain–Barré syndrome, occurring in over 60 per cent (Zochodne 1994). It contributes to the cardiac arrhythmias which are a leading cause of death, particularly in elderly patients (Dalos et al. 1988). Such arrhythmias, sufficient to compromise the circulation, occur in over 10 per cent of those with Guillain–Barré syndrome, and cause or contribute to death in 7 per cent (Winer and Hughes 1988). The presence of autonomic neuropathy cannot be predicted from the severity of the motor and sensory nerve abnormalities. Autonomic dysfunction may manifest either as excessive or as inadequate activity of the sympathetic or parasympathetic nervous systems. Wide fluctuations in blood pressure and heart rate, episodes of facial flushing, pupil abnormalities, patchy anhidrosis, paralytic ileus, or urinary retention may occur. Paroxysmal episodes of increased autonomic activity, causing hypertension, tachycardia, or facial flushing, are associated with a poor prognosis. They can be antecedents of sudden cardiac death in the Guillain–Barré syndrome. The pathophysiological basis of these varied autonomic manifestations is not known, but lymphocytic infiltrations of autonomic ganglia have been described.

Other neurological abnormalities

Other neurological abnormalities occur occasionally in Guillain–Barré syndrome. Papilloedema occasionally develops. If so, it is sometimes associated with headache and raised spinal-fluid pressure and tends to occur after a delay of some weeks (Weiss et al. 1991; Winer et al. 1988a). In some patients, it may reflect altered spinal-fluid hydrodynamics resulting from the high protein content. However, other mechanisms must also be considered, since cases of papilloedema have been documented with normal spinal-fluid protein levels. Optic neuritis and pyramidal tract signs are other rare manifestations which may point to a mild associated acute disseminated encephalomyelitis (Nadkarni and Lisak 1993).

Relapsing forms

Recurrent Guillain–Barré syndrome occurs in up to 3 per cent, often after an interval of many years (Löffel *et al.* 1977). The separate episodes may each be precipitated by new infections, such as recurrent cytomegalovirus exposure (Donaghy *et al.* 1989*a*), or two different infections, such as respiratory syncytial virus and *C. jejuni* (Hayashi *et al.* 1993), or booster vaccinations with tetanus toxoid. Up to six separate episodes have been recorded, each in itself typical of Guillain–Barré syndrome. Relapsing Guillain–Barré syndrome can be distinguished from relapsing forms of chronic idiopathic demyelinating polyneuropathy by the rapidity of onset, the marked degree of recovery, normal CSF protein at the onset of an attack, the high incidence of preceding infections, and the lack of response to immunosuppressant drugs (Grand'Maison *et al.* 1992).

Regional variants

Some patients present without the ascending evolution of areflexic tetraparesis so typical of Guillain–Barré syndrome. However, their time course of deterioration and recovery, acellular spinal fluid with raised protein, and electrophysiological evidence of demyelination, coupled with some otherwise typical clinical features, make these likely to be regional variants of Guillain–Barré syndrome. Those recognized include: bifacial paresis, lateral rectus paresis plus paraesthesiae plus hyporeflexia, areflexic paraparesis, pharyngeal–cervical–brachial weakness, and Miller Fisher syndrome coupled with weakness of bulbar or arm muscles (Ropper 1994). Isolated arm weakness may occur, either as a motor–sensory demyelination or as pure motor axonal involvement with anti-G_{M1} antibodies (Busby and Donaghy 2000). No treatment trials have been undertaken for these rare variants, and it seems wise to treat them according to principles established for Guillain–Barré syndrome.

Cerebrospinal fluid

In 80 per cent of cases the spinal fluid characteristically shows 'dissociation albumino-cytologique' in which the protein content is elevated, often exceeding 2 g/l, with a normal cell count. Normal spinal-fluid protein concentration is most common when the spinal tap is performed during the first few days of neurological symptoms. This limits the diagnostic value of lumbar puncture in early cases. About 10 per cent of patients have a lymphocytic spinal fluid, which should raise consideration of Lyme disease or HIV infection (Cornblath *et al.* 1987). Some patients develop a reduced serum sodium, possibly due to resetting of osmoreceptor responses.

Nerve-conduction studies

Nerve-conduction studies can be surprisingly normal early in the Guillain–Barré syndrome, despite severe paralysis. This reflects the purely radicular location of early demyelination or conduction block in many patients; conventional conduction studies merely measure motor conduction over the distal segments of peripheral nerves. Sometimes many peripheral nerves must be studied before diagnostic abnormalities are detected. Within the first 2 weeks, the most common findings are of mildly prolonged distal motor latencies and of conduction block in which the amplitude of the compound muscle action potential progressively diminishes with more proximal sites of nerve stimulation (Cornblath *et al.* 1988). F-waves may be absent or prolonged. As the disease progresses, the sensory nerve action potentials are usually lost, and motor slowing may become more evident distally. Permanent disability is predicted by electrical inexcitability of nerves early on, and tends to be associated with electrophysiological evidence of axonal degeneration.

Differential diagnosis

The Guillain–Barré syndrome usually presents a distinctive clinical picture (Asbury and Cornblath 1990). The potential range of differential diagnosis of acutely evolving paralysis is enormous: spinal cord disease; neuromuscular transmission disorders; myopathy; vasculitic neuropathy; porphyria; malignant meningitis; infective neuropathies such as diphtheria, borreliosis, or poliomyelitis; biological toxins such as tick paralysis or botulism; drug and chemical toxins; metabolic abnormalities; critical illness polyneuropathy; and psychologically determined weakness (Ropper *et al.* 1991).

Acute spinal-cord lesions pose the most common diagnostic difficulty, and spinal MRI needs to be undertaken in cases of doubt. However, the distinction is usually simple because of the extensor plantar responses, sensory level, prominent sphincter involvement, and the cellular spinal fluid encountered in acute ascending or transverse myelitis. It is rare for acute inflammatory myopathies to be confused with the Guillain–Barré syndrome. Pointers to primary muscle disease include the absence of sensory symptoms, preserved reflexes, normal spinal-fluid protein, abnormal electromyogram, and raised serum creatine kinase levels.

Three rare acute neuropathies should be distinguished from the Guillain–Barré syndrome because they require different approaches to therapy. *Borrelia* infection causing Lyme disease or Bannwarth's syndrome (Section 12.14.3) is suggested by prominent unilateral or bilateral facial paralysis, radicular pain, and a cellular CSF. Porphyric polyneuropathy (Section 12.8.6) is associated with early neuropsychiatric abnormalities, abdominal pain, a purely motor syndrome, and preservation of the ankle jerks despite loss of the knee jerks. Diphtheritic polyneuropathy (Section 12.14.4) is now rare in Western countries, although resurgent in eastern Europe, and should be considered in patients with descending demyelinating polyneuritis starting as bulbar palsy (Logina and Donaghy 1999).

Treatment

Survival in the Guillain–Barré syndrome depends primarily upon meticulous attention to intensive care during the acute paralytic phase. Feeding by nasogastric tube should be instituted in those with bulbar dysfunction. Subcutaneous heparin (5000 units four times daily) and elastic stockings provide prophylaxis against deep venous thrombosis and pulmonary embolism. Vigilant electrocardiographic monitoring allows prompt recognition and treatment of cardiac arrhythmias which may be provoked by endotracheal suctioning or suxamethonium administration (Zochodne 1994). β-Blockers may be required for those with hypertensive crises. Patients with Guillain–Barré syndrome are particularly susceptible to hypotensive side-effects of drugs, including thiopentone (thiopental), frusemide (furosemide), and morphine (Dalos *et al.* 1988). Nursing care will prevent decubitus ulcers. Regular physiotherapy and careful limb positioning will prevent muscle contractions in patients with prolonged paralysis. The gastrocnemius and soleus muscles are particularly prone to such contractures, which may lead to permanent walking disability even if muscle power returns.

Ventilation

Patients likely to deteriorate to the point of needing assisted ventilation should be alerted to this probability beforehand, while they can still ask questions, in a manner of calm planning. Endotracheal intubation and ventilation should be instituted without delay either if respiratory muscle failure is imminent or if paralysis of bulbar and laryngeal muscles places the patient at risk of choking. Assisted ventilation is usually required when the vital capacity has fallen to 15 ml/kg body weight; that is, a vital capacity of approximately 1 litre for a 65 kg adult. Nasal endotracheal tubes are well tolerated by conscious patients and should be replaced by temporary tracheostomy if, as is usually the case, the period of ventilation is likely to exceed 1 week. Pulmonary atelectasis and infection are common in intubated patients and should be treated promptly with antibiotics and physiotherapy.

Steroids

A randomized trial of oral prednisolone therapy in Guillain–Barré syndrome showed no benefit; and, indeed, suggested that steroids might increase the subsequent relapse rate (Hughes *et al.* 1978). Neither oral steroids nor intravenous high-dose steroids have a place in treating the Guillain–Barré syndrome (Guillain–Barré Syndrome Steroid Trial Group 1993).

Plasma exchange

Plasma exchange (Section 12.3.3) shortens the time taken for patients with Guillain–Barré syndrome to start to improve, to regain functional abilities such as walking, and reduces their requirement for assisted ventilation (Guillain–Barré Syndrome Study Group 1985; French Cooperative Group on Plasma Exchange in Guillain–Barré Syndrome 1987; McKhann *et al.* 1988). Plasma exchange enabled the median patient to walk independently at 53 days compared to 85 days for controls, and allowed 82 per cent to walk independently at 6 months compared to 71 per cent of controls. It is unclear whether plasma

exchange improves survival or reduces the number of patients unable to walk at 1 year. Subgroup analysis suggests that those patients with acute motor axonal forms associated with diarrhoea and campylobacter infection have a better outcome following IvIg than plasma exchange (Visser *et al.* 1999). To be maximally effective, plasma exchange needs to be started within the first week of neurological symptoms. It is unlikely to be effective if given after 2 weeks of neurological symptoms. Plasma exchange is recommended for those patients approaching inability to walk or with impairment of bulbar or respiratory function. Plasma-exchange schedules vary, but four or five 4-litre exchanges using a continuous-flow technique, given on sequential days, are recommended. The plasma may be replaced by either albumin or fresh frozen plasma; the risk of non-A, non-B hepatitis being greater with the latter (French Cooperative Group 1987). About 10 per cent of patients treated by plasma exchange will subsequently undergo a mild relapse between 5 and 42 days later, which may be treated by a further course of plasma exchange (Ropper *et al.* 1988). The factors determining poor outcome, such as advanced age or low compound muscle action potential amplitudes, appear to be the same for those receiving plasma exchange as for those receiving conservative therapy (McKhann *et al.* 1988).

Intravenous immunoglobulin

Intravenous immunoglobulin (IvIg) (Section 12.3.3), given at 0.4 g/kg body weight/day for 5 days, is at least equally effective as plasma exchange (van der Meché *et al.* 1992; Plasma exchange/Sandoglobulin Guillain–Barré syndrome Trial Group 1997). IvIg has become the treatment of choice because it is immediately available, does not require cannulation of a major vessel, has fewer side-effects than plasma exchange, and doesn't carry the same risks of exacerbating circulatory disturbances due to autonomic neuropathy. Also, IvIg may be more effective than plasma exchange for the motor axonal subgroup resulting from diarrhoeal campylobacter infections (Visser *et al.* 1999). There is concern that the easy availability of IvIg in district general hospitals may lead to Guillain–Barré syndrome being treated in intensive care units lacking expertise in the disease, with resultant increased death due to complications. As with plasma exchange, IvIg-treated patients may deteriorate secondarily within 2 weeks of treatment (Irani *et al.* 1993). It is unclear whether this simply reflects the natural history of underlying Guillain–Barré syndrome only temporarily modified by IvIg, or some specific IvIg effect, or indeed whether secondary deterioration is an indication for a second course of IvIg. Large-scale trials of IvIg or plasma exchange have not been undertaken in children, but it seems logical to expect similar benefits to those seen in adults, with IvIg being preferable to plasma exchange, particularly given the problem of vascular access in small children.

Prognosis

Most patients with the Guillain–Barré syndrome will make a good spontaneous recovery if they receive competent supportive treatment. Even when general intensive care facilities are available, up to 10 per cent of patients may die in the acute phase of the disease. These patients are usually elderly and generally succumb to cardiac disease, pulmonary embolism, or chest infection (Winer *et al.* 1988a; Lawn and Wijdicks 1999). The mortality is 4–5 per cent even for patients treated in specialist neurological units with plasma exchange or IvIg (Plasma Exchange/ Sandoglobulin Guillain-Barré syndrome Trial Group 1997). Of the survivors, nearly 60 per cent make a full recovery but the other 40 per cent show some permanent residual symptoms and signs, usually weakness of distal leg muscles, absent ankle jerks, or distal sensory loss (Löffel *et al.* 1977). Even after IvIg or plasma exchange therapy, 16.5 per cent are unable to walk at 48 weeks (Plasma Exchange/ Sandoglobulin Guillain-Barré syndrome Trial Group 1997). The factors predictive of poor outcome with slow recovery or permanent disability, include age over 60 years, a preceding diarrhoeal illness, development of severe paralysis within 5 days of the onset, respiratory failure requiring ventilation, and mean distal compound muscle action potentials of less than 20 per cent of normal (McKhann *et al.* 1988; Winer *et al.* 1988a; Visser *et al.* 1999).

12.10.2 Acute motor axonal neuropathy

Acute motor axonal neuropathy (AMAN) is a distinct subtype of Guillain–Barré syndrome which involves axonal degeneration or conduction block affecting motor fibres alone rather than the usual demyelination of both sensory and motor fibres (Section 12.10.1). AMAN was originally recognized in large summer epidemics in China, but is known to occur sporadically worldwide (Hafer-Macko *et al.* 1996). When compared to others with Guillain–Barré syndrome, AMAN patients have purely motor symptoms and signs, are more likely to have a more rapid evolution of limb weakness, plateau earlier on average at 6 days, have predominantly distal weakness, and are less likely to have cranial nerve involvement (Visser *et al.* 1995). Neurophysiology does not show the usual degree of motor slowing and prolongation of distal motor latencies, sensory nerve action potentials are generally preserved, motor nerves may be inexcitable, and electromyography often shows acute denervation changes. The differential diagnosis is similar to Guillain–Barré syndrome (Section 12.10.1), with particular consideration of poliomyelitis where that is still endemic. Subgroup analysis points to a better 6-month outcome if AMAN is treated with IvIg rather than plasma exchange (Visser *et al.* 1995, 1999). AMAN is more likely to be associated with long-term or permanent disability. However, many patients make substantial improvement in the early weeks after IvIg, suggesting that reversible conduction block, rather than axonal degeneration, underlies much of the disability.

The pathogenesis of AMAN is of considerable interest given its clear association with preceding diarrhoeal illness caused by *Campylobacter jejuni* and the frequent development of anti-G_{M1} ganglioside antibodies (Visser *et al.* 1995). AMAN is particularly likely after infection with the Penner 0:19 serotype of *C. jejuni*; campylobacter lipopolysaccharides have ganglioside-like moieties, raising the likelihood of antibodies cross-reacting with nerve (Sheikh *et al.* 1998). Presumably some host susceptibility factor determines whether a campylobacter-infected patient goes on to develop AMAN. This immunopathogenic mechanism is supported by demonstration of IgG and complement deposits on the axolemma at the nodes of Ranvier of motor fibres in fatal cases (Hafer-Macko *et al.* 1996).

12.10.3 Acute sensory neuropathy

Occasional patients with acute polyneuritis show profound limb sensory loss, particularly affecting joint, position, and vibration sensation, with severe ataxia. There may be little or no weakness although motor conduction is often slowed (Oh *et al.* 2000). Autopsies in such patients show lymphocytic infiltration and demyelination in the dorsal roots and sensory peripheral nerves (Dawson *et al.* 1988). This rare sensory form of polyneuritis should be distinguished from acute sensory neuronopathy, in which the limb sensory loss affects all modalities and often starts asymmetrically in the upper limbs, extends on to the trunk and face, there is no motor loss, recovery is unusual, and the pathology primarily involves loss of dorsal root ganglion neurons with lymphocytic infiltration (Windebank *et al.* 1990; Hainfellner *et al.* 1996).

12.10.4 Acute autonomic neuropathy

Rarely, patients present acutely with symptoms of autonomic neuropathy. Their symptoms are varied and reflect failure of the sympathetic and parasympathetic systems: postural hypotension, blurred vision, ptosis, pupillary abnormalities, dry mouth and eyes, anhidrosis, erectile failure, and constipation. Some patients may have varying degrees of associated thermal and pain sensory disturbances in the limbs. Spontaneous neuropathic pain may be prominent. Peripheral neuropathy may not be suspected initially because the sparing of larger myelinated fibres results in preserved tendon reflexes and normal sensory nerve action potentials (Suarez *et al.* 1994). Spontaneous recovery is the rule but is often incomplete. Prompt response to IvIg has been recorded (Mericle and Triggs 1997).

12.10.5 Miller Fisher syndrome

This distinctive syndrome comprises total external ophthalmoplegia, severe ataxia, and generalized tendon areflexia, which all develop over a few days (Fisher 1956). The spinal-fluid protein is elevated and patients recover over a matter of weeks. Some patients have combined features of Guillain–Barré and Miller Fisher syndromes, in which the oculomotor disturbance and limb weakness occur within a few days of one another. There has been debate as to the existence of a central nervous system component to Miller Fisher syndrome. Indeed, some have considered the syndrome to be a form of brainstem encephalitis (Al-Din *et al.* 1982). Although brainstem encephalitis may present a similar clinical picture to the Miller Fisher syndrome, it usually alters consciousness while tendon reflexes are preserved. Serial neurophysiological studies have shown clear evidence of peripheral-nerve involvement in the Miller Fisher syndrome, with prolonged peripheral conduction in the blink reflex arc and subsequent recovery of motor nerve and F-wave conduction velocities (Jamal and Ballantyne 1988). The serum of most patients contains antibodies against the GQ_{1b} gangliosides of both peripheral and central nervous systems, and the titre of this antibody declines commensurate with clinical improvement (Yuki *et al.* 1993). IgG fractions enriched in anti-GQ_{1b} induce both pre-and post-synaptic neuromuscular blockade (Buchwald *et al.* 2001). Patients seem to respond promptly to either plasma exchange or intravenous immunoglobulin.

12.11 Chronic idiopathic polyneuropathies

Significant reversal of severe disability can be achieved with immunosuppressive treatment for many patients with this varied group of neuropathies. Although the sensorimotor demyelinating and axonal forms are the most commonly encountered, the relative degrees of motor and sensory fibre involvement and the relative balance between demyelination, conduction block, and axonal degeneration vary considerably in the different clinical subtypes. It is not yet known whether this reflects fundamentally different underlying pathogenic mechanisms, or whether the various clinical syndromes simply represent noteworthy peaks in a continuum. Distinction of these different syndromes is of practical importance because it influences the approach to treatment. For instance, steroids are usually highly effective in chronic inflammatory demyelinating sensorimotor polyneuropathy, whereas they often cause deterioration, or at best are ineffective, in multifocal motor neuropathy with conduction block. As a general rule, intravenous immunoglobulin seems best effective when much of the disability is due to conduction block, whereas steroids and plasma exchange seem most effective when the disability is associated with histological demyelination, as evidenced by slowed nerve-conduction velocities.

12.11.1 Chronic inflammatory demyelinating sensorimotor polyneuropathy

Chronic inflammatory demyelinating sensorimotor polyneuropathy (CIDP) is a slowly progressive, sometimes relapsing, steroid-dependent, demyelinating sensorimotor polyneuropathy, primarily affecting the limbs. It is also known as chronic relapsing polyneuritis, chronic idiopathic demyelinating poly(radiculo)neuropathy, relapsing corticosteroid-dependent polyneuritis, or relapsing hypertrophic neuritis. Its recognition is of great importance because of the excellent response to immunosuppressant therapy in most patients.

Aetiology

The prevalence of CIDP increases with age from infancy to senescence, with a mean of onset in the fifth decade. It is more common in males. Accurate estimates of its incidence are not available, the overall prevalence is about 2 per 100 000, reaching 6.7 per 100 000 in the eighth decade in Australia (McLeod *et al.* 1999). Up to half the patients have a relapsing and remitting course, in which the initial deterioration can be rapid, resembling the Guillain–Barré syndrome. However, unlike the Guillain–Barré syndrome, patients subsequently progress downhill over more than 2 months. This deterioration may be steady, or relapsing and remitting. In women, relapses are particularly associated with the third trimester of pregnancy or the immediate postpartum period (McCombe *et al.* 1987a). Up to a third of patients give a history of antecedent viral infection or vaccination. Serological evidence of previous cytomegalovirus infection is found in about half, although a directly causative relationship has not been established (McCombe *et al.* 1987b).

Various features point to an immunological mechanism for chronic inflammatory demyelinating polyneuropathy, which might be considered as the chronic counterpart of Guillain–Barré syndrome. Nerve biopsies often show T-lymphocyte cell infiltrates, which may be slight, with early myelin stripping by macrophages. HLA antigen studies showed an increased frequency of the A3, B7, and DR2 antigens, and an association with specific GM haplotypes in a population of Australian patients (Feeney *et al.* 1990). A single causative autoantibody has not been identified.

Pathology

The histological features in sural nerve biopsies are often indistinguishable from those of the Guillain–Barré syndrome. Teased fibres show segmental demyelination and thinly re-myelinated internodes. Inflammatory infiltrates may be found in the endoneurium. Axonal loss may particularly affect large myelinated fibre populations. Some nerve biopsies show hypertrophic (onion-bulb) formations, raising difficulties in distinguishing chronic forms from hereditary motor and sensory neuropathy type I (Section 12.4.2).

Clinical features

Three-quarters of patients present with a mixed sensorimotor neuropathy which is relatively symmetrical. Less commonly, asymmetrical or predominantly motor or sensory forms are encountered. Paraesthesiae are a common early feature and may be painful. Loss of vibration and joint-position senses is usually demonstrable and Rombergism is a common early symptom. Limb weakness is generally distributed both proximally and distally. Usually, all the reflexes are lost. The rate of deterioration varies but progression over more than 8 weeks is a distinguishing criterion from the Guillain–Barré syndrome (McCombe *et al.* 1987b). The cranial nerves are affected in about 15 per cent of patients, usually to a mild degree. Dysphagia, dysarthria, weakness of facial or masticatory muscles, and diplopia are the most common cranial nerve manifestations. Papilloedema occasionally occurs. A coarse, irregular action tremor may occur, seemingly unrelated to the mild degrees of proprioceptive loss or weakness, and resembles that seen in patients with paraproteinaemic neuropathy. This may reflect mismatch of muscle spindle afferent information from agonist and antagonist muscles due to severely slowed peripheral-nerve conduction.

Associated central nervous system abnormalities

Some patients with chronic inflammatory demyelinating polyneuropathy also have a clinical history of a relapsing multifocal central nervous system disorder. Cerebral magnetic resonance imaging may show periventricular plaques of demyelination, and evoked responses may be prolonged (Thomas *et al.* 1987). A prospective study of patients with chronic inflammatory demyelinating polyneuropathy showed that subclinical abnormalities of the central nervous system were present in a third to a half (Ormerod *et al.* 1990). These findings pose questions of overlap with multiple sclerosis. They also raise the possibility that tremor in some patients with chronic inflammatory demyelinating polyneuropathy could be due to associated central nervous system involvement.

Nerve-conduction studies

The mainstay of diagnosis is the demonstration of slowed motor-nerve conduction, often with a degree of conduction block, in a patient with a chronically or subacutely progressive acquired peripheral neuropathy (Ad Hoc Subcommittee 1991). Electrophysiological criteria have been proposed for the diagnosis of chronic inflammatory demyelinating polyneuropathy (Section 2.5.3): motor conduction velocities of less than 75 per cent of the lower limit of normal, distal motor latencies exceeding 130 per cent of the upper limit of normal, temporal dispersion or conduction block following proximal stimulation, and prolonged F-wave latencies. Activity-dependent motor conduction block may be directed after maximal voluntary contraction (Cappelan-Smith *et al.* 2000). Sensory-nerve action potentials are usually diminished or lost. Diagnostic difficulty may arise in patients, usually with early and mild disease, in whom the motor conduction velocity is insufficiently slow to be sure that the neuropathy is primarily demyelinating. In such patients, motor conduction velocities only just below the normal range are not uncommon (McCombe *et al.* 1987b).

Cerebrospinal fluid

CSF protein is usually elevated above 1 g/l, although the level can be normal (McCombe *et al.* 1987b). Although sural nerve biopsy is frequently undertaken, it rarely adds diagnostic information in patients with a characteristic clinical and electrophysiological picture with raised spinal-fluid protein. Histological demonstration of segmental demyelination in nerve biopsy can be valuable if the clinical and electrophysiological picture is not diagnostic.

Differential diagnosis

Differential diagnosis most frequently causes difficulty in the distinction of chronic inflammatory demyelinating polyneuropathy from hereditary motor and sensory neuropathy type I (Section 12.4.2), particularly if molecular genetic tests have been negative for the latter. Pointers favouring chronic inflammatory demyelinating polyneuropathy are a subacute rate of deterioration, relapsing–remitting progression of motor weakness, positive sensory symptoms such as paraesthesiae, raised spinal-fluid protein, absence of a family history, and the absence of onion-bulb formations in a sural nerve biopsy. Motor-nerve conduction studies tend to show multifocal slowing and conduction block in chronic inflammatory demyelinating polyneuropathy, whereas the slowing is more uniform, without focal block, in hereditary motor and sensory neuropathy type I (Lewis and Sumner 1982). Associated deafness and pigmentary retinopathy should raise the possibility of Refsum disease, a rarely encountered possibility confirmable by blood phytanic acid measurement (Section 12.8.1).

MRI-proven hypertrophy of cervical roots, brachial plexus, or the cauda equina may be noted in chronic inflammatory demyelinating polyneuropathy and Guillain–Barré syndrome (Duggins *et al.* 1999). This raises the question of a relationship to focal hypertrophic neuropathies (Section 13.6.6). Sometimes these MRI findings raise the question of a diffuse nerve root infiltrative process, but the presence of electrophysiologically proven demyelinating polyneuropathy is strong evidence against that, and should forestall nerve root biopsy. Hypertrophied roots and nerves may be more vulnerable to compression by stenosis of the lumbar spinal canal, in root exit foramina, and at common entrapment sites.

Chronic inflammatory demyelinating polyneuropathy is not usually a paraneoplastic phenomenon, except in the sense of its common association with paraproteinaemia (Section 12.12.1). One should be suspicious of an underlying lymphoma, carcinoma (Section 12.13.2) or Castleman's disease (Section 12.12.3) in two circumstances. First, when the neuropathy evolves relatively rapidly and there are unusual features, such as extensive cranial nerve involvement or neuropathic pain. Secondly, when the patient relentlessly deteriorates despite immunosuppressant therapy.

Treatment

A proven diagnosis of chronic inflammatory demyelinating polyneuropathy means that there is an excellent chance of recovery with immunosuppressant therapy. Without treatment, chronic inflammatory demyelinating polyneuropathy is eventually fatal in up to 10 per cent of patients (Bouchard *et al.* 1999). Untreated, many of the remainder suffer protracted and serious disability. The degree of associated axonal loss may determine the chance of a good recovery, and may be lessened by prompt and early treatment.

Occasionally immunosuppressant treatment must be started in severe weakness to prevent further decline, before it is clear whether the patient has Guillain–Barré syndrome, which would plateau by 4–6 weeks, or chronic inflammatory demyelinating polyneuropathy, which should progress beyond 8 weeks. Usually it is preferable to give such patients a course of intravenous immunoglobulin or plasma exchange, rather than start steroids, since a secondary deterioration when the treatment effect wears off at 6–10 weeks will indicate that the underlying neuropathy continues to evolve, thus requiring more definitive long-term immunosuppressant therapy. An unusual intermediate form evolving over 4–8 weeks, called subacute idiopathic demyelinating neuropathy, is described (Hughes *et al.* 1992).

Oral steroid therapy is the mainstay of treatment and often produces noteworthy improvements within 3 weeks. The results of therapy can be dramatic; bed-bound patients may regain almost normal motor function. Unfortunately, not all patients respond to steroid therapy (Dyck *et al.* 1982). It is elderly patients, or those with a significant degree of axonal degeneration, who tend to respond less well. Prednisolone administration schedules vary. An initial daily dosage of 60 mg is recommended, falling to 45 mg daily after 2 weeks, and converting to 45 mg on alternate days over the next 2–3 months. Steroid therapy may need to be continued for years, and protection against osteoporosis should be prescribed (Section 12.3.3). Patients frequently relapse within a few months of withdrawing prednisolone.

Other immunosuppressant drugs are sometimes useful. Azathioprine is often added as a steroid-sparing agent, although there is no controlled evidence that it is beneficial in this condition (Dyck *et al.* 1985). None the less, remission does seem to be maintainable by azathioprine in some patients, particularly young women, who may relapse some months after the drug is stopped. Cyclosporin A can induce improvement in some steroid-resistant patients (Hodgkinson *et al.* 1990). Interferon α-2a is effective in some patients resistant to other immunomodulatory therapy (Gorson *et al.* 1998).

Plasma exchange (Section 12.3.3) produces substantial improvement in 80 per cent of patients with either progressive or relapsing forms of chronic inflammatory demyelinating polyneuropathy (Hahn *et al.* 1996a). Given that steroids remain the mainstay of treatment in most patients, plasma exchange is recommended in the following circumstances:

(1) those who fail to respond promptly or adequately to steroids;

(2) those in whom high initial steroid dosages pose contraindications, such as steroid-induced psychosis or brittle diabetes;

(3) to 'kick-start' an improvement in the elderly, who are notoriously slow responders to steroids;

(4) if there is severe disability at the outset;

(5) to reverse a relapse promptly so as to avoid the need for reinstituting very high steroid dosages.

The neuropathy relapses some 4–10 weeks after a successful course of plasma exchange, and definitive long-term therapy should be commenced simultaneously unless repeated plasma exchange is envisaged as maintenance therapy.

Intravenous immunoglobulin (Section 12.3.3) produces significant improvement in about 65 per cent of chronic inflammatory demyelinating neuropathy patients (Hahn *et al.* 1996b).

It can improve conduction block in peripheral nerves. The benefit of a 5-day course usually lasts for 4–10 weeks, and the general indications are identical to plasma exchange. Because it is easier to administer, it provides a better option for maintenance therapy.

Strategies for immunomodulatory treatment vary in different clinical situations. Some patients have such mild forms of chronic inflammatory demyelinating polyneuropathy that the risks of treatment far outweigh the small benefits which could accrue. Usually a patient can be maintained on prednisolone 15–30 mg on alternate days, often in conjunction with azathioprine. For inadequate responses, immunoglobulin then plasma exchange should be tried, and as a last resort, cyclosporin or interferon α-2a. Infantile and childhood chronic inflammatory demyelinating neuropathy responds to steroids or immunoglobulin (Sladky *et al.* 1986; Vedanarayanan *et al.* 1991). The elderly can be slow to begin what may be an ultimately useful response, and plasma exchange or immunoglobulin should be considered with steroids from the outset. Withdrawal of immunomodulatory treatment is only likely to be successful in those unusual patients who fully remit, often children, adolescents, or young women. In these patients azathioprine offers the chance of maintaining steroid-free remission once a good steroid response has been obtained. Relapses on stopping or reducing therapy should be treated promptly, since such patients seem to become less completely responsive due to accumulated axonal damage.

Objective monitoring of therapy is important for judging its effectiveness (Section 12.13.2). Nerve-conduction velocities are of little help in monitoring the ongoing severity of any patient's neuropathy, although quantifiable foci of conduction block can provide useful guidance. Ultimately it is the clinical assessment of reliable parameters such as walking speeds, stair-climbing ability, manipulatory tasks such as buttons, Rombergism, and ability to stand on tiptoe or hop, which provides the best index of any patient's response to treatment.

12.11.2 Chronic ataxic polyneuropathy with ocular palsy

The onset of chronic relapsing polyneuropathy can be preceded by ocular palsies occurring several weeks earlier (Donaghy and Earl 1985). These ocular palsies may be unilateral or bilateral, usually consisting of partial paralysis of ocular abduction. The polyneuropathy may be asymmetrical, markedly ataxic, worse in the arms, and include dysphagia. Nerve-conduction studies usually point to a primarily demyelinating disorder. Ataxic neuropathy and eye movement disorder is often associated with antibodies to GD_{1b} or GQ_{1b}, IgM paraproteins, and cold agglutinins (Willison *et al.* 1993). Rombergism and pseudoathetosis (Fig. 12.16) are prominent and often outweigh the degree of demonstrable joint-position sense loss. Paraesthesiae are a less common symptom than ataxia. This syndrome has become known by the acronym CANOMAD (Chronic Ataxic Neuropathy with **O**phthalmoplegia, **M**-proteins, cold **A**gglutinins and

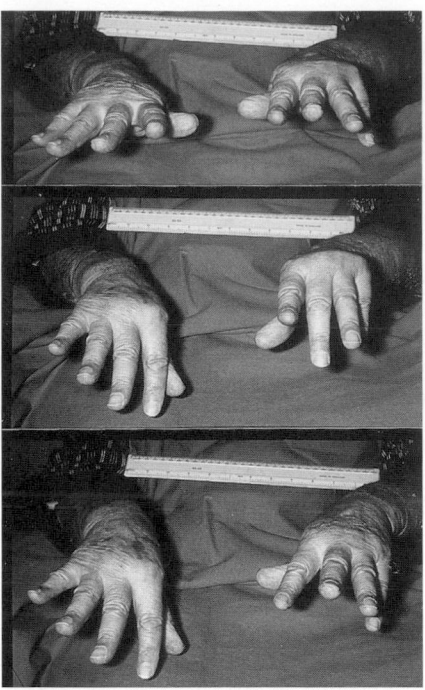

Fig. 12.16. Pseudoathetosis in a patient with sensory ataxic polyneuropathy. Frame intervals at 30 seconds.

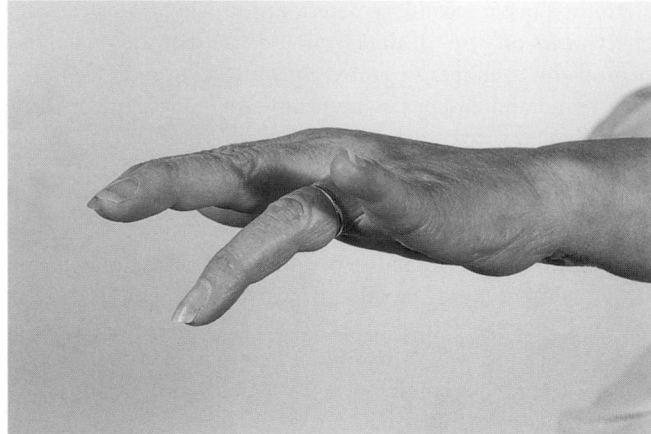

Fig. 12.17. Weakness of extension of a single finger: a common early symptom of multifocal motor neuropathy with conduction block.

anti-Disialated ganglioside antibodies). Many patients do not exhibit the full syndrome at presentation, although many or all of the missing features appear with time; however, the anti-GQ_{1b} antibody seems to be ubiquitous. The eye movement disorder can be symptomatic only intermittently. The same immunomodulatory approach to treatment should be taken as for normal chronic inflammatory demyelinating polyneuropathy (Section 12.11.1).

12.11.3 **Multifocal motor neuropathy with conduction block**

Many patients with multifocal motor neuropathies used to be diagnosed as suffering from benign forms of motor neuron disease solely affecting lower motor neurons. These patients may present at any age in adult life with symptoms that may have progressed slowly for 20 years or more.

Clinical picture

This varies immensely (Pestronk *et al.* 1990). Weakness is usually maximal distally, is often notably asymmetrical, and is more likely to start and predominate in the arms. In retrospect, often the first symptom has been inability to fully extend a single finger (Fig. 12.17), probably reflecting the onset of conduction block in a terminal branch of the posterior interosseous nerve. Muscle atrophy occurs with time. Occasionally a weakened muscle may be hypertrophied (Fig. 12.18). Fasciculations are observed only rarely by comparison with amyotrophic lateral sclerosis. Cranial nerve involvement can occur, affecting bulbar muscles, causing difficulty in differentiation

from amyotrophic lateral sclerosis (Kaji *et al.* 1992; Donaghy *et al.* 1994). Reflex loss is usually restricted to the affected muscles, although it can be more generalized.

Motor-nerve conduction studies

Motor-nerve conduction studies show varying combinations of multifocal motor conduction block, prolonged or absent F-waves, prolonged distal latencies, reduced motor-nerve conduction velocities, or motor axonal loss with electromyographic evidence of denervation (Katz *et al.* 1997). The crucial electrodiagnostic feature is conduction block restricted to a nerve's motor fibres, at a site not vulnerable to compression (Fig.

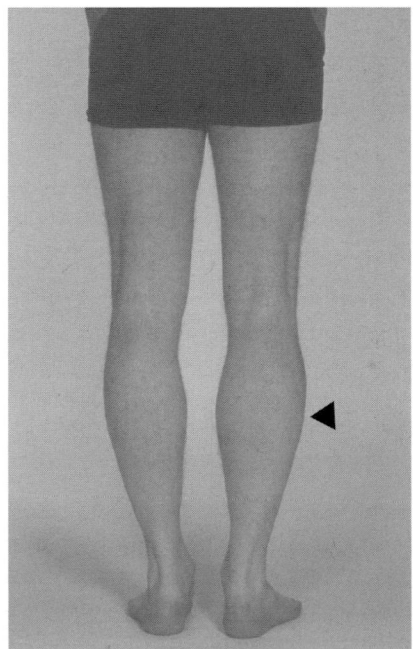

Fig. 12.18. Hypertrophy of the right and weakened calf muscles (arrowed), in a patient with multifocal motor neuropathy with conduction block.

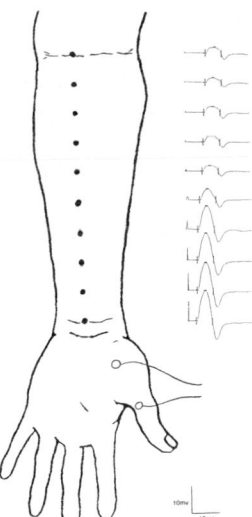

Fig. 12.19. Focal motor conduction block in a mid-forearm segment, demonstrated by inching the stimulating electrode along the median nerve in a patient with multifocal motor neuropathy with conduction block. Sensory conduction was normal throughout this same segment. The compound muscle action potential amplitudes from abductor pollicis brevis are shown to the right (Courtesy of Dr M. Busby.)

12.19); unfortunately this often occurs in electrophysiologically inaccessible segments of an affected nerve. Under such circumstances one should place considerable diagnostic weight upon demonstrating significant weakness in muscles which are not wasted; this clinical sign correlates with conduction block in the afferent nerve. Serum antibodies to G_{M1} gangliosides are present in approximately a third of patients with multifocal motor neuropathy with conduction block. It remains to be established whether anti-G_{M1} plays a pathogenic role in multifocal motor neuropathy (Willison 1994). It binds to nodes of Ranvier in peripheral nerves (Santoro et al. 1990). Focal deposition of immunoglobulins, and demyelination associated with inflammation, have been observed in the motor roots (Oh et al. 1995). The spinal fluid is usually normal.

Sensory function

Usually there are no sensory symptoms and sensory nerve conduction is normal. A few patients report focal paraesthesiae but it is rare to demonstrate underlying abnormal sensory signs. Despite the purely motor features, minor involvement of sensory nerve fibres has been noted on biopsy (Donaghy et al. 1994; Corse et al. 1996). Rare patients are encountered with multifocal conduction block neuropathies involving both motor and sensory nerve fibres, and with MRI evidence of brachial plexus hypertrophy (van den Berg-Vos et al. 2000).

Treatment

Untreated, multifocal motor neuropathy usually deteriorates steadily or in a stepwise fashion over many years. Occasionally it evolves subacutely, causing severe disability within months. Some patients may stabilize with extremely minor degrees of motor

involvement. It is uncertain whether true spontaneous remissions occur. Steroid treatment should be avoided since it is ineffective and often causes substantial motor deterioration (Donaghy et al. 1994). Cyclophosphamide is effective (Feldman et al. 1991) but is not advisable as first-line therapy because of the serious side-effect profile (Section 12.3.3). It is best reserved for patients unresponsive to, or intolerant of, immunoglobulin, or in those rare instances where it is helpful as adjunctive therapy when the beneficial effect of immunoglobulin alone only lasts 2 or 3 weeks. Intravenous immunoglobulin (IvIg) is the mainstay of treatment, often producing a clear clinical response within 36 hours, usually maximal at 10–14 days, and wearing off at 6–12 weeks (Chaudhry et al. 1993; Nobile-Orazio et al. 1993; Donaghy et al. 1994; van den Berg et al. 1995; Frederico et al. 2000). The first treatment with immunoglobulin should be designed to determine whether the response reverses disability sufficiently to make regular treatment worthwhile; up to a third of patients show poor responses (Bouche et al. 1995). Self-infused home therapy at 2–3-weekly intervals is effective, time saving, and convenient, and it can be scheduled to avoid treatment-related fluctuations (Sewell et al. 1997). The long-term benefits of IvIg are unknown and cases of continued downhill deterioration have been recorded (Bouche et al. 1995; van den Berg et al. 1998). However, many patients continue responding well to IvIg for years, with no evidence of background deterioration of the disorder, once a regular programme of maintenance therapy has been established which avoids intermittent relapses. A preliminary report suggests that interferon β-1a may be effective if IvIg or cyclophosphamide treatment has failed (Martina et al. 1999).

12.11.4 Pure motor demyelinating neuropathy

Occasionally patients are encountered with reasonably symmetrical and purely motor polyneuropathy. Although this may involve arms more than legs, usually all four limbs are affected to a similar extent, particularly the distal muscles. The weakness lacks the asymmetry normally associated with multifocal motor neuropathy. It tends to present with deterioration over weeks to months rather than the very slow deterioration normally occurring in typical multifocal motor neuropathy with conduction block. Motor conduction studies show widespread slowing with variable degrees of conduction block. Anti-G_{M1} antibodies may be associated (Pestronk et al. 1990). The implications for choice of treatment underline the importance of differentiating pure motor demyelinating neuropathy from sensorimotor demyelinating neuropathy. Pure motor demyelinating neuropathy often deteriorates with steroids, whereas it responds well to intravenous immunoglobulin (Donaghy et al. 1994). The likelihood of eventual remission is unknown, although natural remission can be observed after patients with young onset pass through adolescence. Even in patients with a similar clinical picture and anti-G_{M1} antibodies, where the electrophysiological picture reflects axonal degeneration rather than demyelination or conduction block, strength may improve over 6–24 weeks following cyclophosphamide and plasma exchange therapy (Pestronk *et al.* 1994).

12.11.5 Chronic idiopathic sensory neuropathy

Chronic ataxia may be due occasionally to a purely sensory form of chronic inflammatory demyelinating polyneuropathy affecting large myelinated kinaesthetic fibres. Patients present with limb ataxia, and sometimes numbness or pain, and are found to have profound loss of proprioceptive sensation which may even affect proximal joints. Muscle strength is normal and there is generalized areflexia. Despite this, motor-nerve conduction is often slowed. Sensory-nerve action potentials are absent (Oh *et al.* 1992). Demyelination may be present on sural nerve biopsy. The spinal fluid protein can be raised. The condition usually deteriorates progressively over months or years. Improvement may follow a trial of immunomodulatory therapy, including intravenous immunoglobulin (van Dijk *et al.* 1996).

Chronic idiopathic neuropathy with purely sensory symptoms presents a difficult differential diagnostic problem. If associated with an eye movement disorder and anti-GQ$_{1b}$ antibodies, the CANOMAD syndrome (Section 12.11.2) will be obvious. Paraneoplastic sensory neuropathy (Section 12.13.1) will be associated with small cell lung cancer or ovarian cancer, usually with subacute progression, involvement of all sensory fibre types, antineuronal antibodies (anti-Hu), a mildly lymphocytic CSF, or other associated features of encephalomyelitis (Griffin *et al.* 1990; Graus *et al.* 1994). The sensory ganglionitis associated with Sjögren's syndrome may or may not be associated with clear-cut symptoms of dry eyes and mouth, usually occurs in women, ataxia due to large fibre loss predominates, and there may be autonomic symptoms, including Adie's pupil. An associated trigeminal neuropathy can occur, antinuclear antibody may be present, and the CSF may be normal (Griffin *et al.* 1990; Sobue *et al.* 1993). A similar neurological picture may occur either acutely or chronically without Sjögren's syndrome (Griffin *et al.* 1990). Vitamin E deficiency (Section 12.21.4) can also produce a sensory ataxic neuropathy. Purely sensory presentations of chronic idiopathic axonal polyneuropathy also occur, usually in late adulthood, often with troublesome pain (Wolfe *et al.* 1999).

12.11.6 Chronic idiopathic axonal polyneuropathy

This disorder usually starts in the sixth decade of life, with clinical evidence of a mild sensorimotor, or less often a purely sensory, polyneuropathy, worse in the legs. All modalities of sensation may be impaired but paraesthesias are uncommon. Neurophysiological and nerve biopsy studies point to axonal degeneration. Progression is slow, and eventual severe disability is rare (Notermans *et al.* 1993). By definition an underlying cause is not discovered; a similar disorder in patients with paraproteinaemia tends to produce more severe arm involvement and worse disability (Notermans *et al.* 1996). Type II hereditary motor and sensory neuropathy (Section 12.4.3) can usually be differentiated by the positive family history, the predominance of motor involvement, the earlier age of onset, and the likelihood of pes cavus (Teunissen *et al.* 1997). The relationship to painful chronic cryptogenic sensory neuropathy with prominent pain (Wolfe *et al.* 1999) or to the painful burning foot syndrome (Periquet *et al.* 1999) is unclear. If abnormalities are limited to the legs, the potentially treatable lumbar canal stenosis syndrome should be sought by MRI (Section 21.3.2). There is no curative treatment for chronic idiopathic axonal polyneuropathy. A chronic relapsing axonal polyneuropathy with unusually severe motor involvement has responded promptly to intravenous immunoglobulin, presumably by reversal of widespread conduction failure (Katirji 1999), but this is not a likelihood in the majority of patients. Rapidly progressive axonal polyneuropathy, usually with subtle multifocal features, can occur occasionally in vasculitis (Section 12.15.2).

12.12 Neuropathies associated with lymphoproliferative disorders

12.12.1 Benign paraproteinaemia

An increased incidence of peripheral neuropathy occurs in patients found to have monoclonal paraproteins on serum electrophoresis. Such paraproteins only have an incidence of 0.1 per cent in the third decade of life, rising to 3 per cent in the eighth decade, yet they are found in 10 per cent of patients with idiopathic peripheral neuropathy (Latov 1995). Diverse neuropathies are encountered. Only a proportion of paraproteinaemic proteins are likely to be directly causative of neuropathy. Thus in many cases the paraprotein is merely a coincidental finding, and a trial of treatment should be considered along the usual lines for the idiopathic equivalent of that particular type of neuropathy (Section 12.11). A wide variety of peripheral neuropathies are encountered, mostly demyelinating. Amyloid neuropathy (Section 12.9.2) may result from immunoglobulin light-chain deposition in patients with paraproteinaemia. Vasculitic neuropathy (Section 12.15) is occasionally associated with cryoglobulins containing monoclonal rheumatoid factors.

CIDP-like polyneuropathy

Demyelinating neuropathies indistinguishable from idiopathic chronic inflammatory demyelinating polyneuropathy (CIDP) are usually associated with IgG or IgA paraproteins and may respond well to immunosuppressant drugs, plasma exchange, or intravenous immunoglobulin. As a group, these paraprotein-associated, CIDP-like neuropathies are more likely to progress slowly, cause less severe disability, and have prominent sensory involvement than idiopathic CIDP (Simmons *et al.* 1995). Paraproteinaemia or other lymphoproliferative disorders can develop, or at least become evident, after the initial diagnosis of chronic demyelinating polyneuropathy (Section 12.11.1). Slowly progressive demyelinating polyneuropathy occurs in about 5 per cent of patients with Waldenström's macroglobulinaemia, a disorder characterized by IgM hyperglobulinaemia, hyperviscosity, lymphadenopathy, hepatosplenomegaly, and lymphocytic infiltration of the bone marrow, and may antedate the systemic illness by some years (Dellagi *et al.* 1983).

Anti-MAG activity

Some chronic sensorimotor demyelinating neuropathies are associated with IgM paraproteins possessing anti-myelin-associated glycoprotein (MAG) activity. Such patients usually develop sensory signs before motor, all go on to develop arm tremor and ataxia and usually stabilize at 2–5 years (Smith 1994). Nerve biopsies from such patients may show characteristic widely spaced myelin lamellae; similar morphological changes occurring in chicks after passive transfer of the IgM paraprotein (Tatum 1993). The IgM paraproteins fix complement at the sites of separation of myelin lamellae (Monaco *et al.* 1990). IgM paraproteinaemic demyelinating polyneuropathy with anti-MAG antibodies may show an unusually distal pattern of weakness (Katz *et al.* 2000). Unlike chronic inflammatory demyelinating polyneuropathy, such neuropathies often respond poorly over the longer term to immunomodulation (Nobile-Orazio *et al.* 2000).

Anti-ganglioside activity

Purely motor neuropathies, often multifocal with conduction block, can be associated with paraproteins showing antibody activity against G_{M1} and G_{D1b} gangliosides (Section 12.11.3). Predominantly sensory neuropathies due to combined axonal degeneration and demyelination are associated with paraproteins with antisulphatide activity (Lopate *et al.* 1997; Ponsford *et al.* 2000). Chronic ataxic neuropathies associated with anti-GQ_{1b} antibodies and intermittent ophthalmoplegia are often also associated with IgM paraproteinaemia, the CANOMAD syndrome (Section 12.11.2).

Anti-chondroitin sulphate activity

Predominantly sensory axonal degeneration neuropathy occasionally occurs in patients with IgM-κ or IgM-λ paraproteins recognizing chondroitin sulphate. The first symptoms are usually peripheral numbness, paraesthesiae, or pain. Abnormalities of all modalities of sensation may be demonstrable. In some patients the disorder is associated with the skin condition, epidermolysis (Sherman *et al.* 1983). In others there may be nerve thickening with features of focal entrapment neuropathy (Yee *et al.* 1989).

Treatment

Treatment of paraproteinaemic polyneuropathies can be difficult and relatively ineffective compared to idiopathic demyelinating neuropathies. Initially steroids, and plasma exchange or immunoglobulin, should be tried, along the lines outlined for chronic inflammatory demyelinating polyneuropathy (Section 12.11.1). If this is insufficiently effective, the first decision concerns whether the patient has a sufficient degree of disability to warrant use of potentially dangerous chemotherapy. If so trials, first of the alkylating agents cyclophosphamide or chlorambucil, and secondly of fludarabine, can be undertaken (Latov 1995). Preliminary studies point to the effectiveness of rituximab, a monoclonal antibody against the β-lymphocyte antigen CD20 (Levine and Prestronk 1999).

12.12.2 Myelomatous neuropathy

Symptomatic neuropathies occur in about 5 per cent of patients with osteolytic multiple myeloma, although electrophysiological evidence of neuropathy may be present in up to 40 per cent of such patients. A wide range of neuropathies is encountered. The chronic demyelinating and amyloid neuropathies are probably a direct effect of paraproteins. A paraneoplastic sensory neuronopathy of the same type most usually associated with small cell lung cancer can occur in myeloma (Kelly *et al.* 1981). Conventional chemotherapy of the underlying myeloma has little effect on the amyloid neuropathy or the sensory neuronopathy. However, patients with demyelinating sensorimotor neuropathy can improve substantially with steroid therapy and plasma exchange given in addition to chemotherapy for their underlying myeloma. Pronounced improvement can occur after ablation therapy for a localized plasmacytoma.

Neuropathy is a common feature of osteosclerotic forms of myeloma, which are rare by comparison to osteolytic forms (Kelly *et al.* 1983). The neuropathy associated with osteosclerotic myeloma, and the accompanying systemic illness, are identical to that seen in Castleman's disease, the POEMS syndrome, and the Crow–Fukase syndrome (Section 12.12.3). If solitary, the osteosclerotic lesion may be treated by localized irradiation or resection, leading to substantial improvement in the neuropathy over subsequent months (Kelly *et al.* 1983).

12.12.3 Castleman's disease, POEMS syndrome

Progressively disabling, predominantly motor neuropathies may occur in association with elements of a characteristic syndrome: papilloedema, gynaecomastia, impotence, glucose intolerance, oedema, hepatosplenomegaly, and paraproteinaemia, usually IgA-λ. The skin changes are particularly characteristic and include diffuse cyanotic discolouration, poor capillary reperfusion after blanching, hypertrichosis, and diffuse non-dependent oedema. This constellation of features is particularly common in Japan where it is known as the Crow–Fukase syndrome (Nakanishi *et al.* 1984). It is otherwise known as the POEMS syndrome (Polyneuropathy, Organomegaly, Edema, M band, Skin changes) (Bardwick *et al.* 1980). Either osteosclerotic myeloma, or angiofollicular lymph-node hyperplasia (Castleman's disease) may underlie this clinical syndrome (Kelly *et al.* 1983; Donaghy *et al.* 1989*b*). The neuropathy may be predominantly motor with severely reduced conduction velocities, or it may be sensorimotor with evidence of both demyelination and axonal loss. Roughly half show a good neurological response some months after the initiation of cyclophosphamide and prednisolone therapies (Donaghy *et al.* 1989*b*) or melphalan and prednisolone therapies (Kuwabara *et al.* 1997). The remainder are relatively unresponsive, and in some a remorseless downhill progression occurs, with eventual death despite chemotherapy for the underlying lymphoproliferative disorder.

12.12.4 Lymphomatous peripheral neuropathy

Five distinct types of polyneuropathy occur as an occasional remote accompaniment of lymphoma. The Guillain–Barré syndrome and chronic relapsing inflammatory demyelinating neuropathy probably reflect disordered immune regulation, and should be treated according to standard principles (Sections 12.10.1, 12.11.1) (Lisak *et al.* 1977; Vallat *et al.* 1995). Paraneoplastic sensory neuronopathy occasionally complicates lymphoma, although this is a rare association by comparison to its incidence in small cell carcinoma of the lung (Section 12.13.1) (Henson and Urich 1982). A subacute motor neuropathy may complicate Hodgkin's disease and other lymphomas, and resolves spontaneously in most patients (Schold *et al.* 1979). Diffuse infiltration of nerves by non-Hodgkin's lymphoma can produce a progressive, painful, asymmetric polyneuropathy (van den Bent *et al.* 1999).

12.13 Carcinomatous neuropathy

Three types of peripheral neuropathy may occur as remote, or paraneoplastic, effects of carcinoma: sensory neuronopathy, sensorimotor polyneuropathy, and, less frequently, vasculitic neuropathy. Small cell carcinoma of the lung is the most common tumour to underlie paraneoplastic neuropathy. Carcinoma of the breast, ovary or gastrointestinal tract, myeloma, or lymphoma occur less frequently. Patients frequently present with neuropathy before experiencing symptoms from the underlying cancer itself. Although symptomatic paraneoplastic neuropathy is relatively uncommon, prospective studies in patients with lung and breast cancer reveal clinical evidence of polyneuropathy in up to 5 per cent, with subclinical electrophysiological abnormalities in another 20 per cent (Hughes *et al.* 1996).

12.13.1 Paraneoplastic sensory neuronopathy

This sensory neuropathy occurs more commonly in women, usually preceding tumour symptoms by 6–15 months and occasionally by as long as 3 years. It usually develops subacutely over a period of weeks before stabilizing spontaneously. Less often it continues to deteriorate inexorably. This distinctive neuropathy

may predominate in the arms and can be asymmetrical. Patients develop sensory ataxia due to loss of kinaesthetic sensation and may experience uncomfortable paraesthesiae. All modalities of sensation are impaired. The gait ataxia may prevent walking. Sensory loss can extend to the trunk and may contribute to impaired sphincter function. Muscle weakness does not occur because motor fibres are spared. The reflexes are usually lost (Horwich *et al.* 1977). Occasionally such paraneoplastic sensory neuropathy runs a slowly progressive course without severe disability (Graus *et al.* 1994). Other forms of paraneoplastic encephalomyelitis frequently coexist, particularly limbic encephalitis (Section 30.6).

Nerve-conduction studies show reduced or absent sensory-nerve action potentials, while motor-nerve conduction is normal. The spinal fluid is usually lymphocytic and proteinaceous. Neuropathologically, there is profound loss of dorsal root ganglion neurons with lymphocytic infiltration; a 'dorsal root ganglionitis'. The serum or spinal fluid may contain high titres of an autoantibody directed against neuronal nucleoproteins of molecular weight 35–40 kDa, known as anti-Hu antibodies (Section 30.6) (Dalmau *et al.* 1992). Anti-Hu antibody also occurs in patients with other forms of paraneoplastic encephalomyelitis. It may also be detected in low titre in some patients with small cell lung cancer who do not have an associated neurological disorder. Detection of this anti-Hu antibody should always provoke careful search for an underlying tumour, which should be repeated after an interval if initially negative. Neither treatment nor removal of the underlying tumour, nor immunosuppression, is known to reverse the sensory neuronopathy. However, the underlying carcinoma should be staged carefully in case of the rare possibility of curative treatment.

Sjögren's syndrome

A similar sensory neuronopathy may occur in women with Sjögren's syndrome or the isolated sicca complex of dry eyes and dry mouth (Griffin *et al.* 1990; Grant *et al.* 1997). This disorder can develop in patients without underlying cancer or Sjögren's syndrome and can be associated with Adie's pupil (Griffin *et al.* 1990). The cases associated with Sjögren's syndrome usually have predominantly kinaesthetic sensory loss, dry eyes on Schirmer testing, a positive antinuclear factor, and they lack other features of paraneoplastic encephalomyelitis. Their sensory disturbance may stabilize or improve slightly.

No treatment is known to alter the natural history of any of these sensory neuropathy syndromes.

12.13.2 Paraneoplastic sensorimotor neuropathy

The presence of muscle weakness distinguishes this from the purely sensory neuronopathy described above. Such neuropathies are a heterogeneous collection; they can be acute, subacute, or chronic in presentation, and primarily demyelinating or axonal in nature. They are not usually associated with other paraneoplastic neurological disorders and they can be associated with a wide range of underlying carcinomas. They may precede or follow tumour symptoms. Mild sensorimotor neuropathy may be detected in up to a quarter of patients with lung cancer (Hughes *et al.* 1996). Most usually the onset is subacute with limb weakness, sensory disturbance, and areflexia. Nerve-conduction studies and electromyography may reveal axonal degeneration, in which case attempts at treatment with steroids are likely to be unsuccessful. Demyelinating neuropathies are occasionally encountered, although more commonly with underlying lymphoma than with carcinoma. Typical Guillain–Barré syndrome or chronic inflammatory relapsing demyelinating polyneuritis may occur, and the latter is often steroid responsive. Nerve biopsies show variable combinations of axonal loss, segmental demyelination and remyelination, and perivascular lymphocytic infiltration.

12.13.3 Paraneoplastic vasculitic neuropathy

Mononeuritis multiplex due to vasculitis occasionally occurs with cancer of the prostate or lung, or lymphoma. Neuropathic symptoms may precede those due to the underlying tumour. Nerve and muscle biopsies allow histological diagnosis of microvasculitis. Cyclophosphamide therapy may lead to stabilization or improvement of the neuropathy (Oh *et al.* 1991).

12.14 Neuropathy due to infections

Peripheral neuropathy is a central clinical feature of some infections: leprosy, diphtheria, human immunodeficiency virus (HIV) infection, borreliosis, and herpes zoster. This section does not cover those peripheral neuropathies, such as the Guillain–Barré syndrome, which are infrequent and indirect manifestations of common infections with a wide variety of viruses and bacteria, all of which may share the common property of disturbing immune regulation or evoking antibodies which cross-react with nerves (Section 12.10). Demyelinating neuropathy is a rare accompaniment of Creutzfeldt–Jakob disease, both in the sporadic and inherited forms (Esiri *et al.* 1997).

12.14.1 Leprosy

Aetiology

Leprosy (Hansen's disease) is due to infection of the skin, mucosal membranes, and peripheral nerves by *Mycobacterium leprae*, an acid-fast bacillus stainable by Ziehl–Neelsen's method. Infection is only likely after prolonged contact with patients suffering from bacillus-rich forms of the disease, especially if being shed in nasal secretions. The skin is the most common portal of entry. Leprosy is common in the Asian subcontinent but may be encountered anywhere in the world. In the Western world it is usually encountered in migrants from endemic areas.

Pathology

The histopathological and clinical picture varies widely in different individuals. This reflects different degrees of cell-mediated immunity. Three general forms may be distinguished within what is, in reality, a continuum, which can be subclassified further (Jacobson and Krahenbuhl 1999). Patients with high immunity develop tuberculoid leprosy, which is not progressive, and is usually associated with a single granulomatous skin lesion containing few bacilli and which may involve an underlying peripheral nerve. Patients with low or absent immunity develop lepromatous leprosy, in which copious bacilli multiply extensively in the cooler tissues in the body, with progressive and extensive involvement of skin and nerves. Most commonly, patients manifest the intermediate or dimorphous forms which occupy the borderland between the tuberculoid and lepromatous varieties.

The exact pathogenetic mechanisms underlying nerve damage in leprosy are not clear. The advanced nerve damage in established tuberculoid leprosy may reflect the compressive and ischaemic consequences of the infiltrating cells forming the granuloma. Nerves in advanced lepromatous leprosy contain vast accumulations of bacilli which may disrupt nerve fibres by virtue of their sheer size (Pedley *et al.* 1980). It is unlikely that early leprous neuropathy reflects primary infection of Schwann cells, because segmental demyelination is not prominent (Jacobs *et al.* 1987). In early leprous neuropathy, the bacilli are most prominent in macrophages and Remak cells, the supporting cells of unmyelinated fibres (Shetty *et al.* 1988).

Clinical features

Early diagnosis is crucial since antibiotic therapy will prevent further irreversible nerve damage. The combination of skin and peripheral-nerve lesions is the hallmark of leprosy. In tuberculoid forms, sharply demarcated, hairless, anaesthetic erythematous plaques, or hypopigmented macules, are associated with sensory and motor loss in the distribution of one or two damaged peripheral nerves. The nerve is often palpably enlarged. The greater auricular and superficial peroneal nerves are the most commonly affected. Occasionally tuberculoid leprosy affects nerves without an associated skin lesion.

In lepromatous leprosy, there is extensive skin involvement with erythematous macules, papules, or nodes. Skin thickening produces the characteristic leonine faces, with thickening of the nose and ear lobes and eventual perforation of the nasal septum. Nerves are diffusely and progressively involved, leading to mononeuritis multiplex. Nerve thickening is rare.

In dimorphous or intermediate forms of leprosy, the skin and neuropathic changes lie between the tuberculoid and lepromatous forms, and poorly defined hypopigmented skin lesions are characteristic. Sensory loss in leprosy tends to spare warm areas of the body, such as the palms, and preferentially affects the skin of cold areas. Patients with advanced leprous neuropathy develop profound pain and temperature loss, leading to acromutilation with trophic ulcers, Charcot joints, and autoamputations.

Diagnosis

The clinical picture is usually characteristic, and failure to prove the diagnosis histologically should not deter the physician from advising drug therapy. The simplest method of proving the diagnosis of leprosy is to take skin biopsies or smears from both the centre and edge of a lesion, and to demonstrate acid-fast bacilli by Ziehl–Neelsen staining. Bacilli are most prominent within dermal nerves. Nerve biopsy is particularly valuable in suspected cases without skin lesions and demonstrates bacilli or characteristic granulomatous reaction and inflammation (Chimelli *et al.* 1997). The lepromin skin test is only positive in tuberculoid forms.

Treatment

Leprosy is the world's most common treatable neuropathy. Adequate early therapy prevents the development of disfiguring disability but will not allow recovery of nerves which are already severely damaged. The following chemotherapeutic regimens are currently recommended (Jacobson and Krahenbuhl 1999). Borderline and lepromatous leprosy should be treated for a minimum of 2 years until skin scrapings and biopsies are negative for bacilli. Daily self-administration of dapsone (100 mg) and clofazimine (50 mg) orally should be accompanied by supervised administration of once-monthly of clofazimine (300 mg) and rifampicin (600 mg). Patients with tuberculoid leprosy should receive daily dapsone (100 mg) with supervised monthly rifampicin (600 mg) for 6 months; single-dose combination therapy of rifampicin, ofloxacin, and minocycline (ROM) may also be effective. Some physicians recommend that rifampicin be administered daily, rather than monthly, for both multi-bacillary and pauci-bacillary leprosy. Following chemotherapy, nerve grafting may restore sensation in patients with severe mononeuritic sensory loss causing acrodystrophic changes. Steroids are recommended to prevent treatment reactions in patients with hypersensitivity phenomena, such as erythema nodosum or iritis. Steroids are advised if a silent neuropathy develops after the initiation of chemotherapy, whether or not associated with systemic evidence of a reaction (Croft *et al.* 1997). Vasculitic neuropathy can develop years after effective treatment in nerves containing persisting leprosy antigen; steroid treatment is effective (Bowen *et al.* 2000).

12.14.2 Human immunodeficiency virus

A wide spectrum of peripheral neuropathy occurs in HIV infection and the acquired immune deficiency syndrome (AIDS). It includes the Guillain–Barré syndrome and chronic inflammatory demyelinating neuropathy developing early in the course of the disease. Later in the disease, the symmetrical distal sensory neuropathy of AIDS must be differentiated from that caused by zalcitabine (ddC) or didanosine (ddI) antiviral therapy (Section 12.18.9). A rapidly progressive multifocal motor and sensory polyradiculopathy due to cytomegalovirus or infiltrative lymphocytosis may occur (So and Olney 1994; Gherardi *et al.* 1998). Necrotizing arteritic neuropathy can also occur in HIV-infected patients (Bradley and Verma 1996).

Possible underlying HIV infection must be considered in a patient with undiagnosed polyneuropathy.

Guillain–Barré syndrome

Typical Guillain–Barré syndrome (Section 12.10.1) occurs early in the course of HIV infection, often around the time of primary infection. HIV antibodies may not be present, and P24 antigen assays may be required to diagnose the infection. A clue to underlying HIV infection comes from finding a spinal-fluid pleocytosis, generally 20–30 cells/mm^3 (Cornblath *et al.* 1987). The usual treatment of the Guillain–Barré syndrome is recommended, including intravenous immunoglobulin administration, with particular care to avoid exposure to body fluids.

Chronic inflammatory demyelinating neuropathy

This occurs regularly in HIV-infected patients, often at a relatively early stage before the development of the acquired immunodeficiency syndrome (de la Monte *et al.* 1988). It should be treated in the usual way (Section 12.11.1). It should be recognized that steroid administration may augment the existing defect in cell-mediated immunity that occurs in HIV infection. Thus, immunoglobulin infusion may be particularly required in HIV-infected chronic inflammatory demyelinating polyneuropathy patients so as to minimize the use of immunosuppressive drugs.

Cytomegalovirus polyradiculoneuropathy

In patients with established HIV infection, cytomegalovirus causes a subacute polyradiculoneuropathy. Some patients may present with a sacral sensory loss and acute urinary retention, and progress to flaccid paraparesis within a few weeks (So and Olney 1994). Cytomegalovirus may be cultured from the spinal fluid and should be sought by polymerase chain reaction. Other patients develop a rapidly progressive multifocal sensory motor neuropathy affecting the limbs, in which dysaesthesiae and pain may be prominent from the outset. Cytomegalovirus may be detected by immunostaining within biopsied peripheral nerves or autopsied spinal-nerve roots. These nerves may contain gigantic cells with inclusions typical of cytomegalovirus infection. Without treatment, death soon follows the development of this neuropathy. Early therapy with ganciclovir or cidofovir can produce improvement (Cohen *et al.* 1993).

Sensory polyneuropathy

A predominantly sensory, symmetrical polyneuropathy affects up to 30 per cent of patients with the acquired immunodeficiency syndrome. This neuropathy becomes increasingly common in the later stages of the illness (Cornblath and McArthur 1988). The initial complaint is of painful paraesthesiae in the feet, and the ankle jerks are usually lost. Electrophysiology shows diminished or absent sensory-nerve action potentials, without slowing of motor-nerve conduction. The neuropathy progressively worsens in the feet. It should be differentiated from the painful sensory neuropathy caused by ddI or ddC antiretroviral drugs (Section 12.18.9), which is likely to develop within months of starting the drug and then tends to deteriorate more rapidly (Berger *et al.* 1993).

12.14.3 Borreliosis

Infection with the tick-borne spirochaete *Borrelia burgdorferi* causes Lyme disease, a multisystem disorder comprising a characteristic expanding annular skin lesion (erythema chronicum migrans), oligoarthritis, carditis, meningoencephalitis, cranial neuritis, polyradiculopathy, and peripheral neuropathy (Halperin *et al.* 1996). Incomplete forms of the disease are frequent and should be recognized because of their impressive response to antibiotic therapy. Neurological features occur in about 15 per cent of patients, starting a few weeks to several months after the tick bite. Human infection usually follows tick bites during the summer. It is most common in patients who have been in woodland areas populated by rodents, squirrels, or deer, the animal reservoirs for *Borrelia burgdorferi*. Infection is frequent in North America and mainland Europe, and also occurs less frequently in Britain, Australia, and Asia. The Bannwarth syndrome of lymphocytic meningoradiculitis is a form of Lyme disease, described in Europe before it was recognized that there was an underlying *Borrelia* infection.

Cranial neuritis

Facial palsy of acute onset, either unilateral or bilateral, commonly occurs in the early weeks of *Borrelia* infection. About a quarter of cases of Bell's palsy may be due to *Borrelia* infection in endemic areas (Halperin *et al.* 1992). The palsy is often incomplete and may be accompanied by subjective facial sensory disturbance. Facial nerve paralysis may be the only neurological feature of Lyme disease. It usually recovers without treatment but may be treated with oral antibiotics and a short course of oral prednisolone if seen within 24 hours of onset.

Polyradiculopathy

Shooting pains in the territories of affected nerve roots are sometimes accompanied by reflex loss or sensorimotor abnormalities in the limbs. Sharp chest-wall pains reflect involvement of thoracic nerve roots. Half the patients with polyradiculopathy also have facial palsy. The polyradiculopathy of borreliosis may last some months, but usually resolves spontaneously.

Peripheral neuropathy

Mononeuritis multiplex, polyneuropathy, and acute brachial neuralgia may all occur in Lyme disease. Any of these neuropathies may accompany polyradiculitis and facial palsy. Mononeuritis multiplex and acute brachial plexus neuropathy tend to occur within the first few months of infection. Up to half of patients with untreated late Lyme disease develop a chronic polyneuropathy with intermittent limb paraesthesiae (Logigian and Steere 1992). Few neuropathic abnormalities are generally found on examination of such patients: mild distal glove-and-stocking sensory loss with preserved reflexes and motor function are the general rule. Nerve-conduction studies show reduced and slowed sensory-nerve action potentials, and, sometimes, increased distal motor latencies. Neurophysiological abnormalities are multifocal in nature, and there is no generalized motor slowing. Sural nerve biopsies may show mild axonal loss, with some perivascular lymphocytic infiltration; necrotizing vasculitis is not encountered.

Central nervous system involvement

Central nervous system involvement may be chronic and take a variety of forms, resembling multiple sclerosis, other infective meningoencephalitides, stroke, or tumour (Oksi *et al.* 1996). MRI can show single or multiple enhancing brain lesions and pathologically these involve demyelination, lymphocytic blood vessel involvement, and detectable *Borrelia* DNA, indicative of direct infection.

Investigations

The demonstration of elevated serum or spinal-fluid IgM or IgG antibody titres to *Borrelia burgdorferi* has been the traditional diagnostic investigation. However, antibody assays are of low diagnostic sensitivity early in infection, and do not discriminate between active and inactive infection later on. The spinal fluid contains a striking white cell pleocytosis of up to 700 cells/mm^3 in patients with polyradiculitis, but may be normal if isolated facial palsy or peripheral neuropathy are the only neurological features. *Borrelia burgdorferi* may be cultured from about 50 per cent of skin lesions but only 5 per cent of CSF specimens. Amplification of small amounts of borrelial DNA in CSF or urine by the polymerase chain reaction (PCR) holds promise as the most specific means to prove infection, but current tests are negative in up to 50 per cent of patients, depending upon the particular clinical manifestations and the stage of the disease (Schmidt 1997).

Treatment

The peripheral neuropathy or radiculopathy of Lyme disease responds well to intravenous benzylpenicillin (2.4 g 6-hourly for 10 days), ceftriaxone (2 g/day for 14 days), or doxycycline (Halperin *et al.* 1987).

12.14.4 Diphtheria

Polyneuropathy is the most common and most important neurological complication of diphtheria; the exotoxin of *Corynebacterium diphtheriae* has an affinity for peripheral nerves. Polyneuropathy is more common in childhood than in adult infections. Paralysis is more likely to follow severe local infections, which are usually faucial but may be extrafaucial. Antitoxin is given to reduce the incidence of paralysis, particularly in patients who can receive it early in the illness.

Palatal paralysis reflects the action of locally produced toxin upon the nerves to the bulbar musculature. Involvement of nerves by locally produced toxin accounts for localized paralysis following a cutaneous infection, the muscles paralysed being those supplied by the spinal segment from which the infected region is innervated. Localized neuropathy in one or more extremities was often seen after diphtheritic infection of limb wounds in the Middle East in the Second World War. Paralysis of accommodation, generalized polyneuropathy, and cardiac toxicity are due to blood-borne dissemination of the toxin to the ciliary muscles, peripheral nerves, and heart.

Diphtheria remains endemic in the Third World but is now rare in Western countries due to improved living conditions and childhood immunization programmes. Occasional outbreaks of clinical diphtheria do occur in previously immunized adults, although the clinical severity is generally reduced. At least 10 per cent of adults vaccinated in childhood have insufficient residual immunity to protect against infection once diphtheria returns to a population (Kjeldson *et al.* 1985). This reduced immunity in adults resulted in a spectacular return of diphtheria to Russia and other eastern European countries after 1993 (Rakhmanova *et al.* 1996; Logina and Donaghy 1999). Overall about 15 per cent of patients diagnosed with diphtheria develop polyneuropathy.

Pathology

The primary lesion in the peripheral nerves is segmental demyelination accompanied by typical slowing of motor-nerve conduction, which may persist for some time after clinical recovery (Solders *et al.* 1989). The neuropathic effects of the toxin are dose-dependent. Once bound to cells, the toxin becomes unavailable for inactivation by antitoxin.

Symptoms and signs

Paralysis of the palate is usually the earliest neurological symptom and appears a median of 10 days after the onset of localized throat diphtheria, generally as the typical palatal pseudomembrane. It is generally bilateral but may be unilateral. The voice becomes nasal, there is regurgitation of fluids through the nose on swallowing, and the larynx becomes paralysed, allowing inhalation and choking. The palatal reflex is usually lost. Twenty per cent of patients develop ventilator-dependent respiratory failure. Improvement of bulbar symptoms occurs at median 30 days from onset. Secondary deterioration of bulbar function, sometimes enough to require ventilation for the first time, occurs in over a third at a median 40 days from initial onset (Logina and Donaghy 1999).

Paralysis of accommodation due to ciliary muscle involvement produces blurred vision for near objects. The pupillary reactions to light and on convergence are unimpaired. Paresis of the face or external ocular muscles may occur.

Generalised sensorimotor polyneuropathy affecting the limbs occurs in 90 per cent, at a median of 37 days from onset. It always occurs after the bulbar symptoms, and sometimes when the bulbar symptoms are already improving. About 50 per cent of patients become unable to walk unaided; 30 per cent develop impaired bladder control. Blood pressure swings or cardiac arrhythmia reflect either autonomic neuropathy or cardiomyopathy (Logina and Donaghy 1999).

Diphtheritic hemiplegia is fortunately rare and is usually due to either embolism or thrombosis of a cerebral artery, or to acute post-infective encephalitis. Its effects are similar to those of other acquired forms of infantile hemiplegia. Meningism was once common in the acute stage, with cervical rigidity or opisthotonos and rigidity of the limbs, so-called 'spasmodic diphtheria'. The CSF in such cases of presumed encephalopathy is usually normal in composition. Permanent bulbar palsy is a rare sequel.

Diagnosis

The chief differential diagnosis of diphtheria is from Guillain–Barré syndrome, which is an ascending, rather than descending, polyneuropathy (Section 12.10.1). Diphtheria is favoured by the high prevalence of bulbar and respiratory dysfunction at a time of little or no limb involvement, by the evolution for longer than 4 weeks, by the preceding sore throat rather than catarrhal illness, and by the simultaneous involvement of other organs, particularly the heart (Logina and Donaghy 1999). The CSF protein tends to be elevated in both conditions. Throat cultures are positive in 98 per cent of those with diphtheria, and 8 per cent have the highly toxic 'bull-neck' form of the disease (Rakhmanova *et al.* 1996).

Prognosis

The prognosis of the paralysis is usually good now that endotracheal intubation prevents death due to bulbar or respiratory muscle failure. Nevertheless, some limb symptoms persist in 80 per cent at 1 year, while 6 per cent are still unable to walk. Sixteen per cent of diphtheria patients die, but usually from cardiac or other organ involvement rather than paralysis (Logina and Donaghy 1999). Hemiplegia is a serious complication, especially in children, as it may not only be fatal, but in patients who survive, recovery is usually incomplete, and epilepsy and dementia may follow.

Treatment

The treatment of diphtheria includes antibiotic therapy and injection of adequate doses of antitoxin as early as possible. Benzylpenicillin (1.2 g 6-hourly intravenously), should be given for 14 days, converting to oral penicillin when the patient can swallow normally. Erythromycin (500 mg four times daily) is an alternative for patients with penicillin allergy. Diphtheria antitoxin should be given intravenously or intramuscularly; serum sickness may occur in up to 10 per cent of patients. It is unclear for how long antitoxin will be beneficial after the onset of diphtheria. In the absence of any formal clinical trials, retrospective evidence suggests little benefit on the incidence of paralysis or death if antitoxin is administered after the second day of the throat infection (Logina and Donaghy 1999). General nursing care, and indications for assisted ventilation, are similar to those in Guillain–Barré syndrome (Section 12.10.1). Tracheostomy may be required early if paralysis of the pharynx or larynx leads to choking while feeding or drinking.

12.14.5 Herpes zoster

Herpes zoster is a reactivation of varicella zoster virus which had been primarily acquired during chickenpox infection.

Zoster is particularly likely in the elderly and the immunosuppressed, and may affect a fifth of all adults at some time in the life. Few patients have more than one attack. Following primary chickenpox infection, the varicella zoster virus becomes latent in the sensory ganglia and motor neurons. During zoster eruptions there is inflammation and haemorrhagic necrosis, destroying neurons of the affected dorsal root ganglion, with a shingles eruption in the skin of the corresponding dermatome.

Clinical features

An attack of shingles is usually heralded by tingling in the dermatome or lancinating pains. These generally precede the visible rash by 2 or 3 days. Erythematous macules and papules rapidly become vesicular, and the lesions accumulate over 3–5 days. Scabbing occurs 3–7 days later, and then dry by 2 weeks. The intensity of the vesicular eruption varies immensely, from a few vesicles only in mildly affected patients, to a dense oedematous rash covering the entirety of one or more dermatomes in more severely affected patients

(Fig. 12.20). When zoster affects the ophthalmic division of the trigeminal nerve, conjunctivitis and keratitis can occur, associated with periorbital oedema (Section 11.1.4). Electromyographically detectable motor involvement is associated with the skin eruption in 50 per cent of patients, and sometimes produces clinically evident muscular paralysis affecting the diaphragm, limb muscles, external ocular, or facial muscles (Haanpaa *et al.* 1997). Zoster eruptions in sacral dermatomes may produce paralysis of the bladder, with haemorrhagic cystitis, and bowel ileus, confusable with an acute abdomen. Clinical evidence of meningoencephalitis is uncommon (Section 34.6.2). However, subclinical evidence of brainstem or spinal-cord involvement at the relevant level is evident on MRI in over 50 per cent, and the CSF is lymphocytic, often with detectable varicella zoster virus DNA in 60 per cent (Haanpaa *et al.* 1998).

Although the diagnosis of shingles can be confirmed by isolation of the varicella zoster virus from vesicular fluid, or immediate demonstration by electron microscopy, the rash is usually sufficiently characteristic to allow unequivocal clinical diagnosis. However, if seeing a patient after resolution of a rash

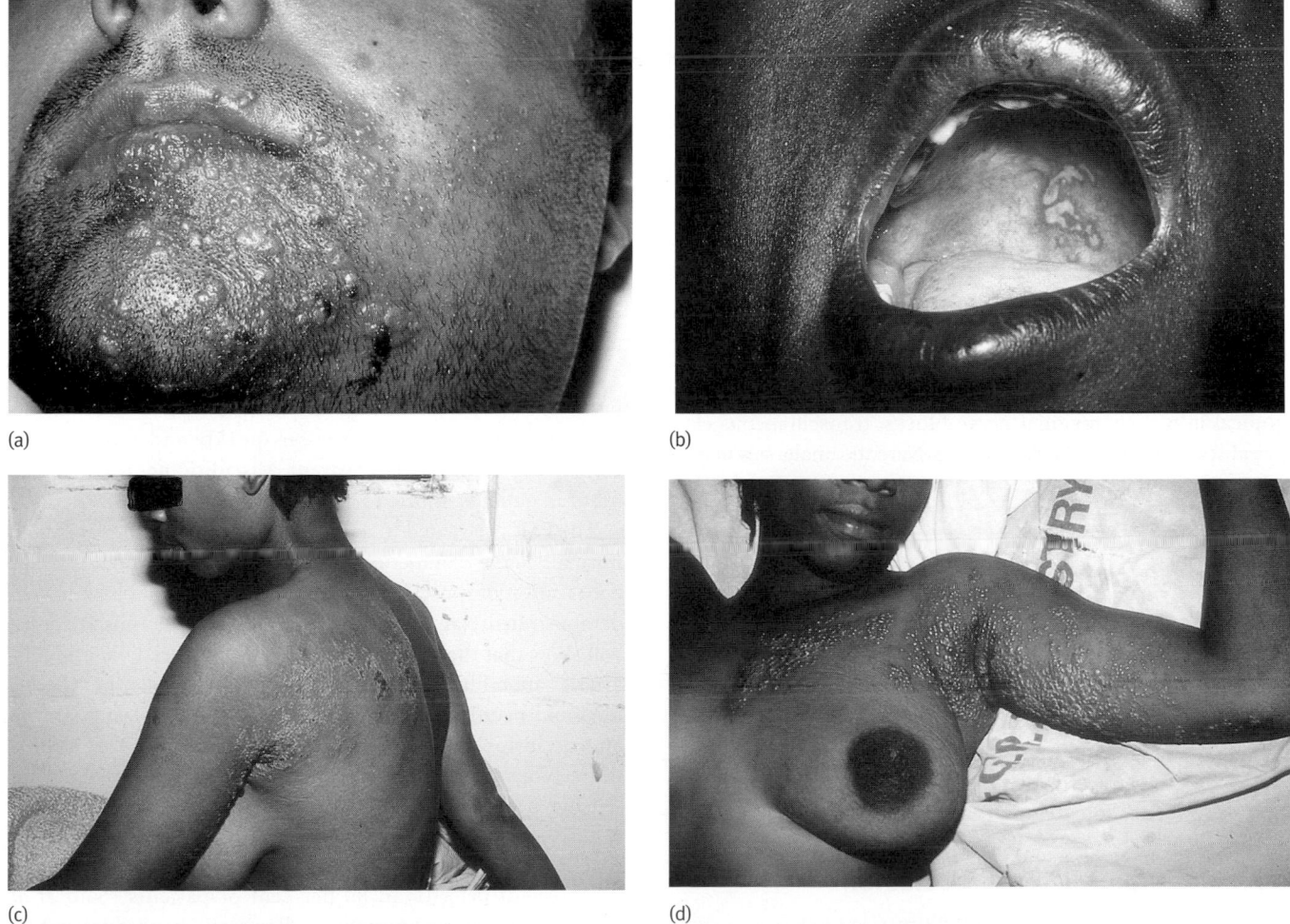

(a)

(b)

(c)

(d)

Fig. 12.20. Herpes zoster eruptions (a) in the mandibular division of the trigeminal nerve; (b) on the tongue and palate, the 'Ramsay Hunt syndrome'; (c) T2 and T3 dermatomes posteriorly; and (d) anteriorly. (Courtesy of Dr C. Conlon).

attributed to zoster, it is advisable to take a clear history concerning the distribution and vesicular character of the eruption, to confirm the likely diagnosis when a patient is seen after resolution of the rash. Sometimes patients self-diagnose other skin disorders as having been attacks of zoster.

Treatment

Treatment of the acute attack should be with analgesics sufficiently potent to relieve pain. Antiviral drugs (acyclovir (aciclovir), valaciclovir, famciclovir) speed resolution of the acute eruption and may reduce the risk of prolonged pain. Oral antiviral drugs are often prescribed for immunocompetent patients with uncomplicated zoster eruptions, although the extent of their value is unclear. Antiviral drugs are clearly indicated in patients displaying clinical evidence of central nervous system involvement, or who are immunocompromised, and should be administered intravenously in more serious clinical situations (Cohen et al. 1999).

Post-herpetic neuralgia

Post-herpetic neuralgia is the feared long-term complication of shingles. It is defined as pain persisting beyond 1 month. Quantification of sensory nerve fibres in skin biopsies from affected dermatomes show a more severe nerve fibre loss in those with post-herpetic neuralgia than in those without (Oaklander et al. 1998). Post-herpetic neuralgia is more likely in the elderly, those who have had a severe rash with significant pain, and those with ophthalmic involvement (Dworkin 1999). Such patients merit antiviral therapy during the acute zoster eruption so as to try and reduce the risk of subsequent post-herpetic neuralgia. Once established, post-herpetic neuralgia can be disturbingly resistant to local and systemic pain-relieving measures. Amitriptyline may be beneficial, particularly if given from an early stage. Topical capsaicin ointment may relieve pain in some, but cause burning in others. Carbamazepine or gabapentin may be tried. Local measures may include topical lidocaine, regional nerve blocks, transcutaneous electrical stimulation, and acupuncture. Narcotic analgesics may be necessary if other measures fail.

12.15 Vasculopathic neuropathy

Ischaemia may produce focal damage to peripheral nerves, causing mononeuropathy or mononeuritis multiplex. This is most familiar in the context of necrotizing vasculitis or diabetic microvascular disease (Section 12.17.1) affecting the vasa nervorum. Patients with a possible diagnosis of vasculitic neuropathy should be investigated urgently so that treatment can be started to forestall further peripheral nerve damage.

12.15.1 Major arterial occlusion

It is unusual for blockage of medium-sized arteries to cause obvious clinical features of neuropathy because of the rich longitudinal anastomosis of the peripheral nerve vasculature. None

the less, axonal loss is demonstrable histologically in nerves from limbs affected by chronic peripheral vascular disease (Nukada et al. 1996). In general, myelinated fibres seem more vulnerable to ischaemia than unmyelinated (Fujimura et al. 1991).

Acute embolic, thrombotic, or traumatic occlusion of a major artery to a limb may cause peripheral nerve dysfunction, but the neuropathic symptoms and signs are usually overshadowed by the prominent effects of associated acute ischaemia of skin and muscle. Prompt restoration of blood flow, for instance by embolectomy, may lead to full recovery of peripheral nerve function. Prolonged ischaemia leads to irreversible peripheral nerve damage, which may be associated with ischaemic contractures of muscles. Multifocal neuropathy resembling vasculitis may occur in the cholesterol emboli syndrome which may be precipitated by arterial catheterization procedures; muscle or nerve biopsy may demonstrate cholesterol clefts within small arteries (Bendixen et al. 1992). The creation of arteriovenous fistulae in the arm for haemodialysis can cause a distal axonal neuropathy, probably due to a vascular steal syndrome (Bolton et al. 1979).

12.15.2 Non-systemic vasculitis

In some patients, necrotizing vasculitis is confined to the peripheral nervous system (Davies et al. 1996). Most patients with non-systemic vasculitic neuropathy develop multiple mononeuropathies affecting the limbs, thoracic roots, or the cranial nerves. Each mononeuropathy evolves over a few hours or days, producing muscle weakness, paraesthesiae and pain, and global sensory disturbance in the territory of the affected nerve. Tendon reflexes may be retained if the damage is restricted to the more distal segments of nerves. A minority of patients present with a symmetrical or asymmetrical distal polyneuropathy which may be sensorimotor or purely sensory. Thus, the potentially treatable condition of vasculitic neuropathy should be considered in patients with a distal axonal polyneuropathy which progresses quickly and for which no convincing diagnosis is apparent. Vasculitic neuropathy may occur in patients infected with HIV (Said et al. 1988).

The ESR is elevated in a minority. The spinal fluid is usually normal. Nerve-conduction studies show focal axonal loss and denervation of muscles. Occasionally conduction block may be demonstrated (Jamieson et al. 1991). Nerve or muscle biopsy will show that the walls of epineurial, perineurial, or muscular arteries are infiltrated by polymorphonuclear cells, and there is fibrinoid necrosis, destruction of the internal elastic lamina, and occlusion of the vessel lumen (Fig. 12.21). The yield of nerve biopsy is greatest if an electrophysiologically abnormal sensory nerve is chosen and biopsied to full thickness (Wees et al. 1981). Superficial peroneal nerve biopsy is positive in just over 50 per cent of patients, whereas muscle biopsy proves the diagnosis of arteritis in 80 per cent of patients (Said et al. 1988). Thus the recommended diagnostic procedure is full-thickness biopsy of a sural or superficial radial nerve if electrophysiologically abnormal and, otherwise, a muscle biopsy.

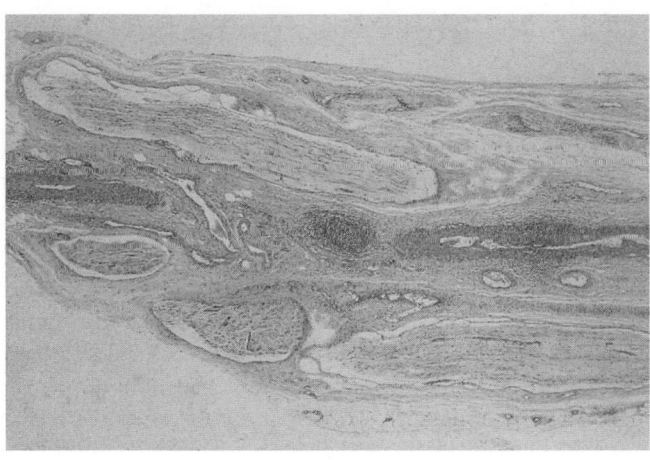
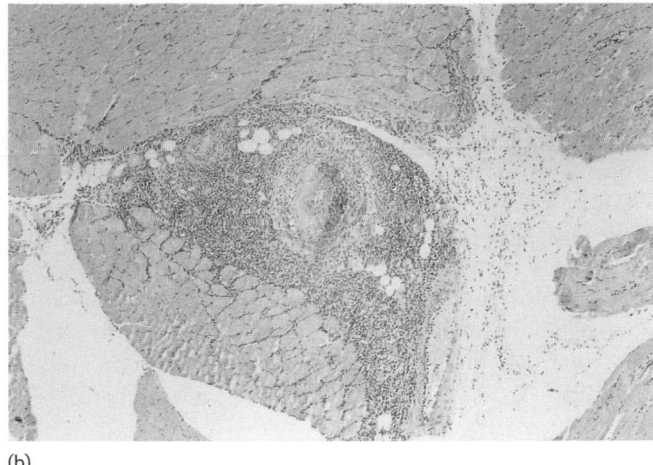

(a)   (b)

Fig. 12.21. Histological features in vasculitic neuropathy. (a) Nerve biopsy, showing inflammatory cell infiltration of an epineural artery (longitudinal section, haematoxylin and eosin); (b) muscle biopsy showing inflammatory cells surrounding and infiltrating the wall of a small artery, with occlusion of the lumen (haematoxylin and eosin).

There have been no controlled studies comparing different therapies for neuropathy in non-systemic or systemic vasculitis. Many consider that prednisolone alone provides adequate therapy for non-systemic vasculitis restricted to the peripheral nervous system. There are no clear guidelines as to the duration of steroid therapy, whether alternate-day steroids are effective as maintenance therapy, and whether relapses are common on cessation of steroid therapy. If steroids incompletely suppress the underlying vasculitis, thereby allowing worsening of the neuropathy, cyclophosphamide therapy should be considered. If the neuropathy is rapidly progressive and destructive, cyclophosphamide should be considered from the outset, given either orally or as intravenous pulses. Given the potential side-effects of immunosuppressive drugs, it is desirable to obtain unequivocal histological proof of vasculitis before starting therapy. The benefits of therapy are: first, to prevent further peripheral nerve damage and, secondly, to allow the moderate degree of recovery of neurological function which occurs during the year after suppressing the vasculitis (Davies *et al.* 1996).

12.15.3 Systemic vasculitis

The majority of patients with vasculitic neuropathy have underlying vasculitic involvement of systemic organs (Said *et al.* 1988; Hawke *et al.* 1991)). The neurological features resemble those of non-systemic vasculitic neuropathy, but often evolve more aggressively. The electrophysiological and nerve biopsy findings are identical to those in non-systemic vasculitic neuropathy (Section 12.15.2).

Neuropathy is a common feature of the systemic necrotizing vasculitides, which include polyarteritis nodosa, microscopic polyarteritis, Churg–Strauss syndrome, and Wegener's granulomatosis (Said *et al.* 1988; Hawke *et al.* 1991; Hattori *et al.* 1999). The various patterns of neuropathy which have been identified in the systemic necrotizing vasculitides include mononeuritis multiplex, involvement of small cutaneous sensory nerves in the fingers or feet, symmetrical distal sensorimotor neuropathy,

brachial plexopathy, and radiculopathy. Antineutrophil cytoplasmic antibodies may present in serum early on in Wegener's granulomatosis and polyarteritis nodosa (Kafka *et al.* 1994). Often the choice of therapy is dictated by systemic manifestations such as renal involvement. Steroids alone are often effective in the Churg–Strauss syndrome, which is diagnosable by the distinctive eosinophilia and late-onset asthma. In patients with progressive vasculitic neuropathy, therapy should be instituted at the earliest opportunity to prevent progressive irreversible nerve damage. Cyclophosphamide can produce dramatic remissions and cures in severe systemic necrotizing vasculitis, to an extent that would be unlikely with steroids alone. However, considerable morbidity and mortality is associated with cyclophosphamide therapy, and it should be supervised by physicians familiar with the drug. It is recommended that cyclophosphamide should only be prescribed for patients with clear histological proof of systemic necrotizing vasculitis, or in whom the clinical syndrome is sufficiently distinctive to be beyond doubt.

Vasculitic neuropathy may occur in patients with nodular rheumatoid arthritis who may develop either mononeuritis multiplex, digital sensory neuropathy, or sensorimotor polyneuropathy. Vasculitic neuropathy also occurs in lupus erythematosus, Sjögren's syndrome, scleroderma, and in up to 14 per cent of patients with giant cell (temporal) arteritis (Peyronnard *et al.* 1982; Caselli *et al.* 1988; Schady *et al.* 1991; Stefurak *et al.* 1999).

12.15.4 Cryoglobulinaemia

Neuropathy occurs in over 50 per cent of patients with essential mixed cryoglobulinaemia (Gemignani *et al.* 1992). Symmetrical sensorimotor polyneuropathy is more common than mononeuritis multiplex. Nerve biopsies may show necrotizing vasculitis, but diffuse endoneurial vessel damage and non-specific axonal loss is a more common pathological finding (Cavaletti *et al.* 1990). Most often the neuropathy produces painful dyaesthesias and sensory loss in a stocking distribution, with prominent symptoms of restless legs, burnings, or formication (Gemignani *et al.* 1992). Prominent vasculitic purpura and Raynaud's phenomenon should suggest the possibility of cryoglobulinaemia. The diagnosis is proven by looking for immune precipitates in the serum of blood allowed to clot at 37 °C. Plasma exchange, steroids, and cyclophosphamide have all been used therapeutically, with occasional success. Indeed, if a patient has been diagnosed with vasculitic neuropathy and continues to progress despite such treatment, the possibility of cryoglobulinaemia should be entertained. Hepatitis C infection commonly underlies essential mixed cryoglobulinaemia, and improvement in the neuropathy has been reported with interferon-α therapy (Khella *et al.* 1995).

12.16 Sensory perineuritis and migrant sensory neuritis

12.16.1 Sensory perineuritis

This rare mononeuropathy causes pain and numbness in the territories of individual cutaneous nerves (Logigian *et al.* 1993). Patients may present with severe pain in the feet induced by standing or walking. Tinel's sign may be produced by percussion along the course of affected nerves. Initially the disorder may be relapsing and remitting, but symmetrical distal sensory loss may eventually appear. Mixed motor and sensory nerve involvement has been described with perineuritis. Unlike the migrant sensory neuritis of Wartenberg, stretching of peripheral nerves does not produce electric shock sensations in sensory perineuritis. Biopsy of affected nerves shows a chronic inflammatory infiltrate in the perineurium surrounding some fascicles but not others. Endoneurial blood vessels are spared. Similar histological findings have been described in the peripheral neuropathy of the Spanish toxic rapeseed oil syndrome (Ricoy *et al.* 1983). The disorder often responds to steroids.

12.16.2 Migrant sensory neuritis of Wartenberg

Patients with this disorder develop sudden pains in the territory of cutaneous nerves; the pain is induced by movements of a limb which stretch or distort the nerve. After repeated episodes of pain, cutaneous sensation may be lost in the nerve's territory for about 6 weeks. The relapsing and remitting nature of the sensory disturbance may initially suggest multiple sclerosis. Migrant sensory neuritis is probably more common than generally appreciated and usually affects patients in middle life (Matthews and Esiri 1983). It has occurred in members of a family with dominantly inherited brachial plexus neuropathy (Thomas and Ormerod 1993). Nerve-conduction studies may show diminished sensory-nerve action potentials in affected nerves. The condition follows a benign course.

12.17 Neuropathy due to systemic medical disorders

12.17.1 Diabetic neuropathy

Diabetes mellitus is one of the most common causes of disabling polyneuropathy. Two types of polyneuropathy are recognized and may coexist: symmetrical sensorimotor and autonomic. Various focal neuropathies occur, including diabetic proximal neuropathy, mononeuropathies of cranial and peripheral nerves, and truncal neuropathies (Watkins 1990; Said 1996). Two or more of these neuropathies commonly coexist within the same patient. Furthermore, many patients with established insulin-dependent diabetes mellitus have subclinical or electrophysiological evidence of sensory or autonomic polyneuropathy, despite being asymptomatic. In a population-based cohort study, neuropathy was present in 66 per cent of insulin-dependent diabetics (polyneuropathy, 54 per cent; carpal tunnel syndrome, 11 per cent; visceral autonomic, 7 per cent) and 59 per cent of non-insulin-dependent diabetics (polyneuropathy, 45 per cent; carpal tunnel syndrome, 6 per cent; visceral autonomic, 5 per cent). However, only about 20 per cent of diabetics have symptoms, and only 6 per cent of insulin-dependent, and 1 per cent of non-insulin-dependent, diabetics had more severe forms of neuropathy (Dyck *et al.* 1993*b*). Neuropathy is significantly associated with diabetic retinopathy or nephropathy.

Diabetic polyneuropathy

This is most prevalent in insulin-dependent diabetics of more than 20 years' standing, and in those with hypertension or poor glycaemic control. Sensory fibres are mainly involved, often accompanied by a variable degree of autonomic neuropathy.

Sensory symptoms usually commence in the legs. The common initial symptoms are paraesthesiae, and burning or lancinating pains. The sensory loss usually reflects abnormalities of unmyelinated fibres, with impaired pain and temperature sensations in a stocking distribution. The hands are also involved in more severe cases. In established cases vibration and joint-position sensations are impaired at the toes. These patients may have a sensory gait ataxia and a positive Romberg's sign. Tall diabetics are at greatest risk of sensory neuropathy, probably by virtue of their longer nerves (Sosenko *et al.* 1986). The ankle jerks are usually lost but generalized areflexia is less common. Involvement of autonomic fibres impairs sweating and prevents skin blood-flow regulation distally in the limbs, leading to a warm, dry foot with hard skin vulnerable to cracking. The combination of pain insensitivity and autonomic denervation predisposes the foot to skin ulceration. Neuropathic joints may develop. Motor loss is less common in diabetic polyneuropathy in comparison with the degree of sensory loss. Distal muscle weakness and wasting may be encountered in long-standing cases. However, marked motor involvement should provoke consideration of other possible contributing causes to the neuropathy apart from diabetes. Chronic inflammatory demyelinating polyneuropathy can occur in diabetics (Krendel *et al.* 1995). The diagnosis of sensory or autonomic poly-neuropathy poses few difficulties in patients with recognized diabetes mellitus. The blood sugar should be checked in all patients presenting with sensory neuropathy, since neuropathy may be the first symptom of diabetes.

Nerve-conduction studies generally show diminished or absent sensory-nerve action potentials, with normal or only mildly impaired motor-nerve conduction velocity. These electrophysiological findings occur in some diabetics before neuropathic symptoms develop (Lamontagne and Buchthal 1970). Electromyography often shows chronic denervation of distal muscles. Sensory-nerve action potentials, which reflect conduction in large myelinated fibres, may be remark-ably normal in those patients with selective loss of pain and temperature sensation.

Sural nerve biopsies usually show axonal loss and Wallerian degeneration affecting both myelinated and unmyelinated fibres. Less frequently, diabetic nerves show segmental demyelin-ation and remyelination, which is likely to be merely a second-ary consequence of primary axonal atrophy (Said 1996). Painful forms of diabetic neuropathy show regenerative sprouting of unmyelinated fibres, possibly the pain results from abnormal discharges in the sprouts (Llewelyn *et al.* 1986). Degeneration of the distal portions of dorsal column axons in the spinal cord is found at autopsy in patients with diabetic neuropathy (Dolman 1963). Thus both the central and peripheral branches of sensory neurons are vulnerable to hyperglycaemia. This observation, considered together with the greater vulnerability of sensory rather than motor neurons, suggests that it may be the perikarya of dorsal root ganglion neurons, rather than axons, which are primarily affected by hyperglycaemia. Fur-thermore, because central nervous axonal branches of sensory neurons are unable to regenerate, full recovery of function is unlikely to result from treatments that merely promote periph-eral nerve regeneration. Epineurial arteriolar walls may be thickened and endoneurial capillary lumens reduced in periph-eral nerves, suggesting an ischaemic contribution to some cases of diabetic polyneuropathy. Morphometric examination of the entire length of nerves from elderly diabetics shows that multifocal ischaemic axonal loss may summate distally and contribute to the polyneuropathy (Dyck *et al.* 1986).

The abnormality of neuronal cell biology responsible for dia-betic polyneuropathy is not known. It is likely that multiple pathogenetic mechanisms interact to varying degrees in pro-ducing a clinical picture of neuropathy which differs from patient to patient. Multifocal ischaemic neuropathy with distal summation of axonal loss may be a factor in elderly patients. However, it is likely that diffuse consequences of the metabolic disturbance are more prominent in causing the polyneuropathy of younger patients. Trials of therapies have been based on the notion that persistent hyperglycaemia may activate the polyol pathway in nerves, causing sorbitol accumulation as a result of enhanced aldose reductase activity. Proposals that this might inhibit myoinositol uptake by nerve fibres, resulting in altered impulse conduction due to reduced axolemmal Na^+,K^+-ATPase activity, have been contradicted by the demonstration that myoinositol is not decreased in diabetic nerve. Levels of glucose and fructose are increased in diabetic nerves and correlate with morphometric estimates of the severity of neuropathy (Dyck *et al.* 1988). Accumulation of these sugars can promote non-enzymatic glycosylation of peripheral-nerve proteins, probably altering their function and irreversibly cross-linking them by advanced glycosylation end-products (Ryle and Donaghy 1995). The slow phase of axonal transport of microtubule and neurofilament cytoskeletal proteins to the distal axon is reduced in experimental diabetes. This could alter the structural integrity of the distal axon and account for the axonal length-related neuropathy of diabetes (Medori *et al.* 1988).

Treatment

Strict control of glycaemia provides the best hope of reducing the occurrence and progression of diabetic polyneuropathy (Diabetes Control and Complications Trial Research Group 1993). Optimal control of glycaemia improves vibration sens-ation in diabetic polyneuropathy (Holman *et al.* 1983). Restora-tion of glycaemia by pancreas transplantation halts the downhill progression of diabetic neuropathy and a minor degree of recovery is apparent 3.5 years after transplantation (Kennedy *et al.* 1990). It should be noted that protracted or recurrent hypoglycaemia due to overzealous insulin treatment may cause a predominantly motor peripheral neuropathy, which is distal and symmetrically distributed, and may particu-larly affect the arms (Jaspan *et al.* 1982). A similar motor neu-ropathy may be seen in the hyperinsulinism of islet-cell tumours. Treatment of established diabetics with the aldose reductase inhibitor, sorbinil, does not significantly improve the clinical or electrophysiological outcome over more than 3 years' follow-up (Sorbinal Retinopathy Trial Research Group 1993). Preliminary evidence suggests that sensory function in symptomatic diabetics with polyneuropathy is improved by recombinant human nerve growth factor (Apfel *et al.* 1998).

Acutely painful diabetic polyneuropathy can be severely disabling and difficult to treat. It usually improves after some months of strict glycaemic control. In newly diagnosed diabet-ics, pain can be precipitated or augmented by insulin therapy (Llewelyn *et al.* 1986). Carbamazepine, phenytoin, or gaba-pentin therapy may help to relieve shooting or stabbing pains. Constant deep, aching pain may respond to amitriptyline within a few days, but this drug may exacerbate a coexisting autonomic neuropathy, causing urinary hesitancy or erectile failure. Skin care is essential so as to prevent chronic ulceration; cuts and abrasions should be treated promptly. Regular advice should be sought from a chiropodist, and the insides of shoes inspected daily for small stones and other irregularities.

Diabetic autonomic neuropathy

Abnormal autonomic function is detectable in a sixth of all patients with insulin-dependent diabetes, although symptoms of autonomic peripheral neuropathy occur only in relatively few (O'Brien *et al.* 1986). Autonomic neuropathy usually co-exists with a small-fibre sensory peripheral neuropathy. The main symptoms are abnormal sweating or diarrhoea. Less frequently, patients are troubled by postural hypotension, vomiting from gastroparesis, micturition difficulties, bladder infection due to atony, sexual impotence, and retrograde ejaculation. Symptomatic autonomic neuropathy predisposes patients to sudden death during anaesthesia, to cardiac arrhythmias, and it may reduce awareness of hypoglycaemia due to failure of catecholamine release. Although notably intermittent in severity, symptoms of autonomic disturbance tend to continue with little change in severity for many years (Sampson *et al.* 1990). A wide variety of autonomic function abnormalities may be measured in diabetic patients (Said 1996). Dry, warm feet, miosis, reduced pupil light reflexes, and ptosis may be observed. Iritis is associated with autonomic neuropathy in diabetics (Watkins 1990). The simplest reliable bedside tests consist of measuring postural hypotension, which reflects failure of sympathetic fibres, and measuring variability of the heart rate during deep breathing (the sinus arrhythmia, which reflects the parasympathetic innervation of the heart) (Section 1.8.2). Tight control of glycaemia by continuous subcutaneous insulin infusion or pancreatic transplantation produces only minor improvements in autonomic function (Kennedy *et al.* 1990). Diarrhoea can be particularly troublesome at night and may respond to codeine phosphate, clonidine, or one or two doses of tetracycline. Oral erythromycin can improve gastric emptying, possibly by mimicking the effects of motilin on gastrointestinal motility, and can be tried in patients disabled by serious vomiting due to diabetic gastroparesis (Janssens *et al.* 1990).

Diabetic proximal neuropathy

This disorder ranges from the familiar extreme of acute asymmetrical painful proximal leg muscle weakness developing over a few days or weeks, to the less familiar extreme of symmetrical painless proximal muscle weakness developing over many weeks or months. Diabetic proximal neuropathy has been termed diabetic myelopathy, polyradiculopathy, amyotrophy, lumbar plexopathy, mononeuropathy multiplex, femoral neuropathy, myopathy, or neuropathic cachexia. It is most common in non-insulin-dependent diabetics, generally in their sixth or seventh decade. Previously unrecognized diabetes may present with proximal neuropathy. Proximal neuropathy is seldom accompanied by diabetic retinopathy or nephropathy (Bastron and Thomas 1981).

Anterior thigh muscle pain is the usual first symptom. Proximal leg muscle weakness, mainly involving the quadriceps muscle, develops over the next few days or weeks. The knee jerks are lost in most patients. Despite the unilateral onset, bilateral weakness eventually occurs in over half of all patients. Occasionally the plantar responses are extensor, hence the original term 'diabetic myelopathy'. The neuropathy is usually accompanied by profound weight loss. Femoral nerve conduction is delayed (Chokroverty *et al.* 1977). The spinal-fluid protein is slightly elevated in most patients, indicating involvement of nerve roots.

Most patients improve neurologically after some months, and this is generally attributed to improved control of hyperglycaemia by insulin or oral hypoglycaemic agents (Coppack and Watkins 1991). Pain is the first symptom to resolve. The return of muscle power is usually substantial but is complete in only 20 per cent of patients. Recovery takes place over a period of 6–18 months. Up to one-fifth of patients may experience recurrence (Bastron and Thomas 1981; Coppack and Watkins 1991). Although common sense requires that hyperglycaemia should be strictly treated in diabetic proximal neuropathy, there is no conclusive evidence that hypoglycaemic therapy promotes recovery over and above that which will occur spontaneously (Donaghy 1991).

The pathogenetic mechanism(s) responsible for diabetic proximal neuropathy remain unclear. The absence of associated diabetic retinopathy or glomerulopathy, the frequent bilaterality, and the relatively slow neurological deterioration in diabetic proximal neuropathy, have argued against vascular occlusion due to diabetic microangiopathy as the primary cause. Epineurial microvasculitis or inflammation is observed in some patients in biopsies of the intermediate cutaneous nerve of the thigh, a cutaneous branch of the femoral nerve (Said *et al.* 1994; Dyck *et al.* 1999). This raises the question of treating severe or enduring cases of diabetic proximal neuropathy with steroids or other immunomodulatory drugs (Krendel *et al.* 1995). It also suggests a relationship to idiopathic lumbosacral plexopathy (Section 13.7.1).

Diabetic mononeuropathy

Diabetics are particularly vulnerable to a wide range of mononeuropathies affecting peripheral or cranial nerves. Nerves vulnerable to compression are most commonly affected, such as the median in the carpal tunnel, the ulnar in the cubital groove, the radial at the humerus, the common peroneal at the fibular head, and the lateral cutaneous nerve of the thigh at the inguinal ligament (Fraser *et al.* 1979). Painful oculomotor nerve palsies, often sparing the pupil, are common in older diabetics and resolve spontaneously. It is likely that pre-existing diabetic microvascular disease makes nerves unusually vulnerable to compression. These mononeuropathies may improve spontaneously, or with surgical release if at sites of compression. However, permanent residual abnormalities are common.

Diabetic truncal neuropathy

Attacks of truncal pain and sensory disturbance occur in diabetic patients. They may be recurrent, of variable severity, and may affect more than one thoracic nerve root territory. Truncal neuropathy typically affects non-insulin-dependent diabetics in their fifth to seventh decades. It is often accompanied by considerable weight loss, similar to that occurring in diabetic proximal neuropathy. The pain may not be strictly localized to the territory of a discrete dermatome. A sensory deficit is usually demonstrable on the trunk and can be restricted to the territory of a single anterior or posterior ramus (Stewart 1989). Abdominal protuberance may result from focal paralysis of abdominal wall muscles. Electromyography often shows denervation of paraspinal muscles. Skin nerve fibres are reduced in biopsies from affected compared to unaffected sensory territories (Lauria *et al.* 1998). The differential diagnosis includes multiple sclerosis and lesions affecting vertebral bones. Spontaneous recovery is usual but may take some months. Carbamazepine or amitriptyline can control the pain.

12.17.2 **Chronic renal failure**

Clinical or electrophysiological evidence of polyneuropathy is present in over 50 per cent of patients with end-stage renal disease. Uraemic neuropathy develops very gradually and is uncommon if the glomerular filtration rate exceeds 10 ml/min. Although uraemia itself is responsible for the neuropathy in many patients with chronic renal failure, it should be recognized that neuropathy may be an independent feature of the underlying disease which has caused the chronic renal failure: diabetes mellitus, systemic vasculitis, myelomatosis, amyloidosis, and systemic lupus erythematosus. The neuropathies caused by these diseases are often focal or demyelinating in nature, unlike the axonal degeneration polyneuropathy of uraemia.

A restless leg syndrome is the most common early symptom of uraemic polyneuropathy: crawling, pricking, and itching sensations occur at night. Burning paraesthesiae may develop. Muscle cramps and fatigability are followed by distal weakness and muscle atrophy. An autonomic neuropathy may cause sexual impotence and contribute to difficulties in intravascular fluid volume regulation, making postural hypotension a particular problem following fluid removal by dialysis. The earliest physical signs are loss of vibration sensation at the toes and absent ankle jerks. A mixed motor, autonomic, and multimodal sensory neuropathy eventually develops (Thomas *et al.* 1971).

Nerve-conduction studies reflect axonal degeneration of motor and sensory fibres. Nerve biopsy shows loss of all sizes of nerve fibres, particularly large, myelinated fibres. Less commonly, there is evidence of segmental demyelination or remyelination which may be secondary to axonal changes (Thomas *et al.* 1971). Autopsy studies show degeneration of the dorsal columns of the spinal cord, representing the central axons of dorsal root ganglion cells. It is presumed that uraemic polyneuropathy results from the accumulation of neurotoxic waste products, but the causative compounds have not been identified.

Renal replacement therapy normally prevents the neuropathy from deteriorating and may allow considerable recovery. The greatest improvement occurs in patients receiving renal transplants rather than those maintained by dialysis. Following successful renal transplantation, clinical and electrophysiological improvement starts after some months and continues slowly (Bolton 1976). However, full recovery of the neuropathy is unusual unless it was initially mild. A carpal tunnel syndrome may develop in patients receiving long-term dialysis, due to deposition of β_2-microglobulin amyloid in the flexor retinaculum (Benz *et al.* 1988). Acute or subacute neuropathy has occurred occasionally in patients treated by peritoneal dialysis. Such patients may have co-existing diabetes mellitus, the neuropathy has demyelinating features, and sometimes improves (Ropper 1993).

12.17.3 **Hypothyroidism**

Paraesthesiae, lancinating limb pains, or muscle cramps occur in half of all patients with established myxoedema. Sensory symptoms in the limbs may be the presenting feature of hypothyroidism. There are few neuropathic signs on examination; minor distal sensory changes are usually the only abnormalities. Although characteristically slowly relaxing, the tendon reflexes are usually retained. Nerve biopsies may show segmental demyelination (Meier and Bischoff 1977). The sensory symptoms may resolve on thyroid hormone replacement therapy. Carpal tunnel syndrome is common, and tarsal tunnel syndrome less common, in myxoedema. Acroparaesthesiae due to the former often resolve with thyroid hormone replacement therapy, but if not, surgical decompression may be required (Murray and Simpson 1958; Schwartz *et al.* 1983).

12.17.4 **Acromegaly**

Both polyneuropathy and the carpal tunnel syndrome are common in patients with acromegaly and are not thought to be due to the associated diabetes mellitus. The polyneuropathy is of insidious onset, causing distal paraesthesiae, depressed reflexes, distal muscle weakness, and multimodal sensory disturbance. The peripheral nerves may be clinically enlarged. Nerve conduction is slightly slowed. Nerve biopsies show axonal loss with some demyelination and remyelination. The fascicular cross-sectional area is increased, with accumulation of tissue subperineurially and endoneurially (Low *et al.* 1974). It is unclear whether the neuropathy improves significantly with treatment of the underlying growth hormone excess. Symptomatic carpal tunnel syndrome should be treated by surgical decompression.

12.17.5 **Primary biliary cirrhosis**

A distal sensory polyneuropathy may develop in patients with primary biliary cirrhosis. Sural nerve biopsy shows perineurial xanthomatous deposits distorting the normal architecture (Thomas and Walker 1965).

12.17.6 **Systemic lupus erythematosus**

A wide variety of peripheral neuropathies occur in systemic lupus erythematosus and should be treated according to principles already outlined. Some evidence of polyneuropathy occurs in 20 per cent, although often mild or even asymptomatic (Omdal *et al.* 1991). Demyelinating neuropathies of the acute Guillain–Barré type (Section 12.10.1) or steroid-responsive chronic inflammatory demyelinating polyneuropathy (Section 12.11.1) may occur (Rechthand *et al.* 1984). Chronic sensorimotor axonal degeneration neuropathies may be encountered. Focal neuropathy due to necrotizing arteritis or carpal tunnel syndrome may be the presenting features of systemic lupus erythematosus (Stefurak *et al.* 1999).

12.17.7 Sarcoidosis

A small proportion of patients with sarcoidosis have peripheral neuropathy. Cranial nerve palsies are most often encountered; these are often multiple, of variable severity, and particularly affecting the facial nerve. Mononeuropathy may affect any peripheral nerve, including the sensory nerves of the trunk. Sensorimotor polyneuropathy is less common and may take acute multifocal or purely sensory forms (Zuniga *et al.* 1991). Sensorimotor polyneuropathy may be associated with multiple small granulomas within biopsied nerves (Gainsborough *et al.* 1991).

12.17.8 Eosinophilia–myalgia syndrome

This disorder followed months or years after ingestion of contaminated L-tryptophan, a component of some body-building food supplements. There was associated eosinophilia and brawny induration of the skin. Some patients developed a painful inflammatory myopathy. Sensorimotor axonal degeneration neuropathies or multifocal neuropathies may occur. The combination of neuropathy and myopathy could result in respiratory failure requiring ventilation (Smith and Dyck 1990). A more chronic demyelinating neuropathy has also occurred (Freimer *et al.* 1992). The neuropathy of the eosinophilia–myalgia syndrome should be distinguished from other neuropathies associated with eosinophilia: hypereosinophilic syndrome (Section 12.17.9), necrotising arteritis of the Churg–Strauss type (Section 12.15.3), and Hodgkin's disease (Section 12.12.4).

12.17.9 Hypereosinophilic syndrome

Symmetrical sensorimotor peripheral neuropathy due to axonal degeneration occurs in about one-tenth of patients with idiopathic hypereosinophilia (Monaco *et al.* 1988). Increased numbers of degranulated eosinophils are found in the blood. The systemic disorder may include a restrictive cardiomyopathy due to endomyocardial fibrosis.

12.17.10 Critical illness polyneuropathy

Sensorimotor polyneuropathy can develop in patients being ventilated for cardiorespiratory disease who develop multiorgan failure or sepsis. The compound muscle action potentials and sensory-nerve action potentials are reduced in amplitude, and needle electrodes show evidence of limb muscle denervation (Zochodne *et al.* 1987). This neuropathy usually comes to light when patients fail to wean from the ventilator. The mortality in such patients is high, but those who recover neurologically do so over 3–6 months. This rapidity of recovery is faster than might be expected from a dense axonal degeneration polyneuropathy, and suggests a degree of potentially reversible conduction failure. The disorder should be distinguished from Guillain–Barré syndrome by normal spinal-fluid protein levels and the electrophysiological characteristic of axonal degeneration rather than demyelination. In a critically ill patient in the intensive care setting, the principal differential diagnosis is a critical illness myopathy, occurring most commonly in acute respiratory disorder, such as asthma treated with non-depolarizing neuromuscular blocking agents or high-dose steroids. Critical illness polyneuropathy and myopathy may coexist, and given that the creatine kinase level often remains normal, muscle biopsy is the only reliable way to diagnose the myopathy (Gutmann and Gutmann 1999).

12.18 Drug-induced polyneuropathy

12.18.1 Alcohol

Alcoholics may develop either polyneuropathy or focal compressive peripheral nerve lesions. Pressure palsies often follow periods of stuporous immobility and generally affect the radial, ulnar, or common peroneal nerves (Kemppainen *et al.* 1982). Polyneuropathy may develop insidiously in long-standing alcoholics. It usually presents with symmetrical burning dysaesthesiae or paraesthesiae distally, or with sensory ataxia. Physical signs of a symmetrical sensorimotor polyneuropathy are often restricted to the legs. Nerve-conduction studies reflect axonal degeneration predominantly affecting sensory axons (Behse *et al.* 1977). Autonomic neuropathy may be present, and is associated with an increased risk of cardiovascular death (Johnson and Robinson 1988). Alcoholic polyneuropathy may be caused either by nutritional deficiency or by direct toxicity of ethanol or its metabolites. Nutritional deficiency polyneuropathies are common in patients with associated Wernicke–Korsakoff syndrome (Section 26.5) and particularly reflect vitamin B_1 (thiamine) deficiency (Section 12.21.1). Ethanol, or its metabolites such as acetaldehyde, may have direct neurotoxic effects; this mechanism may be a particularly important cause of neuropathy in those alcoholics who are not malnourished.

Neuropathy is often ascribed erroneously to alcohol in any patient with moderately high consumption. In practice, neuropathy is unlikely until a lifetime of alcohol consumption of 15 kg ethanol/kg bodyweight is reached; this equates for a 70 kg man to drink 300 ml whisky daily for 25 years (Monforte *et al.* 1995). Occasionally rapidly progressive polyneuropathy resembling Guillain–Barré syndrome, but without raised CSF protein or slowed nerve conduction, has occurred in alcoholics (Wohrle *et al.* 1998). Vitamin B_1 replacement therapy should be given to all patients with alcoholic polyneuropathy. Gradual improvement in the clinical and electrophysiological aspects of peripheral neuropathy occurs in those alcoholics who achieve long-term abstinence (Hillbom and Wennberg 1984). Disulfiram (Antabuse®) therapy may itself produce neuropathy in alcoholics (Section 12.18.10).

12.18.2 Almitrine

Almitrine bismesylate (Vectarion®) caused purely or predominantly sensory polyneuropathy with an onset of symptoms 9–25 months after initiation of therapy in patients with chronic obstructive pulmonary disease or cerebrovascular disease (Bouche *et al.* 1989). The neuropathy presents with distal paraesthesiae or burning pain in the legs, or less often in the hands. All modalities of sensation are impaired in a stocking distribution, gait ataxia may be evident, and the ankle tendon reflexes are usually lost. Weakness or more generalized areflexia are uncommon. Nerve-conduction studies and nerve biopsies show axonal degeneration, chiefly affecting large myelinated fibres. Symptoms generally improve on withdrawing the drug. It should be noted that mild, often subclinical, neuropathy can occur independently of drug therapy in patients with chronic obstructive pulmonary disease (Valli *et al.* 1984).

12.18.3 Amiodarone

This iodine-containing anti-arrhythmic drug causes symmetrical distal sensorimotor polyneuropathy after prolonged administration in 6 per cent of patients (Charness *et al.* 1984). The neuropathy develops some months after starting treatment, can produce severe weakness, and is often associated with a raised spinal-fluid protein level. Sural nerve biopsies show loss of myelinated fibres with lipid-laden lysosomes in Schwann cells; demyelination rather than axonal degeneration is thought to be the primary event. Approximately 70 per cent of patients taking 800 mg of amiodarone daily develop a reversible syndrome of tremor and ataxia which occurs independently of peripheral neuropathy.

12.18.4 Chloroquine

Chloroquine is used to treat malaria, amoebiasis, and chronic discoid lupus erythematosus. A combination of sensorimotor peripheral neuropathy with myopathy, or myopathy alone, may occur in patients taking doses of at least 500 mg daily for a year or more (Whisnant *et al.* 1963). The neuromyopathy improves steadily on stopping the drug.

12.18.5 Cisplatin

Cisplatin is an important drug in treating ovarian, testicular, and bladder tumours. A predominantly sensory peripheral neuropathy, characterized by distal paraesthesiae, develops in almost all patients given a cumulative dose of 300–600 mg/m^2 cisplatin, often accompanied by *Adriamycin*® (LoMonaco *et al.* 1992). Sensory ataxia may be severe. Sensory-nerve conduction is abnormal, motor conduction is normal. Symptoms of neuropathy may start some weeks after the last dose of cisplatin has been administered, and may subsequently worsen for a few

months. Partial or complete recovery of the neuropathy may occur after cessation of cisplatin therapy, usually taking more than a year. Simultaneous treatment with an ACTH analogue prevents or attenuates cisplatin neuropathy (Hovestadt *et al.* 1992).

12.18.6 Clioquinol

Consumption of this antidiarrhoeal agent was associated with subacute myelo-optic neuropathy (SMON) in Japan in the 1960s. Sensory disturbance in the legs was the usual first symptom, followed by muscle weakness. Optic atrophy was commonly associated, and could occur in isolation. The weakness and sensory disturbance in the limbs were probably due mainly to a myelopathy, which produced brisk knee jerks and extensor plantar responses. However, a mild peripheral neuropathy was thought to be present too, as evidenced by absent ankle jerks (Baumgartner *et al.* 1979).

12.18.7 Colchicine

Mild neuromyopathy may be common in patients receiving colchicine as treatment for gout (Kuncl *et al.* 1987). Neuromyopathy is particularly likely to occur if there is associated mild chronic renal impairment. The myopathic element may involve severe proximal muscle weakness, electromyographic features resembling those of polymyositis, elevated serum creatine kinase levels, and electron-microscopic evidence of accumulation of lysosomes and autophagic vacuoles in biopsies of proximal muscles. Creatine kinase levels return to normal within days of stopping colchicine, and proximal muscle strength improves over subsequent weeks. The neuropathic element is less pronounced than the myopathy, with distal limb sensory loss, tendon areflexia, and evidence of axonal degeneration on nerve-conduction studies and sural nerve biopsies.

12.18.8 Dapsone

Motor neuropathy may complicate long-term therapy with dapsone 200–500 mg daily (Guttman *et al.* 1975). Such doses are generally used for the treatment of dermatological conditions, usually dermatitis herpetiformis, and dapsone neuropathy is less likely to complicate leprosy treatment. Weakness and wasting are most prominent distally in the limbs. Motor conduction velocities are normal or only slightly slowed, and evoked muscle action potentials reduced. Tendon reflexes tend to be preserved, although hypoactive. Muscle strength improves following withdrawal of dapsone.

12.18.9 Didanosine

Polyneuropathy occurs regularly in patients with HIV infection treated by the nucleoside analogue drugs didanosine (ddI), zalcitabine (ddC), and stavudine (d4T) and is a dose-limiting side-effect. This neuropathy is painful, purely or predominantly sensory, and often of explosive onset. The most common signs are hyporeflexic ankle jerks, impaired pinprick and vibration sensation in the feet, and gait unsteadiness (Berger *et al.* 1993; Moyle *et al.* 1993). The chance of neuropathy is dosage dependent, and it develops on average 8 weeks after starting high-dose therapy but develops later with contemporary lower-dose therapy. After stopping the drug, the neuropathy may 'coast' with worsening symptoms, before stabilizing and improving. It can be difficult to differentiate this toxic neuropathy from the painful sensory neuropathy which occurs in patients with established HIV infection (Section 12.14.2). However, these drug toxic neuropathies differ in that they occur during the months after starting therapy, the painful symptoms usually evolve abruptly, and the hands are uninvolved. If in doubt, the drug should be withdrawn for some months to see if improvement occurs.

12.18.10 Disulfiram

An axonal degeneration sensorimotor neuropathy may develop after disulfiram (Antabuse®) therapy for alcoholism. Symptoms improve after stopping the drug (Mokri *et al.* 1981). Axonal neurofilament accumulations can be found in the sural nerve on electron microscopy. It is noteworthy that disulfiram is enzymatically converted to carbon disulphide, which itself is known to cause a distal axonopathy with neurofilament accumulations (Section 12.20.2) (Ansbacher *et al.* 1982). Prospective studies suggest that peripheral nerve damage occurs at disulfiram doses of 250 mg/day, but not at 125 mg/day (Palliyath *et al.* 1990).

12.18.11 Ethambutol

Predominantly sensory neuropathy is an occasional consequence of treatment with the antituberculous drug ethambutol (Nair *et al.* 1980). Optic neuropathy is a more common complication of long-term ethambutol administration.

12.18.12 FK506

Subacute demyelinating sensorimotor polyneuropathy has been noted 2 weeks to 6 months after starting FK506 (tacrolimus) immunosuppression in transplant recipients (Bronster *et al.* 1995). It resembles chronic inflammatory demyelinating polyneuropathy and responds to plasma exchange or IvIg treatment. Recovery has been reported following substitution of FK506 by cyclosporin.

12.18.13 Gold

Acute or subacute sensorimotor neuropathy can occur in patients some months after commencing gold therapy for rheumatoid arthritis (Katrak *et al.* 1980). Partial recovery occurs over the months following cessation of gold administration. Myokymia of limb muscles is a distinctive finding. Gold neuropathy should be distinguished from the mononeuritis multiplex that can occur in patients with aggressive rheumatoid disease with vasculitic features (Section 12.15.3).

12.18.14 Isoniazid

Patients with inherited slow drug-acetylation status may develop peripheral neuropathy when they receive long-term isoniazid therapy. Paraesthesiae and numbness are the initial symptoms and neuropathic pain may be prominent. Muscle weakness usually only appears in the later stages. Hyperalgesia and muscle cramping are distinctive features in many patients (Ochoa 1970). Isoniazid antagonizes the actions of vitamin B_6 (pyridoxine) and the neuropathy can be prevented by simultaneous administration of pyridoxine during isoniazid therapy. In patients who develop neuropathy, isoniazid therapy may be interrupted, vitamin B_6 given parenterally (100–200 mg/day), and other antituberculous drugs continued. Variable degrees of improvement in the neuropathy follow these measures.

12.18.15 Lithium

Occasional cases of peripheral neuropathy have been associated with lithium carbonate therapy for depression. Toxic levels of lithium were deemed responsible for a severe generalized sensorimotor neuropathy which shows electrophysiological and nerve biopsy evidence of axonal loss. Recovery can occur following drug cessation (van Hooren *et al.* 1990).

12.18.16 Metronidazole

Sensory neuropathy may follow prolonged administration of the antibacterial drug metronidazole (Coxon and Pallis 1976). Paraesthesiae or numbness of the toes have usually been recorded only in patients who have received a total dose of at least 30 g. Sensory-nerve action potentials are diminished in amplitude but of normal latency. Neuropathic symptoms resolve during the months after stopping the drug. Occasionally convulsions, encephalopathy, and cerebellar ataxia have been associated with metronidazole therapy.

12.18.17 Misonidazole

The drug misonidazole was given as an adjuvant to radiotherapy in the treatment of solid tumours. It produced a severe subacute sensory neuropathy with features of axonal degeneration. Large myelinated sensory fibres are particularly affected (Melgaard *et al.* 1982). A maximum total dose of 11 g/m^2 has been recommended to avoid neurological toxicity (Dische 1978). Partial recovery of the neuropathy occurs after stopping the drug.

12.18.18 Nitrofurantoin

An axonal degeneration sensory neuropathy may follow administration of large doses of the antibiotic, nitrofurantoin. Total dosages usually exceed 20 g, although neuropathy can occur after lower dosage in patients with impaired renal excretion (Lindholm 1967). Partial recovery may follow cessation of the drug.

12.18.19 Perhexiline

Subacute sensorimotor neuropathy followed weeks to years after initiating treatment for angina or cardiac arrhythmias with perhexiline. The spinal-fluid protein content was elevated, nerve-conduction velocities markedly slowed, and nerve biopsies showed segmental demyelination. Electron microscopy showed membrane-bound lysosomal structures within Schwann cells. Improvement occurred over months following withdrawal of the drug (Said 1978).

12.18.20 Phenytoin

Peripheral neuropathy is demonstrable in up to 20 per cent of epileptic patients on long-term anticonvulsant therapy. It is usually relatively mild, involving sensory diminution in a stocking distribution and reduced ankle-tendon reflexes. Although commonly attributed to phenytoin, the evidence relates this neuropathy to a wide range of anticonvulsants. It is most common in patients receiving multiple drugs (Swift et al. 1981).

12.18.21 Pyridoxine

Sensory neuropathy with prominent ataxia may follow self-medication with megadoses of pyridoxine (vitamin B$_6$). The normal human daily pyridoxine requirement is approximately 0.004 g. Sensory neuropathy has usually followed daily oral ingestion of 2–6 g of pyridoxine (Schaumburg et al. 1983) or single massive parenteral doses (2 g/kg) in the treatment of mushroom poisoning (Albin et al. 1987). Neuropathy has also been recorded following long-term chronic consumption of lower doses (0.2 g daily) (Parry and Bredesen 1985). The rate of onset of symptoms is proportional to the magnitude of the daily dosage. The sensory neuropathy probably reflects damage to dorsal root ganglion neurons, and the potential for recovery is limited.

12.18.22 Sodium cyanate

Sensorimotor neuropathy developed in some patients treated with sodium cyanate to prevent sickle-cell crisis (Ohnishi et al. 1975). It is possible that the neuropathy of chronic renal failure might be due in part to cyanate since this compound accumulates in chronic uraemia.

12.18.23 Suramin

Either distal axonal, or subacute demyelinating, sensorimotor polyneuropathies have been noted in more than 80 per cent of patients receiving suramin doses sufficient to achieve plasma levels of 350 µg/ml or more during attempted treatment of hormone-refractory metastatic prostate cancer (Chaudhry et al. 1997).

12.18.24 Taxol

The drugs docetaxel and paclitaxel, derived from yew tree needles, promote microtubule polymerization. They are valuable antitumour drugs but peripheral neuropathy is a dose-limiting side-effect. Sensory neuropathy can occur in humans within days of high-dose paclitaxel therapy or more slowly at lower dosage regimens. Initially, tingling and numbness affect the feet before spreading to the hands. Limb weakness can be present both distally and proximally. Nerve conduction studies show features of both axonal degeneration and demyelination. Symptoms and signs can progressively 'coast' after stopping taxols, but recovery usually starts by 8 weeks (New et al. 1996).

12.18.25 Thalidomide

Sensorimotor neuropathy, with prominent paraesthesiae and muscle cramps, followed the use of thalidomide as a hypnotic in the 1960s. Muscle strength recovers well after cessation of the drug, but sensory symptoms and signs may persist unchanged for years (Fullerton and O'Sullivan 1968).

12.18.26 Vincristine

Vincristine disrupts microtubules and is used chiefly for treating lymphoma or leukaemia. The peripheral neuropathy initially develops after cumulative dosage of 4–19 mg/m^2 and causes paraesthesiae, areflexia, and mild autonomic symptoms. If the drug is continued, severe muscle weakness and sensory loss develop. Autonomic neuropathy may be severe, with paralytic ileus, features of acute abdomen, impotence, or postural hypotension. Laryngeal nerve palsies have been attributed to vincristine therapy. Nerve-conduction studies point to a dying back axonal degeneration neuropathy (Casey et al. 1973). Mild neurotoxicity inevitably occurs with therapeutically effective doses of vincristine. When patients develop numbness or mild manipulatory difficulties, it should be a warning to reduce or stop the drug. Vincristine should be stopped immediately if significant weakness or paralytic ileus develop. Functional recovery is usual if the drug is stopped before the advent of significant toxicity (Donaghy 1996). Permanently absent ankle-tendon jerks are commonly noted in otherwise asymptomatic patients who have received courses of vincristine therapy. Patients with hereditary motor and sensory neuropathy may be unusually sensitive to vincristine neuropathy.

12.19 Metal-poisoning polyneuropathy

This section considers peripheral neuropathies attributable to arsenic, lead, mercury, and thallium poisoning. Neuropathies due to therapy with cisplatin, lithium, and gold are considered in Section 12.18.

12.19.1 Arsenic

Neuropathy due to inorganic arsenic poisoning may develop insidiously in arsenic smelting workers (Feldman et al. 1979). If it occurs acutely after single-dose poisonings (Le Quesne and McLeod 1977) it develops 2–3 weeks later in victims who survive the initial shock and gastrointestinal disturbance of acute intoxication. Numbness and paraesthesiae are the initial symptoms, and abnormalities of vibration and position sensation are demonstrable. Distal leg muscle weakness may develop subsequently. The ankle-tendon reflexes are invariably lost, those at the knee are sometimes lost, and the arm reflexes are generally preserved. White lines across the nails (Mee's lines) develop later. Sensory-nerve action potentials are absent and motor conduction is mildly slowed initially before electrophysiological features of axonal degeneration supervene (Donofrio et al. 1987). Sural nerve biopsies show axonal degeneration. Slow improvement occurs over a period of years but permanent abnormalities are usual (Le Quesne and McLeod 1977).

Chronic arsenical exposure in industrial workers may produce an asymptomatic sensorimotor neuropathy, detectable only by nerve-conduction studies and unaccompanied by neuropathic signs on examination (Feldman et al. 1979). The arsenic level may be elevated in the blood, urine, or hair, depending upon the recency of exposure. Hyperkeratosis of the hands and feet may be noted. Gastrointestinal symptoms are not usually a feature of chronic arsenical poisoning. Chronic poisoning may cause anaemia with basophilic stippling of erythrocytes. Chelation therapy may be indicated, particularly in patients seen soon after the ingestion of a single dose.

12.19.2 Lead

Peripheral neuropathy due to inorganic lead poisoning usually occurs in metal smelting or battery manufacture workers. Organic lead intoxication has not been associated clearly with peripheral neuropathy. Abdominal crampings are a common initial manifestation. Classically a purely motor peripheral neuropathy develops, particularly affecting much-used muscles, such as the wrist extensors of manual workers. Prominent wrist or foot drop are characteristic. Muscle weakness can be profound, causing respiratory failure. The degree of tendon reflex loss varies. Sensory loss is unusual (Cullen et al. 1983). Children with lead neuropathy frequently have an associated encephalopathy (Section 5.7.3). Motor-nerve conduction velocities may be slowed. Sural nerve biopsies show loss of the large myelinated axons with noteworthy paranodal demyelination.

Lead interferes with porphyrin metabolism, which may explain the similarity between the symptoms of lead poisoning and those of porphyric neuropathy (Section 12.8.6): abdominal pain, motor neuropathy, and behavioural disturbance occur in both. In addition, there is a rare inherited condition known as plumboporphyria, due to δ-aminolaevulinic acid dehydratase deficiency, in which porphyric neuropathy may be precipitated by occupational exposure to lead within accepted safety limits (Dyer et al. 1993). The blood lead level reflects recent exposure. The free erythrocyte protoporphyrin level is the best guide to chronic lead exposure. Basophilic stippling of erythrocytes is seen on blood smear. Treatment involves identifying and removing the source of exposure, and using chelating agents. It is unclear whether lead intoxication can cause polyneuropathy

independently of its provocation of porphyria. Certainly it is noteworthy that sensory features, which are absent in classical descriptions of lead neuropathy, are prominent in all other polyneuropathies caused by heavy-metal poisoning.

12.19.3 Mercury

Chronic exposure to inorganic or elemental mercury produces a mild peripheral neuropathy. Mild sensorimotor neuropathy has been noted following long-term exposure of industrial workers to inorganic mercury vapour and in dentists using mercury amalgam. Previously asymptomatic polyneuropathy may be demonstrable many years after occupational elemental mercury exposure (Albers et al. 1988). Elemental mercury poisoning occasionally resembles motor neuron disease (Adams et al. 1983).

Organic mercury poisoning typically causes the combination of paraesthesiae, sensory ataxia, and visual-field constriction. Organic mercury poisoning has occurred after exposure to methyl mercury dust, after eating seafood which has accumulated methyl mercury from industrial effluent (Minamata disease), and after inadvertent consumption of seed grain treated with mercurial fungicides (Bakir et al. 1973). Patients with mercurial neuropathy develop paraesthesiae in and around the mouth and in the fingers and the toes. Nerve-conduction studies may be normal in patients with organic mercury toxicity, suggesting that the sensory loss can be due to central nervous system involvement. Extensive cerebellar involvement is evident at autopsy (Nierenberg et al. 1998).

The diagnosis of mercury poisoning may be confirmed by measuring blood, urine, and hair levels, which are differentially elevated depending upon the type and rate of exposure. The treatment involves identification and elimination of the source of exposure. Chelating agents such as dimercaprol or penicillamine are mainly effective against inorganic and elemental, rather than organic, mercury poisoning. It is unlikely that chelating agents remove mercury that is already bound to neural tissue.

12.19.4 Thallium

Polyneuropathy due to thallium normally follows suicidal or homicidal poisoning attempts with this tasteless, colourless, rodenticide. High doses cause shock due to gastroenteritis and dehydration. If the victim survives, sensorimotor neuropathy becomes evident within a few days. Sensory symptoms occur first and consist of painful paraesthesiae, particularly affecting the feet. The neuropathy may progress rapidly to involve the respiratory and bulbar muscles, thus resembling the Guillain–Barré syndrome. An associated autonomic neuropathy can result in tachycardia and hypertension. Central nervous system involvement occurs in severe poisoning, producing ataxia, optic neuropathy, confusional psychoses, and involuntary movements. Systemic features include dark pigmentation at the hair roots (Fig. 12.22) followed by alopecia; dry, scaly skin; and Mee's lines on the nails. Neuropathological studies show axonal

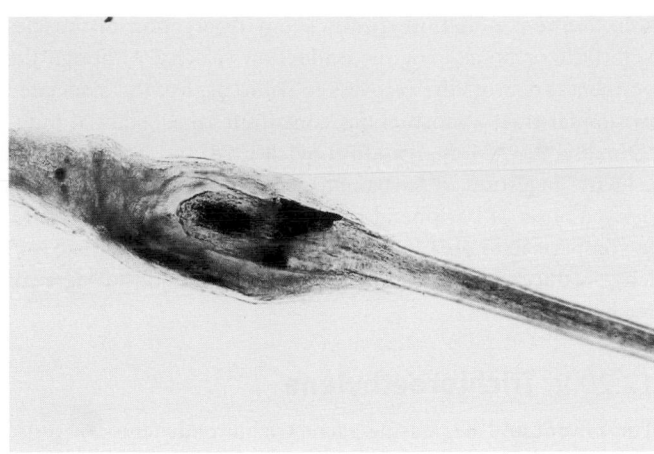

Fig. 12.22. Thallium poisoning: characteristic dark pigmentation at the root of a plucked hair (courtesy of Dr M. Schwartz).

degeneration of fibres in peripheral nerves and dorsal columns. Electron microscopy reveals swollen axons containing large vacuoles and distended mitochondria (Davis *et al.* 1981). Although the neuropathy may eventually recover partially, permanent abnormalities are the rule unless the patient is seen early enough to undertake effective gastric decontamination. Chelating agents have not been effective. Haemoperfusion has been recommended for severe poisoning. Oral Berliner-Blue may promote faecal excretion of thallium (Moeschlin 1980).

12.20 Polyneuropathy due to industrial and agricultural chemicals

12.20.1 Acrylamide

Acrylamide monomer is catalytically polymerized in order to stabilize soil during mining and other earthworkings. The monomer is neurotoxic. High-dose intoxication, as may occur after drinking contaminated well-water, causes a subacute encephalopathy followed some days later by signs of mild polyneuropathy (Igisu *et al.* 1975). Chronic low-dose intoxication generally occurs in construction workers following skin and inhalational exposure. Polyneuropathy may occur following exposure for as little as 4 weeks. The neuropathy involves both sensory and motor fibres. Positive sensory symptoms, such as paraesthesiae, are unusual. Diffuse areflexia is an early finding. Ataxia may be prominent. Contact dermatitis, blistering, and hyperhidrosis of the palms and soles may occur. Sensory-nerve action potentials are small or absent, and only a mild degree of motor slowing occurs. Sural nerve biopsy shows degeneration and regeneration of axons. Electron microscopy shows accumulations of disorganized neurofilaments in occasional axons, but giant axonal swellings are not seen (Davenport *et al.* 1976). In mild or subclinical cases, good recovery follows removal from exposure. Only partial recovery occurs from the more severe neuropathies.

The related compound, methyl methacrylate monomer, is used by dental prosthetic technicians and by orthopaedic surgeons carrying out joint replacements. This monomer penetrates rubber gloves and causes finger paraesthesiae in both occupational groups (Rajaniemi 1986). Generalized sensorimotor neuropathy starting in the hands, and involving neurofilament accumulations in sural nerve axons, has been described in a dental prosthetic technician with more than 20 years of intense skin and inhalational exposure (Donaghy *et al.* 1991).

12.20.2 Carbon disulphide

Peripheral neuropathy has been noted in workers using carbon disulphide in poorly ventilated conditions, in the rubber vulcanization or viscose rayon manufacturing industries. Distal sensorimotor loss and areflexia are usually restricted to the legs, but may involve the arms in severe cases. Electrophysiologically, the neuropathy is due to axonal degeneration (Vasilescu 1976). It is sometimes accompanied by encephalopathy with psychotic features.

12.20.3 Dimethylaminopropionitrile

Dimethylaminopropionitrile was used as a catalyst in the manufacture of polyurethane. Exposed workers developed an axonal degeneration sensorimotor neuropathy with noteworthy involvement of bladder control and sexual dysfunction. The initial symptoms were generally urinary hesitancy and impotence (Keogh *et al.* 1980; Kreiss *et al.* 1980).

12.20.4 Ethylene oxide

Ethylene oxide gas is used both as a precursor for industrial chemicals and for sterilizing heat-sensitive devices used in healthcare. Industrial exposure to the gas has caused both encephalopathy and sensorimotor polyneuropathy (Gross *et al.* 1979).

12.20.5 Herbicides

Peripheral neuropathy has followed intense or repeated skin exposure to derivatives of the weed killer 2,4-D (2,4-dichlorophenoxyacetic acid). Nausea, vomiting, and diarrhoea occur during the days immediately following exposure. First symptoms of peripheral neuropathy develop some days later and consist of painful paraesthesiae in the fingers and toes. Severe motor and sensory disability develop subsequently and recover incompletely. Once the neuropathy is established, motor-nerve conduction velocities are moderately slowed (Goldstein *et al.* 1959).

12.20.6 Hexacarbons

n-Hexane and methyl *n*-butyl ketone (MNBK) are used as solvents in glues and in flexographic printing. They are metabolized to the neurotoxic compound 2,5-hexanedione. Sensorimotor neuropathy has occurred in workers using such glues in shoe or furniture manufacture and following inhalational solvent abuse ('glue-sniffing') (Altenkirch et al. 1977). The neurotoxic potency of hexacarbons is enhanced by simultaneous exposure to methylethylketone (MEK), which is often present in solvent mixtures but is not in itself neurotoxic. The peripheral neuropathy starts with numbness of the digits and may develop into severe symmetrical distal sensory and motor loss. Severe weakness may develop subacutely in 'glue-sniffers' and be misdiagnosed as the Guillain–Barré syndrome. Even after removal from exposure to the toxin, the neuropathy may continue to worsen for 2 or 3 months before stabilization and partial recovery take place. Electron microscopic examination of nerve biopsies shows giant axonal profiles swollen by accumulations of disorganized neurofilaments. Motor-nerve conduction velocities are substantially slowed once the neuropathy is established. This may reflect the marked paranodal demyelination and myelin thinning that occur in relation to giant axonal change; since the neuropathy is not primarily demyelinating in nature.

12.20.7 Methylbromide

Sensorimotor peripheral neuropathy has been reported following chronic low-dose intoxication with methylbromide, a gas used as a fumigant and in fire extinguishers (Kantarjian and Shaheen 1963). Complete recovery of the neuropathy was reported within a year of removal from exposure.

12.20.8 Pesticides

Peripheral neuropathy has occurred following exposure to both organophosphorous and carbamate pesticides. In both cases, the symptoms of peripheral neuropathy develop after a delay of a few days or weeks following a single exposure. This delayed onset of neuropathy follows the earlier cholinergic phase of poisoning, in which acute paralysis, overwhelming bronchial secretions, bradycardia, and seizures may occur (Section 5.8).

In organophosphorus poisoning, symptoms of a predominantly motor neuropathy have been reported 1–3 weeks after acute exposure to the pesticides tricresylphosphate, mipafox, leptophos, trichlorphon, trichlornate, and methamidophos (Senanayake and Johnson 1982; Lotti et al. 1984). Not all organophosphates induce delayed peripheral neuropathy, and it has been proposed that this capacity relates to their propensity to inhibit neurotoxic esterase (Lotti et al. 1984). It is uncertain whether neuropathy can follow chronic low-dose pesticide exposure, or whether it might follow acute intoxication by nerve gases intended for warfare. The initial symptoms of neuropathy consist of cramping in distal leg muscles accompanied by distal paraesthesiae and numbness. Progressive distal leg muscle weakness and hyporeflexia develop, followed by similar weakness of the arms. The severity varies, but severe quadriplegia may occur. Demonstrable sensory signs are mild or absent. Superimposed pyramidal-tract abnormalities may be

seen. Nerve-conduction studies show denervation of muscles with little or no slowing of conduction velocity. Although the peripheral neuropathy recovers to some degree, the associated pyramidal-tract abnormalities contribute to substantial long-term disability (Morgan and Penovich 1978).

Acute ingestion of carbamate pesticides may also produce delayed onset of peripheral neuropathy (Umehara et al. 1991). In comparison to organophosphorus poisoning, carbamate toxicity produces more prominent sensory signs and the degree of recovery is greater.

12.20.9 Trichloroethylene

The solvent and degreasing agent trichloroethylene can cause selective numbness of the facial skin, or polyneuritis cranialis in severe exposures (Feldman et al. 1992).

12.21 Vitamin deficiency polyneuropathy

Many nutritional neuropathies reflect the multiple vitamin deficiencies that occur during malnutrition due to starvation, chronic gastrointestinal disease, and malnourished alcoholism (Section 5.2). Such patients often develop neurological illnesses which do not conform to the classic descriptions of dry beriberi (thiamine deficiency) or pellagra (pyridoxine deficiency). Multiple vitamin deficiencies may produce the combination of predominantly sensory peripheral neuropathy with burning feet, amblyopia, sensorineural deafness, dizziness, myelopathy, and orogenital dermatitis, which is sometimes known as Strachan's syndrome. During the past century, this state has been described in malnourished native West Indians, jail inmates, sugar plantation labourers, and prisoners of war, particularly those held captive in the Far East during the Second World War (Cockerel and Ormerod 1993). Although the symptoms recover in some patients, they are permanent in many, despite reinstitution of a balanced diet. The 'burning feet syndrome' is another permanent sequel of nutritional deprivation.

12.21.1 Vitamin B$_1$ deficiency

Dry or neuropathic beriberi results from thiamine deficiency in malnourished alcoholics or in patients receiving a diet of milled rice without vitamin B supplementation. The latter group of patients are often physically active and consuming large amounts of carbohydrate. Sensorimotor polyneuropathy, leg oedema, and cardiomegaly usually develop simultaneously. The neuropathy is predominantly motor, initially affecting distal leg muscles, and may prevent walking. Neuropathic limb pains or paraesthesiae may occur. The neuropathy can follow a relapsing course prior to the institution of vitamin B$_1$ replacement therapy. Sural nerve biopsies show axonal degeneration predominantly affecting the larger myelinated fibres, with a degree of secondary demyelination (Ohnishi et al. 1980). Motor-nerve conduction is mildly slowed and sensory-nerve action potentials diminished. Measurement of blood or urine thiamine levels is of limited value in making the diagnosis. The red cell transketolase activity is a more sensitive index, but does not distinguish between acute and chronic thiamine deficiency. After supplementation with vitamin B_1, strength and motor-nerve conduction steadily improve and nerve biopsies show extensive regenerative activity.

12.21.2 Vitamin B₆ deficiency

The full-blown syndrome of pellagra is only rarely encountered. It consists of a red-brown hyperkeratotic rash affecting exposed skin, gastrointestinal symptoms, neuropsychiatric features, and peripheral neuropathy. Approximately 50 per cent of pellagrins have sensorimotor peripheral neuropathy with noteworthy paraesthesiae, pain, and tenderness of distal leg muscles (Bomb et al. 1977). The peripheral neuropathy associated with isoniazid therapy is due to this drug's antagonism of vitamin B_6 (Section 12.18.14).

12.21.3 Vitamin B₁₂ deficiency

Sensory peripheral neuropathy is occasionally encountered as the sole neurological manifestation of vitamin B_{12} deficiency, usually caused by underlying pernicious anaemia. It is normally overshadowed by the associated spinal-cord lesion known as subacute combined degeneration (Hemmer et al. 1998) (Section 20.6.3). The peripheral neuropathy contributes to paraesthesiae in the feet and distal loss of all modalities of sensation. The ankle jerks are absent. Nerve-conduction studies show diminished or absent sensory-nerve action potentials. Motor-nerve conduction studies generally show axonal neuropathy, but demyelinating features can occur. Symptoms usually improve over the months following initiation of vitamin B_{12} replacement injections.

12.21.4 Vitamin E deficiency

Long-standing vitamin E deficiency causes a sensory peripheral neuropathy associated with prominent ataxia, resembling a spinocerebellar degeneration (Section 31.7.4). Vitamin E deficiency occurs in patients with fat malabsorption due to cholestatic liver disease, short-bowel syndrome, or cystic fibrosis, and in abetalipoproteinaemia (Brin et al. 1986). Familial vitamin E deficiency is due to mutations of the α-tocopherol transfer protein (Hentati et al. 1996). Chronic vitamin E deficiency can also cause a pigmentary retinopathy. Abnormalities of somatosensory evoked potentials indicate an abnormality of central nervous system axons in the dorsal columns of the spinal cord. The diagnosis is proven by demonstrating a plasma tocopherol level reduced out of proportion to any reduction in plasma lipoprotein levels. The vitamin E content of the sural nerve is reduced, and this deficiency may precede the development of peripheral neuropathy (Traber et al. 1987). Vitamin E supplementation prevents further downhill progression of the neurological disorder (Sokol et al. 1985).

References

Adams, C. R., Ziegler, D. K., and Lin, J. T. (1983). Mercury intoxication simulating amyotrophic lateral sclerosis. *JAMA*, **250**, 642–3.

Adams, D., Didier, S., Goulon-Goeau, C. et al. (2000). The course and prognostic factors of familial amyloid polyneuropathy after liver transplantation. *Brain*, **123**, 1495–504.

Ad Hoc Subcommittee of the American Academy of Neurology AIDS Task Force (1991). Research criteria for diagnosis of chronic inflammatory demyelinating polyneuropathy (CIDP). *Neurology*, **41**, 617–18.

Albers, J. W., Kallenbach, L. R., Fine, L. J. et al. (1988). Neurological abnormalities associated with remote occupational elemental mercury exposure. *Ann. Neurol.*, **24**, 651–9.

Albin, R. L., Albers, J. W., Greenberg, H. S. et al. (1987). Acute sensory neuropathy—neuronopathy from pyridoxine overdose. *Neurology*, **37**, 1729–32.

Al-Din, A. N., Anderson, M., Bickerstaff, E. R. et al. (1982). Brainstem encephalitis and the syndrome of Miller Fisher. *Brain*, **105**, 481–95.

Altenkirch, H., Mager, J., Stoltenburg, G. et al. (1977). Toxic polyneuropathies after sniffing a glue thinner. *J. Neurol.*, **214**, 137–52.

Amato, M. P., Pracucci, G., Ponziani, G. et al. (1993). Long-term safety of azathioprine therapy in multiple sclerosis. *Neurology*, **43**, 831–833.

Andersson, P.-B., Yuen, E., Parko, K. et al. (2000). Electrodiagnostic features of hereditary neuropathy with liability to pressure palsies. *Neurology*, **54**, 40–4.

Andrade, C. (1952). A peculiar form of peripheral neuropathy: familial atypical generalised amyloidosis with special involvement of the peripheral nerves. *Brain*, **75**, 408–27.

Ang, C. W., Yuki, N., Jacobs, B. C. et al. (1999). Rapidly progressive, predominantly motor Guillain–Barré syndrome with anti-GalNAc-GD1a antibodies. *Neurology*, **53**, 2122–7.

Ansbacher, L. E., Bosch, E. P., and Cancilla, P. A. (1982). Disulfiram neuropathy: a neurofilamentous distal axonopathy. *Neurology*, **32**, 424–8.

Apfel, S. C., Kessler, J. A., Adornato, B. T. et al. (1998). Recombinant human nerve growth factor in the treatment of diabetic polyneuropathy. NGF Study Group. *Neurology*, **51**, 695–702.

Asbury, A. K. and Cornblath, D. R. (1990). Assessment of current diagnostic criteria for Guillain–Barré syndrome. *Ann. Neurol.*, **27**, 521–4.

Asbury, A. K., Arnason, B. G., and Adams, R. D. (1969). The inflammatory lesion in idiopathic polyneuritis. *Medicine (Baltimore)*, **48**, 173–215.

Auer-Grumbach, M., Wagner, K., Timmerman, V. *et al.* (2000). Ulcero-mutilating neuropathy in an Austrian kinship without linkage to hereditary motor and sensory neuropathy IIB and hereditary sensory neuropathy loci. *Neurology*, **54**, 45–52.

Axelrod, F. B. and Abularrage, J. J. (1982). Familial dysautonomia: a prospective study of survival. *J. Pediatr.*, **101**, 234–6.

Bakir, F., Damluji, S., Amin-Zaki, L. *et al.* (1973). Methyl mercury poisoning in Iraq. *Science*, **181**, 230–41.

Bardwick, P. A., Zvaifler, N. J., Gill, G. N. *et al.* (1980). Plasma cell dyscrasia with polyneuropathy, organomegaly, endocrinopathy, M protein and skin changes: the POEMS syndrome. *Medicine*, **59**, 311–22.

Bastron, J. A. and Thomas, J. E. (1981). Diabetic polyradiculopathy. Clinical and electromyographic findings in 105 patients. *Mayo Clin. Proc.*, **56**, 725–32.

Baumgartner, G., Gawel, M. J., Kaeser, H. E. *et al.* (1979). Neurotoxicity of halogenated hydroxyquinolones: clinical analysis of cases reported outside Japan. *J. Neurol. Neurosurg. Psychiat.*, **42**, 1073–83.

Behse, F., Buchthal, F., Carlsen, F. *et al.* (1972). Hereditary neuropathy with liability to pressure palsies. *Brain*, **95**, 777–94.

Behse, F. and Buchthal, F. (1977). Alchoholic neuropathy: clinical, electrophysiological, and biopsy findings. *Ann. Neurol.*, **2**, 95–110.

Bejaoui, K., McKenna-Yasek, D., Hosler, B. A. *et al.* (1999). Confirmation of linkage of type I hereditary sensory neuropathy to human chromosome 9q22. *Neurology*, **52**, 510–515.

Bendixen, B. H., Younger, D. S., Hair, L. S. *et al.* (1992). Cholesterol emboli neuropathy. *Neurology*, **42**, 428–30.

Ben Hamida, M., Hentati, F., and Ben Hamida, C. (1990). Giant axonal neuropathy with inherited multisystem degeneration in a Tunisian kindred. *Neurology*, **40**, 245–50.

Benz, R. L., Siegfried, J. W., and Teehan, B. P. (1988). Carpal tunnel syndrome in dialysis patients: comparison between continuous ambulatory peritoneal dialysis and haemodialysis population. *Am. J. Kidney Dis.*, **11**, 473–6.

Berger, A. R., Arezzo, J. C., Schaumburg, H. H. *et al.* (1993). 2′, 3′-Dideoxycytidiine (ddc) toxic neuropathy: a study of 52 patients. *Neurology*, **43**, 358–62.

Birouk, N., Leguern, E., Maisonobe, T. *et al.* (1998). X-linked Charcot–Marie–Tooth disease with Connexin 32 mutations. Clinical and Electrophysiologic study. *Neurology*, **50**, 1074–82.

Blanch, L. C., Meaney, C., Morris, C. P. (1996). A sensitive mutation screening strategy for Fabry Disease: detection of nine mutations in the alpha-galactosidase A gene. *Hum. Mutat.*, **8**, 38–43.

Blumenfeld, A., Slaugenhaupt, S. A., Axelrod, F. B. *et al.* (1993). Localisation of the gene for familial dysautonomia on chromosome 9 and definition of DNA markers for genetic diagnosis. *Nature Genet.*, **4**, 160–4.

Bolton, C. F. (1976). Electrophysiologic changes in uremic neuropathy after successful renal transplantation. *Neurology*, **26**, 152–61.

Bolton, C. F., Driedger, A. A., and Lindsay, R. M. (1979). Ischaemic neuropathy in uraemic patients caused by bovine arterio-venous shunt. *J. Neurol. Neurosurg. Psychiat.*, **42**, 810–14.

Bomb, B. S., Bedi, H. K., and Bhatnagar, K. (1977). Postischaemic paraesthesiae in pellagrins. *J. Neurol. Neurosurg. Psychiat.*, **40**, 265–7.

Bosch, E. P., Pierach, C. A., Bossenmaier, I. *et al.* (1977). Effect of haematin in porphyric neuropathy. *Neurology*, **27**, 1053–6.

Bouchard, C., Lacroix, C., Planté, V. *et al.* (1999). Clinicopathologic findings and prognosis of chronic inflammatory demyelinating polyneuropathy. *Neurology*, **52**, 498–503.

Bouche, P., Lacomblez, L., Leger, J. M. *et al.* (1989). Peripheral neuropathies during treatment with almitrine: report of 46 cases. *J. Neurol.*, **236**, 29–33.

Bouche, P., Cattelin, F., Saint-Jean, O. *et al.* (1993). Clinical and electrophysiological study of the peripheral nervous system in the elderly. *J. Neurol.*, **240**, 263–8.

Bouche, P., Moulonguet, A., Younes-Chennoufi, A. B. *et al.* (1995). Multifocal motor neuropathy with conduction block: a study of 24 patients. *J. Neurol. Neurosurg. Psychiat.*, **59**, 38–44.

Bowen, J. R. C., McDougall, A. C., Morris, J. H. *et al.* (2000). Vasculitic neuropathy in a patient with inactive treated lepromatous leprosy. *J. Neurol. Neurosurg. Psychiat.*, **68**, 496–500.

Bradley, W. G. and Verma, A. (1996). Painful vasculitic neuropathy in HIV-1 infection. *Neurology*, **47**, 1446–51.

Brin, M. F., Pedley, T. A., Lovelace, R. E. *et al.* (1986). Electrophysiologic features of abetalipoproteinaemia: functional consequences of vitamin E deficiency. *Neurology*, **36**, 669–73.

Bronster, D. J., Yonover, P., Stein, J. *et al.* (1995). Demyelinating sensorimotor polyneuropathy after administration of FK506. *Transplantation*, **59**, 1066–8.

Buhwald, B., Bufler, J., Carpo, M. *et al.* (2001). Combined pre- and postsynaptic action of IgG antibodies in Miller Fisher syndrome. *Neurology*, **56**, 67–74.

Busby, M. and Donaghy, M. (2000). Predominant arm weakness in acute idiopathic polyneuritis: a distinct regional variant. *J. Neurol.*, **247**, 343–5.

Cappelen-Smith, C., Kuwabara, S., Lin, S.-Y. *et al.* (2000). Activity-dependent hyperpolarization and conduction block in chronic inflammatory demyelinating polyneuropathy. *Ann. Neurol.*, **48**, 826–32.

Caruso, G., Santoro, L., Perretti, A. *et al.* (1987). Friedreich's ataxia: electrophysiologic and histologic findings in patients and relatives. *Muscle Nerve*, **10**, 503–15.

Caselli, R. J., Daube, J. R., Hunder, G. G. *et al.* (1988). Peripheral neuropathic syndromes in giant cell (temporal) arteritis. *Neurology*, **38**, 685–9.

Casey, E. B., Jelliffe, A. M., Le Quesne, P. M. *et al.* (1973). Vincristine neuropathy: clinical and electrophysiological observations. *Brain*, **96**, 69–86.

Cavaletti, G., Petruccioli, M. G., Crespi, V. *et al.* (1990). A clinico-pathological and follow up study of 10 cases of essential type II cryoglobulinaemic neuropathy. *J. Neurol. Neurosurg. Psychiat.*, **53**, 886–9.

Cavanagh, N. P. C., Eames, R. A., Galvin, R. J. *et al.* (1979). Hereditary sensory neuropathy with spastic paraplegia. *Brain*, **102**, 79–94.

Chalk, C. H., Mills, K. R., Jacobs, J. M. *et al.* (1990). Familial multiple symmetric lipomatosis with peripheral neuropathy. *Neurology*, **40**, 1246–50.

Chance, P. F., Bird, T. D., Matsunami, N. *et al.* (1992). Trisomy 17p associated with Charcot–Marie–Tooth neuropathy type 1A phenotype. *Neurology*, **42**, 2295–9.

Chance, P. F., Alderson, M. K., Leppig, K. A. *et al.* (1993). DNA deletion associated with hereditary neuropathy with liability to pressure palsies. *Cell*, **72**, 143–51.

Charness, M. E., Morady, F., and Scheinman, M. M. (1984). Frequent neurologic toxicity associated with amiodarone therapy. *Neurology*, **34**, 669–71.

Chaudhry, V., Corse, A. M., Cornblath, D. *et al.* (1993). Multifocal motor neuropathy: response to human immune globulin. *Ann. Neurol.*, **33**, 237–42.

Chaudhry, V., Eisenberger, M. A., Sinibaldi, V. J. *et al.* (1996). A prospective study of surmin-induced peripheral neuropathy. *Brain*, **119**, 2039–52.

Chimelli, L., Freitas, M., and Nascimento, O. (1997). Value of nerve biopsy in the diagnosis and follow-up of leprosy. *J. Neurol.*, **244**, 318–23.

Chokroverty, S., Reyes, M. G., Rubino, F. A. *et al.* (1977). The syndrome of diabetic amyotrophy. *Ann. Neurol.*, **2**, 181–94.

Cockerell, O. C. and Ormerod, E. C. (1993). Strachan's syndrome: variation on a theme. *J. Neurol.*, **240**, 315–18.

Cohen, A. S., Rubinow, A., Anderson, J. J. *et al.* (1987). Survival of patients with primary (AL) amyloidosis: cases treated with colchicine from 1976–1983 compared with cases seen in previous years (1961–1973). *Am. J. Med.*, **82**, 1182–90.

Cohen, B. A., McArthur, J. C., Grohman, S. *et al.* (1993). Neurologic prognosis of cytomegalovirus polyradiculomyelopathy in AIDS. *Neurology*, **43**, 493–9.

Cohen, J. I., Brunell, P. A., and Strauss, S. E. (1999). Recent advances in varicella-zoster virus infection. *Ann. Int. Med.*, **130**, 922–32.

Comenzo, R. L., Sanchorawala, V., and Fisher, C. (1999). Intermediate-dose intravenous melphalan and blood stem cells mobilized with sequential GM + G-CSF or G-CSF alone to treat AL (amyloid light chain) amyloidosis. *Br. J. Haematol.*, **104**, 553–9.

Coppack, S. W. and Watkins, P. J. (1991). The natural history of diabetic femoral neuropathy. *Quart. J. Med.*, **79**, 307–13.

Cornblath, D. and McArthur, J. C. (1988). Predominantly sensory neuropathy in patients with AIDS and AIDS-related complex. *Neurology*, **38**, 794–6.

Cornblath, D. R., McArthur, J. C., Kennedy, P. G. E. *et al.* (1987). Inflammatory demyelinating peripheral neuropathies associated with human T-cell lymphotrophic virus type III infection. *Ann. Neurol.*, **21**, 32–40.

Cornblath, D. R., Mellits, E. D., Griffin, J. W. *et al.* (1988). Motor conduction studies in Guillain–Barré syndrome: description and prognostic value. *Ann. Neurol.*, **23**, 354–9.

Cornblath, D. R., Chaudhry, V., Carter, K. *et al.* (1999). Total neuropathy score. Validation and reliability study. *Ann. Neurol.*, **53**, 1660–4.

Corse, A. M., Chaudhry, V., Crawford, T. O. *et al.* (1996). Sensory nerve pathology in multifocal motor neuropathy. *Ann. Neurol.*, **39**, 319–25.

Coxon, A. and Pallis, C. A. (1976). Metronidazole neuropathy. *J. Neurol. Neurosurg. Psychiat.*, **39**, 403–5.

Croft, R. P., Richardus, J. H., and Smith, W. C. S. (1997). Field treatment of acute nerve function impairment in leprosy using a standardized corticosteroid regimen—first year's experience with 100 patients. *Leprosy Rev.*, **68**, 316–25.

Cullen, M. R., Robins, J. M., and Eskenazi, B. (1983). Adult inorganic lead intoxication: presentation of 31 new cases and a review of recent advances in the literature. *Medicine*, **62**, 221–47.

Dalmau, J., Graus, F., Rosenblum, M. K. *et al.* (1992). Anti-Hu associated paraneoplastic encephalomyelitis sensory neuropathy: a clinical study of 71 patients. *Medicine*, **71**, 59–72.

Dalos, N. P., Borel, C., and Hanley, D. F. (1988). Cardiovascular autonomic dysfunction in Guillain–Barré syndrome. *Arch. Neurol.*, **45**, 115–17.

Davenport, J. G., Farrell, D. F., and Sumi, S. M. (1976). 'Giant axonal neuropathy' caused by industrial chemicals. *Neurology*, **26**, 919–23.

Davies, L., Spies, J. M., Pollard, J. D. *et al.* (1996). Vasculitis confined to peripheral nerves. *Brain*, **119**, 1441–8.

Davis, L. E., Standefer, J. C., Kornfeld, M. *et al.* (1981). Acute thallium poisoning: toxicological and morphological studies of the nervous system. *Ann. Neurol.*, **10**, 38–44.

Dawson, D. M., Samuels, M. A., and Morris, J. (1988). Sensory form of acute polyneuritis. *Neurology*, **38**, 1728–31.

De Gasperi, R., Sosa, M. A. G., Sartorato, E. L. *et al.* (1996). Molecular heterogeneity of late-onset forms of globoid-cell leucodystrophy. *Am. J. Hum. Genet.*, **59**, 1233–42.

De Jonghe, P., Timmerman, V., Fitzpatrick, D. *et al.* (1997). Mutilating neuropathic ulcerations in a chromosome 3q13–q22 linked Charcot–Marie–Tooth disease type 2B family. *J. Neurol. Neurosurg. Psychiat.*, **62**, 570–3.

De Jonghe, P., Timmerman, V., Ceuterick, C. *et al.* (1999*a*). The Thr124 Met mutation in the peripheral myelin protein zero (MPZ) gene is associated with a clinically distinct Charcot–Marie–Tooth phenotype. *Brain*, **122**, 281–90.

De Jonghe, P., Timmerman, V., Nelis, E. *et al.* (1999*b*). A novel type of hereditary motor and sensory neuropathy characterized by a mild phenotype. *Arch. Neurol.*, **56**, 1283–8.

de la Monte, S. M., Gabuza, D. H., Ho, D. D. *et al.* (1988). Peripheral neuropathy in the acquired immunodeficiency syndrome. *Ann. Neurol.*, **23**, 485–92.

Dellagi, K., Dupouey, P., Brouet, J. C. *et al.* (1983). Waldenström's macroglobulinaemia and peripheral neuropathy: a clinical review. *Blood*, **62**, 280–5.

Denny-Brown, D. (1951). Hereditary sensory radicular neuropathy. *J. Neurol. Neurosurg. Psychiat.*, **14**, 237–52.

De Veber, G. A., Schwarting, G. A., Kolodny, E. H. *et al.* (1992). Fabry disease: immunocytochemical characterization of neuronal involvement. *Ann. Neurol.*, **31**, 409–15.

Diabetes Control and Complications Trial Research Group (1993). The effect of intensive treatment of diabetes on the development and progression of long-term complications in insulin-dependent diabetes mellitus. *N. Engl. J. Med.*, **329**, 977–86.

Dische, S. (1978). The neurotoxicity of Misonidazole: pooling of data from five centres. *Br. J. Radiol.*, **51**, 1023–4.

Dodd, A., Rowland, S. A., Hawkes, S. L. J. *et al.* (1997). Mutations in the adrenoleucodystrophy gene. *Hum. Mutat.*, **9**, 500–11.

Dolman, C. L. (1963). The morbid anatomy of diabetic neuropathy. *Neurology*, **13**, 135–42.

Donaghy, M. (1991). Diabetic proximal neuropathy: therapy and prognosis. *Quart. J. Med.*, **79**, 287–8.

Donaghy, M. (1996). Vincristine and neuropathies. *Prescriber's J.*, **36**, 116–19.

Donaghy, M. and Earl, C. J. (1985). Ocular palsy preceding chronic relapsing polyneuropathy by several weeks. *Ann. Neurol.*, **17**, 49–50.

Donaghy, M. and Kennett, R. (1999). Varying occurrence of vocal cord paralysis in a family with autosomal dominant hereditary motor and sensory neuropathy. *J. Neurol.*, **246**, 552–5.

Donaghy, M., Hakin, R. N., Bamford, J. M. *et al.* (1987). Hereditary sensory neuropathy with neurotrophic keratitis. Description of an autosomal recessive disorder with a selective reduction of small unmyelinated nerve fibres and a discussion of the classification of the hereditary sensory neuropathies. *Brain*, **110**, 563–83.

Donaghy, M., Brett, E. M., Ormerod, I. E. *et al.* (1988). Giant axonal neuropathy: observations on a further patient. *J. Neurol. Neurosurg. Psychiat.*, **51**, 991–4.

Donaghy, M., Gray, J. A., Squier, W. *et al.* (1989*a*). Recurrent Guillain–Barré syndrome after multiple exposures to cytomegalovirus. *Am. J. Med.*, **87**, 339–41.

Donaghy, M., Hall, P., Gawler, J., *et al.* (1989*b*). Peripheral neuropathy associated with Castleman's Disease. *J. Neurol. Sci.*, **89**, 253–67.

Donaghy, M., King, R. H. M., McKeran, R. O. *et al.* (1990). Cerebrotendinous xanthomatosis: clinical, electrophysiological and nerve biopsy findings, and response to treatment with chenodeoxycholic acid. *J. Neurol.*, **237**, 216–19.

Donaghy, M., Rushworth, G., and Jacobs, J. (1991). Generalized peripheral neuropathy in a dental technician exposed to methyl methacrylate monomer. *Neurology*, **41**, 1112–16.

Donaghy, M., Mills, K. R., Boniface, S. J. *et al.* (1994). Pure motor demyelinating neuropathy: deterioration after steroid treatment and improvement with intravenous immunglobulin. *J. Neurol. Neurosurg. Psychiat.*, **57**, 778–83.

Donaghy, M., Sisodiya, S. M., Kennett, R. P. *et al.* (2000). Steroid-responsive polyneuropathy in a family with a novel myelin protein zero mutation. *J. Neurol. Neurosurg. Psychiat.*, **69**, 799–805.

Donofrio, P. D., Wilbourn, A. J., Albers, J. W. *et al.* (1987). Acute arsenic intoxication presenting as Guillain–Barré-like syndrome. *Muscle Nerve*, **10**, 114–20.

Draghia, R., Letourneur, F., Drugan, C. *et al.* (1997). Metachromatic leucodystrophy: identification of the first deletion in axon 1 and nine novel point mutations in the arylsulfatase gene. *Hum. Mutat.*, **9**, 234–42.

Duggins, A. J., McLeod, J. G., Pollard, J. D. *et al.* (1999). Spinal root and plexus hypertrophy in chronic inflammatory demyelinating polyneuropathy. *Brain*, **122**, 1383–90.

Duston, M. A., Skinner, M., Anderson, J. *et al.* (1989). Peripheral neuropathy as an early marker of AL amyloidosis. *Arch. Intern. Med.*, **149**, 358–60.

Dworkin, R. H. (1999). Prevention of post-herpetic neuralgia. *Lancet*, **353**, 1636–7.

Dyck, P. J., O'Brien, P. C., Oviatt, K. *et al.* (1982). Prednisone improves chronic inflammatory demyelinating polyradiculoneuropathy more than no treatment. *Ann. Neurol.*, **11**, 136–41.

Dyck, P. J., Mellinger, J. F., Reagan, T. J. *et al.* (1983). Not 'indifference to pain' but varieties of hereditary sensory and autonomic neuropathy. *Brain*, **106**, 373–90.

Dyck, P. J., O'Brien, P., Swanson, C. *et al.* (1985). Combined azathiaprine and prednisone in chronic inflammatory demyelinating polyneuropathy. *Neurology*, **35**, 1173–6.

Dyck, P. J., Lais, A., Karnes, J. L. *et al.* (1986). Fiber loss is primary and multifocal in sural nerves in diabetic polyneuropathy. *Ann. Neurol.*, **19**, 425–39.

Dyck, P. J., Zimmerman, B. R., Vilen, T. H. *et al.* (1988). Nerve glucose, fructose, sorbitol, myo-inositol, and fibre degeneration and regeneration in diabetic neuropathy. *N. Engl. J. Med.*, **319**, 542–8.

Dyck, P. J., Chance, P., Lebo, R. *et al.* (1993a). Hereditary motor and sensory neuropathics. In *Peripheral neuropathy*, (3rd edn), (ed. P. J. Dyck, P. K. Thomas, J. Griffin *et al.*), Chapter 57. W. B. Saunders, Philadelphia.

Dyck, P. J., Kratz, K. M., Litchy, W. J. *et al.* (1993*b*). The prevalence of staged severity of various types of diabetic neuropathy, retinopathy, and nephropathy in a population based cohort. *Neurology*, **43**, 817–24.

Dyck, P. J., Litchy, W. J., Minnerath, S. *et al.* (1994). Hereditary motor and sensory neuropathy with diaphragm and vocal cord paresis. *Ann. Neurol.*, **35**, 608–15.

Dyck, P. J. B., Norell, J. E., and Dyck, P. J. (1999). Microvasculitis and ischaemia in diabetic lumbosacral radiculoplexus neuropathy. *Neurology*, **53**, 2113–21.

Dyer, J., Garrick, D. P., Ingus, A., and Pye, I. F. (1993). Plumboporphyria (ALAD deficiency) in a lead worker: a scenario for potential diagnostic confusion. *Br. J. Indust. Med.*, **50**, 1119–21.

Earl, C. J., Fullerton, P. M., Wakefield, G. S. *et al.* (1964). Hereditary neuropathy, with liability to pressure palsies. *Quart. J. Med.*, **33**, 481–98.

Enzi, G., Angelini, C., Negrin, P. *et al.* (1986). Sensory, motor and autonomic neuropathy in patients with multiple symmetric lipomatosis. *Medicine*, **64**, 388–93.

Esiri, M. M., Gordon, W. I., Collin, G. E. J. *et al.* (1997). Peripheral neuropathy in Creutzfeldt–Jakob disease. *Neurology*, **48**, 784.

Feasby, T. E., Gilbert, J. J., Brown, W. F. *et al.* (1986). An acute axonal form of Guillain–Barré polyneuropathy. *Brain*, **109**, 1115–26.

Feeney, D. J., Pollard, J. D., McLeod, J. G. *et al.* (1990). HLA antigens in chronic inflammatory demyelinating polyneuropathy. *J. Neurol. Neurosurg. Psychiat.*, **53**, 170–2.

Feldman, E. L., Bromberg, M. B., Albers, J. W. *et al.* (1991). Immunosuppressive treatment in multifocal motor neuropathy. *Ann. Neurol.*, **30**, 397–401.

Feldman, R. G., Niles, I. A., Kelly-Hayes, M. *et al.* (1979). Peripheral neuropathy in arsenic smelter workers. *Neurology*, **29**, 939–44.

Feldman, R. G., Niles, C., Proctor, S. P., and Jabre, J. (1992). Blink reflex measurement of effects of trichloroethylene exposure on the trigeminal nerve. *Muscle Nerve*, **15**, 490–5.

Fisher, M. (1956). An unusual variant of acute idiopathic polyneuritis (syndrome of ophthalmoplegia, ataxia and areflexia). *N. Engl. J. Med.*, **255**, 57–65.

Fraser, D. M., Campbell, I. W., Ewing, D. J. *et al.* (1979). Mononeuropathy in diabetes mellitus. *Diabetes*, **28**, 96–101.

Frederico, P., Zochodne, D. W., Hahn, A. F. *et al.* (2000). Multifocal motor neuropathy improved by IV1g. *Neurology*, **55**, 1256–62.

Freimer, M. L., Glass, J. D., Chaudhry, V. *et al.* (1992). Chronic demyelinating polyneuropathy associated with eosinophilia-myalgia syndrome. *J. Neurol. Neurosurg. Psychiat.*, **55**, 352–8.

French Cooperative Group on Plasma Exchange in Guillain–Barré Syndrome (1987). Efficiency of plasma exchange in Guillain–Barré syndrome: role of replacement fluids. *Ann. Neurol.*, **22**, 753–61.

Frith, J. A., McLeod, J. G., Nicholson, G. A. *et al.* (1994). Peroneal muscular atrophy with pyramidal tract features (hereditary motor and sensory neuropathy type V): a clinical, neurophysiological and pathological study of a large kindred. *J. Neurol. Neurosurg. Psychiat.*, **57**, 1343–6.

Fujimura, H., Lacroix, C., and Said, G. (1991). Vulnerability of nerve fibres to ischaemia. *Brain*, **114**, 1929–42.

Fullerton, P. M. and O'Sullivan, D. J. (1968). Thalidomide neuropathy: a clinical, electrophysiological, and histological follow-up study. *J. Neurol. Neurosurg. Psychiat.*, **31**, 543–51.

Gabreëls-Festen, A. A. W. M., Hoogendijk, J. E., Meijerink, P. H. S. *et al.* (1996). Two divergent types of nerve pathology in patients with different Po mutations in Charcot–Marie–Tooth disease. *Neurology*, **47**, 761–5.

Gabreëls-Festen, A., van Beersum, J., Eshuis, L. *et al.* (1999). Study on the gene and phenotypic characterization of autosomal recessive demyelinating motor and sensory neuropathy (Charcot–Marie–Tooth disease) with a gene locus on chromosome 5q23–q33. *J. Neurol. Neurosurg. Psychiat.*, **66**, 569–74.

Gabriel, C. M., Howard, R., Finsella, N. *et al.* (2000). Prospective study of the usefulness of sural nerve biopsy. *J. Neurol. Neurosurg. Psychiat.*, **69**, 442–6.

Gainsborough, N., Hall, S. M., Hughes, R. A. C. *et al.* (1991). Sarcoid neuropathy. *J. Neurol.*, **238**, 177–80.

Garcia, A., Combarros, O., Calleja, J. *et al.* (1998). Charcot–Marie–Tooth disease Type IA with 17p duplication in infancy and early childhood. A longitudinal clinical and electrophysiologic study. *Neurology*, **50**, 1061–7.

Gemignani, F., Pavesi, G., Fiocchi, A. *et al.* (1992). Peripheral neuropathy in essential mixed cryoglobulinaemia. *J. Neurol. Neurosurg. Psychiat.*, **55**, 116–20.

Gherardi, K., Chrétien, F., Delfau-Larue, M.-H. *et al.* (1998). Neuropathy in diffuse infiltrative lymphocytosis syndrome. An HIV neuropathy not a lymphoma. *Neurology*, **50**, 1041–4.

Glenner, G. G. and Murphy, M. A. (1989). Amyloidosis of the nervous system. *J. Neurol. Sci.*, **94**, 1–28.

Goebel, H. H., Bardosi, A., Friede, R. L. *et al.* (1986). Sural nerve biopsy studies in Leigh's subacute necrotising encephalomyelopathy. *Muscle Nerve*, **9**, 165–73.

Goldstein, N. P., Jones, P. H., and Brown, J. R. (1959). Peripheral neuropathy after exposure to an ester of dichlorophenoxyacetic acid. *JAMA*, **171**, 1306–9.

Gorson, K. C., Ropper, A. H., Clark, B. D. *et al.* (1998). Treatment of chronic inflammatory demyelinating polyneuropathy with interferon-α 2A. *Neurology*, **50**, 84–7.

Grand' Maison, F., Feasby, T. E., Hahn, A. F. *et al.* (1992). Recurrent Guillain–Barré syndrome. Clinical and laboratory features. *Brain*, **115**, 1093–106.

Grant, I. A., Hunder, G. G., Homburger, H. A. *et al.* (1997). Peripheral neuropathy associated with sicca complex. *Neurology*, **48**, 855–62.

Graus, F., Bonaventura, I., Uchuya, M. *et al.* (1994). Indolent anti-Hu-associated paraneoplastic sensory neuropathy. *Neurology*, **44**, 2258–61.

Griffin, J. W., Cornblath, D. R., Alexander, F. *et al.* (1990). Ataxic sensory neuropathy and dorsal root ganglionitis associated with Sjögren's syndrome. *Ann. Neurol.*, **27**, 304–15.

Gross, J. A., Haas, M. L., and Swift, T. R. (1979). Ethylene oxide neurotoxicity. Report of four cases and review of the literature. *Neurology*, **29**, 978–83.

Guarantors of Brain (1996). *Aids to the examination of the peripheral nervous system*. Ballière Tindall, London.

Guillain, G., Barré, J. A., and Strohl, A. (1916). Sur un syndrome de radiculo-névrite avec hyperalbuminose du liquide céphalorachidien sans réaction cellulaire. Remarques sur les caracteres clinique et graphiques des réflexes tendineux. *Bull. Soc. Méd. Hôp., Paris*, **40**, 1462–70.

Guillain–Barré Syndrome Steroid Trial Group (1993). Double-blind trial of intravenous methylprednisolone in Guillain–Barré syndrome. *Lancet*, **341**, 586–90.

Guillain–Barré Syndrome Study Group (1985). Plasmapheresis and acute Guillain–Barré syndrome. *Neurology*, **35**, 1096–104.

Gutmann, L. and Gutmann, L. (1999). Critical illness neuropathy and myopathy. *Arch. Neurol.*, **56**, 527–8.

Gutmann, L., Martin, J. D., and Watson, W. (1975). Dapsone motor neuropathy—an axonal disease. *Neurology*, **26**, 514–16.

Guzzetta, F., Ferriere, G., and Lyon, G. (1982). Congenital hypomyelination polyneuropathy: pathological findings compared with polyneuropathies starting in later life. *Brain*, **105**, 395–416.

Haanpaa, M., Hakkinen, V., and Nurmikko, T. (1997). Motor involvement in acute herpes zoster. *Muscle Nerve*, **20**, 1433–8.

Haanpaa, M., Dastidar, P., Weinberg, A. *et al.* (1998). CSF and MRI findings in patients with acute herpes zoster. *Neurology*, **51**, 1405–11.

Hafer-Macko, C., Hsieh, S. -T., Li, C. Y. *et al.* (1996). Acute motor axonal neuropathy: an antibody-mediated attack on axolemma. *Ann. Neurol.*, **40**, 635–44.

Hahn, A. F., Gordon, B. A., Feleka, V. *et al.* (1982). A variant form of metachromatic leucodystrophy without arylsulfatase deficiency. *Ann. Neurol.*, **12**, 33–6.

Hahn, A. F., Brown, W. F., Koopman, W. J. *et al.* (1990). X-linked dominant hereditary motor and sensory neuropathy. *Brain*, **113**, 1511–25.

Hahn, A. F., Bolton, C. F., Pillay, N. *et al.* (1996a). Plasma-exchange therapy in chronic inflammatory demyelinating polyneuropathy. A double-blind, sham-controlled, cross-over study. *Brain*, **119**, 1055–66.

Hahn, A. F., Bolton, C. F., Zochodne, D. *et al.* (1996b). Intravenous immunoglobulin treatment in chronic inflammatory demyelinating polyneuropathy. A double-blind, placebo-controlled, cross-over study. *Brain*, **119**, 1067–77.

Hainfellner, J. A., Kristoferitsch, W., Lassmann, H. *et al.* (1996). T cell-mediated ganglioitis associated with acute sensory neuropathy. *Ann. Neurol.*, **39**, 543–7.

Hall, S. M., Hughes, R. A. C., Atkinson, P. F. *et al.* (1992). Motor nerve biopsy in severe Guillain–Barré syndrome. *Ann. Neurol.*, **31**, 441–4.

Halperin, J. J., Little, B. W., Coyle, P. K. *et al.* (1987). Lyme disease: Cause of a treatable peripheral neuropathy. *Neurology*, **37**, 1700–6.

Halperin, J. J., Golightly, M. and the Long Island Neuroborreliosis Collaborative Study Group (1992). Lyme Borreliosis in Bell's Palsy. *Neurology*, **42**, 1268–70.

Halperin, J. J., Logigian, E. L., Finkel, M. F. *et al.* (1996). Practice parameters for the diagnosis of patients with nervous system Lyme borreliosis (Lyme disease). *Neurology*, **46**, 619–27.

Hanyu, N., Ikeda, S., Nakadai, A. *et al.* (1989). Peripheral nerve pathological findings in familial amyloid polyneuropathy: a correlative study of proximal sciatic nerve and sural nerve lesions. *Ann. Neurol.*, **25**, 340–50.

Harari, D., Gibberd, F. B., Dick, J. P. R. *et al.* (1991). Plasma exchange in the treatment of Refsum disease (heredopathia atactica polyneuritiformis). *J. Neurol. Neurosurg. Psychiat.*, **54**, 614–17.

Hardie, R., Harding, A. E., Hirsch, N. *et al.* (1990). Diaphragmatic weakness in hereditary motor and sensory neuropathy. *J. Neurol. Neurosurg. Psychiat.*, **5**, 348–50.

Harding, A. E. and Thomas, P. K. (1980*a*). Hereditary distal spinal muscular atrophy. A report on 43 cases and a review of the literature. *J. Neurol. Sci.*, **45**, 337–48.

Harding, A. E. and Thomas, P. K. (1980*b*). The clinical features of hereditary motor and sensory neuropathy types I and II. *Brain*, **103**, 259–80.

Harding, A. E. and Thomas, P. K. (1980*c*). Autosomal recessive forms of hereditary motor and sensory neuropathy types I and II. *J. Neurol. Neurosurg. Psychiat.*, **43**, 669–78.

Hartung, H. -P., Pollard, J. D., Harvey, G. K. *et al.* (1995*a*). Immunopathogenesis and treatment of the Guillain–Barré syndrome. Part I. *Muscle Nerve*, **18**, 137–53.

Hartung, H. -P., Pollard, J. D., Harvey, G. K. *et al.* (1995*b*). Immunopathogenesis and treatment of the Guillain–Barré syndrome. Part II. *Muscle Nerve*, **18**, 154–64.

Hattori, N., Ichimura, M., Nagamatsu, M. *et al.* (1999). Clinicopathological features of Churg–Strauss syndrome-associated neuropathy. *Brain*, **122**, 427–39.

Hawke, S. B., Davies, L., Pamphlett, R. *et al.* (1991). Vasculitic neuropathy. A clinical and pathological study. *Brain*, **114**, 2175–90.

Hayashi, H., Park-Matsumoto, Y.-C., Yuki, N. *et al.* (1993). A case of recurrent Guillain–Barré syndrome preceded by different infections. *J. Neurol.*, **240**, 196–7.

Hemmer, B., Glocker, F. X., Schumacher, M. *et al.* (1998). Subacute combined degeneration: clinical, electrophysiological, and magnetic resonance imaging methods. *J. Neurol. Neurosurg. Psychiat.*, **65**, 822–7.

Henson, R. A. and Urich, H. (1982). *Cancer and the nervous system*. Blackwell, Oxford.

Hentati, A., Deng, H. -X., Hung, W. -Y. *et al.* (1996). Human α-tocopherol transfer protein: gene structure and mutations in familial vitamin E deficiency. *Ann. Neurol.*, **39**, 295–300.

Herrmann, D. N., Griffin, J. W., Hauer, P. *et al.* (1999). Epidermal nerve fibre density and sural nerve morphometry in peripheral neuropathies. *Neurology*, **53**, 1634–40.

Hillbom, M. and Wennberg, A. (1984). Prognosis of alcoholic peripheral neuropathy. *J. Neurol. Neurosurg. Psychiat.*, **47**, 699–703.

Hodgkinson, S. J., Pollard, J. D., McLeod, J. G. (1990). Cyclosporin A in the treatment of chronic demyelinating polyradiculoneuropathy. *J. Neurol. Neurosurg. Psychiat.*, **53**, 327–30.

Holman, R. R., White, V. M., Orde-Peckar, C. *et al.* (1983). Prevention of deterioration of renal and sensory-nerve function by more intensive management of insulin-dependent diabetic patients. A two-year randomised prospective study. *Lancet*, **1**, 204–8.

Horoupain, D. S. (1989). Hereditary sensory neuropathy with deafness: a familial multisystem atrophy. *Neurology*, **39**, 244–8.

Horwich, M. S., Cho, L., Porro, R. S. *et al.* (1977). Subacute sensory neuropathy: a remote effect of carcinoma. *Ann. Neurol.*, **2**, 7–19.

Hovestadt, A., Van der Burg, M. E. L., and Verbiest, H. B. C. (1992). The course of neuropathy after cessation of Cisplatin treatment, combined with org 1766 or placebo. *J. Neurol.*, **239**, 143–6.

Hughes, R. A. C. (1990). *Guillain–Barré syndrome*. Springer-Verlag, Berlin.

Hughes, R. A. C., Newsom-Davis, J. M., Perkin, G. D. *et al.* (1978). Controlled trial of prednisolone in acute polyneuropathy. *Lancet*, **2**, 750–3.

Hughes, R. A. C., Sanders, E., Hall, S. *et al.* (1992). Subacute idiopathic demyelinating Polyradiculoneuropathy. *Arch. Neurol.*, **49**, 612–16.

Hughes, R. A. C., Sharrack, B., and Rubens, R. D. (1996). Carcinoma and the peripheral nervous system. *J. Neurol.*, **243**, 371–6.

Igisu, H., Goto, I., Kawamura, Y. *et al.* (1975). Acrylamide neuropathy due to well water pollution. *J. Neurol. Neurosurg. Psychiat.*, **38**, 581–4.

Indo, Y., Tsuruta, M., Hayashida, Y. *et al.* (1996). Mutations in the TRKA/NGF receptor gene in patients with congenital insensitivity to pain with anhidrosis. *Nature Genet.*, **13**, 485–8.

Ionasescu, V. A., Searby, C., Sheffield, V. C. *et al.* (1996). Autosomal dominant Charcot–Marie–Tooth axonal neuropathy mapped on chromosome 7p. *Hum. Mol. Genet.*, **5**, 1373–5.

Irani, D. N., Cornblath, D. R., Chaudhry, V. *et al.* (1993). Relapse in Guillain–Barré syndrome after treatment with human immunoglobulin. *Neurology*, **43**, 872–5.

Jacobs, B. S., Rothbarth, P. H., van der Meché, F. G. A. *et al.* (1998). The spectrum of antecedent infections in Guillain–Barré syndrome. *Neurology*, **51**, 1110–15.

Jacobs, J. and Love, S. (1985). Qualitative and quantitative morphology of human sural nerve at different ages. *Brain*, **108**, 897–924.

Jacobs, J. M., Shetty, V. P., and Antia, N. H. (1987). Teased fibre studies in leprous neuropathy. *J. Neurol. Sci.*, **79**, 301–13.

Jacobson, R. R. and Krahenbuhl, J. L. (1999). Leprosy. *Lancet*, **353**, 655–60.

Jamal, G. A. and Ballantyne, J. P. (1988). The localization of the lesion in patients with acute ophthalmoplegia, ataxia and areflexia (Miller Fisher syndrome). *Brain*, **111**, 95–114.

Jamieson, P. W., Giuliani, M. J., and Martinez, A. J. (1991). Necrotising angiopathy presenting with multifocal conduction blocks. *Neurology*, **41**, 442–4.

Janssens, J., Peters, T. L., Vantrappen, G. *et al.* (1990). Improvement of gastric emptying in diabetic gastroparesis by erythromycin. *N. Engl. J. Med.*, **322**, 1028–31.

Jaspan, J. B., Wollman, R. L., Bernstein, L. *et al.* (1982). Hypoglycaemic peripheral neuropathy in association with insulinoma: implications of glucopenia rather than hyperinsulinism. *Medicine*, **61**, 33–44.

Jestico, J. V., Urry, P. A., and Efphimiou, J. (1985). An hereditary sensory and autonomic neuropathy transmitted as an X-linked recessive trait. *J. Neurol. Neurosurg. Psychiat.*, **48**, 1259–64.

Johnson, R. H. and Robinson, B. J. (1988). Mortality in alcoholics with autonomic neuropathy. *J. Neurol. Neurosurg. Psychiat.*, **51**, 476–80.

Joy, J. L. and Oh, S. J. (1989). Tomaculous neuropathy presenting as acute recurrent polyneuropathy. *Ann. Neurol.*, **26**, 98–100.

Kafka, S. P., Condemi, J. J., Marsh, D. O. *et al.* (1994). Mononeuritis multiplex and vasculitis. Association with anti-neutrophil cytoplasmic autoantibody. *Arch. Neurol.*, **51**, 565–8.

Kaji, R., Shibasaki, H., and Kimura, J. (1992). Multifocal demyelinating motor neuropathy: cranial nerve involvement and immunoglubulin therapy. *Neurology*, **42**, 506–9.

Kalaydjieva, L., Gresham, D., Goding, R. *et al.* (2000). N-myc downstream-regulated gene 1 is mutated in hereditary motor and sensory neuropathy-lom. *Am. J. Hum. Genet.*, **67**, 47–58.

Kantarjian, A. D. and Shaheen, A. S. (1963). Methyl bromide poisoning with nervous system manifestations resembling polyneuropathy. *Neurology*, **13**, 1054–8.

Katirji, B. (1999). Chronic relapsing axonal neuropathy responsive to intravenous immunglobulin. *Neurology*, **48**, 1690–4.

Katrak, S. M., Pollock, M., O'Brien, C. P. *et al.* (1980). Clinical and morphological features of gold neuropathy. *Brain*, **103**, 671–93.

Katz, J. S., Wolfe, G. I., Bryan, W. W. *et al.* (1997). Electrophysiologic findings in multifocal motor neuropathy. *Neurology*, **48**, 700–7.

Katz, J. S., Saperstein, D. S., Gronseth, G. *et al.* (2000). Distal acquired demyelinating symmetric neuropathy. *Neurology*, **54**, 615–20.

Kelly, J. J., Kyle, R. A., O'Brien, P. C. *et al.* (1979). The natural history of peripheral neuropathy in primary systemic amyloidosis. *Ann. Neurol.*, **6**, 1–7.

Kelly, J. J., Kyle, R. A., Miles, J. M. *et al.* (1981). The spectrum of peripheral neuropathy in myeloma. *Neurology*, **31**, 24–31.

Kelly, J. J., Kyle, R. A., Miles, J. M. *et al.* (1983). Osteosclerotic myeloma and peripheral neuropathy. *Neurology*, **33**, 202–10.

Kemppainen, R., Juntunen, J., and Hillbom, M. (1982). Drinking habits and peripheral alcoholic neuropathy. *Acta Neurol. Scand.*, **65**, 11–18.

Kennedy, W. R., Navarro, X., Goetz, F. C. *et al.* (1990). Effects of pancreatic transplantation on diabetic neuropathy. *N. Engl. J. Med.*, **322**, 1031–7.

Keogh, J. P., Pestronk, A., Wertheimer, D. *et al.* (1980). An epidemic of urinary retention caused by dimethylaminopropionitrile. *JAMA*, **243**, 746–9.

Khella, S. L., Frost, S., Hermann, G. A. *et al.* (1995). Hepatitis C infection, cryoglobulinaemia, and vasculitic neuropathy. Treatment with interferon alfa: case report and literature review. *Neurology*, **45**, 407–11.

Kjeldsen, K., Simonsen, O., and Heron, I. (1985). Immunity against diptherhia 25–30 years after primary vaccination in childhood. *Lancet*, **i**, 900–2.

Klopstock, T., Naumann, M., Schalke, B. *et al.* (1994). Multiple symmetric lipomatosis: abnormalities in Complex IV and multiple deletions in mitochondrial DNA. *Neurology*, **44**, 862–6.

Kreiss, K., Wegman, D. H., Niles, C. A. *et al.* (1980). Neurological dysfunction of the bladder in workers exposed to Dimethylaminopropionitrile. *JAMA*, **243**, 741–5.

Krendel, D. A., Costigan, D. A., and Hopkins, L. C. (1995). Successful treatment of neuropathies in patients with diabetes mellitus. *Arch. Neurol.*, **52**, 1053–61.

Krivit, W., Shapiro, E., Kennedy, W. *et al.* (1990). Treatment of late infantile metachromatic leucodystrophy by bone marrow transplantation. *N. Engl. J. Med.*, **322**, 28–32.

Kuncl, R. W., Duncan, G., Watson, D. *et al.* (1987). Colchicine myopathy and neuropathy. *N. Engl. J. Med.*, **316**, 1562–8.

Kuwabara, S., Hattori, T., Shimoe, Y. *et al.* (1997). Long term melphalan–prednisolone chemotherapy for POEMS syndrome. *J. Neurol. Neurosurg. Psychiat.*, **63**, 385–7.

Kyle, R. A., Greipp, P. R., Garton, J. P. *et al.* (1985). Primary systemic amyloidosis: comparison of melphalan/ prednisolone versus colchicine. *Am. J. Med.*, **79**, 708–16.

Lamontagne, A. and Buchthal, F. (1970). Electrophysiological studies in diabetic neuropathy. *J. Neurol. Neurosurg. Psychiat.*, **33**, 442–52.

Landrieu, P., Said, G., and Allaire, C. (1990). Dominantly transmitted congenital indifference to pain. *Ann. Neurol.*, **27**, 574–8.

Latov, N. (1995). Pathogenesis and therapy of neuropathies associated with monoclonal gammopathies. *Ann. Neurol.*, **37**, S32–42.

Lauria, G., McArthur, J. C., Haver, P. E. *et al.* (1998). Neuropathological alterations in diabetic truncal neuropathy: evaluation by skin biopsy. *J. Neurol. Neurosurg. Psychiat.*, **65**, 762–6.

Lawn, N. D. and Wijdicks, E. F. M. (1999). Fatal Guillain–Barré syndrome. *Neurology*, **52**, 635–8.

Lenssen, P. P. A., Gabreëls-Festen, A. A. W. M., Valentijn, L. J. *et al.* (1998). Hereditary neuropathy with liability to pressure palsies. Penotypic differences between patients with the common deletion and a PMP22 frame shift mutation. *Brain*, **121**, 1451–8.

Le Quesne, P. M. and McLeod, J. G. (1977). Peripheral neuropathy following a single exposure to arsenic. *J. Neurol. Sci.*, **32**, 437–51.

Levine, T. D. and Pestronk, A. (1999). IgM antibody-related polyneuropathies: B-cell depletion chemotherapy using Rituximab. *Neurology*, **52**, 1701–4.

Lewis, R. A. and Sumner, A. J. (1982). The electrodiagnostic distinctions between chronic familial and acquired demyelinative neuropathies. *Neurology*, **32**, 592–6.

Lindholm, T. (1967). Electromyographic changes after nitrofurantoin (furantoin) therapy in non-uraemic patients. *Neurology*, **17**, 1017–20.

Lisak, R. P., Mitchell, M., Zweiman, B. *et al.* (1977). Guillain–Barré syndrome and Hodgkin's disease: three cases with immunological studies. *Ann. Neurol.*, **1**, 72–8.

Llewelyn, J. G., Thomas, P. K., Fonseca, V. *et al.* (1986). Acute painful diabetic neuropathy precipitated by strict glycaemic control. *Acta Neuropath.*, **72**, 157–63.

Löffel, N. B., Rossi, L. N., Mumenthaler, M. *et al.* (1977). The Landry–Guillain–Barré syndrome: complications, prognosis, and natural history in 123 cases. *J. Neurol. Sci.*, **33**, 71–9.

Logigian, E. L. and Steere, A. C. (1992). Clinical and electrophysiological findings in chronic neuropathy of Lyme disease. *Neurology*, **42**, 303–11.

Logigian, E. L., Shefner, J. M., Frosch, M. P. *et al.* (1993). Nonvasculitic, steroid-responsive mononeuritis multiplex. *Neurology*, **43**, 879–83.

Logina, I. and Donaghy, M. (1999). Diphtheritic polyneuropathy: a clinical study and comparison with Guillain–Barré syndrome. *J. Neurol. Neurosurg. Psychiat.*, **67**, 433–8.

LoMonaco, M., Milone, M., Batocchi, A. P. *et al.* (1992). Cisplatin neuropathy: clinical course and neurophysiological findings. *J. Neurol.*, **239**, 199–204.

Lopate, G., Parks, B. J., and Goldstein, J. M. (1997). Polyneuropathies associated with high titre antisulphatide antibodies: characteristics of patients with and without serum monoclonal proteins. *J. Neurol. Neurosurg. Psychiat.*, **62**, 581–5.

Lotti, M., Becker, C. E., and Aminoff, M. J. (1984). Organophosphorus polyneuropathy: pathogenesis and prevention. *Neurology*, **34**, 658–62.

Low, P. A., McLeod, J. G., Turtle, J. R. *et al.* (1974). Peripheral neuropathy in acromegaly. *Brain*, **97**, 139–52.

Lu, J. L., Sheikh, K. A., Wu, H. S. *et al.* (2000). Physiologic–pathologic correlation in Guillain–Barré syndrome in children. *Neurology*, **54**, 33–9.

Lynch, D. R., Hara, H., Yum, S. W. *et al.* (1997). Autosomal dominant transmission of Déjérine–Sottas disease (HMSN III). *Neurology*, **49**, 601–3.

Madrid, R. and Bradley, W. G. (1975). The pathology of neuropathies with focal thickening of the myelin sheath (tomaculous neuropathy). *J. Neurol. Sci.*, **25**, 415–48.

Magy, L., Birouk, N., Vallat, J. M. *et al.* (1997). Hereditary thermosensitive neuropathy: an autosomal dominant disorder of the peripheral nervous system. *Neurology*, **49**, 1684–90.

Martin, J. J., Ceuterick, C., Mercelis, R. *et al.* (1982). Pathology of peripheral nerves in metachromatic leucodystrophy: a comparative study of ten cases. *J. Neurol. Sci.*, **53**, 95–112.

Martina, I. S. J., van Doorn, P. A., Schmitz, P. I. M. *et al.* (1999). Chronic motor neuropathies: response to interferon-β1a after failure of conventional therapies. *J. Neurol. Neurosurg. Psychiat.*, **66**, 197–201.

Matthews, W. B. and Esiri, M. (1983). The migrant sensory neuritis of Wartenberg. *J. Neurol. Neurosurg. Psychiat.*, **46**, 1–4.

McCombe, P., McManis, P. G., Frith, J. A. *et al.* (1987a). Chronic inflammatory demyelinating polyradiculoneuropathy associated with pregnancy. *Ann. Neurol.*, **21**, 102–4.

McCombe, P. A., Pollard, J. D., and McLeod, J. G. (1987b). Chronic inflammatory demyelinating polyradiculopathy. A clinical and electrophysiological study of 92 cases. *Brain*, **110**, 1617–30.

McFaul, R., Cavanagh, N., Lake, B. D. *et al.* (1982). Metachromatic leucodystrophy: review of 38 cases. *Arch. Dis. Child.*, **57**, 168–75.

McKhann, G. M., Griffin, J. W., Cornblath, D. R. *et al.* (1988). Plasmapheresis and Guillain–Barré syndrome: analysis of prognostic factors and the effect of plasmapheresis. *Ann. Neurol.*, **23**, 347–53.

McLeod, J. G., Pollard, J. D., Macaskill, P. *et al.* (1999). Prevalence of chronic inflammatory demyelinating polyneuropathy in New South Wales, Australia. *Ann. Neurol.*, **46**, 910–13.

Meadows, J. C. and Marsden, C. D. (1969). A distal form of chronic spinal muscular atrophy. *Neurology*, **19**, 53–8.

Medori, R., Autilio-Gambetti, L., Jenich, H. *et al.* (1988). Changes in axon size and slow axonal transport are related in experimental diabetic neuropathy. *Neurology*, **38**, 597–601.

Meier, C. and Bischoff, A. (1977). Polyneuropathy in hypothyroidism. Clinical and nerve biopsy study of four cases. *J. Neurol.*, **215**, 103–14.

Meiner, V., Meiner, Z., Reshef, A. *et al.* (1994). Cerebrotendinous xanthomatosis: molecular diagnosis enables presymptomatic detection of a treatable disease. *Neurology*, **44**, 288–90.

Melgaard, B., Hansen, H. S., Zamieniecka, Z. *et al.* (1982). Misonidazole neuropathy: a clinical, electrophysiological, and histological study. *Ann. Neurol.*, **12**, 10–17.

Mericle, R. A. and Triggs, W. J. (1997). Treatment of acute pandysautonomia with intravenous immunoglobulin. *J. Neurol. Neurosurg. Psychiat.*, **62**, 529–31.

Mitchell, G., Larochelle, J., Lambert, M. *et al.* (1990). Neurologic crises in hereditary tyrosinemia. *N. Engl. J. Med.*, **322**, 432–7.

Mersiyanova, I. V., Perepelov, A. V., Polyakov, A. V. *et al.* (2000). A new variant of Charcot-Marie-Tooth disease type 2 is probably the result of a mutation in the neurofilament-light gene. *Am. J. Hum. Genet.*, **67**, 37–46.

Misu, K., Yoshihara, T., Shikama, Y. *et al.* (2000). An axonal form of Chariot-Marie-Tooth disease showing distinctive features in association with mutations in the peripheral myelin protein zero gene (Thr124Met or Asp75Val). *J. Neurol. Neurosurg. Psychiat.*, **69**, 806–11.

Moeschlin, S. (1980). Thallium poisoning. *Clin. Toxicol.*, **17**, 133–46.

Mokri, B., Ohnishi, A., and Dyck, P. J. (1981). Disulfiram neuropathy. *Neurology*, **31**, 730–5.

Monaco, S., Lucci, B., Laperchia, N. *et al.* (1988). Polyneuropathy in hypereosinophilic syndrome. *Neurology*, **38**, 494–6.

Monaco, S., Bonetti, B., Ferrari, S. *et al.* (1990). Complement-mediated demyelination in patients with IgM monoclonal gammopathy and polyneuropathy. *N. Engl. J. Med.*, **322**, 649–52.

Monforte, R., Estruch, R., Valls-Sole, J. *et al.* (1995). Autonomic and peripheral neuropathies in patients with chronic alcoholism. *Arch. Neurol.*, **52**, 45–51.

Morgan, J. P. and Penovich, P. (1978). Jamaica ginger paralysis: 47-year follow-up. *Arch. Neurol.*, **35**, 530–2.

Moyle, G. J., Nelson, M. R., Hawkins, D. *et al.* (1993). The use and toxicity of didanosine (ddI) in HIV antibody-positive individuals intolerant to zidovudine (AZT). *Quart. J. Med.*, **86**, 155–63.

Muller, D. P. R., Lloyd, J. K., and Wolff, O. H. (1985). The role of vitamin E in the treatment of neurological features of abetalipoproteinaemia and other disorders of fat absorption. *J. Inherit. Metab. Dis.*, **8** (Suppl. 1), 88–92.

Murray, I. P. C. and Simpson, J. A. (1958). Acroparaesthesiae in myxoedema. *Lancet*, **1**, 1360–3.

Nadkarni, N. and Lisak, R. P. (1993). Guillain–Barré syndrome (GBS) with bilateral optic neuritis and central white matter disease. *Neurology*, **43**, 842–3.

Nair, V. S., LeBrun, M., and Kass, I. (1980). Peripheral neuropathy associated with ethambutol. *Chest*, **77**, 98–100.

Nakanishi, T., Sobue, I., Toyokura, Y. *et al.* (1984). The Crow–Fukase syndrome: a study of 102 cases in Japan. *Neurology*, **34**, 712–20.

Nelis, E., Haites, N., and Van Broeckhoven, C. (1999). Mutations in the peripheral myelin genes and associated genes in inherited peripheral neuropathies. *Hum. Mutat.*, **13**, 11–28.

New, P. Z., Jackson, C. E., Rinaldi, D. *et al.* (1996). Peripheral neuropathy secondary to docetaxel (taxotene). *Neurology*, **46**, 108–11.

Nichols, W. C., Dwulet, F. E., Liepnieks, J. *et al.* (1988). Variant apolipoprotein A1 as a major constituent of a human hereditary amyloid. *Biochem. Biophys. Res. Commun.*, **156**, 762–8.

Nierenberg, D. W., Nordgren, R. E., Chang, M. B. *et al.* (1998). Delayed cerebellar disease and death after accidental exposure to dimethylmercury. *N. Engl. J. Med.*, **338**, 1672–6.

Nobile-Orazio, E., Meucci, N., Barbieri, S. *et al.* (1993). High-dose intravenous immunoglobulin therapy in multifocal motor neuropathy. *Neurology*, **43**, 537–44.

Nobile-Orazio, E., Meucci, N., Baldini, L. *et al.* (2000). Long-term prognosis of neuropathy associated with anti-MAG IgM M-proteins and its relationship to immune therapies. *Brain*, **123**, 710–17.

Notermans, N. C., Wokke, J. H. J., Franssen, H. *et al.* (1993). Chronic idiopathic polyneuropathy presenting in middle or old age: a clinical and electrophysiological study of 75 patients. *J. Neurol. Neurosurg. Psychiat.*, **56**, 1066–71.

Notermans, N. C., Wokke, J. H. J., Van den Berg, L. H. *et al.* (1996). Chronic idiopathic axonal polyneuropathy. Comparison of patients with and without monoclonal gammopathy. *Brain,* 119, 421–7.

Nukada, H., Pollock, M., and Haas, L. F. (1982). The clinical spectrum and morphology of type II hereditary sensory neuropathy. *Brain,* 105, 647–65.

Nukada, H., Van Rij, A. M., Packer, G. K. *et al.* (1996). Pathology of acute and chronic ischaemic neuropathy in atheroscherotic peripheral vascular disease. *Brain,* 119, 1449–60.

Numakura, C., Lin, C., Oka, N. *et al.* (2000). Hemizygous mutation of the peripheral myelin protein 22 gene associated with Charcot–Marie–Tooth disease type 1. *Ann. Neurol.,* 47, 101–3.

Oaklander, A. L., Romans, K., Horasek, S. *et al.* (1998). Unilateral postherpetic neuralgia is associated with bilateral sensory neuron damage. *Ann. Neurol.,* 44, 789–95.

O'Brien, I. A. D., O'Hare, J. P., Lewin, I. G. *et al.* (1986). The prevalence of autonomic neuropathy in insulin-dependent diabetes mellitus: a controlled study based on heart rate variability. *Quart. J. Med.,* 61, 957–67.

Ochoa, J. (1970). Isoniazid neuropathy in man: quantitative electron microscope study. *Brain,* 93, 831–50.

Oh, S. J., Slaughter, R., and Harrell, L. (1991). Paraneoplastic vasculitic neuropathy: a treatable neuropathy. *Muscle Nerve,* 14, 152–6.

Oh, S. J., Joy, J. L., and Kuruoglu, R. (1992). 'Chronic sensory demyelinating neuropathy'. Chronic inflammatory demyelinating neuropathy presenting as a pure sensory neuropathy. *J. Neurol. Neurosurg. Psychiat.,* 55, 677–80.

Oh, S. J., Claussen, G. C., Odabasi, Z. *et al.* (1995). Multifocal demyelinating motor neuropathy: pathologic evidence of 'inflammatory demyelinating Polyradiculoneuropathy'. *Neurology,* 45, 1828–32.

Oh, S. J., La Gauke, C., and Claussen, C. G. (2001). Sensory Guillain-Barré syndrome *Neurology,* 56, 82 6.

Ohnishi, A., Petersen, C. M., and Dyck, P. J. (1975). Axonal degeneration in sodium cyanate-induced neuropathy. *Arch. Neurol.,* 32, 530–4.

Ohnishi, A., Tsuji, S., Igisu, H. *et al.* (1980). Beriberi neuropathy. Morphometric study of sural nerve. *J. Neurol. Sci.,* 45, 177–90.

Ohta, M., Ellefson, R. D., Lambert, E. H. *et al.* (1973). Hereditary sensory neuropathy, type II: clinical, electrophysiologic, histologic and biochemical studies of a Quebec kinship. *Arch. Neurol.,* 29, 23–37.

Oksi, J., Kalimo, H., Marttila, R. J. *et al.* (1996). Inflammatory brain changes in Lyme borreliosis. A report on three patients and review of the literature. *Brain,* 119, 2143–54.

Omdal, R., Henriksen, O. A., Mellgren, S. I. *et al.* (1991). Peripheral neuropathy in systemic lupus erythematosus. *Neurology,* 41, 808–11.

Ormerod, I, E. C., Waddy, H. M., Kermode, A. G. *et al.* (1990). Involvement of the central nervous system in chronic inflammatory demyelinating polyneuropathy: a clinical, electrophysiological and magnetic resonance imaging study. *J. Neurol. Neurosurg. Psychiat.,* 53, 789–93.

Othmane, K., Middleton, L. T., Loprest, L. J. *et al.* (1993). Localisation of a gene (CMT 2a) for autosomal dominant Charcot–Marie–Tooth disease, Type 2, to chromosome 1p and evidence of genetic heterogeneity. *Genomics,* 17, 370–5.

Ouvrier, R. A., McLeod, J. G., and Conchin, T. E. (1987). The hypertrophic forms of hereditary motor and sensory neuropathy. A study of hypertrophic Charcot–Marie–Tooth disease (HMSN type I) and Dejerine–Sottas disease (HMSN type III) in childhood. *Brain,* 110, 121–48.

Palliyath, S. K., Schwartz, B. D., and Gant, L. (1990). Peripheral nerve functions in chronic alcoholic patients on disulfiram: a six month follow up. *J. Neurol. Neurosurg. Psychiat.,* 53, 227–30.

Parrilla, P., Ramirez, P., Andreu, L. F. *et al.* (1997). Long-term results of liver transplantation in familial amyloidotic polyneuropathy type 1. *Transplantation,* 64, 646–9.

Parry, J. G. and Bredesen, D. E. (1985). Sensory neuropathy with low-dose pyridoxine. *Neurology,* 35, 1466–8.

Paunio, T., Sunada, Y., Kiuru, S. *et al.* (1995). Haplo type analysis in gelsolin-related amyloidosis reveals independent origin of identical mutation (G654A) of gelsolin in Finland and Japan. *Hum. Mutat.,* 6, 60–5.

Pedley, J. C., Harman, D. J., Waudby, H. *et al.* (1980). Leprosy in peripheral nerves: histopathological findings in 119 untreated patients in Nepal. *J. Neurol. Neurosurg. Psychiat.,* 43, 198–204.

Periquet, M. I., Novak, V., Collins, M. P. *et al.* (1999). Painful sensory neuropathy. Prospective evaluation using skin biopsy. *Neurology,* 53, 1641–7.

Pestronk, A., Chaudhry, V., Feldman, E. L. *et al.* (1990). Lower motor neuron syndromes defined by patterns of weakness, nerve conduction abnormalities, and high titres of antiglycolipid antibodies. *Ann. Neurol.,* 27, 316–26.

Pestronk, A., Lopate, G., Kornberg, A. J. *et al.* (1994). Distal lower motor neuron syndrome with high-titre serum IgM anti-GM$_1$, antibodies. *Neurology,* 44, 2027–31.

Pettit, R. E. and Berdal, K. G. (1984). The Che'diak-Higashi syndrome: neurologic appearance. *Arch. Neurol.,* 41, 1001–2.

Peyronnard, J. M., Charron, L., and Bandet, R. (1982). Vasculitic neuropathy in rheumatoid disease and Sjögren's syndrome. *Neurology,* 32, 839–45.

Phelps, M., Aicardi, J., and Vanier, M.-T. (1991). Late onset Krabbe's leucodystrophy: a report of four cases. *J. Neurol. Neurosurg. Psychiat.*, **54**, 293–6.

Pietrini, V., Rizzuto, N., Vergani, C. *et al.* (1985). Neuropathy in Tangier disease: a clinicopathologic study and a review of the literature. *Acta Neurol. Scand.*, **72**, 495–505.

Planté-Bordeneuve, V., Lalu, T., Misrahi, M. *et al.* (1998). Genotypic–phenotypic variations in a series of 65 patients with familial amyloidotic polyneuropathy. *Neurology*, **51**, 708–14.

Plasma Exchange/Sandoglobulin Guillain–Barré syndrome Trial Group (1997). Randomised trial of plasma exchange, intravenous immunoglobulin, and combined treatments in Guillain–Barré syndrome. *Lancet*, **349**, 225–30.

Pollock, M., Nukadah, H., Taylor, P. *et al.* (1983*a*). Comparison between fascicular and whole sural nerve biopsy. *Ann. Neurol.*, **13**, 65–8.

Pollock, M., Nukada, H., Frith, R. W. *et al.* (1983*b*). Peripheral neuropathy in Tangier disease. *Brain*, **106**, 911–28.

Ponsford, S., Willison, H., Veitch, J. *et al.* (2000). Long-term clinical and neurophysiological following of patients with peripheral neuropathy associated with benign monoclonal gammopathy. *Muscle Nerve*, **23**, 164–74.

Prineas, J. (1981). Pathology of the Guillain–Barré syndrome. *Ann. Neurol.*, **9**, S06–S19.

Rajaniemi, R. (1986). Clinical evaluation of occupational toxicity of methylmethacrylate monomer to dental technicians. *J. Soc. Occup. Med.*, **36**, 56–9.

Rakhmanova, A. G., Lumio, J., Groundstroem, K. *et al.* (1996). Diphtheria outbreak in St Petersburg: clinical characteristics of 1860 adult patients. *Scand. J. Infect. Dis.*, **28**, 37–40.

Rechthand, E., Cornblath, D. R., Stern, B. J. *et al.* (1984). Chronic demyelinating polyneuropathy in systemic lupus erythematosus. *Neurology*, **34**, 1375–7.

Rees, J. H., Soudain, S. E., Gregson, N. A. *et al.* (1995). *Campylobacter jejuni* infection and Guillain–Barré syndrome. *N. Engl. J. Med.*, **333**, 1374–9.

Refsum, S., Stokke, O., Eldjarn, L. *et al.* (1984). Heredopathia atactica polyneuritisformis (Refsum disease). In *Peripheral neuropathy*, (2nd edn), (ed. P. J. Dyck, P. K. Thomas, E. H. Lambert, and R. P. Bunge). WB Saunders, Philadelphia.

Reilly, M. M., Adams, D., Booth, D. R. *et al.* (1995). Transthyretin gene analysis in European patients with suspected familial amyloid polyneuropathy. *Brain*, **118**, 849–56.

Richardson, E. P. and De Girolami, U. (1995). *Pathology of the peripheral nervous system*. W. B. Saunders, Philadelphia.

Ricoy, J. R., Cabello, A., Rodriguez, J. *et al.* (1983). Neuropathological studies on the toxic syndrome related to adulterated rapeseed oil in Spain. *Brain*, **106**, 817–35.

Ridley, A. (1969). The neuropathy of acute intermittent porphyria. *Quart. J. Med.*, **38**, 307–33.

Ropper, A. H. (1986). Severe acute Guillain–Barré syndrome. *Neurology*, **36**, 429–32.

Ropper, A. H. (1993). Accelerated neuropathy of renal failure. *Arch. Neurol.*, **50**, 536–9.

Ropper, A. H. (1994). Further regional variants of acute immune polyneuropathy. *Arch. Neurol.*, **51**, 671–5.

Ropper, A. H., Albert, J. W., and Addison, R. (1988). Limited relapse in Guillain–Barré syndrome after plasma exchange. *Arch. Neurol.*, **45**, 314–15.

Ropper, A. H., Wijdicks, E. F. M., and Truax, B. T. (1991). *Guillain–Barré syndrome*. F. A. Davis, Philadelphia.

Ryle, C. and Donaghy, M. (1995). Non-enzymatic glycation of peripheral nerve proteins in human diabetics. *J. Neurol. Sci.*, **129**, 62–8.

Said, G. (1978). Perhexiline neuropathy: a clinicopathological study. *Ann. Neurol.*, **3**, 259–66.

Said, G. (1996). Diabetic neuropathy: an update. *J. Neurol.*, **243**, 431–40.

Said, G., Lacroix-Ciaudo, C., Fujimara, H. *et al.* (1988). The peripheral neuropathy of necrotising arteritis: a clinicopathological study. *Ann. Neurol.*, **23**, 461–5.

Said, G., Goulon-Goeau, C., Lacroix, C. *et al.* (1994). Nerve biopsy findings in different patterns of proximal diabetic neuropathy. *Ann. Neurol.*, **35**, 559–69.

Sampson, M. J., Wilson, S., Karagiannis, P. *et al.* (1990). Progression of diabetic autonomic neuropathy over a decade in insulin dependent diabetics. *Quart. J. Med.*, **75**, 635–46.

Samuels, M. A., Shahani, B. T., and Sealfon, S. C. (1984). Case 39–1984: A 29-year-old woman with abdominal pain, myalgia and muscle weakness. *N. Engl. J. Med.*, **311**, 839–47.

Santoro, M., Thomas, F. P., Fink, M. E. *et al.* (1990). IgM deposits at nodes of Ranvier in a patient with amyotrophic lateral sclerosis, anti-GM1 antibodies and multifocal motor conduction block. *Ann. Neurol.*, **28**, 373–7.

Schady, W. and Ochoa, J. (1984). Ehlers–Danlos in association with tomaculous neuropathy. *Neurology*, **34**, 1270.

Schady, W., Sheard, A., Hassell, A. *et al.* (1991). Peripheral nerve dysfunction in scleroderma. *Quart. J. Med.*, **292**, 661–75.

Schaumburg, H., Kaplan, J., Widebank, A. *et al.* (1983). Sensory neuropathy from pyridoxine abuse. *N. Engl. J. Med.*, **309**, 445–8.

Schmidt, B. L. (1997). PCR in laboratory diagnosis of human *Borrelia burgdorferii* infections. *Clin. Microbiol. Rev.*, **10**, 185–201.

Schold, S. C., Cho, E.-S., Somasundaram, M. *et al.* (1979). Subacute motor neuronopathy: a remote effect of lymphoma. *Ann. Neurol.*, **5**, 271–87.

Schonberger, L. B., Hurwitz, F. S., Katona, P. *et al.* (1981). Guillain–Barré syndrome: its epidemiology and associations with influenza vaccination. *Ann. Neurol.*, **9** (Suppl.), 31–8.

Schwartz, M. S., Mackworth-Young, C. G., and McKeran, R. O. (1983). The tarsal tunnel syndrome in hypothyroidism. *J. Neurol. Neurosurg. Psychiat.*, **46**, 440–2.

Seddon, H. J. (1975). *Surgical disorders of peripheral nerves*, (2nd edn). Churchill Livingstone, Edinburgh.

Senanayake, N. and Johnson, M. K. (1982). Acute polyneuropathy after poisoning by a new organophosphate insecticide. *N. Engl. J. Med.*, **306**, 155–7.

Sewell, W. A. C., Brennan, V. M., Donaghy, M. *et al.* (1997). The use of self-infused intravenous immunoglobulin home therapy in treatment of acquired chronic demyelinating neuropathies. *J. Neurol. Neurosurg. Psychiat.*, **63**, 106–9.

Sheikh, K. A., Namchamkin, I., Ho, T. W. *et al.* (1998). *Campylobacter jejuni* lipopolysaccharides in Guillain–Barré syndrome: molecular mimicry and host susceptibility. *Neurology*, **51**, 371–8.

Sherman, W. H., Latov, N., Hays, A. P. *et al.* (1983). Monoclonal IgM$_k$ antibody precipitating with chondroitin sulfate C from patients with axonal polyneuropathy and epidermolysis. *Neurology*, **33**, 192–201.

Shetty, V. P., Antia, N. H., and Jacobs, J. M. (1988). The pathology of early leprous neuropathy. *J. Neurol. Sci.*, **88**, 115–31.

Shy, M. E., Arroyo, E., Sladky, J. *et al.* (1997). Heterozygous Po knockout mice develop a peripheral neuropathy that resembles chronic inflammatory demyelinating polyneuropathy (CIDP). *J. Neuropath. Exp. Neurol.*, **56**, 811–21.

Silburn, P. A., Nicholson, G. A., Tch, B. T. *et al.* (1998). Charcot–Marie–Tooth disease and Noonan syndrome with giant proximal nerve hypertrophy. *Neurology*, **50**, 1067–73.

Simmons, Z., Albers, J. W., Bromberg, M. B. *et al.* (1995). Long term follow up of patients with chronic inflammatory demyelinating polyradiculoneuropathy, without and with monoclonal gammopathy. *Brain*, **118**, 359–68.

Sladky, J. T., Brown, M. J., and Berman, P. H. (1986). Chronic inflammatory demyelinating polyneuropathy of infancy: a corticosteroid-responsive disorder. *Ann. Neurol.*, **20**, 76–81.

Smith, B. E. and Dyck, P. J. (1990). Peripheral neuropathy in the eosinophilia–myalgia syndrome associated with L-tryptophan ingestion. *Neurology*, **40**, 1035–40.

Smith, I. S. (1994). The natural history of chronic demyelinating neuropathy associated with benign IgM paraproteinaemia. A clinical and neurophysiological study. *Brain*, **117**, 949–57.

So, Y. T. and Olney, R. K. (1994). Acute lumbosacral polyradiculopathy in acquired immunodeficiency syndrome: experience in 23 patients. *Ann. Neurol.*, **35**, 53–8.

Sobue, G., Mukai, E., Fujii, K. *et al.* (1986). Peripheral nerve involvement in familial chorea–acanthocytosis. *J. Neurol. Sci.*, **76**, 347–56.

Sobue, G., Yasuda, T., Kachi, T. *et al.* (1993). Chronic progressive sensory ataxic neuropathy: clinicopathological features of idiopathic and Sjogren's syndrome-associated cases. *J. Neurol.*, **240**, 1–7.

Sobue, G., Ueno-Natsukari, I., Okamoto, H. *et al.* (1994). Phenotypic heterogeneity of an adult form of adrenoleucodystrophy in monozygotic twins. *Ann. Neurol.*, **36**, 912–15.

Sokol, R. J., Guggenheim, M., Iannaccone, S. T. *et al.* (1985). Improved neurologic function after long-term correction of vitamin E deficiency in children with chronic cholestasis. *N. Engl. J. Med.*, **313**, 1580–6.

Solders, G., Nennesmo, I., and Persson, A. (1989). Diphtheritic neuropathy, an analysis based upon muscle and nerve biopsy and repeated neurophysiological and autonomic function tests. *J. Neurol. Neurosurg. Psychiat.*, **52**, 876–80.

Sorbinal Retinopathy Trial Research Group (1993). The Sorbinal retinopathy trial: neuropathy results. *Neurology*, **43**, 1141–9.

Sosenko, J. M., Gadia, M. T., Fournier, A. M. *et al.* (1986). Body stature as a risk factor for diabetic sensory neuropathy. *Am. J. Med.*, **80**, 1031–4.

Stangel, M., Toyka, K. V., and Gold, R. (1999). Mechanisms of high-dose intravenous immunoglobulins in demyelinating diseases. *Arch. Neurol.*, **56**, 661–3.

Stefurak, T. L., Midroni, G., and Bilbao, J. M. (1999). Vasculitic polyradiculopathy in systemic lupus erythematosus. *J. Neurol. Neurosurg. Psychiat.*, **66**, 658–61.

Steiner, T., Wirguin, I., and Abramsky, O. (1986). Appearance of Guillain–Barré syndrome in patients during corticosteroid treatment. *J. Neurol.*, **233**, 221–3.

Stewart, J. D. (1989). Diabetic truncal neuropathy: topography of the sensory deficit. *Ann. Neurol.*, **25**, 233–8.

Stögbauer, F., Young, P., Kuhlenbäumer, G. *et al.* (2000). Hereditary recurrent focal neuropathies; clinical and molecular features. *Neurology*, **54**, 546–51.

Stojkovic, T., Latour, P., Vandenberghe, A. *et al.* (1999). Sensorineural deafness in X-linked Charcot–Marie–Tooth disease with Connexin-32 mutation (RI42Q). *Neurology*, **52**, 1010–14.

Suarez, G. A., Fealey, R. D., Camilleri, M. *et al.* (1994). Idiopathic autonomic neuropathy: clinical, neurophysiologic, and follow-up studies on 27 patients. *Neurology*, **44**, 1675–82.

Suarez, J. I., Cohen, M. L., Larkin, J. *et al.* (1997). Acute intermittent porphyria: clinicopathologic correlation. *Neurology*, **48**, 1678–83.

Swanson, A. G., Buchan, G. C., and Alvord, E. C. (1965). Anatomic changes in congenital insensitivity to pain: absence of small primary sensory neurons in ganglia, roots and Lissauer's tract. *Arch. Neurol.*, **12**, 12–18.

Swift, T. R., Gross, J. A., Ward, L. C. *et al.* (1981). Peripheral neuropathy in epileptic patients. *Neurology*, **31**, 826–31.

Tatum, A. H. (1993). Experimental paraprotein neuropathy, demyelination by passive transfer of human IgM anti-myelin-associated glycoprotein. *Ann. Neurol.*, **33**, 502–6.

Teunissen, L. L., Notermans, N. C., Franssen, H. *et al.* (1997). Differences between hereditary motor and sensory neuropathy type 2 and chronic idiopathic axonal neuropathy. *Brain*, **120**, 955–62.

Thomas, P. K. and Ormerod, I. E. C. (1993). Hereditary neuralgic amyotrophy associated with a relapsing multifocal sensory neuropathy. *J. Neurol. Neurosurg. Psychiat.*, **56**, 107–9.

Thomas, P. K. and Walker, J. G. (1965). Xanthomatous neuropathy in primary biliary cirrhosis. *Brain*, **88**, 1079–88.

Thomas, P. K., Hollinrake, K., Lascelles, R. G. *et al.* (1971). The polyneuropathy of chronic renal failure. *Brain*, **94**, 761–80.

Thomas, P. K., Walker, R. W. H., Rudge, P. *et al.* (1987). Chronic demyelinating peripheral neuropathy associated with multifocal central nervous system demyelination. *Brain*, **110**, 53–76.

Thomas, P. K., Marques, W., Davis, M. B. *et al.* (1997). The phenotypic manifestations of chromosome 17p11.2 duplication. *Brain*, **120**, 465–78.

Timmerman, V., Nelis, E., Van Hul, W. *et al.* (1992). The peripheral myelin protein gene PMP-22 is contained within the Charcot–Marie–Tooth disease type 1A duplication. *Nature Genet.*, **1**, 171–5.

Traber, M. G., Sokol, R. J., Ringel, S. P. *et al.* (1987). Lack of tocopherol in peripheral nerves of vitamin E deficient patients with peripheral neuropathy. *N. Engl. J. Med.*, **317**, 262–5.

Traynor, A. E., Gertz, M. A., and Kyle, R. A. (1991). Cranial neuropathy associated with primary amyloidosis. *Ann. Neurol.*, **29**, 451–4.

Tyson, J., Ellis, D., Fairbrother, U. *et al.* (1997). Hereditary demyelinating neuropathy of infancy. A genetically complex syndrome. *Brain*, **120**, 47–63.

Umehara, F., Izumo, S., Arimura, K. *et al.* (1991). Polyneuropathy induced by *m*-tolyl methyl carbamate intoxication. *J. Neurol.*, **238**, 47–8.

Vallat, J. M., De Mascarel, H. A., Bordessoule, D. *et al.* (1995). Non-Hodgkin malignant lymphomas and peripheral neuropathies—13 cases. *Brain*, **118**, 1233–45.

Valli, G., Barbieri, S., Sergi, P. *et al.* (1984). Evidence of motor neuron involvement in chronic respiratory insufficiency. *J. Neurol. Neurosurg. Psychiat.*, **47**, 1117–21.

Van den Bent, M. J., de Bruijn, H. G., Bos, G. M. J. *et al.* (1999). Negative sural nerve biopsy in neurolymphomatosis. *J. Neurol.*, **246**, 1159–63.

Van den Berg, L. H., Kerkhoff, H., Oey, P. L. *et al.* (1995). Treatment of multifocal motor neuropathy with high dose intravenous immunoglobulins: a double blind, placebo controlled study. *J. Neurol. Neurosurg. Psychiat.*, **59**, 248–52.

Van den Berg, L. H., Franssen, H., and Wokke, J. H. J. (1998). The long-term effect of intravenous immunoglobulin treatment in multifocal motor neuropathy. *Brain*, **121**, 421–8.

Van den Berg-Vos, R. M., Van den Berg, L. H., Franssen, H. *et al.* (2000). Multifocal inflammatory demyelinating neuropathy. A distinct clinical entity? *Neurology*, **54**, 26–32.

Van der Meché, F. G. A. and van Doorn, P. A. (1997). The current place of high-dose immunoglobulins in the treatment of neuromuscular disorders. *Muscle Nerve*, **20**, 136–47.

Van der Meché, F. G. A., Schmitz, P. I. M. and the Dutch Guillain–Barré Study Group (1992). A randomized trial comparing intravenous immune globulin and plasma exchange in Guillain–Barré syndrome. *N. Engl. J. Med.*, **326**, 1123–9.

Van Dijk, G. W., Notermans, N. C., Franssen, H. *et al.* (1996). Response to intravenous immunoglobulin treatment in chronic inflammatory demyelinating polyneuropathy with only sensory symptoms. *J. Neurol.*, **243**, 318–22.

Van Geel, B. M., Koelman, J. M. T. M., Barth, P. G. *et al.* (1998). Peripheral nerve abnormalities in adrenomyeloneuropathy. *Neurology*, **46**, 112–18.

Van Hooren, G., Dehaene, I., Van Zandkycke, M. *et al.* (1990). Polyneuropathy in lithium intoxication. *Muscle Nerve*, **13**, 204–8.

Vasilescu, C. (1976). Sensory and motor conduction in chronic carbon disulphide poisoning. *Eur. Neurol.*, **14**, 447–57.

Vedanarayanan, V. V., Kandt, R. S., Lewis, D. V. *et al.* (1991). Chronic inflammatory demyelinating polyradiculopathy of childhood: treatment with high-dose intravenous immunoglobulin. *Neurology*, **41**, 828–30.

Visser, L. H., van der Meché, F. G. A., Van Doorn, P. A. *et al.* (1995). Guillain–Barré syndrome without sensory loss (acute motor neuropathy). *Brain*, **118**, 841–7.

Visser, L. H., van der Meché, F. G. A., Meulstff, J. *et al.* (1996). Cytomegalovirus infection and Guillain–Barré syndrome. *Neurology*, 47, 668–73.

Visser, L. H., Schmitz, P. I. M., Meulstff, J. *et al.* (1999). Prognostic factors of Guillain–Barré syndrome after intravenous immunoglobulin or plasma exchange. *Neurology*, 53, 598–604.

Vital, C., Pautrizel, B., and Lagueny, A. (1985). Hypermyélinisation dans un cas de neuropathie périphérique avec gammopathie monoclonale bénigne à IgM. *Rev. Neurol.*, 141, 729–34.

Vogel, P., Gabriel, M., and Dyck, P. J. (1985). Hereditary motor sensory neuropathy type II with neurofilament accumulation: new finding or new disorder? *Ann. Neurol.*, 17, 455–61.

Warner, L. E., Mancias, P., Butler, I. J. *et al.* (1998). Mutations in the early growth response 2 gene are associated with hereditary myelinopathies. *Nature Genet.*, 18, 382–4.

Watkins, P. J. (1990). Natural history of the diabetic neuropathies. *Quart. J. Med.*, 77, 1209–18.

Wees, S. J., Sunwood, L. N., and Oh, S. J. (1981). Sural nerve biopsy in systemic necrotising vasculitis. *Am. J. Med.*, 71, 525–32.

Weiss, G. B., Bajwa, Z. H., and Mehler, M. F. (1991). Co-occurrence of pseudotumour cerebri and Guillain–Barré syndrome in an adult. *Neurology*, 41, 603–4.

Wetterau, J. R., Aggerbeck, L. P., Bouma, M.-E. *et al.* (1992). Absence of microsomal triglyceride transfer protein in individuals with abetalipoproteinaemia. *Science*, 258, 999–1001.

Whisnant, J. P., Espinosa, R. E., Kierland, R. R. *et al.* (1963). Chloroquine neuromyopathy. *Proc. Mayo Clin.*, 38, 501–13.

Willison, H. J. (1994). Antiglycolipid antibodies in peripheral neuropathy: fact or fiction? *J. Neurol. Neurosurg. Psychiat.*, 57, 1303–7.

Willison, H. J., Paterson, G., Veitch, J. *et al.* (1993). Peripheral neuropathy associated with monoclonal IgM anti-Pr₂ cold agglutinins. *J. Neurol. Neurosurg. Psych.*, 56, 1178–83.

Windebank, A. J., Blexrud, M. D., Dyck, P. J. *et al.* (1990). The syndrome of acute sensory neuropathy. *Neurology*, 40, 584–91.

Winer, J. B. and Hughes, R. A. C. (1988). Identification of patients at risk of arrhythmia in Guillain–Barré syndrome. *Quart. J. Med.*, 68, 735–9.

Winer, J. B., Hughes, R. A. C., and Osmond, C. (1988a). A prospective study of acute clinical idiopathic neuropathy. I Clinical features and their prognostic value. *J. Neurol. Neurosurg. Psychiat.*, 51, 605–12.

Winer, J. B., Hughes, R. A. C., Anderson, M. J. *et al.* (1988b). A prospective study of acute idiopathic neuropathy. II Antecedent events. *J. Neurol. Neurosurg. Psychiat.*, 51, 613–18.

Wohrle, J. C., Szpengos, K., Steinke, W. *et al.* (1998). Alcohol-related acute axonal polyneuropathy. *Arch. Neurol.*, 55, 1329–34.

Wokke, J. H. J., Morris, J. H., and Donaghy, M. (1996). Lymphoma, paraproteinaemia and neuropathy. *J. Neurol. Neurosurg. Psychiat.*, 60, 684–9.

Wolfe, G. I., Baker, N. S., Amato, A. A. *et al.* (1999). Chronic cryptogenic sensory polyneuropathy. *Arch. Neurol.*, 56, 540–7.

Yamada, M., Tsukagoshi, H., and Hatakeyama, S. (1988). Skeletal muscle amyloid deposition in AL-(primary or myeloma associated), AA-(secondary), and prealbumin type amyloidosis. *J. Neurol. Sci.*, 85, 223–32.

Yee, W. C., Hahn, A. F., Hearn, S. A. *et al.* (1989). Neuropathy in IgM_λ paraproteinemia. Immunoreactivity in neural proteins and chondroitin sulfate. *Acta Neuropathol.*, 78, 57–64.

Yiannikas, C., McLeod, J. G., Pollard, J. D. *et al.* (1986). Peripheral neuropathy associated with mitochondrial myopathy. *Ann. Neurol.*, 20, 249–57.

Yuki, N., Sato, S., Tsuji, S. *et al.* (1993). Frequent presence of anti-GQ1B antibody in Fisher's syndrome. *Neurology*, 43, 414–17.

Zochodne, D. W. (1994). Autonomic involvement in Guillain–Barré syndrome. A review. *Muscle Nerve*, 17, 1145–55.

Zochodne, D. W., Bolton, C. F., Wells, G. A. *et al.* (1987). Critical illness polyneuropathy: a complication of sepsis and multiple organ failure. *Brain*, 110, 819–42.

Zuniga, G., Ropper, A. H., and Frank, J. (1991). Sarcoid peripheral neuropathy. *Neurology*, 41, 1558–61.

CHAPTER 13

Focal peripheral neuropathy

Michael Donaghy

13.1 Clinical diagnosis of focal neuropathy

13.1.1 Causes of focal neuropathy

Some causes of focal peripheral-nerve damage are self-evident, such as involvement at sites of trauma, tissue necrosis, infiltration by tumour, or damage by radiotherapy (Table 13.1). Focal compressive and entrapment neuropathies are particularly valuable to identify in civilian practice, since recovery may follow relief of the compression. Leprosy is a common global cause of focal neuropathy, which involves prominent loss of pain sensation with secondary acromutilation, and requires early antibiotic treatment. Mononeuritis multiplex due to vasculitis requires prompt diagnosis and immunosuppressive treatment to limit the severity and extent of peripheral-nerve damage. Various other medical conditions, both inherited and acquired, can present with focal neuropathy rather than polyneuropathy, the most common of which is diabetes mellitus. A purely motor focal presentation should raise the question of multifocal motor neuropathy with conduction block, which usually responds well to high-dose intravenous immunoglobulin infusions.

13.1.2 Differentiating root, plexus, and peripheral nerve lesions

A mononeuropathy is a lesion restricted to one single peripheral nerve, producing the characteristic motor sensory and reflex abnormalities distal to the site of the lesion. Multifocal neuropathy or mononeuritis multiplex are the terms used to describe the coexistence of two or more separate mono-

Table 13.1. Causes of focal peripheral neuropathy

Trauma (13.2.1)
Compression
   Entrapment (13.2.3)
   Nerve sheath tumours (13.5.1)
   Hereditary liability to pressure palsies (12.5)
   Mucopolysaccharidoses (12.8)
Infiltration
   Tumour (13.5.2)
   Leprosy (12.14.1)
   Sensory perineuritis (12.16.1)
   Sarcoidosis (12.17.7)
   Amyloidosis (12.9)
Ischaemic
   Vasculitis (12.15)
   Diabetes mellitus (12.17.1)
   Infarction (12.15.1)
   Irradiation (13.5.3)
Unknown mechanism
   Focal hypertrophic neuritis (13.6.6)
   Multifocal motor neuropathy (12.11.3)
   Tangier disease (12.8.7)
   Wartenberg's migrant sensory neuralgia (12.16.2)

neuropathies and these most usually occur in diabetes mellitus and vasculitis. When a patient harbours multiple mononeuropathies, the clinical picture may resemble a polyneuropathy, and the multifocal nature of the condition can be appreciated only from the history of separate onsets of symptoms in different peripheral-nerve territories, and by careful motor and sensory examination to reveal differing densities of clinical involvement in adjacent nerve territories.

Clinical features are crucial to the often difficult distinction between lesions of the roots, plexuses, and peripheral nerves. A lesion of the brachial or lumbosacral plexus is suggested by a pattern of muscle weakness, reflex loss, and sensory disturbance which is not attributable to a lesion of a single nerve root or a single peripheral nerve. Not surprisingly, many early plexus lesions are so anatomically restricted that they fail to satisfy this criterion. Furthermore, the plexus, roots, and peripheral nerves can all be involved simultaneously by pathological processes such as diabetes mellitus, vasculitis, or tumour infiltration. Familiarity with the skin sensory territories and patterns of muscular innervation are crucial to the distinction between root lesions and peripheral-nerve lesions (Fig. 13.1). Discrimination between plexus and multiple root lesions may be impossible on clinical grounds; however, the involvement of autonomic nerve fibres in plexus lesions tends to produce a warm, red, and dry hand or foot. Furthermore, sensory nerve action potentials are preserved in root lesions because the dorsal root ganglion or the peripheral branches of the sensory axons are not affected. Proximal limb muscle weakness tends to be a feature of lesions involving the plexus or roots, rather than of lesions restricted to peripheral nerves.

13.1.3 Double crush lesions

Electrophysiologically proven compression of the median nerve in the carpal tunnel, and of the ulnar nerve at the elbow, are often associated with coexisting radiculopathy due to cervical spondylosis. This led to the proposal that proximal axonal compression might impair the distal axon's ability to resist otherwise subclinical compressive lesions (Upton and McComas 1973). Thus a coexisting, but in itself subclinical, distal compression might become clinically obvious in the presence of a more proximal lesion. This notion of a double crush syndrome has gained popular acceptance despite a relative paucity of experimental support. However, in motor neuron disease, nerve conduction studies have shown that motor nerve fibres are not more vulnerable to focal compression at the elbow than are the healthy sensory nerve fibres (Chaudhry and Clawson 1997). A careful consideration of the various strands of evidence surrounding the double crush hypothesis has concluded that it rarely, if ever, significantly determines clinical symptoms and signs (Wilbourn and Gilliatt 1997). Of course, that does not exclude simple summation of the separate deficits caused by two clinically significant compressions of nerve fibres at two different levels, for instance a C6 radiculopathy combined with carpal tunnel syndrome. In such situations it can be difficult to

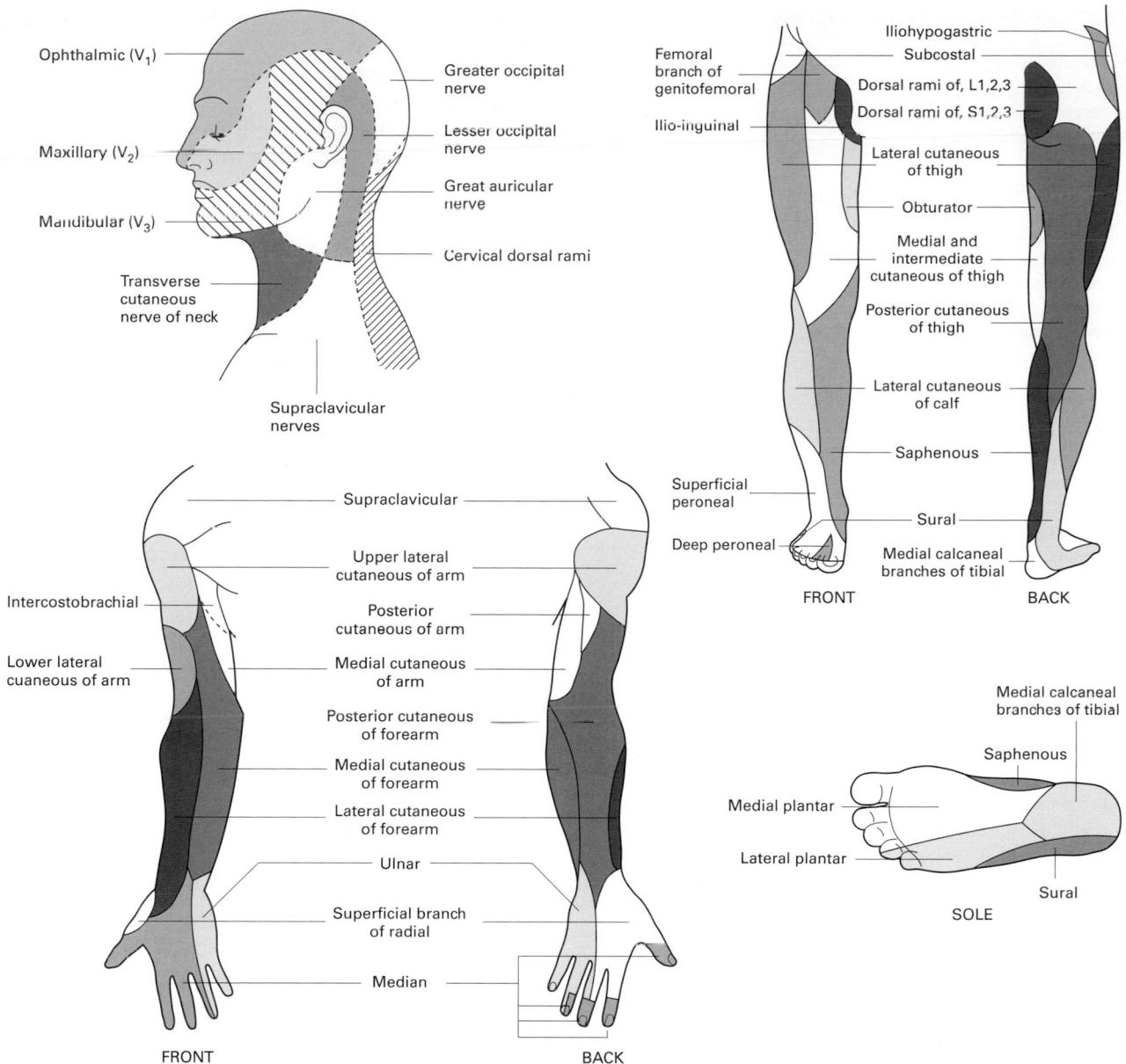

Fig. 13.1. Cutaneous territories supplied by individual peripheral nerves.

decide which of the two lesions is the major determinant of clinical symptoms and thereby merits treatment.

13.1.4 **Small hand muscle wasting**

Wasting and weakness of intrinsic hand muscles is a common differential diagnostic problem which always raises the question of focal neuropathy affecting the median or ulnar nerves, but includes a wide range of other disorders (Table 13.2). These muscles are innervated by the anterior horn cells of the first thoracic segment of the spinal cord, with an occasional minor contribution from the eighth cervical. The causes of wasting, therefore, include lesions of the lower motor neurons at any point between this spinal segment and the muscles, together with certain other conditions in which primary muscular

degeneration or secondary muscular wasting occurs. Electrophysiological assessment and, if necessary, magnetic resonance imaging of the cervical spinal cord and nerve roots, are of particular value in diagnosis.

Acute anterior horn cell lesions

Nowadays, acute anterior horn cell lesions are relatively rare. The most common causes are acute poliomyelitis and related viral infections. These are usually easily distinguished by the acute onset, the non-progressive nature of the subsequent weakness and wasting, and the absence of sensory loss. *Herpes zoster* is a rare cause, but here the pain, rash, and sensory loss are distinctive. Acute postinfective polyradiculopathy (the Guillain–Barré syndrome) usually affects proximal limb

Table 13.2. Causes of wasting of the small hand muscles

Mononeuropathy
    Median nerve (abductor pollicis brevis) (13.10.1)
    Ulnar nerve (dorsal interosseous) (13.10.3)
Polyneuropathy (Chapter 12)
Anterior horn cell diseases
    Amyotrophic lateral sclerosis (14.2)
    Poliomyelitis (14.5)
    Distal spinal muscular atrophy (14.3.4)
    Segmental spinal muscular atrophy (14.6)
Spinal-cord lesions
    Syringomyelia (20.6.2)
    Ischaemia (20.4.8)
    Spinal-cord tumour (20.5.8)
    Traumatic haematomyelia (6.3.2)
    Multiple sclerosis (29.4)
Spinal nerve root lesions
    Vertebral body collapse
    Infiltrating vertebral tumour
    Syphilitic meningomyelitis (34.17)
    Trauma (Klumpke paralysis) (13.6.2)
Central nervous system
    Parietal lobe lesions
    Foramen magnum lesions
Medial cord of brachial plexus
    Cervical rib (13.6.3)
    Irradiation plexopathy (13.5.3)
    Trauma (13.6.2)
Muscular dystrophy
    Distal myopathy (15.2.9)
    Myotonic dystrophy (15.3)
Trophic disorders
    Chronic arthritis
    Shoulder–hand syndrome
    Ischaemic contracture

muscles more severely than distal, at least at first, and like other forms of polyneuropathy (see below) it usually affects all four limbs. The acute motor axonal neuropathy variant of Guillain–Barré syndrome can produce small hand muscle weakness and wasting (Section 12.10). *Vascular lesions of the spinal cord* are a rare cause. Thrombosis of a branch of the anterior spinal artery can destroy anterior horn cells, but in such cases the corticospinal and spinothalamic tracts are usually damaged simultaneously. *Haematomyelia* or cord contusion following acute hyperextension injuries of the neck may also damage anterior horn cells in the cervical enlargement. Wasting is not usually confined to muscles innervated by the first thoracic segment and is generally associated with extensive sensory loss over the upper limbs and with involvement of long ascending and descending tracts of the cord.

Slow-onset anterior horn cell lesions

The most common chronic lesion is *amyotrophic lateral sclerosis*, which often begins with wasting of the small muscles in one or both hands. This condition is distinguished by its progressive course, the presence of fasciculation, and wasting of other muscle groups, the coexistence of corticospinal-tract degenera-

tion, and the absence of sensory loss. Inherited *spinal muscular atrophy* of the distal type can begin in the small muscles of the hands, and often in the feet as well. Segmental spinal muscular atrophies often remain restricted to one arm. In *syringomyelia* wasting of the hand muscles is often an early symptom. The diagnosis depends upon the characteristic associated analgesia and thermo-anaesthesia, trophic lesions, and the frequent involvement of the corticospinal tracts. In *intrinsic tumour of the spinal cord* the signs of a progressive focal lesion at the cervical enlargement are usually accompanied by pain and evidence of involvement of long ascending and descending tracts. The ventral roots are occasionally involved in localized *syphilitic meningomyelitis*, or in *arachnoiditis* in which the cord substance usually also suffers. Such ventral root lesions can be distinguished from a lesion of the anterior horn cells only when the dorsal roots are also involved, giving root pain and impairment of sensation over the affected segmental cutaneous areas.

Lesions of the spinal nerves

The spinal nerve is formed from a fusion of the ventral and dorsal roots. For example, a lesion of the first thoracic nerve causes pain and often sensory loss in a radicular distribution along the ulnar border of the forearm, in addition to wasting of the small muscles of the hand. Although any spinal nerve may be compressed by a vertebral lesion, this is rarely the case for the first thoracic nerve, since intervertebral disc disease or spondylosis are unusual at that level. Indeed, contrary to widespread misconception, wasting of small hand muscles due to a TI root lesion is exceptional, apart from occasions when presumed ischaemia in the first thoracic segment follows cord compression at a higher level. The first thoracic nerve can be compressed as a result of vertebral body collapse or extradural deposits due to malignancy. A traumatic lesion of the first thoracic spinal nerve is responsible for the *Dejerine–Klumpke type of birth palsy*. Lesions involving the first dorsal segment of the spinal cord, its ventral roots and spinal nerve, usually cause loss of the cervical sympathetic innervation, as its preganglionic fibres leave the cord at this level.

Lesions of the medial cord of the brachial plexus

Lesions of the medial cord of the plexus, for example the pressure of a *cervical rib*, cause wasting of some or all of the muscles supplied by the ulnar nerve, including those in the forearm, in addition to the small hand muscles supplied by the median. The weakness and wasting may be confined to the hand. The distribution of pain and sensory loss often involves the eighth cervical and first thoracic segmental areas, that is, roughly, the supply of the ulnar nerve, together with part of the ulnar border of the forearm and arm.

Lesions of the median or ulnar nerves, and polyneuropathy

All lesions situated between the anterior horn cells of the first thoracic segment and the medial cord of the brachial plexus cause wasting of the small hand muscles. Distally to the medial cord of the plexus the innervation of these muscles is divided between the median and ulnar nerves. Lesions of these nerves are distinguished by the characteristic distribution of muscular wasting and sensory loss (Sections 13.10.1 and 13.10.3). Apart from localized lesions of these nerves, wasting in the hand may occur in various forms of *polyneuropathy*, in which a glove pattern of sensory loss is usually present with similar clinical features in the legs.

Central nervous system lesions

Small hand muscle wasting may occur in atrophy of the cervical spinal cord in advanced multiple sclerosis, but the underlying diagnosis will be obvious. Wasting of the contralateral body musculature, often starting in the thenar and hypothenar eminences, is a well-recognized, although rare, occurrence in parietal lobe lesions (Critchley 1953). Compression of the spinal cord above C4, or in the region of the foramen magnum occasionally leads to hand muscle wasting, possibly secondarily to vascular involvement (Symonds and Meadows 1937).

Muscular dystrophy

Wasting of the small hand muscles is found in some forms of *muscular dystrophy*, especially the *distal* type of *myopathy*. Less often it occurs in *myotonic dystrophy*, in which muscles of the forearm are wasted but not so much those of the hands. The diagnosis depends upon the age of onset, the symmetrical character, distribution, and progressive course of the wasting. Fasciculation, sensory loss, or signs of involvement of the central nervous system will be absent. The familial nature of the disorder and the electrophysiological findings provide additional evidence for the muscular dystrophy.

Trophic disorders

Muscular wasting secondary to disuse in *arthritis* of the joints of the hand must not be overlooked. It is easily recognized on account of pain, swelling, and bony changes in the joints, and particularly affects the dorsal interosseous muscles in rheumatoid arthritis. In the so-called *shoulder–hand syndrome*, or *algodystrophy*, pericapsulitis of the shoulder joint is initially associated with painful swelling of the hand, with subsequent occurrence of atrophy of the small hand muscles and demineralization of bones (Sudeck's atrophy). *Ischaemic contracture* caused by major arterial blockage, for instance by fractures in the region of the elbow, leads to paralysis, wasting, and contracture of the muscles of the forearm and hand, with or without sensory loss.

13.2 Traumatic, compressive, and ischaemic mononeuropathy

13.2.1 Trauma

Traumatic nerve injury can produce differential damage to the various elements of a peripheral nerve. These have been classified in a manner that allows some prediction of possible recovery (Seddon 1944). *Neurotmesis* (Section 13.2.4) is complete anatomical division of the axons and connective tissue of a nerve; it includes complete transection. *Axonotmesis* (Section 13.2.5) refers to loss of continuity of the axons without disruption of their connective tissue sheath; Wallerian degeneration of the distal axon occurs over 3–5 days, followed by axonal regeneration from the proximal stump at the rate of approximately 1 mm/day. *Neurapraxia* (Section 13.2.6) is a segmental block of conduction without axonal disruption; this usually involves paranodal or segmental demyelination, or mechanical damage to the myelin sheath, and conduction is restored following myelin repair.

13.2.2 Ischaemia

Nerve ischaemia and infarction due to narrowing or occlusion of vasa nervorum accounts for isolated cranial nerve lesions (usually of a third or sixth nerve) in diabetes, and for mononeuritis multiplex or more diffuse polyneuropathy in diabetes and vasculitis. Ischaemia of the lumbosacral plexus has also been described following inadvertent intravascular injection of vasotoxic drugs into the buttock (Stöhr *et al.* 1980). Ischaemic neuropathy is an important complication of embolic peripheral vascular disease or of vascular surgery on limb arteries (Wilbourn *et al.* 1983). The common peroneal nerve is especially vulnerable. Compression of a nerve for up to 20–30 minutes while unconscious or immobile, or tourniquet application above systolic pressure, produce paralysis and tingling which are immediately reversed by restoring nerve perfusion. More prolonged compression causes disruption of the myelin sheath by a combination of mechanical and ischaemic factors, and ultimately causes disruption of axons.

Ischaemic lesions involving both nerves and muscles may occur as a result of arterial occlusion or injury in closed limb fractures. An example is *Volkmann's ischaemic paralysis* of the arm and hand. Within a few hours of injury, painful sensory disturbance, paralysis, swelling, and cyanosis develop in the limb. Eventual fibrosis of muscles leaves the limb useless and neuropathic pain may ensue. The *anterior tibial syndrome* is a form of ischaemic paralysis of the anterior tibial muscles occurring after unaccustomed exertion (see Section 15.11.6). The muscles swell within their tight fascial compartment and may undergo partial or complete infarction. Early surgical decompression must be considered in both conditions to prevent permanent tissue damage, including infarction of the nerve.

13.2.3 Compression

Repeated or prolonged compression of a nerve causes a combination of ischaemia and mechanical deformation of the myelin sheath with local oedema (Rudge *et al.* 1974). Initially this produces a neurapraxia subsequently proceeding to axonotmesis. If the pressure is not relieved, perineurial fibrosis eventually develops and prevents regeneration. This is the sequence whereby lesions evolve in the neuropathies caused by herniated intervertebral disc, narrowed intervertebral foramen, cervical rib, median nerve compression in the carpal tunnel, ulnar nerve compression at the elbow, meralgia paraesthetica, and other so-called entrapment neuropathies.

13.2.4 Neurotmesis

Neurotmesis occurs as a result of open wounds, direct blunt injuries, severe traction upon a nerve during displaced fractures, and other forms of disruptive local damage such as misplaced injections. Retrograde degeneration occurs in the proximal stump for 2 or 3 cm and the severed distal axonal segment undergoes Wallerian degeneration over 3–5 days. Subsequently, sprouting occurs from axons of the proximal stump. If damage to the connective tissue of the nerve is extensive, axonal regeneration towards the previous target may prove impossible, resulting in a neuroma formed on the proximal stump composed of nerve fibres and scar tissue. Complete division of a mixed peripheral nerve causes motor, sensory, vasomotor, sudomotor, and trophic manifestations corresponding anatomically to the territory supplied by the divided nerve.

Motor symptoms

Interruption of a nerve denervates its muscles, causing flaccid paralysis, wasting developing after 2 weeks, and loss of the tendon reflex. Loss of muscle power in the affected nerve's territory may be compensated by trick movements from the muscles innervated by an intact neighbouring nerve. Electromyography helps identify the denervated muscles from about 4 days after the injury. Nerve conduction in the nerve distal to the lesion slows soon after injury and is lost completely by 3–5 days.

Sensation

Division of a nerve causes complete loss of skin sensation only over the area exclusively supplied by the nerve, the *autonomous zone*. This is surrounded by an *intermediate zone*, which is the area of the nerve's skin territory overlapped by the supply of adjacent nerves. The autonomous and intermediate zones together constitute the *maximal zone*, which is the full extent of the nerve's distribution. The cutaneous area over which light touch appreciation is lost is usually larger than that over which pinprick is lost. The appreciation and localization of pressure, of the pain induced by deep pressure, and the recognition of posture and passive movements at the joints, may be impaired as a result of nerve division. However, these lost sensations are generally confined to a less extensive area than that which is anaesthetic to light touch.

Trophic change

Vasomotor and trophic disturbances which follow destruction of a motor or a mixed nerve are probably due, at least in part, to the interruption of efferent sympathetic fibres concerned in vasoconstriction. Such changes are most marked after injuries of the median, ulnar, and sciatic nerves. After complete division the analgesic area of skin becomes warm and dry. Later, this skin becomes scaly and inelastic owing to retarded desquamation. The limb becomes oedematous when dependent. The analgesic area is liable to suffer injury, and heals slowly after damage, so that ulcers may develop. Growth of the nails and hair is usually slowed, although hypertrichosis occasionally occurs. Adhesions between tendons and their sheaths, and fibrous changes in the muscles and joints eventually set in, but can be offset by repeated passive movements of the joints from early on. Pericapsulitis of the shoulder joint, or 'frozen shoulder', can be very difficult to prevent.

13.2.5 Axonotmesis

This is the type of lesion produced experimentally by crushing a peripheral nerve with forceps, severing all or most of the axons but leaving intact the connective tissue sheath of the nerve. It may result from advanced compression by entrapment, direct blunt injuries such as fractures, dislocations, and traction. Wallerian degeneration occurs after 3 to 5 days in the axon distal to the injury. In acute cases axonal regeneration occurs at a rate of approximately 1 mm/day. A strongly positive Tinel sign over the lesion soon after injury, consisting of paraesthesiae evoked by percussing the nerve, indicates severance of axons, rather than neurapraxia. This positive Tinel sign will move peripherally along the nerve as axons regenerate distally, either through the intact nerve connective tissues in axonotmesis, or after successful nerve suture. Functional recovery is more rapid, complete, and accurate after axonotmesis than after suture repair of a complete division. The early clinical and electrophysiological effects are the same as those of neurotmesis.

13.2.6 Neurapraxia

Neurapraxia is a focal conduction block of intact axons produced by segmental myelin damage. Although nerve function is temporarily impaired or lost, recovery occurs too quickly to be explained by axonal regeneration. Neurapraxic lesions occur in various forms of nerve entrapment, compression, or traction, provided the axons are not actually severed. Mechanical damage to the myelin sheath, which may simply consist of paranodal demyelination, seems to be the most important pathophysiological mechanism (Dawson *et al.* 1999). Although local ischaemia may play a role, it tends to produce axonal degeneration rather than demyelination. The following clinical features are typical of a neurapraxia:

(1) the loss of function is predominantly motor;

(2) there is little wasting, and the EMG shows a reduced or absent interference pattern;

(3) sensory symptoms of numbness, tingling, or burning are common;

(4) sensory loss is often minimal, particularly for modalities transmitted by unmyelinated fibres such as pain, temperature sensations and touch. By contrast, loss of position

and vibration sensations transmitted by myelinated fibres are common;

(5) loss of sweating is unusual;

(6) nerve conduction distal to the lesion is preserved; an observation that rules out axonal degeneration if performed 7 or more days after an acute lesion.

Recovery is fairly rapid, usually beginning after a few days or weeks, and becoming complete within 9–12 weeks (Shyu *et al.* 1993). Occasionally, complete restoration of function may be delayed until 6 months. The recovery progresses irregularly and follows no anatomical order, but is always complete as long as the lesion was purely neurapraxic.

13.3 **Surgical treatment**

The techniques of peripheral-nerve surgery do not fall within the scope of this book, but it is important for neurologists to be aware of the general indications for surgical treatment and its potential. The purpose of surgical intervention consists of one or more of the following (Birch *et al.* 1998). First, to visualize whether a nerve has actually been severed or ruptured; this is most accurately determined within the first 3 days after injury. Secondly, to restore continuity of a severed or ruptured nerve. Thirdly, to remove anything compressing or distorting a nerve, such as bone fragments or sutures.

Peripheral-nerve repair aims to approximate the severed ends so as to allow topographically accurate and unimpeded axonal regeneration. Thus scarring, contamination, infection, haematoma, or excessive instability of the adjacent skeleton should be treated before secondary suture of a nerve is undertaken 3–4 weeks later. Primary repair is suitable for nerves which have been cleanly lacerated by sharp items, such as glass; this accounts for the majority of peacetime injuries. Direct surgical repair may restore the continuity of the epineurium with sutures, a suitable method for small nerves, such as digital nerves, with little non-neural tissue. Alternatively, it may use the operating microscope to restore the continuity of groups of fascicles separately, which is more suitable for large mixed motor and sensory nerves, particularly for partial injuries (Urbaniak 1990).

After closed injuries with fractures, it can be difficult to tell whether the underlying nerve lesion is a neurotmesis, with no potential for regeneration, or an axonotmesis, which will recover. Under these circumstances enough time should be allowed to permit regenerating nerve fibres to reach the most proximal muscle supplied by the nerve, calculating the rate of regeneration at 1 mm/day and allowing a slight margin. After this time has elapsed, if there is no recovery of function in that muscle, consideration should be given to exploring the nerve. However, it is unlikely that motor recovery will occur in adults if the operation is delayed for more than a year. Apart from surgical technique, the age of the patient and the site of the nerve injury are the most important determinants of outcome.

Children may regain normal motor and sensory functions; the elderly rarely do so. Recovery often occurs after such repairs at distal sites, such as the ulnar nerve at the wrist, but is rare after repair to the brachial plexus.

For many years nerve grafting has been used to bridge large gaps in peripheral nerves. Grafting is of use when a segment of nerve has been lost and excessive tension would result from direct apposition of the cut ends. Autologous grafting material is obtained by sacrifice of nerves elsewhere, such as the sural nerve (Narakas 1991).

There are no rigorously established rules governing whether to operate on a peripheral nerve. Indications that commonly arise include the following (Birch *et al.* 1998):

(1) severe paralysis after a wound over the course of a nerve, or after a closed injury associated with tissue damage;

(2) a nerve lesion associated with a bone fracture which required early internal fixation;

(3) paralysis after closed traction injury of the brachial plexus;

(4) no beginnings of recovery from a neurapraxic lesion at 6 weeks, or from an axonotmesis after the calculated interval has elapsed; and

(5) in entrapment neuropathy.

Additionally, surgical inspection of the nerve can be considered when there is persistent pain long after injury or if there is an associated arterial lesion.

13.4 **Causalgia and reflex sympathetic dystrophy**

Causalgia and *reflex sympathetic dystrophy* are the terms used traditionally to describe the chronic burning pain set off by trauma to a limb, coupled with various autonomic and trophic changes in the latter case. The definition and use of these terms has been controversial. Recently there has been a proposal to subsume both entities within the umbrella term of 'complex regional pain syndrome' (CRPS) with the subclassification of CRPS type I being broadly equivalent to reflex sympathetic dystrophy and CRPS type II corresponding to causalgia (Stanton-Hicks *et al.* 1995). Criticisms of the traditional terminology include doubts about whether the syndrome should be regarded as a reflex response to an insult, uncertainty about the pathophysiological role of the sympathetic nervous system, and the varying occurrence and severity of dystrophy. Although the following account uses the familiar headings of causalgia and reflex sympathetic dystrophy, the reader should be aware of these recent proposals for reclassification.

13.4.1 **Causalgia**

The term 'causalgia' describes the enduring burning pain which sometimes follows nerve injury. This continuous pain is often accompanied by *hyperalgesia* (exaggerated sensitivity to painful stimuli) and *dysaesthesia* (pain after light touch of the abnormal area). Because it may be accompanied by increased sweating, skin reddening, or reduced skin temperature, some have defined causalgia more broadly as 'a syndrome of sustained burning pain after a traumatic nerve lesion combined with vasomotor and sudomotor dysfunction and later trophic changes'. However, Schott (1986) points out that this wider definition of causalgia merely serves to amalgamate the condition with reflex sympathetic dystrophy and algodystrophy, and excludes those frequent patients with burning pain yet little or no vasomotor or sudomotor disturbance. Pain indistinguishable from causalgia may also occur in polyneuropathy, most notably in diabetes mellitus. In what follows, the term causalgia simply refers to neuropathic burning pain following a definable peripheral nerve lesion without necessarily being accompanied by skin changes.

Symptoms

Causalgia is a distressing symptom, usually associated with incomplete lesions of a peripheral nerve. Though it may follow a lesion of any nerve, it is most often seen when the inner cord of the brachial plexus or the median or sciatic nerves are damaged. It is an intense and persistent burning pain, subject to paroxysmal exacerbations which may be elicited both by physical contact and by emotional reactions. The pain usually begins a week or two after the injury. Tenderness may be evoked either by superficial or by deep stimuli, less frequently by the latter. Superficial tenderness usually extends over the whole cutaneous area innervated by the nerve. The affected nerve may be tender throughout the whole length of the limb, even as high as the brachial plexus. There may be little or no associated muscular paralysis. Owing to the extreme tenderness of the affected part, the patient makes every effort to protect the limb from all forms of external stimulation. This can make it impossible to carry out a rigorous neurological examination of the limb. Similar symptoms may be referred to the stump following amputation.

Pathophysiology

Many attempts have been made to explain causalgia without a convincing mechanism appearing. One possible explanation has been elaborated on the basis of the 'gate control theory' of sensation (Melzack and Wall 1965). If large-diameter sensory fibres are selectively damaged by injury, the 'gate' mechanism would be biased in favour of small-fibre influences so that all somatic input from the affected area of skin produces hyperalgesia. This theory seems unlikely given that causalgia tends to occur in polyneuropathies selectively affecting small fibres, such as diabetes. A second notion proposes that impulses travel peripherally from the site of injury in the nerve and alter the vasomotor state of the skin, thereby exciting afferent discharges in pain fibres. A third view proposes that efferent sympathetic fibres form artificial synapses which activate sensory afferent fibres at the level of the nerve injury. Schott (1986) questioned the view that causalgia results from involvement of peripheral sympathetic nerve fibres. He drew attention to the occurrence

of causalgia in diseases confined to the central nervous system and in phantom limb states and proposed an important role for central nervous system mechanisms in causalgia. Various pathogenic mechanisms might be responsible in different clinical situations. It remains unclear whether the pathogenesis of pain in pure causalgia is the same as in the similar pain of reflex sympathetic dystrophy.

Treatment

Initially attempts should be made to suppress causalgic pain using carbamazepine or amitriptyline, followed by other anticonvulsant drugs if these measures are ineffective. Mexiletine, a structural analogue of lignocaine, is reputedly effective (Chabal *et al.* 1992). If oral medications proved ineffective, the traditional treatment was sympathetic block with local anaesthetic, followed by sympathectomy if the pain was relieved. But this is not often effective and may generate a separate post-sympathectomy pain (Schott 1998). Surgical excision of the affected segment of nerve followed by resuturing and/or procaine block of somatic afferents, and even cordotomy, are generally ineffective. Seven patients have been reported who suffered chronic pain after partial peripheral-nerve lesions (with causalgia representing the most extreme variety) in whom neurolysis, local anaesthesia, sympathetic block, guanethidine, percutaneous electrical stimulation, and powerful analgesics had all failed to give relief; all underwent resection of the affected nerve segment followed by grafting, and in all pain of similar intensity, character, and distribution recurred (Noordenbos and Wall 1981). Consequently it was suggested that peripheral nerve damage may produce pathophysiological changes in the central nervous system which are not reversed by treatment directed at the site of the original injury. On the other hand, guanethidine block of one limb, or sympathetic chain block, have been shown to be effective in some patients with causalgia due to central nervous system lesions (Loh *et al.* 1981). However, no reliable criteria allow identification of that minority of patients whose pain might benefit from interrupting the sympathetic nervous system. There are some cases in which repetitive percutaneous electrical stimulation of large sensory fibres does give relief, as does sympathectomy. Overall, it must be acknowledged that no single form of treatment is invariably successful, and that some unfortunate patients receive little or no benefit from any of the various treatments that are tried.

Symptoms resembling those of causalgia sometimes develop in amputation stumps, associated with painful neuromata on the distal ends of severed nerves. In such cases, the pain can be reproduced by pressure upon the neuroma. Excision of this neuroma or repeated injection of local anaesthetic or phenol may give relief, although this is unpredictable.

13.4.2 Reflex sympathetic dystrophy

Reflex sympathetic dystrophy (algodystrophy, shoulder–hand syndrome, Sudek's atrophy) can arise as a complication of a wide range of painful conditions affecting the limbs: soft-tissue

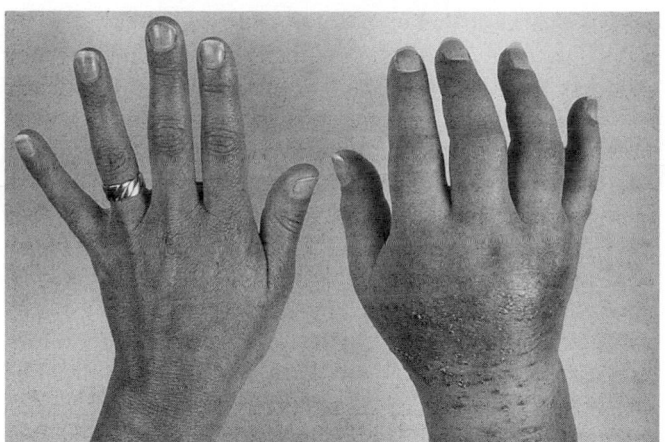

Fig. 13.2. Reflex sympathetic dystrophy affecting the right hand, showing swelling, discolouration, and skin changes. (Courtesy of Dr. C. Glynn.)

injuries, trauma, surgery, arthritis, plexopathy, radiculopathy, tenosynovitis, as well as after myocardial infarction or stroke and other central nervous system disease. Symptoms commence from hours to weeks after injury. In addition to diffuse causalgic pain, which is not limited to the territory of any particular nerve, the early symptoms consist of oedema (Fig. 13.2), altered skin temperature, and increased nail and hair growth. Subsequently, dystrophic changes occur: indurated, cool, sweaty skin, hair loss, and brittle deformities of nails (Sudek's atrophy). Radiography reveals diffuse osteoporosis of the affected limb. Radio-isotope bone scans may show increased periarticular uptake in the affected limb prior to changes seen on radiograms. Eventually, permanent disability and deformity result from contractures of fascia and tendons and ankylosis of joints (Schwartzman and McLellan 1987). The shoulder–hand syndrome is a variant of reflex sympathetic dystrophy accompanied by 'frozen shoulder' which may follow myocardial infarction, cerebrovascular accident, cervical radiculopathy, or primary pericapsulitis of the shoulder joint. A fixed dystonia may become associated with reflex sympathetic dystrophy after a peripheral injury, and this can spread from its initial site to become more generalized (Bhatia *et al.* 1993). Some patients with reflex sympathetic dystrophy recover spontaneously within weeks or months. However, many other instances last for years with chronic invalidism, psychiatric features, or drug addiction. Although these seem likely to be a direct emotional consequence of this chronic state of pain, they can lead physicians to believe that the patient is displaying a primarily psychogenic condition.

The trigger for the development of reflex sympathetic dystrophy is not known. In many it is likely that damage to peripheral-nerve tissue is responsible, including the very distal axonal twigs in soft tissues, but occasional cases are clearly due to central nervous system lesions. Pathological studies of peripheral nerve and muscle in amputation specimens from patients with reflex sympathetic dystrophy have shown abnormalities of unmyelinated nerve fibres with normal myelinated and efferent nerve fibres, and non-specific changes in muscle fibres (van der

Laan *et al.* 1998). Demonstrable autonomic abnormalities in affected limbs are almost universal, affecting resting sweat output, skin temperature, and the sudomotor axon reflex test (Chelimsky *et al.* 1995). Detailed study of a patient with complete loss of skin sympathetic vasoconstriction in early reflex sympathetic dystrophy, which recovered fully, suggested that an underlying defect in central sympathetic control was responsible (Wasner *et al.* 1999). Overall, the evidence points to reduced, rather than augmented, sympathetic efferent activity in reflex sympathetic dystrophy. This has implications for understanding the frequent ineffectiveness of therapeutic approaches based upon interrupting sympathetic outflow, which have been fashionable until recently. Procedures such as destructive sympathectomy and local anaesthetic or regional guanethidine infusion sympathetic blockade provide no lasting benefit for the majority, and the more permanent procedures can themselves generate pain states (Schott 1998). This contrasts with the frequent effectiveness of such measures to block visceral nerves in malignant diseases causing pain states. A reliably effective treatment for reflex sympathetic dystrophy remains to be developed, and current practice centres around treating pain by the methods outlined for causalgia (Section 13.4.1) and using physiotherapy to minimize joint contractures.

13.5 Peripheral nerve tumours and irradiation neuropathy

13.5.1 Primary tumours

Single neurofibromas and schwannomas may arise from nerve roots, from the brachial or lumbosacral plexuses, or from peripheral nerves. Multiple neurofibromas occur in von Recklinghausen's disease, the peripheral type of neurofibromatosis (type 1) (Section 19.2). These tumours often produce no neurological deficit, merely being discovered on inspection or palpation (Fig. 13.3). When they develop in restricted spaces, such as intervertebral exit foramina, they cause progressive neurological dysfunction due to nerve compression. Nerve-sheath tumours hidden within the pelvis may attain an enormous size before detection; CT or MR imaging usually reveals them before palpation. Often, nerve-sheath tumours may be removed surgically with little or no increase in the pre-existing nerve damage. Occasionally focal peripheral-nerve lesions are encountered in patients with neurofibromatosis type 2 (the central form). In such patients no responsible neurofibroma is uncovered despite extensive MRI imaging of the relevant nerve, plexus, and roots, and the causative pathology is not known (Trivedi *et al.* 2000).

Occasionally nerve-sheath tumours undergo malignant transformation, most commonly to neurofibrosarcoma. Such transformation produces a painfully enlarging tumour mass with dysfunction of the affected nerve. Malignant nerve-sheath tumours can follow 2–30 years after therapeutic irradiation of the site, particularly in patients with a personal or family history of neurofibromatosis (Foley *et al.* 1980). Malig-

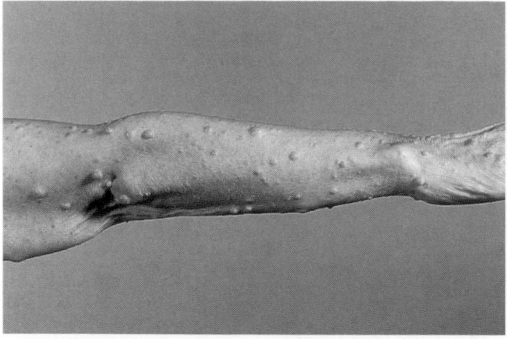

(a)

nant nerve-sheath tumours have a poor prognosis even with aggressive treatment using chemotherapy and radiotherapy.

Rarely, tumours arise from the neural elements themselves: neuroblastomas, ganglioneuroblastomas, and ganglioneurofibromas. Other rare tumours include the paraganglioma or chromaffinoma (which usually grows from the carotid body, glomus jugulare, or the adrenal or retroperitoneal tissues) and the rare granular-cell tumour (usually solitary but rarely multifocal and occasionally malignant) which can arise from the perineurium and may be derived from Schwann cells. Perineuroma, which causes a localized hypertrophic mononeuropathy, is a rare benign peripheral-nerve tumour of perineurial cell origin (Bilbao *et al.* 1984).

Traumatic neuromas, or reactive pseudotumours, can cause pain. They can be excised with variable benefit to the patient. Morton's neuroma of the interdigital nerve of the foot is a distinctive example (Section 13.11.2).

13.5.2 Secondary tumour invading nerves or plexuses

Malignant tumours of non-neural tissue may invade peripheral nerves directly, causing profound pain and loss of neurological function. This occurs commonly in the brachial or lumbosacral plexus due to metastases or by direct extension of tumours which have arisen in nearby structures. Multifocal neuropathy occasionally occurs as a result of direct infiltration of nerves by large cell lymphoma, which can be of the angiotrophic type (Krendel *et al.* 1991; Levin and Lutz 1996). The clinical course of this lymphomatous neuropathy can be subacute with increasingly widespread nerve involvement, so that Guillain–Barré syndrome or a paraneoplastic neuropathy are suspected unless an affected nerve is biopsied. Valuable improvement may follow chemotherapy.

Malignant infiltration of the *brachial plexus* usually results from carcinoma of the breast or bronchus, or malignant lymphoma (Fig. 13.4). Progressive sensorimotor dysfunction

(b)

Fig. 13.3. (a) Multiple neurofibromas on the arm of a patient with no neurological abnormalities. (b) MRI of ulnar nerve neurofibroma (arrowed) 10 cm above elbow: T1 weighted (top), T1 + Gd (middle), and STIR (bottom) sequences.

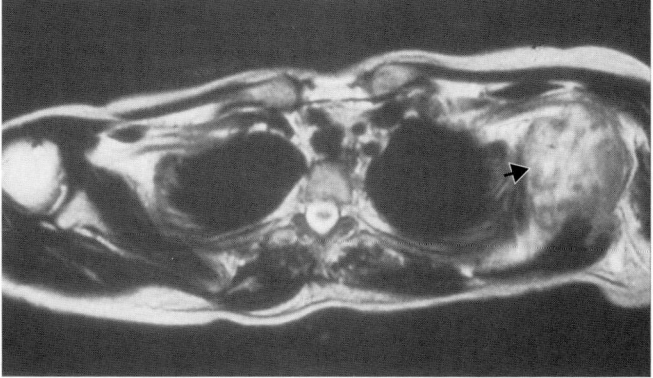

Fig. 13.4. MRI showing a non-Hodgkin's lymphoma in the peripheral portion of the brachial plexus adjacent to the shoulder joint (arrowed) (courtesy of Dr N. Moore).

develops in one arm; over 80 per cent of patients experience severe pain. Tumour infiltration may be palpable in the supraclavicular or axillary regions; and over 50 per cent of patients exhibit Horner's syndrome (Harper *et al.* 1989). Pancoast's tumour refers to infiltration of the lower brachial plexus and the lower cervical sympathetic chain by invasive carcinoma of the apex of the lung. If no tumour is palpable in a patient with painful plexopathy, CT or MRI will reveal the infiltrating tumour in most patients (Thyagarajan *et al.* 1995). Otherwise, diagnostic surgical exploration of the supraclavicular fossa may be required.

Malignant tumour infiltration of the *lumbosacral plexus* commonly results from direct spread from carcinoma of the colon, rectum, uterus, prostate, or ovary, and less frequently by metastatic spread from other tumours. Persistent severe unilateral local or radicular pain is followed by a predominantly proximal motor disturbance progressively worsening over weeks or months. Pelvic CT is abnormal in the majority at initial presentation (Thomas *et al.* 1985). The mode of therapy for tumours invading nerve plexuses is determined by the known responsiveness of the tumour type in question. Pain relief may be achieved by local radiotherapy. The prognosis is poor, with over 80 per cent of patients dying within a year of diagnosis.

13.5.3 Irradiation plexopathy

Brachial plexopathy typically presents more than 6 months after supraclavicular irradiation treatment for breast cancer (Harper *et al.* 1989). Lumbosacral plexopathy presents more than 1 year after external or internal cavity irradiation of the pelvis for lymphoreticular, testicular, uterine, or ovarian malignancies. The threshold radiation dosages have not been clearly established. Slowly progressive arm or leg weakness develops, sometimes bilaterally, and there is relatively little pain compared to that experienced with tumour infiltration. In lumbosacral plexopathy, pelvic CT or MRI has enormously simplified the differential diagnosis between tumour infiltration and radiation-induced plexopathy (Thomas *et al.* 1985). Electromyography of weakened muscles shows low-frequency myokymic discharges in roughly half of patients with irradiation plexopathy. The differential diagnosis between radiation and tumour plexopathy is based on the features given in Table 13.3.

Table 13.3. Differential diagnosis between radiation and tumour plexopathy

	Radiation plexopathy	Tumour plexopathy
Initial symptom	Weakness	Pain
Distribution	Often bilateral	Unilateral
Site of weakness	Distal	Proximal
CT or MRI	Normal	Tumour mass
Myokymic discharges	50%	No

13.6 Brachial plexus lesions

13.6.1 Anatomy

The brachial plexus (Figs 13.5, 13.6) is formed from the anterior primary divisions of the fifth, sixth, seventh, and eighth cervical (C5–C8) and the first thoracic (T1) spinal nerves. It sometimes receives a contribution from the fourth cervical (C4) or the second thoracic nerve (T2). Variations in the composition of the plexus are not uncommon. In the so-called *prefixed* type there is a contribution from C4; C5 is large and there may be no branch from T2. In the *postfixed* type there may be no branch from C4, and that from C5 is comparatively small, whereas the T2 contribution is quite substantial. The spinal segmental representation of muscles may be slightly higher or lower than normal, according to whether the plexus is prefixed or postfixed.

The contributions to the plexus from the anterior primary divisions soon divide into anterior and posterior trunks, and from these its three cords are formed as shown diagrammatically in Fig. 13.5:

◆ *The lateral cord* is formed by a union of anterior trunks of the C5, C6, and C7 nerves. From it arise the lateral pectoral and musculocutaneous nerves and the lateral head of the median nerve.

◆ *The medial or inner cord* is formed by a combination of the anterior trunk of C8 with the contribution of the T1 to the plexus. It gives origin to the medial head of the median nerve, the ulnar nerve, the medial cutaneous nerves of the arm and forearm, and the medial pectoral nerve.

◆ *The posterior cord* is formed by the union of the posterior trunks from the C5, C6, C7, C8, and sometimes the T1 nerves. It gives rise to the axillary and radial nerves, the two subscapular nerves, and the nerve to teres major.

Some proximal muscles are innervated by nerves which leave the plexus before the formation of the three cords. The most important nerves are:

◆ *The dorsal scapular nerve* (C5) supplies the levator scapulae and rhomboid muscles.

◆ *The long (or posterior) thoracic nerve* (C5, C6, C7) supplies the serratus anterior muscle.

◆ *The suprascapular nerve* (C5, C6) supplies the supraspinatus and infraspinatus muscles.

The brachial plexus is vulnerable to damage at many sites from many causes. Knowledge of its anatomical relationships is crucial to understanding these (Fig. 13.6). One or more spinal nerves may be involved by a lesion of the cervical spine, including congenital abnormality such as fusion of vertebrae in the Klippel–Feil syndrome, fracture dislocations, prolapsed intervertebral disc, spondylosis, malignant deposits, neurofibromas, and occasionally tuberculous, syphilitic, or fungal infection.

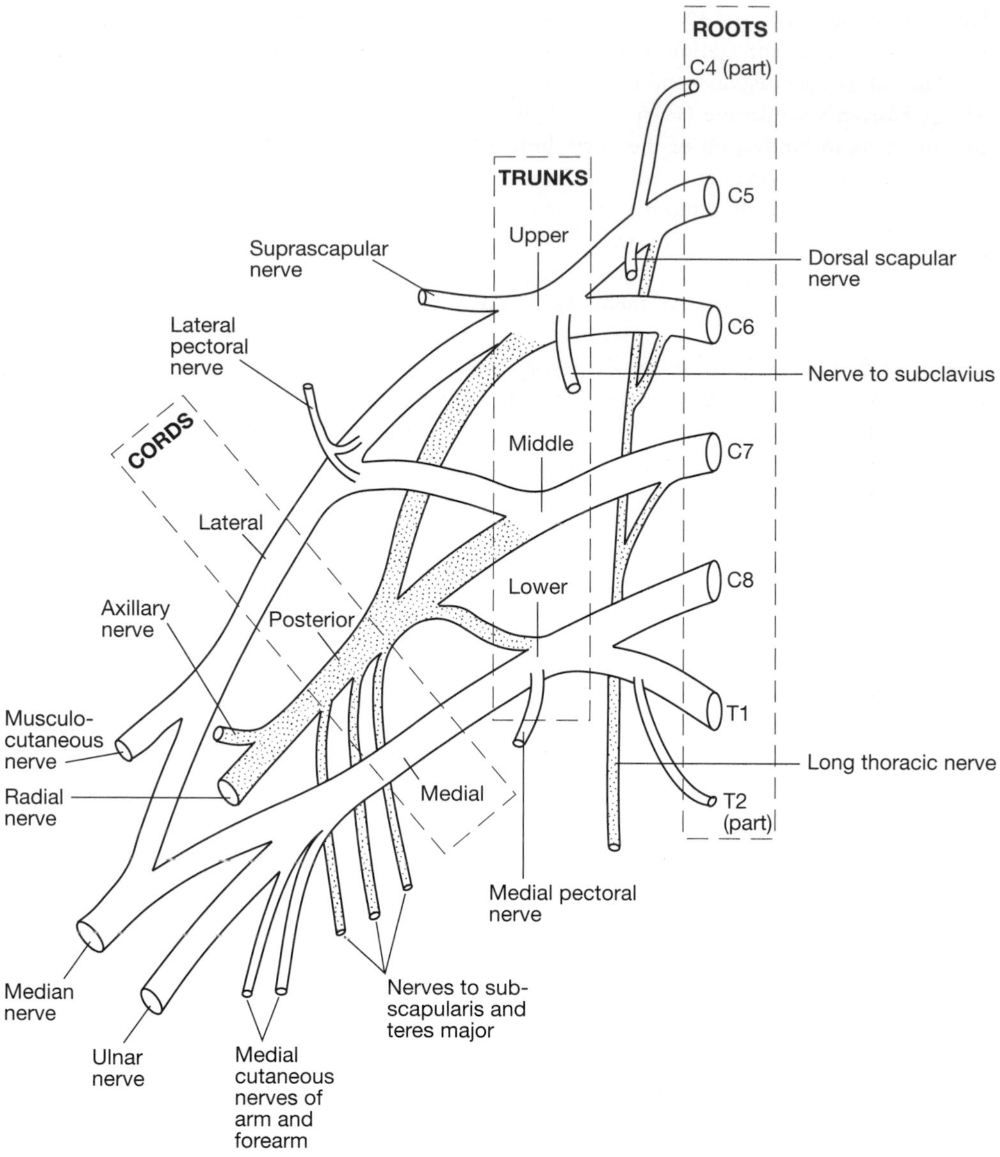

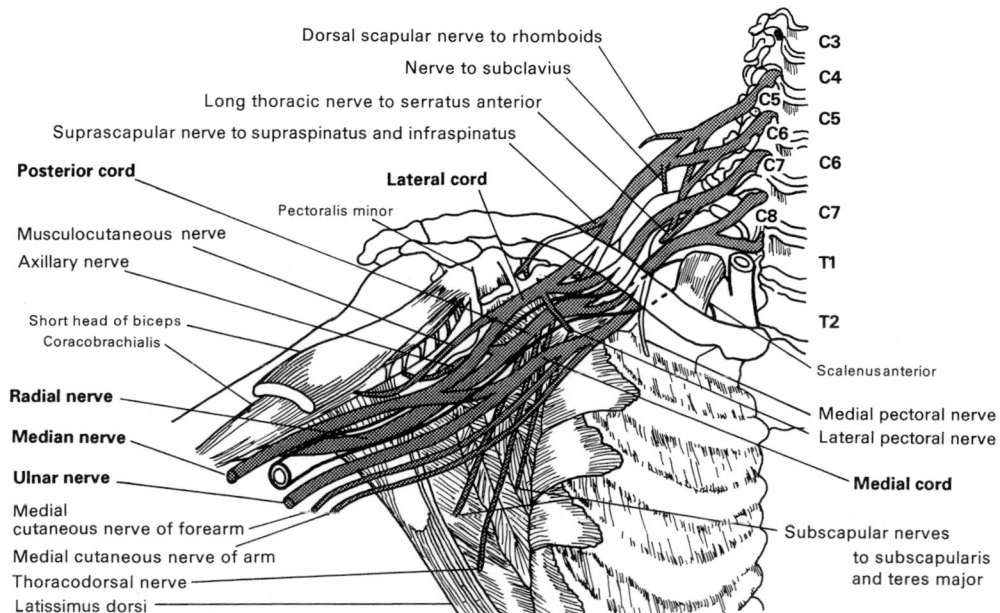

Fig. 13.5. Diagram showing how the trunks and cords of the brachial plexus are formed from the roots, and how they give rise to the peripheral nerves (modified from MacKinnon, P. and Morris, J. (1994). *Oxford textbook of functional anatomy*, Vol 1, Oxford University Press, Oxford).

Fig. 13.6. The anatomical relationships of the brachial plexus and its derivative nerves (from *Aids to the examination of the peripheral nervous system*, Ballière Tindall, London, 1986).

The plexus itself may be injured by surgical, stab, or gunshot wounds, by fracture of the clavicle, or by dislocation of the shoulder joint. Traction injuries of the upper plexus may follow forcible separation of the head and shoulder, and of the lower plexus by forced abduction of the arm. The plexus may be compressed by abnormalities such as cervical ribs in the thoracic outlet (the space between the clavicle and first rib), the plexus can be invaded by metastases, by malignant lymph nodes, or by apical pulmonary neoplasm (Pancoast's tumour), or it can be compressed by a neurofibroma. The character of the resultant motor and sensory disturbances depends upon the location of the lesion within the plexus. Complete lesions of the entire plexus are rare.

Nerve-conduction studies help discriminate between root, plexus, and peripheral-nerve lesions. Sensory-nerve action potentials are only lost if the lesion is distal to the dorsal root ganglion, but their usefulness tends to be restricted to diagnosis of lesions affecting fibres derived from the C6, C7, and C8 roots. The axon response to histamine and the reflex vasodilatation to cold can also help in diagnosis: being absent when the lesion is distal to the dorsal root ganglion and present when it is proximal. MRI or CT scanning may help localize compressive lesions of the nerve roots or plexus.

13.6.2 Traumatic lesions of the brachial plexus

Total plexus paralysis

Total plexus paralysis is rare. When the lesion is close to the vertebral column, all the muscles supplied by the plexus are paralysed and the cervical sympathetic may be involved too. When the plexus is involved at the level of the cords, the spinati, rhomboids, serratus anterior, pectorals, and cervical sympathetic supply may escape. Appreciation of light touch, pain, and temperature is lost over the forearm and hand and over the outer surface of the arm in its lower two-thirds, and sparing the T2 innervation over the upper inner arm and axilla. Joint position sense is lost in the fingers. All upper-limb tendon reflexes are absent.

Upper plexus paralysis (Erb's palsy)

This is due to a lesion of the branch from C5 to the brachial plexus. Occasionally the C6 contribution is also involved. Upper plexus paralysis is usually the result of indirect violence, the nerve being torn by undue separation of the head away from the shoulder. It was once a common form of birth injury due to traction on the head when there was difficulty in delivering one shoulder. It may occur in adults as a result of a fall on the shoulder forcing the head to one side, as on falling violently from a motorcycle. It occasionally follows general anaesthesia in a patient whose arm has been held abducted and externally rotated. The muscles paralysed as a result of interruption of the C5 component are the biceps, deltoid, brachialis, supraspinatus, infraspinatus, and the rhomboids. When the C6 component is also involved there may be partial weakness of brachioradialis,

serratus anterior, latissimus dorsi, triceps, pectoralis major, and extensor carpi radialis. The position of the limb is characteristic. It hangs at the side internally rotated at the shoulder, with the elbow extended and the forearm pronated in the 'waiter's tip' position. There is wasting of the paralysed muscles. Paralysis of the deltoid renders abduction at the shoulder impossible. The elbow cannot be flexed because of paralysis of its flexors. External rotation at the shoulder is lost owing to paralysis of the spinati. Movements of the wrist and fingers are unaffected. The biceps and supinator jerks are lost. There is usually no sensory loss, except for a small area of anaesthesia and analgesia overlying the deltoid. The 'flare' response following local scratching of the skin is an axon reflex which is lost in lesions distal to the ganglia.

The principal determinant of a good outcome is a plexus lesion which is postganglionic rather than preganglionic, thereby affecting peripheral nerves rather than roots. Operative treatment can be beneficial and expert surgical intervention should be considered early on, especially when the upper plexus has been injured by a stab or gunshot wound. Surgery for closed traction injuries is not so successful if the lesion is shown to be proximal to the dorsal root ganglia and involves root avulsion, but results are improving (Birch *et al.* 1998). The prognosis is poor if the 'flare' response is present, and particularly if myelography or MRI demonstrate a traumatic meningocele (Fig. 13.7) or a pattern of root-sleeve filling which indicates that the C5 root or spinal nerve has been torn from the spinal cord. Neurophysiological studies will not reveal axonal degeneration reliably until a week after the injury. The use of splints and physiotherapy is paramount so as to prevent the development of irreversible muscle and joint contrac-

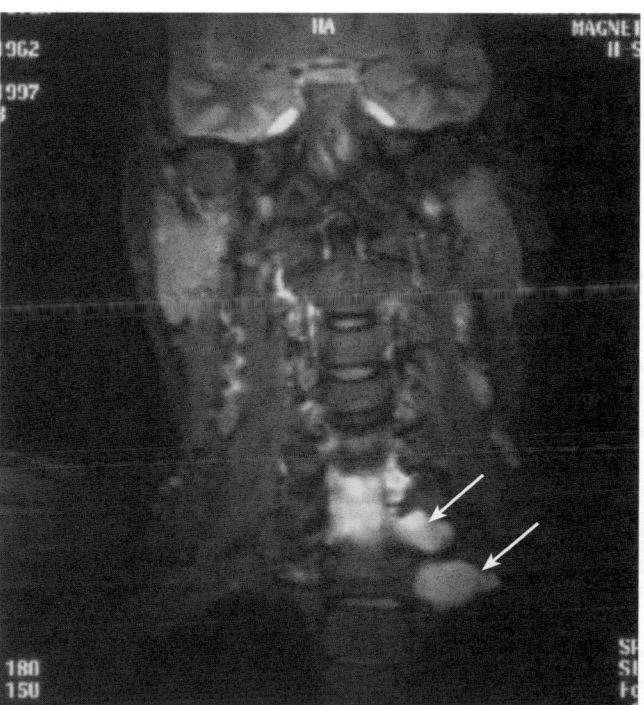

Fig. 13.7. MRI (T2 weighted) showing cerebrospinal fluid accumulation at the sites of traumatic avulsion of the C8 and T1 roots (arrowed) due to brachial plexus traction in a motorbike injury.

tures while awaiting neurological recovery. Aberrant reinnervation may give rise to synkinetic movements of shoulder girdle muscles and one-half of the diaphragm.

Lower plexus paralysis (Klumpke type)

The contribution of T1, and sometimes C8, to the brachial plexus may be torn as a result of traction on the abducted arm. Lower plexus paralysis may result from birth injury, from dropping falls during which the patient endeavours to clutch onto something overhead, or during sliding falls from motorcycles with the arm outstretched. The resulting paralysis and wasting involve all the small hand muscles, since these receive a T1 innervation. A claw-hand results from the unopposed action of the long flexors and extensors of the fingers. When C8 is involved too there is wasting and weakness of the ulnar wrist flexors and the long finger flexors. Cutaneous anaesthesia and analgesia are present in a narrow zone along the ulnar border of the hand and for a variable distance up the forearm. Horner's syndrome due to associated cervical sympathetic paralysis is common when the more proximal T1 contribution to the plexus is damaged. The principles of investigation and treatment are similar to those from upper plexus lesions.

Birth lesions of the brachial plexus

Birth lesions of the infant's brachial plexus were common until the mid-twentieth century. They have since declined dramatically, with recent estimates of less than 0.05 per cent for vertex deliveries but more than a 100-fold increase in occurrence for breech deliveries, which often produce bilateral plexus injury (Birch *et al.* 1998). Heavy babies born by the vertex are more at risk; in such cases shoulder dystocia is common and the upper trunk of the brachial plexus tends to be damaged by traction separating the head away from the shoulder. This produces the Erb type of paralysis. An associated diaphragm palsy due to phrenic nerve involvement is common. In contrast, breech deliveries tend to produce traction injuries of the lower brachial plexus, producing the Klumpke type of paralysis, often associated with a Horner syndrome. Occasionally the whole plexus is involved and this has been termed the Erb–Duchenne– Klumpke type. Overall, roughly 30 per cent make a complete recovery and 60–90 per cent eventually develop useful arm movement. Full recovery is much more likely with the upper plexus lesions. Poor recovery is subsequently associated with reduced limb bone growth in the affected arm. Despite satisfactory reinnervation, some children with previous plexus birth lesions never develop fully functional arm usage. This may represent a developmental apraxia resulting from defective motor programming in early infancy (Brown *et al.* 2000). There is a growing tendency to advise surgical repair of the plexus when the neurophysiology shows severe axonal degeneration and there is a severe lower plexus injury, or when an upper plexus injury involves the phrenic nerve, or there is no recovery of proximal muscle power by 3 months postnatally (Birch *et al.* 1998).

Lesions of the cords of the plexus

The effects of lesions of the cords of the plexus can readily be deduced from Fig. 13.5:

- ◆ *The lateral cord* is occasionally injured in dislocations of the humerus. This causes paralysis of the biceps, coracobrachialis, and of all the muscles supplied by the median nerve, except those of the thenar eminence. Sensation is affected to a variable extent on the radial aspect of the forearm.

- ◆ *The posterior cord* is rarely damaged, but if so there is paralysis of the muscles supplied by the axillary and radial nerves, and loss of sensation in their cutaneous territories. *Middle plexus paralysis* is also rare and is equivalent to interruption of the posterior cord with additional paralysis of the latissimus dorsi, teres major, and subscapularis as a result of involvement of the thoracodorsal and subscapular nerves.

- ◆ *The medial (inner) cord* is most often injured by subcoracoid dislocation of the humerus. This causes paralysis of the muscles supplied by the ulnar nerve, and of those intrinsic hand muscles supplied by the median. Sensory loss occurs along the ulnar border of the hand, forearm, and upper arm in the territories of the ulnar, medial cutaneous of the forearm and arm, nerves.

13.6.3 Thoracic outlet syndromes

Anatomy

The term 'thoracic outlet syndrome' refers to the symptoms and signs resulting from compression of the neurovascular bundle (brachial plexus, subclavian artery or vein) by anomalies of the bones or soft tissues during its course between the neck and axilla. Usually thoracic outlet syndrome has a neurogenic presentation with symptoms of brachial plexus compression. By comparison, syndromes due to subclavian, arterial, or venous compromise are relatively uncommon. The anatomical anomalies which have been associated with thoracic outlet syndromes are:

(1) an extra 'cervical' rib articulating with the seventh cervical vertebrae;

(2) a fibrous band in the same position as a cervical rib and emanating from an elongated C7 transverse process;

(3) healed clavicular or rib fractures with callus formation;

(4) abnormalities of the first thoracic rib;

(5) anomalies of positioning and insertion of the scalenus anterior or medius muscles;

(6) various other fibrous bands within the supraclavicular fossa (Wood *et al.* 1988).

It should be noted that such anomalies, particularly cervical ribs, are common in the general population, few of whom develop thoracic outlet syndromes. It is hypothesized that variations in body segmentation may contribute to the likelihood of developing thoracic outlet syndrome. In an incompletely prefixed brachial plexus the contribution of the T1 spinal nerve to the lower trunk ascends angulating across the developing cervical rib. In incomplete postfixation of the brachial plexus the augmented T2 spinal nerve contribution ascends to join the lower trunk and angulates over the normal first (thoracic) rib. Pedantics will note that the term 'thoracic outlet syndrome' is a misnomer because anatomically the thoracic outlet is bounded by the twelfth rib and closed by the diaphragm. More correct would be the term 'thoracic inlet syndrome' since it is this area of the supraclavicular fossa through which the brachial plexus passes. None the less, the term 'thoracic outlet syndrome' has passed into general acceptance and it will continue to be used here.

Diagnosis

Controversy has surrounded the diagnosis of thoracic outlet syndromes. A definite diagnosis is relatively straightforward in the patient with weakness and wasting of the small hand muscles, particularly in the thenar eminence (Fig. 13.8a); sometimes with forearm flexor compartment wasting too (Fig. 13.8b); a radiographic cervical rib; and neurophysiological studies confirming chronic postganglionic axonal loss and excluding a focal mononeuropathy (Gilliatt *et al.* 1970). Some such patients may have pain and sensory disturbance, predominantly in the ulnar forearm and sometimes in the ulnar side of the hand. This may be aggravated by use of the affected limb, particularly by carrying

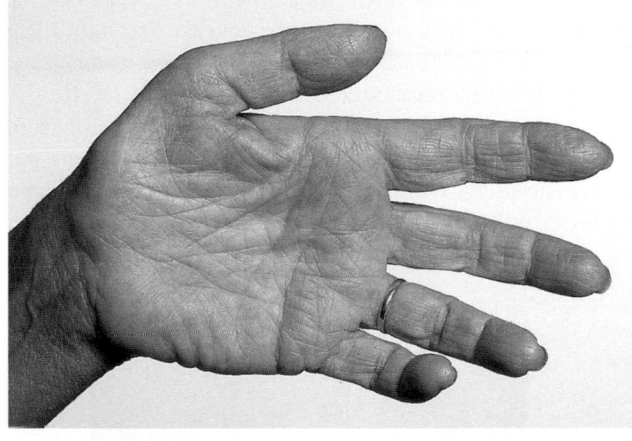

(a)

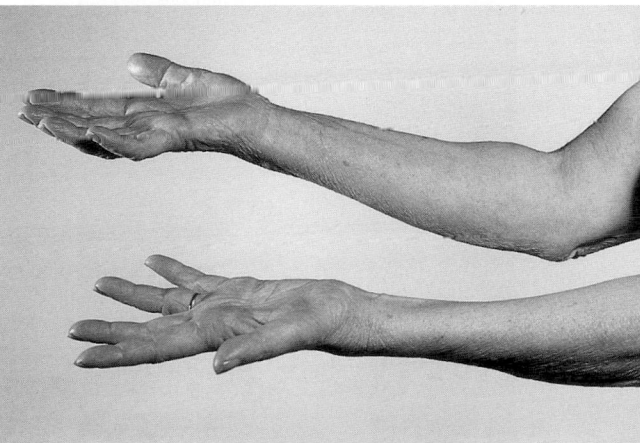

(b)

Fig. 13.8. Wasting of (a) the thenar eminence and (b) the forearm flexor compartment in a patient with a cervical rib and left thoracic outlet syndrome.

heavy objects or working with the arms above the head. Thoracic outlet syndrome is more common in women, with an age of onset ranging from the second to the eighth decade, peaking during the thirties (Gilliatt 1984).

Patients with definite thoracic outlet syndrome have harboured an asymptomatic cervical rib, or some other musculoskeletal anomaly, throughout life before eventually developing symptoms which gradually evolve into full-blown thoracic outlet syndrome over a period of years during adulthood. Thus, it is self-evident that intermediate or incomplete forms of thoracic outlet syndromes must exist as part of the natural history of thoracic outlet syndrome associated with cervical rib. Moreover, given the variable propensity for cervical ribs to cause thoracic outlet syndromes at all, it is likely that many patients will remain with intermediate forms for years, if not forever.

Unsurprisingly, such intermediate, or incomplete forms of thoracic outlet syndrome are harder to diagnose. Patients in this category should be regarded as having 'suspected' rather than 'definite' thoracic outlet syndrome. Sensory symptoms altered by arm usage, are particularly likely to occur in suspected thoracic outlet syndrome. Sensory loss in the T1 and C8 dermatomes, aggravation of pain and paraesthesia by using the affected arm, absence of nocturnal symptoms, and the occurrence of hand colour changes due to vascular involvement are common in this group. Wasting of the thenar eminence and the long finger flexors may not be evident, but these muscles are usually weakened if tested in a suitably sensitive manner to detect mild weakness. For instance, the examiner should use his own flexor digitorum profundus or dorsal interosseous muscles to test the patient's terminal interphalangeal joint flexion and finger abduction respectively. Considerable diagnostic importance accrues from reproducing or precipitating sensory symptoms in the ulnar forearm by manually rolling the brachial plexus in the supraclavicular fossa from behind when the patient is standing with the arms hanging. Also, cervical ribs or other supraclavicular anomalies may be palpated by this manoeuvre. Tendon reflexes are usually preserved. Complaints of pain in the upper arm or shoulder are quite common in such patients, but are not a specific feature useful in diagnosis. Radial pulse obliteration by Wright's manoeuvre (hyperabduction and elevation of the arm) or Adson's test (lateral rotation of the neck and hyperinflation of the chest) is not very reliable as a diagnostic test because 'positive' results occur in many normal asymptomatic people. However, if present only on the symptomatic side, such vascular occlusion signs contribute to the level of diagnostic suspicion. In summary, three groups of patients who present are: first, those with advanced denervation of the small hand and forearm muscles without sensory symptoms; secondly, the patient with a combination of motor and sensory symptoms; and, thirdly, patients with sensory symptoms alone.

Investigations

Radiography of the cervical spine and electrophysiology are the most useful investigations for supporting the diagnosis of thoracic outlet syndrome. Radiographic demonstration of a cervical rib contributes importantly to the diagnosis in a patient with a suitable clinical syndrome. Even if a patient is reputed to have had a 'normal' cervical spine radiograph, this should be inspected since sometimes the anomalous rib emanating from the C7 vertebral transverse process has been mistakenly identified as the 'normal' first thoracic rib. Apart from careful counting of the cervical vertebra, which can be difficult when the skull bones obscure the top of the neck, the key is to note that the seventh cervical vertebra has downturned transverse processes, compared to the upturned transverse processes of the T1 vertebra (Fig. 13.9a). If the transverse process of C7 is unusually elongated and downturned, one should be suspicious that it is the origin of a radiographically invisible fibrous band (Fig. 13.9b). In patients with suspected thoracic outlet syndrome, blinded analysis of volumetrically acquired magnetic resonance images of the brachial plexus detected deviation of the brachial plexus on about 80 per cent of symptomatic sides (Panegyres *et al.* 1993). MRI also detects instances of plexus distortion by post-traumatic callus of the first rib, by a hypertrophied serratus anterior muscle or tumour compression.

Neurophysiological studies are important in diagnosing thoracic outlet syndrome. They exclude alternative diagnoses of common entrapment neuropathies such as carpal tunnel syndrome or ulnar nerve palsy. Electromyography shows denervation of forearm flexors and small hand muscles, and loss of sensory-nerve action potentials confirms that the underlying lesion is postganglionic (Smith and Trojaborg 1987; Wilbourn 1993). Occasionally patients with suspected thoracic outlet syndrome will show normal nerve-conduction studies. While this should be regarded as evidence against brachial plexus compression, it should be noted that an ulnar sensory-nerve action potential which lies within the normal range could have decreased from a higher premorbid level and should be compared with the potential in the unaffected arm. Also, it is the ulnar sensory-nerve action potential, representing the C8 spinal nerve fibres, which is usually measured. However, the less conventional procedure of measuring the amplitude of the sensory action potential of the medial cutaneous nerve of the forearm, which represents the T1 spinal nerve, is a more pertinent test for lower brachial plexus compression. Measurement of somatosensory evoked potentials, or of motor conduction through the supraclavicular fossa following magnetic stimulation of the roots, has not proved to be useful diagnostically. No investigation has absolute diagnostic power for thoracic outlet syndrome, particularly in the milder suspected syndromes. The eventual diagnostic judgement must take into account both clinical features and investigations.

Management

The only definitive treatment for thoracic outlet syndrome is operative removal of the structure which is compressing or distorting the brachial plexus, usually a cervical rib or band. However, despite its extensive history, the surgical treatment of thoracic outlet syndrome is controversial for two reasons. First, the degree of certainty of the diagnosis has a crucial bearing upon whether an operation should be advised. Secondly, there is no consensus as to the most suitable type of operation.

Operation for thoracic outlet syndrome seems to be effective for relieving pain and sensory disturbance in 90 per cent of patients. It improves muscle weakness in some 50 per cent, but produces no useful reinnervation of severely denervated hand muscles in full-blown and advanced cases of thoracic outlet

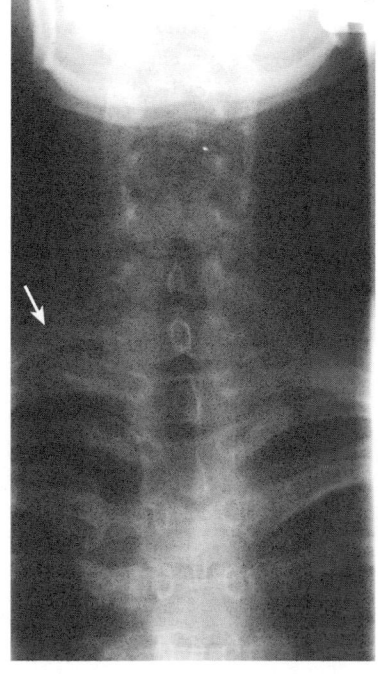

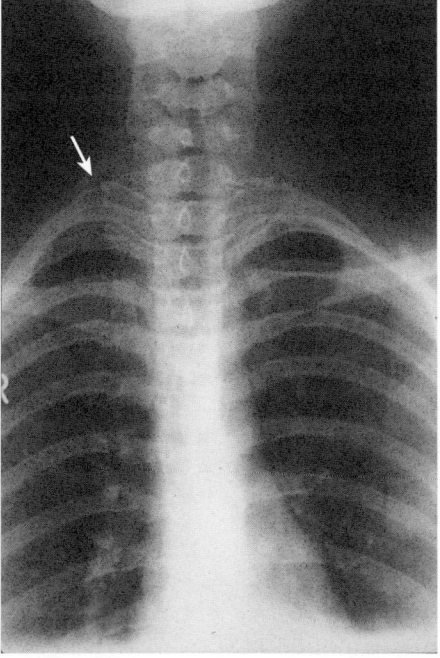

Fig. 13.9. Plain X-ray of the cervical spine in a patient with thoracic outlet syndrome (a) due to right cervical rib (arrowed). Note that this articulates with the C7 vertebra transverse process which is downturned by contrast with the upturned transverse processes of T1. (b) An elongated downturned transverse process (arrowed) of the C7 vertebra, found at operation to give rise to a fibrous band.

(a)   (b)

syndrome (Gilliatt *et al.* 1970; Donaghy *et al.* 1999). This raises an important question concerning the earliness of diagnosis and surgery so as to forestall permanent loss of hand muscle function. It is of little value to undertake an operation in a patient with severe wasting and weakness of hand muscles but without a troublesome sensory disturbance, because no benefit usually results. On the other hand, to operate early so as to forestall irreversible hand muscle denervation carries the risk that some patients will receive an unwarranted operation because the diagnosis of suspected thoracic outlet syndrome is incorrect. When advising upon possible surgery in suspected thoracic outlet syndrome, one should take account of whether the symptoms are disabling, and whether conservative methods aimed at altering posture and arm usage have failed. The patient should be cognisant of possible surgical complications, and, particularly if there is no cervical rib, the exploratory nature of such an operation. The risk of complications depends upon the experience of the surgeon and may be higher if the trans-axillary route has been used (Cherington *et al.* 1986; Donaghy *et al.* 1999). Noteworthy complications include traction injuries to the brachial plexus causing increased symptoms which usually resolve spontaneously, phrenic nerve injury resulting in diaphragm paralysis, reflex sympathetic dystrophy, long thoracic nerve palsy, and cosmetic dissatisfaction with the supraclavicular scar.

Operative procedures

Various operative approaches to decompressing the brachial plexus have been advocated for thoracic outlet syndrome. The anterior supraclavicular approach is probably the operation of choice since it provides the best exposure of the neurovascular bundle, cervical ribs, or fibrous bands, and can be used for first rib resection. Its disadvantages include the risk of damage to the long thoracic or phrenic nerves and the presence of a cosmetically undesirable scar. The trans-axillary route is popular, particularly in the United States, since it leaves a small, hidden scar and requires little dissection, but it does involve strenuous abduction of the arm, leaving the brachial plexus vulnerable to traction injury, and haemostasis may prove difficult if there is intraoperative vascular damage. The infraclavicular approach is not commonly employed because it does not allow the anatomical abnormality to be visualized, despite providing excellent access to the anterior two-thirds of the first rib. It is particularly difficult to compare the effectiveness of these different operations because of the varying criteria which have been em-ployed for preoperative selection and postoperative assessment (Donaghy *et al.* 1999).

Differential diagnosis

Thoracic outlet syndrome is generally distinguished from motor neuron disease by the presence of pain and sensory loss in the former, and by the more malignantly progressive and generalized muscle weakness of the latter. However, focal or segmental spinal muscular atrophies (Section 14.6) and multifocal motor neuropathy (Section 12.11.3) should be considered. In syringomyelia, wasting of the small hand muscles is associated with analgesia and thermo-anaesthesia, but the sensory loss is usually much more extensive than that associated with a cervical rib, deep tendon reflexes are lost, and signs of corticospinal-tract degeneration may be present (Section 20.6.2). Radiographic demonstration of a cervical rib must not be taken as sole proof that it is the cause of the patient's symptoms. Tumour of the lung apex will usually be visible radiographically. Other infiltrating tumours of the brachial plexus may be evident on CT scan or MRI. Entrapment of the median or ulnar nerves may be confused with cervical rib, but these diagnoses are established by the characteristic distribution of the motor and sensory symptoms of lesions of these nerves and the diagnostic nerve-conduction abnormalities. However, some patients with thoracic outlet syndrome do have electrophysiological evidence of additional lesions of the median nerve at the wrist, or of the ulnar nerve at the elbow. For other causes of wasting in the hands see Section 13.1.4.

13.6.4 Acute brachial neuritis

The essence of acute brachial neuritis consists of severe pain in the region of the shoulder, soon followed by weakness of upper limb muscles, usually those of the shoulder girdle. It is also known as shoulder girdle neuritis, neuralgic amyotrophy, cryptogenic brachial plexus neuropathy, or the Parsonage–Turner syndrome.

Pain is the initial symptom in most patients, often of sudden onset, generally severe and unilateral and centred on the shoulder girdle (Tsairis *et al.* 1972). Only occasionally do patients develop muscle weakness without pain (Schott 1983). The pain subsides over a few hours to a few weeks, during which time muscle weakness develops on the same side. The weakness and subsequent muscle wasting usually affect the spinatus and deltoid muscles. Less frequently, the serratus anterior, trapezius, triceps, biceps, or diaphragmatic muscles may be affected. Forearm muscles are occasionally involved, most notably flexor pollicis longus causing weakness of thumb-tip flexion. Each of the above muscles may be involved in isolation, but multiple muscular involvement is more usual. Sensory symptoms are rarely prominent. Some patients experience paraesthesiae at the onset, and occasionally develop patches of skin sensory loss, most frequently over the shoulder in the territory of the axillary (circumflex) nerve.

The symptoms of acute brachial neuritis are usually unilateral. Occasionally bilateral involvement does occur, sometimes sequentially, although it is rarely symmetrical. Electrophysiological studies point to subclinical involvement of the muscles of the asymptomatic limb in up to 25 per cent of patients. Careful clinical and electrophysiological studies show patchy involvement of upper-limb nerves, principally within the brachial plexus and its immediate branches, but sometimes affecting nerves more distally within the arm, such as the anterior interosseous nerve (England and Sumner 1987). The right arm is more frequently affected than the left. The prognosis is good for shoulder muscle involvement, but less good for forearm weakness. Full symptomatic recovery of strength occurs in 90 per cent of patients by 3 years. Fewer than 10 per cent of patients have long-term weakness sufficient to cause disability. Recurrences occasionally occur but are generally not as severe as the initial attack.

The histopathology of affected nerves has not been studied in the acute stage. The underlying cause of acute brachial neuritis is rarely identified. Occasionally it follows serum sickness or inoculations, particularly with tetanus toxoid. It occurs more often in pregnancy and postpartum than can be accounted for by chance (Lederman and Wilbourn 1996). It may follow viral infections, particularly cytomegalovirus or Epstein–Barr virus, and it has been reported following intravenous injection of adulterant heroin mixtures (Challenor et al. 1973). It has occurred in patients with Hodgkin's disease, within days to weeks of radiotherapy treatment (Malow and Dawson 1991). The pathogenic mechanisms underlying acute brachial neuritis are unknown, but it is thought to be immune mediated.

The diagnosis is based on the clinical picture, and investigations are chiefly of help in excluding alternative diagnoses. The differential diagnosis includes hereditary recurrent brachial plexus neuropathy, vasculitic neuropathy, and prolapsed cervical intervertebral disc. In its early stages, acute brachial neuritis is often misdiagnosed as a painful shoulder joint. No treatment is known to affect the long-term outcome; some consider that steroid or adrenocorticotrophic hormone (ACTH) therapy diminishes the severity of pain in the early stages.

13.6.5 Hereditary neuralgic amyotrophy

A tendency to recurrent attacks of brachial neuritis may be inherited as an autosomal dominant trait (Goudier et al. 1994). Individual attacks are indistinguishable from those of neuralgic amyotrophy, as described above. Complete recovery from each attack is usual, although cumulative disability may develop with repeated attacks. Two distinct clinical courses are recognised with only one type occurring in any particular family: a classic relapsing-remitting and a chronic undulating type with exacerbations (van Allen et al. 2000). Attacks may develop puerperally in genetically susceptible women. Apart from the family history, the features suggestive of a familial tendency to brachial neuritis include a prior history of unexplained vocal cord paralysis or, occasionally, of lumbosacral plexus lesions. Affected patients from some families display a distinctive facial asymmetry with close-set eyes, epicanthic folds, dwarfism, or cleft palate. Teased sural nerve fibres may show sausage-shaped swellings of the myelin sheath, the so-called 'tomaculous change' similar to those seen in hereditary liability to pressure palsies (Bradley et al. 1975) (see Section 12.5). However, unlike hereditary liability to pressure palsies, families with hereditary neuralgic amyotrophy do not show deletions, duplications, or point mutations of the PMP22 gene on chromosome 17, electrophysiology does not show a mild background polyneuropathy, and prominent pain occurs during attacks (Goudier et al. 1994). The two conditions are distinct genetic entities, and hereditary neuralgic amyotrophy shows linkage to a separate locus on chromosome 17 (17q25) (Stögbauer et al. 2000).

13.6.6 Chronic brachial plexopathy

Slowly progressive brachial plexus lesions are occasionally encountered in neurological practice. The majority involve a relatively painless progressive motor deficit with mild degrees of sensory loss, and are usually unilateral. Generally, no firm diagnosis is established. However, some of these patients may suffer from focal hypertrophic neuritis, in which fusiform segmental enlargement of peripheral nerves, mimicking peripheral nerve tumours, may be palpated or visualized on CT (Cusimano et al. 1988). Chronic plexopathy due to tumour infiltration or irradiation should be distinguished in patients with known cancer (Section 13.5.3). Brachial plexopathy due to tumour infiltration is generally profoundly painful; it is particularly likely to occur in patients with lymphoma or carcinoma of the breast or lung, is rarely bilateral, and is associated with palpable supraclavicular masses or CT evidence of a mass within the brachial plexus. On the other hand, irradiation-induced brachial plexopathy is usually painless, is more likely to be bilateral, and is often associated with characteristic myokymic discharges on electromyography of affected muscles (Harper et al. 1989).

13.7 Lumbosacral plexus lesions

Most of the lumbosacral plexus lies protected within the bony ring of the pelvis, in contrast to the more exposed location of the brachial plexus. This shields the lumbosacral plexus from direct trauma, unless this is severe enough to fracture–dislocate the pelvic ring. However, tumours of the lumbosacral pelvis are relatively concealed from palpation compared to those of the brachial plexus. The introduction of CT and MRI of the retroperitoneum has greatly simplified the differential diagnosis of lumbosacral plexus lesions. A similar spectrum of disease affects both the lumbosacral and brachial plexuses, although idiopathic lumbosacral plexitis is encountered much less frequently than acute brachial neuralgia, its counterpart in the arm. Differentiation of plexus lesions from those of roots or peripheral nerves is discussed in Section 13.1.2. It is important to recognize that lesions of the lumbosacral plexus, particularly when due to tumours or aneurysms, may induce radiating 'sciatica' pain, worsened by straight-leg-raising, leading to an initial diagnosis of a root lesion (Donaghy 1993). A number of major disease entities affecting the lumbosacral plexus or the intrapelvic segments of nerves derived from it are discussed individually below, and the sites of some important lesions are shown in Fig. 13.10. Other important causes of lumbosacral plexus neuropathy are discussed elsewhere: diabetic proximal neuropathy (Section 12.17.1) and vasculitic neuropathy (Section 12.15), and tumour infiltration (see Fig. 13.11a) (Section 13.5.2).

13.7.1 Idiopathic lumbosacral plexopathy

This is the counterpart in the leg of acute brachial neuritis (Section 13.6.4). It may affect all age groups. Although uncommon, its frequency is probably underestimated because its very existence is under-recognized and because the symptoms may resemble those of prolapsed intravertebral disc. Patients experience an abrupt onset of unilateral severe pain in the anterior thigh if involvement of the lumbar plexus predominates,

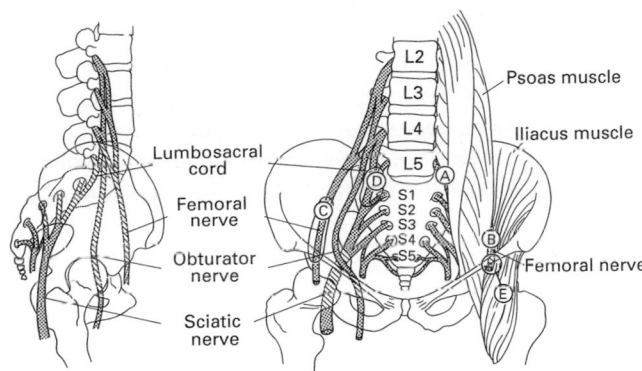

Fig. 13.10. Diagram of the lumbosacral plexus, showing the usual locations of lesions caused by different mechanical factors. (A) Lumbosacral cord compression at the pelvic brim by the fetal head or mid-pelvic forceps, causing maternal obstetric paralysis. (B) Compression of the femoral nerve by surgical retractor blades in the gutter between the iliacus and psoas muscles. (C) Compression of the femoral nerve by haematoma within the iliacus fascia. (D) Lumbosacral trunk damage by fracture–dislocation of the sacroiliac joint. (E) Angulation of the femoral nerve under the inguinal ligament during prolonged flexion and abduction of the hips in the lithotomy position.

or in the buttock and posterior thigh if sacral plexus involvement is predominant (Evans *et al.* 1981). Muscle weakness is noted within 10 days of the onset of pain and may progressively worsen for some weeks before stabilizing. The pain resolves as the weakness develops. The condition most commonly involves the upper portion of the plexus, producing an absent knee-jerk, tenderness on palpation of a femoral nerve, and a positive femoral nerve stretch test. Symptoms of lower plexus involvement may closely resemble those of prolapsed intervertebral disc and the straight-leg-raising test may be positive. All patients experience muscle weakness in varying patterns but objective sensory disturbance occurs only in the minority. Spontaneous recovery occurs over months or years and is often incomplete, although the residual disability is rarely severe. It is not known whether steroid therapy influences the evolution of the weakness, or the extent of the subsequent recovery. Occasionally the syndrome is relapsing or progressive and immunosuppressant therapy or high-dose intravenous immunoglobulin may be effective (Verma and Bradley 1994). It has been associated with Epstein–Barr virus (Sharma *et al.* 1993), *Borrelia burgdorferii* and *Schistosoma japonicum* infections. Like acute brachial neuritis, the syndrome has been reported following intravenous injection of adulterant heroin mixtures. The differential diagnosis includes prolapsed intervertebral disc, which is not associated with such widespread weakness; vasculitic neuropathy, which more commonly affects more peripheral segments of nerves; diabetic proximal neuropathy; and tumour infiltration of the plexus, which is not associated with spontaneous remission of the pain.

13.7.2 Haemorrhagic lumbosacral plexopathy

There are two distinct syndromes of nerve compression by retroperitoneal haemorrhage. Large haematomas may diffusely compress the lumbar plexus within the psoas muscle, leading to weakness in both obturator and femoral nerve territories (Zarranz *et al.* 1981). More frequently, the intrapelvic portion of the femoral nerve is compressed by relatively smaller haematomas within the iliacus muscle and its indistensible fascia (Fig. 13.10C) (Taysvaer 1982). These syndromes usually occur during anticoagulant therapy but also in other bleeding diatheses, most notably haemophilia.

Femoral nerve compression by iliacus haematoma presents with pain in the groin or iliac fossa which radiates to the antero-medial thigh and medial calf. Hip extension exacerbates the pain and patients characteristically assume a hip-flexed posture. The quadriceps muscle is weak, the knee jerk depressed, and there is a variable degree of sensory loss in the femoral and long saphenous nerve territories. The haematoma may be palpable in the lower iliac fossa or visible at the groin. The condition should be distinguished from septic arthritis or haemarthrosis of the hip joint, both of which cause pain during passive rotation at the hip joint.

In contrast, lumbar plexus involvement in psoas muscle haematoma is not associated with pain on forced hip extension, the hip is not held flexed, no haematoma is palpable, and the thigh adductors are weakened, indicating involvement of the obturator nerve territory.

The diagnosis is confirmed by CT scan or MRI of the pelvis, showing haematoma of the psoas or iliacus muscles, thereby differentiating the condition from pelvic abscess. Restoration of normal blood coagulation is the mainstay of therapy and usually allows good recovery. However, some patients with iliacus haematoma develop prolonged neurological disability. To avoid this, some have advocated early surgical drainage to improve the chances of complete neurological recovery (Taysvaer 1982).

13.7.3 Trauma

In civilian practice, traumatic lumbosacral plexus lesions usually result from double vertical fracture–dislocation of the pelvic ring due to motor vehicle accidents (Huttinen and Slatis 1972). The lumbosacral cord is the most commonly affected portion of the plexus (Fig. 13.10D), leading to weakness of muscles innervated by L5 and S1. Less frequently, the obturator or superior gluteal nerves or the L5, S1, S2, and S3 anterior roots may be involved. Lumbosacral plexus lesions are generally overlooked immediately following trauma because of the overwhelming nature of the other injuries. They are generally diagnosed only once it is recognized that recovery of limb movements is unusually delayed following pelvic fractures or fracture dislocations of the hip joint. Significant recovery of neurological function rarely occurs. There is little experience of surgical treatment of lumbosacral plexus injuries.

13.7.4 Intra-arterial injections

Buttock injections can cause ischaemia of the lumbosacral plexus, as well as producing the more familiar problem of direct needle trauma to the sciatic nerve. Vasotoxic or crystalline drugs may be inadvertently introduced into the inferior gluteal artery in the medial aspect of the buttock, particularly if the aspiration test is omitted prior to injection. Toxic vasospasm, or vascular obstruction by crystals, is thought to be responsible for such ischaemic lesions of the sciatic nerve or lumbar plexus (Stöhr *et al.* 1980). In addition to neurological disturbance, the buttock skin develops a characteristic painful, cyanosed swelling which may progress to gangrene, so-called 'embolia cutis medicamentosa'. Only partial recovery of the neurological lesion occurs and persistent severe pain is common. Immediate administration of papaverine, heparin, and sympathetic blockade are recommended on suspicion of the diagnosis (Stöhr *et al.* 1980), but these measures are of unproven value.

13.7.5 Obstetric injuries

Postpartum footdrop occurs most commonly after labour which has been protracted, involved cephalopelvic disproportion or a mid-pelvic forceps delivery (Feasby *et al.* 1992). The lumbosacral cord is directly compressed at the pelvic brim, or as it overlies the sacroiliac joint, most commonly by the infant's brow during an occiput anterior presentation (Fig. 13.10A). Weak ankle dorsiflexion and eversion are generally noticed only once the woman tries walking after delivery. Comprehensive neurophysiological studies localize the lesion to the expected site at the pelvic bone where it is crossed by the lumbosacral trunk (L4, L5) before it joins the S1 root (Feasby *et al.* 1992). Complete spontaneous recovery within 3 months is usual. The recommended management of subsequent deliveries in women with a previous episode of peripheral pelvic nerve compression depends upon whether full recovery had occurred from the previous episode (Donaldson 1988). If there is residual neurological damage indicating axonal degeneration, elective Caesarean section is advised. If full recovery had occurred, a trial of labour should be undertaken but the use of mid-pelvic forceps avoided. When an established lumbosacral plexus lesion develops during labour, it is recommended that labour should be allowed to continue normally since Caesarean section is unlikely to reverse the neurological damage; however, mid-pelvic forceps should be avoided (Gonik *et al.* 1984). Postpartum sacral plexepathy causing persistent perineas, skin sensory loss, either unilateral or bilateral, and associated impairment of sphincter control and sexual finctioning, can occur in multiparous women, or following mid-forceps delivery (Ismael *et al.* 2000).

13.7.6 Catamenial sciatica

The unusual developmental anomaly of implantation of endometriosis in the sciatic nerve at the sciatic notch may cause progressive sensorimotor sciatic nerve palsies in women of childbearing age. These may be associated with perimenstrual pain in the buttock or posterior aspect of the thigh (Salazar-Grueso and Roos 1986). Computed tomography shows a contrast-enhancing mass in the sciatic notch. Pain may be relieved by danazol or progesterone, or by induction of an artificial menopause (Donaldson 1988). Alternatively, the endometriosis may be removed microsurgically, particularly if fertility must be preserved (Salazar-Grueso and Roos 1986).

13.7.7 Surgical conditions

The intrapelvic portion of the femoral nerve may be damaged by laterally placed self-retaining retractor blades in the lower pelvis during abdominal hysterectomy or renal transplantation (Fig. 13.10B). The femoral nerve may also be damaged by prolonged and excessive angulation at the level of the inguinal ligament during operations under anaesthesia in the lithotomy position (Fig. 13.10E). Up to 70 per cent of recipients of hip prostheses display evidence of damage to the sciatic, femoral, or obturator nerves, although this is only a presenting symptom in a minority of about 1 per cent (Weber *et al.* 1976). Aneurysms of the iliac or hypogastric arteries may compress the lumbosacral plexus. In such cases, there is an abrupt onset of sciatic pain and impaired

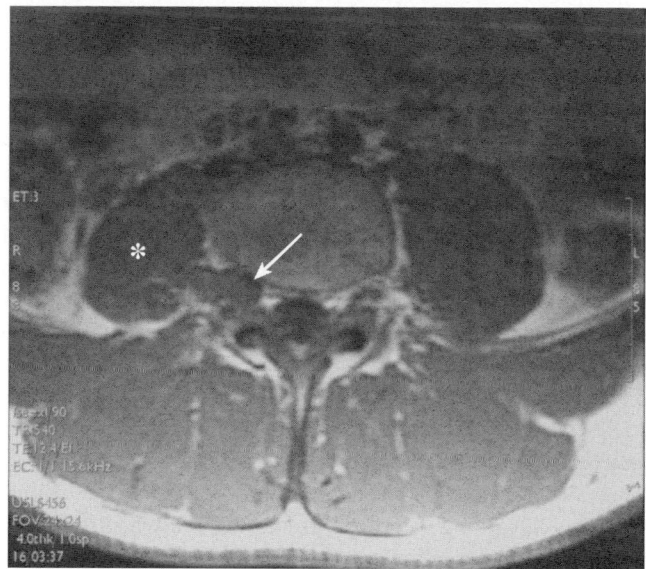

(a)

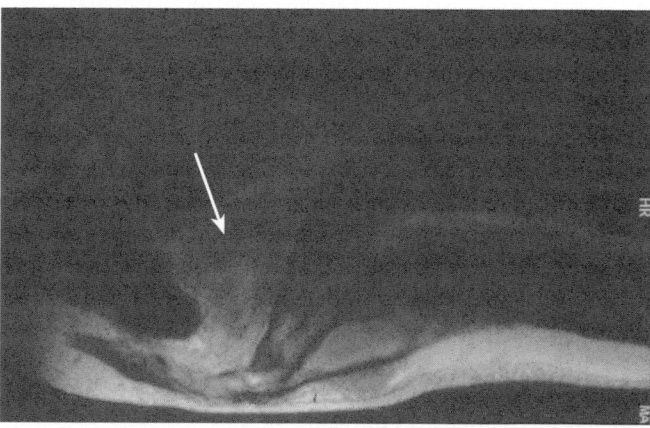

(b)

Fig. 13.11. MRI in the diagnosis of lumbosacral plexus lesions. (a) Tumour (arrowed) involving the lumbar plexus on the postero-medial border of the psoas muscle(*). Note the wasting of the psoas muscle on the affected side. (b) A staphylococcal abscess in the Pouch of Douglas (arrowed) tracking posteriorly to the subcutaneous tissues in a patient with bilateral leg weakness and loss of sphincter control.

straight-leg-raising, suggestive of prolapsed intervertebral disc. On rectal examination, a firm, pulsatile mass is palpable and there is radiological evidence of curvilinear calcification in the aneurysm wall (Chapman *et al.* 1964). Patients with a pelvic abscess may develop leg weakness, which is often bilateral and associated with a variable severity of sensory symptoms, and sphincter involvement if the coccygeal plexus is also affected. The patient will usually be constitutionally unwell, with fever and leucocytosis and MRI demonstrates the abscess (Fig. 13.11b).

13.8 Sacrococcygeal plexus lesions

Locally infiltrative tumours, principally derived from the rectum, prostate, and uterine cervix, may affect the sacrococcygeal plexus. These may involve the sacrum, with evidence of bone erosion on MRI. Pelvic abscess (Fig. 13.11b) or sacral osteomyelitis can also affect the sacrococcygeal plexus and will be revealed by MRI.

Sacral herpes zoster eruptions may lead to urinary retention and are usually associated with mild lymphocytosis of the cerebrospinal fluid (Meyer *et al.* 1959). Aciclovir therapy is generally recommended for this condition, although most patients do make complete or partial recoveries of motor function without this drug.

Acute ano-genital infection with the herpes simplex virus type 2 may produce neuralgia, numbness, and paraesthesiae of the perineum, buttocks, and posterior thighs, followed by urinary reten-

tion, constipation, or erectile failure (Hemrika *et al.* 1986). Reduced anal tone, impaired anal and bulbocavernosus reflexes, and sacral dermatome sensory loss are usually encountered in such patients. Sacrococcygeal plexopathy due to primary genital herpes occurs most commonly in anally receptive homosexual males with herpetic proctitis (Goodell *et al.* 1983). It is less frequent in women with herpetic vulvovaginitis and only rarely follows penile herpes in heterosexual males. Mild meningism and a spinal fluid lymphocytosis are usual in such patients. Herpes simplex virus type 2, rather than type 1, is the usual isolate. Aciclovir therapy is recommended. Even without aciclovir therapy, full recovery generally occurs; neurological symptoms generally last about 10 days and rarely more than 21 days.

Urinary retention and ano-genital sensory loss have been reported during primary infection with human immunodeficiency virus (Zeman and Donaghy 1991). This was associated with spinal-fluid lymphocytosis, and neurological recovery was only partial despite treatment with zidovudine.

13.9 Phrenic and intercostal nerve lesions

13.9.1 The phrenic nerve

Dyspnoea, on exertion or lying flat, is the usual clinical symptom of phrenic nerve palsy. However, this cause is usually overlooked initially because pulmonary and cardiac conditions come to mind. The dyspnoea is partially relieved by standing

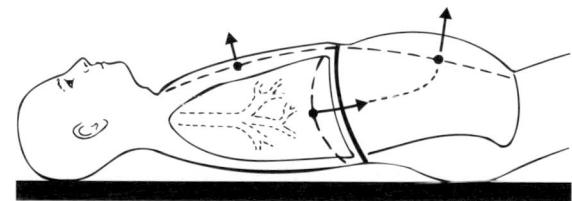
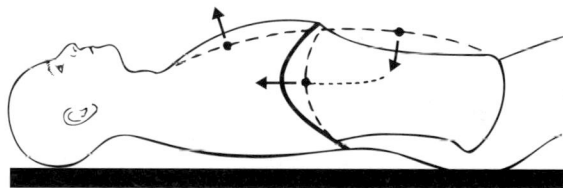

(a) Normal inspiration

(b) Inspiration with a weak diaphragm

(a)

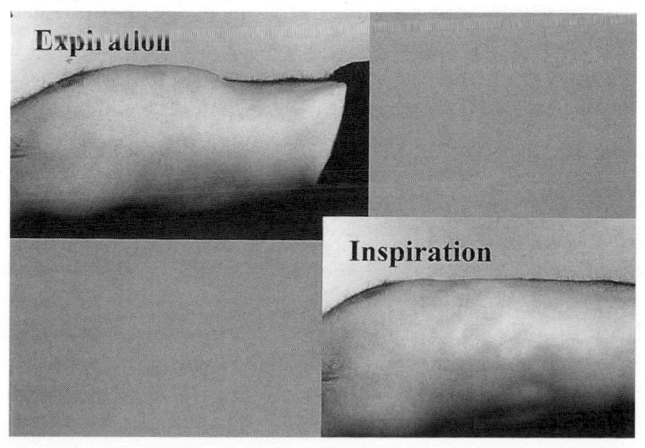

(b)

Fig. 13.12. (a) Diagram illustrating (left) how the diaphragm moves downwards into the abdomen during normal inspiration with the resultant outward movement of the abdominal wall, and (right) how the diaphragm is sucked upwards into the chest, with resultant indrawing of the upper abdominal wall, during inspiration when the diaphragm is weak. (Adapted from Donaghy, M. (1997). *Neurology*. Oxford University Press, Oxford.) (b) Normally the abdominal wall moves outwards during inspiration due to diaphragmatic descent.

because descent of the diaphragm during inspiration is assisted by the weight of the liver attached to its underside. Unilateral diaphragmatic paralysis may be symptomless. Diaphragm paralysis may be confirmed by clinical observation of paradoxical indrawing of the upper abdomen during inspiration with the patient supine (Fig. 13.12), by radiological screening of the diaphragm while the patient sniffs, by enhancement of the vital capacity when measured standing compared to lying, or by trans-diaphragmatic pressure measurement using balloons in the oesophagus and stomach.

The phrenic nerve derives mainly from the C3 and C4 roots, with an insignificant C5 contribution. It may be damaged at any stage in its course by trauma, by surgical procedures, or by tumours of the neck, mediastinum, or thorax. Conduction studies show that it is frequently involved in polyneuropathies (Newsom-Davis 1967). This is most familiar clinically in the context of respiratory failure due to the Guillain–Barré syndrome, in hereditary motor and sensory neuropathy, and in motor neuron disease. Phrenic nerve involvement can occur in acute brachial neuritis, and a syndrome of recurrent isolated alternating phrenic nerve palsies is thought to be a variant of brachial neuritis (Gregory *et al.* 1990). Diaphragm paralysis may also occur as an isolated phenomenon in patients with hereditary recurrent brachial neuropathy (Section 13.6.5). Sometimes the cause of unilateral diaphragmatic paralysis cannot be established. The differential diagnosis of diaphragm paralysis is wide (Laroche *et al.* 1989) and includes lesions of the brainstem or spinal cord above the level of the phrenic outflow, traumatic lesions of the upper brachial plexus, disorders of neuromuscular transmission such as myasthenia gravis or the Lambert–Eaton myasthenic syndrome, and a wide range of primary muscle diseases, of which acid maltase deficiency most notably involves the diaphragm relatively selectively.

13.9.2 Intercostal and truncal nerves

Intercostal neuralgia is a rare and ill-defined disorder which is diagnosed probably more often than it occurs. It is characterized by paroxysmal pain throughout the distribution of an intercostal nerve, frequently associated with cutaneous tenderness in the area it supplies, especially at the point of emergence of its lateral cutaneous branch. Before diagnosing this condition, care must be taken to exclude the many other disorders that may be associated with similar pain due to inflammation, including syphilis or arachnoiditis, or by compression of spinal dorsal roots by neoplasms of the spinal cord, nerve roots, or vertebrae. It may precede or follow an attack of herpes zoster. Notalgia paraesthetica is a rare syndrome of localized burning pain over the scapula thought to be due to compression of the dorsal branches of the thoracic roots passing through the paraspinal muscles. A spinal nerve may be compressed as a result of localized collapse of the vertebral column, most often due to secondary carcinoma, trauma, or tuberculous caries. Spondylosis is often associated with root pains, which may also be produced by scoliosis. Pleurisy, both tuberculous and neoplastic, is sometimes mistakenly diagnosed as inter-

costal neuralgia. The thorax is a common site of referred pain in visceral disease, especially diseases of the upper abdominal viscera, including cholecystitis and carcinoma of the body or tail of the pancreas. Radicular pain or truncal neuropathy may also occur in diabetes mellitus or porphyria. Pain in the distribution of an intercostal nerve is also seen in some patients after thoracotomy, and may be intractable. Truncal muscle involvement is not usually evident clinically, but flaccid bulging of a portion of the abdominal wall can be seen with lower thoracic root or intercostal nerve lesions.

Intercostal neuropathy should be treated with analgesics. Local anaesthetic injections may give temporary relief. If all else fails, the nerve may be injected with alcohol or phenol, care being taken that the needle does not penetrate the pleura. In occasional cases, surgical division of two or three intercostal nerves close to the spine has been tried but even after this operation pain may recur after a few months. Even posterior rhizotomy does not always afford permanent relief.

13.10 Upper-limb mononeuropathy

13.10.1 The median nerve

Anatomy

The median nerve (Fig. 13.13) is derived from C6, C7, C8, and T1 spinal nerves. It is formed by the union of two heads from the medial and lateral cords of the brachial plexus. It runs on the medial aspect of the upper arm and passes through the antecubital fossa anterior to the elbow joint. It usually passes between the two heads of the pronator teres in the upper forearm, before running down the anterior forearm deep to flexor digitorum superficialis. After passing under the transverse carpal ligament at the wrist, which forms the roof of the carpal tunnel, it enters the hand. There are no branches to muscles in the upper arm. In the forearm it supplies the following muscles, with branches given off in the order named: pronator teres (C6, C7), flexor carpi radialis (C6, C7), and palmaris longus. Also, it supplies flexor digitorum superficialis (C7, **C8**, T1) via its anterior interosseous. Sometimes the anterior interosseous branch supplies flexor digitorum profundus to the index and middle fingers (C7, **C8**), flexor pollicis longus (C7, **C8**), and pronator quadratus (C7, **C8**). In the hand the median nerve usually supplies the two radial lumbricals, opponens pollicis, abductor pollicis brevis, and the outer head of the flexor pollicis brevis, all of which are predominantly supplied by the T1 root with a small contribution from C8. Sometimes it supplies the first dorsal interosseous. Anomalies of median nerve innervation most commonly involve the thenar muscles; for instance opponens pollicis may receive pure ulnar nerve innervation. These generally reflect anastomoses between the ulnar and median nerves in the forearm. The most common of these is the Martin–Gruber anastomosis, which occurs in up to 15 per cent of people, in which fibres destined for the thenar eminence lie in the ulnar nerve at the wrist but run in the median nerve at the elbow. This can be a source of clinical and electrophysiological confusion in carpal tunnel syndrome.

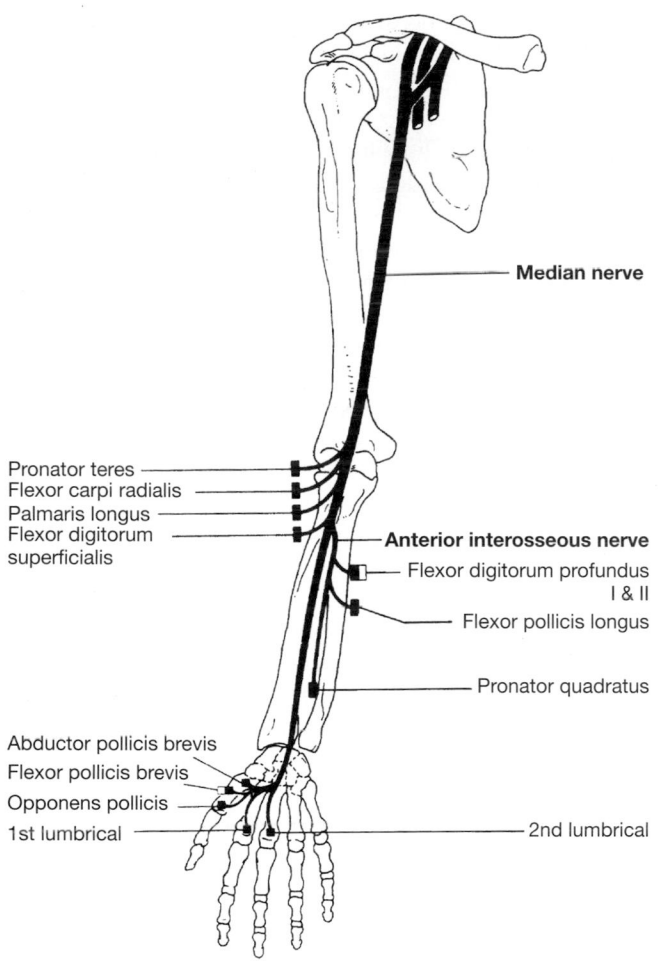

Median nerve

Pronator teres
Flexor carpi radialis
Palmaris longus
Flexor digitorum
superficialis

Anterior interosseous nerve
Flexor digitorum profundus
I & II
Flexor pollicis longus

Pronator quadratus

Abductor pollicis brevis
Flexor pollicis brevis
Opponens pollicis
1st lumbrical

2nd lumbrical

Fig. 13.13. Diagram of the median and anterior interosseous nerves, showing the muscles they innervate. Note that the innervation of flexor digitorum profundus and flexor pollicis brevis is shared with the ulnar nerve.

Trauma

The median nerve may be injured at any point of its course by stab or gunshot wounds. It is occasionally damaged by dislocation of the shoulder joint or by humerus fractures. The most common acute traumatic lesion in civilian practice is a cut at the wrist, usually the result of the hand having been put through a window pane; in such cases the ulnar nerve may be damaged also. Painful lesions of the median nerve and/or of the medial and lateral cutaneous nerves of the forearm are an occasional complication of venepuncture in the antecubital fossa (Berry and Wallis 1977), or of arterial cannulation or axillary block anaesthesia.

Proximal median neuropathy

Proximal median neuropathy is uncommon and is normally associated with ulnar or radial palsy in cases of crutch paralysis, overlong use of surgical tourniquets, or compression during sleep or stupor. Other causes of high median nerve palsy include falls on the shoulder or arm, or hyperextension of the forearm. Not infrequently the cause remains obscure. Occasionally the median nerve is trapped by a *ligament of Struthers*,

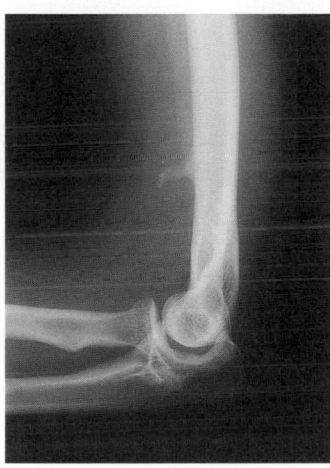

Fig. 13.14. Medial nerve compression by a ligament of Struthers. X-ray showing the bony spur on the shaft of the humerus from which the ligament originates before inserting into the medial epicondyle.

a fibrous band arising from a bony spur on the humerus about 5 cm above the medial epicondyle, to which it runs. Exploration and division of this band are indicated if its presence is suggested radiologically (Fig. 13.14).

In high median nerve lesions the radial flexor of the wrist is paralysed, so that when the wrist is flexed against resistance, the hand deviates to the ulnar side. The terminal phalanx of the thumb and the phalanges of the index finger cannot be flexed. There may be weakness of flexion of the phalanges of the remaining fingers, but not complete paralysis. Since the ulnar half of the flexor digitorum profundus is supplied by the ulnar nerve, the ring and little fingers are usually spared completely. Flexion at the metacarpophalangeal joints is carried out by the interossei and lumbricals, of which only the two lumbricals for the index and middle fingers are innervated by the median. Paralysis of the muscles of the thenar eminence supplied by the median nerve leads to weakness of thumb opposition and abduction; this latter movement must be tested in a plane at right angles to the palm. In established lesions there is wasting of the paralysed muscles, especially conspicuous in the outer half of the thenar eminence, rendering the first metacarpal bone unduly prominent (Fig. 13.15). Superficial sensory loss following a median nerve lesion above the wrist is somewhat variable, especially in regard to the appreciation of pinprick (Fig. 13.16).

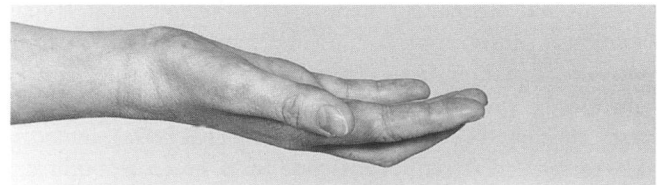

Fig. 13.15. Wasting of abductor pollicis brevis in a median nerve lesion. Note the concave appearance of the muscle at the base of the thumb along the first metacarpal bone when viewed from the side.

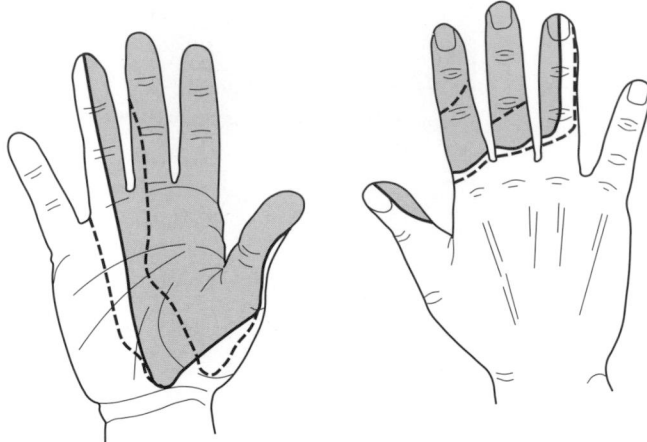

Fig. 13.16. The area of superficial sensory loss after a median nerve lesion above the wrist. This includes the territory supplied by the superficial palmar branch (—— usual boundary; ‑‑‑‑‑‑‑ variations). (Based on Head and Sherren 1905.)

The pronator syndrome

This presumed entrapment syndrome affecting the median nerve in the vicinity of pronator teres is held to be caused by hypertrophy of that muscle or by a variety of tendonous bands within pronator teres or the nearby origin of flexor digitorum superficialis. The characteristic symptom is aching and tenderness in the upper flexor forearm exacerbated by repetitive arm usage, especially in pronation (Morris and Peters 1976). Sometimes there are paraesthesiae in the median nerve distribution, but clear-cut weakness or wasting seems rare. Although electrophysiological studies are usually normal, they sometimes show denervation or loss of sensory-nerve action potentials. The indications for, and results of, surgical exploration, with a view to decompression, are unclear (Dawson *et al.* 1999).

Median nerve compression at the wrist (carpal tunnel syndrome)

Compression of the median nerve in the carpal tunnel is generally an idiopathic phenomenon, occurring spontaneously, usually in middle-aged women. It is often bilateral, although more symptomatic in the dominant hand. Often symptoms develop with repetitive hand movements. Usually the causes involve a reduction in the size of the carpal tunnel (Dawson *et al.* 1999). It occurs after fractures and arthritis involving the wrist joint, in tenosynovitis, in rheumatoid arthritis and gout, in association with ganglia, and in pyogenic infections of the hand. Endocrine disorders (myxoedema, acromegaly, diabetes mellitus and pregnancy) predispose to the condition. It may result from infiltrations with sarcoid or myeloma, or from amyloid deposition in and around the ligament in primary amyloidosis with light-chain deposition, familial amyloidosis with transthyretin deposition (Murakami *et al.* 1994), and possibly in renal dialysis patients due to β_2-microglobulin deposition. It has been described after the surgical establishment of a forearm fistula in patients undergoing repeated haemodialysis (Harding and Le Fanu 1977).

Pain and tingling occur in the hand and fingers, typically awakening the patient at night or occurring on bunching up the hand for tasks such as writing. Many patients with carpal tunnel syndrome seem to think that tingling affects all their fingers, including the little finger; presumably this is because it can be so difficult to localize tingling and pain accurately. Carpal tunnel syndrome is the most common cause of acroparaesthesiae. Often pain and paraesthesiae may be the only symptoms for many months or years. If cutaneous sensory loss develops on the digits, it causes difficulty in handling small objects. Neurological examination is often completely normal. The most common abnormal sign is some blunting of pinprick sensation on the tip of the index compared to the little finger. Less often abductor pollicis brevis is weak, or occasionally wasted. It should be noted that the area of sensory loss is limited to the distal palmar surface of the fingers (Fig. 13.17), which are innervated by the deep palmar branch of the median nerve, rather than its superficial palmar branch, which arcs over the transverse carpal ligament. Tinel's sign of evoking tingling by percussing over the carpal tunnel, and Phalen's test of inducing paraesthesiae by flexing the wrist, are both unreliable.

Nerve-conduction studies usually confirm the diagnosis reliably and should be performed whenever surgical release in envisaged. A prolonged distal motor latency on stimulating the nerve at the wrist and recording the muscle action potential from abductor pollicis brevis is diagnostic in moderate and severe carpal tunnel syndrome. The forearm motor conduction velocity will be normal. If a Martin–Gruber anastomosis between the median and ulnar nerves is present, the motor latency to abductor pollicis brevis will be preserved following proximal stimulation despite being prolonged after stimulation at the wrist (Iyer and Fenichel 1976). In mild cases, a more sensitive index of carpal tunnel syndrome is reduced amplitude of sensory-nerve action potentials when median nerve branches

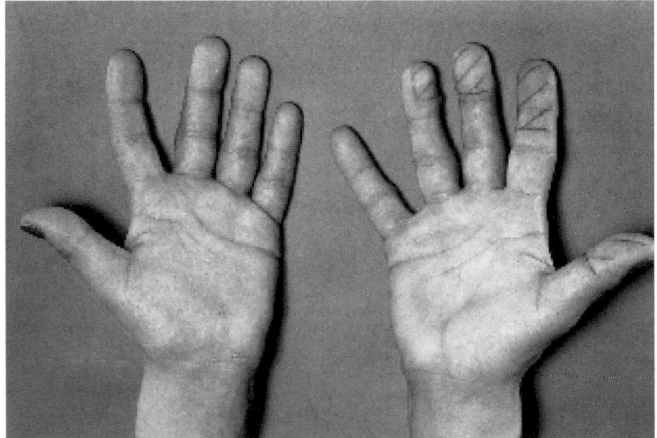

Fig. 13.17. The area of sensory loss in carpal tunnel syndrome. Sensation on the palms and proximal fingers in preserved because the superficial palmar branch of the median nerve does not traverse the carpal tunnel. These apparently masculine hands belong to a woman with acromegaly, the underlying cause of her carpal tunnel syndrome.

are stimulated in the fingers or palm, compared to the normality of sensory conduction in the ulnar nerve.

Mild carpal tunnel symptoms can be treated conservatively, often with wrist splinting. If associated with pregnancy, it will resolve after delivery, and if with hypothyroidism, after endocrine correction. Symptoms which constitute a considerable nuisance or disability by interfering with hand usage or sleep can be treated either by steroid injection of the carpal tunnel, or by surgical decompression. Injection of 15 mg of methylprednisolone into the carpal tunnel by an experienced physician benefits over 95 per cent, with 50 per cent relapsing by 6 months and 90 per cent by 18 months (Girlanda *et al.* 1993). Surgical decompression is the only reliable long-term cure and is mandatory if conservative measures have failed or there is evidence of denervation. Many use surgery as primary treatment for carpal tunnel syndrome, using a variety of approaches and techniques under local anaesthesia (Dawson *et al.* 1999).

13.10.2 The anterior interosseous nerve

This nerve is purely motor, branching from the main trunk of the median nerve just after its emergence from pronator teres in the upper forearm. It supplies flexor pollicis longus (C7, **C8**), flexor digitorum profundus to the index and middle fingers (C7, **C8**), and pronator quadratus (C7, C8) (Fig. 13.13). Isolated lesions of this nerve, developing apparently spontaneously, are quite common, usually causing paralysis of flexion of the terminal phalanges of the thumb and index finger, with disabling loss of pincer grip (Kiloh and Nevin 1952). It may be damaged by fractures and stab wounds around the elbow. Compression by fibrous bands and anomalous muscles occurs much as for the pronator syndrome affecting the median nerve. It is recognized increasingly that spontaneous isolated anterior interosseous nerve lesions, preceded by acute pain in the upper arm or forearm, probably represent a localized variant of acute brachial neuritis (Goulding and Schady 1993); it has been well-recognized as a particular nerve to be involved in more extensive forms of acute brachial neuritis (England and Sumner 1987). Generally such patients start to improve by 10 months; virtually complete recovery takes up to 24 months if it is to occur. This raises doubts about the surgical practice of exploring the nerve for constricting fibrous bands if no recovery is evident by 3 months. Sometimes no cause can be established for acute and painless anterior interosseous nerve palsies. The diagnosis can be confirmed electrophysiologically by demonstrating prolonged latency of motor conduction from the elbow to pronator quadratus (Nakano 1978). The median sensory-nerve action potential is unaffected, in contrast to lesions involving the median nerve itself.

13.10.3 The ulnar nerve

Anatomy

The ulnar nerve (Fig. 13.18) is derived from the C7, C8, and T1 spinal roots. It gives off no branches above the elbow, where it

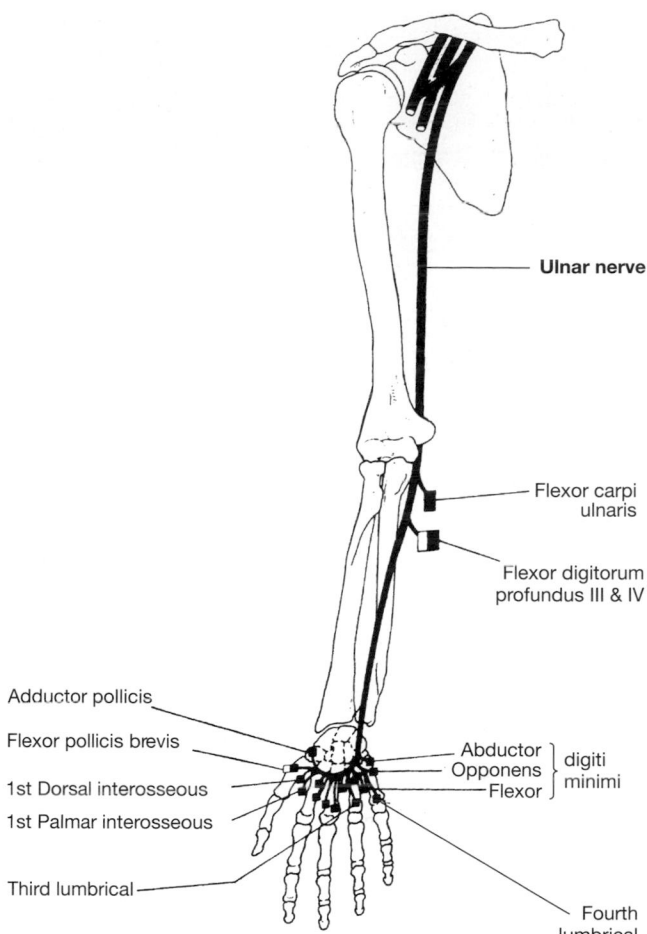

Fig. 13.18. Diagram of the ulnar nerve and its muscular innervation. Note that the innervation of flexor digitorum profundus and flexor pollicis brevis is shared with the anterior interosseous and median nerves, respectively.

lies behind the medial epicondyle of the humerus before entering the cubital tunnel. In the forearm it supplies branches to flexor carpi ulnaris (C7, **C8**, T1) and the portion of flexor digitorum profundus (C7, **C8**) flexing the distal phalanx of the ring and little fingers. Although the nerves to these two muscles usually arise distal to the elbow, the anatomy varies enough to confound clinical localization; sometimes power in these muscles remains normal despite a proven ulnar nerve lesion at the elbow. The dorsal ulnar sensory branch, supplying the back of the hand, is given off a few centimetres above the wrist. In the hand the ulnar nerve usually supplies palmaris brevis, the muscles of the hypothenar eminence, the two medial lumbricals, the palmar and dorsal interossei, the transverse and oblique heads of the adductor pollicis, and the medial head of the flexor pollicis brevis, all of which predominantly receive a T1 root supply with a lesser C8 contribution. The first dorsal interosseous muscle is sometimes supplied by the median nerve. The ulnar nerve enters the hand through Guyon's canal, composed of ligaments between the hamate hook and pisiform bones, where it splits into a superficial terminal sensory branch and a deep motor branch.

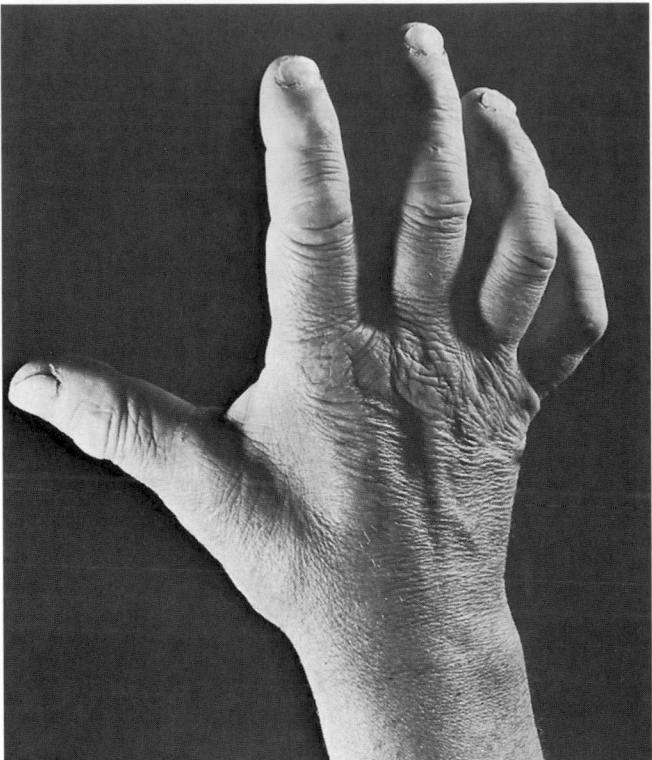

(a)

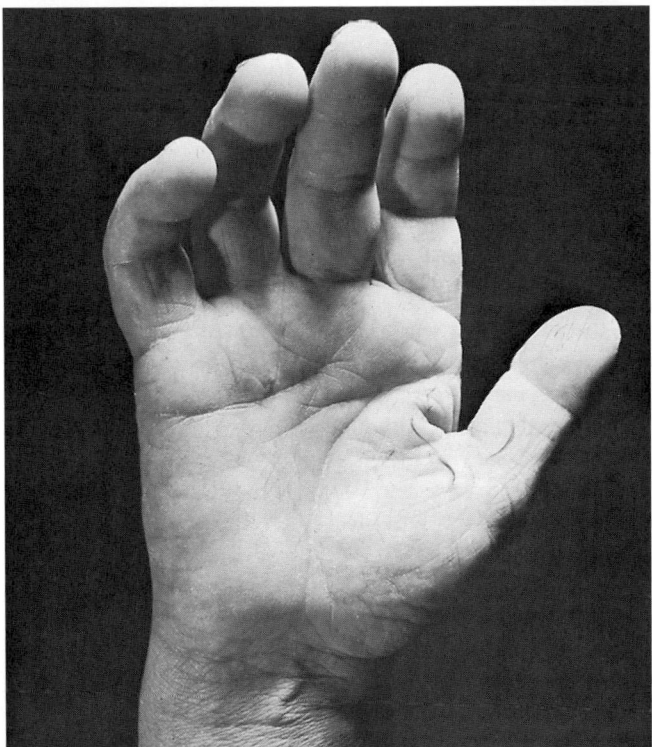

(b)

Fig. 13.19. An ulnar nerve palsy, showing (a) wasting of the first dorsal interosseous muscle, with (b) the typical claw hand appearance due to hyperextension at the metacarpophalangeal joints of the little and ring fingers associated with inability to extend these interphalangeal joints.

Lesions above the elbow

These cause paralysis of all the muscles supplied by the ulnar nerve. Lesions of the ulnar nerve above the elbow are rare, but may be due to direct trauma or compression, as for the median nerve (Section 13.10.1). Paralysis of flexor carpi ulnaris causes the hand to deviate to the radial side on flexion of the wrist against resistance. Paralysis of the ulnar half of the flexor digitorum profundus abolishes flexion of the little and ring fingers at the distal interphalangeal joints. Paralysis of the hypothenar eminence abolishes abduction of the little finger, and impairs flexion of this finger at the metacarpophalangeal joint. Paralysis of the interossei abolishes abduction and adduction of the fingers. When the interossei and lumbricals are paralysed, the fingers cannot be held with the metacarpophalangeal joints flexed and the interphalangeal joints extended. Paralysis of the transverse and oblique heads of the adductor pollicis weakens adduction of the thumb, most evident when the patient attempts to press the thumb flatly against the index finger. Wasting of the paralysed muscles is evident on the ulnar side of the front of the forearm, in the hypothenar eminence, the interosseous spaces, and the ulnar half of the thenar eminence (Fig. 13.19a). Paralysis of the small muscles of the hand causes 'claw-hand' (Fig. 13.19b). This posture is produced by the unopposed action of the long finger extensor muscles in the presence of weakness of the lumbricals of the ring and little fingers.

After a lesion of the ulnar nerve at or above the elbow, the area of altered pinprick sensation varies, but usually covers the little finger, the ulnar border of the palm, and often the ulnar half of the ring finger (Fig. 13.20).

Lesions at the elbow

At the elbow, the ulnar nerve may be affected by fractures and dislocations involving the lower end of the humerus and the

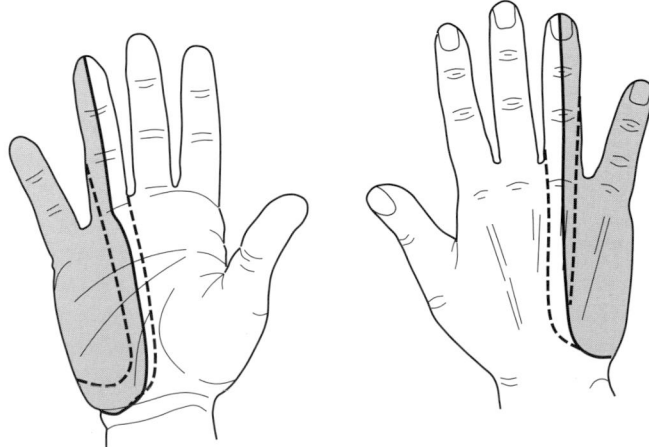

Fig. 13.20. The area of superficial sensory loss after an ulnar nerve lesion above the wrist. This territory includes the dorsal ulnar sensory branch, which supplies the back of the hand and fingers, and arises up to 10 cm proximal to the wrist; this territory is spared by a lesion of the ulnar nerve below the wrist (——— usual boundary; ------- variations)

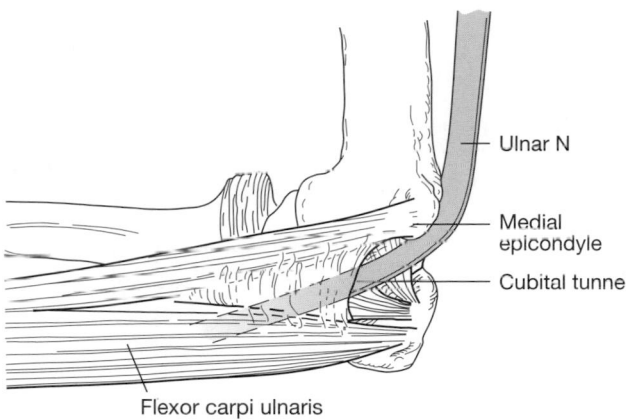

Fig. 13.21. Ulnar nerve compression at the elbow. Medial view of the nerve's passage through the condylar groove behind the medial epicondyle, where it can dislocate from the groove, or be compressed by bony abnormalities. The usual site of compression occurs in the cubital tunnel under the aponeurotic origin of flexor carpi ulnaris. (After Kincaid 1988.)

elbow joint. Such injury to the nerve is usually immediate. Occasionally it becomes involved years later if such an injury has led to cubitus valgus ('tardy ulnar palsy'). Similarly, the nerve may be damaged in the condylar groove by osteophytic outgrowths from arthritis of the elbow joint, by a ganglion, or by a Charcot elbow joint. If the nerve dislocates from the condylar groove when the elbow flexes, it may be damaged during anaesthesia or prolonged recumbency. The most common site of chronic compression lies within the cubital tunnel just distal to the condylar groove, where the nerve is constricted beneath the aponeurotic origin of flexor carpi ulnaris (Fig. 13.21). The earliest symptoms are pain and paraesthesiae referred to the cutaneous distribution of the nerve, often first apparent only when the patient awakens in the morning after sleeping with the elbow flexed. Motor involvement is variable and often not symptomatic. It is surprising how rarely patients notice wasting of the first dorsal interosseous muscle, even when quite advanced.

Neither nerve-conduction studies nor clinical examination can distinguish reliably between condylar groove and cubital tunnel compression. Electrophysiology merely shows motor conduction block or axonal degeneration localized to the segment of the ulnar nerve at the elbow and associated with a diminished sensory-nerve action potential. Management of compressive ulnar nerve lesions at the elbow has been confused, and the following approach is recommended (Stewart 1993; Dawson *et al.* 1999). In general, a 3-month trial of conservative measures is advised so that surgery can be avoided if spontaneous recovery starts after neurapraxic lesions. Conservative therapy consists of avoiding resting on the elbows and padding the elbows. If the patient has a bony deformity of the condylar canal, and the neuropathy does not respond to conservative measures, it should be transposed anteriorly. If the nerve recurrently dislocates from the condylar groove, and the neuropathy fails to respond to elbow padding and avoiding leaning on the elbows, medial epicondylectomy should be considered.

In the most common situation of presumed idiopathic compression in the cubital tunnel, the simplest operation is to decompress the aponeurotic roof of the tunnel, which minimizes the risk of operative nerve damage. However, many authorities recommend as primary procedure. Medial epicondylectomy or anterior transposition of the nerve. Both of these can be considered as secondary procedures if the neuropathy continues to progress, or at the time of surgical inspection if other abnormalities are found unexpectedly.

Lesions at the wrist

Damage at the wrist proximal to Guyon's canal produces paralysis which is confined to those small muscles of the hand supplied by the nerve. Flexor carpi ulnaris and the ulnar half of flexor digitorum profundus escape. Sensory loss is as shown in Fig. 13.20, except that the territory may be spared on the dorsum of the hand and fingers, which are supplied by the dorsal ulnar sensory branch. Lesions in and around Guyon's canal produce a bewildering array of sensory and motor deficits, depending upon the combinations of involvement of the superficial terminal sensory branch and the deep palmar motor branch before and after it subdivides to the hypothenar and thenar muscles. When only the deep palmar branch is involved well distal to Guyon's canal, sensory loss does not occur and the hypothenar muscles escape, weakness being most marked in the first dorsal interosseous muscle.

At the wrist, the ulnar nerve may be injured by cuts, and the median nerve may be involved simultaneously. The entire palmar branch of the ulnar nerve, including its superficial sensory component, is occasionally compressed or injured on the anterior aspect of the wrist in Guyon's canal. A pressure neuropathy of the deep palmar branch of the ulnar nerve sometimes occurs in individuals whose occupation or recreation involves prolonged or recurrent pressure upon the outer part of the palm, for instance in cyclists. Rarely, benign tumours or ganglia may compress the main trunk or the deep branch. Measurement of the sensory-nerve action potential from the little finger, and comparison of the distal motor latencies to abductor digiti minimi and the first dorsal interosseous, are helpful in pinpointing the precise level of ulnar nerve lesions in the wrist or hand. The choice of treatment for ulnar nerve lesions in the wrist and hand depends upon the cause. For instance, lesions of the deep palmar branch that are due to repetitive palm trauma require a change in the use of the hand. Small ganglia or tumours may prove visible on magnetic resonance imaging of the palm.

13.10.4 **The radial nerve**

Anatomy

The radial nerve (Fig. 13.22) continues from the posterior cord of the brachial plexus and is derived from the C5, C6, C7, and C8 spinal nerves. It innervates the following muscles in the upper arm, where it winds posteriorly in the spiral groove of the humerus deep to the triceps muscle: triceps (C6, C7, C8), brachioradialis (C5, C6), and extensor carpi radialis longus

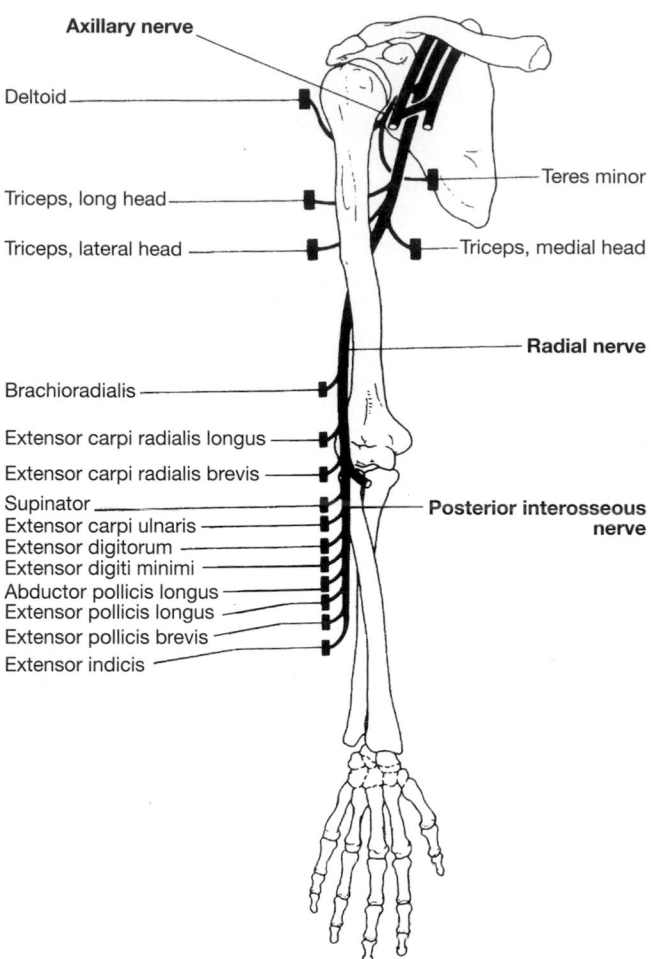

Fig. 13.22. Diagram of the radial, posterior interosseous, and axillary nerves, showing the muscles they innervate.

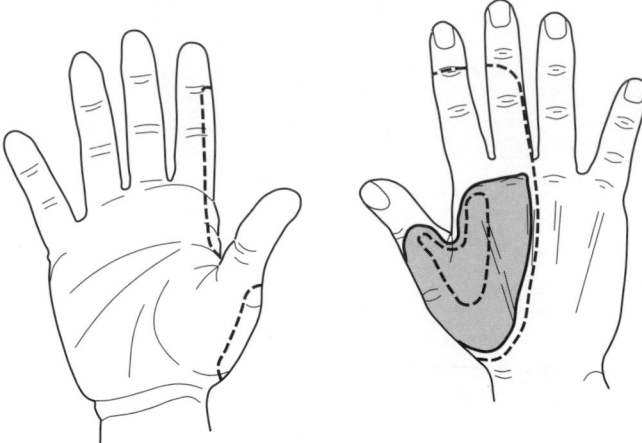

Fig. 13.23. The area of superficial sensory loss in a radial nerve lesion below the origin of the posterior cutaneous nerve of the forearm in the axilla. This skin territory corresponds to the area innervated by the superficial radial nerve (——— usual boundary; -------- variations).

(C5, C6). In the lateral aspect of the upper forearm it divides into the superficial radial nerve, which is purely sensory, and the posterior interosseous nerve, which is purely motor. The posterior interosseous nerve innervates supinator (C6, C7), extensor digitorum (**C7**, **C8**), extensor carpi ulnaris (**C7**, **C8**), and the three extensors of the thumb (C7, C8).

The radial nerve above the origin of the posterior cutaneous nerve of the forearm in the axilla carries sensation from the lower half of the radial aspect of the arm, from the middle of the posterior aspect of the forearm, and also from a variable area on the dorsum of the hand. This area on the hand corresponds to the territory supplied by the superficial radial nerve (Fig. 13.23).

Lesions

Compression of the radial nerve in or above the axilla by crutch palsies or during stupor causes paralysis and wasting of all the muscles it supplies. There is wrist and finger drop and the triceps weakness localizes the high level of this lesion. The triceps and brachioradialis reflexes are lost and the sensory loss involves both posterior cutaneous nerve of the forearm and superficial radial nerve territories.

The nerve is most vulnerable to damage in the upper arm in the spiral groove of the humerus, in which case the triceps power and reflex will be preserved and the main feature is wrist and finger drop accompanied by loss of the brachioradialis reflex. Such lesions are most familiar as a 'Saturday night paralysis' in which the nerve is compressed when the patient, often intoxicated, falls asleep with the arm extended over the arm of a chair. Following a pressure palsy of the radial nerve, sensory loss is variable, and may be absent, but is found usually on the dorsum of the hand between the thumb and index finger. Less frequently, radial nerve lesions of the upper arm follow blunt trauma, misplaced deep intramuscular injections, fractures of the humerus, and careless positioning of the arm during general anaesthesia.

Radial nerve conduction studies may be helpful in determining the site of the lesion. Following compressive lesions, recovery can be anticipated in 9–12 weeks if nerve conduction studies show a neurapraxic lesion with preservation of the radial sensory action potential, no denervation changes on sampling the brachioradialis or the forearm extensors, and evidence of focal conduction block on stimulating the radial nerve in the upper arm (Shyu *et al.* 1993). A light cockup splint may be used to maintain extension of the wrist, thereby allowing the hand to be used while awaiting recovery. The prognosis of lesions of the radial nerve is often good, as most are simple neurapraxias. Even after complete division and suture, signs of returning muscular function are usually evident within 8 months, according to the level of the lesion.

The purely sensory superficial radial nerve may be compressed during an aberrant route through the forearm extensor musculature, or by radius fractures, tight bindings on the wrists, or ruptured synovial effusions from the elbow joint. The nerve lies superficially, especially in the distal forearm, and often tenderness or a Tinel sign can be evoked at the site of the lesion. The area of sensory loss is shown in Fig. 13.23.

13.10.5 **The posterior interosseous nerve**

This purely motor nerve arises from the radial nerve at the elbow and passes through the supinator muscle in the arcade of Frohse. Lesions result in weakness of supinator (C6, C7), extensor digitorum (C7, C8), extensor carpi ulnaris (C7, C8), and the three extensors of the thumb (C7, C8) (Fig. 13.22). This results in wrist and finger drop without sensory loss. The posterior interosseous nerve may be compressed by various masses such as lipomas, or by abnormalities arising from the elbow joint, or by fibrous anomalies of the arcade of Frohse as it passes through the supinator muscle adjacent to the lateral epicondyle. Repetitive pronation–supination of the forearm, such as using a screwdriver, may precede posterior interosseous nerve palsy, which may be accompanied by local aching; some patients with 'resistant tennis elbow' may be suffering from such compression (Stewart 1993). Surgical exploration should be considered if there is no sign of recovery after 9–12 weeks; occasionally fibrous compressive bands will be found.

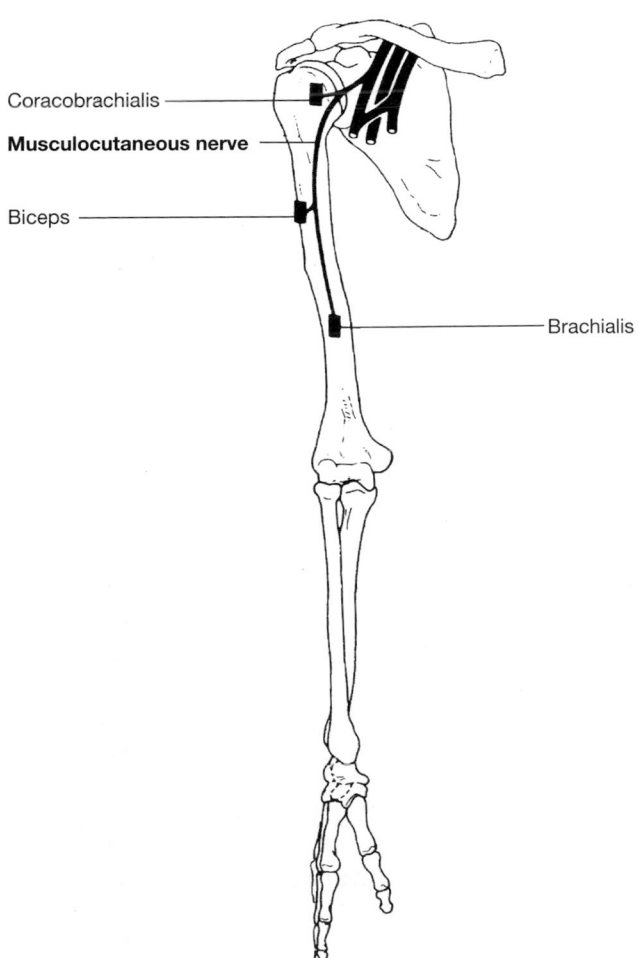

Fig. 13.24. Diagram of the musculoskeletal nerve, showing the muscles it innervates.

13.10.6 **The musculocutaneous nerve**

The musculocutaneous nerve is a branch of the lateral cord of the brachial plexus, its fibres being derived from the C5 and C6 spinal nerves (Fig. 13.24). It supplies the biceps and part of the brachialis, the two principal flexors of the elbow. Its sensory distribution is to the radial border of the forearm as low as the carpometacarpal joint of the thumb, a territory also known as the lateral cutaneous nerve of the forearm (Fig. 13.1).

Division of the musculocutaneous nerve causes weakness of flexion of the elbow joint, although some flexion can still be carried out by brachioradialis and that part of the brachialis which is innervated by the radial nerve. Sensation is impaired over the radial forearm. The musculocutaneous nerve is rarely injured alone, but may be damaged by upper brachial plexus injury, dislocation of the head of the humerus, or by penetrating wounds. Temporary paralysis of the biceps has been known to occur in a man falling asleep with his wife's head lying across his upper arm. The differential diagnosis is from a C6 root lesion, in which case the power and tendon reflex of the brachioradialis would also be lost, and the sensory disturbance would extend below the wrist to the thumb and index finger.

13.10.7 **The axillary (circumflex) nerve**

The axillary nerve arises from the C5 and C6 spinal nerves and the posterior cord of the brachial plexus (Fig. 13.22). It innervates the deltoid muscle (**C5**, **C6**) and its cutaneous branch supplies sensation to an area extending from the acromion process to halfway down the outer aspect of the upper arm (Fig. 13.1). Injury to the axillary nerve causes wasting and weakness of the deltoid, with paralysis of abduction at the shoulder and numbness in the sensory territory (Fig. 13.25). In clinical practice the actual area of sensory loss is often no more than a small area near the insertion of the deltoid. The axillary nerve may be involved by injuries in the region of the neck of the humerus, including dislocation of the shoulder joint, fractures of the upper humerus, and deep intramuscular injections into the deltoid. It may be injured by attempts to reposition a dislocated shoulder, and checking the sensory territory is advised beforehand. It is the nerve most often involved in acute brachial neuritis, in which case there is usually severe and persistent pain in the shoulder region for several hours, or even a few weeks, before the paralysis is noted (Section 13.6.4). Other non-traumatic causes are rare, but it does occur in volleyball players (Paladini *et al.* 1996). In cases due to trauma or compression, operative inspection of the nerve is advised if there is no evidence of recovery at 6 weeks (Mumenthaler 1991).

13.10.8 **The suprascapular nerve**

This nerve is derived from the upper trunk of the brachial plexus and supplies the infraspinatus (**C5**, **C6**) and supraspinatus (**C5**, **C6**) muscles, which respectively externally rotate, and initiate abduction at, the shoulder. There is no sensory component, and weakness, if noticed at all, presents with

(a)

(b)

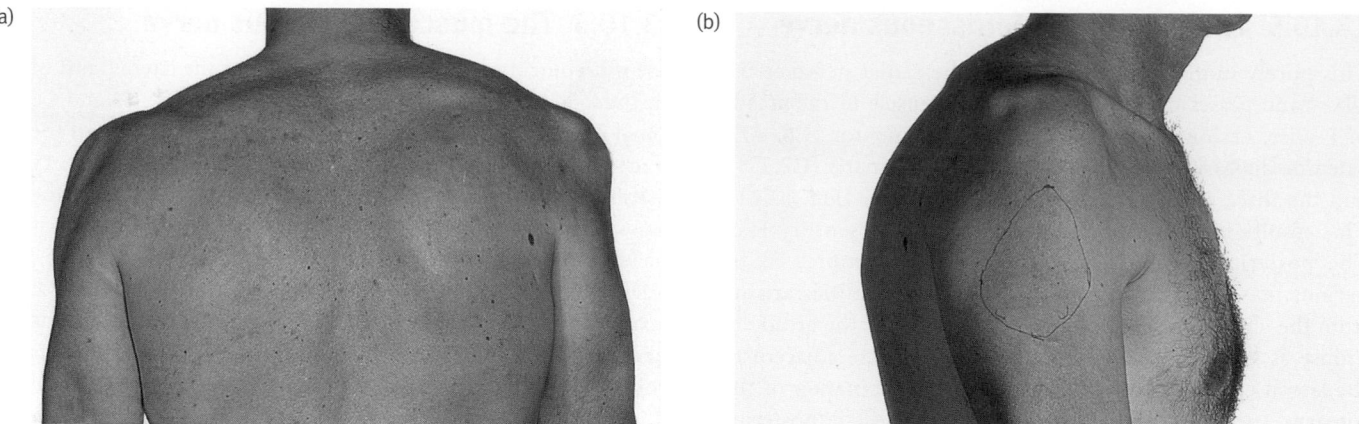

Fig. 13.25. An axillary (circumflex) nerve lesion, showing (a) wasting of the right deltoid muscle (left) and (b) the area of sensory loss on the upper outer arm (right).

inability to initiate shoulder abduction when the arm is hanging at the side, or with difficulty in externally rotating the arm while attempting to write across the page (Mumenthaler 1991). Isolated traumatic lesions of this nerve are rare, although it is occasionally damaged as a sequel of scapular fracture. The nerve may suffer entrapment by a hypertrophied inferior transverse scapular ligament as it passes through the suprascapular foramen in sportsmen, such as fencers (Aiello *et al.* 1982). This may be an unrecognized source of shoulder pain following injury. The spinatus muscles are commonly involved in acute brachial neuritis, often in conjunction with deltoid (Section 13.6.4).

13.10.9 The long thoracic nerve

The long thoracic nerve is derived from the C5, C6, and C7 spinal roots before the formation of the brachial plexus (Fig. 13.6). It supplies the serratus anterior muscle and has no sensory territory. Serratus anterior fixes the scapula to the chest

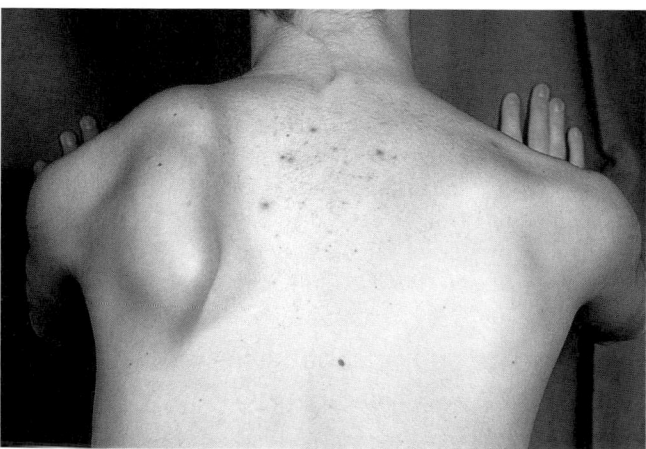

Fig. 13.26. A long thoracic nerve lesion, causing winging of the left scapula when the outstretched arm is pushed forwards against the wall.

wall when the arm is pushed forward in front of the body such as when doing press-ups. Weakness of the muscle causes characteristic winging of the scapula during such movements (Fig. 13.26). Although this weakness may be noted on shoulder movements, equally often the shoulder blade protrusion is first noticed in the bathroom mirror or by others on the beach, or when its protrusion interferes with squeezing through tight spaces. The long thoracic nerve is injured alone most frequently as a result of direct pressure upon the shoulder during carrying, from blows to the shoulder, and during surgical procedures in the axilla. Commonly it is involved in acute brachial neuritis, in which case other muscles are usually also involved (Section 13.6.4). It is occasionally involved in inflammation secondary to apical pleurisy. Autosomal dominantly inherited familial long thoracic nerve palsy is probably a form of hereditary brachial plexus neuropathy (Section 13.6.5) (Phillips 1986). Occasionally the palsy follows pneumonia or other infective illnesses, or arises spontaneously. Compression of the *dorsal scapular nerve* by scalenus medius (Fig. 13.6) is a rare cause of winging of the scapula on wide abduction of the arm (Nakano 1978). Conduction velocity can be measured along the long thoracic nerve and assists in assessing possible lesions. Relatively few isolated lesions recover. Then the question arises as to whether to undertake orthopaedic surgical fixation of the lower angle of the scapula to the ribcage. However, fixation reduces the overall range of shoulder movements and is rarely permanently effective. Dynamic repairs are preferred, such as transposing the insertion of part of pectoralis major onto the lower scapula (Mumenthaler 1991).

13.11 Lower-limb mononeuropathy

13.11.1 The sciatic nerve

Anatomy

The sciatic nerve (Fig. 13.27) is derived from the sacral plexus, which is formed by a fusion of the ventral primary divisions of the L4 and L5 and the S1, S2, and S3 spinal nerves. The nerve is

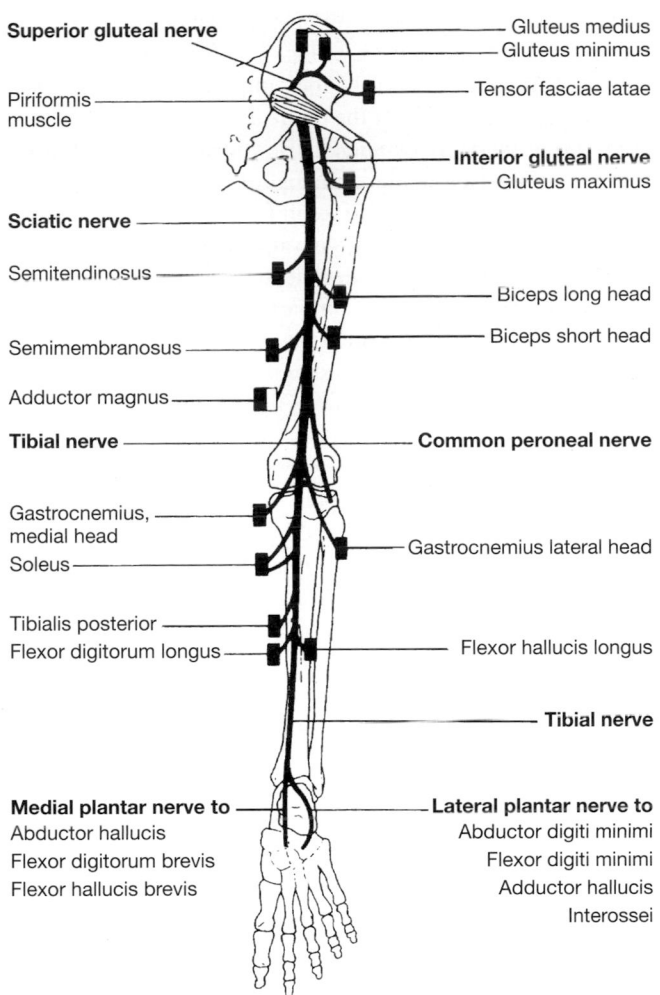

Superior gluteal nerve

Piriformis
muscle

Sciatic nerve

Semitendinosus

Semimembranosus

Adductor magnus

Tibial nerve

Gastrocnemius,
medial head

Soleus

Tibialis posterior
Flexor digitorum longus

Medial plantar nerve to
Abductor hallucis
Flexor digitorum brevis
Flexor hallucis brevis

Gluteus medius
Gluteus minimus

Tensor fasciae latae

Interior gluteal nerve
Gluteus maximus

Biceps long head

Biceps short head

Common peroneal nerve

Gastrocnemius lateral head

Flexor hallucis longus

Tibial nerve

Lateral plantar nerve to
Abductor digiti minimi
Flexor digiti minimi
Adductor hallucis
Interossei

Fig. 13.27. Diagram of the sciatic, tibial, gluteal, and plantar nerves, viewed posteriorly, showing the muscles they innervate.

composed of two trunks, a medial (ventral divisions of L4, L5, S1, S2, and S3) which is destined to form the tibial (medial popliteal) nerve and a lateral (dorsal divisions of L4, L5, S1, and S2) which gives rise to the common peroneal (lateral popliteal) nerve. These two trunks, although bound together by connective tissue, are distinct structures from the moment of their formation in the sacral plexus. This separation of the tibial and peroneal divisions of the nerve means that buttock trauma, such as misplaced injections, may affect either division separately, more usually the more superficially located, common peroneal. The sciatic nerve leaves the pelvis by passing through the great sciatic notch in company with the superior gluteal nerve to gluteus medius and minimus (**L4, L5,** and **S1**), inferior gluteal nerve to gluteus maximus (**L5, S1,** and **S2**), and the posterior cutaneous nerve of the thigh. It enters the buttock, running behind the hip joint, where it usually lies deep to the piriformis muscle. However, anatomical variations occur in this relationship to piriformis, ignorance of which can lead to damage during hip joint surgery: the two trunks can pass on separate sides of this muscle, through the muscle, or anterior to it. Then it enters the back of the thigh, lying midway between

the great trochanter of the femur and the ischial tuberosity, before descending deep to the hamstring muscles. The sciatic nerve terminates at a variable point between the sciatic notch and the popliteal fossa by separating into the common peroneal and tibial nerves. The sciatic nerve supplies the following muscles in the thigh: semitendinosus, semimembranosus and biceps (all L5, S1, and S2) and part of the adductor magnus. Through its terminal branches of the posterior tibial (Section 13.11.2) and common peroneal nerves (Section 13.11.3), the sciatic nerve supplies all muscles below the knee.

Effects of lesions

After complete interruption of the sciatic nerve there is paralysis of flexion of the knee, which is carried out by the hamstrings, and of all the muscles below the knee. Foot-drop occurs as a result of paralysis of the anterior tibial group of muscles and the peronei. The patient can stand and walk, but drags the toes of the affected foot and is unable to stand on his toes or heel on the paralysed side. The skin sensory territory of the sciatic nerve lies entirely below the knee on the lateral half of the calf and dorsum of the foot (common peroneal territory) and the sole and outer border of the foot (posterior tibial territory) (Fig. 13.1). In sciatic nerve lesions the saphenous nerve territory is spared since this is a branch of the femoral nerve which supplies the medial aspects of the calf and the instep. The ankle jerk and plantar reflex are lost, but the knee jerk is retained. Vasomotor and trophic changes are usually conspicuous after complete division: oedema, dry skin, loss of foot sweating, and sometimes ulcers on the sole.

Causes of lesions

The sciatic nerve, or one of its trunks, is usually damaged as a result of fractures and dislocations of the hip joint, pelvis or femur, penetrating wounds of the buttock and thigh, and hip joint replacement surgery (Section 13.7.7) (Yuen *et al.* 1994). Sciatic nerve pressure palsies in the buttock can occur during coma, anaesthesia, enforced recumbency, or meditation. A noteworthy cause of a sciatic nerve lesion is a misplaced injection given too far medially in the buttock rather than in the upper outer quadrant. In such cases, it is usually the common peroneal division of the nerve which is damaged because it lies more superficially. The question of entrapment by the piriformis muscle is debated; this syndrome is said to involve buttock pain radiating down the leg like sciatica, but it is rarely associated with significant clinical or electrophysiological deficits, and the importance of the syndrome remains unclear. The nerve may be compressed within the pelvis by neoplasms, or by deposits of endometriosis at the sciatic notch (Section 13.7.6). Complete division of the nerve is rare. Radiographs of the pelvis and hip joint are necessary in cases resulting from trauma. CT or MRI scans will show lesions within the lower pelvis or sciatic notch. Lack of denervation of paraspinal muscles on EMG will help distinguish sciatic nerve lesions from root compression. Nerve-conduction studies are generally unhelpful in localizing the precise site of a proximal lesion (Dawson *et al.* 1999).

Treatment of sciatic and peroneal nerve lesions

Relatively few sciatic nerve lesions are amenable to surgical correction. It is important to prevent contracture of the Achilles tendon, and the foot should be splinted in dorsiflexion day and night and the ankle moved through its full range passively. Recovery is always slow after suturing a completely divided nerve. In compressive or traction lesions, return of voluntary power is rarely complete, cannot be expected over less than 12–18 months, and usually takes 2–3 years (Yuen *et al.* 1994).

13.11.2 The tibial nerve

Anatomy

The tibial nerve (Fig. 13.27) is an end branch of the sciatic nerve, from which it separates at any point between the sciatic notch and the popliteal fossa. It travels deep to the gastrocnemius muscle and enters the foot via the 'tarsal tunnel' roofed by the flexor retinaculum on the medial aspect of the ankle (Fig. 13.28). It then divides into the calcaneal sensory branches and medial and lateral plantar nerves which supply sensation to the sole of the foot and innervate the intrinsic foot muscles. The tibial nerve supplies gastrocnemius and soleus (S1, S2), tibialis posterior (L4, L5), flexor digitorum longus (L5, S1, S2), and flexor hallucis longus (L5, S1, S2). It gives rise to the medial and lateral plantar nerves supplying the small muscles of the foot (S1, S2).

Effects of lesions

After division of the tibial nerve above gastrocnemius the calf and sole muscles are paralysed and wasted and the foot assumes a position of talipes calcaneovalgus. The ankle jerk is lost, and the plantar reflex may also be inelicitable. Skin sensation is lost over the sole, including the plantar aspect of the toes and the dorsal aspect of their terminal phalanges (Fig. 13.1).

Causes of lesions

The tibial nerve can be compressed in the popliteal fossa by knee-joint cysts, arterial aneurisms, and nerve sheath tumours.

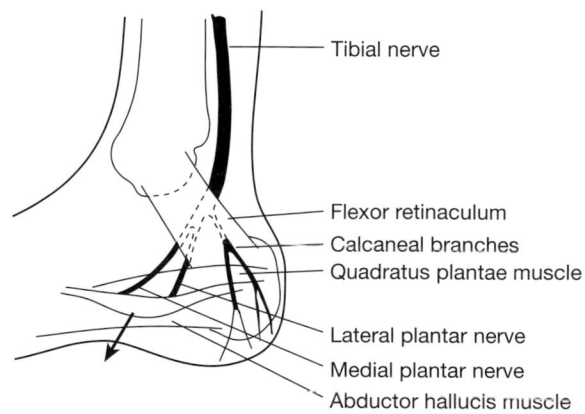

Fig. 13.28. The tarsal tunnel through which the tibial nerve enters the foot (from Stewart 1993).

Occasionally, the posterior tibial nerve may be compressed at the ankle in the tarsal tunnel (Fig. 13.28). This gives rise to burning pain in the sole of the foot and toes and paraesthesiae or sensory loss over almost the entire sole of the foot (the 'posterior' tarsal tunnel syndrome). This syndrome is sometimes a true entrapment by tendon, analogous to carpal tunnel syndrome. More often it seems to result from tight shoes or plaster casts, rheumatoid arthritis, swellings or tenosynositis in the tarsal tunnel, and has been described in hypothyroidism and acromegaly (Stewart 1993). Comparison of motor latency and of sensory-nerve action potentials in the medial and lateral plantar nerves both help in diagnosis, but are somewhat unreliable (Dawson *et al.* 1999).

Occasionally interdigital nerves may be compressed by the adjacent metatarsal heads as they enter the medial aspect of the sole of the foot. This produces pain locally, with numbness and tingling in adjacent toes, worsened by walking or squeezing the forefoot. It usually occurs in the third interspace and is sometimes associated with fusiform neuroma formation, a so-called Morton's neuralgia. Surgical excision of this neuroma may cure the pain (Guiloff *et al.* 1984).

13.11.3 The common peroneal (lateral popliteal) nerve

Anatomy

The common peroneal nerve (Fig. 13.29) is an end branch of the sciatic nerve, from which it separates anywhere between the sciatic notch and the popliteal fossa. It should not be forgotten that pure common peroneal nerve palsies can result from lesions high in the thigh or buttock. Then it winds laterally round the neck of the fibula bone to enter the anterior tibial compartment by passing through the 'fibular tunnel' in the superficial head of peroneus longus. It divides into the superficial and deep peroneal nerves. The superficial nerve supplies the peroneal muscles (L5, S1) and then supplies sensation to the skin of the lower lateral calf and dorsum of the foot (Fig. 13.1). The deep nerve runs deep in the anterior tibial compartment, supplying tibialis anterior (L4, L5), extensor digitorum longus (L5, S1), extensor hallucis longus (L5, S1), and extensor digitorum brevis (L5, S1), and its terminal branch supplies the skin between the first and second toes and the adjacent dorsum of the foot (Fig. 13.1).

Effects of lesions

After division of the common peroneal nerve there is paralysis of dorsiflexion of the foot and toes and of eversion of the foot; foot-drop results. Inversion is lost when the foot is dorsiflexed, but weak inversion is possible in plantar-flexion. When the nerve is divided above the point of origin of the superficial peroneal nerve, sensation is impaired over the dorsum of the foot, including the first two toes, and over the antero-lateral aspect of the lower half of the calf. When the lesion lies below the origin of the superficial peroneal nerve, sensory loss is restricted to the first two toes and adjacent dorsum of the foot.

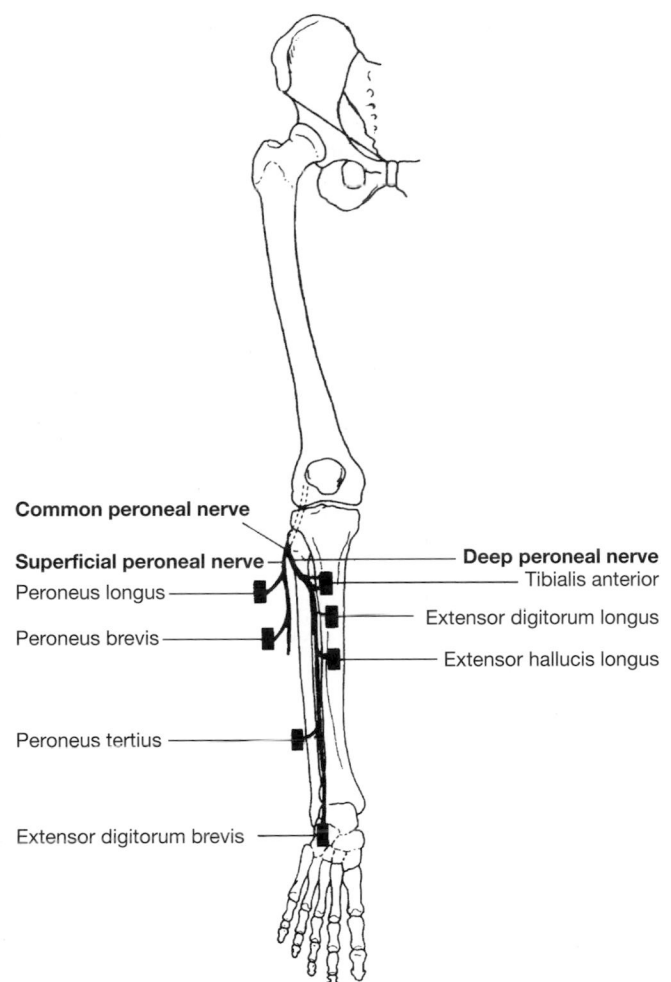

Common peroneal nerve

Superficial peroneal nerve —

Peroneus longus —

Peroneus brevis —

Peroneus tertius —

Extensor digitorum brevis —

Deep peroneal nerve

— Tibialis anterior

— Extensor digitorum longus

— Extensor hallucis longus

Fig. 13.29. Diagram of the common peroneal nerve showing the muscles it innervates.

Causes of lesions

The common peroneal nerve may be injured by penetrating wounds around the knee joint, or by upper fibular fractures. Selective deep peroneal branch injury can occur with arthroscopic knee surgery (Esselman *et al.* 1993). External compression is common, causes including tight bandages or plaster casts applied to the knee, pressure during sleep, and habitual sitting with crossed legs. Emaciated patients are particularly vulnerable, especially those with cancer (Koehler *et al.* 1997). The popliteal fossa should be palpated carefully for bursae, cysts, or tumours; MRI can reveal such lesions compressing the nerve (Fig. 13.30). Prolonged kneeling or squatting can compress the nerve; for instance, in slaters working on roofs with one leg flexed and lying under the other with its outer aspect against the roof surface. Occasionally the nerve is entrapped by a tight fibrous band in the fibular tunnel, relieved by surgery. In cases of entrapment or compression neuropathy, the muscles innervated by the nerve do not always suffer equally. The peronei are usually less severely affected than the anterior tibial group, and the area of sensory loss is often less than that found after complete division (Sourkes and Stewart 1991). Rarely, the

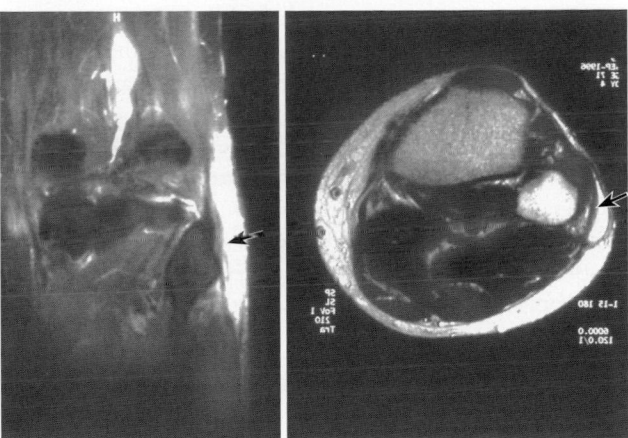

Fig. 13.30. MRI of the knee longitudinally (left) and transversely (right) in a patient with common peroneal nerve palsy caused by a biceps tendon bursa (arrowed).

deep peroneal nerve is selectively compressed by oedema in the anterior compartment syndrome following trauma, ischaemia, or exercise of the lower leg (Section 5.11.6). Terminal sensory branches of the superficial peroneal nerve may be entrapped where they pierce the fascia above the ankle, becoming symptomatic after minor ankle trauma (Styf 1989).

Spontaneously occurring common peroneal nerve palsies of uncertain cause are quite common. They often recover in 2 or 3 months with avoidance of leg crossing or kneeling. Sometimes surgical inspection of the nerve at the fibular neck is required in those for whom there was no convincing explanation for the mononeuropathy, and in whom no spontaneous recovery occurs by 3 months. For it is only at operative inspection that entrapment by fibrous band can be identified. The diagnosis of a common peroneal palsy can be confirmed by measurements of nerve-conduction velocity in the nerve, which may show conduction block across the head of the fibula, particularly if a more proximal stimulation point is used and recordings made from a range of muscles (Sourkes and Stewart 1991). Slowing of sensory conduction across that segment of the nerve localized the lesion accurately in 64 per cent of a series of 47 patients (Singh *et al.* 1974). Sometimes the amplitude of the compound muscle action potential recorded by surface electrodes over the extensor digitorum brevis muscle during supramaximal stimulation of the nerve may be larger on stimulation at the knee than at the ankle. This is due to an anomalous branch of the superficial peroneal nerve, the accessory deep peroneal nerve, which passes alongside the peroneus brevis muscle and behind the lateral malleolus, and supplies the lateral part of the extensor digitorum brevis (Dessi *et al.* 1992).

13.11.4 **The sural nerve**

The sural nerve normally arises from the tibial nerve in the upper calf. It attains a superficial route halfway down the calf and runs lateral to the Achilles' tendon, where it usually receives a contribution from the common peroneal nerve. It passes behind the lateral malleolus to enter the foot and supply sensation to the outer border of the foot from the heel to the fourth and fifth toes (Fig. 13.1). Lesions cause numbness and paraesthesiae in this area. There is no motor component. The most common lesion is total or partial transection for the purposes of diagnostic nerve biopsy, and uncomfortable dysaesthesiae may result (Section 12.2). Otherwise, sural mononeuropathy is rare, but described following local trauma, surgery, lacerations, and external compression at the ankle (Reisin *et al.* 1994). Lesions can result from compression by a Baker's cyst at the knee.

13.11.5 The femoral nerve

Anatomy

The femoral nerve (Fig. 13.31) is derived from the lumbar plexus in the psoas major muscle, arising from the dorsal parts of the L2, L3, and L4 spinal nerves, posterior to the obturator nerve. After passing through the pelvis, where it is vulnerable to compression in the gutter between iliacus and psoas (Section 13.7), it enters the femoral triangle of the thigh beneath the inguinal ligament, lateral to the femoral sheath and vessels. In the abdomen it sends a branch to iliacus. In the femoral triangle it divides into terminal branches which include the supply to the quadriceps (L2, L3, L4). It gives articular branches to the hip and knee joints. The intermediate and medial cutaneous branches supply the anterior and medial aspects of the lower two-thirds of the thigh (Fig. 13.1). The saphenous nerve supplies sensation to the inner aspect of the calf and instep (Fig. 13.1).

Effects of lesions

Proximal lesions of the femoral nerve produce slight weakness of hip flexion due to paralysis of iliacus, but the principal motor disturbance is weakness of knee extension, owing to paralysis of quadriceps. In consequence the leg gives way in walking and climbing stairs, and arising from sitting is difficult. The knee jerk is lost. Sensation is lost over the cutaneous area innervated by the nerve. Usually the clinical picture is unmistakable. It is distinguished from a lumbar plexus lesion by the preservation of thigh adductor power supplied by the obturator nerve. Causalgia may occur in the distribution of the saphenous nerve after partial lesions.

Causes of lesions

The intrapelvic femoral nerve may be damaged by pelvic surgery, psoas abscess, pelvic neoplasia, or iliacus haematoma (Section 13.7). It may be injured in fractures of the pelvis or of the femur, or by hip dislocation or hip replacement. Lesions of this nerve are rarely seen as a result of penetrating wounds of the thigh, as the proximity of the femoral artery renders most such injuries rapidly fatal. Femoral neuropathy may be induced by the lithotomy position. The most common lesion is diabetic proximal neuropathy. Measurement of femoral nerve conduction velocity and terminal latency are valuable in localization by narrowing down muscular involvement to the femoral nerve distribution, but rarely help localize the level of the nerve injury. CT scan or MRI is essential for the diagnosis of intrapelvic femoral nerve lesions.

13.11.6 The saphenous nerve

This long and superficial sensory branch of the femoral nerve is usually damaged by penetrating injuries or surgery. Occasionally it is compressed by stirrups at the inner knee during surgery or childbirth. It supplies sensation to the medial calf and instep (Fig. 13.1). An entrapment syndrome at the exit from Hunter's canal, some 10 cm proximal to the medial femoral condyle, has been postulated. However, there is generally insufficiently clear evidence of sensory loss to make definite this diagnosis of entrapment mononeuropathy (Stewart 1993).

13.11.7 The lateral cutaneous nerve of the thigh

The lateral cutaneous nerve of the thigh is purely sensory and derived from the dorsal divisions of the L2 and L3 spinal

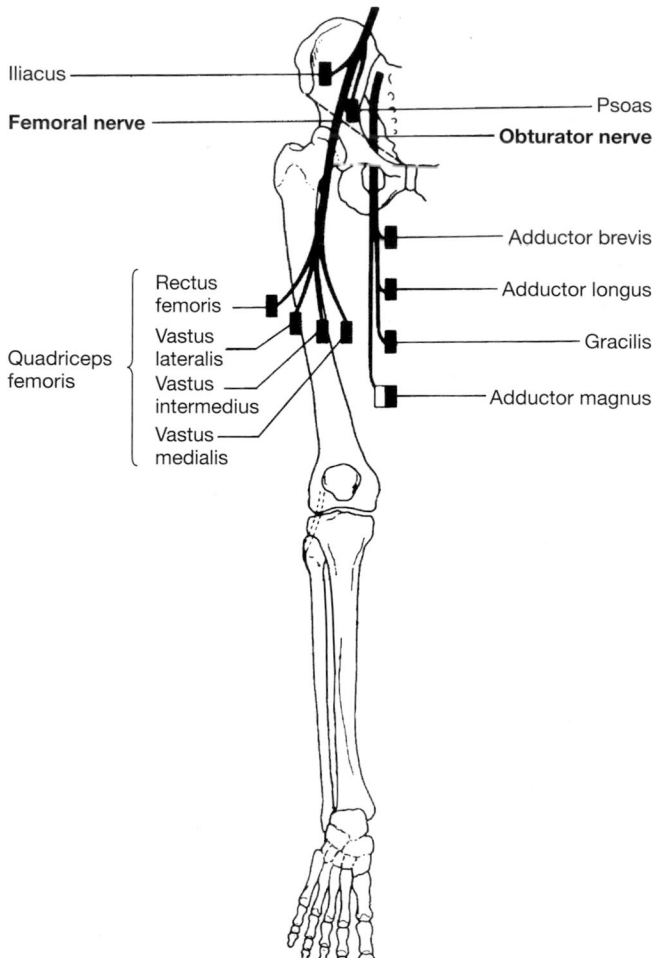

Iliacus

Femoral nerve

Psoas

Obturator nerve

Adductor brevis

Adductor longus

Rectus femoris

Vastus lateralis

Vastus intermedius

Vastus medialis

Quadriceps femoris

Gracilis

Adductor magnus

Fig. 13.31. Diagram of the femoral and obturator nerves, showing the muscles they supply.

nerves. After passing through psoas major and winding round the lateral wall of the pelvis, it enters the thigh beneath the lateral end of the inguinal ligament. It emerges superficially from fascia lata of the thigh about 10 cm distal to the anterior superior iliac spine. Then it divides into an anterior and a posterior branch which carry sensation from the lateral and anterolateral aspects of the thigh from the buttock almost down to the knee (Fig. 13.1). Lesions are usually thought to be due to entrapment and kinking where the nerve passes through the inguinal ligament. This is most common in obese or pregnant patients, who experience uncomfortable paraesthesiae in the lateral thigh, particularly on walking, a syndrome known as 'meralgia paraesthetica'. Numbness is demonstrable in the nerve's territory. Evidence of subclinical entrapment at the inguinal ligament is a common autopsy finding (Jefferson and Eames 1979). Meralgia paraesthetica often resolves spontaneously. When pain is more troublesome, repeated infiltration of local anaesthetic around the lateral half of the inguinal ligament may relieve symptoms. If this is unsuccessful, operative decompression of the nerve just medial to the anterior superior iliac spine may be indicated. Occasionally intrapelvic causes underlie isolated lesions of the lateral cutaneous nerve of the thigh; these are similar to causes of intrapelvic femoral nerve lesions (Sections 13.7, 13.11.5), and some will be revealed by pelvic MRI. They may present with similar symptoms to lesions at the inguinal ligament, although walking-induced pain is less likely.

13.11.8 **The obturator nerve**

Anatomy

The obturator nerve (Fig. 13.31) is derived from the L2, L3, and L4 spinal nerves by branches anterior to those forming the femoral nerve. The union of these roots occurs in the psoas muscle and the nerve emerges from the pelvis by the obturator foramen to supply the thigh adductors (**L2, L3,** L4). It gives branches to the knee and hip joints. Its skin territory is variable, generally comprising a small area on the upper medial thigh (Fig. 13.1).

Lesions

Injury to the obturator nerve causes paralysis of the thigh adductors, except for the flexor fibres of the adductor magnus, which are innervated by the sciatic nerve. Sensory loss is often not detected. Isolated lesions are rare, but can occur with hip and pelvic fractures or hip joint surgery, obstructed labour, abdominal or pelvic surgery, or pelvic cancers (Rogers *et al.* 1993). Occasionally the nerve may be compressed in the obturator canal by an obturator hernia or as a result of osteitis pubis following genito-urinary surgery. If the cause remains undiagnosed, CT or MRI of the pelvis is necessary to detect an occult tumour. In obturator neuropathy, the knee jerk and quadriceps power are normal, thereby excluding a lumbar root lesion or plexopathy.

13.11.9 **The ilioinguinal nerve**

This nerve, derived from the L1 and L2 roots, passes round the abdominal wall in the region of the pelvic rim and through the inguinal canal, to provide sensation to a narrow band of skin across the upper thigh, inguinal region, iliac crest, and the base of the scrotum (or labium majoris) (Fig. 13.1). It contributes motor fibres to the lower abdominal muscles. It is occasionally affected by direct injury, by herniorrhaphy repair, or by other surgical and invasive procedures on the lower abdomen or iliac crest (Stulz and Pfeiffer 1982). Entrapment in abdominal wall muscles near to the anterior superior iliac spine has been described. Pain in the groin, sometimes causing the patient to adopt a flexed posture, is the usual manifestation, and injection of local anaesthetic around the nerve, or division of it, usually affords relief (Stewart 1993).

13.11.10 **The genitofemoral nerve**

The genitofemoral nerve derives from the L1 and L2 spinal roots and is formed from the lumbar plexus in the psoas muscle. It runs down that muscle to separate into the genital and femoral branches. The genital supplies the scrotal cremaster muscle and sensation to the scrotum, labium majoris, and upper medial thigh. The femoral branch supplies skin in the femoral triangle on the upper anterior thigh. This nerve may be entrapped by intra-abdominal adhesions (especially after appendicectomy) or may be damaged by injury to the groin (Nakano 1978). The genital branch can be involved by inguinal hernia surgery. Genitofemoral nerve lesions also follow the wearing of excessively tight jeans (O'Brien 1979). There is pain in the internal inguinal ring, relieved by hip flexion, and there may be sensory impairment in the skin of the femoral triangle. The cremasteric contraction reflex evoked by scratching the inner upper thigh may be lost on the affected side. Surgical decompression is occasionally needed.

13.11.11 **The pudendal nerve**

The pudendal nerve is derived from the S2, S3, and S4 spinal nerve contributions to the sacral plexus. It leaves the pelvis through the sciatic notch, then passing anteriorly into the perineum. It supplies sensation to the scrotum, perineal skin, bladder, rectum, lower vagina and labium, and innervates the erectile tissue of the clitoris or penis. Its dorsal nerve of the penis or clitoris transmits erotic sensations from these organs. Surgical trauma and mass lesions within the pelvis can damage the pudendal nerve. Once outside the pelvis, it can be compressed by prolonged bicycle riding using a hard seat, or by the perineal posts used during hip joint surgery to allow traction for reducing hip fractures (Stewart 1993). Lesions seem to be more commonly symptomatic in men, who complain of perineal pain and numbness of half of the penis, sometimes with mild erectile failure.

References

Aiello, I., Serra, G., Traina, G. C. *et al.* (1982). Entrapment of the suprascapular nerve at the spinoglenoid notch. *Ann. Neurol.*, **12**, 314–16.

Berry, P. R. and Wallis, W. E. (1977). Venepuncture nerve injuries. *Lancet*, **I**, 1236–37.

Bhatia, K. P., Bhatt, M. H., and Marsden, C. D. (1993). The causalgia–dystonia syndrome. *Brain*, **116**, 843–51.

Bilbao, J. M., Koury, N. J. S., Hudson, A. R. *et al.* (1984). Perineuroma (localised hypertrophic neuropathy). *Arch. Pathol. Lab. Med.*, **108**, 557–60.

Birch, R., Bonney, G., and Wynn Parry, C. B. (1998). *Surgical disorders of the peripheral nerves*. Churchill Livingstone, Edinburgh.

Bradley, W. G., Madrid, R., Thrush, D. C. *et al.* (1975). Recurrent brachial plexus neuropathy. *Brain*, **98**, 381–98.

Brown, T., Cupido, C., Scarfore, H. *et al.* (2000). Developmental apraxia arising from neonatal brachial plexus palsy. *Neurology*, **55**, 24–30.

Chabal, C., Jacobson, L., Mariano, A. *et al.* (1992). The use of oral mexilitine for the treatment of pain after peripheral nerve injury. *Anaesthesiology*, **76**, 513–17.

Challenor, Y. B., Richter, R. W., Bruun, B. *et al.* (1973). Nontraumatic plexitis and heroin addiction. *JAMA*, **225**, 958–61.

Chapman, E. M., Shaw, R. S., and Kubik, C. S. (1964). Sciatic pain from arteriosclerotic aneurysm of pelvic arteries. *N. Engl. J. Med.*, **271**, 1410–11.

Chaudhry, V. and Clawson, L. L. (1997). Entrapment of motor nerves in motor neuron disease: does double crush occur? *J. Neurol. Neursurg. Psychiat.*, **62**, 71–6.

Chelimsky, T. C., Low, P. A., Noessens, J. M. *et al.* (1995). Value of autonomic testing in reflex sympathetic dystrophy. *Mayo Clinic Proc.*, **70**, 1029–40.

Cherington, M., Happer, I., Machanic, B. *et al.* (1986). Surgery for thoracic outlet syndrome may be hazardous to your health. *Muscle and Nerve*, **9**, 632–4.

Critchley, M. (1953). *The parietal lobes*. Edward Arnold, London.

Cusimano, M. D., Bilbao, J. M., and Cohen, S. M. (1988). Hypertrophic brachial plexus neuritis: a pathological study of two cases. *Ann. Neurol.*, **24**, 615–22.

Dawson, D. M., Hallett, M., and Wilbourn, A. J. (1999). *Entrapment neuropathies*, (3rd edn). Lippincott-Raven, Philadelphia.

Dessi, F., Durand, G., and Hoffman, J.-J. (1992). The accessory deep peroneal nerve: a pitfall for the electromyographer. *J. Neurol. Neurosurg. Psychiat.*, **55**, 214–15.

Donaghy, M. (1993). Lumbosacral plexus lesions. In *Peripheral neuropathy*, (3rd edn), (ed. P. K. Thomas and P. J. Dyck). W. B. Saunders, Philadelphia.

Donaghy, M., Matkovic, Z., and Morris, P. (1999). Surgery for suspected neurogenic thoracic outlet syndromes: a follow up study. *J. Neurol. Neurosurg. Psychiat.*, **67**, 602–6.

Donaldson, J. O. (1988). *Neurology of pregnancy*, (2nd edn). W. B. Saunders, London.

England, J. D. and Sumner, A. J. (1987). Neuralgic amyotrophy: an increasingly diverse entity. *Muscle Nerve*, **10**, 60–8.

Esselman, P. C., Tanski, M. A., Robinson, L. R. *et al.* (1993). Selective deep peroneal nerve injury associated with arthroscopic knee surgery. *Muscle Nerve*, **16**, 1188–92.

Evans, B. A., Stevens, J. C., and Dyck, P. J. (1981). Lumbosacral plexus neuropathy. *Neurology*, **31**, 1327–30.

Feasby, T. E., Burton, S. R., and Hahn, A. F. (1992). Obstetrical lumbosacral plexus injury. *Muscle Nerve*, **15**, 937–40.

Foley, K. M., Woodruff, J. M., Ellis, F. T. *et al.* (1980). Radiation-induced malignant and atypical peripheral nerve sheath tumours. *Ann. Neurol.*, **7**, 311–18.

Gilliatt, R. W. (1984). Thoracic outlet syndromes. In *Peripheral neuropathy*, (2nd edn), (ed. P. J. Dyck, P. K. Thomas, E. H. Lambert *et al.*). W. B. Saunders, Philadelphia.

Gilliatt, R. W., Le Quesne, P. M., Logue, V., and Sumner, A. J. (1970). Wasting of the hand associated with a cervical rib or band. *J. Neurol. Neurosurg. Psychiat.*, **33**, 615–24.

Girlanda, P., Dattola, R., Venuto, C. *et al.* (1993). Local steroid treatment in idiopathic carpal tunnel syndrome: short- and long-term efficacy. *J. Neurol.*, **240**, 187–90.

Gonik, B., Stringer, C. A., Cotton, D. B. *et al.* (1984). Intrapartum maternal lumbosacral plexopathy. *Obstet. Gynecol.*, **63**, 45–46S.

Goodell, S. E., Quinn, T. C., Mkrtichian, E. *et al.* (1983). Herpes simplex proctitis in homosexual men—clinical, sigmoidoscopic and histopathologic features. *N. Engl. J. Med.*, **308**, 868–71.

Goudier, R., Leguern, E., Emle, J. *et al.* (1994). Hereditary neuralgic amyotrophy and hereditary neuropathy with liability to pressure palsies. *Neurology*, **44**, 2250–2.

Goulding, P. J. and Schady, W. (1993). Favourable outcome in non-traumatic anterior interosseous nerve lesion. *J. Neurol.*, **240**, 83–6.

Gregory, R. P., Loh, L., and Newsom-Davis, J. (1990). Recurrent isolated alternating phrenic nerve palsies: a variant of brachial neuritis? *Thorax*, **45**, 420–1.

Guiloff, R. J., Scadding, J. W., and Klenerman, L. (1984). Morton's neuralgia. *J. Bone Joint Surg.*, **66B**, 586–91.

Harding, A. E. and Le Fanu, J. (1977). Carpal tunnel syndrome related to antebrachial Cimino–Brescia fistula. *J. Neurol. Neurosurg. Psychiat.*, **40**, 511–13.

Harper, C. M., Thomas, J. E., Cascino, T. L. *et al.* (1989). Distinction between neoplastic and radiation-induced brachial plexopathy, with emphasis on the role of EMG. *Neurology*, **39**, 502–6.

Head, H. and Sherren, J. (1905). The consequences of injury to the peripheral nerves in man. *Brain*, **28**, 116–338.

Hemrika, D. J., Schutte, M. F., and Bleker, O. P. (1986). Elsberg syndrome: a neurologic basis for acute urinary retention in patients with genital herpes. *Obstet. Gynecol.*, **68**, 37–39S.

Huttinen, V.-M. and Slatis, P. (1972). Nerve injury in double vertical pelvic fractures. *Acta Chir. Scand.*, **138**, 571–5.

Ismael, S. S., Amarenco, G., Bayle, B. *et al.* (2000). Postpartum lumbosacral plexopathy limited to autonomic and perineal manifestations: clinical and electrophysiological study of 19 patients. *J. Neurol. Neurosurg. Psychiat.*, **68**, 771–3.

Iyer, V. and Fenichel, G. M. (1976). Normal median nerve proximal latency in carpal tunnel syndrome: a clue to coexisting Martin–Gruber anastomosis. *J. Neurol. Neurosurg. Psychiat.*, **39**, 449–52.

Jefferson, D. and Eames, R. A. (1979). Subclinical entrapment of the lateral femoral cutaneous nerve: an autopsy study. *Muscle Nerve*, **2**, 145–54.

Koehler, P. J., Buscher, M., Rozeman, C. A. M. *et al.* (1997). Peroneal nerve neuropathy in cancer patients: a paraneoplastic syndrome? *J. Neurol.*, **244**, 328–32.

Kiloh, L. G. and Nevin, S. (1952). Isolated neuritis of the anterior interosseous nerve. *BMJ*, **i**, 850–1.

Kincaid (1988). *Muscle Nerve*, **11**, 1005–15.

Krendel, D. A., Stahl, R. L., and Chan, W. C. (1991). Lymphomatous polyneuropathy. Biopsy of clinically involved nerve and successful treatment. *Arch. Neurol.*, **48**, 330–2.

Laroche, C. M., Moxham, J., and Green, M. (1989). Respiratory muscle weakness and fatigue. *Quart. J. Med.*, **71**, 373–97.

Lederman, R, I, and Wilhourn, A. J. (1996). Postpartum neuralgic amyotrophy. *Neurology*, **47**, 1213–19.

Levin, K. H. and Lutz, G. (1996). Angiotropic large-cell lymphoma with peripheral nerve and skeletal muscle involvement. *Neurology*, **47**, 1009–11.

Loh, L., Nathan, P., and Schott, G. D. (1981). Pain due to lesions of central nervous system removed by sumpathetic block. *BMJ*, **282**, 1026–8.

Malow, B. A. and Dawson, D. M. (1991). Neuralgic amyotrophy in association with radiation therapy for Hodgkin's disease. *Neurology*, **41**, 440–1.

Melzack, R. and Wall, P. D. (1965). Pain mechanisms: a new theory. *Science*, **150**, 971–9.

Meyer, R., Brown, H. P., and Harrison, J. H. (1959). Herpes zoster involving the urinary bladder. *N. Engl. J. Med.*, **260**, 1062–5.

Morris, H. H. and Peters, B. H. (1976). Pronator syndrome: clinical and electrophysiological features in seven cases. *J. Neurol. Neurosurg. Psychiat.*, **39**, 461–4.

Mumenthaler, M. (1991). Lesions of individual nerves in the shoulder and arm region. In *Peripheral nerve lesions: diagnosis and therapy,* (ed. M. Mumenthaler and H. Schliack). Thieme, New York.

Murakami, T., Tachibana, S., Endo, Y. *et al.* (1994). Familial carpal tunnel syndrome due to amyloidogenic transthyretin His 114 variant. *Neurology*, **44**, 315–18.

Nakano, K. K. (1978). The entrapment neuropathies. *Muscle Nerve*, **1**, 264–79.

Narakas, A. (1991). Principles of the operative treatment of peripheral nerve lesions. In *Peripheral nerve lesions: diagnosis and therapy,* (ed. M. Mumenthaler and H. Schliack). Thieme, New York.

Newsom-Davis, J. (1967). Phrenic nerve conduction in man. *J. Neurol. Neurosurg. Psychiat.*, **30**, 420–6.

Noordenbos, W. and Wall, P. D. (1981). Implications of the failure of nerve resection and graft to cure chronic pain produced by nerve lesions. *J. Neurol. Neurosurg. Psychiat.*, **44**, 1068–73.

O'Brien, M. D. (1979). Genitofemoral neuropathy. *BMJ*, **1**, 1052.

Paladini, D., Dellantonio, R., Cinti, A. *et al.* (1996). Axillary neuropathy in volleyball players: report of two cases and literature review. *J. Neurol. Neurosurg. Psychiat.*, **60**, 345–7.

Panegyres, P. K., Moore, N., Gibson, R. *et al.* (1993). Thoracic outlet syndromes and magnetic resonance imaging. *Brain*, **116**, 823–41.

Phillips, L. H. (1986). Familial long thoracic nerve palsy: a manifestation of brachial plexus neuropathy. *Neurology*, **36**, 1251–3.

Reisin R, Pardal A, Ruggieri V, *et al.* (1994). Sural neuropathy due to external pressure: report of three cases. *Neurology* **44**: 2408–09.

Rogers LR, Borkowski GP, Alberts JW, *et al.* (1993). Obturator mononeuropathy caused by pelvic cancer. *Neurology* **43**: 1489–92.

Rudge, P., Ochoa, J., and Gilliatt, R. W. (1974). Acute peripheral nerve compression in the baboon. *J. Neurol. Sci.*, **23**, 403–20.

Salazar-Grueso, E. and Roos, R. (1986). Sciatic endometriosis: a treatable sensorimotor mononeuropathy. *Neurology*, **36**, 1360–3.

Schott, G. D. (1983). A chronic and painless form of idiopathic brachial plexus neuropathy. *J. Neurol. Neurosurg. Psychiat.*, **46**, 555–7.

Schott, G. D. (1986). Mechanisms of causalgia and related clinical conditions. *Brain*, **109**, 717–38.

Schott, G. D. (1998). Interrupting the sympathetic outflow in causalgia and reflex sympathetic dystrophy. *BMJ*, **316**, 792–3.

Schwartzman, R. J. and McLellan, T. L. (1987). Reflex sympathetic dystrophy. A review. *Arch. Neurol.*, **44**, 555–61.

Seddon, H. J. (1944). Three types of nerve injury. *Brain*, **66**, 237–88.

Sharma, K. R., Sriram, S., Fries, T., and Bevan, H. J. (1993). Lumbosacral radiculoplexopathy as a manifestation of Epstein–Barr virus infection. *Neurology*, **43**, 2550–4.

Shyu, W.-C., Lin, J.-C., Chang, M.-K., and Tsao, W.-L. (1993). Compressive radial nerve palsy induced by military shooting training: clinical and electrophysiological study. *J. Neurol. Neurosurg. Psychiat.*, **56**, 890–3.

Singh, N., Behse, F., and Buchthal, F. (1974). Electrophysiological study of peroneal palsy. *J. Neurol. Neurosurg. Psychiat.*, **37**, 1202–13.

Smith, T. and Trojaborg, W. (1987). Diagnosis of thoracic outlet syndrome. Value of sensory and motor conduction studies and quantitative electromyography. *Arch. Neurol.*, **44**, 1161–3.

Sourkes, M. and Stewart, J. D. (1991). Common peroneal neuropathy: a study of selective motor and sensory involvement. *Neurology*, **41**, 1029–33.

Stanton-Hicks, M., Janig, W., Hassenusch, S. *et al.* (1995). Reflex sympathetic dystrophy: changing concepts and taxanomy. *Pain*, **63**, 127–33.

Stewart, J. D. (1993). Compression and entrapment neuropathies. In *Peripheral neuropathy*, (3rd edn), (ed. P. J. Dych, P. K. Thomas, J. W. Griffin, *et al.*). W. B. Saunders, Philadelphia.

Stögbauer, F., Young, P., Kuhlenbäumer, G. *et al.* (2000). Hereditary recurrent focal neuropathies: clinical and molecular features. *Neurology*, **54**, 546–51.

Stöhr, M., Dichgans, J., and Dorstelmann, D. (1980). Ischaemic neuropathy of the lumbosacral plexus following intragluteal injection. *J. Neurol. Neurosurg. Psychiat.*, **43**, 489–94.

Stulz, P. and Pfeiffer, K. M. (1982). Peripheral nerve injuries resulting from common surgical procedures in the lower portion of the abdomen. *Arch. Surg.*, **117**, 324–7.

Styf, J. (1989). Entrapment of the superficial peroneal nerve. *J. Bone Joint Surg.*, **71B**, 131–5.

Symonds, C. P. and Meadows, S. P. (1937). Compression of the spinal cord in the neighbourhood of the foramen magnum. *Brain*, **60**, 52–84.

Taysvaer, A. T. (1982). Computerised tomography and surgical treatment of femoral compression neuropathy. *J. Neurosurg.*, **57**, 137–9.

Thomas, J. E., Cescino, T. L., and Earle, J. D. (1985). Differential diagnosis between radiation and tumour plexopathy of the pelvis. *Neurology*, **35**, 1–7.

Thyagarajan, D., Cascino, T., and Harms, G. (1995). Magnetic resonance imaging in brachial plexopathy of cancer. *Neurology*, **45**, 421–7.

Trivedi, R. A., Byrne, J., Huson, S. M. *et al.* (2000). Focal amyotrophy in neurofibromatosis type 2. *J. Neurol. Neurosurg. Psychiat.*, **69**, 257–61.

Tsairis, P., Dyck, P. J., and Mulder, D. W. (1972). Natural history of brachial plexus neuropathy. *Arch. Neurol.*, **27**, 109–17.

Upton, A. R. and McComas, A. J. (1973). The double crush in nerve entrapment syndromes. *Lancet*, **2**, 359–62.

Urbaniak, J. R. (1990). Direct repair. In *Controversies in hand surgery*, (ed. R. J. Neviaser). Churchill Livingstone, New York.

Van Alfen, N., Van Engelen, B. G. M., Reinders, J. W. C. *et al.* (2000). The natural history of hereditary neuralgic amyotrophy in the Dutch population. Two distinct types? *Brain*, **123**, 718–23.

Van der Laan, L., ter Laak, H. J., Gabreels-Festen, A. *et al.* (1998). Complex regional pain syndrome type 1 (RSD). Pathology of skeletal muscle and peripheral nerve. *Neurology*, **51**, 20–5.

Verma, A. and Bradley, W. G. (1994). High dose intravenous immunoglobulin therapy in chronic progressive lumbosacral plexopathy. *Neurology*, **44**, 248–50.

Wasner, G., Heckmann, K., Maier, C. *et al.* (1999). Vascular abnormalities in acute reflex sympathetic dystrophy (CRPS 1): complete inhibition of sympathetic nerve activity with recovery. *Arch. Neurol.*, **56**, 613 20.

Weber, E. R., Daube, J. R., and Coventry, M. B. (1976). Peripheral neuropathies associated with total hip arthroplasty. *J. Bone Joint Surg.*, **58**, 66–9.

Wilbourn, A. J. (1993). Brachial plexus disorders. In *Peripheral neuropathy*, (3rd edn), (ed. P. J. Dyck, P. K. Thomas, J. W. Griffin, *et al.*). W. B. Saunders, Philadelphia.

Wilbourn, A. J. and Gilliatt, R. W. (1997). Double-crush syndrome: a critical analysis. *Neurology*, **49**, 21–9.

Wilbourn, A. J., Furlan, A. J., Hulley, W., and Ruschhaupt, W. (1983). Ischaemic monomelic neuropathy. *Neurology*, **33**, 447–51.

Wood, V. E., Twito, R., and Verska, J. M. (1988). Thoracic outlet syndrome. The results of first rib resection in 100 patients. *Orthop. Clin. North Am.*, **19**, 131–46.

Yuen, E. C., Olney, R. K., and So, Y. T. (1994). Sciatic neuropathy: clinical and prognostic features in 73 patients. *Neurology*, **44**, 1669–74.

Zarranz, J. J., Simon, R., and Salisachs, P. (1981). Acute anticoagulant-induced compressive lumbar plexus neuropathy. *Eur. Neurol.*, **20**, 469–72.

Zeman, A. and Donaghy, M. (1991). Acute infection with human immunodeficiency virus presenting with urinary retention. *Genitourin. Med.*, **67**, 345–7.

CHAPTER 14

The motor neuron diseases

Michael Donaghy

14.1 Introduction

14.1.1 Classification

The term 'motor neuron disease' is used ambiguously. Patients, the general public, and many doctors use the term synonymously with amyotrophic lateral sclerosis, the gravest and most frequent of all the motor neuron diseases. However, 'motor neuron disease' is best employed as an umbrella term defining all those diseases that involve selective loss of function of the upper and/or lower motor neurons innervating the voluntary musculature of the limbs and bulbar regions. Precise diagnosis within this group of diseases is essential for advising about prognosis, possible genetic implications, and for identifying those with acquired lower motor neuron syndromes who may benefit from immunomodulation. Table 14.1 classifies the various motor neuron disorders according to whether the upper motor neuron, the lower, or both is affected.

14.1.2 Differential diagnosis

In any patient with a motor neuron disease, precise differential diagnosis requires clinical and electrophysiological classification as to whether the disease involves the upper motor neurons, or the lower, or both. This anatomical differentiation is augmented by age of onset, rate of deterioration, any inheritance, and the anatomical distribution of clinical features, so as to make a

Table 14.1. Classification of the motor neuron diseases

Combined upper and lower motor neuron involvement:
  Amyotrophic lateral sclerosis
    sporadic (A, E)
    familial adult onset (A) [ad]
    familial juvenile onset (c) [ar]

Pure lower motor neuron involvement:
  Proximal hereditary motor neuronopathy
  Acute infantile form (Werdnig–Hoffmann; I) [ar]
  Chronic childhood form (Kugelberg–Welander; I, C) [ar]
  Adult onset forms (A) [ar] [ad]
  Hereditary bulbar palsy
    with deafness (Brown–Violetta–Van Laere; C, A) [?]
    without deafness (Fazio–Londe; C) [ar]
  X-linked bulbospinal neuronopathy (A, E) [slr]
  Hexosaminidase deficiency (C, A) [ar]
  Multifocal motor neuropathies (A, E)
  Postpolio syndrome (E)
  Postirradiation syndrome (A, E)
  Monomelic, focal, or segmental spinal muscular atrophy (A)

Pure upper motor neuron involvement:
  Primary lateral sclerosis (A, E)
  Hereditary spastic paraplegia (A, E) [ar]
  Lathyrism (A)
  Konzo (A)

Age of onset: I, infantile; C, childhood; A, adult (15–50 years); E, elderly (more than 50 years).
Inheritance: ad, autosomal dominant; ar, autosomal recessive; slr, sex-linked recessive.

precise diagnosis (Table 14.1). As a general rule, somatosensation and cognition are normal on clinical examination in the motor neuron diseases. Sphincter control and sexual function are usually preserved in motor neuron diseases, although trunk and abdominal wall weakness may make these activities slow and awkward.

The clinical features of lower motor neuron involvement are muscle wasting, fasciculations, and flaccid weakness. Tendon reflexes are usually retained until profound denervation or fibrous replacement have affected the muscle. In amyotrophic lateral sclerosis the upper motor neuron involvement helps to preserve reflexes. Motor neuron diseases usually produce notable denervation atrophy of weakened muscles; if muscle bulk is relatively preserved in a weak muscle it should raise the question of motor neuropathy with conduction block (Section 12.11.3) rather than denervation. Fasciculations are visible flickerings within the muscle belly which are insufficient to produce movement at the joint. They are usually visualized in large power muscles such as the deltoid or quadriceps, where the size of the motor units is large compared to that in muscles for finer motor control, such as the intrinsic hand muscles. Invisible fasciculations can be detected electromyographically. Fasciculations can only be regarded as pointers to a motor neuron disease if associated with other clinical and electrophysiological evidence of denervation. Muscle cramps are common in motor neuron diseases, and may respond favourably to quinine bisulphate, carbamazepine or verapamil.

Nerve conduction studies will rule out sensorimotor polyneuropathy, and pure motor demyelinating or conduction block neuropathies in patients with suspected motor neuron disease. Maximal motor conduction velocity is often reduced in nerves supplying severely denervated muscles, due to degeneration of large motor axons. However, in amyotrophic lateral sclerosis the motor conduction velocity rarely falls below 80 per cent of the lower limit of normal, and F-waves or distal motor latencies rarely exceed 1.25 times the upper limit of normal; results beyond these limits should raise the possibility of a primarily demyelinating neuropathy (Cornblath et al. 1992). Surface or needle electromyography helps distinguish denervation from myopathy, and may also detect subclinical denervation in clinically normal limbs in patients with early amyotrophic lateral sclerosis. Muscle biopsy may be required to rule out myopathy, particularly in patients with slowly progressive proximal weakness.

The signs of upper motor neuron involvement in motor neuron diseases are familiar: spasticity, clonus, extensor plantar responses, and weakness. In many patients with amyotrophic lateral sclerosis the presence of extensor plantar responses and clonus are masked by profound denervation of the distal leg musculature, thereby obscuring the clinically confirmatory physical signs of upper motor neuron involvement. The superficial abdominal reflexes are usually preserved in motor neuron diseases, thus rarely providing evidence for upper motor neuron involvement. Central motor conduction following transcranial electromagnetic stimulation of the motor cortex offered the attractive prospect of providing electrophysiological evidence for a clinically invisible upper motor neuron lesion. Yet, although altered thresholds to cortical magnetic stimulation have been observed in some patients with amyotrophic lateral sclerosis, it is generally concluded that the technique is not sensitive for diagnostic purposes (Claus *et al.* 1995). This group of patients with amyotrophic lateral sclerosis who do not display clear clinical evidence of upper motor neuron involvement pose a particular diagnostic uncertainty, which is only resolved when the typically brisk rate of deterioration becomes apparent.

The usual diagnostic problem in adults is to distinguish amyotrophic lateral sclerosis from other motor neuron diseases carrying a better prognosis, particularly if evidence of upper motor neuron involvement is lacking. Deterioration in the postpolio syndrome is extremely slow by comparison, causing relatively slight further loss of limb or bulbar function some decades after an earlier attack of acute poliomyelitis. X-linked bulbospinal neuronopathy should be suspected in patients apparently suffering from bulbar forms of amyotrophic lateral sclerosis but who do not deteriorate with the usual speed. Gynaecomastia, grimace-evoked sustained contractions of the lower face, diabetes, and reduced sensory action potentials are typical of X-linked bulbospinal neuronopathy. Multifocal motor neuropathy with conduction block (Section 12.11.3) usually develops over many years, predominates in the arms, may have presented with inability to extend a finger or fingers, is asymmetrical, and associated with electrophysiological evidence of motor nerve conduction slowing or conduction block, and antiganglioside antibodies may be present. Adult-onset proximal hereditary spinal muscular atrophy is only slowly progressive with prominent proximal muscle involvement early on, and rarely, if ever, involves the bulbar musculature.

14.1.3 Benign fasciculations

Spontaneous fasciculations occur in over half of normal healthy people, often occurring in the calves after exercise. They are most likely to be brought to a neurologist's attention by those associated with medicine who fear motor neuron disease, and by those with a close relative who had motor neuron disease. Neurological examination of the muscle in question is normal and electromyography demonstrates no denervation. Benign fasciculations often occur in rather metronomic bursts, unlike the random occurrence of pathological fasciculations. Furthermore, patients themselves can sense the occurrence of benign fasciculations, whereas pathological fasciculations often occur unbeknown to the patient until they have been observed or pointed out by a spouse or a doctor. A syndrome of benign fasciculations, which are excessive and confirmed electromyographically, is recognized and may follow an acute viral infection. Such patients do not go on to develop motor neuron disease (Blexrud *et al.* 1993). Benign fasciculations should be distinguished from neuromyotonia (Section 14.9) in which the twitchings are often evoked by trying to use the muscle and the myotonic discharges are very high frequency, often with characteristic doublets and triplets.

14.1.4 Dysphagia

Before they die, most amyotrophic lateral sclerosis patients experience dysphagia, dribbling, choking, and dysarthria. These same symptoms, often milder and for a duration of several years, can occur in other motor neuron diseases, such as X-linked bulbospinal neuronopathy or bulbar forms of primary lateral sclerosis. Specialist speech therapists are helpful in pinpointing the particular neuromuscular problem responsible for a dysphagia. Weak masseter muscles may prevent grinding of food. There may be difficulty in forming a food bolus within the mouth due to an immobile tongue or weakness of lip closure; this is often signalled by dribbling. A weak spastic tongue may be unable to transport the bolus to the back of the mouth. Soft palate paralysis can lead to nasal regurgitation, or to inadequate elevation of the larynx and epiglottal closure; which is signalled by choking. Obstruction due to a spastic cricopharyngeal sphincter will be shown by videofluoroscopy and may be helped by ice before meals, or by cricopharyngotomy.

In the earlier stages of dysphagia, much can be done to help by altering the consistency of food, and by tongue control exercises, lip-seal strategies, palatal-lift dental plates, and preprandial use of ice. As dysphagia becomes more severe, patients may become malnourished. Embarrassment about slow and messy eating may lead to reclusive eating or even to depression. At this stage, and preferably well before, the defective swallowing musculature should be bypassed by nasogastric tube feeding or percutaneous gastrostomy. Nasogastric tubes are a constantly visible and intrusive reminder, liable to displacement, can cause oesophageal erosions, and may lead to aspiration pneumonia from gastric backspill. Percutaneous endoscopic gastrostomy feeding avoids these disadvantages and is increasingly replacing nasogastric tube feeding. Its complications, such as peritoneal spillage and abdominal wall infection, have been minimized by developments in technique and equipment, and prophylactic antibiotics during insertion. Endoscopic placement of percutaneous gastrostomy tube is safer if performed before severe respiratory failure occurs, but can be undertaken safely in such patients using simultaneous positive pressure ventilation by face mask (Boitano *et al.* 2001). The tube feed regimen should be supervised by a dietician. To connect feed 'giving-sets' requires good hand function from the patient or spouse.

14.1.5 Speech disturbances

Serious speech disturbance is most frequently a problem in amyotrophic lateral sclerosis. Dysarthria due to a weak or spastic tongue is most common and causes 'hot potato speech'. Dysphonia due to laryngeal weakness also occurs, in which case the cough will be bovine rather than explosive. Inability to sound labial consonants such as 'b' or 'p' results from lip muscle weakness. Eventually speech may become completely unintelligible, which is a profoundly distressing and isolating problem especially if the hands have become incapable of writing too.

Depending upon the extent of hand weakness, various appliances can be used to preserve communication when speech has been lost. Simple alphabet charts can be surprisingly effective. Electronic pointers can be controlled by keyboard, mouse-switch, or even by head pointing sensors or a blowing-tube. Inevitably these methods of communication are slow and the listener must deliberately make enough time available.

14.1.6 Respiratory failure

Respiratory failure is the main cause of eventual death in motor neuron diseases. This is not just due to ventilatory respiratory muscle failure. Aspiration and inability to cough lead to aspiration pneumonia. Associated bulbar weakness makes patients prone to choking, which can cause sudden death by asphyxiation.

Usually respiratory failure occurs in the wake of severe limb or bulbar weakness in amyotrophic lateral sclerosis. Very occasionally phrenic motor neurons are severely affected at an otherwise early phase in the disease, and the patient presents with symptoms of respiratory failure. Such patients complain of exertional dyspnoea, orthopnoea, or of symptoms of carbon dioxide retention such as fatigue, concentration difficulties, morning headache or dizziness. Examination with the patient supine may show reduced chest wall expansion due to intercostal muscle weakness. More often, diaphragmatic weakness will be revealed by a paradoxical movement inwards, rather than outwards, of the upper abdominal wall during the second half of inspiration or upon sniffing (Fig. 13.12). In diaphragm weakness the vital capacity will be greater when measured standing, compared to lying, because the weight of the liver assists diaphragmatic descent when upright. Nocturnal monitoring of oxygen saturation by transcutaneous electrodes will document chronic or episodic hypoxaemia.

Assisted ventilation should be considered in those symptomatic patients who retain reasonably good limb power. In principle, tracheostomy and a portable ventilator could prolong life indefinitely in amyotrophic lateral sclerosis. However, such a life is hardly likely to be fulfilling, dignified, or comfortable when the limbs and bulbar muscles have also failed, and it would place a severe psychological burden on other family members. In addition, it would be massively expensive and create subsidiary procedural difficulties to do with living wills and the question of ultimately turning off the ventilator. In practice, doctors don't tend to offer positive pressure ventilation via tracheostomy and patients don't request it; if they do, the implications of initiating such respiratory support must be starkly clarified for each patient. A particular difficulty arises when intubation has been carried out as a life-saving procedure when neither the emergency physician, the patient, nor the relatives are sufficiently informed about the disease and its poor prognosis. Avoidance of this fraught occurrence is one benefit of early education of the patient and relatives about the likely course of the disease.

Symptomatic respiratory failure can be very satisfactorily relieved by other methods of ventilation which do not involve tracheostomy and are usually administered intermittently (Howard *et al.* 1989). Initially, negative pressure ventilation devices were used: cuirasses, jackets, or iron lungs. These have generally fallen out of favour because they are cumbersome to use, skilful and experienced fitters are rare, and the method may provoke upper airway collapse and obstruction if there is coincidental bulbar weakness. None the less, negative pressure ventilation can be preferable to positive pressure ventilation via mask if a facial mask proves intolerably claustrophobic or if positive pressure methods are impractical for other reasons.

Positive pressure ventilation via nasal mask, usually given intermittently at night, is the generally preferred method of respiratory support in motor neuron diseases. It avoids upper airway collapse if there is coexisting bulbar weakness, but it can lead to stomach distension because some air is forced down the gullet. The nasal mask can cause facial skin problems, be insolubly uncomfortable, or produce claustrophobia. The noise of the pump can drive the spouse to sleep in another room.

Respiratory and bulbar muscle failure poses other management questions in motor neuron diseases. Spouses and carers should be taught to apply a forceful bear-hug to the patient's upper abdomen, from behind, when it is necessary to assist coughing or to expel an inhaled foreign body. Chest infections have a poor implication, and although they can usually be treated satisfactorily, a time comes when the overall disability is so severe that the patient and relatives may indicate that 'nature should take its course'. Eventually morphine should be used to palliate the distress of troublesomely symptomatic dyspnoea when the patient has lost the broad range of useful muscular ability and accepts the inevitably terminal nature of his or her state.

14.1.7 Immobility

When limbs start to become weak in motor neuron disease, there is often notable fatigue. At this stage acetylcholinesterase inhibitors occasionally produce short-lived improvements in strength but rarely have any sustained value. With greater degrees of leg weakness, walking aids and eventually a wheelchair will maintain mobility. Difficulties in using the arms for activities such as feeding can be offset by arm supports or by foot-operated manipulators. The need for alterations to the home can be predicted and enacted so they are ready in time for the patient's needs. Cramps and spasticity can be severe. Simple medications include quinine bisulphate or carbamazepine for cramps and Baclofen or diazepam for spasticity. However, as the legs weaken, a degree of spasticity is often desirable so as to maintain weightbearing ability.

14.1.8 Pastoral care

Patients are naturally anxious while their muscle weakness is under in investigation before a definite diagnosis has been made. It is rarely helpful to discuss an evocative diagnosis such as motor neuron disease while it is still only a possibility. Once the doctor is sure of the diagnosis, most patients seem keen for it to be named so as to resolve the anxiety of uncertainty. In deciding how much to say about the diagnosis of motor neuron disease, and its progression and complications, one treads a narrow dividing line between brutal honesty and humane economy of truth. Any problems likely to occur in a particular individual patient's disease should be put in perspective before the patient becomes upset by the summary information so readily available from popular sources, such as journalism. Often it is valuable to discuss the diagnosis in stages with the patient, preferably in the presence of a close relative. Well-meaning relatives may try to prevent doctors from telling the patient that they have amyotrophic lateral sclerosis. But patients ultimately detect this conspiracy of secrecy at a time when death looms, thereby undermining trust and confidence just when these qualities are of inestimable value.

Many patients become angry with their neurologist soon after hearing the diagnosis. This is particularly the case in those too young to have become philosophical about their own mortality. Indeed, doctors may bear the brunt of this anger as though they were somehow responsible for the disease's occurrence. But anger should be understood sympathetically as a natural phase in patients' adjustments to incurable or fatal illness. It usually follows an early phase of denial and isolation before being succeeded by bargaining, then depression, and ultimately by acceptance (Kübler-Ross 1969). During the stages of anger and bargaining, the doctor–patient relationship is vulnerable and can only be preserved by patience and understanding, thereby laying the foundations of confidence which enable patients to trust their doctor's advice when miserable problems arise later in the disease.

Patients greatly appreciate the involvement of those who can provide advice and practical help to offset the various disabilities of motor neuron disease. Consultants in neurological disability and rehabilitation should be involved at the first sign of a needy disability, together with care teams of speech therapists, occupational therapists, physiotherapists, and social workers. Charitable organizations, such as the Motor Neurone Disease Association, can provide valuable equipment and devices with minimal delay, and often provide psychological support and practical advice to patients.

Uncontrollable bouts of tearfulness, or less commonly of laughter, may occur in upper motor neuron lesions affecting the bulbar musculature. Such incontinence of the emotions greatly embarrasses patients in social situations, and contributes to their sense of social estrangement. These outbursts should be distinguished from depression, because the patient knows that they occur without an underlying emotion of sadness, or of jollity. Amitriptyline usually helps such symptoms.

14.2 Amyotrophic lateral sclerosis

14.2.1 Clinical features

Amyotrophic lateral sclerosis is the most feared motor neuron disease of adults, usually causing death within a few years. The first symptoms generally appear in the limbs but are bulbar in a quarter. Definite diagnosis requires the presence of both upper and lower motor neuron signs in the bulbar, arm, and leg musculature, with clear evidence of progression. But earlier on, particularly at the time of initial presentation, the disease is often more focal, only affecting one of these three regions of the body musculature.

Bulbar involvement causes dysphagia, drooling of saliva, dysphonia, or inhalation of foodstuffs due to varying combinations of weakness of the tongue, pharynx, or larynx. Lower motor neuron degeneration affecting the tongue shows as atrophy, fasciculation, and weakness. The tongue should be observed resting in the floor of the mouth, since attempts at protrusion produce pseudofasciculations in many normal people. Less frequently, weakness of the facial or trigeminal muscles causes leakage from the mouth or difficulty in chewing, respectively. Predominantly upper motor neuron lesions cause spasticity of the tongue and dysarthria, resulting in 'hot potato speech'. Such patients may show other evidence of a pseudobulbar palsy, such as a brisk jaw jerk or incontinence of emotional expression, with bouts of laughter or tearfulness. Eventually these bulbar symptoms lead to anarthria, aphagia, choking, and aspiration. Death eventually results from malnutrition, unless alternative routes for feeding are established, or from respiratory failure, asphyxiation, or pneumonia.

The early symptoms of limb muscle denervation are usually cramps and fatigue, associated with observable fasciculations. Frequently such symptoms are ignored until symptomatic weakness and wasting of one hand or foot develops. Wasted small hand muscles or a foot drop are common early features. It is less common for proximal muscles, such as the shoulders, to be involved initially (Fig. 14.1). Usually this first symptomatic limb remains that most severely affected until late in the disease. In the early stages of monomelic involvement, the patient may be investigated for alternative diagnoses, such as focal compressive neuropathy or a root lesion. However, clinical or electrophysiological evidence of denervation in muscles of other limbs is often detectable even in the very early

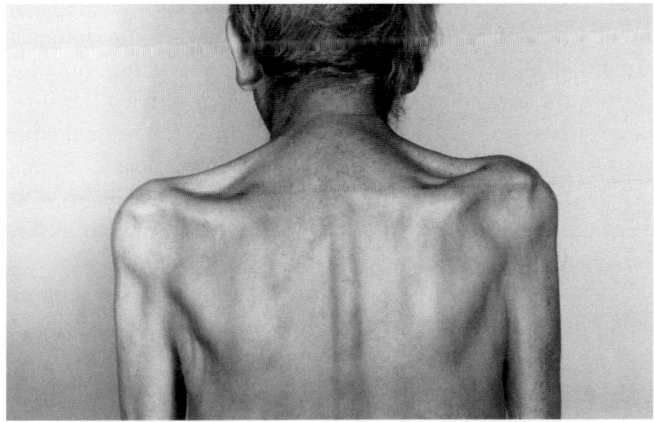

Fig. 14.1. Shoulder girdle muscle wasting in a patient with amyotrophic lateral sclerosis presenting with predominantly proximal muscle involvement.

stages. Over months, obvious weakness spreads to the opposite limb and eventually to remaining limbs and to the bulbar musculature. Eventually the patient becomes wheelchair- or bed-bound, or unable to use the arms for grooming or feeding.

It is rare for spastic weakness due to upper motor neuron loss to be the dominant early symptom in the limbs. None the less, signs of upper motor neuron involvement, such as extensor plantars, hyperreflexia, or spastic catches, are often detectable early on. They are particularly valuable diagnostically if they coexist in a muscle, or a part of a limb, also affected by obvious lower motor neuron degeneration. In general, the tendon reflexes are retained until a muscle is almost completely denervated or the uncommon complication of fibrous replacement has supervened. An extensor plantar response cannot be elicited in severe extensor hallucis longus denervation, thereby sometimes masking the upper motor neuron involvement so necessary for diagnosing amyotrophic lateral sclerosis.

Respiratory muscle failure usually occurs in the wake of noteworthy bulbar muscle failure. Early and selective diaphragm involvement may occur in amyotrophic lateral sclerosis, occasionally as the presenting feature, and often merits ventilatory assistance in such cases. Exertional dyspnoea, orthopnoea, or difficulty in coughing out chest secretions are the common symptoms. Less commonly symptoms such as concentration difficulty, headache, or giddiness occur from carbon dioxide retention due to ventilatory failure. Diaphragm weakness is signalled by orthopnoea, and the forced vital capacity is lower when lying down compared to standing, because the weight of the liver no longer aids diaphragm descent when supine. Less frequently, respiratory symptoms are due to intercostal muscle weakness which may be associated with severe weakness of other axial muscles. If there is weakness of neck extension the chin drops onto the sternum with resultant dysphagia, dysarthria, and visual difficulties. Weakness of the abdominal wall leads to distension, difficulty in coughing powerfully, and inability to build up intra-abdominal pressure for defecation.

Other neuronal systems apart from motor neurons are commonly involved in amyotrophic lateral sclerosis, although generally subclinically. Paraesthesia or other short-lived minor somatosensory phenomena are noted in the early stages in up to 10 per cent of patients. Longitudinal electrophysiological studies show progressive loss of sensory nerve fibre function during the course of the disease, but none the less sensory-nerve action potentials usually remain within the normal range (Gregory et al. 1993). Autopsy studies show loss of spinocerebellar tract neurons from Clarke's nucleus (Williams et al. 1990), but one can only conclude that any corresponding clinical effects are overshadowed by the more severe limb weakness (Williams et al. 1990). Neuropsychological and positron emission tomography studies show impairments of cognitive function in up to 50 per cent of patients (Kew et al. 1993). However, these are rarely sufficient to produce thought deficits of everyday significance, nor indeed to blunt the patient's distressing awareness of being imprisoned within a body that can no longer move. Occasionally, rapidly progressive dementia occurs

in association with motor neuron disease (Neary et al. 1990); or Parkinsonian features may develop simultaneously. Micturition, defecation, and sexual function are not affected in amyotrophic lateral sclerosis, except in so far that trunk and limb muscle weakness may make such activities awkward or impractical. Despite this evidence of other neuronal involvement on detailed investigation, as a general rule, any clear clinical evidence of neuronal involvement outside the motor system should raise questions about the validity of a diagnosis of amyotrophic lateral sclerosis.

14.2.2 Differential diagnosis and investigation

The diagnosis of amyotrophic lateral sclerosis is usually depressingly obvious on simple clinical grounds by the time the patient sees a neurologist, and often nothing needs to be considered in the differential diagnosis. The usual diagnostic problem lies in differentiating amyotrophic lateral sclerosis from other motor neuron diseases, polyneuropathies, or myopathies. Electrophysiological investigation is necessary to confirm denervation rather than myopathy, to detect clinically inapparent denervation in asymptomatic limbs, and to rule out a potentially treatable demyelinating or conduction block neuropathy (Section 12.11). Patients presenting with the combination of arm muscle denervation coupled with upper motor neuron signs in the legs, require magnetic resonance imagining of the cervical spinal cord to rule out a compressive lesion, most usually spondylitic radiculomyelopathy.

Paraproteinaemia is found in up to 5 per cent of motor neuron diseases (Shy et al. 1986), sometimes raising the question of an underlying lymphoid neoplasm. However, most paraproteinaemia-related motor neuron diseases are pure lower motor neuron disorders, often motor neuropathies, rather than amyotrophic lateral sclerosis. An amyotrophic lateral sclerosis-like disorder is seen occasionally to accompany underlying lymphoproliferative disorders, treatment of which does not seem to help the neurological disease (Gordon et al. 1997). Thyrotoxicosis or hyperparathyroidism are reported to simulate motor neuron disease occasionally, but this rarely proves to be an issue in everyday neurological practice. The serum creatine kinase level is often measured because of the question of myopathy, particularly in predominantly proximal and symmetric weakness, but it should be noted that moderate rises in this enzyme level often accompany the denervation of amyotrophic lateral sclerosis. If the question of myopathy persists, muscle biopsy should be undertaken; this can be particularly valuable where the presence of mild bulbar symptoms in patients with proximal weakness raises the question of an inclusion body myositis (Section 15.7.3). Examination of the spinal fluid is rarely helpful in diagnosing motor neuron disease, and slight rises in the protein content occur in a few patients with amyotrophic lateral sclerosis. However, spinal fluid protein levels exceeding 1 g/l, especially if accompanied by lymphocytosis, should raise the question of an underlying tumour.

14.2.3 **Inherited forms**

Five to 10 per cent of amyotrophic lateral sclerosis is inherited, generally displaying autosomal dominance (Mulder *et al.* 1986). There are no particular clinical features, or differences in survival, which distinguish the inherited forms. Usually the clinical phenotype is constant through the generations, but occasional pedigrees show mixtures of amyotrophic lateral sclerosis with spinal muscular atrophy or primary lateral sclerosis (Appelbaum *et al.* 1992). Roughly 20 per cent of familial amyotrophic lateral sclerosis is associated with the 40 different missense mutations of the Cu/Zn superoxide dismutase (*SOD1*) gene on chromosome 21, which catalyses conversion of toxic superoxide anion radicals to hydrogen peroxide (Rosen *et al.* 1993). The disease associated with various *SOD1* mutations shows varying degrees of penetrance and a variable phenotype. A slowly progressive form of amyotrophic lateral sclerosis occurs in Tunisia, with onset at 12 years of age (range 3–25 years), autosomal recessive inheritance, and usually with prominent bulbar involvement, (Ben Hamida *et al.* 1990). It bears similarities to an early onset and relatively benign form seen in India, the so-called Madras form. A similar autosomal dominant form of juvenile onset amyotrophic lateral sclerosis, without significant bulbar or respiratory muscle weakness and only slowly progressive, has been described in a large Maryland family and linked to chromosome 9, whereas the autosomal recessive forms have been linked to chromosome 2 or 15 (Rabin *et al.* 1999).

14.2.4 **Pathology and aetiology**

The most striking neuropathological change is loss of large motor neurons from the anterior horns of the cervical and lumbar enlargements of the spinal cord (Fig. 14.2). Similar loss occurs from the hypoglossal and other motor nuclei of the brainstem but the ocular motor nuclei are rarely affected.

Spheroids, composed of interwoven bundles of disorganized neurofilaments, are evident in the proximal axons of motor neurons in the anterior horn in two-thirds of sporadic cases (Hirano *et al.* 1984). These spheroids within the proximal axon are a distinctive feature, appearing as an early pathological change in motor neurons. Intracytoplasmic inclusions in motor neurons, known as Bunina bodies, are also characteristic. Loss or shrinkage of giant Betz cells from the precentral gyrus of the cerebral cortex is associated with fibre loss from the pyramidal tracts, particularly obviously in the spinal cord and lower brainstem. At autopsy of advanced cases there is often evidence of a lesser degree of neuronal loss from other areas of the nervous system, including dorsal root ganglia and the dorsal (Clarke's) nuclei of the spinal cord (Section 14.2.1).

The cause of sporadic amyotrophic lateral sclerosis is unknown. There is evidence for various risk factors, but none are invariably associated and it is possible that motor neuron degeneration is a singular expression of diverse aetiological factors. Particular associations with rural populations and with trauma have been noted (Román 1996). Many have searched inconclusively for a viral cause for amyotrophic lateral sclerosis; recent tantalizing evidence, yet to be confirmed, showed enterovirus nucleic acid sequences in anterior horn neurons in 88 per cent of affected spinal cords, compared to only 3 per cent of controls (Berger *et al.* 2000). Given the superoxide dismutase (*SOD1*) mutation underlying some cases of hereditary amyotrophic lateral sclerosis, it will be interesting to discover whether acquired disorders of free-radical detoxication underlie the sporadic form of the disease. A motor neuron degeneration occurs in transgenic mice expressing human mutant *SOD1* (Gurney *et al.* 1994); such models provide the potential for screening new therapies. Transgenic mice overexpressing a neurofilament subunit develop progressive weakness with massive accumulations within motor neurons of neurofilaments resembling spheroids (Côté *et al.* 1993). Synaptosomes derived from affected regions of spinal cord in amyotrophic lateral sclerosis show defective uptake of the potentially toxic excitatory amino-acid neurotransmitter, glutamate (Rothstein *et al.* 1992). This observation led to the glutamate excitotoxicity hypothesis from which the drug riluzole was developed.

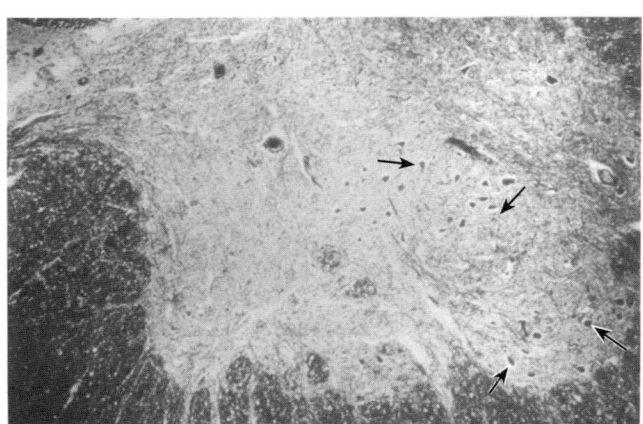

(a)

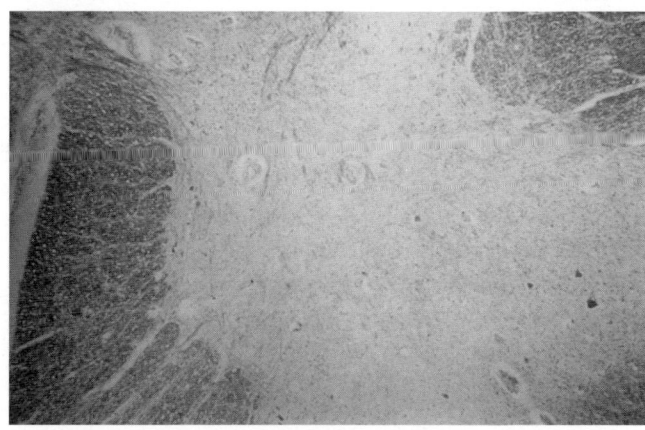

(b)

Fig. 14.2. Loss of motor neurons from the anterior horn of the spinal cord in amyotrophic lateral sclerosis. (a) Normal, showing numerous motor neuron cell bodies in the anterior horn (some arrowed). (b) Amyotrophic lateral sclerosis, showing almost complete absence of motor neuron perikarya. (Courtesy of Professor M. Esiri.)

14.2.5 Epidemiology

Amyotrophic lateral sclerosis occurs throughout the world. Traditionally the incidence has been considered to lie between 0.4 and 1.8 per 100 000, and the prevalence 4–6 per 100 000 (Tandan and Bradley 1985). More contemporary studies with more confident ascertainment note that many elderly patients are diagnosed often outside neurology departments, and that there is an increasing incidence with age, leading to incidences of 2.25–2.6 per 100 000 in Denmark and Scotland (Christensen *et al.* 1990; Chancellor and Warlow 1992). Case-control studies do not identify any ubiquitous risk factor, although the odds ratios are increased by previous long-bone fractures, manual work, and occupational exposures to lead, solvents, or chemicals (Chancellor *et al.* 1993). Men are up to twice as commonly affected as women.

On the Pacific island of Guam, the incidence of motor neuron disease, often associated with parkinsonism and dementia, has fallen from 87 per 100 000 in 1962 to 5 per 100 000 in 1985 (Rodgers-Johnson *et al.* 1986). The reasons for the previous high incidence in Guam are unknown, speculation has centred around the possible role of a dietary excitotoxin found in the locally consumed *Cycas circinalis* flour and upon dietary consumption of calcium and aluminium.

14.2.6 Prognosis and treatment

The severity and extensiveness of muscular weakness progress remorselessly in amyotrophic lateral sclerosis. Death results generally from ventilatory respiratory failure; inhalational pneumonia, or choking and malnutrition may contribute. Bedsores are relatively infrequent despite the immobility of many patients. There is an increased vulnerability to long-bone fractures. The general principles of physical and psychological support for patients with advanced amyotrophic lateral sclerosis are outlined in Section 14.1.

Patients with a bulbar onset have the worst prognosis. Their median survival is approximately 20 months from the onset of bulbar symptoms, with only 5 per cent surviving at 5 years. Median survival for those with spinal onset is somewhat better, at 29 months, with nearly 15 per cent surviving at 5 years (Christensen *et al.* 1990). It seems that mortality has increased in recent decades and that this cannot be explained solely by the increasing age of the population (Seljeseth *et al.* 2000). Alternative diagnoses, such as X-linked bulbospinal neuronopathy (Section 14.4.1), should be considered in those patients surviving for an unexpectedly long time. Occasional patients have a subacute and reversible syndrome resembling the spinal form of amyotrophic lateral sclerosis without bulbar involvement, and recover spontaneously within 5–12 months of symptom onset (Tucker *et al.* 1991). Such cases are so extraordinarily rare that they should not affect the physician's prognostication.

Trials of drug therapy have concentrated upon slowing the downhill progression of disability or improving survival. The antiglutamate agent riluzole, administered orally, has been licensed for treatment of amyotrophic lateral sclerosis (Lacomblez *et al.* 1996). The 100 mg dosage improved the chance of tracheostomy-free survival at 18 months by an extra 35 per cent, although there was no significant benefit on muscle function. Criticisms of this study have included the nature of the Cox model statistical adjustment (Drug and Therapeutics Bulletin 1997), and it should be noted that more of the placebo group had bulbar features at entry to the study. Riluzole is generally well tolerated by patients; nausea, gastrointestinal upset, and raised transaminase enzyme levels may occur, and usually resolve with dosage reduction. Ineffective therapeutic trials have included mixtures of branched-chain amino acids, dextromethorphan, total lymphoid irradiation, and the free-radical scavenger, acetylcysteine.

14.3 Inherited spinal muscular atrophies

Some of this group of motor neuron diseases are also known as hereditary motor neuronopathies. The inherited spinal muscular atrophies are a heterogeneous group. Classification is based principally upon features such as age of onset, mode of inheritance, and pattern of muscular involvement. Reclassification can be expected in coming years based upon identification of the responsible genetic mutations.

14.3.1 Acute infantile spinal muscular atrophy (Werdnig–Hoffmann disease; type I SMA)

This severe infantile form is the second most common fatal autosomal recessive disorder of childhood and occurs about once in every 20 000 births in England. In almost all it is fatal by age 3 years, with delayed motor milestones being a cause of concern to the parents before 6 months of age (Pearn *et al.* 1973). Mothers report that fetal movements were absent in a third and diminished in others. Most are born normally, but deformity, contracture, or dislocations affect the limbs at birth in some cases. Within an affected family there is high concordance for the age at which symptoms become evident, and the age of onset correlates with the age of death. The more severe cases will be hypotonic and weak from birth with poor sucking, and normally die within a year. Such children may never roll over and show no intercostal muscle contribution to respiration, giving the chest a rather bell-shaped appearance. Less severely affected infants show delayed motor abilities within a few months of birth, having particular weakness of trunk, limb girdle, and proximal limb muscles, such that they lie relatively immobile in a frog-like position. The limbs are areflexic, but it is often difficult to appreciate wasting because of subcutaneous fat. The face is usually spared, but the tongue is involved; indeed this is the only site at which fasciculations are observable, usually with difficulty. Eye movements, responses to sensory stimuli, and social responsiveness are normal. With progressive weakness the cry and feeding both become feeble, the child lies immobile, and respiratory infection is the usual eventual agent of death.

The condition needs to be distinguished from other causes of hypotonia in infancy. Polyneuropathy, particularly the steroid-responsive chronic idiopathic demyelinating polyneuropathy of infants (Section 12.11.1) can be excluded by demonstrating normal motor nerve conduction velocity and spinal fluid protein. Muscle biopsy will show the grouped atrophy of fibres, typical of denervation, and helps in the distinction from congenital myopathy (Section 15.4).

Acute infantile spinal muscular atrophy has been linked to chromosome 5q11.2–13.3. Within this region two candidate genes have been isolated, *SMN* (survival motor neuron) and *NAIP* (neuronal apoptosis inhibitory protein). Mutations in these genes occur in up to 98 per cent (*SMN*) and 20–50 per cent (*NAIP*) of patients (Le Febvre *et al.* 1998). Although a valuable aid to diagnosis, and potentially for prenatal diagnosis, it should be noted that *SMN* gene mutations occasionally occur in healthy relatives of an affected proband, and that these mutations, particularly *SMN*, are also found in milder or later-onset forms of spinal muscular atrophy, including Kugelberg– Welander disease. Occasional cases of acute infantile spinal muscular atrophy have a separate, X-linked genetic basis.

14.3.2 Intermediate-onset and chronic childhood forms (including Kugelberg–Welander disease)

Although Werdnig–Hoffmann disease (type I SMA) is a reasonably clearly defined entity, there is debate about the classification of later-onset forms of chronic childhood spinal muscular atrophy. Overall, they appear to be of similar incidence to type I SMA. Two separate forms are often recognized, types II and III, and *SMN* mutations are present in over 90 per cent of these. However, associated *NAIP* mutations are uncommon in these forms compared to type I SMA.

Type II SMA, or the intermediate form, is similar to Werdnig–Hoffmann disease (type I SMA) but with onset after age 6 months, and with lesser severity, such that the child may learn to sit but will not be able to stand or walk. The bulbar and respiratory muscles are less severely affected, scoliosis may develop, and the tendon reflexes may be preserved. Progressive deterioration is not inevitable; the disease appears to arrest spontaneously in some. Death may occur between childhood and early adulthood, with wide variation within an affected family.

Type III SMA, or Kugelberg–Welander disease causes slowly progressive proximal muscle weakness, which can be initially mistaken for a muscular dystrophy, particularly since calf-muscle hypertrophy occurs in a quarter of patients. Proximal leg muscle weakness is prominent, leading to difficulty in rising from the floor and a waddling gait. Proximal arm muscle weakness, trunk muscle involvement resulting in neck weakness and mild kyphoscoliosis, and sometimes facial weakness, occur later. Fasciculations are evident in limb muscles in roughly a half, sometimes provoked by contraction. Respiratory or bulbar involvement is unusual and life expectancy normal, albeit with chronic disability.

14.3.3 Adult-onset proximal forms (type IV SMA)

Proximal motor neuropathy developing between ages 15 and 60 years is a rare disorder of either autosomal recessive or dominant inheritance. It is often mistaken either as a limb girdle muscular dystrophy or as the progressive muscular atrophy variant of amyotrophic lateral sclerosis. Bulbar involvement is unusual. Progressive deterioration is the rule, and is more severe in the dominantly inherited form. Nonetheless many patients can still walk with aids until their fifties.

14.3.4 Distal spinal muscular atrophy

Distal spinal muscular atrophy is one cause of the peroneal muscular atrophy syndrome affecting the distal legs, of which hereditary motor and sensory neuropathy (Charcot–Marie–Tooth disease) (Section 12.4) is the more common cause. Unlike this inherited neuropathy, the nerve conductive studies, including sensory-nerve action potentials, are normal in distal spinal muscular atrophy, particularly for sensory axons. Also clinical examination of sensation is normal, and the tendon reflexes are usually retained, even at the ankle. Distal spinal muscular atrophy is genetically heterogeneous with both autosomal recessive and dominant forms, and the age of onset is variable, although many dominant cases develop before the age of 20 years (Harding and Thomas 1980). Altogether eight different forms of hereditary distal spinal muscular atrophy are recognised, so far, linked to different genetic loci (Auer-Grumbach *et al.* 2000; Christodoulou *et al.* 2000).

Patients with distal spinal muscular atrophy show atrophy of muscles below the knees, with prominent flaccid footdrop. The arms and hands are usually less severely involved than the legs. Occasional pedigrees have been reported in which the arm muscles were predominantly affected (Lander *et al.* 1976), and which have been mapped to chromosome 7 (Christodoulou *et al.* 1995). Another distinctive distal spinal muscular atrophy is associated with vocal cord paralysis (Young and Harper 1980) and should be distinguished from type IIc HMSN (Section 12.4.3). The level of disability varies, but most patients remain able to walk without aid. Apart from the distinction from hereditary motor and sensory neuropathy, the rare autosomal recessive distal muscular dystrophy affecting the legs (Section 15.2.9) should be considered: onset of this is between ages 15 and 25 years, the gastrocnaemius muscles are preferentially involved rather than the peroneal and anterior tibial muscles, and the creatinine kinase level is elevated tenfold (Barohn *et al.* 1991).

14.3.5 **Scapuloperoneal spinal muscular atrophy**

This rare syndrome usually develops between 15 and 25 years of age. Distal leg muscle weakness followed some years later by shoulder girdle weakness (Ricker *et al.* 1968). Notably, the intrinsic muscles of the feet are spared. The disorder is genetically heterogeneous and the age of onset and pattern of muscle weakness vary. Some patients with scapuloperoneal spinal muscular atrophy develop sensory abnormalities. Differentiation from muscular dystrophies may be difficult despite electrophysiological and muscle biopsy study. If cardiomyopathy is present in patients with this pattern of muscle involvement, Emery–Dreifuss muscular dystrophy (Section 15.2.3) is likely.

One North American kindred with autosomal dominant neurogenic scapuloperoneal amyotrophy variably exhibited congenital absence of some muscles or laryngeal palsy. Males were more severely affected and the disease more severe in successive generations (DeLong and Siddique 1992).

14.3.6 **Hexosaminidase deficiency**

Autosomal recessive GM_1 gangliosidosis presents a variable neurological picture, occasionally as a pure motor neuron syndrome due to lower and, rarely, upper motor neuron involvement. More usually these are combined with other neurological abnormalities, such as cerebellar ataxia or dementia. Hexosaminidase assays should be reserved for those patients with early onset of unusual motor neuron disorders, particularly if the parents are consanguineous or Ashkenazi Jews.

14.4 **Hereditary bulbar palsy**

The most common form of inherited bulbar palsy, X-linked bulbospinal neuronopathy, presents in adulthood and occurs in men only. Two rare forms of inherited bulbar palsy occur in childhood or adolescence: of these Brown–Violetto–van Laere syndrome is associated with deafness, whereas hearing is preserved in the other, Fazio–Londe disease. The differential diagnoses include structural disease of the brainstem, myopathies, myasthenia, and other cranial nerve disorders.

14.4.1 **X-linked bulbospinal neuronopathy (Kennedy syndrome)**

This only occurs in men, normally with onset in the third to fifth decades (Kennedy *et al.* 1968; Harding *et al.* 1982; Olney *et al.* 1991). The initial symptom is cramping of limb muscles. Limb weakness predominates in the legs, often of relatively mild severity. Eventually the most severe weakness is bulbar, with a severely wasted tongue, but the dysphagia and dysarthria may not become evident until 20 years after limb symptoms, if at all (Olney *et al.* 1991). Fasciculations are often marked, espe-

cially in the face and tongue. A noteworthy physical sign is the occurrence of grimace-evoked contractions of the lower facial muscles; these contractions characteristically persist for some seconds after relaxing the grimace (Fig. 14.3). In retrospect such facial contractions have often been noted by patients' wives many years before.

In the later stages of the disease patients are prone to aspiration pneumonia. None the less, life expectancy doesn't seem seriously affected, with most surviving to the seventh or eighth decade, although occasionally there is rapid onset of more severe disability (Amato *et al.* 1993). Indeed, X-linked bulbospinal neuronopathy is often misdiagnosed initially as amyotrophic lateral sclerosis until that diagnosis is questioned because of unusually slow deterioration.

There are no signs of upper motor neuron involvement in patients with X-linked bulbospinal neuronopathy and central motor conduction studies are normal (Kachi *et al.* 1992). Often the sensory-nerve action potentials are absent or diminished despite normal clinical examination of sensation. Diabetes mellitus occurs in about a quarter of patients.

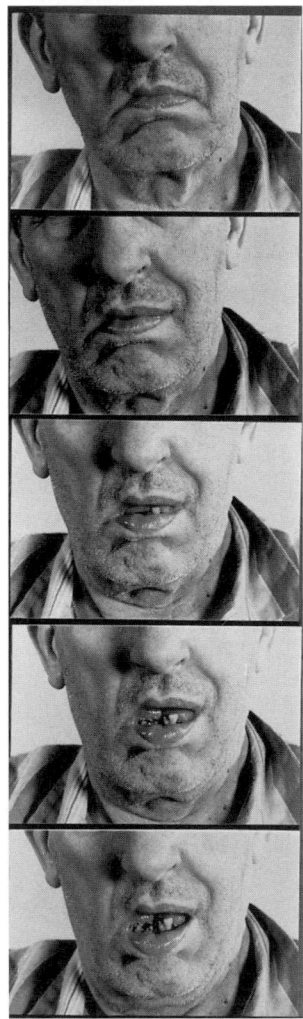

Fig. 14.3. X-linked bulbospinal neuronopathy. Persistence of lower facial muscular contractions in succession time frames after grimacing.

This X-linked disorder is caused by the mutation of an increased-length CAG triplet repeat sequence within the androgen receptor gene (La Spada *et al.* 1991). Molecular genetic analysis of the length of this CAG repeat sequence is a reliable diagnostic test which can also be used for detecting female carriers and affected fetuses (Amato *et al.* 1993). The clinical severity of the disorder varies within families and does not appear to relate to the size of the mutation (Amato *et al.* 1993). However, a relationship of longer CAG repeat sequences to earlier onset of muscle weakness has been noted (Igarashi *et al.* 1992). Some patients with X-linked bulbospinal neuronopathy show altered androgen receptor function on cultured fibroblasts (Warner *et al.* 1992) or diminished androgen receptor populations (Matsuura *et al.* 1992). This explains the common occurrence of impotence and gynaecomastia in the condition. Indeed, gynaecomastia is usually detectable if sought by palpating for glandular breast tissue between the thumb and index finger, rather than by using the flat of the hand. Exactly the same clinical syndrome, including gynaecomastia, has been reported to occur without an expanded CAG repeat in the androgen receptor gene (Ikezoe *et al.* 1999).

14.4.2 **Brown–Violetto–van Laere syndrome**

The essence of this syndrome is progressive bulbar palsy, sensorineural deafness, and progressive palsies of the lower six cranial nerves (Davenport and Mumford 1994). Onset of dysphagia, dysarthria, and facial weakness in the second decade of life has usually been prefaced by progressive deafness a few years earlier.

Respiratory muscle involvement may lead to sleep apnoea and respiratory failure, usually leading to death by the thirties. The precise genetic basis is not understood, and the severity may differ between affected family members. Furthermore, there is clinical heterogeneity, with instances of associated limb muscle denervation, upper motor neuron features, ataxia, and optic atrophy. There is no specific treatment. Respiratory supportive therapy is the mainstay of management.

14.4.3 **Fazio–Londe disease**

This very rare bulbar paralysis develops in children within the first 5 years of life (McShane *et al.* 1992). Stridor is a prominent early symptom, often leading to an initial diagnosis of croup. Dysphagia and dysarthria then develop. Over the next 2 years the limb muscles become involved, respiratory failure develops, and death usually occurs within 2 years of onset. Occasional later onset and longer survival is described, and may reflect the genetic heterogeneity of Fazio–Londe disease; autosomal recessive inheritance is usual, but an even rarer dominant form also exists (McShane *et al.* 1992).

14.5 **Poliomyelitis**

Poliomyelitis is an acute motor neuron disease caused by polio virus infection. Vaccination programmes started in the mid-

1950s have virtually eradicated acute sporadic poliomyelitis from much of the world now, particularly the Americas and western Europe. However, there are still occasional cases related to oral live vaccine strains. Furthermore, there is a syndrome of slow deterioration in neuromuscular function decades after an attack of acute poliomyelitis, which enters into the differential diagnosis of motor neuron syndromes in elderly patients.

14.5.1 **Acute poliomyelitis**

Acute poliomyelitis is due to infection with an enterovirus, the poliovirus, which has three antigenic types. Transmission is usually person-to-person via the alimentary route. The virus multiplies in nasopharyngeal and intestinal lymphoid tissue. Infection tends to occur in late summer and autumn in temperate regions, and throughout the year in the tropics. Overall only 1–2 per cent of those infected develop paralytic forms of poliomyelitis; the infection usually taking the form of an uncomplicated febrile enteritis. Tonsillectomy, physical exertion, pregnancy, and immunodeficiency are all suspected of predisposing to the paralytic form of poliomyelitis, or influencing its severity. The susceptibility to paralytic disease is tenfold higher in adults than young children (Price and Plum 1978).

It remains uncertain whether the neural infection occurs along nerves, or more likely, haematogenously. In paralytic cases, motor neurons are affected in the anterior horns of the spinal cord and the brainstem motor nuclei. Many other areas of the brain are involved histologically in acute attacks, but usually in clinical silence. The white matter tracts are spared. Virus accumulates in affected neurons, inflammatory infiltrates develop, and neuronophagia occurs (Fig. 14.4). Diminished populations of motor neurons are evident in the anterior horns at autopsy of those who have survived an earlier acute attack.

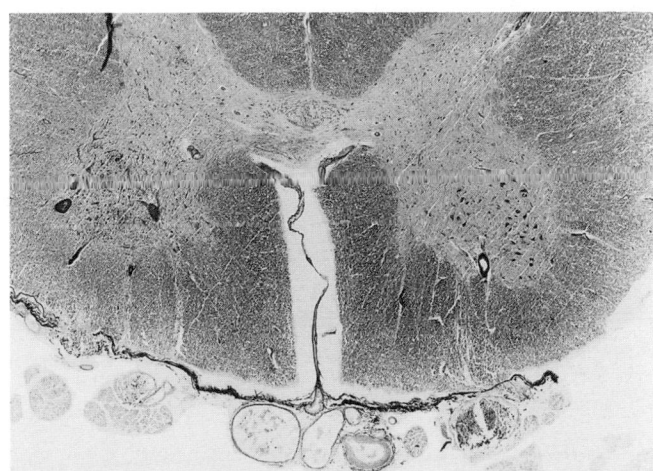

Fig. 14.4. Acute poliomyelitis. Transverse section of the cervical spinal cord, showing intense perivascular inflammatory cell cuffing in both anterior horns. There is parenchymal inflammation with loss of large motor neurons on the left, whereas the motor neuron population is preserved on the right. (Low power (×14) luxol fast blue/cresyl violet.) (Courtesy Professor M. M. Esiri and Blackwell Science Ltd.)

Approximately 5 per cent of those infected by poliovirus develop a preparalytic, meningitic phase, and only 1–2 per cent eventually develop paralysis 2–5 days later (Wood and Anderson 1988). If paralysis occurs, it is usually asymmetrical, predominantly involves proximal muscles with pain and tenderness, and is most likely to affect the leg. The extent of the weakness can vary from a single muscle group to complete tetraparesis. An affected limb is typically weak, flaccid, and areflexic. Wasting commences within a week and fasciculations are prominent. Up to 15 per cent of patients also develop respiratory muscle failure, disturbances of respiratory control, dysphagia, dysphonia, or dysarthria, due to involvement of the lower cranial nerve motor nuclei. Cardiovascular, sweating, and gut motility disturbances may occur. Reduced consciousness can reflect reticular formation involvement. The inflammation can extend to dorsal root ganglia, and, occasionally, sensory loss is a feature.

Acute poliomyelitis is a distinctive condition with marked spinal fluid pleocytosis, usually polymorphonuclear, and a relatively normal spinal fluid protein. Stool viral cultures are usually positive, and serology confirms the diagnosis. Guillain–Barré syndrome (Section 12.10) has a slower evolution, is symmetrical, usually involves sensation, and the spinal fluid is acellular but with a raised protein level. Occasionally, coxsackie infections, acute hepatic porphyrias, tetanus, myasthenia, diphtheria, and brainstem encephalitis enter the differential diagnosis. Tick-borne central European encaphilitis (Section 34.7.4) occasionally causes a poliomyelitic-type of illness with bulbar and arm predominance and a poor prognosis (Schellinger et al. 2000). Treatment of acute poliomyelitis follows the same principles of caring for paralysed patients as given under Guillain–Barré syndrome (Section 12.10), paying particular attention to preventing muscle contractures and avoiding the potentially catastrophic effects of bulbar and respiratory muscle failure by intubating and ventilating. With more modern treatment the mortality is well under 10 per cent, although many are left with severe permanent

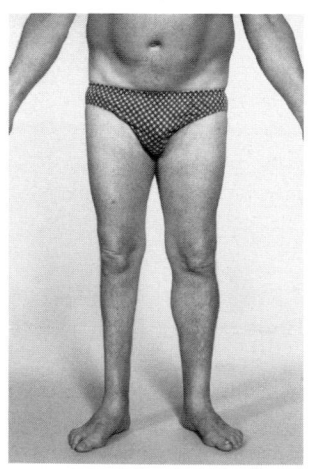
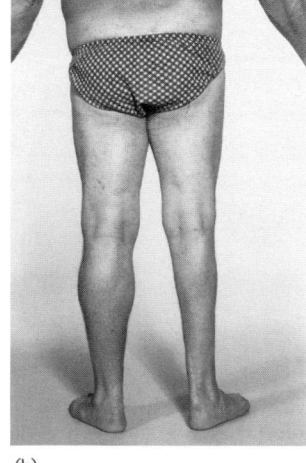

(a)   (b)

Fig. 14.5. Old poliomyelitis: wasting of the right leg musculature following acute poliomyelitis 26 years earlier.

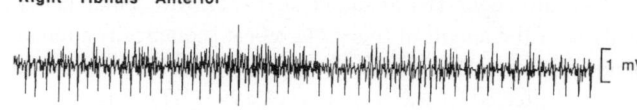

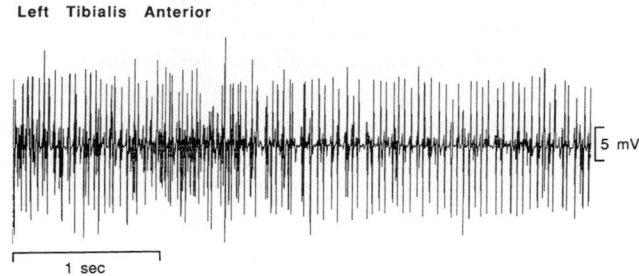

Fig. 14.6. Electromyogram showing giant motor units in a left tibialis anterior muscle previously affected by paralytic poliomyelitis many years earlier. The motor units in the unaffected right tibialis anterior muscle are normal (note the difference in amplification between left and right). (Courtesy of Professor K. R. Mills.)

paralysis and wasting of affected muscles (Price and Plum 1978) (Fig 14.5).

After recovery, affected limb muscles show giant motor nits on electromyography, typical of reinnervation from a diminished population of surviving motor neurons (Fig. 14.6).

14.5.2 Vaccine-related poliomyelitis

Since the mid-1950s paralytic poliomyelitis has been preventable by immunization with inactivated poliovirus (Salk) or live attenuated poliovirus (Sabin) vaccines. Although the live attenuated vaccine has generally gained favour, being orally administered in a single dose, it does occasionally cause poliomyelitis. This can occur in vaccine recipients themselves, or more frequently in those contacts who become secondarily infected by the vaccine strain, which may have reverted partially to the wild-type virus (Nathanson 1982). Those with immunodeficiency are at particular risk (Wyatt 1973) and should be given the inactivated Salk vaccine rather than live vaccine for the purpose of vaccination.

14.5.3 Postpolio weakness

Extremely slowly progressive weakness can affect muscles previously affected by acute paralytic poliomyelitis two or more decades earlier (Dalakas et al. 1986). Although limb muscles are predominantly affected, half of these patients experience mild choking or dysphagia too (Sonies and Dalakas 1991). Increased intrathecal synthesis of poliovirus antibodies is detectable in two-thirds (Sharief et al. 1991). The slow rate of deterioration, the lack of upper motor neuron involvement, the previous history of poliomyelitis, and the huge motor units in affected

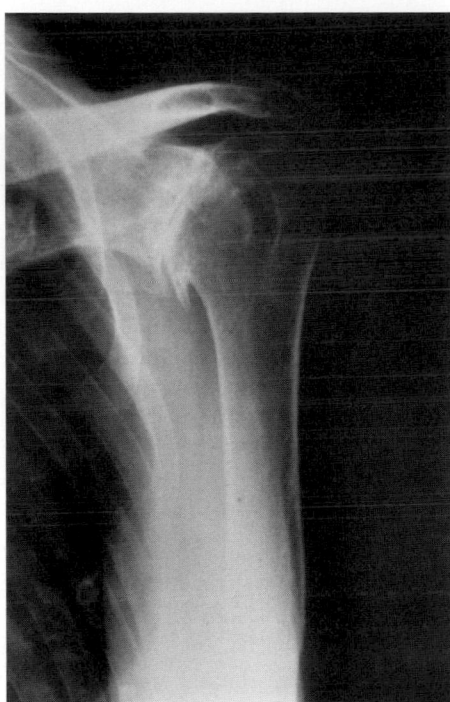

Fig. 14.7. Degenerative arthritis of the shoulder joint, typical of that in prolonged users of arm crutches.

muscles serve to distinguish this from amyotrophic lateral sclerosis.

A specific postpolio syndrome of progressive motor neuron loss is not the only cause of late deterioration in polio survivors. Indeed, some question the true frequency of the neuromuscular syndrome when the superimposed factors of ageing, secondary mechanical disorders affecting joints, and fibromyalgia are taken into account (Trojan and Cashman 1995; Windebank *et al.* 1996; Kidd *et al.* 1997). Degenerative arthritis of the shoulder joint can cause diminished mobility in those who have been critically dependent upon arm crutches (Fig. 14.7). Decisions about the advisability of orthopaedic surgical measures are often difficult. Treatment of fibromyalgic pain, fatigue, and weakness with local measures and low-dose amitriptyline or non-steroidal anti-inflammatory drugs may help.

14.6 Monomelic, focal, and segmental spinal muscular atrophies

This is a heterogeneous group of disorders which are also known as focal motor neuronopathies, or monomelic motor neuron disease. Generally, they are sporadic rather than genetic. Although usually reported from Japan and Asia, these disorders do occur regularly elsewhere in the world, including the United Kingdom and North America. The most usual presentation

occurs in young men, who develop distal wasting and weakness of one hand or forearm (Sobue *et al.* 1978) or, less often, a leg (Uncini *et al.* 1992). As a rule, the condition stabilizes or its evolution slows down after steady progression for up to 2 years. Any later progression tends to involve more proximal muscles. Although the hand can be rendered useless in some patients, in others the eventual loss of manipulatory ability can be fairly mild, such that disability is limited to refined manipulations such as playing the piano. In two-thirds the syndrome is unilateral and in a third it is bilateral, although generally asymmetrically so (Sobue *et al.* 1978). Half the patients lose tendon reflexes from the affected limb. Fasciculations occur, proximal limb muscles are occasionally the main site of involvement, and occasionally there is mild hyperaesthesia. Initially there is concern about amyotrophic lateral sclerosis, but the anticipated bulbar and upper motor neuron involvements fail to materialize, and spread to other limbs is unusual.

The focal spinal muscular atrophies raise a wide range of differential diagnoses apart from the obvious initial question about amyotrophic lateral sclerosis. Syringomyelia (Section 20.6.2) or other structural disorders of the spinal cord will be detected by magnetic resonance imaging. Multifocal motor neuropathy with conduction block (Section 12.11.3) is an important alternative diagnosis to consider, because of the potential for treatment. However, that disorder usually produces relatively little wasting by comparison with the degree of weakness, at least in the first few years, and motor-nerve conduction studies usually show conduction block, slowing or delayed F-waves. The hereditary distal motor neuronopathies (Section 13.3.4) often affect all four limbs, usually start in the legs, are either autosomal recessive or dominant in type, and tend to commence by adolescence (Harding and Thomas 1980).

14.7 Post-irradiation lumbosacral radiculopathy

A predominantly motor disorder can affect the legs following irradiation of the lumbar spinal canal as part of treatment for testicular or other neoplasms. Weakness usually commences between 3 and 25 years after the radiotherapy. The radiotherapy doses exceeded 40 Gy, which is above the current treatment recommendation of 35 Gy fractionated over 4 weeks for testicular tumours. The leg muscle involvement is often distal and asymmetrical and associated with areflexia. Despite the purely motor nature of this disorder early on, all patients develop mild sensory symptoms eventually, although sensory-nerve action potentials remain normal. Half eventually develop mild sphincter disorders, with lack of appreciation of bladder fullness, dribbling, or occasional incontinence (Bowen *et al.* 1996). In most patients the leg weakness slowly progresses, albeit with periods of stabilization for a year or more, and severe disability can result. With improved safety of radiotherapy schedules, and the substitution of chemotherapy for radiotherapy in treating testicular cancer, the incidence of this unusual disorder can be expected to lessen.

It was not known whether this disorder reflected irradiation damage to the cauda equina nerve roots, or alternatively to the motor neurons of the conus medullaris (Bowen *et al.* 1996). However, a recent neuropathological autopsy study showed a radiation-induced vasculopathy of the proximal spinal roots within the cauda equina, whereas the spinal cord architecture and motor neuronal cell bodies were preserved (Fig. 14.8) (Bowen *et al.* 1996). Magnetic resonance imaging shows gadolinium enhancement of the cauda equina in some patients, but this is a relatively non-specific finding.

The differential diagnosis includes neural infiltration by recurrent neoplasm or radiation-induced nerve sheath tumours, for both of which pain, unilaterality, and predominantly proximal weakness are to be expected. Apart from the slow evolution, spinal fluid cytology excludes malignant meningitis. Myokymia may be noted on electromyography, but does not serve to distinguish radiation-induced plexopathies (Section 13.5.3) from radiculopathies.

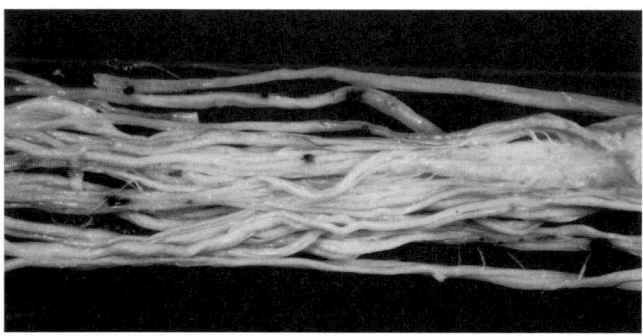

(a)

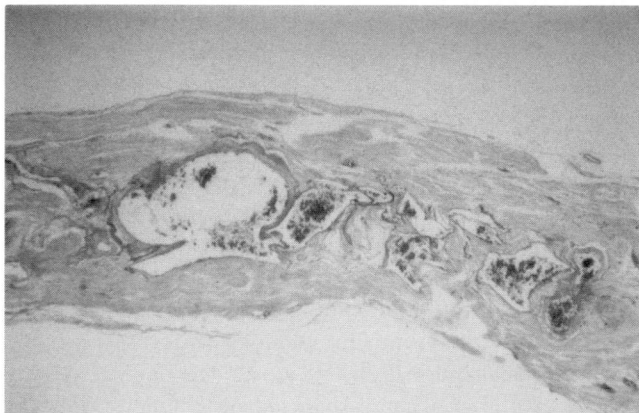

(b)

Fig. 14.8. Radiation-induced lumbosacral radiculopathy. (a) Cauda equina with several thickened roots, some showing focal haemorrhages. (b) Longitudinal section of nerve root, showing clusters of dilated vascular channels with thick hyalinized walls. The nerve is fibrosed and distorted by these vessels. (Elastic van Giesen Stain) (Reproduced from Bowen *et al.* (1997).)

14.8 Pure upper motor neuron disorders

These are the rarest forms of motor neuron disease. They should be considered only after magnetic resonance imaging has excluded structural or demyelinating disease of the spinal cord or brain or abnormalities at the foramen magnum. Spasticity often predominates over weakness in pure upper motor neuron disorders, yet anti-spasticity medications are often surprisingly ineffective. Pure upper motor neuron syndromes are also said to be rare manifestations of borreliosis, *Treponema pallidum*, and human T-cell leukaemia (HTLV-1) (Section 20.6.4) infections.

14.8.1 Primary lateral sclerosis

The nosological identity of this rare form of motor neurone disease has been disputed, but now is generally accepted as a distinct entity. The average age of onset is 50 years, with slow progression thereafter for an average of 15 years (Pringle *et al.* 1992). All the clinical manifestations are attributable to degeneration of the upper motor neurons destined for the bulbar and/or spinal lower motor neuron pools. Spasticity and weakness usually start insidiously in the legs, ultimately ascending to the arms and bulbar muscles, and are associated with hyperreflexia and extensor plantars. Sometimes patients present with a spastic dysarthria causing 'hot potato speech', due to pseudobulbar palsy. Pseudobulbar emotional lability may be distressing for these patients, given their normal insight and intellect, and it often responds well to amitriptyline. Sphincter control is generally preserved, although mild micturition abnormalities can develop late on. The absence of a family history distinguishes primary lateral sclerosis from hereditary spastic paraplegia.

Magnetic resonance imaging of the brain can show atrophy of the motor cortex of the precentral gyrus, reflecting the histopathological observation of loss of the Betz cells giving rise to the pyramidal tract. Central motor conduction is notably delayed following transcranial electromagnetic stimulation of the motor cortex (Pringle *et al.* 1992). Electromyography does not reveal the muscle denervation to be expected in those forms of amyotrophic lateral sclerosis with predominant upper motor neuron involvement.

14.8.2 Hereditary spastic paraplegia

Usually hereditary spastic paraplegia is autosomally dominantly inherited, with linkage to loci on either chromosome 2, 8, 10, 12, 14, or 15 (Reid *et al.* 1999; McDermott *et al.* 2000). The form associated with chromosome 2 is the most common and is associated with mutations of a candidate gene encoding 'spastin' (Hazan *et al.* 1999). Occasionally the inheritance is autosomal recessive (Harding 1981; Nielson *et al.* 1998) with loci identified on chromosomes 8, 15, and 16 (McDermott *et al.* 2000). It is often difficult to date symptom onset precisely, a factor which may account for the apparent variation within families. Symptoms are usually noted in early adulthood, but their onset ranges from childhood to the seventh decade of life.

The most common symptoms of this uncommon disorder are stiff legs and awkward walking. Examination usually shows a degree of spasticity out of proportion to the degree of weakness, which can be minimal. Backache is common and reflects many years of awkward and stiff gait. The arms are usually minimally involved, if at all, and bulbar dysfunction is rare. Somatosensation is usually normal but can be mildly impaired later in the disease. Sphincter function is generally well preserved, although urinary frequency may develop later on (Harding 1981). Examination of asymptomatic family members can reveal upper motor neuron signs, thereby proving the inherited nature of a patient's disorder. Central motor conduction is only minimally prolonged in hereditary spastic paraplegia, unlike the pronounced slowing reported in primary lateral sclerosis. Hereditary spastic paraplegia may be symptomatic for over 30 years in many patients, and life expectancy only slightly reduced.

Sometimes varying combinations of other clinical features have been associated with hereditary spastic paraplegia, particularly with recessively inherited forms: distal amyotrophy, mental retardation, dementia, pigmentary retinopathy, optic atrophy, extrapyramidal features, sensory neuropathy, or ataxia (Harding 1981; Webb *et al.* 1997; White *et al.* 2000). Some complex forms are X-linked, involving mutations of the gene encoding neural cell adhesion molecule L1, occurring in families also showing mental retardation or hydrocephalus (Jouet *et al.* 1994), or mutations in myelin proteolipid protein (Saugier-Veber *et al.* 1994).

14.8.3 Neurolathyrism

Daily oral consumption of the chickling pea vetch (*Lathyrus sativus*) for some months causes a spastic paraparesis known as neurolathyrism. Neurolathyrism is endemic in areas of India, and is also recorded from elsewhere in Asia, China, southern Europe, and North Africa (Ludolph *et al.* 1987). It is most common and most severe in young adult males. Neurolathyrism may be epidemic at times of famine and has occurred in prisoner-of-war and concentration camps. It is thought to be due to an 'excitotoxic' non-protein amino-acid constituent of the chickling pea, β-N-oxalylamino-L-alanine (BOAA) (Ludolph *et al.* 1987). Animal models of the neurological disease have not yet been produced. Osteolathyrism is an animal disease resulting from a different species of *Lathyrus* which contains β-aminopropionitrile; this interferes with collagen cross-linking, thus provoking skeletal deformity and aortic aneurysms.

Neurolathyrism presents a relatively stereotyped clinical picture and may develop either subacutely or chronically. A spastic paraparesis with extensor plantar responses and markedly increased muscle tone in the quadriceps and gastrocaemius leads to a scissoring gait with the weight taken upon the balls of the feet. Patients often require a stick, and some are unable to walk at all. Sensory and sphincter abnormalities are rarely, if ever, present. Little or no recovery occurs, even after eliminating the chickling pea from the diet.

14.8.4 Konzo

Konzo is a form of tropical myelopathy which can occur in epidemics at times of famine in several parts of Africa, including Zaire. It seems to be due to dietary cyanide exposure resulting from insufficient soaking of the cassava roots used to produce flour (Tylleskär *et al.* 1992). There is an abrupt onset of symmetric spastic paraparesis which is non-progressive but permanent. Blood cyanide levels are raised at the onset of the disease.

14.9 Neuromyotonia

Neuromyotonia (see also Section 32.10.5) is a rare syndrome of spontaneously occurring muscle activity triggered by voluntary

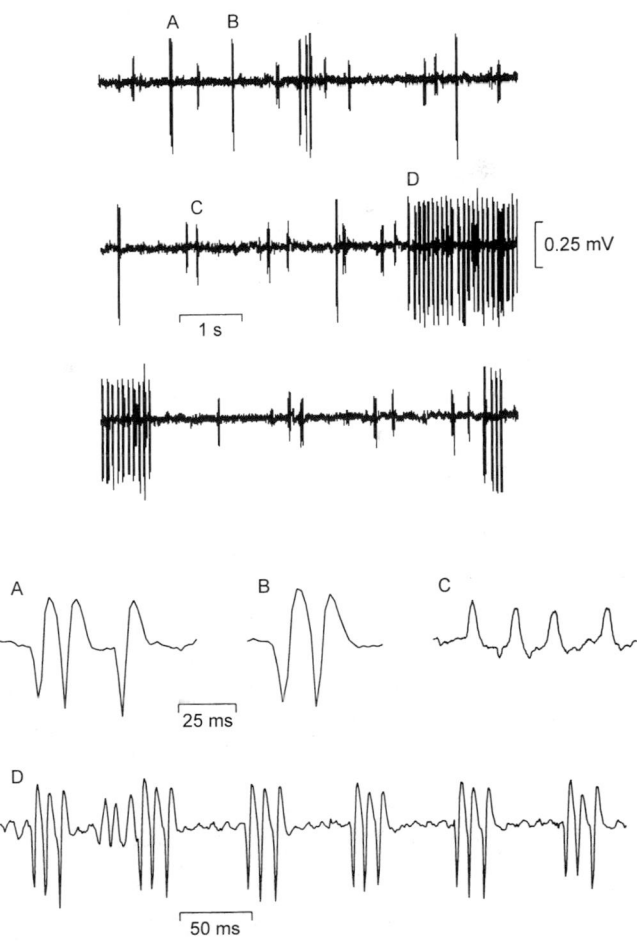

Fig. 14.9. Neuromyotonia. The upper traces are of a 25-second continuous needle EMG recording from medial gastrocnemius muscle in a patient with acquired neuromyotonia. Motor units are seen to fire spontaneously and irregularly as doublets (B), triplets (A) and multiplets (C), with intraburst frequencies of up to 120 Hz. The prolonged discharge seen in the middle of the recording consists of rapidly firing triplets of more than one motor unit (D). (Courtesy of Dr Paul Maddison.)

muscle contraction (Newsom-Davis and Mills 1993). This results in stiffness and cramping on attempts to use muscles. Slow relaxation of muscles, known as pseudomyotonia, and increased sweating may also occur. The underlying power of muscles is usually normal, apart from in those situations where the neuromyotonia is secondary to an underlying neuropathy.

Neuromyotonia is a manifestation of a heterogeneous group of underlying disorders. Most cases are acquired, and some of these are associated with underlying acute idiopathic polyneuritis, myasthenia gravis, raised antiacetylcholine antibody titres, or penicillamine administration (Newsom-Davis and Mills 1993). Neuromyotonia can be associated with underlying tumours in up of a fifth of all cases, usually thymoma or small cell lung cancer (Caress *et al.* 1997). Neuromyotonia also occurs occasionally in hereditary neuropathies (Hahn *et al.* 1991).

Electromyography serves to distinguish true myotonia from neuromyotonia. In neuromyotonia doublet or triplet motor unit discharges occur, or there may be continuous unit discharges at frequencies exceeding 40 per second, which are blocked by pharmacological blockade of neuromuscular transmission (Fig. 14.9).

Neuromyotonia must be considered in the differential diagnosis of visible myokymia, which is restricted to the muscles innervated by injured motor axons; from the stiff man syndrome (Section 32.10.3), in which high-frequency discharges are not seen and the increased muscle activity is abolished by sleep; and from the syndrome of benign camps and fasciculations, although the precise distinction from that disorder is unclear (Newsom-Davis and Mills 1993). Symptoms of neuromyotonia may improve dramatically with carbamazepine or phenytoin treatment. Some patients with acquired neuromyotonia benefit from plasma exchange. This, and the finding of antibodies to voltage-gated potassium channels (Hart *et al.* 1997), point to an antibody-mediated autoimmune pathogenesis.

References

Amato, A. A., Prior, T. W., Barohn, R. J. *et al.* (1993). Kennedy's disease: a clinicopathologic correlation with mutations in the androgen receptor gene. *Neurology*, **43**, 791–4.

Appelbaum, J. S., Roos, R. P., Salazar-Gruezo, E. F. *et al.* (1992). Intrafamilial heterogeneity in hereditary motor neurone disease. *Neurology*, **42**, 1488–92.

Barohn, R. J., Miller, R. G., and Griggs, R. C. (1991). Autosomal recessive distal dystrophy. *Neurology*, **41**, 1365–70.

Ben Hamida, M., Hentati, F., and Ben Hamida, C. (1990). Hereditary motor system diseases (chronic juvenile amyotrophic lateral sclerosis): conditions conducing a bilateral pyramidal syndrome with limb and bulbar amyotrophy. *Brain*, **113**, 347–63.

Berger, M. M., Kopp, N., Vital, C. *et al.* (2000). Detection and cellular localisation of enterovirus RNA sequences in spinal cord of patients with ALS. *Neurology*, **54**, 20–5.

Blexrud, M. D., Windebank, A. J., and Daube, J. R. (1993). Long-term follow up of 121 patients with benign fasciculations. *Ann. Neurol.*, **34**, 622–5.

Boitano, J., Jordan, T. and Benditt, O. (2001). Noninvasive ventilation allows gastrostomy tube placement in patients with advanced ALS. *Neurology*, **56**, 413–14.

Bowen, J., Gregory, R. P., Squier, M. *et al.* (1997). The post-irradiation lower motor neurone syndrome. Neuronopathy or radiculopathy? *Brain*, **119**, 1429–39.

Caress, J. B., Abend, W. K., Preston, D. C. *et al.* (1997). A case of Hodgkin's lymphoma producing neuromyotonia. *Neurology*, **49**, 258–9.

Chancellor, A. M. and Warlow, C. P. (1992). Adult onset motor neuron disease: worldwide mortality, incidence and distribution since 1950. *J. Neurol. Neurosurg. Psychiat.*, **55**, 1106–15.

Chancellor, A. M., Slattery, J. M., Frazer, M. *et al.* (1993). Risk factors for motor neuron disease: a case-control study based upon patients from the Scottish Motor Neuron Disease register. *J. Neurol. Neurosurg. Psychiat.*, **56**, 1200–6.

Christensen, P. B., Højer-Pedersen, E., and Jensen, N. B. (1990). Survival of patients with amyotrophic lateral sclerosis in 2 Danish counties. *Neurology*, **40**, 600–4.

Christodoulou, K., Kyriakides, T., Hristova, A. H. *et al.* (1995). Mapping of a distal form of spinal muscular atrophy with upper limb predominance to chromosome 7p. *Human Mol. Genet.*, **4**, 1629–32.

Christodoulou, K., Zamba, E., Tsingis, M. *et al.* (2000). A novel form of distal hereditary motor neuronopathy maps to chromosome 9p21.1-p12. *Ann. Neurol.*, **48**, 877–84.

Claus, D., Brunhölzl, C., Kerling, F. *et al.* (1995). Transcranial magnetic stimulation as a diagnostic and prognostic test in amyotrophic lateral sclerosis. *J. Neurol. Sci.*, **129** (Suppl.), 30–4.

Cornblath, D. R., Kuncl, R. W., Mellits, E. D. *et al.* (1992). Nerve conduction studies in amyotrophic lateral sclerosis. *Muscle Nerve*, **15**, 1111–15.

Côté, F., Collard, J.-F., and Julien, J.-P. (1993). Progressive neuronopathy in transgenic mice expressing the human neurofilament heavy gene: a mouse model of amyotrophic lateral sclerosis. *Cell*, **73**, 35–46.

Dalakas, M. C., Elder, G., Hallett, M. *et al.* (1986). A long-term follow-up study of patients with post-poliomyelitis neuromuscular symptoms. *N. Engl. J. Med.*, **314**, 959–63.

Davenport, R. J. and Mumford, C. J. (1994). The Brown–Violetto–Van Laere syndrome: a case report and literature review. *Eur. J. Neurol.*, **1**, 51–4.

DeLong, R. and Siddique, T. (1992). A large New England kindred with autosomal dominant neurogenic scapuloperoneal amyotrophy with unique features. *Arch. Neurol.*, **49**, 905–8.

Drug and Therapeutic Bulletin (1997). Riluzole for amyotrophic lateral sclerosis. *Drug Ther. Bull.*, **35**, 11–12.

Gordon, P. H., Rowland, L. P., Younger, D. S. *et al.* (1997). Lymphoproliferative disorders and motor neurone disease. *Neurology*, **48**, 1671–8.

Gregory, R. P., Mills, K. R., and Donaghy, M. (1993). Progressive sensory nerve dysfunction in amyotrophic lateral sclerosis: a prospective clinical and neurophysiological study. *J. Neurol.*, **140**, 309–14.

Gurney, M. E., Pu, H., Chiu, A. Y. *et al.* (1994). Motor neuron degeneration in mice that express a human Cn, Zn superoxide dismutase mutation. *Science*, **164**, 1772–5.

Hahn, A. F., Parkes, A. W., Bolton, C. F. *et al.* (1991). Neuromyotonia in hereditary motor neuropathy. *J. Neurol. Neurosurg. Psychiat.*, **54**, 230–5.

Harding, A. E. (1981). Hereditary 'pure' spastic paraplegia: a clinical and genetic study of 22 families. *J. Neurol. Neurosurg. Psychiat.*, **44**, 871–83.

Harding, A. E. and Thomas, P. K. (1980). Hereditary distal spinal muscular atrophy. A report on 34 cases and a review of the literature. *J. Neurol. Sci.*, **45**, 337–48.

Harding, A. E., Thomas, P. K., Baraitser, M. *et al.* (1982). X-linked recessive bulbospinal neuronopathy: a report of ten cases. *J. Neurol. Neurosurg. Psychiat.*, **45**, 1012–19.

Hart, I. K., Waters, C., Vincent, A. *et al.* (1997). Autoantibodies detected to expressed K$^+$ channels are implicated in neuromyotonia. *Ann. Neurol.*, **41**, 238–46.

Hazan, J., Fonknechten, N., Mavel, D. *et al.* (1999). Spastin, a new AAA protein, is altered in the most frequent form of autosomal dominant spastic paraplegia. *Nature Genet.*, **23**, 296–303.

Hirano, A., Donnenfeld, H., Sasaki, S. *et al.* (1984). Five structural observations of neurofilamentous changes in amyotrophic lateral sclerosis. *J. Neuropath. Exp. Neurol.*, **43**, 461–70.

Howard, R. S., Wiles, C. M. and Loh, L. (1989). Respiratory complications and their management in motor neuron disease. *Brain*, **112**, 1155–70.

Igarashi, S., Tanno, Y., Onodera, O. *et al.* (1992). Strong correlation between the number of CAG repeats in androgen receptor genes and the clinical onset of features of spinal and bulbar muscular atrophy. *Neurology*, **42**, 2300–2.

Ikezoe, M. D., Yoshimura, M. D., Taniwaki, T. *et al.* (1999). Autosomal dominant familial spinal and bulbar muscular atrophy with gynaecomastia. *Neurology*, **53**, 2187–9.

Jouet, M., Rosenthal, A., Armstrong, G. *et al.* (1994). X-linked spastic paraplegia (SPG1), MASA syndrome and X-linked hydrocephalus result from mutations in the L1 gene. *Nature Genet.*, **7**, 402–7.

Kachi, T., Sobue, G. and Sobue, I. (1992). Central motor and sensory conduction in X-linked recessive bulbospinal neuronopathy. *J. Neurol. Neurosurg. Psychiat.*, **55**, 394–7.

Kennedy, W. R., Alter, M., and Sung, J. H. (1968). Progressive proximal spinal and bulbar muscular atrophy of late onset. *Neurology*, **18**, 671–80.

Kew, J. J. M., Goldstein, L. H., Leigh, P. N. *et al.* (1993). The relationship between abnormalities of cognitive function and cerebral activation in amyotrophic lateral sclerosis. *Brain*, **116**, 1399–423.

Kidd, D., Howard, R. S., Williams, A. J. *et al.* (1997). Late functional deterioration following paralytic poliomyelitis. *Q. J. Med.*, **90**, 189–96.

Kübler-Ross, E. (1969). *On death and dying.* Tavistock/Routledge, London.

Lacomblez, L., Bensimon, G., and Leigh, P. N. (1996). Dose-ranging study of Riluzole in amyotrophic lateral sclerosis. *Lancet*, **347**, 1425–31.

Lander, C. M., Eadie, M. J., and Tyrer, J. H. (1976). Hereditary motor peripheral neuropathy predominantly affecting the arms. *J. Neurol. Sci.*, **28**, 389–94.

La Spada, A. R., Wilson, E. M., Lubahn, D. B. *et al.* (1991). Androgen receptor gene mutations in X-linked spinal and bulbar muscular atrophy. *Nature*, **352**, 77–9.

Le Febvre, S., Bürglen, L., Frézal, J. *et al.* (1998). The role of the SMN gene in proximal spinal muscular atrophy. *Hum. Mol. Genet.*, **7**, 1531–6.

Ludolph, A. C., Hugon, J., Dwivedi, M. P. *et al.* (1987). Studies on the aetiology and pathogenesis of motor neuron diseases. Lathyrism: clinical findings in established cases. *Brain*, **110**, 149–66.

Matsuura, T., Demura, T., Aimoto, Y. *et al.* (1992). Androgen receptor abnormality in X-linked spinal and bulbar muscular atrophy. *Neurology*, **42**, 1724–6.

McDermott, C. J., White, K., Bushby K. *et al.* (2000). Hereditary spastic paraperisis: a review of new developments. *J. Neurol. Neurosurg. Psychiat.*, **69**, 150–60.

McShane, M. A., Boyd, S. B., Harding, B. *et al.* (1992). Progressive bulbar paralysis of childhood. A reappraisal of Fazio-Londe disease. *Brain*, **115**, 1889–900.

Mulder, D. W., Kurland, L. T., Offord, K. P. *et al.* (1986). Familial adult motor neuron disease: amyotrophic lateral sclerosis. *Neurology*, **36**, 511–17.

Nathanson, N. (1982). Eradication of poliomyelitis in the United States. *Rev. Infect. Dis.*, **4**, 940–50.

Neary, D., Snowden, J. S., Mann, D. M. A. *et al.* (1990). Frontal lobe dementia and motor neurone disease. *J. Neurol. Neurosurg. Psychiat.*, **53**, 23–32.

Newsom-Davis, J. and Mills, K. R. (1993). Immunological associations of acquired neuromyotonia (Isaacs' syndrome). *Brain*, **116**, 453–69.

Nielsen, J. E., Krabbe, K., Jennum, P. *et al.* (1998). Autosomal dominant pure spastic paraplegia: a clinical, paraclinical, and genetic study. *J. Neurol. Neurosurg. Psychiat.*, **64**, 61–6.

Olney, R. K., Aminoff, M. J., and So, Y. T. (1991). Clinical and electrodiagnostic features of X-linked recessive bulbospinal neuronopathy. *Neurology*, **41**, 823–8.

Pearn, J. M., Carter, C. O., and Wilson, J. (1973). The genetic identity of acute infantile spinal muscular atrophy. *Brain*, **96**, 463–70.

Price, R. W. and Plum, F. (1978). In *Handbook of clinical neurology*, Vol. 34, (ed. P. J. Vinken and G. W. Bruyn), pp. 93–132. Elsevier, Amsterdam.

Pringle, C. E., Hudson, A. J., Munoz, D. G. *et al.* (1992). Primary lateral sclerosis. Clinical features, neuropathology and diagnostic criteria. *Brain*, **115**, 495–520.

Rabin, B. A., Griffin, J. W., Crain, B. J. *et al.* (1999). Autosomal dominant juvenile amyotrophic lateral sclerosis. *Brain*, **122**, 1539–50.

Reid, E., Dearlovea, A. M., and Whiteford, M. L. (1999). Autosomal dominant spastic paraplegia. Refined SPG8 locus and additional genetic heterogeneity. *Neurology*, **53**, 1844–9.

Ricker, K., Mertens, H.-G., and Schimrigk, K. (1968). The neurogenic scapulo-peroneal syndrome. *Eur. Neurol.*, **1**, 257–74.

Rodgers-Johnson, P., Garruto, R. M., Yanagihara, R. *et al.* (1986). Amyotrophic lateral sclerosis and parkinsonism-dementia on Guam. *Neurology*, **36**, 7–13.

Román, G. C. (1996). Neuroepidemiology of amyotrophic lateral sclerosis: clues to aetiology and pathogenesis. *J. Neurol. Neurosurg. Psychiat.*, **61**, 131–7.

Rosen, D. R., Siddique, T., Patterson, D. *et al.* (1993). Mutations in Cu/Zn superoxide dismutase gene are associated with familial amyotrophic lateral sclerosis. *Nature*, **362**, 59–62.

Rothstein, J. D., Martin, L. J., and Kuncl, R. W. (1992). Decreased glutamate transport by the brain and spinal cord in amyotrophic lateral sclerosis. *N. Engl. J. Med.*, **326**, 1464–8.

Saugier-Veber, P., Munnich, A., Bonneau, D. *et al.* (1994). X-linked spastic paraplegia and Pelizaeus–Merzbacher disease are allelic disorders at the proteolipid protein locus. *Nature Genet.*, **6**, 257–62.

Seljeseth, Y., Vollset, S. E. and Tysnes, O. (2000). Increasing mortality from amyotrophic lateral sclerosis in Norway? *Neurology*, **55**, 1262–6.

Sharief, M. K., Hentges, R., and Ciardi, M. (1991). Intrathecal immune response in patients with the post-polio syndrome. *N. Engl. J. Med.*, **325**, 749–55.

Sky, M. E., Rowland, L. P., Smith, T. *et al.* (1986). Motor neuron disease and plasma cell dyscrasia. *Neurology*, **36**, 1429–36.

Sobue, I., Saito, N., Iida, M. *et al.* (1978). Juvenile type of distal and segmental muscular atrophy of upper extremities. *Ann. Neurol.*, **3**, 429–37.

Sonies, B. C. and Dalakas, M. C. (1991). Dysphagia in patients with the post-polio syndrome. *N. Engl. J. Med.*, **324**, 1162–7.

Tandan, R. and Bradley, W. G. (1985). Amyotrophic lateral sclerosis: Part 1. Clinical features, pathology, and ethical issues in management. *Ann. Neurol.*, **18**, 271–80.

Trojan, D. A. and Cashman, N. R. (1995). Fibromyalgia is common in a postpoliomyelitis clinic. *Arch. Neurol.*, **52**, 620–4.

Tucker, T., Layzer, R. B., Miller, R. G. *et al.* (1991). Subacute, reversible motor neuron disease. *Neurology*, **41**, 1541–4.

Tylleskär, T., Banea, M., Bikangi, N. *et al.* (1992). Cassava cyanogens and Konzo, an upper motor neuron disease found in Africa. *Lancet*, **339**, 208–11.

Uncini, A., Servidei, S., Delli Pizzi, C. *et al.* (1992). Benign monomelic amyotrophy of lower limb: report of three cases. *Acta Neurol. Scand.*, **85**, 397–400.

Warner, C. L., Griffin, J. E., Wilson, J. D. *et al.* (1992). X-linked spinomuscular atrophy: a kindred with associated abnormal androgen receptor binding. *Neurology*, **42**, 2181–4.

Webb, S., Patterson, V., and Hutchinson, M. (1997). Two families with autosomal recessive spastic paraplegia, pigmented maculopathy, and dementia. *J. Neurol. Neurosurg. Psychiat.*, **63**, 628–32.

White, K. D. Ince, P. G., Lusher, M. *et al.* (2000). Clinical and pathological findings in hereditary spastic paraparesis with spastic mutation. *Neurology*, **55**, 89–94.

Williams, C., Kozlowski, M. A., Hinton, D. R. *et al.* (1990). Degeneration of spinocerebellar neurons in amyotrophic lateral sclerosis. *Ann. Neurol.*, **27**, 215–25.

Windebank, A. J., Litchy, W. J., Daube, J. R. *et al.* (1996). Lack of progression of neurologic deficit in survivors of paralytic polio. *Neurology*, **46**, 80–4.

Wood, M. and Anderson, M. (1988). *Neurological infections.* W. B. Saunders, London.

Wyatt, H. V. (1973). Poliomyelitis in hypogammaglobulinaemics. *J. Infect. Dis.*, **128**, 802–6.

Young, I. and Harper, P. (1980). Hereditary distal spinal muscular atrophy with vocal cord paralysis. *J. Neurol. Neurosurg. Psychiat.*, **43**, 413–18.

CHAPTER 15

Muscle diseases

David Hilton-Jones

15.1 Introduction

This chapter is concerned with those disorders in which the primary pathological process affects skeletal muscle, and in everyday clinical practice the term 'myopathy' is a convenient shorthand. However, it must be stressed that diseases of the motor nerves and neuromuscular junction can produce an identical clinical picture to several of the myopathies, and this will be emphasized many times throughout the chapter when considering differential diagnosis. Indeed sometimes, despite one's best efforts, one is left uncertain as to whether the primary disease process is in the nerves or muscles—it may be that in some conditions the disease process directly affects both nerves and muscles. The intimate relationship, both structural and functional, between nerves and the muscles they innervate means that disease of one may have a profound effect on the other—the most striking example is the change that occurs in skeletal muscle fibre-type distribution when it is denervated.

Huge advances have been made in our understanding of neuromuscular disorders (i.e. diseases of nerve, neuromuscular junction, and skeletal muscle) over the past two decades, but as yet not all of these have been translated into effective therapy. Myasthenia gravis and many of the idiopathic inflammatory myopathies are treatable, by relatively crude immunosuppressive regimens, but eventually it is to be hoped that more detailed knowledge of their immunopathogenesis will lead to specific, and safer, therapies. The genetic and molecular bases of several forms of muscular dystrophy are now known. This aids diagnosis in individual cases and should, in the future, lead on to specific therapies, either through genetic engineering methods or by strategies that replace a defective protein or ameliorate the effects of the accumulation of a non-functional protein. Diseases associated with abnormal ion-channel function (the so-called channelopathies) are appearing throughout neurology, and the myopathies provide several interesting examples. Primary metabolic disorders, although relatively rare, are a topic of considerable interest, none more so than the mitochondrial cytopathies.

At present, no specific therapies are available for the majority of the myopathies, particularly those that are likely to present to neurological clinics. This increases, rather than decreases, the burden on the clinician. An enormous amount can be done to help the patient and family, and in many countries specialist clinics are now available that aim to provide an integrated approach to management. In addition, for many of these disorders, genetic issues are of enormous importance, but may be overlooked by the non-specialist. If a case of an X-linked disorder is diagnosed, then counselling should be offered to appropriate female family members. In the case of myotonic dystrophy, failure to identify an asymptomatic female carrier of the gene, who then goes on to have a congenitally affected child, is tragic.

This introductory section will cover aspects of the structure and function of the neuromuscular system, and the clinical and laboratory approach to diagnosis. Thereafter, individual disorders will be discussed, with the extent of coverage reflecting the commonness or otherwise of the disorder, rather than the degree of research interest.

15.1.1 Structure and function

It is not necessary to have an in-depth knowledge of the anatomy, physiology, and biochemistry of the neuromuscular system in order to understand, diagnose, and treat most of the conditions to be discussed in this chapter. However, some understanding of the basic processes involved is undoubtedly advantageous. This section covers aspects of structure and function. Biochemical processes are discussed in Section 15.6.

From the practising clinician's point of view, the neuromuscular system can be considered to have three major components: the lower motor neuron, the neuromuscular junction, and muscle fibres. The cell bodies of the *lower motor neurons* are situated in the brainstem motor nuclei and in the grey matter of the anterior horns of the spinal cord (hence their alternative name, anterior horn cells). The motor neuron axons travel in the cranial nerves and the spinal ventral roots. The latter contribute to the brachial and lumbosacral plexuses from which the peripheral nerves arise, which are generally mixed nerves in that they also convey sensory fibres. In terms of differential diagnosis, disorders of anterior horn cells and motor neurons (e.g. spinal muscular atrophy) are of considerable importance because clinically they may closely mimic myopathies. Thus, we now know that some patients previously diagnosed as having Becker muscular dystrophy in fact had chronic spinal muscular atrophy.

A more detailed description of the structure and functioning of the *neuromuscular junction* is given in Section 15.10. In brief, the arrival of a nerve impulse opens voltage-gated calcium channels in the nerve terminal. This leads to an influx of calcium ions, which triggers the release of many quanta of acetylcholine (ACh). The ACh diffuses across the synaptic cleft to interact with ACh receptors on the postsynaptic (muscle) membrane. This leads to an influx of cations, mainly sodium, which causes transient depolarization of the muscle-fibre membrane (the end-plate potential) which, in turn, activates voltage-gated sodium channels, producing an action potential in the muscle fibre. Neuromuscular junction disorders, like anterior horn cell disorders discussed above, are not associated with sensory symptomatology, and may also mimic conditions in which the primary pathology is at muscle fibre level.

Skeletal muscle is composed of numerous *muscle fibres* grouped together in fasciculi (Fig. 15.1). Each fibre is a multinucleate cell containing numerous myofibrils (the contractile proteins), sarcoplasm (equivalent to the cytoplasm of mononuclear cells), mitochondria, and the sarcotubular system (Fig. 15.2). The muscle fibre membrane is called the sarcolemma, and in normal muscle the nuclei lie just beneath it. In clinical practice we recognize diseases that affect the muscle fibre membrane (several types of muscular dystrophy, the channelopathies), biochemical processes occurring in the sarco-

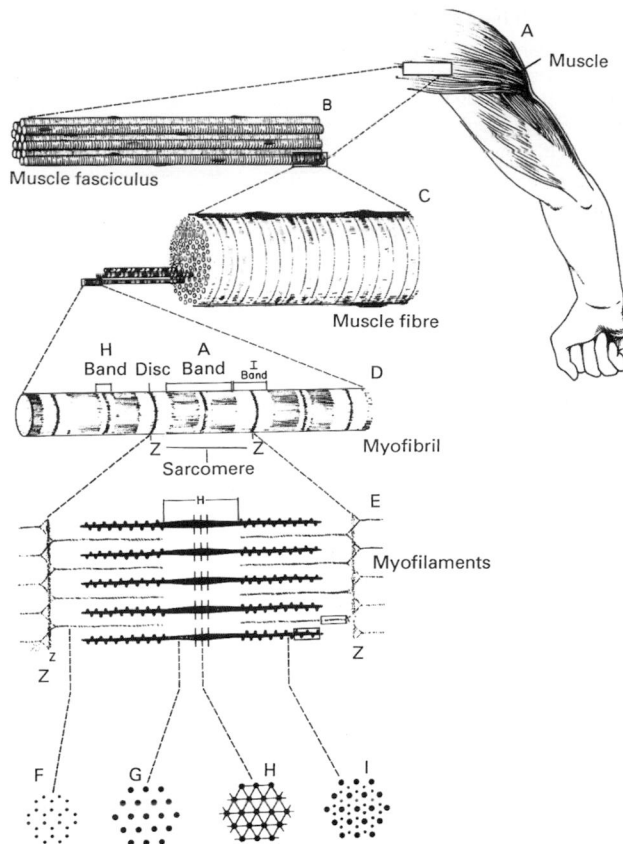

Fig. 15.1. Histological and molecular structure of skeletal muscle. (Reproduced from Patton *et al.* (1976) and modified from Bloom and Fawcett (1970), by kind permission of the authors and publisher.)

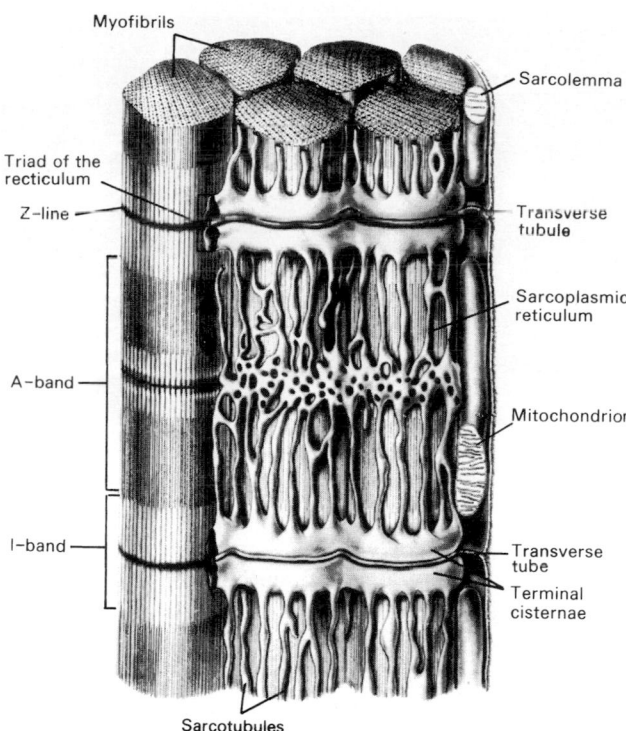

Fig. 15.2. Muscle structure, showing relation of endoplasmic reticulum and of transverse tubular system to fibrils. (Reproduced from Patton *et al.* (1976) and previously published in Bloom and Fawcett (1970), by kind permission of the authors and publisher.)

plasm and mitochondria (the primary metabolic myopathies and mitochondrial cytopathies, myotonic dystrophy, some forms of muscular dystrophy), the sarcotubular system (Brody's syndrome, tubular aggregate myopathy), the microvascular system (dermatomyositis), and inflammatory/immune proesses that destroy muscle fibres (polymyositis), as well as conditions that involve the interstitial tissues.

The muscle fibre action potential is propagated deep into each fibre by the T-tubular system (Fig. 15.2). The T-tubules are intimately associated with the sarcoplasmic reticulum (SR) and depolarization of this leads to release of calcium ions which, in turn, activate the contractile proteins (actin, myosin, and others), an intensely energy-consuming process fuelled by adenosine triphosphate (ATP). Relaxation is achieved through re-uptake of calcium ions into the SR, which is also an energy-dependent process, mediated by SR Ca^{2+}-ATPase.

The *motor unit* is an important concept physiologically and when interpreting the results of clinical neurophysiological studies and muscle biopsy. Each muscle fibre is innervated by only one axon. But each motor neuron undergoes terminal axonal branching and innervates many muscle fibres. These fibres are scattered randomly throughout the muscle, lying between fibres supplied by other motor neurons. Another important, and related, concept is that of *fibre types*. In many

animals two types of muscle are recognized, red and white. Red muscle is composed of type I muscle fibres which are rich in myoglobin (giving the red colour) and mitochondria, are relatively slow to contract, but resistant to fatigue. White muscle, on the other hand, is composed of type II fibres, which have fewer mitochondria and greater glycolytic capacity. It has fast-twitch characteristics and fatigues relatively rapidly. Human muscles in health are composed of a mixture of both fibre types, which gives the characteristic chequerboard appearance

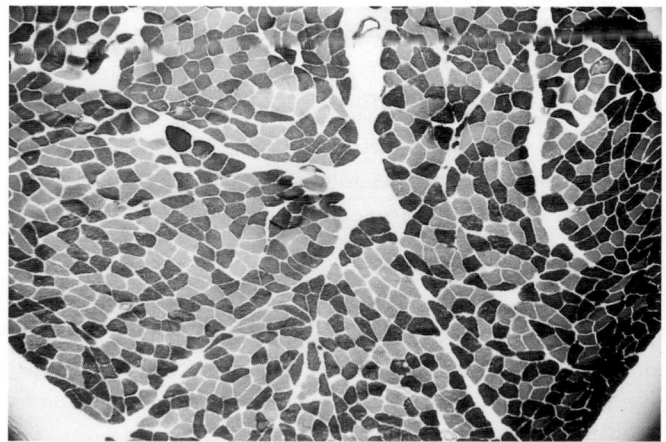

Fig. 15.3. Normal muscle fibre-type distribution. ATPase stain at pH 9.6. Type I fibres pale, type II fibres dark. (Courtesy of Dr Waney Squier.)

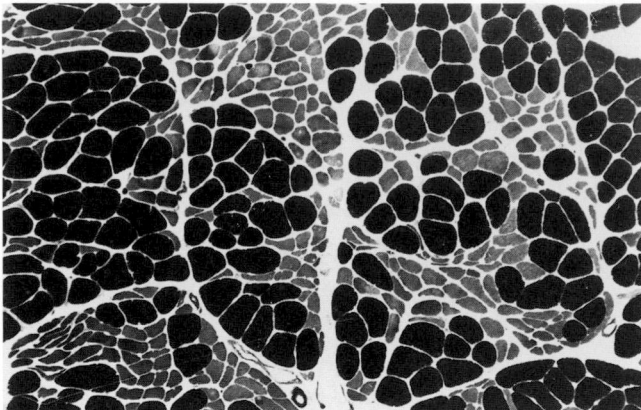

Fig. 15.4. Fibre-type grouping in denervation/reinnervation. Compare with Fig. 15.3. (Courtesy of Dr Waney Squier.)

Table 15.1. Inherited and acquired myopathies

Inherited
    Muscular dystrophies
    Myotonic dystrophy
    Congenital myopathies
    Channelopathies
    Primary metabolic disorders
    Congenital myasthenic syndromes[a]
Acquired
    Drug and toxin induced
    Endocrine
    Secondary metabolic
    Inflammatory
    Paraneoplastic
    Myasthenia gravis[a]
    Lambert–Eaton myasthenic syndrome[a]

*Arguably, these disorders might be classified as channelopathies with there being a primary, inherited, ion-channel abnormality in some of the congenital myasthenic syndromes and secondary, acquired, ion-channel dysfunction or destruction in myasthenia gravis and Lambert–Eaton syndrome.

to a cross-sectional muscle biopsy stained to differentiate between fibre types (Fig. 15.3). A number of histochemical reactions applied to muscle biopsy specimens allow differentiation between different fibre types. The most important technique is myofibrillar ATPase staining. Pre-incubation in acid or alkaline buffers allows distinction between type I and II fibres. In fact, various other subtypes can be identified, notably type II into types IIA, B, and C. Identification of these is of limited diagnostic value in certain pathological states. Considering again the motor unit, there is now overwhelming evidence that the innervating neuron determines the fibre type. Thus, we should think in terms of type I motor neurons, which will make any muscle fibre they innervate have the characteristics of type I muscle fibres, as described above. Similarly for type II motor neurons. Returning to the chequerboard appearance (Fig. 15.3), the distribution of the different fibre types is due to the random innervation of fibres scattered throughout the muscle by individual motor neurons. In pathological conditions that are associated with denervation and subsequent reinnervation this random pattern changes. Surviving neurons sprout and innervate several adjacent previously denervated fibres, converting them all to the same fibre type. The resulting appearance on a cross-sectional muscle biopsy is of fibre-type grouping (Fig. 15.4).

15.1.2 Classification

There is no universally accepted approach to the classification of neuromuscular disorders. Important recent contributions in terms of comprehensive cataloguing of disorders include ICD10-NA (the World Health Organization's *Application of the International Classification of Diseases to neurology*) and *Classification of neuromuscular disorders* (Rowland and McLeod 1994). These comprehensive listings are valuable for coding and other purposes, but in everyday clinical practice what is needed is a simpler classification that helps in focusing investigations (and also in focusing the clinician's mind).

The first major division is between acquired and inherited myopathies (Table 15.1). Subclassification within each of the

categories listed will be discussed in the corresponding section. As a general observation, at the time of writing, no specific therapy is available for any of the inherited conditions listed in Table 15.1, although symptomatic treatment can be very helpful in some, notably the channelopathies (primary periodic paralyses and myotonia congenita) and some forms of congenital myasthenia. Genetic counselling, and in some cases the provision of an antenatal diagnostic service, is of major importance. The particular importance of recognizing acquired myopathies is that many of them are treatable. This may be by correcting the primary underlying disorder, such as an endocrinopathy or metabolic abnormality, by removal of a causative drug or toxin, or by immune modulation (as with the idiopathic inflammatory myopathies, myasthenia gravis, or Lambert–Eaton myasthenic syndrome). It bears stressing that at the bedside even the most experienced neuromuscular clinician may not be able to distinguish between a form of muscular dystrophy, a chronic inflammatory myopathy, and a metabolic disorder—misdiagnosis may have far-reaching consequences, not just for the patient but also for family members in the present and future generations.

15.1.3 Clinical approach

Some disorders are so characteristic that a confident specific diagnosis may be made at the bedside. Further investigation can then be limited to a confirmatory test. For example, classical myotonic dystrophy is confirmable by demonstrating the specific gene abnormality. Even if clinical assessment does not give a specific diagnosis, it will often point to the nature of the problem (e.g. a dystrophy, inflammatory myopathy, or metabolic disorder) and thus to the course of further investigations. This section reviews certain aspects of the history and physical examination as they relate to myopathic disorders, and is followed by further sections detailing particular investigative methods. Muscle has a limited range of responses to a wide range of disease, so the symptoms and signs associated with myopathies are relatively few.

Weakness

Weakness is the most common presenting symptom of muscle disease. The distribution, date of onset, and rate of progression must be determined. Fluctuating weakness is seen in myasthenic syndromes, and in some of the channelopathies and metabolic myopathies.

Considering the cranial nerve territory, variable ptosis and diplopia are characteristic of myasthenia gravis. Constant ptosis is seen in mitochondrial chronic progressive external ophthalmoplegia (CPEO), myotonic dystrophy, oculopharyngeal muscular dystrophy, and several congenital myopathies. Limitation of eye movements, with or without diplopia, is seen in mitochondrial CPEO, myasthenic syndromes, oculopharyngeal muscular dystrophy, and thyroid ophthalmopathy. Constant or fluctuating ptosis and diplopia may be seen with thyroid ophthalmopathy.

Facial weakness in myopathic disorders is usually bilateral and symmetrical, and mild weakness is easily overlooked. Classical symptoms include difficulty whistling, sucking through a straw, and blowing-up balloons. Facial weakness can be striking in myasthenia gravis, myotonic dystrophy, and facioscapulohumeral muscular dystrophy. If present at all, it is usually mild in other dystrophies and inflammatory myopathies. Bulbar weakness, causing dysarthria and dysphagia, is common in myasthenia gravis. Dysphagia may be the presenting symptom in oculopharyngeal muscular dystrophy. It is seen in severe cases of idiopathic inflammatory myopathy and occasionally as a relatively early feature in inclusion-body myositis.

Selective involvement of limb muscles may provide a powerful clue as to the diagnosis. In most of the acquired myopathies (Table 15.1) the selectivity is in the form of proximal greater than distal weakness. A similar distribution may be seen in certain neuropathies, particularly the inflammatory demyelinating polyradiculoneuropathies (Sections 12.10 and 12.11), and in myasthenic syndromes. It is with the dystrophies (including myotonic dystrophy) that the most remarkable selectivity may be seen, and as yet no satisfactory explanation for this phenomenon has been advanced. Individual disorders are discussed later. Particularly striking examples include facioscapulohumeral (FSH) muscular dystrophy, oculopharyngeal muscular dystrophy, and myotonic dystrophy. In FSH dystrophy the scapular and humeral (biceps and triceps) muscles may be profoundly weak and wasted, but, sitting between them, the deltoid appears normal. A few disorders characteristically have distal weakness as an early feature, the most common examples being myotonic dystrophy and inclusion-body myositis.

Respiratory muscle weakness may be seen in the late stages of many neuromuscular disorders, and is often the major factor contributing to the patient's demise (e.g. in Duchenne muscular dystrophy, rigid spine syndrome). Importantly, respiratory failure may be the presenting feature of a number of disorders,

most notably adult-onset acid maltase deficiency and amyotrophic lateral scleroris (Section 14.1.6) motor neuron disease. The earliest symptoms of respiratory insufficiency include nightmares, early-morning headache, and excessive daytime sleepiness. Only later does the patient complain of breathlessness on exertion and orthopnoea. Bedside testing should include vital capacity measurement and looking for paradoxical abdominal movement indicative of diaphragmatic weakness (on inspiration, with the patient lying flat, the upper abdomen is drawn inwards) (Fig. 13.12).

Pain

Pain is perhaps the next most common symptom in a neuromuscular clinic. It is worth noting that if pain is the sole complaint and physical examination is normal, then a specific diagnosis is often not achieved. Pain may be very localized or widespread (Table 15.2), or it may be exercise induced (Table 15.3).

Table 15.2. Disorders causing localized or generalized muscle pain

Localized
Trauma
Ischaemia
Infection
bacterial
parasitic
Acute alcoholic myopathy
Some glycogenoses (e.g. McArdle's disease)
Inflammation: sarcoidosis, eosinophilic fasciitis
Neuralgic amyotrophy
Generalized
Idiopathic inflammatory myopathies (if acute)
Infections
viral
toxoplasmosis
Drug-induced myopathies
Metabolic myopathies
metabolic bone disease
hypothyroid myopathy
carnitine palmitoyltransferase deficiency
Polymyalgia rheumatica
Connective tissue disorders
Guillain–Barré syndrome
Porphyria

Table 15.3. Causes of exercise-induced muscle pain

Metabolic myopathies
Glycogenoses
Mitochondrial cytopathies
Carnitine palmitoyltransferase deficiency
Muscular dystrophies
Duchenne
Becker
Tubular aggregate myopathy
Dermatomyositis
Ischaemia (claudication)

Cramps

Patients may mean one of several things when they complain of muscle cramps. Ordinary cramps are neurogenic in origin; motor nerve hyperactivity causes painful muscle contraction, and electromyography (EMG) shows high-frequency motor unit discharges. They are usually benign but predisposing factors include metabolic disturbances and hypothyroidism. Pathological states associated with neurogenic hyperactivity include neuromyotonia and stiff-man syndrome. However, cramp may also be used to describe problems arising at muscle fibre level. *Myotonia* is caused by recurrent muscle fibre membrane depolarization. The patient complains of delayed relaxation of grip, or jaw stiffness when chewing. The most common cause is myotonic dystrophy, but the phenomenon may be much more severe in the rarer condition of myotonia congenita. Grip and percussion myotonia are readily demonstrated at the bedside (Fig. 15.5). Electrically silent *contractures* are a feature of some metabolic disorders, notably glycogenoses such as myophosphorylase deficiency (McArdle's disease), and the extremely rare conditions of Brody's syndrome and rippling muscle disease.

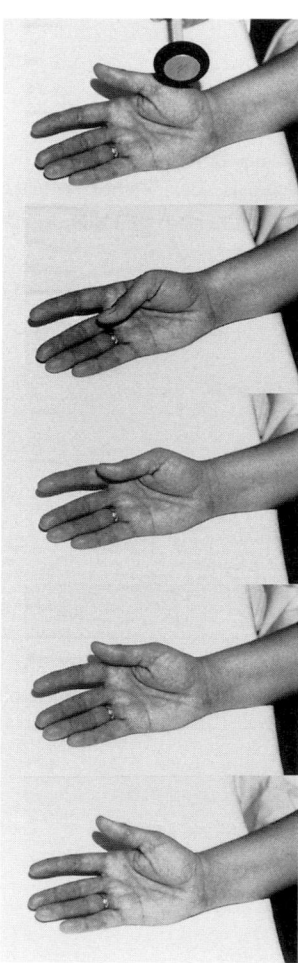

Fig. 15.5. Percussion myotonia. Sequential photographs taken at approximately 3-second intervals, after a sharp tap to the thenar eminence.

The term 'contracture' is also used to describe the shortening of muscles and associated inability to passively stretch them caused by progressive fibrosis of the muscle. This is seen as a late feature in many myopathies and neurogenic disorders, but is also an important early symptom and sign in Emery–Dreifuss muscular dystrophy, Bethlem myopathy, and rigid spine syndrome.

Wasting

Wasting is not a common presenting symptom. In myopathies weakness tends to precede wasting, whereas in neurogenic disorders the two processes tend to occur in parallel. Muscle *pseudohypertrophy* (probably due to fatty and fibrous tissue infiltration) is seen in Duchenne and Becker muscular dystrophy and less commonly in autosomal limb-girdle dystrophies. True *hypertrophy* (a form of work-hypertrophy) is seen in myotonia congenita and neuromyotonia.

Myoglobinuria

Myoglobinuria is noted by the patient as passage of dark urine and is due to extensive muscle damage that allows the release of myoglobin into the bloodstream. It poses a risk of renal failure from acute tubular necrosis. Commoner causes are noted in Table 15.4.

Tendon reflexes

Tendon reflexes tend to be preserved in myopathic disorders, in contrast to neurogenic conditions in which they are depressed or lost at an early stage. In the Lambert–Eaton myasthenic syndrome the reflexes are reduced or absent, but show striking post-contraction potentiation.

Table 15.4. Causes of myoglobinuria

Intensive exercise in normal individuals

Inherited myopathies
  metabolic (glycogenoses, lipid storage disorders, malignant hyperthermia)
  dystrophic (Duchenne and Becker muscular dystrophy)

Acquired myopathies
  inflammatory (dermatomyositis and polymyositis)
  infections (viral and bacterial)

Ischaemia

Trauma
  crush injury
  electric shock
  status epilepticus

Drugs
  opiates
  clofibrate

Toxins
  alcohol
  animal venoms

Others
  neuroleptic malignant syndrome
  metabolic disorders
  heat stroke

Table 15.5. Skeletal myopathies associated with heart involvement

Dysrhythmias
  Myotonic dystrophy
  Emery–Dreifuss muscular dystrophy
  Mitochondrial cytopathies
Cardiomyopathy
  Duchenne and Becker muscular dystrophy
  Emery–Dreifuss muscular dystrophy
  Limb-girdle muscular dystrophy
  Dermatomyositis
  Debranching enzyme deficiency
  Alcoholism
  Endocrine myopathies

The history-taking and examination must extend beyond the neuromuscular system. Important aspects in the history include family history, current or recent drug and toxin exposure (including anaesthetics), past medical history, and systematic review of all other body systems (many myopathies are part of a multisystem disorder, or a purely myopathic condition may lead to secondary effects elsewhere, such as the symptoms associated with respiratory failure). Similarly, physical examination must include a fairly detailed general medical assessment (don't forget respiratory function), as well as assessment of the central nervous system (CNS) and peripheral nervous system (for evidence of sensory nerve dysfunction). Cardiomyopathy and dysrhythmias, which may be either subclinical or which may dominate the clinical picture, are seen in association with a number of skeletal myopathies (Table 15.5). CNS involvement is common in mitochondrial cytopathies (e.g. pigmentary retinopathy, ophthalmoplegia, deafness, cognitive impairment). Sensory symptoms and signs point away from a disorder affecting the anterior horn cell, neuromuscular junction, or muscle, but be aware that compressive neuropathies (e.g. ulnar nerve at the elbow, common peroneal nerve at the knee) may be a secondary consequence of immobility.

15.1.4 Biochemical investigations

The most familiar biochemical test for investigation of a suspected myopathy is estimation of the serum *creatine kinase* (CK) level. Muscle damage, from whatever cause, leads to release of CK into the bloodstream. The specific skeletal muscle isoform is CK MM, in contrast to cardiac muscle CK MB, but

Table 15.6. Causes of an elevated creatine kinase (CK) level in 'normal' individuals

Hypothyroidism
Female carriers of Duchenne/Becker muscular dystrophy gene
Male with Becker muscular dystrophy
Susceptibility to malignant hyperthermia
Drug-induced subclinical myopathy
Strenuous physical exercise

generally only the total CK activity is measured. Serum CK is always elevated in Duchenne, Becker, and Emery–Dreifuss muscular dystrophy. It is usually elevated in inflammatory myopathies, glycogenoses, congenital muscular dystrophy, autosomal limb-girdle muscular dystrophies. Mildly elevated CK levels occur in amyotrophic lateral sclerosis (Section 14.2.2) and Kennedy syndrome (Section 14.4.1). It is often normal in myotonic dystrophy, facioscapulohumeral muscular dystrophy, mitochondrial cytopathies, and drug-induced myopathies (especially steroid myopathy). An elevated CK in an apparently normal individual is a teasing clinical problem with several causes (Table 15.6).

In mitochondrial cytopathies, serum and spinal fluid *lactate* and *pyruvate* levels may be elevated. Serum levels are measured in exercise tests, described below. In disorders of lipid metabolism, blood and urine *carnitine* and *acyl-carnitine* levels and ratios may be altered.

Exercise tests are used to investigate suspected metabolic myopathies. The *forearm exercise test* is used to screen for disorders of glycogenolysis, and glycolysis and biochemical considerations are discussed further in Section 15.6.1. In brief, venous blood from the forearm is assayed after vigorous use of the flexor muscles (typically by repeatedly squeezing a rubber bulb). The normal response is a rise in lactate and ammonia levels. The former is blunted or absent, and the latter accentuated, with defects of the glycogenolytic/glycolytic pathway.

Aerobic exercise is most easily performed on a static bicycle. In mitochondrial disorders there is an excessive rise in serum lactate and in the lactate/pyruvate ratio. This is mainly a research procedure.

Phosphorus magnetic resonance spectroscopy is a powerful tool for investigating aspects of muscle energy metabolism *in vivo*, but availability is very limited. It allows measurement of the phosphorus-containing molecules ATP, phosphocreatine, phosphomonoesters, and inorganic phosphate in muscle, all of which play a vital role in normal energetic processes (Hilton-Jones *et al.* 1995). Intracellular pH can also be determined. It can replace, and indeed give additional information over, the forearm and aerobic exercise protocols described above.

Prolonged fasting may be used to assess disorders of lipid metabolism, but is potentially very hazardous and its use should be restricted to specialist units.

For most of the primary metabolic myopathies the diagnosis is proven by *enzyme assay*, most frequently on a sample of muscle frozen and stored at –70 °C at the time of biopsy. In some conditions assay may be on blood cells, urine, cultured fibroblasts, or liver biopsy.

15.1.5 Neurophysiological studies

These are discussed in Section 2.5, but a brief review of their value in studying suspected myopathies is appropriate here. Nerve-conduction studies are an essential part of the evaluation. As noted, primary neurogenic disorders may clinically mimic a myopathy. Nerve conduction is normal in diseases that affect only muscle, but may be abnormal in conditions in which nerve and muscle pathology may coexist, such as the mitochondrial cytopathies. Similar comments apply to somatosensory evoked potential studies.

Electromyography

The most useful technique for studying primary muscle disease is concentric needle electrode electromyography (EMG), with a modification of this technique (single-fibre EMG) being a major tool for the study of neuromuscular junction disorders. Four particular features can be documented.

Insertional activity

Insertional activity describes the electrical response seen when the EMG needle first enters the muscle or is subsequently moved, and is probably the result of muscle fibre damage. Increased activity is typical of denervation but may also be seen in inflammatory myopathies. Decreased activity is seen in atrophic and fibrotic muscle and during attacks of periodic paralysis.

Spontaneous activity

Spontaneous activity may be seen once any insertional activity has settled. Fibrillation potentials and positive sharp waves are typical of denervation but are also seen in inflammatory myopathies and active muscular dystrophies (Figs. 2.20 and 2.21). Fasciculation potentials indicate anterior horn cell disease but may rarely be seen in thyrotoxic myopathy. Myotonic discharges are most frequently encountered in myotonic dystrophy and the less common condition of myotonia congenita, more rarely in acid maltase deficiency and hypothyroidism.

Motor unit potentials

Motor unit potentials may be analysed in terms of amplitude, duration, number of phases, and the stability of the waveform. The characteristic appearance in myopathic disorders is of polyphasic potentials with reduced amplitude and duration. Instability of the waveform has the same significance as increased jitter (see below) and is seen in neuromuscular junction disorders, denervation, and some inflammatory myopathies.

Interference pattern

The interference pattern is more complex and develops at a lower force of contraction in myopathic disorders. This reflects early recruitment of the surviving muscle fibres.

Single-fibre electromyography

In single-fibre EMG a special electrode is positioned in such a way that it detects the potentials from two muscle fibres, each innervated by a terminal branch of the same axon. In response to nerve stimulation or voluntary contraction the two fibres fire nearly, but not quite, simultaneously. The slight difference between the potentials is called the interpotential difference, and reflects the difference in conduction times of the two ter-

minal pathways. *Jitter* is measured as the mean consecutive difference of successive interpotential intervals. The main source of jitter is neuromuscular transmission and thus it is increased in myasthenic disorders. It is also increased in mitochondrial cytopathies and in denervation.

Compound muscle action potential

Repetitive nerve stimulation and measurement of the evoked compound muscle action potential (CMAP) is also useful for the study of neuromuscular transmission. Myasthenia gravis is associated with a decremental response at 3 Hz stimulation (Fig. 2.22), whereas in the Lambert–Eaton syndrome the resting CMAP is small but increases in amplitude following brief voluntary contraction or with repetitive stimulation at 20 Hz.

15.1.6 Imaging methods

There is considerable variability in the use of muscle imaging, some specialist units not offering it at all, whilst others place great value in it. Potential information that can be obtained includes assessing the distribution and severity of muscle involvement, assessment of disease progress, and selection of a suitable muscle, or region within one muscle, for biopsy. With respect to the latter, ultrasound has been fairly widely used, particularly in paediatric practice and by those who prefer needle to open biopsy. Distribution of muscle involvement may sometimes give a powerful clue towards the diagnosis. Thus, magnetic resonance imaging (MRI) demonstration of involvement of the forearm flexor muscles before finger flexion weakness is clinically evident is typical of inclusion body myositis (Sekul *et al.* 1997). MRI will probably replace CT, not least because of safety considerations.

15.1.7 Muscle biopsy

Although muscle biopsy is of considerable importance in the investigation of myopathies, it must be remembered that muscle has a limited repertoire of responses to a wide range of pathological insults, and that the appearances in a small biopsy specimen may not be representative of the underlying disease process. In other words, the biopsy findings must be interpreted within the context of the clinical evaluation and the results from other tests. This section discusses the biopsy procedure, specimen handling and preparation, and a brief review of major pathological features. There are excellent monographs on the subject of muscle biopsy (Carpenter and Karpati 1984; Dubowitz 1985).

In general, the muscle selected for biopsy should be moderately weak. Very weak muscles often just show end-stage changes of fibrosis and fat replacement. It is important that normal statistics for the chosen muscle are available—for example, certain muscles normally show predominance of a particular fibre type. For this reason only a limited number of muscles are normally used for biopsy, the most common being deltoid and quadriceps (vastus lateralis). It is largely a matter of personal preference and experience as to whether the muscle

Table 15.7. Routine muscle biopsy dyes and stains, and their uses

Dye or stain	Use
Tissue dyes	
Haematoxylin and eosin	Histology
Modified Gomori trichrome	Histology
Periodic acid–Schiff	Demonstrating excess glycogen
Oil red O	Demonstrating excess lipid
Histochemistry	
ATPase (at pH 4.3, 4.6, and 9.4)	Fibre typing
NADH	Myofibrillar architecture
Succinate dehydrogenase	Mitochondrial distribution
Cytochrome oxidase	Mitochondrial function
Acid phosphatase	Lysosomal activity

sample is obtained through an open approach or by the use of a biopsy needle. Both are performed under local anaesthesia (except sometimes in small children). Needle biopsy leaves a smaller scar but less material is obtained—this can cause problems with orientation and, if pathological changes are patchy, as they often are in inflammatory myopathies, they may be missed.

The specimen for light microscopy is orientated under a dissecting microscope and snap frozen by immersion in cooled isopentane. Sections (6 μm) are cut in a cryostat and mounted on coverslips, ready for staining. A panel of routine histological and histochemical stains is applied to each specimen (Table 15.7). Additional histochemical stains may be indicated, such as myophosphorylase staining in suspected McArdle's disease. Immunocytochemistry is a particularly valuable technique for the study of muscular dystrophies and idiopathic inflammatory myopathies. The sections are incubated with an antibody directed against a specific antigen, and the antibody is visualized by use of a coloured tag. Specific examples are considered when discussing individual disorders.

Electron microscopy is of limited value in routine practice. Notable exceptions include the demonstration of filamentous inclusions in inclusion-body myositis and the characterization of ultrastructural abnormalities in several of the congenital myopathies.

Major pathological features

In *denervation*, features include small, angular fibres and fibre-type grouping (reflecting re-innervation) (Fig. 15.4). *Muscular dystrophies* of limb girdle and Xp21 (Duchenne and Becker) type show an increase in the normal variability of fibre size, necrosis, regenerating fibres, fibre splitting, increased numbers of central nuclei, and an increase in fibrous tissue (Fig. 15.8). In myotonic dystrophy and facioscapulohumeral muscular dystrophy, the biopsy is often normal or shows only non-specific features, and biopsy does not form part of their routine assessment. Immunocytochemistry shows dystrophin to be absent in Duchenne and reduced in Becker muscular dystrophy. In the autosomal recessive limb-girdle dystrophies, one or more of the sarcoglycans may be reduced or absent. The *idiopathic inflammatory myopathies* are characterized by the presence of inflammatory infiltrates, composed mainly of lymphocytes,

necrotic fibres, and, in dermatomyositis, capillary loss, infarcts, and perifascicular atrophy (Figs. 15.24 and 15.25). Immunocytochemistry permits identification of lymphocyte subtypes, and the demonstration of major histocompatability complex type I antigen expression on muscle fibres. Many *congenital myopathies* are associated with ultrastructural abnormalities, either affecting fibre architecture (e.g. central-core disease) or in the form of abnormal structures or accumulations within fibres (e.g. nemaline myopathy). In *metabolic myopathies* the appearances are often unremarkable. Excess glycogen and lipid accumulation may be seen in the glycogenoses and lipid metabolism disorders, respectively, but are not invariable. In *mitochondrial cytopathies* the classical finding is of ragged-red fibres seen on Gomori's modified trichrome stain and reflecting aggregations of mitochondria (Fig. 15.22), but these are not always present. NADH and succinate dehydrogenase staining is often abnormal and there may be cytochrome-oxidase-negative fibres. Electron microscopy is not essential, but shows accumulations of structurally abnormal mitochondria, which may contain inclusions.

15.1.8 Molecular genetic studies

The rate of development in this area is so rapid that even specialists in the neuromuscular field have difficulty keeping up to date. Increasing use is being made of Web-site accessible databases (e.g. http://www.path.cam.ac.uk/emd/ for an Emery–Dreifuss muscular dystrophy database). The traditional approach to gene identification was by working backwards from the mutated protein. That approach is not possible when the gene product is not known. Positional cloning (also known as 'reverse genetics') allows us to move in the opposite direction—by studying polymorphic markers in large informative families the chromosomal position of the relevant gene can be identified, and then finer mapping techniques can be used to find its exact position. Expressed transcripts from that area are assessed for possible candidate genes. Once the gene has been identified, the protein product can be deduced.

At present, the ability to identify a specific gene defect aids precise diagnosis and carrier detection, allows accurate genetic counselling and prenatal diagnosis, and may sometimes indicate the likely severity of the phenotype. In the future, knowledge of the gene defect will presumably be essential if genetic engineering approaches to therapy are to be considered. Alternatively, a detailed understanding of the structure and function of the protein product may lead to therapeutic approaches by biochemical means. The types of mutation seen in the more common inherited myopathies are shown in Table 15.8.

15.1.9 Genetic counselling

This is a major issue when considering inherited neuromuscular disorders, but one that is sometimes neglected. Whoever provides counselling must have a detailed understanding not only of the genetic issues but also of the disease itself. The affected individual will want to know not only the

Table 15.8. Gene mutations in myopathic disorders

Type of mutation	Disorders
Large deletion	Duchenne and Becker dystrophy (~70% patients)
Small deletions and point mutations	Duchenne and Becker dystrophy (~30% patients)
Deletion	Mitochondrial cytopathies (mitochondrial DNA)
Point mutations	Many metabolic myopathies
	Limb-girdle dystrophies (e.g. sarcoglycanopathies)
	X-linked Emery–Dreifuss syndrome
	Channelopathies
	Myotonia congenita
	Congenital myasthenic syndromes
	Mitochondrial cytopathies (mitochondrial DNA)
Trinucleotide repeat expansions	Myotonic dystrophy
	Oculopharyngeal muscular dystrophy
Deletion of repeat units	Facioscapulohumeral muscular dystrophy

statistical risk of their offspring being affected, but also the possible severity in those that are. This is a straightforward matter for those conditions that follow simple Mendelian rules, but is very much more difficult for those that do not, such as the trinucleotide repeat expansion disorders and mitochondrial cytopathies. These issues are discussed further when considering individual disorders.

Asymptomatic relatives of affected individuals provide a particular challenge. The counselling issues for women in families carrying an X-linked disorder (e.g. Duchenne/Becker) are well understood. For autosomal dominant disorders, a relative may be asymptomatic because they do not carry the relevant gene. Alternatively, they may carry the gene but not show its manifestations because they are too young to do so, or because there is variability of expression for that disorder. Gene testing in asymptomatic individuals needs considerable care and thought. Carrier and presymptomatic testing is generally not performed in childhood. It can never be assumed that a relative is unaffected on hearsay evidence, but there are difficulties in seeing individuals who believe themselves to be normal and then demonstrating abnormalities, relating to the disease in question, on examination. On the other hand, it is a tragedy if an asymptomatic woman in a family known to suffer from myotonic dystrophy, gives birth to a child with the severe congenital form of the disease when, given appropriate counselling, she might have opted for gene testing, prenatal diagnosis, and selective termination of pregnancy.

15.2 Muscular dystrophies

An early, and still generally useful, definition of these conditions is that they are primary, inherited, progressive, degenerative disorders of muscle. In practice, a few are non-progressive and, in some, degenerative changes are slight or absent. Reclassification may be appropriate when the molecular basis of each form has been determined, but this is still a little way off. Much experimental evidence had suggested that the muscle fibre membrane might be the major site of pathology in the dystrophies, and this appeared to be borne out when dystrophin was identified—its absence causes Duchenne muscular dystrophy, but if it is present in reduced quantity or in a truncated form, the phenotype is that of Becker dystrophy. Subsequently, it was shown that absence of proteins (sarcoglycans) functionally related to dystrophin is responsible for some forms of limb-girdle dystrophy. However, we now know that some dystrophies are due to a defect of a sarcoplasmic protein (calpain-3 in one form of limb-girdle dystrophy, a protein kinase in myotonic dystrophy), and that one, X-linked Emery–Dreifuss muscular dystrophy, is related to deficiency of a nuclear protein (emerin).

Because genetic counselling (discussed above) is such an important aspect of management, a classification based on the Mendelian pattern of inheritance, combined with phenotypic description, is particularly useful in everyday practice (Table 15.9). Despite its name, myotonic dystrophy is usually considered separately (Section 15.3).

15.2.1 Dystrophinopathies

This term encompasses those conditions in which there is a primary abnormality of dystrophin. The clinical phenotype of Duchenne dystrophy is stereotyped and had been well characterized before the discovery of dystrophin. Becker dystrophy was known to have a more variable phenotype, but quite how variable has only become apparent over the past decade. At its most severe, Becker dystrophy is indistinguishable from Duchenne. A less severe form presents in late middle age. In yet another form, weakness may be absent and the picture is that of cramps and episodic rhabdomyolysis and myoglobinuria.

Table 15.9. Classification of the muscular dystrophies

X-linked
  Duchenne
  Becker
  Emery–Dreifuss

Autosomal dominant
  Facioscapulohumeral
  Oculopharyngeal
  Scapuloperoneal
  Limb-girdle (uncommonly)
  Distal myopathies

Autosomal recessive
  Limb-girdle (commonly)
  Congenital
  Distal myopathies

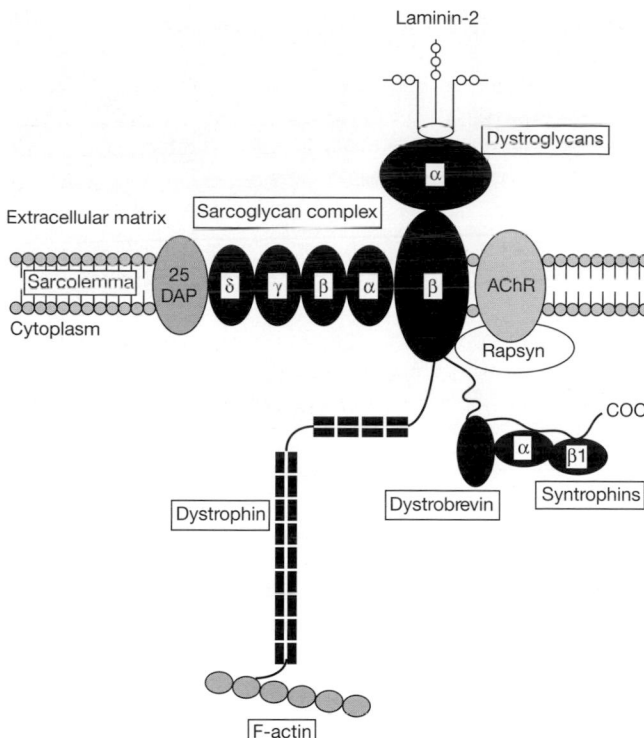

Fig. 15.6. The dystrophin-associated protein complex (courtesy of Rosie Fisher).

Dystrophin and associated proteins

After dystrophin came the identification of other related proteins (Fig. 15.6). Although the precise function of this protein complex remains much debated, the most favoured opinion is that it acts to stabilize the inherently fragile muscle fibre membrane during the rigours of contraction and relaxation. The complex links intracellular actin to proteins in the extracellular matrix.

Duchenne muscular dystrophy

This is the most common form of muscular dystrophy (Emery 1993). Being X-linked, it principally affects boys. Rarely, girls are affected, severely, as a result of chromosomal abnormalities (Turner's syndrome, translocations).

The incidence is 20–30/100 000 live-born males. One-third are known to have a previous family history, one-third are new mutations, and one-third are born to an unknowing carrier. These figures emphasize the difficulties associated with genetic counselling for this disorder.

Clinical features

The principle clinical picture is of progressive weakness, affecting limbs and respiratory muscles, but important additional features include muscle hypertrophy, speech delay, intellectual impairment, and cardiac involvement. These boys appear normal at birth and in the first year of life. Walking is clumsy and delayed, with about one-half still not walking at 18 months. They do not achieve the ability to run, hop, and jump. As the lower-limb weakness progresses, the gait becomes more and

more waddling and the abdomen protuberant because of increasing lumbar lordosis. Climbing stairs is difficult and the child rises from the floor in a characteristic fashion (Gower's manoeuvre)—first turning prone and then placing their hands on their knees and thighs to push themselves erect. Symptomatic shoulder-girdle weakness develops within 2–3 years but is evident on examination much earlier. Ambulation is lost at about 10 years of age. During adolescence the weakness progresses, spinal deformity increases, and contractures, which first involved the hip flexors and Achilles tendons, progress rapidly, particularly affecting elbows and knees. Deformity may prevent comfortable seating in a wheelchair and should be a major target for the physiotherapist. Residual power in finger and wrist flexor muscles allows the boy to use a keyboard and to control an electric wheelchair. Mild facial weakness is evident in the late stage. Particularly in the early stages, muscle hypertrophy (and later pseudohypertrophy due to fatty replacement of muscle) develops in most boys. It is most evident in the calves, quadriceps, and muscles of mastication. It is not pathognomonic and, for example, may also be seen in spinal muscular atrophy. Overall, the increasing weakness is associated with progressive muscular atrophy and loss of tendon reflexes.

Respiratory muscle weakness develops early (as shown by forced vital capacity measurement) and respiratory function is later further compromised by the spinal deformity. The cough becomes weak, leading to aspiration and increased risk of chest infection. Death, which occurs in the late second or early third decade, is usually due to respiratory failure. In the later stages of the disease, carbon dioxide retention may cause excessive daytime sleepiness, early morning headache, and, commonly, a fear of sleeping.

Cardiac involvement is an inevitable feature of the disease, but is not commonly symptomatic, perhaps because of the boys' limited physical activity and thus demand on the heart. The ECG changes early, with a characteristic appearance of tall R waves in the right precordial leads and deep, narrow Q waves in the left precordial and limb leads. Echocardiographic changes appear later and are usually not gross (more severe changes may be seen in Becker dystrophy)—a small proportion of boys develop symptomatic cardiac failure, which is occasionally the cause of death.

Delayed speech development is a common but underrecognized feature—the wise clinician presented with a boy with this symptom checks the serum creatine kinase level, even in the absence of other abnormality. As a group, the average IQ is reduced to about 80, but many individuals are of normal or above-average intelligence.

Diagnosis

A highly confident diagnosis can be made on the basis of the clinical picture and the finding of a very high serum creatine kinase (CK) level. Up to the age of 5 years (including at birth) the CK activity is typically in the order of 100 times the upper limit of normal, and is never within the normal range. As the disease progresses and muscle mass is lost, the CK activity falls.

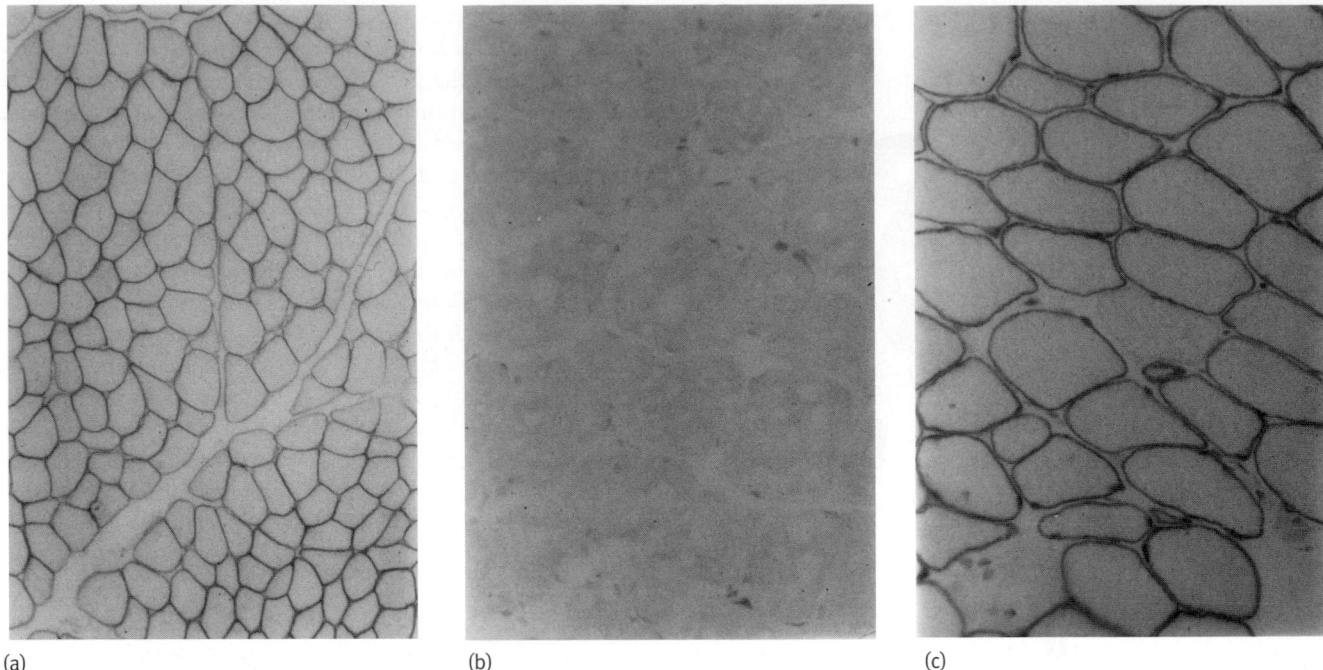

(a) (b) (c)

Fig. 15.7. Dystrophin staining. (a) Normal muscle, note the regular staining around the periphery of each muscle fibre. (b) Duchenne dystrophy, note the complete absence of staining. (c) Becker dystrophy, note irregular staining and a single central fibre with almost absent staining. (Courtesy of Dr Waney Squier.)

A definitive diagnosis depends upon demonstration of an appropriate gene defect. In about two-thirds this consists of a large deletion, easily detected in the laboratory. In the other one-third the gene defect is currently (due to technical and cost considerations) not readily demonstrated—it may consist of a small deletion or duplication, or of a point mutation. In these patients the diagnosis is based upon demonstration, by immuno-cytochemistry and Western blotting, of absence or severe deficiency of dystrophin in a muscle biopsy specimen (Fig. 15.7). The classical histological features of muscular dystrophy are present, consisting of increased variability of fibre size, rounding of fibres, fibre splitting, increased numbers of central nuclei, hyaline fibres, muscle fibre necrosis, phagocytosis and regeneration, and replacement by fat and fibrous tissue (Fig. 15.8).

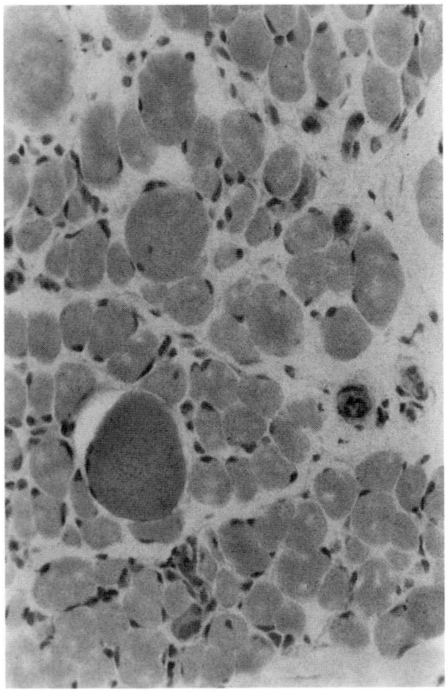

Fig. 15.8. Duchenne muscular dystrophy. Haematoxylin and eosin stain. Note the increased variability in fibre size, roundness of fibres, hypercontracted/hyaline fibre, and increased connective tissue. (Courtesy of Dr Waney Squier.)

Management

The management of Duchenne muscular dystrophy exemplifies the management of most neuromuscular disorders. Genetic counselling issues have already been discussed (Section 15.1.9). Currently there is considerable debate concerning the use of steroids in the treatment of Duchenne muscular dystrophy (Dubrovsky *et al.* 1998). Although there is good evidence that they slow progression of the disease process, as determined by physical measurement, it is not yet clear that any functional gains outweigh the obvious side-effects (e.g. weight gain, psychological effects, fracture risk, cataracts, and infection risk). There is huge interest in the potential for gene therapy, but practical realization is still likely to be some time away. Overall, current management involves physical approaches and dealing with the profound psychological problems associated with a relentlessly progressive debilitating, and eventually fatal, disorder.

Regular exercise is important and can continue even after the boy becomes wheelchair-bound. Bed rest for intercurrent illnesses must be avoided because it is associated with rapid and irreversible further muscle deterioration. Contractures can be delayed, and to some extent reversed, by regular passive exercises—these should be taught to the family by a suitably experienced physiotherapist. Additional techniques include splinting and the use of calipers and other walking aids. The role of surgery for contractures is complicated and controversial. Any such surgery should never be performed without very detailed assessment by an appropriately experienced physician, physiotherapist, and orthotist, in conjunction with a similarly experienced surgeon. This should be done in very close collaboration with the patient and family. Sometimes, although such procedures may prolong walking, the boy decides that he would rather opt for wheelchair existence.

Once wheelchair-bound, spinal curvature rapidly increases. It can be helped by very careful attention to the seating arrangement and the use of a spinal orthosis (e.g. jacket). Spinal fusion, by one of several procedures, may be of value, but by the time it is required there are substantial risks from anaesthesia and surgery relating to the respiratory muscle and cardiac involvement. Rhabdomyolysis and a malignant hyperthermia-like reaction are additional complications. As described above, close liaison between all interested parties is required.

Occupational therapy has a major role to play, and constant reassessment, as the disease progresses and needs change, is required. Dietary advice is needed, to avoid obesity. Emotional support comes from many sources—the Family Care Officer system developed by the Muscular Dystrophy Campaign in Britain is an excellent example of how this can be provided. There are numerous issues relating to schooling (most will go to a mainstream school) and the potential for social isolation. In the early stages the boy should be encouraged towards hobbies and pastimes that he will be able to continue when his disability increases. Parental guilt and depression are common.

Ventilatory failure is inevitable and, typically, associated with intercurrent infection, the most common cause of death. In some boys quality of life is impaired in the last stages of the disease by the symptoms of respiratory failure (e.g. insomnia, excessive daytime sleepiness, morning headache, depression, apathy)—these may be alleviated by assisted ventilation, usually nocturnal positive-pressure assistance using a face mask. Such treatment is not required or requested by all boys.

Becker muscular dystrophy

The incidence of Becker muscular dystrophy (BMD) is about 5/100 000. Originally delineated clinically as a milder phenotype of Duchenne muscular dystrophy, we now know that its basis is either a reduced amount of dystrophin or the presence of dystrophin of lower than normal molecular weight, and that the phenotype varies in severity from a condition indistinguishable from Duchenne, to a late adult-onset proximal myopathy, and to a disorder characterized by cramps, myalgia, and myoglobinuria without weakness (Bushby and Gardner-Medwin 1993; Bushby et al. 1993). At a genetic level, BMD is usually associated with an 'in-frame' deletion. The most common picture is a deletion starting at exon 45 and extending up to

exon 59, associated with a clinical disorder which might be called typical BMD.

In typical BMD, weakness is first evident between the ages of 5 and 20 years. A rather common history is that of an adolescent who has been at the bottom of the class for several years with respect to sporting success, particularly in running. As the lower limb weakness progresses, activities such as climbing stairs and rising from a chair become increasingly difficult.

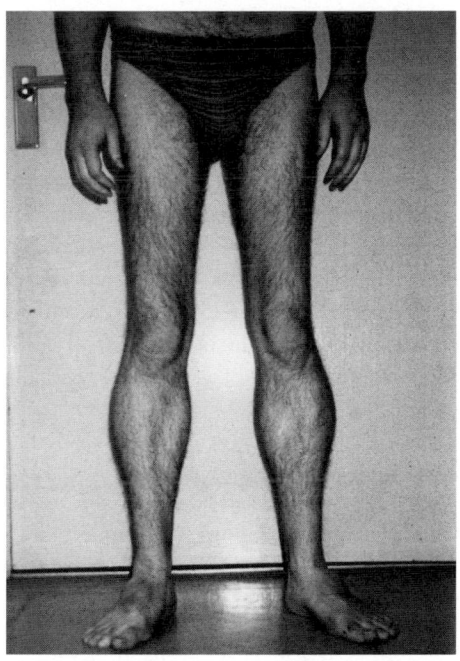

(a)

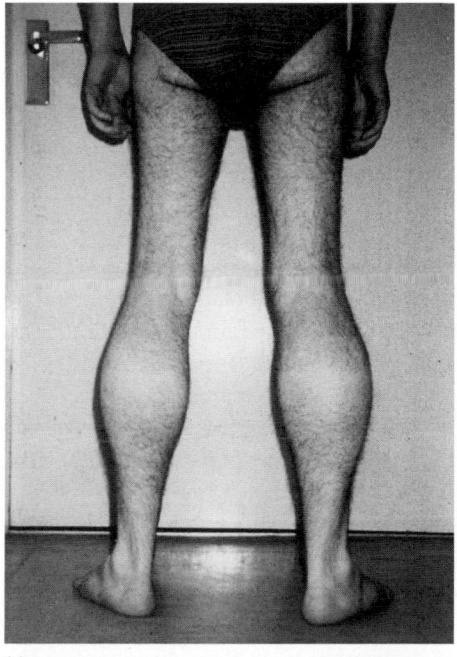

(b)

Fig. 15.9. Becker muscular dystrophy. Note the quadriceps wasting (a) and asymmetrically enlarged calves, so-called pseudohypertrophy (b).

Upper-limb weakness may not be symptomatic for many years, but is often evident earlier on examination. Other common early features are exercise-induced calf cramps, toe-walking, and calf hypertrophy (Fig. 15.9). The pattern of muscle weakness parallels that seen in Duchenne, with early involvement of hip flexors and extensors, quadriceps, pectoralis major, latissimus dorsi, and brachioradialis. The age of loss of ambulation is very variable and many remain ambulant, albeit with an ungainly gait, into late middle age.

Cardiac involvement is underestimated (Hoogerwaard *et al.* 1997). At presentation patients should have an ECG and echocardiogram. These should be repeated periodically, at intervals depending on previous findings and symptomatology. Rapid progression, from being asymptomatic to death from cardiac failure, may occur. Optimal management remains controversial, but may involve the use of diuretics, β-blockers, angiotensin-converting enzyme (ACE) inhibitors, and, rarely, cardiac transplantation.

Rarer cases of very late onset (60 years and later), often presenting with quadriceps weakness, have been described. Another characteristic phenotype is of exercise-induced myalgia and cramps, sometimes with episodes of rhabdomyolysis (Gospe *et al.* 1989) which may initially suggest a metabolic myopathy.

Diagnosis

The principles are as given for diagnosing Duchenne muscular dystrophy. In the one-third of patients who do not have a readily demonstrable gene abnormality, confirmation is easy if Western blotting shows dystrophin of reduced molecular weight or a severe reduction in quantity. Lesser reductions may be more difficult to interpret, and there is overlap with the sarcoglycanopathies (limb-girdle dystrophies), in which there may be secondary reduction of dystrophin. Immunocytochemistry is very suggestive if it shows patchy dystrophin staining (Fig. 15.7) but can never alone exclude the diagnosis. As in Duchenne, the serum creatine kinase is invariably elevated in early stages. Electromyography shows changes consistent with primary muscle disease, with the additional presence of fibrillation potentials and positive sharp waves.

Management

Surgical intervention is rarely required. Contractures are a late feature, following loss of ambulation. The general principles of management are as discussed for Duchenne muscular dystrophy. Particular attention needs to be paid to the heart (noted above) and to ventilatory function. Respiratory failure and its associated symptoms occurs only in late stages, long after ambulation has been lost—nocturnal positive-pressure ventilation with a mask affords symptomatic relief.

Female carriers

Up to 10% of female carriers may show evidence of muscle disease (weakness or hypertrophy) and prior to the identification of dystrophin were often diagnosed as having limb-girdle dystrophy—the basis is skewed X-inactivation (Yoshioka *et al.* 1998). It has been known for some time that occasional carriers present with cardiomyopathy, even in the absence of skeletal muscle involvement, and recent studies have shown that sub-clinical cardiomyopathy is relatively common. It is recommended that all carriers undergo cardiological assessment at diagnosis and at intervals thereafter (Grain *et al.* 2000).

15.2.2 Limb-girdle muscular dystrophies

The term limb-girdle muscular dystrophy (LGMD) acquired widespread usage in the 1950s and has been the subject of much debate ever since. It was used to separate a group of disorders, that had in common limb-girdle weakness and absence of early facial weakness, from the X-linked dystrophies and autosomal dominant facioscapulohumeral muscular dystrophy. Autosomal dominant, autosomal recessive, and sporadic forms were included. Some patients so classified were subsequently shown to have Becker muscular dystrophy, to be manifesting female carriers of the Duchenne/Becker gene abnormality, to have spinal muscular atrophy, or one of a variety of metabolic myopathies (e.g. acid maltase deficiency). Recent genetic and molecular studies (Bushby 1999) have allowed us to re-evaluate the whole concept of LGMD (Table 15.10). It is currently possible to reach a molecular/genetic diagnosis in about 30 per cent of patients presenting with this type of clinical syndrome—implying that there are still many more genes to be identified. Recessive forms are much more common than dominant forms (Bushby 1996).

After the discovery of dystrophin, the dystrophin-associated proteins were identified (Fig. 15.6) and these seemed a likely candidate for other forms of muscular dystrophy, as subsequently proved to be the case (Duggan and Hoffman 1996). Deficiency of each of the four sarcoglycans has been associated with a form of autosomal recessive muscular dystrophy. Another form of recessive LGMD is caused by deficiency of a muscle-specific calcium-activated neutral protease, calpain-3 (Topaloglu *et al.* 1997), and a sixth type with deficiency of a novel protein of unknown function, dysferlin (Liu *et al.* 1998). Other recessive families have shown linkage to particular chro-

Table 15.10. Classification of the limb-girdle muscular dystrophies

	Gene location	Protein	Locus symbol
Autosomal dominant			
LGMD 1A	5q	?	
LGMD 1B	1q11–q21	Lamina/c	
LGMD 1C	3p25	Caveolin-3	
Autosomal recessive			
LGMD 2A	15q15.1–q15.3	Calpain-3	CAPN3
LGMD 2B	2p	Dysferlin	
LGMD 2C	13q12	γ-Sarcoglycan	SGCC
LGMD 2D	17q21	α-Sarcoglycan[a]	SGCA
LGMD 2E	4q12	β-Sarcoglycan	SGCB
LGMD 2F	5q33	δ-Sarcoglycan	SGCD
LGMD 2G	17q11–q12	?	

[a]The naming of the sarcoglycans has changed: α-sarcoglycan was previously known as adhalin and that term is still in common usage.

mosomes, but the relevant genes and their products are not yet known. There is a very considerable interfamilial, and even intrafamilial, variability with respect to phenotype. The sarcoglycanopathies tend to present early—the term severe childhood autosomal recessive muscular dystrophy (SCARMD) has been used to describe a phenotype of similar severity to Duchenne muscular dystrophy. Like those with Becker dystrophy, these patients may present later and, like Becker, a form with predominant myalgia has been described. The phenotype of dysferlin deficiency (LGMD 2B) varies from a limb-girdle syndrome to a form which presents with gastrocnemius weakness (previously called Miyoshi-type distal myopathy). Calpain-3 deficiency can present from early childhood to middle age—the clinical picture is never as severe as in Duchenne muscular dystrophy and may be very mild.

Autosomal dominant LGMD is much less common. Loci have been identified for two forms, one of which is associated with severe cardiomyopathy (LGMD 1B) (van-der-Kooi *et al.* 1997) and has recently been shown to be allelic to autosomal dominant Emery–Dreifuss syndrome (see below). A third form (LGMD 1C), in which there is severe deficiency of the protein caveolin-3, has been described (Minetti *et al.* 1998).

Diagnosis

This is still mainly within the preserve of specialist and research laboratories. Loss of any one component of the sarcoglycan complex leads to secondary loss (or at least lack of proper localization) of the other three. α-Sarcoglycan immunocytochemistry on a muscle biopsy specimen is therefore a useful screening process, supplemented by Western blotting, looking at each of the four sarcoglycans. Calpain-3 deficiency is identified by Western blotting. Diagnosis in all cases can be confirmed by genetic studies, but these are not yet widely available.

15.2.3 Emery–Dreifuss muscular dystrophy

This highly distinctive syndrome is characterized by the triad of early contractures, humero-peroneal distribution of weakness, and cardiac conduction defects (Tsuchiya and Arahata 1997). It is a syndrome because, although the majority of cases are X-linked, autosomal dominant cases which are clinically indistinguishable have been described (see above). The X-linked form is caused by a mutation in the gene encoding the novel protein, emerin (Bione *et al.* 1994), which is located in the nuclear membrane in muscle and is related to the intercalated discs in cardiac muscle. The dominant form is caused by a mutation in the lamin A/C gene (Bonne *et al.* 1999)—the two proteins, lamins A and C, are components of the nuclear lamina and thus presumed to be physically and functionally closely related to emerin

Clinical features

Contractures typically affect the neck, elbows, and ankles (Fig. 15.10). They may predate any demonstrable weakness. Limited neck flexion and elbow extension are usually noted first, from about 2 years of age, followed by toe-walking. Weakness is

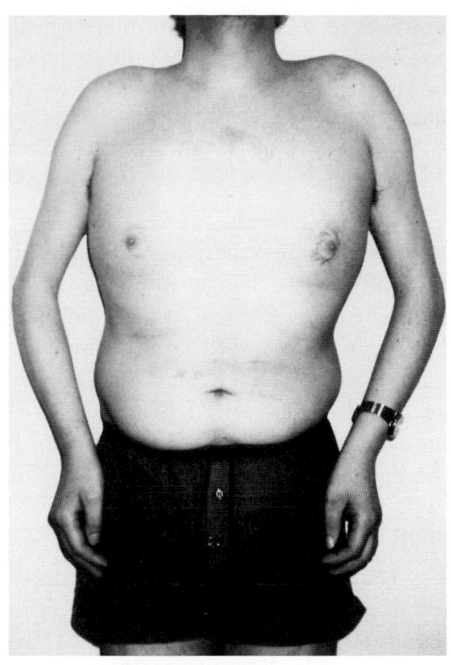

(a)

(b)

Fig. 15.10. Emery–Dreifuss syndrome. Note the humeral muscle wasting and elbow contractures (a), and the Achilles tendon contractures, causing toe-walking (b).

initially in a humero-peroneal distribution, but later spreads to involve the periscapular muscles and proximal lower-limb muscles. Severe weakness is uncommon and most patients remain mobile. Cardiac involvement is usually in the form of conduction abnormalities, ranging from first-degree to complete heart block, and, if untreated, is a major cause of death (Bialer *et al.* 1991). A dilated cardiomyopathy is much less common.

Female carriers of the X-linked form are usually asymptomatic, but rarely may develop severe cardiac conduction problems in the absence of skeletal muscle involvement (Fishbein *et al.* 1993). Therefore, screening of at-risk relatives and periodic review appears appropriate.

Diagnosis

The serum creatine kinase activity is almost invariably elevated. Electromyography shows changes indicating primary muscle disease, and light microscopy of skeletal muscle shows dystrophic changes. In the X-linked form, immunocytochemistry shows absence of emerin in skeletal muscle and skin, and skin biopsy may be used to identify female carriers (Mora *et al.* 1997). Numerous mutations have been identified within the emerin gene. Emerin is normal in autosomal dominant cases.

Management

By far and away the most important aspect is identification and management of cardiac involvement. There is a high incidence of sudden death (Pinelli *et al.* 1987). Regular ECG monitoring is required and the patient should be made aware of the need to report immediately symptoms such as palpitation and dizziness. Pacemaker insertion is often required but may not remove all risk of arrhythmia. The progression of contractures may be reduced by physiotherapy, and Achilles tenotomies are often helpful.

15.2.4 Facioscapulohumeral muscular dystrophy

Facioscapulohumeral (FSH) muscular dystrophy is another condition in which recent genetic advances have led to a better understanding of the extent of phenotypic variability (Tawil *et al.* 1998). It is inherited as an autosomal dominant disorder, with a prevalence of about 5/100 000, and gains its name from the characteristic early pattern of muscle involvement. New mutations are not uncommon. The relevant gene and gene product are unknown—the disease is associated with deletion of an integral number of 3.3 kb repeats in the subtelomeric region of chromosome 4q35. The current view is that this rearrangement has a position effect on one or more genes proximal to the repeat.

Clinical features

Onset is usually in the second decade, and by age 20 years the penetrance is 95 per cent. Uncommonly, onset may be in the first year of life; the parent typically has a much milder form of the disease and this probably reflects somatic mosaicism. Rare examples of non-penetrance by age 60 years mean that occasional cases are seen where the transmitting parent may not manifest the disease. Furthermore, up to one-third of gene carriers are asymptomatic, although examination is abnormal. Thus, a negative family history cannot be taken at face value, and even after examination genetic studies may be necessary. Penetrance is lower in females than males.

The first symptoms, although often not recognized by the patient, relate to facial weakness; poor whistle, difficulty

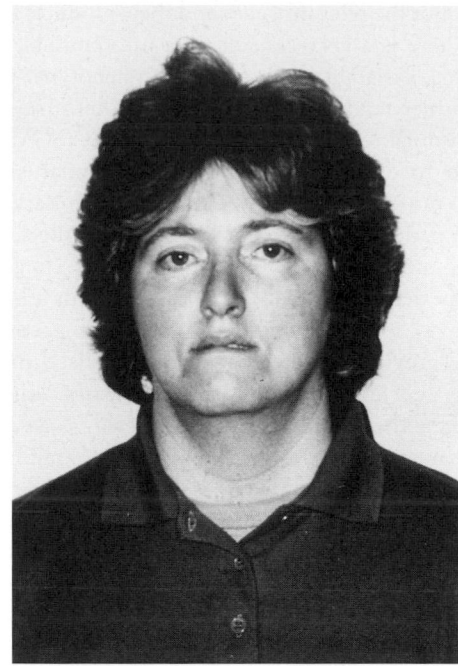

(a)

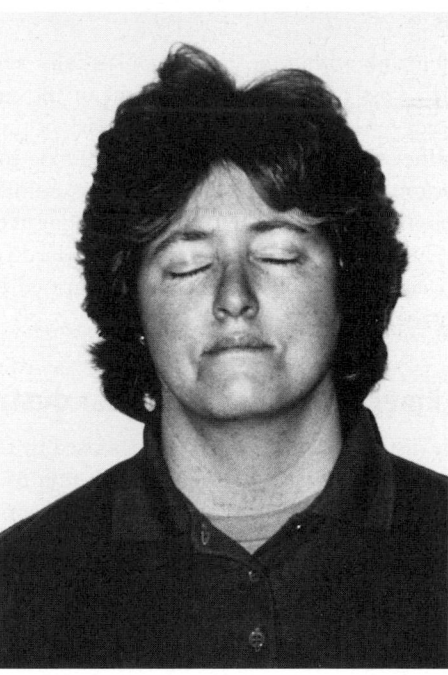

(b)

Fig. 15.11. Facioscapulohumeral muscular dystrophy. The facial weakness may not be striking because it is symmetrical (a). On attempted forceful eye-closure there is incomplete burying of the eyelashes (b).

sucking on a straw and blowing-up balloons. At presentation, 90 per cent have demonstrable facial weakness (Fig. 15.11).

As the name implies, there is selective weakness and wasting of muscles around the shoulder girdle, affecting serratus anterior, rhomboids, and the lower part of trapezius (the scapular

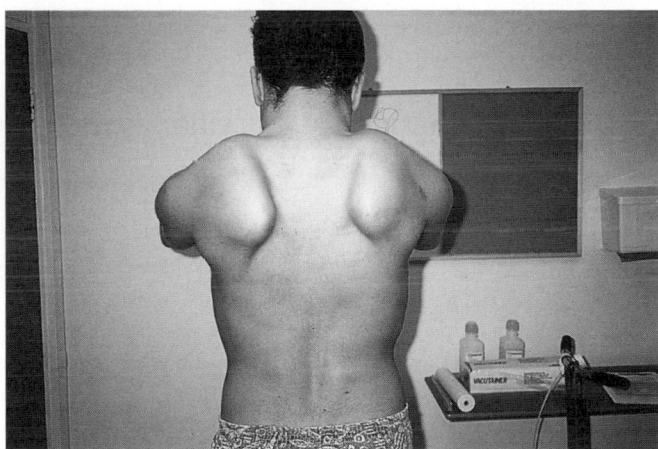

Fig. 15.12. Facioscapulohumeral muscular dystrophy. Classical scapular winging.

Table 15.11. The stages of facioscapulohumeral muscular dystrophy (after Padberg 1998)

Stage 0	Facial weakness
Stage 1	Periscapular weakness and wasting (scapular winging)
Stage 2	Tibialis anterior weakness
Stage 3	Pelvic girdle weakness
Stage 4	Difficulty on stairs and rising from a chair
Stage 5	Wheelchair outdoors
Stage 6	Wheelchair indoors

fixator muscles) and pectoralis major, but with preservation of deltoid. Often scapular winging is noted before weakness (Fig. 15.12). Weakness causes the patient difficulty abducting his or her arms and performing tasks above shoulder height. On examination, the inability to abduct the arms to more than about 60° and the elevation of the scapulae due to the pull of the unaffected deltoid produces a highly characteristic appearance (Fig. 15.13). Unusually for a myopathy, the picture may be quite markedly asymmetric (Fig. 15.14).

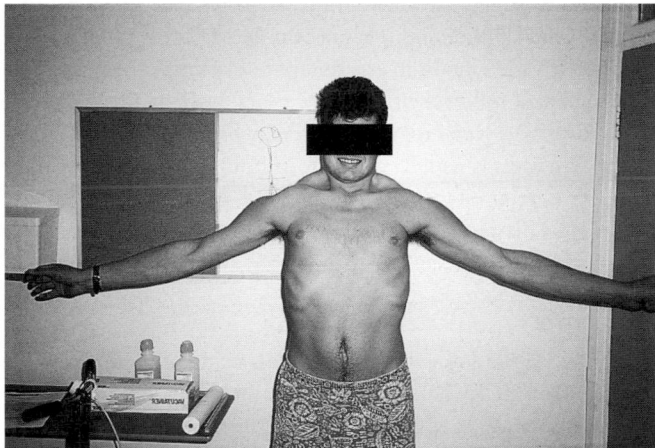

Fig. 15.13. Facioscapulohumeral muscular dystrophy. The patient is attempting to elevate his hands above shoulder height, but is unable to do so.

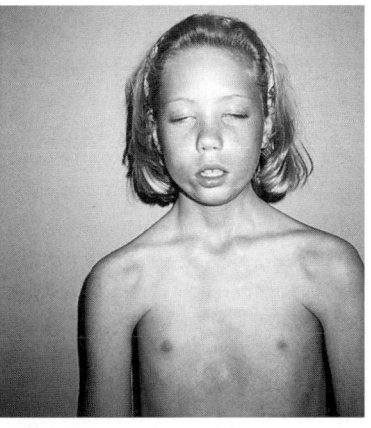

(a)

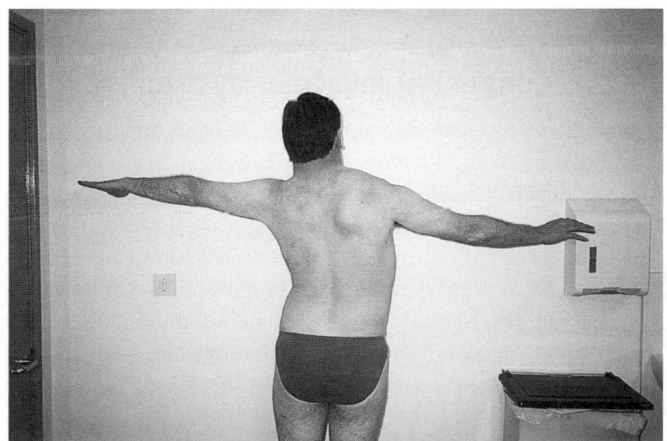

Fig. 15.14. Facioscapulohumeral muscular dystrophy. Compare with Fig. 15.13—the weakness in FSH dystrophy is often asymmetrical.

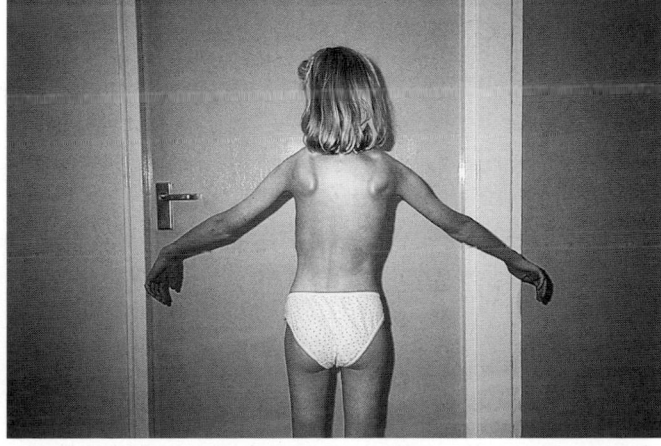

(b)

Fig. 15.15. Facioscapulohumeral muscular dystrophy. Severe, early onset form. Note the profound facial weakness (a) and inability to fully abduct at the shoulders (b).

Weakness of tibialis anterior is evident in most patients at presentation and, rarely, footdrop is a presenting symptom. Similarly, upper arm weakness (biceps more than triceps) may be demonstrated. Padberg (1998) has described seven stages in the progression of the disease (Table 15.11)—progression from one stage to the next may take decades and abortive cases occur. About 20 per cent of patients over the age of 50 years require a wheelchair. Spinal and pelvic girdle weakness may lead to marked lumbar lordosis. The rare, early onset form is associated with severe facial weakness (Fig. 15.15), which may be misdiagnosed as Möbius' syndrome (Section 8.10.7).

Mild sensorineural deafness can be detected in many adults but is rarely symptomatic. It may be more evident in early onset cases. Retinal vascular disease (Coats' disease) may be demonstrated by fluorescein angiography, but routine eye examination is normal and visual symptoms very rare. Pain is common, and under-recognized. It is largely mechanical in origin.

The extraocular and pharyngeal musculatures are not involved. Apart from occasional tightening of the Achilles tendons, contractures are not a major feature.

Diagnosis

This is now based on DNA studies. If these are negative, neurophysiological studies and muscle biopsy may be needed to exclude other disorders that may mimic the condition (although these are extremely rare)—polymyositis, mitochondrial cytopathy, and possibly neurogenic disorders. The serum creatine kinase is quite often normal and is most likely to be elevated in more severe and rapidly progressive cases. EMG findings are those associated with primary muscle disease. Depending on the muscle selected, biopsy findings are sometimes minimal. In a clinically affected muscle there are dystrophic changes and, a subject of much debate, inflammatory infiltrates.

Management

No drugs have been demonstrated to be unequivocally effective and none can be recommended. Pain management is important and usually revolves around physiotherapy and analgesics/anti-inflammatory drugs. Scapula fixation surgery is generally disappointing.

15.2.5 Scapuloperoneal syndrome

The clinical features of this rare syndrome are indicated by the title: periscapular wasting and weakness with associated scapular winging, and wasting and weakness of tibialis anterior, causing weakness of ankle dorsiflexion. In other words, the phenotype of FSH muscular dystrophy without the facial weakness. Indeed, it is likely that many cases represent a forme fruste of FSH dystrophy—this is not true for all cases (Tawil et al. 1995) and further genetic studies are needed. A similar phenotype may be seen in Emery–Dreifuss syndrome and probably in several autosomal dystrophies. Neurogenic cases have been described (a form of spinal muscular atrophy) but few have

been subjected to modern diagnostic methods. One shows linkage to chromosome 12 (Isozumi et al. 1996).

15.2.6 Oculopharyngeal muscular dystrophy

Striking features of this condition include its late onset, typically in the fifth or sixth decade, and the highly selective pattern of muscle involvement. Recent evidence has shown the disease to be associated with a trinucleotide repeat expansion in a gene (the *PABP2* gene) on chromosome 14 (Brais et al. 1998). In the common autosomal dominant form, one of the alleles is expanded from the normal six repeats to eight or more. In a rarer autosomal recessive form, both alleles contain seven repeats. The differential diagnosis includes myasthenia gravis, mitochondrial cytopathy, and dysthyroid eye disease.

Clinical features

The first feature is usually ptosis (often asymmetric), less often dysphagia. As the disease progresses the ptosis may obscure vision (Fig. 15.16). Slight external ophthalmoplegia may develop, but is rarely severe, and diplopia is uncommon. There is often striking overactivity of frontalis in an attempt to overcome the ptosis.

Dysphagia follows within a few years, initially for solids and later for fluids. Nasal regurgitation may occur. At this stage mild facial weakness is usually evident. Although not included in the name, in later stages proximal limb-girdle weakness may develop. This is usually mild and affects the shoulder girdle more often than the pelvic girdle.

Diagnosis

Diagnosis should now be based on DNA analysis (it has not yet been established whether the condition shows genetic heterogeneity). Muscle biopsy will become unnecessary—the characteristic finding is of 8.5 nm intranuclear tubular filaments.

Management

If the ptosis interferes with vision, corrective surgery is appropriate (Fig. 15.16). Dysphagia is managed as for other neuromuscular disorders that impair swallowing. Options include advice from a speech therapist, cricopharyngeal myotomy, and gastrostomy.

15.2.7 Congenital muscular dystrophy

Congenital muscular dystrophy (CMD) is an area of intense research activity, and a comprehensive classification is not yet possible (Voit 1998). These are autosomal recessive disorders and the essential clinical features are of early onset (not always congenital) hypotonia, delayed motor milestones, contractures, and variable central nervous system involvement. Progression is very variable.

Classical (occidental) CMD can be subdivided into two groups. Merosin (laminin-2) is a glycoprotein and an important constituent of the basement membrane. Merosin-negative CMD is associated with a defect of the merosin gene on chromosome 6 (Hillaire et al. 1994; Tome et al. 1994). Children with this defect do not achieve independent standing. Although their mental development is usually normal, MRI shows white-

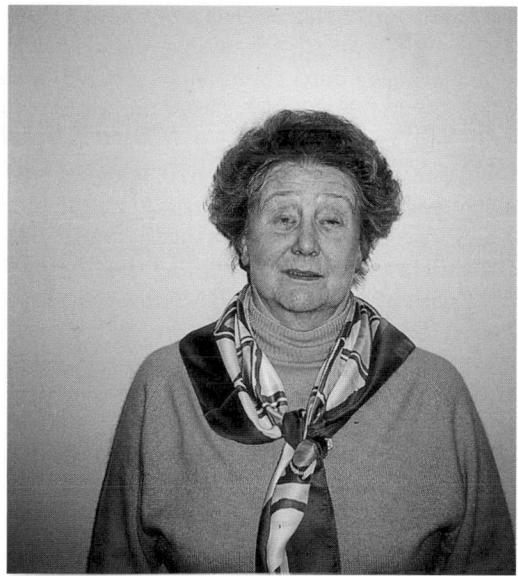

(a)

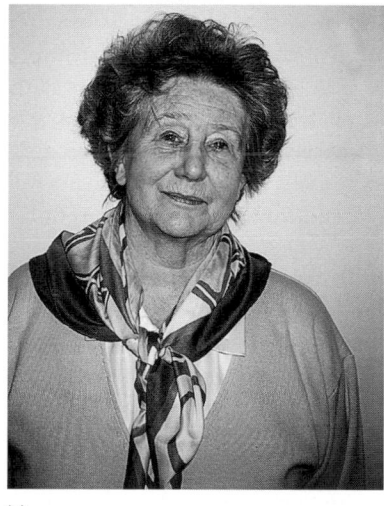

(b)

Fig. 15.16. Oculopharyngeal muscular dystrophy. (a) Before and (b) after ptosis correction surgery.

matter changes. Merosin-positive CMD is genetically and clinically heterogeneous. The course is generally milder, and white-matter changes are not present.

Fukuyama (oriental) CMD, which is rare outside Japan, is due to a defect of the recently identified fukutin gene on chromosome 9 (Kobayashi *et al.* 1998). It is a severe disorder involving the CNS as well as skeletal muscle. Most children do not achieve independent ambulation, are mentally retarded, and die late in the first decade. MRI and CT show cerebral abnormalities.

The eyes, brain, and skeletal muscle are involved in muscle–eye–brain (MEB) disease and in the Walker–Warburg syndrome. Their genetic basis is unknown, but they do not appear to be linked to chromosomes 6 or 9.

15.2.8 Bethlem myopathy

This rare condition is due to a mutation of the collagen VI gene, this collagen being a component of the extracellular matrix protein (Mohire *et al.* 1988; Jobsis *et al.* 1996). It does not merit the term 'muscular dystrophy' but is included here because it resembles clinically other conditions under discussion.

It is inherited as an autosomal dominant trait. The age of onset varies from infancy to adolescence. Proximal lower-limb weakness leads to a Gower's sign, which tends to disappear in adolescence and to reappear in early adult life. Thereafter there is slow progression, and most patients remain ambulant. In the upper limbs there is mild proximal weakness. There is general-ized slimness of the muscles. A characteristic feature is the development of contractures involving the interphalangeal joints, elbows, ankles, and often other joints. The serum crea-tine kinase may be slightly elevated and EMG shows myopathic changes. Diagnosis is established by DNA analysis.

15.2.9 Distal myopathies

Like the congenital muscular dystrophies, the distal myopathies are currently the subject of intensive research, genetic discovery, and reclassification (Barohn *et al.* 1998). Like Bethlem myopathy, they do not all fall readily into the category of the muscular dys-trophies. Their basic feature is early involvement of distal muscles, more often in the lower than the upper limbs, although later widespread weakness may occur. They must be distinguished from other conditions in which there is substantial distal weak-ness, including hereditary motor and sensory neuropathy (Section 12.4), distal spinal muscular atrophy (Section 14.3.4), myotonic dystrophy, inclusion-body myositis, and scapuloper-oneal syndrome. Several type have been described, most fre-quently in certain ethnic populations.

The first type to be defined clearly, and the most common, was the autosomal dominant, late-onset, distal myopathy of Welander (Borg *et al.* 1998). Initially reported in Sweden, it has now been reported in other countries, but usually in people with Swedish ancestors. Weakness is first noted in the hands in the fourth to sixth decade, and appears later in the distal lower limbs. It progresses slowly, but remains confined to the distal muscles.

Two autosomal dominant, late-onset forms, starting in the lower legs (anterior compartment), have been described (Markesbery–Griggs and Udd) and are sometimes referred to as tibial muscular dystrophy. The Markesbery–Griggs form later causes distal upper-limb weakness (Barohn *et al.* 1998). The Udd form appears to be confined to Finns (Udd *et al.* 1998).

Nonaka described an autosomal recessive form in Japan, with anterior compartment weakness developing in early adult life with additional involvement of iliopsoas and neck flexor muscles, and the presence of rimmed vacuoles on muscle biopsy (Nonaka *et al.* 1998).

Miyoshi and others described an early onset, autosomal recessive, myopathy affecting particularly the gastrocnemius, and causing difficulty climbing stairs and hopping. Serum creatine kinase levels were massively elevated. It is now known that this is a phenotypic variant of limb-girdle muscular dystrophy type 2B, which involves a mutation of the dysferlin gene (Liu *et al.* 1998).

15.3 Myotonic dystrophy

This is by far the most common inherited myopathy seen in adult life (Harper 1989). The exact prevalence is uncertain, but is in the order of 5–10/100 000. Clinically it can be considered to exist as one of three main phenotypes: the classical adult form, a late-onset type that may be without symptoms and abnormal signs, and a severe congenital form. It is a multisystem disease for which the term dystrophy is not entirely appropriate, but which is retained mainly for historical reasons. The genetic basis is an unstable trinucleotide (CTG) repeat expansion, and age of onset and severity relate to the size of the expansion (Anonymous 1998). Anticipation, in which the disease is more severe in subsequent generations, is often striking and relates to a marked increase in the size of the repeat, which is more likely to occur when the mother is the transmitting parent (Fig. 15.17). Despite identification of the responsible gene, which codes for a protein kinase, the molecular basis remains uncertain.

Clinical features

The *classical adult form* typically presents in late adolescence or early adult life. Later onset may occur, and a proportion of patients are asymptomatic but are identified during family screening studies. The distribution of muscle involvement is highly characteristic and difficult to confuse with other myopathies. The characteristic facial appearance (Fig. 15.17) is the result of ptosis and wasting and weakness of the facial muscles and muscles of mastication, together with premature balding. In the limbs there is distal weakness, affecting the hands and wrists more than the feet and ankles. Patients complain of difficulties with activities such as unscrewing the lid of a bottle and wringing out a cloth. Tripping due to footdrop is usually later. As the disease progresses, the weakness spreads proximally and, in late middle age, a small proportion of patients become wheelchair-bound, although most retain some independent ambulation. Also characteristic is the presence of wasting and weakness of sternomastoid and other neck flexor muscles—patients have difficulty lifting their head from the pillow, and when in a car their head is thrown backwards when the driver accelerates too rapidly.

Myotonia describes delayed muscle relaxation following voluntary contraction or percussion. It is due to repetitive discharge of the muscle fibre membrane and is rarely absent in myotonic dystrophy, even though the patient might not be aware of it. If symptomatic, the patient may complain of stiffness of the hands causing difficulty relaxing the grip, or of stiffness of the tongue or jaw when chewing and swallowing. Contrary to some reports, it is not always worse in cold weather, and inability to let go after shaking the examiner's hand is seen only in very severe cases. It is best demonstrated by showing slowness of grip relaxation or by percussion of the thenar eminence or extensor digitorum communis muscle (Fig. 15.5). 'Warm-up' occurs so that the myotonia becomes less evident with repeated contractions. Myotonia diminishes as weakness advances.

Respiratory muscle, including diaphragm, weakness develops in later stages and, together with aspiration, contributes to chest infections, which are a common terminal event. Hypoventilation with associated features may occur, but excessive daytime sleepiness, which is common, is usually due to central mechanisms.

Myotonic dystrophy is a multisystem disease with important manifestations outside skeletal muscle (Table 15.12). Foremost amongst these is cardiac involvement (Barnes and Hilton-Jones 1992). This takes the form of conduction problems and rhythm disturbances (typically atrial flutter or fibrillation) and is undoubtedly a major cause of sudden death in these patients.

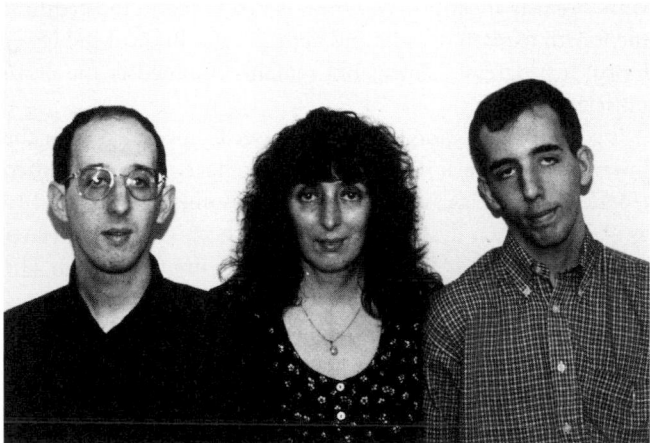

Fig. 15.17. Myotonic dystrophy in mother and sons. Anticipation—the disease is more severe in her two sons.

Table 15.12. Non-skeletal-muscle manifestations of myotonic dystrophy

Heart	Conduction problems
Eyes	Cataracts
CNS	Mental retardation
	Excessive daytime sleepiness
Endocrine	Testicular atrophy
	Reduced fertility
	Male-pattern baldness
Smooth muscle	Dysphagia and aspiration
	'Irritable-bowel-like symptoms'
	Constipation
	Faecal soiling
	Incoordinate uterine contractions
Peripheral nerve	Rarely symptomatic
Pilomatrixomas	

The patient should have an annual ECG and 24-hour ECG monitoring if new abnormalities appear or symptoms (e.g. presyncope, palpitation) develop. In many, but not all, patients the ECG changes evolve from normality, to minor intraventricular conduction abnormalities, to first degree block, and then to higher forms of block. In a few, sudden death occurs even when a recent ECG was normal. Anaesthesia is a particularly hazardous time, with the added risk of respiratory failure.

Excessive daytime sleepiness is present in about three-quarters of patients and may be very disabling. It is rarely due to hypoventilation and appears to be a primary cerebral problem. Smooth-muscle involvement is also underdiagnosed. A particular problem in childhood is faecal soiling. In adults irritable-bowel-like symptoms and constipation are common. Megacolon occurs rarely.

Cataracts are common. The earliest changes, which develop in early adult life, are of polychromatic dots in the anterior and posterior subcapsular regions. Late-stage cataracts are, at the bedside, indistinguishable from ordinary senile cataracts.

As a group, IQ tends to be lower than average, but many individuals are of normal intelligence.

The *late-onset* form, associated with only a small CTG trinucleotide expansion, may be asymptomatic. Commonly the patient develops cataracts at a relatively young age, and myotonic dystrophy should be considered in all patients who develop early cataracts. Myopathic features may be absent or limited to mild facial and hand weakness. There may be premature balding.

The *congenital form* is the most dramatic. The absence of myotonia and the fact that the mother may be asymptomatic means that the diagnosis is sometimes missed. This form is associated with a very large CTG expansion and the prognosis is poor (Reardon *et al.* 1993). Many affected fetuses are aborted spontaneously. Third-trimester polyhydramnios is common. Talipes may be present. At birth there is marked hypotonia, respiratory insufficiency, and feeding difficulties. The facial appearance at birth, with a tented upper lip reflecting muscle weakness, is striking but not pathognomonic. Later, the jaw hangs down due to weakness of the masticatory muscles. The feeding and respiratory problems settle and the hypotonia gradually resolves. Motor milestones are somewhat delayed and there is invariably mental retardation, which eventually results in the need for special schooling. Dysarthria is often marked. As the child reaches adolescence the features of the classical adult form start to become evident.

Diagnosis

The diagnosis is established on the basis of DNA analysis and, in the vast majority of patients, no other diagnostic tests are required. The differential diagnosis for the classical adult form is not wide, but includes the genetically unrelated proximal myotonic myopathy (PROMM) syndrome (Moxley 1996; Ranum *et al.* 1998). The nomenclature concerning myotonic dystrophy and related disorders, and guidelines for DNA testing, have been reviewed recently (International Myotonic Dystrophy Consortium 2000). Paediatricians must be aware of the congenital form, and ophthalmologists should consider the diagnosis in all younger patients presenting with cataract.

Management

There are many strands to successful management. Genetic counselling, not only for the patient but also for at-risk relatives, is vitally important. It must be remembered that a female carrying the gene may be asymptomatic but still be at risk of having a child with the severe congenital form of the disease. It is negligent to fail to offer such people counselling. Antenatal diagnosis, based on chorionic villus sampling, is readily available.

Regular ECGs are important and the patient must be instructed to report symptoms such as dizziness, fainting, and palpitation. Ambulatory 24-hour ECG monitoring should be performed if the ECG changes or symptoms develop. A proportion of patients will eventually require a pacemaker.

Chest infections may be reduced by influenza and pneumococcus vaccinations. Hypoventilation-related symptoms are relatively uncommon, but must be considered. The patient must be aware of the cardiac and respiratory hazards of anaesthesia and many carry a warning card or wear a bracelet or medallion.

Cataracts are treated surgically when vision is sufficiently impaired. Bowel complaints are treated symptomatically. There is no specific treatment for excessive daytime sleepiness. Taking a nap after meals and at other chosen times may limit inappropriate periods of sleep.

Myotonia rarely requires treatment. Drugs that are effective (mexiletine, procainamide, and phenytoin) are theoretically contraindicated because of their potential action on cardiac conduction. The effects of weakness may be, in part, ameliorated by appropriate advice from an occupational therapist and physiotherapist. Speech therapy may help swallowing problems and dysarthria, which is often a major problem for children with congenital myotonic dystrophy.

15.4 Congenital myopathies

Although many of these conditions present in early life with hypotonia, the term 'congenital' is not entirely appropriate as some are not evident at birth and some may not present until adulthood. This is yet another area in which genetic and molecular developments are leading to reclassification and new understanding (Goebel 1996; Sewry 1998). The common features of these disorders include frequent presentation as a 'floppy infant'; morphological changes such as high-arched palate, long face, and skeletal deformity; generalized muscle slimness and weakness; slow or non-progression; normal or only slightly elevated serum creatine kinase; and specific structural changes within muscle (indeed, they are sometimes called ultrastructural myopathies). They may be sporadic, autosomal recessive or dominant, or X-linked, and some individual disorders may show more than one pattern of inheritance. There is an important association between central-core disease and malignant hyperthermia.

15.4.1 Central-core disease

Presentation of central-core disease (CCD) is most often in infancy, but asymptomatic adult cases are recognized. The weakness is usually mild and is either generalized, also affecting the face, or affects mainly proximal lower-limb muscles. Scoliosis and contractures are occasional features. Respiratory failure is unusual. Progression, if it occurs, is slow. There is a complex association with malignant hyperthermia (MH) (Loke and MacLennan 1998). About one-third of patients with CCD are MH susceptible. Conversely, most patients with MH have normal muscle histology. The relationship to mutations affecting the ryanodine receptor is discussed elsewhere (Section 15.6.5). CCD is usually inherited as an autosomal dominant trait, but sporadic cases are reported—the significance of this awaits identification of the genetic basis.

The pathological features include type I fibre predominance and centrally placed cores which run the length of affected fibres, best seen using the NADH-tetrazolium reductase reaction.

15.4.2 Nemaline myopathy

The major pathological feature of this condition is the presence of nemaline rods (of uncertain constitution) in the sub-sarcolemmal region—these appear red using the Gomori trichrome method. They arc not pathognomonic, in that they may be seen as a secondary phenomenon in other disorders. An autosomal dominant form is caused by mutations in a tropomyosin gene, *TPM3* (Laing *et al.* 1995). The most common recessive form is associated with mutations in the gene encoding the giant muscle protein, nebulin (Pelin *et al.* 1999). Less commonly, mutations in the muscle α-actin gene may cause both dominant and recessive forms of nemaline myopathy, as well as a condition called actin myopathy (Nowak *et al.* 1999).

Most cases present at birth as floppy infants, but later onset can occur. There is facial and proximal weakness. Dysmorphic features (long face, high-arched palate, and chest deformity) reflect intrauterine and congenital weakness. Respiratory failure, probably indicating diaphragmatic involvement, is relatively common, and respiratory function must be monitored throughout life. It can be managed by nocturnal mask positive-pressure assisted ventilation. Typically, progression of weakness is very slow.

15.4.3 Congenital fibre-type disproportion

There is a strong suspicion that this is not a single entity but, rather, is a heterogeneous syndrome, in which a particular histological pattern may be caused not only by primary muscle disease but also by neurogenic disorders. The phenotype, as described, is that of a relatively benign condition, whereas the differential diagnosis includes the invariably fatal Werdnig–Hoffmann syndrome.

The characteristic pathological feature is disproportion between the sizes of type I and type II muscle fibres. Normally they are approximately equal in size, but in this condition, due to type II fibre hypertrophy, the difference exceeds 25 per cent.

The typical presentation is as a floppy infant. Contractures and congenital dislocation of the hip are common. There is a wide range of severity, but marked weakness is uncommon. There is no further progression, and indeed often improvement, after 2 years of age. Sporadic and autosomal recessive and dominant patterns of inheritance have been reported.

15.4.4 Minicore (multicore) disease

This is usually a relatively mild condition with onset of generalized weakness in early infancy with very slow or no progression. As in nemaline myopathy, diaphragmatic weakness and respiratory failure can occur. Sporadic cases and autosomal recessive and dominant inheritance have been described.

The name is derived from the appearance of multiple cores, devoid of mitochondria, within muscle fibres, which, unlike those in central-core disease, only run for short lengths along fibres.

15.4.5 Myotubular (centronuclear) myopathy

The name myotubular myopathy was proposed because it was thought that the abnormal fibres, with central nuclei, resembled myotubes, and that the cause might be arrested maturation. This is now doubted; the two names are used interchangeably in the literature and, once again, proper classification awaits further genetic developments.

The cause of the severe X-linked form is a mutation in the *CG2* gene (*MTM1* gene) at Xq28 (Laporte *et al.* 1997). There is often a history of miscarriages and neonatal male deaths. Those males born alive have severe weakness and respiratory insufficiency, and most die in early infancy. Autosomal forms, for which no genes have yet been identified, are of lesser severity. Onset is usually in infancy or early childhood, rarely in early adult life. Weakness is predominantly proximal and some have facial weakness, ptosis, and external ophthalmoplegia. Progression is usually slow or absent.

15.4.6 Other ultrastructural myopathies

There are many reports, often of single cases, of childhood-onset myopathies without specific clinical features but with disturbance of muscle ultrastructure, reflected in the names given to these conditions: cytoplasmic-body myopathy, hyaline-body myopathy, zebra-body myopathy, fingerprint myopathy, sarco-tubular myopathy, reducing-body myopathy, tubular-aggregate myopathy, desmin-storage myopathy, cap disease. Many of these changes may simply be epiphenomena of the basic, currently unknown, disease process. In other children, the biopsy shows minor, non-specific changes, to which the term 'minimal change myopathy' has been applied.

15.5 Non-dystrophic myotonias and periodic paralysis

Many of the conditions to be discussed in this section are caused by an inherited defect of a membrane-bound ion channel (Ptacek 1998; Lehmann-Horn and Jurkatt-Rott 1999). Arguably, they could have been included in a section entitled 'Channelopathies' which, in the neuromuscular field, might also have included malignant hyperthermia and various congenital myasthenic syndromes, as well as the acquired conditions of myasthenia gravis, Lambert–Eaton syndrome, and neuromyotonia. Considering neurology as a whole, other channelopathies include epilepsy, migraine, and certain ataxias (Ptacek 1997). Thus, the channelopathies are clinically a disparate group but represent a newly defined class of disorders, and they are currently the focus of considerable research activity. They may be subdivided on the basis of whether the involved channel is voltage-dependent/gated (the sodium, calcium, and chloride channelopathies, and indirectly the ryanodine receptor), or ligand-dependent (acetylcholine receptor).

The term non-dystrophic myotonias serves to distinguish the conditions accompanied by myotonia described in this section from myotonic dystrophy (Section 15.3), which in turn is now considered separate from the muscular dystrophies (Section 15.2). Further reclassification is likely in the near future, as the genetic and molecular causes of the inherited neuromuscular disorders are identified.

The periodic paralyses are characterized by episodic weakness. Often there is a change in the serum potassium level during an attack; this led to the original classification of hyper-, hypo-, and normo-kalaemic forms. Primary forms are inherited channelopathies, and are now classified upon the basis of the ion channel involved; whereas secondary forms are due to systemic metabolic disturbance. Primary hyperkalaemic periodic paralysis may be accompanied by myotonia.

15.5.1 Myotonia congenita

Although first described (by Thomsen, who himself had the disease) as an autosomal dominant disorder, it was shown later (by Becker) that it is very much more frequently an autosomal recessive condition. Different mutations of the same gene (*CLCN1*) are responsible for each (Zhang *et al.* 1996). The chloride channel has an important role in membrane repolarization.

Clinical features

The recessive and dominant forms are very similar, but with the recessive type tending to be more severe. The characteristic feature is generalized myotonia, first evident in childhood,

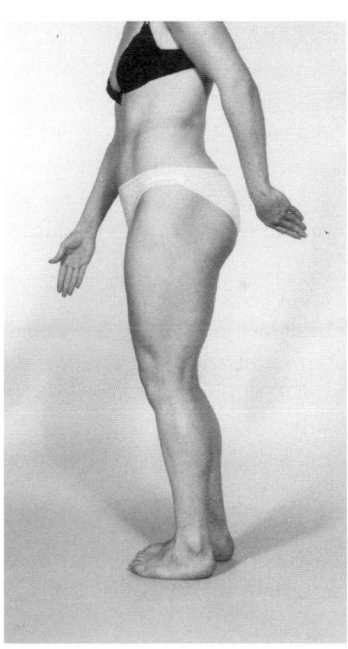

Fig. 15.18. Myotonia congenita. Note the muscle hypertrophy.

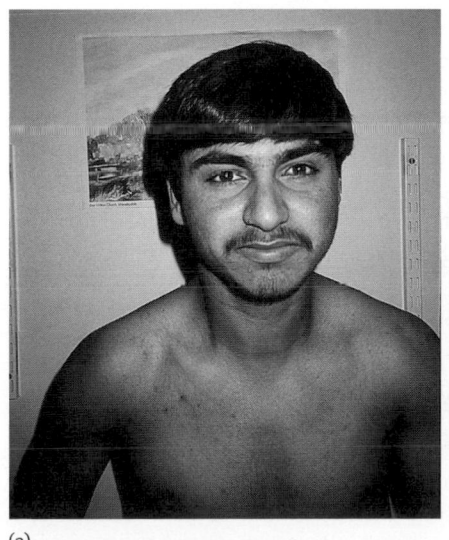 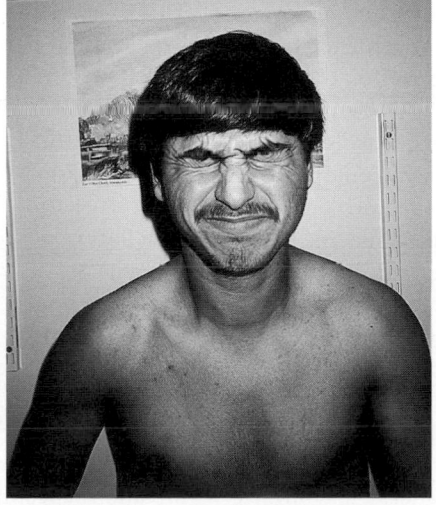 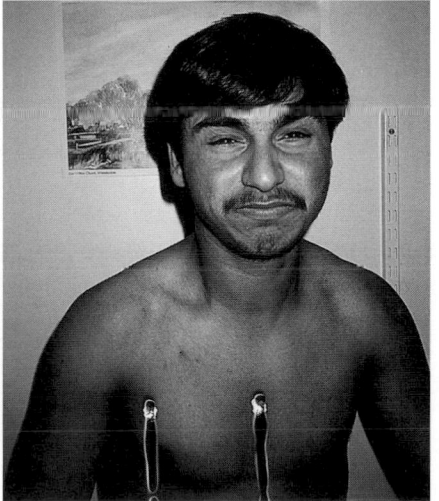

(a)   (b)   (c)

Fig. 15.19. Myotonia congenita. At rest (a), during forceful eye-closure (b), and 5 seconds after relaxing (c).

without persistent weakness. The myotonia eases with repetitive contractions ('warm-up'). In the cranial nerve territory, myotonia can cause difficulty chewing, and in early childhood there may be striking slowness of relaxation of the periorbital muscles (looking a little like blepharospasm) when crying. Grip myotonia causes problems similar to those seen in myotonic dystrophy, but without the additional problem of weakness. In the lower limbs the stiffness may cause patients to fall as they start to walk, and this is most evident after a period of rest—one of my patients regularly fell after having been standing to attention and then ordered to march, to the irritation of the sergeant-major! Transient weakness, lasting several seconds only, may be seen in the recessive form, for example when first making a forceful fist. In some patients there is striking muscle hypertrophy (Fig. 15.18), which represents a form of work hypertrophy consequent upon the myotonia.

At the bedside, myotonia is easily demonstrated on muscle percussion and as slowness of relaxation of grip. Facial muscle myotonia may be seen as lid-lag (the patient looks upwards for several seconds, and then suddenly down towards the ground—the upper lids lag behind the downward eye movement), or as delayed relaxation following forceful eye-closure (Fig. 15.19).

Diagnosis

Electromyography shows generalized myotonia. Serum creatine kinase is normal or mildly elevated. The diagnosis is confirmed by DNA studies. The differential diagnosis, which does not usually cause many difficulties, includes myotonic dystrophy, proximal myotonic myopathy, and sodium channelopathies.

Management

Many patients cope without treatment. For those that require relief from the myotonia, mexiletine is the drug of choice.

15.5.2 Primary hypokalaemic periodic paralysis

This form of periodic paralysis is caused by one of several mutations affecting the *CACLN1A3* gene, which encodes the dihydropyridine receptor (DHPR) (Boerman *et al.* 1995). Skeletal muscle has two, functionally linked, types of calcium channel related to the T-tubular/sarcoplasmic reticular system, which are involved in excitation–contraction coupling. The DHPR is an L-type voltage-gated calcium channel located in the T-tubular membrane. It is coupled to the ryanodine receptor, which is the second calcium channel and which itself is not voltage dependent. The disease is inherited as an autosomal dominant with reduced penetrance in women.

Clinical features

The severity varies enormously. Some carriers are asymptomatic, some have only a handful of attacks in their lifetime, and some have daily episodes. Individual attacks may involve one or a few muscles, or cause generalized paralysis, but even in these respiratory failure is unusual. The bulbar musculature is usually spared and it is easy to see how somebody complaining of total inability to move, but still able to speak, move their head, and to breathe, may be labelled as hysterical.

Most cases present in childhood or adolescence, a few not until the third decade. Typically, the patient wakes in the morning with the paralysis and the weakness resolves during the course of the day. Rarely, attacks last several days. Precipitants include high-carbohydrate food and emotional upset. Gentle exercise may abort an attack.

Many patients develop a slowly progressive proximal myopathy and this is largely independent of the occurrence of paralytic attacks.

Diagnosis

Increasingly, this will become DNA based. Demonstration of a low serum potassium level during a spontaneous attack is very helpful. Provocative tests should only ever be performed by a suitably experienced clinician—they are potentially very dangerous. In these tests, the serum potassium is lowered by glucose loading, either alone or in combination with insulin. During an attack the muscle compound action potential is reduced or absent. Muscle biopsy is not part of the routine diagnostic process, but it patients with permanent weakness it shows a vacuolar myopathy.

Management

Patients should be advised to avoid high-carbohydrate meals and excessive physical exercise. Infrequent mild attacks may not require treatment. More troublesome attacks usually respond to oral potassium chloride (up to 10 g) given as an unsweetened aqueous solution. For prevention of frequent attacks, acetazolamide is the drug of choice. Low doses (e.g. 125 mg on alternate days) may be sufficient. There is no specific treatment for the permanent myopathy.

15.5.3 Thyrotoxic periodic paralysis

This is an important differential diagnosis from primary hypokalaemic periodic paralysis. It is usually sporadic, is much commoner in males, and the majority of cases occur in Orientals (Ober 1992; Ko *et al.* 1996). Features of thyrotoxicosis may be absent. The clinical and biochemical features, and precipitating factors to paralytic attacks, are indistinguishable from those associated with primary hypokalaemic periodic paralysis, with the exception that onset is typically in adult life. In a male over the age of 21 years developing periodic paralysis, the thyrotoxic form is far more likely than the primary form.

15.5.4 Primary hyperkalaemic periodic paralysis and related disorders

Three different conditions are known to be associated with mutations affecting the skeletal muscle sodium-channel gene (SCN4A); hyperkalaemic periodic paralysis, paramyotonia congenita, and potassium-aggravated myotonia (Cannon 1997).

Different clinical expression may be seen within members of the same family and, arguably, all three could be grouped together under the term sodium channelopathy. Inheritance is autosomal dominant, usually with full penetrance.

Hyperkalaemic periodic paralysis

The clinical presentation is similar to the hypokalaemic (calcium channel) form, with episodic weakness in childhood and attacks often occurring before breakfast. They are often fairly brief and may be accompanied by muscle aching. Precipitants include cold, fasting, rest after exercise, emotional stress, pregnancy, alcohol, and potassium-loading. Patients may find out for themselves that intake of a carbohydrate, such as a sweet drink, may abort an attack. The attacks tend to reduce in frequency in later life but, independent of acute episodes, a progressive proximal myopathy may develop.

Emphasizing the relationship to the other two conditions, myotonia may be evident clinically (most often of the facial musculature) or electromyographically, and there may be features of paramyotonia.

The diagnostic approach is similar to that for the hypokalaemic form. Ideally, investigations are performed during spontaneous attacks. An attack can be precipitated by potassium-loading but this is not without hazard. DNA-based diagnosis is becoming more widely available. The form previously classified as normokalaemic, on the basis of no change in serum potassium level during an attack, is now know to be caused by sodium-channel gene mutations.

Treatment consists of avoiding precipitating factors, frequent carbohydrate-rich meals and drug therapy if the attacks are frequent and disabling. Low-dose thiazide diuretics are first choice but acetazolamide also works, although with greater risk of side-effects. Inhalation of a β-adrenergic stimulant, such as salbutamol, may abort attacks.

Paramyotonia congenita

The overlap with hyperkalaemic periodic paralysis was noted above. The characteristic feature of this condition is paramyotonia, which describes myotonia precipitated and exacerbated by exercise and cold. In other forms of myotonia repeated use of a muscle leads to reduction in myotonia ('warm-up' phenomenon) but in this condition the reverse applies. The facial and distal upper-limb muscles are most affected. There is marked cold sensitivity, which not only exacerbates the myotonia but may also induce weakness that can last for hours. Onset is in early infancy. Later, some patients develop paralytic attacks.

Diagnosis is based on the clinical picture, demonstration of cold-exacerbated myotonia, and DNA studies. Treatment is often not required, but mexiletine is effective.

Potassium-aggravated myotonia

This is currently the preferred term for disorders previously labelled as myotonia fluctuans, myotonia permanens, and acetazolamide-responsive myotonia. Features include fluctuating myotonia, sometimes severe, which is exacerbated by exercise (and, as the name implies, potassium loading) but not by cold, and the absence of weakness. New mutations, affecting the sodium-channel gene, appear to be common. They are an important differential diagnosis from myotonia congenita.

15.5.5 Andersen's syndrome

The genetic basis of this condition (Sansone *et al.* 1997) is not yet known but it has been shown not to be linked to the skeletal muscle sodium channel. The three major clinical elements are potassium-sensitive periodic paralysis, cardiac dysrhythmia (bidirectional ventricular tachycardia), and dysmorphic features (face and hands). Partial manifestations, including long-QT syndrome, are common.

15.5.6 Secondary periodic paralyses

Any disease or drug that changes the total body potassium level can induce weakness, which is usually persistent but may be periodic. Weakness is common if the serum potassium level drops below 2.5 mmol/l. In severe cases the respiratory muscles may be involved and rhabdomyolysis can occur. Generalized weakness may develop with serum levels above 6 mmol/l but is rarely severe and the main risk is cardiac dysfunction. Weakness responds rapidly to correction of the serum potassium level.

15.5.7 Schwartz–Jampel syndrome

The major clinical features of this rare syndrome are muscle stiffness, particularly affecting the face and giving a characteristic appearance with blepharospasm, short stature, and bone dysplasia. It is genetically heterogeneous and no specific gene defects have yet been identified, although a patient with a sodium channel mutation producing a similar clinical picture has been described, and some families show linkage to chromosome 1 (Fontaine *et al.* 1996).

15.6 Primary metabolic myopathies

This section is concerned with primary, genetically determined, metabolic disorders of skeletal muscle (Hilton-Jones *et al.* 1995). Many of these are multisystem disorders, reflecting the widespread distribution of some of the enzymes involved; others are confined to muscle. In many, the basic problem is disruption of normal energy-generating processes. In some, the accumulation of lipid and glycogen may disrupt muscle-fibre function. A brief overview of normal energetic processes is followed by discussion of individual disorders. In everyday clinical practice the mitochondrial cytopathies are the most frequently encountered of the metabolic myopathies.

Normal energetic processes

Although individual pathways of energy metabolism, and the relationships between them are complex, they can be simplified

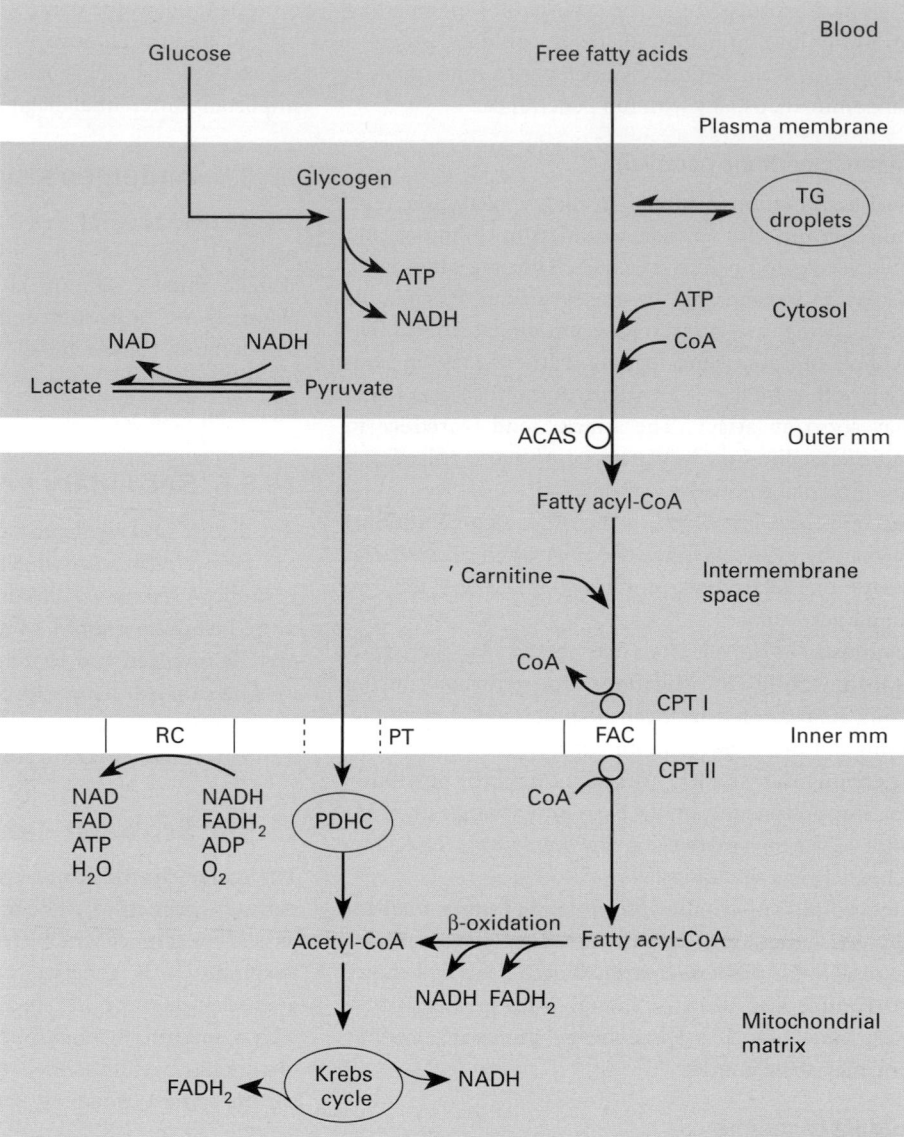

Fig. 15.20. Major metabolic pathways in skeletal muscle. ACAS, acyl-CoA synthetase; ADP, adenosine diphosphate; ATP, adenosine triphosphate; CoA, coenzyme A; CPT, carnitine palmitoyltransferase; FAC, fatty acyl carnitine; FAD, flavine adenine dinucleotide; FADH$_2$, reduced FAD; mm, mitochondrial membrane; NAD, nicotinamide adenine dinucleotide; NADH, reduced NAD; PDH, pyruvate dehydrogenase complex; PT, pyruvate translocase; RC, respiratory chain; TG, triglyceride. (Reproduced with kind permission from the *Oxford Textbook of Medicine*, Oxford University Press).

to allow ready understanding of the metabolic myopathies (Fig. 15.20). Adenosine triphosphate (ATP) is the major immediate energy source. It provides the energy for essential housekeeping metabolic functions as well as providing energy for contraction. Resting muscle uses very little energy, but vigorous exercise can increase ATP utilization by more than two orders of magnitude. Muscle is well adapted to meet this demand. ATP can be re-synthesized through three major pathways: the creatine kinase reaction, glycolysis, and oxidative phosphorylation (Fig. 15.20). The relative contribution from each depends upon the state of nutrition and, more importantly, the level and duration of exercise.

At rest the major fuel source is circulating free fatty acids. These are transported into mitochondria, across the inner mitochondrial membrane by the carnitine transport system, into the matrix, and then undergo β-oxidation. The latter generates the energy-rich electron carriers—reduced nicotinamide

adenine dinucleotide (NADH) and reduced flavine adenine dinucleotide (FADH2). Transfer of their electrons to molecular oxygen in the electron transport (respiratory) chain releases energy, via the pumping of protons, for the generation of ATP (the process being known as oxidative phosphorylation). Circulating glucose entering muscle may undergo glycolysis, with the product pyruvate then being further metabolized within mitochondria, but the contribution to energy generation is small and much of the glucose is stored as glycogen for future use.

During early strenuous exercise, the oxidative pathways cannot cope with the demand for ATP generation—the resting blood flow provides inadequate delivery of oxygen and substrate. The creatine kinase reaction provides a short-term buffer, but then glycogenolysis becomes critical. This produces ATP (but much less efficiently than oxidative metabolism), NADH, and pyruvate. Because of the relative lack of oxygen, pyruvate can not undergo further oxidative metabolism. The increasing NADH/NAD ratio would inhibit glycolysis and is prevented by the reduction of pyruvate to lactate. This explains the lactic acidosis seen in disorders of oxidative metabolism (e.g. the mitochondrial cytopathies) and the failure to generate lactate in disorders of glycogenolysis and glycolysis.

As exercise continues, muscle blood flow increases, the respiratory rate rises, and fatty acids are mobilized from fat stores. Glycogen stores are depleted. Thus, in sustained exercise, fatty acids and oxidative metabolism again become the main energy source.

Observations in clinical practice bear out these simplifications. Disorders of glycogen and glucose metabolism typically produce symptoms in early, particularly intense, exercise, but if activity is sustained a 'second-wind' develops due to the return to fatty acid metabolism. Defective fatty acid metabolism, insufficient to produce symptoms at rest, are exposed by sustained exercise and fasting (which limits carbohydrate metabolism in muscle). Mitochondrial disorders affecting respiratory chain function are often symptomatic at rest, and multisystem in their manifestations, reflecting the critical central role of oxidative phosphorylation.

15.6.1 Disorders of carbohydrate metabolism

The major steps in glycogenolysis are shown in Fig. 15.21, together with those enzymes known to be associated with metabolic myopathies. Acid maltase deficiency differs from the other glycogenoses in that it involves a pathway not directly involved in energy generation. These are autosomal recessive disorders, with the exception of phosphoglycerate kinase deficiency which is X-linked. Although the genetic basis of many of these conditions has been identified, routine DNA based diagnosis is not yet readily available. Diagnosis is based on metabolic investigations. The serum creatine kinase level is usually elevated. In many, forearm exercise is associated with impaired venous lactate production. This information, and more, can be obtained more safely by phosphorus magnetic resonance spectroscopy studies, but these are not widely available. In some cases enzyme deficiency may be demonstrated by histochemical methods applied to a muscle biopsy specimen. Muscle biopsy typically shows glycogen accumulation. Diagnosis is confirmed by enzyme assay. Increasingly, DNA diagnosis will become available.

Myophosphorylase deficiency (type V glycogenosis, McArdle's disease)

The classical presentation is with exercise intolerance in childhood. Exercise induces pain and stiffness. More extreme activity may produce electrically silent cramps and myoglobinuria (Section 15.6.4). Patients often discover the 'second-wind' phenomenon for themselves. Progressive proximal weakness often develops and may be the mode of presentation in later-onset cases (who in retrospect often have a history of mild

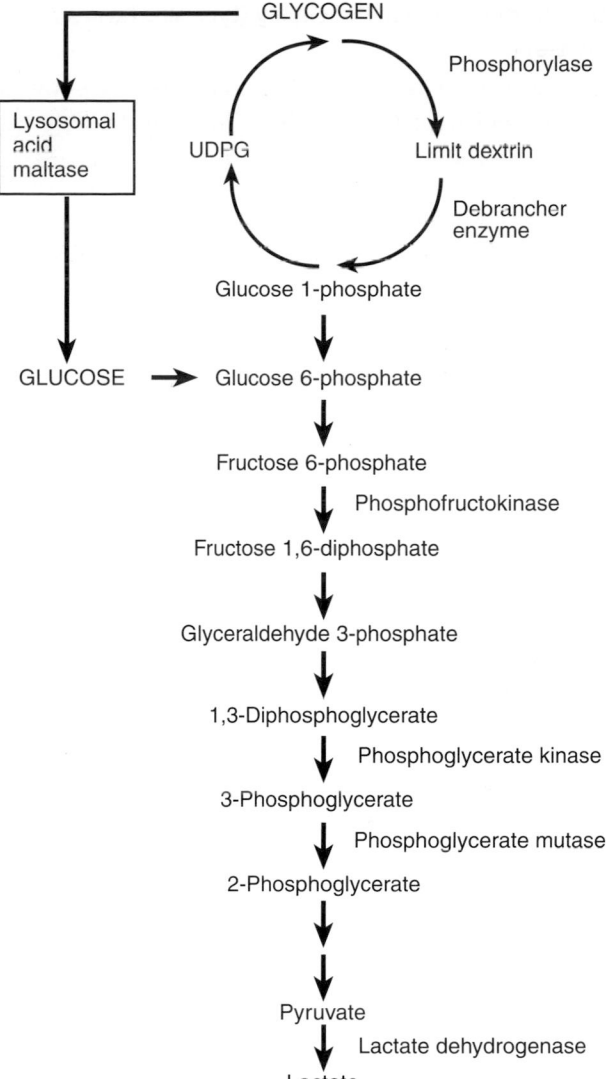

Fig. 15.21. Glycogenolysis and glycolysis (reproduced with kind ermission from the *Oxford Textbook of Medicine*, Oxford University Press).

exercise intolerance). Myophosphorylase is a muscle-specific enzyme and so clinical manifestations are restricted to skeletal muscle.

Debranching enzyme deficiency (type III, Cori–Forbes disease)

The most common form presents in early infancy with hypoglycaemia, seizures, failure to thrive, and hepatomegaly. Myopathic features may be slight. During childhood the liver problems tend to settle but the myopathy progresses, and in adult life a significant cardiomyopathy may develop. Less commonly, presentation is in adulthood with a progressive proximal, less frequently distal, myopathy. A history of a protuberant abdomen in childhood and mild exercise intolerance may be obtained. Overall, exercise intolerance is less prominent than in phosphorylase deficiency.

Phosphofructokinase deficiency (type VII, Tarui's disease)

This is much rarer than the conditions described above, with less than 50 cases having been described. The myopathic features are similar to myophosphorylase deficiency. Most patients have laboratory evidence of increased haemolysis (increased bilirubin and raised reticulocyte count, hyperuricaemia) but clinical accompaniments (jaundice, gallstones, gout) are uncommon.

Other glycogenoses

Deficiencies of phosphoglycerate kinase, phosphoglycerate mutase, and lactate dehydrogenase cause exercise intolerance with myalgia and myoglobinuria. Only a handful of cases have been described. Branching enzyme is required for glycogen synthesis. Deficiency usually causes progressive hepatosplenomegaly (with death by 4 years if untreated by transplantation) and over one-half of these patients have a myopathy. Very rare presentations with cardiac and/or skeletal myopathy, but without liver disease, have been described.

Acid maltase deficiency (type II, Pompe's disease)

This condition differs in many ways from the other glycogenoses (Reuser *et al.* 1995). The functional role of the enzyme is not clear, but it is not apparently involved in energy-generating pathways and deficiency is not associated with exercise intolerance. Three main clinical forms are recognized: infantile (IIa), childhood (IIb), and adult (IIc). The infantile form was the type described by Pompe and is a multisystem disorder causing progressive generalized weakness, failure to thrive, organomegaly (including tongue enlargement), and death by 2 years due to cardiac or respiratory failure. The childhood form presents later, but by age 15 years. There is a progressive proximal myopathy and later cardiomyopathy. Death occurs in the second or third decade from cardiorespiratory failure.

The adult form, which may not present until the seventh decade, is usually restricted to skeletal muscle. It usually presents as a proximal myopathy, clinically indistinguishable from many other causes of 'limb-girdle syndrome'. Diaphragmatic involvement is common and up to one-third of patients present with respiratory failure, although in retrospect there may have been symptoms of limb weakness, and limb weakness is usually evident on examination (Trend *et al.* 1985). With nocturnal ventilatory support many patients can lead active lives for many years before progressive limb weakness causes increasing disability. Muscle biopsy shows glycogen accumulation in vacuoles of lysosomal origin. Diagnosis is confirmed by enzyme assay, usually on the muscle biopsy specimen. Lymphocytes also show glycogen storage, and an air-dried blood film treated with periodic acid–Schiff reagent provides a quick and reliable diagnostic test.

15.6.2 Disorders of lipid metabolism

These rare conditions are sometimes referred to as 'lipid storage myopathies' but this term obscures the fact that, in many cases, lipid accumulation (as shown by fat stains applied to muscle biopsy samples) is not evident. Multisystem features may be more striking than myopathy. Fatty acids entering muscle are activated by acyl-CoA synthetase at the outer mitochondrial membrane (Fig. 15.20). The fatty acyl-CoA is converted to an acyl-carnitine, which is then transported across the inner mitochondrial membrane by the carnitine-dependent transporter system involving carnitine palmitoyltransferase I and II. In the mitochondrial matrix, fatty acyl-CoA is reformed and then undergoes β-oxidation, as described above. Lipid disorders may involve the carnitine system or β-oxidation.

The importance of fatty acid oxidation to muscle energy metabolism has already been discussed. In addition, fatty acids are the substrate for hepatic ketogenesis; ketone bodies are a major auxilliary fuel source for the central nervous system. Further, fatty acids are required for hepatic gluconeogenesis. These latter two observations explain the multi-organ involvement that may occur with these disorders.

Carnitine deficiency

This remains an area of controversy (Kerner and Hoppel 1998). Secondary carnitine deficiency is common. Causes include many defects of intermediary metabolism, notably defects of fatty acid β-oxidation, mitochondrial cytopathies, and haemodialysis. Primary carnitine deficiency, if it exists, is rare. In some cases reported there may be a defect of carnitine transport into muscle.

Carnitine palmitoyltransferase deficiency

This rare condition presents with myalgia, rhabdomyolysis, and myoglobinuria, precipitated by long-sustained exercise (classically an army route march or similar exercise) or by fasting. During an attack, muscle biopsy may show some lipid accumulation, but often not. Diagnosis is by enzyme assay. Mutations in the *CPT II* gene have been identified (Taroni *et al.* 1993).

β-oxidation disorders

The investigation of these conditions is complex (Pourfarzam *et al.* 1994). The most common is medium-chain acyl-CoA dehydrogenase (MCAD) deficiency, and this usually presents in childhood with Reye-like episodes (encephalopathy and hypoketotic hypoglycaemia) and sudden death. Rare cases present later with recurrent rhabdomyolysis. A common point mutation allows DNA diagnosis in about 90 per cent of patients. Many other disorders of β-oxidation have been described, but all are rare—they usually present in infancy with multisystem disease but myopathy may predominate. Correct diagnosis is important in determining therapy. Fasting must be avoided. Diet supplementation with medium-chain fatty acids may help in cases where the metabolic block affects enzymes responsible for long-chain fatty acid metabolism. Carnitine deficiency can be corrected by dietary supplementation but this is of uncertain benefit.

15.6.3 Mitochondrial cytopathies

Although it was myopathy that first led to the identification of this disease group, they are now recognized to be multisytem

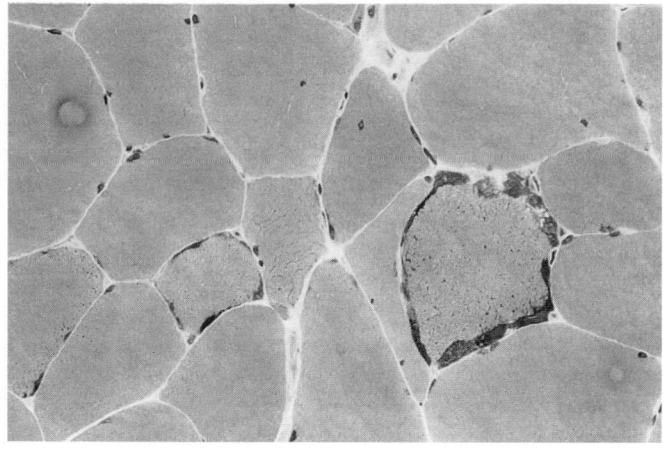

(a)

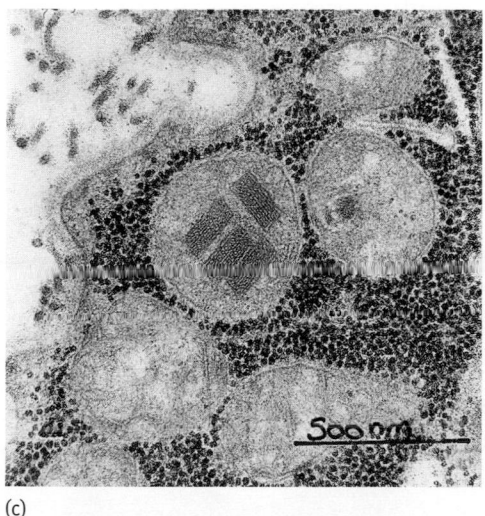

(b)

(c)

Fig. 15.22. Mitochondrial cytopathy. (a) Modified Gomori trichrome stain showing ragged-red fibres. Electron microscopy: (b) morphologically abnormal mitochondria; and (c) paracrystalline inclusions.

disorders affecting not only the central and peripheral nervous systems (Sections 12.7.6 and 27.4.7) but also every other organ system in the body. They were defined initially at a morphological level; light and electron microscopy demonstrated accumulations of mitochondria which often showed structural abnormalities (Fig. 15.22). We now know that morphological changes such as ragged-red fibres are not always present, or are more subtle (such as some fibres showing deficient cytochrome oxidase staining). The next stage involved isolation of mitochondria from such patients and investigation of metabolic pathways, particularly the respiratory chain. It soon became clear that there was a poor correlation between the phenotype and identification of a particular metabolic defect. In 1988 it was shown that some cases were associated with an abnormality of the mitochondrial genome (Holt *et al.* 1988) and subsequent studies have shown a broad correlation between genotype and phenotype. Within this somewhat recherché field there is continuing friendly debate as to whether mitochondrial disorders should be lumped together or split into specific syndromes; in practice, both approaches can be useful. This section will consider basic aspects of mitochondrial biology, genetics, clinical features, characteristic syndromes, diagnosis, and treatment. It will only deal with conditions in which muscle involvement is usually present, and will thus exclude conditions such as Leber's hereditary optic neuropathy and non-neurological disorders such as Pearson syndrome.

Mitochondrial biology

Many of the biochemical functions of mitochondria have been discussed above. The respiratory chain, vital to oxidative phosphorylation, consists of five complexes. Each of these is composed of many subunits. Most of these are encoded by nuclear DNA, but some of the subunits in four of the five complexes are encoded by mitochondrial DNA.

Mitochondrial DNA (mtDNA) is a 16.5 kb, circular, double strand of DNA. A number of properties are important when considering mitochondrial diseases (Section 2.8.3):

1. It is exclusively maternally inherited.

2. It encodes some of the subunits of four of the five respiratory chain complexes (13 subunits in total), as well as 22 tRNAs and two ribosomal RNAs.

3. Each mitochondrion contains several copies of mtDNA and normally these are all the same (homoplasmy).

4. In diseases with mtDNA mutations there is a mixture of both normal (wild-type) and mutated mtDNA (heteroplasmy).

5. There is a threshold effect—symptoms are only manifest if the mutant : wild-type ratio is above a certain level. The critical ratio may vary from organ to organ, depending upon the metabolic demands of that tissue.

6. Nuclear genes influence mitochondrial biogenesis and thus nuclear genetic abnormalities, which will be autosomally inherited, may cause secondary mtDNA abnormalities.

Genetics

An understanding of this is vital, particularly with respect to genetic counselling. Most cases are sporadic, some show classical maternal inheritance, and some show an autosomal pattern of inheritance. Different types of mtDNA mutation tend to be associated with particular inheritance patterns. Mutation types include *major rearrangements* with deletions (typically a length of about 5 kb is deleted) or, less commonly, duplications of a stretch of mtDNA. In most such cases there is a single type of mutation. There will thus be heteroplasmy with two populations—wild type and mutant. Patients with these types of mutation are generally sporadic and their offspring at little risk. Clinically, such patients most frequently have chronic external ophthalmoplegia (CPEO).

The next most common type of mutation is a *point mutation*, typically affecting a tRNA. Such mutations are maternally inherited and are typically associated with multisystem disease, particularly with CNS involvement.

Some patients show *variable deletions*, meaning that there are several populations of mutated mtDNA, each with a different-sized deletion. The usual clinical presentation is with CPEO and inheritance is autosomal dominant. With *mitochondrial depletion* there is a reduced amount of wild-type mtDNA. Inheritance is autosomal dominant or recessive.

Table 15.13. Organ involvement in mitochondrial cytopathies

Organ	Involvement
Muscle	Chronic external ophthalmoplegia
	Proximal myopathy
	Exercise intolerance
Eyes	Pigmentary retinopathy
	Optic atrophy
	Cataracts
Brain	Encephalopathy
	Stroke-like episodes
	Epilepsy
	Dementia
	Extrapyramidal/movement disorders
	Ataxia
	Deafness
	Leigh's syndrome
	Raised CSF protein
Peripheral nerve	Neuropathy (typically subclinical and axonal)
Heart	Cardiac conduction problems
	Cardiomyopathy
Gut	Hypomotility/pseudo-obstruction
Liver	Failure
Endocrine	Diabetes mellitus
	Hypoparathyroidism
	Short stature
Kidney	Fanconi syndrome
Blood	Sideroblastic anaemia
	Folate deficiency
Skin	Multiple lipomatosis

Clinical features

The principal clinical features of the mitochondrial cytopathies are shown in Table 15.13. Such a list makes it clear why these disorders are so often considered in differential diagnosis. The most commonly encountered and significant clinical features include chronic external ophthalmoplegia, asymptomatic retinal pigmentation, proximal myopathy, epilepsy, encephalopathy, deafness, ataxia, cardiac conduction abnormalities, short stature, and diabetes (Petty *et al.* 1986). A number of characteristic syndromes are discussed below, but it must be remembered that presentation of mitochondrial cytopathy may be with any one, or combination, of the features listed in Table 15.13.

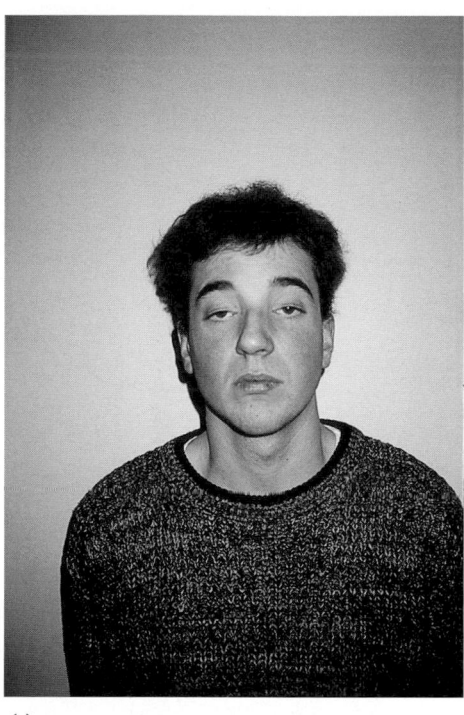

(a)

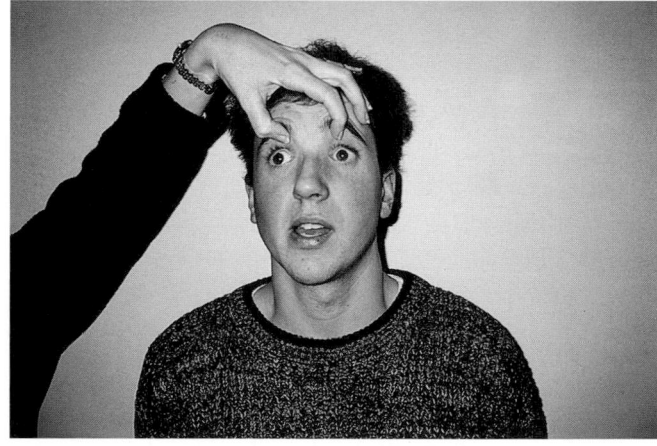

(b)

Fig. 15.23. Mitochondrial chronic progressive external ophthalmoplegia. Note the ptosis (a), and failure of eye movement on attempting to look fully to the right (b).

Characteristic syndromes

There are three relatively stereotyped syndromes which present little diagnostic difficulty.

Chronic external ophthalmoplegia

This is the most frequently encountered phenotype and is seen at all ages. Ptosis and progressive limitation of eye movements develop over many years (Fig. 15.23). Diplopia is uncommon. There is often an asymptomatic peripheral pigmentary retinopathy. In adult life it may occur in isolation, with deafness, with proximal limb weakness, and with diabetes. In childhood the combination of CPEO with, variably, retinopathy, heart block, ataxia, and elevated CSF protein is referred to as Kearns–Sayre syndrome. Some use this eponym loosely to describe all cases of CPEO. Most cases are sporadic and muscle mtDNA shows a single deletion. Autosomal dominant CPEO is rare and is associated with multiple mtDNA deletions. The important differential diagnoses in adult life include myasthenia gravis, oculopharyngeal muscular dystrophy, and thyroid ophthalmopathy.

MELAS syndrome

This acronym is derived from *m*itochondrial myopathy, *e*ncephalopathy, *l*actic *a*cidosis, and *s*troke-like episodes (Pavlakis *et al.* 1984). It is most frequently related to a point mutation (at base point 3243-tRNA$^{Leu(UUR)}$ A→G) but the same phenotype may be seen with other point mutations and, conversely, the 3243 mutation may cause other phenotypes, including CPEO. Presentation is in childhood with stroke-like episodes, often affecting the occipital cortex. Initially recovery from such episodes may be good, but with time major deficits develop. Epilepsy and encephalopathic episodes are common. Exercise may precipitate lactic acidosis with associated systemic upset. Other clinical features may be present, including short stature and deafness. MELAS is inherited maternally, but penetrance appears to be low and it is relatively uncommon to see two people in the same family with the full syndrome, but restricted features, such as deafness and diabetes, are common in many family members.

MERRF syndrome

Myoclonic epilepsy develops in late adolescence or early adult life and later may be accompanied by generalized tonic–clonic convulsions (Wallace *et al.* 1988). Dementia and ataxia are common associated features. Muscle biopsy shows *ragged red fibres* but symptomatic myopathy is unusual. It is most frequently associated with the 8344-tRNA^{Lys} A→G mutation but, as with MELAS, there is genetic and phenotypic heterogeneity. Inheritance is maternal but, also as with MELAS, many individuals carrying the mutation are asymptomatic or oligosymptomatic.

Diagnosis

Many laboratories now offer mtDNA analysis for major rearrangements (deletions and duplications) and the more common point mutations, and this may be all that is required if the phenotype is one of the three characteristic syndromes described above. A practical point to note is that point mutations can be identified in a blood sample, whereas deletions require a sample of muscle. In other situations, investigation is complex and requires specialist facilities, including exercise testing, magnetic resonance spectroscopy, and biochemical studies on extracted mitochondria (Hilton-Jones *et al.* 1995).

Treatment

This is very much in its infancy and, arguably, no specific therapies yet exist. Anecdotal reports of benefit from vitamins, cofactors, and co-enzyme Q have not been substantiated by formal trials. Prednisolone seems to help some children with MELAS. Careful attention must be paid to potentially treatable complications such as heart involvement, diabetes, and epilepsy.

15.6.4 **Myoglobinuria**

Myoglobin is a haem protein which transfers oxygen from the muscle fibre membrane to mitochondria. Membrane damage leads to release of the protein into the bloodstream (myoglobinaemia) and excretion into the urine (myoglobinuria), causing darkening of the urine from pale brown to black. Myoglobinuria is accompanied by massive elevation of the serum creatine kinase level. The principle danger is acute tubular necrosis, and forced alkaline diuresis is often advised to reduce the risk of this, although it is of unproven benefit. Some of the principle causes of myoglobinuria are listed in Table 15.14.

15.6.5 **Malignant hyperthermia**

The relationship between malignant hyperthermia (MH) and central-core disease was mentioned in Section 15.4.1. The central event in this condition is disturbed calcium homoeostasis in the sarcoplasmic reticulum; sudden influx of calcium causes hypermetabolism and muscle contracture (Denborough

Table 15.14. Causes of myoglobinuria

Intense exercise in normal individuals
Inherited myopathies
Glycogenoses
Disorders of lipid metabolism
Malignant hyperthermia
Duchenne/Becker muscular dystrophy
Acquired myopathies
Dermatomyositis/polymyositis
Viral and bacterial infections
Ischaemia and trauma
Drugs and toxins
Alcohol
Opiates
Clofibrate
Venoms
Others
Neuroleptic malignant syndrome
Fever and heat stroke

1998). Attacks are triggered by succinylcholine and, more potently, volatile inhalational anaesthetic agents, notably halothane. The incidence is about 1 in 50 000 anaesthetics and is probably the most common cause of death during anaesthesia. The mortality rate is greatly reduced by prompt recognition and treatment with intravenous dantrolene. Affected individuals may show persistent elevation of the serum creatine kinase and MH is one cause of idiopathic hyperCKaemia.

The clinical features are of rigidity, which may be localized (typically to the masseter) or generalized, accompanied by rapidly increasing body temperature and tachycardia. Metabolically there is acidosis, elevation of the serum creatine kinase, and myoglobinuria.

Whether or not associated with central-core disease, MH is inherited as an autosomal dominant disorder. There is clear evidence of genetic heterogeneity. In pigs the equivalent condition, which is inherited as an autosomal recessive, is invariably related to a mutation in the ryanodine receptor. In man, although some families show mutations in this gene (which may also be associated with central-core disease), many others do not. Some families show linkage to other chromosomes. This means that DNA-based diagnosis is not yet feasible in routine practice.

Susceptible individuals may be assessed by *in vitro* contracture testing; a muscle biopsy sample is exposed to caffeine, halothane, and ryanodine—MH-susceptible individuals show a lower contractile threshold. False-positive and false-negative results may occur. Many clinicians do not use this test but simply advise all at-risk individuals to assume that they are susceptible and to carry documentation/pendants/bracelets to that effect.

15.7 Inflammatory myopathies

Inflammatory myopathies are defined by the presence of inflammatory infiltrates within muscle. There are many unrelated causes and there is no entirely satisfactory classification (Table 15.15). The most common are the idiopathic inflammatory myopathies. Dermatomyositis (DM) and polymyositis (PM) are particularly important, partly because they can mimic many other muscle disorders but mainly because they are treatable. Inclusion-body myositis (IBM) is the most common acquired myopathy in older men. Despite the presence of inflammatory infiltrates, it is doubtful if it is a true inflammatory myopathy and, unlike the other two conditions mentioned, it rarely responds significantly to immunosuppression. However, it is conveniently retained in this category because of clinical similarities with DM and PM. The annual incidence of each of these three disorders is roughly similar and in the order of 1/100 000. This section will concentrate almost exclusively on the idiopathic inflammatory myopathies (Dalakas 1991). Until fairly recently DM and PM were assumed to have a similar pathogenetic basis, with the main clinical difference being the presence or absence of skin involvement. There is now overwhelming evidence that, despite their clinical similarities,

they have different pathogeneses (Dalakas and Sivakumar 1996) and a few specific clinical differences. Their immunopathogenesis is reviewed briefly below. As yet, this information has not translated into specific immunotherapies. Although IBM shares pathological similarities with PM, it is probable that these are secondary.

15.7.1 Immunopathogenesis of the idiopathic inflammatory myopathies

Accumulated evidence indicates that DM is a humorally mediated autoimmune disorder. Complement-dependent attack leads to destruction of capillaries in muscle and skin. In muscle, the resulting microangiopathy leads to the characteristic pathological features of infarction and perifascicular atrophy (Fig. 15.24). Whether it is deposition of circulating immune complexes or the binding of an antibody to an endothelial antigen which triggers the lytic complement pathway is unknown. Immunocytochemical studies, which now form part of the routine assessment of muscle biopsies from patients with these disorders, show deposition of the complement C5b-9 membrane attack complex in capillaries. Inflammatory

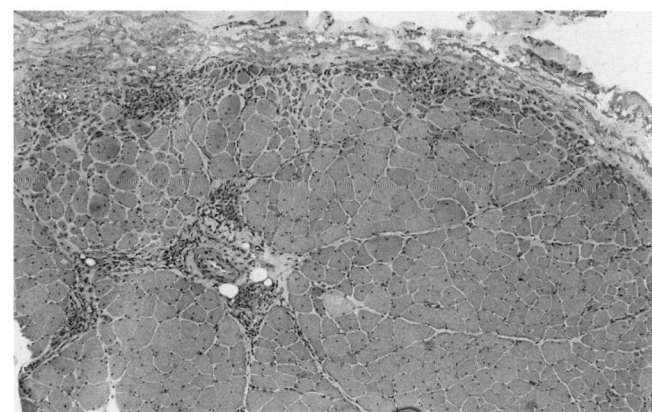

Fig. 15.24. Dermatomyositis. Note the perifascicular atrophy and perivascular inflammation. (Courtesy of Dr Waney Squier.)

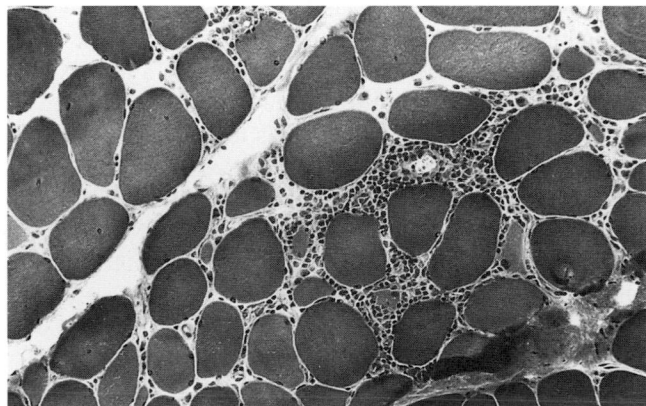

Fig. 15.25. Polymyositis. Note that the inflammatory infiltration is endomysial. (Courtesy of Dr Waney Squier.)

infiltrates are predominantly perivascular, with a predominance of B lymphocytes over T lymphocytes, and a high CD4/CD8 ratio.

Conversely, PM relates to cell-mediated immunity. A characteristic feature is partial invasion of non-necrotic muscle fibres by CD8+ cytotoxic T cells. Inflammatory infiltrates tend to be within fascicles (Fig. 15.25) and T cells predominate over B cells. Invaded and non-invaded fibres show major histocompatability complex (MHC) class I expression.

DM and PM are associated with a number of autoantibodies, the pathological significance of which remains uncertain. Some are particularly seen in so-called overlap cases in which myositis coexists with a connective tissue disorder such as Sjögren's syndrome, scleroderma, systemic lupus erythematosus (SLE), CREST syndrome, and mixed connective tissue disease. A number of myositis-specific antibodies have been described (Love *et al.* 1991), one of which (anti-Jo) correlates strongly with the presence of interstitial lung disease. Anti-Jo and other antisynthetase antibodies are also associated with arthritis, Raynaud's disease, and 'mechanic's hands'—thickening and cracking of the skin of the hands and fingers. Apart from anti-Jo, these antibodies are not yet used widely in clinical practice.

The immunopathological features of IBM are very similar to those of PM but additional strands of evidence suggest that these may be secondary. One view is that the primary disease process leads to destruction of myonuclei.

15.7.2 Dermatomyositis and polymyositis

There is considerable clinical overlap between these conditions (and between PM and IBM) and also potential for confusion at a pathological level. Major clinical and pathological features in DM, PM, and IBM are summarized in Table 15.16.

Table 15.15. The inflammatory myopathies

Idiopathic
Dermatomyositis
Polymyositis
Inclusion-body myositis
Associated with collagen vascular diseases
Systemic lupus erythematosus
Mixed connective tissue disease
Scleroderma
Sjögren's syndrome
Rheumatoid arthritis
Infective
Viral (coxsackie, Epstein–Barr, adeno-, flu, HIV, HTLV-I)
Parasitic
Bacterial
Fungal
Miscellaneous
Eosinophilic myositis
Associated with vasculitis
Granulomatous
Orbital myositis
Graft-versus-host disease

Clinical features

Rash is present in about 90 per cent of patients with DM (in its absence the diagnosis can still be made on pathological grounds). The most common appearances are of erythema of the face and exposed-V of the upper chest (the rash is photosensitive, hence the distribution), red/purple discolouration of the skin over the knuckles, and dilatation of the nail-bed capillaries. Characteristic, but less common, is the violaceous/purple discolouration of the eyelids. Rash may precede or follow the onset of muscle weakness, which in some cases may be trivial. In DM the weakness comes on subacutely, over a matter of weeks, whereas in PM the course is much more protracted and weakness may have been evolving for a year or more before the patient seeks help. With acute onset, the muscles are often painful, tender, and swollen, but otherwise significant discomfort in the idiopathic inflammatory myopathies is uncommon. The weakness is proximal. When severe, the respiratory and bulbar muscles may also be involved.

Extramuscular manifestations are common in DM and include Raynaud's disease and arthralgia. Cardiac involvement, with conduction and contractile abnormalities, is one cause of death. In both DM and PM interstitial pulmonary fibrosis may occur and is associated with the presence of anti-Jo antibody.

Up to 20 per cent of patients with DM, more in the older population, have an associated malignancy, the detection of which may precede or follow the diagnosis of DM (Hilton-Jones and Squier 1992; Sigurgeirsson *et al.* 1992). Appropriate screening includes chest X-ray (CT or MRI scan in a smoker), abdominal imaging, mammography, rectal and vaginal examination, and basic blood tests. Consideration should be given to repeating these after 1 year.

Diagnosis

Standard 'inflammatory' markers such as erythrocyte sedimentation rate (ESR) and C-reactive protein (CRP) are often normal and must not be relied upon. Serum creatine kinase is often, but not always, elevated. Generally it is high in acute cases and often normal, or only minimally elevated, in chronic cases. Electromyography typically shows spontaneous activity (fibrillation potentials and positive sharp waves) and a myopathic pattern of motor unit potentials. The gold standard for diagnosis is muscle biopsy (Table 15.16 and Figs 15.24 and 15.25). The pathological changes are patchy and a single biopsy, particularly if small, may be normal and will have to be repeated.

Treatment

Despite a lack of controlled trials, prednisolone is accepted as the initial treatment of choice, typically at a dose of 1 mg/kg body weight. This is frequently combined with azathioprine (2.5 mg/kg body weight) as a 'steroid-sparing' agent. Some clinicians automatically use it from the outset, others only later if it is clear that the patient is going to need a relatively high dose of prednisolone. After a month or so of high-dose daily prednisolone treatment the dose is gradually reduced on an

Table 15.16. Major clinical and pathological features in the idiopathic inflammatory myopathies

	Dermatomyositis	Polymyositis	Inclusion-body myositis
Clinical features			
Sex	F > M	M = F	M >> F
Age of onset	Any	20 years +	50 years +
Onset	Subacute/acute	Chronic	Chronic
Distribution of weakness	Proximal	Proximal	Proximal + distal + asymmetric (typically quadriceps + finger flexors)
Muscle pain/swelling	In acute cases	No	No
Skin involvement	Often	No	No
Raynaud's, arthralgia	Frequent	Infrequent	No
Dysphagia	In severe cases	Infrequent	Occasional
Association with cancer	Up to 20%	Probably not	No
Cardiac involvement	Yes	No	No
Interstitial lung disease	Associated with anti-Jo	Associated with anti-Jo	No
Pathological features			
Scattered necrotic fibres	–/+	++	++
Infarcts	++	–	–
Scattered atrophic fibres	+	++	++
Perifascicular atrophy	++	–	–
Zonal myofibrillar loss	++	–	–
Capillary loss	++	–	–
Rimmed vacuoles	–	–	++
15 nm filaments	–	–	++
Partial invasion	–	++	++
Perivascular inflammation	++	–	–
Endomysial inflammation	+	++	++

alternate day basis. The rate of reduction depends upon the clinical response and, to some extent, the serum creatine kinase. It is much easier to determine the response in patients who presented acutely than in those with grumbling onset of disease. Particularly in this latter group, azathioprine may be useful as it is very difficult to judge the appropriate dose of prednisolone, with the danger of giving too little, and losing benefit, or too much and inducing a secondary steroid-myopathy.

Alternatives to azathioprine include methotrexate, cyclosporin, and cyclophosphamide. Intravenous immunoglobulin is effective but not demonstrably superior to cheaper drug regimes. Plasma exchange has been less well assessed but, theoretically, may be helpful in DM. None of these treatments has been evaluated in controlled trials.

Appropriate advice should be given with respect to osteoporosis prophylaxis. Adequate nutrition is important, as is encouragement of physical activity. Skin rashes respond to topical steroids and are helped by sun-blocking creams.

Prognosis is difficult to determine accurately in a given individual. Poor prognostic factors include advanced age, longstanding weakness at time of initiation of therapy, associated malignancy, and lung and heart involvement. Most patients require treatment for at least 2 years, many for 5 years, and some remain treatment-dependent. Most patients show some response to therapy. In younger patients with a short history, one generally hopes to return them to normal or near-normal strength. In an older patient with long-standing weakness, one

may prevent progression but gain little improvement in strength.

15.7.3 Inclusion-body myositis

In its most characteristic form this is a readily recognizable condition. The diagnosis is sometimes first made when a patient diagnosed as having PM fails to respond to therapy. As noted, its pathogenesis is still much argued. It is currently the subject of much research interest (Askanas *et al.* 1998).

Clinical features

Onset is unusual before the age of 50 years. It is much more common in men. Rarely, otherwise typical cases of sporadic IBM are seen to be familial. This is not the same as hereditary inclusion-body myopathy, which occurs in younger patients and in which different pathological features are seen. Progression of weakness is slow. Typically the quadriceps are involved early, and IBM is the most common cause of 'isolated quadriceps myopathy'. Also involved early and highly selectively are the finger flexor muscles, causing profound weakness of grip. Together, these two features are virtually pathognomonic. Overall, and in contrast to DM and PM, distal weakness is common and there is often asymmetry between the two sides. Dysphagia is usually a late feature, rarely early. Extramuscular clinical features are absent, but associations with connective tissue diseases and autoantibodies have been noted.

Diagnosis

Serum creatine kinase is normal or modestly elevated. Electromyography shows features similar to those seen in DM and PM but, in addition, 'neurogenic' changes in the form of large-amplitude, long-duration motor unit potentials are often seen. Diagnostic confirmation is by muscle biopsy (Table 15.16), particularly by the demonstration of 15 nm intranuclear and cytoplasmic filaments.

Treatment

Immunosuppression is generally ineffective, or at best shows only a very modest transient benefit. It is arguable whether a trial of such therapy is justified. Intravenous immunoglobulin has proved ineffective (Dalakas *et al.* 2000). The disease is very slowly progressive, but in some patients does become profoundly disabling. Orthoses (at wrists, knees, and ankles) may be helpful.

15.7.4 Other inflammatory myopathies

Associations with other autoimmune/connective tissue diseases have been discussed. Sometimes the term 'overlap syndrome' is used to describe such cases—this simply reflects our incomplete understanding of the pathogenesis of these disorders.

There are important associations between AIDS and inflammatory myopathy (Dalakas 1993). The most common is a PM-like condition virtually indistinguishable from idiopathic PM clinically and pathologically. Retrovirus is present in interstitial cells but does not appear to invade muscle fibres. Patients with AIDS are at risk of opportunistic muscle infections (e.g. microsporidia, toxoplasmosis). Zidovudine can cause mitochondrial depletion and a myopathy in which myalgia predominates over weakness (Arnaudo *et al.* 1991). HTLV-I can also cause a myositis, either alone or in association with tropical spastic paraparesis (Douen *et al.* 1997).

Granulomata in muscle are probably not that uncommon in sarcoidosis, but clinically evident myopathy is rare.

15.8 Endocrine myopathies

Weakness, usually proximal and affecting the pelvic girdle earlier than the shoulder girdle, is a common feature of many endocrinopathies (Ruff and Weissmann 1988). It resolves upon correction of the underlying disorder. Muscle biopsy shows non-specific type II muscle fibre atrophy. The most common is glucocorticoid excess in the form of iatrogenic steroid myopathy, but the clinical features parallel those of Cushing's disease. The most frequently encountered primary endocrine myopathies are those associated with thyroid disease.

15.8.1 Steroid myopathy

Some two-thirds of cases of Cushing's syndrome are due to an ACTH-producing pituitary adenoma, one-sixth due to ectopic ACTH production by a tumour, and one-sixth due to a cortisol-secreting tumour of the adrenal cortex. Weakness is present in about 60 per cent of patients with Cushing's syndrome. Iatrogenic steroid myopathy is most frequently seen in association with the use of 9-α fluorinated steroids, which include dexamethasone, triamcinolone, and betamethasone. Topical application can also cause myopathy. Individuals vary in their susceptibility to developing myopathy, and women are more at risk than men.

Clinical features

Weakness, which is often accompanied by myalgia, starts in a pelvi-femoral distribution and later spreads to the trunk and shoulder girdle. Atrophy is common. It is rare to develop myopathy without other features of glucocorticoid excess being apparent.

Diagnosis

This is predominantly clinical. Serum creatine kinase is usually normal, EMG is often normal or may show non-specific myopathic features, and muscle biopsy shows type II fibre atrophy. An occasional clinical dilemma is distinguishing between increasing weakness due to reactivation of disease and that due to steroids in a patient being treated for an inflammatory myopathy. EMG, serum creatine kinase, and muscle biopsy may help, but sometimes all one can do is alter the dose of steroids and monitor the clinical response.

Treatment

Stopping steroids, or correcting the underlying endocrine disorder, is usually followed by full recovery of the myopathy. If steroid therapy cannot be stopped, then a non-fluorinated drug, such as prednisolone, should be used at the lowest possible dosage and preferably on an alternate-day regime.

15.8.2 Acute steroid myopathy

This iatrogenic condition merits separate mention. It was first clearly delineated in patients with asthma being given a combination of high-dose parenteral steroids and a neuromuscular blocking agent, but it has now been described in a patient receiving steroids alone (Panegyres *et al.* 1993). Weakness, which may be profound and associated with respiratory failure, develops acutely or subacutely. Recovery occurs over 6–12 months. The pathological features are of small, angular fibres and selective loss of myosin filaments.

15.8.3 Thyroid-associated myopathies

The muscle disorders associated with thyroid disease (Table 15.17) show the greatest clinical variability of all of the endocrine myopathies. In myasthenia gravis there is an increased incidence of autoimmune thyroid disease and thyroid function should form part of the routine assessment of such patients.

Hypothyroidism

Although weakness is common, it is less striking than in hyperthyroidism and is very rarely the presenting symptom

Table 15.17. Thyroid-associated muscle disorders

Hypothyroid myopathies
Thyrotoxic myopathy
Thyroid ophthalmopathy (Graves' disease)
Thyrotoxic periodic paralysis
Myasthenia gravis

(Mastaglia *et al.* 1988). In both, it is proximal in distribution. A combination of hypothyroidism, muscle hypertrophy and weakness, and slowness of movement, is sometimes referred to as the Kocher–Debré–Semelaigne syndrome in childhood, and Hoffman's syndrome in adulthood. The serum creatine kinase is almost invariably elevated and occult hypothyroidism is an important cause of otherwise idiopathic elevation of serum CK and of aspartate transaminase (AST)—the latter sometimes leads to a spurious search for liver disease. Muscle features recover after restoring a euthyroid state.

Hyperthyroidism

Weakness is present in about one-half of thyrotoxic patients, usually becoming apparent shortly after the onset of other thyrotoxic symptoms, but in up to 10 per cent it may be the presenting feature. The shoulder girdle may be affected before the pelvic girdle and in some patients early distal weakness is apparent. Atrophy is usually slight. Severe weakness raises the possibility of coexistent myasthenia gravis. The serum creatine kinase is typically normal. Recovery of the myopathy follows successful treatment of the endocrine disorder (Olson *et al.* 1991).

Thyroid ophthalmopathy (Graves' disease)

Although most frequently associated with hyperthyroidism, this can occur in hypothyroid and, clinically most challenging, euthyroid patients (Weetman 1992) (Section 8.12.2). Eyelid lag and retraction are common in hyperthyroidism. Thyroid ophthalmopathy refers to those patients in whom the ocular involvement is much more severe. Conjunctival injection and swelling is followed by diplopia and proptosis due to enlargement of the extraocular muscles and orbital soft tissues. In later stages, vision is further threatened by papilloedema and optic nerve compression. All of these changes may be unilateral. An important clinical subgroup is those patients with diplopia only, in whom the diagnosis is often missed.

Diagnosis is easy if there is obvious clinical or laboratory evidence of thyroid disease. If the thyroxine (T_4), tri-iodothyronine (T_3), and thyroid-stimulating hormone (TSH) are normal, further investigations include antimicrosomal and antithyroglobulin antibodies and a thyrotropin-releasing hormone (TRH) stimulation test. Thyroid-stimulating immunoglobulins are present in many patients. Indirectly, the diagnosis may be supported by demonstrating extraocular muscle swelling by ultrasound, CT, or MRI.

The patient should be made euthyroid. Lid-lag and retraction may respond to topical application of guanethedine 10 per cent. For severe disease, treatment options include surgical decompression of the orbit, orbital irradiation, and high-dose prednisolone (Weetman and Wiersinga 1998).

Thyrotoxic periodic paralysis

Clinically, this resembles hypokalaemic periodic paralysis, but is genetically distinct. Attacks typically start in early adult life. The incidence is very much higher in Orientals than other races and there is a very strong male predominance. Attacks cease when the underlying thyroid disorder is corrected.

15.8.4 Disorders of vitamin D and calcium metabolism

There is a complex relationship between vitamin D metabolism, calcium and phosphate homoeostasis, and parathyroid hormone activity. In clinical practice the most commonly encountered disorders include osteomalacia and metabolic bone disease associated with renal failure.

Osteomalacia

Pelvic girdle weakness is the presenting symptom in about one-third of patients. However, bone pain tends to dominate the clinical picture with particular involvement of the pelvis, femora, and ribs. The gait is typically waddling and Gower's manoeuvre may be present. The diagnosis of osteomalacia can usually be confirmed by demonstrating reduced bone density, low blood calcium and phosphate levels, and elevated serum alkaline phosphatase activity. Bone pain responds quickly to treatment but weakness may take much longer to recover.

Renal failure

The term 'renal osteodystrophy' refers to the disturbed vitamin D metabolism and secondary hyperparathyroidism complicating chronic uraemia. It is often associated with pelvic girdle weakness which responds favourably to dialysis, transplantation, or vitamin D therapy. Dialysis osteodystrophy was due to aluminium toxicity arising from high levels of the metal in water used to prepare the dialysate.

Parathyroid gland dysfunction

Symptomatic weakness is uncommon in hypo- and hyperparathyroidism.

15.8.5 Other endocrine myopathies

Weakness, usually predominantly proximal, may also be seen in acromegaly, hypopituitarism, ACTH excess, primary aldosteronism, and Addison's disease.

15.9 Toxic, nutritional, and drug-induced myopathies

The most important toxic myopathies are those associated with ethanol consumption. Although malnutrition causes muscle wasting, specific nutritional myopathies are rare. Drug-induced myopathies are of considerable importance and are probably under-recognized.

15.9.1 Ethanol-related myopathies

Up to two-thirds of chronic alcoholics have evidence of proximal weakness and muscle wasting, most evident around the pelvic girdle (Sacanella *et al.* 1995) (Section 5.2.10). It is painless and rarely severe. It improves with abstinence. Clinically the picture may be complicated by coexistent alcoholic neuropathy.

More dramatic is acute alcoholic myopathy, which typically develops in a chronic alcoholic following a binge. It may be restricted to a single muscle or be generalized. Cramps precede muscle swelling, which may be dramatic, and weakness. In the lower limb the picture may mimic deep-vein thrombosis. Swelling may induce a compartment syndrome necessitating surgery. There is extensive muscle fibre breakdown (rhabdomyolysis) with gross elevation of the serum creatine kinase, myoglobinuria, posing a risk of renal failure, and sometimes hyperkalaemia. Recovery, which may be incomplete, occurs over several weeks.

15.9.2 Other toxic myopathies

Eosinophilia–myalgia syndrome

This condition was due to a contaminant (called 'peak E') in a batch of L-tryptophan made by a single manufacturer. Early features included myalgia, skin rash, dyspnoea, arthralgia, fever, and weight loss. Several months later some patients developed scleroderma-like skin infiltration, persistent myalgia and weakness (Anonymous 1996).

Toxic oil syndrome

This condition, which affected many thousands of people in Spain in the early 1980s, bears close similarities to the eosinophilia–myalgia syndrome (Kaufman *et al.* 1995). It was due to ingestion of an illegally imported, reprocessed, denatured rapeseed oil. Features included myalgia, eosinophilia, respiratory distress, scleroderma-like skin changes, wasting, and weakness.

Snake venoms

Many are myotoxic (Harris and Cullen 1990).

15.9.3 Nutritional myopathies

Osteomalacia is discussed above. Vitamin E deficiency may be seen in chronic cholestasis, malabsorption syndromes, and abetalipoproteinaemia. Myopathy is one feature of a multifaceted neurological disorder associated with vitamin E deficiency (Sections 12.21.4 and 31.7.4).

Nutritional carnitine deficiency is uncommon but may be caused by prolonged parenteral nutrition and is occasionally seen in patients on renal dialysis and in pregnancy (Duran *et al.* 1990). It causes proximal weakness.

Table 15.18. Drug-induced myopathies[a]

Focal myopathy	IM injections
Acute/subacute painful myopathy	Cholesterol-lowering drugs
	Opiates
	ε-Aminocaproic acid
	Amiodarone
	Cyclosporin
	Emetine
	β-Blockers
	Zidovudine
	Vincristine
Acute rhabdomyolysis	Opiates
	Cocaine
	Amphetamines
	Phencyclidine
Chronic painless myopathy	Corticosteroids
	Chloroquine
	Colchicine
	Perhexiline
	Amiodarone
Hypokalaemia	Diuretics
	Purgatives
	Amphotericin B
	Carbenoxolone
	Liquorice
Inflammatory myopathy	D-penicillamine
	Procainamide

[a] This table lists only the more commonly implicated drugs. For a fuller discussion see Argov and Mastaglia (1994).

15.9.4 Drug-induced myopathies

The mechanisms of drug-induced myotoxicity are many and varied and, in many cases, poorly understood (Argov and Mastaglia 1994). They include direct toxicity, immune mechanisms and electrolyte disturbance. Some also have a neurotoxic effect. For practical purposes a classification based on the clinical presentation is most useful (Table 15.18). This table by no means includes all drugs reported to cause myotoxicity, but lists those most commonly implicated.

15.10 Disorders of the neuromuscular junction

The clinical conditions relating to dysfunction at the neuromuscular junction (NMJ) are myasthenia gravis (by far the most common), the Lambert–Eaton myasthenic syndrome, congenital myasthenic syndromes, and acquired neuromyotonia (Isaacs' syndrome). Each of these relates to disturbed ion-channel function. This is immune-mediated in myasthenia gravis, the Lambert–Eaton syndrome, and neuromyotonia, and due to a genetic defect in the congenital myasthenic syndromes. The relevant major functional components of the NMJ are illustrated schematically in Fig. 15.26. In myasthenia gravis, antibodies are directed against the acetylcholine receptors, in

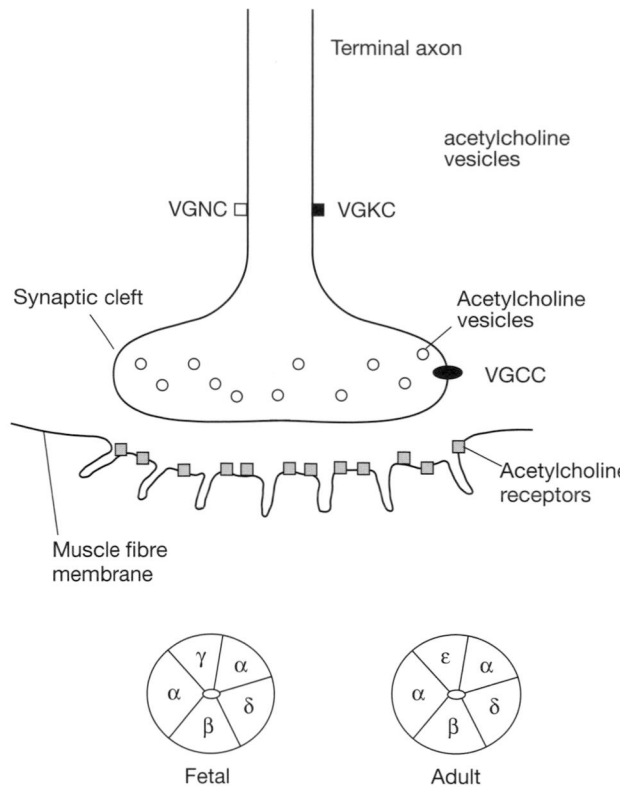

Fig. 15.26. Major functional features of the neuromuscular junction (for discussion see text).

Lambert–Eaton syndrome against the voltage-gated calcium channels (VGCC), and in neuromyotonia against the voltage-gated potassium channels (VGKC).

Two classes of ion channel are involved: the voltage-gated sodium, potassium, and calcium channels, and the ligand-gated acetylcholine receptors. Depolarization of the nerve terminal membrane, which depends on voltage-gated sodium channels (VGNC) opens the calcium channels (VGCC); influx of calcium triggers release of quanta of acetylcholine. Acetylcholine binds to the α-subunits of the receptors on the muscle fibre membrane, which allows influx of sodium ions; this generates the end-plate potential which, in turn, activates muscle fibre membrane voltage-gated sodium channels to create the action potential. This subsequently triggers muscle contraction. Acetylcholine in the synaptic cleft is destroyed by acetylcholinesterase. Nerve terminal repolarization, and closure of the calcium channels, is dependent upon inactivation of the VGNCs and opening of the voltage-gated potassium channels (VGKC). The acetylcholine receptor is a pentameric structure, with a central ion channel, composed of four subunits and has fetal (α_2, β, δ, γ) and adult (α_2, β, δ, ϵ) forms.

15.10.1 Myasthenia gravis

The prevalence of myasthenia gravis is in the order of 5–10/100 000 population. The major clinical features are of weakness and, characteristically, excessive fatiguability (Beekman

et al. 1997). It is associated with an increased incidence of other autoimmune diseases, notably thyroid dysfunction, rheumatoid arthritis, and other connective tissue disorders. Penicillamine may induce myasthenia which is clinically indistinguishable from the idiopathic variety, and in which anti-acetylcholine receptor (anti-AChR) antibodies are present (Kuncl *et al.* 1986). It resolves following drug withdrawal.

Myasthenia may present at any age. Four major groups of patients can be identified:

1. Onset in early adult life. Female preponderance. Anti-AChR antibody titres are high. The thymus shows medullary hyperplasia.

2. Later onset. Male preponderance. Anti-AChR antibody titres tend to be low. The thymus is atrophic.

3. Later onset. Equal sex ratio. Intermediate levels of anti-AChR antibodies. Thymoma present.

4. Any age. Male predominance. Anti-AChR antibodies not detectable by standard assay (seronegative myasthenia). Thymus atrophy. Often restricted to ocular involvement.

As will be noted, the presence or absence of anti-AChR antibodies and the state of the thymus gland influence therapeutic approaches. *Neonatal myasthenia* describes the condition of transient weakness in the newborn due to transplacental transfer of anti-AChR antibody from an affected mother (Morel *et al.* 1988). Symptoms resolve within a few weeks.

Clinical features

Although any muscle may be involved, those most commonly affected at presentation are the extraocular muscles, causing ptosis and diplopia. Facial and bulbar muscle weakness causes dysarthria and dysphagia. Proximal limb weakness exceeds distal. Respiratory muscle weakness severe enough to cause ventilatory embarrassment usually develops only in the presence of substantial limb weakness. Selective weakness of the neck extensors is a rather common feature in older, typically male, patients and causes head-drop. The most characteristic feature of myasthenia gravis is excessive fatiguability. This may be demonstrated on examination, for example showing the development of ptosis on attempted sustained up-gaze, but is evident in the history. Weakness varies during the course of the day and during activity, and is eased by rest. Dysarthria increases the longer the patient speaks. Weakness is exacerbated by emotion, heat, menstruation, and intercurrent infection.

In a small proportion of patients the disease remains confined to the extraocular muscles. If the disease has not spread beyond the eyes within 2 years of onset it is unlikely to do so later. Patients with ocular myasthenia often do not have anti-AChR antibodies.

Untreated, the condition gradually spreads to involve more muscles and, when severe, may cause respiratory failure. The spontaneous remission rate is low.

Diagnosis

The diagnosis is confirmed by demonstrating the presence of anti-AChR antibodies. False-positive results are exceedingly rare. Sensitivity is limited to about 50 per cent in purely ocular myasthenia and about 85 per cent in generalized myasthenia.

If antibodies are not detected, the next most useful investigation is electromyography. The traditional, and simplest, test is to stimulate a nerve at 3 Hz and to measure the compound muscle action potential—a decrement of more than 10 per cent when comparing the fifth to the first response is abnormal. More sensitive, but technically more difficult, is single-fibre electromyography. Studies of orbicularis oculi are particularly valuable in cases of ocular myasthenia.

The thymus is imaged by X-ray computed tomography or magnetic resonance imaging. Most patients with thymoma have anti-striated muscle antibodies in their serum. Thyroid function should also be assessed.

Although well known, discussion of the edrophonium (Tensilon®) test is left until last for several reasons. The principle is that edrophonium, a short-acting anticholinesterase, given intravenously produces a transient improvement in strength in patients with myasthenia gravis. Although this is generally true, it must be noted that:

(1) false-negative results may occur;

(2) false-positive results undoubtedly occur and are seen in myasthenic syndromes, motor neuron disease, mitochondrial myopathies (including chronic external ophthalmoplegia, a major differential diagnosis of ocular myasthenia), and other neuromuscular disorders; and

(3) rarely, cardiorespiratory collapse may occur.

For these reasons, this test should only be done by experienced personnel, when indicated during the diagnostic process. Generally, it is not required.

Treatment

If a thymoma is present, it should be removed because it may be locally invasive (if removal is impossible or incomplete, radiotherapy and chemotherapy should be considered); however, this will not benefit the myasthenia.

Most patients will show some response to the anticholinesterase drug pyridostigmine, given orally in a dose of up to 60 mg six times daily, but this will satisfactorily control only relatively mild disease.

In patients with purely ocular myasthenia, those over the age of about 50 years with generalized disease, and patients without anti-AChR antibodies, the next approach to treatment is alternate-day prednisolone. This is introduced slowly, to prevent acute deterioration, up to a dose of 1.5 mg/kg body weight/alternate day. Following remission, the dose is gradually reduced and the minimum effective dose determined. Azathioprine (at a dose of 2.5 mg/kg body weight/day) is frequently added as a steroid-sparing agent (Palace *et al.* 1998) and it may be possible eventually to withdraw prednisolone and to maintain the patient on azathioprine alone. The maximum benefit of azathioprine is not seen for at least 6 months. Regular monitoring of liver function is required. For patients intolerant of azathioprine, other useful, but potentially more toxic, immunosuppressants include methotrexate, cyclosporin, and cyclophosphamide.

In patients under the age of about 50 years with generalized myasthenia and anti-AChR antibodies, thymectomy (Bulkley *et al.* 1997) is likely to induce remission in about one-third and to lead to improvement in about one-half of patients. Morbidity from trans-sternal thymectomy is low in specialized hands and when patients are given optimal medical management prior to surgery. Such medical management includes the immunosuppressant regimes described above and the use of plasma exchange and intravenous immunoglobulins. These latter two treatments are equally efficacious and give symptomatic improvement for up to 6 weeks. They are useful during the initiation of prednisolone treatment, which in itself can cause transient worsening of the myasthenia, as well as prior to thymectomy. Immunosuppressant therapy should be continued following removal of a benign hyperplastic thymus gland but is gradually tapered as the patient's condition permits.

Prednisolone therapy is likely to be long term, and appropriate consideration must be given to potential side-effects, particularly the risk of osteoporosis.

Immunopathogenesis

Although numerous important observations relating to immune system function in myasthenia gravis have been made, many fundamental questions remain unanswered. Anti-AChR antibodies are of IgG class, although in cases that are seronegative using the standard assay there is evidence that IgM-class antibodies may be involved. Antibodies, which bind to the α-subunit, cause acetylcholine receptor dysfunction in one of several ways: (1) complement-mediated lysis; (2) modulation of turnover; and (3) blocking. Antibody titres correlate with disease activity in an individual patient, but not between patients.

The thymus in seropositive patients typically shows medullary hyperplasia. Anti-AChR antibody is produced by thymic cells, AChR-reactive T cells are present, and myoid cells within the thymus express AChR.

It is hoped that when the afferent and efferent limbs of the immune pathways are better understood it will be possible to develop more selective immunotherapies.

15.10.2 Lambert–Eaton myasthenic syndrome

This is a pre-synaptic disorder in which the quantal release of acetylcholine is reduced as a result of antibodies directed against voltage-gated calcium channels (Motomura *et al.* 1997). It is very much less common than myasthenia gravis. In about 60 per cent of cases it is associated with small cell lung cancer, and up to 3 per cent of patients with this type of tumour may develop Lambert–Eaton myasthenic syndrome (LEMS), although the diagnosis is probably not infrequently missed.

Clinical features

Presentation is usually with gait disturbance (O'Neill *et al.* 1988). This may be attributed directly to weakness but sometimes the description may be less specific, such as one patient who said 'my legs get in the way when I am walking'. There may be mild ptosis, but extraocular signs are much less evident than in myasthenia gravis. Autonomic features are common and include impotence, in males, and dryness of the mouth. On examination, strength and tendon reflexes may augment transiently following forceful voluntary contraction of the relevant muscle.

Diagnosis

The characteristic electromyographic finding is of a small compound muscle action potential that shows marked increase in amplitude following voluntary contraction or high-frequency nerve stimulation. Anti-voltage-gated calcium channel antibodies can be detected in most patients. An underlying small cell lung cancer must be sought (e.g. CT scan) at presentation and, in smokers, at intervals thereafter.

Treatment

Tumour treatment often improves the neurological disorder. Symptomatic relief is obtained from 3,4-diaminopyridine, which blocks voltage-gated potassium channels and thus delays nerve repolarization (Maddison *et al.* 1998). In the absence of tumour, treatment with prednisolone and azathioprine, as for myasthenia gravis, often induces remission. Plasma exchange and intravenous immunoglobulin provide transient benefit and supplement other forms of treatment.

15.10.3 Congenital myasthenic syndromes

This is an extremely rare group of conditions (Engel *et al.* 1999) with an overall prevalence in the order of 1/1 000 000. They are genetically determined, non-autoimmune disorders. The common features are onset in infancy, fatiguable weakness, and a decremental response to repetitive nerve stimulation. There is as yet no entirely satisfactory clinical or genetic system of classification. The most common are postsynaptic disorders in which there is a mutation affecting one of the AChR subunits (commonly the ϵ), which alters the kinetics of the receptor. Also recognized are presynaptic disorders and congenital end-plate acetylcholinesterase deficiency. Apart from the postsynaptic slow-channel syndrome, which is dominant, these various disorders are autosomal recessive conditions.

Therapeutic options are limited. Anticholinesterase drugs offer symptomatic benefit, except in patients with end-plate acetylcholinesterase deficiency. Immune therapies, such as those used in myasthenia gravis are of no value.

15.10.4 Acquired neuromyotonia

Previously known as Isaacs' syndrome of continuous muscle fibre activity, this rare condition is characterized by hyperexcitability of nerves, leading to muscle twitching (myokymia), cramps, paraesthesia, and sweating (Hart and Newsom-Davis 1996) (Section 14.9). Electromyography shows high-frequency bursts of continuous motor unit discharges (Fig. 14.9), or multiplet discharges. It may be seen in association with a number of acquired (myasthenia gravis, demyelinating polyneuropathy, carcinoma) and inherited (neuropathies, spinal muscular atrophy) disorders. Some acquired cases are autoimmune in origin and relate to the presence of antibodies directed against voltage-gated potassium channels (Vincent *et al.* 1998). In these patients immunosuppressant drugs (e.g. prednisolone and azathioprine) may be of benefit, and in severe cases plasma exchange may give transient benefit. Most patients gain symptomatic benefit from carbamazepine or phenytoin.

15.10.5 Botulism

Botulism is caused by a powerful neurotoxin produced by the anaerobic organism *Clostridium botulinum*. The toxin binds to specific acceptors on the cholinergic nerve terminal, is internalised via endocytosis, and then cleaves one of the proteins involved in exocytosis (Humeau *et al.*, 2000). The net result is paralysis and parasympathetic blockade due to inhibition of calcium-mediated release of acetylcholine.

Three clinical forms of botulism are recognised—the figures in brackets give the median number of cases per annum reported to the North American Centers for Disease Control and Prevention from 1973 (Shapiro *et al*, 1998): Food-borne (24); Infant botulism (71); Wound (3).

Food borne

The toxin is ingested in tainted food. It tends to occur in outbreaks and the foodstuffs most commonly implicated include vegetables, fruits, fish, and the products of home-preservation methods. The typical time lag from ingestion to onset of symptoms is 6–36 hours. Symptoms of parasympathetic blockade may develop before or concurrently with paralytic symptoms. Features include blurred vision, mydriasis, abdominal pain, vomiting, diarrhoea, constipation, fever and dry mouth. Paralysis starts in the cranial nerve territory with ptosis, diplopia, dysphagia, dysphonia, and facial weakness. This is followed by increasing fatiguability and weakness in the limbs, loss of the tendon reflexes and respiratory impairment, progressing to the need for ventilatory support in about one-quarter. Progression may occur for up to a week, followed by gradual resolution over many months. Recovery depends upon axonal sprouting and the development of new end-plates and new synapses.

Diagnosis is difficult outside a recognised outbreak. Neurophysiological studies show changes similar to those seen in Lambert-Eaton syndrome. *Cl. botulinum* may be cultured from the contaminated food or from the faeces, or the toxin may be identified in the serum or faeces.

Management is primarily supportive and major issues include ventilatory failure and secondary infection. Attempts at specific therapy have included use of antitoxins and drugs such as diaminopyridine to enhance the release of acetylcholine. These appear to be of limited benefit and take second place to excellent nursing (the similarity to Guillain-Barré synrome is readily evident).

Infant botulism

This usually presents within the first six months of life and is caused by over-colonization of the gastrointestinal tract by *Cl. botulinum*. The onset of symptoms is less acute than for food-borne botulism. The infant presents with constipation, a feeble cry and feeding difficulties, and the signs include hypotonia, ophthalmoplegia, generalised weakness and, in some, respiratory failure. The diagnosis is established by demonstration of *Cl. botulinum* and toxin in faeces.

Management again involves general supportive measures and specific treatment in the form of sterilisation of the gut with antibiotics.

Wound botulism

This is the least common form and is caused by toxin release from a wound contaminated by *Cl. botulinum*. The clinical picture is similar to food-borne botulism. The organism can be recovered from the wound.

15.11 Miscellaneous muscle disorders

This section deals with those conditions which do not fit readily into any of the aforementioned categories, or in which there is debate as to whether or not there is primary involvement of skeletal muscle.

15.11.1 Chronic fatigue syndrome

Of the many symptoms associated with this syndrome the most prominent are fatigue, myalgia, impaired concentration, poor memory, sleep disturbance, and emotional lability. Functional studies have failed to demonstrate clear evidence of a peripheral disorder to explain the patients' perceived neuromuscular difficulties (Lloyd *et al.* 1991). Early claims for persistent viral infection proved to be unfounded (Miller *et al.* 1991), but at least in some cases enteroviral RNA may be detected in muscle (Bowles *et al.* 1993). Metabolic studies in muscle have given conflicting results (Lane *et al.* 1998). Despite some reports suggesting otherwise (Behan *et al.* 1991), muscle biopsy is usually either normal or shows changes reflecting reduced physical activity. It is probable that in the vast majority of patients with chronic fatigue syndrome that there is no primary disorder affecting peripheral nerves, the neuromuscular junction, or skeletal muscle.

15.11.2 Polymyalgia rheumatica

It is doubtful if there is primary muscle involvement in this condition, but it is important in the present context because it may be confused with the idiopathic inflammatory myopathies. In practice, there should rarely be difficulty distinguishing between them. Polymyalgia rheumatica (PMR) is characterized by pain and stiffness (early morning), around the neck and shoulder girdle, less frequently around the pelvic girdle, and the absence of weakness, although this may seem to be present because of the discomfort (Pountain and Hazleman 1995). It is

rare before the age of 55 years and the ESR is almost invariably elevated. There is a prompt clinical response to prednisolone. Some patients go on to develop giant cell (temporal) arteritis. The aetiology of these two conditions is unclear, but there is evidence of vascular involvement and much of the pain and stiffness may relate to chronic synovitis (O'Duffy *et al.* 1980).

Electromyography is usually normal, as is the serum creatine kinase. Muscle biopsy may show type II fibre atrophy, probably reflecting disuse.

15.11.3 Neoplastic disorders

Primary muscle tumours are rare and their classification has caused difficulty (Newton *et al.* 1995). Embryonal rhabdomyomas in early childhood affect the head and neck region and the genito-urinary tract (sarcoma botryoides). In adults they typically involve the head, neck, and throat region. Cardiac rhabdomyomas are seen in tuberous sclerosis. In adults, rhabdomyosarcomas arise in the legs. They are highly aggressive, metastasize early, and respond poorly to radiotherapy.

Apart from the result of local invasion (e.g. breast carcinoma invading pectoralis), secondary tumours in skeletal muscle are rare. Other tumours that may arise in muscle, but not from the muscle itself, include angiomata, dermoid tumours, and neurofibromata.

15.11.4 Paraneoplastic disorders

The most important, and best defined, paraneoplastic disorders affecting skeletal muscle and the neuromuscular junction are dermatomyositis (Section 15.7.2) and the Lambert–Eaton myasthenic syndrome (Section 15.10.2). The term 'carcinomatous neuromyopathy' is widely used to describe a syndrome of symmetrical proximal weakness, often with depressed tendon reflexes (Elrington *et al.* 1991). Many such cases are probably neurogenic in origin (Sections 12.13.2 and 14.2.2), but such patients are, understandably, not always investigated in detail. Endocrine gland tumours causing increased or decreased hormone production may produce weakness, as may tumours that cause metabolic derangement. Weakness in association with cancer may be due to the rather non-specific effect of a number of factors, including cachexia, malnutrition, infection, and inactivity.

15.11.5 Myositis ossificans

This term is used to describe two unrelated conditions, in neither of which is muscle inflammation (myositis) a major feature.

Localized myositis ossificans

This is an acquired disorder and in many, but not all, cases it arises as a result of trauma, either minor repeated trauma or a single substantial injury. Repeated trauma in sportsmen or women is a well-recognized cause. Initially there is localized swelling and tenderness which is followed by bone formation. Small lesions may resolve spontaneously. Larger areas of calcification, impairing movement, may need to be resected.

Fibrodysplasia ossificans progressiva

This is an autosomal dominant condition often caused by a new mutation (Smith 1997). The genetic defect is unknown. Congenital malformation (shortening) of the great toe is present almost invariably, with the thumb being affected less frequently. Endochondral ossification of skeletal muscles occurs in a specific order and the patients are described as developing a second skeleton. It causes profound immobility and most patients are wheelchair-bound by the third decade of life. No treatment has been shown to be of benefit.

15.11.6 Compartment syndromes

Some muscle are contained within semi-rigid fibro-osseous compartments, the most important examples being the anterior tibial compartment and the volar compartment of the forearm. If the muscles within these compartments swell, the pressure rises rapidly. Causes of swelling include ischaemia due to arterial problems (e.g. compression due to displaced fracture, tourniquet pressure, clamping during surgery, haematoma), direct trauma, and drugs that induce rhabdomyolysis (e.g. alcohol, heroin). The rising pressure further impedes capillary blood flow and thus a vicious circle of increasing ischaemia develops (Mars and Hadley 1998). Nerves within the compartment become ischaemic and, if the pressure is sufficient, infarction may occur.

The clinical features are of pain and swelling, and sensory and motor involvement relating to the peripheral nerves compressed within the compartment. Extensive muscle necrosis may lead to myoglobinuria sufficient to cause renal failure (crush syndrome). Clinical assessment may be aided by pressure measurements using a wick-catheter inserted into the compartment. Treatment is surgical—subcutaneous fasciotomy.

The contracture that may arise as a result of fibrosis of the damaged muscle is known as Volkmann's ischaemic contracture.

A chronic form of compartment syndrome is also recognized and the most common example involves the anterior tibial compartment in athletes, less frequently in more sedentary individuals (Schepsis and Lynch 1996). Local pain develops on exercise and resolves with rest. The symptoms may be shown to parallel an increase in pressure within the compartment during exercise. The problem may respond to prolonged rest, but in some patients fasciotomy is required.

References

Anonymous (1996). Proceedings of the Eosinophilia–Myalgia Syndrome: Review and Reappraisal of Clinical, Epidemiologic and Animal Studies Symposium, 7–8 December 1994, Washington, DC, USA. *J. Rheumatol. Suppl.*, **46**, 1–110.

Anonymous (1998). AFM/MDA 1st International Myotonic Dystrophy Consortium Conference 30 June–1 July 1997, Paris, France. *Neuromuscul. Disord.*, **8**, 432–7.

Argov, Z. and Mastaglia, F. L. (1994). Drug-induced neuromuscular disorders in man. In *Disorders of voluntary muscle*, (6th edn), (ed. J. Walton, G. Karpati, and D. Hilton-Jones). Churchill Livingstone, Edinburgh.

Arnaudo, E., Dalakas, M., Shanske, S. *et al.* (1991). Depletion of muscle mitochondrial DNA in AIDS patients with zidovudine-induced myopathy. *Lancet*, **337**, 508–10.

Askanas, V., Serratrice, G., and Engel, W. K. (1998). *Inclusion-body myositis and myopathies*, (1st edn). Cambridge University Press, Cambridge.

Barnes, P. J. and Hilton-Jones, D. (1992). Managing the heart in myotonic dystrophy. *Lancet*, **339**, 528–9.

Barohn, R. J., Amato, A. A., and Griggs, R. C. (1998). Overview of distal myopathies: from the clinical to the molecular. *Neuromuscul. Disord.*, **8**, 309–16.

Beekman, R., Kuks, J. B., and Oosterhuis, H. J. (1997). Myasthenia gravis: diagnosis and follow-up of 100 consecutive patients. *J. Neurol.*, **244**, 112–18.

Behan, W. H. M., More, A. R., and Behan, P. O. (1991). Mitochondrial abnormalities in the postviral fatigue syndrome. *Acta Neuropathol.*, **83**, 61.

Bialer, M. G., McDaniel, N. L., and Kelly, T. E. (1991). Progression of cardiac disease in Emery–Dreifuss muscular dystrophy. *Clin. Cardiol.*, **14**, 411–16.

Bione, S., Maestrini, E., Rivella, S. *et al.* (1994). Identification of a novel X-linked gene responsible for Emery–Dreifuss muscular dystrophy. *Nature Genet.*, **8**, 323–7.

Bloom, W. and Fawcett, D. W. (1970). *A textbook of histology*, (10th edn). Saunders, Philadelphia.

Boerman, R. H., Ophoff, R. A., Links, T. P. *et al.* (1995). Mutation in DHP receptor alpha 1 subunit (CACLN1A3) gene in a Dutch family with hypokalaemic periodic paralysis. *J. Med. Genet.*, **32**, 44–7.

Bonne, G., Di Barletta, M. R., Varnous, S. *et al.* (1999). Mutations in the gene encoding lamin A/C cause autosomal dominant Emery–Dreifuss muscular dystrophy. *Nature Genet.*, **21**, 285–8.

Borg, K., Ahlberg, G., Anvret, M. *et al.* (1998). Welander distal myopathy—an overview. *Neuromuscul. Disord.*, **8**, 115–18.

Bowles, N. E., Bayston, T. A., Zhang, H. Y. *et al.* (1993). Persistence of enterovirus RNA in muscle biopsy samples suggests that some cases of chronic fatigue syndrome result from a previous, inflammatory viral myopathy. *J. Med.*, **24**, 145–60.

Brais, B., Bouchard, J. P., Xie, Y. G. *et al.* (1998). Short GCG expansions in the PABP2 gene cause oculopharyngeal muscular dystrophy. *Nature Genet.*, **18**, 164–7.

Bulkley, G. B., Bass, K. N., Stephenson, G. R. *et al.* (1997) Extended cervicomediastinal thymectomy in the integrated management of myasthenia gravis. *Ann. Surg.*, **226**, 324–35.

Bushby, K. (1996). Towards the classification of the autosomal recessive limb-girdle muscular dystrophies. *Neuromuscul. Disord.*, **6**, 439–41.

Bushby, K. M. D. (1999). Making sense of the limb-girdle muscular dystrophies. *Brain*, **122**, 1403–20.

Bushby, K. M. and Gardner-Medwin, D. (1993). The clinical, genetic and dystrophin characteristics of Becker muscular dystrophy. I. Natural history. *J. Neurol.*, **240**, 98–104 [published erratum appears in *J. Neurol.* (1993), **240** (7), 453].

Bushby, K. M., Gardner-Medwin, D., Nicholson, L. V. *et al.* (1993). The clinical, genetic and dystrophin characteristics of Becker muscular dystrophy. II. Correlation of phenotype with genetic and protein abnormalities. *J. Neurol.* **240**, 105–12.

Cannon, S. C. (1997). From mutation to myotonia in sodium channel disorders. *Neuromuscul. Disord.*, **7**, 241–9.

Carpenter, S. and Karpati, G. (1984). *Pathology of skeletal muscle*, (1st edn). Churchill Livingstone, New York

Dalakas, M. C. (1991). Polymyositis, dermatomyositis, and inclusion-body myositis. *N. Engl J. Med.*, **325**, 1487–98.

Dalakas, M. C. (1993). Retroviruses and inflammatory myopathies in humans and primates. *Baillieres Clin. Neurol.*, **2**, 659–91.

Dalakas, M. C. and Sivakumar, K. (1996). The immunopathologic and inflammatory differences between dermatomyositis, polymyositis and sporadic inclusion body myositis. *Curr. Opin. Neurol.*, **9**, 235–9.

Dalakas, M. C., Koffman, B., Fuji, M. *et al.* (2001). A controlled study of intravenous immunoglobulin combined with prednisone in the treatment of IBM. *Neurology*, **54**, 323–7.

Denborough, M. (1998). Malignant hyperthermia. *Lancet*, **352**, 1131–6.

Douen, A. G., Pringle, C. E., and Guberman, A. (1997). Human T-cell lymphotropic virus type 1 myositis, peripheral neuropathy, and cerebral white matter lesions in the absence of spastic paraparesis. *Arch. Neurol.*, **54**, 896–900.

Dubowitz, V. (1985). *Muscle biopsy. A practical approach*, (2nd edn). Bailliere Tindall, London.

Dubrovsky, A. L., Angelini, C., Bonifati, D. M. *et al.* (1998). Steroids im muscular dystrophy: where do we stand? *Neuromuscul. Disord.*, **8**, 380–4.

Duggan, D. J. and Hoffman, E. P. (1996). Autosomal recessive muscular dystrophy and mutations of the sarcoglycan complex. *Neuromuscul. Disord.*, **6**, 475–82.

Duran, M., Loof, N. E., Ketting, D. *et al.* (1990). Secondary carnitine deficiency. *J. Clin. Chem. Clin. Biochem.*, **28**, 359–63.

Elrington, G. M., Murray, N. M., Spiro, S. G. *et al.* (1991). Neurological paraneoplastic syndromes in patients with small cell lung cancer. A prospective survey of 150 patients. *J. Neurol. Neurosurg. Psychiatry*, **54**, 764–7.

Emery, A. E. H. (1993). *Duchenne muscular dystrophy*, (2nd edn). Oxford University Press, Oxford.

Engel, A. G., Ohno, K., and Sine, S. M. (1999). Congenital myasthenic syndromes. *Arch. Neurol.*, **56**, 163–7.

Fishbein, M. C., Siegel, R. J., Thompson, C. E. *et al.* (1993). Sudden death of a carrier of X-linked Emery–Dreifuss muscular dystrophy. *Ann. Intern. Med.*, **119**, 900–5.

Fontaine, B., Nicole, S., Topaloglu, H. *et al.* (1996). Recessive Schwartz–Jampel syndrome (SJS): confirmation of linkage to chromosome 1p, evidence of genetic homogeneity and reduction of the SJS locus to a 3-cM interval. *Hum. Genet.*, **98**, 380–5.

Goebel, H. H. (1996). Congenital myopathies. *Semin. Pediatr. Neurol.*, **3**, 152–61.

Gospe, S. M., Lazaro, R. P., Lava, N. S. *et al.* (1989). Familial X-linked myalgia and cramps. *Neurology*, **39**, 1277–80.

Grain, L., Cortina-Borja, M., Forfar, C. *et al.* (2001). Cardiac abnormalities and skeletal muscle weakness in carriers of Duchenne and Becker muscular dystrophies and controls. *Neuromuscular disorders* (In press).

Harper, P. S. (ed.) (1989). *Myotonic dystrophy*, Vol. 21, (2nd edn). W. B. Saunders, London.

Harris, J. B. and Cullen, M. J. (1990). Muscle necrosis caused by snake venoms and toxins. *Electron Microsc. Rev.*, **3**, 183–211.

Hart, I. K. and Newsom-Davis, J. (1996). Neuromyotonia. In *Handbook of muscle disease*, (ed. R. J. M. Lane). Marcel Dekker, New York.

Hillaire, D., Leclerc, A., Faure, S. *et al.* (1994). Localization of merosin-negative congenital muscular dystrophy to chromosome 6q2 by homozygosity mapping. *Hum. Mol. Genet.*, **3**, 1657–61.

Hilton-Jones, D. and Squier, M. V. (1992). Risk of cancer in dermatomyositis or polymyositis [letter]. *N. Engl J. Med.*, **327**, 207–8.

Hilton-Jones D., Squier M., Taylor D. *et al.* (1995). *Metabolic Myopathies*. Saunders, WB, London (Y)

Holt I. J., Harding A. E., and Morgan-Hughes, J. A. (1988). Deletions of muscle mitochondrial DNA in patients with mitochondrial myopathies. *Nature*, **331**, 717–19

Hoogerwaard, E. M., de-Voogt, W. G., Wilde, A. A. *et al.* (1997). Evolution of cardiac abnormalities in Becker muscular dystrophy over a 13-year period. *J. Neurol.*, **244**, 657–63.

Humeau, Y., Dousseau, F., Grant, N. J. *et al.* (2000). How botulism and tetanus neurotoxins block neurotransmitter release. *Biochemie*, **82**, 427–46.

International Myotonic Dystrophy Consortium (2000). New nomenclature and DNA testing guidelines for myotonic dystrophy type 1 (DM1). *Neurology*, **54**, 1218–21.

Isozumi, K., DeLong, R., Kaplan, J. *et al.* (1996). Linkage of scapuloperoneal spinal muscular atrophy to chromosome 12q24.1–q24.31. *Hum. Mol. Genet.*, **5**, 1377–82.

Jobsis, G. J., Keizers, H., Vreijling, J. P. *et al.* (1996). Type VI collagen mutations in Bethlem myopathy, an autosomal dominant myopathy with contractures. *Nature Genet.*, **14**, 113–15.

Kaufman, L. D., Izquierdo-Martinez, M., Serrano, J. M., and Gomez-Reino, J. J. (1995). 12-year followup study of epidemic Spanish toxic oil syndrome. *J. Rheumatol.*, **22**, 282–8.

Kerner, J. and Hoppel, C. (1998). Genetic disorders of carnitine metabolism and their nutritional management. *Annu. Rev. Nutr.*, **18**, 179–206.

Ko, G. T., Chow, C. C., Yeung, V. T *et al.* (1996). Thyrotoxic periodic paralysis in a Chinese population. *QJM*, **89**, 463–8.

Kobayashi, K., Nakahori, Y., Miyake, M. *et al.* (1998). An ancient retrotransposal insertion causes Fukuyama-type congenital muscular dystrophy. *Nature*, **394**, 388–92.

Kuncl, R. W., Pestronk, A., Drachman, D. B. *et al.*(1986). The pathophysiology of penicillamine-induced myasthenia gravis. *Ann. Neurol.*, **20**, 740–4.

Laing, N. G., Wilton, S. D., Akkari, P. A. *et al.* (1995). A mutation in the alpha tropomyosin gene TPM3 associated with autosomal dominant nemaline myopathy. *Nature Genet.*, **9**, 75–9 [see comments] [published erratum appears in *Nature Genet.* (1995), **10** (2), 249].

Lane, R. J., Barrett, M. C., Taylor, D. J. *et al.* (1998). Heterogeneity in chronic fatigue syndrome: evidence from magnetic resonance spectroscopy of muscle. *Neuromuscul. Disord.*, **8**, 204–9.

Laporte, J., Guiraud-Chaumeil, C., Vincent, M. C. *et al.* (1997). Mutations in the MTM1 gene implicated in X-linked myotubular myopathy. ENMC International Consortium on Myotubular Myopathy. European Neuro-Muscular Center. *Hum. Mol. Genet.*, **6**, 1505–11.

Lehmann-Horn, F. and Jurkat-Rott, K. (1999). Voltage-gated ion channels and hereditary disease. *Physiol. Rev.*, **79**, 1317–72.

Liu, J., Aoki, M., Illa, I. *et al.* (1998). Dysferlin, a novel skeletal muscle gene, is mutated in Miyoshi myopathy and limb girdle muscular dystrophy. *Nature Genet.*, **20**, 31–6.

Lloyd, A. R., Gandevia, S. C., and Hales, J. P. (1991). Muscle performance, voluntary activation, twitch properties and perceived effort in normal subjects and patients with the chronic fatigue syndrome. *Brain*, **114**, 85.

Loke, J. and MacLennan, D. H. (1998). Malignant hyperthermia and central core disease: disorders of Ca^{2+} release channels. *Am. J. Med.*, **104**, 470–86.

Love, L. A., Leff, R. L., Fraser, D. D. *et al.* (1991). A new approach to the classification of idiopathic inflammatory myopathy: myositis-specific autoantibodies define useful homogeneous patient groups. *Medicine Baltimore*, **70**, 360–74.

Maddison, P., Newsom-Davis, J., and Mills, K. R. (1998). Effect of 3,4-diaminopyridine on the time course of decay of compound muscle action potential augmentation in the Lambert–Eaton myasthenic syndrome. *Muscle Nerve*, **21**, 1196–8.

Mars, M. and Hadley, G. P. (1998). Raised intracompartmental pressure and compartment syndromes. *Injury*, **29**, 403–11.

Mastaglia, F. L., Ojeda, V. J., Sarnat, H. B. *et al.* (1988). Myopathies associated with hypothyroidism: a review based upon 13 cases. *Aust. N Z J Med.*, **18**, 799–806.

Miller, N. A., Carmichael, H. A., Calder, B. D. *et al.* (1991). Antibody to coxsackie B virus in diagnosing postviral fatigue syndrome. *BMJ*, **302**, 140–3.

Minetti, C., Sotgia, F., Bruno, C. *et al.* (1998). Mutations in the caveolin-3 gene cause autosomal dominant limb-girdle muscular dystrophy. *Nature Genet.*, **18**, 365–8.

Mohire, M. D., Tandan, R., Fries, T. J. *et al.* (1988). Early-onset benign autosomal dominant limb-girdle myopathy with contractures (Bethlem myopathy). *Neurology*, **38**, 573–80.

Mora, M., Cartegni, L., Di-Blasi, C. *et al.* (1997). X-linked Emery–Dreifuss muscular dystrophy can be diagnosed from skin biopsy or blood sample. *Ann. Neurol.*, **42**, 249–53.

Morel E, Eymard B, Vernet-der-Garabedian B. *et al.* (1988) Neonatal myasthenia gravis: a new clinical and immunologic appraisal on 30 cases. Neurology 38: 138–142

Motomura, M., Lang, B., Johnston, I. *et al.* (1997). Incidence of serum anti-P/O-type and anti-N-type calcium channel autoantibodies in the Lambert–Eaton myasthenic syndrome. *J. Neurol. Sci.*, **147**, 35–42.

Moxley, R. T. 3rd (1996). Proximal myotonic myopathy: mini-review of a recently delineated clinical disorder. *Neuromuscul. Disord.*, **6**, 87–93.

Newton, W. A. Jr, Gehan, E. A., Webber, B. L. *et al.* (1995). Classification of rhabdomyosarcomas and related sarcomas. Pathologic aspects and proposal for a new classification—an Intergroup Rhabdomyosarcoma Study. *Cancer*, **76**, 1073–85.

Nonaka, I., Murakami, N., Suzuki, Y. *et al.* (1998). Distal myopathy with rimmed vacuoles. *Neuromuscul. Disord.*, **8**, 333–7.

Nowak, K. J., Wattanasirichaigoon, D., Goebel, H. H. *et al.* (1999). Mutations in the skeletal muscle *a*-actin gene in patients with actin myopathy and nemaline myopathy. *Nature Genet.*, **23**, 208–12.

Ober, K. P. (1992). Thyrotoxic periodic paralysis in the United States. Report of 7 cases and review of the literature. *Medicine Baltimore*, **71**, 109–20.

O'Duffy, J. D., Hunder, G. G., and Wahner, H. W. (1980). A follow up study of polymyalgia rheumatica: evidence of chronic axial synovitis. *J. Rheumatol.*, **7**, 685.

Olson, B. R., Klein, I., Benner, R., Burdett, R. *et al.* (1991). Hyperthyroid myopathy and the response to treatment. *Thyroid*, **1**, 137–41.

O'Neill, J. H., Murray, N. M., and Newsom-Davis, J. (1988). The Lambert–Eaton myasthenic syndrome. A review of 50 cases. *Brain*, **111** (Jun Pt 3), 577–96.

Padberg, G. W. (1998). Facioscapulohumeral muscular dystrophy. In *Neuromuscular disorders: clinical and molecular genetics*, (ed. A. E. H. Emery). J. Wiley and Sons, Chichester.

Palace, J., Newsom-Davis, J., and Lecky, B. (1998). A randomized double-blind trial of prednisolone alone or with azathioprine in myasthenia gravis. Myasthenia Gravis Study Group. *Neurology*, **50**, 1778–83.

Panegyres, P. K., Squier, M., and Newsom-Davis, J. (1993). Acute myopathy associated with large parenteral dose of corticosteroid in myasthenia gravis. *J. Neurol. Neurosurg. Psychiatry*, **56**, 702–4.

Patton, H. D., Sundsten, J. W., Crill, W. E. *et al.* (1976). *Introduction to basic neurology*. Saunders, Philadelphia.

Pavlakis, S. G., Phillips, P. C., DiMauro, S. *et al.* (1984). Mitochondrial myopathy, encephalopathy, lactic acidosis, and strokelike episodes: a distinctive clinical syndrome. *Ann Neurol.*, **16**, 481–8.

Pelin, K., Hilpela, P., Donner, K. *et al.* (1999). Mutations in the nebulin gene associated with autosomal recessive nemaline myopathy. *Proc. Natl Acad Sci.*, *USA*, **96**, 2305–10.

Petty, R. K. H., Harding, A. E., and Morgan-Hughes, J. A. (1986). The clinical features of mitochondrial myopathy. *Brain*, **109**, 915–38.

Pinelli, G., Dominici, P., Merlini, L., Di-Pasquale, G. *et al.* (1987). [Cardiologic evaluation in a family with Emery–Dreifuss muscular dystrophy]. *G. Ital. Cardiol.*, **17**, 589–93.

Pountain, G. and Hazleman, B. (1995). ABC of rheumatology. Polymyalgia rheumatica and giant cell arteritis [see comments]. *BMJ*, **310**, 1057–9.

Pourfarzam, M., Schaefer, J., Turnbull, D. M. *et al.* (1994). Analysis of fatty acid oxidation intermediates in cultured fibroblasts to detect mitochondrial oxidation disorders. *Clin. Chem.*, **40**, 2267–75.

Ptacek, L. J. (1997). Channelopathies: ion channel disorders of muscle as a paradigm for paroxysmal disorders of the nervous system. *Neuromuscul. Disord.*, **7**, 250–5.

Ptacek, L. (1998). The familial periodic paralyses and nondystrophic myotonias. *Am. J. Med.*, **105**, 58–70.

Ranum, L. P., Rasmussen, P. F., Benzow, K. A. *et al.* (1998). Genetic mapping of a second myotonic dystrophy locus. *Nature Genet.*, **19**, 196–8.

Reardon, W., Newcombe, R., Fenton, I. *et al.* (1993). The natural history of congenital myotonic dystrophy: mortality and long term clinical aspects. *Arch. Dis. Child.*, **68**, 177–81.

Reuser, A. J., Kroos, M. A., Hermans, M. M. *et al.* (1995). Glycogenosis type II (acid maltase deficiency). *Muscle Nerve*, **3**, S61–S69.

Rowland, L. P. and McLeod, J. G. (1994). Classification of neuromuscular disorders. *J. Neurol. Sci.*, **124** (Suppl.), 109–30.

Ruff, R. L. and Weissmann, J. (1988). Endocrine myopathies. *Neurol. Clin.*, **6**, 575–92.

Sacanella, E., Fernandez-Sola, J., Cofan, M. *et al.* (1995). Chronic alcoholic myopathy: diagnostic clues and relationship with other ethanol-related diseases. *QJM*, **88**, 811–17.

Sansone, V., Griggs, R. C., Meola, G. *et al.* (1997). Andersen's syndrome: a distinct periodic paralysis. *Ann. Neurol.*, **42**, 305–12.

Schapiro, R. L., Hatheway, C., and Swerdlow, D. L. (1998). Botulism in the United States: a clinical and epidemiological review. *Ann. Int. Med.*, **129**, 221–8.

Schepsis, A. A. and Lynch, G. (1996). Exertional compartment syndromes of the lower extremity. *Curr. Opin. Rheumatol.*, **8**, 143–7.

Sekul, E. A., Chow, C., and Dalakas, M. C. (1997). Magnetic resonance imaging of the forearm as a diagnostic aid in patients with sporadic inclusion body myositis. *Neurology*, **48**, 863–6.

Sewry, C. A. (1998). The role of immunocytochemistry in congenital myopathies. *Neuromuscul. Disord.*, **8**, 394–400.

Sigurgeirsson, B., Lindelof, B., Edhag, O. *et al.* (1992). Risk of cancer in patients with dermatomyositis or polymyositis. A population-based study. *N. Engl J. Med.*, **326**, 363–7.

Smith, R. (1997). 49th ENMC-Sponsored International Workshop: fibrodysplasia (myositis) ossificans progressiva (FOP). 14–16 February 1997, Naarden, The Netherlands. *Neuromuscul. Disord.*, **7**, 407–10.

Taroni, F., Verderio, E., Dworzak, F. *et al.* (1993). Identification of a common mutation in the carnitine palmitoyltrans-ferase II gene in familial recurrent myoglobinuria patients. *Nature Genet.*, **4**, 314–20.

Tawil, R., Myers, G. J., Weiffenbach, B. *et al.* (1995). Scapuloperoneal syndromes. Absence of linkage to the 4q35 FSHD locus. *Arch. Neurol.*, **52**, 1069–72.

Tawil, R., Figlewicz, D. A., Griggs, R. C. *et al.* (1998). Facioscapulohumeral dystrophy: a distinct regional myopathy with a novel molecular pathogenesis. FSH Consortium. *Ann. Neurol.*, **43**, 279–82.

Tome, F. M., Evangelista, T., Leclerc, A. *et al.* (1994). Congenital muscular dystrophy with merosin deficiency. *C. R. Acad. Sci. III*, **317**, 351–7.

Topaloglu, H., Dincer, P., Richard, I. *et al.* (1997). Calpain-3 deficiency causes a mild muscular dystrophy in childhood. *Neuropediatrics*, **28**, 212–16.

Trend, P. S. J., Wiles, C. M., Spencer, G. T. *et al.* (1985). Acid maltase deficiency in adults. *Brain*, **108**, 845–60.

Tsuchiya, Y. and Arahata, K. (1997). Emery–Dreifuss syndrome. *Curr. Opin. Neurol.*, **10**, 421–5.

Udd, B., Haravuori, H., Kalimo, H. *et al.* (1998). Tibial muscular dystrophy—from clinical description to linkage on chromosome 2q31. *Neuromuscul. Disord.*, **8**, 327–32.

van-der-Kooi, A. J., van-Meegen, M., Ledderhof, T. M. *et al.* (1997). Genetic localization of a newly recognized autosomal dominant limb-girdle muscular dystrophy with cardiac involvement (LGMD1B) to chromosome 1q11–21. *Am. J. Hum. Genet.*, **60**, 891–5.

Vincent, A., Jacobson, L., Plested, P. *et al.* (1998). Antibodies affecting ion channel function in acquired neuromyotonia, in seropositive and seronegative myasthenia gravis, and in antibody-mediated arthrogryposis multiplex congenita. *Ann. NY Acad. Sci.*, **841**, 482–96.

Voit, T. (1998). Congenital muscular dystrophies: 1997 update. *Brain Dev.*, **20**, 65–74.

Wallace, D. C., Zheng, X. X., Lott, M. T. *et al.* (1988). Familial mitochondrial encephalomyopathy (MERRF): genetic, pathophysiological, and biochemical characterization of a mitochondrial DNA disease. *Cell*, **55**, 601–10.

Weetman, A. P. (1992). Thyroid-associated ophthalmopathy. *Autoimmunity*, **12**, 215–22.

Weetman, A. P. and Wiersinga, W. M. (1998). Current management of thyroid-associated ophthalmopathy in Europe. Results of an international survey [see comments]. *Clin. Endocrinol. (Oxf.)*, **49**, 21–8.

Yoshioka, M., Yorifuji, T., and Mituyoshi, I. (1998). Skewed X inactivation in manifesting carriers of Duchenne muscular dystrophy. *Clin. Genet.*, **53**, 102–7.

Zhang, J., George, A. L. Jr, Griggs, R. C. *et al.* (1996). Mutations in the human skeletal muscle chloride channel gene (CLCN1) associated with dominant and recessive myotonia congenita. *Neurology*, **47**, 993–8.

Structural disease affecting brain, spinal cord, and nerve roots

Head injury

David Mendelow

16.1 Introduction

Trauma remains the most common cause of death under the age of 35 years in most developed countries, and head injury is the most common cause of these accidental deaths (Gennarelli *et al.* 1989). Head injury results in a million patients attending Accident and Emergency (A & E) Departments in the United Kingdom, leaving more than 5000 dead and 1500 with permanent brain damage each year (Jennett 1986). The same pattern has been confirmed in North America (Marshall *et al.* 1991). Many of these injuries result from severe primary brain damage sustained at the moment of impact, and these numbers are unlikely to fall unless vigorous accident prevention campaigns are initiated. Hypoxic and ischaemic brain damage can be minimized by effective and earlier resuscitation. This would have to involve further improvements in paramedical and ambulance services, as well as better education of junior hospital doctors in resuscitation techniques.

Computed tomography (CT) and magnetic resonance imaging (MRI) have become more readily available so that haematomas and other acute complications of head injury are detected before they cause neurological deterioration. However, the distribution of imaging services is uneven, so that the number of head-injured patients with access to imaging varies—in the UK, Hewer and Wood (1989) reported that the availability of CT scanners in health regions varied from 19 to 67 per cent. Undoubtedly this has improved with time, but similar variation can be applied throughout the world. Not only does imaging increase the yield of haematomas, but it also increases our understanding of the pathophysiology of head injury. In particular, MRI displays lesions that were not visible on CT (Jenkins *et al.* 1986; Gentry *et al.* 1988; Ebisu *et al.* 1989). MRI is a useful research tool which is yielding important information about the pathophysiology of brain injury and oedema, although MRI still remains a second-line investigation in most units (Sklar *et al.* 1992).

Intensive care facilities for head-injured patients lead to better resuscitation and management of patients, and, in general, there is considerable optimism about intensive care management. Studies from Sweden (Nordstrom *et al.* 1989, Sundberg *et al.* 1989*a,b*) suggest that the provision of intensive care facilities does improve outcome. Reservations have been expressed about the validity of such conclusions, particularly from the cost–benefit point of view (Jennett 1989). The controversy about aggressive treatment is not new, with advocates of such management having observed better results for some years now (Becker *et al.* 1977), with controversy still apparent (von Wild *et al.* 1998). Another important aspect of management relates to the rehabilitation of head-injured patients. Specialization in all aspects of rehabilitation (physiotherapy, speech therapy, and occupational therapy) is taking place in many centres, and a greater understanding of the special problems of head-injured patients is leading to better results. The important subject of rehabilitation of head injuries is covered in Chapter 6.

16.2 Epidemiology of head injury

Although Rowbotham (1949) published data about head-injured patients many years ago, the first accurate epidemiological data were provided by Jennett and Macmillan (1981), who gave figures per 100 000 population. This is critically important when comparing data from different series. There are very few studies of head injury in A & E departments, but it is clear that many patients with head injury attend such departments. Most of these have minor injuries, although any one could have the potential to develop an intracranial haematoma (less than 1 in 100 of all A & E attendees with head injury). The difficulty is to decide which of these patients with minor head injuries is at risk of developing a serious, reversible complication such as an intracranial haematoma. Quantification of risk has been based on the sort of epidemiological studies first reported by Jennett and Macmillan (1981). The development of a haematoma must remain the most serious complication that doctors in A & E need to exclude. The risk of developing such a haematoma in adult patients in A & E was first reported in 1983 (Mendelow *et al.* 1983*b*). Subsequently, risks were calculated in children (Teasdale *et al.* 1990). These risks are summarized in Table 16.1 and are for patients in A & E, but they have also been calculated for patients in primary surgical wards. The different levels of risk depend on the selection criteria that have been applied, the incidence of haematomas rising as the patient passes down the referral chain to the neurosurgical unit (Table 16.2).

Deaths from head injury are also related to the sample population. The overall mortality from head injury amongst A & E attendees is relatively small, because most of these patients have minor head injuries. The level of consciousness is a major factor in determining outcome and is best measured using the Glasgow Coma Scale (Teasdale and Jennett 1974). Coma is defined as not obeying commands with no verbal response and no eye opening (corresponding to a Glasgow Coma Sum of less

Table 16.1. The estimated number of patients attending hospital in the UK with head injury/year/million total population and the absolute risk of traumatic intracranial haematoma (from Teasdale *et al.* 1990)

	Adults		Children	
	Number attending	Risk (1: *n*)	Number attending	Risk (1: *n*)
No fracture				
Conscious	10700	7866	8100	12599
Impaired consciousness	630	180	280	580
Coma	75	27	26	65
Fracture				
Conscious	10	4	110	157
Impaired consciousness	49	5.1	19	25
Coma	46	3.6	12	12

Table 16.2. Incidence of acute traumatic intracranial haematomas in different populations after head injuries (modifed from Bullock and Teasdale 1990)

Population	Sample Size	Incidence (%)
Accident and Emergency attenders:		
Scotland	3568	0.2
Admissions to general hospitals:		
Scotland	1181	1
Admission to neurosurgery with primary care:		
Edinburgh	1919	4
Hull	4011	2
Transfers to neurosurgery unit:		
Liverpool	448	39
Glasgow: pre-CT	223	34
Glasgow: post-CT	492	26
Oxford	119	19
Patients in coma in neurosurgery unit:		
USA	366	39
Three centres (Rotterdam, Glasgow, Los Angeles)	366	39
USA	1107	42
Italy: pre-CT	1000	35
Italy: post-CT	385	33
USA	746	37

Table 16.3. Classification of mechanisms of brain damage following trauma

Extracranial mechanisms
  Hypoxia
  Hypotension
Intracranial mechanisms
  Primary brain damage
    diffuse axonal injury
    lacerations
    contusions
  Secondary brain damage
    haemorrhage
      extradural
      intradural
    brain swelling
      venous congestion
      oedema: vasogenic
            cytotoxic
            interstitial
    infection
      meningitis
      abscess

per cent. The goal of head-injury management should be to reduce such unacceptably high rates to almost zero.

16.3 Pathophysiology

Brain damage following trauma results from a variety of different mechanisms (Table 16.3).

16.3.1 Extracranial mechanisms of damage

Such insults are still responsible for the global damage that occurs, particularly in fatal injuries, where Graham *et al.* (1978, 1989) have found consistently that more than 90 per cent of patients who die have ischaemic damage at autopsy. This is

than 8). The mortality is high for severe head injuries in coma from the time of the impact. Mortality for extradural haematomas varies from 5 per cent (Bricolo and Pasut 1984) to 44 per cent (Devaux *et al.* 1986), with an average of 24 per cent based on 2654 cases reviewed by Bullock and Teasdale (1990). The mortality from intradural haemorrhage is higher, ranging from 33 per cent (Vigourou and Guillerman 1983) to 76 per cent (Stening *et al.* 1986a,b) with the average being 36 per cent, based on a summary of 3664 cases reviewed by Bullock and Teasdale (1990). The mortality in relation to North American Trauma Centres was described by Gennarelli *et al.* (1989), who reported on nearly 50 000 patients from 95 trauma centres. The mortality in trauma patients with head injury (18.2 per cent) was three times higher than those without head injury (6.1 per cent). In two-thirds of the head-injured patients who died, death was considered to be a direct result of the head injury.

In the UK there are half a million trauma admissions per year and 14 500 of these die (Court-Brown 1990). Of the deaths related to the central nervous system, 7 per cent were considered to be preventable. This underlies the importance of auditing the 'talk and die' rate for head injury as was originally proposed by Rose *et al.* (1977). Since no head-injured patient who talks after the injury should die, the 'talk and die' rate (like the maternal mortality rate) should be close to zero. Many UK units have now accepted this as a standard for the purposes of medical audit of the quality of head-injury services.

In a series of children with head injuries treated prior to 1986. Sharples *et al.* (1990) reported a 'talk and die' rate of 15

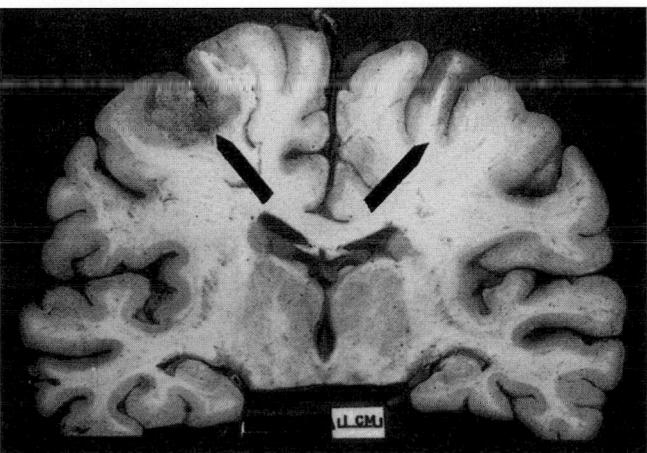

Fig. 16.1. Coronal section of brain showing bilateral boundary zone infarcts (arrowed) in a patient with prolonged hypoxia and hypotension. See also colour Plate 20.

largely the result of hypoxia and hypotension and is often found in the arterial boundary or watershed zones (Fig. 16.1). The causes of extracranial insults are multiple, and active resuscitation of the acutely injured patient should go a long way towards reducing the morbidity and mortality from this mechanism. Modern advanced trauma life support (ATLS) training is directed towards minimizing such extracranial brain damage.

16.3.2 Intracranial mechanisms of damage

It is still clinically useful to divide brain damage into primary and secondary types. Primary, or impact, damage occurs at the time of the insult and the effects are largely immediate. By contrast, secondary brain damage occurs some time after the insult, and is therefore potentially preventable and treatable.

Primary brain damage

In its mildest form this manifests as concussion. There is some evidence that concussion is due to a form of diffuse axonal injury of a minor nature (Oppenheimer 1968). This may explain why even the most minor injury may produce long-term effects (Cartlidge and Shaw 1981). Diffuse axonal injury (DAI) is now well recognized as a cause of primary brain damage (Adams *et al.* 1989, 1991). Shearing injuries of white matter were first described by Strich in 1956. The axons of neurons become disrupted and this may be recognized microscopically by the presence of axonal retraction balls (Strich 1961). Later, microglia surround the area of disruption and form microglial stars. As the white matter degenerates, Wallerian degeneration takes place. Large white-matter tracts may be disrupted primarily and the corpus callosum may be torn (Fig. 16.2). This has now been recognized with increasing frequency in living patients with severe head injury: Gentry *et al.* (1988) found lesions of the corpus callosum in 47 per cent of their patients using MRI. The mechanism of production of DAI has been demonstrated experimentally to be due to angular acceleration (Gennarelli *et al.* 1982), thus confirming

that DAI is a direct consequence of primary impact damage. The microcellular mechanisms of damage in DAI have now been recognized and patterns indicate that there may be a therapeutic window even with DAI (Fitzpatrick *et al.* 1998).

Other types of primary brain damage are lacerations and contusions. Lacerations follow penetrating head injuries; particularly those associated with high-velocity missiles. In these, there is often a surrounding zone of damage caused by release of kinetic energy. Contusions occur on the banks of the sharp sphenoid wings, thus explaining the high frequency of this abnormality on the inferior surface of the frontal lobes and in the tips of the temporal lobes. Bifrontal contusions are well-recognized clinical entities, which often give rise to secondary brain damage with late deterioration (Statham *et al.* 1989).

By and large, primary brain damage produces an immediate effect on the level of consciousness, while secondary brain damage produces a late deterioration in the level of consciousness, with the development of focal neurological signs.

Secondary brain damage

The importance of the classification into primary and secondary damage is to recognize when secondary damage is occurring and that it is treatable. The three main causes of secondary brain damage are haemorrhage, brain swelling, and infection.

Haemorrhage

A subdivision into extradural and intradural haemorrhage is useful. It has become accepted that subdural haemorrhage is very often associated with intracerebral haemorrhage and that therefore they should be classified together, as intradural haemorrhage (Galbraith and Teasdale 1982).

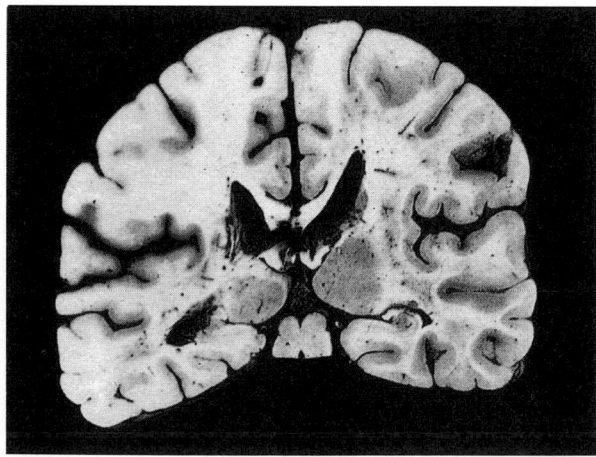

Fig. 16.2. Coronal section of brain showing a corpus callosum tear in a patient with severe diffuse axonal injury.

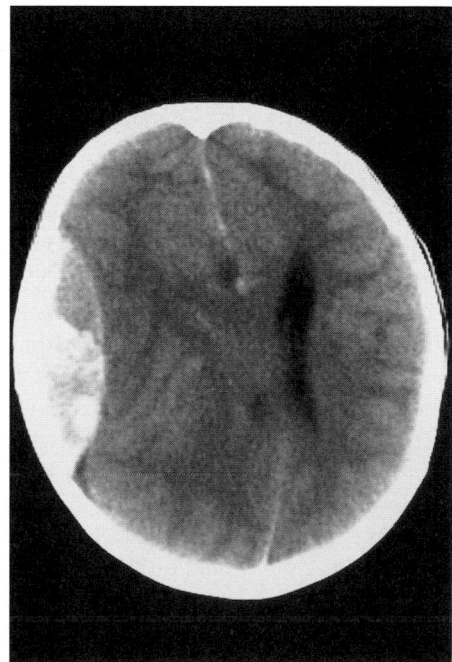

Fig. 16.3. Large extradural haematoma shown by CT scan.

Extradural haemorrhage

Extradural haemorrhage often occurs in patients with minimal primary brain damage (Fig. 16.3). Usually the bleeding is from the middle meningeal artery, which is damaged by a fracture that crosses the middle meningeal groove on the inside of the skull. However, venous bleeding may produce extradural haemorrhage, often in relation to the venous sinuses (Stevenson *et al.* 1964; Bullock and Van Dellen 1982). The vast majority of extradural haematomas are associated with fractures of the skull, even in children, in whom it was thought once that fractures were uncommon.

Intradural haemorrhage

Acute subdural haematomas (Fig. 16.4) are usually associated with underlying brain contusions or intracerebral haemor-

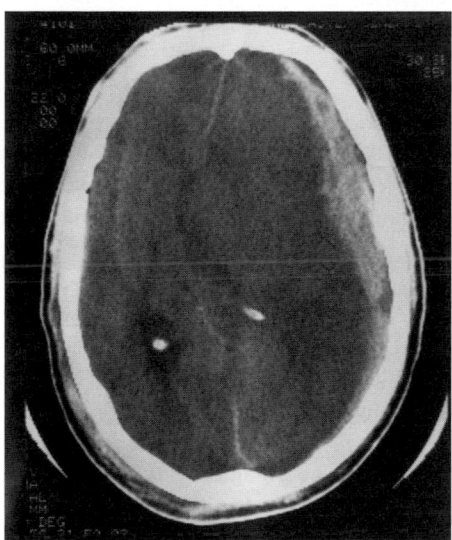

(a)

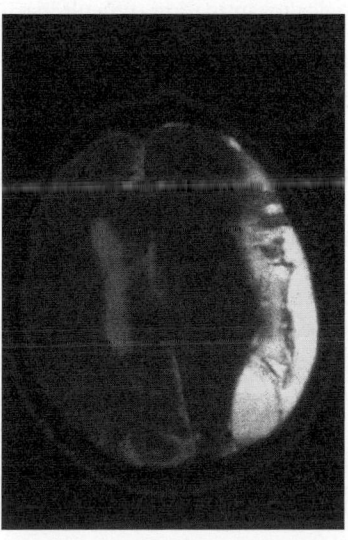

(b)

Fig. 16.4. (a) Acute subdural haematoma shown by CT scan. (b) Chronic (8-week) subdural haematoma shown by MRI.

rhage. Continuing or increasing compression of the brain will lead to ischaemia of the underlying hemisphere, and tentorial or subfalcine herniation (Section 17.1.3). The chronic subdural haematoma is usually associated with minimal primary brain damage, and in one-third of cases there is no history of trauma (Cameron 1978). The longer that a chronic subdural haematoma has been present, the more likely are there to be chronic inflammatory membranes surrounding the clot.

A large intracerebral haematoma is rare in isolation, most often being associated with smaller haemorrhages or contusions. When associated with severe primary brain damage, the contusions may be a component of a 'burst lobe', which subsequently swells and expands further because of haemorrhage from damaged vessels.

Occasionally a delayed haematoma may develop in an area of damaged brain where there was no haematoma on the initial CT scan. This was first recognized by Bollinger in 1891, and accounts for fewer than 2 per cent of surgically significant haematomas (Gentleman *et al.* 1989).

With expanding intradural haemorrhages, a surrounding area of ischaemia can be demonstrated experimentally (Mendelow *et al.* 1984). These studies showed that intracranial haematomas produce a larger ischaemic zone (or penumbra) than an equivalent-sized lesion produced with a balloon (Kingman *et al.* 1987). The effects of such haematomas may be lessened by their removal (Nehls *et al.* 1990). Similarly, in experimental subdural haematomas there is a large zone of cortical ischaemia, which underlies the haemorrhage (Chen *et al.* 1991). In clinical studies, single-photon emission computed tomography (SPECT) scanning has also demonstrated a profound reduction in blood flow around an intracerebral haemorrhage (Bullock *et al.* 1989). With contusions and intradural haemorrhage, clinical studies with MRI have also demonstrated increased blood–brain barrier (BBB) permeability 3–10 days after head injury (Lang *et al.* 1992). This may account for the delayed onset of brain oedema in many of these patients.

Brain swelling

Initially, venous congestion may cause brain swelling, but later brain oedema becomes more common. Acute brain swelling due to venous engorgement may occur within minutes of injury. It may occur at any age, but is best-recognized in children. Brain oedema takes longer to develop and is classically divided into three forms: vasogenic oedema is associated with disruption of the blood (BBB) and results from exudation of proteins into the interstitial space. Cytotoxic oedema is the result of ischaemia with dysfunction of the sodium–potassium pump caused by depletion of high-energy phosphates. The cells themselves swell, hence the term cytotoxic oedema. There is a view that the terms 'vasogenic' and 'cytotoxic' oedema should be replaced by 'open-barrier oedema' and 'closed-barrier oedema', respectively (Betz *et al.* 1989). The third type of oedema occurs with hydrocephalus and is characterized by exudation of fluid from the ventricle across the ependymal lining. This is known as interstitial oedema and may be recognized on

CT as periventricular lucency. The oedema that follows ischaemia is therefore initially cytotoxic, but vasogenic (or open-barrier) oedema may develop later. Ischaemia may also follow direct injury to intracranial or extracranial vessels. Morgan *et al.* (1987) described six patients who developed infarction following intracranial damage to the internal carotid artery. They have suggested that this injury may occur more commonly than was previously thought. Such cases present with marked but unexplained focal brain oedema on CT scan, often corresponding to known patterns of infarction that are well recognized in stroke.

Diffusion-weighted imaging (DWI) with magnetic resonance has helped to characterize the different types of oedema. In cytotoxic oedema, apparent diffusion coefficients (ADCs) are reduced, while they are increased in vasogenic oedema (Ito *et al.* 1995). In the rat acceleration model, DAI with cytotoxic oedema follows secondary insults (Vink 1995).

Infection

Infective causes of secondary brain damage usually present several days after the injury and are due to mechanical disruption of the dura, either of the vault (with compound depressed fractures) or of the base of the skull. In that case patients may present with cerebrospinal fluid (CSF) leaks (rhinorrhoea or otorrhoea). The common presentation is with meningitis (Section 33.2.6), although a brain abscess (Section 34.14) may develop after compound depressed fractures, particularly if there has been a penetrating injury.

16.4 Symptoms and signs

The variability of clinical features makes descriptive neurology impossible in the acute stages of head injury. Almost any feature or features may be observed at different times following the injury, so that it is not possible, or advisable, to describe a 'classical' clinical picture of a specific type of head injury or

Table 16.4. The Glasgow Coma Scale (Teasdale and Jennett 1974)

Eye-opening response
  4 Spontaneous
  3 To speech
  2 To painful stimulus
  1 None

Best motor response in upper limbs
  6 Obeys commands
  5 Localizes
  4 Withdraws (normal flexion)
  3 Flexes abnormally (spastic flexion)
  2 Extends
  1 None

Verbal response
  5 Oriented
  4 Confused
  3 Inappropriate words
  2 Incomprehensive sounds
  1 None

Table 16.5. Adelaide modification of the Glasgow Coma Scale for children (Simpson and Reilly 1982)

Eye response
  4 Spontaneously
  3 To speech
  2 To pain
  1 None

Best motor response in upper limbs (score highest appropriate for age)
  6 Obeys commands   > 2 years
  5 Localizes to pain   6 months–2 years
  4 Normal flexion to pain   > 6 months
  3 Spastic flexion to pain   < 6 months
  2 Extension to pain   < 6 months
  1 none

Best verbal response (score highest appropriate for age)
  5 Oriented to place   > 5 years
  4 Words   > 12 months
  3 Vocal sounds   > 6 months
  2 Cries   < 6 months
  1 None

its complications. The best quantification of the severity of brain damage is the level of consciousness, as expressed by the score on the Glasgow Coma Scale (Teasdale and Jennett 1974). The precise, explicit, and simple language that has become universally accepted in the Glasgow Coma Scale is summarized in Table 16.4.

This has been modified for children by Simpson and Reilly (1982) in what has become known as the Adelaide modification of the Glasgow Coma Scale (Table 16.5). This has now been validated and found to reliable in terms of interobserver variability.

A full and detailed neurological examination is not appropriate when examining a head-injured patient, because it takes too long and may delay the initiation of urgent diagnostic measures and treatment. Furthermore, the unconscious patient makes neurological examination difficult, particularly if pharmacologically paralysed and being ventilated. However, detailed neurological examination does become important in the later stages after head injury when assessment of the residual disability is essential, particularly in assessing the quantum of damage for compensation purposes. The progression of the clinical picture from the moment of impact is the single most important observation to make following head injury. This information may need to be obtained from ambulance personnel and those doctors who first assessed the patient. Once again, use of the Glasgow Coma Scale makes it possible to use a common language understood by many different grades of healthcare personnel from paramedics to surgeons.

It is useful to perform a rapid initial assessment, prior to instituting emergency treatment, and then to perform a more detailed examination at a later stage.

16.4.1 Initial examination

The first priority in examining any head-injured patient is to assess the *airway*. The assessment may lead immediately to the

Table 16.6 The effect of extracranial insults on the outcome from head injury; poor outcome (%) with and without extracranial insults

	Hypoxia and hypotension	Hypotension alone	Hypoxia alone	Neither insult
Kohi et al. (1984)	100	88	71	27
Gentleman and Jennett (1981)	100	75	59	34
Miller and Becker (1982)		65	65	36
Chesnut et al. (1993)	94	74	55	49

institution of treatment, if for example, there is blood or vomitus causing airway obstruction. Every unconscious patient with a head injury should receive oxygen. The respiratory rate and pattern should be observed, and cyanosis or any abnormal respiratory pattern or chest movement, as may occur with a flail chest or tension pneumothorax, should be sought. Because this initial assessment may lead the clinician to intubate and ventilate the patient, it is critically important to assess and record the best verbal response at the earliest stage, because subsequent intubation may prevent the patient from speaking and will thus invalidate any subsequent assessments of verbal communication.

Pulse, blood pressure, and any pallor should then be recorded and corrected, because failure to correct for hypoxia and hypotension results in a morbidity and mortality of almost 100 per cent. If neither of these is present, the morbidity and mortality are reduced to 1 in 3 or 1 in 4 (Table 16.6).

The sequence of events following trauma is important, not only to determine the contribution of primary brain damage

and secondary brain damage, but also to assess the level of consciousness in relation to these extracranial insults. This sequence is best recorded on a chart (Fig. 16.5), on which pupillary reactions and size should also be recorded. The consensual pupil-light reflex helps to differentiate a third-nerve palsy from an injury to the optic nerve.

It also important at this stage to assess and record the motor-response pattern from each limb. It is useful to use the same nursing chart (Fig. 16.5) that is used to record the Glasgow Coma Scale. Finally, in the rapid initial assessment, other injuries should be documented carefully and treated.

16.4.2 **Subsequent examination**

In due course a more detailed neurological examination to assess the effects of injury becomes appropriate, but in the early stages this is often impossible because of the treatment priorities and also because the patient may be paralysed and ventilated in the intensive care unit (ITU). As the patient recovers it becomes more important to document the full effects of the injury. Once again the level of consciousness predominates, but, as recovery takes place, higher intellectual function becomes easier to evaluate. This includes all aspects of language (including speech) which, if disordered, usually reflects left-hemisphere damage. Almost any focal neurological sign may occur following head injury and reflects the structures affected by the injury.

Cranial nerve palsies are quite common after head injury. In particular, anosmia may be the only residual deficit. About two-thirds of such patients may recover their sense of smell, sometimes as long as 5 years later (Sumner 1964).

Loss of vision may result from direct optic nerve or chiasmal damage, or may follow raised intracranial pressure with

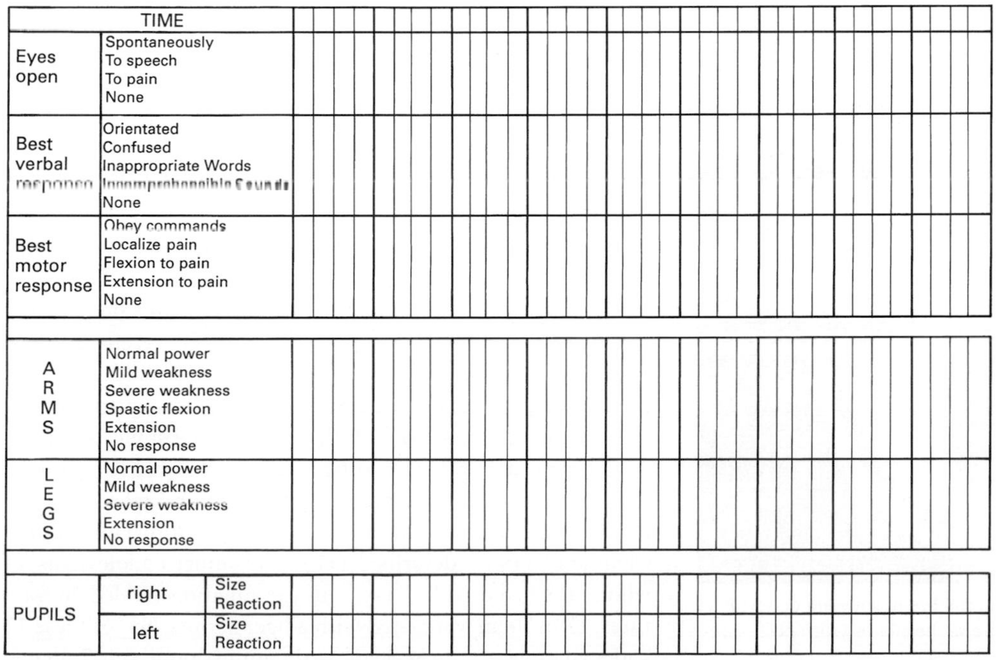

Fig. 16.5. Glasgow Coma Scale: nursing chart with the motor response pattern and pupillary changes to be recorded.

papilloedema. Similarly, abnormalities of eye movements may follow direct injury to cranial nerves III, IV, or VI, or may be due to primary damage to the brainstem. Tentorial herniation may result in a third-nerve palsy which, if unrelieved, is often associated with a contralateral homonymous hemianopia due to a medial occipital infarct resulting from occlusion of the posterior cerebral artery at the site of the tentorial hernia (Fig. 16.6). Other abnormalities of eye movement may include a sixth nerve palsy due to hydrocephalus or Parinaud's syndrome, which is usually due to damage to the tectum of the midbrain. Other injuries of the brainstem may produce internuclear ophthalmoplegias, conjugate lateral gaze palsies, and nystagmus.

Facial nerve injury must be differentiated from the upper motor neuron facial paralysis associated with cerebral hemisphere damage. Direct damage to the facial nerve is of the lower motor neuron type and is quite common, occurring in between 1.7 and 4.1 per cent of all hospital admissions with head injury (Jacobi et al. 1986). A facial nerve palsy may be immediate or delayed in onset, the importance being that delayed lesions are much more likely to recover (Laubert and Schultz-Coulon 1986). Vestibulocochlear injuries cause considerable long-term morbidity and sometimes are the only residual complication of minor head injury. They may take the form of deafness, or vestibular symptoms such as dizziness, ataxia, tinnitus, and vertigo. They may represent trauma to the semicircular canals (Cannalis et al. 1987) or to the vestibular pathways central to Scarpa's ganglion (Sanner and Plikosky 1983). Finally, CSF leaks may develop from the ear (otorrhoea) or from the nose (rhinorrhoea). These are often accompanied by haemorrhage (epistaxis) in the first hours after injury, but are recognized days later when clear fluid is observed. CSF rhinorrhoea often leads to anosmia, while otorrhoea may herald deafness.

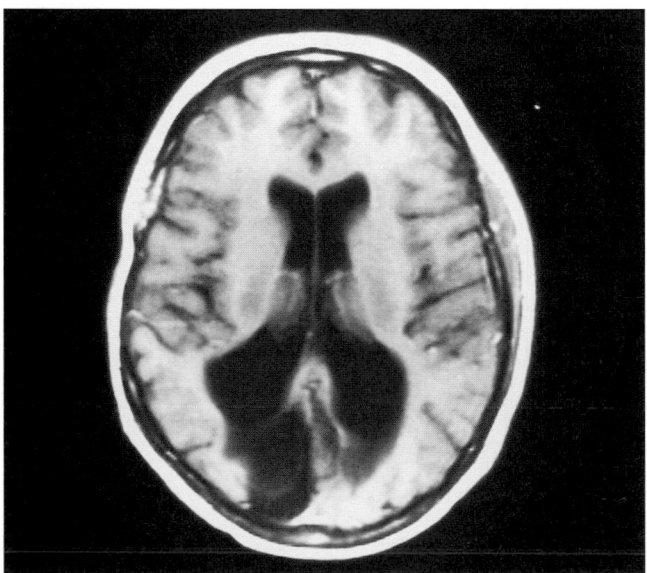

Fig. 16.6. Magnetic resonance image of the brain, showing occipital infarction in a patient who survived tentorial herniation with occlusion of the posterior cerebral artery.

16.4.3 **Clinical features of haematomas**

Because of the varied patterns of injury, which may be associated with intracranial blood clots, there is no single picture that adequately describes a post-traumatic haematoma. The change in the level of consciousness with the passage of time is of paramount importance in recognizing a haematoma, and clearly any patient whose level of consciousness *deteriorates* should be considered to have a haematoma until proved otherwise. However, many patients with haematomas will not have the classical history of deterioration. For this reason, risk factors for haematomas (Table 16.1) are used to select patients for CT scanning before deterioration takes place. In this way haematomas can be detected at a much earlier stage. Prompt treatment is required to minimize the increased morbidity and mortality that occurs with delayed evacuation of clots (Mendelow et al. 1979; Seelig et al. 1981).

16.5 **Investigations**

16.5.1 **The role of CT, MRI, and radiology**

Today most District General Hospitals have CT scanners but still too few can provide an immediate 24-hour scanning facility. Because most head injuries occur out of normal working hours, these patients will not have easily available access to CT scanning in most hospitals. The choice of investigation is usually determined by the resources available. In some parts of the world there are sufficient CT scanners to make routine scanning of all head-injured patients a real possibility. Indeed, in the advanced trauma life support (ATLS) course run by the American College of Surgeons it is suggested that 'all head injured patients will require C.T. scanning' (American College of Surgeons 1997). While this may be possible in some parts of America, it is certainly not possible in many parts of the world. In the UK, Hewer and Wood (1989) estimated that 27 million people in the UK (half of the population) lived in health districts with no CT scanners. Even today, many radiology departments do not provide the 24-hour emergency service that the colleges recommend. Clearly, therefore, the ATLS recommendation cannot be implemented throughout most of the UK, nor in many other parts of the world.

An alternative is to use skull radiography and the level of consciousness as factors for triage of head injury (Mendelow 1991). That skull radiography is important (as was suggested in the Glasgow data) is supported by three recent studies: Rosenthal and Bergman (1989) described 459 children with a brief history of loss of consciousness and a subsequent normal neurological examination. Of these, 358 had a skull X-ray, and 52 (14 per cent) of them had fractures. There were five patients with extradural haematomas and one with bifrontal contusions: all these six patients had a skull fracture. From Hong Kong, Chan et al. (1990) described 1178 head-injured adolescents, of whom 418 had a skull X-ray. This examination yielded 26 fractures, 13 of them associated with a haematoma. Ten of these 13 had a Glasgow Coma Scale of 15 on admission. From Bologna,

Pozzati *et al.* (1989) reported 32 patients with posterior fossa extradural haematomas—six had a lucid interval. There was an occipital fracture in 24, and five had multiple fractures. Each of these three reports refers to patients with apparently minor head injury who had skull fractures, potentially indicative of serious underlying haematoma. The need to scan all patients with skull fractures has thus gained universal acceptance, where CT scanning resources are sufficient to allow all patients at risk to be so examined. If CT resources are sufficient, it may not be necessary to X-ray the skull if the patient has any other indication to proceed directly to CT. There would then appear to be a reduced need for skull radiography if comprehensive and speedy imaging is available. Similar arguments may be applied to MRI in the future, because in some institutions MRI is replacing CT as the primary investigation. The organization of regional neurotrauma services, with *guidelines* for use in referring district general hospitals, has been shown to increase the diagnosis of haematomas (Deogaonkar *et al.* 1997). The other technological advance which aids the decision-making process is the use of image linking between hospitals.

In comparative studies with CT, MRI reveals many more lesions (Jenkins *et al.* 1986; Gentry *et al.* 1988; Ebisu *et al.* 1989). However, it is doubtful whether MRI reveals any more lesions that are likely to require surgery than CT (Zimmerman *et al.* 1986; Levin *et al.* 1987). MR spectroscopy allows the non-invasive measurement of lactate, choline, and aspartate in selected regions of brain and may become useful in helping our understanding of the pathophysiology in human brain injury. MRI is therefore likely to remain a valuable research tool (Vink 1995), but with limited clinical application in routine head-injury management. Similarly, positron emission tomography (PET) scanning can demonstrate cerebral blood flow (CBF) and metabolism in patients with head injury in a way that should shed light on our understanding of the dynamic events which take place in patients in the intensive care unit. Such investigations are also likely to remain important, but limited, research tools.

Table 16.7. Diagnostic categories for severe head injury based upon CT scanning (Marshall *et al.* 1991).

Diffuse injury I	No visible pathology seen on CT scan
Diffuse injury II	Cisterns are present with shift 0–5 mm; no high- or mixed-density lesion >25 ml; may include bone fragments and foreign bodies
Diffuse injury III (swelling)	Cisterns compressed or absent; shift 0–5 mm; no high- or mixed-density lesion >25 ml
Diffuse injury IV (shift)	Shift >5 mm; no high- or mixed-density lesion >25 ml
Evacuated mass lesion	Any lesion evacuated surgically
Non-evacuated mass lesion	High- or mixed-density lesion >25 ml not evacuated surgically

The Traumatic Coma Data Bank (TCDB) classification of severe head injury, based on CT scanning, has now been generally accepted (Table 16.7) (Marshall *et al.* 1991) and is useful when comparing different series of head injury.

16.5.2 Intracranial pressure and cerebral perfusion pressure measurement

While many units use intracranial pressure (ICP) monitoring as a routine, there are others that manage head injuries without such measurement. Its increasing use has made it possible to monitor the cerebral perfusion pressure (CPP) continuously. Routine automated monitoring avoids undetected secondary insults when compared to routine nursing observation (Jones *et al.* 1994). There is now evidence to suggest that maintenance of a CPP in excess of 60 mmHg is associated with a better outcome (Mendelow *et al.* 1992). Recently it has been shown that perfusion pressures of 70 or 80 mmHg may be even better than 60 mmHg (McGraw 1989; Rosner and Rosner 1992). In a recent prospective randomized controlled trial, Robertson *et al.* (1998) have shown that secondary insults, as determined by jugular venous oxygen (JvO2) desaturation, were reduced with CPP-directed therapy as compared with ICP-directed therapy. If CPP and ICP are to be measured, it is important that the method by which ICP is measured is very accurate. The 'gold standard' of ICP has traditionally been via the intraventricular route, but modern catheter-tipped transducers inserted via a screw into the subdural space are now accepted as being as reliable as ventricular catheters (Chambers *et al.* 1990). By contrast, fluid-filled subdural catheters and fluid-filled subdural screws are unreliable (Mendelow *et al.* 1983*a*; Barlow *et al.* 1985; Miller *et al.* 1986). The main benefits of ICP measurement are:

1. To allow the early diagnosis and detection of delayed haematomas, particularly in patients who are not accessible for clinical examination because they are on ventilators. A value in excess of 30 mmHg would indicate a haematoma that should be removed (Galbraith and Teasdale 1981).

2. The maintenance of an adequate perfusion pressure serves to maintain the cerebral blood flow above oligaemic or ischaemic thresholds.

16.5.3 Cerebral blood flow measurement

Cerebral blood flow (CBF) has been measured extensively using a variety of measurement techniques in patients with head injury who have been stabilized in the intensive care environment. Xenon-133 studies have not shown the expected high incidence of oligaemia or ischaemia that was predicted by autopsy reports of head-injured patients, where ischaemic brain damage was seen in more than 90 per cent of cases (Graham *et al.* 1978, 1989). Nevertheless, such studies have tended to show reduced autoregulation of CBF, such that the CBF becomes passively dependent on CPP (Mendelow *et al.* 1985; Muizelaar *et al.* 1989*a,b*). Studies within the first 4 hours of trauma (Shroder *et al.* 1996) have now demonstrated that there is a reduction in CBF which occurs soon after the injury. There is also a group of patients (especially children) where hyper-aemia, caused by increased CBF, may be responsible for brain swelling and elevated ICP (Bruce *et al.* 1981; Uzzell *et al.* 1986).

Clinical studies with stable xenon can be achieved reliably with a 3-minute 'wash-in' time (Fatouros *et al.* 1997), but additional work is required to determine their role in the management of head injury. The potential advantage of such studies is that they could be undertaken at the time of the initial CT scan.

Clinical evidence is emerging that focal reductions in CBF occur in the brain surrounding intracerebral haematomas (ICHs) (Bullock *et al.* 1989). This confirms earlier experimental work, which suggested that an ischaemic penumbra surrounded an ICH, and that the hemisphere beneath an acute subdural haematoma was ischaemic (Bullock *et al.* 1984; Mendelow *et al.* 1984; Bullock and Teasdale 1990). These studies suggest that in focal ischaemia following head injury, treatment designed to minimize ischaemic brain damage may prove valuable. Any agent that proves to be neuroprotective in cerebral ischaemia may therefore be expected to prevent ischaemic brain damage in relation to intracerebral and subdural haematomas.

16.5.4 Brain tissue metabolites (microdialysis)

Measurement of CBF makes it possible to calculate the cerebral metabolic rate of oxygen ($CMRO_2$) if the cerebral arteriovenous difference of oxygen is known. Lower levels of $CMRO_2$ correlate with a poorer outcome (Muizelaar *et al.* 1989*a*; Jaggi *et al.* 1990) (Fig. 16.7).

The levels of glutamate in brain can now be measured directly using microdialysis. With this technique, a number of microcatheters are inserted into the brain tissue (often through the same port as the ICP catheter). A few microlitres of fluid are dialysed and collected for 'on-line' analysis of glutamate (as an index of ischaemia), lactate (as an index of anaerobic glycolysis), and glycerol (as an index of phospholipid membrane

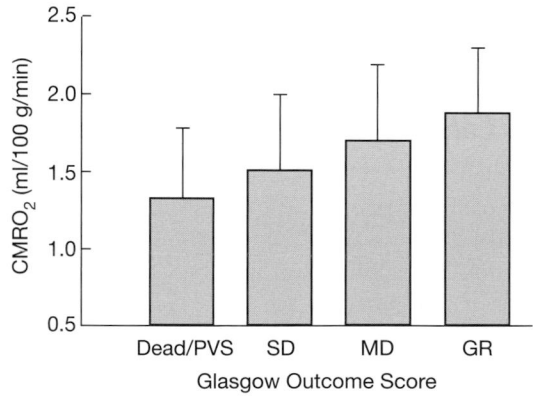

Fig. 16.7. $CMRO_2$ and outcome from head injury (from Jaggi *et al.* 1990). PVS, persistent vegetative state; SD, severe disability; MD, moderate disability; GR, good recovery.

damage). The levels of glutamate have been shown to rise substantially following head injury in humans (Bullock *et al.* 1995). Microdialysis is also useful in determining the pharmacokinetics of drugs that inhibit glutamate activation of receptor-operated calcium channels. For example D-CPP-ene has been shown to penetrate the blood–brain barrier sufficiently well to make it a potentially useful neuroprotective drug in head injury.

Brain tissue metabolism can be measured directly using oxygen-sensitive electrodes placed on the surface of the brain (Maas *et al.* 1992), but the value of such techniques in routine clinical use has yet to be determined.

16.5.5 Jugular venous oxygen saturation

Jugular venous oxygen (J_vO_2) saturation has been used as an index of $CMRO_2$, and preliminary results have indicated that this may be a useful way of monitoring cerebral function (Chan *et al.* 1992). When used frequently in the ITU management of head injury, continuous J_vO_2 monitoring provides a useful warning of impending secondary ischaemia (Cruz 1993).

16.5.6 Near infrared spectroscopy

Near infrared spectroscopy (NIRS) measures light attenuation from oxyhaemoglobin and deoxyhaemoglobin concentrations in the cerebral cortex, skull, and scalp. NIRS has been shown to correlate well with cerebrovascular reactivity during carotid clamping (Smielewski *et al.* 1997). Although attractive as a concept for non-invasive brain monitoring, it is unlikely to be useful unless the systemic changes in arterial blood pressure can be overcome. Also there is the problem of scalp trauma which may alter the contribution from extracranial tissue in such a way that even the most sophisticated algorithms for its correction will fail.

16.5.7 Cerebrospinal fluid metabolites

Biochemical markers in the cerebrospinal fluid (CSF) may indicate the severity of brain damage, although CSF is less frequently available now that ICP measurement is made from catheter-tipped transducers on the brain surface or in the parenchyma. Nevertheless, creatine kinase BB isoenzyme (CKBB) levels correlate with changes in the severity of brain damage (Rabow *et al.* 1986; Hans *et al.* 1987). Noradrenaline and lactate levels in the CSF also become elevated and are an indication of poor outcome (Rabow *et al.* 1986; Woolf *et al.* 1987). Brain tissue metabolism can be measured directly using oxygen-sensitive electrodes placed on the surface of the brain (Maas *et al.* 1992), but the value of such techniques in routine clinical use has yet to be determined.

16.5.8 Transcranial Doppler monitoring

Transcranial Doppler (TCD) utilizes ultrasound to measure flow velocity (FV) in large cerebral arteries as an indirect way of determining CBF, but it is critically dependent on vessel diameter. Vasoconstriction with constant flow will result in increased velocity, while increased flow with a constant diameter also results in a higher velocity: unless both diameter and velocity are known, CBF cannot be inferred. Nevertheless, some useful information has been collected with TCD. When correlated with CPP in patients with severe head injury, a critical 'breakpoint' for FV can be determined for the individual patient (Chan *et al.* 1993). In general, this appeared to be just below 70 mmHg CPP on average, but this may vary from patient to patient. The advantage of TCD is that it is non-invasive, but unfortunately it is poorly tolerated in the restless patient. The headbands are also quite painful for the patient with prolonged use.

16.5.9 Comprehensive monitoring in the ITU

The problem with each of the techniques described above is that no single monitoring method is ideal. Measurement of CBF or oxygen metabolism with imaging techniques is not a practical method for *continuous* monitoring. Continuous monitoring with the existing methods represents indirect determination of cerebral function and metabolism. More direct methods are being developed at present. One solution is the simultaneous use of several probes that can be inserted via a multilumen port, similar to the ICP probes that are currently in use. A combined oxygen, pH, CO2, and temperature probe can be used alongside a microdialysis catheter and an ICP sensor. While the feasibility of such multimodality monitoring has been addressed (Zauner *et al.* 1995; Hutchinson *et al.* 2000), any beneficial effect on outcome has yet to be proven.

16.6 Management and treatment of head injury

16.6.1 Organization of services

The greatest impact on outcome from head injury has been shown to occur through proper organization of services for all patients with such injuries. The adoption of liberal policies for transfer, investigation, and referral of patients reduces the

morbidity and mortality from intracranial haematoma (Mendelow *et al.* 1982; Teasdale *et al.* 1982). The appearance of more CT scanners in those district general hospitals that do not have neurosurgical services has made it necessary to recommend policies based on the predictive risks of the presence of a haematoma (referred to previously), and a more liberal scanning policy has been advocated (Fig. 16.8).

The intensive care management of patients with cardiovascular or respiratory problems due to their injury is sensible but expensive (Nordstrom *et al.* 1989). However, it is difficult to be sure that such management improves outcome (Jennett 1989). Guidelines for the management of head injury have been agreed by the Society of British Neurosurgeons (Teasdale *et al.* 1998) and the training of all doctors that deal with trauma is now commonly implemented with the ATLS methodology. Disappointingly, the development of a dedicated trauma centre alone does *not* appear to improve outcome in the UK (Nicholl and Turner 1997), despite previous optimistic reports from the USA (Shackford *et al.* 1986). Rather, better organization of care and triage using guidelines may yield more traumatic haematomas (Fig. 16.9).

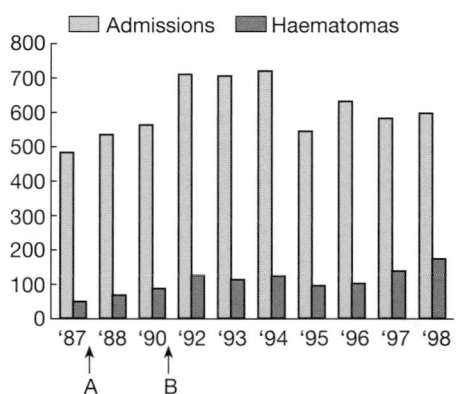

Fig. 16.9. Impact of guidelines for head injury management on admissions and detection of haematomas (updated from Deogaonkar *et al.* 1997).

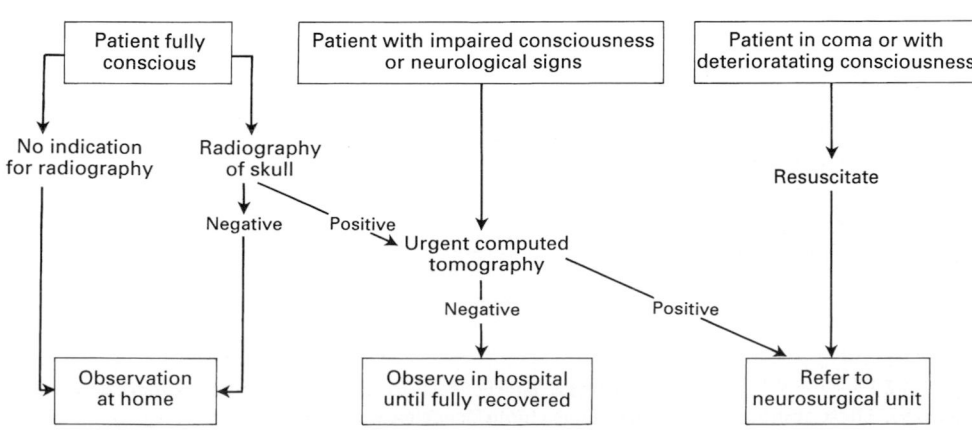

Fig. 16.8. Algorithm for management of head-injured patients in a district general hospital with a CT scanner (from Teasdale *et al.* 1990).

16.6.2 **Pharmacological treatment**

The American Association of Neurological Surgeons (1997) has published guidelines for the management of severe head injuries. These have indicated that no class I evidence exists for the pharmacological treatment of head injuries. Randomized controlled trials of a variety of pharmacological agents have been disappointing so far. In particular, barbiturate treatment has been shown not to improve outcome (Ward *et al.* 1985). Similarly, dexamethasone (Braakman *et al.* 1983), calcium antagonists (Bailey *et al.* 1990), and other high-dose steroids (Gaab and Dietz 1989) have not, at the time of writing, been shown to be of any value in head injury. However, in all these situations new trials (the CRASH trial) are currently in progress.

Antibiotics are prescribed for most patients with compound depressed skull fractures, but their routine use in basal skull fractures with CSF leakage has been questioned (Klastersky *et al.* 1976). The need for prescription of anticonvulsants in head-injured patients has also been studied in randomized controlled trials. Any beneficial effect of prophylactic treatment on the long-term risk of epilepsy is doubtful. However, in high-risk cases (e.g. compound depressed fractures with focal neurological signs) anticonvulsants are used by most neurosurgeons. Mannitol to reduce ICP is useful when waiting to get the patient into the operating theatre or during transfer, but its regular use in head-injured patients does not appear to improve outcome (Jennett and Teasdale 1981).

Mannitol given in a rationalized protocol at times of elevated ICP has also been shown not to benefit patients (Smith *et al.* 1986). Also, regular use of this agent produces an osmotic diuresis, which tends to reduce the circulating blood volume, and this may lead to a drop in cerebral perfusion pressure. Similar arguments against fluid restriction have also been accepted now in many neurosurgical units. In fact, the reverse has been shown to improve outcome, in that plasma volume expansion leads to maintenance of CPP above 80 mmHg and this does result in improved outcome (McGraw 1989; Rosner and Rosner 1992). Similarly, CPP-directed therapy (as compared to ICP-directed therapy) has been shown to reduce secondary insults significantly in a prospective randomized controlled trial (Robertson *et al.* 1998).

16.7 **Prediction of outcome**

Prediction of outcome in head-injured patients is important, not only for their relatives but also for the planning and rationing of services. Of greater value is the ability to use such predictive systems when 'new' or 'different' treatments or policies are instituted. One of the largest databases available comes from the Glasgow unit and this has now been computerized to allow rapid analysis and prediction in any individual patient (Barlow *et al.* 1987). One of the most important factors is age: it is well known that younger patients do better than older individuals (Teasdale *et al.* 1979). These results have

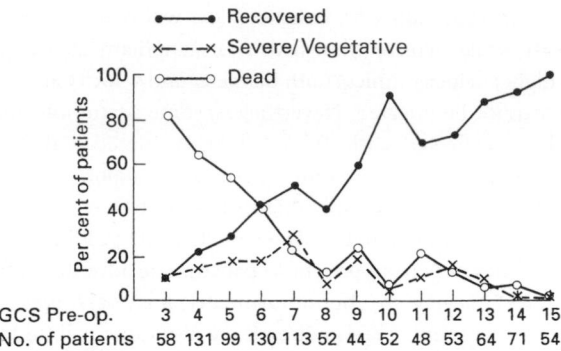

Fig. 16.10. Prediction of outcome at 6 months in patients with traumatic intracranial haematomas (from Bullock and Teasdale 1990). GCS, Glasgow Coma Scale.

now been confirmed by others (Gibson and Stephenson 1989; Howard *et al.* 1989). Recent studies in the UK have indicated that intensive care may be of value in younger patients under the age of 55 years (Teasdale, personal communication). Other systems can be used to predict outcome (Choi *et al.* 1983) but are probably less accurate, even if easier to use. MRI may help to predict which patients in coma at 6–8 weeks may go on to survive in the persistent vegetative state (Kampfl *et al.* 1998). Patients with intracranial haematomas are a special group, and have been studied extensively. Data from Glasgow have also demonstrated that the outcome in patients with intracranial haematomas can be predicted accurately from the Glasgow Coma Scale just before operation (Fig. 16.10).

There is also a relationship between the speed of evacuation of haematomas and outcome in cases of extradural haematoma: a delay of more than 2 hours from the time of deterioration in the level of consciousness to operation is associated with a worse outcome (Fig. 16.11).

Similarly, in cases of acute subdural haematoma a delay of more than 4 hours from injury to operation has an adverse

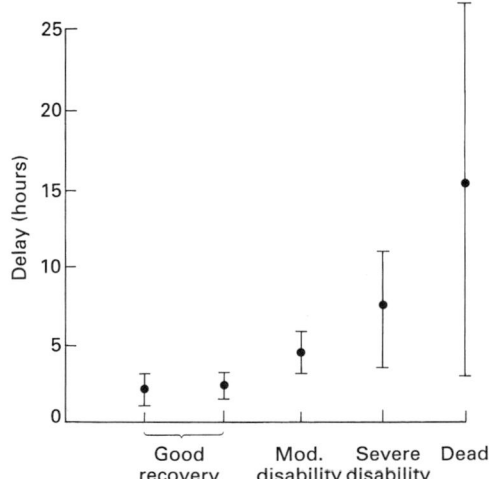

Fig. 16.11. Effect of delayed surgery upon outcome from extradural haematoma (from Mendelow *et al.* 1979).

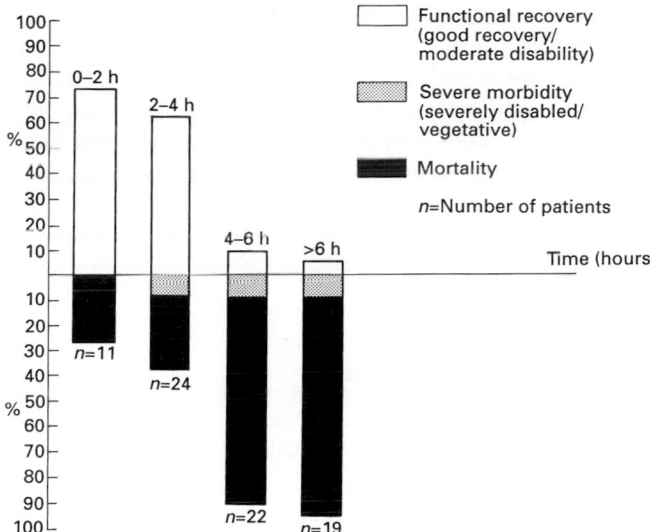

Fig. 16.12. Effect of delayed surgery upon outcome from acute subdural haematomas (from Seelig *et al.* 1981).

Table 16.8. Incidence of late epilepsy after compound depressed fractures in patients with different combinations of risk factors (where three of these are known) (from Jennett 1975)

PTA >24 h	Dural tear	Focal signs	Early epilepsy	Late epilepsy (%)
+	+		+	64
+		+	I	60
+		o	+	60
+	o		+	50
	+	o	+	40
+	+	+		39
	+	+	o	34
	o	+	+	33
	+	+	+	33
+		+	o	33
+	+		o	32
+	o	o		29
+	+	o		29
+		o	o	25
o	+		+	23
o	+	+		23
+	o		o	23
o		+	o	17
	+	o	o	1/
o	+	o		16
o	+		o	16
o		o	+	14
+	o	+		13
o		+	+	9
o		o	o	8
	o	o	+	7
	o	o	o	6
	o	+	o	S
o	o		+	4
o	o	+		4
o	o	o		3
o	o		o	3

o, Sign absent. PTA , post-traumatic amnesia.

16.8 Late complications of head injury

16.8.1 Epilepsy

In those patients who survive following head injury, epilepsy is one of the most feared complications. This is particularly true of minor head injury where the risk is, fortunately, very low, although the consequences are serious for those few who do develop seizures. The analysis of large datasets by Jennett (1975) has made it possible to calculate the risks of epilepsy in any individual patient with a non-missile head injury. Also, those patients with compound depressed fractures may be particularly at risk and this can be determined from Jennett's data (Table 16.8). Similarly, the prognosis for continuing epilepsy can be calculated, the greatest risk being in the first year following trauma. The risk of epilepsy has also been calculated from population-based studies at the Mayo Clinic: 4541 patients were followed up for up to 30 years and the standardized incidence ratios for mild, moderate, and severe injuries were 1.5, 2.9, and 17.0, respectively (Annegers *et al.* 1998). However, after a fit-free interval of a year following injury, the risk of developing a seizure diminishes further. The life expectancy for patients with post-traumatic epilepsy is probably reduced when compared with those without epilepsy (Walker 1989).

16.8.2 Cerebrospinal fluid leaks

CSF rhinorrhoea or otorrhoea indicates that there is a basal skull fracture and these patients are at risk of developing meningitis, often recurrently (Section 33.2.6). Most such leaks stop spontaneously, but if rhinorrhoea persists for more than 7 days or otorrhoea for more than 21 days, most surgeons would recommend craniotomy and dural repair. The localization of CSF leakage is best achieved by means of contrast cisternography combined with CT scanning.

16.8.3 Chronic subdural haematoma

About one-third of patients with chronic subdural haematomas give no history of trauma (Cameron 1978). A subdural haematoma becomes chronic and liquid about 2–3 weeks after it forms. The CT appearances may be misleading during the interim phase when a large chronic subdural haematoma may become isodense on CT scan can be mistaken for an alternative lesion or even overlooked. Similarly, intracerebral haemorrhage may become chronic, also passing through a subacute phase when the CT scan can again be misleading. In both these situations, MRI will differentiate a chronic haematoma from

effect on outcome (Fig. 16.12). In general, patients with extradural haematomas will do better than patients with acute subdural haematomas.

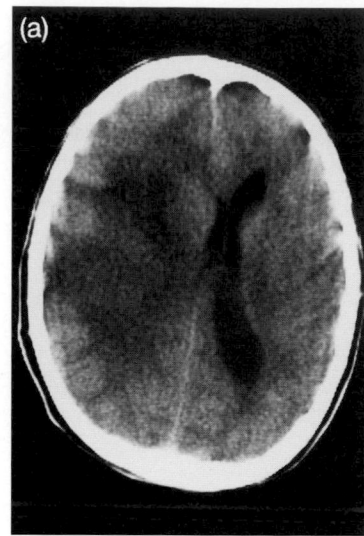

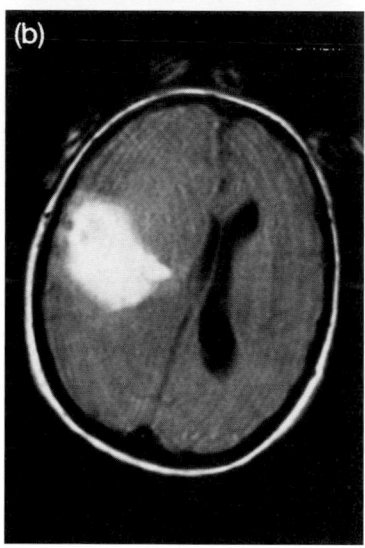

Fig. 16.13. Isodense intracranial contusion on CT scan (a) shown more easily on MRI scan (b).

infarction or other lesions (Fig. 16.13). Large, chronic, subdural haematomas are best treated with burrhole drainage (Markwalder 1981), although small lesions without a major midline shift in patients with a relatively well-preserved level of consciousness may respond well to dexamethasone (Bender and Christoff 1974). Chronic subdural haematomas are common in the elderly, but there is no reason to regard their clinical presentation, treatment, or outcome as being any different from those in younger patients (Nath *et al.* 1985).

16.8.4 Diffuse axonal injury

Although initially recognized by neuropathologists at autopsy, diffuse axonal injury (DAI) is now being recognized with modern imaging techniques with increasing frequency during life (Gentry *et al.* 1988). It is a major cause of morbidity as well as mortality and is responsible for much of the brain damage in patients who survive in the persistent vegetative state (Adams

et al. 1991). Regrettably, there is little that can be done to minimize the damage due to diffuse axonal injury, although neuroprotective agents such as calcium antagonists may have a role to play if administered early. Thus prevention of calcium influx into damaged cells is being studied in patients with head injury. This can be achieved by blocking the voltage-operated calcium channels of the cell membranes with calcium antagonists or the receptor-operated calcium channels with *N*-methyl-D-aspartate (NMDA) receptor antagonists, but clinical trials have yet to demonstrate any benefit.

16.8.5 Hydrocephalus

On CT scan, ventricular enlargement from hydrocephalus is difficult to differentiate from DAI with atrophy. By contrast, late hydrocephalus is a definite entity, which responds well to ventriculo-peritoneal or lumbo-peritoneal shunting. There is also a group of patients with normal-pressure hydrocephalus in whom clinical manifestations may be precipitated by minor trauma. The active hydrocephalus that responds to treatment can be differentiated from *ex vacuo* hydrocephalus with cerebral atrophy in a number of ways. These include MRI, ICP monitoring, or a therapeutic lumbar tap, provided there is no evidence of intracranial mass or CSF pathway obstruction on the scan.

16.8.6 The post-concussional syndrome

Although a patient may recover consciousness rapidly and completely from a head injury, persistent disabling symptoms are common. The three cardinal late symptoms are headache, giddiness, and mental disturbances, which usually develop out of the symptoms of the acute stage. Headache tends to be severe and occurs in paroxysms, which may last several hours, often against a background of continuous pain (Section 3.5). It is brought on or exacerbated by stooping, sneezing, physical exertion, noise, and excitement. The giddiness is not always a sense of rotation, but a feeling of instability, though true vertigo and staggering on sudden head movement are common. Post-traumatic vertigo induced by change of posture is probably due to damage to the utricle and saccule of the internal ear and is accompanied by nystagmus, which can be recorded in the electronystagmogram (Cartlidge and Shaw 1981). Vertigo and nystagmus usually resolve in up to 3 years.

The most common mental symptoms are inability to concentrate, fatigability, and impairment of memory, together with nervousness and anxiety, and intolerance of alcohol. All grades are encountered between the common milder cases and the less frequent more severe examples. In the latter, the patient may develop profound disorientation and confusion, with defects of perception and disorganization of speech. The final picture depends on many factors, especially the psychological constitution of the patient. Residual intellectual impairment is common: severe dementia uncommon. Moods of excitement or depression are not infrequent in cyclothymic individuals while, after severe head injury or prolonged unconsciousness, paranoid and other psychotic manifestations have been reported (Fahy *et al.* 1967).

There has been considerable dispute as to whether the so-called post-concussional or post-traumatic syndrome as described above, when occurring in a setting which may involve financial compensation (e.g. in industrial or road accidents), is largely an organ disorder or an 'accident neurosis' (Miller 1966). Unquestionable headache, giddiness, impaired concentration, and the other symptoms described above occurring after moderate or severe head injury are the result of organic brain damage and may take between 1 and 3 years to recover, if indeed they ever do so (Cartlidge and Shaw 1981). These symptoms tend to be directly proportional in severity and duration to the duration of the post-traumatic amnesia (Steadman and Graham 1970), but may sometimes occur after relatively minor head injury (Gronwall and Wrightson 1974). However, neurotic and hysterical manifestations may cloud the clinical picture, especially when prolonged disability follows minimal, or even trivial injury, and even frank malingering may be difficult to recognize (Miller and Cartlidge 1972). Considerable experience is necessary in the assessment of such cases; detailed psychometric testing may be needed, but reliable objective measures are few and it may only be possible to talk of 'the balance of probabilities'. Gronwall and Wrightson (1981) found no clear correlation between tests of memory and information-processing on the one hand and the duration of post-traumatic amnesia on the other, although Brooks (1976) had found a correlation between the latter and memory defects as demonstrated on the Wechsler scale.

'Punch-drunkenness' is a chronic traumatic encephalopathy that may occur in professional boxers. It leads to deterioration of the personality, impairment of memory, dysarthria, tremor, parkinsonian features, and ataxia (Critchley 1957; Neubuerge et al. 1959; Royal College of Physicians 1969; Jennett 1973). Absence or cavitation of the septum pellucidum can often be demonstrated radiologically. Even in young amateur boxers acute intracranial haemorrhage may occur (Cruikshank et al. 1980). CT scans performed after a knockout in professional boxers commonly reveal unexpected cerebral atrophy (Casson et al. 1982). A chronic traumatic encephalopathy comparable to that found in boxers can occur in steeplechase jockeys after repeated head injury (Foster et al. 1976).

16.9 Rehabilitation

Rehabilitation is one of the most important aspects of head-injury management, particularly in those patients with severe head injuries (Chapter 6). However, the importance of counselling and guidance for patients with minor head injury who develop the post-concussional syndrome (Section 3.5) should not be underestimated. This important aspect of head-injury care must involve many disciplines.

References

Adams, J., Doyle, D., Ford, I. *et al.* (1989). Diffuse axonal injury in head injury: definition, diagnosis and grading. *Histopathology*, 15, 49–59.

Adams, J., Graham, D. I., Gennarelli, T. A. *et al.* (1991). Diffuse axonal injury in non-missile head injury. *J. Neurol. Neurosurg. Psychiat.*, 54, 481–3.

American College of Surgeons (1997). *Advanced trauma life support course for physicians*, p. 133. American College of Surgeons, Chicago.

Annegers, J. F., Hauser, W. A., Coan, S. P. *et al.* (1998). A population based study of seizures after traumatic brain injuries. *N. Engl. J. Med.*, 338, 20–4.

Bailey, I., Bell, A., Gray, J. *et al.* (1990). The effect of Nimodipine on outcome after head injury: a prospective randomised control trial. In *Proceedings of the 2nd International Symposium on Nimodipine, Miami*. Springer, New York.

Barlow, P., Mendelow, A. D., Lawrence, A. E. *et al.* (1985). Clinical evaluation of two methods of subdural pressure monitoring. *J. Neurosurg.*, 63, 578–82.

Barlow, P., Murray, L., and Teasdale, G. M. (1987). Outcome after severe head injury—the Glasgow model. In *Medical applications of microcomputers*, (ed. W. A. Corbett). John Wiley, New York.

Bartlett, J., Kett-White, R., Mendelow, A. D. *et al.* (1998). Guidelines for the initial management of head injuries. Recommendations from the Society of British Neurological Surgeons (members of the working party of the Society of British Neurological Surgeons). *Br. J. Neurosurg.*, 12, 349–52.

Becker, D. P., Miller, J. D., Ward, J. D. *et al.* (1977). The outcome from severe head injury with early diagnosis and intensive treatment. *J. Neurosurg.*, 47, 491–502.

Bender, M. B. and Christoff, N. (1974). Non-surgical treatment of subdural haematomas. *Arch. Neurol.*, 31, 73–9.

Betz, A. L., Iannotti, F., and Hoff, J. T. (1989). Brain oedema: a classification based on blood–brain barrier integrity. *Cerebrovasc. Brain Metab. Rev.*, 1, 133–54.

Braakman, R., Schouten, H. J. A., Blaan-Van Dishock, M. (1983). Megadose steroids in severe head injury: results of a prospective double blind clinical trial. *J. Neurosurg.*, 58, 326–30.

Bricolo, A. P. and Pasut, L. N. (1984). Extradural haematoma: towards zero mortality. A prospective study. *Neurosurgery*, 14, 8–12.

Brooks, D. N. (1976). Wechsler memory scale performance and its relationship to brain damage after severe closed head injury. *J. Neurol. Neurosurg. Psychiat.*, 39, 593–601.

Bruce, D. A., Alavi, A., Bilaniuk, L. *et al.* (1981). Diffuse cerebral swelling following head injury in children: a syndrome of 'malignant brain oedema'. *J. Neurosurg.*, 54, 170–8.

Bullock, R. and Teasdale, G. M. (1990). Surgical management of traumatic intracranial haematomas. In *Handbook of clinical neurology.* Vol. 13 (57): *Head injury,* (ed. R. Braakman). Elsevier, Amsterdam.

Bullock, R. and Van Dellen, J. R. (1982). Chronic extradural haematoma. *Surg. Neurol.,* **18,** 300–2.

Bullock, R., Mendelow, A. D., Teasdale, G. M. *et al.* (1984). Intracranial haemorrhage induced at arterial pressure in the rat. 1: Description of technique, ICP changes and neuropathological findings. *Neurol. Res.,* **6,** 184–8.

Bullock, R., Teasdale, G. M., Wyper, D. *et al.* (1989). Tomographic mapping of CBF and blood–brain barrier changes after focal head injury using SPECT: mechanism for late deterioration. In *Proceedings, VIIth international symposium on intracranial pressure and brain injury, Ann Arbor,* (ed. J. Hoff). Springer, Berlin.

Bullock, R., Zauner, A., Myseros, J. C. *et al.* (1995). Excitatory amino acid release patterns after severe human head injury—experience with microdialysis in 30 patients. *J. Neurotrauma,* **12,** 372.

Cameron, M. M. (1978). Chronic subdural haematoma: a review of 114 cases. *J. Neurol. Neurosurg. Psychiat.,* **41,** 834–9.

Canalis, R. F., Gussen, R., Ebemeyore, E. *et al.* (1987). Surgical trauma to the lateral semi-circular canal with preservation of hearing. *Laryngoscope,* **97,** 575–81.

Cartlidge, N. E. F. and Shaw, D. A. (1981). *Head injury.* Saunders, London.

Casson, I. R., Sham, R., Campbell, E. A. *et al.* (1982). Neurological a CT evaluation of knocked-out boxers. *J. Neurol. Neurosurg. Psychiat.,* **45,** 170–4.

Chambers, I. R., Mendelow, A. D., Sinar, E. J. *et al.* (1990). A clinical evaluation of the Camino subdural screw and ventricular monitoring kits. *Neurosurgery,* **26,** 421–4.

Chan, K. H., Mann, K. S., Yue, C. P. *et al.* (1990). The significance of skull fracture in acute traumatic intracranial heematomas in adolescence. *J. Neurosurg.,* **72,** 189–94.

Chan, K. H., Dearden, N. M., and Miller, J. D. (1992). Multi-modality monitoring of intracranial pressure therapy after severe brain injury. In *ICP and craniospinal dynamics,* (ed. C. J. J. Avezaat). Springer, Berlin.

Chan, K. H., Dearden, N., Miller, J. *et al.* (1993). Multimodality monitoring as a guide to treatment of intracranial hypertension after severe brain injury. *Neurosurgery,* **32,** 547–52.

Chen, M. H., Bullock, R., Graham, D. I. *et al.* (1991). Ischaemic brain damage after acute subdural haematoma in the rat: effects of pretreatment with a glutamate antagonist. *J. Neurosurg.,* **74,** 944–50.

Chestnut, R. L., Marshall *et al.* (1993). The role of secondary brain injury in determining outcome from severe head injury. *J. Trauma,* **34,** 216–22.

Choi, S., Ward, J. D., and Becker, D. P (1983). Chart for outcome prediction in severe head injury. *J. Neurosurg.,* **59,** 294–7.

Court-Brown, C. M. (1990). The treatment of the multiple injured patient in the United Kingdom. *J. Bone Joint Surg.,* **72,** 345–6.

Critchley, M. (1957). Medical aspects of boxing. *BMJ,* **1,** 357–62.

Cruikshank, J. K., Higgens, C. S., and Gray, J. R. (1980). Two cases of acute intracranial haemorrhage in young amateur boxers. *Lancet,* **i,** 626–7.

Cruz, J. (1993). On-line monitoring of global cerebral hypoxia in acute brain injury: relationship to intracranial hypertension. *J. Neurosurg.,* **79,** 228–33.

Deogoankar, M., Treadwell, L., Chambers, I. R. *et al.* (1997). Improved identification of traumatic intracranial haematomas: the impact of patient management guidelines for head injury (1987–1995). *J. Neurol. Neurosurg. Psychiat.,* **63,** 129.

Devaux, B., Rouex, F. X., and Chodkienicz, J. P. (1986). L'hematome extra-dural a l'ere du SAMU et du scanner. Comparison de deux series du Centre Hospitalier Saint-Anne. *Neurochirurgie,* **32,** 221.

Ebisu, T., Yamaki, T., Kobori, N. *et al.* (1989). Magnetic resonance imaging of brain contusion. *Surg. Neurol.,* **31,** 261.

Fahy, T. J., Irving, M. H., and Millac, P. (1967). Severe head injuries. *Lancet,* **ii,** 475.

Fatouros, P., Muizelaar, J. P., and Schroder M. L. (1997). A new method for quantitative regional cerebral blood flow measurements using computer tomography. *Stroke,* **28,** 1998–2005.

Fitzpatrick, M., Maxwell, W., Graham, D. *et al.* (1998). The role of axolemma in the initiation of traumatically induced axonal injury. *J. Neurol. Neurosurg. Psychiat.,* **64,** 285–7.

Foster, J. B., Leiguarda, R., and Tilley, P. J. B. (1976). Brain damage in National Hunt jockeys. *Lancet,* **i,** 981–3.

Gaab, M. R. and Dietz, H. (1989). Ultra-high, short-term dexamethasone therapy in craniocerebral trauma. Rationale and design of a multicentre study. *Neurochirurgia,* **32,** 93–100.

Galbraith, S. and Teasdale, G. M. (1981). Predicting the need for operation in the patient with an occult traumatic intracranial haematoma. *J. Neurosurg.,* **55,** 75–81.

Galbraith, S. and Teasdale, G. M. (1982). Head injuries. In *Recent advances in surgery,* (ed. R. C. G. Russell). Churchill Livingstone, Edinburgh.

Gennarelli, T. A., Thibault, L. E., Adams, J. H. *et al.* (1982). Diffuse axonal injury and traumatic coma in the primate. *Ann. Neurol.,* **12,** 564–74.

Gennarelli, T. A., Champion, H. R., Sacco, J. et al. (1989). Mortality of patients with head injury and extra-cranial injury treated in trauma centres. J. Trauma, 29, 1193–201.

Gentleman, D. and Jennett, B. (1981). Hazards of inter-hospital transfer to comatose head injured patients. Lancet, ii, 853.

Gentleman, D., Nath, F., and Macpherson, P. (1989). Diagnosis and management of delayed traumatic intercerebral haematoma. Br. J. Neurosurg., 3, 367–72.

Gentry, L. R., Thompson, B., and Godersky, J. C. (1988). Trauma to the corpus callosum: MR features. AJNR, 9, 1129–38.

Gibson, M. and Stephenson, G. L. (1989). Aggressive management of severe closed head trauma: time for re-appraisal. Lancet, ii, 369–71.

Graham, D. I., Adams, J. H., and Doyle, D. (1978). Ischaemic brain damage in fatal non-missile head injuries. J. Neurol. Sci., 39, 213–34.

Graham, D. I., Ford, I., Adams, J. H. et al. (1989). Ischaemic brain damage is still common in fatal non-missile head injury. J. Neurol. Neurosurg. Psychiat., 52, 346–50.

Gronwall, D. and Wrightson, P. (1974). Delayed recovery of intellectual function after minor head injury. Lancet, ii, 605–9.

Gronwall, D. and Wrightson, P. (1981). Memory and information processing capacity after closed head injury. J. Neurol. Neurosurg. Psychiat., 44, 889–95.

Hans, P., Born, J. D., and Albert, A. (1987). Extrapolated creatine kinase-BB isoenzyme activity in assessment of initial brain damage after severe head injury. J. Neurosurg., 66, 714–17.

Hewer, R. L. and Wood, V. A. (1989). Availability of computed tomography of the brain in the United Kingdom. BMJ, 298, 1219–20.

Howard, M. A., Gross, A. S., Dacey, R. G. et al. (1989). Acute subdural haematomas: an age-dependent clinical entity. J. Neurosurg., 71, 858–63.

Hutchinson, P., Al-Rawi, P., O'Connell, M. et al. (2000). Onative monitoring of substrate delivery and brain metabolism in head injury. Acta Neurochir., Suppl. 76.

Ito, J., Barzo, P. et al. (1995). Characterisation of edema by diffusion weighted imaging following closed head injury and secondary insult in the rat. J. Neurotrauma, 12, 475.

Jacobi, G., Ritz, A., and Emrich, R. (1986). Cranial nerve damage after paediatric head trauma: a long-term follow-up study of 741 cases. Acta Paediat. Hung., 27, 173–87.

Jaggi, J. L., Obrist, W. D., Gennarelli, T. A. et al. (1990). Relationship of early cerebral blood flow and metabolism to outcome in acute head injury. J. Neurosurg., 72, 176–82.

Jenkins, A., Teasdale, G., Hadley, D. M. et al. (1986). Brain lesions detected by magnetic resonance imaging in mild and severe head injuries. Lancet, ii, 445–6.

Jennett, B. (1973). Boxing brains. Lancet, ii, 1064.

Jennett, B. (1975). Epilepsy after non-missile head injuries, (2nd edn). Heinemann, London.

Jennett, B. (1986). High technology medicine—costs and benefits. Oxford University Press, Oxford.

Jennett, B. (1989). Severe head injuries: Swedish style. Brain Inj., 3, 215.

Jennett, B. and Macmillan, R. (1981). Epidemiology of head injury. BMJ, 282, 101–4.

Jennett, B. and Teasdale, G. M. (1981). Management of head injuries. F. A. Davis, Philadelphia.

Jones, P. A., Andrews, P. J. D., Midgley, S. et al. (1994). Measuring the burden of secondary insults in head injured patients during intensive care. J. Neurosurg. Anaesthetics, 6, 4–14.

Kampfl, A. P., Fauster, B., Denchev, D. et al. (1997). Near infrared spectroscopy in patients with severe brain injury and elevated intracranial pressure. Acta Neurochir., 70, 112–14.

Kingman, T. A., Mendelow, A. D., Graham, D. I. et al. (1987). Experimental intracerebral mass: time-related effects on local cerebral blood flow. J. Neurosurg., 67, 732–8.

Klastersky, J., Sadeghi, M., and Brihaye, J. (1976). Antimicrobial prophylaxis in patients with rhinorrhoea and otorrhoea: a double blind study. Surg. Neurol., 6, 111–14.

Kohi, Y. M., Mendelow, A. D., Teasdale, G. M. et al. (1984). Extra-cranial insults and outcome in patients with acute head injury—relationship to the Glasgow Coma Scale. Injury, 16, 25–9.

Lang, D. A., Hadley, D. M., Teasdale, G. M. et al. (1992). Gadolinium DTPA enhanced magnetic resonance imaging in human head injury. Acta Neurochir., 51, 293.

Laubert, A. and Schultz-Coulon, H. J. (1986). Prognosis of facial paralysis caused by fracture of the petrous bone. HNO, 34, 412–16.

Levin, H. S., Amparo, E., Eisenberg, H. M. et al. (1987). Magnetic resonance imaging and computerised tomography in relation to the neurobehavioural sequelae of mild and moderate head injuries. J. Neurosurg., 66, 706–13.

Maas, A. I. R., Fleckenstein, W., and de Jong, D. A. (1992). Brain tissue monitoring in severe head injury. In ICP and craniospinal dynamics, (ed. C. J. J. Avezaat). Springer, Berlin.

Markwalder, T. M. (1981). Chronic subdural haematomas: a review. J. Neurosurg., 54, 637–45.

Marshall, L. F., Marshall, S. B., Klauber, M. R. et al. (1991). A new classification of head injury based on computerised tomography. J. Neurosurg., 75, S14–S20.

McGraw, C. P. (1989). A cerebral perfusion pressure of greater than 80 mm Hg is more beneficial. In *Intracranial pressure VII*, (ed. J. T. Hoff and A. L. Betz). Springer, Berlin.

Mendelow, A. D. (1991). The early management of head injury. *Curr. Opin. Neurol. Neurosurg.*, 4, 5–11.

Mendelow, A. D., Karmi, M., Paul, K. *et al.* (1979). Extradural haematoma—effect of delayed treatment. *BMJ*, 1, 1240–2.

Mendelow, A. D., Campbell, D. A., Jeffrey, R. R. *et al.* (1982). Admission after mild head injury: benefits and costs. *BMJ*, 285, 1530–2.

Mendelow, A.D, Rowen, J. D., Murray, L. *et al.* (1983*a*). A clinical comparison of subdural screw measurements with ventricular pressure. *J. Neurosurg.*, 58, 45–50.

Mendelow, A. D., Teasdale, G. M., Jennett, S. *et al.* (1983*b*). Risks of intracranial haematoma in head injured adults. *BMJ*, 287, 1173–6.

Mendelow, A. D., Bullock, R., Teasdale, G. M. *et al.* (1984). Intracranial haemorrhage induced at arterial pressure in the rat. Part 2: Short-term changes in local cerebral blood flow measured by autoradiography. *Neurol. Res.*, 6, 189–93.

Mendelow, A. D., Teasdale, G. M., Russell, T. *et al.* (1985). Effect of mannitol on cerebral blood flow and cerebral perfusion pressure in human head injury. *J. Neurosurg.*, 63, 43–8.

Mendelow, A. D., Allcutt, D. A., Chambers, I. *et al.* (1992). Intracranial and cerebral perfusion pressure monitoring in the head injured patient: which index? In *ICP and cranio-spinal dynamics*, (ed. C. J. J. Avezaat). Springer, Berlin.

Miller, H. (1966). Mental after-effects of head injury. *Lancet*, 1 (7750), 580–5.

Miller, H. and Cartlidge, N. (1972). Simulation and malingering after injuries to the brain and spinal cord. *Lancet*, i, 580–5.

Miller, J. D. and Becker, D. P. (1982). Secondary insults to the injured brain. *J. R. Coll. Surg. Edin.*, 27, 292–8.

Miller, J. D., Bobo, H., and Capp, J. P. (1986). Inaccurate pressure readings from subarachnoid bolts. *Neurosurgery*, 19, 253–5.

Morgan, M. K., Besser, M., Johnston, I. *et al.* (1987). Intracranial carotid artery injury in closed head trauma. *J. Neurosurg.*, 66, 192–7.

Muizelaar, J. P., Marmarou, A., DeSalles, A. A. F. *et al.* (1989*a*). Cerebral blood flow and metabolism in severely head injured children. Part I: Relationship with GCS score, outcome, ICP and PVI. *J. Neurosurg.*, 71, 63–71.

Muizelaar, J. P., Ward, J. D., Marmarou, A. *et al.* (1989*b*). Cerebral blood flow and metabolism in severely head injured children. Part II: Autoregulation. *J. Neurosurg.*, 71, 72–6.

Nath, F., Mendelow, A. D., Wu, C.-C. *et al.* (1985). Chronic subdural haematoma in the CT scan era. *Scott. Med. J.*, 30, 152–5.

Nehls, D. G., Mendelow, A. D., Graham, D. I. *et al.* (1990). Experimental intracerebral haemorrhage: early removal of a spontaneous mass lesion improves late outcome. *Neurosurgery*, 27, 675–82.

Neubuerger, K. T., Sinton, D. W., and Denst, J. (1959). Cerebral atrophy associated with boxing. *Arch. Neurol. Psychiat.*, 81, 403.

Nicholl, J. and Turner, J. (1997). Effectiveness of a regional trauma system in reducing mortality from major trauma: before and after study. *BMJ*, 315, 1349–54.

Nordstrom, C.-H., Messeter, K., Sundberg, G. *et al.* (1989). Severe traumatic brain lesions in Sweden. Part 1: Aspects of management in non-neurosurgical clinics. *Brain Inj.*, 3, 247–306.

Oppenheimer, D. R. (1968). Microscopic lesions in the brain following head injury. *J. Neurol. Neurosurg. Psychiat.*, 31, 299–306.

Pozzati, E., Tognetti, F., Cavallo, M. *et al.* (1989). Extradural haematomas of the posterior cranial fossa. *Surg. Neurol.*, 32, 300–3.

Rabow, L., DeSalles, A. A. F., Becker, D. P. *et al.* (1986). CSF brain creatine kinase levels and lactic acidosis in severe head injuries. *J. Neurosurg.*, 65, 625–9.

Robertson, C. S., Valadka, A. B., Gopinath, S. P. *et al.* (1998). Prevention of secondary insults after head injury. *Acta Neurochir. Suppl.*, 71, 378.

Rose, J., Valtonen, S., and Jennett, B. (1977). Avoidable factors contributing to death after head injury. *BMJ*, 2, 616–18.

Rosenthal, B. W. and Bergman, I. (1989). Intracranial injury after moderate head trauma in children. *J. Pediat.*, 115, 346–50.

Rosner, M. J. and Rosner, S. D. (1992). Cerebral perfusion pressure management of head injury. In *ICP and craniospinal dynamics*, (ed. C. J. J. Avezaat). Springer, Berlin.

Rowbotham, G. F. (1949). *Acute injuries of the head. Their diagnosis, treatment, complications and sequels*, (3rd edn). Livingstone, Edinburgh.

Royal College of Physicians (1969). *Report on the medical aspects of boxing*. RCP, London.

Sanner, M. and Plikosky, J. (1983). Vestibular neurectomy for dizziness after head trauma. *ORL*, 45, 216.

Seelig, J. N., Becker, D. P., Miller, J. D. *et al.* (1981). Traumatic acute subdural haematoma: major mortality reduction in comatose patients treated within four hours. *N. Engl. J. Med.*, 304, 1511–18.

Shackford, S., Hollingsworth-Fridland, P., Cooper, G. *et al.* (1986). The effect of regionalisation upon the quality of trauma care as assessed by concurrent audit before and after the institution of a trauma system: a preliminary report. *J. Trauma*, **26**, 812–20.

Sharples, P. M., Storey, A., Aynsley-Green, A. *et al.* (1990). Avoidable factors contributing to death of children with head injury. *BMJ*, **300**, 87–91.

Shroder, M., Muizelaar, J., Kuta, A. *et al.* (1996). Thresholds for cerebral ischaemia after severe head injury: relationship with late CT findings and outcome. *J. Neurotrauma*, **13**, 17–23.

Simpson, D. and Reilly, P. (1982). Paediatric coma scale. *Lancet*, **ii**, 450.

Sumner, D. (1964). Post-traumatic anosmia. *Brain*, **87**, 107.

Sklar, M. L., Quencer, R. M., Bowen, B. C. *et al.* (1992). Magnetic resonance applications in cerebral injury. *Radiol. Clin. North Am.*, **30**, 353–66.

Smielewski, P., Czosnyka, M., Pickard, J. *et al.* (1997). Clinical evaluation of near-infrared spectroscopy for testing cerebrovascular reactivity in patients with carotid artery disease. *Stroke*, **28** (2), 331–8.

Smith, H. P., Kelly, D. L., McWhorter, J. M. *et al.* (1986). Comparison of mannitol regimens in patients with severe head injury undergoing intracranial monitoring. *J. Neurosurg.*, **65**, 820–4.

Statham, P. F., Johnston, R. A., and MacPherson, P. (1989). Delayed deterioration in patients with traumatic frontal contusions. *J. Neurol. Neurosurg. Psychiat.*, **52**, 351–4.

Steadman, J. H. and Graham, J. G. (1970). Head injuries: an analysis and follow-up study. *Proc. R. Soc. Med.*, **63**, 23–8.

Stening, W. A., Berry, G., Dan, N. G. *et al.* (1986a). Experience with acute sub-dural haematomas in New South Wales. *Aust. N.Z. J. Surg.*, **56**, 549–56.

Stening, W. A., Berry, G., Dan, N. G. *et al.* (1986b). Experience with multiple intracranial haematomas in New South Wales. *Aust. N.Z. J. Surg.*, **56**, 543–8.

Stevenson, G. C., Brown, H. A., and Hoyt, W. F. (1964). Chronic venous epidural haematomas at the vertex. *J. Neurosurg.*, **21**, 887.

Strich, S. J. (1956). Diffuse degeneration of cerebral white matter in severe dementia following head injury. *J. Neurol. Neurosurg. Psychiat.*, **19**, 163–85.

Strich, S. J. (1961). Shearing of nerve fibres as a cause of brain damage due to head injury. A pathological study of 20 cases. *Lancet*, **ii**, 443–8.

Sundbarg, G., Messeter, K., and Schalen, W. (1989a). Severe traumatic brain lesions in Sweden. Part II: Impact of aggressive neurosurgical intensive care. *Brain Inj.*, **3**, 267–81.

Sundbarg, G., Norlund, A., Nordstrom, C.-H. *et al.* (1989b). Severe traumatic brain lesions in Sweden. Part III: Economic aspects of aggressive neurosurgical intensive care. *Brain Inj.*, **3**, 283–93.

Teasdale, G. M. and Jennett, B. (1974). Assessment of coma and impaired consciousness: a practical scale. *Lancet*, **ii**, 81–4.

Teasdale, G. M., Skene, A., Parker, K. *et al.* (1979). Age and outcome of severe head injury. *Acta Neurochir.*, **28**, 140–3.

Teasdale, G. M., Galbraith, S., Murray, L. *et al.* (1982). Management of traumatic intracranial haematoma. *BMJ*, **285**, 1695–7.

Teasdale, G. M., Murray, G., Anderson, E. *et al.* (1990). Risks of acute traumatic intracranial haematoma in children and adults: implications for managing head injuries. *BMJ*, **300**, 363–7.

Uzzell, B. P., Obrist, W. E., Dolinskas, C. A. *et al.* (1986). Relationship of acute CBF and ICP findings to neuropsychological outcome in severe head injury. *J. Neurosurg.*, **65**, 630–5.

Vigourou, R. D. and Guillerman, P. (1983). Surgical indicators in pastrami brain contusions and lacerations. In *Advances in neurotraumatology*, (ed. R. Villani, I. Pappo, S. M. Giovanelli, *et al.*). Excerpta Medica, Amsterdam.

Vink, R. (1995). Functional magnetic resonance characterisation of the injured brain: can MR provide clinically relevant information beyond conventional imaging? *J. Neurotrauma*, **12**, 351.

Von Wild, K. R. H., Nordstrom, C.-H., and Hernandez-Meyer, F. (1998). *Pathophysiological principles and controversies in neurointensive care.* W. Zuckscherdt Verlag, Munchen.

Walker, A. E. (1989). Post-traumatic epilepsy in World War II survivors. *Surg. Neurol.*, **32**, 235–6.

Ward, J. D., Becker, D. P., Miller, J. D. *et al.* (1985). Failure of prophylactic barbiturate coma in the treatment of severe head injury. *J. Neurosurg.*, **62**, 383–8.

Woolf, P. D., Hamill, R. W., Lee, L. A. *et al.* (1987). The predictive value of catecholamines in assessing outcome in traumatic brain injury. *J. Neurosurg.*, **66**, 875–82.

Zauner, A., Bullock, R., and Young, H. F. (1995). Continuous brain oxygen, CO_2, pH, and temperature monitoring in neurosurgery patients. *Neurosurgery*, 37–570.

Zimmerman, R. A., Bilamiuk, L. T., Hackney, D. P. *et al.* (1986). Head injury: early results of comparing CT and high-field MR. *Am. J. Neuroradiol.*, **147**, 1215–22.

CHAPTER 17

Raised intracranial pressure, cerebral oedema, and hydrocephalus

David Mendelow

17.1 Raised intracranial pressure

17.1.1 Pathophysiology

Intracranial pressure (ICP) may become pathologically elevated from diffuse swelling of the brain (cerebral oedema or venous congestion), hydrocephalus, or from other intracranial space-occupying lesions, including tumours, haematoma, or abscess. The brain is unique among the viscera in being confined within the rigid case, the cranium. The total volume of the intracranial contents, namely the brain and its coverings, the blood vessels, and the blood and CSF is normally constant, so that an expansion of any one of these can only occur at the expense of the others. However, the intracranial contents do not respond passively to changes in their volume or pressure, but react in a number of complicated ways, depending mainly on the rate at which they expand.

As an intracranial mass lesion increases in size, there is initially a compensatory reduction in the volume of intracranial blood and CSF and, only when this compensatory process is exhausted, does the intracranial pressure increase. This compensation is best when the rate of expansion is very slow. In this first, or compensated, stage there is little change in the clinical condition of the patient but, in the second stage, as the compensatory process becomes increasingly ineffective, headache and a depressed level of consciousness develop. The third stage of increasing intracranial pressure is characterized by further depression of consciousness, increased systemic arterial blood pressure (SABP), bradycardia, and irregular respiration. In the fourth or terminal stage there is deep coma, a progressive fall in systemic arterial blood pressure and the pupils become fixed and dilated (Plum and Posner 1980). The rise of intracranial pressure at this stage results in a fall in cerebral perfusion pressure (CPP) (CPP = SABP − ICP), with reduction in cerebral blood flow (CBF). The fall in cerebral perfusion pressure that accompanies a rise in intracranial pressure is recognized as being just as important as the rise in intracranial pressure itself.

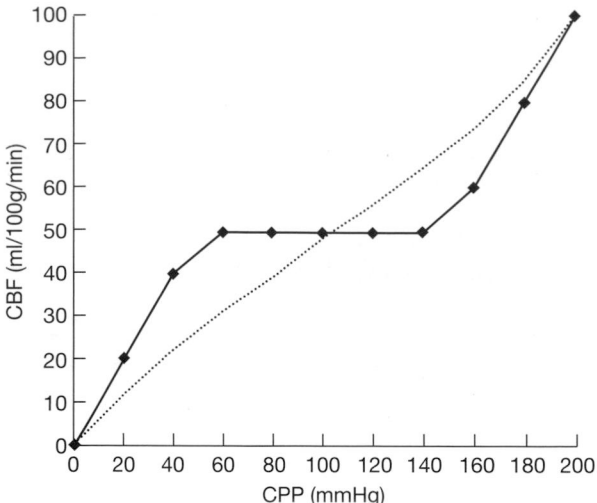

Fig. 17.1. Autoregulation of cerebral blood flow. Cerebral blood flow remains constant over a range of cerebral perfusion pressure from 50 to 150 mmHg. When normal autoregulation is lost, cerebral blood flow becomes passively dependent on cerebral perfusion pressure (dotted line).

This fall in cerebral perfusion pressure will be particularly dangerous if autoregulation of cerebral blood flow is lost (Fig. 17.1). For these reasons the management of cerebral perfusion pressure is now considered to be more important than the management of intracranial pressure alone (Robertson *et al.* 1998). Evidence from randomized controlled trials shows that cerebral perfusion pressure should be maintained above 60 mmHg if secondary insults to the brain are to be avoided.

17.1.2 The general effects of mass lesions

Initially, a slowly growing mass plays a relatively small part in raising intracranial pressure. Because of the partial division of the cranial cavity into compartments by the falx and tentorium, the local rise of pressure is partly confined to the cranial compartment; this is in contrast to the increased pressure throughout

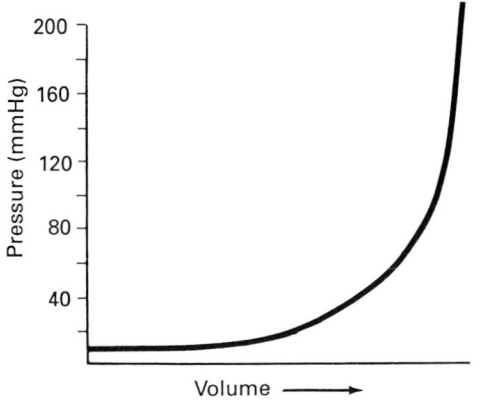

Fig. 17.2. Relationship between intracranial pressure and the volume of a space-occupying lesion (Reproduced from Miller and Adams (1972) by kind permission of the authors, editors, and publisher.)

the craniospinal axis, which is usually produced by diffuse cerebral oedema, or to that which can be produced, for instance, following intracerebral haemorrhage (ICH) or subarachnoid haemorrhage (SAH). A rapid rise in intracranial pressure follows a simulated intracerebral haemorrhage (Bullock *et al.* 1984). The rate of expansion of the mass determines the effectiveness of the compensatory mechanisms. A very slow-growing mass (e.g. a meningioma) reaches a large size without altering cerebral perfusion pressure or intracranial pressure, while a rapidly expanding mass (e.g. a haematoma) produces a large rise in intracranial pressure and a fall in cerebral perfusion pressure. Nevertheless, as compensation fails and the mass of the lesion increases, a volume/pressure curve can be derived, confirming the initial slight rise in intracranial pressure followed by an exponential increase, as it grows larger (Fig. 17.2). As the intracranial pressure rises, cerebral perfusion pressure falls: maintenance of higher levels of cerebral perfusion pressure is associated with a better outcome in patients with head injury (Rosner and Rosner 1991; Chambers 1998). The intracranial pressure waveform is a function of the arterial pressure waveform. Spectral analysis of these waves has shown six harmonic components; amplitude transfer functions can be clearly separated into four types, which reflect the degree of vascular compliance of the cerebral circulation (Piper and Miller 1995). The recognition of the importance of cerebral perfusion pressure has made it possible to correlate marginally reduced cerebral perfusion in head-injured patients with transcranial Doppler and jugular venous oxygen measurements (Chan *et al.* 1993).

Brain herniation

Progressive expansion of the mass leads to herniation of brain tissue from the compartment in which the mass lesion lies. The principal herniation sites are: of the cingulate gyrus beneath the falx cerebri (subfalcine herniation); of the medial temporal lobe through the tentorial hiatus (tentorial herniation); or of the cerebellar tonsils into the foramen magnum (the cerebellar pressure cone). In these circumstances, pressure gradients develop between the various intracranial compartments, depending upon that in which the mass lesion lies. The effects of these lesions will be considered later. Thus an early effect of a mass lesion is to displace CSF from the cranial cavity. Lumbar puncture carries grave risks in any tumour suspect, as the removal of fluid with resultant reduced pressure in the lumbar theca may induce herniation. Additionally, it must be noted that mass lesions, depending upon their situation, can also obstruct the outflow of CSF from one lateral ventricle (due to pressure occlusion of the foramen of Monro), from the third ventricle (due to occlusion of the aqueduct), or from the fourth ventricle, giving rise to hydrocephalus with dilatation of one or more of the ventricles, thus causing an even greater increase in intracranial pressure.

Circulatory effects

The effect of intracranial pressure upon the cerebral circulation is also important. Compression of venous sinuses and cortical veins increases venous pressure, thus contributing to the rise in intracranial pressure. Also, it is one factor responsible for inducing cerebral oedema, an important complication of intracranial mass lesions, which is often most severe in the neighbourhood of the tumour. Thus, brain swelling may be due either to vascular mechanisms (Bouma *et al.* 1993) or to brain oedema (Marmarou *et al.* 1993). Compression of arteries may reduce blood flow focally or generally (if there is a fall in cerebral perfusion pressure) and infarction may result. A fall in cerebral perfusion pressure below 50 mmHg has been shown to reduce cerebral blood flow (CBF).

However, in head injury, subarachnoid haemorrhage, and intracerebral haemorrhage, normal autoregulation is lost (Fig. 17.1) and higher levels of cerebral perfusion pressure may be needed to maintain cerebral blood flow. Arterial hypertension may develop as a compensatory mechanism, the Cushing response, partially in attempted compensation for the increased cerebral arterial resistance and so as to increase cerebral perfusion pressure (Cushing 1902; Fitch and McDowall 1977; Fitch *et al.* 1977). There may also be electrocardiographic abnormalities such as prominent V-waves, ST–T segment changes, notched T-waves, and prolonged (or shortened) Q–T intervals (Jachuck *et al.* 1975). Any arrhythmia may develop, particularly if there is associated haemorrhage. The rise in systemic arterial blood pressure, and perhaps the electro-cardiographic changes, are thought to result, at least in part, from medullary ischaemia due to stretching of perforating branches of the basilar artery, induced in turn by downward brainstem displacement (Fitch *et al.* 1977). The situation may also be influenced by the cerebral vasodilatation induced by hypercapnia or hypoxia. These, in turn, may be a consequence of the respiratory irregularities induced by intracranial pressure. However, these factors, like volatile anaesthetic agents, also increase intracranial pressure. Conversely, hyperventilation and consequent hypocapnia reduce it, as do hypothermia, hyperbaric oxygen, and some drugs.

Skull rigidity

The effects of the rigidity of the skull must also be considered. That of the adult is rigid and unyielding. So, as the intracranial pressure rises, an important consequence visible radiologically is that chronic downward pressure, sometimes of a dilated third ventricle, upon the sella turcica may initially cause decalcification and later erosion of the posterior clinoid processes. Sometimes the sella enlarges, occasionally resulting in an empty sella syndrome (Foley and Posner 1975), occasionally with clinical manifestations of hypopituitarism.

By contrast, non-union of the cranial sutures in infants provides a partial safety valve, so that increased intracranial pressure leads to increased head circumference. This often occurs in hydrocephalus. In children a rise in intracranial pressure may lead to separation of the cranial sutures. Premature union of the sutures (craniostenosis) causes a marked increase in intracranial pressure because skull growth is arrested while a normal brain is still increasing in size.

Symptoms

Symptoms of chronic elevation of intracranial pressure are headache, vomiting, papilloedema, and depression of con-

sciousness. The headache associated with an increased intracranial pressure, especially when resulting from mass lesions, is mainly due to compression or distortion of the dura mater and of the pain-sensitive intracranial blood vessels. It is often paroxysmal, at first worse on waking or after recumbency, throbbing in character, corresponding with the arterial pressure wave. Exertion, coughing, sneezing, vomiting, straining, or sudden changes in posture accentuate it. Such headache is often frontal or occipital or both. Its distribution is of little localizing value, though it is occasionally unilateral, occurring upon the side of the mass lesion. Lesions in the posterior fossa often give suboccipital headache, and may give warning of the presence of a cerebellar pressure cone if there is associated neck stiffness or if pain is increased by attempted neck flexion. The vomiting that accompanies increased intracranial pressure often occurs in the mornings when the headache is at its height. It is generally attributed to compression or ischaemia of the vomiting centre in the medulla oblongata. Similarly, the bradycardia, which is also common, results from dysfunction in the cardiac centre but, in some patients with infratentorial lesions, tachycardia eventually develops.

Papilloedema (Section 8.4.3) develops more rapidly with mass lesions in the posterior fossa because of their especial tendency to cause sudden obstructive hydrocephalus. In contrast, it often appears late in patients with prefrontal lesions. Obstruction of CSF flow in the subarachnoid space and impaired absorption both appear to be important factors in patients with tumours (Van Crevel 1979). Papilloedema is sometimes worse on one side, but it is rarely unilateral, except in the uncommon Foster Kennedy syndrome in which a subfrontal neoplasm on one side, often a meningioma, may compress the ipsilateral optic nerve, giving optic atrophy on that side and papilloedema on the other.

Breathing control is often impaired. Slow and deep respiratory movements often accompany a sudden rise in intracranial pressure sufficient to impair consciousness. Later, breathing may become irregular, Cheyne–Stokes respiration, and periods of apnoea then alternate with phases during which breathing waxes and wanes in amplitude. Central neurogenic hyperventilation, or so-called apneustic or ataxic breathing, are less common effects of brainstem compression or distortion but, in terminal coma, breathing is often rapid or shallow. These abnormalities of respiratory rate and rhythm may be due to compression or distortion of the brainstem. More often they result from median raphe haemorrhages or infarcts in the midbrain and pons, themselves resulting from tentorial herniation.

'False localizing signs' may also arise as a consequence of a sustained rise in intracranial pressure. These include unilateral or bilateral sixth-nerve palsies due to compression of the trunks of one or both nerves as they cross the apex of the petrous temporal bone, and bilateral extensor plantar responses or grasp reflexes resulting from ventricular dilatation in hydrocephalus, a third-nerve palsy. Less common false localizing signs include facial pain or sensory loss due to compression of the Gasserian ganglion in tentorial herniation; an ipsilateral

extensor plantar response due to compression of the opposite cerebral peduncle against the free tentorial edge in tentorial herniation (Kernohan's sign); signs of cerebellar dysfunction rarely resulting from a massive frontal lesion and due to downward displacement of the brainstem; and bilateral, fixed, dilated pupils or defects of upward conjugate gaze due to a central cerebellar lesion displacing the midbrain upwards.

17.1.3 Cerebral herniations

Subfalcine herniations

Subfalcine herniations, that is herniation of the cingulate gyrus beneath the free edge of the falx cerebri, can be identified by angiography or magnetic resonance imaging (MRI). The ipsilateral lateral ventricle is often reduced in size. Usually there are no specific clinical features. Focal necrosis may affect the cingulate gyrus, or extensive frontal infarction may result from compression of the pericallosal arteries.

Tentorial herniation

Tentorial herniation most often develops as a consequence of lesions in the temporal lobe but may complicate any supratentorial mass lesion. As the herniated medial temporal lobe descends in the tentorial hiatus, the midbrain is pushed to the opposite side and downwards, and the opposite cerebral peduncle is compressed against the free edge of the contralateral tentorium. As a result, the aqueduct becomes compressed, and the ipsilateral third nerve is compressed against the tentorial edge, giving first a dilated, fixed pupil and later other signs of a third-nerve palsy. There may be grooving of the uncus and hippocampal gyrus with focal necrosis or infarction.

As herniation increases, there is further downward displacement of the brainstem. The principal complications of this process are: paresis or paralysis of upward conjugate gaze due to compression of the tectal plate; pressure upon one or both posterior cerebral arteries, giving unilateral or bilateral occipital-lobe infarction with consequent hemianopia or cortical blindness; and, most importantly, median raphe haemorrhages or infarction in the brainstem, due to venous obstruction or more often to shearing effects upon perforating branches of the basilar artery, so that irreversible coma results from necrosis of the reticular substance (Zulch *et al.* 1974; Plum and Posner 1980).

Tonsillar herniation

Tonsillar herniation, a cerebellar pressure cone through the foramen magnum, may complicate supratentorial, or particularly infratentorial, lesions. It produces haemorrhagic infarction of the cerebellar tonsils and also compression of the medulla with respiratory and/or cardiac arrest and death, when there is associated downward displacement of the brainstem.

17.1.4 Infratentorial lesions

Infratentorial lesions tend to cause obstructive hydrocephalus because of tonsillar herniation and the effects upon the brain-

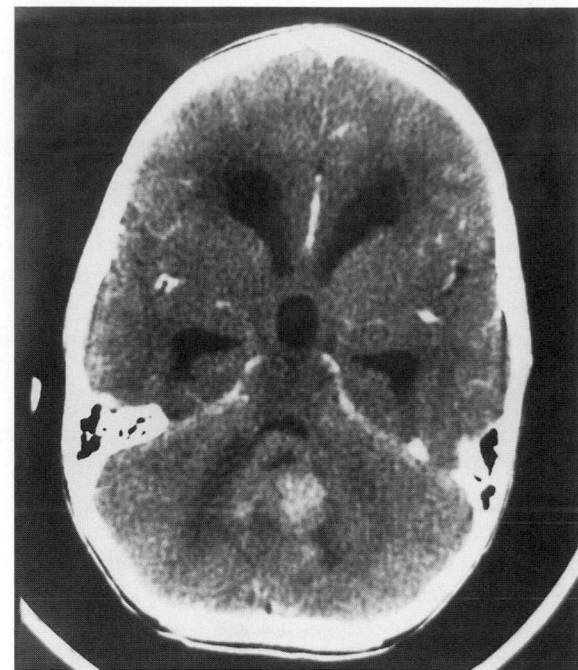

Fig. 17.3. CT scan showing obstructive hydrocephalus due to a posterior fossa tumour in the roof of the fourth ventricle (with contrast enhancement). Note the periventricular lucencies surrounding the frontal horns of the lateral ventricles representing interstitial oedema.

stem, aqueduct, and fourth ventricle (Fig. 17.3). Medullary or cerebellar infarction may occur due to compression of the medulla in the foramen magnum or compression of the posterior inferior cerebellar arteries. Sometimes reversed tentorial herniation occurs, with upward displacement of the brainstem and of the posterior fossa contents. This causes infarction of the superior aspects of the cerebellar hemispheres due to compression of the superior cerebellar arteries. Distortion of the hippocampal gyri due to upward pressure is rarely seen.

17.1.5 Benign intracranial hypertension

This disorder was recognized in the pre-CT scan era as one in which there was high intracranial pressure with no mass lesion, initially called pseudotumour cerebri. It was sometimes known as 'otitic hydrocephalus' because of its association with chronic ear disease. The term 'benign intracranial hypertension' (Section 3.6.3) was used to describe a persistent rise of CSF pressure in the absence of a space-occupying lesion and with ventricles of normal or even reduced size (Foley 1955). Usually it occurs in women, with a peak incidence in the third and fourth decades. They are often obese, and there is an association with oral contraceptive usage, pregnancy, and miscarriage. In a smaller group, affecting the sexes equally, there is a previous history of middle-ear disease, non-specific infection, or mild head injury. The condition may occur in children (1/100 000 annually) and girls are three times more likely to be affected than boys (Gordon 1997). It has been suggested that benign intracranial hypertension is associated with brain swelling, possibly related to increased venous pressure from raised intra-abdominal pressure (Sugerman *et al.* 1997). Many other patho-

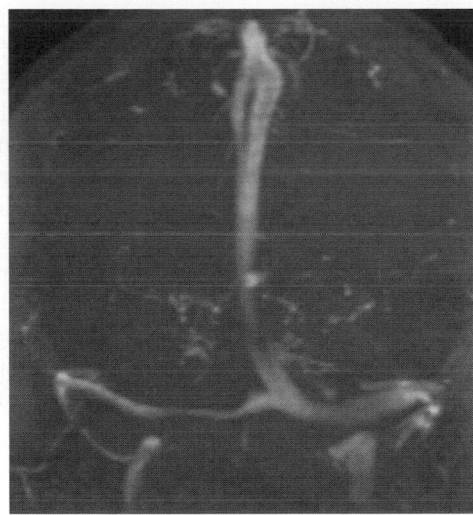

Fig. 17.4. MR angiogram showing unilateral stenosis of the transverse sinus.

genetic associations have been postulated to explain this brain swelling, including hypervitaminosis A (Feldman and Schlezinger 1970), the administration of a variety of antibiotics, an abnormality of the cerebral microvasculature with increased water content of the brain (Raichle *et al.* 1978), increased CSF production associated with an increase in circulating oestrogen (Donaldson 1981), and increased CSF outflow resistance (Johnston and Paterson 1974; Aisenberg and Rottenberg 1980). The CT scan has shown that the ventricles are usually small (Reid *et al.* 1980). The brain swelling in benign intracranial hypertension is not associated with any MRI evidence of a structural abnormality, white matter oedema, or cerebral venous sinus thrombosis. The cerebrospinal fluid (CSF) is acellular and usually has a slightly low protein content. Other causes of raised intracranial pressure without an intracranial mass lesion or ventricular enlargement include venous thrombosis of the transverse or sigmoid sinus (Section 27.11), chronic infective or neoplastic meningitis, or other causes of high protein in the CSF (Chapter 33). These conditions can usually be distinguished by anatomic MRI or MR angiography (Fig. 17.4) and CSF analysis. Head injury with a depressed fracture over a venous sinus may also produce intracranial hypertension.

Headache is the most commonest complaint, and often having a vascular character or the classical headache of raised intracranial pressure (Section 3.6.3). It is sometimes associated with postural obscuration of vision and occasional vomiting. There can be facial numbness or diplopia related to a sixth-nerve palsy. However, apart from tinnitus, other cranial nerve abnormalities are uncommon. By definition, papilloedema is expected, but there may be cases of headache with documented raised intracranial pressure without papilloedema. In the acute stage papilloedema may constitute a serious threat to vision, due either to associated peripapillary haemorrhages or to enlargement of the blind spot, which eventually may encroach on the macula. Blindness or permanent central scotomas occur.

Usually the condition is benign if appropriately treated, with a good prognosis (Bulens *et al.* 1979).

Imaging with CT or MRI shows no abnormality and MR angiography helps to exclude any sinus thrombosis that may require treatment with anticoagulants. Full blood count, and a hypercoagulable tendency should be checked. Frequent monitoring of the visual acuity and documentation of the visual fields is important to assess the response to treatment.

The mainstay of treatment in obese patients is weight reduction, and can be successful (Johnson *et al.* 1998). Weight reduction after gastric surgery has been reported to be very successful in resistant cases, all showing resolution of cranial nerve dysfunction (Sugerman *et al.* 1999). Oral contraception should be stopped. However, if vision is threatened, emergency reduction of intracranial pressure is essential: this can be achieved simply by doing a lumbar puncture, a series of lumbar punctures, or by inserting a lumbar drain or lumbar–subcutaneous shunt. More permanent CSF diversion can be achieved with lumbar–peritoneal or ventricular–peritoneal shunting, although the latter may be difficult because of the very small ventricles in some cases. Treatment of any underlying cause is important. Acetazolamide has also been used with some success (Johnson *et al.* 1998). In severe benign intracranial hypertension, treatment with lumbar puncture and high doses of the steroid dexamethasone (4 mg four times a day) will rapidly reduce intracranial pressure, cerebral oedema, and the threat to vision. In occasional cases with severe papilloedema leading to rapidly failing vision, additional shunting procedures may be needed as an emergency measure. Surgical treatments include optic nerve sheath fenestration (Sallomi *et al.* 1998) and subtemporal decompression (Kessler *et al.* 1998). The more radical surgical interventions are for refractory cases with threatened vision when less invasive interventions have failed.

17.2 Cerebral oedema

Knowledge about brain oedema has changed dramatically with recent developments in MRI (Marmarou *et al.* 1997; Kuroiwa *et al.* 2000). Cerebral oedema accompanies many brain pathologies and contributes to the resultant morbidity and mortality (Katzman *et al.* 1977; Marmarou *et al.* 2000). It plays a major role in head injury, stroke, and brain tumour, brain abscess, encephalitis, meningitis, lead encephalopathy, hypertensive encephalopathy, hypoxia, hypo-osmolality, dialysis dysequilibrium, diabetic ketoacidosis, and obstructive hydrocephalus. Brain oedema can now be measured accurately *in vivo* with MRI (Marmarou *et al.* 2000). The distribution of water in neurons, glia, endothelial cells, and in the interstitial spaces can be determined with diffusion-weighted imaging (DWI). The oscillation of water molecules depends upon the space available within and between cells: when space is limited, movement of molecules is limited and this 'squeeze' can be measured with MRI and expressed as activated diffusion coefficients (ADC). So, if cells fill with water (*cytotoxic oedema*), they swell and reduce the interstitial space, thus reducing the activated diffusion coefficient. This ability to oscillate determines the diffusion of water molecules, so that diffusion-weighted imaging measures the interstitial water content. When the interstitial space becomes filled with water, for example around a brain tumour, the activated diffusion coefficient increases because water molecules are free to oscillate and diffuse over greater distances. This type of intercellular oedema is known as *vasogenic oedema* and is associated with an increased activated diffusion coefficient.

Brain oedema must be distinguished from engorgement due to an increase in the blood volume of the brain due to venous obstruction or vasodilatation. However, prolonged venous engorgement may lead to brain oedema. If localized or mildly generalized, oedema produces few symptoms and signs. If severe, it may cause major focal signs if it is localized to one cerebral hemisphere, and if generalized, it can give rise to the brain herniation described above.

Cerebral oedema was subclassified initially into vasogenic, cellular or cytotoxic, and interstitial (or hydrocephalic) types (Klatzo 1967; Fishman 1980). A better understanding also comes from classifying brain oedema as open-barrier (vasogenic) and closed-barrier (cytotoxic) oedema (Betz *et al.* 1989).

17.2.1 Vasogenic (open-barrier) oedema

The vasogenic variety of oedema, associated with increased capillary permeability and an open blood–brain barrier (BBB), is the most common form observed in clinical practice. It occurs in conditions such as tumour, abscess, haemorrhage, infarction, contusion, and purulent meningitis. The oedema is usually localized around the primary lesion. This produces focal symptoms and signs that are often more due to the oedema than to the primary lesion. It is associated with increased activated diffusion coefficients on diffusion-weighted imaging. Open-barrier oedema is much more likely to respond to intervention with steroids such as dexamethasone than the other types of cerebral oedema that are considered below.

17.2.2 Cytotoxic (closed-barrier) oedema

Cellular, or cytotoxic, oedema is characterized by swelling of all the cellular elements of the brain—neurons, glia, and endothelial cells—with an associated reduction in extracellular fluid but with an intact blood–brain barrier. It resembles that due to water intoxication in experimental animals, or that induced experimentally by triethyl tin, in which, however, there are also vacuoles and clefts in the cerebral white matter. It is characterized by swelling of all the cellular elements of the brain, with an associated reduction in extracellular fluid but with an intact blood–brain barrier. The activated diffusion coefficient on diffusion-weighted imaging is reduced. It occurs clinically in diffuse brain hypoxia, acute hypo-osmolality due to dilutional hyponatraemia, sodium depletion, or excess antidiuretic hormone (ADH) secretion, or in osmotic disequilibrium syndromes, such as in haemodialysis or diabetic ketoacidosis. The clinical manifestations are usually more generalized than in vasogenic oedema, and include drowsiness, stupor or coma, and sometimes convulsions. In ischaemic states a combination

of vasogenic and cytotoxic oedema is often seen. The ultrastructural and molecular mechanisms occurring in the cell membrane are now becoming understood. Ischaemia results in the release of lactate and excitatory amino acids, glutamate and aspartate, which open receptor-activated calcium channels. In contrast, lactate does not rise very much or very early in traumatic oedema, which may therefore be different from ischaemic oedema (Eriskat *et al.* 2000). The influx of calcium leads to the activation of α-amino-hydroxyl-methyl proprionic acid (AMPA) and metabotropic receptors, with upregulation of genes, which may activate lysozymes, with resultant apoptosis. Massive increases in calcium lead to mitochondrial dysfunction, energy failure, cell membrane rupture, and necrosis. In Reye's syndrome, the oedema is cytotoxic and resembles that of triethyl tin intoxication.

17.2.3 Interstitial oedema

Interstitial or hydrocephalic oedema simply identifies the increased water content of the periventricular brain (largely extracellular), which is seen in hydrocephalus. The main site of accumulation of water is periventricular and manifests itself on CT scan as periventricular lucency (Fig. 17.3).

Recognition of the type of oedema has implications with respect to treatment. High doses of steroids (dexamethasone, betamethasone) are of proven efficacy in most forms of vasogenic oedema but not in cytotoxic oedema. In cytotoxic oedema, osmotherapy with hypertonic mannitol or diuretics such as frusemide may be useful. While neuroprotective drugs appear to protect animals from the most severe effects of cerebral ischaemia, their role in the management of brain oedema is still uncertain. This applies particularly to the oedema seen with head injury, where prospective randomized controlled trials of steroids, barbiturates, *N*-methyl-D-aspartate (NMDA) receptor antagonists, and calcium antagonists have been shown not to improve outcome (Ward *et al.* 1985; European Study Group on Nimodipine 1994; Yates *et al.* 1999; Iannotti 2000).

17.3 Hydrocephalus

Hydrocephalus literally means water on the brain (Greek). As a definition, this is non-specific because atrophic dementia results in a passive increase in the volume of CSF in the head and such patients also have large ventricles but do not have hydrocephalus. Rather, hydrocephalus should be defined as an increase in the volume of the CSF within the skull due to an abnormality in its production, circulation, or absorption. This definition embraces those conditions in which there is at some stage an increased volume, and usually pressure, of CSF within the cranial cavity.

17.3.1 Aetiology

Hydrocephalus may be due to:

(1) increased formation of CSF;

(2) obstruction to the flow of fluid at some point between the choroid plexuses of the lateral ventricles from which it is secreted and the arachnoidal villi in the sagittal sinus through which it is reabsorbed; and

(3) impaired absorption of the fluid due to inflammation of the arachnoid (as in meningitis) or to thrombosis of the sagittal sinus.

Normal-pressure hydrocephalus is a clinical syndrome characterized by dementia, gait apraxia, and urinary incontinence (Section 17.3.8).

Increased formation of CSF

Increased formation of CSF occurs with a choroid plexus papilloma (Guthkelch and Riley 1969). In such cases, removal of the tumour is usually curative, but occasionally hydrocephalus persists despite successful removal (McDonald 1969). Another rare syndrome of overproduction of CSF with deficient absorption is due to squamous metaplasia of the arachnoid villi (Davson et al. 1986) but whether it occurs in humans remains undecided.

Obstruction

Obstruction to the CSF circulation may occur at any point of its course. Within the ventricles the most common cause is a neoplasm compressing one or both interventricular foramina or filling the third ventricle. The cerebral aqueduct may be obstructed by a tumour arising in the third ventricle, midbrain, or pineal body, or may be congenitally narrowed or even absent. Owing to its small calibre, slight swelling of its ependymal lining may lead to aqueduct obstruction, and cases have been reported in which hydrocephalus has been due to gliosis caused by ependymitis in this region. Aqueduct stenosis is a cause of infantile hydrocephalus but may give rise to increased intracranial pressure for the first time in adult life (Harrison et al. 1974).

Posterior fossa tumours

Posterior fossa tumours may obstruct the fourth ventricle. Its foramina may be blocked by a congenital septum (the Dandy–Walker syndrome), by adhesions following meningitis, or by displacement of the medulla into the foramen magnum by the pressure of a tumour. The Dandy–Walker syndrome may be due to atresia of the foramina of Magendie and Luschka or to dysplasia of the cerebellum developing early in fetal life, as the cerebellar vermis is often absent or vestigial in such cases (Hart et al. 1972). The malformation may be accompanied by extra-axial leptomeningeal cysts in the posterior fossa (Haller et al. 1971), while such cysts alone may give a similar clinical and radiological picture. Within the subarachnoid space, obstruction may again be due to tumour, to traumatic adhesions, parasitic cysts (Kuper et al. 1958; Allcutt and Coulthard 1991), inflammation, haemorrhage, or to congenital abnormalities such as basilar impression or the Arnold–Chiari malformation.

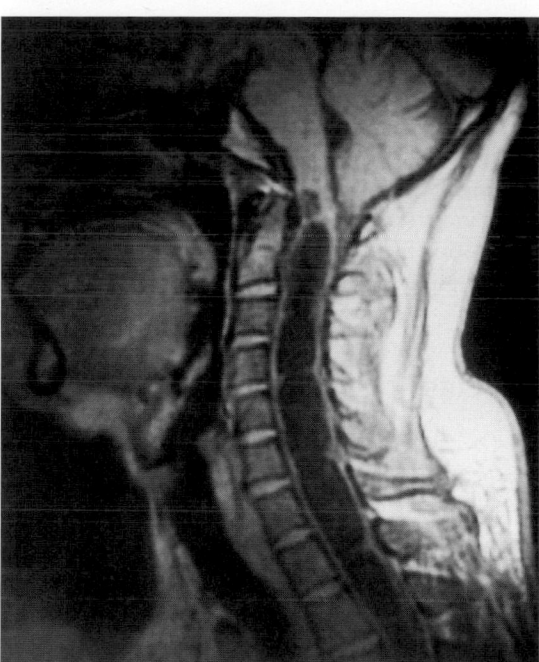

Fig. 17.5. Magnetic resonance image showing a sagittal section of the nervous system in a case of the Arnold–Chiari malformation. Note the abnormally low cerebellar tonsils and the syrinx within the cervical cord.

The Arnold–Chiari malformation

The Arnold–Chiari malformation (Section 4.5.5) consists of congenital displacement of the cerebellar tonsils and of an elongated medulla oblongata downwards into the cervical canal (Fig. 17.5; see also Fig. 4.2). It prevents the egress of CSF from the fourth ventricle into the subarachnoid space. It is sometimes associated with lumbosacral spina bifida and with meningocele or meningomyelocele. When the caudal displacement of the cerebellar tonsils, fourth ventricle, and medulla into the cervical canal is associated with myelodysplasia, they may extend down to the mid-cervical region, and this anomaly is known as a Chiari type II. The Chiari type I anomaly is a simple ectasia of the cerebellar tonsils (down to C1) without any other primary malformation of the neuraxis. Congenital narrowing of the cerebral aqueduct sufficient to cause hydrocephalus was found in 10 of 20 such cases. MacFarlane and Maloney (1957) suggested that a Chiari malformation or, less often, the Dandy–Walker syndrome may result in dilatation of the central canal of the spinal cord early in life (hydromyelia) and that this is probably the most common mechanism causing syringomyelia (Gardner 1965).

The arachnoid villi

The arachnoid villi may be obstructed by inflammatory, neoplastic, or leukaemic cells in infective or neoplastic meningitis. Obstruction of the subarachnoid space and the arachnoid villi by blood accounts for the hydrocephalus seen with subarachnoid haemorrhage and head injury. Absorption of fluid from the arachnoid villi may also be restricted by a rise in the intracranial venous pressure, by compression of venous sinuses by an intracranial tumour, or by impairment of venous drainage from the head due to raised intrathoracic pressure in cases of intrathoracic neoplasm or pulmonary hypertension. In general, venous obstruction results in brain swelling with a reduction in the size of the ventricles. Thrombosis of the superior sagittal sinus (Section 27.11), caused by extension of inflammation from the transverse sinus, is one cause of the condition 'otitic hydrocephalus', in which symptoms of hydrocephalus complicate otitis media or mastoiditis (Symonds 1937).

17.3.2 Classification

Hypertensive hydrocephalus can be further subdivided into:

1. *Obstructive hydrocephalus* (once called internal hydrocephalus, and also known as non-communicating hydrocephalus), in which there is an obstruction to the circulation of the CSF, either within the ventricles or aqueduct, or at the outlet from the fourth ventricle. It prevents free communication between the ventricles and the subarachnoid space.

2. *Communicating hydrocephalus* (once called external hydrocephalus, and also known as non-obstructive hydrocephalus), in which hydrocephalus is due either to disturbance in the formation and absorption of CSF, or to an obstruction to its circulation in the subarachnoid space itself.

Congenital abnormalities are the most common cause of obstructive hydrocephalus in autopsy series, especially in neonates and perinatally (Pinar *et al.* 1998). In 100 consecutive post-mortem examinations, malformation was the sole cause in only 14 per cent of cases, but in association with infection or trauma it accounted for 46 per cent (Laurence 1969). Inflammatory reaction due to infection or haemorrhage but without malformation accounted for another 50 per cent, the remaining 4 per cent being due to tumours.

In the past, a distinction was often made between 'congenital' and 'acquired' hydrocephalus, but this distinction is artificial. A congenital abnormality alone is the most likely cause of hydrocephalus developing before birth, but congenital and acquired factors often both contribute to hydrocephalus in infancy. Nor do congenital factors cease to operate later, since hydrocephalus developing in adult life may be the late result of aqueduct stenosis or Chiari malformation.

The more common causes of hydrocephalus developing in the absence of congenital abnormality are meningeal adhesions following meningitis or haemorrhage, arachnoiditis of obscure origin, thrombosis of intracranial venous sinuses, and intracranial tumour. Chronic inflammatory meningitis or arachnoiditis following tuberculosis are rare causes. Obstruction within the third or fourth ventricle or in the subarachnoid space, may be due occasionally to parasitic cysts.

17.3.3 Incidence

The incidence of all neural malformations, including hydrocephalus, varies considerably between different countries, being much higher, for instance, in Scotland and Ireland than in Japan. In the United States, between 1958 and 1995, 12.4 per cent of all congenital malformations of the central nervous system were due to hydrocephalus (Pinar *et al.* 1998). The incidence is higher in the east, and especially the north-east, than elsewhere (Kurtzke *et al.* 1973). In China the incidence was 0.89 per 1000 births (Hu *et al.* 1996). In Sweden the rate increased from the 1970s to the 1980s, partly due to an increase in ventricular haemorrhage among preterm infants, but declined again in the 1990s (6.99, 25.37, 13.69 per 1000, respectively) (Fernell and Hagberg 1998). The incidence is lower in Eastern Europe (0.44/1000) (Sipek *et al.* 1998) and higher in the Middle East (Rajab *et al.* 1998).

17.3.4 Pathophysiology

The rate of at which hydrocephalus develops determines the ventricular size. Acute obstructive hydrocephalus produces high intracranial pressure with only slight ventricular enlargement. Chronic obstruction may produce massive ventricles with only slightly elevated ICP. When obstruction occurs in the aqueduct, only the lateral and third ventricles are distended. When the obstruction is more caudal, the aqueduct and fourth ventricle may also be enlarged. Ventricular distension causes thinning of the cerebral hemispheres which, in severe cases, may be extreme, and is associated with marked atrophy of the white matter and loss of cortical ganglion cells. The ventricular ependyma is normal, except in inflammatory cases, when a localized or diffuse ependymitis may be present. Meningeal adhesions indicate previous meningitis. Distension of the ventricles leads to pressure upon the calvarium, which becomes thin, especially over the cerebral gyri. Separation of the sutures occurs when hydrocephalus develops in early life, but is not seen, as a rule, after adolescence. Compression of the base of the skull causes erosion of the clinoid processes and excavation of the sella turcica. The olfactory tracts and optic nerves are often atrophic.

17.3.5 Symptoms and signs

These are so dependent upon age and the deformability of the skull that it is useful to divide symptoms and signs into infantile and post-infantile. Nevertheless, infants with hydrocephalus may grow up with or without neurological and cognitive impairment, depending on the effectiveness and timeliness of treatment. The features of infantile hydrocephalus may therefore manifest in later life; leading to a degree of overlap when it comes to long-term disability.

17.3.6 Infantile hydrocephalus

Enlargement of the head is the most conspicuous sign in infantile hydrocephalus (Fig. 17.6) (Section 4.3.4). It is being diagnosed with increased frequency before birth. The disorder becomes evident during the first few weeks of life owing to the large head, prominent scalp veins, and down-turning of the

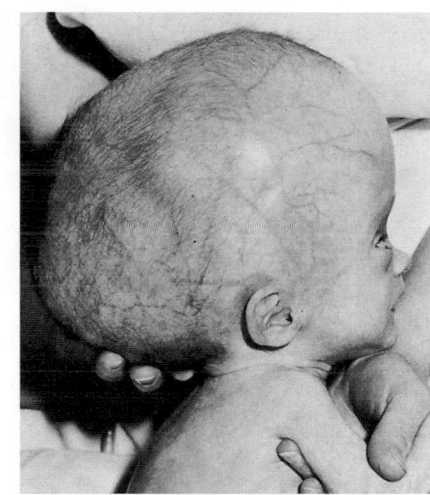

(a)

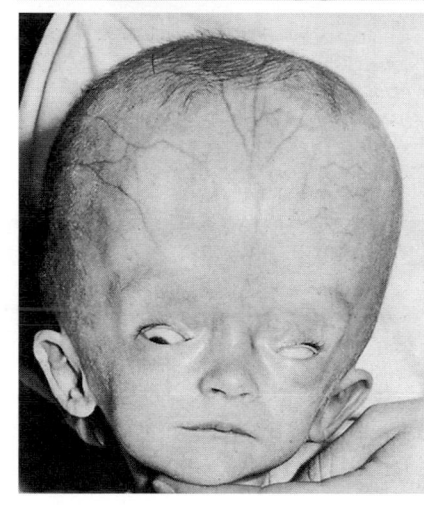

(b)

Fig. 17.6. (a) and (b) Gross enlargement of the head in an infant with obstructive hydrocephalus associated with lumbar meningomyelocele and an Arnold–Chiari malformation. (Photographs originally supplied by Mr L. P. Lassman.)

eyes, 'sun-setting sign'. It is slowly progressive. If untreated, the head may attain a huge size with a circumference of 75 cm or even more. The cranial sutures are widely separated and the anterior fontanelle is much enlarged. There is marked congestion of scalp veins. Enlargement of the head occurs in all diameters and in extreme cases it is translucent. The frontal region bulges forwards, and downward pressure upon the orbital plates causes the eyes to be protruded forwards and downwards. Fortunately such cases are rare today.

Owing to expansibility of the skull in infancy, symptoms of increased intracranial pressure are slight or absent. Hydrocephalic children seem little troubled by headache and rarely vomit. Convulsions are common. In neglected cases bilateral anosmia may occur. Optic atrophy due to pressure upon the nerves is usually present, but in rare cases there is papilloedema. Visual acuity may be progressively reduced until the child becomes blind. Paralysis of other cranial nerves may occur, and squint is not uncommon. Nystagmus may be present. In the limbs there are usually weakness and incoordination, generally more marked in the lower than in the upper limbs. Spasticity

with exaggeration of tendon reflexes is common in the lower limbs, although sometimes tendon reflexes are lost. The plantar reflexes are usually extensor. There may be little or no disturbance of sensibility. The mental state varies. In severe cases there is usually reduced cognitive function and poor memory, but in milder cases this is slight or absent. Intelligence in later life may be surprisingly unimpaired in some cases, even when ventricular dilatation has progressed such that only 1 cm thickness of cerebral substance remains between the ventricles and the inner skull table. In milder cases there may be obesity and/or diabetes insipidus, due to compression of the hypothalamus and pituitary, and, in more severe cases, wasting. Cerebrospinal fluid rhinorrhoea is a rare complication. A unique hydrocephalic 'bobble-head doll syndrome' is characterized by two to four oscillations of the head per minute with psychomotor retardation and results from obstructive lesions in or near the third ventricle or aqueduct (Tomasovic *et al.* 1975; Menkes 1980).

17.3.7 **Hydrocephalus after infancy**

The clinical picture of hydrocephalus developing after infancy varies according to its cause. In obstructive hydrocephalus, symptoms of increased intracranial pressure are conspicuous. Headache and vomiting are early symptoms and are often followed by the development of papilloedema. The headache is initially paroxysmal, but later becomes constant; there are sometimes intense exacerbations characterized by severe headache radiating down the neck associated with head retraction and even with opisthotonos, vomiting, and impairment of consciousness. Giddiness is a common symptom. Some mental deterioration usually occurs after a time, especially in later life. Hallucinations, delusions, and mood changes may occur. Convulsions are less common than in the infantile variety, and enlargement of the head does not occur after the age of 3 years, although slight separation of the sutures may occur until teenage years. In older children this slight separation of the cranial sutures yields a 'cracked-pot sound' on percussion and may be associated with venous congestion of the scalp. The skull remains of normal size following onset in adulthood, for instance in delayed presentation of cerebral aqueduct stenosis (Fig. 17.7). Cranial-nerve palsies may occur, especially paresis of the sixth and seventh nerves, and symptomatic trigeminal neuralgia or facial sensory loss have been reported (Maurice Williams and Pilling 1977). Slight exophthalmos is not uncommon. Gross weakness of the limbs is absent, though clumsiness and slight incoordination are common. The tendon reflexes may be exaggerated or diminished. The plantar reflexes are often extensor. There is usually no sensory loss. Symptoms of hypopituitarism, obesity, and genital atrophy are common in children and adolescents.

17.3.8 **Normal-pressure hydrocephalus**

A form of late-onset communicating hydrocephalus is called 'low-pressure hydrocephalus' since, although the ventricles are

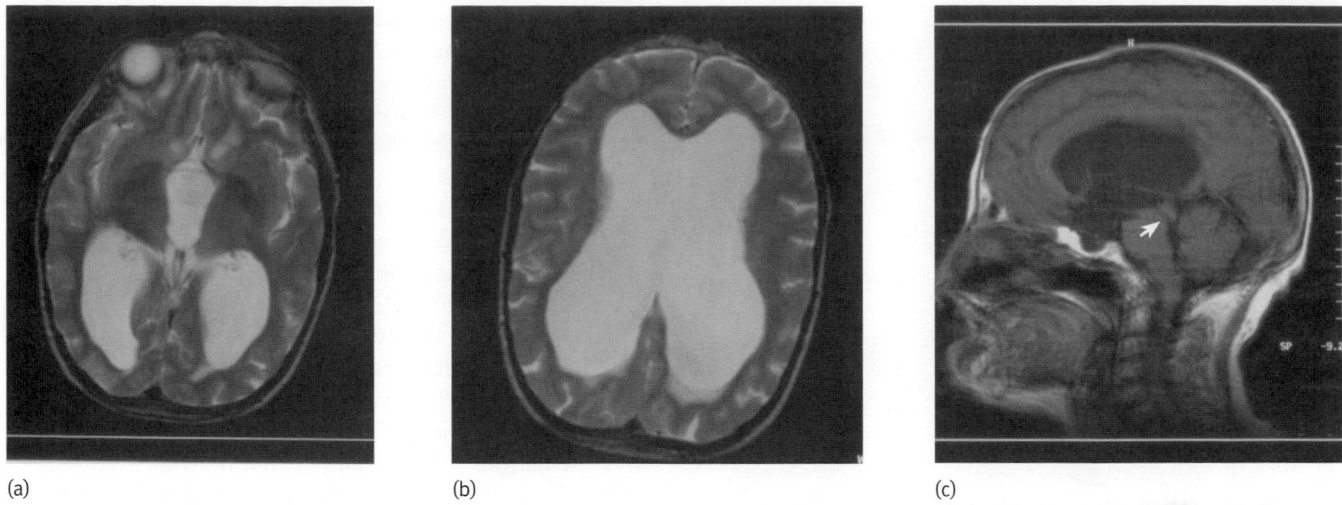

(a)   (b)   (c)

Fig. 17.7. Obstructive hydrocephalus due to aqueduct stenosis in a 50-year-old. (a) Enlargement of lateral and third ventricles (axial T2-weighted MRI). (b) Enlargement of lateral ventricles with some periventricular transudation (axial T2-weighted MRI). (c) Stenotic cerebral aqueduct (arrowed) causing distortion of the third ventricle with depression of the hypothalamic floor, widening of the chiasmatic and infundibular recesses, and erosion of the dorsum sella (midline sagittal T1-weighted MRI). (Courtesy of Dr P. Anslow.)

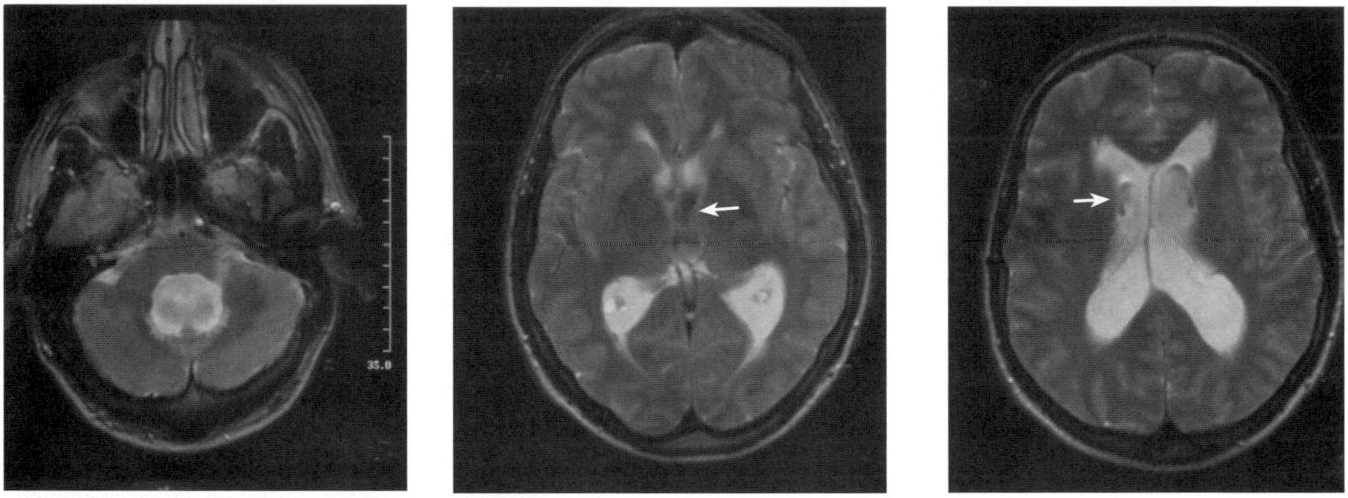

(a)   (b)   (c)

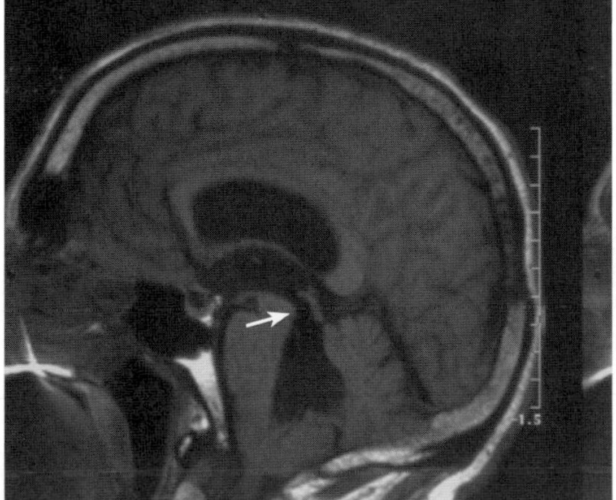

(d)

Fig. 17.8. Communicating or 'normal-pressure' hydrocephalus in a 50-year-old. (a) Enlargement of the fourth ventricle with turbulent CSF flow (axial T2-weighted MRI). (b) Enlargement of the lateral and third ventricles, with turbulent CSF in the third ventricle (arrow) (axial T2-weighted MRI). (c) Enlargement of the lateral ventricles with turbulent flow related to the interventricular foramina (arrow) axial T2-weighted MRI). (d) Distension of the third and fourth ventricles, and the cerebral aqueduct (arrow) (midline sagittal T1-weighted MRI). Note that MRI of communicating hydrocephalus shows distension of the cerebral aqueduct and fourth ventricle, and sometimes turbulent, flowing CSF. These are not features seen in obstructive hydrocephalus due to aqueduct stenosis (see Fig. 17.7). (Courtesy of Dr P. Anslow.)

dilated, the pressure within them at the time of measurement was either normal or only slightly raised (Hakim and Adams 1965). The clinical syndrome is characterized by the triad of progressive dementia, gait apraxia, and urinary incontinence. The CT scan has proved helpful but the findings are not invariably conclusive (Jacobs and Kinkel 1976). Large ventricles and small sulci shown on the CT or MRI, however, are suggestive of this condition (Fig. 17.8) and continuous intracranial monitoring has shown significant B waves for at least 2 hours a day (Symon et al. 1972; Crockard et al. 1977). This has been helpful in identifying patients who may benefit from surgery. Thus, while CSF pressure is usually normal or low, transient episodes of raised pressure occur in many cases. With MRI scanning it is possible to measure the volume of the ventricular CSF and to compare it with the volume of CSF in the subarachnoid spaces and fissures (Grant et al. 1987). In a large prospective study, the most reliable predictive feature of a good response to shunting was the absence of white matter changes on MRI scan (Pickard et al. 1992). The most widely accepted test by neurologists and neurosurgeons is the CSF tap test, where there is clinical improvement following a lumbar puncture (Wikkelso et al. 1982). Of all the tests available, the response to lumbar puncture is thought to be the most reliable (Vanneste and van Acker 1990). Serial psychometric tests are useful in assessing the response to treatment. These, together with a simple walking test, should be documented carefully before and after lumbar puncture (Singh and Crockard 1999).

The condition usually presents in middle or late life, sometimes with dementia alone (Crowell et al. 1973) or with the clinical picture of the parkinsonism–dementia complex (Sypert et al. 1973) and 'drop' attacks may occur (Botez et al. 1977). The cause of the communicating hydrocephalus is unexplained in most such cases, although it may follow subarachnoid haemorrhage or may develop many years after recovery from meningitis or head injury. Differential diagnosis from cerebral atrophy in dementia is clearly important, as shunting operations are of no value in the latter condition; however, no single method provides an absolutely reliable distinction.

17.3.9 **Radiological diagnosis**

Radiographs of the skull in hydrocephalus may show enlargement of the calvarium, with suture diastasis, thinning, and exaggeration of convolutional markings. However, this latter finding alone may be normal and is an unreliable guide to raised intracranial pressure. Separation of the sutures may be present in children. The clinoid processes are often eroded and the sella turcica is deepened and expanded anteroposteriorly. CT and MR imaging give a clear picture of the ventricular size, and often the underlying cause is identified (Figs. 17.7 and 17.8). MRI is superior to CT in identifying posterior fossa causes (Teasdale et al. 1989). The use of three-dimensional fast asymmetric spin-echo (FASE) MR imaging sequences strongly predicts a good response to shunting (Yoshihara et al. 1998). Other MRI techniques to evaluate CSF flow have yielded conflicting results (Bradley et al. 1996; Hakim and Black 1998).

17.3.10 **Monitoring/compliance**

The most frequent form of monitoring is measurement of the head circumference in infants. This is routine in most hospitals and in primary care. Deviation from the percentile for a particular child should trigger referral for further assessment. Also, regular measurement of head circumference allows the efficacy (or otherwise) of treatment to be monitored over time.

Intracranial pressure monitoring may be useful when there is uncertainty about the need for CSF diversion. This may take place via the chamber of a shunt or reservoir inserted specifically for this purpose. In normal-pressure hydrocephalus, intracranial pressure monitoring may be helpful, particularly if pressure waveform analysis is undertaken (Williams et al. 1998). Non-invasive intracranial pressure monitoring is possible via the fontanelle in infants or with the tympanic membrane displacement test in adults (Madan et al. 1998).

Compliance (the reciprocal of elastance) may reflect the reserve capacity to withstand small changes in volume. It can now be measured directly with a continuous compliance monitor (Piper et al. 2000).

17.3.11 **Prognosis**

It has been recognized for many years that untreated infantile hydrocephalus is fatal during the first few years of life, on average a hydrocephalic alive at 3 months has a 26 per cent chance of reaching adult life without surgery, and survival to between 1 and 2 years is associated with a 50 per cent chance of reaching adulthood (Macnab 1966). Some who survive have mental retardation, epilepsy, or blindness. Even with underlying aqueduct stenosis, the hydrocephalic process often arrests spontaneously (Laurence 1969). In 41 per cent of 70 cases without spina bifida the IQ after 6 years was over 85, in 29 per cent below 50. The severity of hydrocephalus bears a close relationship to IQ and physical disability such as spasticity and ataxia. In the past many children with the Arnold–Chiari malformation and myelomeningocele died from infection of the sac or hydrocephalus.

The introduction of ventricular diversion procedures reduced the mortality of hydrocephalus with myelomeningocele to 30 per cent at the end of 2 years, and that of uncomplicated hydrocephalus to less than 20 per cent. Two-thirds of such cases treated surgically had an IQ of 75 or more (Milhorat 1972). More recent figures have claimed IQs of more than 100 in 31 per cent and greater than 70 in 85 per cent. The prognosis of hydrocephalus after infancy depends upon its cause and how far this is amenable to treatment. In non-tumorous hydrocephalus, IQs were greater than 90 in 32 per cent and greater than 70 in 60 per cent (Hoppe-Hirsch et al. 1998). Also, adults who were treated for hydrocephalus due to spina bifida had poorer verbal and visuospatial memory performance than those with aqueduct stenosis (Hommet et al. 1999).

17.3.12 **Treatment by drainage**

In an emergency, obstructive hydrocephalus can be treated by ventricular drainage through a burrhole or twistdrill. Drainage is usually maintained for up to 5 days via a closed system with a fixed-height drip-chamber. By contrast, communicating hydrocephalus can be treated by lumbar puncture or via a lumbar drain, provided that imaging has excluded any intracranial mass or tonsillar herniation. This is often the case with subarachnoid haemorrhage or meningitis. Because they can be set-up under local anaesthesia, such drainage methods may be used in emergency situations and in patients unfit for general anaesthesia. Permanent CSF diversion requires a general anaesthetic.

17.3.13 **CSF diversion and shunts**

In the past many operations, including excision of the choroid plexus, Torkildsen's ventriculo-cisternostomy, ventriculo-subdural, ventriculo-ureteric, ventriculo-atrial and ventriculo-pleural drainage, were used, with varying degrees of success. Now there is general agreement that the treatment of choice is use of various shunts inserted into the lateral ventricle, with catheter drainage into the peritoneum. These shunts have differing hydrodynamic properties, which have been carefully evaluated (Czosnyka *et al.* 1998). Most of them have low hydrodynamic resistance so that flow increases due to a siphoning effect when connected to a long distal catheter. Some shunts are programmable but they are all susceptible to siphoning. Colonization of the valves with *Staphylococcus albus* or diphtheroids may be asymptomatic for some time. The UK shunt registry has documented varying infection and revision rates in the 44 UK units. Revision rates ranged from 18 to 70 per cent and infection rates from 0 to 21 per cent (Pickard 2000).

The appropriate treatment of hydrocephalus after infancy depends upon its cause. A causative intracranial tumour must receive appropriate surgical treatment whenever possible. When there is a tumour in the third ventricle or midbrain or in some other area that is causing obstruction but cannot be removed or treated effectively by radiotherapy, temporary improvement may result from a shunting operation with insertion of a ventriculo-peritoneal (VP) shunt.

While early reports of ventriculo-peritoneal shunting in cases of low-pressure hydrocephalus were encouraging, with about two-thirds of all patients showing early intellectual as well as physical improvement, after 3 years less than half demonstrated continuing benefit (Greenberg *et al.* 1977; Gustafson and Hagberg 1978). In yet another series of patients, only a third were improved, and 50 per cent of a similar group of patients not operated upon failed to deteriorate over a 3-year period; the surgical group also showed a high incidence of complications (Hughes *et al.* 1978). Thus early optimism has not been borne out by good long-term results in all cases. In some longstanding cases, there are irreversible neuropathological changes somewhat similar to those of Alzheimer's disease (Ball 1976), although this is an inevitable occurrence in any large group of patients presenting with mild dementia. With good clinical diagnostic criteria and a positive CSF tap test, shunting undoubtedly leads to improvement in many patients (Vanneste and van Acker 1990).

17.3.14 **Other treatments**

Third ventriculostomy has been reintroduced with advances in endoscopic techniques. It is particularly useful when hydrocephalus is due to aqueduct stenosis

Lumbo-peritoneal shunting is as successful as VP shunting in communicating hydrocephalus, normal-pressure hydrocephalus, and benign intracranial hypertension, and has the advantage of not requiring ventricular cannulation through brain tissue.

Rare underlying causes need to be considered in all cases of hydrocephalus and may need prolonged treatment in their own right. Examples include antituberculous treatment for tuberculous meningitis (Section 33.2.3) or praziquantel for parasitic cysts (Section 34.15.10).

References

Aisenberg, R. M. and Rottenberg, D. A. (1980). The pathogenesis of pseudotumor cerebri: a mathematical analysis. *J. Neurol. Sci.*, **48**, 51–60.

Allcutt, D. A. and Coulthard, A. (1991). Neurocysticercosis: regression of a fourth ventricular cyst with praziquantel. *J. Neurol. Neurosurg. Psychiat.*, **54**, 461–2.

Avezaat, C. J. J., Eijndhoven, J. H. Mv., Mass, A. I.R . *et al.* (1993). Cerebral perfusion pressure management of head injury. *Intracranial Pressure VIII; 1991 1993*. Springer Verlag, Rotterdam.

Ball, M. J. (1976). Neurofibrillary tangles in the dementia of normal pressure hydrocephalus. *Can. J. Neurol. Sci.*, **3**, 227–35.

Betz, A. L., Iannotti, F., and Hoff, J. T. (1989). Brain oedema: a classification based on blood–brain barrier integrity. *Cerebrovasc. Brain Metab. Rev.*, **1**, 133–54.

Botez, M. I., Ethier, R., Leveille, J. *et al.* (1977). A syndrome of early recognition of occult hydrocephalus and cerebral atrophy. *QJM*, **46**, 365–80.

Bouma, G. J., Muizelaar, J. P., Schuurman, R. *et al.* (1993). Cerebral blood volume in acute head injury: relationship to CBF and ICP. *Intracranial Pressure VIII*, pp. 529–34. Springer Verlag, Rotterdam.

Bradley, W. G. J., Scalzo, D., Queralt, J. *et al.* (1996). Normal pressure hydrocephalus: evaluation with cerebrospinal fluid flow measurements at MR imaging. *Radiology*, **198**, 523–9.

Bulens, C., de Vries, W. A., and Van Crevel, H. (1979). Benign intracranial hypertension: a retrospective and follow-up study. *J. Neurol. Sci.*, **40**, 147–57.

Bullock, R., Mendelow, A. D., Teasdale, G. M. *et al.* (1984). Intracranial haemorrhage induced at arterial pressure in the rat: Part 1. Description of technique, ICP changes and neurological findings. *Neurol. Res.*, **6**, 184–8.

Chambers, I. R. (1998). Outcome in head injured patients: ICP and CPP. Ph.D. thesis, University of Newcastle.

Chan, K., Dearden, N., Miller, J. *et al.* (1993). Multimodality monitoring as a guide to treatment of intracranial hypertension after severe brain injury. *Neurosurgery*, **32**, 547–52.

Crockard, H. A., Hanlon, K., Duda, E. E. *et al.* (1977). Hydrocephalus as a cause of dementia: evaluation by computerised tomography and intracranial pressure monitoring. *J. Neurol. Neurosurg. Psychiat.*, **40**, 736–40.

Crowell, R. M., Tew, J. M., and Mark, V. H. (1973). Aggressive dementia associated with normal pressure hydrocephalus. Report of two unusual cases. *Neurology*, **23**, 461–4.

Cushing, H. (1902). Some experimental and clinical observations concerning states of increased intracranial tension. *Am. J. Med. Sci.*, **124**, 375–400.

Czosnyka, Z., Czosnyka, M., Richards, H. *et al.* (1998). Hydrodynamic properties of hydrocephalus shunts. *Acta Neurochir.*, *Suppl.*, **71**, 334–9.

Davson, H. (1986). *The physiology and pathology of the cerebrospinal fluid.* Churchill Livingstone, Edinburgh.

Donaldson, J. O. (1981). Pathogenesis of pseudotumor cerebri syndromes. *Neurology*, **31**, 877–80.

Eriskat, J., Stoffel, M., Plesxilla, A. *et al.* (2000). Interstitial lactate in the peritraumatic penumbra of rat brain. *Acta Neurochir.*, **Suppl. 76.**

European Study Group on Nimodipine in Severe Head Injury (1994). A multicentre trial of the efficacy of Nimodipine on outcome after severe head injury. *J. Neurosurg.*, **80**, 797–801.

Feldman, M. H. and Schlezinger, N. S. (1970). Benign intracranial hypertension associated with hypervitaminosis A. *Arch. Neurol.*, **22**, 1–7.

Fernell, E. and Hagberg, G. (1998). Infantile hydrocephalus: declining prevalence in preterm infants. *Acta Paediat.*, **87** (4), 392–6.

Fishman, R. A. (1980). *Cerebrospinal fluid in diseases of the nervous system.* Saunders, Philadelphia.

Fitch, W. and McDowall, D. G. (1977). Systemic vascular responses to increased intracranial pressure. 1. Effects of progressive epidural balloon expansion on intracranial pressure and systemic circulation. *J. Neurol. Neurosurg. Psychiat.*, **40**, 833–42.

Fitch, W., McDowall, D. G., Keaney, N. P. *et al.* (1977). Systemic vascular responses to increased intracranial pressure. 2. The 'Cushing' response in the presence of intracranial space-occupying lesions: systemic and cerebral haemodynamic studies in the dog and the baboon. *J. Neurol. Neurosurg. Psychiat.*, **40**, 843–52.

Foley, J. (1955). Benign forms of intracranial hypertension in 'toxic' and 'otitic' hydrocephalus. *Brain*, **78**, 1–41.

Foley, K. M. and Posner, J. B. (1975). Does pseudotumor cerebri cause the empty sella syndrome? *Neurology*, **25**, 565–9.

Gardner, W. J. (1965). Hydrodynamic mechanism in syringomyelia: its relationship to myelocele. *J. Neurol. Neurosurg. Psychiat.*, **28**, 247–59.

Gordon, K. (1997). Pediatric pseudotumor cerebri: descriptive epidemiology. *Can. J. Neurol. Sci.*, **24** (3), 219–21.

Grant, R., Condon, B., Lawrence, A. *et al.* (1987). Human cranial CSF volumes measured by MRI: sex and age influences. *Magn. Reson. Imaging*, **5**, 465–8.

Greenberg, J. O., Shenkin, H. A., and Adam, R. (1977). Idiopathic normal pressure hydrocephalus: a report of 73 patients. *J. Neurol. Neurosurg. Psychiat.*, **40**, 336–41.

Gustafson, L. and Hagberg, B. O. (1978). Recovery in hydrocephalic dementia after shunt operation. *J. Neurol. Neurosurg. Psychiat.*, **41**, 940–7.

Guthkelch, A. N. and Riley, N. A. (1969). Influence of aetiology in prognosis in surgically treated infantile hydrocephalus. *Arch. Dis. Child.*, **44**, 29–35.

Hakim, S. and Adams, R. D. (1965). The special clinical problem of symptomatic hydrocephalus with normal cerebrospinal fluid pressure. *J. Neurol. Sci.*, **2**, 307–27.

Hakim, R. and Black, P. M. (1998). Correlation between lumbo-ventricular perfusion and MRI–CSF flow studies in idiopathic normal pressure hydrocephalus. *Surg. Neurol.*, **49**, 14–19.

Haller, J. S., Wolpert, S. M., Rabe, E. F. *et al.* (1971). Cystic lesions of the posterior fossa in infants: a comparison of the clinical, radiological, and pathological findings in Dandy–Walker syndrome and extra-axial cysts. *Neurology*, **21**, 494–506.

Harrison, M. J., Robert, C. M., and Uttley, D. (1974). Benign aqueduct stenosis in adults. *J. Neurol. Neurosurg. Psychiat.*, **37**, 1322–8.

Hart, M. N., Malamud, N., and Ellis, W. G. (1972). The Dandy–Walker syndrome. A clinico-pathological study based on 28 cases. *Neurology*, **22**, 771–80.

Hommet, C., Billard, C., Gillet, P. *et al.* (1999). Neuropsychologic and adaptive functioning in adolescents and young adults shunted for congenital hydrocephalus. *J. Child Neurol.*, **14**, 144–150.

Hoppe-Hirsch, E., Laroussinie, F., Brunet, L. *et al.* (1998). Late outcome of surgical treatment of hydrocephalus. *Childs Nerv. Syst.*, **14**, 97–9.

Hu, Y. H., Li, L. M., and Li, P. (1996). A five years surveillance on neural system birth defects in rural areas of China. *Chin. J. Epidemiol.*, 17, 20–4.

Hughes, C. P., Siegel, B. A., Coxe, W. S. *et al.* (1978). Adult idiopathic communicating hydrocephalus with and without shunting. *J. Neurol. Neurosurg. Psychiat.*, 41, 961–71.

Iannotti, F. (2000). Trial of the NMDA receptor antagonist D-CPP-ene in head injured patients. *Br. J. Neurosurg.*, (in press).

Jachuck, S. J., Ramani, P. S., Clark, F. *et al.* (1975). Electrocardiographic abnormalities associated with raised intracranial pressure. *BMJ*, 1, 242–4.

Jacobs, L. and Kinkel, W. (1976). Computerized axial transverse tomography in normal pressure hydrocephalus. *Neurology*, 26, 501–7.

Johnson, L. N., Krohel, G. B., Madsen, R. W. *et al.* (1998). The role of weight loss and acetazolamide in the treatment of idiopathic intracranial hypertension. *Ophthalmology*, 105, 2313–17.

Johnston, I. and Paterson, A. (1974). Benign intracranial hypertension II. CSF pressure and circulation. *Brain*, 97, 301–12.

Katzman, R., Clasen, R., Klatzo, I. *et al.* (1977). Report of a Joint Committee for Stroke Resources. IV. Brain edema in stroke. *Stroke*, 8, 512–40.

Kessler, L. A., Novelli, P. M., and Reigel, D. H. (1998). Surgical treatment of benign intracranial hypertension—subtemporal decompression revisited. *Surg. Neurol.*, 50, 73–6.

Klatzo, I. (1967). Neuropathological aspects of brain oedema. *J. Neuropath. Exp. Neurol.*, 26, 1–14.

Kuper, S., Mendelow, H., and Proctor, N. S. F. (1958). Internal hydrocephalus caused by parasitic cysts. *Brain*, 81, 235–42.

Kuroiwa, T., Nagaoka, T., Miyasaka, N. *et al.* (2000). Time course of diffusion tensor [Trace (D)] and histology in brain oedema. *Acta Neurochir.*, in press.

Kurtzke, J. F., Goldberg, I. D., and Kurland, L. T. (1973). The distribution of deaths from congenital malformations of the nervous system. *Neurology*, 23, 483–96.

Laurence, K. M. (1969). Neurological and intellectual sequelae of hydrocephalus. *Arch. Neurol.*, 20, 73–81.

MacFarlane, A. and Maloney, A. F. J. (1957). The appearance of the aqueduct and its relationship to hydrocephalus in the Arnold–Chiari malformation. *Brain*, 80, 479–91.

Macnab, G. H. (1966). The development of the knowledge and treatment of hydrocephalus. In *Hydrocephalus and spina bifida*, pp. 1–9.

Madan, S., Marchbanks, R. J., and Burge, D. M. (1998). A review of the management and current methods of investigating intracranial pressure in shunted hydrocephalics and an introduction to the tympanic membrane displacement test. In *Intracranial and inner ear physiology and pathophysiology*, (ed. A. Reid, R. J. Marchbanks, and A. Ernst), pp. 90–107. Whurr Publishers Ltd. London.

Marmarou, A., Fatouros, P., Yoshihara, M. *et al.* (1993). The contribution of brain oedema to brain swelling. In *Intracranial Pressure VIII; 1991 1993*, pp. 525–8. Springer Verlag, Rotterdam.

Marmarou, A., Barzo, P., Fatouros, P. *et al.* (1997). Traumatic brain swelling in head injured patients: brain oedema or vascular engorgement? *Acta Neurochir.*, 70, 68–70.

Marmarou, A., Portella, G., Barzo, P. *et al.* (2000). Distinguishing between cellular and vasogenic edema in head injured patients using magnetic resonance spectrosopy. *Acta Neurochir.*, **Suppl. 76.**

Maurice Williams, R. S. and Pilling, J. (1977). Trigeminal sensory symptoms associated with hydrocephalus. *J. Neurol. Neurosurg. Psychiat.*, 40, 641–4.

McDonald, J. V. (1969). Persistent hydrocephalus following the removal of papillomas of the choroid plexus of the lateral ventricles. *J. Neurosurg.*, 30, 736–40.

Menkes, J. H. (1980). *Textbook of child neurology*, (2nd edn). Lea and Febiger, Philadelphia.

Milhorat, T. H. (1972). *Hydrocephalus and the cerebrospinal fluid*. Williams and Wilkins, Baltimore .

Miller, D. and Adams, H. (1972). In *Scientific foundations of neurology*, (ed. M. Critchley, J. L. O'Leary, and W. B. Jennett). Heinemann, London.

Pickard, J. D. (2001). *UK Hydrocephalus shunt registry*. (Personal communication).

Pickard, J. D., Newton, H., Greene, A. *et al.* (1992). A prospective study of idiopathic normal pressure hydrocephalus—guidelines for outpatient investigation. *J. Neurol. Neurosurg. Psychiat.*, 55, 517–18.

Pinar, H., Tatevosyants, N., and Singer, D. B. (1998). Central nervous system malformations in a perinatal/neonatal autopsy series. *Pediatr. Develop. Pathol.*, 1, 42–8.

Piper, I. R. and Miller, J. D. (1995). The evaluation of the wave-form analysis capability of a new strain-gauge intracranial pressure microsensor. *Neurosugery*, 36, 1142–5.

Piper, I., Dunn, L., Contant, C. *et al.* (2000). Multi-centre assessment of the Spiegelberg compliance monitor: preliminary results. *Acta Neurochir.*, **Suppl. 76.**

Plum, F. and Posner, J. B. (1980). *The diagnosis of stupor and coma*, (3rd edn). Blackwell, Oxford.

Raichle, M. E., Grubb, R. L., Phelps, M. E. *et al.* (1978). Cerebral hemodynamics and metabolism in pseudotumor cerebri. *Ann. Neurol.*, **4**, 104–11.

Rajab, A., Vaishnav, A., Freeman, N. V. *et al.* (1998). Neural tube defects and congenital hydrocephalus in the Sultanate of Oman. *J. Trop. Pediatr.*, **44**, 300–3.

Reid, A. C., Matheson, M. S., and Teasdale, G. (1980). Volume of the ventricles in benign intracranial hypertension. *Lancet*, **ii**, 7–8.

Robertson, C. S., Valadka, A. B., Gopinath, S. P. *et al.* (1998). Prevention of secondary insults after head injury. *Acta Neurochir.*, **71**, 378.

Rosner, M. J. and Rosner, S. D. (1991). Cerebral perfusion pressure management of head injury. In *Intracranial Pressure VIII*, pp. 540–3, Springer Verlag, Rotterdam.

Sallomi, D., Taylor, H., Hibbert, J. *et al.* (1998).The MRI appearance of the optic sheath following fenestration for benign intracranial hypertension. *Eur. Radiol.*, **8**, 1193–6.

Singh, A. and Crockard, H. A. (1999). Quantitative assessment of cervical spondylotic myelopathy by a simple walking test. *Lancet*, **354**, 370–3.

Sipek, A., Gregor, V., Horacek, J. *et al.* (1998). Occurrence of congenital hydrocephalus in the Czech Republic 1961–1995. *Ceska Gynekol.*, **63** (3), 207–10.

Sugerman, H. J., DeMaria, E. J., Felton, W. L. *et al.* (1997). Increased intra-abdominal pressure and cardiac filling pressures in obesity-associated pseudotumor cerebri. *Neurology*, **49**, 507–11.

Sugerman, H. J., Felton, W. L., Sismanis, A. *et al.* (1999). Gastric surgery for pseudotumor cerebri associated with severe obesity. *Ann. Surg.*, **229**, 634–40.

Symon, L., Dorsch, N. W., and Stephens, R. J. (1972). Pressure waves in so-called low-pressure hydrocephalus. *Lancet*, **ii**, 1291–2.

Symonds, C. P. (1931). Otitic hydrocephalus. *Brain*, **54**, 55–71.

Symonds, C. P. (1937). Hydrocephalic and focal cerebral symptoms in relation to thrombophlebitis of the dural sinuses and cerebral veins. *Brain*, **60**, 531–50.

Sypert, G. W., Leffman, H., and Ojemann, G. A. (1973). Occult normal pressure hydrocephalus manifested by parkinsonism-dementia complex. *Neurology*, **23**, 234–8.

Teasdale, G. M., Hadley, D. M., and Lawrence, A. (1989). Comparison of magnetic resonance imaging and computed tomography in suspected lesions in the posterior cranial fossa. *BMJ*, **299**, 349–55.

Tomasovic, J. A., Nelhaus, G., and Moe, P. G. (1975). The bobble-head doll syndrome: an early sign of hydrocephalus. *Develop. Med. Child Neurol.*, **17**, 777–83.

Van Crevel, H. (1979). Papilloedema, CSF pressure and CSF flow in in cerebral tumours. *J. Neurol. Neurosurg. Psychiat.*, **42**, 493–500.

Vanneste, J. and van Acker, R. (1990). Normal pressure hydrocephalus: did publications alter management? *J. Neurol. Neurosurg. Psychiat.*, **53**, 564–8.

Ward, J. D., Becker, D. P., Miller, J. D. *et al.* (1985). Failure of prophylactic barbiturate coma in the treatment of severe head injury. *J. Neurosurg.*, **62**, 383–8.

Wikkelso, C., Andersson, H., Blomstrand, C., and Lindqvist, G. (1982). The clinical effect of lumbar puncture on normal pressure hydrocephalus. *J. Neurol. Neurosurg. Psychiat.*, **45**, 64–9.

Williams, M. A., Razumovsky, A. Y., and Hanley, D. F. (1998). Comparison of P (CSF) monitoring and controlled CSF drainage diagnose normal pressure hydrocephalus. *Acta Neurochir.*, **71**, 328–30.

Yates, D., Farrell, B., Teasdale, G. *et al.* (1999). Corticosteroids in head injury: the CRASH trial. *J. Accid. Emerg. Med.*, **16**, 83–4.

Yoshihara, M., Tsunoda, A., Sato, K. *et al.* (1998). Differential diagnosis of NPH and brain atrophy assessed by measurement of intracranial and ventricular CSF volume with 3D FASE MRI. *Acta Neurochir.*, **71**, 371–4.

Zulch, K. J., Mennel, H. D., and Zimmermann, V. (1974). Intracranial hypertension. In *Handbook of clinical neurology*, (ed. P. J. Vinken and G. W. Bruyn), Chapter 3. North Holland, Amsterdam.

CHAPTER 18

Tumours of the brain and skull

Robert Grant

18.1 Introduction and terminology

Over the past decade, there has been a tremendous growth of knowledge about tumour biology and molecular genetics. Improved neurosurgical techniques, safer methods of directing radiotherapy, new chemotherapy approaches, and novel modalities of therapy provide optimism that there will eventually be improvements in treatment-related morbidity and survival. However, the current literature in neuro-oncology is still heavily influenced by publication bias and 'gearing', where papers are published only when they match or exceed the best of those that are already published. The results of treatment of, for example, glioblastoma multiforme, single metastasis, or malignant meningitis appear therefore to be constantly improving, regardless of what is being achieved by the average clinician. Despite this, there are occasional well-conducted randomized controlled trials which act as a foundation on which to base management. There is increasing rigour in phase II and phase III trial methodology and governmental and private health insurance financial constraints are putting pressure on clinicians not only to prove efficacy, but also to demonstrate improved quality of life and cost-effectiveness. This trend towards evidence-based medicine and randomized controlled trials is being eroded by claims of success of new treatments on the internet, which falsely increase patient expectation and lead to difficulties with patient accrual into randomized studies. It will be interesting to see how research develops over the next decade.

Histological grading is crucial to the understanding of brain tumours and their eventual management. The World Health Organization has recently reclassified and graded brain tumours (Table 18.1) (Kleihues et al., 1993a). The WHO classification recognizes that tumours develop via different pathways and that the behaviour of some grades of malignancy are quite distinct. The classification also allows standardization of reporting for epidemiological studies. The World Health Organization has also revised its grading system of central nervous system tumours to take into account newly defined histological entities (e.g. pleomorphic xanthoastrocytoma and dysembryoplastic neuroepithelial tumours (DNET)) (Table 18.2).

18.2 Epidemiology of brain tumours

18.2.1 Mortality

Brain tumours are the second most common cause of death from neurological disease, surpassed only by stroke. Neuroepithelial brain tumours are the fifth most common cause of death from malignancy under the age of 65 years (Scottish Office 1991). If other intrinsic brain tumours (e.g. metastases and primary central nervous system lymphomas) are included, it is very likely that intracranial tumours are one of the three most common causes of death from cancer in the working population (Registrar General for Scotland 1993).

18.2.2 Incidence and prevalence

Information from cancer registry statistics show that neuro-epithelial tumours are the most common solid malignancy in children, the fourth most common in the under 45 age group, and the eighth most common under the age of 65 years. However, cancer registries frequently do not reliably record incidence data on all primary intracranial tumours (e.g. meningiomas, acoustic neuromas, pituitary adenomas, and primary CNS lymphoma) (Counsell et al. 1997).

Meningiomas, acoustic neuromas, and pituitary tumours account for almost 25 per cent of all intracranial tumours (Table 18.3) and there is evidence that more tumours are being identified, although this may reflect the wider availability of brain imaging. Primary CNS lymphomas, associated with AIDS, have also increased over the past 10 years. Brain metastases account for over 50 per cent of all intrinsic brain tumours and affect 20 per cent of patients with cancer. The incidence of intracranial metastases may also be increasing, as the brain will also act as a 'sanctuary site' for metastases as treatment of the systemic tumour improves.

In a recent study, the incidence of any intracranial tumour was found to be approximately 30 cases per 100 000 population each year (Counsell et al. 1996) (Table 18.3). Assuming no demographic or regional differences, one would expect approximately 200 000 new cases of intracranial tumour each year in Europe and 100 000 new cases each year in North America. Over the past 50 years the incidence of intracranial tumours in developed countries has increased (Davis et al. 1990; Muir et al. 1994). The increase is predominantly in the elderly population and may be due to better case ascertainment because of wider availability of CT and MRI scanning and improved health care for the elderly (Radhakrishnan et al. 1995).

Studies produce a wide range of incidences for neuroepithelial tumours (2.5–$9.1/10^5$/yr), but most recent studies with good case ascertainment are at the higher figure (Kaye et al. 1993; D'Alessandro et al. 1995). The age-specific incidence of primary brain tumours has a small peak in early childhood ($3.5/10^5$/yr), dips in the 15–24-year age range ($2.9/10^5$/year) and then progressively climbs to its highest incidence in the 65–74-year age range ($24/10^5$/yr) before falling off a little to $9.6/10^5$/yr in the above 85 age range (Counsell et al. 1996). Cerebral metastases are rare in the under 25 age group ($1/10^5$/yr) but increase gradually to 53.7 cases/10^5/yr in the 65–74-year age group (confidence interval (CI) 41.6–68.2/10^5/yr). Meningeal tumours are also very rare under 25 years of age ($0.4/10^5$/yr) and increase steadily to a peak incidence of $9.0/10^5$/yr in the age range 75–85 (CI 3.6–18.5/10^5/yr). A recent meta-analysis of incidence studies suggests that the differences could be accounted for by methods of identifying patients, inclusion criteria for what represented primary intracranial tumours, and the scanning techniques used to identify cases. Methodological guidelines for future incidence studies in brain tumours have been suggested, in order to standardize future incidence studies to allow meaningful analysis (Counsell and Grant 1998).

Table 18.1. World Health Organization (WHO) typing of CNS tumours

1. Tumours of neuroepithelial tissue

1.1. Astrocytic tumours

1.1.1 Astrocytoma

1.1.2 Anaplastic (malignant) astrocytoma

1.1.3 Glioblastoma

1.1.4 Pilocytic astrocytoma

1.1.5 Pleomorphic xanthoastrocytoma

1.1.6 Subependymal giant cell astrocytoma

1.2 Oligodendroglial tumours

1.2.1 Oligodendroglioma

1.2.2 Anaplastic (malignant)

1.3 Ependymal tumours

1.3.1 Ependymoma

1.3.2 Anaplastic (malignant)

1.3.3 Myxopapillary ependymoma

1.3.4 Subependymoma

1.4 Mixed gliomas

1.4.1 Oligo-astrocytoma

1.4.2 Anaplastic (malignant)

1.4.3 Other

1.5 Choroid plexus tumours

1.5.1 Choroid plexus papilloma

1.5.2 Choroid plexus carcinoma

1.6 Neuroepithelial tumours

1.6.1 Astroblastoma

1.6.2 Polar spongioblastoma

1.6.3 Gliomatosis cerebri

1.7 Neuronal and mixed neuronal-glial tumours

1.7.1 Gangliocytoma

1.7.2 Dysplastic gangliocytoma of cerebellum

1.7.3 Desmoplastic neuroepithelial tumour

1.7.4 Dysembryoplastic neuroepithelial tumour

1.7.5 Ganglioglioma

1.7.6 Anaplastic (malignant) ganglioglioma

1.7.7 Central neurocytoma

1.7.8 Paraganglioma of the filum terminale

1.7.9 Olfactory neuroblastoma

1.8 Pineal parenchymal tumours

1.8.1 Pineocytoma

1.8.2 Pineoblastoma

1.8.3 Mixed/transitional pineal tumours

1.9 Embryonal tumours

1.9.1 Medulloepithelioma

1.9.2 Neuroblastoma

1.9.3 Ependymoblastoma

1.9.4 Primitive neuroectodermal tumours

2. Tumours of cranial and spinal nerves

2.1 Schwannoma (neurinoma)

2.2 Neurofibroma

2.3 Malignant peripheral nerve sheath tumour

3. Tumours of the meninges

3.1 Tumours of meningothelial cells

3.1.1 Meningioma

3.1.2 Atypical meningioma

3.1.3 Papillary meningioma

3.1.4 Anaplastic (malignant) meningioma

3.2 Mesenchymal, non-meningothelial

Benign neoplasms

3.2.1 Osteocartilaginous tumours

3.2.2 Lipoma

3.2.3 Fibrous histiocytoma

3.2.4 Others

Malignant neoplasms

3.2.5 Haemangiopericytoma

3.2.6 Chondrosarcoma

3.2.7 Malignant fibrous histiocytoma

3.2.8 Rhabdomyosarcoma

3.2.9 Meningeal sarcomatosis

3.2.10 Others

3.3 Primary melanocytic lesions

3.3.1 Diffuse melanosis

3.3.2 Melanocytoma

3.3.3 Malignant melanoma

3.4 Tumours of uncertain histogenesis

3.4.1 Haemangioblastoma

4. Lymphoma and haemopoietic tumours

4.1 Malignant lymphoma

4.2 Plasmocytoma

4.3 Granulocytic sarcoma

4.4 Other

5. Germ cell tumours

5.1 Germinoma

5.2 Embryonal carcinoma

5.3 Yolk sac tumour

5.4 Choriocarcinoma

5.5 Teratoma

5.6 Mixed germ cell tumour

6. Cysts and tumour-like lesions

7. Tumours of the sellar region

7.1 Pituitary adenoma

7.2 Pituitary carcinoma

7.3 Craniopharyngioma

8. Local extensions of regional tumours

8.1 Paraganglioma

8.2 Chordoma

8.3 Chondroma/chondrosarcoma

8.4 Carcinoma

9. Metastatic tumours

10. Unclassified tumour

Table 18.2.　World Health Organization (WHO) grading system (malignancy scale) of CNS tumours

Tumour group	Tumour type	Grade I	Grade II	Grade III	Grade IV
Astrocytic tumours	Subependymal giant cell	*			
	Pilocytic	*			
	Low grade		*		
	Pleomorphic xanthoastrocytoma		*	*	
	Anaplastic			*	
	Glioblastoma				*
Oligodendrogliomas	Low grade		*		
	Anaplastic			*	
Oligo-astrocytomas	Low grade		*		
	Anaplastic			*	
Ependymal tumours	Subependymoma	*			
	Myxopapillary	*			
	Low grade		*		
	Anaplastic			*	
Choroid plexus	Papilloma	*			
	Carcinoma			*	*
Neuronal/glial cell	Gangliocytoma	*			
	Ganglioglioma	*	*		
	Desmoplastic infantile ganglioglioma	*			
	Dysembryoplastic neuroepithelial	*			
	Central neurocytoma	*			
Pineal tumours	Pineocytoma		*		
	Pineocytoma/pineoblastoma			*	*
	Pineoblastoma				*
Embryonal tumours	Medulloblastoma				*
	Other PNET				*
	Medulloepithelioma				*
	Neuroblastoma				*
	Ependymomblastoma				*
Cranial/spinal nerve	Schwannoma	*			
	Malignant peripheral nerve sheath			*	*
Meningeal tumours	Meningioma	*			
	Atypical meningioma		*		
	Papillary meningioma		*	*	
	Haemangiopericytoma		*	*	
	Anaplastic meningioma			*	

Medulloblastomas and ependymomas occur most frequently in childhood or early adolescence, grade 2 astrocytomas and oligodendroglioma in early adulthood (20–40 years), and grade 3 and 4 astrocytomas (malignant gliomas) most commonly in the over-40 age range, although they can occur at any age.

18.2.3　Referral pattern

Intracranial tumours can present to a variety of clinicians. In a recent study looking at the referral pattern in south-east Scotland, the majority of patients with primary intracerebral tumours were referred by their primary care physician to general physicians (57 per cent) or neurologists (23 per cent); patients with acoustic neuromas were referred to physicians (42 per cent), ENT specialists (36 per cent), or neurologists (16 per cent); those with pituitary tumours were referred to obstetricians and gynaecologists (52 per cent), physicians (30 per cent), or neurologists (10 per cent); and patients with metastases were referred predominantly to general physicians (54 per cent) or oncologists (27 per cent) (Grant *et al.* 1996).

Table 18.3. Incident cases of different intracranial tumours diagnosed in south–east Scotland: and expected UK frequency (assuming similar demographics to south–east Scotland)

	Crude incidence (per 10^5)(95% CI)	Expected UK cases/yr
1. Neuroepithelial	8.2 (6.8–9.8)	4641
2. Tumours of cranial (and spinal) nerves	0.7 (0.3–1.2)	396
3. Tumours of the meninges	3.0 (2.6–4.0)	1698
4. Lymphoma and haemopoietic tumours	0.7 (0.3–1.2)	396
5. Germ cell tumours	0.1 (0.0 0.4)	57
6. Cysts and tumour-like lesions	0.1 (0.0–0.5)	57
7. Tumours of the sellar region	2.5 (1.7–3.3)	1415
8. Local extensions from regional tumours	0.1 (0.0–0.4)	57
9. Metastatic tumours	14.3 (12.4–16.3)	8093
10. Unclassified	0.5 (0.1–0.9)	283
Total intracranial tumours	30.2	17093

Following imaging diagnosis, further specialist referral was almost always the rule. Referral occurs at a time of great uncertainty for the patient and family, and close collaboration between clinicians is essential to reduce anxiety. A clear explanation to the patient and family and a simple, well-constructed management plan must be given, and should be consistent between specialists. Communication with patient, family, and general practitioner should be unambiguous and supportive (Davis and Hopkins 1997a).

18.2.4 Geographical, racial, and social influences

Males are 1.1–1.7 times more likely than females to develop primary intracerebral brain tumours (Wrench et al. 1993; Counsell et al. 1996) and females are about 2.2 times more likely to develop meningiomas (Counsell and Grant 1998). There do not appear to be any specific geographical factors that influence the incidence of primary brain tumours, although a dramatic difference in incidence of primary intracranial tumours was identified between two neighbouring regions of northern Italy (Valle d'Aosta and Trento) (Lovaste et al. 1986; D'Alessandro et al. 1995). Some studies report that white Americans have a higher incidence of brain tumours than African-Americans, Hispanics, and Japanese Americans (Leibowitz et al. 1971; SEER 1991). However, others have shown a higher incidence in African-American children than whites (Bunin 1987) and have not found a higher incidence in whites compared with Hispanics (Young et al. 1981).

The level of affluence is associated with the likelihood of developing neuroepithelial brain tumours in adults and children (Sharp et al. 1993; McKinney et al. 1994). The incidence of neuroepithelial tumours is approximately 2.3 times greater in areas of south-east Scotland with the greatest affluence (category 1 and 2 of Carstairs deprivation score) (McLoone 1993) than with the least affluent (categories 6 and 7). The relationship between deprivation category and incidence of neuro-

epithelial tumours is linear (Counsell et al. 1996). The incidence of metastases was about twice as high in the least affluent groups as the most affluent (χ^2 trend 6.18, $P = 0.01$). The relationship between neuroepithelial tumours and social deprivation is very unlikely to be due to inequality of access to care in the health service, because of the existence of the National Health Service and also because the inverse relationship is seen with cerebral metastases.

18.2.5 Risk factors

Several factors have been implicated in the development of intracranial malignancies, although none have been reported consistently as strong risks and some conclusions may be confounded by methodological problems or publication bias. The strongest possible risk factor is therapeutic cranial irradiation. In two studies of neuroepithelial brain tumours, 7–17 per cent of cases had received previous therapeutic irradiation; however, this finding may be confounded by the known increased risk of second malignancies in patients treated for other cancers (about 5–10 per cent) or by genetic predisposition to cancer (Salvati et al. 1991; Hodges et al. 1992). Therapeutic irradiation for scalp ringworm was associated with a fourfold increase in the risk of brain tumour (Ron et al. 1988). A Japanese study of atomic bomb survivors failed to demonstrate any increased risk of brain tumours in children exposed to radiation in utero (Kato et al. 1989). Certain chemicals, such as polycyclic aromic hydrocarbons and nitroso-compounds, can induce brain tumours in experimental animals, but their role in human brain tumours remains unproven (Maekawa and Mitsumori 1990). Vinyl chloride can cause brain tumours in rats, and a Swedish study showed that workers in a vinyl chloride plant were twice as likely to die from brain tumours (Hagmar et al. 1990).

Electromagnetic fields have been suggested as a possible risk factor, however laboratory and clinical studies have failed to demonstrate a direct link. A cohort study of 36 000 electric

Table 18.4. Genes responsible for familial cancer predisposition

Chromosome region	Gene/locus symbol	Familial cancer
3p14	RCC1	von Hippel–Lindau disease
9q22.3	NBCCS	Gorlin syndrome
9q34	TSC1	Tuberous sclerosis
11q22–q23	ATM	Ataxia telangiectasia
13q14	RB1	Retinblastoma
16p13.3	TSC2	Tuberous sclerosis
17p13	p53	Li–Fraumeni syndrome
17q11	NF1	Neurofibromatosis type 1
22q	NF2	Neurofibromatosis type 2

utility employees did not demonstrate any increase in risk of astrocytoma (Mack *et al.* 1991) and a mortality study of 138 905 men employed in the same industry showed only a modest elevation in brain tumour mortality (Savitz and Loomis 1995). There is no good evidence that cellular telephones are associated with brain tumours (Grant 1999, Inskip *et al.* 2001).

Dietary and other chemical exposures, maternal birth characteristics, head trauma, infections, vaccinations, and various medications, including antinauseants during pregnancy, have been suggested as risk factors, but none have shown strong enough correlations to confirm a link (Bondy and Wrensch 1996).

Immunodeficiency states are definitely a risk factor for developing primary CNS lymphoma.

18.2.6 Genetic factors

Many different genes have been associated with familial cancer predisposition and have associations with CNS tumours (Table 18.4). Several genes have been localized on the genome and many have been isolated and characterized. There is a genetic predisposition to brain tumours in patients with the family cancer syndrome described by Li and Fraumeni (1969). Li–Fraumeni syndrome has been linked to a mutation in *p53* on chromosome 17p (Malkin *et al.* 1990). *p53* mutations have been found frequently in all grades of astrocytoma and probably represent an early event in malignant transformation of astrocytic cells (Ohgaki *et al.* 1993).

In hereditary syndromes with linked gene mutations, such as tuberous sclerosis (9q32–34), about 5 per cent of cases will develop cerebral gliomas. In neurofibromatosis type 1 (17q12–22), cerebral or optic nerve glioma will develop in between 4 and 45 per cent of patients, and in neurofibromatosis type 2 (22q), schwannomas, ependymomas, and meningiomas are found more frequently than in the general population. Other rare syndromes, such as Gorlin's syndrome, Turcot's syndrome, and Gardner's syndrome, are associated with brain tumours. Gorlin's syndrome is an autosomal dominant condition with naevoid basal cell carcinoma and is associated with medulloblastoma. Turcot's syndrome and familial polyposis is

associated with an increased incidence of glioma, and Gardner's syndrome with medulloblastoma.

18.3 Biological basis

Our knowledge of cellular and molecular biology has expanded exponentially over the past 10 years. The developments have been used to confirm the histological nature of tumours, determine the proliferating potential of malignant cells, and provide insight into the control mechanisms behind tumour cell proliferation and tumour suppression. Three classes of genes have been implicated in the pathogenesis of cancer: oncogenes, tumour suppressor genes, and mismatch repair genes. Oncogenes are derived from normal cellular genes (proto-oncogenes) which function as growth stimulators. However, if activated, uncontrolled cellular proliferation occurs. Tumour suppressor genes normally restrain cellular proliferation but when inactivated by gene mutation, will result in uncontrolled cellular proliferation. Knudsen proposed the 'Two-hit hypothesis' which suggested that the loss of both alleles of the tumour suppressor gene was necessary before a cancer could develop. Patients with a germline mutation in one of these alleles require a somatic change in the other allele before a tumour develops. Mismatch repair genes are the third class of genes important to the development of tumours. The products of these genes identify mismatches that occur at point mutations in the genome and repair these. If there is a problem, with failure to identify mismatches, gene repair and control are affected.

Carcinogenesis may be initiated by a mutation or alteration in certain genes (e.g. deletion or rearrangement of DNA) or by several different changes in several genes. The mutation can be random, inherited, or induced by radiation, chemicals, or other insult.

18.3.1 Growth factors

Growth factors are usually under the control of proto-oncogenes and tumour suppressor genes. Several proto-oncogenes have been associated with the development of malignant gliomas (e.g. c-*erbB-1*, c-*sis*, c-*myc*, *ras*, c-*fos*, and *ros* oncogenes). *ErbB* encodes an epidermal growth factor receptor (EGFR) and c-*sis* encodes a platelet-derived growth factor (PDGF). The most common growth factor in malignant glioma is EGFR. EGFR is overexpressed in about 40–60 per cent of malignant gliomas but expression is uncommon in astrocytoma. This suggests that the EGFR occurs as a late feature of deregulation of cell division and not an initiating factor of tumorigenesis. There is not a close relationship between overexpression of EGFR and survival in tumours of the same grade. Several other growth factors, such as transforming growth factors (TGF-α, TGF-β), fibroblast growth factor, and insulin-like growth factor, are also overexpressed in some glioblastomas. TGF-α is a polypeptide growth factor that has sequence homology for EGF and binds to EGFR. It is frequently amplified in anaplastic astrocytoma and glioblastoma multiforme, and may act as a growth factor ligand for EGFR and form an autocrine growth loop, leading to proliferation of glioma cells. The amplification and overexpression of TGF-α might be an earlier event in a gradual process of tumorigenesis. TGF-β stimulates astrocytoma cells to migrate and invade (Yamada *et al.* 1995).

18.3.2 Tumour suppressor factors

Several different chromosomes have been reported as having possible loci for tumour suppressor genes. Low-grade brain tumours frequently demonstrate loss of genetic material on chromosomes 6, 13, 17p, or 22. The p53 gene is the most well-known tumour suppressor gene and is situated on chromosome 17p (17p13.1). Mutations of the p53 gene are implicated in many cancers. The loss of wild-type alleles of p53 is an early finding in astrocytomas (most commonly loss of one and mutation in the other), and are found commonly in glioblastomas that have progressed from low-grade tumours. p53 abnormalities are seen much less commonly in *de novo* glioblastomas. Allelic loss of chromosome 19q is found in 46 per cent of grade 3 gliomas but only 11 per cent of grade 2 tumours (von Deimling *et al.* 1994). The most common chromosomal abnormality, present only in glioblastoma, is loss of chromosome 10. A region on chromosome 10 probably acts as a tumour suppressor gene. In primitive neuro-ectodermal tumours (PNET; medulloblastomas and PNET variants) deletions of the short arm of chromosome 17 occur in a high percentage of cases and there is frequently also loss of information on chromosomes 10, 11, and 22. Seventy per cent of meningiomas have a loss on chromosome 22. Despite the large number of potential tumour suppressor genes, there are no specific losses of genetic material that are unique to a particular histological group of tumours, and no specific deletion or other genetic alteration is found in all tumours.

18.4 Clinical features and imaging diagnosis

From a clinical and imaging viewpoint, brain tumours are most easily divided by site and relationship to the cranial fossae:

(1) extracranial but involving neural tissue (e.g. head and neck lesions);

(2) intracranial but extracerebral;
    (a) anterior cranial fossa (e.g. olfactory groove),
    (b) middle cranial fossa (e.g. pituitary region and sphenoid wing),
    (c) posterior cranial fossa (e.g. cerebello-pontine angle, and craniocervical junction);

(3) within the brain substance (e.g. primary or secondary intracerebral tumours).

This simple clinical and anatomical approach can narrow the differential diagnosis and direct more specific investigations.

18.4.1 Head and neck lesions

Patients with tumours of the head and neck most commonly present with headache, lower cranial neuropathies, or facial pain. Where the involvement is in the nasopharynx one should consider nasopharyngeal carcinoma, adenoid cystic carcinoma, and metastatic tumours. Where there is involvement of the carotid body region, glomus jugulare should be considered. Patients with glomus jugulare tumours commonly present with lower cranial nerve palsies, e.g. dysphonia, dysphagia with wasted tongue or weak palate, but, if extensive, it can also cause pulsatile tinnitus, headaches, and hearing loss. Glomus jugulare tumours are usually large when eventually discovered. Plain radiographs (submento-vertex view) will best demonstrate the enlargement of the jugular foramen. CT scanning shows the strongly enhancing tumour mass with erosion of the adjacent bone. MRI will demonstrate the 'salt and pepper' appearance caused by the flow voids within the tumour. Gadolinium-enhanced coronal MRI scan is particularly useful to delineate the extent of the tumour and the relationship to the brainstem. Where there is occipital headache, and lower cranial neuropathies, tumour involvement of the skull base should be considered. In the midline, chordoma, chondroma, and chondrosarcoma are all possible. Imaging of the head/neck by CT scan or MRI scan may demonstrate a lesion with or without soft-tissue involvement. CT scanning is superior when bony involvement is present (e.g. skull osteomas, Paget's disease, fibrous dysplasia) and MRI, with its multiplanar capabilities, is superior for soft-tissue visualization (e.g. nasopharyngeal carcinoma, metastases, and glomus jugulare tumours). Contrast enhancement will better delineate blood vessels from surrounding soft-tissue structures, and ENT opinion, angiography, and simple blood tests (e.g. alkaline phosphatase and myeloma screen) may also be helpful.

18.4.2 Intracranial extracerebral lesions

Anterior cranial fossa

Patients with olfactory groove meningiomas usually present late when the tumour is large enough to cause headache, seizures, or personality changes. Anosmia is rarely complained of in the absence of other symptoms, being usually unilateral.

Middle cranial fossa including pituitary region

Pituitary tumours may present because of endocrine effects (hormone excess or hypopituitarism) or mass effect. Women with prolactinomas commonly present with amenorrhoea and galactorrhoea and are referred to gynaecologists. Men with prolactinomas usually present later than women and may complain of headache, reduced sexual function, and visual field defects. The presence of acromegaly or steroid excess will point to a diagnosis of a growth-hormone- or ACTH-secreting macro-adenoma, respectively, and should stimulate a request for imaging of the pituitary region. Plain lateral skull radiographs may show a 'double floor' or erosion of the sella tursica in the

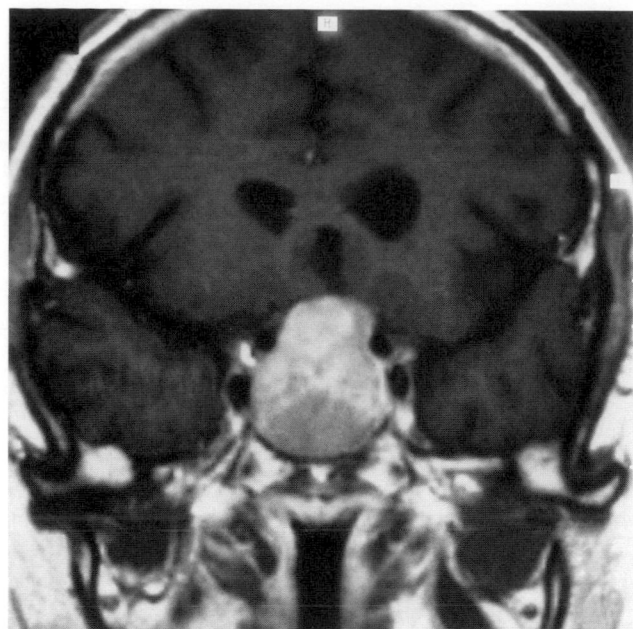

Fig. 18.1. Coronal gadolinium-enhanced MRI, showing a pituitary macroadenoma (non-functioning radiological grade IV) with suprasellar extension in a male who was referred following his third minor road traffic accident in 3 months, where he hit parked cars on his left side. Examination revealed a classical bitemporal homonymous hemianopia and optic nerve pallor. He was found to have panhypopituitarism. He was treated with hydrocortisone, thyroxine, and DDAVP®, and a transphenoidal hypophysectomy was performed with almost complete resection. He elected to have a 'wait and watch' policy rather than pituitary radiotherapy.

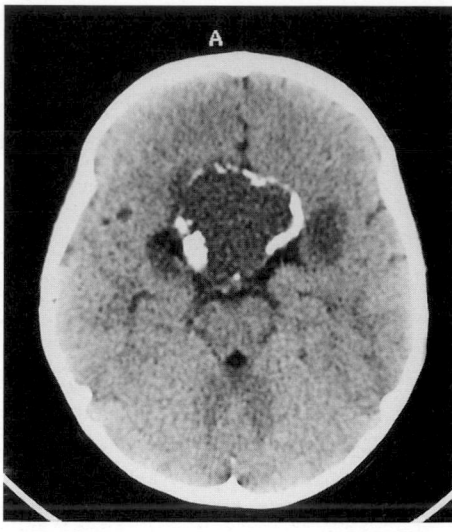

Fig. 18.2. Axial non-contrast CT scan, showing craniopharyngioma with cysts and calcification. As in this case, it can be difficult to distinguish this from an exophytic intracerebral tumour, such as an oligodendroglioma. Further imaging in the coronal plane by MRI with gadolinium contrast can be helpful.

presence of a pituitary macroadenoma. Skull radiography, however, may be entirely normal in macroadenoma and is always normal in microadenomas, and is insufficient to exclude any intracranial tumour. Investigations for hormone-secreting pituitary tumour include prolactin levels, growth hormone levels, and serum or urinary cortisols, plus imaging of the pituitary gland by multiplanar, contrast-enhanced MRI, or contrast-enhanced coronal CT with fine cuts through the pituitary gland (Fig. 18.1).

Craniopharyngiomas commonly present with symptoms and signs of mild hypopituitarism or diabetes insipidus. Almost 90 per cent of men complain of impotence, while most women complain of amenorrhoea. Children present with short stature, and 40 per cent of patients will be hypothyroid at presentation while 25 per cent have adrenal insufficiency. Fifty per cent of patients will have diabetes insipidus and headache. Craniopharyngiomas are usually a complex combination of cysts and solid tumour with calcification (Fig. 18.2). There is generally no surrounding oedema in the brain. Craniopharyngiomas can be difficult to differentiate from dermoid or epidermoid tumours or Rathke's pouch cysts but they generally have more complex cysts than epidermoids, thicker irregular walls, and more calcification on CT scan. Hypopituitarism is also found in 20 per cent of patients with epidermoid and dermoid cysts in the suprasellar or parasellar areas (Fonari *et al.* 1990).

Patients with visual-field loss due to optic nerve or chiasm compression and will be referred to ophthalmologists, physicians, or neurologists. The visual impairment may be due to pathology in the nerve (e.g. glioma), or pressure on the nerve from a tumour (pituitary tumour, craniopharyngioma, meningioma, metastasis) or cyst (dermoid, epidermoid, Rathke's pouch cyst). Symptoms will lead to imaging of the anterior visual pathway. Multiplanar gadolinium-enhanced MRI imaging is the investigation of choice. The coronal images will provide useful information about expansion of the optic nerves consistent with an optic nerve glioma or meningioma, and about the parasellar region and the relationship with any extrinsic pressure on the optic chiasm. Pituitary macroadenomas usually cause expansion of the pituitary fossa and displace the optic chiasm upwards, producing a bitemporal field loss which starts in the superior temporal quadrants (Section 8.6). The visual-field defects with pituitary macroadenomas will vary, depending on whether the optic chiasm is prefixed or postfixed. Craniopharyngiomas expand downwards from the hypothalamus and cause a bitemporal hemianopia, most frequently involving the inferior temporal quadrants, but can also cause a variety of visual field defects, depending on where the tumour presses on the visual apparatus. Epidermoid and dermoid cyst generally appear on CT scanning as well-circumscribed lesions with low density, between that of CSF and brain, due to cholesterol or keratin granules. The wall of epidermoid cysts may be thinly calcified, and since the contents are avascular they do not enhance with contrast. Dermoids are more heterogeneous, have a thicker wall, rarely enhance, and more commonly demonstrate calcification. There is generally no surrounding oedema in the brain. On T1-weighted MRI sequences, epidermoids exhibit a variable signal (white when the lipid content is high or black if the lipid content is low). Classically, epidermoids have low signal on T1-weighted images and very high signal on T2-weighted images. Dermoids give high signal on T1-weighted images in areas containing fat and variable signal where there is a combination of fat, muscle, and bone, and they may be mistaken for a craniopharyngioma or mixed germ cell tumour (teratoma). Mixed germ cell tumours are more heterogeneous than germ cell tumours (germinomas) because they contain a variety of tissues, including bone, cartilage, hair, and fatty tissue. Enhancement following contrast is common in germ cell tumours. Tumours such as hypothalamic astrocytomas and oligodendrogliomas can also extend downwards to cause chiasmal or optic nerve compression and hypopituitarism. These tumours are usually solid with areas of calcification but can also sometimes be exophytic. Rathke's cleft cysts are simple intrasellar cysts containing CSF. Meningiomas are usually easily differentiated from cysts and other tumours; however, en plaque meningioma of the optic nerve may be difficult to visualize, even with gadolinium-enhanced MRI, and should always be considered as a potential diagnosis in patients with progressive optic nerve disease even in the absence of a clear mass lesion on MRI.

Patients who present with periorbital pain, ocular muscle paralysis, or ptosis may have tumours in the orbit (e.g. metastases, lymphoma, lacrimal gland carcinoma) or tumours of the sphenoid wing (e.g. meningioma, carcinoma, dermoid, epidermoid or large pituitary tumours, or craniopharyngioma). Differential diagnosis will depend on the speed of onset of symptoms and the imaging appearance.

Posterior fossa

If the presenting complaint is facial numbness or weakness, or deafness, tinnitus or vertigo, patients are likely to be sent by their family practitioners to see a physician or ENT surgeon. The differential diagnosis includes acoustic neuroma, meningioma, haemangioblastoma, meningioma, dermoid, epidermoid, lipoma, and metastasis.

The most common tumour of the cerebellopontine angle is an acoustic neuroma (Fig. 18.3). Patients most commonly present with deafness, tinnitus, or vertigo (Sections 9.3.6 and 9.7.5). Patients with meningiomas less commonly have acoustic nerve symptoms and more commonly present with other cranial nerve involvement (especially facial numbness and facial weakness); however, differentiating on clinical grounds is unreliable. MRI is the most sensitive imaging technique to delineate lesions of the middle or posterior cranial fossae. Acoustic neuromas usually expand the acoustic nerve and may cause expansion of the internal auditory meatus. Small tumours enhance uniformly and are usually easy to distinguish from other tumours; however, if acoustic neuromas are very large, it may be difficult to identify the origin of the tumour and distinguish it from a meningioma. Meningiomas strongly enhance uniformly on CT, reflecting the vascularity of these tumours, but necrosis, cysts, and calcification can alter the signal characteristics on MRI, making differentiation from dermoids or even haemangioblastomas rather difficult. Cholesteatomas and

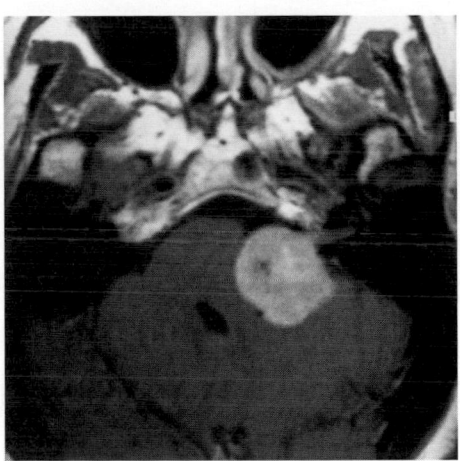

Fig. 18.3. Axial gadolinium-enhanced MRI, showing an acoustic neuroma with distortion of the pons and some midline shift. This 53-year-old woman was fit but presented with moderate unilateral deafness and slight unsteadiness. Examination revealed unilateral sensorineural deafness, horizontal jerk nystagmus, and (in retrospect) a diminished corneal reflex. There were no signs of neurofibromatosis. Management and even surgical approach is debatable (Section 18.7.3) but she had complete surgical resection and was left with unilateral profound deafness, partial lower motor neuron facial weakness, and an anaesthetic cornea.

epidermoids can commonly be differentiated from meningiomas and acoustic neuromas by their relative lack of enhancement.

If the lower cranial nerves are involved, it is imperative to get good imaging of the base of the skull, neural exit foramina, and extracranial soft tissues in the neck.

18.4.3 Intracerebral lesions

Headache, memory or personality changes, and seizures are the most common initial symptoms in patients with primary intracerebral tumours; however, patients are commonly referred to hospital only when focal symptoms or signs become obvious (e.g. seizures, hemiparesis papilloedema, dysphasia, or hemianopia). Hemiparesis or hemisensory loss are the most common symptoms at hospital presentation (Table 18.5).

Table 18.5. Common signs found at first hospital presentation in patients with intracerebral tumours

Sign	High-grade glioma (%)	Low-grade glioma (%)	Other primary (%)	Metastasis (%)	All tumours
Nil	13.2	44.7	5.6	12.4	14.4
Hemiparesis/ hemisensory	53.8	23.4	16.7	45.4	42.7
Cognitive/ personality	32.1	17.0	25.0	26.9	26.9
Papilloedema	23.6	14.9	22.2	9.2	14.4
Dysphasia	20.7	8.5	11.1	13.2	14.4
Hemianopia	18.9	6.4	11.1	6.0	9.6

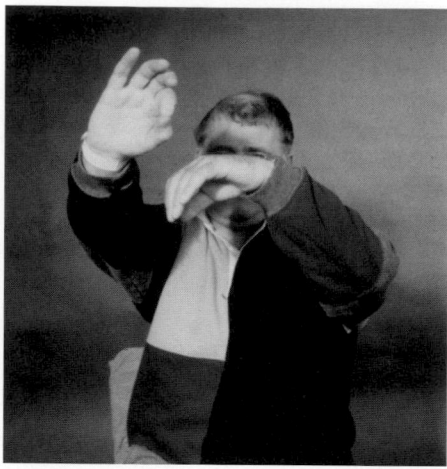

Fig. 18.4. Patient with a right frontal astrocytoma (treated by radiotherapy) with mild to moderate distal weakness of his left hand and leg which led to problems with manipulation and speed of walking. Response to treatment was followed clinically using the timed nine-hole peg test and the timed 10-m walk.

Nearly all patients who have weakness or numbness complain of these symptoms, thus directing the clinician to the abnormality on examination. Only 7 per cent of patients with malignant glioma complain of visual symptoms, yet over 20 per cent have signs of visual field loss and 23 per cent have papilloedema, therefore, careful examination of the visual fields and fundi is important in anyone complaining of headaches or symptoms suggestive of disturbance of higher mental function. Most commonly the upper motor neuron weakness is mild initially and affects fine manipulation first and mild progressive lower limb weakness (hip flexion, knee flexion, and ankle dorsiflexion) (Fig. 18.4). Clinical follow-up using quick, sensitive, simple tests such as the timed nine-hole peg test, timed 10 m walk, and a test of memory and grading of dysphasia are usually sufficient to assess clinical response to treatment (Grant *et al.* 1994*a*; Clyde *et al.* 1998). The Barthel Activities of Daily Living Index may be a useful measure in elderly patients or in patients with metastases where the weakness is commonly severe, but it is insensitive, and its 'ceiling effect' precludes its use in trials of glioma in general and it does not record cognitive disability or dysphasia. The Karnofsky Performance Scale is useful for grading patients for entry into studies, but in practice a three-point grading scale (>60, 60–50, <50) rather than an 11-point scale (100, 90, 80 ... 10, 0) is usually used. It can be used to follow individual patients, although intra-observer and inter-observer errors limit its usefulness.

Stroke-like onset or collapse with coma, occurs in about 5 per cent of patients with intracerebral tumours and is most commonly related to haemorrhage into a malignant brain tumour (malignant glioma or metastasis). Stroke-like presentations and subacute presentations with cognitive deficits, visual-field disorders, or dysphasia are more common in the elderly, and most commonly suggest a poor prognosis. Late-onset

epilepsy (first seizure after age 18) is a common presentation in patients who have low-grade gliomas and meningiomas. It has been estimated that between 3 and 10 per cent of patients with late-onset epilepsy have an underlying tumour of some form (Hopkins *et al.* 1988; Young *et al.* 1982). Seizures are the first presenting symptom in 54 per cent of low-grade gliomas, 50 per cent of anaplastic astrocytomas, 26 per cent of meningiomas, 19 per cent of glioblastomas, 15 per cent of metastases, and 11 per cent of primary CNS lymphomas. Over a follow-up period of 3 years, the prevalence of seizures rises to 70 per cent in low-grade glioma, 56 per cent in anaplastic astrocytoma, 48 per cent in glioblastoma, 44 per cent in meningioma, 39 per cent in primary CNS lymphoma, and 31 per cent in metastases. Tumour-associated epilepsy is partial (focal) in approximately 50 per cent of patients, partial epilepsy with secondary generalization in 25 per cent, and tonic–clonic seizures without warning in 25 per cent of patients. Children are more likely to have posterior fossa, or deep thalamic region tumours and present with cerebellar symptoms or, more frequently, symptoms of raised intracranial pressure.

CT and MRI brain scanning have improved the management of patients with brain tumours dramatically, but diagnostic interpretation is not without its difficulties. The addition of MRI spectroscopy may increase the specificity of diagnostic imaging, although this requires further prospective study. The three levels of diagnosis are:

1. Is it a tumour?

2. What type of tumour is it?

3. If it is a glioma, what grade of glioma is it?

Is it a tumour?

Neuroradiologists will correctly predict an intracerebral tumour in about 90–95 per cent of cases. However, approximately 10 per cent of patients will have had a previous CT or MRI scan that has been reported as either normal or an alternative pathology. In these cases, MRI will usually demonstrate an abnormality but the aetiology of the lesion may not be clear. Even in the best centres 5–10 per cent of CT scans reported by a radiologist as being an intracerebral tumour will later be found to have non-malignant pathologies. The differential diagnosis of non-contrast-enhancing lesions, with standard doses of contrast, include demyelination, encephalitis, infarct, post-traumatic, and non-specific changes. The differential diagnosis in patients with contrast-enhancing lesions includes demyelination, arteriovenous malformation, haemorrhagic stroke, and cerebral abscess. In some cases who present with a stroke-like onset, it may not be evident that the haemorrhage has occurred into an existing mass lesion. The common tumours to present with intratumoural haemorrhage are glioblastoma, metastatic lung cancer, melanoma, and choriocarcinoma.

What type of tumour is it?

Errors in reporting of CT or MRI are even more common when attempts are made to predict the type of malignancy. The main

Table 18.6. Imaging characteristics and pointers towards diagnosis of common intrinsic brain tumours

	Pilocytic astrocytoma	Astrocytoma	Oligodendro-glioma	Medullo-blastoma	Malignant glioma	Metastasis	Primary CNS	Germ cell
Peak age	10–30 yr	20–40 yr	20–50 yr	1–20 yr	40–70 yr	50–80 yr	50–70 yr	10–30 yr
Site	Usually cerebral or midline cerebellar	Adult cerebral; child cerebellar	Fronto-temporal	Cerebellum, IV ventricle	Cerebral	Anywhere	Periventricular, anywhere	Pineal, suprasellar
Single/multiple	Single	Single	Single	Single/CSF	95% single	33% single	60% single; CSF >20%; Vitreous >20%	90% single; CSF >20%
Usual characteristics								
Borders	Well demarcated	Diffuse/infiltrating	Well defined	Well defined	Serpiginous	Well defined	Indistinct	Distinct
Cysts	Common	Uncommon	Uncommon	Uncommon	Occ. necrotic	Occasionally	Nil	Occasionally
Calcification	10–40%	5–10%	50%	Nil	<5%	<3%	Nil	10–15%
Peritumoral oedema	Nil or mild	Mild	Mild	Moderate	Moderate	Moderate/severe	Mild/severe	Nil/mild
Mass effect	Nil or mild	Mild	Mild/moderate	Moderate	Moderate	Moderate/severe	Mild/severe	Nil/mild
CT	Low density; Enhancing nodule	Low density; No enhancement	Low density; No enhancement	Occ. high density; Enhancement	Low density; Border enhances	Low density; Uniform/border	Occ. high density; Uniform/border	Low density; Uniform
MRI								
T1	Iso/hyperintense	Hypointense	Hypointense	Hypointense	Hypointense	Hypointense	Hyper/isointense	Iso/hypointense
T1 Gad	Enhancing nodule	No enhancement	No enhancement	Enhancement	Border enhances	Uniform/border	Uniform/border	Uniform
T2	Hyperintense	Hyperintense	Hyperintense	Hyperintense	Hyperintense	Hyperintense	Hyperintense	Hyperintense
Other helpful tests	–	–	–	MRI spine; CSF	–	Chest/abdo. CT; Tumour markers	Slit-lamp (eyes); CSF	CSF; Tumour markers
Differential diagnosis	Abscess, Malig. glioma, Ganglioglioma, Craniopharyngioma, Germinoma	Multiple sclerosis, Infarct, Oligodendroglioma, Malig. glioma	Meningioma, AVM, Astrocytoma, Craniopharyngioma, Malig. glioma	Astrocytoma, Malig. glioma, Lymphoma, Germinoma	Abscess, Stroke, Metastasis, Oligodendroglioma, Lymphoma	Stroke, Abscess, Malig. glioma, Lymphoma	Multiple sclerosis, Sarcoid, Metastasis, Malig. glioma, Toxoplasmosis	Meningioma, PNET, Malig. glioma, Metastasis

abdo., Abdominal; AVM, arterio-venous malformation; CSF, cerebrospinal fluid; Gad, gadolinium; Malig., malignant; Occ., occasional(ly); PNET, primitive neuro-ectodermal tumour.

areas of difficulty are where tumours have an exophytic extension with involvement of the meninges, intense contrast enhancement, or sometimes calcification of meningeal/vascular origin (e.g. meningioma/haemangiopericytoma) or of glial origin (e.g. glioblastoma or oligodendroglioma). In these cases it may be very difficult to say whether the tumour is extracerebral and invading the brain, or intrinsic and becoming exophytic.

It has been estimated that 5 per cent of brain images reported as multiple metastases by experienced neuroradiologists will actually turn out to be primary brain tumours (glioma or primary CNS lymphoma) (Patchell *et al.* 1990). In one study of single brain metastasis, 11 per cent of patients with known systemic malignancy with a solitary brain lesion thought on imaging to be a metastasis turned out to have a different pathology (in some cases the pathology was not a tumour at all) (Patchell *et al.* 1990). Primary CNS lymphoma can be unifocal (60 per cent) or multifocal (40 per cent). Cells are densely packed and generally homogeneously enhance and thus are commonly mistaken for metastases.

If it is a glioma, what grade of glioma is it?

There are some characteristics on imaging that are more common in a particular histology, but no single characteristic is specific (Table 18.6). Astrocytomas and oligodendrogliomas are commonly homogeneous, may be cystic or show areas of calcification, and usually do not enhance, whereas anaplastic astrocytoma and glioblastoma multiforme are generally heterogeneous with cysts or necrosis, commonly demonstrating shift of midline structures with significant oedema and contrast enhancement. Algorithms have been suggested, based on contrast enhancement, space occupation, cyst formation, necrosis, and oedema, to help predict the grade of malignancy; however, these only predict about 60 per cent of cases correctly. In a recent study, at a time when CT and MRI were readily available, 45 per cent of patients who were suspected of having an astrocytoma had an anaplastic astrocytoma and 5 per cent had a non-malignant histology following biopsy (Kondziolka *et al.* 1993). These figures are in keeping with a more recent (1998–99) prospective audit of everyday practice in three neuroscience centres in Scotland, which revealed that radiologists have a positive predictive value of 0.78 and an accuracy of 0.61, for diagnosing malignant glioma (Grant *et al.* 2000). Pilocytic astrocytomas, subependymal giant cell astrocytoma, myxopapillary ependymoma, and desmoplastic neuro-epithelial tumours can show contrast enhancement and may be misdiagnosed as malignant gliomas or metastases.

Histopathological correlation has proved that enhancing areas on post-contrast CT and MRI scans correspond to densely cellular, hypervascular tissue of viable tumour (Fig. 18.5) (Burger *et al.* 1983; Whelan *et al.* 1988). A consistent finding from stereotactic biopsy studies is of a variable zone of microscopic tumour infiltration outside the enhancing area, extending at least as far as the abnormal signal on the T2-weighted images. There may be even greater extension of isolated tumour cells beyond these

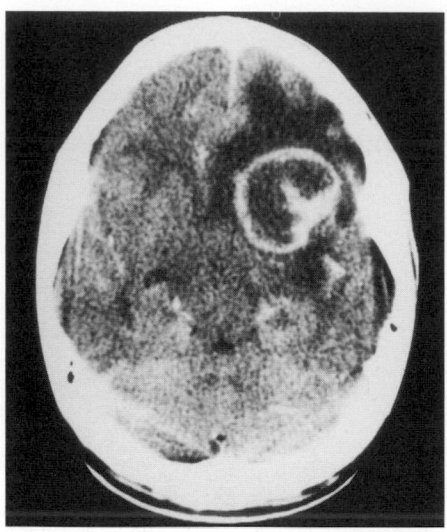

Fig. 18.5. Axial contrast-enhanced CT scan, showing glioblastoma multiforme. Differential diagnosis would include metastasis or even abscess (e.g. toxoplasmosis), depending on the clinical story. Histological confirmation (e.g. stereotactic biopsy or resection) is usually advisable. Freehand biopsy has a high risk–benefit ratio and should be avoided.

radiologically defined boundaries (Kelly *et al.* 1987; Burger *et al.* 1988). This sort of detailed histopathological correlative work will have to be repeated to truly assess the value of newer imaging modalities that purport to better identify the limits of the tumour (e.g. magnetization transfer weighted FLASH (fast, low-angle shot) MR pulse sequences, MRI spectroscopy, and radionuclide SPECT or positron emission tomography).

The small, uniform cells of a primary CNS lymphoma are densely packed together and these tumours are commonly more radiodense than surrounding brain on non-contrast-enhanced CT scan, giving the appearance that some contrast has been given (Fig. 18.6a). When contrast is given, they can

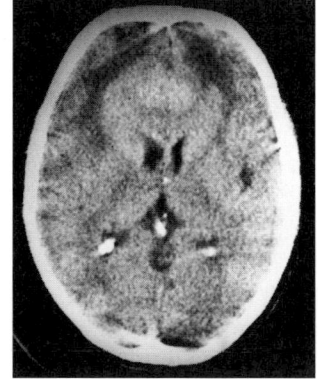
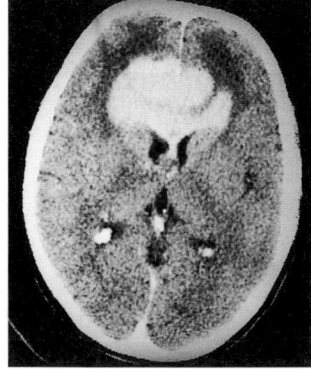

(a)   (b)

Fig. 18.6. Primary CNS lymphoma. (a) Axial non-contrast CT scan, demonstrating periventricular and corpus callosal tumour with pseudo-enhancement due to densely packed, small cells (occasionally found with other small cell tumours, e.g. medulloblastoma and small cell lung cancer). (b) Profound uniform contrast enhancement.

enhance intensely (Fig. 18.6b). These features are non-specific for primary CNS lymphoma and can be seen in other tumours comprised of tightly packed cells (e.g. some metastases, some small cell malignant gliomas, and medullobastomas). Frequently, in AIDS, patients' CNS lymphoma can demonstrate ring enhancement similar to an abscess. Primary CNS lymphomas are commonly located in a periventricular distribution deep in the white matter, and approximately two-thirds occur in the cerebral hemispheres and one-third infratentorially.

The pineal gland lies between the splenium of the corpus callosum above and the superior colliculus below. Numerous tumour types can arise in the pineal region (germ cell tumours, pineocytomas, gliomas, metastases, cysts). Patients commonly present with Parinaud's syndrome with limitation of upgaze and convergence, and impaired pupillary reaction to light and accommodation. Eyelid retraction (Collier's sign) or ptosis can also occur. Some patients will have diabetes insipidus and if there is a β-human chorionic gonadotrophin (β-hCG) secreting germinoma, precocious puberty can occur. CT or MRI scan with gadolinium will demonstrate the lesion, which is generally causing an obstructive hydrocephalus. The most common tumours in this area are teratomas or germinomas. Pineocytomas are less common and arise from the pineal parenchymal cells. Gliomas can arise in the pineal region and metastases to the pineal region also occur. In addition to these solid tumours, pineal region cysts can occur and can be simple, filled with CSF, or can be epidermoid or dermoid cysts. Germinomas are usually solid, enhance uniformly, and may be surrounded by calcium. Teratomas also enhance but are heterogeneous, with multiloculated cysts. Non-germinomatous germ cell tumours are heterogeneous and may enhance irregularly or not at all. Choriocarcinoma bleeds frequently and intratumoural haemorrhage or bleeding into a cyst may occur. Pineocytomas have low signal on T1-weighted images and high signal on T2-weighted images and enhance uniformly, but there can be calcification within the tumour, or haemorrhage if there are any pineoblastoma elements. Pineal gliomas can vary on imaging, depending on whether they are low- or high-grade tumours. Tumours at this site quite commonly seed to the spinal CSF, therefore spinal imaging is also important. Serum and CSF (in the absence of hydrocephalus) analysis for germ cell markers can be valuable. Malignant teratoma, germinoma with syncytioblastic cells, embryonal carcinoma, and endodermal sinus tumours may have elevated levels of α-fetoprotein. Choriocarcinoma and embryonal carcinoma may have elevated levels of β-hCG, whereas only germinomas and germinomas with syncytiotrophoblastic cells have elevated levels of placental alkaline phosphatase. Non-germ cell tumours are negative for all these markers. CSF histology is usually negative. In the presence of these hormones, the most likely diagnosis is a teratoma or choriocarcinoma. If the CSF is negative for these markers, then biopsy of the pineal tumour is recommended. Shunting of the ventricles may be necessary prior to definitive operation or at the time of operation.

18.5 Importance of histological confirmation

The classification scheme used to type tumours is the WHO classification (Table 18.1). Histological classification and grading are important, because management strategies and prognosis are considerably changed depending on the tumour type and tumour grade. For example, diagnostic work-up and management of certain tumours (e.g. primary CNS lymphoma, medulloblastoma, germinoma) are completely different from others (e.g. glioma, meningioma, metastasis). Some tumour types are very sensitive to radiation (e.g. germinoma, lymphoma) while others (e.g. glioma, teratoma) are strongly resistant to radiation. Some tumours are chemosensitive (lymphoma, germinoma, anaplastic oligodendroglioma) while others are relatively chemoresistant (glioblastoma, meningioma).

Various grading systems for glial neoplasms have been proposed. Most current grading systems divide astrocytic neoplasms into three (Ringertz 1950; Zulch 1979; Nelson *et al.* 1983; Burger *et al.* 1985) or four levels of anaplasia (Kernohan and Sayre 1952; Dumas-Duport *et al.* 1988).

The main histological characteristics used to grade primary malignancy are: increased cellularity, increased number and atypical appearance of mitotic activity, pleomorphism or anaplasia, proliferation of the vascular endothelium, and tissue necrosis. Grading systems, e.g. Dumas-Duport, have been validated by correlation between the level of anaplasia and survival after diagnosis (Kim *et al.* 1991).

Until recently, a key diagnostic criterion for glioblastoma multiforme (GBM) has been the presence or absence of necrosis, but the revised World Health Organization system (WHO-2) and the Dumas-Duport systems do not require necrosis for classification as GBM (Kleihues *et al.* 1993b; Dumas-Duport *et al.* 1988). In a recent histological review of glial tumours at University of California, San Francisco, necrosis did predict a shorter survival; however, the magnitude of the survival difference between patients with and without necrosis was small (median survival 10.9 months versus 12.5 months, respectively) and the authors suggested that their data support the WHO-2 classification of endothelial proliferation without necrosis as sufficient to make a diagnosis of GBM (Barker *et al.* 1996). If different centres use different pathological grading systems, it is difficult to determine what is the effect of treatment on survival and what is the effect of the grading system used in the particular department. Most centres now use either the WHO system or the Dumas-Duport system.

The heterogeneous nature of some tumours means that insufficient sampling of the tumour (e.g. by inadequate sampling by stereotactic biopsy) can lead to undergrading of tumours and result in inappropriate treatment planning. The use of image-directed stereotactic techniques have led to a 95 per cent diagnostic success rate (even in small tumours in sites with difficult access) and allows several samples from representative areas of the tumour to be taken, so that grading is more reliable (Revesz *et al.* 1993; Bernstein and Parrent 1994).

18.6 Head, neck, and skull tumours

Tumours of the head and neck can be divided based on their position in relation to the skull and, if biopsied, by their cell type. Extracranial tumours of the head and neck are usually due to carcinoma of the paranasal sinuses, nasopharynx, oral cavity, or oropharynx, or are as a result of tumours arising from local structures, e.g. blood vessels (glomus jugulare) or bone (chordoma, chondroma). These tumours commonly produce cranial neuropathies.

18.6.1 Carcinoma

Head and neck cancer usually affects patients in the fifth and sixth decades. The most common primary tumours are carcinoma of:

(1) the nasal cavity and paranasal sinuses;

(2) nasopharynx;

(3) oral cavity; and

(4) oropharynx.

Squamous cell carcinoma is the most common cell type. Risk factors are smoking and possibly alcohol. Up to 10 per cent of patients with head and neck tumours have second malignancies, which also tend to be cancers associated with tobacco or alcohol (e.g. lung, oesophagus, stomach).

The nasal cavity and paranasal sinuses

Tumours of the nasal cavity and sinuses have an incidence of less than $1/10^5$/year, affect men twice as often as women, and usually occur in patients over 60 years. Higher incidences are found in Japan and South Africa. Occupational factors include nickel or chromium exposure, radium, and isopropyl alcohol. The frequencies of nasal and paranasal cancers are higher in the furniture, shoe, and textile industries (Roush 1979). Tumours in this region are commonly squamous cell carcinomas, but esthesioneuroblastomas and adenoid cystic tumours can also be aggressive and invade the cranial cavity. Tumours are frequently far advanced by the time of diagnosis, because the symptoms of nasal blockage or discharge are frequently ignored. Extension to the orbit may cause diplopia and proptosis, and extension upwards may result in direct invasion of the cribriform plate and frontal lobes, with anosmia and headache. Surgery usually involves a combined approach from a skull base team (e.g. neurosurgeon, ENT surgeon, and faciomaxillary surgeon). Factors that make surgical resection difficult, or sometimes impossible, include the involvement of the base of skull, nasopharynx, or sphenoid sinus. In inoperable patients, local disease can be controlled in a substantial proportion of patients by use of radiation therapy.

Nasopharynx

Nasopharyngeal carcinoma is endemic in China and North Africa. Dietary factors such as nitrosomines in salt-cured food and viral factors (Epstein–Barr virus) have been implicated in the malignant transformation into nasopharyngeal cancer. These tumours usually occur predominantly in 40–60-year-olds, and males are twice as likely to be affected. Nasopharyngeal carcinoma most commonly presents as a lump in the neck, but can also cause nasal blockage and deafness from blockage of the Eustachian tube, or invade the skull base or cavernous sinus, causing cranial nerve palsies. Surgical biopsy confirms the diagnosis and radiation therapy is the treatment of choice. At recurrence, surgery has a limited role. Chemotherapy can be helpful to treat widespread metastatic disease, which occurs in a high proportion of patients with this tumour. Cisplatin, methotrexate, and epirubicin all have some palliative effect. Five-year survival rates of 50–60 per cent can be achieved with combinations of these treatment modalities.

Oral cavity

Tumours of the oral cavity are typically squamous and a close link with smoking has been identified. Alcohol may also be implicated in the aetiology. Diagnosis is usually earlier than other head and neck tumours and neural involvement is less common. These tumours can, however, cause the 'numb-chin syndrome' due to involvement of the mental nerve, a branch of the mandibular division of the trigeminal nerve.

Oropharynx

Tumours of the oropharynx usually occur in patients older than 50 years and, again, are more common in males (4 : 1). Smoking and alcohol are the most common risk factors. Presentation is commonly quite late and lymph node spread and neural involvement are frequently found. Bulbar palsy or isolated involvement of the lower cranial nerves are not uncommon. Surgery and radiation therapy are the mainstays of treatment and survival depends on the site, extent, and staging of the tumour. Laryngeal and hypopharyngeal carcinomas cause local pain or referred pain to the ear and lymphadenopathy in the neck. Dysarthria and swallowing difficulties and recurrent laryngeal nerve palsy can also occur.

In general, if patients with head and neck tumours have early disease, radical resection and postoperative radiotherapy can be curative, although the cosmetic and functional result of treatment may affect quality of life. In advanced disease, where cure is not possible, it may be best to treat the primary site by radiation and any locoregional lymph nodes by surgical resection and radiotherapy. The 5-year survival for nasal and sinus carcinoma is approximately 60 per cent, but depends on the extent of primary disease at presentation. Chemotherapy in the initial treatment regime can lead to significant tumour regression in 60–90 per cent of cases, but does not extend overall survival compared the surgery and chemotherapy alone (Lefebvre *et al.* 1996).

18.6.2 Chordoma

Chordomas are very rare, slow-growing tumours that arise from remnants of the notocord and generally occur in the midline in the region of the clivus at the base of the skull. They are locally invasive and usually present late because of the nondescript nature of the chronic headache or neck pain. They may present with intermittent diplopia, facial numbness if the upper clivus is involved, or as a nasopharyngeal mass with multiple lower cranial neuropathy (glossopharyngeal, vagus, accessory, and hypoglossal nerves) if the lower clivus is involved. Most clivus chordomas produce destruction of the clivus and have extradural extension. CT scan best demonstrates bone destruction, but MRI better demonstrates the tumour margins and soft-tissue structures and blood vessels. MRI demonstrates low signal intensity on T1-weighted scans. Chordomas rarely calcify or enhance. Imaging alone cannot adequately differentiate between chordoma, chondroid chordoma, and chondrosarcoma; however, chondrosarcomas usually arise along the petrooccipital fissure and more commonly calcify. Occasionally chondrosarcomas can arise in the midline in the region of the clivus. Because of the approximation of the tumour to sensitive neural and vascular tissues, complete surgical removal is not usually possible, but surgery is required to make the diagnosis and to reduce bulk disease. Care should be taken try and keep the dura intact when performing trans-sinus surgery because of the risk of postoperative meningitis; however, since 50 per cent of these tumours have already breached the dura by the time of diagnosis, careful postoperative packing with fat and muscle grafts is essential. Radical resection of anterior skull-base tumours has improved in the hands of teams of surgeons specializing in skull-base surgery (Lawton *et al.* 1995), but the advice is to follow surgical removal with local radiation therapy. There are no randomized studies of the effect of radiation, and conventional photon irradiation has shown no dose–response relationship (Tai *et al.* 1995). Even using multiple agents, chemotherapy is only rarely effective (Scimeca *et al.* 1996). The natural history of chordoma is minimally affected by surgery and radiotherapy, although symptom control can be achieved adequately. Five-year survival rates range from 10 to 58 per cent in different series, but most series suggest that less than 50 per cent of patients are alive at 5 years.

18.6.3 Glomus tumours

Glomus tumours arise from the glomus jugulare and can spread medially to involve the middle ear or skull base, and therefore can present with hoarseness and dysphagia due to lower cranial nerve palsies. In some cases these tumours can cause pulsatile tinnitus and deafness and the tumour can be seen behind the tympanic membrane. CT or MRI scan is usually sufficient to make the diagnosis, but angiography is also valuable to define the blood supply to the tumour and to embolize the tumour preoperatively. Surgery can be hazardous and usually involves a skull-base team. It requires mastoid and suboccipital craniectomy and can be complicated by meningitis or facial nerve palsy. The place of radiation therapy is debatable. The tumour is benign, but complete resection is often not possible. Local control can be achieved by radiation therapy alone in approximately 90 per cent of patients with inoperable glomus tumours (Springate and Weichselbaum 1990).

18.6.4 Fibrous dysplasia

Fibrous dysplasia is a benign fibrous process that can involve the skull vault or the base of the skull. The condition can present in isolation or as part of the McCune–Albright syndrome (fibrous dysplasia, café-au-lait spots, endocrinopathy (e.g. precocious puberty, thyrotoxicosis, primary hyperparathyroidism, hyerprolactinaemia)). McCune–Albright syndrome is due to postzygotic somatic mutations in the gene encoding $G_{S\alpha}$ proteins (*GNAS1*) (Ringel *et al.* 1996). Pathologically, the bone is replaced by fibrous tissue composed of collagen and fibroblasts. It can be difficult to distinguish fibrous dysplasia from an ossifying fibroma. Headaches or cranial nerve involvement are the common presenting symptoms. Craniobasal fibrous dysplasia can produce progressive visual loss due to extradural optic nerve compression if it affects the bones of the orbit, or conductive and sensorineural hearing loss if the disease affects the temporal bone. A canal cholesteatoma is found in 40 per cent of patients with temporal bone involvement with fibrous dysplasia. Surgical resection is usually the treatment of choice. Radiation therapy may also be beneficial in relieving symptoms. Malignant transformation to a fibrosarcoma is rare, but can occur.

18.6.5 Skull osteomas

Cranial osteomas are common and not usually symptomatic, but occasionally, because of their size or site, they can cause cosmetic disfigurement, headache, cranial neuropathies, or seizures. Rarely, they are associated with Gardner's syndrome. A new classification for cranial osteomas has been suggested (Haddad *et al.* 1997). The classification divides osteomas into parenchymal, dural, skull base, and skull vault, with the latter being divided into enostotic and exostotic variants. CT scan is the imaging technique of choice. Indications for surgery include progressive ophthalmoplegia, neurological signs, and significant cosmetic deformity.

18.6.6 Paget's disease

Cranial Paget's disease (osteitis deformans) can be monoostotic or polyostotic. Paget's disease involves the cranial vault and temporal bones in 30–40 per cent of cases. It is characterized by excessive and disorganized bone formation and resorption. Patients may present with headaches, hearing loss, tinnitus and vertigo, or hemifacial spasm. The bone alkaline phosphatase is almost always elevated and is a useful marker, but the best marker with which to follow cranial involvement with Paget's is the serum carboxy-terminal propeptide of type 1 procollagen for new bone formation and the urinary C-terminal telopeptide of type 1 collagen for bone resorption (Alvarez *et al.* 1997). Calcitonin and etidronate and newer bisphosphonates (e.g. alendronate) can help control the turnover of new bone and help control pain and prevent neurological or orthopaedic complications.

18.7 Intracranial extracerebral tumours

Intracranial extracerebral tumours arise from pituitary gland (pituitary adenoma), meninges (meningioma), nerves (neuroma), or neuroepithelial remnants (dermoid, epidermoid), and are usually benign. Metastases directly to the dural space do occur (especially with breast cancer and lymphoma) but frequently they are a late complication in patients with widespread systemic involvement or as part of a malignant meningitic process where they can produce mass lesions.

18.7.1 Pituitary tumours

Pituitary tumours can arise from any cell in the anterior pituitary gland and account for 10 per cent of intracranial tumours. They are most commonly benign adenomas, although pituitary carcinomas and metastasis to the pituitary do occur. Tumours can produce symptoms and signs through hypersecretion of hormones, or related to the mass effect of the tumour on the optic nerves or structures adjacent to the pituitary gland. Tumours generally have to be greater than 1 cm in diameter before they cause any symptoms of neural or vascular compression. When the tumour expands the pituitary gland, it can cause hypofunction of certain hormones and produce hypothyroidism, amenorrhoea, or Addison's disease. Involvement of the neurohypophysis can rarely result in diabetes insipidus. When the tumour extends laterally it can involve the cavernous sinus and result in cranial neuropathies. Haemorrhage into the pituitary gland can cause pituitary apoplexy.

The most common type of pituitary adenoma is the microadenoma. Microadenomas by definition are less than 10 mm in diameter, do not expand the pituitary fossa, and usually secrete prolactin. About 70 per cent of prolactin-secreting tumours are microadenomas. Prolactin-secreting microadenomas are more common in women, and women present earlier because of secondary amenorrhoea, infertility, or galactorrhoea. Prolactinomas in men probably present at a later stage and are more commonly macroadenomas. Headache, loss of libido, and visual failure or visual field defect are the usual symptoms. Prolactinomas commonly cause hyperprolactinaemia with blood levels of greater than 100–200 μg/l, although prolactinomas can not be excluded at lower levels of prolactin. Occasionally prolactin levels of more than 100 μg/l are found in idiopathic hyperprolactinaemia and this may lead to diagnostic uncertainty. Other causes of hyperprolactinaemia include drugs, hypothyroidism, and renal failure. To differentiate between a prolactinoma and hyperprolactinaemia from other causes, thyrotrophin response to a dopamine receptor antagonist may be used, since only prolactinomas may have an increased response.

Non-functioning tumours slowly expand, causing upward displacement of the optic chiasm and a characteristic bitemporal hemianopia with headache and sometimes panhypopituitarism. Most clinically non-functioning adenomas express gonadotrophin hormone subunits *in vitro* or, occasionally, *in vivo*. By the time of diagnosis by clinical, radiological, and hormonal studies symptoms have usually been present for some years. Cushing's disease can occur and is associated with elevated adrenocorticotrophin hormone. The clinical features of central obesity, 'moon' facies, buffalo hump, abdominal striae, and hypertension usually make the condition obvious. Some patients do not have the classical appearance but instead complain of depression and lethargy. Thyrotrophin (TSH) secreting pituitary adenomas are commonly macroadenomas and are usually associated with thyrotoxicosis. Occasionally longstanding primary hypothyroidism can result in pituitary hyperplasia with elevated TSH levels and enlargement of the pituitary gland. TSH-secreting pituitary adenomas will require surgical intervention. Growth-hormone-secreting adenomas are rare but present with giantism during puberty and acromegaly after fusion of the epiphyses.

Pituitary metastases are infrequent and usually occur in the context of known systemic cancer with metastatic spread to other sites, but occasionally can be the only manifestation of metastatic spread. Most cases present with headache or diabetes insipidus. Panhypopituitarism and visual field impairment is demonstrated in about 25 per cent (Sioutos *et al.* 1996).

Pituitary tumours can be classified radiologically, based on their size and growth characteristics. Grade 0 tumours are where there are no imaging abnormalities; grade I tumours show minor changes in the pituitary but are less than 1 cm in diameter; grade II shows diffuse enlargement but no focal sellar destruction, grade III shows focal involvement of the sellar, and grade IV tumours show extensive destruction of the sella. Further subclassification will depend on the extent and direction of supra- or parasellar extension. Coronal and sagittal MRI scan with gadolinium contrast gives high-definition information about the pituitary, parapituitary region, and adjacent soft tissues; however, it is not as good as CT at demonstrating bone erosion. High-resolution, contrast-enhanced coronal CT scan with 1.5 mm contiguous slices will also provide information about the homogeneity of the pituitary gland and relationship to surrounding structures. CT of a microadenoma will characteristically show low density within the gland; however, small cysts in the pituitary occur in normal people and therefore the diagnosis of microprolactinoma should not be made on radiological grounds alone. Characterization of the tumour by MRI scan plus or minus MR angiography is usually sufficient to plan surgery (Fig. 18.1). Formal arterial angiography is not usually required.

There is general agreement that bromocriptine is the treatment of choice in prolactin-secreting adenomas. Bromocriptine is a dopamine agonist that directly stimulates specific pituitary cell membrane dopamine receptors (D_2) and inhibits prolactin synthesis and secretion. Treatment will usually cause a reduction in size of any macroadenoma and reduce or normalize prolactin levels in blood. There have been reports of macroadenomas enlarging despite treatment with bromocriptine, and close review of visual acuity and fields is recommended. If patients are unable to tolerate bromocriptine because of side-effects, other dopamine agonists can be tried (e.g. pergolide, cabergoline, lisuride). During pregnancy there can be enlargement of the normal pituitary gland by up to 70 per cent and therefore special care has to be taken during pregnancy in patients with pituitary tumours, especially macroadenomas. During pregnancy bromocriptine can be discontinued if the tumour is a microadenoma. Ideally, it is advisable to wait until any macroadenoma has been adequately treated before a planned pregnancy is attempted. Bromocriptine should be restarted after pregnancy or during pregnancy if there is neurological deterioration.

Prolactin-secreting macroadenomas can also be treated by surgical resection if the tumour does not shrink with bromocriptine, there is serious visual compromise, or side-effects with medical treatment. Visual improvement occurs in 80 per cent of cases but prolactin levels frequently do not reduce to normal. The recurrence rate of macroadenomas after surgery ranges from 25 to 75 per cent, therefore radiotherapy after surgical resection may be necessary if drug therapy is not possible. Neurosurgery or radiotherapy are sometimes recommended before pregnancy, particularly for macroadenomas that have not responded to bromocriptine.

Non-functioning adenomas are usually macroadenomas. Drugs are ineffective at reducing the tumour size. Surgery is the treatment of choice and most can be dealt with via a transphenoidal approach. Surgery will confirm the diagnosis and relieve compression by the tumour on surrounding structures. About 75 per cent of patients with visual field defects will have some recovery of field postoperatively (Ebersold *et al.* 1986). Despite this, it is uncommon to achieve complete resection in macroadenomas because most have invaded the dura or surrounding structures. Close follow-up by MRI scan will usually identify which patients may benefit from radiotherapy.

If there is good endocrine evidence of a pituitary ACTH-secreting adenoma, transphenoidal surgery will result in cure in over 80 per cent and a low recurrence rate (5 per cent). These tumours are frequently microadenomas and MRI scan is commonly normal. ACTH-secreting macroadenomas have a poorer response to surgery and postoperative radiotherapy is commonly required.

Growth-hormone-secreting adenomas can be treated with somatostatin analogues; however, surgery is usually required (Barkan *et al.* 1988). Bromocriptine can also lower growth hormone levels in up to 75 per cent of cases, but it is rare to achieve normal growth hormone levels, treatment must be life-long, and there may not be any shrinkage of macroadenomas. Surgery or radiotherapy is usually required. The growth hormone response to transphenoidal resection is not as good as the endocrine response to surgery for ACTH-secreting tumours. Postoperative radiotherapy is frequently required. Radiotherapy is moderately effective and may be used as the primary treatment or as an adjunct to surgery. It may take many years to achieve normal growth hormone levels, and usually a combination of surgery and radiotherapy, or radiotherapy and drugs, is required (Bloom *et al.* 1984).

18.7.2 Meningeal tumours

Meningiomas are benign, slow-growing intracranial extracerebral tumours, which account for 15–20 per cent of all intracranial tumours. Only 25 per cent of meningiomas are symptomatic at presentation and the frequency of meningiomas increases with age (Radhakishnan *et al.* 1995). Risk factors include gender (women are more commonly affected, female : male ratio 2.2 : 1), previous ionizing radiation, and type 2 neurofibromatosis. In neurofibromatosis there is clear evidence of a genetic predisposition, and the probable cause is deletion of a tumour suppressor gene on chromosome 22q. The WHO histological classification and grading system selects characteristics that predict an aggressive behaviour of the tumour and the risk of early recurrence (Kleihues *et al.* 1993*b*). Proliferation indices identified by immunohistochemical methods on pathological specimens may also predict an aggressive nature. Meningiomas express progesterone and oestrogen receptors and receptors for platelet-derived growth factor (Black *et al.* 1996).

Eighty-five per cent of meningiomas are supratentorial. The most common sites are over the convexities of the skull, the falx or tentorium, followed by the sphenoid ridge, suprasellar areas, and olfactory groove. CT and MRI scanning will demonstrate a well-demarcated enhancing lesion with a dural base that may involve or displace adjacent nerves, or produce significant brain oedema in adjacent brain (Fig. 18.7). Angiography is not usually necessary; however, it may be helpful to identify the feeding vessels and allow immediate preoperative embolization to reduce the potential for severe haemorrhage from the tumour during operation. If the pathologist is not informed

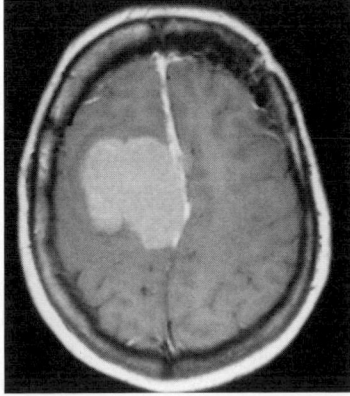

Fig. 18.7. Axial gadolinium-enhanced MRI, showing meningioma.

that preoperative embolization has been performed, an incorrect diagnosis of malignant meningioma may be made because of the necrosis in the specimen. In symptomatic meningiomas with brain oedema, dexamethasone (2–4 mg three times a day) will usually produce speedy relief of symptoms. Although meningiomas are benign tumours, operation is not always straightforward. Asymptomatic meningiomas, especially in the elderly, are best left alone. Large, symptomatic meningiomas will usually require surgery. Surgical mortality can be as high as 14 per cent and the 10-year survival can range from 43 to 77 per cent. Convexity, parasagittal, lateral sphenoid, and olfactory groove meningiomas can usually be resected completely with low morbidity. Suprasellar, cavernous sinus, clivus, tentorial, and posterior fossa meningiomas are more difficult, although improved surgical techniques have resulted in more radical resection. Morbidity is much higher in these areas and there can be a high recurrence rate. It has been estimated that the 10-year risk of recurrence is 9–20 per cent where the surgeon feels there has been a complete resection, and 18–50 per cent recurrence where subtotal resection has been performed. Meningiomas at the base of the skull involving the sphenoid ridge may require a joint surgical approach by both faciomaxillary and neurosurgeons.

In symptomatic meningiomas in the elderly, or at sites that increase operative risk, stereotactic radiation therapy or radiosurgery, as sole treatment, may reduce the size of the tumour or slow the growth rate. Radiosurgery is usually only considered for relatively small tumours (<3 cm in diameter) that do not impinge on structures such as the pituitary/optic nerves or abut the ventricles or where operation would be hazardous. In these selected situations, up to 50 per cent of patients will have some reduction in tumour size and 50 per cent will be alive at 10 years. Following subtotal resection, radiation therapy may be considered. Postoperative radiation reduces the recurrence rate from 60 to 32 per cent and gives a longer time to recurrence (Barbara et al. 1987).

Antiprogesterones have been used with some apparent success in some patients with meningioma (Black 1993). Antioestrogens such as tamoxifen (40 mg/m^2 twice daily for 4 days followed by 10 mg twice daily) may produce a reduction in size of the tumour in 15 per cent of patients (Goodwin et al. 1995).

18.7.3 Neural tumours

Acoustic neuromas (schwannoma) account for approximately 80 per cent of extra-axial lesions in the region of the cerebellopontine angle and 4–10 per cent of intracranial tumours overall (Mahaley et al. 1990; Grant et al. 1996). Other tumours in the region of the cerebellopontine angle include meningiomas (10 per cent), primary cholesteatoma (5–10 per cent), glomus jugulare tumours (1 per cent), facial or trigeminal neuroma (1–2 per cent), and metastasis (1–5 per cent). The incidence of acoustic neuroma is approximately 1/100 000/yr. The acoustic nerve is the most common site for a neuroma (85 per cent) (Section 9.3.6), although they can also arise from the trigeminal

nerve (1–8 per cent), facial nerve (0.5–1 per cent), and spinal roots (10–15 per cent). Schwannomas arise from the junction between the peripheral Schwann cell nerve sheath and the central glial nerve sheath. Ninety five per cent of acoustic neuromas are sporadic and 5 per cent are dominantly inherited as part of neurofibromatosis type 1 (NF1) or type 2 (NF2) (Section 19.2). Karyotype analysis in sporadic schwannomas may be normal. The most common abnormality is monosomy of chromosome 22 and there may be deletions in the long arm of this chromosome (22q). The gene for NF2 has been isolated to a 6 Mb region of the q12 band of the long arm of chromosome 22, and it is highly likely that the relevant area on this chromosome involves a tumour suppressor gene. Mutations to the NF2 gene are also likely to be an important step in the pathogenesis of sporadic unilateral acoustic neuroma and have been found in 40–70 per cent of cases.

The majority of acoustic neuromas arise from the vestibular branch of the nerve (85–90 per cent). Acoustic neuromas present with unilateral slowly progressive hearing loss (95 per cent), sometimes associated with non-specific unsteadiness (77 per cent), tinnitus (71 per cent), or vertigo. Commonly, the sensorineural deafness (90 per cent) is associated with facial sensory loss (50 per cent) or facial weakness (10 per cent). Hydrocephalus due to obstruction of CSF pathways can lead to raised intracranial pressure. MRI is the scanning procedure of choice (Fig. 18.3).

The tumours are very slow growing. Almost half of the tumours do not grow perceptibly over a 5-year follow-up. Of those that do enlarge, in 75–80 per cent of cases the growth rate is only 1–2 mm/year (Bederson et al. 1991). There may therefore be a case for conservative management with careful follow-up rather than intervention, especially in the elderly or those in poor general health, or where the tumour is small or there is contralateral deafness and retained hearing in the affected ear. Growth rate apparently doesn't correlate with the age of the patient, the size of the tumour, or the duration of symptoms (Bederson et al. 1991).

Surgical management has a high morbidity, particularly in patients with retained hearing. A suboccipital approach has the advantage of possibly retaining any existing hearing, but may require cerebellar traction and can cause postoperative headaches and cerebellar symptoms. The translabyrinthine approach has the advantage of requiring little in the way of cerebellar retraction and, because the surgery is largely extradural, complications of meningitis and headache are less; however, hearing is always lost postoperatively. The middle fossa approach is useful for small tumours and may spare hearing; however, there are increased complication rates from facial nerve paresis and possibly temporal lobe sequelae (e.g. seizures, dysphasia, etc.) from temporal lobe traction. Monitoring brainstem auditory evoked potentials (BAEPs) intraoperatively can significantly decrease the morbidity of surgery, especially when trying to preserve hearing. Prolongation of the latency of wave V of the BAEPs is usually an early sign that the acoustic nerve is being compromised. Acoustic neuromas may require a joint surgical approach by both ENT and neurosurgeons. Surgery should aim to remove the tumour completely and to preserve facial nerve function and, where possible, preserve hearing. Neurosurgery for acoustic neuroma has a postoperative mortality of approximately 5 per cent. Mortality is related to the size of the tumour and age of patient (Hardy *et al.* 1989). These percentages are heavily affected by selection of patients, experience of the surgeon, and possibly surgical approach. Mortality using the translabyrinthine approach is probably not significantly different from the suboccipital or middle fossa approaches when patient characteristics are taken into account. There is a view that small tumours are better approached by a translabyrinthine approach whereas large tumours are best approached suboccipitally or by middle fossa approach. Translabyrinthine surgery results in complete hearing loss but this is not a problem if hearing is already lost preoperatively, and there may be slightly more chance of preserving facial nerve function. Anatomical preservation of the facial nerve can be achieved in about 80–90 per cent of cases, but anatomical preservation is not always associated with good facial nerve function. It is exceptionally rare for postoperative hearing to be better than preoperative hearing, using either the suboccipital or middle fossa approaches. Where hearing preservation is the main aim, for instance if there is already contralateral deafness and the affected ear has maintained hearing, a suboccipital approach has advantages. In selected centres it has been shown that with experienced neurosurgeons, using the retromastoid route and evoked potential monitoring, complete resection of the tumour can be accomplished with preservation of hearing in 50 per cent of patients with tumours smaller than 2 cm and more than 80 per cent of patients who have a tumour of less than 1 cm diameter (Post *et al.* 1995). Indeed, if preoperative hearing loss is slight, then the retromastiod approach is preferred for small tumours. However, in a recent review of the literature it is clear that only a few patients have truly normal hearing after surgery (Sanna *et al.* 1995). Delayed deterioration in hearing, years after successful operation, is well recognized in up to 50 per cent of patients, although the cause remains uncertain (Shelton *et al.* 1990; Ogunrinde *et al.* 1994). Attempts at maintaining hearing by minimizing resection can be complicated by recurrence of the tumour.

In some cases, where hearing is preserved and the tumour is small, stereotactic radiosurgery or streotactic radiotherapy using a linear accelerator can be effective. Stereotactic radiosurgery uses a single fraction of high dose but small volume radiation to the tumour. Conformal-beam stereotactic radiotherapy, using a linear accelerator and fractionating the treatment over several days and reducing the dose of each fraction, has potential advantages in that radiation-induced neural side-effects are reduced by reducing the fraction size. Radiation therapy is not usually advised for tumours larger than 3 cm because of the increased risks of central nervous system side-effects. The aim of radiation therapy is to prevent growth of acoustic neuroma . Tumours smaller than 3 cm in diameter commonly show shrinkage (35 per cent) or 'stabilization' (60 per cent) at 2 years after stereotactic radiosurgery (Ogunrinde *et al.* 1994). This apparent success has to be compared with the natural history of acoustic neuroma. One study of conservative management demonstrated that 71 per cent of acoustic neuromas do not enlarge over 3.4 years (Deen *et al.* 1996). Short-term complications from stereotactic radiosurgery or stereotactic radiotherapy using a linear accelerator are infrequent; however, it will be some years before one can fully ascertain the effect of radiation on the acoustic nerve and surrounding structures, particularly in patients with normal preradiation hearing. Hearing is very likely to become impaired with time: only 50 per cent of patients with preserved hearing following radiation therapy will maintain this at 6 months, and only 45 per cent at 1–2 years (Ogunrinde *et al.* 1994). Two years after stereotactic radiosurgery, preserved facial nerve function was achieved in 90 per cent and trigeminal nerve function in 75 per cent of cases who had no deficit immediately postradiotherapy. The results of conformal-beam stereotactic radiotherapy are as good as stereotactic radiosurgery, but long-term side-effects appear to be less, probably reflecting the fractionation schedule and reduction in fraction size. Where surgery is contraindicated because of poor health or poor risk–benefit ratio, radiosurgery or conformal stereotactic radiotherapy should be considered the treatment of choice, and there is adequate evidence that these treatments have a therapeutic role. The role of radiotherapy in the treatment of small acoustic neuromas remains controversial.

18.8 Primary intracerebral tumours

18.8.1 Gliomas

Cerebral gliomas are the most common primary intrinsic brain tumours. Gliomas are locally invasive and, even after apparently successful macroscopic resection, they recur at the same site in 95 per cent of cases. They rarely spread outwith the central nervous system (<1 per cent), although it has been estimated that CSF spread occurs in up to 5 per cent of cases.

For practical purposes they can be divided into low-grade gliomas (WHO or Dumas-Duport grade 1 and 2) and high-grade gliomas (WHO or Dumas-Duport grade 3 and 4).

Low-grade gliomas

Low-grade gliomas account for approximately 20 per cent of all cerebral gliomas. Symptoms will depend on the site of the tumour. Prognosis depends on age at diagnosis, length of preoperative symptoms, epilepsy, and extent of resection (Salcman 1995; Piepmeier *et al.* 1996). WHO grade 1 gliomas include rare entities like pilocytic astrocytoma and subependymal giant cell astrocytoma, and are potentially curable if they can be completely resected. Postoperative radiotherapy is not required. If there is suboptimal resection, these tumours grow so slowly that it is unlikely that early cranial radiotherapy has any advantage over a wait and watch policy, particularly since radiation-induced side-effects increase with the passage of time and there

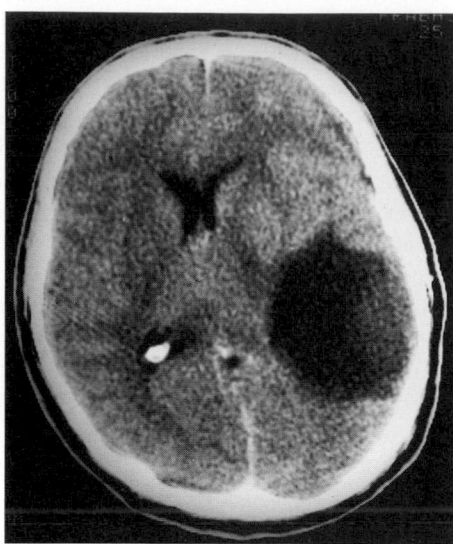

Fig. 18.8. Fibrillary astrocytomas demonstrated by stereotactic biopsy of a 32-year-old male with late onset epilepsy (axial CT scan with contrast). The patient elected not to enter the EORTC low-grade study and adopted a 'watch and wait' policy.

can be extended survival, even in the group with subtotal resection. In symptomatic cases where the risks of resective surgery are considered too great, radiation therapy can produce long-term symptomatic benefit. Approximately 80 per cent of patients with pilocytic astrocytomas are alive at 15 years (Shaw 1995; Shaw *et al.* 1997).

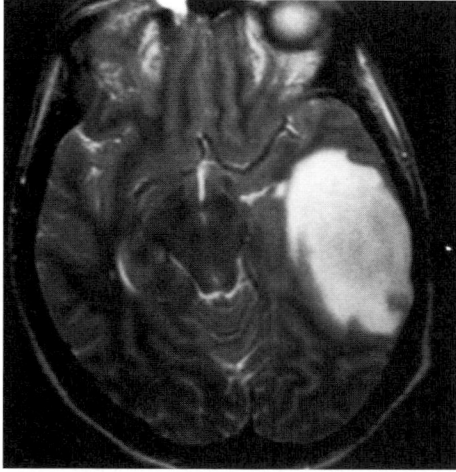

Fig. 18.9. Axial T2-weighted MRI, showing fibrillary astrocytomas in the same patient as in Fig. 18.8, but 2 years later. Seizures remained reasonably controlled but the patient developed occasional predominantly left-sided throbbing headaches, without diurnal variation or any other features. MRI shows slight but further space-occupying effect with displacement of the middle cerebral anteriorly. Interestingly, migraine with or without aura develops in a proportion of patients with brain tumours (of any type), irrespective of whether there is mass effect on the scan. The aura commonly corresponds to the site of the tumour. It responds usually to standard antimigrainous drugs but occasionally steroids are useful. This patient was given steroids and was then treated with radiation (60 Gy in 30 fractions over 6 weeks).

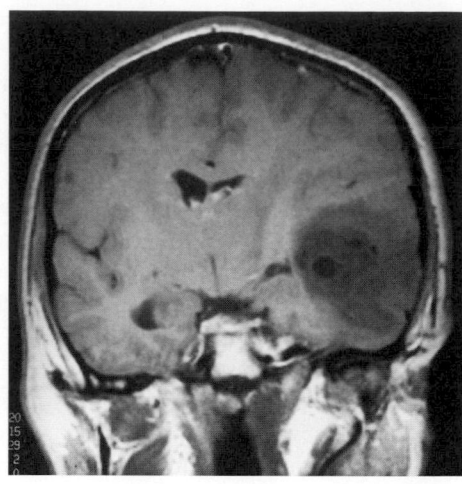

Fig. 18.10. Coronal gadolinium-enhanced MRI, showing fibrillary astrocytomas in the same patient as in Figs 18.8 and 18.9, taken at the same time as Fig. 18.9. This demonstrates the mass effect, with displacement of the temporal horn medially and upwards and the lack of contrast enhancement. The tumour probably remains low grade since the patient remains well with occasional seizures and infrequent 'migraine headaches' 2 years after this MRI. Recent scans reveal little change other than slightly less mass effect.

WHO grade 2 gliomas (fibrillary or protoplasmic astrocytomas, oligoastrocytomas, and oligodendrogliomas) commonly present with seizures without neurological deficit. Age and grade are important prognostic factors (Eyre *et al.* 1993). Patients under the age of 40 years have a median survival of 8 years, compared with 5.5 years for patients aged between 40 and 50 years and 1.6 years if older than 50 years. If patients have a good performance status, the median survival is 7.4 years, compared with 1.6 years if they have a poor performance status (Eyre *et al.* 1993). Most tumours are situated in the fronto-temporal regions and are frequently diffuse, extending throughout a lobe at presentation (Figs 18.8, 18.9, and 18.10). The diffuse infiltrating astrocytomas clearly can not be resected. In the more focal, low-grade astrocytomas in non-eloquent areas, resection may be feasible. There is uncertainty of how best to treat patients with low-grade gliomas. It is probably advisable to biopsy lesions suggestive of low-grade glioma because there can be foci of higher grade despite the lack of enhancement. However, if seizures are the only symptom, a wait and watch policy is preferred by some clinicians and patients. There are no randomized controlled trials of resection versus biopsy in low-grade glioma, and it is unlikely that such a study would see completion because of the excellent survival with astrocytomas (46 per cent 5-year survival) and oligodendroglioma (73 per cent 5-year survival) (Shaw 1995; Shaw *et al.* 1997). There is also uncertainty whether early radiation therapy has any advantage over radiation therapy at the time of change in size of the tumour, new enhancement, or development of neurological signs. Radiation can reduce the size of a tumour but, because of the good survival, this has to be balanced with the increased likelihood of developing delayed radiation-induced toxicity. A European randomized controlled trial of early versus delayed radiotherapy for low-grade gliomas accrued more than 280 patients with a median follow up of 5 years. Early radiotherapy delayed time to progression but survival was identical (Karim *et al.* 1998). A randomized study of radiation versus radiation plus CCNU, (N-(2 chloroethyl)-N-cyclohexyl-N-nitorsourea demonstrated more radiological responses in the radiation-alone group (79 versus 54 per cent), failed to demonstrate any survival advantage with adjuvant chemotherapy, and there were significant haematological toxicities in the chemotherapy-treated group (Eyre *et al.* 1993). Chemotherapy therefore has no proven place in initial treatment. At the time of recurrence most tumours have changed to higher grades of malignancy and chemotherapy may then have something to offer (Muller *et al.* 1977).

High-grade glioma

High-grade gliomas (anaplastic astrocytoma, glioblastoma multiforme, and anaplastic oligodendroglioma) account for approximately 80 per cent of all cerebral gliomas. Prognosis depends on age, grade, performance status, and possibly the extent of remaining disease after surgery. Age is the most important independent prognostic variable at presentation, followed by grade. Performance status is usually recorded using the Karnofsky Performance Scale or the WHO Scale (Zubrod *et al.* 1960; Karnofsky and Burchenal 1989). Patients with poor performance status are less likely to be offered treatment. In randomized trials of treated patients with malignant glioma, patients with poor performance status invariably have shorter survival, even accounting for age and grade (Scanlon and Taylor 1979; Walker *et al.* 1980; Nelson *et al.* 1985). Site of tumour and

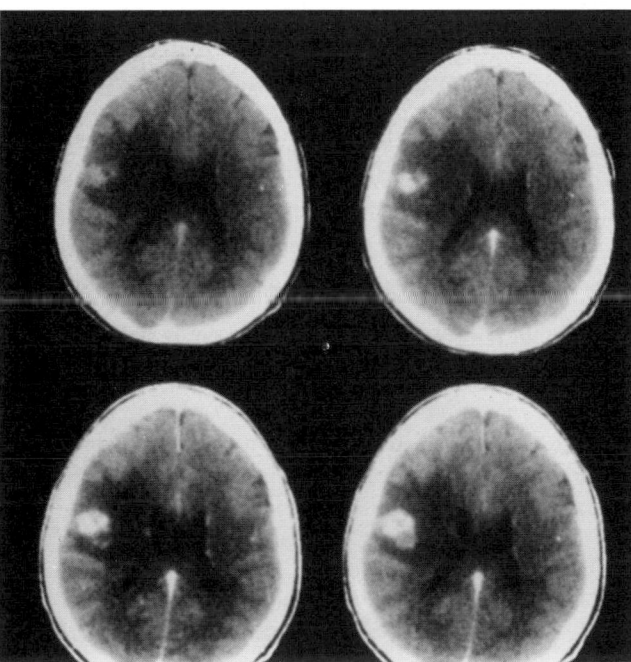

Fig. 18.11. CT scan with contrast in a patient with a right hemisphere tumour taken at different 5-minute intervals after contrast enhancement was given. (By kind permission of Dr P. Warnke.)

volume of tumour on preoperative CT/MRI does not seem to be prognostically important.

Some studies suggest that the amount of peritumoural oedema is associated with a worse prognosis, while others suggest that extensive contrast enhancement, or the volume of tumour remaining on a scan performed at 48–72 hours post-operatively, is associated with poor outcome (Muller *et al.* 1977; Hammoud *et al.* 1996; Piepmeier *et al.* 1996). Care must be taken when interpreting enhanced images with respect to timing of injection of contrast and the time of performance of the scan. Warnke has demonstrated that tumours can significantly alter in their enhancement on dynamic scanning depending on the delay between contrast injection and performance of imaging (Fig. 18.11).

Surgery

It is not certain whether the type of surgery performed (biopsy versus resection) has any survival benefit other than in patients who are on the verge of coning or who have hydrocephalus (Devaux *et al.* 1993; Kreth *et al.* 1993). There is a place for a randomized controlled trial of biopsy versus resection in patients with glioblastoma multiforme. If biopsy is done, this should be by stereotactic technique rather than freehand, because of the higher complication rate associated with the latter. The goal of resective neurosurgery should be as complete resection as possible along its macroscopic boundaries. If achieved without complications, this provides reliable histological diagnosis, potentially improves the patient's neurological status, and may make the tumour more sensitive for additional therapies (e.g. chemotherapy) (Salcman 1987; Shapiro *et al.* 1989). The degree of tumour removal in most studies has been determined by the intraoperative perception of the neurosurgeon. With the increasing availability of neuro-imaging, it has become clear that the surgeon's opinion at the time of operation of what represents a total resection bears little resemblance to the postoperative MRI appearances. Postoperative enhancement on CT scan performed before the fifth postoperative day reflects residual tumour (Jeffries *et al.* 1981; Cairncross *et al.* 1985). Examination of serial postoperative MRI scans has demonstrated that postoperative imaging during days 1–3 after resection of a high-grade glioma avoids artefacts due to postoperative enhancement, and the delineation of tumour was vastly superior to postoperative CT (Albert *et al.* 1994). MRI studies have suggested that postoperative residual tumour was a more important prognostic variable than age or performance status, and the incidence of tumour recurrence is directly related to the volume of residual tumour after initial resection (Albert *et al.* 1994; Berger 1995). However, these results must be interpreted with caution since the selection of patients for aggressive resection based on tumour location and demarcation from surrounding normal tissue may introduce selection bias.

Radiotherapy

Malignant glioma is one of the most aggressive tumours in humans. It rarely spreads outwith the central nervous system, is highly radioresistant, and has a predilection to locoregional recurrence. Each of these three factors has led to particular approaches to primary treatment and management of 'recurrence'. There is good randomized controlled evidence from the early 1970s and 1980s that radiation therapy improves survival in patients with high-grade gliomas (Walker *et al.* 1978, 1980). Radiation therapy increases the median survival from 4 to 5 months to about 9 months. A randomized controlled trial has demonstrated that 60 Gy (in 30 fractions over 6 weeks) was superior to 45 Gy (in 20 fractions over 4 weeks) and resulted in a prolongation of survival by 3 months in the group treated with 60 Gy. (Bleehen and Stenning 1991). The current standard practice is to give 60 Gy in 30 fractions over 6 weeks. Radiation therapy is usually directed at the area of the enhancing tumour plus at least a 2 cm margin of peritumoural oedema. Focal radiation (40 Gy in 20 fractions) over 4 weeks to the tumour and peritumoural oedema is usually followed by a further 20 Gy boost to the enhancing tumour and 1–2 cm margin over 2 weeks. The wide margins are because tumour cells can be found 2 cm (or more) from the apparent radiological boundary of the tumour, in areas that simply look 'oedematous' on CT or MRI, and most studies demonstrate that relapse occurs within 2 cm of the enhancing rim of the tumour in 80 per cent of cases (Halperin *et al.* 1989; Wallner *et al.* 1989). Boosting the radiation dose to the centre of the tumour is now standard practice in most centres. Dose escalation of radiation, using conformal-beam therapy or stereotactic radiation, aims to treat the centre of the tumour maximally and spare normal tissue outwith the 2 cm margin, to reduce long-term morbidity from radiation damage. Whether either of these approaches will extend survival remains to be seen.

The effect of radiation is greater in the young (under 60 years). In the over-60 age group the effect of radiation therapy remains controversial.

Chemotherapy

Numerous chemotherapy agents (nitrosoureas, procarbazine, platinum derivatives, etc.) have been shown to reduce tumour size in about one-third of patients in phase II studies (Mahaley 1991). The beneficial effect of chemotherapy has to be balanced with potentially serious side-effects. The risk–benefit ratio will depend on individual patient factors. It may be helpful to re-examine the current evidence of the effectiveness of chemotherapy in the form of answering some questions.

How much better is chemotherapy than supportive care?

A randomized controlled trial demonstrated that chemotherapy with a nitrosourea extends survival beyond what can be expected from supportive care, but the difference in median survival was only 4.5 weeks in the valid study group (Walker *et al.* 1978). Both groups received similar corticosteroid use during the trial (about 2 weeks on average). Chemotherapy produced an 8 per cent absolute increase in survivors at 6 months and a 10.6 per cent absolute increase in survivors at 1 year. This represented twice as many survivors at 6 months

and four times as many at 1 year with chemotherapy (Walker *et al.* 1978, 1980).

Is chemotherapy superior to supportive care plus regular steroids?

A randomized controlled trial has looked at methylprednisolone given for 1 week each month, compared with chemotherapy (procarbazine or 1, 3-bis [2-chloroethyl]i-nitrosourea; BCNU) (Green *et al.* 1983). Both groups also had radiation therapy. In this study chemotherapy with BCNU or procarbazine was superior to methylprednisolone; however, the survival difference was only really noticeable 12 months after treatment, and treatment with procarbazine only extended survival by a median of 2 weeks for the total randomized population (7 weeks for the 'valid study group'). With BCNU, median survival increased by 9 weeks for the total randomized population (10 weeks for the 'valid study group').

What is the likelihood of responding to chemotherapy?

The likelihood of response is related to the age of the patient at the start of chemotherapy and grade of tumour (Nelson *et al.* 1988). A recent retrospective study suggests that nitrosoureas produce a partial response in almost 40 per cent of patients with high-grade glioma under the age of 40, 17 per cent of patients between 40 and 59 years, but only 5 per cent of patients over 60 years (Grant *et al.* 1995). Median survival from the time of starting chemotherapy is approximately 43 weeks in younger patients (<60 years) and 24 weeks in patients over the age of 60 years. Differences in response rate, time to progression, and survival, related to age, persist following adjustment for grade of tumour. The risk of myelosuppressive complications requiring admission to hospital is approximately 16 per cent in patients younger than 60 years of age but 35 per cent in patients over 60 years of age. Patients older than 60 years are therefore at a greater risk from chemotherapy and have less chance of a response or prolonged survival (Grant *et al.* 1995). It would seem reasonable to consider chemotherapy either adjuvantly or on recurrence in patients with high-grade glioma who are young, but careful thought should be given when suggesting chemotherapy to patients over the age of 60 years (Nelson *et al.* 1988).

Is the imaging response to chemotherapy related to time to progression or survival?

Although one might reasonably think that magnitude of response would be related to duration of response or survival, this has only been demonstrated in patients with anaplastic oligodendroglioma who have achieved a greater than 90 per cent imaging response (Cairncross and Eisenhauer 1995). Magnitude of tumour response has not been demonstrated to be related to duration of response or survival in high-grade glioma (Grant *et al.* 1997). It has been estimated that therapy must be effective in more than 70 per cent of patients before one would see a significant effect on survival. Imaging may show little change, although there is a profound clinical change.

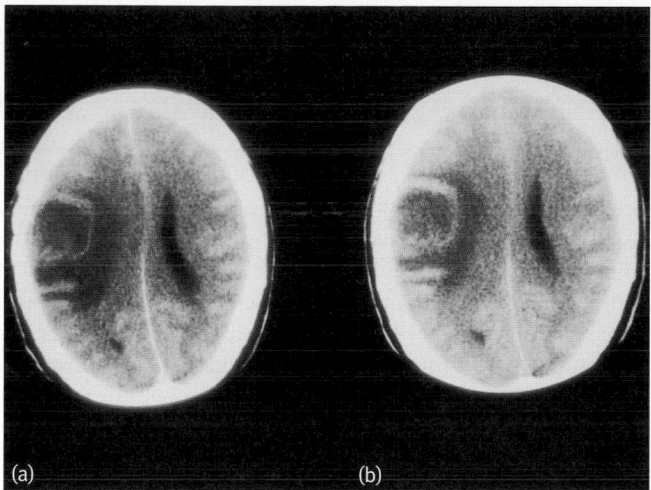

Fig. 18.12. Right parietal glioblastoma in an asymptomatic 54-year-old man. (a) CT scan with contrast. (b) CT scan with contrast taken 1 week later when he presented to the emergency department with headache and 'central cone'. Despite steroids and mannitol he died within 40 minutes of the CT scan. CT shows virtually no change in the degree of enhancement or space occupation.

Figure 18.12 shows an extreme example of this, where clearly the patient 'progressed' with no perceptible change in imaging. Response must take into account clinical, imaging, and steroid information. In addition, some patients appear to respond quickly to chemotherapy on imaging but then progress rapidly despite chemotherapy (presumably as a result of acquired resistance). Other patients respond slowly to chemotherapy, but have more prolonged responses despite discontinuation of chemotherapy (Grant *et al.* 1997). In patients who do respond to chemotherapy, speed of response is not associated with duration of response. However, in one study where serial measures of tumour volume following chemotherapy were taken, the likelihood of achieving a response was associated with the size of tumour in glioblastoma multiforme, with only small-volume tumours having a response. Tumour volume did not seem to influence the likelihood of achieving an imaging response in patients with anaplastic astrocytoma (Grant *et al.* 1999).

Does chemotherapy increase survival?

The main aim of chemotherapy is to prevent disease progression and extend survival. In a meta-analysis of randomized trials of radiotherapy and adjuvant chemotherapy, the addition of chemotherapy increases the absolute number of 1-year survivors by 10.1 per cent (95 per cent confidence intervals (CI) 6.8, 13.3 per cent) and of 2-year survivors by 8.6 per cent (95 per cent confidence intervals 5.2, 12 per cent) (Fine *et al.* 1993). These figures represent a relative increase of 23.4 per cent (CI 15.8, 30.9 per cent) at 1 year and 52.4 per cent (CI 31.7, 73.2 per cent) at 2 years, but studies have failed to demonstrate any major effect on median survival (0–2 months) (Stenning *et al.* 1987; Fine *et al.* 1993).

A meta analysis of individual patient data of randomized controlled trials of chemotherapy for malignant glioma has recently been performed (L. Stewart (personal communication) 2000). Results in 2,368 patients showed an absolute increase in median survival of 2 months (confidence interval 1–3 months). Recurrence free survival was significantly prolonged ($p = 0.00003$) with a hazard ratio of 0.8 (0.72–0.90) and a 6% increase in recurrence free survival from 10% to 16% at two years.

Should chemotherapy be given adjuvantly after radiation therapy or at the time of recurrence?

The term 'recurrence' in the European literature, generally means that there has been resolution of the tumour, or at least a period of stability before the tumour relapses. However, 'recurrence' in the North American literature is frequently used when describing any disease persistence (e.g. on an image performed shortly after surgery and radiation therapy). This distinction has led to different approaches to primary management in North America as compared with Europe. In North America the trend has been toward primary treatment with surgery, radiation therapy, and adjuvant chemotherapy, and in Europe the trend has been for primary treatment with surgery and radiation therapy, with chemotherapy at the time of disease progression. Studies suggest that the moderate effect of chemotherapy can be achieved whether chemotherapy is given adjuvantly with radiation therapy or at the time of clinical or radiological relapse after radiation therapy (Walker *et al.* 1978; European Organization for Research and Treatment of Cancer (EORTC) Brain Tumor Group, 1981).

Is combination chemotherapy superior to single-agent nitrosourea?

Most phase III studies have not shown any survival advantage with combination chemotherapy (PCV) versus single-agent nitrosourea (e.g. BCNU) (Levin *et al.* 1985; Mahaley *et al.* 1987; Shapiro *et al.* 1989). In a subgroup analysis of a randomized study, a doubling of time to progression (TTP) and survival at the 50th and 25th percentile was demonstrated in patients with anaplastic astrocytoma, a Karnofsky Performance Scale of ≥ 70, who had completed radiotherapy and more than one course of chemotherapy (Levin *et al.* 1990). This was an interesting exploratory analysis which may be important, but it was a *post hoc* analysis and may simply reflect a chance finding. A recent meta-analysis of nine randomized controlled trials of multidrug versus single-agent chemotherapy for high grade glioma indicated that patients treated with multi-drug regimes may have a 22% decreased one year survival (Huncharek *et al.* 1998). In addition, high-dose oral procarbazine is probably every bit as effective as nitrosoureas, and has been shown to produce a significant number of partial responses in patients who have progressed while taking nitrosureas (Green *et al.* 1983; Newton *et al.* 1990). It has not been demonstrated that combination therapy (PCV) is superior to sequential single-agent chemotherapy (e.g. BCNU followed by high-dose procarbazine).

When considering the lack of long-term efficacy from chemotherapy, and methods to overcome this, one has to examine primary mechanisms for drug resistance. First, the drug must be able to be delivered to the site of the tumour in sufficient concentration to have an effect. Secondly, the drug must be able to pass through the blood–brain barrier at the 'advancing' edge of the tumour, which may not be well vascularized. Chemotherapy penetration at the necrotic centre or enhancing nidus will not prevent tumour progression at the margin. Thirdly, intracellular mechanisms of drug resistance, such as lack of intracellular drug activation, drug inactivation (e.g. by glutathione-S-transferases), DNA enzyme repair (e.g. by O^6-alkylguanine-DNA-alkyltransferase), and active removal of chemotherapy from the cell by P-glycoprotein, an energy-dependent drug efflux pump (mediated through multidrug resistance gene overexpression), must be overcome. Increasing drug delivery by intra-arterial chemotherapy, can reduce systemic effects of chemotherapy, while maintaining the local concentration of chemotherapy to the tumour; however, the potential benefits are limited by local toxicity to the brain (encephalopathy, seizures) and eye (optic neuropathy) and randomized studies have shown no benefit in terms of survival over systemic chemotherapy (Mahaley *et al.* 1986; Green *et al.* 1989).

What (if anything) should be done after failure of radiation therapy and chemotherapy?

On second relapse, the effects of steroids on neurological impairments are less impressive than when given at initial diagnosis. Most patients will have a poor performance status and little realistic likelihood of responding to any treatment. In young patients with a good performance status, re-operation is frequently necessary to debulk the mass, to exclude radiation necrosis, confirm any change in the tumour grade, and allow time for any further treatment to have a chance of being effective. An alternative approach would be to forget re-operation and concentrate on empirical focal re-irradiation or further chemotherapy.

If the decision is for operation, then this allows the potential for resection and further experimental therapies, e.g. interstitial chemotherapy or radiotherapy, or gene therapy. Various chemotherapy regimes (eg. Temozolomide, BCNV polymer wafers for intestitial use), radiosurgical procedures, gene therapy, immunotherapies, and boron neutron capture have been tried in recurrent malignant glioma and response rates seem encouraging (20–30 per cent), although duration of effect of response is limited, side-effects (e.g. marrow toxicity) are encountered sooner, and good information on quality of life data is not available.

A recent randomized controlled trial of Temozolomide versus oral procarbazine in malignant glioma showed a slight survival benefit and fewer side effects with Temozolomide. Quality of life may have been better with Temozolomide but the low quality of life questionnaire response rate limited interpretation of results (Osoba *et al.* 2000). BCNU impregnated wafers (Gliadel) placed in the resection cavity have been shown to be superior to placebo in a recent randomised controlled trial. The trial has not yet been published but extended survival by approximately 6 weeks. Several trials of interstitial brachytherapy with radioisotope seeds placed directly into tumour have demonstrated a slight survival advantage of about two months, however, about one third of patients require reoperation for radiation induced necrosis (Suh and Barnett 1999). Gene therapy with herpes simplex thymidine kinase gene has been found to be ineffective in a randomized controlled trial completed in approximately 1999. The formal results have never been published in full. Results from studies using immunotherapy and Boron Neutron Capture therapy (BNCT) are yet to demonstrate any significant effect in malignant glioma but research continues.

Anaplastic oligodendroglioma may be a special case. Although malignant glioma continues to have a poor prognosis, anaplastic oligodendroglioma can be responsive to chemotherapy for prolonged periods, and chemotherapy prior to radiation therapy may prove to be more effective. Studies suggest that PCV chemotherapy produces a 75 per cent response rate, with 17 per cent with stable disease, and only 8 per cent with progressive disease (Macdonald *et al.*1990, Kritis *et al.* 1993; Macdonald 1994). In this moderately chemoresponsive tumour, where a large proportion of patients will respond (even those older than 60 years), there is some evidence that patients who have a 'major response' (>90 per cent reduction in contrast-enhancing area) have better survival than those with partial response/stable disease (Macdonald 1994; Cairncross and Eisenhauer 1995).

18.8.2 Medulloblastomas

Medulloblastoma is the most common childhood central nervous system tumour, but is a relatively rare tumour in adults. About 25 per cent of all medulloblastomas occur in adults (age >16 years). The cell of origin of this tumour remains uncertain, but is probably of embryonic origin, with the possibility of taking different lines of differentiation (primitive neuro-ectodermal tumour; PNET). Medulloblastomas usually arise in the midline and are most commonly found in the cerebellum. Presentation is usually either related to a cerebellar ataxia, or raised intracranial pressure related to obstructive hydrocephalus. Cranial nerve presentations (especially diplopia) also occur. The tumour has low signal on T1-weighted MRI scans and high signal on T2-weighted scans and there is usually gadolinium enhancement on T1-weighted images.

There is a risk of any tumour of the posterior fossa or a tumour that abuts the ventricle seeding into the cerebrospinal fluid. This is particularly common with medulloblastoma. Staging of the tumour is therefore important but can wait until after the definitive surgical procedure. Because of the possible contamination of CSF at the time of surgery, it is probably best to defer CSF analysis till 10–14 days after the operation;

however, the MRI scan of the spine to look for gadolinium-enhancing nodules can be performed any time after surgery. Thirty to 40 per cent of children will have CSF dissemination, although this may be greater in children under 5 years of age (Deutsch 1988). The bad prognostic features for medulloblastoma appear to be age less than 3 years, CSF dissemination, and, possibly, extent of resection (Evans *et al.* 1990).

The management of acute obstructive hydrocephalus is controversial. Some surgeons suggest steroids and tumour resection, while others suggest steroids and external ventricular drainage, or steroids and ventriculo-peritoneal shunting, prior to a definitive operation. Surgery for medulloblastoma is performed in the prone position, to avoid the risks of air embolus and pneumocephalus or systemic hypotension when operating in the seated position. A repeat MRI scan at 48 hours may be helpful for assessing the extent of tumour resection.

Radiotherapy to the tumour improves survival in children with medulloblastoma. In addition, there is good evidence that craniospinal irradiation (CSI) reduces the risk of recurrence from CSF dissemination. A randomized prospective trial demonstrated improved disease control using 36 Gy of cranio-spinal irradiation with a posterior fossa boost to 54 Gy, compared with 23.4 Gy with a posterior fossa boost to 54 Gy in 30 fractions (Deutsch *et al.* 1996). This study was closed prematurely after an interim analysis at 16 months demonstrated a significant number of relapses in the low-dose CSI treatment group. Craniospinal irradiation also improves the number of 10-year survivors (Castro-Vita *et al.* 1980; Landverg *et al.* 1980). Radiation therapy to the craniospinal axis can have serious long-term toxicities: neuropsychological, neuroendocrine (e.g. growth retardation and hypothyroidism), bone marrow toxicity, and second neoplasms in long-term survivors (e.g. thyroid and other CNS neoplasms). In attempts to try and reduce these toxicities and to try to improve survival, chemotherapy has been used. Medulloblastoma is a relatively chemosensitive tumour. Randomized studies have compared radiation with radiation and CCNU, vincristine chemotherapy. The overall survival was 53 per cent at 5 years and 45 per cent at 10 years. Although an early analysis demonstrated a significantly better disease-free survival with the addition of chemotherapy, there were subsequently late relapses in the chemotherapy group and no statistically significant effect on disease-free survival is apparent. In *post-hoc* subgroup analyses, chemotherapy was thought to benefit patients with subtotal resection, brainstem involvement, and more extensive disease at presentation (Tait *et al.* 1990). A further randomized controlled study of the same agents in North America came to the same conclusions but also noted a survival advantage in patients with extensive disease in a subgroup analysis (Evans *et al.* 1990).

Currently, there is a vogue for chemotherapy in addition to CSI, with a boost to the primary site for patients with a high risk of progression, in an attempt to improve survival and reduce the dose of CSI (Cohen and Packer 1996). Approximately 10–20 per cent of patients will eventually have metastatic spread outwith the central nervous system (especially lungs and bone).

With treatment, approximately 33–66 per cent of children are alive at 5 years and 25–50 per cent are alive at 10 years, depending on the patient selection for the survival analyses (Bloom *et al.* 1991). Although it was previously thought that adults did less well, a review of cases treated between 1971 and 1981 suggests that survival is no different, or perhaps slightly better (76 per cent alive at 10 years) (Bloom and Bessell 1990).

18.8.3 Primary CNS lymphomas

Primary central nervous system lymphomas account for approximately 1 per cent of all primary intracerebral tumours and are almost always B cell in origin. They occur in higher frequencies in patients with some form of immunosuppression. Approximately 2–6 per cent of patients with AIDS and 0.5–1 per cent of patients following transplantation (Section 5.6.2) will develop a primary CNS lymphoma. Primary CNS lymphomas are also found in association with Wiskott–Aldrich syndrome, systemic lupus, idiopathic thrombocytopenic purpura, Sjögren's syndrome, and sarcoidosis (Remick *et al.* 1990; Ling *et al.* 1997) Despite the association with immunosuppressive states, primary CNS lymphoma more commonly occurs sporadically in the immunocompetent. Epstein–Barr virus (EBV) can be detected in all AIDS-related primary CNS lymphomas, raising the possibility of a direct EBV-related cause (MacMahon *et al.* 1991; Guterman *et al.* 1996).

Clinically, primary CNS lymphoma is classified as an extranodal lymphoma (stage 1_E) and it most commonly presents as single or multiple contrast-enhancing space-occupying lesion(s) within the brain, or as cells in the eye (vitreous lymphoma) or CSF (leptomeningeal lymphoma). Primary CNS lymphoma is most commonly confined to central nervous system or eye, and even at post-mortem only 10 per cent of patients are found to have disease outwith the CNS. The tumour is commonly in a periventricular site and this may explain the high incidence of CSF involvement. Approximately, 20 per cent of patients will have cerebrospinal fluid involvement at the time of presentation, and a further 20 per cent will have had, or develop, a uveitis with 'floaters' and progressive loss of vision due to lymphoma of the vitreous (Hochberg and Miller 1988). The diagnosis may be suspected if the CT/MRI scan is typical, but biopsy is essential. There is no evidence that resection is superior to stereotactic biopsy. The tumours frequently lose their enhancement when steroids are given and it is not uncommon for the tumour to 'disappear' on CT scan after steroids, making stereotactic biopsy difficult (Fig. 18.13a, b). Anecdotally, these tumours have an increased propensity to bleed when biopsied compared with other intracerebral tumours.

Staging of primary CNS lymphoma is important. Slit-lamp examination of the eyes and fundoscopy must be performed to identify uveitis due to vitreous involvement, retinal detachment or haemorrhages, optic neuropathy, or papilloedema. CSF examination should be performed, looking for lymphomatous

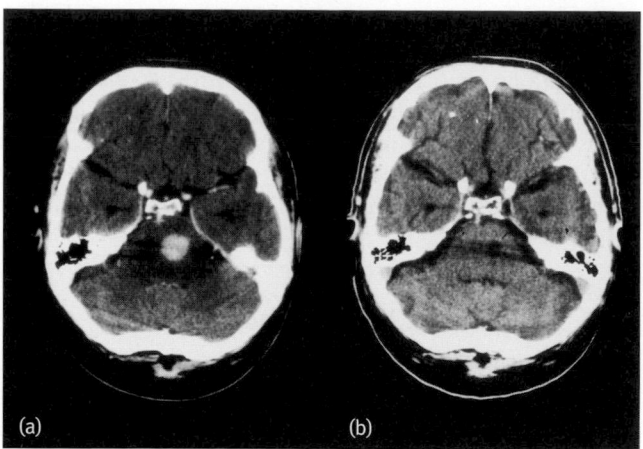

Fig. 18.13. Primary CNS lymphoma involving the pons. (a) Axial CT scan with contrast. (b) Same patient admitted for stereotactic biopsy 1 week after starting steroids ('disappearing tumour'). Steroids were discontinued and the tumour 'returned' on imaging when rescanned 3 weeks later. Biopsy confirmed a primary CNS lymphoma.

cells. The pathologists may have difficulty identifying lymphomatous cells from chronic inflammatory cells and both populations can coexist. Immunohistochemical techniques for cell typing can be helpful. The CSF protein is usually increased and one-third of patients have CSF glucose levels below the lower limit of the accepted range. An HIV test is advisable. CT/MRI scan of the chest and abdomen is almost always negative and bone-marrow biopsy is not required (Hochberg and Miller 1988).

In patients who do not have HIV/AIDS, biopsy and steroids confirm the diagnosis and usually produce a reasonable clinical and radiological response. Corticosteroids are cytotoxic to lymphocytes and prolonged remissions with steroids have been reported. The relative roles of radiation therapy and chemotherapy have not yet been researched adequately. Young patients (<60 years), treated with more than 40 Gy to the whole brain and a boost to 50 Gy to the tumour bed, along with chemotherapy, appear to have a better survival, with a median of around 2–3 years (Reni *et al.* 1997). Escalating the boost to 60 Gy does not appear to produce any survival advantage (Nelson *et al.*, 1992). Chemotherapy used to be kept in reserve for relapsed primary CNS lymphoma; however, more recently chemotherapy with high-dose methotrexate or CHOP (cyclophosphamide, doxorubicin, vincristine, and prednisolone) has been found to be effective, and possibly has better CSF penetration if given prior to radiation (Glass *et al.* 1994; Lachance *et al.* 1994). It is now a common trend to give chemotherapy before radiotherapy, or split before and after the radiation therapy. These protocols have not yet been compared in randomized controlled trials. CSF disease can be treated by intrathecal methotrexate given via an Ommaya reservoir twice weekly, or by giving high-dose systemic methotrexate with leucovorin rescue, since there is some evidence that high-dose methotrexate results in good cerebrospinal fluid penetration.

Ocular disease can be treated symptomatically by steroids, and frequently is misdiagnosed as non-lymphomatous-related uveitis. Steroids usually only have a temporary effect, and radiation to the posterior two-thirds of the eye or chemotherapy with high-dose cytosine arabinoside or methotrexate can be useful.

Radiation therapy plus or minus chemotherapy certainly produces a clinical and radiological response in most cases, and the median survival is in the region of 2–3 years in non-immunocompromised patients. The median survival of AIDS patients with primary CNS lymphomas treated with radiation plus or minus chemotherapy is approximately 3 months.

18.8.4 Pineal region tumours

Pineal region tumours can arise from a number of cell types. The most common tumours in this area are teratomas or germinomas. Pineocytomas are less common and arise from the pineal parenchymal cells, and gliomas can also arise in the pineal region. Occasionally metastases can spread to the pineal region. In addition to these solid tumours, pineal region cysts can occur and can be simple, filled with CSF, or can be epidermoid or dermoid cysts. It can be difficult to distinguish with any certainty by imaging characteristics whether a pineal region tumour is a pineal glioma, an ependymoma, a pineocytoma, germinoma, or teratoma. Serum and CSF analysis can be helpful. If germ cell markers (α-fetoprotein (AFP) and β-human chorionic gonadotropin (β-hCG)) are positive, biopsy of the lesion is not required. Elevated germ cell markers indicate a malignant germ cell tumour. These patients can be treated with radiation therapy and chemotherapy, and can be followed by measuring the tumour markers. If the lesion enlarges but markers reduce, surgical debulking may be necessary (Lee *et al.* 1995). In the absence of tumour markers, surgical confirmation is strongly advised. Hydrocephalus may have to be dealt with first, either by external drainage or placement of a ventriculo-peritoneal shunt. In the presence of mild hydrocephalus, some surgeons prefer performing a definitive resection and placing a ventricular drain at the time of surgery, which later can be clamped and removed, or changed into a ventriculo-peritoneal shunt. Other authors have suggested performing a third ventricular ventriculostomy (Goodman 1993).

If the frozen section reveals germinoma, then there is no need to proceed to resection because this tumour is so radiosensitive (control rates of 90 per cent) and chemosensitive. If the biopsy confirms a benign pineal region tumour (dermoid, epidermoid, pilocytic astrocytoma, ependymoma, or pineocytoma) maximum resection should be attempted, and is generally the only treatment necessary. If the biopsy demonstrates a malignant pineal region tumour (e.g. a non-germinomatous germ cell tumour, choriocarcinoma, embryonal cell carcinoma, immature teratoma or endodermal sinus tumour, malignant glioma), then maximum resection is probably advisable, especially if the patient is young and has a good performance status. Complications of surgery include disorders of eye movement, ataxia, and cognitive problems. If a supratentorial approach to the tumour is taken, there is a higher incidence of visual field defects and hemiparesis. Surgical complications for pineal region tumours range up to 12 per cent and mortality up to 8 per cent (Bruce and Stein 1993). Preoperative or 12-day postoperative spinal MR imaging may identify spinal seeding from the pineal region tumour. Standard radiation schedules for germinoma consist of 4000 cGy to the whole brain and a boost to 5500 cGy to the pineal region. Radiation therapy dosages of less than 5000 cGy are associated with increased risk of recurrence (Schild et al., 1993). The need for craniospinal irradiation is uncertain, but most centres only suggest this for documented CSF metastases. Germinomas are also chemosensitive, and this treatment has been advocated in young patients in order to delay radiation or possibly reduce the dosage of radiation given. Germinomas and non-germinomatous germ cell tumours are sensitive to cisplatinum (plus or minus etoposide) and to cyclophosphamide, and preradiation chemotherapy is now being advocated by some centres (Patel et al. 1992). Pineoblastomas only respond partially to radiation and less well to chemotherapy. Various chemotherapy regimes have been tried with only limited success.

18.8.5 Craniopharyngiomas

Craniopharyngiomas are benign tumours that usually present in childhood or early adulthood. They arise from the embryological remnants of Rathke's pouch in the suprasellar area or pituitary region. Symptoms usually present in adolescence or early adulthood. In children the most common symptom is growth failure, and in adults sexual dysfunction in men and amenorrhoea in women. The tumour can present with hypopituitarism (25–40 per cent), diabetes insipidus (50 per cent), visual failure from pressure on the optic chiasm or optic nerves (40–70 per cent), raised intracranial pressure from hydrocephalus from obstruction of the third ventricle (20–40 per cent), or personality and memory problems. The tumour is usually a mixture of cysts and solid components, where the cysts contain thick fluid (like engine oil) containing cholesterol crystals. Skull radiography may demonstrate calcification in the suprasellar region, but MRI scan is the most valuable investigation (Fig. 18.2). The sagittal and coronal scans provide invaluable information to the surgeon. Differential diagnosis includes meningioma, optic nerve glioma, teratoma, dermoid or epidermoid cyst, metastasis, or sarcoidosis.

After correction of any endocrinopathy, definitive operation can be performed in relative safety. The mainstay of treatment is resection of the tumour, although this has to be tempered by its tendency to be adherent to surrounding structures. Total resection is frequently impractical and attempts at aggressive resection have resulted in high morbidity and mortality (up to 20 per cent) and recurrence rates of 30–40 per cent (Weiss et al. 1989; Wen et al. 1989; Yasergil et al. 1990). Most authors suggest safe subtotal resection and either postoperative radiotherapy to the residual disease or radiotherapy at the time of recurrence,

depending on the age of the patient (Weiss et al. 1989; Wen et al. 1989). Some still suggest attempted complete removal as the best approach (Yasergil et al. 1990). There are no randomized studies of safe subtotal resection (± radiation therapy) versus maximum possible resection (± radiation therapy), and no randomized studies of early radiation versus delayed radiation. If radiation is given after resection, the usual advised dose is at least 5400 cGy. At recurrence, it is not uncommon to get enlargement of one of the cysts. Cystic recurrences can be treated by placement of a reservoir and aspiration of the cyst intermittently (Gutin et al. 1980). A different approach is to instil ^{32}P—a β-emitting isotope with limited penetrance. This has been reported to result in cyst regression in more than 80 per cent of cases, with good symptomatic relief (Pollock et al. 1995). Twenty-year survival for craniopharyngioma approaches 60 per cent, but recurrence is common and morbidity is significant (Regine and Kramer 1992). Craniopharyngiomas probably have a better prognosis when diagnosed in adults than when diagnosed in childhood.

18.9 Metastatic intracerebral tumours

Improved treatment of systemic malignancies has led to an increase in the frequency of brain metastases, possibly because the brain may act as a 'sanctuary site' for cancer cells during systemic chemotherapy (Greig et al. 1990). The incidence of intracerebral metastases is approximately $14/10^5$/yr, therefore each year in the UK one would expect approximately 8000 new cases. Metastases account for 45 per cent of all intracranial tumours and 60 per cent of intracerebral tumours. The frequency of brain metastases varies, depending on the primary tumour, but ranges from 12 to 35 per cent of all cancer patients (Posner and Chernik 1978; Galicich et al. 1996). Brain metastasis are generally a late manifestation of cancer, and systemic metastases frequently coexist; however, 36 per cent of patients do not have a past history of cancer at initial presentation. It has been estimated that only 19 per cent of patients do not have metastases at other sites at the time of presentation, but this was based on a cancer hospital population (Cairncross et al. 1980). The frequency of isolated brain metastases is likely to be higher in a general hospital population study. Lung cancer, cancer of unknown origin, breast cancer, and melanoma account for 90 per cent of brain metastases (Grant et al. 1996). It is very unusual for patients with breast or gastrointestinal tract malignancies to present with brain metastases as the initial manifestation of cancer. If there is no history of malignancy at presentation with brain metastases, the primary site is most commonly lung (55 per cent) or the primary tumour is not identified prior to death (40 per cent) (Grant et al. 1996).

Seizures are the presenting symptom in about 16 per cent and will eventually occur in up to 40 per cent of patients at some stage (Posner 1980). A randomized controlled trial has failed to show any advantage to prophylactic prescription of anticonvulsants in patients with brain metastases (Glantz *et al.* 1996). Anticonvulsants should not be given prophylactically in patients with metastases, but they are helpful in controlling frequency of seizures.

Patients with cancer are at an increased risk of developing deep venous thrombosis (DVT), because of immobility and possibly as a result of hypercoagulation related to cancer (Dhami *et al.* 1993). This risk may be increased by hemiparesis as a result of a brain metastasis. It would seem appropriate to manage patients at risk of DVT with multiple risk factors (e.g. hemiparesis, cancer, operation) with elastic stockings and sub-cutaneous heparin (Monreal *et al.* 1996). A literature study of patients with cancer who had either DVT prophylactic therapy or treatment following a DVT or pulmonary embolus showed that prophylactic anticoagulation or vena caval filter did not improve quality-adjusted life expectancy, but anticoagulant therapy provided a 9 per cent gain in quality-adjusted life expectancy for patients with acute DVT, and a 16 per cent gain for patients who survived a pulmonary embolus, and vena caval filter yielded an 11 per cent and 18 per cent gain, respectively (Sarasin and Eckman 1993).

Symptomatic management of brain metastases, with steroids for headache, focal neurological deficit, or cognitive problems, is very effective in the short term in reducing the effect of brain oedema. The mechanism of action of steroids remains uncertain. Steroids do reduce the amount of oedema around the tumour and repair a leaky blood–brain barrier, but the symptomatic relief (6–24 hours after starting) antedates any obvious change on CT scan or MRI scan. Approximately 70 per cent of patients improve with steroids. A reasonable starting dose would be 4 mg of dexamethasone intravenously four times a day, then changing onto oral medication and altering the timing to give the last dose before 6 p.m., because insomnia is a particularly common side-effect of treatment. Steroids usually reach their maximal effect by 7 days and a gradual reduction in dose is advised by then, whether or not there has been an improvement in neurological deficit. Steroids almost certainly will provide a slight survival benefit, although this has never been proved in any randomized controlled trial and probably never will be. Their long-term use, however, is limited by the growth of the tumour, and the systemic side-effects of long-term treatment.

Prognosis in patients with cerebral metastases will depend on the age, primary tumour type and responsiveness to treatment, site of cerebral metastasis (supratentorial versus infratentorial; resectable versus irresectable), presence of systemic metastases, and performance status at diagnosis.

18.9.1 Single metastases

Single brain metastasis refers to a single metastasis from a systemic tumour irrespective of the extent of spread to other organs. The term 'solitary brain metastasis' refers to the brain being the only site of systemic spread. Solitary brain metastasis is uncommon but has a better prognosis, if the brain disease can be controlled. Approximately 30–40 per cent of cerebral

metastases are single (Delattre *et al.* 1988). Metastases from colon, kidney, and breast are more frequently single than metastases from lung or melanoma, but because lung cancer has a higher incidence than colon or kidney, lung cancer remains the most likely cause.

There is no evidence that operation for a single brain metastasis extends survival in patients with active cancer at other sites. Nevertheless, most patients with known cancer and a presumed single brain metastasis should be considered for resection because of the higher radiological diagnostic error rate for single brain lesions. In one study of patients with known systemic cancer and a CT brain scan suggestive of single metastasis, 11 per cent were found to have a different histological diagnosis (frequently non-malignant) (Patchell *et al.* 1990). If patients are being considered for surgical resection of a single brain metastasis, it is usually advisable to perform an MRI brain scan, to determine whether there are actually multiple micro-metastases not identified on CT scanning (Fig. 18.14). Surgical resection of a cerebral metastasis is feasible in selected patients. A surgically accessible lesion can be defined as one that is superficial (close to the brain surface or abutting a fissure or sulcus) and can be operated on with minimal parenchymal resection. This type of metastasis can frequently be resected even in eloquent areas of the brain. Surgery has the benefit of removing the lesion, reducing the need for long-term steroids, potentially improving quality of life, and providing a small survival gain in certain situations. Because of the high risk of new cerebral metastatic lesions developing in the brain, it should be followed by cranial radiation. Three randomized controlled studies have examined the place of resection of a single brain metastasis in patients with stable disease elsewhere. Two have demonstrated that resection improves survival (40 weeks versus 15 weeks, and 10 months versus 6 months, respectively) (Patchell *et al.* 1990; Vecht *et al.* 1993). The third failed to demonstrate any difference (Mintz *et al.* 1996). The duration of functional independence was better in the surgically treated group and there were fewer deaths from neurological disease.

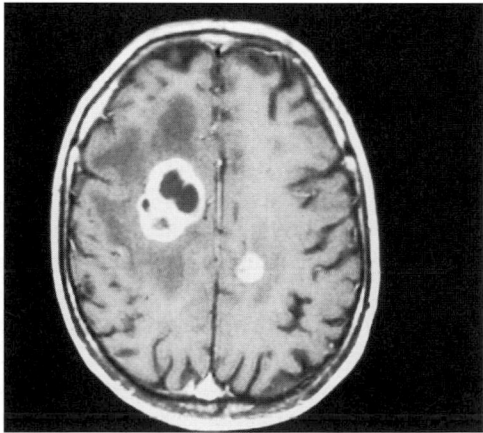

Fig. 18.14. Axial gadolinium-enhanced MRI, showing multiple cerebral metastases.

The postoperative mortality rate was 4 per cent in each group in one study where biopsy and radiation was compared with resection and radiation (Patchell *et al.* 1990), and 9 per cent in the second study in the group treated by resection and radiation versus 0 per cent in the group that received radiation therapy only (Vecht *et al.* 1993). Despite the evidence of benefit of resection followed by radiotherapy, the majority of patients with single brain metastasis will not be suitable for surgery (e.g. tumour inaccessible, systemic disease, or other health-related factors) and radiation remains the accepted palliative treatment for most patients. There is no doubt that certain patients can have a symptomatic and imaging response to radiation. These patients are usually young (age <60 years), have a good Karnofsky Performance Score (>70), radiosensitive tumours, and controlled primary tumour and metastatic disease confined to the brain. Failure of radiation to have any clinical or imaging response is more commonly seen elderly patients and patients with a Karnofsky Performance Scale of less than 70 (Deiner-West *et al.*, 1989). The optimal dose fractionation schedule for treatment of brain metastases remains uncertain and varies widely (e.g. 2000 cGy given over 1 week to 5000 cGy over 4 weeks). Conventional whole-brain radiation is thought to increase median survival in patients with brain metastasis by 3–6 months (Cairncross *et al.* 1980); however, this is based on retrospective non-randomized matched controlled series and is probably optimistic.

Technical advances in radiotherapy have re-opened the debate about the value of surgery for single brain metastasis. Stereotactic radiotherapy (SRT), using a linear accelerator with capability for three-dimensional conformal external radiation and a non-invasive removable frame which allows fractionated treatments, or stereotactic radiosurgery (SRS), using multiple cobalt-60 sources and a fixed, rigid, surgically attached stereotactic frame (gamma knife) for single-session treatment, may be as effective as surgical resection for single brain metastasis. Radiosurgery is high-dose, single-fraction external irradiation of a stereotactically well-defined target. For technical reasons the metastasis must be less than 3 cm in diameter and ideally should not border the ventricles, brainstem, or cranial nerves. Radiosurgery is an option for treatment in patients with single metastasis who are unfit for surgery or have a metastasis in a surgically inaccessible site. Highly selected series have demonstrated local control in 80 per cent of treated cases and an incidence of radiation necrosis of approximately 5–10 per cent (Flickinger *et al.* 1994; Alexander *et al.* 1995). Stereotactic radiosurgery using the conventional LINAC system or gamma knife has probably superseded the use of interstitial brachytherapy, which requires the placement of radioactive implants into the bed of the tumour after surgical resection or by stereotactic implantation and has a high incidence of radionecrosis. Because of the possibilities of treating single brain metastasis with surgical resection or stereotactic radiosurgery, there is now debate whether there is any need to treat the whole brain, if the metastasis is truly single. Randomized controlled trials to examine surgical resection versus radiosurgery alone are under way.

18.9.2 **Multiple metastases**

Management of young patients with multiple brain metastases is different from those with single metastasis. First, there is less of a chance of misdiagnosis on CT/MRI scan; secondly, there is less of a chance of having two or three metastases at surgically resectable sites, and, thirdly, there is usually less opportunity for stereotactic radiotherapy because the metastases are multiple. Conventional whole-brain radiation without histological confirmation is almost always the management of choice. In patients with multiple brain metastases but stable systemic disease, there is no evidence that surgery and cranial radiation is superior to radiation alone. There are highly selected reported cases of good symptom control and extended survival from operation on multiple metastases (two or three brain metastases) at surgically accessible sites, although such cases are few and far between. However, the effectiveness of surgery for multiple cranial metastases remains highly debatable and survival is probably poorer than that of patients with single brain metastasis (Hazuka *et al.* 1993). The series suggesting an advantage to surgery for multiple brain metastases were poorly matched, naturally highly selective, did not compare with patients treated with whole-brain radiotherapy alone, and it is difficult to determine whether resections were complete or not (Bindal *et al.* 1993; Hazuka *et al.* 1993).

Systemic chemotherapy in a very selected patient group with potentially chemoresponsive tumours (e.g. breast, small cell lung, germ cell tumours) may be offered and may improve systemic disease, but usually the blood–brain barrier will limit the efficacy in patients with brain metastases (Kristjansen and Hansen 1988; Boogerd *et al.* 1992). Attempts to overcome the effect of the blood–brain barrier by using fat-soluble chemotherapeutic agents or by giving a bradykinin analogue (e.g. RMP-7) to increase the permeability of the blood–brain barrier and allow chemotherapy (e.g. carboplatin) to cross the blood–brain barrier have been tried with very limited success.

Management of elderly patients with multiple brain metastases and active systemic disease is palliative, with aims being symptomatic control and supportive care. There is no good evidence that radiation extends survival in the elderly.

18.10 **Malignant meningitis**

Malignant meningitis is defined as diffuse or widespread multifocal neoplastic involvement of the subarachnoid space. It can be due to spread from primary CNS tumours, metastatic spread from systemic malignancies, or due to haematological malignancies (Table 18.7) (Grossman and Moynihan 1991; Recht 1991; Walker 1991). The pathogenesis is probably multifactorial. Haematogenous spread via the choroid plexus is considered to be the most common route of spread, especially for haematogenous malignancies, although rupture of cerebral metastases or spread along perivascular spaces of perforating vessels is very likely in cases related to primary CNS malignancies and a percentage of cases with intraparenchymal metas-

Table 18.7. Causes of malignant meningitis

Primary CNS tumours	Systemic tumours	Haematological malignancies
Overall 1–32%	Overall 4–15%	Overall 5–15%
Medulloblastoma, 30–50%	Breast, 12–34%	Acute lymphocytic leukaemia, 40%
Ependymoma, 10–20%	Lung, 10–26%	Acute myelocytic leukaemia, 7%
Glioblastoma, 1–5%	Melanoma, 17–25%	Lymphoma, 7–30%
Primary CNS lymphoma, 20–30%	Gastrointestinal tract, 4–14%	
Oligodendroglioma, 5%	Unknown, 1–7%	

tases. In one study, 50 per cent of patients with malignant meningitis from solid systemic malignancies had previously had intraparenchymal metastases (Grant *et al.* 1994*b*). A further, but less common, possibility is spread from deposits in the subdural space or associated with epidural spinal cord compression and spread along the nerve roots. The dura is thick and acts as a strong physical barrier to direct spread, but about 5 per cent of patients with epidural spinal cord compression have coexisting malignant meningitis.

Primary CNS malignancies that abut the ventricles or lie close to the surface of the brain are most likely to spread to the CSF. CSF spread occurs in 30–50 per cent of cases with medulloblastoma, 10–20 per cent of cases with ependymoma, and 1–5 per cent of cases with glioblastoma. This CSF spread is most commonly asymptomatic, but 'dropped' metastases, especially from tumours in the posterior fossa (e.g. ependymoma and medulloblastoma), can result in cauda equina syndrome or spinal cord compression, and imaging of the spinal canal is an important investigation to consider prior to planning radiation therapy or further management.

Malignant meningitis is seen in 4–8 per cent of autopsied cases dying with systemic cancer. Approximately 5–10 per cent of patients with breast or lung primaries will develop malignant meningitis and these are the two most common primary sites in most series. Nevertheless, the frequency of malignant meningitis is higher in rare malignancies such as melanoma (10–15 per cent) and systemic lymphoma (especially non-Hodgkin's lymphoma—30 per cent). In haematological malignancies, such as acute lymphocytic leukaemia, 40 per cent of patients have malignant cells in the CSF, and in acute myelocytic leukaemia 7 per cent of patients have CSF involvement (Walker 1991).

Macroscopically, there is opacification of the meninges, usually at the base of the brain but also over the convexities or cauda equina region. The pathological changes are similar to infective meningitis. Diffuse or multifocal tumour infiltrates occur with reactive fibrosis and lymphocytosis. It is not uncommon for the reactive lymphocyctosis found in the CSF to cause confusion between systemic malignancy and reactive lymphocytosis, lymphoma, or even infective meningitis. These

infiltrates are commonly at the ventral surface of the brain and in the cerebral and cerebellar sulci. Tumour can encase the basal meningeal vessels, causing ischaemia and infarction of the perforating vessels, or encase the perineurium of the cranial or spinal nerves, causing ischaemia and then degeneration. Occasionally tumour will invade nerves.

The pathophysiology of malignant meningitis can be predicted from the pathology. Hydrocephalus as a result of obliteration of the foramina of Magendie and Luschka rarely occurs, but slowed egress of CSF via the arachnoid villi can produce a communicating hydrocephalus with raised intracranial pressure. Interference with the blood supply to the parenchyma causes infarction. Metabolic competition between tumour and nerves may be the reason for the gradual onset of cranial neuropathy or radiculopathy, although direct invasion of the nerves and parenchyma undoubtedly also occurs. Malignant meningitis is usually a late complication of cancer and often presents at the same time as advancing disease at other sites. Patients will often have already had intraparenchymal disease. The diagnosis of malignant meningitis should be considered particularly in patients with neurological symptoms or signs affecting a combination of cranial nerve, spinal root, or cerebral cortex (Grossman and Moynihan 1991; Recht 1991; Walker 1991). It has been estimated that 50 per cent of patients have mild memory impairment at diagnosis, and dementia occurs in 30 per cent. Headache is a presenting feature in 40 per cent and usually comes on gradually but becomes increasingly severe and intractable. The characteristics of the headache may be those of raised intracranial pressure or meningeal or vascular headache. Focal or generalized seizures occur in 5–10 per cent of cases. Neurological signs are frequently asymptomatic (e.g. absent reflexes, mild weakness, or subtle sensory signs). The single most common feature is a cranial neuropathy (80 per cent). The extraocular muscles are most commonly affected (75 per cent), followed by the facial nerve (47 per cent) or acoustic nerve (40 per cent). The optic nerve is involved in about 38 per cent (papilloedema, 19 per cent; reduced visual acuity, 17 per cent). Spinal root disease is the presenting symptom in about 25 per cent of cases and can be associated with back pain, limb pain, numbness, or weakness. Commonly there is a mixture of upper and lower limb spinal root symptoms, present at the same time. On examination at the time of diagnosis, 80 per cent have weakness in one or more roots and 60 per cent will have absent reflexes at some level. Occasionally cauda equina symptoms occur with sensory deficits from L1 downwards.

Investigations depend on the site of involvement and the differential diagnosis (Section 33.1.4), but the two most useful investigations are an imaging investigation at the appropriate level (e.g. gadolinium-enhanced MRI scan (Fig. 18.15) or myelography) and CSF analysis. T1-weighted MRI with gadolinium enhancement will reveal an abnormality in 30–70 per cent of cases (depending on the case series reported). Myelography may show multiple nodules or spinal block in 27–67 per cent of cases in selected series. CSF analysis will reveal an elevated intracranial pressure of greater than 160 mm CSF in 45–65 per

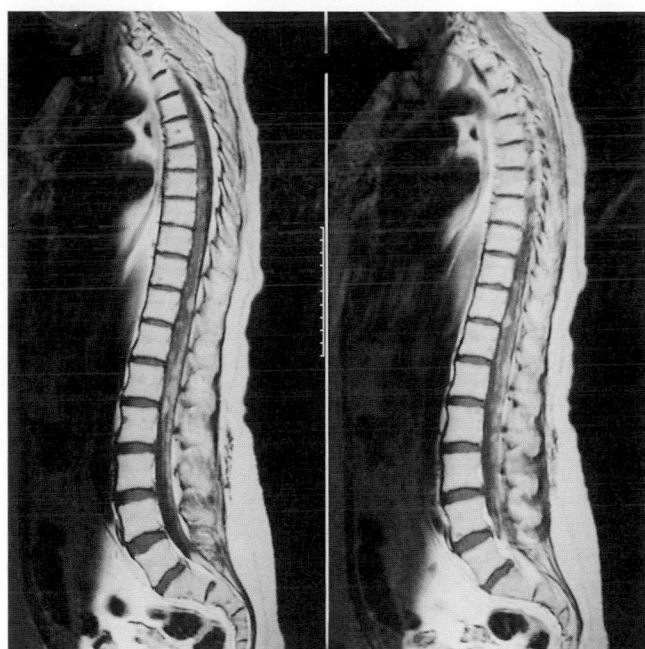

Fig. 18.15. Sagittal gadolinium-enhanced MRI, showing leptomeningeal metastases in a patient with carcinomatous meningitis.

cent of cases. CSF may also reveal an elevated protein (>0.5 g/l) in 81–89 per cent, low CSF glucose (<2.5 mmol/l) in 31–41 per cent, and 'lymphocytosis' (>5 cells/mm^3) but negative cultures in 54–72 per cent (Wasserstrom *et al.* 1982). It is important to send at least 5 ml of fresh CSF quickly to the laboratory or the likelihood of obtaining a diagnostic sample may be impaired. The first CSF sample will be positive for malignant cells in about 54 per cent of cases. This is substantially higher in diffuse cellular malignant meningitis (75 per cent) than multifocal nodular meningeal disease (38 per cent). Repeated lumbar puncture will identify a further 30 per cent of cases missed on the first. If two lumbar punctures do not demonstrate malignant cells, the likelihood of a positive cytological diagnosis reduces dramatically, with only 1 per cent subsequently being positive (Wasserstrom *et al.* 1982).

In the presence of repeated negative cytological specimens, the diagnosis can sometimes be made by cisternal puncture (2 per cent) or from sampling from ventricular CSF if there is a shunt or a ventricular access device (2 per cent). Approximately 10 per cent of cases will persistently have negative cytological CSF examinations, even in the presence of multinodular deposits in the subarachnoid space. It is highly likely that the natural history, management plan, and response to treatment will be different in diffuse highly cellular malignant meningitis compared with the predominantly multinodular form. It may be possible to improve on the diagnostic accuracy and specificity of tumour type by using immunohistological staining methods on cytospun preparations of CSF. Epithelial membrane antigen, cytokeratins, CAM 5.2, prostate-specific antigen, and thyroglobulin can confirm the diagnosis and give clues to site of the primary if previously unknown. B- and T-cell markers may be supportive of lymphoma, HMB 45 is a relatively specific marker for melanoma, and placental alkaline phosphatase may confirm germinoma. Glial fibrillary, acidic-protein-positive staining of cells demonstrates that the cells are of glial origin. α-Fetoprotein estimation and human chorionic gonadotrophin may support a diagnosis of teratoma or choriocarcinoma.

The management of malignant meningitis is controversial. In most cases CSF disease is a late pre-terminal manifestation of widespread disease. Treatment will depend on tumour type (lymphoma and breast more responsive than melanoma and lung), extent of tumour spread (CSF only versus disseminated disease), symptomatic site (cranial versus spinal), raised intracranial pressure with hydrocephalus (ventriculo-peritoneal shunt or not), previous treatment (e.g. cranial radiotherapy for cerebral metastasis, intravenous chemotherapy), effectiveness of systemic chemotherapy, and meningeal deposits versus diffuse CSF pleocytosis. Most commonly, symptom control is all that can be reasonably offered (e.g. steroids, anticonvulsants, analgesia). If there is hydrocephalus, this can be shunted. It is uncertain how effective intra-reservoir treatment is in the presence of shunted hydrocephalus and anecdotally the frequency of encephalopathy is higher. If there are symptomatic solid leptomeningeal metastases, radiation therapy occasionally stops progression or helps symptoms, although relief is usually short lived. If there are no solid leptomeningeal metastases, systemic disease is potentially treatable, and the patient is not severely impaired, then treatment of the CSF may be worthwhile. This is usually best given after placement of a Ommaya reservoir, since the distribution of chemotherapy is probably better than by using the lumbar route (Shapiro *et al.* 1975). Nevertheless, placement of a reservoir and intra-reservoir treatment is not without complications. From a personal review of the literature, technical problems with placement occur in 6.5–28 per cent of cases, infection in 4.9–50 per cent, toxic complications of treatment in 1.7–20 per cent, and the mortality in reported series range from 0.5 to 8.3 per cent.

The only drugs routinely used are methotrexate, cytosine arabinoside, or thiotepa. In practice, if the systemic tumour is not sensitive to these agents, then the CSF disease will not be sensitive. Methotrexate is given at a dose of 8–10 mg/day twice per week until disappearance of tumour cells from the CSF. If CSF disease comes under control and malignant cells disappear from the CSF, the methotrexate can be reduced to once/week or discontinued, and clinical and CSF follow-up will determine whether further treatment is necessary. Intrathecal methotrexate should be given with preservative-free saline, and treatment with leucovorin (folinic acid) should be started (15 mg orally every 12 hours on the day of treatment and for the following 24 hours). Leucovorin reverses the peripheral side-effects and can prevent mucositis and marrow suppression. Methotrexate should be withheld if the white blood cell count falls below 3000/mm^3 or platelets below 100 000/mm^3. If leucoencephalopathy develops, methotrexate should probably be replaced by cytosine arabinoside (40 mg intraventricularly). There are approximately 5 per cent toxic deaths from treatment and 15 per cent of patients develop confusion, disorientation, headache, nausea, or vomiting within 48 hours of methotrexate treatment, although this usually resolves after 48 hours. Arachnoiditis and transverse myelitis can occur with methotrexate. The late complications of treatment with methotrexate include leucoencephalopathy and a necrotizing encephalopathy. In certain situations, systemic chemotherapy may be valuable in treating the CSF disease or extending survival (e.g. high dose intravenous methotrexate for primary CNS lymphoma, breast carcinoma) (Ackland and Schilsky 1987; Grant *et al.* 1994*b*).

The prognosis for treated malignant meningitis varies from series to series, and one suspects that this is an area where 'gearing' of results and publication bias plays a large role in the apparent effectiveness of treatment. There have been no randomized controlled trials. CSF becomes negative for malignant cells in approximately 40 per cent of cases. In general, 25 per cent of patients have symptomatic improvement, 50 per cent remain stable for short periods of several weeks, and 25 per cent progressively decline and die in 6 weeks. Periods of stability and improvement range from 1 week to 2.5 years (median 3 months). Median survival for untreated malignant meningitis is approximately 4–6 weeks. With aggressive treatment one-third are dead in 6 weeks, median survival ranges from 9 to 24 weeks and 10 per cent survive for more than 1 year. In selected cases where there is no systemic disease, two-thirds of patients will remain stable or improve (median survival 10 months), and 20 per cent are alive at 1 year.

18.11 Complications of treatment

18.11.1 Surgery

The complications of surgery for brain tumours will depend on the site of the tumour (e.g. intracerebral versus intracranial extracerebral versus head and neck/skull), surrounding important structures (e.g. nerves, endocrine or vascular structures), the radiological appearance of the tumour (e.g. size and uniformity (e.g. homogeneous versus necrotic)), tumour pathology (e.g. primary versus metastasis), the experience of the neurosurgeon, and the state of general health of the patient.

It is unlikely that the frequency of side-effects recorded in the literature reflects the day-to-day frequency of side-effects in general neurosurgery units (Maurice-Williams 1997). The complications of neurosurgery can be divided into non-surgical and surgical complications.

Non-surgical complications

Patients with cancer are at an increased risk of deep venous thrombosis and pulmonary embolus. The additional risks of a surgical operation with bedrest and possible intratumoural bleeding make perioperative management difficult. Deep venous thrombosis and pulmonary embolus is a serious risk, and prophylaxis with support stockings and subcutaneous heparin are usually indicated (Frim *et al.* 1992). Electrolyte disturbances secondary to diabetes insipidus or syndrome of inappropriate antidiuretic hormone can lead to a stormy perioperative course. Patients may be systemically unwell as a result of malignancy or super-added chest or urinary tract infections. Endocrine deficiencies should be treated prior to neurosurgery on the pituitary gland and close attention paid to any perioperative endocrine complications.

Surgical complications

Postoperative haematomas at the operative site occur in approximately 5 per cent of patients. This frequency is probably higher in patients with malignant melanoma, choriocarcinoma, lung carcinoma, glioblastoma, and lymphoma. This higher risk of bleeding may influence the decision on whether stereotactic biopsy or an open procedure is performed in some cases. In operations for an intracerebral tumour, a transient neurological deficit will occur in approximately 10 per cent of patients postoperatively, slightly less with stereotactic operations. There is recovery of the neurological deficit in approximately 50 per cent of cases. There is also a risk of seizures as a result of operation in those who have no prior history of seizures, and sometimes a flurry of seizures in the postoperative period. Intraoperative stroke will occur in less than 1 per cent (depending on selection). Tumours in the region of the Sylvian fissure are probably best operated on by an open procedure, because of the moderately high risk of damaging one of the branches of the middle cerebral artery, with catastrophic results. Postoperative infective meningitis and cerebral abscess are rare complications of craniotomy, but still occur. Postoperative hydrocephalus is also uncommon, but occurs particularly in patients undergoing posterior fossa surgery, where hydrocephalus is probably due to postoperative brain swelling or contamination of the CSF by blood or debris. Operations in the region of the temporal lobe can result in significant memory deficits, which are sometimes not appreciated because preoperative cognitive assessments are commonly not performed and postoperative bedside assessments more commonly concentrate on focal weakness or sensory impairments (personal communication). Operations on the head and neck may damage cranial nerves (e.g. facial nerve in parotid surgery, infraorbital nerve in maxillary surgery, palatal and vocal cord paralysis due to damage to branches of the vagus in radical neck dissections or ipsilateral Horner's syndrome).

Mortality from craniotomies for malignant glioma or metastasis approach 5 per cent, and for stereotactic neurosurgery they are approximately 1 per cent (depending on the selection of patients and the experience of the surgeon) (Cabantog and Bernstein 1994). However, minimally invasive approaches with cranial nerve monitoring now offer lower morbidity with high chances of successful total excision of benign tumours in the posterior fossa.

18.11.2 **Radiation therapy**

The toxic side-effects of cranial radiation can be divided into local effects and central nervous system effects. The side-effects of radiation therapy depend on the dose fractionation schedule used, the natural history of the underlying disease, and the likelihood of having a radiotherapeutic response.

Local effects

Some people will feel nauseated about 30 minutes to 1 hour after treatments, and find that small meals with a low fat content are usually preferable to a large lunch or dinner. Patients will develop alopecia, but the degree and likelihood of recovery will depend on the dose and fractionation schedule used. Hair loss starts about 2–3 weeks into treatment, and maximum regrowth has occurred by 6 months. Frequently the hair that returns in the irradiated area is fine and curly and may be of a slightly different colour. Skin can become dusky red, dry, and itchy about 3 weeks into treatment and slight deafness can occur due to wax build-up. Most people feel tired and sleepy at the end of a course of radiation and some feel sick.

Some years after cranial irradiation there may be further local neuroendocrine or neural complications. Pituitary failure can occur if the pituitary has received a moderately large dosage directly (for pituitary adenoma) or is in the treatment field (e.g. frontotemporal low-grade glioma). Radiation usually affects the prolactin and sex hormones first (prolactin rises, luteinizing hormone and follicle-stimulating hormone fall) and causes problems with periods or infertility, then the thyroid stimulating hormone (TSH) falls and produces secondary hypothyroidism. If the optic nerve is in the treatment field, one commonly finds an afferent pupillary defect with optic neuropathy, which is usually asymptomatic or only produces mild visual acuity disturbance. Years after temporal lobe or posterior fossa irradiation one may find mild sensorineural hearing loss.

Central nervous system effects

The most serious central nervous system complications of radiation to the nervous system are: acute encephalopathy, subacute (early delayed) demyelination, delayed cerebral radiation necrosis, and chronic leucoencephalopathy (Section 5.9.1).

Acute encephalopathy is rare, but comes on usually within 24 hours of cranial irradiation. Symptoms consist of headache, nausea, vomiting, fever, or worsening of neurological deficits. Occasionally, swelling causes cerebral herniation. The likelihood of developing the acute encephalopathy is related to dose and whether the patient is pre-treated with steroids prior to radiation. It can be difficult in some patients with brain tumours to know whether the deterioration is attributable to radiation or to progression of the underlying tumour. The treatment is steroids and to consider reducing the fraction size of radiation.

Early delayed reaction is common and is seen 4 weeks to 3 months after completion of cranial radiation. In patients with cerebral tumours the symptoms are indistinguishable from those of tumour progression, except that there is commonly a feeling of excessive tiredness and nausea. In cases who have died with early delayed subacute radiation reaction and who have had a post-mortem, there are changes due to demyelination in the white matter of the brainstem and cerebrum, similar to those of multiple sclerosis. The treatment is to re-institute steroids for a period of 4–8 weeks and then gradually to reduce and discontinue them.

Delayed cerebral radiation necrosis is infrequent and can start months or years after cerebral irradiation. In patients who have cerebral tumours, the clinical and radiological appearances mimic tumour recurrence. MRI can not adequately distinguish active tumour from radiation necrosis. Positron emission tomography and single photon emission tomography can sometimes give an indication of whether there is increased radio-isotope uptake, consistent with active tumour, or reduced uptake related to an avascular mass, consistent with radiation necrosis, but neither technique is infallible and the only sure way to find out is to resect the necrotic mass. In patients with malignant glioma, it is common to see areas of necrosis within the tumour consistent with radiation damage and other areas of active tumour. Radiation necrosis is characterized by fibrinoid necrosis, luminal narrowing or occlusion, medial fibrosis, and adventitial proliferation in small arteries. There may also be bizarre, multinucleated astrocytes and foci of necrosis. The necrosis is thought to be due to ischaemia secondary to changes in the small and medium-sized vessels. Other hypotheses for the necrosis are that radiation-induced changes in the glia produce demyelination and white matter damage, or that the radiation causes release of cytokines, etc. into surrounding brain, which results in tissue damage. Necrosis as a result of tumour progression does not have the same degree of small vessel occlusive and fibrotic changes, but has significant endothelial proliferation.

Chronic leucoencephalopathy is usually only found in long-term survivors of cranial irradiation. Ten per cent of patients who survive for more than 1 year after radiotherapy for cerebral metastases will develop cognitive problems. Relatives notice that the patient may lack motivation, there is psychomotor retardation, memory impairment, and ataxia or apraxia of gait. As time passes there may be urinary incontinence, marked dementia, inability to walk due to apraxia or ataxia, and cortical myoclonus. High dose and large fractionation schedules are thought to be associated with a higher incidence of radiation-induced leucoencephalopathy (DeAngelis et al. 1989). The CT/MRI scan shows diffuse changes in the cortical white matter, and ventricular dilatation. The clinical picture is similar to that of normal pressure hydrocephalus, or basal ganglia disease. Patients do not improve with lumbar puncture or ventricular shunting.

18.11.3 **Chemotherapy**

Side-effects of chemotherapy may be a property of the mode of delivery or of the agent itself. Modes of delivery of chemotherapy include direct chemotherapy into the tumour bed at the time of surgery, intra-arterial chemotherapy (where the tumour is confined to an area supplied by one artery, usually the internal carotid), or systemic chemotherapy, either intravenously or orally. Intra-arterial chemotherapy requires arterial catheterization and commonly a general anaesthetic, since there can be severe pain in the distribution supplied by the sensory fibres within the artery. This is a direct toxic effect on the artery. In addition, even with supra-ophthalmic instillation of chemotherapy, there can be significant optic nerve toxicity due to turbulence and back flow along the ophthalmic artery. This can result in unilateral visual loss or ocular necrosis. Intravenous chemotherapy must be given cautiously in a fast-flowing arm vein. If chemotherapy gets into the soft tissues of the arm it can result in a severe local thrombophlebitis.

The other effects of systemic chemotherapy (intra-arterial, intravenous, or oral) relate to the toxic effect of the individual drugs. Nitrosoureas (e.g. BCNU) cause nausea that starts about 2 hours after starting an infusion and may persist for 24–48 hours. Facial flushing or dizziness may occur during infusion; this is rate dependent and resolves on stopping the drug. Bone-marrow suppression occurs with almost all agents and is maximal 4–6 weeks after receiving the drug and usually settles by 8 weeks. Risks of infection, bleeding, and tiredness are greatest around 4 weeks after treatment. Lung toxicity usually starts after a total dose of 1 g. A restrictive ventilatory defect is found and it is valuable to monitor vital capacity regularly in patients who receive more than 1 g total dose. Renal function should also be monitored. Procarbazine can also cause haematological and gastrointestinal symptoms, but in addition can cause flu-like symptoms, rash, and neurological symptoms (ataxia, headaches, paraesthesia, dizziness). Procarbazine can cause hypertensive crisis and severe gastrointestinal symptoms if given with antidepressants, alcohol, or tyramine-rich foods (e.g. cheese, bananas). Vincristine causes neurotoxicity (neuropathy, myopathy, and autonomic disturbance), gastrointestinal symptoms, and sometimes alopecia. Haematological toxicity is mild. Steroid use can result in weight gain, oedema, electrolyte problems, diabetes, osteoporosis, thinning of skin, and predisposition to infections and peptic ulcers. Cisplatinum derivatives cause neurotoxicity (peripheral neuropathy and deafness), renal toxicity, and bone-marrow suppression. High-dose cytosine arabinoside and 5-fluorouracil can cause reversible cerebellar ataxia, in addition to bone-marrow suppression and gastrointestinal and liver toxicity. Alopecia and infertility can occur with any of these drugs. Methotrexate can cause bone-marrow suppression, mucositis and, rarely, pneumonitis. It is nephrotoxic and hepatotoxic and can cause an encephalopathy if given in high doses. The toxic effects of intrathecal methotrexate are mentioned in the section on malignant meningitis.

18.12 Recovery and rehabilitation

Recovery and rehabilitation from a diagnosis of brain tumour, or from medical treatment of a brain tumour, may involve many specialists and support services. The first step is often coming to terms with the diagnosis and this can be eased by accurate, understandable medical information about the disease and its treatment options. This is best done by a doctor experienced in managing patients with brain tumours (Richards 1990). The Royal College of Physicians has produced guidelines regarding breaking bad news to the patients with malignant glioma and their relatives (Davis and Hopkins 1997b). Written information can often be a helpful reminder to patients and relatives, particularly where there are cognitive difficulties. There are also helpful general informational leaflets about different sorts of brain tumours from charitable organizations (see Appendix). Occasionally, patients with brain tumours will have disabling anxiety or will become clinically depressed, and may require special counselling or antidepressant medication. Neuropsychological symptoms may be related to the disease (e.g. seizures, fronto-limbic involvement with tumour), the treatment (anticonvulsants, steroids, radiation therapy, chemotherapy), or fear of the future (e.g. loss of health, independence, work, family position, relationships). Neurocognitive support from psychologists, psychiatrists, support groups, and self-help groups may all play a role in neuropsychological recovery, by providing information, enhancing personal control, and teaching coping mechanisms.

Physical rehabilitation involves improvement of neurological impairment (e.g. by steroids, anticonvulsants, painkillers, speech therapy), coping with physical disability (e.g. walking aids, eating aids, adaptation of home), and maximizing physical independence thus reducing handicap by encouraging re-integration into home, work, and past-times where feasible, and minimizing unnecessary hospital contact. In the early post-operative period physical rehabilitation usually progresses alongside medical therapy in hospital; however, there may be a feeling of active treatment for the tumour grinding to a halt after radiation and this is paradoxically sometimes a period of despair and anxiety while they await 'what's next'. Patients should be made aware of possible early delayed effects, to allay the fear of early recurrence, and should have a target-directed plan for recovery, which includes their own programme for rehabilitation and for periods of rest.

References

Ackland, S. and Schilsky, R. (1987). Review article—High dose methotrexate: A critical reappraisal. *J. Clin. Oncol.*, **5**, 2017–31.

Albert, F. K., Forsting, M., Sartor, K. *et al.* (1994). Early post-operative magnetic resonance imaging after resection of malignant glioma: Objective evaluation of residual tumor and its influence on regrowth and prognosis. *Neurosurgery*, **34** (1), 45–61.

Alexander, E., Moriarty, T. M., Davis, R. B. *et al.* (1995). Sterotactic radiosurgery for the definitive noninvasive treatment of brain metastases. *J. Natl Cancer Inst.*, **87**, 34–40.

Alvarez, L., Peris, P., Pons, F. *et al.* (1997). Relationship between biochemical markers of bone turnover and bone scintigraphic indices in assessment of Paget's disease activity. *Arth. Rheum.*, **40** (3), 461–8.

Barbara, N. M., Gutin, P. H., Wilson, C. B. *et al.* (1987). Radiation therapy in the treatment of partially resected meningiomas. *Neurosurgery*, **20**, 525–8.

Barkan, A. L., Lloyd, R. V., Chandler, W. F. *et al.* (1988). Pre-operative treatment of acromegaly with long acting sandostatin: shrinkage of invasive pituitary macroadenomas and improved surgical remission rate. *J. Clin. Endocrinol. Metab.*, **67**, 1040–8.

Barker, F. G., Davis, R. L., Chang, S. M. *et al.* (1996). Necrosis as a prognostic factor in glioblastoma multiforme. *Cancer*, **77**, 1161–6.

Bederson, J. B., von Ammon, K., Wichmann, W. W. *et al.* (1991). Conservative treatment of patients with vestibular tumors. *Neurosurgery*, **28**, 646–51.

Berger, M. S. (1995). Role of surgery in diagnosis and management. In: *Benign cerebral glioma*, (ed. M. L. J. Appuzzo), pp. 293–307. American Association of Neurological surgeons (AANS), Park Ritdge, USA.

Bernstein, M. and Parrent, A. G. (1994). Complications of CT-guided stereotactic biopsy of intra-axial brain lesions. *J. Neurosurg.*, **81**, 165–8.

Bindal, R. K., Sawaya, R., Leavens, M. E. *et al.* (1993). Surgical treatment of multiple brain metastases. *J. Neurosurg.*, **79**, 210–16.

Black, P. M. (1993). Meningiomas. *Neurosurgery*, **32** (4), 643–57.

Black, P. M., Carroll, R., and Zhang, J. (1996). The molecular biology of hormone and growth factor receptors in meningiomas. *Acta Neurochir. (Suppl.)*, **65**, 50–3.

Bleehen, N. M. and Stenning, S. P. on behalf of the Medical Research Council Brain Tumour Working Party (1991). A Medical Research Council trial of two radiotherapy doses in the treatment of grades 3 and 4 astrocytoma. *Br. J. Cancer*, **64**, 769–74.

Bloom, B. and Kramer, S. (1994). Conventional radiation therapy in the management of acromegaly. In: *Secretory tumors of the pituitary gland*, (ed. P. M. Black, N. T. Zervas, E. C. Ridgeway, and J. B. Martin), pp. 179–90. Raven, New York.

Bloom, H. J. G. and Bessell, E. M. (1990). Medulloblastoma in adults: A review of 47 patients treated between 1952 and 1981. *Int. J. Radiat. Oncol. Biol. Phys.*, **18**, 763–72.

Bloom, H. J. G., Glees, J., and Bell, J. (1991). The treatment and long term prognosis of children with intracranial tumors: a study of 610 cases, 1950–1981. *Int. J. Radiat. Oncol. Biol. Phys.*, **18**, 723–45.

Bondy, M. L. and Wrensch, M. R. (1996). Epidemiology of primary malignant brain tumours. In *Balliere's clinical neurology*, Vol. 5 (2) (Cerebral gliomas), (ed. W. K. A. Yung), pp. 251–70. Balliere Tindall, London.

Boogerd, W., Dalesio, O., Bais, E. M. *et al.* (1992). Response of brain metastases from breast cancer to systemic chemotherapy. *Cancer*, **69**, 972–80.

Bruce, J. N. and Stein, B. M. (1993). Complications of surgery for pineal region tumors. In Postoperative complications in intracranial neurosurgery, (ed. K. D. Post, E. D. Friedman, and P. C. McCormick), pp. 74–86. Thième Medical Publishers, New York.

Bunin, G. (1987). Racial patterns of childhood brain cancer by histologic type. *J. Natl Cancer Inst.*, **78**, 875–80.

Burger, P. C., Dubois, P. J., Schold, S. C. *et al.* (1983). Computerised tomographic and pathologic studies of untreated, quiescent, and recurrent glioblastoma multiforme. *J. Neurosurg.*, **58**, 159–69.

Burger, P. C., Vogel, F. S., Green, S. B. *et al.* (1985). Glioblastoma multiforme and anaplastic astrocytoma. Pathologic criteria and prognostic implications. *Cancer*, **56**, 1106–11.

Burger, P. C., Heinz, E. R., Shibata, T. *et al.* (1988). Topographic anatomy and CT correlations in untreated glioblastoma multiforme. *J. Neurosurg.*, **68**, 698–704.

Cabantog, A. M. and Bernstein, M. (1994). Complications of first craniotomy for intra-axial brain tumour. *Can. J. Neurol. Sci.*, **21**, 213–18.

Cairncross, J. G. and Eisenhauer, E. A. (1995). Response and control: lessons from oligodendroglioma. *J. Clin. Oncol.*, **13**, 2475.

Cairncross, J. G., Kim, J.-H., and Posner, J. B. (1980). Radiation therapy for brain metastases. *Ann. Neurol.*, **7**, 529–41.

Cairncross, J. G., Pexman, J. H. W., Rathbone, M. P. *et al.* (1985). Post-operative contrast enhancement in patients with brain tumor. *Ann. Neurol.*, **17**, 570–2.

Castro-Vita, H., Salazar, O. M., Scarantino, C. *et al.* (1980). Medulloblastomas. *Rev. Int. Radiol.*, **5**, 77–82.

Clyde, Z., Chataway, J., Slattery, J. *et al.* (1998). Significant change in tests of neurological impairment in patients with brain tumours. *J. Neurooncol.* **39**, 81–90.

Cohen, B. H. and Packer, R. J. (1996). Chemotherapy for medulloblastomas and primitive neuroectodermal tumors. *J. Neurooncol.*, **29** (1), 55–68.

Counsell, C. E., Collie, D. A., and Grant, R. (1996). Incidence of intracranial tumours in Lothian Region of Scotland, 1989–90. *J. Neurol. Neurosurg. Psychiat.*, **61**, 143–50.

Counsell, C., Collie, D., and Grant, R. (1997). Limitations of using a cancer registry to identify incident primary intracranial tumours. *J. Neurol. Neurosurg. Psychiat.*, **63** (1), 94–7.

Counsell, C. E. and Grant, R. (1998). A systematic review of the methodology and results of the studies of the incidence of intracranial tumors. *J. Neurooncol.*, **37** (3), 241–50.

D'Alessandro, G., Di Giovanni, M., Iannizzi, L. *et al.* (1995). Epidemiology of primary intracranial tumors in the Valle d'Aosta (Italy) during the 6-year period 1986–1991. *Neuroepidemiology*, **14**, 139–46.

Davis, D. L., Hoel, D., Percy, C. *et al.* (1990). Is brain cancer mortality increasing in industrial countries? *Ann. NY Acad. Sci.*, **609**, 191–204.

Davis, E. and Hopkins, A. (1997*a*). *Improving care for patients with malignant cerebral glioma*. Royal College of Physicians, London.

Davis, E. and Hopkins, A., on behalf of a Working Group (1997*b*). Good practice in the management of adults with malignant cerebral glioma: clinical guidelines. *Br. J. Neurosurg.*, **11** (4), 318–30.

DeAngelis, L. M., Delattre, J. Y., and Posner, J. B. (1989). Radiation induced dementia in patients cured of brain metastases. *Neurology*, **39**: 789–96.

Deen, H. G., Ebersold, M. J., Harner, S. G. *et al.* (1996). Conservative management of acoustic neuroma: an outcome study. *Neurosurgery*, **39** (2), 260–6.

Deiner-West, M., Dobbins, T. W., Phillips, T. L. *et al.* (1989). Identification of an optimal subgroup for treatment evaluation of patients with brain metastases using RTOG study 7916. *Int. J. Radiat. Oncol. Biol. Phys.*, **16**, 669–73

Delattre, J. Y., Krol, G., Thaler, H. T. *et al.* (1988). Distribution of brain metastases. *Arch. Neurol.*, **45**, 741–4.

Deutsch, M. (1988). Medulloblastoma: staging and treatment outcome. *Int. J. Radiat. Oncol. Biol. Phys.*, **14**, 1103–7.

Deutsch, M., Thomas, P. R., Krischer, J. *et al.* (1996). Results of a prospective randomized trial comparing standard dose neuraxis irradiation (3,600 cGy/20) with reduced neuraxis irradiation (2,340 cGy/13) in patients with low-stage medulloblastoma. A combined Children's Cancer Group–Pediatric Oncology Group Study. *Pediatr. Neurosurg.*, **24** (4), 167–76.

Devaux, B. C., O'Fallon, J. R., and Kelly, P. J. (1993). Resection, biopsy, and survival in malignant glial neoplasms. *J. Neurosurg.*, **78**, 767–75.

Dhami, M. S. and Bona, R. D. (1993). Thrombosis in cancer patients. *Postgrad. Med.*, **93** (8), 131–3, 137–40.

Dumas-Duport, C., Scheithauer, B., O'Fallon, J. *et al.* (1988). Grading of astrocytomas. A simple and reproducible method. *Cancer*, **62**, 2152–65.

Ebersold, M. J., Quast, L. M., Laws, E. R. *et al.* (1986). Long term results in transsphenoidal removal of non functioning pituitary adenomas. *J. Neurosurg.*, **64**, 713–19.

EORTC Brain Tumor Group (1981). Evaluation of CCNU, VM-26 plus CCNU, and procarbazine in supratentorial brain gliomas. *J. Neurosurg.*, **55**, 27–31.

Evans, A., Jenkin, D., Sposto, R. *et al.* (1990). The treatment of medulloblastoma: results of a prospective randomized trial of radiation with and without CCNU, vincristine and prednisone. *J. Neurosurg.*, **72**, 575–82.

Eyre, H. J., Crowley, J. J., Townsend, J. J. *et al.* (1993). A randomized trial of radiotherapy versus radiotherapy plus CCNU for incompletely resected low grade gliomas: a Southwest Oncology Group study. *J. Neurosurg.*, **78**, 909–14.

Fine, H. A., Dear, K. B., Loeffler, J. S. *et al.* (1993). Meta-analysis of radiation therapy with and without adjuvany chemotherapy for malignant gliomas in adults. *Cancer*, **71** (8), 2585–97.

Flickinger, J. C., Kondziolka, D., Lunsford, L. D. *et al.* (1994). A multi-institutional experience with steroetactic radiosurgery for solitary brain metastasis. *Int. J. Radiat. Oncol. Biol. Phys.*, **28**, 797–802.

Fonari, M., Solero, C. L., Lasio, G. *et al.* (1990). Surgical treatment of intracranial dermoid and epidermoid cysts in children. *Childs Nerv Syst*, **6**, 66–70.

Frim, D. M., Barker, F. G., Poletti, C. E. *et al.* (1992). Post-operative low-dose heparin decreases thromboembolic complications in neurosurgical patients. *Neurosurgery*, **30**, 830–3.

Galicich, J. H., Arbit, E., and Wronski, M. (1996). Metastatic brain tumours. In: *Neurosurgery*, (2nd edn), (ed. R. H. Wilkins and S. S. Rengachary), pp. 807–12. McGraw-Hill, New York.

Glantz, M. J., Cole, B. F., Friedberg, M. H. *et al.* A randomised, blinded, placebo controlled trial of divalproex sodium prophalaxis in adults with newly diagnosed brain tumors. *Neurology*, **46** (4), 985–91.

Glass, J., Gruber, M. L., Cher, L. *et al.* (1994). Pre-irradiation methotrexate chemotherapy of primary central nervous system lymphoma: long-term outcome. *J. Neurosurg.*, **81**, 188–95.

Goodman, R. (1993). Magnetic resonance imaging-directed stereotactic endoscopic third ventriculostomy. *Neurosurgery*, **32**, 1043–7.

Goodwin, J. W., Crowley, J., Eyre, H. J. *et al.* (1995). A phase II evaluation of tamoxifen in unresectable or refractory meningiomas: a south west oncology group study. *J. Neurooncol.*, **15**, 75–7.

Grant, R. (1999). Mobiles on the brain. *BMJ*, **318**, 1495.

Grant, R., Slattery, J., Gragor, A. *et al.* (1994). Recording neurological impairment in clinical trials of glioma. *J. Neurooncol.*, **19**, 37–49.

Grant, R., Naylor, B., Greenberg, H. S. *et al.* (1994). Clinical outcome in aggressively treated meningeal carcinomatosis. *Arch. Neurol.*, **51**, 457–61.

Grant, R., Liang, B. C., Page, M. S. *et al.* (1995). Age influences chemotherapy response in astrocytomas. *Neurology*, **45**, 929–33.

Grant, R., Whittle, I. R., Collie, D. et al. (1996). Referral pattern and management of patients with malignant brain tumours in South East Scotland. Health Bull., 54 (3), 212–22.

Grant, R., Liang, B. C., Slattery, J. et al. (1997). Chemotherapy response criteria in malignant glioma. Neurology, 48, 1336–40.

Grant, R., Hadley, D., Barton, T., and Osborn, C. (1999). Glioma patients who are slow responders to chemotherapy have no worse prognosis than fast responders. Neurooncol., Abstr. issue, 2: S112.

Grant, R., Whittle, I. R., Gregor, A. et al. (2001). Scottish Audit of the Royal College of Physicians Clinical Guidelines for Good Practice in the management of malignant glioma. Scottish Office Report., HMSO, Edinburgh.

Green, S. B., Byar, D. P., Walker, M. D. et al. (1983). Comparisons of carmustine, procarbazine and high dose methylprednisolone as additions to surgery and radiotherapy for the treatment of malignant glioma. Cancer Treat. Rep., 67, 121–32.

Green, S. B., Shapiro, W. R., Burger, P. C. et al. (1989). Randomized comparison of intra-arterial (IA) cisplatinum and intravenous (IV) PCNU for the treatment of primary brain tumours (BTCG study 8420A). Proc. Am. Soc. Clin. Oncol., 8, 26.

Greig, N. H., Ries, L. G., Yancik, R. et al. (1990). Increasing annual incidence of primary malignant brain tumors in the elderly. J. Natl Cancer Inst., 82, 1621–4.

Grossman, S. and Moynihan, T. (1991). Neoplastic meningitis. Neurol. Clin., 9, 843–56.

Guterman, K. S., Hair, L. S., and Morgello, S. (1996). Epstein–Barr virus and AIDS-related primary central nervous system lymphoma. Viral detection by immunohistochemistry, RNA in situ hybridization, and polymerase chain reaction. Clin. Neuropath., 15 (2), 79–86.

Gutin, P. H., Klemme, W. M., Lagger, R. L. et al. (1980). Management of the unresectable cystic craniopharyngioma by aspiration through an Ommaya reservoir drainage system. J. Neurosurg., 52, 36–40.

Haddad, F. S., Haddad, G. F., and Zaatari, G. (1997). Cranial osteomas: their classification and management. Report on a giant osteoma and review of the literature. Surg. Neurol., 48 (2), 143–7.

Hagmar, L., Akesson, B., Nielsen, J. et al. (1990). Mortality and cancer morbidity in workers exposed to low levels of vinyl chloride monomer at a polyvinyl chloride processing plant. Am. J. Indust. Med., 17, 553–65.

Halperin, E. C., Bentel, G., Heinz, E. R. et al. (1989). Radiation therapy treatment planning in supratentorial glioblastoma multiforme: An analysis based on post mortem topographic anatomy with CT correlations. Int. J. Radiat. Oncol. Biol. Phys., 17, 1347–50.

Hammoud, M. A., Sawaya, R., Shi, W. et al. (1996). Prognostic significance of pre-operative MRI scans in glioblastoma multiforme. J. Neurooncol., 27, 65–73.

Hardy, D. G., Macfarlane, R., Baguley, D. et al. (1989). Surgery for acoustic neuroma: an analysis of 100 translabyrinthine operations. J. Neurosurg., 71, 799–804.

Hazuka, M. B., Burleson, W., Stroud, D. N. et al. (1993). Multiple brain metastases are associated with poor survival in patients treated with surgery and radiotherapy. J. Clin. Oncol., 11, 369–73.

Hochberg, F. H. and Miller, D. H. (1988). Primary central nervous system lymphoma. J. Neurosurg., 68, 835–53.

Hodges, L. C., Smith, J. L., Garrett, A. et al. (1992). Prevalence of glioblastoma multiforme in subjects with prior therapeutic irradiation. J. Neurosci. Nurs., 24, 79–83.

Hopkins, A., Garman, A., and Clarke, C. (1988). The first seizure in adult life: Value of clinical features, electro-encephalography and computerised tomographic scanning in the prediction of seizure recurrence. Lancet, i, 721–6.

Huncharek, M., Muscat, J., and Geschwind, J. F. (1998). Multidrug versus single agent chemotheraphy for high grade astrocytoma; results of a meta-analysis. Anticancer Res., 18, 4693–7.

Inskip, P. O., Tarone, R. D., Hatch, E. E. et al. (2001) Cellular-telephone use and brain tumours. N. Engl. J. Med., 344, 79–86.

Jeffries, B. F., Kishore, P. R. S., Singh, K. S. et al. (1981). Contrast enhancement in the post-operative brain. Radiology, 139, 409–13.

Karim, A. B. M. F., Cornu, P., Bleehen, N. et al. (1998). Immediate post-operative radiotherapy in low grade glioma improves progression free survival, but not overall survival. Preliminary results of an EDRTC/HRC randomized phase III study. Proc. Am. Soc. Clin. Oncol., 17, 400a, (abstract).

Karnofsky, D. and Burchenal, J. H. (1989). Clinical evaluation of chemotherapeutic agents in cancer. In: Evaluation of chemotherapy agents, (ed. C. M. Macleod). Columbia University Press, New York.

Kato, H., Yoshimoto, Y., and Schull, W. J. (1989). Risk of cancer among children exposed to atomic bomb irradiation in utero: a review 1989; In: Perinatal and mutational carcinogenesis, (ed. N. P. Napalkov, J. M. Rice, L. Tomatis, and H. Yamasaki), pp. 365–74. International Agency for Research on Cancer, Lyon.

Kaye, A. H., Giles, G. G., and Gonzales, M. (1993). Primary central nervous system tumors in Australia: a profile of clinical practice from the Australian brain tumor registry. Aust. N Z J. Surg., 63, 33–8.

Kelly, P. J., Dumas-Duport, C., Kispert, D. B. et al. (1987). Imaging based stereotaxic serial biopsies in untreated intracranial glial neoplasms. J. Neurosurg., 66, 865–74.

Kernohan, J. W. and Sayre, G. P. (1952). *Tumors of the central nervous system*. Armed Forces Institute of Pathology, Washington, DC.

Kim, T. S., Halliday, A. L., Hedley-White, E. T. *et al.* (1991). Correlates of survival and the Dumas-Duport grading system for astrocytomas. *J. Neurosurg.*, **74**, 27–37.

Kleihues, P., Burger, P. C., and Scheithauer, B. W. (1993*a*). World Health Organisation. Histological typing of tumours of the central nervous system, (2nd edn). Springer Verlag, Berlin.

Kleihues, P., Burger, P. C., and Scheithauer, B. W. (1993*b*). The new WHO classification of brain tumours. *Brain Pathol.*, **3**, 255–68.

Kondziolka, D., Lunsford, L. D., and Martinez, A. J. (1993). Unreliability of contemporary neurodiagnostic imaging in evaluating suspected adult supratentorial (low grade) astrocytoma. *J. Neurosurg.*, **79**, 533–6.

Kreth, F. W., Warnke, P. C., Scheremet, R. *et al.* (1993). Surgical resection and radiation therapy versus biopsy and radiation therapy in the treatment of glioblastoma multiforme. *J. Neurosurg.*, **78**, 762–6.

Kristjansen, P. E. and Hansen, H. H. (1988). Brain metastases from small cell lung cancer treated with combination chemotherapy. *Eur. J. Cancer Clin. Oncol.*, **24**, 545–9.

Kritis, A. P., Yung, W. K. A., Bruner, J. *et al.* (1993). The treatment of anaplastic oligodendrogliomas and mixed gliomas. *Neurosurgery*, **32** (3), 365–70.

Lachance, D. H., Brizel, D. M., Gockerman, J. P. *et al.* (1994). Cyclophosphamide, doxorubicin, vincristine and prednisone for primary central nervous system lymphoma: short duration response and multifocal intracerebral recurrence preceeding radiotherapy. *Neurology*, **44**, 1721–7.

Landverg, T. G., Lindgren, M. L., Cavalin-Stahl, E. K. *et al.* (1980). Improvements in the radiotherapy of medulloblastoma 1946–1975. *Cancer*, **45**, 670–8.

Lawton, M. T., Hamilton, M. G., Beals, S. P. *et al.* (1995). Radical resection of anterior skull base tumors. *Clin. Neurosurg.*, **42**, 43–70.

Lee, A., Chan, G., Fung, C. *et al.* (1995). Paradoxical response of a pineal immature teratoma to combination chemotherapy. *Med. Pediatr. Oncol.*, **24**, 53–7.

Lefebvre, J. L., Chevalier, D., Lubornski, B. *et al.* (1996). Larynx preservation in hypopharynx and lateral epilarynx cancer: preliminary results of EORTC randomised phase 3 trial 24891. *J. Natl Cancer Inst.*, **88**, 890.

Leibowitz, U., Yablonsky, M., Alter, M. *et al.* (1971). Tumors of the nervous system: incidence and population selectivity. *J. Chron. Dis.*, **23**, 707–21.

Levin, V. A., Wara, W. M., Davis, R. L. *et al.* (1985). Phase III comparison of chemotherapy with BCNU and the combination of procarbazine, CCNU, and vincristine administered after radiation therapy with hydroxyurea to patients with malignant gliomas. *J. Neurosurg.*, **63**, 218–23.

Levin, V. A., Silver, P., Hannigan, J. *et al.* (1990). Superiority of post radiotherapy adjuvant chemotherapy with CCNU, procarbazine, and vincristine (PCV) over BCNU for anaplastic gliomas: NCOG 6G61. Final report. *Int. J. Radiat. Oncol. Biol. Phys.*, **18**, 321–4.

Li, F. P. and Fraumeni, J. F. Jr (1969). Soft tissue sarcoma, breast cancer and other neoplasms. A family syndrome? *Ann. Int. Med.*, **71**, 747–52.

Ling, S. M., Roach, M., Larson, D. A. *et al.* (1997). Radiotherapy of primary central nervous system lymphoma in patients with and without human immunodeficiency virus. Ten years experience at the University of California San Francisco. *Cancer*, **73** (10), 2570–82.

Lovaste, M. G., Ferrari, G., and Rossi, G. (1986). Epidemiology of primary intracranial tumors in the province of Bolzano 1980–1984. *Ital. J. Neurol. Sci.*, **9**, 237–41.

Macdonald, D. R. (1994). Low grade gliomas, mixed gliomas and oligodendrogliomas. *Semin. Oncol.*, **21** (2), 236–48.

Macdonald, D. R., Gaspar, L. E., and Cairncross, J. G. (1990). Successful chemotherapy for newly diagnosed aggressive oligodendroglioma. *Ann. Neurol.*, **27**, 573–4.

Mack, W., Preston-Martin, S., and Peters, J. M. (19991). Astrocytoma risk related to job exposure to electric and magnetic fields. *Bioelectromagnetics*, **12**, 57–66.

MacMahon, E. M. E., Glass, J. D., Harris, N. L. *et al.* (1991). Epstein–Barr virus in AIDS-related primary central nervous system lymphoma. *Lancet*, **338**, 969–73.

Maekawa, A. and Mitsumori, K. (1990). Spontaneous occurrence and chemical induction of neurogenic tumours in rats—influence of host factors and specificity of chemical structure. *Crit. Rev. Toxicol.*, **20**, 287–310.

Mahaley, M. S. (1991). Neuro-oncology index and review (adult brain tumours): Radiotherapy, chemotherapy, immuno-therapy, photodynamic therapy. *J. Neurooncol.*, **11**, 85–147.

Mahaley, M. S., Whaley, R. A., Blue, M. *et al.* (1986). Central neurotoxicity following intracarotid BCNU chemotherapy for malignant glioma. *J. Neurooncol.*, **3**, 297–314.

Mahaley, M. S., Whaley, R. A., Krigman, M. R. *et al.* (1987). Randomized phase III trial of single versus multiple chemotherapeutic treatment following surgery and during radiotherapy for patients with anaplastic gliomas. *Surg. Neurol.*, **27**, 430–2.

Mahaley, M. S., Mettlin, C., Natarajan, N. *et al.* (1990). Analysis of patterns of care of brain tumor patients in the United States: A study of the Brain Tumor Section of the AANS and CNS, and the Commission on Cancer of the ACS. *Clin. Neurosurg.*, **36**, 347–52.

Malkin, D., Li, F. P., Strong, L. C. *et al.* (1990). Germ line p53 mutations in a familial syndrome of breast cancer, sarcoma and and other neoplasms. *Science*, **250**, 1233–8.

Maurice-Williams, R. S. (1997). The notes in the cupboard: the question of intellectual honesty in neurosurgery. *Br. J. Neurosurg.*, **11** (4), 277–9.

McKinney, P. A., Ironside, J. W., Harkness, E. F. *et al.* (1994). Registration quality and descriptive epidemiology of childhood brain tumours in Scotland. *Br. J. Cancer*, **70**, 973–9.

McLoone, P. (1993). *Cartstairs codes for Scottish postcode sectors from the 1991 census.* Public Health Research Unit, University of Glasgow, Glasgow.

Mintz, A. H., Kestle, J., Rathbone, M. P. *et al.* (1996). A randomized trial to assess the efficacy of surgery in addition to radiotherapy in patients with a single intracerebral metastasis. *Cancer*, **78** (7), 1470–6.

Monreal, M., Alastrue, A., Rull, M. *et al.* (1996). Upper extremity deep venous thrombosis in cancer patients with venous access devices—prophalaxis with a low molecular weight heparin (Fragmin). *Thromb. Haemost.*, **75** (2), 251–3.

Muir, C. S., Storm, H. H., and Polednak, A. (1994). Brain and other nervous system tumours. In: *Trends in cancer incidence and mortality (cancer surveys)*, 19/20, (ed. R. Doll, J. F. Fraumeni, and C. S. Muir), pp. 369–91. Cold Spring Harbor Laboratories Press, New York.

Muller, W., Afra, D., and Schroder, R. (1977). Supratentorial recurrences of gliomas: Morphological studies in relation to time intervals with astrocytomas. *Acta Neurochir.*, **37**, 75–91.

Nelson, D. F., Nelson, J. S., Davis, D. R. *et al.* (1985). Survival and prognosis of patients with astrocytoma with atypical or anaplastic features. *J. Neurooncol.*, **3**, 99–103.

Nelson, D. F., Diener-West, M., Horton, J. *et al.* (1988). *Combined modality approach to treatment of malignant gliomas: Re-evaluation of RTOG 7401/ECOG 1374 with long term follow-up: A joint study of the Radiation Therapy Oncology Group and Eastern Cooperative Oncology Group.* National Cancer Institute monograph No. 6, pp. 279–84. GPO, Washington, DC.

Nelson, D. F., Martz, K. L., Bonner, H. *et al.* (1992). Non Hodgkin's lymphoma of the brain: can high dose, large volume radiation therapy improve survival? Report of a prospective trial by the Radiation Therapy Oncology Group (RTOG): RTOG 8315. Int. J. Radiat. Oncol. Biol. Phys., **23**, 9–17.

Nelson, J. S., Tsukada, Y., Schoenfeld, D. *et al.* (1983). Necrosis as a prognostic criterion in malignant supratentorial astrocytic gliomas. *Cancer*, **52**, 550–4.

Newton, H., Junck, L., Bromberg, J. *et al.* (1990). Procarbazine chemotherapy in the treatment of recurrent malignant astrocytomas after radiation and nitrosourea failure. *Neurology*, **40**, 1743–6.

Ogunrinde, O. K., Lunsford, L. D., Flickinger, J. C. *et al.* (1994). Stereotactic radiosurgery for acoustic nerve tumors in patients with useful pre-operative hearing: results at 2 year follow-up examination. *J. Neurosurg.*, **80**, 1011–17.

Ohgaki, H., Eibl, R. H., Schwab, M. *et al.* (1993). Mutations of the p53 tumor supressor gene in neoplasms of the central nervous system. *Mol. Carcinog.*, **8**, 74–80.

Osoba, D., Brada, M., Yung, W. K. *et al.* (2000). Health-related quality of life in patients treated with Temozolomide versus procarbinzine for recurrent glioblastoma multiforme. *J. Clin. Oncol.*, **185**, 1481–91.

Patchell, R. A., Tibbs, P. A., Walsh, J. W. *et al.* (1990). A randomized trial of surgery in the treatment of single metastases to the brain. *N. Engl J. Med.*, **322**, 494–500.

Patel, S. R., Buckner, J. C., Smithson, W. A. *et al.* (1992). Cisplatinum based chemotherapy in primary central nervous system germ cell tumours. *J. Neurooncol.*, **12**, 47–52.

Piepmeier, J., Christopher, S., Spencer, D. *et al.* (1996). Variations in the natural history and survival of patients with supratentorial low grade astrocytomas. *Neurosurgery*, **38** (5), 872–9.

Pollock, B. E., Lunsford, L. D., Kondziolka, D. *et al.* (1995). Phosporus-32 intracavity irradiation of cystic craniopharyngiomas: current technique and long term results. *Int. J. Radiat. Oncol. Biol. Phys.*, **33**, 1944–52.

Posner, J. B. (1980). Clinical manifestations of brain metastasis. In: *Brain metastasis*, (ed. L. Weiss, H. A. Gilbert, and J. B. Posner), pp. 189–207. GK Hall, Boston.

Posner, J. B. and Chernik, N. L. (1978). Intracranial metastases from systemic cancer. *Adv. Neurol.*, **19**, 579–87.

Post, K. D., Eisenberg, M. B., and Catalano, P. J. (1995). Hearing preservation in vestibular schwannoma surgery: What factors affect outcome? *J. Neurosurg.*, **83**, 191–6.

Radhakrishnan, K., Molri, B., Puriui, J. E. *et al.* (1995). The trends in incidence of primary brain tumors in the population of Rochester, Minnesota. *Ann. Neurol.*, **37**, 67–73.

Recht, L. (1991). Neurological complications of systemic lymphoma. *Neurol. Clin.*, **9**, (4), 1001–15.

Regine, W. F. and Kramer, S. (1992). Pediatric craniopharyngiomas: Long term results of combined treatment with surgery and radiation. *Int. J. Radiat. Oncol. Biol. Phys.*, **24**, 611–17.

Registrar General for Scotland (1993) *Annual Report 1992.* Governmental Statistical Services Publishers No. 138, General Register Office, Edinburgh.

Remick, S. C., Diamond, C., Migliozzi, J. A. *et al.* (1990). Primary central nervous system lymphoma in patients with and without the acquired immune deficiency syndrome: a retrospective analysis and review of the literature. *Medicine*, **69**, 345–60.

Reni, M., Ferreri, A. J., Garancini, M. P. *et al.* (1997). Therapeutic management of primary central nervous system lymphoma in immunocompetent patients: results of a critical review of the literature. *Ann. Oncol.*, **8** (3), 227–34.

Revesz, T., Scaravelli, F., Coutinho, L. *et al.* (1993). Reliability of histological diagnosis including grading in gliomas biopsied by image guided stereotactic techniques. *Brain*, **116**, 781–93.

Richards, T. (1990). Chasms in communication. *BMJ*, **301**, 1407–8.

Ringel, M. D., Schwindinger, W. F., and Levine, M. A. (1996). Clinical implications of genetic defects in G proteins. The molecular basis of McCune–Albright syndrome and Albright hereditary osteodystrophy. *Medicine*, **75** (4), 171–84.

Ringertz, N. (1950). Grading of gliomas. *Acta Pathol. Microbiol. Scand.*, **27**, 51–64.

Ron, E., Modan, B., Boice, J. D. Jr *et al.* (1988). Tumours of the brain and nervous system after radiotherapy in childhood. *N. Engl. J. Med.*, **319**, 1033–9.

Roush, G. C. (1979). Epidemiology of cancer of the nose and paranasal sinuses. *Head Neck Surg.*, **2**, 3–11.

Salcman, M. (1987). Surgical decision making for malignant brain tumours. *Clin. Neurosurg.*, **35**, 285–313.

Salcman, M. (1995). The natural history of low grade gliomas. In: *Benign cerebral glioma*, (ed. M. L. J. Apuzzo), pp. 213–29. AANS, Park Ridge.

Salvati, M., Artico, M., Caruso, R. *et al.* (1991). A report on radiation induced gliomas. *Cancer*, **67**, 392–7.

Sanna, M., Karmarkar, S., Landolfi, M. (1995). Hearing preservation in vestibular schwannoma surgery: fact or fantasy? *J. Laryngol. Otol.*, **109** (5), 374–80.

Sarasin, F. P. and Eckman, M. H. (1993). Management and prevention of thromboembolic events in patients with cancer-related hypercoagulable states: a risky business. *J. Gen. Int. Med.*, **8** (9), 476–86.

Savitz, D. A. and Loomis, D. P. (1995). Magnetic field exposure in relation to leukemia and brain cancer mortality among electric utility workers. *Am. J. Epidemiol.*, **141**, 123–34.

Scanlon, P. W. and Taylor, W. F. (1979). Radiotherapy of intracranial astrocytomas: analysis of 417 cases treated from 1960 through 1969. *Neurosurgery*, **5**, 301–8.

Schild, S. E., Scheithauer, B. W., Schomberg, P. J. *et al.* (1993). Pineal parenchymal tumors: clinical, pathologic, and therapeutic aspects. *Cancer*, **72**, 870–80.

Scimeca, P. G., James-Herry, A. G., Black, K. S. *et al.* (1996). Chemotherapy treatment of malignant chordoma in children. *J. Pediatr. Hem. Oncol.*, **18** (2), 237–40.

Scottish Office (1991). *Health in Scotland 1990*. The Scottish Office, Home and Health Department. HMSO, Edinburgh.

SEER (1991). Surveillance, epidemiology and end result registry data provided by the Cancer Statistics Branch, Bethesda, MD.

Shapiro, W. R., Young, D. F., and Mehta, B. M. (1975). Methotrexate: distribution in cerebrospinal fluid after intravenous, ventricular and lumbar injections. *N. Engl. J. Med.*, **293**, 161–6.

Shapiro, W. R., Green, S. B., Burger, P. C. *et al.* (1989). Randomized trial of three chemotherapy regimens and two radiotherapy regimens in postoperative treatment of malignant glioma. BTSG Trial 8001. *J. Neurosurg.*, **71**, 1–9.

Sharp, L., Black, R. J., Harkness, E. F. *et al.* (1993). Cancer Registration statistics in Scotland: 1981–1990. ISD Publications, Edinburgh.

Shaw, E. (1995). The low grade glioma debate: evidence defending the position of early radiotherapy. *Neurosurg. Clin.*, **42**, 488–94.

Shaw, E. G., Scheithauer, B. W., and O'Fallon, J. R. (1997). Supratentorial gliomas: a comparative study by grade and histologic type. *J. Neurooncol.*, **31** (3), 273–8.

Shelton, C., Hitselberger, W. E., House, W. F. *et al.* (1990). Hearing preservation after acoustic tumor removal: long term results. *Laryngoscope*, **100**, 115–19.

Sioutos, P., Yen, V., and Arbit, E. (1996). Pituitary gland metastases. *Ann. Surg. Oncol.*, **3** (1), 94–9.

Springate, S. C. and Weichselbaum, R. R. (1990). Radiation or surgery for chemodectoma of the temporal bone: a review of local control and complications. *Head Neck*, **12**, 303–7.

Stenning, S. P., Freedman, L. S., and Bleehen, N. H. (1987). An overview of published results from randomized studies of nitrosoureas in primary high grade malignant glioma. *Br. J. Cancer*, **56** (1), 89–90.

Suh, J. H. and Barnett, G. H. (1999). Brachytherapy for brain tumours. *Hermatol. Oncol. Clin. North Am.*, **13**, 635–50.

Tai, P. T., Craighead, P., and Bagdon, F. (1995). Optimization of radiotherapy for patients with cranial chordoma. A review of dose response ratios for photon techniques. *Cancer*, **75** (3), 749–56.

Tait, D. M., Thornton-Jones, H., Bloom, H. J. *et al.* (1990). Adjuvant chemotherapy for medulloblastoma: the first multicentre controlled trial of the International Society of Paediatric Oncology (SIOP 1). *Eur. J. Cancer*, **26** (4), 464–9.

Vecht, C. J., Haaxma-Reiche, H., Noordijk, E. M. *et al.* (1993). Treatment of single brain metastasis: radiotherapy alone or combined with neurosurgery? *Ann. Neurol.*, **33**, 583–90.

von Deimling, A., Bender, K. B., Jahnke, R. *et al.* (1994). Loci associated with malignant progression in astrocytomas: a candidate on chromosome 19q. *Cancer Res.*, **54**, 1397–401.

Walker, M. D., Alexander, E. Jr, Hunt, W. E. *et al.* (1978). Evaluation of BCNU and/or radiotherapy in the treatment of anaplastic gliomas: a co-operative clinical trial. *J. Neurosurg.*, **49**, 333–43.

Walker, M. D., Green, S. B., Byar, D. P. *et al.* (1980). Randomized comparisons of radiotherapy and nitrosoureas for the treatment of malignant glioma after surgery. *N. Engl. J. Med.*, **303**, 1323–9.

Walker, R. (1991). Neurologic complications of leukaemia. *Neurol. Clin.*, **9**, 989–99.

Wallner, K. E., Galicich, J. H., Krol, G. *et al.* (1989). Patterns of failure following treatment for glioblastoma multiforme and anaplastic astrocytoma. *Int. J. Radiat. Oncol. Biol. Phys.*, **16**, 1405–9.

Wasserstrom, W., Glass, J., and Posner, J. (1982). *Cancer*, **49**, 759–72.

Weiss, M., Sutton, L., Marcial, V. *et al.* (1989). The role of radiation therapy in the management of childhood craniopharyngioma. *Int. J. Radiat. Oncol. Biol. Phys.*, **17**, 1313–21.

Wen, B. C., Hussey, D. H., Staples, J. *et al.* (1989). A comparison of roles of surgery and radiation therapy in the management of craniopharyngiomas. *Int. J. Radiat. Oncol. Biol. Phys.*, **16**, 17–24.

Whelan, H. T., Clanton, J. A., Wilson, R. E. *et al.* (1988). Comparisons of CT and MRI brain tumor imaging using a canine glioma model. *Pediatr. Neurol.*, **4**, 279–83.

Wrench, M. R., Bondy, M. L., Wiencke, J. *et al.* (1993). Environmental risk factors for primary malignant brain tumors: a review. *J. Neurooncol.*, **17**, 47–64.

Yamada, N., Kato, M., Yamashita, H. *et al.* (1995). Enhanced expression of transforming growth factor-beta and its type I and type II receptors in human glioblastoma. *Int. J. Cancer*, **62**, 386–92.

Yasergil, M. G., Curic, M., Kis, M. *et al.* (1990). Total removal of craniopharyngiomas. Approaches and long term results in 144 patients. *J. Neurosurg.*, **73**, 3–11.

Young, A. C., Costanzi, J. B., Mohr, P. D. *et al.* (1982). *Lancet*, **1**, 1446–7.

Young, J. L., Percy, C. L., and Assire, A. J. (1981). *Is routine computerised axial tomography in epilepsy worthwhile? Cancer Incidence and mortality in the US 1973–77*. National Cancer Institute Monograph No. 57. GPO, Washington DC.

Zimmerman, R. A. (1991). Imaging of adult central nervous system primary malignant gliomas. Staging and follow-up. *Cancer*, **67**, 1278–83.

Zubrod, C. G., Schneiderman, M., Frei, R. *et al.* (1960). Appraisal of methods of study of chemotherapy in cancer in man: Comparative therapeutic trial of nitrogen mustard and triethylene thiophosphoramide. *J. Chronic. Dis.*, **11**, 7–33.

Zulch, K. J. (1979). *Histological typing of tumours of the central nervous system*. World Health Organization, Geneva.

CHAPTER 19

Neurocutaneous syndromes

Robert Grant

19.1 Tuberous sclerosis

19.1.1 Introduction

Tuberous sclerosis (synonyms: epiloia, Bournville's disease) is an autosomal dominant multisystem disease that usually presents in childhood with a characteristic facial rash (adenoma sebaceum) and seizures or learning difficulties. Other organs (e.g. heart and kidney) are less commonly involved. Because the condition has very variable clinical expression, and two-thirds of cases are thought to be new mutations, it is important to examine and screen relatives. Central nervous system lesions in tuberous sclerosis are due to a developmental disorder of neurogenesis and neuronal migration. Management may involve many specialists and close co-operation between specialists is essential.

19.1.2 Incidence and prevalence

The incidence of tuberous sclerosis (TS) is uncertain but the point prevalence is between 1 in 10 000 and 1 in 6000 (Hunt and Lindenbaum, 1984).

19.1.3 Genetic factors

The sites of genetic mutation in tuberous sclerosis are now well established. There is locus heterogeneity with one gene on chromosome 9q34 (*TSC1*) and a second gene on chromosome 16p13.3 (*TSC2*). The *TSC2* gene has been cloned. Most of the *TSC2* mutations are subtle, and somatic and germline mosaicism could explain the phenotypic heterogeneity and possibly non-penetrance. The protein produced by the gene has been termed 'tuberin'. The TS gene may be a tumour suppressor gene which would account for the high incidence of tumours in TS patients, and allelic losses of the tuberous sclerosis genes in the tumours have also been found (Short *et al.* 1995).

19.1.4 Clinical features and imaging diagnosis

Adenoma sebaceum (facial angiofibromas) is the most common outward manifestation of this disorder (Fig. 19.1). Other skin changes include hypopigmented macules, café-au-lait

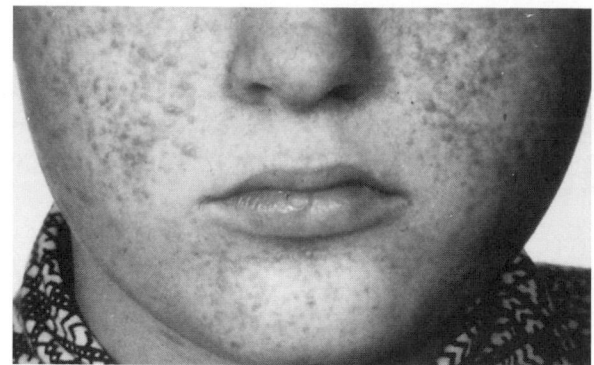

Fig. 19.1. Facial angiofibromas (adenoma sebaceum) in tuberous sclerosis.

spots and 'shagreen patches'. Facial angiofibromas are most commonly seen over the cheeks and nasolabial folds. The rash can extend to the chin and forehead. The angiofibromas are rather greasy and can be mistaken for acne. Hypopigmented macules are frequently shaped like an ash leaf, are 1–3 cm in diameter, and are most easily identified by shining ultraviolet

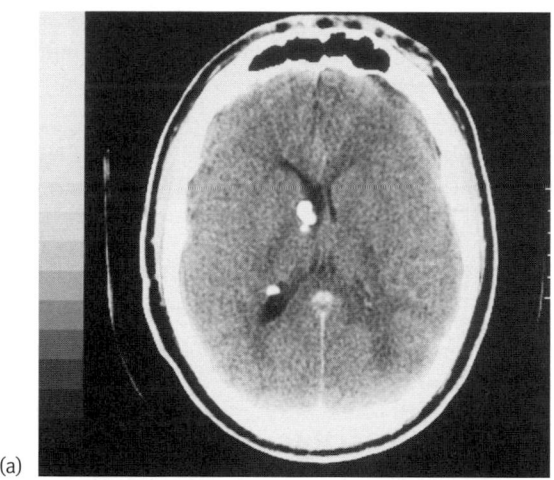

(a)

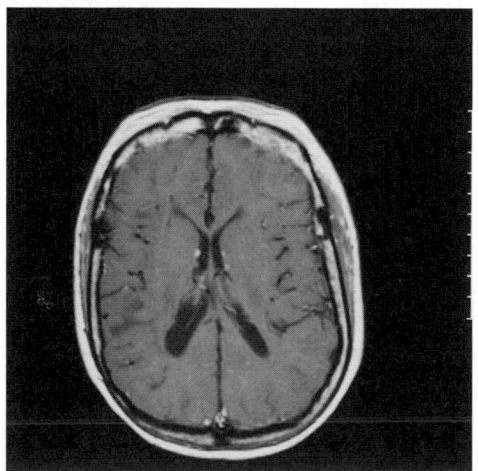

Fig. 19.2. (a) Axial CT brain scan and (b) axial MRI brain scan in patients with tuberous sclerosis.

light over the skin. Subungal fibromas are found in approximately 50 per cent of cases. Seizures are common and can be partial (focal), multifocal, or generalized. Seizure type is commonly related to the site of cortical tubers. The cortical dysplastic lesions are hamartomatous and may calcify (Fig. 19.2a). Sometimes clinically, and even histologically, it can be difficult to differentiate cortical dysplasia from well-defined ganglionic tumours. The most common tumours associated with tuberous sclerosis are subependymal giant-cell astrocytomas. However, immunohistochemical staining may be negative for glial acidic fibrillary protein (GFAP) and there can be evidence of neuronal differentiation, with positivity with neuronal specific enolase (NSE). Tuberous sclerosis can also be associated with gangliogliomas and pleomorphic xanthoastrocytomas. These are categorized as WHO grade 1 astrocytomas and typically alter little in size over several years. MRI with gadolinium enhancement is the investigation of choice for patients with neurocutaneous syndromes. Subependymal nodules and cortical and white matter tubers characteristic of tuberous sclerosis are readily identified by MRI (Fig. 19.2b).

Patients with tuberous sclerosis are at a higher risk of renal disease associated with angiomyolipomas of the kidneys and renal cysts. The gene that accounts for 85 per cent of polycystic kidney disease is situated on chromosome 16p13.3, adjacent to the tuberous sclerosis gene (*TSC2*), and children with large deletions of this region can present with tuberous sclerosis and severe childhood-onset polycystic kidney disease (Harris *et al.* 1995). Renal cysts and angiomyolipomas become increasingly common with the passage of time and can progressively enlarge, as demonstrated by serial renal imaging (O'Hagan *et al.* 1996). Although bilateral renal angiomyolipomas are commonly found, chronic renal failure in the absence of cystic disease is uncommon. The imaging appearances of tuberous-sclerosis-related cystic disease of the kidney resemble those of autosomal dominant polycystic kidney disease; however, the histopathological findings are quite different, with hypertrophic, hyperplastic lining to the renal cysts. Hepatic angiomyolipomas are commonly asymptomatic but can occur and present with abdominal pain followed by malaise and possibly hepatomegaly. The tumour is hyperechoic on ultrasound and has low density (<20 Houndsfield units) by CT and increased vascularity on angiography. There is also an increase in the number and size of retinal hamartomas and cardiac rhabdomyomas with increasing age.

The diagnostic criteria are outlined in Table 19.1 (Osbourne and Fryer 1991).

19.1.5 **Management**

The epilepsy can be severe and resistant to the usual anticonvulsant medications. Carefully selected patients with refractory epilepsy may be suitable for neurosurgical intervention. The success of surgery depends on the clear identification of an epileptogenic focus and identification of a structural abnormality at a corresponding site. Children may be found to have learning difficulties and may require special schooling or assistance (Curatolo 1996).

Table 19.1. Diagnostic criteria for tuberous sclerosis (from Osbourne, J. P. and Fryer, A. E. (1991). Tuberous sclerosis (epiloia, Bourneville's disease). In *Clinical neurology*, (ed. M. Swash and J. Oxbury), p. 1256. Churchill Livingstone, Edinburgh)

One major or two minor criteria:

Major criteria:

1. Definite shagreen patch
2. Ungal fibroma
3. Retinal hamartomas
4. Adenoma sebaceum
5. Bilateral multiple renal angiomyolipomas
6. Subependymal glial nodules on CT/MRI

Minor criteria:

1. Atypical shagreen patch
2. Hypomelanocytic macules
3. Gingival fibromas
4. Bilateral polycystic kidneys
5. Single renal angiomyolipoma
6. Cardiac rhabdomyoma
7. Histological evidence of a cortical tuber
8. Honeycomb lung on X-ray
9. Infantile spasms
10. Forehead fibrous plaques
11. Giant cell astrocytoma
12. A first-degree relative with tuberous sclerosis

If headaches or focal neurological signs develop, CT or MRI scanning of the head is advisable. This may identify cortical tubers or tumours. If a symptomatic cerebral tumour is identified, the best plan of management is to debulk the tumour and follow up by serial MRI scanning annually or if new neurological symptoms develop. The place of radiation therapy is uncertain. Radiation can reduce the size of these tumours but, because of the excellent long-term survival and the frequency of late radiation-induced side-effects, such as radiation-induced dementia and leucoencephalopathy, the optimal time for radiation therapy remains uncertain. Occasionally anaplastic variants can occur and in this situation early radiation therapy is probably advisable. Close monitoring of renal function in tuberous sclerosis is advisable as chronic renal insufficiency is a cause of morbidity and mortality.

Families should have access to genetic counselling and genetic testing for *TSC1* and TSC2. Genetic counselling includes explanation of the risk of a disorder being inherited, the consequences of that risk, the probability of developing or transmitting the disease, and the ways in which transmission can be prevented. Parents and other family members should be examined clinically, including examination under Wood's light (ultraviolet light) and ophthalmoscopic examination of the eyes for retinal phakomas. Chest radiography, CT or MRI brain scan, and renal ultrasound should also be performed. CT scans of parents and sibs of apparently sporadic cases will sometimes demonstrate asymptomatic cortical tubers. Even mildly affected parents can have severely affected children. Once any genetic tests or investigative tests have been performed, further counselling about the results is usually necessary.

19.1.6 Prognosis and complications of treatment

Severe infantile spasms and other severe forms of epilepsy have a poor prognosis because this is usually a sign of severe brain disease and treatment of the seizures is frequently ineffective and status epilepticus is common. There is a high mortality rate in infants with infantile spasms, either due to the seizures or as a result of complications occurring during treatment for status. In the absence of severe epilepsy and significant cognitive impairment, prognosis is good, with most patients having a normal life span. If cerebral tumours develop, these are slow growing and have an excellent prognosis if complete removal can be performed. In most cases, however, partial resection is all that is possible and the median survival is approximately 10–20 years (Nagib *et al.* 1984). Adenoma sebaceum can be treated with laser therapy.

19.1.7 Recovery and rehabilitation

Children will require a great deal of medical support when epilepsy is prominent, and school or learning support during periods when seizures are quiescent. Advice regarding anticonvulsant medication and pastimes to avoid should be openly discussed with the patient and family members. Counselling and support helps re-integration into school and society (Curatolo 1996).

19.2 Neurofibromatosis

19.2.1 Introduction and classification

The neurofibromatoses (NFs) are autosomal dominant neurocutaneous disorders that can be divided into 'peripheral' and 'central' types, although there is significant overlap. The most common type of neurofibromatosis is NF1 (von Recklinghausen's disease or 'peripheral' neurofibromatosis). Less commonly one encounters NF2 ('bilateral acoustic neuromas' or 'central' neurofibromatosis) or a localized form of the disease ('segmental neurofibromatosis') (Miller and Sparks 1977). Segmental neurofibromatosis is characterized by localized cutaneous neurofibromas and café-au-lait spots limited to one segment of the body, but which can include underlying intrathoracic or intra-abdominal neurofibromas.

Diagnostic criteria for NF1 have been developed by the Neurofibromatosis National Institutes of Health Consensus Conference (Table 19.2) (National Institutes of Health Consensus Development Conference 1988). Although not specifically mentioned in this diagnostic categorization, it is well recognized that 100 per cent of patients with NF1 will develop Lisch nodules in the iris. A grading system has also been devised for neurofibromatosis type 1 (Table 19.3)

Table 19.2. Diagnostic criteria for Neurofibromatosis type 1 (from National Institutes of Health Consensus Development Conference (1988). Neurofibromatosis conference statement. *Arch. Neurol.*, **45**, 575–8)

Two or more of:

1. Six or more café-au-lait macules measuring ⟶5 mm in greatest diameter in prepubertal individuals and ⟶15 mm in greatest diameter in post-pubertal individuals
2. Axillary or inguinal freckling
3. Two or more dermal neurofibromas
4. A plexiform neurofibroma
5. A first-degree relative with NF1 (by the NIH consensus statement criteria)
6. Optic nerve glioma
7. Two or more Lisch nodules
8. A distinctive osseous lesion (e.g. sphenoid dysplasia or thinning of the long bone cortex)
    (a) with or without pseudoarthrosis

(Riccardi and Kleiner 1977). Neurofibromatosis type 2 (NF2) is also known as 'bilateral acoustic neurofibromatosis' or 'central neurofibromatosis', because of the predisposition to develop tumours of the nervous system. Diagnostic criteria for NF2 are: bilateral acoustic neuromas; or a first-degree relative with NF2 and either a unilateral acoustic neuroma, neurofibroma, glioma, meningioma, schwannoma, or early onset lens opacity. The severity of phenotypes can be defined by age of onset of symptoms (<20 years versus >20 years), number of associated intracranial tumours (<2 tumours versus >2 tumours), and whether spinal tumours are present or absent (Evans *et al.* 1992*a*; Parry *et al.* 1994).

Table 19.3. Grading system for neurofibromatosis type 1

Grade 1	Minimal	Café-au-lait spots only, or with unobtrusive cutaneous neurofibromas
Grade 2	Mild	Numerous neurocutaneous neurofibromas but without facial disfigurement; small plexiform neurofibromas with no associated problems; asymptomatic osseous lesions; learning difficulties with normal IQ
Grade 3	Moderate	Numerous neurocutaneous neurofibromas with facial disfigurement; plexiform neurofibromas with modest localized hypertrophy; visceral neurofibromas; mild retardation; scoliosis or pseudoarthrosis requiring surgery; controlled epilepsy
Grade 4	Severe	Disease complications leading to major health impairment, often requiring surgical intervention; for example, large plexiform neurofibromas with severe secondary problems, CNS tumours, malignancy, aqueduct stenosis, severe mental retardation, phaeochromocytoma, and renal artery stenosis

19.2.2 Incidence and prevalence

Neurofibromatosis affects all races and has an estimated frequency of approximately 1 in 3000 of live births and a mutation rate of 1×10^4 per gamete per generation (Crowe *et al.* 1956). The point prevalence of NF1 is at least 1 in 4950 ($20.2/10^5$) and NF1 accounts for 90 per cent of cases of NF (Huson *et al.* 1989*a*). The incidence and prevalence of NF2 is uncertain, but is thought to occur in approximately 1 in 40 000 live births (Evans *et al.* 1992*b*; NIH Consensus Statement 1991).

19.2.3 Genetic factors

Neurofibromatosis type 1 is an autosomal dominant condition, but about 50 per cent of all cases are new mutations. The gene for NF1 (von Recklinghausen's disease) was isolated in 1991 and is situated on chromosome 17 (17q11.2). The NF1 gene spans over 350 kb of genomic DNA and encodes a protein of 2818 amino acids ('neurofibromin'). One role of neurofibromin is as a GTPase activating protein (GAP), probably in the same pathway of signal transduction as *ras* proto-oncogene and involved in the regulation of cell growth. It is likely that neurofibromin is important in the formation of neurofibrosarcomas (von Deimling *et al.* 1995). It is very likely that tumorigenesis in NF1 is a multistep phenomenon, with the 'second hit' in the NF1 gene as the initiating event.

Both the NF1 and NF2 genes have a high penetrance, which is virtually 100 per cent by the age of 5 years. There is no evidence of locus heterogeneity within NF1 families, therefore tightly linked polymorphic markers can help determine the risk of a child aged less than 5 years developing NF1 in the presence of equivocal clinical signs (Goldgar *et al.* 1989). Where the mother has NF1, offspring are more likely to be severely affected, but there does not appear to be a definite parental-age effect or birth-order effect (Huson *et al.* 1989*b*).

The NF2 tumour suppressor gene is on chromosome 22q12 and encodes for a protein ('merlin' or 'schwannomin') of the 4.1 family of cytoskeletal-associated proteins, which may link the cytoskeleton and cell membrane. Most NF2 alterations result in a truncated, inactivated merlin protein. Specific NF2 mutations do not always correlate with phenotypic severity but, in general, mutations that lead to premature termination of translation are associated with more aggressive disease. Most of the tumours associated with NF2 are benign (e.g. schwannomas, meningiomas, ependymomas). These tumours also occur sporadically in the general population. In sporadic cases of acoustic neuroma and some cases of meningioma NF2, there are also aberrations at the NF2 locus, strongly suggesting that there is a tumour suppressor gene at this site. DNA-based diagnostic testing is now available for neurofibromatosis. Presymptomatic diagnosis is possible in multigeneration NF2 families using tightly linked DNA markers and mutational analysis (Bijlsma *et al.* 1995). In at-risk individuals who do not carry the NF2 mutation, DNA testing can exclude the condition and prevent needless clinical investigations (Baser *et al.* 1996). The NF2 gene is a tumour suppressor gene, and mutation studies have demonstrated that the NF2 gene is also mutated in sporadic acoustic neuromas and meningiomas (Kley and Seizinger 1995).

19.2.4 Clinical features and imaging diagnosis

Neurofibromatosis type 1

The characteristic features of NF1 are café-au-lait spots, neurofibromas (Fig. 19.3), Lisch nodules, osseous lesions, macrocephaly, short stature and mental retardation, axillary freckling, and can be associated with several different types of tumours. Café-au-lait spots tend to increase in number and size in the first and second decades. Two spots or more occur in only 0.75 per cent of normal children under the age of 5 years, but the presence of five spots with a diameter greater than 0.5 cm is suggestive of the diagnosis of NF1. Nearly all children with NF1 have developed café-au-lait spots by the age of 5 years (Huson 1994) Children of patients with NF1 should be examined annually for cutaneous signs of NF1. If by age 5 years there are no apparent signs, follow-up can be discontinued. In children below 5 years of age with equivocal signs, where confirmation is sought of whether the child is either unaffected or affected, and where there are two or more affected family members are available for study, intragenic polymorphic markers can be used to determine the risks of disease. In adults, the presence of six café-au-lait spots larger than 1.5 cm is almost always abnormal. Freckling in the axilla, groin, under the breasts, and on the neck is also a helpful associated sign of NF1, as are cutaneous or subcutaneous neurofibromas. Cutaneous neurofibromas are soft, violet-coloured lesions, varying from 0.1 cm to several centimetres in diameter. Subcutaneous neurofibromas commonly appear after the age of six and are present in all affected cases by age 17. They are firm nodules in the distribution of the trunks

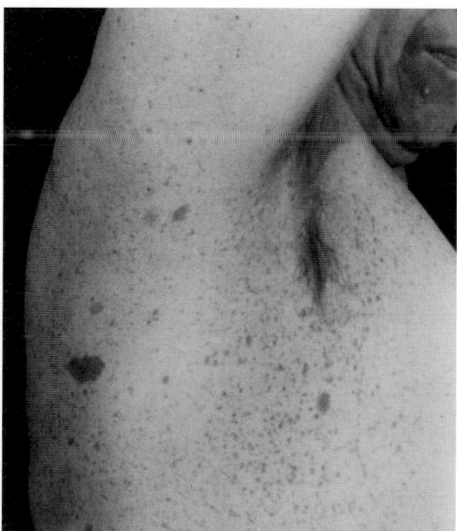

Fig. 19.3. Café-au-lait macules, axillary freckling, and neurofibromas in NF type 1.

of peripheral nerves. They increase in number and size, especially during pregnancy or with use of the oral contraceptive pill. Lisch nodules are melanocytic hamartomas of the iris (brown nodules), which develop in early childhood and are seen by slit-lamp examination in 93–100 per cent of patients with NF1 by the age of 20 years (Huson *et al.* 1989a; Lubs *et al.* 1991).

Plexiform schwannomas are benign peripheral nerve sheath tumours that generally arise in the dermis or subcutaneous tissues (Section 13.5.1). They may be single or multiple, focal or diffuse. Plexiform neurofibromas of the eyelid are frequently associated with glaucoma. Malignant schwannomas occur in almost 30 per cent of patients, and sarcomatous degeneration in neurofibromas occurs in 1–5 per cent of patients (Brasfield and Das Gupta 1972; Huson *et al.* 1988). Sudden enlargement of plexiform neurofibromas or the occurrence of pain should lead to urgent investigation for evidence of malignant peripheral nerve sheath tumour. Complete resection of complex lesions is frequently not possible, and treatment by an interdisciplinary team, including oncologists, surgeons and paediatricians, is probably desirable (Gutman *et al.* 1997).

It has been suggested that there is a fourfold increase in relative risk of cerebral tumours (Sorensen *et al.* 1986). Intracerebral tumours occur in 1.5–8 per cent of cases of NF1 (Brasfield and Das Gupta 1972; Huson *et al.* 1989b). These are commonly optic nerve or brainstem gliomas or gliosarcomas. Optic nerve glioma associated with neurofibromatosis accounts for almost 10 per cent of all patients with optic nerve gliomas, and approximately 1.5 per cent of patients with NF1 will develop an optic nerve glioma. These tumours are commonly bilateral or involve the optic chiasm (Font and Ferry 1972; Listernick *et al.* 1989). Occasionally, optic nerve gliomas extend into the hypothalamus and cause precocious puberty. Optic nerve gliomas are commonly low grade and may not progress for many years (Listernick *et al.* 1994). There appears to be an association between plexiform eyelid neurofibromas and optic nerve glioma. There is also a high frequency of second malignancies (40 per cent of patients).

The frequency of aqueduct stenosis is increased in NF1 (Senveli *et al.* 1989). Ventriculo-peritoneal shunting or ventriculo-atrial shunting should only be contemplated in symptomatic patients (Spadero 1986). Up to 40 per cent of patients with NF1 have mild learning difficulties and 6–10 per cent have epilepsy, which may be associated with minor abnormalities such as gliosis, neuronal heterotopia, and ependymal overgrowth (Carey *et al.* 1979; Riccardi 1981). Children should be tested to detect any learning difficulty prior to school entry. Neurocognitive deficits may be subtle (Eldridge *et al.* 1989). Bony anomalies, such as scoliosis, bone cysts, bone hypertrophy, or skull and facial deformities, occur in 40–60 per cent of patients with NF1. Orthopaedic complications such as scoliosis and pseudoarthrosis of the tibia or fibula occur in about 9 per cent of patients (Akbarnia *et al.* 1992). Gastrointestinal neurofibromas are usually asymptomatic but can cause abdominal pain. Renal hypertension occurs in 1.5 per

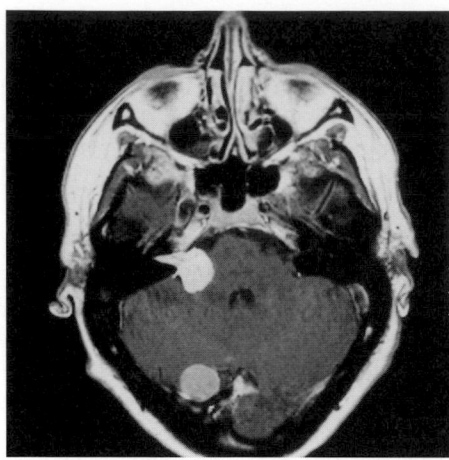

Fig. 19.4. MRI brain scan demonstrating an acoustic neuroma anteriorly and meningioma abutting the cerebellum posteriorly in a patient with NF type 2.

cent of affected individuals, sometimes as a result of renal artery stenosis. Phaeochromocytoma affects less than 1 per cent of all cases (Huson 1994). Screening non-hypertensive patients for phaeochromocytoma is not cost effective (Riccardi and Eichner 1986).

MRI with gadolinium enhancement is the investigation of choice because it provides better soft-tissue contrast. In NF1, optic nerve gliomas, astrocytomas, plexiform neurofibromas, and 'unidentified bright objects' may only be identified by MR. Prenatal risk assessment is only possible in NF1 families if two or more suitable family members are available for blood donation, for study of intragenic polymorphic markers. There is usually no increased risk during pregnancy, but if there is significant kyphoscoliosis labour can be difficult and, rarely, there may be pelvic neurofibromas that can obstruct labour.

Neurofibromatosis type 2

In NF2 typical tumours are benign schwannomas of the vestibular portion of the acoustic nerves (Fig. 19.4), although meningiomas frequently coexist. Ninety-five per cent of patients with an acoustic neuroma do not have NF2. Most commonly, patients with NF2 have few or no cutaneous manifestations of neurofibromatosis; however, café-au-lait spots, axillary freckling, and subcutaneous neurofibromas do rarely occur. Multiple cutaneous plexiform schwannomas can also occur occasionally in NF2. There may be a family history of acoustic neuroma. More than 95 per cent of people with the NF2 gene develop bilateral vestibular nerve tumours. Presentation is generally with deafness or tinnitus (Sections 9.3.6 and 9.7.5), although headache, vertigo, or unsteadiness related to cerebellar involvement can occur. The characteristic hearing-loss pattern is sensorineural hearing loss with impairment of speech discrimination more so than pure tone loss. There is delayed conduction on brainstem auditory evoked potentials. Bilateral acoustic neuromas of NF2 are likely to be identified earlier by MRI than by CT. Most tumours are hypointense (66 per cent) or isointense (33 per cent) with brain on T1-weighted images. All enhance with

gadolinium, either homogeneously (66 per cent) or patchily (33 per cent). The coexistence of NF and tuberous sclerosis or von Hippel–Lindau disease is well recognized.

19.2.5 **Management**

Neurofibromatosis type 1

Assessment of new patients with NF1 should include: general physical examination for evidence of spinal deformity or any painful neurofibromas, neuropsychological assessment in children to look for IQ or mild cognitive impairment, and examination of the eye for Lisch nodules (slit-lamp examination if necessary). Although CNS tumours, aqueduct stenosis, and high-signal lesions on T2-weighted MRI scans are more commonly found in patients with NF1, MRI brain scans are not justified in the absence of symptoms or signs. MRI is the most useful diagnostic investigation in patients with cognitive or focal symptoms. High-signal areas on T2-weighted MRI scans are common in neurofibromatosis type 1 (approximately 50 per cent) but are of no direct relevance in the absence of cognitive or focal symptoms or signs (Duffner *et al.* 1989; Sevick *et al.* 1992). MRI of the brain should include orbits and optic nerves if there is any visual field defect, new visual acuity problem, cognitive problem, or focal neurological signs suggestive of an intracranial cause. If asymptomatic lesions are identified, it would seem reasonable to follow up these patients clinically and by MRI, and to intervene by biopsy or radiation only if there is clinical or radiological progression. Symptomatic lesions should at least be biopsied to confirm diagnosis and determine the grade. It is uncertain whether radical resection followed by radiation therapy is superior to biopsy and radiation. Optic nerve gliomas virtually never develop after age 30.

Appropriate neurological imaging of any symptomatic peripheral neurofibromas should be performed. If hypertension is found, a renal cause or phaeochromocytoma should be actively sought. Measurement of catecholamines or catecholamine derivatives in a 24-hour urine collection and renal imaging should be performed. Surgery for phaeochromocytoma offers a good chance of cure of the hypertension and the tumour (Ferner 1994).

Children with abnormal angulation of the long bones should be referred to an interested orthopaedic surgeon for further investigation and management (Morrissy 1982). Patients should be examined for evidence of spinal deformity at follow-up visits, particularly during the adolescent growth spurt. If there is evidence of spinal deformity, specialist orthopaedic follow-up is desirable. However, spinal surgery is not without its complications (Crawford 1989).

Although CNS tumours, aqueduct stenosis, and high-signal lesions on T2-weighted MRI scans are more commonly found in patients with NF1, MRI brain scans are not justified in the absence of symptoms or signs. MRI is the most useful diagnostic investigation in patients with cognitive or focal symptoms. High-signal areas on T2-weighted MRI scans are common in neurofibromatosis type 1 (approximately 50 per cent) but are of no direct relevance in the absence of cognitive or focal symptoms or signs. (Duffner *et al.* 1989; Sevick *et al.* 1992). It is advisable that patients with NF1 have regular ophthalmological assessment as part of their annual paediatric assessment with particular attention paid to any visual field defects (which are commonly asymptomatic). If there is a history of deterioration of visual acuity, or any visual field or visual acuity abnormality is found by examination, a cranial MRI scan with optic nerve views is indicated.

Neurofibromatosis type 2

The defining feature of NF2 is bilateral vestibular schwannomas (acoustic neuromas). A treatment algorithm has been suggested, based on age, hearing status, tumour size, and symptoms (Silverstein *et al.* 1993). There would be a place for considering screening sibs and offspring of patients with acoustic neuroma. This could be done clinically and by audiometry. If there are any signs to suggest NF2, then MRI would be the most sensitive investigation. Increasingly, small asymptomatic acoustic neuromas are being identified. It is uncertain what the best form of management is, and some centres favour a wait-and-see approach, while others advise early stereotactic radiosurgery or even neurosurgery. Treatment options are as for sporadic acoustic neuroma (Chapter 18).

19.2.6 Prognosis and complications of treatment

Malignant neoplasms or benign central nervous system tumours occur in 45 per cent of probands. This provides a relative risk of 4.0 (95 per cent confidence intervals, 2.8–5.6) compared with expected. The prognosis in patients with tumours affecting the nervous system depends on the age of the patient, the type of tumour, the site of the tumour, and the level of disability at the time of presentation. The complication rate from treatment of these tumours appears to be no higher than in patients with these tumours but without neurofibromatosis. Epilepsy is well controlled with medication in approximately 50–70 per cent of patients.

Hypertension will increase the risk of cerebrovascular disease and there is possibly a higher incidence of cerebral aneurysm and stenosis of intracranial major arteries. Scoliosis and thoracic neurofibromas may lead to thoracic pain, chest infections, and reduced lung volumes. Hydronephrosis due to neurofibromas can lead to renal failure and abdominal pain.

19.2.7 Recovery and rehabilitation

In general, the follow-up of patients with neurofibromatosis should be co-ordinated by one interested clinician. Annual follow-up is recommended, with regular blood pressure measurement and physical, cognitive, and ophthalmological evaluation. Neuropsychological assessment should be performed prior to school entry and perhaps every 3–4 years until 12 years of age, to detect subtle learning difficulties and to allow early

educational support, if appropriate. Physiotherapy, pain relief, and psychological support are important, particularly in the early postoperative stages. Cosmetic advice and, very occasionally, cosmetic surgery may be necessary. However, over medicalization can be psychologically damaging, by increasing anxiety, and, where possible, should be avoided.

19.3 Sturge–Weber syndrome

Sturge–Weber syndrome involves a characteristic 'port-wine' facial naevus or angioma associated with an underlying leptomeningeal angioma or other vascular anomaly. There can be seizures, low IQ, and underlying cerebral hemisphere atrophy, as a result of a chronic state of reduced perfusion and increased oxygen extraction. Patients may present with focal seizures, which are generally resistant to anticonvulsant medication, and can develop glaucoma. Ninety-eight per cent of people with Sturge–Weber syndrome have a cranial port-wine naevus, and 52 per cent have extracranial involvement. At least 60 per cent of patients will develop glaucoma; 83 per cent, seizures; and 65 per cent have neurological difficulties. Seizures usually start in the first two decades; over 40 per cent of these patients will have developmental delay and up to 85 per cent will have emotional and behavioural problems. In cases without epilepsy, developmental delay is rare and behavioural problems are less common (58 per cent). MRI with gadolinium enhancement is more sensitive than CT, and the characteristic features are leptomeningeal angiomatosis, hemiatrophy, cortical calcification and patchy parenchymal gliosis, and demyelination (Adamsbaum *et al.* 1996). Figure 19.5 demonstrates an angiomatous malformation with enlarged draining vein between the

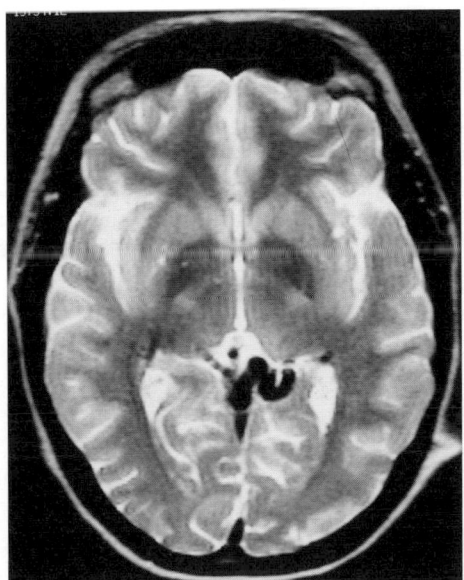

Fig. 19.5. MRI T2-weighted axial image demonstrating an angiomatous malformation with an enlarged draining vein between the cerebral hemispheres, extending posteriorly to the occipital horn of the lateral ventricle.

cerebral hemispheres, extending posteriorly to the occipital horn of the lateral ventricle.

19.4 Von Hippel–Lindau disease

Von Hippel–Lindau disease is one of the most common autosomal dominant inherited genetic diseases that cause familial cancers, and is characterized by certain types of central nervous system tumours (cerebellar and spinal haemangioblastomas and retinal angiomas), in conjunction with bilateral renal carcinomas and phaechromocytoma (Neumann and Wiestler 1991). The prevalence is approximately 1 in 40 000. Von Hippel described angiomas of the retina in 1904 and Lindau described cerebellar and spine angiomas in 1926.

Von Hippel–Lindau (VHL) disease is caused by loss of a tumour suppressor gene situated on the short arm of chromosome 3 (3p25–26) proximal to the locus for the *RAF-1* oncogene (Seizinger *et al.* 1988). The gene for von Hippel–Lindau disease has been cloned (Latif *et al.* 1993). Tumour suppressor genes work on the 'two-hit' hypothesis, that tumours will only develop after both copies of the VHL gene are damaged. In families with VHL, one damaged gene has been inherited. So far more than 140 different mutations have been identified in the VHL gene. The second 'hit' to the allele with the normally functioning gene can occur anytime during life. Recent mutation studies have demonstrated that the tumour suppressor genes are also mutated in the more common sporadic haemangioblastoma and renal carcinoma (Gnarra *et al.* 1994; Kanno *et al.* 1994). Mutations are identified in approximately 80 per cent of VHL families. Certain mutations seem to be predictive for the development of phaeochromocytoma (especially 505 point mutations). Deactivation of the VHL gene seems to be associated with an increase in vascular endothelial growth factor (VEGF), which in turn stimulates new blood vessel formation (angiogenesis). Increased levels of VEGF are found in the vitreal fluid and in renal cysts in patients with von Hippel–Lindau disease. In addition, there are high concentrations of vascular endothelial growth factor receptors and VEGF in haemangioblastomas. Retinal angiomas are histologically similar to cerebellar haemangioblastomas except that they do not have cysts. Haemangioblastomas are benign tumours composed of endothelial cells, pericytes, and stromal cells.

Patients with VHL are at risk of retinal haemangioblastomas (angiomas) (57 per cent), central nervous system haemangioblastomas, renal cell carcinoma (23 per cent), phaeochromocytomas (19 per cent), or simple cysts of the kidney, pancreas liver, etc. Retinal angiomas (haemangioblastomas) occur in one-quarter to one-half of patients, and are bilateral in one-third of patients with retinal haemangioblastoma. Retinal haemangioblastomas can cause progressive unilateral or bilateral blindness, from glaucoma, haemorrhage, retinal detachment, or sympathetic ophthalmitis. Symptoms and signs can occur in infancy or in late life. On ophthalmoscopy haemangioblastomas appear as red masses of any size, fed by dilated tortuous arteries. Central nervous system haemangioblastomas can occur in the cerebellum (54 per cent), brainstem (20 per cent), spinal cord (15 per cent), or, rarely, in the cerebrum. Haemangioblastomas account for 1–2.5 per cent of all intracranial tumours and 10 per cent of posterior fossa tumours in children. Central nervous system haemangioblastomas may be multiple and imaging of the whole of the CNS is recommended. Approximately 30–40 per cent of patients with haemangioblastoma have VHL, while the remainder have sporadic haemangioblastoma. However, the likelihood of haemangioblastoma being associated with VHL approaches 50–60 per cent if diagnosis is made in children or young adults (<30 years of age) and where the haemangioblastoma is of the spinal cord (>80 per cent associated with VHL). These tumours are commonly associated with secondary polycythaemia due to secretion of erythropoietin by the tumour.

Renal lesions are frequently asymptomatic, but may present with haematuria, fever, or pain. Renal carcinoma will develop in 20–25 per cent of patients. Pancreatic lesions can cause abdominal pain and may be associated with diabetes mellitus. Phaeochromocytomas are associated with cerebellar haemangioblastomas and may be unilateral or bilateral. They usually are associated with systemic hypertension.

Diagnostic criteria for VHL are:

(1) evidence of more than one haemangioblastoma in the central nervous system or retina;

(2) two types of tumours commonly found in VHL in the same patient (e.g. cerebellar haemangioblastoma and renal carcinoma); or

(3) a typical tumour related to VHL and a family history of VHL.

Indirect ophthalmoscopy and fluorescein angiography can detect lesions before they are symptomatic. Cerebellar tumours are usually well defined, with a cystic or multiloculated component with a mural nodule, and the wall enhances with contrast on cranial CT or MRI. Magnetic resonance imaging is the best technique to examine the posterior fossa and the spine. Spinal and cerebellar tumours are commonly solid and enhance with contrast. Renal, adrenal, and pancreatic lesions are best identified by MRI of the abdomen. Urinary catecholamines and metadrenaline are elevated in phaeochromocytoma. Cerebellar haemangioblastomas may resemble renal clear-cell metastasis on histology. The diagnosis is usually clarified by immunohistochemical studies which are positive for epithelial membrane antigen in renal cell carcinoma and negative in haemangioblastoma (neuron-specific enolase and GFAP positive).

DNA-based diagnostic testing is now available for von Hippel–Lindau disease in cases where there is diagnostic doubt or in cases where early presymptomatic diagnosis is desired in VHL families (Kley *et al.* 1995). There is an ethical debate at present about the timing of DNA testing. Some favour DNA testing of patients before the age of 5 years, since symptomatic disease (especially retinal angiomas) may start occurring around that age. Others favour regular screening of patients from the age of 5 years, but to wait until the patient has reached the age of legal consent before offering the test. Genetic counselling should be performed prior to DNA testing in patients with possible VHL or asymptomatic family members. This is best done by a trained counsellor.

Following the diagnosis it is important to screen the patient for other associated tumours and to counsel and screen the family members who are at risk. Mutations are detected in approximately 80 per cent of VHL families. Family members who are not gene carriers on DNA testing can be discharged from regular follow-up. In families where the mutation is not detected, genetic linkage studies can be used to predict carrier status in many cases. Screening of patients and at-risk relatives includes

(1) annual clinical assessment, including indirect ophthalmoscopy, from the age of 5 years (with fluorescein angiography if there are any suspicious areas);

(2) annual urinary metadrenaline from the age of 10 years;

(3) biennial cranial imaging (MRI ideally) from the age of 15 years; and

(4) biennial abdominal scanning (CT or MRI) to examine, adrenals, kidneys, and pancreas.

The identification of an intracranial haemangioblastoma should stimulate the search for spinal haemangioblastomas, even in patients without spinal symptoms. Before surgery is contemplated in patients with possible haemangioblastoma, blood and urine tests to exclude a phaeochromocytoma, and abdominal CT or MRI scanning to look for renal or adrenal tumours or cysts, should be performed.

Prognosis depends on the site and size of the haemangioblastomas or other associated tumours. Peripheral lesions in patients with retinal haemangioblastoma will usually be treated at an early stage by photocoagulation or cryotherapy (Annesley *et al.* 1977). Small lesions may be best treated with argon laser. Larger lesions, greater than one optic disc diameter, will respond to a combination of cryotherapy and photocoagulation with xenon arc or argon laser. Angiomas in the central part of vision are difficult to treat, since the tareatment itself can cause some surrounding damage.

Surgical intervention for haemangioblastoma involving the central nervous system is not usually advisable for lesions less than 3 cm in diameter. Tumours of the brainstem and spinal cord carry a high postoperative morbidity from haemorrhage. Haemangiomas of the cerebellum are more easily accessible, and sometimes preoperative embolization can reduce the risk of haemorrhage. Operations on cystic cerebellar lesions appear to have fewer complications than operations on solid lesions (Lamiell *et al.* 1989). Complete resection of the haemangioblastoma can be curative; however, recurrences or new tumours are common.

Renal tumours in VHL grow at a slower rate and are less aggressive than those with sporadic renal small cell carcinoma. Most surgeons practice renal-sparing surgery because there is a very high chance that further tumours will develop in the same kidney or the opposite kidney at a later date. It is uncertain when surgery for renal carcinoma should be carried out. Some

favour operating only when the tumour reaches approximately 4 cm in diameter, while others support early intervention when the tumour is only 2–3 cm in diameter. The difficulty is that metastases are more likely to occur with larger tumours. Most surgeons do not operate for simple renal cysts.

Phaeochromocytomas should be resected when diagnosed.

19.5 Ataxia telangiectasia

Ataxia telangiectasia is an autosomal recessive trait in which affected individuals have a progressive cerebellar ataxia, oculocutaneous telangiectasia, radiosensitivity, predisposition to lymphoid malignancies, and immunodeficiency (Shiloh and Rotman 1996).

The gene is on chromosome 11 (11q22–q23) and has been cloned (ataxia telangiectasia mutated gene, *ATM*). The defective gene encodes an enzyme (very like phosphoinositol 3-kinase) which is responsible for repair of DNA damage and cell control. About 1 per cent of the population are heterozygotes for this gene, and have a two- to sixfold greater risk of developing cancer (Morrell *et al.* 1990; Swift *et al.* 1991). Homozygotes are 100 times more likely to develop cancer than age-matched controls (Morrell *et al.* 1990). The ataxia telangiectasia gene is associated with a sensitivity to ionizing radiation and homozygotes can develop tissue necrosis when exposed to conventional therapeutic doses of radiation. It is thought that diagnostic or occupational exposure to radiation increases the risk of cancer in these individuals.

Ataxia telangiectasia is the common cause of progressive ataxia in childhood, and usually manifests itself by the age of 3 years, when most cases have some element of truncal ataxia (Section 31.5.1). By the teens sufferers are significantly ataxic and may have developed choreo-athetosis, facial hypokinesia, and sialorrhoea, and are usually wheelchair bound. Reflexes are usually reduced or lost by the late teens and there may be some large-fibre neuropathy and spinal muscular atrophy. Telangiectasia may not appear until adolescence, and are found in the conjunctiva, nose, ears, neck, and antecubital fossae. Other skin changes such as hypopigmentation or hyperpigmentation and premature greying of hair are commonly found. There is commonly an ocular dyspraxia, with nystagmus and frequent blinking. There is an increased incidence of sinus infections and respiratory infections, with bronchiectasis and lung abscesses related to deficiencies in serum immunoglobulins (especially IgA). Hypogonadism, growth failure with normal growth hormone levels, and diabetes mellitus, which may be insulin resistant, also occur (Woods and Taylor 1992).

Diagnosis is usually evident on clinical grounds, although the telangiectasias may appear after the ataxia has been present for some time. Serum α-fetoprotein is increased in 90 per cent and some patients also have elevated carcinoembryonic antigen (Woods and Taylor 1992). Serum immunoglobulins (IgA, IgE, IgG2) are decreased or absent, while IgM is normal or elevated. Genetic linkage studies may be helpful if many family members are available.

Management involves treatment of intercurrent infections with physiotherapy and antibiotics and being aware that, if cancers are found, conventional doses of radiation will be highly toxic and are contraindicated. Vaccination with live virus vaccines are also to be avoided (Pohl *et al.* 1992).

19.6 Other neurocutaneous syndromes

19.6.1 Hypomelanosis of Ito

Hypomelanosis of Ito (synonym: incontinentia pigmenti achromians) is a rare, sporadic, multisystem disorder, but is the third most common neurocutaneous syndrome after neurofibromatosis type 1 and tuberous sclerosis. About 50 per cent of

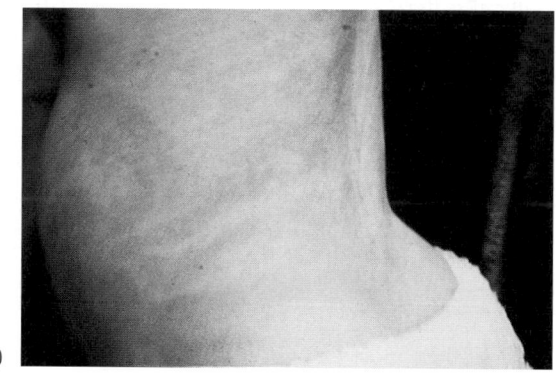

(a)

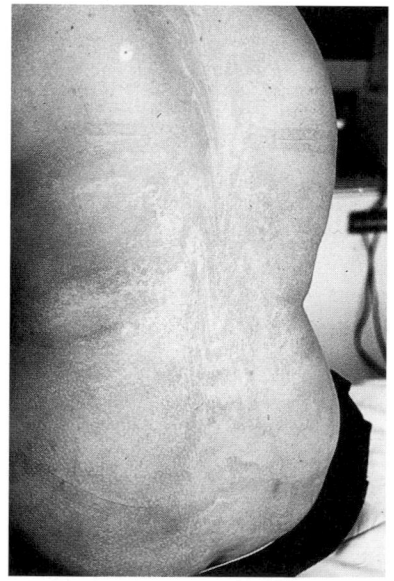

(b)

Fig. 19.6. (a) Hypopigmented streaks in the skin of the back along the lines of Blaschko; (b) depigmented streaks or whorls in the skin of the back, along the lines of Blaschko (courtesy of Professor D, Donnai, Regional Genetic Service, St Mary's Hospital, Manchester).

patients show chromosomal abnormalities, most commonly mosaicisms or translocations, but also trisomies, translocations, and point mutations (Sybert 1994). In families where there are sufficient numbers of affected individuals, genetic linkage analysis may be possible, using markers from the Xq28 region of the X chromosome (Jouet *et al.* 1997).

The term has been used to describe a condition where there are hypopigmented or depigmented streaks or whorls in the skin along the lines of Blaschko (Fig. 19.6a, b). The skin changes are present within the first year of life in 70 per cent of cases and the hypopigmented areas in Caucasians are best seen using Wood's light. The extent of skin changes does not correlate with the severity of the systemic disease. Over 50 per cent of patients have neurological, skeletal, or ocular abnormalities. The neurological problems are due to cerebral and cerebellar developmental abnormalities, arteriovenous malformations, or tumours (e.g. choroid plexus papilloma, medulloblastoma). The most frequent neurological abnormalities are mental retardation and seizures, thought to be related to neuroblast migrational disorders. Oral abnormalities include dental dysplasia and conical teeth. Alopecia and changes in hair colour (grey-white hair) may appear prematurely.

Diagnosis rests on possible genetic linkage analysis of the blood, or karyotyping of blood and affected skin may detect mosaicism (frequently X:autosomal translocation) (Boon *et al.* 1996), and the recognition of skin, nervous system, musculoskeletal, and other anomalies. EEG and MRI findings are common but non-specific. MRI abnormalities can occur in the absence of neurological signs (Steiner *et al.* 1996).

Management is symptomatic: anticonvulsants for seizures, perhaps steroids for infantile spasms, physiotherapy for motor difficulties, educational support for those with learning difficulties, and specialist opinion for ocular, dental, and skeletal problems. First-degree relative should be examined and genetic counselling offered to appropriate family members

19.6.2 Gorlin syndrome

Gorlin syndrome (naevoid basal cell carcinoma syndrome) is a rare autosomal dominant disorder characterized by multiple naevoid basal cell carcinomas (Fig. 19.7), odontogenic keratocysts of the mandible, anomalies of the eye, skeleton, and reproductive system, and medulloblastomas and other neoplasms. Patients usually present with characteristic skin lesions and seizures in childhood. The diagnostic criteria are the presence of two major, or one major and one minor, criteria from the following:

(1) major criteria: more than two basal cell carcinomas in someone under the age of 30 years, odontogenic keratocyst, palmar pits, falx calcification, positive family history;

(2) minor criteria: rib or vertebral abnormalities, macrocrania, fibroma, medulloblastoma, lymphomesenteric cysts.

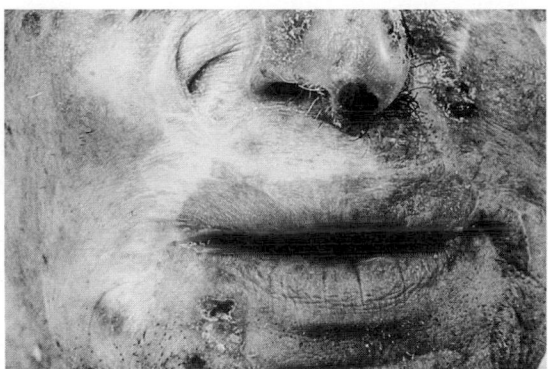

Fig. 19.7. Multiple facial naevoid basal cell carcinomas (courtesy of Professor D. Donnai, Regional Genetic Service, St Mary's Hospital, Manchester).

19.6.3 Sjögren–Larsson syndrome

Sjögren–Larsson syndrome is an autosomal recessive disorder, mapped to chromosome 17p. The condition is associated with deficiency of fatty aldehyde dehydrogenase (De Laurenzi *et al.* 1996), an enzyme involved in long-chain fatty alcohol oxidation. The cDNA encoding this enzyme has been cloned and several different mutations have been found (Lacour 1996). The clinical manifestations of this deficiency are: congenital ichthyosis, mental retardation, speech abnormalities, and spasticity. The skin condition is present in infancy as red, scaly skin which becomes thickened and darker as the sufferer grows older. Half of the children have a degeneration of the pigment of the retina. MRI frequently shows deep white matter changes.

19.6.4 Proteus syndrome

Proteus syndrome (multiple hamartomas) is a condition where there is partial, usually asymmetrical, enlargement of the hands (Fig. 19.8) or feet, hemiatrophy on one side of the face body or limbs, pigmented naevi, tumours (lipomas, lymphangiomas), skull abnormalities (e.g. cranial exostosis, exostosis of the external auditory meatus and nasal bridge, macrocephaly or asym-

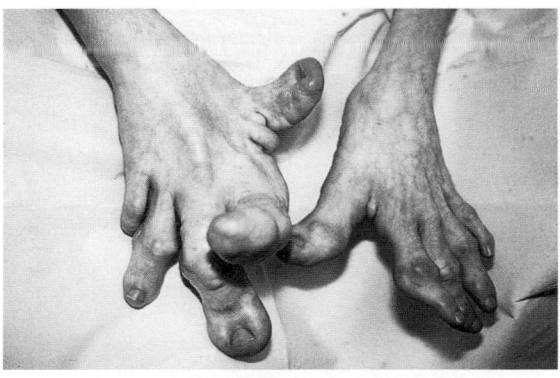

Fig. 19.8. Asymmetrical enlargement of the hands (courtesy of Professor D. Donnai, Regional Genetic Service, St Mary's Hospital, Manchester).

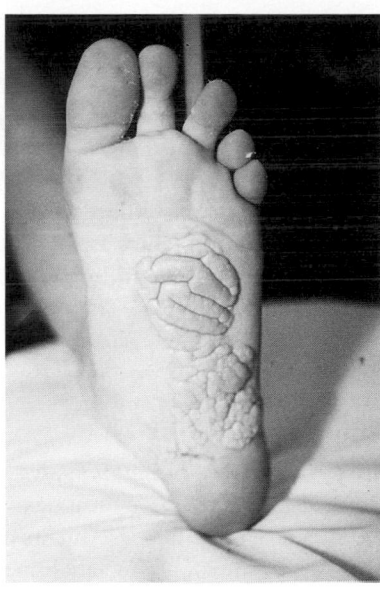

Fig. 19.9. Plantar hyperplasia (overgrowth of the subcutaneous tissues of the soles of the feet) (courtesy of Professor D. Donnai, Regional Genetic Service, St Mary's Hospital, Manchester).

metry of the skull), and plantar hyperplasia (overgrowth of the subcutaneous tissues of the soles of the feet (Fig. 19.9). There may be macrodactyly or syndactyly. Pulmonary and renal abnormalities, such as nephrogenic diabetes insipidus, have been described. Neurological manifestations may include spinal cord compression from tumour infiltration, cerebral malformations, or spinal stenosis as a result of kyphoscoliosis.

The condition may not be hereditary, although Goodship *et al.* (1991) reported a possible case in a father and a son, and a somatic mosaic inheritance has been suggested. Proteus syndrome affects both sexes equally and does not have a particular racial or geographical pattern. It is distinct from neurofibromatosis but certain features may be similar. Clinical features may be very mild or severe. It is thought that the 'elephant man', Joseph Merrick, had Proteus syndrome.

19.6.5 Hemiatrophy and hemihypertrophy

Facial hemiatrophy (synonym: Parry–Romberg syndrome) is a hereditary condition that usually starts in the teens and produces progressive atrophy of the skin and connective tissues of one side of the face, or occasionally one side of the body (Malandrini *et al.* 1997). There may be associated atrophy of the eye and bone and hemicortical atrophy in the ipsilateral cerebral hemisphere. Childhood cases have been described, as have cases starting in the elderly. The cause is unknown. Vitiligo, Horner's syndrome, and loss of hair on the same side of the scalp are recognized associations. Seizures, hemianaesthesia, hemianopia aphasia, migraine, and syringomyelia have also been described. The condition may halt spontaneously and the degree of cosmetic severity varies from case to case. There is no treatment that halts the disease, but symptomatic relief of seizures and pain may be helpful. MRI changes may include unilateral focal infarctions in the corpus callosum, cortex thickening, subcortical white matter changes, and ipsilateral leptomeningeal enhancement or calcification (Cory *et al.* 1997).

Hemihypertrophy (synonym: Klippel–Trenaunay–Weber syndrome) is a rare condition which is the result of hypertrophy of the connective tissues and long bones, cutaneous haemangiomas, and varicose veins. The cause is unknown. Neurological manifestations include seizures.

19.6.6 **Menke's syndrome**

Menke's syndrome (synonyms: trichopoliodystrophy, kinky-hair disease) is an X-linked recessive focal neurodegenerative condition that affects 1 in 35 000 live births and probably results from problems with copper metabolism. The Menke's locus is mapped to Xq13.3 and the defective gene has been isolated, thus allowing the diagnosis to be made by DNA-based tests (Tumer and Horn 1996). The gene is thought to encode for a copper-binding protein that transports copper intracellularly (Harris and Gitlin 1996). Levels of serum copper and caeruloplasmin are reduced, the copper content of the liver is low, but copper content of the fibroblasts is increased. There is a problem with dietary copper absorption; however, patients can utilize copper given intravenously, although this does not prevent or treat the clinical and neurological manifestations.

The appearance of the infant usually points to the diagnosis. Clinically, the hair is colourless, friable, and kinked, curly, and has split shafts (Fig. 19.10). There is focal grey matter damage in the brain and tortuous arteries with damage to the intima. Neurological symptoms appear in the neonatal period, with failure to thrive and hypothermia. Seizures are common and progressive neurological deterioration occurs. Diagnosis is confirmed by copper studies. Increased copper content in the fibroblasts allows intrauterine diagnosis in those with previously affected family members.

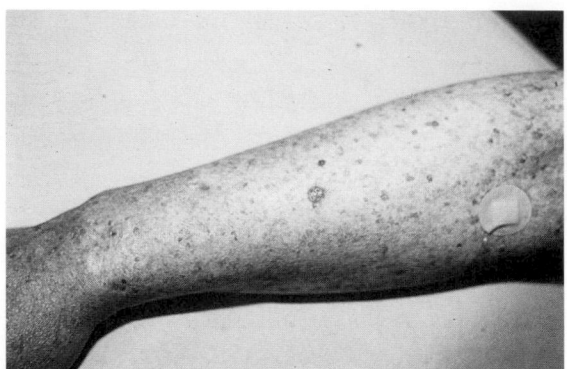

Fig. 19.11. Photosensitivity and skin cancer on the forearm of patient with xeroderma pigmentosum (courtesy of Professor D. Donnai, Regional Genetic Service, St Mary's Hospital, Manchester).

19.6.7 **Xeroderma pigmentosum**

Xeroderma pigmentosum is a rare autosomal recessive disorder which is associated with abnormalities of DNA repair enzymes. The genes affected are probably involved in nucleotide excision repair and RNA transcription. At least eight different genetic defects in DNA repair have been identified in xeroderma pigmentosum (Copeland *et al.* 1997). These defects in DNA repair result in increased sensitivity to ultraviolet light and chemical carcinogens. Patients present with photosensitivity of the skin and skin malignancies (Fig. 19.11). Lid freckling and atrophic skin are seen in nearly all cases. There is a 1000-fold increase in the risk of developing non-melanomatous skin cancers. There is an associated neurological syndrome, with learning difficulties progressing to a dementia, deafness, cerebellar ataxia, seizures, chorea, dystonia, spasticity, and sensory neuropathy (Lambert *et al.* 1995). Prenatal diagnosis is possible by analysing fetal skin fibroblasts (Cleaver *et al.* 1994).

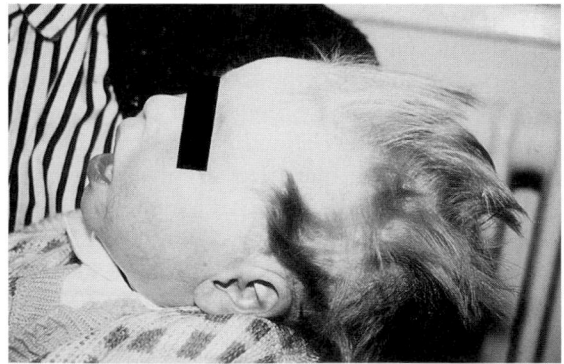

Fig. 19.10. Colourless, friable, and kinked, curly hair with split shafts characteristic of Menke's syndrome (courtesy of Professor D. Donnai, Regional Genetic Service, St Mary's Hospital, Manchester).

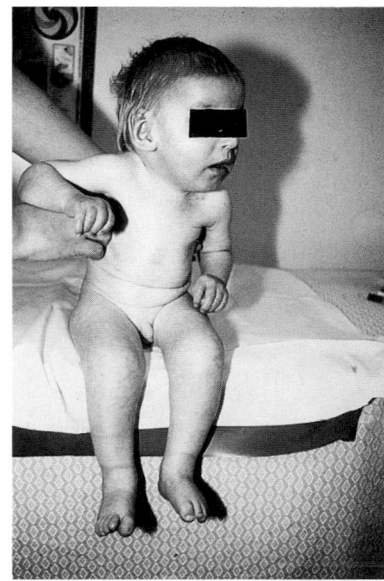

Fig. 19.12. Characteristic facial and general appearance of a child with Cockayne's syndrome.

19.6.8 Cockayne's syndrome

Cockayne's syndrome is another neurocutaneous autosomal recessive condition that is associated with impaired DNA repair. There is frequently a history of consanguinity. The skin manifestations consist of photosensitivity (84 per cent) and the neurological problems are related to learning difficulties, progeroid appearance, retinopathy ('salt and pepper'), ataxia, short stature, and neuropathy (Ozdirim *et al.* 1996) (Fig. 19.12). There is frequently slowing of conduction on nerve conduction studies and brainstem auditory evoked potentials are abnormal (70 per cent), reflecting a disorder of peripheral and central dysmyelination. Prenatal diagnosis is possible by analysing fetal skin fibroblasts (Cleaver *et al.* 1994).

References

Adamsbaum, C., Pinton, F., Rolland, Y. *et al.* (1996). Accelerated myelination in early Sturge–Weber syndrome: MRI-SPECT correlations. *Pediatr. Radiol.*, **26** (11), 759–62.

Akbarnia, B. A., Gabriel, K. R., Beckman, E. *et al.* (1992). Prevalence of scoliosis in neurofibromatosis. *Spine*, **17** (Suppl. 8), S244–8.

Annesley, W. H., Leonard, B. C., Shields, J. A. *et al.* (1977). Fifteen-year review of treated cases of retinal angiomatosis. *Trans. Am. Acad. Ophthalmol. Otolaryngol.*, **83**, 446–53.

Baser, M. E., Mautner, V. F., Ragge, N. K. *et al.* (1996). Pre-symptomatic diagnosis of neurofibromatosis 2 using linked genetic markers, neuroimaging, and ocular examinations. *Neurology*, **47**, 1269–77.

Bijlsma, E. K., Merel, P., Fleury, P. *et al.* (1995). Family with neurofibromatosis type 2 and autosomal dominant hearing loss: identification of carriers of the mutated NF2 gene. *Hum. Genet.*, **96** (1), 1–5.

Boon, C., Markello, T., Jackson-Cook, C. *et al.* (1996). Partial trisomy 10 mosaicism with cutaneous manifestations: report of a case and review of the literature. *Clin. Genet.*, **50** (5), 417–21.

Brasfield, R. D. and Das Gupta, T. K. (1972). Von Recklinghausen's disease: a clinicopathological study. *Ann. Surg.*, **175**, 86–104.

Carey, J. C., Laub, J. M., and Hall, B. D. (1979). Penetrance and variability in neurofibromatosis: a genetic study of 60 families. *Birth Defects*, **15**, 271–281.

Cleaver, J. E., Volpe, J. P., Charles, W. C. *et al.* (1994). Prenatal diagnosis of xeroderma pigmentosum and Cockayne's syndrome. *Prenatal. Diag.*, **14** (10), 921–8.

Copeland, N. E., Hanke, C. W., and Michalak, J. A. (1997). The molecular basis of xeroderma pigmentosum. *Dermatol. Surg.*, **23** (6), 447–55.

Cory, R. C., Clayman, D. A., Faillace, W. J. *et al.* (1997). Clinical and radiological findings in progressive facial hemiatrophy (Parry–Romberg syndrome). *Am. J. Neuroradiol.*, **18** (4), 751–7.

Curatolo, P. (1996). Neurological manifestations of tuberous sclerosis complex. *Childs Nerv. Syst.*, **12** (9), 515–21.

Crawford, A. H. (1989). Pitfalls of spinal deformities associated with neurofibromatosis in children. *Clin. Ortho. Rel. Res.*, **245**, 29–42.

Crowe, F. W., Schull, W. J., and Neel, J. V. (1956). *A clinical, pathological and genetic study of multiple neurofibromatosis.* Charles C Thomas, Springfield, Illinois.

De Laurenzi, V., Rogers, G. R., Hamrock, D. J. *et al.* (1996). Sjogren–Larsson syndrome is caused by mutations in the fatty acid dehydrogenase gene. *Nature Genet.*, **12** (1), 52–7.

Duffner, P. K., Cohen, M. E., Seidel, F. G. *et al.* (1989). The significance of MRI abnormalities in children with neurofibromatosis. *Neurology*, **39**, 373–8.

Eldridge, R., Denckla, M. B., Bien, E. *et al.* (1989). Neurofibromatosis type 1 (Recklinghausen's disease): Neurologic and cognitive assessment with sibling controls. *Am. J. Dis. Child.*, **143**, 833–7.

Evans, D. G. R., Huson, S. M., Donnai, D. *et al.* (1992*a*). A clinical study of type 2 neurofibromatosis. *Q. J. Med.*, **84**, 603–18.

Evans, D. G. R., Huson, S. M., Donnai, D. *et al.* (1992*b*). A genetic study of type 2 neurofibromatosis in the United Kingdom. Prevalence, mutation rate, fitness and confirmation of maternal transmission effect on severity. *J. Med. Genet.*, **29**, 841–6.

Ferner, R. E. (1994). Neurofibromatosis I: A pathogenic and clinical overview. In *The neurofibromatoses: A pathogenic and clinical overview*, (ed. S. M. Huson and R. A. C. Hughes), pp. 316–30. Chapman & Hall, London.

Font, R. L. and Ferry, A. P. (1972). Ocular and adenexal tumours. *Int. Ophthalmol. Clin.*, **12**, 1–50.

Gnarra, J. R., Tory, K., Weng, Y. *et al.* (1994). Mutations of the VHL tumour suppressor gene in renal carcinoma. *Nature Genet.*, **7** (1), 85–90.

Goldgar, D. E., Green, P., Parry, D. M. *et al.* (1989). Multipoint linkage analysis in neurofibromatosis type I: an international collaboration. *Am. J. Hum. Genet.*, **44** (1), 6–12.

Goodship, J., Redfearn, A., Milligan, D. *et al.* (1991). Transmission of Proteus syndrome from father to son? *J. Med. Genet.*, **28**, 781–5.

Gutmann, D. H., Aylsworth, A., Carey, J. C. *et al.* (1997). The diagnostic evaluation and multidisciplinary management of neurofibromatosis 1 and neurofibromatosis 2. *JAMA*, **278** (1), 51–7.

Harris, P. C., Ward, C. J., Peral, B. *et al.* (1995). Polycystic kidney disease. 1: Identification and analysis of the primary defect. *J. Am. Soc. Nephrol.*, **6** (4), 1125–33.

Harris, Z. L. and Gitlin, J. D. (1996). Genetic and molecular basis for copper toxicity. *Am. J. Clin. Nutr.*, **63** (5), 836–41.

Hunt, A. and Lindenbaum, R. H.(1984). Tuberous sclerosis: a new estimate of prevalence within the Oxford region. *J. Med. Genet.*, **21**, 272–7.

Huson, S. M. (1994) In *Neurofibromatosis 1: A pathogenic and clinical overview.* (ed. S. M. Huson and R. A. C. Hughes), pp. 160–203. Chapman & Hall Medical, London.

Huson, S. M., Harper, P. S., and Compston, D. A. (1988). Von Recklinghausen's neurofibromatosis: a clinical and population study in SE Wales. *Brain*, **111** (6), 1355–81.

Huson, S. M., Compston, D. A. S., Clark, P. *et al.* (1989a). A genetic study of von Recklinghausen's neurofibromatosis in south east Wales. 1 Prevalence, fitness, mutation rate, and effect of parental transmission on severity. *J. Med. Genet.*, **26**, 704–11.

Huson, S. M., Compston, D. A. S., Clark, P. *et al.* (1989b). A genetic study of von Recklinghausen's neurofibromatosis in south east Wales. II Guidelines for genetic counselling. *J. Med. Genet.*, **26**, 712–21.

Jouet, M., Stewart, H., Landy, S. *et al.* (1997). Linkage analysis in 16 families with Incontinentia Pigmenti. *Eur. J. Hum. Genet.*, **5**, 168–70.

Kanno, H., Kondo, K., Ito, S. *et al.* (1994). Somatic mutations of the von Hippel–Lindau tumor suppressor gene in sporadic central nervous system hemangioblastoma. *Cancer Res.*, **54**, 4845–7.

Kley, N. and Seizinger, B. R. (1995). The neurofibromatosis 2 (NF2) tumour suppressor gene: implications beyond the hereditary tumour syndrome?. *Cancer Surv.*, **25**, 207–18.

Kley, N., Whaley, J., and Seizinger, B. R. (1995). Neurofibromatosis type 2 and von Hippel–Lindau disease: from gene cloning to function. *Glia*, **15** (3), 297–307.

Lacour, M. (1996). Update on Sjogren–Larsson syndrome. *Dermatology*, **193** (2), 77–82.

Lambert, W. C., Kuo, H. R., and Lambert, M. W. (1995). Xeroderma pigmentosum. *Dermatol. Clin.*, **13** (1), 169–209.

Lamiell, J. M., Salazar, F. G., and Hsia, E. (1989). Von Hippel–Lindau disease affecting 43 members of a single kindred. *Medicine*, **68**, 1–29.

Latif, F., Tory, K., Gnarra, J. R. *et al.* (1993). Identification of the von Hippel–Lindau disease tumor suppressor gene. *Science*, **260**, 1317–20.

Listernick, R., Charrow, J., Greenwald, M. J. *et al.* (1989). Optic nerve gliomas in children with neurofibromatosis type 1. *J. Pediatr.*, **114**, 788–92.

Listernick, R., Charrow, J., Greenwald, M. *et al.* (1994). Natural history of optic pathway tumors in children with neurofibromatosis type 1: A longitudinal study. *J. Pediatr.*, **125**, 63–6.

Lubs, M. L. E., Bauer, M. S., Formas, M. E. *et al.* (1991). Lisch nodules in neurofibromatosis type 1. *N. Engl. J. Med.*, **324**, 1264–6.

Malandrini, A., Dotti, M. T., and Federico, A. (1997). Selective ipsilateral neuromuscular involvement in a case of facial and somatic hemiatrophy. *Muscle Nerve*, **20** (7), 890–2.

Miller, R. M. and Sparkes, R. S. (1977). Segmental neurofibromatosis. *Arch. Dermatol.*, **113**, 837–8.

Morrell, D., Chase, C. L., and Swift, M. (1990). Cancers in 44 families with ataxia telangiectasia. *Cancer Genet. Cytogenet.*, **50**, 119–23.

Morrissy, R. T. (1982). Congenital pseudoarthrosis of the tibia. Factors that affect results. *Clin. Orthop. Rel. Res.*, **166**, 21–7.

Nagib, M. G., Haines, S. J., Erickson, D. L. *et al.* (1984). Tuberous sclerosis. A review for the neurosurgeon. *Neurosurgery*, **14**, 93–8.

National Institutes of Health Consensus Development Conference (1988). Neurofibromatosis conference statement. *Arch. Neurol.*, **45**, 575–8.

National Institutes of Health Consensus Statement (1991). *Acoustic neuroma.* Vol 9. NIS, Bethesda.

Neumann, H. P. H. and Wiestler, O. D. (1991). Clustering of features of Von Hippel–Lindau syndrome: evidence for a complex gene locus. *Lancet*, **337**, 1052–4.

O'Hagan, A. R., Ellsworth, R., Secic, M. *et al.* (1996). Renal manifestations of tuberous sclerosis complex. *Clin. Pediatr.*, **35** (10), 483–9.

Osbourne, J. P. and Fryer, A. E. (1991). Tuberous sclerosis (epiloia, Bourneville's disease). In *Clinical neurology*, (ed. M. Swash and J. Oxbury), p. 1256. Churchill Livingstone, Edinburgh.

Ozdirim, E., Topcu, M., Ozon, A. *et al.* (1996). Cockayne syndrome: review of 25 cases. *Pediatr. Neurol.*, **15** (3), 312–16.

Parry, D. M., Elridge, R., Kaiser-Kupfer, M. I. *et al.* (1994). Neurofibromatosis 2 (NF2): clinical characteristics of 63 affected individuals and clinical evidence for heterogeneity. *Am. J. Med. Genet.*, **52**, 450–61.

Pohl, K. R.., Farley, J. D., Jan, J. E. *et al.* (1992). Ataxia telangiectasia in a child with vaccine associated paralytic poliomyelitis. *J. Pediatr.*, **121**, 405–7.

Riccardi, V. M. (1981). Von Recklinghausen neurofibromatosis. *N. Engl. J. Med.*, **305** (27), 161–27.

Riccardi, V. M. and Eichner, J. E. (1986). *Neurofibromatosis: Phenotype, natural history and pathogenesis.* Johns Hopkins University Press, Baltimore.

Riccardi, V. M. and Kleiner, B. (1977). Neurofibromatosis: a neoplastic birth defect with two age peaks of severe problems. *Birth Defects*, **12** (3C), 131–8.

Seizinger, B. R., Roulleau, G. A., Ozelius, L. J. *et al.* (1988). Von Hippel–Lindau disease maps to the region of chromosome 3 associated with renal cell carcinoma. *Nature*, **332**, 268–9.

Senveli, E., Altinors, N., Kars, Z. *et al.* (1989). Association of von Recklinghausen's neurofibromatosis and aqueductal stenosis. *Neurosurgery*, **24** (1), 99–101.

Sevick, R. J., Barkovich, A. J., Edwards, M. S. *et al.* (1992). Evaluation of white matter lesions in neurofibromatosis Type I. *Am. J. Roentgenol.*, **159**, 171–5.

Short, M. P., Richardson, E. P. Jr, Haines, J. L. *et al.* (1995). Clinical, neuropathological and genetic aspects of the tuberous sclerosis complex. *Brain Pathol.*, **5** (2), 173–9.

Shiloh, Y. and Rotman, G. (1996). Ataxia-telangiectasia and the ATM gene: linking neurodegeneration , immunodeficiency and cancer to cell cycle checkpoints. *J. Clin. Immunol.*, **16** (5), 254–60.

Silverstein, H., Rosenberg, S. I., Flanzer, J. M. *et al.* (1993). An algorithm for the management of acoustic neuromas regarding age, hearing loss, tumor size, and symptoms. *Otolaryngol. Head Neck Surg.*, **108**, 1–10.

Sorensen, S. A., Mulvihill, J. J., and Nielsen, A. (1986). Long term follow up of von Recklinghausen's neurofibromatosis: Survival and malignant neoplasms. *N. Engl. J. Med. Genet.*, **314**, 1010–15.

Spadero, A. (1986). Non-tumoral aqueductal stenosis in children affected by von Recklinghausen's disease. *Surg. Neurol.*, **26**, 487–95.

Steiner, J., Adamsbaum, C., Desguerres, I. *et al.* (1996). Hypomelanosis of Ito and brain abnormalities: MRI findings and literature review. *Pediatr. Radiol.*, **26** (11), 763–8.

Swift, M., Morrell, D., Massey, R. B. *et al.* (1991). Incidence of cancer in families affected by ataxia telangiectasia. *N. Engl. J. Med.*, **325**, 1831–6.

Sybert, V. P. (1994). Hypomelanosis of Ito: a description, not a diagnosis. *J. Invest. Dermatol.*, **103**, S141–3.

Tumer, Z. and Horn, N. (1996). Menke's disease: recent advances and new insights into copper metabolism. *Ann. Med.*, **28** (2), 121–9.

von Deimling, A., Krone, W., and Menon, A. G. (1995). Neurofibromatosis type 1: pathology, clinical features and molecular genetics. *Brain Pathol.*, **5** (2), 153–62.

Woods, C. G. and Taylor, A. M. (1992). Ataxia telangiectasia in the British Isles: the clinical and laboratory features of 70 affected individuals. *Q. J. Med.*, **82**, 169–79.

CHAPTER 20

Spinal cord disorders

David Miller

20.1 An introduction to spinal cord, cauda equina, and nerve root lesions

This chapter and Chapter 21 will deal with non-traumatic pathological disorders involving the spinal cord, cauda equina, and nerve roots within the vertebral canal (traumatic spinal cord disorders are discussed in Section 6.3). Because they share a common location, there is an introductory section in this chapter on the anatomy of these neural structures. The innervation of the bladder, rectum, corpora cavernosa, and seminal vesicles is reviewed in Chapter 21, but pathological disorders outside of the vertebral canal which affect sphincter function are discussed in Section 13.8.

20.2 Anatomy of the spinal cord and cauda equina

The spinal cord lies within the vertebral canal, extending from the foramen magnum, where it joins the medulla oblongata, to the level of the first or second lumbar vertebra. It is oval in shape, being flattened in the antero-posterior axis, and has two enlargements in the cervical and lumbar regions corresponding to the outflow of nerves to the limbs. At its lower end, it terminates in the conus medullaris, from the end of which a delicate filament, the filum terminale, continues downwards to the posterior surface of the coccyx.

The surface of the cord shows several longitudinal grooves, the deep anterior median fissure and the shallower posterior median sulcus, while on the lateral aspect are two sulci, the antero-lateral and postero-lateral. From each of the latter, a series of root filaments emerges on each side. At intervals several filaments from the postero-lateral sulcus unite to form a dorsal root, upon which is situated the dorsal root ganglion; similarly, those from the antero-lateral sulcus unite to form a ventral root. One ventral and the corresponding dorsal root on each side join together just distal to the dorsal root ganglion to form the spinal nerve. Thus there arise a series of spinal nerves, and the spinal cord is regarded as being organized into segments, one corresponding to each pair of spinal nerves. There are 8 cervical, 12 dorsal or thoracic, 5 lumbar, 5 sacral segments, and 1 coccygeal. Since the spinal cord ends at the first or second lumbar vertebra, all the spinal nerves below the first lumbar descend to their respective foramina in a bundle of nerves known as the cauda equina.

The spinal cord, like the brain, is surrounded by three meninges. The pia mater, a fibrous membrane, forms the intermediate covering of the cord, and from it fine septa penetrate into the cord substance. The arachnoid is a delicate, transparent membrane, which lies superficially to the pia mater, from which it is separated by the subarachnoid space; this contains cerebrospinal fluid (CSF) and is bridged by numerous trabeculae. The arachnoid extends as low as the second sacral vertebra. Outside the arachnoid lies the dura mater, which lines the vertebral canal, from which it is separated by the epidural space, containing fat and a thin-walled venous plexus. The dura extends a little lower than the arachnoid, to the second or third sacral vertebra. The spinal cord is suspended within its dural sheath by a series of ligamenta denticulata, which extend laterally from each side to terminate in tooth-like attachments to the inner aspect of the dura.

On the transverse section the cord substance is seen to be divided into the central grey and peripheral white matter. The grey matter is composed of ganglion cells and nerve fibres, and the white matter of fibres and their myelin sheaths. The grey matter forms an H-shaped mass, composed of an anterior and posterior horn on each side, united by the grey commissure, in the middle of which lies the central canal. The anterior horns contain ganglion cells, the axons of which enter the anterior roots and form the lower motor neurons. The cells which innervate the skeletal muscles (alpha motor neurons) measure between 30 and 70 μm in diameter and show certain histological characteristics which usually render their differentiation from the gamma motor neurons comparatively easy, as most of the latter are less than 30 μm in diameter. The large anterior horn cells (motor neurons) are arranged in definite groups (in transverse section) and columns (in longitudinal sections), and specific groups and columns of cells in the cervical and lumbar enlargements consistently innervate various muscle groups and some individual muscles. The total number of limb motor neurons in the lumbosacral cord is remarkably consistent, not only on the two sides of the cord but also in different individuals (Tomlinson et al. 1973). In the cervical spinal cord, motor neurons destined for the lumbosacral segments run lateral to those destined for the cervical segments. A similar relationship exists for ascending fibres in the spinothalamic tracts, but the converse arrangement holds for sensory fibres travelling in the posterior columns (where fibres from the lower limbs lie medial to those from the upper limbs).

The white matter, consisting of longitudinal bundles of nerve fibres, is regarded as being divided into three columns. The anterior column lies between the anterior fissure and the anterior horn of grey matter with its emerging roots. The lateral column lies lateral to the grey matter, between the ventral and dorsal roots, that is, between the antero-lateral and postero-lateral sulci. The posterior column lies between the posterior median septum and the posterior horn of grey matter and its dorsal root. Descending sympathetic autonomic fibres travel in the intermedio-lateral columns of the grey matter on each side in the thoracic cord and upper lumbar segments, while parasympathetic neurons can be identified in the anterior horns of the grey matter of sacral segments.

20.2.1 The blood supply of the spinal cord

Arteries

The spinal cord is richly supplied with blood. There are two posterior spinal arteries, each derived from the corresponding vertebral or posterior inferior cerebellar artery, which pass downwards lateral to the medulla oblongata and throughout the whole length of the cord, where they lie either in front of, or behind, the dorsal nerve roots. The single anterior spinal artery is formed by the union of a branch from each vertebral artery, and descends throughout the whole length of the cord in the anterior median fissure. The spinal arteries are reinforced by segmental arteries, which enter the intervertebral foramina and are derived from the vertebral costocervical trunk, intercostal, and lumbar arteries. The two most important of these are one in the lower cervical region, commonly at C6, and one, the great anterior radicular artery of Adamkiewicz, which usually enters the spinal cord between the T5 and T8 segments but may do so at any level from T5 to L4. The cord is also surrounded in each segment by scanty circumferential vessels that run over its surface and form anastomoses between the anterior and posterior spinal vessels, sending some horizontal branches inwards to supply the white matter and part of the posterior horns of the grey matter.

The direction of blood flow in the anterior spinal artery may not be the same throughout. Bolton (1939) suggested that blood flows downwards in both the anterior and posterior spinal arteries as far as the lower cervical region; he also suggested that in the dorsal and lumbar regions flow was often upwards. Studies with spinal cord angiography in animals and humans have confirmed that flow is often in a rostral direction, even in the lower cervical region, but is variable from one individual to another and may be modified by vascular disease. Methods of measuring spinal cord blood flow have been devised in animals, and experimental work has shown that motor and sensory activity causes temporary vasodilatation and increased blood flow in the relevant portions of the cord and cauda equina (Blau and Rushworth 1958). Within the cord, the anterior spinal artery supplies all but the posterior part of the posterior columns and posterior horns, which are supplied by the posterior spinal arteries. Descending branches from the spinal arteries also supply the cauda equina. The vessels in the lowest segments of the cord and the roots and cauda equina receive tributaries from the iliolumbar and lateral sacral branches of the internal iliac arteries.

Veins

The spinal veins derived from the spinal cord substance terminate in a plexus in the pia mater, in which six longitudinal channels have been described. These pass upwards into the corresponding veins of the medulla oblongata and so drain into the intracranial venous sinuses. The posterior half of the cord is drained by posterior medullary veins; the anterior medullary group has one lateral and two medial groups and the anatomical pattern helps to explain the clinical features of venous infarction of the cord (Hughes 1971; see also Section 20.4.3). Venous drainage through the intervertebral foramina is relatively unimportant, but thrombophlebitis may reach the spinal veins by this route.

20.3 Clinical manifestations

This section discusses the general features of spinal cord lesions and specific findings according to the segmental level of the cord lesion (for full details of the sensory changes according to the level of the lesion, refer to Figs 1.32 and 21.1). The clinical picture of segmental lesions described in Sections 20.3.7 to 20.3.10 may occur with lesions of the conus medullaris (see Section 20.6) and the clinical features described in Sections 20.3.9 and 20.3.10 may also be produced by lesions in the cauda equina (see Chapter 21) .

20.3.1 General features

The signs and symptoms of spinal cord disorders are dependent on the level, longitudinal and transverse extent, and pathological nature of the underlying cause. Because there are many potentially treatable causes of spinal cord dysfunction, and because delays in diagnosis may have an adverse effect on outcome, a thorough knowledge of the clinical manifestations is essential.

Sensory, motor, and sphincter manifestations are each common and classical features of spinal cord disease, although partial lesions may involve only one or two of these functions. Symptoms include weakness below the level of the lesion, with difficulties in walking or upper-limb function. The gait may be described as stiff, dragging, or unsteady. Some patients complain of painful muscle spasms in the lower limbs. Sensory symptoms include numbness, tingling, pins and needles, dermal hypersensitivity, burning sensations, altered temperature sensation, and tight-band-like feelings below the level of the lesions. Loss of all voluntary movements and sensation will occur below the level of a complete cord lesion. Pain may occur at the level of the lesions, especially when there is spinal cord compression from extrinsic disease involving the vertebral column.

The most common sphincter disturbances resulting from spinal cord disease are urgency, frequency, and urge incontinence; less commonly hesitancy or retention occur, except in acute transverse lesions where retention is the rule. Constipation is common and faecal incontinence occurs, though less often. In males, erectile dysfunction is a common symptom. Other autonomic changes may also be seen, e.g. excessive sweating or vasomotor disturbances below the site of the lesion, or a Horner's syndrome with lesions in the cervical cord.

The clinical signs may be divided into those occurring at the level of the lesion and those below due to interruption of long tracts. At the level of a lesion there may be lower motor neuron signs, with focal muscle wasting, fasciculations, and hypo- or areflexia due to involvement of anterior horn cells. This pattern of motor involvement will be focal or segmental. Radicular pain or dermatomal sensory loss may result from damage to sensory roots.

The interruption of long tracts is usually the most serious consequence of spinal cord disease. Damage to the lateral and anterior columns, especially the former, will result in upper motor neuron signs below the level of the lesion, with a pyramidal pattern of weakness (i.e. greater in the antigravity muscles—shoulder abduction, elbow extension, wrist and finger extension, finger abduction, hip flexion, knee flexion, ankle and toe dorsiflexion, and ankle eversion), spasticity, and deep tendon hyperreflexia with absent abdominal reflexes and extensor plantar responses. Mild wasting may occur in patients with longstanding upper motor neuron weakness. Acute severe cord lesions produce a flaccid paraplegia with a temporary phase of hypotonia and areflexia before appearance of more characteristic upper motor neuron signs. In this setting, the differential diagnosis of acute inflammatory polyneuropathy may be considered, and sensory findings (a sensory level with cord disease versus distal limb or non-prominent sensory changes with Guillain–Barré syndrome) along with an assessment of sphincter function (commonly disturbed in cord lesions but less frequently in Guillain–Barré syndrome) are especially helpful in making the distinction.

A complete cord syndrome will result in loss of all sensory modalities below the level of the lesion. Partial syndromes will produce variable findings—posterior column involvement leads to loss of joint position sense, vibration, and two-point discrimination, with a positive Romberg's sign and an ataxic gait. Pseudoathetoid movement may occur in the upper limbs. Contralateral loss of pain and temperature sensation occur with lesions involving spinothalamic pathways.

20.3.2 Upper cervical cord

Upper and lower limbs will be involved with sensory and motor abnormalities, the latter resulting in tetraparesis or tetraplegia. Lesions above C4 may also compromise diaphragm function. Sensory impairment involves the trunk and all four limbs. Lesions in the region of the foramen magnum (e.g. Arnold–Chiari malformation) may also exhibit down-beating nystagmus and cerebellar ataxia.

20.3.3 The fifth and sixth cervical segments

There is atrophy and weakness of the muscles innervated by these segments, namely the rhomboids, deltoids, spinati, biceps, and brachioradialis. There is spastic paralysis of the remaining muscles of the upper limb and of the trunk and lower limbs. The biceps and radial jerks are diminished or lost, but are often also inverted. Sensory signs are found in the lower limbs, trunk, and medial aspects of the upper limbs, including the medial three or four digits.

20.3.4 The eighth cervical and first thoracic segments

Weakness and atrophy involve the flexors of the wrists and fingers and the small hand muscles. A Horner's syndrome is rarely seen. The tendon reflexes of the upper limbs are preserved. There is spastic paralysis of the trunk and lower limbs. There is sensory abnormality in the lower limbs, trunk, medial arm, forearm, and sometimes little finger.

20.3.5 The mid-thoracic region

Atrophic paralysis is confined to the intercostals innervated by the segments involved. Movements of the diaphragm are normal. There is spastic paralysis of the muscles of the abdomen and lower limbs. A sensory level is found on the trunk.

20.3.6 The ninth and tenth thoracic segments

The lower halves of the abdominal recti are paralysed; the upper halves are normal. Consequently, the umbilicus is drawn upwards when the patient raises his head against resistance. The upper abdominal reflexes are preserved, while those of the lower segments are lost. There is spastic paralysis of the lower limbs. Sensory signs are found below the level of the umbilicus.

20.3.7 The twelfth thoracic and first lumbar segments

The abdominal recti are normal, but the lower fibres of obliquus internus and transversus abdominis are paralysed. The abdominal reflexes are preserved, but the cremasteric reflexes are diminished or lost. There is spastic paralysis of the lower limbs. Sensation is impaired throughout the lower limbs.

20.3.8 The third and four lumbar segments

Flexion of the hip is preserved. There is weakness and wasting of the quadriceps and of the hip adductors, with diminution and loss of knee jerks, and spastic paralysis of the remaining muscles of the lower limbs, with exaggeration of the ankle jerks and extensor plantar responses. Sensory loss is found below the knees, on the posterior aspect of the thighs, the buttocks, and perineum.

20.3.9 The first and second sacral segments

Flexion of the hip, adduction of the thigh, extension of the knee, and dorsiflexion of the foot are preserved. There is atrophic paralysis of the intrinsic muscles of the foot and those of the calf, with weakness of knee flexion and hip abduction and extension. The knee jerks are preserved; the ankle jerks and plantar reflexes are lost. The anal and bulbocavernosus reflexes are retained. Sensory impairments involve the buttocks, perineum, and posterior aspects of the lower limbs, including the soles of the feet.

20.3.10 The third and fourth sacral segments

The large bowel and bladder are paralysed with retention of urine and faeces, due to the uninhibited action of the sympathetic nerve supply. The external sphincters are paralysed and the anal and bulbocavernosus reflexes are lost. There is usually sensory loss in the perineum and buttocks in a 'saddle' distribution. The motility and reflexes of the lower limb are normal.

20.3.11 Differential diagnosis

The possible causes of non-traumatic spinal cord disease include compressive, neoplastic, inflammatory, infectious, metabolic, vascular, and degenerative conditions. Many important diagnostic clues will be elicited from the clinical assessment: the patient's age, the tempo of the disease, the severity of the deficits, the pattern of motor and sensory involvement, the presence and nature of pain, the occurrence of sphincter symptoms, are all important pieces of information. Investigations will inevitably be required to secure a diagnosis, and of these magnetic resonance imaging (MRI) is of paramount value, having largely replaced myelography. In some circumstances additional investigations such as CSF examination, evoked potentials, and specific blood tests will be required.

The body of this chapter (Sections 20.4 to 20.6) will consider specific disorders, with respect to their pathology, clinical presentation, investigation, and management. Since the differential diagnosis is quite different when one considers acute or chronic syndromes, these are discussed in separate sections. Because they are a clinically distinctive subgroup, disorders that primarily involve the conus medullaris are reviewed briefly in Section 20.7.

20.4 Acute myelopathies

There could hardly be a more pressing circumstance in the practice of clinical neurology than the need to rapidly establish the diagnosis of acute spinal cord compression and to differentiate it from non-compressive myelopathies (Table 20.1). When the acute cord compression is due to a surgically remediable

Table 20.1. Causes of acute myelopathy

Spinal cord compression
  Intervertebral disc prolapse
  Subdural/epidural haematoma
  Spinal epidural abscess
  Vertebral fracture or dislocation (see Chapter 6)
Inflammatory and demyelinating
  Multiple sclerosis
  Transverse myelitis
  Acute necrotic myelopathy
  Devic's neuromyelitis optica
  Sarcoidosis
Ischaemia
  Anterior spinal artery occlusion
  Fibrocartilaginous embolism
  Dissecting aortic aneurism
  Decompression sickness
Haematomyelia
Infective
  Spinal-cord abscess
  Viral myelitis
  Schistosomiasis
  Brucellosis
  Syphilis

lesion, e.g. a disc protrusion or epidural haematoma, the prognosis for recovery is directly related to the time delay between symptom onset and relief of the compression. The severity of compression and age of patient also influence prognosis.

20.4.1 Compression by intervertebral disc prolapse

This is most common in the cervical region and, if centrally located, can result in acute or subacute cord compression. Much more commonly, cervical disc prolapses occur laterally and result in upper limb pain and signs of a cervical radiculopathy (see Chapter 21). Thoracic disc protrusions, although less common, are a well recognized cause of subacute or chronic cord syndromes, with paraparesis or a Brown-Séquard syndrome when the compression is asymmetrical. A clear-cut sensory level is usual. Sometimes, the neurological symptoms fluctuate over time. MRI readily demonstrates cord compression due to disc prolapse (Fig. 20.1): sagittal and axial views should always be obtained. Occasionally, marked cord compression may be found radiologically in the absence of clinical deficits.

Acute central disc protrusion of a cervical intervertebral disc should be treated immediately by immobilizing the neck in a plastic collar; if cord compression is severe and is resulting in a significant clinical deficit, surgical decompression may be needed. When surgery is carried out sufficiently early, the prognosis is good. Operative treatment is also indicated as a rule in symptomatic cord compression due to a prolapsed thoracic disc, but the operation is more risky, recovery is often incomplete, and irreversible paraplegia due to cord infarction is a more likely complication than is the case for cervical disc surgery.

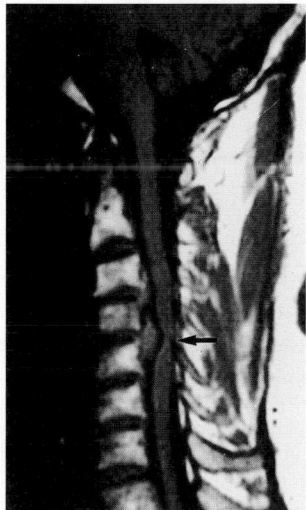

Fig. 20.1. Cord compression from cervical intervertebral disc protrusion. T1-weighted sagittal image shows marked cord compression (arrow) from a prolapsed C4–5 intervertebral disc. (Courtesy of Dr J. Stevens, Neuroradiology Department, National Hospital for Neurology and Neurosurgery.)

20.4.2 **Compression by subdural/epidural haematoma**

Spinal subdural haematoma due to trauma, or occurring as a result of lumbar puncture in patients who are anticoagulated or thrombocytopaenic, are rare causes of acute cord compression. Spontaneous epidural haematoma, usually occurring in the thoracic region (Hernandez *et al.* 1982) is also rare, but is a surgical emergency; sometimes bleeding is due to a vascular malformation and sometimes no cause is ever discovered. Haematomas more than a few days old produce a characteristic high signal on T1-weighted MR images due to the paramagnetic effects of methaemoglobin.

20.4.3 **Spinal epidural abscess**

This disorder is a neurosurgical emergency; if untreated, irreversible paraplegia develops as a result of cord compression and interference with its blood supply. The most common infectious agent is *Staphylococcus aureus*; other organisms include anaerobes, streptococci, and Gram-negative bacilli. The initial source of infection may be a skin lesion or endocarditis with bacteraemia or other cases of septicaemia, with haematogenous spread to the vertebra, intervertebral discs, or directly to the epidural space (vertebral or intervertebral disc infections may spread to the epidural space). Blood-borne spread to the epidural space may sometimes occur in intravenous drug abusers. The presentation is usually with pyrexia and localized back pain, radicular pain at the level of the infection, and the rapid development of a transverse cord syndrome with sensory,

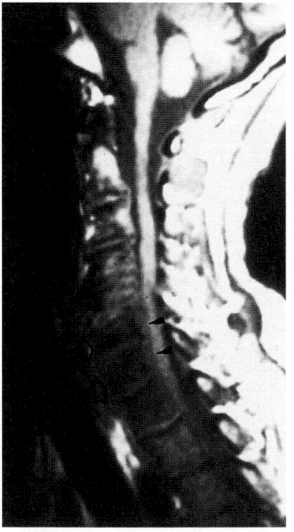

Fig. 20.2. Spinal epidural abscess. Gadolinium-enhanced sagittal T1-weighted image in the cervical region shows a diffuse extradural tissue mass anterior to the cord in the lower cervical region (small closed arrows) with associated cord compression; in addition there is signal abnormality in the adjacent C6, C7, and T1 vertebrae (open arrows), indicating associated vertebral body infection. (Courtesy of Dr J. Stevens, Neuroradiology Department, National Hospital for Neurology and Neurosurgery.)

motor, and sphincter deficits below the level of the lesion. Sometimes the picture emerges more slowly. Helpful pointers towards an infectious cause (although not always present) include an elevated erythrocyte sedimentation rate (ESR) and peripheral white blood cell count, and focal tenderness to palpation of the spinal column at the level of the infection. MRI should be obtained immediately and will reveal the extradural compressive lesion, and also may show signal changes due to infection in the adjacent vertebra (Fig. 20.2); gadolinium enhancement of the abscess may be prominent, with a ring shape. The CSF, if examined, will usually reveal a mild pleocytosis, moderately elevated protein, and a normal glucose, which is the typical pattern when there is a parameningeal focus of infection. However, MRI should be performed first, and the findings of an epidural lesion causing acute cord compression demands immediate neurosurgical intervention—in this situation, a lumbar puncture before surgery is neither necessary nor wise. In addition to immediate laminectomy and abscess drainage, intravenous antibiotics should be given in large doses. The prognosis for recovery is uncertain, but a good outcome is more likely when there has been a rapid surgical and medical intervention. Although less common, spinal subdural abscesses may occur; the presentation and management is as that for extradural abscess.

20.4.4 **Multiple sclerosis**

The spinal cord is frequently involved pathologically and clinically in multiple sclerosis (Section 29.4.3). In about 50 per cent of patients, the first presentation is the onset, over a matter of hours or days, of symptoms suggestive of a spinal cord disturbance. Sensory, motor, and sphincter symptoms may all occur in any combination. Typically, the symptoms indicate only a partial disturbance of spinal cord function, which is readily understood when one considers the pathological findings: focal demyelinating lesions almost always occupy only a part of the cross-section of the spinal cord (Oppenheimer 1978). Common sensory symptoms include tingling, numbness, dysaesthesia, loss of temperature sensitivity, or tight elastic-band-like sensations. The sensations may be unilateral or bilateral, may involve the lower limbs only, or ascend to an upper level in the trunk, or involve upper and lower limbs, or sometimes just the upper limbs alone. A Lhermitte's symptom—tingling or electrical shooting sensations down the back and into the limbs upon neck flexion—is a common manifestation of demyelinating lesions which involve the posterior columns in the cervical cord, and is rarely a manifestation of a thoracic cord lesion; it may occur in isolation or in association with other cord symptoms. Motor symptoms include limb weakness or heaviness, unsteadiness on walking, and dragging or stiffness of the lower limbs. As with sensory symptoms, the motor manifestations can be unilateral or bilateral, and if the latter, they may be symmetrical or asymmetrical. Sphincter disturbance usually manifests as increased frequency and urgency of micturition, sometimes with urge incontinence. Constipation may occur, and rarely, there may be faecal urgency or incontinence. Sexual dysfunction is a common symptom of cord demyelination in males.

The symptoms of the initial relapse will normally stabilize after a few days and then resolve over the next few weeks. Examination subsequently may well be entirely normal, although sometimes residual signs (e.g an extensor plantar response or loss of vibration sense in the lower limbs) may persist. Examination during an acute episode will usually point to the existence of a partial cord lesion. Examples of commonly found patterns of sensory disturbance include unilateral loss of pain and temperature sensation below a segmental level on the trunk (due to involvement of the contralateral spinothalamic tract), deafferentation of one hand due to a lesion in the ipsilateral posterior column in the cervical cord, or bilateral, partial loss of several sensory modalities (e.g. vibration, pain) below a segmental level on the trunk or in the upper limbs. Motor signs include a pyramidal pattern of weakness in the lower and/or upper limbs, spasticity, deep tendon hyperreflexia, loss of abdominal reflexes, and extensor plantar responses.

The investigation of patients, if seen during an acute episode, will usually entail an urgent spinal MRI, not only to confirm the presence of demyelinating lesions, but also to exclude alternative pathology, especially compression. Typical demyelinating lesions of multiple sclerosis are seen as small areas of high signal on T2-weighted images, usually not more than one segment in length (Fig. 20.3); there may be gadolinium enhancement with focal swelling during the acute phase, but these features resolve with follow-up, although persistent swelling may be seen for several weeks or even months. A number of patients will exhibit more than one focal cord lesion,

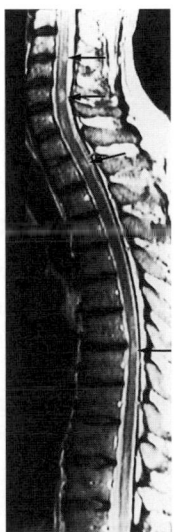

Fig. 20.3. Multiple sclerosis. Sagittal T2-weighted MRI using a phased array coil to cover the whole spinal cord. There are multiple small areas of high signal in the cervical and thoracic cord (arrowed). The lesions are less than one segment in length and occupy only a part of the anteroposterior diameter of the cord.

indicating dissemination in space. If cord imaging suggests demyelination, it may be considered appropriate to obtain additional brain imaging—in about 50 per cent of cases, this will reveal additional cerebral white matter lesions typical of demyelination. Such lesions are prognostically important—their presence indicates a substantial risk of developing clinically definite multiple sclerosis over the next 5–10 years (O'Riordan et al. 1998). On the other hand, the risk of recurrent relapses leading to a diagnosis of multiple sclerosis is much lower in those with normal brain imaging at presentation. A recent trial has demonstrated that treatment with β-interferon in patients with clinically isolated syndromes and an abnormal brain MRI can delay the development of clinically definite MS (Jacobs et al. 2000). The longer term effects of such therapy are unkown at this stage.

Another investigation of diagnostic value is examination of the CSF for intrathecally produced oligoclonal IgG bands (i.e. not matched by serum bands), which are present in about 50 per cent with an isolated cord syndrome suggestive of demyelination, and in over 90 per cent with clinically definite multiple sclerosis. A mild mononuclear pleocytosis and mild elevation of the CSF protein is not uncommon. CSF examination is, however, not required if the classical clinical and MRI features of demyelination are present. Evoked potentials may be used to demonstrate dissemination in space, e.g. a delayed visual evoked potential in a patient with a spinal cord syndrome, but their sensitivity in this regard is much lower than that of MRI. In patients with symptoms or signs which provide only equivocal clinical evidence for a spinal cord lesion, the demonstration of an abnormal somatosensory evoked potential provides useful, objective evidence for a disturbance of central sensory pathways. Positive spinal MRI findings, especially in older patients where brain white matter abnormalities have a lower aetiological specificity, can also be very helpful in such instances.

Recurrent acute spinal cord relapses are also common during the course of multiple sclerosis. In many patients, relapses implicating structures above the foramen magnum will also occur, and such clinical evidence for dissemination in space and time will of course greatly assist a secure diagnosis. While remission is the rule, mild or occasionally more severe residual deficits can occur, and some patients with recurrent relapses will accumulate a stepwise increase in disability over a number of years.

A number of treatments may be helpful in relieving the symptoms of spinal cord demyelination should they become persistent, e.g. baclofen, tizanidine or dantrolene for spasticity; carbamazepine for paraesthesia or a prominent Lhermitte's symptom; amitriptyline or gabapentin for painful dysaesthesia; oxybutynin or detrusitol for urgency of micturition; and sildenafil for erectile dysfunction in males. A short course of high-dose intravenous methylprednisolone has been shown to shorten the duration of relapses in multiple sclerosis, but there is no evidence that the final outcome is altered. Such an intervention is appropriate when relapses cause significant functional impairment, e.g. loss of ability to walk independently due to pyramidal weakness. Patients with frequent relapses, who are in the relapsing-remitting phase of the disease and who are ambulant, should also be considered for long-term treatment with a β-interferon preparation—double-blind, placebo-controlled trials of three different β-interferon preparations in such patient cohorts has revealed a 30 per cent reduction in relapse rate over a 2-year period. Some of the trials have also suggested a beneficial effect in reducing the severity of relapses and the residual disability that results.

20.4.5 Transverse myelitis

The syndrome of acute or subacute and usually complete spinal cord dysfunction may be due to a non-infectious inflammatory process, whence it is known as transverse myelitis (Section 29.3.3). Most cases are preceded by an infectious illness 1–3 weeks earlier, and are considered likely to have an immuno-pathogenic basis. In a few instances, transverse myelitis follows vaccination, while a sizeable number of cases have no antecedent event (idiopathic). A small number of cases occur in association with collagen vascular disorders, most notably systemic lupus erythematosus and the primary antiphospholipid syndrome (Section 28.2); in these instances, the pathological basis may be inflammatory or vasculitic, but may also relate to a non-inflammatory vasculopathy. In the majority of instances, transverse myelitis is a monophasic disorder, but occasional cases are described in whom there were multiple, recurrent episodes.

In the most common setting, post-infectious transverse myelitis, the preceding infection may be identifiable from either the clinical or serological features (e.g. varicella, Epstein–Barr virus, mycoplasma, and, rarely, *Campylobacter* sp.), or it may have been a non-specific upper respiratory or gastrointestinal tract infection. All ages can be affected, and presentation is common in childhood as well as in adults. The neurological onset may be accompanied by pain in the spine, but this is usually not prominent. Weakness and paraesthesia develop in the lower limbs and early urinary retention or incontinence is common. Symptoms rapidly evolve and typically reach their peak within hours to days. Either the cervical or thoracic cord may be affected and the upper level of the symptoms and signs will vary accordingly. Sometimes, after a complete transverse lesion has emerged clinically, evidence of ongoing activity of the disorder is manifested by a progressively ascending level of motor and sensory loss. Spinal MRI reveals swelling and signal change (high signal on T2-weighted images) which is typically extensive, involves several cord segments and the whole antero-posterior diameter on sagittal images. In the acute phase there is patchy gadolinium enhancement. CSF examination usually exhibits a moderate mononuclear pleocytosis, although occasionally it is acellular. The protein is moderately elevated but the glucose is normal. Oligoclonal bands are sometimes, but not always, present, and with follow-up may disappear. Pathologically, the affected cord will reveal perivascular inflammation, sometimes with demyelination; more severe cases exhibit more intense and widespread inflammation and

necrotic changes. Brain MRI occasionally reveals disseminated white matter lesions, suggesting a more diffuse, albeit asymptomatic, inflammatory/demyelinating process; more often, brain imaging is normal. Other investigation should include microbiological work-up to exclude infectious causes of myelitis, and serological investigations for collagen vascular disease.

Therapy for post-infectious transverse myelitis in the acute stage normally includes a short course of high-dose corticosteriods, e.g. intravenous meythylprednisolone, 1 gm/day for 3 days with or without an oral taper. Although there is anecdotal experience with plasma exchange and intravenous immunoglobulin, some apparently favourable, the role of these therapies remains uncertain. The prognosis is variable—some cases make an excellent recovery in spite of a complete paraplegia during the acute stage; others are left with severe residual deficits.

In the acute transverse myelopathy associated with systemic lupus erythematosus, vigorous immunosuppression with high-dose steroids and pulse cyclophosphamide is often employed, but if the neurological deficit is already established, recovery may not occur. In cases of systemic lupus or primary antiphospholipid syndrome where coagulopathy is thought to be contributing to spinal cord disorder, anticoagulation first with heparin and then warfarin may be recommended.

20.4.6 Acute necrotic myelopathy

This relatively rare disorder is characterized by the development of an acute complete transverse myelopathy, followed by a permanent severe disability with flaccid paraplegia or quadriplegia, areflexia, and an atonic bladder. Pathologically there is widespread necrotic change over a number of segments of the spinal cord, involving both white and grey matter. Such a process is recognized in some cases of post-infectious or lupus-related myelopathy, and other cases are seen where there has been a previous history of pulmonary tuberculosis; in the latter cases, the tuberculosis has usually been treated successfully, there is no evidence for active infection within the spinal cord or meninges, and it is thought that the condition has an immuno-pathogenic mechanism (Hughes and Mair 1973).

20.4.7 Devic's neuromyelitis optica

The nosological status of Devic's neuromyelitis optica is controversial, and this relates partly to differences in the way that it is defined (Section 29.3.4). The clinical occurrence of inflammatory lesions in the spinal cord and optic nerves is of course not uncommon in multiple sclerosis. The term 'Devic's syndrome' has usually been applied in the context of there being severe, more-or-less complete episodes of transverse myelitis, in conjunction with episodes of optic neuritis, the episodes occurring in either a monophasic or multiphasic fashion. A complete transverse myelitis is uncommon in multiple sclerosis. Given this definition of Devic's syndrome, there are a few cases in whom a specific underlying disease association is found. These include systemic lupus erythematosus, acute disseminated encephalomyelitis (presenting as simultaneous and monophasic transverse myelitis and bilateral optic neuritis), and Behçet's disease. In many instances, however, a specific aetiology is not found. Two recent series of such cases have been reviewed (Mandler *et al.* 1993, O'Riordan *et al.* 1996), and a number of features have emerged which point to a rather characteristic syndrome distinct from classical relapsing-remitting multiple sclerosis:

(1) a preponderance of non-Caucasians;

(2) a relatively high frequency of poor recovery from the relapses, which often result in severe paraparesis and visual loss in the acute stages;

(3) a low frequency of CSF oligoclonal bands, but often a marked pleocytosis acutely, sometimes with a neutrophil predominance;

(4) brain MRI is often normal;

(5) spinal cord MRI shows extensive swelling and signal change over multiple segments in the acute stage (Fig. 20.4), an appearance like that seen in post-infectious transverse myelitis but unlike the smaller lesions that more commonly manifest in multiple sclerosis;

(6) a high frequency of organ-specific antibodies.

Post-mortem data are more limited and sometimes difficult to interpret in the absence of sufficient clinical details, but in a number of cases, extensive changes, including necrosis, have been seen in the spinal cord, with demyelination in the optic nerves but sparing of the brain.

Taken together, the data suggest that in many cases, Devic's neuromyelitis optica can be regarded as a clinicopathological entity distinct from multiple sclerosis. Although immuno-

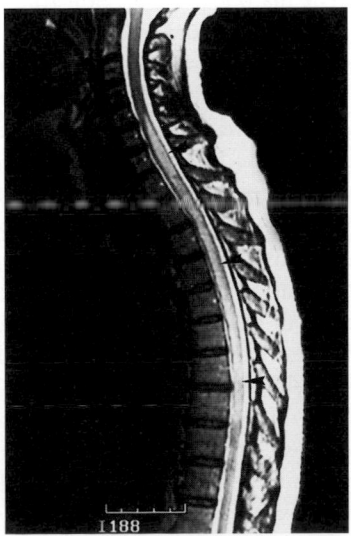

Fig. 20.4. Devic's syndrome. Sagittal T2-weighted MRI using a phased array coil (to survey the whole cord in a single image) during an episode of acute transverse myelitis reveals increased signal from the low cervical to low thoracic cord (arrows), with slight swelling of the cord in addition.

pathogenic mechanisms are likely to be important, the aetiology in these cases remains obscure. Treatment of acute disabling episodes will usually consist of a short course of high-dose steroids, although their use is empirical, as controlled trials demonstrating their efficacy are lacking. If there are repeated episodes of optic nerve and spinal cord relapse, some, but not all, neurologists may use some form of immunosuppression; again, there have been no controlled trials to determine the efficacy of such an approach.

20.4.8 Ischaemia/infarction

Spinal cord ischaemia and infarction may result from embolism or occlusion of the anterior spinal artery due to atheroma, aortic disease, or a drop in perfusion pressure, and may complicate aortography. Posterior spinal artery occlusion due to intrathecal phenol injection has also been described. The motor neurons and central grey matter are generally more vulnerable to ischaemia than white matter.

Occlusion of the anterior spinal artery in the cervical region was shown by Spiller (1909) to produce infarction of the anterior and lateral columns of the cord from the fourth cervical to the third thoracic segments. Clinically the onset is abrupt, often with pain in the neck and back and paraesthesia in the upper limbs, followed by flaccid paralysis of both arms with loss of pain and temperature sensation below a variable level in the cervical region but with preservation of light touch, vibration, and joint-position sense. Initially, there is also flaccid paralysis of both lower limbs (spinal shock) but, if the patient survives, spastic weakness of the lower limbs develops with increased reflexes and extensor plantar responses. There is usually retention of urine and faeces in the early stages but autonomic bladder and bowel control may eventually be achieved. In severe cases, paralysis remains complete and prognosis is poor, but when infarction is less extensive the lower limbs may show a variable degree of recovery.

Anterior spinal artery occlusion in the thoracic region is often a complication of dissecting aneurysm of the aorta, but may result from embolism as a result of disintegration of an atheromatous plaque in the aorta or from a drop in perfusion pressure, from transient cardiac arrest, or as a rare complication of spinal angiography. Other rare causes include surgical correction of aortic coarctation, inadvertent injection of contrast into the thyocervical trunk during cerebral angiography, fibrocartilaginous emboli from intervertebral disc degeneration entering bone marrow, atrial myxoma, sickle-cell anaemia, and non-compressive Paget's disease giving a spinal artery steal phenomenon reversible with calcitonin (Herzberg and Bayliss 1980). The central grey matter seems especially vulnerable to the effects of ischaemia.

Fibrocartilaginous embolism usually presents in healthy children or adults with abrupt pain in the neck or back followed by rapid development of a severe transverse myelopathy or a syndrome of anterior spinal artery occlusion. There is often a history of physical exertion or sometimes injury, e.g. a blow to the back during sports, within a day or so of the neurological event. Post-mortem has revealed occlusion of multiple small arteries and veins within the cord by fibrocartilage, infarction of the cord, and herniation of the nucleus pulposus of an intervertebral disc into an adjacent vertebral body. It is thought that pressure forces the disc material into vessels within the bone marrow of the vertebra with subsequent embolization to the spinal cord (Tosi *et al.* 1996).

When dissecting aneurysm is the cause of spinal cord infarction, and occasionally in other cases, there is severe pain in the back followed by total and permanent flaccid paralysis of the lower limbs, sphincter paralysis, and loss of pain and temperature up to a sensory level at about the umbilicus (corresponding to the T10 segment of the cord), but with preservation of some light touch sensation, and of vibration and joint-position sense. Thrombosis of the posterior spinal arteries complicating intrathecal injection of phenol has been described, as has venous infarction of the cord (Hughes 1971). Venous infarction may be seen as the consequence of an underlying spinal arteriovenous malformation (see Section 20.6.5). Infarction of the upper cervical cord, presumed to be due to spasm of spinal arteries, has been reported as a sequel of minor spinal trauma in childhood.

While the syndrome of anterior spinal artery occlusion is well known, infarction of the cord may be more restricted, perhaps due to occlusion of one posterior spinal artery or of one or more feeding or radicular arteries. In such cases, weakness and sensory impairment may be restricted to one limb or may be asymmetrical in the two lower limbs, and considerable or even complete recovery may take place after such a localized infarct. A rarer manifestation of spinal cord vascular disease is that of recurrent transient attacks of spinal ischaemia, with transient weakness and paraesthesia in the lower limbs, which may sometimes precede infarction.

Other rarer causes of spinal cord embolism or infarction include collagen vascular disorders (e.g. systemic lupus erythematosus, polyarteritis nodosa), bacterial endocarditis, and air embolism due to decompression (Caisson disease). The latter disorder usually manifests in underwater divers; with decompression, nitrogen bubbles can form in spinal vessels, especially in the upper thoracic cord. Symptoms may be mild and transient or may be devastating with a complete transverse myelopathy. The patients should be immediately treated with recompression in a hyperbaric chamber; when the acute deficit is severe, prognosis is variable.

The diagnosis of spinal cord infarction is made largely from the clinical features but should always be supported by spinal MRI, in order to rule out alternative pathology, and in many, but not all instances, to demonstrate the area of infarction. The latter is seen as a high-signal region within the cord on T2-weighted images, sometimes with swelling, extending over a variable number of segments. In patients with anterior spinal artery occlusion, the lesion is seen predominantly in the anterolateral cord; signal change is sometimes seen in adjacent vertebra as a result of ischaemia.

Management of spinal cord infarction includes searching for sources of embolization. If there is evidence for a coagulation disorder, or for venous infarction secondary to thrombosis within an arteriovenous malformation, anticoagulation may be indicated.

20.4.9 Spinal cord abscess

Intramedullary pyogenic spinal abscess is a rare disorder (Candon and Frerebeau 1994), but it is important as it may be difficult to diagnose, and prompt treatment may prevent irreversible paraplegia. The source of infection may be blood borne from bacteraemia or septicaemia, or from a local skin infection with spread through contiguous structures to the spinal cord. The most common infecting organism is *Staphylococcus aureus*. Presentation may be acute, with fever, elevated peripheral blood white cell count, focal spinal pain, and a rapidly developing transverse cord lesion. Other cases may develop a more subacute neurological syndrome and may not display systemic manifestations of infection. MRI reveals a focal high-signal intramedullary lesion on T2-weighted images with gadolinium enhancement, classically in a ring pattern; the radiological appearances may be indistinguishable from primary intraspinal tumour, intraspinal metastasis, or an acute demyelinating lesion. CSF reveals a mild pleocytosis, moderate elevation of the protein and a normal glucose. A high index of clinical suspicion of abscess supported by compatible MRI findings will suggest the need for surgery to both achieve a diagnosis and to drain the abscess. High-dose intravenous antibiotics are also required.

20.4.10 Spinal cord haemorrhage (haematomyelia)

Bleeding into the spinal cord occurs much less often than does bleeding into the brain. It may occur as a result of trauma (see Section 6.3.2). The main identifiable non-traumatic causes are an underlying vascular malformation, bleeding into an intramedullary metastasis, a primary coagulation disorder, or the use of anticoagulants. In other cases, no underlying cause is found. The presentation is of a sudden spinal cord syndrome, usually with pain at the level of the haemorrhage, followed quickly by the development of a transverse cord syndrome with loss of motor and sensory function below the level of the lesion. The clinical symptoms may therefore be indistinguishable from those due to epidural or subdural haemorrhage or from those of acute infarction of the spinal cord, although if the latter is due to anterior spinal artery occlusion, there will be sparing of posterior column sensation.

The diagnosis will be made from MRI, which should be obtained immediately; the cord will be swollen at the level of the haemorrhage and signal loss on T2-weighted sequences due to the effects of deoxyhaemoglobin is apparent if the haemorrhage is more than a few hours old. Surgical evacuation of a discrete haematoma may be performed, although the benefits of this approach are uncertain.

20.4.11 Viral myelitis

Viral causes of myelitis include poliomyelitis, coxsackie viruses, herpes zoster, herpes simplex, human immunodeficiency virus (HIV), Epstein–Barr virus (EBV), cytomegalovirus (CMV), and HTLV-1. The latter produces a characteristic chronic syndrome and is dealt with in Section 20.6.4. Although a number of the former viruses cause an acute infective myelitis, they may also be associated with a post-infectious myelitis, which is likely not to be the result of viral infection but rather to an immune-mediated response triggered by the viral antigens.

Poliomyelitis and coxsackie viruses produce an acute inflammatory meningomyelitis with cord involvement predominantly affecting the anterior horn cells, leading to patchy, multifocal, or sometimes extensive muscle weakness and wasting, with corresponding reflex loss but no sensory abnormality. Acutely, there is a CSF mononuclear pleocytosis and elevation of protein. Varicella zoster usually produces a sensory dermatomal deficit, often with marked pain, due to predominant involvement of the dorsal root ganglion. The associated dermatomal vesicular rash will normally establish the diagnosis. More extensive involvement of the adjacent cord or roots can lead to features of myelopathy or segmental myotomal deficits.

A transverse myelitis due to viral infections such as those above, although much rarer, may be indistinguishable from a post-infectious transverse myelitis. Such infections are more likely to occur in immunocompromised states, including those with HIV infection. The diagnosis is confirmed by the isolation of portions of viral antigen from the CSF by polymerase chain reaction. High-dose aciclovir is indicated for cord infections due to herpes simplex or zoster.

In patients with AIDS, a vacuolar myelopathy sometimes develops. The tempo is subacute with symptoms typically evolving over a number of weeks. Motor, sensory, and sphincter abnormalities all appear, sometimes asymmetrical and predominantly in the legs, although the arms may also be involved. Pathologically, there is vacuolation in the spinal cord white matter which is most marked in the thoracic region. As this manifestation is seen in patients with AIDS rather than in asymptomatic HIV-positive individuals, its appearance should be delayed or prevented by the use of effective antiretroviral therapies.

20.4.12 Schistosomiasis

Schistosomiasis is an important cause of spinal cord disease in Africa, South America, and the Far East (section 34.15.11). The most common cause of myelitis is *Schistosoma mansoni*, but infection may be seen with *Schistosoma haematobium* or *S. japonicum*. The thoracolumbar cord is most likely to be involved, either from a localized granulomatous process or from ova in the arteries and veins leading to ischaemic damage. An acute necrotic myelitis has also been reported (Queiroz *et al.* 1979). MRI reveals a high-signal intrinsic cord lesion on T2-weighted MRI, and gadolinium enhancement on T1-weighted images (Fig. 20.5). The cord may be swollen. CSF may reveal

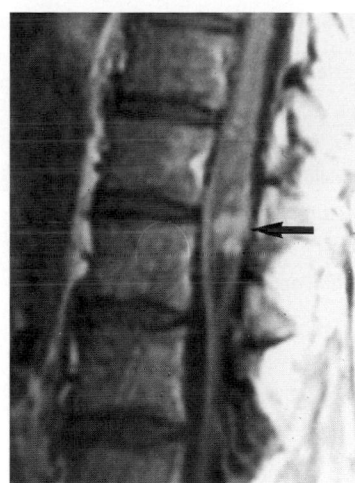

Fig. 20.5. Schistosomiasis. Gadolinium-enhanced T1-weighted MRI at the level of the conus reveals a region of swelling with mixed areas of low signal and gadolinium enhancement (arrow). (Courtesy of Dr J. Stevens.)

pleocytosis and an elevated protein. The diagnosis is supported by the identification of schistosome ova in the faeces or tissue, or by demonstrating a positive serological response to schistosome in the CSF. Treatment with praziquantel should arrest the disease, but existing neurological deficits may not reverse.

20.4.13 Sarcoidosis

Granulomatous intramedullary masses due to sarcoidosis (section 28.15) can result in presentation with an acute, subacute, or chronic myelopathy. Leptomeningeal involvement may also coexist and gadolinium-enhanced MRI may reveal enhancing granulomatous tissue within either the meninges or cord. Any level of the cord may be involved, as may the conus and cauda equina. In some patients, other parts of the central nervous system are affected, e.g. optic nerve, facial nerve, other cranial nerves, hypothalamus, brainstem, and cerebral hemispheres. Most, but not all, patients will have evidence of sarcoidosis outside of the nervous system.

The mainstay of treatment is corticosteroids, initially in high doses. Long-term maintenance steroids may be required to prevent a relapse of cord or other central nervous system involvement. In patients who appear to be dependent on at least moderate doses of long-term maintenance steroids, some authorities recommend additional immunosuppressive therapy (e.g. methotrexate).

20.4.14 Miscellaneous acute myelopathies

Although neurological involvement occurs in only a minority of patients with brucellosis, a meningitis or meningoencephalitis is sometimes seen. Intrinsic cord lesions may be apparent

Table 20.2. Causes of chronic spinal cord compression

Diseases of the vertebral column
   Common
      Metastatic carcinoma
      Cervical spondylosis/disc protrusion
      Traumatic fracture dislocation (see Chapter 6)
   Less common
      Primary vertebral neoplasms
      Sarcoma
      Myeloma
      Osteoma
      Chordoma
      Haemangioma
      Vertebral infections
      Tuberculosis
      Staphylococcal osteomyelitis
      Syphilitic osteitis
      Craniocervical junction abnormalities
      Rheumatoid atlantoaxial subluxation/pannus
      Paget's disease
   Rare
      Achondroplasia
      Mucopolysaccharidosis
      Juvenile osteochondritis
      Thalassaemia
Other causes
   Extradural abscess
      Metastatic infection
      Vertebral osteitis
   Arachnoiditis
      Syphilis
      Tuberculosis
      Sarcoidosis
   Meningeal infiltration
      Lymphoma
      Leukaemia
   Arachnoidal cysts
   Parasitic cysts
      Hydatid
      Cysticercus
   Extramedullary tumours
   Intramedullary tumours
   Dural herniation of the spinal cord

on MRI. Diagnosis is established by positive brucella serology in the CSF. Though nowadays rare, syphilis can result in acute or chronic spinal cord syndromes. Toxic causes of myelopathy are very rare, but one instance of such an event was the syndrome of subacute myelo-optic neuropathy associated with the use of clioquinol to treat traveller's diarrhoea.

20.5 Chronic spinal cord compression

20.5.1 Differential diagnosis

Chronic compression of the spinal cord may be considered in two categories: diseases of the vertebral column and other causes (Table 20.2).

Diseases of the vertebral column

The two most common vertebral column conditions leading to chronic spinal compression are: (1) carcinoma metastases and (2) cervical spondylosis with protrusion of intervertebral discs. Less frequent causes include primary neoplasms arising from the vertebra, such as sarcoma, myeloma, osteoma, chordoma, and haemangioma. Vertebral infections due to tuberculosis, staphylococcal osteomyelitis, or syphilitic osteitis may compress the cord. The osteitis deformans of Paget's disease may lead to cord compression. Rarely, achondroplasia, mucopolysaccharidoses, and severe kyphoscoliosis due to juvenile osteochondritis may have the same effect. Cord compression is also a rare complication of thalassaemia, resulting from massive extension of bone marrow from vertebral bodies into the epidural space. The cord is occasionally compressed by prolapse of an intervertebral disc elsewhere than in the neck, i.e. in the thoracic cord, or as a result of erosion of the vertebrae from without by sarcoma or by aneurysm of the aorta. High cervical cord compression may result from bony and other anomalies at the craniocervical junction and by atlantoaxial subluxation in patients with rheumatoid arthritis. Traumatic cord compression and injury is dealt with in Section 6.3.

Other causes of chronic compression

These include extradural abscess due either to metastatic infection or vertebral osteitis; arachnoiditis due to syphilis, tuberculosis, sarcoidosis, or other granulomatous processes; infiltration of the meninges with lymphoma or leukaemic deposits; arachnoidal cysts and parasitic cysts such as hydatid and cysticercus. The cord may be compromised by extramedullary and intramedullary tumours. Dural herniation of the spinal cord is a more recently described condition which can result in a progressive cord deficit.

20.5.2 Cervical spondylosis

The development during adult life of chronic disc protrusions, combined with osteophyte formation on the vertebral bodies and soft-tissue changes in the paravertebral tissues, frequently cause compression of the cervical cord and/or roots. This slowly progressive degenerative process is known as cervical spondylosis and becomes increasingly common with age. The widespread use of MRI has confirmed that it has a high prevalence in the normal population, albeit usually in a milder form and without symptoms. Spondylitic changes are most common in the mid to lower cervical cord, with the maximal frequency and

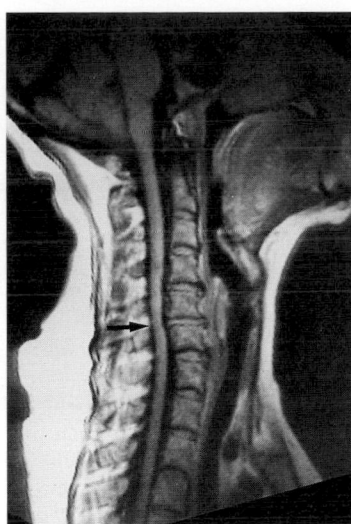

Fig. 20.6. Cervical spondylosis. Sagittal T1-weighted MRI reveals narrowing of the spinal canal with mild compression of the cord at the C5/6 level (arrow).

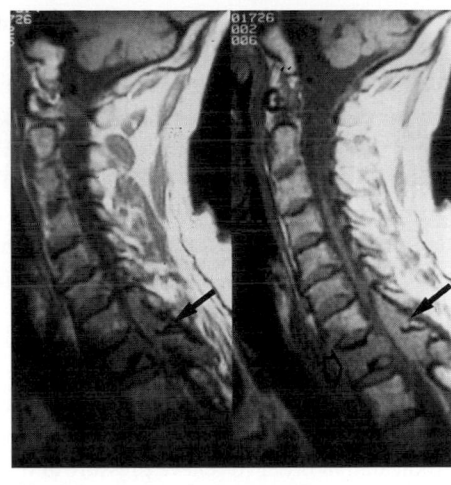

(a)

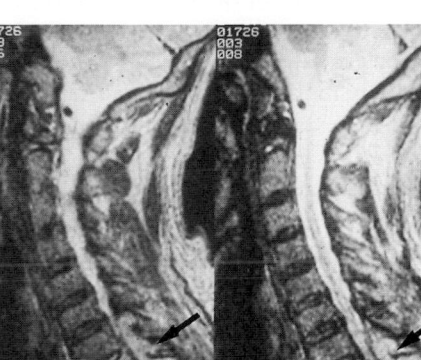

(b)

Fig. 20.7. Cord compression due to vertebral column metastasis. (a) T1- and (b) T2-weighted sagittal images show collapse and abnormal signal in the first thoracic vertebra (open arrows) with an associated soft-tissue mass anterior and posterior (closed arrows) to the cord leading to marked cord compression. (Courtesy of Dr J. Stevens.)

severity of involvement at the C5/6 level. The effect of progressive cervical spondylosis on the cord is complex: in addition to compressing it directly, the protruding discs may interfere with its blood supply; while, owing to tethering of the cord by the ligamenta denticulata and of the spinal roots by narrowing of the intervertebral foramina, ordinary neck movements may produce cumulative trauma. The result is a condition of patchy degeneration—cervical myelopathy (Wilkinson 1973).

The clinical picture of cervical spondylosis may sometimes be indistinguishable from the progressive spastic paraplegia seen in multiple sclerosis, and as the former is such a common condition radiologically, it is not uncommon to find these two disorders coexisting. The additional presence of radicular signs in the upper limbs is seen in some cases of cervical spondylosis, and sometimes extensive lower motor neuron signs in the arms (wasting, reflex loss, and fasciculation) may cause difficulties in the distinction from motor neuron disease. MRI is the diagnostic investigation of choice. However, it should be remembered that many *healthy* older individuals display moderate spondylitic changes, with mild cord indentation or compression (Fig. 20.6); cord compression is likely to be at least moderate, and usually marked, if it is to result in a serious myelopathic functional deficit. There is sometimes high signal in the cord on T2-weighted images at the level of compression, which indicates structural damage to the cord parenchyma by the spondylitic compression. Myelography is almost never needed nowadays unless MRI is contraindicated or unavailable.

In cervical myelopathy due to spondylosis, the natural tendency of the disorder is to become arrested, but in some patients disability increases remorselessly, and most are left with a varying degree of residual disability. In some cases, immobilization of the neck in a soft or hard collar has seemed to arrest clinical progression but the value of this treatment is less certain in contrast to its confirmed beneficial effects in patients with acute cervical disc prolapse. In rapidly progressive cases, especially

when the patient is relatively young, surgical decompression may be necessary. This is particularly so when there is evidence of severe compression radiologically. The choice between posterior decompression by laminectomy or laminoplasty, anterior removal of the discs with spinal fusion (Cloward 1980), or simple discectomy, is a matter of controversy.

20.5.3 Vertebral metastases

Secondary carcinoma is the most common vertebral neoplasm (Fig. 20.7). It is rare before the age of 35. The primary is most often situated in the lung, breast, thyroid or prostate, and less frequently in the uterus, stomach, kidney, or elsewhere (Stark *et al.* 1982). Although the vertebral metastasis may be blood borne, the spine is sometimes involved at the same segmental level as the primary growth, which in such cases may reach it via the perineurial lymphatics. The carcinomatous deposits erode the spongy portions of the vertebral bodies, which finally collapse. The spinal cord may be compressed as a result of the spinal deformity or by an extradural extension of the growth. Usually the spinal roots are compressed earlier than the cord itself so that root and back pain may be present for some time before vertebral collapse gives acute cord compression.

When multiple vertebrae are involved, treatment may only be palliative, and in such circumstances, adequate analgesia with opiates will be needed. Chemotherapy appropriate to the particular form of cancer will sometimes be indicated, e.g. tamoxifen for breast carcinoma. In many cases of acute compression at a single level, emergency laminectomy and decompression is indicated in order to relieve pressure and to obtain a surgical biopsy of the tumour as a preliminary to radiotherapy and chemotherapy. Decompression by an anterior approach is sometimes used. The question as to whether the lesion should be irradiated depends upon the general condition of the patient and the situation and prognosis of the primary lesion, when known. Many patients have relief of pain as a result and, in some, cord compression is relieved; hence this treatment is usually indicated if the lesion is radiosensitive and unless the patient is *in extremis* as a result of the primary growth or metastases elsewhere. Powerful analgesics and, in selected cases, surgical methods of pain relief (cordotomy, stereotactic thalamotomy) may rarely be required.

20.5.4 Other vertebral neoplasms

Sarcomas can arise from a vertebra or invade the spinal column from neighbouring tissues. Cavernous haemangioma is a rare vertebral tumour but can cause spinal cord or nerve root compression and the radiological changes (prominent vertical striation or a honeycomb pattern on radiography, and patchy high signal on unenhanced T1-weighted images with enhancement on post-contrast images) are sometimes distinctive. Myeloma usually arises simultaneously in several vertebral bodies and often also in other bones, especially the ribs, but solitary myelomas of the spine giving cord compression are not uncommon. Osteomas are rare tumours which usually arise from the posterior part of a vertebral body and hence compress the cord anteriorly. So-called chondromas are usually intervertebral disc protrusions associated with spondylosis. Chordomas arise from remnants of the notochord, and arise most commonly in the sacrococcygeal region or from the clivus, but can rarely arise in the cervical or thoracic region and result in cord compression. Deposits of lymphoma or leukaemic metastases usually infiltrate the dura mater extensively on its outer surface but may occasionally invade the cord itself. In such cases pain and symptoms and signs of cord and root compression may occur without any abnormality on plain radiographs; such a malignant meningeal infiltrative process also occurs with other carcinomas and is usually diagnosed from CSF examination, especially cytology, and gadolinium-enhanced MRI (see Section 21.3.1).

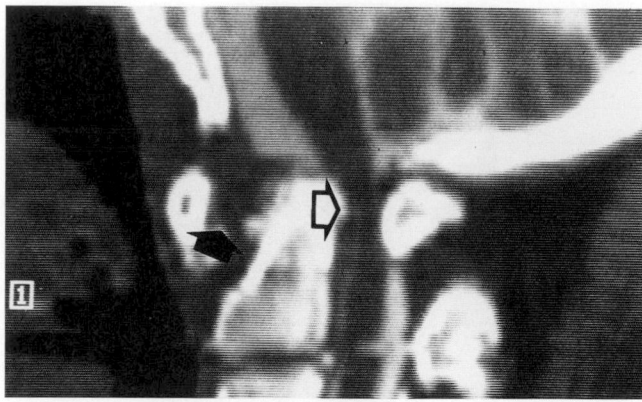

Fig. 20.8. Atlantoaxial subluxation. CT myelogram with sagittal image reconstruction in a patient with rheumatoid arthritis, shows atlantoaxial subluxation (closed arrow) with moderate cord compression (open arrow). (Courtesy of Dr J. Stevens, Neuroradiology Department, National Hospital for Neurology and Neurosurgery.)

20.5.5 Atlantoaxial subluxation

Separation of the odontoid process of the axis, occurring either as a congenital abnormality or as a result of trauma or rheumatoid arthritis may, by permitting abnormal movement of the atlas on the axis, lead in time, sometimes gradually after many years (less often more acutely), to a myelopathy from compression of the cord (Stevens *et al.* 1971). The subluxation can be demonstrated using CT myelography (Fig. 20.8) or MRI (Fig. 20.9). Whereas atlantoaxial subluxation is the most common lesion in rheumatoid cervical myelopathy, some patients have subaxial subluxation alone and others have subluxation in addition between other cervical vertebrae. The preferred treatment is occipitocervical fusion; operative decompression of the upper cervical cord in such cases is sometimes complicated by haematomyelia.

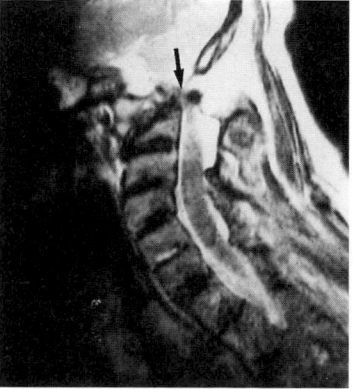

Fig. 20.9. Atlantoaxial subluxation. Sagittal T2-weighted MRI in a patient with rheumatoid arthritis shows an extreme example of atlantoaxial subluxation which results in marked compression of the cord (arrow) at C1. (Courtesy of Dr J. Stevens, Neuroradiology Department, National Hospital for Neurology and Neurosurgery.)

20.5.6 Tuberculous spinal osteitis

This usually occurs in children and young adults, but no age is exempt. It is now much less common in developed countries than in the past, in part as a result of pasteurization of milk, since many cases of skeletal tuberculosis were at one time due to the bovine bacillus, and partly due to the reduction in the frequency of the human bacillus infection. Tuberculous spinal infection is still common in less developed regions of the world. The thoracic cord is most commonly affected. The infective process generally begins in the vertebral body and spreads to adjacent bodies, leading to their collapse and an angular deformity of the spine. It is rare for the deformity as such to be a major factor in compressing the cord, which is more often affected by an extradural tuberculous abscess or tuberculous meningomyelitis. In addition to actual cord compression, which may, however, be absent, interference with the vascular supply of subjacent segments, either by compression of radicular arteries or by endarteritis, is an important factor in producing paraplegia. These considerations probably explain the good outcome that can be achieved by conservative treatment using antituberculous chemotherapy rather than surgical decompression, even in severe cases. *Syphilitic spinal osteitis* is now a very rare cause of spinal compression and produces effects similar to those of tuberculous caries.

20.5.7 Paget's disease

Paget's disease (also known as osteitis deformans) is a primary systemic bone disease in which there is both resorption of normal bone and abnormal formation of new bone. It is of unknown cause. Diagnosis is established on the basis of characteristic radiographic findings, supplemented by an elevated serum alkaline phosphatase. Neurological symptoms result from bony overgrowth in the skull (Section 18.6.6) and vertebral column, leading to compression of adjacent neural structures. Sarcomatous change may occasionally occur. The highly vascular abnormal bone may also reduce blood supply to adjacent neural structures. Spinal cord or cauda equina compression can occur at any level but is most common in the upper thoracic region. Pain may also be prominent. Atlantoaxial fractures and dislocations may occur, leading to neurological problems. Myelopathic features have sometimes been seen without compression where the deficit is thought to be due to a vascular steal phenomenon. When there is cord compression, medical treatment with agents including calcitonin, mithramycin, and diphosphonates have sometimes reduced pain and improved neurological function. Surgical decompression may be indicated in some circumstances.

20.5.8 Spinal tumour

Spinal tumours are conveniently divided into extradural and intradural growths, the latter being further divided into those arising outside the spinal cord (extramedullary tumours) and those from within the cord (intramedullary tumours). About 20 per cent of spinal tumours are primarily extradural, 60 per cent extramedullary, and 20 per cent intramedullary, although some involve more than one location. Extradural tumours have been dealt with in the preceding sections on vertebral neoplasms.

The most common extramedullary, intradural tumours are meningiomas and neurofibromas. Published figures of relative incidence vary, but meningiomas seem to be slightly more common than neurofibromas (Alter 1975), while the two together are between two and three times more common than spinal intramedullary gliomas. Neurofibromas usually arise from the spinal roots, the posterior more frequently than the anterior. They may be single or multiple, and may or may not be associated with generalized neurofibromatosis. Exceptionally, an extramedullary neurofibroma grows out through the intervertebral foramen, thus adopting a dumb-bell shape. The extraspinal portion may be palpable. Meningiomas may arise from arachnoid covering the roots or the cord. While neurofibromas develop at any level of the spinal canal and occur equally in the two sexes, meningiomas almost always lie in the thoracic region and affect females much more often than males. Sarcomatous changes in spinal meningiomas and primary extramedullary sarcomas are rare. Lipomas occasionally occur, but usually in relation to occult spina bifida and spinal dysraphism. Other developmental anomalies, not strictly tumours, but which may mimic growths in causing cord compression, include dorsal neurenteric cysts and congenital extradural cysts (intraspinal meningoceles). It has been suggested that intraspinal epidermoid cysts may follow several years after lumbar puncture due to implantation if fragments of epidermis into the spinal canal. Chordomas are rare malignant tumours arising from a remnant of the notochord. Spinal chordomas are almost invariably situated in the sacrococcygeal region. Dermoid cysts and other forms of teratomatous growth may also develop within the spinal canal.

Kernohan *et al.* (1931), who investigated the histology of intramedullary spinal tumours, claimed to have recognized varieties corresponding to most of the cerebral gliomas. Ependymomas were most common, accounting for 42 per cent of tumours. The next most common intramedullary tumour is astrocytoma. Other tumour types include medulloblastoma, oligodendroglioma, ganglioneuroma, haemangioblastoma, and, rarely, intramedullary carcinoma metastases. Leukaemic and lymphoma deposits may sometimes occur in the cord, as may tuberculomas. Systemic metastases from primary spinal neoplasm are rare, but have been described in ependymoma of the filum terminale. By contrast, intra- and extramedullary spinal deposits resulting from intracranial gliomas, especially medulloblastomas, are not uncommon, particularly in children.

Both sexes are equally liable to spinal tumour (except for meningioma, which is much more common in elderly females), and tumour may develop at any age, although in over 80 per cent symptoms first appear between the ages of 20 and 60. There is no significant difference in incidence in different races, but meningiomas are relatively rare in childhood, as indeed are all spinal neoplasms in comparison to intracranial neoplasms.

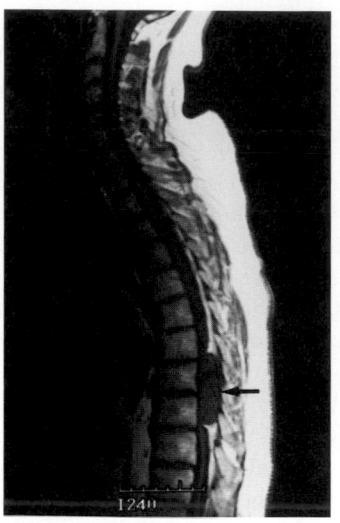
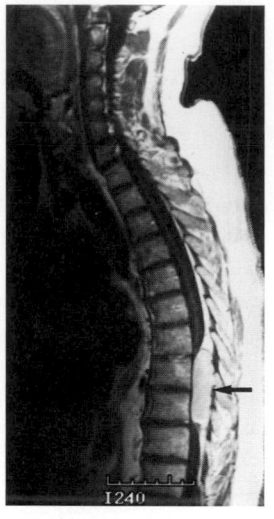

(a)   (b)

Fig. 20.10. Meningioma in the mid-thoracic region (arrows). T1-weighted sagittal MRI (a) pre- and (b) post-injection of gadolinium-DTPA. The tumour is extramedullary and causing marked cord compression. It is isointense with spinal cord on the unenhanced images and shows marked contrast enhancement.

The thoracic cord is the most common site of extradural and extramedullary tumours. Approximately two-thirds of extramedullary tumours are situated on the dorsal or dorsolateral aspects of the cord and approximately one-third on the ventral or ventrolateral aspects.

MRI is the investigation of choice for the diagnosis of all forms of spinal tumour. Neurofibromas are usually hyperintense on T2-weighted images. Meningiomas may be isointense with respect to the spinal cord on T1- and T2-weighted images, but display prominent gadolinium enhancement (Fig. 20.10). Lipomas produce a characteristic high signal on unenhanced T1-weighted images. As a rule, intramedullary tumours display swelling of the cord (Figs 20.11 and 20.12) and gadolinium enhancement.

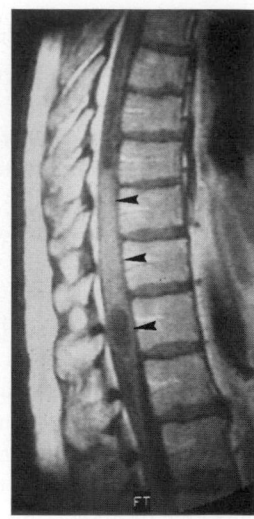

Fig. 20.12. Spinal cord ependymoma. T1-weighted sagittal MRI through the lower thoracic region reveals an intrinsic cord lesion which exhibits mass effect and extends over several segments (arrows). A region of low signal is seen within the lesions at the level of the conus. (Courtesy of Dr J. Stevens.)

Benign extramedullary tumours causing cord compression, resulting in a progressive spastic paraplegia, should be removed surgically, and a generally good prognosis can be expected if the diagnosis is made promptly and the presurgical deficit is not severe. Intramedullary gliomas or ependymomas may be extremely indolent, with a history evolving over many years or even decades. Surgical debulking of ependymomas may be possible in some instances and some cases of intramedullary glioma may benefit from radiotherapy.

20.5.9 Arachnoid cysts

These cysts, of presumed developmental origin, which differ from the neurenteric cyst in not being associated with spina bifida, are an occasional cause of cord compression in children, adolescents, and young adults. Commonly they give episodes of radicular pain with signs of spinal cord dysfunction which develop in a step-like manner. Most lie in the dorsal region pos-

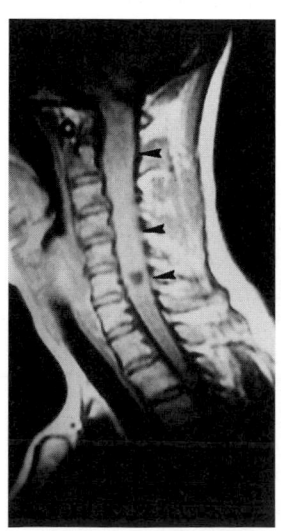

Fig. 20.11. Spinal cord astrocytoma. Sagittal T1-weighted MRI through the cervical cord shows diffuse swelling of the entire cervical cord (arrows); the small area of low signal suggests a cystic component. (Courtesy of Dr J. Stevens.)

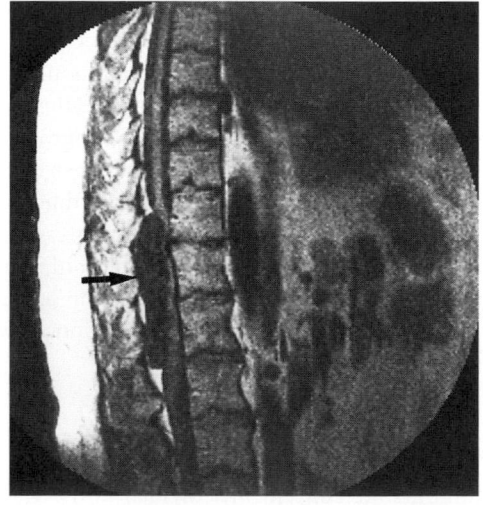

Fig. 20.13. Meningeal cyst (arrow). On a T1-weighted sagittal MRI, the lesion is extramedullary, has low signal, similar to that of CSF, suggesting a cystic lesion, and is causing marked cord compression.

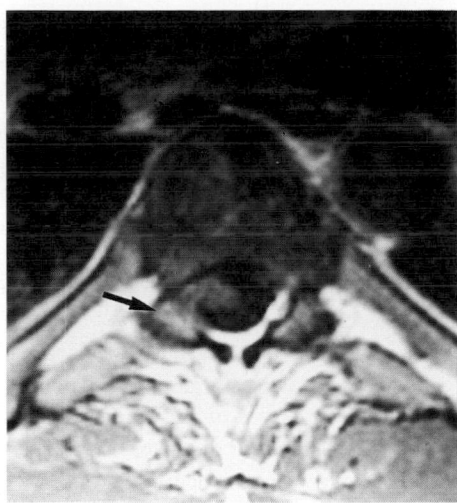

Fig. 20.14. Dural herniation of the spinal cord. Axial T1-weighted MRI through the mid-thoracic region reveals a posterolateral herniation of part of the cord through the dura (arrow); the remaining intradural portion of the cord has an eccentric location within the spinal canal.

terior to the cord and communicate with the subarachnoid space by a narrow orifice which, when myelography was the principal investigation, used only to be easily demonstrable by supine examination. MRI, using T1- and T2-weighted images, usually readily demonstrates the cyst-like structure, which has the signal characteristics of CSF; this is also seen in other meningeal cysts (Fig. 20.13). Arachnoid cysts may be particularly common in cases of Marfan's syndrome. Surgical decompression and excision of the cyst is indicated when there is a progressive clinical deficit.

20.5.10 **Cord herniation through a dural tear**

Rare cases are seen in which there has been herniation of the spinal cord through a dural tear. The cause of the tear has been unclear, there usually being no prior history of trauma. The dural defect occurs most often in the upper or mid thoracic region, and is on the ventral aspect of the cord. Herniation of

Table 20.3. Causes of chronic non-compressive myelopathy

Multiple sclerosis
Syringomyelia
Subacute combined degeneration
HTLV-1 infection
Arteriovenous malformation
Lathyrism
Hereditary spastic paraplegia
Amyotrophic lateral sclerosis
Primary lateral sclerosis
Radiation myelopathy
Adrenomyeloneuropathy
Progressive encephalomyelitis with rigidity
Paraneoplastic myelitis

the cord through the defect into the extradural space occurs. The clinical presentation is with a progressive thoracic cord syndrome with motor and sensory features, often asymmetrical and not leading to complete paraplegia. MRI reveals a characteristic abnormality with the extradural cord herniation being apparent (Fig. 20.14) (Housmann and Moseley 1996). Surgical treatment aims to return the cord to its correct location and to close the dural defect.

20.6 **Chronic non-compressive myelopathies**

The differential diagnosis is summarized in Table 20.3.

20.6.1 **Multiple sclerosis**

A progressive spastic paraplegia is the presenting manifestation of multiple sclerosis in about 5–10 per cent of patients (Section 29.4). When multiple sclerosis presents as a slowly progressive neurological disorder, it is known as primary progressive multiple sclerosis—a small number of patients in this clinical subgroup have other progressive syndromes, such as optic neuropathy, cerebellar ataxia, and dementia, but a progressive myelopathy is by far the most common syndrome. The age of onset is older than the more common relapsing-remitting form of the disease (mean 40 versus 30 years) and it is not unusual to see patients presenting in their 50s. Whereas in relapsing-remitting disease there is a 2 : 1 predominance of females, there is an equal gender prevalence for the primary progressive form of multiple sclerosis. The syndrome may be purely motor (in about half of the cases), or admixed with sensory deficits, of which the most common are paraesthesia, dysaesthesia, and loss of vibration sense in the lower limbs. Sphincter dysfunction is frequent, the most usual symptoms being urgency and incontinence and, in males, erectile dysfunction. Some patients will develop clinical features indicating lesions above the foramen magnum, e.g. optic atrophy, internuclear ophthalmoplegia, or cerebellar ataxia. The majority exhibit cerebral white matter abnormalities on MRI, but often there are strikingly few lesions. The paucity of cerebral change in many cases (and a completely normal brain in a few) limits the diagnostic value of brain MRI in this patient cohort, and contrasts with the larger lesion load seen in most patients who have an initial relapsing-remitting course but subsequently develop a progressive phase (secondary progressive multiple sclerosis), often also with prominent myelopathic features. High-resolution spinal MRI is very helpful in excluding compression and in detecting intrinsic demyelinating cord lesions—the latter are found in most cases. The great majority of patients have oligoclonal IgG bands in the CSF but not serum, indicating intrathecal synthesis. Abnormal visual and brainstem auditory evoked potentials are useful in demonstrating dissemination in space but are less often abnormal than MRI or CSF examination.

The pathological basis of progressive spastic paraplegia due to multiple sclerosis includes both focal and diffuse pathological changes. Thus, multiple focal areas of demyelination are found throughout the spinal cord, mainly involving white matter tracts but also not uncommonly extending into central grey matter. There is a variable degree of axonal loss in such focal lesions and, when marked, this probably contributes in an important way to progressive, irreversible deficits. Diffuse, microscopic changes may also occur in normal-appearing white matter in the brain and cord (e.g areas of gliosis or perivascular inflammation), and the cord frequently becomes atrophic. Sensitive MRI techniques, based on three-dimensional sequences, can be used to detect and monitor atrophic changes; these are most marked in the progressive forms of multiple sclerosis (Stevenson et al. 1998).

The treatment of progressive spastic paraparesis due to multiple sclerosis is largely symptomatic. Baclofen, tizanidine, and dantrolene may all alleviate spasticity and flexor spasms—of these baclofen is the first-choice therapy. The advice of a multi-disciplinary neurorehabilitation team, including a physiotherapist, is also indicated when there are significant functional difficulties. Severe spasticity in chair-bound patients may be helped by intrathecal baclofen, which can be delivered long term via a subcutaneous reservoir and pump. Bed-bound patients with severe spasticity and contractures may be helped by intrathecal phenol. A short course of high-dose corticosteroids (e.g. intravenous methylprednisolone 1 g/day for 3 days) is sometimes given if there has been fairly rapid clinical progression (over months), although convincing evidence of efficacy is lacking, and the side-effects of such a treatment should always be borne in mind. Interferon β-1b has recently been shown, in a single placebo-controlled trial, to modestly slow the progression in disability in secondary progressive multiple sclerosis over a 2–3-year period, although two subsequent β-interferon trials were negative. The effect of β-interferon on patients with primary progressive multiple sclerosis is not yet known. Immunosuppression with agents such as azathioprine, mitoxantrone, and methotrexate have sometimes been used in patients with progressive forms of multiple sclerosis, but evidence for efficacy from large placebo-controlled trials is lacking. A small study which included patients with both primary and secondary progressive multiple sclerosis has suggested that low-dose methotrexate may favourably modify the progression of upper-limb deficits but not ambulation.

20.6.2 Syringomyelia

Syringomyelia is a chronic disorder characterized pathologically by the presence of long cavities, surrounded by gliosis, situated in the central part of the spinal cord and sometimes extending up into the medulla (syringobulbia). The principal clinical features are cutaneous analgesia and thermoanaesthesia, often with preservation of light touch and postural sensibility, but with muscular wasting and trophic changes, especially in the upper limbs, and symptoms of corticospinal-tract dysfunction in the lower limbs. The term syringomyelia was first used by Ollivier in 1824.

Pathology

The typical pathological changes are most frequently found in the lower cervical and upper thoracic regions of the cord. Extension to the medulla is common and, rarely, the process may reach the pons or even as high as the internal capsule. Thoracolumbar and lumbosacral syringomyelia is rare and is usually due to a true hydromyelia associated with developmental anomalies, although ascending cavitation following traumatic transverse lesions of the cord, in association with cord tumours, is also seen.

The affected region of the cord may be enlarged, mainly in the transverse plane. In rare cases, the enlargement is sufficient to cause erosion of the bones of the spinal canal, or at least widening of its antero-posterior diameter. Transverse section of the cord reveals a cavity surrounded by a zone of translucent gelatinous material which, microscopically, contains glial cells and fibres. The protein content of the fluid in the cavity is high. Barnett et al. (1973) distinguished between 'communicating' and 'non-communicating' syringomyelia; the pathogenesis of these two varieties is considered below. There is usually little difference, however, in the pathological characteristics of the cord cavities in the two varieties; the differences lie in the nature of the associated lesions.

The expanding cavity and surrounding gliosis, affecting the less-resistant grey matter more severely than the dense white matter, at least in the first instance, invade the anterior horns of the grey matter, thus causing atrophy of anterior horn cells, and degeneration of their axons in the ventral roots and peripheral nerves. Extension to the brainstem (syringobulbia) usually occurs first in the postero-lateral medulla near the spinal nucleus of the trigeminal nerve and the nucleus ambiguus, so that the earliest signs of brainstem dysfunction are usually due to the involvement of such nuclei. Compression of the long ascending and descending tracts of the cord or brainstem occurs rather later, giving secondary degeneration, most marked first in the corticospinal tracts, later in the spinothalamic tracts, and later still in the posterior columns. Haemorrhage into a syringomyelic cavity constitutes one uncommon form of haematomyelia.

Aetiology and pathogenesis

For many years, it was thought that syringomyelia was due to a congenital abnormality, perhaps causing abnormal closure of the central canal of the spinal cord in the embryo. Others took the view that the condition was a degenerative disorder of unknown cause. It is now evident that 'communicating syringomyelia' is the more common variety (Barnett et al. 1973) and Gardner (1965) was among the first to stress the relationship of the condition to congenital anomalies and other lesions in the neighbourhood of the foramen magnum, including the Chiari type I anomaly (congenital extension of the cerebellar tonsils below the foramen magnum), craniovertebral developmental abnormalities with or without occult hydrocephalus, and basal arachnoiditis. Gardner suggested that abnormalities of this type (as well as the Dandy–Walker syndrome of closure of the foramina of Magendie and Luschka) prevented, perhaps intermittently, the egress of CSF from the fourth ventricle into the subarachnoid space, with the result that pressure waves of fluid were forced down into the central canal of the cord which thus became dilated (hydromyelia).

This view is now generally accepted, although opinions differ as to the exact nature of the hydrodynamic mechanisms involved. The fact that a syringomyelic cavity is sometimes found to lie alongside an apparently normal spinal canal can be accounted for by the fact that, with dilatation of the canal, its ependymal lining quickly disappears and diverticula may form which dissect downwards (or sometimes upwards) alongside the canal in the central grey matter. In several large series of cases, the Chiari type I anomaly has been the most common congenital anomaly to be found, but basal arachnoiditis, developing as a sequel to previous trauma, subarachnoid haemorrhage, or meningitis, or without evident cause, accounts for about a quarter of these cases. Arachnoiditis produced by cisternal injections of kaolin in dogs has been shown to produce experimental syringomyelia. It has also been suggested that perinatal trauma may either produce the cerebellar tonsillar ectopia or may induce the syringomyelia in the presence of such a developmental anomaly. However, it is also clear that primary cerebellar ectopia can be present without causing syringomyelia but with other neurological signs, such as hydrocephalus, paraparesis, or a cerebellar syndrome. True communicating syringomyelia has also been described as a complication of midbrain glioma.

In non-communicating syringomyelia, by contrast (Barnett *et al.* 1973), the condition is more often due to, or associated with, spinal injury, with or without paraplegia, spinal arachnoiditis, or spinal tumour. In these cases, the cavity may develop in the thoracic or lumbar cord first; indeed, except in cases of spina bifida (with which hydromyelia may be associated), the discovery of a lumbar syrinx in a patient without a history of injury should always raise the possibility of a spinal glioma or ependymoma, although intramedullary metastases or extramedullary tumours are less common associations. In cases of traumatic paraplegia or arachnoiditis, the cavities usually ascend from the site of the lesion, but in upper cervical lesions downwards cavitation is sometimes found. The cavitation has been attributed to a combination of factors, including venous obstruction, exudation of protein, and ischaemia, and oedema may be another factor.

Brewis *et al.* (1966) found the prevalence of syringomyelia to be 8.4 per 100 000 in an English city. The pathological condition is probably more common, since the widespread availability of MRI has identified that some individuals can have asymptomatic syrinxes; these are usually small in size. The condition has been described in more than one member of a family and other congenital malformations, including spina bifida, have been found in families containing affected members. It is more common in males than in females and symptoms can appear at any age between 10 and 60 years, but usually do so between the ages of 25 and 40.

Mode of onset

The symptoms of syringomyelia are readily interpreted as the outcome of the progressive lesion in the central region of the spinal cord. The onset is usually insidious, but rarely develops rapidly over the course of a few weeks. Occasionally indeed, the first symptoms may follow an episode of coughing, sneezing, or straining. Wasting and weakness of the small muscles of the hands are common early symptoms, but, alternatively, the patient may notice loss of feeling in the hands or the resulting injuries. Less often, pain or trophic lesions first attract attention. Attention may be drawn to the disorder by the appearance of scoliosis in childhood.

Sensory symptoms and signs

At the earliest stage there is an elongated cavity in the central grey matter, extending longitudinally through several segments, usually in the lower cervical and upper thoracic cord segments. The lesion is often predominantly unilateral at first and therefore interrupts on one side of the cord decussating sensory fibres derived from several consecutive dorsal roots. Since the fibres which decussate shortly after entering the cord are those which conduct impulses concerned in the appreciation of pain, heat, and cold, these forms of sensibility are impaired while others are preserved. This is the dissociated sensory loss described by Charcot, and usually appears first along the ulnar border of the hand, forearm, and arm, and on the upper part of the chest and back on one side, in a 'half-cape' distribution, with a horizontal lower border across the chest wall, ending sharply at the midline. Sometimes, however, sensation is impaired in a 'glove' area. When the lesion is situated centrally, or has extended from one side of the cord to the other, the area of dissociated sensory loss is bilateral. As it extends upwards and downwards in the cord, the area of sensory impairment extends to the radial sides of the upper limbs and neck and downward over the thorax, exhibiting at this stage a distribution 'en cuirasse'. When the lesion reaches the upper cervical segments, it begins to involve the spinal tract and nucleus of the trigeminal nerve, which receives fibres conducting impulses concerned in the appreciation of pain, heat, and cold from the face. Progressive destruction of these fibres causes extension of the area of dissociated sensory loss in a concentric manner from behind forwards on the face, sensibility on the tip of the nose and the upper lip sometimes being last affected. Exceptionally, the disorder begins in the medulla, in which case sensory loss appears first on the face.

The progressive extension of the spinal lesion later causes compression of the lateral spinothalamic tracts on one or both sides, leading to loss of appreciation of pain, heat, and cold over the lower parts of the body. There is sometimes an area of normal sensibility over the abdomen intervening between the area of thoracic anaesthesia due to interruption of the decussating fibres and the area of sensory loss on one or both lower limbs due to compression of the spinothalamic tracts. When the spinothalamic tract is compressed at the level of the medulla, appreciation of pain, heat, and cold is impaired or lost over the whole of the opposite half of the body. The posterior columns are usually the last of the sensory pathways to suffer, but in the late stages appreciation of posture, passive movement, and vibration is likely to be impaired, especially in the lower limbs, and there may even be extensive anaesthesia to light touch.

Thermo-anaesthesia may be detected by the patient, since hot water no longer feels hot over the affected parts, and analgesia exposes the patient to injuries, especially burns to the fingers, which, being painless, are not noticed at the time. Spontaneous pains, though by no means invariable, are sometimes troublesome, and the patient may describe burning, aching, or shooting pains which rarely resemble the lightning pains of tabes; more often the pain is continuous and may then cause considerable distress. Such pains in one side of the face or in the upper limb may be the first symptom. When the lesion begins in the thoracolumbar or lumbosacral regions of the cord, the dissociated loss has an appropriate distribution. In non-communicating cases, secondary to spinal cord trauma or other lesions, an ascending sensory level after months or years during which the neurological condition has been static will suggest the presence of an ascending syrinx.

Motor symptoms and signs

The earliest motor manifestations are usually muscular weakness and wasting, due to compression or destruction of the anterior horn cells. Since the lesion usually begins in the cervicothoracic cord, muscular wasting usually first appears in the small hand muscles. It may be bilateral from the beginning, or one hand may suffer before the other. As the lesion extends, the wasting spreads to involve forearms and later the arms, shoulder girdles, and upper intercostals. It is often slight, and is never as severe as that seen in advanced motor neuron disease. Fasciculation is uncommon. Contractures may develop, especially in hand and forearm muscles. Extension of the lesion to the posterolateral medulla often involves the nucleus ambiguus, causing paresis of the soft palate, pharynx, and vocal cord, occasionally giving laryngeal stridor. The other motor functions of the cranial nerves are less often affected, although Brain observed paralysis of the mandibular muscles, lateral rectus, facial muscles, and soft palate on one side as a result of haemorrhage into a syringomyelic cavity in the pons and medulla. The tongue is commonly involved and nystagmus is also common. It is variable in character, sometimes being phasic and present on lateral gaze, but may be dissociated in type, while vertical nystagmus on upward gaze is often seen; it has been ascribed to involvement of the cerebellar tonsils or of vestibular and cerebellar connections in the brainstem. Paralysis of the ocular sympathetic on one or both sides may be present, giving Horner's syndrome. The reaction to light is preserved.

Compression of the corticospinal tracts in the spinal cord causes weakness, with slight spasticity and extensor plantar responses in most cases in the later stages. The loss of power, however, is rarely severe. The tendon reflexes are exaggerated in

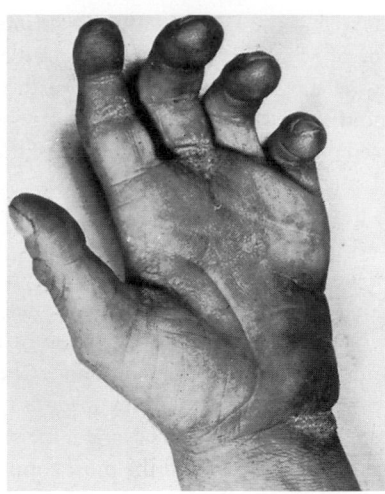

Fig. 20.15. The hand in syringomyelia, showing muscular wasting and fleshy fingers with scars of burns.

the lower limbs, but are diminished and lost early in the upper limbs, particularly on the side of the dissociated anaesthesia, due to interruption of the reflex arc; only very rarely are they exaggerated in the arms, depending on the predominance of the upper motor neuron lesion. The sphincters are usually little affected. As with the sensory findings, ascending weakness of lower or upper motor neuron type, or both, is an important feature of non-communicating syringomyelia, extending upwards from a spinal lesion.

Trophic symptoms and signs

Trophic symptoms may sometimes be conspicuous. True hypertrophy involving all tissues may be present in one limb or one half of the body or even the tongue. Loss of sweating or excessive sweating may occur, usually over the face and upper limbs. Excessive sweating may be spontaneous or may be excited reflexly when the patient takes hot or highly seasoned food. Twenty per cent of patients exhibit osteoarthropathy—Charcot's joints. The shoulders, elbows, and cervical spine are most often affected, less often the joints of the hands, the temporomandibular joint, the sternoclavicular and acromioclavicular joints, and the joints of the lumbar spine and lower limbs. Atrophy and decalcification of bones around joints, with erosion of joint surfaces and subsequent bony destruction, are the usual radiographic findings. The joint changes are not usually associated with pain. The affected joint is often enlarged, and movement evokes loud crepitus but is generally painless. The long bones are often brittle. Trophic changes in the skin include cyanosis, hyperkeratosis, and thickening of the subcutaneous tissues, leading to a swelling of the fingers described as 'la main succulente'. The analgesia, as already described, renders the patient exceptionally liable to repeated minor injuries, and healing is often slow. Ulceration, whitlows, and necrosis of bone are not uncommon. Gangrene rarely occurs. The scars of former injuries are usually evident upon the palmar surface of the fingers (Fig. 20.15).

Syringobulbia

The medulla may be involved by upward extension from the cord or may be the primary site of the disorder, when the onset of symptoms may be sudden or gradual. Trigeminal pain, vertigo, facial, palatal, or laryngeal palsy, or wasting of the tongue may each be the presenting symptom. The physical signs of syringobulbia are described above.

Morvan's syndrome

This title has been applied to cases in which there is progressive loss of pain sensation, ulceration, loss of soft tissue, and resorption of the phalanges with muscular atrophy, not only in the hands, but sometimes also in the feet, with perforating ulcers. While such changes in the hands do rarely occur in syringomyelia, a similar syndrome may occur in leprosy, and when all four extremities are involved, the most common cause is hereditary sensory neuropathy (Section 12.6).

Associated abnormalities

Many developmental and other abnormalities have been described in association with syringomyelia, occurring either in affected individuals or in members of their families. In 1926, Bremer drew attention to the following: deformities of the sternum, kyphoscoliosis, a difference in the size of the breasts, increase in the ratio between arm and body length, acrocyanosis of the hands, curved fingers, enuresis, and anomalies of the hair and ears. Common abnormalities which may be added to this list include cervical rib, spinal bifida, basilar impression of the skull, fusion of cervical vertebrae (the Klippel–Feil syndrome) with shortening of the neck, and other craniovertebral anomalies, hydrocephalus, and pes cavus (Barnett *et al.* 1973). Light

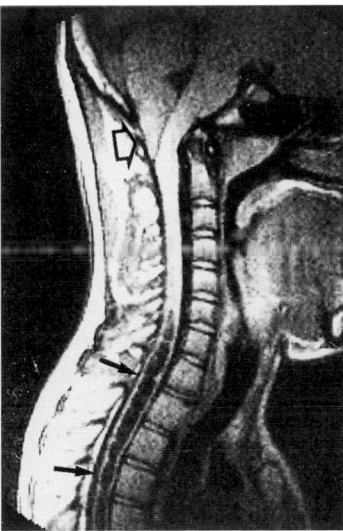

Fig. 20.16. Arnold–Chiari malformation with syringomyelia. Sagittal T1-weighted MRI reveals descent of the cerebellar tonsils through the foramen magnum to C1 (open arrow) with associated distortion of the medulla. In addition, a syrinx cavity is seen extending from C6 downwards (closed arrows) and is associated with expansion of the cord.

brown pigmentation, either in spots or diffuse sheets, often in a segmental distribution, is occasionally seen, especially on the shoulders.

Imaging

MRI is the diagnostic investigation of choice; its widespread availability has enabled a rapid and non-invasive diagnosis, which is often made earlier than in the past. T1-weighted sagittal and axial spin-echo images reveal the low-signal central cavity in the spinal cord (Fig. 20.16), the longitudinal extent of which is highly variable. Cord expansion is usually apparent. When the syrinx is associated with a Chiari malformation, the latter is also readily demonstrated on sagittal T1-weighted images which include the level of the foramen magnum (Fig. 20.16). Where the differential diagnosis includes intrinsic spinal cord tumour, gadolinium enhancement may identify enhancing tumour tissue (enhancement is not seen in syrinxes). Myelography, followed by immediate and delayed CT scanning, the previous 'gold standard' diagnostic investigation, has now been rendered obsolete, except where MRI is contraindicated or unavailable.

Other investigations

The CSF usually shows no abnormality unless the cavity is large enough to cause a block, when the protein content of the fluid is then raised. Single-fibre electromyogram (EMG) studies have shown a relatively constant pattern of involvement of the cervical anterior horn cells in this condition.

Diagnosis

There is little difficulty making the clinical diagnosis of syringomyelia in advanced cases, since the association of wasting and trophic lesions of the hands with extensive dissociated sensory loss, and with signs of long-tract dysfunction in the lower limbs, is distinctive. A clinically based diagnosis is more difficult in the early stages, and must be made then if treatment is to be more effective; however, MRI now allows an early and accurate diagnosis in almost all cases.

Intramedullary tumour of the spinal cord (especially ependymoma) may closely simulate this condition clinically. As a rule, however, it progresses more rapidly, and blockage of the subarachnoid space, with resulting CSF changes, soon occurs. The same is true of extramedullary spinal tumours, while pain is usually a more prominent symptom of these lesions than of syringomyelia. Haematomyelia, although it may produce similar signs, develops acutely; however, haemorrhage into a syringomyelic cavity constitutes one rare form of haematomyelia. Cervical spondylosis, although it may cause wasting of the proximal upper limb muscles and paraesthesia in the hands as well as spastic weakness of the lower limbs, does not cause dissociated sensory loss in the arms and hands. Motor neuron disease may simulate syringomyelia when it begins with wasting of the small hand muscles, especially when corticospinal fibres to the lower limbs are simultaneously involved. Sensory loss, however, is absent, and muscular wasting develops more rapidly, while fasciculation is almost constantly present and usually widespread, whereas in syringomyelia it is less common. Cervical rib may cause symptoms which resemble those of early syringomyelia, and the distinction between the two is rendered difficult by the fact that they may coexist. Pain along the ulnar border of the hand and forearm is a common result of cervical rib, but rare in syringomyelia, and it is usual for the latter to become clinically overt when sensory loss is much more extensive than could be attributed to a cervical rib. Hereditary sensorimotor neuropathy is distinguished from syringomyelia by the fact that muscle wasting usually appears first in the lower limbs, and a distal glove-and-stocking sensory loss is more usual. The trophic symptoms of Raynaud's disease may simulate syringomyelia, but dissociated sensory loss is absent in the former, while in the latter attacks of blanching of the fingers seen in Raynaud's disease do not occur. Hereditary sensory neuropathy is distinguished by its early onset and by the distal loss of pain sensation in all four limbs.

Syringobulbia presents little diagnostic difficulty when it occurs as an upward extension of cervical syringomyelia. When it occurs alone, however, it must be distinguished from other medullary lesions. Thrombosis of the posterior inferior cerebellar artery, which may produce sensory loss similar to that found in syringobulbia, is distinguished by its acute onset. Tumours of the medulla may closely simulate syringobulbia, especially as symptoms of increased intracranial pressure may be slight or absent, but the onset is more rapid, and extension to the pons, leading to paralysis of the lateral rectus or conjugate ocular deviation and to facial paresis, is common in medullary tumours and rare in syringobulbia. Progressive bulbar palsy is distinguished by the lack of sensory loss. The diagnosis of basilar impression, which may closely simulate or be associated with syringomyelia, can be established only by imaging. Indeed, as in the spinal cord, MRI through the foramen magnum and posterior fossa will usually readily allow a diagnosis of syrinx or other structural disorders in this region.

Prognosis

The course of syringomyelia, if untreated, is progressive, though progress is frequently slow, and prolonged arrest may occur, sometimes lasting for many years. A sudden intensification of symptoms may occur following coughing, straining, or minor trauma, or be produced by haemorrhage into a syringomyelic cavity, and exceptionally distension of the spinal cord may become so marked as to produce a complete transverse lesion, leading to paraplegia. These events, however, are exceptional, and sufferers often live for many years, death occurring either from bulbar paralysis, leading to bronchopneumonia, or from some independent disease.

Treatment

Symptomatic treatment for pain and spasticity may be required. Protection of analgesic areas and early treatment of cutaneous lesions in order to promote healing are also essential. In non-communicating cases secondary to spinal tumour or arach-

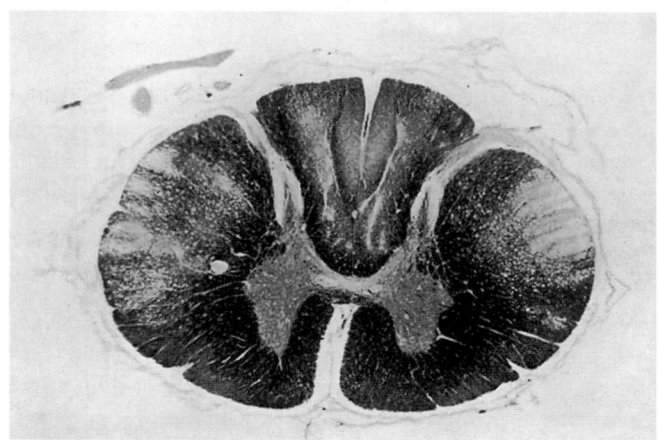

Fig. 20.17. Vitamin B$_{12}$ deficiency causing subacute combined degeneration of the spinal cord. Section at C$_3$ level of cord showing loss of myelin staining of the dorsal columns and corticospinal tracts.

noiditis, laminectomy with partial or complete removal of the causal tumour, decompression, the drainage of arachnoidal cysts or the tumour itself, or the division of fibrous bands tethering the cord have all been helpful in some cases. When ascending cavitation follows a complete traumatic transverse lesion of the cord, the process may be arrested by total excision of a segment of spinal cord at and just above the level of the injury (Barnett et al. 1973). With incomplete post-traumatic myelopathy and syrinx, syringostomy (i.e. shunting the cavity) may relieve pain.

In cases with an associated Chiari malformation, decompression of the foramen magnum and upper cervical cord is sometimes performed. The results are variable (Stevens et al. 1993); there may be relief of head and neck pain, or sometimes reduction in long-tract signs, but less often is there a beneficial effect on the segmental sensory and motor deficits. The response may be better if surgery is performed earlier in the course of the disease. The value of syringostomy in cases of communicating syringomyelia is uncertain. This procedure may also be considered in patients with isolated syringomyelia of uncertain cause, where there is progressive pain or neurological deficit.

20.6.3 Subacute combined degeneration of the cord

Vitamin B$_{12}$ deficiency produces a characteristic subacute myelopathic syndrome, and although rare, it is very important to diagnose and treat promptly in order to minimize the extent of permanent neurological deficit.

Pathology

Macroscopic changes in the nervous system are slight. Slight cerebral atrophy may be seen, and on section of the spinal cord, demyelination is evident from the greyish appearance of the white matter. The principal pathological change is one of focal demyelination in localized areas scattered throughout the white matter, giving a 'spongy' appearance (Fig. 20.17); this is associated with an accumulation of lipid-filled macrophages and gemistocytic astrocytes. The lesions, which closely resemble those seen in experimental vitamin B_{12} deficiency in animals, are most striking in the heavily myelinated fibres of the posterior columns, but also involve the lateral columns. Secondary degeneration of the long tracts, especially involving the posterior columns and corticospinal tracts, follows. In the most severely affected regions, both the myelin sheaths and axon cylinders disappear, leaving vacuolated spaces separated by a fine glial meshwork. Similar areas of degeneration may be found in the cerebral white matter, with degenerative changes especially in association fibres. Peripheral nerve lesions are also invariable, with loss of the larger myelinated fibres in distal sensory nerves and evidence of axonal degeneration in teased single fibres, although in experimental vitamin B_{12} deficiency in monkeys, segmental demyelination predominates (Section 12.21.3).

Pathological changes of pernicious anaemia are usually found in fatal cases, now extremely rare. These include glossitis, anaemia, hyperplasia of bone marrow in the long bones, slight or moderate enlargement of the spleen, excess iron in the reticuloendothelial system, and profound atrophy of all coats of the stomach wall.

Aetiology

Vitamin B_{12} myelopathy is usually seen in middle life, the average age of onset being about 50 years. It can begin in the 20s or as late as 70. The sexes are affected equally. Familial occurrence is uncommon, but is nevertheless described. Although most cases of vitamin B_{12} myelopathy are associated with megaloblastic anaemia, the association is not inevitable: anaemia may be slight or absent altogether in spite of severe spinal degeneration, and only 10–15 per cent of patients with pernicious anaemia suffer from the neurological disorder. Symptoms of confusion, depression, and dementia have been reported due to vitamin B_{12} deficiency with normal blood and bone marrow findings. Some cases of tobacco–alcohol amblyopia have been linked to traces of cyanide in tobacco smoke which interfere with the utilization of vitamin B_{12}; thus hydroxycobalamin, but not cyanocobalamin, is given to treat this condition.

The importance of gastric achylia lies in the lack of an intrinsic factor, secreted by the normal stomach, which facilitates the absorption of vitamin B_{12}. The only function of intrinsic factor is to make possible the absorption of vitamin B_{12} in the terminal ileum via specific receptors on ileal mucosal cells. The fact that the absence of intrinsic factor is often associated with circulating serum antibodies to gastric parietal cells which normally produce it, is one of several facts which suggest that pernicious anaemia is an autoimmune disease. There is also considerable evidence that methyl-group transfer, necessary in the metabolism of myelin, requires the presence of both vitamin B_{12} and methyltetrahydrofolic acid via the methionine synthetase reaction which is dependent upon B_{12}; methionine may possibly have a protective effect (Reynolds 1981). While failure of the stomach to secrete intrinsic factor is the usual fault, impaired absorption may also cause vitamin B_{12} deficiency; so too may inadequate intake, as in vegans, a strict vegetarian group who do not eat any animal products.

In addition to lack of intrinsic factor due to autoimmune disease, vitamin B_{12} deficiency may also follow partial or total gastrectomy, intestinal disease causing malabsorption syndromes, including coeliac disease, Crohn's disease, tropical sprue, bowel resections, diverticulosis, and fistulae of the small intestine. In such cases a megaloblastic anaemia may be due to either folic acid or vitamin B_{12} deficiency. Any folic acid given for the anaemia may aggravate the neurological symptoms of vitamin B_{12} deficiency. Malabsorption due to biologically inert intrinsic factor, to pancreatic disease, or to the effects of drugs has also been described; colchicine is one drug known to interfere with intestinal absorption of this vitamin. It is also of interest that chronic addiction to nitrous oxide inhalation can, after prolonged exposure, produce a myeloneuropathy indistinguishable from that due to B_{12} deficiency (So and Simon 1991). The serum B_{12} and Schilling tests (see below) are almost always normal in such cases, and megaloblastic anaemia has also been reported in infancy due to hereditary transcobalamin deficiency (Thomas *et al.* 1982); even though the serum B_{12} was normal, improvement followed the administration of large doses of vitamin B_{12}.

Neurological manifestations

The clinical picture is usually due to combined features of posterior column, corticospinal tract, and peripheral nerve degeneration, but involvement of the optic nerves and brain is not uncommon.

The onset of symptoms is usually gradual, but can rarely be remarkably rapid. The first symptoms are generally paraesthesia, with tingling sensations, first in the tips of the toes, and later the fingers. Less often, both upper and lower extremities are involved together, or both hands may be first affected. Other paraesthesiae often described include sensations of numbness, coldness and tightness, while sharp, stabbing pains occasionally occur and many patients describe feelings as if the extremities were swollen or encased in tight bandages or constricting bands. The paraesthesiae, which usually begin in the feet and legs, tend to spread slowly up the trunk, and a sense of constriction around the chest or abdomen is common. Motor weakness and ataxia come later. The patient may first notice that he tires easily when walking, or that he walks unsteadily or tends to stumble.

Objective sensory changes are almost always present, involving first the forms of sensibility mediated by the posterior columns. Postural sense and appreciation of passive movement and of vibration sense are impaired first in the lower, and later in the upper limbs. Cutaneous sensation to light touch, pinprick, heat, and cold is impaired at first in the periphery, leading to the characteristic 'glove-and-stocking' distribution of superficial sensory loss. The calves may be tender on pressure. The proximal border of the anaesthetic areas may then ascend gradually.

In some cases weakness and spasticity, in others sensory ataxia, predominate in the lower limbs, but both weakness and sensory ataxia are usually present in all four limbs, and are most severe in the lower, with a positive Romberg's sign. Moderate muscular wasting, especially in the peripheral muscles, may develop later due to peripheral neuropathy.

The reflexes vary considerably. In about 50 per cent of cases the ankle jerks are absent when the patient is first seen; the knee jerks are lost rather less often; in other cases both are exaggerated. The plantar reflexes are flexor at first in about half the cases, but later become extensor in all but a few. When the degeneration is confined to the posterior columns, sensory ataxia throughout predominates. Conversely, spastic paraparesis may alone be present while in yet other cases signs of peripheral neuropathy predominate.

Sphincter disturbances develop late; they first give difficult or precipitate micturition, and later retention of urine or incontinence. Impotence sometimes occurs early.

Bilateral primary optic atrophy with some visual impairment is observed in about 5 per cent of cases and may even be the presenting feature, with central scotomata; nystagmus is relatively common. The pupils may be small, but react normally. Otherwise the cranial nerves are normal, although dysarthria occurs rarely.

Mental changes are common and their importance has been stressed by several investigators. They may be present without anaemia or signs of spinal cord disease. There may be a mild dementia without impaired memory and intellectual capacity, or a confusional psychosis with disorientation and paranoid tendencies, or Korsakoff's syndrome; or the mental disorder may be predominantly affective, manifesting itself in irritability or severe depression. The CSF is normal. In pernicious anaemia, with or without symptoms and signs of involvement of the brain or spinal cord, the EEG may show diffuse activity, and returns to normal after appropriate treatment. MRI may reveal high signal in the spinal cord white matter tracts, especially the posterior columns (Hemmer et al. 1998) and, less often, there may be diffuse signal abnormalities in cerebral white matter; the imaging changes in both the cord and the cerebral white matter have shown striking resolution after starting vitamin B_{12} therapy.

Associated manifestations

Gastric achlorhydria is constantly present in pernicious anaemia, but free acid may be present in the gastric juice when the deficiency is due to low dietary intake or malabsorption. There is usually macrocytic anaemia with a high mean cell volume, megalocytes or even megaloblasts in the circulating blood, poikilocytosis, anisocytosis, polychromatophilia, and leucopenia with a relative lymphocytosis. Even when the peripheral blood count is normal, the bone marrow may be abnormal. Glossitis is common, but may be slight or absent when the anaemia is not severe. Other symptoms may be present if the anaemia is severe, and include dyspnoea, the characteristic lemon tint of the skin, cardiac dilatation, haemic murmurs, and oedema, most marked in the lower limbs. The spleen is rarely palpable. Gastrointestinal symptoms are common, especially anorexia, flatulence, and diarrhoea, particularly when the neuropathy is secondary to intestinal disease.

Diagnosis

The neurological picture must be distinguished from tabes, multiple sclerosis, spinal cord compression, other intrinsic myelopathies, and other causes of polyneuropathy. Reflex iridoplegia is usually present in tabes and the plantars are flexor (except in taboparesis), while in most cases the VDRL (Venereal Disease Research Laboratory) and other serological reactions are positive in either the blood or CSF, if not in both.

In multiple sclerosis, there is often evidence of multiple lesions with pallor of the optic discs and nystagmus. The ankle jerks are usually exaggerated and very rarely diminished. Difficulty in diagnosis is most likely to arise in those cases developing a progressive spastic paraparesis, as is common in middle-aged patients. Multiple sclerosis, however, usually runs a much more chronic course than subacute combined degeneration, while anaemia is absent and the serum B_{12} level normal.

Spinal cord compression may lead to an ataxic paraplegia of gradual onset. Careful examination, however, often indicates a well-defined upper level of motor disability and sensory loss, a finding which is rare in B_{12} deficiency; MRI is, of course, of crucial importance in detecting compressive lesions. Cervical spondylitic myelopathy can produce signs closely resembling those of B_{12} myeloneuropathy, and cervical spondylosis and B_{12} deficiency may coexist, in which case careful investigation of both will be required to assess their relative importance. When peripheral neuropathy due to B_{12} deficiency is associated with symptoms and signs of spinal cord disease, distinction from other forms of neuropathy is not difficult, but when neuropathy is the sole or predominant manifestation, this distinction may be wholly dependent upon estimation of the serum B_{12} and other diagnostic tests. Rarely there may be co-existent deficiency of vitamin B_1. Usually, in B_{12} deficiency, the sensory manifestations are more severe than motor; the electrophysiological findings are predominantly those of an axonal neuropathy with evidence of partial denervation of distal limb muscles. Visual evoked potentials may also show significant conduction delay.

When vitamin B_{12} deficiency is suspected on neurological grounds and, indeed, in any case in which this possibility exists, a blood count should be made and serum B_{12} should be estimated. Chlorpromazine and some other drugs may interfere with the estimation of the serum B_{12}, giving falsely low levels. The present technique of radio-immunoassay involves measuring the competitive binding of radiolabelled vitamin B_{12} to intrinsic factor. False-negative results due to the binding of B_{12} to impurities in intrinsic factor preparations appear to have been eliminated, but the assay may still occasionally be complicated, for example in myeloprolifcrative and hepatic disorders, by variable binding of the cobalamins to various transport proteins (transcobalamins I, II, and III) (see So and Simon 1991). Another useful test is the investigation of vitamin B_{12} absorption using radioactive B$_{12}$. In pernicious anaemia the absorption is almost nil, but if intrinsic factor is given as well it becomes almost normal. When doubt remains as to whether a low serum B$_{12}$ is due to pernicious anaemia or some other cause, the Schilling test (measurement of the urinary output of radioactive vitamin B$_{12}$ after oral administration with and without intrinsic factor) is diagnostic; the presence of elevated titres of gastric parietal cell antibodies in serum gives useful confirmatory evidence.

Prognosis

The average survival of patients with pernicious anaemia before the introduction of liver treatment was about 2 years. Now it is possible with hydroxycobalamin to restore the blood to normal and maintain the patient in good health indefinitely. Such patients should never develop neurological complications. When myeloneuropathy is already present, it can be arrested by introducing vitamin B$_{12}$ therapy, but the degree of recovery depends on the stage which the disease has reached. The peripheral nerves can regenerate; this is not possible in the spinal cord, but some remyelination is possible. Striking improvement may therefore be expected in the symptoms of polyneuropathy, with disappearance of paraesthesiae and pains in the limbs, sensory loss of the 'glove-and-stocking' distribution, and muscular wasting if present, and with return of the deep tendon reflexes and improvement in coordination. However, extensor plantar responses and spastic weakness and gross loss of postural sensibility usually improve much less, and, if severe, may persist unchanged. Even when the disease has been arrested by treatment, intercurrent infection may lead to an exacerbation.

Treatment

Vitamin B$_{12}$ must be given intramuscularly; oral treatment requires very large doses and even when intrinsic factor is given, the results are inconsistent.

Treatment should be begun with 1000 μg of vitamin B$_{12}$ given every 2 or 3 days for five doses to restore the tissue stores. After this, 100 μg should be given weekly for 6 months, after which 100 μg per month is usually sufficient, but may need to be increased if infection or renal insufficiency develops. Vitamin B$_{12}$ must be given for the rest of the patient's life. Folic acid is not only ineffective in treating vitamin B$_{12}$ deficiency but may be deleterious as the administration of a folate load can produce a secondary B$_{12}$ deficiency with exacerbation of neurological symptoms.

Where there are severe residual disabilities, appropriate symptomatic management will be needed, e.g. physiotherapy, antispasticity medication.

20.6.4 **HTLV-1-associated myelopathy**

A progressive paraparesis not due to compression is a common condition in both tropical and temperate regions, but unlike temperate zones, multiple sclerosis is rarely the cause of such a presentation in tropical areas. Rather, many such cases have been proven in the past decade to be due a chronic infection of the spinal cord by the retrovirus HTLV-1 (Section 34.11.1).

HTLV-1-associated myelopathy has been described in the Caribbean, southern United States, southern Japan, South America, and Africa; it is also reported in Afro-Caribbean migrants to the UK, and may emerge a number of year after their migration, but it does not occur in their offspring born in the UK (Cruickshank *et al.* 1989). Patients develop a gradually progressive spinal cord syndrome, evolving over a number of years with increasing paraparesis, spasticity, and increased deep tendon reflexes in the lower limbs, along with extensor plantar responses. Sphincter disturbance is early and prominent. Paraesthesia occurs in the lower limbs and pain is even more prominent in many patients. It often radiates from the buttocks to the feet, and is variously described as aching, tingling, burning, and sharp in character, and sometimes made worse by activity. In some patients it is accompanied by low back pain. Sensory signs are, however, usually mild or absent altogether; the main positive findings are reductions in pinprick, light touch, and vibration in the distal lower limbs. Upper-limb symptoms and signs are uncommon, and clinical involvement above the foramen magnum is very uncommon. MRI reveals cord atrophy in established cases, most marked in the thoracic region. A few patients exhibit mild abnormalities in cerebral hemisphere white matter, but some of this may be non-specific, age-related changes; infratentorial lesions are not encountered. The CSF often shows a mild mononuclear pleocytosis (5–50 cells/mm^3) and a normal protein and glucose but with local oligoclonal IgG bands (not matched by bands in serum). All patients have antibodies to HTLV-1 in the CSF and serum.

The pathological brunt of the disease is in the spinal cord, with perivascular and meningeal inflammation, and areas of demyelination, gliosis, and necrosis. Central grey matter, posterior columns, and corticospinal tracts are all involved. It has been proposed that HTLV-1 infection of lymphocytes may elicit an immune response which is responsible for the chronic inflammatory spinal cord damage that develops. The discovery of HTLV-1-associated myelopathy has excited interest in the possible role of other viral infections in the aetiology of other progressive inflammatory diseases such as multiple sclerosis; however, no viral aetiology for multiple sclerosis has yet been identified.

20.6.5 **Spinal cord arteriovenous malformations**

Arteriovenous malformations are most often found over the surface of the spinal cord (dural), and are less often intramedullary. They have a rather characteristic clinical presentation. The most common age of onset is late middle age or older, although presentation in young adults does also occur. Males are affected far more often than females. The great majority of dural arteriovenous malformations are found in the mid to lower thoracic cord, sometimes extending to the conus and, less often, more rostrally, into the cervical region. A typical arteriovenous malformation extends over a number of segments.

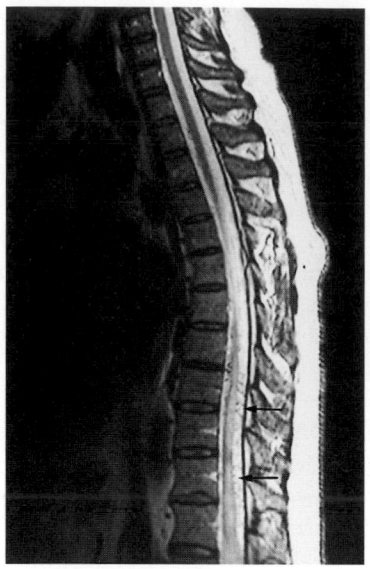
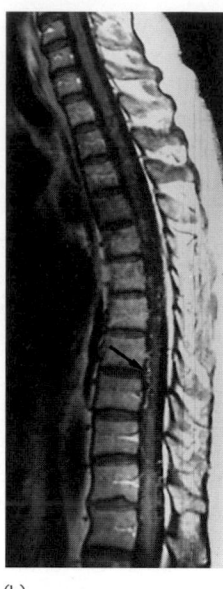

(a)   (b)

Fig. 20.18. Spinal cord arteriovenous malformation. (a) Sagittal
T2-weighted MRI shows increased signal in the lower thoracic cord with
associated cord swelling; in addition, multiple small signal voids are
seen on the surface of the cord (arrows), due to dilated veins.
(b) Gadolinium-enhanced T1-weighted sagittal image reveals patchy
enhancement over the surface of the lower thoracic cord (arrow).

Macroscopically, large tortuous veins are found on the dorsal
aspect of the cord. The feeding artery is usually either the artery
of Adamkiewicz, or one or several of the dorsal segmental
branches from the aorta which feed into the posterior spinal
artery system.

Clinically, a late middle-aged male develops a slowly progressive thoracic cord syndrome. There is often a history of exercise
intolerance, with weakness and sensory disturbance in the
lower limbs and difficulties with sphincter control. Examination reveals upper motor neuron signs in the lower limbs but,
in addition, it is common to find some lower motor neuron
signs involving upper lumbar segments, e.g. wasting, fasciculation, and weakness of quadriceps with reduced or absent knee
jerks. This reflects the commonly found caudal extension of the
malformation into the conus. It is extremely rare to find a
spinal bruit.

The aetiology of dural arteriovenous malformations is
uncertain. A minority of cases may develop as a secondary consequence of venous thrombosis in the paravertebral venous
network; it is rare, however, to identify an underlying coagulation abnormality.

Supine myelography used to be required in order to demonstrate the abnormal vessels over the dorsal surface of the cord.
However, this has now been superseded by MRI; high-
resolution studies reveal a characteristic and, indeed, diagnostic
combination of abnormalities in almost all cases (Fig. 20.18).
There is increased signal with swelling of the cord on T2-
weighted images, usually involving several segments in the
lower thoracic region. Patchy gadolinium enhancement is often

present. The pathognomonic finding is that of multiple, serpiginous, small signal voids which are closely applied to the dorsal
surface of the cord at the same level as the intrinsic cord signal
changes; these represent the dilated and tortuous dorsal veins.
MR angiography or rapid MR imaging after a bolus of gadolinium reveals the lesion more directly. Spinal angiography is still
required to determine the level of the fistula, and to determine
the suitability of the lesion for embolization.

The natural history for dura arteriovenous malformations is
one of gradual progression in clinical deficits, typically over a
matter of years. Acute decompensation is less common, and
when it does occur is probably due to venous infarction; haemorrhage is a very rare complication. Given the poor prognosis,
therapeutic intervention is recommended once a significant
neurological deficit has developed. The main aim of active
treatment is to prevent further deterioration, although occasionally there may be a reversal of existing symptoms. Many
cases are considered suitable for embolization, an important
criterion being that there is adequate alternative arterial supply
to the cord apart from the artery that is catheterized for the
embolization procedure. The results of embolization in experienced hands are generally very good, with partial or complete
obliteration of the malformation, although there is a measura-
ble risk of inducing cord infarction acutely, and later recurrences of the malformation are sometimes seen. Surgical
extirpation of the malformation can also be achieved in many
cases, but is usually chosen only when embolization is unsuccessful or unsuitable, given the greater morbidity of the surgical procedure.

In some cases, where an underlying coagulation disorder is
found, or where it is thought that there has been venous infarction in the cord secondary to thrombosis within the vascular
malformation, anticoagulation may be used; care is needed,
however, as there may also be an increased risk of haemorrhage
from the malformation.

20.6.6 Lathyrism

This disease (Section 14.8.3) is common in some regions of
Africa and India. It is thought to be caused by a toxin in the
chickling pea (*Lathyrus sativus*). During times of famine, when
there is a shortage of wheat and other grains, the diet may
involve the regular ingestion of chickling pea vetch over several
months. In such circumstances a characteristic subacute or
chronic spinal cord syndrome develops, with weakness and
spasticity of the lower limbs, along with paraesthesia and
numbness. Urinary urgency or incontinence and erectile dysfunction are frequently found. Tremor and other involuntary
movements may occur in the upper limbs. Pathologically,
degeneration of the white matter tracts in the spinal cord has
been found. The likelihood that the disease is due to a toxin is
supported by experimental studies in which a neuroexcitatory
amino acid, β-N-oxalylaminoalanine, extracted from chickling
peas, was associated with corticospinal tract degeneration when
fed to monkeys (Spencer *et al.* 1986).

20.6.7 **Hereditary spastic paraplegia**

Several types of hereditary spastic paraplegia are recognized, which vary according to the age of onset and the mode of inheritance (Section 14.8.2). The pure forms of hereditary spastic paraplegia develop as chronic syndromes with almost purely motor involvement. Autosomal dominant and recessive forms exist, the former presenting usually in young adults, the latter more often in childhood. In the absence of a positive family history, it may be difficult to differentiate hereditary spastic paraplegia from other progressive, predominantly or entirely upper motor neuron syndromes, including the primary progressive form of multiple sclerosis. One useful feature is that in hereditary spastic paraplegia, there is often disproportionately severe spasticity in the face of little or no underlying pyramidal weakness. As well, the gait is very spastic and there is often a marked lumbar lordosis.

In hereditary spastic paraplegia, the CSF is acellular and does not contain oligoclonal bands, although a mild elevation in protein may be present. MRI of the spinal cord does not reveal focal signal changes (as are commonly found in multiple sclerosis) and the cord size may be normal or show evidence of diffuse atrophy. Brain imaging is usually normal. There are as yet no specific genetic markers for the diagnosis of hereditary spastic paraplegia. Genetic counselling should be offered to the patient and his or her family. The course is one of slow progression, although patients typically remain ambulant for many years. Spasticity may be helped by the use of baclofen or tizanidine, as well as physiotherapy.

20.6.8 **Radiation myelopathy**

Radiation injury to the central nervous system (Section 5.9.1) can result in a delayed pathological process in which there is vascular hyalinization and occlusion, degeneration of fibre tracts, and necrosis involving both white and grey matter. In a small proportion of patients, a delayed myelopathy follows radiation treatment for tumours in the chest or neck, where the spinal cord was included in the radiation field. The vascular changes found at post-mortem could potentially lead to cord ischaemia and some authorities consider that this is the major mechanism of clinical dysfunction.

Three types of spinal cord syndrome have been described as a consequence of radiation. The first is a transient and benign disorder manifesting limb paraesthesiae and a positive Lhermitte's sign, usually appearing about 2–6 months after radiotherapy. Fortunately, the symptoms subside spontaneously after a few months. The pathological basis of this syndrome is unclear.

The second, most common, and most serious problem is that of a steadily progressive myelopathy, which appears after a somewhat longer interval from the time of radiotherapy; the most common latent period is between 12 and 15 months, but it may range from 6 months to 5 years or even longer. Either the thoracic or cervical cord can be affected, depending on the level of the preceding radiotherapy. Symptoms develop gradually with paraesthesia, dysaesthesia, weakness and stiffness of the lower, and in the case of cervical cord involvement, upper limbs; sphincter disturbance also develops. The initial symptoms and signs can be asymmetrical but eventually there is progression over weeks to months to a more-or-less complete paraplegia with sensory loss below the level of the lesion. Pain at the level of the lesion is not usual.

The third post-radiation syndrome is rare, and presents as a segmental lower motor neuron disorder (with weakness, wasting, and reflex loss), suggesting that there has been degeneration of anterior horn cells in the irradiated part of the cord.

In progressive radiation myelopathy, MRI reveals an area of high signal on T2-weighted images, often with swelling, at the level of the previous irradiation. In the early clinical stages, there may be gadolinium enhancement. The radiological appearances may be indistinguishable from other inflammatory or neoplastic lesions within the cord; however, the exact correspondence of the lesion level with that of the previous radiation and the presence of radiation-induced changes in the adjacent vertebral bodies are valuable diagnostic features. CSF may be normal or show a mild increase in protein.

A review of the literature has led to suggested limits in radiation exposure below which myelopathy should not occur (Kagan *et al.* 1980). These were a total dose below 6000 cGy given over 30–70 days, with a daily fraction not more than 200 cGy and a weekly fraction not more than 900 cGy. Radiation myelopathy should therefore be largely avoidable. In patients with progressive radiation myelopathy, corticosteroids or anticoagulation have both been employed; although there is no proof of efficacy, some patients have appeared to stabilize on steroids and a trial of this therapy would seem reasonable.

20.6.9 **Adrenomyeloneuropathy**

This X-linked peroxisomal disorder most often manifests as a progressive cerebral disorder in boys, whence it has a uniformly poor prognosis (Section 29.6.3). However, some individuals present with a slowly progressive myelopathy during adult life. Onset is usually in young adulthood, between the ages of 20 and 40; males are more frequently affected, although a progressive spastic paraparesis can also occur in heterozygous females. The affected individual slowly develops a spastic paraparesis over a number of years; conjoined with upper motor neuron signs, there may be loss of ankle jerks reflecting coexisting peripheral nerve involvement, and sensory manifestations including paraesthesia, and reduction in the appreciation of light touch, pain, vibration sense, or joint-position sense. The lower limbs are predominantly involved. More generalized central nervous system involvement is occasionally suggested by the presence of cerebellar signs or mild cognitive changes. MRI of the spinal cord reveals no signal abnormality, but there may be generalized cord atrophy, especially in the thoracic region. Brain MRI is normal in some, while in others there are symmetrical cerebral white matter signal abnormalities; these are most often seen in the posterior regions around the trigone and occipital horns, but rarely may be more extensive or involve cerebellar peduncle as well. Some patients have coexisting Addison's disease, with skin hyperpigmentation, a low serum cortisol, and an abnormal synacthen test. The diagnostic investigation is an elevation in plasma very-long-chain fatty acids. It is possible to correct the biochemical abnormality of fatty acids with dietary supplementation with erucic acid, but in patients with established symptoms, there is as yet no convincing evidence that the natural history of the neurological disorder is altered.

An adult presentation with progressive spastic paraparesis and cerebral MRI white matter abnormalities has also been described in Krabbe's globoid-cell leucodystrophy.

20.6.10 Motor neuron disease

Amyotrophic lateral sclerosis

This is the usual form of motor neuron disease, manifesting with both upper and lower motor neuron features in at least three limbs, and in some cases with involvement of bulbar musculature also being apparent (Section 14.2). Once the full clinical picture of upper and motor neuron involvement is apparent, there is little difficulty with the diagnosis. This section is confined to a consideration of cases in which diagnostic difficulty may be encountered.

A few patients present with an initial phase in which the symptoms and signs are largely, if not entirely, attributable to upper motor neuron involvement. In this situation, the differential diagnosis includes other causes of progressive spastic paraparesis, especially multiple sclerosis, cervical spondylosis, or primary lateral sclerosis. The presence of sensory symptoms and signs clearly point towards an alternative diagnosis, but these are not always present in either multiple sclerosis or cervical spondylosis. In general, the tempo of amyotrophic lateral sclerosis is somewhat more rapid than that for patients with progressive spastic paraparesis due to multiple sclerosis or cervical spondylosis.

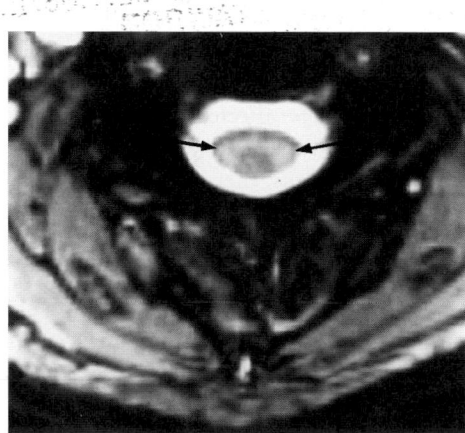

Fig. 20.19. Motor neuron disease. Axial T2-weighted MRI through the upper cervical cord reveals bilateral high signal in the lateral columns (arrows), consistent with corticospinal tract degeneration.

Additional investigations often help clarify the diagnosis. In multiple sclerosis, MRI reveals high-signal lesions in the cerebral white matter and spinal cord, the CSF contains oligoclonal bands, and in some patients the visual evoked potentials are delayed. In amyotrophic lateral sclerosis, brain and axial spinal cord images reveal symmetrical, high signal in the corticospinal tracts on T2-weighted images in two-thirds of patients (Thorpe et al. 1996; Fig. 20.19), a characteristic finding when present and entirely different from the multifocal and asymmetrical lesions found in multiple sclerosis; the CSF may show an elevated protein but there are no oligoclonal bands, and the visual evoked potentials are normal. Although there may be no clinical signs of lower motor neuron involvement in the early stages of amyotrophic lateral sclerosis, EMG may reveal evidence of denervation, and serial EMG studies over several months may show that anterior horn cell involvement is becoming more widespread. EMG may show also denervation in cervical spondylosis, but this is restricted to upper limb muscles and shows little spread in myotome involvement with follow-up. MRI is required to demonstrate cervical spondylosis, but it should be remembered that a degree of spondylosis will frequently coexist in middle-aged patients who develop either multiple sclerosis or amyotrophic lateral sclerosis: careful judgement of all available clinical and investigative data is needed to determine the relative importance of the spondylosis and the underlying neurological disease in contributing to the patient's clinical state. The management of amyotrophic lateral sclerosis is discussed in Section 14.2.6.

Primary lateral sclerosis

This is a rare progressive syndrome in which, even after many years, the clinical syndrome is entirely confined to the upper motor neuron (Section 14.8.1). It is generally regarded as a form of motor neuron disease. The presentation is usually in middle age with a slowly progressive spastic paraparesis. Sensory features are absent, and the tempo is slower than that of amyotrophic lateral sclerosis, with patients often surviving for 10 or 15 years or more. Although symptoms first involve lower-limb function, with weakness, stiffness, and difficulty in walking, the upper limbs and bulbar muscles are subsequently, and eventually markedly, involved; in the fully developed syndrome, there is spastic quadriparesis with pseudobulbar palsy. Cognition remains intact and eye movements are not affected. Bladder dysfunction does occur, but usually at a relatively late stage. MRI does not reveal the signal changes in the corticospinal tract seen in amyotrophic lateral sclerosis, but sagittal T1-weighted brain images may reveal focal atrophy of the precentral gyrus (Pringle et al. 1992). Motor evoked potentials reveal a prolonged central motor conduction time, and CSF examination is normal except for a mildly elevated protein in some patients. Treatment of spasticity may be of symptomatic benefit. There is no therapy known to modify the underlying course of the disease; while modest beneficial effects have been seen with riluzole in amyotrophic lateral sclerosis, it has not been investigated in primary lateral sclerosis.

20.6.11 Progressive encephalomyelitis with rigidity

A syndrome is sometimes encountered in which there is increasing limb tone with rigidity, myoclonic jerking, and deep tendon hyperreflexia, evolving over several months. Muscle spasms may be elicited by a variety of sensory stimuli, and evidence of brainstem abnormalities may also appear. Spinal MRI is normal, but the CSF reveals a mononuclear pleocytosis, elevated protein, and oligoclonal bands. Pathologically, changes are most obvious in the cervical region, with loss of interneurons but preservation of anterior horn cells. Inflammatory changes with perivascular lymphocytes and activated microglia are present. Some patients have antibodies to glutamic acid decarboxylase (GAD); the syndrome has features in common with the stiff man syndrome, in which there is a more gradual development of rigidity of the muscles of the trunk and limbs, and in which 50 per cent of patients have anti-GAD antibodies.

Treatment includes drugs to diminish myoclonus (clonazepam, sodium valproate) and rigidity (baclofen, gabapentin). An autoimmune basis to the disease has been suspected and steroids or other immunosuppression may be tried, although evidence for efficacy is lacking; there are occasional reports of a beneficial response to plasma exchange.

20.6.12 Paraneoplastic myelitis

A myelopathy is one of the less common manifestations of paraneoplastic disease; it is seen less often than the better known cerebellar, brainstem, limbic, and sensory ganglionic paraneoplastic syndromes (Section 30.6.5). Nevertheless, a subacute progressive cord syndrome has been described in association with malignancy. The clinical presentation is with motor, sensory, and sphincter deficits evolving over a matter of weeks to months, and has been in association with lung carcinoma and lymphoma. MRI of the cord may be normal, or may reveal gadolinium enhancement over several segments (Mokri *et al.* 1998). CSF reveals a mild mononuclear pleocytosis and protein elevation with oligoclonal bands. As with other paraneoplastic syndromes, treatment may involve two approaches: one to deal with the primary malignancy, the other to use immunosuppression on the grounds that the paraneoplastic syndrome has an immunopathogenic basis. Usually, however, the latter approach is ineffective, and unless the primary tumour can be effectively treated, the prognosis is poor.

20.7 Conus medullaris syndrome

20.7.1 General features

Lesions predominantly involving the conus medullaris are relatively uncommon but are important as they result in a rather characteristic syndrome. Involvement of this lowest part of the cord results in upper motor neuron signs in the lower limbs (e.g. pyramidal weakness from hip flexors downwards, brisk tendon reflexes, and extensor plantar responses), but additional involvement of numerous lumbosacral roots, as they exit the conus in close proximity as the beginning of the cauda equina, will result in lower motor neuron signs such as loss of ankle reflexes and atrophic paralysis of distal lower limb muscles. Sphincter dysfunction is prominent, with urinary incontinence or retention. The sensory disturbance may vary from a predominant lower sacral loss (involving predominantly perianal regions and buttocks in a saddle-shaped distribution) to more extensive loss with a sensory level up to L1. Low back pain may be prominent, especially with infiltrating or bony lesions. The clinical features of conus lesions may be indistinguishable from those involving the cauda equina, and when myelography was the investigation of choice, were sometimes missed because the conus was not properly examined. With lumbosacral MRI studies, both the conus and cauda equina can be readily examined in a single sagittal field of view.

20.7.2 Causes

The conus may be involved by tumours which also frequently involve the cauda equina, especially ependymoma. A secondary metastasis sometimes occurs in this region of the cord. Dural arteriovenous malformations are most often found in the lower thoracic cord and extend to the conus. Inflammatory myelitides, including post-infectious myelitis and schistosomiasis, may predominantly affect the conus.

20.7.3 Management

The management of conus lesions is the same as that for the same pathological process when it occurs elsewhere in the spinal cord or cauda equina (see other sections in this chapter and Chapter 21).

References

Alter, M. (1975). Statistical aspects of spinal cord tumours. In *Handbook of clinical neurology*, (ed. P. J. Vinken and G. W. Bruyn), vol. 19. North Holland, Amsterdam.

Barnett, H. J. M., Foster, J. B., and Hudgson, P. (1973). Syringomyelia. In *Major problems in neurology series*, (ed. J. N. Walton). Saunders, London.

Blau, J. N. and Rushworth, G. (1958). Observations on the blood vessels of the spinal cord and their response to motor activity. *Brain*, **81**, 354–63.

Bolton, B. (1939). The blood supply of the spinal cord. *J. Neurol. Psychiatry*, **2**, 137–48.

Bremer, F. W. (1926). Klinische untersuchungen zur Atiologie der Syringomyelie, der 'Status dysraphicus'. *Deutsch z. Nervenheilkd.*, **95**, 103.

Brewis, M., Poskanzer, D. C., Rolland, C., and Miller, H. G. (1966). Neurological disease in an English city. *Acta Neurol. Scand.*, **42**, Suppl. 24.

Candon, E. and Frerebeau, P. (1994). Abces bacteriens de la moelle epiniere. *Rev. Neurol.*, **150**, 370–6.

Cloward, R. B. (1980). Acute cervical spine injuries. *CIBA Clinical Symposia*, **31**, 1.

Cruickshank, J. K., Rudge, P., Dalgleish, A. G. *et al.* (1989). Tropical spastic paraparesis and human T cell lymphotropic virus type I in the United Kingdom. *Brain*, **112**, 1057–90.

Gardner, W. J. (1965). Hydrodynamic mechanism of syringomyelia: its relationship to myelocoele. *J. Neurol. Neurosurg. Psychiatry*, **28**, 247–59.

Hemmer, B., Glocker, F. X., Schumacher, M. *et al.* (1998). Subacute combined degeneration: clinical, electrophysiological, and magnetic resonance imaging findings. *J. Neurol. Neurosurg. Psychiatry*, **65**, 822–7.

Hernandez, D., Vinuela, F., and Feasby, T. E. (1982). Recurrent paraplegia with total recovery from spontaneous spinal epidural hematoma. *Ann. Neurol.*, **11**, 623–4.

Herzberg, L. and Bayliss, E. (1980). Spinal cord syndrome due to non-compressive Paget's disease. *Lancet*, **ii**, 13–15.

Housmann, O. N. and Moseley, I. F. (1996). Idiopathic dural herniation of the thoracic spinal cord. *Neuroradiology*, **39**, 503–10.

Hughes, J. T. (1971). Venous infarction of the spinal cord. *Neurology*, **21**, 794–800.

Hughes, R. A. C. and Mair, W. G. P. (1973). Acute necrotic myelopathy with pulmonary tuberculosis. *Brain*, **100**, 223–38.

Jacobs, L. D., Beck, R. W., Simon, J. H. *et al.* (2000). Intramuscular inteferon β-1a therapy initiated during a first demyelinating episode in multiple sclerosis. *N. Engl. J. Med.*, **343**, 898–904.

Kagan, R. A., Wollin, M., Gilbert, H. A. *et al.* (1980). Comparison of the tolerance of the brain and spinal cord to injury by radiation. In: *Radiation damage to the nervous system*, (ed. H. A. Gilbert and R. A. Kagan). Raven Press, New York.

Kernohan, J. W., Woltman, H. W., and Adson, A. W. (1931). Intramedullary tumours of the spinal cord. *Arch. Neurol. Psychiatry*, **25**, 679–701.

Mandler, R. N., Davis, L. E., Jeffery, D. R., and Kornfeld, M. K. (1993). Devic's neuromyelitis optica: a clinicopathological study of 8 patients. *Ann. Neurol.*, **34**, 162–8.

Mokri, B., Weinshenker, B. G., Goudreau, J. L. *et al.* (1998). Long tract myelopathy: a novel paraneoplastic syndrome. *Ann. Neurol.*, **44**, 486.

Oppenheimer, D. R. (1978). The cervical cord in multiple sclerosis. *Neuropathol. Appl. Neurobiol.*, **4**, 151–62.

O'Riordan, J. I., Gallagher, H. L., Thompson, A. J. *et al.* (1996). Clinical, CSF, and MRI findings in Devic's neuromyelitis optica. *J. Neurol. Neurosurg. Psychiatry*, **60**, 382–7.

O'Riordan, J. I., Thompson, A. J., Kingsley, D. P. E. *et al.* (1998). The prognostic value of brain MRI in clinically isolated syndromes of the CNS. A 10-year follow-up. *Brain*, **121**, 495–503.

Pringle, C. E., Hudson, A. J., Munoz, D. G. *et al.* (1992). Primary lateral sclerosis. Clinical features, neuropathology and diagnostic criteria. *Brain*, **115**, 495–520.

Quieroz, L. de S., Nucci, A., Facure, N. O., and Facure, J. J. (1979). Massive spinal cord necrosis in schistosomiasis. *Arch. Neurol.*, **36**, 517–19.

Reynolds, E. H. (1981). Pathogenesis of subacute combined degeneration. *Lancet*, **ii**, 1109.

So, Y. T. and Simon, R. P. (1991). Deficiency diseases of the nervous system. In *Neurology in clinical practice*, (ed. W. G. Bradley, R. B. Daroff, G. M. Fenichel, and C. D. Marsden). Butterworth-Heinemann, Boston.

Spencer, P. S., Roy, D. N., Ludolph, A. *et al.* (1986). Lathyrism: evidence for role of the neuroexcitatory amino acid BOAA. *Lancet*, **ii**, 1066–7.

Spiller, W. G. (1909). Thrombosis of the cervical anterior median spinal artery: syphilitic acute anterior poliomyelitis. *J. Nerv. Ment. Dis.*, **36**, 601–13.

Stark, R. J., Henson, R. A., and Evans, S. J. W. (1982). Spinal metastases. A retrospective survey from a general hospital. *Brain*, **105**, 189–213.

Stevens, J. M., Cartlidge, N. E. F., Saunders, M. *et al.* (1971). Atlantoaxial subluxation and cervical myelopathy in rheumatoid arthritis. *QJM*, **40**, 391–408.

Stevens, J. M., Serva, W. A., Kendall, B. E. *et al.* (1993). Chiari malformation in adults: relation of morphological aspects to clinical features and operative outcome. *J. Neurol. Neurosurg. Psychiatry*, **56**, 1072–7.

Stevenson, V., Leary, S. M., Losseff, N. A. *et al.* (1998). Spinal cord atrophy and disability in MS. A longitudinal study. *Neurology*, **51**, 234–8.

Thomas, P. K., Hoffbrand, A. V., and Smith, A. S. (1982). Neurological involvement in hereditary transcobalamin II deficiency. *J. Neurol. Neurosurg. Psychiatry*, **45**, 74–7.

Thorpe, J. W., Moseley, I. F., Hawkes, C. H. *et al.* (1996). Brain and spinal cord MRI abnormalities in motor neurone disease. *J. Neurol. Neurosurg. Psychiatry*, **61**, 314–17.

Tomlinson, B. E., Irving, D., and Rebeiz, J. J. (1973). Total numbers of limb motor neurones in the human lumbosacral cord and an analysis of the accuracy of various sampling procedures. *J. Neurol. Sci.*, **20**, 313–27.

Tosi, L., Rigoli, G., and Beltramello, A. (1996). Fibrocartilaginous embolism of the spinal cord : a clinical and pathogenetic consideration. *J. Neurol. Neurosurg. Psychiatry*, **60**, 55–60.

Wilkinson, M. (1973). *Cervical spondylosis*, (2nd edn). Heinemann, London.

CHAPTER 21

Cauda equina, spinal roots, and sphincter control

David Miller

21.1 The innervation of the bladder, rectum, corpora cavernosa, and seminal vesicles

21.1.1 Anatomy and physiology: bladder

The parasympathetic nerve supply from the second and third sacral nerves (the nervi erigentes) joins the vesical plexuses. It is doubtful if there is a separately innervated internal sphincter. When the parasympathetic is stimulated, the longitudinal fibres of the detrusor pull the bladder neck open and the circular fibres exert pressure on the bladder contents. The physiology of micturition is discussed by Pearman and England (1976), and the pathophysiology of incontinence by Swash (1985).

The sympathetic fibres to the bladder arise chiefly from the first and second lumbar ganglia, with contributions from the third and fourth. These fibres unite to form the presacral nerve or superior hypogastric plexus, which lies in front of the aortic bifurcation. From this plexus come the two hypogastric nerves, each ending in the vesical plexuses on the lateral aspect of the bladder.

In the 1950s it was concluded by several workers that because so little effect upon bladder function was noted in humans following sympathetic stimulation, the parasympathetic innervation of the detrusor alone was important. However, it was later recognized that there are indeed functional α- and β-adrenergic sympathetic fibres innervating the muscle of the bladder wall. β-Receptors predominate in the bladder wall and stimulation of these allows the bladder to fill; α-receptors are more profuse in the neck of the organ, and stimulation of these causes the internal sphincter to contract. Phenoxybenzamine, which blocks α-receptors, will open the bladder neck; it also has an effect in blocking muscarinic cholinergic receptors and so increases functional bladder capacity. These ideas have been modified by careful analysis of the effects of electrical stimulation of the hypogastric plexus and sacral nerve roots in paraplegic men and women (Brindley 1986, 1988), suggesting that the sympathetic system is much less important in humans than the parasympathetic system in the control of micturition.

In infancy, bladder evacuation occurs reflexly, the reflex arc running through the sacral cord segments. The development of control over bladder evacuation is associated with increasing ability to inhibit the evacuation reflex. Control of the inhibitory impulses lies in the sympathetic system, which maintains closure of the sphincter and inhibits contraction of the detrusor muscles. At the same time it becomes possible voluntarily to overcome this inhibition and so to initiate the act of micturition, which is then completed reflexly. Thus there are three nervous mechanisms controlling bladder function—the sacral reflex arc for evacuation; the inhibitory influence of the sympathetic; and voluntary control which overcomes the latter and initiates micturition. Voluntary control of the autonomically innervated musculature is supported by the actions of the muscles of the pelvic floor and rhabdosphincters of the urethra and anus innervated by the pudendal nerve. These help to maintain continence, and when they are relaxed and the voluntary abdominal wall muscles contract, intra-abdominal pressure increases and the acts of micturition and defecation are assisted. Weakness of these muscles thus potentiates any failure of the autonomic control system.

Bladder sensation, giving a feeling of fullness and a desire to micturate, travels centrally in the second and third sacral nerve roots and the spinothalamic tracts, as does that concerned with urethral pain, while urethral touch and pressure travel in the posterior columns.

The part of the postcentral gyrus lying at the vertex of the cerebral hemisphere is the cortical centre for bladder sensation, and the corresponding area of the precentral gyrus is probably the site of origin of motor impulses initiating the act of micturition. It is well recognized that parasagittal lesions which affect this region bilaterally can cause urinary retention. Unilateral or, more often, bilateral lesions in the superior frontal gyrus may give urgency and frequency of micturition and incontinence, or sometimes retention, and the sensation giving rise to the desire to micturate is diminished or absent. There is also evidence to suggest a probable micturition control centre in the pons in humans and other mammalian species (Griffiths et al. 1990, Blok et al. 1997), which may explain why lesions in this region are occasionally associated with urinary hesitancy or retention.

The voluntary initiation of micturition usually occurs in response to an awareness of bladder distension. The descending motor pathway concerned with voluntary bladder evacuation lies in the lateral columns of the spinal cord on an equatorial plane passing through the central canal.

21.1.2 Disturbances of bladder function involving the sacral reflex arc

Since the sacral reflex arc is concerned in the evacuation of the bladder, its interruption usually causes retention of urine, due to the unopposed action of the sympathetic. In tabes dorsalis, the reflex is interrupted on its afferent side, because of degeneration of the afferent neurons. Lesions of the conus medullaris interrupt the central fibres of the reflex. Lesions of the cauda equina, if they destroy the second and third sacral nerves, interrupt both the afferent and efferent paths of the reflex and hence usually cause retention of urine. Even after severe but incomplete lesions of the conus or cauda equina, however, 'reflex' evacuation of the bladder may occasionally develop. However, in cauda equina lesions and in tabes the bladder is more usually atonic, that is, it accepts a very large volume of urine and slowly distends without contracting reflexly to raise the intravesical pressure.

21.1.3 Disturbances of bladder function due to spinal cord lesions

Incomplete lesions of the spinal cord above the conus medullaris may affect principally either inhibitory fibres destined for the sympathetic outflow, or descending fibres concerned in the voluntary initiation of micturition. In the former case, the patient has difficulty in holding urine and micturition is precipitate. This so-called urgency is a common symptom in the early stages of multiple sclerosis. Moderately severe but still incomplete lesions of the cord tend to impair voluntary control over micturition, so that urinary retention develops, owing to uninhibited action of the sympathetic. A combination of loss of both voluntary control and sympathetic inhibition will result in both retention (revealed as an increase in amount of urine remaining in the bladder immediately after voluntary micturition) and urgency/urge incontinence (due to loss of sympathetic inhibition); such a combination is a common finding in cord disorders such as multiple sclerosis, and the resulting pathophysiological abnormality of the bladder muscles is known as detrusor-sphincter-dyssynergia.

After complete interruption of conduction in the spinal cord, either by transection or by severe transverse lesions above the conus, there is initially retention during the phase of spinal shock, but subsequently enhancement of reflex activity develops in the distal portion, and reflex evacuation of the bladder then occurs through the sacral reflex arc. It may be facilitated by stimuli applied to the sacral cutaneous areas. After some massive lesions of the sacral segments or cord, the bladder remains atonic, presumably because of destruction of the sacral reflex arc in the conus or adjacent cauda equina.

21.1.4 Disturbances of bladder function due to cerebral lesions

The fibres concerned in the voluntary initiation of micturition may be interrupted above the spinal cord, and retention of urine may then develop, usually in association with severe bilateral corticospinal tract signs. Lesions involving the vertical region of the precentral cortex on both sides may also cause retention. Dysfunction of this part of the cerebral cortex or of pathways that descend from it probably account for retention of urine, or for urgency and incontinence, which are not uncommon symptoms of intracranial tumour, anterior communicating artery aneurysm, normal pressure hydrocephalus, or of diffuse cerebral disorders, including Alzheimer's disease and other dementing processes.

Nocturnal enuresis in otherwise normal children probably arises in the first place as a result of delay in developing inhibition of reflex bladder evacuation. Later, for psychological reasons, the child acquires abnormal conditioned reflexes whereby bladder evacuation continues to occur during sleep. Rarely, however, enuresis in childhood can be due to spinal cord or cauda equina lesions associated with spina bifida occulta.

21.1.5 Myotonia of the urethral sphincter

Urinary retention in young women in the absence of overt neurological disease was, for many years, a disorder of uncertain cause, although psychogenic mechanisms were often thought to be important. In the past decade, many such individuals have been discovered to exhibit abnormal electromyogram (EMG)

activity in the urethral sphincter. Typically, abnormal discharges of a myotonic type, with complex repetitive discharges and decelerating bursts, are described (Fowler 1999). The aetiology is uncertain. The condition manifests only in pre-menopausal women, and has been associated with polycystic ovaries, raising the possibility that the myotonia is in some way related to a hormonal abnormality. Clinical neurological examination is normal, as is imaging of the brain, spinal cord, and cauda equina. Treatment has been unsatisfactory, and voiding difficulties may persist for months or years. Recently, sacral nerve stimulation has been helpful for some patients.

21.1.6 The rectum and abnormalities of defecation

The nerve supply of the rectum is similar to that of the bladder, and micturition and defecation are physiologically comparable except that in the rectum voluntary control is exerted over the external sphincter only and the rectum lacks voluntary inhibition.

After destruction of the sacral innervation of the rectum, automatic activity, dependent upon a parasympathetic plexus in its wall, develops, the rectum contracting and the sphincter relaxing in response to a rise of tension within the viscus. This reflex activity is much more complete when the sacral innervation is intact, e.g. after complete transverse division of the spinal cord above the sacral enlargement. Owing to the relatively limited force of rectal contraction, however, it is at best not very efficient and there is a tendency for all disturbances of rectal innervation to cause constipation, although after complete transverse division of the spinal cord, reflex defecation sometimes occurs and may be facilitated by cutaneous stimuli applied to the sacral cutaneous areas. Although less common than constipation, some patients with spinal cord disease develop faecal urgency and incontinence. In most patients with complete spinal cord or cauda equina lesions, satisfactory control of the bowels is eventually achieved by means of twice-weekly enemas or suppositories or by manual evacuation of faeces.

21.1.7 The innervation of the seminal vesicles and corpora cavernosa

The seminal vesicles are innervated from the hypogastric plexus. The corpora cavernosa also receive a sympathetic supply from the hypogastric plexus and, in addition, a parasympathetic supply from S2. In higher mammals, stimulation of the hypogastric plexus may cause either erection or shrinkage of the penis, but in man only erection has been observed, accompanied by seminal emission (Brindley 1988). Erection has also been obtained in man by stimulation of the second sacral nerve root.

21.2 Signs of spinal-nerve root lesions

Dermatomal topography is shown in Fig. 21.1.

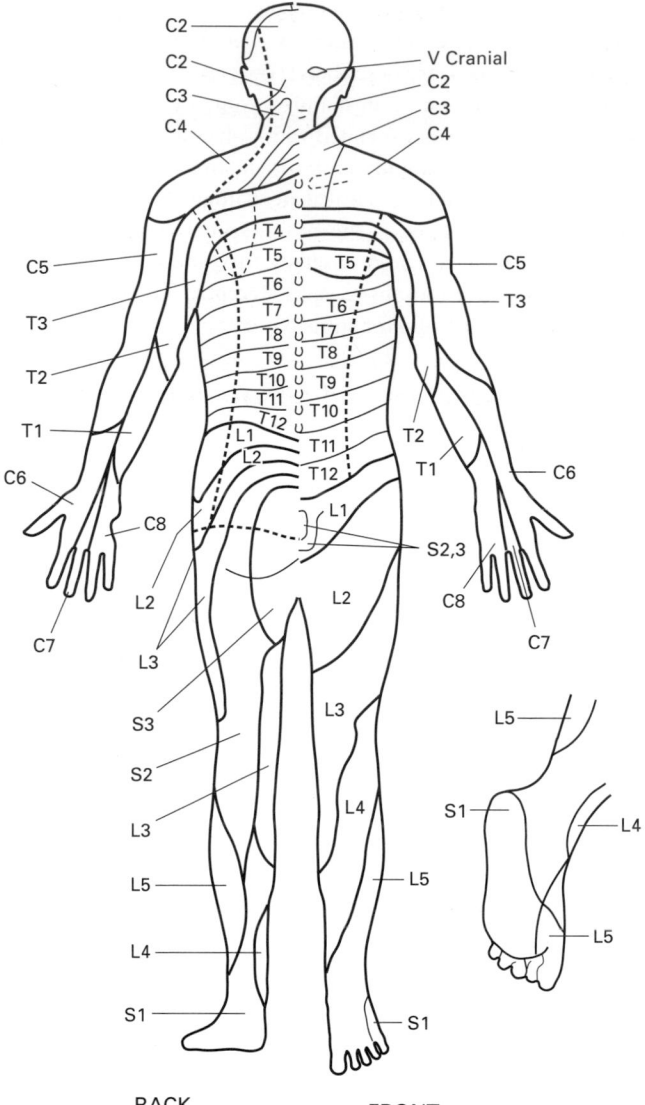

Fig. 21.1. The dermatomes.

21.2.1 Cervical root lesions

C1–3 Sensory loss is found over the back (C2) and side (C3) of the neck; motor supply to a number of neck muscles is interrupted but is not usually clinically apparent.

C4 There is sensory loss in a cape distribution between the side of the neck and the top of the shoulder. Unilateral lesions cause weakness of rhomboids. Bilateral lesions of C2–4 may cause bilateral diaphragm paralysis, manifested as dyspnoea and a reduced vital capacity, especially pronounced on lying flat.

C5 Sensory loss extends from the outer surface of the shoulder down into the lateral arm and forearm. There is weakness and wasting of deltoids, spinati, and pectorals, with loss of the pectoral reflex.

C6 Sensory loss involves the distal lateral forearm and hand, the thumb, and sometimes the index finger. There is weakness

and wasting of biceps brachii, brachioradialis, forearm flexors, and pronator teres. The biceps jerk is absent. The triceps jerk may also be reduced or absent.

C7 Sensory loss involves the index, middle and ring fingers, and a strip in the middle of the hand both on the palmar and dorsal surface. There is weakness and wasting of triceps, wrist and sometimes finger extensors and supinator. The triceps jerk is absent.

C8 Sensory loss involves the little finger, and medial aspect of the hand and forearm. There is wasting and weakness of intrinsic hand muscles, especially interossei, and hypothenar eminence, and sometimes weakness of finger extension. The finger flexion reflex is lost.

21.2.2 Thoracic root lesions

T1 Sensory loss involves the medial aspect of the proximal forearm and upper arm. There is weakness and wasting of the muscles of the thenar eminence

T2–T12 There is a band of sensory loss unilaterally at a level on the trunk according to each nerve. It is helpful to remember that there is an interface of the C4 and T2 dermatomes at the upper chest level, the nipple is approximately T4 and the umbilicus is at approximately T10. Although the muscle supply to intercostal muscles or abdominal wall muscles may be interrupted, there are usually no clinical motor signs of a unilateral lesion, except for a loss of abdominal reflex at the appropriate level (T9–10 for upper abdominal reflexes, T11–12 for lower abdominal reflexes).

21.2.3 Lumbar root lesions

L1 Sensory loss is found in the groin and upper buttock, and there is weakness of iliopsoas.

L2 Sensory loss occurs over the proximal anterior and medial thigh. There is weakness of hip flexion and adduction.

L3 Sensation is lost over distal anterior and medial thigh and medial aspect of the knee. There is weakness of hip flexors and may be mild weakness of quadriceps.

L4 Sensory loss occurs over the anterior and medial shin. There is weakness and wasting of quadriceps, and some weakness of tibialis anterior and ankle inversion. The knee jerk is absent.

L5 The loss of sensation is most apparent on the dorsum and inner aspect of the foot. There is weakness and wasting of the anterior tibial muscles, leading to footdrop and weakness of toe dorsiflexion and eversion. Hip abduction is also weak due to involvement of gluteal muscles.

21.2.4 Sacral root lesions

S1 Sensory loss occurs on the sole and outer aspects of the foot, as well as the calf. There is weakness of plantar flexion of the foot and toes. The ankle jerk is absent. Hip abduction and extension may be weak.

S2–S5 The main findings are of sensory loss, involving the back of the thigh (S2) the buttocks (S3–5) in a saddle-shaped distribution, and the perineum (S5). Bladder retention is the rule with bilateral lesions involving multiple sacral roots in the cauda equina.

21.3 Cauda equina syndromes

21.3.1 Neoplasms compressing the cauda equina

Compression of the cauda equina is most often due to a neoplasm (usually ependymoma or neurofibroma, rarely chordoma, lymphoma, or meningioma), but the nerves may be compressed by an associated lipoma in cases of spina bifida occulta, by a constricting fibrous band, or by chronic arachnoiditis. Ependymomas and neurofibromas are almost equally common, occurring more often in men than in women. Perineurial cysts on the posterior sacral roots are often asymptomatic but may cause sciatic pain; rarely, if ever, do they give rise to other manifestations of cauda equina compression.

The clinical picture is variable, depending upon the site and extent of the source of compression. It may be virtually impossible clinically to distinguish between a neoplasm arising in the cauda equina itself and one arising in the conus medullaris and extending into the cauda. A small tumour may, for a long time, compress only one or two roots on one side. A large and massive growth may involve the whole of the cauda. For anatomical reasons, the lower roots are more likely to be compressed than the upper, since they suffer alone when a growth is situated in the lowest part of the spinal canal, but are also implicated, together with the upper roots, by tumours at a higher level.

In many cases of cauda equina tumour, pain is the earliest symptom (Fearnside and Adams 1978). It is usually felt in the lumbar or sacral regions as a dull, aching pain which is liable to be exacerbated by jerky movements, coughing, or sneezing. Less often it is referred to one or both lower limbs in the distribution of the lower spinal nerves, or it may be referred to the bladder, rectum, or testis.

Motor symptoms consist of weakness and wasting, in a distribution depending on which nerve is affected. Most often there is paralysis of the muscles below the knee (although the tibialis anterior may escape) and of the hamstrings and glutei. In such cases, the ankle jerks are diminished or lost, and the plantar responses may be absent; but the knee jerks are often preserved.

The distribution of sensory loss also depends on which spinal nerves are involved. Compression of the lower sacral dorsal roots or nerves gives a characteristic saddle-shaped area of anaesthesia and analgesia, extending over the perineum, buttocks, and back of the thighs. Compression of the upper sacral and fifth lumbar nerves produces an area of sensory loss over the foot and over the posterior and outer aspect of the leg. When the lowest sacral segments are involved, although the external genitals are anaesthetic, and the patient may be unaware of the passage of a catheter, some bladder sensation usually remains, so that the patient is aware when it distends.

Disturbance of sphincter control is usual but may be unexpectedly late in developing. Compression of the third and fourth ventral and dorsal sacral roots interrupts the reflex arc upon which evacuation of the bladder and rectum depends. The result is retention of urine and faeces due to the unopposed contraction of the internal sphincters, even though the external sphincters are paralysed. Erectile dysfunction occurs in the male. When the lowest sacral nerves are compressed, the anal and bulbocavernosus reflexes are lost.

Trophic changes may occur in the lower limbs, which are often cold and cyanosed, and tend to become oedematous. Slight injuries in analgesic areas can lead to sores which are slow to heal.

The investigation and management of tumours in the cauda equina is similar to that described for spinal cord tumours (see Chapter 20).

21.3.2 Degenerative lumbosacral disease and cauda equina syndromes

Compression of the cauda equina may occur acutely as a result of a central intervertebral disc protrusion. This usually involves one of the lower lumbar discs. Bladder retention is a prominent early symptom and sensory findings characteristically show a saddle-shaped sensory loss over the buttocks or perineum. MRI will readily display the disc protrusion. This condition is a neurosurgical emergency—the prognosis for recovery of bladder function is related to the delay between symptom onset and surgical decompression.

Chronic degenerative changes, such as disc protrusion and osteophytic hypertrophy of the lumbar vertebrae and facet joints, can lead to stenosis of the lumbar canal. This is especially likely if there is pre-existing congenital narrowing of the canal. A striking symptom of lumbar canal stenosis is a poor exertional tolerance, with the development of weakness or pain in the lower limbs on walking. This symptom of spinal claudication may be confused with the claudicating symptoms of peripheral vascular disease. MRI reveals degenerative vertebral column changes and narrowing of the lumbosacral canal, often at multiple levels, especially mid to lower lumbar (Fig. 21.2). Decompressive laminectomy may be performed, especially in the presence of a progressing neurological deficit.

21.3.3 Non-compressive disease of the cauda equina: arachnoiditis

Arachnoiditis can involve any level in the spinal column but is nowadays most commonly found in the lumbosacral region, thus causing a cauda equina syndrome. Pachymeningitis involving both the dura and the arachnoid, and resulting from meningovascular syphilis or from the spread of a staphylococcal

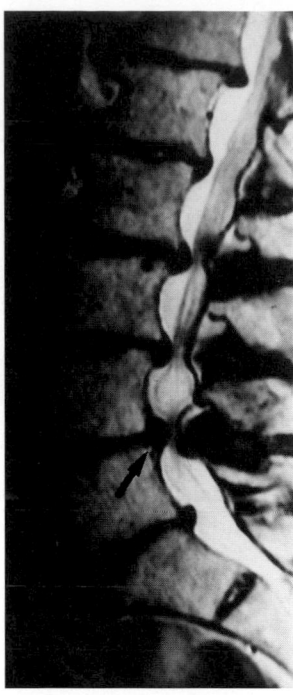

Fig. 21.2. Sagittal T2-weighted MRI in a patient with lumbar canal stenosis. There is narrowing at multiple levels with marked canal stenosis at the L4–5 level (arrow). (Courtesy of Dr J. Stevens.)

or tuberculous infection of the vertebra, was once common but is now very rare. Localized or diffuse arachnoiditis of variable aetiology is now seen more often, although it is still comparatively uncommon. Sometimes the arachnoidal adhesions enclose encysted collections of CSF. Meningococcal, pneumococcal, and viral meningitis have all been known to be followed by arachnoiditis, but granulomatous meningeal processes such as syphilis, cryptococcosis, tuberculosis, or sarcoidosis are more common, although the latter condition more often produces extra- and intramedullary mass lesions. Trauma has also been implicated as a cause, and there is evidence that lumbar intervertebral disc prolapse is sometimes responsible; perhaps, in consequence, lumbosacral arachnoiditis causing a cauda equina syndrome is substantially more common than cervical or thoracic involvement giving paraparesis (Shaw *et al.* 1978). In many cases, despite full investigation, the aetiology remains obscure, and the idiopathic condition is, on rare occasions, familial.

Tuberculous meningitis limited to the spinal cord is a cause of adhesive arachnoiditis in some tropical countries, but tuberculous meningomyelitis is also seen in Britain. Other occasional causes include epidural and spinal anaesthesia, and symptomatic arachnoiditis has also been described as a sequel to myelography using oil-based contrast media. Blood in the theca and intrathecal injections of steroids or methotrexate have been implicated. Although arachnoiditis can interfere with function of the cord as well as the cauda equina and spinal roots, cord compression probably plays comparatively little part in its ill

effects, and interference with the blood supply to the cord seems to be more important.

The cauda equina syndrome which sometimes complicates ankylosing spondylitis (Matthews 1968), is of uncertain pathogenesis but may sometimes be due to arachnoiditis, or more often to associated arachnoid cysts.

MRI in arachnoiditis of the cauda equina shows loss of the normal homogeneous high-signal CSF on T2-weighted images, with clumping of nerve roots and distortion of their passage through the thecal sac. In idiopathic cases, there is no satisfactory treatment.

21.4 Cervical radiculopathy

21.4.1 Spondylitic radiculopathy

Cervical spondylitic changes affect almost all individuals with advancing age, but in many remain only an asymptomatic radiological finding. The changes seen include loss of the disc space, sclerosis of disc margins and facet joints, and osteophytic lipping of vertebrae. Myelopathy occurs when there is significant narrowing of the spinal canal with cord compression. Radiculopathy occurs when the spondylitic process encroaches on the nerve root canal. A combination of radiculopathy and myelopathy often coexists.

Spondylosis most often involves the fifth, sixth, and seventh cervical vertebra and the roots most often compromised are C6 and C7. Pain and sensory loss in the appropriate dermatome may be seen along with segmental weakness, wasting, and reflex loss affecting the relevant myotome (Section 21.2). Neck pain is sometimes, but not always, a feature.

Treatment of radiculopathy may be conservative, with the use of a collar and adequate analgesia, and such an approach is sometimes successful in reducing pain and motor signs. Surgery is often effective in reducing symptoms; the nerve root canal is enlarged either via an anterior or posterior approach. The latter approach, although technically easier, leaves the diseased space mobile with a higher risk of continued spondylitic pain.

21.4.2 Acute cervical disc prolapse

The nucleus pulposus of cervical discs may degenerate and then rupture through the posterior annulus into the spinal canal, resulting in compressions of roots if, as is most common, the prolapse is lateral, or of the cord if the protrusion is central. Disc prolapse can occur at any level, but is most common in the mid to lower cervical region (i.e. C4–5, C5–6, and C6–7). Either radiculopathy or myelopathy. or both, may result, but the former is more common. Acute disc prolapse is often intensely painful, with aggravation by neck movement, coughing, or sneezing, and radicular pain which is aggravated by similar factors is usually present. Sometimes pain is the only manifestation; in other instances it is conjoined with sensory and motor symptoms and signs pointing to a root lesion. The nature of the neurological manifestations depends on the root involved (see Section 21.2).

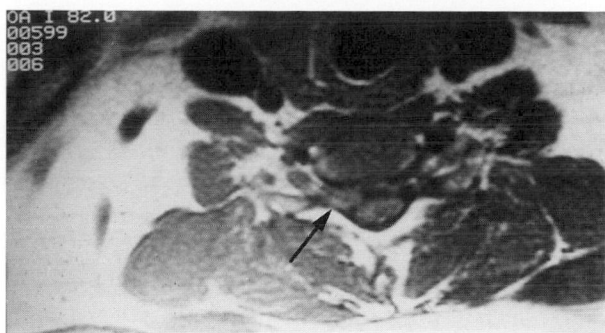

Fig. 21.3. Axial T1-weighted MRI through the cervical cord in a patient with a right-sided lateral C5–6 disc prolapse (arrow), causing a right C6 radiculopathy (courtesy of Dr J. Stevens).

Lateral plain cervical spine radiography may reveal narrowing of the intervertebral disc space, but the main investigation is MRI, which will reveal protrusion of the disc (Fig. 21.3); in the usual instance of lateral protrusion with compression of the root in the intervertebral foramen, this is best appreciated on axial T2-weighted images (Fig. 21.4); the high-signal cuff of CSF surrounding the root as it passes into the foramen is reduced or obliterated and the soft-tissue mass of the protruding disc is visible.

Many disc protrusions may be treated conservatively, especially if pain is the predominant symptom. Large prolapses with clear radicular deficits usually require surgery, and this may be needed urgently when deficits are acute. A central disc prolapse leading to myelopathy needs to be decompressed by an anterior route; a lateral disc prolapse causing radiculopathy may be treated successfully by posterior foraminal decompression.

21.4.3 Other causes of cervical radiculopathy

Inflammatory, infective, or infiltrative processes involving the meninges can involve one or more nerve roots at any level of the spinal cord. Disorders to consider in this regard include infections such as tuberculosis, syphilis, Lyme disease, cytomegalovirus (in immuncompromised patients with HIV the latter typically causes a painful lumbosacral radiculopathy), sarcoidosis, and a malignant meningitis due to carcinoma, lymphoma, or leukaemia. The carcinomas that most often disseminate to the meninges are those of lung and breast. Non-enhanced MRI may be normal but gadolinium-enhanced studies will usually demonstrate diffuse, patchy, multifocal or nodular meningeal enhancement around the spinal cord and in the cauda equina (Fig. 21.5), and also extending to involve the intracranial meninges in many instances. CSF examination is of crucial value; an increase in mononuclear white cells and protein is usual, and glucose may be reduced, especially in malignant or tuberculous meningitis. Appropriate microbiological investigations should be undertaken to detect infective aetiologies. Cytology is required to look for malignant cells; sometimes repeat lumbar puncture and the collection of a larger than usual sample is necessary before the malignant cells are detected. In a few patients with meningoradiculopathy, in whom all other central nervous system and systemically

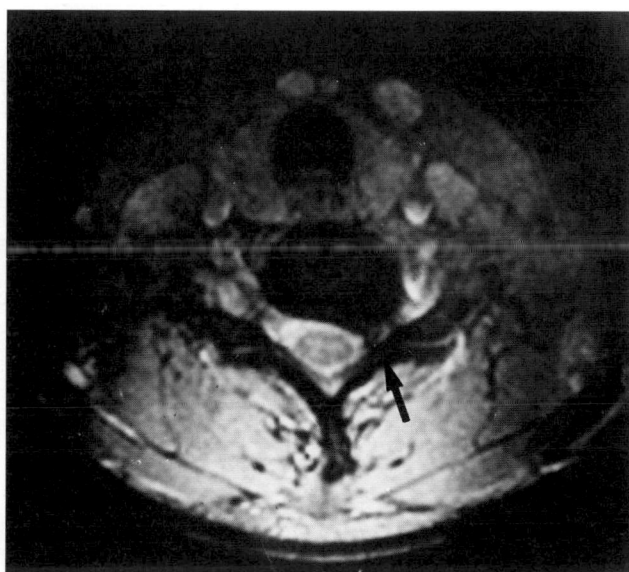

Fig. 21.4. Axial T2-weighted MRI through the cervical canal in a patient with a left C5–6 disc prolapse, causing a left C6 radiculopathy. The lateral protrusion is compressing the root in the intervertebral foramen, where there is loss of the normal sleeve of high signal from CSF surrounding the nerve (arrow). (Courtesy of Dr J. Stevens.)

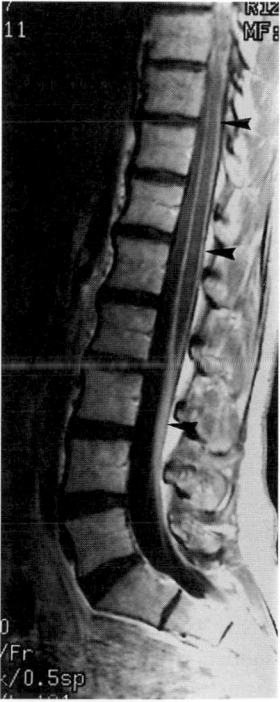

Fig. 21.5. Sagittal gadolinium-enhanced T1-weighted MRI through the thoracolumbar region in a patient with Lyme disease and meningoradiculitis. There is diffuse enhancement of the meninges surrounding the thoracic cord and of the nerve roots in the cauda equina (arrows). (Courtesy of Dr J. Stevens)

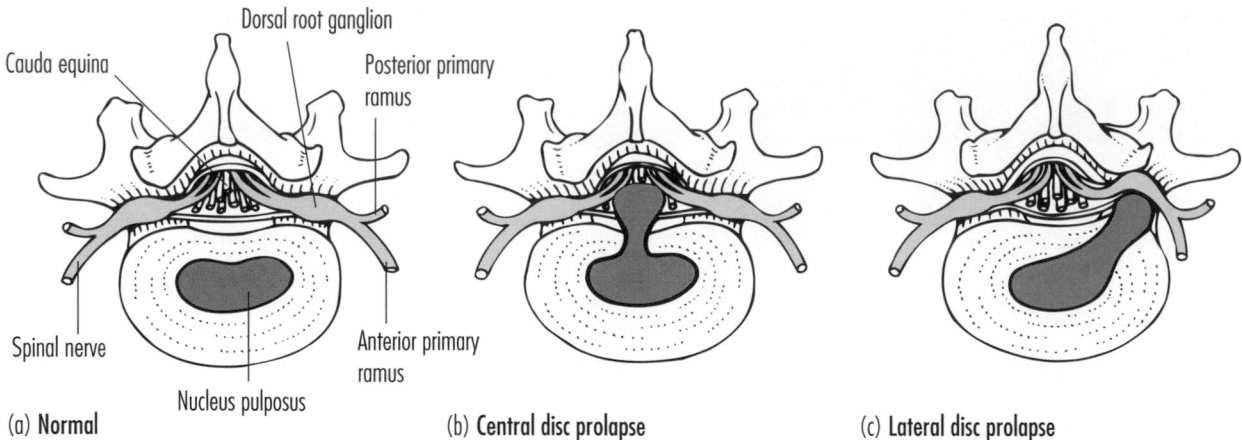

(a) Normal   (b) **Central disc prolapse**   (c) **Lateral disc prolapse**

Fig. 21.6.   (a) The normal relationship between the lumbar intervertebral discs and the nerve roots. (b) Central and (c) lateral prolapse of a lumbar intervertebral disc, causing compression of (b) the cauda equina and (c) the exiting nerve root, respectively (from Donaghy, M. (1997). *Neurology.* Oxford University Press).

directed investigations are non-diagnostic, meningeal biopsy is required; this is most appropriately directed towards an area of meninges that displays gadolinium enhancement on MRI.

21.5 Lumbosacral radiculopathy

21.5.1 Lumbosacral disc degeneration and prolapse

By far the most common cause of lumbosacral radiculopathy is lumbar disc degeneration and prolapse. As in the cervical spine, some degeneration in the lumbosacral region is an almost universal feature of ageing. Degenerative changes of the intervertebral discs become increasingly common with increasing age, occurring most frequently at the L4–5 and L5–S1 levels, where movements of the spine are perhaps greater. Thus L5 or S1 radiculopathy is by far the most common seen in clinical practice. The nucleus pulposus of the disc becomes extruded through a weakened annulus fibrosis. The most common direction of the protrusion is posterolateral, leading to compression of the nerve root and radicular symptoms and signs; less often a large central protrusion leads to an acute cauda equina syndrome (see Section 21.3) (Fig. 21.6).

The most common symptom is low back pain, which may be chronic and of variable severity or which may develop as a severe sudden pain due to acute disc prolapse. Low back pain due to disc prolapse may be difficult to distinguish from other non-specific musculoskeletal disorders. However, acute prolapse may present in a very characteristic way. The ictus may be precipitated by heavy lifting, and sudden severe back pain is typically associated with sciatica, the pains being aggravated by bending, walking, coughing, sneezing, and even sitting. Pain from an L4–5 or L5–S1 radiculopathy radiates from the buttock down the back or side of the leg to the ankle or foot, and may be associated with paraesthesia or numbness in a similar distribution.

Examination will reveal limitation of straight leg raising due to sciatic pain in the case of lower lumbar disc prolapses, or limitation of hip extension in the less common situation of upper lumbar root compression. The motor and sensory signs will depend on the root or roots involved (Section 21.2); the signs are normally unilateral and indicate involvement of only one, or sometimes two, roots.

MRI is now the preferred diagnostic investigation, with sagittal views being complemented by axial views through the level of the intervertebral foramina where the prolapse is thought to exist. On sagittal images, signal change of the intervertebral disc (reduced signal on T2-weighted images) and reduction of the height of the intervertebral space indicate the presence of disc

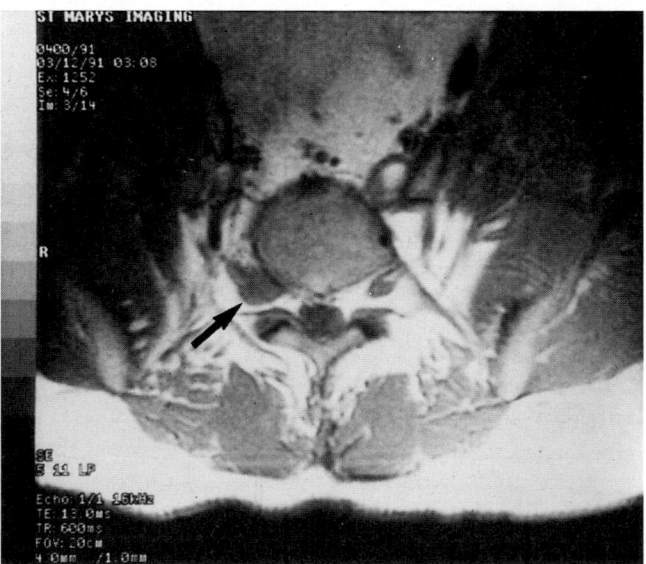

Fig. 21.7. Axial T1-weighted MRI of a patient with an L4-5 intervertebral disc prolapse, resulting in a right L5 radiculopathy. Note the right-sided posterolateral herniation of the disc (arrow) which is compromising the exiting L5 root. (Courtesy of Dr J. Stevens.)

degeneration and dehydration. Axial images are required to demonstrate the posterolateral protrusion with compromise of the nerve root in the region of the intervertebral foramen (Fig. 21.7). CT scanning with axial images will also demonstrate the majority of disc prolapses, but has largely been superceded by MRI given the better soft-tissue discrimination and multiplane imaging that is possible with the latter modality; sagittal imaging also allows views of the conus, an important fact given that a clinical picture of lumbosacral radiculopathy can sometimes be a manifestation of a conus lesion.

Management depends on the duration and severity of symptoms. When pain is the major symptom, conservative treatment with bed rest and analgesia frequently leads to remission. The decision on whether to treat surgically should take into account the severity of signs and length of history. Acute motor weakness, e.g. footdrop from an L5 root lesion, is usually treated surgically, and in the majority of cases with good results in the short term. A not infrequent longer-term complication is fibrosis around the operative site of disc removal, which may lead to recurrent radicular pain and neurological signs. Repeat gadolinium-enhanced MRI assists the distinction from recurrent disc prolapse, the fibrotic reaction being seen as an area of enhancing tissue in the region of the nerve root and canal. Post-surgical fibrosis is treated symptomatically.

21.5.2 Spondylolisthesis

Congenital abnormalities of the facet joints may lead to slipping of the L4 vertebra on L5, or the L5 vertebra on S1. In this situation, the upper vertebra of the pair moves forwards. This results in pain and, if the slip is large, there is occasionally a neurological syndrome as a result of trapping of nerve roots. The resulting syndrome may be one of an isolated lower lumbar radiculopathy or of a more widespread cauda equina syndrome. In such circumstances, surgical procedures may be used to stabilize the vertebrae and relieve the neural compression.

21.5.3 Lumbosacral radiculitis or infiltration

A number of inflammatory disorders produce a syndrome in which there is prominent involvement of several lumbosacral nerve roots. Occasional cases may be due to herpes simplex type 2 infection. This form of herpes virus, which causes genital herpes, may in a few patients be associated with attacks of recurrent aseptic meningitis, or with an acute lumbosacral radiculitis. The latter manifests as urinary retention, weakness of distal lower limb muscles with loss of ankle or knee jerks, and sensory loss, mainly in a sacral or lower lumbar distribution. The neurological episode may be in association with, or separate from, an episode of genital herpes. CSF reveals a mononuclear pleocytosis, and the polymerase chain reaction for herpes simplex type 2 virus DNA is positive. Treatment should be started promptly with intravenous acyclovir.

Cytomegalovirus infection is a recognized cause of a lumbosacral radiculopathy in patients with AIDS, and may be treated with ganciclovir and foscarnet.

Chronic inflammatory demyelinating polyneuropathy is sometimes associated with enlargement of nerve roots in the cauda equina and peripheral nerves elsewhere; the former may be depicted on MRI as demonstrating gadolinium enhancement. The enlargement is due to onion-bulb formation due to repeated efforts at Schwann-cell-mediated remyelination. There may rarely be clinical evidence of a cauda equina syndrome; treatment is that for the underlying polyneuropathy. Another non-inflammatory demyelinating neuropathy which occasionally manifests with local mass effect due to enlarged lumbosacral nerve roots is hereditary motor and sensory neuropathy type III, also sometimes known as hypertrophic polyneuropathy or Dejerine–Sottas syndrome.

Other infiltrative or inflammatory meningeal processes that may involve the lumbosacral roots, predominantly or in conjunction with more widespread disease, include sarcoidosis, lymphoma, leukaemia, and carcinomatous meningeal infiltration (especially breast and lung).

References

Blok, B., Willemsen, T., and Holstege, G. (1997). A PET study of brain control of micturition in humans. *Brain*, **129**, 111–21.

Brindley, G. S. (1986). Sacral root and hypogastric plexus stimulators and what these models tell us about autonomic actions of the bladder and urethra. *Clin. Sci.*, **70** (Suppl. 14), 41S.

Brindley, G. S. (1988). The actions of parasympathetic and sympathetic nerves in human micturition, erection and seminal emission, and their restoration in paraplegic patients by implanted electrical stimulation. *Proc. R. Soc. Med.*, **235**, 111.

Fearnside, M. R. and Adams, C. B. T. (1978). Tumours of the cauda equina. *J. Neurol. Neurosurg. Psychiatry*, **41**, 24–31.

Fowler, C. J. (1999). Neurological disorders of micturition and their treatment. *Brain*, **122**, 1213–31.

Griffiths, D., Holstege, C., de Wall, H. *et al.* (1990). Control and coordination of bladder and urethral function in the brainstem of the cat. *Neurourol. Urodynamics*, **9**, 63–82.

Matthews, W. B. (1968). Neurological complications of ankylosing spondylitis. *J. Neurol. Sci.*, **6**, 561–73.

Pearman, J. W. and England, E. J. (1976). The urinary tract. In *Handbook of clinical neurology*, (ed. P. J. Vinken and G. W. Bruyn), Vol. 26, p. 409. North-Holland, Amsterdam.

Shaw, M. D. M., Russell, J. A., and Grossart, K. W. (1878). The changing pattern of spinal arachnoiditis. *J. Neurol. Neurosurg. Psychiatry*, **41**, 97–107.

Swash, M. (1985). New concepts of incontinence. *BMJ*, **290**, 4–5.

Seizures, and alterations of consciousness and thought

CHAPTER 22

Epilepsy and other paroxysmal disorders in children

Brian Neville

22.1 Non-epileptic attacks of childhood

Children are subject to a large number of paroxysmal events which may be mistakenly diagnosed as epilepsy (Stephenson 1990). Some are specific to childhood and will be described briefly.

22.1.1 Childhood-specific paroxysmal events

Blue 'breath-holding attacks'

Simple blue 'breath-holding attacks' are quite common in children under the age of 5 years. The child starts to cry but then stops breathing in expiration, goes blue, and loses consciousness. Although alarming and sometimes followed by brief stiffening, or even, in some, jerks, the child recovers. The attacks are harmless. The occurrence of many blue breath-holding attacks raises the possibility of psychosocial deprivation. A rare, and apparently different, syndrome of severe prolonged expiratory apnoea has been described (Southall *et al.* 1985), which begins in young babies and appears to risk brain damage and death. The onset is before 6 months, which distinguishes it from the simple attacks described above.

White 'breath-holding attacks'

White 'breath-holding attacks' or, more accurately, reflex asystolic attacks, are also quite common and easily mistaken for epileptic seizures. A strong clue to their nature is their provocation by minor injury. The sequence is therefore of a painful minor injury followed by pallor, rapid coma, stiffening with opisthotonos and sometimes incontinence, and then recovery. The pathophysiology of blue breath-holding attacks appears to be a Valsalva manoeuvre and, by contrast, in white attacks a period of vagally mediated asystole occurs, followed by flattening of the electroencephalogram (EEG). These latter attacks can be induced in susceptible individuals by firm, but not painful, eyeball compression, but the history is usually sufficiently clear for this to be an unnecessary diagnostic test (Stephenson, 1980).

Benign paroxysmal vertigo

Benign paroxysmal vertigo is a syndrome of attacks of pure vertigo, which are clearly described by the affected child: provided, of course, that the child has sufficient command of speech. The attacks occur between the ages of 18 months and 5 years and cause characteristic episodes of panic, rapidly holding on to a fixed object if available, frequently vomiting, and then recovering over a few minutes. The condition, which is ascribed to a peripheral vestibular defect, is self-limiting and without sequelae (Koenigsberger *et al.* 1970).

Benign paroxysmal torticollis of infancy

Benign paroxysmal torticollis of infancy is probably closely related to paroxysmal vertigo. It starts in the first year with prolonged episodes of torticollis and asymmetry of tone and posture with distress and vomiting in a fully conscious baby. Familial paroxysmal extrapyramidal and paralysing disorders usually start later in childhood.

Benign myoclonus of early infancy

Benign myoclonus of early infancy consists of repeated jerks of the limbs in sleep in the first few months of life in an otherwise normal baby.

Dominantly inherited hyperekplexia

The severe form of dominantly inherited hyperekplexia may cause diagnostic confusion. In addition to the startle and provoked stiffening and falling in older children, babies with this condition may be generally hypertonic and have marked axial and limb jerks on falling asleep and attacks of apnoea secondary to muscle spasm.

Sleep phenomena

A range of phenomena are reported in drowsiness and sleep but sudden panic and screaming (night terrors) in young children, and walking, without any of the motor components of epilepsy in older children, who are otherwise normal, are the main clinical indicators that such episodes are not epileptic in origin.

Occasionally, parents and other carers report attacks which are either fabricated or even occasionally induced by the parent. This form of child abuse is being recognized increasingly (Meadow 1984). The clues to this diagnosis are: the reports always come from one parent; the child is usually otherwise completely normal, and investigations fail to reveal any abnormality. However, these latter features are also shared with the other forms of non-epileptic paroxysmal events which can be mistaken for epilepsy. As a general rule, children who have insistent early onset epilepsy which is unresponsive to drug treatment, also tend to have evidence of more widespread neurological disease, and if they are clearly neurologically normal, it should be strongly suspected that they do not have epilepsy. If they do not conform to a recognized condition, it is wise to attempt in-patient monitoring and more detailed verification

of the attacks. Parentally induced episodes, particularly those caused by suffocation, carry a high morbidity and mortality.

Syndrome of alternating hemiplegia

The syndrome of alternating hemiplegia in infancy is rare but important. It is not helpful to regard it as a variant of migraine, because of its serious consequences for cognitive and motor function. The paroxysmal features of the condition, which start in the first year of life, are episodes of hemiplegia, tonic seizures, nystagmus, vasomotor, and respiratory disturbances (including apnoea), which may persist for up to 3 days, occurring separately either side or sometimes bilaterally. Interestingly, the paroxysmal motor phenomena are not present in sleep or for the first 20–30 minutes after waking (Aicardi 1987). Hemiplegia may pass to the opposite side, with a phase of bilateral involvement, in a single episode. Persistent learning and extrapyramidal motor deficits are acquired during the course of these episodes. There is evidence that flunarazine may help to reduce the intensity and frequency of the episodes, but their underlying mechanisms remain unknown (Caesar *et al.* 1987; Andermann *et al.* 1995).

22.2 Epilepsy in childhood

About two-thirds of all attacks of epilepsy begin in childhood. The delineation of benign syndromes with good outcome and 'malignant' ones in which there is strong evidence of cognitive deterioration, coincident with a severe phase of the epilepsy, has mainly arisen from paediatric studies (Aicardi 1986). Epilepsy is also a very common concomitant of acute brain illness and chronic brain syndromes, in which the underlying pathology may be static or progressive. Increasingly, surgical treatment is being extended into childhood, and the range of surgical procedures has increased.

The genetic localization of seizure syndromes is separable into pure lesionless conditions that have epilepsy as their only initial manifestation, and conditions with lesions that commonly cause epilepsy but which have additional primary manifestations. The primary pure genetic epilepsies with simple Mendelian inheritance and gene localization are benign familial neonatal convulsions, benign familial infantile conclusions, partial epilepsy with auditory symptoms, autosomal dominant nocturnal frontal lobe epilepsy, and progressive epilepsy with mental retardation (Northern epilepsy). Possible localizations are proposed for three epilepsies with complex inheritance: febrile convulsions, juvenile myoclonic epilepsy, idiopathic generalized epilepsy (Elmslie and Gardiner 1996).

22.2.1 Benign and malignant syndromes of epilepsy

The benign syndromes of epilepsy are usually age limited, stereotyped, often provoked or provokable, and occur in otherwise normal children. Genetic predisposition is common. They include febrile convulsions (Section 22.2.2), neonatal seizures

(Section 22.2.3), and benign Rolandic epilepsy, benign occipital epilepsy, benign myoclonic epilepsy of infancy, and petit mal epilepsy (all described in Section 22.2.4).

The malignant syndromes of epilepsy include infantile spasms or West syndrome (Section 22.2.5), severe myoclonic or polymorphic epilepsy of infancy (Section 22.2.6), Lennox–Gastaut syndrome (Section 22.2.7), complex partial seizures of temporal lobe origin (Section 22.2.8), the Landau–Kleffner syndrome (Section 22.2.9), tuberous sclerosis (Section 19.1), and Sturge–Weber syndrome (Section 19.3).

The delineation of benign and malignant syndromes of childhood epilepsy generates a set of general rules or trends:

1. Attacks which are of single type, infrequent, or easily controlled by antiepileptic drugs in an otherwise normal child, are likely to be of good outcome. After a year of freedom from attacks in this setting, withdrawal of treatment should be considered on the assumption that the child is in natural remission.

2. Insistent partial seizures imply focal pathology and if no remission has occurred in the first year of attempted treatment, surgical treatment should be considered. The supposition is that an accumulating series of disabilities, which include cognitive, psychiatric, and social problems, may be avoided or minimized by early intervention. In particular, the effects on adolescence that has been dominated by severe epilepsy cannot be reversed.

The adverse factors for outcome of childhood epilepsy in the absence of known progressive disease are: learning disorders, either primary or acquired; multiple seizure types; a high rate of seizures; and episodes of status epileptus, particularly nonconvulsive status.

22.2.2 Febrile convulsions

Febrile convulsions are epileptic seizures that are provoked by fever of extracranial infective origin and occur in approximately 3 per cent of children aged 6 months to 5 years. Any child with fever and seizures deserves clinical investigation for the source of infection and, in a minority, there may be direct involvement of the brain, or the fever may reveal an underlying epileptogenic pathology. The seizures are usually brief, bilateral, clonic or tonic–clonic attacks. A minority of attacks, designated as complex, are prolonged or lateralized and require emergency treatment. Hemiplegia following very prolonged febrile seizures is now very uncommon (Aicardi and Chevrie 1976). The reported proportion of such complex seizures has varied in different studies, and figures of 5 per cent for population-based studies and 15 per cent for those admitted to hospital are reasonable working indications from the published work.

The lowest reported risk of subsequent non-febrile seizures came from the North American Collaborative Childhood Perinatal Project (Nelson and Ellenberg 1981, 1990). The three adverse factors for outcome were a family history of febrile seizures, pre-existing neurological abnormality (particularly slow development), and complicated initial seizures. Even in the presence of all three factors, the later epilepsy rate was only 10 per cent. There is strong circumstantial evidence for linking prolonged febrile seizures with the later development of mesial temporal sclerosis and intractable complex partial seizures of temporal origin. This evidence comes particularly from surgically treated series (Falconer and Taylor 1968) and animal work (Meldrum *et al*. 1974).

Prospective studies, even the very large collaborative study reported abroad, could not produce sufficient numbers of complex febrile convulsions to test the hypothesis of a causal relationship between febrile status and mesial temporal damage, and specifically they could not exclude that pathogenic sequence. Since a very large number of children have febrile seizures this remains an important question, because even if only a small proportion of children suffered this serious outcome, it would be a significant health problem. The usual treatment offered for recurrences, if there has been a prolonged attack, is rectal diazepam. Phenobarbital (Wolf *et al*. 1981), primidone (Wallace 1975), and sodium valproate (Ngwane and Bower 1980) have been shown to reduce the frequency of recurrent attacks, but only a minority of children are treated with these drugs. Barbiturates have a high rate of unacceptable behavioural side-effects and there is a general unwillingness to prescribe valproate for what is, in the main, a benign condition. There is a strong genetic basis to febrile convulsions, which may be separated into some that are clearly polygenic (Rich *et al*. 1987) and others demonstrating dominant inheritance in those who have a great number of attacks (Anderson *et al*. 1988).

22.2.3 Neonatal seizures

Seizures occurring in the first 2 weeks of life have overall a very poor prognosis, but that varies widely for individual conditions within the group. Outcomes are summarized in Table 22.1. This indicates the primary pathological basis for the poor outcome in that the seizures are often merely a marker for pre-existing brain damage. However, the full range of outcomes is seen within the neonatal seizure group. Apparently totally benign, dominantly inherited neonatal seizures occur mostly on the second or third day of life, but are rare. A number of studies have pointed out a peak of unexplained seizures in otherwise normal babies at around the fifth day of life, hence the term 'fifth-day seizures' (Pryor *et al*. 1981). Although these syndromes are defined by their good outcome, this is relative to other seizures in babies and children with evidence of neurological damage, and careful follow-up of most benign syndromes of epilepsy shows that, in general, there is a slight increase in the later rate of epilepsy. The finding of gene marker localization to chromosome 20 for benign familial neonatal convulsions adds conviction to the existence of this syndrome (Leppert *et al*. 1989). Seizures after the seventh day associated with hypocalcaemia are now uncommon but also have a benign outcome. At least 85 per cent of babies with early onset neonatal seizures associated with subarachnoid haemorrhage with focal parenchymal haemorrhage also have a normal outcome,

Table 22.1. Prognosis of neonatal seizures in relation to aetiology (after Aicardi 1986)

Aetiology	Normal development (%)
Hypoxic–ischaemic encephalopathy	16–50
Haemorrhage	
Intraventricular	0–10
Subarachnoid	85–90
Bacterial meningitis	25–65
Developmental defect	0–5
Hypocalcaemia	
Early onset	42–50
Late onset	94–100
Hypoglycaemia	25–50
Unknown	55–62

which contrasts with the very high morbidity and mortality associated with hypoxic ischaemic encephalopathy.

Recessively inherited pyridoxine-dependent epilepsy is very rare. Seizures may begin at any time from the last trimester *in utero* to the second year of life. It is therefore mandatory that a baby with unexplained intractable seizures is given pyridoxine as a therapeutic trial (Clarke *et al.* 1979).

22.2.4 Other benign epilepsy syndromes

Benign epilepsy with Rolandic (centro-temporal interictal) foci

The age of onset is 2–12 years and is maximal at 7–10 years and stops by 13 years. The attacks are clonic, partial motor,

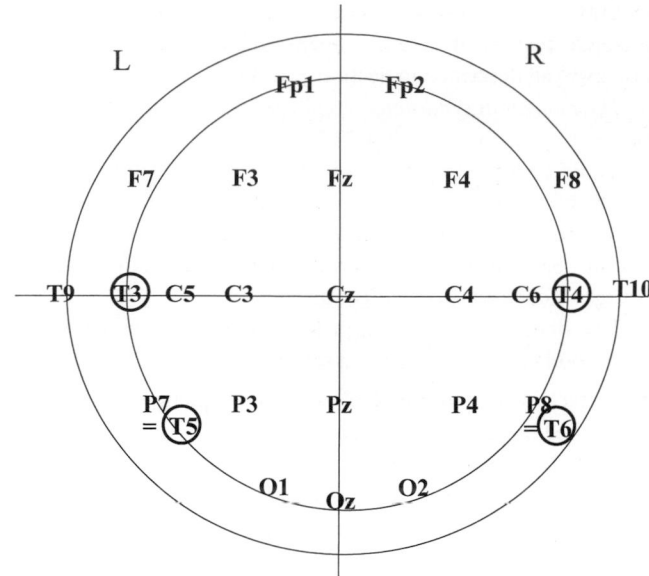

Fig. 22.1. Diagram of electrode positions used in the EEG illustrations in this chapter. The designations are those of the '10–10 system', an extended version of the traditional '10–20 system'. Those electrodes which have different designations under the '10–20 system' are circled.

involving face, bulbar muscles, and arm, and they occur particularly on waking from sleep. The EEG shows centro-temporal discharges (Figs 22.1, 22.2). In one of the largest studies (264 patients with epilepsy who had the appropriate studies seeking EEG abnormality), 43 had neuropsychiatric abnormalities and were therefore excluded from the analysis (Beaussart 1972).

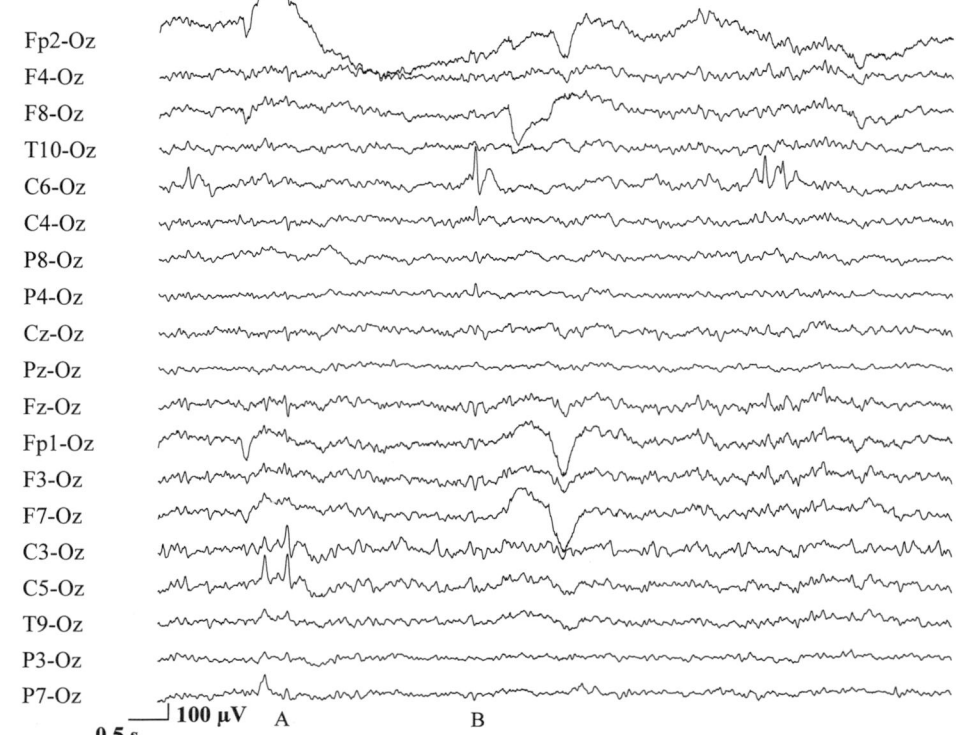

Fig. 22.2. Benign Rolandic epilepsy. EEG from an 8-year-old with a typical history of right facial jerking in the early part of the night, sometimes followed by jerking of the right arm, without loss of consciousness. Note the sharp waves seen independently over the central/Sylvian areas C3/C5 and C4/C6 over both left (A) and right (B). Bilateral discharges are seen in around 40 per cent of cases. (Courtesy of Dr Stewart Boyd.)

Benign occipital epilepsy with sharp and slow wave activity suppressed by eye opening

The attacks are partial seizures consisting of visual phenomena, which may suggest complex migraine. The onset is usually at about 6 years of age and 92 per cent have stopped by the age of 19 years (Gastaut 1982; Aicardi 1986).

Benign myoclonic epilepsy of infancy

The attacks are myoclonic jerks, sometimes resembling infantile spasms but with a different EEG pattern, consisting of 3 Hz spike-waves or polyspikes (Aicardi 1980).

Simple typical absence seizures (petit mal)

Simple typical absence seizures (petit mal) are relatively uncommon despite the wide use of the term. The attacks consist of loss of awareness and responsiveness, lasting for 5–15 seconds with only minor motor phenomena of some eyelid fluttering and sagging of tone in the face, jaw, and sometimes of the limbs and trunk. Onset and offset are abrupt with no aura or post-ictal confusion. In childhood the main differential diagnosis is from daydreaming. Children may have periods of looking blank when they are not engaged. Absence seizures are a clear interruption in activity, such as eating, writing, or speaking. The outcome in terms of tonic–clonic seizures in adult life is predicted by the number of adverse factors (low IQ, tonic–clonic seizures in childhood, and a family history of seizures)—with no (or one) adverse factors only 10 per cent have continuing seizures, but with all adverse factors

the chances of remission from seizures are very low. Thus only a proportion of patients with absence seizures have a benign outcome. The EEG consists of symmetrical, bilateral synchronous bursts of 2.5–3.5 spike-wave activity, which can usually be provoked by hyperventilation (Fig. 22.3). Ethosuximide, sodium valproate and lamotrigine are effective drugs for treating simple absence seizures.

Atypical absences are usually longer with variable disturbance of consciousness (Fig. 22.4). They are often part of multiple-seizures-type syndromes, particularly Lennox–Gastaut syndrome.

22.2.5 Infantile spasms or West syndrome

This syndrome may be symptomatic of a wide range of mostly non-progressive cerebral cortical pathology, occurring prenatally or in the early postnatal period. It is remarkably consistent in its phenomenology. The baby develops characteristic runs of spasms that occur usually at 5–10-second intervals and may continue for many minutes. The most common spasms are episodes of sudden flexion which range from slight neck flexion to violent flexion of the trunk with adduction of the extended arms and hip flexion with the legs extended at the knees. Extensor and mixed types of spasms are also seen, which may show marked asymmetry (Hrachovy and Frost 1989) and focality (Ohtsuka *et al.* 1996). The attacks may start at any time in the first year of life but the peak age of onset is at about 4 months. Quite often the attacks are not recognized as a form

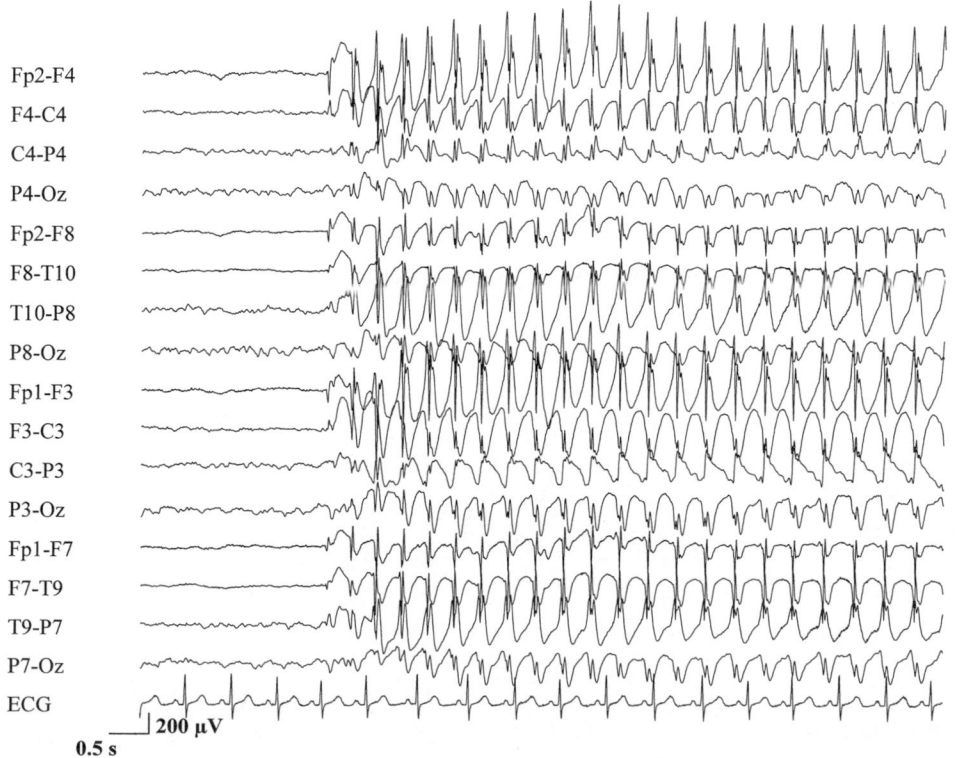

Fig. 22.3. Simple typical absence seizures (petit mal). EEG from a 6-year-old with an 8-month history of episodes of staring for 2–5 seconds, several times per day. Note the typical EEG features of an absence seizure, with an abrupt onset of generalized 3/s spike-wave complexes, of higher amplitude over the frontal regions, slowing to around 2/s as the attack continues. (Courtesy of Dr Stewart Boyd.)

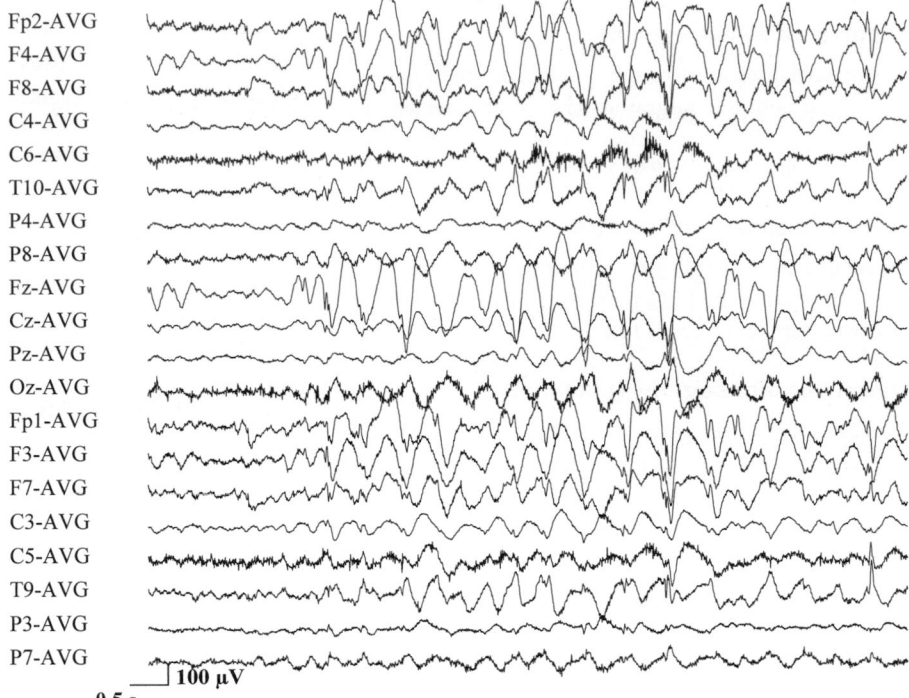

Fig. 22.4. Atypical absence seizures. EEG from a 10-year-old boy with atypical absences and drop attacks. Note the variable and poorly formed spike-wave complexes at around 2/s over the frontal regions. (Courtesy of Dr Stewart Boyd.)

of epilepsy for some time. Parents commonly notice social regression and an alarming lack of developmental progress once the attacks have started. This developmental complaint may well be the presenting symptom. The EEG characteristically shows a gross abnormality, with disorganized high-voltage slow activity, with multifocal spikes and sharp waves. Periods of slow activity occur alternating with polyspikes in sleep. This

EEG abnormality is sometimes referred to as hypsarrhythmia (Fig. 22.5). Somewhat milder EEG abnormalities with some preservation of background rhythms are quite compatible with the syndrome, particularly in its earlier phases. The distinction between those with pre-existing brain pathology and those previously normal has been useful in predicting a better, and occasionally normal, outcome in the latter group. However, with

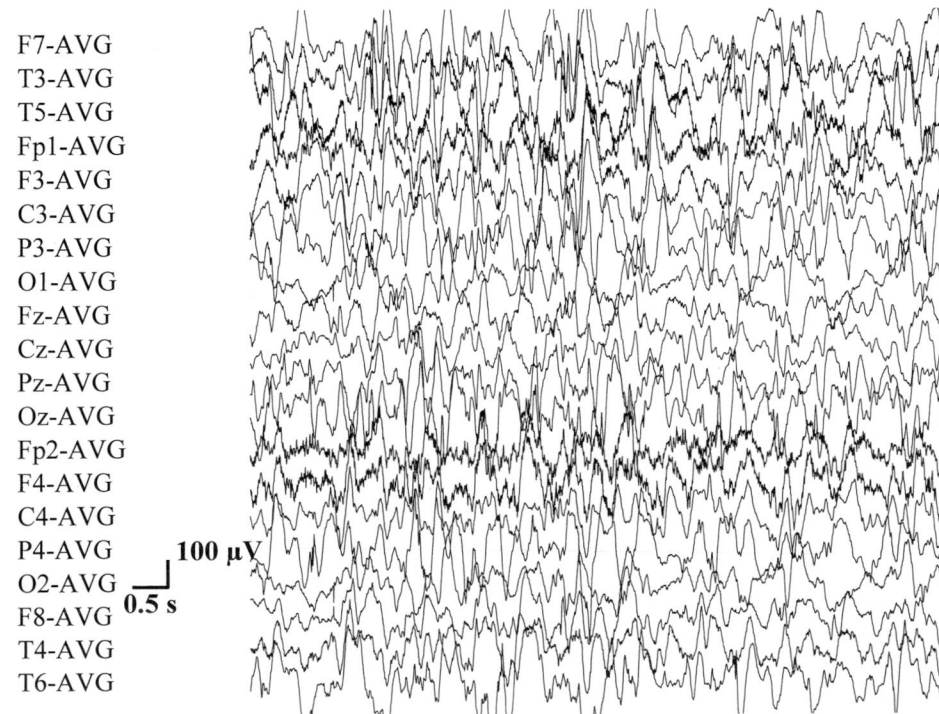

Fig. 22.5. Infantile spasms or West syndrome showing EEG features of hypsarrhythmia. Note the high-amplitude slow activity and multifocal spikes, together with the apparent lack of organization. (Courtesy of Dr Stewart Boyd.)

more detailed examination it is now clear that only about 10 per cent of cases can be presumed to be previously entirely normal, i.e. without a discoverable cause and with previously normal development (Riikonen and Donner 1979; Singer *et al.* 1982).

Treatment has been dominated by corticosteroid drugs (ACTH or analogue or prednisolone) until the efficacy of vigabatrin emerged. In doses of about 100 mg/kg a 68 per cent response rate was observed within 7 days (Aicardi *et al.* 1996) and, in doses of 150 mg/kg, there was a compelling advantage over corticosteroids in the treatment of infantile spasms secondary to tuberous sclerosis (Chiron *et al.* 1997). Corticosteroids tend to be used in short courses, often with long-term positive effects.

A notion that West's syndrome is an unusual form of bilateral epilepsy arising from a focal lesion has partly arisen from positron emission tomography (PET) work, showing 'cold' lesions which have been excised with apparent relief of seizures (Chugani *et al.* 1990). This work clearly needs to be replicated, but focal pathology is quite common in this group. The disastrous outcome for this syndrome, with a mortality of approximately 20 per cent, cerebral palsy in 30–50 per cent of cases, and mental retardation in 70–85 per cent, has prompted the use of a large number of other treatments.

A very important advance was made by Chevrie and Aicardi (1978) in recognizing that early onset (i.e. the first year) spontaneous seizures (i.e. not precipitated by fever, trauma, or metabolic upset) carried a similarly poor outcome to that of classical West's syndrome. If, for example, focal motor seizures begin at a few months of age, infantile spasms or some other form of intractable epilepsy frequently follow. Thus, from the point of view of management and prognosis, early onset spontaneous seizures and infantile spasms can be combined.

An interesting example of the behavioural and cognitive phenotype associated with early onset seizures, particularly infantile spasms, is seen in tuberous sclerosis, in which the outcome is much poorer if such seizures occur, particularly because of the high incidence of autistic features (Gomez 1988). Autistic features are not confined, of course, to tuberous sclerosis and can occur in any child with infantile spasms.

22.2.6 **Severe myoclonic or polymorphic epilepsy of infancy**

This condition begins between 4 and 10 months, often as a prolonged partial clonic seizure associated with fever with recurrences of similar attacks within a few weeks. Later multiple seizure types develop, including complex partial seizures, atypical absences, myoclonic attacks, and sometimes alarming episodes of apnoea. Developmental regression with the onset of multiple seizure types is often dramatic with very severe learning disorder as the usual outcome. The interictal EEG may be normal at an early stage but later characteristically shows fast spike-wave complexes. Approximately 25 per cent of cases show photosensitivity. This condition accounts for some of the worst outcomes of childhood epilepsy. It is not very uncommon and

its pathogenesis is unknown (Cavazzuti *et al.* 1984; Aicardi 1992).

22.2.7 **Lennox–Gastaut syndrome**

This syndrome of severe epilepsy generally starts in the first 7 or 8 years of life (Niedermeyer and Degen 1988). It may be heralded by a variety of types of other seizure, e.g. infantile spasms in the first year, but its full development occurs later. Seizures characteristically include tonic attacks, particularly in sleep, atonic and myoclonic attacks, atypical absences, and episodes of non-convulsive status. This latter phenomenon may dominate the clinical picture with much of the child's life spent in a groggy state with poor memory and variable communication. The characteristic interictal EEG is of bilateral variable slow (1–2 Hz) spike-wave pattern. Mental functioning is delayed in up to half of the children before the onset, and in the majority after 5 years or more of the condition. At the most, 10 per cent make a full recovery and, in the remainder, moderate to severe disability with epilepsy persists. Although intractability to antiepileptic drugs is the rule, benzodiazepines, sodium valproate, corticosteroids, and a ketogenic diet have been thought to be effective to a degree. Felbamate is sometimes used, but is limited by concern about side-effects. For these reasons there is a high risk of intoxication by polytherapy.

The pathological basis of Lennox–Gastaut epilepsy, if found, is usually of a structural brain lesion of early onset, showing a major overlap with the pathologies that cause infantile spasms. Sometimes there is an overlap in the clinical syndromes as well. In general, the lesions are of lesser severity than in infantile spasms and sometimes clearly unilateral; they may be amenable to surgical removal, suggesting that this is, at least in a proportion of cases, a secondary bilateral syndrome of epilepsy.

Although the yield of progressive pathology, structural or biochemical, is low, it is important that all children with regression in association with epilepsy are investigated.

22.2.8 **Complex partial seizures of temporal lobe origin**

The majority of seizures of temporal lobe origin begin in childhood and adolescence. In the seminal work of the Oxford group on 100 children with 'temporal lobe epilepsy' studied for 38 years (Ounsted *et al.* 1987) and the detailed neuropsychiatric studies of Taylor (1972), the following points emerge.

1. There is a significant mortality of 5 per cent in childhood and a further 11 per cent in adults.

2. Approximately one-third recovered, one-third were independent with continued epilepsy and often very significant problems, and one-third were totally dependent. This poor prognosis spread through all aspects of the person's life.

3. A poor outcome was predicted by a number of early factors, including aetiology (i.e. clear evidence of early

brain damage), early age of onset, low IQ, severity of grand mal, severity of partial attacks, and very severe behavioural disorder. The prediction was possible at a relatively early age, i.e. before or early in adolescence.

4. Only 15 per cent of patients were regarded as psychiatrically normal.

5. A strong case for early surgery in those with clear lesions and poor predictions emerges from this study.

6. Because of the range and severity of the problems in this group, total relief of seizures may not be the sole aim of surgery, and a 'Taylored' procedure to provide some amelioration of the person's predicament may be appropriate.

In childhood, dysembryoplastic tumours, particularly of the temporal lobe, may cause massive regression if seizures start in the first year of life, and they require urgent surgical consideration (Neville *et al.* 1997).

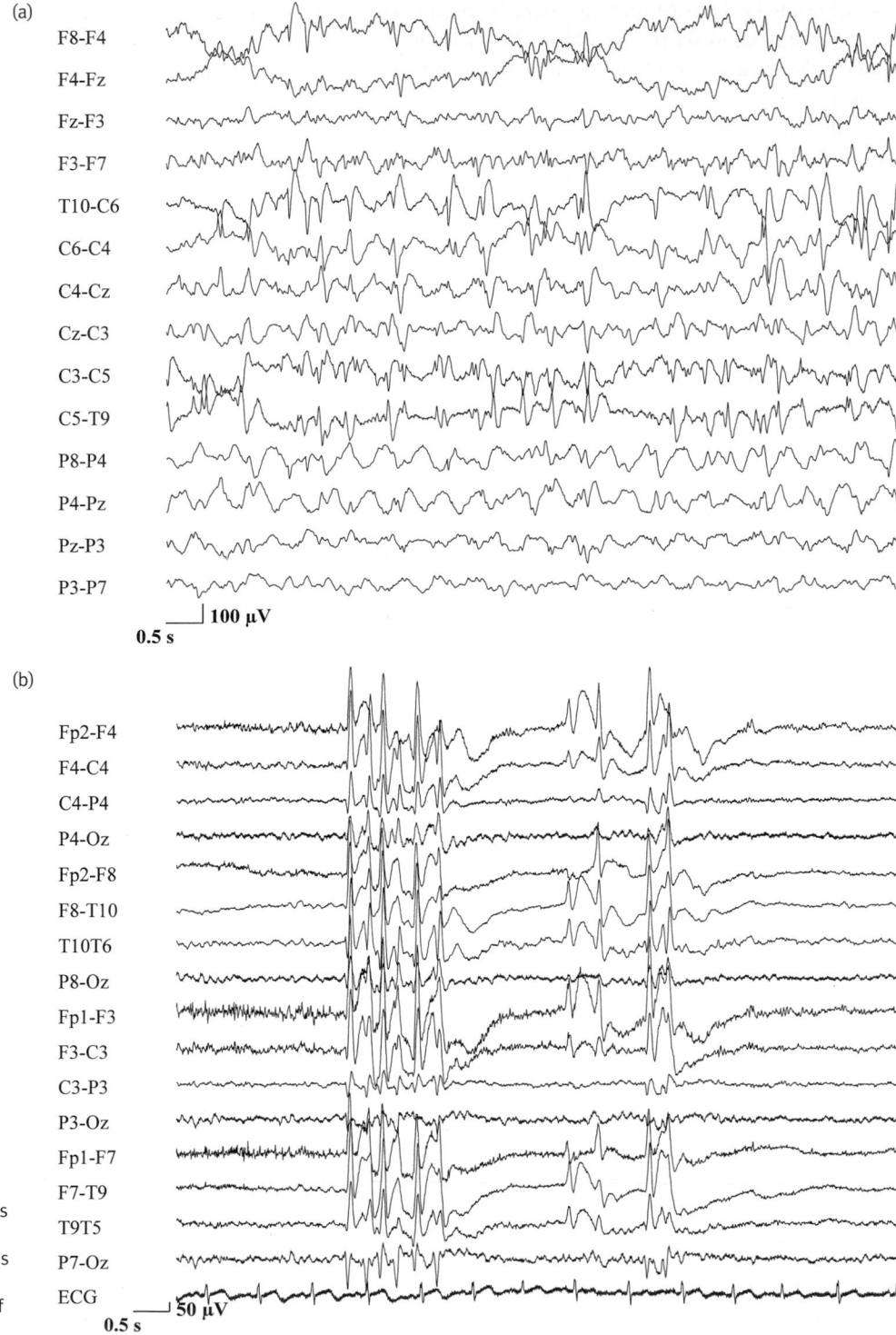

Fig 22.6. EEG features in Landau–Kleffner syndrome. (a) Note the runs of discharges over central and posterior temporal regions during sleep. (b) Some children show more widespread bursts of discharges during drowsiness and sleep. Note that in this case, the spikes are of highest amplitude over the frontal regions. (Courtesy of Dr Stewart Boyd.)

22.2.9 The Landau–Kleffner syndrome

This unusual condition presents either with seizures or aphasia (Beaumanoir 1985) and approximately 20 per cent of patients never have obvious seizures. The typical history is of a child whose development is normal for several years and then, either suddenly or in a fluctuating manner, loses comprehension of speech and the ability to use speech to communicate. The seizures are of no specific type and are mostly mild and infrequent partial or atypical absences. The EEG abnormality is usually bilateral, or of changing lateralization, showing spikes or spike-wave complexes in temporal and parietal regions (Fig. 22.6a). It is intensified in sleep and may amount to non-convulsive sleep status (Fig. 22.6b). Although the typical cognitive deficit is in auditory comprehension, it may be wider and behavioural abnormalities may occur which include problems in social communication which fulfil the criteria for the diagnosis of autism. Motor phenomena are also seen, particularly focal and global apraxia (Neville and Boyd 1995).

In general, imaging is normal. Treatment with antiepileptic drugs, including corticosteroids, is worth trying but is often unsuccessful; therefore communication support is required, sometimes into adult life. There are reports of the surgical treatment of this condition from, as yet, a limited number of centres, the procedure used being one of multiple subpial transections (Morrell *et al.* 1989).

References

Aicardi, J. (1980). Course and prognosis of certain childhood epilepsies with predominantly myoclonic seizures. In *Advances in epileptology: The Xth Epilepsy International Symposium*, (ed. J. A. Wada and J. K. Penry), pp. 159–63. Raven Press, New York.

Aicardi, J. (1986). *Epilepsy in children*. Raven Press, New York.

Aicardi, J. (1987). Alternating hemiplegia of childhood. *Int. Pediatr.*, **2**, 115–19.

Aicardi, J. (1992). *Diseases of the nervous system in childhood*. MacKeith Press with Blackwell Scientific Oxford and Cambridge VP, New York.

Aicardi, J., Mumford, J. P., Sabril IS investigator and Peer Review Groups *et al.* (1996).

Andermann, F., Aicardi J., and Vigevano, F. (ed.) (1995). *Alternating Hemiplegia of Childhood*. Raven Press, New York.

Anderson, V. E., Wilcox, K. J., Hauser, W. A. *et al.* (1988). A test of autosomal dominant inheritance in febrile convulsions. *Epilepsia*, **29**, 705–6.

Beaumanoir, A. (1985). The Landau–Kleffner syndrome. In *Epileptic syndromes in infants, childhood and adolescence*, (ed. J. Roger, C. Dravet, M. Bureau, F. E. Dreifuss, and P. Wolf), pp. 181–91. John Libbey, London.

Beaussart, M. (1972). Benign epilepsy of children with rolandic (centro-temporal) paroxysmal foci: A clinical entity. Study of 221 cases. *Epilepsia*, **13**, 795–811.

Caesar, P., Aicardi, J., Curatolo, P. *et al.* (1987). Flunarazine in alternating hemiplegia in childhood: An international study in 12 children. *Neuropaediatrics*, **18**, 191–5.

Cavazzuti, G. B., Ferrari, P., and Lalla, M. (1984). Follow-up of 482 cases with convulsive disorders in the first year of life. *Dev. Med. Child Neurol.*, **26**, 425–37.

Chevrie, J. J. and Aicardi, J. (1978). Convulsive disorders in the first year of life: Neurological and mental outcome and mortality. *Epilepsia*, **19**, 67–74.

Chiron, C., Dumas, C., Jambaque, I. *et al.* (1997). Randomized trial comparing vigabatrin and hydrocortisone in infantile spasms due to tuberous sclerosis. *Epilepsy Res.*, **26**, 389–95.

Chugani, H. T., Shields, W. D., Shewmon, D. A. *et al.* (1990). Infantile spasms. I: PET identifies focal cortical dysgenesis in cryptogenic cases for surgical treatment. *Ann. Neurol.*, **27**, 406–13.

Clarke, T. A., Saunders, B. S., and Feldman, B. (1979). Pyridoxine-dependent seizures requiring high doses of pyridoxine for control. *Am. J. Dis. Child.*, **133**, 963–5.

Elmslie, F. and Gardiner, M. (1996). The epilepsies. In *Emery and Rimoin's principles and practice of medical genetics*, (ed. D. L. Rimoin, J. M. Connor, and R. E. Pyeritz), pp. 2177–96. Churchill Livingstone, New York.

Falconer, M. A. and Taylor, D. C. (1968). Surgical treatment of drug resistant epilepsy due to mesial temporal sclerosis. *Arch. Neurol.*, **19**, 353–61.

Gastaut, H. (1982). L'epilepsie benigne de l'enfant a pointe-ondes occipitales. *Rev. Electroencephalogr. Neurolphysiol. Clin.*, **12**, 179–201.

Gomez, M. R. (ed.) (1988). *Tuberous sclerosis*, (2nd edn). Raven Press, New York.

Hrachovy, R. A. and Frost, J. D. (1989). Infantile spasms. *Pediatr. Clin. North Am.*, **36**, 311–30.

Koenigsberger, M., Chritonian, A. M., Gold, A. P. *et al.* (1970). Benign paroxysmal vertigo of childhood. *Neurology*, **20**, 1108–13.

Leppert, M., Anderson, V. E., Quattelbaum, T. *et al.* (1989). Benign familial neonatal convulsions linked to genetic markers on chromosome 20. *Nature*, **337**, 647–8.

Meadow, R. (1984). Fictitious epilepsy. *Lancet*, **2**, 25–8.

Meldrum, B. S., Horton, R. W., and Brierly, J. B. (1974). Epileptic brain damage in adolescent baboons following seaizures induced by allylglycins. *Brain*, **97**, 407–18.

Morrell, F., Whistler, W. W., and Bleck, T. P. (1989). Multiple subpial transection: a new approach to the surgical treatment of focal epilepsy. *J. Neurosurg.*, **70**, 231–9.

Nelson, K. B. and Ellenberg, J. H. (ed.) (1981). *Febrile seizures.* Raven Press, New York.

Nelson, K. B. and Ellenberg, J. H. (1990). Prenatal and perinatal antecedents of febrile seizures. *Ann. Neurol.*, **27**, 127–31.

Neville, B. G. R. and Boyd, S. G. (1995). Selective epileptic gait disorder. *J. Neurol. Neurosurg. Pychiat.*, **58**, 371–3.

Neville, B. G. R., Harkness, W. J. F., Cross, J. H. *et al.* (1997). Surgical treatment of autistic regression in childhood epilepsy. *Paediatr. Neurol.*, **16** (2), 137–40.

Ngwane, E. and Bower, B. (1980). Continuous sodium valproate or phenobarbitone in the prevention of 'simple' febrile convulsions. *Arch. Dis. Child.*, **55**, 171–4.

Niedermeyer, E. and Degen, D. (ed.) (1988). The Lennox–Gastaut Syndrome. Alan R. Liss, New York.

Ohtsuka, Y., Murashima, I., Asano, T. *et al.* (1996). Partial seizures in West Syndrome. *Epilepsia*, **37**, 1060–7.

Ounsted, C., Lindsay, J., and Richards, P. (1987). *Temporal lobe epilepsy 1948–1986: A biographical study.* MacKeith Press with Blackwell Scientific, Oxford and Lippincott, Philadelphia.

Pryor, D. S., Don, N., and Macourt, D. C. (1981). Fifth day fits: A syndrome of neonatal convulsion. *Arch. Dis. Child.*, **56**, 753–8.

Rich, S. S., Annegers, J. F., Hauser, W. A. *et al.* (1987). Complex segregation analysis of febrile convulsions. *Am. J. Hum. Genet.*, **41**, 249–57.

Riikonen, R. and Donner, M. (1979). Incidence and aetiology of infantile spasms from 1960 to 1976: a population study in Finland. *Dev. Med. Child Neurol.*, **21**, 333–43.

Singer, W. D., Haller, J. S., Sullivan, L. R. *et al.* (1982). The value of neuroradiology in infantile spasms. *J. Pediatr.*, **100**, 47–50.

Southall, D. P., Talbert, D. G., Johnson, P. *et al.* (1985). Prolonged expiratory apnoea: a disorder resulting in episodes of severe arterial hypoxcaemia in infants and young children. *Lancet*, **2**, 571–7.

Stephenson, J. B. P. (1980). Reflex anoxic seizures and ocular compression. *Dev. Med. Child Neurol.*, **22**, 380–6.

Stephenson, J. B. P. (1990). Fits and faints. *Clin. Develop. Med.*, **109**.

Taylor, D. C. (1972). Mental state and temporal lobe epilepsy: a correlative account of 100 patients treated surgically. *Epilepsia*, **13**, 727–66.

Wallace, S. J. (1975). Continuous prophylactic anti-convulsants in selected children with febrile convulsions. *Acta Neurol. Scand.*, **60** (Suppl. 75), 62–6.

Wolf, S. M., Forsythe, A., Stunden, A. A. *et al.* (1981). Long-term effect of phenobarbital on cognitive function in children with febrile convulsion. *Paediatrics*, **68**, 820–3.

CHAPTER 23

Seizures, epilepsy, and other episodic disorders in adults

David Chadwick

23.1 Causes of blackouts

23.1.1 Definition of seizures and epilepsy

Epilepsy, or more correctly a seizure, is most easily defined in physiological terms, being 'the name for occasional sudden, excessive, rapid and local discharges of grey matter' (Jackson 1873). It is more difficult to offer a comprehensive clinical definition of epileptic seizures and epilepsy because of the varied clinical manifestations produced by cerebral neuronal discharge. However, an epileptic seizure can be defined as an intermittent, stereotyped, disturbance of consciousness, behaviour, emotion, motor function, or sensation that, on clinical grounds, is believed to result from cortical neuronal discharge. Epilepsy can then be defined as a condition in which seizures recur, usually spontaneously.

The differential diagnosis of epilepsy is large because of the enormous range of symptoms that can occur during seizures. Inevitably, the differential diagnosis for tonic–clonic seizures is very different from that for simple partial seizures with autonomic symptoms.

23.1.2 Syncope

Syncope is common and occurs for a wide variety of reasons (Table 23.1). The majority of people who faint are young and have no serious underlying pathology. Such vaso-vagal syncope is precipitated by unpleasant sights or pain, standing for prolonged periods, or after exposure to heat, hunger, dehydration, and alcohol excess. It is posture dependent: symptoms can start while sitting, but loss of consciousness usually occurs when the individual stands. The mechanisms leading to fainting have been studied extensively using nitrites associated with tilt (Weissler *et al.* 1957) and tourniquets and venesection (Barcroft and Edholm 1945). The characteristic changes appear to be a widespread loss of peripheral resistance without any change in cardiac output because of reduced venous return. Pre-syncopal symptoms appear before hypotension and bradycardia and persist after the blood pressure returns to normal.

The subject usually has a feeling of warmth with a dry mouth and a desire for fresh air or a drink of water. Nausea can develop quickly, along with deep, sighing respiration, blurring of vision with spots in front of the eyes and loss of colour vision, noises in the ears, vertigo, and depersonalization. The onset of these symptoms is usually gradual and eye-witnesses comment on pallor and sweating. The subject will collapse if they remain standing. The collapse may be rigid or flaccid and some form of clonic or other positive motor phenomena are common (Lempert *et al.* 1994), raising the spectre of epilepsy for the inexperienced. The EEG shows only generalized slow activity at this time, without any epileptiform features. Reflex anoxic seizures may occur if individuals faint and are maintained in an upright position by either collapsing between a wall and toilet or being supported by well-meaning bystanders.

Loss of consciousness is brief and on recovery the subject is usually nauseated and tremulous with continued pallor and sweating. He or she is rarely confused. Crucially, syncopal individuals recall recovery at the site of their collapse, while those with tonic–clonic seizures have their first recall on the way to hospital.

No single feature will categorically allow a clinical differentiation between syncope and tonic–clonic seizures. The major differences are summarized in Table 23.2. Some complex partial seizures are described as 'temporal-lobe syncope' (Delgado-Escueta *et al.* 1982). In these, sudden falls occurred without warning, but were followed by amnesia and gradual recovery. They are, however, exceptionally rare as a new seizure type in adults, and are often accompanied by other seizure

Table 23.1. Causes of syncope

Reflex syncope
   Postural
   'Psychogenic'
   Micturition syncope
   Cough syncope
   Valsalva
   Swallow syncope
   Glossopharyngeal neuralgia

Cardiac syncope
   Dysrhythmias (heart block, tachycardias, etc)
   Valvular disease (particularly aortic stenosis)
   Atrial myxoma
   Cardiomyopathies
   Shunts
   Pulmonary hypertension

Perfusion failure
   Hypovolaemia
   Syndromes of autonomic failure
   Subclavian steal

Related to head posture
   Carotid sinus sensitivity
   Atlanto-axial subluxation
   Syringomyelia/syringobulbia

Table 23.2. The differences between syncope and seizures characterized by collapse

	Syncope	Seizures
Posture	Upright	Any posture
Pallor and sweating	Invariable	Uncommon
Onset	Gradual	Sudden/aura
Injury	Unusual	Not uncommon
Convulsive jerks	Not uncommon	Common
Incontinence	Rare	Common
Unconsciousness	Seconds	Minutes
Recovery	Rapid	Often slow
Post-ictal confusion	Rare	Common
Frequency	Infrequent	May be frequent
Precipitating factors	Crowded places Lack of food Unpleasant circumstances	Rare

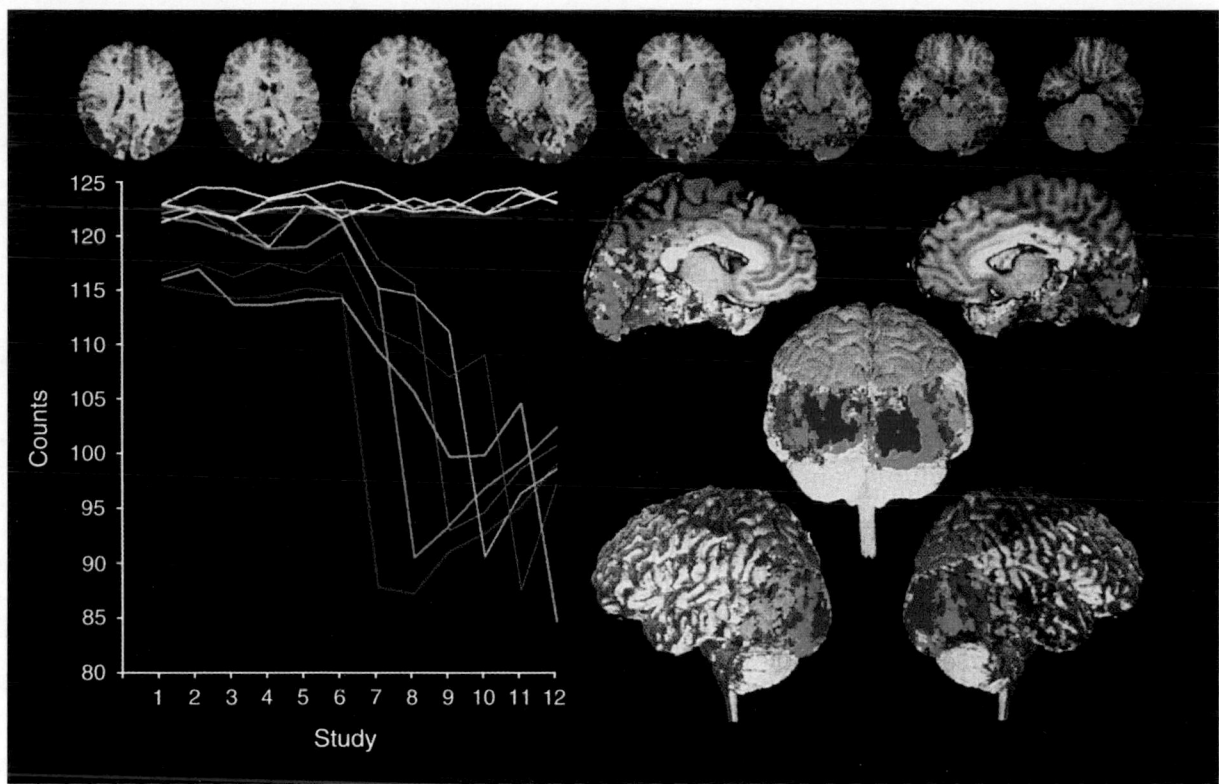

Plate 1 Spreading oligenia in a young woman during a spontaneous migraine attack demonstrated by positron emission tomography. (Reproduced with permission from Woods, R. P. *et al.* (1994). Bilateral spread cerebral hypoperfusion during spontaneous migraine headache. *N. Engl. J. Med.*, 331, 1689–1692, Figure 1.) (See also Fig. 3.2.)

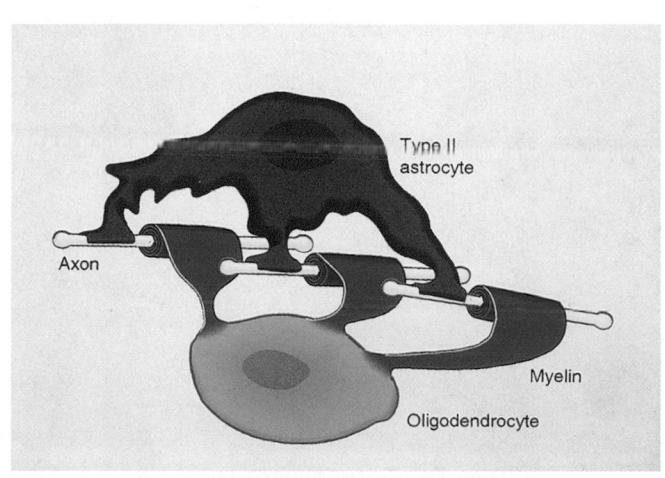

(a)

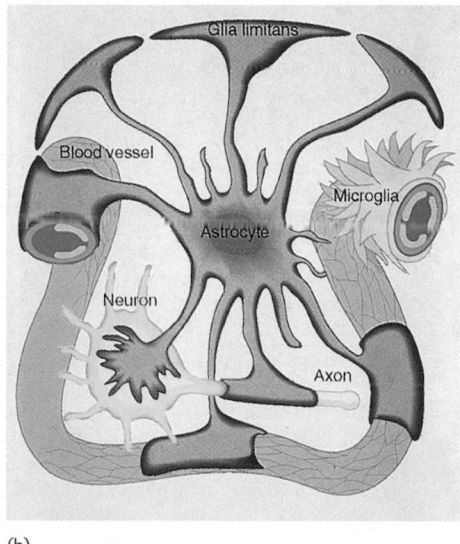

(b)

Plate 2 (a) The cellular architecture of myelinated axons. (b) The functions of astrocytes in the central nervous system. (Reproduced with permission from Compston, D. A. S. (1998) In *McAlpine's multiple sclerosis*, (ed. D. A. S. Compston, G. C. Ebers, H. Lassmann *et al.*), pp. 283–321. Churchill Livingstone, London.) (See also Fig. 7.1.)

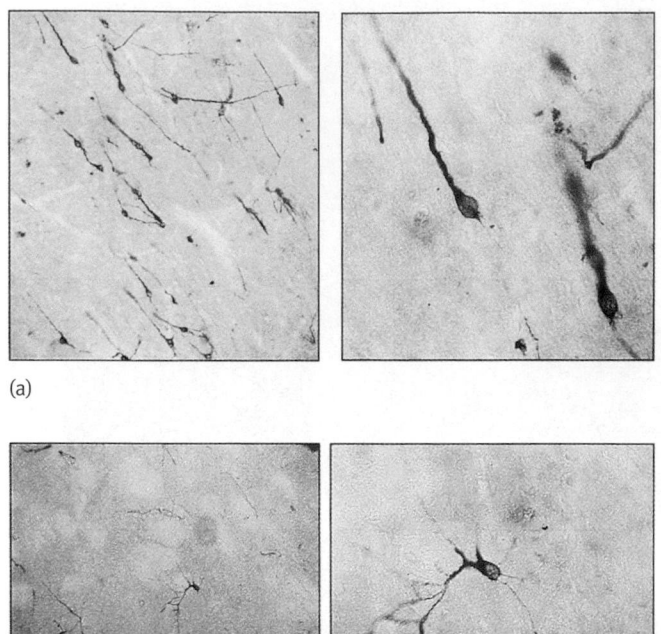

(a)

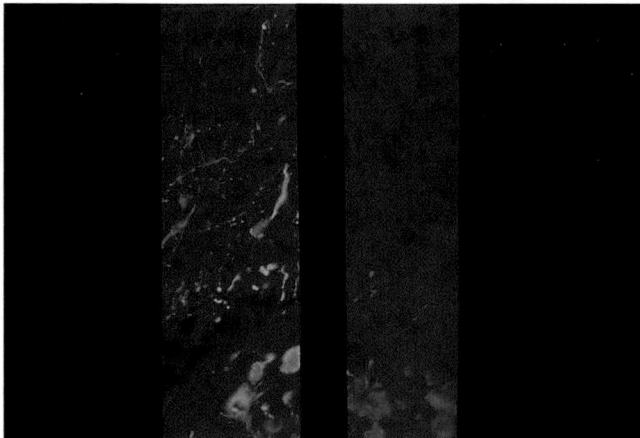

(b)

Plate 3 (a) Morphological features of cortical neurons, shown by human neurosphere cells implanted into the neocortex.
(b) Morphological features of striatal neurons, shown by identical human neurosphere cells implanted into the striatum. (Kindly provided by Dr Anne Rosser.) (See also Fig. 7.2.)

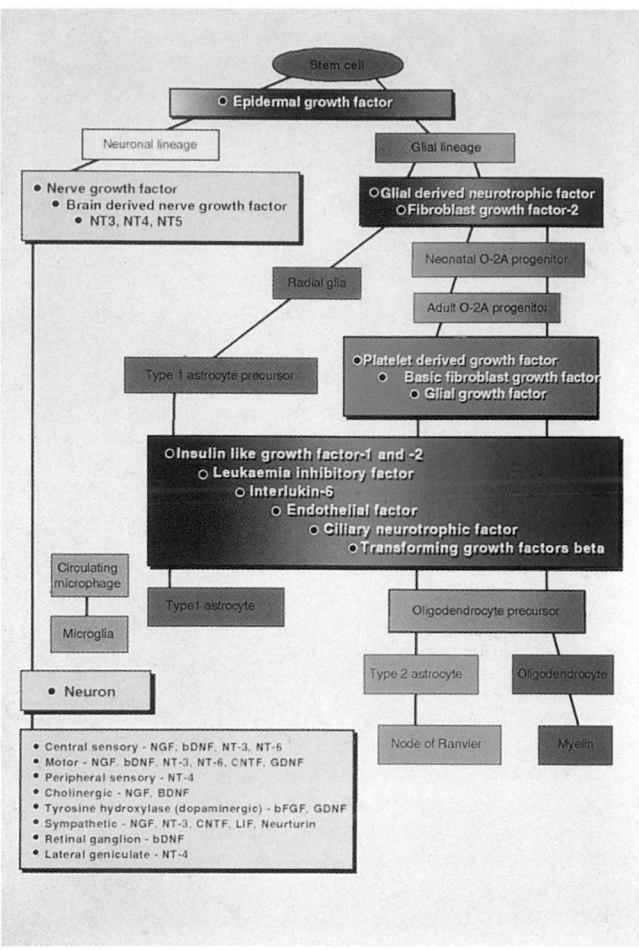

Plate 4 Growth factors which influence proliferation, migration, differentiation, or survival of neurons and glia are shown; most have effects on more than one cell type. (See also Fig. 7.3.)

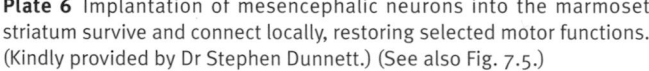

Plate 5 Axonal processes of neurons (shown in yellow) grow through a three-dimensional culture of Schwann cells (left); failure of rat axons to penetrate oligodendrocytes in culture (right). (Kindly provided by Dr James Fawcett.) (See also Fig. 7.4.)

Plate 6 Implantation of mesencephalic neurons into the marmoset striatum survive and connect locally, restoring selected motor functions. (Kindly provided by Dr Stephen Dunnett.) (See also Fig. 7.5.)

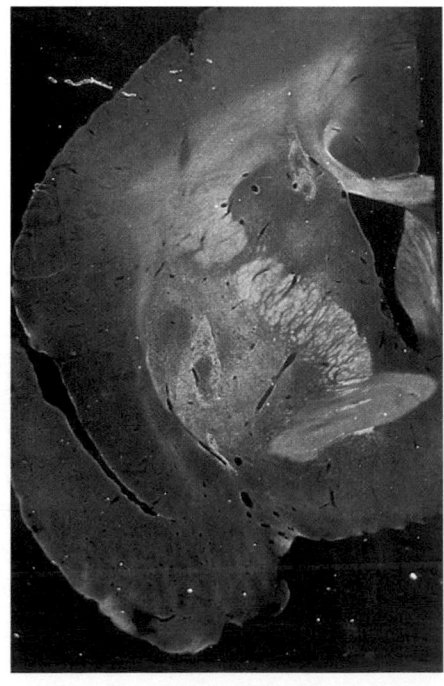

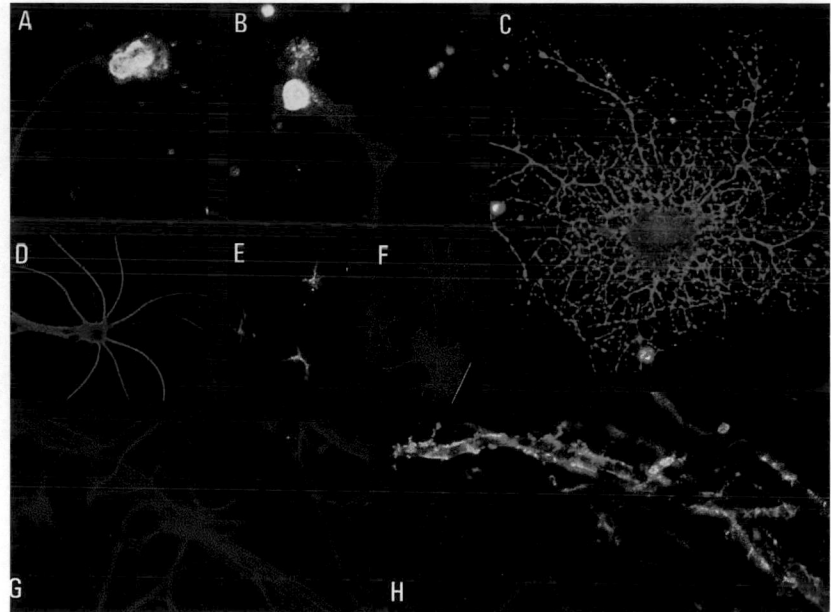

Plate 7 The rodent glial lineage. (a) A bipolar A2B5 positive rat cortex neonatal progenitor undergoing division (bromdeoxyuridine uptake shown in yellow). (b) A unipolar (rat hindbrain) adult progenitor undergoing division. (c) A differentiated oligodendrocyte stained for galactocerebroside. Astrocyte subtypes: (d) the type-1 astrocyte stained for GFAP; (e) the type-2 astrocyte stained for GFAP; (f) the type-2 astrocyte stained for A2B5; (g) the type-2 astrocyte stained with GFAP seen contacting a bundle of axons. (h) Triple staining for axons (blue), asytocytes (red), and oligodendrocytes (green/yellow) to show the interactions of O-2A progenitor progeny and nerve fibres. (Originals kindly provided by Dr John Zajicek.) (See also Fig. 7.6.)

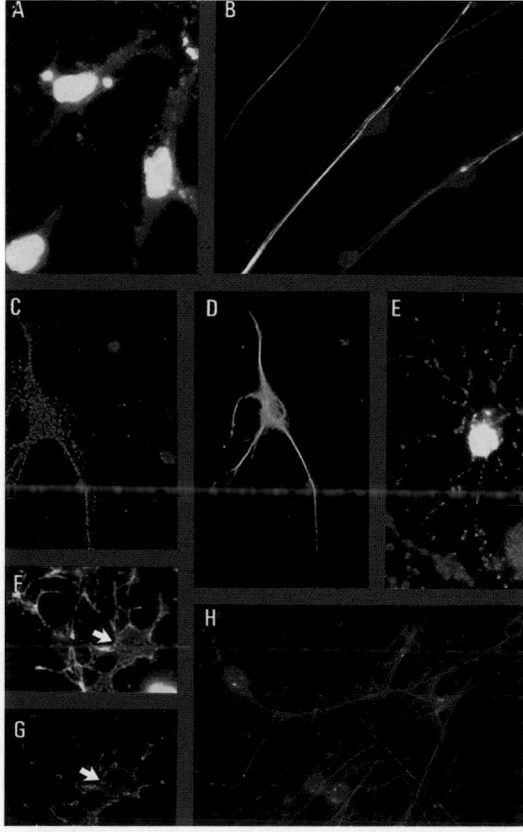

Plate 8 The adult human oligodendrocyte lineage. (a) The oligodendrocyte progenitor stained red with A2B5 proliferates in response to astrocyte-derived factors. (b) The bipolar oligodendrocyte progenitor associates with (rat) dorsal root ganglion neurons stained blue for neurofilament. (c) The progenitor differentiates into an astrocyte stained red with A2B5. (d) The progenitor differentiates into an astrocyte stained green with GFAP. (e) The O4-positive pro-oligodendrocyte stained red with O4 and showing BrdU uptake is considered to have divided as a progenitor and then differentiated. (f) The progenitor differentiates into an oligodendrocyte stained green with antibody for galatocerebroside. (g) The differentiating progenitor stains red with A2B5. (h) Differentiated human glial oligodendrocytes (stained red with galactocerebroside) develop processes which associate with several (rat) dorsal root ganglion axons. (Originals kindly provided by Dr Neil Scolding and Dr Christopher Shaw.) (See also Fig. 7.7.)

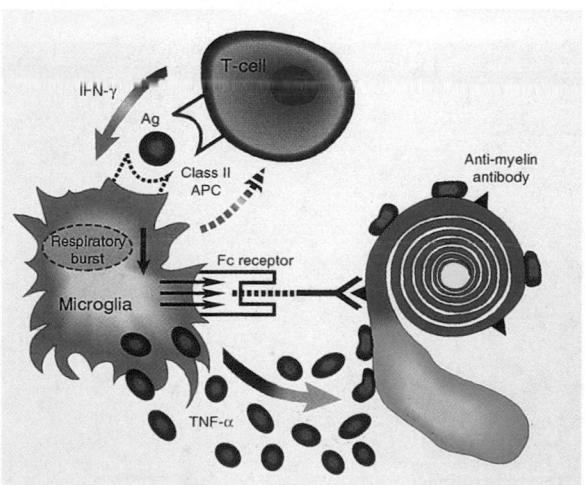

Plate 9 Representation of the T-cell–microglia interaction in the central nervous system. (Reproduced with permission from Compston 1998.) (See also Fig. 7.10)

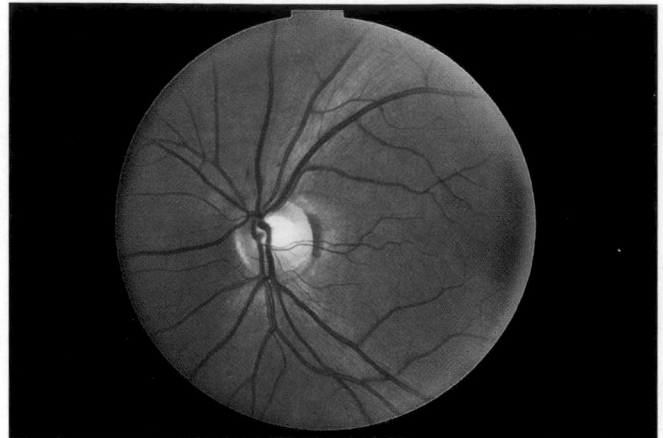

Plate 10 A normal fundus and optic disc. (See also Fig. 8.3.)

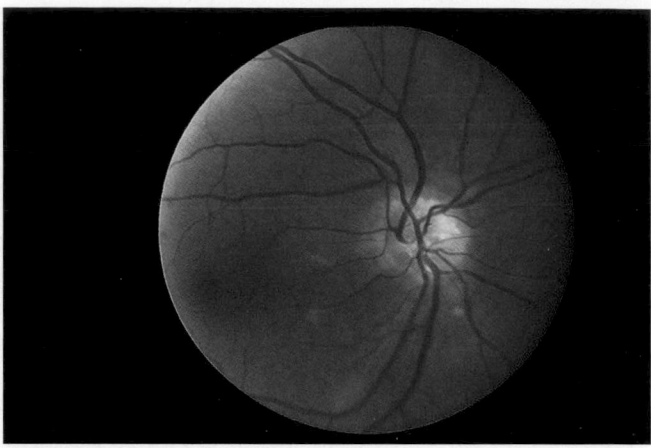

Plate 13 Pseudopapilloedema showing optic nerve head drusen. (See also Fig. 8.6.)

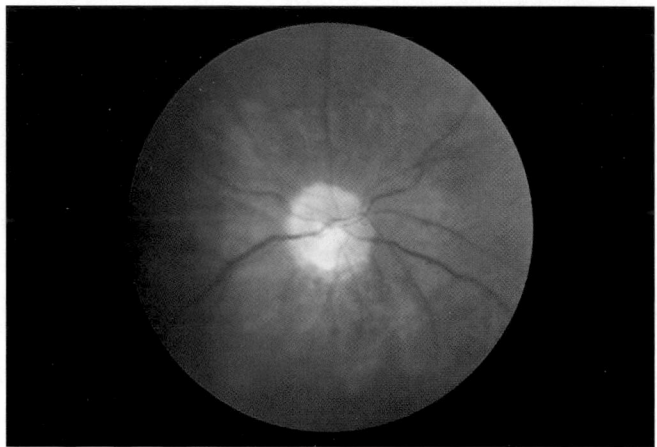

Plate 11 Central retinal artery occlusion. (See also Fig. 8.4.)

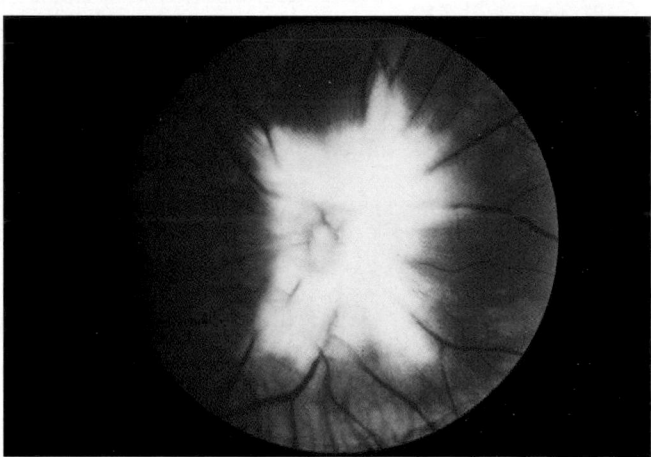

Plate 14 Myelinated retinal nerve fibres. (See also Fig. 8.7.)

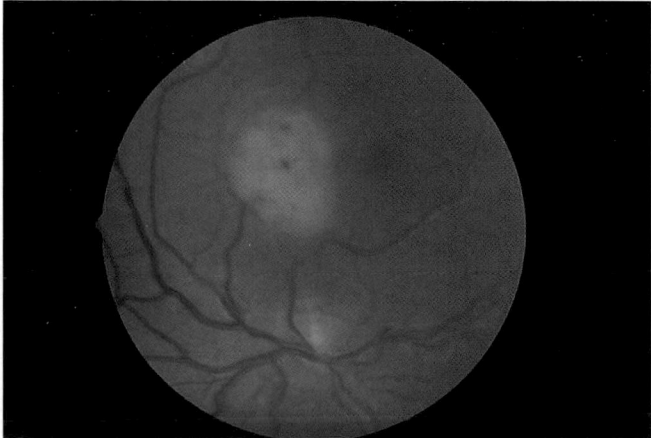

Plate 12 Fundus, showing retinal haematoma associated with tuberous sclerosis. (See also Fig. 8.5.)

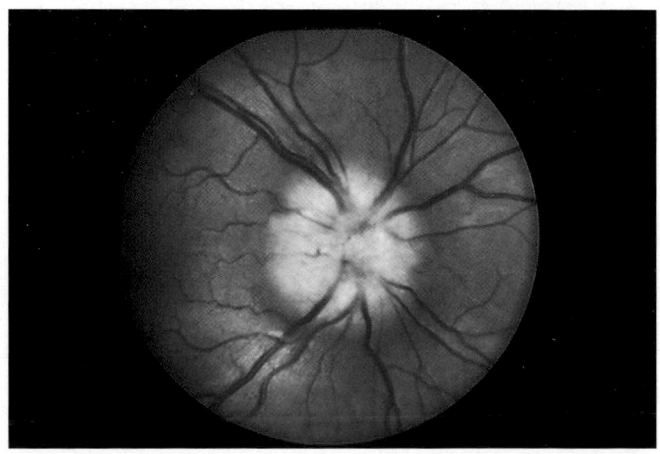

Plate 15 Papilloedema due to raised intracranial pressure. (See also Fig. 8.8.)

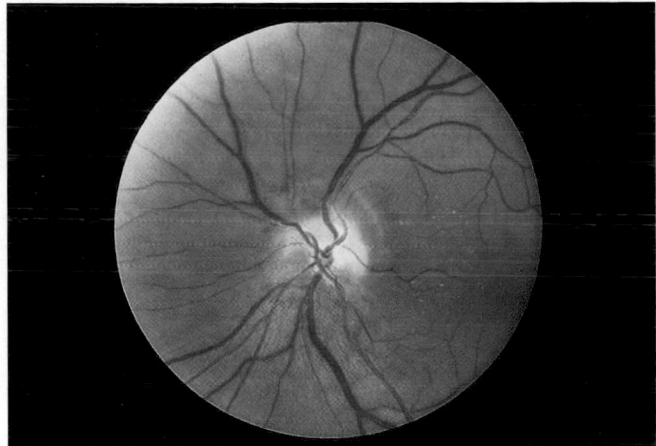

Plate 16 Anterior ischaemic optic neuropathy. (See also Fig. 8.9.)

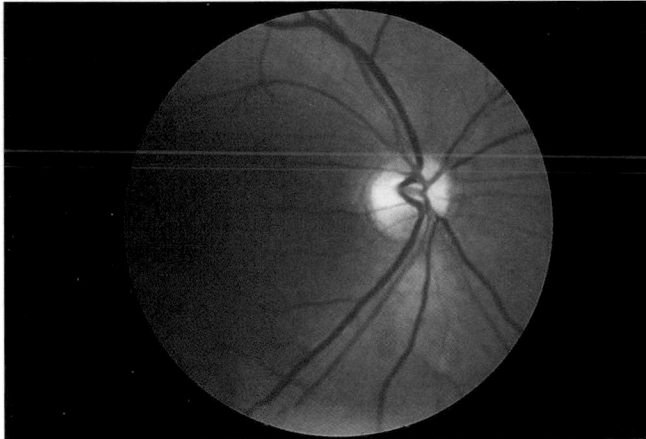

Plate 17 Optic atrophy. (See also Fig. 8.10.)

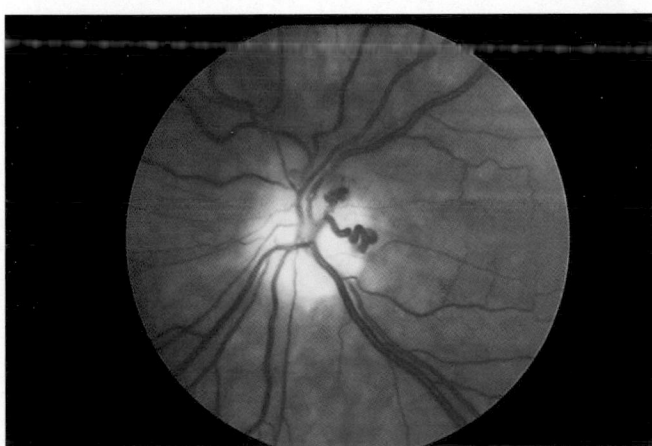

Plate 18 Optociliary shunts due to an optic nerve sheath meningioma. (See also Fig. 8.11.)

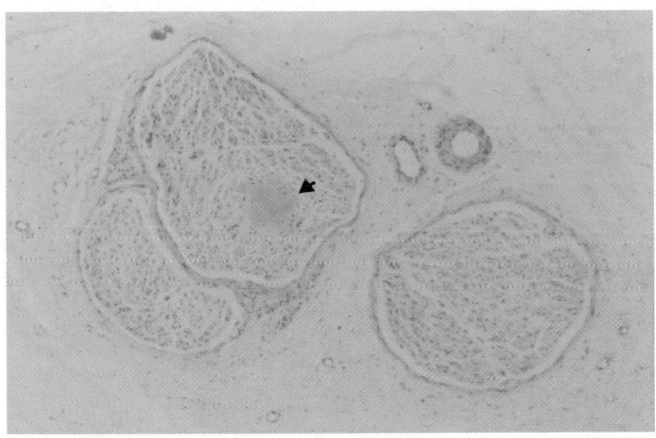

(a)

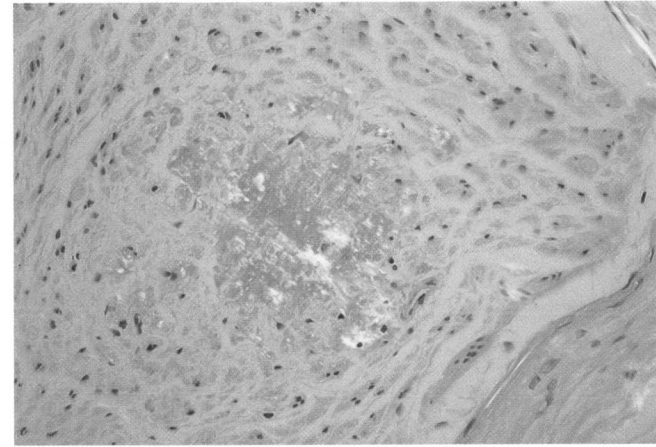

(b)

Plate 19 Amyloid due to immunoglobulin light-chain deposition in peripheral nerve. (a) Eosinophilic deposit within a nerve fascicle (low power, haematoxylin and eosin); (b) apple-green birefringence of the amyloid deposit in polarized light (Congo red, higher power). (See also Fig. 12.1.4.)

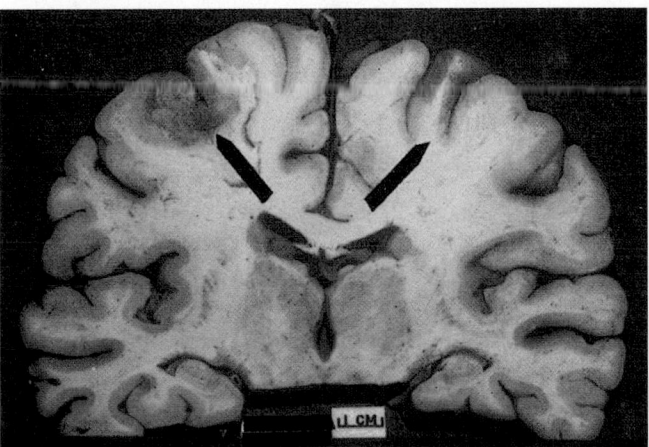

Plate 20 Coronal section of brain showing bilateral boundary zone infarcts (arrowed) in a patient with prolonged hypoxia and hypotension. (See also Fig. 16.1.)

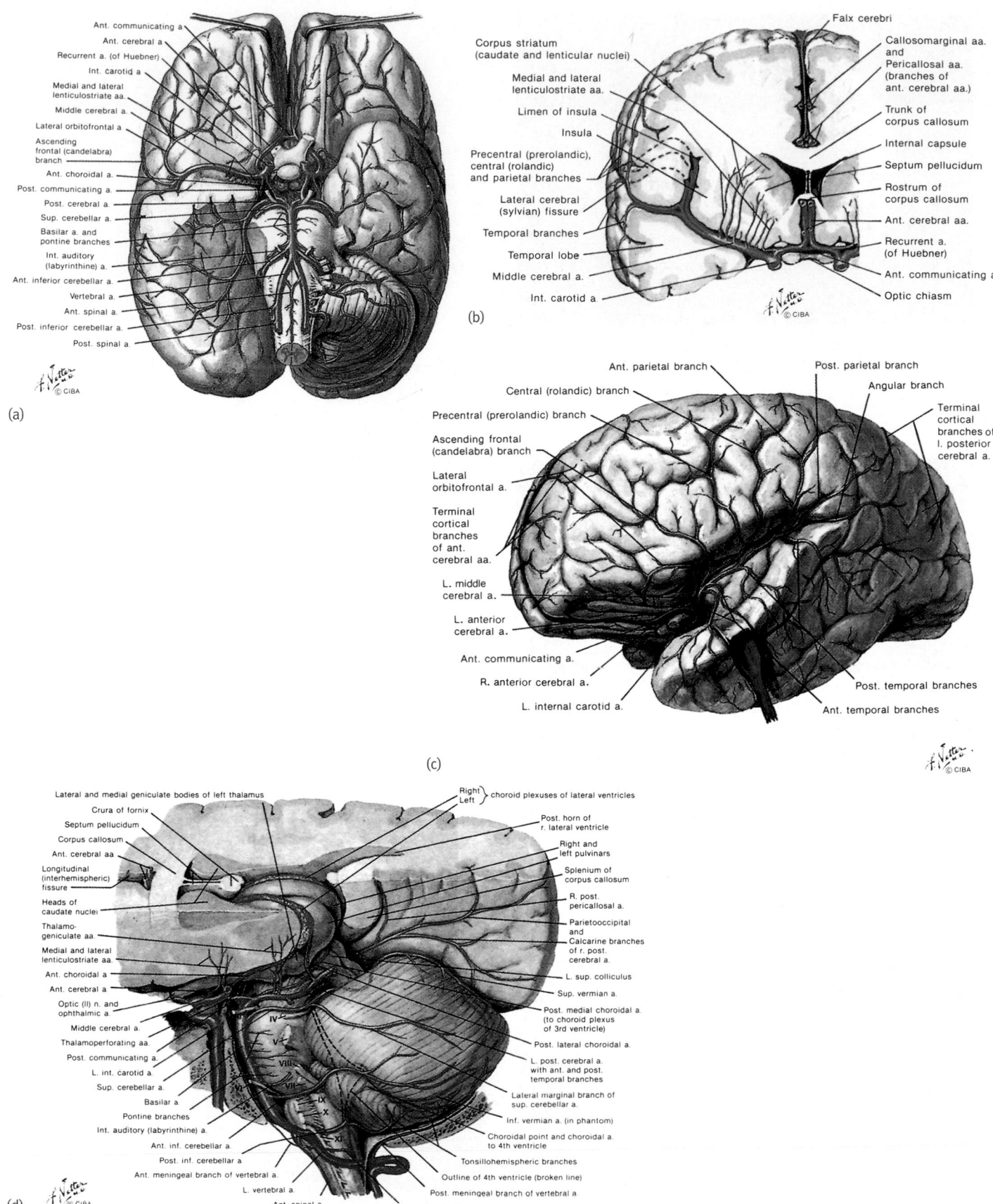

(a)

Ant. communicating a
Ant. cerebral a
Recurrent a. (of Huebner)
Int. carotid a
Medial and lateral lenticulostriate aa.
Middle cerebral a.
Lateral orbitofrontal a
Ascending frontal (candelabra) branch
Ant. choroidal a.
Post. communicating a.
Post. cerebral a.
Sup. cerebellar a.
Basilar a. and pontine branches
Int. auditory (labyrinthine) a.
Ant. inferior cerebellar a.
Vertebral a.
Ant. spinal a.
Post. inferior cerebellar a.
Post. spinal a.

(b)

Corpus striatum (caudate and lenticular nuclei)
Medial and lateral lenticulostriate aa.
Limen of insula
Insula
Precentral (prerolandic), central (rolandic) and parietal branches
Lateral cerebral (sylvian) fissure
Temporal branches
Temporal lobe
Middle cerebral a.
Int. carotid a.

Falx cerebri
Callosomarginal aa. and Pericallosal aa. (branches of ant. cerebral aa.)
Trunk of corpus callosum
Internal capsule
Septum pellucidum
Rostrum of corpus callosum
Ant. cerebral aa.
Recurrent a. (of Huebner)
Ant. communicating a.
Optic chiasm

(c)

Ant. parietal branch
Central (rolandic) branch
Precentral (prerolandic) branch
Ascending frontal (candelabra) branch
Lateral orbitofrontal a.
Terminal cortical branches of ant. cerebral aa.
L. middle cerebral a.
L. anterior cerebral a.
Ant. communicating a.
R. anterior cerebral a.
L. internal carotid a.

Post. parietal branch
Angular branch
Terminal cortical branches of l. posterior cerebral a.
Post. temporal branches
Ant. temporal branches

(d)

Lateral and medial geniculate bodies of left thalamus
Crura of fornix
Septum pellucidum
Corpus callosum
Ant. cerebral aa.
Longitudinal (interhemispheric) fissure
Heads of caudate nuclei
Thalamo-geniculate aa.
Medial and lateral lenticulostriate aa.
Ant. choroidal a
Ant. cerebral a.
Optic (II) n. and ophthalmic a.
Middle cerebral a.
Thalamoperforating aa.
Post. communicating a.
L. int. carotid a.
Sup. cerebellar a.
Basilar a
Pontine branches
Int. auditory (labyrinthine) a.
Ant. inf. cerebellar a.
Post. inf. cerebellar a
Ant. meningeal branch of vertebral a.
L. vertebral a.
Ant. spinal a.

Right Left } choroid plexuses of lateral ventricles
Post. horn of r. lateral ventricle
Right and left pulvinars
Splenium of corpus callosum
R. post. pericallosal a.
Parietooccipital and Calcarine branches of r. post. cerebral a.
L. sup. colliculus
Sup. vermian a.
Post. medial choroidal a. (to choroid plexus of 3rd ventricle)
Post. lateral choroidal a.
L. post. cerebral a. with ant. and post. temporal branches
Lateral marginal branch of sup. cerebellar a.
Inf. vermian a. (in phantom)
Choroidal point and choroidal a. to 4th ventricle
Tonsillohemispheric branches
Outline of 4th ventricle (broken line)
Post. meningeal branch of vertebral a
L. post. spinal a.

Plate 21 (a) A view of the base of the brain to show the circle of Willis, vertebrobasilar arterial system, middle and anterior cerebral arteries. (b) A coronal section of the brain through the optic chiasm to show the penetrating lenticulostriate branches of the main stem of the middle cerebral artery. (c) A lateral view of the brain to show the cortical branches of the middle cerebral artery. (d) Lateral view of the brain to show the vertebral, basilar, and posterior cerebral arteries and their branches in the posterior fossa. (Figures (a)–(d) Copyright 1990 CIBA–GEIGY Corporation. Reprinted with permission from CLINICAL SYMPOSIA, illustrated by Frank N. Netter, MD. All rights reserved.). (See also Fig. 27.7.)

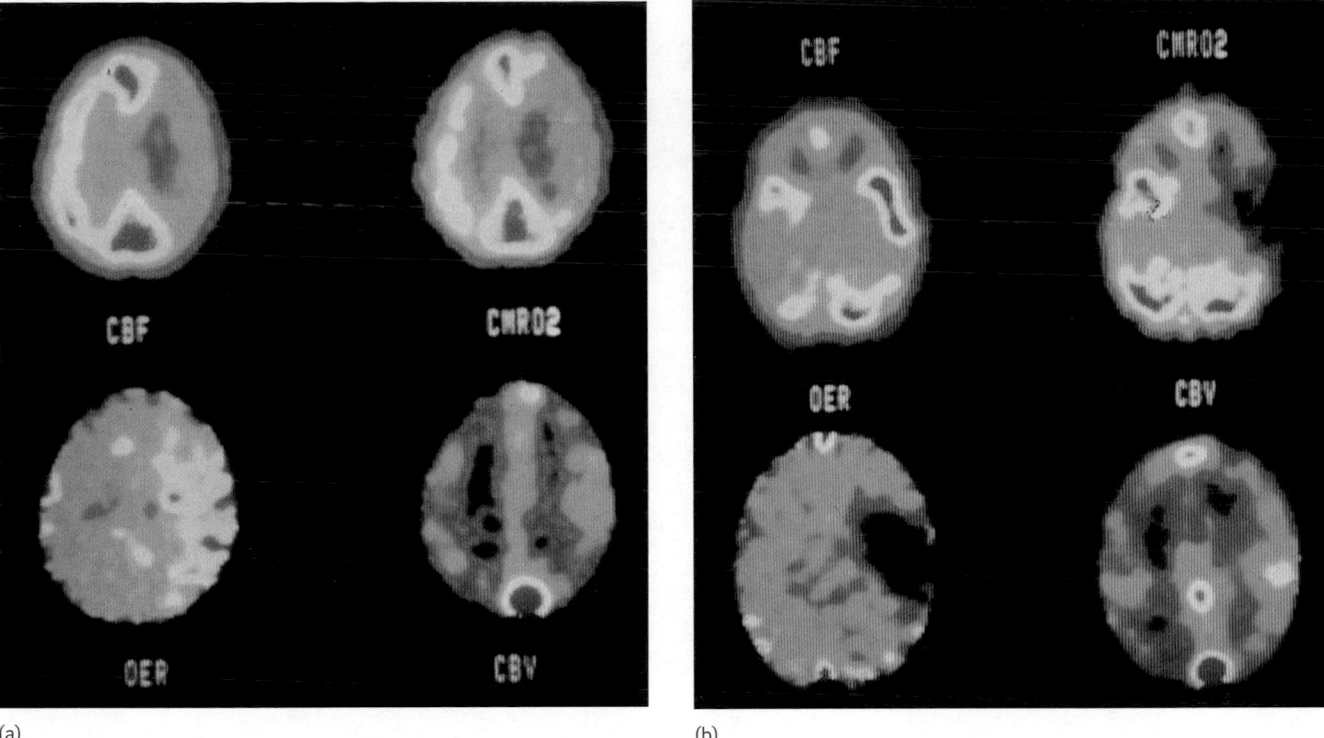

(a) (b)

Plate 22 PET scan 90 minutes after acute left middle cerebral artery occlusion: (a) cerebral blood flow (CBF) is low, cerebral metabolic rate for oxygen ($CMRO_2$) is low, but the oxygen extraction ratio (OER) (fraction) is maximal (i.e. ischaemia). (b) PET scan a week later to show increased CBF and cerebral blood volume (CBV), despite low $CMRO_2$ and OER (i.e. absolute luxury perfusion). (Scans kindly provided by Professor Richard Frackowiak, MRC Cyclotron Unit, London.) (See also Fig. 27.12.)

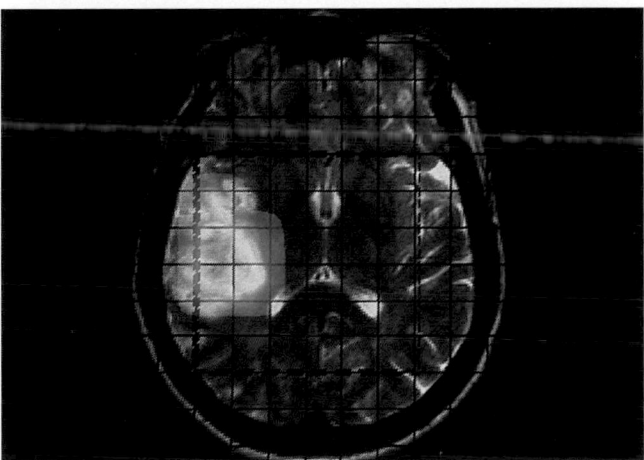

Plate 23 A metabolic 'map' of lactate in the brain by MR spectroscopy (colour coded from blue up to red), superimposed on a structural MR scan. There is an obvious excess of lactate in the infarcted area in the distribution of a branch of the right middle cerebral artery. (Supplied by Dr Joanna Wardlaw.) (See also Fig. 27.13(b).)

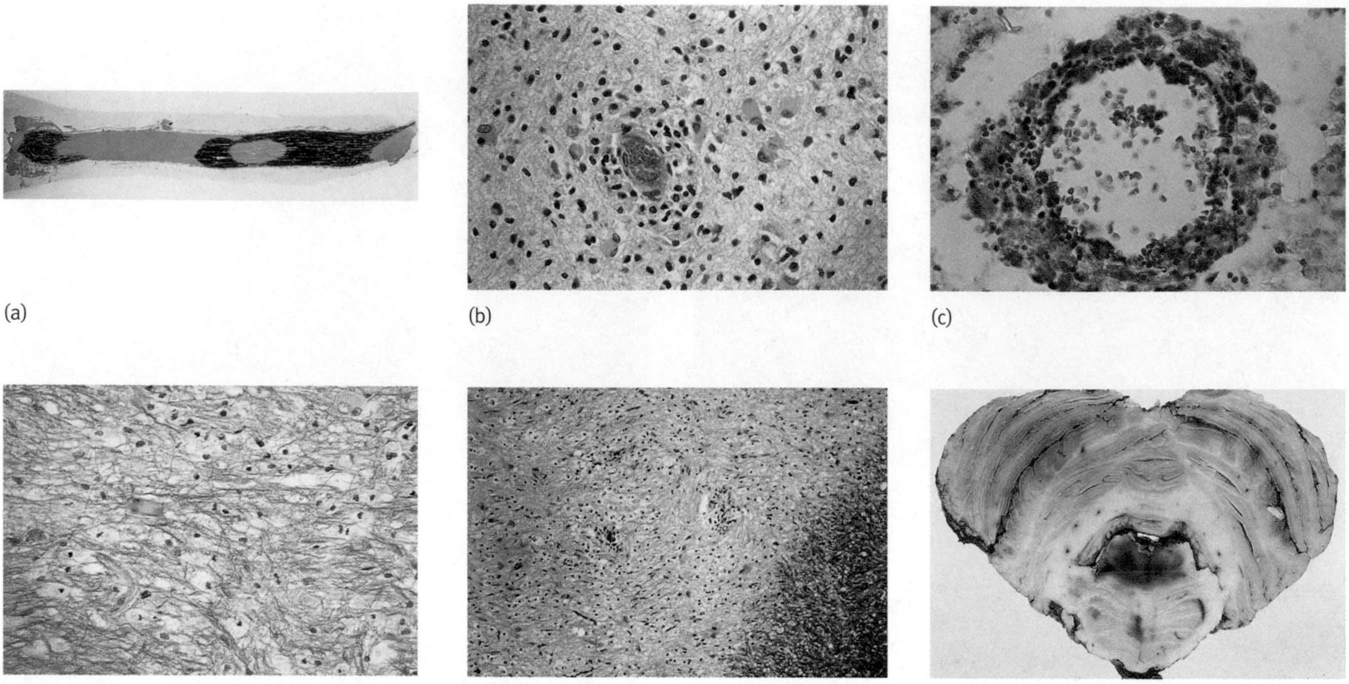

(a)

(b)

(c)

(d)

(e)

(f)

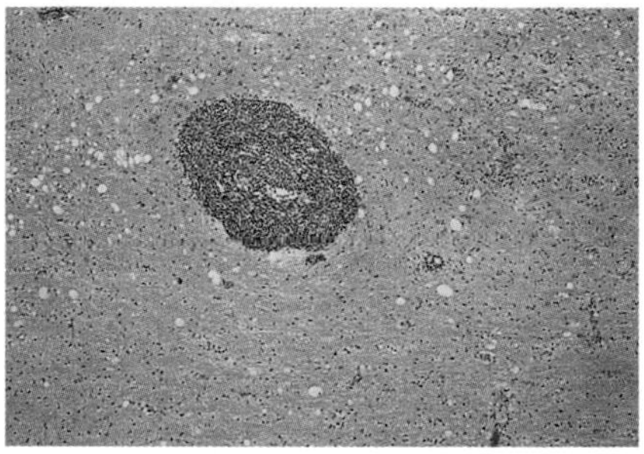

Plate 24 The evolution of demyelination. (a) Macroscopic areas of demyelination in the optic nerve. (b) Perivascular infiltration by activated lymphocytes. (c) Microglial removal of myelin debris. (d) Astrocytosis. (e) Persistent demyelination showing a sharp boundary between normal appearing and demyelinated white matter. (f) Macroscopic appearance of the brain in a patient dying from acute disseminated encephalomyelitis in an illness lasting 10 days, showing diffuse midbrain damage with a combination of demyelination and tentorial herniation due to cerebral oedema. (g) Acute perivascular infiltration in the same patient. (a)–(e) Reproduced with permission from Hall *et al.* (1997*a*); (f) and (g) kindly provided by Dr Janice Anderson and reproduced with permission from Matthews (1998*b*). (See also Fig. 29.1.)

(g)

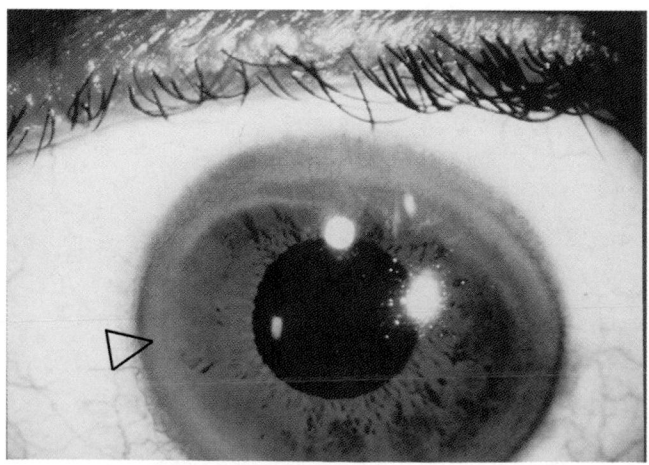

Plate 25 A corneal Kayser–Fleischer ring (arrowed) in Wilson's disease. The patient presented with writer's cramp, mild parkinsonism, and a recent history of depression. (See also Fig. 32.19.)

types in keeping with a frontal onset. A carefully taken history is the most important step and it must always be regarded as unwise to diagnose epilepsy where there is evidence of any of the precipitating factors that are strongly associated with syncope.

Cardiac syncope

Cardiac syncope may have somewhat different characteristics as onset is usually rapid and often instantaneous (Ross 1988).

Atrio-ventricular block or other cardiac dysrhythmias are the most common causes of cardiac syncope (Friedberg 1971). Although bradycardia as low as 30 beats per minute is often better tolerated than tachycardias in excess of 150 per minute, dysrhythmias causing bradycardia or asystole most commonly cause syncope.

Adelman and Wigle (1969) described a syndrome of sino-atrial syncope resulting from sino-atrial block and brady-cardia in addition to supraventricular tachycardias (atrial fibrillation and flutter). It results from bradycardia combined with failure of the usual atrio-ventricular junctional escape mechanisms. Coronary artery disease, cardiomyopathy, and neuromuscular disorders are often associated with this brady-tachy syndrome.

The sick sinus syndrome (Lown 1967) presents with sinus bradycardia and sinus arrest, often associated with pre-syncopal and syncopal symptoms (Rubenstein et al. 1972). Syncope resulting from bradycardia and asystole (Adams–Stokes attacks) often develops suddenly and can lead to injury (Sutton and Perrins 1979). Recovery is usually swift, initial pallor being followed by flushing with recovery. Some clonic movements may be seen. On occasions bradycardia may result in prolonged syncope (Sutton and Perrins 1979).

Tachycardias less commonly cause syncope, and may only do so when patients stand up during an episode. Their presence may be suggested by the symptom of palpitation associated with other pre-syncopal symptoms. Whereas the insertion of a fixed rate or demand pacemaker is the treatment of choice for syncope associated with bradycardias and asystole, appropriate antidysrhythmic drugs may be used for the treatment of paroxysmal tachycardia.

Obstructive heart disease represents another cardiac disorder causing syncope. Aortic stenosis has been recognized as a cause of syncope associated with exercise (Schwartz et al. 1969). Syncope may occur in up to 30 per cent of patients with idio-pathic hypertrophic subaortic stenosis (Schamroth 1971), a condition which may be associated with Friedreich's ataxia and myotonic dystrophia. Atrial myxoma, more commonly of the left atrium, can result in episodes of syncope related to postural changes.

Differentiating between cardiac syncope and seizures may demand 24-hour ambulatory monitoring with the capture of symptomatic events. While cardiac dysrhythmias may be mis-diagnosed as epilepsy, primary cerebral dysrhythmias may also lead to secondary cardiac dysrhythmia. For this reason simultaneous monitoring of ECG and EEG may be necessary (Blumhardt et al. 1986).

Syncope with autonomic failure

Syncope in progressive autonomic failure develops slowly over several minutes. The usual pallor, sweating, and bradycardia may be absent.

A large number of central and peripheral nervous system disorders are associated with symptoms of autonomic failure in which syncope is prominent (Section 1.8.3). Syncope occurs on standing, beginning with a feeling of light-headedness which progresses slowly. Visual obscurations may occur with other central symptoms of cerebral hypoperfusion, but patients show an absence of sweating, bradycardia, or pallor.

The treatment of syncope in autonomic failure may be difficult. Elastic stockings may be helpful (Sheps 1976) and some patients may tolerate a G-suit with good effect. Significant improvement can be produced if the patient sleeps with a head-up tilt, which increases plasma volume and blood pressure (Bannister et al. 1969). α-Fludrocortisone has similar effects and is a useful addition. Other drugs may be helpful, including indomethacin, ephedrine, and pindolol.

Carotid sinus syncope

Whereas compression of the carotid sinus in young people rarely causes any symptoms, in the elderly, particularly those with heart disease, it can cause bradycardia and syncope. Most commonly this is due to reflex vagal inhibition of the heart (Thomas 1969). However, more rarely it may be caused by a vasopressor effect, leading to a fall in blood pressure independent of heart rate. Very rarely, pressure on one carotid can lead to almost immediate loss of consciousness if there is a grossly stenotic or occluded contralateral artery so that ipsilateral carotid compression, in effect, leads to a standstill in much of the cerebral circulation (Ross 1988).

Carotid sinus syncope is most commonly seen in patients with arteriosclerosis and hypertension, but may sometimes occur with local neoplastic disease in the neck or aneurysmal dilatation of the sinus (Ross 1988). The usual precipitant in all cases is a sudden turn of the head inducing dizziness and fainting. The treatment of choice for carotid sinus syncope is a demand cardiac pacemaker but some patients may respond to carotid sinus denervation (Trout et al. 1979).

Pulmonary disorders and syncope

Cough syncope is the most common respiratory cause of syncope. It is seen in middle-aged, usually male, smokers, who are usually overweight and have chronic obstructive airways disease. Fainting is precipitated by a paroxysm of continuous coughing. The individual experiences light-headedness followed by unconsciousness, usually with a quick recovery. The prolonged bout of coughing elevates intrathoracic pressure and thereby impedes venous return and cardiac output. At the same time increased thoracic pressure may be transmitted to the subarachnoid space, further reducing cerebral blood flow (Kerr and Eich 1961). It is doubtful that people with normal respiratory function can cough for a sufficiently long period to induce cough syncope (Pederson et al. 1966). More rarely, cough syncope, as well as cough headache, have been associated with cerebellar ectopia (Larson *et al.* 1974) and syringomyelia (Hampton *et al.* 1982).

Primary or secondary pulmonary hypertension may be associated with syncope because of a failure of the right ventricle to increase output on demand. Syncope may therefore occur during effort in a similar fashion to that seen with aortic stenosis (Ross 1988). Syncope may also occur with pulmonary embolus (Soloff and Rodman 1967).

Oesophageal syncope

Syncope may occur as a reflex response to sensory stimuli within the territories of the glossopharyngeal or vagus nerves. This can lead to vagal discharge with bradycardia and slowed atrioventricular conduction (Levin and Posner 1972). Guberman and Catching (1986) described 29 patients with syncope associated with swallowing. Almost all patients had some form of cardiac disease (ischaemic heart disease or heart block) or oesophageal disorder. In patients with cardiac disease treated with digitalis, high pressures produced within the oesophagus or oesophageal stretching may produce a sufficient stimulus to increase heart block and lead to syncope.

MacDonald *et al.* (1983) described 17 patients who had syncope associated with head and neck cancer. In most, the syncope was spontaneous but could be due to an abnormal carotid sinus reflex. However, Tomlinson and Fox (1975) described a patient with syncope only while eating or drinking. He had a carcinoma of the oesophagus and resection of this stopped the syncope.

Syncope in the period after eating may not be uncommon, particularly in the elderly or in patients with autonomic failure (Fisher 1979). Syncope, as an accompaniment of glossopharyngeal neuralgia, was first described by Riley *et al.* (1942). The pain is precipitated by stimulation or movement of the oropharynx during chewing, swallowing, or coughing, and precedes syncope (Jamshidi and Masroor 1976). Carbamazepine can be used, although microvascular decompression has also been successful (Tsuboi *et al.* 1985). Rarely, syncope may occur with trigeminal neuralgia (Kapoor and Jannetta 1984).

Pelvic syncope

Syncope during and immediately after micturition is a not uncommon phenomenon. It seems to occur in two different groups of people: young, healthy men and older people of either sex who have concurrent medical problems (Kapoor *et al.* 1985). In the first group, syncope usually occurs at the end of voiding after the patient has got out of bed in the middle of the night. It seems to be predisposed to by sleep deprivation, hunger, and intercurrent infection. Alcohol ingestion is also likely to be particularly important (Lyle *et al.* 1961). Bladder dissention may be one means of reflexly precipitating fainting (Whitteridge 1960), which can also occur following the decompression of a painful distended bladder (Maclean *et al.* 1944). The role of the valsalva manoeuvre during voiding is uncertain.

Kapoor *et al.* (1985) described 25 patients with an average age of 60 in whom micturition syncope occurred. The majority were taking diuretics and some had been confined to bed for a prolonged period or had intercurrent illness or cardiac disease. Syncope may, on occasions, occur with defaecation in older patients (Pathy 1978). Other pelvic examinations and interventions are rarely associated with syncopal episodes. Bilbro (1970) described eight episodes of syncope or pre-syncope during 2500 prostatic examinations, and syncope can occur with the insertion of intra-uterine devices (Conrad *et al.* 1973).

23.1.3 Psychogenic alteration in consciousness

Psychogenic non-epileptic attacks (pseudoseizures)

The misdiagnosis of epilepsy is common, and psychogenic attacks mimicking most commonly tonic–clonic seizures, but also, more rarely, non-convulsive seizures, cause the greatest diagnostic difficulty. Their incidence in the community is difficult to ascertain, but could represent 3 per cent of all cases of epilepsy. The incidence increases dramatically as more selected and apparently refractory populations are examined. Thus up to 20 per cent of referrals to tertiary centres are misdiagnosed, and up to 50 per cent of cases of drug-refractory status epilepticus are due to psychogenic non-epileptic attacks (NEAs) (Howell *et al.* 1989).

Table 23.3. The differences between tonic-donic seizures and pseudoseizures

	Epileptic seizure	Pseudoseizure
Onset	Sudden	May be gradual
Retained consciousness in prolonged seizure	Very rare	Common
Pelvic thrusting	Rare	Common
Flailing, thrashing, asynchronous limb movements	Rare	Common
Rolling movements	Rare	Common
Cyanosis	Common	Unusual
Tongue biting and other injury	Common	Less common
Stereotyped attacks	Usual	Uncommon
Duration	Seconds or minutes	Often many minutes
Gaze aversion	Rare	Common
Resistance to passive limb movement or eye opening	Unusual	Common
Prevention of hand falling on to face	Unusual	Common
Induced by suggestion	Rarely	Often
Post-ictal drowsiness or confusion	Usual	Often absent
Ictal EEG abnormality	Almost always (except with simple and some complex partial seizures)	Almost never
Post-ictal EEG abnormal (after seizure with impairment of consciousness)	Usually	Rarely

The diagnosis of pseudoseizures may be difficult (King *et al.* 1982), particularly when they occur in patients who also have a history of true epileptic seizures. Eyewitness accounts and videotapes of events can raise suspicions, but no single clinical feature differentiates NEAs from epilepsy, although a number of factors may be of value (Table 23.3). The most useful clinical feature of attacks is resistance to eye opening in pseudoseizures and the absence of pupillary dilatation, which is an invariable feature of tonic–clonic seizures.

The temporal pattern of attacks should, however, alert the clinician to the possibility of NEAs. They are refractory to anti-convulsant therapy, in contrast to epilepsy, where convulsive seizures in particular are likely to be well controlled. Failure to control apparent tonic–clonic seizures in a patient who develops attacks after the first decade of life, in whom there is no identifiable cerebral disease, and in who interictal EEG recordings have never shown significant epileptiform abnormalities is almost pathognomonic of NEAs. With modern antiepileptic drugs very few patients continue to have frequent tonic–clonic seizures, and those who do, have preceding severe cerebral insults resulting in intellectual and neurological impairments. In short they have 'bad brains'; evidence of which is strikingly absent in people most with NEAs.

Some positive features allow identification of subjects at risk. NEAs occur most commonly in women, with onset most commonly in the second or third decades of life (Roy 1979; Howell *et al.* 1989). Individuals often have a significant history of self-poisoning and self-injury, and previous episodes of un-explained physical symptoms. They come from dysfunctional families, and there is often a history of physical and sexual abuse.

The management of NEAs is more difficult than the diagnosis. Symptomatic events will usually need to be recorded by video-telemetry and be shown to be characteristic of the usual attacks. An open discussion of the non-epileptic nature is necessary, after which antiepileptic drugs can be withdrawn, usually with the advice that this alone will often result in an improvement in attacks. The psychological and psychiatric background needs to be explored by people with experience of the area and an ongoing programme of treatment and support instituted. It is said that the prognosis is good, with remission in over 50 per cent of cases (French *et al.* 1988), although other non-physical symptoms commonly occur in the long term. There is controversy about the incidence of epilepsy in people with NEAs. It is probably low, but those with both problems are exceptionally difficult to manage.

Hyperventilation

Hyperventilation is common and the bulk of cases may go unrecognized but some may be misdiagnosed as epilepsy (Riley 1982). Common manifestations include dizziness, detachment, blurred vision, tingling, muscle spasm, tetany, palpitation, dysp-noea and chest pain, heartburn, epigastric pain, muscle cramps, and fatigue. Some form of alteration in consciousness is common and up to 15 per cent of patients may lose consciousness during attacks (Pincus 1978). The wide variety of symp-toms experienced by patients with hyperventilation will most commonly be confused with complex partial seizures.

The most useful factors allowing differentiation are that hyperventilation attacks are commonly precipitated by stressful circumstances, and that they lack a stereotypic nature, with different types of symptoms referable to different systems occurring on different occasions. A simple diagnostic test is to ask the patient to re-breathe from a paper bag held over the mouth and nose during attacks.

Panic attacks

Panic attacks can be mistaken for complex partial seizures (Harper and Roth 1962). They often include hyperventilation but also commonly encompass abdominal discomfort, a choking feeling, fear, autonomic symptoms, and sometimes even loss of consciousness. The episodes, however, are usually clearly precipitated and often more prolonged than seizures. Panic attacks are most likely to occur in association with phobic anxiety states and patients usually have considerable insight into the nature of their attacks.

Rage outbursts

There are common misconceptions that violent behaviour is common in people with epilepsy and that it may occur during the course of complex partial seizures. In fact it is extremely rare. In spite of this, it is common for individuals who describe sudden outbursts of violent behaviour with minimal provoca-tion, often with some associated patchy amnesia, to be referred for neurological evaluation with a presumptive diagnosis of a seizure disorder. It is striking that individuals are invariably young men from deprived backgrounds who have often them-selves been abused. Violence occurs in response to minimal stimuli and is often directed against a specific family member. This is clearly distinct from epilepsy and the term 'episodic dyscontrol' has been used (Maletzky 1973). The issues are always somewhat complicated by the EEG, as non-specific abnormalities are extremely common in psychopathic indivi-duals (StaffordClark and Taylor 1949). Strict guidelines must be applied before ever accepting that aggressive or violent behav-iour is part of a seizure disorder (Treiman and Delgado-Escueta 1983).

An epileptic basis to such attacks should only be accepted where definite seizures occur at other times and where violent behaviour is a consistent feature of that individual's seizures. Violence can only be accepted as seizure-related where it is brief and poorly directed.

Fugue states

States of psychogenic wandering are prolonged, usually with sudden recovery of awareness. It is often impossible to obtain a clear account of behaviour during such attacks but this usually appears to have been quite normal. Subjects have a dense amnesia for the period for time concerned and individuals usually have an associated depression and the need to escape from some stressful life situation (Stengel 1943). Such episodes may be confused with complex partial status or other forms of non-convulsive status epilepticus (Mayeux and Lender 1978; Mayeux *et al.* 1979), but here there is usually evidence of abnormal behaviour during the amnesia.

23.1.4 Focal cerebral ischaemia

It may sometimes be difficult to differentiate between focal seizures and focal ischaemia due to either migraine or thromboembolic disease.

Transient ischaemic attacks will rarely be confused with seizures because they develop more slowly and last for longer. They are virtually never accompanied by altered consciousness, and motor and sensory phenomena that comprise them are almost uniformly negative. Although focal seizures may rarely be accompanied by predominantly negative motor or sensory problems (Lesser *et al.* 1987), the greatest difficulties occur in rare haemodynamic transient ischaemic attacks (TIAs) in which weakness may be accompanied by some shaking and tremor (Yanagihara *et al.* 1985).

Migraine occurring in a younger population is more likely to lead to confusion with seizures. Loss of consciousness is not uncommon in migraine, although usually it takes the form of syncope associated with nausea and hypotension (Risser 1985). The complex relationship between migraine and epilepsy has been reviewed (Andermann 1987). On occasions migrainous episodes may induce frank seizures and arteriovenous malformations may cause both seizures and migraine-like phenomena. It does seem that migraine and benign Rolandic and occipital epilepsies commonly coexist, as they may do in some mitochondrial disorders (e.g. MELAS).

23.1.5 Transient global amnesia

The syndrome of transient global amnesia (TGA) describes an abrupt onset of amnesia, usually accompanied by repetitive questioning, in an individual who remains alert and communicative (Fisher and Adams 1958). The amnesia lasts for hours and attacks rarely recur. The aetiology of this syndrome remains controversial but it is highly likely that it has different causes, which may include thrombo-embolic disease, migraine, and epilepsy (Hodges and Warlow 1990). The latter authors suggest that up to 7 per cent of patients with TGA are likely to have an epileptic basis to their attacks. These can usually be identified by attacks that are brief and which recur over a short period of time. They are common on wakening, and individuals may have some partial recall. Sometimes such individuals will also describe some features at the start of the attacks, which would support focal seizure onset, for example, olfactory hallucination. Other types of simple or complex partial seizures occur, although transient amnesia can be the sole manifestation (Zeman *et al.* 1998).

23.1.6 Sleep phenomena

These are discussed in greater detail in Chapter 24, but a number of sleep phenomena may be confused with seizures. Hypnic jerks are usually single jerks that occur in the very early stages of sleep. They usually lead to arousal and may be accompanied by a feeling of falling, a cry, or some other kind of brief sensory disturbance. Periodic movements of sleep are rhythmic and repetitive leg movements more commonly seen in later life. They usually consist of jerking movements, usually dorsiflexion of the foot and extension of the toes that can occur repetitively during non-REM sleep (Coleman *et al.* 1980).

Sleepwalking is a form of automatic behaviour occurring during deep non-REM sleep and is much more common in children than in adults. It usually ceases by the mid-teens. In adults it must be distinguished from post-ictal automatism following sleep seizures or from complex partial seizures resulting in automatic behaviour (Pedley and Guilleminault 1977).

Abnormalities of sleep can also lead to confusion with seizures because of daytime disturbances. Narcolepsy should not lead to significant confusion. However, cataplexy, in which there may be sudden collapse with loss of postural tone triggered by emotion or startle or loud noise, could potentially be confused with atonic drop attacks. However, the age of onset of such episodes precludes real confusion, as atonic seizures most commonly occur during the first decade of life and symptoms of the narcoleptic syndrome rarely begin before the second or third decades of life (Parkes 1982). Some subjects with narcolepsy can also exhibit automatic behaviour when they appear to be only half-awake. Such individuals appear drowsy and absent-minded, although they may be capable of carrying on relatively complex tasks for which they are subsequently amnesic.

Sleep apnoea, which is most commonly obstructive in nature and associated with obesity and night-time snoring, leads to daytime drowsiness. Occasionally episodes of daytime sleepiness may be associated with respiratory obstruction and jerks that can lead to referral with the suggestion of a seizure disorder.

23.1.7 Movement disorders

Some unusual movement disorders may, on occasion, cause confusion with seizures. Non-epileptic myoclonus must be differentiated from epileptic myoclonus. Paroxysmal kinesogenic choreoathetosis is a rare disorder in which short-lasting tonic spasms with writhing movements occur, usually affecting an arm or a leg (Kertesz 1967). The onset is usually in adolescence and there is a strong male predominance, and often a family history. The attacks are precipitated by sudden movement after a period rest and are often preceded by a peculiar sensation in the limb before the movement commences. They can occur frequently but respond readily to antiepileptic drugs, although there is no evidence to suggest that they are epileptic in nature. The syndrome is so striking that it should not easily be confused with a seizure disorder, although rarely some patients with movement-induced seizures and abnormal ictal EEGs have been described (Whitty *et al.* 1964).

Mount and Reback (1940) also describe a non-kinesigenic form with very similar movements but usually of much longer duration. This is clearly familial with onset in infancy or childhood, and there is no male predominance. Similar tonic spasms induced by movement can occur in multiple sclerosis, as may paroxysmal episodes of dysarthria and ataxia (Matthews 1975).

23.1.8 Metabolic events

A number of metabolic disturbances may result in acute symptomatic seizures (see below). Hypoglycaemia is unusual in that it may be recurrent and give rise to diagnostic confusion with epilepsy. It is most commonly seen in diabetics receiving insulin or oral hypoglycaemic agents. Diabetics may be particularly sensitive to hypoglycaemia and can experience symptoms at higher blood glucose levels than non-diabetic subjects. Marks (1981) describes different types of neuroglycopenia, the most common of which is acute. As blood sugar falls, pallor, sweating, and tachycardia develop, associated with confusion, collapse, and occasionally coma. True seizures may occur during the course of hypoglycaemia, further complicating diagnosis. Hypoglycaemia must always be considered in the differential diagnosis of epilepsy in a diabetic population, but perhaps the greatest diagnostic difficulty will arise in the rare cases of insulin-secreting tumours in non-diabetic patients. Here, hypoglycaemia is most likely to occur during the course of the night. (Marks 1981) describes a syndrome of 'subacute neuroglycopenia' characteristic of insulinoma. Subjective symptoms are not marked but there is mild confusion and clumsiness. There may be disinhibition, suggesting intoxication with ataxia and slurred speech. This confused behaviour of hypoglycaemia may be difficult to differentiate from complex partial seizures occurring during sleep.

23.1.9 Other miscellaneous events

A negative motor phenomenon that may sometimes be confused with epilepsy is the syndrome of cryptogenic or benign drop attacks of middle-aged women (Stevens and Matthews 1973). These result in a sudden fall, usually onto the knees, without any clouding of consciousness. The episodes tend to be infrequent and the outcome seems to be quite benign. It must be emphasized that while atonic, tonic, and myoclonic seizures can cause brief episodes of falling with rapid recovery in children and occasionally in adolescence, such attacks do not commence in adult life.

McCrory et al. (1997) drew attention to concussive convulsions as a non-epileptic phenomenon. These occur within seconds of impact and are dramatic events, usually occurring in public view, and receiving heroic attention from first aiders. While these events have been widely assumed to represent a form of post-traumatic epileptic seizure, there is now considerable evidence to the contrary. Follow-up of subjects with such events by Jennett (1975) indicated that immediate convulsions were not a predictor of late post-traumatic epilepsy, in contradistinction to other seizures occurring in the first post-traumatic week, and that, on the whole, they tended to be associated with relatively mild concussive head injury. McCrory et al. (1997) identified 22 concussive convulsions in Australian footballers and rugby league players. Convulsions began within 2 seconds of the head injury and usually consisted of a brief tonic phase followed by bilateral myoclonic jerks. Some versive head movements and asymmetric posturing was seen in some

individuals. No convulsion lasted for more than 150 seconds and none of the players had any behavioural or neuropsychological features that suggested anything other than a mild concussion. The authors refer to a rugby league player in an international match who sustained a concussive convulsion in the opening minute of the game. After recovery he returned to the field to win the man of the match award! Follow-up of the group again showed no evidence of a risk from post-traumatic epilepsy. Similar events can occur during other sports, such as flat and National Hunt racing (Chadwick 1998). It is important that they are recognized as non-epileptic in order that inappropriate restrictions are avoided.

23.2 Physiological nature of epilepsy

In humans, spikes and sharp waves are the electroencephalographic hallmarks of interictal recordings of patients with epilepsy. Such activity appears to be due to a hypersynchronization of electrical activity within an abnormal pool of neurons, and they are rarely seen in the EEGs of non-epileptic patients (see below). Simplistically, epileptic seizures occur when excitatory influences in the cerebral hemispheres outweigh inhibitory influences. Study of the basic mechanisms of the human epilepsies is, of course, fraught with ethical and practical difficulty. Knowledge has therefore been accumulated from a number of animal models of seizures and epilepsy. While the direct relevance to the human epilepsies remains in some doubt, it seems likely that knowledge gained in this way will be highly informative.

There is considerable evidence that the fundamental building-block of most seizure disorders is the paroxysmal depolarization shift (PDS) and an associated high-frequency burst firing of neurons (Prince 1978). This phenomenon, illustrated schematically in Fig. 23.1, is one that can be observed in isolated cells, within simple neuronal circuits, in animal models of epilepsy and, indeed, in human postoperative material. PDS may occur normally as part of the spontaneous activity of CA3 hippocampal pyramidal neurons (Wong and Prince 1979, 1981), and in pyramidal cells of layers 4 and 5 of the neocortex (Connors et al. 1982; Gutnick et al. 1982). While PDS and burst firing can be intrinsic properties of neurons, the propagation and synchronization of this kind of activity to produce either interictal spikes or seizures, requires a contribution from neuronal circuits, which may themselves exhibit abnormalities, predisposing neurons within them to behave in an abnormal fashion (Traub and Jefferys 1998). The concept of PDS and burst firing underlies not only our understanding of the basic mechanisms underlying epilepsy, but also the mechanisms of antiepileptic drug action (White 1997).

23.2.1 Molecular and cellular factors

A number of factors control neuronal excitability. These include voltage-gated ion channels, neurotransmitter-activated ion

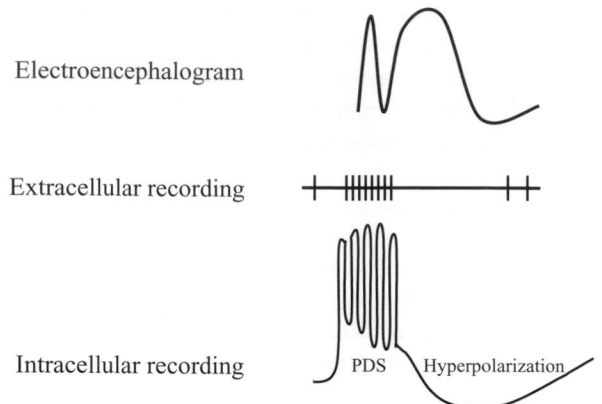

Fig. 23.1.   Epileptiform activity in the EEG and its relationship to intracellular events. Surface spikes are generated by synchronous paroxysmal depolarizations (PDS) in large groups of neurons.

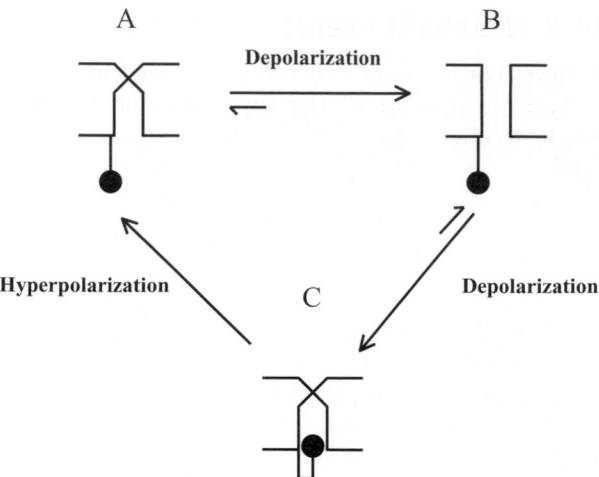

Fig. 23.2.   Different states in which the voltage-sensitive Na⁺ channel may exist: (A) closed but able to be activated; (B) open, allowing entry of Na⁺ ions; (C) closed and not able to be activated, a state that prevents repetitive firing and is made more probable by antiepileptic drugs such as phenytoin, etc.

channels, neuromodulators, and second-messenger systems (Schofield *et al.* 1987). Ligand-gated ion channels are responsible for communication between cells, while voltage-gated channels determine how inhibitory and excitatory influences are integrated in a way that determines the propagation of impulses to other neurons.

Voltage-gated channels

Neuronal membranes are usually polarized to a potential of -90 mV by the activity of Na⁺,K⁺-ATPase transporter systems. Voltage-gated ion channels are membrane-spanning proteins, composed of different subunits, which, when open, permit the passage of ions. Openings may be transient or persistent, depending on the nature of the channel. Most channels will

open on depolarization of the membrane, but some open when the membrane is hyperpolarized. Channels may exhibit a number of different states, as shown schematically in Fig. 23.2.

Voltage-gated sodium channels are intimately involved in the propagation of action potentials, the rapid upstroke being due to an opening of fast transient channels at about -60 mV (Cohen and Barchi 1993). Toxins that prolong sodium-channel opening cause seizures (Garber and Miller 1987). These channels are sensitive to tetrodotoxin, and appear to be a potent site of action for antiepileptic drugs. It has been known for some

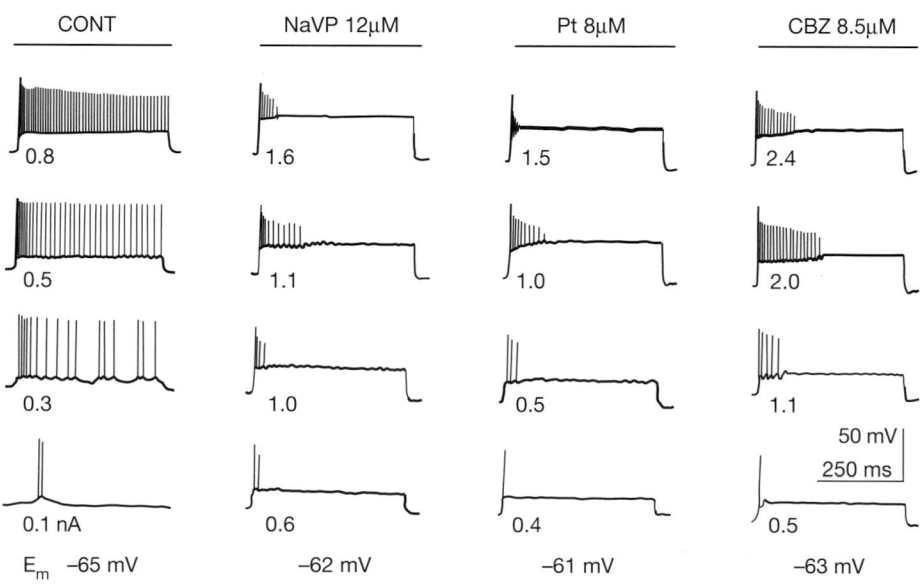

Fig. 23.3.   The effects of increasing depolarizing current pulses on intracellular membrane potentials of spinal neurons in culture. With increasing current there is more prolonged depolarization and burst firing in control (CONT) medium. Sodium valproate (NaVP), phenytoin (PT), and carbamazepine (CBZ) all block repetitive firing, the blockade increasing with increasing applied currents. (Reproduced from Macdonald (1996) with permission.)

time that phenytoin and carbamazepine are able to block repetitive firing of neurons. It appears that they do so by an effect on voltage-gated sodium channels that is both use-dependent and voltage-dependent (Willow *et al.* 1985), as demonstrated in Fig. 23.3 (which also demonstrates that sodium valproate has a similar action). Of the newer drugs, lamotrigine, topiramate, remacemide, and zonisamide may also utilize this mechanism of action. For a number of reasons, this mechanism of action may be seen as having ideal properties. It will tend to block pathological neuronal activity (repetitive firing) with relatively little effect on more physiological patterns of activity, and would also be predicted to be highly effective in preventing the spread of seizure activity.

Voltage-dependent calcium channels contribute to dendritic spikes, slow somatic depolarizations, and associated burst discharges (Scott *et al.* 1991) and, by doing so, trigger neuro-transmitter release. Six subclasses of calcium channels are known to exist: L, N, T, P, Q, and R. T channels have a low threshold of activation at around −70 mV. They inactivate relatively rapidly. These channels are found in high concentrations in thalamic neurons and play an important role in the generation of generalized spike-wave discharges (see below). They appear sensitive to anti-absence drugs such as ethosuximide, methadione derivatives, and sodium valproate (Coulter *et al.* 1989, 1990). Other types of calcium channel have higher thresholds and may open between −30 mV and −10 mV. They may also be involved in the mechanism of action of some antiepileptic drugs (Stefani *et al.* 1997).

Voltage-gated potassium channels are very diverse in their nature. Delayed rectifying potassium currents (I_k) activate at potentials more positive than −40 mV and seem to contribute to spike repolarization (Storm 1987). Fast transient currents activate at −45 mV to −60 mV and they appear to play an important role in the regulation of repetitive firing by prolonging after-spike hyperpolarization and slowing down firing rate (Connor and Stevens 1971). Inward rectifying potassium currents activate in response to hyperpolarization, and help to regulate resting membrane potentials. Potassium currents can be blocked with tetraethylammonium (TEA) and 4-aminopyridine (4-AP) (Jones and Heinemann 1987). Both these are active as convulsant agents but 4-AP seems the more potent (Jones and Heinemann 1987). The potentiation of voltage-dependent potassium currents is currently being explored as a potential role for new antiepileptic drugs.

Inhibitory neurotransmission: γ-aminobutyric acid

γ-Aminobutyric acid (GABA) is the major fast inhibitory neurotransmitter in the forebrain, being present at approximately 30 per cent of all synapses in the central nervous system. The majority of GABAergic neurons are short-axon interneurons, forming local inhibitory loops. Two distinct types of GABA receptor are recognized: GABA$_A$ receptors are post-synaptic receptors linked to chloride ion channels; GABA$_B$ receptors may be pre- or postsynaptic and are coupled to calcium or potassium ion channels via GTP proteins (Bowery

1993; Macdonald and Olsen 1994). GABA$_A$ receptors are large molecular weight proteins that contain a number of binding sites, not only for GABA but also for barbiturates, benzodiazepines, picrotoxin, and anaesthetic steroids. Binding of GABA leads to an opening of the chloride ion channel and resultant hyperpolarization. The openings tend to occur in bursts that can be facilitated in their frequency and duration in different ways by barbiturates and benzodiazepines. The receptor has been cloned and five different subunit families isolated. Most receptors appear to be composed of two α, two β, and one γ subunit (Schofield *et al.* 1987). Receptors constructed from different combinations of subunits appear to exhibit differing pharmacological properties, although binding sites for GABA and barbiturates appear to be highly conserved.

It has long been recognized that drugs such as allylglycine (which prevents the synthesis of GABA), picrotoxin and bicucculine (which block GABA receptors), as well as penicillin, are all potent convulsant agents (Meldrum 1975). The activity of benzodiazepines and barbiturates at GABA$_A$ receptor appears to be responsible for their antiepileptic activity (White 1997). Vigabatrin, a new antiepileptic drug, is a suicidal inhibitor of GABA transaminase, the enzyme responsible for GABA metabolism (Schechter *et al.* 1977). Another new drug, tiagabine, potentiates GABAergic activity by blocking the re-uptake of GABA into neurons and glia (Braestrup *et al.* 1990). The interaction between antiepileptic drugs and the GABA receptor is illustrated in Fig. 23.4. Involvement of the GABA$_B$ receptor in causing epilepsy is somewhat less well established. Loss of GABAergic interneurons may be important in the epilepsies seen after kainate and perforant pathway hippocampal stimulation in animals (Franck and Schwartzkroin 1985; Sloviter 1991). On the

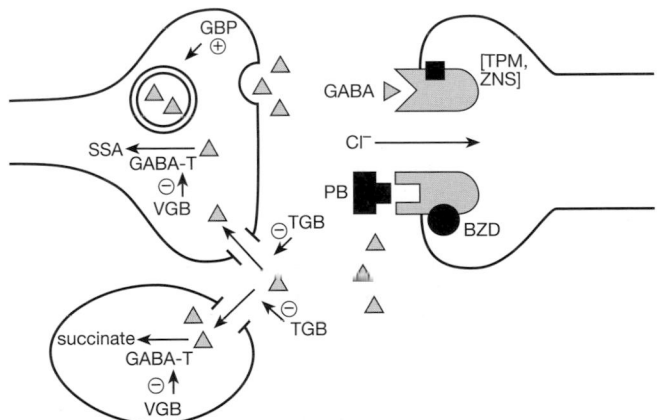

Fig. 23.4. Schematic representation of a GABAergic synapse to illustrate the interactions with antiepileptic drugs. Binding of GABA at GABA$_A$ receptors allows chloride entry and hyperpolarization of membranes. Benzodiazepines (BZD) and topiramate (TPM) increase channel opening and burst frequency, pnemobarbitone (PB) increases burst duration. GABA-mediated inhibition can also be enhanced by blocking re-uptake into neurons and glia (tiagabine (TGB)) or by irreversibly inhibiting GABA aminotransferase (vigabatrin (VGB)) which metabolizes GABA to succinic acid semialdehyde (SSA). Gabapentin (GBP) increases GABA turnover by poorly understood mechanisms. (Reproduced from White (1997), with permission.)

other hand, enhanced GABA-ergic inhibition appears to worsen absence seizures in humans and experimental animals (Snead 1995). It seems likely that this is mediated via a GABA$_B$ receptor effect in enhancing thalamic low-threshold calcium currents (Coulter *et al.* 1989). Conversely, spike-wave discharges can be blocked by GABA$_B$ receptor antagonists.

Excitatory neurotransmission

The major excitatory neurotransmitters are the amino acids L-glutamate and L-aspartate. They exert their synaptic influences by interacting with a number of different types of receptors, which are identified because of specificity for binding different molecules (Hollman and Heinemann 1994). Binding at the DL-α-amino-3-hydroxy-5-methyl-isoxazolepropionic acid (AMPA) receptor makes its associated ion channel permeable to both sodium and potassium. It desensitizes rapidly (Tang *et al.* 1989) and is probably responsible for the majority of rapid excitatory neurotransmission. Four glutamate receptors (GluRs1–4) have now been cloned and appear to be subunits that can express the known electrophysiology and pharmacology of the AMPA receptor. The kainate receptor is also coupled to a channel permeable to sodium and potassium. It does not, however, appear to desensitize at the same rate as the AMPA receptor. Both these channels differ strikingly from the *N*-methyl-D-aspartate (NMDA) receptor. This appears to be a much more complex receptor site, which has an absolute requirement for the presence of a co-agonist, glycine, in order to result in channel opening (Johnson and Ascher 1987). Magnesium, zinc, polyamines, and steroids can also modulate the site. When membranes are hyperpolarized the channel is blocked by magnesium, a blockade that is reversed when the membrane depolarizes. Opening of the channel allows the entry of both sodium and calcium. This acts as an amplification mechanism that leads to prolonged activation of already excited neurons and associated burst firing (Williamson and Wheal 1992). Calcium entry may also result ultimately in excitotoxicity and cell death. Like the AMPA and kainate receptor, the NMDA receptor exists as a number of subfamilies.

Excitatory amino acids are also able to interact with metabotropic receptors that activate second-messenger systems to influence biochemical pathways and ion channels. These receptors are found both pre- and postsynaptically. Activation usually results in presynaptic inhibition and postsynaptic excitation. These receptors may have an important role in supporting epileptic activity (Arvanov *et al.* 1995). There is no doubt that drugs impairing excitatory neurotransmission are potentially potent antiepileptic drugs (Meldrum 1984). However, direct NMDA antagonists have considerable cognitive and behavioural side-effects. Felbamate may possess antiepileptic properties by interacting with the glycine receptor site of NMDA receptors (White *et al.* 1995). Remacemide may also possess some of its antiepileptic properties because of a weak affinity for binding to the NMDA channel (Subramaniam *et al.* 1996).

23.2.2 Epileptic activity in neuronal systems

This can be studied in a wide variety of experimental situations from brain slices through to intact animals. There are a large number of acute seizure models and more chronic models of epilepsy available for study. While acute seizure models have been widely used in screening for antiepileptic drug effects, it is more likely that chronic models will be informative about the basic mechanisms of the epilepsies.

Focal epileptogenesis

One model that has greatly aided understanding of the paroxysmal depolarization shift and the communication of burst firing from one group of neurons to another is the hippocampal brain slice (Bernardo and Pedley 1985). Normal spontaneous activity of CA3 pyramidal neurons consisted of paroxysmal depolarization shifts and associated burst firing of the cell body and apical dendrites (Wong and Prince 1979, 1981). Normal CA1 neurons rarely exhibited such firing patterns.

The paroxysmal depolarization shift in CA3 neurons appears to be calcium dependent. When calcium entry into the cell is blocked by high concentrations of manganese, paroxysmal depolarization shifts and burst firing no longer occur in CA3 neurons (Wong and Prince 1978). A long lasting after-hyperpolarization follows bursting in CA3 neurons (Wong and Prince 1978), which is not seen when calcium entry is impeded (Hotson and Prince 1981). As it is well recognized that most spontaneous synaptic activity is dependent on membrane calcium channels, this represents a major argument for the importance of synaptic mechanisms in focal epileptogenesis.

It is now possible to suggest that similar mechanisms may be involved in focal epileptogenesis in the neocortex. Here 'pacemaker' cells with the ability to produce intrinsic burst firing may be concentrated at the border between layers IV and V of the cortex. These cells may be able to produce burst firing in other cortical layers when inhibitory mechanisms are reduced (Connors *et al.* 1982). While these observations of the synaptic interactions important in focal epileptogenesis are sufficiently plausible to lead to sophisticated computer modelling that can explain cellular bursting and synchronous population discharge in the hippocampus in the presence of impaired post-synaptic inhibition (Wong *et al.* 1984), there is evidence from other sources that other factors may have a role to play.

The function of the hippocampal brain slice can be studied in material from normal animals exposed to a variety of chemical manipulations, as well as in slices from animals expressing a chronic model of epilepsy (Traub and Jefferys 1998). In normal brain material, bursting activity in CA3 neurons has about a 30 per cent chance of evoking bursts in connected neurons. This probability increases when the pyramidal cell is excited by many inputs simultaneously. However, repetitive bursting is made less likely by the inhibitory connections of CA3 neurons.

A number of manipulations, including GABA$_A$ blockade and high extracellular potassium, will generate repeated and long-lasting bursting activity. This primitive epileptic activity clearly depends both on intrinsic properties of hippocampal-slice neurons as well as their synaptic connections.

A number of animal models of focal epilepsy are now well studied, including the topical application of aluminium hydroxide and systemic use of tetanus toxin, kainic acid, and pilocarpine. Most of these models share the characteristic of producing acute seizures followed, often after a latent period, by the development of a chronic epilepsy with seizures and behaviours that are not dissimilar to complex partial seizures in humans. While early seizures may arise from different mechanisms, including impairment of GABA-mediated inhibition or augmentation of glutamate- and acetylcholine-mediated excitation, the chronic models seem to be dependent largely on consequent neuropathological change, which includes gliosis and neuronal loss along with mossy fibre sprouting in the hippocampus and consequent excitatory synaptic reorganization (Avanzini *et al.* 1998).

Similar changes are also seen in the kindling model of epilepsy that perhaps best matches forms of temporal-lobe epilepsy in humans. In this model, repeated subconvulsive electrical stimulation, usually to the amygdala, leads to increasing after-discharge and ultimately to behavioural seizures (Goddard *et al.* 1969). Repeated focal applications of convulsant agents can lead to a similar phenomenon. It appears that limbic structures are particularly sensitive to the development of kindling when compared to neocortex, a situation that is reflected in humans, where the temporal lobe is by far the most common site of seizure onset (see below). It is also of interest that the immature animal seems much more sensitive than is the adult (Moshe 1981).

At a pathological level, kindled animals show evidence of neuronal loss in the hippocampus accompanied by sprouting of the mossy fibre axons of the dentate granule cells (Sutula *et al.* 1988). It seems that sprouting probably requires the death of neurons and that the sprouting fibres take up synaptic sites that are thereby vacated. If new synaptic connections are made to other excitatory cells, this would represent a process potentially contributing to the hyperexcitability of the kindled brain. One factor in mediating this may be NMDA receptors, as it can be shown that antagonists inhibit the kindling process (McNamara *et al.* 1988). The kindling model creates a large number of hypotheses and possible explanations of great clinical relevance. A number of human epilepsies are characterized by a latent period between the development of a particular pathology and a first clinical seizure. Could vascular abnormalities and slowly growing neoplasms induce the clinical hyperexcitability which, over a period of time, begins to express itself as clinical seizures? Could kindling explain the rare phenomenon of secondary epileptogenesis in which a remote cortical site gradually develops independent epileptiform activity over a period of time (Morrell 1985)?

Generalized epilepsies

Here the sudden onset, the bilateral synchrony, and, in the case of simple absences and myoclonus, the non-evolving pattern of electrical activity, clearly suggests some very generalized disturbance of neuronal activity in both hemispheres. Historically, there have been two schools of thought that would explain such a phenomenon. Gibbs and Gibbs (1952) suggested that generalized spike wave discharge was dependent on a primary cortical process. Penfield and Jasper (1954) developed the concept of an unspecified 'centrencephalic' system, in which structures of the upper brainstem and thalamus were responsible for generating the spike wave discharge and driving a cortical synchrony. Gloor (1968) has pointed out that these two hypotheses are not mutually exclusive and has developed a 'generalized cortico-reticular' hypothesis. However, considerable progress has been made since the discovery that the intramuscular injection of 500 000 IU of penicillin in a cat leads, within an hour, to the development of generalized spike wave discharge in the EEG accompanied by some behavioural changes similar to human absence (Prince and Farrell 1969). The spike wave activity tends to increase greatly with sleep and, on occasion, may evolve into a tonic–clonic seizure discharge (Avoli *et al.* 1981). Photosensitivity is also a feature of feline generalized penicillin epilepsy.

In the cat, generalized spike wave discharges can be recorded both at the cerebral cortex and in the thalamus, and they appear to involve both these levels in a synchronous fashion (Avoli and Gloor 1982). Recordings from individual neurons at both levels show that they have a high probability of firing during spike components of the spike wave complex, while the probability of firing is greatly reduced during the slow wave component. Depressing neuronal excitability at either the cortical or thalamic level (with KCl-induced spreading depression) will lead to the disappearance of the spike wave discharge. There is good evidence that the initiation comes from the cortex and that the thalamic neuron may only become involved after two or more cycles (Avoli *et al.* 1983).

The cellular substrate for these phenomena is now well understood (Fig. 23.5). It is dependent on a thalamocortical circuit that includes the nucleus reticularis thalami. The circuits involve excitatory (glutaminergic) synapses and inhibitory GABAergic synapses. The behaviour of thalamic neurons and the circuit is largely determined by the presence of a high density of calcium T channels, which has already been discussed (see above).

In the awake animal, thalamic neurons are maintained at a resting potential of approximately −50 mV because of the effects of normal afferent activity of brainstem activating systems. In this state, calcium T channels are not activated. During drowsiness and sleep, however, thalamic neurons hyperpolarize and begin to exhibit typical repetitive burst firing that contributes to sleep spindles in the EEG (Hirsch *et al.* 1983). Hyperpolarization and burst firing is greatly facilitated by GABAergic activity via GABA$_B$ mechanisms. Thus, classical

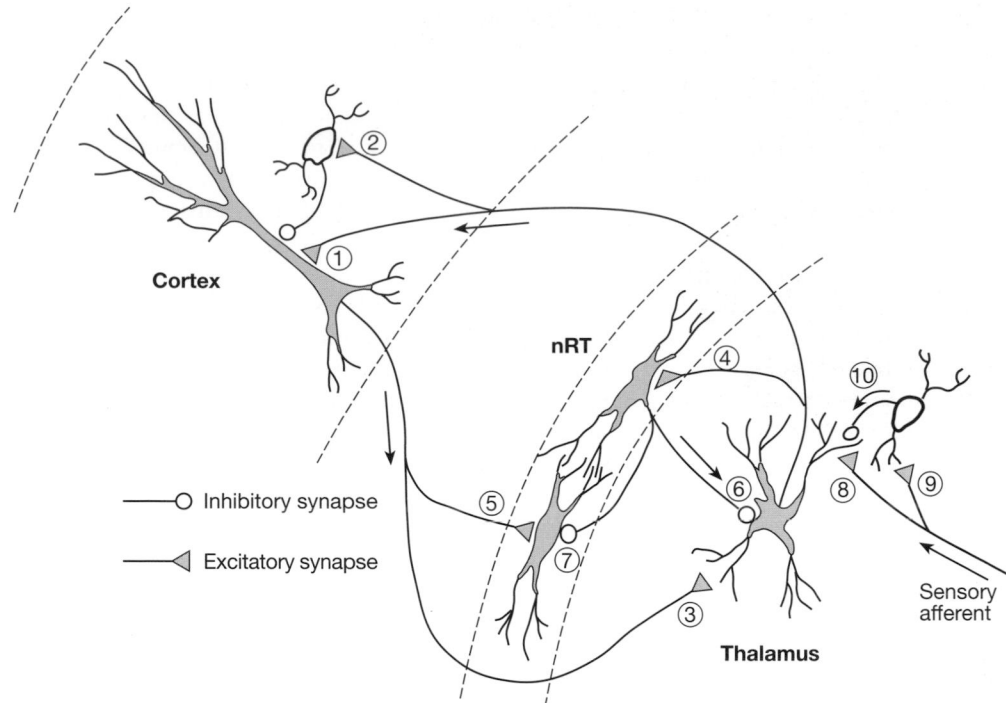

Fig. 23.5. The thalamocortical circuit. Thalamic neurons in the primary sensory relay nuclei project to layers III/IV and V/VI of the cerebral cortex. This projection terminates on both pyramidal neurons (synapse 1) and inhibitory interneurons (synapse 2) in the cortex. Layer VI pyramidal neurons reciprocally innervate the same area of the thalamus from which an ascending afferent is received (synapse 3). Both the thalamocortical and corticothalamic projections send an axon collateral to nucleus reticularis thalami (NRT; synapses 4 & 5). NRT provides inhibitory (GABAergic) innervation to the thalamus (synapse 6) and to other NRT neurons (synapse 7). The major sensory afferents to the thalamus synapse onto the dendrites of both thalamic relay neurons (synapse 8) and inhibitory interneurons (synapse 9). The dendrites of inhibitory interneurons can function as both pre-and postsynaptic elements and can provide inhibitory innervation of thalamic relay dendrites (synapse 10), as well as conventional axonal synaptic connections. (From Coulter (1997), with permission.)

anti-absence drugs reduce low-threshold calcium currents (Coulter *et al.* 1989) while GABA$_B$ receptor agonists exacerbate absence and GABA$_B$ antagonists have anti-absence properties in animal models (Hosford *et al.* 1992; Liu *et al.* 1992). These phenomena probably also explain the effects of vigabatrin in exacerbating absence seizures (Gibbs *et al.* 1992).

23.3 Epidemiology of seizures and epilepsy

Despite problems with differing definitions of epilepsy and case ascertainment methods, there is remarkable agreement about the epidemiology of epilepsy in different populations in the developed world (Sander and Shorvon 1987). Incidence rates vary between approximately 20–55/100 000 per year, whereas the prevalence for active epilepsy is in the range of 4–10/1000. Age-specific incidence prevalence and cumulative incidence are described in Fig. 23.6 for a population in Rochester, Minnesota, but this has been replicated in other populations. It can be seen that the incidence of epilepsy is highest at the extremes of life, but that there are significant differences between the cumulative incidence and prevalence of epilepsy, indicating that the majority of patients who develop epilepsy do not suffer from a

chronic disorder. The cumulative incidence of epilepsy by the age of 70 may be as high as 2–3 per cent of the population. There is evidence that the incidence in children may be falling

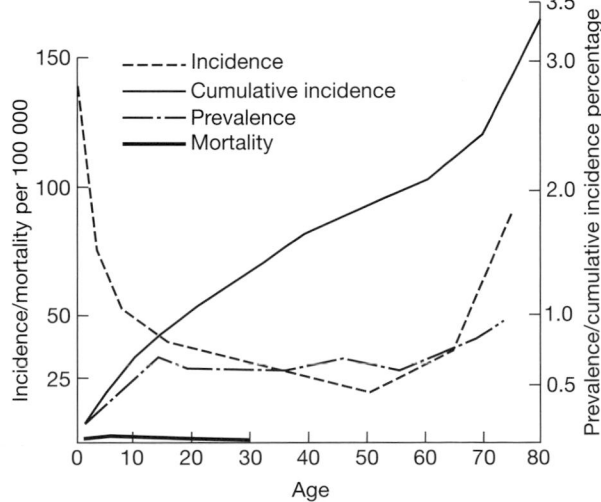

Fig. 23.6. Age-specific incidence, prevalence, and cumulative incidence rates for epilepsy in Rochester, Minnesota 1935–74 (reproduced from Anderson *et al.* (1986), with permission).

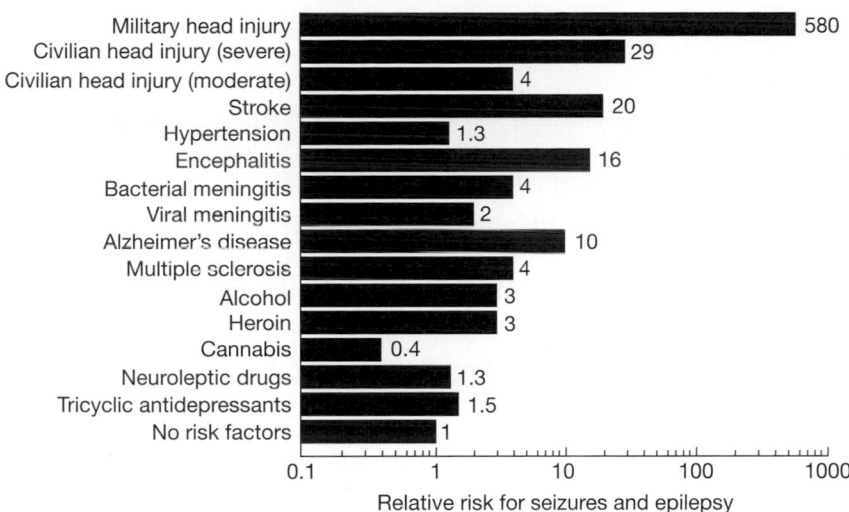

Fig. 23.7. Relative risks for specific risk factors (adapted from Hauser and Hesdorffer (1990), with permission).

with time, although it may be rising in the elderly (Hauser *et al.* 1993). Incidence, though possibly not prevalence, is higher in Third World countries than the West, with rates of 77/100 000 reported from Tanzania (Rwiza *et al.* 1992) and 114/100 000 reported from Chile (Lavados *et al.* 1992).

Most studies suggest a slightly higher incidence and prevalence in men than women, with approximately two-thirds of cases being partial epilepsies and approximately one-third generalized. Epidemiological studies identify a wide range of risk factors for the development of epilepsy. Risk ratios are summarized in Fig. 23.7.

23.3.1 **The prognosis of epilepsy**

Many problems exist in the interpretation of data on this subject, not least the varying minimum period required as a definition of remission, and the period of follow-up. The majority of studies have been hospital based, which has an adverse effect on outcome, patients with more severe and refractory epilepsy being more likely to be referred to specialist centres. In this respect the studies of Annegers *et al.* (1979) and the National General Practice Survey of Epilepsy (NGPSE) (Cockerell *et al.* 1997) are of particular importance in being community, rather than hospital, based. In Rochester, Minnesota, 457 patients were identified with a history of two or more non-febrile seizures, and were followed for at least 5 years (for 20 years in the case of 141). The probability of being in a remission lasting for 5 years or more was 61 per cent at 10 years, and as high as 70 per cent at 20 years (Fig. 23.8). Similarly in the NGPSE, 68 per cent of patients achieved a 5-year remission by 9 years of follow-up. Further support for such high rates of remission is obtained from studies of patients followed prospectively from diagnosis and the commencement of therapy, which show that between 50 and 77 per cent of such patients are 'controlled', depending on how 'control' is defined (Turnbull *et al.* 1985; Reynolds 1987). In contrast, the majority of hospital-based studies are striking in that remission rates are

consistent at between 20 and 30 per cent, despite the fact that they include periods before the advent of modern anticonvulsant therapy. Annegers *et al.* (1979) were unable to show major changes in remission rates for patients diagnosed with epilepsy between the years of 1935 and 1959 and those diagnosed between 1960 and 1974.

The converse of the above information is that 20–30 per cent of patients with epilepsy never achieve remissions; they have a refractory epilepsy that is associated with psychosocial handicap (Jacoby *et al.* 1996). Relatively few patients switch between seizure and seizure-free states, indicating that epilepsy is bimodal in its outcome. The question then arises as to what determines prognosis?

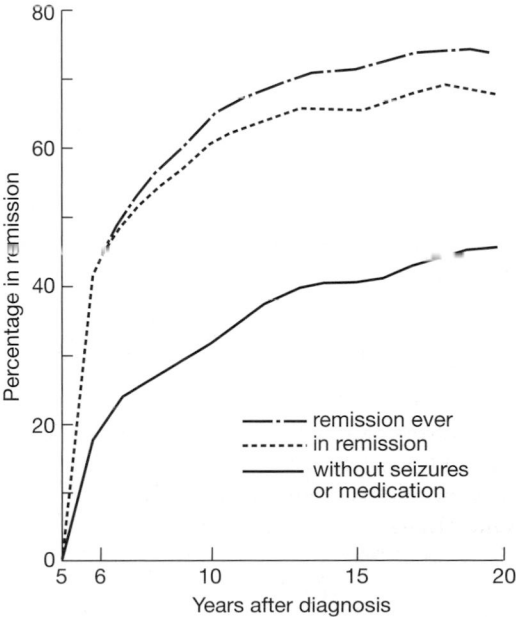

Fig. 23.8. Prognosis for 5-year remission of epilepsy following diagnosis in a cohort from Rochester, Minnesota (from Annegers *et al.* 1979).

The type of epilepsy or epilepsy syndrome is of considerable importance and is dealt with subsequently (see below). Thus, juvenile myoclonic epilepsy is lifelong, but benign Rolandic epilepsy never recurs during adult life. However, many children and adults with epilepsy cannot be classified by epilepsy syndrome (Berg *et al.* 1996*b*) and even within many syndromes there may be considerable variation in outcome. In West's syndrome, follow-up for up to 35 years showed that 30 per cent had died, but 24 per cent survived with normal intelligence and 35 per cent were seizure-free (Riikonen 1996). In general, partial epilepsies have a poorer prognosis than generalized epilepsy (Annegers *et al.* 1979; Cockerell *et al.* 1997). The combination of different seizure types also has an adverse effect on outcome (Collaborative Group for the Study of Epilepsy 1992).

The age of onset of epilepsy is perhaps one of the most important factors affecting outcome. The commencement of seizures within the first year of life (when it is usually symptomatic of cerebral pathology and indicative of one of the malignant childhood epilepsies), carries a particularly adverse prognosis (Kiorboe 1961; Sofijanov 1982). In childhood, the risk of intractability falls strongly with each additional year of age of onset (Berg *et al.* 1996*a*). The same effect of age is seen in studies that include adults, although the effect is weaker (Cockerell *et al.* 1997).

Whatever the age of onset, the long-term outcome of epilepsy can usually be predicted around the time of diagnosis. The outcome is worse the more seizures that occur before diagnosis (Cockerell *et al.* 1997). Annegers *et al.* (1979) showed that most patients who achieve remission do so early during the course of treatment. With continuing seizures it becomes progressively less likely that an individual patient will enter remission (Reynolds 1987). Thus, there is a plateau in the number of patients in remission 15–20 years after the onset of epilepsy. The possible importance of the early course and treatment of epilepsy on its long-term outcome has been discussed in detail by Reynolds (1987), using data from a number of sources to argue that early treatment may reduce the risk of intractability. This view remains controversial, and there is more evidence to suggest that the timing of treatment has little effect on outcomes (Shinnar and Berg 1996).

Epilepsy of unknown aetiology has a better prognosis than symptomatic epilepsy (Annegers *et al.* 1979; Juul-Jensen and Foldspang 1983). In keeping with this, epilepsy complicated by an associated neurological or psychiatric deficit carries an adverse prognosis (Sofijanov 1982).

There is a considerable volume of literature on EEG findings and their prognostic value. It provides no clear indication that any specific EEG abnormalities, either in historical EEGs or at a particular point in time when prognosis is to be predicted, are of great value (Rowan and French 1988).

There is evidence that the way in which factors affecting the prognosis of epilepsy interact may vary between childhood- and adult-onset epilepsy. Shafer *et al.* (1988) examined the prognosis of 306 patients diagnosed between 1935 and 1978 to investigate the factors determining the likelihood of achieving a 5-year seizure-free period and a 5-year seizure-free period off drugs. Prognostic factors included the absence of early brain damage, never having had a tonic–clonic seizure, and the absence of generalized spike waves from a number of EEGs. Similar factors were also predictive of 5-year seizure-free periods off antiepileptic drugs. In children, early age at onset, remote symptomatic, as opposed to idiopathic, epilepsy, and a history of infantile spasms and status epilepticus, all predicted intractability (Berg *et al.* 1996*a*).

23.3.2 Mortality from epilepsy

All available studies show an increased mortality ratio for epilepsy of between 2 and 3 times the expected (Hauser and Hesdorffer 1990; Cockerell *et al.* 1997). A number of factors appear to contribute to this excess mortality. The greatest excess seems to occur in the early years of life (Hauser *et al.* 1980) and to be more obvious in men. The risk of mortality is greatest in the early years following diagnosis, and is highest for patients with tonic–clonic seizures, seizures that recur frequently, and for those with remote symptomatic epilepsy.

Much of the excess mortality seems to be associated with the underlying aetiology of an epilepsy rather than the occurrence of seizures themselves. The risk is higher for patients with a symptomatic epilepsy than for those with idiopathic epilepsy (Hauser *et al.* 1980). The association of epilepsy with cerebrovascular disease in later life probably accounts for the excess mortality associated with the diagnosis of epilepsy in the elderly. The association with mental handicap and cerebral palsy in younger age groups seems to be of considerable importance (Satishchandra *et al.* 1988). Both neoplasms and arteriovenous malformations contribute to the excess mortality from symptomatic epilepsies.

Some controversy surrounds the role of sudden unexpected death in people with epilepsy (SUDEP). A number of studies have highlighted cases in which people with epilepsy are found dead, usually in bed (Leestma *et al.* 1984; Neuspiel and Kuller 1985). It is usually assumed that deaths are related to seizures and possibly to associated cardiorespiratory abnormalities. Certainly the risk of SUDEP increases dramatically with the severity of epilepsy, from 1 : 2500 patient years in patients in remission (Medical Research Council Antiepileptic Drug Withdrawal Study Group 1991, [see comments]) to 1 : 200 patient years for patients with frequent seizures (Nashef *et al.* 1995*a*,*b*). While status epilepticus continues to be associated with mortality, its rarity means that it does not contribute significantly to the excess mortality associated with epilepsy.

Accident is a not uncommon cause of death in epilepsy, accounting for up to 10 per cent of all deaths (Krohn 1963), drowning being responsible for the great majority (Blisard and McFeeley 1988). Accidents are also a common cause of injury. In a community-based study in the UK, 24 per cent of those with active epilepsy reported head injuries within the previous year, and 16 per cent, burns (Buck *et al.* 1997).

23.4 Classification of seizures

The great heterogeneity of clinical phenomena that can be associated with seizure discharge necessitates some system of

Table 23.4. Classification of seizures (Commission on Classification and Terminology of the International League Against Epilepsy 1981)

Partial seizures (seizures beginning locally)
  Simple (consciousness not impaired)
    with motor symptoms
    with somatosensory or special sensory symptoms
    with autonomic symptoms
    with psychic symptoms
  Complex (with impairment of consciousness)
    beginning as simple partial seizures (progressing to complex seizure)
    impairment of consciousness at onset
      (1) impairment of consciousness only
      (2) with automatism
  Partial seizures becoming secondarily generalized
Generalized seizures
  Absence seizures
    simple (petit mal)
    complex
  Myoclonic seizures
  Clonic seizures
  Tonic seizures
  Tonic–clonic seizures
  Atonic seizures

Table 23.5. Iternational classification of epilepsies, epileptic syndromes, and related seizure disorders (Commission on Classification and Terminology of the International League against Epilepsy 1989)

1 Localization-related (focal, local, partial)
  Idiopathic (primary)
  1.1 Benign childhood epilepsy with centro-temporary spike
      Childhood epilepsy with occipital paroxysms
      Primary reading epilepsy
  Symptomatic (secondary)
  1.2 Temporal lobe epilepsies
      Frontal lobe epilepsies
      Parietal lobe epilepsies
      Occipital lobe epilepsies
      Chronic progressive epilepsia partialis continua of childhood
      Syndromes characterized by seizures with specific modes of precipitation
  Cryptogenic
  1.3 Defined by:
      seizure type (see ICES)
      clinical features
      aetiology
      anatomical localization
2 Generalized
  2.1 Benign neonatal familial convulsions
      Benign neonatal convulsions
      Benign myoclonic epilepsy in infancy
      Childhood absence epilepsy (pyknolepsy)
      Juvenile myoclonic epilepsy (impulsive petit mal)
      Epilepsies with grand mal seizures (GTCS) on wakening
      Other generalized idiopathic epilepsies
      Epilepsies with seizures precipitated by specific modes of activation
  Cryptogenic symptomatic
  2.2 West's syndrome (infantile spasms, Blitz–Nick–Salaam Krampfe)
      Lennox–Gastaut syndrome
      Epilepsy with myoclonic–astatic seizures
      Epilepsy with myoclonic absences
  2.3.1 Non-specific aetiology
      Early myoclonic encephalopathy
      Early infantile epileptic encephalopathy with suppression bursts
      Other symptomatic generalized epilepsies
  2.3.2 Specific syndromes
      Epileptic seizures may complicate many disease states
3 Undetermined epilepsies
  3.1 With both generalized and focal seizures
      Neonatal seizures
      Severe myoclonic epilepsy in infancy
      Epilepsy with continuous spike wave during slow-wave sleep
      Acquired epileptic aphasia (Landau–Kleffner syndrome)
      Other undetermined epilepsies
  3.2 Without unequivocal generalized or focal features
4 Special syndromes
  4.1 Situation-related seizures
      Febrile convulsions
      Isolated seizures or isolated status epilepticus
      Seizures occurring only when there is an acute or toxic event due to factors such as alcohol, drugs, eclampsia, non-ketotic hyperglycaemia

classification. An international classification of epileptic seizures was proposed in 1981 and is summarized in Table 23.4 (Commission on Classification and Terminology of the International League Against Epilepsy 1981). This classification divides seizures broadly into those which begin locally (partial seizures), which may spread or evolve into secondarily generalized tonic–clonic seizures, and generalized seizures in which the onset is sudden and in which both cerebral hemispheres are involved in the discharge from a very early point in the seizure. The classification makes use of both clinical and electro-encephalographic (EEG) information. However, similar seizures may occur at different ages and have very different implications. Conversely, a patient may experience differing seizures during the course of his or her life, so that a classification of different epileptic syndromes based on seizure types occurring within the syndrome, age of onset, and aetiology will also be of vital importance in the management of patients with epilepsy. A proposed classification of epilepsy syndromes is presented in Table 23.5 (Commission on Classification and Terminology of the International League Against Epilepsy 1989).

23.4.1 Simple partial seizures

Classical neurological teaching has suggested that motor and sensory phenomena may be used to infer precise localizing value. This has been questioned increasingly as more detailed intracranial recording has become available to correlate with observed clinical phenomena. Thus, the clinical phenomena of seizures reflect not only the site of origin, but also the structures through which seizure discharge spreads during the seizure.

Simple motor seizures

Simple partial seizures with motor signs may give rise to clonic or tonic movements involving any part of the body. Seizures most often involve the face or hand area, because of the disproportionate amount of the motor cortex occupied by the somatotopic representation of these parts of the body. Although clonic seizures involving an arm or a leg may be taken as a reasonably satisfactory indication of seizures involving the motor strip, movements of the eye or facial muscles around the eye can be produced by occipital discharge, and clonic movements of the mouth, tongue, or pharynx by temporal discharge (Lesser *et al.* 1987). True Jacksonian 'march', with a slow spread of clonic activity from one muscle group to another, is uncommon (Mauguiere and Courjon 1978) but, when seen, does seem to imply relatively specific localization to the pre-central gyrus.

It is evident that tonic motor seizures resulting in adversion or dystonic posturing of limbs have considerably less localizing value than was previously understood. They may arise from involvement of wider areas of cortex that include the premotor region and supplementary motor area (SMA). However, versive movement can occur in seizures arising in temporal, parietal, and occipital lobes, as well as in generalized seizures (Ajmone-Marsan and Goldhammer 1973). Ipsilateral head-turning can be as common as contralateral head-turning (Ochs *et al.* 1984). However, version occurs earlier in seizures with frontal onset than in those with temporal onset (Chee *et al.* 1993).

Negative motor phenomena may occur during simple partial seizures. Speech arrest may be the most common manifestation. While speech arrest with a preserved ability to understand speech suggests a seizure in the dominant inferior frontal gyrus (Geier *et al.* 1977), less specific forms of speech arrest can occur with seizure onset in the supplementary motor areas of the dominant or non-dominant hemisphere (Geier *et al.* 1977). Very rarely, inhibition of movement has been described as part of simple partial seizures (Lesser *et al.* 1987). Post-ictal paralysis (Todd's paralysis) seems specific for seizures involving the contralateral motor strip at some point. Versive seizures tend not to be followed by such paralysis.

Simple sensory seizures

These are rare and occur in no more than 2 per cent of patients with epilepsy. Somatosensory seizures usually arise in the postcentral area, but almost always spread to the pre-motor strip at an early stage, so that motor phenomena dominate the seizure semiology. They most commonly affect the face or hand, and may occasionally spread as do Jacksonian seizures. Sensations are usually those of paraesthesiae or numbness (Mauguiere and Courjon 1978). Rarely, disturbing or painful sensations can occur (Young and Blume 1983). Post-ictal numbness similar to Todd's phenomena may occur.

Primitive visual symptoms, including spots, flashes of light, or patterns in one visual field, are most commonly associated with occipital seizures. On occasion, occipital seizures may produce visual symptoms that involve both half visual fields. More complex visual hallucinations are less likely to have an occipital onset (see below).

Although non-specific 'dizziness' is often described by patients as part of a simple partial seizure, it usually seems that this term is used because of difficulties in describing complex sensory disturbances. True vertigo must be exceptionally uncommon (Smith 1960). Buzzing, hissing, whistling, and ringing noises can be experienced most commonly with involvement of the lateral parts of the temporal lobe.

Olfactory and gustatory symptoms are commonly associated with medial temporal involvement or involvement of the frontal orbital regions. Smells and tastes are usually unpleasant but may be difficult to characterize further than this. Such symptoms are sometimes described as uncinate seizures, and although it has been suggested that they are more likely to be associated with temporal tumours, this seems unlikely (Howe and Gibson 1982).

Visceral symptoms form one of the most common components of simple partial seizures. They are most often associated with involvement of limbic structures of the temporal and frontal lobes. Most common is an epigastric sensation, sometimes described as butterflies or nausea, which tends to rise characteristically into the throat or mouth. More rarely stomach pain, belching, or even vomiting can occur (Van Buren 1963). Autonomic symptoms can include pallor, flushing and sweating, pupillary dilatation, and increases in heart rate (Blumhardt *et al.* 1986). Sexual arousal may also occur (Lesser *et al.* 1987). Involuntary micturition or defaecation, while not uncommon in seizures associated with loss of consciousness, is extremely rare in simple partial seizures (Maurice-Williams 1974).

Complicated psychic symptoms are not uncommon during simple partial seizures. Again, they usually indicate involvement of mesial temporal or frontal limbic structures. Psychic symptoms are often associated with other olfactory, gustatory, or autonomic disturbances. Dysmnesic symptoms are perhaps the most common, with sensations of familiarity (*déjà vu*) or strangeness (*jamais vu*). Memory flashbacks or playbacks may occur and may merge into rather non-specific symptoms of dream-like states, unreality, and depersonalization on the one hand, and more formed illusions and hallucinations combining visual and auditory aspects on the other. A variety of perceptual changes may occur during seizures, with objects appearing larger or smaller or changing in shape or being perseverated (Gloor *et al.* 1982). Emotional experiences are often described, the most frequent being intense fear (Williams 1956). Pleasurable sensations are much rarer but laughter can occur (Gumpert *et al.* 1970). Anger or rage is extremely rare as a true ictal disturbance.

23.4.2 Complex partial seizures

Complex partial seizures in adults are of considerable importance. They are the predominant seizure-type in approximately 40 per cent of patients with epilepsy (Gastaut *et al.* 1975; Juul-Jensen and Foldspang 1983). They tend to be more resistant to antiepileptic drug treatment, with at best only 50 per cent of patients attaining long-term remissions (Annegers *et al.* 1979). Patients with this seizure type commonly present additional psychological or psychiatric handicap, which greatly adds to the complexity of the management problems that they present. Additionally, it is in this group of patients that a surgical approach to the treatment of epilepsy is likely to be most successful.

The international classification of seizures emphasizes that complex partial seizures must include some impairment of consciousness and amnesia. They may or may not be preceded by symptoms of a simple partial seizure and they may or may not be associated with automatism. The site of origin for complex partial seizures is most commonly in the medial temporal lobes (70 per cent of cases) and the frontal lobes in 20 per cent of cases. By the onset of the complex partial seizure it is inferred that seizure discharge has involved the limbic system bilaterally. It is important to emphasize that complex partial seizures are not identical or synonymous with temporal-lobe seizures and that there is no absolute correlation between the phenomenology of complex partial seizures and their site of origin.

The most typical form of temporal complex partial seizure will start with a visceral aura or simple partial seizure. There is then an arrest of activity and a motionless stare followed by a phase of stereotyped automatism. Such automatisms occur in a similar fashion in most of an individual patient's seizures, and most commonly consist of lip smacking, chewing or swallowing, or picking at clothes or fidgeting with objects (Delgado-Escueta *et al.* 1982). Walking or running or verbal automatisms are less frequent. Dystonic asymmetrical posturing is common. Stereotyped automatisms are usually followed by a phase of confusion associated with reactive automatisms. In these, the patient may continue with a previous activity or begin some form of activity that may be considerably influenced by the patient's immediate environment. Restraint during this phase of a seizure may sometimes give rise to reactive violent behaviour. It is probable that the majority of such typical complex partial seizures arise from the hippocampus (Delgado-Escueta and Walsh 1985), but by no means all do so (Williamson *et al.* 1985). Patients with this seizure type often have well-localized anterior temporal spikes and sharp waves that may be unilateral or bilateral.

Complex partial seizures, arising from the frontal regions, are more likely to exhibit some of the following phenomena: they are usually frequent, brief and less commonly followed by post-ictal confusion; the onset of seizures is without warning and automatisms begin immediately without a preceding motionless stare; automatisms tend to be bilateral and include thrashing, rolling, kicking or bicycling movements; sexual automatism with pelvic thrusting may be more common with seizures of frontal onset. There is a marked predominance of sleep seizures, and complex partial status seems to be more common with frontal seizures (Williamson *et al.* 1985; Quesney 1986). Inter-ictally the EEG may be unremarkable or show apparently generalized epileptiform abnormalities.

A third type of complex partial seizure is sometimes described in which there is a sudden loss of postural tone that has been described as temporal-lobe syncope (Caffi 1973). This seizure type must be rare, the author never having seen one in his experience of video-telemetry. Complex partial seizures should not enter into the differential diagnosis of sudden collapse with onset in adult life.

23.4.3 **Partial seizures evolving to secondarily generalized seizures**

Secondarily generalized seizures are relatively uncommon and may only contribute approximately 9 per cent of seizures in adults, compared to approximately 16 per cent in children (Gastaut *et al.* 1975). Furthermore, they are particularly amenable to antiepileptic drug treatment and the majority of patients developing partial epilepsy in adult life have very few secondarily generalized seizures, even though their partial seizures remain a management problem (Turnbull *et al.* 1985). In adults, secondarily generalized seizures not infrequently occur during sleep. Late-onset tonic–clonic seizures occurring during sleep must be regarded as having a focal onset until proved otherwise.

23.4.4 **Generalized seizures**

Although typical absence, myoclonus, and generalized tonic–clonic seizures may begin in adolescence and early adult life, other forms of generalized seizures, such as atypical absence, tonic, and atonic seizures, are features of age-related childhood epilepsies (Section 22.2). While they may persist into adult life, they rarely, if ever, commence in adult life. However, many children with severe childhood epilepsies tend to develop more typical partial seizures (particularly complex partial seizures) or may expect remission when they enter adult life (Huttenlocher and Hapke 1990).

23.4.5 **Status epilepticus**

Almost all seizures are self-limiting events, although the mechanisms leading to termination of seizures are poorly understood. Status epilepticus can be defined as two or more seizures occurring without full recovery of function, or as more continuous seizure activity for 30 minutes or more. While it is true that there are as many types of status epilepticus as there are types of seizures, it is increasingly apparent that status has a dynamic of its own that goes beyond the semiology of seizures themselves. At a simplified level, status may be classified into generalized convulsive status epilepticus, non-convulsive status epilepticus (including complex partial and absence status), and simple partial status (Treiman and Delgado-Escueta 1980).

Generalized convulsive status epilepticus (GCSE) is most common. Best estimates of its incidence lie between 200 and 300/1 000 000 (Shorvon 1994). It probably makes up about 70 per cent of all cases of status and is associated with the highest morbidity and mortality. Mortality rates for GCSE remain high, with most series demonstrating rates of 10–20 per cent (Treiman and Delgado-Escueta 1980). It is more common in children than in adults.

GCSE may have many different causes. The number of cases with a previous history of chronic epilepsy may be falling and less than 5 per cent of people with epilepsy ever experience GCSE. In this group, discontinuation of antiepileptic drugs is by far the most common provocative factor. Other causes of status in those without epilepsy include drug abuse (particularly alcohol), metabolic disorders, cerebral hypoxia, stroke, trauma, tumour, and CNS infection. The outcome is determined largely by the aetiology and by the speed at which effective treatment is instituted.

At onset of GCSE, typical and relatively discreet tonic–clonic seizures may be observed. However, with progression, convulsive activity commonly becomes less marked and may eventually be confined to myoclonic jerks of the head, eyes, and face. At this stage, the usual EEG characteristics may be lost and more periodic activity is seen (Treiman *et al.* 1990). This has been called 'subtle convulsive status' and may represent a terminal state. It is most frequently described in series that include large numbers of cases of status following cardiorespiratory arrest during anoxic coma, and it remains somewhat controversial whether it really represents an anoxic rather than a seizure-related state.

Early in GCSE there is immediate catecholamine release, resulting in tachycardia, hypertension, and hyperglycaemia (Walton 1993). Pulmonary oedema may occur as may a combined respiratory and metabolic acidosis. Hyperpyrexia commonly occurs and appears important in determining poor outcomes (Meldrum and Horton 1973). This, combined with blood and CSF leucocytosis, can suggest the presence of infection, when they are, in fact, the result of the status. Late in GCSE the blood pressure and heart rate begin to fall, hypoglycaemia may occur, and renal failure may be caused by rhabdomyolysis.

Few conditions should be confused with GCSE, although it is not unusual for recurrent pseudoseizures to be managed by the inexperienced as true status epilepticus (Howell *et al.* 1989). Acute encephalopathies due to hypoxia, uraemia, or other metabolic causes, which are associated with multifocal myoclonus, may also be confused with true status epilepticus on occasions.

The incidence of complex partial status epilepticus (CPSE) is uncertain, largely because it is underdiagnosed (Shorvon 1994). Probably one-third of cases occur without a previous history of epilepsy and often start with one or two discrete tonic–clonic seizures. It may well be that the condition is more common in subjects with frontal than temporal-lobe epilepsy. The typical picture is of a twilight state with varying degrees of confusion. Typical automatisms of complex partial seizures may or may not be seen. The EEG is crucial for a diagnosis but a variety of changes occur, from localized seizure discharges, through periodic lateralized epileptiform discharges (PLEDs), to generalized patterns of disturbance. Episodes vary in length, some examples lasting months are documented (Roberts and Humphrey 1988; Shorvon 1994).

The differential diagnosis of CPSE is exceptionally wide and includes a variety of psychiatric disorders as well as any unexplained confusional state or alteration of consciousness.

There may be surprisingly little morbidity to even prolonged episodes of CPSE, and there are very few case reports of significant memory impairment following such episodes.

Simple partial status epilepticus (SPSE) is probably even rarer and commonly takes a somatomotor form. In adults, stroke, tumour, and non-ketotic hypoglycaemia are probably the most common causes.

23.5 Epilepsy syndromes in adult life

A systematic classification of epilepsy syndromes has been proposed (Commission on Classification and Terminology of the International League Against Epilepsy 1989) (Table 23.5). Most epilepsy syndromes are age-related and occur in childhood, while the majority of the epilepsies of adult life are symptomatic partial epilepsies. For this reason the classification has less relevance to adults, in whom accurate localization of the onset of partial seizures and determination of their aetiology is of greater importance (see below).

Some reference does, however, need to be made to those specific epilepsy syndromes where seizures have a predilection to continue into adult life.

23.5.1 Idiopathic generalized epilepsies

This is a relatively well-defined group of syndromes with age-specific onsets and generalized spike wave abnormality in the EEG. They are primarily genetic, although the mode of inheritance is likely to be complex and heterogeneous (see Section 22.2).

Childhood absence epilepsy

This syndrome probably accounts for about 8 per cent of epilepsy in school-age children (Cavazzuti 1980). It is certainly genetic, with 75 per cent concordance for monozygotic twins (Metrakos and Metrakos 1972; Hauser and Anderson 1986). The prognosis is said to be excellent, with anywhere between 33 per cent (OllerDaurella and Sanchez 1981) and 80 per cent (Dalby 1969) achieving long-term remission. Figures at the lower range of these estimates include patients followed up for longer periods. Only about 6 per cent of patients with this seizure disorder have absences that persist into adult life (OllerDaurella and Sanchez 1981). Tonic–clonic seizures commonly develop between 5 and 10 years after the onset of absences (Loiseau *et al.* 1983), in between 40 per cent (Loiseau *et al.* 1983) and 60 per cent of patients (OllerDaurella and Sanchez 1981). Again, there may be significant effects of varying lengths of follow-up of patients on the proportion developing tonic–clonic seizures.

Children with best outlook seem to be those with absence commencing early in childhood, whose absences are not associated with myoclonus, and who do not have tonic–clonic seizures preceding or coinciding with the onset of absences. In those with absence persisting into adult life, Panayiotopoulos *et al.* (1992) found atypical features suggesting alternative diagnoses, such as eyelid or perioral myoclonus with absence, or that the absences were part of a juvenile myoclonic or absence epilepsy.

When tonic–clonic seizures occur in subjects with this syndrome in adult life, they occur without an aura and have a tendency to occur within 1–2 hours of wakening. Sodium valproate is undoubtedly the drug of choice for the treatment of persisting seizures in adults with this syndrome (Loiseau 1985). Lamotrigine also appears to be effective, and the combination with valproate in those unusual patients refractory to a single drug is often strikingly effective (Richens 1992).

Juvenile absence epilepsy

This syndrome is less common than childhood absence epilepsy and may account for 20 per cent of patients with typical absence. Absence seizures begin between the ages of 7 and 16 years, but tend to be much less frequent than those of childhood absence epilepsy, while a greater proportion (80 per cent) have tonic–clonic seizures, 75 per cent of which occur on awakening (Janz 1969). Myoclonic seizures can also occur in this syndrome, perhaps in as many as 16 per cent of patients (Wolf and Inoue 1984). The EEG shows a high incidence of polyspike and wave and photosensitivity.

Valproate is again the drug of choice, with remission in 85 per cent of patients (Wolf and Inoue 1984). Lamotrigine alone or in combination with valproate also seems to be effective. In distinction from childhood absence epilepsy, the syndrome is probably lifelong (Bouma et al. 1996).

Other absence epilepsies

Eyelid myoclonia with absences (EMA) has been well described by Panayiotopoulos (Giannakodimos and Panayiotopoulos 1996). Onset is in childhood and the seizures begin with rhythmic, fast, brief jerking of the eyelids and upward jerking of the eyeballs, followed by brief mild absence. They mainly occur on eye closure. The EEG shows 3–6 Hz generalized polyspike and wave, and all patients are photosensitive. Most patients experience occasional tonic–clonic seizures with sleep deprivation. Myoclonus of the lower face may be associated with absence (perioral myoclonia with absence: PMA). Here there are rhythmic contractions causing protrusion of the lips and twitching of the corners of the mouth with mild absence (Panayiotopoulos et al. 1994). These seizures may build to absence status and then a tonic–clonic seizure. Both EMA and PMA seem likely to persist into adult life.

Juvenile myoclonic epilepsy

This is a common epilepsy syndrome, which was first described comprehensively by Janz and Christian (1957). It is a genetic disorder and up to 25 per cent of patients have a family history (Janz 1969). In some pedigrees the gene encoding for this disorder has been shown by linkage analysis to lie on the short arm of the chromosome 6 (Greenberg et al. 1988), while in others linkage to this region has been excluded (Whitehouse et al. 1993), suggesting that genetic heterogeneity exists.

It accounts for approximately 5–10 per cent of epilepsies. Seizures can begin between 8 and 26 years, but 80 per cent commence between the ages of 12 and 18 (Janz 1969). Myoclonic jerks are usually symmetric and mostly affect the upper limbs. Myoclonus can, on occasion, be associated with absence, or typical absence seizures can occur independently. Seizures most commonly occur after wakening, but there may also be a second peak in seizure susceptibility during the evening. Sleep deprivation appears to be a potent provocative factor.

Ninety per cent of patients have generalized tonic–clonic seizures and 10 per cent of patients have absence seizures (Janz 1969). It is, however, the tonic–clonic seizures that precipitate medical referral, and patients may not recognize the important association with jerks, which may have preceded the first tonic–clonic seizure by some time. It is therefore important in identifying this syndrome to ask specifically for a history of myoclonus.

The EEG typically shows polyspike and spike wave activity at a more rapid rate than the classic three cycle per second spike wave (Janz 1969). Photosensitivity is extremely common and is usually identified in about 30 per cent of patients, although frequently this phenomenon may be blocked by treatment with valproate (Goosses 1984). There can be no doubt that valproate is the drug of choice in this syndrome, although lamotrigine is also effective. Remission may be uncommon if patients are treated with other antiepileptic drugs (Delgado-Escueta and Enrile-Bacsal 1984) and carbamazepine and vigabatrin may exacerbate myoclonus. Remissions of this syndrome are drug-dependent and 90 per cent of patients will relapse if drugs are withdrawn (Janz et al. 1983).

Tonic–clonic seizures on awakening

Tonic–clonic (or clonic–tonic–clonic) seizures predominate in this syndrome, although the presence of occasional myoclonus or absence does not preclude the diagnosis. Janz (1962) examined the timing of tonic–clonic seizures in 2825 patients: 33 per cent had tonic–clonic seizures on awakening, compared to 44 per cent occurring during sleep and 23 per cent occurring at random. There was a strong association between tonic–clonic seizures occurring on wakening and generalized spike wave activity in the EEG. The syndrome has the widest range of age at onset of the idiopathic generalized epilepsies, from 5 to 30 years, with peak onset at 17–20 years.

Precipitating factors include sleep deprivation, sudden arousal, and alcohol intake, but catamenial exacerbations are also prominent. Avoidance of precipitating factors is important in management, and valproate and lamotrigine are the drugs of choice for this syndrome. The history of seizures on wakening seems to increase the risk of relapse in patients in whom drugs are withdrawn after a period of remission (Janz et al. 1983; Medical Research Council Antiepileptic Drug Withdrawal Study Group 1991; Chadwick 199?).

Generalized epilepsy with febrile seizures plus

Generalized epilepsy with febrile seizures plus (GEFS+) has recently been described by Berkovic and colleagues (Scheffer and Berkovic 1997; Wallace et al. 1998). They have identified a number of large pedigrees with an epilepsy beginning around the age of 1 year with apparent febrile seizures, which however, continue with afebrile tonic–clonic seizures through childhood. Some affected individuals can exhibit absence, myoclonus, and, most severely, myoclonic astatic epilepsy. Seizures often remit before puberty. In one family linkage to 19q13.1 was found and an abnormality demonstrated in a $\beta1$ subunit of the voltage-gated sodium channel.

23.5.2 Symptomatic generalized epilepsies

These childhood epilepsies are frequently malignant (see Section 22.2.1) and are associated with a significant mortality. However, many children with such epilepsies will survive into the adult age-range. They are frequently mentally handicapped and may also have motor disability (cerebral palsy). In adult life there is often a change in the nature of seizures with myoclonic, tonic, atonic, and atypical absence seizures becoming less frequent. More typical simple partial and complex partial seizures become evident. The characteristic of these seizures is often that they appear to be multifocal from a clinical and electro-encephalographic point of view. While such patients may continue to have a severe epilepsy during adult life, seizure frequency tends to be less than in childhood.

23.5.3 Idiopathic partial epilepsies

Some idiopathic age-related syndromes (e.g. benign Rolandic epilepsy) are not seen in adult life as they have an early age of onset in childhood and a uniformly excellent prognosis and do not continue into adult life. However, the range of genetically determined partial epilepsies seen in adults is increasing.

Autosomal dominant nocturnal frontal lobe epilepsy has been described in a number of families from Australia, the UK, and Canada (Scheffer et al. 1995). Many patients previously diagnosed as having paroxysmal nocturnal dystonia probably have this seizure disorder. Seizures begin in childhood and persist into adult life. They occur during sleep, often in clusters and are typical frontal lobe seizures that are brief, associated with vocalization, and include varieties of motor activity, including thrashing, tonic stiffening, and clonic jerks. Occasional secondarily generalized tonic–clonic seizures occur. The interictal EEG is usually normal, as can be ictal EEG recording. Most patients are responsive to carbamazepine. Some families show linkage to markers on chromosome 20q. A missense mutation has been demonstrated in the gene encoding the α-4 subunit of the nicotinic acetylcholine receptor (Steinlein et al. 1995). Other families do not show this linkage and there may be genetic heterogeneity.

Other genetically determined partial epilepsies probably occur in adult life. Berkovic et al. (1994) described a twin study in which 19 monozygotic twins were concordant for a temporal-lobe epilepsy with a very benign course. Similar cases have been reported in non-twin families. The age of onset was anywhere between 10 and 60 years. Seizures tended to be brief simple or complex partial temporal-lobe seizures, which were very easily controlled with carbamazepine or phenytoin.

Ottman et al. (1995) reported a family with characteristic temporal-lobe seizures associated with an auditory aura. There was evidence of linkage to chromosome 10q.

23.5.4 Cryptogenic partial epilepsy

Mesial temporal lobe epilepsy

The syndrome of mesial temporal-lobe epilepsy (MTLE) may still best be described as a cryptogenic epilepsy in spite of increasing understanding of its aetiological and pathological mechanisms. There are no good epidemiological data about its incidence and prevalence, but information from surgical series would suggest that it is probably a major contributor to the total number of cases of temporal-lobe epilepsy. Up to two-thirds of cases have a history of prolonged febrile convulsions in childhood (Cendes et al. 1993; Williamson et al. 1993) and in others there may be a history of trauma or infection (Mathern et al. 1995). A case controlled study has suggested that complicated febrile seizures during childhood may be the aetiological factor in up to 20 per cent of all patients with complex partial seizures (Rocca et al. 1987). The pathology shows neuronal loss and gliosis in the hippocampus (hippocampal sclerosis) associated with synaptic reorganization resulting in functional hyper-synchronization and hyperexcitability. This type of pathological change can be seen following seizures in experimental animals (Sutula et al. 1988) and is also seen, on occasion, associated with hamartomas and cortical dysplasias in humans.

The most striking clinical feature of MTLE is its progressive nature. Typical temporal-lobe seizures may be noted as early as the first decade of life. However, when they begin they are often simple partial seizures that are brief, and they may continue for years before the diagnosis is made. When recognized in childhood, seizures are often suppressed, only to return in adolescence or early adult life (French et al. 1993). By this time, the seizures are more severe and commonly are typical temporal-lobe complex partial seizures, and some episodes of secondary generalization start to appear. Ninety per cent of subjects describe an aura, including, most commonly, visceral sensations, olfactory hallucination, and memory disturbance. There is then a typical progression to complex partial seizures, beginning with motor arrest and staring, oro-alimentary automatisms, and fumbling and picking automatisms of the hands. Versive symptoms may occur, either early or late. There is also evidence of a progressive disturbance of cognitive function, particularly memory (Selwa et al. 1994). There is some evidence that the severity of MRI changes of hippocampal sclerosis increases with the duration of disease (Salmenpera et al. 1998).

Investigations may show a normal interictal EEG or, alternatively, characteristic anterior temporal sharp waves which are bilaterally independent in up to a third of patients. High-resolution T1-weighted MR imaging shows hippocampal atrophy that is most commonly unilateral but can be bilateral (Fig. 23.9). T2-weighted images and FLAIR sequences show high signal in the affected hippocampus.

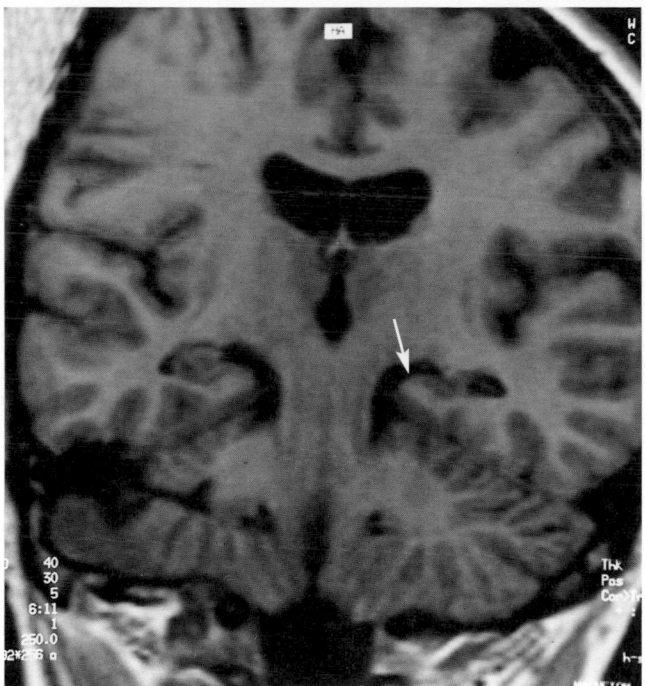

Fig. 23.9.   Coronal T1-weighted images, showing marked left mesial temporal sclerosis and atrophy (arrow).

While antiepileptic drug treatment reduces or may abolish secondarily generalized tonic–clonic seizures, complex partial seizures are most refractory and many patients exhibit considerable psychosocial disadvantage. Surgical treatment will usually abolish disabling seizures in about 80 per cent of subjects. For this reason, it is extremely important that the syndrome is recognized early so that the impact of the disorder can be minimized (see Section 23.11).

Rasmussen's encephalitis

This is a, fortunately, rare syndrome that is usually seen in children but which can occur in adults. It comprises epilepsia partialis continua, slowly progressive hemiplegia and intellectual impairment with progressive atrophy of one cerebral hemisphere. Histological examination reveals a low grade inflammatory response (Rasmussen *et al.* 1958). While various viruses have been suggested as an aetiological agent, there are no consistent findings in this area. Recently some cases have demonstrated GluR3 antibodies (Rogers *et al.* 1994) and immunosuppression can be helpful (Hart *et al.* 1994). Some cases will come to hemispherectomy (see below).

23.6 Factors precipitating seizures

A number of factors may appear to precipitate seizures in susceptible individuals. These may be classified as either specific sensory stimuli or actions (reflexly induced seizures), or non-specific precipitants.

23.6.1 Reflexly induced seizures

Although the term 'reflex epilepsy' has been widely applied, two-thirds of patients who have reflexly induced seizures may also have apparently spontaneous seizures occurring at other times. Photosensitive epilepsy is the most common reflex epilepsy, accounting for about 5 per cent of patients with epilepsy (Jeavons and Harding 1975). The crudest visual stimulus to evoke seizures is flicker or flash, a factor that is made use of in the routine recording of most EEGs. This form of sensitivity is most common in childhood and juvenile absence epilepsy, juvenile myoclonic epilepsy, and some forms of progressive myoclonic epilepsy. It is a much rarer accompaniment of symptomatic generalized epilepsies and is rarely seen in partial epilepsy. Flicker stimuli may be produced in the environment by television and video games, stroboscopic illumination, or sunlight passing through trees or railings or other regularly spaced objects. Most individuals are maximally sensitive between 15 and 20 Hz (Jeavons and Harding 1975). Maximum sensitivity often occurs just after the eyes are closed or when the eyes are open. Stimulation of one eye rather than both eyes reduces sensitivity. The greater the visual field taken up by stimuli and the greater the luminance then the greater the potential for photosensitivity and, in many individuals, patterned flash is a potent stimulus.

The electrophysiological correlate of photosensitivity is the photoconvulsive response. This is most commonly seen in females during adolescence and may disappear in adult life. A photoconvulsive response consists of bilaterally synchronous spike wave activity, which persists for a second or more after the cessation of the flash stimulus. It must be differentiated clearly from photic following and photomyoclonic responses, which have no significant association with photically induced seizures.

About a third of flash-sensitive patients exhibit sensitivity to patterns, the most potent of which are strong stripes, and 70 per cent do so if the pattern oscillates (Wilkins *et al.* 1980). The most important practical implication of pattern sensitivity is television epilepsy. A television picture is created by variations in the brightness of a spot that scans the screen repeatedly from left to right. The pattern that is generated in this way is similar to a vibrating pattern, which is a very potent stimulus to pattern-sensitive individuals.

Seizures can be prevented in susceptible individuals by maintaining a satisfactory distance from the television set and using a remote control to adjust the picture. More complex methods involve viewing the screen through polarized spectacles so as to produce only monocular stimulation (Wilkins and Lindsay 1985). Most antiepileptic drugs block photic sensitivity, but valproate seems to be the treatment of choice, although lamotrigine and benzodiazepines may also be effective.

Particular interest has been aroused by the occurrence of seizures with computer games (Fish *et al.* 1994). The incidence has been estimated as approximately 1.5 per 100 000 of the population between 7 and 19 years. Most subjects show sensitivity to flicker or pattern, but in some cases it may be absent, suggesting a contribution from more complex visual or cognitive stimuli (Maeda *et al.* 1990).

Primary reading epilepsy can be viewed as a form of visually induced epilepsy. The characteristic seizures in this disorder are myoclonic jerks of the jaw, which may proceed to tonic–clonic seizures. Both focal and paroxysmal EEG abnormalities have been described in this condition (Wilkins and Lindsay 1985). A number of different mechanisms may be involved in producing seizures with reading. In some patients, the lines of print may act as patterns (Mayersdorf and Marshall 1970). In others, eye movements may potentially provoke the seizures (Alajouanine *et al.* 1959). In some patients neither pattern sensitivity nor eye movements appear important, and in these comprehension of the written material may be the important provocative factor (Forster 1977).

Sudden noise or other startle may give rise to seizures, particularly in mentally handicapped patients (Anderman and Andermann 1986). More complex auditory stimuli can also provoke seizures in musicogenic epilepsy (Critchley 1937; Poskanzer *et al.* 1962), where seizures are usually complex partial in nature. A variety of other complex reflex epilepsies have been described including eating epilepsy, which gives rise to complex partial seizures, and writing epilepsy, producing jerking of the writing hand. Other cognitive functions, such as arithmetic (Ingvar and Nyman 1962) and listening to spoken language (Tsuki and Kasuga 1978) can evoke seizures in rare cases.

Touch or muscle stretch may occasionally provoke seizures, but more commonly evokes myoclonic jerking in patients with progressive myoclonic or post-hypoxic myoclonus. Immersion in hot or cold water can act as a seizure precipitant, particularly in the Indian subcontinent (Gururaj and Satishchandra 1992). Rarely, seizures may be provoked by movement (Lishman *et al.* 1962), although many of the patients described in this paper probably had paroxysmal choreoathetosis.

23.6.2 Non-specific precipitants

The sleep–waking cycle can have a profound influence on the occurrence of seizures in susceptible individuals (Baldy-Moulinier 1986). Many patients have tonic–clonic seizures only during sleep (Gibberd and Bateson 1974). A number of epilepsy syndromes show a predilection for seizures during non-REM sleep, including the idiopathic partial epilepsies, electrical status epilepticus during slow wave sleep, and temporal and frontal lobe epilepsies. Sleep may enhance focal epileptogenic discharges, and tonic–clonic seizures limited to sleep in the adult should usually be regarded as having a partial onset until proved otherwise (Janz 1962).

Seizures occurring shortly after wakening are common in the idiopathic generalized epilepsies: juvenile myoclonic epilepsy, tonic–clonic seizures on awakening, and childhood and juvenile absence epilepsy (see above). Such individuals seem particularly sensitive to sleep deprivation or to sudden rousing from deep sleep. The symptomatic generalized epilepsies are characterized by occurrence of seizures that are independent of the sleep–waking cycle.

Many women with epilepsy are subject to catamenial exacerbation of seizures, although it is uncommon to see women who only have seizures corresponding to such a pattern (Newmark and Penry 1980). The time of greatest susceptibility seems to be in the few days preceding the onset of menstruation. Although it has been suggested that water retention is an important factor in the mechanisms precipitating such seizures, the evidence for this is weak and diuretics seem to have little effect in suppressing such seizures. There is, however, evidence that oestrogens may be potentially epileptogenic and progestogens potentially anticonvulsant (Backstrom 1976). In spite of this, regulation of periods using oral contraceptive preparations has not shown any benefit in suppressing seizures. Where periods are regular, the prescription of a benzodiazepine, such as clobazam, for a number of days around the period of maximum risk can be beneficial (Feely *et al.* 1982). The effects of pregnancy on seizure control in women with epilepsy are unpredictable. In some individuals seizures may increase in frequency, in some they may decrease, but in the majority there is no significant change in seizure frequency.

Psychological stress is often claimed by patients to precipitate seizures. Emotional stress precipitated fits in 21 per cent of patients with temporal-lobe epilepsy (Currie *et al.* 1971). The mechanisms involved may, in some circumstances, include alterations in sleep–waking cycle which commonly accompany stress, and the role of psychotropic drugs in increasing seizure susceptibility must always be remembered (see below).

Finally, poor compliance with antiepileptic drug regimes must represent one of the most common precipitants of seizures.

23.7 Causes of seizures in adults

The great majority of seizures and epilepsies developing in adult life will be regarded as and, with the advent of modern MR imaging, shown to be symptomatic. It may be useful to divide causes of seizures and epilepsy in adult life into acute symptomatic seizures occurring in response to systemic illness or cerebral insult, and remote symptomatic epilepsies in which epilepsy develops in relationship to a persisting cerebral lesion or damage. Some aetiologies, such as head injury, stroke, and intracranial infections may cause both acute symptomatic seizures and remote symptomatic epilepsy. The presence of the one is not necessarily associated with the other. Sander *et al.* (1990*a*) found that the most common remote symptomatic causes of epilepsy were vascular disease (15 per cent) and tumour (6 per cent). Remote symptomatic epilepsy was most common in the elderly, where vascular disease accounted for 49 per cent of cases. Tumour was a rare cause of epilepsy below 30 (1 per cent), but accounted for 19 per cent of cases between 50 and 59 years of age. Trauma caused 3 per cent of cases, infection 2 per cent. Acute symptomatic seizures occurred in 15 per cent, and alcohol was the most common single cause (6 per cent), its incidence being highest between 30 and 39 years (27 per cent).

23.7.1 **Causes of acute symptomatic seizures**

The term 'acute symptomatic seizure' was suggested by Hauser *et al.* (1982). These seizures occur commonly: in a series of 1758 patients admitted to an intensive care unit, 217 exhibited neurological complications, of whom 61 had seizures (Bleck *et al.* 1993). When they occur as a result of systemic disorders, they are associated with an acute encephalopathy and, most commonly, seizures are of a tonic–clonic type. Patients will often exhibit tremor, asterixis, and multifocal myoclonus. Their occurrence is determined more by the rate of metabolic change or drug exposure than by the absolute disturbance. They are particularly common in the elderly, where they may account for as much as 77 per cent of the incidence of seizures (Loiseau *et al.* 1990). Focal seizures are more likely to be seen in association with acute cerebral insults, when they are usually recognized as focal motor seizures, sometimes as epilepsia partialis continua. It is suggested that complex partial seizures rarely occur as acute symptomatic seizures, but such seizures could be difficult to recognize when accompanied by an acute confusional state or coma.

Although acute symptomatic seizures may be suppressed by short-acting antiepileptic drugs (e.g. benzodiazepines) they do not usually require longer-term antiepileptic drug treatment. On occasion, acute symptomatic seizures may be resistant to benzodiazepines and other antiepileptic drugs, and correction of the underlying metabolic abnormality may be necessary to suppress seizures.

Disorders of fluid and electrolyte balance

Hypernatraemia may occur in gastroenteritis, fever, sweating, burns and diabetes, and due to gross fluid restriction or excessive salt intake. Neurological signs are seen in 50 per cent of patients with serum sodium concentrations above 151 mmol/l. (Swanson 1976). Altered consciousness is common, and focal or generalized tonic–clonic seizures occur most commonly in patients who are also uraemic or acidotic (Stephenson 1971). They are also seen during rehydration, which should be undertaken cautiously with dextrose–saline solutions (Bruck *et al.* 1968).

Hyponatraemia is more common than hypernatraemia and may be seen with congestive cardiac failure, liver disease, nephrotic syndrome, water overload, and diuretic misuse, as well as with renal disease and inappropriate antidiuretic hormone (ADH) syndromes which can be caused by neurological disorders. Tonic–clonic seizures occur with occasional status. Convulsions were noted in 9 per cent of 65 patients with serum sodium concentrations of less than 125 mmol/l (Arieff *et al.* 1976). Hyponatraemia is associated with a high mortality, and too rapid a correction by the overenthusiastic use of hypertonic saline has been associated with the occurrence of central pontine myelinolysis (Norenberg *et al.* 1982).

Hypocalcaemia may be seen in hypoparathyroidism, vitamin D deficiency, acute pancreatitis, and pseudohypoparathyroidism. Up to 70 per cent of patients with hypoparathyroidism may have seizures associated with tetany, altered consciousness and abnormal behaviour, and dyskinesia (Frame 1976). Both tonic–clonic and focal motor seizures are described.

Hypercalcaemia occurs most commonly in disseminated malignant disease and hyperparathyroidism. It results in weakness, drowsiness and confusion, and occasionally seizures, which can be generalized (Bauermeister *et al.* 1967) or focal motor seizures (Herishanu *et al.* 1970). *Hypomagnesaemia* may be seen in inflammatory bowel disease, bowel resection, and other malabsorption syndromes, and is often associated with other electrolyte disturbance. Neurological syndromes may be seen with levels below 1.3 mmol/l, and the clinical state (with startle, tremor and myoclonus, and Chvostek's sign) may be indistinguishable from that of hypocalcaemia (Hanna *et al.* 1960), although tetany may be less common (Fishman 1965). Hypomagnesaemic seizures may be resistant to antiepileptic drug therapy and may only respond to the administration of magnesium. This fact should be remembered as hypomagnesaemia not infrequently accompanies hypocalcaemia. Hypomagnesaemia needs to be considered if seizures continue in a treated hypocalcaemic patient.

Hypophosphataemia may occur in association with long-duration, intensive therapy or parenteral feeding. Tonic–clonic seizures may occur with serum phosphate levels below 1 mg/100 ml (Knochel 1977). Most hypophosphataemic patients will also required potassium and magnesium replacement.

Metabolic disorders

Diabetes

Seizures seem particularly common in association with non-kerotihyperglycaemia (Venna and Sabin 1981). They may occur in up to a quarter of patients, and simple partial motor seizures account for approximately 80 per cent of seizures. Epilepsy partialis continua can occur. In about 6 per cent of patients focal motor seizures were the initial symptom of the disorder (Aquimno and Gabor 1980). Such seizures may be very resistant to antiepileptic drug treatment but seem to respond rapidly to the correction of the hyperglycaemia. In contrast, seizures seem to be very rare in ketoacidotic coma (Messing and Simon 1986).

Hypoglycaemia

Hypoglycaemia is usually seen in diabetic patients using insulin or hypoglycaemic drugs. It occurs more rarely with insulinoma, other neoplasms, or severe liver disease. Seizures, usually tonic–clonic seizures without an aura, may occur in 7 per cent of patients (Malouf and Brust 1985).

Thyroid disease

Seizures appear to be extremely uncommon in hyperthyroidism but they do occasionally occur (Korczyn and Bechar 1976). They can form a prominent feature of Hashimoto's encephalopathy that sometimes precedes other manifestations of thyrotoxicosis (Thrush and Boddie 1974). Myoclonic seizures may occur along with tonic–clonic seizures (Ghika-Schmid *et al.* 1996). Seizures appear to be more common in patients with hypothyroidism and may occur in as many as a quarter of patients with myxoedema coma (Jellinek 1962). Patients would not seem to be at risk of continued seizures after the underlying thyroid abnormality has been corrected.

Porphyria

Seizure may occur in approximately 15 per cent of patients during episodes of acute intermittent porphyria, and may be a presenting feature (Reynolds and Miska 1976). Control of seizures can be a significant management problem as hydantoins, barbiturates, and carbamazepine can all induce attacks of porphyria. Benzodiazepines may be used with caution, but it has also been suggested that magnesium sulphate may be effective in controlling seizures (Taylor 1981). Of the new antiepileptic drugs, gabapentin may be safe.

Liver disease

Seizures are a feature of acute hepatic failure but not of chronic hepatic dysfunction. Seizures may be focal but are more commonly tonic–clonic seizures, often preceded by multifocal myoclonus. Their incidence varies greatly in different series. Adams and Foley (1953) reported convulsions in a third of patients, but only 1 of 83 patients reported by Plum and Posner (1980) had fits. Some differences may arise from the aetiology of hepatic failure, alcohol being much more common in the former series. Hypoglycaemia complicating acute liver failure may be a further factor affecting the incidence of seizures (Plum and Hindfelt 1968).

Renal failure

Acute uraemic encephalopathy commonly presents with motor excitability, including tremors, asterixis, multifocal myoclonus, chorea, and dystonia. Convulsions occur in as many as a third of patients (Raskin and Fishman 1976). Again, most are tonic–clonic seizures but focal motor seizures and epilepsia partialis continua can occur (De Deyn et al. 1992). Seizures have also been reported during dialysis (dialysis disequilibrium syndrome) and as part of dialysis encephalopathy, a subacute progressive disorder in which speech disorders, dementia, and myoclonus are prominent (Lederman and Henry 1978). This disorder seems to be related to levels of aluminium in water used for dialysis medium (Dunea et al. 1978).

The use of antiepileptic drugs in patients with chronic renal failure presents some difficulties. Protein-bound antiepileptic drugs such as phenytoin may have a relatively high free fraction relative to total estimated plasma levels. Similar problems may exist for carbamazepine, which also tends to be excreted in the urine, and dosage reduction may be necessary (Bennett et al. 1980).

Drug-related seizures

Drugs, and particularly alcohol, are a common cause of seizures (Chadwick 1983; Messing et al. 1984), and many different drugs have been associated with seizures (Table 23.6). The Boston Collaborative Drugs Surveillance Program (1972) reported 26 cases of drug-induced convulsions in approximately 33 000 in-

patients (an incidence of 0.08 per cent). The most commonly involved drugs were penicillin, hypoglycaemic drugs, lignocaine, and psychotropic agents. Messing et al. (1984) reviewed case records of over 3000 patients presenting with seizures, and found that they were drug-related in 1.7 per cent, the most common drugs involved being isoniazid, psychotropic drugs, bronchodilators, hypoglycaemic agents, lignocaine, and penicillin. The majority of seizures were tonic–clonic, but whereas most began without an aura, there was a simple partial (motor) onset in nine patients.

Seizures may be provoked in two ways: there may be specific CNS excitatory effects for some drugs or, alternatively, there may be non-specific effects resulting from high doses of drugs, often administered during self-poisoning. Most drug-induced seizures are dose related and particular care must be exercised when drugs are administered parenterally or intrathecally. Patients with renal or hepatic failure may be at risk because of inability to metabolize potentially convulsant drugs, and individuals with a previous history of epilepsy or pre-existing brain disease may be particularly at risk.

Antibiotics

Penicillin is a potent epileptogenic substance in animals and has been widely used as a model for both focal and generalized epilepsies. It appears to act as a GABA antagonist and may also bind to benzodiazepine receptors (Curtis et al. 1972; Antoniadis et al. 1980). Benzylpenicillin is probably the most potent antibiotic in causing seizures, but ampicillin and cephalosporins carry some risk. Newer quinalone antibiotics may interfere similarly with GABAergic mechanisms, and isoniazid may cause seizures because of its action in antagonizing pyridoxine, a coenzyme required for the synthesis of GABA (Blakemore 1980).

Table 23.6. Drugs associated with seizures

Anaesthetics	Antibiotics	Antipsychotic agents
Ether	Benzylpenicillin	Chlorpromazine
Halothane	Carbenicillin	Lithium
Ketamine	Oxacillin	
Methohexitone	Ampicillin	**Radiographic contrast media**
Propanidid	Cycloserine	
Althesin	Isoniazid	Meglumine
	Nalidixic acid	carbamate
Analeptics	Quinalone	Meglumine
Nikethamide		iothalamate
Aminophylline	**Antiepileptic drugs** (in	Metrizamide
Amphetamines	overdosage)	
Ephedrine	Phenobarbitone	**Miscellaneous**
	Phenytoin	D-Penicillamine
Analgesics	Vigabatrin	Baclofen
Cocaine	Carbamazepine	Hyperbaric oxygen
Pethidine		Folate
Dextropropoxyphene	**Antidepressants**	Piperazine
	Amitriptyline	Cyclosporin
Antidysrhythmics	Imipramine	Interferon
Disopyramide	Mianserin	
Lignocaine	Maprotiline	

Psychotropic drugs

Tricyclics are particularly likely to cause myoclonus and convulsions when taken in overdose, but seizures may occur in up to 1 per cent of patients taking therapeutic dosages (Lowry and Dunner 1980). Amitriptyline is probably the drug with the highest risk, but monoamine oxidase inhibitors and selective serotonin uptake inhibitors appear to be relatively safe (Dailey and Naritoku 1996) and may even possess antiepileptic properties at therapeutic dosage (Favale *et al.* 1995). Antipsychotic use may be complicated by seizures. Phenothiazines, particularly chlorpromazine, are associated with a 1–2 per cent incidence of seizures (Logothetis 1967). Pimozide and sulpiride are relatively safe. Lithium toxicity may be associated with seizures.

Analeptic drugs

Most CNS stimulant drugs are capable of causing seizures and problems most commonly arise with theophylline and its derivatives, which significantly lower the seizure threshold, possibly by elevating cyclic GMP levels in brain (Walker 1981).

Drugs of abuse

Cocaine, amphetamines, narcotics, and phencyclidine have been associated with seizures (Holland *et al.* 1993; Kuniasaki and Augenstein 1994). They have stimulant actions on the central nervous system and lower seizure threshold (Gawin and Ellinwood 1988). Cocaine presents the most frequent problem, with tonic–clonic seizures occurring in 5 per cent of Accident and Emergency attendances with acute toxicity (Pascual-Leone *et al.* 1990). Organic solvents have been reported to cause epilepsy (Jacobsen *et al.* 1994).

Transplantation and immunosuppressants

Seizures can occur in up to 20 per cent of children undergoing renal transplantation (McEnery *et al.* 1989), but only 4 per cent of liver transplants (Wijdicks *et al.* 1996). Cyclosporin and some other immunosuppressant drugs give rise to seizures. Inevitably, drug effects may interact with other factors, such as metabolic disturbance and infection. Cyclosporin-induced seizures may occur in 1–2 per cent of renal transplants and 5 per cent of bone-marrow transplants (Wijdicks *et al.* 1995).

Withdrawal seizures

The withdrawal of chronically administered sedative drugs which show tolerance is a well-recognized cause of seizures, and may occur with alcohol, barbiturates, and benzodiazepines (Chadwick 1983). The best studied of withdrawal seizures are those that occur with alcohol and which may be a part of the delirium tremens syndrome. The abuse of alcohol is an important cause of seizures in the community (Sander *et al.* 1990*a*) and it must be considered in adults developing tonic–clonic seizures for the first time (Hillbom 1980). The risk is clearly related to the dose of alcohol consumed (Ng *et al.* 1988; Lechtenberg and Worner 1992). It seems that abrupt, absolute, or relative withdrawal of alcohol is most commonly responsible for causing seizures. Alcohol can be shown to have short-term antiepileptic properties in rodents, and a similar effect has been

suggested in humans (Mattson *et al.* 1975). The studies of Victor and Adams (1953) and Victor and Brausch (1967) showed a clustering of seizures between 7 and 48 hours after the withdrawal of alcohol. Sixty per cent of patients had more than one seizure, but status epilepticus occurred in less than 5 per cent of patients. During the withdrawal period photomyoclonic and photoconvulsive responses may be seen in the EEG.

On occasion, seizures do seem to occur in patients while intoxicated with alcohol. This has been explained conventionally by suggesting a relative withdrawal of alcohol as being responsible (Simon 1988), but Ng *et al.* (1988) cast some doubt on this assertion. An alternative explanation may be that alcohol has different effects at different doses, in the same way as do the antiepileptic drugs, phenytoin and phenobarbital (Chadwick 1983).

It is well recognized that non-compliance with antiepileptic drug medication is a common cause of seizures in people with epilepsy, and indeed is an important cause of status epilepticus (Aminoff and Simon 1980). Abuse of barbiturates and subsequent withdrawal in non-epileptics has been an important cause of seizures. This effect is dose related and seizures occur with other withdrawal symptoms, such as insomnia, tremor, anorexia, and autonomic overactivity (Fraser *et al.* 1958). The EEG of patients undergoing barbiturate withdrawal shows features of both photomyoclonic and photoconvulsant responses (Essig 1967). Benzodiazepines have also, on occasion, been associated with presumed withdrawal seizures. Narcotic drug withdrawal has also been associated with seizures (Wijdicks and Sharbrough 1993).

23.8 Causes of remote symptomatic epilepsy

It is well recognized that a number of cerebral insults and pathologies predispose to the development of epilepsy. Where such insults also lead to acute symptomatic seizures, the importance of the latter will be discussed in this section.

23.8.1 Hypoxic ischaemic cerebral insults

Mental and motor handicap present from birth as a static encephalopathy are commonly associated with seizure disorders. Some, but by no means all, may be caused by cerebral hypoxia. Zielinski (1974) found 20 per cent of the epileptic population to be retarded or dull, and Gudmundsson (1966) found a similar proportion of mentally handicapped individuals to have epilepsy in Iceland. Cerebral palsy is also strongly associated with epilepsy and as many as 50 per cent of individuals with both mental handicap and cerebral palsy have a seizure disorders (Hauser *et al.* 1987). The more severe the mental and physical handicap, the higher the risk of epilepsy (Blomquist *et al.* 1981; Edebol-Tysk 1989).

The great majority of individuals with mental handicap and cerebral palsy develop seizures early in life, but up to 15 per cent of patients may have a seizure disorder that starts after the age of 15 years (Forsgren *et al.* 1990). Whereas generalized seizures, including myoclonus, tonic and atonic seizures, and infantile spasms, as part of a symptomatic generalized epilepsy, are common in childhood, as individuals mature partial seizures and secondarily generalized tonic–clonic seizures predominate (Forsgren *et al.* 1990). In this population the outcome for epilepsy is poor, only a third achieving seizure remissions of a year or more, and a third having at least one seizure per month. Early brain damage is one of the strongest factors predicting a poor outcome of epilepsy (Shafer *et al.* 1988).

Generalized cerebral hypoxia during adult life seems much less likely to result in seizures. Acute hypoxia is commonly associated with convulsions and multifocal myoclonus (Wardrope *et al.* 1991). In patients with post-hypoxic coma following an anoxic insult, seizures seem to be much rarer (Bates *et al.* 1977) and when they occur they may be associated with an adverse prognosis. Seizures seem to be relatively rare in adults surviving post-hypoxic coma, but action myoclonus can be disabling in such individuals (Lance and Adams 1963).

23.8.2 Head injury

The relationship between head injury, acute symptomatic seizures (within the first week of injury), and late post-traumatic epilepsy represents perhaps the best studied of all causes of epilepsy (Section 16.8.1). Head injury as a cause of epilepsy is well known to every member of the public and most patients developing epilepsy will recall a minor head injury sometime before the development of seizures. However, it is clear that only specific types of head injury carry a significant risk of post-traumatic epilepsy.

Although perhaps 2 per cent of all concussive head injuries result in epilepsy (Annegers *et al.* 1980), head trauma was the cause of seizures in 3 per cent of patients registered in the National General Practitioners Survey of Epilepsy (Sander *et al.* 1990*a*). There can be no doubt that the more severe the head injury, the higher the risk of post-traumatic epilepsy (Jennett 1975; Annegers *et al.* 1980).

Missile injuries and epilepsy

Brain injuries caused by missiles provide a well-defined and relatively homogeneous group of injuries that, fortunately, are rare in civilian life. They have, however, been fully studied in cohorts of patients from the First World War through to the Vietnam War. In many, the localization and the extent of the injury are known to be anatomically precise and the relationship between the incidence of epilepsy and factors such as retention of foreign bodies, haematoma, brain infection, and the extent of the cerebral injury can be determined. Overall, it would seem that 50 per cent of patients surviving such injuries will develop post-traumatic epilepsy, and that the relative risk of developing epilepsy will initially be 580 times higher than that of a general age-matched population during the first year, falling to 25 times higher after 10 years (Salazar *et al.* 1985).

The site of the injury may be important, wounds of the motor and pre-motor cortex having a higher risk of epilepsy than wounds elsewhere (Russell and Whitty 1952). There is no doubt that the extent of the cerebral injury and the amount of brain loss, which may also be determined by surgical intervention, is an important factor. An association between the risk of epilepsy and the extent of the wound has been reported, as judged by surface and depth measurements (Walker and Jablon 1961) and, more recently, CT scan assessment of the extent of the injury (Salazar *et al.* 1985). Almost certainly correlated with the extent of the injury is the presence of persisting neurological deficit, which has consistently been associated with a high risk of epilepsy (Russell and Whitty 1952; Salazar *et al.* 1985).

Walker and Jablon (1961) did not find that the removal of intracranial metal and bone fragments affected the incidence of epilepsy, although Ascroft (1941) noted a higher incidence of epilepsy when metal had been removed than when it was left indwelling, indicating another possible effect of surgical intervention.

Infection probably exerts an important influence on the incidence of epilepsy. After abscess formation, the incidence of late epilepsy may rise to 73 per cent (Walker and Jablon 1961), and even higher risks of epilepsy are associated with complicating fungal infections (Caveness *et al.* 1979). Salazar *et al.* (1985) suggested that 75 per cent of patients develop seizures with a partial onset, although 70 per cent have at least one tonic–clonic seizure. Persistence of seizures in the face of treatment was more common in patients with simple partial than complex partial seizures. Seizure frequency during the first year seems to predict the duration and frequency of subsequent epilepsy, although the characteristics of the wound and persisting neurological deficit did not seem to determine persistence. Fifteen years after injury 53 per cent of patients with epilepsy had had at least one seizure in the previous 2 years (28 per cent of all head-injured subjects; Salazar *et al.* 1985). Only 8 per cent of patients had a single seizure.

Blunt injuries to the head

The most satisfactory unselected population of patients developing post-traumatic epilepsy has been studied by Annegers *et al.* (1980, 1998). This study utilized the records-linkage system of the Mayo Clinic to identify 4541 patients with head injuries between 1935 and 1984. The minimal clinical criterion for inclusion in the study was an injury resulting in loss of consciousness, post-traumatic amnesia, or evidence of skull fracture. Patients were excluded if they died within 1 month of injury or had epilepsy pre-dating the index head injury. The head injuries were classified as:

- severe: brain contusion, intracerebral or intracranial haematoma, or 24 hours of unconsciousness or amnesia;

- moderate: skull fracture or 30 minutes to 24 hours of unconsciousness or post-traumatic amnesia;

- mild: briefer periods of unconsciousness or amnesia.

While mild and moderate head injuries may carry a small increased risk for the development of epilepsy in subsequent years (standardised incidence ratios of 1.5 and 2.9 respectively), more severe head injuries are accompanied by a considerably increased risk (standardised incidence ratio 17.0) for the development of epilepsy that extends for over ten years following an injury. Within the neurosurgical population studied by Jennett[2], three factors had the greatest influence on the risk of post-traumatic epilepsy. These were the presence of a compound depressed fracture, the presence of intracranial haemorrhage and the occurrence of early (within the first post-traumatic week) acute symptomatic seizures. In those few subjects with all three risk factors, the likelihood of post-traumatic epilepsy could be as high as 50–80%. Anneggers et al[1] found the most important risk factors were brain contusion, subdural haematoma and skull fractures.

The significance of early seizures has been further elucidated. Jennett recognised that seizures occurring immediately on impact do not seem to carry any subsequent excess risk of epilepsy and indeed characterise relatively mild concussive injuries. McCrory et al[3] studied such immediate "concussive convulsions" in Australian sportsmen and came to the same conclusions. They questioned whether these events are seizures rather than a form of acute temporary decerebration. Anneggers et al. have further clarified the importance of early, as opposed to immediate, seizures in predicting late post-traumatic epilepsy by showing, in multivariate analyses, that early seizures have no independent effect on the risk of late post-traumatic epilepsy, but merely act as a marker of injuries of sufficient severity to cause late epilepsy.

Studies that have included CT scanning also emphasize the contribution of intracerebral haematoma to risk (D'Alessandro et al. 1988), a view supported by experimental evidence for the role of haemosiderin in producing seizures (Willmore et al. 1978).

The prognosis for post-traumatic epilepsy following blunt injuries is variable. All series agree that once a late seizure has occurred, the risk of further seizures is high (65–90 per cent). Prolonged follow-up for at least 15 years showed that approximately 50 per cent of patients had no seizures for at least 5 years, 25 per cent were experiencing between 1 and 6 seizures per year, and the other 25 per cent, more than 6 seizures per year (Walker and Erculei 1968).

Management of post-traumatic epilepsy

The ability to identify patients with a high prospective risk of post-traumatic epilepsy, as well as early uncontrolled reports (Servit and Musil 1981), persuaded many neurosurgeons to recommend prophylactic anticonvulsant drugs after head injuries carrying a high prospective risk of epilepsy (Rapport and Penry 1973). Subsequent prospective randomized studies, however, have failed to show any significant effects of prophylaxis in the longer term (Young et al. 1983; Temkin et al. 1990), although phenytoin may reduce the incidence of seizures within the first week following a head injury (Temkin et al.

1990). A systematic review of all relevant rates showed that, while the relative risk for seizures in the first week after injury was reduced by a third, there was no reduction in mortality or late seizures (Schierhout and Roberts 1998).

These disappointing findings, coupled with the difficulty in maintaining compliance in head-injured patients given prophylaxis (McQueen et al. 1983), mean that routine prophylaxis in head-injured patients cannot be recommended with currently available antiepileptic drugs. However, the debate about prophylactic treatment will continue, as it can be argued that those antiepileptic drugs studied to date (phenytoin in particular) do not have significant effects in suppressing kindling in animals. Valproate has some effects in this model of epilepsy and may be a more rational drug with which to attempt prophylaxis (Hauser 1990). However, a large randomized controlled trial investigating the effects of valproate was stopped because of an unexpected increase in early mortality associated with the use of the drug (Temkin et al. 1999).

Post-craniotomy seizures and epilepsy

These can, to a degree, be viewed as a type of head injury, although the underlying pathology contributes significantly to risk. The overall incidence of seizures occurring after supratentorial craniotomy has been estimated at 17 per cent during a follow-up period of at least 5 years (Foy et al. 1981a). The incidence varied from 3 to 92 per cent, depending on the condition for which the craniotomy was undertaken.

Approximately one-fifth of patients undergoing aneurysm surgery develop postoperative seizures (Cabral et al. 1976b; North et al. 1983). The incidence varies according to the site of the aneurysm. Thus, approximate risks may be 7.5 per cent from internal carotid aneurysm, 21 per cent from anterior communicating aneurysm, and 39 per cent for a middle cerebral artery aneurysm (Cabral et al. 1976a; Foy et al. 1981a). Additional factors influencing the incidence may be the presence of an intracerebral haematoma, cortical damage, splitting the Sylvian fissure, cerebral swelling and perioperative aneurysmal rupture, and the length of surgery (Foy et al. 1981a, b). That at least part of the risk of epilepsy associated with aneurysm is associated with a surgical procedure is suggested by the 8.3 per cent incidence in 261 conservatively managed survivors following aneurysmal subarachnoid haemorrhage reported by Storey (Storey 1967). Arteriovenous malformations and spontaneous intracerebral haematoma from other causes carry risks of epilepsy of 50 per cent and 20 per cent, respectively, and surgical treatment does seem to be an additional risk factor for these conditions (Crawford et al. 1986). Cavernous angiomas probably represent 10–20 per cent of all CNS vascular malformations, and seizures are the only symptom in up to 70 per cent (Farmer et al. 1988). The MR changes, with high T2 signal core and a halo of low signal due to haemosiderin, suggest that many may bleed asymptomatically. Here surgery seems to be highly effective in seizure control.

The incidence of epilepsy following tumour surgery is more difficult to assess, because of the usually progressive nature of the underlying pathology. However, surgery may play a role, as Cabral *et al.* (1976*b*) found that postoperative seizures only occurred in patients with acoustic neuroma who underwent a transtentorial approach, and by the fact that burrhole biopsy carries a lower risk of seizures than craniotomy (Foy *et al.* 1981*a*).

The incidence of seizures commencing *de novo* following meningioma surgery is of the order of 20 per cent (North *et al.* 1983). The incidence is higher for parasagittal lesions than for convexity or basal tumours. Some 44 per cent of patients who have preoperative seizures do not have any further seizures postoperatively. The incidence of seizures following frontal surgery for pituitary adenomas and craniopharyngiomas may be as high as 15 per cent (Cast and Wilson 1981; Smith *et al.* 1991). Surgery for supratentorial abscess carries a very high risk. With sufficiently long follow-up, virtually all patients develop epilepsy (Legg *et al.* 1973). Ventricular shunting procedures can be associated with a 24 per cent risk of seizures (Copeland *et al.* 1982) and multiple shunt revisions and shunt infections significantly increase the risks.

Thirty-seven per cent of all patients who experience postoperative seizures do so within the first week, and 40 per cent of this group continue to have later seizures. By the time 1 year has elapsed, 77 per cent of those who will develop seizure disorders will have done so, and by 2 years, 92 per cent will have had their first seizure (Foy *et al.* 1981*b*). Those with the highest continuing risk after 2 years are patients with supratentorial abscess. In patients with early seizures, the risk of developing further seizures is high. Only 5 per cent of patients developing seizures later than 1 week postoperatively have a single seizure (Foy *et al.* 1981*b*).

The possible effects of prophylaxis in high-risk patients has been studied by a number of authors (Smith *et al.* 1991). There is no evidence that phenytoin or carbamazepine significantly reduce the incidence of post-craniotomy seizures in high-risk groups of patients, nor do they seem to effect the likelihood of persistence of the seizure disorder over a period of time. This use of prophylactic antiepileptic drugs can be associated with a high incidence of adverse effects, particularly drug-induced rash (Chadwick *et al.* 1984). For this reason prophylactic treatment does not seem to be justified.

23.8.3 **Intracranial tumours**

The relationship between intracranial tumours and epilepsy is well recognized and results in a considerable pressure to image all patients presenting with epilepsy. In fact, brain tumours are responsible for late-onset epilepsy in only about 10 per cent of cases from many series. The incidence of tumours rises steeply where seizures are clearly focal in nature (Raynor *et al.* 1959; Sumi and Teasdall 1963). Tumours of the frontal, parietal, and occipital lobes seem to carry the highest risk of epilepsy (Penfield and Jasper 1954; Mauguiere and Courjon 1978). The incidence of tumours causing complex partial seizures is lower (about 15 per cent) (Currie *et al.* 1971). Gastaut found that

16 per cent of 1702 epileptic patients with epilepsy beginning over the age of 20 had tumours on CT scanning (Gastaut 1976).

These early studies can, of course, be criticized as showing a falsely low frequency of tumour epilepsies, having been undertaken in the era before modern neurological imaging. In less selected populations of patients, the incidence of tumours found on CT scanning is even lower. They were found in 6 per cent of patients registered with the National General Practitioner Survey of Epilepsy (Sander *et al.* 1990*a*) and only 3 per cent of patients investigated following a first seizure (Hopkins *et al.* 1988). The combination of focal seizures, focal slowing on the EEG, and focal neurological signs predicts the presence of a tumour on CT scanning in a high proportion of cases (Young *et al.* 1982).

In general, about 40 per cent of those with seizures due to tumour have seizures as the first symptom (Penfield and Jasper 1954). In the past, the interval between the first seizure, the diagnosis of the tumour, and the development of further neurological problems has often been prolonged (Douglas 1971; Smith *et al.* 1991). This reflects the fact that the majority of tumours that present only with epilepsy tend to be benign. Thus, oligodendrogiomas are complicated by epilepsy in 80–90 per cent of cases, meningioma in 40–60 per cent of cases, and astrocytoma in 60–70 per cent of cases, compared to 60 per cent of malignant glioma or glioblastoma (Lund 1952; Penfield and Jasper 1954; Moots *et al.* 1995). Indeed, presentation with the first symptom of epilepsy is one of the most powerful prognostic factors indicating a good prognosis (Smith *et al.* 1991). Such intracerebral tumours are most commonly shown to be low density, non-enhancing lesions on initial CT scans and to be relatively low-grade astrocytomas or oligodendrogliomas. The incidence of seizures with cerebral metastases is lower, probably about 20 per cent at the time of presentation (Cohen *et al.* 1988)

The prognosis for tumour epilepsies is poor. Only 11 of 164 patients achieved a 1-year remission of epilepsy with antiepileptic drug treatment (Smith *et al.* 1991) and 50 per cent of patients with tumour epilepsies in adult life die within 4 years. However, 20–30 per cent show prolonged survival.

There is considerable dilemma about the management of intracerebral tumours. Meningiomas and other well-defined intracerebral lesions should be treated surgically where this is practical and where the patient is not old or infirm. Seizures will be suppressed in about 40 per cent of patients with meningiomas (Foy *et al.* 1981*a*) and up to 80 per cent of other patients undergoing lesionectomy (Cascino *et al.* 1990). In contrast, many neurologists find it difficult to recommend aggressive treatment with biopsy or tumour debulking and radiotherapy in a patient with a low-grade infiltrative tumour whose only symptom is epilepsy and in whom there is a good prospect of good-quality survival for many years. In this case tumours are rarely fully resectable and the risk–benefit for early surgical treatment remains uncertain.

Cerebral tumours are another area in which prophylactic treatment with antiepileptic drugs has been advocated, even before the first seizure. Two randomized controlled trials have, to date, failed to show any benefit in preventing the first seizure (Weaver *et al.* 1995; Glantz *et al.* 1996). Given that antiepileptic drugs have a considerable propensity to interact with chemotherapeutic agents and steroids, and that tumour-related epilepsies tend to be drug resistant, there seems to be no justification for this approach.

23.8.4 Cerebrovascular disease

Cerebrovascular disease and stroke become an increasingly common cause of epilepsy in the later years of life (Loiseau *et al.* 1990; Sander *et al.* 1990a). It has been estimated that cerebrovascular disease may account for 15 per cent of new cases of epilepsy (Sander *et al.* 1990a) and more than 50 per cent of new cases in the elderly. A community-based study of stroke showed a 5-year actuarial risk of seizures of 11.5 per cent, over 30 times that expected. The risk was highest for subarachnoid haemorrhage (30 per cent) and primary intracerebral haematoma (25 per cent), while the risk in ischaemic stroke (9 per cent) was restricted to survivors of large anterior circulation stokes. Seizures within 24 h of stroke onset were a risk factor for late seizures, which occurred in 35 per cent of such patients (Burn *et al.* 1997). Other studies have emphasized that embolic or haemorrhagic strokes carry the highest risk (Lesser *et al.* 1985). However, asymptomatic carotid occlusion (Cocito *et al.* 1982) and asymptomatic cerebral infarction (Shorvon *et al.* 1984) may be found in patients presenting with epilepsy in later life and seizures may also precede a stroke (Shinton *et al.* 1987; Burn *et al.* 1997).

Venous sinus thrombosis (Section 27.11) is increasingly recognized as an important type of stroke in younger people. Seizures commonly complicate the acute illness, but the long-term prognosis appears good, with few survivors developing epilepsy. In a series of 77 patients, 28 had acute symptomatic seizures, but only four had late seizures and epilepsy, all of whom had acute seizures (Preter *et al.* 1996).

Arteritic disorders can be accompanied by seizures as part of stroke-like syndromes or acute encephalopathies. Anywhere between 17 and 50 per cent of patients with systemic lupus erythematosis and CNS involvement have seizures (Bennett *et al.* 1972). Seizures may also complicate, to a lesser degree, involvement in polyarteritis nodosa, Behçet's disease, and mixed connective tissue disease (Shannon and Goetz 1989). Seizures can occur in hypertensive encephalopathy and in subacute bacterial endocarditis.

A rare cerebrovascular cause of seizures is the hyper-reperfusion syndrome occurring after carotid endarterectomy, where seizures can occur during the first postoperative day. It is doubtful that this has a significant risk for late epilepsy (Nielsen *et al.* 1995).

23.8.5 CNS infections and infestations

A wide range of viral, bacterial, opportunistic, and parasitic infestations can be associated with seizures. Infections accounted for 3 per cent of seizure disorders in the epidemiological study in Rochester, Minnesota (Hauser and Kurland 1975). Annegers *et al.* (1988) examined the risks of unprovoked seizures following common CNS infections in 714 survivors of encephalitis and meningitis. Overall, the 20-year risk of developing unprovoked seizures was 6.8 per cent, almost seven times the expected rate. Increased incidence of seizures was highest during the 5 years after a CNS infection, but continued to be elevated for as long as 15 years. The risk was highest (22 per cent) for patients with a viral encephalitis associated with acute symptomatic seizures, and 10 per cent for patients with viral encephalitis without early seizures. For bacterial meningitis associated with early seizures, the risk was 13 per cent, but only 2.4 per cent for patients with bacterial meningitis without early seizures. The risk of seizures for aseptic meningitis was not increased over that of the general population.

Seizures commonly occur during acute viral encephalitis (Section 34.3.1), and they may be most common with herpes simplex encephalitis (Section 34.6.1) when the seizures are frequently focal in nature. Prenatal infection with cytomegalovirus, rubella, and herpes can produce retardation associated with late epilepsy (Forsgren *et al.* 1990). Seizures can also occur with subacute measles encephalitis (Chadwick *et al.* 1982) and subacute rubella encephalitis, as well as with 'slow virus infections' including subacute sclerosing panencephalitis and Creutzfeldt–Jakob disease, but in both these conditions myoclonus tends to dominate the picture. More recently it has been recognized that infection with HIV can be associated with seizures, not only because of an increased risk of opportunistic infections, but also because the direct neurotropic effects of the virus (Wong *et al.* 1990) (Section 34.11.2). In 100 patients who were HIV positive and had seizures, 45 had evidence of opportunistic infection or CNS lymphoma, 24 evidence of the AIDS-dementia complex, but 23 had no identifiable cause (Holtzman *et al.* 1989).

Bacterial infections causing meningitis are occasionally associated with seizures, particularly if complicated by cortical vein or sinus thrombosis or cerebral abscess (see above). Chronic meningitis due to tuberculosis may present with seizures, and in the Indian subcontinent tuberculomas may be a common cause of epilepsy associated with disappearing, ring-enhancing CT lesions (Goulatia *et al.* 1987) (Section 34.15.1). Other causes of chronic meningitis are not infrequently associated with seizures, e.g. *Cryptococcus* sp., *Candida* sp. Perhaps the most common infestation associated with seizures is cysticercosis (Section 34.15.10), which may account for 50 per cent of incident cases in adults in developing countries (Medina *et al.* 1990). Others include schistosomiasis, hydatidosis, malaria, and toxoplasmosis (Bittencourt *et al.* 1988).

23.8.6 Disorders of cortical development

The introduction of modern high-resolution MR scanning has shown that these are important and common causes of epilepsy (Section 4.6). A series from Norway found that 13 of

Table 23.7. Classification of cortical dysplasias

Diffuse cortical dysplasias	Focal cortical dysplasias
Lissencephaly	Isolated focal cortical dysplasia
Polymicrogyria	Schizencephaly
Pachygyria	Microdysplasia
Hemimegalencephaly	Heterotopia
Tuberous sclerosis	
Band heterotopia/XLIS	
Periventricular nodular dysplasia	

XLIS, X-linked lissencephaly.

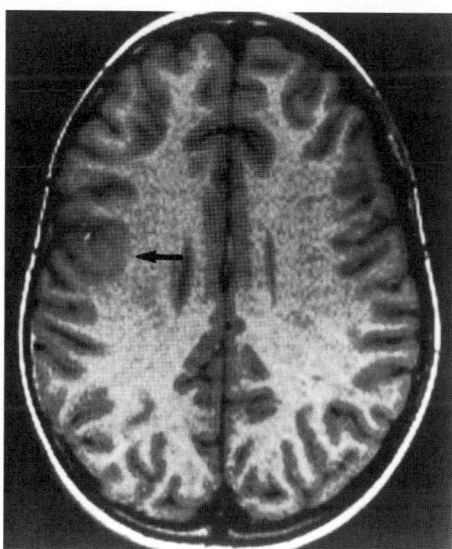

Fig. 23.10. Focal cortical dysplasia shown in axial MRI (reproduced from Kuzniecky and Jackson (1997), with permission).

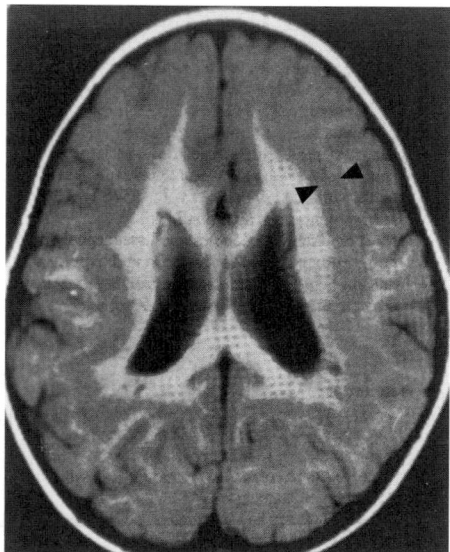

Fig. 23.11. Subcortical-band heterotopia on MRI T1-weighted images (reproduced from Kuzniecky and Jackson (1997), with permission).

303 patients had such developmental anomalies (Brodtkorb *et al.* 1992), while 16 of 222 patients with temporal lobe epilepsy had developmental abnormalities in another series (Lehericy *et al.* 1995). Cortical dysplasias may be generalized, when they are usually associated with developmental delay and a static encephalopathy from birth, as well as a severe epilepsy, or they may be focal, when seizures may be the only symptom. Focal dysplasias may account for 15–20 per cent of the adult population with intractable epilepsy (Kuzniecky and Jackson 1995). A classification of the cortical dysplasias is presented in Table 23.7. Of 100 patients with dysplasia, 39 had abnormalities of gyration, 28 had heterotopias, 5 had tuberous sclerosis, 7 had focal cortical dysplasias, and 21 had dysembrioplastic neuroepithelial tumours (DNET) (Raymond *et al.* 1995). Many cortical dysplasias have a genetic basis and some form a part of other well-recognized symptom complexes, such as the neuro-cutaneous syndromes (for example, tuberous sclerosis). They may also be environmental and related to congenital causes, infection, toxins, and radiation.

Focal cortical dysplasia is usually extratemporal, with MR findings of abnormal gyral thickening often associated with abnormalities of the underlying white matter (Fig. 23.10) (Section 4.6.9). On occasions, the abnormality may be 'trans-mantle', extending from the ventricle to the cortical surface. The heterotopias are, by definition, normal cells present in an abnormal location. *Subcortical-band heterotopia* is seen in women, and consists of MR changes with a circumferential band of subcortical grey matter (Palmini *et al.* 1991) (Fig. 23.11). Patients usually have evidence of developmental delay and, in some cases, pyramidal signs (Palmini *et al.* 1991). There is evidence that the condition forms part of an X-linked lissencephaly, in which the males exhibit classical lissencephaly and heterozygous females have subcortical-band heterotopia (Dobyns *et al.* 1996). *Periventricular or subependymal nodular heterotopias* are probably the most common developmental disorders seen in patients with epilepsy (Barkovich and Kjos 1992). MR appearances are of multiple, smooth nodules of grey matter lining the lateral ventricles, which may be associated with other focal subcortical heterotopias (Fig. 23.12). On rare occasions, focal subcortical heterotopia can be seen in the absence of subependymal heterotopia. Most patients have relatively normal development, but perhaps 80 per cent of patients with the disorder have epilepsy.

Polymicrogyria refers to the presence of an area with many abnormally small gyri (Section 4.6.8). When diffuse, it can be associated with severe developmental delay; when localized, epilepsy may be the only symptom. *Schizencephaly* describes the presence of grey-matter-lined clefts that extend from the cortical surface to the ependymal lining (Section 4.6.5). The condition can be unilateral or bilateral. Developmental delay and contralateral hemiparesis are common.

The importance of the recognition and accurate diagnosis of cortical dysplasia lies in the potential for surgical treatment in some patients. Cortical dysplasias of the temporal lobe seem to have by far the best outcome, with up to 50 per cent being seizure-free (Kuzniecky and Jackson 1997). Unfortunately, the

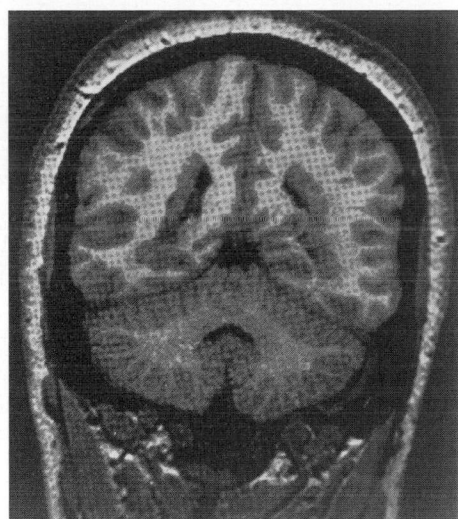

Fig. 23.12. Periventricular nodular heterotopia on MRI T1-weighted images (reproduced from Kuzniecky and Jackson (1997), with permission).

majority of cortical dysplasias are extratemporal, and here lower seizure-free rates are seen when localized resection of focal dysplasias is attempted.

Dysembrioplastic neuroepithelial tumours (DNETs) have only recently been recognized (Daumas-Duport *et al.* 1988). Undoubtedly, many patients diagnosed as having low-grade temporal gliomas or hamatomas in old series probably have this condition. The lesions are usually seen within areas of dysplastic cortex and seem to have a predilection for the temporal lobes, although they may also occur in the frontal lobes. They may make up between 5 and 10 per cent of the pathology found in temporal lobectomy series (Wolf *et al.* 1993).

23.8.7 Other causes of symptomatic seizures and epilepsy

Neurodegenerative disorders can be associated with epilepsy. In Alzheimer's disease, seizures occur usually late in the illness in up to 15 per cent of patients (Romanelli *et al.* 1990). Hauser *et al.* (1986) calculated a relative risk of 10 for autopsy-proven causes of Alzheimer's disease (Section 26.6.2). Myoclonus is also evident, particularly in patients with familial Alzheimer's disease (Jacob 1970) and with Alzheimer's change complicating Down syndrome. In contrast, seizures appear to be rare in Pick's disease.

Several authors have noted an increased incidence of seizures in association with multiple sclerosis, the usual figure being quoted as around 5 per cent of cases (Muller 1949). It may be that seizures are particularly likely to occur as an acute symptomatic phenomenon related to plaque formation (Kinnunen and Wikstrom 1986). More chronic epilepsy can be seen in severely disabled patients with frontal lobe syndromes and numerous frontal subcortical plaques (Moreau *et al.* 1998).

23.9 The diagnosis of epilepsy

The diagnosis of epilepsy in the adult is essentially clinical, and based on a detailed description of events experienced by the patient before, during, and after a seizure, and, more importantly, on an eyewitness account. In view of the social and economic implications, diagnostic errors must be avoided at all costs. Thus, the first rule about diagnosing epilepsy is never to make the diagnosis without incontrovertible clinical evidence. If there is any doubt, the clinician should resist the temptation to attach a label and should rely on the passage of time and the further description of symptomatic events, in order to reach a firm conclusion. Few people with epilepsy will come to harm from a delay in diagnosis, whereas a false-positive diagnosis is always gravely damaging.

However, it is not enough simply to decide that a patient's attacks are epileptic in nature. Other considerations must be addressed in the diagnostic process:

◆ Are the attacks acute symptomatic seizures, requiring treatment of the underlying condition only, or are they part of an epilepsy?

◆ If the seizures are thought to be part of an epilepsy, an adequate classification of seizures and of the epilepsy syndrome must be attempted, because of the important prognostic, therapeutic, and aetiological implications.

◆ Wherever possible, a cause should be identified, because this might require treatment in its own right, and so that the patient can be informed fully about his or her condition.

While the differentiation of seizures from other episodic events is made on clinical grounds, investigations have particular importance in answering the subsequent diagnostic questions.

23.9.1 The electroencephalogram

The EEG may rarely provide information that adds weight to the clinical diagnosis but, more importantly, it aids the classification of epilepsy (Section 2.3). Routine interictal EEG recording is one of the most abused investigations in clinical medicine and is unquestionably responsible for great human suffering. The diagnostic value of an interictal EEG is widely misunderstood (Binnie 1997). EEGs are often requested either to exclude or to prove a diagnosis of epilepsy—something that can seldom, if ever, be done. Erroneous interpretation of the EEG is probably the most common reason for non-epileptic events being diagnosed as seizures. Misinterpretation of non-epileptiform sharp transients, such as 6 and 14 per second positive spikes and benign epileptiform transients of sleep, and responses to hyperventilation and photic stimulation cause particular problems.

Ajmone Marsan and Zivin (1970) showed that in a population of patients with definite epilepsy from a tertiary referral centre, 30 per cent exhibited epileptiform activity in every routine interictal record, while 11 per cent never did. Binnie (1997) obtained similar results in newly diagnosed patients. He emphasized that sleep recording may increase sensitivity, by showing, in an audit of 3000 patients with epilepsy, that epileptiform abnormalities occurred in 63 per cent of 51 per cent of subjects without discharges in an initial awake record. When it is recognized that simple partial and brief complex partial seizures can occur without detectable changes at scalp electrodes in ictal records, the sensitivity of interictal EEG recording will always be poor. It must be remembered that the figures quoted apply to populations with clinically definite epilepsy, and considerably overestimate the value of the EEG in populations for whom there is diagnostic uncertainty. King *et al.* (1998) found interictal epileptiform features in 39 per cent of adults with a first presentation of seizures or epilepsy, many of whom had recordings within 24 hours of a first seizure. This rate was increased by subsequent sleep-deprived recording.

The specificity of the interictal EEG is best demonstrated by series that screened military personnel (Robin *et al.* 1978; Gregory *et al.* 1993). In a total of 21 000 individuals, epileptiform abnormalities were found in only 2.4 per 1000.

The interictal EEG is potentially important in two clinical settings. In patients with seizures occurring without an aura that are characterized by a brief period of absence with or without automatism, it may be difficult to differentiate absence seizures from complex partial seizures. The finding of generalized spike wave or focal spike activity, respectively, will clarify the diagnosis. The differentiation has important implications for treatment and prognosis. In patients with tonic–clonic seizures without an aura, especially when these occur during sleep, the EEG can again differentiate between generalized epilepsies (characterized by generalized spike waves) and seizures with a focal onset (in which there may be localized abnormalities).

Ictal EEG, using ambulatory or, more satisfactorily, videotelemetry techniques, is important in distinguishing epileptic seizures from pseudoseizures. Even here, movement and other artefacts may complicate interpretation. Identifying tonic–clonic seizures should, however, present no problems because of the post-ictal changes. Differentiating between non-convulsive pseudoseizures and complex partial seizures, particularly those of frontal origin, can still be difficult.

23.9.2 Neurological imaging in the diagnosis of epilepsy

Over the past decade the role of neurological imaging in the diagnosis and management of epilepsy has changed considerably. On the one hand, CT scanning is universally available; on the other, MR scanning has become enormously sophisticated and capable of demonstrating many abnormalities not previously recognized by CT. The debate is no longer about which patients with epilepsy need CT scanning, but rather, in which patients is imaging unnecessary and should CT be abandoned in favour of MRI?

The frequency of abnormalities in CT scans of patients with epilepsy varies greatly. In surveys of patients with established epilepsy from tertiary centres, 60–80 per cent may have abnormal CT scans, but most of these abnormalities are atrophic in

nature (Gastaut 1976). Tumours may be identified in approximately 10 per cent of patients (see above). In patients who present with either a first seizure or early epilepsy, the frequency is lower—abnormalities are detected in less than 20 per cent of cases—but again atrophic abnormalities predominate. CT scan abnormalities are very strongly predicted by the presence of focal rather than generalized seizures, focal neurological signs, and focal EEG abnormalities (Young *et al.* 1982). Where all three are present, CT abnormalities may be found in up to 70 or 80 per cent of cases.

Magnetic resonance imaging is more sensitive for most cerebral pathologies that are associated with chronic epilepsy, with the exception of calcification, which is not well demonstrated by this modality. Mesial temporal sclerosis, low-grade neoplasia, vascular lesions (particularly cavernomas), and developmental abnormalities are all likely to be missed on CT, but readily demonstrated by MRI (Franceschi *et al.* 1989; Kilpatrick *et al.* 1991). In the elderly, however, MRI shows a high incidence of lesions, the clinical relevance of which may be difficult to determine. In a series of 300 children and adults presenting with seizures for the first time, MRI identified epileptogenic lesions in 17 per cent of 154 patients with definite partial epilepsy and 18 per cent with unclassified epilepsy, but was normal in all patients with clinical and EEG evidence of a generalized epilepsy syndrome (King *et al.* 1998). MRI scanning was more sensitive than CT in the early detection of causative lesions. Indeed, CT detected only half the 17 tumours found, but how many of these would have been optimally treated by surgery at diagnosis was uncertain.

At present a reasonable approach is to undertake CT scanning at the point of diagnosis in all adults except those who can be identified clinically and neurophysiologically as having one of the syndromes of idiopathic generalized epilepsy. This should identify all of the more aggressive tumours causing epilepsy, but could miss some of the most indolent of gliomas. MRI scanning should be undertaken in all patients with epilepsy who appear to be refractory to pharmacological treatment. Here investigation should be tailored to the individual, but will usually include high-definition T1 thin-slice scans, often with hippocampal volumetry (Cook *et al.* 1992), T2-weighted, and FLAIR images.

Other technologies that produce 'functional' images, such as positron emission tomography (PET), single-photon emission computed tomography (SPECT), and functional MR imaging and spectroscopy, are largely experimental and to date have usually been used in the assessment of patients for surgical treatment of their epilepsy.

23.10 Pharmacological treatment of epilepsy

23.10.1 General principles

At a time when there is a sudden and dramatic increase in the number and choice of drugs to treat epilepsy, it is perhaps important to begin by considering some broad principles that need to be applied to the treatment of an individual patient.

1. The diagnosis of seizures or epilepsy should be secure. There is no place for a therapeutic trial when the diagnosis is uncertain. Acute symptomatic seizures must be differentiated from seizures occurring spontaneously as a part of epilepsy. The former will rarely need anything other than acute treatment of seizures together with a treatment of the underlying cause (e.g. alcohol withdrawal, acute metabolic disorders).

2. An initiation or change in antiepileptic drug therapy needs a full and adequate discussion with the patient. He or she needs to be fully aware of the aims of treatment, the benefits, and potential adverse effects. Many of the decisions to be made in treatment of epilepsy are not of a black-and-white nature, but are varying shades of grey. The individual's personal circumstances and views therefore become important in ensuring compliance with regimes. In many circumstances the doctor should be a provider of relevant information rather than a decision-taker. Compliance is a major issue in the long-term management of epilepsy and poor compliance does not identify the 'bad' patient, it identifies a poor doctor–patient relationship and an inadequately informed patient.

3. The ultimate aim of treatment of epilepsy will be no seizures and no drugs. Unfortunately, this may not be readily achievable for many patients with epilepsy who have a chronic disorder. The first step in treating epilepsy will always be to choose the minimum effective dose of an appropriate antiepileptic drug. In practice, this means initiating treatment, usually at a low dose of an antiepileptic drug, and slowly increasing this dose if and when further seizures occur. This approach, using a single antiepileptic drug (monotherapy), will usually be successful in 50–80 per cent of new patients presenting with epilepsy. Alternative monotherapies, or combined treatments (polytherapy) will only be necessary in the minority with more severe epilepsies. In this group of patients a law of diminishing returns will apply. Briefly stated, the longer that seizures remain poorly controlled, the less the likelihood of remission of epilepsy. This has two consequences. The first is that some agreement will often need to be reached with the patient, as to an acceptable compromise between a reduced seizure frequency and the severity of unwanted side-effects of antiepileptic drugs. The second is that non-pharmacological treatments may demand serious consideration at a relatively early stage (see below).

4. In choosing between different drugs, a number of issues will demand careful consideration. These include judgements about the efficacy of the drug for an individual patient and its tolerability and safety. Both these factors will contribute to the overall effectiveness of an antiepileptic drug. In the current age of 'evidence-based medicine' it is implicit that comparative judgements of efficacy, tolerability, and effectiveness are best based on the results of appropriate randomized clinical trials (Marson et al. 1996). In addition to these fundamental principles, it is helpful if antiepileptic drugs are simple for patients to use, needing no more than twice-daily dosing and not requiring troublesome antiepileptic blood level monitoring.

There is now very good evidence from many studies (see below) that the chief factor determining relative effectiveness is likely to be the spectrum of adverse effects of antiepileptic drugs. Thus, it has proved difficult to detect significant differences in efficacy outcomes in comparative monotherapy studies, but differences are often apparent in the proportion of patients who withdraw from studies because of adverse effects (Mattson et al. 1985; Brodie et al. 1995). Antiepileptic drugs possess dose-related, largely CNS, adverse effects as well as idiosyncratic side-effects. In addition, because of the long periods of time for which they may be taken, these drugs have also been associated with chronic toxicity, as well as teratogenicity (as they may be taken through the childbearing years). All these issues need to be taken into account in choosing drug treatment (see below).

23.10.2 Starting therapy

In the past, antiepileptic treatment has been advocated before seizures occur. Such prophylactic treatment has been recommended for patients with a high prospective risk of epilepsy after head injury and craniotomy for various neurosurgical conditions. Because no clear evidence exists that antiepileptic treatment is effective in preventing late epilepsy (see above), it seems better to delay treatment until seizures have occurred, rather than to adopt a policy of treatment of all those at risk— particularly as there may be a high incidence of side-effects with prophylactic treatment (Chadwick et al. 1984) and poor compliance (McQueen et al. 1983) .

When two or more unprovoked seizures have occurred within a short interval, antiepileptic therapy is usually indicated. However, problems do arise in defining a short interval. Most would include periods of 6 months to 1 year within the definition. Even where seizures occur close together, the identification of specific precipitating factors may make it more important to counsel patients than to commence drug therapy. The most common examples are photically induced and alcohol-withdrawal seizures in adults.

23.10.3 The choice of drug

There is agreement that patients with newly diagnosed epilepsy should be treated with a single drug. The key issue in the choice of a first drug at diagnosis is an accurate and adequate diagnosis of seizure type and, if possible, epilepsy syndrome. By no means all drugs are effective against all seizure types. The spectrum of efficacy of drugs is represented graphically in Fig. 23.13. It is particularly important to avoid the use of drugs that may exacerbate seizures. Hence, there is evidence that carbamazepine and vigabatrin (Perucca et al. 1998) may both exacerbate absence and myoclonic seizures in the generalized epilepsy syndromes. It is perhaps here that syndromic classification of epilepsy becomes most important, as a drug should be chosen that would be effective against all seizure types known to occur in that syndrome, rather than only those that have occurred in an individual patient to date.

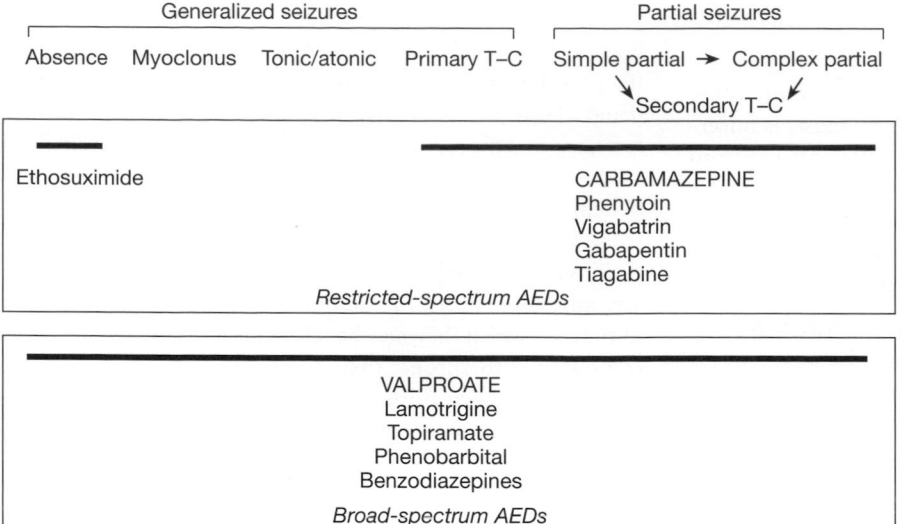

Fig. 23.13. Spectrum of activity of antiepileptic drugs (AEDs) by seizure type. Drugs in upper case are current first-choice agents. secondary T–C: secondary tonic–clonic.

The improvements in the clinical classification of both seizures and epilepsy syndromes in the past 20 years has also occurred at a time when we have developed a clearer understanding of the mechanism of action of antiepileptic drugs. It is now becoming possible to associate particular antiepileptic mechanisms with effects against different seizure types and different adverse effects. Inevitably, many antiepileptic drugs (AEDs), particularly valproate, lamotrigine, and topiramate, may have multiple mechanisms of action, some of which are not fully understood. Table 23.8 summarizes different mechanisms of action for antiepileptic drugs. Several drugs modify ionic sodium conductance across membranes, binding to ion channels in order to maintain them in an inactivated state, thereby blocking repetitive neuronal firing. Drugs that possess this property include phenytoin, carbamazepine, lamotrigine, topiramate, and valproate (White 1997). All are effective in preventing partial seizures and both generalized and second-

arily generalized tonic–clonic seizures. Most of these drugs (with the exception of valproate) can be associated with dose-related neurotoxicity syndromes that include ataxia, nystagmus, and diplopia. The second direct membrane effect is displayed by drugs such as ethosuximide and possibly valproate, which modify slow or calcium T currents in the thalamus. This mechanism seems particularly effective against spike wave mechanisms and absence seizures. These same calcium conductances can be enhanced by GABAergic inputs to the thalamus via $GABA_B$ receptors (Crunelli and Leresche 1991), which may explain the exacerbation of absences by vigabatrin.

A number of antiepileptic drugs exert their properties through modulation of the $GABA_A$ receptor/chloride ionophore. Thus, both benzodiazepines and barbiturates bind close to this site to increase chloride-ion conductance and maintain membrane hyperpolarization. Newer drugs, such as vigabatrin

Table 23.8. Mechanism of action of antiepileptic drugs

	Na+ channels	Ca2+ channels	GABA receptor	GABA turnover	GABA T'ase	GABA uptake	NMDA receptor	AMPA receptor
Older drugs								
Carbamazepine	++							
Valproate	+	+ (T)		+				
Phenytoin	++							
Barbiturates	+		+					
Ethosuximide		+ (T)						
Benzodiazepines			+					
Newer drugs								
Vigabatrin					+			
Lamotrigine	++	? (T)						
Gabapentin		+		+				
Felbamate							+	
Topiramate	++		+					+
Tiagabine						+		
Oxcarbazepine	++							
Zonisamide	+	+ (T)	+					

Table 23.9. Efficacy and toxicity of antiepileptic drugs

Structure	Indications	Contraindications	Dosage in adults	Optimal plasma levels	Adverse effects			Teratogenicity
					Dose related	Idiosyncratic	Chronic	
Carbamazepine	Drug of Choice: Partial epilepsy	Idiopathic Generalized Epilepsy	600–1600 mg/day with gradual introduction because of autoinduction	4–10 µg/ml, but very variable upper limit to tolerability	Dizziness, diplopia & unsteadiness	Rash & acute hypersensitivity reactions Aplastic anaemia (1:200 000)	Few that are well documented (hyponatraemia & neutropenia)	Spina bifida in 1% of pregnancies
Clobazam	Second choice drug: Probable broad spectrum AED. Useful for treating clusters of seizures		20–60 mg/day Therapeutic and adverse effects may show tolerance		Drowsiness & sedation, but less than other benzodiazepines			
Ethosuximide	Second choice drug: Absence persisting into adult life	Partial epilepsy & generalized tonic–clonic seizures	0.5–2.0 G/day	40–100 µg/ml	Nausea, drowsiness & dizziness	Rash & acute hypersensitivity reactions. SLE-like syndromes		Little information
Felbamate	Occasional use: Lennox–Gastaut syndrome		1200–4800 mg/day		Insomnia & GI intolerance	Aplastic anaemia (1:3000–5000) Hepatic failure	Weight loss	
Gabapentin	Second choice drug: Partial epilepsies		900 mg – 4.8 G/day		Drowsiness & sedation	None known	Possible weight gain	
Lamotrigine	First choice drug: Broad spectrum for partial epilepsy & possibly generalized syndromes		100–800 mg/day		Diplopia, dizziness, & sedation	Rash & acute Hypersensitivity reactions (particularly with valproate comedication)		
Lorazepam	First choice drug: Status epilepticus	Drug of choice: Status epilepticus	0.1mg/kg					
Oxcarbazepine	Drug of Choice: Partial epilepsy – broadly epilepsy comparable with carbamazepine	Idiopathic generalized	600–3000 mg/day	50–150 µmol/L	Dizziness, diplopia, & unsteadiness,	Rash, but less frequent than carbamazepine; 25% of patients sensitive to CBZ will also be sensitive to OXP	Hyponatraemia	

Table 23.9. *(continued)*

Structure	Indications	Contraindications	Dosage in adults	Optimal plasma levels	Adverse effects			
					Dose related	Idiosyncratic	Chronic	Teratogenicity
Phenobarbitone	Occasional use in partial and generalized epilepsies (excepting absence) & status		60–200mg/day	15–35 µg/ml but limits often modified by tolerance	Drowsiness, sedation, & unsteadiness, adverse effects on cognition and behaviour	Rash	Tolerance & habituation. Dupuytrens contracture & connective tissue disorders	Hare-lip/cleft palate & cardiological abnormalities
Phenytoin	Second choice drug: Partial epilepsy and generalized tonic–clonic seizures		200–600 mg/day	10–20 µg/ml. Monitoring is indicated whenever there is poor control of seizures or side effects	Drowsiness, ataxia, & dysarthria. Rarely abnormal movements	Rash & acute hypersensitivity reactions	Gum hypertrophy, coarsening of facial features, hirsutism & acne. SLE-like syndromes	Hare-lip/cleft palate & cardiological abnormalities
Primidone	Rarely used: probable efficacy as phenobarbital		500–1500 mg/day	As phenobarbital to which it is metabolized	Drowsiness, sedation & unsteadiness, adverse effects on cognition and behaviour	Rash	Tolerance & habituation. Dupuytrens contracture & connective tissue disorders	Hare-lip/cleft palate & cardiological abnormalities
Tiagabine	Second choice drug: Partial epilepsy	Idiopathic generalized epilepsy	15–60 mg/day		Dizziness, depression, tremor. May be exacerbation of partial seizures at higher doses.			
Topiramate	Second choice: Broad spectrum AED		100–800 mg/day		Sedation, cognitive difficulty		Renal calculi	
Valproate (Sodium)	First choice broad spectrum drug: may be less effective in partial epilepsy than carbamazepine		1–3 G/day	Of no value	Tremor, irritability, & occasional confusion	Gastric intolerance. Hepatotoxicity (rare in adults). Pancreatitis	Weight gain, alopecia, insulin resistance, polycystic ovarian syndrome	Spina bifida in 2–3% of pregnancies. Fetal valproate syndrome
Vigabatrin	Final choice drug for partial epilepsies. May be useful in adult survivors of West's syndrome	Idiopathic generalized epilepsy	1.5–6.0 G/day	Of no value	Depression	Psychosis	Weight gain, and visual field constriction.	

AED, antiepileptic drug; CBZ, carbamazepine; GI, gastrointestinal; OXP, oxcarbazepine; SLE, systemic lupus erythematosus.

and tiagabine may have more direct effects in prolonging the synaptic action of GABA. To date evidence suggests that these drugs are effective against partial and secondarily generalized seizures but may exacerbate spike wave epilepsies. They are less likely to cause sedation and ataxia but may have a higher risk of psychiatric disorder, including depression (Marson *et al.* 1997). Drugs that interfere with excitatory neurotransmission via glutamate and aspartate receptors may yet prove to be valuable antiepileptic drugs. Some of the antiepileptic properties of felbamate may be due to its ability to interfere with the action of glycine in facilitating glutaminergic activity, and a number of drugs with potential glutaminergic activity have entered clinical trial programmes, with varying success.

Actions, common side-effects and indications for use are summarized briefly in Table 23.9, a detailed discussion being beyond the scope of this chapter. Further details of the pharmacokinetics of these drugs are also presented later in this chapter.

Partial (localization-related) epilepsies

Currently, a large number of drugs can be considered for treating patients with cryptogenic and symptomatic partial epilepsies. These include both older and newer drugs, including those with a spectrum of efficacy limited to the partial epilepsies and those with a broader spectrum of effects (see Fig. 23.13). An increasing number of studies are available, which have compared individual drugs in monotherapy regimes. There is a consensus that carbamazepine is, to date, the drug of first choice in these epilepsies. None of the larger monotherapy studies has demonstrated a drug with greater efficacy (Mattson *et al.* 1985; Richens *et al.* 1994), and Mattson *et al.* (1992) showed some advantages over valproate in some measures of efficacy. Mattson *et al.* (1985) showed that both phenytoin and carbamazepine were better tolerated than barbiturate antiepileptic drugs (phenobarbital and primidone). Brodie *et al.* (1995), comparing the first of the newer antiepileptic drugs to be studied in a monotherapy design, showed that lamotrigine was better tolerated than carbamazepine.

Phenytoin is no longer considered a first-line AED in partial epilepsy in the UK, because of its complex pharmacokinetics, which demand blood-level monitoring; its untoward cosmetic chronic effects, its enzyme-inducing properties that result in a drug–drug interactions, and its teratogenicity. However, US clinicians take a different view.

The place of new AEDs is largely limited to add-on therapy of the partial epilepsies in the absence of adequate randomized controlled trials that compare their effects directly to those of carbamazepine (Chadwick 1998).

The generalized epilepsies

The management and treatment of the cryptogenic and symptomatic generalized epilepsies is more relevant to childhood epilepsy and will not be discussed further here. However, the choice of drug therapy in the idiopathic generalized epilepsies is a major issue, as collectively these may represent between 20 and 30 per cent of all human epilepsy. There is a general consensus that valproate is the most effective in the treatment of these epilepsies, possessing a broad spectrum of activity that includes all the seizure types occurring in these syndromes. The place of newer antiepileptic drugs in these syndromes has yet to be defined. There is evidence from open studies that lamotrigine is effective (Richens 1997). As valproate use may be limited by an increased incidence of weight gain and polycystic ovarian syndrome (Isojarvi *et al.* 1993, 1996), as well as concerns about potential teratogenicity (see below), there is an urgent need for comparative monotherapy studies of valproate versus lamotrigine.

Unclassified epilepsy

Decisions about starting antiepileptic drug treatment often have to be made in the face of some uncertainty concerning a syndromic classification. While the clinician may be certain that seizures have occurred, there may be insufficient information available from a few poorly witnessed events to provide a definite syndrome diagnosis. Common situations in which this occurs are the patient with witnessed tonic–clonic seizures during sleep, and infrequent daytime trance-like episodes (absence or complex partial seizures). Where this uncertainty exists, it is relatively unusual for the EEG or other investigations to provide definitive information. In these circumstances, a broad-spectrum AED, such as valproate or lamotrigine, would be preferred.

When prescribing AEDs, it is important that patients are counselled about the possible adverse effects and their significance.

Acute dose-related toxicity

Most AEDs, including phenytoin, carbamazepine, lamotrigine, barbiturates, and benzodiazepines, give rise to a non-specific encephalopathy associated with high blood concentrations. Patients exhibit sedation and nystagmus and, with increasing blood levels, ataxia, dysarthria, and ultimately confusion and drowsiness (Schmidt 1982). In some instances seizure frequency may increase with high blood levels, and occasionally involuntary movements are seen, particularly with phenytoin (Chadwick *et al.* 1976). Phenytoin is especially likely to result in dose-related toxicity because of its unusual pharmacokinetics (see below). Carbamazepine may cause similar symptoms if the dose is not built up slowly, because of its ability to autoinduce liver microsomal enzymes. Valproate does not appear to be associated with this typical syndrome of neurotoxicity, but some patients with high blood levels may exhibit restlessness and irritability, sometimes with a frank confusion state. Postural tremor is a common accompaniment (Turnbull *et al.* 1983).

All antiepileptic drugs can have adverse effects on cognitive function and behaviour with increasing dose and blood concentrations, although there is little evidence that these effects are common in patients using therapeutic doses as monotherapy (Meador *et al.* 1990). While carbamazepine and valproate may have smaller risks of this type than barbiturates and phenytoin, the newer generation of drugs may be even better tolerated (Chadwick 1998).

Drug interactions may increase the risk of dose-related toxicity. Thus valproate may greatly prolong the half-life of lamotrigine, making dosage reduction necessary during co-medication (Richens 1997).

Acute idiosyncratic toxicity

Most antiepileptic drugs, particularly phenytoin, carbamazepine, and lamotrigine, may cause a delayed hypersensitivity reaction, consisting of a maculopapular erythematous eruption which, in more severe cases, may be associated with fever, lymphadenopathy, and hepatitis. The incidence of the allergic skin reaction with phenytoin may be as high as 10 per cent, and with carbamazepine up to 15 per cent (Chadwick *et al.* 1984). Lamotrigine is also associated with similar problems in up to 5 per cent of new prescriptions (Marson *et al.* 1997). It may be possible to avoid such reactions with a cautious build-up of initial dosage. Marrow aplasia is a rare complication of carbamazepine, but is more common with felbamate (Kaufman *et al.* 1997). Reports of fatal cases of liver failure in association with valproate therapy largely concern children under the age of 2 years, who are often multiply handicapped and receiving many different antiepileptic drugs. It may be that they have an underlying error of metabolism that predisposes them to liver failure (Dreifuss *et al.* 1987). Vigabatrin has been associated with behaviour disorders, depression, and psychosis, particularly in patients with a previous psychiatric history (Sander *et al.* 1990b). The potential for rare idiosyncratic side-effects of topiramate and gabapentin is currently uncertain, but probably small.

Chronic toxicity

Antiepileptic drugs are unusual in that they may be administered to patients over a long period as treatment for chronic epilepsy. This may lead to the development of a wide variety of syndromes of chronic toxicity (summarized in Table 23.9). A number of factors seem to predispose to the development of these disorders, including the use of polypharmacy, the dosage used, and the length of therapy. While valproate and carbamazepine may have fewer chronic toxic effects than barbiturates and phenytoin, the length of time that elapsed before quite common chronic toxic effects were recognized with the older agents should warn us that continued vigilance is needed in the use of the newer antiepileptic drugs. It has emerged that some patients exposed to long-term treatment with vigabatrin have developed severe irreversible concentric visual-field loss (Eke *et al.* 1997), and that quantitative visual-field assessment can reveal asymptomatic, usually nasal, visual-field constriction, associated with electroretinographic changes in keeping with retinal cone system dysfunction (Krauss *et al.* 1998) in larger numbers of patients treated with vigabatrin. Further follow-up of 32 patients continuing monotherapy with vigabatrin and 19 patients continuing carbamazepine from the randomized controlled trial reported by Kalviainen *et al.* (1998) showed that 41 per cent of vigabatrin-treated patients had visual-field con-

striction, compared to no carbamazepine-treated patients, indicating a causal relationship between long-term vigabatrin exposure and visual-field loss.

Teratogenicity

All antiepileptic drugs must be regarded as potentially teratogenic, making adequate preconceptual counselling essential. The way in which this risk compares to that from seizures during pregnancy is uncertain, but the optimal policy seems to be to suppress seizures with the lowest effective dose of a single AED. Phenytoin and barbiturate antiepileptic drugs may increase the risk of major fetal malformation by two to three times, the most common malformations being hare-lip, cleft palate, and cardiovascular anomalies. The risks are higher with polytherapy than with monotherapy. There is an association between neural tube defects and exposure to valproate or carbamazepine (Lindhout and Schmidt 1986; Rosa 1990). There is little evidence to compare the relative risks of different AEDs to pregnancy, and the interpretation of that available is inevitably confounded by factors such as the type of epilepsy and its severity. A pooled analysis of 1221 exposed pregnancies found a relative risk for major congenital malformations of 4.9 for both valproate and carbamazepine monotherapy compared to unexposed pregnancies. A clear dose effect was evident for valproate, with a threshold at 1 g/day (Samren *et al.* 1997). Early screening for neural tube defects, using ultrasound and amniocentesis, and testing for α-fetoprotein, therefore seems to be indicated in women becoming pregnant while taking these drugs. It is now good practice to prescribe folate supplements to women taking AEDs who are sexually active (Morrell 1997).

In addition to major abnormality, dysmorphic syndromes have been described with a number of AEDs. Phenytoin may be associated with epicanthic folds, hypertelorism, broad flat nasal bridges, and distal digital hypoplasia (Hanson and Smith 1975). Valproate has been associated with inferior epicanthic folds, flat nasal bridges with upturned nasal tips, a shallow philtrum and down-turned mouths (DiLiberti *et al.* 1984). These abnormalities can be associated with radial ray dysplasia. Carbamazepine has been associated with similar features, with microcephaly in addition (Jones *et al.* 1989). The main concern with all these syndromes is the possible association with growth retardation and developmental delay. Unfortunately, the risk for these syndromes is uncertain and therefore counselling is difficult.

The role of newer AEDs in pregnancy has yet to be determined. Topiramate has been shown to possess the typical teratogenicity of carbonic anhydrase inhibitors in animal species. Other new drugs do not appear to possess animal teratogenicity but human experience is limited.

23.10.4 Long-term management of drug therapy

The majority of patients developing epilepsy achieve a long-lasting remission soon after the start of therapy. For these patients drug withdrawal may be considered after 2, 3, or more years (see below). Some 20 per cent of patients developing epilepsy have a chronic disorder, never completely controlled by drugs. Of patients who are not controlled, but comply with, maximal tolerated doses of a single antiepileptic drug, about 30 per cent may respond to an alternative monotherapy (Hakkarainen 1980), particularly if the reason for a first failure is intolerance. In this same study, 5 of the original 100 patients with newly diagnosed epilepsy required two drugs for seizure control, compared with 28 who remained uncontrolled even after being exposed to the combination of carbamazepine and phenytoin. A policy of polytherapy, however, inevitably increases the risks of dose-related, idiosyncratic, and chronic toxicity (Beghi *et al.* 1986). In essence, a law of diminishing returns applies. Thus, for this group of patients an appropriate aim may not be complete remission of seizures but a compromise of reduced seizure frequency with less severe seizures, to be achieved with one or, at most, two drugs.

Some patients may continue to have seizures but are not disabled by them; they may have very infrequent seizures, or seizures that are minor in their symptomatology, or which are confined to sleep. In such patients, assuming that a single drug has been used appropriate to the seizure type and epilepsy syndrome, there is usually little to be gained from alternative drugs or additional drugs.

Patients who continue to be disabled by the occurrence of seizures, despite treatment with a single drug in optimal dosage, demand further careful consideration. In particular, it is important to consider whether there are factors that would explain an unsatisfactory response to therapy, such as unidentified structural pathology, the presence of complex partial seizures, or poor compliance. If this is not the case, then it is important to review the diagnosis: a common reason for failure of therapy is that the patient does not have epilepsy.

Where none of these conditions applies, it may be reasonable to try alternative drugs as monotherapy, and then to undertake a trial of the addition of a second drug. However, this demands careful discussion with the patient and the understanding that the second drug will be withdrawn in the absence of a satisfactory sustained response.

Refractory epilepsy and rational polytherapy

We are currently entering an era in which the importance of polytherapy and drug combinations will need to be re-examined. In the 1970s and 1980s a dogma of monotherapy was established, with the recognition that large numbers of patients with epilepsy respond well to a single antiepileptic drug and that polytherapy may be complicated by an increasing frequency of adverse events, poor compliance, and the necessity for antiepileptic drug monitoring. This was seen as being a far greater problem than any minimal improvement in seizure control.

There are no randomized clinical trials that compare alternative monotherapy with add-on therapy in groups of patients with poorly controlled epilepsy. However, Mattson *et al.* (1985) placed 82 patients failing on monotherapy on two-drug regimes; 40 per cent of these were judged to be improved and 11 per cent became seizure free. Marson *et al.* (1997), in reviewing placebo-controlled add-on studies of new antiepileptic drugs in partial epilepsy, concluded that the odds of a reduction in seizure frequency of 50 per cent or greater were two to five times that of placebo. Empirically, all those experienced in treating patients with epilepsy recognize that most patients with refractory epilepsy will receive combinations of therapy and that it will be extremely difficult to reduce therapy to achieve treatment with a single drug. Thus, at present the weight of evidence suggests that drug combinations can possess greater efficacy in patients failing on monotherapy. Remaining issues are the degree of benefit and the extent to which it may be offset by an increased risk of adverse events.

There are many examples of polytherapy leading to problems with dose-related neurotoxicity. Thus, the ability of sulthiame to inhibit the metabolism of phenytoin, and that of valproate to inhibit the metabolism of lamotrigine, can both result in symptoms of intoxication. However, the ability of patients to tolerate given blood levels of carbamazepine and lamotrigine may be strongly influenced by whether or not they are taking other drugs with actions on sodium conductances. Thus, the incidence of ataxia and diplopia in placebo-controlled add-on studies of lamotrigine is strikingly higher than that for GABAergic drugs such as vigabatrin and tiagabine (Marson *et al.* 1997).

While acute idiosyncratic adverse events are not usually thought to be influenced by pharmacokinetic parameters, there is considerable evidence to the contrary (Chadwick *et al.* 1984). In particular co-medication with valproate greatly increases the risk of acute drug-related rash due to lamotrigine (Richens 1997).

The impact of polytherapy on the incidence of chronic toxicity and teratogenicity in patients with epilepsy is more difficult to assess. There is a consensus that chronic toxicity is more commonly seen in patients exposed to long-term polytherapy, and that the incidence of teratogenicity rises strikingly with the number of antiepileptic drugs administered during pregnancy. Thus, three-drug pregnancies may be associated with anything up to a 50 per cent incidence of major fetal malformations (Nakane *et al.* 1980).

Consideration of the above evidence leads to two conclusions: that there is an urgent need for pragmatic clinical trials to examine the benefits of combination therapy, and that when polytherapy is used, it should embrace a number of principles suggested by Ferrendelli (1995):

♦ It is best to combine AEDs with different mechanisms of action than to prescribe combinations of AEDs that have similar mechanisms of action. (The additional efficacy will be limited but, in the latter, the incidence of adverse events would be expected to be multiplied.)

♦ It is best to select AEDs with relatively little potential for pharmacokinetic interaction.

♦ Patients treated with polytherapy demand more intensive monitoring, both clinically and of antiepileptic drug levels.

A remaining issue is to determine the drug combinations that may carry with them particular benefits in effectiveness. A number of hypotheses remain to be examined. Perhaps the most pressing is the belief that combining valproate and lamotrigine has a particular synergistic effect in both the control of generalized seizures and the production of tremor as a side-effect. Could the combination of gabergic and glutaminergic antiepileptic drugs have particular benefits? Is the best balance between efficacy and tolerability achieved through highly specific, limited mechanisms of action within the nervous system, or through broader, multiple mechanisms of action?

Administering and monitoring drug therapy

Pharmacokinetic data (Table 23.10) define drug absorption, distribution, metabolism, and elimination. One clinical application of pharmacokinetics is therapeutic drug monitoring (TDM) in serum or plasma.

There is a non-linear relation between the dose and the serum concentration of phenytoin (Richens and Dunlop 1975). This results in a narrow therapeutic window, and monitoring is

Table 23.10. Pharmacokinetics of antiepileptic drugs

	Absorption[a] (hours)	Protein-binding (%)	Active metabolites	Metabolism (half-life in hours)	Important interactions
Carbamazepine	4–24	75	10,11-epoxide	8–30	Enzyme inducer, reducing blood levels of phenytoin, barbiturates, lamotrigine, topiramate, tiagabine and oral contraceptives. Its own metabolism shows auto-induction and is induced by other enzyme-inducing AEDs
Clobazam	1–3	90	N-desmethyl	10–50	
Ethosuximide	2–6	–		40–70	
Felbamate	2–6	25		12–24	Reduces carbamazepine levels, but increases epoxide. Increases phenytoin, valproate, and phenobarbitone levels. Its levels are reduced by enzyme-inducing AEDs but slightly increased by valproate
Gabapentin	2–3	–		5–7	Not metabolized and no interactions
Lamotrigine	2–3	50		12–48	Is not an enzyme inducer, but its metabolism may be induced by other AED enzyme inducers, and inhibited by valproate
Oxcarbazepine	2–6	40		8–10	Less enzyme induction than carbamazepine, but usual precautions with oral contraceptives
Phenobarbital	1–6	45		50–160	Enzyme inducer, reducing blood levels of phenytoin, carbamazepine, lamotrigine, topiramate, tiagabine, and oral contraceptives. Its metabolism is induced by other-inducing AEDs
Phenytoin	4–12	90		9–140	Enzyme inducer, reducing blood levels of carbamazepine, barbiturates, lamotrigine, topiramate, tiagabine, and oral contraceptives. Its metabolism and is induced by other enzyme-inducing AEDs
Primidone	2–5	20	Phenobarbital; phenylethyl-malonamide	4–12	Enzyme inducer, reducing blood levels of phenytoin, carbamazepine, lamotrigine, topiramate, tiagabine, and oral contraceptives. Its metabolism is induced by other enzyme-inducing AEDs
Tiagabine	1–2	95		4–9	Is not an enzyme inducer, but its metabolism is induced by other AED enzyme inducers
Topiramate	1.5–4	15		12–24	Is not an enzyme inducer, but its metabolism may be induced by other AED enzyme inducers
Valproate (sodium)	1–4	90		8–20	Enzyme inhibitor of lamotrigine metabolism
Vigabatrin	1–2	–		5–7	Phenytoin levels may fall, but mechanism is uncertain

[a] Time (hours) to peak plasma concentration after oral dose.

necessary to avoid neurotoxicity in patients taking an increased dose. The concept of the 'therapeutic' or 'optimal' range for phenytoin has been extended to other antiepileptic drugs, and many laboratories now routinely estimate serum concentrations of drugs other than phenytoin. This is a somewhat questionable practice.

A single measurement will give a good approximation of the steady-state concentration for drugs with long half-lives (phenytoin and phenobarbitone) but not for drugs with short half-lives. Measurements of sodium valproate concentrations from specimens taken at random during the day are impossible to interpret, as they may represent peak, trough, or intermediate concentrations. Collecting early morning specimens for measuring troughs is, however, rarely practicable.

Even when concentrations of free drugs and their metabolites in the blood are known, important pharmacodynamic considerations may alter the relationship between the blood concentration and therapeutic effect. Thus, for sodium valproate the onset of action is slower and longer lasting than can be explained by the pharmacokinetics of the drug (Rowan *et al.* 1979). Similarly, tolerance to the neurotoxic and therapeutic effects of benzodiazepines and barbiturate drugs is not explained by pharmacokinetic changes and must be due to drug–receptor interactions. There are further fundamental biological reasons for doubting the value of routine monitoring of blood concentrations of antiepileptic drugs. The upper limit of a therapeutic range may be defined as the concentration of the drug at which toxic effects are likely to appear. The most consistent relationship between the serum concentration and toxic effect is for phenytoin, but even with this drug some patients may tolerate, and indeed require, serum concentrations above 20 μg/ml (Gannaway and Mawer 1981). For sodium valproate, phenobarbital, and carbamazepine there is a wide variation in individual tolerance of serum concentrations.

The lower limit of the therapeutic range is even more difficult to define, and most patients have epilepsy that is controlled by antiepileptic serum concentrations well below the optimal range (Turnbull *et al.* 1985). Unquestioning acceptance of therapeutic ranges creates problems: patients with satisfactory control of seizures and low blood concentrations of drugs may have their doses needlessly increased, and patients who tolerate and need high blood concentrations may have their doses reduced. Treating patients is much more important than treating blood concentrations.

Routine monitoring is a valuable aid in the management of certain categories of patients:

(1) those receiving phenytoin or multiple drug treatment in whom dosage adjustment is necessary because of dose-related toxicity or poor seizure control;

(2) mentally retarded patients in whom the assessment of toxicity may be difficult;

(3) patients with renal or hepatic disease; and

(4) patients who may not be complying with treatment.

The place of AED monitoring in the use of new AEDs remains uncertain, although the simplicity of the pharmacokinetics of gabapentin and vigabatrin probably means that it will be of little value in their case. The ability of enzyme inducers (carbamazepine) and inhibitors (valproate) to interfere with the metabolism of lamotrigine may indicate that TDM may be helpful here.

Antiepileptic drug withdrawal

Both population and cohort studies have demonstrated that 70–80 per cent of patients diagnosed and treated for epilepsy will attain long-term remission in excess of 2 years (see above). The decision to start a trial of drug withdrawal should be made by the patient after appropriate advice. This needs to cover difficult areas, which include an individual assessment of risk of relapse on withdrawal of treatment and, indeed, on continued treatment, the timing of any trial of withdrawal, and the outlook if seizures recur.

Most commonly, seizure-free periods of 2 years or more are generally considered necessary before consideration of withdrawal. It is usually suggested that longer seizure-free periods result in a lower risk of recurrence. This is most likely to be due to selection bias, patients who relapse while still on medication after shorter periods of time being excluded.

Recent randomized controlled trials have examined policies of differing lengths of treatment prior to stopping medication. Peters *et al.* (1998) randomized children who entered remission within 2 months of starting treatment to stop medication after 6 months or 12 months. Six months after the first follow-up, 22 per cent still on AEDs had relapsed despite treatment, compared to 37 per cent who had been withdrawn from their drugs. However, by 24 months after randomization the risk of relapse was 49 per cent and 48 per cent respectively. The shape of the relationship between the time elapsed seizure-free and the risk

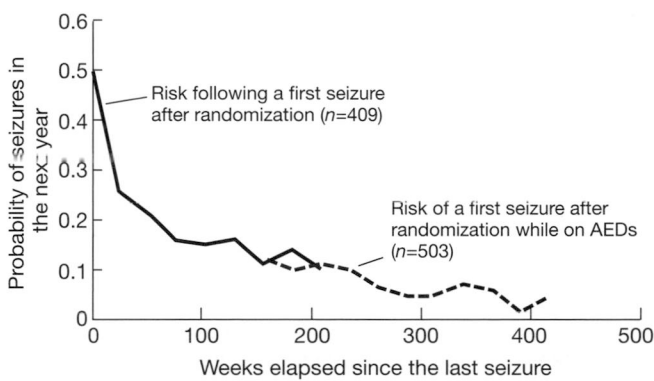

Fig. 23.14. The probability of a further seizure in a following year, while on drug therapy, and its relationship to the passage of time. Data is derived from the MRC study of antiepileptic drug (AED) withdrawal. Early risk is calculated from those patients who experienced a seizure following randomization, and who were thereafter treated. Later risk is calculated from the group of patients randomized to continued therapy, whose median duration of remission was 3 years.

of seizures in the following year on treatment is illustrated in Fig. 23.14, using data from the Medical Research Council Antiepileptic Withdrawal Study (1991), from those patients who had a recurrence of seizures during the course of the study, all of whom were on treatment after such a seizure, and all those patients randomized to continue treatment at the outset of the study. The risk of a seizure in the next year is about 50 per cent immediately after a seizure and approximately 20 per cent after 1 year seizure-free. By 4–5 years, the risk of a seizure in the next year falls to about 10 per cent. The risk for seizures after this time changes relatively little so that a policy of considering discontinuation of AEDs after 2–5 years in adults seems reasonable.

Studies that include a broad mix of patients and that require 2 years' seizure remission before stopping treatment, on average show a risk of relapse of 25 per cent in the first year and 29 per cent after 2 years (Berg and Shinnar 1994). Eighty per cent of all recurrences occur within the first year and 90 per cent within the first 2 years. Many factors have been identified that appear to influence the degree of risk.

Some epilepsy syndromes are very clearly associated with particular levels of risk of relapse after stopping treatment. Absence epilepsy has an uncertain prognosis for remission. Although, in the short term, most become seizure-free on treatment, about 25 per cent relapse when medications are withdrawn. Juvenile myoclonic epilepsy has an excellent response to treatment, but relapses occur in almost all patients when medications are stopped. The partial epilepsies are less well defined with respect to both response to treatment and the prognosis following withdrawal. However, epilepsy syndromes may be difficult to identify, particularly in patients with mild epilepsies characterized by only a few seizures responding immediately to treatment. Because of this, most studies have examined the outcome of particular types of seizures rather than syndromes. Because a single seizure type may be a characteristic of very differing syndromes, the results of such analyses are, not surprisingly, in some conflict.

Most studies find a favourable prognosis for epilepsy with onset in childhood. Studies including both childhood- and adolescent-onset epilepsy usually find a substantially increased risk of relapse in those with adolescent onset. Childhood onset of epilepsy is usually associated with a risk of relapse of approximately 20 per cent, compared to 35–40 per cent for adolescent-onset epilepsy. Adult-onset epilepsy, on the other hand, is about 30 per cent more likely to relapse than childhood-onset epilepsy (Berg and Shinnar 1994).

Individuals with an identifiable aetiology associated with their epilepsy (remote symptomatic epilepsy) are less likely to enter remission than those with idiopathic or cryptogenic epilepsy. Once in remission, they are about 50 per cent more likely to relapse if medication is stopped. Learning disability may be a stronger predictor of relapse than motor impairments or other neurological disorders that are not associated with impairment of cognitive function (Shinnar et al. 1994). The impact of remote symptomatic epilepsy on prognosis for adult-onset epilepsy is rather less dramatic than in children, and was not found to be an important factor in the MRC Antiepileptic Drug Withdrawal Study (1991), which was essentially a study of adults in remission.

There is considerable controversy over the value of the EEG in predicting the prognosis for relapse after stopping treatment. Some studies have examined the amount of 'improvement' in the EEG from starting treatment to the time of its cessation. Most studies examine the correlation between an EEG immediately prior to withdrawal and relapse. Overall, the data suggest that the EEG is of greater prognostic significance in children than in adults. It is uncertain to what degree EEG abnormalities are independent prognostic variables and to what degree they are simply more common in individuals already identified at high risk by clinical factors such as having a symptomatic epilepsy or other adverse clinical prognostic factors. Because of considerable variation amongst the studies, we cannot say with any certainty which aspects of the EEG are most important. Certainly, in a multivariate model predicting outcomes, the EEG added little to other more important clinical factors (Medical Research Council Antiepileptic Drug Withdrawal Study Group 1993).

A number of different clinical features that may reflect the severity of epilepsy have been studied and reported in the literature. They include a history of status epilepticus, the duration of epilepsy and its treatment, the number of seizures before remission, the requirement for two or more antiepileptic drugs for remission, and previous failed attempts to stop medication. Most studies indicate that these surrogate measures all adversely affect the risk of recurrence (Berg et al. 1998). However, no single indicator or set of indicators of severity is clearly superior to the others as a marker of prognosis after stopping AEDs.

The MRC Antiepileptic Drug Withdrawal Study (1991), was sufficiently large to develop and test a predictive model for relapse in patients continuing or stopping their medication. The model gives decreasing weight to the following factors: whether or not treatment is withdrawn, period of time seizure-free, taking two or more antiepileptic drugs, being 16 or older at the time of withdrawal, having myoclonic seizures, and having tonic–clonic seizures of any type. The final factor was an abnormal EEG. The resulting predictive equation was well calibrated for risks between 10 and 80 per cent and would correctly identify juvenile myoclonic epilepsy as having a high risk of relapse. Table 23.11 outlines the use of this model.

Most evidence indicates that the majority of patients who relapse when medication is stopped will regain acceptable control when treatment is re-introduced. In the MRC Study, 95 per cent of those who relapsed experienced at least a 1-year remission within 3 years of the initial relapse. By 5 years, 90 per cent had experienced a remission of at least 2 years' duration (Chadwick et al. 1996). If a decision is taken to withdraw treatment, clear advice should be offered about the speed of withdrawal. Tennison et al. (1994) found no difference in recurrence rates when antiepileptic drugs were tapered over 6 weeks as

Table 23.11. Factors for the calculation of a prognostic index for seizure recurrence by 1 and 2 years following continued treatment or slow withdrawal of antiepileptic drugs, in patients with a minimum remission of seizures lasting for 2 years while on treatment

Factor	Value to be added to score
1. Starting score for all patients	−175
Age ----> 16years	45
Taking more than 1 AED	50
Seizures occuring after the start of treatment	35
History of any tonic–clonic seizure (generalized or partial in onset)	35
History of myoclonic seizures	50
Electroencephalogram while in remission	
Not done	15
Abnormal	20
Duration of seizure-free period (years) = **D**	200/**D**
2. Total score	**T**
3. Exponentiate T/100 (Z = $e^{T/100}$)	**Z**

	Probability of seizure recurrence	
	By 1 year	By 2 years
On continued treatment	$1-0.89^Z$	$1-0.79^Z$
On slow withdrawal of treatment	$1-0.69^Z$	$1-0.60^Z$

opposed to 9 months. From a practical point of view, it seems reasonable to taper most regimes gradually over a 2–3-month period. For most adults a seizure recurrence will require the prompt re-institution of the antiepileptic drug regime that was previously successful.

23.10.5 **The management of status epilepticus**

Status epilepticus is a medical emergency because of the mortality and morbidity that can result both from the systemic

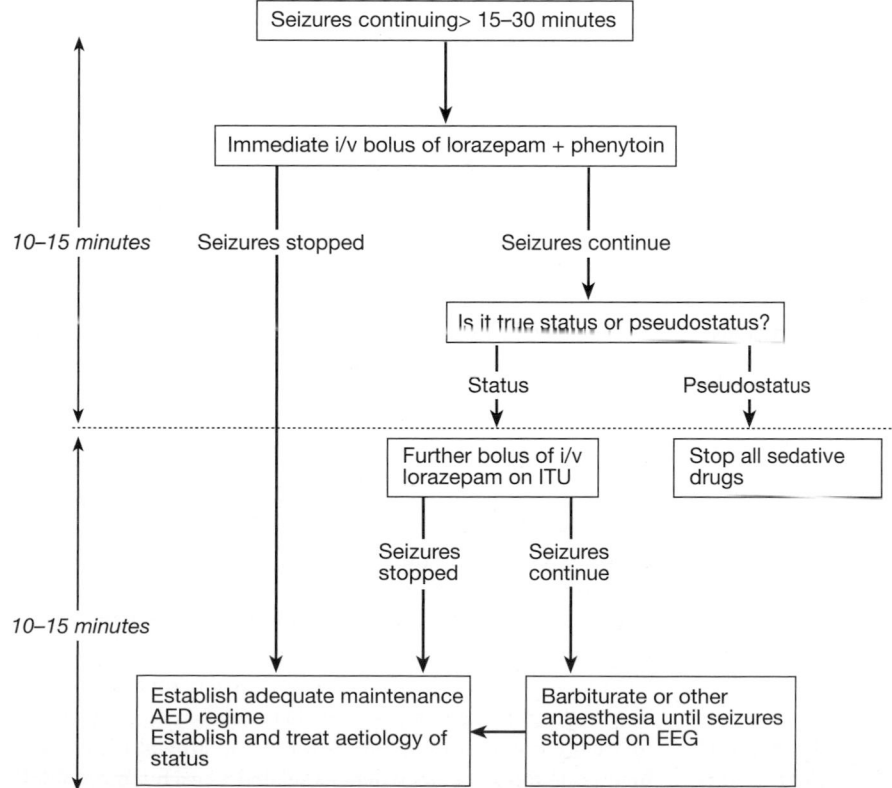

Fig. 23.15. Flow diagram of the management of status epilepticus.

complications and from the continuing epileptic activity, which itself may result in neuronal damage and loss. The satisfactory management of convulsive status epilepticus demands aggressive treatment with rapidly acting antiepileptic drugs aimed at abolishing motor and electrical evidence of status, as well as all the necessary cardiovascular, respiratory, and metabolic support. This will not easily be available outside an intensive therapy setting. An approach to management is outlined in Fig. 23.15. Early suppression of seizures must be combined with adequate investigation to disclose the cause of status and institution or maintenance of satisfactory longer-term anticonvulsant therapy.

The choice of antiepileptic drug lies between those that are available for intravenous use, which enter the brain rapidly and have an immediate mode of action. Thus benzodiazepines, barbiturates, and phenytoin can all be considered. Data comparing different drugs is sparse and is from small numbers of patients, with the exception of a large Veterans Affairs Cooperative study comparing phenobarbital, lorazepam, phenytoin, and diazepam plus phenytoin. The only regime shown to be different was phenytoin alone, which was less successful than lorazepam (Treiman *et al.* 1998). Certainly lorazepam should now be preferred to diazepam in view of its longer action. It should be administered as a loading dose of 0.1 mg/kg. It is still worthwhile combining this with phenytoin (20 mg/kg) to allow a seamless transfer to oral administration at a future date.

23.11 The surgical treatment of epilepsy

Although the surgical treatment of epilepsy was pioneered in the UK over 100 years ago, it has never been made widely available to patients with epilepsy. However, the increasing sophistication of EEG investigation, neurological imaging, and neuropsychology means that this form of treatment can be highly successful in large numbers of patients. It has been estimated that between a half and a quarter of all medically intractable patients, or 5–10 per cent of all patients with epilepsy, may benefit from surgery (NIH Consensus Conference 1990). Given a cumulative incidence of 135/100 000 for intractability (Juul-Jensen and Foldspang 1983), it can be seen that surgery is grossly under-utilized.

The philosophy of surgical treatment requires either the accurate identification of a localized site of seizure onset, with the aim of a curative resection, or the disconnection of epileptogenic zones so as to interrupt seizure spread in a palliative procedure (callosotomy or multiple pial resections). Inevitably, excisions of epileptogenic lesions and zones will also involve interruption of their connections to some degree. Engel (1987) reviewed the varying procedures undertaken at centres worldwide: 68 per cent of operations involve some form of temporal-lobe surgery, whereas extratemporal cortical excisions accounted for 24 per cent of operations; 2 per cent were hemispherectomies and 6 per cent corpus callosotomy.

To be considered for any of these procedures, patients need to demonstrate a history of medically refractory epilepsy. There may be some controversy about a precise definition of refractory epilepsy, but this will usually be established within 2 years of onset if appropriate antiepileptic drugs have been administered singly or in combination in optimal doses. Most patients exhibit epilepsy syndromes with poor prognoses at presentation so that, thereafter, there can be little optimism that the manipulation of drug therapy is likely to radically alter the outcome of epilepsy in such a patient (see above). Patients should be sufficiently disabled by their epilepsy to warrant the risks of the necessary presurgical evaluation and surgical treatment (which are approximately 0.5 per cent mortality and 5 per cent morbidity). There should be a high probability that an improvement in seizure control will lead to a significant improvement in the individual's quality of life. Other factors determining suitability of treatment will include the type of procedure to be performed, but the above criteria may be relaxed when neurological imaging shows the presence of a lesion, such as a low-grade tumour, that would demand surgical treatment in its own right. The timing of surgical treatment is important, given that it is rare for individuals over the age of 30 years to radically improve their psychosocial status even if they become seizure-free at this age (Crandall 1987).

A number of different epilepsy syndromes may be considered for surgery.

Mesial temporal lobe epilepsy

There is no doubt that patients with mesial temporal epilepsy due to hippocampal sclerosis can expect excellent results of surgery, with 70–80 per cent of patients becoming seizure free (Oxbury and Adams 1989), but other foreign-tissue lesions in this region have equally good outcomes.

A detailed clinical history will usually identify the clinical features of this syndrome (see above), and the history of febrile seizures is always a helpful marker. The interictal EEG may show anterior temporal spikes or sharp waves in a high proportion of cases. Modern, high-quality MRI has revolutionized investigation, with its ability to demonstrate hippocampal atrophy with T1 volumetry, abnormal T2 signal, and FLAIR (Kuzniecky and Jackson 1995). In specialist centres, functional imaging using positron emission tomography (PET) or single-photon emission tomography (SPECT) may also be of some value. Epileptogenic zones are characteristically hypometabolic and hypoperfused during the interictal state but may become hypermetabolic and hyperperfused ictally, or immediately post-ictally (Engel *et al.* 1982; Fish 1989). The role of more modern techniques, such as MR spectroscopy and functional imaging, remain to be defined.

Neuropsychological assessment is essential. An overall IQ of less than 70 would tend to indicate diffuse cerebral damage which reduces the likelihood of a good outcome to surgery. Particular evaluation of verbal and visual memory can be important in lateralizing deficits that are likely to be ipsilateral to seizure onset. Testing after intracarotid amytal is helpful in further defining memory deficits related to each temporal lobe and lateralizing speech. Where a well-lateralized memory deficit is found, the likelihood of a good outcome is high. Amytal testing is also important in ensuring that memory function in the temporal lobe contralateral to that on which surgery is being considered is adequate to sustain memory postoperatively. If there is agreement between ictal semiology, MRI, interictal EEG, and neuropsychology, no further investigations may be necessary, although some centres undertake ictal recording in all cases.

Invasive EEG monitoring is now only necessary in those patients in whom the MRI changes are bilateral, or in whom there is disagreement between non-invasive tests. The technique of foramen ovale recording has proved invaluable in several centres, in providing high-quality intracranial recording without craniotomy (Wieser *et al.* 1985). More extensive recordings can be obtained following the insertion of subdural electrodes and stereotactically implanted depth electrodes, or a combination of the two (Hahn and Luders 1987).

The most common surgical procedure is the *en bloc* anteriotemporal lobectomy pioneered by Falconer *et al.* (1955). More recently amygdalo-hippocampectomy has been pioneered for patients in whom it can be shown that there is a definite medial temporal onset to seizures (Yasargil and Wieser 1987). Potentially, this procedure may offer results as good as classical *en bloc* resection, with potentially better preservation of memory (Oxbury and Adams 1989), but the resection is potentially more technically demanding and the two operations have not been compared in a randomized controlled trial.

Lesional neocortical epilepsy

Partial epilepsies caused by tumour, vascular malformation, or localized cortical dysplasia constitute another, not uncommon, surgically treatable group of epilepsies. Where lesions are well circumscribed and away from functionally important areas, complete resection will be associated with a high success rate (Fish *et al.* 1993). More difficulties may arise from lesions close to eloquent areas, where more detailed neurophysiological and functional mapping may be necessary to define the extent of the epileptogenic zone. This is particularly the case with focal cortical dysplasia, where the extent of the lesion may be difficult to define purely from structural imaging.

Non-lesional neocortical epilepsy

The results of surgery in this group of patients are significantly poorer than for mesial temporal and lesional neocortical epilepsy, but surgery may still be considered where seizure semiology and well-localized interictal spiking suggest a satisfactory localization. Ictal SPECT may have a particular value in the investigation of patients (Harvey *et al.* 1993; Ho *et al.* 1995), allowing satisfactory planning of subdural or intracerebral ictal recording. Surgery will usually consist of extensive resection away from eloquent areas. In eloquent areas multiple sub-pial transections may provide palliation (Morrell *et al.* 1989).

Hemispheric epilepsy syndromes

Hemispherectomy may be suitable for patients with intractable epilepsy and an infantile hemiplegia with a useless hand and

hemianopia. Such epilepsy may occur with Sturge–Weber syndrome, Rasmussen's encephalitis, and childhood stroke. Overall, 70–80 per cent of patients become seizure free following this operation, and behavioural abnormalities can also improve. However, the operation fell into disrepute as up to 25 per cent of those undergoing hemispherectomy developed delayed complications (Oppenheimer 1966). Most suffered from recurrent subdural haemorrhage from the subdural membrane lining the hemipherectomy cavity. Adams (1983) modified the hemispherectomy procedure to eliminate the large extradural space and to isolate the ventricular system from the subdural cavity. Hemispherectomy should probably now be restored to its previous position in children with infantile hemiplegia and epilepsy, and also in those rare children and adults with chronic progressive focal encephalitis (Rasmussen *et al.* 1958; Hart *et al.* 1994).

Other partial epilepsy syndromes

Gelastic seizures associated with hypothalamic hamartomas are rare. The success of surgical treatment is controversial, some series suggesting poor results (Cascino *et al.* 1993), others suggesting success (Valdueza *et al.* 1994).

Symptomatic/cryptogenic generalized epilepsy

Section of the corpus callosum and hippocampal commissure is an accepted palliative procedure for uncontrolled secondarily generalized seizures (Spencer *et al.* 1987). The procedure seeks to prevent the generalization of seizures, particularly those that generalize rapidly, resulting in falls (tonic and atonic seizures). Early procedures were often complicated by ventriculitis, meningitis, and hydrocephalus, by more severe and frequent focal seizures immediately postoperatively, and by a characteristic disconnection syndrome of mutism, apraxia of the nondominant limbs, agnosia, apathy, confusion, and infantile behaviour. Refinements of the surgical procedure and the introduction of anterior and two-stage operations have reduced the morbidity. In some series up to 80 per cent of patients have had a complete cessation of generalized seizures with falls, although about 25 per cent may have more intense partial seizures than previously. It also seems that a callosotomy may reduce the incidence of status epilepticus.

The selection criteria for corpus callosotomy are more poorly defined than for other surgical procedures. The operation will be most commonly considered in children and adolescents with very severe epilepsy with generalized or multifocal origin to seizures, or with seizures of sudden onset resulting in falls.

References

Adams, C. B. T. (1983). Hemispherectomy—a modification. *J. Neurol. Neurosurg. Psychiatry*, **46**, 617–19.

Adams, R. D. and Foley, J. M, (1953). The neurological disorder associated with liver disease. In *Metabolic and toxic diseases of the nervous system*, (ed. H. H. Merritt and C. C. Hare), pp. 198–237. Williams and Wilkins, Baltimore.

Adelman, A. G. and Wigle, E. D. (1969). The bradycardia, tachycardia, asystole syndrome: treatment by pacemaker. *Can. Med. Assoc. J.*, **100**, 75–7.

Ajmone-Marsan, C. and Goldhammer, L. (1973) Clinical ictal patterns and electrographic data in cases of partial seizures of frontal central parietal origin. In *Epilepsy, its phenomenon in Man*, (ed. M. A. B. Brazier), pp. 235–58. Academic Press, New York.

Ajmone-Marsan, C. and Zivin, L. S. (1970). Factors related to the occurrence of typical paroxysmal abnormalities in the EEG records of epileptic patients. *Epilepsia*, **11**, 361–8.

Alajouanine, T., Nehil, J., and Gabersek, V. (1959). A propos d'un cas d'epilepsie declenche par la lecture. *Rev. Neurol. (Paris)*, **101**, 463–7.

Aminoff, M. J. and Simon, R. P. (1980). Status epilepticus: causes, clinical features and consequences in 98 patients. *Am. J. Med.*, **69**, 657–66.

Andermann, F. (1987). Migraine–epilepsy relationships. *Epilepsy Res.*, **1**, 213–25.

Anderman, F. and Andermann, E. (1986). Excessive startle syndromes: startle disease, jumping and startle epilepsy. *Adv. Neurol.*, **43**, 321–38.

Anderson, V. E., Hauser, W. A. , and Rich, S. S. (1986). Genetic heterogeneity in the epilepsies. *Adv. Neurol.*, **44**, 000–00.

Annegers, J. F., Hauser, W. A., and Elverback, L. R. (1979). Remission of seizures and relapse in patients with epilepsy. *Epilepsia*, **20**, 729–37.

Annegers, J. F., Grabow, J. D., Groover, R. V. *et al.* (1980). Seizures after head trauma: a population study. *Neurology*, **30**, 683–9.

Annegers, J. F., Hauser, W. A., Beghi, E. *et al.* (1988). The risk of unprovoked seizures after encephalitis and meningitis. *Neurology*, **38**, 1407–10.

Annegers, J. F., Hauser, W. A., Coan, S. P. *et al.* (1998). A population based study of seizures after traumatic brain injuries. *N. Engl. J. Med.*, **338**, 20–4.

Antoniadis, A., Mueller, W. E., and Wollert, U. (1980). Benzodiazepine receptor interactions may be involved in the neurotoxicity of various penicillin derivatives. *Ann. Neurol.*, **8**, 71–3.

Aquimno, A. and Gabor, A. J. (1980). Movement induced seizures in nonketotic hypoglycaemia. *Neurology*, **30**, 600–4.

Arieff, A. I., Llach, F., and Massry, S. G. (1976). Neurological manifestations and morbidity of hyponatraemia: correlation with brain water and electrolytes. *Medicine*, **55**, 121–9.

Arvanov, V., Holmes, K., Keele, N. *et al.* (1995). The functional role of metabotropic glutamate receptors in epileptiform activity induced by 4-aminopyridine in the rat amygdala slice. *Brain Res.*, **669**, 140–4.

Ascroft, P. B. (1941). Traumatic epilepsy after gunshot wounds of the head. *BMJ*, **1**, 739–44.

Avanzini, G., Moshe, S. L., Schwartzkroin, P. A. *et al.* (1998). Animal models of localization-related epilepsy. In *Epilepsy: a comprehensive textbook*, (ed. J. Engel and T. A. Pedley), pp. 427–42. Lippincott-Raven, New York.

Avoli, M. and Gloor, P. (1982). Role of the thalamus in generalized penicillin epilepsy: observations on decorticated cats. *Exp. Neurol.*, **77**, 386–402.

Avoli, M., Siatitsas, I., Kostopoulos, G. *et al.* (1981). Effects of postictal depression on experimental spike and wave discharges. *Electroencephalogr. Clin. Neurophysiol.*, **52**, 373–4.

Avoli, M., Gloor, P., Kostopoulos, G. *et al.* (1983). An analysis of penicillin-induced generalized spike and wave discharges using simultaneous recordings of cortical and thalamic single neurons. *J. Neurophysiol.*, **50**, 819–37.

Backstrom, T. (1976). Epileptic seizures in women related to plasma oestrogen and progesterone during the menstrual cycle. *Acta Neurol. Scand.*, **54**, 321–47.

Baker, G. A., Jacoby, A., and Chadwick, D. W. (1996). The associations of psychopathology in epilepsy: a community study. *Epilepsy Res.*, **25** (1), 29–39.

Baldy-Moulinier, M. (1986). Interrelationships between sleep and epilepsy. In *Recent advances in epilepsy*, Vol. 3, (ed. T. A. Pedley and B. S. Meldrum), pp. 37–57. Churchill Livingstone, London.

Bannister, R., Ardill, L., and Fentem, P. (1969). An assessment of various methods of treatment of idiopathic hypotension. *QJM*, **38**, 377–95.

Barcroft, H. and Edholm, O. G. (1945). On the vasodilatation in human skeletal muscle during posthaemorrhagic fainting. *J. Physiol.*, **104**, 161–75.

Barkovich, A. J. and Kjos, B. O. (1992). Gray matter heterotopias: MR characteristics and correlation with developmental and neurologic manifestations. *Radiology*, **182**, 493–9.

Bates, D., Caronna, J. J., Cartlidge, N. E. F. *et al.* (1977). A prospective study of nontraumatic coma: methods and results in 310 patients. *Ann. Neurol.*, **2**, 211–20.

Bauermeister, D., Jennings, E. R., Crusc, D. *et al.* (1967). Hypercalcaemia with seizures. a clinical paradox. *JAMA*, **201**, 132–4.

Beghi, E., Di Mascio, R., and Tognoni, G. (1986). Drug treatment of epilepsy. outline, criticisms and perspectives. *Drugs*, **31**, 249–65.

Bennett, R., Hughes, G. R. V., Bywaters, E. G. L. *et al.* (1972). neuropsychiatric problems in systemic lupus erythematosis. *BMJ*, **1**, 342–4.

Bennett, W. M., Muther, R. S., Parker, R. A. *et al.* (1980). Drug therapy in renal failure: dosing guidelines for adults. *Ann. Intern. Med.*, **93**, 323–5.

Berg, A. T. and Shinnar, S. (1994). Relapse following discontinuation of antiepileptic drugs: a meta-analysis. *Neurology*, **44**, 601–8.

Berg, A. T., Levy, S. R., Novotny, E. J., *et al.* (1996*a*). Predictors of intractable epilepsy in childhood: a case-control study. *Epilepsia*, **37** (1), 24–30.

Berg, A. T., Shinnar, S. , and Chadwick, D. (1998). Discontinuing antiepileptic drugs. In *Epilepsy: a comprehensive text*, (ed. J. Engel and T. A. Pedley), pp. 1275–84. Lippincott-Raven, New York.

Berkovic, S. F., McIntoch, A., Howell, R. A. *et al.* (1994). Familial temporal lobe epilepsy: a benign, unrecognised and common disorder. *Epilepsia*, **35** (Suppl. 8), 109.

Bernardo, L. A. and Pedley, T. A. (1985). Cellular mechanisms of focal epileptogenesis. In *Recent advances in epilepsy*, Vol. 2, (ed. T. A. Pedley and B. S. Meldrum), pp. 21–36. Churchill Livingstone, London.

Bilbro, R. H. (1970). Syncope after prostatic massage. *N. Engl. J. Med.*, **282**, 167–8.

Binnie, C. D. (1997). The electroencephalogram: advances and pitfalls. in *The epilepsies 2*, (ed. R. J. Porter and D. Chadwick), pp. 111–40. Butterworth-Heinemann, Boston.

Bittencourt, P. R. M., Gracia, C. M., and Lorenzana, P. (1988). Epilepsy and parasitosis of the central nervous system' In *Recent advances in epilepsy* , Vol. 4, (ed. T. A. Pedley and B. S. Meldrum), pp. 123–60. Raven Press, New York.

Blakemore, W. F. (1980). Isoniazid. In *Experimental and clinical neurotoxicology*, (ed. P. S. Spencer and H. H. Schaumburg), pp. 476–89. Williams and Wilkins, Baltimore.

Bleck, T. P., Smith, M. C., Pierre-Louis, S. J.-C. *et al.* (1993). Neurologic complications of critical medical illnesses. *Crit. Care Med.*, **21**, 98–103.

Blisard, K. S. and McFeeley, P. J. (1988). The spectrum of neuropathological findings in deaths associated with seizure disorders. *J. Forensic Sci.*, **22**, 910–14.

Blomquist, H. K., Gustavson, K. H., and Holmgren, G. (1981). Mild mental retardation in children in a northern Swedish county *J. Ment. Defic. Res.*, **25**, 169–86.

Blumhardt, L. D., Smith, P. E. M., and Owen, L. (1986). Electrocardiographic accompaniments of temporal lobe epileptic seizures. *Lancet*, **1**, 1051–5.

Boston Collaborative Drug Surveilllance Program (1972). Drug-induced convulsions. *Lancet*, **2**, 677–9.

Bouma, P. A., Westendorp, R. G., van Dijk, J. G. *et al.* (1996). The outcome of absence epilepsy: a meta-analysis. *Neurology*, **47**, 802–8.

Bowery, N. G. (1993). GABA$_B$ receptor pharmacology. *Annu. Rev. Pharmacol. Toxicol.*, **33**, 109–47.

Braestrup, C., Nielsen, E. B., Sonnewald, U. *et al.* (1990). NO-328 binds with high affinity to the brain GABA uptake carrier. *J. Neurochem.*, **54**, 639.

Brodie, M. J., Richens, A., and Yuen, A. W. C. (1995). Double-blind comparison of lamotrigine and carbamazepine in newly diagnosed epilepsy. *Lancet*, **345**, 476–9.

Brodtkorb, E., Nilsen, G., and Smevik, O. (1992). Epilepsy and anomalies of neuronal migration: MRI and clinical aspects. *Acta Neurol. Scand.*, **86**, 24–32.

Bruck, E., Abal, G., and Aceto, T. Jr (1968). Therapy of infants with hypertonic dehydration due to diarrhoea. *Am. J. Dis. Child.*, **115**, 281–301.

Buck, D., Baker, G. A., Jacoby, A. *et al.* (1997). Patients' experiences of injury as a result of epilepsy. *Epilepsia*, **38** (4), 439–44.

Burn, J., Dennis, M., Bamford, J. *et al.* (1997). Epileptic seizures after a first stroke: the Oxfordshire Community Stroke Project. *BMJ*, **315**, 1582–7.

Cabral, R. J., King, T. T., and Scott, D. F. (1976*a*). Epilepsy after two different neurological approaches to the treatment of ruptured intracranial aneurysm. *J. Neurol. Neurosurg. Psychiatry*, **39**, 1052–6.

Cabral, R. J., King, T. T., and Scott, D. F. (1976*b*). incidence of postoperative eplspey after a transtentorial approach to acoustic nerve tumours. *J. Neurol. Neurosurg. Psychiatry*, **39**, 663–5.

Caffi, J. (1973). Zur Frage Klinischer Anfallformen Bei Psychomotorischer Epilepsie. *Schweiz. Med. Wochenschr.*, **103**, 469–75.

Cascino, G. D., Kelly, P. J., Hirschorn, K. A. *et al.* (1990). Stereotactic resection of intra-axial cerebral lesions in partial epilepsy. *Mayo Clin. Proc.*, **65**, 1053–60.

Cascino, G. D., Andermann, F., Berkovic, S. F. *et al.* (1993). Gelastic seizures and hypothalamic hamartomas: evaluation of patients undergoing chronic intracranial EEG monitoring and outcome of surgical treatment. *Neurology*, **43**, 747–50.

Cast, I. P. and Wilson, P. J. E. (1981). Pituitary tumours (Abstract). *J. Neurol. Neurosurg. Psychiatry*, **44**, 371.

Cavazzuti, G. B. (1980). Epidemiology of different types of epilepsy in school-age children of Modena, Italy. *Epilepsia*, **21**, 57–62.

Caveness, W. F., Meirowsky, A. M., Rish, B. C. *et al.* (1979). The nature of post-traumtic epilepsy. *J. Neurosurg.*, **50**, 545–53.

Cendes, F., Andermann, F., Gloor, P. *et al.* (1993). Atrophy of mesial structures in patients with temporal lobe epilepsy: cause or consequence of related seizures? *Ann. Neurol.*, **34**, 795–801.

Chadwick, D. (1983). Drug-induced convulsions. In *Recent progress in epilepsy*, (ed. F. C. Rose), pp. 151–60. Pitman, London.

Chadwick, D. (1998). Do new antiepileptic drugs justify their expense? *Arch. Neurol.*, **55** (8), 1140–2.

Chadwick, D., Reynolds, E. H., and Marsden, C. D. (1976). Anticonvulsant induced dyskinesias: a comparison with dyskinesias induced by neuroleptics. *J. Neurol. Neurosurg. Psychiatry*, **39**, 1210–18.

Chadwick, D., Martin, S., Buxton, P. H. *et al.* (1982). Measles virus and subacute neurological disease: an unusual presentation of measles inclusion body encephalitis. *J. Neurol. Neurosurg. Psychiatry*, **45**, 680–4.

Chadwick, D., Shaw, M. D., Foy, P., *et al.* (1984). Serum anticonvulsant concentrations and the risk of drug induced skin eruptions. *J. Neurol. Neurosurg. Psychiatry*, **47** (6), 642–4.

Chadwick, D., Taylor, J., and Johnson, A. (1996). Outcomes after seizure recurrence in people with well controlled epilepsy and the factors that influence it. *Epelepsia*, **37**, 1043–50.

Chee, M. L., Kotagal, P. Van Ness, P. C. *et al.* (1993). Lateralizing value in intractable partial epilepsy: blinded multiple-observer analysis. *Neurology*, **43**, 2519–25.

Cocito, L., Favle, E., and Reni, L. (1982). Epileptic seizures in cerebral arterial occlusive disease. *Stroke*, **13**, 189–95.

Cockerell, O. C., Johnson, A. L., Sander, J. W. A. S. *et al.* (1997). Prognosis of epilepsy: a review and further analysis of the first nine years of the British National General Practice Study of Epilepsy, a prospective population-based study. *Epilepsia*, **38** (1), 31–46.

Cohen, N., Strauss, G., Lew, R. *et al.* (1988). Should prophylactic anticonvulsants be administered to patients with newly diagnosed cerebral metastases. A retrospective analysis. *J. Clin. Oncol.*, **6**, 1621–4.

Cohen, S. A. and Barchi, R. I. (1993). Voltage-dependent sodium channels. *Int. Rev. Cytol.*, **137C**, 55–103.

Coleman, R. M., Pollak, C. P., and Weitzman, E. D. (1980). Periodic movements in sleep (nocturnal myoclonus): relation to sleep disorders. *Ann. Neurol.*, **8**, 416–21.

Collaborative Group for the Study of Epilepsy (1992). Prognosis of epilepsy in newly referred patients: a multicenter prospective study of the effects of monotherapy on the long-term course of epilepsy. *Epilepsia*, **33** (1), 45–51.

Commission on Antiepileptic Drugs of the International League against Epilepsy (1989). Guidelines for clinical evaluation of antiepiletic drugs. *Epilepsia*, **30** (4), 400–8.

Commission on Classification and Terminology of the International League Against Epilepsy (1981). Proposal for revised clinical and electroencepahlographic classification of epileptic seizures. *Epilepsia*, **22**, 489–501.

Commission on Classification and Terminology of the International League Against Epilepsy (1989). Proposal for revised classification of epilepsies and epileptic syndromes. *Epilepsia*, **30**, 389–99.

Connor, J. A. and Stevens, C. F. (1971). Voltage clamp studies of a transient outward current in gastropod neural somata. *J. Physiol. (Lond.)*, **213**, 21–30.

Connors, B. W., Gutnick, M. J., and Prince, D. A. (1982). Electrophysiological properties of neocortical neurons in vitro. *J. Neurophysiol.*, **48**, 1321–35.

Conrad, C. C., Ghazi, M., and Kitay, D. Z. (1973). Acute neurovascular sequelae of intrauterine device insertion or removal. *J. Reprod. Med.*, **11**, 211–12.

Cook, M. J., Fish, D. R., Shorvon, S. D. *et al.* (1992). Hippocampal volumetric and morphometric studies in frontal and temporal lobe epilepsy. *Brain*, **115**, 1001–15.

Copeland, G. P., Foy, P., and Shaw, M. D. M. (1982). The incidence of epilepsy after ventricular shunting operations. *Surg. Neurol.*, **17**, 279–81.

Coulter, A. (1997). Thalamocortical anatomy and physiology. In *Epilepsy: a comprehensive textbook*, Vol. 1, (ed. J. Engel Jr and T. A. Pedley), pp. 341–51. Lippincott-Raven, New York.

Coulter, D. A., Huguenard, J. R., and Prince, D. A. (1989). Specific petit mal anticonvulsants reduce calcium currents in thalamic neurons. *Neurosci. Lett.*, **98**, 74–8.

Coulter, D. A., Huguenard, J. R. , and Prince, D. A. (1990). Differential effects of petit mal anticonvulsants on thalamic neurones: calcium current reduction. *Br. J. Pharmacol.*, **100**, 800–6.

Crandall, P. H. (1987). Cortical resections. in Surgical treatment of epilepsies, (ed. J. Engel), pp. 377–404. Raven Press, New York.

Crawford, P. M., West, C. R., Chadwick, D. W. *et al.* (1986). Arteriovenous malformations of the brain: natural history in unoperated patients. *J. Neurol. Neurosurg. Psychiatry*, **49** (1), 1–10.

Critchley, M. (1937). Musicogenic epilepsy. *Brain*, **60**, 13–27.

Crunelli, V. and Leresche, N. (1991). A role for $GABA_B$ receptors in excitation and inhibition of thalamocortical cells. *Trends Neurol. Sci.*, **14**, 16–21.

Currie, S., Heathfield, K. W. G., Henson, R. A. *et al.* (1971). Clinical course and prognosis of temporal lobe epilepsy. *Brain*, **94**, 173–90.

Curtis, D. R., Game, C. J. A., Johnston, G. A. R. *et al.* (1972). Convulsant action of penicillin. *Brain Res.*, **43**, 242–5.

Dailey, J. W. and Naritoku, D. K. (1996). Antidepressants and seizures: clinical anecdotes overshadow neuroscience. ‘ *Biochem. Pharmacol.*, **52** (9), 1323–9.

Dalby, M. A. (1969). Epilepsy and 3 per second spike and wave rhythms. A clinical, electroencephalographic and prognostic analysis of 346 patients. *Acta Neurol. Scand.*, **45** (Suppl. 40), 000–00.

D'Alessandro, R., Ferrara, R., Benassi, G. *et al.* (1988). Computed tomographic scans in post-traumatic epilepsy. *Arch. Neurol.*, **45**, 42–3.

Daumas-Duport, C., Scheithauer, B. W., Chodkiewicz, J. P. *et al.* (1988). Dysembryoplastic neuroepithelial tumor: a surgically curable tumor of young patients with intractable partial seizures. *Neurosurgery*, 23, 545–56.

De Deyn, P. P., Saxena, V. K., Abts, H. *et al.* (1992). Clinical and pathphysiological aspects of neurological complications in renal failure. *Acta Neurol. Belg.*, 92, 191–206.

Delgado-Escueta, A. V. and Enrile-Bacsal, F. (1984). Juvenile myoclonic epilepsy of Janz. *Neurology*, 34, 285–94.

Delgado-Escueta, A. V. and Walsh, G. O. (1985). Type I complex partial seizures of hippocampal origin: excellent results of anterior temporal lobectomy. *Neurology*, 35, 143–54.

Delgado-Escueta, A. V., Bascal, F. E., and Treiman, D. M. (1982). Complex partial seizures on closed circuit television and EEG: a study of 691 attacks in 79 patients. *Ann. Neurol.*, 57, 292–300.

DiLiberti, J. H., Farndon, P. A., Dennis, N. R. *et al.* (1984). The fetal valproate syndrome. *Am. J. Genet.*, 19, 473–81.

Dobyns, W., Andermann F. *et al.* (1996). X-linked malformations of neuronal migration. *Neurology*, 47, 331–9.

Douglas, D. B. (1971). Interval between first seizure and diagnosis of brain tumour. *Dis. Nerv. Syst.*, 32, 255.

Dreifuss, F. E. *et al.* (1987). Valproic acid fatalities: a retrospective review. *Neurology*, 37, 379–85.

Dunea, G., Mahurkar, S. D., Mamdani, B. *et al.* (1978). Role of aluminium in dialysis dementia. *Ann. Intern. Med.*, 88, 502–4.

Edebol-Tysk, K. (1989). Epidemiology of spastic tetraplegic cerebral palsy in Sweden. I. Impairments and disabilities. *Neuropediatrics*, 20, 41–5.

Eke, T., Talbot, J. F., and Lawden, M. C. (1997). Severe persistent visual field constriction associated with vigabatrin. *BMJ*, 314, 180–1.

Engel, J. (1987). Outcome with respect to epileptic seizures. In Surgical treatment of the epilepsies, (ed. J. Engel), pp. 553–72. Raven Press, New York.

Engel, J., Kuhl, D., Phelps, M. E. *et al.* (1982). Comparative localisation of epileptic foci in partial epilepsy by PET and EEG. *Ann. Neurol.*, 12, 529–72.

Essig, C. F. (1967). Clinical and experimental aspects of barbiturate withdrawal convulsions. *Epilepsia*, 8, 21–30.

Falconer, M. A., Hill, D., Meyer, A. *et al.* (1955). Treatment of temporal lobe epilepsy by temporal lobectomy. A survey of findings and results. *Lancet*, 1, 827–35.

Farmer, J.-P., Cosgrove, J. R., Villemure, J.-G. *et al.* (1988). Intracerebral cavernous angiomas. *Neurology*, 38, 1699–704.

Favale, E., Rubino, V., Mainardi, P. *et al.* (1995). Anticonvulsant effect of fluoxetine in humans. *Neurology*, 45, 1926–7.

Feely, M., Calvert, R., and Gibson, J. (1982). Clobazam in catamenial epilepsy. A model for evaluating anticonvulsants. *Lancet*, 10 (2), 71–3.

Ferrendelli, J. A. (1995). Rational polypharmacy. *Epilepsia*, 36 (2), 5115–18.

Fish, D. (1989). CT and PET in drug resistant epilepsy. In Chronic epilepsy, its progress and management, (ed. M. R. Trimble), pp. 59–72. Wiley, Chichester.

Fish, D. R., Smith, S. J., Quesney, L. F. *et al.* (1993). Surgical treatment of children with medically intractable frontal or temporal lobe epilepsy: results and highlights of 40 years experience. *Epilepsia*, 34, 244–7.

Fish, D. R., Quirk, J. A., Smith, S. J. M. *et al.* (1994). *National Survey of Photosensitivity and Seizures Induced by Electronic Screen Games*. Department of Trade and Industry, London.

Fisher, C. M. (1979). Syncope of obscure nature. *Can. J. Neurol. Sci.*, 6, 7–20.

Fisher, C. M. and Adams, R. D. (1958). Transient global amnesia. *Trans. Am. Neurol. Assoc.*, 83, 143–6.

Fishman, R. A. (1965). Neurological aspects of magnesium metabolism. *Arch. Neurol.*, 12, 562–9.

Forsgren, L., Edvinsson, S. O., Blomquist, H. K. *et al.* (1990). Epilepsy in a population of mentally retarded children and adults. *Epilepsy Res.*, 6, 234–48.

Forster, F. M. (1977). *Reflex epilepsy, behavioural therapy and conditional reflexes*. Thomas, Illinois.

Foy, P. M., Copeland, G. P., and Shaw, M. D. M. (1981a). The incidence of postoperative seizures. *Acta Neurochir.*, 55, 253–64.

Foy, P. M., Copeland, G. P., and Shaw, M. D. M. (1981b). The natural history of postoperative seizures. *Acta Neurochir.*, 57, 15–22.

Frame, B. (1976). Neuromuscular manifestations of parathyroid disease. In *Handbook of clinical neurology*, Vol. 27, (ed. P. J. Vinken and G. W. Bruyn), pp. 283–320. Elsevier North Holland, Amsterdam.

Franceschi, M., Triulzi, F., Ferini-Srambi, L. *et al.* (1989). Focal cerebral lesions found by magnetic resonance imaging in cryptogenic nonrefractory temporal lobe epilepsy patients. *Epilepsia*, 30, 540–5.

Franck, J. E. and Schwartzkroin, P. A. (1985). Do kainate-lesioned hippocampi become epileptogenic? *Brain Res.*, 329, 309–13.

Fraser, H. F., Wikler, A., Essig, C. F. *et al.* (1958). Degree of physical dependence induced by secobarbital or pentobarbital. *JAMA*, 166, 126–9.

French, J. A., Rosenbaum, D. H., and Rowan, A. J. (1988). Outcome in 55 patients with documented psuchogenic seizures: clinical and EEG correlates. *Epilepsia*, 29, 653–7.

French, J. A., Williamson P. D., Thadani V. M. *et al.* (1993). Characteristics of medial temporal lobe epilepsy I. Results of history and physical examination. *Ann. Neurol.*, **34**, 774–80.

Friedberg, C. K. (1971). Syncope. Pathological physiology: differential diagnosis and treatment (I) and (II). *Mod. Concepts Cardiovasc. Dis.*, **XL**, 55–63.

Gannaway, D. J. and Mawer, G. E. (1981). Serum phenytoin concentrations and clinical response in patients with epilepsy. *Br. J. Clin. Pharmacol.*, **12**, 833–9.

Garber, S. S. and Miller, C. (1987). Single Na$^+$ channels activated by veratridine and batrachotoxin. *J. Gen. Physiol.*, **89**, 459–80.

Gastaut, H. (1976). Conclusions: computerized transverse axial tomography in epilepsy. *Epilepsia*, **17**, 337–8.

Gastaut, H., Gastaut, J. L., Gonclaves e Silva, G. E. *et al.* (1975). Relative frequency of different types of epilepsy: a study employing the classification of the International League Against Epilepsy. *Epilepsia*, **16**, 457–61.

Gawin, F. H. and Ellinwood, E. H. (1988). Cocaine and other stimulants. *N. Engl. J. Med.*, **318**, 1173–82.

Geier, S., Bancaud, J., Talairach, J. *et al.* (1977). The seizures of frontal lobe epilepsy. *Neurology*, **27**, 951–8.

Ghika-Schmid, F., Ghika, J., Regli, F. *et al.* (1996). Hashimoto's myoclonic encephalopathy: an undiagnosed treatable condition? *Mov. Disord.*, **11**, 555–62.

Giannakodimos, S. and Panayiotopoulos, C. P. (1996). Eyelid myoclonia with absences: a clinical and video-EEG study in adults. *Epilepsia*, **37**, 36–44.

Gibberd, F. B. and Bateson, M. C. (1974). Sleep epilepsy: its pattern and prognosis. *BMJ*, **2**, 403–5.

Gibbs, F. A. and Gibbs, E. L. (1952). *Atlas of electroencephalography*, Vol. 2: *Epilepsy*. Addison-Westley, Cambridge, MA.

Gibbs, J. M., Appleton, R. E., and Rosenbloom, L. (1992). Vigabatrin in intractable childhood epilepsy: a retrospective study. *Ped. Neurol.*, **8**, 338–40.

Glantz, M. J., Cole, B. F., Friedberg, M. H. *et al.* (1996). A randomised, blinded, placebo-controlled trial of divalproex sodium prophylaxis in adults with newly diagnosed brain tumors. *Neurology*, **46**, 985–91.

Gloor, P. (1968). Generalized corticoreticular epilepsies. Some considerations on the pathophysiology of generalized bilaterally synchronous spike and wave discharge. *Epilepsia*, **9**, 249–63.

Gloor, P., Olivier, A., Quesney, L. F. *et al.* (1982). The role of the limbic system in experential phenomena of temporal lobe epilepsy. *Ann. Neurol.*, **12**, 129–44.

Goddard, G. V., McIntyre, D. C., and Leech, C. K. (1969). A permanent change in brain function resulting form daily electrical stimulation. *Exp. Neurol.*, **25**, 295–330.

Goosses, R. (1984). *Die Beziehung Der Fotosensibilitat Zu Den Verschiedenen Epileptischen Syndromen*. West Berlin.

Goulatia, R. K., Verma, A., Mishra, N. K. *et al.* (1987). Disappearing CT lesion in epilepsy. *Epilepsia*, **28**, 523–7.

Greenberg, D. A., Delgado-Escuata, A. V., Widelitz, H. *et al.* (1988). Juvenile myoclonic epilepsy (JME) may be linked to the BF and HLA loci on human chromosome 6. *Am. J. Med. Genet.*, **31**, 185–92.

Gregory, R. P., Oates, T., and Merry, R. T. G. (1993). Electroencephalogram epileptiform abnormalities in candidates for aircrew training. *Electroencephalogr. Clin. Neurophysiol.*, **86**, 75–81.

Guberman, A. and Catching, J. (1986). Swallow syncope. *Can. J. Neurol. Sci.*, **13**, 267–9.

Gudmundsson, G. (1966). Epilepsy in Iceland. *Acta Neurol. Scand.*, **43** (Suppl. 25), 72–3.

Gumpert, J., Hanisota, P., and Upton, A. (1970). Gelastic epilepsy. *J. Neurol. Neurosurg. Psychiatry*, **33**, 479–83.

Gururaj, G. and Satishchandra, P. (1992). Correlates of hot water epilepsy in Rural South India: a descriptive study. *Neuroepidemiology*, **11**, 173–9.

Gutnick, M. J., Connors, B. W., and Prince, D. A. (1982). Mechanisms of neocortical epileptogenesis in vitro. *J. Neurophysiol.*, **48**, 1321–35.

Hahn, J. F. and Luders, H. (1987). Placement of subdural grid electrodes at the Cleveland Clinic. In *Surgical treatment of the epilepsies*, (ed. J. Engel), pp. 621–7. Raven Press, New York.

Hakkarainen, H. (1980). Carbamazepine vs diphenylhydantoin vs their combination in adult epilepsy (Abstract). *Neurology*, **30**, 354.

Hampton, F., Williams, B., and Loizou, L. A. (1982). Syncope as a presenting feature of hindbrain herniation with syringomyelia. *J. Neurol., Neurosurg. Psychiatry*, **45**, 919–22.

Hanna, S., Harrison, M., MacIntyre, I. *et al.* (1960). The syndrome of magnesium deficiency in Man. *Lancet*, **2**, 172–6.

Hanson, J. W. and Smith, D. W. (1975). The fetal hydantoin syndrome. *J. Paediatr.*, **87**, 285–90.

Harper, M. and Roth, M. (1962). Temporal lobe epilepsy and the phobic anxiety depersonalization syndrome. Part 1. A comparative study. *Compr Psychiatry*, **3**, 129–51.

Hart, Y. M., Cortez, M., Andermann, F. *et al.* (1994). Medical treatment of Rasmussen's syndrome (chronic encephalitis and epilepsy): effect of high dose steroids and immunoglobulins in 19 patients. *Neurology*, **44**, 1030–6.

Harvey, A. S., Hopkins, I. J., Bowe, J. M. *et al.* (1993). Frontal lobe epilepsy: clincial seizure chercteristics and localization with ictal ^{99m}Tc HMPOA SPECT. *Neurology*, **43**, 1966–9.

Hauser, W. A. (1990). Prevention of posttraumatic epilepsy. *New Engl. J. Med.*, **323**, 540–2.

Hauser, W. A. and Anderson, V. E. (1986). Genetics of epilepsy. In *Recent advances in epilepsy*, Vol. 3, (ed. T. A. Pedley and B. S. Meldrum), pp. 21–36. Churchill Livingstone, Edinburgh.

Hauser, W. A. and Hesdorffer, D. C. (1990). *Epilepsy: frequency, causes and consequences*. Demos Publications, New York.

Hauser, W. A. and Kurland, L. T. (1975). The epidemiology of epilepsy in Rochester, Minnesota, 1935 through 1967. *Epilepsia*, **16**, 166–82.

Hauser, W. A., Annegers, J. F., and Elveback, L. R. (1980). Mortality in patients with epilepsy. *Epilepsia*, **21**, 339–41.

Hauser, W. A., Anderson, V. E., Loewenston, R. B. *et al.* (1982). Seizure recurrence after a first unprovoked seizure. *N. Engl. J. Med.*, **307**, 525–8.

Hauser, W. A., Morris, M. L., Heston, L. L. *et al.* (1986). Seizures and myoclonus in patients with Alzheimer's disease. *Neurology*, **36**, 1226–30.

Hauser, W. A., Shinnar, S., Cohen, H. *et al.* (1987). Clinical predictors of epilepsy among children with cerebral palsy and/or mental retardation. *Neurology*, 37 (Suppl. 1), 150–65.

Hauser, W. A., Annegers, J. F., and Kurland, L. T. (1993). Incidence of epilepsy and unprovoked seizures in Rochester, Minnesota: 1935–1984. *Epilepsia*, **34** (3), 453–68.

Herishanu, Y., Abramsky, O., and Lavy, S . (1970). Focal neurological manifestations in hypercalcaemia. *Europ. Neurol.*, **4**, 283–8.

Hillbom, M. E . (1980). Occurrence of cerebral seizures provoked by alcohol abuse. *Epilepsia*, **21**, 459–66.

Hirsch, J. C., Fourment, A., and Marc, M. E. (1983). Sleep-related variations of membrane potential in the lateral geniculate body relay neurons of the cat. *Brain Res.*, **259**, 308–12.

Ho, S. S., Berkovic, S. F., Newton, M. R. *et al.* (1995). Parietal lobe epilepsy: clinical features and seizure localization by ictal SPECT. *Neurology*, 44, 2277–80.

Hodges, J. R. and Warlow, C. P. (1990). Syndromes of transient amnesia: towards a classification. A study of 153 cases. *J. Neurol. Neurosurg. Psychiatry*, **53**, 834–43.

Holland, R. W., Marx, J. A., Earnest, M. P., *et al.* (1993). Grand mal seizures temporally related to cocaine use: clinical and diagnostic features. *Emerg. Med.*, **22**, 758.

Hollman, M. and Heinemann, S. (1994). Cloned glutamate receptors. *Annu. Rev. Neurosci.*, **17**, 31–108.

Holtzman, D., Kaku, D., and So, Y. (1989). New-onset seizures associated with HIV infection: causation and clinical features in 100 cases. *Am J Med.*, **87**, 173–7.

Hopkins, A., Garman, A., and Clarke, C. (1988). The first seizure in adult life. *Lancet*, **1**, 721–6.

Hosford, D. A., Clark S., Cao Z. *et al.* (1992). The role of GABAB receptor activation in absence seizures of lethargic (Lh/Lh) mice. *Science*, **257**, 398–400.

Hotson, R. J. and Prince, D. A. (1981). Penicillin and barium-induced bursting in hippocampal neurons: actions on calcium and potassium potentials. *Ann. Neurol.*, **10**, 11–17.

Howe, J. G. and Gibson, J. D. (1982). Uncinate seizures and tumours, a myth reexamined. *Ann. Neurol.*, **12**, 227–31.

Howell, S. J. L., Owen, L., and Chadwick, D. W . (1989). Pseudostatus epilepticus. *QJM*, **266**, 507–19.

Huttenlocher, P. R. and Hapke, R. J. (1990). A followup study of intractable seizures in childhood. *Ann. Neurol.*, **28**, 699–705.

Ingvar, D. H. and Nyman, G. E. (1962). Epilepticus arithmetices. A new psychologic trigger mechanism in a case of epilepsy. *Neurology*, **12**, 282–7.

Isojarvi, J. I., Laatikainen, T. J., Pakarinen, A. J. *et al.* (1993). Polycystic ovaries and hyperandrogenism in women taking valproate for epilepsy. *N. Engl. J. Med.*, **329** (19), 1383–8.

Isojarvi, J. I., Laatikainen, T. J., Knip, M. *et al.* (1996). Obesity and endocrine disorders in women taking valproate for epilepsy [see comments]. *Ann. Neurol.*, **39** (5), 579–84.

Jackson, J. H. (1873). On the anatomical, physiological and pathological investigation of epilepsies. *West Riding Lunatic Asylum Medical Reports* 3 (3.5). Reprinted in Taylor, J. (ed.) *Selected writings of John Hughlings Jackson*, pp. 90–111. Hodder and Stroughton, London.

Jacob, H. (1970). Muscular twitchings in Alzheimer's disease. In *Alzheimer's disease and related conditions*, (ed. G. E. W. Wolsteholme and M . O'Connor), pp. 758–9. J & A Churchill, London.

Jacobsen, M., Baelum, J., and Bonde, J. P. (1994). Temporal epileptic seizures and occupational exposure to solvents. *Occup. Environ. Med.*, **00**, 429–30.

Jacoby, A., Baker, G. A., Steen, N. *et al.* The clinical course of epilepsy and its psychosocial correlates: findings from a UK community study. *Epilepsia*, 37 (2), 148 61.

Jamshidi, A. and Masroor, M. A. (1976). Glossopharyngeal neuralgia with cardiac syncope. Treatment with a permanent pacemaker and carbamazepine. *Arch. Int. Med.*, **136**, 843–6.

Janz, D. (1962). The grandmal epilepsies and the sleepingwaking cycle. *Epilepsia*, **3**, 69–109.

Janz, D. (1969). *Die Epilepsien*. Thième, Stuttgart.

Janz, D. and Christian, W. (1957). Impulsiv—petit mal. *J. Neurol.*, **176**, 346–86.

Janz, D., Kern, A., Mossinger, H. J. *et al.* (1983). Ruckfallprognose Nach Reduktion Der Medikamente Hei Epilepsiebehandlung. *Nervenarzt*, **54**, 525–9.

Jeavons, P. M. and Harding, G. F. A . (1975). *Photosensitive epilepsy*. Heinemann, London.

Jellinek, E. H. (1962). Fits, faints, coma and dementia in myxoedema. *Lancet*, **2**, 1010–12.

Jennett, W. B. (1975). *Epilepsy after nonmissle head injuries*. Heinemann Medical Books, London.

Johnson, J. W. and Ascher, P. (1987). Glycine potentiates the NMDA response in cultured mouse brain neurons. *Nature*, **325**, 529–31.

Jones, K. L., Lacro, R. V., Johnson, K. A. *et al.* (1989). Pattern of malformations in the children of women treate with carbamazepine during pregnancy. *N. Engl. J. Med.*, **320**, 1661–6.

Jones, R. S. G. and Heinemann, U. (1987). Pre- and post-synaptic K^+ and Ca^{2+} fluxes in area CA1 of the rat hippocampus in vitro: effects of Ni^{2+}, TEA and 4-AP. *Exp. Brain Res.*, **68**, 205–9.

Juul-Jensen, P. and Foldspang, A . (1983). Natural history of epileptic seizures. *Epilepsia*, **24**, 297–312.

Kalviainen, R., Nousiainen, I., Mantyjarvi, M. *et al.* (1998). Initial vigabatrin montherapy is associated with increased risk of visual field constriction. *Epilepsia*, **39** (Suppl. 6), 72.

Kapoor, W. N. and Jannetta, P. J. (1984). Trigeminal neuralgia associated with seizure and syncope. *J. Neurosurg.*, **61**, 594–5.

Kapoor, W. N., Peterson, J. R., and Karpf, M. (1985). Micturition syncope: a reappraisal. *JAMA*, **253**, 796–8.

Kaufman, D. W., Kelly, J. P., Anderson, T. *et al.* (1997). Evaluation of case reports of aplastic anemia among patients treated with felbamate. *Epilepsia*, **38** (12), 1265–9.

Kerr, A. and Eich, R. H. (1961). Cerebral concussion as a cause of cough syncope. *Arch. Int. Med.*, **108**, 248–52.

Kertesz, A. (1967). Paroxysmal kinesigenic choreoathetosis. *Neurology*, **17**, 680–90.

Kilpatrick, C. J., Tress, B. M., O'Donnell, C. *et al.* (1991). Magnetic resonance imaging of late onset epilepsy. *Epilepsia*, **32**, 358–62.

King, D. W., Gallagher, B. B., Murvin, A. J. *et al.* (1982). Pseudoseizures: diagnostic evaluation. *Neurology*, **32**, 18–23.

King, M. A., Newton, M. R., Jackson, G. D. *et al.* (1998). Epileptology of the first-seizure presentation: a clinical, electroencephalographic, and megnetic resonance imaging study of 300 consecutive patients. *Lancet*, **352**, 1007–11.

Kinnunen, E. and Wikstrom, J. (1986). Prevalence and prognosis of epilepsy in patients with multiple sclerosis. *Epilepsia*, **27**, 729–33.

Kiorboe, E. (1961). The prognosis of epilepsy. *Acta Neurol. Scand.*, **36** (Supp. 150), 166–78.

Knochel, J. P. (1977). The pathophysiology and clinical characteristics of severe hypophosphataemia. *Arch. Int. Med.*, **137**, 203–20.

Korczyn, A. D. and Bechar, M. (1976). Convulsive fits in thyrotoxicosis. *Epilepsia*, **17**, 33–4.

Krauss, G. L., Johnson, M. A., and Miller, N. R. (1998). Vigabatrin-associated retinal cone system dysfunction: electroretinogram and ophthalmologic findings. *Neurology*, **50**, 614–18.

Krohn, W. (1963). Causes of death among epileptics. *Epilepsia*, **38**, 439–44.

Kuniasaki, T. A. and Augenstein, W. L. (1994). Drug and toxin-induced seizures. *Emerg. Med. Clin. North Am.*, **12**, 1027–56.

Kuzniecky, R. and Jackson, G. (1995). Neuroimaging in epilepsy. In *Magnetic resonance in epilepsy*, pp. 27–48. Raven Press, New York.

Kuzniecky, R. I. and Jackson, G. D. (1997). Developmental disorders. In *Epilepsy: a comprehensive textbook*, Vol. 3, (ed. J. Engel Jr and T. A. Pedley), pp. 2517–32. Lippincott-Raven, New York.

Lance, J. W. and Adams, R. D. (1963). The syndrome of intention or action myoclonus as a sequel to hypoxic encephalopathy. *Brain*, **86**, 111–36.

Larson, S. J., Sances, A., Baker, J. B. *et al.* (1974). Herniated cerebellar tonsils and cough syncope. *J. Neurosurg.*, **40**, 524–8.

Lavados, J., Germain, I., Morales, A. *et al.* (1992). A descriptive study of epilepsy in the district of El Salvador, Chile, 1984–1988. *Acta Neurol. Scand.*, **91**, 718–29.

Lechtenberg, R. and Worner, T. M. (1992). Seizure incidence enhancement with increasing alcohol intake. *Ann. NY Acad. Sci.*, **654**, 474–6.

Lederman, R. J. and Henry, C. E . (1978). Progressive dialysis encephalopathy. *Ann. Neurol.*, **4**, 199–204.

Leestma, J. E., Kalelkar, M. B., Teas, S. S. *et al.* (1984). Sudden unexpected death associated with seizures: analysis of 66 cases. *Epilepsia*, **25**, 84–8.

Legg, N. J., Gupta, P. C., and Scott, D. F. (1973). Epilepsy following cerebral abscess: a clinical and EEG study of 70 patients. *Brain*, **96**, 259–68.

Lehericy, S., Dormont, D., Semah, F. *et al.* (1995). Developmental abnormalities of the medial temporal lobe in patients with temporal lobe epilepsy. *Am. J. Neuroradiol.*, **16**, 617–23.

Lempert, T., Bauer, M., and Schmidt, D. (1994). Syncope: a videometric analysis of 56 episodes of transient cerebral hypoxia. *Ann. Neurol.*, **36**, 233–7.

Lesser, R. P., Luders, H., Dinner, D. S. *et al.* (1985). Epileptic seizures due to thrombotic and embolic cerebrovascular disease in older patients. *Epilepsia*, **26**, 622–30.

Lesser, R. P., Luders, H., Dinner, D. S. *et al.* (1987). Simple partial seizures in epilepsy. In *Electroclinical syndromes*, (ed. H. Luders and R. P. Lesser), pp. 223–78. SpringerVerlag, London.

Levin, B. and Posner, J. B . (1972). Swallow syncope report of a case and review of the literature. *Neurology*, 22, 1086–93.

Lindhout, D. and Schmidt, D. (1986). In-utero exposure to valproate and neural tube defects. *Lancet*, 1, 1392–3.

Lishman, W. A., Symonds, P., Whitty, C. W. M. *et al.* (1962). Seizures induced by movement. *Brain*, 85, 93–108.

Liu, Z., Vergnes, M., Depaulis, A. *et al.* (1992). Involvement of intrathalamic GABAB neurotransmission in the control of absence seizures in the rat. *Neuroscience*, 48, 87–93.

Logothetis, J. (1967). Spontaneous epileptic seizure and electroencephalographic changes in the course of phenothiazine therapy. *Neurology*, 17, 869–77.

Loiseau, J., Loiseau, P., Duche, B. *et al.* (1990). A survey of epileptic disorders in Southwest France: seizures in elderly patients. *Ann. Neurol.*, 27, 232–7.

Loiseau, P. (1985). Childhood absence epilepsy. In *Epileptic syndromes in infancy, childhood and adolescence*, (ed. J. Roger, C. Dravet, M. Bureau, F. E. Dreifuss, and P. Wolf), pp. 106–20. John Libbey, London.

Loiseau, P., Pestre, M., Dartigues, J. F. *et al.* (1983). Longterm prognosis in two forms of childhood epilepsy; typical absence seizures and epilepsy with Rolandic (centrotemporal) EEG foci. *Ann. Neurol.*, 13, 642–8.

Lown, B . (1967). Electrical reversion of cardiac arrhythmias. *Br Heart J.*, 29, 469–89.

Lowry, M. R. and Dunner, F. J. (1980). Seizures during tricyclic therapy. *Am. J. Psychiatry*, 137, 1461–2.

Lund, M . (1952). Epilepsy associated with intracranial tumours. *Acta Psych. Neurol. Scand. Suppl.*, 81.

Lyle, C. B., Monroe, J. T., Finn, D. E. *et al.* (1961). Micturition syncope. Report of 24 cases. *N. Engl. J. Med.*, 265, 982–6.

Macdonald, D. R., Strong, E., Nielson, S. *et al.* (1983). Syncope from head and neck cancer. *J. Neurol.*, 1, 257–67.

Macdonald, R. L. and Olsen, R. W. (1994). GABA$_A$ receptor channels. *Annu. Rev. Neurosci.*, 7, 569–602.

Maclean, A. E., Allen, E. V., and Magrath, T. B. (1944). Orthostatic tachycardia and orthostatic hypotension: defects in return of venous blood to the heart. *Am. Heart Assoc.*, 27, 145–63.

Maeda, Y., Kurokawa, T., Sakamoto, K. *et al.* (1990). Electroclinical study of video-game epilepsy. *Dev. Med. Child Neurol.*, 32, 493–500.

Maletzky, B. M. (1973). The episodic dyscontrol syndrome. *Dis. Nervous Syst.*, 34, 178–85.

Malouf, R. and Brust, J. C. M. (1985). Hypoglycaemia: causes, neurological manifestations and outcome. *Ann. Neurol.*, 17, 421–30.

Marks, V. (1981). Symptomatology. In *Hypoglycaemia*, (2nd edn), (ed. V. Marks and F. C. Rose), pp. 458–63. Blackwell Scientific Publications, Oxford.

Marson, A. G., Beghi, E., Berg, A. *et al.* (1996). The Cochrane Collaboration and its relevance to epilepsy. *Epilepsia*, in press.

Marson, A. G., Kadir, Z. A., Hutton, J. L. *et al.* (1997). The new antiepileptic drugs: a systematic review of their efficacy and tolerability. *Epilepsia*, 38 (8), 859–80.

Mathern, G. W., Pretorius, J. K., and Babb, T. L. (1995). Influence of the type of initial precipitating injury and at what age it occurs on course and outcome in patients with temporal lobe seizures. *J. Neurosurg.*, 82, 220–7.

Matthews, W. B. (1975). Paroxysmal symptoms in multiple sclerosis. *J. Neurol. Neurosurg. Psychiatry*, 36, 617–23.

Mattson, R. H., Sturman, J. K., Gronowski, M. L., and Goico, H. (1975). Effect of alcohol intake in nonalcoholic epileptics. *Neurology*, 25, 361–2.

Mattson, R. H., Cramer, J. A., Collins, J. F. *et al.* (1985). Comparison of carbamazepine, phenobarbital, phenytoin, and primidone in partial and secondarily generalized tonic–clonic seizures. *N. Engl. J. Med.*, 313 (3), 145–51.

Mattson, R. H., Cramer, J. A., and Collins, J. F. (1992). A comparison of valproate with carbamazepine for the treatment of complex partial seizures and secondarily generalised tonic clonic seizures in adults. *N. Engl. J. Med.*, 327 (11), 765–71.

Mauguiere, F. and Courjon, J. (1978). Somatosensory epilepsy: a review of 127 cases. *Brain*, 101, 307–32.

Maurice-Williams, R. M. (1974). Micturition symptoms in frontal tumours. *J. Neurol. Neurosurg. Psychiatry*, 37, 431–6.

Mayersdorf, A. and Marshall, C. (1970). Pattern activation in reading epilepsy: a case report. *Epilepsia*, 2, 423–6.

Mayeux, R. and Lender, H. (1978). Complex partial status epilepticus: case report and proposal for diagnostic criteria. *Neurology*, 00, 957–61.

Mayeux, R., Alexander, M. P., Benson, D. F. *et al.* (1979). Poriomania. *Neurology*, 00, 1616–19.

McCrory, P. R., Bladin, P. F., and Berkovic, S. F. (1997). Retrospective study of concussive convulsions in elite Australian Rules and Rugby League footballers: phenomenology, aetiology, and outcome. *BMJ*, 314, 171–4.

McEnery, P. T., Nathan, J., Bates, S. R. *et al.* (1989). Convulsion in children undergoing renal transplantation. *J. Paediatr.*, 00, 532–6.

McNamara, J. O., Russell, R. D., Rigsbee, L. *et al.* (1988). Anticonvulsant and antiepileptogenic actions of MK-801 in the kindling and electroshock models. *Neuropharmacology*, 27, 563–8.

McQueen, J. K., Blackwood, D. H., Harris, P. *et al.* (1983). Low risk of late posttraumatic seizures following severe head injury: implications for clinical trials of prophylaxis. *J. Neurol., Neurosurg. Psychiatry*, 46, 899–904.

Meador, K. J., Loring, D. W., Huh, K. *et al.* (1990). Comparative cognitive effects of anticonvulsants. *Neurology*, 40 (3, Pt 1), 391–4.

Medical Research Council Antiepileptic Drug Withdrawal Study Group (1991). Randomised study of antiepileptic drug withdrawal in patients in remission. *Lancet*, 337, 1175–80.

Medical Research Council Antiepileptic Drug Withdrawal Study Group (1993). Prognostic index for recurrence of seizures after remission of epilepsy. *BMJ*, 306, 1374–8.

Medina, M. T., Rosas, E., Rubio-Donnadieu, F. *et al.* (1990). Neurocysticercosis as the main cause of late-onset epilepsy in Mexico. *Arch. Int. Med.*, 150 (2), 325–7.

Meldrum, B. S. (1975). Epilepsy and gamma-aminobutyric acid inhibition. *Int. Rev. Neurobiol.*, 17, 1–25.

Meldrum, B. S. (1984). Amino acid neurotransmitters and new approaches to anticonvulsant drug action. *Epilepsia*, 25 (Suppl. 2), 140–6.

Meldrum, B. S. and Horton, R. W. (1973). Physiology of status epilepticus in primates. *Arch. Neurol.*, 28, 1–9.

Messing, R. O. and Simon, R. P. (1986). Seizures as a manifestation of systemic disease. *Neurologic Clin.*, 4, 563–84.

Messing, R. O., Closson, R. G., and Simon, R. P. (1984). Drug-induced seizures: A 10 year experience. *Neurology*, 34, 1582–6.

Metrakos, J. D. and Metrakos, K. (1972). Genetic factors in the epilepsies. In *The epidemilogy of epilepsy: a workshop*, Vol. 14, (ed. R. Alter and W. A. Hauser), pp. 97–102. NINDS Monograph. US Government Printing Office, Washington DC.

Moots, P. L., Maciunas, R. J., Eiscrt, D. R. *et al.* (1995). The course of seizure disorders in patients with malignant gliomas. *Arch. Neurol.*, 52, 717–24.

Moreau, Th., Sochurova, D., Lemesle, M. *et al.* (1998). Epilepsy in patients with multiple sclerosis: radiologocal-clinical correlations. *Epilepsia*, 39, 893–6.

Morrell, F. (1985). Secondary epileptogenesis in Man. *Arch. Neurol.*, 42, 318–35.

Morrell, F., Whisler, W. W., and Bleck, T. P. (1989). Multiple sub-pial transection: a new approach to the surgical treatment of focal epilepsy. *J. Neurosurg.*, 70, 231–9.

Morrell, M. (1997). Pregnancy and epilepsy. In *The Epilepsies 2*, (ed. R. J. Porter and D. Chadwick), pp. 313–46. Butterworth-Heinemann, Boston.

Moshe, S. L. (1981). The effects of age on the kindling phenomenon. *Dev. Psychobiol.*, 14, 75–81.

Mount, L. A. and Reback, J. (1940). Familial paroxysmal choreoathetosis: preliminary report on a hitherto undescribed clinical syndrome. *Arch. Neurol.*, 44, 841–6.

Muller, R. (1949). Studies on disseminated sclerosis with special reference to symptomatology, course and prognosis. *Acta Med. Scand.*, 133 (Suppl. 222), 11–24.

Nakane, Y., Okuma, T., Takashi, R. *et al.* (1980). Multi-institutional study on the teratogenicity and fetal toxicity of antiepileptic drugs. a report of a collaborative study group in Japan. *Epilepsia*, 21, 663–80.

Nashef, L., Fish, D. R., Garner, S. *et al.* (1995a). Sudden death in epilepsy: a study of incidence in a young cohort with epilepsy and learning difficulty. *Epilepsia*, 36 (12), 1187–94.

Nashef, L., Fish, D. R., Sander, J. W. *et al.* (1995b). Incidence of sudden unexpected death in an adult outpatient cohort with epilepsy at a tertiary referral centre. *J. Neurol. Neurosurg. Psychiatry*, 58 (4), 462–4.

Neuspiel, D. R. and Kuller, L. H. (1985). Sudden and unexpected natural death in childhood and adolescence. *JAMA*, 254, 1321–5.

Newmark, M. E. and Penry, J. K. (1980). Catamenial epilepsy: a review. *Epilepsia*, 21, 281–300.

Ng, S. K. C., Hauser, W. A., Brust, J. C. M. *et al.* (1988). Alcohol consumption and withdrawal in new onset seizures. *N. Engl. J. Med.*, 319, 666–73.

Nielsen, T. G., Sillesen, H., and Schroeder, T. V. (1995). Seizures following carotid endarterectomy in patients with severely compromised cerebral circulation. *Eur. J. Vasc. Endovasc. Surg.*, 9 (1), 53–7.

NIH Consensus Conference (1990). Surgery for epilepsy. *JAMA*, 264, 729–33.

Norenberg, M. D., Leslie, K. O., and Robertson, A. S. (1982). Association between rise in serum sodium and central pontine myelinolysis. *Ann. Neurol.*, 11, 128–35.

North, J. B., Penhall, R. K., Hanieh, A. *et al.* (1983). Phenytoin and postoperative epilepsy: a double blind study. *J. Neurosurg.*, 58, 672–7.

Ochs, R., Bloor, P., Quesney, F. *et al.* (1984). Does headturning during a seizure have lateralising or localising significance? *Neurology*, 34, 884–90.

OllerDaurella, L. and Sanchez, M. E. (1981). Evolucion De Las Ausencias Tipicas. *Rev. Neurol. (Barcelona)*, 9, 81–102.

Oppenheimer, H. B. (1966). Persistent intracranial bleeding as a complication of hemispherectomy. *J. Neurol. Neurosurg. Psychiatry*, 29, 229–40.

Ottman, R., Risch, N., Hauser, W. A. *et al.* (1995). Localization of a gene for partial epilepsy to chromosome 10q. *Nature Genetics*, 10 (1), 56–60.

Oxbury, J. M. and Adams, C. B. T. (1989). Neurosurgery for epilepsy. *Br. J. Hosp. Med.*, **41**, 372–7.

Palmini, A., Andermann, F., Aicardi, J. *et al.* (1991). Diffuse cortical dysplasia, or the 'double cortex' syndrome: the clinical and epileptic spectrum in 10 patients. *Neurology*, **41** (10), 1656–62.

Panayiotopoulos, C. P., Chroni, E., Daskalopoulos, C. *et al.* (1992). Typical absence seizures in adults: clinical, EEG, video-EEG findings and diagnostic/syndromic considerations. *J. Neurol. Neurosurg. Psychiatry*, **55**, 1002–8.

Panayiotopoulos, C. P., Ferrie, C. D., Giannakodimos, S. *et al.* (1994). Perioral myoclonia with absences: a new syndrome? In *Epileptic seizures and syndromes*, (ed. P. Wolf), pp. 143–53. John Libbey, London.

Parkes, J. D. (1982). Narcolepsy. In *Pseudoseizures*, (ed. T. L. Riley and A. Roy), pp. 62–8. Williams & Wilkins, Baltimore.

Pascual-Leone, A., Dhuna, A., Altafullah, I. *et al.* (1990). Cocaine-induced seizures. *Neurology*, **40** (3 Pt 1), 404–7.

Pathy, M. S . (1978). Defaecation syncope. *Age and Ageing*, 7, 233–6.

Pederson, A., Sandoe, E., Hvidberg, E. *et al.* (1966). Studies on the mechanism of tussive syncope. *Acta Med. Scand.*, **179**, 653–61.

Pedley, T. A. and Guilleminault, C. (1977). Episodic nocturnal wanderings responsive to anticonvulsant drug therapy. *Ann. Neurol.*, **2**, 30–5.

Penfield, W. and Jasper, H. (1954). *Epilepsy and the functional anatomy of the human brain*. Little, Brown, Boston.

Perucca, E., Gram, L., Avanzini, G. *et al.* (1998). Antiepileptic drugs as a cause of worsening of seizures. *Epilepsia*, **39** (1), 5–17.

Peters, A. C. B., Brouwer, O. F., Geerts, A. T. *et al.* (1998). Randomised prospective study of early discontinuation of antiepileptic drugs in children with epilepsy: Dutch study of epilepsy in childhood. *Neurology*, **50**, 724–30.

Phillips, G . (1954). Traumatic epilepsy after closed head injury. *J. Neurol. Neurosurg. Psychiatry*, **17**, 110 24.

Pincus, J. H. (1978). Disorders of conscious awareness: hyperventilation syndrome. *Br. J. Hosp. Med.*, **19**, 312–13.

Plum, F. and Hindfelt, B. (1968). The neurological complications of liver disease. In *Handbook of clinical neurology*, Vol. 27, (ed. P. J. Vinken and G. W. Bruyn), pp. 349–77. Elsevier, Amsterdam.

Plum, F. and Posner, J. B. (1980). *The diagnosis of stupor and coma*, (3rd edn). F. A. Davis, Philadelphia.

Poskanzer, D. C., Brown, A. E., and Miller, H. (1962). Musicogenic epilepsy caused only be a discrete frequency band of church bells. *Brain*, **85**, 77–92.

Preter, M., Tzourio, C. T., Ameri, A. *et al.* (1996). Long-term prognosis in cerebral venouis thrombosis. *Stroke*, **27**, 243–6.

Prince, D. A. (1978). Neurophysiology of epilepsy. *Annu. Rev. Neurosci.*, **1**, 395–415.

Prince, D. A. and Farrell, D. (1969). 'Centrencephalic' spikewave discharges following parental penicillin injection in the cat. *Neurology*, **19**, 309–10.

Quesney, L. F. (1986). Seizures of frontal lobe origin. In *Recent advances in epilepsy*, Vol. 3, (ed. T. A. Pedley and B. S. Meldrum), pp. 81–110. Churchill Livingstone, Edinburgh.

Rapport, R. L. and Penry, J. K . (1973). A survey of attitudes towards the pharmacological prophylaxis of posttraumatic epilepsy. *J. Neurosurg.*, **38**, 159–66.

Raskin, N. H. and Fishman, R. A. (1976). Neurologic disorders in renal failure. *N. Engl. J. Med.*, **294**, 204–10.

Rasmussen, T., Olszewski, J., and LloydSmith, D. (1958). Focal seizures due to localized chronic encephalitis. *Neurology*, **8**, 435–48.

Raymond, A. A., Fish, D. R., Sisodiya, S. M. *et al.* (1995). Abnormalities of gyration, heteratopias, tuberose sclerosis, focal cortical dysplasia, microdysgenesis, dysembryoplastic neuroepithelial tumour and dysgenesis of the archicortex in epilepsy. *Brain*, **118**, 629–41.

Raynor, R. B., Paine, R. S., and Carmichael, E. A. (1959). Epilepsy of late onset. *Neurology*, **9**, 111–17.

Reynolds, E. H. (1987). Early treatment and prognosis of epilepsy. *Epilepsia*, **28**, 97–106.

Reynolds, N. C. and Miska, R. M. (1976). Safety of anticonvulsants in hepatic porphyrias. *Neurology*, **31**, 480–4.

Richens, A. (1992). Lamotrigine. In *Recent advances in epilepsy*, Vol. 5, (ed. T. A. Pedley and B. S. Meldrum), pp. 197–210. Churchill Livingstone, Edinburgh.

Richens, A. (1997). Vigabatrin and lamotrigine. In *The epilepsies 2*, (ed. R. J. Porter and D. Chadwick), pp. 201–22. Butterworth Heinemann, New York.

Richens, A. and Dunlop, A. (1975). Serum phenytoin levels in the management of epilepsy. *Lancet*, **2**, 247–9.

Richens, A., Davidson, D. L., Cartlidge, N. E. *et al.* (1994) A multicentre comparative trial of sodium valproate and carbamazepine in adult onset epilepsy. Adult EPITEG Collaborative Group. *J. Neurol. Neurosurg. Psychiatry*, **57** (6), 682–7.

Riikonen, R. (1996). Long-term outcome of West syndrome: a study of adults with a history of infantile spasms. *Epilepsia*, **37** (4), 367–72.

Riley, H. A., German, W. J., Wortis, H. *et al.* (1942). Glossopharyngeal neuralgia initiating or associated with cardiac arrest. *Trans. Am. Neurol. Assoc.*, **68**, 28–30.

Riley, T. L. (1982). Syncope and hyperventilation. In *Pseudoseizures*, (ed. T. L. Riley and A. Roy), pp. 34–61. Williams & Wilkins, Baltimore.

Risser, W. L. (1985). Syncope in adolescents. *Am. Fam. Physician*, **32**, 117–23.

Roberts, M. A. and Humphrey, P. R. D. (1988). Prolonged complex partial status epilepticus: a case report. *J. Neurol. Neurosurg. Psychiatry*, **51**, 586–92.

Robin, J. J., Tolan, G. D., and Arnold, J. W. (1978). Ten year experience with abnormal EEG's in asymptomatic adult males. *Aviat. Space Environ. Med.*, **49**, 732–40.

Rocca, W. A., Sharbrough, F. W., Hauser, W. A. *et al.* (1987). Risk factors for complex partial seizures: a population-based casecontrol study. *Ann. Neurol.*, **21**, 22–31.

Rogers, S. W., Andrew, P. I., Gahring, L. C. *et al.* (1994). Autoantibodies to glutamate receptor GluR3 in Rasmussen's encephalitis. *Science*, **265**, 648–51.

Romanelli, M. F., Morris, J. C., Ashkin, K. *et al.* (1990). Advanced Alzheimer's disease is a risk factor for late onset seizures. *Arch. Neurol.*, **47**, 847–50.

Rosa, F. H. (1990). Spina bifida in maternal carbamazepine exposure cohort data. *Teratology*, **41**, 587–8.

Ross, R. T. (1988). *Syncope*. W. B. Saunders, London.

Rowan, A. J. and French, J. A. (1988). The role of the electroencephalogram in the diagnosis and management of epilepsy. In *Recent advances in epilepsy*, Vol. 4, (ed. T. A. Pedley and B. S. Meldrum), pp. 63–92. Raven Press, New York.

Rowan, A. J., Binnie, C. D., Warfield, C. A. *et al.* (1979). The delayed effect of sodium valproate on the photoconvulsive response in man. *Epilepsia*, **20**, 618–24.

Roy, A. (1979). Hysterical seizures. *Arch. Neurol.*, **36**, 447–54.

Rubenstein, J. J., Schulman, C. L., Yurchak, P. M. *et al.* (1972). Clinical spectrum of the sick sinus syndrome. *Circulation*, **46**, 513–25.

Russell, W. R. and Whitty, C. W. M. (1952). Studies in traumatic epilepsy, Part I Factors influencing the incidence of epilepsy after brain wounds. *J. Neurol. Neurosurg. Psychiatry*, **15**, 93–8.

Rwiza, H. T., Kilonzo, G. P., Haule, J. *et al.* (1992). Prevalence and incidence of epilepsy in Ulanga, a rural Tanzanian district: a community-based study. *Epilepsia*, **33**, 1051–6.

Salazar, A. M., Jabbari, B., Vance, S. C. *et al.* (1985). Epilepsy after penetrating head injury: I. Clinical correlates. *Neurology*, **35**, 1406–14.

Salmenpera, T., Kalviainen, R., Partanen, K. *et al.* (1998). Hippocampal damage caused by seizures in temporal lobe epilepsy [Letter; see Comments]. *Lancet*, **351** (9095), 35.

Samren, E. B., van Duijn, C. M., Koch, S. *et al.* (1997). maternal use of antiepileptic drugs and the risk of major congenital malformations: a joint European study of human teratogenesis associated with maternal epilepsy. *Epilepsia*, **38**, 981–90.

Sander, J. W. A. S. and Shorvon, S. D. (1987). Incidence and prevalence studies in epilepsy and their methodological problems: a review. *J. Neurol. Neurosurg. Psychiatry*, **50**, 829–39.

Sander, J. W. A. S., Hart, Y. M., Johnson, A. L. *et al.* (1990*a*). National General Practice Study of Epilepsy: newly diagnosed seizures in a general population. *Lancet*, **336**, 1267–71.

Sander, J. W. A. S., Trevisol-Bittencourt, P. C., Hart, Y. M. *et al.* (1990*b*). Evaluation of vigabatrin as an add-on drug in the management of severe epilepsy. *J. Neurol. Neurosurg. Psychiatry*, **53**, 1008–10.

Satishchandra, P., Chandra, V., and Schoenberg, B. S. (1988). Case control study of associated conditions at the time of death in patients with epilepsy. *Neuroepidemiology*, **7**, 109–14.

Schamroth, L. (1971). *The disorders of cardiac rhythm*. Blackwell Scientific Publications, Oxford.

Schechter, P. J., Tranier, Y., Jung, M. J. *et al.* (1977). Audiogenic seizure protection by elevated brain GABA concentration in mice: effects of gamma-acetylenic GABA and gamma-vinyl GABA, two irreversible GABA-T inhibitors. *Eur. J. Pharmacol.*, **45**, 319.

Scheffer, I. E. and Berkovic, S. F. (1997). Generalized epilepsy with febrile seizures plus. A genetic disorder with heterogeneous clinical phenotypes. *Brain*, **120** (Pt 3), 479–90.

Scheffer, I. E., Bhatia, K. P., Lopes-Cendes, I. *et al.* (1995). Autosomal dominant nocturnal frontal lobe epilepsy—a distinctive clinical disorder. *Brain*, **118**, 61.

Schierhout, G. and Roberts, I. (1998). Prophylactic antiepileptic agents after head injury: a systematic review. *J. Neurol. Neurosurg. Psychiatry*, **64**, 108–12.

Schmidt, D. (1982). *Adverse effects of antiepileptic drugs*. Raven Press, New York.

Schofield, P. R., Darlison, M. G., and Fujita, N. (1987) Sequence and functional expression of the GABA_A receptor shows a ligand-gated receptor super-family. *Nature*, **328**, 221–7.

Schwartz, L. S., Goldfischer, J., Sprague, G. J. *et al.* (1969). Syncope and sudden death in aortic stenosis. *Am. J. Cardiol.*, **23**, 647–58.

Scott, R. H., Pearson, H. A., and Dolphin, A. C. (1991). Aspects of vertebrate neuronal voltage-activated calcium currents and their regulation. *Prog. Neurobiol.*, **36**, 485–520.

Selwa, L. M., Berent, S., Giordani, B. *et al.* (1994). Serial cognitive testing in temporal lobe epilepsy: longitudinal changes with medical and surgical therapies. *Epilepsia*, **35**, 743–9.

Servit, Z. and Musil, F. (1981). Prophylactic treatment of posttraumatic epilepsy; results of a longterm followup in Czechoslovakia. *Epilepsia*, **22**, 315–20.

Shafer, S. Q., Hauser, W. A., Annegers, J. F. *et al.* (1988). EEG and other early predictors of epilepsy remission: a community study. *Epilepsia*, **29**, 590–600.

Shannon, M. and Goetz, G. (1989). Connective tissue diseases and the nervous system. In *Neurology and general medicine*, (ed. M. Aminoff), pp. 389–412. Churchill Livingstone, New York.

Sheps, S. G. (1976). The use of an elastic garment in the treatment of idopathic orthostatic hypotension. *Cardiology*, **61**, 271–9.

Shinnar, S. and Berg, A. T. (1996). Does antiepileptic drug therapy prevent the development of 'chronic' epilepsy? *Epilepsia*, **37** (8), 701–8.

Shinnar, S., Berg, A. T., Mooke, S. L. *et al.* (1994). Discontinuing antiepileptic drugs in children with epilepsy: a prospective study. *Ann. Neurol.*, **35**, 534–45.

Shinton, R. A., Zezulka, A. V., Gill, J. S. *et al.* (1987). The frequency of epilepsy preceding stroke. *Lancet*, **1**, 1113–16.

Shorvon, S. D. (1994). *Status epilepticus. Its clinical features and treatment in children and adults.* Cambridge University Press, Cambridge.

Shorvon, S. D., Gilliat, R. W., Cox, T. C. S. *et al.* (1984). Evidence of vascular disease from CT scanning in late onset epilepsy. *J. Neurol., Neurosurg. Psychiatry*, **47**, 225–30.

Simon, R. P. (1988). Alcohol and seizures. *N. Engl. J. Med.*, **309**, 715–16.

Sloviter, R. S. (1991). Permanently altered hippocampal structure, excitability and inhibition after experimental status epilepticus in the rat; the 'dorman basket cell' hypothesis and its possible relevance to temporal lobe epilepsy. *Hippocampus*, **1**, 41–66.

Smith, B. H. (1960). Vestibular disturbance in epilepsy. *Neurology*, **10**, 465–9.

Smith, D. F., Hutton, J. L., Sandemann, D. *et al.* (1991). The Prognosis of primary intracerebral tumours presenting with epilepsy: the outcome of medical and surgical management. *J. Neurol. Neurosurg. Psychiatry*, **54** (10), 915–20.

Snead, O. C. (1995). Basic mechanisms of generalized absence seizures. *Ann. Neurol.*, **37**, 146–57.

Sofijanov, N. G. (1982). Clinical evolution and prognosis of childhood epilepsies. *Epilepsia*, **23**, 61–9.

Soloff, L. A. and Rodman, T. (1967). Acute pulmonary embolism. II. Clinical features. *Am. Heart J.*, **74**, 710–24.

Spencer, S. S., Gates, J. R., Reeves, A. R. *et al.* (1987). Corpus callosum section. In *Surgical treatment of the epilepsies*, (ed. J. Engel), pp. 425–44. Raven Press, New York.

StaffordClark, D. and Taylor, F. H. (1949). Clinical and electroencephalographic studies of prisoners charged with murder. *J. Neurol., Neurosurg. Psychiatry*, **12**, 325–30.

Stefani, A., Spadoni, F., and Bernardi, G. (1997). Voltage-activated calcium channels: targets of antiepileptic drug therapy. *Epilepsia*, **38**, 959–65.

Steinlein, O. K., Mulley, J. C., Propping, P. *et al.* (1995). A missense mutation in the neuronal nicotinic receptor *a*4 subunit is associated with autosomal dominant nocturnal frontal lobe epilepsy. *Nature Genet.*, **11**, 201.

Stengel, E. (1943). Further studies on pathological wandering (fugue with the impuse to wander). *J. Mental Sci.*, **89**, 224–41.

Stephenson, J. B. P. (1971). Uraemia as a determinant of convulsions in acute infantile hypernatraemia. *Arch. Dis. Child.*, **46**, 676–79.

Stevens, D. L. and Matthews, W. B. (1973). Cryptogenic drop attacks. An affliction of women. *BMJ*, **1**, 439–42.

Storey, P. B. (1967). Psychiatric sequelae of subarachnoid haemorrhage. *BMJ*, **3**, 261–6.

Storm, J. F. (1987). Action potential repolarisation and a fast after-hyperpolarisation in rat hippocampal pyramidal cells. *J. Physiol. (Lond.)*, **385**, 733–59.

Subramaniam, S., Donevan, S. D., and Rogawski, M. A. (1996) Block of the *N*-methyl-D-aspartate receptor by remacemide and its des-glycine metabolite. *J. Pharmacol. Exp. Ther.*, **276**, 161.

Sumi, S. M. and Teasdall, R. D. (1963). Focal seizures. A review of 150 cases. *Neurology*, **13**, 582–6.

Sutton, R. and Perrins, E. J. (1979). Neurological manifestations of the sick sinus syndrome. In *Cerebral manifestations of episodic cardiac dysrhythmias*, (ed. E. Busse), pp. 174–81. Excerpta Medica, Amsterdam.

Sutula, T., He, X. X., Cavazos, J. *et al.* (1988). Synaptic reorganization in the hippocampus induced by abnormal functional activity. *Science*, **239**, 1147–50.

Swanson, P. D. (1976). Neurological manifestations of hypernatraemia. In *Handbook of Clinical Neurology*, Vol. 28, (ed. P. J. Vinken and G. W. Bruyn), Elsevier, Amsterdam.

Tang, C.-M., Dichter, M., and Morad, M. (1989). Quisqualate activates a rapidly inactivating high conductance ionic channel in hippocampal neurons. *Science*, **243**, 1474–7.

Taylor, R. L. (1981). Magnesium sulphate for AIP seizures. *Neurology*, **31**, 1371–2.

Temkin, N. R., Dikmen, S. S., Wilensky, A. J., *et al.* (1990). A randomized, doubleblind study of phenytoin for the prevention of posttraumatic seizures. *N. Engl. J. Med.*, **323**, 497–502.

Tennison, M. B., Greenwood, R. S. Lewis, D. V. *et al.* (1994). Rate of taper of antiepileptic drugs in children with epilepsy: a comparison of six-week and nine-month taper periods. *N. Engl. J. Med.*, **330**, 1407–10.

Thomas, J. E. (1969). Hyperactive carotid sinus reflex and carotid sinus syncope. *Mayo Clin. Proc.*, **44**, 127–39.

Thrush, D. C. and Boddie, H. G. (1974). Episodic encephalopathy associated with thyroid disorders. *J. Neurol. Neurosurg. Psychiatry*, 37, 696–700.

Tomlinson, J. W. and Fox, K. M. (1975). Carcinoma of the oesophagus with 'swallow syncope. *BMJ.*, 2, 315–16.

Traub, R. D. and Jefferys, J. G. R. (1998). Epilepsy in vitro: electrophysiology and computer modeling. In *Epilepsy: a comprehensive textbook*, (ed. J. Engel and T. A. Pedley), pp. 405–18. Lippincott-Raven, New York.

Treiman, D. M. and Delgado-Escueta, A. V. (1980). Status epilepticus. In *Critical care of neurological and neurosurgical emergencies*, (ed. R. A. Thomson and J. R. Green), pp. 53–99. Raven Press, New York.

Treiman, D. N. and Delgado-Escueta, A. V. (1983). Violence in epilepsy: a critical review. In *Recent advances in epilepsy*, (ed. T. A. Pedley and B. S. Meldrum), pp. 179–209. Churchill Livingstone, Edinburgh.

Treiman, D. M., Walton, N. Y., and Kendrick, C. (1990). A progressive sequence of electroencephalographic changes during generalised convulsive status epilepticus. *Epilepsy Res.*, 5, 49–60.

Treiman, D. M., Meyers, P. D., Walton, N. Y. *et al.* (1998). A comparison of four treatments for generalized convulsive status epilepticus. Veterans Affairs Status Epilepticus Cooperative Study Group. *N. Engl. J. Med.*, 339 (12), 792–8.

Trout, H. H., Brown, L. L., and Thompson, J. E. (1979). Carotid sinus syndrome: treatment by carotid sinus denervation. *Ann. Surg.*, 189, 575–80.

Tsuboi, M., Suzuki, K., Nagao, S. *et al.* (1985). Glossopharyngeal neuralgia with cardiac syncope. A case successfully treated with microvascular decompression. *Surg. Neurol.*, 24, 279–83.

Tsuki, H. and Kasuga, I. (1978). Paroxysmal discharges triggered by hearing spoken language. *Epilepsia*, 19, 147–54.

Turnbull, D. M., Rawlins, M. D., Weightman, D. *et al.* (1983). Plasma concentrations of sodium valproate: their clinical value. *Ann. Neurol.*, 14, 38–42.

Turnbull, D. M., Howell, D., Rawlins, M. D. *et al.* (1985). Which drug for the adult epileptic patient: phenytoin or valproate? *BMJ*, 290, 815–19.

Valdueza, J. M., Cristante, L., Dammann, O. *et al.* (1994). Hypothalamic hamartomas with special reference to gelastic epilepsy and surgery. *Neurosurgery*, 34, 949–58.

Van Buren, J. M. (1963). The abdominal aura: a study of abdominal sensations occurring in epilepsy and produced by depth stimulation. *Electroencephalogr. Clin. Neurophysiol.*, 15, 119–23.

Venna, N. and Sabin, T. D. (1981). Tonic focal seizures in nonketotic hyperglycaemia of diabetes mellitus. *Arch. Neurol.*, 38, 512–14.

Victor, M. and Brausch, C. (1967). The role of abstinence in the genesis of alcoholic epilepsy. *Epilepsia*, 8, 120–5.

Walker, J. E. (1981). Effect of aminophylline on seizure thresholds and brain regional cyclic nucleotides in the rat. *Exp. Neurol.*, 74, 299–304.

Walker, A. E. and Erculei, F. (1968). *Head-injured men 15 years later*. Charles C. Thomas, Springfield, Illinois.

Walker, A. E. and Jablon, S. (1961). *A followup study of head wounds in World War II*. Veterans Association Medical Monographs. US Government Printing Office, Washington DC.

Wallace, R. H., Wang, D. W., Singh, R. *et al.* (1998). Febrile seizures and generalized epilepsy associated with a mutation in the Na$^+$-channel beta-1 subunit gene *SCN1B*. *Nature Genet.*, 19 (4), 366–70.

Walton, N. Y. (1993). Systematic effects of convulsive status epilepticus. *Epilepsia*, 34 (Supp. 1), S54–S58.

Wardrope, J., Ryan, F., Clark, G. *et al.* (1991). The Hillsborough Tragedy [see Comments]. *BMJ*, 303 (6814), 1381–5.

Weaver, S., Forsyth, P., Fulton, D. *et al.* (1995). A prospective randomised study of prophylactic anticonvulsants (AC) in patients with primary brain tumors (PBT) or metastatic brain tumors (MBT) and without prior seizures (Sz): a preliminary analysis of 67 patients. *Neurology*, 45 (Suppl. 4), A263.

Weissler, A. M., Warren, J. V., Estes, E. H. *et al.* (1957). Vasodepressor syncope factors influencing cardiac output. *Circulation*, 15, 875–82.

White, H. S. (1997). Mechanisms of antiepileptic drugs. In *The epilepsies 2*, (ed. R. J. a. C. D. Porter), pp. 1–30. Butterworth-Heinemann.

White, H. S., Harmsworth, W. L., Sofia, R. D. *et al.* (1995). Felbamate modulates the strychnine-insensitive glycine receptor. *Epilepsy Res.*, 20, 41.

Whitehouse, W. P., Rees, M., Curtis, D. *et al.* (1993). Linkage analysis of idiopathic generalized and marker loci on chromosome 6p in families of patients with juvenile myoclonic epilepsy: no evidence for an epilepsy locus in the HLA region. *Am. J. Hum. Genet.*, 53, 652.

Whitteridge, D. (1960). Cardiovascular reflexes initiated from afferent sites other than the cardiovascular system itself. *Physiol. Rev.*, 30, 198–215.

Whitty, C. W. M., Lishman, W. A., and Fitzgibbon, J. P. (1964). Seizures induced by movement: a form of reflex epilepsy. *Lancet*, 1, 1403–5.

Wieser, H. G., Elger, C. E., and Stodieck, S. R. G. (1985). The 'foramen ovale electrode' a new recording method for the preoperative evaluation of patients suffering from mediobasal temporal lobe epilepsy. *Electroencephalogr. Clin. Neurophysiol.*, 61, 314–22.

Wijdicks, E. F. M. and Sharbrough, F. W. (1993). New-onset seizures in critically ill patients. *Neurology*, **43**, 1042–4.

Wijdicks, E. F., Wiesner, R. H., and Krom, R. A. (1995) Neurotoxicity in liver transplant recipients with cyclosporine immunosuppression. *Neurology*, **45** (11), 1962–4.

Wijdicks, E. F. M., Plevak, D. J., Wiesner, R. H. *et al.* (1996). Causes and outcome of seizures in liver transplant recipients. *Neurology*, **47**, 1523–5.

Wilkins, A. and Lindsay, F. (1985). Common forms of reflex epilepsy: physiological mechanisms and techniques for treatment. In *Recent advances in epilepsy*, Vol. 2, (ed. B. S. Meldrum and T. A. Pedley), pp. 239–72. Churchill-Livingstone, Edinburgh.

Wilkins, A. J., Binnie, C. D., and Darby, C. E. (1980). Visually-induced seizures. *Prog. Neurobiol.*, **15**, 85–117.

Williams, D. (1956). The structure of emotions reflected in epileptic experiences. *Brain*, **79**, 29–35.

Williamson, P. D., Spencer, D. D., Spencer, S. S. *et al.* (1985*a*). Complex partial seizures of frontal lobe origin. *Ann. Neurol.*, **18**, 497–504.

Williamson, P. D., Spencer, D. D., Spencer, S. S. *et al.* (1985*b*). Complex partial status epilepticus: a depth-electrode study. *Ann. Neurol.*, **18**, 647–54.

Williamson, P. D., French, J. A., Thadani, V. M. *et al.* (1993). Characteristics of medial temporal lobe epilepsy II. Interictal and ictal scalp electroencephalography, neuropsychological testing, neuroimaging, surgical results and pathology.' *Ann. Neurol.*, **34**, 781–7.

Williamson, R. and Wheal, H. V. (1992). The contribution of AMPA and NMDA receptors to graded bursting activity in the hippocampal CA1 region in an acute in vitro model of epilepsy. *Epilepsy Res.*, **12**, 179–88.

Willmore, L. J., Sypert, G. W., and Munson, J. B. (1978). Recurrent seizures induced by cortical iron injection: a model of post-traumatic epilepsy. *Ann. Neurol.*, **4**, 329–36.

Willow, M., Gonoi, T., and Catterall, W. A. (1985). Voltage clamp analysis of the inhibitory actions of diphenylhydatoin and carbamazepine on voltage-sensitive sodium channels in neuroblastoma cells. *Mol. Pharmacol.*, **27**, 549.

Wolf, H. K., Zentner, J., Hufnage, A. *et al.* (1993). Surgical pathology of temporal lobe epilepsy. Experience with 216 cases. *J. Neuropathol. Exp. Neurol.*, **52**, 499–506.

Wolf, P. and Inoue, Y. (1984). Therapeutic response of absence seizures in patients of an epilepsy clinic for adolescents and adults. *J. Neurol.*, **231**, 225–9.

Wong, M. C., Suite, N. D. A., and Labar, D. R. (1990). Seizures in human immunodeficiency virus infection. *Neurology*, **47**, 640–2.

Wong, R. K. S. and Prince, D. A. (1978). Participation of calcium spikes during intrinsic burst firing in hippocampal neurons. *Brain Res.*, **159**, 385–90.

Wong, R. K. S. and Prince, D. A. (1979). Dendritic mechanisms underlying penicillin induced epileptiform activity. *Science*, **204**, 1228–31.

Wong R. K. S and Prince D. A. 1981. 'Afterpotential Generation in Hippocampal Pyramidal Cells.' *Journal of Neurophysiology* 45:86–97.

Wong, R. K. S., Traub, R. D, and Miles, R. (1984). Epileptogenic mechanisms as revealed by studies of the hippocampal slice. In *Electrophysiology of epilepsy*, (ed. P. A. Schwartzkroin and H. V. Wheal), pp. 253–75. Academic Press, London.

Yanagihara, T., Piepgras, D. G., and Klass, D. W. (1985). Repetitive involuntary movements associated with episodic cerebral ischaemia. *Ann. Neurol.*, **18**, 244–50.

Yasargil, M. G. and Wieser, H. G. (1987). Selective amygdalohippocampectomy at the University Hospital, Zurich. In *Surgical treatment of the epilepsies*, (ed. J. Engel), pp. 653–8. Raven Press, New York.

Young, A. C., Bog Costanzi, J., Mohr, P. D. *et al.* (1982). Is routine computerised axial tomography in epilepsy worthwhile? *Lancet*, **ii**, 1446–7.

Young, B., Rapp, R. P., Norton, J. A. *et al.* (1983). Failure of prophylactically administered phenytoin to prevent late posttraumatic seizures. *J. Neurosurg.*, **58**, 236–41.

Young, G. B. and Blume, W. T. (1983). Painful epileptic seizures. *Brain*, **106**, 537–54.

Zeman, A. Z., Boniface, S. J., and Hodges, J. R. (1998). Transient epileptic amnesia: a description of the clinical and neuropsychological features in 10 cases and a review of the literature. *J. Neurol. Neurosurg. Psychiatry*, **64** (4), 435–43.

Zielinski, J. J. (1974). *Epidemiology and medical social problems of epilepsy in Warsaw*. Warsaw Psychoneurological Institute, Warsaw.

Sleep and sleep disorders

David Chadwick

Approximately a third of a person's life is spent in sleep. Although the requirement for sleep varies considerably with age, sleep deprivation has immediate effects on function. It causes sleepiness, poor performance, vigilance, attention and concentration, and reaction time increases. All these problems may be due to brief 'micro-sleeps' in which the EEG shows patterns of stage I non-REM sleep.

While disorders of sleep are common, they have been somewhat ignored by neurology, perhaps because they are rarely life-threatening. They are, however, a significant source of complaint and a number of sleep-related phenomena enter into the differential diagnosis of many neurological conditions. While this chapter will deal primary disorders of sleep, sleep disturbance is commonly seen in neurological disorders such as coma, encephalitis, head injury, and dementia.

24.1 Normal sleep architecture

Sleep has long been regarded as a largely negative phenomenon in which consciousness and vigilance are switched off. However, it is now clear that sleep includes different phases, during which there may be considerable neurophysiological activity within various brain regions. A normal period of sleep may last for between 6 and 10 hours, during which a number of clinical and neurophysiological changes identify different stages of sleep, including the electroencephalography (EEG), electromyography (EMG), eye movements, and autonomic changes. The criteria for sleep staging were described by (Rechtschaffen and Kales 1968); it is readily divisible on behavioural and physiological grounds into non-rapid eye movement (NREM) and rapid eye movement (REM) sleep.

24.1.1 NREM sleep

NREM sleep accounts for 75–80 per cent of sleeping time in adults. Stage I NREM sleep accounts for up to 10 per cent of sleep time and comprises a state of drowsiness in which there may be slow fluctuation of pupillary size and slow random eye movements. The eyes close and posture and tone are reduced. It begins with the diminution of alpha waves in the EEG and their replacement by theta rhythms. Within a few minutes, 12–16 Hz sleep spindles may be seen intermixed with 'K' complexes and vertex sharp waves. Stage II sleep, which accounts for about 50 per cent of total sleep time, is usually achieved within 10–15 minutes in a comfortable, darkened environment. Body movement is diminished and the changes of position that may occur in stage I sleep largely disappear. The threshold for arousal increases. Some dreaming may occur in stage II sleep, but recall is more difficult than from REM sleep. Muscle tone decreases further and the EEG starts to show theta and delta waves, with fronto-central 'sleep spindles', 'K' complexes, and vertex sharp waves in response to sudden noises or other stimuli. Stages III and IV make up approximately 15–20 per cent of sleep time in adults, but up to 50 per cent in children, and are characterized by increasing time with delta waves, which in stage IV constitute more than 50 per cent of activity. They will usually be reached within 30–45 minutes in adults. They may last from a few minutes to an hour.

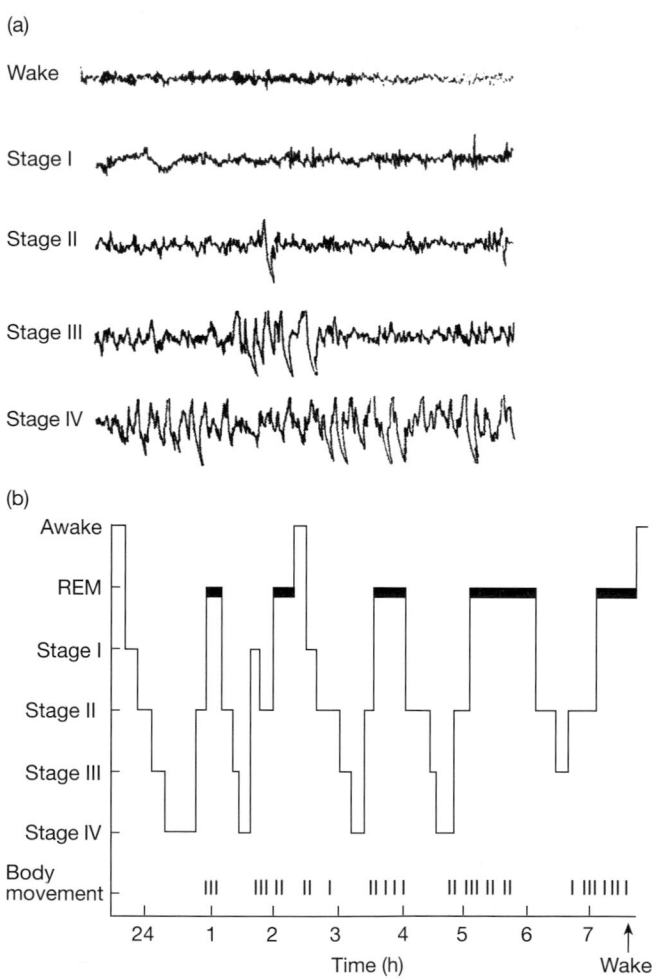

Fig. 24.1. EEG patterns associated with wakefulness and sleep (A) and the time course of normal sleep (B). (Adapted from McCarley, R. W. (1995). Sleep, dreams and states of consciousness. In *Neuroscience in medicine*, (ed. P. N. Conn), p. 537. Lippincott, Philadelphia.)

24.1.2 **REM sleep**

REM sleep accounts for 20–25 per cent of total sleep time. It comprises two stages, tonic and phasic. In the tonic phase the EEG becomes desynchronized and there is profound atonia of muscles. In the phasic stage events are marked by bursts of rapid eye movements and myoclonic twitches of facial and limb muscles. The occurrence of REM sleep is cyclical. A full cycle consists of a sequence of NREM and REM sleep lasting between 90 and 120 minutes. Generally, 4–6 sleep cycles occur during a night's sleep, with the amount of REM tending to increase progressively (see Fig. 24.1). It is believed that most dreams occur on wakening from REM sleep, but they may also occur on wakening from NREM sleep.

Disorders of sleep occur in a wide range of clinical settings. A simplified version of the International Classification of Sleep Disorders (American Sleep Disorders Association 1997) is presented in Table 24.1.

24.2 **Dyssomnias**

24.2.1 **Narcolepsy**

Narcolepsy may be viewed as a primary sleep disorder in which there is an imbalance between wakefulness, NREM sleep, and REM sleep. Individuals with narcolepsy show very short latency to the onset of sleep and REM sleep tends to occur at the beginning of a period of sleep rather than later (Howard 1985). The

Table 24.1. Classification of sleep disorders

Dyssomnias
  Intrinsic sleep disorders
    Narcolepsy
    Obstructive sleep apnoea
    Central sleep apnoea syndrome
    Restless legs syndrome
    Periodic limb movement disorder
  Extrinsic sleep disorders
    Environmental
    Altitude insomnia
    Alcohol
    Stimulant drugs
  Circadian disorders
    Jet-lag
    Shift working

Parasomnias
  Sleep–wake transition disorders
    Hypnic jerks
  Arousal disorders
    Confusional arousals
    Sleep walking
    Sleep terrors
  Parasomnias associated with REM sleep
    Nightmares
    Sleep paralysis
    Rapid eye movement sleep behaviour disorder

Sleep disorders associated with medical or psychiatric disorder term 'narcolepsy' was first used by Gelineau (1880) to describe irresistible episodes of sleep that were of short duration and recurring in nature. Others emphasized the association with cataplexy, sleep paralysis, and hypnagogic hallucination in a clinical tetrad (Yoss and Daly 1960).

Prevalence rates are usually quoted of around 0.05 per cent of the population, with men and women being equally affected. Age of onset varies between childhood and the fifth decade, with maximum incidence in the second and third decades. A genetic basis for narcolepsy has now been widely explored. (Honda *et al.* 1983) found that 100 per cent of Japanese narcoleptic patients expressed the haplotype DR15 DQw6. Oligotyping has further demonstrated that DQb1–0602 is the most common haplotype associated with narcolepsy. In spite of this, familial occurrence of narcolepsy is not frequent, and up to 10 per cent of narcoleptics are negative for DQb1–0602 (Singh *et al.* 1990). Monozygotic twin pairs discordant for narcolepsy have been observed (Montplaisir and Poirier 1988). Furthermore, only a small proportion of people with the DQb1–0602 haplotype suffer from excessive daytime sleepiness or narcolepsy.

Clinical features

Brief episodes of daytime sleepiness and sleeping can recur several times a day, most obviously under favourable circumstances, such as during monotonous activity or after a heavy meal, but also when the patient may be fully involved in a task. They are usually more frequent in the afternoon. Sleeping may last from a few minutes up to an hour, but the person usually feels refreshed and there may be a refractory period of an hour or more before the next episode of sleepiness.

Cataplexy is an abrupt loss of muscle tone, usually for a few seconds but occasionally for several minutes. The attacks are usually triggered by emotion, shock, or fatigue. Severe attacks may be associated with falls, but milder episodes may be barely noticeable to observers. Sleep paralysis can occur during the process of falling asleep or awakening. Patients are unable to move their extremities, speak, open their eyes, or breathe deeply. It may be associated with hallucinations. Attacks may be terminated either spontaneously or due to some kind of external stimulus, such as a noise.

Hypnagogic hallucinations consist of a variety of visual hallucinations, some formed and some unformed. Symptoms of excessive daytime sleepiness usually predominate in any individual. There may be a latent period between the onset daytime sleepiness and other clinical features. Once established, the course of the condition is chronic, although there may be fluctuations in the severity of symptoms over the years. It should also be noted that cataplexy, sleep paralysis, and hypnagogic hallucination can occur as individual symptoms without any other features of the narcoleptic syndrome.

The role of investigation in reaching a diagnosis of narcoleptic syndrome is somewhat controversial. The multiple sleep latency test can certainly be helpful (Carskadon and Dement 1982). It consists of four or five scheduled naps in quiet surroundings at 2-hourly intervals during polygraphic monitoring. Mean scores under 8 minutes are generally considered to be pathological, those over 10 minutes being considered normal. Multiple sleep latency testing confirms the presence of narcolepsy if, in addition, there are two or more sleep-onset REM periods.

Treatment of the narcoleptic syndrome

Most individuals with narcolepsy can be helped by some adaptation of their life and work patterns. One or two planned periods of sleep during the day are usually helpful. Shift work may be difficult. It is not uncommon for narcoleptics to have sleep attacks while driving (Roth 1980), therefore all sufferers need counselling about driving, and people with narcolepsy should be advised not to drive if they are off treatment, or on treatment but are poorly controlled (Parkes 1983).

An enormous range of drugs has been recommended as treatment for the narcoleptic syndrome (Parkes 1985), indicating that none are very successful. These include virtually any kind of CNS stimulant, including caffeine, ephedrine, and amfetamines. Most have sympathomimetic side-effects, produce tolerance, and have a potential for misuse. It may be reasonable to start treating narcolepsy with a less potent compound such as mazindol, 3–8 mg/day (Parkes and Schachter 1979). More potent stimulants, such as methylphenidate (10–60 mg/day) or dexamfetamine (10–60 mg/day) can be used for those who do not respond to less potent alternatives. The treatment of choice for cataplexy seems to be clomipramine (Hishikawa *et al.* 1966), which is capable of abolishing cataplexy in over two-thirds of narcoleptics.

24.2.2 Idiopathic hypersomnolence

This condition, of unknown cause, is probably rarer than narcolepsy and appears to be a primary disorder of non-REM sleep. Individuals have long episodes of daytime sleeping for 1–2 hours at a time. Daytime sleeping is probably more resistible than in the narcoleptic syndrome, but often the most difficult problems are morning waking. The condition may again be familial, with up to 35 per cent of patients having an affected family member. On occasion, daytime drowsiness may not be responsive to stimulant drugs (Parkes 1981).

24.2.3 Sleep apnoea

An apnoea may be defined as a cessation of breathing for 10 seconds or more, hypopnoea being a reduction in ventilation for a similar period of time. Classically, it has been divided into the central sleep apnoeas associated with neurological disorders and obstructive sleep apnoeas.

Central sleep apnoea

Central sleep apnoea can be associated with a variety of brainstem disorders, including tumour or infarction, multiple sclerosis, or primary autonomic failure. It is also a common feature of myopathic disorders and dystrophy (Fulmer and Jackson 1982).

It is seen in Ondine's curse, in which there is a primary insensitivity of the respiratory centre, with loss of automatic respiratory drive.

Obstructive sleep apnoea

Obstructive sleep apnoea (OSA) is due to upper airways obstruction, most commonly during slow-wave sleep (McCoy *et al.* 1981). Movement at the air or mouth ceases but those of the thorax and diaphragm continue (Guilleminault *et al.* 1978). While up to 10 per cent of the male population may exhibit significant periods of sleep apnoea (Young *et al.* 1993) the incidence of symptomatic OSA is probably 1–2 per cent of the middle-aged male population. The prevalence increases with age and REM obesity, and it occurs more frequently in men than in women (Stradling and Crosby 1991). The condition is associated with pulmonary and systemic hypertension, but there is currently insufficient evidence to indicate that this is associated with increased vascular morbidity and mortality (Wright *et al.* 1997).

Patients complain of daytime somnolence more prominently than of the disturbed sleep, which is accompanied by snoring of sufficient severity to persuade the conjugal partner to sleep in a separate room. Daytime sleeps can last for 1–2 hours at a time, but they are rarely refreshing. The condition may be associated with a greatly increased risk of accident on the road and in the workplace (Findley *et al.* 1988).

Treatment

For some individuals with obstructive sleep apnoea, sleeping with a head-up tilt, weight loss, and daytime exercise may be sufficient treatment. For others, continuous positive airway pressure (CPAP) is the treatment of choice, two randomized controlled trials having shown improvements in symptoms, cognitive function, and mood (Engleman *et al.* 1994, 1997). Surgical interventions short of tracheostomy are probably not indicated, but intra-oral devices that advance the mandible may be helpful (Ferguson *et al.* 1996).

24.2.4 Periodic limb movements in sleep and the restless legs syndrome

The restless legs syndrome was recognized by Ekbom (1960). Most patients with this syndrome exhibit periodic limb movements in sleep (Section 32.10.1). However, periodic limb movements in sleep are common and only a third of people exhibiting them have restless legs syndrome.

Periodic limb movements in sleep are repetitive rather stereotyped movements, often occurring periodically during non-REM sleep. They usually involve the legs with extension of the great toe and fanning of the other toes, resembling a Babinski reflex, with a general withdrawal and flexion of the leg. Movements tend to recur, often with a periodicity of 20–40 seconds, in clusters going on for several minutes. These are often terminated with a shift in body position and some alerting. The prevalence of periodic limb movements in sleep

increases with age, but they are probably asymptomatic in the majority of people exhibiting them. Patients in which they are symptomatic frequently complain of difficulty maintaining sleep and excessive daytime sleepiness. In the past, some families have been described with this disorder, who have subsequently been shown to have frontal lobe seizures, indicating that the differential diagnosis can present difficulties.

Restless legs syndrome describes characteristic sensory and motor symptoms that are very much evoked by rest, attempts to sleep, and drowsiness. They may be described as tingling or burning sensations associated with restlessness and an urge to move. The patients use voluntary movements to ease these symptoms. They primarily complain of difficulty getting to sleep, but associated periodic limb movements in sleep may lead to difficulty in maintaining sleep.

Both restless legs syndrome and periodic limb movements of sleep may be associated with a wide range of neurological and medical disorders, including neuropathies, radiculopathies, Parkinson's disease, anaemia, and uraemia.

Many treatments have been suggested to be effective in both conditions. These include benzodiazepines, opioids, dopaminergic drugs, antiepileptic drugs including gabapentin, and clonidine. Much of the evidence supporting these treatments is at best anecdotal.

24.2.5 The Kleine–Levin syndrome

Kleine (1925) and Levin (1936) described a rare disorder characterized by periodic attacks of profound sleepiness associated with excessive appetite. A considerable number of cases ascribed to this syndrome have appeared subsequently in the literature (Fresco *et al.* 1971), but most of the cases are atypical and many authorities have never seen a case corresponding to the classical picture (Parkes 1985).

In the rare typical cases there is a marked male preponderance, with onset in adolescence. Episodes of hypersomnia occur, lasting from a few days to several weeks (on average 5–7 days). Attacks may occur at monthly to yearly intervals, with great variability, but the disorder seems benign and usually disappears in adult life. Overeating is common during attacks and is often associated with rapid weight gain. Recovery from attacks is often associated with mood changes of depression and disgust, and hypersexuality may occur in about one-fifth of cases.

The cause of attacks is uncertain and some have doubted the organic basis of the syndrome. This may, however, be due to the inclusion of atypical cases with psychological aetiology within the case literature on this subject.

24.2.6 Fatal familial insomnia

This is an unusual prion disorder in which progressive derangement of sleep and saccadian rhythms occurs in association with ataxia, myoclonus, and dementia. It exhibits an autosomal dominant pattern of inheritance. The mutation in this condition is identical to a recognized familial form of Creutzfeldt–

Jakob disease (CJD), with asparagine substitution for aspartic acid at locus 178 (Section 26.6.5 and 34.12). The phenotype expressed depends on which polymorphism occurs at locus 129. Methionine results in fatal familial insomnia, whereas alanine gives rise to a more typical CJD phenotype.

24.3 Parasomnias

A variety of sleep-related behaviours (parasomnias) and confusional episodes not uncommonly present diagnostic problems to neurologists. *Hypnic jerks* occur during sleep onset and are asymmetric, most commonly affecting the legs but also on occasions the arms and head, and are associated with a feeling of falling. They are most often spontaneous but can also be evoked by stimuli. They can be associated with vertex sharp waves in the EEG (Oswald 1959). They are entirely benign and should not be confused with the wakening myoclonic jerks of juvenile myoclonic epilepsy, or with frontal seizures during sleep.

Sleep terrors consist of the individual usually suddenly sitting up and screaming, with obvious distress and agitation. They arise from deep slow-wave sleep and are usually self-limiting, the individual returning to sleep without arousal or subsequent recall. They are more common in children than in adults.

Confusional arousals usually occur with arousal from deep slow-wave sleep during the early parts of the night. There is evidence of confusion and slowed mental processes, although somewhat purposeful activity can occur. Many junior hospital staff may have experienced episodes during which they have given advice by phone in the middle of the night, but been unable to recall the event the next day.

Sleep walking also occurs during deep slow-wave sleep, and consists of walking and other automatic behaviours lasting for up to 5 minutes. It is difficult to wake the individual, who may well be confused and subsequently amnesic if wakened. It is much more common in children than in adults, and those adults who exhibit it usually did so as children.

It is possible to view sleep walking, confusional arousal, and sleep terrors as a spectrum of parasomnias of slow-wave sleep. On rare occasions they may assume a medico-legal significance, as they have been used as a defence against conviction for crimes of violence (Broughton *et al.* 1994; Broughton and Shimizu 1995). Such extreme behaviour may be more likely after sleep deprivation or the use of psychotropic drugs (Mahowald and Schenck 1999).

Rapid eye movement sleep behaviour disorder

Individuals with this condition usually describe vivid dreaming states during which there are excessive movements that are occasionally violent and cause injury to the subject or their bed partner. It appears that the incidence increases with age and may be more common in those with degenerative disorders such as Parkinson's disease and multisystem atrophy. During polysonography, tonic or phasic abnormalities in muscle tone occur during REM sleep. Benzodiazepines, particularly clonazepam, may be effective in suppressing this violent sleep behaviour.

References

American Sleep Disorders Association (1997). *The international classification of sleep disorders: Diagnostic and coding manual* (revised). American Sleep Disorders Association, Rochester, Minnesota.

Broughton, R. and Shimizu, T. (1995). Sleep-related violence: a medical and forensic challenge. *Sleep*, **18**, 727–36.

Broughton, R., Billings, R., Cartwright, R. *et al.* (1994). Homicidal sonambulism: a case report. *Sleep*, **17**, 235–8.

Carskadon, M. A. and Dement, W. C. (1982). The multiple sleep latency test: what does it measure? *Sleep*, **5**, 67–72.

Ekbom, K. A. (1960). Restless leg syndrome. *Neurology*, **10**, 868–73.

Engleman, H. M., Martin, S. E., Deary, I. J. *et al.* (1994). Effect of continuous positive airway pressure treatment on daytime function in sleep apnoea/hypnoea syndrome. *Lancet*, **343**, 572–5.

Engleman, H. M., Martin, S. E., Deary, I. J., *et al.* (1997). Effect of CPAP therapy on daytime function in patients with mild sleep apnoea/hypopnoea syndrome. *Thorax*, **52**, 114–19.

Ferguson, K. A., Ono, T., Lowe, A. A., *et al.* (1996). A cross-over study of an oral appliance vs nasal CPAP in the treatment of mild-moderate obstructive sleep apnoea. *Chest*, **109**, 1269–75.

Findley, L. J., Unverzagt, M. E., and Suratt, P. M. (1988). Automobile accidents involving people with obstructive sleep apnoea. *Am. Rev. Respir. Dis.*, **138**, 337–41.

Fresco, R., Guidicelli, S., Poinso, Y. *et al.* (1971). Le syndrome de Kleine Levin. *Ann. Med. Psychol.*, **129**, 625–68.

Fulmer, J. and Jackson, L. (1982). Hypoxemia: a peril of sleep. *South Med. J.*, **75**, 1.

Gelineau, J. B. (1880). De la narcolepsie. *Gaz. Hop. (Paris)*, **53**, 626–8, 635–7.

Guilleminault, C., van den Hoed, J., and Miller, M. (1978). Clinical overview of the sleep apnea syndromes. In *Sleep apnea syndromes*, (ed. C. Guilleminault and W. Dement), p. 1. Alan R. Liss, New York.

Hishikawa, Y., Ida, H., Nakai, K. *et al.* (1966). Treatment of narcolepsy with imipramine (Tofranil) and desmethylimipramine. *J. Neurol. Sci.*, **3**, 453–61.

Honda, Y., Asaka, A., Tanaka, Y. *et al.* (1983). Discrimination of narcolepsy by using genetic markers. *Sleep Res.*, **12**, 254–60.

Howard, G. (1985). Laboratory assessment of sleep and related functions. In *Clinical aspects of sleep and sleep disturbance*, (ed. T. Riley), pp. 197–217. Butterworths, Stoneham MA.

Kleine, W. (1925). Penodische Schlafsuchr. *Mschr. Psychial. Neurol.* **57**, 285–320.

Levin, M. (1936). Periodic Somnolence and morbid hunger. *Brain*, **59**, 494–515.

Mahowald, M. W. and Schenck, C. H. (1999). Sleep-related violence and forensic medicine issues. In *Sleep disorders medicine: basic science, technical and clinical aspects*, (2nd edn), (ed. S. Chokrovery), pp. 729–39. Butterworth Heinemann, Boston.

McCoy, K., Koopmann, C., and Tausigg, J. (1981). Sleep related breathing disorders. *Am. J. Otolaryngol.*, 3, 228–37.

Montplaisir, J. and Poirier, G. (1988). HLA in narcolepsy in Canada. In *HLA in narcolepsy*, (ed. Y. Honda and T. Juji), pp. 97–105. Springer, Berlin.

Oswald, I. (1959). Sudden bodily jerks on falling asleep. *Brain*, 82, 92–103.

Parkes, J. D. (1981). Day time drowsiness. *Lancet*, 2, 1213–18.

Parkes, J. D. (1983). The sleepy driver. In *Driving and epilepsy and other causes of impaired consciousness*, Vol. 25, (ed. R. B. Godwin-Austen and M. L. E. Espir). Royal Society of Medicine, London.

Parkes, J. D. (1985). *Sleep and its disorders*. W. B. Saunders, London.

Parkes, J. D. and Schachter, M. (1979). Mazindol in the treatment of narcolepsy. *Acta Neurol. Scand.*, 60, 250–4.

Rechtschaffen, A. and Kales, A. (1968). *A manual of standardized terminology: techniques and scoring for sleep studies of human subjects*. National Institutes of Health, Bethesda.

Roth, B. (1980). *Narcolepsy and hypersomnia*. S. Karger, Basel.

Singh, S., George, C. F., Kryger, M. H. *et al.* (1990). Genetic heterogeneity in narcolepsy. *Lancet*, 335 (8691), 726–7.

Stradling, J. R. and Crosby, J. H. (1991). Predictors and prevalence of obstructive sleep apnoea and snoring in 1001 middle-aged men. *Thorax*, 46, 85–90.

Wright, J., Johns, R., Watt, I. *et al.* (1997). Health effects of obstructive sleep apnoea and the effectiveness of continuous positive airways pressure: a systematic review of the research evidence. *BMJ*, 314, 851–60.

Yoss, R. E. and Daly, D. D. (1960) Hereditary aspects of narcolepsy. *Trans. Am. Neurol. Assoc.*, 85, 239–40.

Young, T., Palta, M., Dempsey, J. *et al.* (1993). Occurrence of sleep disordered breathing among middle-aged adults. *N. Engl. J. Med.*, 328, 1230–5.

Coma

Martin Rossor

25.1 Introduction

25.1.1 Neural basis of consciousness

We all have an intuitive sense of what is meant by consciousness generally and what it is to be conscious ourselves. However, since, in a sense, consciousness is a primary element in experience, it cannot be readily defined in terms of anything else.

Although a simple definition of consciousness remains elusive, a number of components, relevant neurologically, can be considered to contribute: wakefulness, perceptual awareness, and concept of self and of experience of awareness (Zeman *et al.* 1997). The neurology of sleep and awake states is the best understood and is covered in Chapter 3. Awareness of visual and auditory stimuli enrich our consciousness. However, the example of blindsight in patients and in monkeys (Cowey and Stoerig 1995), in which the subject will respond correctly to visual stimuli but without being aware, suggests that particular areas of cortex are required for the awareness of a sensory stimulus. Awareness of self—for example, recognition in a mirror, which emerges in children at around 18 months and may be evident in chimpanzees—might also be considered an important component. Whether this concept of self survives in patients with dementia, in which 'consciousness' is considered to be present, is unclear.

These studies would suggest that, with improved understanding, consciousness as a neurobiological phenomenon is likely to be fractionated into a number of discrete components. Nevertheless, at present a distinction of value to the clinical neurologist is that between the content of consciousness and the state of consciousness itself. The content of consciousness depends upon the activities of the cerebral cortex, the thalamus, and their interrelationship; lesions of these structures will diminish the content of consciousness without, as a rule, changing the state of consciousness as such. By contrast, the ascending reticular activating system, which extends from the lower border of the pons to the ventromedial thalamus, profoundly influences the state of consciousness or arousal. The cells of origin of this system occupy a paramedian area in the brainstem, extending from the lower part of the pons to a rostral level that includes the posterior hypothalamus, the thalamic intralaminar nuclei, and the septal area (Fig. 25.1). The landmark studies of Magoun and his collaborators (Magoun 1952) demonstrated that there are two broad inputs to the cerebral cortex, namely those that alter the activity of the

greater part, or the whole, of the cerebral cortex, and those that activate very specific cortical projection areas, such as the visual or the primary sensory cortices. Destruction of the reticular system does not interfere with the action of the sensory impulses on a specific projection area, but it eliminates the tonic impulses from the hypothalamic–reticular system to the cortex as a whole. The reticular activating system is now seen as a complex system which subsumes noradrenergic and cholinergic projections to the cortex. Drugs that tend to produce unconsciousness, such as anaesthetics and hypnotics, selectively depress the ascending reticular activating system, while those that cause wakefulness have the opposite, facilitatory effect.

A further observation that supports the distinction between content and state of consciousness is the observation that sleep is a separate active physiological process and not merely a feature of arousal. Moreover, sleeping and waking can occur in humans even after total bilateral destruction of the cerebral hemispheres, as in the vegetative state (see below). Thus to cause coma, as defined as a state of unconsciousness in which the eyes are closed and sleep–wake cycles absent (Plum and Posner 1980), a lesion of the cerebral hemispheres needs to be extensive and bilateral; lesions of the brainstem must be above the lower third of the pons and destroy both sides of the paramedian reticulum.

Many pathological processes can thus be responsible for stupor or coma, for example head injury, tumour, vascular and inflammatory lesions, and, most commonly, toxic and metabolic states which usually lead to unconsciousness primarily through their effect upon the brainstem. In the series of Plum and Posner (1980) of 500 cases of stupor or coma, initially of unknown aetiology, 101 proved to be due to supratentorial lesions (probably producing their effects by indirect action upon the brainstem), 65 to subtentorial lesions, and 326 to diffuse or metabolic brain dysfunction, while there were eight cases of psychiatric 'coma'.

25.1.2 Terminology

Between full consciousness and pathological complete unconsciousness or coma, there is a continuum of severity, but, in addition, there exist many states which differ not only in degree, but also in quality, and especially in the nature of impairment of consciousness and, by implication, the content of such consciousness as remains (Giacino 1997). In an attempt to distinguish states of impaired consciousness that differ in degree, a number of terms have been introduced. An early definition of coma required that the patient could not be aroused by any stimulus, however vigorous and painful. Semicoma was then defined as complete loss of consciousness with a response only at the reflex level, while less severe degrees of impairment of consciousness were entitled severe, moderate, and mild confusion (Medical Research Council 1941). The term 'semicoma' is now obsolete. Stupor has been applied to the situation wherein the subject can only be aroused by vigorous and continuous external stimulation; as previously defined, the

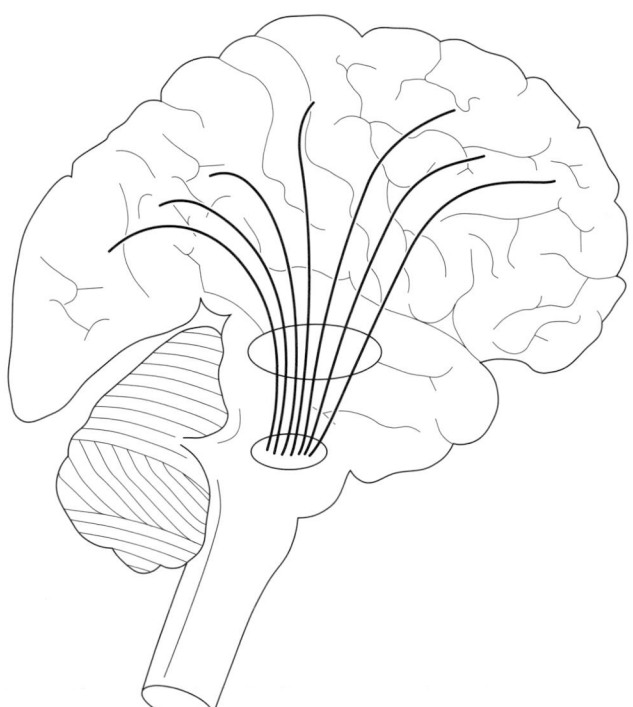

Fig. 25.1. The reticular activating system extends from the lower third of the pons to the thalamus, and lesions disrupting this system, as well as extensive lesions of the cerebral cortex, will lead to coma.

patient in coma elicits no response to any external stimulus or inner need (Plum and Posner 1980). More recently, the term 'minimally conscious state' has been introduced for the patient who demonstrates inconsistent but reproducible evidence of awareness of the environment or self (Giacino 1997).

The terms 'clouding of consciousness', 'obtundation', and 'lethargy' all imply mild disturbances of arousal, but are too imprecise to be of clinical value. The use of terms other than coma and stupor to indicate the degree of impairment of consciousness is beset with difficulties and more important is the use of coma scales, such as the Glasgow Coma Scale, which indicate the severity of coma using a number of easily identifiable behavioural features (Teasdale and Jennett 1974; Teasdale *et al.* 1978).

Patients who survive coma (i.e. in a state of unresponsiveness to external stimuli with eyes closed) do not remain in this state for more than 2–3 weeks, but rather develop a persistent unresponsive state in which sleep–wake cycles return. This is seen after severe brain injury, and the implication is that brainstem function returns with sleep–wake cycles, eye opening in response to verbal stimuli, and normal respiratory control. However, such patients show no apparent understanding or behavioural responses that would allow one to infer that they are truly conscious (Zeman 1997). There are no verbal responses and no discrete localizing motor responses. The term proposed by Teasdale and Jennett (1974) is the 'vegetative state', which has now replaced the terms 'coma vigil' and 'apallic syndrome'.

Akinetic mutism, described by Cairns (1952) in a patient with an epidermoid cyst of the third ventricle, resembled sleep, in being associated with general muscular relaxation, but differed from sleep in that, although the patient's eyes remained apparently alert to moving objects, strong afferent stimuli were necessary to achieve arousal. The state has been described as one of 'motionless, mindless wakefulness' and, despite the patient's immobility, there are few signs of damage to descending motor pathways. Most cases are caused by bilateral lesions of the orbitomesial frontal cortex, limbic system, or diencephalic reticular system (Nemeth *et al.* 1986; Marin 1990). Akinetic mutism is suggested to be classified within the minimally conscious state (Anonymous 1995).

Also different is the so-called de-efferented state or 'locked-in' syndrome, in which the patient is fully aware of his surroundings, being conscious and alert but usually tetraplegic, aphonic, and anarthric, so that he can communicate only through blinking or by vertical eye movements (Bauer *et al.* 1979). It is therefore most important to distinguish this state in which the patient can hear, respond, and, indeed, display complex ideas despite extensive paralysis, from akinetic mutism and the chronic vegetative state.

Functional neuroimaging has compared cerebral metabolism in these states. The lowest level metabolism comparable to that seen with general anaesthesia, is seen in the persistent vegetative state (PVS), only minor reductions are seen in the locked-in state (Levy *et al.* 1987).

25.1.3 Approaches to differential diagnosis

General examination

The patient in coma requires the most detailed and systematic examination, as the clue to the cause of the unconsciousness may lie in any system. However, on arrival in an Accident and Emergency department, immediate attention will need to be given to appropriate resuscitation measures. Thus the airway will need to be protected and, if necessary, intubation and assisted respiration instituted. Attention then needs to be given to the circulation, and on establishing intravenous access blood should be withdrawn and stored for estimation of glucose, other biochemical parameters, and possible drug screening. Attention is then directed towards the assessment of the patient in terms of the severity of the coma and to diagnostic evaluation. Although the patient is unable to provide a history, it is essential that this is not neglected. All possible information should be gathered, particularly about the mode of onset, which can be obtained from relatives, paramedics, ambulance personnel, or bystanders. Previous medical history, including epilepsy, diabetes, and drug history, is of great importance, and the patient's general practitioner may need to be contacted. Clues may also be obtained from the patient's clothing or handbag.

The general examination is as important as the neurological examination, and careful examination for rigors or trauma requires complete exposure and 'log roll' to examine the back. Needle marks should also be specifically looked for.

A careful neurological examination will inevitably need to await stabilization of the patient. If head trauma is suspected, the examination must await adequate stabilization of the neck. Documentation of the severity of coma is essential for subsequent management. The Glasgow Coma Scale (see below) provides a widely understood scale of proven value and should be assessed at the outset. Following this, particular attention should be paid to brainstem and motor function.

Pupils

The pupils must be assessed for size, any inequality, and the reaction to a bright light. Particular care should be taken with small pupils or the pinpoint pupils of pontine haemorrhage, and to assess the light response a magnifying glass may be necessary. An important general rule is that coma due to metabolic disturbance is associated with preservation of the pupillary light response, and most metabolic encephalopathies give small pupils with preserved light reflex. Drugs such as atropine, and cerebral anoxia tend to dilate the pupils, and opiates will constrict them. Structural lesions are more commonly associated with pupillary asymmetry and with loss of light reflex. Midbrain tectal lesions give round, regular, medium-sized pupils, which do not react to light but may show hippus; nuclear midbrain lesions also, as a rule, give medium-sized pupils, fixed to all stimuli, which are often irregular and unequal. A third-nerve lesion distal to the nucleus gives a fixed, dilated pupil on the side of the lesion. Tegmental lesions in the pons give bilaterally small pupils which, in pontine haemorrhage, may be pinpoint, although reactive. A lateral medullary lesion can give an ipsilateral Horner's syndrome, while the pupil on the side of an occluded carotid artery causing cerebral infarction is often small.

Ocular movements

The position of the eyes at rest and the presence of spontaneous eye movement should be assessed and then the reflex responses to oculocephalic and oculovestibular manoeuvres determined. In the unconscious patient with diffuse cerebral disturbance but intact brainstem function, slow roving eye movements can be observed. A frontal lobe lesion may cause deviation of the eyes towards the side of the lesion while, conversely, a lateral pontine lesion can cause conjugate deviation to the opposite side. Conjugate deviation downwards indicates a midbrain lesion, and disconjugate ocular deviation will also indicate a structural brainstem lesion.

The oculocephalic (doll's head) response can be tested by rotating the head from side to side and observing the position of the eyes. If the eyes move conjugately in the opposite direction to that of head movement, the response is positive and indicates an intact pons mediating a normal vestibulo-ocular reflex. However, cervical trauma will need to have been excluded before undertaking this test, and the caloric oculovestibular responses may be more reliable. These are tested by the installation of ice-cold water into the external auditory meatus, having confirmed that there is no tympanic rupture. A normal response in a conscious patient is the development of nystagmus with the quick phase away from the stimulated side. This requires intact cerebropontine connections. In an unconscious patient with an intact brainstem, a tonic response occurs without the correcting fast phase of nystagmus, with the tonic movement towards the stimulated side. With both the oculocephalic and oculovestibular responses, disconjugate movement of the eyes, for example that occurring with damage to the medial longitudinal fasciculus causing an internuclear ophthalmoplegia, may be observed. Complete absence of these brainstem ocular reflexes indicates severe brainstem involvement. The corneal response is normally well preserved until late.

Respiration

Cheyne–Stokes respiration, in which hyperpnoea alternates with apnoea, is commonly found in comatose patients, often in association with cerebral disease, but is relatively non-specific. Rapid, regular respiration is also common in comatose patients (Leigh and Shaw 1976) and is often found with pneumonia or acidosis. Central neurogenic hyperventilation (Plum and Swanson 1958) has been described in patients with dysfunction of the brainstem tegmentum. It is a rare syndrome, comprising elevated arterial oxygen tension (PO_2), decreased arterial carbon dioxide tension (PCO_2), and respiratory alkalosis in the absence of any evidence of pulmonary disease. Most such patients have brainstem tumours, and most, but not all, are in a coma (Rodriguez *et al.* 1982). Sometimes the condition may compli-

cate hepatic encephalopathy (Plum 1982). Brainstem lesions may also give apneustic breathing with a pause at full inspiration (Plum and Alvord 1964), or ataxic, irregular respiration with random deep and shallow breaths—a pattern that is seen particularly with medullary lesions (Plum and Swanson 1958).

Motor function

With the examination of the motor system, particular attention should be directed towards asymmetry of tone or movement. The plantar responses are usually extensor, but asymmetry is again important. The tendon reflexes are less useful. The motor response to painful stimuli should be assessed carefully and forms part of the Glasgow Coma Scale (see below).

The most commonly used painful stimuli are supraorbital nerve pressure and nailbed pressure. Rubbing of the sternum should be avoided as this can cause bruising and distress to the relatives. Patients may localize or exhibit a variety of responses. Flexion of the upper limb with extension of the lower limb (decorticate response) and extension of the upper and lower limb (decerebrate response) may be observed. Again asymmetry is important. In general, extensor responses (decerebrate pattern) indicate a more severe disturbance and prognosis.

Head and neck

The head should be examined carefully for evidence of injury and the skull should be palpated for depressed fractures. The ears and nose should be examined for haemorrhage and leakage of CSF, and examination of the fundi may demonstrate papilloedema or subhyaloid or retinal haemorrhages. In the presence of trauma to the head, associated trauma to the neck should be assumed until proven otherwise. If established as safe to do so, the cervical spine should be gently flexed and a positive Kernig's sign sought, which may indicate a meningitis or subarachnoid haemorrhage. However, neck stiffness may occur with raised intracranial pressure and incipient tonsillar herniation.

Investigation of coma

At presentation blood will be taken for determination of glucose, electrolytes, liver function, calcium, osmolality, and blood gases. Blood should also be stored for a subsequent drug screen if needed. Following the clinical examination, a broad distinction between a metabolic cause, with preserved pupillary responses, or a structural cause of coma is likely to have been established. Although most patients with coma will require CT scanning, or indeed all with persisting coma, clearly this is of greater urgency when a structural lesion is suspected. In the absence of focal signs, but with evidence of meningitis, a lumbar puncture may need to be performed before scanning, as a matter of clinical urgency. In other situations, lumbar puncture should be delayed until after the brain scan because of the risk of precipitating a pressure cone secondary to a cerebral mass lesion. All patients will require chest radiography and ECG, and more detailed investigations of systemic disease will be directed by the clinical examination. The EEG can be of value in the diagnosis of coma, but it is relatively limited. It is of

Table 25.1. The Glasgow Coma Scale (derived from Teasdale and Jennett 1974)

	Score
Eye-opening	
Nil	1
To pain	2
To voice	3
Spontaneously (with blinking)	4
Motor response	
Nil	1
Extension	2
Flexion	3
Withdrawal	4
Localizing	5
Voluntary	6
Verbal response	
Nil	1
Groans	2
Words (expletive)	3
Disorientated	4
Orientated	5

value in identifying the occasional patient with subclinical status epilepticus, and is clearly of value in assessing the patient who has been admitted following an unsuspected seizure. Fast activity is commonly found with drug overdose and slow wave abnormalities with metabolic and anoxic coma. An isoelectric EEG may occur with drug-induced comas, but otherwise indicates severe cerebral damage.

25.1.4 **Measurement of coma**

It is most important that the level of coma should be documented from the earliest opportunity. Subsequent records will indicate whether the level of consciousness is improving, when clearly decisions concerning further investigation and therapy are less urgent. The Glasgow Coma Scale (Table 25.1) provides an easy clinical assessment and is now widely used (Teasdale and Jennett 1974).

25.1.5 **Management of the unconscious patient**

The management of the unconscious patient will consist of treatment of the underlying cause where possible, and the maintenance of the normal physiology in terms of respiration, circulation, and nutrition while the patient is unconscious. Improvements in intensive care have been so dramatic recently, as a result of improved technology, that patients in a comatose state can be maintained in a condition of adequate health.

In the short term, the unconscious patient should be nursed on his or her side without a pillow, and attention will clearly need to be paid to the airway, requiring an oral airway as a minimum, although usually patients will require intubation and, if coma is prolonged, tracheostomy. The unconscious patient will have retention or incontinence of urine and will

require catheterization. Intravenous fluid is necessary and, if coma persists, adequate nutrition is required. Disturbances of electrolytes, particularly sodium, are common in the intensive care situation and need scrupulous monitoring. The nursing and medical techniques of the intensive care of unconscious patients are covered in a number of texts (Ropper and Kennedy 1988).

25.1.6 **Prognosis in coma**

In general, coma carries a serious prognosis. Nevertheless, this is dependent to a large extent on the underlying cause. Coma due to depressant drugs carries an excellent prognosis provided that resuscitative and supportive measures are available and no anoxia has been sustained. Thus coma from depressant drugs, even that persisting for days, can be associated with a full and complete recovery. In general, metabolic causes, apart from anoxia, carry a better prognosis than structural lesions and head injury. A number of factors contribute to predicting the outcome, and recently considerable work has been directed towards identifying these. Many studies have now been published on the outcome of coma, and they show broad agreement. Early studies tended to differ in the outcome measures used, but, following the lead of Jennett and Bond (1975), five simple outcome measures are now widely used. 'Good recovery' indicates patients who return to their normal life; 'moderate disability' indicates patients who achieve independence in daily living, but do not resume their previous level of function; 'severe disability' refers to patients who regain some cognitive functions but are dependent on others for daily support; in the 'vegetative state' (see above) patients awaken but give no sign of cognitive awareness; and with 'no recovery' patients remain in coma until death. In general, the length of coma is of poor prognostic significance, as is increasing age. Whether the underlying cause is metabolic or structural, the brainstem reflexes early in the coma are an important predictor of outcome. For example, in Jennett's series of head injuries (Jennett et al. 1979), if the pupils were fixed at 24 hours, 91 per cent of 1000 patients died and only 4 per cent made satisfactory recovery. A similar pattern is found with non-traumatic coma. Thus only 2 per cent of patients made a moderate or good recovery with absent brainstem reflexes at 1 day, and there were no recoveries, other than to a vegetative state or severe disability, if reflexes were absent at 3 days (Levy et al. 1981).

Neurologists are often asked to give a prognosis on patients arriving in the intensive care unit following cardiopulmonary arrest, and, in general, the absence of pupillary light and corneal reflexes 6 hours after the onset of coma is very unlikely to be associated with survival (Snyder et al. 1981). The chronic vegetative state usually carries a uniformly poor prognosis, although a partial return of cognition, or even restoration to partial independence, has been reported very rarely (Rosenberg et al. 1977; Shuttleworth 1983). Although unassociated with coma, the 'locked-in' syndrome also carries a poor prognosis, with only rare recoveries reported (McCusker et al. 1982).

25.2 **Metabolic causes of coma**

25.2.1 **Renal coma**

Uraemic coma may occur in acute or chronic renal failure, but with the more widespread use of haemodialysis and peritoneal dialysis, unsuspected renal failure as a cause of coma is encountered only rarely. It more commonly enters the differential diagnosis where there are a number of potential causes of coma. The metabolic changes produced in renal failure are complex, and a raised blood urea alone cannot be responsible for the loss of consciousness, although the blood urea concentration does provide a useful index of severity of the renal failure. There is usually metabolic acidosis, accompanied by complex electrolyte disturbances. Water intoxication, due to fluid retention, with a serum osmolality of less than 260 mOsm/l, is a factor in some cases. As is general with cerebral insults, the speed of metabolic disturbance may dictate the severity of the disturbance of consciousness. Although the clinical features are similar with both acute and chronic renal failure, acute metabolic disturbance may result in an impairment of consciousness that would not occur with the more gradual change encountered in chronic renal failure. Headache, vomiting, dyspnoea, mental confusion, drowsiness or restlessness, and insomnia are early symptoms, and later muscular twitchings, asterixis, myoclonus, and generalized convulsions are likely to precede the coma. The raised blood urea or creatinine establishes the diagnosis, but differentiation from hypertensive encephalopathy, often accompanied by signs of renal impairment, can be difficult (Bolton and Young 1990).

Patients undergoing dialysis may develop iatrogenic causes of impaired consciousness. The dialysis disequilibrium syndrome, which is more common in children and during rapid changes in blood solutes, is a temporary, self-limiting disorder, but it can be fatal. Animal studies indicate that rapid osmotic shift of water into the brain is the main problem, which can be corrected by careful control. The dialysis disequilibrium syndrome is usually accompanied by headache, nausea, vomiting, and restlessness before drowsiness and marked somnolence. It can occur during or just after dialysis treatment, but resolves in 1 or 2 days at the most.

Whereas the dialysis disequilibrium syndrome is self-limiting, dialysis encephalopathy results in progressive dysarthria, mental changes, and progression to seizures, myoclonus, asterixis, and focal neurological signs. Terminally, there may be coma. Characteristically, the EEG reveals paroxysmal bursts of irregular, generalized spike and wave activity. Dialysis encephalopathy (or the dialysis dementia syndrome) has been attributed to the neurotoxic effects of aluminium, arising both from the use of aluminium-containing antacids and a high aluminium content in the water (Dunea *et al.* 1978). Dialysis dementia reached its peak prevalence in the mid 1970s, before preventive action was taken. However, rare cases are still seen occasionally.

25.2.2 **Hepatic coma**

The cause of hepatic coma is still incompletely understood. The diagnosis is not usually difficult when the patient is known to be suffering from liver failure, but stupor and coma may supervene in patients with chronic liver failure and portosystemic shunting. In these cases jaundice may be absent. Such patients are also particularly vulnerable to precipitation of hepatic coma by gastrointestinal haemorrhage, infection, the use of certain diuretics, sedatives, and analgesics, general anaesthesia, and the ingestion of high-protein food or ammonium compounds. Hepatic coma is usually of subacute onset, although it can be sudden, with an initial confusional state often accompanied by bilateral asterixis or flapping tremor. Asterixis, considered a negative myoclonus jerk, results in sudden loss of a maintained posture. It can be elicited readily by asking the subject to maintain extension at the wrist; asterixis will be seen as a sudden loss of posture (Fig. 25.2). As coma supervenes, there is often decerebrate and/or decorticate posturing with extensor plantar responses. The diagnosis rests upon the presence of physical

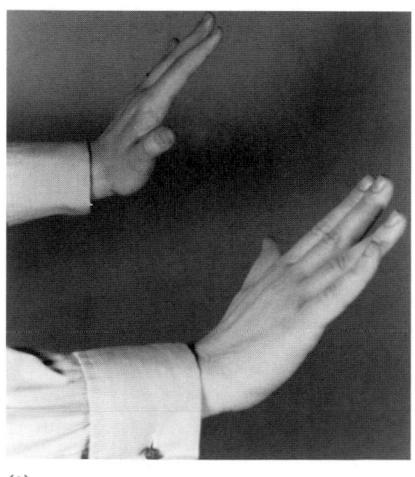 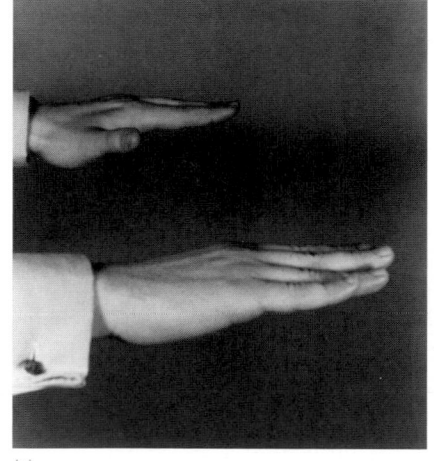 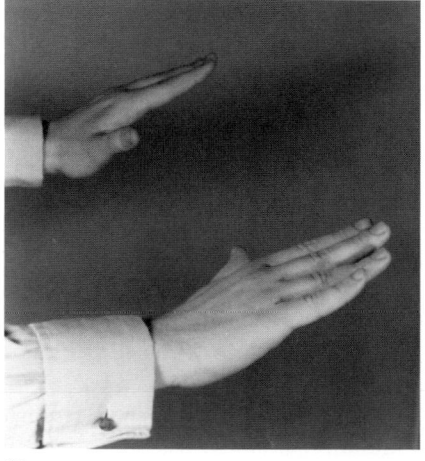

(A)   (B)   (C)

Fig. 25.2. Asterixis is best elicited by asking the patient to extend the wrists with the arms outstretched (A); asterixis is seen as a sudden loss of posture with momentary flexion (B) and (C).

signs of liver disease, including hepatic fetor, and biochemical evidence of disturbed liver function. The EEG is characteristically abnormal, with paroxysms of bilaterally synchronous slow waves in the delta range or with occasional triphasic waves.

The disturbance of consciousness has traditionally been considered to be due to raised ammonia, and indeed treatments to reduce ammonia (e.g. avoidance of high-protein foods, chemical cleansing of the bowel, etc.) are effective (reviewed by Cooper and Plum 1987). More recently, however, attention has been directed towards the GABA$_A$ receptor, which is modulated by benzodiazepines and barbiturates. There is evidence that endogenous benzodiazepine ligands may contribute to the hepatic coma (Mullen et al. 1988). The beneficial use of the benzodiazepine antagonist, flumazenil, in hepatic coma would support this view.

25.2.3 Pancreatic encephalopathy

The biochemical cause of pancreatic encephalopathy is unclear. It can rarely occur with acute pancreatitis, but is more commonly seen as episodic stupor or coma in chronic relapsing pancreatitis. The impairment of consciousness usually begins between the second and fifth day, is characterized by an acute confusional state with hallucinations, followed by focal or generalized convulsions, and there may be corticospinal-tract dysfunction (Pallis and Lewis 1974; Menza and Murray 1989). Patchy demyelination and perivascular haemorrhages have been found at autopsy (Estrada et al. 1979).

25.2.4 Salt and water imbalance

Since sodium is the principal serum cation, hypo-osmolality is largely equivalent to hyponatraemia (Kumar and Berl 1998). It is an important cause of confusional states and, if severe, stupor and coma. Low sodium is usually due to impaired water excretion attributable to renal insufficiency, chronic sodium depletion (which can often be diuretic induced), or to the syndrome of inappropriate antidiuretic hormone (ADH) secretion. This is often seen in neurological practice, for example with infections, head injury, a variety of drugs, and following surgery. Lesions within the region of the hypothalamus are also an important neurological cause. Very rarely some psychiatrically disturbed patients may be compulsive water drinkers, giving rise to hyponatraemia.

The speed of change in sodium concentration is critical as to whether neurological features emerge. Certainly the diagnosis should be considered with sodium concentrations below 120 mmol/l, but even concentrations up to 128 mmol/l may be implicated if there has been a sudden fall. Conversely, patients with chronic sodium depletion may survive concentrations down to 110 mmol/l with little to find neurologically. Hyponatraemia is associated with seizures and can be associated with focal neurological deficits. Although hyponatraemia with neurological disturbance represents a medical emergency, sudden correction can give rise to central pontine myelinolysis, and the sodium levels should probably be raised by no more than 0.5 mmol/l/h (Anonymous 1990).

Hypernatraemia may also cause confusional states and lethargy, but less often coma. It may be seen in children with severe diarrhoea, with adults with diabetes insipidus, and is common in patients with coma who are unable to drink normally or when parenteral fluids have been inadequate. Very rarely, it may be seen in neurological disease with diencephalic involvement, when there is an impaired thirst response. This has been reported with tumours and with infections (Maxwell et al. 1987).

Hypo-osmolar states can also be seen with hyperglycaemia (Section 25.2.6).

25.2.5 Inborn errors of metabolism

A vast array of hereditary disorders of metabolism can result in episodic stupor or coma, as well as occurring as a terminal feature. The majority are very rare and usually present in childhood (Section 4.10). Associated biochemical disturbance can provide clues; for example, inherited disorders of the urea cycle, resulting in hyperammonaemia in children (Walter and Leonard 1987). Porphyria can present with disturbance of consciousness in adults, particularly after the administration of a variety of drugs. Mitochondrial disorders can also present for the first time in adults as an encephalopathy (Howard et al. 1995).

25.2.6 Disturbance of glucose metabolism

The classic presentation of diabetic coma is of subacute onset with late development of coma. There is a marked ketoacidosis, a blood sugar that is usually above 40 mmol/l, together with ketonuria. There is often a secondary lactic acidosis which needs to be distinguished from the lactic acidosis that can follow severe anoxia or methyl alcohol or paraldehyde poisoning. Patients are dehydrated, there is rapid, shallow breathing, and occasionally acetone can be detected on the breath. The plantar responses are usually flexor until coma supervenes.

Hyperglycaemic non-ketotic diabetic coma is important to consider and is more commonly seen in the elderly. Coma is more common than with ketoacidosis. There is profound cellular dehydration and patients are at risk of developing cerebral venous thrombosis, which may contribute to the disturbance of consciousness. In addition to diabetes, hyperglycaemic non-ketotic coma may be induced by drugs, acute pancreatitis, burns, and heat stroke (Section 25.4).

By contrast to diabetic coma, hypoglycaemic coma is of much more rapid onset. Symptoms appear with blood sugars of less than 2.5 mmol/l; initially autonomic disturbance with sweating and pallor, and then symptoms of inattention and irritability before progressing to stupor, coma, and frequent seizures. Some patients may present with a focal onset, for example with a hemiparesis (Malouf and Brust 1985). Plantar responses are frequently found to be extensor. Patients may be hypothermic.

The diagnosis is relatively straightforward if the patient is known to be taking insulin. Spontaneous hypoglycaemia may be more difficult to diagnose, and patients with insulinomas are usually diagnosed late. There may be a long history of intermittent symptoms and the history often suggests that these occur in relation to fasting or exercise. Hypoglycaemia may also be precipitated by hepatic disease, alcohol intake, hypopituitarism, and Addison's disease. Treatment is with glucose, which should be administered together with thiamine if there is any doubt as to the diagnosis.

Unless treated promptly, hypoglycaemia results in irreversible brain damage. Cerebellar Purkinje cells, the cerebral cortex, and particularly the hippocampus and basal ganglia are affected, in a pattern similar to that of anoxia. Dementia and a cerebellar ataxia are the clinical sequelae of inadequately treated hypoglycaemia.

25.2.7 Other endocrine causes of coma

Pituitary failure is a rare cause of coma and is the result of a number of factors, including hypoglycaemia, hypotension, hypothermia, and impaired adrenocortical function (Section 25.2.8). There is usually a history of fatigue, occasionally depression and loss of libido, but, because of the slow onset of symptoms, these are often missed. Patients with hypopituitarism are very sensitive to infections and to sedative drugs, which often precipitate impaired consciousness. Acute onset of hypopituitarism occurs with haemorrhagic infarction in pre-existing tumours, 'pituitary apoplexy'; patients present with impaired consciousness, meningism, and opthalmoplegia.

Mental symptoms are common in hypothyroidism, together with headaches, poor concentration, and apathy; this is frequently diagnosed as depression. With progression there is increasing somnolence and, as with hypopituitarism, patients become sensitive to drugs and infections. These and cold weather, particularly in the elderly, may precipitate myxoedemic coma. Myxoedemic coma has a high mortality and is associated with hypoglycaemia and hyponatraemia. The diagnosis may be missed if not thought of, and to detect hypothermia a low-reading thermometer is required. Treatment is with support of ventilation and blood pressure and cautious correction of the thyroid deficiency with tri-iodothyronine (Blum 1972).

Similarly, hyperthyroidism can cause mild mental symptoms, usually of anxiety, restlessness, and reduced attention. Rarely, patients may develop a 'thyroid storm' with agitated delirium, which can progress to coma. Such patients may have an associated bulbar paralysis (Newcomer *et al.* 1983). By contrast, some patients, particularly the elderly, may develop an apathetic form of thyrotoxicosis, with depression leading to apathy, confusion, and coma without any signs of hypermetabolism (Thomas *et al.* 1970). As with myxoedema coma, the diagnosis is easily missed if not considered.

25.2.8 Adrenocortical failure

Mental changes are common in Addison's disease and secondary hypoadrenalism. Undiagnosed Addison's disease is frequently associated with behavioural changes and fatigue. Intercurrent infection or trauma may cause the precipitation of coma and associated metabolic disturbances of hypotension,

hypoglycaemia, and dehydration. Tendon reflexes are often absent, and raised intracranial pressure with papilloedema can occur (Jefferson 1956). Acute adrenal failure due to meningococcal septicaemia (the Friedrichsen–Waterhouse syndrome) is now rarely seen as a cause of sudden coma in infants. However, acute adrenal failure due to HIV infection can occur.

25.2.9 Disturbance of calcium and magnesium metabolism

Hypercalcaemia is an important cause of mental confusion and apathy, often with headache. If severe, this can progress to stupor and even coma. Causes of hypercalcaemia are numerous and are probably seen most commonly with metastatic bone disease, including multiple myeloma (Bushinsky and Monk 1998). Hypocalcaemia primarily affects the peripheral nervous system, with tetany and sensory disturbance. Only very rarely will it cause disturbance of consciousness, although it can be associated with intracranial hypertension and papilloedema (Grant 1953).

Hypomagnesaemia occurs with inadequate intake and is usually seen in patients with prolonged parenteral feeding. It is often overshadowed by other metabolic disturbances, including hypocalcaemia, but can give rise to a similar clinical picture. Hypermagnesaemia can occur due to renal insufficiency, although rarely at a clinically significant level. Overzealous replacement of magnesium and its use clinically (for example, in the treatment of eclampsia) can give rise to magnesium intoxication, with major CNS depression.

25.2.10 Drugs

Poisoning, drug abuse, and alcohol intoxication are the major causes of coma, accounting for up to 30 per cent of those presenting through Accident and Emergency departments. Despite its frequency, the majority, perhaps as high as 80 per cent, require only simple observation in their management. The most commonly encountered drugs in suicide attempts are benzodiazepines, paracetamol, and antidepressants. Narcotic overdoses can occur, particularly with purchase of street supplies of heroin of variable purity. Characteristic pinpoint pupils and shallow respirations provide the diagnosis and may be aided by obvious needle marks. However, some addicts use mydriatics to mask the pupillary changes. The coma is easily reversible with naloxone but, in view of its short half-life, this may need to be continued as an infusion. Solvent abuse and glue sniffing should be considered in the undiagnosed patient with coma. Drugs may also result in disturbed consciousness due to secondary metabolic derangement; for example, the acidosis associated with ethylene glycol and with carbon monoxide poisoning (Balzan *et al.* 1996). Blood for subsequent toxicology is important to consider, although the results are rarely available quickly enough to influence acute management.

Coma due to alcohol intoxication is often apparent from the history, flushed face, rapid pulse, and low blood pressure. This can be aided by the smell of alcohol on the breath, but this should never be assumed to be the cause of coma. Due to the widespread use of social alcohol, this is a common finding in patients with coincidental illness. Moreover, patients who are intoxicated are at increased risk of hypothermia and of head injury, both of which can be the primary cause of coma. At low plasma concentrations of alcohol, mental changes are common, and at higher levels, coma ensues. In non-alcoholics levels above 350 mg/dl may prove fatal.

25.3 Hypoxia and hypercarbia

Hypoxia has devastating effects on the brain. It occurs in a whole variety of settings, including high altitude, suffocation, drowning, cardiac arrest and pulmonary disease, and ventilatory failure. Anoxia following cardiac and respiratory arrest are very common causes of coma in patients on intensive care units. The dysfunction depends upon the rate. Acute hypoxia is much more devastating, and patients may maintain function with chronically lowered oxygen tensions and associated hypercarbia with relatively modest symptoms, which if they were to occur acutely would result in neurological dysfunction. Arterial oxygen tensions of 40–50 mmHg are associated with a decline in cognitive function, and at pressures below 30 mmHg consciousness is usually lost. Ventilatory failure and pulmonary disease lead to associated hypercarbia with respiratory acidosis as well as hypoxia. Clinical features are asterixis, myoclonus, obtundation, conjunctival injection, and papilloedema. Chronic bronchitic patients often have markedly impaired blood gases but lack dyspnoea. Such patients are at risk because their resistance to hypercarbia means that they require a hypoxic drive to maintain ventilation. The injudicious administration of oxygen can result in marked deterioration with resulting stupor or coma.

Cerebral malaria due to *Plasmodium falciparum* is rare in Europe but is an important cause of hypoxic encephalopathy worldwide (Section 34.13.4).

Recovery from hypoxic coma is uncommon in patients who have been comatose for 6 hours or longer and a persistent vegetative state is a common outcome (Section 25.13) (Levy *et al.* 1981). Rarely, a delayed post-anoxic encephalopathy may occur following a period of apparent recovery. The patient deteriorates with progressive impairment of consciousness and motor disturbance after a period of some 5–10 days. This is associated with widespread leucoencephalopathy.

25.4 Disturbance of thermoregulation

Loss of thermoregulation giving rise to hyperthermia or heat stroke is a clinical emergency. This may be encountered after prolonged exertion in a hot environment; for example, in endurance sports such as cycle racing and marathon running. The initial rise in body temperature with profuse sweating is followed by hyperpyrexia, an abrupt cessation of sweating, and

then the rapid onset of coma, convulsions, and death (Section 5.9.2). This may be exacerbated by certain drugs and can be seen with 'Ecstasy' abuse—involving a loss of the thirst reaction in individuals engaged in prolonged dancing. Tetanus, pontine haemorrhage, and lesions in the floor of the third ventricle may also give rise to hyperpyrexia, as may neuroleptics in the neuroleptic malignant syndrome, and malignant hyperpyrexia with anaesthetics. Survivors of heat stroke may be left with permanent neurological sequelae of paraparesis, cerebellar ataxia, and, rarely, dementia (Salem 1966).

Hypothermia may also give rise to impairment of consciousness. This may be seen with hypopituitarism and hypothyroidism, and also induced by certain drugs (commonly seen previously with chlorpromazine). However, there is always a risk of hypothermia in the elderly with inadequately heated rooms, and this may be exacerbated by immobility, for example in those with Parkinson's disease. It will also occur in patients exposed to low temperature environments or cold-water immersion. In these situations the history is clear. There is usually generalized rigidity and muscle fasciculation but true shivering may be absent. Hypoxia and hypercarbia are common. Gradual warming is necessary and may require peritoneal dialysis with warm fluids. It is important to establish the diagnosis (a low-reading rectal thermometer is required).

Spontaneous periodic hypothermia (Shapiro's syndrome) is a rare syndrome of recurrent hypothermia, often associated with agenesis of the corpus callosum, polydipsia, polyuria, and hyponatraemia (Mooradian *et al.* 1984).

25.5 Cerebrovascular causes of coma

Cerebrovascular disease is a frequent cause of coma. A common mechanism is the impairment of perfusion of the reticular activating system, as occurs with hypotension, brainstem herniation due to parenchymal haemorrhage, or swelling from infarct, or more rarely, extensive brainstem infarction.

25.5.1 Subarachnoid haemorrhage

Loss of consciousness is common with subarachnoid haemorrhage (see also Section 27.7) and only about one-half of patients recover from the initial effects of the haemorrhage. Contributing causes to coma are the acute rise in intracranial pressure and, later, the emergence of vasospasms. Secondary metabolic effects may also contribute and hyponatraemia is a common finding. This may occur with renal salt loss and volume contraction, so-called 'cerebral salt wasting'. It is proposed that this is due to the increased release of brain natriuretic peptide, resulting in an increase in urine volume and sodium excretion (Berendes *et al.* 1997). The diagnosis is made on the history and, in patients in whom there is loss of consciousness, blood is normally apparent on neuroimaging.

25.5.2 **Parenchymal haemorrhage**

A large parenchymal haemorrhage may cause a rapid decline in consciousness, either from rupture into the ventricles or from subsequent herniation and brainstem compression. Of particular importance is the diagnosis of a cerebellar haemorrhage or of a cerebellar infarct with subsequent oedema and direct brainstem compression. Diagnosis and early decompression can be lifesaving.

25.5.3 **Hypotension**

The critical blood flow in humans required to maintain effective cerebral activity is about 20 ml/100 g/min and any fall below this leads rapidly to cerebral insufficiency. The causes are legion, and include syncope in younger patients and, commonly, cardiac disease in older patients. These are covered elsewhere.

25.5.4 **Hypertensive encephalopathy**

Hypertensive encephalopathy is now rare with better control of blood pressure. Patients could present with impaired consciousness and a grossly raised blood pressure with papilloedema. Neuropathologically, fibrinoid necrosis, arteriolar thrombosis, microinfarction, and cerebral oedema result. The latter appears to relate to failure of autoregulation.

25.6 **Raised intracranial pressure**

Raised intracranial pressure *per se*, as occurs with benign intracranial hypertension, does not cause coma. Rather, mass effects such as tumours, abscesses, haemorrhage, subdural, and extradural haematomata will cause impairment of consciousness due to distortion of the reticular activating system. This is the classical feature of brainstem herniation (Section 17.1.3). The clinical development and pattern depends on a number of features, such as normal variation in the tentorial aperture, site of lesion, and the speed of development. Lesions located deeply, laterally, or in the temporal lobes will have a greater tendency to herniation and loss of consciousness than those located at a distance, such as the frontal and occipital lobes (Andrews *et al.* 1988). The speed of development of a mass is also important. Slowly growing tumours may achieve a substantial size and distortion of cerebral structure without impairment of consciousness, in contrast to small rapidly expanding lesions.

Classically, two patterns of downward movement of the brainstem have been recognized, although typically these may coincide. Central herniation involves downward displacement of the upper brainstem, in contrast to uncal herniation in which the medial temporal lobe herniates through the tentorium. In the former, small pupils are followed by midpoint pupils, and irregular respiration gives way to hyperventilation as coma deepens. With uncal herniation there is classically a unilateral dilated pupil, due to compression of the third nerve, and asymmetric motor signs. As coma deepens, the opposite pupil loses the light reflex and may constrict briefly before enlarging (Ropper 1990). Rarely, upward herniation can occur with posterior fossa masses (Cuneo *et al.* 1979).

25.7 **Head injury**

Trauma is the leading cause of death below the age of 45, and head injury accounts for half of all trauma deaths (see also Chapter 16). It is also a major cause of patients presenting with coma. A history is usually available and, if not, signs of injury such as bruising of the scalp or skull fracture lead one to the diagnosis. However, as with assuming that alcohol on the breath provides a direct clue to a cause of coma, evidence of head injury need not necessarily imply that this is the cause. Other causes of impaired consciousness, for example epileptic seizure, may have resulted in a subsequent head injury.

Impact damage can be diffuse or focal. Rotational forces of the brain cause surface cortical contusions and even lacerations. These are most obvious frontotemporally because of the irregular sphenoidal wing and orbital roof. Tearing of veins may give rise to subdural bleeding. This is less important than the damage to nerve fibres. This is not apparent macroscopically but diffuse axonal injury is now seen as the major consequence of head injury and associated coma (Adams *et al.* 1982). Mild degrees of axonal injury also occur with concussion and brief loss of consciousness.

Secondary damage can occur from parenchymal haemorrhage, brain swelling due to oedema, and vascular dilatation, all of which will lead to raised intracranial pressure. This will reduce perfusion pressure, which can be accentuated by systemic hypoxia and blood loss. The specific instances of subdural and extradural haematomata which may cause impairment of consciousness following apparent recovery are important to diagnose, as they are readily treatable surgically.

25.8 **Infections**

Systemic infections may result in coma as an event secondary to metabolic and vascular disturbance or seizure activity. However, direct infections of the CNS, as with meningitis and encephalitis, can all be associated with coma. When meningitis causes coma, the onset of symptoms is usually subacute, before losing consciousness the patient complains of intense headache, associated with fever and neck stiffness (Section 33.1.4). However, meningococcal meningitis may be fearfully rapid in onset. The diagnosis is confirmed by identifying the characteristic changes in the CSF, from which it may be possible to isolate the causative organism. Prompt treatment of acute meningitis is, however, imperative and may, of necessity, precede diagnostic confirmation. The onset of encephalitis is also usually subacute, and often associated with fever and/or seizures, although herpes simplex encephalitis may be explosive at onset, leading to coma within a matter of hours (Section 34.3.1). Treatment with aciclovir, by necessity, precedes definitive diagnosis.

A number of parasitic infections may give rise to coma, of which by far the most important is cerebral malaria (Section 34.13.4). Cerebral malaria, which carries a 25 per cent mortality rate, is associated with 2–10 per cent of cases of infection with *Plasmodium falciparum*. There is an acute profound mental obtundation or psychosis, leading to coma with extensor plantar responses. Although the CSF may show increased protein, characteristically there is no pleocytosis. Patients often develop hypoglycaemia and lactic acidosis, which may contribute to the coma. Treatment is with intravenous quinine. Steroids, which were at one time prescribed widely for oedema, are now contraindicated as they prolong the coma (Warrell *et al.* 1982).

Independently of direct infections of the CNS, septic patients commonly develop an encephalopathy (Section 35.2). In some patients this can be severe, with a prolonged coma. Lumbar puncture in such patients is usually normal or only associated with a mildly elevated protein level. The EEG is valuable and is abnormal, ranging from diffuse theta through to triphasic waves and suppression or burst-suppression. Although there is a high mortality, there is the potential for complete reversibility, and so the presence of coma should not prevent an aggressive approach to management of such patients including, for example, haemodialysis to deal with acute renal failure (Bolton *et al.* 1993).

25.9 Miscellaneous causes of coma

Seizures are a common cause of coma, with a period of unconsciousness following a single generalized seizure commonly lasting between 30 and 60 minutes. Following status epilepticus, there may be a prolonged period of coma (Section 23.4.5). If the history is unavailable, clues may be provided from trauma to the tongue or inside of the mouth. Seizures secondary to metabolic disturbances may have a longer period of coma.

Extensive neurological disease may also result in impaired consciousness, for example progressive multifocal leucoencephalopathy (Section 34.10) and severe end-stage multiple sclerosis (Section 29.4). Prion disease may lead to coma over a short period of 6–8 weeks, but this is following a progressive course of widespread neurological disturbance (Section 34.12).

25.9.1 Eclampsia

Eclampsia presents in the second half of pregnancy and represents a failure of autoregulation, with raised blood pressure. Since the upper limit of autoregulation is directly related to the individual's normal blood pressure, the level at which eclampsia occurs may be very variable. Neuropathologically there are ring haemorrhages around occluded small vessels with fibrinoid deposits. The clinical characteristics are those of seizures, cortical blindness, and coma. Management is the control of convulsions and raised blood pressure. Parental magnesium is commonly employed, particularly in the US

(Weisinger and Bellorin-Font 1998) and this itself may give rise to hypermagnesaemia.

Postpartum complications of pregnancy, including cerebral angiitis and venous sinus thrombosis (Section 27.11), may also lead to coma.

25.10 Coma in children

The basic principles of the approach to coma in children are the same as for adults. However, the Glasgow Coma Scale (Teasdale and Jennett 1974), originally intended for use in adults with closed head injury, cannot be applied without modification in the very young, principally because the motor and verbal components require adjustment for age. A number of special coma scales have since been devised, the Paediatric Coma Scale having the highest interobserver reliability (Simpson *et al.* 1991). To overcome the difficulty of assessing verbal ability in the intubated patient, a grimace score has been proposed as a surrogate measure, also with moderately good interobserver reliability (Kirkpatrick 1997). A fundamental problem in assessing coma in children is that, whereas a GCS of 8 or less in adults signifies a high probability of intracranial hypertension and need for intensive care, no such correlative data are available in children (Gemke and Tasker 1998), making evaluation of interventions and prognosis difficult.

The major causes of coma in children are accidental and non-accidental injury, infection, hypoxia, and epilepsy (Seshia *et al.* 1977, 1983). Inborn errors of metabolism as causes of coma are relatively more common in children, for example those arising from urea cycle disorders, disorders of glycogen storage, pyruvate metabolism, respiratory chain disorders, and medium-chain acyl-CoA dehydrogenase deficiency, only rarely seen in adult neurology. Inborn errors of metabolism may also mimic the features of birth asphyxia in neonates. Reye syndrome is now seen very rarely in Western countries, since the association with aspirin use has been recognized and prevented. Occasional cases are associated with varicella and influenza B infection. The initial stage starts 3–6 days after the appearance of the varicella rash and may progress rapidly from vomiting to increasing coma, metabolic disturbance, liver failure, and cerebral oedema with herniation. Hypertonic dehydration, usually secondary to gastroenteritis in small children, may cause subdural haematomas or venous sinus thrombosis as water is drawn out of the brain. Too rapid correction of dehydration may precipitate cerebral oedema and seizures.

Head injury may be caused by non-accidental means, and a history of trauma is not always available. It should be suspected if there are signs of other injuries (Caffey 1972), fractures of differing ages, or if there is discrepancy between the account of the injury and that expected from the clinical examination. Coma precipitated by trauma may develop after a longer lucid interval than in adults. In infants, the relative elasticity of the skull, along with the presence of open fontanelles and unfused sutures, can lead to a different pattern of intracranial pathology with haematomas, dural and tentorial tears, and oedema

(Zimmerman and Bilaniuk 1981). It is important to recognize that child abuse may also result in coma through asphyxia or poisoning.

Cardiovascular causes of coma are rare in children outside the context of cyanotic congenital heart disease complicated by cerebral venous thrombosis or abscess, or after circulatory bypass cardiac surgery. It may be difficult clinically to decide whether a young child who has, for example, had complex cardiac surgery or cardiorespiratory arrest and is requiring intensive care is in a coma or not. It is usual that intracranial pressure, cerebral perfusion pressure, and EEG are monitored in these situations, so that measures for the management of reduced cerebral perfusion pressure and of subclinical status epilepticus can be instituted, in an effort to minimize the subsequent impairments.

There are relatively fewer data on the prognosis of coma in children than in adults. In non-traumatic coma, infants have a higher mortality (44 per cent) compared to older children (24 per cent) (Seshia 1983; Johnston and Seshia 1984). All patients who died had internal or external ophthalmoplegia or problems in regulating body temperature. Children with anoxic injuries (e.g. cardiac arrest) have the highest mortality. Duration of coma best predicts disability in survivors (Johnston and Seshia 1984). Slow, poorly reactive EEG patterns at day 10 of coma also predict neurological impairment (Bricolo et al. 1978). In general, children with traumatic head injury fare better than adults, with the opportunity for substantial recovery (Berger et al. 1985).

In young children the potential for apparent 'recovery' includes the process of normal development. It is thus inappropriate to use the term chronic vegetative state in very young children. Certainly it should not be used under the age of 1 year. In older children, although the adult definitions appear to apply in the short to medium term, there is a very common tendency for some recovery of awareness and responsiveness, albeit with very severe disability. Modern neonatal care allows the survival of some very severely cerebrally damaged babies, in whom the brainstem is sufficiently robust to support vegetative functions.

There is now an increasing population of chronically ventilated children whose predicament follows acute cerebral and spinal cord injuries and illnesses. This is now becoming a significant issue for families and health providers.

In general, the criteria for brain death are as in adults, but with caution being exercised in neonates. Ashwal and Schneider (1989) suggest that up to 2 months of age there should be two examinations and EEGs 48 hours apart; that up to 1 year these two examinations and EEGs can be 24 hours apart; and that over a year, the usual prior criteria and two examinations 12–24 hours apart may suffice. Under a year they suggested that some form of angiographic demonstration of lack of cerebral blood flow was a useful adjunct and, in another study, use of middle cerebral artery pulsed Doppler ultrasound was found to be extremely helpful as an adjunct to this diagnosis (Kirkham et al. 1987).

25.11 Psychogenic unresponsiveness

In psychogenic unresponsiveness, the patient, although apparently unconscious (Plum and Posner 1980), usually shows some response to external stimuli. For example, an attempt to elicit the corneal reflex may cause a vigorous contraction of the orbicularis oculi. Marked resistance to passive movement of the limbs may be present, and signs of organic disease are absent. The caloric and optokinetic responses and the EEG are all generally normal. It is not possible to mimic the roving eye movements of coma, nor is it possible to mimic the slow closure that is seen after the eyelids are raised by the examiner. However, the diagnosis of catatonic stupor as a cause of psychogenic unresponsiveness is more difficult, as in such cases the EEG may be abnormal. Catatonia, in which the limbs maintain a posture passively imposed by the examiner, may be a helpful sign in such cases.

25.12 The locked-in state

The de-efferented state or 'locked-in' syndrome occurs with lesions of the medulla or anterior pons, with sparing of the tegmentum and thus preservation of consciousness. It is most commonly seen with basilar artery infarcts. The patient, despite being tetraplegic and anarthric, is fully aware of his or her surroundings, as tragically and eloquently described by J. D. Bauby in *The diving bell and the butterfly'* (Bauby 1997). The EEG shows a reactive alpha rhythm consistent with consciousness, and event-related potentials are normal (Onofrj et al. 1997). So-called alpha coma, in which an alpha rhythm is found in association with coma, is seen usually with brainstem infarcts, but is usually unresponsive to stimuli, although rarely this can occur with drug intoxication, when the alpha rhythm may be more responsive (Carroll and Mastaglia 1979). In the classical locked-in syndrome, there is preservation of vertical eye movements, which can provide a means of communication. Total locked-in syndrome may occur with lesions of the cerebral peduncles, in which there is a complete ophthalmoplegia (Karp and Hurtig 1974). Although most commonly occurring in association with basilar territory infarct, it can occur with demyelination, as in central pontine myelinolysis, and a similar syndrome can occur with peripheral disorders with severe polyneuropathies, myasthenia, and neuromuscular blocking agents. Even with infarcts, patients can make good recoveries, justifying aggressive treatment in the early stages (Patterson and Grabois 1986).

25.13 Persistent vegetative state

Patients who survive in coma, i.e. are in a state of unresponsiveness to external stimuli with eyes closed, do not remain in this state for more than 2–3 weeks, but rather develop a persistent unresponsive state in which sleep–wake cycles return. There is, however, no evidence of consciousness; they are awake but not aware. Jennett and Plum (1972) proposed the term 'the persistent or chronic vegetative state' which has now replaced the earlier terms of 'coma vigil' and 'apallic syndrome' (Zeman 1997).

25.13.1 Diagnosis

By definition, the vegetative state is a clinical condition of complete unawareness of the self and the environment, which is accompanied by sleep–wake cycles and complete or partial preservation of hypothalamic and brainstem autonomic functions. There should be no evidence of sustained, reproducible, purposeful, or voluntary behavioural responses to visual, auditory, tactile, or noxious stimuli, and no evidence of language comprehension or expression. The Multi-Society Task Force on PVS defined the persistent vegetative state as one that is present 1 month after acute traumatic or non-traumatic brain injury, or lasting for at least 1 month in patients with degenerative or metabolic disorders or developmental malformations (Multi-Society Task Force on PVS 1994). The Royal College of Physicians Working Group (1996) defined the vegetative state as a 'clinical condition of unawareness of self and environment in which the patient breathes spontaneously, has a stable circulation and shows cycles of eye closure and eye opening which may simulate sleep and waking'. They go on to define the continuing vegetative state (CVS) as being when the vegetative state continues for more than 4 weeks. It then becomes increasingly unlikely that the condition is part of the recovery phase from coma and the diagnosis for CVS can be made. The permanent vegetative state (PVS) can be made when the diagnosis of irreversibility has been established with a high degree of clinical certainty. It is considered a reasonable diagnosis when a patient has been in a CVS following head injury for more than 12 months, or following other causes of brain damage for more than 6 months.

The vegetative state needs considerable skill to diagnose and requires assessment over a period of time to ensure that indeed there is no purposeful response to external stimuli. Thus, Andrews and co-workers, in a study of 40 patients with a referral diagnosis of vegetative state, found that 43 per cent did not fulfil the criteria. Most of the misdiagnosed patients were blind or severely visually impaired (Andrews *et al.* 1996).

It is assumed that there is relative presentation of brainstem structures and that the main site of pathology is in the cerebral cortex, and indeed cortical laminar necrosis may be found. However, the neuropathological features of a patient who suffered a cardiopulmonary arrest in 1975 and died 10 years later (The Quinlan case) confirmed a relatively intact brainstem but profound bilateral and extensive thalamic damage, more so than the cerebral cortex (Kinney *et al.* 1994).

25.13.2 Management and prognosis

The management of PVS has attracted considerable debate (Howard and Miller 1995). Until the diagnosis of PVS has been made beyond doubt, full nursing support and nutrition, usually by gastrostomy, should be provided. In patients in whom an undoubted diagnosis has been made, recovery of consciousness for a post-traumatic PVS is unlikely after 12 months, and for a non-traumatic PVS, extremely rare after 3 months. The life span in PVS is reduced and, for most patients, life expectancy ranges from 2 to 5 years, although survival beyond 10 years is reported. When a diagnosis has been established, an application may be made, often involving a court of law and depending upon national guidelines, for withdrawal of tube feeding.

25.14 Brainstem death

This problem has assumed considerable importance in recent years, first because of the increasing difficulty of deciding whether it is justifiable to maintain life indefinitely with artificial support in patients with severe brain damage, and secondly because of the difficult question of deciding when a cerebral lesion is irreversible and death is imminent, so that viable organs for donation may be removed.

25.14.1 Definition

Many different criteria have been developed, but all are broadly similar (Halevy and Brody 1993). The diagnosis of brain death is equated with functional death of the brainstem, and when brainstem death has occurred, there is no possible chance of recovery (Pallis 1982). Although there are some national variations, most criteria include the same conditions for diagnosing brain death and similar tests for confirming brainstem death. The following are the UK criteria (Conference of Medical Royal Colleges and their Faculties in the United Kingdom 1976).

25.14.2 Criteria for diagnosis

Conditions for considering diagnosis of brain death

All of the following should coexist:

1. The patient must be deeply comatose. There should be no suspicion that this is due to CNS depressant drugs, primary hypothermia must have been excluded, and any metabolic or endocrine contribution or cause of the coma carefully assessed.

2. The patient must be maintained on a ventilator because spontaneous respiration had previously become inadequate or ceased altogether. Neuromuscular blocking agents must have been excluded as a cause of respiratory failure. The failure of neuromuscular transmission from other causes may need to be excluded by use of a nerve stimulator.

3. There should be no doubt that the patient's condition is due to irremediable structural brain damage and the diagnosis of the underlying cause of brain death should have been fully established.

Tests for confirming brain death

All brainstem reflexes should be absent, as follows:

(1) The pupils are fixed in diameter and do not respond to sharp changes in the intensity of incident light.

(2) There is no corneal reflex.

(3) The vestibulo-ocular reflexes are absent. These are absent when no eye movement occurs during or after the slow infusion by syringe of 20 ml of ice-cold water into each external auditory meatus in turn, clear access to the tympanic membrane having been established by direct inspection. This test may be contraindicated on one or other side by local trauma.

(4) No motor responses within the cranial nerve distribution can be elicited by adequate stimulation of any somatic area.

(5) There is no gag reflex or reflex response to bronchial stimulation by a suction catheter passed down the trachea.

(6) No respiratory movements occur when the patient is disconnected from the mechanical ventilator for long enough to ensure that the arterial carbon dioxide tension rises above the threshold for stimulating respiration—that is the $Paco_2$ must normally reach 6.7 kPa (50 mmHg). (Hypoxia during disconnection should be prevented by delivering oxygen at 6 litres/min through a catheter into the trachea.)

Criteria in other countries may vary, particularly as to whether an isoelectric EEG is added to the criteria. This is not necessary in the UK. It is well established that spinal cord function can persist in the absence of brainstem function, and the presence of such reflexes do not preclude a diagnosis of brainstem death.

The tests should be repeated, to ensure that there is no observer error, by two independent clinicians. The timing of the two tests is not fixed, and will depend to some extent on the underlying cause. It may be as long as 24 hours. It is important that experienced clinicians, one of whom is a consultant, perform the tests.

The British criteria have been found reliable in clinical practice; for example, of 1003 survivors of severe head injury, none would have been suspected of being brainstem dead on the above criteria (Jennett *et al.* 1981).

References

Adams, J. H., Graham, D. I., Murray, L. S. *et al.* (1982). Diffuse axonal injury due to nonmissile head injury in humans: an analysis of 45 cases. *Ann. Neurol.*, **12**, 557–63.

Andrews, B. T., Chiles, B. W., Olsen, W. L. *et al.* (1988). The effect of intracerebral hematoma location on the risk of brain-stem compression and on clinical outcome. *J. Neurosurg.*, **69**, 518–22.

Andrews, K., Murphy, L., Munday, R. *et al.* (1996). Misdiagnosis of the vegetative state: retrospective study in a rehabilitation unit [see comments]. *BMJ*, **313**, 13–16.

Anonymous (1990). Severe symptomatic hyponatraemia: dangers in lack of therapy. *Lancet*, **335**, 825–6.

Anonymous (1995). Recommendations for use of uniform nomenclature pertinent to patients with severe alterations in consciousness. American Congress of Rehabilitation Medicine [see comments]. *Arch. Phys. Med. Rehabil.*, **76**, 205–9. [Published erratum appears in *Arch. Phys. Med. Rehabil.* (1995) **76** (4), 397.]

Ashwal, S. and Schneider, S. (1989). Brain death in the newborn. *Paediatrics*, **84**, 429–37.

Balzan, M. V., Agius, G., and Galea, D. A. (1996). Carbon monoxide poisoning: easy to treat but difficult to recognise [see comments]. *Postgrad. Med. J.*, **72**, 470–3.

Bauby, J.-D. (1997). *The diving-bell and the butterfly*. Fourth Estate, London.

Bauer, G., Gerstenbrand, F., and Rumpl, E. (1979). Varieties of the locked-in syndrome. *J. Neurol*, **221**, 77–91.

Berendes, E., Walter, M., Cullen, P. *et al.* (1997). Secretion of brain natriuretic peptide in patients with aneurysmal subarachnoid haemorrhage. *Lancet*, **349**, 245–9.

Berger, M. S., Pitts, L. H., Lovely, M. *et al.* (1985). Outcome from severe head injury in children and adolescents. *J. Neurosurg.*, **62**, 194–9.

Blum, M. (1972). Myxedema coma. *Am. J. Med. Sci.*, **264**, 432–43.

Bolton, C. F. and Young, G. B. (1990). *Neurological complications of renal disease*. Butterworth–Heinemann, Stoneham, MA.

Bolton, C. F., Young, G. B., and Zochodne, D. W. (1993). The neurological complications of sepsis. *Ann. Neurol.*, **33**, 94–100.

Bricolo, A., Turazzi, S., Faccioli, F. *et al.* (1978). Clinical application of compressed spectral array in long-term EEG monitoring of comatose patients. *Electroencephalogr.Clin. Neurophysiol.*, **45**, 211–25.

Bushinsky, D. A. and Monk, R. D. (1998). Calcium. *Lancet*, **352**, 306–11.

Caffey, J. (1972). On the theory and practice of shaking infants. Its potential residual effects of permanent brain damage and mental retardation. *Am. J. Dis. Child.*, **124**, 161–9.

Cairns, H. (1952). Disturbances of consciousness with lesions to the brain stem and diencephalon. *Brain*, **75**, 109.

Carroll, W. M. and Mastaglia, F. L. (1979). Alpha and beta coma in drug intoxication uncomplicated by cerebral hypoxia. *Electroencephalogr. Clin. Neurophysiol.*, **46**, 95–105.

Conference of Medical Royal Colleges and their Faculties in the United Kingdom (1976). Diagnosis of brain death. Statement issued by the honorary secretary of the Conference of Medical Royal Colleges and their Faculties in the United Kingdom on 11 October 1976. *BMJ*, **2**, 1187–8.

Cooper, A. J. and Plum, F. (1987). Biochemistry and physiology of brain ammonia. *Physiol. Rev.*, **67**, 440–519.

Cowey, A. and Stoerig, P. (1995). Blindsight in monkeys [see comments]. *Nature* **373**, 247–9.

Cuneo, R. A., Caronna, J. J., Pitts, L. *et al.* (1979). Upward transtentorial herniation: seven cases and a literature review. *Arch. Neurol.*, **36**, 618–23.

Dunea, G., Mahurkar, S. D., Mamdani, B. *et al.* (1978). Role of aluminum in dialysis dementia. *Ann. Intern. Med.*, **88**, 502–4.

Estrada, R. V., Moreno, J., Martinez, E. *et al.* (1979). Pancreatic encephalopathy. *Acta Neurol. Scand.*, **59**, 135–9.

Gemke, R. J. and Tasker, R. C. (1998). Clinical assessment of acute coma in children. *Lancet*, **351**, 926–7.

Giacino, J. T. (1997). Disorders of consciousness: differential diagnosis and neuropathologic features. *Semin. Neurol.*, **17**, 105–11.

Grant, D. K. (1953). Papilloedema and fits in hypoparathyroidism. *QJM*, **22**, 243.

Halevy, A. and Brody, B. (1993). Brain death: reconciling definitions, criteria, and tests. *Ann. Intern. Med.*, **119**, 519–25.

Howard, R. S. and Miller, D. H. (1995a). The persistent vegetative state. *BMJ*, **310**, 341–2.

Howard, R. S., Russell, S., Losseff, N. *et al.* (1995b). Management of mitochondrial disease on an intensive care unit. *QJM*, **88**, 197–207.

Jefferson, A. (1956). Clinical correlation between encephalopathy and papilloedema in Addison's disease. *J. Neurol. Neurosurg. Psychiatry*, **19**, 21.

Jennett, B. and Bond, M. (1975). Assessment of outcome after severe brain damage. *Lancet*, **1**, 480–4.

Jennett, B. and Plum, F. (1972). Persistent vegetative state after brain damage. A syndrome in search of a name. *Lancet*, **1**, 734–7.

Jennett, B., Teasdale, G., Braakman, R. *et al.* (1979). Prognosis of patients with severe head injury. *Neurosurgery*, **4**, 283–9.

Jennett, B., Gleave, J., and Wilson, P. (1981). Brain death in three neurosurgical units. *BMJ Clin. Res. Ed.*, **282**, 533–9.

Johnston, B. and Seshia, S. S. (1984). Prediction of outcome in non-traumatic coma in childhood. *Acta Neurol. Scand.*, **69**, 417–27.

Karp, J. S. and Hurtig, H. I. (1974). 'Locked-in' state with bilateral midbrain infarcts. *Arch. Neurol.*, **30**, 176–8.

Kinney, H. C., Korein, J., Panigrahy, A. *et al.* (1994). Neuropathological findings in the brain of Karen Ann Quinlan. The role of the thalamus in the persistent vegetative state [see comments]. *N. Engl. J. Med.*, **330**, 1469–75.

Kirkham, R. J., Levin, S. D., Padayachee, R. S. *et al.* (1987). Transcranial pulsed Doppler ultrasound findings in brain stem death. *J. Neurol. Neurosurg. Psychiatry*, **50**, 1504–13.

Kirkpatrick, P. J. (1997). On guidelines for the management of the severe head injury [see comments]. *J. Neurol. Neurosurg. Psychiatry*, **62**, 109–11.

Kumar, S. and Berl, T. (1998). Sodium. *Lancet*, **352**, 220–8.

Leigh, R. J. and Shaw, D. A. (1976). Rapid regular respiration in unconscious patients. *Arch. Neurol.*, **33**, 356–61.

Levy, D. E., Bates, D., Caronna, J. J. *et al.* (1981). Prognosis in nontraumatic coma. *Ann. Intern. Med.*, **94**, 293–301.

Levy, D. E., Sidtis, J. J., Rottenberg, D. A. *et al.* (1987). Differences in cerebral blood flow and glucose utilization in vegetative versus locked-in patients. *Ann. Neurol.*, **22**, 673–82.

Magoun, H. W. (1952). The ascending reticular activating system. *Res. Publ. Ass. Res. Nerv. Ment. Dis.*, **30**, 480.

Malouf, R. and Brust, J. C. (1985). Hypoglycemia: causes, neurological manifestations, and outcome. *Ann. Neurol.*, **17**, 421–30.

Marin, R. S. (1990). Differential diagnosis and classification of apathy. *Am. J. Psychiatry*, **147**, 22–30.

Maxwell, M. H., Kleeman, C. R., and Narins, R. G. (1987). *Clinical disorders of fluid and electrolyte metabolism*, (4th edn). McGraw Hill, New York

McCusker, E. A., Rudick, R. A., Honch, G. W. *et al.* (1982). Recovery from the 'locked-in' syndrome. *Arch. Neurol.*, **39**, 145–7.

Medical Research Council (1941). *A glossary of psychological terms commonly used in cases of head injury.* HMSO, London.

Menza, M. A. and Murray, G. B. (1989). Pancreatic encephalopathy. *Biol. Psychiatry*, **25**, 781–4.

Mooradian, A. D., Morley, G. K., McGeachie, R. *et al.* (1984). Spontaneous periodic hypothermia. *Neurology*, **34**, 79–82.

Mullen, K. D., Martin, J. V., Mendelson, W. B. *et al.* (1988). Could an endogenous benzodiazepine ligand contribute to hepatic encephalopathy? *Lancet*, **1**, 457–9.

Multi-Society Task Force on PVS (1994). Medical aspects of the persistent vegetative state (1). *N. Engl. J. Med.*, **330**, 1499–508.

Nemeth, G., Hegedus, K., and Molnar, L. (1986). Akinetic mutism and locked-in syndrome: the functional–anatomical basis for their differentiation. *Funct. Neurol.*, 1, 128–39.

Newcomer, J., Haire, W., and Hartman, C. R. (1983). Coma and thyrotoxicosis. *Ann. Neurol.*, 14, 689–90.

Onofrj, M., Thomas, A., Paci, C. *et al.* (1997). Event related potentials recorded in patients with locked-in syndrome. *J. Neurol. Neurosurg. Psychiatry*, 63, 759–64.

Pallis, C. (1982). ABC of brain stem death. From brain death to brain stem death. *BMJ Clin. Res. Ed.*, 285, 1487–90.

Pallis, C. and Lewis, P. D. (1974). *The neurology of gastrointestinal disease.* W. B. Saunders, London.

Patterson, J. R. and Grabois, M. (1986). Locked-in syndrome: a review of 139 cases. *Stroke*, 17, 758–64.

Plum, F. (1982). Mechanisms of 'central' hyperventilation. *Ann. Neurol.*, 11, 636.

Plum, F. and Alvord, E. C. Jr (1964). Apneustic breathing in man. *Arch. Neurol. Psychiatry, Chicago*, 10, 101.

Plum, F. and Posner, J. B. (1980). *Stupor and coma*, (3rd edn). Davis, Philadelphia.

Plum, F. and Swanson, A. G. (1958). Abnormalities in the central regulation of respiration in acute and convalescent poliomyelitis. *Arch. Neurol. Psychiatry, Chicago*, 80, 267.

Rodriguez, M., Baele, P. L., Marsh, H. M. *et al.* (1982). Central neurogenic hyperventilation in an awake patient with brainstem astrocytoma. *Ann. Neurol.*, 11, 625–8.

Ropper, A. H. (1990). The opposite pupil in herniation. *Neurology*, 40, 1707–9.

Ropper, A. H. and Kennedy, S. K. (1988). *Neurological and neurosurgical intensive care.* Asten Publishers, Frederick, Maryland.

Rosenberg, G. A., Johnson, S. F. and Brenner, R. P. (1977). Recovery of cognition after prolonged vegetative state. *Ann. Neurol.*, 2, 167.

Royal College of Physicians Working Group (1996). The permanent vegetative state. Review by a working group convened by the Royal College of Physicians and endorsed by the Conference of Medical Royal Colleges and their faculties of the United Kingdom. *J. R. Coll. Physicians,London*, 30, 119–21.

Salem, S. N. (1966). Neurological complications of heat stroke in Kuwait. *Ann. trop. Med. Parasitol.*, 60, 393.

Seshia, S. S., Seshia, M. M., and Sachdeva, R. K. (1977). Coma in childhood. *Dev. Med. Child. Neurol.*, 19, 614–28.

Seshia, S. S., Johnston, B., and Kasian, G. (1983). Non-traumatic coma in childhood: clinical variables in prediction of outcome. *Dev. Med. Child. Neurol.*, 25, 493–501.

Shuttleworth, E. (1983). Recovery to social and economic independence from prolonged postanoxic vegetative state. *Neurology*, 33, 372–4.

Simpson, D. A., Cockington, R. A., Hanieh, A. *et al.* (1991). Head injuries in infants and young children: the value of the Paediatric Coma Scale. Review of literature and report on a study. *Childs Nerv. Syst.*, 7, 183–90.

Snyder, B. D., Gumnit, R. J., Leppik, I. E. *et al.* (1981). Neurologic prognosis after cardiopulmonary arrest: IV. Brainstem reflexes. *Neurology*, 31, 1092–7.

Teasdale, G. and Jennett, B. (1974). Assessment of coma and impaired consciousness. A practical scale. *Lancet*, 2, 81–4.

Teasdale, G., Knill, J. R., and van-der, S. J. (1978). Observer variability in assessing impaired consciousness and coma. *J. Neurol. Neurosurg. Psychiatry*, 41, 603–10.

Thomas, F. B., Mazzaferri, E. L., and Skillman, T. G. (1970). Apathetic thyrotoxicosis: A distinctive clinical and laboratory entity. *Ann. Intern. Med.*, 72, 679–85.

Walter, J. H. and Leonard, J. V. (1987). Inborn errors of the urea cycle. *Br. J. Hosp. Med.*, 38, 176–83.

Warrell, D. A., Looareesuwan, S., Warrell, M. J. *et al.* (1982). Dexamethasone proves deleterious in cerebral malaria. A double-blind trial in 100 comatose patients. *N. Engl. J. Med.*, 306, 313–19.

Weisinger, J. R. and Bellorin-Font, E. (1998). Magnesium and phosphorus. *Lancet*, 352, 391–6.

Zeman, A. (1997). Persistent vegetative state. *Lancet*, 350, 795–9.

Zeman, A. Z., Grayling, A. C., and Cowey, A. (1997). Contemporary theories of consciousness [editorial]. *J. Neurol. Neurosurg. Psychiatry*, 62, 549–52.

Zimmerman, R. A. and Bilaniuk, L. T. (1981). Computed tomography in pediatric head trauma. *J. Neuroradiol.*, 8, 257–71.

CHAPTER 26

Neuropsychological disorders, dementia, and behavioural neurology

Martin Rossor

26.1 Introduction

26.1.1 General principles

The diseases that disrupt the cerebral cortex and its subcortical connections result in a wide variety of clinical features, which include the classical syndromes of higher cortical dysfunction, such as the dysphasias, dyspraxias, amnesias, and agnosias, together with a wide variety of behavioural and emotional disturbances. Clinical investigation of such disorders frequently overlaps with the disciplines of clinical psychology and psychiatry. Historically there has been a broad split between those diseases that are seen by neurologists and those that are seen by psychiatrists. To some extent the distinction reflects the different clinical approaches employed; neurologists concentrate on the generality of disease caused by lesions in defined areas, whereas psychiatrists often deal with diseases that show a greater interaction with the individual's own personal history and place in society (Lishman 1987). In this chapter, disturbances of higher cortical function, the dementias, and behavioural aspects of neurological lesions are discussed. Awareness of the occasional presentation of psychiatric disease to the neurologist is important, and further details are available in textbooks of psychiatry. A review of clinical syndromes referable to identified areas of the cerebral cortex is followed by a functional approach, which discusses the main neuropsychological syndromes. The more generalized cognitive impairment seen with the dementias, such as Alzheimer's and Pick's diseases, are then reviewed, followed by areas of neuropsychiatric overlap.

26.1.2 Anatomy and physiology of the cerebral cortex

The human cerebral cortex consists of six laminae, comprising in total some 28×10^9 neurons and approximately the same number of glial cells: from the external surface, these are the molecular layer, the external granular, the external pyramidal, the internal granular, the internal pyramidal, and the multiform or fusiform layer. The interconnection of the neurons comprises a staggering 10^{12} synapses. Despite this dramatic development, the basic structural organization of the cerebral cortex in modular terms is the same across species. The basis of the modular organization is the minicolumn, representing some 80–100 neurons connected vertically, and within each minicolumn are all of the major cortical neuronal types. Two broad categories of neuronal cell types can be distinguished: the large pyramidal cells, which are the origin of the main outflow tracts and which utilize glutamate as the main neurotransmitter; and the smaller, non-pyramidal cells, which have predominantly local connections and primarily utilize the inhibitory amino acid γ-aminobutyric acid, together with a variety of coexistent neuropeptides. There is an increasing subcategorization of the small non-pyramidal cells, and an increasing understanding of the intrinsic connectivity of these cells within the minicolumns. Cortical columns are minicolumns bound together by horizontal connections over a short range, which share physiological features based in part upon shared input and output characteristics. Layers 2 and 3 project to other cortical areas and layers 5 and 6 are primarily subcortical projections. Columns vary only from 300 to 600 μm in diameter across a very wide range of species. The expansion of the human brain is due to the increase of the total number of modular units rather than a difference in their size (Rakic 1995).

The organization of the cerebral cortex, in terms of the functional characteristics of the cortical columns, was established using single-cell recording for the somatic sensory cortex by Mountcastle, and the visual cortex by Hubel and Wiesel (reviewed by Mountcastle 1997). The response characteristics of a somatic sensory column depend both upon modality and topography of the receptive fields. Similarly, in the visual cortex, columns can be defined by various properties of increasing complexity from ocularity and place through to orientation. This modular organization in anatomical and functional terms accords with the general view from cognitive psychology of modular processing (Fodor 1983). As the modular processing becomes more complex, the defining characteristics of the cortical column become the inputs from other columns, the outputs of which represent a further level of cortical processing. This achieves greatest complexity in the association cortices or homotypical cortical areas.

There is regional specialization within the cerebral cortex, which is reflected to some extent in architectonic differences, such as that originally identified by Brodmann (1909). However, particularly at the higher level of cortical processing, as represented by the association areas, cortical operations are also distributed. Evidence for distributed networks is provided both by functional brain imaging (Section 26.2) and by anatomical evidence of enormous convergent and reciprocal connections, for example those between the parietal and frontal cortex (Goldman 1988).

26.2 Clinical syndromes associated with specific areas of the cerebral cortex

A number of clinical syndromes are recognized as characteristic of lesions in specific areas of the cerebral cortex. The syndromes largely, but not invariably, involve loss of function, although in some instances loss of inhibition may present as release phenomena. The descriptions of many of these clinical syndromes were derived from patients with discrete lesions due to ischaemic infarcts or tumours, and formerly required follow-up to post-mortem to determine the location. Modern neuroimaging has considerably improved the power of such studies and there has been a spate of reports that locate specific syndromes to precise brain regions.

However, it should be emphasized that the observed associations are between clinical syndromes and brain areas and do not necessarily locate function to a specific brain region. Although a specific function may be lost following damage at a given site, the function itself is more likely to depend upon successful integration of a neural network. The particular area would be part of such a network and assumed to be of central importance.

In addition to the location of clinical syndromes to specific cortical areas, some syndromes may be better interpreted as representing disconnections of one area from another. The concept of disconnection syndromes was originally postulated by Dejerine and other early neurologists, and re-explored in considerable detail by Geschwind (1965). Some of the clinical syndromes arising from damage to the corpus callosum are most easily explained in terms of disconnection.

Functional imaging has contributed further to our knowledge of localization of function. Baseline measures of blood flow or cerebral glucose metabolism with positron emission tomography (PET scanning) can identify areas of reduced basal function when abnormalities on structural imaging may not be readily apparent. This has been most valuable in patients with frontal lobe degeneration. Activation studies can provide information on changes in cerebral blood flow, or deoxygenation of haemoglobin, and thus regions which are activated during a specific cognitive task relative to another. Such functional imaging studies have revealed that activation is often widely distributed, indicating that distributed networks are involved in such cognitive tasks. However, as with structure–function relationships, caution has to be exercised in their interpretation. Although lesion studies show areas which may be necessary for a particular function, they can only localize deficits and it cannot be inferred that the specific function occurs in that area. They will show areas and structures that are necessary, but not sufficient, for that function. Similarly, activation may occur in areas that are not necessarily essential to a function. For example, activation studies of language may show areas of increased blood flow in the right hemisphere and yet lesion studies indicate that dysphasia does not occur with lesions in the same area.

The most widely used activation studies involve subtraction paradigms, as developed by Petersen *et al.* (1988). A baseline task is compared with an activation task that engages the cognitive component of interest. When the baseline data are subtracted, then areas that are activated are believed to relate directly to the particular cognitive component under study. More sophisticated models have been used to deal, for example, with language function, where it may be difficult to identify an appropriate baseline task. In these paradigms, referred to as cognitive conjunctions, areas of common activation rather than areas of different activation are sought (Price and Friston 1997). Functional imaging has provided valuable insights into the distributive networks involved in many cognitive processes, such as language (reviewed by Gabrieli 1998; Price 1998). It does, however, remain a research tool and as yet has had limited impact on routine neurological management.

26.2.1 The frontal lobes

The frontal lobes lie rostral to the central sulcus and superior to the Sylvian fissure. They show the greatest development in humans, compared with other primates. Within the frontal lobes are the primary motor cortices, located within the precentral area, together with the supplementary motor areas and the frontal eye fields. The dominant frontal lobe encompasses Broca's area and the adjacent area of the motor cortex is involved with the motor control of the oropharynx, lesions of which result in impairment of articulation and phonation. However, the prefrontal cortex, Brodmann areas 9, 10, 11, 12 and 45, 46 and 47, is particularly developed in humans and yet has a less clearly defined function.

The frontal cortex has widespread connections with other areas of the brain. The pyramidal cells of the motor cortex form the major fronto-striatal outflow tract and, similarly, there are extensive projections from subcortical structures into the frontal cortex, notably the dopaminergic, noradrenergic, and cholinergic cortical projection systems.

Early studies with experimental frontal lobe lesions in non-human primates revealed impaired performance on a number of tasks which suggested perseverative responses and difficulty in switching between preferred modes of response. These difficulties with switching cognitive sets were explored further using the Wisconsin card-sorting test (Milner 1963). Patients tend to perseverate on these tasks and yet on other tasks, such as cognitive estimates, patients may be quite impulsive and unable to monitor their performance.

The combination of perseverative responses, lack of initiative, and impulsivity has been brought together in the hypothesis of a supervisory attentional system for the frontal lobes (Norman and Shallice 1980). In this model, the frontal lobes have an important role in both selecting appropriate behavioural responses and inhibiting inappropriate ones. This can explain the paradoxical combination of both aspontaneity and lethargy together with impulsivity, even within the same patient. Breakdown in such a system results in markedly impaired social behaviour and adaptability, and yet formal testing shows that intelligence may often be spared (Shallice 1982). One of the most distinctive features of the frontal lobe syndrome is a change in personality, most commonly towards disinhibition. The effect upon personality of massive bifrontal lesions was well demonstrated by the celebrated case of Phineas Gage who, in 1848, had a crowbar driven through the front of his skull. He was described as 'fitful, irreverent, indulging at times in the greatest profanity … manifesting but little deference for his fellows, impatient of restraint or advice when it conflicts with his desires, at times pertinaciously obstinate, yet capricious and vacillatory'. Thus a frontal lobe syndrome has come to be recognized: an affected individual previously capable of judgement and sustained application and organization of his life, may become aimless and improvident, with loss of tact, sensitivity, and self-control, and with impulsiveness and a failure to appreciate the consequences of reckless behaviour.

The disinhibited behaviour may result in childish excitement (moria) or joking and pathological punning (*Witzelsucht*); there may in addition be sexual indiscretions and exhibitionism. Alternatively, the syndrome may present with lack of initiative and profound psychomotor slowing (abulia). This may be accompanied, particularly with bifrontal lesions, by urinary incontinence (Andrew and Nathan 1964), which can occasionally be seen with unilateral lesions. This incontinence is commonly associated with lack of concern and social awareness, which is a useful clinical clue since this type of incontinence is rarely found with generalized dementing conditions such as Alzheimer's disease.

The behavioural disturbance can be striking, and can precede changes on formal tests of frontal lobe function by many years (Selai *et al.* 1999). A distinction has been drawn between dorsolateral frontal lesions, which may be associated with cognitive decline and apathy, and/or orbitomedial lesions with prominent behavioural change (Devinsky *et al.* 1995; Blair and Cipolotti 2000). Often the changes in behaviour are most apparent to the spouse, who may feel that they are married to somebody entirely different.

Clinical examination may be less revealing than the history, and often patients perform relatively well on formal tests of intelligence. However, specific tasks, such as the Wisconsin card sorting test, the Weigl sorting test, cognitive estimates, verbal fluency, and bimanual motor tasks, will show impairment, but even this may be patchy and inconsistent. The patient's appearance may be clearly abnormal, appearing unkempt, unwashed, and lacking all spontaneity. Neurological examination may reveal primitive reflexes, such as the rooting reflexes, both tactile and oral, and sucking reflexes, if severe. Grasp reflexes are easily elicited by running the hand across the palm and may be elicited from the foot (Seyffarth and Denny-Brown 1948). The grasp reflex and instinctive grasp reaction can be seen as part of a more generalized magnetic behaviour, elicited as utilization behaviour (Lhermitte 1983; Shallice *et al.* 1989). This is a striking example of environmental dependency, in which presentation of an object will elicit a behavioural response regardless of whether or not it is appropriate. Patients offered spectacles, for example, may place them on their nose, followed by further pairs, until three or four are stacked upon one another, the inappropriateness of this completely eluding the patient.

As lesions extend more posteriorly in the dominant frontal lobe, there may be an associated non-fluent anterior dysphasia and impairment of speech production. Lesions in relation to the orbital surface may result in unilateral visual failure and anosmia. The latter will rarely be found unless specifically sought and is a characteristic feature of olfactory groove meningiomas (Fig. 26.1). On examination, prominent changes in tone may be found which increase in response to the stimulus, so-called paratonia or *Gegenhalten*. More posteriorly placed lesions may result in mild pyramidal signs, but most striking are bifrontal medial lesions causing prominent gait impairment with truncal instability, often referred to as gait apraxia (Meyer and Barron 1960). With the availability of CT and MRI scanning, frontal lobe tumours are far more readily diagnosed.

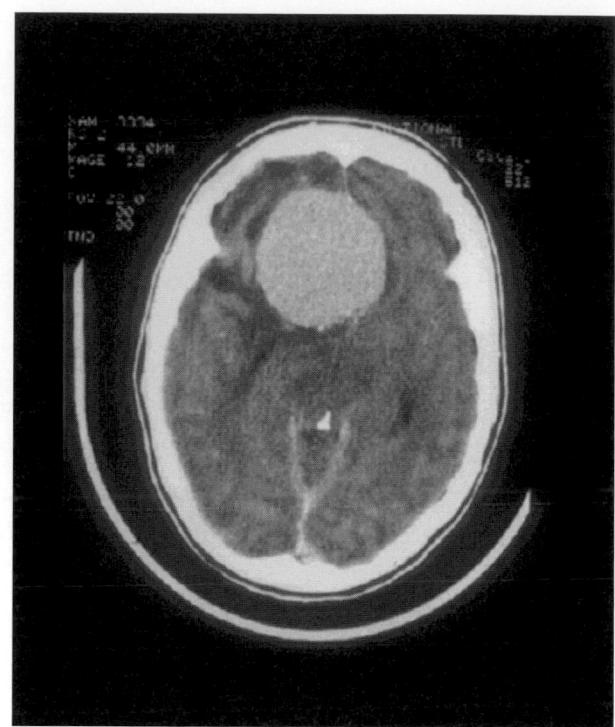

Fig. 26.1. CT scan reveals an olfactory groove meningioma in a patient with anosmia and a frontal lobe syndrome.

However, with the gradual onset of personality changes, many cases are still missed until late. In general, frontal lobe syndromes are seen more commonly with tumours and degenerative disease than with vascular disease (Bogousslavsky 1994).

26.2.2 The temporal lobes

The Sylvian fissure separates the temporal lobe from the frontal lobe and rostral part of the parietal lobe. There is, however, no clear boundary between the posterior temporal lobe and the parietal and occipital lobes. The temporal lobes have easily discernible gyri—the superior, middle, and inferior temporal gyri—and also the parahippocampal and hippocampal convolutions. The hippocampus demonstrates a three-layered cortical structure, in contrast to the six-layered neocortex. Heschl's gyrus in the Sylvian fissure represents the primary auditory receptive area, and fibres terminating here do so in a tonotopic arrangement. Deep within the temporal lobe is the amygdala.

Discrete lesions of the anterior temporal poles may be clinically silent and, in general, lesions of the non-dominant temporal lobe are less obvious clinically; sometimes the only clue on neurological examination being a superior quadrantic visual field defect or behavioural change. However, bitemporal lesions and those of the dominant temporal lobe may result in profound functional impairments. The predominant lesion of the dominant temporal lobe is that of a language impairment, classically a Wernicke's aphasia (Section 26.4.4) or, rarely, a pure word deafness or auditory verbal agnosia.

Unilateral lesions of the dominant temporal lobe can be shown to result in impairment of memory for verbal material, by contrast to impaired visual memory with non-dominant lesions (Milner 1971). Unilateral lesions of Heschl's gyrus rarely result in deafness, but careful binaural testing reveals subtle abnormalities in the area contralateral to the lesions. The inability to recognize faces, prosopagnosia, is usually seen with bilateral lesions but has also been described with unilateral non-dominant temporoparietal lesions (Warrington and James 1967). Patients with prosopagnosia may have a variety of deficits, ranging from an inability to recognize the face through to loss of familiarity and inability to match faces. This can sometimes be so severe that patients are incapable of recognizing members of their own family but can do so immediately on hearing their voices.

Very rarely, lesions of the temporal lobe can result in a true auditory agnosia. Simple perception of sound and pure tone is intact but the interpretation of complex sounds is severely impaired. In pure auditory agnosia recognition of all noises, for example the sound of a bell, dogs barking, or running water, is lost (Hecaen 1962). More common is the loss of appreciation of music, or amusia, seen with right temporal lobe lesions. The patient's appreciation of melody, timbre, and rhythm all tend to be impaired and they may also have difficulty in musical recognition.

Bilateral temporal lobe lesions are far more devastating. These cases are rare and occur after herpes encephalitis or in the later stages of frontotemporal degeneration. They are normally associated with a dysphasia and, in addition, profound memory impairments (Section 26.4.7) (Milner 1958; Milner *et al.* 1968). Bilateral removal of the temporal lobes in the monkey produces a striking behavioural state referred to as the Kluver–Bucy syndrome. The monkeys show increased exploratory behaviour, in which they will examine objects by oral and manual manipulation with apparent inability to recognize them visually. They are usually placid but with hypersexuality. Similar cases have been described with herpes encephalitis and with frontotemporal degenerations (Cummings and Duchen 1981; Lilly *et al.* 1983). The frontotemporal degenerations encompass a variety of disease processes, including Pick's disease. They are often associated with obsessional behaviour, change in eating habits, hypereligiosity, and both hypo- and hypersexuality. Some of these features may reflect involvement of the amygdala.

A variety of episodic symptoms may be found with temporal lobe lesions, which are usually on an epileptic basis and range from auditory hallucinations to disruption of time perception and disturbances of sexual behaviour. In addition, however, chronic bilateral lesions, particularly those of the medial temporal lobes, may cause profound disintegration of personality and behaviour. In its extreme form patients react to any stimulus by excessive rage with screaming, biting, and spitting. This distressing clinical picture is seen most commonly in survivors of herpes encephalitis.

26.2.3 **The parietal lobes**

The parietal lobes lie behind the central sulcus and above the Sylvian fissure, but the posterior boundaries with the occipital and temporal lobes are not clearly defined. Immediately behind the central sulcus is the primary sensory cortex, which is delineated posteriorly by the post central sulcus. The superior temporal sulcus curves upwards posteriorly into the inferior parietal lobule in relation to the angular gyrus. This is adjacent to the posterior extremity of the Sylvian fissure, which also curves up into the inferior parietal lobule in relation to the supramarginal gyrus. The supramarginal and angular gyri, together with the posterior third of the superior temporal gyrus, constitute the Wernicke speech area. The parietal lobes are well developed in humans and continue to develop until about the seventh year of life. There are extensive connections with other association areas.

Lesions within the parietal lobes can present with an enormous variety of disturbances of higher cortical function, some of which are quite dramatic in their presentation. Dominant parietal lobe lesions are often associated with dysphasia. This may be predominantly a motor or sensory dysphasia, depending upon the antero-posterior location. More posterior lesions are associated with dyslexia, dysgraphia, and dyscalculia, and ideational apraxia is a consistent feature of dominant parietal lobe lesions. Gerstmann's syndrome refers to the association of finger agnosia, dyscalculia, right–left disorientation, and agraphia. Although this is commonly seen with lesions of the dominant angular gyrus (Gerstmann 1940), this particular clustering of deficits is no more common than other patterns. Lesions of either parietal lobe may result in visuospatial disturbance and topographical disorientation. Similarly, both parietal lobes are involved with selective attention (Mesulam 1982). However, it is with lesions of the non-dominant parietal lobe that the most striking disturbances of visuospatial function and disturbances of body image are seen. Patients with non-dominant parietal lesions have marked impairment of selective attention which will affect both right- and left-sided space, but most commonly left-sided space. This may be so severe that they will ignore the left side of the body, resulting in problems in dressing, and in shaving only one half of their face. If this is associated with a left hemiplegia, they may be unaware of the deficit (anosognosia) and indeed deny that the paralysed limb has anything to do with them.

On examination, patients with parietal lobe lesions may show the obvious neglect of the left side, with an arm hung loosely at the side or out of the sleeve of their jacket, with the left face unshaven, and associated pyramidal signs. Field defects are most commonly inferior quadrantanopias. Gaze impersistence, an inability to sustain lateral gaze on testing eye movements, is seen quite commonly and can be very frustrating for the examiner. Cortical sensory loss may be found in the contralateral limbs, which can be most readily picked up by testing two-point discrimination, which is impaired together with astereognosis (inability to recognize objects by their shape), or alternatively inability to recognize figures written on the hand (agraphesthesia). Neglect can be unmasked by simultaneous tactile or visual stimuli, when the patient may only recognize one of the two simultaneously presented stimuli, ignoring that contralateral to the lesion. The sensory testing may be difficult, with patients showing considerable variability and being easily fatigued (Critchley 1953). Simple bedside tests of visuospatial function that can be helpful include drawing a cube or clock face, when patients will often ignore features to the left-hand side. Dressing apraxia can be assessed by watching the patient put on clothing, and the task made more difficult by inverting one sleeve.

26.2.4 The occipital lobes

The occipital lobes are separated on the medial surface from the parietal lobes by the parieto-occipital fissure, but there are no clearly defined margins between the parietal and temporal lobes on the lateral surface. The occipital lobes subsume the termination of the visual pathways, and the primary visual cortex, Brodmann area 17, lies on either side of the calcarine fissure, which runs from the occipital pole to the splenium of the corpus callosum. It has the histological characteristic that its fourth layer is divided into two granular cell layers by a thickened band of heavily myelinated fibres, the external band of Baillarger. This band is visible to the naked eye, hence the name of striate cortex. The classical findings with lesions of the occipital cortex are homonymous visual field defects; a homonymous hemianopia when confined to one occipital lobe. Bilateral lesions may cause altitudinal defects, since the termination of the optic radiation is topographically arranged, with lower retinal fibres terminating in the cortex below the calcarine fissure. Superior quadrantic defects are found with inferior lesions and vice versa.

With extensive bilateral lesions various abnormalities are found, ranging from complete cortical blindness, through to subtle visual disturbances. With complete cortical blindness, the pupillary responses are preserved, as is visual imagery in dreams, but cortical evoked responses and the alpha rhythm on the EEG are both lost. Strikingly, patients with complete cortical blindness may develop a visual anosognosia (Anton's syndrome) with denial of their loss of sight. These patients may walk around as if they can see but will bump into objects and often explain their difficulties by complaining about the light or their loss of glasses. With partial recovery from cortical blindness, or with lesions involving the visual association areas, there may be a variety of disturbances of higher visual processing. These may fractionate into distinct syndromes such as visual disorientation, in which the ability to locate objects within the visual field is considerably impaired and patients may be effectively blind. This forms a major component of Balint's syndrome (Hecaen and Ajuriaguerra 1954), in which patients have an inability to direct gaze into the peripheral field despite full eye movements, a visual inattention affecting the periphery of the visual field, and prominent optic ataxia, in which there is failure to grasp or touch an object under visual guidance. Other syndromes involve selective loss of colour, achromatopsia, and (very rarely) impairment of movement perception (Zihl et al. 1983; Shipp et al. 1994). Rarely patients may develop genuine visual object agnosia if the lesion involves the occipitotemporal areas. These patients are unable to recognize objects by sight, but can do so on palpation or by sound.

The lesions are usually bilateral but may be found with dominant lesions.

Patients may complain of a variety of visual hallucinations and illusions, more commonly with bilateral or non-dominant lesions. Many of these are associated with epileptic phenomena, such as elementary unformed hallucinations and flashes of light, colours, or geometric forms. They may be seen within the setting of a hemianopic disturbance. Striking visual illusions may occur with metamorphopsias and marked changes in shape. In addition polyopia (multiple images) may be seen, or the striking disturbance of palinopsia, in which perserveration of visual images occurs and colour may spread outside the geometric confines of the object.

26.3 Subcortical syndromes

Although the cerebral cortex is viewed as the main seat of cognitive behaviour, it is becoming increasingly recognized that damage to subcortical structures can give rise to profound behavioural and cognitive disturbance. In many instances, these may mimic deficits arising from lesions within the cerebral cortex, for example the dysphasia and dyspraxia which may be seen with dominant thalamic lesions (Graff et al. 1984). These may share characteristics with cortical lesions by virtue of the extensive neural interconnections; an interpretation supported by observed changes in metabolism within connected areas of the cerebral cortex demonstrated on SPECT scanning subsequent to subcortical infarcts (Perani et al. 1987). Many of the behavioural disturbances are discussed elsewhere under the appropriate sections, but some structures are particularly notable. The importance of the amygdalae in behaviour has already been referred to, and rare instances of a Kluver–Bucy syndrome have been described (Cummings and Duchen 1981). In addition, bilateral damage to the amygdalae can result in disturbance of memory as well as disturbed social behaviour (Tranel and Hyman 1990) and impaired recognition of emotional facial recognition (Adolphs et al. 1999); the latter may contribute to some of the social behavioural disturbances seen in frontotemporal degeneration (Lavenu et al. 1999).

Disease of the basal ganglia can give rise to prominent cognitive and conative dysfunction, most commonly observed with massive destructions following haemorrhage, infarcts, or intoxications. Bilateral thalamic infarcts are dominated by disturbances of attention, but fluctuating aphasia is characteristic of left-sided lesions, whereas right thalamic infarcts can result in the 'left neglect' syndromes which mimic non-dominant parietal lesions (Castaigne et al. 1981; Graff et al. 1984). Thalamic haemorrhages tend to be more dramatic in their presentation and usually cause a relatively fluent aphasia with marked fluctuation and superimposed hypophonia (Luria 1977). Caudate lesions are more commonly associated with behavioural disturbances, usually abulia, than with motor syndromes (Bhatia and Marsden 1994). A syndrome of dysphasia with dysarthria and orofacial dyspraxia can occur with dominant head of caudate infarcts (Naeser et al. 1982), and dysphasic syndromes can also occur with lesions of the adjacent white matter or internal capsule (Damasio *et al.* 1982). Apraxia is very rare with lesions confined to basal ganglia, but can be seen more commonly with lesions of the thalamus (Pramstaller and Marsden 1996). Bilateral lesions of the basal ganglia can result in profound behavioural disturbance. Marked apathy, similar to a frontal lobe syndrome, can occur with bilateral lesions of the globus pallidus, so called pure psychic akinesia (Laplane *et al.* 1984). Bilateral infarction of the head of caudate has resulted in severely aggressive and criminal behaviour (Richfield *et al.* 1987). Occlusions of the basilar artery at the bifurcation, the so-called 'top of the basilar' syndrome, result in complex disorders of eye movement, with convergent spasm, retraction nystagmus, and skew deviation. It is commonly accompanied by memory disturbance and an agitated confusional state with prominent visual hallucinations, so-called peduncular hallucinosis (Caplan 1980).

26.4 Neuropsychological syndromes

In the preceding section clusters of neuropsychological deficits which are characteristic of damage to particular areas of cerebral cortex were described. Often relatively pure deficits may present to neurologists, and more detailed understanding of the precise nature of the functional impairment, over and above the localizing significance, can be helpful in diagnosis and management.

26.4.1 Disorders of perception and the agnosias

In 1890, Lissauer introduced the terms apperceptive and associative 'mind blindness' to distinguish between patients whose abilities to perceive and discriminate an object are impaired, and those patients who are unable to recognize the object having correctly perceived it. The following year, Freud introduced the term agnosia, which subsequently replaced the term 'mind blindness'.

Visual agnosias have been most widely studied and Lissauer's original analysis has subsequently proved useful in the analysis of neurological patients. In order to perceive an object, a number of features must be analysed and processed, such as shape, colour, location within space, and movement; these may each be selectively damaged. Shape discrimination can be assessed by asking the patient to discriminate between rectangles and squares of increasing similarity (Efron 1968). Preservation of shape and location but with loss of colour (achromatopsia) is rare (Zeki 1990), and is usually seen with bilateral damage to the fusiform and lingual gyri. There is commonly an associated superior altitudinal field defect (Meadows 1974a). Impairment of visual location, visual disorientation (Holmes 1918), can cause great impairment and render the patient functionally blind. Finally, patients have very rarely been described with inability to detect movement, indicating a further dimension of early visual processing (Zihl *et al.* 1983).

These abnormalities of early visual processing are most commonly seen with bilateral occipital and occipitoparietal lesions, but can be seen with unilateral lesions, in which case the deficit is found in the contralateral field of vision. In these instances the functional impairment may be less prominent and patients less likely to present with a specific history. These disorders of visual processing are usually due to ischaemic lesions, but visual disorientation can be found in degenerative lesions of the occipital and parietal cortex, sometimes referred to as posterior cortical atrophy, which can be a presenting feature of Alzheimer's disease (Benson *et al.* 1988).

In apperceptive agnosia there is impairment of the generation of a structured percept of an object despite adequate initial processing of shape, colour, and location. This impairment can be demonstrated in patients who have difficulty coping with perceptually difficult visual stimuli, such as incomplete line drawings, overlapping line drawings (De *et al.* 1969), fragmented letters (Warrington and James 1967a), and unusual views (Warrington and Taylor 1973). Unlike the retinotopic organization of early visual processing, the entire visual field is involved in patients with apperceptive agnosia, and the minimal lesion is usually found in the posterior non-dominant parietal lobe.

Associative visual agnosia is very rare (Hecaen and Angelergues 1963). Patients can describe an object very well and copy drawings of it precisely but it has no meaning for them. They are, however, able to recognize the object immediately through other sensory channels. Patients with visual agnosia usually have bilateral lesions, but these can occur with unilateral left posterior parietal lesions. Classically, visual agnosia has been interpreted as a disconnection of the percept from a central meaning system, but an alternative interpretation is the existence of modality-specific meaning systems, and visual agnosia would thus be seen as a loss of the specific meaning system associated with the visual domain, i.e. a visual semantic memory impairment (McCarthy and Warrington 1990).

Within the overall category of visual agnosias, some defects have been singled out for particular consideration because they present as striking clinical deficits. Examples include the inability to recognize colour (colour agnosia) and inability to recognize faces (prosopagnosia). Colour agnosia (Hecaen and Albert 1978) implies intact colour perception and semantic knowledge of colour, but the majority of cases appear to have an associated impairment of colour naming. Faces present a perceptually difficult visual task and, clearly, problems in visual processing and perception will result in difficulty in face recognition. However, some patients present with a relatively selective impairment of facial recognition. Such cases can present a striking clinical picture, in that patients may be unable to recognize those very close to them, but can immediately do so when they hear them speak, or by looking for other clues in their dress or mannerisms. Prosopagnosia is usually associated with right occipitotemporal lesions and is commonly associated with a left homonymous superior quadrantanopia (Meadows 1974b). Prosopagnosia can be analysed in a similar way to object recognition-employing tests to assess perceptual analysis, such as matching pictures of faces and matching facial expressions. Some patients may have normal performance on face-matching tasks but be quite unable to recognize familiar faces (Warrington and James 1967b; De 1986). Others may show intact face matching but be unable to match facial expression (Etcoff 1984). These theoretical aspects of prosopagnosia have generated a number of information-processing models of face recognition (Bruce and Young 1986).

Agnosias in other sensory domains have been far less well studied and have a less secure theoretical basis. Cortical deafness can occur with bilateral temporal lesions which result in deficits of discrimination, temporal sequencing, and spatial localization of sound. Pure word deafness as an isolated agnosia for speech sounds (Goldstein 1974) usually overlaps with Wernicke's aphasia. Auditory agnosia is extremely rare and refers to patients with intact hearing and intact language comprehension but who are unable to recognize meaningful nonverbal sounds. Following Lissauer's original terminology, these have also been divided into apperceptive and associative agnosias (Vignolo 1982).

Tactile agnosia is even less secure as a distinct syndrome. Patients with parietal lesions will often have difficulty with the appreciation of size, texture, and shape of objects held in the hand, and astereognosis, which is more strictly referred to as stereoanasthesia or stereohypoasthesia. These patients will have impairment of two-point discrimination and sometimes subtle proprioceptive changes. Strictly speaking, astereognosis should exist when shape and discrimination is intact, as evidenced by the patient's description, but recognition impaired. Astereognosis, however, may occur as a disconnection syndrome in patients with callosal lesions (Geschwind and Kaplan 1962). In such patients objects can be recognized in the right hand but not in the left; they can, however, be correctly identified from a visual array. This is interpreted as disconnection of the sensory information from the right parietal cortex reaching the left hemisphere language area.

26.4.2 Disorders of spatial awareness and the body image

We are aware of the existence of our bodies, their position in space, and the relation of their parts to one another because we receive data through numerous sensory channels; these include vision, cutaneous sensibility, and proprioceptive information from the muscles, joints, and labyrinths. The somatic impulses pass via the ventral nucleus of the thalamus to the supramarginal gyrus, which is thus concerned with awareness of the opposite side of the body. This concept of the body in consciousness is known as the body image or body schema.

Symptoms of disorders of the body image may be positive or negative. The chief positive symptom is the phantom—an illusion of the persistence of a part of the body lost by amputation, e.g. a phantom limb, or an illusory awareness of a part from which sensation has been lost through interruption of afferent pathways. Phantom limbs after amputation may be painless or painful (Riddoch 1941). The painless phantom soon becomes less obtrusive, and gradually shortens, eventually to disappear. Painful phantoms may persist indefinitely and cause much distress.

Impairment of spatial sense together with neglect is most commonly seen following right parietal lesions and can present a dramatic clinical picture. Such patients frequently manifest spatial disorientation both for external space and for the body image, and, within hospital, mislocate their bed. These patients often have an associated left hemiparesis, again indicating a relationship with the non-dominant parietal lobe (Benson et al. 1976). Patients with right hemisphere lesions exhibit neglect that is most obvious to the left side of the body and left space, and these patients may not shave the left side of their face, may eat food only on the right side of the dinner plate, and may demonstrate neglect dyslexia. Most striking is inattention to left-sided deficits, such as left hemiparesis, so called anosognosia (Babinski 1914). In a less severe degree of negelect, patients may recognize their left hemiparesis but are unconcerned, a complication which can make rehabilitation extremely difficult (Denes et al. 1982).

There are two main theories of spatial neglect in association with lesions of the non-dominant parietal lobe. One proposes that there is a central representation of space, which is damaged; the other proposes that there is a defect of selective attention, a function for which the right hemisphere is dominant.

26.4.3 Apraxia

Apraxia may be defined as the inability to carry out a purposive movement, the nature of which the patient understands, in the absence of severe motor weakness or paralysis, sensory loss, or ataxia. For example, a patient who is asked to protrude his tongue is unable to do so on request, although he may carry out inappropriate movements such as opening his mouth. A moment later he spontaneously protrudes his tongue to lick his lips. Apraxia may involve any movement that is normally initiated voluntarily—movements of the eyes, face, muscles of articulation, chewing and swallowing, manipulation of objects, gestures with the upper limb, walking, or sitting down. Apraxia is seen most commonly with left hemisphere lesions, and is then found in association with dysphasia.

The terminology of apraxia is particularly confusing since it includes a number of conditions that are not genuinely apraxic and, additionally, employs terms that are derived from the theoretical framework developed by Liepmann at the turn of the century. He defined three types of apraxia, namely limb-kinetic, ideomotor, and ideational. These were based upon a theoretical neuroanatomical model similar to those that have been developed for speech. Limb-kinetic apraxia is rarely used and probably reflects a mild pyramidal lesion. Ideomotor dyspraxia refers to the poor performance of a motor act in response to a verbal command. This is most commonly explored at the bedside by asking patients to mime. It has been interpreted in terms of disconnection, although the most secure disconnection model for ideomotor dyspraxia is seen in patients with lesions of the anterior corpus callosum, who have difficulty with performing tasks to command using the left hand, i.e. the 'praxis centre' in the left hemisphere is disconnected from the right motor cortex which controls the left hand (Geschwind 1965). This is sometimes referred to as callosal apraxia and is commonly seen with anterior cerebral artery infarcts.

Ideational apraxia was defined by Liepmann as an inability to perform a sequential motor act, even though each could be carried out separately. However, this is relatively non-specific and may be a feature of frontal lobe lesions, reflecting a difficulty of programming rather than of dyspraxia. De Renzi *et al.* (1968) have defined ideational apraxia as an impairment in manipulation of actual objects. Subsequently, De Renzi has postulated that these patients have an agnosia for tool usage (De Renzi and Lucchelli 1988) which, in this context, is associated with lesions of the posterior dominant parietal lobe. Patients with clinically obvious apraxia are relatively rare but severely disabled. They have considerable difficulty using a knife and fork and with many other common tasks which require manual dexterity, and they will often look at their hands in a bemused way. By contrast, patients who demonstrate ideomotor dyspraxia at the bedside may not be functionally disabled, representing merely a feature of a specific neurological examination.

In addition to the syndromes described above, which relate to manual dexterity, other body-part dyspraxias have been described. A dissociation between limb apraxia and an axial dyspraxia, demonstrated by difficulty with adopting truncal postures such as a boxer's stance, has been described. Patients with gait apraxia show severe impairment of walking and often of standing, with additional truncal instability (Meyer and Barron 1960). Orofacial dyspraxia is found with dominant frontal lesions and often associated with a cortical dysarthria (Nathan 1947); such patients show a characteristic inability to make oral movements to command but with sparing of eye movements. When asked to cough they will frequently repeat the word 'cough'; however, they will be observed to carry out such motor acts spontaneously. This may be seen on a degenerative basis (Tyrrell *et al.* 1991). Dressing apraxia is associated with non-dominant parietal lobe lesions and is normally seen in a context of spatial impairment and left-sided neglect.

Constructional apraxia (Kleist 1922) refers to a disorder of the spatial disposition of an action and is illustrated at the bedside by inability to copy a cube or to make a simple arrangement of matches. This was originally identified as a disconnection syndrome between spatial analysis and voluntary action. This remains to be proven, and apparent constructional apraxia may be due to more than one defect. Patients with left hemisphere lesions may make dyspraxic errors and commonly they will retain the spatial organization but simplify a diagram, whereas those with right hemisphere lesions show impairment of the spatial organization and will often neglect the left side (Arrigoni and De Renzi 1964; Warrington *et al.* 1966).

26.4.4 Dysphasias

Since so much of the complexity of human behaviour depends upon language, impairment in this domain often presents early and with striking features. Historically the language disorders were also the first to be associated with precise focal brain lesions. The terms 'dysphasia' and 'aphasia' are often used interchangeably. American usage favours 'dysphasia' for developmental or congenital language disorders, reserving 'aphasia' for the acquired disorders of language. In Europe 'dysphasia' has been applied in the strict sense of a partial acquired language disorder, with 'aphasia' referring to complete absence of language. However, this is rarely adhered to strictly.

Aphasias are disturbances of language and not simply motor speech dysfunctions, thus a patient with aphasia will also have impairment of other aspects of language, such as writing. The term 'aphemia' is reserved for patients with impaired speech but with intact writing. 'Dysarthrias' refer to impaired speech sound production, and 'dysphonia' to local disturbances of the larynx and pharynx. Different terms have been used to describe the clinical spectrum of language disturbance. Many of these arose out of the early descriptions of neurologists, which were based on a variety of theoretical constructs, for example conduction, transcortical motor, and transcortical sensory aphasias were terms introduced to describe syndromes based upon theoretical models of language developed by Wernicke and Lichtheim. These models implied precise localization of function with fibre tracts connecting them. These were assumed to have an anatomical basis. Subsequently considerable advances were made in analysing individual components of speech comprehension and production, using information-processing models. The theoretical models and diagrams in these instances relate to individual components of the process without implying any anatomical correlates. However, in some instances the information-processing models can be correlated with the earlier theoretical and neurological models (Shallice 1981*a*). With improved techniques of neuro-imaging, and particularly the opportunities of functional neuroimaging with activation paradigms on PET scanning, considerable advances in the anatomical correlates of the individual processes in language can be anticipated.

A broad distinction between fluent and non-fluent aphasias is followed here, as this can provide a useful starting point for the clinician (Goodglass *et al.* 1964; Benson 1967), and within this framework the broad distinction between disturbances of production and comprehension are considered. Disturbances of reading, the dyslexias; of writing, the dysgraphias; and of calculation, the dyscalculias, are often associated but are considered separately.

Many of the clinical language syndromes can be identified by simple bedside testing, although detailed neuropsychological assessment is required both for quantitation and careful dissection of the individual components of language failure. Examination should include careful observation of the patient's spontaneous speech, which can be assisted by the use of picture description. The fluency should be noted and the occurrence of paraphasias documented. These may be phonemic paraphasias, in which one or two of the syllables of the word are mistaken or substituted, for example 'stable' for 'table', a pattern more commonly found with anterior lesions. By contrast, semantic paraphasias, the substitution of semantically similar words, for example 'chair' for 'table', are found more commonly with posterior lesions. Comprehension can be tested at the single-word and at the sentence level, and a variety of neuropsychological tests are available for this, such as the Peabody test. For bedside testing, word comprehension can be assessed by giving the patient verbal instructions, but care has to be exercised both in patients in whom intellect may be impaired and in patients with dyspraxia, if the task is motor dependent. Individual word comprehension can be tested by verbal definition and confrontational naming, which can also assess word retrieval. Repetition can provide evidence of dissociations between errors in spontaneous speech and repetition, and serves to distinguish the clinical syndromes of conduction aphasias and the transcortical aphasias. Finally, both reading and writing should be assessed.

Aphasias are most commonly encountered in the setting of strokes and neoplasms, i.e. focal lesions, and patients will often have associated neurological signs such as hemiparesis or visual field defects. More difficult to assess are patients with aphasia as part of a more generalized cognitive impairment, such as occurs with degenerative dementias. In addition, patients with psychosis or with acute confusional states can create problems, although the language process itself is preserved if carefully observed. Thus paraphasic errors are rare in the psychoses, although the rare schizophrenic 'word salad' can create diagnostic difficulty. However, other evidence of disturbed behaviour is apparent, whereas the patient with jargon aphasia as part of a Wernicke's dysphasia is seen to behave normally in the realm of non-language behaviour. The mute patient presents a particular diagnostic challenge. Patients may be mute because of a severe dysphasia, but more commonly are anarthric, in which case writing will be preserved. Alternatively, mutism may be associated with disturbances in attention, such as occurs with frontal and subfrontal disease and may be seen in akinetic mutism (Chapter 25).

Clearly, any assessment of a patient requires knowledge of handedness. The vast majority of people have language represented in the left hemisphere. Very rarely (less than 1 per cent) of right-handed individuals may develop aphasia with right hemisphere lesions (crossed aphasia in dextrals) (Zangwill 1979). In approximately half of patients who are left-handed language also resides in the left hemisphere.

Non-fluent and Broca's aphasia

In 1861 Broca described the case of Monsieur Leborgne, who had sustained a stroke with damage to the left inferior frontal gyrus and underlying white matter. The patient was initially mute and was then left with a severe non-fluent aphasia. Broca's original terminology for this, aphemia, has subsequently been confined to patients with impairment of speech but preservation of writing, usually with lesions of the dominant inferior

motor cortex. The term aphasia, introduced by Trousseau, supplanted the term aphemia (Schiff *et al.* 1983). The striking feature of Broca's aphasia is that the speech is non-fluent, being both slow and reduced in output, and patients are often mute initially. The content of the speech may be impaired, with frequent phonemic errors, and is usually agrammatic, with the omission of prepositions, adjectives, and adverbs. Repetition and confrontation naming (see below) are normally impaired, although the patients are often helped by cueing. Writing is faulty, both in morphology and in terms of spelling and grammar.

One of the clinically distinguishing features of Broca's aphasia is that the impairment is largely confined to language expression, with relative preservation of comprehension. Indeed, auditory comprehension of individual words is very well preserved, although performance on tests used to explore sentence comprehension is usually impaired (Goodglass and Kaplan 1972); similar subtle impairment of comprehension can be found in reading.

The traditional Broca's area, established in the original cases, is the posterior part of the inferior frontal gyrus. An associated ideomotor apraxia of the non-dominant hand may be found, depending upon the extent of subcortical damage. Some patients will show quite striking dysarthria and associated orofacial dyspraxia.

Two distinct clinical patterns of Broca's aphasia have been described (Mohr *et al.* 1978), depending on the size of the lesion. Lesions confined to Broca's area and subcortical white matter are usually due to embolic strokes in the anterior branches of the left middle cerebral artery, and are associated with rapid recovery of expressive speech. Patients with occlusions of the middle cerebral artery, sparing the territory of the inferior division which supplies the temporal lobe, or patients with occlusion of the internal carotid, have a more widespread lesion, which renders them globally aphasic initially, and often unable to comprehend, together with a dense hemiparesis. However, over the subsequent months of recovery, comprehension improves and a residual Broca's aphasia is left.

The majority of patients with Broca's aphasia have suffered strokes, but the syndrome may also be found with tumours, although in a less pure form. Some cases of selective left hemisphere degeneration may also present with a non-fluent speech, as in primary progressive aphasia (Mesulam 1982), and some patients with degeneration of the frontal lobe, such as occurs in Pick's disease, may develop a striking orofacial dyspraxia with speech impairment (Tyrrell *et al.* 1991).

Lichtheim had originally proposed a model of cortical concept centres for words, which were connected with the motor centre or word sound centre by transcortical pathways. Theoretical syndromes based on this model and involving disconnections between the centres were postulated for conduction (see below), transcortical motor and transcortical sensory aphasias. In transcortical motor aphasia, patients make frequent errors of speech production with a very low output and frequent phonemic paraphasias. However, repetition is intact.

Transcortical motor aphasia is seen most commonly with anterior cerebral artery lesions, with an associated ideomotor apraxia of the left hand and a right hemiparesis affecting the leg more than the arm.

By contrast with transcortical motor aphasia, patients with conduction aphasia have a profound impairment of repetition with frequent phonemic paraphasias. This was explained as a disconnection between intact comprehension and intact motor centres which would allow for relatively normal spontaneous speech. Anatomically, this was attributed to lesions of the arcuate fasciculus which, indeed, are often associated with conduction aphasias.

Speech production requires the correct selection and ordering of phonemes, impairment of which gives rise to the characteristic phonemic errors seen with a conduction aphasia. A pattern of deficit has also been recognized due to impairment of the motor coordination required for phoneme production, so-called kinetic speech production impairment. This is often associated with lesions in the inferior precentral gyrus (Lecours 1976). These disturbances of phoneme selection and expression can be distinguished from dysarthrias, in which there are characteristic impairments in swallowing and generation of meaningless sounds, which require the same motor apparatus.

Nominal dysphasia

Intact speech is dependent upon appropriate word retrieval. Patients with impaired word retrieval may be relatively fluent but their speech appears empty with frequent circumlocutions. Clinically this can be tested by confrontational naming, when abnormalities may be apparent, particularly for low-frequency words, that are less obvious in spontaneous speech. Word-finding difficulties are found quite frequently in neurological practice, but can occur as a relatively isolated finding in patients with left temporal lobe lesions. The study of word retrieval has proved to be a fertile area for theoretical modelling and a number of important clinical observations have been made. First, naming may be modality specific; for example, patients may be unable to name when presented with the object visually but are able to do so when presented to touch, so called optic aphasia. In addition, patients have been described in whom a tactile naming impairment is confined to the left hand, and such cases are most easily interpreted as disconnection syndromes involving lesions of the corpus callosum (Geschwind and Kaplan 1962). Another distinction has been drawn between patients whose failure at naming is consistent, and patients in whom the failure varies between different testing sessions and appears to be sensitive to the precise timing of confrontation. Different names are failed on different occasions and an object may be correctly named, but not if immediately shown again. The latter has been interpreted as an impairment of access to the word store, so called semantic access dysphasia (Warrington and McCarthy 1983). This syndrome of impaired access can be contrasted with patients in whom confrontational naming is impaired because they have lost their verbal semantic memory;

in these instances the same words tend not to be named and patients can quite often verbalize their loss of comprehension.

One of the striking clinical features of word-finding difficulty is the phenomenon of category specificity, namely that certain categories of words are more impaired than others (Goodglass *et al.* 1966). In some instances, the specificity is so striking as to have been recognized as a distinct syndrome, for example, colour anomia in patients who are unable to name but can adequately match colours; letter naming or letter anomia, and body part naming, or autotopagnosia. Many additional dissociations have been demonstrated, for example, between action naming and object naming, living and inanimate objects, etc. These category-specific dysphasias provide important theoretical insights into language organization and have been proposed to depend upon the association of the word with various attributes at the time meaning is acquired. Thus, for example, words which are associated with a strong visual component, of which colour would be the most striking, can be contrasted with those, such as tools and manipulable objects, which would depend on a major proprioceptive input when the word acquires its meaning (Warrington and McCarthy 1987). Such an account would accord well with current concepts of parallel distributed processing across neural networks.

Wernicke's aphasia

Shortly after Broca's description, Karl Wernicke outlined the features of a fluent aphasia which, in many respects, provided the clinical counterpart of a Broca's aphasia. The striking feature is that such patients speak fluently but the speech is often empty of meaning with frequent semantic paraphasias. At times the paraphasias may be profound with frequent neologisms, so called jargon aphasia. Comprehension is invariably impaired, as is reading. Writing reflects the language impairment, with frequent semantic paraphasias and spelling errors. Repetition, as with Broca's aphasia, is impaired. Wernicke's aphasia is commonly due to a vascular lesion and the acute onset of a jargon aphasia is usually due to an embolus to the inferior division of the middle cerebral artery. The area involved is the posterior superior temporal gyrus, often extending into the inferior parietal area. By contrast to Broca's aphasia, Wernicke's aphasia is often unaccompanied by neurological deficit on examination, which to the unwary can lead to faulty diagnosis of a psychotic disturbance. A right superior quadrantanopia may be found if carefully sought.

Intact comprehension requires intact speech perception, and patients may be seen with so-called pure word deafness. A number of these patients, with bilateral temporal lobe lesions, have been shown to have impairment of auditory temporal acuity (Auerbach *et al.* 1982). However, some patients have impairment of phoneme discrimination which can be associated with left temporal lobe lesions.

As the counterpart to transcortical motor aphasia, Lichtheim proposed the syndrome of transcortical sensory aphasia, in which patients are able to repeat, and whose speech is fluent, but is associated with impaired comprehension and paraphasias. The model postulated that the word recognition centre was intact, as shown by an intact repetition, but dissociation from a central meaning system resulted in impaired comprehension. This syndrome is now interpreted as an impairment of verbal semantic memory. It can be seen with posterior border zone infarcts but more commonly in frontotemporal degeneration, where it is the major feature of the clinical syndrome of semantic dementia (Section 26.6.4). Rarely, patients may be seen with isolation of the speech area who are neither able to speak nor to understand, but are able to repeat (Geschwind *et al.* 1968).

Dysprosody

Patients with Broca's aphasia often have impairment of the normal rhythm of speech, so-called dysprosody. Sometimes this may be so pronounced as to be referred to as the 'foreign accent syndrome' (Blustein *et al.* 1987). Impairment of the emotional expression and comprehension of speech is often found with right hemisphere lesions, and attempts have been made to seek comparable dysphasia syndromes to those found with left hemisphere lesions (Ross 1981).

Subcortical aphasias

Dysphasias are classically associated with cortical lesions, but subcortical damage is increasingly being recognized as a cause of dysphasia. To some extent these mimic the classical dysphasia syndromes, depending upon their location, for example, anterior lesions resulting in a non-fluent aphasia. In many instances reduced metabolism can be demonstrated on PET scanning in the appropriate cortical area, and is presumed to reflect impaired projection systems. Other syndromes have been described; for example, ischaemic lesions of the head of the caudate nucleus and associated internal capsule present with striking orofacial dyspraxia, dysarthria, and non-fluent dysphasia (Naeser *et al.* 1982). Left thalamic haemorrhages frequently give rise to an aphasia, often with fluctuations in arousal with concomitant fluctuation in language function.

26.4.5 Disorders of speech production and dysarthria

Dysarthria as a disorder of articulation does not involve any disturbance in the proper construction and use of words. In the dysarthric patient, symbolic verbal formulation is normal: only the mechanism of verbal sound production is faulty. When so severely affected that the patient is totally unable to articulate, it is referred to as anarthria. Dysphonia is applied to local disturbance of the larynx and may also render the patient mute. As well as structural abnormalities of the larynx, impaired innervation of laryngeal muscles can lead to dysphonia. A 'bovine cough' is a simple clinical sign of inability to close the larynx.

The articulatory muscles on each side appear to be innervated by both cerebral hemispheres. Hence a unilateral corticospinal lesion, for example in the internal capsule, may cause temporary but not permanent dysarthria. However, an extensive unilateral lesion involving the motor cortex may cause persistent dysarthria, especially when the dominant hemisphere is involved; in this case the dysarthria is often associated with some degree of Broca's aphasia. However, dysarthria is consistently produced by bilateral corticospinal lesions, due, for example, to congenital diplegia, vascular lesions of both internal capsules, degeneration of both corticospinal tracts (as in motor neuron disease), and lesions such as tumours involving both corticospinal tracts together in the midbrain. With such lesions, the articulatory muscles are weak and spastic and the tongue appears smaller, firmer, and less mobile than normal. The jaw-jerk and the palatal and pharyngeal reflexes are exaggerated. Speech is slurred and often explosive, production of consonants, especially labials and dentals, being severely affected. Spastic dysarthria is usually associated with dysphagia and often with impairment of voluntary control over emotional expression, the syndrome of 'pseudobulbar palsy'.

With lesions of the corpus striatum, articulation is impaired, partly, at least, as a result of muscular rigidity. Thus in hepatolenticular degeneration and in parkinsonism, articulation is slow and slurred, owing to immobility of the lips and tongue, and the pitch of the voice is monotonous. In the dystonias and Huntington's disease, dysarthria is common; indeed in severe cases speech may be unintelligible. In these diseases irregular respiration may also contribute to the dysarthria.

The co-ordination of articulation suffers severely when the cerebellar vermis is damaged and also when lesions involve the cerebellar connections in the brainstem. Speech in such cases is often explosive, with slurring and undue separation of individual syllables—scanning or syllabic speech. Ataxic dysarthria of this character is seen after acute cerebellar lesions and in multiple sclerosis and the hereditary ataxias.

Lower motor neuron lesions cause wasting and weakness, and often fasciculation, of the muscles of articulation (true bulbar palsy). In the early stages, the pronunciation of labials suffers most. Later, progressive weakness of the tongue impairs the production of dentals and gutterals, and weakness of the soft palate gives the voice a nasal quality. There is often associated dysphonia and finally total anarthria. Motor neuron disease is the most common cause, but paresis of the bulbar muscles may also be seen in syringobulbia, bulbar poliomyelitis, cranial polyneuritis, and brainstem tumours.

Combinations of these varieties of dysarthria are common; for example, in multiple sclerosis the articulatory muscles may be both spastic and ataxic, and in motor neuron disease a combination of upper and lower motor neuron lesions may be present.

Diseases of the muscles, such as myasthenia gravis, polymyositis, and muscular dystrophy involving facial muscles, lead to a dysarthria similar to that resulting from lesions of the lower motor neurons. In myasthenia, fatigability may cause increased slurring if the patient is asked to count aloud. In the myotonias, impaired muscular relaxation may add a spastic quality to the speech.

Palilalia

Palilalia is a rare disorder of speech which, as its name implies (from the Greek *palin*, again; *lalein*, to chatter), is characterized by repetition of a phrase which the patient reiterates with increasing rapidity. Palilalia most frequently occurs in postencephalitic parkinsonism, in general paresis, frontotemporal degenerations, and in pseudobulbar palsy due to vascular lesions. In echolalia the patient repeats or echoes words or brief phrases spoken by the examiner. It is usually seen in frontotemporal degenerations.

26.4.6 **Agraphia, alexia, and acalculia**

The majority of aphasic syndromes are associated with impairment of writing or dysgraphia. This is such a frequent association clinically that sparing of writing with impaired speech usually indicates that the speech impairment is due to a disruption of speech production rather than a pure dysphasic syndrome. Similarly, some patients may demonstrate dysgraphia with intact speech. Agraphias have been broadly divided into those that affect the processes of spelling and those that affect writing. The latter can be seen as a particular type of ideational dyspraxia, although patients are described in whom praxis is otherwise preserved. Disorders of spelling as such have also been subdivided, and have allowed the generation of theoretical models similar to the informational processing models for reading (Shallice 1981*b*). Dysgraphias are typically associated with posterior dominant parietal lesions.

Acquired disorders of reading, or dyslexias, are commonly found with dysphasias but can present in isolation. These were originally classified by Dejerine into two broad groups: those with and those without dysgraphia. In clinical terms this distinction has stood the test of time. Dyslexia with dysgraphia is commonly seen with lesions of the left angular gyrus. This type of dyslexia is often seen together with agraphia, acalculia, and anomia, and has been described as a distinct syndrome by Gerstmann, although this is only an observed clustering and each of these is not dependent on the others (Benton 1961). In the syndrome of alexia without agraphia, patients are unable to read but are able to write, even though they cannot read their own writing. This is often found with colour anomia, and patients usually have a right hemianopia. It is most commonly seen with lesions of the left parieto-occipital area, often involving the splenium of the corpus callosum. The classical interpretation of this syndrome has been that of a disconnection of visual information in the intact left field from the left angular gyrus. However, this does not explain readily a striking feature of these patients, which is the ability to read using a letter by letter strategy. Information-processing models have now largely replaced the neurological models of reading (Marshall and Newcombe 1966). Using these models, alexia without agraphia can be interpreted as a word-form dyslexia, supported by the fact that these patients are more impaired on reading script than print (Warrington and Shallice 1980). It is argued that following initial word-form recognition, analysis may proceed either by a phonological route or by a sight vocabulary route. For further discussion of the information-processing models see McCarthy and Warrington (1990).

Impairment of arithmetic ability is relatively common and is seen frequently with aphasia. However, it can be recognized as a selective lesion and is found most commonly with left parietal lesions. The dyscalculia commonly arises as a consequence of dyslexia or dysgraphia and so-called spatial acalculia due to visuospatial disorganization when written arithmetic calculations are performed. Amusia, an inability to produce and appreciate music is seen most commonly with non-dominant hemisphere lesions (Brust 1980), although the reading and writing of music notation may be seen with left hemisphere lesions.

26.4.7 **Disorders of memory**

Memory is the ability to store and subsequently retrieve past experience and is central to many cognitive functions, and the maintenance of an autobiographical memory is central to personal identity.

It is clear that memory is not a unitary function and there is a profusion of different terms. However, it is usual to draw a distinction between short-term (or primary) and long-term (or secondary) memory. Short term, primary, or immediate memory can be tested at the bedside as the digit span. A normal person can usually retain a maximum of seven or eight digits, with rapid forgetting over some 30 seconds unless rehearsed. Although less commonly tested at the bedside, patients may also have a selective impairment of short-term visual memory. The original simple model that memory involved entry into the short-term store before consolidation into a long-term store, secondary memory is no longer tenable, as patients with impaired digit span may have normal learning and secondary memory. Current theories of the role of primary memory range from a component of the working memory model of Baddeley (1986), to involvement in language fluency, or as a safety back-up resource (Shallice and Warrington 1970). From the neurologist's point of view, reduced digit span is commonly seen with impairment of attention, but as an isolated finding can be related to lesions of the inferior dominant parietal lobe, where it often occurs with dyscalculia.

Disabling memory impairments arise when individuals lose the ability to maintain an autobiographical memory. This can occur in a variety of clinical situations, such as dementia and confusional states, but it is the patients with otherwise intact cognition who have provided the main basis for study. Such patients typically have two components to their impairment: an anterograde amnesia (i.e. a deficit in acquiring new memories following the illness) and a retrograde amnesia (i.e. a loss of recall for events prior to the illness). The patient H.M., who had bilateral medial temporal lobe resections extending back some 8 cm from the temporal poles, has been studied intensively and provided important insights into amnesia. These studies demonstrate a profound impairment of both verbal and non-verbal learning with intact immediate recall, as evidenced by normal digit span (Scoville and Milner 1957; Milner *et al.* 1968). Subsequent similar cases of amnesia have followed this pattern. The status of remote memories has been less secure. Ribot's law states that there is a direct relationship between the strength of a memory and its recency, i.e. old memories being better preserved, and indeed this is often observed at the bedside. However, there are problems of interpretation since it is difficult to match the saliency of the remembered events. Despite the profound memory loss in H.M. and other similar cases, there is preservation of certain types of learning, for example improved performance on the recognition of fragmented letters can be demonstrated and, most strikingly, a retained ability to acquire new motor skills, often without recollection of having done so.

In the case of H.M., impaired learning of both verbal and visual material was found, but these can be selectively impaired. Group studies indicate that patients with left hemisphere damage have impaired verbal memory and the converse for non-verbal or visual memory. Often these material-specific memory impairments do not present clinically, but rather are found on specific testing. On occasions, however, some do present to the neurologist, the most striking being a topographical memory impairment in patients who are unable to recall familiar routes or buildings (Patterson and Zangwill 1945).

Studies of amnesia had focused previously on failure at various putative stages of memory, in terms of input, storage, and retrieval. Impairments of input and consolidation suggested that the strength and endurance of a memory depends on the extent of processing and thus consolidation (Craik and Lockhart 1972). This interpretation of amnesia in terms of impaired storage had argued that consolidation and retrieval mechanisms were intact, but that there was an increased rate of forgetting. More recently, however, attention has focused on the dissociations between preserved and impaired memory functions, observations which cannot easily be accommodated within a simple unitary model of memory with consolidation and retrieval models. Cohen and Squire (1982) contrasted procedural learning, i.e. 'knowing how', and declarative knowledge, 'knowing that', memory. This describes the situation of patients acquiring new motor skills often without explicit knowledge of having done so. One patient for example, was able to learn a new piano tune without any recollection of having done so, and replay if prompted with the initial bars (Starr and Phillips 1970). However, the dimension of declarative memory does not easily explain the deficits seen in patients such as H.M. in whom memory for words, part of declarative knowledge, is well preserved. Tulving (1973) drew attention to the difference between episodic, i.e. memory for day-to-day events, and semantic memory. Other approaches have looked at the dynamic processes involved rather than observed dichotomies, for example the processes involved in implicit and explicit learning, i.e. those which are variably dependent upon the degree of conscious recall.

A large variety of diseases may be associated with amnesia. Most commonly, memory impairment is seen with confusional states or dementia, but in these instances the amnesia is part of a wider spectrum of cognitive impairment (see below). Diseases affecting the medial temporal lobes and other structures on the limbic circuit may cause amnesia. Thus midline tumours in the region of the third ventricle, such as craniopharyngiomas, colloid cysts, massive pituitary tumours (Williams and Pennybacker 1954), thalamic gliomas, and tumours of the splenium of the corpus callosum, believed to be due to involvement of the fornix (Rudge and Warrington 1991), can all cause a severe amnesia. Inflammatory disorders, such as sarcoidosis and other granulomatous lesions in the same areas and limbic encephalitis as a paraneoplastic phenomenon (Henson and Urich 1982), are also associated with amnesia. A profound memory impairment is also commonly seen with herpes encephalitis, due to the selective involvement of the medial temporal cortex. Vascular events of the posterior cerebral artery, which supplies the medial temporal lobe and hippocampus, can cause amnesia (Benson *et al.* 1974). This often occurs with bilateral damage in association with basilar artery syndromes, but can occur with unilateral cerebral artery occlusions, particularly in the elderly, which may be due to pre-existing contralateral hippocampal damage.

The Korsakoff syndrome is a striking amnesia which usually follows a Wernicke's encephalopathy (Section 26.5). Patients present with a profound amnesia and are quite unable to remember events even within the last half an hour, but may be shown to have implicit learning, of motor skills for example. Other tests of cognitive function are well preserved in the pure form of Korsakoff's syndrome, but in clinical practice a spectrum may be seen, with the more generalized cognitive impairment of alcoholic dementia at one end and patients with a pure Korsakoff syndrome at the other (Cutting 1978). It is, however, the striking contrast between the profound amnesia and the relatively minor additional cognitive defects that characterizes Korsakoff's syndrome. There is often striking confabulation, when a patient may provide imaginary accounts of his actions to create what, at times, can be a plausible autobiographical memory.

Transient loss of memory is also a common clinical problem with both anterograde and retrograde amnesia, the latter shrinking on recovery, leaving a gap in memory for the period of anterograde memory impairment subsequent to the onset. Temporary memory loss may occur with a variety of conditions which result in either generalized cerebral dysfunction or with selective disturbance of the medial temporal lobe and diencephalon. These include epilepsy, most commonly temporal lobe epilepsy, and in some patients there may be no obvious disturbance of consciousness. Cerebral tumours may cause episodic memory loss which may also be on an epileptic basis (Lisak and Zimmerman 1977). Head injury, drugs, especially alcohol (Goodwin *et al.* 1969), and benzodiazepines are common causes. Transient memory impairment may also occur as a feature of transient ischaemic episodes in posterior cerebral territory. A picture resembling transient global amnesia may also occur with migraine but this is usually with a clinical history of previous migraine attacks and the episodes are normally followed by headache (Caplan *et al.* 1981). Psychogenic amnesia and hysterical fugue states, a not infrequent topic of newspaper stories, are discussed below.

Transient global amnesia

This is a striking syndrome affecting the middle aged and the elderly. The history is obtained of sudden onset of impairment of episodic or autobiographical memory (Hodges and Ward 1989). The attacks are frequently reported to have been triggered by sexual intercourse or sudden cold, winter bathing in the elderly being a classic history (Fisher, 1982). The attacks last from 1–24 hours and the patients may repeatedly ask questions and appear anxious, but otherwise able to drive home, and there have been reports of virtuoso musical performances during an attack. Investigations are usually normal and a full recovery can be anticipated, although some patients are left with mild memory impairment (Mazzucchi *et al.* 1980). Recurrences are rare but do occur in a small proportion (Shuping *et al.* 1979). A vascular cause may underlie the syndrome of transient global amnesia (Fisher and Adams 1958), although supportive evidence has been difficult to establish and epidemiological studies have suggested a closer link to migraine (Hodges and Warlow 1990).

Paramnesias

Confabulation, the production of memories without any basis in real events, can accompany amnesia and is most commonly observed in Korsakoff's syndrome. However, confabulation can be seen in patients with adequate performance on routine memory testing and is therefore more appropriately considered as a paramnesia (Stuss *et al.* 1978). Two classes of confabulation have been distinguished (Berlyne 1972). Momentary or provoked confabulation occurs in response to questions and requests for specific information that the patient might reasonably be expected to know. More florid is fantastic confabulation, in which the patient will spontaneously produce bizarre accounts, often far in excess of what might be required in response to the situation. Confabulation is found most commonly in association with frontal-lobe lesions, particularly in medial frontal-lobe lesions (Stuss *et al.* 1978; Damasio *et al.* 1985).

Reduplicative paramnesia (Pick 1903) describes a behavioural disturbance in which the patient transposes or reduplicates places. For example he might claim that his home is not his normal home but a very similar building in which he is staying, or alternatively that the hospital in which he has been admitted is in his home town. Such patients usually have bifrontal or right frontal lesions (Kapur *et al.* 1988). A similar syndrome is the Capgras syndrome in which patients refuse to recognize people, often close relatives who are familiar to them, claiming them to be impostors. The Capgras syndrome is usually seen in association with right hemisphere lesions (Alexander *et al.* 1979).

26.5 Wernicke–Korsakoff syndrome

In 1887, Korsakoff reported a syndrome of mental changes, predominantly of memory impairment in association with polyneuropathy. The tendency to confabulate was noted, as was the link with alcohol abuse, but it was also reported with typhoid fever and prolonged vomiting. Six years earlier, Wernicke had described an acute illness of ataxia, ophthalmoplegia, polyneuropathy, and a confusional state. It was later observed that these syndromes often occurred sequentially in the same patient. The majority of cases are now associated with alcohol abuse, and thiamine deficiency plays a key role in Wernicke's encephalopathy.

Wernicke's encephalopathy presents with an acute or subacute confusional state, together with oculomotor disturbance and ataxia. The confusional state involves inattention and disorientation but can progress to drowsiness and even to coma and death if the underlying thiamine deficiency is not recognized and treated. The examination may reveal nystagmus, VIth nerve palsies, conjugate gaze palsies, and ataxia. Criteria reflecting the classic triad of encephalopathy, oculomotor disturbance, and ataxia have been developed (Caine *et al.* 1997). The occurrence of any two of the following—dietary deficiency, oculomotor palsies, cerebellar dysfunction, and altered mental state—can provide high diagnostic accuracy.

Korsakoff's syndrome emerges as Wernicke's encephalopathy resolves, and the confusional state clears to reveal a profound amnesia with both an inability to recall recent events and to learn new facts (Kopelman 1995). However, it may emerge gradually without a prominent preceding encephalopathic stage. The key component is the impairment of memory out of proportion to other cognitive domains. The deficit relates to event or episodic memory with sparing of semantic memory, and implicit learning can be demonstrated. Early lifetime memories are preserved, with a steeper temporal gradient than is typically seen in Alzheimer's disease (Kopelman 1995). Classically, patients also confabulate and will easily confuse the temporal sequence of memories that are recalled; this is believed to relate to additional frontal damage and, indeed, many patients lack insight and initiative, indicative of a frontal syndrome. However, more widespread cognitive deficits may be seen, and a clinical picture which merges with 'alcohol dementia' (Cutting 1978). Some have suggested that Korsakoff's syndrome and alcohol dementia are all part of the same spectrum, but the memory impairment of the former does set it apart, as does involvement of diencephalic structures. Bilateral haemorrhagic lesions in the areas of the third and fourth ventricle and aqueduct are characteristic of Wernicke's encephalopathy, and the diencephalic lesions are critical to the emergent amnesia of Korsakoff's syndrome. The original proposal that damage to the dorsal medial nucleus of the thalamus was the minimal lesion (Victor *et al.* 1989) has been considered too specific, and anterior and medial thalamic and mammillary body involvement are also implicated. Shrinkage of the mammillary bodies is also seen in non-Korsakoff alcoholic cognitive impairment. Thiamine deficiency is believed to underlie the pathogenesis of the disorder, and explains its occurrence in other disorders such as prolonged vomiting, nutritional deficiency, and hyperemesis gravidarum. In patients who abuse alcohol, there is considerable variability in susceptibility to Wernicke–Korsakoff syndrome, suggesting not only subtle differences in diet but also potential genetic factors.

The key to the treatment is to make the diagnosis, which should be considered in all patients presenting acutely with unexplained cognitive impairment or coma. Treatment is with intravenous thiamine, at least 100 mg daily. In the acute situation it is important to give thiamine before intravenous glucose (Heye *et al.* 1994).

26.6 Dementia

26.6.1 Approaches to a differential diagnosis

The term 'dementia' refers to the clinical syndrome of impairment in multiple domains of cognitive function, which must include memory, in a patient who remains alert with normal arousal. This serves to distinguish patients with dementia from those with confusional states or delirium, who have abnormal arousal, and from those with a single discrete cognitive deficit such as a dysphasia. This definition has been used to create operational criteria, such as those of the diagnostic and statistical manual (DSM-IV) of the American Psychiatric Association (American Psychiatric Association 1994) and the ICD-10 (World Health Organization 1992). An important feature of these definitions is that the dementia must be sufficiently severe to interfere with social and occupational function. There is clearly no simple cut-off from normality, and whether this criterion is met will depend upon premorbid function and on the patient's social and occupational demands. This is particularly relevant to the elderly, in whom some decline of cognitive function, particularly memory, is commonplace. Attempts have been made to distinguish patients with a progressive dementia, normally due to Alzheimer's disease, from less severe memory impairment associated with ageing. The terms 'benign senescent forgetfulness' (Kral 1962), 'age-associated memory impairment' (Crook *et al.* 1986), and 'age-associated cognitive decline' have largely been superseded by the term 'mild cognitive impairment' or MCI (Tierney *et al.* 1996). The MCI group will include patients with a mild, non-progressive memory impairment as well as those in the early stages of Alzheimer's disease or other progressive disorder. The annual rate of progression to dementia is approximately 15 per cent per year (Tierney *et al.* 1996).

The definition of dementia is a broad one, and it is not surprising, therefore, that the syndrome can be associated with a large variety of diseases (Table 26.1). All of these may be associated with widespread cognitive impairment, but the clinical patterns vary and can lead to characteristic features. A broad distinction has been drawn between subcortical and cortical dementias (Albert *et al.* 1974; Cummings 1986). The term 'subcortical dementia' was originally applied to the cognitive deficits seen in progressive supranuclear palsy and Huntington's disease, and is characterized by a marked slowness in cognition with additional impairments of motivation and attention. Indeed, if the patient is allowed time, then performance on routine neuropsychological testing may improve, but performance in everyday life remains severely compromised. The diseases that are most commonly found with this type of dementia are those affecting the basal ganglia and frontal connections. Dysphasia, dyspraxia, and agnosia are not prominent in these patients, by contrast to those with cortical dementia, in whom the memory impairment is generally not improved by cues, and the speed of cognition is relatively normal. The prototypic cortical dementia is Alzheimer's disease and the characteristic clinical pattern reflects damage to the cortical association areas (Table 26.2).

Of the many diseases listed in Table 26.1, some are very rare, and in others dementia is only an occasional clinical feature. The cognitive impairment may vary from minor deficits found only on specific testing, to a more prominent dementia. Vascular dementia, for example, subsumes a large variety of different pathological entities, with a variable cognitive profile.

A significant minority of patients with dementia have been found to have a treatable disease in published series (Clarfield 1988), the most common being the subcortical dementia of depressive illness, but other treatable diseases include benign neoplasms, infections, vitamin deficiencies, and normal-pressure hydrocephalus. However, the proportion of patients with reversible dementia seen by neurologists has lessened with earlier and better assessment (Walstra *et al.* 1997). In view of the profound consequences of dementia, a comprehensive approach to investigation is justified, although clearly the extent of investigations will be determined by the clinical features and age of the patient. Both European (Waldemar *et al.* 2000) and US (Corey Bloom *et al.* 1995; Small *et al.* 1997; Anonymous 1999) guidelines on investigation and management of patients with dementia have been published. It would be inappropriate to undertake intensive investigation in a very elderly patient with multiple systemic illnesses and cognitive impairment; by contrast, the young or atypical patient requires exhaustive investigation. All patients presenting with dementia should undergo a careful neuropsychological assessment. This will establish whether the patient does indeed have a generalized cognitive impairment and will help to detail the pattern of deficits. Routine biochemical and haematological determinations, which should include an ESR, thyroid function, syphilis and *Borrelia* serology and autoantibody screen, will identify many of the potentially remediable causes. Vitamin B12 is often found to be low, but rarely implicated as a cause of dementia. At-risk individuals with a subcortical dementia may require HIV testing. Chest radiography and ECG complete the general assessment, which will also serve to identify co-morbid illnesses

Table 26.1. Illustrative causes of adult-onset dementia

Primary cerebral degenerations	Cerebral infections and inflammatory disorders
Alzheimer's disease	Neurosyphilis
Down syndrome and Alzheimer histopathology	Viral encephalitis especially herpes simplex
Pick's disease	HIV infection
Progressive supranuclear palsy	Progressive multifocal leucoencephalopathy
Corticobasal degeneration	Subacute sclerosing panencephalitis
Frontal lobe degeneration	Subacute rubella encephalitis
Dementia with motor neuron disease inclusions	Viral, bacterial, and fungal meningitides
Parkinsonism-dementia complex of Guam	Whipple's disease
Parkinson's disease and dementia	Behçet's syndrome
Dementia with Lewy bodies	Disseminated encephalomyelitis
Thalamic degeneration	Multiple sclerosis
Calcification of the basal ganglia with neurofibrillary tangles	Sarcoidosis
Huntington's disease	
Spinocerebellar degenerations	
Progressive myoclonic epilepsy	

Prion dementias	Cerebrovascular disease
Sporadic and familial Creutzfeldt-Jakob disease	Multiple cortical infarcts
Gerstmann-Straussler-Schenke syndrome	Multiple lacunar infarcts
Kuru	Binswanger's disease
Iatrogenic Creutzfeldt-Jakob disease	Congophilic angiopathy including hereditary Dutch amyloid angiopathy
Variant Creutzfeldt-Jakob disease	Cerebral autosomal dominant arteriopathy with subcortical infarcts and leucoencephalopathy (CADASIL)
Familial fatal insomnia	Cranial arteritis
	Cerebral arteritides inc PAN, SLE, thromboangiitis obliterans, and granulomatous angiitis
	Thrombotic thrombocytopenic purpura
	Subacute diencephalic angioencephalopathy
	Subdural haematoma
	Giant aneurysms
	Arteriovenous malformations
	Hyperviscosity syndromes

Inherited metabolic and storage disorders	Metabolic and toxic causes (the majority more commonly present as confusional states)
Porphyria	Hypothyroidism
Wilson's disease	Hyper- and hypocalcaemia
Mitochondrial cytopathies	Hypoglycaemia
Kuf's disease	Hypo- and hypernatraemia
Metachromatic and adrenoleucodystrophy	Uraemia
Membranous lipodystrophy	Dialysis dementia
Cerebrotendinous xanthomatosis	Chronic hepatic encephalopathy
	Hashimoto's encephalopathy
	Wernicke-Korsakoff syndrome
	Alcoholic dementia
	Marchiafava-Bignami disease
	Hypoxia
	Drugs, poisons, heavy metals
	Vitamin B_{12} deficiency
	Pellagra
	Malabsorption syndrome and coeliac encephalopathy

Neoplasms	Miscellaneous
Meningiomas	Aqueduct stenosis
Gliomas especially callosal	Normal pressure hydrocephalus
Parapituitary tumours	Open and closed head injuries
Pineal and midbrain tumours	Dementia pugilistica
Cerebral lymphoma	Post-cerebral irradiation
Cerebral metastases	
Carcinomatous meningitis	
Paraneoplastic syndromes including limbic encephalitis	

Table 26.2. Cortical and subcortical dementias (derived in part from Cummings 1986)

	Subcortical dementia	Cortical dementia
Severity	Mild to moderate	More severe earlier in course
Speed of cognition	Slow	Normal but frequent errors
Neuropsychology	Memory impairment, recall aided by cues	More severe memory impairment unaided by cues
Mood	Apathy, depression	Depression less common
Motor abnormalities	Extrapyramidal, dysarthria	Uncommon, *Gegenhalten*
Neuropathology	Prominent changes in striatum and thalamus	Prominent changes in cortical association areas

which may contribute to the cognitive impairment. Other blood tests, for example, genotyping, will depend upon the clinical features.

All patients should have neuroimaging, either CT scanning or MRI. Tumours and hydrocephalus can be excluded by both imaging modalities, but MRI has the additional advantage of more detailed imaging of white matter disease in demyelination and vascular disease. Increasingly, MRI can also provide information on regional atrophy, e.g. selective atrophy of hippocampi in Alzheimer's disease, of value in differential diagnosis (Jack *et al.* 1999). Serial MRI may also demonstrate rates of atrophy in degenerative disease outside the normal range (Fox *et al.* 1999*a, b*). Positron emission tomography (PET) can also identify regional deficits of blood flow and cerebral metabolism in degenerative dementia, using either oxygen-15 or fluoro-deoxyglucose scanning. Thus, a characteristic feature of Alzheimer's disease is posterior biparietal bitemporal hypometabolism (Frackowiak *et al.* 1981), which can be contrasted with frontal deficits in the frontotemporal degenerations. The use of single photon emission computed tomography (SPECT) is more readily available and, although it lacks the quantitative information provided by PET scanning, can also contribute to the identification of regional deficits, most useful in frontal degeneration, where atrophy may be difficult to identify on structural images (reviewed by Kennedy 1998). The EEG may identify patients with subclinical seizure activity and the characteristic changes of the spongiform encephalopathies; in addition it can assist in the distinction of patients with Alzheimer's disease, with early slow wave changes, from patients with frontotemporal degenerations, in whom the EEG is relatively well preserved (Stigsby *et al.* 1981). Examination of the cerebrospinal fluid is important in patients in whom one suspects an inflammatory or infective cause, and increasingly CSF markers such as $A\beta_{1-42}$ and tau are being sought in Alzheimer's disease (Hulstaert *et al.* 1999). A relatively specific protein marker, P14–3–3 is found in cerebrospinal fluid in Creutzfeldt–Jakob disease (CJD) (Hsich *et al.* 1996). Tissue biopsy, e.g. muscle (mitochondrial cytopathy), skin (Kuf's disease) and tonsil (variant CJD; Hill *et al.* 1999) may be diagnostic. In rare instances, meningeal and cerebral tissue biopsy will be necessary, and may be the only way to establish a diagnosis of isolated cerebral vasculitis.

The majority of the diseases causing dementia which are listed in Table 26.1 are discussed elsewhere. In general, most cause a largely subcortical picture. In many of these instances there will be other clinical clues. The primary degenerative dementias give rise to a dementia with few other neurological findings in the early stages, and these are dealt with in detail here.

26.6.2 Alzheimer's disease

In 1906, Alois Alzheimer described a 51-year-old lady with dementia, and senile plaques and neurofibrillary tangles at autopsy. Originally Alzheimer's disease was viewed as a rare pre-senile dementia. However, clinicopathological studies in the 1960s demonstrated an overall relationship between dementia and the presence of senile plaques in both young and elderly demented patients (Blessed *et al.* 1968), and the view emerged that Alzheimer's disease and senile dementia of the Alzheimer type was a single disease. Nevertheless, within the broad group of Alzheimer's disease cases, clinical and pathological heterogeneity can be observed. This originally focused on the age at onset, with subtle distinctions being made between early and late onset disease. At a neuropathological level, distinctions have been drawn between cases that consist predominantly of neurofibrillary tangles and those that consist predominantly of senile plaques. However, the most robust biological categorization relates to cases with a clear family history. Up to 40 per cent have a family history of an affected first-degree relative (Farrer *et al.* 1990); rarely there is a clear autosomal dominant history. Pathogenic mutations in three different genes have been identified in this group, namely presenilin 1 and 2 and amyloid precursor protein (APP) genes, which account for up to 50 per cent of the autosomal dominant familial Alzheimer's disease cases described (Cruts *et al.* 1998). Inheritance of an E4 allele of the apolipoprotein E gene is associated with an increased risk of developing Alzheimer's disease (Corder *et al.* 1993).

It is now recognized that Alzheimer's disease is the major cause of dementia. Epidemiological studies indicate a doubling of the prevalence of dementia with each decade above 65 years to a prevalence of nearly 50 per cent in those aged 85 and above (Evans *et al.* 1989). Approximately 70 per cent of cases of dementia will be due to Alzheimer's disease, either alone or in combination with vascular disease. Estimates suggest a global figure of approximately 15 million people with dementia as we enter the next millennium.

Clinical features

Alzheimer's disease is a disorder of middle and late life. Early onset cases are described in the fourth and fifth decade but these are rare and almost exclusively familial. The clinical features of familial Alzheimer's disease associated with mutations in the APP and presenilin genes are broadly similar to sporadic disease, apart from the age at onset. However, cases with mutation at *APP* 692 have more amyloid angiopathy with cerebral haemorrhages and, thus, share similarities to hereditary cerebral haemorrhage with amyloidosis of the Dutch type due to mutations at *APP* 693.

The classical presentation of Alzheimer's disease is with memory impairment and, in some patients, there may be a relatively prolonged course, with isolated memory deficits until late into the disease. Patients who fulfil the criteria for MCI (Section 26.6.1) with an isolated memory impairment are often subsequently found to have Alzheimer's disease (Tierney *et al.* 1996). The memory impairment primarily affects episodic and autobiographical memory, the patient forgets appointments and mislays objects. Procedural memory and learning may be relatively preserved and, as with Korsakoff's syndrome, patients may demonstrate procedural learning without apparent parallel declarative learning (Knopman and Nissen 1987). It is often stated that remote memory is preserved, but if specifically investigated, remote memory is also disrupted. Language impairment can occur relatively early, and emergence of verbal semantic memory impairment implicates involvement of temporal lobe structures, extending beyond the hippocampus. Some patients present with a relatively focal dysphasia with low

progression (Kirshner *et al.* 1984). Dyspraxia is generally a late feature (Della *et al.* 1987), although ideomotor dyspraxia is often found if specifically sought. Visuospatial and visuoperceptual deficits are also prominent and, in some patients, may be the presenting feature. Patients are quite often unaware of their cognitive deficits, often being brought to the attention of doctors by their relatives. The denial or anosognosia is not related to severity (Feher *et al.* 1991).

The general neurological examination is relatively normal in Alzheimer's disease at presentation, although motor abnormalities of extrapyramidal type emerge in up to 60 per cent in some series (Sulkava 1982). Increased muscle tone or *Gegenhalten* is the main feature and appears unrelated to the nigrostriatal deficit seen in Parkinson's disease (Tyrrell *et al.* 1990a), although many patients with additional bradykinesia are found to have dementia with Lewy bodies (Perry *et al.* 1996). Primitive reflexes such as the instinctive grasp reaction, rooting, and sucking occur late. Generalized seizures occur in 10–20 per cent over the total course of the disease, and myoclonus is seen in approximately 10 per cent of younger cases, and in some it may be a prominent feature (Faden and Townsend 1976).

Structural neuroimaging characteristically shows medial temporal lobe atrophy which can be seen on CT scan (Jobst *et al.* 1992) or, more specifically, hippocampal atrophy on MRI (Kennedy 1998) (Fig. 26.2). Functional imaging with SPECT or PET reveals a posterior biparietal bitemporal pattern of hypometabolism. EEG shows slowing and loss of alpha rhythm relatively early in the disease. Many CSF markers have been sought, and increased tau and decreased $A\beta_{1-42}$ is claimed to

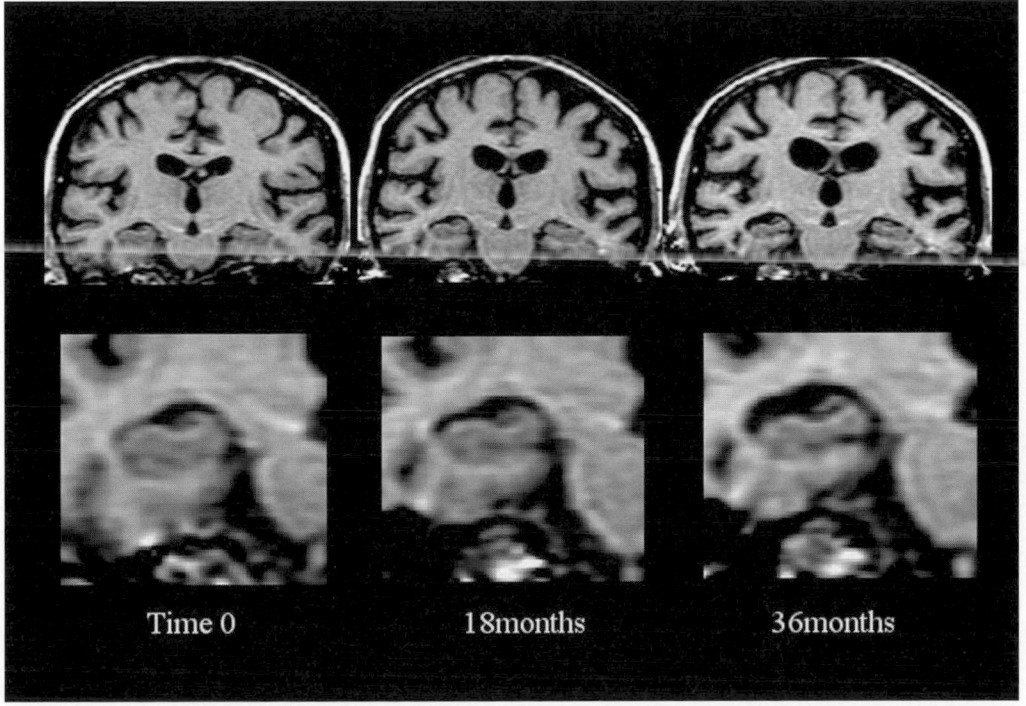

Fig. 26.2. Coronal T1-weighted MRI, showing progressive hippocampal atrophy in a patient with Alzheimer's disease.

be of value (Hulstaert *et al.* 1999) but is not yet in routine clinical practice. The NINCDS ADRDA criteria for diagnosis of Alzheimer's disease provide levels of probable and possible diagnosis; definite Alzheimer's disease is reserved for those in whom histological confirmation of plaques and tangles is available (McKhann *et al.* 1984). Clinical diagnosis has steadily improved and, using NINCDS criteria, accuracies in the region of 80–90 per cent are commonly reported (Tierney *et al.* 1988; Kukull *et al.* 1990).

Neuropathology

The histopathological hallmarks of the disease are neurofibrillary tangles and senile plaques. Neurofibrillary tangles are intraneuronal and found predominantly in the allocortex and temporoparietal neocortex (Fig. 26.3). There is a predilection for pyramidal cells to be involved, particularly in layers 3 and 5 of the neocortex, the CA1 layer of the hippocampus, subiculum, and layers 2 and 5 of the entorhinal cortex. Braak and Braak (1991) quantified regional tangle formation in normal elderly and mild to severe Alzheimer's disease cases, and suggested a staging system with progression of the disease from entorhinal cortex and hippocampus to neocortex. Neurofibrillary tangles consist of paired helical filaments which can be seen under electron microscopy (Kidd 1963), with a filament diameter of 10 nm wound in a double helix with a periodicity of 160 nm. Neurofibrillary tangles are also found within the dystrophic neurites of senile plaques. The major component of the paired helical filament has been shown to be the microtubule-associated protein, tau, which is abnormally phosphorylated (Lee *et al.* 1991). All six tau isoforms are deposited in Alzheimer's disease (Goedert *et al.* 1992), which distinguishes the tau pathology from that found in progressive supranuclear palsy (PSP), Pick's disease, and the other tauopathies.

Senile plaques are also found predominantly in neocortical association areas and consist of glial processes, abnormal nerve endings or dystrophic neurites, and a central core of β-amyloid; they vary between 25 and 200 μm in diameter. β-Amyloid is also deposited in cerebral blood vessels. The β-amyloid protein has been isolated and shown to be derived from a much larger transmembrane molecule, the amyloid precursor protein (Kang *et al.* 1987). Diffuse plaques are not associated with dystrophic neurites and are believed to precede the classical mature plaque.

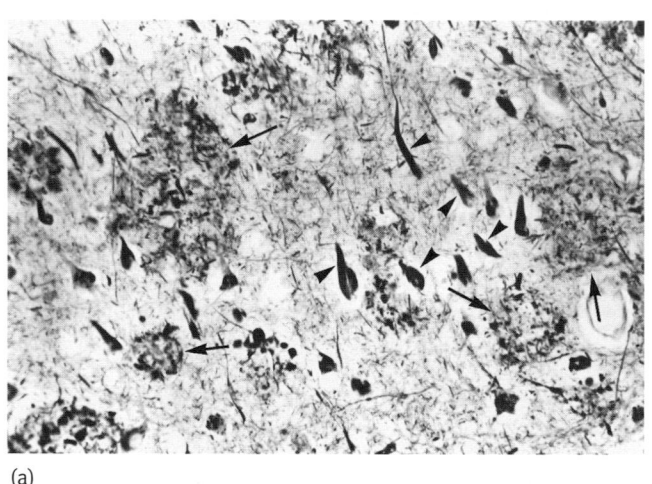

(a)

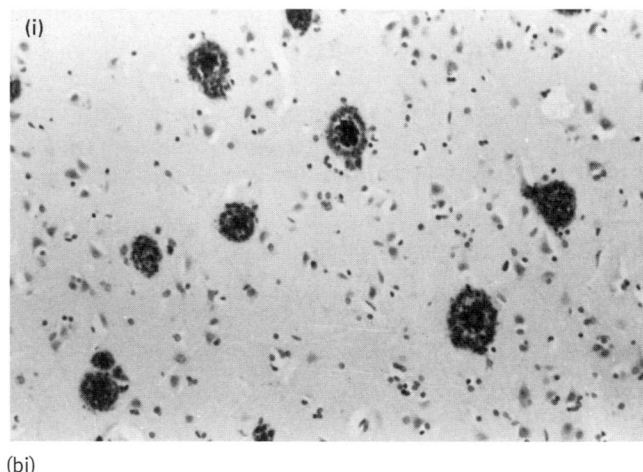

(bi)

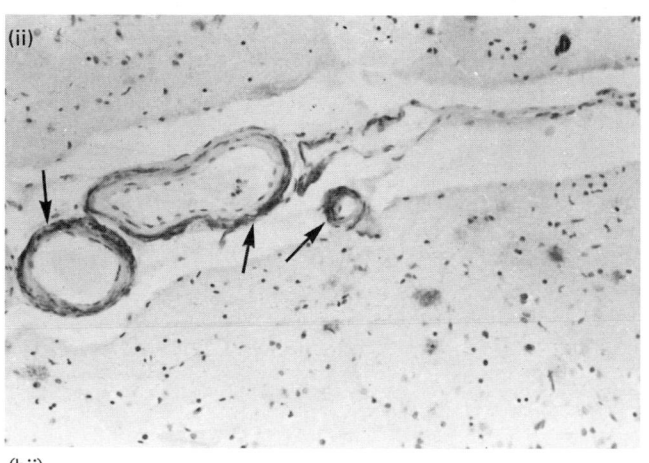

(bii)

Fig. 26.3. (a) Senile plaques (arrows) and neurofibrillary tangles (arrowheads) in the hippocampus in Alzheimer's disease (modified Bielschowsky silver impregnation; 300). (b) Positive immunostaining of (i) plaques (250) and (ii) blood vessels (250), with an antibody to A4 protein. Avidinbiotin complex method. (Antibody to A4 kindly provided by Professor B. H. Anderton, Department of Neuroscience, Institute of Psychiatry, London; the micrographs were kindly provided by Professor P. L. Lantos, Department of Neuropathology, Institute of Psychiatry, London; the photographic assistance of Mr A Brady, Department of Neuropathology is acknowledged.)

The central amyloid core consists predominantly of the Aβ1–42 species (see below), which may act as a nidus for subsequent fibrillary amyloid deposition (Iwatsubo *et al.* 1995).

Neuronal cell loss is also maximal in the hippocampus and association areas of the neocortex. Cell loss also occurs in sub-cortical nuclei, which include the amygdala and the origins of the subcortical projection systems, the nucleus basalis of Meynert, the nucleus raphe, and the locus ceruleus. The damage to the nucleus basalis and septal nuclei results in the cholinergic deficit, a consistent but not specific feature of Alzheimer's disease. Replacement of the cholinergic deficit is the basis of current symptomatic treatment. There is an overall association between cell loss and the histological features of plaques and tangles, and it is assumed that cells that contain neurofibrillary tangles are degenerating. Other histological changes found predominantly in the hippocampus include eosinophilic Hirano bodies and vacuolar changes in cytoplasm referred to as granulovacuolar degeneration. The severity of the histological changes of senile plaques and neurofibrillary tangles shows an overall association with severity of dementia. They are not, however, specific to Alzheimer's disease and neurofibrillary tangles in the hippocampus are found commonly in normal old age, as are limited numbers of senile plaques throughout the cortex. This has led to quantitative criteria for diagnosis (Khachaturian 1985) which have largely been superseded by the CERAD (Consortium to Establish a Registry of Alzheimer's Disease) criteria, based on numbers of neuritic plaques irrespective of neurofibrillary tangles (Mirra *et al.* 1991).

The cause of Alzheimer's disease is still not established, but considerable advances have been made which identify a central role for amyloid deposition. This is best understood in patients with autosomal dominant familial Alzheimer's disease. The rare mutations in the *APP* gene either increase the total amount of β-amyloid produced or alter the processing to favour amyloid deposition. The *APP* 670–671 mutation increases the total amount of β-amyloid peptide produced from the precursor protein, and is similar in this regard to Down syndrome, where there is an increased amount of amyloid produced due to a gene dosage effect arising from the trisomy 21. The amyloid precursor protein is normally cleaved at putative β- and γ-secretase sites to release the 40-amino-acid Aβ peptide, whose physiological function is unclear. It can be measured as a soluble peptide in both plasma and CSF but will form fibrillary aggregates of β amyloid in senile plaques. Mutations at *APP* 717, close to the putative γ-secretase site, result in a subtle increase in the proportion of molecules extended at the C terminus of Aβ1–42 (Fig. 26.4). Aβ1–42 has a greater propensity to fibril formation and can act as a nidus for subsequent Aβ1–40 deposition. The familial Alzheimer's disease cases associated with mutations in the presenilin 1 and 2 genes (Cruts and Van Broeckhoven 1998a) also result in altered metabolism of APP and a relative increase in Aβ1–42; there has even been speculation that presenilin 1 may be the γ-secretase. ApoE4, also known to be an important genetic risk factor, is associated with enhanced amyloid deposition and may stabilize fibril formation.

These lines of evidence all support a central role for amyloid deposition and the 'amyloid cascade' hypothesis (Hardy and Higgins 1992). This model predicts that the neuronal loss and neurofibrillary tangle formation are secondary events, but as yet, it is not known why amyloid is neurotoxic. Recent evidence for this central role is provided by transgenic mouse models arising from overexpression of a human mutated *APP* gene, which result in senile plaque formation which can be prevented by immunization with Aβ1–42 (Schenk *et al.* 1999). The secondary role for neurofibrillary tangles in this pathogenic cascade does not diminish their potential importance as a final common pathway. Moreover, in some of the hereditary tauopathies presenting with frontotemporal degeneration (Section 26.6.4), mutations in the tau gene are the key pathogenic event.

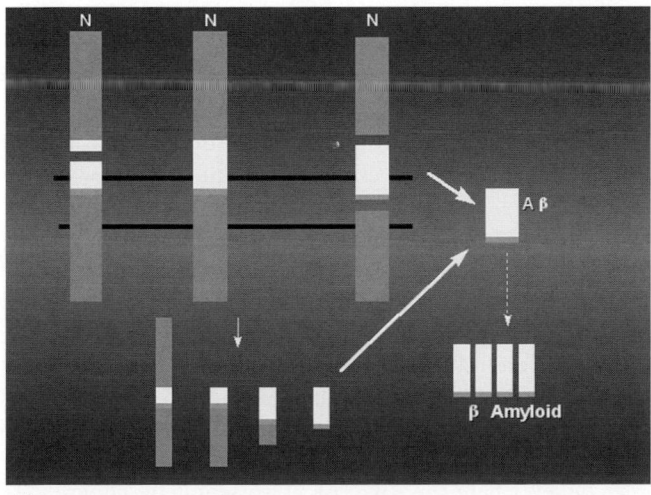

(a)

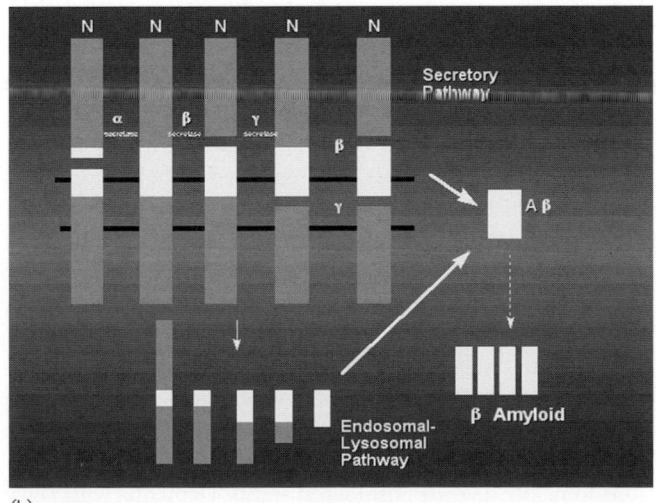

(b)

Fig. 26.4. (a) Metabolism of APP. (b) Metabolism of APP with extension at the C terminus.

Treatment

Advice, support and a sensible prognosis for the carer should be available, and information can be obtained from national Alzheimer's Disease Societies and Alzheimer's Disease International. Treatment of systemic disease such as infections and heart failure are important as these may cause further deterioration in cognition, and patients with dementia are very sensitive to the cognitive side-effects of drugs. Agitation and delusional symptoms may need to be treated, but neuroleptic medication should be kept to an absolute minimum (McShane et al. 1997). Depression is a common early feature of Alzheimer's disease and a trial of a selective serotonin re-uptake inhibitor (SSRI) is indicated if there is a clinical suspicion of depressive symptomology. Tricyclics should be avoided because of anticholinergic side-effects. Patients who hold a driving licence should inform the national driving authority at the time of diagnosis, according to national guidelines, but the decision of when to stop driving will depend upon their cognitive function (Waldemar et al. 2000).

There is no treatment to affect the progression of Alzheimer's disease. A trial of selegiline and vitamin E, both alone and in combination, suggested a possible delay in progression (Sano et al. 1997). Although this trial has not been replicated and there were methodological problems, many patients are prescribed vitamin E in doses of up to 2000 units daily. Inhibition of cholinesterase activity in the brain will enhance levels of acetylcholine and thus ameliorate the cholinergic deficit arising from degeneration of the ascending projections from basal forebrain to hippocampus and the neocortex. Tacrine (Cognex®) has been largely superseded by donepezil (Aricept®) and rivastigmine (Exelon®). The symptomatic effects are modest, but improvement in cognitive measures and clinical global impression is seen in 20–25 per cent of patients over and above a placebo response (therapeutic gain) (Rogers et al. 1998; Rosler et al. 1999). There is no evidence of any effect on disease progression.

26.6.3 Dementia with Lewy bodies

Terminological confusion has surrounded the group of patients with Parkinsonian features and dementia. It has been known for a long time that patients with Parkinson's disease may develop cognitive impairment, and such patients are found to have Lewy bodies, the pathological hallmark of Parkinson's disease, throughout the cerebral cortex. With systematic autopsy studies, such cases have emerged as being common, perhaps constituting as many as 15–20 per cent in some series of older patients (Klatka et al. 1996; Perry et al. 1996). Series based on clinical diagnosis would suggest a similar proportion. However, there are overlaps in terms of both the clinical and pathological features with Alzheimer's disease, for example, senile plaques are found in dementia with Lewy bodies and Lewy bodies are found in classical Alzheimer's disease, making assessment difficult. However, it is now sufficiently clear that there is a distinct clinical picture with management implications to justify its own nosological status. Dementia with Lewy bodies is now the preferred term, but this condition has previously been, and still is, referred to as cortical Lewy body disease, Lewy body dementia, senile dementia of the Lewy body type, and Lewy body variant of Alzheimer's disease.

The characteristic clinical picture is that of a cognitive impairment which precedes or follows closely a symmetrical Parkinsonian syndrome. Tremor is rare compared with classical brainstem Lewy body Parkinson's disease. The cognitive impairment is similar to Alzheimer's disease, except that visual memory and visuoperceptual and visuospatial impairments are more prominent. The additional striking feature is marked fluctuation of cognitive function which can appear as a confusional state with impairment of attention. Reduplicative paramnesias and hallucinations complete the picture. In between these periods of worsening cognition, caregivers will often report episodes of lucidity. Hallucinations also occur late in Alzheimer's disease, however, if present at an early and mild stage, this is a strong indicator of an underlying diagnosis of dementia with Lewy bodies (Ballard et al. 1999). The features have been formalized into criteria in which two out of three of a Parkinsonian syndrome, fluctuations, and hallucinations are required to be present (McKeith et al. 1996). Sleep disturbance is common and myoclonus may be observed. In some patients, the disorder is of an apparent subacute onset with rapid deterioration. A characteristic feature is marked sensitivity to neuroleptics.

The EEG usually shows slowing. Magnetic resonance imaging may show atrophy with relative greater involvement of the parahippocampal gyrus than hippocampus in contrast to Alzheimer's disease (O'Brien et al. 1997). Functional imaging shows the biparietal bitemporal pattern of Alzheimer's disease, but in addition, more prominent occipital changes which may reflect the visuoperceptual problems and hallucinations (Albin et al. 1996).

The Lewy body in dementia with Lewy bodies is identical to that found in brainstem Lewy body Parkinson's disease, consisting of eosinophilic inclusions on haematoxylin and eosin staining. Recently, α-synuclein has been shown to be a major component of Lewy bodies (Spillantini et al. 1997) and immunohistochemistry not only shows the widespread distribution of Lewy bodies but also neuritic change in affected cells, so-called Lewy neurites (Fig. 26.5). Lewy bodies are found predominantly in the parahippocampal and entorhinal cortex. Many cases have associated β-amyloid plaques, but typically without the extensive tau-positive neuritic change found in Alzheimer's disease. However, 50 per cent of cases will have neurofibrillary tangles, and although the distribution is somewhat different from Alzheimer's disease, there is clearly overlap of these disorders.

Management is notoriously difficult. Treatment of the Parkinsonian syndrome will worsen the confusional state. Patients are exquisitely sensitive to neuroleptics, which not only precipitate a profound extrapyramidal syndrome but also result in worsening cognition. There is some evidence that the atypical neuroleptics such as olanzapine and risperidone may be safer, but even here, there is a risk of worsening the clinical state and, in general, all such drugs should be avoided if at all

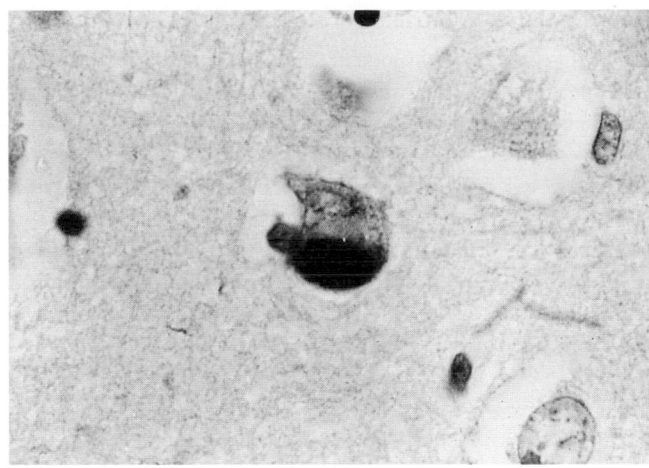

Fig. 26.5. Photomicrograph showing a Lewy body in the insular cortex; α-synuclein immunohistochemistry (antibody by courtesy of Professor BH Anderton), magnification 900. (Courtesy of Dr T. Revesz.)

possible. In early trials of acetylcholinesterase inhibitors, there was a suggestion that patients with dementia with Lewy bodies may respond. Autopsy studies have demonstrated a cholinergic deficit comparable to or even greater than that found in Alzheimer's disease. A recent preliminary report of the acetylcholinesterase inhibitor rivastigmine suggests that this may prove to be a useful line of treatment for managing the hallucinations and confusional state.

26.6.4 Frontotemporal degenerations

The frontotemporal degenerations are a group of disorders which are considered together as they all share the characteristic feature of a degenerative process affecting the frontal and/or temporal lobes (Snowden *et al.* 1996). The anatomical distribution determines the clinical features, which may often be asymmetric. These disorders are characterized by disturbances of language, speech production, frontal dysexecutive, and behavioural features. Clinical descriptions of the prototypic syndromes, frontotemporal dementia, progressive non-fluent aphasia, and semantic dementia, have been published (Neary *et al.* 1998), but other presentations, for example, primary progressive prosopagnosia (Tyrrell *et al.* 1990*b*) also occur. The neuropathological processes underlying these diseases are variable and include Pick's disease, non-specific frontal-lobe degeneration, hereditary tauopathies, corticobasal degeneration, and ubiquitin-positive tau-negative motor neuron disease type inclusions. The difficulty in predicting the underlying neuropathology from the clinical features demands a clinical descriptive approach to the frontotemporal degenerations before considering the potential diseases defined neuropathologically. The nosology surrounding these disorders is confused further by the terminology relating to Pick's disease. Originally, Pick described cases of focal atrophy with the clinical features of dysphasia and/or a frontal-lobe syndrome. This purely descriptive clinical terminology has been championed by some who suggest the term 'Pick syndrome' (Kertesz and Munoz 1998), but in parallel, the development started by Alzheimer, who observed the swollen Pick cells and argentophilic inclusions (Pick bodies), has defined a particular type of neuropathology. More recently, our understanding of the molecular pathology of Pick's disease has further defined its nosological status.

The term 'asymmetrical cortical degeneration' is another term that was introduced by Caselli and Jack (1992) to refer to the group of slowly progressive focal degenerations. In a sense, all degenerative dementias start as a focal syndrome, even including Alzheimer's disease, which initially is that of a memory impairment. Most of these focal cortical degenerations are subsumed within the frontotemporal degenerative group, but primary progressive apraxia, often associated with corticobasal degeneration and posterior cortical atrophy (Benson *et al.*, 988), usually associated with Alzheimer's disease, fall outside the general rubric of the frontotemporal degenerations.

Typically, the frontotemporal degenerations show structural or functional imaging changes indicative of frontotemporal degeneration. The EEG is characteristically normal by contrast to Alzheimer's disease (Stigsby *et al.* 1981). Cerebrospinal fluid examination is usually unremarkable.

Frontotemporal dementia

Although the term 'frontotemporal dementia' has been retained as one of the prototypic clinical syndromes of frontotemporal degeneration (Neary *et al.* 1998), the clinical features are those of a frontal syndrome, although the disease process does extend into the temporal lobes with time. It is, however, the behavioural change, as opposed to language or speech impairment, which characterizes this group of patients. Social skills deteriorate early, with difficulties at work, and the change in personality can be particularly distressing for the spouse. Some patients become disinhibited and overactive, reflecting predominant involvement of the orbitomedial frontal cortex, whereas others become apathetic, reflecting dorsolateral involvement. Patients who are at first overactive and at times aggressive, may become quieter as the disease progresses.

Other behavioural features include changes in food preference, usually towards sweet foods, ritualistic behaviours, and daily routines. Preservation of other cognitive skills means that the patient can go off walking on a stereotyped route, without ever getting lost. Dramatic failures on tests sensitive to frontal lobe function are apparent, although some patients may do well even on these tests, but fail on those of social cognition (Blair and Cipolotti 2000). Utilization behaviour may be observed. In some, speech gradually reduces with the features of a dynamic aphasia.

Some patients can develop a frontotemporal degeneration in association with motor neuron disease. Characteristically, this involves the anterior horn cells as opposed to long tracts, and fasciculation is seen characteristically in the proximal upper limb (Kew and Leigh 1992).

Progressive non-fluent aphasia

A non-fluent aphasia with relative preservation of comprehension was originally referred to as primary progressive aphasia (Mesulam 1982). Speech is non-fluent and effortful, although writing may be preserved early on. Comprehension is relatively preserved even as the disease progresses to mutism. At this stage, patients may travel alone or even drive a car without difficulty. Social skills are preserved early, but with disease progression, behavioural changes do emerge. Structural imaging shows left perisylvian atrophy, which can also be seen on functional imaging.

Semantic dementia

The third commonly encountered syndrome is referred to as semantic dementia and describes patients whose presenting feature is that of a verbal semantic memory impairment (Snowden *et al.* 1989; Hodges *et al.* 1992). Speech is fluent, and on first encounter the disorder may be missed. However, more detailed examination soon reveals the naming and comprehension deficit. At no time is speech production impaired, but it does become progressively more empty and communication more difficult. Regularization errors occur on reading aloud, indicative of a surface dyslexia. As the disease progresses, the semantic memory deficit may extend into the visual domain (rarely this can be the presenting feature) with the appearance of a visual associative agnosia. Behavioural changes with altered eating and ritualistic stereotypes occur. The disease starts with language impairment, reflecting left temporal lobe involvement, but with involvement of the right temporal lobe, patients can develop a prosopagnosia and an inability to recognize emotional expressions, impairing further their ability to communicate. The MRI and functional imaging reveal asymmetric left anterior temporal lobe atrophy (Fig. 26.6). In some patients, right temporal lobe atrophy predominates, with more florid behavioural changes, and, in some, prosopagnosia is the presenting feature (Tyrrell *et al.* 1990b; Hodges *et al.* 1992).

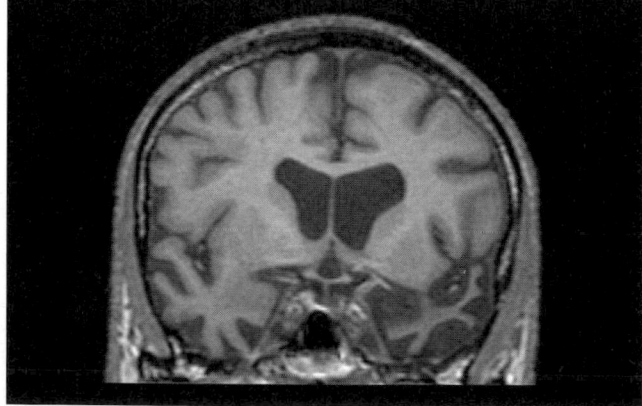

Fig. 26.6. Coronal T1-weighted MR image of a patient with semantic dementia, showing left temporal lobe atrophy.

Neuropathology of the frontotemporal degenerations

A variety of neuropathological changes are associated with the frontotemporal degenerations. Although particular syndromes tend to be associated with certain pathologies, there is considerable overlap, such that the underlying disease process cannot at present be predicted reliably from the clinical presentation. Moreover, it is not yet clear whether the apparent neuropathological entities do indeed represent distinct nosological entities or merely a spectrum of patterns of neuronal degeneration. Recent advances in molecular pathology are helping to clarify this complex group of disorders.

Pick's disease

At a macroscopic level, there is striking asymmetric focal atrophy, usually with a distinct border. Affected gyri may be very thin with a 'knife-edged' appearance. The anterior temporal and frontal lobes are predominantly involved, with the superior temporal gyrus characteristically spared, particularly posteriorly. Astrocytic gliosis is variable. The hallmark lesion is the presence of tau-positive, ubiquitin-positive argentophilic inclusions (Pick bodies), which are widespread and typically prominent in the dentate gyrus; there may in addition, be ballooned neurons (Pick cells) (reviewed by Binetti *et al.* 1998). Recent studies have demonstrated that the tau inclusions consist only of tau isoforms which contain the three repeat microtubule binding domains ('three-repeat tau'); this now distinguishes Pick's disease from the other tauopathies (Delacourte *et al.* 1996). A wider neuropathological substrate has been attributed to Pick's disease in the past. Constantinidis *et al.* (1974) considered three types of Pick's disease. Type A included Pick bodies together with Pick cells, and this would now be considered as typical Pick's disease. Type B cases were associated only with Pick cells in the absence of Pick bodies, and such cases would now be diagnosed as corticobasal degeneration. The balloon cells are tau positive and Aβ crystallin positive, and can be identified in a number of cases of frontotemporal degeneration as well as in typical cases of corticobasal degeneration. Pick's disease type C had no specific inclusion bodies, although gliosis was often present, and this group includes a variety of disorders.

Pick's disease is now seen as a very rare sporadic disorder. Criteria have been developed but are yet to be validated (ECAPD Consortium *et al.* 1998). The cases considered as familial Pick's disease in the past usually have a different neuropathological phenotype and many are now known to have mutations in the tau gene.

Hereditary tauopathies

Families with apparent autosomal dominant inheritance of frontotemporal degeneration have long been recognized. Many, but by no means all, are now linked to mutations in the tau gene (Hutton *et al.* 1998; Poorkaj *et al.* 1998). Neuropathologically these are associated with glial tau inclusions, tau-positive ballooned neurons (Pick cells), and atypical Pick bodies. The clinical phenotype is variable and often includes an extrapyramidal syndrome and amyotrophy. Before the discovery of tau mutations, these cases were referred to as 'frontotemporal dementia with Parkinsonism linked to chromosome 17' (Foster *et al.* 1997).

Frontal lobe degeneration

Frontal lobe degeneration of the non-Alzheimer type (Brun 1993) lacks inclusion bodies or other hallmark features, and has also been referred to as 'dementia lacking distinctive histology', (Knopman *et al.* 1990) and non-specific dementia (Kim *et al.* 1981). Atrophy tends to be symmetrical, in contrast to the asymmetry of Pick's disease, but can be severe, affecting the frontal lobes. There is microvacuolation or mild spongiosis and astrocytic gliosis, particularly in laminae 1–3. There is no abnormal tau immunoreactivity or inclusions. This type of histology underlies many of the cases of progressive non-fluent aphasia.

Frontotemporal degeneration with motor neuron disease

This shows similar changes in the frontal lobe to those described under frontal lobe degeneration but with additional loss of motor neurons in the spinal cord. In addition, ubiquitin-positive, tau-positive inclusion bodies are found, particularly in layer 2 of the frontal and temporal cortex. Moreover, ubiquitin-positive, tau-negative inclusions have been reported in prototypical cases of semantic dementia without anterior horn cell disease involvement of motor neurons (Rossor *et al.* 2000).

Rarely, cases with a phenotype of frontal lobe degeneration are reported in whom the underlying histopathology is that of Alzheimer's disease or prion disease.

26.6.5 Prion diseases

The prion diseases, also referred to as the spongiform encephalopathies, comprise Creutzfeldt–Jakob disease (CJD), variant CJD, Gerstmann–Straussler–Schenker syndrome, kuru, and familial fatal insomnia; diseases that are now grouped together because they share a common disease mechanism involving aberrant protein folding (Prusiner *et al.* 1998). The novel disease mechanism which results in a disorder that can be both hereditary and transmissible, together with a threat of an epidemic of variant CJD consequent upon the bovine spongiform encephalopathy (BSE) crisis in Europe, has focused considerable attention on these diseases, despite their rarity.

The transmission of kuru, the spongiform encephalopathy found amongst the Fore highlanders of Papua New Guinea, to non-human primates by Gajdusek led to the concept of a 'slow virus', although the transmissible agent remained elusive (Section 34.12). Ultimately this was shown to be a protein devoid of nucleic acid—the prion protein (PrP) (Prusiner 1991). The transmissible prion protein (PrP^{sc}) is derived from a normal cellular protein (PrPC) by post-translational modification, resulting in a high β-sheet content; the mechanism of the subsequent cellular degeneration is not established. The abnormal isoform of the protein (PrP^{sc}) has the ability to induce aberrant folding of the host protein, hence the transmission, which can occur either through cannibalism, as in kuru,

or iatrogenically, as with growth hormone derived from cadaveric pituitary glands and surgical interventions. Species differences in the PrP sequence make transmission of the disease across species inefficient (species barrier) but this can occur experimentally and is now believed to have occurred with variant CJD following the BSE epidemic. Mutations in the PrP gene are believed to facilitate the aberrant protein folding and underlie familial CJD, familial fatal insomnia, and Gerstmann–Straussler–Schenker syndrome. A common methionine/valine polymorphism at PrP 129 is a genetic risk factor for the disease (Palmer *et al.* 1991).

Prion diseases (Section 34.12) are multisystem central nervous system disorders with variable degrees of dementia, cerebellar, pyramidal, and extrapyramidal features. CJD occurs worldwide, with an annual incidence of about 1 per million. It is invariably fatal. The classical triad of dementia, myoclonus, and abnormal EEG with periodic or pseudoperiodic complexes is seen typically in patients between the ages of 50 and 70 years. It has a subacute onset; rarely, the disease can be extremely rapid with death within 2 months, whereas in others there is a slower progression of the disease over 1–2 years (Brown *et al.* 1986). The different clinical phenotypes in terms of progression have been related to different isoforms of the aberrant prion protein (PrP^{sc}) (Parchi *et al.* 1996). About 10 per cent of cases of prion disease are familial, with autosomal dominant transmission due to mutations in the PrP gene. The phenotype can be varied, some mimicking Alzheimer's disease and others Huntington's disease; cases with the 144 bp insert tend to have a slow progression with a variable phenotype (Collinge *et al.* 1992). Patients with a prominent cerebellar component were originally described as Gerstmann–Straussler-Schenker syndrome, and the recently described familial fatal insomnia (Lugaresi *et al.* 1986) is characterized by insomnia with loss or dramatic reduction of slow wave and REM sleep, together with autonomic disturbance.

Iatrogenic cases have been associated with corneal grafting, dura mater grafts, and in-depth electrode recording. The majority of iatrogenic cases have been associated with cadaveric pituitary derived growth hormone treatment, a practice which was discontinued in the mid 1980s. These cases have more cerebellar features and less dementia (Fradkin *et al.* 1991). A variant of CJD has emerged in the UK and France in the past 5 years and is believed to have resulted from ingestion of contaminated food from BSE-infected cattle. It is associated with a characteristic PrP^{sc} isoform (Collinge *et al.* 1996). The cases of variant CJD are younger than classical CJD, some even in their teens, with early depression and anxiety. Cerebellar and basal ganglia features are more prominent than cognitive impairment early in the disorder (Will *et al.* 1996).

The characteristic histopathology is the spongiform change, although this is variable; it is associated with neuronal intracytoplasmic vacuolation together with astrocytosis and gliosis. The abnormal prion protein (PrP^{sc}) can be demonstrated on immunohistochemistry and can form plaques, especially in the cerebellum in Gerstmann–Straussler–Schenker syndrome. Variant CJD is also associated with PrP plaques reminiscent of kuru (Will *et al.* 1996).

Blood tests are usually normal in prion disease, although there can be mildly abnormal liver function tests. PrP genotyping will identify mutations in the familial cases and cases of variant CJD reported to date have all been methionine homozygous at PrP 129. Magnetic resonance imaging may show signal changes on T2-weighted images in the basal ganglia and characteristic posterior thalamic signal change in variant CJD. Cerebrospinal fluid is unremarkable, although P14–3–3, which probably reflects rapid neuronal disintegration, is found in classical CJD cases (Hsich *et al.* 1996). The EEG may be normal or non-specific early in the disease, but in classical CJD pseudoperiodic or periodic complexes are seen. Tonsillar biopsy in variant CJD can reveal the specific PrP^{sc} isoform (Hill *et al.* 1999).

At present there is no specific treatment for the prion diseases. The PrP^{sc} is highly resistant to degradation and thus instruments cannot be routinely sterilized. Neurosurgical instruments must be quarantined and if the diagnosis confirmed, destroyed. There is no need to barrier-nurse patients but disposable instruments should be used for invasive procedures, and all samples should indicate the suspected diagnosis clearly (Health Service Circular 1999).

26.6.6 Vascular dementia

Impairment of blood supply to the brain used to be considered to be the main cause of dementia in the elderly, until it was recognized that such a mechanism is rarely, if ever, implicated. Multiple small strokes, referred to as multi-infarct dementia, were subsequently identified as the principal mechanism, both clinically and at autopsy (Hachinski *et al.* 1974). In most neuropathological and clinical series, vascular dementia is the most common cause after Alzheimer's disease, accounting for some 10–20 per cent of dementia cases alone, and an important concomitant of Alzheimer's disease or other degenerative dementias. The incidence of vascular dementia may be falling with better management of vascular risk factors. It is also believed that many cases of dementia with Lewy bodies were previously diagnosed clinically as vascular dementia. If cases of dementia where there is a vascular component are considered, then there is no doubt that vascular disease is a major cause or contributor to cognitive impairment (Hachinski and Bowler 1993). The term 'vascular dementia' is preferable to 'multi-infarct dementia' as it reflects the considerable heterogeneity of the condition and includes cases due to haemorrhage, small lacunar infarcts, large cortical infarcts, and vasculitides. In comparison to Alzheimer's disease, there is a paucity of epidemiological data on vascular dementia. In part, this is due to the fact that patients with major strokes are often excluded, and yet, in one study, up to 25 per cent of patients 3 months after a stroke were considered to have dementia using DSM-IV criteria, and up to 60 per cent had cognitive impairment (Pohjasvaara *et al.* 1997).

Clinical criteria for the diagnosis of vascular dementia have been dominated by the development of criteria for Alzheimer's disease. Thus, memory remains as a key component and yet may be relatively less important in vascular dementia (Bowler *et al.* 1997). Early criteria assumed that stepwise deterioration and motor abnormalities would be characteristic, and from this was developed the Hachinski score. Patients with a score of 4 or less were considered likely to be degenerative by contrast to those with a score of 7 or more, who were thought to have a multi-infarct dementia. This remains a useful guide, and series have been verified pathologically (Moroney *et al.* 1997). More recently, the NINCDS-AIREN criteria (Roman 1998) have been developed, which require the appearance of cognitive impairment within 3 months of a stroke, or sudden onset and fluctuation of cognitive impairment. In view of the potential contribution of focal neuropsychological deficits from a discrete stroke, the cognitive criteria for dementia are that there should be memory impairment plus at least *two* other domains. There should also be relevant vascular changes on imaging which are thought to be directly related. However, very different proportions of cases are diagnosed as vascular dementia, depending upon the use of NINCDS-AIREN, DSM-IV, or ICD-10 criteria. (Wetterling *et al.* 1996).

Three main vascular pathologies are believed to be associated with vascular dementia; namely, single discrete cortical infarcts, multiple infarcts (multi-infarct dementia), and subcortical arteriosclerotic encephalopathy (Binswanger's disease). In reality, these may overlap.

Single discrete infarcts, for example, in right middle cerebral and posterior cerebral artery territories and thalamic infarcts, can present with a picture suggestive of dementia. Much more common, however, is the accumulation of deficits from multiple single cortical and/or subcortical infarcts. Men are more commonly affected than women, and there is usually a vascular history, particularly of hypertension. There is a gradual accumulation of cognitive deficits with episodes of confusion or focal neurology. If there are mainly subcortical infarcts, patients tend to have a subcortical pattern of cognitive deficit with cognitive slowing and additional motor features. Some may develop an extrapyramidal syndrome, and in others a pseudobulbar palsy can be prominent with pathological laughing and crying. Neuropathologically, multiple small subcortical infarcts appear to be more important in vascular dementia than single large infarcts (Esiri *et al.* 1997).

Subcortical arteriosclerotic encephalopathy (Binswanger's disease)

Binswanger originally described eight cases of periventricular demyelination and dementia. This was considered a rarity until the advent of neuroimaging, and many patients with white matter changes on scanning acquired this diagnosis. Clinically, the features are very similar to those seen in patients with multiple subcortical infarcts, namely frontal and subcortical cognitive features, dysarthria, and pseudobulbar palsy. Gait impairment may occur early and is characterized by a wide-based shuffling gait, in contrast to the narrower base seen in Parkinson's disease (Thompson and Marsden 1987). Criteria have been suggested for the diagnosis of Binswanger's disease (Bennett *et al.* 1990).

Much confusion has arisen from attempts to diagnose Binswanger's disease from neuroimaging. Non-specific periventricular white matter abnormalities are common both in patients with dementia and in the non-demented elderly, and the term leuko-araiosis has been proposed (Hachinski *et al.* 1987). Leuko-araiosis appears as low attenuation on CT scan, particularly around the frontal and occipital horns, and as increased signal on T2-weighted MRI. Neuropathologically, there is demyelination, gliosis, and hyalinosis, with fibrinoid necrosis of small blood vessels, similar to that seen in hypertension. Minor degrees of white matter disease are also seen in pure Alzheimer's disease.

Treatment is primarily that of management of vascular disease risk factors such as hypertension, smoking, diabetes, carotid stenosis, and heart disease. There have been few control trials of management of risk factors and its affect on cognition, but treatment of isolated systolic hypertension in the elderly may reduce the incidence of dementia (Forette *et al.* 1998).

Other causes of vascular dementia

Significant cognitive impairment, sufficient to justify the criteria of dementia, can occur after subarachnoid haemorrhage, subdural haematomas, and global ischaemia following cardiac arrest with laminar necrosis and hippocampal cell loss. A variety of vasculitides can also be associated with the early development of cognitive impairment and even present as a dementia; these include systemic lupus erythematosus (SLE) and primary cerebral angiitis, which is usually accompanied by headaches. Sneddon's syndrome (Rebollo *et al.* 1983) is the association of livedo reticularis with cerebrovascular disease, and can present with cognitive impairment. A number, but not all, are associated with anticardiolipin antibodies.

The rare cases of hereditary cerebral amyloidosis, both of the Icelandic and the Dutch and the Flemish type, can be associated with cognitive impairment, although the salient clinical feature is that of recurrent cerebral haemorrhage. Cerebral autosomal dominant arteriopathy with subcortical infarcts and leucoencephalopathy (CADASIL) (Dichgans *et al.* 1998) is characterized by recurrent subcortical ischaemic events with the subsequent development of a pseudobulbar palsy and cognitive impairment. Early symptoms include migraine-like headache and psychiatric disturbance. The MRI scan shows a striking leucoencephalopathy in addition to multiple small infarcts. This condition, which is increasingly recognized, is linked to mutations in the *Notch 3* gene (Joutel *et al.* 1996).

26.6.7 Miscellaneous causes of dementia

Since cognition is so easily disrupted by diseases affecting the cortex and its subcortical connections, cognitive impairment or dementia is very common in neurological practice. In the majority of cases the other clinical features provide the diagnostic clues. These dementia plus syndromes are numerous and include Huntington's disease (Section 32.5.2), some spinocerebellar ataxias (Chapter 31), and a variety of inherited metabolic disorders, such as metachromatic leucodystrophy, Kuf's disease, lysosomal storage disorders, and mitochondrial cytopathies. Normal-pressure hydrocephalus can present as the classic triad of dementia, incontinence, and gait disturbance, but has tended to be overdiagnosed (Section 17.3.8). The cognitive impairment is very much that of a subcortical impairment with cognitive slowing. Patients with prominent cognitive impairment are more likely to have a coexisting degenerative disease, and rarely, if ever, respond to shunting. Multiple sclerosis patients will often develop cognitive impairment, and in some this can be a prominent, and even presenting, feature.

Syphilis is the classic infection which can be associated with dementia (Section 34.17.2). However, late cases of *Borrelia burgdorfei* (Lyme disease) can also be associated with dementia (Krupp *et al.* 1991) (Section 34.17.4) and Whipple's disease can rarely involve the cerebral cortex, with cognitive impairment that responds to antibiotic treatment (Singer 1998) (Section 34.13.7). The other major infection associated with dementia is HIV encephalopathy, and dementia can be a presenting feature (Janssen *et al.* 1992) (Section 34.11.2). There is evidence that this is becoming less common with treatment with zidovudine (Melton *et al.* 1997). Progressive multifocal leucoencephalopathy is frequently associated with cognitive impairment and occurs in a variety of immunosuppressed patients as well as those with HIV (Section 34.10).

One of the main reasons for neuroimaging of patient with dementia is to identify tumours, the treatment of which can result in cognitive improvement. However, with malignant tumours, irradiation itself may give rise to late cognitive impairment (Keime-Guibert *et al.* 1998). The paraneoplastic phenomenon of limbic encephalitis, usually associated with carcinoma of the bronchus, can result in a memory impairment that precedes diagnosis of the tumour by a number of years and can mimic Alzheimer's disease (Section 30.6.2). However, examination of the CSF usually reveals oligoclonal bands and occasionally pleocytosis (Bakheit *et al.* 1990). Drugs, particularly barbiturates, can lead to cognitive slowing, as can heavy metals, such as lead, arsenic, manganese, and mercury. Workers in the felt hat industry who were exposed to mercury frequently developed a confusional state with cognitive impairment, hence the term 'mad as a hatter'. Dementia pugilistica, arising from recurrent head injury, particularly in boxers, is associated with tangles and presents as a cognitive impairment with dysarthria and an extrapyramidal syndrome.

A variety of rare degenerative dementias are gradually being delineated, although some, such as argyrophilic grain dementia (Braak *et al.* 1989) are really only diagnosed at autopsy. Kosaka (1994) described a series of patients with basal ganglia calcification on neuroimaging, with neurofibrillary tangles but no senile plaques. The rare Worster–Drought syndrome, a familial disorder with dementia and spastic paraparesis, is now recognized as a novel amyloidosis due to a stop codon mutation in the *BRI* gene (Vidal *et al.* 1999).

26.7 Acute confusional states

Acute confusional states are extremely common, especially in the elderly, and may occur in up to 25 per cent of those admitted to medical and surgical wards (Lipowski 1983; Taylor and Lewis 1993); this figure may be even higher in those admitted to geriatric wards. By contrast to dementia, confusional states are usually short-lived and reversible, with prominent impairments of attention and arousal (Lipowski 1990). The term 'acute confusional state' tends to be most commonly used in Europe and the term 'delirium' to be used in the US. The terms 'toxic psychosis', 'acute brain syndrome', 'acute encephalopathy', and 'transient cognitive disorder' are all synonymous (Lipowski 1990). Patients are likely to be elderly, although the very young are also vulnerable. The condition is often seen within the setting of systemic disease or multiple drug therapy. Disruption of attention, i.e. the ability to focus on specific stimuli, is a key feature. This consists of impairment of selective attention, with the patient unable to attend to the examiner and being continually distracted by irrelevant environmental stimuli (Geschwind 1982). Arousal may be impaired, with somnolence and descent into stupor, or, alternatively, agitation may occur. However, attention is impaired even if arousal is enhanced. These disturbances of selective attention and arousal result in marked disorientation in place and time, particularly of a sense of time of day, but, as with dementia, personal identity is normally preserved. The sleep–wake cycle is disrupted, with patients being awake at night, leading to the familiar feature of the patient wandering into the street in their nightclothes. Memory is impaired, in particular short-term memory, as assessed by the digit span, is greatly disrupted by the impairment of attention. However, this is not specific to confusional states. There are frequent paramnesias, such as reduplicative paramnesia and the Capgras syndrome (Section 26.4.7). Misperceptions, particularly with visual hallucinations, are prominent, whereas auditory hallucinations should raise the suspicion of a functional psychosis. Patients may have bizarre and very frightening hallucinations, often with metamorphopsia, and these can occur particularly with drugs and toxins. Language is relatively preserved, although the content is abnormal. Errors may relate to the disrupted thought processes, and errors on naming may reflect visual misperceptions or reflect paramnesic errors; these disturbances on confrontational naming have been referred to as non-aphasic misnaming (Weinstein and Kahn 1952). Dysgraphia is very frequent, with prominent spatial errors in addition to disturbances of spelling and syntax (Chedru and Geschwind 1972). As might be predicted, judgement is grossly impaired, particularly since anosognosia is the rule rather than the exception, and may result in patients being combative and aggressive when being examined or if any attempt is made to restrain them. Mood lability is common, and fluctuations in the cognitive state are frequent, such that the patient may be seen in a lucid interval when examined. The onset of a confusional state is acute or subacute over hours or days, in contrast to the common dementias, and fluctuation characteristic.

In addition to the cognitive features, clinical examination commonly reveals autonomic disturbance with tachycardia, hypertension, sweating, fever, and tachypnoea. Asterixis, myoclonus, increased tone, and carphologia, or plucking at the bedclothes, are often found. There may be evidence of systemic disease, such as cardiac failure, respiratory failure, or infections, and these should be sought carefully.

Common difficulties with differential diagnosis include the functional psychoses (Lishman 1987). In general, patients with functional psychoses are orientated in time and place and not overtly dysphasic, although there may be a bizarre content. An abrupt onset in an older patient without a psychiatric history would be most unusual for functional psychosis. Similarly, any clouding of consciousness or disorientation suggests an acute confusional state, as does the predominance of visual over auditory hallucinations.

The distinction from dementia may be difficult with chronic confusional states. Moreover, the two often coexist; acute confusional states may evolve into dementia, and patients with a dementia are very prone to acute confusional states due to infections or drugs. Dementia with Lewy bodies (Section 26.6.3) may also present with features of a confusional state. Patients with dementia may also develop confusion with reduced or unfamiliar environmental cues, so called 'sundowning' at night. In general, when a patient presents with cognitive impairment suggestive of an acute confusional state with rapid onset and fluctuation, the more aggressive should be the investigation for reversible underlying causes.

The disturbance of arousal in acute confusional states can be attributed to dysfunction of the reticular activating system, and patients will have associated disturbances of the sleep–wake cycle and may deteriorate into stupor or even coma. Abnormalities of arousal, however, are not necessary to make a diagnosis of an acute confusional state in those instances in which impaired attention is prominent. Attention requires both disregard of irrelevant environmental stimuli and sustained attention on relevant stimuli. The association cerebral cortices provide the anatomical substrate of selective attention (Mesulam 1981) with particular involvement of the non-dominant parietal lobe, as evidenced by the occurrence of acute confusional states with right middle cerebral artery infarcts (Mesulam et al. 1976). However, a disturbance of selective attention may also occur with frontal lobe lesions.

The disturbances that cause acute confusional states tend to be generalized, and it has been proposed that the selective vulnerability of the systems that subserve arousal and selective attention is due to their polysynaptic characteristics. It has also been suggested that the ascending cholinergic system may be particularly vulnerable because of the prominent confusional state that can occur with anticholinergic drugs; but drug-induced confusional states are by no means specific to anticholinergic drugs (Tune et al. 1981).

The causes of acute confusional states are legion. Acquired metabolic disturbances, particularly hypoxia and hypoglycaemia, are common and require prompt treatment. Thiamine deficiency should always be considered in patients who are admitted to Accident and Emergency departments without a clear history, since the administration of glucose can precipitate a Wernicke's encephalopathy. Drugs are a very common cause, particularly in patients on multiple drug regimens (Carter *et al.* 1996). Anticholinergics, anti-Parkinsonian, and benzodiazepine drugs, as causes of confusional states, are commonly encountered in neurological patients (Foy *et al.* 1995). Recreational drugs including alcohol, cocaine, 'crack', amphetamines, and LSD are all well-recognized causes. Acute confusional states commonly occur following surgery and are often due to a combination of drugs, hypoxia, electrolyte disturbance, and infection, but may also be exacerbated by fragmented sleep. Confusional states are common after cataract surgery in the elderly and may relate to sensory deprivation (Summers and Reich 1979). Approximately 30 per cent of patients undergoing open-heart surgery or coronary artery bypass grafting develop confusional states (Smith and Dimsdale 1989): recognition of a confusional state in the setting of an intensive care unit can be diagnostically challenging. Cerebrovascular disease can cause acute confusional states, particularly right middle cerebral artery infarcts (Mesulam *et al.* 1976), but also occur with posterior cerebral artery infarcts (Medina *et al.* 1974). Migraine attacks may rarely be associated with a confusional state, particularly in children, and epilepsy is a common cause, both during the seizure and as a post-ictal phenomenon.

Investigation should be thorough and will, in part, be directed by the general medical examination. Not only will this include screening of blood sugar, electrolytes, liver function tests, and a search for infection, but where necessary a drug screen. Neuroimaging, EEG (diffuse slowing or low-voltage fast activity), and examination of CSF may all be necessary.

Management depends upon treatment of the underlying cause, and symptomatic measures should be directed towards the maintenance of constant environmental stimuli so as to avoid over- and understimulation; a night-light may be valuable. Drug therapy should be kept to an absolute minimum, but patients may rarely require a neuroleptic for marked agitation.

In general, the prognosis is good, although caution is necessary in the elderly, many of whom may have underlying degenerative disease which renders them vulnerable to confusional states, and in whom a stable cognitive deficit may emerge as the confusional state clears (Levkoff *et al.* 1992).

26.8 Hallucinosis

Hallucinations are a common accompaniment of confusional states, but they can also occur in a variety of other disorders. An hallucination may be defined as a sensory perception occurring without an external stimulus, but appearing to be located, or to possess a cause located, outside the subject. An illusion is defined as a misinterpretation of an external stimulus and can occur in normal people, particularly with fatigue. A delusion, by contrast, is an idea or thought (such as a false concept of persecution) which has no substance in fact; in contrast to visual and auditory hallucinations, it is purely a thought process with no sensory content. Hallucinations and delusions may occur together in various toxic or confusional states and in psychotic illnesses, such as schizophrenia.

The principal circumstances in which hallucinations may occur are: (1) in dreaming and the hypnagogic state; (2) in pathological disorders of sleep; (3) as a result of disease of the peripheral sense organs; (4) focal disturbance of the central nervous system; (5) drug-induced hallucinations; and (6) in certain psychoses. Hallucinations are not uncommon in states of drowsiness and will occur in hypnagogic (falling asleep) and hypnopompic (awakening from sleep) states, but to an exaggerated extent in patients suffering from narcolepsy. Visual hallucinations can occur particularly in the elderly with reduced visual acuity, and can occur with lesions anywhere along the visual pathway. Auditory hallucinations may also occur following acquired deafness, and again may be more common in the elderly (Hammeke *et al.* 1983). Hallucinations involving various sensory modalities, together with perceptual illusions and other disorders of consciousness, are particularly liable to occur as a result of lesions of the temporal lobes. These may frequently occur as epileptic phenomena. The perceptual illusions include disordered visual perception; for example, macropsia or micropsia, and a similar alteration in auditory perception, feelings of unreality of the self or the surroundings, and disturbances of awareness of the body. Visual hallucinations have been described in which the individual feels that he is observing his own body from outside his physical self; this unusual phenomenon has some affinity with sensations of intense depersonalization or unreality. Visual hallucinations also sometimes occur as a result of epileptic discharge arising in the posterior part of the temporal lobe or in the parieto-occipital region. Agitated delirium and visual impairment may, for example, result from medial temporo-occipital infarction (Medina *et al.* 1977). Lhermitte described peduncular hallucinosis with lesions of the upper part of the brainstem, which was interpreted as a dissociation of the state of sleep. Hallucinations may also result from brainstem compression (Dunn *et al.* 1983) and elementary auditory hallucinations may occur with pontine lesions, so-called 'pontine auditory hallucinosis'.

A variety of drugs may result in hallucinations, mescaline and lysergic acid being notorious. However, withdrawal of alcohol can result in hallucinosis, which may become permanent, particularly in established alcoholics. Hallucinations are an important diagnostic feature of the psychoses. They may occur with severe affective disorders, such as depression, in which they are often associated with morbid features. Auditory hallucinations occurring in clear consciousness which are mood incongruent are very suggestive of schizophrenia. It is characteristic that these auditory hallucinations involve argument about the patient in the third person.

26.9 Psychiatric disorders in neurological practice

26.9.1 Disturbance of mood

Affective disturbances commonly involve the neurologist, either because patients with a primary diagnosis of depression present with neurological symptoms, because the patient develops a depressive reaction to their neurological disability, or, less commonly, a depressive illness arises directly as a result of central nervous system disease.

A depressive illness is the most common psychiatric diagnosis to be found in neurological practice (Kirk and Saunders 1977). The most common presentations are headache, dizziness, and memory impairment. A careful history may unearth depressive symptomatology, such as persistent dysphoria, loss of appetite and libido, and disturbed sleep patterns, with early morning waking. Suicidal ideation should be specifically sought. However, patients may not volunteer or may minimize mood symptoms, focusing instead on somatic complaints. Depressive pseudodementia (Caine 1981) is an important diagnosis since it is the main cause of a reversible dementia. The term 'pseudodementia' is not ideal, as these patients do have impaired cognition and probably share some of the neurochemical disturbances found in other dementias, namely deficits in the ascending monoaminergic projections to cerebral cortex. The clinical features are those of a subcortical dementia with marked slowing of cognition. The patients often complain of their memory disturbance and are clearly distressed by it. Patients give many 'don't know' answers to questions, in contrast to patients with Alzheimer's disease who will give incorrect or circumlocutory refutable answers. Effortful, as opposed to implicit memory function, is particularly affected. As a general rule, patients who spontaneously complain of memory should always raise the possibility of a depressive illness. Depression is, however, common early in Alzheimer's disease and requires appropriate treatment.

A depressed mood as a reaction to neurological disability is commonplace and can be difficult to distinguish from persistent depression, which may be more intimately related to the neurological disturbance itself. Diseases of the basal ganglia and connections to frontal lobe are particularly liable to cause depressive illness. Thus, frontal meningiomata were commonly misinterpreted as depressive illness, particularly in the pre-scanning days. Depression is a common accompaniment of Parkinson's disease that is not relieved by improvement in motor function following drug treatment (Mindham *et al.* 1976; Santamaria *et al.* 1986); this may indicate an overlap in the underlying biochemical disturbance of monoamine systems. Cerebrovascular disease is a frequent cause of mood changes, with up to a third of patients developing depression after stroke. It is important for management, since many patients may become depressed some

months after their stroke and appropriate follow-up is essential (Wade *et al.* 1987). Some studies have suggested a high prevalence of depression with dominant hemisphere infarcts, particularly with more anteriorly located lesions (Starkstein and Robinson 1993). This has not been confirmed in other studies, although the high prevalence of depression is recognized (House *et al.* 1990). Hypomania and euphoria are much less common, but can occur with cerebral infarcts and with Huntington's disease. It is often stated that patients with multiple sclerosis develop a euphoria, and although this may be observed, depressive illness is still the major mood change (Schiffer 1987).

26.9.2 Anxiety

Both DSM-IV and ICD-10 classify anxiety disorders into a number of categories; the most relevant to neurological practise are generalized anxiety disorder, panic disorder, specific phobias, and post-traumatic stress disorder. As with depression, patients may develop anxiety in response to their neurological illness and, in addition, patients with anxiety may present to the neurologist by virtue of their symptoms. Generalized anxiety may result in a number of symptoms of nervousness, fatigue, loss of concentration, and vertigo. These are generally non-specific symptoms, and the key features are the additional acute attacks of anxiety. These attacks are associated with nervousness and increasing panic which, if severe, as in phobic-anxiety attacks, may result in intense sensations of depersonalization and fear of impending death. There may be a sense of being smothered, together with dyspnoea and frequently palpitations, both of which may result in referrals to a cardiologist. Nausea, urinary frequency, and vertigo during attacks are common. Hyperventilation, which by virtue of the reduction in $P\text{CO}_2$, will itself contribute to the sense of vertigo and result in paraesthesiae, classically affecting the fingers and circumoral region. If sufficiently severe, this may result in tetany.

Panic attacks may occur in relation to obvious precipitating factors, particularly in relation to specific phobias, such as open spaces or heights. They are quite frequent following trauma, and caffeine may precipitate anxiety in normal people and panic attacks in those who are susceptible. However, they may occur in apparently unprovoked situations. Diagnostic confusion occurs with epilepsy, labyrinthine disturbance, essential tremor, and cognitive impairment. Anxiety and panic attacks usually present in patients in their twenties and are rare as an initial presentation after the age of 40. Forced hyperventilation for a period of 2–3 minutes may reproduce many of the symptoms aiding diagnosis, but care should be taken in the interpretation since many of the symptoms of paraesthesiae, vertigo, and derealization can be precipitated as a normal concomitant of forced hyperventilation.

Post-traumatic stress disorder is usually associated with both anxiety and depression. Key diagnostic features are flashbacks to the original trauma, which may be triggered by relevant stimuli. Patients characteristically avoid situations which might be associated with the original trauma. Such symptoms are common immediately after a traumatic event but are considered abnormal if persisting for more than a month.

26.9.3 Obsessive–compulsive disorders

Obsessions are recurrent, intrusive thoughts or images that are often repulsive to the individual. Compulsions are repetitive and stereotyped behaviours that are found in association with obsessions, are usually performed according to certain rules, and may be used to neutralize obsessional thoughts. Commonest amongst the obsessive–compulsive disorders are ritual washing and cleaning, and ritual checking. Pure obsessive disorder with stereotyped thoughts, which are often of an illicit sexual or sacrilegious nature, are less common. Primary obsessive slowness (Rachman 1974), in which patients suffer severe slowness in the execution of even the simplest of daily tasks, such as dressing or eating, is rare. A close association of obsessive–compulsive disorders with neurological disease has been recognized, since the development of obsessive–compulsive behaviour was observed in association with post-encephalitic Parkinsonism, especially with oculogyric crisis. There is also a high prevalence of obsessive–compulsive disorder in Gilles de la Tourette syndrome (Robertson et al. 1988) and in patients with Sydenham's chorea (Swedo et al. 1989). Neurological abnormalities are frequently found on examination in patients with obsessional slowness, and include speech and gait abnormalities, cogwheel rigidity and tics, together with frontal neuropsychological deficits (Hymas et al. 1991). This suggests dysfunction within the fronto-striatal connections, a view supported by focal hypometabolism on oxygen-15 PET scanning in the orbital frontal, pre-motor, and mid-frontal cortex (Sawle et al. 1991).

26.10 Somatoform and conversion disorders

Patients without a clear diagnosis are common in neurological practice. In many, an anatomical diagnosis is made with some precision even if the cause is elusive. In many, careful follow-up will reveal the correct diagnosis. In a minority, no diagnosis emerges of a neurological illness which is sufficient to explain the symptoms in their entirety. Indeed, there may be features that are inconsistent with our current concepts of neurobiological function.

The diagnosis and management of this group of patients has been hampered by a confusion of terms, some of which, such as hysteria, carry with them an implication of an underlying mechanism. Hysteria, in particular, carries conceptual baggage, from the wandering womb of ancient medicine to the Freudian concepts of primary and secondary gain. While the concept of primary gain in hysteria, i.e. the conversion of psychic disturbance into physical symptoms in order to ease distress, has not proved useful, attention has been focused on secondary gain. The secondary gain reflects the potential advantages in financial, social, and relationship terms from continuing illness,

Table 26.3. Classification of somatoform disorders (American Psychiatric Association 1994; Trimble 2000)

1. Somatization disorder (Briquet's syndrome): many physical complaints, beginning before age 30, patients usually female

2. Conversion disorder: one or more symptoms or deficits affecting motor or sensory function, not fully explained by a general or medical condition

3. Hypochondriasis: preoccupation and fears of having a serious disease in spite of appropriate medical evaluation and reassurance

4. Body dysmorphic disorder: preoccupation with an imagined defect in appearance

5. Pain disorder: pain is the predominant focus of the clinical presentation, and psychological factors are judged to have the important role of maintaining it

6. Undifferentiated somatoform disorder: one or more physical complaints that are unexplained by a known medical condition, leading to considerable impairment in social functioning; or when related to a known medical condition, there is social impairment grossly in excess of what would be expected from the physical findings

7. Somatoform disorder not otherwise specified: those that do not fit the above; includes fatigue, pseudocyesis

and this new emphasis has led to the introduction of terms such as 'sick role' and 'abnormal illness behaviour', which are as much sociological constructs as neurobiological (Crimlisk and Ron 1999).

There have been recent attempts to classify these disorders, although this implies an unrealistic understanding of underlying disease mechanisms. There are inconsistencies between the major disease classification systems; for example, in the DSM-IV, conversion disorder (hysteria) is classified with the somatoform disorders, in contrast to dissociative symptoms such as hysterical fugue states which are classified under the dissociative disorders. The ICD-10 classification groups them all together under neurotic, stress-related, and somatoform (Table 26.3) disorders. The term 'hysteria', while still widely used in practice, has been dropped from the DSM-IV and ICD-10. In view of the ambiguity of the term and the pejorative associations, this is no bad thing. In neurological practice, it is easy to imagine that many of these disorders are part of a spectrum rather than distinct diseases.

26.10.1 Somatization disorders

Somatic symptoms arising in relation to psychological distress are very common (Smith et al. 1986); many such patients are managed in primary care and will never reach the neurologist. Somatization may take many forms and potentially involve many different specialists, such as gastroenterologists for those with recurrent abdominal discomfort and cardiologists for those with dyspnoea. Somatization disorder, also referred to as Briquet's syndrome, is a long-standing disorder rather than acute, with the behaviour pattern being established early in life. Patients are predominantly female and acquire voluminous sets of hospital notes involving many different departments. The prognosis is poor, but good communication between primary care and hospital departments can help to limit overinvestigation. However, the clinician must remain vigilant as patients with Briquet's syndrome are as entitled to neurological disease as any other patient.

Another disorder classified under the somatoform disorders is body dysmorphic disorder or dysmorphophobia, which is similar to monosymptomatic delusional hypochondriases such as delusional parasitosis. These patients occasionally present to neurologists in a dramatic fashion with delusions of changing body shape. They require careful assessment as parietal lobe lesions can give rise to distorted body image.

26.10.2 Conversion disorder and fugue states

A central feature to the diagnosis of conversion disorder or hysteria is that the somatic symptoms and signs develop in the absence of a neurological illness that is sufficient to explain them in their entirety. There should also be an associated psychological stressor, but this may as much depend upon the interpretation of the examining doctor. The negative, as opposed to positive, feature of the diagnosis, i.e. the absence of a neurological disease, has always been a major concern, as it may only reflect current conceptual thinking and available technology for investigation. The influential study by Slater reviewed patients at The National Hospital for Neurology and Neurosurgery (Slater 1965) diagnosed with hysteria, and found at follow-up that 50 per cent had developed a significant neurological or psychiatric diagnosis. More recent follow-up studies suggest a much lower emergence of alternative diagnoses (Crimlisk et al. 1998). This change reflects both improved diagnostic techniques and improved understanding of a number of disorders, such as spastic dysphonia and writer's cramp, which had previously been considered within the conversion hysteria group and are now firmly established as neurological diseases.

Are there positive, as opposed to merely negative, features to the diagnosis of a conversion syndrome? The most common manifestations involve the motor system, particularly weakness; the next most common is sensory. Examination will often reveal clear inconsistencies, such as co-contraction of antagonist and agonist muscles, or sensory deficits which are inconsistent, such as loss of vibration sense on either side of the sternal midline. 'Belle indifference' was often said to be a key feature, but this has not been found to be of predictive value (Sharma and Chaturvedi 1995). A consistent observation has been that conversion symptoms are more common on the left than the right, with the suggestion that the underlying pathophysiology may involve disturbed attentional mechanisms. In this regard, there would be some overlap with the anosagnosia that can arise with right parietal lesions. Positron emission tomography in one patient with a hysterical hemiplegia revealed that, on attempts to move the paralysed limb, pre-motor areas known to be involved in movement preparation and execution were activated, but not the primary motor cortex. By contrast, significant activation in cingular and orbital frontal and anterior cingular cortices suggested an inhibitory effect of these regions (Marshall et al. 1997).

Disorders of cognition present a particularly difficult challenge, and amnesia, on either an hysterical or a malingering basis, is not uncommon. The Ganser syndrome describes patients with apparent gross disturbance of cognition who appear to be unable to answer even the simplest of questions. They often give approximate answers or 'answer past the point' (Vorbeireden), examples being 'five' in answer to the question, 'How many legs does a cow have?' Although classically considered to be on a 'hysterical' basis, some cases are found following head trauma, and others are found in association with a depressive illness (Lishman 1987). In patients with functional retrograde amnesia, there may be a sharp cut-off chronologically (Schacter et al. 1982) and memory testing is very variable (reviewed by Kopelman 1987).

Psychiatric co-morbidity is common with conversion disorder and, in particular, depression. It is essential that this is recognized, as not only is the treatment of the depression associated with improved prognosis, but failure to recognize this leads to a significant suicide risk. Management of patients requires close collaboration with a psychiatrist experienced in this area.

Fugue states, in which patients wander away from home and on recovery have amnesia for the event, may occur in a number of conditions. Wandering may occur as a post-ictal phenomenon, but in this instance it is usually short lived, and the patient will appear confused and will have had difficulty with travelling and negotiating roads or public transport. The same comments apply to the rare instances of somnambulism in which people may leave the home. Transient global amnesia (Section 23.1.4) may involve travelling away from home with amnesia for the event, but in most instances patients travel only familiar routes since they have well-preserved topographical memories. They will often appear perplexed during the attacks. By contrast, there are patients who disappear from home to turn up many hours or even days later. They will have successfully negotiated the period of travel and will not have drawn attention to themselves by virtue of their confused behaviour. They have amnesia for the event and often a retrograde amnesia which extends back prior to the period of travel, and in some instances appears to be lifelong. In these situations it is often accompanied by amnesia for personal identity. Such behaviour may be associated with depressive illness, and these patients present a suicide risk; in other instances these fugue states are considered as part of the spectrum of conversion disorder.

26.10.3 Simulated neurological disease

Simulation and malingering can be difficult to distinguish from conversion disorders, but is often encountered in medico-legal practice, and private investigators employed by insurance companies may be instrumental in the diagnosis. In studies in which medical students were asked to simulate cognitive impairment, there was a gradual improvement in performance with continuous testing, which is in striking contrast to patients with genuine cognitive impairment in whom performance gradually worsens and in whom, indeed, it may precipitate a catastrophic reaction (Lishman 1987).

A particularly florid instance of simulation of disease is to be seen in patients with the 'Münchausen syndrome' (Asher 1951), who may simulate a whole variety of disorders, including neurological disease. Such patients move from hospital to hospital, cleverly feigning physical illness, including cardiac infarction, renal colic, perforated peptic ulcer or even cerebrovascular accidents. One well-known British patient, an ex male nurse, cleverly feigned a pontine lesion by using eye drops to dilate one pupil and constrict the other, while demonstrating convincing evidence of a hemiplegia and hemianalgesia with an extensor plantar response on the affected side. Many other such cases have been reported. While some such individuals are addicted to morphine or pethidine and simply seek injections of the appropriate drugs, and others seek nothing more than a bed for the night, most undertake these activities for complex psychological reasons (Mayer-Gross et al. 1960). While conversion disorder is more common in young women, those with Münchausen syndrome are nearly always men, often with a lifelong pattern of social maladjustment (Bayliss 1984).

26.11 Disorders of sexual behaviour

Disturbances of sexual behaviour, as opposed to disturbance of the mechanics of sexual activity arising from disease to the spinal cord and peripheral nerves, is seen predominantly with diseases of the basal ganglia and frontal and temporal lobes. Sexual imagery may form part of the obsessive–compulsive disorder, and disturbed behaviour may arise in association with post-encephalitic Parkinson's disease (Section 32.3.6). Similarly, cases of increased libido and paraphilia have been found in patients on treatment for Parkinson's disease (Quinn et al. 1983) (Section 32.3.1). Disturbances in sexual behaviour in patients with frontal lobe lesions probably reflect disinhibition. Lesions of the temporal lobes are frequently associated with disturbances in sexual behaviour, found most commonly as part of the spectrum of temporal lobe epilepsy. Reduced libido with impotence as an inter-ictal phenomenon is common, but hypersexuality can occur as an immediate post-ictal phenomenon (Blumer 1970). In addition to hyper- or hyposexuality, the development of paraphilias can occur with temporal-lobe lesions or temporal-lobe epilepsy. The most famous case was that described by Mitchell et al. (1954) of a 38-year-old man who had experienced pleasure in looking at, and imagining, safety pins, since adolescence. Increasingly this would be associated with sexual arousal and on occasions would result in the precipitation of temporal-lobe seizures. As the attacks became more frequent, he developed impotence. Post-ictally, he would occasionally dress in his wife's clothing. He was found to have a left temporal-lobe focus with increased EEG activity on looking at safety pins. He underwent left temporal lobectomy and, at operation, gliosis was found. Following surgery, there was a resolution of his attacks, restoration of potency, and cessation of the paraphilia.

Finally, side-effects of a variety of drugs in neurological practice may alter sexual behaviour. Neuroleptics, antihypertensives, and anticonvulsants may reduce libido. L-DOPA can be associated with increased libido and, rarely, with emergence of paraphilias.

26.12 Eating disorders

Neuroendocrine control of feeding behaviour is carefully balanced, and an increasing number of neurotransmitters, hormones, and receptors are now known to be involved, including neuropeptide Y, corticotrophin releasing factor, leptins, and insulin (Woods et al. 1998). These are primarily under hypothalamic control, and eating disorders are commonly found with hypothalamic lesions. Anorexia and bulimia nervosa, classically considered psychiatric disorders, may relate to hypothalamic disturbance. These disorders are seen primarily in adolescent and young women. Anorexia nervosa is associated with a distorted body image and the fear of gaining weight, and individuals have increased physical activity, reduced caloric intake, and, at times, dramatic weight loss. Bulimia nervosa involves episodic gorging followed by self-induced vomiting, laxative, and diuretic abuse.

The Kleine–Levin syndrome is rare and originally described in males, but can rarely be seen in females (Section 24.2.5). It typically starts in adolescence and may resolve with time. It is characterized by episodes, typically lasting from 4 to 7 days, of hypersomnia, hypersexuality, hyperphagia, and altered mood. The hyperphagia may herald the onset of an attack, with the individual eating raw and cooked food with a voracious appetite (Critchley 1962). The same clinical syndrome has been reported with a localized diencephalic encephalitis.

Sleep-related eating disorder, first reported in 1955 as 'night eating syndrome' (Stunkard et al. 1955), is linked to somnambulism. Patients develop nocturnal hyperphagia, insomnia, and subsequent obesity. It is more common in women than men, and there is commonly partial or complete amnesia for the event.

Changes in eating behaviour can also be seen with frontotemporal degenerations (Section 26.6.4) and a variety of drugs in neurological practice; for example, sodium valproate and steroids can lead to enhanced appetite.

References

Adolphs, R., Tranel, D., Hamann, S. et al. (1999). Recognition of facial emotion in nine individuals with bilateral amygdala damage. Neuropsychologia, 37, 1111–17.

Albert, M. L., Feldman, R. G., and Willis, A. L. (1974). The 'subcortical dementia' of progressive supranuclear palsy. *J. Neurol. Neurosurg. Psychiatry*, **37**, 121–30.

Albin, R. L., Minoshima, S., D'Amato, C. J. *et al.* (1996). Fluoro-deoxyglucose positron emission tomography in diffuse Lewy body disease. *Neurology*, **47**, 462–6.

Alexander, M. P., Stuss, D. T. and Benson, D. F. (1979). Capgras syndrome: a reduplicative phenomenon. *Neurology*, **29**, 334–9.

American Psychiatric Association (1994). *Diagnostic and statistical manual of mental disorders (DSM-IV)*, (4th edn). APA, Washington DC.

Andrew, J. and Nathan, P. W. (1964). Lesions of the anterior frontal lobes and disturbances of micturition and defaecation. *Brain*, **87**, 233–62.

Anonymous (1999). Swedish consensus on dementia diseases. *Acta Neurol. Scan. Suppl.*, **90**, 1–31.

Arrigoni, G. and De Renzi, E. (1964). Constructional apraxia and hemispheric locus of lesion. *Cortex*, **1**, 170.

Asher, R. (1951). Munchausen's syndrome. *Lancet*, **1**, 339–41.

Auerbach, S. H., Allard, T., Naeser, M. *et al.* (1982). Pure word deafness. Analysis of a case with bilateral lesions and a defect at the prephonemic level. *Brain*, **105**, 271–300.

Babinski, J. (1914). Contribution a l'étude des trouble mentaux dans l'hemiplégie organique cérébral (anosognosie). *Rev. Neurol.*, **27**, 845–52.

Baddeley, A., Bressi, S., Della Sala, S. *et al.* (1986). Dementia and working memory. *Q.J. Exp.Psychol.*, **38 A**, 603–18.

Bakheit, A. M. O., Kennedy, P. G. E., and Behan, P. O. (1990). Paraneoplastic limbic encephalitis: clinico-pathological correlations. *J. Neurol. Neurosurg. Psychiatry*, **53**, 1084–8.

Ballard, C., Holmes, C., McKeith, I. *et al.* (1999). Psychiatric morbidity in dementia with Lewy bodies: a prospective clinical and neuropathological comparative study with Alzheimer's disease. *Am. J. Psychiatry*, **156**, 1039–45.

Bayliss, R. I. (1984). The deceivers [editorial]. *BM J, Clin. Res.Edn*, **288**, 583–4.

Bennett, D. A., Wilson, R. S., Gilley, D. W. *et al.* (1990). Clinical diagnosis of Binswanger's disease. *J. Neurol. Neurosurg. Psychiatry*, **53**, 961–5.

Benson, D. F. (1967). Fluency in aphasia: Correlation with radioactive scan localisation. *Cortex*, **3**, 373–94.

Benson, D. F., Marsden, C. D., and Mcadows, J. C. (1974). The amnesic syndrome of posterior cerebral artery occlusion. *Acta Neurol. Scand.*, **50**, 133–45.

Benson, D. F., Gardner, H., and Meadows, J. C. (1976). Reduplicative paramnesia. *Neurology*, **26**, 147–51.

Benson, F., Davis, J., and Snyder, B. D. (1988). Posterior cortical atrophy. *Arch. Neurol.*, **45**, 789–93.

Benton, A. L. (1961). The fiction of the 'Gerstmann Syndrome'. *J. Neurol. Neurosurg. Psychiatry*, **24**, 176–81.

Berlyne, N. (1972). Confabulation. *Br. J. Psychiatry*, **120**, 31–9.

Bhatia, K. P. and Marsden, C. D. (1994). The behavioural and motor consequences of focal lesions of the basal ganglia in man. *Brain*, **117**, 859–76.

Binetti, G., Growdon, J. H., and Vonsattel, J. P. (1998). Pick's disease. In *The dementias*, (ed. J. H. Growdon and M. N. Rossor), pp. 7–44. Butterworth-Heinemann, Newton.

Blair, R. J. R. and Cipolotti, L. (2000). Impaired social response reversal: A case of 'acquired sociopathy'. *Brain*, **123**, 321–5.

Blessed, G., Tomlinson, B., and Roth, M. (1968). The association between quantitative measures of dementia and of senile change in the cerebral grey matter of elderly subjects. *Br. J. Psychiatry*, **114**, 797–811.

Blumer, D. (1970). Hypersexual episodes in temporal lobe epilepsy. *Am. J. Psychiatry*, **126**, 1099–106.

Blumstein, S. E., Alexander, M. P., Ryalls, J. H. *et al.* (1987). On the nature of the foreign accent syndrome: A case study. *Brain Lang.*, **31**, 215–44.

Bogousslavsky, J. (1994). Frontal stroke syndromes. *J. Europ. Neurol.*, **34**, 306–15.

Bowler, J. V., Eliasziw, M., Steenhuis, R. *et al.* (1997). Comparative evolution of Alzheimer disease, vascular dementia, and mixed dementia. *Arch. Neurol.*, **54**, 697–703.

Braak, H. and Braak, E. (1991). Neuropathological staging of Alzheimer-related changes. *Acta Neuropathol.*, **82**, 239–59.

Braak, H., Braak, E., Bohl, J. *et al.* (1989). Alzheimer's disease—amyloid plaques in the cerebellum. *J. Neurol. Sci.*, **93**, 277–87.

Brodmann, K. (1909). *Vergleichende Lokalisationslehre der Grosshirnrinde in ihren Prizipien dargestellt auf Grund des Zellenbauer*. J.A. Basth, Leipzig.

Brown, P., Cathala, F., Castaigne, P. *et al.* (1986). Creutzfeldt–Jakob disease: clinical analysis of a consecutive series of 230 neuropathologically verified cases. *Ann. Neurol.*, **20**, 597–602.

Bruce, V. and Young, A. (1986). Understanding face recognition. *Br.J. Psychol.*, **77**, 305–27.

Brun, A. (1993). Frontal-lobe degeneration of non-Alzheimer type revisited. *Dementia*, **4**, 126–31.

Brust, J. C. (1980). Music and language: musical alexia and agraphia. *Brain*, **103**, 367–92.

Caine, D., Halliday, G. M., Kril, J. J. *et al.* (1997). Operational criteria for the classification of chronic alcoholics: identification of Wernicke's encephalopathy. *J. Neurol. Neurosurg. Psychiatry*, **62**, 51–60.

Caine, E. D. (1981). Pseudodementia. Current concepts and future directions. *Arch. Gen. Psychiatry*, **38**, 1359–64.

Caplan, L. R. (1980). 'Top of the basilar' syndrome. *Neurology*, **30**, 72–9.

Caplan, L., Chedru, F., Lhermitte, F. *et al.* (1981). Transient global amnesia and migraine. *Neurology*, **31**, 1167–70.

Carter, G. L., Dawson, A. H., and Lopert, R. (1996). Drug-induced delirium. Incidence, management and prevention. *Drug Saf.*, **15**, 291–301.

Caselli, R. J. and Jack, C. R. (1992). Asymmetric cortical degeneration syndromes—a proposed clinical classification. *Arch. Neurol.*, **49**, 770–80.

Castaigne, P., Lhermitte, F., Buge, A. *et al.* (1981). Paramedian thalamic and midbrain infarct: clinical and neuropathological study. *Ann. Neurol.*, **10**, 127–48.

Chedru, F. and Geschwind, N. (1972). Writing disturbances in acute confusional states. *Neuropsychologia*, **10**, 343–53.

Clarfield, A. M. (1988). The reversible dementias: do they reverse? *Ann. Intern. Med.*, **109**, 476–86.

Cohen, N. J. and Squire, L. R. (1980). Preserved learning and retention of pattern analysing skill in amnesia: Dissociation of 'knowing how' and 'knowing that'. *Science*, **210**, 207–10.

Collinge, J., Brown, J., Hardy, J. *et al.* (1992). Inherited prion disease with 144 base pair gene insertion. 2. Clinical and pathological features. *Brain*, **115**, 687–710.

Collinge, J., Sidle, K. C. L., Meads, J. *et al.* (1996). Molecular analysis of prion strain variation and the etiology of new variant CJD. *Nature*, **383**, 685–90.

Constantinidis, J., Richard, J., and Tissot, R. (1974). Pick's disease: Histological and clinical correlations. *Europ. Neurol.*, **11**, 208–17.

Corder, E. H., Saunders, A. M., Strittmatter, W. J. *et al.* (1993). Gene dose of apolipoprotein E type 4 allele and the risk of Alzheimer's disease in late onset families. *Science*, **261**, 921–3.

Corey Bloom, J., Thal, L. J., Galasko, D. *et al.* (1995). Diagnosis and evaluation of dementia. *Neurology*, **45**, 211–18.

Craik, F. I. M. and Lockhart, R. S. (1972). Levels of processing: a framework for memory research. *J. Verb. Learning Verb. Behaviour*, **11**, 671–84.

Crimlisk, H. L. and Ron, M. A. (1999). Conversion hysteria: History, diagnostic issues and clinical practice. *Cogn. Neuropsychiatry*, **4**, 165–80.

Crimlisk, H. L., Bhatia, K., Cope, H. *et al.* (1998). Slater revisited: 6 year follow up study of patients with medically unexplained motor symptoms. *BMJ*, **316**, 582–6.

Critchley, M. (1953). *The parietal lobes*. Arnold, London.

Critchley, M. (1962). Periodic hypersomnia and megaphagia in adolescent males. *Brain*, **85**, 627–56.

Crook, T., Bartus, R., Ferris, S. *et al.* (1986). Age associated memory impairment: Proposed diagnostic criteria and measures of clinical change. Report of a National Institute of Mental Health work group. *Dev. Neuropsychol.*, **2** (4), 261–76.

Cruts, M. and Van Broeckhoven, C. (1998*a*). Molecular genetics of Alzheimer's disease. In *The dementias*, (ed. J. H. Growdon and M. N. Rossor), pp. 155–70. Butterworth–Heinemann, Boston.

Cruts, M., Van, D. C., Backhovens, H. *et al.* (1998*b*). Estimation of the genetic contribution of presenilin-1 and -2 mutations in a population-based study of presenile Alzheimer disease. *Hum. Mol. Genet.*, **7**, 43–51.

Cummings, J. L. (1986). Subcortical dementia. Neuropsychology, neuropsychiatry, and pathophysiology. *Br. J. Psychiatry*, **149**, 682–97.

Cummings, J. L. and Duchen, L. W. (1981). Kluver–Bucy syndrome in Pick disease: Clinical and pathologic correlations. *Neurology*, **31**, 1415–22.

Cutting, J. (1978). The relationship between Korsakoff's syndrome and 'alcoholic dementia'. *Br. J. Psychiatry*, **132**, 240–51.

Damasio, A. R., Damasio, H., Rizzo, M. *et al.* (1982). Aphasia with nonhemorrhagic lesions in the basal ganglia and internal capsule. *Arch. Neurol.*, **39**, 15–24.

Damasio, A. R., Graff, R. N., Eslinger, P. J. *et al.* (1985). Amnesia following basal forebrain lesions. *Arch. Neurol.*, **42**, 263–71.

De, R. E. (1986). Prosopagnosia in two patients with CT scan evidence of damage confined to the right hemisphere. *Neuropsychologia*, **24**, 385–9.

De, R. E., Scotti, G., and Spinnler, H. (1969). Perceptual and associative disorders of visual recognition. Relationship to the side of the cerebral lesion. *Neurology*, **19**, 634–42.

Delacourte, A., Robitaille, Y., Sergeant, N. *et al.* (1996). Specific pathological Tau protein variants characterize Pick's disease. *J. Neuropathol. Exp. Neurol.*, **55**, 159–68.

Della, S. S., Lucchelli, F., and Spinnler, H. (1987). Ideomotor apraxia in patients with dementia of Alzheimer type. *J. Neurol.*, **234**, 91–3.

Denes, G., Semenza, C., Stoppa, E. *et al.* (1982). Unilateral spatial neglect and recovery from hemiplegia: a follow-up study. *Brain*, **105**, 543–52.

De Renzi, E. and Lucchelli, F. (1988). Ideational apraxia. *Brain*, **111**, 1173–88.

De Renzi, E., Pieczuro, A. C., and Vignolo, L. A. (1968). Ideational apraxia: a quantitative study. *Neuropsychologia*, **6**, 41–52.

Devinsky, O., Morrell, M. J., and Vogt, B. A. (1995). Contributions of anterior cingulate cortex to behaviour. *Brain*, **118**, 279–306.

Dichgans, M., Mayer, M., Uttner, I. *et al.* (1998). The phenotypic spectrum of CADASIL: clinical findings in 102 cases. *Ann. Neurol.,* **44,** 731–9.

Dunn, D. W., Weisberg, L. A., and Nadell, J. (1983). Peduncular hallucinations caused by brainstem compression. *Neurology,* **33,** 1360–1.

ECAPD Consortium, Alvarez, X. A., Barker, S. *et al.* (1998). Provisional clinical and neuroradiological criteria for the diagnosis of Pick's disease. *Europ. J. Neurol.,* **5,** 519–20.

Efron, R. (1968). What is perception? In *Boston studies in the philosophy of science,* (ed. R. S. Cohen and M. Wartofsky), pp. 137. Humanities Press, New York.

Esiri, M. M., Wilcock, G. K., and Morris, J. H. (1997). Neuropathological assessment of the lesions of significance in vascular dementia. *J. Neurol. Neurosurg. Psychiatry,* **63,** 749–53.

Etcoff, N. L. (1984). Selective attention to facial identity and facial emotion. *Neuropsychologia,* **22,** 281–95.

Evans, D. A., Funkenstein, H. H., Albert, M. S. *et al.* (1989). Prevalence of Alzheimer's disease in a community population of older persons. Higher than previously reported. *JAMA,* **262,** 2551–6.

Faden, A. I. and Townsend, J. J. (1976). Myoclonus in Alzheimer disease. A confusing sign. *Arch. Neurol.,* **33,** 278–80.

Farrer, L. A., Myers, R. H., Cupples, L. A. *et al.* (1990). Transmission and age-at-onset patterns in familial Alzheimer's disease: evidence for heterogeneity. *Neurology,* **40,** 395–403.

Feher, E., Mahurin, R., Inbody, S. *et al.* (1991). Anosognosia in Alzheimer's Disease. *Neuropsychiat. Neuropsychol. Behav. Neurol.,* **4,** 136–146.

Fisher, C. M. (1982). Transient global amnesia. Precipitating activities and other observations. *Arch. Neurol.,* **39,** 605–8.

Fisher, C. M. and Adams, R. D. (1958). Transient global amnesia. *Trans. Am. Neurol. Assoc.,* **83,** 143–6.

Fodor, J. (1983). *The modularity of mind.* MIT Press, Cambridge, MA.

Forette, F., Seux, M. L., Staessen, J. A. *et al.* (1998). Prevention of dementia in randomised double-blind placebo-controlled Systolic Hypertension in Europe (Syst-Eur) trial. *Lancet,* **352,** 1347–51.

Foster, N. L., Wilhelmsen, K., Sima, A. A. *et al.* (1997). Frontotemporal dementia and parkinsonism linked to chromosome 17: a consensus conference. Conference Participants. *Ann. Neurol.,* **41,** 706–15.

Fox, N. C., Scahill, R. I., Crum, W. R. *et al.* (1999*a*). Correlation between rates of brain atrophy and cognitive decline in AD. *Neurology,* **52,** 1687–9.

Fox, N. C., Warrington, E. K., and Rossor, M. N. (1999*b*). Serial magnetic resonance imaging of cerebral atrophy in preclinical Alzheimer's disease. *Lancet,* **353,** 2125.

Foy, A., O'Connell, D., Henry, D. *et al.* (1995). Benzodiazepine use as a cause of cognitive impairment in elderly hospital inpatients. *J. Gerontol. A Biol. Sci. Med. Sci.,* **50,** M99–106.

Frackowiak, R. J., Pozzilli, C., Legg, N. J. *et al.* (1981). Regional cerebral oxygen supply and utilization in dementia. A clinical and physiological study with oxygen-15 and positron tomography. *Brain,* **104,** 753–78.

Fradkin, J. E., Schonberger, L. B., Mills, J. L. *et al.* (1991). Creutzfeldt–Jakob disease in pituitary growth hormone recipients in the United States. *JAMA,* **265,** 880–4.

Gabrieli, J. D. (1998). Cognitive neuroscience of human memory. *Annu.Rev Psychol* **49,** 87–115.

Gerstmann, J. (1940). Syndrome of finger agnosia, disorientation for right and left: agraphia and acalculia. *Arch. Neurol. Psychiatry, Chicago,* **44,** 398–408.

Geschwind, N. (1965). Disconnexion syndromes in animals and man. *Brain,* **88,** 585–641.

Geschwind, N. (1982). Disorders of attention: a frontier in neuropsychology. *Philos. Trans. R. Soc.Lond. B. Biol. Sci.,* **298,** 173–85.

Geschwind, N. and Kaplan, E. (1962). A human cerebral deconnection syndrome. *Neurology,* **12,** 675–85.

Geschwind, N., Quadfasel, F. A., and Segarra, J. M. (1968). Isolation of the speech area. *Neuropsychologia,* **6,** 327–40.

Goedert, M., Spillantini, M. G., Cairns, N. J. *et al.* (1992). Tau-proteins of Alzheimer paired helical filaments—abnormal phosphorylation of all 6 brain isoforms. *Neuron,* **8,** 159–68.

Goldman, R. P. (1988). Topography of cognition: parallel distributed networks in primate association cortex. *Annu. Rev. Neurosci.,* **11,** 137–56.

Goldstein, M. (1974). Auditory agnosia for speech ('pure-word deafness'): A historical review with current implications. *Brain Lang.,* **1,** 195–204.

Goodglass, H. and Kaplan, E. (1972). *The assessment of aphasia and related disorders.* Lea and Febiger, Philadelphia.

Goodglass, H., Quadfasel, F. A., and Timberlake, W. H. (1964). Phrase length and the type of severity of aphasia. *Cortex,* **1,** 133–53.

Goodglass, H., Klein, B., Carey, P. *et al.* (1966). Specific semantic word categories in aphasia. *Cortex,* **2,** 74–89.

Goodwin, D. W., Crane, J. B., and Guze, S. B. (1969). Alcoholic 'blackouts': a review and clinical study of 100 alcoholics. *Am. J. Psychiatry,* **126,** 191–8.

Graff, R. N., Eslinger, P. J., Damasio, A. R. *et al.* (1984). Nonhemorrhagic infarction of the thalamus: behavioral, anatomic, and physiologic correlates. *Neurology,* **34,** 14–23.

Hachinski, V. C. and Bowler, J. V. (1993). Vascular dementia [letter; comment]. *Neurology*, **43**, 2159–60.

Hachinski, V., Lassen, N., and Marshall, J. (1974). Multi-infarct dementia. A cause of mental deterioration in the elderly. *Lancet*, **July 27**, 207–9.

Hachinski, V. C., Potter, P., and Merskey, H. (1987). Leuko-araiosis. *Arch. Neurology*, **44**, 21–3.

Hammeke, T. A., McQuillen, M. P., and Cohen, B. A. (1983). Musical hallucinations associated with acquired deafness. *J. Neurol. Neurosurg. Psychiatry*, **46**, 570–2.

Hardy, J. A. and Higgins, G. A. (1992). Alzheimer's disease: the amyloid cascade hypothesis. *Science*, **256**, 184–5.

Health Service Circular (1999). *Variant Creutzfeldt–Jakob Disease (vCJD): Minimising the risk of transmission. HSC 1999/178*, pp.1–14. Department of Health. London.

Hecaen, H. (1962). Clinical symptomatology in right and left hemispheric lesions. In *Interhemispheric relations and cerebral dominance*, (ed. V. B. Mountcastle), pp. 215. John Hopkins, Baltimore.

Hecaen, H. and Ajuriaguerra, J. (1954). Balint's syndrome (psychic paralysis of visual fixation) and its minor forms. *Brain*, **77**, 373–400.

Hecaen, H. and Albert, M. L. (1978). *Human neuropsychology*. Wiley, New York.

Hecaen, H. and Angelergues, R. (1963). *Le cécité psychique*. Masson, Paris.

Henson, R. A. and Urich, H. (1982). *Cancer and the nervous system*. Blackwell, Oxford.

Heye, N., Terstegge, K., Sirtl, C. *et al.* (1994). Wernicke's encephalopathy–causes to consider. *IntensiveCare Med.*, **20**, 282–6.

Hill, A. F., Butterworth, R. J., Joiner, S. *et al.* (1999). Investigation of variant Creutzfeldt–Jakob disease and other human prion diseases with tonsil biopsy samples. *Lancet*, **353**, 183–9.

Hodges, J. R. and Ward, C. D. (1989). Observations during transient global amnesia. A behavioural and neuropsychological study of five cases. *Brain*, **112**, 595–620.

Hodges, J. R. and Warlow, C. P. (1990). The aetiology of transient global amnesia. A case-control study of 114 cases with prospective follow-up. *Brain*, **113**, 639–57.

Hodges, J. R., Patterson, K., Oxbury, S. *et al.* (1992). Semantic dementia. Progressive fluent aphasia with temporal lobe atrophy. *Brain*, **115**, 1783–806.

Holmes, G. (1918). Disturbances of visual orientation. *Br. J. Ophthalmol.*, **2**, 449–68.

House, A., Dennis, M., Warlow, C. *et al.* (1990). Mood disorders after stroke and their relation to lesion location. A CT scan study. *Brain*, **113**, 1113–29.

Hsich, G., Kenney, K., Gibbs, C. J. *et al.* (1996). The 14–3–3 brain protein in cerebrospinal fluid as a marker for transmissible spongiform encephalopathies. *N. Engl. J. Med.*, **335**, 924–30.

Hulstaert, F., Blennow, K., Ivanoiu, A. *et al.* (1999). Improved discrimination of AD patients using beta-amyloid(1–42) and tau levels in CSF. *Neurology*, **52**, 1555–62.

Hutton, M., Lendon, C., Rizzu, P. *et al.* (1998). Association of missense and 5'-splice-site mutations in tau with the inherited dementia FTDP-17. *Nature*, **393**, 702–5.

Hymas, N., Lees, A., Bolton, D. *et al.* (1991). The neurology of obsessional slowness. *Brain*, **114**, 2203–33.

Iwatsubo, T., Mann, D. M., Odaka, A. *et al.* (1995). Amyloid β protein (Aβ) deposition: Aβ42(43) precedes Aβ40 in Down syndrome. *Ann. Neurol.*, **37**, 294–9.

Jack, C. R., Petersen, R. C., Xu, Y. C. *et al.* (1999). Prediction of AD with MRI based hippocampal volume in mild cognitive impairment. *Neurology*, **52**, 1397–403.

Janssen, R. S., Nwanyanwu, O. C., Selik, R. M. *et al.* (1992). Epidemiology of human-immunodeficiency-virus encephalopathy in the United States. *Neurology*, **42**, 1472–6.

Jobst, K. A., Smith, A. D., Szatmari, M. *et al.* (1992). Detection in life of confirmed Alzheimer's disease using a simple measurement of medial temporal lobe atrophy by computed tomography. *Lancet*, **340**, 1179–83.

Joutel, A., Corpechot, C., Ducros, A. *et al.* (1996). Notch3 mutations in cadasil, a hereditary adult-onset condition causing stroke and dementia. *Nature*, **383**, 707–10.

Kang, J., Lemaire, H.-G., Unterbeck, A. *et al.* (1987). The precursor of Alzheimer's disease amyloid A4 protein resembles a cell-surface receptor. *Nature*, **325**, 733–7.

Kapur, N., Turner, A., and King, C. (1988). Reduplicative paramnesia: possible anatomical and neuropsychological mechanisms. *J. Neurol. Neurosurg. Psychiatry*, **51**, 579–81.

Keime-Guibert, F., Napolitano, M., and Delattre, J. Y. (1998). Neurological complications of radiotherapy and chemotherapy. *J. Neurol.*, **245**, 695–708.

Kennedy, A. M. (1998). Functional neuroimaging in dementia. In *The dementias*, (ed. J. H. Growdon and M. N. Rossor), pp. 219–55. Butterworth–Heinemann, Boston.

Kertesz, A. and Munoz, D. (1998). Pick's disease, frontotemporal dementia, and Pick complex: emerging concepts. *Arch. Neurol.*, **55**, 302–4.

Kew, J. and Leigh, N. (1992). Dementia with motor neurone disease. *Baillieres Clin. Neurol.*, **1**, 611–26.

Khachaturian, Z. S. (1985). Diagnosis of Alzheimer's disease. *Arch. Neurol.*, **42**, 1097–105.

Kidd, M. (1963). Paired helical filaments in electronmicroscopy in Alzheimer's disease. *Nature*, **197**, 192–3.

Kim, R. C., Collins, G. H., Parisi, J. E. *et al.* (1981). Familial dementia of adult onset with pathological findings of a nonspecific nature. *Brain,* **104**, 61–78.

Kirk, C. and Saunders, M. (1977). Primary psychiatric illness in a neurological out-patient department in North East England. An assessment of symptomatology. *Acta Psychiatr. Scand.,* **56**, 294–302.

Kirshner, H. S., Webb, W., Kelly, M. P. *et al.* (1984). Language disturbance. An initial disturbance of cortical degenerations and dementia. *Arch. Neurol.,* **41**, 491–6.

Klatka, L. A., Louis, E. D., and Schiffer, R. B. (1996). Psychiatric features in diffuse Lewy body disease: a clinicopathologic study using Alzheimer's disease and Parkinson's disease comparison groups. *Neurology,* **47**, 1148–52.

Kleist, K. (1922). Die psychomotorischen Storungen und ihr Verhaltnis zu den Motilitatsstorungen bei der Stammganglien. *Mschr. Pychiat. Neurol.,* **52**, 253–302.

Knopman, D. and Nissen, M. (1987). Implicit learning in patients with probable Alzheimer's disease. *Neurology,* **37**, 784–8.

Knopman, D. S., Mastri, A. R., Frey, W. H. *et al.* (1990). Dementia lacking distinctive histologic features: a common non- Alzheimer degenerative dementia. *Neurology,* **40**, 251–6.

Kopelman, M. D. (1987). Amnesia—organic and psychogenic. *Br. J. Psychiatry,* **150**, 428–42.

Kopelman, M. D. (1995). The Korsakoff syndrome. *Br. J. Psychiatry,* **166**, 154–73.

Kosaka, K. (1994). Diffuse neurofibrillary tangles with calcification: a new presenile dementia. *J. Neurol. Neurosurg. Psychiatry,* **57**, 594–6.

Kral, V. A. (1962). Senescent forgetfulness: benign and malignant. *Can. Med. Assoc. J.,* **86**, 257–60.

Krupp, L. B., Masur, D., Schwartz, J. *et al.* (1991). Cognitive functioning in late Lyme borreliosis. *Arch. Neurol.,* **48**, 1125–9.

Kukull, W. A., Larson, E. B., Reifler, B. V. *et al.* (1990). The validity of 3 clinical diagnostic criteria for Alzheimer's disease. *Neurology,* **40**, 1364–9.

Laplane, D., Baulac, M., Widlocher, D. *et al.* (1984). Pure psychic akinesia with bilateral lesions of basal ganglia. *J. Neurol. Neurosurg. Psychiatry,* **47**, 377–85.

Lavenu, I., Pasquier, F., Lebert, F. *et al.* (1999). Perception of emotion in frontotemporal dementia and Alzheimer disease. *Alzheimer Dis. Assoc. Disord.,* **13**, 96–101.

Lecours, A. R. (1976). The 'Pure Form' of the phonetic disintegration syndrome (pure anarthria); anatomo-clinical report of a historical case. *Brain Lang.,* **3**, 88–113.

Lee, V. M. Y., Balin, B. J., Otvos, L. *et al.* (1991). A68—a major subunit of paired helical filaments and derivatized forms of normal-tau. *Science,* **251**, 675–8.

Levkoff, S. E., Evans, D. A., Liptzin, B. *et al.* (1992). Delirium. The occurrence and persistence of symptoms among elderly hospitalized patients. *Arch. Intern. Med.,* **152**, 334–40.

Lhermitte, F. (1983). 'Utilization behaviour' and its relation to lesions of the frontal lobes. *Brain,* **106**, 237–55.

Lilly, R., Cummings, J. L., Benson, D. F. *et al.* (1983). The human Kluver–Bucy syndrome. *Neurology,* **33**, 1141–5.

Lipowski, Z. J. (1983). Transient cognitive disorders (delirium, acute confusional states) in the elderly. *Am. J. Psychiatry,* **140**, 1426–36.

Lipowski, Z. J. (1990). *Acute confusional states,* (2nd edn). Oxford University Press, New York.

Lisak, R. P. and Zimmerman, R. A. (1977). Transient global amnesia due to a dominant hemisphere tumor. *Arch. Neurol.,* **34**, 317–18.

Lishman, W. A. (1987). *Organic psychiatry, the psychological consequences of cerebral disorder,* (2nd edn). Blackwell Scientific, Oxford.

Lugaresi, E., Medori, R., Montagna, P. *et al.* (1986). Fatal familial insomnia and dysautonomia with selective degeneration of thalamic nuclei. *N.Engl. J. Med.,* **315**, 997–1003.

Luria, A. R. (1977). On quasi-aphasic speech disturbances in lesions of the deep structures of the brain. *Brain Lang.,* **4**, 432–59.

Marshall, J. C. and Newcombe, F. (1966). Syntactic and semantic errors in paralexia. *Neuropsychologia,* **4**, 169–76.

Marshall, J. C., Halligan, P. W., Fink, G. R. *et al.* (1997). The functional anatomy of a hysterical paralysis. *Cognition,* **64**, B1–B8.

Mayer-Gross, W., Slater, E., and Roth, M. (1960). *Clinical psychiatry,* (2nd edn). Cassell, London.

Mazzucchi, A., Moretti, G., Caffarra, P. *et al.* (1980). Neuropsychological functions in the follow-up of transient global amnesia. *Brain,* **103**, 161–78.

McCarthy, R. A. and Warrington, E. K. (1990). *Cognitive neuropsychology. A clinical introduction.* Academic Press, London.

McKeith, L. G., Galasko, D., Kosaka, K. *et al.* (1996). Consensus guidelines for the clinical and pathologic diagnosis of dementia with Lewy bodies (DLB): report of the consortium on DLB international workshop. *Neurology,* **47**, 1113–24.

McKhann, G., Drachman, D., Folstein, M. *et al.* (1984). Clinical diagnosis of Alzheimer's Disease: Report of the NINCDS–ADRDA work group under the auspices of Department of Health and Human Services Task Force on Alzheimer's Disease. *Neurology,* **34**, 939–44.

McShane, R., Keene, J., Gedling, K. *et al.* (1997). Do neuroleptic drugs hasten cognitive decline in dementia? Prospective study with necropsy follow up [see comments]. *BMJ*, **314**, 266–70.

Meadows, J. C. (1974*a*). Disturbed perception of colours associated with localized cerebral lesions. *Brain, 97*, 615–32.

Meadows, J. C. (1974*b*). The anatomical basis of prosopagnosia. *J. Neurol. Neurosurg. Psychiatry*, **37**, 489–501.

Medina, J. L., Rubino, F. A., and Ross, E. (1974). Agitated delirium caused by infarctions of the hippocampal formation and fusiform and lingual gyri: a case report. *Neurology*, **24**, 1181–3.

Medina, J. L., Chokroverty, S., and Rubino, F. A. (1977). Syndrome of agitated delirium and visual impairment: a manifestation of medial temporo-occipital infarction. *J. Neurol. Neurosurg. Psychiatry*, **40**, 861–4.

Melton, S. T., Kirkwood, C. K., and Ghaemi, S. N. (1997). Pharmacotherapy of HIV dementia. *Ann. Pharmacother.*, **31**, 457–73.

Mesulam, M. M. (1981). A cortical network for directed attention and unilateral neglect. *Ann. Neurol.*, **10**, 309–25.

Mesulam, M. M. (1982). Slowly progressive aphasia without generalized dementia. *Ann. Neurol.*, **11**, 592–8.

Mesulam, M. M., Waxman, S. G., Geschwind, N. *et al.* (1976). Acute confusional states with right middle cerebral artery infarctions. *J. Neurol. Neurosurg. Psychiatry*, **39**, 84–9.

Meyer, J. S. and Barron, D. W. (1960). Apraxia of gait: a clinico-physiological study. *Brain*, **83**, 261–84.

Milner, B. (1958). Psychological defects produced by temporal lobe excision. *Res. Publ. Ass. Nerv. Ment. Dis.*, **36**, 244–57.

Milner, B. (1963). Effects of different brain lesions on card sorting. *Arch. Neurol.*, **9**, 90.

Milner, B. (1971). Interhemispheric differences in the localization of psychological processes in man. *Br.Med. Bull.*, **27**, 272–7.

Milner, B., Corkin, S., and Teuber, H. L. (1968). Further analysis of the hippocampal amnesic syndrome: 14 year follow up of HM. *Neuropsychologia*, **6**, 215.

Mindham, R. H., Marsden, C. D., and Parkes, J. D. (1976). Psychiatric symptoms during l-dopa therapy for Parkinson's disease and their relationship to physical disability. *Psychol. Med.*, **6**, 23–33.

Mirra, S. S., Heyman, A., McKeel, D. *et al.* (1991). The consortium to establish a registry for Alzheimer's disease (CERAD) . Standardization of the neuropathologic assessment of Alzheimer's disease. *Neurology*, **41**, 479–86.

Mitchell, W., Falconer, M. A., and Hill, D. (1954). Epilepsy with fetishism relieved by temporal lobectomy. *Lancet*, **2**, 626–30.

Mohr, J. P., Pessin, M. S., Finkelstein, S. *et al.* (1978). Broca aphasia: pathologic and clinical. *Neurology, 28*, 311–24.

Moroney, J. T., Bagiella, E., Desmond, D. W. *et al.* (1997). Meta-analysis of the Hachinski Ischemic Score in pathologically verified dementias. *Neurology*, **49**, 1096–105.

Mountcastle, V. B. (1997). The columnar organization of the neocortex. *Brain*, **120**, 701–22.

Naeser, M. A., Alexander, M. P., Helm, E. N. *et al.* (1982). Aphasia with predominantly subcortical lesion sites: description of three capsular/putaminal aphasia syndromes. *Arch. Neurology*, **39**, 2–14.

Nathan, P. W. (1947) Facial apraxia and apraxic dysarthria. *Brain*, **70**, 449–78.

Neary, D., Snowden, J. S., Gustafson, L. *et al.* (1998). Frontotemporal lobar degeneration: a consensus on clinical diagnostic criteria. *Neurology*, **51**, 1546–54.

Norman, D. A. and Shallice, T. (1980). *Attention to action: willed and automatic control of behaviour.* 99, Centre for Human Information Processing, University of California, San Diego.

O'Brien, J. T., Desmond, P., Ames, D. *et al.* (1997). Magnetic resonance imaging correlates of memory impairment in the healthy elderly: Association with medial temporal lobe atrophy but not white matter lesions. *Int. J. Geriatr. Psychiatry*, **374**, 369–74.

Palmer, M. S., Dryden, A. J., Hughes, J. T. *et al.* (1991). Homozygous prion protein genotype predisposes to sporadic Creutzfeldt–Jakob disease. *Nature*, **352**, 340–2.

Parchi, P., Castellani, R., Capellari, S. *et al.* (1996). Molecular basis of phenotypic variability in sporadic Creutzfeldt–Jakob disease. *Ann. Neurol.*, **39**, 767–78.

Paterson, A. and Zangwill, O. L. (1946). A case of topographical disorientation associated with a unilateral cerebral lesion. *Brain*, **68**, 188–212.

Perani, D., Vallar, G., Cappa, S. *et al.* (1987). Aphasia and neglect after subcortical stroke. A clinical/cerebral perfusion correlation study. *Brain*, **110**, 1211–29.

Perry, R. H., McKeith, I. G., and Perry, E. K. (1996). *Dementia with Lewy bodies.* Cambridge University Press, Cambridge.

Petersen, S. E., Fox, P. T., Posner, M. I. *et al.* (1988). Positron emission tomographic studies of the cortical anatomy of single-word processing. *Nature*, **331**, 585–9.

Pick, A. (1903). On reduplicative paramnesia. *Brain, 26*, 260–7.

Pohjasvaara, T., Erkinjuntti, T., Vataja, R. *et al.* (1997). Dementia three months after stroke. Baseline frequency and effect of different definitions of dementia in the Helsinki Stroke Aging Memory Study (SAM) cohort. *Stroke* **28**, 785–92.

Poorkaj, P., Bird, T. D., Wijsman, E. *et al.* (1998). Tau is a candidate gene for chromosome 17 frontotemporal dementia. *Ann. Neurol.*, **43**, 815–25.

Pramstaller, P. P. and Marsden, C. D. (1996). The basal ganglia and apraxia. *Brain*, **119**, 319–40.

Price, C. J. (1998). The functional anatomy of word comprehension and production. *Trends Cognitive Sci.*, **2**, 281–8.

Price, C. J. and Friston, K. J. (1997). Cognitive conjunction: a new approach to brain activation experiments. *Neuroimage*, **5**, 261–70.

Prusiner, S. B. (1991). Molecular biology of prion diseases. *Science*, **252**, 1515–22.

Prusiner, S. B., Scott, M. R., DeArmond, S. J. *et al.* (1998). Prion protein biology. *Cell*, **93**, 337–48.

Quinn, N. P., Toone, B., Lang, A. E. *et al.* (1983). Dopa dose-dependent sexual deviation. *Br. J. Psychiatry*, **142**, 296–8.

Rachman, S. (1974). Primary obsessional slowness. *Behav. Res. Ther.*, **12**, 9–18.

Rakic, P. (1995). A small step for the cell, a giant leap for mankind: a hypothesis of neocortical expansion during evolution. *Trends Neurosci.*, **18**, 383–8.

Rebollo, M., Val, J. F., Garijo, F. *et al.* (1983). Livedo reticularis and cerebrovascular lesions (Sneddon's syndrome). Clinical, radiological and pathological features in eight cases. *Brain*, **106**, 965–79.

Richfield, E. K., Twyman, R., and Berent, S. (1987). Neurological syndrome following bilateral damage to the head of the caudate nuclei. *Ann. Neurol.*, **22**, 768–71.

Riddoch, G. (1941). Phantom limbs and body shape. *Brain*, **64**, 197–22.

Robertson, M. M., Trimble, M. R., and Lees, A. J. (1988). The psychopathology of the Gilles de la Tourette syndrome. A phenomenological analysis. *Br. J. Psychiatry*, **152**, 383–90.

Rogers, S. L., Doody, R. S., Mohs, R. C. *et al.* (1998). Donepezil improves cognition and global function in Alzheimer disease: a 15-week, double-blind, placebo-controlled study. Donepezil Study Group. *Arch. Int. Med.*, **158**, 1021–31.

Roman, G. C. (1998). Diagnostic criteria in cerebrovascular diseases and vascular dementia. *Europ. J. Neurol.*, **5**, S3–S8

Rosler, M., Anand, R., Cicin, S. A. *et al.* (1999). Efficacy and safety of rivastigmine in patients with Alzheimer's disease: international randomised controlled trial [see comments]. *BMJ*, **318**, 633–8.

Ross, E. D. (1981). The aprosodias. Functional–anatomic organization of the affective components of language in the right hemisphere. *Arch. Neurol.*, **38**, 561–9.

Rossor, M. N., Revesz, T., Lantos, P. L. *et al.* (2000). Semantic dementia with ubiquitin-positive tau-negative inclusion bodies. *Brain*, **123**, 267–76.

Rudge, P. and Warrington, E. K. (1991). Selective impairment of memory and visual perception in splenial tumours. *Brain*, **114**, 349–60.

Sano, M., Ernesto, C., Thomas, R. G. *et al.* (1997). A controlled trial of selegiline, alpha-tocopherol, or both as treatment for Alzheimer's disease. The Alzheimer's Disease Cooperative Study. *N. Engl. J. Med.*, **336**, 1216–22.

Santamaria, J., Tolosa, E., and Valles, A. (1986). Parkinson's disease with depression: a possible subgroup of idiopathic parkinsonism. *Neurology*, **36**, 1130–3.

Sawle, G. V., Hymas, N. F., Lees, A. J. *et al.* (1991). Obsessional slowness. Functional studies with positron emission tomography. *Brain*, **114**, 2191–202.

Schacter, D. L., Wang, P. L., Tulving, E. *et al.* (1982). Functional retrograde amnesia: a quantitative case study. *Neuropsychologia*, **20**, 523–32.

Schenk, D., Barbour, R., Dunn, W. *et al.* (1999). Immunization with amyloid-beta attenuates Alzheimer disease-like pathology in the PDAPP mouse. *Nature*, **400**, 173–7.

Schiff, H. B., Alexander, M. P., Naeser, M. A. *et al.* (1983). Aphemia. Clinical–anatomic correlations. *Arch. Neurol.*, **40**, 720–7.

Schiffer, R. B. (1987). The spectrum of depression in multiple sclerosis. An approach for clinical management. *Arch. Neurol.*, **44**, 596–9.

Scoville, W. B. and Milner, B. (1957). Loss of recent memory after bilateral hippocampal lesions. *J. Neurol. Neurosurg. Psychiatry*, **20**, 11–21.

Selai, C. E., Trimble, M. R., Rossor, M. N. *et al.* (1999). Effectiveness of rivastigmine in Alzheimer's disease—patients' view on quality of life should be assessed. *BMJ*, **319**, 641–2.

Seyffarth, H. and Denny-Brown, D. (1948). The grasp reflex and the instinctive grasp reaction. *Brain*, **71**, 109–83.

Shallice, T. (1981*a*). *From neuropsychology to mental structure*. Cambridge University Press, New York.

Shallice, T. (1981*b*). Phonological agraphia and the lexical route in writing. *Brain*, **104**, 413–29.

Shallice, T. (1982). Specific impairments of planning. *Phil. Trans. R. Soc. Lond. B. Biol. Sci.*, **298**, 199–209.

Shallice, T. and Warrington, E. K. (1970). Independent functioning of verbal memory stores: a neuropsychological study. *Q. J. Exp. Psychol.*, **22**, 261–73.

Shallice, T., Burgess, P. W., Schon, F. *et al.* (1989). The origins of utilization behaviour. *Brain*, **112**, 1587–98.

Sharma, P. and Chaturvedi, S. K. (1995). Conversion disorder revisited. *Acta Psychiatr. Scand.*, **92**, 301–4.

Shipp, S., Dejong, B. M., Zihl, J. *et al.* (1994). The brain activity related to residual motion vision in a patient with bilateral lesions of V_5. *Brain*, **117**, 1023–38.

Shuping, J. R., Toole, J. F. and Rollinson, R. D. (1979). Transient global amnesia. *Trans. Am. Neurol. Assoc.*, **104**, 183–6.

Singer, R. (1998). Diagnosis and treatment of Whipple's disease. *Drugs*, **55**, 699–704.

Slater, E. (1965). Diagnosis of hysteria. *BMJ*, **1**, 1395–9.

Small, G. W., Rabins, P. V., Barry, P. P. *et al.* (1997). Diagnosis and treatment of Alzheimer disease and related disorders. Consensus statement of the American Association for Geriatric Psychiatry, the Alzheimer's Association, and the American Geriatrics Society. *JAMA*, **278**, 1363–71.

Smith, G. R., Monson, R. A., and Ray, D. C. (1986). Psychiatric consultation in somatization disorder. A randomized controlled study. *N. Engl. J. Med.*, **314**, 1407–13.

Smith, L. W. and Dimsdale, J. E. (1989). Postcardiotomy delirium: conclusions after 25 years? *Am. J. Psychiatry*, **146**, 452–8.

Snowden, J. S., Goulding, P. J., and Neary, D. (1989). Semantic dementia: a form of circumscribed cerebral atrophy. *Behav. Neurol.*, **2**, 167–82.

Snowden, J. S., Neary, D., and Mann, D. M. A. (1996). *Fronto-temporal lobar degeneration*, Churchill Livingstone, Edinburgh.

Spillantini, M. G., Schmidt, M. L., Lee, V. M. *et al.* (1997). Alpha-synuclein in Lewy bodies [letter]. *Nature*, **388**, 839–40.

Starkstein, S. E. and Robinson, R. G. (1993). Depression in cerebrovascular disease. In *Depression in neurological disease*, (ed. S. E. Starkstein and R. G. Robinson) pp. 28–49. John Hopkins University Press, Baltimore.

Starr, A. and Phillips, L. (1970). Verbal and motor memory in the amnestic syndrome. *Neuropsychologia*, **8**, 75–88.

Stigsby, B., Johannesson, G., and Ingvar, D. H. (1981). Regional EEF analysis and regional cerebral blood-flow in Alzheimer's and Pick's diseases. *Electroencephalogr. Clin. Neurophysiol.*, **51**, 537–47.

Stunkard, A. J., Grace, W. J., and Wolff, H. G. (1955). Night-eating syndrome; pattern of food intake among certain obese patients. *Am. J. Med.*, **19**, 78–86.

Stuss, D. T., Alexander, M. P., Lieberman, A. *et al.* (1978). An extraordinary form of confabulation. *Neurology*, **28**, 1166–72.

Sulkava, R. (1982). Alzheimer's disease and senile dementia of the Alzheimer type. *Acta Neurol. Scand.*, **65**, 636–50.

Summers, W. K. and Reich, T. C. (1979). Delirium after cataract surgery: review and two cases. *Am. J. Psychiatry*, **136**, 386–91.

Swedo, S. E., Rapoport, J. L., Cheslow, D. L. *et al.* (1989). High prevalence of obsessive–compulsive symptoms in patients with Sydenham's chorea. *Am. J. Psychiatry*, **146**, 246–9.

Taylor, D. and Lewis, S. (1993). Delirium. *J. Neurol. Neurosurg. Psychiatry*, **56**, 742–51.

Thompson, P. D. and Marsden, C. D. (1987). Gait disorder of subcortical arteriosclerotic encephalopathy: Binswanger's disease. *Mov. Dis.*, **2**, 1–8.

Tierney, M. C., Fisher, R. H., Lewis, A. J. *et al.* (1988). The NINCDS-ADRDA Work Group criteria for the clinical diagnosis of probable Alzheimer's disease: a clinicopathologic study of 57 cases [see comments]. *Neurology*, **38**, 359–64.

Tierney, M. C., Szalai, J. P., Snow, W. G. *et al.* (1996). Prediction of probable Alzheimer's disease in memory-impaired patients: A prospective longitudinal study. *Neurology*, **46**, 661–5.

Tranel, D. and Hyman, B. T. (1990). Neuropsychological correlates of bilateral amydala damage. *Arch Neurol.*, **47**, 349–55.

Trimble, M. R. (2000). Behaviour and Personality Disturbances. In *Neurology in clinical practice: principles of diagnosis and management*, (ed. W. G. Bradley, R. B. Daroff, G. M. Fenichel, and C. D. Marsden), (3rd edn), pp. 89–104. Butterworth–Heinemann, Boston.

Tulving, E. (1973). Episodic and semantic memory. In *Organization of memory*, (ed. E. Tulving and W. Donaldson), pp. 382. Academic Press, New York.

Tune, L. E., Damlouji, N. F., Holland, A. *et al.* (1981). Association of postoperative delirium with raised serum levels of anticholinergic drugs. *Lancet*, **2**, 651–3.

Tyrrell, P. J., Sawle, G. V., Ibanez, V. *et al.* (1990*a*). Clinical and positron emission tomographic studies in the 'extrapyramidal syndrome' of dementia of the Alzheimer type. *Arch. Neurol.*, **47**, 1318–23.

Tyrrell, P. J., Warrington, E. K., Frackowiak, R. S. J. *et al.* (1990*b*). Progressive degeneration of the right temporal-lobe studied with positron emission tomography. *J. Neurol. Neurosurg. Psychiatry*, **53**, 1046–50.

Tyrrell, P. J., Kartsounis, L. D., Frackowiak, R. S. *et al.* (1991). Progressive loss of speech output and orofacial dyspraxia associated with frontal lobe hypometabolism [see comments]. *J. Neurol. Neurosurg. Psychiatry*, **54**, 351–7.

Victor, M., Adams, R. D., and Collinge, G. H. (1989). *The Wernicke–Korsakoff's syndrome and related disorders due to alcoholism and malnutrition*. FA Davis, Philadelphia.

Vidal, R., Frangione, B., Rostagno, A. *et al.* (1999). A stop-codon mutation in the *BRI* gene associated with familial British dementia. *Nature*, **399**, 776–81.

Vignolo, L. (1982). Auditory agnosia. *Phil. Trans. R. Soc. Lond. B, Biol. Sci.*, **298**, 49–57.

Wade, D. T., Legh, S. J., and Hewer, R. A. (1987). Depressed mood after stroke. A community study of its frequency. *Br. J. Psychiatry*, **151**, 200–5.

Waldemar, G., Dubois, B., Emre, M. *et al.* (2000). Diagnosis and management of Alzheimer's disease and other disorders associated with dementia: The role of neurologists in Europe. *Europ. J. Neurol.*, **7**, 133–44.

Walstra, G. J., Teunisse, S., van Gool, W. A. *et al.* (1997). Reversible dementia in elderly patients referred to a memory clinic. *J. Neurol.,* **244,** 17–22.

Warrington, E. K. and James, M. (1967). An experimental investigation of facial recognition in patients with unilateral cerebral lesions. *Cortex,* **3,** 317–26.

Warrington, E. K. and James, M. (1967a). Disorders of visual perception in patients with localized cerebral lesions. *Neuropsychologia,* **5,** 253–66.

Warrington, E. K. and McCarthy, R. (1983). Category specific access dysphasia. *Brain,* **106,** 859–78.

Warrington, E. K. and McCarthy, R. A. (1987). Categories of knowledge. Further fractionations and an attempted integration. *Brain,* **110,** 1273–96.

Warrington, E. K. and Shallice, T. (1980). Word-form dyslexia. *Brain,* **103,** 99–112.

Warrington, E. K. and Taylor, A. M. (1973). The contribution of the right parietal lobe to object recognition. *Cortex,* **9,** 152–64.

Warrington, E. K., James, M., and Kinsbourne, M. (1966). Drawing disability in relation to laterality of cerebral lesion. *Brain,* **89,** 53–82.

Weinstein, E. A. and Kahn, R. L. (1952). Non-aphasic misnaming (paraphasia) in organic brain disease. *Arch. Neurol. Psychiatry,* **62,** 72–9.

Wetterling, T., Kanitz, R. D., and Borgis, K. J. (1996). Comparison of different diagnostic criteria for vascular dementia (ADDTC, DSM-IV, ICD-10, NINDS-AIREN). *Stroke,* **27,** 30–6.

Will, R. G., Ironside, J. W., Zeidler, M. *et al.* (1996). A new variant of Creutzfeldt–Jakob disease in the UK [see comments]. *Lancet,* **347,** 921–5.

Williams, M. and Pennybacker, J. (1954). Memory disturbance in third ventricle tumours. *J. Neurol. Neurosurg. Psychiatry,* **17,** 115–23.

Woods, S. C., Seeley, R. J., Porte, D. *et al.* (1998). Signals that regulate food intake and energy homeostasis. *Science,* **280,** 1378–83.

World Health Organization (1992). *The ICD-10 classification of mental and behavioural disorders. Clinical descriptions and diagnostic guidelines.* WHO, Geneva.

Zangwill, O. L. (1979). Two cases of crossed aphasia in dextrals. *Neuropsychologia,* **17,** 167–72.

Zeki, S. (1990). A century of cerebral achromatopsia. *Brain,* **113,** 1721–77.

Zihl, J., von Cramon, D. and Mai, N. (1983). Selective disturbance of movement vision after bilateral brain damage. *Brain,* **106,** 313–40.

Vascular, demyelinating, inflammatory, and degenerative disorders of the brain

CHAPTER 27

Stroke, transient ischaemic attacks, and intracranial venous thrombosis

Charles Warlow

27.1 Introduction

27.1.1 Scope and definitions

This chapter is concerned with those diseases of the cerebral and ocular circulation that cause ischaemia or infarction of the brain and eye, or spontaneous haemorrhage into or around the brain. Most of these vascular diseases take many years to develop (e.g. atheroma, saccular aneurysms) and there is a long asymptomatic period before any clinical manifestations occur (e.g. ischaemic stroke, subarachnoid haemorrhage). These manifestations depend on the location, size, intensity, duration, and number of ischaemic or haemorrhagic events. Although the classification of cerebrovascular disease can be made complex, three practical definitions are adequate for most purposes:

A *transient ischaemic attack* (TIA) is an acute loss of focal brain or monocular function with symptoms lasting less than 24 hours and which is thought to be due to inadequate cerebral or ocular blood supply as a result of arterial thrombosis, embolism, or low flow, associated with arterial, cardiac, or haematological disease (Hankey and Warlow 1994). Residual but functionally unimportant neurological signs may persist for longer, and some patients have CT or MR imaging evidence of infarction in the brain area relevant to the symptoms.

A *stroke* (previously known as a cerebrovascular accident) is rapidly developing clinical symptoms and/or signs of focal, and at times global (applied to patients in deep coma and to those with subarachnoid haemorrhage) loss of brain function, with symptoms lasting more than 24 hours or leading to death, with no apparent cause other than that of vascular origin (Hatano 1976). There is a wide range of severity, from recovery in a few days, through persistent disability, to death.

Although arbitrary, separating TIA from stroke on the basis of this 24-hour time limit is helpful because the differential diagnosis of TIA is not quite the same as stroke, the clinical syndrome of TIA is almost never caused by intracerebral haemorrhage, and in any studies of incidence it is best to concentrate on strokes, which are more uniformly defined and more likely to be reported than TIAs. However, there is no qualitative difference between a TIA and an ischaemic stroke: anything that causes a TIA may, if more severe or prolonged, cause an ischaemic stroke, while any cause of ischaemic stroke may, if less severe or prolonged, cause merely a TIA (Sempere *et al.* 1998). Moreover, the investigation of a patient with a TIA and a mild ischaemic stroke is identical, and there is little difference in their long-term management to reduce the similar risk of any further strokes and other serious vascular events such as myocardial infarction.

About 80 per cent of all first-ever-in-a-lifetime strokes are ischaemic, 10 per cent are due to primary intracerebral haemorrhage, about 5 per cent are due to subarachnoid haemorrhage, and in the remainder there is uncertainty. These proportions are rather similar everywhere strokes have been reliably assessed by CT scanning in community-based incidence studies which, at present, is still largely just in white populations (Fig. 27.1) (Section 27.2.4).

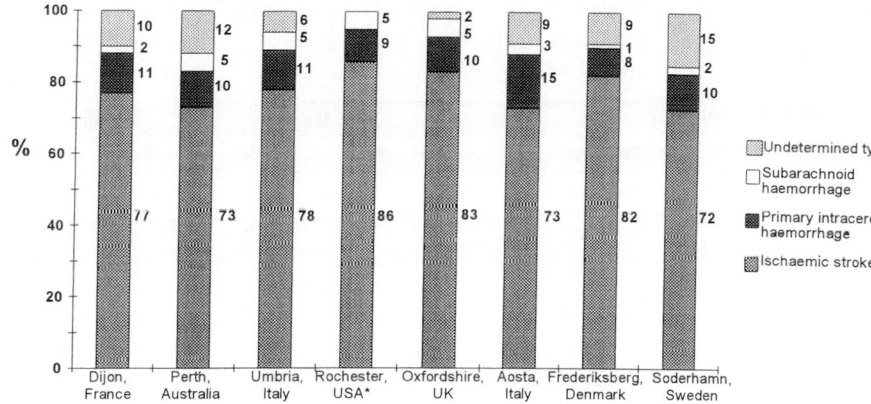

Fig. 27.1. The percentage distribution of the three pathological types of first-ever-in-a-lifetime stroke from age 45 to 84 years in eight comparable community-based studies in the 1980s and 1990s. The numbers by the columns refer to percentages. Undetermined classified as ischaemic stroke.* (Reproduced with permission from Sudlow and Warlow 1997.)

Vascular (so-called arteriosclerotic or multi-infarct dementia) is deterioration in previously normal intellect and/or memory due to repeated clinical or subclinical episodes of cerebral ischaemia, infarction, or haemorrhage (Section 26.6.6). Naturally, after one overt stroke involving the cerebral cortex, a patient may well be left 'demented', but this is not normally what is meant by vascular dementia.

27.1.2 The burden of stroke

After coronary heart disease and all cancers, stroke is the third most common cause of death in the world, causing about 4 million deaths in 1990, three-quarters of them in developing countries (Murray and Lopez 1997). It accounts for 12 per cent of all deaths in England and Wales (Secretary of State for Health 1992), is the most common life-threatening neurological disease (Warlow 1991), and is the most important single cause of severe disability in people living in their own home (Harris 1971). Furthermore, even if the incidence of stroke is declining (Section 27.2.5), the burden will remain substantial for the foreseeable future. If the incidence does not fall, and given the ageing of the population, any increasing burden in the UK, and probably other developed countries, will fall more on the acute hospital services than on rehabilitation facilities, because strokes are more likely to be fatal in very elderly and disabled people than in younger and fitter patients (Malmgren *et al.* 1989).

The cost of stroke is all but impossible to calculate because so much is absorbed by the patients and their families, and much of it is also buried in overall social services budgets. Moreover, very different systems of healthcare incur very different costs, and exchange rates vary. In Scotland, for example, about 7 per cent of all hospital bed days are accounted for by stroke patients, who represent 2 per cent of all hospital discharges; this bed usage is greater than all other conditions with the exception of 'mental disorders' and 'mental handicap'. In financial terms, stroke represents 6 per cent of hospital running costs and 4.6 per cent of all National Health Service costs (Isard and Forbes 1992), and 3 per cent of the Dutch healthcare budget (Evers *et al.* 1997). The average hospital cost for each stroke in Scotland in 1988 was about £6000. Of course, many stroke patients and most transient ischaemic attack patients are not

admitted to hospital or even seen as outpatients, particularly in the UK, and the cost of their care is unknown (Bamford *et al.* 1986; Anderson *et al.* 1994a). A more realistic lifetime cost, which is dominated by the cost of long-term care, including all healthcare services in the community, was nearer £26 000 at 1991 prices in The Netherlands, and although that did not include the cost to the families, it did include the cost of co-morbid conditions (Bergman *et al.* 1995). If the indirect costs of lost productivity are included, the lifetime cost of a stroke works out at about £70 000 at 1990 prices in the USA (Taylor *et al.* 1996). One must remember that many stroke patients are, or will become, disabled by something else, which is also likely to be costly (e.g. coronary artery disease, osteoarthritis), and they may even already be in nursing homes, so the cost of any stroke has to be seen as an incremental cost over and above any non-stroke costs, about £45 000 in Sweden in 1991 (Terent *et al.* 1994).

27.2 Epidemiology of stroke

Our knowledge of stroke epidemiology has lagged behind that of coronary heart disease because:

1. Strokes are not only less frequent than coronary events but they occur later in life, and so in many cohort studies, even with prolonged follow-up, the number of incident strokes is still relatively small (Khaw 1996).

2. The diagnosis of stroke (versus not stroke) is still a matter of clinical skill, often without the help of many, or any, confirmatory investigations. However, this does have the advantage that the diagnosis is independent of the availability and quality of rapidly changing technology (such as CT scanners), which is often not available at all in developing countries, or even universally available in developed countries.

3. Stroke is a disorder of late middle age and the elderly, where other diseases frequently coexist to confuse the situation.

4. There is a low post-mortem rate in most countries.

5. The inaccuracy of death certificates.

Also, strokes are pathologically more diverse than coronary events, which are mostly due to the thrombotic and embolic complications of atheroma. On the other hand, strokes may be due to intracranial small vessel disease which is different from atheroma, embolism from the heart, primary intracerebral haemorrhage (PICH), and subarachnoid haemorrhage (SAH). Therefore, the incidence and aetiology of the main pathological types of stroke should ideally be considered separately, but in many large epidemiological studies this has been impossible, due to lack of CT scanning to reliably separate PICH from ischaemic stroke during life and a low post-mortem rate in fatal cases, and because of the difficulty ascribing a reasonably precise cause for stroke in many patients (e.g. definitely due to atherothromboembolism versus definitely due to intracranial small vessel disease, etc.).

27.2.1 Mortality

Stroke mortality rises rapidly with age (Bonita and Beaglehole 1992). The age-standardized death rate attributed to stroke varies sixfold between developed countries, while very little is known about the developing world (Inzitari *et al.* 1995) (Table 27.1). There is also substantial variation within countries (Pocock *et al.* 1980; Wing *et al.* 1988; He *et al.* 1995) (Table 27.2), and even within cities such as London (Franks *et al.* 1991). Part of the variation arises because stroke mortality is declining so quickly in many countries (Section 27.2.5) that differences may be overestimated if different years are compared. More problematical is that variation in mortality could be due to differences, both in time and place, in how death certificates are completed and coded, as well as uncertainties about the population denominators in terms of both age and sex. The rate of both over- and under-reporting of stroke on death certificates is depressingly high, even in well-organized places such as Framingham (Corwin *et al.* 1982). Fortunately, sudden death is seldom caused by stroke and is, therefore, usually attributed to coronary heart disease, even when no post-mortem is done, and this is correct much more often than not (Thomas *et al.* 1988). Whether, in certain places, some sudden deaths were certified or coded in the past as a stroke rather than a coronary death is unclear. The few relatively sudden stroke deaths that do occur are much more likely to be due to intracranial haemorrhage than ischaemic stroke (Phillips *et al.* 1977).

Naturally, any comparisons in mortality must be age-standardized or, perhaps better, restricted to certain age groups where the diagnosis of stroke is most likely to be correct (age 55–64 years) or where the number of strokes is largest (65–74 years). Of course, a stroke subtype with a very low case fatality (e.g. lacunar infarction) hardly contributes to mortality statistics at all because they reflect only those subtypes with a high case fatality (e.g. total anterior circulation infarction). Therefore, little is known of the relative distribution of stroke subtype mortality between different countries.

Table 27.1. Age-standardized stroke mortality (per 100 000 population) between 40 and 69 years of age in 27 countries in 1985 (Bonita *et al.* 1990)

Country	Men		Women	
	Rank	Rate	Rank	Rate
Bulgaria	1	249	1	156
Hungary	2	229	2	130
Czechoslovakia	3	177	4	103
Romania	4	172	3	129
Yugoslavia	5	145	5	101
Singapore	6	136	6	92
Japan	7	107	11	60
Scotland	8	99	7	77
Finland	9	98	13	57
Poland	10	96	10	62
Hong Kong	11	94	9	64
Austria	12	90	16	48
Northern Ireland	13	84	8	67
Ireland	14	72	12	59
England and Wales	15	71	14	54
Germany	16	68	19	39
Belgium	17	64	18	41
New Zealand	18	62	15	50
France	19	60	26	28
Australia	20	60	17	45
Denmark	21	55	20	38
Norway	22	55	22	35
Sweden	23	48	24	30
Netherlands	24	47	23	31
United States	25	45	21	35
Canada	26	39	25	28
Switzerland	27	38	27	21

Despite these difficulties, very large differences in stroke mortality are probably real, with particularly high rates reported in eastern Europe and Japan, and particularly low rates in North America and some, but not all, western European countries (Table 27.1). These differences seem unlikely to be due to differences in the treatment of acute stroke because, apart from fairly recently introduced stroke units, none are very effective (Section 27.8). Also, one would expect similar early case fatality (death within 30 days) in different countries, any reported differences being more to do with variation in methodology than reality. On the other hand, increasing long-term survival after stroke (Garraway *et al.* 1983), so that later death is attributed to something other than stroke-related disability, such as pneumonia, or is actually due to another dis-

Table 27.2. Cerebrovascular disease mortality in the regions of England and Wales, 1975–79 (Haberman 1984)

Region	Standardized mortality ratio	
	Males	Females
North	121	111
Wales	116	116
North-west	116	111
Yorkshire/Humberside	106	101
East Midlands	104	101
West Midlands	104	101
East Anglia	100	103
South-west	98	103
South-east	84	89

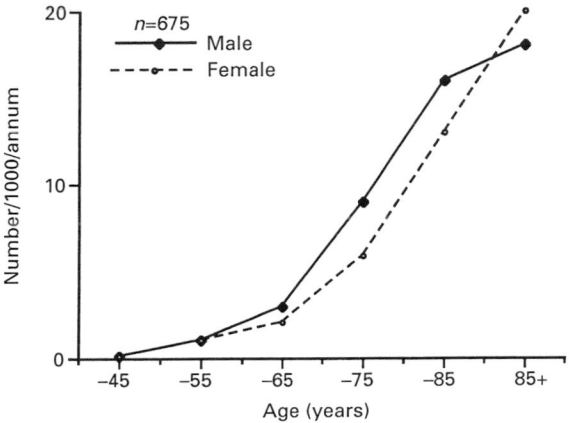

Fig. 27.2. Age- and sex-specific annual incidence of first-ever-in-a-life-time stroke per 1000 population in Oxfordshire in the mid 1980s (with permission from Bamford *et al.* 1988).

order, such as coronary heart disease, may be part of the explanation of mortality differences (Corwin *et al.* 1982). Another reason might be that the strokes most likely to be fatal (e.g. intracranial haemorrhage) are more frequent in countries with high stroke mortality; but there are no good data to substantiate this, particularly since the diagnosis of pathological type of stroke, other than subarachnoid haemorrhage, from death certificates is very unreliable (Florey *et al.* 1969). Finally, differences in mortality might reflect differences in incidence but, at least where incidence has been measured, any differences are not so extreme and cannot be the entire explanation (Section 27.2.2).

27.2.2 **Incidence**

The incidence of new cases of first-ever-in-a-lifetime stroke, usually expressed per 1000 population per annum, can only be reliably assessed in prospective community-based studies using obsessional methodology to identify all possible patients (Sudlow and Warlow 1996). Hospital-based studies are subject to referral bias, and claims that 'all stroke patients are admitted' have seldom, if ever, been substantiated; both very mild and rapidly fatal strokes are the least likely to be represented in hospital statistics. The incidence in the UK is approximately 2/1000/year (Bamford *et al.* 1988); about 100 000 patients have a first stroke every year, one every 5 minutes or so. As is already clear from general experience, stroke incidence rises rapidly with age; about a quarter occur below the age of 65, and about a half below the age of 75 (Fig. 27.2).

Curiously, there is much less between-country difference in stroke incidence than in mortality (Section 27.2.1). However, reasonably accurate and comparable estimates of incidence are only really available in a few white populations (Fig. 27.3) and, even where they are, the sample sizes are often too small for satisfactory precision (Lemesle *et al.* 1996). None the less,

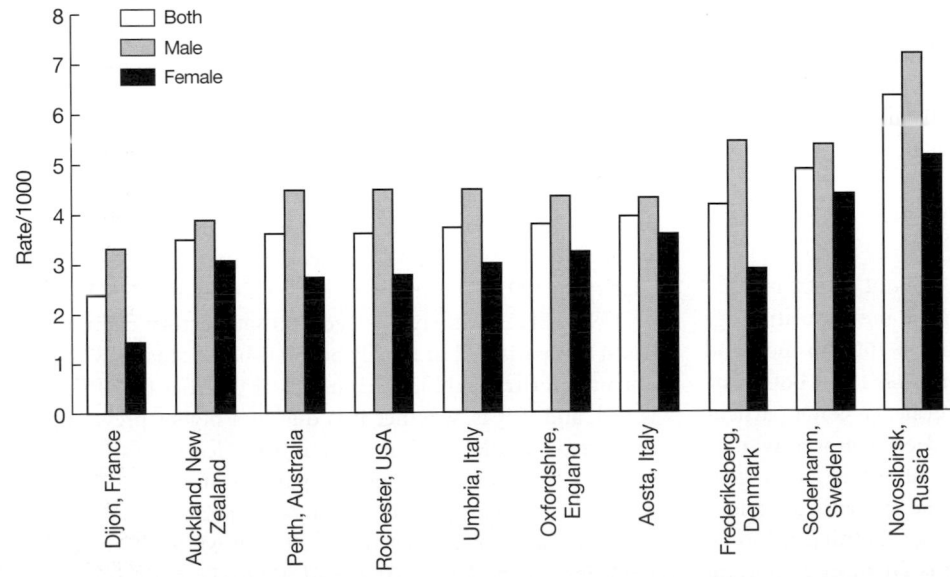

Fig. 27.3. Age- and sex-standardized annual incidence of first-ever-in-a-lifetime stroke per 1000, aged 45–84 years, males and females considered separately and together, in 10 'ideal' community-based studies in the 1980s and 1990s (with permission from Sudlow and Warlow 1997).

stroke incidence does seem to be about twice as common in Novosibirsk in Russia compared with Dijon, but not Avallon, in France, notwithstanding a much larger difference in stroke mortality between the two countries.

Like mortality, the interpretation of different incidence rates depends on when the study was done, because, in some countries at least, the incidence is changing (Section 27.2.5). If there really are large geographical variations in stroke incidence, we clearly need to find out how much can be explained by differences in risk-factor prevalence (and the causes of any differences such as diet) and by differences in the prevalence of direct causes of stroke, such as rheumatic heart disease, and how these relate to racial and genetic factors. The WHO MONICA study is examining these issues for both coronary heart disease and stroke, but will not provide as much information on the latter because of the considerable difficulties in measuring, monitoring, and comparing stroke incidence overall, let alone by stroke type (Sudlow and Warlow 1996), and also because patients over the age of 65, where about 75 per cent of strokes occur, are mostly not accounted for (Asplund *et al.* 1995). On the whole, the MONICA results are similar to others, with the highest stroke incidence in Russia, eastern Europe, and China, but the very large variation in case fatality does suggest that there were problems with case ascertainment, something so difficult to avoid in one place, let alone in almost 20 (Thorvaldsen *et al.* 1995).

Apart from subarachnoid haemorrhage, it is impossible to separate strokes reliably during life into pathological types without CT scanning, so until recently no study could provide much information on incidence for each type separately. Indeed, an apparent increase in incidence, but fall in case fatality, of primary intracerebral haemorrhage was readily explained by the more sensitive diagnosis of small, non-fatal haemorrhages after CT scanning was introduced (Drury *et al.* 1984). Also, because ischaemic stroke accounts for the vast majority of strokes (Fig. 27.1), the rates for primary intracerebral and subarachnoid haemorrhage are less robust since they are based on small numbers. None the less, the incidence of all three main pathological types of stroke increases with age; the small decline of primary intracerebral and subarachnoid haemorrhage incidence in the very elderly may be due to diagnostic difficulties in this group of people (Bamford *et al.* 1990*a*).

27.2.3 Prevalence

A typical estimate of stroke prevalence is about 5/1000 population, but clearly the exact figure depends on the population age and sex structure, and becomes about 50/1000 in men and 25/1000 in women aged 65–74 (Wyller *et al.* 1994; Bots *et al.* 1996; Geddes *et al.* 1996). However, prevalence is not particularly interesting because incidence, and even mortality, data provide much more useful information about aetiology, geographical distribution, time trends, and the influence of various risk factors. Furthermore, for health service planning purposes, the prevalence of disability in general is far more important than just stroke-related disability, particularly when one comes

to consider elderly populations who have so many additional causes of disability impossible to disentangle from stroke-related disability, such as arthritis, claudication, and dementia. Indeed, prevalence is difficult to measure anyway because a large representative sample of the population has to be identified as the denominator, a large number of people in that sample must be surveyed and perhaps seen and questioned, many past stroke episodes are forgotten by patients, fatal strokes are not included, and there is the ever-present possibility of diagnostic error in retrospective surveys. Also, stroke prevalence depends on incidence and survival, both of which may vary by time and place (Section 27.2.5).

27.2.4 Racial and social influences

Despite the difficulties in defining racial groups, measuring deprivation, and understanding the concept of social class, there are some interesting, and perhaps informative, differences in stroke risk.

Japanese and Chinese populations

Although there have been no absolutely comparable incidence studies, it does seem likely that stroke, particularly primary intracerebral haemorrhage (PICH), is more common in Japan and China than in Western countries (Huang *et al.* 1990). Also there is less extracranial but more intracranial arterial disease in the Japanese and Chinese compared with white populations (Resche *et al.* 1969; Feldman *et al.* 1990; Leung *et al.* 1993).

South Asian populations in the UK

South Asian populations in the UK have a high prevalence of coronary heart disease, central obesity (i.e. high waist-to-hip ratio), insulin resistance, non-insulin-dependent diabetes, and hypertension (McKeigue *et al.* 1991), and a high stroke mortality, but there is no good information on incidence (Balarajan 1991). This seems to be due partly to genetic susceptibility (high serum lipoprotein(a) levels) in these people, potentiated by dietary- and lifestyle-induced changes in lipid levels (Bhatnagar *et al.* 1995).

Black populations

In the USA and the UK, stroke mortality, as well as prevalence and possibly incidence, are higher in black than white populations, and this applies to ischaemic stroke as well as PICH (Balarajan 1991; Howard *et al.* 1994; Giles *et al.* 1995; Pickle *et al.* 1997). Because there has been no satisfactory community-based comparison, but mostly hospital-based studies with their potential for referral bias, it is not clear whether this difference is real, and if it is, whether it is due to a higher prevalence of hypertension, diabetes, obesity, and sickle-cell trait in black patients. Nor is it clear that the pattern of arterial disease is definitely different, with less extracranial and more intracranial occlusive vascular disease compared with whites (Caplan *et al.* 1986; Sacco *et al.* 1995; Wityk *et al.* 1996). Perhaps some of the geographical pattern of stroke mortality in the USA can be explained by the distribution of the black population, but another explanation could be social deprivation in these patients, either at the time of the survey or much earlier during childhood or even neonatal life (Davey Smith *et al.* 1998). Almost nothing is known of stroke rates in Sub-Saharan Africa, where mortality is said to be high.

Maori and Pacific Islands people

Maori and Pacific Islands people in New Zealand have a higher stroke incidence than Europeans, perhaps due to differences in risk factors and health-related behaviours (Bonita *et al.* 1997).

Deprivation

In the UK stroke mortality is greater in deprived than in affluent areas (Carstairs and Morris 1990), amongst the un-employed (Franks *et al.* 1991), and in lower compared with higher social classes (Shaper *et al.* 1991). The situation is similar in other countries (Kunst *et al.* 1998). At least in part, this is due to poverty being associated with adverse health behaviours and risk factors such as smoking (Pekkanen *et al.* 1995). There is also evidence that poor maternal and infant health is associated with increased mortality from stroke some decades later, apparently independently of the confounding effect of adverse circumstances in adult life being so often associated with similar circumstances in early life (Barker 1995; Martyn *et al.* 1996). Possibly this is because adult blood pressure, non-insulin-dependent diabetes, and raised plasma fibrinogen are all related to low birth weight, a marker of fetal growth failure, perhaps itself a consequence of fetal undernutrition. However, this intriguing hypothesis has not gone unchallenged and there is evidence of a cumulative effect of socio-economic deprivation throughout life (Ben-Shlomo and Davey Smith 1991; Paneth and Susser 1995; Davey Smith *et al.* 1997).

27.2.5 Time trends in mortality and incidence

With some striking exceptions in eastern Europe, stroke mortality is declining in those places where it has been measured, and even faster than coronary heart disease mortality (Fig. 27.4). The reality of the reported decline does depend on the proper interpretation of the changes in ICD coding over the years (Schoenberg and Schulte 1989) and on the accuracy of the mortality statistics themselves (Section 27.2.1). If the decline is real, which it almost certainly is, it may reflect: improved survival after stroke, for which there is some evidence, but this can have had little to do with specific treatments because in acute stroke nothing makes very much difference, except stroke units which are a recent development in only a few places (Section 27.8) (Garraway *et al.* 1983; Terent 1989; Bonita *et al.* 1993; Peltonen *et al.* 1998); less misclassification of sudden deaths as stroke; a decline in the incidence of only primary intracerebral or sub-arachnoid haemorrhage, which are more likely to be fatal than ischaemic stroke; or a decline in the incidence of strokes of all severities. Direct evidence of a decline in stroke incidence is hard to come by, because if measuring incidence once in one place is

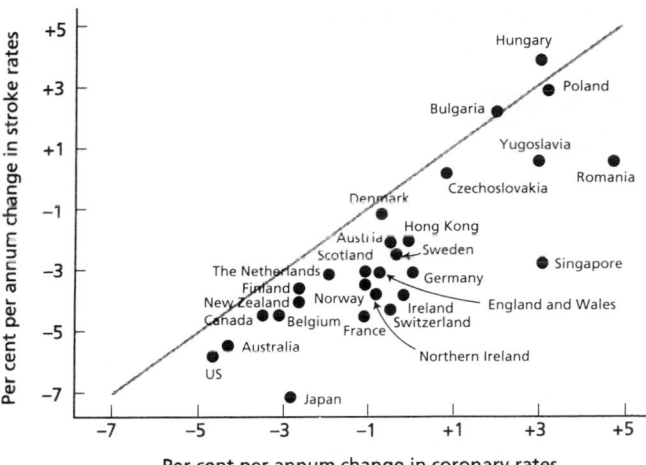

Fig. 27.4. Comparison of the annual percentage decline of age-standardized mortality due to stroke compared with coronary heart disease, in men aged 40–69 years, from 1970 to 1985 in 27 countries with reasonably reliable death certification data (with permission from Bonita *et al.* 1990).

difficult (Section 27.2.2), measuring it accurately over time is even more difficult as definitions and diagnostic technology change (Bonita and Baeglehole 1996). For example, incidence did decline in Rochester, Minnesota, but is now increasing again (Brown *et al.* 1996a) and is declining in Copenhagen (Truelsen *et al.* 1997). However, it seems to be increasing in Novosibirsk (Feigin *et al.* 1995) and in Soderhamn, Sweden (Terent 1988), but not changing in Auckland, New Zealand, perhaps because strokes are getting milder, and milder strokes are getting easier to detect (Bonita *et al.* 1993). The reported decline in stroke incidence in most of the MONICA centres is based on a rather small number of events, an age cut-off at 65 years, and some concerns about accurate case ascertainment, but at least it goes along with the notion that stroke incidence really is on the decline (WHO MONICA Project 1997). CT scanning has not been available for long enough to provide data on time trends for the various pathological types of stroke, although it does not seem that subarachnoid haemorrhage has declined in Rochester, Minnesota (Ingall *et al.* 1989), although it has in New Zealand (Truelsen *et al.* 1998).

If incidence really is declining, the reasons are unclear, but they must be environmental (diet, smoking, etc.), and so potentially modifiable, rather than genetic. Possibly the prevalence of causative risk factors (such as hypertension) or direct causes (such as rheumatic heart disease) is less than it was, but accurate data are hard to come by. Although often assumed, it is most unlikely that the treatment of hypertension is responsible, since the decline in stroke mortality probably started earlier (Whisnant 1983) and, in any event, treatment cannot explain more than 25 per cent of the decline at most (Bonita and Beaglehole 1989). The identification and treatment of TIAs is unlikely to have had much population impact, largely because only a small proportion of strokes are preceded by TIAs (Warlow 1998a).

27.2.6 **Seasonal and diurnal variation**

In most studies, both stroke mortality and hospital admission rates are higher in winter than summer (Douglas *et al.* 1991; Pan *et al.* 1995; Feigin and Weibers 1997). This seasonal variation might be explained by the complications of stroke being more likely to be fatal in the winter (e.g. pneumonia) and because it might be more difficult to look after stroke patients at home in cold weather. It cannot just be assumed to reflect stroke incidence. Indeed, where incidence has been measured in the community, there is little, if any, seasonal variation, at least in temperate climates, although primary intracerebral haemorrhage is somewhat more likely on cold days (Rothwell *et al.* 1996; Jakovljevic *et al.* 1996). There is little doubt that stroke occurs most frequently in the hour or two after waking in the morning, but whether this applies to categories of stroke other than just ischaemic stroke is difficult to say because of the relatively small proportion of intracranial haemorrhages (Kelly-Hayes *et al.* 1995; Elliott 1998). Subarachnoid haemorrhage is very unlikely to occur during sleep and, in general, most likely during strenuous activities (Wroe *et al.* 1992).

27.2.7 **Risk factors**

Risk factors for ischaemic stroke are listed in Table 27.3.

A risk factor (e.g. for ischaemic stroke) is a characteristic of an individual, or of a population, associated with an increased risk of disease (e.g. an ischaemic stroke) compared with an individual, or a population, without that characteristic. This association can be over or underestimated (i.e. confounded) by not taking into account, for example, age, because the prevalence of most vascular risk factors, other than smoking, increases with age, which is itself the strongest determinant of stroke incidence. Therefore, any estimate of excess risk associated with a risk factor must be adjusted, at the very least, for age if those with and those without the risk factor are of different ages.

The *strength* of the association between a risk factor and, for example, stroke is given by a ratio (relative risk or relative odds), the number of times greater the frequency of stroke is in a group of individuals with the risk factor compared with the frequency in those without it (Table 27.4). But, association does not necessarily imply causality, which is inferred more by the strength of the association (high relative risk or relative odds); the consistency of the association in different studies and populations; the presence of a dose–response relationship (the more

Table 27.3. Risk factors for ischaemic stroke: the order is not related to the strength or relevance of their association with stroke and these associations are not necessarily 'causal', or independent from each other

Factors associated with an increased risk of vascular disease

  Age
  Male sex
  Increasing blood pressure
  Cigarette smoking
  Blood lipids*
  Diabetes mellitus
  Increasing plasma fibrinogen
  Raised factor VII coagulant activity*
  Raised tissue plasminogen activator antigen*
  Low blood fibrinolytic activity*
  Raised von Willebrand factor
  Raised haematocrit
  Atrial fibrillation
  Sex hormones
  Excess alcohol consumption
  Obesity and diet*
  Physical inactivity
  Raised white blood cell count
  Recent infection*
  Hyperhomocysteinaemia
  Snoring*
  Corneal arcus*
  Psychological factors*
  Vasectomy*
  Low serum albumin*
  Diagonal earlobe crease*
  Impaired ventilatory function*
  Family history of stroke
  Social deprivation

Evidence of pre-existing vascular disease

  Myocardial infarction/angina
  Cardiac failure
  Left ventricular hypertrophy
  Peripheral vascular disease
  Cervical arterial bruit and stenosis
  Transient ischaemic attacks

* Somewhat uncertain association with stroke

Table 27.4. Calculation of relative risk, relative odds, and absolute risk difference in a longitudinal study of a cohort of individuals, some of whom have a risk factor for stroke at baseline ($a + b$), and some of whom develop a stroke during follow-up ($a + c$)

		Stroke	
		yes	no
Risk factor	yes	a	b
	no	c	d

Risk of stroke in those with the risk factor $(R+) = \dfrac{a}{a+b}$

Risk of stroke in those without the risk factor $(R-) = \dfrac{c}{c+d}$

Relative risk $= \dfrac{(R+)}{(R-)}$ i.e. $\dfrac{ac+ad}{ac+bc}$ **Absolute risk difference** $= (R+) - (R-)$

Odds of stroke in those with the risk factor $(o+) = \dfrac{a}{b}$

Odds of stroke in those without the risk factor $(o-) = \dfrac{c}{d}$

Relative odds (or odds ratio) $= \dfrac{o+}{o-}$ i.e. $\dfrac{ad}{bc}$

When stroke is rare (i.e. if a and c are small compared with b and d) then the relative risk and relative odds are about the same size.

the risk factor, the higher the frequency of the disease); independence from confounding factors; temporal sequence with the risk factor first and then the disease, remembering that the onset of the symptoms of stroke may be years after the onset of the underlying pathology (e.g. atheroma, aneurysm, etc.); biological and epidemiological plausibility; and by the effect of experimental removal of the risk factor in randomized trials or, rather less persuasively, in non-randomized comparisons.

The *relevance* of the association of a risk factor to the incidence of stroke is given by the absolute risk difference between those with and those without the risk factor (Table 27.4). Even if the relative risk high, the relevance will be small if the risk factor is rarely present in the population (Ebrahim 1990). For example, although the relative risk of stroke for patients with rheumatic atrial fibrillation is very high, the fact that rheumatic heart disease is now so rare in developed countries means that it is still a very rare cause of stroke, i.e. it 'explains' only a small proportion of strokes and so has a low attributable risk. On the other hand, a risk factor that is common and yet does not carry a particularly high relative risk (e.g. mild hypertension) will 'explain' a much higher proportion of strokes (compared with severe hypertension, which is rare); indeed, about three-quarters of stroke deaths attributed to hypertension arise in people whose diastolic blood pressure is less than 110 mmHg (Table 27.5). Also, if the background risk of stroke in a population is very low (e.g. in young women), exposure to quite a high relative risk (e.g. by taking oral contraceptives) will not increase the absolute risk of stroke to a high level. The effect of risk factors on subsequent stroke incidence is usually additive or multiplicative, so that the presence of several risk factors puts an individual at particularly high risk. Not surprisingly, therefore, there have been attempts to assign individuals into categories of stroke risk on the basis of their risk-factor profile, but these mathematical models have not yet been validated widely nor used much in clinical practice (D'Agostino *et al.* 1994; Truelsen *et al.* 1994).

Most of the reliable evaluations of stroke risk factors have come from cohort studies, such as in Framingham, where there has been no, or little, division of strokes into ischaemic stroke or primary intracerebral haemorrhage, and even less division into subtypes such as lacunar infarction. Other studies have often only assessed stroke mortality, with the problem that stroke types likely to be fatal are over-represented (e.g. haemor-

rhagic stroke, stroke in diabetes, etc.). Also, because most strokes are ischaemic, most studies have been to do with risk factors for ischaemic rather than haemorrhagic stroke. In case-control studies it is easier to divide strokes into their pathological types, but there is also more potential for various biases in the selection of controls (selection bias), exclusion of cases through death (survival bias), unblinded assessment of risk factors (recall bias), and the possibility that the stroke itself, or changed patient behaviour after the stroke, has changed a risk factor in some way (reverse causality). Recently, studies relating risk factors to carotid stenosis, itself a variable mixture of atheroma and thrombosis, as assessed with ultrasound, have begun to appear, but so far have not led to any new insights or aetiological hypotheses (Fine-Edelstein *et al.* 1994). Even more recently, risk factors have been related to the intima–media thickness of the carotid arterial wall, also assessed with ultrasound, as a possible surrogate for atheroma (Crouse *et al.* 1996).

Although there do seem to be quantitative differences between ischaemic stroke and coronary heart disease risk factors (the sex difference being the most obvious), there is probably no qualitative difference (i.e. a risk factor for one is a risk factor for the other, even if the strength of the association is different). This is not very surprising because a large proportion of strokes are due to the thromboembolic complications of atheroma, as are most clinical manifestations of coronary heart disease.

The vast majority of ischaemic stroke patients have well-recognized risk factors for vascular disease, mostly known about for some time before stroke onset (Table 27.6) (Shaper *et al.* 1991). This suggests it should be possible to make a considerable impact on stroke incidence by reducing the prevalence of causal risk factors in the population and by screening or case finding for 'high-risk' individuals to whom preventive treatment may be offered (Section 27.10.1).

Age

Age is the strongest risk factor for ischaemic stroke, primary intracerebral haemorrhage, and subarachnoid haemorrhage

Table 27.6. Prevalence of vascular risk factors in 244 patients with a first-ever-in-a-lifetime ischaemic stroke in the Oxfordshire Community Stroke Project (Sandercock *et al.* 1989)

	n	(%)
Hypertension (BP >160/90 mmHg × 2 pre-stroke)	126	(52)
Angina and/or myocardial infarction	92	(38)
Current smokers*	66	(27)
Claudication and/or absent foot pulses	60	(25)
Major cardiac embolic source	50	(20)
Transient ischaemic attack	35	(14)
Cervical arterial bruit	33	(14)
Diabetes mellitus	24	(10)
Any of the above	196	(80)

* Unpublished data.

Table 27.5. Population-attributable mortality from stroke in males arising at different levels of blood pressure: the Whitehall Study (Rose 1981)

Diastolic blood pressure (mmHg)	Cumulative % of excess deaths attributable to hypertension
<80	0
<90	14
<100	25
<110	73

(Bamford *et al.* 1990*a*) and almost certainly for the subtypes of ischaemic stroke as well (e.g. lacunar infarction (Fig. 27.2.)). For example, stroke in people aged 75–84 is about 25 times more common than in people aged 45–54.

Sex

There is a small excess of males, which is most prominent in middle to old age, disappearing in the very elderly and probably absent in the young (Fig. 27.2). Even though most strokes are due to infarction, and most infarcts are due to atherothromboembolism, it is curious how the male predominance is so much less than in the other two main clinical manifestations of atheroma—myocardial infarction and peripheral vascular disease.

Blood pressure

In healthy populations, in both sexes and allowing for the association with age, increasing blood pressure is strongly associated with subsequent stroke risk, and probably with all the main pathological types (Whelton 1994; Thrift *et al.* 1998). Although most of the information comes from consideration of the diastolic blood pressure, the relationship with systolic blood pressure is similar and possibly stronger, and even 'isolated' systolic hypertension is associated with increased risk (Shaper *et al.* 1991; Keli *et al.* 1992; Sagie *et al.* 1993; Petrovitch *et al.* 1995). The relationship between usual diastolic blood pressure and stroke is 'log-linear' throughout the normal range, with no evidence of a threshold below which the risk becomes stable, even in patients who have already had cerebrovascular symptoms (Rodgers *et al.* 1996) (Fig. 27.5). The percentage difference in stroke risk associated with a given difference in blood pressure is similar, in males and females, at all levels of blood pressure and about doubles with each 7.5 mmHg

increase in usual diastolic blood pressure in Western populations, and with each 5.0 mmHg in Japanese and Chinese populations (MacMahon *et al.* 1990; Eastern Stroke and Coronary Heart Disease Collaborative Research Group 1998). Studies that have shown a 'J'-shaped curve, with increasing risk of stroke at the lowest blood pressures, have probably been subject to publication bias and almost certainly included patients with prior vascular disease or treated hypertension, which might have led to higher risks at low blood pressures.

Because the strength of the blood pressure/stroke association is so strong, consistent, and biologically plausible (see below), and because treatment of hypertension reduces stroke risk (Collins and MacMahon 1994; Mulrow *et al.* 1994) (Section 27.10.3), one can be sure that hypertension is a causal risk factor, at least for strokes in general, even if not for any one particular type of stroke compared with another. Moreover, the population-attributable risk for mild hypertension is not only greater than for severe hypertension (Table 27.5), but because it is so prevalent in the population at large, it is greater than any other risk factor.

Overall, the association between increasing blood pressure and stroke is less in the elderly than in middle age (Prospective Studies Collaboration 1995). What is not quite so clear is whether hypertension is still a risk factor in the very elderly, where stroke may be associated with low pressures, perhaps because low pressures are a reflection of pre-existing cardiovascular and other disease (Evans 1987; Glynn *et al.* 1995).

Hypertension probably increases stroke risk by increasing the extent and severity of atheroma (Chobanian 1983; Lusiani *et al.* 1987; Reed *et al.* 1988; Fine-Edelstein *et al.* 1994) and the prevalence of small vessel disease in the perforating arteries within the brain (Ross Russell 1975).

Cigarette smoking

Cigarette smoking has been better accepted as a risk factor for coronary heart disease than stroke. However, there is no doubt of an association with stroke (relative risk about 1.5), there is a dose–response relationship, males and females are equally affected, the association seems to become weaker in the elderly, and there is perhaps an association with passive smoking (Shinton and Beevers 1989; Donnan *et al.* 1993; Doll *et al.* 1994; Thrift *et al.* 1999). Although smoking is a strong risk factor for subarachnoid haemorrhage (relative risk about 3.0) and for ischaemic stroke (relative risk about 2.0) there appears to be less association with primary intracerebral haemorrhage. Ex-cigarette smokers have a sustained excess risk of stroke for some years (Shinton and Beevers 1989; Kawachi *et al.* 1993). Smoking has been related to the extent of carotid disease in patients selected for angiography (Homer *et al.* 1991), by ultrasound (Fine-Edelstein *et al.* 1994; Howard *et al.* 1998), and in identical twins discordant for smoking (Haapanen *et al.* 1989). There are no good data linking pipe and cigar smoking with coronary heart disease, let alone with stroke, perhaps because there are not enough people to study in these more than usually anti-social smoking groups.

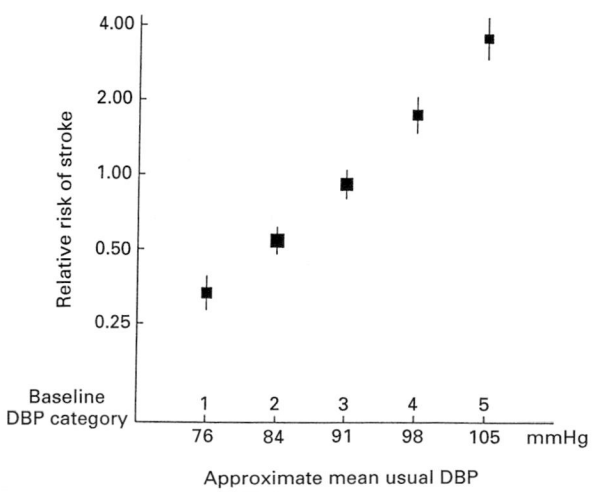

Fig. 27.5. The relative risk of stroke related to the usual diastolic blood pressure (DBP) at baseline from an overview of seven prospective studies in mostly Western populations. The error bars are 95 per cent confidence intervals (with permission from MacMahon *et al.* 1990).

Blood lipids

There is no doubt that increasing levels of total plasma cholesterol and low-density lipoprotein cholesterol, and to a lesser extent decreasing levels of high-density lipoprotein cholesterol, are strong risk factors for coronary heart disease, whereas blood triglyceride levels are less predictive (Law *et al.* 1994*a*; Hokanson and Austin 1996). The relationship with cholesterol is causal, because lowering plasma cholesterol reduces the risk of coronary events; a long-term reduction in plasma cholesterol of 0.6 mmol/l should reduce the risk of coronary events by about 25 per cent, more so in the young than in the elderly. However, any relationship between blood lipids and stroke is much weaker, if it exists at all (Lindenstrom *et al.* 1994; Prospective Studies Collaboration 1995), although perhaps increased serum lipoprotein(a) is predictive (Jurgens *et al.* 1995). Some attempts to relate atheroma in the extra- and intracranial circulation to blood lipid concentrations have suggested an association (Reed *et al.* 1988; Homer *et al.* 1991; Fine-Edelstein *et al.* 1994). Rather surprisingly, therefore, cholesterol lowering does seem to reduce stroke risk, albeit in fairly low-risk (of stroke) populations (Section 27.10.3).

This contrast between cardiovascular and cerebrovascular disease is unexpected, and may be due to lipid levels being less associated with vascular events in elderly people (where most strokes occur) than in younger people (where coronary events are much more common than stroke); loss of stroke-susceptible individuals from populations by prior coronary death; lack of statistical power in cohort studies and randomized trials, which have mostly been concerned with coronary events rather than with the smaller number of strokes; confounding in case-control and cohort studies; the relatively narrow range of blood cholesterol that has been examined in many studies; or, perhaps, because cholesterol is negatively associated with intracranial haemorrhage which obscures any positive association with ischaemic stroke in studies of 'all strokes' (Law *et al.* 1994*b*; Eastern Stroke and Coronary Heart Disease Collaborative Research Group 1998).

Diabetes mellitus

Diabetes mellitus has long been recognized as a risk factor for vascular disease and about doubles the risk of stroke compared with non-diabetics, probably independently of any association with other risk factors such as hypertension (Rosengren *et al.* 1989; Manson *et al.* 1991; Burchfiel *et al.* 1994). However, care must be taken when interpreting any relationship between diabetes and mortality, since strokes in diabetics are more likely to be fatal (Jorgensen *et al.* 1994).

Haemostatic variables

Although there is a relationship between increasing plasma fibrinogen and stroke, it is attenuated by adjusting for cigarette smoking and other confounding variables, such as infections and even social class (Cook and Ubben 1990; Rosengren *et al.* 1990; Qizilbash *et al.* 1991; Ernst and Resch 1993; Brunner *et al.* 1996; Lowe al 1997). Perhaps the adverse vascular effect of ciga-rette smoking is mediated, at least in part, by increasing fibrinogen levels and thus accelerating thrombosis. On the other hand, it is not at all certain that a raised plasma fibrinogen is causally related to stroke, either by increasing plasma viscosity or by promoting thrombosis. It is difficult to lower plasma fibrinogen consistently and no randomized trials have been done.

Raised plasma factor VII coagulant activity, raised tissue plasminogen activator antigen, low blood fibrinolytic activity, and raised von Willebrand factor are all risk factors for coronary heart disease and perhaps also for stroke (Meade *et al.* 1993; Qizilbash *et al.* 1997; Macko *et al.* 1999). Other coagulation, fibrinolytic, and platelet parameters have not been associated consistently with vascular disease, and the literature is bedevilled by the problem that these factors are so often affected by the stroke itself, and the lack of large cohort studies.

Haematocrit

Although cerebral blood flow is strongly related to haematocrit (Section 27.3.4), any association of increasing haematocrit with risk of stroke, or type of stroke, is weak and confounded by cigarette smoking, blood pressure, and plasma fibrinogen (Welin *et al.* 1987).

Atrial fibrillation

The most frequent potential cardiac source of embolism to the brain is atrial fibrillation (AF), by virtue of clot forming in the left atrium and its appendage (Narayan *et al.* 1997. In developed countries, where rheumatic heart disease is now rare, atrial fibrillation is usually 'non-rheumatic' (Table 27.7) (Hart and Halperin 1994). Both 'non-rheumatic' and, more so, rheumatic AF have been associated with stroke from postmortem evidence (Aberg 1969; Yamanouchi *et al.* 1997*b*); case-control studies (Friedman *et al.* 1968); and cohort studies (Wolf *et al.* 1978; Flegel *et al.* 1987; Harmsen *et al.* 1990). The risk of first stroke is about 5 per cent per year in non-rheumatic atrial fibrillation. 'Lone' atrial fibrillation (i.e. no other cardiac disease) seems still to be a risk factor unless so strictly defined that it represents less than 10 per cent of all

Table 27.7. Prevalence of potential cardiac sources of embolism in 244 patients with a first-ever-in-a-lifetime ischaemic stroke in the Oxfordshire Community Stroke Project (Sandercock *et al.* 1989)

	n	(%)
Atrial fibrillation without rheumatic heart disease	28	(11)
Atrial fibrillation with rheumatic heart disease	3	(1)
Any atrial fibrillation	31	(13)
Mitral incompetence	15	(6)
Recent myocardial infarction (previous 6 weeks)	12	(5)
Prosthetic heart valve	3	(1)
Mitral stenosis	2	(1)
Paradoxical embolism	1	(1)
Any of the above	50	(20)
Any minor potential cardiac source of embolism*	28	(11)

* Aortic stenosis/sclerosis, mitral annulus calcification, mitral leaflet prolapse, aortic incompetence, cardiomyopathy.

fibrillators where the embolic risk is then minimal (Close *et al.* 1979; Brand *et al.* 1985; Kopecky *et al.* 1987). Within the fibrillating population, there are individuals at particularly high risk of stroke, for example probably those with a previous embolic event, increasing age, hypertension, diabetes, along perhaps with left ventricular dysfunction and an enlarged left atrium (Stroke Prevention in Atrial Fibrillation Investigators 1992, 1995; Atrial Fibrillation Investigators 1994; Di Pasquale *et al.* 1995).

Some of the association between AF and stroke must be coincidental rather than causal, because AF can be caused by coronary and hypertensive heart disease, both of which may be associated with stroke by mechanisms other than embolism from the fibrillating left atrium, such as carotid stenosis or hypertensive primary intracerebral haemorrhage. Also, apparent intracerebral haemorrhage in AF may be confused with haemorrhagic transformation of an infarct on CT, or the AF may even be a consequence of stroke. Although anticoagulation markedly reduces the risk of first or recurrent stroke (Sections 27.10.1 and 27.10.3), this is not good evidence for causality because this treatment may be working in other ways, such as inhibiting artery-to-artery embolism.

Because AF prevalence is very closely related to age, most strokes associated with AF are in the very elderly, where the proportion attributed to AF is also highest (Wolf *et al.* 1991*a*). However, the population-attributable risk should not be exaggerated, since AF is present in less than 20 per cent of all ischaemic stroke patients who, anyway, may have some other, possibly more likely, cause of stroke, such as carotid stenosis or intracranial small vessel disease (Bogousslavsky *et al.* 1990; Sandercock *et al.* 1992; Kanter *et al.* 1994).

The epidemiological and clinical evidence is insufficient to link either the onset, or the chronicity, of AF with the development of embolic stroke, nor is it clear whether paroxysmal AF is particularly likely or unlikely to cause stroke (Lip 1997; Yamanouchi *et al.* 1997*a*). How often thyrotoxic AF causes embolic stroke is uncertain, but it cannot be very frequently (Parker and Lawson 1973; Petersen and Hansen 1988).

Sex hormones

It is tempting to attribute the lower incidence of ischaemic vascular disorders, including stroke, in women compared with men to differences in their endogenous sex hormones. However, this is difficult to sustain because exogenous high-dose oestrogen given to elderly men with prostatic cancer increases their risk of vascular death (Byar and Corle 1988); if anything, men with coronary heart disease do not have low, but high, levels of female sex hormones; in female survivors, stroke severity is related to oestrogen levels (Jeppesen *et al.* 1996); and oral contraceptives about triple the risk of ischaemic stroke (less for haemorrhagic strokes). Fortunately, the modern oral contraceptive, progestagen-only or with a lower oestrogen content, probably carries a lower risk, and there is no excess risk in ex-users. In fact, only about 10 per cent of strokes in young women are likely to be due to oral contraceptives, even assuming the association is causal (Stampfer *et al.* 1990; WHO

Collaborative Study 1996*a, b*; Heinemann *et al.* 1997). Unless a user of oral contraceptives is also hypertensive, a cigarette smoker, and over the age of about 30, the absolute risk of a serious vascular event is so low that even a tripling of stroke risk does not give great cause for concern. Oral contraceptive users who are also carriers of mutations causing thrombophilias are particularly likely to be affected by intracranial venous thrombosis (Vandenbroucke 1998).

Although there were concerns about postmenopausal oestrogen replacement, it now seems there is no increased risk of stroke or coronary events, indeed there may even be less risk, but the effect of added progestagen is not known (Paganini-Hill *et al.* 1988; Grady *et al.* 1992; Belchetz 1994). On the other hand, there is some increased risk of breast and uterine cancer, and of venous thromboembolism (Davidson 1995; Vandenbroucke and Helmerhorst 1996). However, all this information is based on observational data rather than randomized trials, which are mostly as yet unfinished, and so there is still much controversy about the routine use of this treatment in post-menopausal women (Goldman and Tosteson 1991; Hulley *et al.* 1998). But, if a woman on replacement therapy has a cerebrovascular event, this is probably not a good reason to stop the treatment (Pedersen *et al.* 1997).

The effect of the menopause is difficult to disentangle from confounding by age and cigarette smoking. Probably the natural menopause has no effect on coronary heart disease incidence, although cardiovascular mortality is higher in women who have had an early menopause, while bilateral oophorectomy without oestrogen replacement about doubles the risk (Colditz *et al.* 1987; van der Schouw *et al.* 1996).

Alcohol

While heavy alcohol consumption may be an independent, and in some way causal risk factor, more obviously for haemorrhagic than ischaemic stroke, it seems that modest consumption might even be protective for ischaemic stroke (van Gijn *et al.* 1993; Kiyohara *et al.* 1995; Wannamethee and Shaper 1996; Thun *et al.* 1997). Confusion arises because it is difficult to measure alcohol consumption, particularly over time; uncertainty whether any effect on stroke is due to alcohol *per se* or to the type of alcoholic beverage; different patterns of drinking behaviour may have different effects; groups classified as non-drinking may include high-risk ex-heavy-drinkers; the biases inherent in case-control studies, particularly the selection of an appropriate control group; small numbers in many studies; confounding of the association by cigarette smoking (which is positively related to alcohol consumption), with physical exercise (which is negatively associated with alcohol consumption), and with socio-economic status; and the problem of distinguishing ischaemic and haemorrhagic strokes, if their relationship with alcohol consumption really is different (Marmot and Brunner 1991; Doll 1997). Also it is difficult to disentangle any causal pathway from alcohol consumption to stroke, because alcohol almost certainly raises blood pressure (Malhotra *et al.* 1985; MacMahon and Norton 1986; Marmot *et al.* 1994; Kaplan 1995), affects blood lipids

(Gaziano *et al.* 1993), can cause atrial fibrillation and cardio-myopathy, and, of course, one has to explain the apparent pro-tective effect in modest drinkers compared with heavy and non-drinkers. Equal confusion surrounds the possible causal effect of binge drinking on stroke, although there is no short-age of possible explanations for such a relationship (van Gijn *et al.* 1993).

Obesity

The exact relationship between obesity and stroke has seldom been studied, and that between obesity and coronary heart disease is controversial. Difficulties include inadequate numbers of stroke events for analysis; a possible difference between the relationship for ischaemic versus haemorrhagic strokes; mea-suring obesity satisfactorily (waist-to-hip ratio versus weight for a given height, etc.; Walker *et al.* 1996); confounding by cig-arette smoking, because smokers are lighter than non-smokers (Garrison *et al.* 1983; Wannamethee and Shaper 1989); and the fact that obesity is associated with (probably causally) hyper-tension, diabetes, and hypercholesterolaemia, and is more common in people who take little exercise (VanItallie 1990). However, there is little doubt that the risk of coronary events, in men and women, is greater in the obese, particularly if the weight has been gained in middle age or has fluctuated substan-tially (Manson *et al.* 1990; Lissner *et al.* 1991). Any higher risk of stroke in the obese may be mediated by associated hyper-tension and diabetes (Welin *et al.* 1987; Shinton *et al.* 1995; Rexrode *et al.* 1997).

Diet

Relating various dietary constituents to the risk of vascular disease is fraught with difficulty because not only are dietary questionnaires tricky to construct but diets change with fashion, where people live, with time, and as a result of disease or believing oneself to be at risk of a disease, all of which make both case-control and cohort studies very difficult to interpret. So often, one dietary constituent is associated with another, which makes it impossible to know which is responsible for any difference or change in vascular risk; for example, because coffee is so often drunk with milk, is any association of a disease with coffee actually due to an association with milk? Also people who eat so-called healthy diets often have an inherently healthy lifestyle, which makes confounding an ever-present problem in observational studies. Even 'negative' clini-cal trials can be misleading because it is conceivable that a dietary intervention is simply too late to affect the long-stand-ing underlying vascular disease which is the cause of stroke (Steinberg 1995).

The 'Eskimo diet' is rich in fish which contains more long-chain, omega-3 polyunsaturated fatty acids and less saturated fatty acids than 'Western diets'. This is said to explain the low risk of coronary heart disease in Eskimos. Whether adding fish, or fish oils, to Western diets is likely to, or does, reduce the risk of coronary events is very unclear, and the situation for stroke is even less clear (Katan 1995; Prichard *et al.* 1995; Orencia *et al.* 1996; Daviglus *et al.* 1997).

Excessive and even moderate salt intake may well be respon-sible for increasing the blood pressure, although the food industry says not (Law *et al.* 1991; Frost *et al.* 1991; Midgley *et al.* 1996; Elliott *et al.* 1996; Thelle 1996). Also, a high intake of potassium may possibly reduce stroke risk, perhaps by lowering blood pressure (Khaw and Barrett-Connor 1987; Whelton *et al.* 1997).

Deficiency of fresh fruit and vegetables, vitamin E, vitamin C, beta-carotene and flavonoids have all been proposed as vas-cular risk factors at various times. The unifying hypothesis, that most of these foodstuffs are antioxidants and protect the arter-ial intima from oxidative damage to DNA and lipoproteins, is far from proven (Acheson and Williams 1983; Witztum 1994; Jha *et al.* 1995; Greenberg and Sporn 1996; Rimm *et al.* 1996; Stephens 1997).

Coffee, particularly if boiled or unfiltered, has a small hyper-lipidaemic effect but no independent (of cholesterol and other confounding variables) predictive effect on vascular events (Kawachi *et al.* 1994).

Exercise

Exercise reduces blood pressure, plasma cholesterol, and fibrinogen, and the risk of non-insulin-dependent diabetes mellitus, so perhaps not surprisingly lack of exercise is associ-ated with both coronary heart disease and stroke (Connelly *et al.* 1992; Manson *et al.* 1992; Curfman 1993; Kokkinos *et al.* 1995; Lee *et al.* 1999).

Infections and inflammation

There is increasing interest in the role of both chronic and acute infection in the development and stability of atheromatous plaques (Danesh *et al.* 1997). A raised peripheral white blood cell count has been associated with vascular events for some time (Ernst *et al.* 1987; Kannel *et al.* 1992; Danesh *et al.* 1998) and there is now evidence of an association between stroke and serum C-reactive protein and various immediately preceding and distant infections (Bova *et al.* 1996; Cook and Lip 1996; Maseri 1997; Cook *et al.* 1998).

Homocysteinaemia

Homozygous patients with a rare inherited deficiency of cyst-athionine synthase develop severe homocysteinaemia and homocystinuria and present as children with mental retarda-tion, dislocated lenses, Marfanoid features, and a tendency to venous and arterial thrombosis. Heterozygotes have modestly raised levels of blood homocysteine, as do the much more common heterozygotes for methylenetetrahydrofolate reductase deficiency, and some with methionine synthase deficiency, and patients who are mildly deficient in the co-factors to these enzymes—folic acid, vitamin B_{12}, and pyridoxine. There is enough reasonably consistent observational data linking coro-nary heart disease and stroke (and venous thromboembolism too) with increasing plasma homocysteine (hyperhomo-cyteinaemia) for trials of folic acid and pyridoxine to have been started (Danesh and Lewington 1998; Refsum *et al.* 1998; Welch and Loscalzo 1998; Yoo *et al.* 1998).

Other possible associations

Innumerable other risk factors have been linked with coronary heart disease, if not with stroke, at various times, but data are sparse and there is probably a lot of confounding: adverse life events and difficulties; type A behaviour; phobic anxiety; stress; depression and hopelessness; low job control; sleep apnoea and snoring; large platelets; corneal arcus; vasectomy; high body iron stores; dental disease; low bone density; blood group; low serum albumin; diagonal ear lobe crease; impaired ventilatory function; and family history of stroke (Warlow *et al.* 2000*a*). Risk factorology is clearly still alive and well. Whether 'fishing expeditions' for yet more risk factors will one day turn up any useful aetiological truths, rather than just a jumble of more or less unlikely hypotheses, remains to be seen.

Non-stroke vascular disease

Independent of age, coronary heart disease (i.e. angina or myocardial infarction) is clearly associated with ischaemic stroke, which is hardly surprising because atheroma in one arterial system is so often accompanied by atheroma in other arteries in the same individual (Section 27.4.2). The evidence comes from post-mortems (Kagan 1976; Stemmermann *et al.* 1984); case-control studies (Friedman *et al.* 1968; Di Pasquale *et al.* 1986; Woo *et al.* 1991); cohort studies (Kannel *et al.* 1983, Harmsen *et al.* 1990; Shaper *et al.* 1991; Wolf *et al.* 1991*b*); and the correlation between coronary disease and carotid stenosis in ultrasound studies (Craven *et al.* 1990). ECG abnormalities and cardiac failure, reflecting hypertension or coronary heart disease, are, not surprisingly, associated with stroke, as is left ventricular hypertrophy (Kagan *et al.* 1980; Kannel *et al.* 1983; Knutsen *et al.* 1988; Shaper *et al.* 1991).

Claudicants and people with asymptomatic peripheral vascular disease are at excess risk of both myocardial infarction and stroke, presumably reflecting the association of atheromatous disease in different parts of the circulation in the same (predisposed) individuals (Harmsen *et al.* 1990; Criqui *et al.* 1992; Ogren *et al.* 1993; Bainton *et al.* 1994; Leng *et al.* 1996).

Abdominal aortic aneurysms occur in about 10–20 per cent of patients with cerebrovascular disease but whether this is definitely more than expected is not clear. It is not known if people with aneurysms have more strokes or other vascular events, compared with people without aneurysms (Carty *et al.* 1993; Karanjia *et al.* 1994).

Carotid and supraclavicular arterial (i.e. cervical) bruits are imperfectly related to stenosis of the underlying arteries (Section 27.5.1). Both bruits and stenosis become more prevalent with age and about 5 per cent of the normal elderly have severe carotid stenosis (O'Leary *et al.* 1992). Both bruits and severe stenosis are risk factors for subsequent stroke, but not necessarily in the same arterial territory because disease (usually atherothrombotic) in one artery is likely to be associated with disease in other arteries in the same (predisposed) individual. The risk of stroke increases with the severity of the stenosis and perhaps also with progression of stenosis (Warlow 1996; Mackey *et al.* 1997).

Because *transient ischaemic attacks* are, in a sense, ischaemic strokes which happen to recover within 24 hours, it is not surprising that they are a risk factor for stroke. A TIA patient has an excess risk of stroke about 5–10 times greater than that of a non-TIA patient of the same age (Section 27.10.2).

27.2.8 Genetic factors

A few strokes are clearly 'familial', with a simple Mendelian pattern of inheritance of the underlying cause (e.g. haemophilia) (Table 27.8) (Natowicz and Kelley 1987). Also, there is evidence that parental history of stroke is a risk factor (Liao *et al.* 1997). There is increasing interest in complex genetic disorders thought to be due to multiple gene interactions, perhaps influenced by environmental factors, but how easy it will be to separate shared genes from shared environment in a disease as common as stroke remains to be seen. Of course, it has been clear for some time that many of the classical vascular risk factors are genetically determined in part (e.g. hypertension and hyperlipidaemia) but it is equally clear that envi-

Table 27.8. Some causes of stroke which can be 'familial' (including intracranial venous thrombosis and intracranial haemorrhage)

Vascular anomalies
    Intracranial vascular malformation (Section 27.4.8)
    Saccular aneurysm (Section 27.4.8)
    Hereditary haemorrhagic telangiectasia (Section 27.4.8)

Connective tissue anomalies
    Ehlers–Danlos syndrome (Section 27.4.4)
    Pseudoxanthoma elasticum (Section 27.4.4)
    Marfan's syndrome (Section 27.4.4)
    Fibromuscular dysplasia (Section 27.4.4)
    Polycystic kidney disease (Section 27.4.8)
    Mitral leaflet prolapse (Section 27.4.5)

Haematological diseases
    Haemophilia and other coagulation factor deficiencies (Section 27.4.6)
    Sickle-cell disease/trait (Section 27.4.6)
    Antithrombin III deficiency (Section 27.4.6)
    Protein C deficiency (Section 27.4.6)
    Activated protein C resistance (Section 27.4.6)
    Protein S deficiency (Section 27.4.6)
    Plasminogen abnormality/deficiency (Section 27.4.6)
    Dysfibrinogenaemia (Section 27.4.6)

Others
    Familial hypercholesterolaemia
    Cerebral amyloid angiopathy (Icelandic and Dutch forms) (Section 27.4.8)
    Neurofibromatosis
    Tuberous sclerosis
    Homocysteinaemia (Section 27.4.7)
    Fabry's disease (Section 27.4.7)
    Migraine (Section 27.4.7)
    Cardiac myxoma (Section 27.4.5)
    Cardiomyopathy (Section 27.4.5)
    Von Hippel–Lindau disease
    Mitochondrial cytopathy (Section 27.4.7)
    CADASIL (Section 27.2.8)

ronmental influences can and do modify them (e.g. salt and saturated fat consumption, respectively). The contribution of genetic factors to stroke risk in populations has been difficult to work out, as it has for coronary heart disease (Alberts 1991). A better approach might be to study the genetic determinants of the causal risk factors themselves rather than of stroke in general. Disentangling the interactions, identifying the gene(s) involved, and working out the pathway from genotype to phenotype are monumental tasks (Rastenyte *et al.* 1998).

Cerebral autosomal dominant arteriopathy with subcortical infarcts and leucoencephalopathy (CADASIL) is a recently characterized and quite rare syndrome in which migraine with aura develops in the 30s, recurrent lacunar ischaemic strokes and TIAs start in the 40s, subcortical dementia develops in the 50s, and the patients die in their 60s. Depression is also quite common. Very characteristically, and from the earliest stages, even when the patient is still asymptomatic, brain MRI shows widespread focal, diffuse, and confluent white matter changes, particularly periventricular and subcortical (Chabriat *et al.* 1995, 1998; Hutchinson *et al.* 1995; Dichgans *et al.* 1998). The underlying small vessel arteriopathy is distinct from arteriosclerotic and amyloid angiopathy and can be found in skin biopsies as well as in the leptomeningeal and perforating arteries of the brain (Jung *et al.* 1995). The genetic locus is on chromosome 19q12 (Tournier-Lasserve *et al.* 1993).

27.3 The blood supply to the brain

At rest the brain, which is only 2 per cent of total body weight, receives 20 per cent of the cardiac output of blood and consumes about 20 per cent of the total inspired oxygen. This rich blood supply is delivered by the two internal carotid and two vertebral arteries (Fig. 27.6) which anastomose at the base of

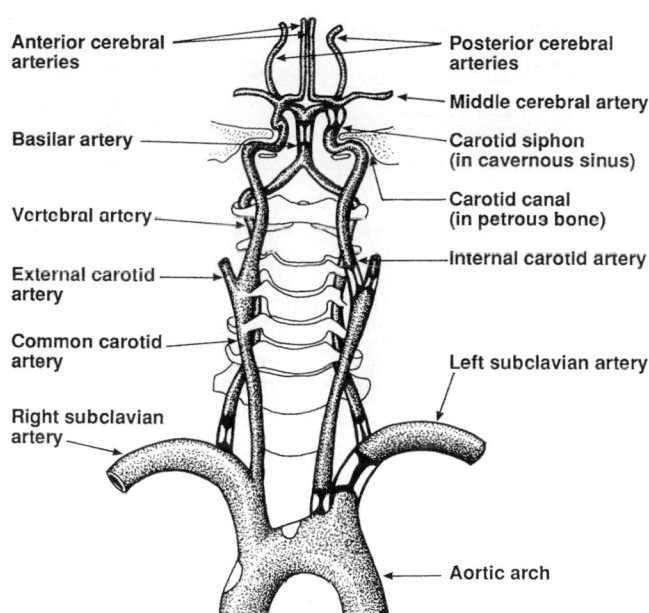

Fig. 27.6. The anatomy of the arterial circulation to the brain and eye. White indentations into the arterial lumen represent sites at which atherothrombosis is particularly common.

the brain to form the circle of Willis (Fig. 27.7a). The carotid arteries supply the anterior, and the vertebrobasilar arterial system supplies the posterior, portions of the brain.

27.3.1 The anatomy of the cerebral circulation

Figure 27.7b shows the anatomy of the cerebral circulation; the detailed anatomy is well described by Sheldon (1981). Not unexpectedly, there is individual variation, particularly in the

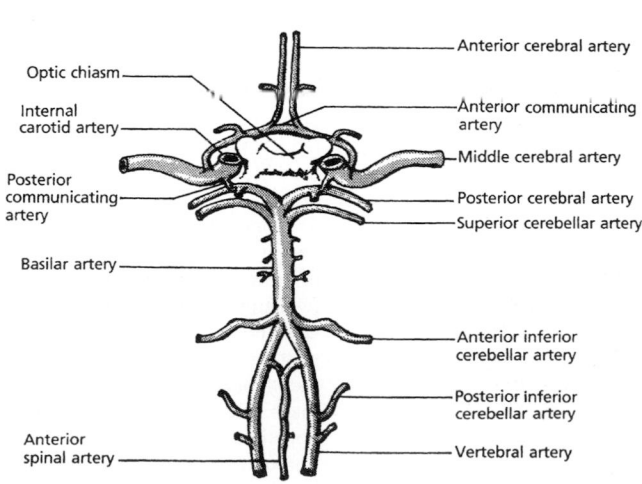

(a)

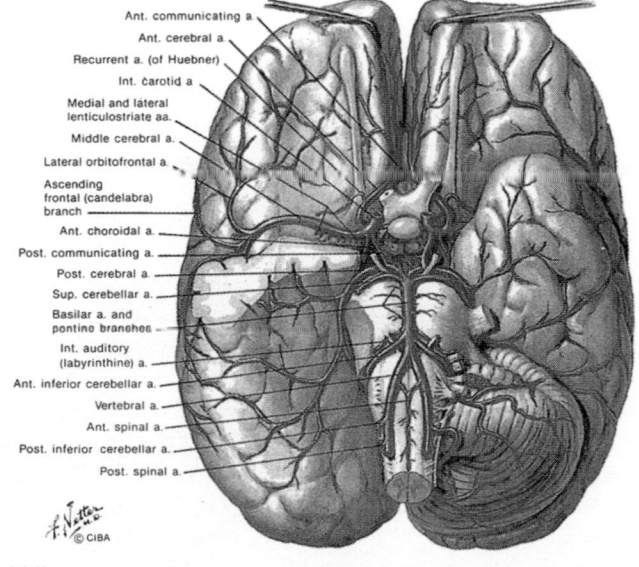

(b)(i)

Fig. 27.7. (a) The circle of Willis at the base of the brain as seen from below. There is considerable anatomical variation and this figure represents but one rather typical arrangement. (b) (i) A view of the base of the brain to show the circle of Willis, vertebrobasilar arterial system, middle and anterior cerebral arteries.

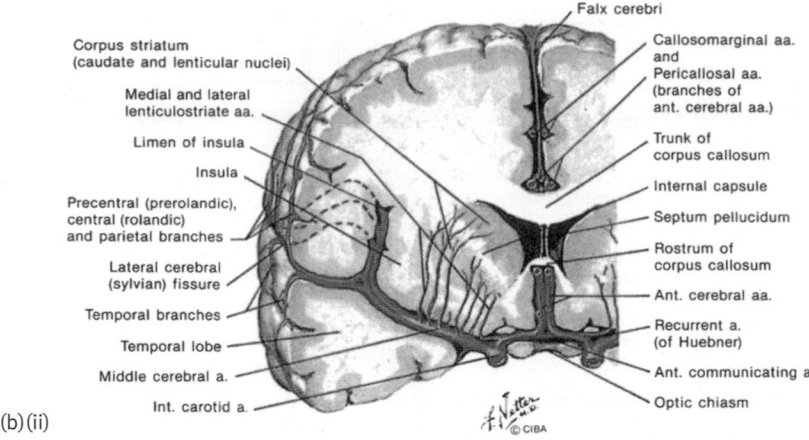

(b)(ii)

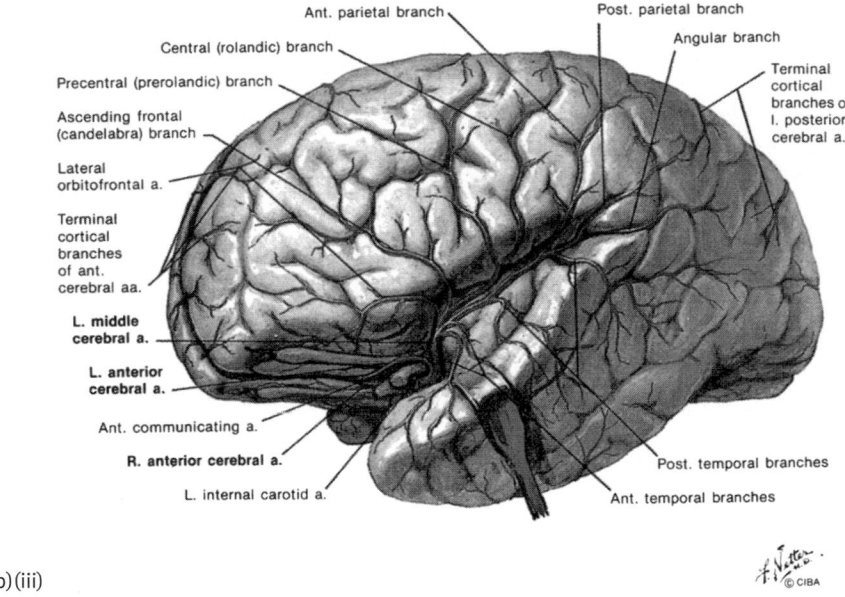

(b)(iii)

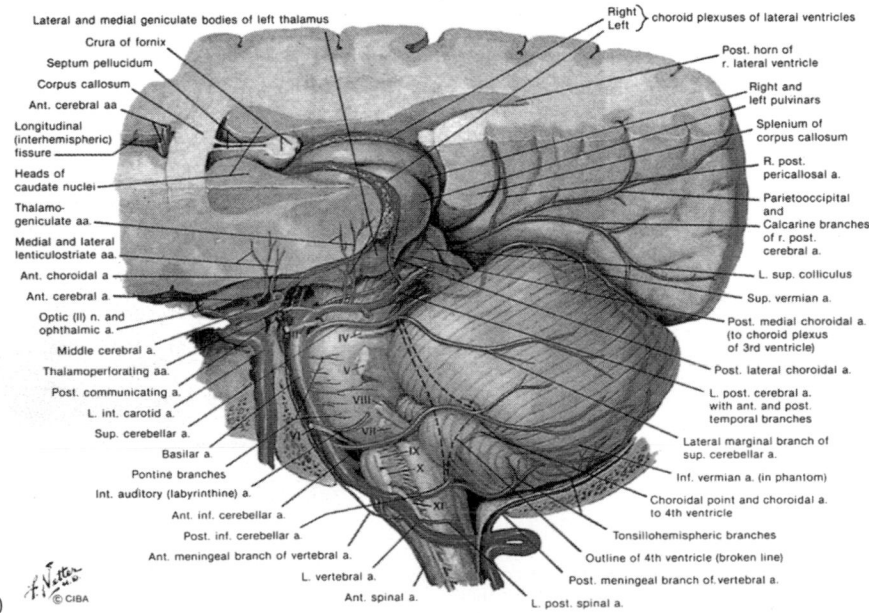

(b)(iv)

Fig. 27.7. (*contd.*) (b) (ii) A coronal section of the brain through the optic chiasm to show the small penetrating lenticulostriate branches of the main stem of the middle cerebral artery.
(iii) A lateral view of the brain to show the cortical branches of the middle cerebral artery.
(iv) Lateral view of the brain to show the vertebral, basilar, and posterior cerebral arteries and their branches in the posterior fossa. (Figures (bi)–(biv) Copyright 1990 CIBA–GEIGY Corporation. Reprinted with permission from CLINICAL SYMPOSIA, illustrated by Frank N. Netter, MD. All rights reserved.) (See also Plate 21.)

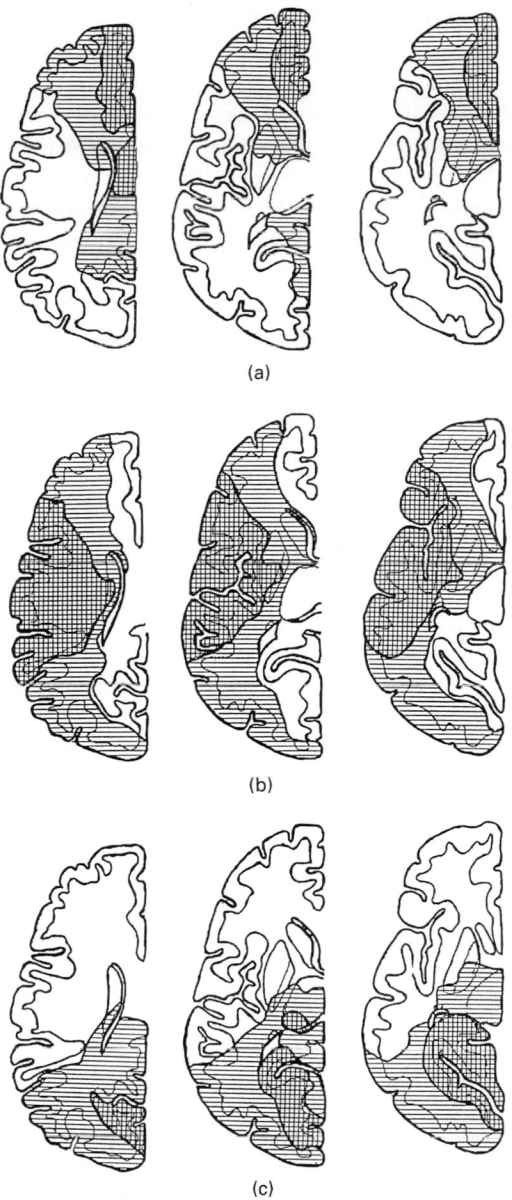

(a)

(b)

(c)

Fig. 27.8. Horizontal sections of the brain to show areas supplied by the anterior (a), middle (b), and posterior (c) cerebral arteries. The vertical lines represent the smallest and the horizontal lines the largest areas of supply in various individuals. (With permission from Dr Albert van der Zwan, University of Utrecht.)

branches of the main cerebral arteries. Well-recognized developmental anomalies include marked inequality in size of the two vertebral arteries; the left vertebral artery arising from the aorta; the right common carotid artery arising from the aortic arch; a combined origin of the left common carotid and innominate arteries; hypoplasia or absence of one (or less often both) posterior communicating artery(ies); hypoplasia or absence of the anterior communicating artery; hypoplasia or absence of the proximal part of one anterior cerebral artery (ACA) so that blood flow to both ACAs comes from one internal carotid artery (ICA); a persistent trigeminal artery joining the ICA with the basilar artery; and a paired basilar artery. Any one description of

arterial anatomy must, therefore, be taken as the usual rather than the invariable pattern. Also it is hardly surprising that there is considerable variation between individuals in the usual brain territories of supply of the various major arteries, and these territories can be asymmetrical and even change with time, depending in part on the availability of functional collaterals (van der Zwan *et al.* 1992) (Fig. 27.8). Any maps of CT/MR-displayed arterial territories should not therefore be taken as a fixed truth for all individuals (Damasio 1983; Tatu *et al.* 1996).

The *internal carotid artery* (ICA) starts as the carotid sinus at the bifurcation of the *common carotid artery* (CCA) at the level of the thyroid cartilage. It runs up the neck, without any branches, to the base of the skull, where it passes through the foramen lacerum to enter the carotid canal of the petrous bone. It then runs through the cavernous sinus in an S-shaped curve (the carotid siphon), pierces the dura, and exits just medial to the anterior clinoid process, and then bifurcates into the anterior cerebral artery and the larger middle cerebral artery.

The *external carotid artery* (ECA) also starts at the CCA bifurcation. Branches supply the jaw, face, scalp, neck, and meninges (superficial temporal, facial, occipital arteries, etc.).

The *ophthalmic artery* is the first major branch of the ICA and arises in the cavernous sinus. It passes through the optic foramen to supply the eye and other structures in the orbit.

The *posterior communicating artery* (PoCA) is the next artery to arise from the ICA. It passes back to join the first part of the posterior cerebral artery, so contributing to the circle of Willis. Tiny branches supply the adjacent optic chiasm, optic tract, hypothalamus, thalamus, and midbrain.

The *anterior choroidal artery* arises from the last section of the ICA, just beyond the PoCA origin, and supplies the optic tract, internal capsule, medial parts of the basal ganglia, the medial part of the temporal lobe, thalamus, lateral geniculate body, proximal optic radiation, and midbrain. Occasionally it arises from the proximal middle cerebral artery or PoCA. Minor twiglets from the distal ICA contribute blood to the pituitary gland, optic chiasm, and nearby structures, including the meninges.

The *anterior cerebral artery* (ACA) passes horizontally and medially to enter the interhemispheric fissure, anastomoses with its counterpart of the opposite side via the anterior communicating artery (ACoA), curves up around the genu of the corpus callosum, and supplies the anterior and medial parts of the cerebral hemisphere. Small branches also supply parts of the optic nerve and chiasm, hypothalamus, anterior basal ganglia, and internal capsule.

The *middle cerebral artery* (MCA) enters the Sylvian fissure and divides into 2–4 branches which supply the lateral parts of the cerebral hemisphere. From its main trunk a medial and lateral group of tiny lenticulostriate arteries and arterioles pass upwards to penetrate the base of the brain and supply the basal ganglia and internal capsule (Marinkovic *et al.* 1985). Some of these small penetrating vessels extend up into the white matter of the corona radiata in the centrum semiovale towards the small medullary perforating branches of the cortical arteries coming down from above.

The *vertebral artery* arises from the proximal subclavian artery and ascends to pass through the transverse foramina of the sixth to second cervical vertebrae, giving off small muscular branches on the way. It then passes posteriorly around the articular process of the atlas to enter the skull through the foramen magnum. It unites with the opposite vertebral artery on the ventral surface of the brainstem at the pontomedullary junction to form the basilar artery. Branches to the meninges arise at the foramen magnum. The vertebral artery gives rise to the anterior and posterior spinal arteries, the posterior inferior cerebellar artery (to inferior vermis and inferior and posterior surfaces of the cerebellar hemispheres, and brainstem), and small penetrating arteries to the medulla.

The *basilar artery* ascends ventral to the pons to the ponto-midbrain junction in the interpeduncular cistern, where it divides into the two posterior cerebral arteries. Numerous small branches penetrate the brainstem and cerebellum. The basilar artery also gives rise to the anterior inferior cerebellar artery (to rostral cerebellum, brainstem, inner ear) and the superior cerebellar artery (to brainstem, superior half of the cerebellar hemisphere, vermis, and dentate nucleus).

The *posterior cerebral artery* (PCA) encircles the midbrain close to the oculomotor nerve at the level of the tentorium and supplies the inferior part of the temporal lobe, and the occipital lobe (Marinkovic *et al.* 1987). Many small perforating arteries arise from the proximal portion of the PCA to supply the midbrain, thalamus, hypothalamus, and geniculate bodies. Sometimes a single perforating artery supplies the medial part of each thalamus, or both sides of the midbrain. In about 15 per cent of individuals the PCA is a direct continuation of the PoCA, its main blood supply then coming from the ICA rather than the basilar artery.

The meninges are supplied by branches of the ECA, ICA, and vertebral arteries. The most prominent branches from the ECA are the middle meningeal artery, and tributaries of the ascending pharyngeal and occipital arteries. Most of the branches from the ICA arise near the cavernous sinus and from the ophthalmic artery in the orbit. Branches from the vertebral artery arise at the foramen magnum. There are numerous meningeal anastomoses between these small arteries.

The scalp is supplied by branches of the ECA, particularly the superficial temporal, occipital, and posterior auricular arteries. Above the orbit there is a contribution from terminal branches of the ophthalmic artery. There is a rich anastomotic network between the various arteries of the scalp.

27.3.2 The collateral blood supply to the brain

This topic is described by Fields *et al.* (1985). Normally the ICA provides blood to the anterior two-thirds of the ipsilateral cerebral hemisphere. There is rather little mixing of blood via the PoCA and so the posterior circulation is usually supplied by the vertebral, basilar, and posterior cerebral arteries. However, there are several ways in which collateral blood supply to the brain can develop distal to occlusion of major arteries in the neck or head.

The actual pattern of collateral blood flow depends on where the major vessels are stenosed or occluded, and on which collateral channels are anatomically available in a particular individual, and free from disease. On the whole, the development of effective collateral channels is more likely if any occlusion develops gradually rather than suddenly. Unlike the normal cerebral blood supply (Section 27.3.4), the functional capacity of the collateral blood supply to respond to changes in perfusion pressure is limited. Collateral blood flow may develop via:

◆ The circle of Willis, which is formed by the proximal part of the two ACAs connected by the ACoA, and the proximal part of the two PCAs, which are connected to the distal ICAs by the PoCAs. However, about 50 per cent of circles have one or more hypoplastic or absent segments (usually one of the communicating arteries). Because atheroma commonly affects the circle of Willis, the potential for collateral flow is not always as good as it might first appear from idealized diagrams of 'normal' anatomy (Fig. 27.7a).

◆ Around the orbit, branches of the ECA anastomose with branches of the ophthalmic artery if the ICA is severely stenosed or obstructed. Collateral flow from the ECA into the orbit then passes retrogradely through the ophthalmic artery to fill the carotid siphon, MCA, and ACA. Sometimes flow may even reach the PCA and vertebrobasilar system.

◆ Muscular branches of the vertebral artery in the neck, distal to a vertebral obstruction, may receive blood retrogradely from occipital and ascending pharyngeal branches of the ECA, or from the deep and ascending cervical arteries. Also, anastomoses can develop between branches of the subclavian artery and ECA to take blood retrogradely down the ECA to the carotid bifurcation and then up the ICA when the common carotid artery is obstructed.

◆ Leptomeningeal anastomoses on the surface of the brain may develop between cortical branches of the anterior, middle, and posterior cerebral arteries, and, to a lesser extent, between pial branches of the cerebellar arteries.

◆ Dural anastomoses can develop between meningeal branches of the ICA, ECA, and vertebral arteries. Occasionally small dural anastomoses develop between cortical leptomeningeal and dural arteries.

◆ Parenchymal anastomoses occasionally develop in the precapillary bed of the penetrating arteries at the base of the brain supplying the basal ganglia (moyamoya syndrome, Section 27.4.4).

◆ The anterior choroidal artery (a branch of the ICA) can anastomose with the posterior choroidal artery (a branch of the PCA).

27.3.3 Venous drainage

The venous anatomy is very variable. In general, venous blood flows centrally via the deep cerebral veins, and peripherally via the superficial cerebral veins into the dural venous sinuses

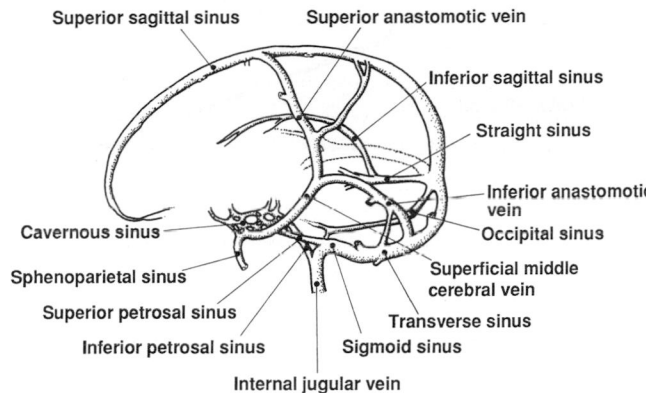

Fig. 27.9. Diagram of the venous drainage of the brain (modified with permission from F. A. Davis and Co.).

(which lie between the endosteal outer and meningeal inner layer of the dura) which drain into the internal jugular veins (Bousser and Ross Russell 1997) (Fig. 27.9). The cerebral veins are thin-walled, have no valves, and the blood flow is often in the same direction as in neighbouring arteries. There are numerous venous connections between the cerebral veins and dural sinuses, as well as with the venous system of the meninges, skull, scalp, and nasal sinuses, so facilitating the propagation of thrombus or spread of infection between these vessels.

27.3.4 **The regulation of cerebral blood flow**

Although it has been possible to measure cerebral blood flow (CBF) for more than 50 years (Kety and Schmidt 1945), and although the methods have become more accurate and reliable, and information on regional as well as global blood flow linked to metabolic demand is now available, it is still not practical nor helpful to measure CBF in routine clinical practice. Nonetheless, increasing knowledge of CBF regulation, and the relationship between CBF and cerebral metabolism, has had a major influence on how we think about the pathophysiology of chronically impaired perfusion reserve and of acute ischaemic stroke (Frackowiak 1986; Baron 1991; Marchal *et al.* 1996*a*).

CBF in normal humans is about 50 ml/100 g of brain/min. Using regional techniques (position emission tomography, PET; Frackowiak *et al.* 1980) it has been shown that CBF, cerebral blood volume (CBV), and cerebral energy metabolism, measured as cerebral metabolic rate of oxygen (CMR_{O_2}) or of glucose (CMR_{glu}), are all coupled, and higher in grey than in white matter. This means that the oxygen extraction fraction (OEF) is about the same (approximately one-third) throughout the brain (Leenders *et al.* 1990). Therefore, in normal resting human brain, CBF (i.e. flow) is a reliable reflection of CMR_{O_2} (i.e. function). There is a gradual fall of CBF, CBV, CMR_{glu} and CMR_{O_2} with age, but they are all still normally coupled, so the OEF remains more or less constant (Blesa *et al.* 1997).

Cerebral blood flow and blood gas tensions

CBF is very influenced by small changes in Pa_{CO_2}; an acute rise of 1 mmHg causes an immediate increase in CBF of about 5 per cent due to dilatation of cerebral resistance vessels. In chronic respiratory failure, however, adaptation occurs and CBF is normal despite the hypercapnia. Modest changes in arterial oxygen tension do not affect CBF, but when the Pa_{O_2} is below about 50 mmHg, and oxygen saturation starts falling, there is a fall in cerebral vascular resistance and CBF rises (Brown *et al.* 1985). Increasing Pa_{O_2} above the normal level has little effect on CBF.

Cerebral blood flow and blood viscosity

In normal health, CBF is inversely related to whole-blood viscosity, which is itself much higher at low than high shear rates (Thomas 1982). The main determinant of whole-blood viscosity is the haematocrit, so that haematocrit and flow are inversely and closely related (Thomas *et al.* 1977; Brass *et al.* 1988; Ameriso *et al.* 1990). However, this is not because the high viscosity of high-haematocrit blood slows flow, at least not in normal vessels, but because the higher oxygen content of high-haematocrit blood reduces flow and so maintains normal oxygen delivery to the tissues to meet normal metabolic demands (Brown and Marshall 1985). Similarly, although reducing whole-blood viscosity by venesection may increase CBF, it does not necessarily mean that more oxygen is delivered, because the oxygen content of the blood is lower (Hino *et al.* 1992). Of course, in ischaemic brain, where vasodilatation is likely to be maximal, the lower oxygen content of the blood after haemodilution might not lead to any increase of CBF at all. Also, at very low shear rates which might be found in ischaemic brain, whole-blood viscosity depends more on plasma fibrinogen than haematocrit (Weaver *et al.* 1969); also, other factors increasing blood viscosity may come in to play to reduce flow, at least locally e.g. platelet aggregation, red cell aggregation, and perhaps increasing red cell fragility as a result of anoxia (Wood and Kee 1985). Under these circumstances lowering blood viscosity might conceivably be helpful. Very high blood viscosity is found in the leukaemias and para-proteinaemias, but because CBF depends more on blood oxygen content, the CBF can be normal, or even high if the patient is anaemic (Brown and Marshall 1985).

Brain activity

Increasing regional functional activity of the brain (e.g. in the motor cortex contralateral to voluntary hand movements) increases regional metabolic activity in the same area (Lassen *et al.* 1977). The increasing CMR_{O_2} and CMR_{glu} are achieved not by increasing OEF or the glucose extraction fraction, but by a very quick response of the cerebral circulation, over seconds; local vasodilatation of the cerebral resistance vessels, increase in CBV and, therefore, in CBF. Conversely, low functional and metabolic demand (e.g. in a cerebral infarct) are associated with a low CBF; therefore, low flow does not necessarily mean that the supplying artery is obstructed, it may simply mean the brain is dead. The normal coupling of flow with metabolism and function has been suspected for over a century (Roy and Sherrington 1890) but the mechanism is still unknown; it may be due to the release of vasodilatory metabolites in metabolically active areas of brain, or neural regulation of the resistance blood vessels (Lou *et al.* 1987).

Perfusion pressure

CBF depends on cerebral perfusion pressure (CPP) and cerebrovascular resistance. The perfusion pressure is the difference between systemic arterial pressure at the base of the brain when in the recumbent position and the venous pressure at exit from the subarachnoid space, the latter being approximated by the intracranial pressure. CPP divided by CBF gives the cerebrovascular resistance. In normal humans, CBF remains almost constant when the mean systemic blood pressure is between about 50 and 170 mmHg which, under normal circumstances when the intracranial venous pressure is negligible, is the same as the CPP (Fig. 27.10).

This homeostatic mechanism to maintain a constant CBF in the face of changes in CPP is known as *autoregulation* (Reed and Devous 1985; Powers 1991). Within the autoregulatory range, as CPP falls there is, within seconds, vasodilatation of the small cerebral resistance vessels, a fall in cerebrovascular resistance, a rise in CBV, and therefore CBF remains constant (Fig. 27.11) (Aaslid *et al.* 1989). Whether myogenic, metabolic, or neurogenic processes are responsible for this response is unknown. When vasodilatation is maximal and CBV can rise no more, and if CPP continues to fall due to a fall in systemic blood pressure or an increase in intracranial pressure, the CBF itself starts to fall; in other words, the cerebral perfusion reserve is exhausted (see below). However, metabolic activity is maintained by increasing OEF and, if the jugular vein is catheterized, an increased arteriovenous oxygen difference is found: this is 'misery' perfusion or oligaemia (Fig. 27.11). Eventually OEF can rise no more and, with further CPP reduction, metabolic activity (i.e. $CMRo_2$) starts to fall, and metabolism becomes limited by perfusion. This is what is normally meant by ischaemia; the perfusion reserve is exhausted and flow is inadequate to meet the metabolic demands of the tissues. At around this point the patient becomes symptomatic (non-focal features such as faintness if the whole brain is involved, or focal features such as hemiparesis if only the motor part of the brain is involved).

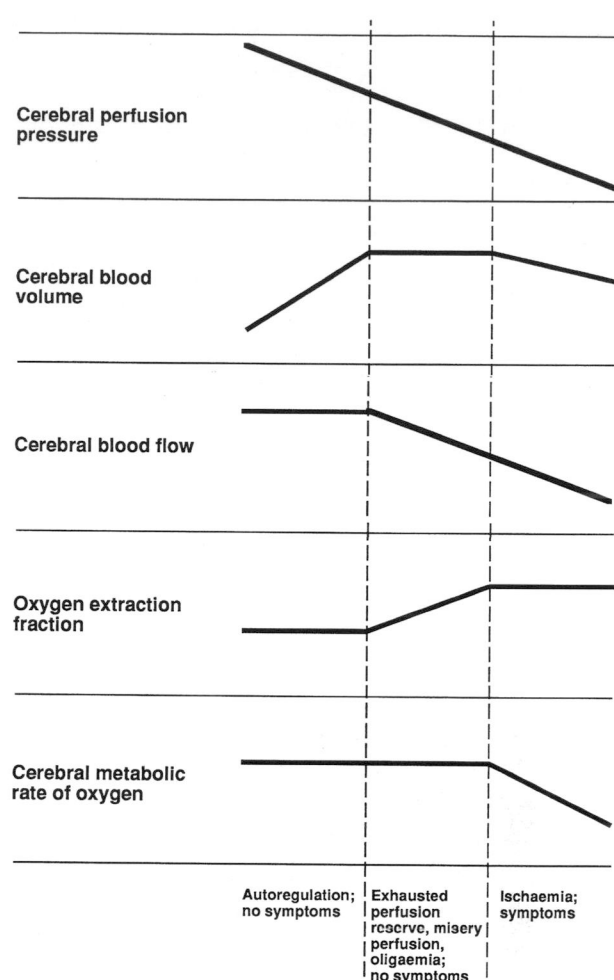

Fig. 27.11. A model to demonstrate the compensatory mechanisms which maintain cerebral metabolic activity as cerebral perfusion pressure falls.

It is possible, but difficult and not really realistic in clinical practice, to assess autoregulation directly in humans by various manipulations to alter the blood pressure while recording middle cerebral artery blood flow with transcranial Doppler (carotid compression, Valsalva manoeuvre, thigh compression cuffs, etc.) (Aaslid *et al.* 1989; Larsen *et al.* 1994; Smielewski *et al.* 1996; Tiecks *et al.* 1996; Panerai *et al.* 1998). Of course, patients who cannot autoregulate as a result of brain injury (i.e. they cannot vasoconstrict or vasodilate in response to CPP) are likely to have impaired cerebral perfusion reserve as well. However, there are some situations where autoregulation is impaired even though CO_2 reactivity is still preserved (White and Markus 1997).

If the perfusion pressure rises above the autoregulatory range, where compensatory vasoconstriction and cerebrovascular resistance return (CVR) are maximal, then hyperaemia occurs, followed by vasogenic oedema, raised intracranial pressure, and the clinical syndrome of hypertensive encephalopathy (Section 25.5.4).

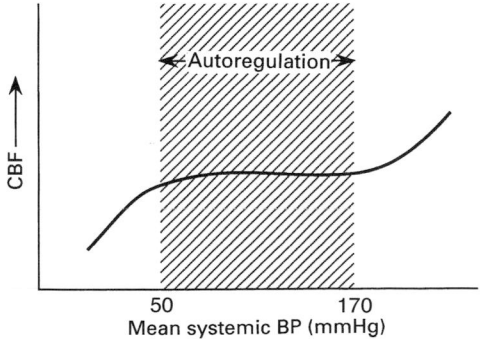

Fig. 27.10. A diagram to illustrate autoregulation of cerebral blood flow (CBF) in normal humans. Between a mean systemic blood pressure (BP) of about 50 and 170 mmHg cerebral blood flow remains roughly constant.

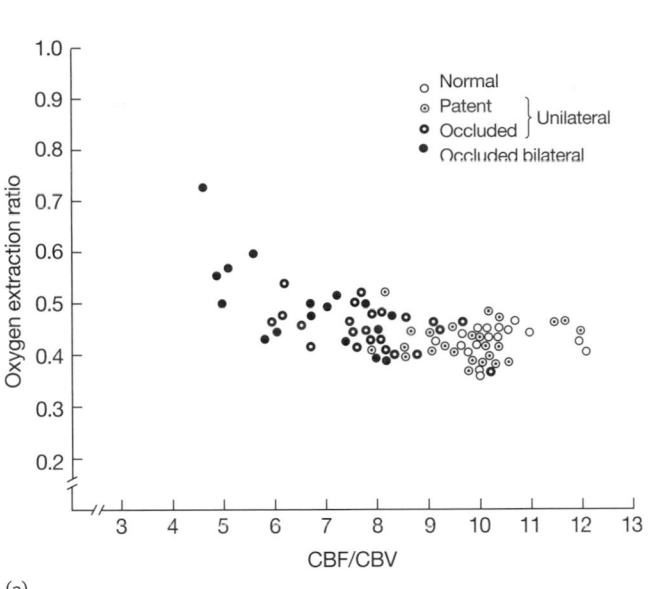

(a)

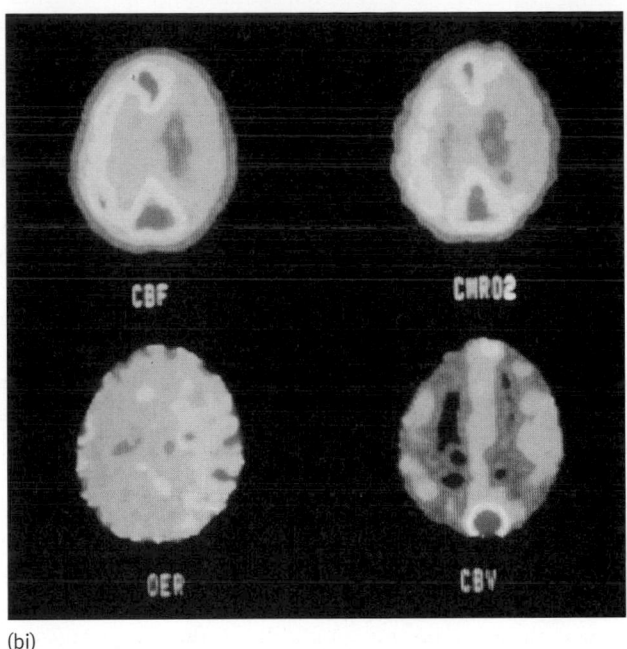

(bi)

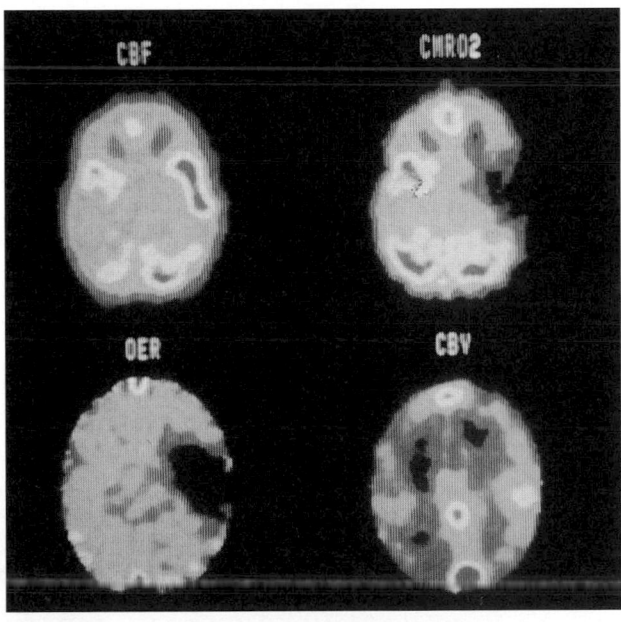

(bii)

Fig. 27.12. (a) Relation between oxygen extraction ratio (or fraction) and cerebral blood flow divided by cerebral blood volume (CBF/CBV) in each of the 82 middle-cerebral artery regions from 32 patients with patent or occluded carotid arteries, and nine normal subjects (with permission from Gibbs *et al.* 1984). (b) PET scan 90 minutes after acute left middle cerebral artery occlusion: (i) cerebral blood flow (CBF) is low, cerebral metabolic rate for oxygen ($CMRo_2$) is low, but the oxygen extraction ratio (OER) (fraction) is maximal (i.e. ischaemia). (ii) PET scan a week later to show increased CBF and cerebral blood volume (CBV), despite low $CMRo_2$ and OER (i.e. absolute luxury perfusion). (Scans kindly provided by Professor Richard Frackowiak.) See also Plate 22.

Perfusion reserve

It follows from the above that the ratio CBF/CBV is a measure of *cerebral perfusion reserve* (Schumann *et al.* 1998). Below about 6.0, even if CBF is still normal, vasodilatation and CBV are maximal and the reserve is exhausted, as shown by a rising OEF on PET scanning (Fig. 27.12).

Chronically impaired perfusion reserve tends to occur when one or both internal carotid arteries are stenosed enough to impair blood flow through the artery and produce a fall in pressure distally, i.e. stenosis of at least 50 per cent of the luminal diameter, often much more (Brice *et al.* 1964; DeWeese *et al.* 1970; Schroeder 1988), or are occluded *and* the collateral circulation is inadequate (Powers *et al.* 1987; Derlon *et al.* 1992). Under

these circumstances of maximal vasodilatation, the brain is vulnerable to any further fall in CPP (e.g. as a consequence of drugs, standing quickly, etc.) and cerebral metabolism is beginning to become impaired, with the appearance of structural abnormalities on MRI (van der Grond *et al.* 1996; Isaka *et al.* 1997).

Indirect assessment of perfusion reserve can be achieved by measuring the response of CBF to hypercapnia during CO_2 inhalation, breath holding, or after intravenous acetazolamide, a carbonic anhydrase inhibitor (Herold *et al.* 1988). It is simpler to use transcranial Doppler monitoring to measure middle cerebral artery (MCA) velocity flow responsiveness as a surrogate for CBF responsiveness. However, there seems little agreement about how these various tests should be standardized and how to define 'normality', given that a continuous variable is being measured (Bishop *et al.* 1986; Markus and Harrison 1992; Dahl *et al.* 1995). Near-infrared spectroscopy to measure the concentration of oxy- and deoxyhaemoglobin non-invasively, and the response of MCA flow to contralateral motor tasks, are other possibilities (Silvestrini *et al.* 1994; Smielewski *et al.* 1997). Also, because CBF/CBV is mathematically equivalent to the reciprocal of the mean cerebrovascular transit time, the direct measurement of the latter might be another practical, if indirect, method of assessing perfusion reserve (Merrick *et al.* 1991; Naylor *et al.* 1991). It should be noted that the indirect methods of measuring perfusion reserve are inaccurate when the normal relationships between CBF, CBV, OEF, and vascular reactivity break down, as they may well do in ischaemic or infarcted brain (Powers 1991).

As yet, the relevance of impaired perfusion reserve to various outcomes (e.g. ipsilateral ischaemic stroke distal to unoperated severe carotid disease, and the risk of carotid endarterectomy or of extra-to-intracranial bypass surgery) is unclear, probably because the tests are not standardized, the sample sizes not large, the impairment can diminish or improve spontaneously with time, and many patients in the published series were operated on irrespective of their perfusion reserve (Derlon *et al.* 1992; Widder *et al.* 1994; Klijn *et al.* 1997). Once oxygen extraction starts to rise, then there may well be an increased stroke risk in patients with carotid occlusion, but monitoring this requires PET availability (Grubb *et al.* 1998).

Cerebral blood flow, hypertension, and brain damage

In chronically hypertensive patients, the autoregulatory range is shifted upwards so that CBF starts falling and ischaemic symptoms occur at a higher systemic blood pressure than normal (Strandgaard *et al.* 1973). It follows that sudden lowering of blood pressure is more likely to cause ischaemic symptoms, and even cerebral infarction, in chronic compared with acute hyper-

tension. This upward shift of autoregulation is partially returned to normal in some patients when hypertension is treated, but very few patients have been studied prospectively (Strandgaard 1976). On the other hand, hypertensive encephalopathy is more likely to occur in acute hypertension because the upper limit of autoregulation is still normal (e.g. toxaemia of pregnancy).

Autoregulation is impaired, or abolished, in damaged areas of brain (e.g. by ischaemia, trauma, etc.) so that CBF becomes 'pressure passive' and follows perfusion pressure (Symon *et al.* 1976; Fieschi and Lenzi 1983; Strandgaard and Paulson 1984; Dearden 1985). Autoregulation is also impaired if the Pa_{CO_2} is high, presumably because further vasodilatation cannot occur as perfusion pressure falls, and the same applies if the perfusion reserve is exhausted (Aaslid *et al.* 1989). Autoregulation is less effective in the elderly, so that postural hypotension is more likely to be symptomatic (Wollner *et al.* 1979).

27.3.5 Pathophysiology of acute cerebral ischaemia

The consequences of ischaemia

The brain normally derives its energy from the oxidative metabolism of glucose. Because there are negligible stores of glucose in the brain, when CBF falls and the brain becomes ischaemic, a series of neurophysiological and functional changes, which are dependent on the oxidative metabolism of glucose to provide energy in the form of ATP, occur at various thresholds of flow before cell death (infarction) (Fig. 27.13). Different mechanisms are responsible for reversible loss of cellular function, and for irreversible cell death, and there are also differences between the mechanisms that cause death of neurons, glia, and endothelial cells, and perhaps between white matter and grey matter (Dearden 1985; Pulsinelli 1992; Hossmann 1994).

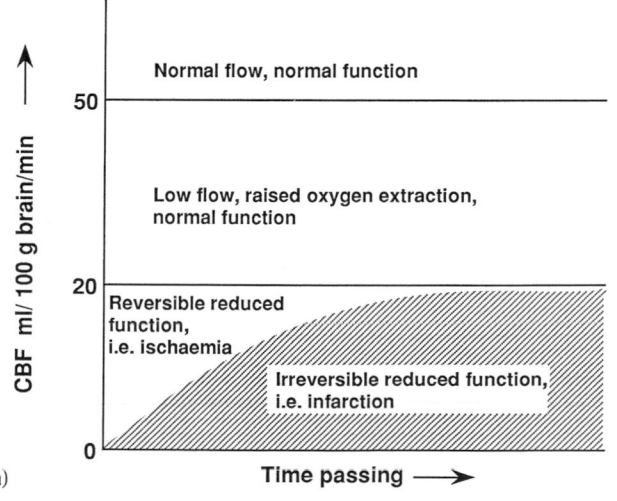
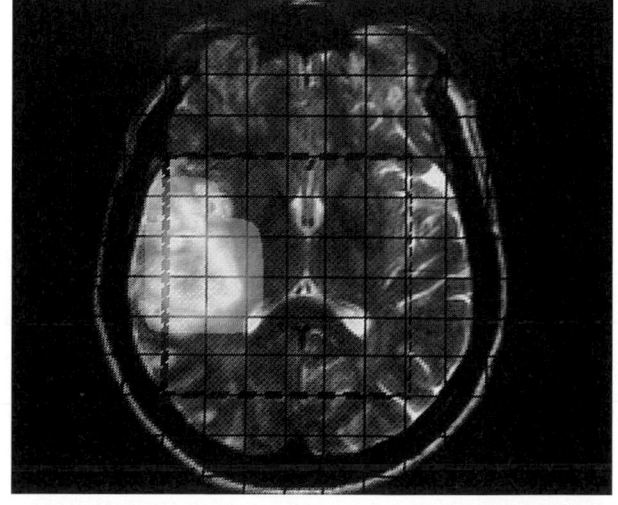

Fig. 27.13. (a) The thresholds of cerebral ischaemia at different levels of cerebral blood flow (CBF) in relation to the duration of ischaemia. (b) A metabolic 'map' of lactate in the brain by MR spectroscopy, superimposed on a structural MR scan. There is an obvious excess of lactate in the infarcted area in the distribution of a branch of the right middle cerebral artery. (Supplied by Professor Joanna Wardlaw). See also Plate 23.

When CBF falls below about 20 ml/100 g brain/min, the oxygen extraction fraction becomes maximal and $CMRo_2$ begins to fall (i.e. ischaemia, Fig. 27.11) (Wise *et al.* 1983). The EEG flattens, evoked responses disappear and neurological signs appear. In fact, a high OEF is only seen early after acute ischaemic stroke, in the first day or so (Plate 23a). If flow is restored, functional recovery is still possible (Fig. 27.13a). With increasing ischaemia, impaired protein synthesis is the earliest detectable metabolic change, followed by the inefficient anaerobic metabolism of glucose which causes a rise in lactate production, fall in intra- and extracellular pH, and impaired phosphocreatine and ATP synthesis, and so energy failure. As flow falls further, the energy-dependent functions of the cell membranes, including ion pumps, become progressively affected; water, sodium, and chloride enter cells (the beginnings of cytotoxic oedema), calcium also enters and is cytotoxic, and potassium leaks out. Cellular transport mechanisms and neurotransmitter systems fail, potentially neurotoxic excitatory transmitters, such as glutamate and aspartate, are released from neurons into the extracellular space; free oxygen radicals, nitric oxide and lipid peroxides are formed, so damaging cells further; proteases are activated and lyse structural proteins; and neurons release platelet-activating factor which may be neurotoxic (Martin 1997; Kristian and Siesjo 1998). An acute inflammatory response, with the migration of neutrophils and then of monocytes and macrophages into the ischaemic area, with activation of microglia, is another possible mechanism of neuronal death, perhaps mediated by the release of cytokines (Becker 1998). At flows below about 10 ml/100 g brain/min infarction occurs, and even if flow is restored, function does not recover. Later on apoptosis rather than necrosis may be responsible for neuronal death (Miles and Knuckey 1998). With MR spectroscopy it may be possible to track some of these metabolic changes in humans with high levels of lactate, indicating anaerobic metabolism, and low *N*-acetyl aspartate, a neuronal marker, being found in large infarcts with a poor prognosis (Fig. 27.13b) (Wardlaw *et al.* 1998a).

At the stage of infarction, $CMRo_2$ is low and CBF is either appropriately low as well, with a normal OEF (pure metabolic depression), or the OEF is low, indicating that CBF is in excess of the low metabolic demands of the infarcted tissue, i.e. luxury perfusion (Fig. 27.12b). In absolute luxury perfusion, CBF is increased (hyperperfusion), while in relative luxury perfusion it is normal or decreased. In either case the CBF is in excess of the prevailing $CMRo_2$ which itself may be normal or reduced, depending on the severity of the ischaemic damage (Baron 1991).

The consequences of the fall in CBF depend not just on the depth of ischaemia, but also on its duration (Fig. 27.13a). When ischaemia is due to an occluded artery, flow is almost never reduced to zero because of the availability of some sort of collateral blood supply which is, therefore, a further factor in determining the metabolic consequences. The local CBF may also be influenced by the development of cerebral oedema and raised intracranial pressure; acid metabolites and increasing extracellular potassium concentration, which cause vasodilata-

tion; the release of vasoconstrictor prostaglandins from aggregating platelets and damaged cell membranes and of other vasoconstrictors such as endothelin-1; whole-blood viscosity (Section 27.3.4); accumulation of leucocytes; aggregation of formed elements of the blood in the sluggish microcirculation and eventually thrombosis; and the local ability of the ischaemic tissues to autoregulate, which will probably be impaired.

A curious phenomenon is the possible ability of brain, like myocardium, to resist ischaemic infarction if it has been 'preconditioned' with brief episodes of ischaemia within the previous few hours. But, at the moment, this observation is confined to animals and doesn't seem very likely to lead to any therapeutic advances (Barone *et al.* 1998).

The ischaemic penumbra

Around, and presumably as islands within infarcted brain, there is an ischaemic penumbra (Astrup *et al.* 1981). Here the blood flow is low, function depressed, and the OEF high. In other words, there is 'viable tissue' with 'misery' perfusion where the metabolic needs of the tissue are not being met. The tissue may die or recover, depending on the speed and extent of restoration of blood flow. This concept immediately opens up the possibility of a 'therapeutic time window' during which restoration of flow and/or neuronal protection from ischaemic damage might prevent both immediate cell death and the recruitment of neurons for apoptosis, a slower process which occurs for some time after stroke onset. Other brain areas may show relative or absolute hyperaemia due to good collateral flow; reperfusion after an occluded artery has been reopened; inflammation; and vasodilatation in response to hypercapnia. Here OEF is low, indicating that flow is in excess of metabolic requirements, perhaps because the tissue has been irreversibly damaged; this is 'luxury' perfusion.

Recently PET studies have demonstrated, in humans, that about one-third of the ultimately infarcted tissue on late CT is in areas where, within hours of stroke onset, there had been potentially viable 'penumbral' tissue (on the basis of $CMRo_2$ levels associated with tissue viability), mostly as one would expect where early OEF was high and CBF somewhat low (Marchal *et al.* 1996a). However, it is still not clear for how long this penumbral region persists in a potentially viable state, nor how functionally important it is, but at least some recovery is possible if flow is restored (Lassen *et al.* 1991; Furlan *et al.* 1996). Unfortunately, accurate information about the ischaemic penumbra, and any areas of luxury perfusion, requires PET, which is neither available nor practical, nor quick enough and easily repeatable, to be very helpful in the *routine* management of acute ischaemic stroke, when flow and metabolism are changing at different rates in different parts of the ischaemic lesion (Baron 1991). Conceivably MR diffusion weighted and perfusion imaging, or some other tool such as spectroscopy, will prove to be more routinely available (Baird *et al.* 1997; Barber *et al.* 1998a). Very recently, a study using xenon-enhanced CT suggested that any ischaemic penumbra was much smaller than had been demonstrated by PET (Kaufmann *et al.* 1999).

Reperfusion and the therapeutic time window

Spontaneous recanalization, at least of MCA occlusion, occurs commonly and quite rapidly—perhaps, in two-thirds or so of patients, within a week, often in the first 48 hours (Fieschi *et al.* 1989; Kaps *et al.* 1992; Zanette *et al.* 1995). But, in humans it is not known exactly how long and how deep focal ischaemia has to be before tissue necrosis occurs and recovery of function is impossible. Any therapeutic window before the damage is irreversible could be minutes or it might be hours, which presumably explains why the consequences of acute arterial occlusion range from nothing, through a TIA, to a fatal ischaemic stroke (Fisher 1954). Nor is it known whether recanalization of an occluded artery and reperfusion is likely to be harmful at particular stages in the evolution of cerebral ischaemia to infarction, by increasing the perfusion pressure to brain with damaged autoregulation and so causing hyperperfusion, cerebral oedema, and haemorrhagic transformation (Toni *et al.* 1998) (Section 27.8.3). Put simply, it is conceivable that early recanalization may be 'good' (less tissue necrosis) while later it may be 'bad' (cerebral oedema and haemorrhage). On the whole, the CT and functional outcomes are both better with recanalization and reperfusion, and even with early hyperperfusion, than if the MCA remains occluded (Wardlaw *et al.* 1993; Marchal *et al.* 1996*b*; Barber *et al.* 1998*b*).

Ischaemic cerebral oedema

Cerebral ischaemia causes not only reversible and then irreversible loss of brain function, but also cerebral oedema (Symon *et al.* 1979; Hossman 1983). Ischaemic oedema is partly 'cytotoxic' and partly 'vasogenic'. Cytotoxic oedema starts early, within minutes of stroke onset, and affects the grey more than the white matter, with damaged cell membranes allowing intracellular water to accumulate. Vasogenic oedema, which starts rather later, within hours of stroke onset, affects the white matter more than the grey; the damaged blood–brain barrier allowing plasma constituents to enter the extracellular space. Ischaemic cerebral oedema reaches its maximum in 2–4 days and then subsides over a week or two. It certainly complicates large infarcts, being visible on CT and at post-mortem, but whether it occurs to any extent in small infarcts (e.g. lacunar) is not known. Reperfusion, only 2 hours after stroke onset, can certainly exacerbate oedema in baboons, but less consistently, it seems, in humans (Bell *et al.* 1985).

Cerebral oedema not only increases local hydrostatic pressure and compromises flow even further (by increasing pressure in the extravascular space and by swelling of the perivascular astroglial cells), but also causes mass effect, brain shift, and eventually transtentorial herniation with compression of the posterior cerebral artery, and brainstem distortion with haemorrhage (Fig. 27.14). Hyperaemia (in response to low CBF, acidosis, and hypoxia), vascular congestion, and any haemorrhagic transformation of the infarct (Section 27.8.3) all contribute to the swelling. A large infratentorial infarct may cause upward herniation through the tentorium or downward medullary coning at the foramen magnum. Death in the first

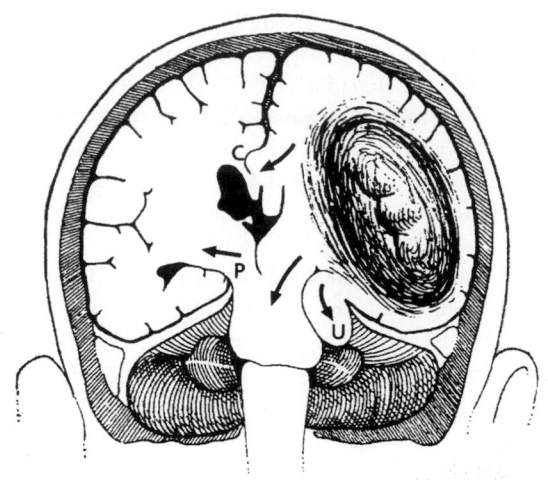

Fig. 27.14. A large oedematous cerebral infarct in the distribution of the middle cerebral artery causes herniation of the cingulate gyrus (c) under the falx cerebri; of the ispsilateral uncus (u) under the tentorium to compress the oculomotor nerve, posterior cerebral artery, and brainstem, and of the contralateral cerebral peduncle (p) to cause ipsilateral hemiparesis. (Reproduced with permission from Plum and Posner, 1985.)

week after cerebral infarction is usually due to these mass effects.

The effect of systemic blood pressure

Ischaemic and infarcted brain cannot autoregulate. Therefore, relatively modest increases in CPP (perhaps by spontaneous or therapeutic recanalization of an occluded artery, or by pharmacologically increasing the systemic blood pressure) can cause hyperaemia, increased CBF, cerebral oedema, and haemorrhagic infarction. All these changes will increase intracranial pressure, which would then tend to reduce the perfusion pressure. On the other hand, a fall in CPP can easily exacerbate cerebral ischaemia. It is not surprising, therefore, that it is not at all clear whether the systemic blood pressure in acute ischaemic stroke should be raised, lowered, or ignored and, if it is altered, by how much, how quickly, with what, for how long, and starting precisely when after stroke onset. This therapeutic dilemma is compounded by the fact that systemic blood pressure tends to be increased in acute stroke anyway, perhaps due to raised catecholamine and corticosteroid levels, and it usually falls spontaneously over the next few days, irrespective of any blood pressure lowering treatment (Bath and Bath 1997).

Secondary insults

Damaged brain may well have impaired responsiveness to $PaCO_2$ and PaO_2 as well as impaired autoregulation (Fieschi and Lenzi 1983). This makes the brain very sensitive to any further insults, such as systemic hypoxia (as a consequence of pneumonia, etc.), hypotension, and raised intracranial pressure (so-called secondary insults) (Cormio *et al.* 1997). However, it is not clear how often, and for how long, this vulnerability persists after the onset of stroke. Hyperglycaemia is undoubtedly associated with a poor outcome after stroke, either because the consequences of ischaemia are exacerbated in the presence of high blood glucose concentrations, perhaps mediated by excess lactate production (Weir *et al.* 1997), or because hyperglycaemia reflects the stress response, and so the severity of the initial stroke (Toni *et al.* 1992; Tracey *et al.* 1993). Clearly, trials of glucose lowering need to be done to sort this out (Scott *et al.* 1998). Fever is associated with a worse outcome and hypothermia with a better outcome in stroke but, like blood sugar, it is not clear whether this association represents a causal relationship, and therefore whether any intervention would be worthwhile (Reith *et al.* 1996). Induced hypothermia is protective in animals, but has not yet been properly tested in humans (Buchan and Pulsinelli 1990). Dehydration, increasing haematocrit, and raised whole-blood viscosity are further potential exacerbating factors.

Diaschisis

Acute or chronic cerebral injury may cause effects in remote areas of brain, so-called 'diaschisis', by reducing neuronal inputs, metabolic activity, and thus blood flow. In practice, this phenomenon is easy to demonstrate in the cerebellum contralateral to a large MCA-territory infarct, but more difficult to show convincingly in the contralateral cerebral hemisphere or in other parts of the ipsilateral cerebral hemisphere, which appear unaffected on CT, and even on MRI (Pappata *et al.* 1987; Andrews 1991; De Reuck *et al.* 1997). The functional consequences, if any, of such metabolic and flow changes at a distance from the primary lesion are not at all clear (Bowler *et al.* 1995).

27.4 The causes of stroke

27.4.1 Cerebral ischaemia and infarction

Cerebral ischaemia and infarction are usually caused by sudden occlusion of an artery supplying the brain or, less often, by low flow distal to an already occluded or highly stenosed artery. Occlusion or stenosis can be the result of disease of the arterial wall; embolism from the heart; haematological disorders; and various rare, but sometimes treatable, conditions which are proportionately more common in young stroke patients (where degenerative arterial disease is unusual) but which can still be a cause of stroke in the elderly (Table 27.9). Venous infarction is considered later (Section 27.11). Ischaemia due to head injury, encephalitis, and other global encephalopathies is beyond the scope of this chapter.

27.4.2 Atherothromboembolism

Atheroma seems to be an almost inevitable accompaniment of ageing, at least in developed countries. It is by far the most common arterial disorder and, when complicated by thrombosis or embolism, is the most frequent, but by no means only, cause of cerebral ischaemia and infarction (Table 27.10).

Table 27.9. The causes of cerebral ischaemia and infarction

Arterial wall disorders
  Atherothromboembolism (Section 27.4.2)
  Intracranial small vessel disease (lipohyalinosis, arteriolosclerosis, microatheroma) (Section 27.4.3)
  Trauma (Table 27.11)
  Dissection (Table 27.12)
  Fibromuscular dysplasia (Section 27.4.4)
  Congenital arterial anomalies (Section 27.4.4)
  Moyamoya syndrome (Section 27.4.4)
  Embolism from arterial aneurysms (Section 27.4.4)
  Inflammatory vascular diseases (Table 27.13)
  Leukoaraiosis (Section 27.4.4)
  Irradiation (Section 27.4.4)
  Infections (Section 27.4.4)

Embolism from the heart (Table 27.14)

Haematological disorders (Table 27.15)

Miscellaneous conditions (Section 27.4.7)
  Pregnancy/puerperium
  Oral contraceptives and other female sex hormones (Section 27.2.7)
  Drug abuse
  Cancer
  Perioperative
  Migraine
  Inflammatory bowel disease
  Homocystinaemia
  Fabry's disease
  Mitochondrial cytopathy
  Hypoglycaemia
  Fibrocartilaginous embolism
  Snake bite
  Fat embolism
  Epidermal naevus syndrome
  Susac's syndrome
  Nephrotic syndrome (Section 27.4.6)
  CADASIL (Section 27.2.8)

Although difficult to prove, atheroma may not have become more prevalent during the period of increasing incidence of ischaemic heart disease and stroke during the first half of the twentieth century, which suggests perhaps that these clinical syndromes may be due to the thrombotic (and embolic) complications of atheroma, rather than to the atheroma itself (Morris 1951*a,b*; Joseph *et al.* 1993). It is, after all, remarkable how widespread atheroma can be in patients with no clinical complications, while fatal stroke and myocardial infarction can occur even when atheroma is relatively restricted and mild; is this back luck, bad atheroma, or bad clotting? Of course, if atheroma itself is actually caused by thrombosis as some believe, any distinction between the two is artificial (Duguid 1976). In this context, it is important to remember that epidemiologically defined vascular risk factors for clinical events such as stroke (Section 27.2.7) are not necessarily associated with atheroma but are perhaps associations, and even the causes, of the complicating thrombosis.

Table 27.10. The approximate relative frequency of the main causes of ischaemic stroke and TIA (summarized from Sandercock *et al.* 1989)

Atherothrombosis affecting large and medium-sized arteries between the heart and the brain	50%
Intracranial small vessel disease (small vessel disease lipohyalinosis/microatheroma, etc.)	25%
Embolism from the heart	20%
Miscellaenous rare disorders	5%

Distribution of atheroma

Atheroma mainly affects large (e.g. aortic arch) and medium-sized arteries at places of arterial branching (e.g. carotid bifurcation), tortuosity (e.g. carotid siphon), and confluence (e.g. basilar artery) (see Fig. 27.6) (Fisher 1951, 1954; Hutchinson and Yates 1957; Schwartz and Mitchell 1961; Cornhill *et al.* 1980; Ross *et al.* 1988). These are sites of haemodynamic sheer stress and thus endothelial trauma; boundary layer separation, blood stagnation, and the accumulation of platelets; and of turbulence, all of which are likely to promote thrombosis (Grady 1984; Reneman *et al.* 1985; Nicholls *et al.* 1989). This might explain the distribution of atheroma in the cerebral circulation if thrombosis is intimately involved with its progression, even if not in its very beginnings. It is remarkable how free of atheroma some sites can be: for example, the internal carotid artery (ICA) between the commonly affected origin and less commonly affected siphon, and the main cerebral arteries distal to the circle of Willis (Lhermitte *et al.* 1970; Miller and Cohen 1987). However, in the same individual, atheroma in one place does tend to be accompanied by atheroma in other parts of the same artery, with atheroma in other arteries to the brain, and in arteries to other organs such as the heart (Mitchell and Schwartz 1962; Miller and Cohen 1987). Presumably this reflects individual susceptibility to atheroma as a result of the presence of causal vascular risk factors (such as hypertension) and genetic predisposition which determines who will develop atheroma, while the arterial anatomy determines where the lesions occur. None the less, it is curious how severely one arterial site can be affected and yet, in the same individual, the mirror-image site on the other side of the body is still normal, perhaps because of subtle asymmetries in arterial geometry (Gnasso *et al.* 1997).

Natural history of atheroma

Atheroma starts in childhood, it is thought in response to endothelial injury (Ross 1999). Intimal fatty streaks appear first. In a gradual process stretching over many years, circulating monocyte-derived macrophages adhere to and invade the arterial wall, there is an inflammatory response with cytokine production and T-lymphocyte activation, intra- and, later, extracellular cholesterol and other lipids are deposited, particularly in macrophages which are then described as foam cells, smooth muscle cells proliferate, fibrosis occurs, and so

fibrolipid plaques are formed (Fuster *et al.* 1992*a*,*b*; Libby 1996). Necrosis and calcification complicate advanced lesions. These atheromatous plaques invade the media, gradually spread around and along the arterial wall, and narrow the lumen, although at times the vessel dilates. The plaques are complicated by platelet adhesion, activation, and aggregation, which initiates blood coagulation and subsequent thrombosis.

Thrombus may be incorporated into the atheromatous plaques which then re-endothelialize; it may grow to obstruct the arterial lumen and then propagate proximally or distally in the stagnant column of blood as far as the next branching point or beyond; it may be lysed by natural fibrinolytic mechanisms in the vessel wall; or it may embolize in whole or in part to occlude a distal artery, usually at a branching point. Such artery-to-artery emboli vary in size and shape, and consist of some combination of cholesterol debris from the atheromatous plaque, platelet aggregates, and fibrin, which may be newly formed and relatively friable, or old and well organized. Depending on local blood flow and on the size, composition, and consistency of the impacted emboli, they may be lysed, fragment, and vanish into the microcirculation, or remain to occlude the artery and promote local thrombosis. Thrombosis is further encouraged by the release from platelets of thromboxane A_2, which is also a vasoconstrictor. However, it is opposed by prostacyclin and nitric oxide, both vasodilators, released from vascular endothelium, as well as by endothelium-derived plasminogen activator (Vane *et al.* 1990). The balance of pro- and antithrombotic factors determines whether a thrombus complicating an atheromatous plaque or an occlusive embolus, grows, is lysed, or is incorporated into the vessel wall.

It is likely that atheromatous plaques become 'active' or 'unstable' from time to time as a result of fissuring and cracking of thin parts of the fibrous cap which covers the rather rigid lesion; of ulceration perhaps; or sometimes of haemorrhage within the plaque, rather than the more commonly found haemorrhage entering via a crack in the endothelial surface (Fisher *et al.* 1987; Svindland and Torvik 1988; Richardson *et al.* 1989; Torvik *et al.* 1989; Gomez 1990; Ogata *et al.* 1990; Davies 1997; Lammie *et al.* 1999). Any of these events exposes the highly thrombogenic necrotic core of the plaque to blood and so causes thrombus to form and then perhaps to embolize. Thus, atherothromboembolism can be regarded as an acute-on-chronic disease; at any one time a plaque may be static and quiescent with a thick fibrous cap, slowly growing but asymptomatic, or active with ongoing thrombosis and embolization, which may or may not be symptomatic depending on the depth and duration of the consequent ischaemia (Section 27.3.5). This concept may explain the tendency for TIAs to cluster, for stroke to occur early after a TIA and to affect the same arterial territory, for presumed artery-to-artery embolic strokes to recur early, and for the risk of stroke to decline with time even distal to a severe symptomatic stenosis (Section 27.10.2).

Complicated atheromatous lesions which eventually become fibrotic and heavily calcified make the whole artery rigid, elongated and so tortuous, and sometimes ectatic. Ectasia and aneurysmal bulging, particularly of the basilar artery, may compress adjacent structures, such as the lower cranial nerves and brainstem. Also, emboli may be released from the atheromatous walls and complicating thrombosis. However, arterial rupture is exceptional (Schwartz *et al.* 1993; Passero and Filosomi 1998).

Atherothrombotic plaques are clearly highly dynamic lesions, progressing and regressing in various parts of the arterial tree at different rates and at different times, usually showing layers of thrombus of different ages. Progression and regression of these atherothrombotic lesions can, to some extent, be followed non-invasively in humans with ultrasound imaging, but it is difficult to distinguish atheroma, which is likely to change only slowly, from thrombus, which may grow or be lysed much faster (Hennerici and Steinke 1991; Beletsky *et al.* 1996). Also, intraplaque haemorrhage presumably may cause quite sudden enlargement of a plaque, followed by fairly rapid shrinkage as the haematoma is absorbed. Recently it has become possible to monitor the release of emboli from carotid plaques, and elsewhere, into the cerebral circulation with transcranial Doppler of the middle cerebral artery, again an indication of plaque 'instability'. Not surprisingly, high-intensity embolic signals are more common distal to symptomatic compared with asymptomatic stenoses, but even then the number is rather low, perhaps because of technical difficulties or insufficient recording time (Del Sette *et al.* 1997; Koennecke *et al.* 1998; Molloy *et al.* 1998; Wijman *et al.* 1998).

Symptoms of focal ischaemia occur as a consequence of reduced blood flow (Section 27.3.5) which, in the context of atheroma, is most commonly due to embolism from a plaque complicated by thrombosis in an extracranial artery (such as the carotid bifurcation) to occlude a smaller intracranial artery (such as the mainstem or branch of the middle cerebral artery (MCA)) (Gunning *et al.* 1964; Lhermitte *et al.* 1970; Caplan and Hennerici 1998) (Fig. 27.15). The notion that the carotid siphon might filter out emboli en route to the brain is interesting but unproven (Hugh 1987). Occasionally emboli may reach the brain via the collateral circulation; for example from a stenosed internal carotid artery (ICA) across the circle of Willis into the MCA distal to an occluded contralateral ICA; from thrombus in the blind proximal stump of an occluded contralateral ICA, a stenosed proximal external carotid artery (ECA), or from more proximal sites of atheroma, but all via the ECA and through the ophthalmic circulation to the carotid siphon and beyond. Also, emboli may arise from the distal end of a thrombus occluding the ICA. Finally, ischaemia may occur due to haemodynamic compromise beyond an occluded ICA (Section 27.3.4) (Hankey and Warlow 1991*a*; Klijn *et al.* 1997). Furthermore, focal ischaemia may occur *between* arterial territories (i.e. in boundary zones) usually due to low flow distal to an occluded artery (Section 27.6.2).

Symptomatic *in situ* atherothrombotic occlusion does not appear to be very common in the anterior cerebral circulation, perhaps because the most commonly affected site for atheroma is in a relatively large artery (i.e. the ICA origin) rather than in smaller arteries, such as the MCA, which are more often occluded by embolism than by *in situ* atherothrombosis (Lhermitte *et al.* 1970; Ogata *et al.* 1990, 1994). Another reason might be the relatively effective collateral circulation distal to any occlusion in the extracranial carotid system (Section 27.3.2). On the other hand, symptomatic atherothrombotic occlusion does appear to be more common in the posterior circulation, particularly in the basilar artery. But even here, embolism from non-occlusive thrombus into smaller arteries supplying the brainstem and elsewhere is well described (Castaigne *et al.* 1973; Schwarz *et al.* 1997; Martin *et al.* 1998).

In an individual patient it is relatively easy to diagnose acute focal ischaemia or infarction but, because angiography is seldom done early, or at all, it is difficult to know what the pattern of any arterial pathology is and exactly how the ischaemia has occurred. Even when angiography, or (increasingly often) ultrasound of the extra- and intracranial circulation, reveals an occluded artery, this does not necessarily mean that the occlusion was recent, or that it was embolic rather than due to *in situ* thrombosis, or whether any embolism had occurred via collaterals or from the distal end of the occluded thrombus, or whether the ischaemia was due to low flow distal to an old occlusion (Ringelstein *et al.* 1983; J. P. H. Wade *et al.* 1987). To confuse matters further, it is now clear that occluded arteries can recanalize spontaneously quite quickly, particularly the mainstem of the MCA. Possibly emboli from the heart are more likely to lyse than those from atheromatous arteries, and thrombotic occlusion of the MCA or ICA is perhaps less likely to open spontaneously. Recanalization rates presumably also depend on the constituents and age of the occluding material. However, whatever the exact cause of the ischaemia, any demonstrated arterial pathology in the aorta, neck, basilar artery, or circle of Willis is usually atherothrombosis and the assumption is then reasonably made that thromboembolism has occurred at some stage and is likely to occur again. If, as is so often the case (Zhu and Norris 1990), little or no arterial pathology is demonstrated by vascular imaging, or macroscopically at post-mortem, then focal ischaemia is most likely due to embolism from the heart (Section 27.4.5) or to intracranial small vessel disease (Section 27.4.3) (Fig. 27.15).

Cholesterol embolization syndrome

This rare disorder seems to be due to the rupture of atheromatous plaques in elderly people with widespread disease, either spontaneously, but perhaps more often as a complication of instrumentation or surgery of large atheromatous arteries such as the aorta, and possibly of anticoagulation or therapeutic thrombolysis. Cholesterol debris is released and embolizes to the microcirculation of many organs throughout the body, including the brain and spinal cord. Hours or days after instrumentation or surgery there is the subacute onset of a syndrome very similar to systemic vasculitis or infective endocarditis: malaise, fever, abdominal pain, proteinuria and renal failure, stroke-like episodes, drowsiness, confusion, skin petechiae, splinter haemorrhages, livedo reticularis, cyanosis of fingers and toes, raised erythrocyte sedimentation rate, neutrophil leucocytosis, and

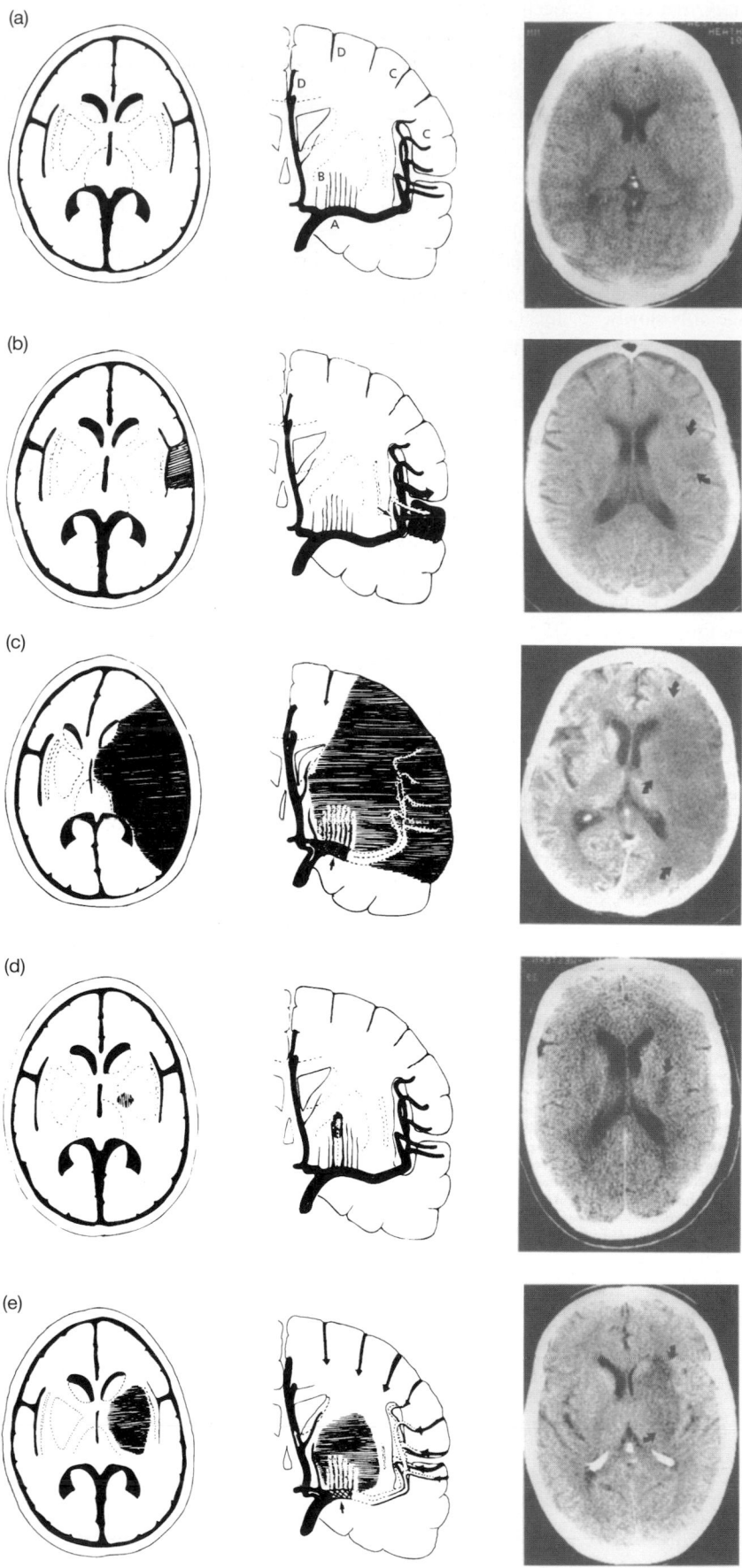

Fig. 27.15. Various patterns of arterial occlusion causing different types of ischaemic stroke. Left-hand column, diagram of axial CT brain scan through the level of the basal ganglia; middle column, diagram of the middle cerebral artery (MCA) and anterior cerebral arteries on a coronal brain section; right-hand column, corresponding axial CT brain scan. (A) main trunk of MCA; (B) lenticulostriate perforating branches of the MCA; (C) cortical branches of the MCA; (D) cortical branches of the anterior cerebral arteries. (a) Normal arterial anatomy and CT scan; (b) occlusion (usually embolic (arrow) from heart, aorta, or internal carotid artery) of a cortical branch of the MCA and restricted cortical infarct on CT (arrows); (c) occlusion (usually embolus (arrow) as in (b) above) of MCA trunk to cause infarction of entire MCA territory (arrows); (d) occlusion of a single lenticulostriate artery to cause a lacunar infarct (arrow); note that the patient has an old lacunar infarct in the opposite hemisphere; (e) occlusion of the MCA trunk with good cortical collaterals from the anterior and posterior cerebral arteries to cause a striatocapsular infarct (arrows).

eosinophilia. The diagnosis is made by finding cholesterol debris in the microcirculation of biopsy material, usually from the kidney but sometimes from skin or muscle (Fine *et al.* 1987; Cross 1991; Rhodes 1996).

27.4.3 Intracranial small vessel disease

The small penetrating arteries of the brain (less than about 500 μm in diameter) are not supported by a good collateral circulation; i.e. the lenticulostriate branches of the middle cerebral artery (MCA), the thalamoperforating branches of the proximal posterior cerebral artery, and the perforating arteries to the brainstem. Therefore, occlusion is rather likely to cause infarction, albeit in a small, restricted area of brain. Such 'lacunar' infarcts comprise about one-quarter of first ischaemic strokes and TIAs (Bamford *et al.* 1987; Sempere *et al.* 1998). Because the case fatality is so low (about 1 per cent), there are few pathological data, but it does seem that these small arteries are much less likely to be occluded by emboli either from the heart or from extracranial sites of atherothrombosis, compared with the trunk or cortical branches of the MCA (Olsen *et al.* 1985; Bamford and Warlow 1988; Orgogozo and Bogousslavsky 1989; Hankey and Warlow 1991*b*; Tegeler *et al.* 1991; Boiten *et al.* 1996; Gan *et al.* 1997). Furthermore, ischaemic lacunar strokes are less often associated with MCA emboli detected with transcranial Doppler (Koennecke *et al.* 1998).

Although not universally accepted, it is generally thought that these small perforating arteries are occluded by thrombus complicating not atheroma but a distinct small vessel arteriopathy variously described as lipohyalinosis, complex small vessel disease, arteriolosclerosis, fibrohyalinosis or microatheroma (Millikan and Futrell 1990; Fisher 1991; Lammie *et al.* 1997). The muscle and elastin in the arterial wall are replaced by collagen, there is subintimal hyalinization, the wall becomes thickened and the lumen narrowed, and the vessel becomes tortuous, possibly with the formation of microaneurysms (Charcot–Bouchard aneurysms) which may rupture (Fig. 27.16b). It is, therefore, conceivable that this small vessel arteriopathy can lead to small, deep haemorrhages as well as lacunar infarcts; indeed, both types of stroke have been described in the same patients (Miyashita *et al.* 1991; Besson *et al.* 1993; Samuelsson *et al.* 1996; Kwa *et al.* 1998). Although hypertension is common in patients with lacunar infarction, it cannot explain every case and, in any event, the risk factors, including hypertension, seem to be rather similar to those in ischaemic stroke patients with presumed atherothrombotic arterial disease (Adams *et al.* 1989; Lodder *et al.* 1990; Sacco *et al.* 1991; Mast *et al.* 1995; You *et al.* 1995; Schmal *et al.* 1998). Perhaps the same individuals are susceptible to both atherothrombosis of large and medium-sized arteries and small vessel disease, but one becomes symptomatic before the other. Or perhaps the concept of a distinct small vessel disease causing lacunar infarction is incorrect. Certainly, at least some small infarcts in the brainstem and internal capsule can be due to atheroma at the mouth of the small penetrating vessels spreading from atheroma of the larger parent artery (Fisher and Caplan 1971; Fisher 1979).

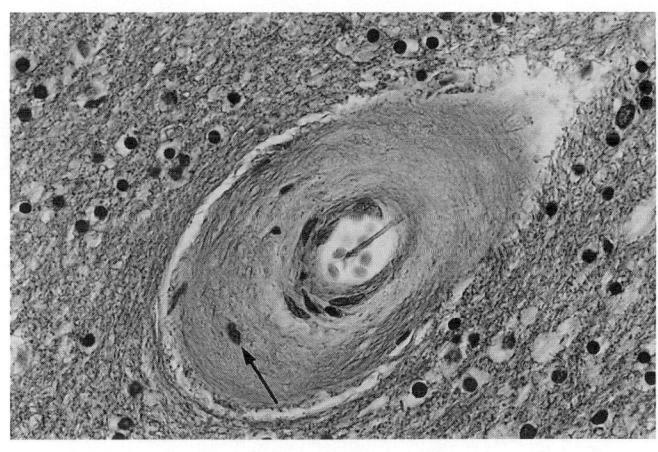

(a)

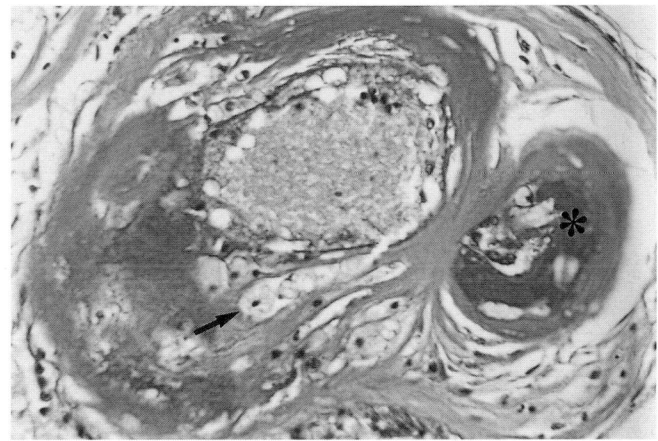

(b)

Fig. 27.16. Photomicrograph of penetrating lenticulostriate artery in the putamen, illustrating two distinctive patterns of vessel pathology. (a) Concentric hyaline wall thickening with a few remaining vascular smooth muscle cell nuclei (arrow). The lumen remains patent. Such 'simple' small vessel disease is an almost invariable feature of elderly brains, most prominent in hypertensives and diabetics. (b) A complex, disorganized vessel segment showing an asymmetric destructive process with focal fibrinoid material (asterix) and mural foam cells (arrow). The lumen is visible cut in two planes of section. This 'complex' vessel lesion corresponds to what C. M. Fisher termed 'lipohyalinosis', and in this case the lesion was adjacent to, and presumably the cause of, a right striatocapsular lacunar infarct. (Haematoxylin and eosin; (a) ×420; (b) ×210. Provided by Dr Alistair Lammie, University of Walts.)

27.4.4 Rare arterial disorders

Trauma

Penetrating neck injuries are more likely to damage the carotid than the better-protected vertebral artery (Table 27.11). Laceration, dissection, and intimal tears may be complicated by thrombosis and then embolism, and therefore ischaemic stroke at the time of, or some days or even weeks after, the injury. Later stroke may be a consequence of the formation of a traumatic aneurysm, arteriovenous fistula, or a fistula between the carotid and vertebral arteries (Davis and Zimmerman 1983).

Table 27.11. Causes of injury of the arteries supplying the brain

Penetrating injury
    Missile wounds
    Neck laceration
    Neck surgery
    Tonsillectomy
    Oral trauma
    Catheter angiography
    Jugular vein cannulation

Non-penetrating injury
    Blow to the neck
    Carotid compression tests
    Attempted strangulation
    Neck injury (fracture, subluxation, dislocation)
    Sudden neck movements (whiplash injury, 'head-banging', ceiling
      painting, head injury, head turning, minor falls)
    Yoga
    Neck manipulation
    Labour
    Tonic–clonic seizure
    Vomiting
    Bronchoscopy
    Atlanto-axial dislocation
    Occipito-atlantal instability
    Fractured base of skull
    Cervical rib
    Fractured clavicle

Table 27.12. Causes of dissection of the extra- and intracranial arteries

Traumatic (Table 27.11)
    Penetrating injury
    Non-penetrating injury

Spontaneous
    Fibromuscular dysplasia
    Cystic medial necrosis
    Marfan's syndrome
    Ehlers–Danlos syndrome
    Pseudoxanthoma elasticum
    Inflammatory arterial disease
    Infective arterial disease (e.g. syphilis)

Non-penetrating neck injury (Table 27.11) is a more subtle cause of ischaemic stroke because the injury does not have to be very severe (at least superficially) to cause intimal tearing or dissection, or it is overshadowed by other injuries. Hours, days, or weeks later stroke occurs as the result of complicating thrombotic occlusion or embolization (Davis and Zimmerman 1983; Thie *et al.* 1993a; Tulyapronchote *et al.* 1994). This can occur at any age, but in young adults it is the most frequent identifiable cause of ischaemic stroke in some series (Hilton-Jones and Warlow 1985). A direct blow to the neck is more likely to injure the carotid than the vertebral artery (Hughes and Brownell 1968). On the other hand, the vertebral artery appears to be more vulnerable to rotational and hyperextension injuries of the neck, particularly at the level of the atlas and axis (Sherman *et al.* 1981; Frisoni and Anzola 1991). The subclavian artery can be damaged by a fractured clavicle or a cervical rib, with later embolization up the vertebral arteries or even up the right common carotid artery (Prior *et al.* 1979).

Traumatic rupture of an atheromatous plaque, or vasospasm, are both most unusual.

Arterial dissection

Arterial dissection is an increasingly recognized but none the less rare cause of ischaemic stroke and TIAs. Sometimes there is a predisposing cause (Table 27.12), particularly neck trauma, but often there is no explanation. Blood tracks along a split within the arterial wall and there may or may not be an intimal tear so that the false lumen is in communication with the true lumen. The artery may become occluded by the wall haematoma itself,

thrombosis and embolism may complicate occlusive or non-occlusive dissections, and aneurysmal bulging of the weakened wall may occur (O'Connell *et al.* 1985). Arterial rupture is unusual.

Before, at the time of, and even without any stroke or TIA complications, internal carotid artery (ICA) dissection frequently causes ipsilateral pain (around the eye, face, and neck), sometimes an ipsilateral Horner's syndrome due to sympathetic nerve involvement in the lesion, and occasionally a cervical bruit which the patient may hear because the lesion can be much more distal than the usual proximal site of atheromatous ICA stenosis. Lower cranial nerve palsies, particularly hypoglossal, occasionally occur as a result of aneurysmal ICA dilatation at the base of the skull, or perhaps of periarterial inflammation and haematoma formation (Sturzenegger and Huber 1993; Silbert *et al.* 1995; Mokri et 1996).

As well as focal brainstem and cerebellar ischaemia, vertebral dissection often causes occipital pain over the site of the arterial lesion, usually at the level of the atlas and axis, and sometimes cervical root lesions due to compression from the distended arterial wall (Caplan and Tettenborn 1992a; Hetzel *et al.* 1996; de Bray *et al.* 1997).

On angiography there is usually a long, tapered, narrow or occluded segment, perhaps with an intimal flap, double lumen, or intraluminal thrombus, and sometimes an associated aneurysm (Fig. 27.17). Intracranial arterial occlusion, presumably embolic, may be seen. Carotid dissection can often be strongly suspected on Duplex scanning (Sturzenegger *et al.* 1993, 1995), and both carotid and vertebral dissection even more strongly suspected by a combination of axial MRI through the lesion, to show the acute haematoma in the arterial wall, with MR angiography (Auer *et al.* 1998).

The radiological appearances of dissection normally resolve within days or weeks. Recurrent dissections in the same, or a different artery, are very infrequent unless the patient has a rare connective tissue abnormality such as the Ehlers–Danlos syndrome (Leys *et al.* 1995).

Intracranial arterial dissection is much rarer, may present with subarachnoid haemorrhage due to rupture of a pseudo-aneurysm, as well as with ischaemic stroke, and is less often diagnosed during life (Farrell *et al.* 1985; de Bray *et al.* 1997).

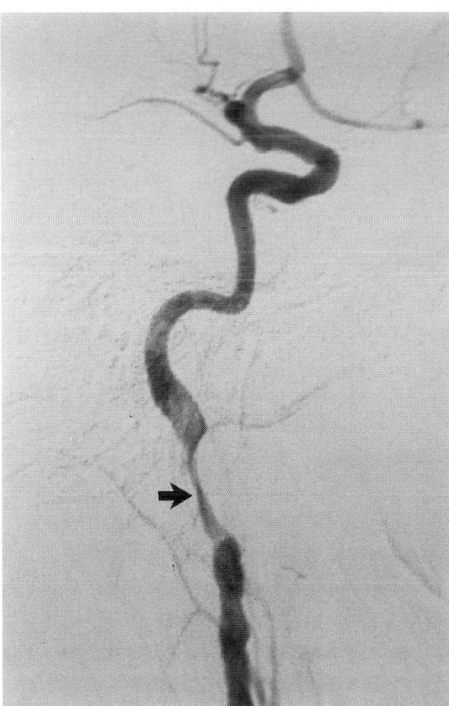

Fig. 27.17. Lateral view of a selective carotid angiogram to show dissection of the internal carotid artery with a smooth narrowing of the lumen (arrow) at the base of the skull well distal to its origin.

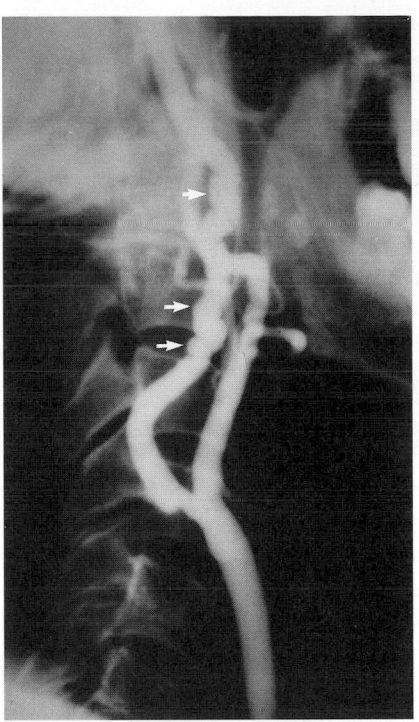

Fig. 27.18. Lateral view of a selective carotid angiogram showing the typical 'string of beads' appearance of fibrous muscular dysplasia (arrows).

Aortic arch dissection causes profound hypotension with global, and sometimes boundary zone, cerebral ischaemia, or focal cerebral ischaemia if the dissection spreads up one of the neck arteries. Clues to this diagnosis are anterior chest or interscapular pain along with diminished, unequal, or absent arterial pulses in the arms or neck; a normal ECG, unlike acute myocardial infarction; acute aortic regurgitation; and pericardial effusion (Gerber *et al.* 1986; Carrel *et al.* 1991, Pretre and von Segesser 1997).

Fibromuscular dysplasia

Fibromuscular dysplasia (FMD) is a rare segmental disorder of small and medium-sized arteries (Luscher *et al.* 1987). The patients are of any age, females are affected more than males, and the cause is unknown. It usually affects more than one artery in the same individual and is most common in the renal arteries, causing hypertension. The mid-cervical portion of the ICA is the most commonly affected artery to the brain. Sometimes the vertebral arteries are affected at the level of the first two cervical vertebrae. Intracranial involvement is exceptional (Arunodaya *et al.* 1997). Histologically there is fibrosis and thickening of the arterial wall alternating with atrophy, so the typical angiographic appearance is likened to a 'string of beads' (Fig. 27.18). In rare cases there is concentric tubular narrowing of the affected segments, or sometimes just a 'web' at the proximal ICA (Morgenlander and Goldstein 1991). FMD is associated with intracranial saccular aneurysms and arteriovenous malformations, and can be complicated by aneurysmal bulging of the atrophic segments as well as by dissection. FMD

of some arteries to the brain may be found in up to 1 per cent of routine post-mortems, so that any association with cerebral ischaemia or infarction may be no more than coincidence. Occasionally, however, it may indeed be complicated by thrombosis and embolism. The natural history is unknown and treatment with anticoagulants or angioplasty is entirely empirical.

Congenital arterial anomalies

Unless fibromuscular dysplasia, saccular aneurysms (Section 27.4.8), and vascular malformations (Section 27.4.8) are regarded as 'congenital', there are few examples of congenital arterial anomalies which become symptomatic. Occasionally the carotid arteries are hypoplastic or even absent, perhaps rendering the brain more vulnerable to ischaemia (Kubis *et al.* 1996). Various degrees of kinking, acute angulation, buckling, tortuosity, and looping of the internal carotid artery are quite often seen on angiograms (Metz *et al.* 1961); such appearances can be due to atheroma or fibromuscular dysplasia, but sometimes a congenital origin is possible, particularly if one remembers that during embryogenesis the carotid artery lengthens and straightens. The difficulty is to distinguish between atheromatous and congenital cases, and there is a tendency to regard anomalies in children and young adults as 'congenital' and those in the middle aged and elderly as 'atherosclerotic'.

Congenital carotid loops may be associated with: aneurysm formation (leading to a pulsatile neck swelling, intraluminal thrombosis, and embolism; possibly with endothelial damage and thrombosis; and exceptionally with focal ischaemia on head movement (Sarkari *et al.* 1970; Desai and Toole 1975). Rarely, these loops may cause hypoglossal nerve lesions or pulsatile tinnitus.

Some inherited disorders of connective tissue can present with (or be complicated by) arterial dissection or even rupture, intra- and extracranial aneurysm formation, carotico-cavernous fistula, and mitral leaflet prolapse, e.g. the *Ehlers–Danlos syndrome* (North *et al.* 1995), *pseudoxanthoma elasticum* (Mayer *et al.* 1994), and *Marfan's syndrome* (Bowen *et al.* 1987; Schievink *et al.* 1994).

Moyamoya syndrome

In Japanese *moyamoya* means a haze, like a puff of smoke, and the term describes a characteristic, but rare, radiologically defined consequence of severe stenosis or occlusion of one or, more often, both distal ICAs, frequently with additional involvement of parts of the circle of Willis and sometimes of the proximal cerebral and basilar arteries. Fine anastomotic collaterals develop from the perforating and pial arteries at the base of the brain, orbital and ethmoidal branches of the external carotid artery, and leptomeningeal and transdural vessels, giving the characteristic 'puff of smoke' appearance on angiography (Chen *et al.* 1988).

The disorder seems to be almost confined to the Japanese and other Asians, and in most cases the cause is unknown (Bruno *et al.* 1988; Chiu *et al.* 1998). Some cases are familial (Kitahara *et al.* 1979), others appear to be due to a generalized fibrous disorder of arteries (Aoyagi *et al.* 1996), and a few may be due to a congenital hypoplastic anomaly affecting arteries at the base of the brain, or associated with Down's syndrome (Cramer *et al.* 1996). Sometimes the arterial narrowing and obstruction is a result of basal meningeal or nasopharyngeal infection, vasculitis, irradiation, trauma, fibromuscular dysplasia, sickle-cell disease, or neurofibromatosis (Tomsick *et al.* 1976). Atheromatous disease of the distal ICA very rarely causes the moyamoya syndrome, perhaps because profuse collateral development is impossible except in children, or perhaps because such distal distribution of atheroma is so uncommon.

The syndrome presents in infancy with recurrent episodes of cerebral ischaemia and infarction, mental retardation, headache, epileptic seizures, and occasionally involuntary movements. In adults the presentation is as, or more, often with subarachnoid or primary intracerebral haemorrhage, because of rupture of the fine collateral system. There have also been a few reports of associated intracranial aneurysms (Iwama *et al.* 1997).

Embolism from intra- and extracranial arterial aneurysms

Embolism from thrombus within the cavity of an aneurysm must be rare and is difficult to prove in an individual case. Such aneurysms may be of the saccular type and intracranial (Fisher *et al.* 1980; Sakaki *et al.* 1980; Przelomski *et al.* 1986; Catala *et al.* 1993), or of the ICA in the neck as the result of trauma, infection, atheroma, carotid surgery, irradiation, or fibromus-

cular dysplasia (Schwartz *et al.* 1962; Nesbit *et al.* 1979; Mokri and Piepgras 1981). Of course, such aneurysms may be innocent bystanders, with symptomatic atherothrombosis elsewhere in the cerebral circulation, or a cardiac source of embolism, thus making any cause-and-effect relationship for ischaemic stroke something of a guess. Imaging the thrombus within the aneurysm by CT, MR, or angiography would, of course, make a causal role somewhat more likely.

It is far more common for an intracranial aneurysm to present with rupture and subarachnoid haemorrhage (Section 27.4.8) and for ICA aneurysms to present as a pulsatile, and maybe painful and tender, mass in the neck or pharynx, perhaps with an ipsilateral Horner's syndrome, or more rarely with compression of the lower cranial nerves at the base of the skull (Rhodes *et al.* 1976; Hommel *et al.* 1984).Extracranial vertebral artery aneurysms may also present with pain in the neck and arm, a mass, spinal cord compression, and upper limb ischaemia (Catala *et al.* 1993).

Leukoaraiosis (Binswanger's disease, chronic progressive subcortical encephalopathy, subcortical arteriosclerotic encephalopathy, periventricular leucoencephalopathy)

The number of alternative titles reflects the confusion between the clinical, radiological, and pathological literature. It is probably best to think first in terms of a radiological appearance, which can, and now should, be uniformly described and graded. On CT there is more-or-less symmetrical but irregular periventricular hypodensity, with or without ventricular dilatation and focal white matter hypodensities (Fig. 27.19). This is better seen as high signal on T2-weighted MR images. In the absence of other causes, such as multiple sclerosis or irradiation, this periventricular radiological appearance is due to demyelination, axonal loss, and gliosis, probably as a consequence of diffuse rather than focal ischaemia in the distribution of the long perforating arteries from the pial surface of the brain. These vessels are rendered sclerotic, it is assumed, by chronic hypertension, and the ischaemia is perhaps exacerbated by periods of hypotension as a result of cardiac failure, brief perturbations in perfusion pressure, and impaired cerebral autoregulation. Vascular occlusion has not been seen (Caplan 1995a; Pantoni and Garcia 1997). This radiological appearance is frequent in the normal elderly but particularly so in patients who are demented, have had ischaemic or haemorrhagic strokes, or who are unsteady. It is more frequent in hypertensive patients and in those with other vascular risk factors, but not with increasing carotid stenosis severity (Bogousslavsky *et al.* 1987; van Swieten *et al.* 1991; Leys *et al.* 1992; Bots *et al.* 1993; Adachi *et al.* 1997; Tell *et al.* 1998). It may be, therefore, that the association with stroke is because hypertension causes leukoaraiosis as well as lacunar and atherothrombotic ischaemic stroke in the same individuals. It is not the cause of the stroke clinical syndrome. The most important differential diagnosis, because it may be treatable, is normal-pressure hydrocephalus (Section 17.3.8).

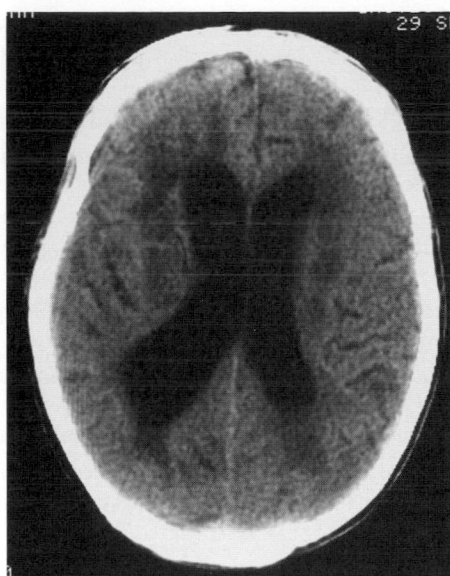

Fig. 27.19. Brain CT to show the typical appearances of leukoaraiosis; periventricular low density.

Inflammatory vascular disease

There are a number of acute, subacute and chronic inflammatory disorders of the arterial (or venous) wall which may cause cerebral ischaemia and haemorrhage (Table 27.13; see also Chapter 28). The inflammation may provoke enough cellular proliferation, necrosis, and fibrosis in the vessel wall to occlude the lumen; to precipitate thrombosis and then embolism; or promote aneurysm formation, dissection, and even rupture of the vessel. These 'vasculitic' disorders may present with, or be complicated during their course by: ischaemic stroke, intracranial haemorrhage, intracranial venous thrombosis, and, more often, by a generalized encephalopathy (Sigal 1987; Berlit *et al.* 1993; Charles and Maini 1993; Futrell 1995; Ostrov and Barron 1995; Jennette and Falk 1997). There is no sensitive or specific angiographic appearance and the diagnosis is made on the basis of the clinical syndrome, systemic features (usually a raised ESR and anaemia), backed up by antibody tests and, if

Table 27.13. Inflammatory vascular diseases causing stroke

Giant-cell arteritis (Sections 3.7.3, 8.4.4)
Takayasu's disease
Systematic lupus erythematosus (Section 28.2.1)
Antiphospholipid antibody syndrome (Section 28.2.2)
Primary systematic vasculitis (Sections 12.15.3, 28.4, 28.5, 28.6)
Rheumatoid disease (Section 28.8)
Sjögren's syndrome (Section 28.9)
Behçet's disease (Section 28.11)
Relapsing polychondritis (Section 28.12)
Progressive systemic sclerosis (Section 28.13)
Sarcoid angiitis (Section 28.15)
Isolated angiitis of the central nervous system (Section 28.16)
Malignant atrophic papulosis (Section 28.19)
Acute posterior multifocal placoid pigment epitheliopathy
Buerger's disease (Section 28.18)

necessary, biopsy (skin, kidney, brain, etc.). The CSF is either normal or shows non-specific inflammatory changes.

Giant-cell arteritis is the most common vasculitic cause of stroke (Sections 3.7.3, 8.4.4, 12.15.3). Medium and large arteries are affected, particularly branches of the external carotid artery, the ophthalmic artery, and the vertebral artery. The patients are elderly. Malaise, polymyalgia, and other systemic symptoms are almost invariable and the ESR is usually raised, often to over 100 mm in the first hour (Wilkinson and Ross Russell 1972; Huston and Hunder 1980; Caselli *et al.* 1988).

Takayasu's disease is a chronic vasculitis, histologically identical to giant-cell arteritis, but affecting only the aorta and large arteries arising from it, mainly in young Oriental women. Systemic features are common (e.g. malaise, weight loss, arthralgia, fever). The neurological complications reflect progressive narrowing and eventual occlusion of the large arteries in the neck: claudication of the jaw muscles, ischaemic oculopathy, syncope, epileptic seizures, confusion, boundary zone infarction, and rather rarely focal ischaemic stroke or TIAs. In addition, there may be ischaemia of the arms, and of the kidneys to cause hypertension, as well as ischaemic necrosis of the lips, nasal septum, and palate (Lupi-Herrera *et al.* 1977; Hall *et al.* 1985).

Other causes of a similar aortic arch syndrome include advanced atheroma, giant-cell arteritis, syphilis, subintimal fibrosis, arterial dissection, trauma, and coarctation (Ross and McKusick 1953; Dalal *et al.* 1971).

Systemic lupus erythematosus (SLE) is more likely to cause a subacute or chronic generalized encephalopathy than symptomatic focal ischaemia (Sections 12.17.6, 28.2). Surprisingly, the underlying vascular pathology, if any is found, appears to be mostly intimal proliferation rather than a vasculitis (Bennett *et al.* 1972; Kitagawa *et al.* 1990; Mills 1994; Hama and Boumpas 1995). The extracranial arteries do not often seem to be affected, but embolism from heart-valve vegetations may be quite common, particularly when there are circulating antiphospholipid antibodies (Haas 1982; Devinski *et al.* 1988; Khamashta *et al.* 1990; Mitsias and Levine 1994; Roldan *et al.* 1996). Intracranial venous thrombosis is rare (Vidailhet *et al.* 1990).

In some patients with little clinical evidence of SLE there is prominent livedo reticularis which, when associated with stroke, is referred to as Sneddon's syndrome, in which antiphospholipid antibodies are particularly common (Burton 1988; Stockhammer *et al.* 1993; Kalashnikova *et al.* 1994; Geschwind *et al.* 1995) (Section 28.2.3).

Antiphospholipid antibody syndrome is a constellation of various recurrent clinical events as well as specific immunological features: recurrent ischaemic stroke/TIA, intracranial venous thrombosis, arterial and venous thrombi elsewhere in the body, migraine-like episodes, recurrent miscarriage, livedo reticularis, cardiac valvular vegetations, thrombocytopenia, false-positive syphilis serology and—the defining feature—persistently and substantially raised (>20 units) circulating IgG anticardiolipin antibodies and/or the circulating lupus anticoagulant, usually detected by prolongation of the activated partial thromboplastin time (Section 28.2.2). It overlaps with

SLE but falls short of the whole syndrome. The same antibodies are found in some normal people, and in SLE (Levine *et al.* 1987; Bick 1993; Hughes 1993; Dahle *et al.* 1995; Feldmann and Levine 1995; Levine *et al.* 1995).

Primary systemic vasculitis is a group of related disorders, including polyarteritis nodosa, Wegener's granulomatosis, the Churg–Strauss syndrome, and various hypersensitivity vasculitides, which have very rare cerebrovascular consequences, similar to those of SLE (Savage *et al.* 1997) (Sections 28.3, 28.4, 28.5, 28.6). However, unlike SLE, it is more common to find underlying vascular pathology (i.e. a necrotizing vasculitis affecting medium and small arteries) while the circulating antibodies so frequently found in SLE are usually absent. More common are haematuria, eosinophilia, and circulating antineutrophil cytoplasmic antibodies (ANCA) (Ford and Siekert 1965; Moore and Fauci 1981; Nishino *et al.* 1993).

Rheumatoid disease is rarely complicated by a systemic vasculitis which can involve the brain (see above) (Watson *et al.* 1977; Beck and Corbett 1983). Occasionally atlanto-axial dislocation causes symptomatic vertebral artery compression (Howell and Molyneux 1988).

Sjögren's syndrome is occasionally complicated by systemic vasculitis (see above) causing focal cerebral ischaemia, global encephalopathy, and aseptic meningitis (Alexander *et al.* 1982; de la Monte *et al.* 1983; Bragoni *et al.* 1994) (Section 28.9).

Neurological complications are well described in *Behçet's disease*, usually with or after the onset of the mucocutaneous manifestations. The vasculitis may affect cerebral arteries, particularly to the brainstem, to cause ischaemic stroke, and possibly intracranial haemorrhage. Intracranial venous thrombosis is another complication (Kawakita *et al.* 1967; Iragui and Maravi 1986; Altinors *et al.* 1987; Wechsler *et al.* 1993; Devlin *et al.* 1995; Akman-Demir *et al.* 1996; Farah *et al.* 1998)

Relapsing polychondritis may be complicated by a generalized encephalopathy, stroke-like episodes, and ischaemic optic neuropathy as a result of systemic vasculitis (Stewart *et al.* 1988) (Section 28.12).

Progressive systemic sclerosis is hardly ever complicated directly by stroke, although a carotid and cerebral vasculopathy has been described (Gordon and Silverstein 1970; Heron *et al.* 1998) (Section 28.13).

Sarcoid angiitis affects the brain rarely, usually causing a generalized encephalopathy rather than focal features due to ischaemia or haemorrhage (Matthews 1979; Stern *et al.* 1985; Libman *et al.* 1997) (Section 28.15).

Isolated angiitis of the central nervous system is a very rare disorder which affects leptomeningeal, cortical, and sometimes spinal cord blood vessels (Section 28.16). It is 'isolated' in the sense that it is confined to the central nervous system. Histologically it is similar to sarcoid angiitis and it can occur in association with herpes zoster and lymphoma. The course is subacute, usually leading to death in weeks or months, with mental confusion and impairment, headache, vomiting, stroke-like episodes, and myelopathy. Systemic symptoms are very uncommon. Diagnosis is only really possible from meningeal/cortical biopsy (Hankey 1991; Vollmer *et al.* 1993).

Malignant atrophic papulosis (Degos' disease) is a very rare syndrome consisting of crops of painless pinkish papules on the trunk and limbs which heal as distinctive circular porcelain-white scars (Section 28.19). It may be complicated by ischaemic gut, brain, spinal cord, and root lesions as a result of endothelial proliferation in small arteries (Sotrel *et al.* 1983; Subbiah *et al.* 1996).

Acute posterior multifocal placoid pigment epitheliopathy is a rare and usually benign and self-limiting chorioretinal disorder with rapidly deteriorating central vision. However, it can be complicated by systemic vasculitis, aseptic meningitis, and stroke (Manto *et al.* 1995; Comu *et al.* 1996)

Buerger's disease (thromboangiitis obliterans) is a rare inflammatory disorder of small and medium-sized arteries and veins, chiefly of the limbs and almost never of the cerebral circulation, much more common in men than women, and in smokers (Drake 1982; Spittell 1983; Berlit *et al.* 1984; Lie 1986) (Section 28.18).

Irradiation

Excessive irradiation of the head and neck can damage intra- and extracranial arteries, both large and small. Within the radiation field, months or years later, a localized, stenotic, and sometimes apparently atheromatous lesion may become symptomatic. There can be considerable fibrosis of the arterial wall and even aneurysm formation (Murros and Toole 1989; Scodary *et al.* 1990; Zuber *et al.* 1993; Bitzer and Topka 1995; Griewing *et al.* 1995).

27.4.5 Embolism from the heart

There is no doubt that emboli arising from within the heart, or passing through it from the venous system, can reach the brain and eye (and elsewhere) to cause ischaemic stroke, retinal infarction, and TIAs (Cerebral Embolism Task Force 1989; Hart 1992; Oppenheimer and Lima 1998). Increasingly sensitive imaging technology is throwing up more and more possible embolic sources, but so often of dubious relevance, such as mitral valve strands (Cohen *et al.* 1997). Fortunately, although there are a large number of potential cardiac sources of embolism (Table 27.14), the vast majority of relevance can be diagnosed easily enough using straightforward clinical examination, ECG, and chest radiography, along with non-invasive echocardiography (Section 27.5.3). The much greater difficulty is in deciding whether an identified embolic source is the source, particularly when it is common in normal people (e.g. mitral leaflet prolapse, patent foramen ovale); or in an elderly person when significant atheroma affecting the cerebral circulation is so commonly found as well; or when the stroke is lacunar and rather unlikely to be caused by embolism from the heart or extracranial arteries (Section 27.4.3) (De Bono and Warlow 1981; Bogousslavsky *et al.* 1986a,b, 1990; Caplan 1995b). Moreover, some embolic sources are much more threatening (e.g. prosthetic valve, rheumatic atrial fibrillation) than others (e.g. mitral leaflet prolapse, patent foramen ovale).

In developed countries, about 20 per cent of ischaemic strokes and TIAs are probably due to embolism from the heart,

Table 27.14. Cardiac sources of embolism (in anatomical sequence)

Paradoxical emoblism from the venous system
    Atrial septal defect
    Ventricular septal defect
    Patent foramen ovale
    Pulmonary arteriovenous fistula

Left atrium
    Atrial fibrillation
    Sinoatrial disease
    Myxoma
    Inter-atrial septal aneurysm

Mitral valve
    Rheumatic stenosis or regurgitation
    Infective endocarditis
    Non-bacterial thrombotic (marantic) endocarditis
    Prosthetic valve
    Mitral annulus calcification
    Mitral leaflet prolapse
    Libman–Sacks endocarditis
    Papillary fibroelastoma

Left ventricular mural thrombus
    Acute myocardial infarction
    Left ventricular aneurysm
    Cardiomyopathy
    Myxoma
    Blunt chest injury
    Mechanical artificial heart

Aortic valve
    Rheumatic stenosis or regurgitation
    Infective endocarditis
    Non-bacterial thrombotic (marantic) endocarditis
    Prosthetic valve
    Calcification and/or sclerosis
    Syphilis
    Congenital cardiac disorders (particularly with right to left shunt)
    Cardiac surgery, catheterization, angioplasty

Others
    primary oxalosis
    hydatid cyst

the most common cause being non-rheumatic atrial fibrillation with presumed, but seldom proven, thrombus in the left atrium (Nishide *et al.* 1983; Kittner *et al.* 1990) (see Table 27.7). Of course, emboli vary in their composition from mostly fibrin (atrial fibrillation) to mostly platelets (mitral leaflet prolapse) to calcium (mitral annulus calcification), tumour (myxoma), or infected vegetations (infective endocarditis). The emboli also vary in size so they may impact in a medium-sized artery to cause a substantial infarct (e.g. middle cerebral artery (MCA) origin, basilar artery) or in a smaller artery to cause merely a restricted defect (e.g. central retinal artery branch, cortical branch of MCA) (Castaigne *et al.* 1973; Caplan 1993). Some emboli, perhaps even most, like other causes of cerebral ischaemia, may be completely asymptomatic.

Although it is becoming much less common, rheumatic valvular disease, mitral far more often than aortic, is well recognized as an embolic source, either because of thrombus in the

left atrium or valvular debris (Daley *et al.* 1951; Coulshed *et al.* 1970). Atrial fibrillation has already been discussed (Section 27.2.7). Some other conditions are worth discussing in detail:

Coronary artery disease: in the pre-thrombolytic era, left ventricular mural thrombus diagnosed echocardiographically occurred within days of an acute myocardial infarction (MI) in about 20 per cent of patients. Those with anterior infarcts are at higher risk than those with inferior infarcts; large infarcts and a dyskinetic wall segment are also risk factors (Meltzer *et al.* 1986). These thrombi may embolize, particularly if protruding or mobile, and are associated with about a fivefold excess risk of stroke in the first few days and weeks after MI (Vaitkus and Barnathan 1993). But most seem to do little harm, since the frequency of clinically evident systemic embolism is well under 5 per cent (Fibrinolytic Therapy Trialists' (FTT) Collaborative Group 1994; Mooe *et al.* 1997). Moreover, at least some, and maybe many, post-MI strokes must be due to hypotension and boundary zone infarction, atrial fibrillation with left atrial thrombus, paradoxical embolism in patients with right ventricular infarction and a patent foramen ovale, coronary and aortic instrumentation (see below), while others are primarily haemorrhagic as a consequence of the increasing use of antithrombotic and thrombolytic drugs (Sloan and Plotnick 1990; Maggioni *et al.* 1992). Sometimes acute stroke and acute myocardial infarction appear to start simultaneously, making it difficult to know which was first, or whether there was some common underlying mechanism (Chin *et al.* 1977; von Arbin *et al.* 1982). Even more rarely, the same non-atheromatous disorder can cause both ischaemic stroke and acute MI (giant cell arteritis, aortic arch dissection, infective endocarditis).

The long-term risk of stroke after acute MI is about 1.5 per cent per annum, 8 per cent in 5 years. Although some strokes may be due to embolization from thrombus in a chronic left ventricular aneurysm, many must be due atrial fibrillation, or coincidental arterial disease affecting the cerebral circulation (Meltzer *et al.* 1986; Martin *et al.* 1993; Loh *et al.* 1997).

Mitral leaflet prolapse (MLP) is a common echocardiographic and even clinical finding in asymptomatic people, particularly if they are tall and thin, and it is sometimes familial (Levy and Savage 1987). It can be complicated by gross mitral regurgitation, infective endocarditis, atrial fibrillation and left atrial thrombus and so embolism to the brain. But although early case-control studies suggested that uncomplicated MLP was more common in ischaemic stroke and TIA patients than expected, this has not been confirmed. Moreover, there is no excess risk of first or recurrent stroke in patients with MLP and there is little pathological confirmation of significant thrombi on the abnormal valve cusps (Geyer and Franzini 1979; Chesler *et al.* 1983; Orencia *et al.* 1995a,b). Therefore, if uncomplicated MLP is discovered in an ischaemic stroke patient, it is most unwise to assume a causal relationship (i.e. embolism from valvular vegetations to the brain) unless echocardiography reveals vegetations and no other cause is found, and even then keeping an open mind.

Calcification (and possibly sclerosis) of the aortic and mitral valves can, rarely, be a cause of embolism of calcific or complicating thrombotic material. However, these 'degenerative' (or perhaps rheumatic) disorders of heart valves are so common, particularly in the elderly, that it has been very difficult to associate them causally with stroke (De Bono and Warlow 1979; Benjamin et al. 1992; Boon et al. 1996). Unless calcific emboli are seen in the retina, or on CT of the brain, it is all but impossible to infer a causal relationship with ischaemic stroke in individuals (Brockmeier et al. 1981; Mouton et al. 1997; Shanmugam et al. 1997). Any associated atrial fibrillation, coronary heart disease, and carotid stenosis just compound the diagnostic problem.

Paradoxical embolism from the venous system (or exceptionally from thrombus in the right side of the heart) is a well-accepted mechanism of ischaemic stroke, based on a number of convincing cases described at post-mortem. However, definitive diagnosis during life is almost impossible because a patent foramen ovale can be found not only in about 25 per cent of unselected post-mortems but, with modern non-invasive technology (transoesophageal echocardiography with intravenous contrast), in about 15 per cent of normal people (Gautier et al. 1991; Jeanrenaud and Kappenberger 1991). In an individual case of ischaemic stroke or TIA with a patent foramen ovale (or an atrial septal defect or ventricular septal defect), suggestive clues to paradoxical embolism are the presence, or high likelihood, of thrombosis in the leg or even pelvic veins, or pulmonary embolism, shortly before the stroke (afterwards it could be a result of the stroke); no other cause of stroke is identified; onset of stroke occurs during likely sustained or transitory elevation of right heart pressure (pulmonary hypertension, Valsalva manoeuvre, right ventricular myocardial infarction, etc.); and thrombus in the right atrium or ventricle is demonstrated or highly likely (Jeanrenaud and Kappenberger 1991). However, these clues are far from specific or sensitive (Petty et al. 1997). The risk of recurrent stroke is very uncertain but probably not particularly high (Bogousslavsky et al. 1996).

A pulmonary arteriovenous fistula (often visible on chest radiography and not necessarily only in patients with hereditary haemorrhagic telangiectasia) is a very rare route by which emboli may reach the brain from the venous system (Dennis 1985).

Sinoatrial disease (sick sinus syndrome) is associated with systemic embolism, particularly if there is bradycardia alternating with tachycardia, or atrial fibrillation (Bathen et al. 1978).

Inter-atrial septal aneurysm is increasingly recognized with echocardiography, and some evidence is emerging that it may be complicated by thrombosis and then embolism to the brain (Silver and Dorsey 1978; Nater et al. 1992; Cabanes et al. 1993). However, it is often associated with other cardiac conditions which have embolic potential (particularly a patent foramen ovale) or which may be associated with atheromatous disease of the cerebral arteries (such as coronary heart disease).

Infective endocarditis, acute or subacute, is complicated by ischaemic stroke or TIA as a result of embolism of infected vegetations in about 20 per cent of cases (Section 35.4). Stroke can be the first symptom but more often occurs at about the time of hospitalization and the diagnosis of the cardiac pathology.

Mycotic aneurysms may form at sites of embolic occlusion (usually on distal branches of the middle cerebral artery) and some rupture to cause intracerebral or subarachnoid haemorrhage, usually during the acute illness and rarely a few weeks later. Intracranial haemorrhage is also caused by pyogenic necrosis of the arterial wall (Jones and Siekert 1989; Hart et al. 1990; Kanter and Hart 1991; Salgado 1991; Masuda et al. 1992).

Non-bacterial thrombotic (marantic) endocarditis: small, friable, and sterile vegetations made of fibrin and platelets can be found on the heart valves of cachectic and debilitated patients, and in the antiphospholipid antibody syndrome, systemic lupus erythematosus, and possibly protein C deficiency (Section 27.4.6). Mostly they are too small to be diagnosed during life, although some can now be picked up on transoesophageal echocardiography (Lopez et al. 1987; Walz et al. 1998).

Prosthetic heart valves, particularly mechanical ones, have long been known to be complicated by thrombosis with embolic potential, and infective endocarditis. There seems to be little difference in this respect between the different mechanical valves, but those in the mitral position are most prone to thrombosis. The overall risk of clinically evident embolism is 1–2 per cent per annum, even on anticoagulants (Vongpatanasin et al. 1996). The very frequent signals on transcranial Doppler probably mostly represent gas cavitation bubbles forming on prosthetic valves, particular mechanical ones, rather than formed emboli, and do not seem to be clinically relevant (Sliwka and Georgiadis 1998).

Cardiac myxomas are rare, occasionally familial, and arise in any heart chamber, but 75 per cent are found in the left atrium (Markel et al. 1987; Reynen 1995). Tumour material, or complicating thrombus, may embolize to the brain, eye, and elsewhere, and very often, but not always, there are additional features of intracardiac obstruction (dyspnoea, cardiac failure, syncope) and constitutional upset (malaise, weight loss, fever, rash, arthralgia, myalgia, anaemia, raised ESR, hypergammaglobulinaemia) (Sandok et al. 1980). Myxomatous emboli impacted in cerebral arteries may also cause aneurysmal dilatation with subsequent intracerebral or subarachnoid haemorrhage (Roeltgen et al. 1981).

Valvular fibroelastoma is an even rarer embologenic cardiac tumour (Giannesini et al. 1999). Other very rare primary and secondary cardiac tumours may embolize (Joynt et al. 1965; Chalmers and Campbell 1987; Reynen 1995).

Dilating cardiomyopathies are well recognized to be complicated by intracardiac thrombus, but this seems to be a remarkably rare cause of embolic stroke. Any atrial fibrillation is likely to exacerbate the tendency (Dec and Fuster 1994).

Cardiac surgery is complicated by stroke or retinal/optic nerve infarction in about 2 per cent of cases, the risk being greater for valve than coronary artery surgery (Lancet 1989; Roach et al. 1996). Early post-operative confusion is much more common, and although cognitive deficits may persist for some weeks or longer, they seldom seem to cause much persistent functional impairment (Shaw et al. 1989; Walzer et al. 1997). Possible mechanisms include embolization during surgery (of platelet aggregates, fibrin, calcific debris from valves, atheromatous debris, fat, air, silicone or particulate matter from the pump-oxygenator system); embolism after surgery (from thrombus on suture lines, prosthetic material, complicating myocardial infarction, endocarditis, or atrial fibrillation); hypotension during or after surgery, causing boundary zone ischaemia; haemodilution during surgery; the cholesterol embolization syndrome; a simultaneous carotid endarterectomy; thrombosis associated with heparin-induced thrombocytopenia; and intracranial haemorrhage due to anticoagulation or thrombocytopenia. The neurological complications are not very clearly related to any particular risk factors, even carotid stenosis, perhaps because studies have been too small to demonstrate them reliably and no systematic reviews have been done.

Instrumentation of the coronary arteries and aorta may be associated with similar neurological complications by dislodging valvular or atheromatous debris (Ayas and Wijdicks 1995) and the cholesterol embolization syndrome (27.4.2).

27.4.6 **Haematological disorders**

A number of quite easily diagnosed haematological disorders, many of which are common, may very occasionally cause ischaemic stroke and TIA (Hart and Kanter 1990; Markus and Hambley 1998) (Table 27.15).

Polycythaemia is usually defined as a haematocrit above 0.50 in males and 0.47 in females, provided the patient is rested and normally hydrated, and blood is taken without venous occlusion. Polycythaemia rubra vera (primary polycythaemia) may be complicated by TIAs, ischaemic stroke, or intracranial venous thrombosis (Silverstein *et al.* 1962; Pearson and Wetherley-Mein 1978). This is both because the platelet count is raised and platelet activity possibly enhanced, and because of increased whole-blood viscosity. Paradoxically there may also be a haemostatic defect as a result of defective platelet function, so causing intracranial haemorrhage. Relative polycythaemia is due to reduced plasma volume (as a result of diuretics, hypertension, alcohol, dehydration, obesity, etc.) and secondary polycythaemia is due to a raised red cell mass (as a result of chronic hypoxia, smoking, congenital cyanotic heart disease, renal tumour, cerebellar haemangioblastoma, etc.); in both, the raised haematocrit may be a weak risk factor for stroke (Section 27.2.7).

Essential thrombocythaemia (idiopathic primary thrombocytosis) is another myeloproliferative disorder. The platelet

Table 27.15. Haematological disorders causing ischaemic stroke

Polycythaemias
Essential thrombocythaemia
Leukaemia
Sickle-cell disease/trait and other haemoglobinopathies
Iron deficiency anaemia
Paraproteinaemias
Paroxysmal nocturnal haemoglobinuria
Thrombotic thrombocytopenic purpura
Disseminated intravascular coagulation
Thrombophilias and other causes of 'hypercoagulability'

count is raised (usually over 1000×10^9/l, but it may be as low as 500) with circulating erythroid and/or megakaryocyte progenitors. Other causes for thrombocytosis include malignancy, splenectomy, hyposplenism, surgery, trauma, haemorrhage, iron deficiency, infections, polycythaemia rubra vera, myelofibrosis, and the leukaemias. There is a tendency for arterial and venous thrombosis and, paradoxically, intracranial haemorrhage because the platelets are haemostatically defective (Preston *et al.* 1979; Murphy *et al.* 1983; Michiels *et al.* 1993; Arboix *et al.* 1995; Harrison *et al.* 1998).

Leukaemia is more commonly a cause of intracranial haemorrhage (because of the haemostatic defect or CNS leukaemic infiltration) than cerebral venous or arterial occlusion due to the increased whole-blood viscosity (Davies-Jones 1995). Intravascular lymphoma is a very rare cause of stroke-like episodes fading into a progressive global encephalopathy (Lennox *et al.* 1989). Asparaginase treatment is another possible cause of ischaemic or haemorrhagic stroke (Feinberg and Swenson 1988).

Sickle-cell disease (and rarely other haemoglobinopathies) may be complicated by ischaemic stroke or, sometimes, intracranial haemorrhage (Adams *et al.* 1988; Pavlakis *et al.* 1988). The patients are usually homozygote children, although sometimes a sickle-cell crisis, provoked in an adult heterozygote by hypoxia, can be responsible (Greenberg and Massey 1985; Feldenzer *et al.* 1987). Small and large arteries, as well as veins, develop a fibrous vasculopathy and are occluded by thrombi as a result of the abnormally rigid red blood cells and raised whole blood viscosity, thrombocytosis and impaired fibrinolytic activity (Adams *et al.* 1997; Steen *et al.* 1998).

Stroke may also complicate haemoglobin SC disease (Fabian and Peters 1984) and maybe thalassaemia (Aessopos *et al.* 1997).

Iron deficiency anaemia, if severe, causes non-specific neurological symptoms (presumably hypoxic in origin) such as faintness, poor concentration, giddiness, tiredness, and general weakness. Just occasionally, TIAs and even ischaemic stroke seem to be provoked by profound anaemia, but usually in association with severe extracranial occlusive arterial disease, or thrombocytosis (Siekert *et al.* 1960; Akins *et al.* 1996).

The *paraproteinaemias*, multiple myeloma and macroglobulinaemia, are associated with anaemia because of defective erythropoesis, and this causes non-specific neurological symptoms (see above). A haemostatic defect due to reduced platelet number, and perhaps reactivity as a result of complicating uraemia, may cause intracranial haemorrhage. However, most of the 'cerebral' features of these patients can be explained by the 'hyperviscosity syndrome' which is characterized by headache, ataxia, diplopia, dysarthria, lethargy, drowsiness, poor concentration, visual blurring, and deafness (the same syndrome can be seen in primary polycythaemia, leukaemia, etc.). Similar symptoms may also be due to complicating hypercalcaemia, uraemia, and lymphoma. The retina shows characteristic changes with dilatation and tortuosity of the veins, venous occlusions, papilloedema, and haemorrhages. The abnormal circulating proteins and tendency to red cell aggregation are responsible for the raised whole-blood viscosity, although to some extent the effects are ameliorated by the low haematocrit. Cerebral infarction may occur (arterial or venous) and at post-mortem the microcirculation is occluded with acidophilic material thought to be precipitates of the abnormal proteins. It is exceptional for patients with neurological involvement not to have a raised ESR, which gives the clue to performing protein electrophoresis, so confirming the diagnosis (Preston *et al.* 1978; Scheithauer *et al.* 1984; Davies-Jones 1995).

Paroxysmal nocturnal haemoglobinuria is a very rare acquired disorder in which haemopoetic stem cells become peculiarly sensitive to complement-mediated lysis. Venous, and perhaps arterial, thrombosis occurs in the brain and elsewhere. Almost always patients are anaemic at neurological presentation and there may be a history of dark urine, evidence of haemolysis, and a low platelet and granulocyte count (Al-Hakim *et al.* 1993; Socie *et al.* 1996).

Thrombotic thrombocytopenic purpura (TTP) is a rare acute or subacute disease in adults, rather similar to the haemolytic-uraemic syndrome in children. Haemorrhagic infarcts due to platelet microthrombi occur in many organs, and in the brain they may cause stroke-like episodes. More commonly, the presentation is with a global encephalopathy on the background of systemic malaise, fever, skin purpura, renal failure, haematuria, and proteinuria. The blood film shows thrombocytopenia, haemolytic anaemia, and fragmented red cells (Ridolfi and Bell 1981; Sheth *et al.* 1986; Kay *et al.* 1991; Oberlander *et al.* 1995; Garrett el al 1996). The differential diagnosis includes systemic lupus erythematosus, infective endocarditis, idiopathic thrombocytopenia, heparin-induced throbocytopenia with thrombosis, non-bacterial thrombotic endocarditis, and disseminated intravascular coagulation.

Disseminated intravascular coagulation: the neurological complications are usually submerged in the features of the underlying serious illness. Widespread haemorrhagic brain infarcts and intracranial haemorrhages tend to cause an acute or subacute global encephalopathy rather than stroke-like episodes. The diagnosis is confirmed by a low platelet count, low plasma fibrinogen, and raised fibrin degradation products and D-dimer (Schwartzman and Hill 1982; Baglin 1996). The differential diagnosis includes non-bacterial thrombotic endocarditis, cerebral hypoxia, hepatic failure, and uraemia.

The *thrombophilias and other causes of 'hypercoagulability'* are very rare causes of any sort of 'stroke' (Greaves 1993; Schafer 1994). Antithrombin III deficiency (Arima *et al.* 1992), protein S deficiency (Koelman *et al.* 1992; Rich *et al.* 1993; Nighoghossian *et al.* 1994), protein C deficiency (Vieregge *et al.* 1989; Kazui *et al.* 1993; Confavreux *et al.* 1994; van Kuijck *et al.* 1994; Blecic *et al.* 1996), activated protein C resistance due to factor V Leiden mutation (Hourihane *et al.* 1997) and plasminogen abnormality or deficiency (Schutta *et al.* 1991; Nagayama *et al.* 1993) can all cause peripheral and intracranial venous thrombosis (usually recurrent and often with a family history). However, they have seldom been convincingly reported to cause arterial thrombosis (but paradoxical embolism must always be considered as an explanation of arterial occlusion). To complicate matters, there are many asymptomatic patients with these deficiencies and to make any causal link it is important to exclude other causes of stroke, for the deficiency to be demonstrated more than once and some months after the stroke to avoid any acute effects of the stroke itself, and preferably in family members as well (Forsyth and Dolan 1995; Munts *et al.* 1998).

The nephrotic syndrome, certain snake bites, the antiphospholipid antibody syndrome, widespread cancer, antifibrinolytic drugs, intravenous immunoglobulin and desmopressin are other occasional causes of 'hypercoagulability' and ischaemic stroke. The role of coagulation proteins as vascular risk factors has already been discussed (Section 27.2.7).

27.4.7 Miscellaneous rare causes of stroke

Stroke complicates *pregnancy and the puerperium* in about 10 per 100 000 deliveries in developed countries, about twice the background rate (Grosset *et al.* 1995; Sharshar *et al.* 1995; Kittner *et al.* 1996; Mas and Lamy 1998). Causes and mechanisms particularly relevant to pregnancy, rather than to young stroke in general, have not been well studied but include intracranial venous thrombosis; cervical arterial dissection during labour; acute middle cerebral or other large artery occlusion, perhaps due to paradoxical embolism from the leg or pelvic veins; low-flow infarction and disseminated intravascular coagulation complicating eclampsia and other obstetric disasters; puerperal angiopathy, perhaps due to ergot-type and other vasoconstricting drugs or dopaminergic agonists such as bromocriptine; infective endocarditis; peripartum cardiomyopathy; sickle-cell crisis; and intracranial haemorrhage(s) due to eclampsia, anticoagulants, rupture of a pre-existing aneurysm or vascular malformation (Wiebers 1985; Wiebers and Mokri 1985; Cantu and Barinagarrementeria 1993; Dyken and Biller 1994; Comabella *et al.* 1996; Drislane and Wang 1997). Metastases of choriocarcinoma can present with stroke-like episodes, and on CT look remarkably like primary intracerebral haemorrhages. The risk of recurrent stroke in any future pregnancy is of crucial interest, but unknown. Presumably if no underlying cause is found for the first stroke, the risk of recurrence is low.

An ever-increasing number of strokes caused by *drug abuse* are being reported, at least from the USA where the problem has been recognized for some years (Caplan *et al.* 1982; McEvoy *et al.* 1998). At present the most commonly implicated drug is cocaine (and its 'crack' form) which causes cerebral infarction, intracerebral and subarachnoid haemorrhage, usually within hours of use. Although a 'vasculitis' has been described, more likely explanations are an acute rise in blood pressure and intracranial haemorrhage; an underlying vascular malformation or aneurysm; cardiac arrhythmia, cardiomyopathy and cerebral embolism; and cerebral vasoconstriction (Cregler and Mark 1986; Krendel *et al.* 1990; Levine *et al.* 1990; Fredericks *et al.* 1991; Daras *et al.* 1991; Kaufman *et al.* 1998).

Amphetamines can cause a small vessel vasculopathy, leading to intracerebral haemorrhage or infarction. Acute hypertension, perhaps with a pre-existing vascular anomaly, is a likely mechanism of intracerebral haemorrhage (Harrington *et al.* 1983; Rothrock *et al.* 1988; Heye and Hankey 1996). Other sympathomimetic drugs such as ephedrine, phenylpropanolamine, fenfluramine and phentermine may cause stroke by similar mechanisms, as may 'Ecstasy' (Glick *et al.* 1987; Kase *et al.* 1987; Harries and De Silva 1992; Henry *et al.* 1992; Bruno *et al.* 1993; Wen *et al.* 1997).

Other causes of stroke in drug abusers should not, of course, be forgotten (infective endocarditis and HIV infection) and nor should the frequent complications of head injury and alcohol abuse.

Stroke in *cancer* patients can easily be a coincidence, but causal possibilities include embolism of non-infected heart valve vegetations (non-bacterial thrombotic—or marantic—endocarditis; Section 27.4.5); infection (fungi, herpes zoster, bacterial endocarditis); tumour emboli, sometimes with secondary aneurysm formation and then rupture; haemorrhage into primary tumours (malignant astrocytoma, oligodendroglioma, medulloblastoma, haemangioblastoma) and metastases (melanoma, germ cell tumours, choriocarcinoma, lung, hypernephroma); haemostatic failure (leukaemia, etc.); hyperviscosity syndrome (Section 27.4.6); 'hypercoagulability'; disseminated intravascular coagulation (Section 27.4.6); and intracranial venous thrombosis (Section 27.11) (Hickey *et al.* 1982; Graus *et al.* 1985). Irradiation damage (Section 27.4.4) or neoplastic compression or invasion of neck arteries are both most unusual causes of ischaemic stroke.

Perioperative stroke complicates well under 5 per cent of non-cardiac surgical procedures (for cardiac surgery, see Section 27.4.5). It can be due to hypotension and boundary zone infarction, trauma to and dissection of neck arteries, paradoxical embolism, fat embolism, infective endocarditis, myocardial infarction, atrial fibrillation, and a haemostatic defect caused by antithrombotic drugs or disseminated intravascular coagulation (Hart and Hindman 1982; Tettenborn *et al.* 1993). It is more common in patients with previous strokes, other manifestations of vascular disease, and chronic obstructive lung disease (Limburg *et al.* 1998).

The relationship between *migraine* and stroke is difficult to disentangle (Olesen *et al.* 1993). For some reason stroke is probably rather more frequent in migraineurs, particularly young women, than in the normal population (Chang *et al.* 1999). However, a 'normal' stroke (with an obvious cause such as carotid atherothromboembolism) may precipitate a migrainous episode of a type previously experienced, or be followed by typically migrainous attacks which have never been experienced before. Or sometimes symptomatic migraine with aura seems to be precipitated by severe carotid stenosis. Also, a 'normal' stroke may start in the midst of a typical migrainous episode for that patient and so appear to be provoked by it. The term 'migrainous stroke' should be reserved for a persisting focal neurological deficit which starts during a typical migrainous aura (with or without headache), *clearly* mimicking the symptomatology of previously experienced auras, and for which there is no better, or even other, explanation (Bousser *et al.* 1985a). Such migrainous strokes usually cause a homonymous

hemianopia or focal sensory deficit, seldom persisting disability, and do not appear to recur very often (Henrich *et al.* 1986; Broderick and Swanson 1987; Hoekstra-van Dalen *et al.* 1996). Sometimes arterial occlusion is demonstrated by angiography and the cause is postulated as 'vasospastic'. No provoking factors are known. Naturally other possible causes of stroke in the context of migraine-like headache must be seriously considered (i.e. carotid dissection, antiphospholipid antibody syndrome, mitochondrial cytopathy, ruptured vascular malformation, CADASIL). When diagnostic mistakes are made, the strokes are seldom truly migrainous in the sense described above (Shuaib 1991; Tietjen 1995). Migraine auras without headache may be confused with TIAs (Section 27.5.2).

Chronic meningitis may involve the arteries at the base of the brain, or the perforating arteries, and so be complicated by ischaemic stroke and intracranial haemorrhage. This has been well described in tuberculous, syphilitic, and fungal infections (Dalal and Dalal 1989; Landi *et al.* 1990; Saez de Ocariz *et al.* 1996). Very occasionally *acute infection* can cause inflammation of, and secondary thrombosis in, the carotid artery in the neck (e.g. tonsillitis, pharyngitis, lymphadenitis; Bickerstaff 1964); in the dural sinuses (otitis media, etc.); and in the cerebral arteries and veins: bacterial meningitis (Igarashi *et al.* 1984), ophthalmic herpes zoster and chicken pox (Bourdette *et al.* 1983; Leopold 1993; Melanson *et al.* 1996), cysticercosis (del Brutto 1992; Bang *et al.* 1997), leptospirosis (Lessa and Cortes 1981), mycoplasma (Mulder and Spierings 1987), AIDS (Park *et al.* 1990; Qureshi *et al.* 1997), cat scratch disease (Selby and Walker 1979), neurotrichinosis (Fourestie *et al.* 1993), and possibly borreliosis (Reik 1993).

Inflammatory bowel disease, both ulcerative and Crohn's colitis, may occasionally be complicated by intracranial venous thrombosis or arterial occlusion (Johns 1991; Jorens *et al.* 1991; M. Jackson *et al.* 1993; Lossos *et al.* 1995). The bowel disease is not necessarily severe at the time. This association has been related to thrombocytosis, hypercoagulability, immobility and paradoxical embolism from the legs, vasculitis and dehydration, but with no very good evidence. *Coeliac disease* can also be complicated by a cerebral vasculitis, but this presents more with an encephalopathy than with stroke (Mumford *et al.* 1996).

Homocystinuria, an autosomal recessive inborn error of metabolism, is complicated by cerebral arterial or venous thrombosis (Schimke *et al.* 1965; Visy *et al.* 1991; Rubba *et al.* 1994). Heterozygotes may have an increased risk of vascular disease (Section 27.2.7).

Fabry's disease is occasionally complicated by ischaemic stroke, particularly in the vertebrobasilar territory, but usually not until after other more common features are well established (Mitsias and Levine 1996) (Section 12.8.5).

Mitochondrial cytopathy may present with stroke-like episodes with hypodensity on CT scan, particularly in the occipital regions, and complicated by epilepsy. There are often other clinical features, such as calcification of the basal ganglia, migraine, episodic vomiting, short stature, sensorineural deafness, diabetes, and learning disability. A particular syndrome is known as MELAS (mitochondrial encephalopathy, lactic acidosis, and strokes). The blood and CSF lactate are usually raised and most patients have an abnormal muscle biopsy (Hasuo *et al.* 1987; Ciafaloni *et al.* 1992; Gilchrist *et al.* 1996).

Hypoglycaemia, almost always as a result of hypoglycaemic drugs rather than an insulinoma, is a well-recognized, but rare, cause of transient focal neurological episodes, particularly right hemiplegia and aphasia masquerading as TIAs. Consciousness is normal and there is a striking absence of the usual systemic manifestations of hypoglycaemia. The episodes tend to occur on waking in the morning, or after exercise. By the time the patient is seen, the blood glucose may well have returned to normal. Persisting focal deficits seem to be unusual (Malouf and Brust 1985; Wallis *et al.* 1985; Service 1995; Shanmugam *et al.* 1997).

Hypercalcaemia (Longo and Witherspoon 1980) and, less convincingly, *hyponatraemia* (Ruby and Burton 1977; Berkovic *et al.* 1984) have been reported to cause TIA-like episodes.

Fibrocartilaginous embolism is a rare and curious disorder where fibrocartilaginous emboli, presumably from degenerative intervertebral disc material, are found in various organs—the spinal cord more often than the brain (Toro-Gonzales *et al.* 1993).

Snake bite with injection of venom may cause intracranial haemorrhage, as a consequence of defibrination and other haemostatic defects, and rarely ischaemic stroke (Bashir and Jinkins 1985).

Fat embolism, which occurs following long bone fracture or surgery, usually causes a global encephalopathy, but on occasion there may be focal features, presumably reflecting focal ischaemia (Jacobson *et al.* 1986; van Oostenbrugge *et al.* 1996).

Epidermal naevus syndrome, a sporadic neurocutaneous disorder, can be complicated by stroke (Dobyns and Garg 1991).

Susac's syndrome is a rare triad of branch retinal artery occlusions, hearing loss, and microangiopathy of the brain, causing a subacute encephalopathy, almost only in women (Ballard *et al.* 1996).

27.4.8 Spontaneous intracranial haemorrhage

Spontaneous intracranial haemorrhage occurs within the brain (primary intracerebral haemorrhage), into the subarachnoid space (subarachnoid haemorrhage), sometimes into the ventricles (intraventricular haemorrhage), and rarely into the subdural space (subdural haemorrhage). The exact site of origin may not necessarily be immediately obvious because, for example, a saccular aneurysm can rupture into the brain as well as into the subarachnoid space, or disruption of a small perforating artery can cause intraventricular haemorrhage as well as a basal ganglia haematoma. Even at post-mortem there may be uncertainty because the source of the haemorrhage may well have been destroyed, particularly if small (e.g. a tiny intracranial vascular malformation). The causes of intracranial haemorrhage are much the same, whatever the primary site of the bleeding, although their relative frequency varies somewhat with the site (Table 27.16).

Table 27.16. Causes of spontaneous intracranial haemorrhage

Hypertension (chronic, acute) (Section 27.4.8)

Aneurysms
    Saccular (Section 27.4.8)
    Atheromatous (Section 27.4.2)
    Mycotic (Section 27.4)
    Myxomatous (Section 27.4.5)
    Dissecting (Section 27.4.4)

Cerebral amyloid angiopathy (Section 27.4.8)

Intracranial vascular malformations (Section 27.4.8)
    Arteriovenous (cerebral, dural)
    Venous
    Cavernous
    Telangiectasis

Haemostatic failure (Section 27.4.6)
    Haemophilia and other coagulation disorders
    Thrombocytopenia
    Thrombotic thrombocytopenic purpura
    Anticoagulation
    Therapeutic thrombolysis
    Antiplatelet drugs
    Polycythaemia rubra vera
    Essential thrombocythaemia
    Paraproteinaemias
    Disseminated intravascular coagulation
    Renal failure
    Liver failure
    Snake bite

Inflammatory vascular disease (Section 27.4.4)

Haemorrhagic transformation of cerebral infarction, venous more often than arterial (Section 27.8.3)

Intracranial venous thrombosis (Section 27.11)

Sickle-cell disease/trait (Section 27.4.6)

Moyamoya syndrome (Section 27.4.4)

Carotid endarterectomy (Section 27.10.3)

Posterior fossa and other intracranial surgery

Delayed post-traumatic 'spat-apoplexie'

Alcoholic binge (Section 27.2.7)

Wernicke's encephalopathy

Vascular tumours
    Melanoma
    Choriocarcinoma
    Malignant astrocytoma
    Oligodendroglioma
    Medulloblastoma
    Haemangioblastoma
    Choroid plexus papilloma
    Hypernephroma
    Endometrial carcinoma
    Bronchogenic carcinoma

Drug abuse (Section 27.4.7)

Infections (Section 27.4.7)
    Herpes simplex
    Leptospirosis
    Anthrax
    Chronic meningitis

Scorpion bite

Silastic dural substitute

Primary intracerebral haemorrhage

Primary intracerebral haemorrhage (PICH) is somewhat more frequent than subarachnoid haemorrhage, the incidence increases with age, and it is probably more common in the Japanese and Chinese than in Whites (Section 27.2.4). It is most commonly due to intracranial small vessel disease associated with hypertension, cerebral amyloid angiopathy, and intracranial vascular malformations, but there is usually a combination of different factors operating in any one individual, e.g. hypertension and cerebral amyloid angiopathy, therapeutic thrombolysis and a vascular malformation, etc. (Warlow *et al.* 2000*b*). Less common causes include saccular aneurysms; haemostatic defects, particularly induced by anticoagulation (Hart *et al.* 1995), therapeutic thrombolysis, perhaps with cerebral amyloid angiopathy (Simoons *et al.* 1993; Fibrinolytic Therapy Trialists' Collaborative Group 1994), and possibly antiplatelet drugs (He *et al.* 1998); cerebral vasculitis (Section 27.4.4); and drug abuse (Section 27.4.7) (Kase 1986; Caplan 1988). The site of PICH, shown on CT, provides some clue to the cause; 'hypertensive' haemorrhages tend to occur slightly more in the basal ganglia, thalamus, and pons, while lobar haemorrhages (i.e. superficial in cerebrum) tend to be somewhat more often due to cerebral amyloid angiopathy, vascular malformations, and haemostatic failure (Schutz *et al.* 1990; Molinari 1993). Occasionally PICHs occur in different parts of the brain simultaneously, or over a short period of time (Table 27.17). Rarely, PICH is familial (see Table 27.8).

It has previously been assumed that bleeding occurs abruptly and is limited, more or less at once, by the increasing pressure in the surrounding brain tissue. Quite commonly, however, continuing or early rebleeding visible on CT does occur within hours of stroke onset, and can cause deterioration (Brott *et al.* 1997). Perhaps the initial haemorrhage sets off an 'avalanche' of surrounding secondary haemorrhages by distorting the microvasculature. In addition, early deterioration can be due to ischaemia and oedema around the haematoma (Mendelow 1991). Some brainstem haemorrhages evolve surprisingly subacutely, particularly those caused by a vascular malformation (O'Laoire *et al.* 1982; Howard 1986).

Any large haematoma may cause brain shift, transtentorial herniation, brainstem compression, and raised intracranial pressure. Haematomas in the posterior fossa are particularly likely to cause obstructive hydrocephalus. Rupture into the ventricles, or on to the surface of the brain is common (so causing blood to appear in the subarachnoid space and lumbar CSF).

Spontaneous subarachnoid haemorrhage

The incidence of spontaneous subarachnoid haemorrhage (SAH) increases with age and is about 5–10/100 000 population/annum, being somewhat more frequent in women than men, and is particularly common in Finland (Linn *et al.* 1996). A ruptured saccular aneurysm is by far the most common cause (Vermeulen *et al.* 1992). Some SAHs are due to bleeding from an intracranial vascular malformation, a few are due to rarities (Table 27.16), and—depending on the intensity of investigation—in about 15 per cent no cause can be identified in life

Table 27.17. Causes of simultaneous and multiple spontaneous intracerebral haemorrhages

Cerebral amyloid angiopathy (Section 27.4.8)
Metastases (Table 27.16)
Haemostatic defect (Section 27.4.6)
Thrombolytic drugs (Section 27.4.6)
Intracranial venous thrombosis (Section 27.11)
Inflammatory vascular disease (Section 27.4.4)
Intracranial vascular malformations (Section 27.4.8)
Malignant hypertension (Section 27.4.8)
Eclampsia (Section 27.4.7)
Multiple haemorrhagic infarcts (usually embolic from the heart)
Occult head injury
Drug abuse (Section 27.4.7)

(Rinkel *et al.* 1993). In about two-thirds of the 'no cause' category there is a characteristic pattern of restricted bleeding around the midbrain, so-called perimesencephalic haemorrhage, where the case fatality and risk of re-bleeding are both so low that there is not even post-mortem information about the cause (van Gijn *et al.* 1985*a*; Rinkel *et al.* 1991). Chronic or repeated subarachnoid bleeding can produce the rare syndrome of superficial haemosiderosis of the central nervous system: sensorineural deafness, cerebellar ataxia, pyramidal signs, dementia, and bladder disturbance (Fearnley *et al.* 1995).

Primary intraventricular haemorrhage is very unusual, except in premature babies. In adults, a cause is not always found. Some may be due to a vascular malformation in the ventricular wall (Gates *et al.* 1986; Darby *et al.* 1988). The clinical features are so similar to SAH that it can only be differentiated on CT, or at post-mortem.

Subdural haemorrhage is more often traumatic, or due to ventricular decompression for hydrocephalus, than spontaneous (but remembering that trauma can so easily be ignored or forgotten). Rupture of a vascular malformation in the dura or of a very peripheral aneurysm (mycotic much more likely than saccular), a haemostatic defect (particularly therapeutic anticoagulation), or a peripheral cerebral tumour can be responsible. It is also a very rare complication of lumbar puncture. Often no convincing cause is found.

Specific causes of intracranial haemorrhage

Chronic hypertension causes thickening and disruption of the walls of the small arteries which perforate the base of the brain, particularly in the region of the basal ganglia (lenticulostriate arteries), along with microaneurysm formation (Charcot–Bouchard aneurysms) (Ross Russell 1975). It is the rupture of these abnormal vessels which is thought to cause hypertensive primary intracerebral haemorrhage (PICH), although it is almost impossible to prove a cause and effect relationship in individuals because the haemorrhage destroys the exact site of the bleeding (Takebayashi and Kaneko 1983). More recently, the very existence of microaneurysms has been challenged as a post-mortem artefact (Challa *et al.* 1992). In practice, the clinical diagnosis of 'hypertensive' PICH is based on the lack of any alternative explanation (bearing in mind angiography is seldom done in elderly patients and those in poor clinical condition) in a patient known to have had hypertension, or clearly has evidence of hypertensive organ damage (e.g. left ventricular hypertrophy, retinopathy, etc.), not just high blood pressure as a consequence of the stroke. However, it seems very likely that other factors, such as cerebral amyloid angiopathy, interact with hypertension to cause PICH in a particular individual. After all, hypertension is neither necessary nor sufficient to explain every case of PICH.

Saccular aneurysms vary from a few millimetres to several centimetres in diameter, can enlarge with time, but not necessarily, and almost certainly are much more often acquired than congenital. Associations for aneurysmal haemorrhage, which may or may not be causal, include polycystic kidney disease, hypertension, smoking, alcohol, oral contraceptives, and possibly coronary heart disease (Longstreth *et al.* 1985; Teunissen *et al.* 1996; Johnston *et al.* 1998; Uehara *et al.* 1998). Sometimes aneurysms are familial (ter Berg *et al.* 1992; Bromberg *et al.* 1995; Ronkainen *et al.* 1998) (Table 27.18). Saccular aneurysms tend to occur at branching points on the circle of Willis and proximal cerebral arteries; about 40 per cent on the anterior communicating artery complex, 30 per cent on the posterior communicating artery or distal internal carotid artery (ICA), 20 per cent on the middle cerebral artery, and 10 per cent in the posterior circulation (basilar, posterior cerebral artery, etc.). About 25 per cent occur at multiple sites. Aneurysms are an incidental finding in about 6 per cent of cerebral angiograms done for various reasons in adults, an almost certain overestimate of the true rate, which may be about 2 per cent (Rinkel *et al.* 1998). They present most commonly in middle life with subarachnoid haemorrhage. Other presentations include primary intracerebral haemorrhage; compression of adjacent structures (e.g. optic nerve from an anterior communicating artery aneurysm; optic chiasm, third, fourth, and fifth cranial nerves from a distal ICA or posterior communicating artery aneurysm; brainstem from a basilar artery aneurysm); seizures due to pressure on adjacent brain; TIA or ischaemic stroke due to embolism of intra-aneurysmal thrombus (Section 27.4.4); and carotico-cavernous fistula from rupture of an intra-cavernous carotid aneurysm (Raps *et al.* 1993).

Cerebral amyloid angiopathy (CAA) is an organ-specific form of amyloid deposition in small and medium arteries, less commonly veins, of the cerebral cortex and meninges, particularly in the elderly. Very often there is additional subcortical small vessel disease and demyelination, very reminiscent of Binswanger's disease (Section 27.4.4). CAA can be associated with Alzheimer's disease, Down's syndrome, cerebral vasculitis, cerebral irradiation, and dementia pugilistica (Venters 1987). It is increasingly presumed—but seldom biopsy or post-mortem proven—to be the cause of lobar haemorrhages in the elderly, often multiple and recurrent, and perhaps very rarely of subarachnoid haemorrhage. Fibrinoid necrosis seems to be a common accompaniment but could be secondary to, rather than the cause of, the haemorrhage (Vonsattel *et al.* 1991). Patients, with or without primary intracerebral haemorrhage

Table 27.18. Associations of intracranial saccular aneurysms

Polycystic kidney disease*
Fibromuscular dysplasia
Cervical artery dissection*
Coarctation of the aorta
Intracranial arteriovenous malformations*
Marfan's syndrome*
Ehlers–Danlos syndrome*
Pseudoxanthoma elasticum*
Neurofibromatosis type 1*
α_1-Antitrypsin deficiency*
Hereditary haemorrhagic telangiectasia*
Moyamoya syndrome
Klinefelter's syndrome
Progeria

* Can be familial.

(PICH), may also have a progressive dementia and a history of minor stroke-like episodes and TIAs, and even focal epileptic seizures, possibly due to small PICHs undetectable except perhaps by MRI (Greenberg *et al.* 1993). Dominantly inherited forms of CAA cause PICH in young adults in Iceland (Jensson *et al.* 1987) and in middle-aged adults in Holland (Bornebroek *et al.* 1997), and a syndrome of progressive dementia, ataxia, and spasticity associated sometimes with stroke in the UK (Plant *et al.* 1990).

Intracranial vascular malformations (IVMs) are uncommon, probably congenital, and sometimes familial. Those in the dura, draining into the sinuses rather than cerebral veins, can be caused by skull fracture, craniotomy, or dural sinus thrombosis (Nabors *et al.* 1987). The overall IVM detection rate is about 3 per 100 000 population per annum and the prevalence is about 20 per 100 000 (Brown *et al.* 1996b). There are four main types (Stein and Mohr 1988), as follows:

Arteriovenous malformations (AVMs) are the most common clinically and consist of an abnormal fistulous connection(s) between one or more hypertrophied feeding arteries and dilated draining veins (Fig. 27.20). The blood supply is derived from one or, more often, several cerebral arteries, perhaps with a contribution from branches of the external carotid artery. AVMs vary from a few millimetres to several centimetres in diameter. About 15 per cent are associated with aneurysms on their feeding arteries. Some grow during life but a few shrink or even disappear, and some multiple (Mendelow *et al.* 1987; Reddy *et al.* 1987).

These fistulae occur in or on the brain, or in the dura of the intracranial sinuses. They present at almost any age, with partial or secondary generalized epileptic seizures due to a cerebral AVM; intracerebral more often than subarachnoid or subdural haemorrhage from the AVM itself or associated aneurysm; as a mass lesion; with a carotico-cavernous fistula due to a dural AVM (see below); with TIA-like episodes, perhaps due to vascular steal or venous thrombosis; or with an audible bruit to the patient, particularly if a dural AVM is near the transverse/sigmoid sinus and petrous bone (Lasjaunias *et al.* 1986); with

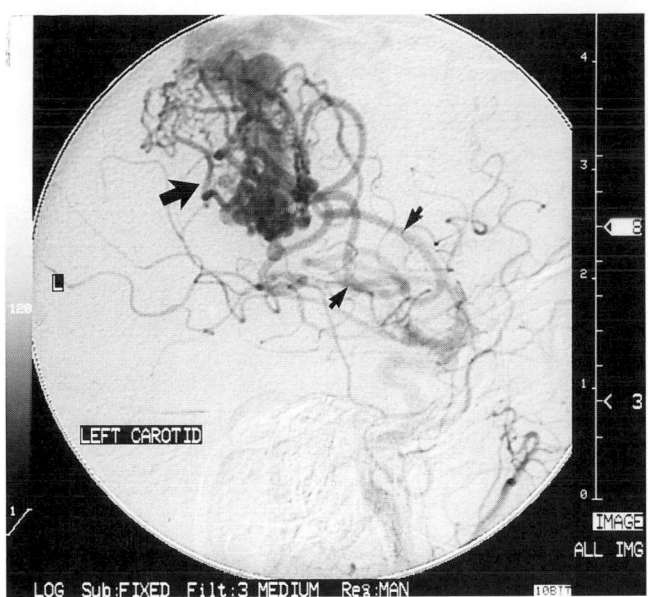

Fig. 27.20. Intracranial view of selective carotid angiogram to show a large arteriovenous malformation (arrow) supplied by branches of the middle cerebral artery (small arrows).

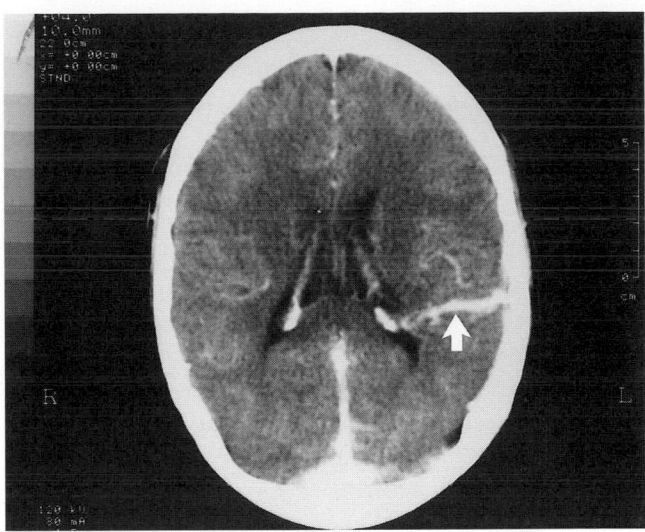

Fig. 27.21. CT scan showing the large draining vein of a venous malformation (arrow).

the syndrome of benign intracranial hypertension due to increased pressure in cerebral draining veins or sinuses (Chimowitz *et al.* 1990; or with high-output cardiac failure in neonates and infants (Davidson and Falconer 1973). Headache, although common, is not by itself diagnostically helpful and may well be a coincidence. Rather rarely, a bruit can be heard over the skull or orbits. A brainstem AVM can present like multiple sclerosis, with fluctuating symptoms and signs of brainstem dysfunction, perhaps due to recurrent haemorrhage (Stahl *et al.* 1980).

The diagnosis can be suspected on CT; a plain scan may show calcification and rather non-specific hypo- or hyperdensity, while an enhanced scan is likely to show the dilated vessels of large malformations. MRI is more sensitive, showing evidence of old haemorrhage and vascular flow voids. Angiography is the definitive investigation but can be normal with small malformations. It is crucial to display all the possible feeding vessels, not forgetting branches from the external carotid artery feeding dural AVMs (Tsitsopoulos *et al.* 1987; Abe *et al.* 1989).

Venous malformations consist of collections of venous channels and a large draining vein. Most are asymptomatic but they can possibly present with haemorrhage into the ventricles, or seizures. On contrast CT the draining vein may appear as a linear enhancing streak, but a flow void on MRI is more sensitive (Fig. 27.21). The definitive diagnosis is made on the venous phase of a cerebral angiogram.

Cavernous malformations (cavernomas) are sharply circumscribed collections of thin-walled sinusoidal vessels lined with a single layer of endothelium without intervening brain parenchyma or identifiable mature vessel wall elements. They are sometimes multiple and occasionally familial. Most are asymptomatic and picked up on MRI being done for an unre-

lated problem. But they can present with seizures, recurrent subacute brainstem syndromes, or even as a mass lesion, but rather seldom with haemorrhage. The angiogram is usually normal but CT can show a hypo- or hyperdense area which may enhance, and perhaps calcification, usually without surrounding oedema or mass effect. The most sensitive imaging is with MRI, revealing sharply circumscribed lesions, typically with evidence of haemosiderin as a result of old but asymptomatic haemorrhage (Fig. 27.22). However, they cannot always be distinguished from small AVMs by imaging (Requena *et al.* 1991; Kattapong *et al.* 1995).

Telangiectasias are collections of dilated capillaries which are usually of no clinical significance (Milandre *et al.* 1987). They may be associated with hereditary haemorrhagic telangiectasia (Osler–Weber–Rendu syndrome) but this is more likely to be associated with neurological complications from a pulmonary AVM with right-to-left shunting (cerebral hypoxia, brain abscess, paradoxical and septic embolism), or from an associated intracranial AVM or aneurysm (Roman *et al.* 1978; Guttmacher *et al.* 1995, McDonald *et al.* 1998).

Carotico-cavernous fistula is an abnormal connection between the carotid arterial system and the cavernous sinus. It occurs as a result of a ruptured dural AVM or intracavernous internal carotid artery aneurysm, closed or penetrating head injury, Ehlers–Danlos syndrome, or pseudoxanthoma elasticum. More often, it seems to be spontaneous, particularly in the elderly. With high-flow, direct fistulae from the carotid artery itself, the onset is dramatic, with unilateral pulsating exophthalmos and an orbital bruit, often audible to the patient. In addition, there may be orbital pain, papilloedema, dilated conjunctival veins and chemosis, glaucoma, monocular visual loss, and involvement of the third, fourth, sixth, and the first and perhaps second sensory division of the trigeminal nerve. The ophthalmoplegia may also be due to hypoxia and swelling within the extraocular muscles. Dural fistulae present more

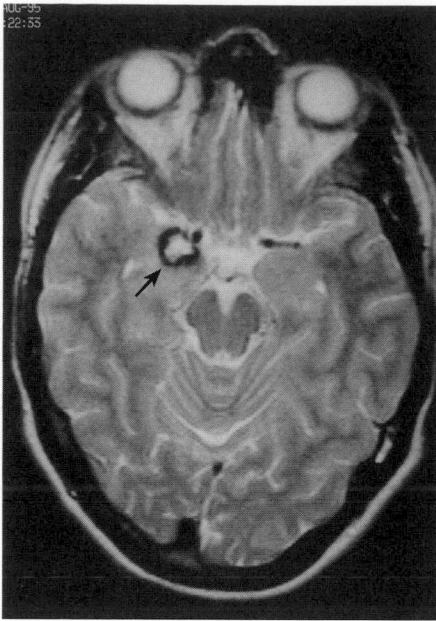

Fig. 27.22. T2-weighted MR brain scan to show a cavernous malformation (arrow). The 'black' halo representing old haemorrhage is very characteristic.

Table 27.19. Causes of transient focal neurological attacks

Focal cerebral ischaemia (i.e. TIA)
Migraine with aura
Partial epileptic seizures

Structural intracranial lesions
    Tumour
    Chronic subdural haematoma
    Vascular malformation
    Giant aneurysm

Multiple sclerosis
Labyrinthine disorders (e.g. Meniere's disease, benign positonal vertigo)
Peripheral nerve or root lesion

Metabolic
    Hypoglycaemia
    Hyperglycaemia
    Hypercalcaemia
    Hyponatraemia

Psychological

insidiously because the blood flow is lower from small meningeal branches of the internal or external carotid arteries in the cavernous sinus (Barrow *et al.* 1985). If there is no spontaneous resolution, it may be possible to obliterate the fistula with balloon catheterization.

27.5 The clinical features and investigation of transient ischaemic attacks

27.5.1 Clinical diagnosis

As far as one can tell, about 15 per cent of first stroke patients have had earlier TIAs, but only about half of them consult a doctor. Therefore, the incidence of TIAs presenting to medical attention (about 0.5 per 1000 population per annum) must be an underestimate of the real situation (Hankey and Warlow 1994; Brown *et al.* 1998). By definition, the symptoms last less than 24 hours, but a few patients have residual neurological signs of no functional significance, e.g. reflex asymmetry. About 25 per cent have focal hypodensity on CT, relevant to the symptoms in about half and therefore perhaps representing recent infarction (Dennis *et al.* 1990*a*). Not surprisingly, an even higher proportion have focal lesions on MRI (Awad *et al.* 1986). However, the diagnosis depends *not* on either neurological signs or imaging but essentially on the nature and duration of the symptoms in the right 'vascular' milieu (elderly, vascular risk factors, absent pulses, and bruits, etc.). Fortunately, in general, there is less interobserver disagreement about symptoms, which are remembered, than signs which are likely to attenuate and

disappear (Tomasello *et al.* 1982). The main use of brain imaging is to rule out the very occasional structural lesion causing 'transient focal neurological attacks' (Table 27.19 and Section 27.5.2).

Symptoms and their explanation

There is seldom a precipitating event. The symptoms start more or less abruptly, and they are 'focal', indicating a disturbance in a particular area of brain, or in one eye (Hankey and Warlow 1994). Motor symptoms are the most common: weakness, clumsiness or maybe heaviness in the upper limb or lower limb or face alone, or in various combinations, usually on just one side of the body (Table 27.20). Unilateral sensory symptoms are described as numbness, tingling, or deadness. If the attacks occur while speaking, the speech may be dysphasic, dysarthric, or both. Transient monocular blindness (amaurosis fugax) affects the upper or lower half of vision, or all the vision of one eye, and is often described like a blind or shutter coming down from above, or up from below. It must be distinguished from transient homonymous hemianopia, which is difficult if the patient has not covered each eye to check, or has only one good eye. Simultaneous bilateral motor (and perhaps sensory) loss is almost always due to brainstem ischaemia. Sudden simultaneous bilateral blindness in elderly patients usually indicates bilateral occipital ischaemia. Vertigo, diplopia, dysphagia, unsteadiness, tinnitus, amnesia, drop attacks, and possibly dysarthria are so often due to global cerebral ischaemia, or non-vascular causes, that if one occurs as an single symptom the diagnosis of TIA is very uncertain, although not impossible (Gomez *et al.* 1996). Transient loss of consciousness is almost unheard of, not surprisingly as it is rare even in an ischaemic stroke unless severe, and can only be accepted during a TIA if there are additional clear-cut focal symptoms of a sort that are

Table 27.20. Clinical features and vascular distribution of transient ischaemic attacks

Symptoms	Vascular distribution		Proportion[b]
	Carotid	Vertebrobasilar	(%)
Unilateral weakness, heaviness, or clumsiness	+	+	50
Unilateral sensory symptoms	+	+	35
Dysarthria[a]	+	+	23
Transient monocular blindness	+	–	18
Dysphasia	+	(+)	18
Unsteadiness/ataxia[a]	(+)	+	12
Bilateral simultaneous blindness	–	+	7
Vertigo[a]	–	+	5
Homonymous hemianopia	(+)	+	5
Diplopia	–	+	5
Bilateral motor loss	–	+	4
Dysphagia[a]	(+)	+	1
Crossed sensory and motor loss	–	+	1

[a] In general if these symptoms are *isolated* it is best not to diagnose definite TIA.

[b] The proportion of TIA patients with various symptoms from the Oxfordshire Community Stroke Project, unpublished: many patients had more than one symptom (e.g. weakness *and* numbness, etc.).

unlikely to be epileptic (Bogousslavsky *et al.* 1986*a*; Landi 1992; Hankey and Warlow 1994).

If more than one body part is involved, the symptoms usually start more or less simultaneously in all parts, persist for a while and then gradually wear off in a few minutes (particularly amaurosis fugax) or an hour or so, sometimes longer. Indeed, if a patient still has symptoms more than an hour after the onset, the chances are that they will persist for more than 24 hours and so the patient will actually have had a stroke (Levy 1988). Further attacks may be identical, or the symptoms may be different if the ischaemia is in a different arterial territory. A mild headache during, and sometimes after, the neurological symptoms is quite common, usually ipsilateral to the affected arterial territory (Loeb *et al.* 1985; Koudstaal *et al.* 1991). If cerebral symptoms are very brief, perhaps less than a minute, and particularly if they are 'sensory', then the diagnosis of TIA is difficult to sustain, and if they are neither due to a partial seizure nor psychogenic causes, they may remain unexplained. On the other hand, symptoms of retinal ischaemia can be, and often are, very brief.

To some extent, the symptoms allow one to categorize attacks as being within the carotid (about 80 per cent) or vertebrobasilar vascular territories (about 20 per cent). However, because the motor and sensory pathways are supplied by both vascular systems at different points in their course, it is not always possible to distinguish which territory is involved, although the carotid circulation is usually assumed if the symptoms are unilateral (Table 27.20). Definite cortical (e.g. dysphasia) or brainstem (e.g. diplopia) symptoms are helpful in this situation, as well as any evidence of *recent* infarction on brain imaging. Ischaemia in the territory of supply of the deep perforating arteries (lacunar TIAs) may be suspected if the patient has a transient lacunar syndrome (Section 27.6.2) and no positive evidence of cortical involvement such as dysphasia (Hankey and Warlow 1991*b*).

Most TIAs are probably due to artery-to-artery or heart-to-artery embolism, or acute arterial thrombosis (Bogousslavsky *et al.* 1986*a*). However, sometimes there is strong circumstantial evidence that the attacks are due to low flow, almost always distal to a severely stenosed or occluded artery in the neck, which makes the patient susceptible to a small drop in blood pressure, perhaps because autoregulation is impaired or cerebral perfusion reserve exhausted (Ross Russell 1988); for example, hours or days after a patient is given blood-pressure-lowering drugs or vasodilators, or the dose is increased (such as calcium blockers, glycerol trinitrate, etc.); or, if attacks occur on standing or sitting up quickly; after a heavy meal; after a hot bath; after exercise; or during a clinically obvious cardiac arrhythmia (Caplan and Sergay 1976; Ruff *et al.* 1981; Ross Russell and Page 1983; Kamata *et al.* 1994). Also, low-flow TIAs may be somewhat atypical and therefore recognizable in the sense that the symptoms may take some minutes to develop. They can consist of irregular shaking or dystonic posturing of the arm or leg contralateral to the cerebral ischaemia; or there is monocular or binocular visual blurring, dimming, fragmentation, or bleaching, often just in bright light (Furlan *et al.* 1979; Yanagihara *et al.* 1985; Wiebers *et al.* 1989; Hess *et al.* 1991). Normally, of course, a sudden fall in systemic blood pressure causes non-focal neurological symptoms, such as dizziness, faintness, loss of consciousness, confusion, imbalance, bilateral visual blurring, generalized weakness, and tingling. Feeling intermittently 'dizzy' is almost universal in elderly people when they move their heads suddenly, particularly when looking up. It is rare indeed to find a patient with clear-cut focal brainstem symptoms due to intermittent obstruction of a vertebral artery by cervical osteophytes, presumably because collateral blood flow to the brainstem is sufficient if the carotid circulation and contralateral vertebral artery are reasonably normal (Sakai *et al.* 1988; Sturzenegger *et al.* 1994). Finally, although 'vasospasm' has been intermittently invoked as a cause for TIAs, there is little current enthusiasm for this hypothesis (Winterkorn *et al.* 1993).

Retrograde flow in the vertebral artery (subclavian steal) is a common angiographic and ultrasound finding when there is stenosis or occlusion of the subclavian artery proximal to the vertebral artery origin, or of the inominate artery. When the ipsilateral arm is exercised, the increased blood flow to meet the metabolic demand may be enough to 'steal' blood down the vertebral artery, away from the brainstem into the axillary artery. If there is poor collateral blood flow to the brainstem, then symptoms may occur, but this is very rare. The subclavian disease is almost always severe enough to be suspected by unequal radial pulses and blood pressures, and often there is a supraclavicular bruit (Fig. 27.23) (Bohmfalk *et al.* 1979; Bornstein and Norris 1986; Hennerici *et al.* 1988).

Signs

Not surprisingly, there is seldom an opportunity to examine patients during a TIA, when focal neurological signs might indicate the site of the lesion, and so of the ischaemic area. Later examination for non-neurological signs can, however, help elucidate the cause of the attacks. For example, the presence of a focal arterial bruit over the carotid bifurcation (Fig. 27.23) is predictive of more than 25 per cent internal carotid artery (ICA) stenosis, although very tight stenosis, or occlusion, may not cause a bruit at all (Hankey and Warlow 1990). Bruits transmitted from the aortic valve become attenuated towards the angle of the jaw, those due to a generally hyperdynamic circulation are diffuse, and venous hums can be obliterated with light pressure over the jugular vein (Sandok *et al.* 1982). Atheromatous carotid stenosis is usually too proximal at the carotid bifurcation for patients to hear their own bruit; self-audible bruits (i.e. pulsatile tinnitus) are more likely to be due to distal ICA stenosis (dissection, fibromuscular dysplasia), a dural arteriovenous fistula near the petrous temporal bone, a glomus tumour, a carotico-cavernous fistula, raised intracranial pressure, or heightened awareness of the normal pulse (Thie *et al.* 1993*b*; Waldvogel *et al.* 1998). Absent common carotid or superficial temporal pulses suggests common carotid or external carotid disease, respectively.

Fibrin-platelet emboli are rarely observed moving through the retinal circulation. On the other hand, cholesterol emboli are more often seen lodged at arteriolar branching points, where they look like glittering yellow bodies which reflect the ophthalmoscope light, but usually do not obstruct blood flow.

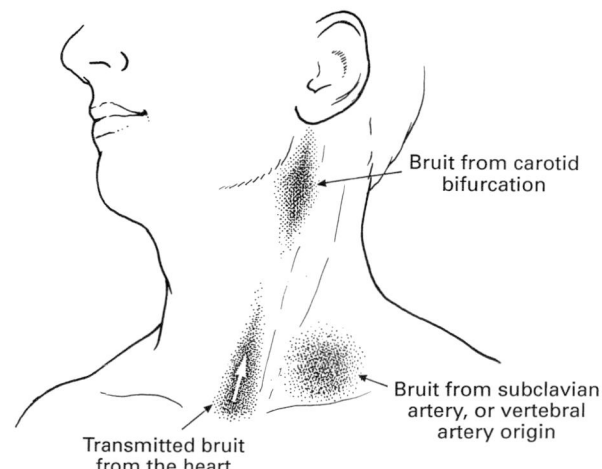

Fig. 27.23. The localization and implications of cervical bruits in various places. Note that a bruit arising from the carotid bifurcation is high up under the angle of the jaw and that supraclavicular bruits can be due to either subclavian or vertebral artery origin stenosis.

Such findings strongly suggest proximal atheroma. 'Calcific' retinal emboli look solid, white, and non-reflective, they tend to impact at the optic disc edge and suggest embolism from aortic or mitral valve calcification (Arruga and Sanders 1982). Later, embolized vessels may become white and 'sheathed' but this appearance eventually disappears. Severe ICA disease, usually with ipsilateral external carotid artery (ECA) involvement as well, may cause such profound retinal ischaemia that venous stasis retinopathy develops with dilated retinal veins, haemorrhages, and microaneurysms. The episcleral arteries may be dilated, because of increased collateral blood flow via branches of the ECA (Countee *et al.* 1978). Worsening ischaemia causes ischaemic oculopathy with pain; impaired vision; 'low pressure' glaucoma; and with light pressure on the globe the retinal arterioles collapse (Ross Russell and Ikeda 1986).

Large artery disease elsewhere (e.g. unequal arm blood pressure/pulses, known coronary artery disease, claudication, femoral bruits, absent foot pulses) suggests that TIAs are due to atherothromboembolism of the extracranial arteries, while a cardiac valvular lesion may suggest embolism from the heart (Section 27.4.5).

27.5.2 Differential diagnosis

TIAs are but one cause of 'transient focal neurological attacks' (Table 27.19) and 'transient monocular blindness' (Table 27.21). Distinguishing the various causes depends essentially on taking a good history, often from a witness as well as the patient, and excluding obvious structural abnormalities in the brain (CT/MRI) and eye (ophthalmoscopy). There is no diagnostic test to confirm a TIA, although a test may reject the diagnosis (e.g. CT scan shows intracranial tumour). Some conditions are particularly frequently misdiagnosed as TIAs and will be discussed in detail.

Migraine with aura

This is not a diagnostic problem if the aura is accompanied by, or followed by, a significant headache with or without nausea and vomiting. Nor is it a problem if one day a migraineur develops a typical aura (for him or her) but no headache. However, occasionally migraine auras start in middle age and, if there is no headache, they can be confused with TIAs. The difference is that migrainous auras come on slowly, spread and intensify over several minutes, and fade in 20–30 minutes. The symptoms tend to begin in one domain (particularly vision), fade and move on to another (e.g. language). Also the symptoms tend to be positive (e.g. flashing lights, tingling) rather than the typically negative symptoms of a TIA (e.g. weakness, visual loss, numbness). With a careful history these 'migraines without headache' or 'transient migrainous accompaniments' can usually be recognized and the patient reassured (Dennis and Warlow 1992). Retinal migraine is a controversial entity but gradually intensifying and spreading, and positive (flashing, scintillations, etc.) visual symptoms in one eye are suggestive (Appleton *et al.* 1988).

Table 27.21. Causes of transient monocular blindness (amaurosis fugax)

Ischaemia (i.e. TIA)
Glaucoma
Uhthoff's phenomenon in retrobulbar neurotis
Raised intracranial pressure with papilloedema
Retinal haemorrhage
Retinal venous thrombosis
Retinal detachment
Macular degeneration
Intra-orbital tumour
Carotico-cavernous fistula
Retinal migraine
Intracranial dural malformation
Paraneoplastic retinopathy
Reversible diabetic cataract
Ureitis–glaucoma–hyphaema syndrome

Epilepsy

This is not a diagnostic problem unless the seizures are partial. Although partial sensory seizures tend to cause positive symptoms like TIAs (e.g. tingling), the symptoms 'march' across a hand or foot, and up the limb in a minute or so and may, eventually, be accompanied by focal motor seizures or secondary generalization. Sudden speech arrest seems to be more often epileptic, not necessarily arising in the dominant hemisphere, than due to ischaemia, which is more likely to cause dysphasic speech (Cascino *et al.* 1991). Transient inhibitory seizures may mimic the focal motor weakness of TIAs, but are most unusual (Kaplan 1993).

Intracranial structural lesions

Just occasionally one can stumble on an intracranial structural lesion causing TIAs, or at least TIA-like episodes. Obviously one has to be alert to their coincidence with a more common vascular explanation such as carotid stenosis. Compression of an intracranial artery is perhaps an explanation of symptoms for those patients with tumours or a chronic subdural haematoma, although focal seizures misdiagnosed as TIAs is a more likely possibility (Auld and Shafey 1976; Welsh *et al.* 1979; UK-TIA Study Group 1993). Intracranial vascular malformations might cause local stealing of blood and so a TIA, or perhaps focal epileptic attacks mimicking TIAs (Gautier *et al.* 1983). Embolism from aneurysms has been mentioned earlier (Section 27.4.4).

Transient global amnesia

Transient global amnesia (TGA) is a characteristic, but uncommon, clinical syndrome, usually in the middle aged or elderly. The onset is more or less sudden, with severe anterograde amnesia accompanied, usually, by retrograde amnesia stretching back weeks, months, or longer. The attack lasts several hours, after which the patient recovers the ability to lay down new memories and recall old ones, but permanently forgets the period of the attack itself. During the attack the patient is fully conscious, has no loss of personal identity, looks normal, if a little subdued and bewildered, and has no other symptoms apart perhaps from some headache and nausea. The patient can perform normal everyday activities, even driving, but typically asks the same question repetitively because of the anterograde amnesia. Naturally a witness is required to differentiate such attacks from hysterical fugues, alcoholic amnesic states, or even complex partial seizures. Normally the prognosis is excellent. Although the attacks may occasionally recur, there is no excessive risk of serious vascular events so that, in general, TGA is not a manifestation of cerebral ischaemia. It seems to be due to some sort of temporary perturbation in the medial temporal lobes bilaterally (Strupp *et al.* 1998). However, if there are additional focal symptoms (e.g. suggesting brainstem involvement), then a vascular cause is more likely. Sometimes epilepsy develops later, usually complex partial seizures, particularly if the TGA has been short (less than an hour), occurred on wakening, and with early recurrence. There are not necessarily other independent episodes more obviously 'temporal lobe' epileptic (Zeman *et al.* 1998). However, in the vast majority of TGA cases no cause is obvious at the time or later (Hodges 1991), although 'stress' has often been considered (Rosler *et al.* 1999).

Cryptogenic drop attacks

These affect middle-aged and elderly women, almost only when walking rather than just standing or sitting. Without any warning, prior or other symptoms, the patient crashes to the ground but without definite loss of consciousness and without any leg weakness. The attacks may recur but then disappear as mysteriously as they came. There is usually no known cause, although carotid sinus syncope and orthostatic hypotension are possibilities (Dey *et al.* 1996). On the whole, there appear to be no serious prognostic implications (Stevens and Matthews 1973; Meissner *et al.* 1986). Sudden weakness of both legs can occur in brainstem ischaemia and, rarely, if both anterior cerebral arteries are supplied from the same (stenosed) internal carotid artery (Ho *et al.* 1986). Bilateral motor, sensory, or visual impairments can also be due to bihemispheric boundary zone ischaemia distal to severe carotid disease (Sloan and Haley 1990). Finally, spinal cord 'TIAs' do occur but are even rarer

Table 27.22. Baseline tests for most TIA and ischaemic stroke patients

Investigation	Treatable disorders detected
Full blood count	Anaemia, polycythaemia, leukaemia, thrombocythaemia
ESR	Vasculitis, infective endocarditis, hyperviscosity, myxoma
Electrolytes	Hyponatraemia or hypokalaemia
Urea	Renal impairment
Plasma glucose	Diabetes, hypoglycaemia
Plasma cholesterol	High cholesterol
Urine analysis	Diabetes, renal disease, vasculitis
Electrocardiogram	Left ventricular hypertrophy, arrhythmia, conduction block, myocardial infarction

Table 27.23. Second-line investigations for selected ischaemic stroke/TIA patients

Investigation	Indications
Blood	
Liver function	Fever, malaise, raised ESR, suspected malignancy
Calcium	Recurrent focal neurological symptoms very rarely due to hypercalcaemia
Thyroid function tests	Atrial fibrillation
Activated partial thromboplastin time, dilute Russell's viper venom time, anticardiolipin antibody[a], antinuclear and other autoantibodies	Young (<50 years) and no other cause found, past history or family history of venous thrombosis, especially if unusual site (cerebral, mesenteric, hepatic veins), recurrent miscarriage, thrombocytopenia, cardiac valve vegetations, livedo reticularis, raised ESR, malaise, etc., positive syphilis serology
Serum proteins, serum protein electrophoresis, plasma viscosity	Raised ESR
Haemoglobin electrophoresis	Afro-Caribbean patients
Protein C and S, antithrombin III, activated protein C resistance, thrombin time[b]	Personal or family history of thrombosis (usually venous, particularly in unusual sites such as hepatic vein) at unusually young age
Blood cultures	Fever, cardiac murmur, haematuria, deranged liver function, raised ESR, malaise, unexplained stroke at any age
HIV serology	Young (<40 years), drug addict, homosexual, blood products transfusion, systemically unwell, lymphadenopathy, pneumonia, CMV retinitis, etc.
Lipoprotein fractionation	Elevated cholesterol or strong family history Hyperlipoproteinaemia
Serum homocysteine (after methionine load)	Marfanoid habitus, high myopia, dislocated lenses, osteoporosis, mental retardation, young patient
Leucocyte α-galactosidase A	Corneal opacities, cutaneous angiokeratomas, paraesthesias and pain, renal failure
Blood/CSF lactate	Young patient, basal ganglia calcification, epilepsy, MELAS/mitochondrial cytopathy, parieto-occipital ischaemia
Syphilis serology	Young patient, high risk of sexually transmitted diseases
Cardiac enzymes	History or ECG evidence of recent myocardial infarction
Drug screen	Young patient, no other obvious cause, cocaine/amphetamine, etc.-induced
Urine	
Amino acids	Marfanoid habitus, high myopia, dislocated lenses, osteoporosis, mental retardation, young patient
Drug screen	Young patient, no other obvious cause, cocaine/amphetamine, etc.-induced
Imaging	
Chest X-ray (CXR)	Hypertension, finger-clubbing, cardiac murmur or abnormal ECG, young patient, ill patient
Brain CT scan	Continuing carotid TIAs of the brain, carotid endarterectomy being considered, thrombolysis being considered, taking or due to take anticoagulants or antiplatelet drugs, deteriorating stroke patient
MRI	Suggestion of arterial dissection, uncertain diagnosis of stroke
Carotid ultrasound with a view to carotid angiography	Carotid TIA or mild ischaemic stroke
Catheter angiography	Carotid ultrasound suggests about <70% stenosis of recently symptomatic internal carotid artery and patient fit and willing for surgery, suspected arterial dissection, arteritis, AVM or aneurysm
Arch aortography	Symptoms of subclavian steel and unequal brachial pulses and blood pressures
Cardiac	
Echocardiography (transthoracic or transoesophageal)	Possible cardiac source of embolism and young (<50 years), or clinical, ECG or CXR evidence of embologenic heart disease, aortic arch dissection
24-hour ECG	Palpitations or loss of consciousness during a suspected TIA, suspicious resting ECG
Others	
EEG	Doubt about diagnosis of TIA or stroke: ?epilepsy
CSF	Positive blood syphilis serology, young patient, ?infective endocarditis, possibility of multiple sclerosis
Body red cell mass	Raised haematocrit
Temporal artery biopsy	Older (<60 years), jaw claudication, headache, polymyalgia, malaise, anaemia, raised ESR

[a] Repeat to ensure persistently raised.

[b] Transient falls occur after stroke, so any low level must be repeated and family members investigated.

than spinal cord infarction (Cheshire *et al.* 1996). Clearly, care has to be taken to pick up the occasional patient with falls due to an extrapyramidal syndrome. Cataplexy is almost invariably precipitated by excitement or emotion and seldom causes the patient to fall over.

Psychogenic attacks

These are usually situational (e.g. open spaces, etc.) but can be confusing if the symptoms consist merely of tingling, particularly if this affects only one side of the body rather than both. Suspicion should be aroused if the patient is young (less than 50); there are no signs of vascular or cardiac disease, or risk factors; if the left rather than right side is affected (Rothwell 1994); there are other features of hyperventilation such as difficulty taking a deep breath or swallowing, and dizziness; there are numerous other medically unexplained symptoms; and obvious non-organic motor or sensory signs.

27.5.3 **Investigation**

Investigations are not much to do with distinguishing a TIA from some other type of 'funny turn' (a difference essentially based on a good history), but are directed at determining the cause of the TIA, particularly if this is likely to influence management. Simple baseline tests should be done in most cases (Warlow *et al.* 1996a) (Table 27.22). Further investigations (Table 27.23) depend on the clinical situation, the age of the patient, and the results of the baseline tests. Because the risk of stroke is highest soon after TIA (Section 27.10.2), it is important to do the investigations quickly, perhaps in 'one-stop' clinics, so that preventive treatments can be started before any stroke occurs (Section 27.10.3). Some investigations require further discussion, as follows.

Imaging the brain

The purpose of non-contrast CT, or MRI, is to exclude the very rare situation when an intracranial space-occupying lesion or vascular malformation presents as a 'TIA' (Section 27.5.2). Scanning does not necessarily have to be routine, particularly if the TIAs have affected only the eye or the brainstem, but is certainly indicated if the TIAs are frequent, or if the patient is being considered for carotid endarterectomy. Finding hypodense lesions (i.e. presumed infarcts), relevant to the symptoms or not, has no impact on management (Dennis *et al.* 1990a). There should be little concern about missing primary intracerebral haemorrhage, which has almost never been reported to cause TIAs with symptoms that really last less than 24 hours, although haemorrhage can cause remarkably trivial strokes (Scott and Miller 1985; Dennis *et al.* 1987; Gunatilake 1998).

Imaging the cerebral circulation in TIA (and mild ischaemic stroke) patients (Section 2.2)

Cerebral catheter angiography

Cerebral angiography is seldom required unless a patient with a carotid ischaemic event is fit for, and prepared to consider,

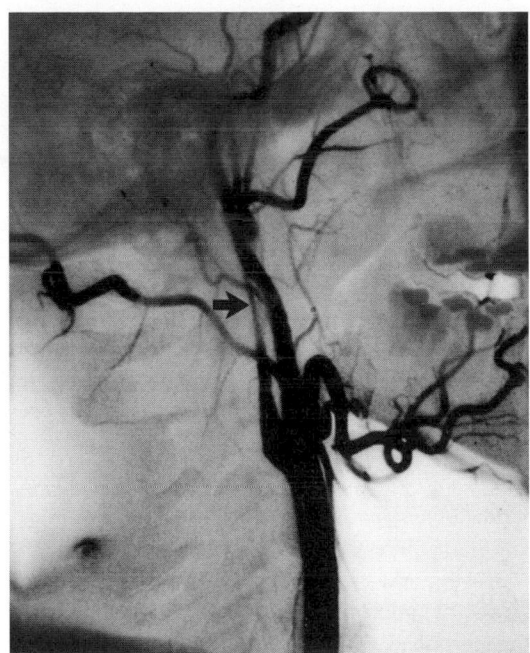

Fig. 27.24. Selective lateral carotid angiogram showing near occlusion of the proximal internal carotid artery (arrow). However, there is a trickle of contrast beyond the stenosis.

carotid endarterectomy (Section 27.10.3); there is suspicion of traumatic arterial dissection (Section 27.4.4) which, if diagnosed, would have medico-legal implications; or in the occasional patient with frequent vertebrobasilar TIAs, particularly in association with subclavian steal which might be amenable to surgery (Sellar 1995). Very rarely, cerebral angiography will show an intracranial giant aneurysm, or vascular malformation, which might have caused the symptoms.

Intra-arterial digital angiography is now universally preferred but may not be that much safer than conventional catheter cerebral angiography (Warnock *et al.* 1993). But it is quicker and the images have better contrast resolution (but rather inferior spatial resolution), and they are easier to manipulate and store. Late views are required to show collateral circulation distal to severe stenosis or occlusion, and to show any trickle of contrast through a very tight stenosis which would otherwise appear like an inoperable occlusion (Fig. 27.24). Neither intravenous digital nor conventional arch angiography are satisfactory by themselves because so often the images are poor, vessels overlap, and there is insufficient intracranial information.

Unfortunately, angiography is uncomfortable and carries about a 4 per cent risk of TIA or stroke, a quarter of which are permanent (Hankey *et al.* 1990a,b; Davies and Humphrey 1993). This is due to: dislodgement of atheromatous plaque or arterial trauma from the catheter tip, or during injection or flushing, particularly if there is severe carotid disease; clots forming in syringes and catheters; and possibly air bubbles during injection. Systemic and allergic adverse effects can also occur, particularly during intravenous digital angiography when large quantities of contrast have to be used; these include

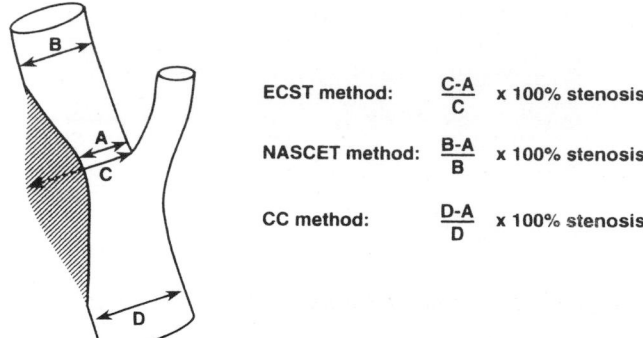

ECST method: $\dfrac{C-A}{C}$ x 100% stenosis

NASCET method: $\dfrac{B-A}{B}$ x 100% stenosis

CC method: $\dfrac{D-A}{D}$ x 100% stenosis

Fig. 27.25. Diagram to show the three methods of measuring stenosis on a carotid angiogram. The CC (common carotid artery) and the ECST (European Carotid Surgery Trial) methods give much the same results (Rothwell *et al.* 1994a). They can be converted to the NASCET (North American Symptomatic Carotid Endarterectomy Trial) method by the formula: NASCET % stenosis = (ECST or CC % stenosis − 40)/0.6.

bradycardia, hypotension, angina, shortness of breath, nausea, vomiting, headache, epileptic seizures, transient bilateral blindness, periorbital oedema, urticaria, bronchospasm, renal failure, and the cholesterol embolization syndrome. Occasionally patients develop a haematoma, aneurysm, or nerve injury at the site of arterial puncture, or ischaemia in the leg distal to a femoral artery puncture.

The image showing the smallest residual lumen is used to calculate the percentage diameter stenosis, selecting for the denominator the normal internal carotid artery distal to the lesion (which underestimates the stenosis), an estimate of the original arterial diameter at the level of the lesion, or the normal portion of the common carotid artery (Fig. 27.25). Despite angiography being the 'gold standard', there is considerable observer variation in measuring stenosis, which can only be regarded as approximate, but none the less it is extremely good in predicting the risk of stroke (Rothwell and Warlow 1996).

Carotid ultrasound

The risks and benefits of carotid endarterectomy are quite finely balanced (Section 27.10.3). Because any preceding catheter angiography can only add to the risk, huge efforts have been made to develop ultrasound techniques to a stage where they can provide the surgeon with enough information about the carotid stenosis that angiography can be abandoned altogether. Techniques are changing so rapidly that any conclusions about their accuracy in defining the severity and morphology of carotid stenosis have to be constantly updated and, more importantly, applied in the context of the ultrasound quality in one's own institution (Ringelstein 1995; Carpenter *et al.* 1996). For example, the standard technique of Duplex sonography, which is a combination of real-time ultrasound imaging and Doppler flow analysis, can now be combined with colour-coded Doppler-derived flow signals and complemented by power Doppler (Fig. 27.26) (Furst *et al.* 1992; Griewing *et al.* 1996). Because ultrasound techniques are so operator-dependent, it is

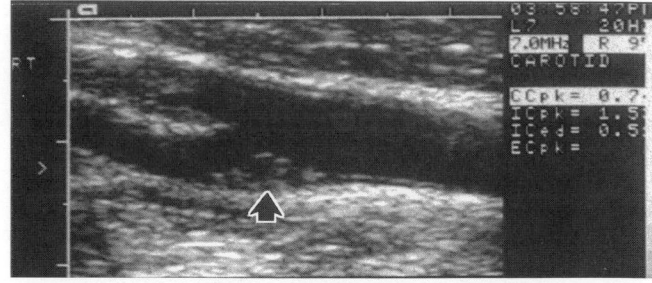

Fig. 27.26. Ultrasound image of the carotid bifurcation showing a plaque on the posterior wall of the internal carotid artery (arrow).

crucial that their local accuracy is kept under constant review, preferably using angiography as the gold standard if possible (Elgersma *et al.* 1998).

However, some surgeons will not operate on the basis of ultrasound imaging alone but still require angiography to display: the length of the symptomatic lesion and position of the bifurcation; any coincidental intracranial aneurysm, or severe intracranial stenosis which might influence the endarterectomy decision; inoperable occlusion which can be confused on ultrasound with operable but very severe stenosis; and the state of the other major arteries in the neck. Furthermore, irregularity and ulceration of a stenotic lesion can only really be shown by angiography, and this may have prognostic, and so management, importance (Section 27.10.3).

Magnetic resonance angiography and CT angiography

Both magnetic resonance angiography (MRA) (Fig. 27.27) and CT angiography (CTA) (Fig. 27.28) are, apart from intravenous

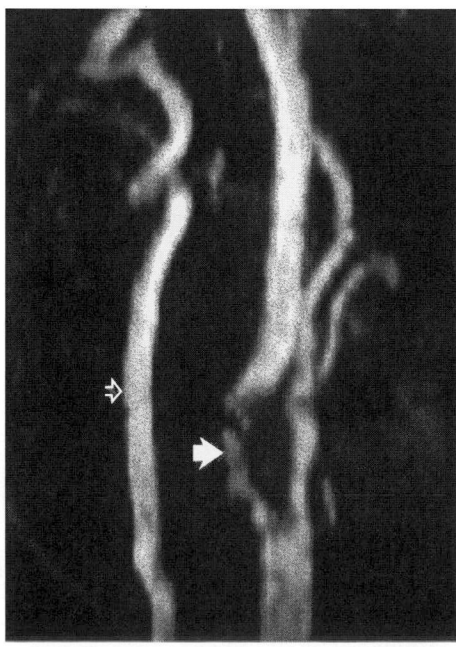

Fig. 27.27. Magnetic resonance angiography to show stenosis of the internal carotid artery origin (closed arrow). The vertebral artery is also seen (open arrow).

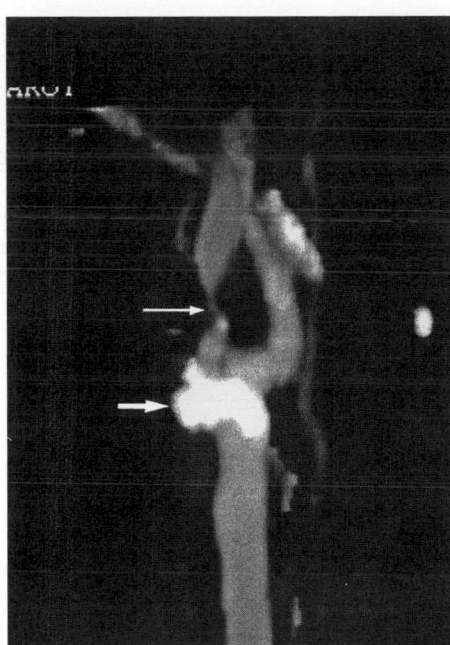

Fig. 27.28. Computed tomographic angiography (CTA) to show stenosis of the internal carotid artery origin (thin arrow). Calcification shows up white in this two-dimensional reconstruction (thick arrow).

contrast injection for the latter, non-invasive and safe. Although they do not provide as much anatomical detail as intra-arterial digital angiography, there may be enough to guide the surgeon planning a carotid endarterectomy, particularly if the results agree with an independent Duplex examination. The main concerns with MRA are: overestimation of stenosis severity; sometimes loss of signal distal to a stenosis and so confusing this with occlusion; inability to image ulceration; and institutions using outdated methods (Siewert *et al.* 1995). Problems with CTA are calcification at the carotid bifurcation and not using the optimal scanning technique (Leclerc *et al.* 1995).

Many now regard the best policy for detecting 'operable carotid stenosis' as Duplex first and, if that shows a stenosis severe enough for surgery, a repeat Duplex by an independent operator, or CTA, or MRA. In the few cases where there is serious disagreement between the two measurements, or some other concern, then selective intra-arterial digital angiography is indicated.

Transcranial Doppler sonography

Transcranial Doppler (TCD) sonography, nowadays with colour coding and if necessary with intravenous contrast, can detect occlusion and stenosis of the largest intracranial vessels as well as gaseous or solid emboli passing through them (middle cerebral, anterior cerebral, posterior cerebral, and basilar arteries). Although at present it is of no routine clinical value, it may become so if it turns out that intracranial collateral flow patterns, or impaired cerebrovascular reserve, should influence the management of severe carotid stenosis or occlusion (Bornstein and Norris 1994). However, TCD is not without problems: the skull is impenetrable to ultrasound in up

to 30 per cent of elderly patients; flow has been detected in vessels found, in some instances, to be occluded on angiography; no flow has been seen when in fact the artery is patent; branches of the middle cerebral artery cannot be insonated; high flow can represent either stenosis or hyperaemia; it is very dependent on operator skill; techniques must be standardized; and the patient has to keep still (Baumgartner *et al.* 1997; Ringelstein *et al.* 1998).

Diagnosis of embolism from the heart to the brain

With improving technology it has become less of a problem to identify potential cardiac sources of embolism (Hart 1992) (see Table 27.14). But, it is still not much easier to assess the embolic *relevance* of what is found. In practice, most cardiac lesions likely to be of embolic relevance can be suspected, and even definitively diagnosed, on the basis of a competent clinical examination, ECG, and chest X-ray. Transthoracic echocardiography will refine the diagnosis and management of many clinically suspected lesions (e.g. mitral stenosis, atrial myxoma), and transoesophageal echocardiography with echocontrast, while somewhat invasive and risky, will provide even more information (e.g. thrombus in left atrium, patent foramen ovale, mitral valve vegetations, spontaneous echo contrast) and display atheromatous plaques in the aortic arch (Tegeler and Downes 1991; Adams and Love 1995; Daniel and Mugge 1995; Leung *et al.* 1995). Unfortunately, the increasing number and variety of lesions that can now be detected by echocardiography has generated more questions than answers and made very little evidence-based impact on patient management. On the whole, echocardiography is not justified unless there is a strong suspicion of embolism from the heart, or the patient is young and so unlikely to have a competing arterial cause (see below).

Long-term monitoring of the ECG is more confusing than helpful unless the history suggests intermittent atrial fibrillation (and therefore perhaps the need for anticoagulation) or the cerebrovascular episodes are thought to be due to a cardiac arrhythmia, which is unusual (i.e. accompanying symptoms of chest pain, palpitations, faintness). Various transient cardiac arrhythmias are so frequently seen in elderly patients that unless they coincide with the symptoms one can almost never be sure of their relevance (De Bono and Warlow 1981).

If there is clinical or ECG suspicion of a recent myocardial infarction, and therefore of embolism from the left ventricle, then the detection of a typical rise in cardiac enzymes may be helpful if it is not too late after the onset.

Because a cardiac source of embolism is so often found in association with other causes of TIA (such as carotid stenosis) (De Bono and Warlow 1981; Bogousslavsky *et al.* 1986a), and it is usually impossible to be sure that a potentially embolic lesion (e.g. atrial fibrillation) really has caused embolization even if thrombus is observed in the heart (e.g. in the left atrium), the diagnosis of embolism has to be made on circumstantial evidence. Indeed, about half the cerebral ischaemia patients with non-rheumatic atrial fibrillation have another equally, or more likely, cause of the ischaemia (Bogousslavsky *et al.* 1990).

The clinical features of the cerebrovascular event are not really distinctive enough to be helpful, although lacunar TIAs (or lacunar ischaemic strokes) are less likely to be due to embolism than those affecting the cerebral cortex or the brainstem (Bogousslavsky *et al.* 1986b; Kittner *et al.* 1990). Detection of emboli by transcranial Doppler examination is not yet practical. Observing intra-arterial calcific particles in the retina, or on a brain CT, is extremely unusual and, anyway, compatible with embolism from atheromatous plaques as well as from a calcific aortic or mitral valve. One can be most confident about embolism from the heart if there is: no competing cause of cerebral ischaemia (e.g. carotid stenosis); no general vascular disease (e.g. angina, claudication, arterial bruits) or risk factors; ischaemic episodes in more than one arterial territory or part of the body; and the patient is young (under the age of about 40). Lack of intracardiac thrombus in patients with atrial fibrillation or a recent myocardial infarction does not necessarily exclude embolism, because the thrombus may have been lysed, or it has all embolized, or it may be too small to be detected. On the other hand, the detection of such thrombi does not necessarily mean that parts have embolized, or will do so again.

In practice, the search for, and relevance of, a cardiac source of embolism is greatest when no other definite cause of TIA can be found, which is usually in younger rather than older patients (Biller *et al.* 1986). If one looks equally hard, these same cardiac lesions can be found in elderly ischaemic stroke patients, albeit in a smaller proportion because there are so many other more common causes (carotid stenosis, etc.). In that situation, determining the actual cause of the stroke, or of any future strokes, is difficult and based on probabilities rather than certainties.

27.6 The clinical features and investigation of acute ischaemic stroke and primary intracerebral haemorrhage

27.6.1 Diagnosis of stroke versus not stroke

The diagnosis of stroke—versus not stroke—is straightforward if there is a clear history of focal brain dysfunction which started suddenly, or was first noticed on waking, particularly if the patient has not had a previous stroke, is over the age of 50, and has vascular risk factors or disorders (see Table 27.6). There may be some progression over the first few minutes or hours, but usually the deficit stabilizes by 12–24 hours and, if the patient survives, recovery starts within a few days in most cases. The severity ranges from a trivial deficit which is gone in a day, through a persistent deficit with or without disability, to death within hours of onset. Of course, if as is increasingly the case, patients are seen within a few hours of onset, one cannot be absolutely certain whether the patient is destined to have a TIA rather than a stroke.

Table 27.24. Differential diagnosis of acute stroke

Intracranial tumour: glioma, meningioma, etc.
Chronic subdural haematoma
Epileptic seizure
Metabolic/toxic encephalopathy: hypoglycaemia, hepatic failure, alcohol intoxication
Cerebral abscess/encephalitis
Hypertensive encephalopathy
Multiple sclerosis
Head injury
Peripheral nerve lesion
Psychogenic: somatization, hysteria
Creutzfeldt–Jakob disease

If the history is clear-cut, the chance of a CT or MR brain scan showing anything other than an infarct or haemorrhage (or being normal if done early in the case of infarction, or the lesion is very small) is under 5 per cent (Sandercock *et al.* 1985). If there is doubt about the speed of onset of a focal deficit, then the diagnosis is rather more likely to be an intracranial mass lesion, such as a tumour or chronic subdural haematoma (Table 27.24). If the onset was clearly sudden, but there was no obvious focal deficit, then brain imaging may show a thalamic or cerebellar infarct or haemorrhage (Section 27.6.2). Clinical clues to an intracranial tumour are recent headaches, seizures, papilloedema, a worsening deficit over days or weeks, and any suggestion of a primary tumour outwith the brain. Clues to a chronic subdural haematoma are head injury in the previous few weeks; more drowsiness, confusion and headache than anticipated from the severity of the neurological deficit; a fluctuating course; and a patient on anticoagulants. Other diagnoses are usually but not necessarily obvious: multiple sclerosis (young age); peripheral nerve or root lesion (clinical signs); post-seizure hemiparesis (history); metabolic encephalopathy (global rather than focal neurological features); somatization and hysteria (young age, signs); encephalitis (fever, clinical symptoms and signs, diffusely abnormal EEG); and intracranial abscess (fever and predisposing cause such as sinusitis, congenital heart lesion, etc.) (Norris and Hachinski 1982). Occasionally head injury causing intracerebral haemorrhage can be missed if the patient is amnesic for the injury itself and has an unmarked scalp; while ischaemic stroke shortly after an obvious head injury may be due to neck artery dissection (Section 27.4.4). Haemorrhagic strokes causing a fall and so head injury can be equally confusing if the CT scan shows 'primary intracerebral haemorrhage' or 'subarachnoid haemorrhage' and the circumstances at the onset are unclear (Berlit *et al.* 1991). If there are persisting signs from a previous stroke, and the patient then falls ill for some other reason such as an infection, or has an epileptic seizure, the old signs may appear to worsen and so mimic stroke recurrence.

27.6.2 Determining the site of the lesion

Having diagnosed 'a stroke', the next step is to decide where in the brain the lesion is. This depends on classical clinico-anatomical correlation, which need not be taken to eponymous extremes, particularly if speed is important (Caplan and Stein 1986; Bogousslavsky 1991). Of course, it is not strictly necessary to localize the lesion at all unless doing so provides useful prognostic information for survival, residual disability, and recurrence; clues to the cause of the stroke and, therefore, some help to select investigations and treatments; and guidance in rehabilitation (Bamford 1992).

A useful, robust, and very simple system, which does not require great neurological skill, divides stroke patients first into four main clinical syndromes: total anterior circulation syndrome (TACS), partial anterior circulation syndrome (PACS), lacunar syndrome (LACS), and posterior circulation syndrome (POCS). Occasionally one has to put the patient in an uncertain category. This division depends entirely and only on the symptoms and signs, which are accessible to everyone, irrespective of the availability or standard of any technology. Next, on the basis of brain CT or perhaps MRI (Section 27.6.3), patients with primary intracerebral haemorrhage are separated off. The rest, where the scan is either normal or shows infarction in a relevant area, can then be divided into: total anterior circulation infarct, about 15 per cent of the total in community-based studies (TACI); partial anterior circulation infarct, 35 per cent (PACI); lacunar infarct, 25 per cent (LACI); and posterior circulation infarct, 25 per cent (POCI) (Bamford et al. 1991; Mead et al. 2000a). These categories provide some prognostic information for survival (Section 27.8.2), residual disability (Section 27.9.1), and recurrence (Section 27.10.2), and an indication of the cause of the stroke (Olsen et al. 1985; Anderson et al. 1994a; Martin and Bogousslavsky 1995).

Of course, like any other system which is simple, practical, and quick, it will not predict the site of the lesion in every case, particularly if there are residual signs from a previous stroke or the patient is not examined when the deficit is maximal (either because the patient is seen very early before the full syndrome has evolved, or rather late after some of the signs have disappeared). Occasionally the CT scan (or MRI) shows a recent infarct in a place which does not 'fit' with the clinical syndrome: if the infarct looks the correct age and is likely to be relevant to the symptoms and signs, then the patient's syndrome should be reclassified on the basis of the scan (Mead et al. 1999).

Total anterior circulation syndrome (TACS)

A large haematoma in one cerebral hemisphere, or an infarct large enough to affect the cortex, basal ganglia, and internal capsule, causes a characteristic clinical syndrome of contralateral hemiparesis, with or without a sensory deficit, involving the whole of at least two of the three body areas (face, upper limb, lower limb), a homonymous visual field defect, and new higher cerebral—or 'cortical'—dysfunction (dysphasia, neglect, visuospatial problems, etc., depending on cerebral dominance). Often the patients are so drowsy that any cognitive or visual field defects have to be assumed. Deviation of the eyes towards the affected hemisphere is common but recovers in a few days (Kelley and Kovacs 1986). A large haematoma may cause midline shift, transtentorial herniation, and coma within 24 hours, whereas these changes take 2 or 3 days to evolve with large infarcts as cerebral oedema develops (see Fig. 27.14).

Total anterior circulation infarcts (TACIs) are usually due to acute occlusion of the internal carotid artery (normally atherothrombotic), or embolic occlusion of the proximal middle cerebral artery from a cardiac or proximal arterial source (Caplan 1993; Lindgren et al. 1994; Wardlaw et al. 1996). Sometimes the cortex is relatively spared (due to good pial collaterals or rapid recanalization of the occluded artery) and infarction is largely subcortical in the distribution of several lenticulostriate arteries; this causes a characteristic area of 'striatocapsular infarction' on CT (see Fig. 27.15). This clinical syndrome is not so severe as a TACI, with less cognitive deficit and often without an homonymous hemianopia (Nicolai et al. 1996).

Partial anterior circulation syndrome (PACS)

A lobar haemorrhage, or a cortical infarct, causes a more restricted clinical syndrome consisting of only two of the three components of the total anterior circulation syndrome; or just isolated higher cortical dysfunction such as dysphasia; or a predominantly proprioceptive deficit in one limb; or a motor/sensory deficit restricted to one body area or part of one body area (out of the face, upper limb, and lower limb) (Boiten and Lodder 1991; Bassetti et al. 1993). If the 'cortical' signs are rather subtle (dressing apraxia, neglect, dysphasia mistaken for dysarthria, etc.), the patient may be misclassified as 'lacunar'.

Partial anterior circulation—or cortical—infarcts (PACIs) are caused by occlusion of a branch of the middle cerebral artery, or rarely the trunk of the anterior cerebral artery, usually as a consequence of embolism from the heart or proximal atherothrombosis, in the same ways as TACIs (see Fig. 27.15). Anterior cerebral artery infarcts cause contralateral weakness, predominantly of the lower limb, perhaps with some cortical sensory loss, and aphasia if in the dominant hemisphere. Left, and rarely right, anterior cerebral infarcts can cause a curious dyspraxia of the left upper limb due to infarction of the corpus callosum disconnecting the right motor centres from the left language centres (McNabb et al. 1988; Kazui et al. 1992). Bilateral leg and even additional bilateral arm weakness has been described when both anterior cerebral arteries are supplied from one stenosed ICA, or both ACAs are occluded by embolism, so mimicking a brainstem or spinal cord syndrome (Ho et al. 1986; Borggreve et al. 1994).

Some anterior circulation syndromes, usually classified as PACS, are caused by boundary zone infarcts (see below). Anterior choroidal artery distribution infarcts, which can be defined only by their CT/MR pattern, are rare, probably due to small vessel disease as well as embolism, and can cause a PACS or lacunar syndrome (Hupperts et al. 1994).

Lacunar syndrome (LACS)

Lacunar syndromes are defined clinically and are highly predictive of small, deep lesions affecting the motor and/or sensory pathways, i.e. in the corona radiata, internal capsule, thalamus, cerebral peduncle, and pons (Bamford and Warlow 1988; Boiten and Lodder 1991; Lodder *et al.* 1994). Although a few patients have a PICH (Bamford *et al.* 1987; Anzalone and Landi 1989), the great majority have small infarcts which are sometimes visible on CT, more often on MRI (Donnan *et al.* 1982; Samuelsson *et al.* 1994). These are caused by presumed occlusion of a small perforating artery affected by degenerative intracranial small vessel disease (Section 27.4.3) (see Fig. 27.15). There is no visual field defect, no new cortical defect (such as dysphasia, visuospatial disturbance, nor predominantly proprioceptive sensory loss), no impairment of consciousness, and nothing to suggest a brainstem syndrome (such as diplopia, crossed motor and sensory deficit, etc.).

The four main lacunar syndromes are most reliably defined if there has been no previous stroke and if the patients are examined at the time of their maximal deficit:

1. *Pure motor stroke* (about 50 per cent of lacunar cases) is a unilateral motor deficit involving two or three areas (face, upper limb, lower limb), including the whole of each area which is affected. There are often sensory symptoms but no sensory signs. The lesion is where the motor pathways are closely packed together, separate from other pathways: usually in the internal capsule or pons, sometimes the corona radiata or cerebral peduncle, rarely the medullary pyramid (Chamorro *et al.* 1991; Norrving and Staaf 1991). There may be a flurry of immediately preceding TIAs, the so-called capsular warning syndrome (Donnan *et al.* 1996).

2. *Pure sensory stroke* (about 5 per cent of cases) has the same distribution as pure motor stroke but the symptoms are of sensory loss, with or without sensory signs affecting all modalities equally, or sparing proprioception. The lesion is usually in the thalamus but can be in the brainstem (Fisher 1982).

3. *Sensorimotor stroke* (about 35 per cent of cases) is the combination of a pure motor stroke with sensory signs in the affected body parts. The lesion is usually in the thalamus or internal capsule, but can be in the corona radiata or pons (Huang *et al.* 1987; Landi *et al.* 1991). Compared with other lacunar syndromes, sensorimotor stroke is more often due to larger cortical and subcortical infarcts (Blecic *et al.* 1993).

4. *Ataxic hemiparesis* (about 10 per cent of cases) is the combination of corticospinal and ipsilateral cerebellar-like dysfunction affecting the arm and/or leg, and includes the syndrome in which there is little more than dysarthria and one clumsy hand. The lesion is usually in the pons, internal capsule or cerebral peduncle (Glass *et al.* 1990; Moulin *et al.* 1995). Dysarthria, with or without upper motor neuron facial weakness, may also be a lacunar syndrome with similar lesion localization as ataxic hemiparesis, but there are other localizing possibilities as well (Kim 1994; Gorman *et al.* 1998).

Centrum semiovale infarcts are small, deep infarcts in the subcortical white matter of the corona radiata. They may be due to small vessel disease affecting the medullary perforating arteries extending down from cortical branches of the middle cerebral artery (MCA), or embolism. In view of this anatomy, it is not surprising that the patients present as either a lacunar syndrome, or occasionally as a partial anterior circulation syndrome with 'cortical' features (Read *et al.* 1998; Lammie and Wardlaw 1999). They are not, however, easy to classify and to distinguish from border zone infarcts deeper in the white matter, between the arterial territories of the deep perforators from the first part of the MCA and the superficial medullary perforators.

Various other lacunar syndromes have been described with rather poor clinico-pathological–anatomical correlation; for example, chorea or hemiballismus usually appears to be due to a small lesion in the contralateral subthalamic nucleus or elsewhere in the basal ganglia, and tends to get better (Orgogozo and Bogousslavsky 1989).

Posterior circulation syndrome (POCS)

Brainstem, cerebellar, thalamic, or occipital lobe signs normally indicate infarction in the distribution of the vertebrobasilar (i.e. posterior) circulation (Castaigne *et al.* 1973; Caplan and Tettenborn 1992*b*; Amarenco and Caplan 1993; Bogousslavsky *et al.* 1993), or a localized haemorrhage (Caplan 1992). A combination of brainstem and occipital lobe signs is highly suggestive of infarction due to thromboembolism within the basilar and posterior cerebral artery (PCA) territories. Just occasionally, proximal PCA occlusion causes enough temporal, thalamic, and perhaps midbrain infarction to cause some contralateral hemiparesis and sensory loss, a marked cognitive deficit such as aphasia, as well as the expected homonymous hemianopia, and so be confused with occlusion of the middle cerebral artery or one of its branches (Argentino *et al.* 1996); this is the so-called 'walking total anterior circulation syndrome (TACS)' because although it fulfils the definition of a TACS, the motor loss is mild.

The causes of infarction in the vertebrobasilar territory are rather heterogeneous and, in individual patients, difficult to sort out, particularly because vertebral angiography is seldom carried out, non-invasive arterial imaging is difficult, and case fatality is relatively low. Some lacunar syndromes are due to small brainstem or thalamic infarcts as a consequence of small vessel occlusion (perhaps intracranial small vessel disease, or perhaps atheroma at the mouth of small perforating arteries). However, both small and large infarcts can be due to embolism from the heart and from atherothrombosis affecting the vertebral and basilar arteries; thrombotic occlusion complicating atheroma of the basilar artery or its major branches; or low flow distal to vertebral and other arterial occlusions.

Although a large number of posterior circulation syndromes have been described, it is difficult to associate any one of them reliably with a unique pattern of arterial occlusion, or with a particular cause, and they do not have much relevance in terms of prognosis. Like any other strokes, these vertebrobasilar syndromes can be mild or severe, and due to infarction or haemorrhage. Therefore, the recognition of the 'top of the basilar' syndrome (Caplan 1980), various other midbrain syndromes (Bogousslavsky *et al.* 1994), the locked-in syndrome (Patterson and Grabois 1986), pontine syndromes (Bassetti *et al.* 1996), and lateral and medial medullary syndromes (Bassetti *et al.* 1997; Kim *et al.* 1998) is more an exercise in clinico-anatomical correlation than being very useful for clinical management. Because thalamic and cerebellar strokes can cause diagnostic confusion, and the latter may require surgical treatment, they are given separate consideration below.

Thalamic stroke

Infarction or haemorrhage in the thalamus is not common and, if the lesion is small, may cause merely a pure sensory stroke or sensorimotor stroke, perhaps with some ataxia in the same limbs. However, some thalamic lesions cause various other deficits in isolation, or in combination: paralysis of upward gaze, small pupils, depressed consciousness, hypersomnolence, disorientation, visual hallucinations, aphasia and impairment of verbal memory (dominant side), visuospatial dysfunction (non-dominant side), and hallucinations (Castaigne *et al.* 1981; Graff-Radford *et al.* 1985; Bogousslavsky and Caplan 1993; Chung *et al.* 1996). Occlusion of a single small branch of the proximal PCA can cause bilateral paramedian thalamic infarction with severe retrograde and anterograde amnesia (Graff-Radford *et al.* 1990). Therefore, thalamic stroke should be considered when there is a sudden onset of one or more of the above deficits. The diagnosis is often missed if there is only somnolence, confusion, or amnesia, but the sudden onset provides the clue.

Cerebellar strokes

Cerebellar strokes are uncommon. They can be mild with sudden vertigo, nausea, imbalance, and horizontal nystagmus which soon recovers, frequently misdiagnosed as 'labyrinthitis' (Huang and Yu 1985). More extensive infarction, or haemorrhage, causes additional ipsilateral limb and truncal ataxia, as well as dysarthria. Even more severe strokes cause occipital headache, vomiting, and depressed consciousness, so making it impossible to detect limb or truncal ataxia (Heros 1982; Dunne *et al.* 1987; Amarenco 1991). There are then additional brainstem signs (such as ipsilateral facial weakness and sensory loss, a gaze palsy to the side of the lesion, ipsilateral deafness and tinnitus, and bilateral extensor plantar responses) because of pressure from a large oedematous infarct or haematoma, or because an occluded artery supplying the cerebellum so often supplies parts of the brainstem as well. Mass effect can obstruct CSF flow from the fourth ventricle to cause acute or subacute hydrocephalus with subsequent coma and meningism which is very easily confused with subarachnoid haemorrhage, particularly if there is no obvious weakness or sensory loss in the limbs, which is usually the case. CT scan will reveal a haematoma but the signs of an infarct are more subtle, with disappearance or shift of the fourth ventricle due to mass effect before the low density of the lesion itself appears. MRI is more sensitive and provides detail of any additional brainstem involvement.

Patients who become acutely or subacutely comatose have a very poor prognosis. However, if there is little evidence of primary brainstem infarction, then drainage of any hydrocephalus and/or decompression of the posterior fossa may sometimes be followed by relatively good-quality survival (van der Hoop *et al.* 1988; Hornig *et al.* 1994; Mathew *et al.* 1995).

Boundary zone (inappropriately named watershed) infarcts

These are infarcts in the border zones between arterial territories, i.e. between the superficial territories of the middle cerebral artery (MCA) and anterior cerebral artery (ACA) in the fronto-parasagittal region (anterior boundary zone); the superficial territories of the MCA and posterior cerebral artery (PCA) in the parieto-occipital region (posterior boundary zone); and the superficial medullary penetrators and deep lenticulostriate territories of the MCA in the paraventricular white matter of the corona radiata (subcortical boundary zone). They probably account for only a small percentage of strokes.

There are two main situations of hypotension—or low flow—which may cause boundary zone infarcts (Bladin and Chambers 1994). First, systemic hypotension which is sudden and profound, as during cardiac arrest, may cause bilateral infarcts usually in the posterior boundary zones, presumably where blood flow is at its most precarious. Clinical features include cortical blindness, visual disorientation and agnosia, and amnesia. Secondly, internal carotid occlusion, or extreme stenosis, may predispose to unilateral boundary zone infarction when there is a relatively small drop in systemic blood pressure, or perhaps just because collateral blood flow is so poor and perfusion reserve is exhausted (Weiller *et al.* 1991). Anterior boundary zone and subcortical boundary zone infarcts are the most common, and cause contralateral weakness of the leg more than the arm with sparing of the face, some impaired sensation in the same areas, and aphasia if in the dominant hemisphere. Unilateral posterior boundary zone infarcts are less common and cause contralateral hemianopia and cortical sensory loss, along with aphasia if in the dominant hemisphere. Curiously, these 'low-flow' infarcts sometimes seem to develop and progress gradually over days or weeks (Bogousslavsky and Regli 1986; Bladin and Chambers 1993). Occasionally, microemboli obstructing the circulation (platelets, cholesterol, tumour), rather than low flow, cause infarction in boundary zones (Torvik 1984).

The diagnosis is difficult to be sure about in an individual case. While it is not too difficult to know where the lesion is, from the clinical picture and brain imaging, and about the state of the cerebral circulation, from arterial imaging, it is far more difficult to be sure of just why a stroke has occurred. The site of the infarct is not a reliable guide to a particular boundary zone because of the variability of the territorial supply of the cerebral arteries (Section 27.3.1). Therefore, to diagnose 'low flow' rather than embolic occlusion one has to depend more on the situational evidence, i.e. when a drop in systemic blood pressure at or just before stroke onset has been likely (Section 27.5.1), or clamping the internal carotid artery during endarterectomy. Internal carotid artery occlusion or severe stenosis is a clue in unilateral cases but, even so, there are many cases of doubt and embolic infarction is still possible, even within a so-called border zone area (Hupperts *et al.* 1997).

Miscellaneous clinical features

Lower cranial nerves: unilateral supratentorial stroke lesions can cause contralateral weakness of the bulbar muscles (e.g. unilateral weakness of the palate and tongue) and forehead muscles, and therefore what looks very much more like a lower motor neuron than an upper motor neuron facial palsy (Willoughby and Anderson 1984). Because all these muscles have a strong bilateral upper motor neuron innervation, this weakness tends to disappear quite quickly in most cases. The bulbar muscle weakness may be enough to cause significant, albeit temporary, dysphagia, which is therefore not only a feature of brainstem strokes (Gordon *et al.* 1987). Dysarthria is common in supratentorial strokes, but usually in proportion to any facial weakness (Ropper 1987). It is also a defining feature of the clumsy hand–dysarthria syndrome, but it can be isolated with no particular localizing value at all (Ichikawa and Kageyama 1991). Any weakness of the sternomastoid muscle is ipsilateral to a supratentorial lesion, so there is difficulty turning the head away from the side of the lesion (Mastaglia *et al.* 1986). Lower cranial nerve lesions ipsilateral to a supratentorial infarct suggest dissection of the internal carotid artery (ICA) (Section 27.4.4). Third, fourth, and sixth cranial nerve lesions have rarely been described ipsilateral to ICA occlusion, presumably due to ischaemia of the nerve trunks (Kapoor *et al.* 1991).

Headache is not uncommon around the time of stroke onset, more often and severe in primary intracerebral haemorrhage than ischaemic stroke, and more often with posterior than anterior circulation strokes. If the headache is localized at all, it tends to be over the site of the lesion. Headache is more common in cortical and posterior circulation than lacunar infarcts (Kumral *et al.* 1995). Severe unilateral neck, orbital, or scalp pain suggests internal carotid artery dissection, particularly if there is an ipsilateral Horner's syndrome. Occipital headache can occur with vertebral artery dissection. Headache is also a particular feature of venous infarcts (Section 27.11.1). Unusual headache in the days before stroke would suggest giant-cell arteritis, or perhaps a mass lesion rather than a stroke.

Movement disorders: acute hemiparkinsonism contralateral to a basal ganglia stroke must be very rare but has been described. Rather more common is contralateral chorea, hemiballismus, and sometimes tremor or dystonia (D'Olhaberriague *et al.* 1995; Scott and Jankovic 1996; Giroud *et al.* 1997). In fact, dystonia more often develops gradually in a hemiplegic limb some weeks after the stroke, particularly in children and young adults. Rather nondescript 'limb-shaking' has been described in 'low flow' TIA patients and can occur in stroke (Section 27.5.1).

Vascular examination is as, or more, important than the neurological examination, i.e. arterial bruits, pulses, heart sounds, etc. (Section 27.5.1).

27.6.3 **Investigation**

The next step, after diagnosing a stroke versus not stroke and using classical clinical rules to predict the site of the lesion, is to determine whether the brain lesion is a primary intracerebral haemorrhage (PICH) or cerebral infarction by CT scanning, or increasingly by MRI (Wardlaw 1994). If the distinction is of no management consequence (perhaps because the patient is very elderly and disabled already), then only routine baseline investigations are required, identical to those after TIAs (see Table 27.22), except that with PICH it is worthwhile doing a coagulation screen if there is no immediately obvious cause.

Intracerebral haemorrhage versus ischaemic stroke

Haemorrhage or infarction in the same part of the brain causes the same clinical deficit. Although primary intracerebral haemorrhage (PICH) tends to be more severe (so that diminished consciousness within hours of onset, bad headache, and meningism are suggestive features), some PICHs can be very mild with recovery in a few days (Scott and Miller 1985). Small haematomas confined to the brain do not cause major neurological deficits and nor does blood enter the CSF. Therefore, it is not surprising that mathematical models based on clinical features alone do not discriminate reliably between PICH and ischaemic stroke (Hawkins *et al.* 1995), nor that lack of blood and altered haemoglobin in the CSF rule out haemorrhage (Allen 1983).

When it is essential to exclude PICH (Table 27.25), there is no alternative to a CT scan, preferably within hours of stroke onset before any haematoma has vanished (Fig. 27.29), or haemorrhagic transformation of an infarct has occurred which can look very similar to a PICH (Fig. 27.30). Care must be taken to avoid confusing PICH with haemorrhagic venous infarction (Section 27.11.2). A normal scan after a few days does not exclude a haemorrhage, which may have resolved by then, and nor does an area of hypodensity, unless it is very wedge-shaped in the cortex in the typical distribution for a major cerebral artery occlusion. Late MRI may reveal old haemorrhage but it is unclear how sensitive this is, and how easy it is

Table 27.25. Non-negotiable indications for brain CT scan in acute stroke

Uncertain diagnosis of stroke versus not stroke
Atypical progression after onset (tumour/subdural haematoma/ haemorrhagic transformation of infarct)
Exclusion of intracerebral haemorrhage: patients taking or requiring anticoagulants/thrombolysis patients taking or requiring antiplatelet drugs patients likely to be suitable for carotid endarterectomy
Cerebellar stroke
Thalamic stroke
Subarachnoid haemorrhage
Young patient (<50 years)

In practice most stroke patients should have a CT scan within hours of onset.

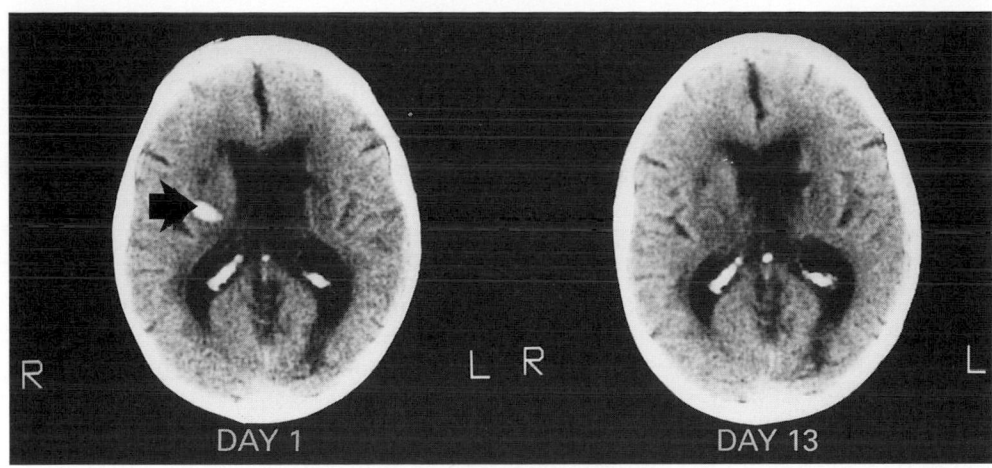

Fig. 27.29. Unenhanced CT brain scan to show rapid disappearance of an intracerebral haemorrhage (arrow) from the region of the right basal ganglia.

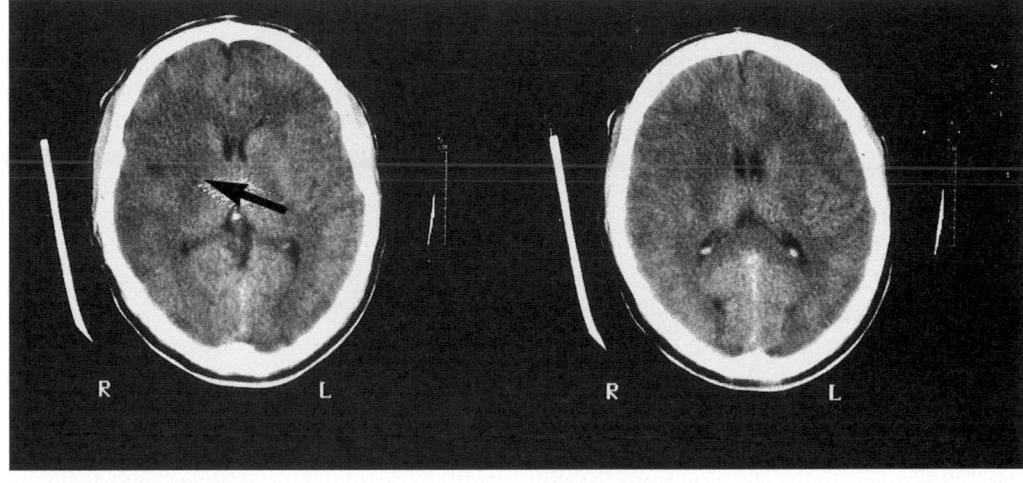

(a)

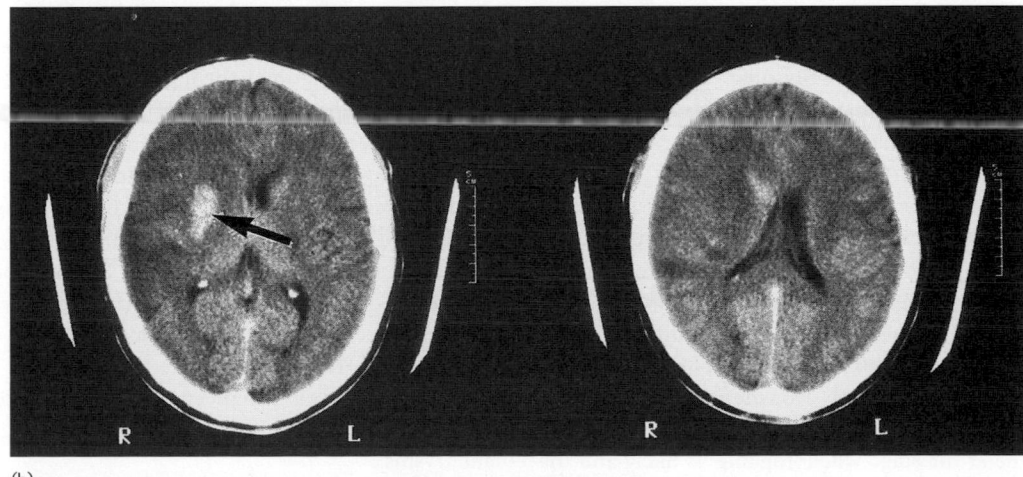

(b)

Fig. 27.30. (a) Unenhanced CT brain scan within 24 hours of an ischaemic stroke with a large middle cerebral artery infarct (arrow). (b) The next day the scan shows haemorrhagic transformation (arrow) which would be very difficult to distinguish from primary intracerebral haemorrhage without knowledge of the first scan.

to differentiate PICH from haemorrhagic transformation of an infarct or a haemorrhagic venous infarct, and so how much MRI can be relied on before starting anticoagulants or even perhaps an antiplatelet drug.

Further investigation does depend somewhat on knowing whether one is attempting to find the cause of an infarct, or the cause of a haemorrhage (see Tables 27.9, 27.16, 27.23).

Imaging the brain

Ischaemic stroke: the CT scan is normal immediately after onset, and if the lesion is small (less than about 0.5 cm in diameter), or in the posterior fossa, the scan may remain normal. With larger infarcts, a diffuse low-density area begins to appear, due to increasing brain water content, within a few hours. This may be accompanied by subtle effacement of sulci and loss of the normal grey–white matter differentiation, loss of the insular ribbon, loss of outline of the lentiform nucleus, and compression of the adjacent ventricle (Horowitz *et al.* 1991; Moulin *et al.* 1996). When the lesion is large, more obvious infarct swelling, brain shift, and herniation may be seen a few days after onset. Also CT can show haemorrhagic transformation, either asymptomatic or symptomatic, and although this tends to occur a few days after stroke onset in large infarcts, it can happen within hours and the haemorrhagic area can look very like a primary haemorrhage (Bogousslavsky *et al.* 1991) (Section 27.8.3, Fig. 27.3.0). Sometimes an acute thrombus or embolus in the middle cerebral artery, or other large intracranial artery, may be visible for a few days as a high-density streak on an unenhanced scan; this can be confused with vascular calcification but then a later scan will show persistence of the hyperdensity. An infarct may become isodense in the second and third weeks (the 'fogging' effect) before reappearing as a well-demarcated low-density area (Skriver and Olsen 1981). Later there may be ipsilateral ventricular dilatation due to loss of brain substance. To some extent, the site of any low density can be related to an arterial distribution, but bearing in mind the variability between and within individuals (Section 27.3.1). A small proportion of first-ever-stroke patients have focal hypodensities on CT in areas irrelevant to the present symptoms, presumably representing previous asymptomatic or undetected infarcts. Others have such widespread diffuse periventicular hypodensity that any new infarcts are difficult, if not impossible, to delineate (Chodosh *et al.* 1988).

Various patterns of contrast enhancement appear a few days to about 4 weeks after onset, particularly during the 'fogging' effect stage, due to hyperaemia and/or disruption of the blood–brain barrier (Skriver and Olsen 1982; Hornig *et al.* 1985). Sometimes this enhancement can cause confusion with a cerebral tumour, but the history is different, and in cases of doubt time will reveal the truth (Masdeu 1983). There is seldom any indication for intravenous contrast, except possibly if the scan is done at the stage when 'fogging' is likely and the unenhanced scan is therefore normal.

MRI is more sensitive but less specific than CT, so that although many more 'lesions' are shown, it is sometimes difficult to decide which one is relevant to the current symp-

toms (Edelman and Warach 1993). It shows acute infarcts best as high-intensity signal on T2-weighted images which persists; this is particularly helpful when the infarcts are small, or in the posterior fossa, and for clinico-anatomical research. T1-weighted images may be normal or show a low signal which tends to persist. Like for CT, there may be fogging in the second week or so. MRI displays swelling of oedematous infarcts. It can also show loss of normal flow voids in occluded cerebral arteries and may sometimes definitively display arterial dissection. However, MRI is less available than CT and patients have to lie still for longer, which for acute stroke makes CT the preferred immediate imaging technique, particularly since it displays intracerebral haemorrhage more reliably (Patel *et al.* 1996). Also, MRI is not necessarily superior to CT in detecting the very earliest signs of cerebral infarction (Mohr *et al.* 1995).

Diffusion-weighted MR imaging (DWI) is being increasingly improved and used. This does show lesions earlier than conventional MRI and, usefully, it also displays the new lesion(s) amongst old areas of infarction, by virtue of the reduced diffusion of water within acute infarcts (Warach *et al.* 1995; van Everdingen *et al.* 1998).

Positron emission tomography (PET) and single-photon emission tomography (SPET) are interesting research tools but, as yet, of no great clinical relevance in acute stroke.

Primary intracerebral haemorrhage (PICH) appears at once on CT as a well-demarcated high-density round or oval area, with or without rupture into the ventricles or on to the surface of the brain. Lesions as small as 0.5 cm in diameter can be picked up. Mixed-density haemorrhages, suggesting blood of different ages, is rather characteristic of amyloid angiopathy, and a blood-fluid level suggests a haemostatic defect of some sort (Pfleger *et al.* 1994). Within a day or so, a low-density halo appears, which may be due to oedema, ischaemic necrosis, or clot retraction. With large haemorrhages, CT may show brain shift, herniation, and hydrocephalus if the CSF pathways are obstructed. As the blood is absorbed and haemoglobin broken down, the area of high intensity shrinks and becomes less dense, then isodense with surrounding brain, and finally—in some patients—hypodense, appearing quite like an old infarct. With small haematomas the high density may be gone in a few days, so to exclude PICH the CT must be done quickly after stroke onset, preferably within hours, if not a day or two (see Fig. 27.29) (Dennis *et al.* 1987). Another reason for speed is because haemorrhagic infarcts can be indistinguishable from PICH, and such transformation can occur within a day of ischaemic stroke onset (see above). Further confusion can be caused by haemorrhagic venous infarction (Section 27.11.2). Resolving haematomas may enhance after intravenous contrast, sometimes with a very marked ring effect, looking like a tumour or abscess. Enhancement may also occur in vascular malformations and their associated enlarged vessels or aneurysms.

MR images go through a series of confusing changes after the onset of PICH as the haemoglobin changes to deoxyhaemoglobin (the T2-weighted image shows a low signal, particularly in the centre of the haematoma, the T1 image is low signal too); to methaemoglobin (the T1-weighted image signal becomes high but the T2 image remains much the same); to haemosiderin in the chronic stage (the T2-weighted image becomes bright in the centre with a very dark rim, the T1 images are similar but less marked). Within the first few hours, the image may be normal or may mimic cerebral infarction with a high signal on T2-weighted images. Exactly when all these changes occur depends not just on the haematoma itself but also on the strength of the magnetic field and the scanning sequence. MRI may also show flow voids in AVMs, haemorrhage into tumour, and dural sinus thrombosis.

The PICH site may give a clue to its cause: hypertensive haemorrhages tend to be in the basal ganglia, pons, and cerebellum, while lobar haemorrhages are rather more likely to be caused by an aneurysm, vascular malformation, haemostatic defect, venous infarction, or amyloid angiopathy. Multiple haemorrhages suggest certain specific causes (see Table 27.17).

Imaging the cerebral circulation in ischaemic stroke

A patient with a mild carotid-territory ischaemic stroke should have similar imaging to patients with carotid TIAs because endarterectomy may be indicated if there is severe carotid stenosis (Section 27.5.3). In more severe strokes, an early angiogram may have some medico-legal relevance if there is any suspicion of carotid or vertebral artery dissection after trauma, because it may reveal the dissection and no other cause such as atherothrombosis (see Fig. 27.17). But, demonstrating an occluded cerebral artery in an ischaemic stroke patient is usually of no more than academic interest, and a normal artery a few days after onset does not preclude the possibility of an occlusion which has recanalized.

Imaging the cerebral circulation in intracerebral haemorrhage

Cerebral angiography to reveal an intracranial vascular malformation (IVM) or aneurysm is only indicated if this might lead to treatment to remove or obliterate it. Therefore, it is seldom done unless the situation of the haematoma makes an aneurysm very likely. Otherwise, bearing in mind the uncertainties surrounding the treatment of IVMs (Section 27.7.4), angiography is reserved for young patients with relatively mild strokes, provided, of course, there is no other likely cause such as anticoagulation, thrombolysis, etc. Vascular malformations and aneurysms are most likely if the cerebral haemorrhage is lobar or intraventricular and there is no hypertension (Zhu et al. 1997). MRI can often be more sensitive than angiography in picking up vascular malformations (particularly cavernomas), and MRA is increasingly able to pick up aneurysms of a size likely to rebleed (Section 27.4.8).

Lumbar puncture

Normally after stroke there is no excess of white blood cells in the CSF, but sometimes there can be up to 100 per mm^3. More than this suggests septic emboli to the brain (Powers 1986). However, *routine* lumbar puncture has no place because it can be dangerous if there is a large intracerebral haematoma, or an oedematous infarct causing brain shift. Also, in anticoagulated patients lumbar puncture can be complicated by spinal haemorrhage. Primary intracerebral haemorrhage (PICH) and ischaemic stroke are much better distinguished by early CT; no red blood cells in the CSF certainly does not rule out PICH. Only if there is diagnostic doubt about stroke might lumbar puncture be useful, especially if the other possibilities include encephalitis or multiple sclerosis. If there is any possibility that ischaemic stroke has been caused by chronic meningitis (e.g. syphilis, tuberculosis) then CSF analysis is required.

Electroencephalography (EEG)

Infarcts, or haemorrhages, involving the cerebral cortex, are likely to cause ipsilateral slowing of the EEG, while lacunar strokes are rather less likely to perturb the surface record. However, this anatomical distinction is better made, and certainly more quickly made, clinically, even when brain imaging is normal (Section 27.6.2). If the diagnosis of stroke is unclear and encephalitis or a generalized encephalopathy is a possibility, then an EEG showing diffuse bilateral slowing would weigh against the diagnosis of stroke. Also, when there is confusion between stroke and epilepsy, either masquerading as stroke or making an old stroke seem worse, focal seizure activity on the EEG is obviously helpful. A routine EEG is certainly not indicated (Faught 1993).

27.7 The recognition and management of spontaneous subarachnoid haemorrhage

27.7.1 Clinical features

Subarachnoid haemorrhage (SAH) is commonly provoked by exertion and very rarely occurs during sleep (Ferro and Pinto 1994; Vermeer et al. 1997). Almost always there is sudden headache, usually severe and generalized, often described like an unexpected blow on the head, and not lasting less than an hour (Vermeulen et al. 1992; Warlow et al. 2000c; Schievink 1997). Loss of consciousness occurs in about half the patients but may only be brief. Nausea and vomiting are less common. Partial or generalized seizures occasionally occur at around the onset (Pinto et al. 1996). Early focal symptoms and signs suggest an associated intracerebral haematoma, or local pressure from an aneurysm (e.g. posterior communicating artery aneurysm causing a third nerve palsy), later they are more likely due to delayed cerebral ischaemia (Section 27.7.4). Meningism takes a few hours to develop and may not do so at all in deeply unconscious patients. In severe cases, however, the whole back becomes painful and stiff, and on occasion the pain radiates down the legs, mimicking sciatica. Preretinal and subhyaloid haemorrhages may occur, probably as a result of the acute rise in intracranial pressure being transmitted to the retinal veins (Keane 1979). There may be a mild fever and reactively raised

Table 27.26. World Federation of Neurological Surgeons' Scale for grading subarachnoid haemorrhage, 1988

Grade	Glasgow coma scale	Motor or language deficit
I	15	Absent
II	14–13	Absent
III	14–13	Present
IV	12–7	Present or absent
V	6–3	Present or absent

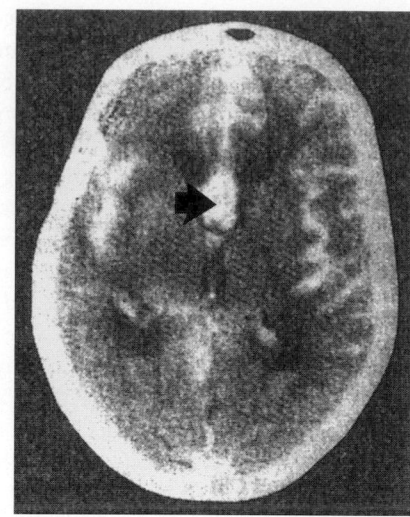

Fig. 27.31. Unenhanced CT brain scan showing blood (white areas) in the subarachnoid space and between the frontal horns of the lateral ventricles (arrow) where an anterior communicating artery aneurysm has ruptured.

blood pressure. Patients are often irritable and photophobic and the headache lasts for days, if not for some weeks. SAH is one cause, albeit an unusual one, of sudden or relatively sudden death, and about 15 per cent of SAH patients die before receiving any medical attention (Bonita and Thomson 1985). The patients' state is usefully graded using the World Federation of Neurological Surgeons' Scale (Table 27.26).

Some patients have experienced similar sudden headaches before, perhaps because of so-called 'warning leaks' from saccular aneurysms, or maybe simply because a previous diagnosable SAH had not been reported or was misdiagnosed as something else (Verweij *et al.* 1988). In the community, of patients presenting with sudden and severe headache lasting more than an hour, about a quarter turn out to have SAH, about an eighth have some other serious neurological disorder, and the rest are a mixture of acute neck pain, migraine, and other benign, if undiagnosable conditions (Linn *et al.* 1994).

27.7.2 **Diagnosis**

Quite often the history of onset is unclear and one cannot be sure that the headache had started all that suddenly, and the differential diagnosis is then quite wide (Table 27.27). But, with a

Table 27.27. Differential diagnosis of sudden unexpected headache

With neck rigidity
 Subarachnoid haemorrhage
 Acute painful neck conditions
 Meningitis/encephalitis
 Cerebellar stroke
 Intraventricular haemorrhage
 Recent head injury

Without neck rigidity
 Migraine
 Thunderclap headache
 Benign orgasmic cephalalgia
 Benign exertional headache
 Pituitary apoplexy
 Reaction while on monoamine oxidase inhibitors
 Phaeochromocytoma
 Expanding intracranial aneurysm
 Carotid or vertebral artery dissection
 Intracranial venous thrombosis
 Occipital neuralgia
 Acute obstructive hydrocephalus

good history of a sudden and unexpected headache, the most likely possibilities other than subarachnoid haemorrhage (SAH) are 'thunderclap headache', cerebellar or intraventricular haemorrhage, benign orgasmic or exertional cephalalgia, and migraine which uncharacteristically can sometimes start suddenly rather than gradually.

Any delay in the diagnosis of aneurysmal SAH can be overtaken by rebleeding, which is potentially disastrous and avoidable (Mayer *et al.* 1996; Neil-Dwyer and Lang 1997). Therefore, in patients with a suggestive clinical syndrome, an urgent unenhanced CT scan must be done which is the quickest, most informative, and cost-effective confirmatory investigation for blood in the subarachnoid space (Warlow *et al.* 2000c). On the first day it will show subarachnoid and/or intraventricular blood in over 90 per cent of cases, but less frequently thereafter (Fig. 27.31); by a week or so the blood is gone, perhaps sooner with very mild SAH (Brouwers *et al.* 1992). Importantly, in addition, CT provides a baseline for the diagnosis of later rebleeding; shows any associated intracerebral, ventricular, or subdural haematoma which may require removal; shows any complicating hydrocephalus which may need treatment; and provides the best clue to which aneurysm has bled if more than one is found on later angiography (Adams *et al.* 1983; Vermeulen and van Gijn 1990). The scan may also show calcification in the rim of an aneurysm or the characteristic pattern of benign perimesencephalic haemorrhage (Rinkel *et al.* 1991) (Fig. 27.32). CT may also show unsuspected evidence of traumatic head injury: brain contusions, soft-tissue swelling of the scalp, and skull fracture. The patient may either have fallen as a result of a spontaneous SAH, or any haemorrhage on the scan might be the result of a head injury (at which point the history must be reviewed to sort out which came first). Just occasionally, in almost brain dead patients, CT may seem to

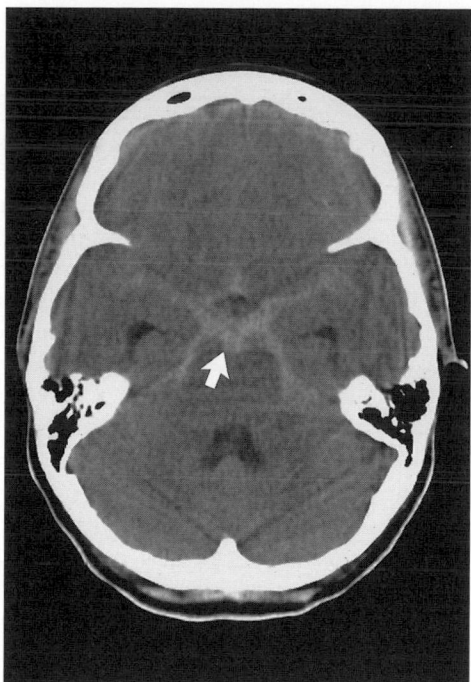

Fig. 27.32. Unenhanced CT brain scan to show perimesencephalic subarachnoid haemorrhage (white area predominantly anterior to the midbrain, arrow).

show SAH but this is probably blood in congested meningeal vessels (Opeskin and Silberstein 1998).

If CT is unavailable, or if it is available but no intracranial blood is visible, then a lumbar puncture must be done to confirm blood in the CSF and exclude bacterial meningitis (van der Wee *et al.* 1995). In fact, bacterial meningitis is unlikely if the headache onset really is sudden, but this may not necessarily be known if the patient is unconscious or confused. It is important to remember that blood, and xanthochromia, may well not appear in the lumbar CSF until about 12 hours after the onset (Vermeulen and van Gijn 1990). Therefore, if the history of sudden onset headache is definite, consciousness is normal, and there are no signs of infection (normal temperature, etc.), it is best to delay lumbar puncture for this period of time. Lumbar puncture can precipitate transtentorial herniation and cerebellar coning, particularly if there is an intracerebral or cerebellar haemorrhage, but this ought to be suspected from the presence of focal signs or coma (Duffy 1982).

As well as frank blood, the CSF must be inspected for xanthohromia, the result of breakdown of haemoglobin to pigments (oxyhaemoglobin, bilirubin) which have been released into the CSF some hours before (Vermeulen 1996; Beetham *et al.* 1998). These colour the supernatant of the spun-down CSF yellow. If the supernatant is clear to the naked eye, then spectrophotometry should probably be done as a more sensitive test for these pigments, but often it isn't. Failing to look for, and therefore missing, xanthochromia is a common cause for the incorrect assumption of a 'traumatic tap' when the CSF is bloody to the naked eye; this cannot be reliably confirmed by the well-worn method of observing clearing of blood across three consecutive tubes of CSF. A bloody CSF *without* xanthochromia (because the blood has entered the CSF at the time of the lumbar puncture) on spectrophotometry is the best indication of a traumatic tap. Red blood cells and xanthochromia clear from the CSF in about 2 weeks, or maybe less if the SAH is mild. In the acute stage the CSF glucose may be low, the protein slightly raised, and not uncommonly there is a slight excess of lymphocytes and polymorphs.

If the history is suggestive of SAH, but an early CT scan and CSF are both normal within days of onset, then SAH is most unlikely and the risk of a true SAH later is negligible (Wijdicks *et al.* 1988; Markus 1991). Therefore, cerebral angiography is not required under these circumstances. Similar headaches may recur (so-called thunderclap headaches) or they may become more obviously migrainous or tension-related. If, on the other hand, a patient presents more than about a week or two after a *typical* SAH story, then four-vessel (both carotid and vertebral arteries) catheter angiography is almost unavoidable, whatever the results of the CT scan and CSF. Despite a very small risk, it is still the definitive investigation to demonstrate saccular aneurysms (Fig. 27.33), arteriovenous malformations (Fig. 27.20) and the very occasional intracranial arterial dissection or mycotic aneurysm, although CT angiography and MR angiography are both improving rapidly and may become preferred. If an aneurysm is found, and angiography is not of all four vessels, then it is not impossible that an asymptomatic unruptured aneurysm has been demon-

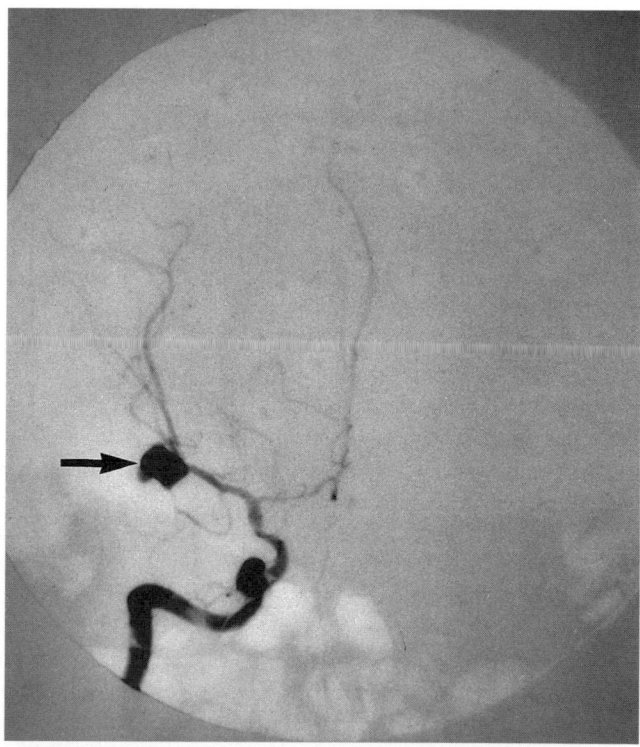

Fig. 27.33. Antero-posterior view of a right carotid angiogram to show a middle cerebral artery aneurysm (arrow).

strated, which would lead to treatment of the wrong lesion. Therefore, unless it is very obvious from CT where an aneurysm has bled, and there is no intention of treating any coincidental unruptured aneurysm, angiography should aim to display all the cerebral vessels and be timed shortly before surgery (or coiling) is contemplated (Section 27.7.4). An aneurysm may not be visualized if it is filled with thrombus, or if there is considerable vasospasm of the aneurysm-bearing artery, and so angiography may have to be repeated later (but not if CT has shown only perimesencephalic haemorrhage, see above).

Spinal subarachnoid haemorrhage is very rare. It is due to a vascular malformation, haemostatic failure, coarctation of the aorta, inflammatory vascular disease, mycotic aneurysm, or a vascular tumour (e.g. ependymoma). There is sudden back or neck pain, radiating often to the head and down the legs, and meningism develops, so making for confusion with intracranial SAH. Complicating haematoma may compress the cord. Suspicion is aroused if the cerebral angiogram is negative and the patient develops spinal cord signs.

27.7.3 Prognosis

In the population at large, about half the patients with aneurysmal SAH die in the first month, of whom half of them die on the first day as a result of the initial bleed. Admitted patients, particularly to neurosurgical centres, do better because those who die very early and often those in coma are not included (Hop *et al.* 1997). Coma on admission, old age, and a large amount of blood on the initial CT scan are all associated with a worse prognosis (Kassel *et al.* 1990*a,b*). But, even after correcting for these adverse prognostic factors, any comparison between the management results of centres, or within centres at different times, is still almost certainly confounded by case mix and chance, and is a fruitless exercise, despite exactly these sorts of comparisons cluttering up the literature.

Early deterioration, sometimes leading to death in the first week or so, may be caused by aneurysmal rebleeding, hydrocephalus, delayed cerebral ischaemia, hyponatraemia, hypoxia, hypotension, seizures, and cardiac failure (Broderick *et al.* 1994; Warlow *et al.* 1996*d*) (Sections 27.7.4 and 27.8.3). Therefore, in a deteriorating patient it is important not only to do an urgent CT scan (to reveal rebleeding, hydrocephalus, infarction) but also to check on the blood pressure, PaO_2, and electrolytes.

Focal neurological deficits and, more commonly, cognitive deficits, behavioural disorders, seizures, anxiety, depression, and poor quality of life are frequent long-term sequelae (Saveland *et al.* 1986; Desantis *et al.* 1989; Hop *et al.* 1998). About 15 per cent of SAH survivors are dependent and 50 per cent disabled to some extent (Hijdra *et al.* 1987*a*; Hop *et al.* 1997).

If no cause for SAH is found, early case fatality and risk of rebleeding are very low (less than 1 per cent per annum). This is probably because the diagnosis is sometimes wrong and the CSF obtained by traumatic tap, and because some patients have a perimesencephalic pattern of bleeding which has an exceptionally good prognosis (Rinkel *et al.* 1993).

27.7.4 The treatment of subarachnoid haemorrhage

The aims of management are to make the diagnosis of subarachnoid haemorrhage (SAH) (Section 27.7.2); identify the cause, usually with angiography; care for the patient and prevent the general complications of stroke (Section 27.8.6); prevent and treat the specific complications of SAH, such as hydrocephalus, delayed cerebral ischaemia, hyponatraemia, and haematoma (Vermeulen *et al.* 1984); and deal with the source of the bleeding as is soon as reasonably possible, to prevent recurrence (Vermeulen *et al.* 1992; Wijdicks 1995).

The patient should be nursed in a quiet, darkened room. Headache, nausea, vomiting, anxiety, irritability, seizures, urinary incontinence, and constipation all require symptomatic treatment on their own merits. As with other stroke types, the management of raised blood pressure is controversial and, on balance, it should probably not be treated, certainly not routinely (Section 27.8.4). Hypovolaemia should be avoided, and between 2 and 3 litres of fluid per day are routinely necessary, sometimes more. Although a variety of cardiac arrhythmias are very common in the first few days, they do not often seem to pose a problem and so seldom need suppressing (Andreoili *et al.* 1987; Brouwers *et al.* 1989). None the less, it is prudent to monitor the ECG. Neurogenic pulmonary oedema is fortunately rare, but can occur very early, sometimes confusing the diagnosis by being more prominent than the headache. It may be due to either increased pulmonary capillary permeability, or cardiogenic dysfunction, and clearly the patient needs intensive cardiovascular monitoring and treatment to normalize the haemodynamic variables (Parr *et al.* 1996). When the headache has resolved the patient can be mobilized (Warlow *et al.* 1996*d*).

Rebleeding

In aneurysmal cases, without clipping or coiling, about 10 per cent rebleed within hours and another 30 per cent within a few weeks, during which there is no particularly high-risk time; no known factors predict further rebleeding, which is more likely to be fatal than the first bleed (Hijdra *et al.* 1987*b*; Hijdra *et al.* 1988). Subsequently, the rebleeding rate is about 2–3 per cent per annum (Winn *et al.* 1977). Deterioration is usually sudden, with reduced conscious level and, like the original bleed, there are few, if any, focal neurological features. But if the patient is being ventilated, these signs will not be seen and the clue is sudden fixed dilatation of the pupils (Hijdra *et al.* 1987*b*). Rebleeding can only be diagnosed by repeat CT scan to show fresh haemorrhage, and even then it can be difficult to be sure. Repeat lumbar puncture is not helpful and sometimes dangerous (i.e. if deterioration is actually due to intracerebral haematoma).

The breakdown of the fibrin clot sealing an aneurysmal leak can be inhibited, and so the risk of rebleeding reduced before the aneurysm is clipped or coiled, by prophylactic antifibrinolytic drugs, such as ϵ-aminocaproic acid and tranexamic acid. Unfortunately these drugs exacerbate delayed cerebral ischaemia and so there is no overall effect on outcome (Roos *et al.* 1999).

Ruptured arteriovenous malformations have a lower case fatality than aneurysmal SAH and are less likely to rebleed, certainly in the early period after the initial haemorrhage and if they have not already bled (Crawford *et al.* 1986; Ondra *et al.* 1990; Mast *et al.* 1997). Exactly which features of the vascular anatomy, or other factors, are associated with particularly high risks of bleeding or epilepsy is not clear (Duong *et al.* 1998).

Definitive treatment for ruptured saccular aneurysms

Provided the patient is in a good clinical state and it is technically feasible, aneurysms are clipped as soon as possible and convenient. This reduces the risk of early rebleeding and makes it safer to increase the blood pressure in the management of delayed cerebral ischaemia. The risk of rebleeding long-term is very low, but not zero (Tsutsumi *et al.* 1998). In fact there is no good evidence that delaying surgery by a few weeks leads to a worse overall outcome, nor is there any randomized controlled trial evidence that any sort of surgery is better than conservative medical management, although few would doubt that it is (Ohman and Heiskanen 1989; Kassell *et al.* 1990*b*). Although the surgical risk declines with time after SAH onset, so does the risk of rebleeding, so the results of surgical series must be interpreted cautiously, and certainly in the light of the overall state of the patient on admission; the earlier the patient is admitted to a neurosurgical ward, the worse the likely clinical grade will be and, therefore, the worse the outcome with or without surgery.

If aneurysms are multiple, it can be difficult to decide which one has bled. The best clue is the main collection of subarachnoid blood, or any haematoma, on early CT. Less useful clues are the localization of any focal deficit, focal vasospasm on the angiogram, unilateral retro-orbital or head pain, an irregular aneurysm, and a large aneurysm on angiography (Nehls *et al.* 1985).

Endovascular treatment, usually with electrically released thrombogenic platinum coils detached from an intra-arterial catheter, to isolate the aneurysm from the circulation, is gaining in popularity, particularly for aneurysms where a surgical approach is too risky (Byrne *et al.* 1995; Nelson *et al.* 1997). Moreover, this technique is applicable very early after SAH onset and may turn out to be safer, and as durable, for aneurysms which are currently clipped. But until the current trials are reported this cannot be certain.

Definitive treatment for intracranial vascular malformations

For arteriovenous malformations (AVMs), other than 'do nothing', there are three options: endovascular treatment with various embolization techniques which obliterate the AVM more or less at once (Deveikis 1998); surgical removal, which again is quickly effective but may be impossible for big lesions in very eloquent brain areas; and stereotactic radiotherapy for small lesions which then take some months to disappear, but this may have long-term adverse consequences for the surrounding areas of normal brain (Flickinger *et al.* 1998). In any one individual, it is extraordinarily difficult to pick the best option because no randomized trials have ever been done; non-randomized case series have so often been of unrepresentative patients; furthermore, case series have commonly been retrospective with an inadequate period of follow-up; imaging advances have made it easier to detect AVMs over time, so that studies are constantly going out of date; the number of cases treated in any one centre is small; the lesions are very heterogeneous in their anatomy; and the natural history is not known clearly (Al-Shahi and Warlow 1999).

Treatment is not usually recommended at all if an AVM has not ruptured, since the bleeding rate is no more than 1 or 2 per cent per annum (Iansek *et al.* 1983; Aminoff 1987). Dural AVMs are usually dealt with by endovascular techniques (Freitag *et al.* 1992). Cavernomas are surgically an easier prospect than AVMs, but whether surgery has any effect on their natural history is unknown. One would like to think that if a cavernoma is the cause of intractable epilepsy that its removal would be helpful.

Complications of subarachnoid haemorrhage and their management

Hydrocephalus, due to blood obstructing CSF flow, occurs within days of onset in about 20 per cent of patients. It may be asymptomatic, but if there is no other reason for clinical worsening and the conscious level is deteriorating, and particularly if the ventricles are enlarging on repeat CT, then temporary external ventricular drainage may lead to dramatic improvement. Ventriculitis, and possibly rebleeding if the aneurysm has not been dealt with first, are complications (van Gijn *et al.* 1985*b*; Hasan *et al.* 1989; Heros 1989). Therefore, in patients who do not have blood obstructing the ventricles or any brain shift, repeated lumbar puncture may possibly be a safer alternative (Hasan *et al.* 1991). Months or years later, organized thrombus and fibrosis in the CSF pathways can lead to the syndrome of normal-pressure hydrocephalus (Section 17.3.8).

Delayed cerebral ischaemia appears 4–14 days after onset in about 25 per cent of cases and has a bad prognosis. Poor initial clinical state, large quantities of subarachnoid or intraventricular blood on CT, hyponatraemia, and the use of antifibrinolytic drugs are all risk factors (Wijdicks *et al.* 1985; Hijdra *et al.* 1986; Adams *et al.* 1987; Hasan *et al.* 1990). Cerebral ischaemia seems to be caused by vasospasm, often with structural changes in the vessel wall, of one or more cerebral arteries, not necessarily the one bearing the ruptured aneurysm. It is a much less frequent phenomenon in non-aneurysmal subarachnoid haemorrhage (Kassell *et al.* 1985). Clinical onset is usually gradual with deteriorating conscious level accompanied, or followed within hours, by evolving focal neurological signs in most cases. To make the diagnosis, there should be no other explanation for deterioration, and in particular a repeat CT should not show any rebleeding (Hijdra *et al.* 1986).

Plasma volume expansion and induced hypertension have been suggested as treatments but are not always effective (Awad *et al.* 1987). Fortunately, the risk of delayed cerebral ischaemia can be reduced and the overall outcome improved by prophylactic calcium blockers, specifically nimodipine, 60 mg 4-hourly, administered orally or by nasogastric tube, for 21 days (Feigin *et al.* 1998). If this causes hypotension, then the dose should be reduced. There is no good evidence to support *intravenous* nimodipine, which is particularly likely to cause unacceptable hypotension.

Hyponatraemia occurs in about one-third of patients in the first week or two after subarachnoid haemorrhage and is related to the severity of the initial presentation. It is not usually due to inappropriate ADH secretion and dilutional hyponatraemia but to 'salt wasting', i.e. excess loss of both salt and water by the kidneys with a decrease in plasma volume. Below a plasma sodium of about 125 mmol/l, correction is necessary, not usually by water restriction, but by plasma volume expansion (using dextrose–saline or plasma) while monitoring central venous or pulmonary wedge pressure (Wijdicks *et al.* 1985; Berendes *et al.* 1997).

Intracerebral haematoma may cause a focal deficit initially, or later, and may be worth removing if there is coma, clinical deterioration, and brain shift, particularly if the ruptured aneurysm or vascular malformation can be dealt with at the same time (Heiskanen *et al.* 1988).

27.7.5 Unruptured saccular aneurysms

Unruptured aneurysms, either discovered while investigating SAH or in some other way, should normally be clipped or coiled if they are symptomatic; for example, eye pain from a posterior communicating artery aneurysm (Raps *et al.* 1993). Unruptured asymptomatic aneurysms are more problematic because their risk of rupture is, on average, perhaps about 4 per cent per annum if over 10 mm in diameter, and rather less than 1 per cent per annum for smaller aneurysms (Rinkel *et al.* 1998). But the rates were much lower in the recent large international series (International Study of Unruptured Aneurysm Investigators 1998). These risks have to be set against the risk of clipping or coiling, about 8 per cent dead or dependent (Raaymakers *et al.* 1998). Also, account must be taken of how long the patient is likely to live with an untreated aneurysm, and how an individual patient feels about the competing risks. The problem of screening high risk of aneurysm populations (such as first-degree relatives of patients with ruptured aneurysms, families with multiple members affected by aneurysmal rupture, and polycystic kidney families), at what age, how often, and with what imaging technology, is even more fraught, and no firm conclusions are possible.

27.8 The treatment of acute stroke

27.8.1 General principles

There is now good evidence that organized care in stroke units is better than care in general medical wards; fewer deaths, fewer dependent survivors, and fewer patients remaining in an institution, all without lengthening hospital stay. The crucial ingredients appear to be not intensive care, but co-ordinated multidisciplinary rehabilitation, education, and training in stroke care, and specialization of staff, including nurses. Although intensive care is seldom needed, ideally patients should be admitted to a designated area of the hospital and their acute care seamlessly integrated with their rehabilitation (Stroke Unit Trialists' Collaboration 1997*a*, *b*). Admission to hospital is generally not necessary for TIA patients, and nor even for mild strokes, provided they can be cared for at home with very rapid back up from a hospital-based stroke service for diagnostic help, neuroradiology (which, apart from catheter angiography, can all be done in outpatient departments), and possibly even for domiciliary rehabilitation. Also elderly and previously dependent people with a severe stroke may be better off out of hospital, particularly if they are already in a nursing home. Clearly, hospital admission rates vary depending on local custom and practice, geography, patient expectations, and how well organized the primary care and hospital-based care are. However, admission rates are likely to be driven up by the increasing realization that not only should stroke patients be treated by experts in their disease, but that emerging new treatments—such as thrombolysis—must be given in hospital and very rapidly indeed to have any chance of success. This will require education of the public to recognize stroke, better organization of emergency services out of hospital, and very fast tracking of stroke patients once they get into hospital.

The general approach to early management is identical whether the stroke is due to cerebral infarction, primary intracerebral haemorrhage, or subarachnoid haemorrhage (van Gijn and Dennis 1998):

◆ Make the correct diagnosis of stroke versus not stroke as rapidly as possible (Section 27.6.1).

◆ Establish the cause of stroke in terms of pathological type (infarct or haemorrhage) (Section 27.6.3) and underlying cause, particularly if directly treatable (atherothromboembolism, cardiogenic embolism, vascular malformation, etc.).

◆ Estimate the prognosis for the individual patient as far as it is possible to do so (Sections 27.8.2 and 27.9.1).

◆ Initiate appropriate specific treatment for acute ischaemic stroke (Section 27.8.4), primary intracerebral haemorrhage (Section 27.8.5), or subarachnoid haemorrhage (Section 27.7.4).

◆ Unless the patient is very elderly, seriously handicapped, or expected to die rapidly, reduce early mortality and later disability by: maintenance of pulmonary, cardiovascular, fluid, electrolyte, and nutritional homeostasis (Section 27.8.6); and avoidance, recognition, and treatment of any cause of neurological deterioration (Section 27.8.3) and of the general complications (Section 27.8.7).

◆ Initiate rehabilitation (Section 27.9.2).

◆ Initiate secondary prevention in patients who might benefit (Section 27.10.3).

◆ Treat coincidental disorders such as cardiac failure, angina, claudication, and abdominal aortic aneurysm.

27.8.2 Survival after stroke

Early death

The prognosis of hospitalized patients tends to be worse than that of patients in the population at large because mild strokes are more likely to be cared for at home. Overall in the whole community, about 20 per cent of all first-ever-in-a-lifetime stroke patients are dead within a month, the prognosis being much better for ischaemic stroke than for intracranial haemorrhage (about 10 per cent versus 50 per cent dead) (Bamford *et al.* 1990*a*). Deaths in the first few days are almost all due to the brain lesion itself: either intracerebral haemorrhage, or large cerebral infarcts with associated oedema, causing brain shift and herniation, or direct disruption of vital brainstem centres by the primary lesion. Sudden, or more-or-less sudden, death only occurs as a consequence of intracranial haemorrhage, as do the majority of any other deaths on the first day (Phillips *et al.* 1977; Silver *et al.* 1984; Bamford *et al.* 1990*b*; Derouesne *et al.* 1993). Deaths after the first week are more likely to be due to the indirect consequences of the brain lesion (e.g. broncho-pneumonia and pulmonary embolism) or coincidental cardiac disease (Fig. 27.34).

Adverse prognostic factors for early death

Immediately after stroke onset the main clinical question is 'Will this patient survive?'. It is not only helpful for relatives and healthcare providers to know who is likely to die and who may survive and require continuing rehabilitation or long-term care but, increasingly, politicians and healthcare purchasers are wanting to compare outcomes from different hospitals, which requires prognostic models for case-mix adjustment (Davenport *et al.* 1996*a*; Weir *et al.* 2001).

Haemorrhagic stroke carries a higher early case-fatality than ischaemic stroke, but the distinction requires early access to CT scanning (Section 27.6.3) (Fig. 27.35). Within the ischaemic stroke category, the readily clinically distinguished subtypes

have very different outcomes; for example, patients with total anterior circulation infarction have just as poor an outcome as those with primary intracerebral haemorrhage (Fig. 27.35). The best single predictor of early death is impaired consciousness, which is easily assessed in every patient. Other predictors reflect, on the whole:

(1) the extent of the brain lesion and so stroke severity: size of any haematoma and intraventricular extension of blood; midline shift; high as well as low blood pressure (Section 27.8.4); atrial fibrillation; fever and high blood glucose; and

(2) the premorbid state of the patient: increasing age; pre-stroke handicap (Section 27.3.5);

(Anderson *et al.* 1994*b*; Jorgensen *et al.* 1995; Arboix *et al.* 1996; Fogelholm *et al.* 1997; Pullicino *et al.* 1997; Castillo *et al.* 1998; De Keyser 1998; Scott *et al.* 1998). Visible infarction on CT adds a little more prognostic information (Wardlaw *et al.* 1998*b*). Of course many of these variables are interrelated (e.g. conscious level, size of haematoma, and midline shift; age, pre-stroke handicap, and atrial fibrillation). However, to predict death, prognostic models based on independent variables do not necessarily provide much more information than an experienced clinician's informal estimate, can be impractical to use in routine practice and, so far, most have not been satisfactorily validated on independent data sets (Counsell *et al.* 2001).

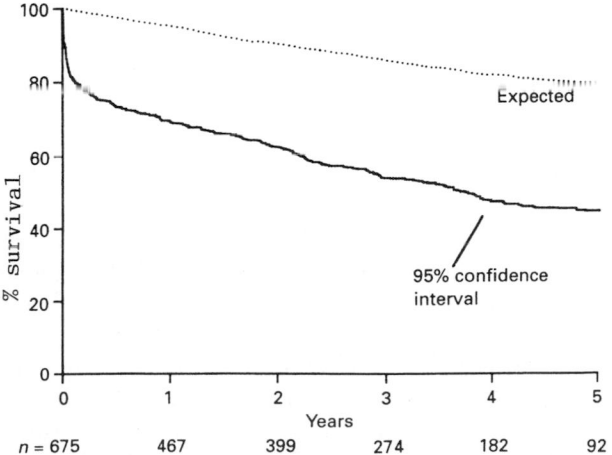

Fig. 27.34. Survival curve to show the probability of survival in the 675 first-ever-in-a-lifetime stroke patients in the Oxfordshire Community Stroke Project, compared with expected survival (with permission from Dennis *et al.* 1993).

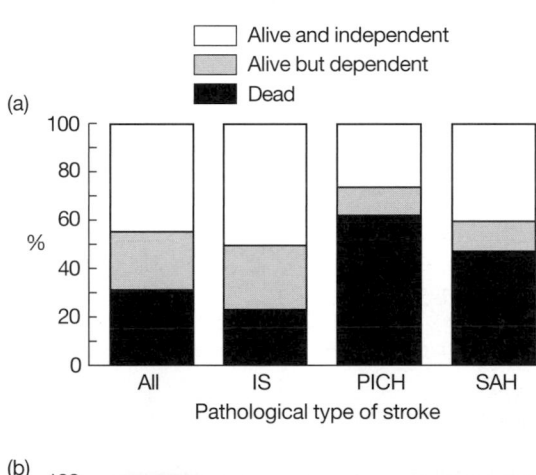

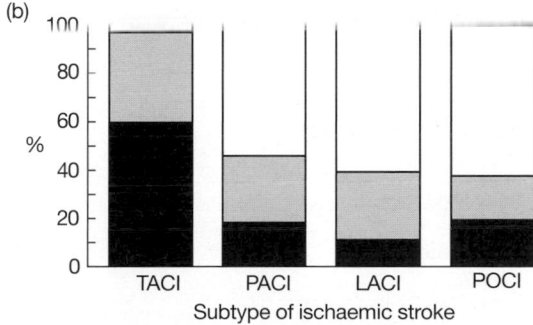

Fig. 27.35. Outcome at 1 year in the 675 first-ever-in-a-lifetime stroke patients in the Oxfordshire Community Stroke Project by (a) pathological type and (b) subtype of ischaemic stroke. IS, ischaemic stroke; PICH, primary intracerebral haemorrhage; SAH, subarachnoid haemorrhage; TACI, total anterior circulation infarct; PACI, partial anterior circulation infarct; LACI, lacunar infarction; POCI, posterior circulation infarction. (From Bamford *et al.* 1990*a*, 1991).

Later death

After the first month, the risk of death becomes much less (about 7 per cent per annum) but it is still about twice that of the background population because stroke patients are particularly likely to die of a further stroke and even more likely to die of the consequences of associated ischaemic heart disease (Fig. 27.34) (Dennis *et al.* 1993).

27.8.3 Early deterioration after acute ischaemic stroke

Although stroke onset is usually abrupt, the neurological deficit often worsens over the following minutes, hours, and sometimes days. It is therefore important to monitor the patient's neurological state. If it deteriorates, there are two immediate questions: 'Why', and then, 'What to do about it?'. Terms such as 'stroke-in-evolution', 'stroke-in-progression', and 'progressing stroke', which hint at knowledge we do not have about the cause of deterioration in most individual cases, are misleading and should be abandoned (Asplund 1992). Systemic factors can certainly cause neurological deterioration: hypoxia, hypotension, infections, and electrolyte imbalance should be easy and fairly quick to diagnose, and are often treatable (Table 27.28). Neurological causes for deterioration are summarized in Table 27.29. Of course, progressive non-stroke pathologies should also be reconsidered in a patient going from bad to worse, e.g. brain tumour, subdural haematoma, etc. (Section 27.6.1). Therefore, as well as a repeat CT brain scan, it is impor-

Table 27.28. Systemic causes of neurological deterioration after stroke

Hypoxia
  Pneumonia
  Pulmonary embolism
  Cardiac failure
  Chronic respiratory disease

Hypotension
  Pulmonary embolism
  Cardiac failure
  Cardiac arrhythmia
  Pneumonia
  Dehydration
  Septicaemia
  Hypotensive drugs/vasodilators
  Bleeding peptic ulcer

Infection and fever
  Pneumonia
  Urinary tract infection
  Septicaemia

Others
  Water and electrolyte imbalance
  Hypo/hyperglycaemia
  Depression
  Sedatives/hypnotics
  Anticonvulsants

Table 27.29. Neurological causes of deterioration after stroke

	Ischaemic stroke	Primary intracerebral haemorrhage	Subarachnoid haemorrhage
Haemorrhagic transformation	+	−	−
Cerebral oedema	+	(+)	(+)
Brain shift (mass effect)	+	+	(+)
'Vasospasm'	−	−	+
Thrombus propagation	+	−	−
Recurrent embolism	+	−	−
Haemorrhage growth/recurrence	−	+	+
Hydrocephalus	(+)	+	+
Epileptic seizures	+	+	+

tant not to forget blood urea, electrolytes, sugar, chest radiography, ECG, blood and urine cultures, possibly an EEG, and a review of any medications.

Haemorrhage into cerebral infarcts (haemorrhagic transformation): at post-mortem, spontaneous petechial haemorrhages are very common in infarcts. During life they are seen on brain CT in perhaps 15 per cent of patients, but case selection and definitions vary, and there is significant interobserver variation in detection and classification of haemorrhage (Motto *et al.* 1997). Confluent haematoma on CT appears in about 5 per cent of patients, usually within 2 weeks of stroke onset but sometimes within 24 hours. It can be extremely easily confused with primary intracerebral haemorrhage unless there is an earlier normal CT scan, or one showing infarction (Hart and Easton 1986; Hornig *et al.* 1986; Bogousslavsky *et al.* 1991).

Haemorrhagic transformation is said to be more common in heart-to-brain than artery-to-artery embolic or thrombotic infarcts, but this may merely reflect the fact that the former are more likely to be large and severe than lacunar, and that the patients are often anticoagulated, factors all associated with haemorrhagic transformation (Hart and Easton 1986; Lodder *et al.* 1986; Okada *et al.* 1989). The conventional, but possibly incorrect, explanation for haemorrhagic transformation is recanalization of the occluded artery and reflow of blood into a damaged and 'leaky' microcirculation (Del Zoppo *et al.* 1998). The same mechanism might explain worsening cerebral oedema, although there is no good evidence that cerebral oedema really is associated with recanalization, rather the reverse in fact (Section 27.3.5).

Haemorrhagic transformation is not often symptomatic unless there is confluent haematoma (Hornig *et al.* 1986; Larrue *et al.* 1997). Clinically obvious haemorrhagic transformation is certainly more common with heparin and thrombolytic treatment, but not aspirin (International Stroke Trial Collaborative Group 1997; Wardlaw *et al.* 1997).

Peri-infarct oedema reduces local cerebral blood flow and causes brain shift and herniation, the latter being the most common 'neurological' cause of death (Section 27.3.5). This complication is a common explanation for worsening over the first few days, and can often be detected by CT brain scan. Intravenous mannitol may reduce the deficit for a while, but is unlikely to make a major impact on outcome. In deteriorating cases with massive swelling, claims for the success of neurosurgical decompression have been made, but convincing trials need to be done (Schwab *et al.* 1998).

Propagating thrombosis (proximal or distal to a thrombotic, embolic or any other type of occlusion, or within collateral vessels) is often assumed to explain neurological deterioration if other causes have been excluded. Direct evidence in individuals is almost impossible to obtain, except perhaps with transcranial Doppler (TCD).

Recurrent embolization is another possibility, but does not necessarily cause identifiable sudden worsening, particularly if it is to the previously affected arterial territory. However, even with angiography, the distinction between propagating thrombosis and embolization is very difficult (Irino *et al.* 1983). Emboli detection with TCD is not helpful either. There is only anecdotal evidence that full anticoagulation with intravenous heparin slows progression and improves outcome if no other cause of deterioration is evident (Slivka and Levy 1990).

Epileptic seizures, partial or generalized, occur for the first time in about 2 per cent of acute strokes at around the time of onset, rising to about 10 per cent at 5 years, more with large cortical infarcts or intracranial haemorrhage (Pohlmann-Eden *et al.* 1996, 1997; Burn *et al.* 1997). Seizures can cause neurological deterioration in the acute phase and be mistaken for recurrent stroke later. Usually this is obvious unless the patient is unconscious or confused for some other reason, or the history is vague. Anticonvulsants are indicated in the usual way, but not as routine prophylaxis for all stroke patients. Intractable epilepsy is distinctly unusual.

27.8.4 Specific treatments for acute ischaemic stroke

The logic is to tip the balance away from thrombosis and continuing embolization towards clot lysis and vascular recanalization, and to prevent ischaemic but still viable neurons from dying. In the last edition, I wrote 'Despite numerous suggestions, some sensible and others absurd, there is still no routine treatment which, given early after acute ischaemic stroke, increases the number of independent survivors. For many treatments no randomized trials have been done and, when they have, the numbers of patients have been too small to provide precise results'. The situation is now more optimistic, some would say transformed (Hill and Hachinski 1998). Randomized trials are bigger and therefore more precise, and even somewhat better, and meta-analysis of similar trials is widely accepted (Bath *et al.* 1998). There is now general agreement that the most important outcome to focus on is independent survival.

Death alone is too insensitive to detect a treatment effect; moreover, reducing case fatality might increase the proportion with residual disability, and survival in an independent state is probably as, or more, important to patients than survival at any cost.

As a result there is now enough information about aspirin, heparin, and perhaps thrombolysis to influence clinical practice. So far there is no definite evidence to support or refute the use of defibrinating drugs, haemodilution, dextran, calcium channel blockers, magnesium, the myriad of so-called neuroprotective drugs, naftidrofuryl, hyperbaric oxygen, glycerol, mannitol, corticosteroids, hypothermia, reducing the blood glucose, emergency carotid endarterectomy with or without embolectomy, and neurosurgical brain decompression. Under such circumstances of 'uncertainty', these interventions are not appropriate in routine clinical practice but only in the context of well-organized randomized controlled trials.

Aspirin

Aspirin (to obtain an immediate full antiplatelet effect 160–300 mg is given by mouth, nasogastric tube, or rectally) has a small but definite benefit, probably because its antiplatelet action reduces the risk of early recurrent ischaemic stroke; for every 1000 patients treated, about nine fewer are dead or have a recurrence at 14 days, and about 13 fewer are dead or dependent in the longer term (International Stroke Trial Collaborative Group 1997; CAST (Chinese Acute Stroke Trial) Collaborative Group 1997; Chen *et al.* 2000). Presumably aspirin will also reduce the few myocardial infarctions that occur in this early period and have a useful impact on reducing the risk of venous thromboembolism. Ideally CT should be done first to exclude intracerebral haemorrhage (PICH), but if any delay is likely and the patient is unlikely to have a PICH (i.e. not in coma), then aspirin can be given and later stopped if the scan shows bleeding; it does not seem to increase the risk of clinically evident intracranial bleeding under these circumstances. In essence, this means that aspirin can be started at once and carried on at a lower dosage of 75 mg daily for secondary prevention (Section 27.10.3).

Heparin

In many countries heparin has been used for years on the assumption that by inhibiting thrombus propagation and recurrent embolization it improves the outcome of acute ischaemic stroke. Furthermore, there is good evidence that it reduces the risk of deep venous thrombosis and perhaps pulmonary embolism as well (Gubitz *et al.* 1999). In the past, the risk of inducing intracranial as well as extracranial bleeding has been rather downplayed. However, it is now very clear that although low (5000 units daily) and medium (25 000 units daily) doses of subcutaneous heparin do reduce the risk of early ischaemic stroke recurrence, this is offset by an increased risk of haemorrhagic stroke, even in patients with atrial fibrillation and presumed embolism from the heart to the brain. There is absolutely no effect on long-term death and dependency, in the presence or absence of aspirin (International Stroke Trial

Collaborative Group 1997). Low molecular weight heparin is similarly disappointing (Publications Committee for the Trial of ORG 10172 in Acute Stroke Treatment (TOAST) Investigators 1998). There is no available randomized evidence for higher doses of unfractionated heparin. Therefore, heparin should not be given routinely, although many will still use it for ischaemic strokes that appear to be deteriorating as a result of continuing thromboembolism. The risk of deep venous thrombosis can best be reduced in other ways (Section 27.8.7)

Thrombolysis

Recanalization and haemorrhagic transformation of the infarct are spontaneous events in some patients, and both may be potentiated by therapeutic thrombolysis. There is, therefore, a balance to be struck between the risk of intracranial haemorrhage and any benefit from recanalization in terms of increased survival free of dependency. In fact, for patients randomized within 3 hours of stroke onset, and possibly even 6 hours, the benefit may well outweigh the risk (Wardlaw et al. 1997). However, it is very unclear whether the same advantage would be found in normal clinical practice outside the controlled environment of clinical trials, and much more needs to be known about which patients are particularly likely to bleed, and which to recanalize. For now, therefore, thrombolysis should be restricted to a very few specialist centres and large pragmatic randomized trials. There is no direct randomized evidence of the relative effects of streptokinase versus tissue plasminogen activator (tPA), but the indirect evidence somewhat favours the latter (alteplase, 0.9 mg/kg, maximum 90 mg, intravenously in 1 hour).

Raised blood pressure

An unresolved dilemma is whether to lower raised blood pressure in acute stroke patients (Powers 1993) (Section 27.3.5). Both high, and to a lesser extent low, pressures are associated with a poor outcome but it is unclear whether this is a cause or an effect of severe stroke (Signorini et al. 1999). There is no adequate randomized trial evidence on which to make evidence-based decisions, and the many non-randomized comparisons are too subject to various forms of bias to be helpful (Chamorro et al. 1998). But, in general, if a patient is taking hypotensive drugs before the stroke, most physicians continue them in the same dose. Moderately raised blood pressure is often 'reactive' in the sense that it falls spontaneously. If it doesn't fall after a week or two, then the normal indications for gradual and permanent blood pressure lowering for secondary prevention apply (Section 27.10.3). Presumably a systolic pressure greater than about 240 mmHg, or a diastolic pressure greater than perhaps 120 mmHg, should be lowered more urgently, but not too quickly for fear of precipitating cerebral ischaemia, particularly in the ischaemic penumbra where autoregulation is likely to be impaired (see hypertensive encephalopathy, Section 25.5.4). Systemic hypotension may exacerbate ischaemia and is best treated by removing the cause (Table 27.28). The neurological state should be monitored carefully during any induced blood pressure change and, if it worsens, the pressure should be restored to what it was.

27.8.5 Specific treatment of primary intracerebral haemorrhage.

Other than the occasional need to relieve acute hydrocephalus, particularly after cerebellar haemorrhage (Section 27.6.2), there are no specific treatments except to remove the haematoma, but this is controversial. In theory, haematoma evacuation should reduce intracranial pressure, at least locally if not generally, and so ameliorate any surrounding brain ischaemia and oedema, and perhaps also reduce secondary bleeding around the haematoma and haematoma growth (Masdeu and Rubino 1984; Brott et al. 1997; Mayer et al. 1998) (Section 27.4.8). Unfortunately, the natural history is very variable (for example, small lobar haemorrhages can leave very little, if any, disability), the literature is dominated by non-randomized and often retrospective case series with all their potential for bias, there have been very few randomized trials, and meta-analysis is inconclusive (Hankey and Hon 1997; Prasad et al. 1999). Not surprisingly, therefore, there is no consensus. In practice, it is probably reasonable to evacuate haematomas causing deterioration not explained by systemic complications (Table 27.28) (i.e. if the conscious level is falling with or without increasing focal signs as a consequence of brain shift, increasing intracranial pressure, or perhaps continuing or recurrent bleeding). Careful histological examination of the clot and any surrounding brain sometimes reveals the cause of the bleeding.

27.8.6 General management of all strokes

If the stroke causes more than mild disability, then good nursing is essential to ensure that the patient is comfortable, hydrated, fed, toileted, and clean; is in a suitable posture and turned regularly; the airway is maintained and swallowing safe; and the patient is monitored reliably (Table 27.30). Oxygen is required if the patient becomes hypoxic, or develops pneumonia or a pulmonary embolus, although it is often given routinely. Headache, nausea, vomiting, and constipation must all be treated on their merits. Attention to even trivial

Table 27.30. Routine monitoring in acute stroke severe enough to require nursing care

Vital signs
Respiratory rate and rhythmn, and blood gases
Heart rate and rhythm (often with ECG monitor)
Blood pressure (normal arm)
Temperature (normal axilla)
Neurological
Conscious level (Glasgow Coma Scale)
Pupils
Limb weakness
Epileptic seizures
General
Fluid balance
Electrolytes and urea
Blood glucose
Haematocrit

details can make a difference, e.g. ensuring the patient has the right spectacles on their nose, correctly fitting false teeth, a properly fitted hearing aid that is switched on, and a bell within reach.

Impaired swallowing with risk of aspiration and so pneumonia is particularly common in drowsy patients with severe hemispheric strokes, and those with brainstem strokes. It almost always gets better in days or weeks (Hamdy *et al.* 1997). Significant difficulty in swallowing is best routinely tested by asking the patient to sip and then swallow some water, observing any tendency to choke in the next minute or so, and for added sensitivity using simple quantification (Mari *et al.* 1997; Hinds and Wiles 1998). If there is a problem, and certainly if the patient has impaired consciousness, then fluids should be given by nasogastric tube or intravenously. Feeding in the first few days may not be all that important but later the patient should be kept well nourished by mouth if possible. For non-swallowers, it is not clear which is the better option—nasogastric tube or percutaneous endoscopic gastrostomy (PEG) tube.

After a severe stroke there is often a stress response which subsides spontaneously in a few days: raised blood pressure, mild fever, leucocytosis, hyperglycaemia and even glycosuria, and 'ischaemic' changes on the ECG. Of course fever should not be ignored as other causes are possible (Table 27.31).

27.8.7 The general non-neurological complications of stroke and their management

The non-neurological complications after acute stroke are more frequent with increasing age, pre-stroke disability, stroke severity, and poor general nursing and other care (Table 27.32). To some extent the site of the lesion may also be relevant, e.g. seizures do not occur in brainstem strokes whereas both obstructive and central sleep apnoea might (Davenport *et al.* 1996a; van der Worp and Kappelle 1998). Although some appear rather trivial, these complications often delay recovery, interfere with rehabilitation, and are occasionally fatal.

Pneumonia is a common complication in any elderly patient who becomes ill and goes to bed. It is particularly likely in stroke because of the risk of inhalation of fluids or food when difficulty in swallowing has not been properly managed; there is

Table 27.31. Causes of fever after stroke

Infection
Urine
Pneumonia
Pressure sores
Septicaemia
Intravenous access site
Deep vein thrombosis and pulmonary embolism
Infective endocarditis
Drug reaction

Table 27.32. General non-neurological complications of acute stroke

Pneumonia
Venous thromboembolism
Urinary incontinence and infection
Pressure sores
Cardiac arrhythmias, failure, myocardial infarction
Fluid imbalance, hyponatraemia
'Mechanical' problems
spasticity
contractures
malalignment/subuxation/frozen shoulder
falls and fractures
osteoporosis
ankle swelling
peripheral nerve pressure palsies
Mood disorders
Gastric 'stress' ulceration and haemorrhage
Central post-stroke ('thalamic') pain

a poor cough reflex due to brainstem disturbance or coma; poor respiratory movement (Houston *et al.* 1995); and pulmonary embolism (see below). The risks can be reduced by good nursing and chest physiotherapy. A pharyngeal airway may be required, particularly in drowsy patients or after a brainstem stroke, but ventilation is seldom needed.

Venous thromboembolism: about 50 per cent of hemiparetic patients in hospital very quickly develop a deep vein thrombosis (DVT) in their paralysed leg, although this is not usually detectable clinically and in most cases seems to cause little problem. However, if the leg does become swollen and painful, then rehabilitation is compromised. Pulmonary embolism is common at post-mortem but it is not clear how often it is the cause, or a contributory cause, of death in patients who are otherwise likely to survive to make a reasonable recovery (Warlow 1978). Non-fatal pulmonary embolism causes hypoxia, encourages pneumonia, and so potentially compromises neurological recovery, but is difficult to diagnose during life (Wijdicks and Scott 1997). There is little doubt that low-dose subcutaneous heparin (5000 units twice a day) substantially reduces the risk of DVT, and possibly of pulmonary embolism as well, although the overall outcome of the stroke is not affected and the risks of intra- and extracranial haemorrhage are too high (Section 27.8.4). Routine heparin prophylaxis is not, therefore, recommended. Compression stockings are a very reasonable alternative, although evidence for efficacy is only available in non-stroke patients. Clinically evident and confirmed DVT or pulmonary embolism should be treated with anticoagulants in the usual way, but probably not if the patient has had any intracranial haemorrhage in the previous few days. Under these circumstances some would use an inferior venous cava filter despite the lack of evidence of overall benefit.

Urinary incontinence is common enough in elderly people, but is much more common after stroke, particularly severe stroke, at least for a matter of days or weeks, but sometimes permanently (Brittain *et al.* 1998). Despite best efforts, catheterization is often required to maintain skin care, at least for a period. Condom-sheath drainage in males is sometimes feasible. Catheterization, as well as general immobility, may cause urinary infection, and perhaps secondary renal infection or even septicaemia, which should be treated with appropriate antibiotics.

Pressure sores are a consequence of being found some time after stroke onset, poor nursing, incontinence, or malnourishment. They may become infected and take months to heal, perhaps causing septicaemia and certainly delaying rehabilitation. They can be avoided by attention to pressure points, using appropriate mattresses and supports, and turning immobile patients every few hours (Effective Health Care 1995).

Cardiac complications: ST depression, T wave flattening and inversion, U waves and a prolonged Q-T interval on the ECG are common but transient after acute ischaemic, and even more after acute haemorrhagic, stroke, but seldom appear to be of serious concern. Some abnormalities were probably present before the stroke, bearing in mind how common cardiac disease is in these 'vascular' patients (Oppenheimer *et al.* 1990). Whether monitoring the ECG improves the prognosis is unknown, but it is often recommended, particularly after subarachnoid haemorrhage (Section 27.7.4). Some patients have a rise in cardiac enzymes as a result of diffuse myocardial damage (presumably related to stress, cardiac failure, or trauma), an epileptic convulsion, or perhaps brain damage (Norris *et al.* 1979). Therefore, the diagnosis of immediately preceding, simultaneous, or complicating acute myocardial infarction depends more on serial ECG changes than cardiac enzymes, particularly if there are no cardiac symptoms (von Arbin *et al.* 1982). Cardiac failure due to ischaemic heart disease, pulmonary oedema, and pulmonary embolism can be problematic and should be treated on its merits.

Fluid imbalance: dehydration is a consequence of either being found late, or poor nursing. Patients require at least 1500 ml of fluid daily from the onset and, if necessary, this must be given by nasogastric tube or intravenously. Hyponatraemia, probably reflecting salt wasting and the stress response, is particularly common after subarachnoid haemorrhage and, in general, should be treated by plasma volume expansion and not fluid restriction (Section 27.7.4). Urinary tract infection and dehydration may cause renal failure.

Mechanical problems: spasticity, muscle contractures, painful shoulder and stiffness in other joints of a paralysed limb, malalignment or subluxation of the shoulder, falls and fractures can all potentially be avoided by good nursing, backed up by expert physiotherapy from day 1, with appropriate advice and aids (Smith *et al.* 1981; Overstall 1995). Osteoporosis developing in a paralysed limb does not seem to cause much of a problem, although presumably it predisposes to fractures; but it may be unavoidable (Sato *et al.* 1998). Ankle swelling, if not due to a deep vein thrombosis or cardiac failure, is most often caused by a poor gait and can be alleviated by elasticated stockings and keeping the feet up. If ignored, it may encourage pressure sores, particularly if footwear is too tight. Peripheral nerve pressure palsies are not common and can be prevented by good nursing.

Acute gastric ulceration, with or without haemorrhage or perforation, is a well-recognized but rare complication in severe stroke which is difficult to avoid. When it occurs it should be treated on its merits. (Davenport *et al.* 1996c).

Mood disorders: major depression is not particularly common in stroke survivors, but other, rather less easily defined, mood disorders are minor depression, anxiety, worry, distress, agoraphobia often related to fears of falling, social withdrawal, apathy, self-neglect, and pathological emotionalism. Their exact frequency depends on both definition and case mix (House 1987; House *et al.* 1991; Andersen *et al.* 1995; Astrom 1996; O'Rourke *et al.* 1998). These mood disorders can certainly impede rehabilitation and contribute to disability and handicap, but usually improve with time. Explanation, support, and counselling should help prevent them, and sometimes antidepressants are required for depression and, in lower doses, for pathological emotionalism, despite their quite common adverse effects.

Central post-stroke (thalamic) pain: very rarely a burning, severe, and paroxysmal pain exacerbated by touch and other stimuli, develops more or less at once, but more often weeks or months, after stroke (Leijon *et al.* 1989; Nasreddine and Saver 1997). There are usually some sensory signs in the affected parts. Although the lesion is often in the contralateral thalamus, it can be elsewhere in the central sensory pathways. Treatment is not very successful with carbamazepine or other anticonvulsants, amitriptyline, and various sorts of counter stimulation.

27.9 Recovery and rehabilitation

27.9.1 Prognosis for functional recovery

The great majority of patients who survive the first month after stroke improve, many back to their pre-stroke level of function which, in elderly patients, may have been far from optimal. About two-thirds of the survivors become independent, with little difference between ischaemic or haemorrhagic strokes (see Fig. 27.35). However, within the ischaemic group, only about 5 per cent of patients with infarction of the whole middle cerebral artery territory are alive and independent at a year post-stroke, compared with 50 per cent of those with more restricted infarcts (Dombovy *et al.* 1987; Wade and Langton Hewer 1987; Bamford *et al.* 1990a). About 90 per cent of stroke survivors get home, leaving only a very small proportion in institutional care but, because stroke is so common, their absolute number is large (Legh-Smith *et al.* 1986).

The rate of recovery of all impairments is maximal in the first few weeks, slows down after 2 or 3 months, and probably stops at about 6–12 months post-stroke (Wade and Langton Hewer 1987; Stone *et al.* 1992; Duncan *et al.* 1994; Pedersen *et al.* 1995). Later improvement in functional abilities, and particularly in social activities, is probably more to do with adaptation to disability and minimizing handicap (suitable housing, aids, social support, etc.) than further recovery of physical impairments. However, one should not underestimate the difficulty of measuring such change, particularly bearing in mind individual variation from day to day; the fact that many patients cannot complete some of the tests at all; the confounding effect of pre-stroke and other non-stroke disabilities; the difficulty developing standardized and simple measurements in elderly people; and also that many of the tests have ceiling effects and so cannot detect improvement in patients who are nearly recovered (e.g. the Barthel Index, Section 27.9.2). Impaired quality of life is very common, even when patients appear to be little disabled; they tend to be concerned with their physical problems while their carers are more concerned with social isolation and restriction of their normal life, and by the mental state and changed personality of the patients (Holbrook 1982; Anderson 1988). Carers themselves may become anxious and depressed, and feel guilty (Dennis *et al.* 1998; Scholte opReimer *et al.* 1998).

Prediction of functional outcome for individuals immediately after stroke onset is difficult but becomes somewhat easier, and more relevant, once it is clear that the patient is likely to survive (i.e. at about 2 weeks post-stroke). At this stage good prognostic signs include young age, initially mild deficit, fully conscious, good sitting balance, normal orientation, no cognitive impairment, urinary continence, and rapid improvement. Independent living is also contingent on a high level of social support. Mathematical models, based on clinical features backed up by various tests to do with the size of the brain lesion and the systemic consequences of stroke severity, cannot predict the outcome with enough accuracy to influence individual patient management very much; there are too many patients who improve unexpectedly, and others who do poorly despite having a good predicted prognosis. Also, very few models have been externally validated (i.e. do they actually work?) and most are simply impractical for routine clinical practice (Kwakkel *et al.* 1996; Pohjasvaara *et al.* 1998). On the other hand, predicting outcome in groups of stroke patients, allowing adjustment for case mix when comparing the outcomes in different hospitals, is rather more accurate but has hardly got beyond looking at case fatality. But even quite large differences in outcome may still be due to chance or residual confounding, and perhaps to the quality of care (Davenport *et al.* 1996a; Weir *et al.* 2001).

27.9.2 Strategies for rehabilitation

Stroke rehabilitation attempts to restore patients to their previous physical, mental, and social capability (Langton Hewer 1990). The most important goals are: first, to maximize the patients' role fulfilment and independence in their environment, all within the limitations imposed by the underlying pathology and impairments and by the availability of resources; and, secondly, to help the patients make the best adaptation possible to any differences between roles achieved and roles desired (Wade 1992). Clearly, this must all be a team effort, involving

Table 27.33. Sources of support and help for stroke patients

Doctor (neurologist, geriatrician, rehabilitationist, vascular surgeon, neurosurgeon, psychiatrist)

Nurse (hospital, community, liaison)

Physiotherapist

Occupational therapist

Speech therapist

Social worker

Clinical psychologist

Dietician

Pharmacist

Chiropodist

Home help

Voluntary worker

Local authority housing department

Meals-on-wheels service

many people as well as the patient and their carer, if there is one (Table 27.33). Demarcation disputes between therapists, arguments over funding between agencies, over specialization, and confusion are potential problems which can be difficult to resolve. Therefore, the stroke team must have a leader with good negotiating skills and awareness of the aspirations and sensitivities of others. The team must be well organized, enthusiastic, optimistic, and professional. It must also meet regularly to discuss the assessment, short-term and long-term goals, interventions, and evaluation for each patient. Non-specialized, but trained 'practical helpers' have been suggested as a cost-effective means of supporting disabled people in the community, particularly if the sheer number of different professionals interacting with each patient could thereby be reduced (Hopkins 1984). Perhaps better, is allowing and encouraging the separate professions to take on enough of each other's skills to keep the rehabilitation process going 24 hours a day.

Rehabilitation should not necessarily be confined to patients admitted to hospital. It can be delivered to patients being nursed at home and probably should be continued for a while for patients discharged home from hospital if there is any continuing disability and handicap. Indeed, vigorous attempts are being made to discharge patients earlier with continuing rehabilitation at home, or in a day-hospital, but it is not yet clear whether this strategy leads to as good an outcome as rehabilitation in hospital (Gladman *et al.* 1995; Rudd *et al.* 1997). In practice, each individual should be assessed on their merits, and where to continue rehabilitation must depend very much on their home conditions, distance from the hospital, and the nature of the available hospital and domiciliary services. Although it seems sensible to support patients through the difficult transition from hospital to home with specialist domiciliary nurses or care workers, it is difficult to demonstrate any definite benefit (Dennis *et al.* 1997a).

Planning (goal setting)

It is important that the rehabilitation team, patient and carer agree on short-term, medium-term, and long-term targets to be achieved. The targets must be neither too easy nor too difficult, a judgement which depends heavily on how predictable any natural recovery is likely to be. Initially, the target is survival, and then changes to recovery from impairments, to getting home, and finally returning to normal work-related and social activities. Unrealistic aims on the part of the patient may well need to be sympathetically modified, but without causing a collapse in morale.

Assessment tools used in rehabilitation

Assessment tools identify, measure, and record impairments, disabilities, handicaps, and quality of life. They are important because assessment is the first step in rehabilitation and measurement of outcome is crucial for clinical trials, audit, and comparing outcomes in different institutions. Depending on the problem, various instruments are available (Warlow *et al.* 2000*e*; Lyden and Hantson 1998). To be useful, any instrument must be relevant, valid, sensitive to change, and reliable. In clinical practice it also has to be simple, practical, and communicable to others. Complicated scoring systems which sum individual scores for various impairments (e.g. aphasia plus weakness plus conscious level, etc.) are about as helpful as adding together the urea, sodium, and potassium concentrations to provide a 'metabolic' score (van Gijn and Warlow 1992). Furthermore, in any assessment it is important to compare the present state of the patient with their premorbid level, and also to try and disentangle the contribution of the stroke morbidity from the numerous co-morbidities likely to be present in the elderly, such as claudication, dementia, and arthritis (Collen and Wade 1991).

The motricity index and trunk control test are useful measures of motor impairment (Collin and Wade 1990), the walking speed is simply measured over a standard distance, with or without a turn, using a stop-watch (D. T. Wade *et al.* 1987; Collen *et al.* 1990), while the Rivermead mobility index is a measure of disability (Collen *et al.* 1991). The abbreviated Hodkinson Mental Test Score is recommended for overall cognitive function (Hodkinson 1972), the Frenchay Aphasia Screening Test for aphasia (Enderby *et al.* 1986), and the Star Cancellation Test for neglect (Jehkonen *et al.* 1998). Mood disorder is difficult to measure simply, there is no good screening technique, and many stroke patients cannot complete the questionnaires anyway (House *et al.* 1989).

The Barthel Activities of Daily Living index is a familiar and good measure of all-round disability, although it does have a floor and ceiling effect and takes no account of vision, hearing, and speaking. The Office of Population Censuses and Surveys (OPCS) instrument might be better (Wade and Collin 1988; Barer and Nouri 1989; Wellwood *et al.* 1995). The modified Rankin Scale (Table 27.34), sometimes called the Oxford Handicap Scale, probably captures overall disability and handicap better than the Barthel Index (Bamford *et al.*

Table 27.34. Oxford Handicap Scale (modified Rankin scale)

Grade	
0	No symptoms
1	Minor symptoms which do not interfere with lifestyle
2	Minor handicap. Symptoms which lead to some restriction in lifestyle but do not interfere with the patients' ability to look after themselves
3	Moderate handicap. Symptoms which significantly restrict lifestyle and prevent totally independent existence
4	Moderately severe handicap. Symptoms which clearly prevent independent existence although not needing constant care and attention
5	Severe handicap. Totally dependent, requiring constant attention day and night

1989). For clinical trial and audit purposes in large samples, three simple questions—face to face, by post, or on the telephone—neatly group patients into those who are completely recovered, those who are still symptomatic but independent, those who are dependent, or dead (Fig. 27.36) (Dennis *et al.* 1997*b*,*c*).

The Frenchay Activity Index can be used for social functioning, although this is very influenced by gender and culture (Wade *et al.* 1985). The importance of 'quality of life' after stroke is widely acknowledged. However, it is not at all clear how this should be measured, how to score patients who cannot complete the questionnaires, and what the scores really 'mean'. The most widely used generic instrument is the Short Form-36, but maybe the EuroQol is marginally better. Neither are reliable enough to monitor individuals over time but they are probably good enough to compare groups of patients (de Haan *et al.* 1993; Dorman *et al.* 1998).

Interventions

It is remarkably difficult to evaluate the various techniques used in rehabilitation, when they should be started, how long they should be continued for, how much should be attempted every day and what are the appropriate outcomes, although many attempts are now being made both in primary research and in systematically reviewing the evidence (Dombovy *et al.* 1986; Ernst 1990; Effective Health Care 1992; Scottish Intercollegiate Guidelines Network 1998). Whatever the difficulties, everyone agrees that some sort of rehabilitation is important for all except mildly affected patients, and those likely to die within hours or days. Also, everyone agrees that even best efforts can be haphazard and unfocused. Many patients in hospital receive remarkably little rehabilitation or other therapeutic activity in a day, particularly outside stroke units (Lincoln *et al.* 1996). Of course patients must be cared for, which may require hospital admission for nursing, while treatments are delivered to improve impairments and disabilities (usually by acting on the patient) and to minimize handicap (usually by manipulating the environment).

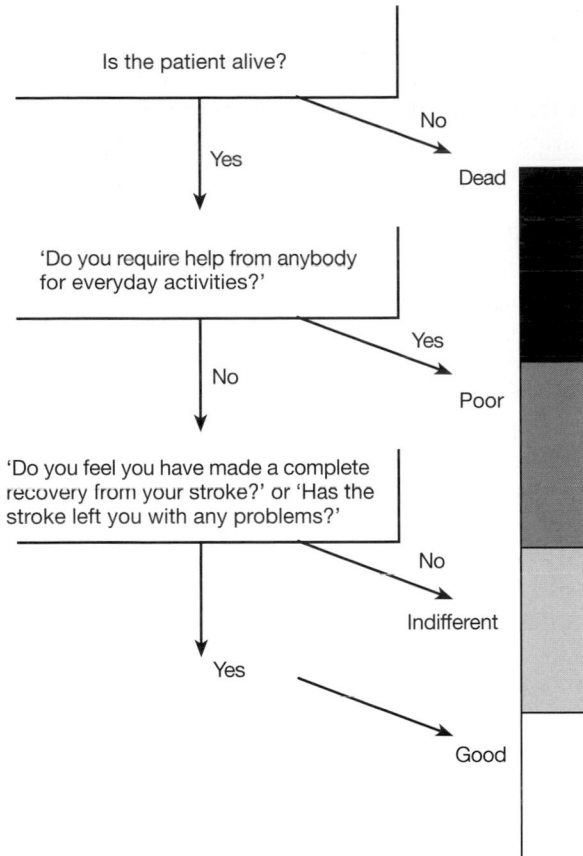

Fig. 27.36. Three simple questions divide stroke patients into four outcome categories (from Lindley *et al.* 1994).

Patients with mobility problems undoubtedly need advice from a physiotherapist about walking, transferring strategies and aids, such as foot-drop splints, sticks, and wheelchairs. Carers need instruction about helping patients with transferring, lifting, walking, and exercises. Despite the difficulties inherent in proper evaluation, there is reasonable evidence that physiotherapy itself really does improve outcome, but systematic reviews are needed to make better sense of the evidence (Smith *et al.* 1981; Wade *et al.* 1992; Dean and Shepherd 1997). Physiotherapists are also well placed to advise on the care of the hemiplegic arm, particularly the shoulder, and may be able to enhance arm function too (Sunderland *et al.* 1994; Feys *et al.* 1998).

Occupational therapists play a valuable role in helping patients minimize handicap and relearn activities of daily living. Spatial and visual neglect can be a major problem but there is no certain way to alleviate it (Edmans and Lincoln 1989).

Much time (patient and professional) can be wasted on speech therapy. While a trained speech therapist is invaluable in patient assessment, counselling relatives, and providing helpful communication strategies, it is unclear that therapy *itself* improves the outcome of aphasia compared with what occurs spontaneously, or with help from motivated volunteers.

But then evaluation in this area is notoriously difficult and the present lack of evidence of benefit must not be mistaken for evidence of lack of benefit. Moreover, many would argue that intensive and appropriately targeted therapy has never been tested, but unfortunately such time-consuming treatment may be unaffordable (Allen 1990; Whurr *et al.* 1992). Speech therapists also have a role in the management of dysarthria (which is seldom a persistent problem post-stroke) and swallowing (Section 27.8.6).

Patients and carers need advice and information about the whole range of available interventions, their availability and likely effects (whether delivered in hospital, day centre, or at home), as well as information about stroke and the problems it may cause. There is evidence that an information leaflet enhances the effect of verbal information (Lomer and McLellan 1987). In addition, specific advice is needed about return to work, driving, finance, benefits, and sexual activity. Potential problems after discharge can be attenuated by help from care attendants (Townsend *et al.* 1988) and counselling of carers improves family adjustment (Evans *et al.* 1988). Information about local stroke clubs and other voluntary organizations should be given to patients and carers.

Elderly stroke survivors often have other impairments and disabilities requiring attention during their rehabilitation, particularly with vision (new spectacles, registration as partially sighted, etc.), hearing (suitable hearing aid), teeth (properly fitting false teeth), and feet (adequate chiropody). 'Medical' problems may also need sorting out (cardiac failure, urinary and chest infections, seizures, and arthritis), while the adverse effects of drugs must be minimized and not forgotten when trying to explain post-stroke problems (e.g. sedation, confusion, constipation, hypotension, etc.).

27.10 Stroke prevention

Stroke must be preventable, at least to some extent. It is clearly not an inevitable accompaniment of ageing, nor just of genetic predisposition, because its frequency is higher in, for example, areas of deprivation (Sections 27.2.4). This hints that improving social conditions should reduce stroke risk, provided any interventions do not increase stroke risk in some way (e.g. anticoagulation may reduce ischaemic stroke risk but increase haemorrhagic stroke risk). Of course, any intervention has to be not just effective but affordable, and acceptable to those involved.

In general, there are two complementary approaches to disease prevention: the 'high-risk' strategy, which identifies people at particularly high risk of the disease in question and treats just them to reduce their risk (e.g. finding and treating TIA patients to prevent them having a stroke), and the 'mass strategy' which seeks to modify disease risk in the whole population by reducing everyone's risk by a small amount (e.g. reducing the salt content of food and so reducing the population mean blood pressure by a few millimetres of mercury) (Rose 1992; Warlow *et al.* 2000*f*). On the whole, the 'high-risk' strategy is to do with doctors finding and treating 'patients' and is particularly pertinent to preventing recurrent stroke, and stroke after TIA, i.e. secondary prevention (Warlow 1998a). The 'mass strategy' is mostly to do with political and fiscal action to modify the exposures and behaviours of whole populations and is more pertinent to preventing stroke before it occurs, i.e. primary prevention.

27.10.1 Primary stroke prevention

Public health campaigns to modify dietary habits and smoking are not the responsibility of most doctors and, however important in reducing the risk of stroke and coronary heart disease, are beyond the scope of this chapter (Marmot and Poulter 1992; Bonita 1994). Likewise, screening for and treating people with hypertension and other vascular risk factors is not the direct concern of neurologists but of primary care physicians and other specialists. However, three specific interventions are of relevance to neurological practice and worth brief mention:

Embolism from the heart: anticoagulation with warfarin is commonly recommended for a wide range of cardiac conditions associated with a high risk of embolism to the brain and elsewhere (e.g. mechanical heart valves, rheumatic atrial fibrillation with mitral stenosis, recent myocardial infarction, dilating cardiomyopathy, etc.) (Hart *et al.* 1996). Also, in recent years it has become very clear from meta-analysis of a number of randomized trials that long-term oral anticoagulation, usually with warfarin, reduces the risk of stroke in patients with non-rheumatic atrial fibrillation, the most common cardiac source of embolism to the brain. Aiming for an International Normalized Ratio (INR) of 2.0–3.0 reduces stroke risk by about two-thirds from 4.5 to 1.5 per cent per annum, without an unacceptable risk of intra- or extracranial bleeding (Hart *et al.* 1996). It is particularly worthwhile in patients at higher absolute risk than this average because reducing their relative risk by two-thirds produces a greater absolute risk reduction and so reduces the 'number-needed-to-treat' to prevent one stroke. Patients with only atrial fibrillation and no other cardiac problem are probably not at high enough risk of stroke to make the risk of anticoagulation worthwhile, and for them aspirin is preferable. Of course, monitoring anticoagulation and ensuring patient compliance is not easy, and there are frequent contraindications in routine practice. Under these circumstances, a safer and easier alternative to anticoagulation is aspirin (150–300 mg daily). Although it only reduces stroke risk by about one-fifth, aspirin may be applicable to more patients and so prevent as many or more strokes as anticoagulation (Atrial Fibrillation Investigators 1994; Lip 1999).

Antiplatelet drugs: long-term aspirin in healthy middle-aged people has nothing to offer because their risk of stroke, and other serious vascular events, is so low. Indeed, it is conceivable that even the low risk of treatment causing intra- and extracranial haemorrhage is, under these circumstances, actually higher than the untreated risk of stroke (Antiplatelet Trialists' Collaboration 1994; Medical Research Council's General Practice Research Framework 1998).

Asymptomatic carotid stenosis may be discovered contralateral to a symptomatic stenosis, in patients being worked up for surgery below the neck, and in people with a carotid bruit. And the greater the stenosis, the higher the risk of later ischaemic stroke ipsilateral to the lesion (European Carotid Surgery Trialists' Collaborative Group 1995). Although carotid endarterectomy to remove a severe asymptomatic stenosis reduces the overall risk of stroke by about 30 per cent (Benavente *et al.* 1998), the operation is hardly sensible because, on average, the unoperated risk of ipsilateral stroke is only about 2 per cent per annum so about 50 people have to have surgery to prevent one having a stroke in 3 years. Surgery will only become worthwhile if some way can be found to pick out and operate just on those patients who have a much higher unoperated risk of stroke (Warlow 1998b).

The rather special situation of patients scheduled for major surgery below the neck and who have severe asymptomatic carotid stenosis is controversial. On balance, most believe that the risk of stroke due to carotid endarterectomy is probably greater than the risk of perioperative stroke if the stenosis is left alone.

At present screening to detect severe asymptomatic stenosis may actually cause more strokes than it prevents, largely because in populations with a low prevalence of stenosis, the number of false positives detected by ultrasound far exceeds the number of true positives, and inappropriate patients may then be subjected to the rigours of catheter angiography and surgery (Whitty *et al.* 1998).

27.10.2 The risk of serious vascular events in TIA patients, and after ischaemic stroke

The long-term risk of stroke in TIA patients is so similar to the risk of recurrent stroke in ischaemic stroke survivors that they can be considered together, with the one exception that TIAs in the eye have a much better prognosis than TIAs in the brain (Dennis *et al.* 1989). It is also important to consider the risk of myocardial infarction and sudden presumed cardiac death, which are both common and potentially preventable by similar strategies to stroke prevention.

Stroke risk

The risk of stroke is greatest early after presentation, within days or weeks, particularly in patients with carotid stenosis, and those with a partial anterior circulation rather than a lacunar infarct (Fig. 27.37) (Dennis *et al.* 1990b; Bamford *et al.* 1991; Sandercock and Tangkanakul 1997). Perhaps the reason is that an atheromatous plaque becomes unstable by fissuring and exposes the thrombogenic core to flowing blood, and this causes mural thrombosis and the release of an embolus, which is soon followed by another one before the plaque 'heals' by endothelial repair. Or perhaps collateral channels develop to restore a reasonable blood supply beyond a stenotic lesion and so the risk of stroke declines. Whatever the explanation, preventive treatments should clearly be started as soon as possible.

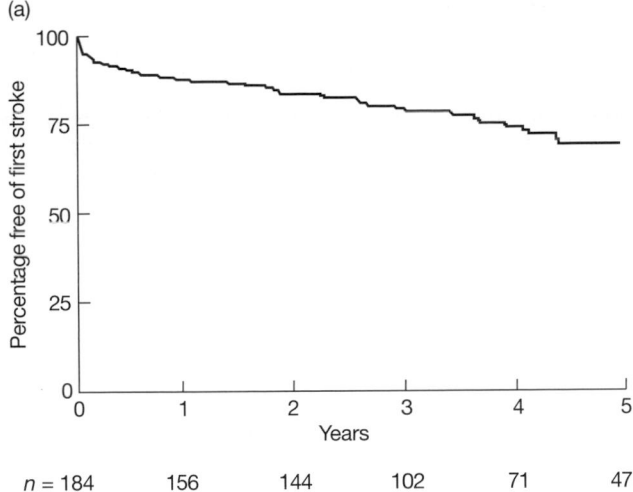

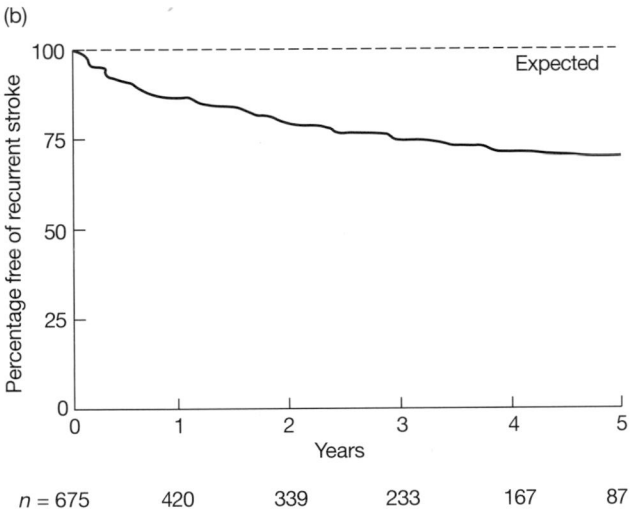

Fig. 27.37. (a) Kaplan–Meier plot to show survival free from first-ever-in-a-lifetime stroke in 184 TIA patients over 5 years in the Oxfordshire Community Stroke Project, censoring the non-stroke deaths; and (b) recurrent stroke in 675 first-ever-in-a-lifetime stroke patients, censoring deaths not due to recurrent stroke and compared with the expected risk of first-ever-in-a-lifetime stroke. (With permission from Dennis *et al.* 1990*b* and Burn *et al.* 1994.)

In community-based studies, the risk of stroke in the first year after TIA, or ischaemic stroke, is about 10 per cent and then settles down to 5 per cent per annum, which is about seven times the expected risk in the background population (Dennis *et al.* 1990*b*; Burn *et al.* 1994; Hankey *et al.* 1998; Petty *et al.* 1998). The risk in hospital-referred series is lower, probably because the patients are younger with fewer vascular risk factors (Hankey *et al.* 1991, 1993*a*). More than half the strokes occur in the same vascular territory as the earlier event, some are mild, and one or two are due to primary intracerebral haemorrhage rather than the anticipated cerebral infarction. Although strokes due to embolism from the heart and proximal arterial sites tend, if they recur, to be of the same type, lacunar strokes are more variable (Hankey *et al.* 1991; Cillessen *et al.* 1993;

Yamamoto and Bogousslavsky 1998). About one-third of TIA patients have further TIAs, which must be an underestimate because such evanescent symptoms may not be reported or recorded (Hankey and Warlow 1994). This is perhaps unimportant, because the main aim of management is to reduce the risk of strokes, particularly disabling ones, and not just to reduce TIA frequency unless it is very high.

Cardiac risk

The risk of a serious cardiac event (i.e. fatal or non-fatal myocardial infarction (MI), sudden presumed cardiac death, etc.) is substantial (about 3–5 per cent per annum), presumably because of the association of atheroma in one artery with atheroma in another artery in the same susceptible individual (Hankey and Warlow 1994; Pop *et al.* 1994). There is no early high-risk period, presumably because the coronary arterial lesion is obviously in a different place and may not be 'unstable' at the same time as the recently symptomatic cerebral arterial lesion. There is, therefore, much sense in considering the risk of all serious vascular events together (i.e. stroke, MI, and other vascular death), because they are almost all potentially preventable by the control of vascular risk factors and antithrombotic drugs. The risk of this combined outcome is about 9 per cent per annum in the community.

In the long term, cardiac death is more frequent than stroke death and, as time goes by, non-vascular deaths, such as cancer, become relatively more frequent (Dennis *et al.* 1990*b*).

Predicting risk in individuals and in groups of patients

The risks quoted so far are very much 'on average'. The actual risk in any series of patients must depend crucially on the prevalence of various vascular risk factors, in other words on 'case mix'. However, it is very difficult to predict reliably those *individuals* who *will* have a stroke and therefore for whom riskier and expensive treatments (e.g. carotid endarterectomy and clopidogrel, respectively) might be indicated as well as, or instead of, low-risk and inexpensive treatments (e.g. aspirin) which can be given to a much wider range of patients who *might* have a stroke. On the other hand, *groups* of patients in strata of increasing risk are identifiable using mathematical models based on independent predictors of risk, and it may even be possible to slim these models down to a simple addition and subtraction process (Hankey *et al.* 1992, 1993*b*; Rothwell *et al.* 1999). Certainly, increasingly severe carotid stenosis increases the risk of ipsilateral ischaemic stroke early after presentation (Fig. 27.38), as does irregularity/ulceration of the lesion on angiography.

Increasing usual blood pressure is another risk factor (Fig. 27.39), and most studies implicate increasing age, frequently recurrent TIAs, and sometimes diabetes mellitus (Warlow *et al.* 2000*g*). Finally, microembolic signals detected by transcranial Doppler may predict risk, but so far this observation is based on tiny numbers and the technique will not be very practical in the near future (Valton *et al.* 1998).

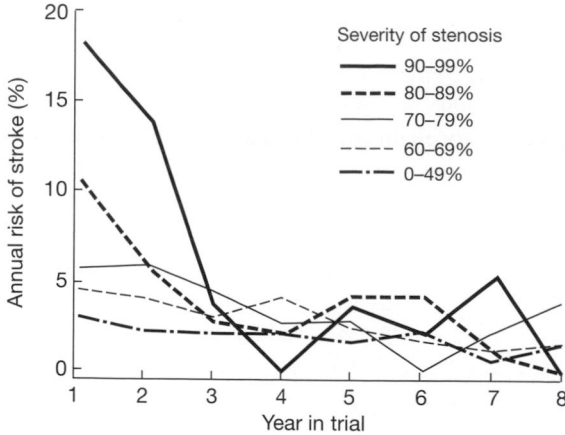

Fig. 27.38. The risk of stroke in various strata of symptomatic stenosis in each year after randomization in the no-surgery group of the European Carotid Surgery Trial. Note that stroke risk is highest with severe degrees of stenosis, but only in the first 2–3 years. (With permission from the European Carotid Surgery Trialists' Collaborative Group 1998.)

27.10.3 Secondary prevention after ischaemic stroke and transient ischaemic attacks

Secondary prevention of stroke depends on the control of vascular risk factors, appropriate antithrombotic drugs, and vascular surgery. The great majority of patients have assumed, or sometimes demonstrated, atherothromboembolism, intracranial small vessel disease, or non-rheumatic atrial fibrillation. Naturally, for the occasional patient with a specific cause of cerebral ischaemia, specific treatment should prevent recurrence (e.g. giant-cell arteritis, cardiac myxoma, etc.). But it is important to realize that treating TIA patients, however effectively for them at the individual level, will prevent only a very small proportion of all strokes, largely because only about 15 per cent of strokes are preceded by TIAs, half of which are not reported anyway (Warlow 1998a).

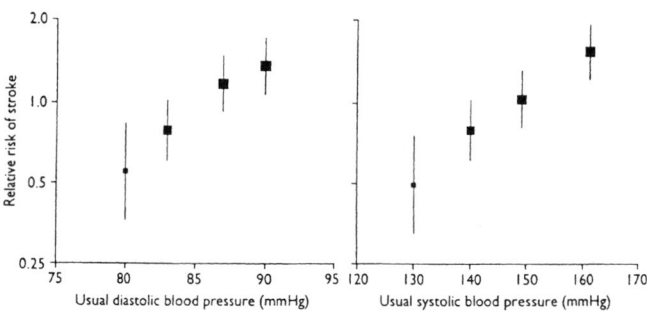

Fig. 27.39. Relative risk of stroke by usual blood pressure in 2435 patients with TIA or mild ischaemic stroke in the UK–TIA Aspirin Trial. The vertical bars indicate 95 per cent confidence intervals and the size of the boxes is proportional to the number of strokes in each category. (With permission from Rodgers et al. 1996.)

Control of vascular risk factors

There have been almost no direct studies of the control of vascular risk factors in TIA or ischaemic stroke patients, even though they are very often present (see Table 27.6). None the less, until directly relevant randomized trails are done, it is reasonable to base treatment on inferences from the results of primary stroke prevention trials, and from coronary prevention trials, because cardiac events are so common in cerebrovascular patients.

Lowering raised *blood pressure* with diuretics or beta-blockers reduces the risk of first-ever stroke by about 40 per cent, even within a few years. The effect on coronary events is less impressive (MacMahon and Rodgers 1993; Psaty et al. 1997). This proportional risk reduction applies essentially to all levels of blood pressure, so that individuals at highest risk (i.e. severely hypertensive with other vascular risk factors) have the most to gain, and the 'numbers-needed-to-treat' to prevent a stroke will not be too big, although more strokes will be prevented by treating mild and moderately hypertensive patients because there are so many more of them (Rose 1981). There is much less direct evidence in TIA patients and stroke survivors, but a very large trial with 6000 patients will report (PROGRESS Management Committee 1996; INDANA Project Collaborators 1997).

For now, it seems reasonable to gradually reduce sustained hypertension to a systolic pressure of about 150 mmHg and a diastolic (phase 5) pressure of about 90 mmHg, although some would be more aggressive; first by non-pharmacological methods (weight reduction, salt reduction, regular moderate exercise, and cutting down excessive alcohol consumption) and then, if necessary, by the addition of drugs (starting with low-dose diuretics and then beta-blockers perhaps) (R. Jackson et al. 1993; Alderman 1994; Kaplan and Gifford 1996). There is seldom any need for urgent and rushed treatment of blood pressure in TIA patients or stroke survivors (Section 27.8.4).

Naturally, treatment should be modified if adverse effects occur: postural hypotension, lethargy, impotence, peripheral oedema, etc. Great care should be taken to avoid overtreatment, particularly if there is severe carotid disease in the neck, for fear of producing low-flow ischaemic stroke. If any TIAs or strokes are thought to be due to low flow in the first place (Sections 27.5.1, 27.6.2), it is probably best to leave the blood pressure alone, at least until any arterial stenosis in the neck has been dealt with surgically (Leira et al. 1997).

The indirect evidence that stopping *smoking* reduces the risk of coronary events and stroke, and generally improves health, is so good that randomized trial evidence is not really required to support treatment of patients and general anti-smoking advice. Large randomized trials with sufficient difference in smoking behaviour between the intervention and control groups to demonstrate a definite reduction in risk of vascular events (or lung cancer) have not been feasible (Rose et al. 1982).

Reduction in plasma *cholesterol* undoubtedly reduces the risk of coronary events and should in theory be helpful in TIA/ischaemic stroke patients with their high risk of myocardial infarction (MI). Of some concern, however, is that this might increase the risk of primary intracerebral haemorrhage because of the possible inverse association with lower cholesterol levels (Section 27.2.7). On the other hand, at least in asymptomatic people and in the survivors of MI, there is very good evidence that cholesterol lowering reduces overall stroke risk, surprisingly in view of the weak association between increasing plasma cholesterol levels and stroke; a mean reduction of total plasma cholesterol of 22 per cent with statins is associated with a 29 per cent reduction in stroke risk (Hebert *et al.* 1997). Whether routine cholesterol lowering, and to what level, should be recommended for stroke survivors and TIA patients will become clearer when the results of directly relevant trials become available. In the meantime, it seems sensible to give dietary advice to all these patients which should reduce their plasma cholesterol by a small amount, and to give statins to those who already have angina or have had an MI, to reduce their plasma cholesterol to less than about 5.0 mmol/l (Drug and Therapeutics Bulletin 1996).

Diabetes mellitus requires treatment in its own right but this does not definitely reduce the risk of serious macrovascular events such as ischaemic stroke or myocardial infarction (UK Prospective Diabetes Study Group 1998).

Coronary event prevention: it is uncertain whether TIA/mild ischaemic stroke patients should have coronary angiography to detect lesions requiring bypass if these are asymptomatic, although the prevalence of coronary atheroma must be high.

Antiplatelet drugs

Antiplatelet drugs given in the long term to TIA or mild ischaemic stroke patients (and to others at high risk of vascular events) reduce the relative risk of 'stroke, myocardial infarction, and vascular death' by about one-quarter (Antiplatelet Trialists' Collaboration 1994). This seems to be much the same in males and females, old and young, diabetics and non-diabetics, and hypertensives as well as non-hypertensives. About 1000 patients have to be treated for 3 years to prevent 40 having a serious vascular event (Fig. 27.40).

Aspirin: until recently most of the evidence on antiplatelet drugs has come from trials of various doses of aspirin versus control, there being very few direct comparisons of different aspirin doses (Dutch TIA Trial Study Group 1991; UK–TIA Study Group 1991; Antiplatelet Trialists' Collaboration 1994). There are, of course, good theoretical reasons for supposing that low-dose aspirin is as effective as higher doses, because platelet cyclooxygenase is irreversibly inhibited, and so thromboxane A_2 production almost completely abolished, by a single 100 mg dose, or after a cumulative daily dose of 30–50 mg for a week or so (Patrono 1994). From the trials it seems that doses between about 30 and 1500 mg daily are equally effective, and the usual recommendation is to use 'paediatric' aspirin, 75 mg daily, which is the lowest dose which has definitely been shown to have a treatment effect (SALT Collaborative Group 1991; Drug and Therapeutics Bulletin 1997). Certainly, the lower the dose, the less the upper gastrointestinal adverse effects such as

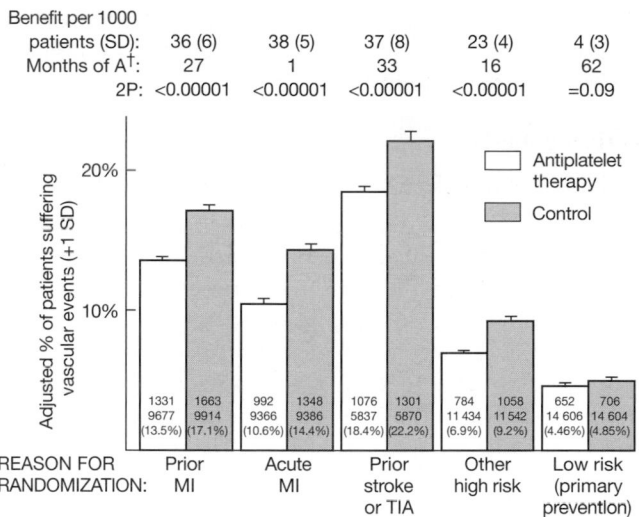

Fig. 27.40. Absolute effects of antiplatelet drugs on the risk of 'stroke, myocardial infarction, and vascular death' (i.e. serious vascular events) in various categories of patient from a systematic review of 145 randomized trials (with permission from the Antiplatelet Trialists' Collaboration 1994).

indigestion. On 300 mg daily the risk of gastrointestinal bleeding is—depending on definitions—up to about 1 per cent per annum (Dickinson and Prentice 1998). This low risk of an alarming, but usually non-fatal complication, is worth taking compared with the risk of stroke. There is some evidence that aspirin increases the risk of intracranial haemorrhage (perhaps 2 per 1000 patients per annum) but, overall, stroke risk is still substantially reduced (Antiplatelet Trialists' Collaboration 1994). The antiplatelet effects of aspirin are probably not attenuated with time, so presumably the drug should be given indefinitely.

Dipyridamole has long been known to have antiplatelet effects as well as being a vasodilator, in part by being an inhibitor of phosphodiesterase (FitzGerald 1987). It reduces the risk of serious vascular events by much the same amount as aspirin. In combination with aspirin it may be better than aspirin alone, particularly for stroke prevention, the dose being 200 mg of the modified release formulation in combination with 25 mg aspirin, given twice daily (Diener *et al.* 1996). A further trial is in progress to clarify this issue and also to explore the possibility that the effect is more to do with blood pressure lowering than platelets. The main adverse effects are headache and hypotension.

Ticlopidine and *clopidogrel* are thienopyridines which block platelet activation by ADP by inhibiting its binding to platelets, so interfering with ADP-dependent activation of the GpIIb–IIIa site, the major receptor for fibrinogen on the platelet surface. In comparison with aspirin, they reduce the risk of serious vascular events by a rather modest 10 per cent, or about five events prevented per 1000 patients treated per annum (CAPRIE Steering Committee 1996; Hankey *et al.* 2001). In view of their high cost, these drugs are probably best restricted to patients who are definitely aspirin intolerant or at very high risk of serious vascular events. Clopidogrel (75 mg daily) is preferred to ticlopidine because it does not cause neutropenia; rash and diarrhoea are the main adverse effects.

Anticoagulants

Patients in sinus rhythm and presumed arterial disease

Long-term oral anticoagulation was once fashionable but the trials were never adequate to show a benefit, if one exists, even when systematically reviewed in a meta-analysis (Liu *et al.* 1999). Furthermore, in comparison with antiplatelet drugs, there is an unacceptable risk of intracranial haemorrhage, at least with a target INR of 3.0–4.5 (Stroke Prevention in Reversible Ischaemia (SPIRIT) Study Group 1997). Lower INR target ranges are being tested in further trials.

Non-rheumatic atrial fibrillation

The situation here is rather different, with the risk of stroke being reduced substantially from about 12 per cent to 4 per cent per annum with a target INR of 2.0–3.0 (European Atrial Fibrillation Trial Study Group 1993, 1995). Although the risk of bleeding was low in the trial, in routine practice it may not be sensible nor safe to anticoagulate a large proportion of fibrillating stroke survivors and TIA patients because of various contraindications or logistical difficulties, and for these patients aspirin 300 mg daily has a small and useful effect (Sudlow *et al.* 1995).

Other cardiac sources of embolism

As for primary prevention (Section 27.10.1), there is little direct evidence from randomized trials, but the same general recommendations apply if there is a major embolic risk. For cardiac sources of embolism of uncertain relevance (e.g. mitral leaflet prolapse, atrial septal aneurysm, mitral annulus calcification, aortic sclerosis, etc.), it is probably best just to use aspirin, particularly as the actual cause of the cerebral ischaemia is rather more likely to be arterial disease if the patient is above the age of about 50.

When to start anticoagulation is controversial. If too late after ischaemic stroke, then further embolism might occur, but if too soon, there is a risk of haemorrhagic transformation of any cerebral infarct. My own practice is to start with aspirin in the usual way (Section 27.8.4) and then gradually substitute warfarin after about a week, longer if there is known haemorrhagic transformation of the infarct. The warfarin can be replaced by aspirin later if the thromboembolic risk declines (for example, maybe 6 months after an acute myocardial infarction), or if there are complications from the anticoagulants. TIA patients can be anticoagulated at presentation.

Carotid endarterectomy for recently symptomatic carotid stenosis

Carotid endarterectomy removes an atherothrombotic plaque from the carotid bifurcation with its potential for embolism and its effect on flow, and so reduces the risk of ischaemic

stroke in the arterial territory ipsilateral to the operation. However, this benefit must be set against the main risk of surgery, which is to cause stroke by several possible mechanisms: interrupting cerebral blood flow during the operation; embolism from the operation site during manipulation of the artery, or shunt insertion; intimal dissection with complicating thrombosis and embolism immediately after surgery; and occasionally intracerebral haemorrhage due to increased perfusion pressure into a damaged area of brain. The other serious complications are very rare, and some others may be more common but they are usually rather mild and temporary (Table 27.35).

To make surgery as cost-effective as possible, it is important to reduce both the risk of surgery by attention to surgical technique and avoiding operating on very high surgical risk patients, and to select patients at particularly high risk of what surgery can prevent, i.e. ipsilateral ischaemic stroke. The most important risk factor for unoperated stroke is increasing severity of stenosis so that, on balance, the immediate risk of surgery (about 5–10 per cent stroke or death in routine practice) is worth taking for long-term benefit in patients with a recent carotid distribution event and more than about 80 per cent stenosis of the symptomatic artery, who have more than a 20 per cent risk of stroke over the next few years (Fig. 27.41)

Table 27.35. Complications of carotid endarterectomy

Ischaemic stroke (almost always ipsilateral to the operated artery) due to:

    Embolism from the operation site during surgery
    Embolism from the operation site after surgery
    Carotid dissection
    Perioperative carotid occlusion
    Low cerebral blood flow during surgery
    Perioperative systemic hypotension

Haemorrhagic stroke (almost always ipsilateral to the operated artery) due to:

    Perioperative hypertension
    Post-endarterectomy cerebral hyperperfusion

Death due to:

    Stroke
    Myocardial infarction
    Pulmonary embolism
    Rupture of arterial operation site

Myocardial infarction

Local complications

    Nerve injury (vagal, hypoglossal, marginal mandibular branch of facial, spinal accessory, greater auricular, transverse, cervical nerves)
    Wound infection
    Neck haematoma
    Aneurysmal dilatation at operation site
    Patch disruption and haemorrhage

Others

    Deep venous thrombosis
    Transhemispheric cerebral oedema
    Headache, focal motor seizures
    Facial (parotid) pain
    Pain at vein donor site after vein patch angioplasty

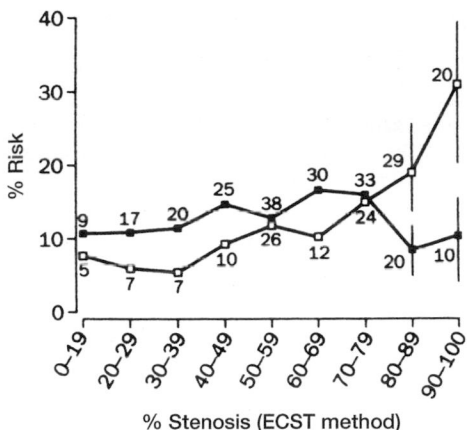

Fig. 27.41. Risk of stroke at 3 years, and all operative deaths, in patients randomized to carotid endarterectomy (closed squares) versus no surgery (open squares) in the European Carotid Surgery Trial, by severity of symptomatic carotid stenosis. The numbers by the curves are the number of patients with an event and the vertical lines are 95 per cent confidence intervals. (From the European Carotid Surgery Trialists' Collaborative Group 1998, with permission.)

(Barnett *et al.* 1998; European Carotid Surgery Trialists' Collaborative Group 1998).Without surgery, the risk of stroke is highest soon after presentation, so for maximum benefit surgery must be done in recently symptomatic patients, i.e. within days or weeks of presentation, not months (Fig. 27.38). However, most surgeons feel that after stroke of any severity it is probably best to wait 2 or 3 weeks to have an acceptably low risk of perioperative stroke. Other independent factors which may increase the risk of stroke in unoperated patients are irregularity and ulceration of the stenosis and ischaemia in the brain rather than the eye. On the other hand, independent patient variables that may increase the risk of surgery are female sex, hypertension, and peripheral vascular disease. Clearly, therefore, advising surgery in an individual requires a balance to be struck between early risk and later benefit, and very much considering the patient's view as well (Rothwell *et al.* 1999).

Whether to advise coronary artery surgery (in cardiac symptomatic patients) before (and risk a perioperative stroke) or after carotid surgery (and risk a perioperative myocardial infarction) is unclear, but both operations should probably not be done under the same anaesthetic. Each individual must be considered on his or her own merits.

Extra- to intracranial (EC–IC) bypass surgery

In theory, anastomosing a branch of the external carotid artery (usually a branch of the superficial temporal artery) with a distal cortical branch of a cerebral artery (usually the middle cerebral artery, MCA) ought to improve blood flow distal to an internal carotid artery (ICA) or MCA occlusion (both of which are inoperable), or distal to an inaccessible (to surgery) ICA stenosis. Perhaps it does, but the overall stroke risk was not reduced in the only randomized trial ever done (EC–IC Bypass Study Group 1985). It is, of course, conceivable that there is a

responsive subgroup of patients, such as those is impaired cerebrovascular reactivity, but this needs to be shown before surgery can be recommended (Warlow 1986).

Vertebrobasilar TIAs and ischaemic strokes

Endarterectomy of the vertebral artery origin is technically difficult and various reconstruction procedures have been devised to bypass a stenosis or occlusion. However, there is no good evidence that surgery improves the prognosis, even when vertebrobasilar TIAs are very frequent. Other possible approaches are an extra- to intracranial bypass, carotid endarterectomy if there is associated severe disease at the carotid bifurcation, and angioplasty; again, there is no evidence of benefit. Frequent and disabling vertebrobasilar TIAs due to definite subclavian steal can perhaps be relieved by surgery to remove or bypass the occlusive lesion (Bohmfalk *et al.* 1979).

Percutaneous transluminal angioplasty

Angioplasty, with or without stenting, of stenosed coronary and peripheral limb arteries is now commonplace. It may also benefit patients with subclavian or proximal vertebral artery stenosis if there is symptomatic subclavian steal, or disabling and frequent vertebrobasilar TIAs, although there is no randomized evidence (Zeumer 1985; Terada *et al.* 1996). For internal carotid artery origin stenosis, there are now an increasing number of non-randomized studies with all their inherent potential biases. Although there are natural concerns about intimal dissection, and of embolization of atherothrombotic material to the brain and eye, it is said that the risk of stroke is no higher than during carotid endarterectomy (Brown 1992; Eckert *et al.* 1996). However, so far the one randomized trial was too small to show whether angioplasty is as safe and as durable as carotid endarterectomy for symptomatic stenosis (CAVATAS 1999). If this does turn out to be the case, angioplasty will certainly be quicker, more comfortable, and free of the consequences of a surgical incision in the neck (cranial nerve injury, haematoma, infection, numbness) and general anaesthesia. But for now, it should only be done in the context of randomized trials and perhaps in the occasional patient who needs carotid surgery but who is thought to be an unacceptable anaesthetic risk.

What to do about frequent TIAs

Very frequent TIAs (several a week) unresponsive to aspirin may be of such concern to the patient (and doctor) that it is worth attempting to stop them, irrespective of whether the treatment also prevents stroke. If there is severe extracranial or intracranial stenotic or occlusive arterial disease, then it is important to first consider the blood pressure which, if too low, may be responsible for frequent low-flow TIAs. If that is not the case, it is reasonable to add dipyridamole to the aspirin (see above) and then, if that is not effective, empirically to try full heparinization followed, if successful, by warfarin for a few weeks and then aspirin indefinitely. In addition, carotid surgery may be indicated. If neither antithrombotic drugs nor surgery are effective, the diagnosis should be reconsidered, particularly if there is little, if any, arterial disease in the neck, and the heart is normal (migraine, epilepsy, multiple sclerosis, and psychogenic causes are the most likely, Section 27.5.2).

27.10.4 Secondary prevention after primary intracerebral haemorrhage

Much less is known of the long-term risk of recurrence after primary intracerebral haemorrhage than ischaemic stroke; who is at particularly high or low risk; what proportion of further strokes are haemorrhagic or ischaemic; and whether any recurrence occurs in the same place or in different parts of the brain. This is because the follow-up studies have either been very small, although prospective and based in the community, or retrospective and based on hospitalized populations, although reasonably large.

The rebleeding risk after rupture of a vascular malformation has been discussed earlier (Section 27.7.4). For patients with a haemostatic defect (e.g. haemophilia) the risk is presumably high. For patients with no obvious cause, the risk of recurrent stroke is about 5 per cent per annum. Less than half of the recurrences are definitely further haemorrhages, many are cerebral infarcts, but often the pathology is not known (Counsell *et al.* 1995; Passero *et al.* 1995). One might imagine that recurrence is more likely with cerebral amyloid angiopathy or severe hypertension, but this is difficult to prove (Neau *et al.* 1997).

Other than attempting to remove the cause (e.g. a vascular malformation) it is sensible to minimize vascular risk factors, particularly hypertension (Section 27.10.3).

27.11 Intracranial venous thrombosis

Thrombosis in the dural sinuses and/or cerebral veins (see Fig. 27.9) is much less common than cerebral arterial thromboembolism, and leads to a number of rather different clinical syndromes which are seldom like 'a stroke' (Bousser and Ross Russell 1997). However, intracranial venous thrombosis shares some of the same causes as ischaemic stroke, which these days are far less frequently 'septic' than in the past (Table 27.36) (Southwick *et al.* 1986). No cause at all is found in something like 20 per cent of cases. Although it was originally regarded as a rare condition which was commonly fatal, nowadays with heightened awareness of mild cases and more sophisticated imaging, it is clearly a more common condition which is rarely fatal.

Thrombosis in a dural sinus can be relatively restricted when it tends to cause raised intracranial pressure and the syndrome of benign intracranial hypertension without any neurological deficit (Section 17.1.4). On the other hand, thrombosis in cerebral veins, with or without dural sinus thrombosis, is more likely to cause widespread and multiple 'venous' infarcts which are congested, oedematous, and often haemorrhagic.

Table 27.36. Causes of intracranial venous thrombosis

Local conditions affecting the cerebral veins and sinuses directly:
    Head injury (with or without fracture)
    Intracranial surgery
    Local sepsis (sinuses, ears, mastoids, scalp, nasopharynx)
    Subdural empyema
    Bacterial meningitis
    Dural arteriovenous fistula (Section 27.4.8)
    Tumour invasion of dural sinus (malignant meningitis, lymphoma, skull base secondary, etc.)
    Catheterization of jugular vein
    Lumbar puncture

Systemic disorders:
    Dehydration
    Septicaemia
    Pregnancy and the puerperium (Section 27.4.7)
    Oral contraceptives (Section 27.2.7)
    Haematological disorders (Table 27.15)
    Inflammatory vascular disorders (Table 27.13)
    Homocysteinuria (Section 27.2.7)
    Congestive cardiac failure
    Inflammatory bowel disease (Section 27.4.7)
    Androgen therapy
    Antifibrinolytic drugs
    Non-metastatic effect of extracranial malignancy
    Nephrotic syndrome

27.11.1 Clinical features

There are several clinical syndromes, so intracranial venous thrombosis enters into the consideration of patients with benign intracranial hypertension, diffuse encephalopathies, sometimes strokes, and rarely subarachnoid haemorrhage (Bousser *et al.* 1985*b*; Enevoldson and Ross Russell 1990).

In perhaps one-quarter of 'benign intracranial hypertension' patients the cause is dural sinus thrombosis, which should be particularly considered in males and non-obese females (Tehindrazanarivelo *et al.* 1992). In these cases, there is seldom propagation of thrombosis into the cerebral veins with venous infarction and focal neurological features. Indeed, the clinical picture seems identical to that of idiopathic benign intracranial hypertension. The prognosis is very good, although a few patients may be left blind due to optic atrophy.

The other common presentation is with an encephalopathy coming on over days, a week or two, or sometimes months. Headache is almost universal and other common features include partial and generalized epileptic seizures, confusion, declining conscious level, papilloedema, and sometimes focal neurological deficits such as hemiparesis and dysphasia. The differential diagnosis is therefore wide, and includes encephalitis, cerebral abscess, subdural empyema, and cerebral vasculitis, as well as metabolic and toxic encephalopathies. In this situation there is widespread and often propagating thrombosis in cerebral veins, as well as, usually, the dural sinuses. Mortality and morbidity are high, although some patients recover spontaneously, even to normal. The main difficulty is to think of the diagnosis at all, often because it may be confused by features which suggest infection (e.g. fever, raised ESR, neutrophil leucocytosis, etc.).

'Strokes' are seldom due to intracranial venous thrombosis, but on occasion a more or less sudden focal neurological deficit can occur as a result of cortical vein thrombosis. There may be progression and fluctuation, more headache than usual for an arterial stroke, rather typically seizures, any infarct on brain imaging is seldom in a typically 'arterial' pattern, and the patients are 'too young' for an ordinary stroke. Migraine and glioma are frequent misdiagnoses. There is a good prognosis (Jacobs *et al.* 1996).

Sudden headache, often with blood in the CSF, is a very rare presentation and clearly can be confused with spontaneous subarachnoid haemorrhage due to aneurysmal rupture (de Bruijn *et al.* 1996). Even isolated cranial nerve palsies have been described with transverse sinus thrombosis (Kuehnen *et al.* 1998).

Cavernous sinus thrombosis is a restricted form of intracranial venous thrombosis, usually due to sepsis spreading from the veins in the face, nose, orbits, or sinuses. In diabetics and immunocompromised hosts, fungal infection can be responsible, particularly mucormycosis. The presentation is with unilateral orbital pain, periorbital oedema, chemosis, proptosis, reduced visual acuity, and papilloedema. The third, fourth, sixth, and upper two divisions of the fifth cranial nerves may be involved. Thrombus may propagate to the other cavernous sinus to cause bilateral signs. Septic meningitis and epidural empyema are occasional complications. The patients are generally severely toxic and ill (Clifford Jones *et al.* 1982; Southwick *et al.* 1986). The differential diagnosis includes severe facial and orbital infection, and carotico-cavernous fistula.

27.11.2 Diagnosis and investigations

Is it intracranial venous thrombosis? So often the diagnosis is not quickly considered but is stumbled on, particularly on brain MRI, after others have been considered and then excluded. The CSF can be normal but usually there is a modest increase in cells (lymphocytes, red blood cells, and perhaps polymorphs) and protein, and almost always an increase in pressure if the venous sinuses are occluded. These changes are, however, very non-specific. There are no oligoclonal bands. The EEG may be slowed bilaterally (even when the clinical picture is unilateral or asymmetrical), with or without epileptic discharges, but again that is hardly specific.

Brain CT is the most helpful initial investigation because, although it can be normal (particularly with the 'benign intracranial hypertension' presentation), there is often evidence of brain swelling, small ventricles, and rarely there is intensification of the dural sinuses or a cerebral vein (Chiras *et al.* 1985). Low-density areas of infarction, but not in the usual arterial territories, may appear and also single or multiple areas of high-density haemorrhagic infarction. There is often a lot of early swelling beyond the boundaries of the hypodense infarct. Sometimes there is subarachnoid blood, which is most unusual in either arterial infarcts or primary intracerebral haemorrhage

(Bakac and Wardlaw 1997). After intravenous contrast there may be gyral, falcine or tentorial enhancement and, occasionally, the 'empty delta' sign (hypodensity in the middle of the posterior part of the superior sagittal sinus representing an area of no filling due to thrombus). Unfortunately, CT is neither sensitive nor specific enough by itself, so if there is any possibility of intracranial venous thrombosis either cerebral angiography or MR must be done, or both.

Cerebral angiography with late venous views is the definitive investigation. There should be total or partial occlusion of at least one dural sinus on two projections (Fig. 27.42). Often there is also occlusion of cerebral veins, late venous emptying, and evidence of venous collateral circulation. A lack of filling of a transverse (lateral) sinus is not due to congenital hypoplasia if there is an appropriate sinus groove and jugular foramen on the plain skull X-ray, or if magnetic resonance venography (MRV) is diagnostic. In obscure subacute encephalopathies, cerebral angiography or MR (see below) should always be done to rule out intracranial venous thrombosis before resorting to brain biopsy.

Magnetic resonance imaging and venography can now provide a definitive diagnosis in most patients, although attention to technique and exclusion of artefacts are essential. MRI can visualize thrombus in the sinuses (Fig. 27.43), less often in the cerebral veins, and is more sensitive than CT in displaying brain parenchymal changes (Bousser and Ross Russell 1997).

What is the cause of the intracranial venous thrombosis? Once the diagnosis of venous thrombosis is made, it is important to consider all the possible causes listed in Table 27.36 and to investigate the patient appropriately. It is probably always worth checking for thrombophilia as a predisposing cause even when a more obvious 'cause' (such as oral contraceptives, pregnancy, etc.) is present (clotting screen, protein C, protein S, antithrombin III, activated protein C resistance (Factor V Leiden), lupus anticoagulant, etc.) (Deschiens *et al.* 1996).

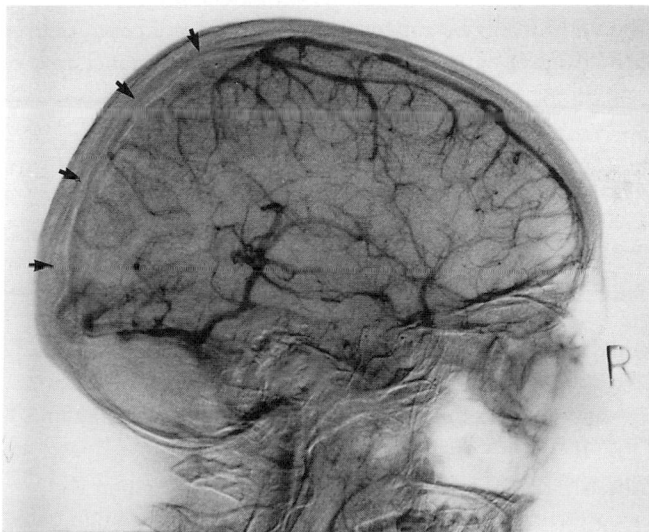

Fig. 27.42. Lateral view of the venous phase of a carotid angiogram showing lack of filling of the superior sagittal sinus (arrows).

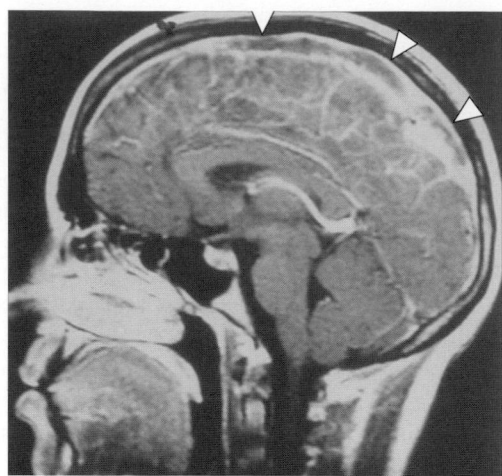

Fig. 27.43. MRI showing venous thrombosis of the sagittal sinus (arrows).

27.11.3 Treatment

The general principles of stroke treatment apply (Sections 27.8.6, 27.8.7). In addition, it seems that immediate and full heparinization is not only surprisingly safe, even in the presence of haemorrhage on brain CT, but also improves the prognosis (Einhaupl *et al.* 1991). However, a recent Dutch trial did not confirm this result (de Bruijn and Stam 1999). Local thrombolytic infusion into the occluded veins is said to be dramatically effective but no real trials have been done and no doubt any disasters have not been published (Kasner *et al.* 1998).

Once the patient is clearly improving, warfarin can be started or substituted for the heparin, and continued for several months. If after withdrawal of warfarin the patient relapses, or has a venous or arterial thrombosis in another site, both of which are unusual, then re-anticoagulation should probably be lifelong. Naturally, any underlying cause should be treated on its merits; for example, patients with a definite thrombophilia should probably be anticoagulated for life, oral contraceptives should never be used again, but a further pregnancy may be safe (Preter *et al.* 1996).

References

Aaslid, R., Lindegaard, K.-F., Sorteberg, W. *et al.* (1989). Cerebral autoregulation dynamics in humans. *Stroke,* **20,** 45–52.

Abbott, R. D., Behrens, G. R., Sharp, D. S. *et al.* (1994). Body mass index and thromboembolic stroke in nonsmoking men in older middle age. The Honolulu Heart Program. *Stroke,* **25,** 2370–6.

Abe, M., Kjellberg, R. N., and Adams, R. (1989). Clinical presentations of vascular malformations of the brain stem: comparison of angiographically positive and negative types. *J. Neurol. Neurosurg. Psychiatry,* **52,** 167–75.

Aberg, H. (1969). Atrial fibrillation. I. A study of atrial thrombosis and systemic embolism in a necropsy material. *Acta Med. Scand.* **185,** 373–9.

Acheson, R. M. and Williams, D. R. R. (1983). Does consumption of fruit and vegetables protect against stroke? *Lancet,* **1,** 1191–3.

Adachi, T., Takagi, M., Hoshino, H. *et al.* (1997). Effect of extracranial carotid artery stenosis and other risk factors for stroke on periventricular hyperintensity. *Stroke,* **28,** 2174–9.

Adams, H. P. and Love, B. B. (1995). Transeosophageal echocardiography in the evaluation of young adults with ischaemic stroke: promises and concerns. *Cerebrovasc. Dis.,* **5,** 323–7.

Adams, H. P., Kassell, N. F., Torner, J. C. *et al.* (1983). CT and clinical correlations in recent aneurysmal subarachnoid haemorrhage: a preliminary report of the Cooperative Aneurysm Study. *Neurology,* **33,** 981–8

Adams, H. P., Kassell, N. F., Torner, J. C. *et al.* (1987). Predicting cerebral ischaemia after aneurysmal subarachnoid haemorrhage: influences of clinical condition, CT results, and antifibrinolytic therapy. A report of the Cooperative Aneurysm Study. *Neurology,* **37,** 1586–91.

Adams, R. J., Nichols, F. T., McKie, V. *et al.* (1988). Cerebral infarction in sickle cell anemia: Mechanism based on CT and MRI. *Neurology,* **38,** 1012–17.

Adams, R. J., Carroll, R. M., Nichols, F. T. *et al.* (1989). Plasma lipoproteins in cortical versus lacunar infarction. *Stroke,* **20,** 448–52.

Adams, R. J., McKie, V. C., Carl, E. M. *et al.* (1997). Long-term stroke risk in children with sickle cell disease screened with transcranial Doppler. *Ann. Neurol.,* **42,** 699–704.

Aessopos, A., Farmakis, D., Karagiorga, M. *et al.* (1997). Pseudoxanthoma elasticum lesions and cardiac complications as contributing factors for strokes in beta-thalassemia patients. *Stroke,* **28,** 2421–4.

Akins, P. T., Glen, S., Nemeth, P. M. *et al.* (1996). Carotid artery thrombus associated with severe iron-deficiency anaemia and thrombocytosis. *Stroke,* **27,** 1002–5.

Akman-Demir, G., Bahar, S., Baykan-Kurt, B. *et al* (1996). Intracranial hypertension in Behcet's disease. *Eur. J. Neurol.,* **3,** 66–70.

Alberts, M. J. (1991). Genetic aspects of cerebrovascular disease. *Stroke,* **22,** 276–80.

Alderman, M. H. (1994). Non-pharmacological treatment of hypertension. *Lancet,* **344,** 307–11.

Alexander, E. L., Provost, T. T., Stevens, M. B. *et al.* (1982). Neurologic complications of primary Sjogren's syndrome. *Medicine,* **61,** 247–57.

Al-Hakim, M., Katirji, M. B., Osorio, I. *et al.* (1993). Cerebral venous thrombosis in paroxysmal nocturnal haemoglobinuria: report of two cases. *Neurology*, **43**, 742–6.

Allen, C. M. C. (1983). Clinical diagnosis of the acute stroke syndrome. *QJM*, **52**, 515–23.

Allen, C. M. C. (1990). Trials and tribulations in speech therapy. At a guess we need more therapists. *BMJ*, **301**, 302–3.

Al-Shahi, R. and Warlow, C. P. (in press). Invited review: A systematic review of the frequency and prognosis of arteriovenous malformations of the brain in adults.

Altinors, N., Senveli, E., Arda, N. *et al.* (1987). Intracerebral haemorrhage and haematoma in Behcet's disease: Case report. *Neurosurgery*, **21**, 582–3.

Amarenco, P. (1991). The spectrum of cerebellar infarctions. *Neurology*, **41**, 973–9.

Amarenco, P. and Caplan, L. R. (1993). Vertebral occlusive disease: review of selected aspects. 3. Mechanisms of cerebellar infarctions. *Cerebrovasc. Dis.*, **3**, 66–73.

Ameriso, S. F., Paganini-Hill, A., Meiselman, H. J. *et al.* (1990). Correlates of middle cerebral artery blood velocity in the elderly. *Stroke*, **21**, 1579–83.

Aminoff, M. J. (1987). Treatment of unruptured cerebral arteriovenous malformations. *Neurology*, **37**, 815–19.

Andersen, G., Vestergaard, K., and Ingeman-Nielsen, M. (1995). Post-stroke pathological crying: frequency and correlation to depression. *Eur. J. Neurol.*, **2**, 45–50.

Anderson, C. S., Taylor, B. V., Hankey, G. J. *et al.* (1994a). Validation of a clinical classification for subtypes of acute cerebral infarction. *J. Neurol. Neurosurg. Psychiatry*, **57**, 1173–9.

Anderson, C. S., Jamrozik, K. D., Broadhurst, R. J. *et al.* (1994b). Predicting survival for 1 year among different subtypes of stroke. Results from the Perth Community Stroke Study. *Stroke*, **25**, 1935–44.

Anderson, D. C., Koller, R. L., Asinger, R. W. *et al.* (1999). Atrial fibrillation and stroke: epidemiology, pathophysiology, and management. *Neurologist*, **4**, 235–58.

Anderson, R. (1988). Quality of life of stroke patients and their carers. In *Living with chronic illness*, (ed. R. Anderson and M. Bury), p. 14. Unwin Hyman, London.

Andreoli, A., di Pasquale, G., Pinelli, G. *et al.* (1987). Subarachnoid haemorrhage: frequency and severity of cardiac arrhythmias. A survey of 70 cases studied in the acute phase. *Stroke*, **18**, 558–64.

Andrews, R. J. (1991). Transhemispheric diaschisis: a review and comment. *Stroke*, **22**, 943–9.

Antiplatelet Trialists' Collaboration (1994). Collaborative overview of randomised trials of antiplatelet therapy I: Prevention of death, myocardial infarction, and stroke by prolonged antiplatelet therapy in various categories of patients. *BMJ*, **308**, 71–2, 81–106.

Antunes, J. L. and Correll, J. W. (1976). Cerebral emboli from intracranial aneurysms. *Surg. Neurol.*, **6**, 7–10.

Anzalone, N. and Landi, G. (1989). Non ischaemic causes of lacunar syndromes: prevalence and clinical findings. *J. Neurol. Neurosurg. Psychiatry*, **52**, 1188–90.

Aoyagi, M., Fukai, N., Yamamoto, M. *et al.* (1996). Early development of intimal thickening in superficial temporal arteries in patients with Moyamoya disease. *Stroke*, **27**, 1750–4.

Appleton, R., Farrell, K., Buncie, J. R. *et al.* (1988). Amaurosis fugax in teenagers. A migraine variant. *Am. J. Dis. Child.*, **142**, 331–3.

Arboix, A., Besses, C., Acin, P. *et al.* (1995). Ischaemic stroke as first manifestation of essential thrombocythemia. Report of six cases. *Stroke*, **26**, 1463–6.

Arboix, A., Garcia-Eroles, L., Massons, J. *et al.* (1996). Predictive factors of in-hospital mortality in 986 consecutive patients with first-ever stroke. *Cerebrovasc. Dis.*, **6**, 161–5.

Argentino C., De Michele M., Fiorelli M. *et al.* (1996). Posterior circulation infarcts simulating anterior circulation stroke: perspective of the acute phase. *Stroke*, **27**, 1306–9.

Arima, T., Motomura, M., Nishiura, Y. *et al.* (1992). Cerebral infarction in a heterozygote with variant antithrombin III. *Stroke*, **23**, 1822–5.

Arruga, J. and Sanders, M. D. (1982). Ophthalmologic findings in 70 patients with evidence of retinal embolism. *Ophthalmology*, **89**, 1336–47.

Arunodaya, G. R., Vani, S., Shankar, S. K. *et al.* (1997). Fibromuscular dysplasia with dissection of basilar artery presenting as 'locked-in-syndrome'. *Neurology*, **48**, 1605–8.

Asplund, K. (1992). Any progress on progressing stroke? *Cerebrovasc. Dis.*, **2**, 317–19.

Asplund, K., Bonita, R., Kuulasmaa, K. *et al.* for the WHO MONICA Project (1995). Multinational comparisons of stroke epidemiology. Evaluation of case ascertainment in the WHO MONICA Stroke Study. *Stroke*, **26**, 355–60.

Astrom, M. (1996). Generalized anxiety disorder in stroke patients. A 3-year longitudinal study. *Stroke*, **27**, 270–5.

Astrup, J., Siesjo, B. K., and Symon, L. (1981). Thresholds in cerebral ischaemia. The ischaemic penumbra. *Stroke*, **12**, 723–5.

Atrial Fibrillation Investigators: Atrial Fibrillation, Aspirin, Anticoagulation Study, Boston Area Anticoagulation Trial for Atrial Fibrillation Study, Canadian Atrial Fibrillation Anticoagulation Study, Stroke Prevention in Atrial Fibrillation Study, and Veterans Affairs Stroke Prevention in Nonrheumatic Atrial Fibrillation Study (1994). Risk factors for stroke and efficacy of antithrombotic therapy in atrial fibrillation. *Arch. Int. Med.*, **154**, 1449–57.

Auer, A., Felber, S., Schmidauer, C. *et al.* (1998). Magnetic resonance angiographic and clinical features of extracranial vertebral artery dissection. *J. Neurol. Neurosurg. Psychiatry*, **64**, 474–81.

Auld, A. W. and Shafey, S. (1976). Transient ischaemic attacks not produced by extracranial vascular disease: a plea to complete and early angiographic investigation. *South. Med. J.*, **69**, 722–4.

Awad, I. A., Carter, P., Spetzler, R. F. *et al.* (1987). Clinical vasospasm after subarachnoid haemorrhage: response to hypervolaemic haemodilution and arterial hypertension. *Stroke*, **18**, 365–72.

Awad, I., Modic, M., Little, J. R. *et al.* (1986). Focal parenchymal lesions in transient ischaemic attacks: correlation of computed tomography and magnetic resonance imaging. *Stroke*, **17**, 399–403.

Ayas, N. and Wijdicks, E. F. M. (1995). Cardiac catherterization complicated by stroke: 14 patients. *Cerebrovasc. Dis.*, **5**, 304–7.

Baglin, T. (1996). Disseminated intravascular coagulation: diagnosis and treatment. *BMJ*, **312**, 683–7.

Bainton, D., Sweetnam, P., Baker, I. *et al.* (1994). Peripheral vascular disease: consequence for survival and association with risk factors in the Speedwell prospective heart disease study. *Br. Heart J.*, **72**, 128–32.

Baird, A. E., Donnan, G. A., Austin, M. C. *et al.* (1995). Early reperfusion in the 'spectacular shrinking deficit' demonstrated by single-photon emission computed tomography. *Neurology*, **45**, 1335–9.

Baird, A. E., Benfield, A., Schlaug, G. *et al.* (1997). Enlargement of human cerebral ischaemic lesion volumes measured by diffusion-weighted magnetic resonance imaging. *Ann. Neurol.*, **41**, 581–9.

Bakac, G. and Wardlaw, J. M. (1997). Problems in the diagnosis of intracranial venous infarction. *Neuroradiology*, **39**, 566–70.

Balarajan, R. (1991). Ethnic differences in mortality from ischaemic heart disease and cerebrovascular disease in England and Wales. *BMJ*, **302**, 560–4.

Ballard, E., Butzer, J. F., and Donders, J. (1996). Susac's syndrome: neuropsychological characteristics in a young man. *Neurology*, **47**, 266–8.

Bamford, J. (1992). Clinical examination in diagnosis and subclassification of stroke. *Lancet*, **339**, 400–2.

Bamford, J. M. and Warlow, C. P. (1988). Evolution and testing of the lacunar hypothesis. *Stroke*, **19**, 1074–82.

Bamford, J., Sandercock, P., Warlow, C. *et al.* (1986). Why are patients with acute stroke admitted to hospital? *BMJ*, **292**, 1369–72.

Bamford, J., Sandercock, P. A. G., Jones, L. *et al.* (1987). The natural history of lacunar infarction: the Oxfordshire Community Stroke Project. *Stroke*, **18**, 545–51.

Bamford, J. M., Sandercock, P. A. G., Dennis, M. *et al.* (1988). A prospective study of acute cerebrovascular disease in the community: the Oxfordshire Community Stroke Project 1981–86. 1. Methodology, demography and incident cases of first-ever stroke. *J. Neurol. Neurosurg. Psychiatry*, **51**, 1373–80.

Bamford, J., Sandercock, P. A. G., Warlow, C. P. *et al.* (1989). Interobserver agreement for the assessment of handicap in stroke patients. *Stroke*, **20**, 828.

Bamford, J., Sandercock, P. A. G., Dennis, M. *et al.* (1990a). A prospective study of acute cerebrovascular disease in the community: the Oxfordshire Community Stroke Project, 1981–86. 2. Incidence, case fatality rates and overall outcome at one year of cerebral infarction, primary intracerebral and subarachnoid haemorrhage. *J. Neurol. Neurosurg. Psychiatry*, **53**, 16–22.

Bamford, J. M., Dennis, M., Sandercock P. A. G. *et al.* (1990b). The frequency, causes and timing of death within 30 days of a first stroke: the Oxfordshire Community Stroke Project. *J. Neurol. Neurosurg. Psychiatry*, **53**, 824–9.

Bamford, J., Sandercock P., Dennis M. *et al.* (1991). Classification and natural history of clinically identifiable subtypes of cerebral infarction. *Lancet*, **337**, 1521–6.

Bang, O. Y., Heo, J. H., Choi, S. A. *et al.* (1997). Large cerebral infarction during praziquantel therapy in neurocysticercosis. *Stroke*, **28**, 211–13.

Barber, P. A., Darby, D. G., Desmond, P. M. *et al.* (1998a). Prediction of stroke outcome with echoplanar perfusion- and diffusion-weighted MRI. *Neurology*, **51**, 418–26.

Barber, P. A., Davis, S. M., Infeld, B. *et al.* (1998b). Spontaneous reperfusion after ischaemic stroke is associated with improved outcome. *Stroke*, **29**, 2522–8.

Barer, D. and Nouri, F. (1989). Measurement of activities of daily living. *Clin. Rehab.*, **3**, 179–87.

Barker, D. J. P. (1995). Fetal origins of coronary heart disease. *BMJ*, **311**, 171–4.

Barnett, H. J. M., Taylor, D. W., Eliasziw, M. *et al.* for the North American Symptomatic Carotid Endarterectomy Trial Collaborators (1998). Benefit of carotid endarterectomy in patients with symptomatic moderate or severe stenosis. *N. Engl. J. Med.*, **339**, 1415–25.

Baron, J. C. (1991). Pathophysiology of acute cerebral ischaemia: PET studies in humans. *Cerebrovasc. Dis.*, **1** (Suppl. 1), 22–31.

Barone, F. C., White, R. F., Spera, P. A. *et al.* (1998). Ischaemic preconditioning and brain tolerance: temporal histological and functional outcomes, protein synthesis requirement, and interleukin-1 receptor antagonist and early gene expression. *Stroke*, **29**, 1937–50.

Barrow, D. L., Spector, R. H., Braun, I. F. *et al.* (1985). Classification and treatment of spontaneous carotid–cavernous sinus fistulas. *J. Neurosurg.*, **62**, 248–56.

Bashir, R. and Jinkins, J. (1985). Cerebral infarction in a young female following snake bite. *Stroke*, **16**, 328–30.

Bassetti, C., Bogousslavsky, J. *et al.* (1993). Sensory syndromes in parietal stroke. *Neurology*, **43**, 1942–9.

Bassetti, C., Bogousslavsky, J., Barth, A. *et al.* (1996). Isolated infarcts of the pons. *Neurology*, **46**, 165–75.

Bassetti, C., Bogousslavsky, J., Mattle, H. *et al.* (1997). Medial medullary stroke: report of seven patients and review of the literature. *Neurology*, **48**, 882–90.

Bath, F. J. and Bath, P. M. W. (1997). What is the correct management of blood pressure in acute stroke? The Blood Pressure in Acute Stroke Collaboration. *Cerebrovasc. Dis.*, **7**, 205–13.

Bath, F. J., Owen, V. E., and Bath, P. M. W. (1998). Quality of full and final publications reporting acute stroke trials: a systematic review. *Stroke*, **29**, 2203–10.

Bathen, J., Sparr, S., and Rokseth, R. (1978). Embolism in sinoatrial disease. *Acta Med. Scand.*, **203**, 7–11.

Baumgartner, R. W., Mattle, H. P., Aaslid, R. *et al.* (1997). Transcranial colour-coded Duplex sonography in arterial cerebrovascular disease. *Cerebrovasc. Dis.*, **7**, 57–63.

Beck, D. O. and Corbett, J. J. (1983). Seizures due to central nervous system rheumatoid meningovasculitis. *Neurology*, **33**, 1058–61.

Becker, K. J. (1998). Inflammation and acute stroke. *Curr. Opin. Neurol.*, **11**, 45–9.

Beetham, R., Fahie-Wilson, M. N., and Park, D. (1998). What is the role of CSF spectrophotometry in the diagnosis of subarachnoid haemorrhage? *Ann. Clin. Biochem.*, **35**, 1–4.

Belchetz, P. E. (1994). Hormonal treatment of postmenopausal women. *N. Engl. J. Med.*, **330**, 1062–71.

Beletsky, V. Y., Kelley, R. E., Fowler, M. *et al.* (1996). Ultrasound densitometric analysis of carotid plaque composition. Pathoanatomic correlation. *Stroke*, **27**, 2173–7.

Bell, B. A., Symon, L., and Branston, N. M. (1985). CBF and time thresholds for the formation of ischaemic cerebral oedema, and effect of reperfusion in baboons. *J. Neurosurg.* **62**, 31–41.

Benavente, O., Moher, D., and Pham, Ba. (1998). Carotid endarterectomy for asymptomatic carotid stenosis: a meta-analysis. *BMJ*, **317**, 1477–80.

Benjamin, E. J., Plehn, J. F., D'Agostino, R. B. *et al.* (1992). Mitral annular calcification and the risk of stroke in an elderly cohort. *N. Engl. J. Med.*, **327**, 374–9.

Bennett, R., Hughes, G. R. V., Bywaters, E. G. L. *et al.* (1972). Neuropsychiatric problems in systemic lupus erythematosus. *BMJ*, **4**, 342–5.

Ben-Shlomo, Y. and Davey Smith, G. (1991). Deprivation in infancy or in adult life: which is more important for mortality risk? *Lancet*, **337**, 530–4.

Berendes, E., Walter, M., Cullen, P. *et al.* (1997). Secretion of brain natriuretic peptide in patients with aneurysmal subarachnoid haemorrhage. *Lancet*, **349**, 245–9.

Bergman, L., van der Meulen, J. H. P., Limburg, M. *et al.* (1995). Cost of medical care after first-ever stroke in the Netherlands. *Stroke*, **26**, 1830–6.

Berkovic, S. F., Bladin, P. F., and Darby, D. G. (1984). Metabolic disorders presenting as stroke. *Med. J. Aust.*, **140**, 421–4.

Berlit, P., Kessler, C., Reuther, R. *et al.* (1984). New aspects of thromboangiitis obliterans (von Winiwarter–Buerger's Disease). *Eur. J. Neurol.*, **23**, 394–9.

Berlit, P., Rakicky, J., and Tornow, K. (1991). Differential diagnosis of spontaneous and traumatic intracranial haemorrhage. *J. Neurol. Neurosurg. Psychiatry*, **54**, 1118.

Berlit, P., Moore, P. M., and Bluestein, H. G. (1993). Vasculitis, rheumatic disease and the neurologist: the pathophysiology and diagnosis of neurologic problems in systemic disease. *Cerebrovasc. Dis.*, **3**, 139–45.

Besson, G., Clavier, I., Hommel, M. *et al.* (1993). Association of lacunar infarcts and intracranial haematomas. *Rev. Neurologique*, **149**, 55–7.

Bhatnagar, D., Anand, I. S., Durrington, P. N. *et al.* (1995). Coronary risk factors in people from the Indian subcontinent living in West London and their siblings in India. *Lancet*, **345**, 405–9.

Bick, R. L. (1993). The antiphospholipid–thrombosis syndromes. Fact, fiction, confusion and controversy. *Am. J. Clin. Pathol.*, **100**, 477–80.

Bickerstaff, E. R. (1964). Aetiology of acute hemiplegia in childhood. *BMJ*, **2**, 82–7.

Biller, J., Johnson, M. R., Adams, H. P. *et al.*. (1986). Echocardiographic evaluation of young adults with nonhaemorrhagic cerebral infarction. *Stroke*, **17**, 608–12.

Bishop, C. C. R., Powell, S., Insall, M *et al.* (1986). Effect of internal carotid artery occlusion on middle cerebral artery blood flow at rest and in response to hypercapnia. *Lancet*, **1**, 710–12.

Bitzer, M. and Topka, H. (1995). Progressive cerebral occlusive disease after radiation therapy. *Stroke*, **26**, 131–6.

Bladin, C. F. and Chambers, B. R. (1993). Clinical features, pathogenesis, and computed tomographic characteristics of internal watershed infarction. *Stroke*, **24**, 1925–32.

Bladin, C. F. and Chambers, B. R. (1994). Frequency and pathogenesis of haemodynamic stroke. *Stroke*, **25**, 2179–82.

Blecic, S. A., Bogousslavsky, J., Van Melle, G. *et al.* (1993). Isolated sensorimotor stroke: a re-evaulation of clinical topographic and aetiological patterns. *Cerebrovasc. Dis.*, 3, 357–63.

Blecic, S., Capel, P., Van Blercom, N. *et al.* (1996). Bilateral posterior cerebral infarction in a young man with a congenital deficit in protein C. *Cerebrovasc. Dis.*, 6, 370–1.

Blesa, R., Mohr, E., Miletich, R. S. *et al.* (1997). Changes in cerebral glucose metabolism with normal aging. *Eur. J. Neurol.*, 4, 8–14.

Bogousslavsky, J. (1991). Topographic patterns of cerebral infarcts: correlation with aetiology. *Cerebrovasc. Dis.*, 1, 61–8.

Bogousslavsky, J. and Caplan, L. R. (1993). Vertebrobasilar occlusive disease: review of selected aspects. 3 Thalamic infarcts. *Cerebrovasc. Dis.*, 3, 193–205.

Bogousslavsky, J. and Regli, F. (1986). Unilateral watershed cerebral infarcts. *Neurology*, 36, 373–7.

Bogousslavsky, J., Hachinski, V. C., Boughner, D. R. *et al.* (1986*a*). Cardiac and arterial lesions in carotid transient ischaemic attack. *Arch. Neurol.*, 43, 223–8.

Bogousslavsky, J., Hachinski, V. C., Boughner, D. R. *et al.* (1986*b*). Clinical predictors of cardiac and arterial lesions in carotid ischaemic attacks. *Arch. Neurol.*, 43, 229–33.

Bogousslavsky, J., Regli, F., and Uske, A. (1987). Leukoencephalopathy in patients with ischaemic stroke. *Stroke*, 18, 896–9.

Bogousslavsky, J., van Melle, G., Regli, F. *et al.* (1990). Pathogenesis of anterior circulation stroke in patients with nonvalvular atrial fibrillation: the Lausanne Stroke Registry. *Neurology*, 40, 1046–50.

Bogousslavksy, J., Regli, F., Uske, A., and Maeder, P. (1991). Early spontaneous haematoma in cerebral infarct: is primary cerebral haemorrhage overdiagnosed? *Neurology*, 41, 837–40.

Bogousslavsky, J., Regli, F., Maeder, P. *et al.* (1993). The aetiology of posterior circulation infarcts: a prospective study using magnetic resonance imaging and magnetic resonance angiography. *Neurology*, 43, 1538–3.

Bogousslavsky, J., Maeder, P., Regli, F. *et al.* (1994). Pure midbrain infarction: clinical syndromes, MRI, and aetiologic patterns. *Neurology*, 44, 2032–40.

Bogousslavsky, J., Garazi, S., Jeanrenaud, X. *et al.* for the Lausanne Stroke with Paradoxal Embolism Study Group (1996). Stroke recurrence in patients with patent foramen ovale: the Lausanne study. *Neurology*, 46, 1301–5.

Bohmfalk, G. L., Story, J. L., Brown, W. E. *et al.* (1979). Subclavian steal syndrome. Part I: Proximal vertebral to common carotid artery transposition in three patients, and historial review. *J. Neurosurg.*, 51, 628–40.

Boiten, J. and Lodder, J. (1991). Lacunar infarcts. Pathogenesis and validity of the clinical syndromes. *Stroke*, 22, 1374–8.

Boiten, J., Rothwell, P. M., Slattery, J. *et al.* for the European Carotid Surgery Trialists' Collaborative Group (1996). Ischaemic lacunar stroke in the European Carotid Surgery Trial. Risk factors, distribution of carotid stenosis, effect of surgery and type of recurrent stroke. *Cerebrovasc. Dis.*, 6, 281–7.

Bonita, R. (1992). Epidemiology of stroke. *Lancet*, 339, 342–4.

Bonita, R. (1994). Epidemiological studies and the prevention of stroke. *Cerebrovasc. Dis.*, 4 (Suppl. 1), 2–10.

Bonita, R. and Beaglehole, R. (1989). Increased treatment of hypertension does not explain the decline in stroke mortality in the United States, 1970–1980. *Hypertension* 13, I-69–73.

Bonita, R. and Beaglehole, R. (1992). Stroke mortality. In *Population based studies of stroke*, (ed. J. P. Whisnant), pp. 1–30. International Medical Review Series, Butterworth, Oxford.

Bonita, R. and Beaglehole, R. (1996). The enigma of the decline in stroke deaths in the United States. The search for an explanation. *Stroke*, 27, 370–2.

Bonita, R. and Thomson, S. (1985). Subarachnoid haemorrhage: epidemiology, diagnosis, management, and outcome. *Stroke*, 16, 591–4.

Bonita, R., Stewart, A., and Beaglehole, R. (1990). International trends in stroke mortality 1970 1985. *Stroke*, 21 989–92.

Bonita, R., Broad, J. B., and Beaglehole, R. (1993). Changes in stroke incidence and case-fatality in Auckland, New Zealand, 1981–1991. *Lancet*, 342, 1470–3.

Bonita, R., Broad, J. B., and Beaglehole, R. (1997). Ethnic differences in stroke incidence and case fatality in Auckland, New Zealand. *Stroke*, 28, 758–61.

Boon, A., Lodder, J., Cheriex, E. *et al.* (1996). Risk of stroke in a cohort of 815 patients with calcification of the aortic valve with or without stenosis. *Stroke*, 27, 847–51.

Borggreve F., De Deyn P. P., Marien P. *et al.* (1994). Bilateral infarction in the anterior cerebral artery vascular territory due to an unusual anomaly of the circle of Willis. *Stroke*, 25, 1279–81.

Bornebroek, M., Westemdorp, R. G. J., Haan, J. *et al.* (1997). Mortality from hereditary cerebral haemorrhage with amyloidosis–Dutch type. The impact of sex, parental transmission and year of birth. *Brain*, 120, 2243–9.

Bornstein, N. M. and Norris, J. W. (1986). Subclavian steal: a harmless haemodynamic phenomenon? *Lancet*, 2, 303–5.

Bornstein, N. M. and Norris, J. W. (1994). Transcranial Doppler sonography is at present of limited clinical value. *Arch. Neurol.*, 51, 1057–9.

Bosma, H., Marmot, M. G., Hemingway, H. *et al.* (1997). Low job control and risk of coronary heart disease in Whitehall II (prosective cohort) study. *BMJ*, **314**, 558–65.

Bots, M. L., van Swieten, J. C., Breteler, M. M. B. *et al.* (1993). Cerebral white matter lesions and atherosclerosis in the Rotterdam study. *Lancet*, **341**, 1232–7.

Bots, M. L., Looman, S. J., Koudstaal, P. J. *et al.* (1996). Prevalence of stroke in the general population. The Rotterdam study. *Stroke*, **27**, 1499–501.

Bourdette, D. N., Rosenberg, N. L., and Yatsu, F. M. (1983). Herpes zoster ophthalmicus and delayed ipsilateral cerebral infarction. *Neurology*, **33**, 1428–32.

Bousser, M.-G. and Ross Russell, R. (1997). *Cerebral venous thrombosis.* Saunders, London.

Bousser, M.-G., Baron, J. C., and Chiras, J. (1985*a*). Ischaemic strokes and migraine. *Neuroradiology* **27**, 583–7.

Bousser, M.-G., Chiras, J., Bories, J. *et al.* (1985*b*). Cerebral venous thrombosis – a review of 38 cases. *Stroke*, **16**, 199–213.

Bova, I. Y., Bornstein, N. M., and Korczyn, A. D. (1996). Acute infection as a risk factor for ischaemic stroke. *Stroke*, **27**, 2204–6.

Bowen, J., Boudoulas, H., and Wooley, C. F. (1987). Cardiovascular disease of connective tissue origin. *Am. J. Med.*, **82**, 481–8.

Bowler, J. V., Wade, J. P. H., Jones, B. E. *et al.* (1995). Contribution of diaschisis to the clinical deficit in human cerebral infarction. *Stroke*, **26**, 1000–6.

Bragoni, M., Di Piero, V., Priori, R. *et al.* (1994). Sjogren's syndrome presenting as ischaemic stroke. *Stroke*, **25**, 2276–9.

Brand, F. N., Abbott, R. D., Kannel, W. B. *et al.* (1985). Characteristics and prognosis of lone atrial fibrillation: 30-year followup in the Framingham study. *J. Am. Med. Assoc.*, **254**, 3449–53.

Brass, L. M., Pavlakis, S. G., DeVivo, D. *et al.* (1988). Transcranial Doppler measurements of the middle cerebral artery. Effect of haematocrit. *Stroke*, **19**, 1466–9.

Brice, J. G., Dowsett, D. J., and Lowe, R. D. (1964). Haemodynamic effects of carotid artery stenosis. *BMJ*, **2**, 1363–6.

Brittain, K. R., Peet, S. M., and Castleden, C. M. (1998). Stroke and incontinence. *Stroke*, **29**, 524–8.

Brockmeier, L. B., Adolph, R. J., Gustin, B. W. *et al.* (1981). Calcium emboli to the retinal artery in calcific aortic stenosis. *Am. Heart J.*, **101**, 32–7.

Broderick, J. P. and Swanson, J. W. (1987). Migraine-related strokes. Clinical profile and prognosis in 20 patients. *Arch. Neurol.*, **44**, 868–71.

Broderick, J. P., Brott, T. G., Duldner, J. E. *et al.* (1994). Initial and recurrent bleeding are the major causes of death following subarachnoid hemorrhage. *Stroke*, **25**, 1342–7.

Bromberg, J. E. C., Rinkel, G. J. E., Algra, A. *et al.* (1995). Subarachnoid haemorrhage in first and second degree relatives of patients with subarachnoid haemorrhage. *BMJ*, **311**, 288–9.

Brott, T., Broderick, J., Kothari, R. *et al.* (1997). Early haemorrhage growth in patients with intracerebral haemorrhage. *Stroke*, **28**, 1–5.

Brouwers, P. J. A.-M., Wijdicks, E. F. M., Hasan, D. *et al.* (1989). Serial electrocardiographic recording in aneurysmal subarachnoid haemorrhage. *Stroke*, **20**, 1162–7.

Brouwers, P. J. A.-M., Wijdicks, E. F. M., and van Gijn, J. (1992). Infarction after aneurysm rupture does not depend on distribution or clearance rate of blood. *Stroke*, **23**, 374–9.

Brown, M. M. (1992). Balloon angioplasty for cerebrovascular disease. *Neurol. Res.*, **14** (Suppl. 1), 59–63.

Brown, M. M. and Marshall, J. (1985). Regulation of cerebral blood flow in response to changes in blood viscosity. *Lancet*, **1**, 604–9.

Brown, M. M., Wade, J. P., and Marshall, J. (1985). Fundamental importance of arterial oxygen content in the regulation of cerebral blood flow in man. *Brain*, **108**, 81–93.

Brown, R. D., Whisnant, J. P., Sicks, J. D. *et al.* (1996*a*). Stroke incidence, prevalence, and survival. Secular trends in Rochester, Minnesota, through 1989. *Stroke*, **27**, 373–80.

Brown, R. D., Wiebers, D. O., Torner, J. C. *et al.* (1996*b*). Incidence and prevalence of intracranial vascular malformations in Olmsted County, Minnesota, 1965 to 1992. *Neurology*, **46**, 949–52.

Brown, R. D., Petty, G. W., O'Fallon, W. M. *et al.* (1998). Incidence of transient ischaemic attack in Rochester, Minnesota, 1985–1989. *Stroke*, **29**, 2109–13.

Brunner, E., Davey Smith, G., Marmot, M. *et al.* (1996). Childhood social circumstances and psychosocial and behavioural factors as determinants of plasma fibrinogen. *Lancet*, **347**, 1008–13.

Bruno, A., Adams, H. P., Biller, J. *et al.* (1988). Cerebral infarction due to moyamoya disease in young adults. *Stroke*, **19**, 826–33.

Bruno, A., Nolte, K. B., and Chapin, J. (1993). Stroke associated with ephedrine use. *Neurology*, **43**, 1313–16.

Buchan, A. and Pulsinelli, W. A. (1990). Hypothermia but not the Nmethyl-D-aspartate antagonist MK-801, attenuates neuronal damage in gerbils subjected to transient global amnesia. *J. Neurosci.* **10**, 311–16.

Burchfiel, C. M., Curb, J. D., Rodriguez, B. L. *et al.* (1994). Glucose intolerance and 22 year stroke incidence. The Honolulu Heart program. *Stroke*, **25**, 951–7.

Burn, J., Dennis, M., Bamford, J. *et al.* (1994). Long-term risk of recurrent stroke after a first-ever stroke. The Oxfordshire Community Stroke Project *Stroke*, **25**, 333–7.

Burn, J., Dennis, M., Bamford, J. *et al.* (1997). Epileptic seizures after a first stroke: the Oxfordshire Community Stroke Project. *BMJ*, **315**, 1582–7.

Burton, J. L. (1988). Livedo reticularis, porcelain-white scars, and cerebral thromboses. *Lancet* 1, 1263–4.

Byar, D. P. and Corle, D. K. (1988). Hormone therapy for prostate cancer: results of the Veterans Administration Cooperative Urological Research Group Studies. *NCI Monographs* 7, 165–70.

Byrne, J. V., Molyneux, A. J., Brennan, R. P *et al.* (1995). Embolisation of recently ruptured intracranial aneurysms. *J. Neurol. Neurosurg. Psychiatry,* **59**, 616–20.

Cabanes, L., Mas, J. L., Cohen, A. *et al.* (1993). Atrial septal aneurysm and patent foramen ovale as risk factors for cryptogenic stroke in patients less than 55 years of age. A study using transoesophageal echocardiography. *Stroke*, **24**, 1865–73.

Candelise, L., Pinardi, G., Morabito, A. *et al.* (1991). Mortality in acute stroke with atrial fibrillation. *Stroke*, **22**, 169–74.

Cantu, C. and Barinagarrementeria, F. (1993). Cerebral venous thrombosis associated with pregnancy and puerperium. Review of 67 cases. *Stroke*, **24**, 1880–4.

Caplan, L. R. (1980). 'Top of the basilar' syndrome. *Neurology*, **30**, 72–9.

Caplan, L. R. (1988). Intracerebral haemorrhage revisited. *Neurology*, **38**, 624–7.

Caplan, L. R. (1992). Intracerebral haemorrhage. *Lancet*, **339**, 656–8.

Caplan, L. R. (1993). Brain embolism, revisited. *Neurology*, **43**, 1281–7.

Caplan, L. R. (1995a). Binswanger's disease – revisited. *Neurology*, **45**, 626–33.

Caplan, L. R. (1995b). Clinical diagnosis of brain embolism. *Cerebrovasc. Dis.*, **5**, 79–88.

Caplan, L. R., Gorelick, P. B., and Hier, D. B. (1986). Race, sex and occlusive cerebrovascular disease: a review. *Stroke*, **17**, 648–55.

Caplan, L. R. and Hennerici, M. (1998). Impaired clearance of emboli (washout) is an important link between hypoperfusion, embolism, and ischaemic stroke. *Arch. Neurol.*, **55**, 1475–82.

Caplan, L. R. and Tettenborn, B. (1992a). Vertebrobasilar occlusive disease: review of selected aspects. 1. Spontaneous dissection of extracranial and intracranial posterior circulation arteries. *Cerebrovasc. Dis.*, **2**, 256–65.

Caplan, L. R. and Tettenborn, B. (1992b). Vertebrobasilar occlusive disease: review of selected aspects 2. Posterior circulation embolism. *Cerebrovasc. Dis.*, **2**, 320–6.

Caplan, L. R. and Sergay, S. (1976). Positional cerebral ischaemia. *J. Neurol. Neurosurg. Psychiatry*, **39**, 385–91.

Caplan, L. R. and Stein R. W. (1986). *Stroke: a clinical approach.* Butterworths, Boston.

Caplan, L. R., Hier, D. B., and Banks, G. (1982). Current concepts of cerebrovascular disease: stroke and drug abuse. *Stroke*, **13**, 869–72.

CAPRIE Steering Committee (1996). A randomised, blinded, trial of clopidogrel versus aspirin in patients at risk of ischaemic events (CAPRIE). *Lancet*, **348**, 1329–39.

Carpenter J. P., Lexa F. J., and Davis J. T. (1996). Determination of duplex Doppler ultrasound criteria appropriate to the North American Symptomatic Carotid Endarterectomy Trial. *Stroke*, **27**, 695–9.

Carrel, T., Laske, A., Jenny, R. *et al.* (1991). Neurological complications associated with acute aortic dissection: is there a place for a surgical approach? *Cerebrovasc. Dis.*, **1**, 296–301.

Carstairs, V. and Morris, R. (1990). Deprivation and health in Scotland. *Hlth Bull.*, **48**, 162–75.

Carty, G. A., Nachtigal, T., Magyar, R. *et al.* (1993). Abdominal duplex ultrasound screening for occult aortic aneurysm during carotid arterial evaluation. *J. Vasc. Surg.*, **17**, 696–702.

Cascino, G. D., Westmoreland, B. F., Swanson, T. H. *et al.* (1991). Seizure-associated speech arrest in elderly patients. *Mayo Clinic Proc.*, **66**, 254–8.

Caselli, R. J., Hunder, G. G., and Whisnant, J. P. (1988). Neurologic disease in biopsy-proven giant cell (temporal) arteritis. *Neurology*, **38**, 352–9.

CAST (Chinese Acute Stroke Trial) Collaborative Group (1997). CAST: randomised placebo-controlled trial of early aspirin use in 20,000 patients with acute ischaemic stroke. *Lancet*, **349**, 1641–9.

Castaigne, P., Lhermitte, F., Gautier, J. C. *et al.* (1973). Arterial occlusions in the vertebro-basilar system. A study of 44 patients with post-mortem data. *Brain*, **96**, 133–54.

Castaigne, P., Lhermitte, F., Buge, A. *et al.* (1981). Paramedian thalamic and midbrain infarcts: clinical and neuropathological study. *Ann. Neurol.*, **10**, 127–48.

Castillo, J., Davalos, A., Marrugat, J. *et al.* (1998). Timing for fever-related brain damage in acute ischaemic stroke. *Stroke*, **29**, 2455–60.

Catala, M., Rancurel, G., Koskas, F. *et al.* (1993). Ischaemic stroke due to spontaneous extracranial vertebral giant aneurysm. *Cerebrovasc. Dis.*, **3**, 322–6.

The CAVITAS Investigators (in press) The carotid and vertebral artery transluminal angioplasty study (CAVITAS): results in patients with carotid artery stenosis randomised between endovascular treatment and surgery. *Lancet.*

Cerebral Embolism Task Force (1989). Cardiogenic brain embolism. The second report of the cerebral embolism task force. *Arch. Neurol.*, **46**, 727–43.

Chabriat, H., Vahedi, K., Iba-Zizen M. T. *et al.* (1995). Clinical spectrum of CADASIL: a study of 7 families. *Lancet*, **346**, 934–9.

Chabriat, H., Levy, C., Taillia, H. *et al.* (1998). Patterns of MRI lesions in CADASIL. *Neurology*, **51**, 452–7.

Challa, V. R., Moody, D. M., and Bell, M. A. (1992). The Charcot–Bouchard aneurysm controversy: impact of a new histologic technique. *J. Neuropath. Exp. Neurol.*, **51**, 264–71.

Chalmers, N. and Campbell, I. W. (1987). Left atrial metastasis presenting as recurrent embolic strokes. *Br. Heart J.*, **58**, 170–2.

Chamorro A., Sacco R. I., Mohr J. P. *et al.* (1991). Clinical-computed tomographic correlations of lacunar infarction in the Stroke Data Bank. *Stroke*, **22**, 175–81.

Chamorro, A., Vila, N., Ascaso, C. *et al.* (1998). Blood pressure and functional recovery in acute ischaemic stroke. *Stroke*, **29**, 1850–3.

Chang, C. L., Donaghy, M., Poulter, N. *et al.* (1999). Migraine and stroke in young women: case-control study. *BMJ*, **318**, 13–18.

Charles, P. J. and Maini, R. N. (1993). The clinical implications of autoantibody detection in rheumatology. *J. R. Coll. Physicians Lond.*, **27**, 358–62.

Chen, S. T., Liu, Y. H., Hsu, C. Y. *et al.* (1988). Moyamoya disease in Taiwan. *Stroke*, **19**, 53–9.

Chen, Z.-M., Sandercock, P.A.G., Pan, H-C. *et al.* on behalf of the CAST and IST Collaborative groups (2000). Indications for early aspirin use in acute ischaemic stroke. A combined analysis of 40,000 randomised patients from the Chinese Acute Stroke Trial and the International Stroke Trial. *Stroke*, **31**, 1240–9.

Cheshire, W. P., Santos, C. C., Massey, E. W. *et al.* (1996). Spinal cord infarction: aetiology and outcome. *Neurology*, **47**, 321–30.

Chesler, E., King, R. A., and Edwards, J. E. (1983). The myxomatous mitral valve and sudden death. *Circulation*, **67**, 632–9.

Chimowitz, M. I., Little, J. R., Awad, I. A. *et al.* (1990). Intracranial hypertension associated with unruptured cerebral arteriovenous malformations. *Ann. Neurol.*, **27**, 474–9.

Chin, P. L., Kaminski, J., and Rout, M. (1977). Myocardial infarction coincident with cerebrovascular accidents in the elderly. *Age Ageing*, **6**, 29–37.

Chiras, J., Bousser, M.-G., Meder, J. F. *et al.* (1985). CT in cerebral thrombophlebitis, *Neuroradiology*, **27**, 145–54.

Chiu, D., Shedden, P., Bratina, P. *et al.* (1998). Clinical features of moyamoya disease in the United States. *Stroke*, **29**, 1347–51.

Chobanian, A. R. (1983). The influence of hypertension and other hemodynamic factors in atherogenesis. *Progr. Cardiovasc. Dis.*, **26**, 177–96.

Chodosh, E. H., Foulkes, M. A., Kase, C. S. *et al.* (1988). Silent stroke in the NINCDS stroke data bank. *Neurology*, **38**, 1674–9.

Chung, C.-S., Caplan, L. R., Han, W. *et al.* (1996). Thalamic haemorrhage. *Brain*, **119**, 1873–86.

Ciafaloni, E., Ricci, E., Shanske, S. *et al.* (1992). MELAS: clinical features, biochemistry, and molecular genetics. *Ann. Neurol.*, **31**, 391–8.

Cillessen, J. P. M., Kappelle, L. J., van Swieten, J. C. *et al.* (1993). Does cerebral infarction after a previous warning occur in the same vascular territory? *Stroke*, **24**, 351–4.

Clifford-Jones, R. E., Ellis, C. J. K., Stevens, J. M. *et al.* (1982). Cavernous sinus thrombosis. *J. Neurol. Neurosurg. Psychiatry*, **45**, 1092–7.

Close, J. B., Evans, D. W., and Bailey, S. M. (1979). Persistent lone atrial fibrillation – its prognosis after clinical diagnosis. *J. R. Coll. General Pract.*, **29**, 547–9.

Cohen, A., Tzourio, C., Chauvel, C. *et al.* for the French Study of Aortic Plaques in Stroke (FAPS) Investigators (1997). Mitral valve strands and the risk of ischaemic stroke in elderly patients. *Stroke*, **28**, 1574–8.

Colditz, G. A., Willett, W. C., Stampfer, M. J. *et al.* (1987). Menopause and the risk of coronary heart disease in women. *N. Engl. J. Med.*, **316**, 1105–10.

Collen, F. M. and Wade, D. T. (1991). Residual mobility problems after stroke. *Int. Dis. Studies*, **13**, 12–15.

Collen, F. M., Wade, D. T., and Bradshaw, C. M. (1990). Mobility after stroke: reliability of measures of impairment and disability. *Int. Dis. Studies*, **12**, 6–9.

Collen, F. M., Wade, D. T., Robb, G. F. *et al.* (1991). The Rivermead Mobility Index: a further development of the Rivermead Motor Assessment. *Int. Dis. Studies*, **13**, 50–4.

Collin, C. and Wade, D. (1990). Assessing motor impairment after stroke: a pilot reliability study. *J. Neurol. Neurosurg. Psychiatry*, **53**, 576–9.

Collins, R. and MacMahon, S. (1994). Blood pressure, antihypertensive drug treatment and the risks of stroke and of coronary heart disease. *Br. Med. Bull.*, **50**, 272–98.

Comabella, M., Alvarez-Sabin, J., Rovira, A. *et al.* (1996). Bromocriptine and postpartum cerebral angiopathy: a causal relationship? *Neurology*, **46**, 1754–6.

Comu, S., Verstraeten, T., Rinkoff, J. S. *et al.* (1996). Neurological manifestations of acute posterior multifocal placoid pigment epitheliopathy. *Stroke*, **27**, 996–1001.

Confavreux, C., Brunet, P., Petiot, P. *et al.* (1994). Congenital protein C deficiency and superior sagittal sinus thrombosis causing isolated intracranial hypertension. *J. Neurol. Neurosurg. Psychiatry*, **57**, 655–7.

Connelly, J. B., Cooper, J. A., and Meade, T. W. (1992). Strenuous exercise, plasma fibrinogen, and factor VII activity. *Br. Heart J.*, **67**, 351–4.

Cook, N. S. and Ubben, D. (1990). Fibrinogen as a major risk factor in cardiovascular disease. *Trends Pharmacol. Sci.*, **11**, 444–51.

Cook, P. J. and Lip, G. Y. H. (1996). Infectious agents and atherosclerotic vascular disease. *QJM*, **89**, 727–35.

Cook, P. J., Honeybourne, D., Lip, G. Y .H. *et al.* (1998). *Chlamydia pneumoniae* antibody titers are significantly associated with acute stroke and transient cerebral ischaemia: the West Birmingham Stroke Project. *Stroke*, **29**, 404–10.

Cormio, M., Robertson, C. S., and Narayan, R. K. (1997). Secondary insults to the injured brain. *J. Clin. Neurosci.*, **4**, 132–48.

Cornhill, J. F., Akins, D., Hutson, M. *et al.* (1980). Localization of atherosclerotic lesions in the human basilar artery. *Atherosclerosis*, **35**, 77–86.

Coronary Drug Project Research Group (1970). The coronary drug project. Initial findings leading to modifications of its research protocol. *J. Am. Med. Assoc.*, **214**, 1303–13.

Corwin, L. E., Wolf, P. A., Kannel, W. B. *et al.* (1982). Accuracy of death certification of stroke: the Framingham study. *Stroke*, **13**, 818–21.

Coulshed, N., Epstein, E. J., McKendrick, C. S. *et al.* (1970). Systemic embolism in mitral valve disease. *Br. Heart J.*, **32**, 26–34.

Counsell, C., Boonyakarnkul, S., Dennis, M. *et al.* (1995). Primary intracerebral haemorrhage in the Oxfordshire Community Stroke Project. 2. Prognosis. *Cerebrovasc. Dis.*, **5**, 26–34.

Counsell, C. and Dennis, M. (in press). Systematic review of prognostic models in patients with acute stroke. *Cerebrovascular Diseases*.

Countee, R. W., Gnanadev, A., and Chavis, P. (1978). Dilated episcleral arteries–a significant physical finding in assessment of patients with cerebrovascular insufficiency. *Stroke*, **9**, 42–5.

Cramer, S. C., Robertson, R. L., Dooling, E. C. *et al.* (1996). Moyamoya and Down syndrome. Clinical and radiological features. *Stroke*, **27**, 2131–5.

Craven, T. E., Ryu, J. E., Espeland, M. A. *et al.* (1990). Evaluation of the associations between carotid artery atherosclerosis and coronary artery stenosis. A case-control study. *Circulation*, **82**, 1230–42.

Crawford, P. M., West, C. R., Chadwick. D. W. *et al.* (1986). Arteriovenous malformations of the brain: natural history in unoperated patients. *J. Neurol. Neurosurg. Psychiatry*, **49**, 1–10.

Cregler, L. L. and Mark, H. (1986). Medical complications of cocaine abuse. *N. Engl. J. Med.*, **315**, 1495–500.

Criqui, M. H., Langer, R. D., Fronek, A. *et al.* (1992). Mortality over a period of 10 years in patients with peripheral arterial disease. *N. Engl. J. Med.*, **326**, 381–6.

Cross, S. S. (1991). How common is cholesterol emoblism? *J. Clin. Pathol.*, **44**, 859–61.

Crouse, J. R., Goldbourt, U., Evans, G. *et al.* for the ARIC Investigators (1996). Risk factors and segment-specific carotid arterial enlargement in the Atherosclerosis Risk in Communities (ARIC) Cohort. *Stroke*, **27**, 69–75.

Curfman, G. D. (1993). The health benefits of exercise: A critical reappraisal. *N. Engl. J. Med.*, **328**, 574–6.

D'Agostino, R. B., Wolf, P. A., Belanger, A. J. *et al.* (1994). Stroke risk profile: adjustment for antihypertensive medication. The Framingham Study. *Stroke*, **25**, 40–3.

Dahl, A., Russell, D., Rootwelt, K. *et al.* (1995). Cerebral vasoreactivity assessed with transcranial Doppler and regional cerebral blood flow measurements. Dose, serum concentration and time course of the response to Acetazolamide. *Stroke*, **26**, 2302–6.

Dahle, C., Vrethem, M., Olsson, J.-E. *et al.* (1995). High level of anticardiolipin antibodies is an unusual finding in an unselected stroke population. *Eur. J. Neurol.*, **2**, 331–6.

Dalal, P. M. and Dalal, K. P. (1989). Cerebrovascular manifestations of infectious disease. In *Handbook of clinical neurology*, (ed. P. J. Vinken, G. W. Bruyn, and H. L. Klawans), pp. 411–41. Elsevier Science Publishers, New York.

Dalal, P. M., Deshpande, C. K., and Daftary, S. G. (1971). Aortic arch syndrome. *Neurology India*, **19**, 155–71.

Daley, R., Mattingly, T. W., Holt, C. L. *et al.* (1951). Systemic arterial embolism in rheumatic heart disease. *Am. Heart J.*, **42**, 566–81.

Damasio, H. (1983). A computed tomographic guide to the identification of cerebral vascular territories. *Arch. Neurol.*, **40**, 138–42.

Danesh, J. and Lewington, S. (1998). Plasma homocysteine and coronary heart disease: systematic review of published epidemiological studies. *J. Cardiovasc. Risk*, **5**, 229–32.

Danesh, J., Collins, R., and Peto, R. (1997). Chronic infections and coronary heart disease: is there a link? *Lancet*, **350**, 430–6.

Danesh, J., Collins, R., Appleby, P. *et al.* (1998). Association of fibrinogen, C-reactive protein, albumin, or leukocyte count with coronary heart disease: meta-analyses of prospective studies. *JAMA*, **279**, 1477–82.

Daniel, W. G. and Mugge, A. (1995). Transeosophageal echocardiography. *N. Engl. J. Med.*, **332**, 1268–79.

Daras, M., Tuchman, A. J., and Marks, S. (1991). Central nervous system infarction related to cocaine abuse. *Stroke*, **22**, 1320–5.

Darby, D. G., Donnan, G. A., Saling, M. A. *et al.* (1988). Primary intraventricular haemorrhage: clinical and neuropsychological findings in a prospective stroke series. *Neurology*, **38**, 68–75.

Davenport, R. J., Dennis, M. S., and Warlow, C. P. (1996*a*). Effect of correcting outcome data for case mix: an example from stroke medicine. *BMJ*, **312**, 1503–5.

Davenport, R. J., Dennis, M. S., Wellwood, I. *et al.* (1996*b*). Complications after acute stroke. *Stroke*, **27**, 415–20.

Davenport, R. J., Dennis, M. S., and Warlow, C. P. (1996*c*). Gastrointestinal hemorrhage after acute stroke. *Stroke*, **27**, 421–4.

Davey Smith, G., Hart, C., Blane, D. *et al.* (1997). Lifetime socioeconomic position and mortality: prospective observational study. *BMJ*, **314**, 547–52.

Davey Smith, G., Neaton, J. D., Wentworth, D. *et al.* for the MRFIT Research Group (1998). Mortality differences between black and white men in the USA: contribution of income and other risk factors among men screened. *Lancet*, **351**, 934–9.

Davidson, N. E. (1995). Hormone replacement therapy – breast versus heart versus bone. *N. Engl. J. Med.*, **332**, 1638–9.

Davidson, S. and Falconer, M. A. (1973). Cerebral arteriovenous malformation causing cardiac enlargement and epilepsy: correction after operation. *BMJ*, **2**, 754–5.

Davies, K. N. and Humphrey, P. R. (1993). Complications of cerebral angiography in patients with symptomatic carotid territory ischaemia screened by carotid ultrasound. *J. Neurol. Neurosurg. Psychiatry*, **56**, 967–72.

Davies, M. J. (1997). The composition of coronary-artery plaques. *N. Engl. J. Med.*, **336**, 1312–14.

Davies-Jones, G. A. B. (1995). Neurological manifestations of haematological disorders. In *Neurology and general medicine*, (2nd edn), (ed. M. J. Aminoff), pp. 219–45. Churchill Livingstone, New York.

Daviglus, M. L., Stamler, J., Orencia, A. J. *et al.* (1997). Fish consumption and the 30-year risk of fatal myocardial infarction. *N. Engl. J. Med.*, **336**, 1046–53.

Davis, J. M. and Zimmerman, R. A. (1983). Injury of the carotid and vertebral arteries. *Neuroradiology*, **25**, 55–69.

Dean, C. M. and Shepherd, R. B. (1997). Task-related training improves performance of seated reaching tasks after stroke. A randomised controlled trial. *Stroke*, **28**, 722–8.

Dearden, N. M. (1985). Ischaemic brain. *Lancet* **2**, 255–9.

De Bono, D. P. and Warlow, C. P. (1979). Mitral-annulus calcification and cerebral or retinal ischaemia. *Lancet*, **2**, 383–5.

De Bono, D. P. and Warlow, C. P. (1981). Potential sources of emboli in patients with presumed transient cerebral or retinal ischaemia. *Lancet*, **1**, 343–5.

De Bray, J. M., Penisson-Besnier, I., Dubas, F. *et al.* (1997). Extracranial and intracranial vertebrobasilar dissections: diagnosis and prognosis. *J. Neurol. Neurosurg. Psychiatry*, **63**, 46–51.

De Bruijn, S. F. T. M. and Stam, J. (1999). Randomised, placebo controlled trial of anticoagulant treatment with low molecular weight heparin for cerebral sinus thrombosis. *Stroke*, **30**, 484–8.

De Bruijn, S. F. T. M., Stam, J. and Kappelle, L. J. for the CVST Study Group (1996). Thunderclap headache as first symptom of cerebral venous sinus thrombosis. *Lancet*, **348**, 1623–5.

Dec, G. W. and Fuster, V. (1994). Idiopathic dilated cardiomyopathy. *N. Engl. J. Med.*, **331**, 1564–75.

De Haan, R., Aaronson, N., Limburg, M. *et al.* (1993). Measuring quality of life in stroke. *Stroke*, **24**, 320–7.

De Keyser, J. (1998). Antipyretics in acute ischaemic stroke. *Lancet*, **352**, 6–7.

de la Monte, S. M., Hutchins, G. M., and Gupta, P. K. (1983). Polymorphous meningitis with atypical mononuclear cells in Sjogren's syndrome. *Ann. Neurol.*, **14**, 455–61.

Del Brutto, O. H. (1992). Cysticercosis and cerebrovascular disease: a review. *J. Neurol. Neurosurg. Psychiatry*, **55**, 252–4.

Del Sette, M., Angeli, S., Stara, I. *et al.* (1997). Microembolic signals with serial transcranial Doppler monitoring in acute focal ischaemic deficit. A local phenomenon. *Stroke*, **28**, 1310–13.

Del Zoppo, G. J., von Kummer, R., and Hamann, G. F. (1998). Ischaemic damage of brain microvessels: inherent risks for thrombolytic treatment in stroke . *J. Neurol. Neurosurg. Psychiatry*, **65**, 1–9.

Dennis, M. S. (1985). Neurological complications of pulmonary arteriovenous malformations. *BMJ*, **289**, 1392–3.

Dennis, M. and Warlow C. P. (1992). Migraine aura without headache: transient ischaemic attack or not? *J. Neurol. Neurosurg. Psychiatry*, **55**, 437–40.

Dennis, M., Bamford, J. M., Molyneux, A. J. *et al.* (1987). Rapid resolution of signs of primary intracerebral haemorrhage in computed tomograms of the brain. *BMJ*, **295**, 379–81.

Dennis, M., Bamford, J., Sandercock, P. *et al.* (1989). A comparison of risk factors and prognosis for transient ischaemic attacks and minor ischaemic strokes. The Oxfordshire Community Stroke Project. *Stroke*, **20**, 1494–9.

Dennis, M., Bamford, J. M., Sandercock, P. *et al.* (1990*a*). Computed tomography in patients with transient ischaemic attacks: when is a transient ischaemic attack not a transient ischaemic attack but a stroke? *J. Neurol.*, **237**, 257–61.

Dennis, M., Bamford, J., Sandercock, P. *et al.* (1990*b*). The prognosis of transient ischaemic attacks in the Oxfordshire community stroke project. *Stroke*, **21**, 848–53.

Dennis, M. S., Burn, J. P., Sandercock, P. A. *et al.* (1993). Long-term survival after first-ever stroke: the Oxfordshire Community Stroke Project. *Stroke*, **24**, 796–800.

Dennis, M. S., O'Rourke, S., Slattery, J. *et al.* (1997*a*). Evaluation of a stroke family care worker: results of a randomised controlled trial. *BMJ*, **314**, 1071–7.

Dennis, M., Wellwood, I., and Warlow, C. (1997*b*). Are simple questions a valid measure of outcome after stroke? *Cerebrovasc. Dis.*, **7**, 22–7.

Dennis, M., Wellwood, I., O'Rourke, S. *et al.* (1997*c*). How reliable are simple questions in assessing outcome after stroke? *Cerebrovasc. Dis.*, **7**, 19–21.

Dennis, M., O'Rourke, S., Lewis, S. *et al.* (1998). A quantitative study of the emotional outcome of people caring for stroke survivors. *Stroke*, **29**, 1867–72.

De Reuck, J., Decoo, D., Jansen, H. *et al.* (1997). Positron emission tomographic study of contralateral hemispheric hypometabolism in middle cerebral artery infarction. *Cerebrovasc. Dis.*, **7**, 43–7.

Derlon, J. M., Bouvard, G., Viader, F. *et al.* (1992). Impaired cerebral hemodynamics in internal carotid occlusion. *Cerebrovasc. Dis.*, **2**, 72–81.

Derouesne, C., Cambon, H., Yelnik, A. *et al.* (1993). Infarcts in the middle cerebral artery territory. Pathological study of the mechanisms of death. *Acta Neurol. Scand.*, **87**, 361–6.

Desai, B. and Toole, J. F. (1975). Kinks, coils, and carotids: A review. *Stroke* **6**, 649–53.

Desantis, A., Laiacona, M., Barbarotto, R. *et al.* (1989). Neuropsychological outcome of patients operated upon for an intracranial aneurysm: analysis of general prognostic factors and of the effects of the location of the aneurysm. *J. Neurol. Neurosurg. Psychiatry*, **52**, 1135–40.

Deschiens, M.-A., Conard, J., Horellou, M. H. *et al.* (1996). Coagulation studies, factor V Leiden, and anticardiolipin antibodies in 40 cases of cerebral venous thrombosis. *Stroke*, **27**, 1724–30.

Deveikis, J. P. (1998). Endovascular therapy of intracranial arteriovenous malformations. Materials and techniques. *Neuroimaging Clin. North Am.*, **8**, 401–24.

Devinsky, O., Petito, C. K., and Alonso, D. R. (1988). Clinical and neuropathological findings in systemic lupus erythematosus: the role of vasculitis, heart emboli, and thrombotic thrombocytopenic purpura. *Ann. Neurol.*, **23**, 380–4.

Devlin, T., Gray, L., Allen, N. B. *et al.* (1995). Neuro–Behcet's disease: factors hampering proper diagnosis. *Neurology*, **45**, 1754–7.

DeWeese, J. A., May, A. G., Lipchik, E. O. *et al.* (1970). Anatomic and haemodynamic correlations in carotid artery stenosis. *Stroke*, **1**, 149–57.

Dey, A. B., Stout, N. R., and Kenny, R. A. (1996). Cardiovascular syncope is the commonest cause of drop attacks in the older patient. *Eur. J. Cardiac Pacing Electrophysiol.*, **6**, 84–8.

Dichgans, M., Mayer, M., Uttner, I. *et al.* (1998). The phenotypic spectrum of CADASIL: clinical findings in 102 cases. *Ann. Neurol.*, **44**, 731–9.

Dickinson, J. P. and Prentice, C. R. M. (1998). Aspirin: benefit and risk in thromboprophylaxis. *QJM*, **91**, 523–38.

Diener, H. C., Cunha, L., Forbes, C. *et al.* (1996). European Stroke Prevention Study. 2. Dipyridamole and acetylsalicylic acid in the secondary prevention of stroke. *J. Neurol. Sci.*, **143**, 1–13.

Di Pasquale, G., Andreoli, A., Pinelli, G. *et al.* (1986). Cerebral ischaemia and asymptomatic coronary artery disease: A prospective study of 83 patients. *Stroke*, **17**, 1098–101.

Di Pasquale, G., Urbinati, S., and Pinelli, G. (1995). New echocardiographic markers of embolic risk in atrial fibrillation. *Cerebrovasc. Dis.*, **5**, 315–22.

Dobyns, W. B. and Garg, B. P. (1991). Vascular abnormalities in epidermal nevus syndrome. *Neurology*, **41**, 276–8.

D'Olhaberriague, L., Arboix, A., Marti-Vilalta, J. L. *et al.* (1995). Movement disorders in ischaemic stroke: clinical study of 22 patients. *Eur. J. Neurol.*, **2**, 553–7.

Doll, R. (1997). One for the heart. *BMJ*, **315**, 1664–8.

Doll, R., Peto, R., Wheatley, K. *et al.* (1994). Mortality in relation to smoking: 40 years' observations on male British doctors. *BMJ*, **309**, 901–11.

Dombovy, M. L., Sandok, B. A., and Basford, J. R. (1986). Rehabilitation for stroke: A review. *Stroke*, **17**, 363–9.

Dombovy, M. L., Basford, J. R., Whisnant, J. P. *et al.* (1987). Disability and use of rehabilitation services following stroke in Rochester, Minnesota, 1975–1979. *Stroke* **18**, 830–6.

Donahue, R. P., Abbott, R. D., Reed, D. M. *et al.* (1986). Alcohol and hemorrhagic stroke, The Honolulu Heart Program. *J. Am. Med. Assoc.*, **255**, 2311–14.

Donnan G. A., Tress B. M., and Bladin P. F. (1982). A prospective study of lacunar infarction using computerised tomography. *Neurology*, **32**, 49–56.

Donnan, G. A., You, R., Thrift, A. *et al.* (1993). Smoking as a risk factor for stroke. *Cerebrovasc. Dis.*, **3**, 129–38.

Donnan, G. A., O'Malley, H. M., Quang, L. *et al.* (1996). The capsular warning syndrome: the high risk of early stroke. *Cerebrovasc. Dis.*, **6**, 202–7.

Dorman, P., Slattery, J., Farrell, B. *et al.* for the United Kingdom Collaborators in the International Stroke Trial (1998). Qualitative comparison of the reliability of health status assessments with the EuroQol and SF-36 questionnaires after stroke. *Stroke*, **29**, 63–8.

Douglas, A. S., Allan, T. M., and Rawles, J. M. (1991). Composition of seasonality of disease. *Scott. Med. J.*, **36**, 76–82.

Drake, M. E. (1982). Winiwarter–Buerger Disease ('Thromboangiitis obliterans') with cerebral involvement. *JAMA*, **248**, 1870–2.

Drislane, F. W. and Wang, A.-M. (1997). Multifocal cerebral haemorrhage in eclampsia and severe pre-eclampsia. *J. Neurol.*, **244**, 194–8.

Drug and Therapeutics Bulletin (1996). Management of hyperlipidaemia. *Drug Ther. Bull.*, **34**, 89–93.

Drug and Therapeutics Bulletin (1997). Which prophylactic aspirin? *Drug Ther. Bull.*, **35**, 7–8.

Drury, I., Whisnant, J. P., and Garraway, W. M. (1984). Primary intracerebral hemorrhage: impact of CT on incidence. *Neurology*, **34**, 653–7.

Duffy, G. P. (1982). Lumbar puncture in spontaneous subarachnoid haemorrhage. *BMJ*, **285**, 1163–4.

Duguid, J. B. (1976). *The dynamics of atherosclerosis.* Aberdeen University Press, Aberdeen.

Duncan, P. W., Goldstein, L. B., Horner, R. D. *et al.* (1994). Similar motor recovery of upper and lower extremities after stroke. *Stroke*, **25**, 1181–8.

Dunne, J. W., Chakera, T., and Kermode, S. (1987). Cerebellar haemorrhage – diagnosis and treatment: A study of 75 consecutive cases. *QJM*, **64**, 739–54.

Duong, D. H., Young, W. L., Vang, M. C. *et al.* (1998). Feeding artery pressure and venous drainage pattern are primary determinants of haemorrhage from cerebral arteriovenous malformations. *Stroke*, **29**, 1167–76.

Dutch TIA Trial Study Group (1991). A comparison of two doses of Aspirin (30 mg vs. 283 mg a day) in patients after a transient ischaemic attack or minor ischaemic stroke. *N. Engl. J. Med.*, **325**, 1261–6.

Dyken, M. E. and Biller, J. (1994). Peripartum cardiomyopathy and stroke. *Cerebrovasc. Dis.*, **4**, 325–8.

Eastern Stroke and Coronary Heart Disease Collaborative Research Group (1998). Blood pressure, cholesterol and stroke in Eastern Asia. *Lancet*, **352**, 1801–7.

Ebrahim, S. (1990). *Clinical epidemiology of stroke.* Oxford University Press, Oxford.

EC-IC Bypass Study Group (1985). Failure of extracranial–intracranial arterial bypass to reduce the risk of ischaemic stroke: results of an international randomised trial. *N. Engl. J. Med.*, **313**, 1191–200.

Eckert, B., Zanella, F. E., Thie, A. *et al.* (1996). Angioplasty of the internal carotid artery: results, complications and follow-up in 61 cases. *Cerebrovasc. Dis.*, **6**, 97–105.

Edelman, R. R. and Warach, S. (1993). Magnetic resonance imaging (first of two parts). *N. Engl. J. Med.*, **328**, 708–16.

Edmans, J. A. and Lincoln, N. B. (1989). Treatment of visual perceptual deficits after stroke: four single case studies. *Int. Dis. Studies*, **11**, 25–33.

Effective Health Care (1992). No. 2: *Stroke rehabilitation.* University of Leeds, Leeds.

Effective Health Care (1995). Vol. 2, No. 1: *The prevention and treatment of pressure sores.* Churchill Livingstone, Edinburgh.

Einhaupl, K. M., Villringer, A., Meister, W. *et al.* (1991). Heparin treatment in sinus venous thrombosis. *Lancet*, **338**, 597–600.

Elgersma, O. E. H., Van Leersum, M., Buijs, P. C. *et al.* (1998). Changes over time in optimal duplex threshold for the identification of patients eligible for carotid endarterectomy. *Stroke*, **29**, 2352–6.

Elliott, P., Stamler, J., Nichols, R. *et al.* for the Intersalt Cooperative Research Group (1996). Intersalt revisited: further anlsyses of 24 hour sodium excretion and blood pressure within and across populations. *BMJ*, **312**, 1249–53.

Elliott, W. J. (1998). Circadian variation in the timing of stroke onset: a meta-analysis. *Stroke*, **29**, 992–6.

Enderby, P. M., Wood, V. A., Wade, D. T. *et al.* (1986). The Frenchay Aphasia Screening Test: a short simple test for aphasia appropriate for non-specialists. *Int. Rehabil. Med.*, **8**, 166–70.

Enevoldson, T. P. and Ross Russell, R. W. (1990). Cerebral venous thrombosis: new causes for an old syndrome? *QJM*, **77**, 1255–75.

Ernst, E. (1990). A review of stroke rehabilitation and physiotherapy. *Stroke*, **21**, 1081–5.

Ernst, E. and Resch, K. L. (1993). Fibrinogen as a cardiovascular risk factor: A meta-analysis and review of the literature. *Ann. Intern. Med.*, **118**, 956–63.

Ernst, E., Hammerschmidt, D. E., Bagge, U. *et al.* (1987). Leukocytes and the risk of ischaemic diseases. *J. Am. Med. Assoc.*, **257**, 2318–24.

European Atrial Fibrillation Trial Study Group (1993). Secondary prevention in non-rheumatic atrial fibrillation after transient ischaemic attack or minor stroke. *Lancet*, **342**, 1255–62.

European Atrial Fibrillation Trial Study Group (1995). Optimal oral anticoagulant therapy in patients with nonrheumatic atrial fibrillation and recent cerebral ischemia. *N. Engl. J. Med.*, **333**, 5–10.

European Carotid Surgery Trialists' Collaborative Group (1995). Risk of stroke in the distribution of an asymptomatic carotid artery. *Lancet*, **345**, 209–12.

European Carotid Surgery Trialists' Collaborative Group (1998). Randomised trial of endarterectomy for recently symptomatic carotid stenosis: final results of the MRC European Carotid Surgery Trial (ECST). *Lancet* **351**, 1379–87.

Evans, J. G. (1987). Blood pressure and stroke in an elderly English population. *J. Epidemiol. Community Hlth*, **41**, 275–82.

Evans, R. L., Matlock, A.-L., Bishop, D. S. *et al.* (1988). Family intervention after stroke: Does counseling or education help? *Stroke*, **19**, 1243–9.

Evers, S. M. A. A., Engel, G. L., and Ament, A. J. H. A. (1997). Cost of stroke in The Netherlands from a societal perspective. *Stroke*, **28**, 1375–81.

Fabian, R. H. and Peters, B. H. (1984). Neurological complications of haemoglobin SC disease. *Arch. Neurol.*, **41**, 289–92.

Farah, S., Al-Shubaili, A., Montaser, A. *et al.* (1998). Behcet's syndrome: a report of 41 patients with emphasis on neurological manifestations. *J. Neurol. Neurosurg. Psychiatry*, **64**, 382–4.

Farrell, B., Godwin, J., Richards, S. *et al.* (1991). The United Kingdom transient ischaemic attack (UK-TIA) aspirin trial: final results. *J. Neurol. Neurosurg. Psychiatry*, **54**, 1044–54.

Farrell, M. A., Gilbert, J. J., and Kaufman, J. C. E. (1985). Fatal intracranial arterial dissection: clinical pathological correlation. *J. Neurol. Neurosurg. Psychiatry*, **48**, 111–21.

Faught, E. (1993). Current role of electroencephalography in cerebral ischaemia. *Stroke*, **24**, 609–13.

Fearnley, J. M., Stevens, J. M., and Rudge, P. (1995). Superficial siderosis of the central nervous system. *Brain*, **118**, 1051–66.

Feigin, V. L. and Wiebers, D. O. (1997). Environmental factors and stroke: a selective review. *J. Stroke Cerebrovasc. Dis.*, **6**, 108–13.

Feigin, V. L., Wiebers, D. O., Whisnant, J. P. *et al.* (1995). Stroke incidence and 30-day case-fatality rates in Novosibirsk, Russia, 1982 through 1992. *Stroke*, **26**, 924–9.

Feigin, V. L., Rinkel, G. J. E., Algra, A. *et al.* (1998). Calcium antagonists in patients with aneurysmal subarachnoid haemorrhage: a systematic review. *Neurology*, **50**, 876–83.

Feinberg, W. M. and Swenson, M. R. (1988). Cerebrovascular complications of L-asparaginase therapy. *Neurology*, **38**, 127–33.

Feldenzer, J. A., Bueche, M. J., Venes, J. L. *et al.* (1987). Superior sagittal sinus thombosis with infarction in sickle cell trait. *Stroke*, **18**, 656–60.

Feldman, E., Daneault, N., Kwan, E. *et al.* (1990). Chinese–white differences in the distribution of occlusive cerebrovascular disease. *Neurology*, **40**, 1541–5.

Feldmann, E. and Levine, S. R. (1995). Cerebrovascular disease with antiphospholipid antibodies: immune mechanisms, significance, and therapeutic options. *Ann. Neurol.*, **37**(S1), S114–S130.

Ferro, J. M. and Pinto, A. N. (1994). Sexual activity is a common precipitant of subarachnoid haemorrhage. *Cerebrovasc. Dis.*, **4**, 375.

Feys, H. M., De Weerdt, W. J., Selz, B. E. *et al.* (1998). Effect of a therapeutic intervention for the hemiplegic upper limb in the acute phase after stroke: a single-blind, randomised, controlled multicenter trial. *Stroke*, **29**, 785–92.

Fibrinolytic Therapy Trialists' (FTT) Collaborative Group (1994). Indications for fibrinolytic therapy in suspected acute myocardial infarction: collaborative overview of early mortality and major morbidity results from all randomised trials of more than 1000 patients. *Lancet*, **343**, 311–22.

Fields, W. S., Bruetman, M. E., and Weibel, J. W. (1985). *Collateral circulation of the brain*. Williams and Wilkins, Baltimore.

Fieschi, C. and Lenzi, G. L. (1983). Cerebral blood flow and metabolism in stroke. In *Vascular disease of the central nervous system*, (ed. R. W. Ross Russell), pp. 101–27. Churchill Livingstone, Edinburgh.

Fieschi, C., Argentino, C., Lenzi, G. L. *et al.* (1989). Clinical and instrumental evaluation of patients with ischaemic stroke within the first six hours. *J. Neurol. Sci.*, **91**, 311–22.

Fine, M. J., Kapoor, W., and Falanga, V. (1987). Cholesterol crystal embolisation: a review of 221 cases in the English literature. *Angiology*, **38**, 769–84.

Fine-Edelstein, J. S., Wolf, P. A., O'Leary, D. H. *et al.* (1994). Precursors of extracranial carotid atherosclerosis in the Framingham Study. *Neurology*, **44**, 1046–50.

Fisher, C. M. (1951). Occlusion of the internal carotid artery. *Arch. Neurol. Psychiatry*, **65**, 346–77.

Fisher, C. M. (1954). Occlusion of the carotid arteries. *Arch. Neurol. Psychiatry*, **72**, 187–204.

Fisher, C. M. (1979). Capsular infarcts – the underlying vascular lesions. *Arch. Neurol. Psychiatry*, **36**, 65–73.

Fisher, C. M. (1982). Pure sensory stroke and allied conditions. *Stroke*, **13**, 434–47.

Fisher, C. M. (1991). Lacunar infarcts – a review. *Cerebrovasc. Dis.*, **1**, 311–20.

Fisher, C. M. and Caplan, L. R. (1971). Basilar artery branch occlusion: A cause of pontine infarction. *Neurology*, **21**, 900–5.

Fisher, M. and Fieman, S. (1990). Geometric factors of the bifurcation in carotid atherogenesis. *Stroke*, **21**, 267–71.

Fisher, M., Davidson, R. I., and Marcus, E. M. (1980). Transient focal cerebral ischaemia as a presenting manifestation of unruptured cerebral aneurysms. *Ann. Neurol.*, **8**, 367–72.

Fisher, M., Sacoolidge, J. C., and Taylor, C. R. (1987). Patterns of fibrin deposits in carotid artery plaques. *Angiology* **38**, 393–9.

FitzGerald, G. A. (1987). Dipyridamole. *N. Engl. J. Med.*, **316**, 1247–57.

Fledmann, E. and Levine, S. R. (1995). Cerebrovascular disease with antiphospholipid antibodies: Immune mechanisms, significance, and therapeutic options. *Ann. Neurol.*, **37**, S114–S130.

Flegel, K. M., Shipley, M. J., and Rose, G. (1987). Risk of stroke in nonrheumatic atrial fibrillation. *Lancet*, **1**, 526–9.

Flickinger, J. C., Kondziolka, D., Pollock, B. E. *et al.* (1998). Radiosurgical management of intracranial vascular malformations. *Neuroimaging Clin. North Am.*, **8**, 483–92.

Florey, C. du V., Senter, M. G., and Acheson, R. M. (1969). A study of the validity of the diagnosis of stroke in mortality data. II Comparison by computer of autopsy and clinical records with death certificates. *Am. J. Epidemiol.*, **89**, 15–24.

Fogelholm, R., Avikainen, S., and Murros, K. (1997). Prognostic value and determinants of first-day mean arterial pressure in spontaneous supratentorial intracerebral haemorrhage. *Stroke*, **28**, 1396–400.

Folsom, A. R., Prineas, R. J., Kaye, S. A. *et al.* (1990). Incidence of hypertension and stroke in relation to body fat distribution and other risk factors in older women. *Stroke*, **21**, 701–6.

Ford, R. G. and Siekert, R. G. (1965). Central nervous system manifestations of periarteritis nodosa. *Neurology*, **15**, 114–22.

Forsyth, P. D. and Dolan, D. (1995). Activated protein C resistance in cases of cerebral infarction. *Lancet*, **345**, 795.

Fourestie, V., Douceron, H., Brugieres, P, *et al.* (1993). Neurotrichinosis. A cerebrovascular disease associated with myocardial infarction and hypereosinophilia. *Brain*, **116**, 603–16.

Frackowiak, R. S. J. (1986). PET scanning: can it help resolve management issues in cerebral ischaemic disease? *Stroke*, **17**, 803–7.

Frackowiak, R. S. J., Jones, T., Lenzi, G. L. *et al.* (1980). Regional cerebral oxygen utilization and blood flow in normal man using oxygen-15 and positron emission tomography. *Acta Neurol. Scand.*, **62**, 336–44.

Franks, P. J., Adamson, C., Bulpitt, P. F. *et al.* (1991). Stroke death and unemployment in London. *J. Epidemiol. Community Hlth*, **45**, 16–18.

Fredericks, R. K., Lefkowitz, D. S., Challa, V. R. *et al.* (1991). Cerebral vasculitis associated with cocaine abuse. *Stroke*, **22**, 1437–9.

Freitag, H., Zeumer, H., Nahser, H. C. *et al.* (1992). Intracranial dural fistulae. Diagnostic and therapeutical considerations. *Cerebrovasc. Dis.*, **2**, 145–51.

Friedman, G. D., Loveland, D. B., and Ehrlich, S. P. (1968). Relationship of stroke to other cardiovascular disease. *Circulation*, **38**, 533–41.

Frisoni. G. B. and Anzola, G. P. (1991). Vertebrobasilar ischaemia after neck motion. *Stroke*, **22**, 1452–60.

Frost, C. D., Law, M. R., and Wald, N. J. (1991). By how much does dietary salt reduction lower blood pressure? II – Analysis of observational data within populations. *BMJ*, **302**, 815–18.

Furlan, A. J., Whisnant, J. P., and Kearns, T. P. (1979). Unilateral visual loss in bright light. An unusual symptom of carotid artery occlusive disease. *Arch. Neurol.*, **36**, 675–6.

Furlan, M., Marchal, G., Viader, F. *et al.* (1996). Spontaneous neurological recovery after stroke and the fate of the ischaemic penumbra. *Ann. Neurol.*, **40**, 216–26.

Furst, H., Hartl, W. H., Jansen, I. *et al.* (1992). Colour-flow Doppler sonography in the identification of ulcerative plaques in patients with high-grade carotid artery stenosis. *Am. J. Neuroradiol.*, **13**, 1581–7.

Fuster, V., Badimon, L., Badimon, J. J. *et al.* (1992*a*). The pathogenesis of coronary artery disease and the acute coronary syndromes (first of two parts). *N. Engl. J. Med.*, **326**, 242–50.

Fuster, V., Badimon, L., Badimon, J. J. *et al.* (1992*b*). The pathogenesis of coronary artery disease and the acute secondary syndromes (second of two parts). *N. Engl. J. Med.*, **326**, 310–18.

Futrell, N. (1995). Inflammatory vascular disorders: diagnosis and treatment in ischaemic stroke. *Curr. Opin. Neurol.*, **8**, 55–61.

Gan, R., Sacco, R. L., Kargman, D. E. *et al.* (1997) Testing the validity of the lacunar hypothesis: The Northern Manhattan Stroke Study experience. *Neurology*, **48**, 1204–11.

Garraway, W. M., Whisnant, J. P., and Drury, I. (1983). The changing pattern of survival following stroke. *Stroke*, **14**, 699–703.

Garrett, W. T., Chang, C. W. J., and Bleck, T. P. (1996). Altered mental status in thrombotic thrombocytopenic purpura is secondary to nonconvulsive status epilepticus. *Ann. Neurol.*, **40**, 245–6.

Garrison, R. J., Feinleib, M., Castelli, W. P. *et al.* (1983). Cigarette smoking as a confounder of the relationship between relative weight and long-term mortality. *JAMA*, **249**, 2199–203.

Gates, G. C., Barnett, H. J. M., Vinters, H. V. *et al.* (1986). Primary intraventricular haemorrhage in adults. *Stroke*, **17**, 872–7.

Gautier, J. C., Awada, A., and Loron, Ph. (1983). A cerebrovascular accident with unusual features. *Stroke*, **14**, 808–10.

Gautier, J. C., Durr, A., Koussa, S. *et al.* (1991). Paradoxical cerebral embolism with a patent foramen ovale. A report of 29 patients. *Cerebrovasc. Dis.*, **1**, 193–202.

Gaziano, J. M., Buring, J. E., Breslow, J. L. *et al.* (1993). Moderate alcohol intake, increased levels of high-density lipoprotein and its subfractions, and decreased risk of myocardial infarction. *N. Engl. J. Med.*, **329**, 1829–34.

Geddes, J. M. L., Fear, J., Tennant, A. *et al.* (1996). Prevalence of self reported stroke in a population in northern England. *J. Epidemiol. Community Hlth*, **50**, 140–3.

Gerber, O., Heyer, E. J., and Vieux, U. (1986). Painless dissections of the aorta presenting as acute neurologic syndromes. *Stroke*, **17**, 644–7.

Geschwind, D. H., FitzPatrick, M., Mischel, P. S. *et al.* (1995). Sneddon's syndrome is a thrombotic vasculopathy: neuropathologic and neuroradiologic evidence. *Neurology*, **45**, 557–60.

Geyer, S. J. and Franzini, D. A. (1979). Myxomatous degeneration of the mitral valve complicated by nonbacterial thrombotic endocarditis with systemic embolisation. *Am. J. Clin. Path.*, **72**, 489–92.

Giannesini, C., Kubis, N., N'Guyen, A. *et al.* (1999). Cardiac papillary fibroelastoma: a rare cause of ischaemic stroke in the young. *Cerebrovasc. Dis.*, **9**, 45–9.

Gibbs, J. M., Wise, R. J. S., Leenders, K. L. *et al.* (1984). Evaluation of cerebral perfusion reserve in patients with carotid-artery occlusion. *Lancet* **1**, 310–14.

Gilchrist, J. M., Sikirica, M., Stopa, E. *et al.* (1996). Adult-onset MELAS. Evidence for involvement of neurons as well as cerebral vasculature in strokelike episodes. *Stroke*, **27**, 1420–3.

Giles, W. H., Kittner, S. J., Hebel, J. R. *et al.* (1995). Determinants of black–white differences in the risk of cerebral infarction. The National Health and nutrition examination survey. Epidemiologic follow-up study. *Arch. Int. Med.*, **155**, 1319–24.

Giroud, M., Lemesle, M., Madinier, G. *et al.* (1997). Unilateral lenticular infarcts: radiological and clinical syndromes, aetiology, and prognosis. *J. Neurol. Neurosurg. Psychiatry*, **63**, 611–15.

Gladman, J., Forster, A., and Young, J. (1995). Hospital- and home-based rehabilitation after discharge from hospital for stroke patients: analysis of two trials. *Age Ageing*, **24**, 49–53.

Glass J. D., Levey A. I., and Rothstein J. D. (1990). The dysarthria-clumsy hand syndrome: a distinct clinical entity related to pontine infarction. *Ann. Neurol.*, **27**, 487–94.

Glick, R., Hoying, J., Cerullo, L. *et al.* (1987). Phenylpropanolamine: an over-the-counter drug causing central nervous system vasculitis and intracerebral haemorrhage. Case report and review. *Neurosurgery*, **20**, 969–74.

Glynn, R. J., Field, T. S., Rosner, B. *et al.* (1995). Evidence for a positive linear relation between blood pressure and mortality in elderly people. *Lancet*, **345**, 825–9.

Gnasso, A., Irace, C., Carallo, C. *et al.* (1997). In vivo association between low wall shear stress and plaque in subjects with asymmetrical carotid atherosclerosis. *Stroke*, **28**, 993–8.

Goldman, L. and Tosteson, A. N. A. (1991). Uncertainty about postmenopausal estrogen. Time for action, not debate. *N. Engl. J. Med.*, **325**, 800–2.

Gomez, C. R. (1990). Carotid plaque morphology and risk for stroke. *Stroke*, **21**, 148–51.

Gomez, C. R., Cruz-Flores, S., Malkoff, M. D. *et al.* (1996). Isolated vertigo as a manifestation of vertebrobasilar ischaemia. *Neurology*, **47**, 94–7.

Gordon, C., Langton Hewer, R., and Wade, D. T. (1987). Dysphagia in acute stroke. *BMJ*, **295**, 411–14.

Gordon, R. M. and Silverstein, A. (1970). Neurologic manifestations in progressive systemic sclerosis. *Arch. Neurol.*, **22**, 126–33.

Gorman, M. J., Dafer, R., and Levine, S. R. (1998). Ataxic hemiparesis: critical appraisal of a lacunar syndrome. *Stroke*, **29**, 2549–55.

Grady, D., Rubin, S. M., Petitti, D. B. *et al.* (1992). Horomone therapy to prevent disease and prolong life in postmenopausal women. *Ann. Int. Med.*, **117**, 1016–37.

Grady, P. A. (1984). Pathophysiology of extracranial cerebral arterial stenosis – a critical review. *Stroke*, **15**, 224–36.

Graff-Radford, N. R., Damasio, H., Yamada, T. *et al.* (1985). Nonhaemorrhagic thalamic infarction. Clinical, neuropsychological and electrophysiological findings in four anatomical groups defined by computerized tomography. *Brain*, **108**, 485–516.

Graff-Radford, N. R., Tranel, D., Van Hoesen, G. W. *et al.* (1990). Diencephalic amnesia. *Brain*, **113**, 1–25.

Graus, F., Rogers, L. R., and Posner, J. B. (1985). Cerebrovascular complications in patients with cancer. *Medicine*, **64**, 16–35.

Greaves, M. (1993). Coagulation abnormalities and cerebral infarction. *J. Neurol. Neurosurg. Psychiatry*, **56**, 433–9.

Greenberg, E. R. and Sporn, M. B. (1996). Antioxidant vitamins, cancer and cardiovascular disease. *N. Engl. J. Med.*, **334**, 1189–90.

Greenberg, J. and Massey, E. W. (1985). Cerebral infarction in sickle cell trait. *Ann. Neurol.*, **18**, 354–5.

Greenberg, S. M., Vonsattel, J. P. G., Stakes, J. W. *et al.* (1993). The clinical spectrum of cerebral amyloid angiopathy. Presentations without lobar haemorrhage. *Neurology*, **43**, 2072–9.

Griewing, B., Guo, Y., Doherty, C. *et al.* (1995). Radiation-induced injury to the carotid artery: a longitudinal study. *Eur. J. Neurol.*, **2**, 379–83.

Griewing, B., Morgenstern, C., Driesner, F. *et al.* (1996). Cerebrovascular disease assessed by colour-flow and power Doppler ultrasonography: comparison with digital subtraction angiography in internal carotid artery stenosis. *Stroke*, **27**, 95–100.

Grosset, D. G., Ebrahim, S., Bone, I. *et al.* (1995). Stroke in pregnancy and the puerperium: what magnitude of risk? *J. Neurol. Neurosurg. Psychiatry*, **58**, 129–31.

Grubb, R. L., Derdeyn, C. P., Fritsch, S. M. *et al.* (1998). Importance of haemodynamic factors in the prognosis of symptomatic carotid occlusion. *JAMA*, **280**, 1055–60.

Gubitz, G., Counsell, C., Sandercock, P. A. G. *et al.* (2000). Anticoagulants for acute ischaemic stroke (in Cochrane Library, Oxford: Update Software 2001).

Gunatilake, S. B. (1998). Rapid resolution of symptoms and signs of intracerebral haemorrhage: case reports. *BMJ*, **316**, 1495–6.

Gunning, A. J., Pickering, G. W., Robb-Smith, A. H. T. *et al.* (1964). Mural thrombosis of the internal carotid artery and subsequent embolism. *QJM*, **33**, 155–95.

Guttmacher, A. E., Marchuk, D. A., and White, R. I. (1995). Hereditary haemorrhagic telangiectasia. *N. Engl. J. Med.*, **333**, 918–24.

Haapanen, A., Koskenvuo, M., Kaprio, J. *et al.* (1989). Carotid arteriosclerosis in identical twins discordant for cigarette smoking. *Circulation*, **80**, 10–16.

Haas, L. F. (1982). Stroke as an early manifestation of systemic lupus erythematosus. *J. Neurol. Neurosurg. Psychiatry*, **45**, 554–6.

Haberman, S. (1984). Geographical variation in cerebrovascular disease mortality in England and Wales. *Neuroepidemiology*, **3**, 207–22.

Hall, S., Barr, W., Lie, J. T. *et al.* (1985). Takayasu arteritis. A study of 32 North American patients. *Medicine*, **64**, 89–99.

Hama, N. and Boumpas, D. T. (1995). Cerebral lupus erythematosus. Diagnosis and rational drug treatment. *CNS Drugs*, **3**, 416–26.

Hamdy, S., Aziz, Q., Rothwell, J. C. *et al.* (1997) Explaining oropharyngeal dysphagia after unilateral hemispheric stroke. *Lancet*, **350**, 686–92.

Hankey, G. J. (1991). Isolated angiitis/angiopathy of the central nervous system. *Cerebrovasc. Dis.*, **1**, 2–15.

Hankey, G. J. and Hon, C. (1997). Surgery for primary intracerebral haemorrhage: is it safe and effective? A systematic review of case series and randomised trials. *Stroke*, **28**, 2126–32.

Hankey, G. J. and Warlow, C. P. (1990). Symptomatic carotid ischaemic events: safest and most cost effective way of selecting patients for angiography, before carotid endarterectomy. *BMJ*, **300**, 1485–91.

Hankey, G. J. and Warlow, C. P. (1991a). Prognosis of symptomatic carotid artery occlusion. An overview. *Cerebrovasc. Dis.*, **1**, 245–56.

Hankey, G. J. and Warlow, C. P. (1991b). Lacunar transient ischaemic attacks: a clinically useful concept? *Lancet*, **337**, 335–8.

Hankey, G. J. and Warlow, C. P. (1994). *Transient ischaemic attacks of the brain and eye*. Saunders, London.

Hankey, G. J., Warlow, C. P., and Molyneux, A. J. (1990a). Complications of cerebral angiography for patients with mild carotid territory ischaemia being considered for carotid endarterectomy. *J. Neurol. Neurosurg. Psychiatry*, **53**, 542–8.

Hankey, G. J., Warlow, C. P., and Sellar, R. J. (1990b). Cerebral angiographic risk in mild cerebrovascular disease. *Stroke*, **21**, 209–22.

Hankey, G. J. Slattery, J., and Warlow, C. P. (1991). The prognosis of hospital referred transient ischaemic attacks. *J. Neurol. Neurosug. Psychiatry*, **54**, 793–802.

Hankey, G. J. Slattery, J., and Warlow, C. P. (1992). Transient ischaemic attacks. Which patients are at high (and low) risk of serious vascular events? *J. Neurol. Neurosurg. Psychiatry*, **55**, 640–52.

Hankey, G. J., Dennis, M. S., Slattery, J. M. *et al.* (1993a). Why is the outcome of transient ischaemic attacks different in different groups of patients? *BMJ*, **306**, 1107–111.

Hankey, G. J., Slattery, J. M., and Warlow, C. P. (1993b). Can the long term outcome of individual patients with transient ischaemic attacks be predicted accurately? *J. Neurol. Neurosurg. Psychiatry*, **56**, 752–9

Hankey, G. J., Jamrozik, K., Broadhurst, R. J. *et al.* (1998). Long-term risk of first recurrent stroke in the Perth Community Stroke Study. *Stroke*, **29**, 2491–500.

Hankey, C. J., Dunbabin D. W., and Sudlow, C. L. M. (1999). Thienopyridine derivatives (ticlopidine, clopidogrel) versus aspirin for secondary prevention of stroke and other important vascular events in high risk patients (Cochrane Review), in preparation.

Harmsen, P., Rosengren, A., Tsipogiannia, A. *et al.* (1990). Risk factors for stroke in middle-aged men in Goteborg, Sweden. *Stroke*, **21**, 223–9.

Harries, D. P. and De Silva, R. (1992). 'Ecstasy' and intracerebral haemorrhage. *Scott. Med. J.*, **37**, 150–2.

Harrington, H., Heller, A., Dawson, D. *et al.* (1983). Intracerebral haemorrhage and oral amphetamine. *Arch. Neurol.*, **40**, 503–7.

Harris, A. I. (1971). *Handicapped and impaired in Great Britain*. The Stationery Office, London.

Harrison, C. N., Linch, D. C., and Machin, S. J. (1998). Desirability and problems of early diagnosis of essential thrombocythaemia. *Lancet*, **351**, 846–7.

Hart, R. G. (1992). Cardiogenic embolism to the brain. *Lancet*, **339**, 589–94.

Hart, R. G. and Easton, J. D. (1986). Haemorrhage infarcts. *Stroke*, **17**, 586–9.

Hart, R. G. and Halperin, J. L. (1994). Atrial fibrillation and stroke. Revisiting the dilemmas. *Stroke*, **25**, 1337–41.

Hart, R. and Hindman, B. (1982). Mechanisms of perioperative cerebral infarction. *Stroke*, **13**, 766–73.

Hart, R. G. and Kanter, M. C. (1990). Haematologic disorders and ischaemic stroke. A selective review. *Stroke*, **21**, 1111–21.

Hart, R. G., Foster, J. W., Lutner, M. F. *et al.* (1990). Stroke in infective endocarditis. *Stroke*, **21**, 695–700.

Hart, R. G., Boop, B. S., and Anderson, D. C. (1995). Oral anticoagulants and intracranial haemorrhage. Facts and hypotheses. *Stroke*, **26**, 1471–7.

Hart, R. G., Talbert, R. L., Kadri, K. *et al.* (1996). Warfarin for prevention of stroke: a practical, clinical review. *Neurologist*, **2**, 319–41.

Hasan, D., Vermeulen, M., Wijdicks, E. F. M. *et al.* (1989). Management problems in acute hydrocephalus after subarachnoid haemorrhage. *Stroke*, **20**, 747–53.

Hasan, D., Wijdicks, E. F. M., and Vermeulen, M. (1990). Hyponatraemia is associated with cerebral ischaemia in patients with aneurysmal subarachnoid haemorrhage. *Ann. Neurol.*, **27**, 106–8.

Hasan, D., Lindsay, K. W., and Vermeulen, M. (1991). Treatment of acute hydrocephalus after subarachnoid haemorrhage with serial lumbar puncture. *Stroke*, **22**, 190–4.

Hasuo, K., Tamura, S., Yasumori, K. *et al.* (1987). Computed tomography and angiography in MELAS (mitochondrial myopathy, encephalopathy, lactic acidosis and stroke-like episodes); report of 3 cases. *Neuroradiology*, **29**, 393–7.

Hatano, S. (1976). Experience from a multicentre stroke register: a preliminary report. *WHO Bull.*, **54**, 541–53.

Hawkins, G. C., Bonita, R., Broad, J. B. *et al.* (1995). Inadequacy of clinical scoring systems to differentiate stroke subtypes in population-based studies. *Stroke*, **26**, 1338–42.

He, J., Klag, M. J., Wu, Z. *et al.* (1995). Stroke in the People's Republic of China. I. Geographic variations in incidence and risk factors. *Stroke*, **26**, 2222–7.

He, J., Whelton, P. K., Vu, B. *et al.* (1998). Aspirin and risk of haemorrhagic stroke. A meta-analysis of randomised controlled trials. *JAMA*, **280**, 1930–5.

Hebert, P. R., Gaziano, J. M., Chan, K. S. *et al.* (1997). Cholesterol lowering with statin drugs, risk of stroke, and total mortality. An overview of randomised trials. *JAMA*, **278**, 313–21.

Heinemann, L. A. J., Lewis, M. A., Thorogood, M. *et al.* (1997). Case-control study of oral contraceptives and risk of thromboembolic stroke: results from international study on oral contraceptives and health of young women. *BMJ*, **315**, 1502–4.

Heiskanen, O., Poranen, A., Kuurne, T. *et al.* (1988). Acute surgery for intracerebral haematomas caused by rupture of an intracranial arterial aneurysm. A prospective randomized study. *Acta Neurochir.*, **90**, 81–3.

Hennerici, M. and Steinke, W. (1991). Carotid plaque developments: Aspects of haemodynamic and vessel wall-platelet interaction. *Cerebrovasc. Dis.*, **1**, 142–8.

Hennerici, M., Klemm, C., and Rautenberg, W. (1988). The subclavian steal phenomenon: a common vascular disorder with rare neurologic deficits. *Neurology*, **38**, 669–73.

Henrich, J. B., Sandercock, P. A. G., Warlow, C. P. *et al.* (1986). Stroke and migraine in the Oxfordshire Community Stroke Project. *J. Neurol.*, **233**, 257–62.

Henry, J. A., Jeffreys, K. J., and Dawling, S. (1992). Toxicity and deaths from 3,4-methylenedioxymethamphetamine ('ecstasy'). *Lancet*, **340**, 384–7.

Herold, S., Brown, M. M., Frackowiak, R. S. J. *et al.* (1988). Assessment of cerebral haemodynamic reserve: correlation between PET parameters and CO_2 reactivity measured by the intravenous ^{133}xenon injection technique. *J. Neurol. Neurosurg. Psychiatry*, **51**, 1045–50.

Heron, E., Fornes, P., Rance, A. *et al.* (1998). Brain involvement in scerloderma. Two autopsy cases. *Stroke*, **29**, 719–21.

Heros, R. C. (1982). Cerebellar haemorrhage and infarction. *Stroke*, **13**, 106–9.

Heros, R. C. (1989). Acute hydrocephalus after subarachnoid haemorrhage. *Stroke*, **20**, 715–17.

Hess, D. C., Nichols, F. T., Sethi, K. D. *et al.* (1991). Transient cerebral ischaemia masquerading as paroxysmal dyskinesia. *Cerebrovasc. Dis.*, **1**, 54–7.

Hetzel, A., Berger, W., Schumacher, M., and Lucking, C. H. (1996). Dissection of the vertebral artery with cervical nerve root lesions. *J. Neurol.*, **243**, 121–5.

Heye, N. and Hankey, G. J. (1996). Amphetamine-associated stroke. *Cerebrovasc. Dis.*, 6, 149–55.

Hickey, W. F., Garnick, M. B., Henderson, I. C. *et al.* (1982). Primary cerebral venous thrombosis in patients with cancer – a rarely diagnosed paraneoplastic syndrome. Report of three cases and review of the literature. *Am. J. Med.*, 73, 740–50.

Hijdra, A., van Gijn, J., Stefanko, S. *et al.* (1986). Delayed cerebral ischaemia after aneurysmal subarachnoid haemorrhage: clinicoanatomic correlations. *Neurology*, 36, 329–33.

Hijdra, A., Braakman, R., van Gijn, J. *et al.* (1987a). Aneurysmal subarachnoid haemorrhage: complications and outcome in a hospital population. *Stroke*, 18, 1061–7.

Hijdra, A., Vermeulen, M., van Gijn, J. *et al.* (1987b). Rerupture of intracranial aneurysms: a clinicoanatomic study. *J. Neurosurg.*, 67, 29–33.

Hijdra, A., van Gijn, J., Nagelkerke, N. J. D. *et al.* (1988). Prediction of delayed cerebral ischaemia, rebleeding, and outcome after aneurysmal subarachnoid haemorrhage. *Stroke*, 19, 1250–6.

Hill, M. D. and Hachinski, V. (1998). Stroke treatment: time is brain. *Lancet*, 352, 10–14.

Hilton-Jones, D. and Warlow, C. P. (1985). Non-penetrating arterial trauma and cerebral infarction in the young. *Lancet*, 1, 1435–8.

Hinds, N. P. and Wiles, C. M. (1998). Assessment of swallowing and referral to speech and language therapists in acute stroke. *QJM*, 91, 829–35.

Hino, A., Ueda, S., Mizukawa, N. *et al.* (1992). Effect of haemodilution on cerebral haemodynamics and oxygen metabolism. *Stroke*, 23, 423–6.

Ho, R. T. K., Harrison, M. J. G., and Earl, C. J. (1986). Transient paraparesis—a manifestation of ischaemic episodes in the anterior cerebral artery territory. *J. Neurol. Neurosurg. Psychiatry*, 49, 101–2.

Hodges, J. R. (1991). *Transient amnesia. Clinical and neuropsychological aspects.* Major Problems in Neurology No. 24. W. B. Saunders, London.

Hodkinson, H. M. (1972). Evaluation of a mental test score for assessment of mental impairments in the elderly. *Age Ageing*, 1, 233–8.

Hoekstra-van Dalen, R. A. H., Cillessen, J. P. M., Kappelle, L. J. *et al.* (1996). Cerebral infarcts associated with migraine: clinical features, risk factors and follow up. *J. Neurol.*, 243, 511–15.

Hokanson, J. E. and Austin, M. A. (1996). Plasma triglyceride level is a risk factor for cardiovascular disease independent of high-density lipoprotein cholesterol level: a meta-analysis of population-based prospective studies. *J. Cardiovasc. Risk*, 3, 213–19.

Holbrook, M. (1982). Stroke: social and emotional outcome. *J. R. Coll. Physicians Lond.*, 16, 100–4.

Homer, D., Ingall, T. J., Baker, H. L., *et al.* (1991). Serum lipids and lipoproteins are less powerful predictors of extracranial carotid artery atherosclerosis than are cigarette smoking and hypertension. *Mayo Clinic Proc.*, 66, 259–67.

Hommel, M., Pollak, P., Gaio, J. M. *et al.* (1984). Paralysies du nerf grand hypoglosse par deux aneurismes et un aneurisme dissequant de l'artere carotide interne. *Revue Neurologique*, 140, 415–21.

Hop, J. W., Rinkel, G. J. E., Algra, A. *et al.* (1997). Case-fatality rates and functional outcome after subarachnoid haemorrhage: a systematic review. *Stroke*, 28, 660–4.

Hop, J. W., Rinkel, G. J. E., Algra, A. *et al.* (1998). Quality of life in patients and partners after aneurysmal subarachnoid haemorrhage. *Stroke*, 29, 798–804.

Hopkins, A. (1984). Practical help. *Lancet*, 1, 1393–6.

Hornig, C. R., Busse, O., Buettner, T. *et al.* (1985). CT contrast enhancement on brain scans and blood–CSF barrier disturbances in cerebral ischaemic infarction. *Stroke*, 16, 268–73.

Hornig, C. R., Dorndorf, W., and Agnoli, A. L. (1986). Haemorrhagic cerebral infarction—a prospective study. *Stroke*, 17, 179–85.

Hornig, C. R., Rust, D. S., Busse, O. *et al.* (1994). Space-occupying cerebellar infarction. Clinical course and prognosis. *Stroke*, 25, 372–4.

Horowitz, S. H., Zito, J. L., Donnarumma, R. *et al.* (1991). Computed tomographic–angiographic findings within the first five hours of cerebral infarction. *Stroke*, 22, 1245–53.

Hossman, K.-A. (1983). Experimental aspects of stroke. In *Vascular disease of the central nervous system*, (ed. R. W. Ross Russell), pp. 73–100. Churchill Livingstone, Edinburgh.

Hossmann, K.-A. (1994). Viability thresholds and the penumbra of focal ischaemia. *Ann. Neurol.*, 36, 557–65.

Hourihane, J. M., Deloughery, T. G., and Clark, W. M. (1997). Homozygous hereditary resistance to activated protein C presenting as cerebral venous thrombosis. *J. Stroke Cerebrovasc. Dis.*, 6, 370–2.

House, A. (1987). Mood disorders after stroke: a review of the evidence. *Int. J. Geriatric Psychiatry*, 2, 211–??.

House, A., Dennis, M., Hawton, K. *et al.* (1989). Methods of identifying mood disorders in stroke patients: experience in the Oxfordshire Community Stroke Project. *Age Ageing*, 18, 371–9.

House, A., Dennis, M., Mogridge, L. *et al.* (1991). Mood disorders in the year after first stroke. *Br. J. Psychiatry*, 158, 83–92.

Houston, J. G., Morris, A. D., Grosset, D. G. *et al.* (1995). Ultrasonic evaluation of movement of the diaphragm after acute cerebral infarction. *J. Neurol. Neurosurg. Psychiatry,* 58, 738–41.

Howard, G., Anderson, R., Sorlie, P. *et al.* (1994). Ethnic differences in stroke mortality between non-Hispanic whites, Hispanic whites, and blacks. The national longitudinal mortality study. *Stroke,* 25, 2120–5.

Howard, G., Wagenknecht, L. E., Burke G. L. *et al.* for the ARIC Investigators (1998). Cigarette smoking and progression of atherosclerosis: the Atherosclerosis Risk in Communities (ARIC) Study. *JAMA,* 279, 119–24.

Howard, R. S. (1986). Brainstem haematoma due to presumed cryptic telangiectasia. *J. Neurol. Neurosurg. Psychiatry,* 49, 1241–5.

Howell, S. J. L. and Molyneux, A. J. (1988). Vertebrobasilar insufficiency in rheumatoid atlanto-axial subluxation: a case report with angiographic demonstration of left vertebral artery occlusion. *J. Neurol.,* 235, 189–90.

Huang, C. Y. and Yu, Y. L. (1985). Small cerebellar strokes may mimic labyrinthine lesions. *J. Neurol. Neurosurg. Psychiatry.,* 48, 263–5.

Huang C. Y., Woo E., Yu Y. L. *et al.* (1987). When is sensorimotor stroke a lacunar syndrome? *J. Neurol. Neurosurg. Psychiatry.,* 50, 720–6.

Huang, C. Y., Chan, F. L., Yu, Y. L. *et al.* (1990). Cerebrovascular disease in Hong Kong Chinese. *Stroke,* 21, 230–5.

Hugh, A. E. (1987). The carotid siphon: A natural arterial filter? *Lancet,* 2, 886–7.

Hughes, G. R. V. (1993). The antiphospholipid syndrome: ten years on. *Lancet,* 342, 341–4.

Hughes, J. T. and Brownell, B. (1968). Traumatic thrombosis of the internal carotid artery in the neck. *J. Neurol. Neurosurg. Psychiatry,* 31, 307–14.

Hulley, S., Grady, D., Bush, T. *et al.* for the Heart and Estrogen/progestin Replacement Study (HERS) Research Group (1998). Randomised trial of eostrogen plus progestin for secondary prevention of coronary heart disease in postmenopausal women. *JAMA,* 280, 605–13.

Hupperts, R. M. M., Lodder, J., Heuts-van Raak, E. P. M. *et al.* (1994). Infarcts in the anterior choroidal artery territory. Anatomical distribution, clinical syndromes, presumed pathogenesis and early outcome. *Brain,* 117, 825–34.

Hupperts, R. M. M., Warlow, C. P., Slattery, J. *et al.* (1997). Severe stenosis of the internal carotid artery is not associated with borderzone infarcts in patients randomised in the European Carotid Surgery Trial. *J. Neurol.,* 244, 45–50.

Huston, K. A. and Hunder, G. G. (1980). Giant cell (cranial) arteritis: a clinical review. *Am. Heart J.,* 100, 99–106.

Hutchinson, E. C. and Yates, P. O. (1957). Carotico-vertebral stenosis. *Lancet,* 1, 2–8.

Hutchinson, M., O'Riordan, J., Javed, M. *et al.* (1995). Familial hemiplegic migraine and autosomal dominant ateriopathy with leukoencephalopathy (CADASIL). *Ann. Neurol.,* 38, 817–24.

Iansek, R., Elstein, A. S., and Balla, J. I. (1983). Application of decision analysis to management of cerebral arteriovenous malformation. *Lancet,* 1, 1132–5.

Ichikawa, K. and Kageyama, Y. (1991). Clinical anatomic study of pure dysarthria. *Stroke,* 22, 809–12.

Igarashi, M., Gilmartin, R. C., Gerald, B. *et al.* (1984). Cerebral arteritis and bacterial meningitis. *Arch. Neurol.,* 41, 531–5.

INDANA (INdividual Data ANalysis of Antihypertensive intervention trials) Project Collaborators, Gueyffier, F., Boissel, J. P., Boutitie, F. *et al.* (1997). Effect of antihypertensive treatment in patients having already suffered from stroke. Gathering the evidence. *Stroke,* 28, 2557–62.

Ingall, T. J., Whisnant, J. P., Wiebers, D. O. *et al.* (1989). Has there been a decline in subarachnoid haemorrhage mortality? *Stroke,* 20, 718–24.

International Stroke Trial Collaborative Group (1997). The International Stroke Trial (IST): a randomised trial of aspirin, subcutaneous heparin, both, or neither among 19,435 patients with acute ischaemic stroke. *Lancet,* 349, 1569–181.

International Study of Unruptured Intracranial Aneurysms Investigators (1998). Unruptured intracranial aneurysms—risk of rupture and risks of surgical intervention. *N. Engl. J. Med.,* 339, 1725–33.

Inzitari, D., Lamassa, M., and Amaducci, L. (1995). Stroke epidemiology in Europe. *Eur. J. Neurol.,* 2, 75–81.

Iragui, V. J. and Maravi, E. (1986). Behcet syndrome presenting as cerebrovascular disease. *J. Neurol. Neurosurg. Psychiatry,* 49, 838–40.

Irino, T., Watanabe, M., Nishide, M. *et al.* (1983). Angiographical analysis of acute cerebral infarction followed by 'Cascade'-like deterioration of minor neurological deficits. What is progressing stroke? *Stroke,* 14, 363–8.

Irwin, P. and Rudd, A. (1998). Casemix and process indicators of outcome in stroke. The Royal College of Physicians minimum data set for stroke. *J. R. Coll. Physicians,* 32, 442–4.

Isaka, Y., Nagano, K., Narita, M. *et al.* (1997). High signal intensity of T2-weighted magnetic resonance imaging and cerebral hemodynamic reserve in carotid occlusive disease. *Stroke,* 28, 354–7.

Isard, P. A. and Forbes, J. F. (1992). The cost of stroke to the National Health Service in Scotland. *Cerebrovasc. Dis.*, 2, 47–50.

Iwama, T., Hashimoto, N., Murai, B. N. *et al.* (1997). Intracranial rebleeding in moyamoya disease. *J. Clin. Neurosci.*, 4, 169–72.

Jabaily, J., Iland, H. J., Laszlo, J. *et al.* (1983). Neurologic manifestations of essential thrombocythaemia. *Ann. Int. Med.*, 99, 513.

Jackson, M., Lennox, G., Jaspan, T. *et al.* (1993). Cerebral venous and systemic thrombosis in resolving ulcerative colitis. *Cerebrovasc. Dis.*, 3, 178–9.

Jackson, R., Barham, P., Bills, J. *et al.* (1993). Management of raised blood pressure in New Zealand: a discussion document. *BMJ*, 307, 107–10.

Jacobs, K., Moulin, T., Bogousslavsky, J. *et al.* (1996). The stroke syndrome of cortical vein thrombosis. *Neurology*, 47, 376–82.

Jacobson, D. M., Terrence, C. F., and Reinmuth, O. M. (1986). The neurological manifestations of fat embolism. *Neurology*, 36, 847–51.

Jakovljevic, D., Salomaa, V., Sivenius, J. *et al.* (1996). Seasonal variation in the occurence of stroke in a Finnish adult population. The FINMONICA Stroke Register. *Stroke*, 27, 1774–9.

Jeanrenaud, X. and Kappenberger, L. (1991). Patent foramen ovale and stroke of unknown origin. *Cerebrovasc. Dis.*, 1, 184–92.

Jehkonen, M., Ahonen, J.-P., Dastidar, P. *et al.* (1998) How to detect visual neglect in acute stroke *Lancet*, 351, 727–8.

Jennette, J. C. and Falk, R. J. (1997). Small-vessel vasculitis. *N. Engl. J. Med.*, 337, 1512–23.

Jensson, O., Gudmundsson, G., Arnason, A. *et al.* (1987). Hereditary cystatin C (γ-trace) amyloid angiopathy of the CNS causing cerebral haemorrhage. *Acta Neurol. Scand.*, 76, 102–14.

Jeppesen, L. L., Jorgensen, H. S., Nakayama, H. *et al.* (1996). Endogenous sex hormones in women with ischaemic stroke. *Cerebrovasc. Dis.*, 6, 288–93.

Jha, P., Flather, M., Lonn, E., Farkouh, M., and Yusuf, S. (1995). The antioxidant vitamins and cardiovascular disease. A critical review of epidemiologic and clinical trial data. *Ann. Int. Med.*, 123, 860–72.

Johns, D. R. (1991). Cerebrovascular complications of inflammatory bowel disease. *Am. J. Gastroenterol.*, 86, 367–70.

Johnston, S. C., Colford, J. M., and Gress, D. R. (1998). Oral contraceptives and the risk of subarachnoid haemorrhage. A meta-analysis. *Neurology*, 51, 411–18.

Jones, H. R. and Siekert, R. G. (1989). Neurological manifestations of infective endocarditis. Review of clinical and therapeutic challenges. *Brain*, 112, 1295–315.

Jorens, P. G., Delvigne, C. R., Hermans, C. R. *et al.* (1991). Cerebral arterial thrombosis preceding ulcerative colitis. *Stroke*, 22, 1212.

Jorgensen, H. S., Nakayama, H., Raaschou, H. O. *et al.* (1994). Stroke in patients with diabetes. The Copenhagen Stroke Study. *Stroke*, 25, 1977–84.

Jorgensen, H. S., Nakayama, H., Raaschou, H. O. *et al.* (1995). Intracerebral haemorrhage versus infarction: stroke severity, risk factors, and prognosis. *Ann. Neurol.*, 38, 45–50.

Joseph, A., Ackerman, D., Talley, J. D., Jonstone, J., and Kupersmith, J. (1993). Mainfestations of coronary atherosclerosis in young trauma victims—An autopsy study. *J. Am. Coll. Cardiol.*, 22, 459–67.

Joynt, R. J., Zimmerman, G., and Khalifeh, R. (1965). Cerebral emboli from cardiac tumours. *Arch. Neurol.*, 12, 84–91.

Jung, H. H., Bassetti, C., Tournier-Lasserve, E. *et al.* (1995). Cerebral autosomal dominant arteripathy with subcortical infarcts and leukoencephalopathy: a clinicopathological and genetic study of a Swiss family. *J. Neurol. Neurosurg. Psychiatry*, 59, 138–43.

Jurgens, G., Taddei-Peters, W. C., Koltringer, P. *et al.* (1995). Lipoprotein(a) serum concentration and apolipoprotein(a) phenotype correlate with severity and presence of ischaemic cerebrovascular disease. *Stroke*, 26, 1841–8.

Kagan, A. R. (1976). Atherosclerosis and myocardial lesions in subjects dying from fresh cerebrovascular disease. *Bull. WHO*, 53, 597–600.

Kagan, A. R., Popper, J. S., and Rhoads, G. G. (1980). Factors related to stroke incidence in Hawaii Japanese men. The Honolulu Heart Study. *Stroke*, 11, 14–21.

Kalashnikova, L. A., Nasonov, E. L., Stoyanovich, L. Z. *et al.* (1994). Sneddon's syndrome and the primary antiphospholipid syndrome. *Cerebrovasc. Dis.*, 4, 76–82.

Kamata, T., Yokata, T., Furukawa, T. *et al.* (1994). Cerebral ischaemic attack caused by postprandial hypotension. *Stroke*, 25, 511–13.

Kannel, W. B., Wolf, P. A., and Verter, J. (1983). Manifestations of coronary disease predisposing to stroke. The Framingham Study. *JAMA*, 250, 2942–6.

Kannel, W. B., Anderson, K., and Wilson, P. W. F. (1992). White blood cell count and cardiovascular disease. Insights from the Framingham Study. *JAMA*, 267, 1253–6.

Kanter, M. C. and Hart, R. G. (1991). Neurologic complications of infective endocarditis. *Neurology*, 41, 1015–20.

Kanter, M. C., Tegeler, C. H., Pearce, L. A. *et al.* on behalf of the Stroke Prevention in Atrial Fibrillation Investigators (1994). Carotid stenosis in patients with atrial fibrillation. *Arch. Intern. Med.*, 154, 1372–7.

Kaplan, N. M. (1995). Alcohol and hypertension. *Lancet*, **345**, 1588–9.

Kaplan, N. M. and Gifford, R. W. (1996). Choice of initial therapy for hypertension. *JAMA*, **275**, 1577–80.

Kaplan, P. W. (1993). Focal seizures resembling transient ischaemic attacks due to subclinical ischaemia. *Cerebrovasc. Dis.*, **3**, 241–3.

Kapoor, R., Kendall, B. E., and Harrison, M. J. G. (1991). Permanent oculomotor palsy with occlusion of the internal carotid artery. *J. Neurol. Neurosurg. Psychiatry*, **8**, 745–6.

Kaps, M., Teschendorf, U., and Dorndorf, W. (1992). Haemodynamic studies in early stroke. *J. Neurol.*, **239**, 138–42.

Karanjia, P. N., Madden, K. P., and Lobner, S. (1994). Co-existence of abdominal aortic aneurysm in patients with carotid stenosis. *Stroke*, **25**, 627–30.

Karunaratne, P. M., Norris, C. A., and Syme, P. D. (1999). Analysis of six months' referrals to a 'one-stop' neurovascular clinic in a district general hospital: implications for purchasers of a stroke service. *Health Bull.*, **57**, 17–28.

Kase, C. S. (1986). Intracerebral haemorrhage: non-hypertensive causes. *Stroke*, **17**, 590–5.

Kase, C. S., Foster, T. E., Reed, J. E. *et al.* (1987). Intracerebral haemorrhage and phenylpropanolamine use. *Neurology*, **37**, 399–404.

Kasner, S. E., Gurian, J. H., and Grotta, J. C. (1998). Urokinase treatment of sagittal sinus thrombosis with venous haemorrhagic infarction. *J. Stroke Cerebrovasc. Dis.*, **7**, 421–5.

Kassell, N. F., Sasaki, T., Colohan, A. R. T., and Nazar, G. (1985). Cerebral vasospasm following aneurysmal subarachnoid haemorrhage. *Stroke*, **16**, 562–72.

Kassell, N. F., Torner, J. C., Haley, E. C. *et al.* (1990*a*). The International Cooperative Study on the Timing of Aneurysm Surgery. Part 1: Overall management results. *J. Neurosurg.*, **73**, 18–36.

Kassell, N. F., Torner, J. C., Jane, J. A. *et al.* (1990*b*). The international cooperative study on the timing of aneurysm surgery. Part 2 Surgical Results. *J. Neurosurg.*, **73**, 37–47.

Katan, M. J. (1995). Fish and heart disease. *N. Engl. J. Med.*, **332**, 1024–5.

Kattapong, V. J., Hart, B. L., and Davis, L. E. (1995). Familial cerebral cavernous angiomas: clinical and radiologic studies. *Neurology*, **45**, 492–7.

Kaufman, M. J., Levin, J. M., Ross, M. H. *et al.* (1998). Cocaine-induced cerebral vasoconstriction detected in humans with magnetic resonance angiography. *JAMA*, **279**, 376–80.

Kaufmann, A. M., Firlik, A. D., Fukui, M. B. *et al.* (1999). Ischaemic core and penumbra in human stroke. *Stroke*, **30**, 93–9.

Kawachi, I., Colditz, G. A., Stampfer, M. J. *et al.* (1993). Smoking cessation and decreased risk of stroke in women. *JAMA*, **269**, 232–6.

Kawachi, I., Colditz, G. A., and Stone, C. B. (1994). Does coffee drinking increase the risk of coronary heart disease? Results from a meta-analysis. *Br. Heart J.*, **72**, 269–75.

Kawakita, H., Nishimura, M., Satoh, Y. *et al.* (1967). Neurological aspects of Behcet's disease. A case report and clinico-pathological review of the literature in Japan. *J. Neurol. Sci.*, **5**, 417–39.

Kay, A. C., Solberg, L. A., Nichols, D. A. *et al.* (1991). Prognostic significance of computed tomography of the brain in thrombotic thrombocytopenic purpura. *Mayo Clinic Proc.*, **66**, 602–7.

Kazui, S., Sawada, T., Naritomi, H. *et al.* (1992). Left unilateral ideomotor apraxia in ischaemic stroke within the territory of the anterior cerebral artery. *Cerebrovasc. Dis.*, **2**, 35–9.

Kazui, S., Kuriyama, Y., Sakata, T., Hiroki, M., Miyashita, K., and Sawada, T. (1993). Accelerated brain infarction in hypertension complicated by hereditary heterozygous protein C deficiency. *Stroke*, **24**, 2097–103.

Keane, J. R. (1979). Retinal hemorrhages. Its significance in 100 patients with acute encephalopathy of unknown cause. *Arch. Neurol.*, **36**, 691–4.

Keli, S., Bloemberg, B., and Kromhout, D. (1992). Predictive value of repeated systolic blood pressure measurements for stroke risk. The Zutphen Study. *Stroke*, **23**, 347–51.

Kelley, R. E. and Kovacs, A. G. (1986). Horizontal gaze paresis in hemispheric stroke. *Stroke*, **17**, 1030–2.

Kelly-Hayes, M., Wolf, P. A., Kase, C. S. *et al.* (1995). Temporal patterns of stroke onset. The Framingham study. *Stroke*, **26**, 1343–7.

Kety, S. S. and Schmidt, C. F. (1945). The determination of cerebral blood flow in man by the use of nitrous oxide in low concentrations. *Am. J. Physiol.*, **143**, 53–66.

Khamashta, M. A., Cervera, R., Asherson, R. A. *et al.* (1990). Association of antibodies against phospholipids with heart valve disease in systemic lupus erythematosus. *Lancet*, **335**, 1541–4.

Khaw, K.-T. (1996). Epidemiology of stroke. *J. Neurol. Neurosurg. Psychiatry*, **61**, 333–8.

Khaw, K..-T. and Barrett-Connor, E. (1987). Dietary potassium and stroke-associated mortality. A 12-year prospective population study. *N. Engl. J. Med.*, **316**, 235–40.

Kim J. S. (1994). Pure dysarthria, isolated facial paresis, or dysarthria-facial paresis syndrome. *Stroke*, **25**, 1994–8.

Kim, J. S., Lee, J. H., and Choi, C. G. (1998). Patterns of lateral medullary infarction. Vascular lesion—magnetic resonance imaging correlation of 34 cases. *Stroke*, **29**, 645–52.

Kitagawa, Y., Gotoh, F., Koto, A. *et al.* (1990). Stroke in systemic lupus erythematosus. *Stroke*, **21**, 1533–9.

Kitahara, T., Ariga, N., Yamaura, A. *et al.* (1979). Familial occurrence of moya-moya disease: report of three Japanese families. *J. Neurol. Neurosurg. Psychiatry*, **42**, 208–14.

Kittner, S. J., Sharkness, C. M., Price, T. R. *et al.* (1990). Infarcts with a cardiac source of embolism in the NINCDS Stroke Data Bank: historical features. *Neurology*, **40**, 281–4.

Kittner, S. J., Stern, B. J., Feeser, B. R. *et al.* (1996). Pregnancy and the risk of stroke. *N. Engl. J. Med.*, **335**, 768–74.

Kiyohara, Y., Kato, I., Iwamoto, H. *et al.* (1995). The impact of alcohol and hypertension on stroke incidence in a General Japanese population. The Hisayama Study. *Stroke*, **26**, 368–72.

Klijn, C. J. M., Kappelle, L. J., Tulleken, C. A. F. *et al.* (1997). Symptomatic carotid artery occlusion. A reappraisal of haemodynamic factors. *Stroke*, **28**, 2084–93.

Knutsen, R., Knutsen, S. F., Curb, J. D., Reed, D. M., Dautz, J. A., and Yano, K. (1988). Predictive value of resting electrocardiograms for 12-year incidence of stroke in the Honolulu Heart Program. *Stroke*, **19**, 555–9.

Koelman, J. H. T. M., Bakker, C. M., Plandsoen, W. C. G. *et al.* (1992). Hereditary protein S deficiency presenting with cerebral sinus thrombosis in an adolescent girl. *J. Neurol.*, **239**, 105–6.

Koennecke, H., Mast, H., Trocio, S. H. *et al.* (1998). Frequency and determinants of microembolic signals on transcranial Doppler in unselected patients with acute carotid territory ischaemia. A prospective study. *Cerebrovasc. Dis.*, **8**, 107–12.

Kokkinos, P. F., Narayan, P., Colleran, J. A. *et al.* (1995). Effects of regular exercise on blood pressure and left ventricular hypertrophy in African–American men with severe hypertension. *N. Engl. J. Med.*, **333**, 1462–7.

Kopecky, S. L., Gersh, B. J., McGoon, M. D. *et al.* (1987). The natural history of lone atrial fibrillation. A population-based study over three decades. *N. Engl. J. Med.*, **317**, 669–74.

Koudstaal, P. J., van Gijn, J., Kappelle, L. J., for the Dutch TIA Study Group (1991). Headache in transient or permanent cerebral ischaemia. *Stroke*, **22**, 754–9.

Krendel, D. A., Ditter, S. M., Frankel, M. R. *et al.* (1990). Biopsy-proven cerebral vasculitis associated with cocaine abuse. *Neurology*, **40**, 1092–4.

Kristian, T. and Siesjo, B. K. (1998). Calcium in ischaemic cell death. *Stroke*, **29**, 705–18.

Kubis, N., Zuber, M., Meder, J. F. *et al.* (1996). CT scan of the skull base in internal carotid artery hypoplasia. *Cerebrovasc. Dis.*, **6**, 40–4.

Kuehnen, J., Schwartz, A., Neff, W. *et al.* (1998). Cranial nerve syndrome in thrombosis of the transverse/ sigmoid sinuses. *Brain*, **121**, 381–8.

Kumral, E., Bogousslavsky, J., Van Melle, G., Regli, F., and Pierre, P. (1995). Headache at stroke onset: the Lausanne Stroke Registry. *J. Neurol. Neurosurg. Psychiatry*, **58**, 490–92.

Kunst, A. E., Del Rios, M., Groenhof, F. *et al.* for the European Union Working Group on Socioeconomic Inequalities in Health (1998). Socioeconomic inequalities in stroke mortality among middle-aged men. An international overview. *Stroke*, **29**, 2285–91.

Kwa, V. I. H., Franke, C. L., Verbeeten, B. *et al.* (1998). Silent intracerebral microhemorrhages in patients with ischaemic stroke for the Amsterdam Vascular Medicine Group. *Ann. Neurol.*, **44**, 372–7.

Kwakkel, G., Wagenaar, R. C., Kollen, B. J. *et al.* (1996). Predicting disability in stroke—a critical review of the literature. *Age Ageing*, **25**, 479–89.

Lammie, G. A. and Wardlaw, J. M. (1999). Small centrum ovale infarcts—a pathological study. *Cerebrovasc. Dis.*, **9**, 82–90.

Lammie, G. A., Brannan, F., Slattery, J. *et al.* (1997). Nonhypertensive cerebral small-vessel disease. An autopsy study. *Stroke*, **28**, 2222–9.

Lammie, G. A., Sandercock, P. A. G., and Dennis, M. S. (1999). Recently occluded intracranial and extracranial carotid arteries: relevance of the unstable atheromatous plaque. *Stroke*, **30**, 1319–25.

Lancet (1989). Brain damage and open-heart surgery. *Lancet*, **2**, 364–6.

Landi, G. (1992). Clinical diagnosis of transient ischaemic attacks. *Lancet*, **339**, 402–5.

Landi, G., Villani, F., and Anzalone, N. (1990). Variable angiographic findings in patients with stroke and neurosyphilis. *Stroke*, **21**, 333–8.

Landi G., Anzalone N., Cella E. *et al.* (1991). Are sensorimotor strokes lacunar strokes? A case-control study of lacunar and non-lacunar infarcts. *J. Neurol. Neurosurg. Psychiatry*, **54**, 1063–8.

Langton Hewer, R. (1990). Rehabilitation after stroke. *QJM*, **76**, 659–74.

Larrue, V., von Kummer, R., del Zoppo, G. *et al.* (1997). Haemorrhagic transformation in acute ischemic stroke. Potential contributing factors in the European Cooperative Acute Stroke Study. *Stroke*, **28**, 957–60.

Larsen, F. S., Olsen, K. S., Hansen, B. A. *et al.* (1994). Transcranial Doppler is valid for determination of the lower limit of cerebral blood flow autoregulation. *Stroke*, **25**, 1985–8.

Lasjaunias, P., Chiu, M., Brugge, K. T. *et al.* (1986). Neurological manifestations of intracranial dural arteriovenous malformations. *J. Neurosurg.*, **64**, 724–30.

Lassen, N. A., Roland, P. E., Larsen, B. *et al.* (1977). Mapping of human cerebral functions: A study of the regional cerebral blood flow pattern during rest, its reproducibility and the activations seen during basic sensory and motor functions. *Acta Neurol. Scand.*, **64**, 262–3.

Lassen, N. A., Fieschi, C., and Lenzi, G. L. (1991). Ischaemic penumbra and neuronal death: Comments on the therapeutic window in acute stroke with particular reference to thrombolytic therapy. *Cerebrovasc. Dis.*, **1**, (Suppl. 1), 32–5.

Law, M. R., Frost, C. D., and Wald, N. J. (1991). By how much does dietary salt reduction lower blood pressure? I— Analysis of observational data among populations. *BMJ*, **302**, 811–15.

Law, M. R., Wald, N. J., Wu, T. *et al.* (1994*a*). Systematic underestimation of association between serum cholesterol concentration and ischaemic heart disease in observational studies: data from the BUPA study. *BMJ*, **308**, 363–6.

Law, M. R., Thompson, S. G., and Wald, N. J. (1994*b*). Assessing possible hazards of reducing serum cholesterol. *BMJ*, **308**, 373–9.

Leclerc X., Godefroy O., Pruvo J. P. *et al.* (1995). Computed tomographic angiography for the evaluation of carotid artery stenosis. *Stroke*, **26**, 1577–81.

Lee, I-M., Hennekens, C. H., Berger, K. *et al.* (1999). Exercise and risk of stroke in male physicians. *Stroke*, **30**, 1–6.

Leenders, K. L., Perani, D., Lammertsma, A. A. *et al.* (1990). Cerebral blood flow, blood volume and oxygen utilisation. Normal values and effect of age. *Brain*, **113**, 27–47.

Legh-Smith, J., Wade, D. T., and Langton-Hewer, R. (1986). Services for stroke patients one year after stroke. *J. Epidemiol. Community Hlth*, **40**, 161–5.

Leijon, G., Boivie, J., and Johansson, I. (1989). Central post-stroke pain-neurological symptoms and pain characteristics. *Pain*, **36**, 13–25.

Leira, E. C., Ajax, T., and Adams, H. P., Jr (1997). Limb-shaking carotid transient ischaemic attacks successfully treated with modification of the antihypertensive regimen. *Arch. Neurol.*, **54**, 904–5.

Lemesle, M., Giroud, M., Menassa, M. *et al.* (1996). Incidence and case-fatality rates of stroke in Burgundy (France). Comparison between a rural (Avallon) and an urban (Dijon) population, between 1989 and 1993. *Eur. J. Neurol.*, **3**, 109–15.

Leng, G. C., Fowkes, F. G. R., Lee, A. J. *et al.* (1996). Use of ankle brachial pressure index to predict cardiovascular events and death: a cohort study. *BMJ*, **313**, 1440–4.

Lennox, I. M., Zeeh, J., Currie, N. *et al.* (1989). Malignant angioendotheliosis—an unusual cause of stroke. *Scott. Med. J.*, **34**, 407–8.

Leopold, N. A. (1993). Chickenpox stroke in an adult. *Neurology*, **43**, 1852–3.

Lessa, I. and Cortes, E. (1981). Cerebrovascular accidents as a complication of leptospirosis. *Lancet*, **2**, 1113.

Leung, D. Y., Black, I. W., Cranney, G. B. *et al.* (1995). Selection of patients for transoesophageal echocardiography after stroke and systemic embolic events. Role of transthoracic echocardiography. *Stroke*, **26**, 1820–4.

Leung, S. Y., Ng, T. H. K., Yuen, S. T. *et al.* (1993). Pattern of cerebral atherosclerosis in Hong Kong Chinese: Severity in intracranial and extracranial vessels. *Stroke*, **24**, 779–86.

Levine, S. R., Kieran, S., Puzio, K. *et al.* (1987). Cerebral venous thrombosis with lupus anticoagulants. Report of two cases. *Stroke*, **18**, 801–4.

Levine, S. R., Brust, J. C. M., Futrell, N. *et al.* (1990). Cerebrovascular complications of the use of the 'crack' form of alkaloidal cocaine. *N. Engl. J. Med.*, **323**, 699–704.

Levine, S. R., Brey, R. L., Sawaya, K. L. *et al.* (1995). Recurrent stroke and thrombo-occlusive events in the antiphospholipid syndrome. *Ann. Neurol.*, **38**, 119–24.

Levy, D. E. (1988). How transient are transient ischaemic attacks? *Neurology*, **38**, 674–7.

Levy, D. and Savage, D. (1987). Prevalence and clinical features of mitral valve prolapse. *Am. Heart J.*, **113**, 1281–90.

Leys, D., Pruvo, J. P., Scheltens, P. *et al.* (1992). Leukoaraiosis: relationship with the types of focal lesions occurring in acute cerebrovascular disorders. *Cerebrovasc. Dis.*, **2**, 169–76.

Leys, D., Moulin, Th., Stojkovic, T. *et al.* (1995). Follow-up of patients with history of cervical artery dissection. *Cerebrovasc. Dis.*, **5**, 43–9.

Lhermitte, F., Gautier, J. C., and Derouesne, C. (1970). Nature of occlusions of the middle cerebral artery. *Neurology*, **20**, 82–8.

Liao, D., Myers, R., Hunt, S. *et al.* (1997). Familial history of stroke and stroke risk. The Family Heart Study. *Stroke*, **28**, 1908–12.

Libby, P. (1996). Atheroma: more than mush. *Lancet*, **348**, s4–s7.

Libman, R. B., Sharfstein, S., Harrington, W. *et al.* (1997). Recurrent intracerebral haemorrhage from sarcoid angiitis. *J. Stroke Cerebrovasc. Dis.*, **6**, 373–5.

Lie, J. T. (1986). Thromboangiitis obliterans (Buerger's disease) in women. *Medicine*, **65**, 65–72.

Limburg, M., Wijdicks, E. F., and Li, H. (1998). Ischaemic stroke after surgical procedures: clinical features, neuroimaging, and risk factors. *Neurology*, **50**, 895–901.

Lincoln, N. B., Willis, D., Philips, S. A. *et al.* (1996). Comparison of rehabilitation practice on hospital wards for stroke patients. *Stroke*, **27**, 18–23.

Lindenstrom, E., Boysen, G., and Nyboe, J. (1994). Influence of total cholesterol, high density lipoprotein cholesterol, and triglycerides on risk of cerebrovascular disease: the Copenhagen city heart study. *BMJ*, **309**, 11–15.

Lindgren, A., Roijer, A., Norrving, B. *et al.* (1994). Carotid artery and heart disease in subtypes of cerebral infarction. *Stroke*, **25**, 2356–62.

Lindley, R. I., Waddell, F. W., Livingstone, M. *et al.* (1994). Can simple questions assess outcome after stroke? *Cerebrovasc. Dis.*, **4**, 314–24

Linn, F. H., Wijdicks, E. F. M., van der Graaf, Y. *et al.* (1994). Prospective study of sentinel headache in aneurysmal subarachnoid haemorrhage. *Lancet*, **344**, 590–3.

Linn, F. H. H., Rinkel, G. J. E., Algra, A. *et al.* (1996). Incidence of subarachnoid haemorrhage. Role of region, year, and rate of computed tomography: a meta-analysis. *Stroke*, **27**, 625–9.

Lip, G. Y. H. (1997). Does paroxysmal atrial fibrillation confer a paroxysmal thromboembolic risk? *Lancet*, **349**, 1565–66.

Lip, G. Y. H. (1999). Thromboprophylaxis for atrial fibrillation. *Lancet*, **353**, 4–6.

Lipton, S. A. and Rosenberg, P. A. (1994). Excitatory amino acids as a final common pathway for neurologic disorders. *N. Engl. J. Med.*, **330**, 613–22.

Lissner, L., Odell, P. M., D'Agostino, R. B. *et al.* (1991). Variability of body weight and health outcomes in the Framingham population. *N. Engl. J. Med.*, **324**, 1839–44.

Liu, M., Counsell, C., and Sandercock, P. A. G. (1999). Anticoagulation for preventing recurrence following ischaemic stroke or transient ischaemic attack. (Cochrane Review). In *The Cochrane Library*, Issue 1. Update Software, Oxford.

Lodder, J., Krijne-Kubat, B., and Broekman, J. (1986). Cerebral haemorrhagic infarction at autopsy: cardiac embolic cause and the relationship to the cause of death. *Stroke*, **17**, 626–9.

Lodder, J., Bamford, J. M., Sandercock, P. A. G. *et al.* (1990). Are hypertension or cardiac embolism likely causes of lacunar infarction? *Stroke*, **21**, 375–81

Lodder, J., Bamford, J., Kappelle, J. *et al.* (1994). What causes false clinical prediction of small deep infarcts? *Stroke*, **25**, 86–91.

Loeb, C., Gandolfo, C., and Dall'Agata, D. (1985). Headache in transient ischaemic attacks (TIA). *Cephalalgia* (Suppl. 2), 17–19.

Loh, E., St John Sutton, M. S., Wun, C-C. *et al.* (1997). Ventricular dysfunction and the risk of stroke after myocardial infarction. *N. Engl. J. Med.*, **336**, 251–7.

Lomer, M. and McLellan, D. L. (1987). Informing hospital patients and their relatives about stroke. *Clin. Rehabil.*, **1**, 33–6.

Longo, D. L. and Witherspoon, J. M. (1980). Focal neurologic symptoms in hypercalcemia. *Neurology*, **30**, 200–1.

Longstreth, W. T., Koepsell, T. D., Yerby, M. S. *et al.* (1985). Risk factors for subarachnoid haemorrhage. *Stroke*, **16**, 377–85.

Lopez, J. A., Ross, R. S., Fishbein, M. C. *et al.* (1987). Nonbacterial thrombotic endocarditis: A review. *Am. Heart J.*, **113**, 773–84.

Lossos, A., River, Y., Eliakim, A. *et al.* (1995). Neurologic aspects of inflammatory bowel disease. *Neurology*, **45**, 416–21.

Lou, H. C., Edvinsson, L., and MacKenzie, E. T. (1987). The concept of coupling blood flow to brain function: revision required? *Ann. Neurol.*, **22**, 289–97.

Lowe, G. D. O., Lee, A. J., Rumley, A. *et al.* (1997). Blood viscosity and risk of cardiovascular events: the Edinburgh Artery Study. *Br. J. Haematol.*, **96**, 168–73.

Lupi-Herrera, E., Sanchez-Torres, G., Marcushamer, J. *et al.* (1977). Takayasu's arteritis. Clinical study of 107 cases. *Am. Heart J.*, **93**, 94–103.

Luscher, T. F., Lie, J. T., Stanson, A. W. *et al.* (1987). Arterial fibromuscular dysplasia. *Mayo Clinic Proc.*, **62**, 931–52.

Lusiani, L., Visona, A., Castellani, V. *et al.* (1987). Prevalence of atherosclerotic involvement of the internal carotid artery in hypertensive patients. *Int. J. Cardiology*, **17**, 51 6.

Lyden, P. D. and Hantson, L. (1998). Assessment scales for the evaluation of stroke patients. *J. Stroke Cerebrovasc. Dis.*, **7**, 113–27.

Mackey, A. E., Abrahamowicz, M., Langlois, Y. *et al.* and the Asymptomatic Cervical Bruit Study Group (1997). Outcome of asymptomatic patients with carotid disease. *Neurology*, **48**, 896–903.

Macko, R. F., Kittner, S. J., Epstein, A. *et al.* (1999). Elevated tissue plasminogen activator antigen and stroke risk. The stroke prevention in young women study. *Stroke*, **30**, 7–11.

MacMahon, S. W., and Norton, R. N. (1986). Alcohol and hypertension: Implications for prevention and treatment. *Ann. Int. Med.*, **105**, 124–6.

MacMahon, S. and Rodgers, A. (1993). The effects of antihypertensive treatment on vascular disease: reappraisal of the evidence in 1994. *J. Vasc. Med. Biol.*, **4**, 265–71.

MacMahon, S,. Peto, R., Cutler, J. *et al.* (1990). Blood pressure, stroke, and coronary heart disease. Part 1, prolonged differences in blood pressure: prospective observational studies corrected for the regression dilution bias. *Lancet*, **335**, 765–74.

Maggioni, A. P., Franzosi, M. G., Santoro, E. *et al.* Studio Della Sopravvivenza nell' Infarto Miocardico II (GISSI-2) and the International Study Group (1992). The risk of stroke in patients with acute myocardial infarction after thrombolytic and antithrombotic treatment. *N. Engl. J. Med.*, **327**, 1–6.

Malhotra, H., Mehta, S. R., Mathur, D. et al. (1985). Pressor effects of alcohol in normotensive and hypertensive subjects. Lancet, 2, 584–6.

Malmgren, R., Bamford, J., Warlow, C. et al. (1989). Projecting the number of patients with first-ever strokes and patients newly handicapped by stroke in England and Wales. BMJ, 298, 656–60.

Malouf, R. and Brust, J. C. M. (1985). Hypoglycaemia: Causes, neurological manifestations, and outcome. Ann. Neurol., 17, 421–30.

Manson, J. E., Colditz, G. A., Stampfer, M. J. et al. (1990). A prospective study of obesity and risk of coronary heart disease in women. N. Engl. J. Med., 322, 882–9.

Manson, J. E., Colditz, G. A., Stampfer, M. J. et al. (1991). A prospective study of maturity-onset diabetes mellitus and risk of coronary heart disease and stroke in women. Arch. Intern. Med., 151, 1141–7.

Manson, J. E., Nathan, D. M., Krolewski, A. S. et al. (1992). A prospective study of exercise and incidence of diabetes among US male physicians. JAMA, 268, 63–7.

Manto, M., Cordonnier, M., Blecic, S. et al. (1995). Acute posterior multifocal placoid pigment epitheliopathy presenting as an aseptic meningitis. Eur. J. Neurol., 2, 181–3.

Marchal, G., Beaudouin, V., Rioux, P. et al. (1996a). Prolonged persistence of substantial volumes of potentially viable brain tissue after stroke A correlative PET-CT study with voxel-based data analysis. Stroke, 27, 599–606.

Marchal, G., Furlan, M., Beaudouin, V. et al. (1996b). Early spontaneous hyperperfusion after stroke. A marker of favourable tissue outcome? Brain, 119, 409–19.

Mari, F., Matei, M., Ceravolo, M. G. et al. (1997). Predictive value of clinical indices in detecting aspiration in patients with neurological disorders. J. Neurol. Neurosurg. Psychiatry, 63, 456–60.

Marinkovic, S. V., Milisavljevic, M. M., Kovacevic, M. S. et al. (1985). Perforating branches of the middle cerebral artery. Micro-anatomy and clinical significance of their intracerebral segments. Stroke, 16, 1022–9.

Marinkovic, S. V., Milisavljevic, M. M, Lolic-Draganic, V. et al. (1987). Distribution of the occipital branches of the posterior cerebral artery. Correlation with occipital lobe infarcts. Stroke, 18, 728–32.

Markel, M. L., Waller, B. F., and Armstrong, W. F. (1987). Cardiac myxoma: a review. Medicine, 66, 114–25.

Markus, H. S. (1991). A prospective follow up of thunderclap headache mimicking subarachnoid haemorrhage. J. Neurol. Neurosurg. Psychiatry, 54, 1117–18.

Markus, H. S. and Hambley, H. (1998) Neurology and the blood: haematological abnormalities in ischaemic stroke. J. Neurol. Neurosurg. Psychiatry, 64, 150–9.

Markus, H. S. and Harrison, M. J. G. (1992). The estimation of cerebrovascular reactivity using transcranial Doppler, including the use of breath-holding as the vasodilatory stimulus. Stroke, 23, 668–73.

Markus, H. S., Thomson, N. D., and Brown, M. M. (1995). Asymptomatic cerebral embolic signals in symptomatic and asymptomatic carotid artery disease. Brain, 118, 1005–11.

Marmot, M. and Brunner, E. (1991). Alcohol and cardiovascular disease: the status of the U shaped curve. BMJ, 303, 565–8.

Marmot, M. G. and Poulter, N. R. (1992). Primary prevention of stroke. Lancet, 339, 344–7.

Marmot, M. G., Elliott, P., Shipley, M. J. et al. (1994). Alcohol and blood pressure: the INTERSALT study. BMJ, 308, 1263–7.

Martin, P. J., Chang, H. M., Wityk, R. et al. (1998). Midbrain infarction: associations and aetiologies in the New England Medical Center Posterior Circulation Registry. J. Neurol. Neurosurg. Psychiatry, 64, 392–5.

Martin, R. L. (1997). Experimental neuronal protection in cerebral ischaemia. Part I: Experimental models and pathophysiological responses. J. Clin. Neurosci., 4, 96–113.

Martin, R. and Bogousslavsky, J. for the Lausanne Stroke Registry Group (1993). Mechanisms of late stroke after myocardial infarct: the Lausanne Stroke Registry. J. Neurol. Neurosurg. Psychiatry, 56, 760–4.

Martin, R. and Bogousslavsky, J. (1995). Embolic versus nonembolic causes of ischaemic stroke. Cerebrovasc. Dis., 5, 70–4.

Martyn, C. N., Barker, D. J .P., and Osmond, C. (1996). Morthers' pelvic size, fetal growth, and death from stroke and coronary heart disease in men in the UK. Lancet, 348, 1264–8.

Mas, J.-L. and Lamy, C. (1998). Stroke in pregnancy and the puerperium. J. Neurol., 245, 305–13.

Masdeu, J. C. (1983). Enhancing mass on CT: neoplasm or recent infarction? Neurology, 33, 836–40.

Masdeu, J. C. and Rubino, F. A. (1984). Management of lobar intracerebral haemorrhage: medical or surgical. Neurology, 34, 381–3.

Maseri, A. (1997). Inflammation, atherosclerosis, and ischaemic events—exploring the hidden side of the moon. N. Engl. J. Med., 336, 1014–15.

Mast, H., Thompson, J. L. P., Lee, S.-H., Mohr, J. P. et al. (1995). Hypertension and diabetes mellitus as determinants of multiple lacunar infarcts. Stroke, 26, 30–3.

Mast, H., Young, W. L., Koennecke, H.-C. et al. (1997). Risk of spontaneous haemorrhage after diagnosis of cerebral arteriovenous malformation. Lancet, 350, 1065–8.

Mastaglia, F. L., Knezevic, W., and Thompson, P. D. (1986). Weakness of head turning in hemiplegia: a quantitative study. *J. Neurol. Neurosurg. Psychiatry*, **49**, 195–7.

Masuda, J., Yutani, C., Waki, R. *et al.* (1992). Histopathological analysis of the mechanisms of intracranial haemorrhage complicationg infective endocarditis. *Stroke*, **23**, 843–50.

Mathew, P., Teasdale, G., Bannan, A. *et al.* (1995). Neurosurgical management of cerebellar haematoma and infarct. *J. Neurol. Neurosurg. Psychiatry*, **59**, 287–92.

Matthews, W. B. (1979). Neurosarcoidosis. In *Handbook of clinical neurology*, Vol. 38, *Neurological manifestations of systemic disease*, (ed. P. J. Vinken and G. W. Bruyn), Part 1, p. 521–42. North-Holland, Amsterdam.

Mayer, P. L., Awad, I. A., Todor, R. *et al.* (1996). Misdiagnosis of symptomatic cerebral aneurysm. Prevalence and correlation with outcome at four institutions. *Stroke*, **27**, 1558–63.

Mayer, S. A., Tatemichi, T. K., Spitz, J. L. *et al.* (1994). Recurrent ischaemic events and diffuse white matter disease in patients with pseudoxanthoma elasticum. *Cerebrovasc. Dis.*, **4**, 294–7.

Mayer, S. A., Lignelli, A., Fink, M. E. *et al.* (1998). Perilesional blood flow and oedema formation in acute intracerebral haemorrhage: a SPECT study. *Stroke*, **29**, 1791–8.

McDonald, M. J., Brophy, B. P., and Kneebone, C. (1998). Rendu–Osler–Weber syndrome: a current perspective on cerebral manifestations. *J. Clin. Neurosci.*, **5**, 345–50.

McEvoy, A. W., Kitchen, N. D., and Thomas, D. G. T. (1998). Intracerebral heamorrhage caused by drug abuse. *Lancet*, **351**, 1029.

McKeigue, P. M., Shah, B., and Marmot, M. G. (1991). Relation of central obesity and insulin resistance with high diabetes prevalence and cardiovascular risk in South Asians. *Lancet*, **337**, 971–3.

McNabb, A. W., Carroll, W. M., and Mastaglia, F. L. (1988). 'Alien hand' and loss of bimanual coordination after dominant anterior cerebral artery territory infarction. *J. Neurol. Neurosurg. Psychiatry*, **51**, 218–22.

Meade, T. W., Ruddock, V., Stirling, Y. *et al.* (1993). Fibrinolytic activity, clotting factors, and long-term incidence of ischaemic heart disease in the Northwick Park Heart Study. *Lancet*, **342**, 1076–9.

Mead, G. E., Lewis, S. C., Wardlaw, J. M. *et al.* (1999). Should CT appearance of lacunar stroke influence patient management *J. Neurol. Neurosurg. Psychiat.*, **67**, 682–4.

Mead, G. E., Lewis, S. C., Wardlaw, J. M. *et al.* (2000). How well does the Oxfordshire Community Stroke Project classification predict the site and size of the infarct on brain imaging *J. Neurol. Neurosurg. Psychiat.*, **68**, 558–62.

Medical Research Council's General Practice Research Framework (1998). Thrombosis prevention trial: randomised trial of low-intensity oral anticoagulation with warfarin and low-dose aspirin in the primary prevention of ischaemic heart disease in men at increased risk. *Lancet*, **351**, 233–41.

Meissner, I., Wiebers, D. O., Swanson, J. W. *et al.* (1986). The natural history of drop attacks. *Neurology*, **36**, 1029–35.

Melanson, M., Chalk, C., Georgevich, L. *et al.* (1996). Varicella-zoster virus DNA in CSF and arteries in delayed contralateral hemiplegia: evidence for viral invasion of cerebral arteries. *Neurology*, **47**, 569–70.

Meltzer, R. S., Visser, C. A., and Fuster, V. (1986). Intracardiac thrombi and systemic embolization. *Ann. Int. Med.*, **104**, 689–98.

Mendelow, A. D. (1991). Spontaneous intracerebral haemorrhage. *J. Neurol. Neurosurg. Psychiatry*, **54**, 193–5.

Mendelow, A. D., Erfurth, A., Grossart, K. *et al.* (1987). Do cerebral arteriovenous malformations increase in size? *J. Neurol. Neurosurg. Psychiatry*, **50**, 980–7.

Merrick, M. V., Ferrington, C. M., and Cowen, S. J. (1991). Parametric imaging of cerebral vascular reserves. 1. Theory, validation and normal values. *Eur. J. Nucl. Med.*, **18**, 171–7.

Metz, H., Murray-Leslie, R. M., Bannister, R. G. *et al.* (1961). Kinking of the internal carotid artery. *Lancet*, **1**, 424–6.

Michiels, J. J., Koudstaal, P. J., Mulder, A. H. *et al.* (1993). Transient neurologic and ocular manifestations in primary thrombocythaemia. *Neurology*, **43**, 1107–10.

Midgley, J. P., Matthew, A. G., Greenwood, C. M. T *et al.* (1996). Effect of reduced dietary sodium on blood pressure. A meta-analysis of randomised controlled trials. *JAMA*, **275**, 1590–7.

Milandre, L., Pellissier, J. F., Boudouresques, G. *et al.* (1987). Non-hereditary multiple telangiectasias of the central nervous system. *J. Neurol. Sci.*, **82**, 291–304.

Miles, A. N. and Knuckey, N. W. (1998). Apoptotic neuronal death following cerebral ischaemia. *J. Clin. Neurosci.*, **5**, 125–45.

Miller, V. T. and Cohen, B. A. (1987). Angiographic comparison of carotid arteries in unilateral cerebral ischaemia. *Neurology*, **37**, 1027–30.

Millikan, C. and Futrell, N. (1990). The fallacy of the lacune hypothesis. *Stroke*, **21**, 1251–7.

Mills, J. A. (1994). Systemic lupus erythematosus. *N. Engl. J. Med.*, **330**, 1871–9.

Mitchell, J. R. A. and Schwartz, C. J. (1962). Relationship between arterial disease in different sites. A study of the aorta and coronary, carotid and iliac arteries. *BMJ*, **1**, 1293–301.

Mitsias, P. and Levine, S. R. (1994). Large cerebral vessel occlusive disease in systemic lupus erythematosus. *Neurology*, **44**, 385–93.

Mitsias, P. and Levine, S. R. (1996). Cerebrovascular complications of Fabry's Disease. *Ann. Neurol.*, **40**, 8–17.

Miyashita, K., Naritomi, H., Nakamura, M. *et al.* (1991). Old cerebral haemorrhages in cases of multiple lacunar infarction found by magnetic resonance imaging. *Cerebrovasc. Dis.*, **1**, 321–6.

Mohr, J. P., Biller, J., Hilal, S. K. *et al.* (1995). Magnetic resonance versus computed tomographic imaging in acute stroke. *Stroke*, **26**, 807–12.

Mokri, B. and Piepgras, D. G. (1981). Cervical internal carotid artery aneurysm with calcific embolism to the retina. *Neurology*, **31**, 211–14.

Mokri, B., Silbert, P. L., Schievink, W. I. *et al.* (1996). Cranial nerve palsy in spontaneous dissection of the extracranial internal carotid artery. *Neurology*, **46**, 356–9.

Molinari, G. F. (1993). Lobar haemorrhages. Where do they come from? How do they get there? *Stroke*, **24**, 523–6.

Molloy, J., Khan, N., and Markus, H. S. (1998). Temporal variability of asymptomatic embolisation in carotid artery stenosis and optimal recording protocols. *Stroke*, **29**, 1129–32.

Mooe, T., Eriksson, P., and Stegmayr, B. (1997). Ischaemic stroke after acute myocardial infarction. A population-based study. *Stroke*, **28**, 762–7.

Moore, P. M. and Fauci, A. S. (1981). Neurological manifestations of systemic vasculitis. A retrospective and prospective study of the clinicopathologic features and responses to therapy in 25 patients. *Am. J. Med.*, **71**, 517–24.

Morgenlander, J. C. and Goldstein, L. B. (1991). Recurrent transient ischaemic attacks and stroke in association with an internal carotid artery web. *Stroke*, **22**, 94–8.

Morris, J. N. (1951*a*). Recent history of coronary disease. *Lancet*, **1**, 1–7.

Morris, J. N. (1951*b*). Recent history of coronary disease. *Lancet*, **1**, 69–73.

Motto, C., Aritzu, E., Boccardi, E. *et al.* (1997). Reliability of haemorrhagic transformation diagnosis in acute ischaemic stroke. *Stroke*, **28**, 302–6.

Moulin T., Bogousslavsky J., Chopard J.-L. *et al.* (1995). Vascular ataxic hemiparesis: a re-evaluation. *J. Neurol. Neurosurg. Psychiatry*, **58**, 422–7.

Moulin, T., Cattin, F., Crepin-Leblond, T. *et al.* (1996). Early CT signs in acute middle cerebral artery infarction: predictive value for subsequent infarct locations and outcome. *Neurology*, **47**, 366–75.

Mouton, P., Biousse, V., Crassard, I. *et al.* (1997). Ischaemic stroke due to calcific emboli from mitral valve annulus calcification. *Stroke*, **28**, 2325–6.

Mulder, L. J. M. M. and Spierings, E. L. H. (1987). Stroke due to intravascular coagulation in mycoplasma pneumoniae infection. *Lancet*, **2**, 1152–3.

Mulrow, C. D., Cornell, J. A., Herrera, C. R. *et al.* (1994). Hypertension in the elderly. Implications and generalizability of randomised trials. *JAMA*, **272**, 1932–8.

Mumford, C .J., Fletcher, N. A., Ironside, J. W. *et al.* (1996). Progressive ataxia, focal seizures, and malabsorption syndrome in a 41 year old woman. *J. Neurol. Neursurg. Psychiatry*, **60**, 225–30.

Munts, A. G., van Genderen, P. J. J., Dippel, D. W. J. *et al.* (1998). Coagulation disorders in young adults with acute cerebral ischaemia. *J. Neurol.*, **245**, 21–5.

Murphy, M. F., Clarke, C. R. A., and Brearley, R. L. (1983). Superior sagittal sinus thrombosis and essential thrombocythaemia. *BMJ*, **287**, 1344.

Murray, C. J. L. and Lopez, A. D. (1997). Mortality by cause for eight regions of the world: Global burden of disease study. *Lancet*, **349**, 1269–76.

Murros, K. E. and Toole, J. F. (1989). The effect of radiation on carotid arteries. A review article. *Arch. Neurol.*, **46**, 449–55.

Nabors, M. W., Azzam, C. J., Albanna, F. J. *et al.* (1987). Delayed postoperative dural arteriovenous malformations. Report of two cases. *J. Neurosurg.*, **66**, 768–72.

Nagayama, T., Shinohara, Y., Nagayama, M. *et al.* (1993). Congenitally abnormal plasminogen in juvenile ischaemic cerebrovascular disease. *Stroke*, **24**, 2104–7.

Narayan, S. M., Cain, M. E., and Smith, J. M. (1997). Atrial fibrillation. *Lancet*, **350**, 943–50.

Nasreddine, Z. S. and Saver, J. L. (1997). Pain after thalamic stroke: right diencephalic predominance and clinical features in 180 patients. *Neurology*, **48**, 1196–9.

Nater, B., Bogousslavsky, J., Regli, F. *et al.* (1992). Stroke patterns with atrial septal aneurysm. *Cerebrovasc. Dis.*, **2**, 342–6.

Natowicz, M. and Kelley, R. I. (1987). Mendelian aetiologies of stroke. *Ann. Neurol.*, **22**, 175–92.

Naylor, A. R., Merrick, M. V., Slattery, J. M. *et al.* (1991). Parametric imaging of cerebral vascular reserve. 2. Reproducibility, response to CO_2 and correlation with middle cerebral artery velocities. *Eur. J. Nucl. Med.*, **18**, 259–64.

Neau, J.-P., Ingrand, P., Couderq, C. *et al.* (1997). Recurrent intracerebral hemorrhage. *Neurology*, **49**, 106–13.

Neil-Dwyer, G. and Lang, D. (1997). 'Brain attack' – aneurysmal subarachnoid haemorrhage: death due to delayed diagnosis. *J. R. Coll. Physicians Lond.*, **31**, 49–52.

Nehls, D. G., Flom, R. A., Carter, L. P. *et al.* (1985). Multiple intracranial aneurysms: determining the site of rupture. *J. Neurosurg.*, **63**, 342–8.

Nelson, P. K., Levy, D., Masters, L. T. *et al.* (1997). Neuroendovascular management of intracranial aneurysms. *Neuroimaging Clin. North Am.*, 7, 739–62.

Nesbit, R. R., Neistadt, A., and May, A. G. (1979). Bilateral internal carotid artery aneurysms. *Arch. Surg.*, 114, 293–5.

Nicholls, S. C., Phillips, D. J., Primozich, J. F. *et al.* (1989). Diagnostic significance of flow separation in the carotid bulb. *Stroke*, 20, 175–82.

Nicolai, A., Lazzarino, L. G., and Biasutti, E. (1996). Large striatocapsular infarcts: clinical features and risk factors. *J. Neurol.*, 243, 44–50.

Nighoghossian, N., Berruyer, M., J.-C., G., and Trouillas, P. (1994) Free protein S spectrum in young patients with stroke. *Cerebrovasc. Dis.*, 4, 304–8.

Nishide, M., Irion, T., Gotoh, M., Naka, M. *et al.* (1983). Cardiac abnormalities in ischaemic cerebrovascular disease studied by two dimensional echocardiography. *Stroke* 14, 541–5.

Nishino, H., Rubino, F. A., DeRemee, R. A. *et al.* (1993). Neurological involvement in Wegener's granulomatosis: an analysis of 324 consecutive patients at the Mayo Clinic. *Ann. Neurol.*, 33, 4–9.

Norris, J. W. and Hachinski, V. C. (1982). Misdiagnosis of stroke. *Lancet*, 1, 328–31.

Norris, J. W., Hachinski, V. C., Myers, M. G. *et al.* (1979). Serum cardiac enzymes in stroke. *Stroke*, 10, 548–53.

Norrving, B. and Staaf, G. (1991). Pure motor stroke from presumed lacunar infarct: incidence, risk factors and initial course. *Cerebrovasc. Dis.*, 1, 203–9.

North, K. N., Whiteman, D. A. H., Pepin, M. G. *et al.* (1995). Cerebrovascular complications in Ehlers–Danlos syndrome Type IV. *Ann. Neurol.*, 38, 960–4.

Oberlander, D. A., Biller, J., and McCarthy, L. J. (1995). Thrombotic thrombocytopenic purpura: a neurological perspective. *J. Stroke Cerebrovasc. Dis.*, 5, 175–9.

O'Connell, B. K., Towfighi, J., Brennan, R. W. *et al.* (1985). Dissecting aneurysms of head and neck. *Neurology*, 35, 993–7.

Ogata, J., Masuda, J., Yutani, C. *et al.* (1990). Rupture of atheromatous plaque as a cause of thrombotic occlusion of stenotic internal carotid artery. *Stroke*, 21, 1740–5.

Ogata, J., Masuda, J., Yutani, C. *et al.* (1994). Mechanisms of cerebral artery thrombosis: a histopathological analysis on eight necropsy cases. *J. Neurol. Neurosurg. Psychiatry*, 57, 17–21.

Ogren, M., Hedblad, B., Isacsson, S.-O. *et al.* (1993). Non-invasively detected carotid stenosis and ischaemic heart disease in men with leg arteriosclerosis. *Lancet*, 342, 1138–41.

Ohman, J. and Heiskanen, O. (1989). Timing of operation for ruptured supratentorial aneurysms: a prospective randomised study. *J. Neurosurg.*, 70, 55–60.

Okada, Y., Yamaguchi, T., Minematsu, K. *et al.* (1989). Haemorrhagic transformation in cerebral embolism. *Stroke*, 20, 598–603.

O'Laoire, S. A., Crockard, A., Thomas, D. G. T. *et al.* (1982). Brain-stem haematoma. A report of six surgically treated cases. *J. Neurosurg.*, 56, 222–7.

O'Leary, D. H., Polak, J. F., Kronmal, A. *et al.* on behalf of the CHS Collaborative Research Group (1992). Distribution and correlates of sonographically detected carotid artery disease in the Cardiovascular Health Study. *Stroke*, 23, 1752–60.

Olesen, J., Friberg, L., Olsen, T. S. *et al.* (1993). Ischaemia-induced (symptomatic) migraine attacks may be more frequent than migraine-induced ischaemic insults. *Brain*, 116, 187–202.

Olsen, T. S., Skriver, E. B., and Herning, M. (1985). Cause of cerebral infarction in the carotid territory. Its relation to the size and the location of the infarct and to the underlying vascular lesion. *Stroke*, 16, 459–66.

Ondra, S. L., Troupp, H., George, E. D. *et al.* (1990). The natural history of symptomatic arteriovenous malformations of the brain: a 24-year follow-up assessment. *J. Neurosurg.*, 73, 387–91.

Opeskin, K. and Silberstein, M. (1998). False positive diagnosis of subarachnoid haemorrhage on computed tomography scan. *J. Clin. Neurosci.*, 5, 382–6.

Oppenheimer, S. M. and Lima, J. (1998). Neurology and the heart. *J. Neurol. Neurosurg. Psychiatry*, 64, 289–97.

Oppenheimer, S. M., Cechetto, D. F., and Hachinski, V. C. (1990). Cerebrogenic cardiac arrhythmias. Cerebral electrocardiographic influences and their role in sudden death. *Arch. Neurol.*, 47, 513–19.

Orencia, A. J., Petty, G. W., Khandheria, B. K. *et al.* (1995*a*). Risk of stroke with mitral valve prolapse in population-based cohort study. *Stroke*, 26, 7–13.

Orencia, A. J., Petty, G. W., Khandheria, B. K. *et al.* (1995*b*). Mitral valve prolapse and the risk of stroke after initial cerebral ischaemia. *Neurology*, 45, 1083–6.

Orencia, A. J., Daviglus, M. L., Dyer, A. R. *et al.* (1996). Fish consumption and stroke in men. 30-year findings of Chicago Western Electric Study. *Stroke*, 27, 204–9.

Orgogozo, J. M. and Bogousslavsky, J. (1989). Lacunar syndromes. In *Handbook of Clinical Neurology*, Vol. 10, (ed. P. J. Vinken, G. W. Bruyn, and H. L. Klawans), pp. 235–69. Elsevier, Amsterdam.

O'Rourke, S., MacHale, S., Signorini, D. *et al.* (1998). Detecting psychiatric morbidity after stroke: comparison of the GHQ and the HAD Scale. *Stroke*, 29, 980–5.

Ostrov, B. E. and Barron, T. F. (1995). Cerebral vasculitis. Diagnosis and current treatment recommendations. *CNS Drugs*, 3, 115–25.

Overstall, P. W. (1995). Falls after strokes. *BMJ*, 311, 74–5.

Paganini-Hill, A., Ross, R. K., and Henderson, B. E. (1988). Postmenopausal oestrogen treatment and stroke: a prospective study. *BMJ*, 297, 519–22.

Pan, W.-H., Li, L.-A., and Tsai, M.-J. (1995). Temperature extremes and mortality from coronary heart disease and cerebral infarction in elderly Chinese. *Lancet*, 345, 353–5.

Panerai, R. B., White, R. P., Markus, H. *et al.* (1998). Grading of cerebral dynamic autoregulation from spontaneous fluctuations in arterial blood pressure. *Stroke*, 29, 2341–6.

Paneth, N. and Susser, M. (1995). Early origin of coronary heart disease (the 'Barker hypothesis'). Hypotheses, no matter how intriguing, need rigorous attempts at refutation. *BMJ*, 310, 411–12.

Pantoni, L. and Garcia, J. H. (1997). Pathogenesis of leukoaraiosis. A review. *Stroke*, 28, 652–9.

Pappata, S., Tran Dinh, S., Baron, J. C. *et al.* (1987). Remote metabolic effects of cerebrovascular lesions: magnetic resonance and positron tomography imaging. *Neuroradiology*, 29, 1–6.

Park, Y. D., Belman, A. L., Kim, T.-S. *et al.* (1990). Stroke in paediatric acquired immunodeficiency syndrome. *Ann. Neurol.*, 28, 303–11.

Parker, J. L. W. and Lawson, D. H. (1973). Death from thyrotoxicosis. *Lancet*, 2, 894–5.

Parr, M. J. A., Finfer, S. R., and Morgan, M. K. (1996). Reversible cardiogenic shock complicating subarachnoid haemorrhage. *BMJ*, 313, 681–3.

Passero, S. and Filosomi, G. (1998). Posterior circulation infarcts in patients with vertebrobasilar dolichoectasia. *Stroke*, 29, 653–9.

Passero, S., Burgalassi, L., D'Andrea, P. *et al.* (1995). Recurrence of bleeding in patients with primary intracerebral haemorrhage. *Stroke*, 26, 1189–92.

Patel, M. R., Edelman, R. R., and Warach, S. (1996). Detection of hyperacute primary intraparenchymal haemorrhage by magnetic resonance imaging. *Stroke*, 27, 2321–4.

Patrono, C. (1994). Aspirin as an antiplatelet drug. *N. Engl. J. Med.*, 330, 1287–94.

Patterson, J. R. and Grabois, M. (1986). Locked-in syndrome: a review of 139 cases. *Stroke*, 17, 758–64.

Pavlakis, S. G., Bello, J., Prohovnik, I. *et al.* (1988). Brain infarction in sickle cell anaemia: Magnetic resonance imaging correlates. *Ann. Neurol.*, 23, 125–30.

Pearson, T. C. and Wetherley-Mein, G. (1978). Vascular occlusive episodes and venous haematocrit in primary proliferative polycythaemia. *Lancet*, 2, 1219–22.

Pedersen, A. T., Lidegaard, O., Kreiner, S. *et al.* (1997). Hormone replacement therapy and risk of non-fatal stroke. *Lancet*, 350, 1277–83.

Pedersen, P. M., Jorgensen, H. S., Nakayama, H. *et al.* (1995). Aphasia in acute stroke: incidence, determinants, and recovery. *Ann. Neurol.*, 38, 659–66

Peery, W. H. (1987). Clinical spectrum of hereditary haemorrhagic telangiectasia (Osler–Weber–Rendu disease). *Am. J. Med.*, 82, 989–97.

Pekkanen, J., Tuomilehto, J., Uutela, A. *et al.* (1995). Social class, health behaviour, and mortality among men and women in eastern Finland. *BMJ*, 311, 589–93.

Peltonen, M., Stegmayr, B., and Asplund, K. (1998). Time trends in long-term survival after stroke: the Northern Sweden Multinational Monitoring of Trends and Determinants in Cardiovascular Disease (MONICA) study, 1985–1994. *Stroke*, 29, 1358–65.

Penney, G. C., Glasier, A., and Templeton, A. (1994). Multicentre criterion based audit of the management of induced abortion in Scotland. *BMJ*, 309, 15–19.

Petersen, P. and Godtfredsen, J. (1986). Embolic complications in paroxysmal atrial fibrillation. *Stroke*, 17, 622–6.

Petersen, P. and Hansen, J. M. (1988). Stroke in thyrotoxicosis with atrial fibrillation. *Stroke*, 19, 15–18.

Petrovitch, H., Curb, D., and Bloom-Marcus, E. (1995). Isolated systolic hypertension and risk of stroke in Japanese–American men. *Stroke*, 26, 25–9.

Petty, G. W., Khandheria, B. K., Chu, C.-P. *et al.* (1997). Patent foramen ovale in patients with cerebral infarction. A transesophageal echocardiographic study. *Arch. Neurol.*, 54, 819–22.

Petty, G. W., Brown, R. D., Jr, Whisnant, J. P. *et al.* (1998). Survival and recurrence after first cerebral infarction: a population-based study in Rochester, Minnesota, 1975 through 1989. *Neurology*, 50, 208–16.

Pfleger, M. J., Hardee, E. P., Contant, C. F. *et al.* (1994). Sensitivity and specificity of fluid-blood levels for coagulopathy in acute intracerebral haematomas. *Am. J. Neuroradiol.*, 15, 217–23.

Phillips, L. H., Whisnant, J. P., and Reagan, T. J. (1977). Sudden death from stroke. *Stroke*, 8, 392–5.

Pickle, L. W., Mungiole, M., and Gillum, R. F. (1997). Geographic variation in stroke mortality in blacks and whites in the United States. *Stroke*, 28, 1639–47.

Pinto, A. N., Canhao, P., and Ferro, J. M. (1996). Seizures at the onset of subarachnoid haemorrhage. *J. Neurol.*, 243, 161–4.

Plant, G. T., Revesz, T., Barnard, R. O., Harding, A. E. *et al.* (1990). Familial cerebral amyloid angiopathy with nonneuritic amyloid plaque formation. *Brain*, 113, 721–47.

Plum, F. and Posner, J. B. (1985). *The diagnosis of stupor and coma*. F. A. Davis Co., Philadelphia.

Pocock, S. J., Shaper, A. G., Cook, D. G. *et al.* (1980). British Regional Heart Study: geographic variations in cardiovascular mortality, and the role of water quality. *BMJ*, **280**, 1243–9.

Pohjasvaara, T., Erkinjuntti, T., Vataja, R. *et al.* (1998). Correlates of dependent living 3 months after ischaemic stroke. *Cerebrovasc. Dis.*, **8**, 259–66.

Pohlmann-Eden, B., Hoch, D. B., Cochius, J. I. *et al.* (1996). Stroke and epilepsy: critical review of the literature Part I: Epidemiology and risk factors. *Cerebrovasc. Dis.*, **6**, 332–8.

Pohlmann-Eden, B., Cochius, J. I., Hoch, D. B. *et al.* (1997). Stroke and epilepsy: critical review of the literature. Part II: risk factors, pathophysiology and overlap syndromes. *Cerebrovasc. Dis.*, **7**, 2–9.

Pop, G. A., Koudstaal, P. J., Meeder, H. J., Algra, A., van Latum, J. C., and van Gijn, J. for the Dutch TIA Trial Study Group (1994). Predictive value of clinical history and electrocardiogram in patients with transient ischaemic attack or minor ischaemic stroke for subsequent cardiac and cerebral ischaemic events. *Arch. Neurol.*, **51**, 333–41.

Powers, W. J. (1986). Should lumbar puncture be part of the routine evaluation of patients with cerebral ischaemia? *Stroke*, **17**, 332–3.

Powers, W. J. (1991). Cerebral hemodynamics in ischaemic cerebrovascular disease. *Ann. Neurol.*, **29**, 231–40.

Powers, W. J. (1993). Acute hypertension after stroke: the scientific basis for treatment decisions. *Neurology*, **43**, 461–7.

Powers, W. J., Press, G. A., Grubb, R. L. *et al.* (1987). The effect of hemodynamically significant carotid artery disease on the hemodynamic status of the cerebral circulation. *Ann. Int. Med.*, **106**, 27–34.

Prasad, K. and Shrivastava, A. (1999). Surgery for primary supratentorial intracerebral haematoma (Cochrane Review). In *The Cochrane Library*, Issue 1. Update Software, Oxford.

Preston, F. E., Cooke, K. B., Foster, M. E. *et al.* (1978). Myelomatosis and the hyperviscosity syndrome. *Br. J. Haematol.*, **38**, 517–30.

Preston, F. E., Martin, J. F., Stewart, R. M. *et al.* (1979). Thrombocytosis, circulating platelet aggregates, and neurological dysfunction. *BMJ*, **2**, 1561–3.

Preter, M., Tzourio, C., Ameri, A. *et al.* (1996). Long-term prognosis in cerebral venous thrombosis: follow-up of 77 patients. *Stroke*, **27**, 243–6.

Pretre, R. and von Segesser, L. K. (1997). Aortic dissection. *Lancet*, **349**, 1461–4.

Prichard, B. N. C., Smith, C. C. T., Ling, K. L. E. *et al.* (1995). Fish oils and cardiovascular disease: beneficial effects on lipids and the haemostatic system. *BMJ*, **310**, 819–20.

Prior, A. L., Wilson, L. A., Gosling, R. G. *et al.* (1979). Retrograde cerebral embolism. *Lancet*, **2**, 1044–7.

PROGRESS Management Committee (1996). Blood pressure lowering for the secondary prevention of stroke: rationale and design for PROGRESS. *J. Hypertens.*, **14** (Suppl. 2), S41–6.

Prospective Studies Collaboration (1995). Cholesterol, diastolic blood pressure, and stroke: 13,000 strokes in 450,000 people in 45 prospective cohorts. *Lancet*, **346**, 1647–53.

Przelomski, M. M., Fisher, M., Davidson, R. I. *et al.* (1986). Unruptured intracranial aneurysm and transient focal cerebral ischaemia: a follow-up study. *Neurology*, **36**, 584–7.

Psaty, B. M., Smith, N. L., Siscovick, D. S. *et al.* (1997). Health outcomes associated with antihypertensive therapies used as first-line agents. A systematic review and meta-analysis. *JAMA*, **277**, 739–45.

Publications Committee for the Trial of ORG 10172 in Acute Stroke Treatment (TOAST) Investigators (1998). Low molecular weight heparinoid, ORG 10172 (Danaparoid), and outcome after acute ischaemic stroke. A randomised controlled trial. *JAMA*, **279**, 1265–72.

Pullicino, P. M., Alexandrov, A. V., Shelton, J. A. *et al.* (1997). Mass effect and death from severe acute stroke. *Neurology*, **49**, 1090–5.

Pulsinelli, W. (1992). Pathophysiology of acute ischaemic stroke. *Lancet*, **339**, 533–6.

Qizilbash, N., Jones, L., Warlow, C. *et al.* (1991). Fibrinogen and lipids as risks factors for transient ischaemic attacks and minor ischaemic strokes. *BMJ*, **303**, 605–9.

Qizilbash, N., Duffy, S., Prentice, C. R. M. *et al.* (1997). Von Willebrand factor and risk of ischaemic stroke. *Neurology*, **49**, 1552–6.

Qureshi, A. I., Janssen, R. S., Karon, J. M. *et al.* (1997). Human immunodeficiency virus infection and stroke in young patients. *Arch. Neurol.*, **54**, 1150–3.

Raaymakers, T. W. M., Rinkel, G. J. E., Limburg, M. *et al.* (1998). Mortality and morbidity of surgery for unruptured intracranial aneurysms: a meta-analysis. *Stroke*, **29**, 1531–8.

Raps, E. C., Rogers, J. D., Galetta, S. L. *et al.* (1993). The clinical spectrum of unruptured intracranial aneurysms. *Arch. Neurol.*, **50**, 265–8.

Rastenyte, D., Tuomilehto, J., and Sarti, C. (1998). Genetics of stroke—a review. *J. Neurol. Sci.*, **153**, 132–45.

Read, S. J., Pettigrew, L., Schimmel, L. *et al.* (1998). White matter medullary infarcts: acute subcortical infarction in the centrum ovale. *Cerebrovasc. Dis.*, **8**, 289–95.

Reddy, K., West, M., and McClarty, B. (1987). Multiple intracerebral arteriovenous malformations. A case report and literature review. *Surg. Neurol.*, **27**, 495–9.

Reed, D. M., Resch, J. A., Hayashi, T *et al.* (1988). A prospective study of cerebral artery atherosclerosis. *Stroke*, **19**, 820–5.

Reed, G. and Devous, M. (1985). Southwestern Internal Medicine Conference: Cerebral blood flow autoregulation and hypertension. *Am. J. Med. Sci.*, **289**, 37–44.

Refsum, H., Ueland, P. M., Nygard, O. *et al.* (1998). Homocysteine and cardiovascular disease. *Annu. Rev. Med.*, **49**, 31–62.

Reik, L. (1993). Stroke due to Lyme disease. *Neurology*, **43**, 2705–7.

Reith, J., Jorgensen, H. S., Pedersen, P. M. *et al.* (1996). Body temperature in acute stroke: relation to stroke severity, infarct size, mortality, and outcome. *Lancet*, **347**, 422–5.

Reneman, R. S., van Merode, T., Hick, P. *et al.* (1985). Flow velocity patterns in and distensibility of the carotid artery bulb in subjects of various ages. *Circulation*, **71**, 500–9.

Requena, I., Arias, M., Lopez-Ibor, L. *et al.* (1991). Cavernomas of the central nervous system: clinical and neuroimaging manifestation in 47 patients. *J. Neurol. Neurosurg. Psychiatry*, **54**, 590–4.

Resche, J. A., Okabe, N., Loewenson, R. B. *et al.* (1969). Patterns of vessel involvement in cerebral atherosclerosis: a comparative study between a Japanese and Minnesota population. *J. Atherosclerosis Res.*, **9**, 239–50.

Rexrode, K. M., Hennekens, C. H., Willett, W. C. *et al.* (1997). A prospective study of body mass index, weight change, and risk of stroke in women. *JAMA*, **277**, 1539–45.

Reynen, K. (1995). Cardiac myxomas. *N. Engl. J. Med.*, **333**, 1610–17.

Rhodes, E. L., Stanley, J. C., Hoffman, G. L. *et al.* (1976). Aneurysms of extracranial carotid arteries. *Arch. Surg.*, **111**, 339–43.

Rhodes, J. M. (1996). Cholesterol crystal embolism: an important 'new' diagnosis for the general physician. *Lancet*, **347**, 1641.

Rich, C., Gill, J. C., Wenick, S. *et al.* (1993). An unusual cause of cerebral venous thombosis in a four-year-old child. *Stroke*, **24**, 603–5.

Richardson, P. D., Davies, M. J., and Born, G. V. R. (1989). Influence of plaque configuration and stress distribution on fissuring of coronary atherosclerotic plaques. *Lancet*, **2**, 941–4.

Ridolfi, R. L. and Bell, W. R. (1981). Thrombotic thrombocytopenic purpura. Report of 25 cases and review of the literature. *Medicine*, **60**, 413–28.

Rimm, E. B., Ascherio, A., Giovannucci, E. *et al.* (1996). Vegetable, fruit, and cereal fiber intake and risk of coronary heart disease among men. *JAMA*, **275**, 447–51.

Ringelstein, E. B. (1995). Skepticism toward carotid ultrasonography: a virtue, an attitude, or fanaticism? *Stroke*, **26**, 1743–6.

Ringelstein, E. B., Zeumer, H., and Angelou, D. (1983). The pathogenesis of strokes from internal carotid artery occlusion. Diagnostic and therapeutical implications. *Stroke*, **14**, 867–75.

Ringelstein, E. B., Droste, D. W., Babikian, V. I. *et al.* (1998). Consensus on microembolus detection by TCD: international consensus group on microembolus detection. *Stroke*, **29**, 725–9.

Rinkel, G. J. E., Wijdicks, E. F. M., Hasan, D. *et al.* (1991). Outcome in patients with subarachnoid haemorrhage and negative angiography according to pattern of haemorrhage on computed tomography. *Lancet*, **338**, 964–8.

Rinkel, G. J. E., van Gijn, J., and Wijdicks, E. F. M. (1993). Subarachnoid haemorrhage without detectable aneurysm. A review of the causes. *Stroke*, **24**, 1403–9.

Rinkel, G. J. E., Djibuti, M., Algra, A. *et al.* (1998). Prevalence and risk of rupture of intracranial aneurysms: a systematic review. *Stroke*, **29**, 251–6.

Roach, G. W., Kanchuger, M., Mangano, C. M. *et al.* for the Multicenter study of Perioperative Ischaemia Research Group and the Ischaemia Research and Education Foundation Investigators (1996). Adverse cerebral outcomes after coronary bypass surgery. *N. Engl. J. Med.*, **335**, 1857–63.

Roberts, L. and Counsell, C. (1998). Assessment of clinical outcomes in acute stroke trials. *Stroke*, **29**, 986–91.

Rodgers, A., MacMahon, S., Gamble, G. *et al.* for the United Kingdom Transient Ischaemic Attack Collaborative Group (1996). Blood pressure and risk of stroke in patients with cerebrovascular disease. *BMJ*, **313**, 147.

Roeltgen, D. P., Weimer, G. R., and Patterson, L. F. (1981). Delayed neurologic complications of left atrial myxoma. *Neurology*, **31**, 8–13.

Roldan, C. A., Shively, B. K., and Crawford, M. H. (1996). An echocardiographic study of valvular heart disease associated with systematic lupus erythematosus. *N. Engl. J. Med.*, **335**, 1424–30.

Roman, G., Fisher, M., Perl, D. P. *et al.* (1978). Neurological manifestations of hereditary haemorrhagic telangiectasia (Rendu–Osler–Weber disease): report of 2 cases and review of the literature. *Ann. Neurol.*, **4**, 130–44.

Ronkainen, A., Miettinen, H., Karkola, K. *et al.* (1998). Risk of harboring an unruptured intracranial aneurysm. *Stroke*, **29**, 359–62.

Roos, Y. B. W. E. M., Rinkel, G. J. E., Vermeulen, M. *et al.* (1999). Antifibrinolytic treatment in aneurysmal subarachnoid haemorrhage (Cochrane Review) In *The Cochrane Library*, Issue 1. Update software, Oxford.

Ropper, A. H. (1987) Severe dysarthria with right hemisphere stroke. *Neurology*, **37**, 1061–3.

Rose, G. (1981). Strategy of prevention: lessons from cardiovascular disease. *BMJ*, **282**, 1847–51.

Rose, G. (1992). *The strategy of preventive medicine*. Oxford Medical Publications, Oxford.

Rose, G., Hamilton, P. J. S., Colwell, L. *et al.* (1982). A randomised controlled trial of anti-smoking advice: 10 year results. *J. Epidemiol. Community Hlth*, **36**, 102–8.

Rosengren, A., Welin, L., Tsipogianni, A. *et al.* (1989). Impact of cardiovascular risk factors on coronary heart disease and mortality among middle aged diabetic men: a general population study. *BMJ*, **299**, 1127–31.

Rosengren, A., Wilhelmsen, L., Welin, L. *et al.* (1990). Social influences and cardiovascular risk factors as determinants of plasma fibrinogen concentration in a general population sample of middle aged men. *BMJ*, **330**, 634–8.

Rosler, A., Mrass, G. J., Frese, A. *et al.* (1999). Precipitating factors of transient global amnesia. *J. Neurol.*, **246**, 53–4.

Ross, R. S. and McKusick, V. A. (1953). Aortic arch syndromes. Diminished or absent pulses in arteries arising from arch of aorta. *Arch. Intern. Med.*, **92**, 701–40.

Ross, R. (1999) Atherosclerosis—an inflammatory disease. *N. Engl. J. Med.*, **340**, 115–26.

Ross, R. T., Morrow, I. M., and Cheang, M. S. (1988). The relationship of brachiocephalic vessel atheroma to transient ischaemia of the brain and retina. *QJM*, **67**, 487–95.

Ross Russell, R. W. (1975) How does blood pressure cause stroke? *Lancet*, **2**, 1283–5.

Ross Russell, R. W. (1988). Cause and treatment of insufficiency in the cerebral circulation. *Clin. Neurol. Neurosurg.*, **90**, 19–24.

Ross Russell, R. W., and Ikeda, H. (1986). Clinical and electrophysiological observations in patients with low pressure retinopathy. *Br. J. Ophthalmol.*, **70**, 651–6.

Ross Russell, R. W. and Page, N. G. R. (1983). Critical perfusion of brain and retina. *Brain*, **106**, 419–34.

Rothrock, J. F., Rubenstein, R., and Lyden, P. D. (1988). Ischaemic stroke associated with methamphetamine inhalation. *Neurology*, **38**, 589–92.

Rothwell, P. M. (1994). Investigation of unilateral sensory or motor symptoms: frequency of neurological pathology depends on side of symptoms. *J. Neurol. Neurosurg. Psychiatry* **57**, 1401–2.

Rothwell, P. M. (1999). Model paper based on ECST. *Lancet*, in press.

Rothwell, P. M. and Warlow, C. P. (1996). Making sense of the measurement of carotid stenosis. *Cerebrovasc. Dis.*, **6**, 54–8.

Rothwell, P. M., Gibson, R. J., Slattery, J. *et al.* for the European Carotid Surgery Trialists' Collaborative Group (1994*a*). Equivalence of measurements of carotid stenosis: a comparison of three methods on 1001 angiograms. *Stroke*, **25**, 2435–9.

Rothwell, P. M., Gibson, R. J., Slattery, J. *et al.* for the European Carotid Surgery Trialists' Collaborative Group (1994*b*). Prognostic value and reproducibility of measurements of carotid stenosis. A comparison of three methods on 1001 angiograms. *Stroke*, **25**, 2440–4.

Rothwell, P. M., Wroe, S. J., Slattery, J., and Warlow, C. P., on behalf of the Oxfordshire Community Stroke Project (1996). Is stroke incidence related to season or temperature? *Lancet*, **347**, 934–6.

Roy, C. W. and Sherrington, C. S. (1890). On the regulation of the blood supply to the brain. *J. Physiol. (London)*, **11**, 85–108.

Royden Jones, H. and Siekert, R. G. (1989). Neurological manifestations of infective endocarditis. Review of clinical and therapeutic challenges. *Brain*, **112**, 1295–315.

Rubba, P., Mercuri, M., Faccenda, F. *et al.* (1994) Premature carotid atherosclerosis: does it occur in both familial hypercholesterolemia and homocystinuria? Ultrasound assessment of arterial intima-media thickness and blood flow velocity. *Stroke*, **25**, 943–50.

Ruby, R. J. and Burton, J. R. (1977). Acute reversible hemiparesis and hyponatraemia. *Lancet*, **1**, 1212.

Rudd, A. G., Wolfe, C. D. A., Tilling, K. *et al.* (1997). Randomised controlled trial to evaluate early discharge scheme for patients with stroke. *BMJ*, **315**, 1039–44.

Ruff, R. L., Talman, W. T., and Petito, F. (1981). Transient ischaemic attacks associated with hypotension in hypertensive patients with carotid artery stenosis. *Stroke*, **12**, 353–5.

Sacco, R. L., Kargman, D. E., Gu, Q. *et al.* (1995). Race-ethnicity and determinants of intracranial atherosclerotic cerebral infarction. The Northern Manhattan Stroke Study. *Stroke*, **26**, 14–20.

Sacco, S. E., Whisnant, J. P., Broderick, J. P. *et al.* (1991). Epidemiological characteristics of lacunar infarcts in a population. *Stroke*, **22**, 1236–41.

Sacz de Ocariz, M. d. M., Nader, J. A., Del Brutto, O. H. *et al.* (1996). Cerebrovascular complications of neurosyphilis: the return of an old problem. *Cerebrovasc. Dis.*, **6**, 195–201.

Sagie, A., Larson, M. G., and Levy, D. (1993). The natural history of borderline isolated systolic hypertension. *N. Engl. J. Med.*, **329**, 1912–17.

Sakai, F., Ishii, K., Igarashi, H. *et al.* (1988). Regional cerebral blood flow during an attack of vertebrobasilar insufficiency. *Stroke*, **19**, 1426–30.

Sakaki, T., Kinugawa, K., Tanigake, T. *et al.* (1980). Embolism from intracranial aneurysms. *J. Neurosurg.*, **53**, 300–4.

Salgado, A. V. (1991). Central nervous system complications of infective endocarditis. *Stroke*, **22**, 1461–3.

SALT Collaborative Group (1991). Swedish Aspirin Low-dose Trial (SALT) of 75 mg aspirin as secondary prophylaxis after cerebrovascular ischaemic events. *Lancet*, **338**, 1345–9.

Samuelsson, M., Lindell, D., and Norrving, B. (1994). Gadolinium-enhanced magnetic resonance imaging in patients with presumed lacunar infarcts. *Cerebrovasc. Dis.*, **4**, 12–19.

Samuelsson, M., Lindell, D., and Norrving, B. (1996). Presumed pathogenetic mechanisms of recurrent stroke after lacunar infarction. *Cerebrovasc. Dis.*, **6**, 128–36.

Sandercock, P. A. G. and Tangkanakul, C. (1997). Very early prevention of stroke recurrence. *Cerebrovasc. Dis.*, **7** (Suppl. 1), 10–15.

Sandercock, P. A. G., Molyneux, A., and Warlow, C. (1985). Value of computed tomography in patients with stroke: Oxfordshire Community Stroke Project. *BMJ*, **290**, 193–7.

Sandercock, P. A. G., Warlow, C. P., Jones, L. N. *et al.* (1989). Predisposing factors for cerebral infarction: the Oxfordshire Community Stroke Project. *BMJ*, **298**, 75–80.

Sandercock, P. A. G., Bamford, J., Dennis, M. *et al.* (1992). Atrial fibrillation and stroke: Frequency in different stroke types and influence on early and long term prognosis. The Oxfordshire community stroke project. *BMJ*, **305**, 1460–5.

Sandok, B. A., von Estorff, I., and Giuliani, E. R. (1980). CNS embolism due to atrial myxoma. *Arch. Neurol.*, **37**, 485–8.

Sandok, B. A., Whisnant, J. P., Furlan, A. J. *et al.* (1982). Carotid artery bruits. Prevalence, surgery and differential diagnosis. *Mayo Clinic Proc.*, **57**, 227–30.

Sarkari, N. B. S., Holmes, J. M., and Bickerstaff, E. R. (1970). Neurological manifestations associated with internal carotid loops and kinks in children. *J. Neurol. Neurosurg. Psychiatry*, **33**, 194–200.

Sato, Y., Kuno, H., Kaji, M. *et al.* (1998). Increased bone resorption during the first year after stroke. *Stroke*, **29**, 1373–7.

Savage, C. O. S., Harper, L., and Adu, D. (1997). Primary systemic vasculitis. *Lancet*, **349**, 553–8.

Saveland, H., Sonesson, B., Ljunggren, B. *et al.* (1986). Outcome evaluation following subarachnoid haemorrhage. *J. Neurosurg.*, **64**, 191–6.

Schafer, A. I. (1994). Hypercoagulable states: molecular genetics to clinical practice. *Lancet*, **344**, 1739–42.

Scheithauer, B. W., Rubinstein, L. J., and Herman, M. M. (1984). Leukoencephalopathy in Waldenstrom's macroglobulinemia. Immunohistochemical and electron micrscopic observations. *J. Neuropathol. Exp. Neurol.*, **43**, 408–25.

Schievink, W. I. (1997). Intracranial aneurysms. *N. Engl. J. Med.*, **336**, 28–40.

Schievink, W. I., Michels, V. V., and Piepgras, D. G. (1994). Neurovascular manifestations of heritable connective tissue disorders. A review. *Stroke*, **25**, 889–903.

Schimke, R. N., McKusick, V. A., Huang, T. *et al.* (1965). Homocystinuria. Studies of 20 families with 38 affected members. *JAMA*, **193**, 711–19.

Schmal, M., Marini, C., Carolei, A., Di Napoli, M., Kessels, F., and Lodder, J. (1998). Different vascular risk factor profiles among cortical infarcts, small deep infarcts, and primary intracerebral haemorrhage point to different types of underlying vasculopathy. A study from the L'Aquila Stroke Registry. *Cerebrovasc. Dis.*, **8**, 14–19.

Schoenberg, B. S. and Schulte, B. P. M. (1989). Cerebrovascular disease: epidemiology and geopathology. In *Handbook of clinical neurology*, (ed. P. J. Vinken, G. Bruyn, and H. L. Klawans), pp. 1–6. Elsevier, Amsterdam.

Scholte op Reimer, W. J. M., de Haan, R. J., Rijnders, P. T. *et al.* (1998). The burden of caregiving in partners of long-term stroke survivors. *Stroke*, **29**, 1605–11.

Schroeder, T. (1988). Hemodynamic significance of internal carotid artery disease. *Acta Neurol. Scand.*, **77**, 353–72.

Schumann, P., Touzani, O., Young, A. R. *et al.* (1998). Evaluation of the ratio of cerebral blood flow to cerebral blood volume as an index of local cerebral perfusion pressure. *Brain*, **121**, 1369–79.

Schutta, H. S., Williams, E. C., Baranski, B. G. *et al.* (1991). Cerebral venous thrombosis with plasminogen deficiency. *Stroke*, **22**, 401–5.

Schutz, H., Bodeker, R.-H., Damian, M., *et al.* (1990). Age-related spontaneous intracerebral haematoma in a German community. *Stroke*, **21**, 1412–18.

Schwab, S., Steiner, T., Aschoff, A. *et al.* (1998) Early hemicraniectomy in patients with complete middle cerebral artery infarction. *Stroke*, **29**, 1888–93.

Schwartz, A., Rautenberg, W., and Hennerici, M. (1993). Dolichoectatic intracranial arteries: review of selected aspects. *Cerebrovasc. Dis.*, **3**, 273–9.

Schwartz, C. J., and Mitchell, J. R. A. (1961). Atheroma of the carotid and vertebral arterial systems. *BMJ*, **2**, 1057–63.

Schwartz, C. J., Mitchell, J. R. A., and Hughes, J. T. (1962). Transient recurrent cerebral episodes and aneurysm of carotid sinus. *BMJ*, **1**, 770–1.

Schwartz, G. L. (1990). Initial therapy for hypertension—individualising care. *Mayo Clinic Proc.*, **65**, 73.

Schwartzman, R. J. and Hill, J. B. (1982). Neurologic complications of disseminated intravascular coagulation. *Neurology*, **32**, 791–7.

Schwarz, S., Egelhof, T., Schwab, S. *et al.* (1997). Basilar artery embolism. Clinical syndrome and neuroradiologic patterns in patients without permanent occlusion of the basilar artery. *Neurology*, **49**, 1346–52.

Scodary, D. J., Twe, J. M., Thomas, G. M. *et al.* (1990). Radiation-induced cerebral aneurysms. *Acta Neurochir.*, **102**, 141–4.

Scott, B. L. and Jankovic, J. (1996). Delayed-onset progressive movement disorders after static brain lesions . *Neurology*, **46**, 68–74.

Scott, J. F., Gray, C. S., O'Connell, J. E. *et al.* (1998). Glucose and insulin therapy in acute stroke; why delay further? *QJM*, **91**, 511–15.

Scott, W. R. and Miller, B. R. (1985). Intracerebral haemorrhage with rapid recovery. *Arch. Neurol.*, **42**, 133–6.

Scottish Intercollegiate Guidelines Network (1998). *Management of patients with stroke. IV: rehabilitation, prevention and management of complications and discharge planning, a national clinical guideline recommended for use in Scotland*. Scottish Intercollegiate Guidelines Network, Edinburgh.

The Scottish Stroke Outcomes Study Group (in press). Towards a national system for monitoring the quality of hospital-based stroke services. *Stroke*.

Secretary of State for Health (1992). *The health of the nation.* HMSO, London.

Selby, G. and Walker, G. L. (1979). Cerebral arteritis in cat-scratch disease. *Neurology*, **29**, 1413–18.

Sellar, R. J. (1995). Imaging blood vessels of the head and neck. *J. Neurol. Neurosurg. Psychiatry*, **59**, 225–37.

Sempere, A. P., Duarte, J., Cabezas, C. *et al.* (1998). Aetiopathogenesis of transient ischaemic attacks and minor ischaemic strokes. A community-based study in Segovia, Spain. *Stroke*, **29**, 40–5.

Service, F. J. (1995). Hypoglycemic disorders. *N. Engl. J. Med.*, **332**, 1144–52.

Shanmugam, V., Chhablani, R., and Gorelick, P. B. (1987). Spontaneous calcific cerebral embolus. *Neurology*, **48**, 538–9.

Shanmugam, V., Zimnowodzki, S., Curtin, J. *et al.* (1997). Hypoglycemic hemiplegia: insulinoma masquerading as stroke. *J. Stroke Cerebrovasc. Dis.*, **6**, 368–9.

Shaper, A. G., Phillips, A. N., Pocock, S. J. *et al.* (1991). Risk factors for stroke in middle aged British men. *BMJ*, **302**, 1111–15.

Sharshar, T., Lamy, C., Mas, J. L. for the Stroke in Pregnancy Study Group (1995). Incidence and causes of stroke associated with pregnancy and puerperium. A study in public hospitals of Ile de France. *Stroke*, **26**, 930–6.

Shaw, P. J., Bates, D., Cartlidge, N. E. F. *et al.* (1989). An analysis of factors predisposing to neurological injury in patients undergoing coronary bypass operations. *QJM*, **267**, 633–46.

Sheth, K. J., Swick, H. M., and Haworth, N. (1986). Neurological involvement in haemolytic-uraemic syndrome. *Ann. Neurol.*, **19**, 90–3.

Sheldon, J. J. (1981). *Blood vessels of the scalp and brain.* CIBA Pharmaceutical Company, New Jersey.

Sherman, D. G., Hart, R. G., and Easton, J. D. (1981). Abrupt change in head position and cerebral infarction. *Stroke*, **12**, 2–6.

Shinton, R. and Beevers, G. (1989). Meta-analysis of relation between cigarette smoking and stroke. *BMJ*, **298**, 789–94.

Shinton, R., Sagar, G., and Beevers, G. (1995). Body fat and stroke: unmasking the hazards of overweight and obesity. *J. Epidemiol. Community Hlth*, **49**, 259–64.

Shuaib, A. (1991). Stroke from other etiologies masquerading as migraine-stroke. *Stroke*, **22**, 1068–74.

Siekert, R. G., Whisnant, J. P., and Millikan, C. H. (1960). Anaemia and intermittent focal cerebral arterial insufficiency. *Arch. Neurol.*, **3**, 386–90.

Siewert, B., Patel, M. R., and Warach, S. (1995). Magnetic resonance angiography. *Neurologist*, **1**, 167–84.

Sigal, L. H. (1987). The neurologic presentation of vasculitic and rheumatologic syndromes. *Medicine*, **66**, 157–80.

Signorini, D. F., Sandercock, P. A. G., and Warlow, C. P. for the IST Collaborative Group (1999). Systolic blood pressure at randomisation and outcome in the International Stroke Trial (abstract). *Cerebrovascular Diseases*, **9** (**suppl. 1**), 34 (abst. 11).

Silbert, P. L., Mokri, B., and Schievink, W. I. (1995). Headache and neck pain in spontaneous internal carotid and vertebral artery dissections. *Neurology*, **45**, 1517–22.

Silver, F. L., Norris, J. W., Lewis, A. J. *et al.* (1984). Early mortality following stroke: a prospective review. *Stroke*, **15**, 492–6.

Silver, M. D. and Dorsey, J. S. (1978). Aneurysms of the septum primum in adults. *Arch. Pathol. Lab. Med.*, **102**, 62–5.

Silverstein, A., Gilbert, H., and Wasserman, L. R. (1962). Neurologic complications of polycythaemia. *Ann. Intern. Med.*, **57**, 909–16.

Silvestrini, M., Troisi, E., Cupini, L. M. *et al.* (1994). Transcranial Doppler assessment of the functional effects of symptomatic carotid stenosis. *Neurology*, **44**, 1910–14.

Simoons, M. L., Maggioni, A. P., Knatterud, G. *et al.* (1993) Individual risk assessment for intracranial haemorrhage during thrombolytic therapy. *Lancet*, **342**, 1523–8.

Skriver, E. B. and Olsen, T. S. (1982). Transient disappearance of cerebral infarcts on CT scan, the so-called fogging effect. *Neuroradiology*, **22**, 61–5.

Sliwka, U. and Georgiadis, D. (1998). Clinical correlations of Doppler microembolic signals in patients with prosthetic cardiac valves. Analysis of 580 cases. *Stroke*, **29**, 140–3.

Sloan, M. A. and Haley, E. C. (1990). The syndrome of bilateral hemispheric border zone ischaemia. *Stroke*, 21, 1668–73.

Sloan, M. A. and Plotnick, G. D. (1990). Stroke complicating thrombolytic therapy of acute myocardial infarction. *J. Am. Coll. Cardiol.*, 16, 541–4.

Smielewski, P., Czosnyka, M., Kirkpatrick, P. *et al.* (1996). Assessment of cerebral autoregulation using carotid artery compression. *Stroke*, 27, 2197–203.

Smielewski, P., Czosnyka, M., Pickard, J. D. *et al.* (1997). Clinical evaluation of near-infrared spectroscopy for testing cerebrovascular reactivity in patients with carotid artery disease. *Stroke*, 28, 331–8.

Smith, D. S., Goldenberg, E., Ashburn, A. *et al.* (1981). Remedial therapy after stroke: a randomised controlled trial. *BMJ*, 282, 517–20.

Socie, G., Mary, J-Y., de Gramont, A. *et al.* for the French Society of Haematology (1996). Paroxysmal nocturnal haemoglobinuria: long-term follow-up and prognostic factors. *Lancet*, 348, 573–7.

Sotrel, A., Lacson, A. G., and Huff, K .R. (1983). Childhood Kohlmeier–Degos disease with atypical skin lesions. *Neurology*, 33, 1146–51.

Southwick, F. S., Richardson, E. P., and Swartz, M. N. (1986). Septic thrombosis of the dural venous sinuses. *Medicine (Baltimore)*, 65, 82–106.

Spittell, J. A. (1983). Thromboangiitis obliterans—an autoimmune disorder? *N. Engl. J. Med.*, 308, 1157–8.

Stahl, S. M., Johnson, K. P., and Malamud, N. (1980). The clinical and pathological spectrum of brain-stem vascular malformations. Long-term course stimulates multiple sclerosis. *Arch. Neurol.*, 37, 25–9.

Stampfer, M. J., Willett, W. C., Colditz, G. A. *et al.* (1990). Past use of oral contraceptives and cardiovascular disease: A meta analysis in the context of the Nurses' Health Study. *Am. J. Obstet. Gynecol.*, 163, 285–91.

Steen, R. G., Langston, J. W., Ogg, R. J. *et al.* (1998). Ectasia of the basilar artery in children with sickle cell disease: relationship to haematocrit and psychometric measures. *J. Stroke Cerebrovasc. Dis.*, 7, 32–43.

Stein, B. M. and Mohr, J. P. (1988). Vascular malformations of the brain. *N. Engl. J. Med.*, 319, 368–9.

Stein, J. H. and Soble, J. S. (1995). Thrombus associated with mitral valve calcification. A possible mechanism for embolic stroke. *Stroke*, 26, 1697–9.

Steinberg, D. (1995). Clinical trials of antioxidants in atherosclerosis: are we doing the right thing? *Lancet*, 346, 36–8.

Stemmermann, G. N., Hayashi, T., Resch, J. A. *et al.* (1984). Risk factors related to ischaemic and hemorrhagic cerebrovascular disease at autopsy: The Honolulu Heart Study. *Stroke*, 15, 23–8.

Stern, B. J., Krumholz, A., Johns, C. *et al.* (1985). Sarcoidosis and its neurological manifestations. *Arch. Neurol.*, 42, 909–17.

Stevens, D. L. and Matthews, W. B. (1973). Cryptogenic drop attacks: an affliction of women. *BMJ*, 1, 439–42.

Stewart, S. S., Ashizawa, T., Dudley, A. W. *et al.* (1988). Cerebral vasculitis in relapsing polychondritis. *Neurology*, 38, 150–2.

Stockhammer, G., Felber, S. R., Zelger, B. *et al.* (1993) Sneddon's syndrome: diagnosis by skin biopsy and MRI in 17 patients. *Stroke*, 24, 685–90.

Stone, S. P., Patel, P., Greenwood, R. J. *et al.* (1992). Measuring visual neglect in acute stroke and predicting its recovery: the visual neglect recovery index. *J. Neurol. Neurosurg. Psychiatry*, 55, 431–6.

Stout, R. W. (1989). Hyperglycaemia and stroke. *QJM*, 73, 997–1004.

Strachan, D. P. (1991). Ventilatory function as a predictor of fatal stroke. *BMJ*, 302, 84–7.

Strandgaard, S. (1976). Autoregulation of cerebral blood flow in hypertensive patients. The modifying influence of prolonged antihypertensive treatment on the tolerance to acute, drug-induced hypotension. *Circulation*, 53, 720–7.

Strandgaard, S. and Paulson, O. B. (1984). Cerebral autoregulation. *Stroke*, 15, 413–16.

Strandgaard, S., Olesen, J., Skinhoj, E. *et al.* (1973). Autoregulation of brain circulation in severe arterial hypertension. *BMJ*, 1, 507–10.

Stroke Prevention in Atrial Fibrillation Investigators (1992). Predictors of thromboembolism in atrial fibrillation: II. Echocardiographic features of patients at risk. *Ann. Int. Med.*, 116, 6–12.

Stroke Prevention in Atrial Fibrillation Investigators (1995). Risk factors for thromboembolism during aspirin therapy in patients with atrial fibrillation: The Stroke Prevention in Atrial Fibrillation Study. *J. Stroke Cerebrovasc. Dis.*, 5, 147–57.

Stroke Prevention in Reversible Ischaemia Trial (SPIRIT) Study Group (1997). A randomised trial of anticoagulants versus aspirin after cerebral ischaemia of presumed arterial origin. *Ann. Neurol.*, 42, 857–65.

Stroke Unit Trialists' Collaboration (1997a). Collaborative systematic review of the randomised trials of organised inpatient (stroke unit) care after stroke. *BMJ*, 314, 1151–9.

Stroke Unit Trialists' Collaboration (1997b). How do stroke units improve patient outcomes? A collaborative systematic review of the randomised trials. *Stroke*, 28, 2139–44.

Strupp, M., Bruning, R., Wu, R. H. *et al.* (1998). Diffusion-weighted MRI in transient global amnesia: elevated signal intensity in the left mesial temporal lobe in 7 of 10 patients. *Ann. Neurol.*, 43, 164–70.

Sturzenegger, M. and Huber, P. (1993). Cranial nerve palsies in spontaneous carotid artery dissection. *J. Neurol. Neurosurg. Psychiatry*, **56**, 1191–9.

Sturzenegger, M., Mattle, H. P., Rivoir, A. *et al.* (1993). Ultrasound findings in spontaneous extracranial vertebral artery dissection. *Stroke*, **24**, 1910–21.

Sturzenegger, M., Newell, D. W., Douville, C. *et al.* (1994). Dynamic transcranial Doppler assessment of positional vertebrobasilar ischaemia. *Stroke*, **25**, 1776–83.

Sturzenegger, M., Mattle, H. P., Rivoir, A. *et al.* (1995). Ultrasound findings in carotid artery dissection: analysis of 43 patients. *Neurology*, **45**, 691–8.

Subbiah, P., Wijdicks, E., Muenter, M. *et al.* (1996). Skin lesion with a fatal neurologic outcome (Degos' disease). *Neurology*, **46**, 636–40.

Sudlow, C. L. M. and Warlow, C. P. (1996). Comparing stroke incidence worldwide. What makes studies comparable? *Stroke*, **27**, 550–8.

Sudlow, C. L. M. and Warlow, C. P. (1997). Comparable studies of the incidence of stroke and its pathological types. Results from an International collaboration. *Stroke*, **28**, 491–9.

Sudlow, C. M., Rodgers, H., Kenny, R. A. *et al.* (1995). Service provision and use of anticoagulants in atrial fibrillation. *BMJ*, **311**, 558–60.

Sunderland, A., Fletcher, D., Bradley, L. *et al.* (1994). Enhanced physical therapy for arm function after stroke: a one year follow up study. *J. Neurol. Neurosurg. Psychiatry*, **57**, 856–8.

Svindland, A. and Torvik, A. (1988). Atherosclerotic carotid disease in asymptomatic individuals. An histological study of 53 cases. *Acta Neurol. Scand.*, **78**, 506–17.

Symon, L., Branston, N. M., and Strong, A. J. (1976). Autoregulation in acute focal ischaemia. An experimental study. *Stroke*, **7**, 547–54.

Symon, L., Branston, N. M., and Chikovani, O. (1979). Ischemic brain edema following middle cerebral artery occlusion in baboons: relationship between regional cerebral water content and blood flow at 1 to 2 hours. *Stroke*, **10**, 184–91.

Takebayashi, S. and Kaneko, M. (1983). Electron microscopic studies of ruptured arteries in hypertensive intracerebral haemorrhage. *Stroke*, **14**, 28–36.

Tatu, L., Moulin, T., Bogousslavsky, J. *et al.* (1996). Arterial territories of human brain: brainstem and cerebellum. *Neurology*, **47**, 1125–35.

Taylor, T. N., Davis, P. H., Torner, J. C. *et al.* (1996). Lifetime cost of stroke in the United States. *Stroke*, **27**, 1459–66.

Tegeler, C. H. and Downes, T. R. (1991). Cardiac imaging in stroke. *Stroke*, **22**, 1206–11.

Tegeler, C. H., Shi, F., and Morgan, T. (1991). Carotid stenosis in lacunar stroke. *Stroke*, **22**, 1124–8.

Tehindrazanarivelo, A., Evrard, S., Schaison, M. *et al.* (1992). Prospective study of cerebral sinus venous thrombosis in patients presenting with benign intracranial hypertension. *Cerebrovasc. Dis.*, **2**, 22–7.

Tell, G. S., Lefkowitz, D. S., Diehr, P. *et al.* (1998). Relationship between balance and abnormalities in cerebral magnetic resonanace imaging in older adults. *Arch. Neurol.*, **55**, 73–9.

Terada, T., Higashida, R. T., Halbach, V. V. *et al.* (1996). Transluminal angioplasty for arteriosclerotic disease of the distal vertebral and basilar arteries. *J. Neurol. Neurosurg. Psychiatry*, **60**, 377–81.

ter Berg, H. W. M., Dippel, D. W. J., Limburg, M. *et al.* (1992). Familial intracranial aneurysms. A review. *Stroke*, **23**, 1024–30.

Terent, A. (1988). Increasing incidence of stroke among Swedish women. *Stroke*, **19**, 598–603.

Terent, A. (1989). Survival after stroke and transient ischaemic attacks during the 1970's and 1980's. *Stroke*, **20**, 1320–6.

Terent, A., Marke, L. A., Asplund, K. *et al.* (1994). Costs of stroke in Sweden. A national perspective. *Stroke*, **25**, 2363–9.

Tettenborn, B., Caplan, L. R., Sloan, M. A. *et al.* (1993). Postoperative brainstem and cerebellar infarcts. *Neurology*, **43**, 471–7.

Teunissen, L. L., Rinkel, G. J. E., Algra, A. *et al.* (1996). Risk factors for subarachnoid haemorrhage. A systematic review. *Stroke*, **27**, 544–9.

Thelle, D. S. (1996). Salt and blood pressure revisited. *BMJ*, **312**, 1240–1.

Thie, A., Hellner, D., Lachenmayer, L. *et al.* (1993a). Bilateral blunt traumatic dissections of the extracranial internal carotid artery: report of eleven cases and review of the literature. *Cerebrovasc. Dis.*, **3**, 295–303.

Thie, A., Goossens-Merkt, H., Freitag, J. *et al.* (1993b) Pulsatile tinnitus: clinical and angiological evaluation. *Cerebrovasc. Dis.*, **3**, 160–7.

Thomas, A. C., Knapman, P. A., Krikler, D. M. *et al.* (1988). Community study of the causes of 'natural' sudden death. *BMJ*, **297**, 1453–6.

Thomas, D. J. (1982). Whole blood viscosity and cerebral blood flow. *Stroke*, **13**, 285–7.

Thomas, D. J., Du Boulay, G. H., Marshall, J. *et al.* (1977). Effect of haemotocrit on cerebral blood-flow in man. *Lancet*, **2**, 941–3.

Thorvaldsen, P., Asplund, K., Kuulasmaa, K. *et al.* for the WHO MONICA Project, (1995). Stroke incidence, case fatality, and mortality in the WHO MONICA Project. *Stroke*, **26**, 361–7.

Thrift, A. G., McNeil, J. J., Forbes, A. *et al.* Melbourne Risk Factor Study Group (1998). Three important subgroups of hypertensive persons at greater risk of intracerebral haemorrhage. *Hypertension*, **31**, 1223–9.

Thrift, A. G., McNeil, J. J., and Donnan, G. A. for the Melbourne Risk Factor Study Group (1999). The risk of intracerebral haemorrhage with smoking. *Cerebrovasc. Dis.*, 9, 34–9.

Thun, M. J., Peto, R., Lopez, A. D. *et al.* (1997). Alcohol consumption and mortality among middle-aged and elderly U. S. adults. *N. Engl. J. Med.*, 337, 1705–14.

Tiecks, F. P., Douville, C., Byrd, S. *et al.* (1996). Evaluation of impaired cerebral autoregulation by the Valsalva Manoeuvre. *Stroke*, 27, 1177–82.

Tietjen, G. E. (1995). Transient focal neurologic events in young adults: TIA, migraine, and their relationship to stroke. *Neurologist*, 1, 248–58.

Tomasello, F., Mariani, F., Fieschi, C. *et al.* (1982). Assessment of inter-observer differences in the Italian multicenter study on reversible cerebral ischaemia. *Stroke*, 13, 32–5.

Tomsick, T. A., Lukin, R. R., Chambers A. A. *et al.* (1976). Neurofibromatosis and intracranial arterial occlusive disease. *Neuroradiology*, 11, 229–34.

Toni, D., Sacchetti, M. L., Argentino, C. *et al.* (1992). Does hyperglycaemia play a role on the outcome of acute ischaemic stroke patients? *J. Neurol.*, 239, 382–6.

Toni, D., Fiorelli, M., Zanette, E. M. *et al.* (1998). Early spontaneous improvement and deterioration of ischaemic stroke patients. A serial study with transcranial Doppler ultrasonography. *Stroke*, 29, 1144–8.

Toro-Gonzalez, G., Navarro-Roman, L., Roman, G. C. *et al.* (1993). Acute ischaemic stroke from fibrocartilaginous emoblism to the middle cerebral artery. *Stroke*, 24, 738–40.

Torvik, A. (1984). The pathogenesis of watershed infarcts in the brain. *Stroke*, 15, 221–3.

Torvik. A., Svindland, A., and Lindboe, C. F. (1989). Pathogenesis of carotid thrombosis. *Stroke*, 20, 1477–83.

Tournier-Lasserve, E., Joutel, A., Melki, J. *et al.* (1993). Cerebral autosomal dominant arteriopathy with subcortial infarcts and leukoencephalopathy maps to chromosome 19q12. *Nature Genet.*, 3, 256–9.

Townsend, J., Piper, M., Frank, A. O. *et al.* (1988). Reduction in hospital readmission stay of elderly patients by a community based hospital discharge scheme: a randomised controlled trial. *BMJ*, 297, 544–7.

Tracey, F., Crawford, V. L. S., Lawson, J. T. *et al.* (1993). Hyperglycaemia and mortality from acute stroke. *QJM*, 86, 439–46.

Truelsen, T., Lindenstrom, E., and Boysen, G. (1994). Comparison of probability of stroke between the Copenhagen City Heart Study and the Framingham Study. *Stroke*, 25, 802–7.

Chen, S. T., Liu, Y. H., Hsu, C. Y. *et al.* (1988). Moyamoya disease in Taiwan. *Stroke*, 19, 53–9.

Truelsen, T., Bonita, R., Duncan, J. *et al.* (1998). Changes in subarachnoid haemorrhage mortality, incidence, and case fatality in New Zealand between 1981–1983 and 1991–1993. *Stroke*, 29, 2298–303.

Tsitsopoulos, P., Andrew, J., and Harrison, M. J. G. (1987). Occult cerebral arteriovenous malformations. *J. Neurol. Neurosurg. Psychiatry*, 50, 218–20.

Tsutsumi, K., Ueki, K., Usui, M., Kwak, S. *et al.* (1998). Risk of recurrent subarachnoid haemorrhage after complete obliteration of cerebral aneurysms. *Stroke*, 29, 2511–13.

Tulyapronchote, R., Selhorst, J. B., Malkoff, M. D., and Gomez, C. R. (1994). Delayed sequelae of vertebral artery dissection and occult cervical fractures. *Neurology*, 44, 1397–9.

Uehara, T., Tabuchi, M., and Mori, E. (1998). High frequency of unruptured intracranial aneurysms in female patients with ischaemic heart disease. *J. Neurol. Neurosurg. Psychiatry*, 64, 536–8.

UK Prospective Diabetes Study (UKPDS) Group (1998). Intensive blood-glucose control with sulphonylureas or insulin compared with conventional treatment and risk of complications in patients with type 2 diabetes (UKPDS 33). *Lancet*, 352, 837–53.

UK-TIA Study Group (1991). The United Kingdom transient ischaemic attack (UK-TIA) aspirin trial: final results. *J. Neurol. Neurosurg. Psychiatry*, 54, 1044–54.

UK-TIA Study Group (1993). Intracranial tumours that mimic transient cerebral ischaemia: lessons from a large multicentre trial. *J. Neurol. Neurosurg.*, 56, 563–6.

Vaitkus, P. T. and Barnathan, E. S. (1993). Embolic potential, prevention and management of mural thrombus complicating anterior myocardial infarction: a meta-analysis. *J. Am. Coll. Cardiol.*, 22, 1004–9.

Valton, L., Larrue, V., Pary le Traon, A. *et al.* (1998). Microembolic signals and risk of early recurrence in patients with stroke or transient ischaemic attack. *Stroke*, 29, 2125–8.

Vandenbroucke, J. P. (1998). Cerebral sinus thrombosis and oral contraceptives. There are limits to predictability. *BMJ*, 317, 483–4.

Vandenbroucke, J. P. and Helmerhorst, F. M. (1996). Risk of venous thrombosis with hormone-replacement therapy. *Lancet*, 348, 972.

van der Grond, J., Eikelboom, B. C., and Mali, W. P. Th. M. (1996). Flow-related anaerobic metabolic changes in patients with severe stenosis of the internal carotid artery. *Stroke*, 27, 2026–32.

van der Hoop, R. G., Vermeulen, M., and van Gijn, J. (1988). Cerebellar haemorrhage: diagnosis and treatment. *Surg. Neurol.*, 29, 6–10.

van der Schouw, Y. T., van der Graaf, Y., Steyerberg, E. W. *et al.* (1996). Age at menopause as a risk factor for cardiovascular mortality. *Lancet*, **347**, 714–18.

van der Wee, N., Rinkel, G. J. E., Hasan, D. *et al.* (1995). Detection of subarachnoid haemorrhage on early CT: is lumbar puncture still needed after a negative scan? *J. Neurol. Neurosurg. Psychiatry*, **58**, 357–9.

van der Worp, H. B. and Kappelle, L. J. (1998). Complications of acute ischaemic stroke. *Cerebrovasc. Dis.*, **8**, 124–32.

van der Zwan, A., Hillen, B., Tulleken, C. A. F. *et al.* (1992). Variability of the territories of the major cerebral arteries. *J. Neurosurg.*, **77**, 927–40.

Vane, J. R., Anggard, E. E., and Botting, R. M. (1990). Regulatory functions of the vascular endothelium. *N. Engl. J. Med.*, **323**, 27–35.

van Everdingen, K. J., van der Grond, J., Kappelle, L. J. *et al.* (1998). Diffusion-weighted magnetic resonance imaging in acute stroke. *Stroke*, **29**, 1783–90.

van Gijn, J. and Dennis, M. S. (1998). Issues and answers in stroke care. *Lancet*, **352**, (Suppl. II), 23–7.

van Gijn, J. and Warlow, C. P. (1992). Down with stroke scales! *Cerebrovasc. Dis.*, **2**, 244–7.

van Gijn, J., van Dongen, K. J., Vermeulen, M. *et al.* (1985*a*). Perimesencephalic haemorrhage: A nonaneurysmal and benign form of subarachnoid haemorrhage. *Neurology*, **35**, 493–7.

van Gijn, J., Hijdra, A., Wijdicks, E. F. M. *et al.* (1985*b*). Acute hydrocephalus after aneurysmal subarachnoid haemorrhage. *J. Neurosurg.*, **63**, 355–62.

van Gijn, J., Stampfer, M. J., Wolfe, C. *et al.* (1993). The association between alcohol and stroke. In *Health issues related to alcohol consumption*, (ed. P. M. Verschuren), pp. 44–79. ILSI Press, Washington.

VanItallie, T. B. (1990). The perils of obesity in middle-aged women. *N. Engl. J. Med.*, **322**, 928–9.

van Kuijck, M. A. P., Rotteveel, J. J., van Oostrom, C. G. *et al.* (1994). Neurological complications in children with protein C deficiency. *Neuropediatrics*, **25**, 16–19.

van Oostenbrugge, R. J., Freling, G., Lodder, J. *et al.* (1996). Fatal stroke due to paradoxical fat embolism. *Cerebrovasc. Dis.*, **6**, 313–14.

van Swieten, J. C., Geyskes, G. G., Derix, M. M. A. *et al.* (1991). Hypertension in the elderly is associated with white matter lesions and with cognitive decline. *Ann. Neurol.*, **30**, 825–30.

Venters, H. V. (1987). Cerebral amyloid angiopathy. A critical review. *Stroke*, **18**, 311–24.

Vermeer, S. E., Rinkel, G. J. E., and Algra, A. (1997). Circadian fluctuations in onset of subarachnoid haemorrhage. New data on aneurysmal and perimesencephalic haemorrhage and a systematic review. *Stroke*, **28**, 805–8.

Vermeulen, M. (1996). Subarachnoid haemorrhage: diagnosis and treatment. *J. Neurol.*, **243**, 496–501.

Vermeulen, M. and van Gijn, J. (1990). The diagnosis of subarachnoid haemorrhage. *J. Neurol. Neurosurg. Psychiatry*, **53**, 365–72.

Vermeulen, M., Van Gijn, J., Hijdra, A. *et al.* (1984). Causes of acute deterioration in patients with ruptured intracranial aneurysm. A prospective study with serial CT scanning. *J. Neurosurg.*, **60**, 935–9.

Vermeulen, M., Lindsay, K. W., and van Gijn, J. (1992). *Subarachnoid haemorrhage*. Saunders, London.

Verweij, R. D., Wijdicks, E. F. M., and van Gijn, J. (1988). Warning headache in aneurysmal subarachnoid haemorrhage. A case-control study. *Arch. Neurol.*, **45**, 1019–20.

Vidailhet, M., Piette, J.-C., Wechsler, B. *et al.* (1990). Cerebral venous thrombosis in systemic lupus erythematosus. *Stroke*, **21**, 1226–31.

Vieregge, P., Schwieder, G., and Kompf, D. (1989). Cerebral venous thrombosis in hereditary protein C deficiency. *J. Neurol. Neurosurg. Psychiatry*, **52**, 135–6.

Visy, J. M., Le Coz, P., Chadefaux, B. *et al.* (1991). Homocystinuria due to 5,10-methylenetetrahydrofolate reductase deficiency revealed by stroke in adult siblings. *Neurology*, **41**, 1313–15.

Vollmer, T. L., Guarnaccia, J., Harrington, W. *et al.* (1993). Idiopathic granulomatous angiitis of the central nervous system. Diagnostic challenges. *Arch. Neurol.*, **50**, 925–30.

von Arbin, M., Britton, M., de Faire, U. *et al.* (1982). Myocardial infarction in patients with acute cerebrovascular disease. *Eur. Heart J.*, **3**, 136–41.

Vongpatanasin, W., Hillis, L. D., and Lange, R. A. (1996). Prosthetic heart valves. *N. Engl. J. Med.*, **335**, 407–16.

Vonsattel, J. P. G., Myers, R. H., Hedley-Whyte, E. T. *et al.* (1991). Cerebral amyloid angiopathy without and with cerebral haemorrhages: a comparative histological study. *Ann. Neurol.*, **30**, 637–49.

Wade, D. T. (1992). Stroke: rehabilitation and long-term care. *Lancet*, **339**, 791–3.

Wade, D. T. and Collin, C. (1988). The Barthel ADL index: a standard measure of physical disability. *International Disability Studies*, **10**, 64–7.

Wade, D. T. and Langton Hewer, R. (1985). Hospital admission for acute stroke: who, for how long, and to what effect? *J. Epidemiol. Community Health*, **39**, 347–52.

Wade, D. T., and Langton Hewer, R. (1987). Functional abilities after stroke: measurement, natural history and prognosis. *J. Neurol. Neurosurg. Psychiatry*, **50**, 177–82.

Wade, D. T., Legh-Smith, J., and Langton Hewer, R. (1985). Social activities after stroke: measurement and natural history using the Frenchay Activities Index. *Int. Rehabil. Med.*, **7**, 176–81.

Wade, D. T., Wood, V. A., Heller, A. *et al.* (1987). Walking after stroke. Measurement and recovery over the first 3 months. *Scand. J. Rehabil. Med.*, **19**, 25–30.

Wade, D. T., Wood, V. A., and Langton Hewer, R. (1988). Recovery of cognitive function soon after stroke: a study of visual neglect, attention span and verbal recall. *J. Neurol. Neurosurg. Psychiatry*, **51**, 10–13.

Wade, D. T., Collen, F. M., Robb, G. F. *et al.* (1992). Physiotherapy intervention late after stroke and mobility. *BMJ*, **304**, 609–13.

Wade, J. P. H., Wong, W., Barnett, H. J. M. *et al.* (1987). Bilateral occlusion of the internal carotid arteries. *Brain*, **110**, 667–82.

Waldvogel, D., Mattle, H. P., Sturzenegger, M. *et al.* (1998). Pulsatile tinnitus – a review of 84 patients. *J. Neurol.*, **245**, 137–42.

Walker, S. P., Rimm, E. B., Ascherio, A. *et al.* (1996). Body size and fat distribution as predictors of stroke among US men. *Am. J. Epidemiol.*, **144**, 1143–50.

Wallis, W. E., Donaldson, I., Scott, R. S. *et al.* (1985). Hypoglycaemia masquerading as cerebrovascular disease (hypoglycaemic hemiplegia). *Ann. Neurol.*, **18**, 510–12.

Walz, E. T., Slivka, A. P., Tice, F. D. *et al.* (1998). Noninfective mitral valve vegetations identified by transesophageal echocardiography as a cause of stroke. *J. Stroke Cerebrovasc. Dis.*, **7**, 310–14.

Walzer, T., Herrmann, M., and Wallesch, C.–W. (1997). Neuropsychological disorders after coronary bypass surgery. *J. Neurol. Neurosurg. Psychiatry*, **62**, 644–8.

Wannamethee, G. and Shaper, A. G. (1989). Body weight and mortality in middle aged British men: impact of smoking. *BMJ*, **299**, 1497–502.

Wannamethee, S. . and Shaper, A. . (1996). Patterns of alcohol intake and risk of stroke in middle-aged British men. *Stroke*, **27**, 1033–9.

Warach, S., Gaa, J., Siewert, B. *et al.* (1995). Acute human stroke studied by whole brain planar diffusion-weighted magnetic resonance imaging. *Ann. Neurol.*, **37**, 231–41.

Wardlaw, J. M. (1994). Is routine computed tomography in strokes unnecessary? *BMJ*, **309**, 1498–500.

Wardlaw, J. M. and Warlow, C. P. (1992). Thrombolysis in acute ischaemic stroke – Does it work? *Stroke*, **23**, 1826–39.

Wardlaw, J. M. and White, P. M. (1999). The detection and management of unruptured intracranial aneurysms. *Brain*, in press.

Wardlaw, J. M., Dennis, M. S., Lindley, R. I. *et al.* (1993). Does early reperfusion of a cerebral infarct influence cerebral infarct swelling in the acute stage or the final clinical outcome? *Cerebrovasc. Dis.*, **3**, 86–93.

Wardlaw, J. M., Merrick, M. V., Ferrington, C. M. *et al.* (1996). Comparison of a simple isotope method of predicting likely middle cerebral artery occlusion with Transcranial Doppler ultrasound in acute ischaemic stroke. *Cerebrovasc. Dis.*, **6**, 32–9.

Wardlaw, J. M., Warlow, C. P., and Counsell, C. (1997). Systematic review of evidence on thrombolytic therapy for acute ischaemic stroke. *Lancet*, **350**, 607–14.

Wardlaw, J. M., Marshall, I., Wild, J. *et al.* (1998*a*). Studies of acute ischaemic stroke with proton magnetic resonance spectroscopy: relation between time from onset, neurological deficit, metabolite abnormalities in the infarct, blood flow, and clinical outcome. *Stroke*, **29**, 1618–24.

Wardlaw, J. M., Lewis, S. C., Dennis, M. S. *et al.* (1998*b*). Is visible infarction on computed tomography associated with an adverse prognosis in acute ischaemic stroke? *Stroke*, **29**, 1315–19.

Warlow, C. P. (1978). Venous thromboembolism after stroke. *Am. Heart J.*, **96**, 283–5.

Warlow, C. P. (1986). Extracranial to intracranial bypass and the prevention of stroke. *J. Neurol.*, **233**, 129–30.

Warlow, C. P. (1991). Introduction. In *Handbook of neurology*. Blackwell, Oxford.

Warlow, C. P. (1996). Surgical treatment of asymtomatic carotid stenosis. *Cerebrovasc. Dis.*, **6** (Suppl. 1), 7–14.

Warlow, C. P. (1998*a*). Can neurologists influence stroke incidence and do they? *J. R. Coll. Physicians Lond.*, **32**, 466–72.

Warlow, C. P. (1998*b*). Carotid endarterectomy for asymptomatic carotid stenosis: better data, but the case is still not convincing. *BMJ*, **317**, 1468.

Warlow, C. P., Dennis, M. S., van Gijn, J. *et al.* (2000*a*). *Stroke: a practical guide to management*, 2nd edn., chapter 6. Blackwell Scientific, Oxford.

Warlow, C. P., Dennis, M. S., van Gijn, J. *et al.* (2000*b*). *Stroke: a practical guide to management*, 2nd edn., chapter 8. Blackwell Scientific, Oxford.

Warlow, C. P., Dennis, M. S., van Gijn, J. *et al.* (2000*c*). *Stroke: a practical guide to management*, 2nd edn., chapter 5. Blackwell Scientific, Oxford.

Warlow, C. P., Dennis, M. S., van Gijn, J. *et al.* (2000*d*). *Stroke: a practical guide to management*, 2nd edn., chapter 13. Blackwell Scientific, Oxford.

Warlow, C. P., Dennis, M. S., van Gijn, J. *et al.* (2000*e*). *Stroke: a practical guide to management*, 2nd edn., chapter 15. Blackwell Scientific, Oxford.

Warlow, C. P., Dennis, M. S., van Gijn, J. *et al.* (2000*f*). *Stroke: a practical guide to management*, 2nd edn., chapter 18. Blackwell Scientific, Oxford.

Warlow, C. P., Dennis, M. S., van Gijn, J. *et al.* (2000*g*). *Stroke: a practical guide to management*, 2nd edn., chapter 16. Blackwell Scientific, Oxford.

Warnock, N. G., Gandhi, M. R., Bergvall, U. *et al.* (1993). Complications of intraarterial digital subtraction angiography in patients investigated for cerebral vascular disease. *BJR*, **66**, 855–8.

Watson, P., Fekete, J., and Deck, J. (1977). Central nervous system vasculitis in rheumatoid arthritis. *Can. J. Neurol. Sci.*, **4**, 269–72.

Weaver, J. P. A., Evans, A., and Walder, D. N. (1969). The effect of increased fibrinogen content on the viscosity of blood. *Clin. Sci.*, **36**, 1–10.

Wechsler, B., Dell'Isola, B., Vidailhet, M. *et al.* (1993). MRI in 31 patients with Behçet's disease and neurological involvement: prospective study with clinical correlation. *J. Neurol. Neurosurg. Psychiatry*, **56**, 793–8.

Weiller, C., Ringelstein, E. B., Reiche, W. *et al.* (1991). Clinical and haemodynamic aspects of low-flow infarcts. *Stroke*, **22**, 1117–23.

Weir, C. J., Murray, G. D., Dyker, A. G. *et al.* (1997). Is hyperglycaemia an independent predictor of poor outcome after acute stroke? Results of a long term follow up study. *BMJ*, **314**, 1303–6.

Weir, N. *et al.* (2001). Case mix and adjustment paper.

Welch, G. N. and Loscalzo, J. (1998). Homocysteine and atherothrombosis. *N. Engl. J. Med.*, **338**, 1042–50.

Welin, L., Svardsudd, K., Wilhelmsen, L., Larsson, B., and Tibblin, G. (1987). Analysis of risk factors for stroke in a cohort of men born in 1913. *N. Engl. J. Med.*, **317**, 521–6.

Wellwood, I., Dennis, M. S., and Warlow, C. P. (1995). A comparison of the Barthel Index and the OPCS disability instrument used to measure outcome after acute stroke. *Age and Ageing*, **24**, 54–7.

Welsh, J. E., Tyson, G. W., Winn, H. R. *et al.* (1979). Chronic subdural haematoma presenting as transient neurologic deficits. *Stroke*, **10**, 564–7.

Wen, P. Y., Feske, S. K., Teoh, S. K. *et al.* (1997). Cerebral haemorrhage in a patient taking fenfluramine and phentermine for obesity. *Neurology*, **49**, 632–3.

Whelton, P. K. (1994). Epidemiology of hypertension. *Lancet*, **344**, 101–6.

Whelton, P. K., He, J., Cutler, J. A. *et al.* (1997). Effects of oral potassium on blood pressure. Meta-analysis of randomised controlled clinical trials. *JAMA*, **277**, 1624–32.

White, R. P. and Markus, H. S. (1997). Impaired dynamic cerebral autoregulation in carotid artery stenosis. *Stroke*, **28**, 1340–4.

Whitty, C. J., Sudlow, C. L. M., and Warlow, C. P. (1998). Investigating individual subjects and screening populations for asymptomatic carotid stenosis can be harmful. *J. Neurol. Neurosurg. Psychiatry*, **64**, 619–23.

Whisnant, J. P. (1983). The role of the neurologist in the decline of stroke. *Ann. Neurol.*, **14**, 1–7.

WHO Collaborative Study of Cardiovascular Disease and Steroid Hormone Contraception (1996*a*). Ischaemic stroke and combined oral contraceptives: results of an international, multicentre, case-control study. *Lancet*, **348**, 498–505.

WHO Collaborative Study of Cardiovascular Disease and Steroid Hormone Contraception (1996*b*). Haemorrhagic stroke, overall stroke risk, and combined oral contraceptives: results of an international, multicentre, case-control study. *Lancet*, **348**, 505–10.

WHO MONICA Project, prepared by Thorvaldsen, P., Kuulasmaa, K., Rajakangas, A.-M. *et al.* (1997). Stroke trends in the WHO MONICA Project. *Stroke*, **28**, 500–6.

Whurr, R., Perlman Lorch, M., and Nye, C. (1992). A meta-analysis of studies carried out between 1946 and 1988 concerned with the efficacy of speech and language therapy treatment for aphasic patients. *Eur. J. Disord. Commun.*, **27**, 1–17.

Widder, B., Kleiser, B., and Krapf, H. (1994). Course of cerebrovascular reactivity in patients with carotid artery occlusions. *Stroke*, **25**, 1963–7.

Widen Holmqvist, L., von Koch, L., Kostulas, V. *et al.* (1998). A randomised controlled trial of rehabilitation at home after stroke in southwest Stockholm. *Stroke*, **29**, 591–7.

Wiebers, D. O. (1985). Ischaemic cerebrovascular complications of pregnancy. *Arch. Neurol.*, **42**, 1106–13.

Wiebers, D. O. and Mokri, B. (1985). Internal carotid artery dissection after childbirth. *Stroke*, **16**, 956–9.

Wiebers, D. O., Swanson, J. W., Cascino, T. L. *et al.* (1989). Bilateral loss of vision in bright light. *Stroke*, **20**, 554–8.

Wiebers, D. O., Whisnant, J. P., Sandok, B. A. *et al.* (1990). Prospective comparison of a cohort with asymptomatic carotid bruit and a population-based cohort without carotid bruit. *Stroke*, **21**, 984–8.

Wijdicks, E. F. M. (1995). Worse-case scenario: management in poor-grade aneurysmal subarachnoid haemorrhage. *Cerebrovasc. Dis.*, **5**, 163–9.

Wijdicks, E. F. M. and Scott, J. P. (1997). Pulmonary embolism associated with acute stroke. *Mayo Clin. Proc.*, **72**, 297–300.

Wijdicks, E. F. M., Vermeulen, M., Hijdra, A. *et al.* (1985). Hyponatraemia and cerebral infarction in patients with ruptured intracranial aneurysms: is fluid restriction harmful? *Ann. Neurol.*, **17**, 137–40.

Wijdicks, E. F. M., Kerkhoff, H., and van Gijn, J. (1988). Long-term follow-up of 71 patients with thunderclap headache mimicking subarachnoid haemorrhage. *Lancet*, **1**, 68–9.

Wijman, C. A. C., Babikian, V. L., Matjucha, I. C. A. *et al.* (1998). Cerebral microembolism in patients with retinal ischaemia. *Stroke*, **29**, 1139–43.

Wilkinson, I. M. S. and Ross Russell, R. W. (1972). Arteries of the head and neck in giant cell arteritis. *Arch. Neurol.*, **27**, 378–91.

Willoughby, E. W. and Anderson, N. E. (1984). Lower cranial nerve motor function in unilateral vascular lesions of the cerebral hemisphere. *BMJ*, **289**, 791–4.

Wing, S., Casper, M., Davis, W. B. *et al.* (1988). Stroke mortality maps, United States whites aged 35–74 years, 1962–1982. *Stroke*, **19**, 1507–13.

Winn, H. R., Richardson, A. E., and Jane, J. A. (1977). The long-term prognosis in untreated cerebral aneurysms: I. The incidence of late haemorrhage in cerebral aneurysm: A 10 year evaluation of 364 patients. *Ann. Neurol.*, **1**, 358–70.

Winterkorn, J. M., Kupersmith, M. J., Wirtschafter, J. D. *et al.* (1993). Brief report: treatment of vasospastic amaurosis fugax with calcium-channel blockers. *N. Engl. J. Med.*, **329**, 396–8.

Wise, R. J. S., Bernardi, S., Frackowiak, R. S. J. *et al.* (1983). Serial observations on the pathophysiology of acute stroke. The transition from ischaemia to infarction as reflected in regional oxygen extraction. *Brain*, **106**, 197–222.

Wityk, R. J., Lehman, D., Klag, M. *et al.* (1996). Race and sex differences in the distribution of cerebral atherosclerosis. *Stroke*, **27**, 1974–80.

Witztum, J. L. (1994). The oxidation hypothesis of atherosclerosis. *Lancet*, **344**, 793–5.

Wolf, P. A., Dawber, T. R., Thomas, E. *et al.* (1978). Epidemiologic assessment of chronic atrial fibrillation and risk of stroke: The Framingham Study. *Neurology*, **28**, 973–7.

Wolf, P. A., Abbott, R. D., and Kannel, W. B. (1991*a*). Atrial fibrillation as an independent risk factor for stroke: the Framingham Study. *Stroke*, **22**, 983–8.

Wolf, P. A., D'Agostino, R. B., Belanger, A. J. *et al.* (1991*b*). Probability of stroke: a risk profile from the Framingham Study. *Stroke*, **22**, 312–18.

Wollner, L., McCarthy, S. T., Soper, N. D. W. *et al.* (1979). Failure of cerebral autoregulation as a cause of brain dysfunction in the elderly. *BMJ*, **1**, 1117–18.

Woo, J., Lau, E., Lam, C. W. *et al.* (1991). Hypertension, lipoprotein (a), and apoliprotein A-I as risk factors for stroke in the Chinese. *Stroke*, **22**, 203–8.

Wood, J. H. and Kee, D. B. (1985). Haemorheology of the cerebral circulation in stroke. *Stroke*, **16**, 765–72.

World Federation of Neurological Surgeons (1988). Report of World Federation of Neurological Surgeons Committee on a universal subarachnoid haemorrhage grading scale. *J. Neurosurg.*, **68**, 985–6.

Wroe, S. J., Sandercock, P., Bamford, J. *et al.* (1992). Diurnal variation in the incidence of stroke: The Oxfordshire Community Stroke Project. *BMJ*, **304**, 155–7.

Wyller, T. B., Bautz-Holter, E., and Holmen, J. (1994). Prevalence of stroke and stroke-related disability in North Trondelag County, Norway. *Cerebrovasc. Dis.*, **4**, 421–7.

Yamamoto, H. and Bogousslavsky, J. (1998). Mechanisms of second and further strokes. *J. Neurol. Neurosurg. Psychiatry*, **64**, 771–6.

Yamanouchi, H., Mizutani, T., Matsushita, S. *et al.* (1997*a*). Paroxysmal atrial fibrillation: high frequency of embolic brain infarction in elderly autopsy patients. *Neurology*, **49**, 1691–4.

Yamanouchi, H., Nagura, H., Mizutani, T. *et al.* (1997*b*). Embolic brain infarction in nonrheumatic atrial fibrillation: a clinicopathologic study in the elderly. *Neurology*, **48**, 1593–7.

Yanagihara, T., Piepgras, D. G., and Klass, D. W. (1985). Repetitive involuntary movement associated with episodic cerebral ischaemia. *Ann. Neurol.*, **18**, 244–50.

Yoo, J.-H., Chung, C.-S., and Kang, S.-S. (1998). Relation of plasma homocyst(e)ine to cerebral infarction and cerebral atherosclerosis. *Stroke*, **29**, 2478–83.

You, R., McNeil, J. J., O'Malley, H. M. *et al.* (1995). Risk factors for lacunar infarction syndromes. *Neurology*, **45**, 1483–7.

Zanette, E. M., Roberti, C., Mancini, G. *et al.* (1995). Spontaneous middle cerebral artery reperfusion in ischaemic stroke. A follow-up study with transcranial Doppler. *Stroke*, **26**, 430–3.

Zeman, A. Z. J., Boniface, S. J., and Hodges, J. R. (1998). Transient epileptic amnesia: a description of the clinical and neuropsychological features in 10 cases and a review of the literature. *J. Neurol. Neurosurg. Psychiatry*, **64**, 435–43.

Zeumer, H. (1985). Vascular recanalizing techniques in interventional neuroradiology. *J. Neurol.*, **231**, 287–94.

Zhu, C. Z. and Norris, J. W. (1990). Role of carotid stenosis in ischaemic stroke. *Stroke*, **21**, 1131–4.

Zhu, X. L., Chan, M. S. Y., and Poon, W. S. (1997). Spontaneous intracranial haemorrhage: which patients need diagnostic cerebral angiography? A prospective study of 206 cases and review of the literature. *Stroke*, **28**, 1406–9.

Zuber, M., Khoubesserian, P., Meder, J.-F. *et al.* (1993). A 34-year delayed and focal postirradiation intracranial vasculopathy. *Cerebrovasc. Dis.*, **3**, 181–2.

CHAPTER 28

Vasculitis and collagen vascular disorders affecting the central nervous system

Charles Warlow

28.1 Introduction

Most of the autoimmune or collagen vascular and related disorders can be complicated by, or occasionally present with, almost any neurological syndrome, such as subacute encephalopathy, aseptic meningitis, stroke, peripheral neuropathy, and myopathy (Sigal, 1987; Ferro, 1998; Moore and Richardson, 1998; Jennekens and Kater, 1999; Scolding, 1999). Often, but certainly not always, the neurological syndrome is due to an acute, subacute, or chronic inflammatory reaction in the arterial and/or venous wall, with or without granuloma formation, so-called vasculitis. The mural cellular proliferation, necrosis, and subsequent fibrosis may be sufficient to occlude the vessel lumen; precipitate thrombosis, which may be complicated by embolism; and promote aneurysm formation, dissection or even wall rupture and haemorrhage. Therefore, vasculitis may cause not just focal and generalized ischaemia in the brain, spinal cord, peripheral nerves, and muscle, either due to arterial or venous occlusion, but also sometimes haemorrhage. In addition, patients may develop neurological symptoms as a result of non-neurological complications of collagen vascular disorders (e.g. hypertension due to renal involvement causing intracranial haemorrhage); adverse effects of immunosuppressive treatment (e.g. opportunistic meningeal and cerebral infections causing cerebral ischaemia or haemorrhage, and cranial nerve palsies); and iatrogenic aseptic meningitis due to non-steroidal anti-inflammatory drugs, azathioprine, intravenous gamma globulin, etc.

28.1.1 Classification

Despite numerous attempts, there is no very satisfactory classification of the various, often eponymous, syndromes which may result from vasculitis (Jennette and Falk, 1997; Savage *et al.* 1997). It may be useful to think in terms of vessel size, even though some conditions affect vessels of varying size (Table 28.1), and to distinguish primary vasculitis where no cause is identified from secondary vasculitis where there is a cause, such as infection, for example. But, a problem with any classification is that not all the features of the disease, or the neurological complications, are due to vasculitis or even anything to do with the vessels (e.g. spinal cord compression in rheumatoid disease). Furthermore, there is an ongoing debate about whether many of these conditions should be 'lumped' together and thought about and treated in the same way, or 'split' as being fundamentally different (e.g. is the antiphospholipid syndrome one form of systemic lupus erythematosus (SLE), or something different, notwithstanding the fact that the same autoantibodies can be found in both?). On balance, it still seems sensible – at least for clinical diagnosis—to think largely in terms of the various different clinical syndromes and what their neurological complications might be, whether due to vasculitis or not. At the same time one must acknowledge that these syndromes, and perhaps their causes, often overlap, and that the mainstay of disease-modifying treatment is almost always immunosuppression.

28.1.2 Diagnosis

In a patient presenting with neurological symptoms, clues to the diagnosis of an underlying vasculitis or collagen vascular disorder, unless it is already diagnosed, are: systemic features such as weight loss, headache, malaise, skin rash, livedo reticularis, arthropathy, renal failure, and fever; the lack of any other obvious cause of the neurological problem; a raised erythrocyte sedimentation rate (ESR) and C-reactive protein (the latter not in SLE), or anaemia, in the routine screening tests; and, when diagnostic suspicion is aroused, more specific immunological abnormalities such as serum anticardiolipin antibodies, antinuclear factor, or antineutrophil cytoplasmic antibodies

Table 28.1. The major categories of vasculitis

Large vessel vasculitis (aorta, arteries to the organs and limbs)
    Giant cell arteritis (Sections 3.7.3, 8.4.4, 12.15.3, 27.4.4)
    Takayasu's arteritis (Section 27.4.4)

Medium-sized vessel vasculitis (main visceral arteries and their branches)
    Classical poyarteritis nodosa (Sections 28.3, 12.15.3)
    Kawasaki's disease (Section 28.7)

Small vessel vasculitis (arterioles, venules and capillaries)
    ANCA-associated small vessel vasculitis (Section 27.4.4)
        Microscopic polyangiitis (Sections 28.4, 12.15.3)
        Churg–Strauss syndrome (Sections 28.5, 12.15.3)
        Wegener's granulomatosis (Sections 28.6, 12.15.3)

    Systemic lupus erythematosus (Sections 28.2, 12.17.6, 27.4.4)
    Rheumatoid disease (Sections 28.8, 12.15.3, 27.4.4)
    Sjögren's syndrome (Sections 28.9, 11.1.5, 27.4.4)
    Henoch–Schönlein purpura (Section 28.10)
    Behçet's disease (Sections 28.11, 27.4.4)
    Systemic sclerosis (Section 28.13)
    Essential cryoglobulinaemia (Sections 28.14, 12.15.14)
    Goodpasture's syndrome
    Primary angiitis of the central nervous system (Sections 28.16, 27.4.4)
    Non-systemic vasculitic neuropathy (Section 12.15.2)
    Cutaneous leucocytoclastic angiitis
    Serum sickness

Miscellaneous
    Relapsing polychondritis (Section 28.12)
    Sarcoidosis (Sections 28.15, 12.17.7)
    Buerger's disease (Section 28.18)
    Intravascular lymphoma (formerly malignant angioendotheliosis) (Section 28.17)
    Malignant atrophic papulosis (Section 28.19)
    Inflammatory bowel disease (Section 27.4.7)
    Coeliac disease (Section 27.4.7)
    Drug-induced (Sections 27.4.7, 28.20)
    Paraneoplastic (Sections 28.21, 12.13.3)
    Acute posterior multifocal placoid pigment epitheliopathy (Section 27.4.4)
    Eales' disease (Section 28.22)
    Cogan's syndrome (Section 28.23)
    Lymphatoid granulomatosis (Section 28.24)
    Infection-induced
        Bacterial meningitis (Section 33.2.2)
        Tuberculous meningitis (Section 33.2.3)
        Meningovascular syphilis (Section 34.17.2)
        Borrelia (Section 34.17.4)
        Herpes zoster (Section 34.6.2)
        Cytomegalovirus (Section 34.6.3)
        Fungal meningitis (Section 33.2.5)

(ANCA). Biopsy is then often required to confirm the diagnosis: of the superficial temporal artery, meninges, cerebral cortex, peripheral nerve, muscle, skin, kidney, etc. A point to watch is that the absence of histopathological proof-positive of vasculitis may be misleading because the vascular lesions can and do heal, and they are so often patchy in distribution. On the other hand, assuming that a patient must have vasculitis on the basis of the clinical syndrome, along perhaps with an abnormal cerebral angiogram, is not much better than guesswork, and dangerous

Table 28.2. Some causes of segmental narrowing, dilatation, and beading of cerebral arteries on angiography

Cerebral vasculitis (Section 28.1)

Tumour emboli (e.g. myxoma) (Section 27.4.5)

Irradiation (Section 27.4.4)

Malignant meningitis (Section 18.10)

Chronic meningeal infection (Section 33.2)

Drug abuse (cocaine, amphetamines, etc.) (Sections 5.3, 27.4.7)

Multiple emboli from proximal arteries or the heart (Sections 27.4.2, 27.4.5)

Idiopathic reversible cerebral vasoconstriction (e.g. puerperal angiopathy) (Section 28.25)

Arterial dissection (Section 27.4.4)

Intravascular lymphoma (Section 28.17)

Malignant hypertension

Phaeochromocytoma

---

guesswork if immunosuppression is contemplated. Any changes in the cerebrospinal fluid are merely a non-specific lymphocytic and occasionally polymorph inflammatory reaction; oligoclonal bands do not really help in differentiating vasculitic disorders from multiple sclerosis because they occur in both (McLean *et al.* 1995). Brain CT, and the more sensitive MRI, may show areas of presumed infarction, and sometimes haemorrhage, in both grey and white matter, sometimes along with diffuse meningeal and subependymal involvement (cf. multiple sclerosis, where the lesions are confined to the periventricular white matter and corpus callosum, but the distinction from vasculitis is impossible in many cases) (Miller *et al.* 1987). There are no *specific* cerebral angiographic criteria for cerebral 'vasculitis': focal narrowing, dilatation and beading of small cerebral arteries, sometimes with aneurysm formation, are seen in many other situations

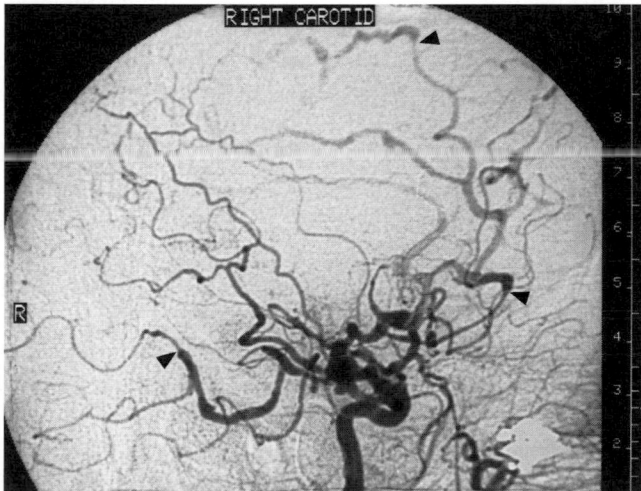

Fig. 28.1. Selective catheter angiogram to show the cerebral circulation (lateral skull view). The medium-sized and small arteries are irregular with areas of narrowing and dilatation (arrows). This is seen in various disorders, including vasculitis (Table 28.2).

(Table 28.2 and Fig. 28.1). Moreover, angiography is often normal in biopsy-proven vasculitis. The electroencephalogram may help in the sense that bilateral diffuse slowing in a patient who clinically seems to have only a single focal cerebral lesion would suggest a diffuse encephalopathic process of some sort.

28.1.3 Treatment

For years, the treatment of vasculitic and collagen vascular disorders has consisted of high-dose steroids, with or without other means of immunosuppression, such as cyclophosphamide and azathioprine. There is a dearth of randomized evidence, and what there is does not apply directly to the management of many neurological complications (Savage *et al.* 1997; Jennekens and Kater 1999). Whatever else, it is important for neurologists to work with rheumatologists when managing the diseases which are unusual in neurological practice but quite common in rheumatological practice (e.g. Sjögren's syndrome, systemic lupus erythematosus, etc).

28.2 Systemic lupus erythematosus and related disorders

28.2.1 Systemic lupus erythematosus

This chronic autoimmune multisystem disease occasionally presents with neurological symptoms, but these occur much more often in the context of well-established active disease with systemic features such as fever, general malaise, arthritis, skin rash and photosensitivity, and nephritis (Mills 1994; Jennekens and Kater 1999; Scolding 1999). Neurological involvement is said to occur in up to 75 per cent of patients but the figure must depend on what is meant by involvement, the stage of the disease, whether a series is cross-sectional or prospective over many years, and case-selection factors. Like other features of systemic lupus erythematosus (SLE), the neurological complications may relapse and remit, and patients may have more than one at any one time.

Cerebrovascular complications: SLE can cause focal ischaemic and sometimes haemorrhagic cerebral episodes, presenting as TIAs or strokes, mostly arterial but sometimes venous in origin (Haas 1982; Devinsky *et al.* 1988; Kitagawa *et al.* 1990; Mitsias and Levine 1994). Scattered cerebral infarcts and haemorrhages of varying size are found in some, but by no means all, cases coming to post-mortem. If any vascular pathology at all *is* found, it is seldom a florid vasculitis but rather bland intimal proliferation involving small vessels, but of course this may represent healed vasculitis. Why the occasional patient has large artery occlusion is unknown, but embolism from heart valves affected by SLE is obviously one possibility. Indeed, embolism from non-infective cardiac valvular vegetations to cerebral arteries is probably quite common (Roldan *et al.* 1996). Eventually the patients may dement.

Subacute encephalopathy with clouding of consciousness, confusion, headache, epileptic seizures and occasional focal neurological features is well recognized but unusual. The CSF contains excess lymphocytes and sometimes polymorphs, and the EEG is diffusely abnormal. Clearly, opportunistic CNS infection must be excluded. The cerebral pathology is probably the same as for the vascular complications described above (Hama and Boumpas 1995).

Neuropsychiatric problems: lupus patients quite frequently have various rather chronic—and sometimes subacute—psychiatric and behavioural disturbances, such as depression, anxiety, agitation, hallucinations, delusions, paranoia, and catatonia. How much all this is due to an organic encephalopathy rather than being psychological or induced by drug treatment, how it overlaps with the subacute encephalopathy above, and what any underlying brain and vascular pathology may be, is very unclear (Lim *et al.* 1988).

Epileptic seizures are common, either in isolation or as part of the subacute or chronic encephalopathy syndrome, or as a result of various other complications such as stroke, renal failure, and opportunistic infections. They may be partial or generalized.

Chorea, and sometimes athetosis and hemiballismus, is a well known but rare complication, more often generalized than focal. It is either isolated or part of the subacute encephalopathy. It often starts suddenly and may be due to some kind of cerebral vascular lesion (Bruyn and Padberg 1984).

Headache is probably more common in those with SLE than in normal people, partly because of associations with migraine, intracranial venous thrombosis, aseptic meningitis, and subacute and chronic encephalopathies.

Aseptic meningitis is rare, with subacute or chronic headache, fever, and a lymphocytic (rarely polymorphic) CSF with a normal glucose level. Other rare complications include *intracranial venous thrombosis* (Vidailhet *et al.* 1990), *cranial neuropathies, optic neuropathy, cerebellar ataxia, spinal cord infarction/myelitis* (Harisdangkul *et al.* 1995), *radiculopathy and peripheral neuropathy* (Section 12.17.6) (Stefurak *et al.* 1999), *autonomic neuropathy*, and *polymyositis* (Jennekens and Kater 1999). Also, neurological complications can arise from the general effects of SLE, such as renal failure, hypertension, thrombocytopenia; CNS opportunistic infections as a consequence of the SLE itself or its treatment with immuno-suppression; and from other adverse effects of treatment (steroid myopathy and depression, etc.).

Diagnosis

The great majority of the 'neurological' patients are already known to have SLE, the ESR is raised (but not necessarily the C-reactive protein), and there are circulating antinuclear autoantibodies of various sorts; antinuclear factor is highly sensitive but not specific at a dilution of at least 1 : 160, while both double-stranded DNA and anti-sm antibodies are more specific but present in less than 50 per cent of cases. A high proportion of patients also have anticardiolipin antibodies (Section

28.2.2), which seem to be particularly associated with cardiac valvular vegetations and arterial thrombosis (Khamashta *et al.* 1990). Lymphopenia, leucopenia, normochromic normocytic anaemia, haemolytic anaemia, and thrombocytopenia may all be present in some cases. A false-positive serological test for syphilis is an occasional and well-known feature. It is clearly crucial to rule out any opportunistic infection, or other complication of treatment, as the cause of the neurological syndrome. Occasionally there can be difficulty in distinguishing multiple sclerosis (MS) from SLE without many, if any, systemic features other than raised antinuclear and anticardiolipin antibodies (Kaarussis *et al.* 1998). In both MS and SLE there may be a lymphocytic CSF with oligoclonal bands and a mildly raised protein. However, MRI in SLE is more likely to show cortical lesions and less likely to show corpus callosum lesions (Miller *et al.* 1992).

Treatment

Treatment to suppress the disease and improve long-term outcome is controversial. In severe cases, high-dose corticosteroids are used, and even cyclophosphamide and azathioprine immunosuppression (Drug and Therapeutics Bulletin 1996). Not surprisingly, both plasma exchange and intravenous immunoglobulin have been tried. Clearly, collaboration with a rheumatologist is essential.

28.2.2 Antiphospholipid syndrome

From 1 to 40 per cent of ischaemic stroke/TIA patients have raised circulating IgG or, probably less relevant, IgM, anticardiolipin autoantibodies, and/or the lupus anticoagulant detected by the activated partial thromboplastin time or the dilute Russell's viper venom time (Montalban *et al.* 1994; Muir *et al.* 1994). The exact proportion must depend on the selection of patients; the timing of the blood sample after symptom onset; the laboratory methods, which are very varied; and what level is deemed 'normal'; and bearing in mind spontaneous fluctuations in titre. However, very few stroke patients have some or all of the constellation of features comprising the antiphospholipid syndrome: recurrent miscarriage, arterial and venous thrombosis in any sized vessel but without vasculitis, and variably livedo reticularis, heart valve vegetations, migraine-like headaches, thrombocytopenia, and false-positive syphilis serology (Feldmann and Levine 1995; Carhuapoma *et al.* 1997; Greaves 1999). If a patient has the typical syndrome but no antibodies, then the test should be repeated because the titres may fall during the acute episode (Drenkard *et al.* 1989). Anticardiolipin antibodies are not specific to the antiphospholipid syndrome (APS) (Table 28.3), particularly if they are not present in high (>40 units) titres on *repeated* testing, and they can occasionally be found in normal people (Tanne *et al.* 1999). The catastrophic antiphospholipid antibody syndrome consists of rapid onset and severe multi-organ failure, including the adult respiratory distress syndrome, abdominal pain, and fulminant encephalopathy, usually in people who are known already to have the APS (Asherson and Piette 1996).

Table 28.3. Causes of raised serum anticardiolipin antibodies

Systemic lupus erythematosus

Antiphospholipid syndrome

Sneddon's syndrome

Malignancy

Lymphoma

Paraproteinaemias

Human immunodeficiency virus (HIV) and other infections

Patients with multiple vascular risk factors

Drugs such as phenothiazines, hydralazine, phenytoin, valproate, procainamide, and quinidine

The cause of thrombosis, the prognosis for recurrent stroke, the nature of the relationship and overlap with SLE, and what, if any, treatment should be (aspirin, anticoagulants, immunosuppression) are all uncertain. But, at least aspirin as an antithrombotic drug is safe. If symptoms recur, anticoagulation is usually recommended (Finazzi *et al.* 1996; Antiphospholipid Antibodies and Stroke Study Group (APASS) 1997; Levine *et al.* 1997; Verro *et al.* 1998).

28.2.3 Sneddon's syndrome

Sneddon's syndrome is the rare combination of widespread and prominent livedo reticularis with ischaemic strokes/TIAs, and sometimes the autoantibodies associated with SLE (particularly anticardiolipin antibodies and the lupus anticoagulant), if not the full-blown syndrome. Clearly, this could be one variety of the antiphospholipid syndrome, itself part of the spectrum of SLE (Burton 1988; Stockhammer *et al.* 1993; Kalashnikova *et al.* 1994; Boortz-Marx *et al.* 1995; Geschwind *et al.* 1995).

28.3 Classical polyarteritis nodosa

Classical polyarteritis nodosa affects medium-sized arteries, and aneurysm formation is rather characteristic. Involvement of the kidneys with secondary hypertension, the gut with perforation and haemorrhage, and the skin with purpura and even gangrene are common clinical manifestations, along with systemic symptoms such as malaise, fever, weight loss, and arthralgia. The most common neurological feature is a peripheral neuropathy due to vasculitic ischaemic damage to nerves; the usual pattern is a painful, subacute mononeuropathy, radiculopathy, or mononeuritis multiplex rather than a symmetrical distal neuropathy (Section 12.15.3). Cerebrovascular complications are less common, but ischaemia and haemorrhage can affect the brain, optic nerve, and spinal cord. One is unlikely to find the serum antibodies characteristic of SLE or antineutrophil cytoplasmic antibodies (ANCA) and more likely to find eosinophilia, and haematuria reflecting the renal involvement (Moore and Fauci 1981). The diagnosis is usually made by biopsy of affected tissue (kidney, nerve, etc.). Sometimes it can be confused with the cholesterol embolization syndrome (Section 27.4.2).

28.4 Microscopic polyangiitis

This small vessel systemic vasculitis affects predominantly the kidneys and to a lesser extent the lungs, gut, joints, and skin. Unlike classical poyarteritis nodosa, serum ANCA antibodies are characteristic. The neurological complications are similar to those of polyarteritis nodosa, although probably less common (Jennette and Falk 1997).

28.5 Churg–Strauss syndrome

This small vessel systemic vasculitis, often with granuloma formation, has a particular predilection for the lungs, causing asthma and frequently pulmonary infiltrates on the chest radiograph. Otherwise, it is similar to polyarteritis nodosa. Mononeuritis multiplex is the most common neurological complication (Section 12.15.3). Other patterns of peripheral neuropathy, ischaemic stroke, ischaemic optic neuropathy, radiculopathy, and trigeminal neuropathy are less common (Sehgal *et al.* 1995; Hattori *et al.* 1999).

28.6 Wegener's granulomatosis

This is another small vessel systemic vasculitis with, in addition, granuloma formation. It tends particularly to affect the upper and lower respiratory tracts, leading to subacute or chronic sinusitis, nasal ulceration and septal perforation, otitis media, tracheal stenosis, haemoptysis, and pneumonitis. The kidneys, eyes, and orbits are also affected and there is eosinophilia. Any neurological complications are similar to those of polyarteritis nodosa; most commonly peripheral neuropathy, particularly mononeuritis multiplex (Section 12.15.3), and cranial nerve palsies (Nishino *et al.* 1993).

28.7 Kawasaki's disease

This systemic vasculitis causes an acute illness in infants and children, with fever, conjunctival injection, fissuring of the lips, cervical lymphadenopathy, rash, and reddening of the palms and soles. Coronary arteritis is the most important complication, but there are occasional neurological features: aseptic meningitis, facial palsy, epileptic seizures, and encephalopathy (Jennekens and Kater 1999).

28.8 Rheumatoid disease

Although mainly a chronic disorder of joints, there can by systemic features and there are several neurological complications: entrapment neuropathies of the ulnar and median nerves; peripheral neuropathy due sometimes to systemic vasculitis

(Section 12.15.3); atlanto-axial dislocation causing spinal cord compression and, very rarely, vertebral artery compression and brainstem stroke; vertical subluxation of the odontoid peg to compress the brainstem; polymyositis; rheumatoid nodules causing brain and spinal cord compression; and, very rarely, cerebral necrotizing vasculitis, causing a global encephalopathy (Nakano 1975; Watson *et al.* 1977; Beck and Corbett 1983; Howell and Molyneux 1988).

28.9 Sjögren's syndrome

Dry eyes and dry mouth due to inflammation and destruction of the lacrimal and salivary glands are the defining features, characteristically with serum anti-Ro antibodies, but antinuclear and rheumatoid factors are also common. It is frequently associated with other autoimmune disorders such as SLE, systemic sclerosis, rheumatoid arthritis, polymyositis, and primary biliary cirrhosis, and may progress to non-Hodgkin's lymphoma. Peripheral neuropathy—symmetrical more often than mononeuritis multiplex—is the most common neurological complication, sometimes as a presenting feature when any sicca symptoms are not at all prominent (Alexander *et al.* 1982; Grant *et al.* 1997; Jennekens and Kater 1999). Trigeminal sensory neuropathy may also occur (Section 11.1.5). Transient or permanent focal neurological deficits, epileptic seizures, aseptic meningitis, global encephalopathy, and spinal cord infarction and haemorrhage can be due to vasculitis or extraglandular extension of the inflammatory lymphoproliferative process (de la Monte *et al.* 1983; Bragoni *et al.* 1994; Li *et al.* 1999). The renal tubular necrosis may cause enough hypokalaemia to lead to severe muscular paralysis (Poux *et al.* 1992).

28.10 Henoch–Schönlein purpura

This small vessel vasculitis, mainly in children, typically involves the skin, gut, and kidneys, and is associated with arthritis. Subacute encephalopathy, perhaps with focal features, and peripheral nerve involvement are all rare (Belman *et al.* 1985). Meningococcal meningitis is an important differential diagnosis.

28.11 Behçet's disease

This is an inflammatory relapsing and remitting syndrome of oro-genital ulceration and uveitis, often along with skin, joint, and gut involvement, and recurrent venous thrombosis (Sakane *et al.* 1999). Both large and small vessel vasculitis is well described, but florid necrotizing vasculitis appears to be distinctly unusual. There are no specific circulating autoantibodies and the diagnosis is made on the clinical manifestations and a positive pathergy test (cutaneous needle prick causes an erythematous nodule 24–48 hours later). Behçet's disease can be complicated by a chronic aseptic meningitis which can cause cranial nerve palsies; occlusion of extra- and intracranial arteries, perhaps most often those supplying the brainstem, to cause

ischaemic stroke/TIA; and primary intracerebral and sometimes subarachnoid haemorrhage. A more global subacute and relapsing encephalopathy is well recognized—perhaps as much to do with low-grade inflammation within the brain as in the vessel walls—while intracranial venous thrombosis is probably the most commonly recognized neurological complication. The spinal cord and peripheral nerves are only exceptionally affected. The neurological symptoms tend to coincide with flare-ups of the mucocutaneo-ocular symptoms, but can antedate them (Farah *et al.* 1998; Serdaroglu 1998). The CSF usually contains an excess of lymphocytes and polymorphs.

28.12 Relapsing polychondritis

Relapsing polychondritis is very rare. It is characterized by recurrent inflammatory episodes affecting cartilage of the ear, nose, trachea, larynx, and ribs, often accompanied by inflammation of the eyes and joints, deafness and vertigo, malaise, fever, anaemia, and high ESR. It is sometimes complicated by a systemic and cerebral vasculitis with subacute aseptic meningitis, global encephalopathy, epileptic seizures, stroke/TIA, cranial nerve palsies, ischaemic optic neuropathy, and aortic arch syndromes (Stewart *et al.* 1988; Kothare *et al.* 1998).

28.13 Systemic sclerosis

This is characterized by widespread and slowly progressive fibrous sclerosis affecting the skin, lungs, kidneys, gut, and heart. It is said to be the least likely collagen vascular disorder to have neurological complications, although it overlaps with polymyositis and SLE and their complications (so-called mixed connective tissue disease). Trigeminal sensory neuropathy, peripheral neuropathies, and myelopathy have all been described, and also perhaps entrapment neuropathies (Hagen *et al.* 1990; Averbuch-Heller *et al.* 1992; Dyck *et al.* 1997). A cerebral arteritis occurs, as well as nondescript intracerebral small vessel disease (Lee and Haynes 1967; Hietaharju *et al.* 1995; Heron *et al.* 1998). Other neurological manifestations may be due to uraemia, malabsorption, and the complications of treatment (corticosteroids, colchicine, penicillamine).

28.14 Essential cryglobulinaemia

Slowly progressive peripheral neuropathy, or a subacute mononeuritis multiplex (Section 12.15.3), are the most common neurological complications of this rather chronic disease, which is manifested by purpura, Raynaud's phenomenon, arthralgia, hepatic dysfunction, and progressive renal failure. The plasma contains cryoglobulins, but there is no other cause for them (such as malignancy or infections), and circulating monoclonal and/or polyclonal immunoglobulins. There is a widespread systemic vasculitis with immune complex deposition. There are occasional reports of polymyositis and cerebral vasculitis (Abramsky and Slavin 1974; Gorevic *et al.* 1980; Voll *et al.* 1993; Monti *et al.* 1995; Apartis *et al.* 1996).

28.15 Sarcoidosis

Sarcoidosis is a systemic and multiorgan non-caseating granulomatous disorder, which mostly affects the lungs, lymph nodes, eyes, and skin. The cause is unknown (Newman *et al.* 1997). The illness may be subacute and self-limiting, it may recur, and occasionally it is chronic. It may even remain subclinical and only be discovered on incidental chest radiography or during abdominal surgery for an unrelated condition.

Neurological complications are rare but well recognized. It is exceptional for the patient not to have non-neurological features as well. The most common neurological syndrome is an aseptic and fairly transitory meningitis, perhaps with cranial nerve involvement, particularly the facial, or sometimes a more indolent chronic meningitis with obstructive hydrocephalus, multiple cranial nerve palsies, and marked meningeal contrast enhancement on CT, or more reliably on MRI (Sharma 1997; Larner *et al.* 1999a; Zajicek *et al.* 1999). Sarcoid granulomas may be found compressing or within the brain, acting as mass lesions; in the spinal cord, or compressing the cord and roots; and they also occur in the hypothalamus, pituitary gland, orbit, optic nerve (causing an atypical optic neuritis-like picture), single or multiple nerve roots, and peripheral nerves (Section 12.17.7) affecting not just the limbs but the torso too, and muscle, where they are usually asymptomatic. Granulomas tend to enhance on both brain and spinal CT and MRI. Very rarely, sarcoid causes a vasculitis of the small arteries and veins of the meninges and brain. This can lead to a chronic or subacute global encephalopathy, focal cerebral ischaemia and haemorrhage, causing stroke and TIAs (Libman *et al.* 1997). Opportunistic infections of the nervous system, such as progressive multifocal leucoencephalopathy, are other complicating issues, even without immunosuppressive treatment

The diagnosis of neurosarcoidosis should be reasonably obvious from the non-neurological features, such as hilar lymphadenopathy, uveitis, malaise, weight loss, fever, etc., and the exclusion of other possible diagnoses. A raised serum (or CSF) angiotensin converting enzyme level is neither sensitive nor specific. The CSF may well contain inflammatory cells, a raised protein level, and oligoclonal bands with or without similar bands in the serum, rarely a low glucose, and is usually needed to exclude opportunistic and other infections as well as meningeal malignancies masquerading as neurosarcoidosis. Sometimes a biopsy of affected tissue is necessary for certain diagnosis or, if this is risky, a skin or transbronchial lung biopsy, remembering that sarcoid is not the only cause of non-caseating granulomas.

The mainstay of treatment is corticosteroids for anything more than mild and resolving disease, both in the short term and long term if the disease relapses as steroids are withdrawn.

28.16 Primary angiitis of the central nervous system

Primary, or isolated, angiitis of the CNS is a rare disorder. Very occasionally it is associated with herpes zoster infection and lymphoma. A granulomatous angiitis, similar to sarcoid, affects the small leptomeningeal, cortical, and spinal cord blood vessels to cause a subacute encephalopathy with headache, confusion, cognitive decline, and epileptic seizures, with or without stroke-like episodes due to ischaemia or sometimes haemorrhage, and sometimes a myelopathy or even radiculopathy. Systemic symptoms are uncommon, but sometimes there is fever, headache, raised ESR, and a raised CSF protein with lymphocytosis. Brain imaging is either normal or non-specific, with one or more ischaemic-looking lesion, which may show mass effect and contrast enhancement, sometimes haemorrhage. The diagnosis can only be made from meningeal/cortical biopsy. Although somewhat risky, this may well be worthwhile if only to stop the continuing search for an alternative diagnosis and for specific immunosuppressive treatment, although this is not particularly successful (Hankey 1991; Vollmer *et al.* 1993; Riche *et al.* 1996; Hunn *et al.* 1998). So-called benign cases with spontaneous resolution have been described, but unless there is confirmatory histopathology, one is always left feeling insecure about the real diagnosis, particularly if it is based largely on cerebral angiography which is so non-specific (Table 28.2) (Woolfenden *et al.* 1998).

28.17 Intravascular lymphoma (formerly malignant angioendotheliosis)

This rare form of B-cell lymphoma, with proliferation of neoplastic lymphocytes within the lumen of small vessels in almost every organ, can present with multi-focal stroke and TIA-like episodes, typically in late middle age. But more often, the cerebral features are diffuse, with global dementia. Spinal cord, roots, and peripheral nerves can also be involved. Characteristically there are skin nodules and plaques, malaise, and a raised plasma lactate dehydrogenase. Brain imaging is non-specific, with infarct-like and mass lesions, and meningeal enhancement. Outside the artificial confines of a clinicopathological conference, where guesswork and gaming are all important, the diagnosis can only be made by biopsy, typically of the skin or brain. The course is relentlessly progressive to death in a few months (Glass *et al.* 1993; Chapin *et al.* 1995; Williams *et al.* 1998; Al-Shahi *et al.* 2001)

28.18 Buerger's disease (thromboangiitis obliterans)

Buerger's disease is a rare, but it seems distinct, inflammatory disorder of mainly distal small and medium arteries and veins, in the lower and upper limbs, to cause digital gangrene, much more often in men than women, and in smokers. It is often associated with migrating thrombophlebitis and Raynaud's phenomenon, but not with the systemic or immunological disturbances so often seen in other forms of vasculitis. Cerebrovascular complications have very occasionally been described, but, without a standardized definition of the vasculopathy, it is difficult to know if the cases described were really all of the same condition (Biller *et al.* 1981; Drake 1982; Lie 1986; Larner *et al.* 1999*b*; Bischof *et al.* 1999).

28.19 Malignant atrophic papulosis (Kohlmeier–Degos disease)

Malignant atrophic papulosis is another very rare vasculopathy. There are crops of painless, but occasionally itchy, umbilicated, pinkish papules on the trunk, which heal to form distinctive, circular, porcelain-white scars. Intimal endothelial proliferation and thrombosis in small arteries can cause ischaemia and haemorrhage in the brain, spinal cord, gut, and other organs. Sometimes muscles and nerves are affected (Subbiah *et al.* 1996).

28.20 Therapeutic drugs

Various therapeutic drugs have been implicated, with varying levels of proof, in hypersensitivity reactions which may include a cerebral vasculitis, e.g. *allopurinol* (Mills 1971) and *deoxycoformycin* (Steinmetz *et al.* 1989).

28.21 Paraneoplastic vasculitis

Vasculitis, sometimes affecting the brain, is recognized as being very rarely associated with various malignant tumours, particularly lymphoproliferative disorders (Fortin 1996; Wooten and Jasin 1996). Peripheral nerves can also be affected (Section 12.13.3).

28.22 Eales' disease

This rare disorder affects predominantly young men, with retinal 'perivasculitis' causing recurrent bilateral retinal and vitreous haemorrhage. Stroke and TIA have been described, and cerebral and leptomeningeal vasculitis (Herson and Squier 1978; Gordon *et al.* 1988).

28.23 Cogan's syndrome

This rare eponymous and subacute syndrome is characterized by interstitial keratitis along with vertigo, tinnitus, and hearing loss in middle age. There are systemic symptoms and aortic regurgitation, and it is probably due to a vasculitis. Occasional cases with cerebral vasculitis are in the literature (Vollertsen *et al.* 1986).

28.24 Lymphomatoid granulomatosis

Lymphomatoid granulomatosis is a rare disorder, possibly lymphomatous, which mostly affects the lungs, with diffuse infiltration and nodules, but also the skin, central, and peripheral nervous system as a result of vascular infiltration by abnormal lymphocytes and plasmacytoid cells. There is a vasculitis and the vessel walls become necrotic. The neurological syndrome is of a subacute encephalopathy, cranial neuropathies, seizures, and stroke (Liebow 1973; Patton and Lynch 1982; Schmidt *et al.* 1984).

28.25 Idiopathic reversible cerebral 'vasoconstriction'

This is a curious and rather poorly characterized syndrome, in apparently healthy adolescents or young adults, of severe headache which can start suddenly, nausea and vomiting, fluctuating and sometimes bilateral focal deficits, cortical visual signs, and sometimes seizures (Call *et al.* 1988; Meschia *et al.* 1998). On angiography there is segmental narrowing and dilatation of cerebral arteries, which is assumed to be due to vasoconstriction (notwithstanding the numerous other causes of this appearance, Table 28.2). These arterial changes, if not the neurological defects, seem to resolve, usually completely, over a matter of weeks. This kind of syndrome has also been described with the use of triptans, and in the puerperium, and is presumably similar to that seen in some drug abusers (Section 27.4.7). Conceivably it could represent a benign form of primary angiitis of the central nervous system (Section 28.16).

References

Abramsky, O. and Slavin, S. (1974). Neurologic manifestations in patients with mixed cryoglobulinaemia. *Neurology*, **24**, 245–9.

Alexander, E. L., Provost, T. T., Stevens, M. B. *et al.* (1982). Neurologic complications of primary Sjögren's syndrome. *Medicine*, **61**, 247–57.

Al-Shahi, R., Warlow, C. P., Jansen, G. H. *et al.* (2000). A 59 year old man with progressive spinal cord and peripheral nerve dysfunction culminating in encephalopathy. *J. Neurol. Neurosurg. Psychiatry*, in press.

Antiphospholipid Antibodies and Stroke Study Group (APASS) (1997). Anticardiolipin antibodies and the risk of recurrent thrombo-occlusive events and death. *Neurology*, **48**, 91–4.

Apartis, E., Leger, J-M., Musset, L. *et al.* (1996). Peripheral neuropathy associated with essential mixed cryoglobulinaemia: a role for hepatitis C virus infection? *J. Neurol. Neurosurg. Psychiatry*, **60**, 661–6.

Asherson, R. A. and Piette, J.-C. (1996). The catastrophic antiphospholipid syndrome 1996: acute multi-organ failure associated with antiphospholipid antibodies: a review of 31 patients. *Lupus*, **5**, 414–17.

Averbuch-Heller, L., Steiner, I., and Abramsky, O. (1992). Neurologic manifestations of progressive systemic sclerosis. *Arch. Neurol.*, **49**, 1292–5.

Beck, D. O. and Corbett, J. J. (1983). Seizures due to central nervous system rheumatoid meningovasculitis. *Neurology*, **33**, 1058–61.

Belman, A. L., Leicher, C. R., Moshe, S. L. *et al.* (1985). Neurologic manifestations of Schoenlein–Henoch purpura: report of three cases and review of the literature. *Pediatrics*, **75**, 687–92.

Biller, J., Asconape, J., Challa, V. R. *et al.* (1981). A case for cerebral thromboangiitis obliterans. *Stroke*, **12**, 686–9.

Bischof, F., Kuntz, R., Melms, A. *et al.* (1999). Cerebral vein thrombosis in a case with thromboangiitis obliterans. *Cerebrovasc. Dis.*, **9**, 295–7.

Boortz-Marx, R. L., Clark, B., Taylor, S. *et al.* (1995). Sneddon's syndrome with granulomatous leptomeningeal infiltration. *Stroke*, **26**, 492–5.

Bragoni, M., Di Piero, V., Priori, R. *et al.* (1994). Sjögren's syndrome presenting as ischaemic stroke. *Stroke*, **25**, 2276–9.

Bruyn, G. W. and Padberg, G. (1984). Chorea and systemic lupus erythematosus. A critical review. *Eur. Neurol.*, **23**, 435–48.

Burton, J. L. (1988). Livedo reticularis, porcelain-white scars, and cerebral thromboses. *Lancet*, **1**, 1263–5.

Call, G. K., Fleming, M. C., Sealfon, S. *et al.* (1988). Reversible cerebral segmental vasoconstriction. *Stroke*, **19**, 1159–70.

Carhuapoma, J. R., Mitsias, P., and Levine, S. R. (1997). Cerebral venous thrombosis and anticardiolipin antibodies. *Stroke*, **28**, 2363–9.

Chapin, J. E., Davis, L. E., Kornfeld, M. *et al.* (1995). Neurologic manifestations of intravascular lymphomatosis. *Acta Neurol. Scand.*, **91**, 494–9.

de la Monte, S. M., Hutchins, G. M., and Gupta, P. K. (1983). Polymorphous meningitis with atypical mononuclear cells in Sjogren's syndrome. *Ann. Neurol.*, **14**, 455–61.

Devinsky, O., Petito, C. K., and Alonso, D. R. (1988). Clinical and neuropathological findings in systemic lupus erythematosus: the role of vasculitis, heart emboli, and thrombotic thrombocytopenic purpura. *Ann. Neurol.*, **23**, 380–4.

Drake, M. E.. (1982). Winiwarter–Buerger disease ('thromboangiitis obliterans') with cerebral involvement. *JAMA*, **248**, 1870–2.

Drenkard, C., Sanchez-Guerrero, J., and Alarcon-Segovia, D. (1989). Fall in antiphospholipid antibody at time of thromboocclusive episodes in systemic lupus erythematosus. *J. Rheumatol.*, **16**, 614–17.

Drug and Therapeutics Bulletin (1996). Systemic lupus erythematosus. *Drug Ther. Bull.*, **34**, 20–3.

Dyck, P. J., Benstead, T. J., Conn, D. L. *et al.* (1987). Nonsystemic vasculitic neuropathy. *Brain*, **110**, 843–54.

Dyck, P. J. B., Hunder, G. G., and Dyck, P. J. (1997). A case-control and nerve biopsy study of CREST multiple mononeuropathy. *Neurology*, **49**, 1641–5.

Farah, S., Al-Shubaili, A., Montaser, A. *et al.* (1998). Behcet's syndrome: a report of 41 patients with emphasis on neurological manifestations. *J. Neurol. Neurosurg. Psychiatry*, **64**, 382–4.

Feldmann, E. and Levine, S. R. (1995). Cerebrovascular disease with antiphospholipid antibodies: immune mechanisms, significance, and therapeutic options. *Ann. Neurol.*, **37** (S1), S114–30.

Ferro, J. M. (1998). Vasculitis of the central nervous system. *J. Neurol.*, **245**, 766–76.

Finazzi, G., Brancaccio, V., Moia, M. *et al.* (1996). Natural history and risk factors for thrombosis in 360 patients with antiphospholipid antibodies: a four-year prospective study from the Italian Registry. *Am. J. Med.*, **100**, 530–6.

Fortin, P. R. (1996). Vasculitides associated with malignancy. *Curr. Opin. Rheumatol.*, **8**, 30–3.

Geschwind, D. H., Fitzpatrick, M., Mischel, P. S. *et al.* (1995). Sneddon's syndrome is a thrombotic vasculopathy: neuropathologic and neuroradiologic evidence. *Neurology*, **45**, 557–60.

Glass, J., Hochberg, F. H., and Miller, D. C. (1993). Intravascular lymphomatosis. A systemic disease with neurologic manifestations. *Cancer*, **71**, 3156–64.

Gordon, M. F., Coyle, P. K., and Golub, B. (1988). Eales' disease presenting as stroke in the young adult. *Ann. Neurol.*, **24**, 264–6.

Gorevic, P. D., Kassab, H. J., Levo, Y. *et al.* (1980). Mixed cryoglobulinaemia: clinical aspects and long-term follow-up of 40 patients. *Am. J. Med.*, **69**, 287–308.

Grant, I. A., Hunder, G. G., Homburger, H. A. *et al.* (1997). Peripheral neuropathy associated with sicca complex. *Neurology*, **48**, 855–62.

Greaves, M. (1999). Antiphospholipid antibodies and thrombosis. *Lancet*, **353**, 1348–53.

Haas, L. F. (1982). Stroke as an early manifestation of systemic lupus erythematosus. *J. Neurol. Neurosurg. Psychiatry*, **45**, 554–6.

Hagen, N. A., Stevens, J. C., and Michet, C. J. (1990). Trigeminal sensory neuropathy associated with connective tissue diseases. *Neurology*, **40**, 891–6.

Hama, N. and Boumpas, D. T. (1995). Cerebral lupus erythematosus. Diagnosis and rational drug treatment. *CNS Drugs*, **3**, 416–26.

Hankey, G. J. (1991). Isolated angiitis/angiopathy of the central nervous system. *Cerebrovasc. Dis.*, **1**, 2–15.

Harisdangkul, V., Doorenbos, D., and Subramony, S. H. (1995). Lupus transverse myelopathy: better outcome with early recognition and aggressive high-dose intravenous corticosteroid pulse treatment. *J. Neurol.*, **242**, 326–31.

Hattori, N., Ichimura, M., Nagamatsu, M. *et al.* (1999). Clinicopathological features of Churg–Strauss syndrome-associated neuropathy. *Brain*, **122**, 427–39.

Heron, E., Fornes, P., Rance, A. *et al.* (1998). Brain involvement in scerloderma. Two autopsy cases. *Stroke*, **29**, 719–21.

Herson, R. N. and Squier, M. (1978). Retinal perivasculitis with neurological involvement. A case report with pathological findings. *J. Neurol. Sci*, **36**, 111–17.

Hietaharju, A., Jaaskelainen, S., Hietarinta, M. *et al.* (1995). Central nervous system involvement and psychiatric manifestations in systemic sclerosis (scleroderma): clinical and neurophysiological evaluation. *Acta Neurol. Scand.*, **87**, 382–7.

Howell, S. J. and Molyneux, A. J. (1988). Vertebrobasilar insufficiency in rheumatoid atlanto-axial subluxation: a case report with angiographic demonstration of left vertebral artery occlusion. *J. Neurol.*, **235**, 189–90.

Hunn, M., Robinson, S., Wakefield, L. *et al.* (1998). Granulomatous angiitis of the CNS causing spontaneous intracerebral haemorrhage: the importance of leptomeningeal biopsy. *J. Neurol. Neurosurg. Psychiatry*, **65**, 956–7.

Jennekens, F. G. I. and Kater, L. (1999). *Neurology of the inflammatory connective tissue diseases*. Saunders, London.

Jennette, J. C. and Falk, R. J. (1997). Small-vessel vasculitis. *N. Engl. J. Med.*, **337**, 1512–23.

Kalashnikova, L. A., Nasonov, E. L., Stoyanovich *et al.* (1994). Sneddon's syndrome and the primary antiphospholipid syndrome. *Cerebrovasc. Dis.*, **4**, 76–82.

Karussis, D., Leker, R. R., Ashkenazi, A. *et al.* (1998). A subgroup of multiple sclerosis patients with anticardiolipin antibodies and unusual clinical manifestations: Do they represent a new nosological entity? *Ann. Neurol*, **44**, 629–34.

Khamashta, M. A., Cervera, R., Asherson, R. A. *et al.* (1990). Association of antibodies against phospholipids with heart valve disease in systemic lupus erythematosus. *Lancet*, **335**, 1541–4.

Kitagawa, Y., Gotoh, F., Koto, A. *et al.* (1990). Stroke in systemic lupus erythematosus. *Stroke*, **21**, 1533–9.

Kothare, S. V., Chu, C. C., VanLandingham, K. *et al.* (1998). Migratory leptomeningeal inflammation with relapsing polychondritis. *Neurology*, **51**, 614–17.

Larner, A. J., Ball, J. A., and Howard, R. S. (1999*a*). Sarcoid tumour: continuing diagnostic problems in the MRI era. *J. Neurol. Neurosurg. Psychiatry*, **66**, 510–12.

Larner, A. J., Kidd, D., Elkington, P., Rudge, P. *et al.* (1999*b*). Spatz–Lindenberg disease: a rare cause of vascular dementia. *Stroke*, **30**, 687–9.

Lee, J. E. and Haynes, J. M. (1967). Carotid arteritis and cerebral infarction due to scleroderma. *Neurology*, **17**, 18–22.

Levine, S. R., Salowich-Palm, L., Sawaya, K. L. *et al.* (1997). IgG anticardiolipin antibody titre > 40 GPL and the risk of subsequent thrombo-occlusive events and death. A prospective cohort study. *Stroke*, **28**, 1660–5.

Li, J-Y., Lai, P-H., Lam, H-C. *et al.* (1999). Hypertrophic cranial pachymeningitis and lymphocytic hypophysitis in Sjogren's syndrome. *Neurology*, **52**, 420–3.

Libman, R. B., Sharfstein, S., Harrington, W. *et al.* (1997). Recurrent intracerebral haemorrhage from sarcoid angiitis. *J. Stroke Cerebrovasc. Dis.*, **6**, 373–5.

Lie, J. T. (1986). Thromboangiitis obliterans (Buerger's disease) in women. *Medicine*, **65**, 65–72.

Liebow, A. A. (1973). The J. Burns Amberson lecture—pulmonary angiitis and granulomatosis. *Am. Rev. Resp. Dis.*, **108**, 1–18.

Lim, L., Ron, M. A., Ormerod, I. E. C. *et al.* (1988). Psychiatric and neurological manifestations in systemic lupus erythematosus. *QJM*, **66**, 27–38.

McLean, B. N., Miller, D., and Thompson, E. J. (1995). Oligoclonal banding of IgG in CSF, blood–brain barrier function, and MRI findings in patients with sarcoidosis, systemic lupus erythematosus, and Behcet's disease involving the nervous system. *J. Neurol. Neurosurg. Psychiatry*, **58**, 548–4.

Meschia, J. F., Malkoff, M. D., and Biller, J. (1998). Reversible segmental cerebral arterial vasospasm and cerebral infarction: possible association with excessive use of sumatriptan and Midrin. *Arch. Neurol.*, **55**, 712–14.

Miller, D. H., Ormerod, I. E. C., Gibson, A. *et al.* (1987). MR brain scanning in patients with vasculitis: differentiation from multiple sclerosis. *Neuroradiology*, **29**, 226–31.

Miller, D. H., Buchanan, N., Barker, G. et al. (1992). Gadolinium-enhanced magnetic resonance imaging of the central nervous system in systemic lupus erythematosus. J. Neurol., 239, 460–4.

Mills, J. A. (1994). Systemic lupus erythematosus. N. Engl. J. Med., 330, 1871–9.

Mills, R. M. (1971). Severe hypersensitivity reactions associated with Allopurinol. JAMA, 216, 799–802.

Mitsias, P. and Levine, S. R. (1994). Large cerebral vessel occlusive disease in systemic lupus erythematosus. Neurology, 44, 385–93.

Montalban, J., Rio, J., Khamastha, M. et al. (1994). Value of immunologic testing in stroke patients. A prospective multicentre study. Stroke, 25, 2412–15.

Monti, G., Galli, M., Invernizzi, F. et al. (1995). Cryoglobulinaemias: a multi-centre study of the early clinical and laboratory manifestations of primary and secondary disease. GISC. Italian Group for the Study of Cryoglobulinaemias. QJM, 88, 115–26.

Moore, P. M. and Fauci, A. S. (1981). Neurologic manifestations of systemic vasculitis. A retrospective and prospective study of the clinicopathologic features and responses to therapy in 25 patients. Am. J. Med., 71, 517–24.

Moore, P. M. and Richardson, B. (1998). Neurology of the vasculitides and connective tissue diseases. J. Neurol. Neurosurg. Psychiatry, 65, 10–22.

Muir, K. W., Squire, I. B., Alwan, W., and Lees, K. R. (1994). Anticardiolipin antibodies in an unselected stroke population. Lancet, 344, 452–6.

Nakano, K. K. (1975). Neurologic complictions of rheumatoid arthritis. Orthop. Clin. North Am., 6, 861–80.

Newman, L. S., Rose, C. S., and Maier, L. A. (1997). Sarcoidosis. N. Engl. J. Med., 336, 1224–34.

Nishino, H., Rubino, F. A., DeRemee, R. A., Swanson, J. W., and Parisi, J. E. (1993). Neurological involvement in Wegener's granulomatosis: an analysis of 324 consecutive patients at the Mayo Clinic. Ann. Neurol., 33, 4–9.

Patton, W. F. and Lynch, J. P. (1982). Lymphomatoid granulomatosis. Clinicopathologic study of four cases and literature review. Medicine, 61, 1–12.

Poux, J. M., Peyronnet, P., Le Meur, Y., Favereau, J. P., Charms, J. P., and Leroux-Robert, C. (1992). Hypokalaemic quadriplegia and respiratory arrest revealing primary Sjogren's syndrome. Clin. Nephrol., 37, 189–91.

Riche, G., Nighoghossian, N., Kopp, N., Froment, J. C., and Trouillas, P. (1996). Pseudobulbar palsy due to isolated angiitis of the central nervous system. Cerebrovasc. Dis., 6, 372–3.

Roldan, C. A., Shively, B. K., and Crawford, M. H. (1996). An echocardiographic study of valvular heart disease associated with systematic lupus erythematosus. N. Engl. J. Med., 335, 1424–30.

Sakane, T., Takeno, M., Suzuki, N. et al. (1999). Behcet's Disease. N. Engl. J. Med., 341, 1284–91.

Savage, C. O. S., Harper, L., and Adu, D. (1997). Primary systemic vasculitis. Lancet, 349, 553–8.

Schmidt, B. J., Meagher-Villemure, K., and Del Carpio, J. (1984). Lymphomatoid granulomatosis with isolated involvement of the brain. Ann. Neurol., 15, 478–81.

Scolding, N. (1999). Immunological and inflammatory disorders of the central nervous system. Butterworth Heinemann, Oxford.

Sehgal, M., Swanson, J. W., DeRemee, R. A. et al. (1995). Neurologic manifestations of Churg–Strauss syndrome. Mayo Clin. Proc., 70, 337–41.

Serdaroglu, P. (1998). Behcet's disease and the nervous system. J. Neurol., 245, 197–205.

Sharma, O. P. (1997). Cardiac and neurologic dysfunction in sarcoidosis. Clin. Chest Med., 18, 813–25.

Sigal, L. H. (1987). The neurologic presentation of vasculitic and rheumatologic syndromes. A review. Medicine, 66, 157–80.

Stefurak, T. L., Midroni, G., and Bilbao, J. M. (1999). Vasculitic polyradiculopathy in systemic lupus erythematosus. J. Neurol. Neurosurg. Psychiatry, 66, 658–61.

Steinmetz, J. C., DeConti, R., and Ginsburg, R. (1989). Hypersensitivity vasculitis associated with 2-deoxycoformycin and allopurinol therapy. Am. J. Med., 86, 498–9.

Stewart, S. S., Ashizawa, T., Dudley, A. W. et al. (1988). Cerebral vasculitis in relapsing polychondritis. Neurology, 38, 150–2.

Stockhammer, G., Felber, S. R., Zelger, B. et al. (1993). Sneddon's syndrome: diagnosis by skin biopsy and MRI in 17 patients. Stroke, 24, 685–90.

Subbiah, P., Wijdicks, E., Muenter, M. et al. (1996). Skin lesion with a fatal neurologic outcome (Degos' disease). Neurology, 46, 636–40.

Tanne, D., D'Olhaberriague, L., Schultz, L. R. et al. (1999). Anticardiolipin antibodies and their associations with cerebrovascular risk factors. Neurology, 52, 1368–73.

Verro, P., Levine, S. R., and Tietjen, G. E. (1998). Cerebrovascular ischaemic events with high positive anticardiolipin antibodies. Stroke, 29, 2245–53.

Vidailhet, M., Piette, J.-C., Wechsler, B. et al. (1990). Cerebral venous thrombosis in systemic lupus erythematosus. Stroke, 21, 1226–31.

Voll, C., Ang, L. C., Sibley, J. *et al.* (1993). Polymyositis with plasma cell infiltrate in essential mixed cryoglobulinaemia. *J. Neurol. Neurosurg. Psychiatry*, **56**, 317–18.

Vollertsen, R. S., McDonald, T. J., Younge, B. R. *et al.* (1986). Cogan's syndrome: 18 cases and a review of the literature. *Mayo Clin. Proc.*, **61**, 344–61.

Vollmer, T. L., Guarnaccia, J., Harrington, W. *et al.* (1993). Idiopathic granulomatous angiitis of the central nervous system. Diagnostic challenges. *Arch. Neurol.*, **50**, 925–30.

Watson, P., Fekete, J., and Deck, J. (1977). Central nervous system vasculitis in rheumatoid arthritis. *Can. J. Neurol. Sci.*, **4**, 269–72.

Williams, R. L., Meltzer, C. C., Smirniotopoulos, J. G. *et al.* (1998). Cerebral MR imaging in intravascular lymphomatosis. *Am. J. Neuroradiol.*, **19**, 427–31.

Woolfenden, A. R., Tong, D. C., Marks, M. P. *et al.* (1998). Angiographically defined primary angiitis of the CNS: is it really benign? *Neurology*, **51**, 183–8.

Wooten, M. D. and Jasin, H. E. (1996). Vasculitis and lymphoproliferative diseases. *Semin. Arth. Rheum.*, **26**, 564–74.

Zajicek, J. P., Scolding, N. J., Foster, O. *et al.* (1999). Central nervous system sarcoidosis—diagnosis and management. *QJM*, **92**, 103–17.

CHAPTER 29

Multiple sclerosis and other demyelinating diseases

Alastair Compston

29.1 Classification of demyelinating disease

The oligodendrocyte–myelin unit subserves saltatory conduction of the nerve impulse in the healthy central nervous system. Several disease processes compromise the structure and function of myelinated axons. Many result from inflammation and autoimmunity (see Chapter 7 for discussion of glial neurobiology and neuroimmunology). Demyelination is the usual explanantion for episodic neurological symptoms and signs suggesting damage to white matter tracts of the optic nerves, brainstem, or spinal cord when this occurs in young people. Neurologists will also consider this explanation in older patients presenting with progressive symptoms implicating these same pathways, even when there is no suggestive past history. Both in its typical and atypical forms, multiple sclerosis is the most common demyelinating disease. This can usually be distinguished from rarer forms of demyelinating disease, but since our understanding of the cause, pathogenesis, and features of each remains incomplete, the present classification of demyelinating disease integrates aetiological, clinical, pathological, and laboratory components (Table 29.1). However, we anticipate that a major part of future studies in multiple sclerosis will be to resolve further the question of disease heterogeneity, leading to a new taxonomy based on mechanisms rather than clinical empiricism. But at present, the variable ages of onset, clinical course, and protean manifestations, and the non-specific laboratory investigations continue to make demyelinating disease one of the more challenging diagnostic areas in neurology.

Pathologically, a simple approach is to distinguish those disorders of myelinated pathways associated with perivascular inflammatory cell infiltration from the non-inflammatory forms of demyelination. Inflammation initially characterizes the focal and multifocal lesions associated with demyelination in optic neuritis, transverse myelitis, multiple sclerosis, acute haemorrhagic (Hurst's disease) and acute disseminated encephalomyelitis, subacute necrotizing myelitis, transverse myelitis, and acute bilateral optic neuritis. Some other conditions, which have at times been separated, are now more often

Table 29.1. The classification of demyelinating disease

Isolated demyelinating syndromes
  Acute haemorrhagic leucoencephalomyelitis—Hurst's disease
  Acute disseminated encephalomyelitis (Section 29.3.1)
  Optic neuritis (Sections 8.5.1, 29.3.2)
  Cord lesions
    acute necrotizing myelitis (Sections 20.4.6, 29.33)
    transverse myelitis (Sections 20.4.5, 29.3.3)
    chronic progressive myelopathy
    radiation myelopathy (Sections 5.9.1, 20.6.8)
    HTLV-I associated myelopathy (Sections 20.6.4, 34.11.1)
  Monophasic isolated demyelination—site unspecified

Multiple sclerosis (Section 29.4)
  Relapsing remitting
  Secondary progressive
  Primary progressive
  Benign
  Malignant or Marburg variant
  Childhood
  Silent multiple sclerosis
  Devic's disease (Section 29.3.4)
  Balo's concentric sclerosis
  Combined central and peripheral demyelination

Central pontine myelinolysis (Section 29.5)
  Pontine
  Extrapontine

Leucodystrophies
  Schilder's disease (Section 29.6.1)
    myelinoclastic diffuse sclerosis
    transitional diffuse sclerosis
  Globoid cell (Krabbe's disease) leucodystrophy (Sections 12.8.3, 29.6.2)
  Adrenoleucodystrophy (Sections 12.8.4, 29.6.3)
    X-linked childhood adrenoleucodystrophy
    X-linked adult onset adrenomyeloneuronopathy
    autosomal recessive neonatal adrenoleucodystrophy
    autosomal recessive Zellweger's syndrome
  Metachromatic leucodystrophy (Sections 12.8.2, 29.6.4)
    late infantile
    juvenile
    adult
    multiple sulphatase deficiency
  Pelizaeus Merzbacher disease (Section 29.6.5)
    classical
    connatal form
    late onset
  Adult-onset leucodystrophies (Section 29.6.6)

considered within the general context of multiple sclerosis; these include Balo's concentric demyelination, neuromyelitis optica (Devic's disease), Marburg-type hyperacute demyelination, and mixed peripheral and central forms of demyelination.

In some young patients with progressive neurological disease, there is widespread demyelination arising from genetically determined disorders of myelin formation. These leucodystrophies are characterized by extensive non-inflammatory confluent areas of demyelination. Because myelin is structurally abnormal in these conditions, they are often referred to as dys-

myelinating disorders. The most common leucodystrophies encountered in paediatric and adult neurological clinical practice are metachromatic leucodystrophy, adrenoleucodystrophy, and Krabbe's disease. As new leucodystrophies are described, and diagnostic acumen and precision improve, many individuals previously classifed as having diffuse sclerosis can now be diagnosed more accurately. However, a proportion of childhood and adult-onset white-matter diseases cannot be classified biochemically, and remain in the heterogeneous group of diffuse sclerosis, also known as Schilder's disease.

Magnetic resonance studies have established the important point (not easily gathered from neuropathological studies) that single patches of demyelination rarely occur. It is now clear that many patients apparently having clinically isolated episodes of demyelination do, in fact, have widespread lesions. Later, they show a high conversion rate to clinically definite multiple sclerosis. The areas of white-matter damage in patients with leucodystrophy can be imaged and appear as diffuse confluent areas of abnormality in the cerebral white matter. These are usually quite distinct from the widespread discrete periventricular lesions seen in multiple sclerosis and other inflammatory demyelinating disorders. Although conventional magnetic resonance protocols do not reliably depict separate components of the pathological process in demyelinating disease, the distribution and appearance of lesions in multiple sclerosis, acute disseminated encephalomyelitis, primary progressive inflammatory demyelination, the leucodystrophies, and central pontine myelinolysis can usually be distinguished.

It is now well recognized that patients developing clinical evidence for extensive brainstem damage in the context of electrolyte imbalance, or following its correction, may develop large areas of pontine myelinolysis. These are not common conditions, but under the heading of central pontine myelinolysis should also be considered the even rarer cases of extrapontine myelinolysis and Marchiafava–Bignami disease, consisting of callosal demyelination associated with injudicious consumption of Italian red wine—a condition faithfully listed in textbooks but never knowingly encountered by their authors (this one included).

29.2 The pathogenesis of demyelination

The hallmark of demyelinating disease in the context of multiple sclerosis is formation of the sclerotic plaque. This represents the end stage of a process which, microscopically, involves inflammation, demyelination, remyelination, oligodendrocyte depletion, astrocytosis, and axon degeneration (Fig. 29.1a–e). Although there is no shortage of opinion, the order and relationship of these separate components remains to be fully resolved (Lassmann 1998). The classical analysis would be that inflammation and demyelination with intact but demyelinated axons predate astroglial scarring with formation of the sclerotic plaque. This interpretation is currently undergoing some

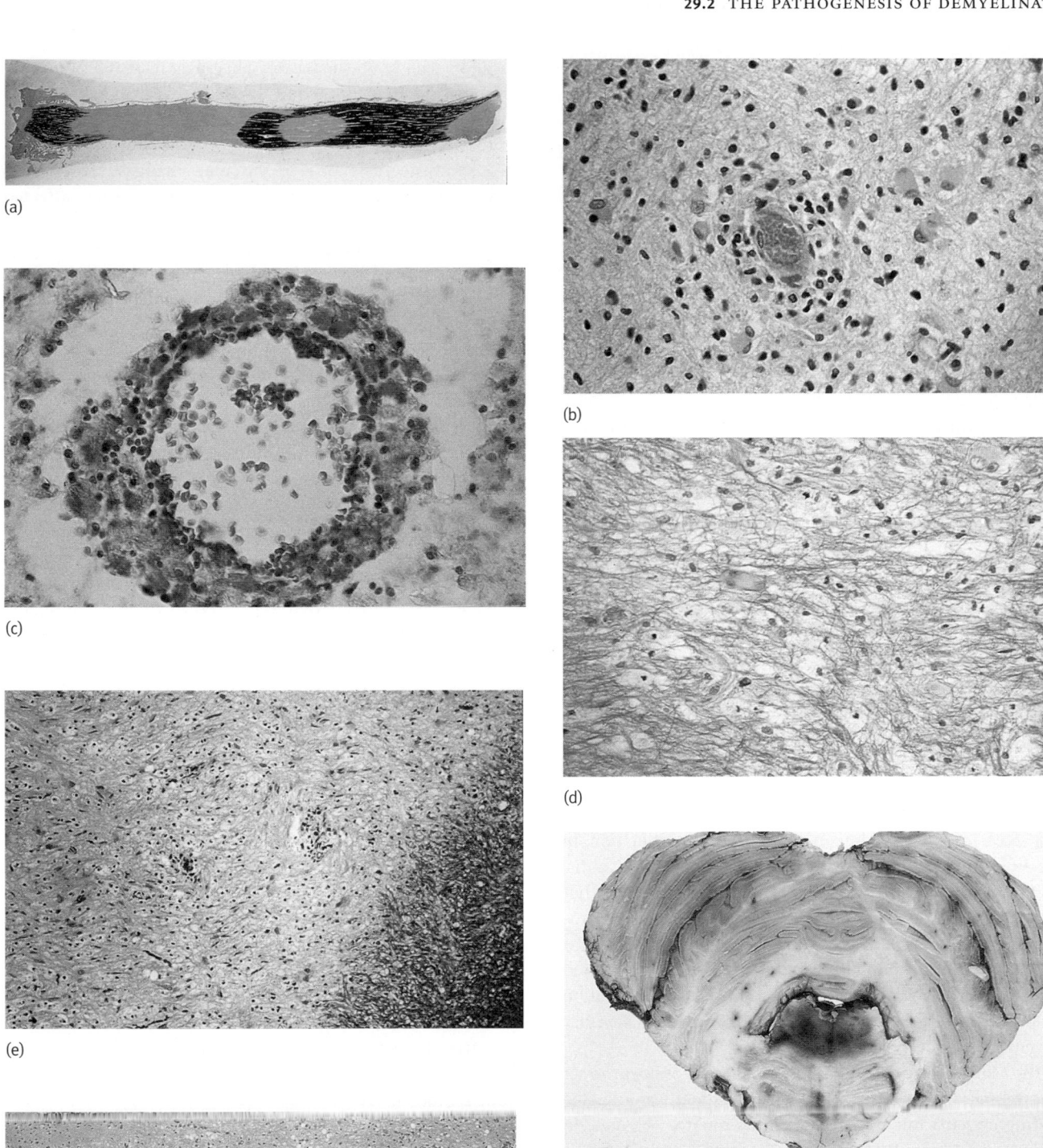

Fig. 29.1. The evolution of demyelination. (a) Macroscopic areas of demyelination in the optic nerve. (b) Perivascular infiltration by activated lymphocytes. (c) Microglial removal of myelin debris. d) Astrocytosis. (e) Persistent demyelination showing a sharp boundary between normal appearing and demyelinated white matter. (f) Macroscopic appearance of the brain in a patient dying from acute disseminated encephalomyelitis in an illness lasting 10 days, showing diffuse midbrain damage with a combination of demyelination and tentorial herniation due to cerebral oedema. (g) Acute perivascular infiltration in the same patient. (a)–(e) Reproduced with permission from Hall *et al.* (1997); (f) and (g) kindly provided by Dr Janice Anderson and reproduced with permission from Matthews (1998*b*). See also Plate 24.

modification in order to accomodate evidence for acute changes in oligodendrocytes and axons, and the role of remyelination.

Demyelination occurs throughout central nervous system white matter but certain zones are preferentially affected, and grey matter is not spared. Plaques are clustered around the lateral ventricles, in the corpus callosum and floor of the aqueduct and fourth ventricle, and in the cortical or subcortical white matter (Kidd et al. 1999). The optic nerve and the brainstem are commonly involved. In the cervical portion of the spinal cord, lesions tend to be subpial and located where the denticulate ligament intermittently makes contact with the dorsal cord. These are to some extent areas containing extensive networks of veins and where the blood–brain barrier is relatively or absolutely defective. These associations emphasize the primary role of vascular permeability in the pathogenesis of demyelinating disease. They have also been used, spuriously in our opinion, to fuel the debate on whether trauma can precipitate demyelination (see below).

Biopsy of acute lesions mistaken radiologically for tumours, and autopsy series in which plaques of varying ages happen to be present, provide an opportunity to characterize the detailed cellular pathology of inflammatory demyelination. The acutely inflamed brain is visibly swollen and oedematous. In cases of acute disseminated encephalomyelitis, the histological appearances may be restricted to intense perivenular mononuclear cell infiltration without demyelination. In the most acute form, acute haemorrhagic encephalomyelitis, there is fibrinoid necrosis and inflammatory infiltration of vessels, oedema, perivenular petechial haemorrhage, and macrophage infiltration around vessels, both in grey and white matter, but no demyelination. In less severe forms of acute disseminated encephalomyelitis, oedema and petechial perivascular haemorrhage may occur, but more conspicuous are the inflammatory infiltrates of neutrophils, lymphocytes, plasma cells, microglia, and foamy myelin-debris containing macrophages, indicating demyelination and phagocytosis. The pathological findings correlate with duration of the illness and show an evolution from diffuse vascular involvement to widespread demyelination.

In the Marburg type of demyelination, large confluent zones of demyelination are seen with extensive axonal loss and surrounding oedema but rather slight inflammatory change. In Schilder's diffuse cerebral sclerosis, changes not dissimilar to the Marburg variant occur, sometimes with central cavitation in the cerebrum, brainstem, and cerebellum. In Balo's concentric sclerosis, symmetrical demyelination surrounded by normal or repaired myelin occurs in rings, not unlike the onion bulb appearance of demyelinating peripheral neuropathies. In Devic's disease, although the brunt of the pathological process and its clinical expression are borne by the optic nerves and spinal cord, more extensive demyelination is usually present, with thinning of the affected parts, gliosis, meningeal thickening, necrosis, and even some remyelination. Demyelination is not confined to the clinically affected sites and the histological features of perivascular infiltration, demyelination, and gliosis

can all be seen in affected areas. This suggests that lesions have formed at different times and implies similarities between the course of Devic's disease and more typical forms of multiple sclerosis. In other cases, white and grey matter in the spinal cord show necrosis due to vascular changes rather than demyelination, although this may coexist in other affected parts.

The principles of neuroimmunology are described in Chapter 7 but summarized here. When the brain is inflamed, lymphocytes cross the blood–brain barrier and accumulate on the abluminal surface of venules. Lymphocytes which are not activated against brain antigen either return to the circulation or (in common with immune cells that have outlived their purpose elsewhere) die by apoptosis. Activated T cells that encounter antigen persist within the nervous system. The cells most probably contributing to local immune responses, in all types of inflammatory demyelination, are initially confined to the perivascular or Virchow–Robin spaces and, with the exception of a few antibody-producing plasma cells, do not contact the myelin sheaths. But as T and B lymphocytes, plasma cells, and macrophages accumulate around the vessels, pro-inflammatory cytokines (especially interferon-γ; [IFN-γ]) drive an amplification of the immune response in which microglia are activated, leading to the release of yet more T-cell derived IFN-γ, and the recruitment of additional naive microglia (Hall et al. 1999). Contact is established between activated microglia and the oligodendrocyte–myelin unit if the latter is opsonized with ligands for receptors activated on the surface of microglia (Fc and complement). Activated microglia deliver a lethal signal to the target oligodendrocyte producing a high concentration of cell-surface-bound tumour necrosis factor-α (TNF-α) (Zajicek et al. 1992). Together, these inflammatory processes lead to disruption of the myelin membrane, with increased spacing, vesicular disruption, splitting, vacuolation, and fragmentation of the lamellae.

It is increasingly clear that the oligodendrocyte undergoes many acute changes in demyelinating disease. In a detailed analysis of acute lesions, Luchinetti et al. (1999) showed consistent variations, either an increase or decrease, in the number of oligodendrocytes within lesions from the same individual, indicating a much more dynamic sequence of injury and recovery of the myelinating cell than has previously been assumed. The implication is of turnover with macrophage-associated loss of healthy oligodendrocytes and recruitment of new progenitors which then undergo differentiation (see Chapter 7).

Recently, much emphasis has been placed on the role of axon degeneration as a pathological feature. Immunohistochemical staining for the amyloid precursor protein shows that axonal injury, which culminates in loss of axons during the chronic progressive phase of the disease, is initiated as part of the acute demyelinating lesion (Ferguson et al. 1997). It is not certain when axons actually die. They may be damaged directly as part of the initial inflammatory disease process, through non-specific exposure to inflammatory mediators after demyelination, as a direct result of an anti-neuronal immune response to previously sequestered antigens on the demyelinated axon, or because nerve fibres have a limited capacity for surviving prolonged demyelination. A partial answer is provided by Trapp *et al.* (1998), who studied acute and chronic lesions and showed extensive damage to axons with transection; this appeared early and the circumstantial evidence suggests that vulnerability of recently demyelinated axons to the inflammatory environment of acute lesions or secondary degenerative effects of demyelination through loss of trophic support are more likely than primary immunological injury to the intact axon by infiltrating mononuclear cells and their mediators. The significant increase in frequency of antiganglioside antibodies in sera from patients with progressive multiple sclerosis compared with those in the relapsing–remitting phase and controls suggest that anti-neuronal antibodies may contribute to axonopathy, but the finding does not directly distinguish between the cause and consequence of axon damage in multiple sclerosis (Tayyebeh Saditpour *et al.* 1998). Although axonopathy is seen in acute plaques, its clinical expression is mostly considered to be the basis for disability during the chronic progressive phase of multiple sclerosis (Davie *et al.* 1995) (see Fig. 29.2 for a summary of the pathogenesis and clinical course). The best imaging surrogate for axonal loss appears to be T1 hypointensity and magnetization transfer ratio (van Waesberghe *et al.* 1999).

It is now accepted that remyelination does occur, especially in the acute lesion, and that this accounts for the appearance of shadow plaques which are seen both in acute and chronic plaques (Prineas *et al.* 1993) and may coexist with areas of active demyelination. Significantly, remyelination is associated with the inflammatory process in which myelin debris is removed by macrophages (or microglia), leaving naked axons ready for remyelination and promoting astrocyte reactivity which, in turn, re-establishes the growth factor environment needed to recruit remyelinating cells. The morphological criteria used as evidence for remyelination are myelin lamellae

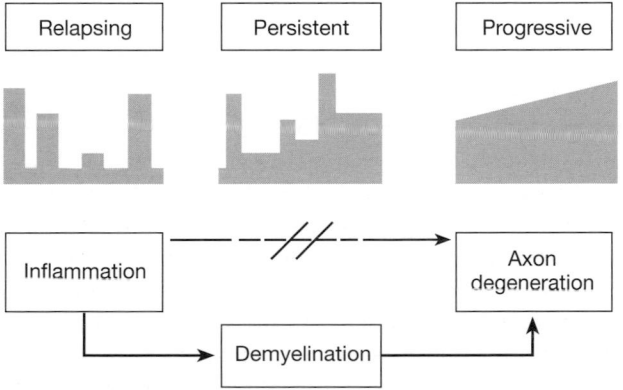

Fig. 29.2. Stages in the clinical course of multiple sclerosis: remitting episodes associated with perivascular cuffs of infiltrating lymphocytes; persistent symptoms due to demyelination with minimal inflammation and limited repair; disease progression—inflammation and active myelin breakdown are no longer apparent, the demyelination is associated with astrocytosis, and there is axonal pathology leading to axon degeneration.

which are inappropriately thin for the corresponding axon, with a short internode, the myelin embedded in a satellite cell with a membrane which is continuous from the surface of the cell around the axon, back to the surface again, and compacted (Gledhill *et al.* 1973).

Myelin injury blocks saltatory conduction through myelinated pathways in the central nervous system. Although function may be preserved by redundancy in individual systems or tracts, strategically placed pathways lose their safety factor for conduction, resulting in neurological symptoms and signs. In large measure, the manifestations of multiple sclerosis are not specific to the disease process or its physiological consequences, but merely reflect the abnormalities to be expected from any process that disrupts physiological performance at that site. However, saltatory conduction may be compromised by partial demyelination in a variety of ways that are characteristic and account for some clinical manifestations of multiple sclerosis (McDonald 1998a).

Partially demyelinated axons cannot transmit fast trains of impulse and this may explain those symptoms that reflect physiological fatigue. Depolarization may traverse the lesion but at reduced velocity. This abnormality does not of itself explain particular symptoms in multiple sclerosis, but it does account for the characteristic delay in arrival of potentials evoked by sensory stimuli and recorded over appropriate cortical receptor zones. Partially demyelinated axons may discharge spontaneously, thus accounting for many unpleasant distortions of sensation reported by a high proportion of patients. Increased mechanical sensitivity manifests as movement-induced symptoms including flashes of light provoked by eye movement, and the electric sensation that spreads down the spine, limbs, or anterior chest wall after neck flexion—Lhermitte's symptom and sign—which has a less common motor counterpart in the spontaneous limb movements sometimes provoked by neck flexion in patients with multiple sclerosis. Spontaneous discharge in brainstem facial nerve neurons probably accounts for myokymia.

Increased temperature sensitivity, with a reduction in the safety factor for conduction in partially demyelinated axons, explains the temporary increase in severity of pre-existing symptoms, experienced by many patients after exercise or immersion in hot water. Conversely, cold may improve performance—some patients even adopting complicated water-cooled systems and others reporting that, for example, vision improves after eating ice-cream. Ephaptic transmission occurs between neighbouring and partially demyelinated axons, giving rise to paroxysmal symptoms of demyelination usually manifesting as trigeminal neuralgia, ataxia, and dysarthria, or tonic brainstem seizures. These are often triggered by touch or movement.

Despite these pathophysiological explanations for the symptoms of multiple sclerosis, there are many enigmatic aspects of the disease. Discrepancies exist between the sites of the nervous system that are necessarily involved from an analysis of the symptoms and signs, and the lesions that can be demonstrated

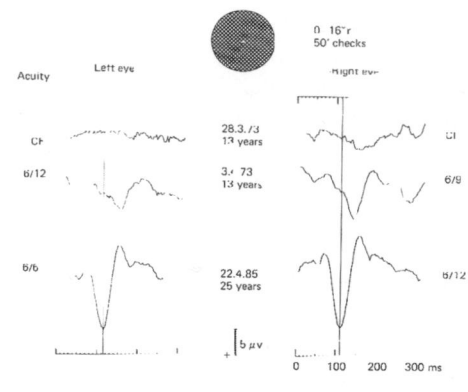

(a)

(b)

Fig. 29.3. (a) Visual evoked potentials recorded at 3 days, 9 days, and 12 years after an episode of acute bilateral optic neuritis in a 13-year-old girl. (b) The effect of a nitric oxide donor (spermine NONOate) on conduction along axons passing through a demyelinating lesion in the rat spinal cord, based on averaging 128 successive records over a recording period of *c.* 4 hours. (Reproduced with permission from (a) McDonald 1998*a*; (b) Redford *et al.* 1997.)

by imaging or at autopsy. It is necessary to conclude that symptoms can arise from areas that are not demyelinated and that, at certain sites, demyelination may be clinically silent.

There are several mechanisms of symptom recovery early in the course of multiple sclerosis. These include the resolution of conduction block in nerve fibres which were never demyelinated, re-establishment of conduction in persistently demyelinated axons, functional reorganization of surviving pathways, and remyelination (Fig. 29.3a). Youl *et al.* (1991) first showed that onset and recovery of conduction block and visual impairment in optic neuritis match the phase of acute inflammation. Symptoms which recover depend on the direct action of cytokines delivered by activated lymphocytes accumulating within the central nervous system as a consequence of alterations in the blood–brain barrier. TNF-α has been suggested as

a candidate for causing this effect, but experimental studies now preferentially implicate nitric oxide as the mediator mainly responsible for reversible conduction block in myelinated axons (Redford *et al.* 1997) (Fig 29.3b). Function may be restored after demyelination by rearrangement of sodium channels providing a variety of alternative patterns of ordered or partially disordered conduction. There is probably also a contribution from the remyelination seen in acute lesions; experimentally, remyelinated axons restore conduction of the nerve impulse and motor function (Jeffrey and Blakemore 1997).

29.3 Isolated demyelinating syndromes

Syndromes resulting from focal demyelination are often the first manifestation of an illness which subsequently recurs, leading to the diagnosis of multiple sclerosis. Alternatively, the symptoms and signs may be truly monophasic and never relapse. Attempts have been made to assess the risk of multiple sclerosis following each type of isolated episode, considered according to the part affected, and basing outcome both on clinical features and laboratory investigations. The natural history varies with the different syndromes, ages of presentation, and duration of follow-up. Clinically definite multiple sclerosis can reliably be diagnosed only when more than one demyelinating episode, separated by at least 1 month and with recovery between attacks, has occurred. The situation is more complex with respect to imaging studies. Although these have established that a high proportion of patients with clinically isolated demyelinating syndromes already have anatomically disseminated lesions at presentation, recent analyses do suggest that patients with no lesion other than that attributable to the presenting episode have a lower conversion rate for multiple sclerosis.

29.3.1 Acute disseminated encephalomyelitis

Acute encephalopathy in children or young adults occurs as part of several specific metabolic and infectious illnesses, which can be identified by laboratory investigations. These are distinct from the acute or subacute encephalomyelitis, simultaneously affecting multiple parts of the nervous system, which follows an exanthematous or infectious illness. The typical features of acute disseminated encephalomyelitis are headache, drowsiness and fits, and one or more focal lesions producing hemisphere syndromes and disturbances of vision. In other cases, the clinical manifestations reflect damage either to the brainstem, optic nerves, or spinal cord, but each may be involved together and the peripheral nervous system is sometimes affected. These cases were more common before the advent of public health programmes which have reduced the frequency of predisposing exanthematous disorders, and fortunately they are seldom seen following vaccination itself, so that nowadays there is no distinct prodromal illness in most incident cases. Therefore, both in children and adults, a presumptive diagnosis of acute disseminated encephalomyelitis often has to be made in the absence of an identifiable cause.

However, a proportion of patients, especially adults, recovering from the initial episode, later relapse and follow a clinical course that is typical of multiple sclerosis. Thus it is important to recognize that multiple sclerosis may present in an encephalopathic form. In others situations, the illness remains monophasic but separate sites are involved sequentially and in a step-wise fashion, giving the appearance of a temporally disseminated illness. For this reason, it is unwise to consider symptoms evolving over several weeks as necessarily signifying a relapsing illness sufficient for the diagnosis of multiple sclerosis.

The hyperacute form of acute disseminated encephalomyelitis (Hurst 1941) is usually preceded by a non-specific respiratory infection 3–10 days before the onset of neurological symptoms. Young adult males are most commonly affected, complaining initially of headache or dizziness and progressing over hours through stages of disorientation, confusion, and drowsiness to coma. The rate of progress is such that events usually overtake the detection of focal signs, and this form of the disease is frequently fatal, although affected individuals may remain in a persistent vegetative state for several weeks and some survive with severe disability following treatments which reduce intracranial pressure (Fig. 29.1f, g). The combination of pyrexia and a marked cerebrospinal fluid pleocytosis with a predominantly neutrophil response mimics pyogenic infection of the central nervous system, but the course is not influenced by antimicrobial treatment. In some cases the clinical and pathological features of acute haemorrhagic leucoencephalitis are entirely focal, mimicking rapidly growing tumour or herpes simplex encephalitis.

In the classical account of acute disseminated encephalomyelitis, Miller *et al.* (1956) reviewed several hundred cases gathered from the literature, but made no attempt to separate diffuse from anatomically restricted forms of parainfectious neurological disease, including polyradiculitis. Some of their cases may have arisen from direct viral infection of the nervous system and related disorders that were not then recognized. The Newcastle experience indicated that about 1 : 1000 children with exanthematous disorders develop acute disseminated encephalomyelitis, the risk being slightly higher with pertussis and scarlet fever than with measles and rubella. Nowadays, the majority of cases are encephalitic or multifocal. Affected individuals develop headache, drowsiness, meningeal irritation, focal or generalized fits, and combinations of lesions indicating damage to the cerebrum, optic nerves, brainstem, or spinal cord about 10–20 days after the prodromal illness. The symptoms and signs evolve over the course of a few days. Cerebrospinal fluid shows a mixed polymophonuclear and lymphocytic or predominantly mononuclear pleocytosis with raised protein and slight reduction in glucose; oligoclonal bands may be present. While there is an appreciable mortality, the majority of patients survive and there is some evidence to suggest that the outcome is influenced by the early use of high-dose steroids, but this has not been formally evaluated. Despite surviving the acute illness, patients may be left with persistent neurological deficits.

Patients with severe post-infectious focal inflammation of the central nervous system are often systemically ill with pyrexia and marked meningism. These features occur both in the encephalitic and myelitic forms of the disease. There are no obvious differences in acute disseminated encephalomyelitis complicating the various childhood exanthematous illnesses. The post-rubella syndrome is less frequent and more severe but does also have a late progressive variant, analogous to subacute sclerosing panencephalitis. Almost 50 per cent of post-varicella cases present with a pure cerebellar syndrome, sometimes associated with involuntary movements. This carries a relatively good prognosis with a low rate of persistent disability.

The symptomatology, course, and prognosis of acute disseminated encephalomyelitis in young adults is clinically similar. A wider range of causative organisms has been implicated, and the individual case more usually develops in the context of a non-specific respiratory infection. New specific causes of acute disseminated encephalomyelitis have been described and these include echovirus, coxsackievirus, and herpes virus, mycoplasma, borreliosis, and cases associated with neoplasia and acquired immunodeficiency syndrome.

The magnetic resonance appearances of cerebral lesions in acute disseminated encephalomyelitis have been well described. In a series of 12 cases, including six adults and six children developing optic nerve, cerebral, brainstem, and cord disease, alone or in combination, following infection by mumps, varicella, mycoplasma, adenovirus, and non-specific respiratory infections, Kesselring *et al.* (1990) showed multifocal asymmetric white matter abnormalities in (generalized and clinically isolated) post-infectious demyelinating syndromes, which were indistinguishable from the lesions of multiple sclerosis, although many cases showed extensive and rather symmetric changes in the cerebral or cerebellar white matter and in the basal ganglia. More discriminating was the transient presence of oligoclonal bands in acute disseminated encephalomyelitis.

Serial or gadolinium–diethylenetriaminepentaacetic acid (DTPA)-enhanced scans are more useful and suggest that, whereas lesions persisting long after the clinical manifestations have resolved do not discriminate, the development of new lesions or the demonstration of areas with enhancement indicates disease activity, typical of multiple sclerosis and excluding acute monophasic demyelination. The interval that should be allowed before conclusions can safely be reached is uncertain. It has been claimed that, in children, new episodes of central nervous system damage may occur 18 months after the initial episode in acute disseminated encephalomyelitis, but this interpretation assumed that multiple sclerosis does not occur in childhood, and cases of this type would not now be included in a series of patients with acute disseminated encephalomyelitis.

One reason for believing that acute disseminated encephalomyelitis arises from immune sensitization to brain antigens is that it has followed the use of vaccines containing central nervous system tissue. In its day, this form of the disease behaved much as other cases of acute disseminated encephalitis and the pathological features were also indistinguishable. Post-vaccinial encephalomyelitis has become a rare disorder following alterations in the preparation of this and other vaccines. The definitive series were collected several decades ago following episodes in which the need arose to vaccinate large numbers of individuals against smallpox as part of public-health measures. The 62 cases studied clinico-pathologically and reported by de Vries (1960) had been collected over 34 years and were necessarily severe. In all, the neurological illness developed within 21 days of vaccination and, in fatal cases, death occurred at, or soon after, 13 days. In these hyperacute cases, the pathological findings mimic transitional forms of acute haemorrhagic or disseminated encephalomyelitis. The clinical illness starts with a vaccinial skin reaction and systemic symptoms which merge with the neurological manifestations, typically affecting the cerebrum but sometimes presenting as a myelitic disorder. Despite having a high mortality, post-vaccinial encephalomyelitis may recover spontaneously and completely.

29.3.2 Optic neuritis

Optic neuritis usually presents with pain on eye movement, followed or accompanied by blurred vision (Section 8.5.1). Many patients first notice the visual loss on waking, or on accidentally closing one eye. Some report selective impairment of central vision with preservation of the peripheral field and awareness of movement. The symptoms usually evolve over hours or days, and the degree of visual loss that accompanies the clinical nadir varies from slight blurring to blindness. A number of other visual symptoms are described. Some patients notice selective loss of colour intensity or perception, usually in the red range. Others describe disturbances of visual perception with persistence of images on re-fixation or flashes of light (phosphenes) provoked by eye movement. The usual pattern is that the pain disappears after a few days. Vision improves, rapidly at first and then more slowly, full recovery often taking several months. About 90 per cent of patients consider themselves to have made a full visual recovery, but more formal assessments indicate that up to 50 per cent have persistent defects of vision, and colour perception frequently remains impaired. In the most recent follow-up series, no difference was observed in the outcome for vision at 5 years between treatment groups, and 6 per cent of all patients had poor visual recovery (Optic Neuritis Study Group 1997a).

The symptoms of bilateral simultaneous optic neuritis do not differ from unilateral disease, but there is usually a marked disparity in the extent to which each eye is affected and the implications for recurrence of the neurological symptoms are not the same. The rate of onset varies, and in some cases the loss of vision is progressive. Particular care needs to be taken in this situation so as to exclude compression of the anterior visual pathway, but it is also the case that structural lesions of the optic nerve can manifest as relapsing visual failure, closely mimicking optic neuritis. The diagnosis is one of exclusion, and ischaemic optic neuropathy needs to be considered in older patients. Relapsing visual loss may be due to optic nerve sarcoidosis or Eales' disease, in young women and men, respectively. A careful family history should be taken, since the onset of visual failure in Leber's hereditary optic neuropathy (Section 8.5.2) can be confused with bilateral sequential optic neuritis in men. Mistakes may also occur in the context of toxic amblyopia. Recently, the syndrome of a multiple sclerosis-like illness associated with mutations of mitochondrial DNA and manifesting as central nervous system demyelination with disproportionate involvement of the optic nerves has been recognized (Harding et al. 1992; Riordan-Eva et al. 1995: this is now designated as Harding's disease). The variable density of the bony orbital walls means that sinus infection may spread to affect the optic nerve directly or as a consequence of local tissue oedema. The lesion responsible for optic neuritis can be imaged, the nerve appearing swollen and showing a focal increase in magnetic resonance signal. Inflammation within the intracanalicular portion of the nerve and long lesions are associated with delayed or incomplete recovery of vision (Miller et al. 1988) (Fig. 29.4a, b).

Optic neuritis is one of the most common presenting features of multiple sclerosis. Clinical involvement of the optic nerve occurs in more than 50 per cent of patients at some time, and the visual pathway is invariably affected at autopsy. These statistics lead to a high level of anxiety in the informed patient that an episode of optic neuritis is likely to be the first manifestation of multiple sclerosis. It has proved difficult to establish statistics for the rate of conversion which can be applied to the individual, since the reported series have varied in their selection criteria and ascertainment biases have inevitably been introduced. Methodological factors and differences in classification almost certainly account for geographical differences in the risk of multiple sclerosis developing after an attack of optic neuritis.

The main factor determining the reported frequency of multiple sclerosis after optic neuritis is the duration of follow-up. The risk is highest in the first 5 years, but the proportion of cases with widespread demyelination increases steadily with time. Several retrospective and prospective series have been treated to life-table analysis in an attempt to compensate for the varying length of follow-up. This approach gives estimates of 38–78 per cent conversion, depending on the location and actuarial time point. Age at presentation influences the risk of multiple sclerosis developing after an attack of optic neuritis. In children, the disorder is commonly bilateral and further symptoms of demyelination affecting the visual pathways or other parts of the nervous system rarely occur. Bilateral simultaneous optic neuritis in adults, although much less common than in children, also carries a low risk of multiple sclerosis, and in both situations the likely explanation is that these are anatomically restricted forms of acute disseminated encephalomyelitis.

Optic neuritis recurred in 28 per cent of patients recruited for a recent treatment trial (Optic Neuritis Study Group 1997*b*). Recurrence carried an increased risk for multiple sclerosis and was also more common in those who did not convert if treated at presentation with oral prednisolone. However, most clinicians would not assign the same diagnostic significance to a second attack of optic neuritis as an episode of demyelination affecting another part of the central nervous system. Other factors reported at one time or another to increase the risk of progression include young age of onset, female sex, and recurrence of optic neuritis.

Parkin *et al.* (1984) reviewed a series of cases with bilateral optic neuritis 25 years after presentation. Of the six adults with acute simultaneous optic neuritis, one had died with Devic's disease and another was thought to have had early probable multiple sclerosis but died from other causes at the age of 76 years. No other patient developed multiple sclerosis. Conversely, 20 patients had bilateral sequential optic neuritis within 3 months and, of these, seven were known to have developed multiple sclerosis. A recent follow-up of 23 cases with acute or subacute simultaneous bilateral optic neuropathy revealed that, after a mean of 71 months, four were shown by genetic analysis to have a mutation in mitochondrial DNA typical of Leber's disease, and another five had developed multiple sclerosis; the rest remained undiagnosed (Morrissey *et al.* 1995).

There is a confused literature on whether the treatment of acute optic neuritis, either with intravenous methylprednisolone or oral prednisolone, influences the risk of conversion to multiple sclerosis. In the most up-to-date analysis, 30 per cent of the 308 patients enrolled between 1988 and 1991 converted to clinically definite multiple sclerosis, but there was no difference in rate between the groups depending on treatment. Lesions on magnetic resonance imaging at presentation were a poor risk factor; all 185 patients with no prior symptoms of imaging abnormalities, lack of pain, relative preservation of acuity, and a swollen disc carried a relatively good prognosis for conversion to multiple sclerosis (Optic Neuritis Study Group 1997*b*).

Given these uncertainties, attempts have been made to determine whether laboratory indices which are characteristic of multiple sclerosis serve to identify patients with optic neuritis who are destined to develop widespread demyelination; the usefulness of each factor depends on the specificity and sensitivity of that marker for the diagnosis of multiple sclerosis (Soderstrom *et al.* 1998). The visual evoked response characteristically shows delay with preserved amplitude once the phase of inflammation has settled, and this feature has the same implications for conversion to multiple sclerosis as a second episode of optic neuritis when it is detected in a clinically unaffected eye. Retinal vascular sheathing, or the presence of inflammatory cells in the ocular vitreous, occur in 30 per cent of patients with optic neuritis and are associated with a slightly increased risk of multiple sclerosis at follow-up (Lightman *et al.* 1987). Periventricular white matter abnormalities demonstrated by magnetic resonance imaging are found in 61 per cent of patients with optic neuritis, more of whom develop multiple sclerosis than those with normal brain scans (O'Riordan *et al.*

1998). HLA DR2 is present in a higher proportion of patients with optic neuritis who subsequently develop multiple sclerosis than isolated cases, but the relative risk is low and HLA typing is not a useful prognostic marker. A higher proportion of patients with optic neuritis shown to have oligoclonal bands on cerebrospinal fluid electrophoresis at presentation subsequently develop multiple sclerosis than those with normal spinal fluid. Fifty-two per cent of patients with oligoclonal bands had developed multiple sclerosis at early follow-up, compared with 24 per cent having normal spinal fluid; however, almost half the patients with abnormal magnetic resonance scans, most of whom had oligoclonal bands from presentation and were HLA DR2 positive, had not developed clinical evidence for widespread demyelination many years after the initial episode of optic neuritis (Sandberg-Wollheim *et al.* 1990). In patients who underwent spinal fluid analysis at presentation as part of the Optic Neuritis Treatment Trial (Optic Neuritis Study Group 1997*b*), the presence of oligoclonal bands slightly increased the relative risk for developing multiple sclerosis within 2 years, but imaging abnormalities were more discriminating predictors of widespread demyelination in this group.

29.3.3 Isolated spinal cord syndromes

The spinal cord is especially vulnerable to inflammatory demyelination. As with more generalized forms of inflammatory central nervous system disease, the relationship of isolated spinal demyelination to multiple sclerosis is complex. Acute or subacute cord involvement in patients with multiple sclerosis is usually partial, sometimes conforming to the Brown–Séquard syndrome, but lesions may occur which exactly mimic transverse myelitis. This term is usually reserved for patients in whom the spinal lesion does not recur but the distinction is only possible in retrospect. Even though a monophasic episode of cord inflammation may result in persistent disability, many patients, including those with severe myelitis, recover fully and without sequelae. The diagnosis of transverse myelitis is often made by exclusion and the precipitating cause not identified, as with acute disseminated encephalomyelitis in adults. However, clinical and laboratory criteria can usefully distinguish the various conditions.

Acute necrotizing myelitis

The original description of necrotizing myelitis was made in men, rather older than most cases of transverse myelitis, with slowly progressive lumbar cord disease occurring in association with chronic respiratory disease (Foix and Alajounanine 1926). The term 'acute necrotizing myelitis' can reasonably be applied to patients developing severe inflammation of the thoracic or spinal cord, in whom flaccid areflexic paraplegia with anaesthesia and loss of sphincter control progresses rapidly over hours (Section 20.4.6). Inflammation is sufficient to cause severe pain with meningism and systemic symptoms, including pyrexia. The clinical presentation suggests compression, and contrast radiology or imaging often reveals a swollen cord with spinal block. Since the cerebrospinal fluid shows a marked polymorphonuclear pleocytosis, raised protein and lowered glucose concentrations, these patients are frequently thought to have pyogenic or tuberculous infection of the central nervous system and are treated with appropriate antimicrobial therapy. In some cases surgical exploration is undertaken to exclude intraspinal abscess. Because of the possibility of infection, there is often a reluctance to use corticosteroids, but the course of acute necrotizing myelitis can be significantly influenced by high-dose intravenous methylprednisolone. Acute necrotizing myelitis has an appreciable mortality, but in survivors the systemic features resolve within weeks, leaving significant handicap and disability. Several organisms have been implicated in the aetiology of acute necrotizing myelitis and it is also described after rabies vaccination, as a complication of acute lymphocytic leukaemias, lymphoma, hypernephroma and other forms of carcinoma, and in acquired immunodeficiency syndrome.

Transverse myelitis

The majority of patients with transverse myelitis are not systemically ill and the neurological disorder usually evolves over a few days (Section 20.4.5). Pain at the site of the lesion may be the initial symptom, followed by weakness in the legs and positive sensory symptoms with sphincter involvement. With time, the weakness increases and may spread to involve one or both arms, usually in an asymmetric pattern and showing the flaccid areflexia characteristic of spinal shock. These features are infrequently seen when cord inflammation occurs in the context of multiple sclerosis, and have been used to distinguish monophasic from relapsing disease. Sensory loss replaces the paraesthesia and there is often a band of unpleasant hyperaesthesia at the upper sensory level; as in other cases of incomplete focal spinal disease, this may not accurately reflect the site of spinal affection, due to lamination of fibres in the spinothalamic pathways. Sphincter control is lost; unlike patients with multiple sclerosis, the patient is usually unable to empty rather than fill the bladder. The need to exclude a structural cause for subacute cord injury occurring as a manifestation of transverse myelitis means that many patients undergo radiological investigation. This may demonstrate mild cord swelling, which is rarely sufficient to cause spinal block, but imaging usually shows a longitudinal rather than transverse area of increased signal (Fig. 29.4c). Lumbar puncture should be carried out in cases investigated by magnetic resonance imaging. The spinal fluid shows an increased mononuclear cell count, numerically intermediate between the marked pleocytosis of acute necrotizing myelitis and the abnormalities seen in patients with multiple sclerosis. The total protein is raised and oligoclonal bands may be present on electrophoresis, but the glucose is usually normal. Multiple sclerosis and transverse myelitis cannot reliably be distinguished on the basis of changes in cerebrospinal fluid, but oligoclonal bands are more frequent and a cell count in excess of 100 lymphocytes/cm less likely in the former.

Some clinical guidelines can be used to distinguish transverse myelitis from multiple sclerosis. The most reliable indicator is the presence of spinal shock in acute monophasic lesions. Scott

et al. (1998) emphasize that symmetry of the motor and sensory manifestations of acute inflammatory spinal cord disease usefully identifies patients with transverse myelitis, whereas spinal involvement in multiple sclerosis is almost invariably asymmetric. Defined in this way, they report a low conversion rate from transverse myelitis to multiple sclerosis. Unlike acute disseminated encephalomyelitis, transverse myelitis is more common in adults than children, and in women than men. Since it is a diagnosis of exclusion, in which laboratory abnormalities and bacteriological findings may be unhelpful, the probability arises that a heterogeneous collection of cases has been included in most large series. Transverse myelitis differs from acute disseminated encephalomyelitis in the peak age of onset and its more frequent occurrence as a manifestation of systemic vasculitis, immunodeficiency, and greater range of specific infectious causes. It has a low rate of conversion to multiple sclerosis, and in this respect resembles bilateral rather than unilateral optic neuritis in adults.

The series reported by Berman *et al.* (1981) is probably representative with respect to prognosis: 22 of 59 (68 per cent) of patients in whom follow-up information was available made an adequate recovery over the ensuing 3 months; 3 died and 14 were left with significant persistent disability. A high proportion of a population-based sample of cases originally designated as transverse myelitis had later to be excluded from their study. In the remainder, incidence peaked in the second and third decades, with a further bimodal increase in patients aged over 70 years. Only one patient subsequently developed multiple sclerosis. Preceding infection was reported in one third of patients, the majority of whom had upper respiratory infection, other causes being herpes zoster or simplex virus infection, hepatitis, and smallpox vaccination. Identifiable infection was more common in young patients, suggesting that cases with spinal stroke, including examples due to collagen vascular disease, are sometimes erroneously diagnosed as having transverse myelitis, and this is especially problematic in patients with sensory signs indicating an anterior cord lesion. Tyler *et al.* (1986) have collated the viral causes of transverse myelitis, listing picornaviruses, togaviruses, retroviruses, orthomyxoviruses, paramyxoviruses, bunyaviruses, arenaviruses, rhabdoviruses, hepatitis viruses, herpes viruses, and poxviruses. More recent single case reports emphasize the occurrence of transverse myelitis after infection with hepatitis A, cytomegalovirus, herpes simplex type 2, toxoplasmosis, and schistosomiasis.

29.3.4 Devic's disease

Neuromyelitis optica (or Devic's disease) is characterized by confluent demyelination in both optic nerves and the chiasm, together with equally severe spinal cord damage. These sites can be affected simultaneously or sequentially and in either order, events usually being separated by several weeks or months (Fig. 29.4d, e). The syndrome may complicate collagen vascular disease, Behçet's disease (Section 28.11), and acute disseminated encephalomyelitis (Section 29.3.1). Opinions differ about whether this form of demyelination is usually an atypical mani-

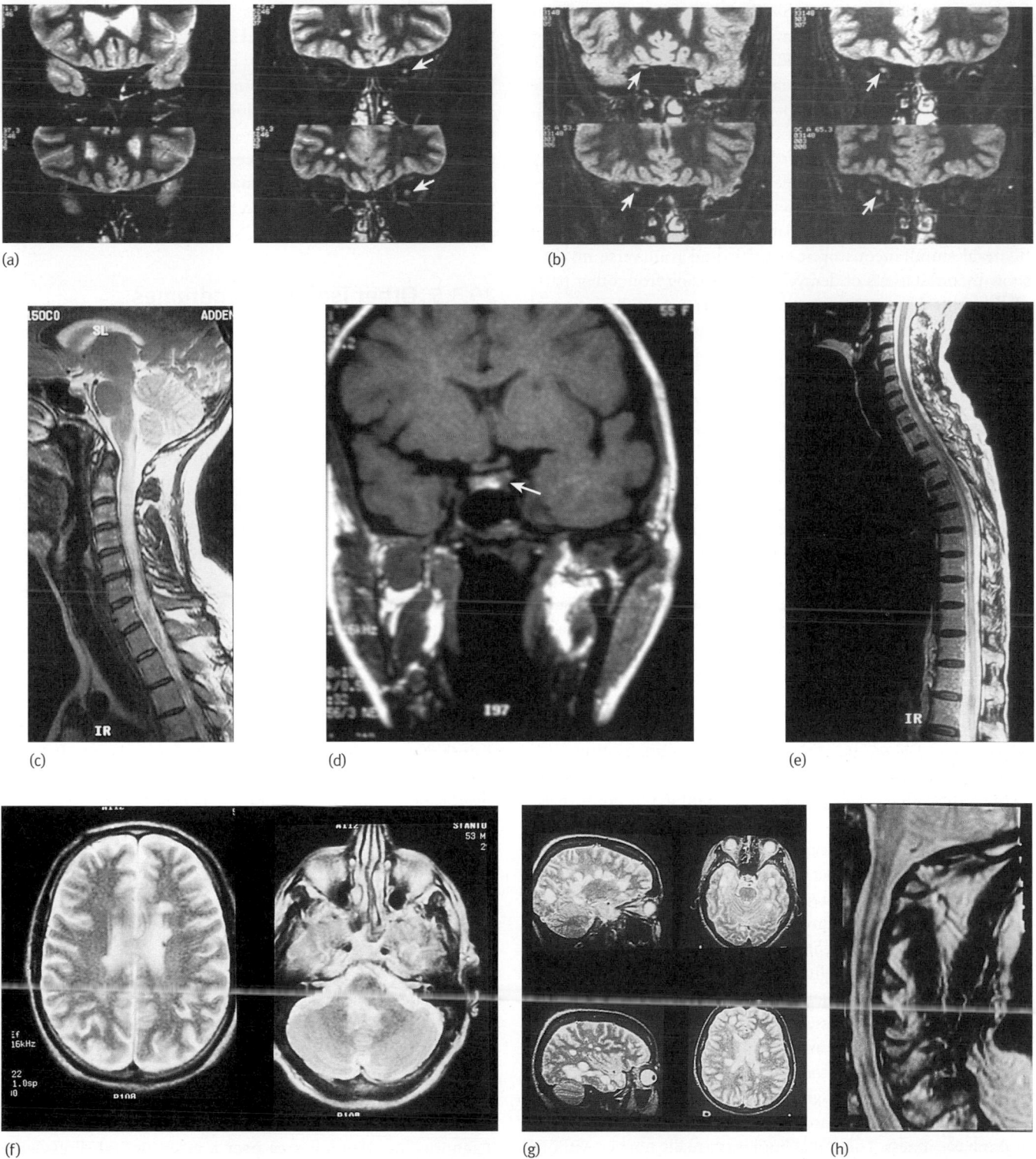

Fig. 29.4. Magnetic Resonance Imaging (MRI) in Multiple Sclerosis and isolated demyelinating syndromes. MRI STIR sequences showing lesions in the optic nerve (arrows): (a) Good prognosis—the lesion does not extend posteriorly into the canal; white matter lesions are also seen in the frontal lobes. (b) Poor prognosis—the optic nerve abnormality is seen in all four slices including the canal (arrows). (c) Swelling and high T2-weighted signal in the cervical cord and medulla from a patient with acute transverse myelitis. (d) MRI showing increased signal of the chiasm (arrow) in a patient with bilateral optic neuritis due to Devic's disease in association with lymphoma. (e) Spinal cord imaging showing extensive abnormality over several segments in the same patient as (d) the cerebral MRI scan shows a single periventricular abnormality. (f) A pontine lesion demonstrated on MRI responsible for the one-and-a-half syndrome. (g) Multiple cerebral white matter MRI abnormalities in multiple sclerosis. (h) Multiple spinal cord lesions in multiple sclerosis. ((a), (b) Kindly provided by Professor David Miller and Dr Raj Kapoor. All images reproduced with permission from Matthews (1998*a, b*) and (c), (d), (e), and (f) kindly provided by Dr Nagui Antoun.)

festation of multiple sclerosis. Similar difficulties arise in distinguishing vasculitic from demyelinating cases, as with other examples of post-infectious inflammatory disease affecting the central nervous system. The fact that demyelinating disease more often follows the Devic pattern in Japanese, where multiple sclerosis is rare, and some series of patients with neuromyelitis optica studied in northern Europe have shown a very low conversion rate to multiple sclerosis, suggesting that they are separate disorders. Conversely, the experience of many clinicians is that the majority of patients with the combination of bilateral simultaneous optic neuritis and transverse myelitis show manifestations of demyelination arising from other parts of the central nervous system and experience multiple events with time. That has usually been our experience of these rare but tragic cases in whom a series of aggressive episodes of demyelination produce severe morbidity and threaten life.

The issue is not settled. Mandler *et al.* (1993) make a strong case for a different aetiology; they describe eight patients, three of whom had optic neuritis and myelitis simultaneously, and the remainder at intervals of 4–24 months. Cerebral magnetic resonance imaging in three cases examined showed no brain lesions. Imaging of the spinal cord showed swelling and cavitation. Oligoclonal bands in the CSF were found transiently in one case and were absent in six. These cases had a high mortality. Silber *et al.* (1990) reported 11 cases of Devic's disease occurring in the Cape coloured population of South Africa. In six, the neurological disorder started soon after the development of pulmonary tuberculosis, and optic nerve damage preceded the spinal lesion, both of which had a poor outcome. The short-term mortality was 25 per cent. Others have reported the occurrence of acute necrotizing myelitis in association with tuberculosis. Taken with the pleocytosis and glycorrhachic changes that often occur in cerebrospinal fluid, it is not surprising that these patients are usually treated with anti-tuberculous therapy, at least until bacteriological results are available.

In contrast to these specific causes of the Devic syndrome, O'Riordan *et al.* (1996) retrospectively reviewed 12 patients from the UK, of whom more than 50 per cent were Asian or African, taking as their definition cases with a rapidly evolving complete transverse myelitis, uni- or bi-lateral optic neuropathy, and no involvement outside these sites. Antecedent causes or coexistent illnesses were present in five. The myelopathy was often relapsing and functional recovery poor despite treatment with corticosteroids; bilateral involvement with recurrence and poor prognosis also characterized the optic neuropathy. Thus, the patients in this series typically had a multiphasic illness. The spinal fluid was usually normal without oligoclonal bands and the cellular reaction involved polymorphonuclear cells more than lymphocytes. When cerebral white matter abnormalities were present (approximately 50 per cent of patients), these tended to be frontotemporal and the spinal cord was often diffusely swollen with extensive or multiple T2-weighted lesions. The most recent and largest series of 71 patients observed over 43 years at the Mayo Clinic adopts strict diagnostic criteria relating to the bilaterality of optic nerve involvement and the interval between defining events, but

usefully demonstrates a pattern of reasonable recovery when the optic nerves and spinal cord are affected in rapid sequence, and a poor prognosis with high mortality in relapsing patients with more than the two defining episodes. As now generally recognized, the spinal lesion is long, extending over several segments, in contrast to the several short lesions which characterize spinal magnetic resonance imaging in multiple sclerosis; cerebral imaging may be normal and there is typically more pronounced pleocytosis of the cerebrospinal fluid (Wingerchuk *et al.* 1999).

29.3.5 Other isolated syndromes

Each part of the central nervous system in which demyelination can occur may manifest isolated syndromes, but of these the most common is the brainstem. These are usually the harbinger of more widespread demyelination, providing sufficient evidence for the diagnosis of multiple sclerosis. The risks and predictors are summarized by O'Riordan *et al.* (1998). Of 16 patients presenting with a brainstem syndrome, 11 had progressed to clinically definite multiple sclerosis; all had abnormal magnetic resonance imaging outside the affected site at presentation, and only one patient with multiple lesions had not developed widespread demyelination at 10 years. Corresponding figures for conversion, with and without magnetic resonance imaging lesions, in patients with clinically isolated optic nerve and spinal cord lesions in this series were 25/28 and 1/14, and 10/15 and 2/8, respectively. The clinical symptoms and signs of isolated brainstem demyelination do not differ from those seen in multiple sclerosis, and typically consist of dysequilibrium, disturbed eye movements, facial numbness, and dysarthria, but there may be severe headache which rightly leads to early investigation in order to exclude a structural lesion.

29.4 Multiple sclerosis

29.4.1 Environmental factors and multiple sclerosis

Epidemiological studies of multiple sclerosis have been used to generate aetiological hypotheses, to assess local needs for the provision of services and the allocation of resources, and to define the natural history of the disease. For northern Europeans, an approximate estimate of lifetime risk for multiple sclerosis is 1 : 400. Incidence measures the number of new diagnoses in a defined area over a given period. Prevalence defines the number of individuals in whom the diagnosis has been made, or those with a particular feature, in a population at-risk on a given occasion. Because it includes all individuals who currently have the disease, irrespective of when this occurred, it is numerically larger than incidence. Mortality describes the number of individuals with multiple sclerosis, as a proportion of the at-risk population dying within a defined area and over a given period. Self-evidently, morbidity statistics are dependent on the precision of case ascertainment. This varies inversely with the size and accessibility of the population at-risk. First surveys underestimate prevalence (and incidence), and higher figures are obtained with second and subsequent assessments due to improved awareness and vigilance amongst both the population at-risk and the investigators. Mortality estimates often fail to distinguish death from, or with, multiple sclerosis. Koch-Henriksen *et al.* (1998) showed prospectively that about 50 per cent patients with multiple sclerosis die from the disease or related infections, with higher rates from cardio-vascular disease, suicide, and accidents.

Incidence, prevalence, and mortality are closely related. Unless aetiological factors have changed, and assuming adequate ascertainment, incidence should equal mortality, and prevalence will be the product of either statistic and disease duration. The factor that makes morbidity statistics for multiple sclerosis most difficult to establish is the range of ages at onset. This obstacle is partially overcome by calculating age- and sex-specific rates, which relate the number of affected individuals to a denominator confined to that proportion of the at-risk population born in the same decade. The usual way of dealing with variations in demography is to derive standardized prevalence ratios and to quote 95 per cent confidence intervals for each statistic.

Methodological factors have limited the value of many epidemiological studies. Most vulnerable have been the comparisons of prevalence between regions, and the serial studies of single places. Kurtzke (1975) collated the estimates for prevalence and suggested that the distribution of multiple sclerosis could broadly be classified into bands of low, medium, and high prevalence. High risk ($>25/10^5$) was found throughout northern Europe, the northern United States, Canada, southern Australia, and New Zealand. Medium risk ($5–25/10^5$) was found in southern Europe, the southern United States, and northern

Australia. Low risk ($<5/10^5$) areas included Asia, South America, and many uncharted regions. Systematic updating of these figures shows that the absolute estimates have almost invariably risen and Kurtzke's original definitions of high-, medium-, and low-frequency bands no longer apply; also, many apparent latitudinal gradients were once overemphasized but the disease does show variations in its distribution over quite small distances, which may be informative (Compston 1998*a*) (Fig. 29.5).

Multiple sclerosis is common in northern Europe, continental North America, and Australasia compared to other places. Within northern Europe, the disease is more frequent in southern Scandinavia, northern Germany, the UK, and parts of Italy, than in northern Scandinavia, France, Spain, and the eastern Mediterranean countries. The areas of highest prevalence in the UK are north-east Scotland, and the Orkney and Shetland islands. In Italy, marked differences in prevalence exist between regions and islands that are geographically close but differ in their genetic and cultural histories. In North America, there is a gradient in frequency, with highest rates in the mid-west and lowest in the Mississippi delta. In Australia, a latitudinal gradient does appear to exist for the white Australian population with higher rates in the south than north.

Migration has influenced the distribution of multiple sclerosis and, taken alone, this evidence defines multiple sclerosis as an acquired exogenous disorder. Dean (1967) showed in South Africa that the age-corrected frequency is relatively high in immigrants from Europe, low in Afrikaners, and intermediate in South African English, both with respect to prevalence and incidence; no cases were found in African blacks but a slightly higher rate was seen in the Cape coloured population, which has mixed African and European ancestry. In English-speaking whites, those moving from northern Europe to southern Africa as adults took with them the high frequency of the country of origin, whereas those migrating below the age of 15 years showed the lower rates characteristic of native-born inhabitants of southern Africa.

The prevalence of multiple sclerosis in the UK-born children of West Indian, African, and Asian immigrants approximates to that seen in similar age groups amongst Caucasians (Elian *et al.* 1990). Another important series of epidemiological studies showed no substantial difference in the frequency of multiple sclerosis amongst Orientals living in Japan, Hawaii, or the west coast of North America, despite more marked variations in the frequencies amongst Caucasians in some of these locations, indicating a protective effect for Orientals irrespective of environment (Detels *et al.* 1977). The recently updated study of multiple sclerosis in Israeli immigrants shows a difference in prevalence between northern Europeans (Ashkenazim) and Asians and Africans (Sephardim). The implication is that racially determined differences in risk for multiple sclerosis are modified by environment (Kahana *et al.* 1994). A study of the military showed that the mortality ratio for United States army veterans depended not on where they were born (southern, middle, or northern states) but from where they entered military service as young adults (Kurtzke 1993).

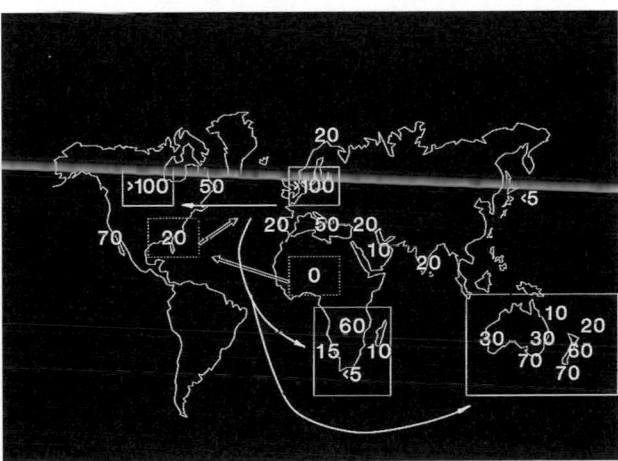

Fig. 29.5. A summary of epidemiological patterns in multiple sclerosis. Figures are estimates for prevalence. Solid lines with arrows represent migration vectors of northern Europeans. Open lines with arrows represent migration routes of Africans to the Caribbean and Mississippi delta and to the UK. In South Africa the numbers refer to English-speaking whites migrating as adults (60), English-speaking whites migrating as children (15), Afrikaners (10), and Cape coloureds (<5). (Reproduced with permission from Compston 1998*a*.)

The first (retrospective) survey of Iceland showing increased quinquennial rates for incidence between 1945 and 1954, during which age-at-onset was also younger. This led to the conclusion that there has been a post-war epidemic of multiple sclerosis in Iceland, but others prefer the interpretation that this was due to improved recognition (Benedicz *et al.* 1994). In the Orkney and Shetland Islands, the incidence and prevalence of multiple sclerosis were at one time higher than anywhere else. Serial estimates of prevalence between 1954 and 1974 showed a systematic rise to $309/10^5$ in Orkney and $184/10^5$ in Shetland (Poskanzer *et al.* 1980). These frequencies have now fallen, but remain higher than in places of comparable latitude. The original observations on multiple sclerosis in the Faeroe Islands showed fewer cases than expected from comparisons with neighbouring Orkney and Shetland. Based on a total of 41 cases with onset between 1943 and 1986, Kurtzke (1993) concluded that the critical factor determining the Faeroes experience of multiple sclerosis was occupation by British troops between 1940 and 1945, the development of multiple sclerosis showing both a temporal and spatial relationship to villages where individuals lived who contributed to the peak of incidence.

Several studies have attempted to correlate exposure to viral illness in childhood with subsequent development of multiple sclerosis (reviewed by Granieri and Casetta 1997). The picture to emerge is that the risk is increased for individuals who develop a variety of exanthematous and other common viral disorders relatively late in childhood; this applies to measles, mumps, rubella, and Epstein–Barr virus (EBV) infection. The studies suggest that a narrow and age-linked period of susceptibility to viral exposure exists in those who are constitutionally at risk of developing the disease. Attempts to provide laboratory evidence implicating a specific environmental agent have used increasingly sophisticated methods of investigation but the results have not come closer to incriminating a particular agent. The long list of suspects includes rabies, herpes simplex viridae, scrapie agent, parainfluenza 1, measles, the Carp and bone marrow agents, cytomegalovirus and coronavirus and, in recent years, human retroviruses. The latest candidate is a multiple sclerosis-associated retrovirus (MSRV) recovered from CSF (Perron *et al.* 1997) and serum from cases but not controls (Garson *et al.* 1998).

Enthusiastic reports based on serology continue, with increased concentrations of human herpes virus (HHV)-6 IgM and DNA recovery from serum samples and brain tissue (Friedman *et al.* 1999), being offered as one putative viral trigger of multiple sclerosis (Soldan *et al.* 1997). Others have not been able to confirm the serological findings or demonstrate disease-specific HHV-6 virus in mononuclear cells (Mayne *et al.* 1998). The most recent candidate is *Chlamydia pneumoniae*, which was isolated in cerebrospinal fluid from 64 per cent of patients with relapsing or progressive multiple sclerosis but only 11 per cent of controls, detected by polymerase chain reaction (97 per cent) and antibody formation (84 per cent), and represented one component of the oligoclonal bands in a proportion of patients (Sriram *et al.* 1999). But these findings are not confirmed; Boman *et al.* (2000)

found no chlamydial DNA in spinal fluid from 48 patients with multiple sclerosis and the frequency of IgG antibodies was no different from that of controls (68 per cent and 82 per cent, respectively).

29.4.2 The genetics of multiple sclerosis

Multiple sclerosis has a familial recurrence rate of approximately 15 per cent and it is usually assumed that this is due to co-inheritance of susceptibility genes (reviewed by Compston 1998*b*). The most comprehensive studies are from Canada, the UK, and Belgium (Sadovnick *et al.* 1988; Robertson *et al.* 1996; Carton *et al.* 1997). Meta-analysis of recurrence risk amongst 44 177 relatives of 2163 probands from these three population-based series shows that the age-adjusted risk is highest for siblings (3 per cent), then parents (2 per cent) and children (2 per cent), with lower rates in second- and third-degree relatives (Fig. 29.6). Overall, the reduction in risk changes from 3 per cent (relative risk 9.2) in first-degree relatives to 1 per cent in second- and third-degree relatives (relative risks 3.4 and 2.9, respectively), compared with a background age adjusted risk in northern European Caucasians of 0.3 per cent. Three recent studies approximate to a population-based series of multiple sclerosis in twins. Two show remarkable consistency in demonstrating a higher clinical concordance rate in monozygotic (approximately 25 per cent) than dizygotic pairs (about 3 per cent) (Sadovnick *et al.* 1993; Mumford *et al.* 1994); and the third is not inconsistent with this result given the wide confidence intervals of reported concordance rates between monozygotic and dizygotic twins (French Research Group on Multiple Sclerosis 1992). The relative risk for multiple sclerosis in the monozygotic twin partner of an affected proband is *c*.190.

Considering individuals with multiple sclerosis who are adopted before the age of 1 year, and affected individuals who, through adoption, have non-biological siblings or children, the frequency of multiple sclerosis in non-biological parents, siblings, and children is more or less identical to the population

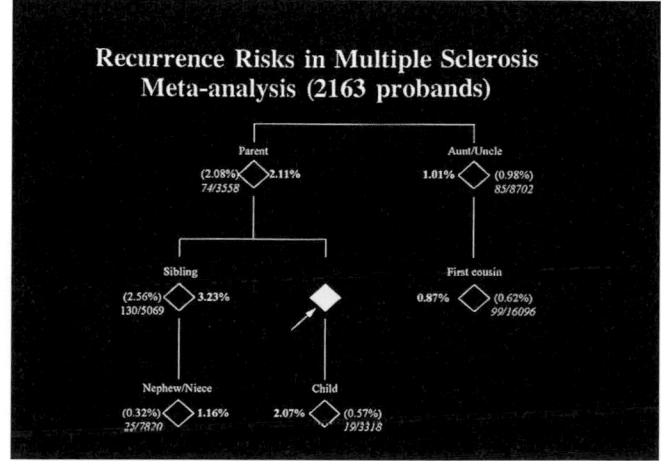

Fig. 29.6. Meta-analysis of recurrence risks for relatives of probands with multiple sclerosis. (Kindly provided by Dr Neil Robertson and reproduced with permission from Compston *et al.* 1998*b*.)

prevalence and lifetime risk for Europeans, and significantly lower than that expected from the study of recurrence risk in the biological relatives of index cases (Ebers *et al.* 1995). The age-adjusted risk for half-siblings is significantly lower than for full siblings, and there is no difference in risk for half-siblings reared together and apart (Sadovnick *et al.* 1996a). The recurrence risk is higher for the children of conjugal than single affected parents (Robertson *et al.* 1997: Ebers *et al.*2000).

Population studies demonstrate an association between the class II MHC alleles DR15 and DQ6 and their corresponding genotypes DRB1*1501, DRB5*0101 and DQA1*0102, DQB2*0602 (Olerup and Hillert 1991). A specifically different association in seen in Mediterranean populations. In Sardinians, multiple sclerosis is associated with DR4 (DRB1*0405-DQA1*0301-DQB1*0302) (Marrosu *et al.* 1992) and the same association occurs in the Canaries and in Turkey. Extensive searches, using association and linkage studies over many years, have only yielded additional putative candidate genes in the VH2–5 (14q32) immunoglobulin heavy chain and the T-cell receptor β (TCR-β) chain (7q32) variable regions. Recent contributions to this aspect of the genetics of multiple sclerosis have tended to illustrate the difficulty which exists in confirming these and other weak associations. Studies of linkage or association with the genes encoding cytokines, chemokines, adhesion molecules, and growth factors and their receptors (IFN-γ, IL-1ra, IL-1β, IL-2, IL-4, IL-4R, IL-10, TGF-β1 and -β2, ICAM-1, CCR5 and 23 separate growth factor genes and their receptors) (He *et al.* 1998; Mertens *et al.* 1998) have all been relatively unrewarding, although IFN-γ (12q24.1), IL-4R (16p12.1), and TGF-β2 (1q41) cannot be fully excluded. Stratification has occasionally yielded subgroups, such as those with more severe disease, who show associations with these candidates, for example IL-1ra and IL-1β alleles in combination (Schrijver *et al.* 1999). Except in the isolated population of Finns, where there is both an association and linkage to the gene for myelin basic protein (Tienari *et al.* 1998), studies of structural genes of myelin have also been uninformative (Rodriguez *et al.* 1997).

Four groups of investigators have undertaken a systematic search of the genome in an attempt to locate additional susceptibility genes using affected family members—usually identity by descent analysis in sibling pairs. Genotyping was completed on cohorts of between 21 and 225 families, together involving in excess of 1000 individuals, for each of between 257 and 443 microsatellite markers chosen to have an average spacing of around 10 centiMorgans and giving enough power to identify regions encoding a major susceptibility gene. These are sufficiently polymorphic to make a high proportion of the available families fully informative. Although linkage analysis has revealed several new genomic regions which may encode genes conferring susceptibility to multiple sclerosis, some will turn out to be true and others false positives. Superficially, the results show a disappointing lack of overlap. In common with most other complex traits, no major susceptibility gene has been identified. The possible reasons are that no such gene exists; it has been missed by all three groups; or genetic complexity (i.e. heterogeneity) has obscured the picture. The

importance of the major histocompatibility complex is confirmed, but of the other new putative susceptibility loci, several are clearly unique to each screen and so may be false positives (Fig. 29.7a). The regions of interest emerging from the UK genome screen (Sawcer *et al.* 1996) are 1cen, 5cen, 6p, 7p, 14q, 17q, 19q, and Xp. They are 2p, 3p, 5p, 11q, and Xp in the Canadian series (Ebers *et al.* 1996). The United States/French consortium identified 6p, 7q, 11p, 12q, and 19q (Multiple Sclerosis Genetics Group 1996). Positive lod scores were obtained for 6p21 (MHC) and 5p14–p12 in a relatively small Finnish screen (Kuokkanen *et al.* 1997); when all 21 families were typed across regions of interest, the highest lod score (2.8) was at 17q22–q24, confirming the previously reported UK screen.

These genetic analyses are predicated on the assumption that multiple sclerosis is one disease. Mutations of mitochondrial DNA are responsible for a multiple sclerosis-like illness, characterized by disproportionate involvement of the anterior visual pathway (Harding *et al.* 1992; Riordan-Eva *et al.* 1995), although mitochondrial genes do not contribute generally to susceptibility in multiple sclerosis. Conditioning the UK genome screen for DR15 (or an extended DR15-linked haplotype also encoding alleles of TNF and the DQ locus) shows that the regions of interest on 1p, 17p, 17q, and X cluster in families which are identical by state for DR15, whereas the non-sharing group associated with 1cen, 3p, 5cen, 7p, 14q, and 22q (Coraddu *et al.* 1999); in addition, new regions of interest are found at 5q and 13p (DR15 sharing) and 16p and 20p (DR15 non-sharing). The contribution to susceptibility made by the genes which have provisionally been identified only accounts for a proportion of the increased risk of multiple sclerosis implicated by family studies. Clearly there is more to be learned concerning susceptibility to multiple sclerosis and the interplay between genes and environmental factors (Fig 29.7b).

29.4.3 Clinical symptomatology

There are many authoritative clinical accounts of multiple sclerosis, drawing on geographically defined population bases, hospital clinics, or extensive personal experience of the disease (Matthews 1998a). The account that follows is organized by system and does not prioritize the relative importance or frequency of individual manifestations in multiple sclerosis.

Cognitive and affective symptoms

Periventricular plaques are almost invariably present in patients with multiple sclerosis from an early stage, but it is usually held that these are not clinically significant. Approximately 60 per cent of patients can be shown to have mental changes, and systematic testing has revealed that impairment of memory and learning ability may occur early in the course. These deficits are, as expected, more severe and prevalent in patients with chronic progressive than relapsing disease and in advanced multiple sclerosis, although significant dementia may occasionally be an early or even the presenting symptom. It has not proved easy to correlate cognitive abnormalities with focal brain lesions. For

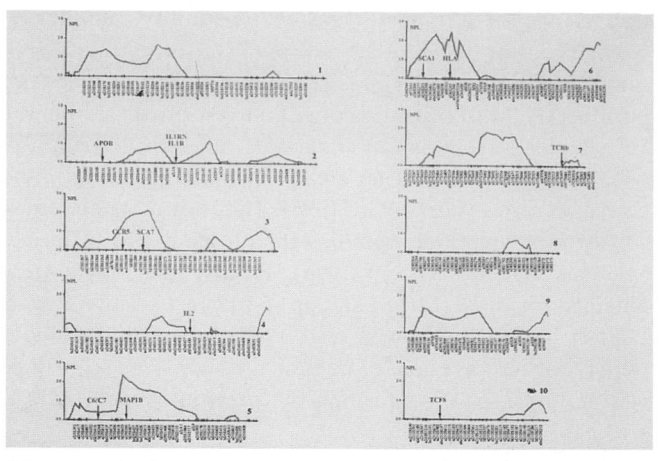
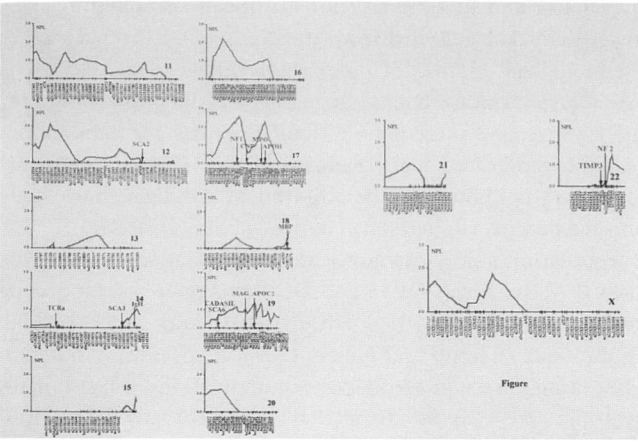

(a)

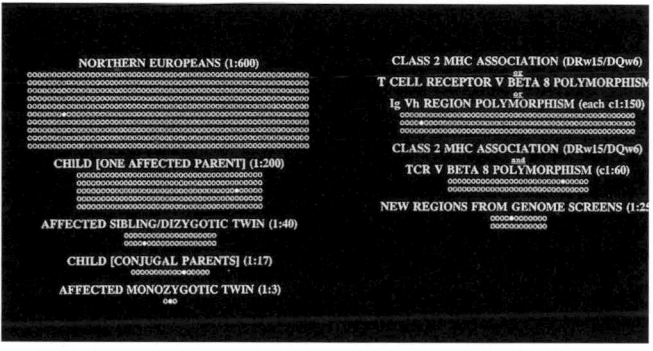

(b)

Fig. 29.7. (a) Regions of interest shown on the meta-analysis of three genome screens in multiple sclerosis involving *c.* 500 families and *c.* 500 markers on the 22 autosomes and X chromosome. Positional candidates are also identified, and are shown as vertical arrows. (b) Scheme to demonstrate the reduction in crude risk for multiple sclerosis depending on relationship to the proband and the presence of defined susceptibility factors. Comparable age-adjusted figures are: children of single affected parents 1 in 50; siblings 1 in 30; children of conjugal pairs 1 in 5; monozygotic twins 1 in 2. ((a) Kindly prepared by Dr Stephen Sawcer. (b) Reproduced with permission from Compston 1997.)

example, Foong *et al.* (1997) were unable to disentangle the contribution from frontal lobe pathology to the general clouding of intellect, and found no correlation with regional magnetic resonance lesions. However, it is claimed that white matter lesions often affect the arcuate fasciculus in patients with prominent depressive symptoms (Pujol *et al.* 1997).

Amato *et al.* (1995) compared cognitive function in 50 patients early in the course of multiple sclerosis and after 4 years, with 70 controls. The patients performed worse at both assessments but, whereas defects of verbal memory and abstract reasoning remained stable, linguistic difficulties emerged in patients over time and there was a poor correlation between cognitive and physical deficits. McIntosh-Michaelis *et al.* (1991) studied a population-based sample of more than 400, stratified for disability, and showed impaired intellect, working memory, or frontal lobe function in over 50 per cent. These findings have been extended to patients with isolated demyelinating lesions, showing impaired cognitive ability due mainly to defects of visual and auditory attention.

The cognitive defects usually occur in the absence of psychiatric symptoms, although depression is more frequent in patients with multiple sclerosis than those with comparable neurological or medical disorders. Although it can be difficult to distinguish affective disease as a manifestation of multiple sclerosis from the reaction to physical deficits and their far-reaching implications, by comparing rates in first-degree rela-

tives and unrelated individuals Sadovnick *et al.* (1996*b*) showed that depression is reactive and not constitutional in patients with multiple sclerosis. The risk of suicide is increased (about sevenfold) in the first few years of diagnosis and in the descent from expectation to reality for the participants of clinical trials (Sadovnick *et al.* 1991). There is seldom much to be gained by confronting functional symptoms and exaggeration of physical deficits in multiple sclerosis, but occasionally hysteria is a major cause of handicap in a patient with otherwise minimally disabling disease. The usual methods of attempting to improve function by physical therapy and exhortation without confrontation may succeed.

Patients are occasionally seen with specific cognitive syndromes due to hypothalamic involvement including a Korsakoff state (Section 26.5) and features of the Klein–Levin syndrome (bulimia, lack of social restraint, mental inertia, and mutism) (Section 24.2.5). Amongst disturbances of mood are included hypomania, psychotic behaviour, the euphoria traditionally associated with multiple sclerosis, pathological laughter and crying arising through loss of central inhibition of facial and pharyngeal reflexes as part of a pseudo-bulbar palsy, and schizophrenia and mania (Feinstein *et al.* 1993).

Special senses

Anosmia has been reported in a high proportion of asymptomatic patients examined with more than usual clinical thoroughness (Pinching 1977). By contrast, involvement of the visual pathway is almost invariable; the manifestations of acute uniocular and bilateral optic neuritis are described above. As with so many manifestations of multiple sclerosis, the episodic visual blurring described by patients early in the course may later evolve to slow visual deterioration. Rather few patients escape noticeable visual symptoms, and many experience difficulties with reading late in the course. Disproportionate visual impairment is unusual except in the special context of associated mutations in mitochondrial DNA (Harding *et al.* 1992). A minority of patients present with progressive loss of vision in one or both eyes—a clinical syndrome requiring special vigilance in the exclusion of other causes of visual failure (Ormerod and McDonald 1984). Apart from the appearances of retinal vessels on ophthalmoscopy, uveitis is reported in association with multiple sclerosis. The frequency is estimated at 1 per cent in a recent large hospital-based survey (Biousse *et al.* 1999). Patchy involvement of the visual pathways and accumulated deficits from separate events, occasionally results in unusual visual field defects. These include bitemporal hemianopia, hemianopic or junctional scotomas, visual slipping and post-fixational blindness, homonymous hemianopia which usually results from diffuse damage and is associated with hemiplegia or aphasia, and visual perceptual defects (Plant *et al.* 1992).

Deafness occurs in multiple sclerosis, usually in established cases but occasionally at presentation. It is usually associated with other clinical and electrophysiological manifestations of brainstem disease, although sudden unilateral or bilateral sequential deafness with tinnitus have been described as the sole presenting symptom, as has cortical deafness. Feelings of unsteadiness are common, sometimes as part of acute vestibular symptoms with severe positional vertigo, vomiting, ataxia and the headache that typifies acute brainstem demyelination. Taste may be subjectively abnormal but genuine aguesia due to involvement of the tractus solitarius has not been studied systematically.

Eye movements

Abnormalities of eye movement are common in multiple sclerosis (Section 0.11). They often occur in the absence of symptoms and so provide one method for detecting widespread demyelination in patients with clinically isolated lesions. The common symptomatic disorders are sixth nerve palsy, internuclear ophthalmoplegia, other horizontal and vertical gaze palsies, and the one-and-a-half syndrome, in which there is horizontal gaze palsy to one side and impaired adduction to the other (Fig. 29.4f and Fig. 29.8a, b, and c). Isolated third and fourth nerve palsies are reported (Barnes and McDonald 1992).

The most common sign is first-degree symmetrical horizontal jerking nystagmus. Bilateral internuclear ophthalmoplegia is always associated with vertical up-beating nystagmus. Down-beating nystagmus has other important causes, which can be confused with multiple sclerosis. Ocular flutter consists of bursts of horizontal saccadic oscillations without an intersaccadic interval. Opsoclonus, in which the movements occur in all directions, is equally disabling. Ocular bobbing consists of an initial rapid downward eye movement followed by slow return to the neutral position, and denotes cerebellar involvement. Abrupt displacement from the primary position during central fixation (square wave jerks) occurs with severe cerebellar deficits.

Involvement of other cranial nerves

Thomke *et al.* (1997) described an isolated cranial nerve palsy in less than 2 per cent of patients (1 third, 1 fourth, 12 sixth, 3 seventh, 6 vestibular, and 1 cochlear portion of the eighth nerve) with definite multiple sclerosis; 5 per cent seen at presentation had an isolated cranial nerve lesion and this was the sole manifestation of a new relapse in a further 0.8 per cent of cases. Other than trigeminal neuralgia, isolated involvement of the fifth nerve is rare. In a large Japanese series, 20 per cent had facial palsy within the first 6 years of the illness and 5 per cent presented with facial weakness, almost always with lesions in the pontine tegmentum ipsilateral to the facial weakness (Fukazawa *et al.* 1997a) (see Fig. 29.8d). Hemifacial spasm and myokymia (diffuse rippling of muscle fibres) are seen and, exceptionally, there may be unilateral involvement of the hypoglossal and recurrent laryngeal nerves.

Other brainstem manifestations

Extensive brainstem demyelination may produce disturbances of consciousness and respiratory failure distinct from the narcolepsy syndrome, which is seen more frequently in patients with multiple sclerosis than expected by chance—an observation of immunogenetic interest in view of the strong HLA-DR2 association with narcolepsy. Rare manifestations include the locked-in state, persistent hiccough, and the lateral medullary syndrome.

Paroxysmal symptoms occurring in multiple sclerosis result from ephaptic transmission in partially demyelinated brainstem pathways (Matthews 1998a). These are invariably brief but repetitive and last a few months before remitting. An individual patient may experience more than one type of attack. Symptomatic trigeminal neuralgia may begin in the first division or bilaterally, at a younger age, and with associated signs of trigeminal involvement, including motor weakness and sensory loss. It is usually associated with lesions of the dorsal root entry zone (Gass *et al.* 1997) but may coexist with compression of the fifth cranial nerve by ectatic vessels (Broggi *et al.* 1999). Paroxysmal dysarthria and ataxia with a clumsy arm, complex disturbances of sensation, and painful tetanic posturing of the limbs lasting 1 or 2 minutes are often triggered by movement and preceded by positive sensory symptoms on the side opposite to the muscular spasm. These are easily recognized and treated. Bursts of pain and paraesthesiae, sensory distortion, itching, cough and hiccough, painful extensor spasm, akinesia, kinesogenic choreoathetosis, and complex gaze palsies—any of which may respond to anticonvulsants, especially carbamazepine—also appear to be paroxysmal manifestations of multiple sclerosis (Fig. 29.9a, b).

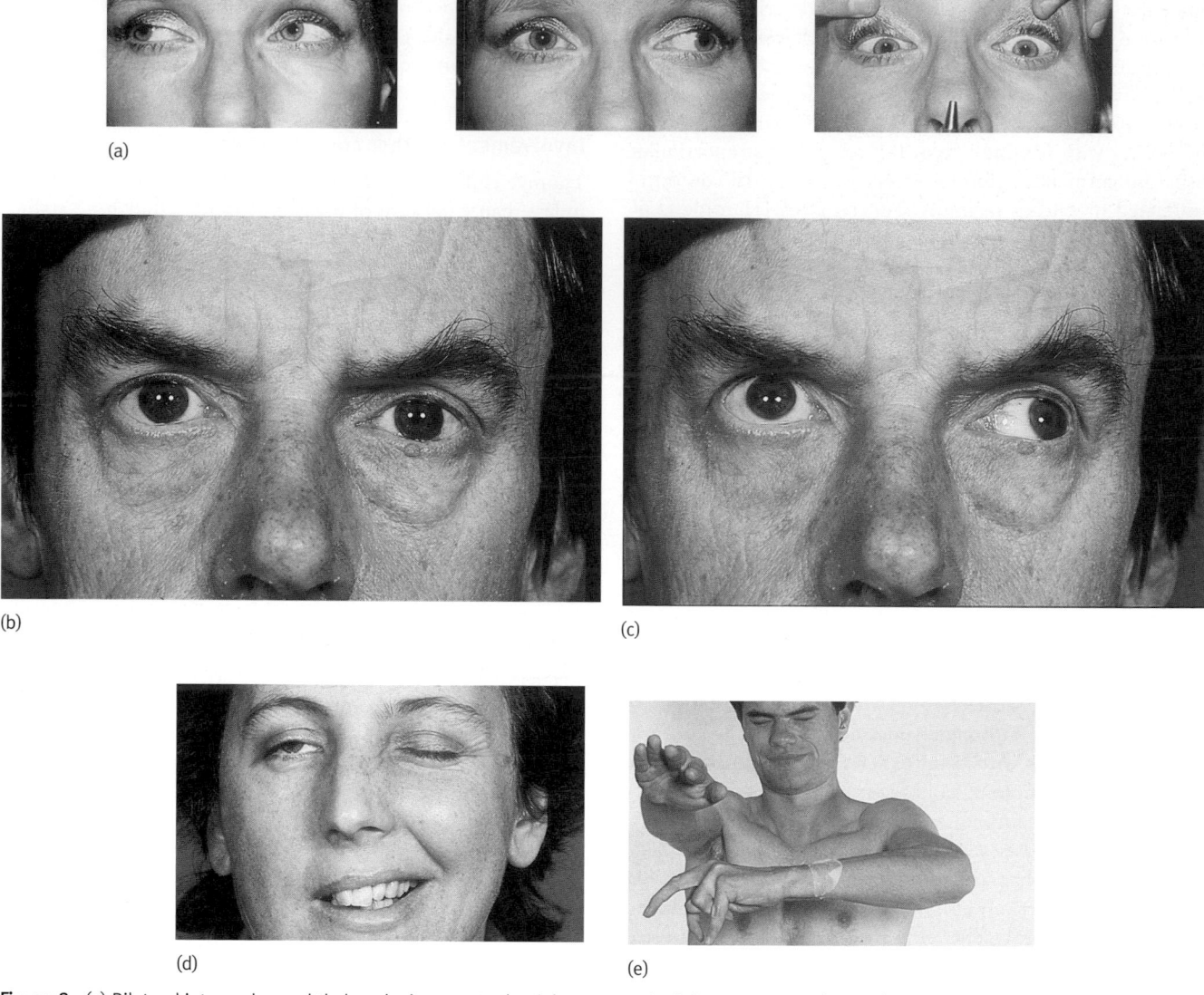

Fig. 29.8. (a) Bilateral internuclear ophthalmoplegia; gaze to the right; gaze to the left; convergence (normal). The one-and-a-half syndrome; (b) gaze to the right (absent). (c) gaze to the left (abduction only). (d) Facial weakness during an acute episode of brainstem demyelination due to multiple sclerosis. (e) On attempting to maintain posture with the eyes closed, the fingers develop 'pseudoathetosis' and the affected arm moves towards the opposite axilla. ((b) and (c) reproduced with permission from Matthews 1998a.)

Hemisphere involvement

Multiple sclerosis may present as a cerebral mass lesion with hemiplegia, focal or generalized fits, and confusion. These are often due to large, confluent, space-taking lesions. Headache is probably more common with acute demyelination in the posterior fossa than the cerebrum. Other rare cerebral manifestations of multiple sclerosis are aphasia, callosal disconnection syndromes, and cortical sensory loss. Epilepsy occurs in 2 per cent of patients with clinically definite multiple sclerosis and may manifest as tonic–clonic attacks with partial or focal seizures, or with epileptic status.

Motor symptoms and signs

Impaired mobility occurs in the majority of patients with multiple sclerosis at some stage, but the pathophysiological basis and severity vary between cases. Weakness may develop gradually in one or more limbs, increasing with use. It is usually described as heaviness or clumsiness. Confusion may arise if the onset is sudden or the distribution hemiparetic, thus mimicking a cerebrovascular episode. Although hemiplegia sometimes results from cord disease, spinal demyelination more usually causes progressive weakness in both legs, especially when multiple sclerosis presents in older patients.

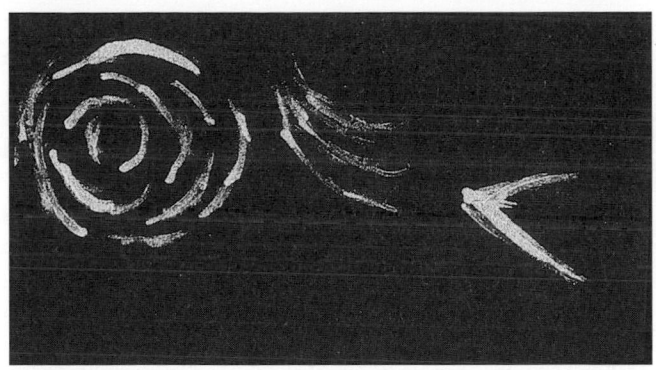

(a)

(b)

Fig. 29.9. (a) Movement induced phosphenes depicted by a patient with multiple sclerosis wishing to explain this 'unexpected' symptom. (b) Transient disturbance of handwriting in (two) patients with multiple sclerosis. '*virus—can it be caught—how long will it last—MRI when?— results of lumbar puncture when?—results of other tests*' (the usual questions of informed patients at the time of investigation). '*Karen ********* Royston Herts ****** Addenbrooke's Hospital AA*'.

Movements are slow, weakness differentially affecting extensors in the arms and flexors in the legs, and there are the expected reflex signs of upper motor neuron lesions. Motor disability in the limbs is often compounded by cerebellar ataxia and tremor, particularly in the arms, and by loss of postural sense and fatigue.

Spasticity forms only one component of the upper motor neuron syndrome but, depending on which descending corticospinal tracts are involved, it may dominate the clinical phenotype associated with damage to central motor pathways. In the progressive stage, increased muscle tone can manifest as painful spasms (flexor and extensor) which disturb sleep and often eject the patient from a wheelchair. As paraplegia in flexion and adduction develops, wheelchair and bladder management become difficult and the pain increases.

Signs of lower motor neuron involvement (wasting and loss of the tendon reflexes) are seen in multiple sclerosis. This occurs either because of associated pressure palsies or extensive demyelination adjacent to the dorsal root entry zones and spinal cord grey matter or conus medullaris. The coexistence of peripheral neuropathy, probably not due to chance, is well recognized (Thomas *et al.* 1987) with either the central or peripheral component dominating the clinical picture.

Equally disabling is fatigue—a poorly understood manifestation of multiple sclerosis which is declared by a high proportion of patients to whom the question is put and is the dominant complaint of a few, often not otherwise disabled, young patients. Using a quantitative index, Djaldetti *et al.* (1996) correlated fatigue with pyramidal tract involvement, implicating a physical rather than psychological mechanism in multiple sclerosis. Based on physiological measurements, Sheean *et al.* (1997) prefer the explanation that fatigue reflects impaired cortical drive despite sustained effort.

Involvement of the cerebellum and its connections interferes with co-ordination of speech, bulbar function, eye movements, the individual limbs or balance, usually in combination with corticospinal damage. Tremor is postural or kinetic, with several additional features which disrupt the rhythm or accuracy of goal-directed movement, but rarely present at rest (Alusi *et al.* 1999). There are few clinical syndromes more disabling for the patient, more distressing for their carers or therapeutically more frustrating for the neurologist than the combination of proximal upper limb tremor, titubation, and violent shaking of the trunk on attempted change in posture. This may result from lesions at several sites, but especially from involvement of the superior cerebellar peduncle.

Involuntary movements are an uncommon feature of multiple sclerosis, but several stereotyped disorders are reported as symptoms rather than chance associations—a tricky distinction since many do not have a firm anatomical substrate. The literature is usefully summarized by Tranchant *et al.* (1995), who describe 14 new cases (nine had dystonia; three, parkinsonism; and two, myoclonus) in the context of 135 listed from other publications. The authors conclude that paroxysmal dystonias (or tonic spasms), ballism or chorea and palatal myoclonus can be manifestations of multiple sclerosis, whereas parkinsonism, dystonia, and other types of myoclonus are co-incidental.

Sensory symptoms and signs

Altered sensation occurs at some stage in nearly every patient with multiple sclerosis. Certain patterns are characteristic but practically any part may be affected, although these symptoms commonly arise from spinal involvement.

Demyelination of the dorsal or lumbar segments of the spinal cord produces paraesthesiae and numbness in the legs, which usually starts distally, ascending to a variable level on the trunk, indicating gradual extension of the evolving lesion through laminated fibres of the sensory pathways. Sacral sparing may occur, but, alternatively, a characteristic sensory syndrome seen in patients with multiple sclerosis is numbness of the perineum and genitalia together with disturbed sphincter function.

Cervical cord lesions tend differentially to affect the posterior columns, producing perversions of normal feelings which are perceived as tight, burning, twisting, tearing, or pulling sensations. These are more or less invariably unpleasant. Pain, frequently described as a manifestation of multiple sclerosis, often represents a complication of disability related to abnormal posture, spasm of the spinal musculature or osteoporosis arising from immobility and repeated courses of corticosteroids. Dysaesthetic limb pain is one of the most difficult problems encountered in pain-relief clinics and is notoriously intractable. More disabling is the loss of proprioception and other forms of discriminative sensation which severely compromise function (Fig. 29.8e). A useful physical sign is pseudoathetosis of the outstretched hand but a better test is the ability to do up buttons.

Lhermitte's symptom and sign consists of an electric feeling in the trunk or limbs provoked by bending the neck, although other movements, such as coughing or laughing, can evoke the same effect. It results from involvement of the posterior columns. Some patients describe involuntary movements of the legs provoked by flexion of the spine or neck. Almost 50 per cent of patients experience the symptom and it may be a presenting feature, alone or in combination.

Features of the Brown–Séquard syndrome are seen with involvement of the spinothalamic tract, the patient noticing loss of thermal and pain sensation, but the diagnosis of multiple sclerosis should be questioned if there are painless burns. Non-specific tingling without accompanying signs is often encountered; and the most common physical sign found in the absence of symptoms is impaired vibration sense in the legs.

Autonomic involvement

Bladder control depends on the ability of upper motor neurons, which originate from the pontine tegmental micturition centre and are set by the inferior frontal micturition centres, to modulate spinal reflexes so as to promote either storage or emptying; curiously, these centres are both right dominant in men and women (Blok *et al.* 1998). With uncoupling of reciprocal arrangements between the detrusor and sphincter, the bladder contracts against a closed sphincter, leading to urgency and frequency, with hesitancy or incomplete emptying and incontinence. In conus lesions, the problem is more of impaired emptying than failure to fill, and urinary hesitancy then occurs in association with retention. In other situations, the mechanisms of bladder filling and emptying become uncoupled, leading to sphincter dyssynergia; attempts to promote filling may then further compromise emptying, and vice versa.

Bladder symptoms are described by 80 per cent patients, often in association with other manifestations of spinal cord disease, but in some patients they are the predominant complaint and constitute the main factor interfering with aspects of daily living. Betts *et al.* (1993) report that of 170 patients with multiple sclerosis referred because of urinary symptoms, 85 per cent had urgency, 82 per cent frequency, 63 per cent urge incontinence, 49 per cent hesitancy, and 14 per cent nocturnal enuresis. Only two patients had acute retention. An unstable bladder is more common in women; bladder symptoms are less prevalent in males in whom sexual impotence is the more frequent complaint.

Failure to control the rectal sphincter is much less of a problem than failure of emptying, and other disturbances of gastrointestinal function rarely occur. Occasional faecal incontinence has probably been underestimated in multiple sclerosis, occurring at least once in the previous 3 months in 51 per cent of a large clinical series (Hinds *et al.* 1990). Persistent incontinence is much less common, but constipation, defined as two or fewer bowel movements a week, is reported in 43 per cent, and can be a major problem in bedridden patients.

The distinction is often made in clinical practice between males who are impotent but retain reflex erections, in which case psychogenic factors are often inferred, and those with erectile failure due to spinal cord demyelination. Assessment of libido may help in making this distinction, which is important since both aspects can usefully be managed. The role of the autonomic nervous system in these problems is shown by the close association with other functional disturbances. Betts *et al.* (1994) found that a complaint of erectile failure in multiple sclerosis was always accompanied by urinary symptoms and by signs indicating disease affecting the spinal cord. Hulter and Lundborg (1995) emphasize that multiple sclerosis also has a profound effect on many aspects of female sexuality.

Other autonomic features in multiple sclerosis include loss of thermoregulatory sweating, hyperthermia, hypothermia, fever, Horner's syndrome, abnormal cardiovascular responses, postural hypotension, atrial fibrillation, acute pulmonary oedema, fatal emaciation, and inappropriate secretion of antidiuretic hormone (Matthews 1998*a*).

Childhood multiple sclerosis

Even though criteria for the diagnosis of multiple sclerosis widely used in clinical practice limit the ages of onset to between 10 and 50 years, symptoms subsequently attributable to demyelination may first occur in childhood. These represent about 5 per cent of prevalent cases. The majority first experience symptoms as teenagers but onset in the first decade also occurs (Duquette *et al.* 1987; Bauer and Hanefeld 1993).

Children with multiple sclerosis are usually girls and, happily, the course is often relatively benign. If there is a special clinical flavour, it is the tendency to present with a subacute encephalopathy. Fever and meningism, impaired conscious level due to cerebral oedema with swollen optic discs, and seizures all occur, and the distinction from acute disseminated encephalomyelitis can often only be made by the later occurrence of remission and relapse. Equally difficult is the separation of childhood multiple sclerosis from restricted forms of acute disseminated encephalomyelitis. In a retrospective series from the Mayo Clinic (1950–88), 13 per cent of 79 children, aged less than 16 years at presentation and reviewed a mean of 19 years later, had developed multiple sclerosis; actuarial analysis indicated conversion rates of 22 and 26 per cent at 30 and 40 years, respectively (Lucchinetti *et al.* 1997) but there were no useful prognostic clinical features.

29.4.4 Clinical course and prognosis

The clinical course of multiple sclerosis is no less variable than the symptoms that may occur, but some patterns can usefully be defined. Eighty per cent of patients present with episodic neurological symptoms, either multifocal or anatomically discrete, which recover fully at first. Further episodes occur at a random frequency and for an unpredictable period but, in the majority of cases, seldom exceeding 1 year, apart from brief bursts of more active disease. With time, recovery from each episode is incomplete and persistent symptoms begin to accumulate. Eventually, a proportion of patients cease to describe episodic manifestations and the course thereafter is slowly progressive. In 20 per cent of patients the illness is progressive from onset (Fig. 29.10). In a prevalent population, approximately one-third of patients are in a quiescent phase of the disease and not significantly disabled. A further third are slowly deteriorating and the remainder stable but disabled having had the disease for many years (Weinshenker *et al.* 1989; Runmarker and Andersen 1993). The duration of disease from onset or presentation is difficult to assess in a representative population but has been estimated at more than 25 years.

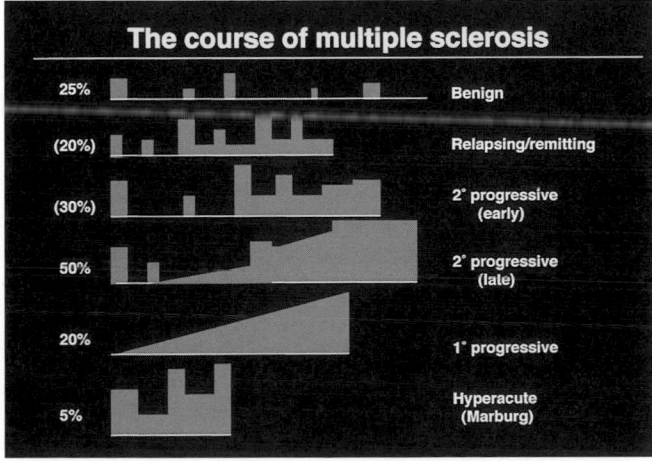

Fig. 29.10. The course of multiple sclerosis; relapsing/remitting with accumulating disability (50%), progressive from onset with or without superimposed relapses (20%), hyperacute (5%), and benign (25%) forms of the disease are depicted.

Relapsing/remitting disease

Many patients report new symptoms on waking; in others, the rate of onset of relapse varies from hours to days with symptoms accumulating in an anatomically coherent way. The most commonly affected sites are the optic nerves, cervical portion of the spinal cord, and the brainstem, and these will be affected in most patients at some stage in the illness. There is a tendency for old symptoms to recur in subsequent relapses, in part reflecting the reduced safety factor for transmission of the nerve impulse in hypomyelinated pathways. The rate of recovery is invariably slower than onset, and several outcome patterns are recognized. Relapse may occur on an asymptomatic background or complicate existing disability. Recovery from an episode is often complete but, after the first few years, many patients experience a step-wise accumulation in disability with each new relapse. Symptoms which last less than 24 hours are not usually categorized as signifying a new relapse; and it is usual to regard those which evolve over a few weeks as part of the same episode. In about 5 per cent of patients, a latent period of more than 20 years occurs after the initial episode.

Multiple sclerosis is not necessarily a disabling disease. Depending on social and personal circumstances, disproportionate handicap may arise from lesions that do not cause impairment, but about 25 per cent of patients have forms of the disease in which disability is minimal even after many years. Benign multiple sclerosis is epitomized by young females with predominantly sensory symptoms and complete recovery from individual episodes. Occasionally, patients with a mild clinical course suddenly deteriorate without useful recovery after a prolonged period of inactive disease (Hawkins and McDonnell 1999). Conversely, patients may die early with medullary involvement causing respiratory failure or massive confluent cerebral demyelination. In a few cases, relapse rate is high and sustained, leading to rapid accumulation of disability producing immobility, lack of protective pharyngeal reflexes, and bladder involvement, all of which expose the patient to potentially fatal complications, including infection and the hazards of immobility. This so-called Marburg variant affects about 5 per cent of patients, but up to 15 per cent become severely disabled and dependent within a short time.

Progressive disease

Approximately 75 per cent of all patients eventually show slow progression of disabilities due to multiple sclerosis and in those who previously experienced episodes, the relapses tend to reduce in frequency or stop altogether. This is designated secondary progressive multiple sclerosis. In 20 per cent, the course is progressive from onset. Primary progressive multiple sclerosis almost invariably manifests as spinal disease but this diagnosis should only be made in patients who have been investigated extensively. It is the most common mode of presentation when multiple sclerosis develops in or after the fifth decade, although relapsing disease is occasionally seen in this age group. The clinical and laboratory features which distinguish primary progressive multiple sclerosis from other forms of the disease are reviewed by Thompson *et al.* (1997). The spinal cord bears the brunt of progressive multiple sclerosis, whether this occurs after a period of relapsing disease or from onset, but syndromes referable to progressive involvement of the optic nerves, cerebrum, and brainstem are also seen. Secondary progressive multiple sclerosis tends to affect whichever system has borne the brunt of the disease earlier in the course, and may more frequently involve the cerebellar system than primary progressive multiple sclerosis. Progression may follow directly upon a severe relapse with partial recovery, be interrupted by further episodes, or occur without these temporary deviations. The comparable age at which primary and secondary progressive cases present raises the possibility that episodic disease activity has been subclinical or neglected in the former, and that progression is nothing more than the expiry of physiological or anatomical redundancy in functional pathways.

Gayou *et al.* (1997) showed that amongst 214 consecutively presenting patients, 12 had transitional multiple sclerosis (in which a single episode is followed some years later by progressive disease) compared to 38 with primary and 55 with secondary progressive disease; serial assessments of clinical activity confirm that magnetic resonance imaging appearances in transitional progressive multiple sclerosis conform more to primary than secondary progressive disease. Confusion arises from the occasional overlap of relapsing and progressive phases of the disease—in either sequence. The preferred classification is now only to distinguish primary and secondary progression, discarding terms such as relapsing–progressive and progressive– relapsing to define subtle variations since the latter two do not usefully distinguish different clinical courses (Kremenchutsky *et al.* 1999).

Prognosis

Every patient, at presentation, is anxious to know how the illness will progress. Since the outcome is variable and largely unpredictable, it is reasonable to err on the optimistic side when discussing prognosis early in the course. Nevertheless, certain clinical features can reliably be used in advising the individual patient on the medium- or long-term outlook. The prognosis is relatively good when the features are exclusively (or mainly) relapsing disturbances of cutaneous sensation. These patients are often young women. Conversely, cases characterized by motor involvement, especially when co-ordination or balance are disturbed, have a less good prognosis. The outlook is also poor in older-onset patients, usually males, compared with those developing multiple sclerosis in their youth. In some patients, a brisk start with several severe attacks settles down into a much more favourable subsequent course, but the large population-based studies have shown that attack rate in the early years is of prognostic value. Frequent, prolonged relapses with incomplete recovery and a short interval between the initial episode and first relapse carry a worse prognosis, but the single most worrying feature in any patient with multiple sclerosis is the development of progressive disease, whether from onset or after a number of relapses (Weinshenker *et al.* 1991). The relatively poor prognosis for disability in primary progressive multiple sclerosis, whether

or not there are associated relapses during the course (as occurs in 28 per cent patients), is further influenced by the rate of early deterioration and the number of systems contributing to the clinical phenotype. The outcome from clinical onset is worse in primary progressive multiple sclerosis, but once it has occurred, the rate of change is actually faster in secondary than primary progressive disease (Cottrell *et al.* 1999).

Factors influencing the clinical course

Prospective surveys indicate that relapse rate is affected by pregnancy. A major confounder in the interpretation of these studies is the decision by women with severe disability not to embark on pregnancy and the corresponding preparedness of those with mild disease to start or extend their families. The evidence suggests approximately a threefold higher risk in the 3–6 months after term than during pregnancy and the attacks may be more severe. Runmarker and Andersen (1995) studied an inception cohort in Goteborg, Sweden and disposed of the hypothesis that the onset of multiple sclerosis is influenced by pregnancy; in fact, there was a conspicuous absence of onset bouts during pregnancy compared with non-pregnant epochs, including the puerperal 8 months. The most recent large prospective study shows, for 222 completed pregnancies, a reduction in the pre-pregnancy relapse rate (per quartile) for each trimester with a subsequent increase in the puerperium. The clinical course is uninfluenced by breastfeeding or epidural anaesthesia, and pregnant women show the expected rate of clinical deterioration (Confavreux *et al.* 1998).

By comparison with the unconfirmed studies on causation, there is unequivocal evidence from prospective studies that new episodes of demyelination are more likely to occur following presumed viral exposure (Sibley *et al.* 1985), especially upper respiratory (adenovirus) and gastrointestinal infections (Andersen *et al.* 1991). Nine per cent of presumed infections are followed by relapse; 27 per cent of new episodes are related to infection; and the relative risk for a new episode in the 4-week period after infection is 1.3. The emerging evidence suggests that disease activity is not increased by vaccination (Zipp *et al.* 1999).

Several lines of evidence are considered relevant to the debate on whether trauma can trigger clinical manifestations of multiple sclerosis in someone who has the disease process, or alter the course in individuals who have already experienced symptoms. Bamford *et al.* (1981) failed to show a relationship between trauma and onset of multiple sclerosis in a retrospective case series, and this was followed by a more systematic study of trauma and disease activity in 170 patients studied prospectively by questionnaire (monthly) and physical examination (3 monthly) for 8 years (Sibley *et al.* 1991). Defining either the 3- or 6-month period following each event as at-risk, only electrical trauma showed an association with new episodes (defined as the occurrence of new manifestations lasting more than 48 hours, in the absence of fever, or an exacerbation of old symptoms if there was a change in neurological examination) and all other forms of trauma were negatively correlated both with clinical exacerbations and disease progression. Most recently, Siva *et al.* (1993) identified trauma in the year preceding onset in only 3/223 incident patients from the Mayo Clinic series; specifically, they failed in prospective studies to show an increased risk after head trauma, limb fracture, and cervical or lumbar disc surgery. Sibley *et al.* (1991) found that patients with multiple sclerosis had more surgical procedures than controls, through complications of the disease, but relapse rate in the period at-risk and rate of progression were uninfluenced.

Against this epidemiological background, further consideration of hypotheses for a causal link between trauma and multiple sclerosis might be considered redundant. Oppenheimer (1978) correlated demyelinating lesions in the cervical region with the regional distribution of spondylitic lesions but Kidd *et al.* (1993) used magnetic resonance imaging to show the maximum distribution of cervical cord lesions at different levels from the sites of compression by spondylitic bars.

Diagnostic and disability scales

A number of diagnostic and descriptive scales based on clinical features have been devised and many clinicians intuitively use these discriminators when discussing the prognosis with individual patients. The Poser criteria (Poser *et al.* 1983) have as their core requirement for the diagnosis of multiple sclerosis two (or more) attacks affecting two (or more) necessarily separate sites within the CNS (including one or other optic nerves). Imaging, electrophysiology, and cerebrospinal fluid examination are used to supplement evidence for the diagnosis in situations where the clinical criteria are not met, either through absence of the second episode or affected site.

The most extensively used descriptive scale for multiple sclerosis is the expanded disability status scale (EDSS) (Kurtzke 1983). It is excessively weighted to motor involvement and is non-linear. It depends on subjective assessments of physical examination, does not assess handicap, provides no information on how the present state has arisen, or what is to be expected. Despite coming in for a good deal of criticism, it has been validated extensively and widely used in clinical trials, so cannot be ignored. The United Kingdom neurological disability scale (Sharrack and Hughes 1999) is a formidable questionnaire which comprehensively explores symptoms but, with practice, can be completed in a reasonably short time. Others have devised standardized protocols and databases for describing the history, current status, disability, and treatments in individual patients; inevitably, these become unwieldy and very few clinicians find them convenient for routine use, but they are essential for describing patients participating in clinical research. Sharrack *et al.* (1999) have methodically rated and compared the scales in common usage, highlighting the merits and emphasizing the unsatisfactory exploration each provides of psychometric performance. The problem of how best to store this information remains unsolved, but any system needs to be versatile without becoming excessively complex; the European database in multiple sclerosis (EDMUS; Confavreux *et al.* 1992) has been adopted in Europe, whereas COSTAR (Paty *et al.* 1994) is preferred in North America.

29.4.5 Investigation of multiple sclerosis

Investigations are used in patients with multiple sclerosis to document the anatomical dissemination of lesions, to confirm the presence of intrathecal inflammation, and to exclude conditions that may mimic demyelinating disease. In many situations the clinical evidence is sufficient to establish the diagnosis, and laboratory studies are superfluous, but, in general, it is right to err on the side of caution. Erroneous diagnoses are identified in all large series of patients considered to have multiple sclerosis and revisions are required in up to 10 per cent of cases placed on population-based registers.

Electrophysiology

The principles of using evoked potentials in clinical neurology are described in Section 2.4. The pathophysiological consequences of demyelination can be used to identify lesions in clinically unaffected pathways (McDonald 1998a). The latency of the potential evoked by sensory or motor stimulation is characteristically delayed in patients with demyelinating disease, whereas the amplitude is unaffected, except in the acute phase (Youl *et al.* 1991). Initially, access was limited to the visual, auditory, and somatosensory systems, but central motor conduction has subsequently been studied using the technique of magnetic brain stimulation, and event-related potentials provide some evidence for cognitive processing. The application of evoked potentials provided the first reliable and non-invasive means of demonstrating widespread involvement of the central nervous system in patients with isolated demyelination, and the techniques correlate with areas of histological damage, but, in this respect, their role has been replaced by imaging techniques. Evoked potentials provide very little additional information in patients with clinical involvement of the pathways under investigation; occasionally, for example in the visual system, they can be useful in distinguishing compressive from demyelinating lesions. However, evoked potentials remain the best method for showing that a demonstrable anatomical lesion has delayed conduction of the nerve impulse and is therefore likely to be demyelinating in nature. In providing this clue to the pathology of the underlying lesion, evoked potentials remain an essential part of the diagnostic kit in multiple sclerosis.

Imaging

Magnetic resonance imaging, which depends on the relaxation time of protons exposed to a magnetic field, demonstrates reliably the lesions of multiple sclerosis (Fig. 29.4g, h). Discrete, focal, or confluent areas of periventricular, callosal, pontine, medullary, or cerebellar white matter demyelination are seen in 98 per cent of patients. Spinal cord abnormalities occur in patients with normal cerebral scans and, unlike the cerebral lesions, these are rarely seen in normal individuals (Thorpe *et al.* 1993). Abnormalities can often be detected in the anterior and posterior visual pathways. The lesions correspond to areas of histological damage but are not specific for any one pathological process or diagnosis. However, characteristic patterns and distributions of proton density and T2-weighted lesions are seen which make the diagnosis of multiple sclerosis highly likely in the right context. These lesions are dynamic, and the element which fades or disappears is explained by alterations in water content due to resolution of oedema. Magnetization transfer imaging and T1-weighted sequences may be preferable for showing parenchymal destruction. Cerebral lesions are perhaps best demonstrated using fluid-attenuated inversion recovery (FLAIR) and this may be more specific for the spinal cord (reviewed by McDonald 1998b).

Gadolinium–DTPA crosses the blood–brain barrier when vascular permeability is increased and image enhancement indicates active inflammation. Serial studies of individual patients have established important principles about the dynamics of plaque formation. The earliest change seen in an evolving lesion is an increase in blood–brain barrier permeability; new lesions are first recognizable as areas of gadolinium enhancement which last for approximately 4 weeks and precede the onset of T2-weighted magnetic resonance changes or symptoms, by up to 2 weeks. As other features of the lesion develop, persistent enhancement is seen to occur as a ring around the edge of the lesion, although a uniform increase in signal also occurs. The lesions may recur in individual lesions and the cycles tend to complete within about 8 weeks. Enhancement is most obvious in the relapsing–remitting phase of the disease. It continues during secondary progression but is less evident in patients with primary progressive multiple sclerosis (Thompson et al. 1991). All serial studies have shown that magnetic resonance lesions occur many times more frequently than new clinical events, especially with the use of triple dose delayed enhancing protocols. Some develop in areas which are strategically placed so as not readily to produce clinical symptoms but an alternative explanation is that many lesions never evolve to the stage at which pathophysiological disruption occurs. The dynamics of lesion formation are further complicated by studies showing that changes in magnetization transfer anticipate, by up to 3 months, areas which later enhance (Filippi et al. 1998). It has proved difficult to account for disability on the basis of conventional magnetic resonance imaging measurements, although lesion load in and around the corticospinal tracts matches scores on the EDSS (Riahi et al. 1998) and there is a much better correlation between disability and imaging abnormalities dependent on axonal loss than white matter involvement both in the cerebrum (De Stefano et al. 1998) and spinal cord (Stevenson et al. 1998). Remarkably, areas of the contralateral cortex homologous to those involved in active demyelination show transient spectroscopic changes consistent with temporary axonal dysfunction, indicating widespread structural or metabolic effects of inflammatory demyelination in the central nervous system (De Stefano et al. 1999). Axonal loss produces atrophy, as may demyelination, but quantitative spectroscopic changes in N-acetyl aspartate are reliably associated with axonal loss both in affected and normal-appearing white matter (Fu et al. 1998).

Isolated enhancing lesions can be detected in most patients with optic neuritis (Youl et al. 1991; Gass et al. 1996). Long intracanalicular lesions are associated with poor visual outcome. Focal abnormalities, correlating with the clinical syndrome, can also be detected in patients with brainstem and spinal cord demyelination. Lesions which do not match the presenting clinical symptoms and signs are often present in patients with isolated demyelination. These are the harbingers of recurrent clinical activity. In a definitive prospective series, 85 per cent of those with additional lesions had developed clinically definite multiple sclerosis at 10 years compared with 11 per cent of patients with no other lesions (O'Riordan et al. 1998).

Cerebrospinal fluid

Cerebrospinal fluid analysis provides qualitatively different but complementary information in patients suspected of having multiple sclerosis. There is an increase in cell count, usually due to a lymphocytic pleocytosis rarely exceeding 50 cells/mm^3, in about 50 per cent of patients and a modest rise in total protein, especially during periods of clinical activity. More sensitive and specific are increases in the immunoglobulin concentration and the presence of oligoclonal bands on protein electrophoresis, after correction for leakage of serum proteins through the blood–brain barrier (Section 2.6.7). Both are evidence for intrathecal immunoglobulin synthesis and are seen in about 85 per cent of patients. Oligoclonal bands are seen in other diseases, many also associated with magnetic resonance abnormalities indistinguishable from the lesions of multiple sclerosis. The specificity of the antibodies appearing in spinal fluid has not been resolved, but some at least are directed against components of the oligodendrocyte cell body or its myelin membranes and extrinsic viruses (Schadlich et al. 1987; Xiao et al. 1991). Molecular techniques provide an opportunity for identifying the antigens represented in these bands by screening against various libraries, and this approach has implicated Epstein–Barr virus nuclear antigen 1 in a small cohort of patients compared with controls (Rand et al. 1998). No treatments have reproducibly been shown to eliminate or reduce the number of oligoclonal bands in patients with multiple sclerosis.

Spinal fluid examination is particularly valuable in older patients who present some years after first developing symptoms, and in those with a late-onset progressive syndrome which may be due to demyelination—situations in which cerebral white matter lesions otherwise suggestive of multiple sclerosis can be age-related; the detection of oligoclonal bands is then highly informative and suggests inflammatory brain disease. The other situation where spinal fluid analysis can prove definitive is when spondylitic myelopathy has to be distinguished from primary progressive multiple sclerosis in patients with a progressive cord syndrome, equivocal changes of cord flattening on magnetic resonance imaging, and no cerebral white matter abnormalities. The presence of oligoclonal bands may then tilt the balance of probabilities in favour of demyelinating disease and spare the patient unrewarding spinal surgery.

Investigation of the individual patient

The patient with episodes disseminated in time, each of which can be attributed to demyelination, requires no investigation prior to establishing the diagnosis of clinically definite multiple sclerosis if presentation occurs between 20 and 50 years of age, separate anatomical sites have been affected, and the clinical phenotype is typical for multiple sclerosis. When these criteria are not met, the appropriate first investigation is cerebral magnetic resonance imaging. If this demonstrates typical abnormalities, no further investigation is necessary, but many neurologists nevertheless advise spinal fluid examination in order to provide evidence for inflammatory brain disease. Multiple sclerosis occasionally occurs in the absence of imaging, spinal-fluid, and evoked potential abnormalities, but the main priority in such cases is to exclude conditions which can mimic the diagnosis.

Structural lesions can present with relapsing symptoms and for this reason imaging directed at the affected site is essential, even in the context of a relapsing history, if the previous events have not involved separate sites in the central nervous system. Even then, errors can occasionally arise from the coexistence of more than one disease. For this reason, the past episodes need to be evaluated carefully before deciding that investigation is unnecessary, even in the patient with a relapsing history. Outside the limits of 20–50 years, the probability of an alternative diagnosis increases and the threshold for investigation of disorders with which multiple sclerosis can be confused should fall. The diagnosis should always be carefully considered in individuals not of Caucasian origin.

The decision to investigate patients with an isolated episode of demyelination and a past history of neurological symptoms, depends on interpretation of the previous event. If this can reasonably be attributed with confidence to demyelination, management is the same as for the patient with disseminated lesions. If the previous episode is of doubtful significance, investigation follows the protocol for patients with a first episode of demyelination. Making the distinction between significant previous episodes and those which can safely be ignored requires clinical experience. Symptoms likely to be relevant in retrospectively establishing the diagnosis of multiple sclerosis include unilateral blurring of vision, numbness in an anatomical distribution, or Lhermitte's symptom, double vision, and inability to use a limb. Symptoms from the past history mentioned by patients but usually turning out not to be important include events lasting for less than 24 hours, patchy numbness relieved by change in posture, giddiness, encephalitis or meningitis, bladder symptoms on straining, psychiatric symptoms, and epilepsy.

Imaging the cerebrum can be misleading in the acute phase of an isolated episode since, although the presence of additional cerebral lesions at presentation is associated with an increased risk of clinical recurrence, multiple lesions do not invariably correlate with further manifestations of demyelination. Conversely, recurrent demyelination undoubtedly does occur in patients with normal imaging at presentation. The erroneous diagnosis of multiple sclerosis, based on magnetic resonance imaging appearances, sometimes has to be reversed in patients with monophasic but anatomically diffuse episodes of demyelination and those with acute disseminated encephalomyelitis. A good case can therefore be made for waiting until further clinical events occur before consolidating the diagnosis of multiple sclerosis. If it proves necessary to resolve this uncertainty more rapidly, the diagnosis of multiple sclerosis can be made by comparing the results of magnetic resonance imaging and spinal fluid electrophoresis at intervals over at least 6 months. If both are transiently abnormal and no further clinical episodes occur, the balance of evidence is in favour of the presenting episode being due to monophasic demyelination. Abnormalities which persist are not in themselves sufficient for the diagnosis of multiple sclerosis but if new lesions are detected on the second scan, or the spinal fluid becomes positive for oligoclonal bands, there is a high probability that further clinical episodes will occur, leading to the diagnosis of multiple sclerosis. The other approach is to delay investigation until several months after the presenting episode and repeat the scan with gadolinium–DTPA enhancement to maximize the probability of showing new lesions.

Thorough investigation is essential in all patients with slowly progressive symptoms referable to a single anatomical site. Some structural abnormalities, such as disc herniation with narrowing of the cervical canal and slight cord compression, are not necessarily significant—the presenting symptoms and signs of demyelination happening to arise at a site of minor but insignificant structural damage. Under these circumstances, and when imaging shows no structural lesion, it is necessary also to carry out cerebral magnetic resonance so as to demonstrate white matter abnormalities indicative of multifocal inflammatory brain disease. Imaging the head before the affected part may show white matter abnormalities, suggestive of multiple sclerosis, when there is a coexisting structural lesion. Where neuroradiological investigation and spinal fluid analysis exclude a structural abnormality but fail to provide evidence sufficient for the diagnosis of multiple sclerosis, the wise clinician will repeat all the investigations after an interval.

In terms of specificity, the detection of spinal cord white matter lesions can reliably be taken as evidence for demyelination, although their presence does not distinguish a monophasic illness from multiple sclerosis. Spinal fluid analysis may resolve a difficult diagnostic situation when imaging both the affected part and the cerebrum fails to provide sufficient information for establishing the diagnosis. Evoked potentials may also be delayed in those disorders which can be confused with multiple sclerosis and present in older patients with progressive disease referable to a single site. Here, the demonstration of oligoclonal bands favours the diagnosis of inflammatory brain disease rather than late-onset genetically determined or degenerative conditions. In each of these situations, additional investigations will be required to exclude the many conditions that can mimic multiple sclerosis but if these are negative, and there are abnormalities both of cerebrospinal fluid and magnetic resonance imaging, then the diagnosis can reliably be made at presentation, even in patients with a single event or relapsing disease at one anatomical site.

29.4.6 Differential diagnosis

Matthews (1998*b*) usefully summarizes the differential diagnosis of multiple sclerosis into the following categories: diseases that may cause multiple lesions of the central nervous system and also often follow a relapsing–remitting course; systematized diseases causing lesions in separate regions of the brain and spinal cord but usually with symmetrical manifestations and a progressive course; single lesions with either a remitting or progressive course; disorders which occur monophasically and at a single site; and non-organic symptoms which mimic the clinical manifestations and course of multiple sclerosis.

Clinical, immunological and imaging abnormalities indistinguishable from those of multiple sclerosis are seen in inflammatory disorders of the central nervous system. The cerebral or myelopathic form of systemic lupus erythematosus (Section 28.2) can occur in the relative absence of systemic manifestations and with only weakly positive serological abnormalities. Karussis *et al.* (1998) identified a group of patients with multiple sclerosis, many of whom had progressive myelopathy or optic neuropathy and an unusual clinical phenotype, in whom white matter lesions were associated with antiphospholipid antibodies. Primary Sjögren's syndrome can mimic multiple sclerosis, and there is evidence that these two conditions coexist more often than expected by chance. Sarcoidosis may present with widespread and relapsing involvement of the central nervous system, showing typical magnetic resonance and cerebrospinal fluid abnormalities, and in the absence of characteristic pulmonary or cutaneous manifestations (Zajicek *et al.* 1999) (Section 28.15). The distinction from multiple sclerosis cannot be made with confidence even in the presence of uveitis. A history of oro-genital ulceration in a patient with the clinical manifestations of multiple sclerosis should suggest the diagnosis of Behçet's disease (Section 28.11).

Racial differences in susceptibility make it necessary to consider alternative diagnoses when multiple sclerosis is diagnosed in individuals of African or Oriental origin. In both groups, the development of a progressive spinal disorder even with visual involvement is more probably due to HTLV-1 associated tropical spastic paraplegia (Sections 20.6.4, 34.11.1). In Orientals, Devic's disease (see above) is more common than multiple sclerosis as a cause of spinal and visual pathway demyelination. Direct infection of the nervous system may mimic the syndromes of acute isolated demyelination or multiple sclerosis; these include tuberculous and other potentially chronic meningitides, the protean neurological manifestations of acquired immunodeficiency syndrome, and Lyme disease. The characteristic painful polyradiculitis and facial palsy that epitomize *Borrelia* infection (Section 12.14.3) in areas where this form of tick-borne spirochaetal infection has hitherto been uncommon, does not cause confusion, but the suggestion that borreliosis may produce a chronic or relapsing disorder of the central nervous system creates genuine diagnostic difficulty.

When considering systematized disorders, care must be taken in the diagnosis of multiple sclerosis if several affected members are identified in the same family. Pedigrees with hereditary spastic paraplegia (Section 14.8.2) mimic familial multiple sclerosis; and this may be the correct diagnosis in isolated cases of progressive spastic paraplegia, especially when the characteristic abnormality of gait occurs in the relative absence of muscle weakness. Other familial disorders that can be confused with multiple sclerosis include the hereditary ataxias (Sections 31.4, 31.8) and adult-onset leucodystrophies (Eldridge *et al.* 1984). Although migraine, episodes of sudden onset indicating a vascular basis, early cognitive deficits, and a family history suggesting dominant inheritance do not immediately suggest multiple sclerosis, that is often the initial diagnosis in patients with CADASIL (cerebral autosomal dominant arteriopathy with subcortical infarcts and leucoencephalopathy), especially when the cerebral white matter cerebral imaging appearances are seen in individuals with only ataxia and an unstable bladder (Dichgans *et al.* 1998); the distinction can be made by detection of the notch 3 gene mutation (encoded on chromosome 19p13) and by skin biopsy. Pedigrees characterized by affected males showing maternal inheritance may be examples of X-linked adrenoleucodystrophy (Moser 1997) (Section 29.6.3). Patients with clinically definite multiple sclerosis occur in families which otherwise manifest the clinical and genetic features of Leber's hereditary optic atrophy (Harding *et al.* 1992; Riordan-Eva *et al.* 1995) (Section 8.5.2). The leucodystrophies are discussed in Section 29.6. Differences in the age and clinical manifestations of subacute combined degeneration of the spinal cord (Section 20.6.3) should prevent confusion with multiple sclerosis, although focal relapsing spinal syndromes, often accompanied by Lhermitte's symptom, may occur in B_{12} deficiency.

Isolated syndromes related to multiple sclerosis are discussed above. The least forgivable error in the context of demyelinating disease is to accept the diagnosis of multiple sclerosis in patients with a progressive history in whom investigations have failed adequately to exclude a structural lesion—those at the foramen magnum being particularly well placed to confuse the unwary through appearing to produce independent spinal and brainstem symptoms. Errors also occur when the progressive or relapsing symptoms of brainstem and spinal arteriovenous malformations are mistaken for multiple sclerosis.

Increased public awareness of multiple sclerosis and its manifestations leads many individuals with predominantly sensory symptoms or dizziness to seek neurological advice. Frequent but brief symptoms not accompanied by physical signs can usually be dismissed, but those who always ignore these complaints may occasionally be surprised by the findings of their more compliant colleagues. This is very different from the fabrication of spurious symptoms by individuals seeking the dignity of a neurological diagnosis in the setting of neurotic or psychiatric disease. Their management requires experience and firm handling. As in the whole of clinical neurology, a clear distinction has to be made between malingering and the tendency for any patient to exaggerate genuine manifestations of demyelinating disease in order to get their symptomatic message across to the busy practitioner or specialist.

29.4.7 The management and treatment of demyelinating disease

When the initial discussion of the diagnosis takes place, it is usually possible to convey the picture of an illness which is not necessarily severe. Although expectant management is appropriate in the early stages, later there may be a need to improve the quality of everyday life in the face of significant disability by masking individual symptoms or achieving temporary improvement at times of recent symptomatic deterioration, and to try and influence the long-term course of the disease. In terms of health economics, the annual cost of multiple sclerosis has been estimated (in Europe) at 9336 ECUs per affected individual (representing 1 per cent of the healthcare budget deployed for 0.1 per cent of the population); the more severe 17 per cent of affected people requires 50 per cent of this budget, with 6.5 per cent of institutionalized patients needing 23 per cent (Carton et al. 1998). In the United States, the annual cost per case is estimated at US$34 000, of which just under 50 per cent is the direct cost of healthcare, or US$2.2 million over the lifetime of each patient (Whetton-Goldstein et al. 1998).

Management of the acute episode

Since corticosteroids are effective in abbreviating acute episodes in multiple sclerosis (Milligan et al. 1987), the issue is not so much the choice of therapy but more the preferred protocol for its administration. Most variations have been compared and the trend has been towards short, high-dose oral regimens with fewer adverse effects, not requiring hospital admission. Thompson et al. (1989) compared methylprednisolone (3 g over 3 days) and corticotrophin (a decremental regimen starting at 80 units over 14 days) in patients who were not spontaneously improving within 4 weeks of an acute relapse. There was no difference in the response between groups of relapsing/remitting and secondary progressive cases. La Mantia et al. (1994) showed that oral high-dose methylprednisolone achieves earlier reduction in the EDSS and more predictably reduces clinical inactivity over 1 year than low-dose methylprednisolone or dexamethasone. As expected, oral high-dose methylprednisolone achieves more rapid improvement in disability after an acute episode than placebo (Sellebjerg et al. 1998) and shows a dose–response effect on new lesion formation (Oliveri et al. 1998). Alam et al. (1993) compared oral and intravenous methylprednisolone (500 mg for 5 days) in patients with acute relapse, but showed no immediate or late (28 days) difference in the EDSS. Since no increase in adverse effects was seen in patients taking high-dose oral corticosteroids, the authors recommend this regimen for future use.

In an increasingly cost-aware medical culture, the expense of hospital admission for intravenous methylprednisolone (estimated in the UK at £500) has prompted a further randomized and masked comparison of the efficacy of oral prednisolone [a decremental dose of 48 mg (equivalent to 60 mg prednisolone) to 12 mg of methylprednisolone daily over 3 weeks (costing £2.80)] and intravenous methylprednisolone (1 g daily for 3 days by slow infusion in dextrose). No difference in response to treatment at 4, 12, and 24 weeks was seen between groups in this trial, using a variety of outcome measures, and the treatment protocols were equally uncomplicated. Perhaps, there was a surprising overall lack of improvement in both groups from the relapse which determined qualified entry into the trial (Barnes et al. 1997). A recent survey of neurologists working in the UK reflects the ambiguities remaining from these comparisons. Methylprednisolone given as 1 g daily for 3 days remains the most popular regimen, given in many but not all acute episodes and to some patients with chronic progressive disease, usually during day-case admissions to hospital, and more usually without than with a tapering course of oral steroids; however, circumstances dictate many variations from this usual practice (Tremlett et al. 1998). There may be role for intravenous immunoglobulin in patients with severe acute deficits which do not respond to corticosteroids; although this has not be subjected to clinical trials, there is evidence that plasma exchange given up to 1 month after onset can usefully reduce persistent severe deficits, although this does not prevent subsequent disease activity (Weinshenker et al. 1999).

The treatment of symptoms

Several manifestations of multiple sclerosis that cause persistent disability can usefully be improved by symptomatic treatment (Table 29.2). Patients who have lost the ability to inhibit reflex bladder emptying and those with sphincter dysynergia often first train themselves to achieve reasonable bladder emptying by abdominal pressure or perineal stimulation. They may tolerate occasional mild incontinence but are helped by drugs which inhibit the detrusor. Drugs with anticholinergic properties, especially oxybutynin (or propantheline), are the mainstay of treatment, since failure to store is the common problem. Other treatments aimed at improving either storage or emptying include flavoxate, dicyclamine, empromium, imipramine, maprotilene, and isoprenaline to inhibit the detrusor; ephedrine, phenylpranolamine, and imipramine to stimulate the urethral sphincter. Drugs which inhibit the urethral sphincter include phenoxybenzamine, prazocin, terazocin, diazepam, baclofen, and dantrium; drugs which stimulate the detrusor are carbachol, bethanecol, and distigmine.

A simple means for reducing the volume of urine in the bladder, and hence the desire to micturate, is to use intranasal desmopressin spray, especially at night. When significant impairment of bladder emptying coexists with failure to fill, the preferred treatment is clean, self-intermittent catheterization. This is taught quickly and adopted easily by motivated patients with adequate vision and arm function. It can be performed discretely at work or at home using a rigid or low friction catheter and ensures complete bladder emptying, with many social advantages and improved sleep. Permanent use of a

Table 29.2.   Treatment of persistent symptoms

	Early	Late
Spasticity	Baclofen Dantrium Intravenous methylprednisolone Benzodiazepines Threonine Tizanidine Vigabatrin Clonidine Mexiletine Ivermectin Cannabinoids	Intrathecal baclofen Botulinum toxin Phenol Tendon surgery Rhizotomy Nerve section Magnetic stimulation
Tremor	Beta-blockers Primidone Glutethamide Clonazepam Isoniazid Ondanestron Hyoscine Carbamazepine Sodium valproate	Stereotactic thalamotomy Thalamic stimulation Physical restraint
Dizziness and nystagmus	Cinnarizine Prochlorperazine	
Fatigue	Amantidine Pemoline Fluoxetine Modefanil	
Strength		4-Aminopyridine 3,4-Diaminopyridine Electrical stimulation
Bladder storage (detrusor)	Oxybutynin Propantheline Imipramine Flavoxate Dicyclamine Maprotilene Isoprenaline Empromium	
Bladder storage (sphincter)	Ephedrine Phenylpranolamine Imipramine Desmopressin	
Bladder emptying (detrusor)	Carbachol Bethanecol Distigmine Abdominal pressure	Local phenol Local capsaicin Local lidocaine Local verapamil
Bladder emptying (sphincter)	Phenoxybenzamine Prazocin Terazocin Diazepam Baclofen Dantrium Perineal stimulation	Electrical stimulation Bladder neck surgery
Combined storage and emptying	Self-catherization ± oxybutynin	Artificial sphincters Permanent catherization Urinary diversion

Table 29.2. (*continued*)

	Early	Late
Bowel	Loperamide Bulk laxatives Enemas	Faecal containment Colostomy
Sexual (males)	Papapaverine Yohimbine Phentolamine Prostaglandin E$_1$ Sildenafil	Mechanical prostheses Electro-ejaculation
Sexual (females)	Artificial lubrication	
Paroxysmal	Carbamazepine Misoprostol	
Pain	Anticonvulsants Anti-depressants	Nerve section Alcohol injection Sympathetic block Cutaneous nerve stimulation (TENS

catheter is preferable to constant dribbling incontinence, which leads to skin excoriation and aggravates other manifestations of spinal cord disease. A short period of self-intermittent catheterization combined with bladder retraining can achieve useful and lasting reduction in residual bladder volume. Intravesicular oxybutynin can be delivered by self-intermittent catheterization (Weese *et al.* 1993). Sub-trigonal phenol, capsaicin, lidocaine, or verapamil have also been used for intravesicular therapy injection (Fowler *et al.* 1994). Alternative measures include urinary diversion through an ileal conduit, insertion of an artificial mechanical sphincter, or electrical stimulation of the spinal nerve roots in an attempt to synchronize sphincter contraction and relaxation (Rudd Bosch and Groen 1996). The use of an ileal conduit remains a treatment option in patients with severe incontinence, and is preferable to an indwelling catheter, although satisfactory management may be achieved using a suprapubic catheter with closure of the lower urinary tract. A few patients require low-dose maintenance antibiotics for recurrent bladder infections; repeated infections promote the development of bladder stones and urinary tract obstruction, with deleterious effects on renal function.

The principle of managing constipation in multiple sclerosis is dietary alteration and the use of bulk laxatives, avoiding agents that act directly on the bowel wall. Loperamide may be useful where the predominant complaint is rectal urge incontinence.

The contribution of psychological factors should be considered in impotent males with multiple sclerosis; but in most cases, even when erections are still occurring, the problem is a direct consequence of spinal demyelination. The use of semi-rigid prostheses and vacuum pump-induced tumescence is likely to be reduced with the availability of oral treatments for impotence. Pharmacological treatments include yomhibine (an α-2 agonist), self-administered cavernous injection of papaverine,

and prostaglandin E$_1$ or phentolamine, which can be applied through the urethra. The licensing of sildenafil (Viagra$^{(r)}$), a phosphodiesterase inhibitor which acts by increasing local production of nitric oxide in response to sexual stimulation, offers an easier method for restoring potency in males (Goldstein *et al.* 1998) including those with spinal cord demyelination. Electrical techniques can be used to achieve ejaculation and achieve fertility, and this can also be applied to management of the urinary sphincter.

The mainstay of pharmacological treatment for tremor is beta-blockers (propranolol, metoprolol, nadolol, and sotalol); alternatives include primidone and its barbiturate parent, clonazepam, carbamazepine, isoniazid, ondansetron (a 5-HT$_3$ antagonist), and hyoscine. Physical restraint is rarely successful. Stereotactic procedures involving stimulation of the ventrolateral nucleus produce results comparable to destructive procedures, but there are practical difficulties and the dividend is small (Hooper and Whittle 1998). Unsteadiness arising from altered vestibular input may improve with the use of a vestibular sedative such as prochlorperazine or cinnarizine.

Amongst the many which have been tried, the only potential drug treatment for symptomatic nystagmus is carbamazepine. Local injection of botulinum toxin has also been used. Fatigue is poorly understood and not explained by increased release of any biological marker of disease activity; improvement has been reported with amantidine (Krupp *et al.* 1995), pemoline (Weinshenker *et al.* 1992) and 3,4-diaminopyridine (Sheean *et al.* 1998). Many years' research experience on the pharmacological approach to increasing conduction properties of demyelinated axons leaves no doubt that use of the aminopyridines is limited by adverse effects, including the risk of convulsions. Although these can improve vision and muscle strength (Schwid *et al.* 1997), they are not in routine clinical use.

Baclofen is still the most widely used effective antispastic agent. Benzodiazepines (diazepam, clonazepam, and tetrazepam) also reduce spasticity by increasing pre-synaptic spinal inhibition. The dose of each requires titration since either may cause muscle weakness and drowsiness. Dantrolene sodium has a direct effect on skeletal muscle and acts by uncoupling excitation–contraction mechanisms in individual fibres. Other drugs tested more recently include vigabatrin, clonidine, threonine, mexiletine, and ivermectin. Different sites of action can be exploited by combining drug use on the same or different occasions. Tizanidine, which indirectly modulates the response to excitatory amino acids, reduces spasticity at an incremental dose of 20 mg daily (United Kingdom Tizanidine Trial Group 1994) but no clear preference emerges from comparative studies with baclofen. Patients report that spasticity improves with the use of cannabis and this has been evaluated in small trials (Greenberg et al. 1994), although a definitive study is awaited. Intrathecal baclofen (Dressnandt and Conrad 1996), which carries the potential advantage of selectively reducing muscle tone in affected muscles while leaving others intact, is mainly appropriate for patients with advanced disease and seems not to have any additional adverse effects compared to systemic administration. Another approach is to use local injection of botulinum toxin, and there may be a role for surgical interruption of the reflex pathways or tenotomy and peripheral nerve block with phenol or alcohol. Magnetic stimulation may relieve spasticity (Nielsen et al. 1996).

The paroxysmal manifestations of multiple sclerosis are amongst the most satisfying to treat. Tonic brainstem attacks stop abruptly with the use of anticonvulsants that increase membrane stability (carbamazepine and phenytoin) and these drugs may also help patients with trigeminal neuralgia or the more refractory forms of pain arising from spinal demyelination. Trigeminal neuralgia also responds to the prostaglandin E_1 agonist misoprostol, presumably by an effect on cytokines which mediate painful inflammation of trigeminal nerve roots. Alternative measures which may prove necessary for pain relief include destruction of nerve fibres using alcohol or phenol and differential nerve root section, cutaneous electrical stimulation of the dorsal spinal cord, transcutaneous nerve stimulation (TENS), or regional sympathetic blockade. An open uncontrolled study suggests that gabapentin may have a role in the management of painful syndromes associated with multiple sclerosis, although adverse effects can limit the perceived benefits in these clinical contexts (Houtchens et al. 1997). All these sensations are coped with less well in the context of impaired mood and can respond usefully to tricyclic antidepressants, especially amitriptyline. This is an easy explanation for the putative effect of cannabis on pain in multiple sclerosis, although its active constituent (delta-9-tetrahydrocannabinol) acts through a brainstem pathway (the rostral ventromedial medulla) that also subserves the analgesic effects of morphine (Meng et al. 1998).

For those who develop significant disabilities and impairments, comprehensive care includes access to physical and occupational therapists, social workers, and other healthcare staff with expertise in the management of chronic neurological illness. Complications are best prevented by awareness and anticipation since they usually develop quickly yet take months to resolve. Minimizing handicap by attention to social, vocational, marital, sexual, and psychological aspects of the illness remains more important to most patients than drug treatment. In situations where the natural history has already led to loss of mobility, the early use of mechanical aids and home adaptations should be encouraged despite the associated stigma.

Measuring these interventions is not straightforward. Disability and handicap, but not impairment, improve for several months in patients with chronic progressive multiple sclerosis participating in a relatively brief programme of in-patient rehabilitation, compared to matched controls who were merely placed on a waiting list or managed by exercises at home (Freeman et al. 1999; Solari et al. 1999). Many of the effects can be attributed to the institution of appropriate treatment for managing symptoms, especially bladder dysfunction.

Immunological treatment in multiple sclerosis

The use of non-specific agents in multiple sclerosis proved the concept that immunosuppression is a valid approach to treatment, even if the magnitude of the effect often failed to establish a role for any one drug, alone or in combination (Fig. 29.11). Based on meta-analysis of seven trials involving 793 participants, Yudkin et al. (1991) showed that the odds ratio for the probability of remaining free from relapse attributable to azathioprine at 2 years is 2.0 (95 per cent CI, 1.4–2.9; $P < 0.001$), whereas reduction in the expanded disability status score (EDSS) is not significant at –0.22 (95 per cent CI, 0.43 to +0.003; $P < 0.06$). Discussion of this reduction in relapse rate with a more modest effect on disability was rightly cautious. The emphasis was on the small effect, conceivably within the errors of clinical observation, of doubtful value to the individual patient, perhaps due to un-blinding, and potentially posing serious long-term risks. As a result, azathioprine has not been used routinely to treat patients with multiple sclerosis.

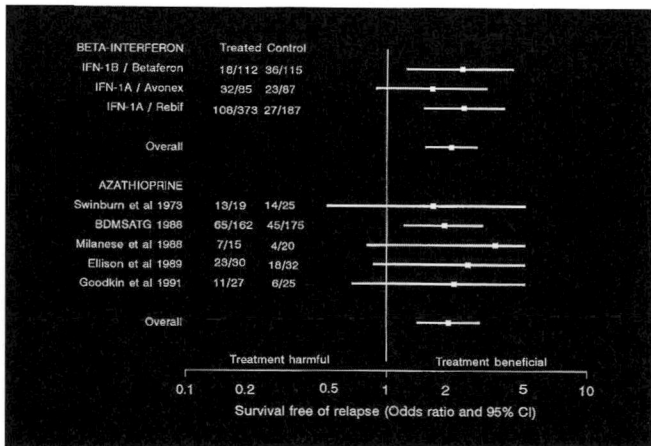

Fig. 29.11. The effect of treatment on the proportion of patients free from relapse at the end of 2 years (odds ratio and confidence intervals) in those randomized controlled trials of β-interferon and azathioprine for which data are available. (Kindly provided by Dr Peter Rothwell.)

Several potential disease-modifying drugs in multiple sclerosis have recently disappeared from interest because of a poor showing in phase III trials or unexpected toxicity. Casualties include linomide, cladribine, anti-TNF-α antibody, oral myelin, and sulfasalazine (Noseworthy *et al.* 1998). Goodkin *et al.* (1995, 1996) assessed the clinical role of methotrexate in chronic progressive multiple sclerosis and the effect on magnetic resonance imaging. Patients and independent observers were equally unimpressed by the results; and, by comparison with the claims of other agents for an effect on surrogate markers of disease activity, methotrexate is relatively unpromising.

Mitoxantrone (mitozantrone; an anthracenedione antineoplastic which intercalates with DNA and inhibits both DNA and RNA synthesis) was well tolerated and achieved a higher conversion to disease inactivity (clinical and gadolinium-enhanced magnetic resonance imaging) in patients with active disease receiving monthly injections of methylprednisolone before randomization to 6 months' treatment with intravenous mitoxantrone (12 mg/m^2/month) or no additional therapy (Edan *et al.* 1997). In another study, differences in disability and relapse rate but not imaging abnormalites were reduced in patients receiving intravenous mitoxantrone for 1 year (Millefiorini *et al.* 1997). Mitoxantrone is now licensed for the treatment of relapsing/remitting multiple sclerosis (in the United States).

Fazekas *et al.* (1997) randomized 150 patients with relapsing multiple sclerosis having clinical evidence for moderate disability to a single monthly infusion of 0.15–0.2 g/kg intravenous immunoglobulin. On an intention-to-treat analysis, the proportions improving, worsening, or unchanged in the treated group were 31 per cent, 16 per cent, and 53 per cent, compared with 14 per cent, 23 per cent, and 63 per cent in placebo patients; the magnitude of the change was small, being –0.2 EDSS points in treated patients and +0.1 in the placebo group (a difference of 0.3; $P = 0.008$). Treated patients had a reduction in baseline relapse rate of –0.8 during the first year which stabilised thereafter at –0.4, compared with reductions of –0.1 and –0.5 in the placebo group, respectively. Based on the logic that immune suppression can be achieved by mimicking the antigenic challenge that initiates the disease process, a large phase III trial of patients randomized to glatiramer acetate (Copolymer 1; 20 mg by daily subcutaneous injection for 2 years) or placebo showed a reduction in relapse rate, more relapse-free patients, and a delay in time to relapse both in the initial analysis and a blinded extension, but there was a less clear-cut effect on disability (Johnson *et al.* 1995, 1998). The clinical effect on relapse rate is associated with a change in serum or peripheral blood mononuclear cell leucocyte cytokine production from a Th-1 (TNF-α) to Th-2/3 (IL-10, TGF-β and IL-4) profile (Miller *et al.* 1998). Glatiramer acetate is licensed for the treatment of relapsing/remitting multiple sclerosis (in the United States and Europe).

Information gathered from a variety of sources shows that IFN-β has both pro- and anti-inflammatory effects. Yong *et al.* (1998) summarize the actions of IFN-β as reducing the peripheral antigen-presenting properties of systemic immune cells, promoting a Th-2 phenotype, reducing the migration of cells across the blood–brain barrier by an effect on adhesion molecules and metalloproteinases, inhibiting the activation of microglia with reduced TNF-α and enhanced IL-10 production, and stimulating astrocytes to produce nerve growth factor (NGF)—thereby protecting axons. Circulating levels of tissue inhibitors of metalloproteinases correlate with disease activity (Lee *et al.* 1999); balancing the relative availability of these proteases and their inhibitors may therefore limit local inflammation and tissue destruction.

The definitive trial of IFN β-1b (Betaseron™/Betaferon™: IFNB Multiple Sclerosis Study Group 1993; IFNB Multiple Sclerosis Study Group and the University of British Columbia MS/MRI Analysis Group 1995) involved 372 patients, each having two relapses in the previous 2 years and with pre-entry scores on the Kurtzke EDSS of less than 5.5. At late follow-up, participants had remained in the study for a median time of just under 4 years. Taking this entire period, the reduction in relapse rate associated with the use of IFN β-1b was maintained throughout the study, although the main effect was achieved in the first year. The trial of IFN β-1a (Avonex™: given as 6 million units intramuscularly on a weekly basis) involved 301 patients with clinically definite multiple sclerosis in the relapsing phase and with disabilities of less than 3.5 on the Kurtzke scale. Each had two or more documented relapses in the preceding 3 years, but none in the previous 2 months, and the pre-treatment exacerbation rate was more than 0.67/year (Jacobs *et al.* 1996). Fewer treated patients had three or more exacerbations during the study than controls; annual exacerbation rates were reduced, as was the proportion free from any relapse at 2 years. This study differed from the trial of IFN β-1b (Betaferon™) in also showing a modest effect on disability and the probability of sustained progression. Conversely, the IFN β-1a (Avonex™) study did not confirm the reduction in magnetic resonance lesion load, claimed for IFN β-1b (Betaferon™: Paty *et al.* 1993), even though the number of lesions was fewer in treated patients and there was a reduction in the number of disease activity. In the subsequent trial of IFN β-1a (Rebif™), 560 patients with relapsing remitting multiple sclerosis having two or more relapses between 2 and 48 months before treatment, and an EDSS score of 0–5, received IFN β-1a (Rebif™) by subcutaneous injection [6 MIU (22 μg) or 12 MIU (44 μg)] or a placebo preparation three times/week for 2 years (PRISMS Study Group 1998). Each dose was associated with a significant reduction in relapse rate compared to controls (1.73, 1.82, and 2.56 over 2 years, respectively: $P < 0.0002$), achieving about a 35 per cent reduction across the study period. The number of patients remaining free from relapse was 32 per cent, 26 per cent, and 15 per cent in the two treated groups and controls ($P < 0.0001$ and 0.002, respectively). The likelihood of remaining exacerbation free increased by 75 per cent and 119 per cent, and there was a delay to the time of first relapse of 69 per cent and 113 per cent, for the two treatment groups, respectively. Each dose was associated with a reduction in the severity of those relapses which did occur. The results are summarized in Fig. 29.12).

Time to confirmed progression of more than 1 Kurtzke EDSS point increased in both treatment groups but, as for the trials of IFN β-1b (Betaferon™) and IFN β-1a (Avonex™), this was less

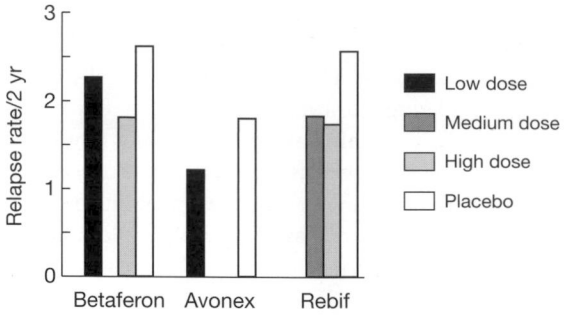

(a)

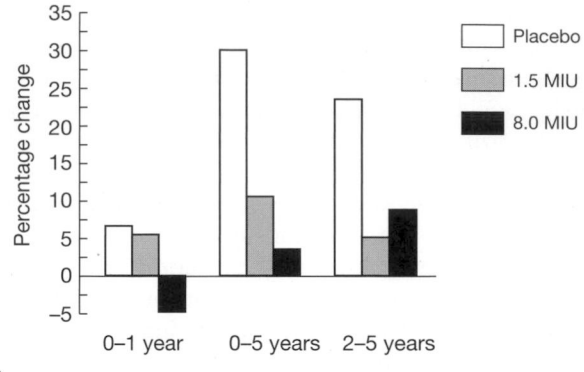

(b)

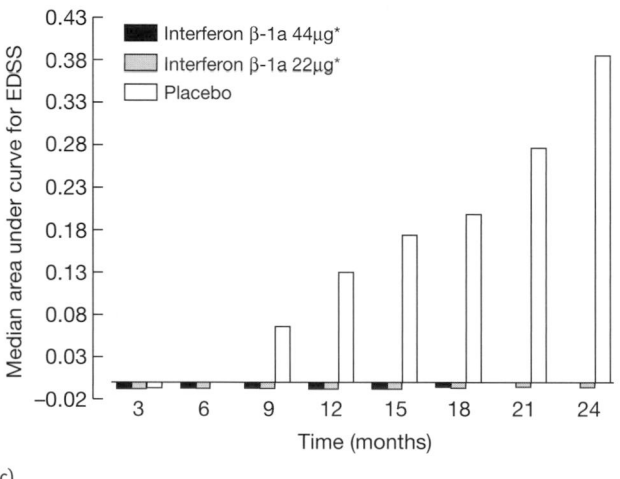

(c)

Fig. 29.12. (a) Relapses rates over 2 years compared to the appropriate control group depending on monthly prescribed doses in the trials of Betaseron™, Avonex™, and Rebif™. (b) Change in MRI disease burden from baseline (o) to year 1 and to year 5, and from years 2–5 in patients receiving high- and low-dose IFN β-1b (Betaseron™). (c) Cumulative disability ('area under the curve') in patients receiving high- and low-dose IFN β-1α (Rebif™). ((a) Reproduced from Compston 1998*c*; (b) adapted from Paty *et al.* (1993) and the IFNB Multiple Sclerosis Study Group (1993, 1995); (c) reproduced with permission from PRISMS Study Group 1998.)

marked than the effect on relapse rate. A novel composite score of integrated disability (amounting to the area under the EDSS curve over time) showed a 77 per cent reduction in accumulated burden of disability during the study period. All patients were studied by magnetic resonance imaging twice during the study and a subgroup had frequent analyses. There was a reduction, by around 70 per cent but higher in the more frequently studied cohort, in median number of active lesions per patient per scan in each treated group compared with controls. Burden of disease increased by 11 per cent in the control patients and decreased by 1 per cent and 4 per cent in the low- and high-dose-treated groups, respectively ($P < 0.0001$) (Li *et al.* 1999).

The magnitude of the reduction in rate of accumulation of disability in patients receiving IFN β-1a (Avonex™ or Rebif™) and IFN β-1b (Betaferon™) compared with their respective placebo controls is rather similar, and the Rebif™ study consolidates the position. Most would now accept that there is reduction of around 30 per cent in relapse rate and a more substantial reduction in accumulation of new imaging lesions (whatever that means for the natural history). The first trial of IFN β-1b in chronic progressive multiple sclerosis was stopped early with placebo patients being switched to active treatment: the European Study Group on Interferon β-1b in Secondary Progressive Multiple Sclerosis (1998) showed that IFN β-1b (Betaferon™)

delays progression by 1 EDSS point for 9–12 months over a 2–3 year period, in patients with secondary progressive multiple sclerosis. This result has led to an alteration in the product licence and extension of the prescibing indications for using IFN β-1b to include patients with secondary progressive multiple sclerosis. Imaging results from this study provide some support for the interpretation that the clinical effects result more from reduction of new inflammatory lesions than other components contributing to secondary progression (Miller *et al.* 1999). But the remaining and, as yet unpublished, results using IFN-β 1a (Avonex™ and Rebif™) and IFN-beta 1b (the United States study) in secondary progressive multiple sclerosis support the view that these treatments have little to offer patients in the secondary progressive phase of multiple sclerosis unless superimposed relapses still dominate the clinical picture. It also remains to be established whether the IFNs influence markers of disability and progression such as brain parenchymal fraction (Rudick *et al.* 1999) and atrophy (Molyneux *et al.* 2000). The most recent emphasis of clinical trials has been to assess the conversion rate to multiple sclerosis in patients with a first episode of demyelination. With some differences in selection criteria, the two completed studies achieve the predictable reduced new episode rate and therefore a delay in meeting existing criteria for the diagnosis of multiple sclerosis (Jacobs *et al.* 2000; Comi *et al.* unpublished).

These studies do not establish that the beta interferons prevent the onset of multiple sclerosis in individuals at risk through having had a single episode of demyelination.

Despite a good deal of public debate, not all considered free from conflicts of interest, what remains unresolved is whether there are useful differences in efficacy or immunogenicity between the three products, dose–response effects, and additive effects of other immunological agents. Apart from local injection-site reactions, the main adverse effects of IFN-β are flu-like symptoms and hyperthermia. These may be related to the production of IFN-γ, TNF-α and IL-6; combination therapy with IFN β-1b and pentoxifylline (oxpentifylline) reduces both the cytokine production and flu-like symptoms (Weber *et al.* 1998). In a study of 29 patients treated with intravenous methylprednisolone, the duration of reduction in gadolinium-enhancing magnetic resonance imaging abnormalities was longer (up to 4 months) in those also receiving IFN-β (Gasperini *et al.* 1998). Concern that release of IFN-γ might also increase relapse frequency in the early phase of treatment is not borne out by retrospective experience (Khan and Hebel 1998). During post-marketing experience in the United States, adverse effects reported to the Food and Drug Administration are noted to develop early, but may be delayed for up to 29 months after starting treatment. Females are preferentially affected and the effects usually consist of injection-site reactions (91 per cent) but stopping short of injection- or non-injection-site necroses (8 per cent and 1 per cent, respectively) (Gaines and Varricchio 1998). Less predictable, but potentially more serious, adverse effects include autoimmune disease, capillary leak syndrome, anaphylactic shock, and thrombocytopenic purpura (reviewed by Walther and Hohlfeld 1999). Probably, not all the long-term adverse effects of IFN-β are yet known.

Up to 45 per cent of patients on high-dose (8 MIU) IFN β-1b (Betaferon™) develop neutralizing activity; this usually occurs in the first year (34/124; 7/124 in year 2, and 2/124 in year 3). The reported rate was lower in the secondary progressive study (28 per cent) but changes in assay and manufacturing process make these observations difficult to compare. In the trial of IFN β-1a (Avonex™), persistent neutralizing anti-interferon activity was seen in 14 per cent of treated individuals by 1 year and 23 per cent at 2 years, compared with 4 per cent of placebo patients (in whom antibody activity disappeared upon repeat testing). Neutralizing antibodies developed in 24 per cent of patients treated with low-dose, and 13 per cent of those receiving high-dose IFN β-1a (Rebif™). Neutralizing antibodies to IFN β-1a and IFN β-1b are immunologically and biologically cross-reactive, suggesting that switching product may not escape the consequences for the immunoreactive individual of exposure to the more immunogenic preparation (Khan and Dhib-Jalbut 1998).

Much effort has gone into the design of treatments in multiple sclerosis which target T cells wherever they are located. The rationale, experimental background, and pharmacological strategies planned or in progress are summarized by Hohlfeld

(1997). Lymphocyte migration involves the loose tethering of cells to the endothelial lining through binding of selectins and their ligands, which strengthens as integrins and immunoglobulin superfamily structures (VLA-4 and ICAM-1) are engaged; penetration follows the involvement of VLA-4 with CD31 (Archelos and Hartung 1997). Migration of lymphocytes into the central nervous system is prevented by antibodies directed at the α4 chain of integrins, with effects on inflammation and demyelination. In a double-blind, placebo-controlled study of a humanized anti-α4 integrin antibody in relapsing–remitting or progressive multiple sclerosis, there were fewer active magnetic resonance lesions in the 24 weeks after two pulses separated by 1 month but no effect on clinical relapses, which continued in the treatment and placebo groups (Turbridy *et al.* 1999).

Chimeric and humanized monoclonal antibodies have been used to remove lymphocytes from the systemic circulation and thus prevent both cell migration and inflammation within the central nervous system. The advantage of using monoclonal antibodies which deplete or block T cells lies in the possibility of prolonged stabilization of disease from pulsed therapy, but there are concerns about the long-term consequences of immune depletion. In practice, many antibodies fail to suppress the systemic lymphocyte count adequately and so do not fully test the hypothesis that immune behaviour can be altered by depletion. But with the adoption of strategies for making these antibodies more innocuous in terms of anti-idiotypic responses, and the introduction of new specificities, greater use of monoclonal antibodies in multiple sclerosis can be anticipated. Several specificities have now been tested and these include murine, chimeric, or humanized anti-CD6, -CD2, and -CD3, but most experience relates to anti-CD4 (Lindsey *et al.* 1994*a,b*; van Oosten et 1997) and -CD52 (Moreau *et al.* 1994, 1996; Coles *et al.* 1999*a, b*) antibodies.

In patients receiving one or more courses of a chimeric anti-CD4 antibody under open uncontrolled conditions, and in doses ranging from 10 to 200 mg given as a single infusion or over 3 days, there was a partial and sustained reduction in CD4 cells (Lindsey *et al.* 1994*a,b*). The treatment was well tolerated but the clinical and imaging effects were modest and seen only in a minority of patients. Subsequently, van Oosten *et al.* (1996) randomized patients with clinical and radiological disease activity to treatment with chimeric anti-CD4 or placebo under double-blind conditions. Although the antibody effectively reduced the circulating CD4 counts, both groups showed persistent radiological disease activity but with fewer clinical episodes in the treated group. Together, these studies do not suggest that the presently available anti-CD4 monoclonals used in isolation have a therapeutic future in multiple sclerosis.

The humanized anti-CDw52 (Campath-1H) has proved to be a much more potent depletor of lymphocytes and is effective in multiple sclerosis (Moreau *et al.* 1994). The first dose provokes a transient rehearsal of previous symptoms, due to release of cytokines that directly or indirectly impede conduction at previously demyelinated sites. Disease activity persists for around 4 weeks but, thereafter, radiological markers of cerebral inflam-

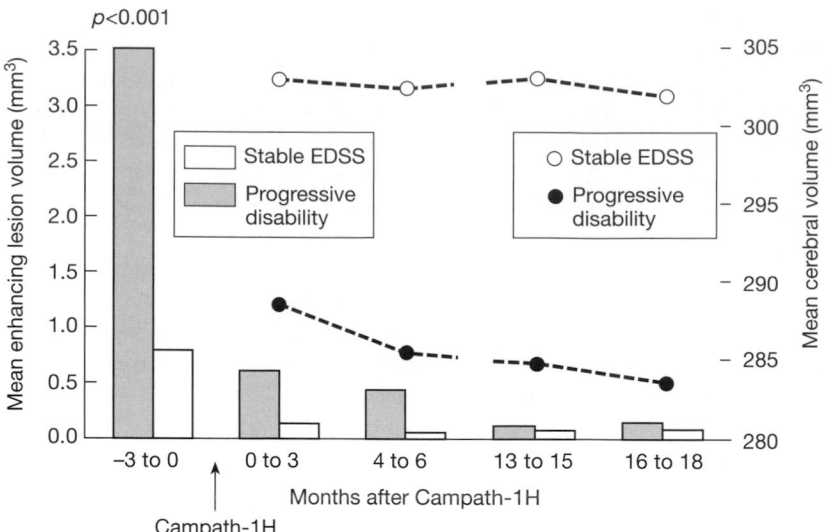

29.13. Gadolinium-enhanced magnetic resonance imaging lesions and mean cerebral volume in patients with multiple sclerosis treated with Campath-1H. (Reproduced with permission from Coles *et al.* (1999*b*) and Compston (1998*c*).)

mation are suppressed, maximally by more than 90 per cent and for at least 18 months during which no new relapses occur. However, 50 per cent of patients become progressively disabled from deficits acquired prior to treatment; these show brain atrophy with evidence for axon degeneration on magnetic resonance spectroscopy, but this subgroup of poor-prognosis patients cannot be distinguished retrospectively from the remainder (Fig. 29.13). Clinical progression and atrophy correlate with the amount of brain inflammation in the pre-treatment phase but occur in the absence of ongoing disease activity. The reduction in brain inflammation is associated with alteration in the immune response from a Th-1 pattern of cytokine release which also lasts for around 18 months. This suppresses disease activity in multiple sclerosis but, unexpectedly, exposes autoimmune thyroid disease in the second year after treatment (Coles *et al.* 1999*a,b*). The acute cytokine release syndrome associated with the use of Campath-1H is uninfluenced by effective removal of TNF-α (Coles *et al.* 1999*a*), suggesting that other mediators of inflammation are responsible. The data relating to TNF-α and multiple sclerosis had not, however, predicted that a fusion protein linked to the soluble TNF-α receptor would be associated with a dose-dependent increased relapse rate, reduced time to relapse, and longer and more severe episodes in those receiving soluble TNF-α receptor (Lenercept Multiple Sclerosis Study Group and the University of British Columbia MS/MRI Analysis Group 1999)—results which probably have their explanation in the complex interacting networks of pro- and anti-inflammatory cytokines, with some having more than one effect, depending on context.

Comparable assaults on the immune system can be achieved with cytotoxic drugs and autologous or allogeneic bone marrow transplantation, and it seems likely that this will be assessed in more formal trials over the next few years. Fassas *et al.* (1997) reported on 15 patients with progressive disease who received haematologic stem cells mobilized with cytokines and drugs, after ablative immunotherapy with BCNU, etoposide, cytosine arabinoside, and melphalan with antilymphocyte globulin given after transplantation. All survived the immediate procedure, despite significant toxicity. At 6 months follow-up, half of the group was deemed to have stabilized or improved.

Taken together, the results of clinical trials support the hypothesis that inflammation is necessary for new lesion formation and conditions axon degeneration. The implication is that immunological therapies will best prevent progression of disability if given early in the course and before the cascade of events leading to axon degeneration is irretrievably established. This may explain the present limitations of immunotherapy in patients with secondary progressive multiple sclerosis. But it raises the dilemma of exposing individuals who may never develop disabilities from multiple sclerosis to the unpredictable hazards of prolonged immunosuppression as the price paid for stabilizing the disease process in those who are destined to do badly.

29.5 Central pontine myelinolysis

Central pontine myelinolysis was first described in four patients in whom autopsy studies revealed a single, sharply outlined focus of myelin destruction in the rostral part of the pons, indiscriminately involving all descending and ascending fibre pathways, with the exception of the ventrolateral tract, but sparing nerve fibres (Adams *et al.* 1959) (Fig. 29.14a, b). The disorder is not rare and much has since been learned concerning the aetiology, pathology, and clinical manifestations. Although the original descriptive term 'central pontine myelinolysis' remains valid, demyelination is often observed outside the pons (Wright *et al.* 1979). A high proportion of the cases first described were metabolically disturbed, often as a result of alcohol abuse (Section 5.2.6), but the condition is now known to occur in association with Wernicke's encephalopathy, liver cirrhosis not due to alcohol, as part of Wilson's disease,

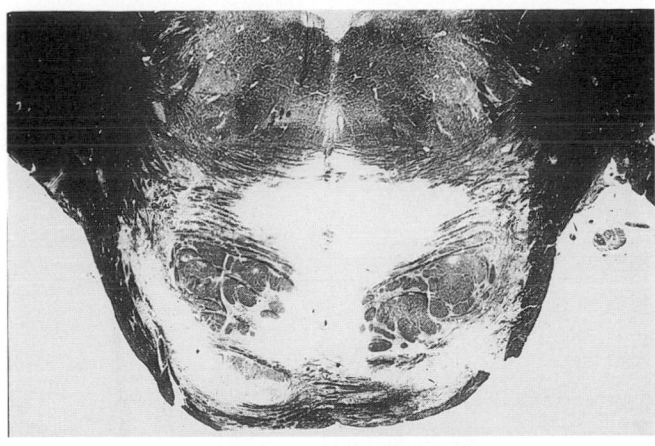

(a)

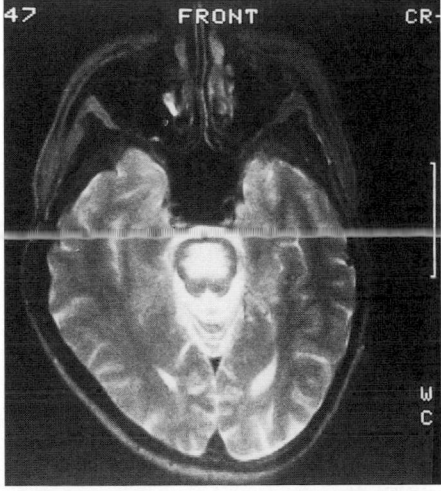

(b)

(c)

Fig. 29.14. (a) An area of confluent demyelination in the central pons which occurred in a patient in whom the serum sodium rose from 112 to 145 mmol/l over 24 hours following liver transplantation (kindly provided by Dr J. Anderson); (b) sagittal MRI (T1-weighted); and (c) horizontal MRI (T2-weighted) of another patient with central pontine myelinolysis.

after hepatic transplantation, and in non-cirrhotic liver disease. Central pontine myelinolysis is also seen as a complication of leukaemia, uraemia and haemodialysis, hyperemesis gravidarum or other causes of prolonged vomiting, following diuretic therapy, and in children. In several of these situations, the diagnosis can be confused with Wernicke's encephalopathy, but an important difference is that patients with central pontine myelinolysis are often hyponatraemic before the onset of neurological symptoms. This observation led to the suggestion that the pons is unusually susceptible to changes in electrolyte balance, but it is now believed that central pontine myelinolysis is caused by overzealous correction of a low serum sodium (Sterns *et al.* 1986). A prospective study of electrolyte correction in patients with hyponatraemia demonstrated that pontine damage correlates both with the degree of hyponatraemia and speed with which it is corrected—starting levels of less than 110 mmol/l or rates of correction above 2 mmol/l/h increasing the risk of pontine damage (Brunner *et al.* 1990). Experimental studies have shown that rapid changes in sodium can better be tolerated when hyponatraemia has arisen acutely than in chronic electrolyte imbalance. Central pontine myelinolysis is occasionally seen as a result of sustained or rapidly corrected hypernatraemia.

Clinically, the process begins with damage to pathways placed centrally within the pons and then spreads centrifugally. The fully evolved clinical picture is of flaccid paralysis with facial and bulbar weakness, disordered eye movements, profound imbalance, and alterations in consciousness. The recent literature highlights movement disorder and other extrapyramidal manifestations of central pontine and extrapontine myelinolysis (Seiser *et al.* 1998). Some manifestations can be attributed to the poor medical condition of affected individuals. Since central pontine myelinolysis tends to occur following therapeutic intervention and correction of the serum sodium, other features of hyponatraemia, such as fits, tend not to be associated. In a series observed in hospitals in New York and Oxford, Ellis (1995) reported only one case of central pontine myelinolysis (with a striatal syndrome) amongst 184 patients presenting with hyponatraemia and managed in a variety of ways, including rapid correction of serum sodium in some instances. Newell and Kleinschmidt-DeMasters (1996) carried out an autopsy-based epidemiological survey of the prevalence and features of central pontine myelinolysis over a period in which management of hyponatraemia was changing, but observed no change in the incidence. Of 15 clinically undiagnosed cases, 5 of 6 with active lesions were associated with overzealous correction of the serum sodium; these correlations could not be made for comparison in those with remote episodes of central pontine myelinolysis.

The prognosis for clinical recovery is largely determined by the underlying metabolic disorder and the extent to which that can be managed; but with stabilization of the serum sodium, management of the bulbar failure and time, the prognosis for neurological recovery is good and the condition does not relapse spontaneously. Menger and Jorg (1999) reviewed retrospectively

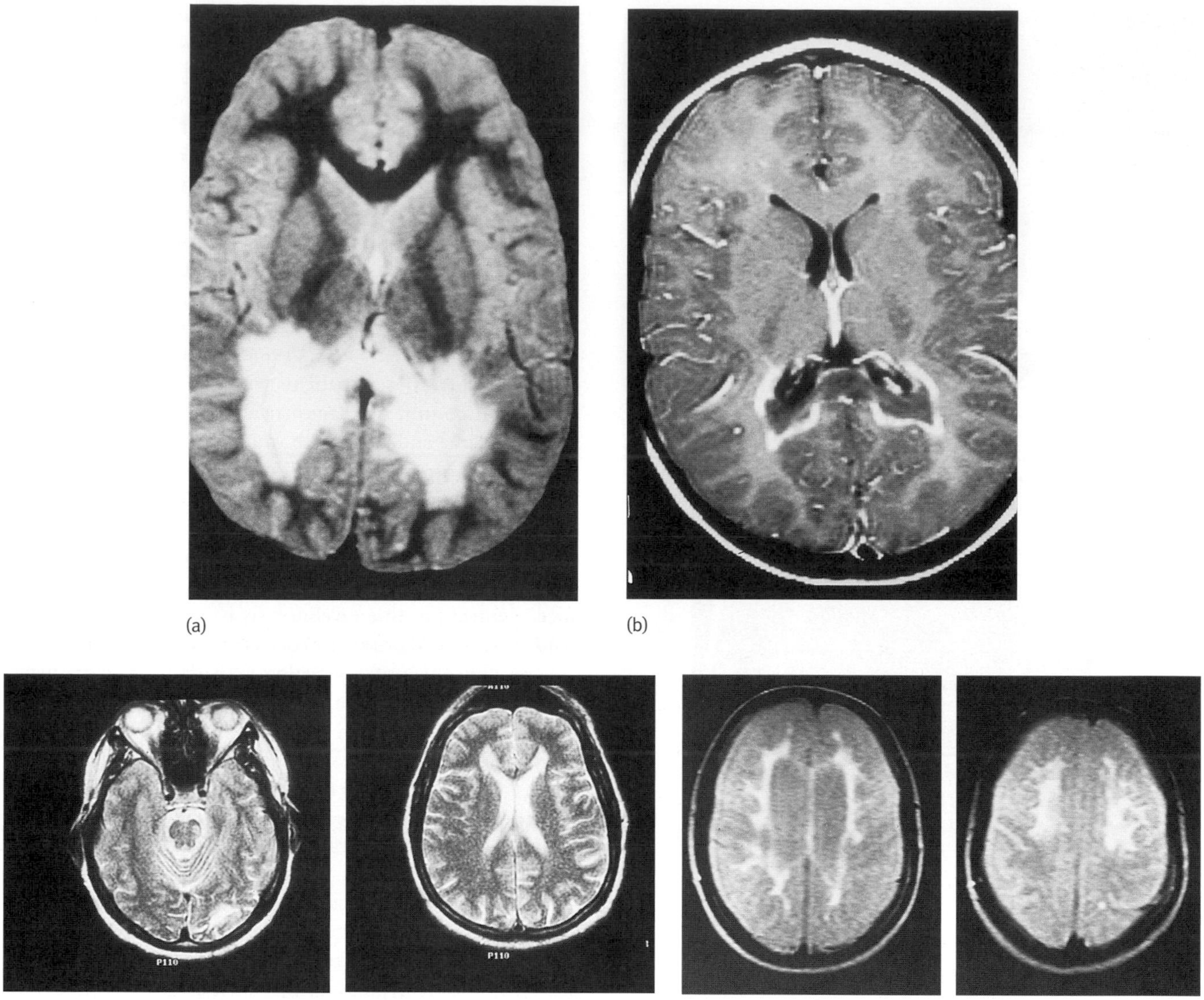

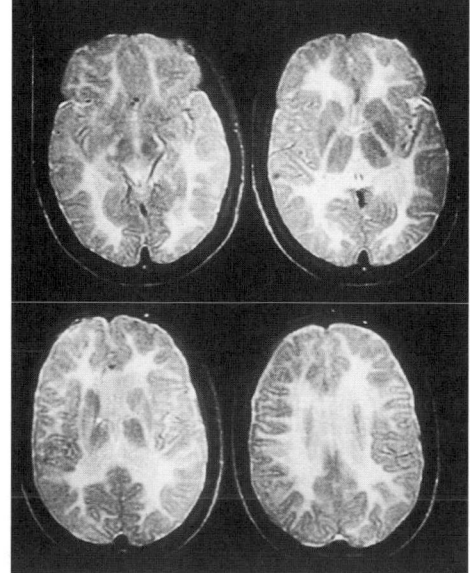

Fig. 29.15. Magnetic resonance imaging in the leucodystrophies: T2-weighted images. (a) Adrenoleucodystrophy in childhood. (b) Same patient as in (a), showing T1-weighted image after injection of gadolinium-DTPA. Note the extensive enhancement around the trigones. (c) Adrenoleucodystrophy in an adult male with a cerebellar syndrome and Addison's disease; high signal abnormality in the corticospinal tract in the pons with atrophy of the cerebellum and midbrain, (d) bilateral high signal intensities adjacent to the anterior peri-ventricular region bilaterally.(e), (f) Metachromatic leucodystrophy; proton-density-weighted image. (g) Pelizaeus–Merzbacher disease. (Reproduced with permission from McDonald 1998a.)

the outcome in 44 patients and concluded that death in two, or poor recovery in 10, with residual deficits not affecting independence in a further 11, hinged on the general medical complications of the more acute illness or its precipitating events, rather than the severity of pontine myelinolysis; they did not identify any radiological or electrophysiological predictors of poor outcome.

The clinical features of brainstem disease occurring in a patient with hyponatraemia are sufficiently distinctive not to cause diagnostic difficulties, but uncertainty may arise if only a small reduction in serum sodium has occurred or the fall has not been documented, in which case brain imaging may be informative. The acute changes can be recognized by computed tomography or magnetic resonance imaging and persistent abnormal signals attributable to astrocytic proliferation and gliosis can be detected long after the clinical features have resolved. Ultrastructural studies support the view that the condition is due to a metabolic process which is directed primarily at oligodendroglia.

29.6 Leucodystrophies

The leucodystrophies are a group of disorders, originally described on the basis of their non-inflammatory demyelinating neuropathology and including an heterogeneous collection of conditions, many of which are now known to result from specific defects affecting genes that determine the synthesis, maintenance, and structure of myelin (Table 29.1). Other disorders originally classified as leucodystrophies have specifically different aetiologies and are no longer included in the group. These are rare conditions even in paediatric practice, but need to be considered in young adults with atypical syndromes combining physical and intellectual deficits, with or without peripheral nerve involvement, in whom imaging shows more confluent lesions confined to white matter (Fig. 29.15).

No attempt is made comprehensively to cover this miscellaneous group of predominantly paediatric developmental and neurodegenerative disorders, but readers are referred to the full clinical, biochemical, and beautifully illustrated imaging descriptions given by van der Knaap and Valk (1995) and other definitive accounts (Moser 1997). Here, the emphasis is mainly on those disorders that may be seen in adult neurological practice and their childhood forms.

29.6.1 Diffuse sclerosis (Schilder's disease)

Earlier editions of this book described, as diffuse sclerosis or Schilder's disease (Schilder 1912), a condition in which a previously healthy child between the ages of 5 and 12 years developed intellectual impairment and a gait disorder. The onset was occasionally rapid but usually insidious. Headache and giddiness occurred, but fever was exceptional. Visual impairment was often an early symptom and sometimes preceded by mental deterioration, epileptic attacks, aphasia, or weakness and incoordination of the limbs. Visual failure was usually due to

destruction of the optic radiations. Homonymous hemianopia occurred when one occipital lobe was first involved, but the remaining visual field was gradually lost as the pathological process spread, and the end result was blindness in most cases. Visual impairment was less often due to bilateral retrobulbar neuritis causing central scotomas. In these cases, disc swelling in the acute stage was followed by optic atrophy. Acute widespread demyelination sometimes caused cerebral oedema, raised intracranial pressure, and papilloedema. Diplopia was usually due to lateral rectus paralysis and accompanied by nystagmus more often than third nerve palsy. Loss of smell and taste, deafness, and tinnitus were described.

The children then developed progressive spastic weakness of the extremities, leading eventually to spastic tetraplegia. Sensory loss of cortical type was common, with loss of postural sensibility, appreciation of passive movement, and tactile discrimination, but cutaneous sensation could also be involved, producing hemi-analgesia. Aphasia was noticeable in the early stages; later, this was masked by spastic dysarthria, and dysphagia due to pseudobulbar palsy eventually supervened. The mental changes were those of progressive dementia. Generalized or focal motor seizures were seen at any stage.

The early onset of blindness with progressive dementia and spastic paralysis was considered to constitute a distinctive clinical picture. This could be confused with intracranial tumour when the symptoms and signs were predominantly unilateral and especially if there was papilloedema. The disease was almost invariably progressive and usually fatal, although temporary remissions and, very rarely, arrest or recovery did occur. It ran an acute course, leading to death within 1 or 2 months. Few patients survived more than 3 years from onset but life occasionally was prolonged for several years.

In describing this condition, we use the past tense because it has since become clear that the term 'diffuse cerebral sclerosis' has been used to identify a heterogeneous group of diseases affecting cerebral white matter. Not all have turned out to be genetically determined disorders of myelin formation and metabolism. Thus, of the diseases originally classified under this heading, familial sudanophilic diffuse sclerosis, Pelizaeus–Merzbacher disease, Krabbe's diffuse sclerosis (globoid cell leucodystrophy), Canavan's diffuse sclerosis (spongy degeneration of the white matter), Alexander's disease, and metachromatic leucodystrophy are all dysmyelinating leucodystrophies. Conversely, Binswager's subcortical encephalopathy is a consequence of diffuse cerebral arteriosclerosis—although the provocative suggestion has since been made that this was an early example of CADASIL (Dichgans et al. 1998); and Balo's concentric sclerosis is considered within the spectrum of multiple sclerosis. Many male cases previously classified as having diffuse sclerosis were probably suffering from adrenoleucodystrophy. Some of the relapsing disorders were almost certainly examples of Leigh's disease associated with mutations of mitochondrial DNA. An extreme interpretation is that diffuse sclerosis was never anything more than an exceptionally severe and generalized variety of childhood multiple sclerosis.

Relatively simple investigations have proved useful in distinguishing some of these childhood encephalomyelopathies. Electroencephalography is of considerable value in making the distinction from subacute sclerosing panencephalitis and the lipidoses; it usually shows diffuse slow activity which is unlike the recurrent bizarre complexes of subacute sclerosing panencephalitis or the irregular spike and wave discharges that characterize Tay–Sachs disease. Imaging demonstrates extensive areas of low attenuation in the white matter of both cerebral hemispheres but these are not specific. Even after separating these specifically different conditions, the nosological status of diffuse sclerosis remains uncertain and some experts consider that, between them, acute multiple sclerosis and adrenoleucodystrophy account for all the cases (Lassmann 1998).

29.6.2 Krabbe's disease

Globoid cell leucodystrophy usually presents during early infancy, and late onset is uncommon—almost all cases present before the age of 5 years and so are almost never confused with (childhood) multiple sclerosis. Grewel *et al.* (1991) describe the onset in a boy of 14, not finally diagnosed until the age of 24 years. The clinical picture is dominated by behavioural changes with light and noise startle, progressive intellectual and motor decline, with pyramidal, extrapyramidal, and cerebellar involvement, and epilepsy, visual failure, and peripheral neuropathy (Section 12.8.3) leading to severe disabilities with pyrexia and other autonomic features prior to the onset of a vegetative state. Visual evoked potentials are delayed and the spinal fluid has a raised protein but does not contain oligoclonal bands. Magnetic resonance imaging shows periventricular lesions and subsequently extensive white matter changes.

Examination of peripheral blood leucocytes or skin fibroblasts shows a deficiency of α-galactocerebrosidase which leads to the accumulation of cerebroside in phagocytes, resulting in the diagnostic feature of globoid cells; these represent the end stage of oligodendrocyte and myelin degradation triggered by psychosine accumulation. Although myelinating cells in the central and peripheral nervous systems are each affected, there seems to be differential susceptibility of oligodendrocytes and Schwann cells.

29.6.3 Adrenoleucodystrophy

The biochemical characterization of a peroxisomal defect separated adrenoleucodystrophy from the other dysmyelinating disorders, although the X-linked pattern of inheritance had always been a distinctive feature. There are several types, each characterized by the accumulation of very-long-chain saturated fatty acids (VLCFAs) in all lipid-containing tissues and body fluids (Moser *et al.* 1981). The various disorders arise from defective very-long-chain fatty acyl coenzyme-A synthetase activity in peroxisomes (Wanders *et al.* 1988) and lead to the accumulation of membrane-like cytoplasmic inclusions in brain tissue. One hypothesis is that the protein product of the adrenoleucodystrophy gene normally anchors very-long-chain

fatty acids into the peroxisomal membrane or translocates these into peroxisomes. The diagnosis may also be made by ultrastructural examination of nerve biopsied from the skin or conjunctiva which show typical curved clefts and leaflets in Schwann cells. Four related syndromes share this biochemical abnormality: childhood adrenoleucodystrophy and adult-onset adrenomyeloneuropathy are sex linked, whereas neonatal adrenoleucodystrophy and Zellweger's syndrome are autosomal recessive disorders (Moser 1997). About 25 per cent of cases are of adult onset with a progressive myelopathy developing in the third or fourth decade.

X-linked adrenoleucodystrophy may present in childhood with behavioural disturbance, dementia, and epilepsy, followed by involvement of the special senses and motor systems and leading to total disability within the first decade. Even though this is a dysmyelinating leucodystrophy, the aggressive childhood cases may show inflammatory demyelination with confluent symmetrical magnetic resonance imaging and spectroscopic (*N*-acetyl aspartate reduced and choline increased) abnormalities. The proposal is that VLCFAs trigger the inflammatory response which is mediated by TNF-α produced by activated microglia. Although a significant proportion of children later develop adrenal insufficiency, Addison's disease may precede the neurological manifestations by several years. Treatment has been proposed with a dietary supplement containing a 4 : 1 mixture of glyceryl trioleate and trierucate, popularly known as Lorenzo's oil. This lowers the plasma levels of VLCFA but appears not to influence the phenotype in individuals with established neurological disease, although there may yet be role in prophylaxis. Bone-marrow transplantation is successful in early symptomatic cases and, in view of the inflammatory reaction, trials of immunosuppression are in progress (reviewed by Moser 1997).

X-linked adrenomyeloneuropathy presents in adult men with spastic paraparesis and sensory loss in the legs; although clinicians may be alerted to unusual causes for this otherwise common neurological problem by the presence of peripheral nerve involvement, the diagnosis may be overlooked if adrenal insufficiency is not clinically or biochemically apparent at the time of presentation and unless VLCFAs are assayed. Some patients show a progressive cerebellar phenotype and intellectual function may be impaired with a subcortical pattern of dementia. The clinical phenotypes of childhood and adult adrenoleucodystrophy, which are usually quite distinct, may both be seen in the same family (Elrington *et al.* 1989). The availability of a biochemical assay that reliably identifies the peroxisomal defect in easily sampled body tissues or fluids, has inevitably led to the demonstration of cases with obscure clinical manifestations; these include focal cerebral lesions with imaging abnormalities, the Kluver–Bucy syndrome, dementia, spinocerebellar degeneration, and olivopontocerebellar atrophy.

About 20 per cent of female heterozygotes develop relatively mild, and occasionally remitting, spastic limb weakness and sensory loss, but cerebellar involvement is rare, as is cerebral or adrenal involvement; the age of onset is usually in the fourth or fifth decade. A higher proportion of manifesting carriers have neurological signs without clinical disabilities. Although adrenal disease is almost never present in carriers, VLCFAs are usually elevated and brain imaging or measurement of the auditory-evoked brainstem responses may help in diagnosis of the carrier state (O'Neill *et al.* 1983). The spinal fluid is usually normal, although oligoclonal bands have been described, and white matter lesions are occasionally seen on magnetic resonance imaging (Ménage *et al.* 1994). Such cases may first be diagnosed as having multiple sclerosis, but the symmetry of the lesions and their diffuseness (even if predominantly placed posteriorly in the early stages) differ from the usual findings in multiple sclerosis. The correct diagnosis can be established on the family history and by finding an excess of VLCFAs in plasma or fibroblasts. Adrenal failure may precede neurological involvement or present as X-linked Addison's disease without nervous system involvement (Josien *et al.* 1993). Biochemical abnormalities include reduced urinary excretion of 17-hydroxy-corticosteroids and 17 oxysteroids, with impaired response to corticotrophin but high basal levels; there may be associated androgen deficiency. All racial groups are affected by the sex-linked adrenoleucodystrophies and the gene has been mapped to the region of Xq28, close to that for glucose 6-phosphate dehydrogenase deficiency and colour blindness (Aubourg *et al.* 1990). It encodes a peroxisomal membrane protein (now known as ALD protein) belonging to the ATP-binding cassette protein family.

Autosomal recessive adrenoleucodystrophy presents in infancy with seizures, hypotonia, retardation, retinal degeneration, and hepatic involvement; females are more commonly affected than males. The pattern of organ involvement and mode of inheritance are similar in neonatal adrenoleucodystrophy and Zellweger's syndrome but these are thought to be separate disorders.

These X-linked recessive disorders can produce a clinical picture which mimics multiple sclerosis; the distinction is most reliably made on the basis that affected patients have or subsequently develop the clinical and biochemical manifestations of Addison's disease.

The sensitivity and specificity of routine assaying of VLCFAs has been reviewed (Moser *et al.* 1999): together, the level of hexacosanoic acid and its ratios to tetrasanoic and docosanoic acids are fully discriminating in homozygote males, irrespective of the clinical phenotype, from the day of birth, if dietary supplements have not been given, providing an opportunity for mass screening; there is a false negative rate of 15 per cent for heterozygotes.

29.6.4 Metachromatic leucodystrophy

The separation of metachromatic leucodystrophy from the heterogeneous group of diffuse sclerosis was first made when metachromatic material was detected in urinary deposits (Austin 1957). It subsequently became clear that the diagnosis can be confirmed by demonstrating increased urinary sulphatide excretion with a deficiency of arylsulphatase A in urine, peripheral blood leucocytes, and skin fibroblasts, or by the demonstration of metachromatic material in peripheral nerve biopsies which show segmental demyelination and remyelination. There is diffuse white matter involvement due to non-inflammatory demyelination with loss of oligodendrocytes, axon preservation, and reactive astrocytes which, together with macrophages, contain the metachromatic material, especially in the most extensively demyelinated areas.

The gene for arylsulphatase A is encoded on chromosome 22 and the clinical phenotype varies with the amount of surviving enzyme, depending on heterozygosity of the mutant allele; pseudo-deficiency refers to those individuals with low but sufficient levels of arylsulfatase A who do not have a clinical phenotype. Some affected individuals have a genetic defect of the arylsulphatase A activator (encoded on chromosome 10) and this is associated with a more complex pattern of sphingomyelin storage, biochemically and in terms of the tissue distribution. The most common form of metachromatic leucodystrophy develops in late infancy, with delayed walking and other motor milestones, due to the neuropathy which may be painful. There are also features of brainstem involvement and the emergence of diffuse upper motor neuron signs with reduced intellectual development, optic atrophy, and death within about 5 years from presentation. In older-onset childhood cases, after several years of normal development, there are behavioural changes with poor school performance, ushering a cerebellar and upper motor neuron pattern of disability which then follows much the same course as in the younger cases, although with less evidence for neuropathy. The early adult form of metachromatic leucodystrophy is rare, or perhaps seldom diagnosed, and tends to present with intellectual or emotional abnormalities; as with many other inherited disorders, onset after the age of 60 years has been described. Onset with dementia and behavioural disorders is usual, with ataxia, paralysis, and optic atrophy only developing at late stages, although the presentation is occasionally with paraparesis or cerebellar ataxia (Hageman *et al.* 1995) and the condition can then more easily be mistaken for multiple sclerosis. Clinical evidence for peripheral neuropathy may be revealed by slowed nerve conduction (Section 12.8.2). The full range of clinical manifestations has probably not yet been fully explored. For example, Sadeh *et al.* (1992) describe an apparently unique case with a relapsing–remitting course; more usually, the disorder is progressive with steady decline into dementia or persistent vegetative state. Treatments have included dietary manipulation with reduced vitamin A and sulphur-containing substances, and bone-marrow transplantation, but the successes are limited.

Multiple sulphatase deficiency combines the features of metachromatic leucodystrophy with mucopolysaccharidosis. It, too, has neonatal, early childhood, and juvenile forms. The pattern of combined motor and mental regression or lack of development reflecting widespread dysmyelination with peripheral neuropathy is associated with dysmorphic features and organomegaly. The more severe phenotype also reflects extensive neuronal loss due to the combination of stored sulphatide, sulphated steroids, and mucopolysaccharides. The enzyme defects are complex, involving many sulphatases other than arylsulphatase A.

29.6.5 Pelizaeus–Merzbacher disease

The three phenotypes of X-linked Pelizaeus–Merzbacher disease usually present in childhood. The clinical features which may distinguish the otherwise ubiquitous motor and developmental delay with epilepsy are abnormal eye movements, dystonia and choreoathetosis, and laryngeal paralysis. Affected individuals often stabilize with severe disabilities and live into early adult life. In the earlier-onset group (connatal), either sex may be affected, with X-linked and autosomal pedigrees; the phenotype has many of the same features but the course is more accelerated. There are also transitional cases of intermediate prognosis. Some cases do not manifest until early adult life but here the blur with specifically different disorders becomes more apparent. Magnetic resonance imaging either fails to show myelin or depicts myelin which is immature with an atrophic brain.

The molecular defect is a mutation of the gene for proteolipid protein (PLP: encoded on X-q21.2) and, in severe cases, this leads to extensive loss of myelin in the central nervous system, with patchy depletion of oligodendrocytes and axons. Proteolipid protein is normally involved in stabilizing the lamellar structure of central myelin. Biochemically, there is a reduction in sulphatide and cerebroside. Over 30 mutations have been described, and novel ones are still being identified, resulting in expression of truncated forms of PLP sufficient to cause extensive oligodendrocyte loss and failure of myelination (Aoyagi et al. 1999), but no one can be detected in most patients. Osaka et al. (1999) found causative mutations in 6 members of 27 families, and correlated severity of the phenotype and closely related X-linked hereditary spastic paraplegia (in which the closely related myelin protein DM20 may substitute for PLP) with these defects. Because more severe genetic mutations of PLP and DM20 are sometimes associated with a relatively mild phenotype, one mechanism for the dysmyelination is an increase in toxicity of mutant PLP through metabolic exertion of the compromised myelinating oligodendrocyte. Almost certainly, another genetic defect explains the non-X-linked families.

29.6.6 Adult-onset dominant leucodystrophies

Forms of dominantly inherited leucodystrophy also occur exclusively in adults and may closely resemble chronic progressive multiple sclerosis (Eldridge et al. 1984; Schwankhaus et al. 1994). Magnetic resonance imaging shows diffuse, non-discrete, white matter disease and there are no oligoclonal bands in the spinal fluid. It remains uncertain whether all the adult-onset dominant leucodystrophies are one and the same disorder, and many are difficult to distinguish from the complicated hereditary spastic paraplegias and CADASIL. The various phenotypes are gradually being classified as their biochemical and genetic defects are characterized. Fukazawa et al. (1997b) described a family with spastic paraparesis, ataxia, and mild dementia, presenting in adulthood but with onset in childhood; diffuse white matter abnormalities were present on cerebral magnetic resonance, whereas pathognomonic features of the other leucodystrophies were absent. The most recent addition to this group involves two siblings with behavioural abnormalities progressing to dementia, with extensive white matter magnetic resonance abnormalities, in whom brain biopsy showed glycolipid inclusions in macrophages unlike any other lysosomal storage disease (Simon et al. 1998).

References

Adams, R. D., Victor, M., and Mancall, E. L. (1959). Central pontine myelinolysis. *Arch. Neurol. Psych.*, **81**, 154–72.

Alam, S. M., Kyriakides, T., Lawden, M. *et al.* (1993). Methylprednisolone in multiple sclerosis: a comparison of oral with intravenous therapy at equivalent high dose. *J. Neurol. Neurosurg. Psychiatry*, **56**, 1219–20.

Alusi, S. H., Glickman, S., Aziz, T. Z. *et al.* (1999). Tremor in multiple sclerosis. *J. Neurol. Neurosurg. Psychiatry*, **66**, 131–4.

Amato, M. P., Ponziani, G., Pracucci, G. *et al.* (1995). Cognitive impairment in early-onset multiple sclerosis. Pattern, predictors, and impact on everyday life in a 4-year follow-up. *Arch. Neurol.*, **52**, 168–72.

Andersen, O., Lygner, P.-E., Berstrom, T. *et al.* (1991). Viral infections trigger multiple sclerosis relapses: a prospective seroepidemiological study. *J. Neurol.*, **240**, 417–22.

Aoyagi, Y., Kobayashi, H., Tanaka, K. *et al.* (1999). A de novo splice donor site mutation causes in-frame deletion of 14 amino acids in the proteolipid protein in Pelizaeus–Merzbacher disease. *Ann. Neurol.*, **46**, 112–15.

Archelos, J. J. and Hartung, H.-P. (1997). The role of adhesion molecules in multiple sclerosis: biology, pathogenesis and therapeutic implications. *Mol. Med. Today*, **3**, 310–21.

Aubourg, P., Feil, R., Guidoux, S. *et al.* (1990). The red–green visual pigment gene region in adrenoleucodystrophy. *Am. J. Hum. Genet.*, **46**, 459–69.

Austin, J. H. (1957). Metachromatic form of diffuse cerebral sclerosis. 1. Diagnosis during life by urine sediment examination. *Neurology*, **7**, 415–26.

Bamford, C. R., Sibley, W. A., Thies, C. *et al.* (1981). Trauma as an etiologic and aggravating factor in multiple sclerosis. *Neurology*, **31**, 1229–34.

Barnes, D. and McDonald, W. I. (1992). The ocular manifestations of multiple sclerosis 2. Abnormalities of eye movement. *J. Neurol. Neurosurg. Psychiatry*, **55**, 863–8.

Barnes, D., Hughes, R. A. C., Morris, R. W. *et al.* (1997). Randomised trial of oral and intravenous methylprednisolone in acute relapses of multiple sclerosis. *Lancet*, **349**, 902–6.

Bauer, H. J. and Hanefeld, F. A. (1993). *Multiple sclerosis: its impact from childhood to old age.* Saunders, London.

Benedikz, J. G., Magnusson, H., and Gudmundsson, G. (1994). Multiple sclerosis in Iceland, with observations on the alleged epidemic in the Faeroe Islands. *Ann. Neurol.*, **36** (Suppl. 2), S175–9.

Berman, M., Feldmann, S., Alter, M. *et al.* (1981). Acute transverse myelitis: incidence and aetiologic considerations. *Neurology*, **31**, 966–71.

Betts, C. D., D'Mellow, M. T., and Fowler, C. J. (1993). Urinary symptoms and the neurological features of bladder dysfunction in multiple sclerosis. *J. Neurol. Neurosurg. Psychiatry*, **56**, 245–50.

Betts, C. D., Jones, S. J., Fowler, C. G. *et al.* (1994). Erectile dysfunction in multiple sclerosis; associated neurological and neurophysical deficits, and treatment of the condition. *Brain*, **117**, 1303–10.

Biousse, V., Trichet, C., Bloch-Michel, E. *et al.* (1999). Multiple sclerosis associated with uveitis in two large clinic-based series. *Neurology*, **52**, 179–81.

Blok, B. F. M., Sturms, L. M., and Holstege, G. (1998). Brain activation during micturition in women. *Brain*, **121**, 2033–42.

Boman, J., Roblin, P. M., Sundstrom, P. *et al.* (2000). Failure to detect *Chlamydia pneumoniae* in the central nervous system of patients with MS. *Neurology*, **54**, 265.

Broggi, G., Ferroli, P., Franzini, A. *et al.* (2000). Microvascular decompression for trigeminal neuralgia: comments on a series of 250 cases, including 1) patients with multiple sclerosis. *J. Neurol. Neurosurg. Psychiatry*, **68**, 59–64.

Brunner, J. E., Redmond, J. M., Haggar, A. M. *et al.* (1990). Central pontine myelinolysis and pontine lesions after rapid correction of hyponatraemia: a prospective magnetic resonance imaging study. *Ann. Neurol.*, **27**, 61–6.

Carton, H., Vlietinck, R., Debruyne, J. *et al.* (1996). Recurrence risks of multiple sclerosis in relatives of patients in Flanders, Belgium. *J. Neurol. Neurosurg. Psychiatry*, **62**, 329–33.

Carton, H., Loos, R., Pacolet, J. *et al.* (1998). Utilisation and cost of professional care and assistance according to disability of patients with multiple sclerosis in Flanders (Belgium). *J. Neurol. Neurosurg. Psychiatry*, **64**, 444–50.

Coles, A. J., Paolili, A., Molyneux, P. *et al.* (1999a). Monoclonal antibody treatment exposes three mechanisms underlying the clinical course in multiple sclerosis. *Ann. Neurol.*, **46**, 296–304.

Coles, A. J., Wing, M. G., Hale, G. *et al.* (1999b). Pulsed monoclonal antibody treatment modulates T cell responses in multiple sclerosis but induces autoimmune thyroid disease. *Lancet*, **354**, 1691–5.

Compston, A. (1997). Genetic epidemiology of multiple sclerosis. *J. Neurol. Neurosurg. Psychiatry*, **62**, 553–61.

Compston, D. A. S. (1998a). The distribution of multiple sclerosis. In *McAlpine's multiple sclerosis*, (ed. D. A. S. Compston, G. C. Ebers, H. Lassmann, W. I. McDonald, W. B. Matthews, and H. Wekerle), pp. 63–100. Churchill Livingstone, London.

Compston, D. A. S. (1998b). Genetic susceptibility to multiple sclerosis. In *McAlpine's multiple sclerosis*, (ed. D. A. S. Compston, G. C. Ebers, H. Lassmann, W. I. McDonald, W. B. Matthews, and H. Wekerle), pp. 100–42. Churchill Livingstone, London.

Compston, D. A. S. (1998c). The neurobiology of multiple sclerosis. In *McAlpine's multiple sclerosis*, (ed. D. A. S. Compston, G. C. Ebers, H. Lassmann, W. I. McDonald, W. B. Matthews, and H. Wekerle), pp. 437–98. Churchill Livingstone, London.

Confavreux, C., Compston, D. A. S., Hommes, O. R. *et al.* (1992). EDMUS, an European database for multiple sclerosis. *J. Neurol. Neurosurg. Psychiatry*, **55**, 671–6.

Confavreux, C., Hutchinson, M., Marie-Hours, M. *et al.* (1998). Rate of pregnancy-related relapse in multiple sclerosis. *N. Engl. J. Med.*, **339**, 285–91.

Coraddu, F., Sawcer, S., Feakes, R. *et al.* (1999). HLA typing in the United Kingdom multiple sclerosis genome screen. *Neurogenetics*, **2**, 24–33.

Cottrell, D. A., Kremenchutzky, M., Rice, G. P. A. *et al.* (1999). The natural history of multiple sclerosis: a geographically based study. 5. The clinical features and natural history of primary progressive multiple sclerosis. *Brain*, **122**, 625–39.

Davie, C. A., Barker, G. J., Webb, S. *et al.* (1995). Persistent functional deficit in multiple sclerosis and autosomal dominant cerebellar ataxia is associated with axon loss. *Brain*, **118**, 1583–92.

Dean, G. (1967). Annual incidence, prevalence and mortality of MS in white South African-born and in white immigrants to South Africa. *BMJ*, **2**, 724–30.

De Stefano, N., Matthews, P. M., Fu, L. *et al.* (1998). Axonal damage correlates with disability in patients with relapsing–remitting multiple sclerosis: results of a longitudinal magnetic resonance spectroscopy study. *Brain*, **121**, 1469–77.

De Stefano, N., Narayanan, S., Matthews, P. M. *et al.* (1999). In vivo evidence for axonal dysfunction remote from focal cerebral demyelination of the type seen in multiple sclerosis. *Brain*, **122**, 1933–9.

Detels, R., Visscher, B., Malmgrem, R. M. *et al.* (1977). Evidence for lower susceptibility to multiple sclerosis in Japanese–Americans. *Am. J. Epidemiol.*, **105**, 303–10.

de Vries, E. (1960). *Postvaccinial perivenous encephalitis.* Elsevier, Amsterdam.

Dichgans, M., Mayer, M., Uttner, I. *et al.* (1998). The phenotypic spectrum of CADASIL: clinical findings in 102 cases. *Ann. Neurol.*, **44**, 731–9.

Djaldetti, R., Ziv, I., Achiron, A., and Melamed, E. (1996). Fatigue in multiple sclerosis compared with chronic fatigue syndrome: a quantitative assessment. *Neurology*, **46**, 632–5.

Dressnandt, J. and Conrad, B. (1996). Lasting reduction of severe spasticity after ending chronic treatment with intrathecal baclofen. *J. Neurol. Psychiatry*, **60**, 168–73.

Duquette, P., Murray, T. J., Pleines, J. *et al.* (1987). Multiple sclerosis in childhood: clinical profile in 125 patients. *J. Pediatr.*, **111**, 359–63.

Ebers, G. C., Sadovnick, A. D., and Risch, N. J. (1995). A genetic basis for familial aggregation in multiple sclerosis. *Nature*, **377**, 150–1.

Ebers, G. C., Kukay, K., Bulman, D. *et al.* (1996). A full genome search in multiple sclerosis. *Nature Genet.*, **13**, 472–6.

Ebers, G. C., Yee, I. M. L., Sadovnick, A. D. *et al.* (2000). Conjugal multiple sclerosis: population-based prevalence and recurrence risks in offspring. *Ann. Neurol.*, **48**, 927–31.

Edan, G., Miller, D. H., Clanet, M. *et al.* (1997). Therapeutic effect of mitoxantrone combined with methylprednisolone in multiple sclerosis: a randomised multi-center study of active disease using MRI and clinical criteria. *J. Neurol. Neurosurg. Psychiatry*, **62**, 112–18.

Eldridge, R., Anayiotos, C. P., Schlesinger, S. *et al.* (1984). Hereditary adult onset leukodystrophy simulating chronic progressive multiple sclerosis. *N. Engl. J. Med.*, **311**, 948–53.

Elian, M., Nightingale, S., and Dean, G. (1990). Multiple sclerosis among United Kingdom-born children of immigrants from the Indian subcontinent, Africa and the West Indies. *J. Neurol. Neurosurg. Psychiatry*, **53**, 906–11.

Ellis, S. J. (1995). Severe hyponatraemia: complications and treatment. *QJM*, **88**, 905–9.

Elrington, G. M., Bateman, D. E., Jeffrey, M. J., and Lawton, N. F. (1989). Adrenoleukodystrophy: heterogeneity in two brothers. *J. Neurol. Neurosurg. Psychiatry*, **52**, 310–13.

European Study Group on Interferon β-1b in Secondary Progressive MS (1998). Placebo-controlled multicentre randomised trial of interferon β-1b in treatment of secondary progressive multiple sclerosis. *Lancet*, **352**, 1491–7.

Fassas, A., Anagnostopolous, A., Kasis, A. *et al.* (1997). Peripheral blood stem cell transplantation in the treatment of progressive multiple sclerosis: first results of a pilot study. *Bone Marrow Transplant.*, **20**, 631–8.

Fazekas, F., Deisenhammer, F., Strasser-Fuchs, S. *et al.* (1997). Randomised placebo-controlled trial of monthly intravenous immunoglobulin therapy in relapsing–remitting multiple sclerosis. *Lancet*, **349**, 589–93.

Feinstein, A., du Boulay, G., and Ron, M. A. (1993). Psychotic illness in multiple sclerosis: a clinical and MRI study. *Br. J. Psychiatry*, **161**, 680–5.

Ferguson, B., Matyszak, M. K., Esiri, M. M. *et al.* (1997). Axonal damage in acute multiple sclerosis lesions. *Brain*, **120**, 393–9.

Filippi, M., Rocca, M. A., Martino, G. *et al.* (1998). Magnetization transfer changes in the normal appearing white matter precede the appearance of enhancing lesions in patients with multiple sclerosis. *Ann. Neurol.*, **43**, 809–14.

Foix, C. and Alajouanine, T. (1926). La myelite necrotique subaigue. *Rev. Neurol.*, **2**, 1–42.

Foong, J., Rozewicz, L., Quaghebeur, G. *et al.* (1997). Executive function in multiple sclerosis: the role of frontal lobe pathology. *Brain*, **120**, 15–26.

Fowler, C. J., Beck, R. O., Gerrard, S. *et al.* (1994). Intravesical capsaicin for treatment of detrusor hyperreflexia. *J. Neurol. Neurosurg. Psychiatry*, **57**, 169–73.

Freeman, J. A., Langdon, D. W., Hobart, J. C. *et al.* (1999). Inpatient rehabilitation in multiple sclerosis. Do the benefits carry over into the community? *Neurology*, **52**, 50–6.

French Research Group on Multiple Sclerosis (1992). Multiple Sclerosis in 54 twinships: concordance rate is independent of zygosity. *Ann. Neurol.*, **32**, 724–7.

Friedman, J. E., Lyons, M. J., Cu, G. *et al.* (1999). The association of the human herpesvirus-6 and MS. *Multiple Sclerosis*, **5**, 355–62.

Fu, L., Matthews, P. M., De Stefano, N. *et al.* (1998). Imaging axonal damage of normal appearing white matter in multiple sclerosis. *Brain*, **121**, 103–13.

Fukazawa, T., Moriwaka, F., Hamada, K. *et al.* (1997a). Facial palsy in multiple sclerosis. *J. Neurol.*, **244**, 483–8.

Fukazawa, T., Sasaki, H., Kikuchi, S. *et al.* (1997b). Dominantly inherited leukodystrophy showing cerebellar deficits, and spastic paraparesis: a new entity? *J. Neurol.*, **244**, 446–9.

Gaines, A. R. and Varricchio, F. (1998). Interferon beta-1b injection site reactions and necroses. *Multiple Sclerosis*, **4**, 70–3.

Garson, J. A., Tuke, P. W., Giraud, P. *et al.* (1998). Detection of virion-associated MSRV-RNA in serum of patients with multiple sclerosis. *Lancet*, **351**, 33.

Gasperini, C., Pozzilli, C. D., Bastianelli, S. *et al.* (1998). Effect of steroids on Gd-enhancing lesions before and during recoombinant beta interferon 1a treatment in relapsing remitting multiple sclerosis. *Neurology*, **50**, 403–6.

Gass, A., Kitchen, N., MacManus, D. C. R. *et al.* (1997). Trigeminal neuralgia in patients with multiple sclerosis: lesion localisation with MRI. *Neurology*, **49**, 1142–4.

Gayou, A., Brochet, B., and Dousset, V. (1997). Transitional progressive multiple sclerosis: a clinical and imaging study. *J. Neurol. Neurosurg. Psychiatry*, **63**, 396–8.

Gledhill, R. F., Harrison, B. M., and McDonald, W. I. (1973). Pattern of remyelination in the CNS. *Nature*, **244**, 443–4.

Goldstein, I., Lue, T. F., Padma-Nathan, H. *et al.* (1998). Oral sildenafil in the treatment of erectile dysfunction. *N. Engl. J. Med.*, **338**, 1397–404.

Goodkin, D. E., Rudick, R. A., VanderBrug Medendorp, S. *et al.* (1995). Low-dose (7.5 mg) oral methotrexate reduces the rate of progression in chronic progressive multiple sclerosis. *Ann. Neurol.*, **37**, 30–40.

Goodkin, D. E., Rudick, R. A., VanderBrug Medendorp, S. *et al.* (1996). Low-dose oral methotrexate in chronic progressive multiple sclerosis: analyses of serial MRIs. *Neurology*, **47**, 1153–7.

Granieri, E. and Casetta, I. (1997). Common childhood and adolescent infections and multiple sclerosis. *Neurology*, **49** (Suppl. 2), S42–54.

Greenberg, H. S., Werness, S. A. S., Pugh, J. E. *et al.* (1994). Short term effects of smoking marijuana on balance in patients with multiple sclerosis and normal volunteers. *Clin. Pharmacol. Ther.*, **51**, 292–6.

Grewel, R. P., Petronas, N., and Barton, N. W. (1991). Late onset globoid cell leukodystrophy. *J. Neurol. Neurosurg. Psychiatry*, **54**, 1011–12.

Hageman, A. T. H., Gabreels, F. J. M., de Jong, J. G. N. *et al.* (1995) Clinical symptoms of adult metachromatic leukodystrophy and arylsulfatase A pseudo deficiency. *Arch. Neurol.*, **52**, 408–13.

Hall, G., Compston, D. A. S., and Scolding, N. J. (1997). Beta interferon and multiple sclerosis. *Trends in Neurosciences*, **20**, 63–7.

Hall, G. L., Girdlestone, J., Compston, D. A. S. *et al.* (1999). Recall antigen presentation by gamma interferon activated microglia results in T cell proliferation, cytokine release and propagation of the immune response. *J. Neuroimmunol.*, **98**, 105–11.

Harding, A. E., Sweeney, M. G., Brockington, M. *et al.* (1992). Occurrence of a multiple sclerosis-like illness in women who have a Leber's hereditary optic neuropathy mitochondrial DNA mutation. *Brain*, **115**, 979–989.

Hawkins, S. A. and McDonnell, G. V. (1999). Benign multiple sclerosis? Clinical course, long term follow up, and assessment of prognostic factors. *J. Neurol. Neurosurg. Psychiatry*, **67**, 148–52.

He, B., Xu, C., Yang, B. *et al.* (1998). Linkage and association analysis of genes encoding cytokines and myelin proteins in multiple sclerosis. *J. Neuroimmunol.*, **86**, 13–19.

Hinds, J. P., Eidelman, B. H., and Wald, A. (1990). Prevalence of bowel dysfunction in multiple sclerosis: a population survey. *Gastroenterology*, **98**, 1538–42.

Hohlfeld, R. (1997). Biotechnical agents for the immunotherapy of multiple sclerosis. principles, problems and perspectives (review). *Brain*, **120**, 865–916.

Hooper, J. and Whittle, I. R. (1998). Long term outcome after thalamotomy for movement disorders in multiple sclerosis. *Lancet*, **352**, 1984.

Houtchens, M. K., Richert, J. R., Sami, A., and Rose, J. W. (1997). Open label gabapentin treatment for pain in multiple sclerosis. *Multiple Sclerosis*, **3**, 250–3.

Hulter, B. M. and Lundborg, P. O. (1995). Sexual function in women with advanced multiple sclerosis. *J. Neurol. Neurosurg. Psychiatry*, **59**, 83–6.

Hurst, E. W. (1941). Acute haemorrhagic leuco-encephalitis, a previously undefined entity. *Med. J. Aust.*, **2**, 1–6.

IFNB Multiple Sclerosis Study Group (1993). Interferon beta-1b is effective in relapsing–remitting multiple sclerosis. 1. Clinical results of a multicenter, randomized, double-blind, placebo-controlled trial. *Neurology*, **43**, 655–61.

IFNB Multiple Sclerosis Study Group and the University of British Columbia MS/MRI Analysis Group (1995). Interferon beta-1b in the treatment of multiple sclerosis: final outcome of the randomised controlled trial. *Neurology*, **45**, 1277–85.

Jacobs, L. D., Cookfair, D. I., Rudick, R. A. *et al.* (1996). Intramuscular interferon beta-1a for disease progression in relapsing multiple sclerosis. *Ann. Neurol.*, **39**, 285–94.

Jacobs, L. D., Beck, R. W., Simon, J. H. *et al.* (2000). Intramuscular interferon β-1a therapy initiated during a first demyelinating event in multiple sclerosis. CHAMPS Study Group. *N. Engl. J, Med.*, **343**, 898–304.

Jeffery, N. D. and Blakemore, W. F. (1997). Locomotor deficits induced by experimental spinal cord demyelination are abolished by spontaneous remyelination. *Brain*, **120**, 27–37.

Johnson, K. P., Brooks, B. R., Cohen, J. A. *et al.* (1995). Copolymer 1 reduces relapse rate and improves disability in relapsing–remitting multiple sclerosis: results of a phase III multicenter, double-blind placebo-controlled trial. *Neurology*, **45**, 1268–76.

Johnson, K., Brooks, B. R., Cohen, J. A. *et al.* (1998). Extended use of glatiramer acetate (Copaxone) is well tolerated and maintains its clinical effect on multiple sclerosis relapse rate and degree of disability. *Neurology*, **50**, 701–8.

Josien, E., Lefebvre, V., Vermesch, P. *et al.* (1993). Adrénoleucomyéloneuropathie de l'adulte. *Rev. Neurol. (Paris)*, **149**, 230–2.

Kahana, E., Zilber, N., Abramson, J. H. *et al.* (1994). Multiple sclerosis: genetic versus environmental aetiology: epidemiology in Israel updated. *J. Neurol.*, **241**, 341–6.

Karussis, D., Leker, R. R., Ashkenazi, A. *et al.* (1998). A subgroup of multiple sclerosis patients with anticardiolipin antibodies and unusual clinical manifestations: do they represent a new nosological entity? *Ann. Neurol.*, **44**, 629–34.

Kesselring, J., Miller, D. H., Robb, S. A. *et al.* (1990). Acute disseminated encephalomyelitis. MRI findings and the distinction from multiple sclerosis. *Brain*, 113, 291–302.

Khan, O. A. and Dhib-Jalbut, S. S. (1998). Neutralising antibodies to interferon β-1a and interferon β-1b in multiple sclerosis are cross reactive. *Neurology*, 51, 1698–702.

Khan, O. A. and Hebel, J. R. (1998). Incidence of exacerbations in the first 90 days of treatment with recombinant human interferon β-1b in patients with relapsing–remitting multiple sclerosis. *Ann. Neurol.*, 44, 138–9.

Kidd, D., Thorpe, J. W., Thompson, A. J. *et al.* (1993). Spinal cord MRI using multi-array coils and fast spin echo. II: Findings in multiple sclerosis. *Neurology*, 43, 2632–7.

Kidd, D., Barkhof, F., McConnell, R. *et al.* (1999). Cortical lesions in multiple sclerosis. *Brain*, 122, 17–26.

Koch-Henriksen, N., Bronnum-Hansen, H. *et al.* (1998). Underlying cause of death in Danish patients with multiple sclerosis: results from the Danish Multiple Sclerosis Registry. *J. Neurol. Neurosurg. Psychiatry*, 65, 56–9.

Kremenchutzky, M., Cottrell, D., Rice, G. *et al.* (1999). The natural history of multiple sclerosis: a geographically based study. 7. Progressive-relapsing and relapsing-progressive multiple sclerosis: a re-evaluation. *Brain*, 122, 1941–9.

Krupp, L. B., Coyle, P. K., Doscher, C. *et al.* (1995). Fatigue therapy in multiple sclerosis: results of a double-blind, randomiscd, parallel trial of amantidine, pemoline and placebo. *Neurology*, 45, 1956–61.

Kuokkanen, S., Gschwend, M., Rioux, J. D. *et al.* (1997). Genomewide scan of multiple sclerosis in Finnish multiplex families. *Am. J. Hum. Genet.*, 61, 1379–87.

Kurtzke, J. F. (1975). A reassessment of the distribution of multiple sclerosis. *Acta Neurol. Scand.*, 51, 110–57.

Kurtzke, J. F. (1983). Rating neurologic impairment in multiple sclerosis. An expanded disability status scale (EDSS). *Neurology*, 33, 1444–52.

Kurtzke, J. F. (1993). Epidemiologic evidence for multiple sclerosis as an infection. *Clin. Microbiol. Rev.*, 6, 382–427.

La Mantia, L., Eoli, M., Milanese, C. *et al.* (1994). Double-blind trial of dexamethasone versus methylprednisolone in multiple sclerosis acute relapses. *Eur. Neurol.*, 34, 199–203.

Lassmann, H. (1998). The pathology of multiple sclerosis. In *McAlpine's multiple sclerosis*, (ed. D. A. S. Compston, G. C. Ebers, H. Lassmann, W. I. McDonald, W. B. Matthews, and H. Wekerle), pp. 323–58. Churchill Livingstone, London.

Lee, M. A., Palace, J., Stabler, G. *et al.* (1999). Serum gelatinase B, TIMP-1 and TIMP-2 levels in multiple sclerosis. A longitudinal clinical and MRI study. *Brain*, 122, 191–7.

Lenercept Multiple Sclerosis Study Group and the University of British Columbia MS/MRI Analysis Group (1999). TNF neutralisation in MS. Results of a randomised, placebo-controlled multicenter study. *Neurology*, 53, 457–65.

Li, D. K. and Paty, D. W. (1999). The UBC MS/MRI Analysis Research Group 1999 magnetic resonance imaging results of the PRISMS trial: a randomized, double-blind, placebo-controlled study of the interferon-β1a in relapsing–remitting multiple sclerosis. *Ann. Neurol.*, 46, 197–206.

Lightman, S., McDonald, W. I., Bird, A. C. *et al.* (1987). Retinal venous sheathing in optic neuritis. Its significance for the pathogenesis of multiple sclerosis. *Brain*, 110, 405–14.

Lindsey, J. W., Hodgkinson, S., Mehta, R. *et al.* (1994a). Phase 1 clinical trial of chimeric monoclonal anti-CD4 antibody in multiple sclerosis. *Neurology*, 44, 413–19.

Lindsey, J. W., Hodgkinson, S., Mehta, R. *et al.* (1994b). Repeated treatment with chimeric anti-CD4 antibody in multiple sclerosis. *Ann. Neurol.*, 36, 183–9.

Lucchinetti, C. F., Kiers, L., O'Duffy, A. *et al.* (1997). Risk factors for developing multiple sclerosis after childhood optic neuritis. *Neurology*, 49, 1413–18.

Luchinetti, C., Bruck, W., Parisi, J. *et al.* (1999). A quantitative analysis of oligodendrocytes multiple sclerosis lesions: a study of 117 cases. *Brain*, 122, 2279–95.

Mandler, R. N., Davis, L. E., Jeffrey, D. R. *et al.* (1993). Devic's neuromyelitis optica: a clinicopathological study of 8 patients. *Ann. Neurol.*, 34, 162–8.

Marrosu, M. G., Muntoni, F., Murru, M. R. *et al.* (1992). HLA-DQB1 genotype in Sardinian multiple sclerosis: evidence for a key role of DQB1.0201 and DQB1.0302 alleles. *Neurology*, 42, 883–6.

Matthews, W. B. (1998a). The symptoms and signs of multiple sclerosis. In *McAlpine's multiple sclerosis*, (ed. D. A. S. Compston, G. C. Ebers, H. Lassmann, W. I. McDonald, W. B. Matthews, and H. Wekerle), pp. 145–90. Churchill Livingstone, London.

Matthews, W. B. (1998b). The differential diagnosis of multiple sclerosis and related disorders. In *McAlpine's multiple sclerosis*, (ed. D. A. S. Compston, G. C. Ebers, H. Lassmann, W. I. McDonald, W. B. Matthews, and H. Wekerle), pp. 223–50. Churchill Livingstone, London.

Mayne, M., Krishnan, J., Metz, L. *et al.* (1998). Infrequent detection of human herpesvirus 6 DNA in peripheral blood mononuclear cells from multiple sclerosis patients. *Ann. Neurol.*, 44, 391–4.

McDonald, W. I. (1998a). The pathophysiology of multiple sclerosis. In *McAlpine's multiple sclerosis*, (ed. D. A. S. Compston, G. C. Ebers, H. Lassmann, W. I. McDonald, W. B. Matthews, and H. Wekerle), pp. 358–78. Churchill Livingstone, London.

McDonald, W. I. (1998b). Diagnostic methods and investigations of multiple sclerosis. In *McAlpine's multiple sclerosis*, (ed. D. A. S. Compston, G. C. Ebers, H. Lassmann,

W. I. McDonald, W. B. Matthews, and H. Wekerle), pp. 251–79. Churchill Livingstone, London.

McIntosh-Michaelis, S. A., Roberts, M. H., Wilkinson, S. M. et al. (1991). The prevalence of cognitive impairment in a community survey of multiple sclerosis. Br. J. Clin. Psychol., 30, 333–48.

Ménage, P., Carreau, V., Tourbah, A. et al. (1994). Les adrénoleucodystrophies hétérozygotes symptomatiques de l'adulte: 10 cas. Rev. Neurol. (Paris), 149, 445–54.

Meng, I. D., Manning, B. H., Martin, W. J. et al. (1998). An analgesia circuit activated by cannabinoids. Nature, 395, 381–3.

Menger, H. and Jorg, J. (1999). Outcome of central pontine myelinolysis (n = 44). J. Neurol., 246, 700–5.

Mertens, C., Brassat, D., Reboul, J. et al. (1998). A systematic study of oligodendrocyte growth factors as candidates for genetic susceptibility to MS. Neurology, 51, 748–53.

Millefiorini, E., Gasperini, C., Pozzilli, C. et al. (1997). Randomized placebo-controlled trial of mitoxanthrone in relapsing–remitting multiple sclerosis: 24 month clinical and MRI outcome. J. Neurol., 244, 153–9.

Miller, A., Shapiro, S., Gershtein, R. et al. (1998). Treatment of multiple sclerosis with Copolymer-1 (Copaxone[R]) implicating mechanisms of Th1 to Th2/3 immune-deviation. J. Neuroimmunol., 92, 113–21.

Miller, D. H., Newton, M. R., and van der Poel, J. C. (1988). Magnetic resonance imaging of the optic nerve in optic neuritis. Neurology, 38, 175–9.

Miller, D. H., Molyneux, P. D., Barker, G. J. et al. (1999). Effect of interferon-β1b on magnetic resonance imaging outcomes in secondary progressive multiple sclerosis: results of a European multicenter, randomised, double-blind placebo-controlled trial. Ann. Neurol., 46, 850–9.

Miller, H. G., Stanton, J. B., and Gibbons, J. L. (1956). Parainfectious encephalomyelitis and related syndromes. QJ M, 25, 427–505.

Milligan, N. M., Newcombe, R., and Compston, D. A. S. (1987). A double blind controlled trial of high dose methylprednisolomne in patients with multiple sclerosis. I. Clinical effects. J. Neurol. Neurosurg. Psychiatry, 50, 511–16.

Molyneux, P. D., Kappos, L., Polman, C., et al. (2000). The effect of interferon β-1b treatment on MRI measures of cerebral atrophy in secondary progressive multiple sclerosis. European Study Group on Interferon β-1b in secondary progressive multiple sclerosis. Brain, 123, 2256–63.

Moreau, T., Thorpe, J., Miller, D. et al. (1994). Reduction in new lesion formation in multiple sclerosis following lymphocyte depletion with CAMPATH-IH. Lancet, 344, 298–301.

Moreau, T., Hale, G., Waldmann, H. et al. (1996). Cytokine release increases conduction block in partially demyelinated pathways due to multiple sclerosis. Brain, 119, 235–7.

Morrissey, S. P., Borruat, F. X., Miller, D. H. et al. (1995). Bilateral simultaneous optic neuritis in adults, clinical, imaging, serological and genetic studies. J. Neurol. Neurosurg. Psychiatry, 58, 70–4.

Moser, A. B., Kreiter, N., Bezman, L. et al. (1999). Plasma very long chain fatty acids in 3000 peroxisome disease patients and 29000 controls. Ann. Neurol., 45, 100–10.

Moser, H. W. (1997). Adrenoleukodystrophy: phenotype, genetics, pathogenesis and therapy. Brain, 120, 1485–508.

Moser, H. W., Moser, A. B., Frayer, K. K. et al. (1981). Adrenoleukodystrophy: increased plasma content of saturated very long chain fatty acids. Neurology, 31, 1241–9.

Multiple Sclerosis Genetics Group (1996). A complete genomic screen for multiple sclerosis underscores a role for the major histocompatibility complex. Nature Genet., 13, 469–71.

Mumford, C. J., Wood, N. W., and Kellar-Wood, H. F. (1994). The British Isles survey of multiple sclerosis in twins. Neurology, 44, 11–15.

Newell, K. L. and Kleinschmidt-Demasters, B. K. (1996). Central pontine myelinolysis at autopsy; a twelve year retrospective analysis. J. Neurol. Sci., 142, 134–9.

Nielsen, J. F., Sinkjaer, T., and Jakobsen, J. (1996). Treatment of spasticity with repetitive magnetic stimulation; a double-blind placebo-controlled study. Multiple Sclerosis, 2, 227–32.

Noseworthy, J. H., O'Brien, P., Erickson, B. J. et al. (1998). The Mayo Clinic–Canadian cooperative trial of sulfasalazine in active multiple sclerosis. Neurology, 51, 1342–52.

Olerup, O. and Hillert, J. (1991). HLA class II associated genetic susceptibility in multiple sclerosis: a critical evaluation. Tissue Antigens, 38, 1–15.

Oliveri, R. L., Valentino, P., Russo, C. et al. (1998). Randomized trial comparing two different high doses of methylprednisolone in MS: a clinical and MRI study. Neurology, 50, 1833–6.

O'Neill, B. P., Moser, H. W., and Saxena, K. M. (1982). Familial X-linked Addison disease as an expression of adrenoleukodystrophy (ALD): elevated C26 fatty acids in cultured skin fibroblasts. Neurology, 32, 543–7.

Oppenheimer, D. (1978). The cervical cord in multiple sclerosis. Neuropathol. and Appl. Neurobiol., 4, 151–62.

Optic Neuritis Study Group (1997a). Visual function 5 years after optic neuritis. Arch. Ophthalmol., 115, 1545–52.

Optic Neuritis Study Group (1997b). The 5-year risk of MS after optic neuritis. Experience of the Optic Neuritis Treatment Trial. Neurology, 49, 1404–13.

O'Riordan, J. I., Gallagher, H. L., Thompson, A. J. *et al.* (1996). Clinical, CSF, and MRI findings in Devic's neuromyleitis optica. *J. Neurol. Neurosurg. Psychiatry*, **60**, 382–7.

O'Riordan, J. I., Thompson, A. J., Kingsley, D. P. E. *et al.* (1998). The prognostic value of brain MRI in clinically isolated syndromes of the CNS. A 10-year follow-up. *Brain*, **121**, 495–503.

Ormerod, I. E. C. and McDonald, W. I. (1984). Multiple sclerosis presenting with progressive visual failure. *J. Neurol. Neurosurg. Psychiatry*, **47**, 943–46.

Osaka, H., Kawanishi, C., Inoue, K. *et al.* (1999). Pelizaeus–Merzbacher disease: three novel mutations and implication for locus heterogeneity. *Ann. Neurol.*, **45**, 59–64.

Parkin, P. J., Hierons, R., and McDonald, W. I. (1984). Bilateral optic neuritis: a long term follow-up. *Brain*, **107**, 951–64.

Paty, D. W., Li, D. K. B., and The IFNB Multiple Sclerosis Study Group (1993). Interferon beta-1b is effective in relapsing–remitting multiple sclerosis. MRI results of a multicenter, randomized, double-blind, placebo-controlled trial. *Neurology*, **43**, 662–7.

Paty, D. W., Studney, D., Redekop, K., *et al.* (1994). MS COSTAR: a computerised patient record adapted for clinical research purposes. *Ann. Neurol.*, **36** (Suppl.), S134–5.

Perron, H., Garson, J. A., Bedin, F. *et al.* (1997). Molecular identification of a novel retrovirus isolated from patients with multiple sclerosis. *Proc. Natl Acad. Sci. USA*, **94**, 7583–8.

Pinching, A. J. (1977). Clinical testing of Olfaction reassessed. *Brain*, **100**, 377–88.

Plant, G., Kermode, A. G., Turano, G. *et al.* (1992). Symptomatic retrochiasmal lesions in multiple sclerosis: clinical features, visual evoked potentials and magnetic resonance imaging. *Neurology*, **42**, 68–76.

Poser, C. M., Paty, D. W., Scheinberg, L. *et al.* (1983). New diagnostic criteria for multiple sclerosis: guidelines for research protocols. *Ann. Neurol.*, **13**, 227–31.

Poskanzer, D. C., Prenney, L. P., Sheridan, J. L., *et al.* (1980). Multiple sclerosis in the Orkney and Shetland Islands. 1. Epidemiology, clinical factors and methodology. *J. Epidemiol. Community Hlth*, **34**, 229–39.

Prineas, J. W., Barnard, R. O., Kwon, E. E. *et al.* (1993). Multiple sclerosis: remyelination of nascent lesions. *Ann. Neurol.*, **33**, 137–51.

PRISMS Study Group (1998). Randomised double-blind placebo-controlled study of interferon β-1a in relapsing/remitting multiple sclerosis. *Lancet*, **352**, 1498–504.

Pujol, J., Bello, J., Deus, J. *et al.* (1997). Lesions in the left arcuate fasciculus region and depressive symptoms in multiple sclerosis. *Neurology*, **49**, 1105–10.

Rand, K. H., Houck, H., Denslow, N. D. *et al.* (1998). Molecular approach to find targets for oligoclonal bands in multiple sclerosis. *J. Neurol. Neurosurg. Psychiatry*, **65**, 48–55.

Redford, E. J., Kapoor, R., Smith, K. J. (1997). Nitric oxide donors reversibly block axonal conduction: demyelinated axons are especially susceptible. *Brain*, **120**, 2149–57.

Riahi, F., Zijbendos, S., Narayanan, S. *et al.* (1998). Improved correlation between scores on the expanded disability status scale and cerebral lesion load in relapsing–remitting multiple sclerosis: results of the application of new imaging methods. *Brain*, **121**, 1305–12.

Riordan-Eva, P., Sanders, M. D., Govan, G. G. *et al.* (1995). The clinical features of Leber's hereditary optic neuropathy defined by the presence of pathogenic mitochondrial DNA mutation. *Brain*, **118**, 319–37.

Robertson, N. P., Fraser, M., Deans, J. *et al.* (1996). Age adjusted recurrence risks for relatives of patients with multiple sclerosis. *Brain*, **119**, 449–55.

Robertson, N. P., O'Riordan, J. I., Chataway, J. *et al.* (1997). Clinical characteristics and offspring recurrence rates of conjugal multiple sclerosis. *Lancet*, **349**, 1587–90.

Rodriguez, D., Della Gaspera, B., Zalc, B. *et al.* (1997). Identification of a Val 145 Ile substitution in the human myelin oligodendrocyte glycoprotein: lack of association with multiple sclerosis. *Multiple Sclerosis*, **3**, 377–82.

Rudd Bosch, J. L. R. and Groen, J. (1996). Treatment of refractory urge urinary incontinence with sacral spinal nerve stimulation in multiple sclerosis patients. *Lancet*, **348**, 717–19.

Rudick, R. A., Fisher, E., Lee, J. C. *et al.* (1999). Use of the brain parenchymal fraction to measure whole brain atrophy in relapsing-remitting MS. Multiple Sclerosis Collaborative Research Group. *Neurology*, **53**, 1698–704.

Runmarker, B. and Andersen, O. (1993). Prognostic factors in a multiple sclerosis incident cohort with twenty-five years of follow-up. *Brain*, **116**, 117–34.

Runmarker, B. and Andersen, O. (1995). Pregnancy is associated with a lower risk of onset and a better prognosis in multiple sclerosis. *Brain*, **118**, 253–61.

Sadeh, M., Kuritsky, A., Ben-David, E., and Goldhammer, Y. (1992). Adult metachromatic leucodystrophy with an unusual relapsing–remitting course. *Postgrad. Med. J.*, **68**, 192–5.

Sadovnick, A. D., Baird, P. A., and Ward, R. H. (1988). Multiple sclerosis; updated risks for relatives. *Am. J. Med. Genet.*, **29**, 533–41.

Sadovnick, A. D., Eisen, K., Ebers, G. C., and Paty, D. W. (1991). Cause of death in patients attending multiple sclerosis clinics. *Neurology*, **41**, 1193–6.

Sadovnick, A. D., Armstrong, H., Rice, G. P. A. *et al.* (1993). A population-based study of multiple sclerosis in twins: update. *Ann. Neurol.*, **33**, 281–5.

Sadovnick, A. D., Ebers, G. C., Dyment, D. A. *et al.* (1996a). Evidence for genetic basis of multiple sclerosis. *Lancet*, **347**, 1728–30.

Sadovnick, A. D., Remick, R. A., Allen, J. *et al.* (1996b). Depression and multiple sclerosis. *Neurology*, **46**, 628–32.

Sandberg-Wollheim, S., Bynke, H., Cronqvist, S. *et al.* (1990). A long term prospective study of optic neuritis: evaluation of risk factors. *Ann. Neurol.*, **27**, 386–93.

Sawcer, S., Jones, H. B., Feakes, R. *et al.* (1996). A genome screen in multiple sclerosis reveals susceptibility loci on chromosome 6p21 and 17q22. *Nature Genetics*, **13**, 464–8.

Schadlich, H.-J., Karber, H., and Felgenhauer, K. (1987). The prevalence of locally synthesised virus antibodies in various forms of multiple sclerosis. *J. Neurol. Sci.*, **80**, 343–9.

Schilder, P. (1912). Zur Kenntnis der sogenannten diffusen Sklerose (uber Encephalitis periaxalis diffusa). *Z. gesamte Neurol. Psychiatrie*, **10**, 1–60.

Schriver, H. M., Crusius, J. B. A., Uitehaag, B. M. J. *et al.* (1999). Association of interleukin-1β and interleukin-1 receptor antagonist genes with disease severity in MS. *Neurology*, **52**, 595–9.

Schwankhaus, J. D., Katz, D. A., Eldridge, R. *et al.* (1994). Clinical and pathological features of an autosomal dominant, adult-onset leukodystrophy simulating chronic progressive multiple sclerosis. *Arch. Neurol.*, **51**, 757–66.

Schwid, S. R., Petrie, M. D., McDermott, M. P. *et al.* (1997). Quantitative assessment of sustained-release 4-aminopyridine for symptomatic treatment of multiple sclerosis. *Neurology*, **48**, 817–21.

Scott, T. F., Bhagavatula, K., Snyder, P. J. *et al.* (1998). Transverse myelitis. Comparison with spinal cord presentations of multiple sclerosis. *Neurology*, **50**, 429–33.

Seiser, A., Schwarz, S., and Aichinger-Steiner, M. M. (1998). Parkinsonism and dystonia in central pontine and extrapontine myelinolyisis. *J. Neurol. Neurosurg. Psychiatry*, **65**, 119–21.

Sellebjerg, F., Frederiksen, J. L., Nielsen, P. M. *et al.* (1998). Double-blind, randomized, placebo-controlled study of oral, high-dose methylprednisolone in attacks of MS. *Neurology*, **51**, 529–34.

Sharrack, B. and Hughes, R. A. C. (1999). The Guy's Neurological Disability Scale. *Multiple Sclerosis*, **5**, 223–33.

Sharrack, B., Hughes, R. A. C., Soudain, S., *et al.* (1999). The psychometric properties of clinical rating scales used in multiple sclerosis. *Brain*, **122**, 141–59.

Sheean, G. L., Murray, N. M. F., Rothwell, J. C. *et al.* (1997). An electrophysiological study of the mechanism of fatigue in multiple sclerosis. *Brain*, **120**, 299–315.

Sheean, G. L., Murray, N. M. F., Rothwell, J. C. *et al.* (1998). An open-labelled clinical and electrophysiological study of 3,4-diaminopyridine in the treatment of fatigue in multiple sclerosis. *Brain*, **121**, 967–75.

Sibley, W. A., Bamford, C. R., and Clark, K. (1985). Clinical viral infections and multiple sclerosis. *Lancet*, **i**, 1313–15.

Sibley, W. A., Bamford, C. R., Clark, K. *et al.* (1991). A prospective study of physical trauma and multiple sclerosis. *J. Neurol. Neurosurg. Psychiatry*, **54**, 584–9.

Silber, M. H., Willcox, P. A., Bowen, R. M. *et al.* (1990). Neuromyelitis optica (Devic's syndrome) and pulmonary tuberculosis. *Neurology*, **40**, 934–8.

Simon, D. K., Rodriguez, M. L., Frosch, M. P. *et al.* (1998). A unique familial leucodystrophy with adult onset dementia and abnormal glycolipid storage: a new lysosomal disease. *J. Neurol. Neurosurg. Psychiatry*, **65**, 251–4.

Siva, A., Radhakrishnan, K., Kurland, L. T. *et al.* (1993). Trauma and multiple sclerosis: a population based cohort study from Olmsted County, Minnesota. *Neurology*, **43**, 1878–82.

Soderstom, M., Ya-Ping, J., Hillert, J., and Link, H. (1998). Optic neuritis. Prognosis for multiple sclerosis from MRI, CSF and HLA findings. *Neurology*, **50**, 708–14.

Solari, A., Filippini, G., Gasco, P. *et al.* (1999). Physical rehabilitation has a positive effect on disability in multiple sclerosis patients. *Neurology*, **52**, 57–62.

Soldan, S. S., Berti, R., Salem, N. *et al.* (1997). Association of human herpes virus 6 (HHV-6) with multiple sclerosis: increased IgM response to HHV-6 early antigen and detection of serum HHV-6 DNA. *Nature Med.*, **3**, 1394–7.

Sterns, R. H., Riggs, J. E., and Schochet, S. S. (1986). Osmotic demyelination syndrome following correction of hyponatraemia. *N. Engl. J. Med.*, **314**, 1535–42.

Stevenson, V. L., Leary, S. M., Losseff, N. A. *et al.* (1998). Spinal cord atrophy and disability in MS: A longitudinal study. *Neurology*, **51**, 234–8.

Tayyebeh Saditpour, B., Greer, J. M., and Pender, M. P. (1998). Increased circulating antiganglioside antibodies in primary and secondary progressive multiple sclerosis. *Ann. Neurol.*, **44**, 980–3.

Thomas, P. K., Walker, R. W. H., Rudge, P. R. *et al.* (1987). Chronic demyelinating peripheral neuropathy associated with multifocal central nervous system demyelination. *Brain*, **110**, 53–76.

Thomke, F., Lensch, E., Ringel, K. *et al.* (1997). Isolated cranial nerve palsies in multiple sclerosis. *J. Neurol. Neurosurg. Psychiatry*, **63**, 682–5.

Thompson, A. J., Kennard, C., Swash, M. *et al.* (1989). Relative efficacy of intravenous methylprednisolone and ACTH in the treatment of acute relapse in MS. *Neurology*, **39**, 969–71.

Thompson, A. J., Kermode, A. G., Wicks, D. *et al.* (1991). Major differences in the dynamics of primary and secondary progressive multiple sclerosis. *Ann. Neurol.*, **29**, 53–62.

Thompson, A. J., Polman, C. H., Miller, D. H. *et al.* (1997). Primary progressive multiple sclerosis (review). *Brain*, **120**, 1085–96.

Thorpe, J. W., Kidd, D., and Kendall, B. E. (1993). Spinal cord MRI using multi-array coils and fast spin echo. I: Technical aspects and findings in healthy adults. *Neurology*, **43**, 2625–31.

Tienari, P., Kuokkanen, S., Pastinen, T. *et al.* (1998). Golli-MBP gene in multiple sclerosis. *J. Neuroimmunol.*, **81**, 158–67.

Tranchant, C., Bhatia, K. P., and Marsden, C. D. (1995). Movement disorders in multiple sclerosis. *Movement Disorders*, **10**, 418–23.

Trapp, B. D., Peterson, J., Ransohoff, R. M. *et al.* (1998). Axonal transection in the lesions of multiple sclerosis. *N. Engl. J. Med.*, **338**, 278–85.

Tremlett, H. L., Luscombe, D. K., and Wiles, C. M. (1998). Use of corticosteroids in multiple sclerosis by consultant neurologists in the United Kingdom. *J. Neurol. Neurosurg. Psychiatry*, **65**, 362–5.

Turbridy, N., Behan, P. O., Capildeo, R. *et al.* (1999). The effect of anti-α4 integrin antibody on brain lesion activity in MS. *Neurology*, **53**, 466–72.

Tyler, K. L., Gross, R. A., and Cascino, G. D. (1986). Unusual viral causes of transverse myelitis: hepatitis A virus and cytomegalovirus. *Neurology*, **36**, 855–8.

United Kingdom Tizanidine Trial Group (1994). A double-blind, placebo-controlled trial of tizanidine in the treatment of spasticity caused by multiple sclerosis. *Neurology*, **44** (Suppl. 9), S70–8.

van der Knaap, M. S. and Valk, J. (1995). *Magnetic resonance of myelin, myelination and myelin disorders*. Springer, Berlin.

van Oosten, B. W., Lai, M., Hodgkinson, S. *et al.* (1997). Treatment of multiple sclerosis with the monoclonal anti-CD4 antibody cM-T412; results of a randomised, double-blind, placebo-controlled, MR monitored phase II trial. *Neurology*, **49**, 351–7.

van Waesberghe, J. H. T. M., Kamphorst, W., De Groot, C. J. A. *et al.* (1999). Axonal loss in multiple sclerosis lesions: magnetic resonance imaging insights into substrates of disability. *Ann. Neurol.*, **46**, 747–54.

Walther, E. U. and Hohlfeld, R. (1999). Multiple sclerosis. Side effects of interferon beta therapy and their management. *Neurology*, **53**, 1622–7.

Wanders, R. J. A., van Roermund, C. W. T., van Wijland, M. J. A. *et al.* (1988). X linked adrenoleukodystrophy: identification of the primary defect at the level of a deficient peroxisomal very long chain fatty acyl CoA synthetase using a newly developed method for the isolation of peroxisomes from skin fibroblasts. *Journal of Inherited and Metabolic Diseases*, **11** (Suppl. 2), 173–7.

Weber, F., Ploak, T., Gunther, A. *et al.* (1998). Synergistic immunomodulatory effects of interferon-β1b and the phosphodiesterase inhibitor pentoxyfilline in patients with relapsing-remitting multiple sclerosis. *Ann. Neurol.*, **44**, 27–34.

Weese, D., Roskamp, D., Leach, G. *et al.* (1993). Intravesical oxybutinin chloride: experience with 42 patients. *Urology*, **41**, 527–30.

Weinshenker, B. G., Bass, B., Rice, G. P. *et al.* (1989). The natural history of multiple sclerosis: A geographically based study. 2. Predictive value of the early clinical course. *Brain*, **112**, 1419–28.

Weinshenker, B. G., Bass, B., Rice, G. P. *et al.* (1991). The natural history of multiple sclerosis: A geographically based study. 3. Multivariate analysis of predictive factors and models of outcome. *Brain*, **114**, 1045–56.

Weinshenker, B. G., Penman, M., and Bass, B. (1992). A double-blind, randomised controlled trial of pemoline in fatigue associated with multiple sclerosis. *Neurology*, **42**, 1468–71.

Weinshenker, B. G., O'Brien, P. C., Petterson, T. M. *et al.* (1999). A randomized trial of plasma exchange in acute central nervous system inflammatory demyelinating disease. *Ann. Neurol.*, **46**, 878–86.

Whetton-Goldstein, K., Sloan, F. A., and Kulas, E. D. (1998). A comprehensive assessment of the cost of multiple sclerosis in the United States. *Multiple Sclerosis*, **4**, 419–25.

Wingerchuk, D. M., Hogancamp, W. F., O'Brien, P. C. *et al.* (1999). The clinical course of neuromyelitis optica (Devic's syndrome). *Neurology*, **53**, 1107–14.

Wright, D. G., Laureno, R., and Victor, M. (1979). Pontine and extrapontine myelinolysis. *Brain*, **102**, 361–85.

Xiao, B.-G., Linington, C., and Link, H. (1991). Antibodies to myelin–oligodendrocyte glycoprotein in cerebrospinal fluid from patients with multiple sclerosis and controls. *J. Neuroimmunol.*, **31**, 91–6.

Yong, V. W., Chabot, S., Stuve, O. *et al.* (1998). Interferon beta in the treatment of multiple sclerosis: mechanism of action. *Neurology*, **51**, 682–9.

Youl, B. D., Turano, G., Miller, D. H. *et al.* (1991). The pathophysiology of acute optic neuritis: an association of gadolinium leakage with clinical and electrophysiological deficits. *Brain*, **114**, 2437–50.

Yudkin, P. L., Ellison, G. W., Ghezzi, A. *et al.* (1991). Overview of azathioprine treatment in multiple sclerosis. *Lancet*, **338**, 1051–5.

Zajicek, J. P., Wing, M., Scolding, N. J. *et al.* (1992). Interactions between oligodendrocytes and microglia, a major role for complement and tumour necrosis factor in oligodendrocyte adherence and killing. *Brain*, **115**, 1611–31.

Zajicek, J. P., Scolding, N. J., Foster, O. *et al.* (1999). Central nervous system sarcoidosis—diagnosis and management. *QJM*, **92**, 103–17.

Zipp, F., Weil, J. G., and Einhaupl, K. M. (1999). No increase in demyelinating diseases after hepatitis B vaccination. *Nature Med.*, **5**, 964–5.

CHAPTER 30

Cancer and the nervous system

Alastair Compston

30.1 Introduction

Primary neoplasms often spread to the central nervous system and in many patients neurological symptoms first draw attention to the presence of an underlying malignancy. Tumours may spread by direct invasion from neighbouring sites or by blood-borne metastasis. As a result, discrete secondary tumours grow within the substance of the brain or spinal cord, compress these tissues by external growth, or infiltrate along nerves and meningeal planes as diffuse sheets of malignant tissue. In other situations, neurological syndromes occur as remote effects of malignant disease. Here, the clinical manifestations are much more stereotyped and only a few tumour types are involved. Several mechanisms are involved in these characteristic paraneoplastic syndromes.

30.2 Invasion of the nervous system by tumour

Primary and secondary tumours affecting the nervous system, skull, and spinal canal are considered in detail elsewhere (Sections 18.6, 18.9, 20.5.3). Those arising from neighbouring structures which directly invade the nervous system are comparatively rare. They include chordomas, osteomas, chondromas, and sarcomas of bone; glomus jugulare tumours; and malignant tumours arising in the orbit, nasal sinuses, and nasopharynx. Granulomatous, vasculitic, and infectious disease of the nasal sinuses can mimic invasive tumour. The most common primary carcinomas likely to produce cerebral metastases arise from the bronchus, breast, kidney, stomach, and thyroid. Not infrequently, symptoms of cerebral metastasis often first bring the patient to medical attention. At the other extreme—especially in the case of breast cancer—there may be a latent interval of many years between the seemingly successful removal of a primary growth and development of a cerebral metastasis. Brain imaging often demonstrates multiple metastases, only one of which is causing clinical symptoms.

In general, the management of multiple cerebral metastases is palliative, but there may be indications for removing the solitary deposit and a strategically placed lesion causing significant morbidity even when multiple metastases have been demonstrated. In general, the dividend from chemotherapy or whole-brain X-irradiation is low, not least because the genuinely isolated secondary deposit is rare. Russell and Rubinstein (1989) found a single secondary cerebral bronchial tumour in 30 per cent of 117 cases but metastases were almost invariably present in other organs.

Peripheral plexuses or nerves are sometimes invaded either by diffuse primary spread or metastatic growth from neighbouring lymph nodes (Section 13.5.2). The brachial plexus and phrenic or recurrent laryngeal nerves are directly involved in tumours arising at the apex of the lung (Pancoast's tumour) but also in carcinoma of the thyroid and breast. Recurrent malignancy can be difficult to distinguish from radiation neuritis in patients who develop painful brachial plexopathies in the context of previous local treatment for apical lung or axillary breast carcinomas (Section 13.5.3). Infiltration of the lumbosacral plexus by pelvic cancer, usually of the uterus or rectum, manifests as lower limb pain, weakness, and sensory loss. Involvement of peripheral nerves by haematogenous metastases is rare, except in lymphoma, although several nerves may be diffusely infiltrated producing a clinical picture that mimics peripheral neuropathy. Isolated metastasis and diffuse infiltration of skeletal muscle are recognized pathologically but usually asymptomatic.

30.3 Carcinomatous meningitis

Deposits in the bones of the skull base often cause intractable headache and cranial nerve palsies. Tumour spread along meningeal planes can lead to the syndrome of carcinomatous meningitis (Section 18.10). The clinical manifestations are of multiple and bilateral lower cranial nerve palsies together with long-tract signs and evidence for meningeal irritation. The cerebrospinal fluid contains a few cells, some of which are reactive lymphocytes, but it may be difficult to confirm that others are malignant unless immunocytochemical methods are used to detect cell-surface markers of tumour antigens, and repeated samples assessed. The glucose concentration is usually reduced. The combination of severely glycorrhachic cerebrospinal fluid with a slight mononuclear pleocytosis should always raise the suspicion of carcinomatous or lymphomatous meningitis. Except in places with a high prevalence of HIV infection, this is a much more common cause of low cerebrospinal fluid glucose than fungal or tuberculous infection of the central nervous system. The prognosis is extremely poor and treatment usually ineffective, other than in providing relief from symptoms.

30.4 Neurological complications of reticuloendothelial malignancies

Lymphoproliferative disorders frequently involve the central and peripheral nervous systems. Several mechanisms other than direct spread may be involved. Malignancies that reduce immune competence expose individuals to opportunistic infection by cryptococcosis and other fungi, protozoa such as toxoplasmosis, unusual manifestations of herpes viridae, measles, and cytomegalovirus, and progressive multifocal leucoencephalopathy (see Henson and Urich 1982). Some haematological malignancies and non-Hodgkin's lymphomas are associated with alterations in blood viscosity which manifest as spontaneous thromboses in cerebral arteries and venous sinuses (Section 27.4.6).

30.4.1 Myeloma and paraproteinaemic disorders

Myeloma may arise within the bones of the skull, orbit, or spine, and may then secondarily invade the nervous system. Headache, nausea, vomiting, and malaise are systemic symptoms sometimes misconstrued as resulting from direct intracranial disease. One or more cranial nerves may be compressed but the optic neuropathy is not necessarily associated with deposits—and may be reversible. Myeloma may compress the spinal cord, cauda equina, or spinal roots. Plasma cells can usually be recovered from the cerebrospinal fluid in the context of meningeal involvement. Symptomatic herpes zoster, hypercalcaemic encephalopathy, and the carpal tunnel syndrome also complicate myelomatosis.

Polyneuropathy, not resulting from compression of nervous structures by tumour tissue, is a common complication of multiple myeloma (Kelly et al. 1981) (Section 12.12.2). Very severe mixed neuropathies may also occur with osteosclerotic metastatic multiple myeloma or plasmacytoma (Read and Warlow 1978; Kelly et al. 1983). In its most extreme form, this syndrome is associated with peripheral neuropathy, organomegaly, endocrine disorders, M protein, and skin disease (POEMS) (Bardwick et al. 1980) (Section 12.12.3). These are usually demyelinating neuropathies in which profound slowing of nerve conduction typically produces postural and intention tremor. However, the neuropathy is sometimes predominantly axonal. Either is characteristically painful. Systemic amyloidosis may complicate multiple myeloma, and amyloid laid down in peripheral nerves may contribute to the neuropathy (Section 12.9.2). Chemotherapy does not usually improve the neuropathy but solitary myelomas respond to irradiation, as does the polyneuropathy that complicates osteosclerotic myeloma (Kelly et al. 1983).

Twenty-five per cent of patients with Waldenström's macroglobulinaemia develop neurological complications. Many are due to increased serum viscosity with vascular occlusion; others result from the increased tendency for intracranial haemorrhage. The principal abnormalities are retinopathy with papilloedema and haemorrhages, and features of encephalopathy. Progressive cerebellar ataxia has been described in the absence of hyperviscosity. Several myelopathic syndromes are associated with macroglobulinaemia but these are probably explained on the basis of one or other vascular mechanisms and merely reflect the location of these complications within the neuraxis. Peripheral neuropathy, usually resulting both from demyelination and axonal degeneration, occurs in about 8 per cent of cases. There may be deposition of macroglobulin and IgM within the myelin sheaths of affected nerve fibres (Julien *et al.* 1978). Symptoms due to increased blood viscosity can be relieved by plasmapheresis.

These neuropathies, and that more typically associated with benign IgM-κ gammopathy (Smith *et al.* 1983; Ilyas *et al.* 1984), have a different pathogenesis from other tumour-associated syndromes (Section 12.12.1). Each is a primary demyelinating neuropathy associated with severe slowing of nerve conduction. In many cases the IgM-κ paraprotein is specific for myelin-associated glycoprotein, a structural component of the myelin sheath that functions as an adhesion molecule at the Schwann cell axonal junction. Since there is an increased prevalence of symptomatic neuropathy in patients with IgM paraproteinaemia having myelin-associated glycoprotein specificity, it is probable that this auto-antibody is directly pathogenic to peripheral myelin.

Typically, paraprotein-associated neuropathy presents with a slowly progressive mixed motor and sensory neuropathy. That associated with IgG gammopathy is perhaps more likely to show a relapsing–remitting course, similar to some otherwise typical cases of chronic inflammatory demyelinating polyneuropathy. The much rarer IgA-associated cases often manifest a pure motor neuropathy. These disorders may respond to corticosteroids and immunosuppression—although the mild course in many makes either unnecessary. A few of these patients later develop myeloma or Waldenström's macroglobulinaemia. Sudden deterioration in the course of the neuropathy should therefore prompt re-evaluation of the status of the underlying monoclonal gammopathy in order to exclude malignant transformation or the development of a discrete plasma cell lesion.

Some paraproteins act as cryoglobulins—precipitating when cooled and dissolving with heat. The syndrome of cryoglobulinaemia may occur alone or as a complication of plasma-cell dyscrasia. Other than the cold-associated peripheral vascular syndromes and strokes, cryoglobulinaemia may be complicated by peripheral neuropathy which progresses in a step-wise fashion following each episode, and may therefore be asymmetric, affecting both cranial and peripheral nerves but soon summating to the picture of a generalized neuropathy (Section 12.15.4).

30.4.2 Leukaemia

Neurological complications of acute leukaemia in childhood have been reported with increasing frequency and are attributed to the longer survival achieved with modern treatment. But central nervous system involvement, either at presentation or during the course of the disease, is a relatively poor prognostic feature. The neurological features are seen most often, but not exclusively, in lymphoblastic leukaemia. This complication manifests as subacute meningitis, multiple cranial nerve palsies, especially affecting the facial nerves, and raised intracranial

pressure. Leukaemic cells reach the nervous system by vascular or lymphatic routes and directly across meningeal barriers. Cerebral involvement has been attributed to the entry of leukaemic cells into the brain at sites of intracranial petechial haemorrhage.

The clinical features are most often attributable to malignant meningitis with headache, drowsiness, neck stiffness, and cranial or nerve root involvement. Diagnosis is confirmed by examination of the spinal fluid after brain imaging to exclude intracranial mass lesions. These can occur in isolation, affecting any part of the central nervous system, manifesting as any other mass lesion at that site. One characteristic mass lesion is the orbital or cerebello-pontine angle (mastoid) syndromes produced by chloromas, solid deposits of acute or chronic myeloid leukaemia—often with evidence for a generalized increase in intracranial pressure. An hypothalamic disorder is also well recognized as a focal syndrome complicating childhood leukaemias. Meningitis occurs typically in acute lymphoblastic leukaemia of childhood but can complicate other types, especially acute myelomonocytic leukaemia associated with abnormalities of chromosome 16. Peripheral nerve involvement is also usually due to diffuse infiltration, or the effects of treatment, but cases of paraneoplastic neuropathy are described.

A variety of vascular syndromes are seen in leukaemia due to increased haemorrhage in association with thrombocytopaenia and disseminated intravascular coagulopathy (Section 27.4.6). Since the outlook is worse when the central nervous system is involved early in children with acute lymphoblastic leukaemia, and relapse rates are lower when effective prophylactic neuraxis treatment is given before neurological symptoms develop, the combination of intrathecal methotrexate and craniospinal irradiation is probably most effective for prophylaxis. However, apart from the well-recognized incidence of peripheral neuropathy, chemotherapy brings a new set of problems for the patient with leukaemia and related disorders. Many of the neurotoxic agents also show effects on the central nervous system (Delattre and Posner 1995): cisplatin is associated with myelopathy, encephalopathy, vestibular symptoms, and optic neuropathy; vincristine with encephalopathy; nitrosoureas with ocular toxicity and encephalopathy; 5-fluorouracil with a cerebellar syndrome; cytosine arabinoside with meningitis, cerebellar disturbance, encephalopathy, and myelopathy; methotrexate with a necrotizing myelopathy and encephalopathy. The neurological features are more likely to result from intrathecal or arterial delivery of the chemotherapeutic agents into the nervous system, and especially when initial treatment also involves cranial radiotherapy. Aside from the acute toxicity, transient encephalopathy can develop within a few months of radiotherapy and there is a late necrotizing white matter disorder which manifests either as recurrence of the initial symptoms or signs for which treatment was given, as a new focal syndrome related to the anatomy of previous restricted therapy, or as a diffuse encephalopathy.

Bone-marrow transplantation is also associated with neurological disease (Section 5.6). The majority of individuals undergoing allogeneic bone-marrow transplantation develop neurological signs or neuropsychological abnormalities at late follow-up, with evidence from brain imaging for atrophy and focal white matter abnormalities. There is a strong association with the development of chronic graft-versus-host disease and prior immunosuppression, perhaps leading to angiitis (Padovan *et al.* 1998, 1999); for this reason, neurological complications are less often seen after autologous bone-marrow transplantation.

30.4.3 Lymphomas

It has long been recognized that intracerebral deposits of Hodgkin's lymphoma, follicular lymphoma, reticulum cell sarcoma, and lymphosarcoma may produce symptoms and signs of a space-occupying lesion, while spinal-cord, cauda equina or root compression, symptomatic herpes zoster, and peripheral nerve or plexus lesions are even more common. Primary lymphoma, previously classified as microglioma, is now routinely diagnosed radiologically and with brain biopsy using immunocytochemical markers which identify the B-cell origin (Section 18.8.3). The tumour is commonly multifocal. Many arise in previously healthy individuals but risk factors include previous immunosuppressive therapy, organ transplantation, HIV infection, and genetically determined abnormalities of immune function. Diagnosis may be possible from cytological analysis of the cerebrospinal fluid. The presentation is similar to that of other tumours of the nervous system, with focal deficits and the symptoms of raised intracranial pressure, but special features include meningeal involvement and uveitis. Given the favourable response to corticosteroids and radiotherapy, detection of central nervous system lymphoma is a major indication for obtaining a tissue diagnosis in patients with space-taking lesions on brain imaging, even when these are multifocal. Although cerebral lymphoma may be complicated by paraneoplastic neuropathy, primary origin in the spinal cord or peripheral nerves is rare.

Mass lesions due to Hodgkin's disease are seen more frequently with the advent of improved imaging and with better survival from initial therapy, but are still more common with non-Hodgkin's lymphoma. Treatment is with radiotherapy for solitary lesions, or chemotherapy if there is evidence for meningeal involvement. All types of lymphoma may be deposited in the epi- or subdural space and this is seen particularly in the spinal column.

Lymphomatous meningitis (Section 18.10) is more common in non-Hodgkin's lymphoma than are intracerebral deposits, and multiple cranial nerve palsies are a well-recognized clinical presentation. Cells gain access to the central nervous system by vascular and lymphatic routes and through direct spread. This syndrome is particularly associated with histologically undifferentiated lymphomas and leukaemia complicating lymphoma. Other risk factors include widespread involvement of solid organs and prior chemotherapy. The clinical features are much as in any other malignant meningitis. Burkitt's lymphoma, associated with Epstein–Barr virus infection, is frequently complicated by neurological involvement of cranial nerves adjacent to the infiltrated mandible or maxilla, but with a significant frequency of metastatic deposits throughout the neuraxis producing the usual range of meningeal, cerebral, spinal, and peripheral nerve-root compressive syndromes.

Polyneuropathy may result from diffuse infiltration of nerves roots or plexuses by lymphoma or from paraneoplastic mechanisms similar to those which complicate carcinoma (Sections 12.12.4, 13.5.2).

Neoplastic angioendotheliosis, in which small arterioles and capillaries are obliterated by malignant cells, causing multifocal infarction throughout the neuraxis, is a rare manifestation of systemic cancer (Dolman *et al.* 1979). It is often confused with the cerebral vasculitides, the correct diagnosis emerging when tissue is available for histological analysis using immunocytochemical markers which identify the infiltrating B lymphocytes (Section 28.17).

The lymphomas and leukaemias are complicated by opportunistic infections arising from immunological consequences of the conditions and their treatments. Thus, clinicians should be alert to the possibility of infection by Listeria monocytogenes, Toxoplasma, Cryptococcus, Candida, and Aspergillus—as well as infections such as tuberculosis, which also manifest without the advantage of the immunocompromised host, and persistent viral infections.

30.5 Progressive multifocal leucoencephalopathy

Progressive multifocal leucoencephalopathy (Section 34.10) is an opportunistic viral infection of the central nervous system characterized by foci of demyelination in the white matter of the cerebral hemispheres, sometimes also involving the brainstem, cerebellum, and the spinal cord (Richardson 1965; Henson and Urich 1982). Progressive multifocal leucoencephalopathy was formerly a rare disorder, usually occurring as a terminal event in patients suffering from the reticuloses and the leukaemias, and occasionally in sarcoidosis, tuberculosis, carcinomatosis, or apparently healthy individuals, but it has emerged as one of the common neurological manifestations of HIV1 infection (Berger *et al.* 1987). The pathological lesions vary in size and usually consist of areas with confluent demyelination and axon preservation. Inflammatory cell infiltration is absent, but the astrocytes are characteristically enlarged, often with bizarre and mitotic nuclei. Oligodendrocytes show pale nuclei and contain inclusion bodies. Brain imaging shows multiple low-attenuation areas. It results from opportunistic invasion of the nervous system in patients with defective immune responses by papovavirus (Zu Rhein and Chou 1965), which can be detected within affected oligodendrocytes; the agent has been characterized as one of the polyoma SV subgroup of papovaviruses, now generally called the JC type, but SV40 and BK viridae have also been implicated. The demyelination results from viral destruction of oligodendrocytes.

Progressive multifocal leucoencephalopathy is characterized by symptoms of massive destruction of cerebral or cerebellar white matter, producing convulsions, quadriplegia, aphasia, visual-field defects including blindness, dysarthria, and ataxia, leading eventually to coma and death. The cerebrospinal fluid is usually normal. Other opportunistic infections (especially cryptococcosis or listerosis) to which immunocompromised patients are also vulnerable sometimes further complicate the clinical picture. The disorder usually terminates fatally in 3–6 months from onset, but treatment with antiviral drugs is occasionally associated with prolonged survival.

30.6 Paraneoplastic diseases of the nervous system

Primary cancers, notably those affecting the lung, breast, and ovary, cause a number of relatively stereotyped syndromes through remote effects (Brain and Norris 1965; Posner 1995; Dalmau and Posner 1996). These are known collectively as the paraneoplastic neurological syndromes. Some tumours secrete bioactive peptides and hormones which directly produce endocrine non-metastatic phenotypes, but these do not affect the central or peripheral nervous system routinely. Most of the paraneoplastic disorders are immunologically mediated (Dropcho 1989). Some result from the synthesis by tumours of antibodies with antineuronal specificity. These tend to involve the peripheral nervous system. In other situations, the tumour expresses an epitope which stimulates an antitumour immune response, having molecular mimicry with normal neurons (Carpentier et al. 1998). These tend to affect the central nervous system and the target antigens are cytoplasmic or nuclear. Whereas previously these conditions required tissue diagnosis, several can now be defined serologically (Anderson et al. 1988a; Posner 1995).

The separate syndromes seen in the context of paraneoplastic disease are described below, but these may occur in clusters. Despite these discrete patterns, the same tumour type may be associated with more than one paraneoplastic disorder and each clinical syndrome may be associated with more than one antineuronal antibody. The list of antibodies used to screen for these disorders is steadily increasing and, in many, the causative antigen is also identified. Anti-*Hu* (antineuronal antibody-1) is usually associated with paraneoplastic encephalomyelitis or sensory neuropathy. Anti-*Yo* (anti-Purkinje cell antibody) is present in 40 per cent of patients with cerebellar degeneration. Anti-*Ri* (antineuronal antibody-2) characterizes opsoclous/myoclonus syndrome in adults. Antibodies against the synaptic vesicle protein amphiphysin are present in most clinical variants of the paraneoplastic stiff-person syndrome, whereas the idiopathic form is more commonly linked to anti-glutamic acid decarboxylase (GAD) antibodies. Circulating anti-*VPS* antibody is detected in patients with cancer-associated retinopathy. Anti-voltage gated calcium channel auto-antibodies are found in the Lambert–Eaton myasthenic syndrome, anti-voltage gated potassium channel antibody in the paraneoplastic myotonic syndromes, and anti-acetylcholine receptor antibodies in thymoma-associated myasthenia gravis. These IgG1 and IgG3 subtype antibodies are relatively specific and have an extremely

low normal prevalence, although they are seen in individuals with cancer who do not appear to have a paraneoplastic complication.

The antibodies are synthesized within the central nervous system in association with lymphocytic and plasma-cell infiltration of affected sites (Dalmau et al. 1991) and are often associated with oligoclonal banding of cerebrospinal fluid proteins. A protein (designated 14–3–3), present in the cerebrospinal fluid of patients with Creutzfeldt–Jakob disease, is also detected in a proportion of individuals with paraneoplastic disease, although these can be distinguished by the banding pattern (Saiz et al. 1999). The target antigens are generally proteins involved in transcription and translation, DNA replication, cell division, or RNA processing. Some progress has been made in defining the immunological pathways involved in paraneoplasia with the demonstration of an antigen-driven oligoclonal cytotoxic T-cell response favouring particular Vβ T-cell receptor families (Voltz et al. 1998) and increased in vitro HuD reactivity of CD4$^+$/CD45RO$^+$ Th1 cells from affected individuals (Benyahia et al. 1999). In turn, epitope specificity of the anti-*Hu* response principally involves the 90–101 or 171–206 amino-acid epitope, with identical reactivity in those individuals with an underlying malignancy whether or not this is complicated by a paraneoplastic disorder (Sodeyama et al. 1999). Some, but not all, of these disorders can be transferred passively to experimental animals.

It is logical to remove the primary tumour where possible, and this may be associated with improvement in those, mainly peripheral nervous system, disorders where antibody directly mediates the paraneoplastic disorder, but it less helpful in the central nervous system conditions where cell-mediated immunity is implicated and antibody merely a marker of immune response to the tumour. Anti-*Hu* antibody does not disappear during chemotherapy in patients without identified paraneoplastic complications of small cell lung cancer; even though its presence correlates with earlier tumour detection and fewer brain metastases, survival does not differ between patients with and without antibody (Verschuren et al. 1999). However, unlike the disorders associated with anti-*Hu* and -*Yo* conditions, the Lambert–Eaton syndrome often responds to cancer therapy. Immunosuppression may be useful (Stark et al. 1995); success has also been claimed for plasmapheresis and intravenous immunoglobulin in patients with a variety of paraneoplastic syndromes and underlying malignancies; immunological treatment sometimes leads to a reduction in the titre of antineuronal antibody (Blaes et al. 1999). However, these treatments do not usually influence the course of the paraneoplastic disorder (Uchuya et al. 1996).

In a consecutive series of 2000 brain autopsies, Peiffer (1987) identified 456 patients with extracerebral primary malignant tumours, of whom 362 had neurological manifestations of malignancy. These were direct or metastatic in 100, non-metastatic in 218, and mixed in 44 cases. After excluding the consequences of therapy, nutrition, and agonal events, remote effects of cancer were thought to be responsible for neurological syndromes in 17 per cent of these 262 patients. Although

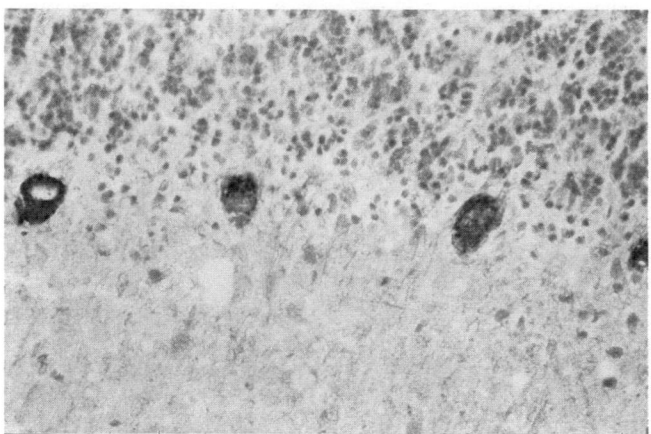

Fig. 30.1. Anti-Purkinje-cell auto-antibody staining with serum from a patient with a progressive cerebellar syndrome (kindly provided by Professor R. A. C. Hughes).

not a population-based survey, this gives some idea of the frequency with which paraneoplastic syndromes occur in neurological practice.

30.6.1 Progressive cerebellar degeneration

Progressive cerebellar degeneration (Section 31.11.3) is one of the most characteristic paraneoplastic syndromes encountered in adult neurological practice, but even this probably only occurs in less than 1 per cent of patients with cancer. The pathological appearances are of diffuse Purkinje cell loss throughout the cerebellum (Fig. 30.1), astrocytic proliferation, some neuronal loss, and demyelination. The changes are usually confined to the peridentate regions, but similar changes may be seen elsewhere in the nervous system.

Neurological symptoms usually predate recognition of the associated malignancy and manifest as acute or subacute ataxia progressing rapidly to produce such severe loss of axial balance that affected individuals often cannot stand or sit unless fully supported (Brain *et al.* 1951; Anderson *et al.* 1988a). The selective disturbance of midline cerebellar function is followed by incoordination of the individual limbs, dysarthria, and disorders of eye movement, especially the presence of downbeating nystagmus, indicating diffuse damage to the brainstem cerebellar connections. In many cases, signs of more widespread disease are apparent, with cognitive decline, other signs of diffuse encephalomyelitis, and, less frequently, peripheral neuropathy. Symptomatic progression is rapid but the condition may arrest at an advanced stage, albeit with severe disability. Cerebellar degeneration may occur in association with other paraneoplastic disorders as part of the subacute sensory neuronopathy–encephalomyelitis syndrome.

Investigation of these patients shows the expected cerebrospinal fluid pleocytosis, elevated immunoglobulins, and presence of oligoclonal bands. Patients with paraneoplastic cerebellar degeneration usually have serum and cerebrospinal fluid antibodies directed against cerebellar Purkinje cells (Anderson

et al. 1988b). Purkinje-cell antigens are selectively expressed in tumour tissue (Furneaux *et al.* 1990) and this is the usual specificity of anti-*Yo*, which serves as a marker for paraneoplastic cerebellar degeneration associated with carcinoma of the ovary, uterus, adnexa, or breast but also described in transitional cell carcinoma of the bladder (Greenlee *et al.* 1999)—generally a rare cause of paraneoplastic syndromes. Anti-*Yo* recognizes two groups of proteins, having molecular weights of 34–38 and 62–64 kDa, respectively (Furneaux *et al.* 1989). It stains the endoplasmic reticulum and Golgi complexes in Purkinje cells and their dendrites. The function of these proteins and the molecular basis of the disease have yet to be defined, although the gene encoding the smaller product is uniquely expressed in cerebellum and in tumour tissue from affected patients (Dropcho *et al.* 1987). In some cases, different antibody staining properties are seen in the presence of an otherwise typical clinical phenotype, but additional antibodies, recognizing different proteins extracted from neurons and not showing the same staining pattern, have also been identified in patients with mixed syndromes of cerebellar degeneration, encephalopathy, neuropathy, and autonomic failure. These seem not to occur in patients with breast or ovarian tumour without paraneoplastic neurological syndromes. Anti-*Tr* is associated with paraneoplastic cerebellar degeneration and Hodgkin's disease (Graus *et al.* 1997).

Most recently, Dalmau *et al.* (1999) identified anti-*Ma*, a novel auto-antibody, in 4/1705 samples, from patients in whom the phenotype was usually cerebellar degeneration due to extensive Purkinje-cell loss but with some variation in the clinical manifestations. *In vitro* studies showed widespread antineuronal nucleus and testis specificity, reacting against 37 and 40 kDa antigens which were also detected on the primary tumour in each case.

In a series of 47 patients with progressive cerebellar degeneration (Anderson *et al.* 1988a), 18 had typical anti-Purkinje-cell antibodies. These cases were all women with ovarian or breast carcinoma in whom cerebellar disease predated recognition of the tumour and tended to follow rapidly upon a systemic illness involving diarrhoea and vomiting. As is usually the case in paraneoplastic disorders of the central nervous system, removal of the primary tumour does not influence the neurological disorder, and treatment with plasmapheresis and immunosuppression are equally unrewarding, even though the antibody titre may fall for a while.

The clinical features of cancer-associated progressive cerebellar degeneration not associated with antineuronal antibodies differ from the antibody-positive cases, in that men are more commonly affected; the neurological symptoms more often complicate lung tumour and more commonly develop after recognition of the primary lesion; and the clinical symptomatology is broadly similar, as are the cerebrospinal fluid findings and the response to treatment.

Symptomatic treatment is generally unrewarding, although there may be some response to clonazepam. Albert *et al.* (2000) suggest that treatment with tacrolimus, which selectively inhibits the activated T cells present in the circulation and spinal fluid of patients with cerebellar degeneration, may benefit the paraneoplastic complication without risking tumour recurrence.

30.6.2 Limbic encephalomyelitis

One stereotyped paraneoplastic syndrome is characterized clinically by subacute loss of memory leading to anxiety, confusion, behavioural changes, and alteration in mood; there is a high frequency of partial complex or generalized seizures (Bakheit *et al.* 1990; Dalmau *et al.* 1992). The encephalitis may extend outside the limbic system, causing motor deficits, cranial nerve palsies, and central respiratory involvement when the brainstem is involved. Not infrequently, the clinical phenotype merges into other forms of paraneoplastic disease. All these features arise from neuronal loss and gliosis, together with diffuse perivenous inflammatory cell infiltration seen in the other paraneoplastic disorders, maximally in CA1 layers of the hippocampus, although this may extend to other parts of the limbic system and associated cortex. The cerebrospinal fluid also shows a mild reactive lymphocytic pleocytosis, raised immunoglobulin, and oligoclonal bands. Anti-*Hu* is the serological marker of this paraneoplastic disorder.

The syndrome usually occurs in patients with small cell carcinoma of the lung, but has been reported in association with germinal tumours (Burton *et al.* 1988) and malignant thymoma (McArdle and Milligen 1988). More recently, Voltz *et al.* (1999) have implicated testicular tumours and antigens in 10 cases of paraneoplastic limbic and brainstem encephalitis, all sharing the presence of anti-*Ta* auto-antibody directed against the Ma2 antigen. As expected, in this series, neurological presentation usually preceded detection of the tumour, often by several months.

It has been suggested that these cases respond to removal of the primary tumour, and that others arrest spontaneously, but this may reflect the small numbers that have been studied in detail by comparison with more frequent cases of progressive cerebellar degeneration. A retrospective review of 51 cases, of whom the majority had small cell lung cancer, indicated that successful tumour therapy is associated with improved outcome of the paraneoplastic syndrome; immunotherapy did not adversely affect tumour outcome, but neither did it favourably influence the features of encephalomyelitis (Keime-Guibert *et al.* 1999). In one anti-*Ta* associated case, the illness was characterized by spontaneous remissions and with a response to radical treatment of the primary tumour Voltz *et al.* (1999).

30.6.3 Optic neuritis and retinal degeneration

Subacute degeneration of the optic nerve, or more commonly the retina, is a rare manifestation of small cell carcinoma of the lung (Section 8.3.2); visual failure, indistinguishable from other causes of retinal or optic nerve disease, develops rapidly due to degeneration of retinal ganglion cells (Fig. 30.2)

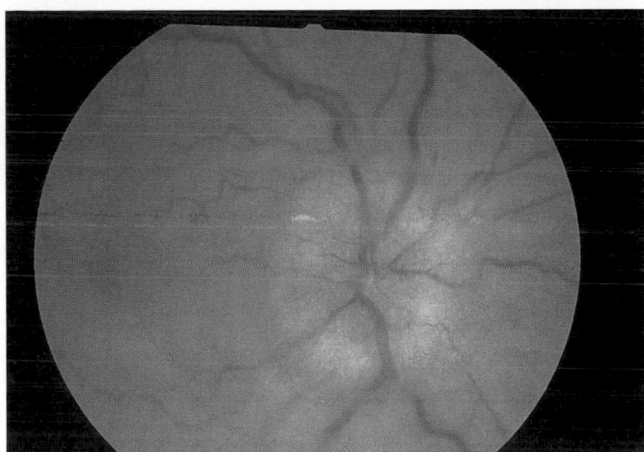

Fig. 30.2. Optic disc appearance in a patient with paraneoplastic bilateral sequential visual failure in association with bronchial cancer.

(Boghen *et al.* 1988; Dropcho 1989). Circulating anti-*VPS* antibody is detected in some patients and this reacts with 20–24, 65, 145, and 205 kDa bands isolated from normal retina. The target antigens in cancer-associated retinopathy have provisionally been identified as recoverin and tubby-like protein 1 (Kikuchi *et al.* 2000).

30.6.4 Opsoclonus

One of the most characteristic paraneoplastic syndromes is opsoclonus associated with neuroblastoma in childhood and with a variety of neoplasms—usually small cell lung, breast, or ovarian carcinoma—in adults (Anderson *et al.* 1988c; Dropcho 1989). Opsoclonus (Section 8.11.5) describes the rapid, chaotic, conjugate, spontaneous, saccadic eye movements that severely distort ocular fixation and are often associated with ataxia, impaired balance, and other manifestations of brainstem disturbance. This eye movement disorder also occurs in adults with encephalitis and in patients with multiple sclerosis. One pathophysiological explanation for the disturbance of eye movement involves the paramedian pontine reticular formation, and the centres responsible for co-ordinating vertical gaze, which contain neurons that initiate (burst and burst tonic), maintain (tonic), and permit (pause) alteration in the steady state of conjugate eye movements. Selective loss of pause cells would, it is argued, disinhibit burst neurons, leading to random saccades. However, this hypothesis is not supported by pathological evidence; pause cells located within the nucleus raphe interpositus seem to be intact (Ridley *et al.* 1987). Histological findings include Purkinje cell loss, neuronal changes in the inferior olives, and diffuse perivascular mononuclear cell infiltration of the leptomeninges and brain parenchyma.

A useful clinical response to treatment with corticosteroids has suggested that opsoclonus arises from humoral immune reactions to tumour antigens cross-reacting with brainstem neurons. Antibodies that react with 53–61 kDa and 79–84 kDa antigens present on neuronal nuclei have been recognized in one patient with opsoclonus associated with breast cancer, but not in several other cases (Budde-Steffen *et al.* 1988*a*); and high titres of the anti-*Ri* antibody, which react with 55 kDa and 80 kDa antigens detected on cortical neurons, have been identified in eight patients with opsoclonus occurring in the context of gynaecological cancer, but not tumour cases without neurological symptoms, or patients with different paraneoplastic neurological syndromes (Luque *et al.* 1991).

Similarities exist between opsoclonus and progressive cerebellar degeneration. Both are associated with impaired balance, perivascular lymphocytic infiltration, cerebrospinal fluid pleocytosis, the presence of ovarian lung or breast cancer, and presentation with the remote effects before identification of the primary tumour. However, by contrast with progressive cerebellar degeneration, opsoclonus is more usually of sudden onset, and associated with generalized myoclonus and encephalopathy but with preserved speech and co-ordination of the individual limbs. In a series of 19 patients, males and females were equally affected; 9 had lung tumours, 7 of which were small cell carcinomas. Opsoclonus was usually associated with impaired balance but not limb co-ordination (18), and with vertigo (14), myoclonus (12), encephalopathy (5), and dysarthria (4). The onset was rapid in 12 cases, progressing to coma or death within weeks in 7 but responding partially to treatment in 12. Pleocytosis was present in 12 and oligoclonal bands in 2; magnetic resonance imaging was invariably normal and Purkinje cell loss rarely observed despite the presence of perivascular lymphocytic infiltration in the majority of autopsied cases (Anderson *et al.* 1988*c*).

30.6.5 Spinal syndromes

Several spinal syndromes have been reported in association with cancer. Necrotizing myelitis is described elsewhere (Section 20.4.6). Segmental spinal myoclonus occurs following radiation of the cord (Section 32.7.4) but has also been described as a remote effect of small cell carcinoma of the lung and lymphoma (Roobal *et al.* 1987). Histologically, there is degeneration of spinal interneurons and alpha motor neurons and the spinal fluid shows similar changes to those seen in other paraneoplastic syndromes. Multisystem disorders, in which conspicuous anterior horn cell loss is associated with focal or diffuse muscle wasting, usually occur in the context of small cell lung carcinoma. More controversial is the issue of whether classical motor neuron disease ever complicates cancer (Brain *et al.* 1965). It is now clear that the clinical phenotype of motor neuron disease includes cases with antibodies directed against gangliosides G_{M1} and G_{D1b}, many of whom conform to the multifocal motor neuropathy phenotype and have electrophysiological evidence for localized conduction block. These are distinct from the pure motor neuropathies (see above) that occur in association with plasma cell dyscrasias and IgM-κ gammopathies, but an association with several other autoimmune and paraneoplastic spinal disorders is recognized. Claims that mixed upper and lower neuron disease without sensory involvement, conforming clinically to the typical case of

motor neuron disease, seem to have been exaggerated, and few would now advocate an extensive search for underlying cancer in these cases.

The disorder of painful spasms, symmetric axial muscle rigidity, and uncontrollable contractions with disturbed posture, summarized as the stiff-person syndrome, includes a proportion of patients with paraneoplastic disease. Stiffness may be confined to one or more limbs. Unlike the localized forms of stiff-person syndrome, the paraneoplastic variant is commonly associated with more extensive neurological involvement implicating several systems, including peripheral nerves, but with an emphasis on the brainstem, including myoclonus and opsoclonus. Antibodies against the synaptic vesicle protein amphiphysin are associated with the paraneoplastic stiff-person syndrome (Folli *et al.* 1993). Amphiphysin is a synaptic-vesicle-associated protein which also localizes to nodes of Ranvier (Butler *et al.* 1997). Anti-GAD may be present and this probably accounts for the increased frequency of diabetes—at least in the non-paraneoplastic variants of the stiff-person syndrome—although the titre and specificities of the anti-GAD antibody differ.

30.6.6 Pure sensory neuropathy

The association between cancer and sensory neuropathy was described before the spectrum of paraneoplastic syndromes affecting the nervous system came to be fully recognized (Denny Brown 1948; Croft *et al.* 1967) (Section 12.13.1). Presentation is with diffuse distal symmetric sensory symptoms, and early involvement of discriminative modalities producing profound incoordination, pseudoathetosis and extreme uselessness of the limbs, and areflexia but with relative preservation of strength suggests an underlying malignancy. A similar syndrome may complicate autoimmune disease, plasma-cell dyscrasias, treatment with pyridoxine, or chemotherapy, and is seen as one variant of acute post-infectious polyneuritis. As with the other prototypic paraneoplastic disorders, sensory neuropathy is often associated with small cell carcinoma of the lung and presents in advance of the underlying cancer, but is more common in women than men. The symptoms and signs arise from selective damage to neurons in the dorsal root ganglia associated with perivascular lymphocytic infiltration. Secondary degeneration then occurs in the posterior nerve roots, dorsal columns, and peripheral nerves. Many patients show more widespread evidence of encephalomyelitis at autopsy and this may be clinically apparent during life. Serum from these patients contains anti-*Hu* antibody binding the 35–40 kDa antigen expressed on small cell lung tumour lines and cross-reacting with dorsal root ganglia (Anderson *et al.* 1988*b*; Budde-Steffen *et al.* 1988*b*; Dropcho 1989). These disorders may occasionally complicate breast and prostatic carcinoma, but anti-*Hu* antibodies rarely, if ever, occur in the absence of one tumour type or another. The list of anti-*Hu*-positive syndromes has now been extended to include cases with more extensive paraneoplastic neurological disorders than pure sensory neuropathy (Fig. 30.3).

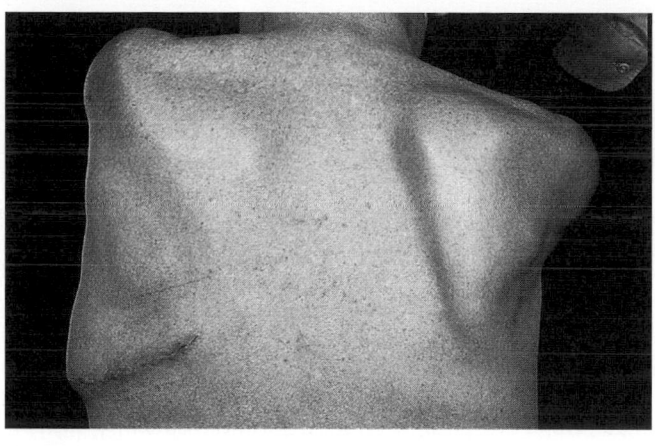

(a)

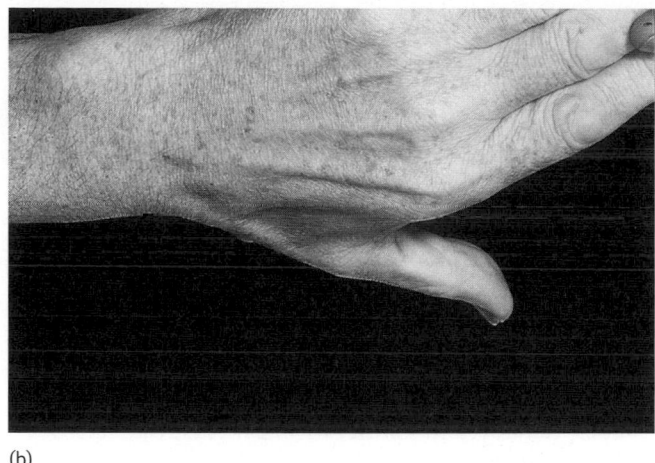

(b)

Fig. 30.3. Proximal (a) and peripheral (b) muscle wasting in a patient with severe paraneoplastic proximal myopathy and neuropathy in association with anti-*Hu* antibody.

Although highly characteristic, the pure sensory neuropathy is far less common in patients with malignancy than mixed forms of peripheral neuropathy. There is considerable clinical, electrophysiological, and histological heterogeneity in these cases. A mixed progressive sensorimotor axonal neuropathy complicating cancer is the form most usually encountered, although this rarely dominates the clinical picture (Section 12.13.2). The onset and course vary considerably and the illness may be indistinguishable from the Guillain–Barré syndrome. Segmental demyelination dominates the histological picture in some cases and in others the mechanism is vasculitic (Section 12.13.3). A subacute motor neuropathy occurs in the context of lymphoma, especially Hodgkin's disease, usually complicating treatment and often unrelated to activity of the underlying disorder; it results from degeneration of anterior horn cells and peripheral nerve fibres—features which suggest an opportunistic viral infection allied to enterovirus. The cause of these syndromes is presumed to be immunological or due to release of toxic substances synthesized by the tumour, but no specific auto-antibody has yet been identified.

The full list of small cell cancer associated syndromes includes autonomic degeneration, and this may cause severe visceral neuropathy due to neuronal loss within the myenteric plexus (Chinn and Schuffler 1988). In other cases, neuronal degeneration is confined to central autonomic pathways. The clinical manifestations vary from pupillary abnormalities to severe generalized dysautonomia. This variant of paraneoplastic neuropathy has also been reported in association with anti-*Hu* antibody.

30.6.7 Disorders of the neuromuscular junction

The Lambert–Eaton syndrome epitomizes the relationship between malignancy, autoimmunity, and paraneoplastic affection of the nervous system (Eaton and Lambert 1957; Brain and Norris 1965) (Section 15.10.2). The diagnosis is often not established at presentation, since symptoms of fatigue tend to outweigh the signs of muscle weakness. The Lambert–Eaton myasthenic syndrome can be confused with myasthenia gravis but differs in several important clinical, physiological, and immunological respects. Fatiguable weakness affects the shoulder and pelvic girdles rather than the ocular, facial, bulbar, respiratory, and shoulder muscle involvement that characterizes the pattern of weakness in myasthenia gravis. Although ophthalmoplegia does not occur, most patients show mild ptosis and there is a high frequency of autonomic disturbance manifesting as dry mouth, sphincter disturbance, and impotence in males. The tendon reflexes are often absent, but can briefly be restored by sustained tetanic muscle contraction (O'Neill *et al.* 1988). This reflects the physiological defect which, unlike myasthenia gravis, depends on impaired presynaptic acetylcholine release. Repetitive stimulation at high frequency overcomes the defect, increasing the amplitude of the evoked muscle potential. Approximately 50 per cent of patients with the Lambert–Eaton syndrome have an underlying small cell carcinoma of the lung, but the condition is sometimes associated with autoimmune diseases; in both categories, there is a response to plasma exchange or immunosuppression. The muscle weakness and physiological defects can be transferred passively to experimental animals using the immunoglobulin fraction of serum from affected patients, thus indicating the presence of a circulating auto-antibody (Fukunuga *et al.* 1983). This is now shown to be an IgG antibody, directed against presynaptic calcium channels, which blocks quantal acetylcholine release by cross-linking and depleting the presynaptic active zone particles and inhibiting potassium-stimulated calcium influx (Motomura *et al.* 1995). There is evidence that cross-reacting epitopes exist on small cell lung tumour lines. Treatment with agents that increase acetylcholine release have not proved useful or practical to administer, so the mainstay of therapy is removal of the underlying tumour and immunosuppression.

Mason *et al.* (1997) assessed the frequency of P/Q and N-type voltage-gated calcium channel antibodies in patients with small cell carcinoma of the lung, alone or complicated by paraneoplastic cerebellar degeneration. Anti-*Hu* antibody was present in 51 per cent of cases with cerebellar degeneration but in none of the patients with uncomplicated small cell carcinoma. Where tissue became available, it was associated with a more intense inflammatory infiltrate in affected parts of the central nervous system. Those with high antibody titres (>1 : 10 000) tended to be female, more disabled, and with extensive paraneoplastic syndromes. Nine patients developed the Lambert–Eaton syndrome, of whom seven had anti-calcium-channel antibodies. By contrast, these were present in 20 per cent of anti-*Hu*-negative patients with cerebellar degeneration and 2 per cent of cases with isolated small cell carcinoma. Treatment influenced the Lambert–Eaton syndrome but not the cerebellar degeneration; this was associated with a worse prognosis than uncomplicated small cell carcinoma and usually determined the cause of death, especially in anti-*Hu*-positive patients.

The 10 per cent of patients with myasthenia gravis (Section 15.10.1) having an associated thymoma can be regarded as having a paraneoplastic syndrome, but in other respects the clinical picture is indistinguishable from routine cases. Immunologically, each is associated with circulating anti-acetylcholine receptor antibodies, but striated muscle antibody may be a serum marker of thymoma. The intratumourous 153 kDa protein having an acetylcholine-receptor-like epitope in paraneoplastic myasthenia gravis is now identified as midsize neurofilament and, unlike all other individuals with myasthenia gravis and uncomplicated thymoma, these patients show selective T-cell responses to this auto-antigen (Schultz *et al.* 1999).

Although the relationship between cancer and polymyositis may have previously been overstated, the presence of dermatomyositis (Section 15.7.2) suggests an underlying malignancy in the context of inflammatory muscle disease. Women are preferentially affected and the tumours commonly involve the breast, lung, ovary, or gastrointestinal tract. Other than the clue from skin involvement, no laboratory or histological feature reliably distinguishes the regular from paraneoplastic variant of polymyositis. A non-inflammatory proximal myopathy is often seen in the context of cancer, alone or as part of the general cachectic state.

A related disorder is neuromyotonia (Section 14.9) characterized by myokymia, cramps, sweating, muscle hypertrophy, and with involvement of the central nervous system, producing hallucinations and mood changes resulting from the presence of anti-voltage-gated potassium channels acting on peripheral nerves (Newsom-Davis and Mills 1993). Isaacs' syndrome is associated with peripheral neuropathy and with abnormalities of the immune system; several cases are described in association with lung carcinoma (reviewed by Newsom-Davis and Mills 1993).

30.6.8 Neurometabolic disorders associated with neoplasms

Tumours of many different kinds produce metabolic disorders leading to neurological symptoms which may bring the patient under observation. The most important symptoms are mental disturbances and muscular weakness. The principal syndromes of this kind are reviewed by Henson and Urich (1982).

The production of hypercalcaemia due to the release of parathormone by a tumour of the parathyroid gland has long been recognized. However, there are several other ways in which hypercalcaemia may occur in association with malignancy. Tumours arising in organs other than the parathyroid gland may produce a parathormone-like substance which leads to hypercalcaemia, while genuine primary hyperparathyroidism has been reported in patients with carcinomas or leukaemia. The hypercalcaemia of sarcoidosis may also cause neurological symptoms but here, too, the mechanism is not understood. In myelomatosis and carcinomatosis of bone, tissue destruction may liberate calcium into the bloodstream faster than it can be excreted, and so cause hypercalcaemia. Hypercalcaemia, however produced, may lead to non-specific symptoms of encephalopathy, such as drowsiness, confusion or stupor, and to muscular weakness.

Various tumours, including bronchial adenoma, bronchogenic carcinoma, thymoma, or pancreatic carcinoma, may secrete corticotrophin and so lead to adrenal hypercorticism. There is evidence that virtually all oat-cell carcinomas of the bronchus and bronchial carcinoids secrete corticotrophin-like materials. This may not lead to the typical symptoms of Cushing's syndrome in the early stages but can result in hypokalaemic alkalosis, the symptoms of Cushing's syndrome developing later. Clinically this syndrome can present with confusional psychosis or dementia and with myopathy (O'Riordan *et al.* 1966).

Tumours other than those arising in the pancreas may produce hypoglycaemia. Kahn (1980) found that mesenchymal tumours were responsible for this complication in 45 per cent of cases, hepatomas in 23 per cent, and adrenocortical carcinoma in 10 per cent. It is thought that in some cases the tumour elaborates a material with insulin-like activity which nevertheless differs in structure from insulin, while in other cases it is possible that rapid consumption of glucose by the tumour is involved in the production of symptoms. The presenting symptoms—enephalopathy characterized by stupor, coma, and convulsions—are typical of hypoglycaemia from other causes (Section 25.2.6).

Apart from the many metastatic and non-metastatic complications of malignant disease, patients with cancer may develop neurological manifestations due to nutritional deficiencies of specific vitamins or chronic malnutrition. In many, there is associated hyponatraemia which is most likely to occur in association with bronchogenic carcinomas or adenomas which secrete a vasopressin-like substance that has antidiuretic hormone activity and results in the syndrome of inappropriate ADH secretion, causing hypo-osmolarity with concentrated urine. The patient usually presents with water intoxication and encephalopathy characterized by coma and convulsions. Treatment depends upon fluid restriction rather than infusion of hypertonic fluids.

References

Albert, M. L., Austin, L. M., and Darnell, R. B. (2000). Detection and treatment of activated T cells in the cerebrospinal fluid of patients with paraneoplastic cerebellar degeneration. *Ann. Neurol.*, **47**, 9–17.

Anderson, N. E., Rosenblum, M. K., and Posner, J. B. (1988*a*). Paraneoplastic cerebellar degeneration: clinical-immunological correlations. *Ann. Neurol.*, **245**, 559–67.

Anderson, N. E., Rosenblum, M. K., Graus, F. *et al.* (1988*b*). Autoantibodies in paraneoplastic syndromes associated with small cell lung cancer. *Neurology*, **38**, 1391–8.

Anderson, N. E., Budde-Steffen, C., Rosenblum, M. K. *et al.* (1988*c*). Opsoclonus, myoclonus, ataxia, and encephalopathy in adults with cancer: a distinct paraneoplastic syndrome. *Medicine*, **67**, 100–9.

Bakheit, A. M. O., Kennedy, P. G. E., and Behan, P. O. (1990). Paraneoplastic limbic encephalitis: clinico-pathological correlations. *J. Neurol. Neurosurg. Psychiatry*, **53**, 1084–8.

Bardwick, P. A., Zvaiffler, N. J., Gill, G. N. *et al.* (1980). Plasma cell dyscrasia with polyneuropathy, organomegaly, endocrinopathy, M protein and skin changes; the POEMS syndrome: report of two cases and a review of the literature. *Medicine*, **59**, 311–22.

Benyahia, B., Liblau, R., Merle-Beral, H. *et al.* (1999). Cell-mediated autoimmunity in paraneoplastic neurological syndromes with anti-Hu antibodies. *Ann. Neurol.*, **45**, 162–7.

Berger, J. R., Kaszpvitz, B., Post, M. J. *et al.* (1987). Progressive multifocal leucoencephalopathy associated with human immunodeficiency virus infection: a review of the literature with a report of 16 cases. *Ann. Int. Med.*, **107**, 78–87.

Blaes, F., Strittmatter, K. M., Merkelbach, S. *et al.* (1999). Intravenous immunoglobulins in the therapy of paraneoplasatic neurological disorders. *J. Neurol.*, **246**, 299–303.

Boghen, J., Sebag, M., and Michaud, J. (1988). Paraneoplastic optic neuritis and encephalomyelitis. *Arch. Neurol.*, **45**, 353–7.

Brain, W. R. and Norris, F. H. (1965). *The remote effects of cancer on the nervous system. Contemporary Neurology Symposia*, Vol. 1, p. 230. Grune and Stratton, New York.

Brain, W. R., Daniel, P. M., and Greenfield, J. G. (1951). Subacute cerebellar degeneration associated with neoplasms. *J. Neurol. Neurosurg. Psychiatry*, **14**, 59–75.

Brain, W. R., Croft, P. B., and Wilkinson, M. (1965). Motor neurone disease as a manifestation of neoplasms. *Brain*, **88**, 479–500.

Budde-Steffen, C., Anderson, N. E., Rosenblum, M. K. *et al.* (1988*a*). An antineuronal autoantibody in paraneoplastic opsoclonus. *Ann. Neurol.*, **23**, 528–31.

Budde-Steffen, C., Anderson, N. E., Rosenblum, M. K., *et al.* (1988*b*). Expression of an antigen in small cell lung carcinoma lines detected by antibodies from patients with paraneoplastic dorsal root ganglionopathy. *Cancer Res.*, **48**, 430–4.

Burton, G. V., Bullard, D. E., Walther, P. J., *et al.* (1988). Paraneoplastic limbic encephalopathy with testicular carcinoma. *Cancer*, **62**, 2248–51.

Butler, M. H., David, C., Ochoa, G. C. *et al.* (1999). Amphiphysin II (SH3P9; BINI) a member of the ampiphysin/Rvs family, is concentrated in the cortical cytomatrix of axon initial segments and nodes of Ranvier in brain and around T tubules in skeletal muscle. *J. Cell Biol.*, **137**, 1355–67.

Carpentier, A. F., Voltz, R. D., Deschamps, T. *et al.* (1998). Absence of Hud gene mutations in paraneoplastic small cell lung cancer tissue. *Clin. Cancer Res.*, **4**, 2818–24.

Chinn, J. S. and Schuffler, M. D. (1988). Paraneoplastic visceral neuropathy as a cause of severe gastrointestinal motor dysfunction. *Gastroenterology*, **95**, 1279–86.

Croft, P. B., Urich, H., and Wilkinson, M. (1967). Peripheral neuropathy of sensorimotor type associated with malignant disease. *Brain*, **90**, 31–66.

Dalmau, J. and Posner, J. B. (1996). Neurological paraneoplastic syndromes. *Springer Semin. Immunopathol.*, **18**, 85–95.

Dalmau, J., Furneaux, H. M., Rosenblum, M. K. *et al.* (1991). Detection of the anti-Hu antibody in specific regions of the nervous system and tumor from patients with paraneoplastic encephalomyelitis/sensory neuropathy. *Neurology*, **41**, 1757–64.

Dalmau, J., Graus, F., Rosenblum, M. K., *et al.* (1992). Anti-Hu-associated paraneoplastic encephalomyelitis/sensory neuropathy—a clinical study of 71 patients. *Medicine (Baltimore)*, **71**, 59–72.

Dalmau, J., Gultekin, S. H., Voltz, R. *et al.* (1999). Ma1, a novel neuron- and testis-specific protein, is recognised by ther serum of patients with paraneoplastic neurological disorders. *Brain*, **122**, 27–39.

Delattre, J.-V. and Posner, J. B. (1995). Neurological complications of chemotherapy and radiation therapy. In *Neurology and general medicine*, (ed. M. Aminoff), pp. 421–45. Churchill Livingstone, Edinburgh.

Denny Brown, D. E. (1948). Primary sensory neuropathy with uscular changes associated with carcinoma. *J. Neurol. Neurosurg. Psychiatry*, **11**, 73–87.

Dolman, C. L., Sweeney, V. P., and Magil, A. (1979). Neoplastic angioendotheliosis; the case of the missed primary? *Arch. Neurol.*, **36**, 5–7.

Dropcho, E. J. (1989). The remote effects of cancer on the nervous system. *Neurol. Clin.*, 7 (3), 579–603.

Dropcho, E. J., Chen, Y.-T., Posner, J. B., *et al.* (1987). Cloning of a brain protein identified by autoantibodies from a patient with paraneoplastic cerebellar degeneration. *Proc. Natl Acad. Sci. USA*, **84**, 4552–6.

Eaton, L. M. and Lambert, E. H. (1957). Electromyography and electrical stimulation in nerves in diseases of the motor unit; observations on a myasthenic syndrome associated with malignant tumours. *JAMA*, **163**, 1117–24.

Folli, F., Solimena, M., Cofiell, R. *et al.* (1993). Autoantibodies to a 128-kd synaptic protein in three women with the stiff-man syndrome and breast cancer. *N. Engl. J. Med.*, **328**, 546–51.

Fukunaga, H., Engel, A. G., Lang, B. *et al.* (1983). Passive transfer of Lambert Eaton myasthenic syndrome with IgG from mouse to man depletes the presynaptic membrane active zones. *Proc. Natl Acad. Sci. USA*, **80**, 7636–40.

Furneaux, H. M., Dropcho, E. J., Barbut, D. *et al.* (1989). Characterisation of a cDNA encoding a 34 kDa Purkinje neuron protein recognised by sera from patients with paraneoplastic cerebellar degeneration. *Proc. Natl Acad. Sci. USA*, **86**, 2873–7.

Furneaux, H. M., Rosenblum, M. K., Dalmau, J. *et al.* (1990). Selective expression of Purkinje-cell antigens in tumor tissue from patients with paraneoplastic cerebellar degeneration. *N. Engl. J. Med.*, **322**, 1844–51.

Graus, F., Dalmau, J., Valdeoriola, F. *et al.* (1997). Immunological characterisation of a neuronal antibody (anti-*Tr*) associated with paraneoplastic cerebellar degeneration and Hodgkin's disease. *J. Neuroimmunol.*, **74**, 55–61.

Greenlee, J. E., Dalmau, J., Lyons, T. *et al.* (1999). Association of anti-Yo (type 1) antiody with paraneoplastic cerebellar degeneration in the setting of transitional cell carcinoma of the bladder: detection of Yo antigen in tumor tissue and fall in antibody titers following tumor remocval. *Ann. Neurol.*, **45**, 805–9.

Henson, R. A. and Urich, H. (1982). *Cancer and the nervous system. The neurological manifestations of systemic malignant disease*. Blackwell, Oxford.

Ilyas, A. A., Quarles, R. H., Macintosh, T. D. *et al.* (1984). IgM in a human neuropathy related to paraproteinaemia binds to a carbohydrate determinant in the myelin associated glycoprotein and to a ganglioside. *Proc. Natl Acad. Sci. USA*, **81**, 1225–9.

Julien, J., Vital, C., Vallat, J.-M. *et al.* (1978). Polyneuropathy in Waldenstrom's macroglobulinaemia: deposition of M component on myelin sheaths. *Arch. Neurol.*, **35**, 423–5.

Kahn, C. R. (1980). The riddle of tumour hypoglycaemia revisited. *Clin. Endocrin. Metab.*, **9**, 335.

Keime-Guibert, F., Graus, F., Broet, P. *et al.* (1999). Clinical outcome of patients with anti-Hu associated encephalomyelitis after treatment of the tumour. *Neurology*, **53**, 1719–23.

Kelly, J. J., Kyle, R. A., Miles, J. M., *et al.* (1981). The spectrum of peripheral neuropathy in myeloma. *Neurology*, **31**, 24–31.

Kelly, J. J., Kyle, R. A., Miles, J. M., *et al.* (1983). Osteosclerotic myeloma and peripheral neuropathy. *Neurology*, **33**, 202–10.

Kikuchi, T., Arai, J., Shibuki, H. *et al.* (2000). Tubby-like protein 1 as an autoantigen in cancer-associated retinopathy. *J. Neuroimmunol.*, **103**, 26–33.

Luque, F. A., Furneaux, H. M., Ferziger, R. *et al.* (1991). Anti-Ri: an antibody associated with paraneoplastic opsoclonus and breast cancer. *Ann. Neurol.*, **29**, 241–51.

McArdle, J. P. and Millingen, K. S. (1988). Limbic encephalitis associated with malignant thymoma. *Pathology*, **20**, 292–5.

Mason, W. P., Graus, F., Lang, B. *et al.* (1997). Small-cell lung cancer, paraneoplastic cerebellar degeneration and the Lambert–Eaton myasthenic syndrome. *Brain*, **120**, 1279–300.

Meucci, N., Baldini, L., Cappellari, A. *et al.* (1999). Anti-myelin associated glycoprotein antibodies predict the development of neuropathy in asymptomatic patients with IgM monoclonal gammopathy. *Ann. Neurol.*, **46**, 119–22.

Motomura, M., Johnston, I., Lang, B. *et al.* (1995). An improved diagnostic assay for Lambert–Eaton myasthenic syndrome. *J. Neurol. Neurosurg. Psychiatry*, **58**, 85–7.

Newsom-Davis, J. and Mills, K. R. (1993). Immunological associations of acquired neuromyotonia (Isaacs' syndrome). Report of five cases and review of the literature. *Brain*, **116**, 453–69.

O'Neill, J. H., Murray, N. M., and Newsom-Davis, J. M. (1988). The Lambert Eaton myasthenic syndrome; a review of 50 cases. *Brain*, **111**, 577–96.

O'Riordan, J. L., Blanshard, G. P., Moxham, A., *et al.* (1966). Corticotrophin-secreting carcinomas. *QJM*, **35**, 137–47.

Padovan, C. S., Yousry, T. A., Schleuning, M. *et al.* (1998). Neurological and neuroradiological findings in long-term survivors of allogeneic bone marrow transplantation. *Ann. Neurol.*, **43**, 627–33.

Padovan, C. S., Bise, K., Hahn, J. *et al.* (1999). Angiitis of thecentral nervous system after allogeneic bone marrow transp[lantation? *Stroke*, **30**, 1651–6.

Peiffer, J. (1987). Encephalomyelopathies associated with extracerebral malignant tumors. *Pathol. Res. Pract.*, **182**, 585–608.

Posner, J. B. (1995). Paraneoplastic syndromes. In *Neurologic complications of cancer*, (ed. J. B. Posner), pp. 353–85. F. A. Davis, Philadelphia.

Read, D. and Warlow, C. P. (1978). Peripheral neuropathy and solitary plasmacytoma. *J. Neurol. Neurosurg. Psychiatry*, **41**, 177–84.

Richardson, E. P. (1965). Progressive multifocal leukoencephalopathy. In *The remote effects of cancer on the nervous system*, (ed. W. R. Brain and F. Norris), pp. 6–16. Grune and Stratton, New York.

Ridley, A., Kennard, C., Scholtz, C. L. *et al.* (1987). Omnipause neurons in two cases of opsoclonus associated with oat cell carcinoma of the lung. *Brain*, **110**, 1699–709.

Roobal, T. H., Kazzaz, B. A., and Vecht, Ch. J. (1987). Segmental rigidity and spinal myoclonus as a paraneoplastic syndrome. *J. Neurol. Neurosurg. Psychiatry*, **50**, 628–31.

Russell, D. A. and Rubinstein, L. J. (1989). *Pathology of tumours of the nervous system*. Arnold. London.

Saiz, A., Graus, F., Dalmau, J. *et al.* (1999). Detection of 14–3–3 brain protein in the cerebrospinal fluid of patients with paraneoplastic neurological disorders. *Ann. Neurol.*, **46**, 774–7.

Schultz, A., Hoffacker, V., Wilisch, A. *et al.* (1999). Neurofilament is an autoantigenic determinant in myasathenia gravis. *Ann. Neurol.*, **46**, 167–75.

Smith, I. S., Kahn, S. N., Lacey, B. W. *et al.* (1983). Chronic demyelinating neuropathy associated with benign IgM paraproteinaemia. *Brain*, **106**, 169–95.

Sodeyama, N., Ishida, K., Jaeckle, K. A. *et al.* (1999). Pattern of epitopic reactivity of the anti-Hu antibody on HuD with and without paraneoplastic syndrome. *J. Neurol. Neurosurg. Psychiatry*, **66**, 97–9.

Stark, E., Wurster, U., Patzold, U. *et al.* (1995). Immunological and clinical response to immunosuppressive treatment in paraneoplastic cerebellar degeneration. *Arch. Neurol.*, **52**, 814–18.

Uchuya, M., Graus, F., Vega, F. *et al.* (1996). Intravenous immunoglobulin treatment in paraneoplastic neurological syndromes with antineuronal antibodies. *J. Neurol. Neurosurg. Psychiatry*, **60**, 388–92.

Voltz, R., Dalmau, J., Posner, J. B., *et al.* (1998). T-cell receptor analysis in anti-Hu associated paraneoplastic encephalomyelitis. *Neurology*, **51**, 1146–50.

Voltz, R., Gultekin, H. S., Posner, J. B. *et al.* (1999). A serological marker of paraneoplastic limbic and brainstem encephalitis in patients with testicular cancer. *N. Engl. J. Med.*, **340**, 1788–95.

Verschuren, J. J., Perquin, M., ten Velde, G. *et al.* (1999). Anti-Hu antibody titre and brain metastases before and after treatment for small cell lung cancer. *J. Neurol. Neurosurg. Psychiatry*, **67**, 353–7.

Zu Rhein, G. and Chou, S. M. (1965). Particles resembling papova viruses in human cerebral demyelinating disease. *Science*, **148**, 1477–9.

CHAPTER 31

Tremor, ataxia, and cerebellar disorders

Nicholas Fletcher

31.1 Tremor

31.1.1 Clinical diagnosis of tremor

Tremors are characterized by rhythmic oscillations of one or more body parts. Although typically seen in the upper limbs, almost any area may be involved including the trunk, head, facial muscles, and legs. Sometimes tremor is not visible at all but may be heard or palpated for example in vocal or orthostatic tremor, respectively. In neurological practice, the diagnosis and treatment of tremor is an everyday problem. A common scenario is the distinction between essential tremor and Parkinson's disease; although this is normally straightforward, diagnostic error and consequently inappropriate medication are surprisingly frequent. The diagnosis of tremor depends crucially on the history, especially duration, exacerbating or relieving factors, associated symptoms, and family history. For example, a tremor that has been present for 20 years, is alleviated by alcohol, occurred in a parent and which is associated with little or no disability is unlikely to be Parkinson's disease. The response of the tremor to alcohol or sometimes to medication is helpful but can be difficult to gauge. It is important to note that anxiety will exacerbate any tremor, leading to the erroneous conclusion that it is psychogenic. Wilson's disease must always be kept in mind in the neurological clinic whenever a younger patient presents with tremor (or indeed almost any other movement disorder) particularly if associated with psychiatric changes, dystonia, parkinsonism, or cerebellar features (see Section 32.8); there should be a low threshold for the use of the appropriate screening tests, especially a search for corneal Kayser–Fleischer rings and measurement of the serum caeruloplasmin. At one time, a tremor of the face, tongue, and hands was seen in association with neurosyphilis (general paresis) (Section 34.17.2); this possibility should still be considered when tremor is seen in conjunction with dementia or psychiatric changes.

On examination, the appearance of the tremor and its relationship to the state of activation of the affected limb is important, along with any associated signs such as parkinsonism, cerebellar dysfunction, or areflexia (see below). Frequency is often emphasized as a means to diagnosis; a slower 4–5 Hz tremor is said to be suggestive of parkinsonism and a faster 8–12 Hz frequency is associated with essential tremor. In fact, there is considerable overlap of frequencies in different forms of tremor and the frequency of any given tremor may vary with age and the body part affected (Bain 1993). Moreover, it is almost impossible to establish the frequency of a tremor clinically. Thus, tremor frequency is often unhelpful.

31.1.2 Clinical and physiological classification of tremor

Having taken an accurate and complete history, the tremor should first be classified by examination of its appearance and relationship to the activity in the affected limb (Table 31.1). This is not always simple or quick and certain difficulties occur repeatedly. It may be difficult to demonstrate a rest tremor if

Table 31.1. Classification of tremor by state of activity

Type of tremor	Features
Rest tremor	Tremor apparent with the limb supported against gravity and with no voluntary activation of muscles
Action tremor	Tremor during any voluntary movement (includes postural, kinetic, isometric, and task-specific tremors)
Postural tremor	Tremor during voluntary maintenance of a posture against gravity
Kinetic tremor	Tremor during any movement
Intention/terminal tremor	Clinically obvious exacerbation of a kinetic tremor at the end of a goal directed movement as the target is approached, e.g. during finger–nose testing
Task-specific tremor	Tremor appearing only or almost exclusively during a particular (usually skilled and precise) movement
Isometric tremor	Tremor appearing when a movement is opposed by a static force or object

Table 31.2. Classification of tremor by aetiology

Physiological tremor

Parkinsonian tremor

Essential tremor

Cerebellar tremor

Midbrain tremor (rubral tremor)

Dystonic tremor (myorhythmia)

Orthostatic tremor

Cortical tremor*

Asterixis (flapping tremor, hepatic tremor)*

Neuropathic tremor

Toxic tremor

Post-taumatic tremor

Task-specific tremor

Site-specific tremor

* Not strictly a tremor but due to positive or negative myoclonus.

the patient cannot relax fully; it may help to rest the affected arm on a pillow or the arm of a chair. Postural tremor may be obvious in one posture of the hands but not others; it is wise to test for this with the arms and hands in several positions, not just with the arms outstretched and hands pronated. Task-specific tremors will only be seen during the relevant activity such as writing or using an instrument or tool. The next step is to combine the data from the history and examination and arrive if possible at an aetiological classification (Table 31.2).

Neurophysiological measurements have not been particularly useful in the classification of tremor but frequency analysis may occasionally help. Examples include primary orthostatic tremor which has a very characteristic fast (14–18 Hz) frequency and hysterical tremor which may reveal marked frequency variation, a feature not seen with organic tremors (Cleeves *et al.* 1994).

31.1.3 Physiological tremor

This tremor is present in normal individuals but is usually asymptomatic. It may become more apparent during very precise delicate movement or in association with anxiety or excitement. It can be very difficult in some individuals to distinguish exaggerated physiological tremor from essential tremor. There are two components to physiological tremor; a constant 8–12 Hz low-amplitude tremor is evident during limb postures and is so constant that it is likely to originate in the central nervous system (CNS). In addition there is a variable *mechanical reflex component* which is a passive mechanical oscillation produced by a complex interaction of the mechanical properties of the limbs, arterial pulsation, tetanic muscle contraction, stretch reflex feedback from muscle spindles, and motor neurone activation patterns. Physiological tremor is exacerbated by increased stimulation of β-adrenoceptors as a consequence of anxiety, thyrotoxicosis, hypoglycaemia, caffeine, and other β-agonists (e.g. salbutamol, amphetamine, or aminophylline); some drugs such as sodium valproate and lithium probably act via a similar mechanism. Enhanced physiological tremor can be treated if necessary, for example in musicians, technicians, and other occupations requiring steadiness and dexterity, with propranolol (Hallett 1984).

31.1.4 Essential tremor

Essential tremor (ET) is one of the most common movement disorders with a population prevalence of 0.3–1.7 per cent in different population surveys. The age of onset is bimodal with peaks at about 15 and 50 years and the sexes are equally affected. Up to 70 per cent of cases have a positive family history and in these families, inheritance is autosomal dominant with full penetrance by the age of 65 years (Bain *et al.* 1994). ET is genetically heterogeneous with two identified loci (ETM1 and ETM2) on chromosomes 2p22–25 and 3q13 (Gulcher *et al.* 1997; Higgins *et al.* 1997). The pathophysiology of ET is poorly understood but seems to involve bilateral cerebellar overactivity (Jenkins *et al.* 1993) and abnormal rhythmic discharges of thalamic neurones (Hua *et al.* 1998).

Clinically, sporadic and familial ET are identical. Onset is typically in one or both arms and the tremor is mainly postural with a typical frequency of 4–12 Hz. In about 20 per cent of cases there may be a mild kinetic or intention component. Although the onset may be unilateral, most cases eventually become bilateral (Bain *et al.* 1994) but often asymmetrical. The tremor slowly deteriorates over many years but is usually confined to the upper limbs. In about a third of cases the legs become affected and in severe ET, there may be involvement of the head (of either yes–yes or no–no type), tongue, voice, jaw, and face in decreasing order of frequency. Isolated tremors of the legs, head, face, or voice do not occur (Bain *et al.* 1994). Mild ataxia of gait is seen in 50 per cent of patients (Singer *et al.*

1994). ET is characteristically relieved by 2–4 units of alcohol but the effect lasts only a few hours, is often incomplete, and is only evident in about a half of cases; accordingly alcohol responsiveness is a useful diagnostic indicator of ET but need not be present in every case. Unfortunately, patients with ET are still diagnosed incorrectly as having Parkinson's disease. Although some patients with Parkinson's disease can have a postural tremor, additional signs of bradykinesia and rigidity should be present; moreover, most patients with ET present to the clinic after many years of shaking and are likely to have a family history, alcohol response, or both. It has to be said that in the majority of patients, Parkinson's disease and ET should be easily differentiated.

Many patients with ET do not require treatment; in these cases an explanation and reassurance are adequate. Many of these patients are referred to the outpatient department with a diagnosis of Parkinson's disease and often, anti-Parkinsonian medication has been administered unsuccessfully for years. These patients are usually greatly relieved by the correct diagnosis but require tactful handling and discontinuation of inappropriate drugs. However, ET is not entirely benign; many patients have significant disability and handicap, especially in terms of employment. Propranolol at a dose of up to 240–320 mg/day will significantly relieve but not abolish tremor in about 70 per cent of cases (Koller and Vetere-Overfield 1989) but is contraindicated in asthma, cardiac disease, or diabetes. Primidone is equally effective but often poorly tolerated due to sedation; it is important to start at very low doses (50 mg once a day) and increase very slowly (e.g. 50 mg every 2 weeks) to a maximum of 750–1000 mg/day. In practice, very few patients can tolerate high doses. Many other drugs have been tried in ET but without success. Gabapentin may be helpful but consistent benefit has not been demonstrated (Gironell et al. 1999; Pahwa et al. 1998). Some patients have been treated with local injections of botulinum toxin (Jankovic et al. 1996); although tremor is reduced, the benefit is temporary and the injections need to be repeated. This form of treatment requires further evaluation but is unlikely to become widespread.

In severe cases of ET, stereotactic Vim nucleus thalamotomy has been effective (Shahzadi et al. 1995). Most series have reported favourable results but large numbers of patients have not been treated, the effect is upon tremor in the contralateral limbs only and the duration of benefit is unclear. Bilateral thalamotomy is best avoided in view of the increased risk of adverse events such as dysarthria. A more promising technique is thalamic (Vim) stimulation (Benabid et al. 1991), which also appears to be effective in suppressing ET but can be carried out bilaterally (Benabid et al. 1996; Pahwa et al. 1999). The duration of benefit in ET is uncertain, but some patients do show a reduced response to Vim stimulation with time.

There have been several reports of possible relationships between ET and other neurological disorders, especially Parkinson's disease (Koller et al. 1994; De Michele et al. 1995) and idiopathic torsion dystonia (ITD) (Fletcher et al. 1991). In Parkinson's disease, the difficulty arises because some patients have an additional postural component to the tremor and in some ET patients, there may be tremor apparently 'at rest'. In addition, there are reports of an increased incidence of ET among the relatives of Parkinson's disease patients. However, a recent detailed clinical analysis of ET showed no convincing evidence of rest tremor or parkinsonism (Bain et al. 1994) and an earlier large study of patients with ET, Parkinson's disease, and controls showed no evidence of any association (Cleeves et al. 1988). Moreover, there is no neuropathological evidence of Parkinson's disease in patients with ET (Rajput et al. 1993) and positron emission tomography (PET) studies show no evidence of nigrostriatal dysfunction in ET (Jenkins et al. 1993). While this issue is not entirely resolved, any association between ET and Parkinson's disease seems tenuous (Pahwa and Koller 1993). In ITD, an upper limb postural tremor similar to ET is often seen with torticollis but can occur with other forms of ITD and may even be the sole clinical abnormality in some ITD gene carriers (see below and Section 32.4.2.3). Despite this clinical overlap between ET and ITD, the two disorders are genetically distinct; there is no genetic linkage between the ITD locus (DYT1) on chromosome 9 and ET (Conway et al. 1993; Durr et al. 1993).

31.1.5 Parkinsonism and tremor

The pathophysiology and clinical features of Parkinsonian tremor are discussed in Sections 32.2.2 and 32.3.1.8 and also in Section 31.1.4 (above). Many patients with Parkinson's disease have a postural tremor in addition to the typical Parkinsonian rest tremor; the former is very similar to ET. In some cases, propranolol may be of benefit but the response is not as clear as that seen in ET and primidone does not seem to be helpful (Cleeves et al. 1994). In multiple system atrophy and drug-induced parkinsonism (see Chapter 32) tremor is less common and usually postural, while tremor is unusual in other forms of parkinsonism. Wilson's disease must again be emphasized as a vitally important diagnosis (Section 32.8).

31.1.6 Rubral (midbrain) tremor

This type of tremor was first described by Gordon Holmes (Holmes 1904) who noted a low-frequency and large-amplitude upper limb tremor, present at rest but exacerbated by posture and movement with an intention (terminal) component. This combination of Parkinsonian and cerebellar features pointed to a lesion of the midbrain tegmentum in the region of the red nucleus and the cerebellothalamic pathway (Section 32.2.2). This localization has been confirmed by neuropathological studies. Midbrain tremor is usually severe and disabling, producing wild and uncontrollable arm tremor. Most cases are due to brainstem trauma, multiple sclerosis, vascular lesions, or cerebellar degenerations; a few are idiopathic and unilateral. Ipsilateral striatal dopamine deficiency due to nigrostrital tract damage has been demonstrated in some cases (Remy et al. 1995). Treatment is notoriously difficult; levodopa, propranolol, and anticholinergic agents may be tried but the response to these drugs is unpredictable. In very severe cases, thalamotomy or thalamic (Vim) stimulation has been tried (Broggi *et al.* 1993; Geny *et al.* 1996).

31.1.7 Cerebellar tremor

Tremor is one of the cardinal features of cerebellar disease, along with dysmetria, dysdiadochokinesis, dysarthria, hypotonia, abnormal eye movement, ataxia, and decomposition of movement. Cerebellar disease produces a slow, high-amplitude *kinetic* tremor, which worsens during a movement leading to a terminal or intention component (Table 31.1). This is seen clinically during finger–nose or heel–knee–shin testing and will usually be accompanied by dysmetria (past pointing) unless quite mild. In addition to the typical kinetic cerebellar tremor there may be a large amplitude postural tremor of the head (titubation) and sometimes the trunk and limbs. A hallmark of cerebellar tremor is that it mainly affects axial or proximal limb muscle groups. Pathology of the midline cerebellar vermis tends to produce ataxia of gait and titubation of the head and trunk while lesions of the lateral cerebellar hemispheres or cerebellar outflow pathways are associated with the kinetic (intention) limb tremor (Gilman *et al.* 1981). There is no specific treatment for cerebellar tremor.

31.1.8 Drug- and alcohol-induced tremor

An action tremor of the hands is commonly seen in alcoholics as a withdrawal symptom ('morning shakes'). This is usually relieved promptly by the first drink of the day. In full-blown withdrawal, the tremor can be severe and associated with prominent mental changes, fever, autonomic instability, and dehydration (delerium tremens). β-Adrenergic agonists such as salbutamol or aminophylline, used in asthma, are a common iatrogenic cause of an action tremor of the hands. In some individuals, a similar phenomenon is seen after caffeine ingestion. Neuroleptic drugs may cause tremor as a feature of drug-induced parkinsonism; this is usually symmetrical and sometimes of action/postural type rather than a resting tremor (Section 32.3.4). In the 'rabbit syndrome', a particular form of drug-induced Parkinsonian tremor, there is a resting 4–6 Hz tremor of the lips. In some patients receiving long-term neuroleptic therapy, a persistent rest and postural tremor appears which is increased by drug withdrawal and improved by dopamine depletion with terabenazine; these similarities to other tardive phenomena have led to the term tardive tremor for this phenomenon (Stacy and Jankovic 1992). Tricyclic antidepressants are prone to cause an action tremor and sometimes parkinsonism or rabbit syndrome (Vandel *et al.* 1997). Other causes of a postural or action tremor of the hands include lithium, sodium valproate, cyclosporin A, and amiodarone.

31.1.9 Orthostatic tremor

This rare condition is seen mostly in older adults in whom there is a fast tremor of the legs and sometimes paraspinal muscles which develops only during standing and not when walking, sitting, or leaning on a support (Heilman 1984; Britton and Thompson 1995). The tremor tends to develop after standing for a minute or so, so that the patient feels increasingly unsteady and is in fear of falling and injury. Orthostatic tremor (OT) is fast and barely visible (Britton *et al.* 1992); it may be detected only by palpation of the legs while the patient is standing. There are no other features and in particular, an upper limb tremor is characteristically absent (but has occasionally been noted) and the gait is normal. The condition tends to worsen over several years and the disorder does not appear to be familial. The tremor is much faster than ET, typically 13–18 Hz (McManis and Sharbrough 1993) and this is one of the rare situations where tremor frequency measurement is diagnostically useful. OT is not affected by peripheral stimuli and is likely to originate in the CNS. The relationship between OT and ET is uncertain but the differences between the two suggest that they are separate disorders (Table 31.3). PET has shown abnormally increased cerebellar activation, similar to that seen in ET, suggesting that cerebellar overactivity may be a consequence of tremor caused by different mechanisms (Wills *et al.* 1996). β-Blockers are not effective in OT but the symptoms are improved with clonazepam (Heilman 1984). Some cases have responded to primidone, given with clonazepam (Poersch 1994) but only small numbers of cases have been described. Some patients have responded to L-dopa or gabapentin (Wills *et al.* 1999; Evidente *et al.* 1998).

31.1.10 Site-specific tremors

In addition to patients who develop a focal onset of well-recognized tremors such as Parkinson's disease (in which tremor may be remarkably localized, even in only one digit, at onset) or the syndrome of painful feet and moving toes (Section 32.10.7), there is a miscellaneous group of disorders in which patients present with spontaneous tremor confined to one body part. It should be noted that focal tremor confined to the head, face, trunk, or legs is highly unusual in ET and in one recent study of familial ET was not seen at all (Bain *et al.* 1994).

Table 31.3. Differences between orthostatic tremor and essential tremor

	Orthostatic tremor	Essential tremor
Age of onset	Late	Bimodal
Main site affected	Legs	Arms
Main symptom	Unsteadiness	Shaking hands
Tremor visible?	No	Yes
Frequency	13–18 Hz	4–12 Hz
Familial	No	Often
Response to alcohol	No	Often
Response to β-blockers	No	Often
Response to primidone	Sometimes	Often
Response to clonazepam	Yes	Variable

◆ Isolated head and trunk tremors are usually dystonic and not due to ET (Rivest and Marsden 1990). Such tremors are not a feature of Parkinson's disease and although cerebellar disease can lead to a slow nodding head tremor (titubation), additional cerebellar signs will be present in this situation. These focal tremors tend to be worse during standing or walking and absent when lying down and there are often subtle dystonic movements of the trunk or neck in addition. A common outpatient situation is the occurrence of tremulous cervical dystonia in which the patient presents with a complex multidirectional head tremor but with slight additional torticollis or laterocollis as a clue to the true nature of the problem. It should be noted that dystonia may be jerky or tremulous and does not always produce fixed abnormal postures or spasms (Section 32.4.1). Patients with isolated head and trunk tremors may be treated with anticholinergics or cervical botulinum toxin injections (Jankovic et al. 1991).

◆ Isolated leg resting tremor is usually due to Parkinson's disease, while focal lower limb tremor developing during standing is suggestive of primary OT (see above).

◆ Focal tremor of the chin (geniospasm) may occur as a hereditary disorder (Danek 1993). Inheritance is autosomal dominant and one gene locus on chromosome 9q13–21 has been identified (Jarman et al. 1997).

31.1.11 Primary writing tremor and other task-specific tremors

In some patients, a focal upper limb tremor develops in association with a particular action. The best known example is primary writing tremor (PWT) (Bain et al. 1995) but similar task-specific tremors have been reported with other activities such as playing golf, throwing darts, shooting, playing a musical instrument, drinking, or using tools (Soland et al. 1996). The cause of PWT and other task-specific tremors is unclear. The striking task specificity is reminiscent of the focal dystonias such as writer's cramp or those of musicians (Section 32.4) leading some to conclude that they are variants of focal dystonia, although studies of reciprocal inhibition are normal (Bain et al. 1995) unlike writer's cramp (Marsden and Rothwell 1987). Others have regarded task-specific tremors as variants of ET. At present the issue is unsettled but a relationship to focal dystonia seems more likely. In terms of response to drug therapy, some patients with focal task-specific tremors respond like ET to propranolol or primidone while others behave like a dystonia and improve with anticholinergic medication (Cleeves et al. 1994). Overall, the response to treatment is poor and most patients are not improved by any medication. Botulinum toxin has been used in a few cases of PWT and the use of thalamotomy has been described (Ohye et al. 1982). Although the occupational handicap in PWT may be considerable, it is difficult to recommend the use of stereotactic neurosurgery for this condition.

31.1.12 Tremor and dystonia

It has long been apparent that some patients with ITD, especially those with cervical dystonia (torticollis) can have a postural tremor of the hands, which is indistinguishable from ET (Jankovic et al. 1991). Other patients with focal dystonias have tremor in addition to dystonic spasms in the affected body part such as in writer's cramp (Sheehy and Marsden 1982) and axial dystonia (Rivest and Marsden 1990). Such tremors are also seen in patients with generalized ITD (Marsden and Harrison 1974) and may be the only clinical manifestation in otherwise asymptomatic ITD gene carriers (Fletcher et al. 1990). The tremor in these patients appears to be a manifestation of ITD and not because of coexistent ET and as mentioned in Section 31.1.4, the genetic loci for ITD and ET are separate. Tremor and dystonia share a number of features, suggesting that they may arise by similar mechanisms. Not only do both sometimes appear in the same patients, but they share a tendency to task specificity (as seen in the task-specific tremors discussed above) and may both develop as a response to peripheral trauma (see below).

In addition to the coexistence of tremor and dystonia in some patients, it should be noted that dystonic movements themselves are sometimes deceptively tremulous, especially when the neck (see Section 31.1.10) or upper limbs are involved, a feature sometimes referred to as myorhythmia (Herz 1944).

31.1.13 Post-traumatic tremor

In addition to the severe midbrain tremor seen after traumatic brain injury (Section 31.1.6) there are rare reports of tremor following mild head injuries (Biary et al. 1989) and also peripheral injury (Jankovic and Van der Linden 1988). The mechanism by which peripheral injuries lead to the onset of a tremor in the affected body part is unclear but a genetic predisposition, suggested by a mild pre-existing tremor or a family history of ET is possible, as suggested for post-traumatic dystonia (Section 32.4.11).

31.1.14 Neuropathic tremor

Tremor may be prominent in patients with peripheral neuropathy (Cleeves et al. 1994) and this possibility must be considered in all patients presenting with tremor. A postural tremor of the hands is the most common type but cases of rest tremor and intention tremor have also been reported. The majority of neuropathic tremors are seen with demyelinating neuropathies such as hereditary motor and sensory neuropathy type I, chronic inflammatory demyelinating polyneuropathy, and dysproteinaemic neuropathy (Sections 12.4, 12.11, 12.12.1). Diabetes, alcoholism, and porphyria have occasionally been responsible (Said et al. 1982). The mechanism of neuropathic tremor is unclear. Treatment with propranolol may be helpful, along with management of the underlying neuropathy if possible.

31.2 **Cerebellar disorders: diagnosis and classification**

The anatomy and physiology of the cerebellum are described in Chapter 32 along with the rest of the motor system and the principal regions of the cerebellum are shown in Fig. 31.1. Clinically, the recognition of cerebellar disease is usually straightforward. A useful practical point is that lesions of the cerebellar vermis (palaeocerebellum) tend to produce ataxia of gait, abnormal eye movement, and axial tremor (titubation) only, whereas more lateral cerebellar lesions of the hemispheres (neocerebellum) are more likely to result in a full range of cerebellar deficits, namely gait ataxia, eye movement abnormalities, decomposition of movement, ataxia, tremor and dysmetria of the limbs, dysdiadochokinesis, and hypotonia (Gilman *et al.* 1981). Dysarthria is seen with a wide range of cerebellar lesions and is of little localizing value.

Disorders of the cerebellum lead to well-recognized symptoms and physical signs. It must be remembered that ataxia, clumsiness, disordered ocular motility, dysarthria, and even kinetic (intention) tremor are not always caused by cerebellar disease. Diagnostic problems do arise in which a cerebellar disorder is suspected initially but it eventually turns out that a different pathology is simulating cerebellar disease. Certain difficulties arise repeatedly in the clinic:

- Patients with peripheral neuropathy, especially hereditary motor and sensory neuropathy type I (HMSN I) (Section 12.4.2), chronic inflammatory demyelinating polyneuropathy (CIDP) (Section 12.11.1), Guillain–Barré syndrome (GBS) (Section 12.10), and the Miller Fisher syndrome (Section 12.10.5) may have prominent ataxia of gait. In early GBS particularly, the abnormal gait may be the presenting feature, before clear signs of peripheral nerve involvement are apparent. The ataxia is a consequence of impaired proprioception and may also lead to clumsiness and inco-ordination of the limbs; sometimes, a neuropathic tremor of the limbs may also resemble that seen in cerebellar disease (Section 31.1.14). The absence of dysarthria, normal eye movements (except for Miller Fisher syndrome), areflexia, and nerve conduction studies will usually lead to the correct diagnosis but not invariably. The distinction between early Friedreich's ataxia (FA) and HMSN I, in which the only early signs may be ataxia and areflexia, can be particularly difficult without nerve conduction studies or, increasingly, DNA analysis.

- Cervical spondylotic myelopathy (Section 20.5.2) often leads to impaired upper limb proprioception because of dorsal column involvement of the cervical cord; this can produce a combination of unsteadiness of gait and ataxic upper limbs. Clear pyramidal signs may not always be detectable, or if present may be attributed to one of the late onset cerebellar degenerations (Sections 31.8, 31.9).

- An unsteady wide based gait is seen with frontal lobe pathlogy, especially hydrocephalus, cerebrovascular disease (Binswanger's encephalopathy), and mass lesions (see Section 32.10.10). Although this 'frontal gait disorder' can usually be identified clinically, the unsteadiness can be so severe (Nutt *et al.* 1993) that the distinction from a cerebellar syndrome is very difficult (frontal ataxia of Bruns).

- In Steele–Richardson–Olzsewski disease (Section 32.3.9), falling and instability of gait may be prominent before other signs such as ophthalmoparesis have developed and a cerebellar disorder may initially be suspected. Even if parkinsonism and abnormal eye movements are present, it can be difficult to exclude a sporadic late onset cerebellar degeneration in the early stages.

- The distinction between cerebellar and pseudobulbar dysarthria is sometimes difficult. Accordingly, motor neurone disease, cerebrovascular disease, or multiple sclerosis may initially be confused with a cerebellar degeneration. Signs of pseudobulbar palsy such as emotional lability, slowing of tongue movement, and a brisk jaw jerk may be helpful.

- Wilson's disease (Section 32.8) may present with unsteadiness and clumsiness suggestive of a cerebellar disorder, the so-called 'pseudosclerotic' presentation. Although very rare, this is an important clinical consideration because the condition is treatable.

- Vitamin B12 deficiency may present with a progressive ataxia due to subacute combined degeneration of the spinal cord and loss of dorsal column proprioceptive function (Section 20.6.3). This is therefore a spinal rather than a cerebellar ataxia (as is FA), but B12 deficiency must always be considered in the ataxic patient if permanent and avoidable neurological damage is to be prevented.

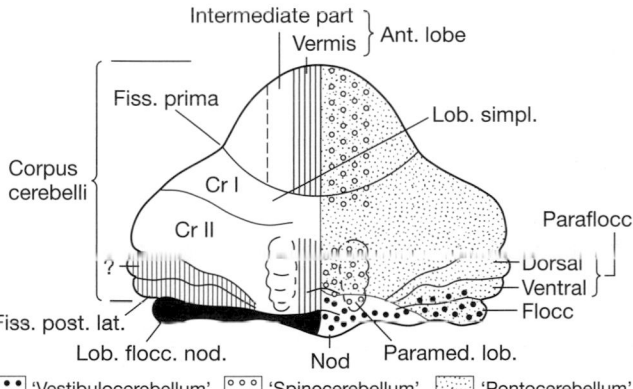

Fig. 31.1. A simplified anatomical representation of thecerebellum. In the left half are the three main subdivisions: the archicerebellum (vestibulocerebellum) comprising the flocculonodular lobe (black); paleocerebellum (spinocerebellum) comprising the anterior and posterior vermis and the paraflocculus (vertical hatching); and the neocerebellum (pontocerebellum) comprising the central vermis and bulk of the hemispheres (white). On the right, the terminations of the vestibulocerebellar (heavy dots), spinocerebellar (open dots) and pontocerebellar (small dots) afferents are shown. (From Brodal A. (1981). *Neurological anatomy in relation to clinical medicine.* Oxford University Press, Oxford.)

The classification of the various causes of cerebellar ataxia has long been a troublesome issue. Cerebellar diseases may be classified in terms of age of onset, aetiology, clinical features, neuropathology, inheritance and, increasingly, molecular genetic abnormalities. None of these approaches is entirely satisfactory for such a heterogeneous group of disorders in which there is a poor correlation between aetiology, clinical features, and neuropathological appearances. A pragmatic clinical approach is to think of the ataxias initially in terms of mode and age of onset and with regard to any detectable underlying cause or inheritance. Aetiology may be suggested by the mode of onset and the age of the patient as shown in Table 31.4. The principal causes of ataxia are shown, with the usual speed and age of onset indicated. This is a helpful clinical classification of ataxia, which is readily applied in the clinic or the acute ward setting. In practice, most cases of acute (or subacute) ataxia are due to toxins (principally drugs and alcohol), vascular lesions (in older adults), or demyelination (in younger patients) while the most common cause of any chronic, slowly progressive ataxia is a degenerative cerebellar or spinal ataxia.

It is important not to overlook a treatable cause of ataxia; the important possibilities are drugs and toxins, deficiency states (thiamine and vitamins B12 and E), posterior fossa mass lesions, hypothyroidism, hydrocephalus, cholestanolosis, and Whipple's disease.

Physical examination may reveal abnormalities which aid diagnosis. Features of the neurological examination are given in Table 31.5 and general examination findings are considered in Table 31.6. The use of special investigations will be determined by the likely diagnostic possibilities. In patients with adult onset cerebellar ataxia, MR scanning, thyroid function tests, a vitamin B12 estimation, and a chest X-ray are usually adequate. If a para-

Table 31.4. Clinical classification of the ataxias by mode of onset, age, aetiology, and inheritance

Mode of onset and cause of ataxia	Inheritance	Childhood	Young adults	Older adults
Congenital ataxia				
Ataxic cerebral palsy		+		
Hereditary congenital ataxias	AD/AR/XL	+		
Acute/subacute onset ataxia				
Infarction/haemorrhage				+
Demyelination (MS)			+	
Demyelination (ADEM)		+	+	
Post-infectious cerebellar ataxia		+	+	
Paraneoplastic		+	+	
Toxins		+	+	+
Thiamine deficiency (Wernicke)			+	+
Abscess/tumour		+	+	+
Basilar migraine		+	+	
Slowly progressive ataxia				
Early onset hereditary degenerative ataxia (<25 years)	AR (AD/XL rarely)	+	(+)	
Late onset hereditary degenerative ataxia (>25 years)	AD (AR/XL rarely)		+	+
Sporadic idiopathic cerebellar degeneration				+
Tumour		+	+	+
Foramen magnum compression			+	+
Alcoholic cerebellar ataxia				+
Hydrocephalus		+	+	+
Hypothyroidism				+
Drugs, e.g. phenytoin				+
Prion disease	(occasionally AD)		+	+
Metabolic ataxias	AR/XL/mitochondrial	+	+	
Vitamin E deficiency	AR		+	
Intermittent ataxia				
Drugs/toxins			+	+
Multiple sclerosis			+	
Transient ischaemic attacks				+
Foramen magnum compression			+	+
Intermittent hydrocephalus			+	+
Metabolic ataxias	AR/XL/mitochondrial	+	+	
Periodic ataxias (hereditary)	AD	+	+	

AD = autosomal dominant; AR = autosomal recessive; XL = X-linked.
MS = multiple sclerosis; ADEM = acute disseminated encephalomyelitis.

Table 31.5. Associated neurological/ocular features in ataxic disease

Sign	Association
Cognitive impairment:	
• Learning disability	Congenital ataxia; ataxic CP; early onset hereditary degenerations; some metabolic ataxias
• Dementia	Late onset hereditary degenerations; idiopathic degenerations; prion disease; hydrocephalus; some metabolic ataxias; paraneoplastic syndromes; hypothyroidism
Ocular features:	
• Retinopathy	Hereditary degenerations; vitamin E deficiency; mitochondrial disease
• Retinal angioma	Von Hippel Lindau disease
• Optic atrophy	MS; hereditary degenerations; alcoholism; some metabolic ataxias; congenital ataxias;
• Aniridia	Gillespie syndrome
• Cataract	Marinesco–Sjogren syndrome; cholestanolosis
• INO	Demyelination; Wernicke's encephalopathy; degenerations; posterior fossa tumour; stroke
• Ophthalmoplegia	Degenerations; some metabolic ataxias; mitochondrial disease; hydrocephalus; Wernicke's encephalopathy
• Ocular apraxia	Ataxia telangiectasia
• Ptosis	Mitochondrial disease; degenerations; stroke
• Downbeating nystagmus	Foramen magnum compression
• Opsoclonus/ocular flutter	Paraneoplastic syndromes; drugs; post-infectious cerebellitis
Extraphyramidal features:	
• Parkinsonism	Degenerations
• Dystonia/chorea	Degenerations; ataxia telangiectasia; some metabolic ataxias
Myoclonus	Ramsay Hunt syndrome; prion disease; drugs
Deafness	Degenerations; some metabolic ataxias
Stupor/coma	Tumour; stroke; abscess; toxins and drugs; basilar migraine; Wernicke's encephalopathy; some metabolic ataxias
Headache	Tumour; stroke/TIA; abscess; basilar migraine
Pyramidal signs	Congenital ataxia; degenerations; demyelination; foramen magnum compression; hydrocephalus; stroke/TIA; some metabolic ataxias
Areflexia	Degenerations (various hereditary forms and idiopathic); vitamin E deficiency; Wernicke's encephalopathy; some metabolic ataxias; neuropathic ataxia (see text); paraneoplastic
Muscle fasciculations/wasting	Degenerations (hereditary or idiopathic); hexosaminidase deficiency; paraneoplastic

neoplastic ataxia is suspected, anti-neuronal antibodies and investigations to reveal a malignancy are indicated (pelvic ultrasound, CT of the thorax and abdomen, and probably mammography); the EEG is helpful in some cases of prion disease and nerve conduction studies may be needed to exclude a neuropathic ataxia along with a cerebrospinal fluid (CSF) examination (if acute GBS or CIDP are suspected). In younger patients, an ECG may be very helpful as it points very strongly to the diagnosis of FA in the clinic without the need for additional tests other than DNA analysis (see below). Additional investigations such as lipids, white cell enzymes, immunoglobulins, α-fetoprotein, caeruloplasmin, slit lamp examination for Kayser–Fleischer rings, muscle biopsy, lactate/pyruvate, very long chain fatty acids, and bone marrow examination are usually indicated in younger patients if a neurometabolic disorder is suspected. The vitamin E level is important in younger patients, especially those with a FA phenotype, even if cardiomyopathy is present. It is essential not to miss vitamin E deficiency which is treatable; a sound clinical tip is to consider the diagnosis and request a vitamin E estimation in patients with ataxia and areflexia. Cholestanolosis is also treatable and although cholestanol estimations are not easily available, tendon xanthomas, cataracts, and a low serum cholesterol level are suggestive clues to the diagnosis.

Increasingly, DNA analysis is applied in the diagnosis of various hereditary cerebellar ataxias (see below). This has led to a tendency to classify the hereditary ataxias, particularly the adult onset dominant ataxias, by their underlying genetic mutations. Although this has an academic and scientific appeal, such an approach is not very helpful in the clinic where the molecular diagnosis is initially unknown and difficult to predict on the basis of the clinical phenotype. This problem is discussed further in Section 31.8 but in this chapter, a clinical classification of the hereditary ataxias (Harding 1984) will be used.

31.3 Congenital ataxia (ataxic cerebral palsy)

The congenital ataxias are a rare group of disorders characterized by a congenital neurological syndrome of which the salient feature is cerebellar ataxia, a static non-progressive course (which is an important distinguishing feature from other hereditary and idiopathic cerebellar degenerations), and variable associated clinical features. Some congenital cerebellar disorders such as Dandy–Walker syndrome and the Chiari malformations do not cause congenital ataxia and are not dealt with in this chapter. The

Table 31.6. Other associations with ataxic disease

Feature	Association
Dysmorphism	Some congenital and metabolic ataxias
Scoliosis	Various congenital and early onset degenerations, especially Friedreich's ataxia
Skin changes:	
• Pigmentation; scanty hair	Adrenoleucodystrophy
• Telengiectasia	Ataxia telangiectasia
• Photosensitivity	Xeroderma pigmentosum; ataxia telangiectasia; Cockayne syndrome; Hartnup disease
• Tendon xanthomas	Cholestanolosis
Malnutrition/cachexia	Wernicke's encephalopathy (alcoholism); malabsorption (acquired vitamin E deficiency); sometimes paraneoplastic ataxia
Cardiac disease	Friedreich's ataxia; sometimes mitochondrial disease and vitamin E deficiency
Hypogonadism	Holmes syndrome; adrenoleucodystrophy; Marinesco–Sjogren syndrome

first signs of congenital ataxia are usually motor delay and hypotonia, followed in due course by cerebellar signs as the child starts to sit and walk. Among the congenital ataxias, there is considerable clinical and pathological heterogeneity. Some patients have a pure cerebellar syndrome of congenital onset while in most cases there are additional features such as learning disability, spasticity, or other abnormalities (Steinlin 1998). Pathologically, there are several recognized forms of cerebellar hypoplasia affecting the hemispheres or confined to the vermis and in some cases the cerebellum is almost totally absent. Similar pathological appearances can be associated with widely different clinical features. For example, cerebellar aplasia may present as a severe neurological disorder of infancy or, surprisingly, as a mild congenital ataxia with clinical presentation in late adult life (Harding 1984). The aetiology of the congenital ataxias is mixed. Probably about 50 per cent are hereditary, mostly autosomal recessive but with occasional examples of X-linked and autosomal dominant inheritance (Bundey 1992). The remainder, which are difficult to distinguish clinically, are of unknown and presumably environmental origin. The high incidence of genetic disorders and usually normal perinatal histories among patients with congenital ataxia means that the term 'ataxic cerebral palsy' is preferably avoided.

31.3.1 Miscellaneous hereditary cerebellar hypoplasias

♦ There are numerous clinically or pathologically defined hereditary congenital ataxia syndromes associated with hypoplasia of the cerebellum (Harding 1984). These conditions are rare and some were described many years ago, before modern neuroimaging and metabolic investigations

were available. Any distinction between the following disorders and the other eponymous congenital ataxias (see below) is somewhat artificial and many patients do not easily fit into any of these diagnostic entities.

♦ Pontoneocerebellar hypoplasia causes cerebellar ataxia, learning disability, spasticity, microcephaly, and sometimes agensis of the corpus callosum. It is likely to be autosomal recessive.

♦ Granule cell layer hypoplasia is associated with congenital cerebellar ataxia of limbs and gait, nystagmus, short stature, and learning disability. It is probably autosomal recessive.

♦ Various forms of mild congenital cerebellar ataxia with hypoplasia of the cerebellar vermis have been described. There are no associated neurological features other than mild learning disability, which is not present in all cases. Inheritance can be autosomal dominant, X-linked, or autosomal recessive. A similar disorder is described as SCA13 (Section 31.8.2).

♦ A more severe syndrome of cerebellar ataxia, learning disability, and spasticity is associated with vermis and cerebellar hemisphere hypoplasia; inheritance is autosomal recessive (al Shahwan et al. 1995).

♦ COACH syndrome (Cerebellar vermis hypoplasia, Oligophrena, congenital Ataxia, Coloboma, Hepatic fibrocirrhosis) presents with hepatic failure in infancy, due to hepatic fibrosis, and a congenital ataxia (Gentile et al. 1996). Inheritance is probably autosomal recessive but could be X-linked in some families.

♦ An X-linked congenital cerebellar ataxia with ophthalmoplegia has been described, with a disease gene mapped to Xq23 (Illarioshkin et al. 1996).

♦ In another severe form of X-linked congenital ataxia with associated learning disability, affected boys later develop myoclonus and retinal degeneration. A gene locus has been identified at Xp22 (des Portes et al. 1996).

31.3.2 Paine syndrome

The original description was of an X-linked congenital ataxia with cerebellar hypoplasia, microcephaly, developmental delay, spasticity, myoclonus, seizures, and optic atrophy (Paine 1960). Harding (1984) cited other examples of this syndrome but a clear distinction from various other X-linked cerebellar hypoplasias (see above) seems uncertain.

31.3.3 Gillespie syndrome

Gillespie syndrome is characterized by partial aniridia, cerebellar ataxia, and mental retardation. The diagnosis is suggested by the discovery of fixed dilated pupils in a hypotonic infant. The ocular findings are specific to this disorder and are apparent from birth. Neurological involvement includes motor delay, hypotonia, disabling ataxia, and learning disability. There is cerebral and cerebellar atrophy and white matter changes may be seen with MR scanning (Nelson *et al.* 1997). Gillespie syndrome seems to be genetically heterogeneous with both autosomal recessive and autosomal dominant forms.

31.3.4 Marinesco–Sjogren syndrome

This is a rare autosomal recessive disorder causing motor delay, cerebellar ataxia, cataract, and learning disability. In addition there is often short stature and reflexes may be absent, normal, or brisk; plantar responses are usually extensor. In addition to the obvious CNS and ocular features, patients may have a peripheral neuropathy (Zimmer *et al.* 1992; Muller-Felber *et al.* 1998) and myopathy with fibre necrosis, atrophy, and rimmed vacuole formation (Sasaki *et al.* 1996). There have also been reports of hypogonadism (McLaughlin *et al.* 1996). MR imaging shows cerebellar atrophy with pituitary hypoplasia and white matter abnormalities. Characteristic changes are seen in conjunctival biopsies (Zimmer *et al.* 1992). This is likely to be a lysosomal disorder and inheritance is autosomal recessive.

31.3.5 Joubert syndrome

In this rare but striking autosomal recessive disorder, cerebellar vermis agenesis is associated with hypotonia and developmental delay, ataxia, severe learning disability, abnormal eye movements, and irregular respiration (Saraiva and Baraitser 1992). The respiratory pattern is intermittent hyperpnoea alternating with apnoea; oculomotor abnormalities include nystagmus, slow saccades, and impaired pursuit movements (Maria *et al.* 1997). In a subgroup of families, the syndrome includes a combination of retinal dystrophy and renal cysts, suggesting possible genetic heterogeneity. Other associations include ocular colobomas, polydactyly, lingual tumours, and hepatic fibrosis (Lewis *et al.* 1994; Pellegrino *et al.* 1997). There are similarities with the COACH syndrome (see above). Cerebellar vermis agenesis and brainstem abnormalities are seen with MR imaging. Affected children may die in infancy with severe respiratory

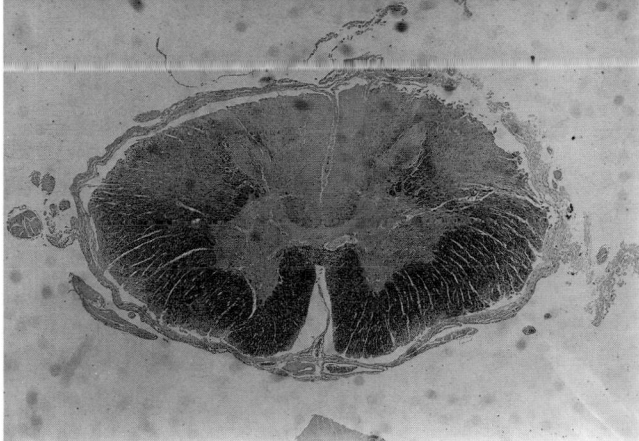

Fig. 31.2. The cervical spinal cord in Friedreich's ataxia (myelin stain) showing degeneration of the posterior columns (courtesy of Dr J. Broome, Liverpool).

abnormalities and developmental failure; others survive into adolescence with variable disability (Steinlin *et al.* 1997).

31.3.6 The dysequilibrium syndrome

This syndrome has been described mainly in Scandinavia (Sanner 1973). Affected children are grossly hypotonic with clumsiness and delayed motor milestones; a disabling congenital ataxia becomes apparent and the child is unable to stand without falling. Walking is eventually achieved by about 10 years but is always abnormal. Speech delay and learning disability are common and cataracts have been described. Neuroimaging studies may reveal cerebellar vermis hypoplasia. Inheritance is autosomal recessive.

31.4 Friedreich's ataxia and other early onset hereditary degenerative ataxias

The early onset hereditary degenerative ataxias are conveniently grouped together because they usually (but not invariably) start in childhood, adolescence, or early adult life, usually before the age of 25 years. They are therefore distinguished from the congenital ataxias and the late onset (usually starting after 25 years) degenerative ataxias. It must be realized that sometimes these conditions present after 25 years and so the age of onset (which can be difficult to gauge) is only an approximate guide to diagnosis. However, even with the advent of molecular genetic classification of these disorders, a clinically based classification remains a useful approach and will be retained here. The term 'early onset cerebellar ataxia' is widely used but is potentially misleading in situations where the ataxia is largely spinal, as in Friedreich's ataxia.

31.4.1 Friedreich's ataxia

Friedreich's ataxia (FA) is an autosomal recessive disorder causing a degenerative ataxia which is principally of spinal origin. It is the most common of the degenerative ataxias with a frequency in the population of approximately 1 in 50 000 (Harding 1984). Although rigorous clinical diagnostic criteria have been established for typical FA, recent molecular genetic studies have shown that clinical variability is actually greater than previously suspected (Montermini *et al.* 1997*b*). The disorder is caused by an unstable trinucleotide (GAA) expansion (or occasionally point mutation) of a gene (*X25*) located on chromosome 9q13. This gene encodes a 210 amino acid mitochondrial protein of uncertain function, frataxin.

Pathology

The major findings are in the spinal cord where there is degeneration of the dorsal columns and spinocerebellar tracts and also of the pyramidal tracts (Harding 1984). The former is worse at cervical level (Fig. 31.2) whereas the latter is more marked at lumbar level. These findings suggest a distal axonopathy. In addition there is loss of dorsal root ganglion cells with depletion of large myelinated fibres in peripheral nerves. The dorsal roots are atrophic. Interestingly, the earliest changes seen in young children are in peripheral nerves where there is large fibre loss, suggesting damage to dorsal root ganglion sensory neurones. Neuropathological changes in the cerebellum, brainstem, or cerebrum are absent or minimal.

Clinical features

In the classical form of FA, onset is usually between 8 and 16 years but the range is wide and one large series reported a mean of 10.5 years with 95 per cent confidence limits of 0–25 years (Harding 1981a). Almost all cases present with progressive gait ataxia but occasionally, scoliosis or cardiac disease precede neurological involvement (Tsao et al. 1992). At presentation there is also lower limb areflexia and electrophysiological evidence of a sensory axonal peripheral neuropathy. Additional signs including generalized areflexia, extensor plantar responses, dysarthria, pyramidal weakness of the legs and loss of joint position and vibration sense appear later, usually within 5 years and almost always by 10 years from onset (Harding 1984). These core features are essential for the diagnosis of the classical form of FA (Table 31.7).

Scoliosis occurs in approximately 80 per cent of cases and can be severe in about 10 per cent of these patients. This tends to worsen at puberty, with increasing growth and can lead to pain and cardiorespiratory complications. Cardiomyopathy is common but not invariable. An abnormal ECG (see Fig. 31.3) is seen in 65 per cent of cases (Harding and Hewer 1983) but single ECG recordings are normal in 25 per cent. Echocardiography reveals hypertrophic changes or dilated cardiomyopathy in approximately 60 per cent of cases (Gunal et al. 1996). In patients who undergo continuous ECG monitoring, echocardiography, and nuclear ventriculography, the incidence of cardiac abnormalities is even higher. In some patients, the ECG becomes abnormal years after onset, even when earlier records have been normal. In contrast to the high frequency of ECG abnormalities, clinically apparent cardiomyopathy with signs of cardiac failure or evidence of arrythmia is uncommon, probably developing in less than 15 per cent of cases (Harding and Hewer 1983).

There are several less common features of FA. Optic atrophy is seen in approximately 25 per cent of cases but in only 5 per cent of patients is visual acuity significantly reduced. Nystagmus is seen in 20 per cent, but other forms of disordered eye movement such as jerky pursuit movements, dysmetric saccades, square wave jerks, and failure of vestibulo-ocular reflex suppression are more common (Moschner et al. 1994). Deafness develops in 10 per cent of cases. Distal wasting is seen in about a half of cases but is usually not associated with weakness. Diabetes develops in 10 per cent of patients and usually requires insulin therapy. In some patients truncal ataxia makes sitting or standing still difficult and there is a motor restlessness which may be mistaken for chorea (Harding 1984); this may occur very early in the disease. Another common feature of advanced FA is the development of cold, cyanosed, and oedematous feet.

The prognosis of classical FA is variable. On average, patients lose the ability to walk after 15 years from onset; over half of cases are so affected by the age of 26 years and 95 per cent by 44 years of age. A few patients continue to walk independently into their 50s but this is unusual. Age at death is also highly variable, depending on associated features such as cardiac disease and diabetes (De Michele et al. 1996); some patients survive into the sixth and seventh decades.

Table 31.7. Clinical features of classical and variant forms of Friedrelch's ataxia (FA)

Classical FA		
Almost all cases	<5 years from onset	Progressive ataxia of gait
		Lower limb areflexia
		Extensor plantar responses
		Sensory axonal neuropathy detected on nerve conduction tests
	5–10 years from onset	Leg weakness
		Reduced vibration and joint position sense in lower limbs
		Dysarthria
		Generalized areflexia
Variable features	(i) in >50% of cases	Cardiomyopathy on ECG
		Scoliosis
	(ii) in <50% of cases	Nystagmus
		Optic atrophy
		Deafness
		Diabetes
		Pes cavus
		Distal weakness and wasting
Variant FA		Late onset disease (25–50 years)
		Mild, slowly progressive (Acadian) FA
		Lower limb spasicity and hyperreflexia in FA
		Chorea at presentation

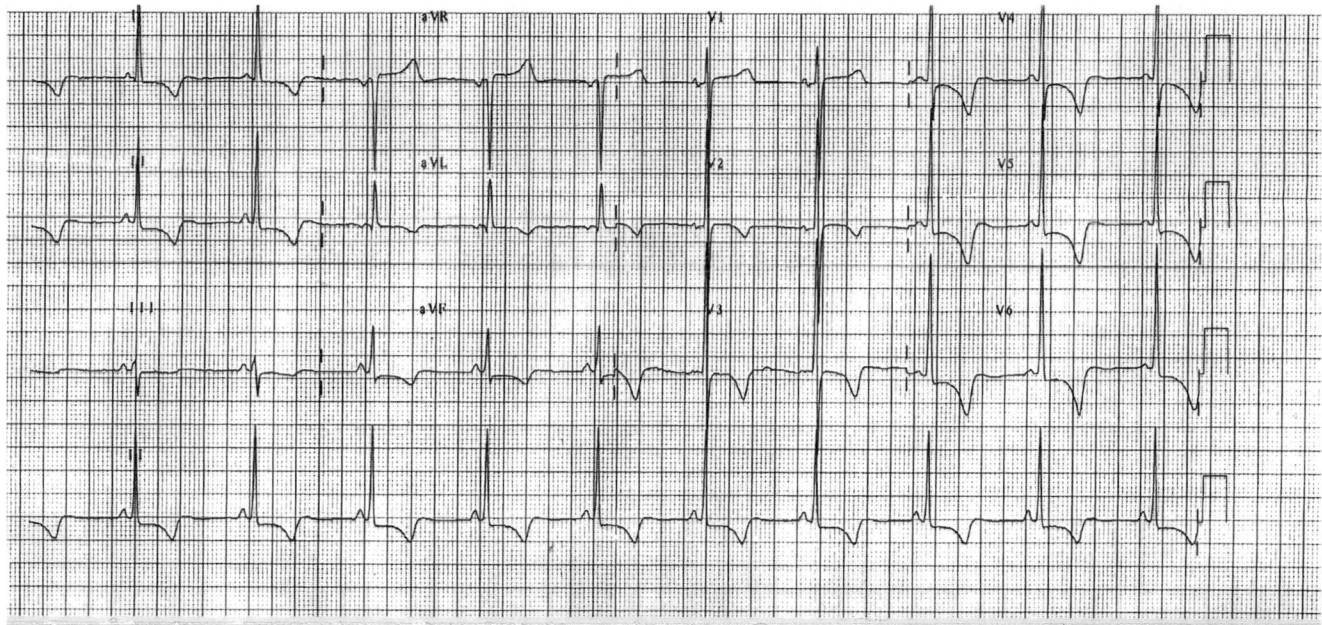

Fig. 31.3. The ECG in a case of Friedreich's ataxia. Note the widespread T-wave abnormalities.

The relationship between cases of atypical FA and the classical phenotype has long been controversial (Harding 1984). Three variant forms have been identified.

◆ Late onset FA develops after the age of 25 years, often in the fourth decade but sometimes as late as 51 years. There is slower progression and a lower incidence of skeletal deformity (De Michele *et al.* 1994). In these families, genetic linkage to the FA locus has been established (Klockgether *et al.* 1993; De Michele *et al.* 1994) and the GAA expansion mutation has now been detected in such patients who tend to have lower repeat numbers (Montermini *et al.* 1997*b*).

◆ FA with retained reflexes (FARR) differs from classical FA because of retained or increased reflexes, lower limb spasticity, and extensor plantar responses. These features were previously regarded as incompatible with a diagnosis of FA, and such patients were thought to have a separate condition, early onset ataxia with retained reflexes (Harding 1984). However, some FARR patients have cardiomyopathy and in some families genetic linkage to the FA 9q13 locus was established (Palau *et al.* 1995; Klockgether *et al.* 1996). These patients also have the FA GAA mutation (Lamont *et al.* 1997) but repeat lengths seem similar to those seen in classical FA (Montermini *et al.* 1997*b*).

◆ Acadian FA is confined to a population of French descent living in the southern USA and Canada. The age of onset is similar but progression is slower, with a lower incidence of cardiomyopathy. These patients sometimes have lower limb spasticity and extensor plantar responses. Linkage to the FA locus has been established (Richter *et al.* 1996) and the GAA repeat expansion has been confirmed in Acadian FA (Montermini *et al.* 1997*b*).

◆ Recently, the FA intron 1 expansion has been detected in patients presenting with generalized chorea (Hanna *et al.* 1998). The frequency of this phenotype of FA is unclear.

Genetics

FA is inherited as an autosomal recessive trait. The carrier frequency is approximately 1 in 110 and parental consanguinity is present in 5–10 per cent of cases (Bundey 1992). Accordingly, the risk to siblings of affected children is 1 in 4. In 1988 the FA gene locus was established on chromosome 9q13 (Chamberlain *et al.* 1988). Subsequently, a gene, *X25*, was identified which contained a homozygous expansion of a GAA trinucleotide repeat sequence within the first intron of the gene in 96–97 per cent of FA patients (Campuzano *et al.* 1996). The few remaining patients were compound heterozygotes with one expanded allele and a point mutation of the other. In normal individuals the gene contains 7–29 GAA repeats, increasing to between 66 and 1700 repeats in affected individuals (Durr *et al.* 1996; Schols *et al.* 1997). Larger GAA repeat numbers are associated with earlier age of onset, more severe areflexia, and increased incidence of cardiomyopathy, optic atrophy, and deafness while smaller expansions are likely to result in milder, later onset disease (Durr *et al.* 1996; Gellera *et al.* 1997; Isnard *et al.* 1997; Montermini *et al.* 1997*b*). Although there is a correlation between repeat size and greater neurological damage (Santoro *et al.* 2000), it is possible for mutations containing large GAA expansions (>800 repeats) to cause very late onset (58 years) FA (Bidichandani *et al.* 2000). The mutation is unstable during meiosis and mitosis leading to variability in repeat size within the same family and in different tissues from the same individual. Somatic mosaicism has been noted within the nervous system but does not appear to explain the pattern of neuropathological changes (Montermini *et al.* 1997*a*). However, one patient with mild neurological features was found to have much smaller repeat sizes in peripheral nerve than in blood (Machkhas *et al.* 1998) indicating that somatic mosaicism might influence the FA phenotype.

The majority of parents of affected children are heterozygous for the GAA expansion but occasionally, one parent carries a premutation, a large allele of intermediate size (40–100 repeats), which has undergone further expansion during meiosis (Cossee *et al.* 1997; Delatycki *et al.* 1998). There are rare reports of patients inheriting FA from an affected parent. Some of these are explained by misdiagnosis but others arise when one parent has FA and the other is a heterozygote. The risk of such pseudodominant transmission to offspring is 1 in 220, based on a heterozygote frequency of 1 in 220 and a 1 in 2 risk of the healthy but heterozygous parent transmitting the expanded rather than the normal allele (Harding and Zilkha 1981). Recently, pseudodominant transmission has been confirmed by direct mutation analysis in some families (McGovern *et al.* 2000) but in others, a very mildly affected parent has been heterozygous for the GAA expansion (Lamont *et al.* 1997). These affected parents had a late onset, after the age of 40, of ataxia and dysarthria but preserved reflexes. Point mutations of *X25* or other ataxia mutations were excluded and it is likely that such mildly affected parents are manifesting carriers of the FA gene.

The gene product, frataxin, is a 210 amino acid protein. In FA the level of frataxin mRNA is reduced, leading to a cellular deficiency of the protein (Bidichandani *et al.* 1998). Frataxin is a mitochondrial protein (Koutnikova *et al.* 1997; Priller *et al.* 1997) which is involved in mitochondrial iron homeostasis (Babcock *et al.* 1997). Frataxin deficiency leads to intramitochondrial iron accumulation (Adamec *et al.* 2000) with abnormal mitochondrial respiration and regulation of mitochondrial DNA (Rotig *et al.* 1997; Wilson *et al.* 1998). In cardiac muscle there is reduced mitochondrial respiratory enzyme activity. With mitochondrial DNA depletion and evidence of oxidative stress, as gauged by lowered aconitase levels (Bradley *et al.* 2000). Skeletal muscle shows slight reduction in mitochondrial function but cerebellar tissue and dorsal root ganglia do not. Abnormal mitochondrial activity can be demonstrated in vivo using (31)P magnetic resonance spectroscopy (Vorgerd *et al.* 2000). The clinical similarities between FA and some of the mitochondrial encephalomyopathies in terms of neurological involvement, cardiomyopathy, and deafness are consistent with the notion of FA as a disorder of mitochondrial function.

It is possible that very occasional patients with otherwise typical FA do not have mutations of the frataxin gene (Schols *et al.* 1997). In these families, no GAA expansion is detected, suggesting either point mutations of both alleles or the involvement of a separate gene.

Investigations and differential diagnosis

FA should be strongly suspected in children, adolescents, or young adults presenting with ataxia, areflexia, and extensor plantar responses. In the light of recent molecular genetic studies (see above) the diagnosis must be considered in those with later age of onset than has hitherto been regarded as typical, as well as patients with lower limb spasticity and retained reflexes. Features against the diagnosis include apparent autosomal dominant inheritance (but see above), dementia, parkinsonism or dystonia, ophthalmoplegia or a congenital onset. In the outpatient clinic, an ECG is both easily available and very useful; if abnormal, with evidence of T wave changes or ventricular hypertrophy, the diagnosis is very likely. It should be noted however, that ataxia due to isolated vitamin E deficiency (Cavalier *et al.* 1998) or mitochondrial disease (Chinnery *et al.* 1997) can be associated with cardiomyopathy and that the ECG may be normal in FA. Nerve conduction studies reveal normal conduction velocities but small or absent sensory nerve action potentials. This is an important means of distinguishing FA in which dysarthria and extensor plantar responses have not yet appeared, from early type I hereditary motor and sensory neuropathy (HMSN I) in which there is also ataxia with areflexia and pes cavus but usually autosomal dominant inheritance and slow conduction velocities (<40 m/s). It is essential to exclude vitamin B12 deficiency in which ataxia, areflexia, and extensor plantar responses are cardinal signs of subacute combined degeneration. Vitamin E deficiency can cause a neurological phenotype indistinguishable from FA but is treatable and must be excluded by vitamin E estimation, especially in patients who appear to have FA (even with cardiomyopathy) but in whom DNA studies do not reveal a FA mutation (Hammans and Kennedy 1998). Visual evoked potentials are frequently abnormal, even in those without clinically obvious optic atrophy and pyramidal tract dysfunction may be revealed by central motor conduction studies (Claus *et al.* 1988). CT and MRI scans usually show normal cerebellar anatomy although slight atrophy of the vermis and medulla may be seen in advanced cases (Ormerod *et al.* 1994). In contrast, the cervical cord is atrophic on MRI scanning (Fig. 31.4). The presence of marked cerebellar atrophy, especially in the early stages of an ataxic illness, makes FA unlikely.

Increasingly, the diagnosis of FA is made by direct mutation screening of DNA samples to detect the GAA trinucleotide expansion (Lamont *et al.* 1997). This prevents the need for neurophysiological and neuroradiological investigations but a negative result should be followed up with additional investigations. These should include MRI scanning, vitamin E and B$_{12}$ levels and alphafetoprotein estimation; further DNA analysis for autosomal dominant SCA mutations (Section 31.8) may also be helpful as there is some overlap between the onset age ranges of these disorders and that of FA. The presence of antigliadin antibodies, with or without coeliac disease can be associated with a very similar spinocerebellar ataxia (Section 31.11.11) and in these patients, antibody estimations and jejunal biopsy may be required. Abnormal eye movements and head thrusting may be seen with ataxia telangiectasia or with a distinct autosomal recessive 'ataxia with oculomotor apraxia' or 'AT-like' syndrome) (linked to a gene on chromosome 9q34) (Nemeth *et al.* 2000).

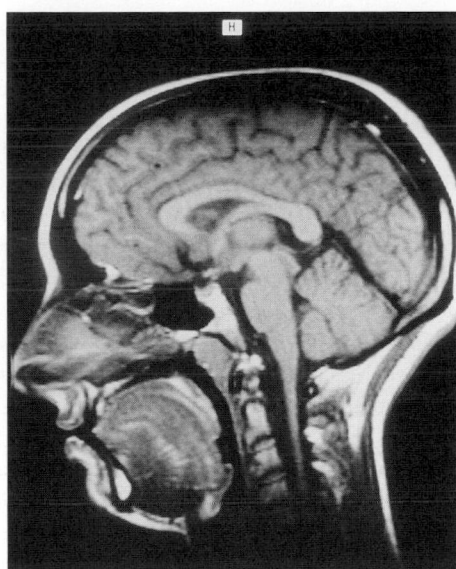

Fig. 31.4. Magnetic resonance scan of a patient with Friedreich's ataxia, showing cervical cord atrophy with preserved cerebellar anatomy.

In some clinically typical FA cases, alternative diagnoses such as vitamin E deficiency, atypical presentation of ataxia telangiectasia or early onset of a dominant ataxia such as SCA3 (Section 31.8.2) may be established (McCabe *et al.* 2000) but in a small number, no alternative explanation is found. If the patient is heterozygous for the GAA repeat with one expanded and one normal length allele, there are several possibilities to consider. The patient may be one of the 3–4 per cent of FA cases who are compound heterozygotes with a GAA expansion and a point mutation of the other frataxin gene. Alternatively, some cases with very late onset of mild ataxia may be manifesting carriers (see above). However, unless compound heterozygosity can be verified, alternative diagnoses should be excluded by appropriate investigation.

Treatment

There is no effective treatment for FA. Various studies have reported negative results with a range of compounds. Recently, slight improvement in co-ordination was reported with levohydroxytryptophan (Trouillas *et al.* 1995) but this was not confirmed in a second study (Wessel *et al.* 1995). The finding of increased intramitochondrial iron in mitochondria with defective frataxin function has led to the suggestion that iron chelation may be effective, but serum iron and ferritin are normal in FA patients (Wilson *et al.* 1998) and the benefits of such an approach seem uncertain. It is important to discuss the prognosis openly with the patient and genetic counselling is vital for both patients and their families. Physiotherapy and occupational therapy are important, along with appropriate seating for those who have lost the ability to walk. Orthopaedic advice is essential for those with scoliosis and foot deformity along with early diagnosis and treatment of cardiac complications and diabetes. Selected patients will require hearing aids and low

visual aids. Dependent oedema and cyanosis of the feet can be very troublesome; elevation of the feet and prevention of secondary contractures are probably more helpful than diuretics. These patients are often worse after a period of bed rest during illness or after surgery; indeed the diagnosis may first become apparent at such a time. It is important to encourage the earliest possible mobilization in these circumstances.

31.4.2 **Early onset ataxia with retained reflexes**

This disorder is probably half as common as FA (Chio *et al.* 1993) from which it has previously been distinguished on clinical criteria (Harding 1984). The age of onset is similar to FA but progression is slower, with patients becoming wheelchair dependent after about 30 years from onset (in contrast to a mean of 15 years in FA). Upper limb and knee reflexes are preserved and there is often lower limb spasticity. Skeletal deformity occurs but is usually mild. Harding (1984) found no evidence of cardiomyopathy, optic atrophy, or diabetes in her series but recent studies have detected these features do occur in some cases (Klockgether *et al.* 1991; Montermini *et al.* 1997*b*). Neurophysiological studies reveal peripheral neuropathy in some but not all patients (Klockgether *et al.* 1991; Santoro *et al.* 1992). The frequency of skeletal deformity, sensory changes, distal wasting, and cardiomyopathy may be lower than in FA (Klockgether *et al.* 1991) but this is uncertain. Cerebellar atrophy is seen with MRI in some patients but is absent in others (Klockgether *et al.* 1991; Ormerod *et al.* 1994). These findings indicate that early onset cerebellar ataxia with retained reflexes is heterogeneous. Clinical genetic studies have suggested autosomal recessive inheritance, with increased parental consanguinity but slightly lower segregation ratios in siblings than the 0.25 expected (Filla *et al.* 1990; Chio *et al.* 1993). On the basis of genetic linkage and direct mutation screening studies, some of these patients have Friedreich's ataxia (Kellett *et al.* 1997) but others do not (Geschwind *et al.* 1997*b*). The aetiology of the non-Friedreich's ataxia cases is unclear. However, the distinction from classical FA is important in terms of prognosis.

31.4.3 **Early onset ataxia with myoclonus**

The combination of cerebellar ataxia with myoclonus is referred to as progressive myoclonic ataxia or the Ramsay Hunt syndrome. This confusing and highly heterogeneous syndrome is discussed fully in Chapter 32. Several neurometabolic disorders may present in this way including mitochondrial disorders, neuronal ceroid lipofuscinosis, and sialidosis. Other cases are due to coeliac disease or Whipple's disease. An autosomal recessive disorder, Unverricht–Lundborg disease (also referred to as Baltic or Mediterranean myoclonus) is probably responsible for most otherwise unexplained cases in children (see Chapter 32) while autosomal dominant dentatorubropallidoluysian atrophy is discussed in Section 31.9.6.

31.4.4 Early onset ataxia with hypogonadism (Holmes ataxia)

This rare autosomal recessive disorder is heterogeneous. Onset is variable up to the age of 40 but usually before 30 years of age. The ataxia is progressive, leading to severe disability after 15–20 years (Holmes 1907). Dysarthria is common, along with variable nystagmus, learning disability, skeletal deformities, tremor, and peripheral neuropathy (De Michele *et al.* 1993); tendon reflexes may be absent or brisk and plantar responses are sometimes extensor (Harding 1984). Pigmentary retinopathy has been described in a few cases. Neuroimaging studies reveal cerebellar atrophy. The hypogonadism is clinically obvious from puberty onwards and is also heterogeneous, with hypogonadotrophic hypogonadism in some cases while others have gonadal failure (De Michele *et al.* 1993). A form of mitochondrial disease has been suspected in one report (De Michele *et al.* 1993). A disorder with similar clinical features has been described as the Boucher–Neuhauser syndrome (Limber *et al.* 1989). Cerebellar ataxia has occasionally been described in the Lawrence–Moon–Barted–Biedl syndrome in which hypogonadism is a major feature, but this disorder is exceptionally rare and the clinical features are distinctive (Green *et al.* 1989). Hypogonadism and ataxia also coexist in some cases of the Marinesco–Sjogren syndrome (McLaughlin *et al.* 1996) (see Section 32.3.4).

31.4.5 Early onset ataxia with retinopathy

There have been several reports of cerebellar ataxia in association with pigmentary retinopathy. Harding (1984) reviewed these and grouped them together as a subtype of early onset ataxia. The group is clearly heterogeneous and the majority of cases are probably autosomal recessive. Additional clinical features have included dementia, deafness, peripheral neuropathy, and pyramidal signs. Many of these cases were described before modern biochemical investigations were available and the diagnosis in some is questionable. Retinopathy is a feature of several metabolic ataxias including abetalipoproteinaemia (Section 31.7.3), hypobetalipoproteinaemia (Matsuo *et al.* 1994) and other forms of acquired vitamin E deficiency (Harding 1987*b*) as well as autosomal recessive ataxia with isolated vitamin E deficiency (Yokota *et al.* 1997) (Section 31.7.4). Retinopathy and ataxia can be prominent features of mitochondrial disease (Chinnery *et al.* 1997), especially the Kearns–Sayre (Holt *et al.* 1989) and NARP syndromes (Holt *et al.* 1990) as discussed in Section 31.7.7. Finally, it should be noted that autosomal dominant cerebellar ataxia type II (due to the *SCA7* mutation) sometimes presents in childhood causing ataxia and retinopathy (see Section 31.8.3).

31.4.6 Early onset ataxia with optic atrophy

This subgroup of early onset ataxia was suggested by Harding (1984) but is highly heterogeneous. Optic atrophy can be associated with classical and variant forms of Friedreich's ataxia

(Section 31.4.1) and may also occur in combination with cerebellar signs in X-linked ataxia (see below), leucodystrophies, various forms of mitochondrial disease, including Leber's disease (Funakawa *et al.* 1995; Murakami *et al.* 1996), biotin deficiency (Rahman *et al.* 1997), neuronal ceroid lipofuscinosis, or demyelinating disease. Ataxia and optic atrophy are also features of the Wolfram syndrome (Scolding *et al.* 1996).

There remain however, otherwise unexplained and apparently autosomal recessive examples of this syndrome (Harding 1984; Bundey 1992). The Behr syndrome comprises cerebellar ataxia, optic atrophy, spasticity, and mild learning disability; other features such as peripheral neuropathy and deafness have also been described. Inheritance is autosomal recessive and similar families have been reported by several authors (see Harding 1984; Bundey 1992). Recently, patients with Behr syndrome have been discovered to have 3-methylglutaconic aciduria (Costeff *et al.* 1993; Elpeleg *et al.* 1994) which may be secondary to an enzyme deficiency or a mitochondrial disorder.

31.4.7 Early onset ataxia with deafness

A few families with ataxia and deafness have been reported (Harding 1984; Bundey 1992) and this is probably a heterogeneous autosomal recessive disorder (Pratap-Chand *et al.* 1995). However, in several reports there have been patients with other features such as cardiomyopathy and retinopathy, suggestive of mitochondrial disease. Deafness and ataxia are common features of several mitochondrial disorders, especially if there are other features such as short stature, retinopathy, ptosis, myopathy, or lactic acidosis (Chinnery *et al.* 1997). The May–White syndrome of ataxia, myoclonus, and deafness (a variant of the MERRF syndrome discussed in Chapter 32) has now been established as a mitochondrial disorder (Vaamonde *et al.* 1992).

31.4.8 Early onset ataxia with extrapyramidal features

In contrast to the later onset ataxias (see below), the combination of ataxia with parkinsonism, dystonia, or chorea is very uncommon. Some overlap in age of onset with the later onset ataxias, such as type I autosomal dominant cerebellar ataxia or DRPLA, accounts for some of these cases but the olivopontocerebellar atrophy variant of multiple system atrophy (see Chapter 32) does not present in childhood or adolescence. Chorea has been described with cerebellar ataxia and other features in mitochondrial disease (Nelson *et al.* 1995).

31.4.9 X-linked early onset ataxia

X-linked cerebellar ataxias are very rare but have been reported by several authors (Harding 1984). Onset is usually in childhood or adolescence and the salient features are a spastic paraparesis, upper limb ataxia, dysarthria, and nystagmus. In some, ankle jerks were absent with neurophysiological evidence of a peripheral neuropathy. There is also a more severe form of childhood onset X-linked ataxia with spastic paraparesis (Apak *et al.* 1989). In other families, the prognosis is better with a slowly progressive pure cerebellar syndrome (Lutz *et al.* 1989). A rapidly fatal childhood onset ataxia is associated with visual loss, deafness, and recurrent infections (Arts *et al.* 1993). Female carriers have ataxia and mild lower limb spasticity (Verhagen *et al.* 1996). It is important to exclude adrenoleucodystrophy in families presenting with an unexplained X-linked ataxic or paraplegic illness; the same applies to sporadic male cases.

31.5 Ataxias caused by DNA repair defects

31.5.1 Ataxia telangiectasia (Louis–Barr syndrome)

Ataxia telangiectasia (AT) is an autosomal recessive condition caused by a variety of mutations of the *ATM* (AT mutated) gene on chromosome 11q23 (Lange *et al.* 1995). The population frequency is 1 in 100 000–300 000. *ATM* is a tumour suppressor gene encoding a large protein kinase with phosphatidyl-inositol 3 kinase activity which is usually truncated in AT with consequent loss of function (Uhrhammer *et al.* 1998), defective DNA repair mechanisms, and increased chromosomal fragility. The normal function of *ATM* is unclear but involves DNA repair and interaction with the cellular protein p53 (Khanna *et al.* 1998). Many different *ATM* gene mutations have been identified and most patients are compound heterozygotes with two different mutations, one on each *ATM* allele (Wright *et al.* 1996).

Ataxia develops in early childhood, usually as walking starts, and is rapidly progressive with the appearance of cerebellar dysarthria and kinetic tremor. Most patients are in wheelchairs by the age of 15 years. There is a characteristic oculomotor apraxia with grossly reduced saccadic eye movements and the use of head thrusts to achieve refixation (Stell *et al.* 1989). Many patients are small and dysmorphic and mild learning disability is seen in a proportion of cases (Bundey 1992). Other neurological features in some patients include myoclonus (de Graaf *et al.* 1995), dystonia (Koepp *et al.* 1994), peripheral neuropathy (McFarlin *et al.* 1972), and anterior horn cell degeneration (Larnaout *et al.* 1998). The characteristic conjunctival telangiectasia (Fig. 31.5) usually appear during early childhood but sometimes later; they may also appear on the face, ears, neck, flexor creases of the limbs, gums, and palate; occasionally they are absent (Friedman and Weitberg 1993). There is impaired immunity with thymic hypoplasia, low circulating levels of IgA, and frequently recurrent sinopulmonary and cutaneous infections. There is an increased risk of malignancy, especially lymphoma and leukaemia in patients and to a lesser extent heterozygous relatives.

Clinically helpful laboratory abnormalities include an elevated α-fetoprotein as well as low serum IgA levels. Neuroimaging typically shows cerebellar atrophy (Farina *et al.*

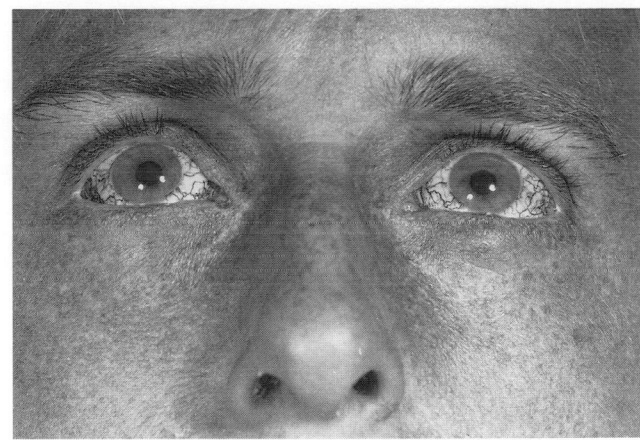

Fig. 31.5. Conjunctival telangiectasia in ataxia telangiectasia.

1994). In addition, chromosomal abnormalities are common, including abnormally increased chromosome fragility after gamma or X-irradiation. DNA diagnosis is difficult due to the high degree of allelic heterogeneity in AT, with a large number of different *ATM* mutations in different families (Wright *et al.* 1996). There is no correlation between the ATM mutation, level of ATM protein, in vitro radiosensitivity or clinical phenotype (Becker-Catania *et al.* 2000).

The prognosis is generally poor although life expectancy is variable, depending on the severity of the immunodeficiency and the development of malignancy. The recurrence risk to siblings is 1 in 4. Symptomatic management of infections and movement disorders is generally possible, while the management of malignancies is complicated by increased sensitivity to radiotherapy.

31.5.2 Xeroderma pigmentosum

This is a rare autosomal recessive disorder with a frequency of 1 in 250 000. It is characterized by severe photosensitive skin disease with cutaneous malignancies including basal and squamous carcinomas and melanomas (Section 19.6.7). Sunlight exposed skin is atrophic and scaly with pigmentary changes, scaling, keratoses, and telangiectasia (Fig. 31.6). Conjunctivitis and keratitis also occur. Neurological features, which only develop in some xeroderma pigmentosum (XP) patients, include peripheral neuropathy (Kanda *et al.* 1990) or more severe multisystem manifestations (de Sanctis–Cacchione syndrome). The latter include ataxia, dementia, deafness, spasticity, and chorea (Mimaki *et al.* 1986). XP is genetically heterogeneous, with seven subtypes (complementation groups) XP-A to XP-G. These are caused by mutations of several genes encoding DNA repair proteins including the *XPAC* gene on chromosome 9 (XP-A), the *ERCC-3* gene on chromosome 2 (XP-B), a DNA repair gene *XPCC* (XP-C), and the *ERCC-2* gene on chromosome 19 (XP-D). Other XP genes have also been identified (Banfi and Zoghbi 1994).

31.5.3 Cockayne syndrome

Cockayne syndrome (CS) is also a rare autosomal recessive condition due to inherited abnormality of DNA repair (Section

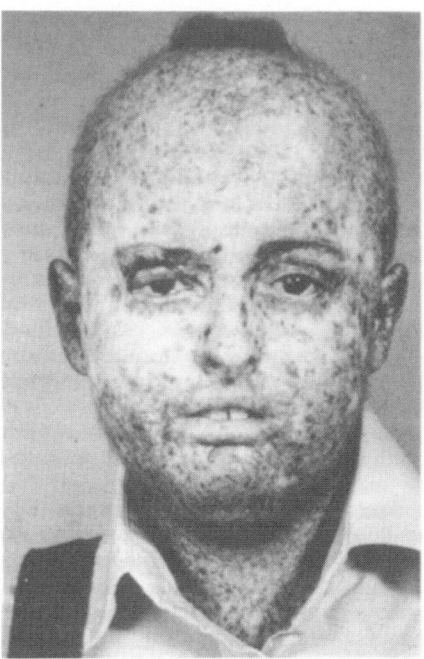

Fig. 31.6. Xeroderma pigmentosum (from Harding 1984).

19.6.8). Clinical features are dwarfism, microcephaly, ataxia, spasticity, retinopathy, deafness, and peripheral neuropathy. There is a characteristic facial appearance, the skin becomes atrophic, and cataracts appear (Nance and Berry 1992). CT scans show intracranial calcification. Like XP, CS is genetically heterogeneous and has been associated with several of the known XP mutations (Banfi and Zoghbi 1994). It appears that mutations of these genes may result in XP, CS, or a mixed picture (Cotella et al. 2000).

31.6 Intermittent metabolic ataxias

31.6.1 Hyperammonaemias

Hyperammonaemia, usually due to metabolic defects of the urea cycle, is the most common cause of intermittent metabolic ataxia. Various enzyme deficiencies may be involved. Ornithine transcarbamylase (OTC) deficiency is an X-linked disorder in which affected boys develop episodes of ataxia and encephalopathy with elevated ammonia levels. Female carriers may also be affected (Pridmore et al. 1995). The other urea cycle defects are autosomal recessive, including argininosuccinate synthetase deficiency, argininosuccinase deficiency (argininosuccinic aciduria) (Gerrits et al. 1993), and arginase deficiency. Hyperammonaemia may also occur in hyperornithinaemia (Tuchman et al. 1990). Ataxia may occur as a feature of the intermittent metabolic encephalopathy (often with cerebral oedema) seen in these patients. Such episodes may be precipitated by infection or intercurrent illness. Periodic hyperammonaemic encephalopathy with ataxia has also been reported after ureterosigmoidoscopy (Cascino et al. 1989). Hyper-

ammonaemia has complex effects on brain function, including GABAergic neurotransmission (Ha and Basile 1996), inhibition of cerebral energy metabolism, and disruption of neurotransmitter function (Butterworth 1998).

31.6.2 Disorders of amino acid metabolism

Hartnup disease is caused by defective intestinal and renal transport of neutral amino acids and is an autosomal recessive inborn metabolic error. Affected children develop a pellagra-like rash and an intermittent neurological syndrome with ataxia. Intermittent ataxia, similar to that seen in the hyperammonaemias, is also seen with nonketotic hyperglycinaemia (Nightingale and Barton 1991), intermittent branched chain ketoaciduria, and isovaleric aciduria (Harding 1984). Clinically, these intermittent metabolic ataxias are similar to the hyperammonaemias. Glutamic aciduria and hydroxyglutaric aciduria are associated with a progressive ataxia (Sawada et al. 1991; de Klerk et al. 1997).

31.6.3 Disorders of pyruvate and lactate metabolism

Intermittent ataxia also occurs in pyruvate dehydrogenase deficiency (Robinson et al. 1996). This condition is genetically and clinically heterogeneous. Most cases are X-linked while a few are autosomal recessive. Clinically, there may be severe infantile lactic acidosis, intermittent acidosis with ataxia (Bindoff et al. 1989; Kinoshita et al. 1997), Leigh's syndrome, or chronic neurological impairment with learning disability, ataxia, spasticity, seizures, and various cerebral malformations (Zeviani and Taroni 1994; Robinson et al. 1996). Intermittent ataxia may also occur in some forms of autosomal recessive pyruvate carboxylase deficiency.

Progressive ataxia is a common feature of mitochondrial diseases and is considered below.

31.7 Progressive metabolic ataxia

Various metabolic disorders are associated with a progressive ataxic syndrome. Often there are prominent additional neurological features which overshadow the ataxic component except for vitamin E deficiency, which resembles a degenerative ataxia.

31.7.1 Cholestanolosis (cerebrotendinous xanthomatosis)

This is a rare autosomal recessive disorder caused by mutations of the sterol 27-hydroxylase (CYP27) gene (Chen et al. 1998). Clinical features are bilateral Achilles tendon xanthomas, cataracts, low intelligence, spastic paraplegia, cerebellar signs, convulsions, peripheral neuropathy, foot deformity, premature cardiovascular disease, EEG abnormality, and increased CSF protein (Berginer et al. 1989) (Section 12.8.9). In some patients, there are xanthomata in other sites or they may be absent and dementia is not invariable. Metabolically, serum cholesterol is reduced and increased levels of cholestanol, the 5α-dihydro derivative of cholesterol, accumulate in xanthomas, the nervous system, and in bile. CT and MR scans reveal brain atrophy and white matter abnormalities (Dotti *et al.* 1994). Progression of cerebrotendinous xanthomatosis may be prevented with chenedeoxycholic acid and pravastatin (Kuriyama *et al.* 1994). In the absence of tendon xanthomas, cerebrotendinous xanthomatosis may resemble the Marinesco–Sjogren syndrome with cataract, ataxia, and spasticity (Siebner *et al.* 1996). In many cases, the spastic paraparesis is more prominent than the cerebellar features. There is considerable allelic heterogeneity with up to 37 different mutations of the CYP27 gene; there is a poor genotype-phenotype correlation (Verrips *et al.* 2000).

31.7.2 Leucodystrophies

Ataxia is a common feature of the complex neurological phenotypes seen in various leucodystrophies, including Krabbe's disease, metachromatic leucodystrophy (MLD), adrenoleucodystrophy (ALD), and Pelizaeus Merzbacher disease (PMD) (Section 29.6). In most cases, cerebellar signs are accompanied by and often overshadowed by other features such as dementia, spasticity, visual loss, and peripheral neuropathy. Occasionally, a slowly progressive cerebellar phenotype occurs, not unlike progressive multiple sclerosis (Klemm and Conzelmann 1989). Diagnosis of leucodystrophy is suggested by certain clinical syndromes (especially in ALD and PMD) and can be confirmed by white matter abnormalities on MR scanning, very long chain fatty acid levels (ALD), white cell enzyme estimations (Krabbe's and MLD), and DNA analysis (PMD).

31.7.3 Abetalipoproteinaemia and hypobetalipoproteinaemia

This disorder is an autosomal recessive trait, characterized by a failure of synthesis of apolipoprotein-B containing lipoproteins (very low density lipoprotein and chylomicrons) (Section 12.8.8). There is a deficiency of microsomal triglyceride-transfer protein (MTP) (Wetterau *et al.* 1992) caused by mutations of the MTP gene on chromosome 4q22–24 (Narcisi *et al.* 1995; Wang *et al.* 2000). The resulting fat malabsorption causes steatorrhoea and malabsorption of the fat soluble vitamins A, D, E, and K. The patients are of small stature, with a pigmentary retinopathy and progressive cerebellar ataxia. Clinically, the neurological disorder is similar to Friedreich's ataxia with areflexia, doral column sensory loss, and peripheral neuropathy (Harding 1987*b*). In some patients, the gastrointestinal symptoms are mild or subclinical. Laboratory investigations reveal peripheral blood acanthocytes, reduced serum cholesterol, and an abnormal lipoprotein electrophoretic pattern. Vitamin E levels are undetectable. Treatment with vitamin replacement, especially vitamin E, can prevent progression of the neurological damage. It is important to measure vitamin E levels regularly; oral doses may need to be large and some patients require intramuscular therapy (Perlmutter *et al.* 1987).

Familial hypobetalipoproteinaemia is a distinct autosomal dominant condition causing less severe abnormalities of low density and very low density lipoprotein assembly due to mutations of the apolipoprotein B-100 gene. Serum cholesterol levels are reduced but neurological function is usually normal. In rare patients who have been homozygous for this disorder, a neurological syndrome similar to that seen in abetalipoproteinaemia has been reported (Harding 1987*b*).

31.7.4 Ataxia with isolated vitamin E deficiency (AVED) and other vitamin E deficiency states

A selective autosomal recessively inherited deficiency of vitamin E has been described without lipid abnormalities, acanthocytosis, or other features of fat malabsorption (Harding 1987*b*). In this disorder, mutations of the α-tocopherol transfer protein (α-TPP) gene on chromosome 8q13 cause a loss of α-TPP function with rapid loss of vitamin E from serum after absorption (Yokota *et al.* 1997). The resulting vitamin E deficiency is associated with a neurological disorder 'ataxia with isolated vitamin E deficiency (AVED)' similar to Friedreich's ataxia with ataxia, dorsal column sensory loss, and peripheral neuropathy affecting large myelinated fibres (Section 12.21.4); some patients also have a cardiomyopathy (Hammans and Kennedy 1998) and although usually absent, retinopathy has occasionally been described (Yokota *et al.* 1997; Usuki and Maruyama 2000). This condition must always be considered in the differential diagnosis of Friedreich's ataxia (Section 31.4.1). AVED may be treated with large doses of vitamin E as in abetalipoproteinaemia. Reversal of the ataxia is unlikely but further deterioration may be prevented.

Occasionally vitamin E deficiency causes neurological damage similar to that seen in AVED or abetalipoproteinaemia as a result of other causes of intestinal malabsorption such as intestinal resection and cholestatic liver disease (usually in children) (Muller *et al.* 1983; Harding 1987*b*).

31.7.5 Partial hypoxanthine guanine phosphoribosyltransferase (HPRT) deficiency

HPRT deficiency is an X-linked disorder in which affected males develop hyperuricaemia with secondary complications. Severe HPRT deficiency leads to the Lesch–Nyhan syndrome of severe learning disability, dystonia, spasticity, and self-mutilation. Partial HPRT deficiency is associated with gouty arthritis, nephrolithiasis and, in about 20 per cent of cases, neurological features (Caskey and Rossiter 1993). There is cerebellar ataxia with mild learning disability and spasticity but no self-mutilation. The variable phenotype of HPRT deficiency is caused by different mutations of the HPRT gene on chromosome Xq26 (allelic heterogeneity). Treatment with allopurinol is helpful for gouty arthritis and nephrolithiasis but not the neurological features.

31.7.6 Neimann–Pick type C (juvenile dystonic lipidosis)

This is an autosomal recessive disorder with a gene locus (NPCI) identified on chromosome 18q11–12. Several different deletion, insertion and missense point mutations of the NPC1 gene have been described (Carstea *et al.* 1997). Intracellular cholesterol metabolism is impaired and there is accumulation of cholesterol in lysosomes (Lossos *et al.* 1997; Sato *et al.* 1998). The clinical features are dementia, vertical supranuclear gaze palsy, ataxia, extrapyramidal signs, spasticity, and sometimes splenomegaly (Fink *et al.* 1989); some patients are severely affected in infancy while in others there is a gradual later onset presentation with dementia or psychosis (Campo *et al.* 1998). Neuroimaging is usually normal but a multiple sclerosis like presentation with prominent dementia has been described (Grau *et al.* 1997). The diagnosis of Niemenn-Pick disease type C can be established by the demonstration of lipid laden macrophages ('sea blue histiocytes') in the bone marrow but this test may be negative, in which case filipin staining of cultured skin fibroblasts may be diagnostic (van de Vlasakker *et al.* 1994).

31.7.7 Hexosaminidase A deficiency

Hexosaminidase A deficiency is usually associated with Tay–Sachs disease but atypical later onset phenotypes exist. One variant is characterized by progressive cerebellar ataxia, ophthalmoparesis, and anterior horn cell disease with neurogenic muscle weakness (Hund *et al.* 1997). Dementia may not be prominent in this form of the condition; inheritance is autosomal recessive.

31.7.8 Mitochondrial diseases

The mitochondrial diseases are a highly heterogeneous group of disorders caused by abnormal mitochondrial energy metabolism. The classification of mitochondrial disorders is complex and the reader is referred to reviews elsewhere (Zeviani and Taroni 1994). The clinical features of mitochondrial diseases are numerous but for the neurologist, the two most important are CNS involvement and a characteristic metabolic myopathy. The latter is often but not invariably associated with characteristic 'ragged red fibres' or cytochrome oxidase (COX) negative fibres seen with different histochemical staining of muscle biopsy specimens. Clinical clues to the existence of a mitochondrial disorder are given in Table 31.8.

Cerebellar ataxia is common in the various neurological syndromes associated with mitochondrial disease, especially those caused by defects of mitochondrial DNA (mtDNA) (Chinnery *et al.* 1997). There are several specific mitochondrial syndromes in which ataxia is prominent:

- Kearns–Sayre syndrome is characterized by ptosis and chronic progressive external ophthalmoplegia, metabolic myopathy, cerebellar ataxia, pigmentary retinopathy, and cardiac conduction defects; some patients have dementia or deafness and the CSF protein is typically raised. Usually, mtDNA analysis reveals large deletions but some cases are

Table 31.8. Clinical features suggestive of mitochondrial disease

Fatiguable proximal myopathy (especially in combination with CNS disease)
Ptosis, progressive ophthalmoplegia or pigmentary retinopathy, optic atrophy
Short stature
Deafness (sensorineural)
Myoclonus, seizures
Diabetes mellitus, hypoparathyroidism
Cardiomyopathy, cardiac conduction defects
Lipomas
Unexplained stroke before 40 years of age
Migraine
Lactic acidosis
Raised CSF protein/lactate
Muscle biopsy (ragged red fibres, COX negative fibres)

Adapted from Chinnery and Turnbull (1997).

due to the 3243 MELAS point mutation (see below) or other mtDNA point mutations (Zeviani and Taroni 1994).

- MERRF syndrome (myoclonic epilepsy with ragged red fibres) is discussed in Section 32.7.8 and is often associated with cerebellar ataxia.

- NARP syndrome comprises neurogenic weakness (due to peripheral neuropathy), cerebellar ataxia, and retinitis pigmentosa; seizures and dementia may also occur. It is associated with the G8993mtDNA point mutation (Holt *et al.* 1990).

- Leber's hereditary optic neuropathy (Section 8.5.2) is occasionally associated with CNS involvement, including progressive cerebellar ataxia (Murakami *et al.* 1996).

In addition to these characteristic syndromes, there are various other presentations of mitochondrial disease. Some patients with a phenotype similar to adult onset idiopathic degenerative cerebellar ataxia (see Section 31.10) have been discovered to have mutations of mtDNA (Truong *et al.* 1990). A spinocerebellar degeneration may also be caused by the 8344 MERRF mtDNA mutation (Howell *et al.* 1996). The 3243 MELAS (mitochondrial encephalomyopathy, lactic acidosis, and stroke-like episodes) mutation may also occasionally cause a progressive cerebellar ataxia (Arai and Ohshima 1997). Moreover, abnormal mitochondrial function has been identified in other ataxias such as Friedreich's ataxia and Holmes ataxia (see above).

31.8 Late onset hereditary cerebellar ataxias

31.8.1 Overview

In contrast to the autosomal recessive ataxias, which usually develop before the age of 25 years, patients with autosomal dominant cerebellar ataxia (ADCA) generally develop symptoms after this age. Although there is some overlap between the two groups, especially with ADCA type II/*SCA7* (see below), this remains a clinically useful generalization when considering the differential diagnosis of hereditary degenerative ataxia. Unfortunately, the classification of the autosomal dominant ataxias is one of the most confusing issues in clinical neurology. Several classifications based on clinical features have been proposed, which have the advantage of being applicable in the clinic, often in advance of any investigation results (Harding 1984). With the discovery of several genes causing autosomal dominant cerebellar ataxia, confusingly referred to as spinocerebellar ataxia (*SCA*) genes, a classification based on genotype has been proposed (Junck and Fink 1996). The clinical classification proposed by Harding (Table 31.9) remains clinically useful but now requires modification to accommodate dentatorubropallidoluysian atrophy and episodic ataxia while the patients in ADCA type IV probably had mitochondrial disease and so this subgroup is obsolete. Unfortunately, one difficulty with any purely clinical classification is that the clinical signs may evolve over time, so that it may be difficult to classify individual patients confidently in the early years of the illness. An alternative genotypic classification based on the *SCA* and other autosomal dominant ataxia genes is shown in Table 31.10. A problem with such a genotypic organization is that while scientifically attractive, it cannot readily be applied in the clinic because the *SCA* gene mutations do not reliably define distinct clinical phenotypes (Subramony and Filla 2001). A revised classification, incorporating Harding's clinical system (ADCA I–III) and recent molecular data is shown in Table 31.11 and will be used in this chapter.

An interesting common feature of several of the recently discovered *SCA* genes (Table 31.10) is that they all involve pathological expansion of a CAG trinucleotide repeat sequence (Figs 31.7 and 31.8). This is the same mechanism of mutation as seen in Huntington's disease, myotonic dystrophy, fragile X syndrome, and X-linked bulbospinal neuronopathy.

31.8.2 **Autosomal dominant cerebellar ataxia type I**

This is a heterogeneous category characterized by progressive cerebellar ataxia with additional features including supra-

Table 31.9. Clinical classification of the autosomal dominant cerebellar ataxias (from Harding 1984)

ADCA type I	Cerebellar ataxia with optic atrophy/ophthalmoplegia/dementia/pyramidal/extrapyramidal features/amyotrophy
ADCA type II	Cerebellar ataxia with pigmentary retinal degeneration +/– ophthalmoplegia/pyramidal/extrapyramidal features
ADCA type III	'Pure' cerebellar ataxia of later onset (+/– pyramidal signs)
ADCA type IV	Cerebellar ataxia with myoclonus and deafness

nuclear ophthalmoplegia, slow eye movements, optic atrophy, dementia, extrapyramidal features, dysphagia, pyramidal signs, amyotrophy, and peripheral neuropathy in various combinations (Harding 1984). Pathologically, most patients have olivopontocerebellar atrophy. In contrast to the olivopontocerebellar atrophy form of multiple system atrophy (Chapter 31), glial and neuronal cytoplasmic inclusions are usually absent (Section 32.3.8). Age of onset is typically between 30 and 49 with a median of 40 years (Klockgether *et al.* 1998) but a minority of cases develop in childhood or old age. The degree of dementia and any visual impairment due to optic atrophy are usually mild. Parkinsonism or dystonia are the usual extrapyramidal manifestations but chorea is occasionally seen. Tendon reflexes may be increased, normal, or absent depending on the degree of pyramidal or peripheral nerve dysfunction. Anterior horn cell involvement is usually manifest as lingual, facial, or limb fasciculation. Bladder dysfunction is common. Progression is relentless and treatment is entirely palliative. Most patients are wheelchair dependent after 17 years and survive up to 25 years after disease onset (Klockgether *et al.* 1998). Several subtypes within ADCA type I have been defined genotypically. Details of these mutations are shown in Table 31.10.

◆ The *SCA1* mutation is present in 13–35 per cent of ADCA type I cases (Giunti *et al.* 1998; Klockgether *et al.* 1998) but the proportion varies considerably among different series (Hammans 1996). As with other trinucleotide repeat expansions, increasing repeat length is associated with earlier age of onset, increased disease severity, and reduced survival (Banfi and Zoghbi 1994; Goldfarb *et al.* 1996) although one series was unable to demonstrate a relationship between repeat length and rate of disease progression (Klockgether *et al.* 1998). *SCA1* families also demonstrate anticipation with increased severity and earlier onset in succeeding generations, especially with paternal transmission of the *SCA1* gene (Genis *et al.* 1995); the molecular basis for this is the tendency for the *SCA1* mutation, like other unstable trinucleotide repeats, to expand during meiosis especially in spermatogenesis (Banfi and Zoghbi 1994). Clinically, *SCA1* patients more commonly have optic atrophy, dysphagia, dysarthria, spasticity, and increased tendon reflexes compared with *SCA2* or *SCA3* cases (Burk *et al.* 1996). Hyporeflexia and ophthalmoplegia are less common. MR scanning reveals cerebellar and brainstem atrophy. The mechanism by which the *SCA1* mutation causes selective neurodegeneration is unknown. In normal alleles, the CAG repeat sequence is usually interrupted, while pathological expansions are continuous and incorporate a polyglutamine sequence into the translated ataxin 1 protein (as seen with the Huntington's disease mutation and the Huntington protein). The function of ataxin 1 is unclear and the regional selectivity of the neuropathology in *SCA1* patients difficult to explain; this does not appear to be due to somatic mosaicism of CAG repeat length within the brain (Lopes-Cendes *et al.* 1996).

◆ The *SCA2* mutation has been reported in 21–40 per cent of ADCA type I cases in two large recent series (Giunti *et al.*

Table 31.10. Autosomal dominant cerebellar ataxia genes

Gene	Locus	Mutation type	Gene product	Trinucleotide repeats (Approximate)
SCA1	6p23	CAG expansion	Ataxin 1	36–68 (normal = 7–34)
SCA2	12q24	CAG expansion	Ataxin 2	35–59 (normal = 14–31)
SCA3	14q32	CAG expansion	Ataxin 3	65–84 (normal = 13–44)
SCA4	16q22	Unknown	Ataxin 4	–
SCA5	11cen	Unknown	Ataxin 5	–
SCA6*	19p13	CAG expansion	a-1A calcium channel	21–27 (normal = 4–16)
SCA7	3p12	CAG expansion	Ataxin 7	38–130 (normal = 7–17)
SCA8	13q21	CTG expansion	Ataxin 8	107–127 (normal = 16–37)
SCA10	22q13	Unknown	Ataxin 10	
SCA11	15q14–21	Unknown	Ataxin 11	
SCA12	5q31	CAG expansion	Ataxin 12	66–78 (normal = 9–28)
SCA13	**19q**	**Unknown**		
SCA14	**19q**	**Unknown**		
SCA15	**?**	**Unknown**		
SCA16	**8q**	**Unknown**		
DRPLA	12p13	CAG expansion	Atrophin 1	49–85 (normal = 5–35)
EA-1	12p13	Point mutations	KCNA1 potassium channel	–
EA-2*	19p13	Point mutations	a-1A calcium channel	–
EA-3	**2q22–23**	**Point mutation**	**CACNB4 calcium channel**	**–**

SCA = spinocerebellar ataxia; EA = episodic ataxia; DRPLA = dentatorubropallidoluysian atrophy;

*SCA6 and EA-2 are allelic, resulting from different mutations of the alpha 1A calcium channel (CACNL1A4) gene

Note SCA9 is currently not utilised

SCA 13-16 are rare mutations described only in single families (see text).

Table 31.11. Clinical and molecular classification of the autosomal dominant cerebellar ataxiasa

Clinical classification	Associated genes identified
ADCA type I	SCA1; SCA2; SCA3; SCA8; SCA12; **SCA13**; ?SCA15; ?SCA16**; others
ADCA type II	SCA7; ? **other loci**
ADCA type III	SCA3; SCA5; SCA6; SCA10*; SCA11; SCA14***; others
Ataxia with sensory neuropathy (Biemond's ataxia)	SCA4
DRPLA	DRPLA gene (atrophin 1)
Episodic ataxia type 1 (with myokymia)	KCNA1
Episodic ataxia type 2 (without myokymia)	SCA6/CACNL1A4
Episodic ataxia type 3 (without myokymia)	**CACNB4**

For ADCA definitions see Table 9; abbreviations are as in Table 10.

SCA10 is associated with epilepsy

**SCA13 develops in early infancy and is more correctly a hereditary congenital ataxia

***SCA14 can cause earlier onset ataxia with myoclonus

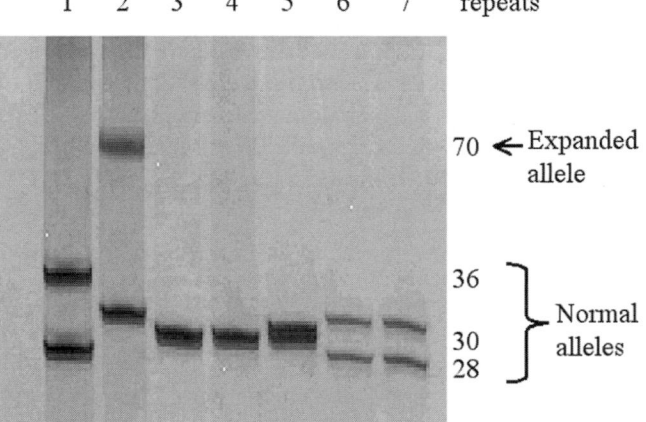

Fig. 31.7. Detection of CAG repeat expansion in the *SCA1* locus by PCR amplification, polyacrylamide gel electrophoresis and silver staining. DNA from different individuals has been electrophoresed in lanes 1–7; the mutant allele is shown in lane 2. (Courtesy of Dr R. Mountford, Regional Molecular Genetics Laboratory, Liverpool.)

1998; Klockgether *et al.* 1998). The effect of repeat length on age of onset (Fig. 31.9) and severity is similar to *SCA1* and large expansions are associated with paternal transmission (Giunti *et al.* 1998); as with *SCA1*, pathological expansions

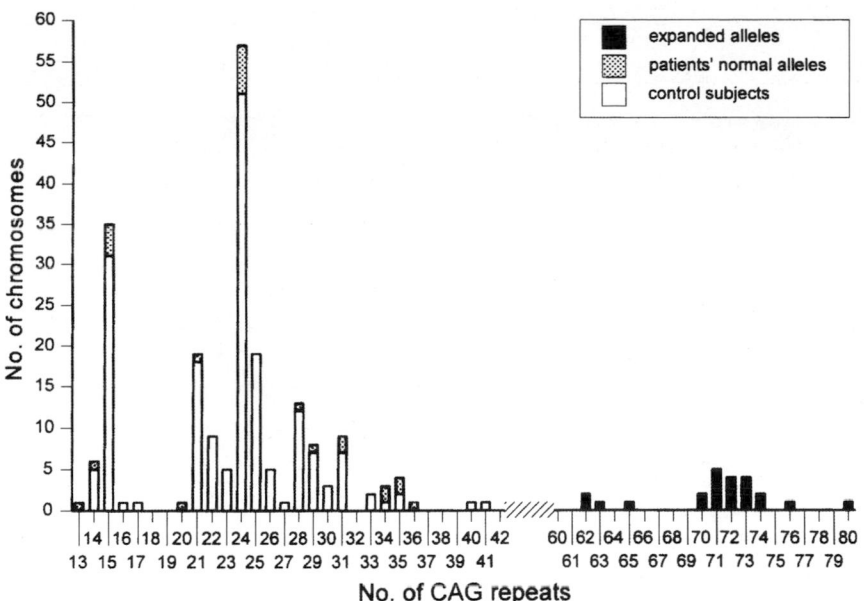

Fig. 31.8. Distributions of CAG repeat lengths in normal chromosomes of 91 control subjects, and normal and expanded alleles of 22 patients with the *SCA3* mutation (from Giunti *et al.* 1995).

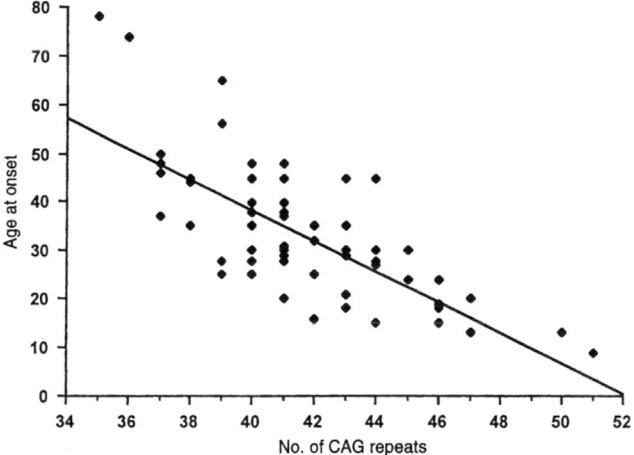

Fig. 31.9. Correlation between the number of *SCA2* CAG repeats and the age of disease onset in years (from Giunti *et al.* 1998).

are continuous while normal alleles often have interruptions within the CAG repeat sequence. As expected, anticipation is observed in *SCA2* kindreds. Neurological deterioration in *SCA2* patients is faster in females and with increasing CAG repeat lengths (Klockgether *et al.* 1998). Clinically, the *SCA2* mutation is consistently more frequently associated with ophthalmoplegia and areflexia (Durr *et al.* 1995; Filla *et al.* 1995; Burk *et al.* 1996; Giunti *et al.* 1998). Dementia and fasciculations have been reported more often than in *SCA1* or *SCA3* by some authors. The rate of progression is probably similar to other forms of ADCA type I. MR scanning reveals cerebellar and brainstem atrophy, the latter tending to be more severe than in *SCA1* or *3* (Burk *et al.* 1996) as shown in Fig. 31.10.

♦ The frequency of the *SCA3* mutation (Fig. 31.8) within ADCA type I is also uncertain, with estimates of 17–40 per cent in different series (Hammans 1996; Silveira *et al.* 1996; Giunti *et al.* 1998; Klockgether *et al.* 1998). CAG repeat size and age of onset are inversely related as with *SCA1* and *2* and anticipation is also observed in *SCA3* families (Giunti *et al.* 1995; Burk *et al.* 1996; Higgins *et al.* 1996) but a clear effect of parental sex on repeat size has not been demonstrated so far. As with *SCA2*, females and those with larger repeat sizes tend to deteriorate more quickly (Klockgether *et al.* 1998). Clinically, ADCA type I patients with a *SCA3* mutation do not differ significantly from those with the *SCA1* gene and MRI appearances are also similar. It is now clear that the *SCA3* mutation is also the genetic basis of Machado–Joseph disease (MJD) (Matilla *et al.* 1995; Higgins *et al.* 1996). This condition, which is especially common among those of Portuguese or Azorean descent, was for many years regarded as a distinct clinical entity although Harding (1984) included MJD within ADCA type I. Progressive cerebellar ataxia was the salient feature of MJD but a high frequency of parkinsonism, dystonia, eyelid retraction, and bulbar fasciculation was considered characteristic (Rosenberg 1992) although all of these features are seen in *SCA1*, *SCA2*, and *SCA3*. Accordingly, MJD does not, after all, appear to be clinically or genetically distinct from *SCA3*. Although the cerebellar syndrome is the most common presentation of the *SCA3* mutation, there is considerable variation between and within families as noted in earlier descriptions of MJD. Some patients have pure cerebellar ataxia without prominent additional features (Ishikawa *et al.* 1996) or 'non-cerebellar' presentations including levodopa responsive parkinsonism with peripheral neuropathy (Tuite *et al.* 1995) (Section 32.3.13),

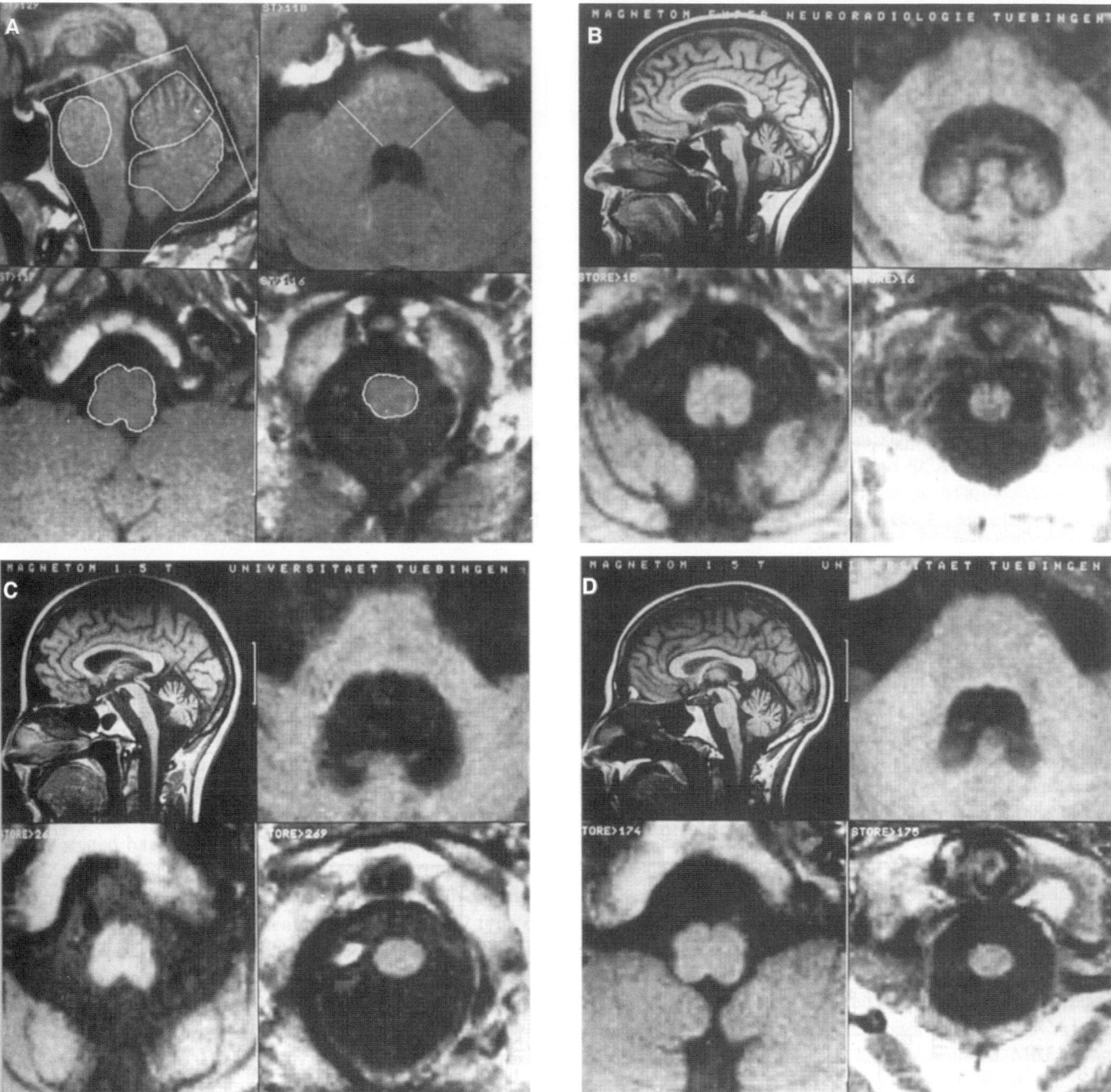

Fig. 31.10. T1-weighted MRI scans of infratentorial brain structures, showing the posterior fossa in the midsagittal plane (upper left) and axial images at the level of the middle cerebellar peduncles (upper right), inferior olive complex (lower left) and cervicomedullary junction (lower right). (A) MRI of 43-year-old healthy male. The areas for comparison are indicated. (B) MRI of a 44-year-old male *SCA1* patient. (C) MRI of a 38-year-old *SCA2* patient. (D) MRI of a 41-year-old male *SCA3* patient. The degree of cerebellar, brainstem, and cervical cord atrophy is evident. (From Burk *et al.* 1996.)

dystonia, and spastic paraplegia (Sakai and Kawakami 1996). It is therefore likely that if the whole *SCA3* phenotype is considered, rather than just the usual cerebellar syndrome, the frequency of extrapyramidal features is greater with *SCA3* than *SCA1* or *2*. The reasons for the phenotypic variability of *SCA3* or the mechanism by which the polyglutamine sequence in ataxin 3 causes neurodegeneration are unclear, but as with *SCA1*, this cannot be accounted for simply by CAG repeat length variability (Lopes-Cendes *et al.* 1996).

Generalized dystonia was the main clinical feature of a patient homozygous for the *SCA3* mutation, suggesting that gene dosage also influences the phenotype (Lang *et al.* 1994).

◆ *SCA8* is a CTG expansion mutation in the 3′ untranslated region of a gene on chromosome 13q21. It is a rare cause of ADCA type I; affected patients have had dysarthria, spasticity, and sensory loss in addition to slowly progressive cerebellar ataxia (Koob *et al.* 1999). However, expanded SCA8 repeats have been described in some normal individuals and in conditions other than cerebellar ataxia. Accordingly, the existence of this gene as a definite ataxia locus is uncertain (Vincent, *et al.* 2000).

♦ *SCA12* is also a rare cause of the ADCA I phenotype; onset ranges from 8 to 55 years but is typically in the 4th decade of life. Tremor of the head and upper limbs is prominent, with mild cerebellar signs, hyperreflexia, parkinsonism and dementia or psychiatric features. Neuroimaging shows cerebral and cerebellar atrophy. In some cases, subtle neurological signs are present in infancy (O'Hearn *et al.* 2001).

♦ SCA13 has been described in a single family with ataxia, learning disability, motor developmental delay and pyramidal features. MR scanning shows cerebellar and pontine atrophy. A gene locus has been mapped to chromosome 19q (Herman-Bert et al. 2000). Although currently classified among the dominant later onset ataxias (Subramony and Filla 2001), this condition is of congenital onset and should probably be included in the congenital ataxias (see section 31.3.1).

♦ SCA15 and SCA16 are also described only in single families; at this stage, detailed clinical features are unclear and their ultimate classification is uncertain (Subramony and Filla 2001).

♦ Some ADCA type I families do not have any of the currently known *SCA* mutations and although the exact proportion is unclear it is probably small. Different reports have quoted various frequencies of *SCA1–3* in ADCA I, probably reflecting differences in ascertainment which has usually not been systematic. Nevertheless, two large recent ADCA type I series demonstrated *SCA1, 2,* or *3* mutations in 74 and 90 per cent of families (Giunti *et al.* 1998; Klockgether *et al.* 1998).

31.8.3 Autosomal dominant cerebellar ataxia type II

This form of ADCA is characterized clinically by the presence of visual loss due to a pigmentary retinopathy (Harding 1984). Pathologically there is olivopontocerebellar atrophy with additional pregeniculate visual pathway involvement but these findings are not unique. ADCA II has recently been mapped to chromosome 3 and the pathogenic mutation (*SCA7*) identified as another unstable CAG trinucleotide repeat expansion (Benomar *et al.* 1995; Lindblad *et al.* 1996) as previously predicted clinically (Enevoldson *et al.* 1994). The *SCA7* CAG repeat is more unstable than any other trinucleotide repeat expansion, especially with paternal transmission; increased repeat size, as in other neurodegenerative CAG repeat disorders, is associated with earlier onset, greater severity, and the phenomenon of anticipation. The age of onset in patients with *SCA7* is wider than in other forms of ADCA and it is with this condition that the approximate guideline of autosomal recessive and autosomal dominant cerebellar ataxia usually developing either side of about 25 years of age is least dependable. Many patients are first affected in their 30s or later but children may be affected with a more severe form of the disorder from infancy onwards.

Occasionally patients develop symptoms in their 60s and there are some asymptomatic gene carriers indicating a gene penetrance of 95 per cent (Enevoldson *et al.* 1994). Patients with later onset show less rapid progression. The usual presenting features are ataxia or visual failure but both are usually present within a few years. Pyramidal signs and ophthalmoplegia are commonly associated while chorea, dementia, amyotrophy, and sensory loss are less common. With this combination of features it is not surprising that misdiagnoses of multiple sclerosis have been reported. The visual failure is due to retinal degeneration with loss of central visual field and eventually severe visual loss in most cases. However, patients are often unaware of the insidious progression of visual loss until quite late in the disease and although ophthalmoscopic examination reveals a pigmentary retinopathy in advanced cases (Fig. 31.11), the fundoscopic appearances may be normal for many years leading to diagnostic difficulty. Careful ophthalmological examination, and especially electroretinogram (ERG) recordings may be needed to reveal the characteristic retinal involvement (Enevoldson *et al.* 1994). In contrast, visual evoked potentials are less sensitive and may be misleadingly normal. Early onset infantile cases are much more severe and rapidly fatal with wasting, weakness, fasciculations, dementia, and blindness; retinal pigmentary changes are usually prominent. ADCA II is probably heterogeneous; at least one family with the phenotype does not have the SCA7 mutation (Giunti *et al.* 1999).

31.8.4 Autosomal dominant cerebellar ataxia type III

This form of ADCA typically has a later onset, after 50 years of age, and slow progression; there may or may not be mild additional pyramidal signs (Harding 1984). Such cases are not

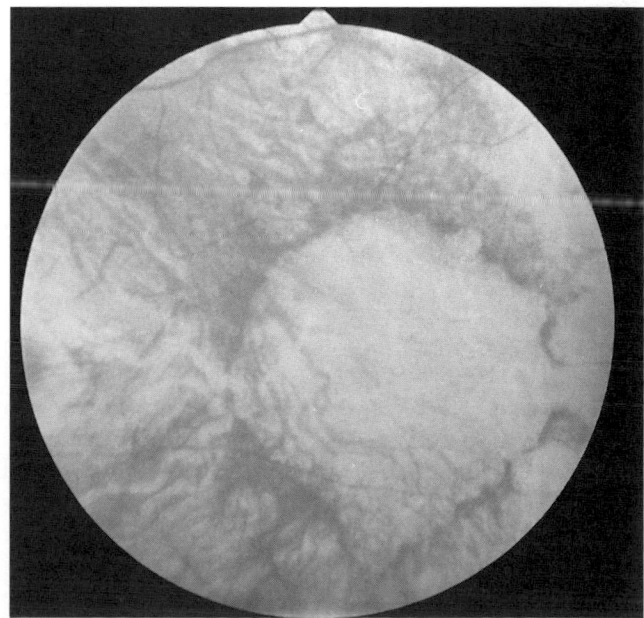

Fig. 31.11. Retinal appearance in ADCA type II (*SCA7*).

common and ADCA III is heterogeneous (Table 31.11). Pathologically, there is cerebellar cortical atrophy which can lead to severe cerebellar atrophy but only very slow clinical deterioration (Frontali *et al.* 1992). One form of mild late onset ataxia has been described in the descendants of President Lincoln (Lincoln ataxia) and a gene locus designated *SCA5* mapped to chromosome 11 (Ranum *et al.* 1994). The *SCA3* mutation may also produce a pure cerebellar phenotype occasionally (see above). Other cases are associated with a small CAG repeat expansion within the alpha 1A calcium channel gene on chromosome 19 (Zhuchenko *et al.* 1997) which has been designated *SCA6* (Table 31.10). Clinically these patients also have late onset, slowly progressive ataxia which is usually not associated with additional signs; cerebellar atrophy is marked on magnetic resonance scans but the brainstem is preserved (Stevanin *et al.* 1997). Two families with an ADCA III phenotype and epilepsy have a gene designated *SCA10* which has been mapped to chromosome 22 (Zu *et al.* 1999). Two other ADCA III families have now been linked to the *SCA11* locus on chromosome 15 (Worth *et al.* 1999); the nature of this mutation is currently unknown. A single family with mild, late onset cerebellar ataxia and cerebellar atrophy on neuroimaging studies has been described with linkage to a gene (SCA14) on chromosome 19q13.4-ter (Yamashita *et al.* 2000). The same family contains patients with younger onset ataxia associated with axial myoclonus.

31.8.5 Autosomal dominant cerebellar ataxia with sensory neuropathy

This is a rare form of autosomal dominant cerebellar ataxia in which there is a prominent sensory peripheral neuropathy; it is likely to be the same disorder previously referred to as Biemond's ataxia (Harding 1984). Pathologically there is degeneration of cerebellar Purkinje cells, dorsal columns, dorsal root ganglion cells, and peripheral nerves (Nachmanoff *et al.* 1997). The sensory symptoms, affecting the face and limbs, and rapid progression of the disorder are unlike ADCA I, II, or III. In one family, linkage to a locus on chromosome 16, designated *SCA4*, has been reported (Flanigan *et al.* 1996).

31.8.6 Dentatorubropallidoluysian atrophy (DRPLA)

This rare autosomal dominant condition was until recently described mainly in Japan (Ilzuka *et al.* 1984) but also occurs in Europe. It has been reported elsewhere as the 'Haw River syndrome'. DRPLA is caused by a CAG repeat expansion mutation of the atrophin 1 gene on chromosome 12 (Koide *et al.* 1994). Pathologically there is degeneration in the dentate nucleus and external segment of the pallidum (Gpe) along with the projections of these areas to the red and subthalamic nuclei (Warner *et al.* 1994). However, the neuropathological findings are variable and may not suggest the diagnosis. Most patients develop symptoms in adult life although earlier onset in childhood may

occur. The phenotype is highly variable both within and between families; some patients have progressive cerebellar ataxia with prominent chorea and dystonia while others have dementia with chorea (pseudo-Huntingtonian type) or a progressive myoclonic epilepsy (Ilzuka *et al.* 1984). Other patients have various combinations of these subtypes and a psychotic presentation has also been described. As expected for a trinucleotide expansion disorder, age of onset is earlier with increased repeat length (Koide *et al.* 1994) and DRPLA families show anticipation and more severe manifestations following paternal transmission (Warner *et al.* 1995). MR scans show cerebellar and brainstem atrophy as well as multiple white matter hyperintensities on T_2 sequences (Koide *et al.* 1997). DRPLA needs to be considered in the differential diagnosis of Huntington's disease (especially if DNA testing is negative), ADCA type I cases with prominent dystonic or choreiform manifestations and progressive myoclonic epilepsy. However, a DRPLA mutation is usually absent in patients without a family history (Warner *et al.* 1995). As with SCA mutations, the regional selectivity of the neuropathology in DRPLA is not due to differences in CAG repeat length or gene expression in different brain regions (Nishiyama *et al.* 1997). There is possibly a defect of mitochondrial respiration in muscle in DRPLA based on results of in vivo magnetic resonance spectroscopy studies (Lodi *et al.* 2000).

31.8.7 Episodic ataxias

In these disorders there are attacks of ataxia, with or without persistent cerebellar signs. The episodic ataxias (EA) are due to defective ion channel function and should be distinguished from the intermittent metabolic ataxias (Section 31.6). An obvious clinical distinction from metabolic ataxia is a family history of autosomal dominant inheritance. There are two main types of EA.

◆ Episodic ataxia with myokymia (EAM/EA 1) develops in early childhood with brief attacks lasting seconds or minutes. These may be triggered by startle or exercise and can be prevented with acetazolamide or phenytoin (Griggs and Nutt 1995). Persistent cerebellar signs or nystagmus do not occur. The myokymia may be subtle and causes fine twitching or flickering in the face and hands. Some patients report episodic stiffening or jerking. EA 1 is caused by point mutations of the potassium channel gene on chromosome 12p (Browne *et al.* 1994; Comu *et al.* 1996).

◆ Episodic ataxia with nystagmus (EAN/EA 2) generally starts later in late childhood or adolescence with more prolonged attacks of ataxia lasting hours or days. Ataxic episodes are associated with stress or exertion but not startle and there is no myokymia (Griggs and Nutt 1995). Between attacks, there may be persistent nystagmus, usually downbeating (Gancher and Nutt 1986) along with a slowly progressive persistent cerebellar syndrome. Some patients with progressive ataxia do not have acute attacks. MRI may show atrophy of the cerebellar vermis. Acetazolamide effectively prevents attacks. EA 2 is caused by point mutations of the alpha 1A calcium channel gene

(*CACNL1A4*) on chromosome 19p (Vahedi *et al.* 1995; Ophoff *et al.* 1996). Interestingly, other point mutations of the same gene cause familial hemiplegic migraine (in which a mild persistent cerebellar ataxia may develop) while a small CAG repeat expansion within the *CACNL1A4* gene (the *SCA6* mutation) causes a slowly progressive ADCA type III phenotype (see above). Some patients who clinically have EA 2 have a *SCA6* mutation rather than a point mutation in *CACNL1A4* (Geschwind *et al.* 1997*a*).

- In EA-3, a missense mutation of the cacium channel beta 4 subunit gene CACNB4 on chromosome 2q22-23 has been described in a family with acetazolamide responsive episodic ataxia (Escayg *et al.* 2000). The same mutation has been associated with epilepsy in another family.

- Periodic vestibulocerebellar ataxia is also an autosomal dominant condition causing attacks of ataxia, diplopia, oscillopsia, and vertigo. A persistent cerebellar syndrome may eventually develop (Damji *et al.* 1996). This disorder is not linked to EA 1 or 2.

31.9 Idiopathic late onset cerebellar ataxias

A common clinical problem is the occurrence of a progressive idiopathic cerebellar syndrome in patients without a family history. In the majority of these cases there is no evidence of an underlying cause for the problem even after investigation (Table 31.4). These patients appear to have an idiopathic neurodegenerative disorder affecting the cerebellum, frequently with additional widespread central and peripheral nervous system involvement (Harding 1984). Neuropathological appearances are variable but most patients have olivopontocerebellar atrophy (OPCA) or cortical cerebellar atrophy. These findings are not specific to idiopathic late onset cerebellar ataxia as similar appearances are seen in various forms of ADCA and multiple system atrophy (see Chapter 32). Accordingly, the tendency to use the term 'OPCA' (a not entirely accurate neuropathological term introduced at the beginning of the century) as a diagnostic label for idiopathic late onset ataxia is misleading (Harding 1987*a*). Unfortunately, the term OPCA does persist as a diagnostic term in patients with the cerebellar presentation of multiple system atrophy (Section 32.3.8).

There has been remarkably little attention paid to this category of adult onset ataxic patients in contrast to the explosion of information about the autosomal dominant cerebellar ataxias. Idiopathic late onset cerebellar ataxia is probably as common as the autosomal dominant forms, but this question has not been addressed specifically. In the series of Harding (1984) there were equal numbers of autosomal dominant and sporadic cases of adult onset ataxia. Age of onset tends to be later than in ADCA, with a mean of 50 years (Harding 1981*b*). Deterioration is relentless but variable; patients lose the ability to walk independently

between 5 and 20 years from onset. An important clinical difference from ADCA is that optic atrophy and retinopathy are not observed and ophthalmoplegia is less common (Burk *et al.* 1997). Three main categories have been suggested (Harding 1981*b*) based on clinical features and similarities to categories of these cases appearing in the earlier literature.

- A 'Marie–Foix–Alajouanine' type presents with gait and lower limb ataxia but little or no upper limb involvement and infrequent dysarthria (Marie *et al.* 1922). Age of onset is usually in the 50s and pathologically there is marked vermian cerebellar atrophy. Extracerebellar degeneration is mild.

- Other patients develop a progressive cerebellar syndrome with very severe postural and intention tremor, similar to the 'dyssynergia cerebellaris progressiva' described by Hunt (1914). Onset is usually around 50 years of age.

- A 'Dejerine–Thomas type' in which a progressive ataxia develops slightly earlier, between 35 and 55 years, and is associated with additional features including dysarthria, pyramidal signs, dementia and sometimes ophthalmoplegia, parkinsonism, or peripheral neuropathy. Bladder dysfunction is not uncommon. These cases are similar to those described previously as 'sporadic olivopontocerebellar atrophy' (Dejerine and Thomas 1900).

Investigation of these patients is usually unrewarding but is important in order to exclude any treatable underlying condition. Neuroimaging is essential in order to exclude hydrocephalus or a posterior fossa mass lesion, which can mimic a cerebellar degeneration (Fig. 31.12). Most patients however, have cerebellar and brainstem atrophy (Wittkamper *et al.* 1993) as shown in Fig. 31.13. It is important to exclude other potential causes of

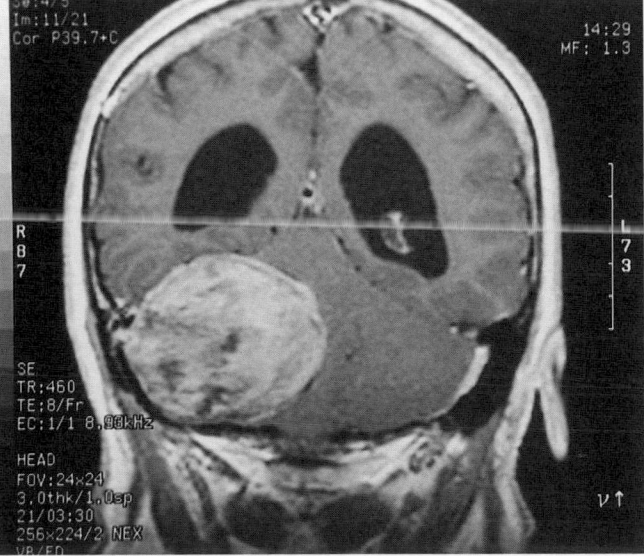

Fig. 31.12. Gadolinium-enhanced magnetic resonance scan showing a large posterior fossa meningioma on the right. The patient presented with a slowly evolving cerebellar ataxia without lateralizing signs or evidence of raised intracranial pressure.

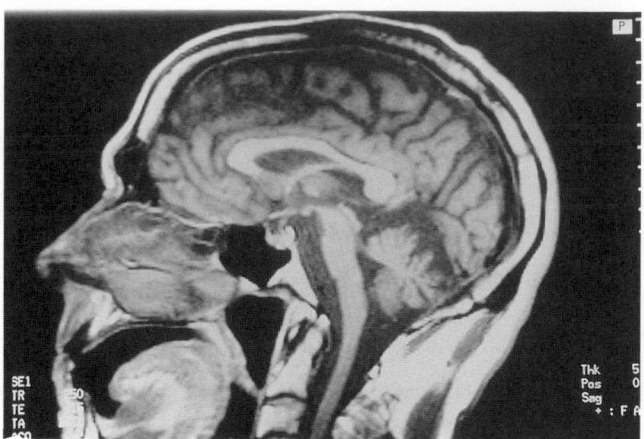

Fig. 31.13. Magnetic resonance scan showing severe cerebellar and brainstem atrophy in a case of idiopathic late-onset cerebellar degeneration (courtesy of Dr T. P. Enevoldson).

slowly progressive ataxia (Table 31.4). An approach to investigations in this situation is discussed in Section 31.2. In most older adults, MR scanning and blood tests for thyroid function, vitamin B12 estimation and basic investigations to exclude bronchial, ovarian, or breast malignancy is adequate unless other possibilities are suggested by the clinical presentation. Nerve conduction tests often show evidence of a peripheral neuropathy, while the EEG and CSF examination are rarely helpful.

A major difficulty in the differential diagnosis of the idiopathic late onset cerebellar ataxias is the distinction, if one exists, from the cerebellar presentation of multiple system atrophy (MSA), now the only condition correctly referred to clinically as OPCA. This is particularly difficult in patients with the Dejerine–Thomas category. This problem is discussed in Section 32.3.8 and it may not be possible to resolve the matter without post-mortem neuropathological examination, which may reveal characteristic glial and neuronal cytoplasmic inclusions in MSA (Gilman and Quinn 1996). Pronounced autonomic impairment, with postural hypotension and bladder dysfunction is suggestive of MSA rather than idiopathic late onset cerebellar ataxia. A fast clinical progression is also more typical of MSA with patients losing independent walking after about 6 years and surviving 9 years from onset (Klockgether *et al.* 1998). It is likely that some patients with late onset idiopathic cerebellar ataxia have MSA but cannot be identified clinically but the degree of overlap between these two diagnostic groups has yet to be analysed in detail. A recent study estimated that over 10 years, perhaps a quarter of Dejerine-Thomas type idiopathic cerebellar ataxia patients develop features of MSA (Gilman *et al.* 2000).

31.10 Genetic counselling and DNA testing in adult onset cerebellar ataxia

Patients with ADCA are faced with a genetic situation not unlike that confronting those with Huntington's disease. The prognosis is poor with slow neurological deterioration and reduced life expectancy. The risk to offspring is 50 per cent and siblings are also at significant risk depending on their ages. The situation is particularly complex in ADCA type II (*SCA7*) families in which mildly affected or even asymptomatic adults may have severely affected children who may die in infancy or early childhood (Enevoldson *et al.* 1994). Patients and family members should be offered genetic counselling so that they are able to make fully informed reproductive decisions. In those patients with a family history of ADCA type I, DNA testing is often positive with most patients carrying one of the *SCA* mutations (Moseley *et al.* 1998). In general, it is often impossible to predict the underlying genetic mutation from the clinical features in ADCA with any confidence. *SCA6* is more likely to be found in those with a mild slowly progressive pure cerebellar ataxia but the early stages of ADCA I or II may be indistinguishable. It is reasonable to include the *SCA7* mutation in DNA analysis in ADCA even in the absence of visual failure or retinopathy which may not be clinically detectable at onset in some cases, thereby making a clinical diagnosis of ADCA II difficult initially. Many laboratories therefore offer screening for *SCA1, 2, 3, 6,* and *7* along with DRPLA which can also produce a mainly cerebellar clinical picture. Although *SCA*/DRPLA gene testing could be used for predictive diagnosis in healthy at-risk relatives and antenatal testing (Nance *et al.* 1994) this has not yet become common practice.

Genetic counselling in sporadic adult onset ataxia is difficult and further studies are needed to clarify this issue. Care is needed when advising patients who have 'negative' but actually incomplete family histories; for example where contact has been lost with relatives whose state of health is therefore uncertain or when a parent died prematurely. Certain clinical features such as optic atrophy, retinopathy, or ophthalmoplegia also increase the likelihood that the patient has autosomal dominant ataxia (see Section 31.9). Harding (1984) proposed that patients were advised that the risk of their ataxic illness being autosomal dominant was approximately 10 per cent, increasing to 20 per cent in the presence of an unreliable family history or the suspicious ophthalmological features already mentioned and 40 per cent with both factors present; risks to offspring are therefore 5, 10, and 20 per cent, respectively. The use of DNA diagnosis in sporadic cases has generally been unhelpful but not yet studied on a large scale. Theoretically, some patients below the age of 50 years may have a late presentation of autosomal recessive Friedreich's ataxia (Section 31.4.1) and testing for the frataxin gene GAA expansion in this situation may be helpful although potentially misleading if a single FA allele is detected given the population carrier frequency of about 1 per cent. In most reports *SCA* mutations have been detected very infrequently in sporadic cases of adult onset ataxia although in another recent study, Friedreich's ataxia or *SCA* mutations were detected in 5 and 4 per cent, respectively, of sporadic cases (Moseley *et al.* 1998). At present it is difficult to give firm advice about the use of DNA analysis in sporadic late onset ataxia but the yield from such investigations is likely to be low unless the clinical features raise suspicion that the patient has ADCA (Section 31.8).

31.11 Other causes of cerebellar ataxia

31.11.1 Toxic and drug-induced ataxia

The most common drug-induced cerebellar syndrome is that seen with anticonvulsant therapy. Phenytoin is usually the cause but carbamazepine and barbiturates may have similar effects and ataxia has been reported with low doses of gabapentin (Steinhoff *et al.* 1997). Patients develop ataxia, nystagmus, dysarthria, and drowsiness, often with serum anticonvulsant concentrations above the therapeutic range but not always. A permanent cerebellar syndrome with cerebellar atrophy and loss of Purkinje cells may develop in patients with chronic phenytoin toxicity; this has been reported in a significant proportion of institutionalized patients with severe epilepsy (Young *et al.* 1994). Other drugs prone to cause cerebellar toxicity include benzodiazepines, piperazine, lithium, cyclosporin A, and cytotoxic drugs especially cytosine arabinoside and 5-flurouracil. Lithium can cause tremor, cerebellar ataxia, or encephalopathy even with normal serum concentrations, and a permanent cerebellar syndrome may also develop (Kores and Lader 1997). In rare cases lithium has produced an encephalopathy with ataxia and myoclonus similar to that seen with Creutzfeldt–Jakob disease (Fear 1992).

A cerebellar syndrome may also occur following the use of illicit drugs including marijuana, phencyclidine, and organic solvents. Usually this is in the context of a toxic encephalopathy but cerebellar atrophy has been detected in young drug abusers suggesting permanent cerebellar damage; this is difficult to separate from the effects of alcohol excess which is also common in this group (Aasly *et al.* 1993). Drug-induced ataxia is a common clinical problem and should always be suspected in any child or young adult presenting with acute cerebellar ataxia; in one series of 40 cases of acute childhood ataxia, 17 out of 35 drug screens were positive (Gieron-Korthals *et al.* 1994). Accidental exposure to organic solvents, acrylamide, and mercury may also produce cerebellar ataxia.

31.11.2 Alcoholic cerebellar ataxia

Ataxia is a cardinal feature of the clinical presentation of acute Wernicke's encephalopathy (Wernicke–Korsakoff syndrome), along with ophthalmoplegia, nystagmus, and confusion (Section 5.2.4). This condition is due to thiamine deficiency in malnourished alcoholics and also occurs in other thiamine deficiency states. Pathologically there is loss of Purkinje cells in the superior cerebellar vermis and a permanent cerebellar ataxia commonly persists after thiamine replacement (Butterworth 1993). Alcoholics also develop a chronic cerebellar ataxia which usually evolves subacutely over weeks or months but sometimes more insidiously. Lower limb and gait ataxia are prominent while upper limb involvement, dysarthria, and nystagmus are rare (Johnson-Greene *et al.* 1997). CT or MR scans typically show vermian atrophy and pathologically the appearances are similar to those seen in Wernicke–Korsakoff syndrome. Improvement with thiamine treatment is rarely complete. The role of a direct toxic effect of alcohol is more controversial but cannot entirely be discounted. Although brain atrophy is seen in well-nourished alcoholics (Nicolas *et al.* 1997), most cases of alcoholic ataxia seem to be nutritional and should be treated urgently with parenteral thiamine.

31.11.3 Paraneoplastic cerebellar degeneration

This condition is rare and mainly occurs with tumours of the lung (small cell carcinoma), breast, female genital tract, and with lymphomas. Pathologically there is severe depletion of cerebellar Purkinje cells with variable additional inflammatory changes (Section 30.6.1). Typically there is a subacute onset over weeks or sometimes months of rapidly progressive severe gait and limb ataxia with vertigo, nystagmus, oscillopsia, and dysarthria. Mental changes are common and there may be evidence of other paraneoplastic syndromes such as opsoclonus, limbic encephalitis, peripheral neuropathy, or Lambert–Eaton myaesthenic syndrome (Anderson *et al.* 1988; Tsukamoto *et al.* 1993; Mason *et al.* 1997). Most patients are severely disabled within weeks or months (Peterson *et al.* 1992) and then stabilize; it is this severity and rapidity of the cerebellar ataxia, unlike most other forms of cerebellar degeneration, that is suggestive of a paraneoplastic aetiology (Bolla and Palmer 1997). It has been suggested that up to 50 per cent of patients over the age of 50 who present with this type of cerebellar syndrome have a paraneoplastic disorder (Henson and Urich 1982) although this is still a small proportion of adult onset ataxic syndromes overall. In most cases the ataxia appears months—but sometimes a few years—before the cancer is apparent. Brain CT and MR scans are often normal but cerebellar atrophy may develop later; a lymphocytic pleocytosis in the CSF is commonly detected along with elevated protein and positive testing for oligoclonal bands. Many patients, especially women with breast, ovarian, or uterine cancer have circulating antineuronal (anti-Hu) or more commonly anti-Purkinje cell (anti-Yo or PCA-1) antibodies (Dropcho 1995) but the role of these is uncertain. Other cases of paraneoplastic cerebellar degeneration have been associated with autoantibodies other than Yo/PCA-1, directed against voltage gated calcium channels (anti VGCC), glutamic acid decarboxylase (anti GAD) and anti-Ri antibodies (Kikuchi *et al.* 2000; Trivedi *et al.* 2000). In most cases, treatment of the underlying neoplasm does not influence the neurological symptoms but there are occasional reports of some improvement with immunosuppression, intravenous immunoglobulin, or plasmapheresis (Moll *et al.* 1993; Dropcho 1995; Stark *et al.* 1995; David *et al.* 1996). Occasionally, a similar syndrome occurs without any underlying malignancy although careful follow up and clinically directed re-investigation of these patients is wise in view of the delay before a malignancy becomes apparent in some cases.

31.11.4 Acute disseminated encephalomyelitis and multiple sclerosis

Cerebellar ataxia is often prominent in these conditions (Sections 29.3.1, 29.4). In acute disseminated encephalomyelitis there is usually an acute onset with depressed consciousness and signs of multifocal neurological involvement. Most cases follow viral illnesses, mycoplasma infection, or vaccination. Multiple sclerosis usually does not present with a progressive cerebellar syndrome but cerebellar features are very common in advanced cases.

31.11.5 Infections and acute cerebellar ataxia of childhood

The most important post-infectious cerebellar syndrome is acute cerebellar ataxia of childhood (Gieron-Korthals et al. 1994). Most cases occur in children aged 1–6 years and follow non-specific viral illnesses or varicella; in the latter the ataxia develops about 3 weeks after the rash. Ataxia develops within hours or days and mainly affects gait with cerebellar tremor, opsoclonus or ocular flutter, and myoclonus. The clinical features are similar to the paraneoplastic myoclonic encephalopathy of childhood associated with neuroblastoma (see below). MR brain scans are normal but the CSF sometimes contains elevated protein and a lymphocytic pleocytosis. The prognosis is excellent but recovery is gradual and takes months. A similar disorder has been reported in older children and young adults. Cerebellar ataxia is also seen in approximately 10 per cent of cases of Legionnaire's disease, sometimes with confusion, cranial neuropathies, headache, and somnolence (Plaschke et al. 1997). Cerebellar ataxia is a recognized feature of mycoplasma infection but this is probably as a result of an immunologically mediated acute disseminated encephalomyelitis (Komatsu et al. 1998). A self-limiting cerebellar syndrome, similar to acute cerebellar ataxia of childhood, has also been described after plasmodium falciparum malaria (Senanayake and de Silva 1994).

Chronic progressive cerebellar ataxia is a feature of prion diseases (Section 31.1.7), subacute sclerosing panencephalitis (Section 34.9), and progressive rubella panencephalitis (see Chapter 34).

31.11.6 Heatstroke

The acute neurological manifestations of heatstroke include confusion, drowsiness, seizures, and focal neurological signs (Section 5.9.2). The majority of patients recover fully but some develop a persistent cerebellar syndrome with cerebellar atrophy suggesting neuronal loss (Biary et al. 1995).

31.11.7 Prion disease

These disorders are discussed in detail in Sections 26.6.5 and 34.12. Cerebellar ataxia is a prominent feature of Creutzfeldt–Jakob disease (CJD), Gerstmann–Straussler–Scheinker syndrome, kuru, and new variant CJD (Zeidler et al. 1997). In about 10 per cent of cases of classical CJD, a cerebellar ataxia is the presenting feature but is soon accompanied by myoclonus and dementia.

31.11.8 Opsoclonus–myoclonus syndrome (myoclonic encephalopathy of infancy; Kinsbourne syndrome)

Although typically seen in infants, this condition may be seen in older children and adults and is heterogeneous. Most patients have a combination of opsoclonus, generalized myoclonus, and cerebellar ataxia. Additional features in some cases include altered mental function, motor and language delay, and behavioural changes (Koh et al. 1994). About 50 per cent of children have an underlying neuroblastoma (although only a small proportion of children with neuroblastoma develop opsoclonus–myoclonus ataxia) while the remainder are idiopathic (Section 30.6.4). Neuroblastoma related cases are more likely to have benign tumour and have a better prognosis; there is also a greater chance of a thoracic neuroblastoma. In idiopathic or neuroblastoma related cases the CSF may show an inflammatory response but brain imaging is usually normal (Mitchell and Snodgrass 1990). Urinary catecholamine excretion may be increased in neuroblastoma cases but this is not consistent and the levels may be normal. In some cases detailed CT scanning of the abdomen and thorax is required to detect a tumour (Mitchell and Snodgrass 1990). The neurological disorder often responds to steroids (or ACTH) and to treatment of an underlying neuroblastoma but many children are left with chronic and persistent symptoms (Koh et al. 1994) requiring long-term steroid therapy. In other children the signs clear up spontaneously and it is likely that these patients have had a post-infectious acute cerebellar ataxia (see above).

A similar disorder occurs in adults. About half of these cases are idiopathic and others are paraneoplastic, associated with anti-Ri antibodies. A favourable response may be seen with steroids or immunoglobulin in paraneoplastic or idiopathic cases (Bataller et al. 2001). As in children, some acute self-limiting cases are likely to be post-infectious acute cerebellar ataxia (Section 31.11.5).

31.11.9 Hypothyroidism

Cerebellar ataxia has been described as a consequence of hypothyroidism (Jellinek and Kelly 1960). Although thyroid function tests are routinely requested as part of the laboratory evaluation of ataxic patients, only a few cases of hypothyroidism related ataxia have ever been reported and usually in association with severe overt myxoedema. One of the patients originally described with ataxia attributed to myxoedema was subsequently found to have multiple system atrophy and a malignancy (Quinn et al. 1992).

31.11.10 Nutritional deficiency

In Europe, nutritional cerebellar ataxia is most commonly seen in chronic malnourished alcoholics (Section 31.11.2). An identical syndrome may be seen in nutritional deficiency for other reasons for example in some haemodialysis patients and those with cachexia due to malignant disease. A seasonal ataxia is also endemic in some parts of the world, which has been shown to be caused by dietary thiamine deficiency (Adamolekun *et al.* 1994). A cerebellar ataxia is seen in pellagra due to deficiency of nicotinic acid but is rare. Vitamin E deficiency has been discussed in Section 31.7.4.

31.11.11 **Gluten ataxia**

It is well recognized that patients with coeliac disease may develop a progressive spinocerebellar degeneration (Cooke and Smith 1966). Other coeliac patients have developed a myoclonic ataxia (Ramsay Hunt syndrome) as discussed in Chapter 32. In some of these cases there has been clinically evident intestinal malabsorption but in others the diagnosis has been made only by small bowel biopsy or the presence of anti-gliadin antibodies (Lu *et al.* 1993; Chinnery *et al.* 1997). Recently, 28 patients with progressive cerebellar ataxia associated with anti-gliadin antibodies have been reported (Hadjivassiliou *et al.* 1998). Some had gastrointestinal symptoms or abnormal duodenal biopsies but in 11 cases neither was present and the only clue to the diagnosis was the anti-gliadin titre. Clinically the mean age of onset was 54 with a progressive gait and lower limb ataxia usually without nystagmus or dysarthria; the cerebellar syndrome was similar to the Marie–Foix–Alajouanine type of idiopathic late onset ataxia (see Section 31.9). It is possible that gluten sensitivity is an important cause of otherwise unexplained cerebellar ataxia but this has not been confirmed. In a recent series of 32 cases of idiopathic cerebellar ataxia, none was associated with antigliadin antibodies (Combarros *et al.* 2000).

References

Aasly, J., Storsaeter, O., Nilsen, G. *et al.* (1993). Minor structural brain changes in young drug abusers. A magnetic resonance study. *Acta Neurol. Scand.*, **87**, 210–4.

Adamec, J., Rusnak, F., Owen, W., *et al.* (2000). Iron-dependent self-assembly of recombinant yeast frataxin: implications for Friedreich ataxia. *Am. J. Hum. Genet.*, **67**, 549–62.

Adamolekun, B., Adamolekun, W. E., Sonibare, A. D. *et al.* (1994). A double-blind, placebo-controlled study of the efficacy of thiamine hydrochloride in a seasonal ataxia in Nigerians. *Neurology*, **44**, 549–51.

al Shahwan, S. A., Bruyn, G. W., and al Deeb, S. M. (1995). Non-progressive familial congenital cerebellar hypoplasia. *J. Neurol. Sci.*, **128**, 71–7.

Anderson, N. E., Budde-Steffen, C., Rosenblum, M. K. *et al.* (1988). Opsoclonus, myoclonus, ataxia, and encephalopathy in adults with cancer: a distinct paraneoplastic syndrome. *Medicine (Baltimore)*, **67**, 100–9.

Apak, S., Yuksel, M., Ozmen, M. *et al.* (1989). Heterogeneity of X-linked recessive (spino)cerebellar ataxia with or without spastic diplegia. *Am. J. Med. Genet.*, **34**, 155–8.

Arai, M. and Ohshima, S. (1997). Maternally inherited diabetes and deafness with cerebellar ataxia: a new clinical phenotype associated with the mitochondrial DNA 3243 mutation [letter]. *J. Neurol.*, **244**, 468–9.

Arts, W. F., Loonen, M. C., Sengers, R. C. *et al.* (1993). X-linked ataxia, weakness, deafness, and loss of vision in early childhood with a fatal course. *Ann. Neurol.*, **33**, 535–9.

Babcock, M., de Silva, D., Oaks, R. *et al.* (1997). Regulation of mitochondrial iron accumulation by Yfh1p, a putative homolog of frataxin. *Science*, **276**, 1709–12.

Bain, P. (1993). A combined clinical and neurophysiological approach to the study of patients with tremor. *J. Neurol. Neurosurg. Psychiatry*, **56**, 839–44.

Bain, P. G., Findley, L. J., Thompson, P. D. *et al.* (1994). A study of hereditary essential tremor. *Brain*, **117**, 805–24.

Bain, P. G., Findley, L. J., Britton, T. C. *et al.* (1995). Primary writing tremor. *Brain*, **118**, 1461–72.

Banfi, S. and Zoghbi, H. Y. (1994). Molecular genetics of hereditary ataxias. *Baillieres Clin. Neurol.*, **3**, 281–95.

Bataller, L., Graus, F., Saiz, A., *et al.* (2001). Clinical outcome in adult onset idiopathic or paraneoplastic opsoclonus. *Brain*, **124**, 437–43.

Becker-Catania, S., Chen, G., Hwang, M., *et al.* (2000). Ataxia-telangiectasia: phenotype/genotype studies of ATM protein expression, mutations, and radiosensivity. *Mol. Genet. Metab.*, **70**, 122–33.

Benabid, A. L., Pollak, P., Gervason, L. *et al.* (1991). Long-term suppression of tremor by chronic stimulation of the ventral intermediate thalamic nucleus. *Lancet*, **337**, 403–6.

Benabid, A. L., Pollak, P., Gao, D. *et al.* (1996). Chronic electrical stimulation of the ventralis intermedius nucleus of the thalamus as a treatment of movement disorders. *J. Neurosurg.*, **84**, 203–14.

Benomar, A., Krols, L., Stevanin, G. *et al.* (1995). The gene for autosomal dominant cerebellar ataxia with pigmentary macular dystrophy maps to chromosome 3p12–p21.1. *Nat. Genet.*, **10**, 84–8.

Berginer, V. M., Salen, G., and Shefer, S. (1989). Cerebrotendinous xanthomatosis. *Neurol. Clin.*, **7**, 55–74.

Biary, N., Cleeves, L., Findley, L. *et al.* (1989). Post-traumatic tremor. *Neurology*, **39**, 103–6.

Biary, N., Madkour, M. M., and Sharif, H. (1995). Post-heatstroke parkinsonism and cerebellar dysfunction. *Clin. Neurol. Neurosurg.*, **97**, 55–7.

Bidichandani, S. I., Ashizawa, T., and Patel, P. I. (1998). The GAA triplet-repeat expansion in Friedreich ataxia interferes with transcription and may be associated with an unusual DNA structure. *Am. J. Hum. Genet.*, **62**, 111–21.

Bidichandani, S., Garcia, C., Patel, P., *et al.* (2000). Very late-onset Friedreich ataxia despite large GAA triplet repeat expansions. *Arch. Neurol;* 57, 246–51.

Bindoff, L. A., Birch-Machin, M. A., Farnsworth, L. *et al.* (1989). Familial intermittent ataxia due to a defect of the E1 component of pyruvate dehydrogenase complex. *J. Neurol. Sci.,* 93, 311–8.

Bolla, L. and Palmer, R. M. (1997). Paraneoplastic cerebellar degeneration. Case report and literature review. *Arch. Intern. Med.,* 157, 1258–62.

Bradley, J., Blake, J., Chamberlain, S., *et al.* (2000). Clinical, bio-chemical and molecular genetic correlations in Friedreich's ataxia. *Hum. Mol. Genet.* 9, 275–82.

Britton, T. C., Thompson, P. D., van der Kamp, W. *et al.* (1992). Primary orthostatic tremor: further observations in six cases. *J. Neurol.,* 239, 209–17.

Britton, T. C. and Thompson, P. D. (1995). Primary orthostatic tremor [editorial]. *BMJ,* 310, 143–4.

Broggi, G., Brock, S., Franzini, A. *et al.* (1993). A case of posttraumatic tremor treated by chronic stimulation of the thalamus. *Mov. Disord.,* 8, 206–8.

Browne, D., Gancher, S., Nutt, J. *et al.* (1994). Episodic ataxia/myokymia syndrome is associated with point mutations in the human potassium channel gene KCNA-1. *Nat. Genet.,* 8, 136–40.

Bundey, S. E. (1992). *Genetics and neurology.* Churchill Livingstone, Edinburgh.

Burk, K., Abele, M., Fetter, M. *et al.* (1996). Autosomal dominant cerebellar ataxia type I clinical features and MRI in families with SCA1, SCA2 and SCA3. *Brain,* 119, 1497–505.

Burk, K., Fetter, M., Skalej, M. *et al.* (1997). Saccade velocity in idiopathic and autosomal dominant cerebellar ataxia. *J. Neurol. Neurosurg. Psychiatry,* 62, 662–4.

Butterworth, R. F. (1993). Pathophysiology of cerebellar dysfunction in the Wernicke–Korsakoff syndrome. *Can. J. Neurol. Sci.,* 20, S123–6.

Butterworth, R. F. (1998). Effects of hyperammonaemia on brain function. *J. Inherit. Metab. Dis.,* 1, 6–20.

Campo, J. V., Stowe, R., Slomka, G. *et al.* (1998). Psychosis as a presentation of physical disease in adolescence: a case of Niemann–Pick disease, type C. *Dev. Med. Child Neurol.,* 40, 126–9.

Campuzano, V., Montermini, L., Molto, M. D. *et al.* (1996). Friedreich's ataxia: autosomal recessive disease caused by an intronic GAA triplet repeat expansion. *Science,* 271, 1423–7.

Carstea, E., Morris, J., Coleman, K., *et al.* (1997). Niemann-Pick C1 disease gene: homology to mediators of cholesterol homeostasis [see comments]. *Science,* 277, 228–31.

Cascino, G. D., Jensen, J. M., Nelson, L. A. *et al.* (1989). Periodic hyperammonemic encephalopathy associated with a ureterosigmoidostomy. *Mayo Clin. Proc.,* 64, 653–6.

Caskey, C. and Rossiter, B. (1993). HPRT deficiency: Lesch–Nyhan syndrome and gouty arthritis. In: *Molecular basis of neurology* (ed. P. Conneally), pp. 129–46. Blackwell, Boston.

Cavalier, L., Ouahchi, K., Kayden, H. J. *et al.* (1998). Ataxia with isolated vitamin E deficiency: heterogeneity of mutations and phenotypic variability in a large number of families. *Am. J. Hum. Genet.,* 62, 301–10.

Caviness, J. N., Forsyth, P. A., Layton, D. D. *et al.* (1995). The movement disorder of adult opsoclonus. *Mov. Disord.,* 10, 22–7.

Chamberlain, S., Shaw, J., Rowland, A. *et al.* (1988). Mapping of mutation causing Friedreich's ataxia to human chromosome 9. *Nature,* 334, 248–50.

Chen, W., Kubota, S., Teramoto, T. *et al.* (1998). Genetic analysis enables definite and rapid diagnosis of cerebrotendinous xanthomatosis. *Neurology,* 51, 865–7.

Chinnery, P. and Turnbull, D. (1997). Clinical features, investigation and management of patients with defects of mitochondrial DNA. *J. Neurol. Neurosurg. Psychiatry,* 63, 559–63.

Chinnery, P. F., Reading, P. J., Milne, D. *et al.* (1997). CSF antigliadin antibodies and the Ramsay Hunt syndrome. *Neurology,* 49, 1131–3.

Chio, A., Orsi, L., Mortara, P. *et al.* (1993). Early onset cerebellar ataxia with retained tendon reflexes: prevalence and gene frequency in an Italian population. *Clin. Genet.,* 43, 207–11.

Claus, D., Harding, A., Hess, C. *et al.* (1988). Central motor conduction in degenerative ataxic disorders: a magnetic stimulation study. *J. Neurol. Neurosurg. Psychiatry,* 51, 790–5.

Cleeves, L., Findley, L. J., and Koller, W. (1988). Lack of association between essential tremor and Parkinson's disease. *Ann. Neurol.,* 24, 23–6.

Cleeves, L., Findley, L. J., and Marsden, C. D. (1994). Odd tremors. In: *Movement disorders,* Vol. 3 (ed. C. D. Marsden and S. Fahn), pp. 434–58. Butterworth Heinemann, Oxford.

Colella, S., Nardo, T., Botta, E., *et al.* (2000). Identical mutations in the CSB gene associated with either Cockayne syndrome or the DeSanctis-cacchione variant of xeroderma pigmentosum. *Hum. Mol. Genet.,* 9, 1171–5.

Combarros, O., Infante, J., Lopez-Hoyos, M., *et al.* (2000). Celiac disease and idiopathic cerebellar ataxia. *Neurology,* 54, 2346.

Comu, S., Giuliani, M., and Narayanan, V. (1996). Episodic ataxia and myokymia syndrome: a new mutation of potassium channel gene Kv1.1. *Ann. Neurol.,* 40, 684–7.

Conway, D., Bain, P. G., Warner, T. T. *et al.* (1993). Linkage analysis with chromosome 9 markers in hereditary essential tremor. *Mov. Disord.*, **8**, 374–6.

Cooke, W. T. and Smith, W. T. (1966). Neurological disorders associated with adult coeliac disease. *Brain*, **89**, 683–722.

Cossee, M., Schmitt, M., Campuzano, V. *et al.* (1997). Evolution of the Friedreich's ataxia trinucleotide repeat expansion: founder effect and premutations. *Proc. Natl Acad. Sci. USA*, **94**, 7452–7.

Costeff, H., Elpeleg, O., Apter, N. *et al.* (1993). 3-Methylglutaconic aciduria in 'optic atrophy plus'. *Ann. Neurol.*, **33**, 103–4.

Damji, K. F., Allingham, R. R., Pollock, S. C. *et al.* (1996). Periodic vestibulocerebellar ataxia, an autosomal dominant ataxia with defective smooth pursuit, is genetically distinct from other autosomal dominant ataxias. *Arch. Neurol.*, **53**, 338–44.

Danek, A. (1993). Geniospasm: hereditary chin trembling. *Mov. Disord.*, **8**, 335–8.

David, Y. B., Warner, E., Levitan, M. *et al.* (1996). Autoimmune paraneoplastic cerebellar degeneration in ovarian carcinoma patients treated with plasmapheresis and immunoglobulin. A case report. *Cancer*, **78**, 2153–6.

de Graaf, A. S., de Jong, G., and Kleijer, W. J. (1995). An early-onset recessive cerebellar disorder with distal amyotrophy and, in two patients, gross myoclonia: a probable ataxia telangiectasia variant. *Clin. Neurol. Neurosurg.*, **97**, 1–7.

de Klerk, J. B., Huijmans, J. G., Stroink, H. *et al.* (1997). L-2-hydroxyglutaric aciduria: clinical heterogeneity versus biochemical homogeneity in a sibship. *Neuropediatrics*, **28**, 314–7.

De Michele, G., Filla, A., Cavalcanti, F. *et al.* (1994). Late onset Friedreich's disease: clinical features and mapping of mutation to the FRDA locus. *J. Neurol. Neurosurg. Psychiatry*, **57**, 977–9.

De Michele, G., Filla, A., Marconi, R. *et al.* (1995). A genetic study of Parkinson's disease. *J. Neural Transm. Suppl.*, **45**, 21–5.

De Michele, G., Filla, A., Striano, S. *et al.* (1995). Heterogeneous findings in four cases of cerebellar ataxia associated with hypogonadism (Holmes' type ataxia). *Clin. Neurol. Neurosurg.*, **95**, 23–8.

De Michele, G., Perrone, F., Filla, A. *et al.* (1996). Age of onset, sex, and cardiomyopathy as predictors of disability and survival in Friedreich's disease: a retrospective study on 119 patients. *Neurology*, **47**, 1260–4.

Dejerine, J. and Thomas, A. (1900). L'atrophie olivo-ponto-cerebelleuse. *Nouvelle iconographie de la Salpetriere*, **13**, 330–76.

Delatycki, M. B., Paris, D., Gardner, R. J. *et al.* (1998). Sperm DNA analysis in a Friedreich ataxia premutation carrier suggests both meiotic and mitotic expansion in the FRDA gene. *J. Med. Genet.*, **35**, 713–6.

des Portes, V., Bachner, L., Bruls, T. *et al.* (1996). X-linked neurodegenerative syndrome with congenital ataxia, late-onset progressive myoclonic encephalopathy and selective macular degeneration, linked to Xp22.33-pter. *Am. J. Med. Genet.*, **64**, 69–72.

Dotti, M. T., Federico, A., Signorini, E. *et al.* (1994). Cerebrotendinous xanthomatosis (van Bogaert–Scherer–Epstein disease): CT and MR findings. *AJNR Am. J. Neuroradiol.*, **15**, 1721–6.

Dropcho, E. (1995). Autoimmune central nervous system paraneoplastic disorders: mechanisms, diagnosis and therapeutic options. *Ann. Neurol.*, **37** (S1), S102–13.

Durr, A., Stevanin, G., Jedynak, C. P. *et al.* (1993). Familial essential tremor and idiopathic torsion dystonia are different genetic entities. *Neurology*, **43**, 2212–4.

Durr, A., Smadja, D., Cancel, G. *et al.* (1995). Autosomal dominant cerebellar ataxia type I in Martinique (French West Indies). Clinical and neuropathological analysis of 53 patients from three unrelated SCA2 families. *Brain*, **118**, 1573–81.

Durr, A., Cossee, M., Agid, Y. *et al.* (1996). Clinical and genetic abnormalities in patients with Friedreich's ataxia [see comments]. *N. Engl. J. Med.*, **335**, 1169–75.

Elpeleg, O. N., Costeff, H., Joseph, A. *et al.* (1994). 3-Methylglutaconic aciduria in the Iraqi-Jewish 'optic atrophy plus' (Costeff) syndrome. *Dev. Med. Child Neurol.*, **36**, 167–72.

Enevoldson, T. P., Sanders, M. D., and Harding, A. E. (1994). Autosomal dominant cerebellar ataxia with pigmentary macular dystrophy. A clinical and genetic study of eight families. *Brain*, **117**, 445–60.

Escayg, A., De Waard, M., Lee, D. D. *et al.* (2000). Coding and non coding variation of the human calcium channel beta (4)-subunit gene CACNB4 in patients with idiopathic generalised epilepsy and episodic ataxia. *Am. J. Hum. Genet.*, **66**, 1531–39.

Evidente, V., Adler, C., Caviness, J. *et al.* (1998). Effective treatment of orthostatic tremor with gabapentin. *Mov. Disord.*, **13**, 829–31.

Farina, L., Uggetti, C., Ottolini, A. *et al.* (1994). Ataxia-telangiectasia: MR and CT findings. *J. Comput. Assist. Tomogr.*, **18**, 724–7.

Fear, C. (1992). Drug induced Creutzfeldt Jacob like syndrome: a review. *Hum. Psychopharmacol.*, **7**, 89.

Filla, A., De Michele, G., Cavalcanti, F. *et al.* (1990). Clinical and genetic heterogeneity in early onset cerebellar ataxia with retained tendon reflexes. *J. Neurol. Neurosurg. Psychiatry*, **53**, 667–70.

Filla, A., De Michele, G., Banfi, S. *et al.* (1995). Has spinocerebellar ataxia type 2 a distinct phenotype? Genetic and clinical study of an Italian family. *Neurology*, **45**, 793 6.

Fink, J. K., Filling-Katz, M. R., Sokol, J. *et al.* (1989). Clinical spectrum of Niemann–Pick disease type C. *Neurology*, **39**, 1040–9.

Flanigan, K., Gardner, K., Alderson, K. *et al.* (1996). Autosomal dominant spinocerebellar ataxia with sensory axonal neuropathy (SCA4): clinical description and genetic localization to chromosome 16q22.1. *Am. J. Hum. Genet.*, **59**, 392–9.

Fletcher, N. A., Harding, A. E., and Marsden, C. D. (1990). A genetic study of idiopathic torsion dystonia in the United Kingdom. *Brain*, **113**, 379–95.

Fletcher, N. A., Harding, A. E., and Marsden, C. D. (1991). A case–control study of idiopathic torsion dystonia. *Mov. Disord.*, **6**, 304–9.

Friedman, J. H. and Weitberg, A. (1993). Ataxia without telangiectasia. *Mov. Disord.*, **8**, 223–6.

Frontali, M., Spadaro, M., Giunti, P. *et al.* (1992). Autosomal dominant pure cerebellar ataxia. Neurological and genetic study. *Brain*, **115**, 1647–54.

Funakawa, I., Kato, H., Terao, A. *et al.* (1995). Cerebellar ataxia in patients with Leber's hereditary optic neuropathy. *J. Neurol.*, **242**, 75–7.

Gancher, S. and Nutt, J. (1986). Autosomal dominant episodic ataxia: a heterogeneous syndrome. *Mov. Disord.*, **1**, 239–53.

Gellera, C., Pareyson, D., Castellotti, B. *et al.* (1997). Very late onset Friedreich's ataxia without cardiomyopathy is associated with limited GAA expansion in the X25 gene. *Neurology*, **49**, 1153–5.

Genis, D., Matilla, T., Volpini, V. *et al.* (1995). Clinical, neuropathologic, and genetic studies of a large spinocerebellar ataxia type 1 (SCA1) kindred: (CAG)n expansion and early premonitory signs and symptoms. *Neurology*, **45**, 24–30.

Gentile, M., Di Carlo, A., Susca, F. *et al.* (1996). COACH syndrome: report of two brothers with congenital hepatic fibrosis, cerebellar vermis hypoplasia, oligophrenia, ataxia, and mental retardation. *Am. J. Med. Genet.*, **64**, 514–20.

Geny, C., Nguyen, J. P., Pollin, B. *et al.* (1996). Improvement of severe postural cerebellar tremor in multiple sclerosis by chronic thalamic stimulation. *Mov. Disord.*, **11**, 489–94.

Gerrits, G. P., Gabreels, F. J., Monnens, L. A. *et al.* (1993). Argininosuccinic aciduria: clinical and biochemical findings in three children with the late onset form, with special emphasis on cerebrospinal fluid findings of amino acids and pyrimidines. *Neuropediatrics*, **24**, 15–8.

Geschwind, D. H., Perlman, S., Figueroa, K. P. *et al.* (1997*a*). Spinocerebellar ataxia type 6. Frequency of the mutation and genotype–phenotype correlations. *Neurology*, **49**, 1247–51.

Geschwind, D. H., Perlman, S., Grody, W. W. *et al.* (1997*b*). Friedreich's ataxia GAA repeat expansion in patients with recessive or sporadic ataxia. *Neurology*, **49**, 1004–9.

Gieron-Korthals, M. A., Westberry, K. R., and Emmanuel, P. J. (1994). Acute childhood ataxia: 10-year experience. *J. Child Neurol.*, **9**, 381–4.

Gilman, S., Bloedel, J. R., and Lechtenberg, R. (1981). *Disorders of the cerebellum*. F. A. Davis, Philadelphia.

Gilman, S. and Quinn, N. P. (1996). The relationship of multiple system atrophy to sporadic olivopontocerebellar atrophy and other forms of idiopathic late-onset cerebellar atrophy. *Neurology*, **46**, 1197–9.

Gilman, S., Little, R., Johanns, J. *et al.* (2000). Evolution of sporadic olivopontocerebellar atrophy into multiple system atrophy. *Neurology*, **55**, 527–32.

Gironell, A., Kulisevsky, J., Barbanoj, M. *et al.* (1999). A randomized placebo-controlled comparative trial of gabapentin and propranolol in essential tremor. *Arch. Neurol.*, **56**, 475–80.

Giunti, P., Sweeney, M. G., and Harding, A. E. (1995). Detection of the Machado–Joseph disease/spinocerebellar ataxia three trinucleotide repeat expansion in families with autosomal dominant motor disorders, including the Drew family of Walworth. *Brain*, **118**, 1077–85.

Giunti, P., Sabbadini, G., Sweeney, M. *et al.* (1998). The role of the SCA2 trinucleotide repeat expansion in 89 autosomal dominant cerebellar ataxia families. *Brain*, **121**, 459–67.

Giunti, P., Stevanin, G., Worth, P. *et al.* (1999). Molecular and clinical study of 18 families with ADCA type II: evidence for genetic heterogeneity and de novo mutation. *Am. J. Hum. Genet.*, **64**, 1594–603.

Goldfarb, L. G., Vasconcelos, O., Platonov, F. A. *et al.* (1996). Unstable triplet repeat and phenotypic variability of spinocerebellar ataxia type 1. *Ann. Neurol.*, **39**, 500–6.

Grau, A. J., Brandt, T., Weisbrod, M. *et al.* (1997). Adult Niemann–Pick disease type C mimicking features of multiple sclerosis [letter]. *J. Neurol. Neurosurg. Psychiatry*, **63**, 552.

Green, J. S., Parfrey, P. S., Harnett, J. D. *et al.* (1989). The cardinal manifestations of Bardet–Biedl syndrome, a form of Laurence–Moon–Biedl syndrome. *N. Engl. J. Med.*, **321**, 1002–9.

Griggs, R. C. and Nutt, J. G. (1995). Episodic ataxias as channelopathies [editorial; comment]. *Ann. Neurol.*, **37**, 285–7.

Gulcher, J. R., Jonsson, P., Kong, A. *et al.* (1997). Mapping of a familial essential tremor gene, FET1, to chromosome 3q13. *Nat. Genet.*, **17**, 84–7.

Gunal, N., Saraclar, M., Ozkutlu, S. *et al.* (1996). Heart disease in Friedreich's ataxia: a clinical and echocardiographic study. *Acta Paediatr. Jpn*, **38**, 308–11.

Ha, J. H. and Basile, A. S. (1996). Modulation of ligand binding to components of the GABAA receptor complex by ammonia: implications for the pathogenesis of hyperammonemic syndromes. *Brain Res.*, **720**, 35–44.

Hadjivassiliou, M., Grunewald, R. A., Chattopadhyay, A. K. *et al.* (1998). Clinical, radiological, neurophysiological, and neuropathological characteristics of gluten ataxia. *Lancet*, **352**, 1582–5.

Hallett, M. (1984). Classification and treatment of tremor. *JAMA*, **266**, 1115–7.

Hammans, S. R. (1996). The inherited ataxias and the new genetics [editorial]. *J. Neurol. Neurosurg. Psychiatry*, **61**, 327–32.

Hammans, S. R. and Kennedy, C. R. (1998). Ataxia with isolated vitamin E deficiency presenting as mutation negative Friedreich's ataxia. *J. Neurol. Neurosurg. Psychiatry*, **64**, 368–70.

Hanna, M. G., Davis, M. B., Sweeney, M. G. *et al.* (1998). Generalized chorea in two patients harboring the Friedreich's ataxia gene trinucleotide repeat expansion. *Mov. Disord.*, **13**, 339–40.

Harding, A. (1981*a*). Friedreich's ataxia: a clinical and genetic study of 90 families with an analysis of early diagnostic criteria and intrafamilial clustering of cases. *Brain*, **104**, 589–620.

Harding, A. (1981*b*). Idiopathic late onset cerebellar ataxia: a clinical and genetic study of 36 cases. *J. Neurol. Sci.*, **51**, 259–71.

Harding, A. (1987*a*). Olivopontocerebellar atrophy is not a useful concept. In: *Movement disorders*, Vol. 2 (ed. C. Marsden and S. Fahn), pp. 269–71. Butterworths, London.

Harding, A. and Zilkha, K. (1981). 'Pseudodominant inheritance' in Friedrcich's ataxia. *J. Med. Genet.*, **18**, 285–7.

Harding, A. and Hewer, R. (1983). The heart disease of Friedreich's ataxia: a clinical and electrocardiographic study of 115 patients, with an analysis of serial electrocardiographic changes in 30 cases. *Q. J. Med.*, **208**, 489–502.

Harding, A. E. (1984). *The hereditary ataxias and related disorders*. Churchill Livingstone, Edinburgh.

Harding, A. (1987*b*). Vitamin E and the nervous system. *CRC Crit. Rev. Neurobiol.*, **3**, 89–103.

Heilman, K. (1984). Orthostatic tremor. *Arch. Neurol.*, **41**, 880–1.

Henson, R. and Urich, H. (1982). *Cancer and the nervous system*. Blackwell Scientific, London.

Herman-Bert, A., Stevanin, G., Netter, J., *et al.* (2000). Mapping of spinocerebellar ataxia 13 to chromosome 19q13.3–q13.4 in a family with autosomal dominant cerebellar ataxia and mental retardation. *Am. J. Hum. Genet.*, **67**, 229–35.

Herz, E. (1944). Dystonia. I. Historical review; analysis of dystonic symptoms and physiologic mechanisms involved. *Arch. Neurol. Psychiatry*, **51**, 305–18.

Higgins, J., Nee, L., Vasconcelos, O. *et al.* (1996). Mutations in American families with spinocerebellar ataxia (SCA) type 3: SCA3 is allelic to Machado–Joseph disease. *Neurology*, **46**, 208–13.

Higgins, J. J., Pho, L. T., and Nee, L. E. (1997). A gene (ETM) for essential tremor maps to chromosome 2p22–p25. *Mov. Disord.*, **12**, 859–64.

Holmes, G. (1904). On certain tremors in organic cerebral lesions. *Brain*, **27**, 327–75.

Holmes, G. (1907). A form of familial degeneration of the cerebellum. *Brain*, **30**, 466–89.

Holt, I. J., Harding, A. E., Cooper, J. M. *et al.* (1989). Mitochondrial myopathies: clinical and biochemical features of 30 patients with major deletions of muscle mitochondrial DNA. *Ann. Neurol.*, **26**, 699–708.

Holt, I. J., Harding, A. E., Petty, R. K. *et al.* (1990). A new mitochondrial disease associated with mitochondrial DNA heteroplasmy. *Am. J. Hum. Genet.*, **46**, 428–33.

Howell, N., Kubacka, M., Smith, R. *et al.* (1996). Association of the mitochondrial 8344 MERRF mutation with maternally inherited spinocerebellar degeneration and Leigh disease. *Neurology*, **46**, 219–22.

Hua, S. E., Lenz, F. A., Zirh, T. A. *et al.* (1998). Thalamic neuronal activity correlated with essential tremor. *J. Neurol. Neurosurg. Psychiatry*, **64**, 273–6.

Hund, E., Grau, A., Fogel, W. *et al.* (1997). Progressive cerebellar ataxia, proximal neurogenic weakness and ocular motor disturbances: hexosaminidase A deficiency with late clinical onset in four siblings. *J. Neurol. Sci.*, **145**, 25–31.

Hunt, J. (1914). Dyssynergia cerebellaris progressiva—a chronic progressive form of cerebellar tremor. *Brain*, **37**, 247–68.

Illarioshkin, S. N., Tanaka, H., Markova, E. D. *et al.* (1996). X-linked nonprogressive congenital cerebellar hypoplasia: clinical description and mapping to chromosome Xq. *Ann. Neurol.*, **40**, 75–83.

Ilzuka, R., Hirayama, K., and Maehara, K. (1984). Dentato-rubro-pallidoluysian atrophy: a clinico-pathological study. *J. Neurol. Neurosurg. Psychiatry*, **47**, 1288–98.

Ishikawa, K., Mizusawa, H., Igarashi, S. *et al.* (1996). Pure cerebellar ataxia phenotype in Machado–Joseph disease. *Neurology*, **46**, 1776–7.

Isnard, R., Kalotka, H., Durr, A. *et al.* (1997). Correlation between left ventricular hypertrophy and GAA trinucleotide repeat length in Friedreich's ataxia. *Circulation*, **95**, 2247–9.

Jankovic, J. and Van der Linden, C. (1988). Dystonia and tremor induced by peripheral trauma: predisposing factors. *J. Neurol. Neurosurg. Psychiatry*, **51**, 1512–9.

Jankovic, J., Leder, S., Warner, D. *et al.* (1991). Cervical dystonia: clinical findings and associated movement disorders. *Neurology*, **41**, 1088–91.

Jankovic, J., Schwartz, K., Clemence, W. *et al.* (1996). A randomized, double-blind, placebo-controlled study to evaluate botulinum toxin type A in essential hand tremor. *Mov. Disord.*, **11**, 250–6.

Jarman, P. R., Wood, N. W., Davis, M. T. *et al.* (1997). Hereditary geniospasm: linkage to chromosome 9q13–q21 and evidence for genetic heterogeneity. *Am. J. Hum. Genet.*, **61**, 928–33.

Jellinek, E. and Kelly, R. (1960). Cerebellar syndrome in myxoedema. *Lancet*, **ii**, 225–7.

Jenkins, I. H., Bain, P. G., Colebatch, J. G. *et al.* (1993). A positron emission tomography study of essential tremor: evidence for overactivity of cerebellar connections. *Ann. Neurol.*, **34**, 82–90.

Johnson-Greene, D., Adams, K. M., Gilman, S. *et al.* (1997). Impaired upper limb coordination in alcoholic cerebellar degeneration. *Arch. Neurol.*, **54**, 436–9.

Junck, L. and Fink, J. (1996). Macado–Joseph disease and SCA3: the genotype meets the phenotype. *Neurology*, **46**, 4–8.

Kanda, T., Oda, M., Yonezawa, M. *et al.* (1990). Peripheral neuropathy in xeroderma pigmentosum. *Brain*, **113**, 1025–44.

Kellett, M. W., Fletcher, N. A., Wood, N. *et al.* (1997). Trinucleotide (GAA)n repeat expansion in two families with Friedreich's ataxia with retained reflexes. *J. Neurol. Neurosurg. Psychiatry*, **63**, 780–3.

Khanna, K. K., Keating, K. E., Kozlov, S. *et al.* (1998). ATM associates with and phosphorylates p53: mapping the region of interaction. *Nat. Genet.*, **20**, 398–400.

Kikuchi, H., Yamada, T., Okayama, A. *et al.* (2000). Anti-Ri-associated paraneoplastic cerebellar degeneration without opsoclonus in a patient with a neuroendocrine carcinoma of the stomach. *Fukuoka Igaku Zasshi*, **91**, 104–9.

Kinoshita, H., Sakuragawa, N., Tada, H. *et al.* (1997). Recurrent muscle weakness and ataxia in thiamine-responsive pyruvate dehydrogenase complex deficiency. *J. Child Neurol.*, **12**, 141–4.

Klemm, E. and Conzelmann, E. (1989). Adult-onset metachromatic leucodystrophy presenting without psychiatric symptoms. *J. Neurol.*, **236**, 427–9.

Klockgether, T., Petersen, D., Grodd, W. *et al.* (1991). Early onset cerebellar ataxia with retained tendon reflexes. Clinical, electrophysiological and MRI observations in comparison with Friedreich's ataxia. *Brain*, **114**, 1559–73.

Klockgether, T., Chamberlain, S., Wullner, U. *et al.* (1993). Late-onset Friedreich's ataxia. Molecular genetics, clinical neurophysiology, and magnetic resonance imaging. *Arch. Neurol.*, **50**, 803–6.

Klockgether, T., Zuhlke, C., Schulz, J. B. *et al.* (1996). Friedreich's ataxia with retained tendon reflexes: molecular genetics, clinical neurophysiology, and magnetic resonance imaging. *Neurology*, **46**, 118–21.

Klockgether, T., Ludtke, R., Kramer, B. *et al.* (1998). The natural history of degenerative ataxia: a retrospective study in 466 patients. *Brain*, **121**, 589–600.

Koepp, M., Schelosky, L., Cordes, I. *et al.* (1994). Dystonia in ataxia telangiectasia: report of a case with putaminal lesions and decreased striatal [^{123}I]iodobenzamide binding. *Mov. Disord.*, **9**, 455–9.

Koh, P. S., Raffensperger, J. G., Berry, S. *et al.* (1994). Long-term outcome in children with opsoclonus–myoclonus and ataxia and coincident neuroblastoma. *J. Pediatr.*, **125**, 712–6.

Koide, R., Ikeuchi, T., Onodera, O. *et al.* (1994). Unstable expansion of CAG repeat in hereditary dentatorubral-pallidoluysian atrophy (DRPLA). *Nat. Genet.*, **6**, 14–8.

Koide, R., Onodera, O., Ikeuchi, T. *et al.* (1997). Atrophy of the cerebellum and brainstem in dentatorubral pallidoluysian atrophy. Influence of CAG repeat size on MRI findings. *Neurology*, **49**, 1605–12.

Koller, W. C. and Vetere-Overfield, B. (1989). Acute and chronic effects of propranolol and primidone in essential tremor. *Neurology*, **39**, 1587–8.

Koller, W. C., Busenbark, K., and Miner, K. (1994). The relationship of essential tremor to other movement disorders: report on 678 patients. Essential Tremor Study Group. *Ann. Neurol.*, **35**, 717–23.

Komatsu, H., Kuroki, S., Shimizu, Y. *et al.* (1998). Mycoplasma pneumoniae meningoencephalitis and cerebellitis with antiganglioside antibodies. *Pediatr. Neurol.*, **18**, 160–4.

Koob, M. D., Moseley, M. L., Schut, L. J. *et al.* (1999). An untranslated CTG expansion causes a novel form of spinocerebellar ataxia (SCA8). *Nat. Genet.*, **21**, 379–84.

Kores, B. and Lader, M. H. (1997). Irreversible lithium neurotoxicity: an overview. *Clin. Neuropharmacol.*, **20**, 283–99.

Koutnikova, H., Campuzano, V., Foury, F. *et al.* (1997). Studies of human, mouse and yeast homologues indicate a mitochondrial function for frataxin. *Nat. Genet.*, **16**, 345–51.

Kuriyama, M., Tokimura, Y., Fujiyama, J. *et al.* (1994). Treatment of cerebrotendinous xanthomatosis: effects of chenodeoxycholic acid, pravastatin, and combined use. *J. Neurol. Sci.*, **125**, 22–8.

Lamont, P. J., Davis, M. B., and Wood, N. W. (1997). Identification and sizing of the GAA trinucleotide repeat expansion of Friedreich's ataxia in 56 patients. Clinical and genetic correlates. *Brain*, **120**, 673–80.

Lang, A. E., Rogaeva, E. A., Tsuda, T. *et al.* (1994). Homozygous inheritance of the Machado–Joseph disease gene. *Ann. Neurol.*, **36**, 443–7.

Lange, E., Borresen, A. L., Chen, X. *et al.* (1995). Localization of an ataxia-telangiectasia gene to an approximately 500-kb interval on chromosome 11q23.1: linkage analysis of 176 families by an international consortium. *Am. J. Hum. Genet.*, **57**, 112–9.

Larnaout, A., Belal, S., Ben Hamida, C. *et al.* (1998). Atypical ataxia telangiectasia with early childhood lower motor neuron degeneration: a clinicopathological observation in three siblings. *J. Neurol.*, **245**, 231–5.

Lewis, S. M., Roberts, E. A., Marcon, M. A. *et al.* (1994). Joubert syndrome with congenital hepatic fibrosis: an entity in the spectrum of oculo-encephalo-hepato-renal disorders. *Am. J. Med. Genet.*, **52**, 419–26.

Limber, E. R., Bresnick, G. H., Lebovitz, R. M. *et al.* (1989). Spinocerebellar ataxia, hypogonadotropic hypogonadism, and choroidal dystrophy (Boucher–Neuhauser syndrome). *Am. J. Med. Genet.*, **33**, 409–14.

Lindblad, K., Savontaus, M. L., Stevanin, G. *et al.* (1996). An expanded CAG repeat sequence in spinocerebellar ataxia type 7. *Genome Res.*, **6**, 965–71.

Lodi, R., Schapira, A., Manners, D. *et al.* (2000). Abnormal in vivo skeletal muscle energy metabolism in Huntington's disease and dentatorubropallidoluysian atrophy. *Ann. Neurol.*, **48**, 72–6.

Lopes-Cendes, I., Maciel, P., Kish, S. *et al.* (1996). Somatic mosaicism in the central nervous system in spinocerebellar ataxia type 1 and Machado–Joseph disease. *Ann. Neurol.*, **40**, 199–206.

Lossos, A., Schlesinger, I., Okon, E. *et al.* (1997). Adult-onset Niemann–Pick type C disease. Clinical, biochemical, and genetic study. *Arch. Neurol.*, **54**, 1536–41.

Lu, C. S., Thompson, P. D., Quinn, N. P. *et al.* (1993). Ramsay Hunt syndrome and coeliac disease: a new association? *Mov. Disord.*, **1**, 209–19.

Lutz, R., Bodensteiner, J., Schaefer, B. *et al.* (1989). X-linked olivopontocerebellar atrophy. *Clin. Genet.*, **35**, 417–22.

Machkhas, H., Bidichandani, S. I., Patel, P. I. *et al.* (1998). A mild case of Friedreich ataxia: lymphocyte and sural nerve analysis for GAA repeat length reveals somatic mosaicism. *Muscle Nerve*, **21**, 390–3.

Maria, B. L., Hoang, K. B., Tusa, R. J. *et al.* (1997). 'Joubert syndrome' revisited: key ocular motor signs with magnetic resonance imaging correlation. *J. Child Neurol.*, **12**, 423–30.

Marie, P., Foix, C., and Alajouanine, T. (1922). De l'atrophie cerebelleuse tardive a predominance corticale. *Rev. Neurol. (Paris)*, **2**, 849–85.

Marsden, C. D. and Harrison, M. G. J. (1974). Idiopathic torsion dystonia (dystonia musculorum deformans). A review of forty-two patients. *Brain*, **97**, 793–810.

Marsden, C. D. and Rothwell, J. C. (1987). The physiology of idiopathic dystonia. *Can. J. Neurol. Sci.*, **14**, 521–7.

Mason, W. P., Graus, F., Lang, B. *et al.* (1997). Small-cell lung cancer, paraneoplastic cerebellar degeneration and the Lambert–Eaton myasthenic syndrome. *Brain*, **120**, 1279–300.

Matilla, T., McCall, A., Subramony, S. H. *et al.* (1995). Molecular and clinical correlations in spinocerebellar ataxia type 3 and Machado–Joseph disease. *Ann. Neurol.*, **38**, 68–72.

Matsuo, M., Nomura, S., Hara, T. *et al.* (1994). A variant form of hypobetalipoproteinaemia associated with ataxia, hearing loss and retinitis pigmentosa. *Dev. Med. Child Neurol.*, **36**, 1015–20.

McCabe, D., Ryan, F., Moore, D. *et al.* (2000). Typical Friedreich's ataxia without GAA expansions and GAA expansion without typical Friedreich's ataxia. *J. Neurol.*, **247**, 346–55.

McFarlin, D., Strober, W., and Waldmann, D. (1972). Ataxia-telangiectasia. *Medicine*, **51**, 281–314.

McGovern, M., Stewart, M., Morrison, P. *et al.* (2000). Early onset of Friedreich's ataxia in a compound heterozygote. *Arch. Dis. Child*, **83**, 74–5.

McLaughlin, J. F., Pagon, R. A., Weinberger, E. *et al.* (1996). Marinesco–Sjogren syndrome: clinical and magnetic resonance imaging features in three children [corrected and republished article originally printed in *Dev. Med. Child Neurol.*, **38** (4), 363–70, 1996]. *Dev. Med. Child Neurol.*, **38**, 636–44.

McManis, P. G. and Sharbrough, F. W. (1993). Orthostatic tremor: clinical and electrophysiologic characteristics. *Muscle Nerve*, **16**, 1254–60.

Mimaki, T., Itoh, N., Abe, J. *et al.* (1986). Neurological manifestations in Xeroderma Pigmentosum. *Ann. Neurol.*, **20**, 70–5.

Mitchell, W. G. and Snodgrass, S. R. (1990). Opsoclonus-ataxia due to childhood neural crest tumors: a chronic neurologic syndrome [published erratum appears in *J. Child Neurol.*, **5** (3), 266, 1990]. *J. Child Neurol.*, **5**, 153–8.

Moll, J. W., Henzen-Logmans, S. C., Van der Meche, F. G. *et al.* (1993). Early diagnosis and intravenous immune globulin therapy in paraneoplastic cerebellar degeneration [letter]. *J. Neurol. Neurosurg. Psychiatry*, **56**, 112.

Montermini, L., Kish, S. J., Jiralerspong, S. *et al.* (1997*a*). Somatic mosaicism for Friedreich's ataxia GAA triplet repeat expansions in the central nervous system. *Neurology*, **49**, 606–10.

Montermini, L., Richter, A., Morgan, K. *et al.* (1997*b*). Phenotypic variability in Friedreich ataxia: role of the associated GAA triplet repeat expansion. *Ann. Neurol.*, **41**, 675–82.

Moschner, C., Perlman, S., and Baloh, R. W. (1994). Comparison of oculomotor findings in the progressive ataxia syndromes. *Brain*, **117**, 15–25.

Moseley, M. L., Benzow, K. A., Schut, L. J. *et al.* (1998). Incidence of dominant spinocerebellar and Friedreich triplet repeats among 361 ataxia families. *Neurology*, **51**, 1666–71.

Muller, D., Lloyd, J., and Wolff, O. (1983). Vitamin E and neurological function. *Lancet*, **i**, 225–8.

Muller-Felber, W., Zafiriou, D., Scheck, R. *et al.* (1998). Marinesco Sjogren syndrome with rhabdomyolysis. A new subtype of the disease. *Neuropediatrics*, **29**, 97–101.

Murakami, T., Mita, S., Tokunaga, M. *et al.* (1996). Hereditary cerebellar ataxia with Leber's hereditary optic neuropathy mitochondrial DNA 11778 mutation. *J. Neurol. Sci.*, **142**, 111–3.

Nachmanoff, D. B., Segal, R. A., Dawson, D. M. *et al.* (1997). Hereditary ataxia with sensory neuronopathy: Biemond's ataxia. *Neurology*, **48**, 273–5.

Nance, M. A. and Berry, S. A. (1992). Cockayne syndrome: review of 140 cases. *Am. J. Med. Genet.*, **42**, 68–84.

Nance, M. A., Sevenich, E. A., and Schut, L. J. (1994). Knowledge of genetics and attitudes toward genetic testing in two hereditary ataxia (SCA 1) kindreds. *Am. J. Med. Genet.*, **54**, 242–8.

Narcisi, T. M., Shoulders, C. C., Chester, S. A. *et al.* (1995). Mutations of the microsomal triglyceride-transfer-protein gene in abetalipoproteinemia. *Am. J. Hum. Genet.*, **57**, 1298–310.

Nelson, I., Hanna, M. G., Alsanjari, N. *et al.* (1995). A new mitochondrial DNA mutation associated with progressive dementia and chorea: a clinical, pathological, and molecular genetic study. *Ann. Neurol.*, **37**, 400–3.

Nelson, J., Flaherty, M., and Grattan-Smith, P. (1997). Gillespie syndrome: a report of two further cases. *Am. J. Med. Genet.*, **71**, 134–8.

Nemeth, A. H., Bochukova, E., Dunne, E., *et al.* (2000). Autosomal recessive cerebellar ataxia with oculomotor apraxia (Ataxia telangiectasia-like syndrome) is linked to chromosome 9q34. *Am. J. Human. Genet.*, **67**, 1320–26.

Nicolas, J. M., Estruch, R., Salamero, M. *et al.* (1997). Brain impairment in well-nourished chronic alcoholics is related to ethanol intake. *Ann. Neurol.*, **41**, 590–8.

Nightingale, S. and Barton, M. E. (1991). Intermittent vertical supranuclear ophthalmoplegia and ataxia. *Mov. Disord.*, **6**, 76–8.

Nishiyama, K., Nakamura, K., Murayama, S. *et al.* (1997). Regional and cellular expression of the dentatorubral-pallidoluysian atrophy gene in brains of normal and affected individuals. *Ann. Neurol.*, **41**, 599–605.

Nutt, J. G., Marsden, C. D., and Thompson, P. D. (1993). Human walking and higher level gait disorders, particularly in the elderly. *Neurology*, **43**, 268–79.

O'Hearn, E., Holmes, S., Calvert, P., *et al.* (2001). Spinocerebellar ataxia type 12 (SCA12): clinical and neuro-radiologic features. *Neurology*, **56**, 299–303.

Ohye, C., Miyazaki, M., Hirai, T. *et al.* (1982). Primary writing tremor treated by stereotactic surgery. *J. Neurol. Neurosurg. Psychiatry*, **45**, 988–97.

Ophoff, R. A., Terwindt, G. M., Vergouwe, M. N. *et al.* (1996). Familial hemiplegic migraine and episodic ataxia type-2 are caused by mutations in the Ca^{2+} channel gene CACNL1A4. *Cell*, **87**, 543–52.

Ormerod, I. E., Harding, A. E., Miller, D. H. *et al.* (1994). Magnetic resonance imaging in degenerative ataxic disorders. *J. Neurol. Neurosurg. Psychiatry*, **57**, 51–7.

Pahwa, R. and Koller, W. C. (1993). Is there a relationship between Parkinson's disease and essential tremor? *Clin. Neuropharmacol.*, **16**, 30–5.

Pahwa, R., Lyons, K., Hubble, J. *et al.* (1998). Double-bind controlled trial of gabapentin in essential tremor. *Mov. Disord.*, **13**, 465–7.

Pahwa, R., Lyons, K., Wilkinson, S. B. *et al.* (1999). Bilateral thalamic stimulation for the treatment of essential tremor. *Neurology*, **53**, 1447–50.

Paine, R. S. (1960). Evaluation of familial biochemically determined mental retardation in children with special reference to aminoaciduria. *N. Engl. J. Med.*, **262**, 658–65.

Palau, F., De Michele, G., Vilchez, J. J. *et al.* (1995). Early-onset ataxia with cardiomyopathy and retained tendon reflexes maps to the Friedreich's ataxia locus on chromosome 9q. *Ann. Neurol.*, **37**, 359–62.

Pellegrino, J. E., Lensch, M. W., Muenke, M. *et al.* (1997). Clinical and molecular analysis in Joubert syndrome. *Am. J. Med. Genet.*, **72**, 59–62.

Perlmutter, D., Gross, P., Jones, H. *et al.* (1987). Intramuscular vitamin E repletion in children with chronic cholestasis. *Am. J. Dis. Childhood*, **141**, 170.

Peterson, K., Rosenblum, M. K., Kotanides, H. *et al.* (1992). Paraneoplastic cerebellar degeneration. I. A clinical analysis of 55 anti-Yo antibody-positive patients. *Neurology*, **42**, 1931–7.

Plaschke, M., Strohle, A., Then Bergh, F. *et al.* (1997). [Neurologic and psychiatric symptoms of legionella infection. Case report and overview of the clinical spectrum]. *Nervenarzt*, **68**, 342–5.

Poersch, M. (1994). Orthostatic tremor: combined treatment with primidone and clonazepam [letter]. *Mov. Disord.*, **9**, 467.

Pratap-Chand, R., Gururaj, A. K., and Dilip-Kumar, S. (1995). A syndrome of olivopontocerebellar atrophy and deafness with onset in infancy. *Acta Neurol. Scand.*, **91**, 133–6.

Pridmore, C. L., Clarke, J. T., and Blaser, S. (1995). Ornithine transcarbamylase deficiency in females: an often overlooked cause of treatable encephalopathy. *J. Child Neurol.*, **10**, 369–74.

Priller, J., Scherzer, C. R., Faber, P. W. *et al.* (1997). Frataxin gene of Friedreich's ataxia is targeted to mitochondria. *Ann. Neurol.*, **42**, 265–9.

Quinn, N., Barnard, R. O., and Kelly, R. E. (1992). Cerebellar syndrome in myxoedema revisited: a published case with carcinomatosis and multiple system atrophy at necropsy. *J. Neurol. Neurosurg. Psychiatry*, **55**, 616–8.

Rahman, S., Standing, S., Dalton, R. N. *et al.* (1997). Late presentation of biotinidase deficiency with acute visual loss and gait disturbance. *Dev. Med. Child Neurol.*, **39**, 830–1.

Rajput, A. H., Rozdilsky, B., Ang, L. *et al.* (1993). Significance of parkinsonian manifestations in essential tremor. *Can. J. Neurol. Sci.*, **20**, 114–7.

Ranum, L. P., Schut, L. J., Lundgren, J. K. *et al.* (1994). Spinocerebellar ataxia type 5 in a family descended from the grandparents of President Lincoln maps to chromosome 11. *Nat. Genet.*, **8**, 280–4.

Remy, P., de Recondo, A., Defer, G. *et al.* (1995). Peduncular 'rubral' tremor and dopaminergic denervation: a PET study. *Neurology*, **45**, 472–7.

Richter, A., Poirier, J., Mercier, J. *et al.* (1996). Friedreich ataxia in Acadian families from eastern Canada: clinical diversity with conserved haplotypes. *Am. J. Med. Genet.*, **64**, 594–601.

Rivest, J. and Marsden, C. D. (1990). Trunk and head tremor as isolated manifestations of dystonia. *Mov. Disord.*, **5**, 60–5.

Robinson, B. H., MacKay, N., Chun, K. *et al.* (1996). Disorders of pyruvate carboxylase and the pyruvate dehydrogenase complex. *J. Inherit. Metab. Dis.*, **19**, 452–62.

Rosenberg, R. (1992). Machado–Joseph disease: an autosomal dominant motor system degeneration. *Mov. Disord.*, **7**, 193–203.

Rotig, A., de Lonlay, P., Chretien, D. *et al.* (1997). Aconitase and mitochondrial iron–sulphur protein deficiency in Friedreich ataxia. *Nat. Genet.*, **17**, 215–7.

Said, G., Bathien, N., and Cesaro, P. (1982). Peripheral neuropathies and tremor. *Neurology*, **32**, 480–5.

Sakai, T. and Kawakami, H. (1996). Machado–Joseph disease: a proposal of spastic paraplegic subtype. *Neurology*, **46**, 846–7.

Sanner, G. (1973). The dysequilibrium syndrome. *Neuropaeditrie*, **4**, 403–13.

Santoro, L., Perretti, A., Filla, A. *et al.* (1992). Is early onset cerebellar ataxia with retained tendon reflexes identifiable by electrophysiologic and histologic profile? A comparison with Friedreich's ataxia. *J. Neurol. Sci.*, **113**, 43–9.

Santoro, L., Perretti, A., Lanzillo, B. *et al.* (2000). Influence of GAA expansion size and disease duration on central nervous system impairment in Friedreich's ataxia: contribution to the understanding of the pathophysiology of the disease. *Clin. Neurophysiol.*, **111**, 1023–30.

Saraiva, J. M. and Baraitser, M. (1992). Joubert syndrome: a review. *Am. J. Med. Genet.*, **43**, 726–31.

Sasaki, K., Suga, K., Tsugawa, S. *et al.* (1996). Muscle pathology in Marinesco–Sjogren syndrome: a unique ultrastructural feature. *Brain Dev.*, **18**, 64–7.

Sato, M., Akaboshi, S., Katsumoto, T. *et al.* (1998). Accumulation of cholesterol and GM2 ganglioside in cells cultured in the presence of progesterone: an implication for the basic defect in Niemann–Pick disease type C. *Brain Dev.*, **20**, 50–2.

Sawada, H., Seriu, N., Udaka, F. *et al.* (1991). Cerebellar ataxia with glutamic aciduria. *Acta Neurol. Scand.*, **84**, 70–2.

Schols, L., Amoiridis, G., Przuntek, H. *et al.* (1997). Friedreich's ataxia. Revision of the phenotype according to molecular genetics. *Brain*, **120**, 2131–40.

Scolding, N. J., Kellar-Wood, H. F., Shaw, C. *et al.* (1996). Wolfram syndrome: hereditary diabetes mellitus with brainstem and optic atrophy. *Ann. Neurol.*, **39**, 352–60.

Senanayake, N. and de Silva, H. J. (1994). Delayed cerebellar ataxia complicating falciparum malaria: a clinical study of 74 patients. *J. Neurol.*, **241**, 456–9.

Shahzadi, S., Tasker, R. R., and Lozano, A. (1995). Thalamotomy for essential and cerebellar tremor. *Stereotact Funct Neurosurg*, **65**, 11–7.

Sheehy, M. P. and Marsden, C. D. (1982). Writer's cramp—a focal dystonia. *Brain*, **105**, 462–80.

Siebner, H. R., Berndt, S., and Conrad, B. (1996). Cerebrotendinous xanthomatosis without tendon xanthomas mimicking Marinesco–Sjoegren syndrome: a case report. *J. Neurol. Neurosurg. Psychiatry*, **60**, 582–5.

Silveira, I., Lopes-Cendes, I., Kish, S. *et al.* (1996). Frequency of spinocerebellar ataxia type 1, dentatorubropallidoluysian atrophy, and Machado–Joseph disease mutations in a large group of spinocerebellar ataxia patients. *Neurology*, **46**, 214–8.

Singer, C., Sanchez-Ramos, J., and Weiner, W. J. (1994). Gait abnormality in essential tremor. *Mov. Disord.*, **9**, 193–6.

Soland, V. L., Bhatia, K. P., Volonte, M. A. *et al.* (1996). Focal task-specific tremors. *Mov. Disord.*, 11, 665–70.

Stacy, M. and Jankovic, J. (1992). Tardive tremor. *Mov. Disord.*, 7, 53–7.

Stark, E., Wurster, U., Patzold, U. *et al.* (1995). Immunological and clinical response to immunosuppressive treatment in paraneoplastic cerebellar degeneration. *Arch. Neurol.*, 52, 814–8.

Steinhoff, B. J., Herrendorf, G., Bittermann, H. J. *et al.* (1997). Isolated ataxia as an idiosyncratic side-effect under gabapentin. *Seizure*, 6, 503–4.

Steinlin, M., Schmid, M., Landau, K. *et al.* (1997). Follow-up in children with Joubert syndrome. *Neuropediatrics*, 28, 204–11.

Steinlin, M. (1998). Non-progressive congenital ataxias. *Brain Dev.*, 20, 199–208.

Stell, R., Bronstein, A. M., Plant, G. T. *et al.* (1989). Ataxia telangiectasia: a reappraisal of the ocular motor features and their value in the diagnosis of atypical cases. *Mov. Disord.*, 4, 320–9.

Stevanin, G., Durr, A., David, G. *et al.* (1997). Clinical and molecular features of spinocerebellar ataxia type 6. *Neurology*, 49, 1243–6.

Subramony, S. H. and Filla, A. (2001). Autosomal dominant spinocerebellar ataxias ad infinitum? *Neurology*, 56, 287–89.

Trivedi, R., Mundanthanam, G., Amyes, E. *et al.* (2000). Autoantibody screening in subacute cerebellar ataxia [letter]. *Lancet*, 356, 565–6.

Trouillas, P., Serratrice, G., Laplane, D. *et al.* (1995). Levorotatory form of 5-hydroxytryptophan in Friedreich's ataxia. Results of a double-blind drug–placebo cooperative study. *Arch. Neurol.*, 52, 456–60.

Truong, D. D., Harding, A. E., Scaravilli, F. *et al.* (1990). Movement disorders in mitochondrial myopathies. A study of nine cases with two autopsy studies. *Mov. Disord.*, 5, 109–17.

Tsao, C. Y., Lo, W. D., and Craenen, J. (1992). Congestive heart failure and cardiac thrombus as first presentations of Friedreich ataxia. *Pediatr. Neurol.*, 8, 313–4.

Tsukamoto, T., Mochizuki, R., Mochizuki, H. *et al.* (1993). Paraneoplastic cerebellar degeneration and limbic encephalitis in a patient with adenocarcinoma of the colon. *J. Neurol. Neurosurg. Psychiatry*, 56, 713–6.

Tuchman, M., Knopman, D. S., and Shih, V. E. (1990). Episodic hyperammonemia in adult siblings with hyperornithinemia, hyperammonemia, and homocitrullinuria syndrome. *Arch. Neurol.*, 47, 1134–7.

Tuite, P. J., Rogaeva, E. A., St George-Hyslop, P. H. *et al.* (1995). Dopa-responsive parkinsonism phenotype of Machado–Joseph disease: confirmation of 14q CAG expansion. *Ann. Neurol.*, 38, 684–7.

Uhrhammer, N., Bay, J. O., and Bignon, Y. J. (1998). Seventh International Workshop on Ataxia-Telangiectasia. *Cancer Res.*, 58, 3480–5.

Usuki, F., Maruyama, K. (2000). Ataxia caused by mutations in the alpha-tocopherol transfer protein gene. *J. Neurol. Neurosurg. Psychiat.*, 69, 254–6.

Vaamonde, J., Muruzabal, J., Tunon, T. *et al.* (1992). Abnormal muscle and skin mitochondria in family with myoclonus, ataxia, and deafness (May and White syndrome). *J. Neurol. Neurosurg. Psychiatry*, 55, 128–32.

Vahedi, K., Joutel, A., and Van Bogaert, P. E. A. (1995). A gene for hereditary paroxysmal ataxia maps to chromosome 19p. *Ann. Neurol.*, 37, 289–93.

van de Vlasakker, C., Gabreels, F., Wijburg, H. *et al.* (1994). Clinical features of Niemann-Pick disease type C. An example of the delayed onset, slowly progressive phenotype and an overview of recent literature. *Clin. Neurol. Neurosurg.*, 96, 119–23.

Vandel, P., Bonin, B., Leveque, E. *et al.* (1997). Tricyclic antidepressant-induced extrapyramidal side effects. *Eur. Neuropsychopharmacol.*, 7, 207–12.

Verhagen, W. I., Huygen, P. L., and Arts, W. F. (1996). Multi-system signs and symptoms in X-linked ataxia carriers. *J. Neurol. Sci.*, 140, 85–90.

Verrips, A., Hoefsloot, L., Steenbergen, G. *et al.* (2000). Clinical and molecular genetic characteristics of patients with cerebrotendinous xanthomatosis. *Brain*, 123, 908–19.

Vincent, J., Neves-Pereira, M., Paterson, A. *et al.* (2000). An unstable trinucleotide repeat region on chromosome 13 implicated in spinocerebellar ataxia: a common expansion locus. *Am. J. Hum. Genet.*, 66, 819–29.

Vorgerd, M., Schols, L., Hardt, C., *et al.* (2000). Mitochondrial impairment of human muscle in Friedreich ataxia in vivo. *Neuromuscul. Disord.*, 10, 430–5.

Wang, J., Hegele, R. (2000). Microsomal triglyceride transfer protein (MTP) gene mutations in Canadian subjects with abetalipoproteinemia. *Hum. Mutat. Online*, 15, 294–5.

Warner, T., Lennox, G., Janota, I. *et al.* (1994). Autosomal dominant dentatorubropallidoluysian atrophy in the United Kingdom. *Mov. Disord.*, 9, 289–96.

Warner, T. T., Williams, L. D., Walker, R. W. *et al.* (1995). A clinical and molecular genetic study of dentatorubropallidoluysian atrophy in four European families. *Ann. Neurol.*, 37, 452–9.

Wessel, K., Hermsdorfer, J., Deger, K. *et al.* (1995). Double-blind crossover study with levorotatory form of hydroxytryptophan in patients with degenerative cerebellar diseases. *Arch. Neurol.*, 52, 451–5.

Wetterau, J. R., Aggerbeck, L. P., Bouma, M. E. *et al.* (1992). Absence of microsomal triglyceride transfer protein in individuals with abetalipoproteinemia. *Science*, 258, 999–1001.

Wills, A. J., Thompson, P. D., Findley, L. J. *et al.* (1996). A positron emission tomography study of primary orthostatic tremor. *Neurology*, **46**, 747–52.

Wills, A., Brusa, L., Wang, H. *et al.* (1999). Levodopa may improve orthostatic tremor: case report and trial of treatment. *J. Neurol. Neurosurg. Psychiat.*, **66**, 681–4.

Wilson, R. B., Lynch, D. R., and Fischbeck, K. H. (1998). Normal serum iron and ferritin concentrations in patients with Friedreich's ataxia. *Ann. Neurol.*, **44**, 132–4.

Wittkamper, A., Wessel, K., and Bruckmann, H. (1993). CT in autosomal dominant and idiopathic cerebellar ataxia. *Neuroradiology*, **35**, 520–4.

Worth, P. F., Giunti, P., Gardner-Thorpe, C. *et al.* (1999). Autosomal dominant cerebellar ataxia type III: linkage in a large British family to a 7.6-cM region on chromosome 15q14–21.3. *Am. J. Hum. Genet.*, **65**, 420–6.

Wright, J., Teraoka, S., Onengut, S. *et al.* (1996). A high frequency of distinct ATM gene mutations in ataxia-telangiectasia. *Am. J. Hum. Genet.*, **59**, 839–46.

Yamashita, I., Sasaki, H., Yabe, I. *et al.* (2000). A novel locus for dominant cerebellar ataxia (SCA14) maps to a 10.2-cM interval flanked by D19S206 and D19S605 on chromosome 19q13.4-qter. *Ann. Neurol.*, **48**, 156–63.

Yokota, T., Shiojiri, T., Gotoda, T. *et al.* (1997). Friedreich-like ataxia with retinitis pigmentosa caused by the His101Gln mutation of the alpha-tocopherol transfer protein gene. *Ann. Neurol.*, **41**, 826–32.

Young, G. B., Oppenheimer, S. R., Gordon, B. A. *et al.* (1994). Ataxia in institutionalized patients with epilepsy. *Can. J. Neurol. Sci.*, **21**, 252–8.

Zeidler, M., Stewart, G. E., Barraclough, C. R. *et al.* (1997). New variant Creutzfeldt–Jakob disease: neurological features and diagnostic tests. *Lancet*, **350**, 903–7.

Zeviani, M. and Taroni, F. (1994). Mitochondrial diseases. *Baillieres Clin. Neurol.*, **3**, 315–34.

Zhuchenko, O., Bailey, J., Bonnen, P. *et al.* (1997). Autosomal dominant cerebellar ataxia (SCA6) associated with small polyglutamine expansions in the alpha 1A-voltage-dependent calcium channel. *Nat. Genet.*, **15**, 62–9.

Zimmer, C., Gosztonyi, G., Cervos-Navarro, J. *et al.* (1992). Neuropathy with lysosomal changes in Marinesco–Sjogren syndrome: fine structural findings in skeletal muscle and conjunctiva. *Neuropediatrics*, **23**, 329–35.

Zu, L., Figueroa, K. P., Grewal, R., and Pulst, S. M. (1999). Mapping of a new spinocerebellar ataxia to chromosome 22. *Am. J. Hum. Genet.*, **64**, 594–9.

CHAPTER 32

Movement disorders

Nicholas Fletcher

32.1 Introduction to movement disorders and the motor system

32.1.1 The clinical approach to a patient with a movement disorder

Almost any neurological disorder can produce a disorder of movement but the 'movement disorders' include the akinetic rigid syndromes, hyperkinesias, and some tremors (Table 32.1). It can sometimes seem, especially with the widespread use of videotape recordings, that diagnosis of movement disorders is mainly a matter of correct visual recognition. Such an approach is not recommended and can lead to mistakes unless, as in other areas of medicine, the history is considered first and the physical signs second. Obvious examples include the family history in Huntington's disease, developmental history in dystonic cerebral palsy, and neuroleptic drug treatment in patients with tardive dyskinesia. In addition, a single disorder may give rise to several different types of involuntary movement. For example, Huntington's disease may give rise to an akinetic rigid state, chorea, myoclonus, tics, or dystonia. Patients with Parkinson's disease taking levodopa may show different types of movement disorder at different times of the day.

In akinetic rigid states the diagnostic issue will be whether the patient has idiopathic Parkinson's disease or one of the other Parkinsonian syndromes. With involuntary movements, the first step in diagnosis is to classify these as dystonia, tics,

Table 32.1. Types of movement disorder

Effect on movement	Movement disorder	Aetiology
Hypokinesia	Akinetic rigid syndromes	Parkinson's disease Other Parkinsonian disorders
Hyperkinesia	Dystonia	Idiopathic torsion dystonia Other forms of hereditary dystonia Secondary dystonia
	Chorea	Huntington's disease Other causes of chorea
	Tics	Tourette's syndrome Other causes of tics
	Myoclonus	Cortical myoclonus Brainstem myoclonus Spinal myoclonus Other forms of myoclonus
	Tremor	Parkinsonian tremor Benign essential tremor Cerebellar tremor Other tremors

tremor, chorea, or myoclonus (Table 32.1). It must be remembered that involuntary movements are merely physical signs, not diagnostic entities, and that they do not always occur in a pure form; for example, patients with dystonia may have additional choreiform movements or tremor. If more than one form of abnormal movement seems to be present, the diagnosis should be based on the most obvious one. The next step is to decide on the cause of the movements and this stage the diagnosis must be based upon an accurate and complete history as noted above.

The movement disorders are often associated with abnormalities of the basal ganglia and, to some extent, vice versa. This is not entirely correct. Disturbances of basal ganglia function certainly have profound effects on movement with the development of bradykinesia, rigidity, tremor, or the various forms of dyskinesia. However, it is not correct when considering the pathophysiology of movement disorders to regard the basal ganglia as an isolated movement control centre. In fact, they are an important but poorly understood component of a much wider motor system. It is also important to remember that the basal ganglia are involved in the processing of limbic and other cognitive processes which may also be disturbed by basal ganglia dysfunction.

32.1.2 A brief overview of the motor system

The spinal cord anterior horn cells are influenced by descending pathways from the cerebral cortex and from brainstem centres. These motor cortical and brainstem outflow areas are regulated by other cortical areas, the basal ganglia and cerebellum. The basal ganglia and the cerebellum are both characterized by parallel processing of inputs from cortical areas and subsequent projection back to cortex via thalamic relay nuclei (Alexander 1997).

Motor cortex

There are several motor cortical areas in the human; these are classified and numbered in a variety of ways but may be classified simply as the primary motor cortex, lateral pre-motor cortex, supplementary motor area (SMA), and motor regions of the cingulate cortex (Dum and Strick 1991).

♦ The primary motor cortex (Brodmann's area 4) pyramidal cells are the principal source of the pyramidal tract but also project to other motor cortical areas and to sensory cortex, the thalamus, the basal ganglia (corpus striatum), the red nucleus, brainstem reticular nuclei, and the cerebellum (via the corticopontine fibres and pontine nuclei). The primary motor cortex shows a somatotopic organization (Lemon 1988) but pyramidal cells may activate more than one muscle and a muscle may be affected by pyramidal cells spread over a wide cortical area. Primary motor cortex cells are activated prior to and during voluntary contralateral movement, as shown by functional imaging and neurophysiological event-related recordings. Lesions of the primary motor cortex are associated principally with deficits of small accurate finger

and hand movements. Such movements require motor cortex outputs not only to agonist muscle spinal motor neurons but also those needed to regulate the activity of antagonists and muscles needed to stabilize proximal joints.

♦ The lateral pre-motor cortex (the lateral part of Brodmann's area 6) is located on the lateral aspect of the frontal lobe, anterior to the primary motor cortex. There are two discreet motor areas (superior and inferior) within the lateral pre-motor cortex with separate motor cortical maps and corticospinal projections. There is a considerable output from the lateral pre-motor cortex to the medial brainstem tegmentum which projects to the spinal cord in the ventromedial descending system (see below). The pre-motor cortex is important for the control of axial and proximal limb movements and also for the control of movements in response to external cues or instructions. The activation of the lateral pre-motor cortex begins prior to the execution of movement, suggesting an important role in preparation for movement, and may be bilateral (Remy et al. 1994). Lesions of the lateral pre-motor area produce proximal limb weakness and impairment of movements requiring use of the whole arm and hand. There is also impaired learning of motor responses to external cues.

♦ The SMA (medial part of Brodmann's area 6) is on the inner aspect of the frontal lobe, anterior to area 4 and continuous with the lateral pre-motor cortex. The SMA receives considerable basal ganglia inputs and has outputs to the primary motor cortex, corticospinal tract, basal ganglia, cerebellum, red nucleus, and reticular formation. Like the lateral pre-motor cortex, the SMA seems to be important for the preparation of movements, particularly internally generated, learned, sequential, or bimanual movements (Passingham 1987; Rothwell 1994). Blood flow experiments indicate that activation of SMA prior to movement may be bilateral (Remy et al. 1994). SMA lesions lead to difficulty initiating speech and movement, impaired bimanual co-ordination, and the 'alien limb' phenomenon where the arm moves spontaneously in response to external stimuli, grasping at objects spontaneously. This may represent a dissociation of externally (lateral pre-motor cortex) and internally (SMA) cued movement.

♦ Cingulate motor areas have been identified in humans and non-human primates (Rothwell 1994; Alexander 1997). They have outputs to spinal cord and the basal ganglia and receive inputs from frontal pre-motor cortex. Cingulate motor neurons are active in internally generated movements and cingulate activation is seen mainly with complex motor tasks. Stimulation of cingulate cortex produces complex motor activity.

Movement-related cortical potentials

Surface scalp recordings in man have revealed bilateral activation of frontal motor cortex beginning about 1.5 s before movement onset. This early phase, the pre-movement or bereitschaftspotential arises from primary motor cortex and the SMA. Following the pre-movement potential, about 500 ms before the movement, a second potential, the negative slope, is detected. This is also bilateral and arises in the SMA and the contralateral primary motor cortex. In the 50–100 ms before movement, a movement potential (MP) occurs and arises from contralateral primary motor cortex (Neshige *et al.* 1988).

The descending pathways

The descending pathways are grouped into two divisions within the spinal cord. A dorso-lateral group contains the lateral corticospinal tract along with the rubrospinal tract and the crossed reticulospinal tract (from the lateral pontine tegmentum). These dorso-lateral pathways are concerned with distal movements. The ventro-lateral group is made up of the ventral corticospinal tract with the interstitiospinal, vestibulospinal, and reticulospinal (from medial pontine and medullary tegmentum) tracts and is involved in the control of proximal movements (Rothwell 1994; Alexander 1997).

The pyramidal tract comprises the corticobulbar and corticospinal tracts and in the human, the latter component contains about one million fibres on each side. About 60 per cent of the fibres in the corticospinal tract originate in the frontal motor areas. The remainder are from parietal and somatosensory cortex. The corticospinal tract influences spinal afferent pathways, inhibitory interneurons, and gamma efferent cells as well as the alpha motor neurons. There is considerable convergence and divergence within the corticospinal tract; cortical pyramidal cells project to several muscles and each muscle can be activated by cells from a large cortical motor field. Direct synapses with alpha motor neurons are particularly dense on cells concerned with finger movements and there is a close association between the corticospinal tract and the execution of fine finger movements. Lesions of the pyramidal tract tend to produce impaired manual dexterity with variable degrees of weakness.

Other descending pathways are poorly understood in man. The reticulospinal pathway appears to be important in the startle reflex (Brown *et al.* 1991*a*). Vestibulospinal pathways are concerned in part with postural control.

The regulation and co-ordination of movement; the cerebellum and basal ganglia

Neither the cerebellum nor the basal ganglia have direct efferent connections to the spinal motor apparatus and yet both are clearly involved in the correct execution and control of movement. This has long been evident from clinicopathological studies of patients with lesions of these structures. Such patients exhibit profound disturbances of movement as their primary symptoms. Anatomically, both structures are characterized by extensive inputs from the cerebral cortex, parallel internal circuitry, and projections back to the cortex via thalamic relay nuclei. Despite much information about the anatomy and cellular neurophysiology of the cerebellum and basal ganglia, their precise functions are not clear.

The cerebellum

The cerebellum is made up of two hemispheres separated by a midline vermis. There are three lobes, the anterior, posterior, and the flocculonodular lobe. There are three deeply situated outflow nuclei in each hemisphere, the fastigial nucleus medially, the interposed (made up of globose and emboliform), and the dentate nucleus laterally. The majority of cerebellar efferents leave via the superior peduncle. The inferior and middle peduncles are largely composed of afferent fibres from the spinal cord and brainstem nuclei. Within the cerebellum there are three phylogenetic regions:

1. The neocerebellum (pontocerebellum) includes the bulk of the cerebellar hemispheres and the central portion of the vermis. It receives the bulk of the pontine inputs via the middle peduncle. The neocerebellum is principally concerned with the co-ordination of the ipsilateral limbs.

2. The paleocerebellum (spinocerebellum) consists of the parafloccular lobes and the remainder of the vermis of the anterior and posterior lobes. It receives direct inputs from the spinal cord via the inferior peduncle and is probably concerned with the regulation of muscle tone.

3. The archicerebellum (vestibulocerebellum) is composed of the flocculonodular lobe only and receives direct vestibular inputs via the inferior peduncle.

In fact, there is considerable overlap in the connections of these three regions and their separation on the basis of their inputs is only approximate. The cerebellum may also be subdivided on the basis of outflow projections. The lateral mass of each hemisphere projects to the dentate nucleus, the vermis projects mainly to the fastigial nucleus and an intermediate zone sends fibres to the interposed nucleus. The flocculonodular lobe, vermis, and certain hemisphere areas also project to the vestibular nuclei. Another interesting feature of cerebellar organization concerns sagittal strips of cortex which share inputs from the same regions of the olivary nuclei.

Afferents

All cerebellar afferents terminate in both the cortex and the cerebellar nuclei. The cerebellar afferent systems are as follows (Brodal 1981; Ito 1984):

♦ The vast majority of cerebellar afferents are from the pontine nuclei, through the middle peduncle. These nuclei relay cortical inputs to the cerebellum from the ipsilateral frontal and parietal lobes. These are not collaterals of motor corticospinal fibres. The pontocerebellar projection is to most areas of the contralateral cerebellum and the interposed and dentate nuclei. Pontocerebellar afferents form mossy fibres within the cerebellum, synapsing in the granule cell layer of the cerebellar cortex and in the cerebellar nuclei.

♦ Direct spinocerebellar input is via the inferior peduncle along with afferents from the vestibular and brainstem reticular nuclei. These also enter the cerebellum as mossy fibres.

◆ The inferior olivary nucleus receives inputs from the spinal cord, cerebral motor cortex, and brainstem. It sends climbing fibres directly to cerebellar Purkinje cells and the cerebellar nuclei.

◆ Direct aminergic inputs arise from the locus coeruleus (noradrenergic), raphe nuclei (5HT), and midbrain ventral tegmentum (dopaminergic). These project directly to Purkinje cells (Ito 1984).

Cerebellar cortex

There is a complex somatotopic representation in the cerebellar cortex which can only be detected in anaesthetized animals. There appear to be two maps, one in the anterior lobe and one in the posterior lobe. Midline structures are represented in the vermis and limbs laterally in the hemispheres.

The circuitry of the cerebellar cortex is located in three cortical layers; the superficial molecular layer, the Purkinje cell layer, and a deep granule cell layer. Afferents arrive as either mossy or climbing fibres (except for the small number of aminergic afferents) and all efferents are Purkinje cell axons which terminate in the cerebellar or vestibular nuclei. There is some evidence that the firing characteristics of the Purkinje cells are altered by the pattern of climbing and parallel fibre activation, and that this may form the basis of cerebellar learning (Ito 1984).

Efferents

The Purkinje cells are the only efferent cells of the cerebellum and they project to the cerebellar and vestibular nuclei; they are inhibitory. The fastigial nucleus, the main outflow of the medial cerebellar structures, projects mainly to the vestibular nuclei, brainstem reticular formation, and the spinal cord. The interposed and dentate nuclei relay efferents from more lateral cerebellar structures to the contralateral red nucleus and thalamus via the superior peduncle. These axons also have descending branches to the lower brainstem reticular formation. In the thalamus, cerebellar efferents reach the VL and VPL nuclei which then project to the primary motor cortex (area 4). Thalamic nucleus X also receives cerebellar efferents and projects to the lateral pre-motor cortex (area 6). Although cerebellar projections via the thalamus reach a wide area of cerebral cortex, the bulk of the output is to frontal motor cortex (Rothwell 1994).

Cerebellar function

The cerebellum receives inputs from the cerebral cortex and also from the spinal cord and vestibular system via the mossy and climbing systems, respectively. This may enable a comparison of the motor command and the actual movement of the body, allowing correction and adjustment of the movement. The cerebellum is also involved in the correct planning of movement. Activation of lateral cerebellar cortical neurons occurs before movement, suggesting that cerebellar input to the frontal motor cortex is an important part of preparation for movement. There is evidence that the cerebellum is involved in the correct timing and force of the agonist and antagonist activation during movement; cerebellar dysfunction leads to delayed and prolonged agonist bursts and delayed antagonist activation, leading to dysmetria and dysdiadochokinesis. The cerebellum is also thought to be involved in the learning of motor tasks (Rothwell 1994).

There are three main theories of cerebellar function in relation to movement (Johnson and Montgomery 1997).

A. A feedback control of the ongoing movement. This assumes continuous monitoring of afferent signals from the periphery by the cerebellum. This allows a continuous correction of the motor cortex activity by the cerebellar outflow (feedback mechanism).

B. A centre for the generation of precise motor plans concerning the timing and amplitude of movements which are then sent to the frontal motor cortex for execution (feedforward mechanism).

C. The efference copy theory integrates feedback and feedforward models and assumes that the cerebellum receives a copy of the movement command from the cerebral cortex and compares it to current and ongoing afferent signals from the periphery. The motor command is then adjusted and refined by the cerebellum to allow for the position and motion of the body prior to movement onset and during the execution of the movement itself.

32.2 The basal ganglia

The basal ganglia are thought to be important for motor control because of their anatomical connections, the neurophysiological properties of their neurons, and the effects of anatomical lesions and alterations in basal ganglia neurotransmitter function on movement. The basal ganglia are made up of the putamen and caudate nucleus (neostriatum), the globus pallidus (paleostriatum), the substantia nigra, and the subthalamic nucleus (STN). The inclusion of other nuclear structures such as the nucleus accumbens and parts of the olfactory tubercle (the ventral striatum) has been emphasized recently.

32.2.1 Anatomy and physiology

The putamen, globus pallidus, and caudate nucleus are large masses of grey matter lateral to the thalamus and separated from it by the internal capsule; anteriorly the internal capsule also separates the putamen from the head of the caudate nucleus (Fig. 32.1). The putamen lies lateral to the globus pallidus and these together form the lentiform nucleus with the head of the caudate nucleus lying anteriorly and the body curving over superiorly and then posteriorly in the floor of the lateral ventricle. The subthalamic nucleus and substantia nigra lie inferiorly and caudally in the diencephalon and rostral midbrain, respectively.

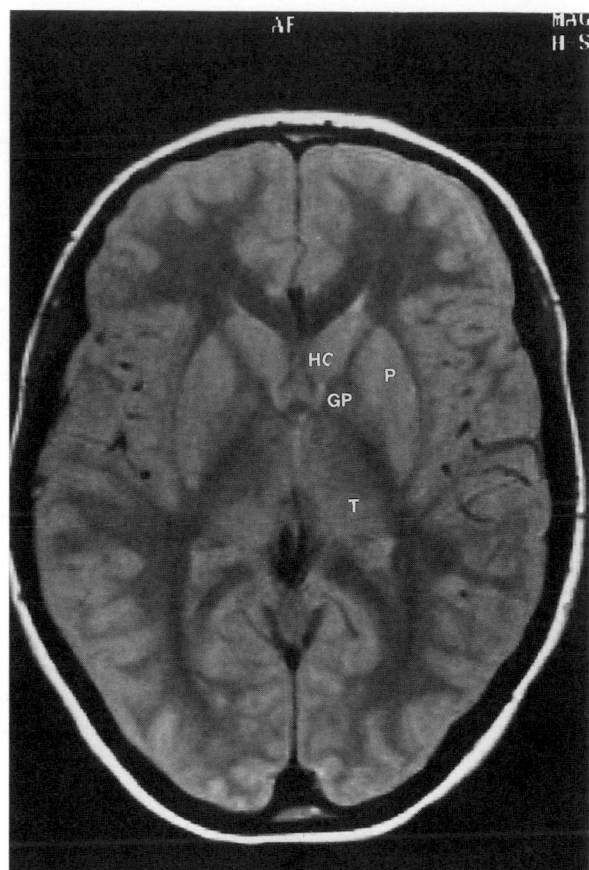

Fig. 32.1. MR brian scan showing the anatomy of the basal ganglia. The head of the caudate nucleus (HC), putamen (P), globus pallidus (GP) and thalamus (T) are indicated.

The striatum takes its name from the histological appearance caused by efferent myelinated fibres (Wilson's pencils) traversing the putamen and caudate. The globus pallidus is subdivided into external (GPe) and internal (GPi) regions which have different connections. The substantia nigra is also divided into a dorsal pars compacta (SNpc) and a ventral pars reticulata (SNpr); the latter is homologous to the GPi.

Connections and functional loops

The striatum is the input region of the basal ganglia and receives excitatory corticostriatal fibres from all areas of the cerebral cortex but mainly the motor and somatosensory areas, prefrontal, and limbic cortex; it also receives the dopaminergic nigrostratal projection. There are two pathways from the striatum to the GPi, the source of the basal ganglia output; a direct pathway and an indirect circuit via Gpe and the STN (Fig. 32.2). The basal ganglia output from GPi (and also SNpr) is inhibitory and is mainly to the thalamus; there is a smaller output to the superior colliculus and the pedunculopontine nucleus. The thalamic output is excitatory and is thought to 'drive' the motor cortical outflow. The input–output connections of the basal ganglia therefore form a loop from cortex to basal ganglia and back to cortex. Several separate and parallel

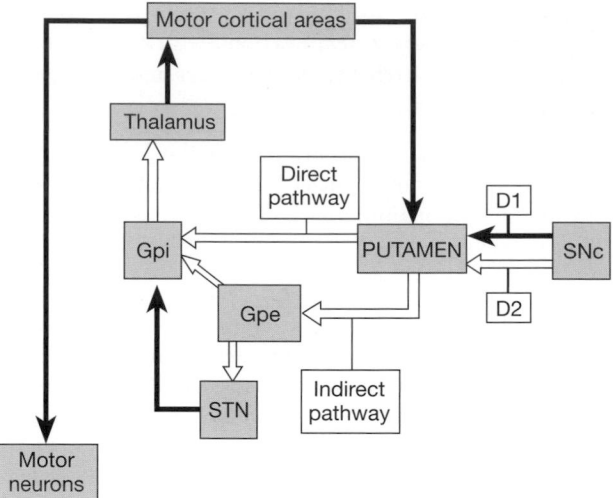

Fig. 32.2. The connections of the basal ganglia showing the direct and indirect pathways. Open arrows are inhibitory, filled are excitatory. For abbreviations see text.

loops through the basal ganglia have been identified (motor, oculomotor, limbic, and prefrontal) depending on the cortical component of the circuit. Different areas of the striatum are involved with different loops (Fig. 32.3); for the motor loop the putamen is the striatal component. Within the striatum there are groups of cells which are more densely packed and contain more substance P, met-enkephalin and opiate receptors but less acetylcholinesterase. These areas 'striosomes' appear to be involved in the processing of the limbic and prefrontal inputs and are seen mainly in the caudate rather than the putamen. The patches also receive most of the dopaminergic afferents from the SNc.

Within the motor loop there are smaller but still separate loops related to different body regions. There is therefore considerable somatotopy within the putamen corresponding to the

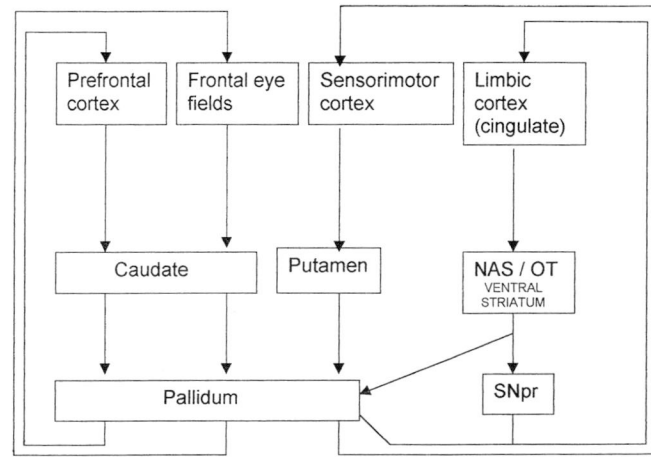

Fig. 32.3. Parallel loop circuits in the basal ganglia. NAS = nucleus accumbens septi; OT = olfactory tubercle; SNpr = substantia nigra pars reticulata

routes of the various parts of the motor loop. Neurophysiological studies indicate that the various loops remain separate during their course through the basal ganglia although the anatomical studies suggest otherwise. The dendritic trees of pallidal neurons are very large, suggesting considerable potential for functional convergence. Moreover, the numbers of neurons within different basal ganglia regions also suggests convergence of 5000 : 1 from cortex to striatum; from striatum to pallidum the ratios are 300 : 1 and 100 : 1 to Gpe and Gpi, respectively (Alexander 1997). Nevertheless there appears to be very little if any functional convergence within the basal ganglia.

With regard to the functions of the direct and indirect pathways from putamen to GPi within the motor loop, it can be seen from Fig. 32.2 that increased activity in the direct pathway will inhibit basal ganglia outflow and therefore increase motor cortex activation whereas indirect pathway activity increases STN activity and therefore GPi outflow with an opposite effect on motor cortex activity.

Transmitters

The corticostriatal projection is excitatory and glutamatergic and these fibres synapse on the GABA containing medium spiny neurons (MSNs) which are the major cell type in the striatum; the remainder are mainly the large aspiny neurons which are cholinergic and inhibitory to the MSNs. The projection from the putamen to the globus pallidus via the direct or indirect pathways is from the inhibitory MSNs which all utilize GABA; the direct pathway MSNs also contain dynorphin and substance P while the indirect MSNs which project initially to the GPe utilize enkephalin as a co-transmitter. All other circuits within the basal ganglia (see Fig. 32.2) are inhibitory (utilizing GABA) with the exception of the glutamatergic subthalamic input to the Gpi which is excitatory.

Dopamine

The role of the dopaminergic nigrostriatal projection is complex. This pathway arises in the SNpc and projects to the striatal MSNs. Dopamine is inhibitory to the indirect pathway MSNs and excitatory to the direct pathway striatal neurons. The effect of dopaminergic input to the striatum is therefore to reduce the inhibitory GPi outflow to the thalamus, thereby releasing the excitatory thalamocortical projection to the motor cortical areas. This differential effect of dopamine on striatal MSNs is mediated via two distinct classes of dopamine receptors, D_1-like (D_1 and D_5) and D_2-like (D_2, D_3, D_4). In the striatum, most receptors are either D_1 or D_2; D_4 may be involved in limbic functions (Van Tol *et al.* 1991). D_1 receptor stimulation leads to activation of adenyl cyclase and excites the direct pathway striatopallidal cells. D_2 receptor binding inhibits adenyl cyclase and suppresses the indirect pathway striatal cells. The effect of dopamine on the basal ganglia is therefore to increase the direct pathway activity and suppress the indirect pathway, thereby facilitating movement (Fig. 32.2). There are some difficulties with this model, which is probably an over-

simplification. In particular, D_1 and D_2 receptor stimulation is synergistic, each potentiating the effects of the other (Carlson *et al.* 1987). There are also D_2 receptors on the presynaptic terminals of the nigrostriatal cells; stimulation of these receptors inhibits dopamine synthesis and release. This is clinically important in terms of the worsening of parkinsonism seen with low brain concentrations of levodopa or dopamine agonists which preferentially activate presynaptic D_2 autoreceptors (Merello and Lees 1992).

Acetylcholine

The role of acetylcholine in the basal ganglia is complex and uncertain. Both nicotinic and muscarinic receptors exist in the brain; the role of nicotinic receptors is unclear but all five (M_1–M_5) muscarinic receptor types are found in the basal ganglia. It is likely that acetylcholine has a differential action on the direct and indirect pathways and interacts with dopaminergic activity. D_1 and D_2 receptor activation is followed by striatal acetylcholine release increasing or decreasing, respectively. Anticholinergic drugs acting at muscarinic receptors are effective in several movement disorders especially dystonia and parkinsonism. The mechanism of such clinical effects is unclear but must involve some degree of local basal ganglia cholinergic overactivity.

32.2.2 Pathophysiology of basal ganglia disorders

Parkinsonism

Loss of dopaminergic input to the striatum follows destruction of the SNpc. The pathophysiological consequences have been studied in the MPTP treated primate model of parkinsonism (DeLong 1990). As the normal effect of dopamine is to activate

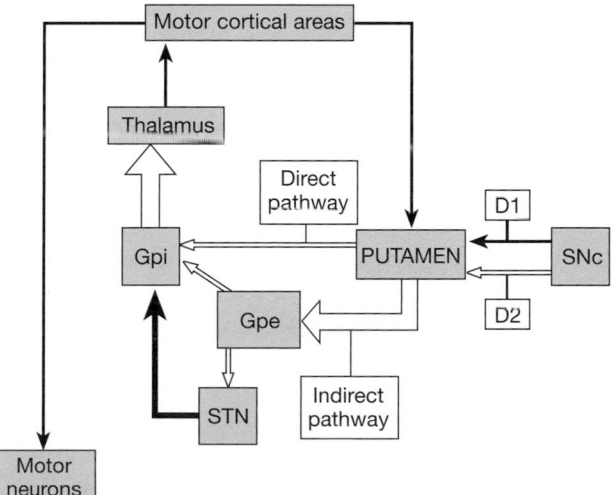

Fig. 32.4. The basal ganglia in Parkinson's disease. The width of the arrow indicates the activity of the relevant pathway. Open arrows are inhibitory, filed are excitatory. For abbreviations see text.

the direct basal ganglia circuit and suppress the indirect pathway, the opposite effect follows striatal dopamine loss (Fig. 32.4). The same result may be produced by pharmacological depletion of brain dopamine or blockade of dopamine receptors. The effect of reduced direct and increased indirect pathway activity is to increase tonic activity in STN and GPi. This inhibits the thalamocortical neurons therefore suppressing motor cortex activity. This in turn leads to akinesia, bradykinesia, and rigidity due to abnormal pre-motor and motor cortex activation. Surface recordings of movement-related cortical potentials and cerebral blood flow studies in Parkinsonian patients tend to support this concept. In addition to altered tonic activity of STN and GPi neurons, the responses of these cells to peripheral movement are also altered, leading to abnormal feedback to the motor and pre-motor cortex. This leads to abnormal preparation and initiation of movement with small initial agonist bursts and prolonged movement times. The rigidity of Parkinson's disease is associated with abnormally increased long latency stretch reflexes, probably due to abnormal central processing of peripheral inputs. The exact mechanism by which the abnormalities of basal ganglia and motor cortex function are translated into bradykinesia and rigidity is poorly understood.

Parkinsonian tremor is more difficult to explain. Intracerebral recordings in animal models and Parkinsonian patients have detected groups of neurons firing in bursts at the same frequency as the rest tremor in the thalamic ventralis intermedius nucleus and motor cortex and lesions of these areas abolish the tremor. This has been documented in Parkinsonian patients after stereotactic thalamic lesions or strokes involving the motor cortex or internal capsule. In animal models however, a rest tremor cannot be produced by a pure nigrostriatal lesion; a midbrain lesion involving nigrostriatal and cerebellothalamic pathways is required. Although a 4–6 Hz rest tremor is a feature of Parkinson's disease, it cannot be assumed that this is the result of damage to the nigrostriatal tract because other brain regions are affected by Parkinson's disease. Moreover, abnormal nigrostriatal function as measured by flurodopa PET correlates reasonably with akinesia and rigidity but not with the severity of tremor (Otsuka *et al.* 1996), and suppression of Parkinsonian tremor is associated with reduced cerebellar activity (Deiber *et al.* 1993). Accordingly, it is not clear whether the thalamocortical oscillations underlying resting tremor are due to thalamic, cerebellar, or basal ganglia abnormalities. Probably all are involved and it may be unrealistic to expect to localize a single tremor generating site. It is likely that the basal ganglia are involved because of the reduction in tremor seen after surgical lesions of the basal ganglia outflow pathways although this is not as impressive as that seen after thalamic lesions (Obeso *et al.* 1997). In addition, basal ganglia pallidal and STN neurons may show rhythmic oscillatory activity in animals and Parkinsonian patients (Wichmann and DeLong 1997).

Ballism

Hemiballismus is closely associated with lesions of the subthalamic nucleus, usually vascular (Lee and Marsden 1994*a*;

Vidakovic *et al.* 1994). This interrupts the indirect pathway so that the GPi is influenced only by the direct inhibitory striatopallidal pathway. Reduced Gpi outflow releases the excitatory thalamocortical projection with increased motor cortical activity and involuntary movement.

Chorea

In Huntington's disease, degeneration of the striatal MSNs will lead to chorea if the source of the indirect GABA/enkephalin pathway is principally affected (Crossman *et al.* 1988). This leads to reduced GPi output and thalamocortical hyperactivity as in hemiballismus. If the direct pathway GABA/substance P containing MSNs are involved later (or in some cases earlier), akinesia and rigidity are observed (Wichmann and DeLong 1997).

Dystonia

Although dystonia is commonly associated with basal ganglia lesions, the underlying mechanism is more difficult to explain on the basis of disordered basal ganglia circuitry. Dystonia is closely associated with putaminal or thalamic lesions (Bhatia and Marsden 1994; Kostic *et al.* 1996; Lehericy *et al.* 1996) but in some patients there are focal abnormalities in the brainstem (Gibb *et al.* 1988; Kulisevsky *et al.* 1988; Zweig *et al.* 1988; Esteban Munoz *et al.* 1996), cerebellum, spinal cord (Cammarota *et al.* 1995), or peripheral nerves. The mechanism by which dystonia occurs is poorly understood, with various levels of the CNS implicated. There is increased excitability of the motor cortex detectable with transcranial magnetic stimulation studies (Ridding *et al.* 1995; Ikoma *et al.* 1996) and PET functional imaging (Eidelberg *et al.* 1995). MRCPs recorded over the pre-motor areas are reduced, suggesting abnormal motor programming, possibly secondary to abnormal basal ganglia output (Deuschl *et al.* 1995; Kaji *et al.* 1995; Van der Kamp *et al.* 1995). Abnormal basal ganglia function has been difficult to detect but a PET study showed metabolic overactivity of the lentiform nucleus, probably due to overactivity of the direct putamenopallidal inhibitory pathway (Eidelberg *et al.* 1995). There is also evidence of increased interneuronal excitability in the brainstem of patients with cranial dystonia (Tolosa *et al.* 1988) and reduced reciprocal inhibition at spinal cord level, reflecting impaired spinal inhibitory circuitry (Marsden and Rothwell 1987). How these abnormalities could be secondary to a primary basal ganglia malfunction is unclear. There is even evidence of abnormal sensory processing in dystonia; vibration applied to an affected limb will activate dystonic postures and this effect can be abolished by intramuscular lignocaine. This must be due to abnormal central processing of Ia muscle spindle afferent inputs. It is possible that this explains the reduction of dystonia by so-called 'sensory tricks' (Section 32.4.1).

32.2.3 Neurosurgical interventions in basal ganglia disorders

It can be seen from Fig. 32.2 that there are several points at which the internal circuitry of the basal ganglia may be altered by surgical lesions. The most commonly used are the globus pallidus and the thalamus but there is increasing interest in the subthalamic nucleus as a surgical target. The main indications for neurosurgical treatment of movement disorders are in Parkinson's disease, dystonia, and tremor. Localized neuronal inactivation may be produced by a destructive electrolytic lesion or implantation of a deep brain neurostimulation electrode.

Parkinson's disease

Parkinson's disease is associated with increased neuronal firing in the STN and GPi. Tremor-related firing patterns are present in thalamic cells as well as the STN and GPi. As might be predicted from these observations, lesions of the GPi (pallidotomy), STN (subthalamotomy or subthalamic stimulation), or thalamus (thalamotomy) all produce useful improvement in Parkinsonian patients (Obeso *et al.* 1997). The relative merits of these procedures, which are shown in Fig. 32.5, in different types of patients are currently under evaluation but it appears that the main value of thalamotomy is in the suppression of medically intractable Parkinsonian tremor and pallidotomy is of greater value in the relief of contralateral rigidity and akinesia. Functional imaging has shown increased activity of motor cortex after pallidotomy (Grafton *et al.* 1995; Eidelberg *et al.* 1996). Some improvement is also seen in ipsilateral akinesia (Dogali *et al.* 1995; Lozano *et al.* 1995). Pallidotomy also leads to impressive suppression of contralateral levodopa-induced dyskinesia. This presumably follows reduction of abnormal pallidal outflow activity caused by alterations in the responses of striatal neurons to dopaminergic stimulation. Subthalamic stimulation (which inhibits subthalamic activity) also leads to reduced inhibitory pallidothalamic outflow and improvement of parkinsonism (Limousin *et al.* 1998). A difficulty with the currently popular direct–indirect pathway model of basal ganglia function is that a thalamic lesion should exacerbate Parkinsonian akinesia rather than lead to clinical improvement.

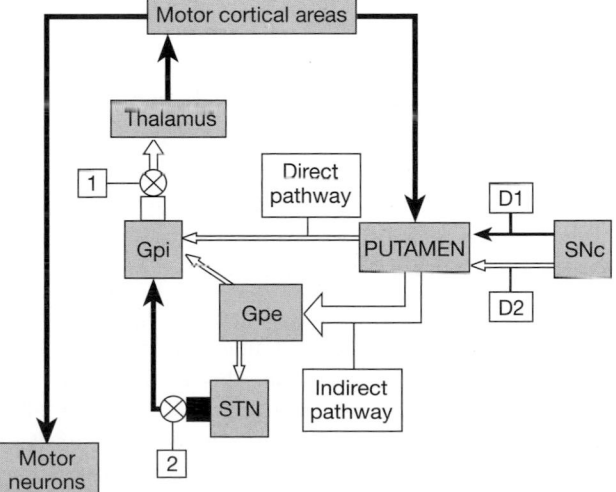

Fig. 32.5. The basal ganglia in Parkinson's disease, showing the effects of pallidal (1) and subthalamic (2) surgical intervention with correction of excessive inhibitory pallidothalamic or excitatory subthalamopallidal activity and restored motor cortical outflow.

This does not appear to be a major problem after thalamotomy leading to the suggestion that the anti-Parkinsonian effect of stereotactic surgery follows the removal of abnormal thalamocortical activity rather than merely a reduction of excessive pallidal outflow (Marsden and Obeso 1994). In fact, there is some evidence that thalamotomy does indeed reduce motor cortex activation and produces subtle impairment of finger dexterity contralaterally. This tends to be overshadowed however by the beneficial effect of tremor reduction (Boecker *et al.* 1997).

Dystonia

Although the nature of the basal ganglia dysfunction in dystonia is less well understood, alteration of the pallidothalamic outflow to the motor cortex is likely. Lesions of the motor thalamus are effective in dystonia, especially of the contralateral distal musculature (Andrew *et al.* 1983). There are few data regarding pallidotomy in dystonia but a recent report of bilateral interruption of pallidal outflow in a case of severe generalized dystonia was encouraging (Iacono *et al.* 1996). The benefits of thalamotomy or pallidal procedures in dystonia are probably due to the removal of abnormal basal ganglia output to the motor cortical areas.

32.3 The akinetic rigid disorders

In these disorders the clinical picture is one of parkinsonism with slowness of movement and muscular rigidity. Usually this clinical presentation is easily recognized but akinetic rigid states are not the only causes of slowness and diminished movements. Depression, catatonic schizophrenia (catalepsy), and frontal lobe dysfunction (abulia) may cause striking immobility. Lesions of the descending corticospinal tracts leading to pseudobulbar palsy and spastic tetraparesis may, if mild, resemble an akinetic rigid state and cause initial diagnostic confusion. Pyramidal lesions may cause only contralateral slowness of fine finger movements. Psychiatric disease, degenerative cerebral disorders, cerebrovascular disease, and motor neuron disease may, on occasions, be mistaken for parkinsonism.

Although the majority of akinetic rigid patients have idiopathic Parkinson's disease, other causes of parkinsonism must be considered before this diagnosis is made (Table 32.2). Careful enquiry must be made regarding exposure to drugs and toxins as well as a family history. The onset and subsequent progression of the condition and, crucially, the response to any dopamine replacement therapy must be reviewed in order to distinguish Parkinson's disease from other Parkinsonian disorders.

32.3.1 Parkinson's disease (paralysis agitans)

Definition

'Involuntary tremulous motion, with lessened muscular power, in parts not in action and even when supported; with a propensity to bend the trunk forward, and to pass from a walking to a running pace: the senses and intellects being uninjured.'

Table 32.2. Akinetic rigid syndromes

Parkinson's disease

Symptomatic parkinsonism	Common	Drug-induced parkinsonism
		Cerebrovascular disease
	Rare	Cerebral trauma
		Toxic parkinsonism
		Hydrocephalus
		Intracranial masses
		CJD
		Post-encephalitic parkinsonism
		Rett syndrome
		Post-anoxic parkinsonism
Other akinetic rigid syndromes		Diffuse Lewy body disease
		Multiple system atrophy
		Steele–Richardson–Olszewski disease
		Corticobasal degeneration
		Hemiparkinsonism–hemiatrophy
		Other non-Lewy body parkinsonism
Metabolic disorders		Basal ganglia calcification
		Chronic hepatocerebral degeneration
Degenerative disorders		Alzheimer's disease
		Pick's disease
		Idiopathic late onset cerebellar degenerations
Hereditary disorders		Dopa responsive dystonia
		Juvenile Huntington's disease
		Hallervorden–Spatz disease
		Hereditary cerebellar ataxias
		Wilson's disease
		X-linked dystonia–parkinsonism
		Pallidal degenerations
		Parkinsonism with hypoventilation
		Neuroacanthocytosis

James Parkinson's original description of this disorder immediately suggests one of the most distinctive conditions in medicine. Parkinson's disease is one of the most frequently encountered neurological conditions and presents an increasing challenge to the health services of developed nations with ageing populations. Clinically, Parkinson's disease may be defined as (a) the presence of two out of the three cardinal features of bradykinesia, rigidity, and tremor, (b) a good clinical response to levodopa, and (c) no 'atypical' features suggestive of another Parkinsonian syndrome. Pathologically there is extensive loss of pigmented dopaminergic substantia nigra neurons and the presence of Lewy bodies.

Epidemiology

Numerous studies have yielded crude prevalence rates of 10–400 cases per 100 000 people (Zhang and Roman 1993). These estimates are difficult to compare mainly due to different methods of case ascertainment. In Europe and North America the prevalence has been estimated to be between 100 and 250 per 100 000. Rates are higher in the Parsi community in India (Bharucha et al. 1988) and lower in China and Africa (Schoenberg et al. 1988) although the reliability of these geographical variations is questionable. In Europe, prevalence rates are similar in all countries and there is no significant difference between men and women (De Rijk et al. 1997) in contrast to some earlier studies which suggested that Parkinson's disease was slightly more common among men. There are many undetected cases and in one study, 24 per cent were diagnosed by the research survey (De Rijk et al. 1997). The usual age of onset is after 50 years with the frequency rising steeply with age. Onset before 40 years is unusual and before 20 is exceptional. Advancing age remains the most powerful predictor of developing Parkinson's disease.

Epidemiological studies have detected a variety of risk factors. These include rural residence, exposure to well water, pesticides and herbicides, farming, wood pulp mills, and iron and steel production (Tanner and Goldman 1996). The significance of these findings is unclear but a common thread is that Parkinson's disease might be due to exposure to an unidentified environmental toxin (see below). A well-known association with non-smokers is unexplained. There is no convincing association between Parkinson's disease and infection but an association with head trauma has been suggested in some studies but this may be an effect of recall bias.

The cause of nigral cell death

The cause of Parkinson's disease is the destruction of the pigmented dopaminergic neurons of the substantia nigra and some other brain regions. The mechanism appears to involve defective mitochondrial respiration and oxidative stress. This in turn may be due to toxic exposure, genetic factors, or an interaction of the two.

◆ Mitochondrial complex 1 is reduced in the substantia nigra of the brain in Parkinson's disease (Schapira et al. 1990; Schapira 1994) but not in other brain regions. Although mitochondrial DNA deletions are seen, these appear similar to those associated with normal ageing. No pathogenic mutations have been detected and so the complex 1 deficiency is likely to be acquired. It is likely that reduction of complex 1 leads to impairment of neuronal energy metabolism, calcium homeostasis, oxidative stress, and ultimately premature cell death (Swerdlow et al. 1996).

◆ Oxidative stress is increased in the substantia nigra. There is increased nigral superoxide dismutase (SOD) activity due to increased superoxide production. This leads to more hydrogen peroxide and hydroxyl radical production, especially in the presence of iron which is concentrated in the substantia nigra. Increased lipid peroxidation has been detected in the substantia nigra in Parkinson's disease (Jenner and Olanow 1996) and there is also a reduction in the level of reduced glutathione, implying increased production of toxic free radicals. There are increased levels of iron in the substantia nigra in Parkinson's disease and this also increases oxidative stress, particularly the production of hydroxyl radicals. The reason for the iron accumulation in the brain is unclear but it is known that iron binds to neuromelanin. Dopamine metabolism by monoamine oxidase (MAO) may also increase oxidative stress because of the production of hydroxyl ions. This raises considerable concern about the safety of levodopa therapy in Parkinson's disease but experimental evidence regarding levodopa toxicity to neurons is conflicting and there is no evidence that the adverse effects of chronic levodopa treatment in Parkinson's disease are related to increased nigral cell death. Oxidative stress damages cell membranes, proteins, and both nuclear and mitochondrial DNA (Jenner and Olanow 1996). Oxidative stress may be associated with animal fat intake which is increased in Parkinson's disease (Logroscino et al. 1996) but there is no association with dietary antioxidants.

◆ It is difficult to know whether oxidative damage or defective mitochondrial respiration is the initiating event in nigral cell depletion as either could cause the other as a secondary effect. Some evidence exists to suggest that oxidative stress may be more obvious in very early Parkinson's disease than mitochondrial dysfunction.

Environmental factors and the toxin hypothesis

The association of Parkinson's disease with certain environmental factors has already been mentioned and suggests a possible role for some as yet unidentified environmental toxin. This has stimulated much interest in possible toxic compounds which might cause Parkinson's disease but the disorder is not new and so an industrial substance is unlikely to be responsible. Nor are these environmental associations consistent. In 1983 however, a number of cases of parkinsonism caused by methylphenyl-tetrahydropyridine (MPTP) attracted considerable attention (Langston et al. 1983). MPTP caused a rapidly progressive form of parkinsonism which was clinically and pathologically very similar to idiopathic Parkinson's disease. MPTP reproduces parkinsonism reliably in experimental animals. Metabolism of the MPTP pro-toxin by monoamine oxidase B yields methylphenylpyridinium ion (MPP$^+$) which is taken up into dopaminergic neuron terminals where it inhibits cellular mitochondrial complex 1 leading to cell death (Tanner 1994). Although the MPTP mechanism fits so well with other data concerning mitochondrial and oxidative factors, no similar toxin has been linked to sporadic Parkinson's disease.

Metabolic and genetic polymorphisms

It has been suggested that Parkinson's disease might be caused by slower detoxification of a pathogenic environmental agent and that the condition might therefore develop in metabolically susceptible individuals. An association between the activity of debrisoquine hydroxylase, a marker of cytochrome P450 function, and certain alleles of the CYP2D6 gene has been reported (Smith et al. 1992) but has not been confirmed and seems unlikely (Plante-Bordeneuve et al. 1994). A recent meta-analysis of the relationship between Parkinson's disease and numerous gene polymorphisms concluded that an association was confirmed only with the genes for monoamine oxidase B, N-acetyltransferase 2, glutathione transferase and the mitochondrial tRNAGlu gene (Tan et al. 2000).

Genetics of Parkinson's disease

Several lines of evidence point to the role of hereditary factors in Parkinson's disease, in addition to the weak genetic associations already mentioned.

◆ The tendency for Parkinson's disease to occur more commonly among the relatives of affected patients than would be expected by chance. This has been noted for many years but the exact proportion of patients with affected relatives has varied depending on the methods used and the definition of an affected relative. Some studies have included patients with postural tremor while others have not. Recent studies have tended to use family history only and suggest that 10–40 per cent of patients have affected relatives. Among families with more than one affected individual, autosomal dominant inheritance with reduced penetrance seems likely with segregation ratios of 20–30 per cent among sibs and parents (Maraganore et al. 1991; Plante-Bordeneuve et al. 1995). A problem with such studies is the late age of onset of Parkinson's disease so that a normal relative may yet become affected with time. Positron emission tomography studies using flurodopa scans have indeed detected relatives with pre-clinical Parkinson's disease (Piccini et al. 1997).

◆ The discovery of a few remarkable families containing many affected individuals and showing autosomal dominant inheritance (Golbe et al. 1990; Markopoulou et al. 1995; Wszolek et al. 1995) shows that clinically and pathologically typical Parkinson's disease may be caused by a genetic mutation of the gene for α-synuclein on chromosome 4q21. (Polymeropoulos et al. 1997; Kruger et al. 1998). The relevance of such unusual families to the generality of patients with Parkinson's disease is uncertain and this genetic mutation is not found in cases of sporadic Parkinson's disease.

◆ A mutation of the ubiquitin-carboxy-terminal hydrolase L1 gene (UCH-L1) on chromosome 4p14 has also been described in autosomal dominant Parkinson's disease (Leroy et al. 1998). The significance of this finding is uncertain.

◆ In a small number of other autosomal dominant Parkinson's disease families, linkage has been detected to loci on chromosomes 2p13 (Gasser et al. 1998), and 4p15 (Farrer et al 1999).

◆ Twin studies have shown very low concordance rates which is not consistent with a significant genetic factor. However, some co-twins only develop Parkinson's disease after many years and follow-up studies have shown slightly higher concordance rates many years later. Such studies are also confounded by co-twins with pre-clinical Parkinson's disease which may be detected by PET scanning (Burn *et al.* 1992). The statistical inaccuracies of the twin method also make exclusion of a genetic contribution difficult.

Pathology of Parkinson's disease

It is likely that Parkinson's disease symptoms are related to impaired nigral cell function and subsequent cellular loss as it is difficult to account for the natural history of the condition in terms of cell losses alone. The basic neuropathological features of idiopathic Parkinson's disease are neuronal loss in the substantia nigra with Lewy bodies in the surviving cells and a normal corpus striatum. The pathological hallmark of Parkinson's disease is the Lewy body (Fig. 32.6), an eosinophilic intracellular inclusion. Typically there is a central core within a less intensely staining body surrounded by a pale halo. The significance of the Lewy body is unclear and the process by which it is formed is unknown. Lewy bodies have a complex composition but contain neurofilament proteins, presumably derived from the neuronal cytoskeleton as well as ubiquitin and synuctein. Lewy bodies are not absolutely specific to Parkinson's disease as is sometimes suggested; they are found in a few other neurological disorders such as ataxia telangiectasia and Hallervorden–Spatz disease. Nor are they found only in the substantia nigra but in many areas of the nervous system including the locus coeruleus, dorsal motor nucleus of the vagus, and other brainstem regions as well as the nucleus basalis of Meynert, thalamus, cerebral cortex, intermediolateral columns of the spinal cord, and within the autonomic nervous system. The pale body is a more homogeneous granular inclusion which is specific to the substantia nigra and locus coeruleus. Lewy bodies are associated with devastating depletion of the melanin containing dopaminergic neurons of the pars compacta of the substantia nigra (SNc) (Fig. 32.7). In symptomatic patients, at least 70 per cent or more of nigral cells

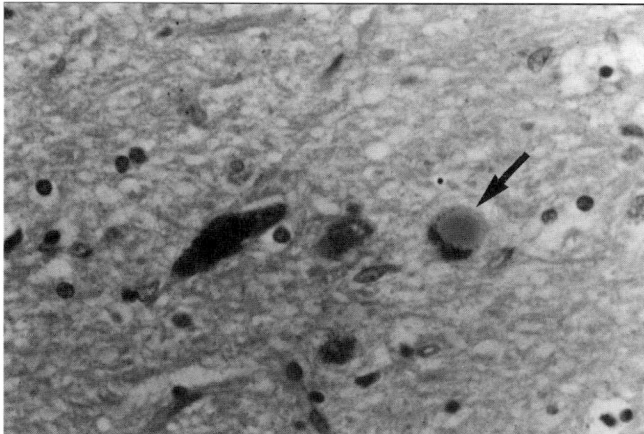

Fig. 32.6. A substantia nigra Lewy body (arrowed) in Parkinson's disease (Courtesy of Dr J. Broome, Consultant Neuropathologist, Walton Centre).

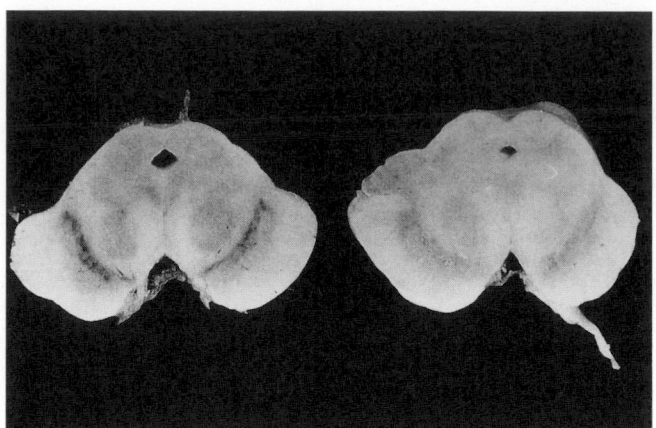

Fig. 32.7. A midbrain section from a normal brain (left) and in Parkinson's disease (right) showing depletion of the pigmented substantia nigra (Courtesy of Dr J. Broome, Consultant Neuropathologist, Walton Centre).

are lost. Cell loss is also seen in other regions in association with Lewy bodies. The nigral cell loss is initially rapid and then slows down later in the disease; there is also preferential cell loss in the ventro-lateral region of the SNc with relative preservation of the dorsal tier (Fearnley and Lees 1991). This differs from the pattern seen in normal ageing where the rate of cell loss is lower, the severity of active cell death appears much less and the emphasis is on the dorsal tier of the SNc (Fearnley and Lees 1991).

The term 'incidental Lewy body disease' has been coined to describe the occurrence of Lewy bodies and other features of Parkinson's disease in the brains of people without clinical evidence of Parkinson's disease during life. The prevalence of incidental Lewy bodies approaches 10 per cent of those aged over 80 years. Such individuals presumably died during the presymptomatic phase of Parkinson's disease.

Clinical features

The onset is insidious and the patient may have difficulty recalling when the first symptom appeared. Some patients mention malaise, tiredness, and a general slowing up of physical activity. Not uncommonly this history may reach back several years and may be clearer to family members. The symptoms are often attributed to depression or 'normal ageing'. The older patient, living alone, may simply start 'not coping' and may seem to relatives to be in a general decline. Writing becomes small and untidy, gradually fading away, leading to problems at work or when signing cheques. Musculoskeletal pain or stiffness especially in an upper limb may be prominent and cause diagnostic confusion. Some mention abnormal sensations such as pain and 'internal' tremor before it is clinically apparent (Shulman *et al.* 1996). Gradually the typical resting tremor, rigidity, and slowness of movement appear.

Parkinson's disease is often regarded as an easy 'end of the bed' diagnosis but is highly variable in presentation and frequently misdiagnosed (Hughes *et al.* 1993*b*). Two principal

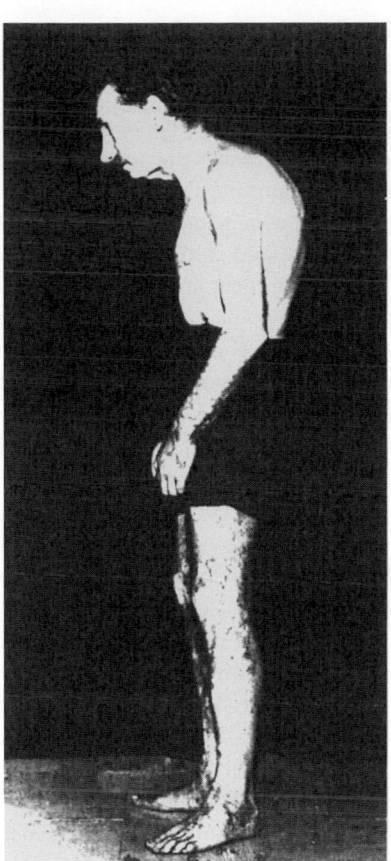

Fig. 32.8. A patient with Parkinson's disease. Note the typical posture with flexion of the elbows.

forms are recognized. In one (tremor dominant), the main feature is tremor, in the other (akinetic rigid), bradykinesia or gait disturbance is more prominent. The appearance of the patient is characteristic and becomes more so with time (Fig. 32.8). Bradykinesia causes a poverty of movement leading to an abnormal stillness and impassive appearance. The posture becomes one of flexion of the neck, spine, elbows, wrists, hips, and knees. The patient stands and walks on a narrow base. Facial expression is reduced with the mouth slightly open, the voice is quiet and monotonous, and later there is a greasy skin. Some patients present with minimal and easily overlooked physical signs such as slightly reduced arm swing on one side while walking with barely noticeable wrist rigidity brought out by synkinesis of the contralateral arm; others present at a surprisingly late stage with gross parkinsonism and considerable disability. The most characteristic presentation is with tremor, bradykinesia, and rigidity of an upper limb. Unilateral onset is typical of Parkinson's disease and yet this often causes diagnostic confusion and the ordering of investigations to exclude a structural lesion of one cerebral hemisphere.

The most reliable diagnostic principle is the presence of two out of the three cardinal features of tremor, bradykinesia, and rigidity. To this could be added the presence of a good response to levodopa therapy which is observed in all but a handful of patients (Hughes *et al.* 1993*b*).

The Parkinsonian tremor is noticeable at rest and is less prominent or absent with action or posture. The frequency is slow, 4–7 Hz, and may involve only the thumb or one finger at first. In some patients the typical 'pillrolling' appearance is seen but this is not invariable. It is more evident with the patient distracted and can be brought out by asking the patient to carry out simple mental arithmetic or counting with the eyes shut and sitting quietly at rest. The tremor is increased by movement of the contralateral limbs or walking. Eventually the tremor spreads to the contralateral limbs but often remains more noticeable on the initially affected side. In some cases, the face and jaw are eventually involved. In addition to the classical rest tremor, there is often a faster postural or action tremor seen in the outstretched hands but this is not as prominent. Patients with a marked postural tremor, especially if this is the principal symptom are not likely to have Parkinson's disease.

Parkinsonian rigidity may be a smooth resistance to passive movement (lead pipe or plastic rigidity) or may have a ratchet-like cogwheel effect due to additional postural tremor. Parkinsonian rigidity is more obvious in the extremities and only later becomes prominent in the axial musculature. It is detectable with slow passive limb movement unlike spasticity which is related to rapid movement. It can be brought out by contralateral limb movement (Froment sign) and a useful point in the out-patient clinic is that the rigidity is often more noticeable at the wrist while the patient is standing or walking about.

Bradykinesia refers to the slowness of movement and is closely related to akinesia or absence of movement. Movement is slow and delayed, initially distally and later in the proximal muscles. There are many manifestations of bradykinesia including reduced facial expression, drooling of saliva, reduced blinking, reduced arm swing while walking, difficulty turning in bed or rising from a chair, slowness of gait, and small shuffling steps. Repetitive movements show slowing and reduced amplitude; finger movements are particularly affected and become clumsy and laboured. Handwriting becomes small and spidery at an early stage (micrographia) and may be a presenting symptom.

Postural instability is often cited as a fourth core feature of Parkinson's disease but it is not often an early symptom. The patient has a tendency to topple forwards or backwards if pushed or pulled (propulsion or retropulsion) and when walking there is a liability to topple forward with faster steps and difficulty stopping (festination). Falls increase and the gait develops into the typical slow shuffling walk with small steps on a narrow base. There is a delay in the initiation of gait and the patient becomes intermittently stuck and unable to move (freezing), usually in confined spaces or at thresholds. Eventually it is impossible to walk unaided and without treatment a bedbound state develops. Postural instability and gait failure are the most disabling features of Parkinson's disease and the most resistant to dopamine replacement therapy although some improvement can be seen with levodopa even in the later stages of the condition. Parkinson's disease rarely presents initially with falling or gait disturbance and other disorders such as Steele–Richardson–Olszewski disease, cerebrovascular disease, or multiple system atrophy should be considered if this is the case.

In addition to the four cardinal features of tremor, bradykinesia, rigidity, and postural instability, a number of other problems develop. Painful off period dystonia of one or both feet is a frequent symptom, especially in the early morning (Poewe *et al.* 1988). The foot locks into a plantar flexed and inverted posture which makes standing or walking difficult; there may also be stiffness of the calf. These spasms may last a few minutes or over an hour until anti-Parkinsonian medication is taken. In some patients the episodes appear later in the day as well, when the effects of medication have worn off before the next dose. Other patients develop dystonic movements of the face, trunk, or limbs as a complication of levodopa therapy and these spasms are seen after medication has been taken.

It is estimated that 20–30 per cent of patients will become demented, the proportion rising with advancing age and longer duration of disease (Aarsland *et al.* 2001). The clinical detection of dementia is sometimes difficult due to depression or the neuropsychiatric side effects of medication. In early Parkinson's disease there are some mild neuropsychological abnormalities, which are consistent with impaired frontal lobe function but these are not clinically obvious; patients who develop dementia as a presenting or early feature of their illness are unlikely to have Parkinson's disease. In those who do develop dementia, cognitive slowing, depression, and prominent memory impairment are typical whereas aphasia and agnosias are rare; this pattern is said to indicate a 'subcortical' dementia. Other patients however, develop a pattern of cognitive impairment similar to Alzheimer's disease and the distinction between subcortical and cortical dementia is not clear cut. The pathological basis of dementia in Parkinson's disease is similarly uncertain. Some patients have cortical Lewy body pathology, some have Alzheimer's disease, and others have both (McKeith *et al.* 1996). In some demented patients, the pathological basis of the dementia is unclear. A characteristic clinical picture is the patient with fluctuating confusion, disorientation and visual hallucinations, and advanced Parkinson's disease. The mental state seems to be exacerbated by anti-Parkinsonian medi-cation, especially dopamine agonists. This pattern of neuropsychological impairment is often attributed to drug side effects whereas it is characteristic of cortical Lewy body dementia (McKeith *et al.* 1996). In other patients, confusion may be precipitated by the use of amantadine or anticholinergic drugs.

Depression is common in Parkinson's disease and may exacerbate both physical and cognitive function. Patients may complain that their Parkinson's disease is worse in a non-specific way or that their medication is not effective. Others complain of memory problems or insomnia. Demented patients are more likely to be depressed and depression can give a misleading impression of dementia. It is important to consider antidepressant treatment in patients who are deteriorating physically or mentally before concluding that this is due to disease progression or dementia. Parkinsonian patients frequently complain of insomnia and this may be an early clue to the presence of depression. On the other hand, the condition itself also predisposes to sleep disturbance due to stiffness and immobility in bed. Patients complain that they cannot get into a comfortable position, adjust the bedclothes, or roll over. This leads to frustration and fatigue and can exacerbate depression. Other patients experience prominent limb pain or restlessness at night which prevents sleep.

In the later stages of the condition, speech becomes quiet and indistinct, and significant dysarthria eventually occurs in about a half of patients. Dysphagia may be prominent in some patients with severe Parkinson's disease when it is usually accompanied by marked dysarthria. Some patients develop urinary frequency and urgency by day as well as nocturia. In older men this may be due to benign prostatic enlargement but Parkinson's disease can be associated with detrusor instability. Autonomic disturbances are seen in advanced disease but are not as severe or early as in multiple system atrophy (Section 32.3.8). Postural hypotension is the most common manifestation but it may be difficult to assess the relative contributions of the disease and medications, especially dopamine agonists. The fall in blood pressure is rarely severe or disabling in idiopathic Parkinson's disease. Impotence is frequently reported and is probably secondary to autonomic involvement, depression, and physical immobility, especially at night. Constipation is very common in Parkinson's disease at most stages of the condition and is sometimes severe, requiring hospital admission. There are several factors underlying this; autonomic dysfunction, reduced exercise, dietary changes, and the effects of anticholinergic drugs all contribute to the problem. Patients often lose weight and this may be considerable in the later stages. The cause of this is unclear. Many patients notice increased sweating; in the later stages of the condition, especially in severe off periods in levodopa treated patients, there may be attacks of drenching sweating with immobility, fear, and often pain.

It is not widely appreciated that Parkinson's disease can be associated with severe pain in some patients (Quinn *et al.* 1986). The cause of the pain is often missed and unnecessary investigations and therapies are deployed to no effect other than the frustration of patient and doctor. The pain may precede the diagnosis for several months or even years, or may appear later in relation to the timing of levodopa doses. There may or may not be associated spasms or dystonia with the pain which may occur at the beginning, middle, or end of the dose, or in the intervening off periods.

Diagnosis and investigations

Parkinson's disease remains a clinical diagnosis. Many cases are straightforward but diagnostic error is surprisingly common (Hughes *et al.* 1992). There are numerous causes of a Parkinsonian syndrome (Table 32.2) but many of these are obvious clinically. In clinical practice, the same diagnostic difficulties arise repeatedly:

◆ In some cases the presenting symptoms may not immediately suggest the diagnosis or even seem neurological. Pain or weight loss may lead to inappropriate tests or treatment before the problem becomes more obvious. Surprisingly few physicians realize that an asymmetric onset is typical. The elderly patient with evolving Parkinson's disease may be placed in residential care due to inability to cope in the community and the diagnosis may be considered only at a very late stage. Patients regularly undergo psychiatric evaluation and treatment for depression or sometimes an anxiety neurosis before a careful physical examination reveals signs of bradykinesia or rigidity. In those who have received neuroleptic drugs, akinetic rigid features may be attributed to medication.

◆ Multiple system atrophy (MSA) poses the greatest difficulty. The striatonigral degeneration form may remain indistinguishable from Parkinson's disease throughout the illness and may only be diagnosed post-mortem (Hughes *et al.* 1993*b*). A poor response to levodopa is the single most reliable indicator of this condition and because of this a diagnosis of Parkinson's disease is always provisional until the response to levodopa has been evaluated at a follow-up clinic visit. Even this is not absolutely reliable as some MSA patients do respond well to levodopa and very occasional patients with a poor response are later found to have Parkinson's disease post-mortem (Hughes *et al.* 1993*b*). In other patients, an atypical or absent tremor, pyramidal signs, cerebellar involvement, early orofacial dyskinesia, autonomic failure, or more rapid progression of disability will suggest MSA.

◆ Benign essential tremor is often misdiagnosed as Parkinson's disease. The postural tremor, length of the history (often many years by which time Parkinson's disease would be very severe), lack of additional neurological impairment, response to alcohol, and family history should all help to avoid this error.

◆ Drug-induced parkinsonism is common. A careful history will identify the offending agent. Although dopamine receptor blocking drugs are well known to cause parkinsonism, others such as fluoxetine, calcium channel blockers, and amiodarone are less obvious culprits.

◆ Patients with a frontal lobe gait apraxia are often thought to have Parkinson's disease and receive inappropriate anti-Parkinsonian drugs. Usually these patients have cerebrovascular disease or normal pressure hydrocephalus. The gait disorder is different to that in Parkinson's disease with small shuffling steps on a wide base with falling and little additional evidence of parkinsonism, especially in the upper body. In some older patients, there may be features of gait apraxia and otherwise typical Parkinson's disease. In this situation, there may be a combination of Parkinson's disease and cerebrovascular disease. This difficulty sometimes requires a therapeutic trial of levodopa to exclude a treatable Parkinsonian component to the patient's disability.

◆ Occasionally, rare akinetic rigid disorders such as Steele–Richardson–Olszewski disease and corticobasal degeneration cause confusion. The early appearance of postural instability and falling, dysarthria and eventually pyramidal signs and a supranuclear downgaze palsy (Litvan *et al.* 1997*b*) are features of the former. The latter is characterized by striking asymmetry throughout the illness with cortical sensory loss, the alien limb phenomenon, supranuclear gaze palsy, and myoclonus. Pallidal degenerations (Jellinger 1968) may also cause an atypical Parkinsonian syndrome.

In order to reduce diagnostic error in Parkinson's disease, diagnostic criteria have been proposed (Hughes *et al.* 1993*b*) and widely accepted (Table 32.3).

Often, the investigations are normal or misleading and must be interpreted in the light of the likely clinical diagnosis. CT brain scans are rarely helpful; in the elderly there may be cerebral atrophy but this is unlikely to be of significance. Although patients with multiple system atrophy may have cerebellar atrophy, ataxia is usually apparent clinically (Wenning *et al.* 1994*b*). CT may be helpful in cases where hydrocephalus or a structural lesion (Section 32.3.13) are suspected clinically or in patients with the hemiparkinsonism–hemiatrophy syndrome. MRI brain scans are particularly liable to cause confusion; many patients over the age of 60 years have subcortical vascular lesions which are unlikely to be relevant to the patient's akinetic rigid state (Section 32.3.11). However, in patients who are thought to have Steele–Richardson–Olszewski (Section 32.3.9) disease the MR scan may show striking brainstem atrophy. Although positron emission tomography (Brooks *et al.* 1992; Burn *et al.* 1994), SPECT (Schwarz *et al.* 1993), and magnetic resonance spectroscopy (Federico *et al.* 1997) may differentiate Parkinson's disease from other akinetic rigid states such as Steele–Richardson–Olszewski disease and multiple system atrophy, they are not widely available.

In younger patients with parkinsonism, where idiopathic Parkinson's disease is unlikely, a more detailed laboratory evaluation is essential. It is particularly important to exclude Wilson's disease by appropriate biochemical and ophthalmological investigations (Section 32.8).

Management

With the exception of a few, usually elderly, patients who present late, most patients are not markedly disabled at the time of diagnosis. Accordingly, immediate drug treatment is often unnecessary. The most important thing at this point is a careful explanation of the diagnosis, treatment options, and prognosis. Many clinics now employ a nurse specialist to provide additional support to the patient at the time of diagnosis and afterwards. Patients are often frightened by the mention of Parkinson's disease and worried that they should have consulted a doctor sooner. They should be reassured that this would not have influenced the situation. It is necessary to explain that no treatment will completely suppress all symptoms; this avoids premature drug therapy and pointless over-

Table 32.3. Diagnosis criteria for Parkinson's disease, Parkinson's disease society brain bank criteria (Gibb 1988)

1. Criteria required to establish the presence of parkinsonism	Bradykinesia Plus one of the following: Rigidity Resting tremor Postural instability
2. Exclusion criteria for Parkinson's disease	Repeated stroke or stepwise progression Repeated head injury Encephalitis Oculogyric crises Recent neuroleptic treatment Relevant toxic exposure >1 affected relative Sustained remission of symptoms Unilateral signs after 3 years Supranuclear gaze palsy Cerebellar signs Severe, early autonomic failure Severe, early dementia Pyramidal signs Mass lesion or hydrocephalus on CT scan No response to levodopa
3. Positive criteria (3 or more required) for Parkinson's disease	Unilateral onset Rest tremor Progressive disorder Persistent asymmetry Excellent (70–100%) response to levodopa Severe levodopa induced dyskinesia Response to levodopa lasting >5 years Clinical course over >10 years

medication which is a common reaction to residual symptoms in treated patients.

Unfortunately, no currently available treatment prevents the progression of Parkinson's disease and the clinical deterioration of the patient. Treatment may therefore be thought of in three stages:

1. neuroprotection in the patient not yet requiring suppression of symptoms;

2. early symptomatic therapy;

3. management of advanced disease with treatment-related complications and drug-resistant features.

Neuroprotection

In recent years there has been great controversy surrounding neuroprotective therapy. The issue is whether any treatment influences the rate of nigral cell death and with it the progression of the disease. To date, no drug has been shown to do this conclusively. There are theoretical reasons to suppose that inhibition of type B monoamine oxidase (MAO-B) might retard the progression of Parkinson's disease. MAO-B was shown to be involved in the conversion of MPTP to MPP^+ (see above) and so might be similarly important in the activation of a theoretical pathogenic pro-toxin in Parkinson's disease and oxidative reactions caused by dopamine metabolism might also be slowed by MAO-B inhibition. If patients with very early Parkinson's disease are treated with the MAO-B inhibitor selegiline (deprenyl), the need for symptomatic treatment with levodopa is indeed delayed, by about 9 months (Parkinson Study Group 1993). This has been interpreted widely as a neuroprotective effect and selegiline has therefore been prescribed widely in early Parkinson's disease, often immediately after diagnosis. Subsequently, the role of selegiline has become highly controversial. It has been argued that the delay in the need for levodopa in early Parkinson's disease is due to a mild reduction in symptoms due to a weak direct anti-Parkinsonian action of selegiline rather than any slowing of disease progression, i.e. a symptomatic rather than a neuroprotective action (Ward 1994). Others have not agreed with this interpretation and continue to propose a neuroprotective effect (Larsen, J. P., Boas, J., Erdal, J. E. (2000). Does selegiline modify the progression of early Parkinson's disease? Results from a five-year study. The Norwegian-Danish study group. *European Journal of Neurology*, 6, 539–47). Whatever the mechanism of selegiline in Parkinson's disease, it has little if any influence on the clinical progression of the disease (Parkinson's Disease Research Group in the United Kingdom 1993; Parkinson Study Group 1996). In addition, there has been concern about increased mortality in patients taking selegiline (Lees 1995) although this finding has not been confirmed (Donnan, *et al.* 2000). Overall, neuroprotection by selegiline is possible but uncertain, a clear effect on disease progression is hard to detect, and safety is questionable. Accordingly, the indiscriminate use of selegiline in early Parkinson's disease cannot be recommended and the role of the drug remains uncertain. Vitamin E is another possible means of reducing nigral oxidative damage but does not appear to have any effect on the progression of Parkinson's disease (Parkinson Study Group 1993).

Early symptomatic treatment

It follows that the use of medication for Parkinson's disease is for the control of symptoms rather than any effect on the disorder itself. Accordingly, there is no point in administering anti-Parkinsonian drugs until the patient's condition warrants this. This point will vary between patients and depends on social, psychological, and employment issues as well as the severity of the parkinsonism. Many drugs are now available for the treatment of Parkinson's disease, with several new agents arriving within the last few years (Table 32.4).

Non-dopaminergic drugs These may be considered in the mildly affected patient with early disease, usually in order to delay or avoid levodopa or a dopamine agonist (see below). Anticholinergics have been used to treat Parkinson's disease since the

Table 32.4. Drugs used in the treatment of Parkinson's disease

Anticholinergics	Benzhexol (trihexphenidyl)
	Procyclidine
	Orphenadrine
	Benztropine
Amantadine	
Levodopa	Levodopa + carbidopa* (co-careldopa) (Sinemet ®)
	Levodopa + benzserazide* (co-beneldopa) (Madopar ®)
	Both in standard and slow release formulations
MAO inhibitor	Selegilene
COMT inhibitors	Entacapone
Dopamine agonists	Bromocriptine
	Pergolide
	Lisuride
	Ropinirole
	Pramipexole
	Cabergoline
	Apomorphine

MAO = monoamine oxidase, COMT = catechol-O-methyltransferase.
* Peripheral decarboxylase inhibitor.

time of Charcot. Modern agents such as orphenadrine or benzhexol (trihexphenidyl) cause a modest reduction in tremor and rigidity but are less active against akinesia. There is little evidence to support the commonly expressed view that anticholinergics are superior to levodopa for the suppression of tremor but they may be helpful in the early stages of Parkinson's disease when tremor rather than akinesia is the main problem. Motor disability is slightly reduced but side effects are common, especially in the elderly in whom they are best avoided. It is worth trying an anticholinergic in patients with tremor dominant disease who are not helped by levodopa but the response is often disappointing. Amantadine is also weakly anti-Parkinsonian (Obeso and Martinez-Lage 1992). Its mode of action is complex. It increases presynaptic dopamine re-uptake and release and is a weak NMDA receptor antagonist, inhibiting the subthalamic glutamatergic output to GPi. It is mildly effective against Parkinsonian symptoms but not in all patients and the effect may wear off within months. Insomnia, agitation, confusion, ankle oedema, and livedo reticularis may occur. Amantadine may be tried in the early stages of Parkinson's disease in younger patients who are more likely to tolerate it.

Dopaminergic therapy For patients with significant disability, dopaminergic treatment will be required. The dilemma at this stage is whether to use levodopa or dopamine agonist monotherapy. This decision is difficult as it may determine the course of the disease in the longer term, especially in younger patients (under 60) who are more vulnerable to the long-term side effects of levodopa and are more likely to tolerate agonist monotherapy.

Levodopa is the most effective anti-Parkinsonian drug available. It is metabolized peripherally to 3-O-methyldopa (3-O-MD) and dopamine by catechol-O-methyltransferase (COMT) and aromatic amino acid decarboxylase (AADC), respectively (Fig. 32.9). Levodopa absorption is reduced by food because of reduced gastric emptying and competition from dietary protein derived large neutral amino acids (LNAA). Residual levodopa crosses the blood–brain barrier (where there is also competition from LNAA and 3-O-MD) where it is converted to dopamine by AADC in surviving dopaminergic nigral neurons and also other non-dopaminergic cells. Interestingly, the ability of the brain to convert levodopa to dopamine is not significantly reduced by progressive loss of residual nigrostriatal cells (Durso *et al.* 1997). Dopamine acts on striatal dopamine receptors and is then metabolized by striatal MAO and COMT (Fig. 32.9). In order to increase the bioavailability of orally administered levodopa it is given with a peripherally acting decarboxylase inhibitor (PDI), either benzserazide (as Madopar) or carbidopa (as Sinemet). This reduces conversion to dopamine outside the brain and permits a lower oral dose with fewer side effects, especially nausea and vomiting.

Levodopa is highly effective against tremor, rigidity, and akinesia and a good response, with a 70 per cent or more improvement in symptoms, is a diagnostic feature of idiopathic Parkinson's disease. The onset of action is rapid, with most patients improving within days or weeks. The dose of levodopa required in early Parkinson's disease is variable, but most patients respond well to 300 mg/day (given with a PDI) and almost all to 600 mg. It is wise to start at 100 mg daily and increase slowly to 300 mg over 2 or 3 weeks. If there is no response to this dose, the diagnosis should be questioned. If there is no improvement on 600 mg daily, the patient is extremely unlikely to have Parkinson's disease. Side effects are unusual. Some patients develop nausea which can be reduced by slow initial dose increases and administration with food (which simply reduces bioavailability). If the problem persists, additional domperidone (20 mg tds) is usually effective.

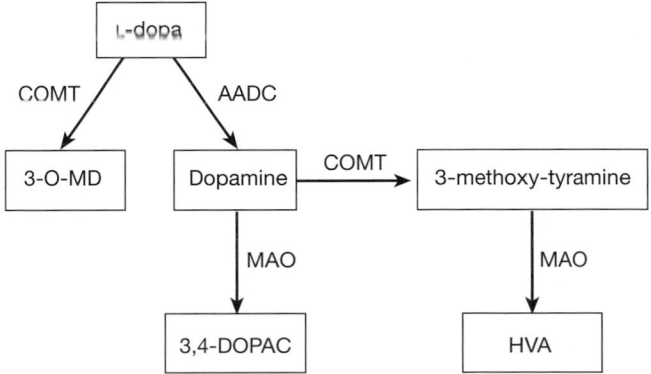

Fig. 32.9. The Metabolism of levodopa. COMT = catechol-o-methyltranferase; MAO = monoamine oxidase; AAAD = aromatic amino acid decarboxylase; 3-0-MD = 3-0-methyldopa; DOPAC = dihydroxyphenylacetic acid; HVA = homovanillic acid.

Postural hypotension, confusion, cardiac arrhythmias, and drowsiness are less common and a haemolytic anaemia is very rare.

At the present time levodopa is a therapeutic paradox. On the one hand it is undoubtedly the most effective treatment for Parkinson's disease and on the other it is associated with such serious long-term problems that there is growing reluctance to use it. The initial dramatic response to levodopa is unfortunately not maintained. Within 5 years, about a half of all patients experience problems due to instability of response and this occurs in almost all within 10 years, especially in younger patients. There is progressive shortening of the response to each dose leading to the 'wearing off effect' or 'end of dose deterioration' with the reappearance of parkinsonism before the next dose is due. These motor fluctuations become increasingly severe and rapid until eventually the patient frequently switches between a mobile 'ON' state and increasingly severe rigid 'OFF' periods. The daily levodopa requirement increases as does the dose frequency. In addition, the on periods are often associated with dyskinetic movements. Initially these are mild choreiform movements after each levodopa dose (peak dose dyskinesia) but later there may be severe dystonic and ballistic movements at the beginning and end of the dose (diphasic dyskinesia). Such dyskinesias may lead to exhaustion and injury. Ultimately the patient hardly seems to derive any benefit from the levodopa but experiences a chaotic roller coaster existence switching from severe dyskinesia to rigid immobility, sometimes within minutes.

The mechanisms underlying the development of fluctuations and dyskinesias are incompletely understood (Nutt and Holford 1996). Disease progression leads to worsening of the underlying parkinsonism thereby increasing the contrast between the medicated and unmedicated states. Increasing nigrostriatal tract destruction reduces presynaptic storage of dopamine reducing the long duration response. The short duration levodopa response (probably reflecting the action of dopamine synthesized and acting outside the nigrostriatal terminals) becomes increasingly evident, shorter and more abrupt due to altered brain handling of levodopa and dopamine receptor activity. The 'negative response' also appears in which low striatal dopamine levels at the beginning and end of each levodopa dose worsen parkinsonism by shutting off residual endogenous dopamine release via presynaptic dopamine autoreceptors. On periods are marred by dyskinesia, the threshold for which moves increasingly close to that for the on response, probably due to alterations in dopamine receptor activity and other mechanisms (Nutt and Holford 1996). Although these problems only occur in levodopa treated patients, there is no agreement about the relative roles of levodopa therapy and disease progression in their production. One view is that motor oscillations and dyskinesias are related to the duration and dosage of levodopa treatment (Rinne 1985, 1987; Hely et al. 1994; Montastruc et al. 1994). This might be due to levodopa inducing alterations in its own pharmacological action and the responses of striatal cells to dopamine or possibly a direct neurotoxic action by increasing dopamine metabolism and oxidative reactions (Fahn 1996). An alternative view is that the changes in the clinical response to levodopa in chronically treated patients are actually due to disease progression (Caraceni 1994). The issue of levodopa toxicity and levodopa-induced acceleration of Parkinson's disease is unresolved.

Whatever the reasons for the problems associated with long-term levodopa treatment, the use of the drug over the last 30 years has led to increasing awareness of these difficulties and questioning of its automatic use as the mainstay of treatment, especially in younger patients who are at much higher risk of fluctuation and dyskinesia.

Dopamine agonist monotherapy is increasingly employed as an alternative to levodopa in order to prevent the onset of long-term levodopa-related problems. Bromocriptine monotherapy relieves parkinsonism (Rinne 1987) but not as well as levodopa which usually has to be added within a few years. Side effects such as nausea, hypotension, and confusion are also common. Although bromocriptine monotherapy is tolerated by only 30–50 per cent of patients (because of inadequate relief of symptoms or side effects) the incidence of fluctuations and dyskinesias among patients taking this treatment is dramatically reduced compared with levodopa (Rinne 1987; Parkinson's Disease Research Group in the United Kingdom 1993). Even among those who start with bromocriptine monotherapy and subsequently take additional levodopa, the incidence of fluctuation and dyskinesia is reduced and their appearance is delayed (Rinne 1987; Hely et al. 1994; Montastruc et al. 1994). Whether this is a protective effect of the dopamine agonist or simply because of delaying or reducing levodopa is unclear. A recent five year study comparing levodopa and ropinirole monotherapy (Rascol et al. 2000) obtained similar results. Of the patients taking ropinirole, 47 per cent were able to continue the drug for five years and 34 percent of theses did not require additional levodopa. The incidence of dyskinesia was much lower with ropinirole compared with levodopa (20 and 45 per cent respectively). Similar results have been obtained with pergolide and pramipexole monotherapy in shorter 2-3 year trials. Overall, dopamine agonist monotherapy is associated with a much lower incidence of dyskinesia and motor fluctuation than is seen with levodopa. In patients who start with an agonist but subsequently take additional levodopa, motor complications are reduced or delayed. Unfortunately, despite these favourable results, monotherapy with the currently available drugs fails in many patients because of side effects or inadequate antiparkinsonian efficacy. Only about a half of patients with early Parkinson's disease are able to tolerate an agonist. Common adverse effects include nauseas (which can usually be avoided by using additional domperidone for the first few weeks), hypotension, oedema, confusion and hallucination. These drugs must be used with caution or not at all in those with a history of cardiac disease, peptic ulceration, psychiatric illness and in the elderly. The newer non-ergot derived agonists (pramipexole and ropinirole) may cause somnolence and daytime sleep attacks (Frucht et al. 1999) which prevent driving. Ergot derivative agonists (especially bromocriptine, cabergoline and pergolide) can

Table 32.5. Characteristics of levodopa treatment compared to dopamine agonist monotherapy

Feature	Levodopa	Agonist monotherapy
Initial anti-Parkinsonian efficacy	Excellent	Moderate
Time to achieve full effect	Weeks	Months
Dose increase	Fast	Slow
Adverse effects	Rare	Common
Overall tolerance	Good	Poor
Fluctuation and dyskinesia	Very common	Very rare
Long-term anti-Parkinsonian effect	Poor	Good
Cost	Low	High

occasionally be associated with erythromelalgia (an uncomfortable erythematous skin induration, usually around the ankles), retroperitoneal fibrosis, pleural effusions and severe inflammatory lung disease. Among patients who successfully tolerate agonist monotherapy, many are unable to obtain adquate relief of parkinsonism and will require the addition of or substitution with levodopa. Accordingly, the choice between levodopa and dopamine agonist monotherapy (see Table 32.5) in early Parkinson's disease remains controversial. In general, younger patients (under 60 years) are more likely to tolerate agonist monotherapy which should be considered seriously in view of the near certainty of severe fluctuation and dyskinesia with levodopa. The patient must be willing to accept reduced short-term relief of symptoms and a greater risk of adverse effects in return for a lower risk of fluctuation and dyskinesia in the longer term. Much will depend on the patient's individual preference and social situation, particularly the extent to which parkinsonism threatens continued employment. If agonist monotherapy is not tolerated, contraindicated, or declined by the patient, levodopa should be used but in as low a dose as possible. It will not be possible to abolish all symptoms completely with either therapy and attempts to do so will be unsuccessful and may lead to side effects. There is no consensus regarding the dose of levodopa to be used but most patients will need at least 300 mg (with a PDI). In some studies, fluctuation and dyskinesia has been less in those taking low dose levodopa combined with a dopamine agonist than in those taking unrestricted doses of levodopa (Rinne 1987; Hely *et al.* 1994; Montastruc *et al.* 1994). It is therefore reasonable to consider the addition of a dopamine agonist in younger patients in whom 300 mg of levodopa is not adequate treatment. In the elderly, the risk of early fluctuation and dyskinesia is lower and agonist monotherapy is less likely to be tolerated. Moreover, older patients are often more disabled by Parkinsonian symptoms and a rapid therapeutic response may be needed to maintain activity and independence.

Stereotactic thalamotomy of the nucleus ventralis intermedius (Vim) continues to have a role in early Parkinson's disease in patients with severe tremor (Obeso *et al.* 1997). Patients with tremor dominant disease sometimes have a dis-

appointing response to medical treatment and this is an exception to the general rule that idiopathic Parkinson's disease always responds to levodopa. Contralateral tremor is abolished in up to 85 per cent of cases but there is little effect on akinesia or rigidity. Complications are uncommon with a unilateral lesion but there is a high risk of dysarthria with bilateral lesions (Hauser *et al.* 1995). Recently thalamic stimulation using an electrode implanted into Vim has been used successfully. The results are comparable to thalamotomy and it has the advantage of being reversible but can be associated with technical difficulties postoperatively (Obeso *et al.* 1997). The relative roles of thalamotomy and thalamic stimulation are unclear but the latter is increasingly favoured due to fewer adverse effects, especially in those who have had an earlier contralateral thalamotomy or who have dysarthria in addition to tremor.

Medical management of advanced Parkinson's disease

Most of the difficulties in advanced Parkinson's disease are caused by levodopa-related complications and emerging drug-resistant features.

Early fluctuations with end of dose deterioration/wearing off effects may be improved in several ways. Levodopa may be increased and given more frequently but this may be only a short-term solution and there is a danger of increasingly frequent fluctuation with higher doses. Controlled release levodopa preparations prolong on periods and reduce the number of levodopa doses required. This is usually successful in mild, early fluctuation but can be associated with a slow onset of action, especially with the first dose of the day. The addition of a small dose of conventional Sinemet or Madopar at this time may provide an initial 'kick in' but this is not always effective. The COMT inhibitor entacapone (100–200 mg tds) reduces the metabolism of levodopa to 3-O-MD thereby prolonging the action of levodopa and reducing end of dose wearing off effects (Rinne, *et al.* 1998). Levodopa requirements are reduced and on time increased in most patients. Side effects include increased dyskinesia and diarrhoea. A third option is to add a dopamine agonist to relieve off periods and fluctuations, preferably before the patient has started to take large doses of levodopa (Rinne 1987; Hely *et al.* 1994; Montastruc *et al.* 1994). A reasonable point at which to consider this is when the fluctuating patient is on 300–600 mg of levodopa. In patients taking larger doses, the addition of an agonist should allow a reduction in levodopa as well as improving control. Several dopamine agonists are available (Table 32.4) with similar clinical effects. There is some evidence that pergolide is more effective than bromocriptine for stabilisation of motor fluctuations (Clarke and Speller 2000) while pramipexole appears to have useful activity against tremor (Kunig *et al.* 1999). The long duration of action of cabergoline is helpful in patients with severe overnight Parkinsonism. Otherwise, there are no major differences between these different agonists. The side effects of dopamine agonists are significant, as discussed above, and they should be used with caution in some patients, particularly the elderly and those with ischaemic heart disease; if there is a history of confusion or hallucination (see below) agonists should be avoided. Nausea and vomiting are very common in those starting agonist therapy and it is sensible to prescribe domperidone (20 mg tds) in the first four to six weeks. Another common difficulty is deterioration of motor function in the first few weeks while the patient is gradually increasing the agonist but has not yet reached a therapeutic dosage (Kellet and Steiger 1999); patients should be warned of this and advised to carry on with the dose escalation until a therapeutic effect is reached. It is a common error to give supplemental agonists at too low a dosage. In most patients, the improvement in fluctuation is considerable when an adequate dosage is achieved.

Severe off periods can be extremely unpleasant with rigidity and immobility, unpleasant limb restlessness, sweating, pain, autonomic abnormalities, and marked psychological distress (Riley and Lang 1993). Such attacks may be reduced if an orally active dopamine agonist is introduced or its dose increased but this may not be effective in advanced cases and very severe attacks. In this situation a more powerful dopamine agonist, apomorphine, is usually effective (Frankel *et al.* 1990; Hughes *et al.* 1993*a*). Apomorphine must be given by subcutaneous injection, acts rapidly and usually relieves such attacks within 10 min of injection and lasts 60–90 min. It is essential to administer domperidone (20 mg tds) to prevent apomorphine-induced vomiting. Many patients manage with a few injections per day but in those requiring more, a continuous subcutaneous infusion may be preferable. Patients often develop skin lesions (nodules and small areas of skin necrosis) at the injection sites, especially in those using subcutaneous infusions. Interestingly, psychosis appears to be less common with apomorphine than with other dopamine agonists and may be tolerated by patients in whom drug-induced psychosis has prevented the use of other agonists. Fluctuating patients are vulnerable to small changes in plasma levodopa concentrations and alterations in levodopa absorption. Taking levodopa without food and restriction of dietary protein often leads to more predictable and effective absorption and improved stability.

Dyskinesias are difficult to treat. In patients taking large doses of levodopa, the introduction of a dopamine agonist and reduction in levodopa dosage is often effective. The aim should be to give as much dopaminergic treatment as possible in the form of the agonist and to reduce the levodopa to the lowest dose possible without an undue increase in off periods. In some cases it may be possible to stop levodopa and use high dose agonist monotherapy but this usually leads to unacceptable parkinsonism. Moreover, some patients are unable to tolerate dopamine agonists because of side effects. In this situation there is little alternative to simply finding a dose of levodopa which provides the best balance between parkinsonism and dyskinesia. Dyskinesias are often worse in the latter part of the day in which case omitting a midday dose of levodopa may be effective. It might be supposed that biphasic dyskinesias occurring at the beginning and end of levodopa doses (see above) might respond to an increase of levodopa but this is not the case; they usually respond in a similar fashion to peak dose dyskinesias to a reduction of levodopa intake. A few other drugs have been tried but without consistent benefit. Recently, amantadine (100–300 mg/day) has proved to be surprisingly effective at reducing dyskinesia, possibly by inhibiting the glutamatergic pathway from the subthalamic nucleus to GPi (Rajput *et al* 1998). In some patients, despite amantadine, a dopamine agonist in high dose and reduced levodopa intake, dyskinesia remains severe and any further levodopa reduction causes a severe off state. No further adjustment of medication is likely to help these patients for whom stereotactic surgery is now probably the treatment of choice (see below and Section 32.2.3). Painful early morning foot dystonia is an off period symptom and responds to oral levodopa or apomorphine on waking, or taking a dopamine agonist or slow release levodopa at night. Baclofen or lithium may help in some cases.

Confusion and psychosis are seen in some cases of advanced Parkinson's disease (especially in older patients) but are an earlier feature in Lewy body dementia. Hallucinations are usually visual and well formed and confusion may become severe with agitation and delirium. Confusion is worse at night and may be precipitated by intercurrent illness, increased anti-Parkinsonian medication (especially dopamine agonists and anticholinergics), or strange surroundings (such as respite care or an unwise hospital admission). The situation may be improved by stopping anticholinergics or dopamine agonists, followed if necessary by a reduction of levodopa. An increase in parkinsonism is inevitable but it is often easier for the patient and carers to manage this than the psychosis. Most neuroleptic drugs worsen parkinsonism due to dopamine receptor blockade but this is not seen with the atypical neuroleptic clozapine which often improves the mental state without a significant increase of parkinsonism. Unfortunately clozapine is associated with a risk of agranulocytosis and regular blood counts are needed. Risperidone is of limited value as it worsens Parkinsonism and, despite initially favourable results in the last few years, it has recently become apparent that this also occurs with olanzapine. At present, the drug of choice is uncertain but quetiapine is a resonable option as this has been associated with the least motor deterioration (Friedman and Factor 2000) but this is based on limited data and further study of this area is badly needed. As mentioned earlier, care is needed in using anticholinergics or dopamine agonists in older Parkinsonian patients or those with any history of confusion or mental illness. Admission of such patients to hospital also requires caution.

Depression may be difficult to detect as the patient often complains of non-specific worsening of parkinsonism, confusion, poor memory, or insomnia. Tricyclic antidepressants such as amitripyline or dothiepin are usually effective and are a useful treatment for insomnia in Parkinson's disease. The anticholinergic effect of tricyclics may also be useful overnight. Serotonin re-uptake inhibitors are best avoided as they may exacerbate Parkinson's disease (Leo 1996).

Gait failure, with freezing, shuffling, and falling is very difficult to treat. Disordered axial movement is often associated and causes immobility in bed. Anti-Parkinsonian medication can improve these problems to some extent but the improvement is usually modest and marked gait failure carries a poor prognosis (Rajput *et al.* 1993). Physiotherapy may help but such patients usually remain disabled and require adaptation of the living environment and mobility aids. Dysarthria and dysphagia are resistant to anti-Parkinsonian drugs and can be managed only with speech therapy and in some cases a percutaneous gastrostomy tube may be needed. Sialorrhoea can be severe and distressing; anticholinergic drugs can help but their propensity to cause adverse effects has already been mentioned. In extreme cases, parotid radiotherapy may be considered. Constipation can be a major problem in all stages of Parkinson's disease and requires attention to diet, the use of laxatives, and awareness of the exacerbating effects of some drugs, especially anticholinergics. Faecal impaction in the rectum with intermittent overflow diarrhoea often causes problems in immobile patients and requires regular manual rectal evacuation rather than inappropriate (and sometimes risky) use of laxatives and antidiarrhoeal drugs. Although significant autonomic dysfunction is not a feature of early Parkinson's disease, this can develop in advanced cases. Bladder dysfunction due to detrusor instability is common in the later stages of Parkinson's disease. It can be difficult to distinguish from prostatism in older men and urodynamic testing may be needed. Anticholinergic drugs and adjustment of fluid intake are partially successful in most cases. Orthostatic hypotension is also seen, especially in those taking dopamine agonists. A head up tilt of the bed at night or oral fludrocortisone is helpful but it is wise to review the patient's medication beforehand.

Neurosurgical treatment of advanced Parkinson's disease

Before the advent of levodopa therapy in the late 1960s, there had been numerous attempts to improve parkinsonism with neurosurgical lesions of the pyramidal and later extrapyramidal system. Initially these were associated with limited improvement and considerable morbidity. Thalamotomy was effective for tremor but had little impact on bradykinesia and rigidity. Pallidal lesions were not as effective for suppression of tremor and although Leksell had reported improved pallidotomy results in the 1960s, this issue was overshadowed by the discovery and introduction of levodopa. There are several reasons for a new wave of enthusiasm for surgical treatment of Parkinson's disease. There is a better understanding of the functional anatomy of the basal ganglia and improved imaging and stereotactic methods allow greater surgical precision and the selection of physiologically logical targets. Most importantly however is the realization that chronic levodopa therapy often leads to intractable motor instability with increasing numbers of patients disabled by fluctuations and, more importantly, dyskinesia.

Stereotactic thalamotomy has already been discussed and is indicated principally for the suppression of contralateral Parkinsonian tremor. This is ideally a procedure to consider in early tremor dominant Parkinson's disease if the response to medical treatment is inadequate.

Stereotactic pallidotomy is increasingly used in fluctuating patients, principally to suppress dyskinesia. Medical measures, especially reduced levodopa intake and a trial of amantadine should, however, be tried first (see above). Pallidotomy is effective in those with severe fluctuation and dyskinesia including elderly patients in whom good results have been reported (Uitti *et al.* 1997). Improved results have followed the selection of the posteroventral lateral pallidum as a target (Leksell's pallidotomy) (Laitinen *et al.* 1992) and several groups have reported excellent results in carefully selected patients (Dogali *et al.* 1995; Iacono *et al.* 1995; Lozano *et al.* 1995; Obeso *et al.* 1996). Overall there is impressive (over 80 per cent) suppression of contralateral and to a lesser degree ipsilateral dyskinesias and overall disability is significantly reduced. Off period parkinsonism is partly improved by 25–30 per cent. The effect on tremor is modest and improvement of ipsilateral parkinsonism is not striking; postural instability, gait failure, dysarthria are not significantly improved. There is controversy concerning the use of microelectrode recordings to localize the sensorimotor area of the pallidum or whether to rely on image-guided anatomical localization (Olanow 1996; Obeso *et al.* 1997). The former is claimed to be more accurate but increases the duration of the surgery. Complications include haemorrhage, hemiparesis, and visual field loss but overall the risk of adverse effects has been 10–15 per cent. The role of bilateral pallidotomy is currently uncertain but is being examined by several groups and may prove valuable in some patients (Obeso *et al.* 1997). Staged bilateral pallidotomy can produce excellent suppression of dyskinesia with a low incidence of adverse effects. There has been some concern about cognitive and beavioural changes after left sided and especially bilateral procedure but these are mild and have not been consistently observed (Counihan *et al.* 2001).

An alternative to stereotactic brain lesions is deep brain stimulation. This has the advantage of reversibility but technical problems are greater than with conventional lesion procedures and postoperative management is intensive and time consuming. The effect of the stimulating electrode is inhibitory at the site of the electrode terminal, which is implanted into the selected brain target and connected to a subcutaneously placed neurostimulator, usually on the anterior chest wall. The results of thalamic Vim stimulation for tremor in Parkinson's disease have already been discussed. In advanced fluctuating disease, impressive results have been observed with bilateral subthalamic stimulation (Limousin *et al.* 1998; Kumar *et al.* 1998). All aspects of Parkinson's disease are improved, including gait, and drug requirements considerably reduced. Improvements in motor scores of 60 per cent are seen in the off state and on time is substantially increased. In contrast to pallidal or thalamic surgery, levodopa intake is reduced by 50 per cent (Hallett *et al.* 1999). Dyskinesias are markedly reduced, probably due to reduction in levodopa requirements. Hemiballismus, which might be expected with subthalamic surgery, is rare, probably due to altered direct pathway basal ganglia function in Parkinsonism (Guridi and Obeso 2001). Complications include weight gain, mild dystonia, eyelid apraxia, haemorrhage, infection and cognitive impairment (Kumar *et al.* 1998; Saint Cyr *et al.* 2000). Initial experience with pallidal stimulation is encouraging (Siegfried and Lippitz 1994; Pahwa *et al.* 1997) but this has not yet been used in many patients.

Another neurosurgical development has been the use of transplanted fetal mesencephalic neurons into the striatum of patients with advanced Parkinson's disease. Several groups have now reported results in small series of patients (Lindvall *et al.* 1994; Peschanski *et al.* 1994; Freeman *et al.* 1995; Defer *et al.* 1996). Over 100 patients have now been treated worldwide but evaluation of the results is impaired by variable methodology and assessment despite more recent attempts to standardize these. Fetal tissue has been unilaterally or bilaterally transplanted as cell suspensions or solid grafts into the host striatum (putamen or caudate). Considerable improvement in all aspects of parkinsonism have appeared 3–6 months after transplantation and have been maintained up to 3 years of follow up. Levodopa requirements have been reduced in some patients. Positron emission tomography has demonstrated striatal flurodopa accumulation and post-mortem examination of the graft site in one patient has shown robust graft survival and re-innervation of the host striatum (Kordower *et al.* 1995). There is uncertainty regarding the optimal method of grafting, the required number of fetal donors per graft, the need for immunosuppression and the use of adjuvant growth factors. At present, technical and ethical issues mean that fetal transplantation remains an experimental approach. A recent study of 20 transplanted patients showed a modest 15 per cent improvement in motor scores but a high incidence of severe dyskinesia appearing over a year postoperatively (Freed *et al.* 2001).

Other aspects of management

Not all these problems are soluble with medical or neurosurgical therapy and advanced Parkinson's disease, even with modern treatment, remains a disabling and progressive condition. Physiotherapy, occupational therapy, and speech therapy are helpful in advanced cases with accumulating disability. Patients require intensive social support in the community and in some cases, residential care may be the only practical option. There is increasing emphasis on the development of specialist multidisciplinary clinics although proof of their value is lacking. Nurse practitioners, ideally working from specialist movement disorder units, provide invaluable additional support to patients, carers, and family doctors, especially those using apomorphine and with severe treatment-related fluctuations. In the UK, patients and their families are assisted by the Parkinson's Disease Society who are able to provide information and support.

32.3.2 Dementia with Lewy bodies (cortical Lewy body disease)

The relationship of this condition to Parkinson's disease is controversial but the two disorders share several clinical and pathological characteristics. Originally, Lewy body dementia

(LBD) was defined pathologically (Kosaka 1993) with Lewy bodies distributed throughout the cerebral cortex in addition to the substantia nigra and other brainstem nuclei. In fact, cortical Lewy bodies occur in Parkinson's disease but not in the numbers seen in DLB. Two forms of DLB are recognized, a common form with additional Alzheimer pathology, and a pure form in which this is absent. Those who regard DLB as a variant of Parkinson's disease have proposed the concept of 'Lewy body disease' incorporating three groups. Type A (diffuse type), type B (transitional or limbic type), and type C (brainstem type, synonymous with Parkinson's disease) (Kosaka 1993; McKeith *et al.* 1996). The frequency of DLB is unknown but 15 cases were identified in a single year at a UK centre, suggesting that this may be one of the more common forms of dementia (Byrne *et al.* 1989).

Clinically, DLB is characterized by dementia and parkinsonism. The Parkinsonian features are similar to idiopathic Parkinson's disease but there is a lower incidence of tremor and the response to levodopa is not as satisfactory. In some patients there may be additional myoclonus (20 per cent of cases). Rare patients have had supranuclear gaze palsies similar to those seen in Steele–Richardson–Olszewski disease (Fearnley *et al.* 1991). The dementia is striking and may precede or follow the development of parkinsonism or sometimes occur alone (especially with the common form). Poor memory is usually the first sign but a key diagnostic clue is prominent fluctuation of the mental state, sometimes day to day and sudden deterioration of cognitive function sometimes suggests some other event such as a stroke or intercurrent infection. Psychotic features such as hallucinations and paranoid delusions are common (Byrne *et al.* 1989).

The diagnosis of DLB may be obvious clinically. Patients who develop Parkinson's disease and then dementia at an unusually early stage with prominent fluctuation in the severity of their confusion and hallucinations are likely to have DLB. So are those with this type of dementia who later develop parkinsonism. The difficulty is with those who have only the dementia (in whom it may be difficult to make the diagnosis in life) and those with atypical features such as myoclonus or supranuclear gaze palsy in whom other diagnoses such as Creutzfeldt–Jakob disease and Steele–Richardson–Olszewski disease may be suspected. A common problem is the patient with what appears to have been typical levodopa responsive Parkinson's disease for years who then develops confusion and hallucinations. Whether these patients have Parkinson's disease with mental changes caused by additional dementia and the effects of anti-Parkinsonian drugs or DLB is usually impossible to determine clinically. Pathologically some but not all of these patients have DLB.

The management of DLB is difficult because of the tendency of dopaminergic treatment to exacerbate the patient's confusion and the obvious potential effects of neuroleptics on parkinsonism. Patients with DLB are often highly sensitive to dopamine receptor blocking drugs. Generally the management is similar to that of confusion and psychosis in Parkinson's disease (Section 32.3.1). The prognosis is poor, but rivastigmine can produce some cognitive improvement and appears well tolerated (McKeith *et al.* 2000).

32.3.3 **Early onset Parkinson's disease**

Early onset Parkinson's disease (EOPD) refers to patients in whom the age of onset is before 40 years. In Europe and North America this accounts for less than 10 per cent of cases but EOPD is more common in Japan. EOPD is heterogeneous; some patients have idiopathic Parkinson's disease presenting at an unusually early age but others do not. Clinically, EOPD patients have typical Parkinsonian rest tremor, rigidity, and bradykinesia but there is an increased incidence of lower limb dystonia (prior to levodopa therapy) and less dementia; autonomic features such as dizziness, abnormal sweating, and urinary frequency are slightly more common. There is also an increased incidence of familial cases compared with older onset Parkinson's disease. A good response to levodopa is seen but fluctuation and dyskinesia is much more common and occurs very early, sometimes within months of starting treatment (Quinn *et al.* 1987; Golbe 1991; Muthane *et al.* 1994). Despite these treatment-related complications in some levodopa treated patients, the progression of EOPD is slower than in older patients. Metabolic studies of cerebrospinal fluid indicate presynaptic dopamine deficiency (Muthane *et al.* 1994). It has been suggested that EOPD can be divided into two groups. Those with onset before 20 years (juvenile parkinsonism—JP) and between 20 and 40 years (young onset Parkinson's disease—YOPD) (Quinn *et al.* 1987). A family history of similarly affected relatives, suggesting autosomal recessive or sometimes dominant inheritance, is more common in JP than YOPD but there are few consistent clinical differences between the two groups (Muthane *et al.* 1994). Pathological studies are confusing; some cases of EOPD have had characteristic neuropathological changes of Parkinson's disease but others have showed atypical nigral degeneration without Lewy bodies. Pathological findings have included neuronal loss without Lewy bodies, ballooned neurons, and neurofibrillary tangles. Neuropathological evidence of idiopathic Parkinson's disease has been more common in YOPD cases than JP. One form of non-Lewy body autosomal recessive JP has been linked to a gene on chromosome 6q25 (Matsumine *et al.* 1997). Recently, this condition has been shown to be a result of mutations of a closely linked gene at this locus. The gene encodes a protein (Parkin) of unknown function (Kitada *et al* 1998). Parkinsonism due to autosomal recessive Parkin gene mutations is associated with early age of onset, usually before 30 but ranging from 7 to 58 years. Progression is usually slow and dyskinesias appear early. Parkin mutations appear to be a common cause of EOPD (Lucking *et al.* 2000). Another form of JP is caused by mutations of the tyrosine hydroxylase gene on chromosome 11p (Ludecke *et al.* 1996).

In all young patients presenting with an akinetic rigid syndrome, it is essential to exclude Wilson's disease by biochemical and ophthalmological investigations. A liver biopsy is indicated if the results of these initial tests are in any way equivocal (Section 32.8). Dopa responsive dystonia must also be considered along with other rare causes of parkinsonism includ-ing rigid Huntington's disease, Hallervorden–Spatz disease, neuroacanthocytosis, and the hereditary cerebellar degenerations.

32.3.4 **Drug-induced parkinsonism**

The most common cause of drug-induced parkinsonism (DIP) is exposure to neuroleptic medication. Clinically overt parkinsonism is seen in 10–15 per cent of patients taking neuroleptic drugs but this is almost certainly an underestimate (Arblaster *et al.* 1993). It should be noted that the atypical limbic selective antipsychotics clozapine, quetiapine, and olanzapine do not appear to cause DIP (Durif *et al.* 1997; Reus 1997; Tran *et al.* 1997). Clinically, DIP is indistinguishable from sporadic idiopathic Parkinson's disease and although a postural rather than resting tremor and asymmetry are more common this is not consistent. Some patients develop a rest tremor of the lips (rabbit syndrome) without other signs of parkinsonism. Obviously, the diagnosis depends on taking a careful history of current and recent medication. In the psychiatric patient on large doses of neuroleptic treatment, the diagnosis is all too clear but some cases are less obvious. Some patients take prochlorperazine for years for dizziness and tablets containing a mixture of a tricyclic antidepressant and a neuroleptic are sometimes used in depression. In cases like these, chronic neuroleptic exposure may not immediately be evident. There is a poor correlation between duration and dosage of neuroleptic therapy and the development of parkinsonism, suggesting that blockade of dopamine receptors is not the only mechanism. Some patients develop parkinsonism rapidly within days of starting a neuroleptic while others tolerate large doses for years without problems. DIP appears to be more common in older patients and females; there is also an association with HLA types (Metzer *et al.* 1989) but the significance of this is unclear.

Several lines of evidence suggest that some patients with DIP probably have sub-clinical Parkinson's disease which has been revealed by interference with dopaminergic neurotransmission. Not all patients obtain a remission after discontinuation of neuroleptics and some develop Parkinson's disease after an initial remission (Goetz 1983; Hardie and Lees 1988). Some patients with DIP have abnormal flurodopa PET scans indicating presynaptic dopamine deficiency and persistence of parkinsonism is more likely in these patients (Burn and Brooks 1993). Moreover, a few patients with DIP have had pathological evidence of Parkinson's disease post-mortem (Rajput *et al.* 1982). However, the frequency of DIP suggests that not all of these patients have Parkinson's disease which is much less common.

A number of other drugs may less commonly cause DIP (Table 32.6). Dopamine depleting agents such as reserpine (no longer available) and tetrabenazine cause parkinsonism by reducing dopamine release at nigrostriatal terminals. Metoclopramide has a dopamine receptor blocking action and is, in this respect, similar to the neuroleptic major tranquillizers. This drug is widely prescribed for nausea and may cause long-lasting DIP especially in the presence of renal impairment (Sethi *et al.* 1989). Calcium channel blockers such as cinnarizine are important as they are widely prescribed and often for long periods. The mechanism by which they induce DIP is unclear. Cinnarizine is commonly prescribed for dizziness and is liable

Table 32.6. Causes of drug-induced parkinsonism

Dopamine receptor blocking drugs	Neuroleptics
	Metoclopramide
	Prochlorperazine
Dopamine depleting drugs	Tetrabenazine
	Reserpine
	α-Methyldopa
Miscellaneous drugs	Cinnarizine
	SSRIs
	Amiodarone
	Lithium

SSRI = selective serotonin re-uptake inhibitor antidepressants.

Table 32.7. Causes of toxic parkinsonism

| MPTP |
| Manganese |
| Carbon monoxide |
| Carbon disulphide |
| Cyanide |
| Methanol |

to cause DIP in the elderly. It is important to note the association of the newer serotonin re-uptake inhibitors (SSRIs) with DIP (Leo 1996). Depression commonly produces psychomotor slowing and so the symptoms of DIP may erroneously be attributed to depression; moreover, depression is common in Parkinson's disease and SSRIs should be avoided in case of exacerbation of physical symptoms.

In most cases, DIP will remit after discontinuation of the causative agent but this may take weeks or months. It is not possible to decide whether parkinsonism is drug induced or due to underlying idiopathic Parkinson's disease until a reasonable period off medication has elapsed. Some remissions have not occurred for years. This remains an area of difficulty but it is reasonable to expect most cases of DIP to show improvement within 6 months of drug withdrawal. Most of those in whom parkinsonism persists are older and likely to have Parkinson's disease but occasionally younger patients fail to improve, suggesting permanent nigrostriatal damage by the medication (Melamed et al. 1991). In some patients, continuing neuroleptic treatment may be unavoidable because of severe psychiatric illness; in these patients, the use of an atypical neuroleptic such as clozapine or olanzapine may be preferable (Reus 1997; Tran et al. 1997). There is no evidence that the use of atypical limbic selective neuroleptics will allow reversal of already established DIP although this might be expected in view of their comparative freedom from extrapyramidal side effects. There is some recent evidence that olanzapine can cause parkinsonism; accordingly quetiapine may be preferable.

In patients with DIP who await remission after withdrawal of the responsible drug or in whom this is not possible, anti-Parkinsonian drugs may be used. Levodopa or anticholinergics may be used but dopamine agonists must be avoided in psychotic patients in case the mental state is made worse. The rabbit syndrome responds to anticholinergics.

32.3.5 Toxic parkinsonism

The possible role of an exogenous toxin in Parkinson's disease and the effects of exposure to MPTP have already been discussed in section 32.3.1. MPTP-induced Parkinson's disease

is no longer seen and only occurred in a few patients but was clinically very similar to sporadic Parkinson's disease (Langston 1996). The response to levodopa was good but fluctuation and dyskinesia occurred very quickly. In some cases the disease slowly progressed as in Parkinson's disease.

Other cases of toxic parkinsonism (Table 32.7) are very rare and do not closely resemble Parkinson's disease. Nevertheless the possibility of toxic parkinsonism is often raised in the clinic by patients who have possibly been exposed to various industrial toxins. Patients with clinically typical Parkinson's disease, with tremor and a good response to levodopa are extremely unlikely to have toxic parkinsonism. Manganese is one of the best-known causes of parkinsonism and enters the differential diagnosis of the Parkinsonian patient with an industrial or mining background from time to time (Section 5.7.4). In manganese miners there is a brief psychotic reaction as a prodrome to the development of parkinsonism but those with chronic lower level exposure do not show this feature. In both groups, parkinsonism appears insidiously but akinesia, rigidity, and gait disturbance are prominent and tremor is usually absent. Lower limb dystonia is common and cerebellar features may be seen. Pathologically, manganese causes degeneration of the globus pallidus and there is little improvement with levodopa (Pahwa 1997). Other toxic causes of parkinsonism are very rare and share some of the salient features of manganism, namely a predominantly rigid and akinetic state with inconspicuous or absent tremor and no response to levodopa. Dystonia and spasticity are also noted frequently along with variable cognitive impairment (Pahwa 1997).

32.3.6 Post-encephalitic parkinsonism

This was most commonly seen after the large epidemic of encephalitis lethargica (Von Economo's encephalitis) which occurred in Europe and North America from 1917 until the 1930s. Many survivors from the epidemic had long-term psychiatric and neurological impairments, most notably oculogyric crises (seen in 20 per cent) and post-encephalitic parkinsonism (in about 50 per cent). Occasional cases of encephalitis lethargica still occur (Howard and Lees 1987) but are extremely rare. Parkinsonism sometimes appeared immediately but could take years to develop, after a latent interval. Bradykinesia and rigidity were prominent but tremor was variably present. Oculogyric crises, with forced vertical deviation of the eyes and accompanying anxiety or depression lasted for several minutes or hours and were characteristic of post-encephalitic parkinsonism. Additional features such as respiratory irregularity, behavioural disturbances, somnolence, ophthalmoparesis, and various hyperkinesias were also seen. Progression was very slow or negligible in many patients but late deterioration, many years later has been described. Pathologically there was severe neuronal loss and gliosis in the substantia nigra and widespread neurofibrillary tangle formation, especially in the brainstem. Anticholinergic treatment was often successful and well tolerated but the response to levodopa was less predictable and side effects were common, mainly dyskinesias and agitation.

32.3.7 Post-traumatic parkinsonism

There are three aspects to the issue of head injury and Parkinson's disease which has been controversial for over a century. These are the roles of acute major brain injury, repeated concussion and head injury without evidence of brain damage.

Occasionally a head injury can induce parkinsonism secondary to direct basal ganglia or substantia nigra damage. Such cases are rare and a confident diagnosis requires evidence of significant brain damage and the early appearance of parkinsonism. There should be radiological or later pathological evidence of basal ganglia or brainstem injury. It is likely that other neurological signs will be present.

Chronic repeated concussion as seen in boxers may result in chronic traumatic encephalopathy (dementia pugilistica or punch drunkenness). This produces akinetic rigid features and associated cognitive decline, ataxia, dysarthria, and neuropsychiatric abnormalities. CT scanning may reveal a cavum septum pellucidum and cerebral atrophy but other investigations are unhelpful. The response of the parkinsonism to levodopa is variable. It will be noted that the akinetic rigid syndrome associated with chronic head injury is quite unlikely to be confused clinically with idiopathic Parkinson's disease.

Head trauma without significant brain injury is more controversial; while some studies have claimed an association with Parkinson's disease others have not and some studies are unreliable. What seems clear, and evident from daily clinical practice, is that the symptoms of Parkinson's disease become worse in association with stress, intercurrent illness, or injury (Goetz and Stebbins 1991) but this is not due to any direct effect on the disease process and is almost always reversible.

32.3.8 Multiple system atrophy

Definition and prevalence

This disorder is marked by considerable clinical variability and causes parkinsonism, cerebellar dysfunction, pyramidal signs, and autonomic failure in various combinations. The aetiology of multiple system atrophy (MSA) is unknown and it does not

Table 32.8. Clinical variants of multiple system atrophy

Clinical type	Major clinical feature	Additional features
OPCA	Ataxia	Pyramidal signs Parkinsonism Autonomic failure
Shy–Drager syndrome	Autonomic failure	Parkinsonism Muscle fasciculation and wasting*
Striatonigral degeneration	Parkinsonism	Pyramidal signs Autonomic failure
Progressive autonomic failure	Autonomic failure	Parkinsonism Pyramidal signs Ataxia

* Observed in one of the two cases only.

appear to be hereditary. Unfortunately, there is widespread confusion regarding the definition of MSA. This is mainly because it was originally described under different diagnostic terms such as olivopontocerebellar atrophy (OPCA), striatonigral degeneration (SND), and the Shy–Drager syndrome (SDS) whose clinical features were dominated by cerebellar ataxia, parkinsonism, or autonomic failure, respectively. However, it is important to note that each of these disorders actually featured all three of the key clinical manifestations of MSA as shown in Table 32.8. The complex and confusing evolution of the MSA concept has been reviewed in detail elsewhere (Quinn 1994) but the constituent disorders (OPCA, SND, SDS) were assembled into a single condition (MSA) by Graham and Oppenheimer (1969) who reported a case of autonomic failure followed by cerebellar signs but not parkinsonism. Pathologically however, there were changes similar to those previously reported as OPCA, SND (despite the lack of clear akinetic rigid features in life), and cell loss in the intermediolateral columns of the spinal cord. This one case therefore combined the pathological features of three previously distinct entities. In retrospect, previous cases reported as OPCA, SND, and SDS also had the pathological changes of MSA. More recently, this concept of MSA as a unitary disorder has been strengthened by the finding of a common neuropathological feature, glial, and neuronal cytoplasmic inclusions (detected with Beilschowsky silver or anti-ubiquitin stains) in patients from each of the different clinical subgroups of MSA (Quinn 1994).

The frequency of MSA is unclear due to incomplete ascertainment and incorrect diagnosis, mainly as Parkinson's disease or sporadic late onset cerebellar degeneration. Based upon neuropathological series, MSA may be the correct diagnosis in 10–20 per cent of patients diagnosed as having parkinsonism in life but such studies are unrepresentative because atypical cases are more likely to be studied post-mortem. In one recent study of patients selected on the basis of a clinical diagnosis of Parkinson's disease in life, 5 per cent actually had MSA (Hughes *et al.* 1992). A recent estimate of prevalence is 4 per 100,000 (Schrag *et al.* 1999).

Pathology

Pathologically, there is neuronal loss and gliosis in the striatum, substantia nigra, locus coeruleus, pontine nuclei, and/or middle cerebellar peduncles, cerebellar Purkinje cells, inferior olivary nuclei and intermediolateral columns and Onuf's nucleus of the spinal cord; not all of these are involved in every case but at least two areas are required for a pathological diagnosis along with the characteristic glial cytoplasmic inclusions (GCIs) common to all forms of MSA (Papp *et al.* 1989). These inclusions, which contain alpha synuclein and ubiquitin (Dickson *et al.* 1999), are also seen in neurons (Papp and Lantos 1994) and may be detected while neuronal loss is still very mild (Wenning *et al.* 1994c). The significance of GCIs is unclear but they are not seen in other neurological conditions (including Parkinson's disease and Steele–Richardson–Olszewski disease) with two exceptions; one case of dominantly inherited cerebellar ataxia (SCA type 1) (Gilman *et al.* 1996) and a previously reported case of adult onset hereditary cerebellar degeneration. GCIs were absent in all other cases of hereditary ataxia studied. Although the pathology of MSA is variable, neuronal loss in the substantia nigra and striatum is usually seen in patients who had significant parkinsonism in life.

Clinical features

The onset of MSA is usually between 40 and 70 years and has not been described before 30. The first symptoms are usually due to parkinsonism (in 46 per cent) and autonomic dysfunction is almost as frequent (in 41 per cent); a few patients present with a cerebellar syndrome (5 per cent) or a mixed picture (7 per cent) (Wenning *et al.* 1994a). Eventually most patients develop parkinsonism, cerebellar dysfunction, pyramidal, and autonomic involvement in various combinations and with differing emphasis. Clinically, the majority of patients (about 80 per cent) have a mainly Parkinsonian picture, with or without additional cerebellar features (SND type). A predominantly cerebellar syndrome (OPCA type) is seen in approximately 20 per cent of cases, usually with additional parkinsonism. Autonomic impairment occurs in the majority of patients in both groups but is occasionally absent (Quinn 1994; Wenning *et al.* 1994a).

Parkinsonism is the dominant clinical feature of MSA, occurring in 90 per cent or more of cases to some degree, and is the dominant clinical feature in about 80 per cent of patients, leading to the SND type of MSA. Usually there are atypical features such as an absent or jerky postural type of tremor, a poor response to levodopa with frequent unusual orofacial dyskinesia (dyskinesia in Parkinson's disease usually involves the limbs initially), symmetrical onset, early falling, and unusually rapid progression. Small myoclonic jerks of the fingers may be

seen (Salazar *et al.* 2000). Pyramidal signs occur in 60 per cent of MSA patients but are usually mild, with exaggerated tendon reflexes, extensor plantar responses, and sometimes spasticity. In most cases of SND type MSA, the additional cerebellar signs, pyramidal or autonomic features will point to the correct diagnosis and not idiopathic Parkinson's disease. However, some MSA patients have levodopa responsive parkinsonism with asymmetrical onset, typical resting tremor, and no additional atypical features. Such cases are clinically indistinguishable from Parkinson's disease and may be detected only at postmortem (Hughes *et al.* 1992).

Autonomic failure develops in the great majority of patients and is often a presenting feature. Urgency and frequency of micturition, impotence, and postural hypotension are the usual features; the latter rarely causes severe hypotension or syncope. Faecal incontinence is occasionally encountered and some patients develop urinary retention. It is rare for autonomic failure to be the only or dominant clinical problem in MSA. It is almost always accompanied by parkinsonism, cerebellar ataxia, or a combination of the two after a few years.

Cerebellar manifestations of MSA include gait ataxia, dysarthria, limb ataxia, and nystagmus. About a half of patients overall have cerebellar involvement clinically but this is rarely the presenting feature and of those patients (about 20 per cent) who have a predominantly cerebellar syndrome (the OPCA type of MSA), careful examination usually reveals evidence of autonomic involvement or parkinsonism (Wenning *et al.* 1997). Although cerebellar involvement may not be evident during life, this is much more commonly detected pathologically (Wenning *et al.* 1995).

Other clinical signs may be seen in some patients. Some patients have an unusually severe and characteristic antecollis (Fig. 32.10), fine myoclonic jerks of the fingers, cold cyanotic extremities, or respiratory irregularities (Quinn 1994). Eye movement abnormalities include nystagmus and mild limitation of eye movement but never to the degree seen in Steele–Richardson–Olszewski disease. Inspiratory stridor is a dramatic and well-recognized manifestation in some patients (Wenning *et al.* 1994a). This is often severe enough to require tracheostomy and is occasionally a presenting symptom. Some patients have a dysarthria which is difficult to classify and is prominent at a much earlier stage than in Parkinson's disease. A rare but curious feature in a few patients has been the emergence of MSA (and sometimes Parkinson's disease) in men with REM sleep behaviour disorder (Schenck *et al.* 1996). In contrast to Parkinson's disease, treatment-related psychosis does not occur in MSA, and although mild frontal lobe cognitive deficits may be detectable, dementia is not seen (Wenning *et al.* 2000). Peripheral nerve involvement is mild and almost always sub-clinical.

Diagnosis

The diagnosis of MSA may be difficult, especially in cases of pure levodopa responsive parkinsonism and in the minority of cases with a cerebellar presentation. The latter group are in

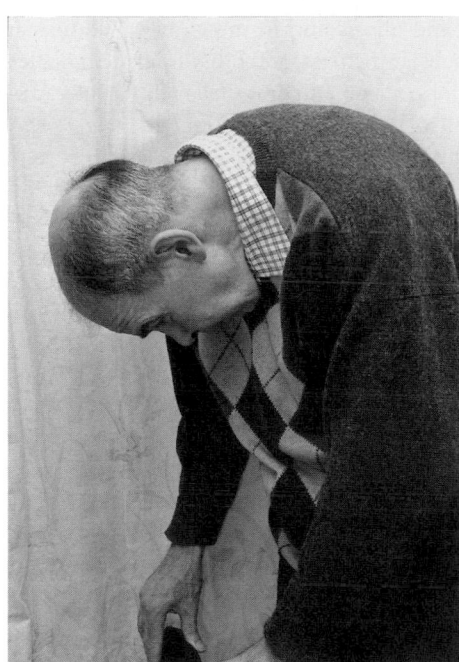

Fig. 32.10. Severe antecollis in a patient with multiple system atrophy (striatonigral degeneration type).

many respects similar to patients with sporadic late onset cerebellar degeneration in which cerebellar ataxia, parkinsonism, and pyramidal signs are common. It is the presence of autonomic impairment and lack of a family history that should suggest MSA rather than other forms of idiopathic or hereditary late onset cerebellar degeneration (Gilman 1996). The features of parkinsonism which should suggest a diagnosis of MSA have already been mentioned. A recurrent difficulty is the presence of mild autonomic problems such as urgency of micturition and postural hypotension in a patient with otherwise typical Parkinson's disease. It may be difficult to exclude MSA in such cases but the autonomic features of MSA tend to be more severe, occur much earlier, and affect younger patients. Obviously the response to levodopa and the clinical features of such patients require careful scrutiny.

Investigations are usually unhelpful in the diagnosis. Although brain CT scanning often reveals cerebellar or brain stem atrophy this is usually apparent clinically (Wenning *et al.* 1994*b*). MRI will detect posterior fossa atrophy more reliably and may show altered putaminal signal, possibly reflecting altered striatal iron levels (Schwarz *et al.* 1996) although this is not yet adequately validated for routine clinical practice. Positron emission tomography (PET) using ^{18}Fdopa has been used to detect reduced nigrostriatal dopaminergic function in MSA including cases with primarily Parkinsonian, cerebellar, or autonomic presentations (Brooks *et al.* 1990; Rinne *et al.* 1995). However, PET studies of nigrostriatal dopaminergic innervation and postsynaptic striatal D$_2$ receptor density, using ^{18}Fdopa and ^{11}C raclopride ligands have not consistently discriminated MSA from Parkinson's disease (Brooks *et al.* 1992; Burn *et al.* 1994). Analysis of postsynaptic striatal opioid recep-

tor density, using ^{11}C diprenorphine seems more promising (Burn *et al.* 1995) as does ^{18}F deoxyglucose PET to detect striatal and cerebellar hypometabolism in MSA (Eidelberg *et al.* 1993*a*). The integrity of the striatal dopamine receptors (which should be intact in Parkinson's disease) can also be studied using ^{131}I-iodobenzamide (IBZM) SPECT scanning. Reduced striatal IBZM binding is suggestive of a diagnosis of MSA rather than Parkinson's disease and has successfully predicted levodopa responsiveness (Oertel *et al.* 1993; Schwarz *et al.* 1993). Neuronal loss in the putamen has also been detected using proton magnetic resonance spectroscopy (MRS) (Davie *et al.* 1995). Although PET, SPECT, and MRS are promising diagnostic techniques, they are not easily available and not reliable enough for widespread application. By contrast, external urethral sphincter EMG is very useful as denervation changes are highly suggestive of MSA (Pramstaller *et al.* 1995). False positive results may occur after pelvic surgery, in multiparous women and in Steele–Richardson–Olszewski disease (Valldeoriola *et al.* 1995). In a few MSA patients, the sphincter EMG is normal. Autonomic dysfunction may be detected by autonomic function tests or urodynamic studies but in patients with significant autonomic failure, this should be evident clinically. The central autonomic dysfunction of MSA can be distinguished from the peripheral autonomic impairment seen in Parkinson's disease by cardiac radionucleotide scanning using [^{123}I]metaiodobenzylguanidine (MIBG). In Parkinson's disease there is reuced cardiac but normal mediastinal uptake whereas in MSA, both are reduced (Braune *et al.* 1999).

Management and prognosis

The management of MSA is difficult. Patients usually deteriorate relentlessly. Median survival is about 10 years and most patients are dead after 15 years. Parkinsonism may improve with levodopa in about a third of cases but rarely as well as in Parkinson's disease; additional dopamine agonists or anticholinergics are usually unhelpful in patients who do not respond well to levodopa. Postural hypotension often responds to a head up tilt of the bed at night, fludrocortisone, or DDAVP at night; elastic stockings are rarely helpful and are uncomfortable. Bladder dysfunction may respond to anticholinergic medication sometimes with additional intermittent or permanent catheterization depending on residual manual dexterity. Stridor may require tracheostomy and intracavernosal papaverine may help male impotence. Like many neurologically disabled patients, those with MSA need access to speech therapy, occupational therapy, social services, continence advisors, and physiotherapy when required.

Differentiation of autonomic failure in MSA from primary autonomic failure (PAF)

In MSA the autonomic failure is caused by central nervous system involvement affecting the brainstem, intermediolateral columns, and Onuf's nucleus of the spinal cord. In these regions there is neuronal loss, gliosis, and GCIs (see above); Lewy bodies are absent. Parkinsonism, cerebellar ataxia, or both develop in all cases within a few years of onset. The progression of MSA is often rapid and the prognosis is poor. The distinction between MSA and Parkinson's disease with autonomic involvement has already been mentioned above. Another point which may cause confusion is the distinction between MSA and primary autonomic failure (PAF), sometimes referred to as idiopathic orthostatic hypotension or the Bradbury Ecclestone syndrome. This is a more slowly progressive (and sometimes static) disorder with slower onset and a better prognosis than MSA. There are no additional CNS features such as parkinsonism, pyramidal involvement, or cerebellar signs and REM sleep disorder does not occur (Plazzi *et al.* 1998). Postural hypotension, defined as a blood pressure reduction of 20 mmHg systolic or 10 mmHg diastolic within 3 min of standing (Consensus Statement 1996), occurs in PAF and MSA but tends to be more severe in PAF with a higher incidence of syn-cope and post-prandial hypotension. Pathologically the main changes are in the autonomic ganglia of the peripheral nervous system, with degeneration of postganglionic sympathetic neurons and the presence of Lewy bodies in the ganglia or the postganglionic neurons. There may be much less conspicuous and asymptomatic pathological involvement, including the presence of Lewy bodies, in brainstem nuclei, substantia nigra, and intermediolateral columns (Hague *et al.* 1997). The supine plasma noradrenaline level is reduced in PAF but not in MSA. Essentially, MSA is characterized by central autonomic dysfunction and PAF by peripheral autonomic impairment. This distinction may be detected by the use of growth hormone measurements after the administration of clonidine (Kimber *et al.* 1997); in normal individuals, Parkinson's disease, and PAF, the level of growth hormone is increased by clonidine but this does not occur in MSA. The cause of PAF is unknown and its relationship to Parkinson's disease and cortical Lewy body disease (or Lewy body dementia; Section 32.3.2) is unclear. In some patients, the distinction between PAF and MSA is very difficult; about 10 per cent of those who initially appear to have PAF go on to develop other neurological features of MSA after several years. The treatment of the autonomic symptoms is similar in the two disorders (see above). Recent develop-ments include the use of the noradrenaline precursor 3,4-DL-*threo*-dihydroxyphenylserine, the α-adrenergic agonist midodrine and erythropoietin to improve postural hypotension.

32.3.9 Steele–Richardson–Olszewski disease (progressive supranuclear palsy)

Definition

This is a progressive degenerative disorder causing early gait instability and falling with axial rigidity, dementia, pseudobulbar palsy, pyramidal signs, and a characteristic eye movement disorder (supranuclear downgaze palsy).

Pathology, frequency, and aetiology

The key feature of Steele–Richardson–Olszewski (SRO) disease is neurofibrillary tangle (NFT) formation, with variable neur-

onal loss and gliosis and in the globus pallidus, subthalamic nucleus, substantia nigra, and other brainstem nuclei, especially the superior colliculi and pretectal areas (involved in eye movement control), pedunculopontine nucleus (PPN), pontine nuclei, and the interstitial nucleus of Cajal. Involvement of the PPN has been linked to the prominent gait instability in SRO disease and the marked axial and neck rigidity may be associated with involvement of the interstitial nucleus of Cajal. Disordered eye movement is probably secondary to the tectal and pretectal lesions as well as the nucleus raphe interpositus (Revesz *et al.* 1996). Cortical involvement, especially of the frontal motor areas is common, in contrast to earlier reports (Verny *et al.* 1996). The NFTs contain abnormally phosphorylated tau protein, similar to that seen in Alzheimer's disease, but the distribution and morphology of NFTs in SRO disease are different. There is no association between SRO disease and the apo-e4 genotype (Tabaton *et al.* 1995).

The aetiology of SRO disease is unknown. Associations with both above and below average education and residence in small towns have been reported but these are of doubtful significance. There is an assoiation between SRO disease and one allele (A0) of the tau gene on chromosome 17 (Morris *et al.* 1999). The presence of the A0 allele is also associated with an earlier age of onset. The majority of cases are sporadic but rare families with an autosomal dominant pattern of inheritance have been described (Rojo et al. 1999); some of these have been associated with mutations of the tau gene (Stanford *et al.* 2000; Delisle *et al.* 1999) but these are absent in sporadic cases and other families with hereditary SRO disease (Hoenicka *et al.* 1999). SRO disease is rare, with a prevalence estimated at 6 per 100 000 but is almost certainly underdiagnosed (Schrag *et al.* 1999).

Clinical features

The onset is always after the age of 40 years and the two most important features are early falling and a characteristic eye movement disorder. These are usually seen with frontal lobe impairment, pseudobulbar palsy, bradykinesia, rigidity, and pyramidal signs. Difficulty walking with the rapid development of falling, typically backwards, within a year of onset is the most common presenting feature. The second salient feature is the development of a supranuclear downgaze palsy, probably due to damage to the substantia nigra pars retriculata. Downgaze may initially be slowed or reduced and optokinetic responses to a downward moving stimulus are impaired. Saccades tend to be lost before pursuit movements. Other eye movement abnormalities such as impaired upward or lateral movements, internuclear ophthalmoplegia, absent Bell's phenomenon, square wave jerks, and impaired suppression of vestibulo-ocular reflexes are common but less specific and are seen in many other neurological disorders. Eventually there is often a severe ophthalmoplegia in all directions but particularly downwards (Lees 1987). This leads to difficulty with eating, reading, and safely coming downstairs. The face has a striking frozen staring expression with reduced blinking, frontalis overaction, and a fixed gaze (Fig. 32.11). Eyelid abnormalities including blepharospasm,

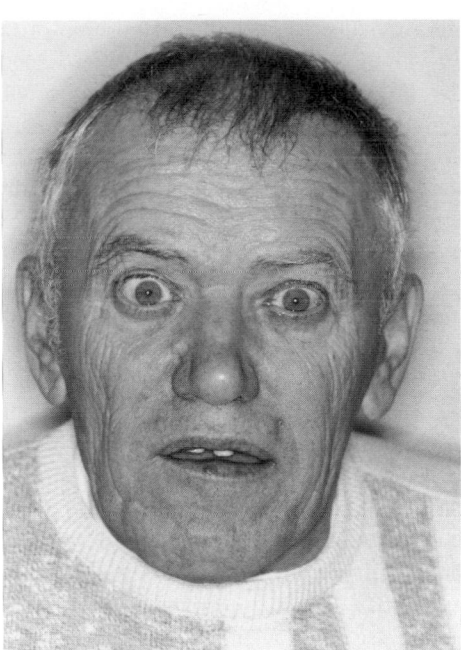

Fig. 32.11. The typical facial appearance of Steele-Richardson-Olszewski disease.

apraxia of eyelid opening (due to blepharospasm of the pretarsal orbicularis oculi), apraxia of eyelid closure, and ptosis are also common and contribute to the facial appearance. Speech is strained and dysarthric due to a pseudobulbar palsy and there may also be palilalia, stuttering, explosive coughing, and intermittent inspiratory sighs and emotional lability (Litvan *et al.* 1996*a–d*). Dysphagia frequently develops and is eventually a major determinant of survival (Litvan *et al.* 1996*c*). The patient develops a severe axial rigidity with extension of the neck and less prominent stiffness and slowness of the limbs. Tremor is usually absent but has been observed in a minority of cases (Masucci and Kurtzke 1989). Pyramidal involvement with brisk limb reflexes and extensor plantar reactions, in addition to the pseudobulbar signs eventually appear in most cases. Cognitive impairment commonly develops (Grafman *et al.* 1990; Litvan *et al.* 1996*d*) typically a frontal lobe syndrome with apathy, disinhibition, mood alterations, anxiety, and psychomotor slowing as well as perseveration and frontal release signs. Aggression and irritability are uncommon and psychiatric features are mild (Menza *et al.* 1995). Autonomic impairment is not a major feature but bladder dysfunction with urinary incontinence may be seen in more severe cases. Sleep disturbance is common.

Although the clinical picture of typical SRO disease is unmistakable, atypical presentations occur. There may be prominent limb dystonia (Barclay and Lang 1997), resting tremor (Masucci and Kurtzke 1989; Collins *et al.* 1995), and an asymmetrical akinetic rigid picture which may resemble Parkinson's disease for years before the characteristic axial rigidity and ophthalmoplegia appear (Lees 1987; Collins *et al.* 1995). Some patients present with a syndrome of pure akinesia with striking slowness of movement affecting gait, speech, and writing but no

other signs of the condition (Matsuo *et al.* 1991; Riley *et al.* 1994). Such patients do not always subsequently develop typical ocular and other SRO disease features. There are also pathologically confirmed cases in which the characteristic ophthalmoplegia was absent during life (Daniel *et al.* 1995).

Diagnosis

The diagnosis often proves difficult initially. There may be vague complaints about vision, a change in speech, altered personality, and a general slowness and stiffness which may erroneously suggest Parkinson's disease. There may be no obvious physical cause for falling or difficulty with balance and walking. It may be several years before the suggestive physical signs develop and permit the correct diagnosis (Maher and Lees 1986).

In order to improve diagnostic accuracy, clinical criteria have been proposed which emphasize the early development of falling within a year of onset and a supranuclear downgaze palsy (Litvan *et al.* 1996*a,d*) as the most important diagnostic features and the diagnosis can scarcely be made without these features. Difficulty may arise in distinguishing SRO from Parkinson's disease, multiple system atrophy, cortical Lewy body disease (CLBD), corticobasal degeneration, and Pick's disease (Litvan *et al.* 1997*a,b*). The axial rigidity, rarity of tremor, lack of response to levodopa, and early falling should avoid confusion with Parkinson's disease but this distinction may not be easy in the first few years of the disease before it has fully developed. Hallucinations and mental fluctuations are not seen in SRO disease in contrast to CLBD. Multiple system atrophy usually begins at an earlier age and is not associated with such a marked ophthalmoplegia. Autonomic impairment is more severe in MSA but an abnormal external urethral sphincter EMG may be noted in either disorder (Valldeoriola *et al.* 1995). Pick's disease is not associated with ophthalmoplegia or falling. There may be difficulty with corticobasal degeneration in which an ophthalmoplegia, gait disorder, and rigidity may occur (Rinne *et al.* 1994*b*). In SRO disease however, the ophthalmoplegia is much more severe, falling is more prominent, and strikingly asymmetrical signs or the alien limb sign are not encountered. In atypical cases, especially those without ophthalmoplegia, the diagnosis may not be possible without prolonged follow up and in some cases may never become so.

On occasions, other conditions such as cerebrovascular disease, progressive subcortical gliosis (Will *et al.* 1988; Foster *et al.* 1992), cortical Lewy body disease (Fearnley *et al.* 1991), Creutzfeldt–Jakob disease (Bertoni *et al.* 1992), cerebral tumour, and basal ganglia calcification (Silbert *et al.* 1993; Saver *et al.* 1994) may closely resemble SRO disease. Hydrocephalus may cause gait impairment, dementia, and sometimes a vertical gaze palsy similar to SRO disease but downgaze is usually spared and axial rigidity is not seen. It may be difficult, especially in advanced cases, to distinguish SRO disease from late onset cerebellar degeneration in which a severe ophthalmoplegia, inability to walk, and pyramidal signs may also occur; in this situation much will depend on the history and physical signs in the earlier years of the illness and the detection of cerebellar atrophy by neuroimaging. Whipples disease may also resemble SRO disease (Averbuch-Heller *et al.* 1999).

Investigations in SRO disease are of limited value. MR scanning may reveal brainstem atrophy but the cerebellum appears normal and hydrocephalus, cerebral infarcts, mass lesions, and other disorders associated with ophthalmoplegia such as Whipple's disease are easily excluded. Neuropsychological evaluation can be helpful in confirming a clinical impression of frontal lobe dysfunction and frontal hypoperfusion may be detected by SPECT blood flow scanning (Neary *et al.* 1987). In more specialized research studies, loss of striatal dopamine receptors detected by SPECT or PET (Brooks *et al.* 1992; Schwarz *et al.* 1993) can help to exclude Parkinson's disease, and striatal neuronal loss may be detected by magnetic resonance spectroscopy (Federico *et al.* 1997). Specialized neurophysiological studies have shown loss of the normal auditory startle response, probably reflecting damaged brainstem reticular formation neurons (Rothwell *et al.* 1994).

Management and prognosis

The course of SRO disease is relentless with a median survival of 6 years (Maher and Lees 1986; Litvan *et al.* 1996c). A few atypical patients have a milder and more protracted illness which may partly resemble Parkinson's disease. Levodopa and other anti-Parkinsonian drugs are of minimal benefit but are often tried (Lees 1987). Tricyclic antidepressants may be helpful in some patients (Newman 1985) but the effect is modest. There is no role for stereotactic surgery. Botulinum toxin may be used for blepharospasm and possibly for rigidity although experience in SRO disease is limited. Speech therapy may improve dysarthria and dysphagia but some patients require gastrostomy feeding eventually. Increasing physical disability may be improved by physiotherapy and occupational therapy. Community services are eventually required in most cases, including personal and respite care. In the UK, the PSP association provides helpful information and support to patients and carers.

32.3.10 Corticobasal degeneration

This is a rare sporadic degenerative disorder of unknown aetiology. It is characterized by the combination of a very asymmetrical akinetic rigid syndrome and localized cortical deficits such as cortical sensory loss, dyspraxia, myoclonus, and the alien limb phenomenon. Pathologically there is asymmetric frontoparietal cortical atrophy which is particularly severe around the Rolandic fissure. Microscopically, there is cerebral cortical degeneration, with neuronal loss, gliosis, and ballooned or achromatic neurons; Pick bodies are not seen. There is also severe degeneration of the substantia nigra and variable involvement of the basal ganglia, brainstem, and cerebellar nuclei. Neurofibrillary tangles (NFTs) are seen in cerebral cortex, basal ganglia, and brainstem, as in SRO disease, but are usually slightly different in appearance. Corticobasal degeneration (CBD) shares some neuropathological features with SRO

disease and Pick's disease including deposition of tau and an association with the Ao tau allele (Di Maria *et al.* 2000).

Typically the onset of CBD is after the age of 60 years. In most patients there is atypical levodopa resistant parkinsonism with striking asymmetry (Riley *et al.* 1990). Rigidity and bradykinesia are often confined to one limb, usually an arm, with additional dystonia and apraxia. The patient may hold the arm in an odd, flexed, and abducted posture with little abnormality in the other limbs (Fig. 32.12). In other cases, one leg is initially affected. Postural instability and falling may occur early and a rest tremor is seen in a third of cases (Watts *et al.* 1997; Wenning *et al.* 1998). The tremor is faster than that seen in Parkinson's disease and is typically jerky and irregular, sometimes with additional focal myoclonus. In a few cases, the initial presentation may resemble idiopathic Parkinson's disease. In addition to the akinetic rigid syndrome, various cortical features occur such as focal cortical sensory loss, stimulus sensitive focal myoclonus (typically in a rigid dyspraxic upper limb), apraxia, and aphasia. The supplementary motor area is often involved giving rise to the 'alien limb sign'. Usually this involves an arm which wanders about, uncontrollably moves and grasps independently, and may interfere with the activity of the other hand (intermanual conflict). Pyramidal signs, dystonia, myoclonus, and abnormal eye movements gradually appear along with increasing asymmetrical parkinsonism. Gradually there is progression of the ipsilateral and later the contralateral limbs but marked asymmetry persists and is characteristic of CBD (Riley *et al.* 1990). A supranuclear eye movement disorder is common and can involve vertical or horizontal movements (Rinne *et al.* 1994b). Cognitive impairment is usually absent in the earlier stages of CBD but a frontoparietal dementia appears

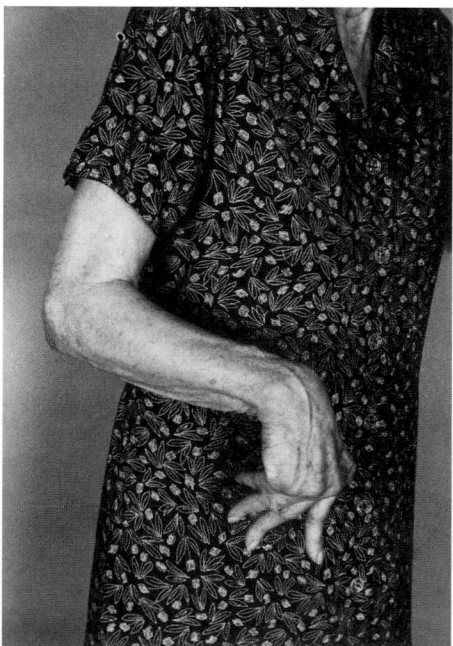

Fig. 32.12. Corticobasal degeneration. Note the appearance of the rigid, flexed arm which is characteristic of the condition.

later in many cases (Rinne *et al.* 1994*b*; Wenning *et al.* 1998) with frontal lobe deficits and apraxia (Pillon *et al.* 1995). In some atypical cases, dementia or dysphasia are presenting features with little motor involvement (Bergeron *et al.* 1996).

The diagnosis of CBD is often difficult and may not be possible without observation of the patient over time. Other conditions such as Alzheimer's disease, SRO disease, Pick's disease and Creutzfeldt-Jacob disease have been diagnosed pathologically in cases of clinically diagnosed CBD (Boeve *et al.* 1999). CBD is distinguished from Parkinson's disease by the lack of response to levodopa and the various additional clinical features. The combination of an akinetic rigid syndrome with a vertical supranuclear gaze palsy will usually suggest SRO disease as the principal diagnosis. Early falling, axial and symmetrical rigidity (rather than in one limb), and ophthalmoplegia affecting downgaze more than horizontal movement are more suggestive of SRO disease but atypical cases of SRO are occasionally indistinguishable from CBD (Case records of the Massachusetts General Hospital 1993). Isolated focal cortical deficits causing apraxia, aphasia, cortical sensory loss, or an alien limb may be caused by structural lesions, Alzheimer's disease, or a focal cortical degeneration but the additional akinetic rigid features or gait disturbance in CBD point to a more diffuse neurological disorder and will usually allow the correct diagnosis. The myoclonus of Creutzfeldt–Jakob disease is usually more widespread and the rate of progression faster than in CBD. Although the typical presentations of CBD and Pick's disease are clearly distinguishable, atypical cases of either may cause difficulty. Pick's disease typically presents with a frontotemporal dementia with prominent conduct disorder and personality change. Some atypical cases may have parkinsonism, gait disturbances, and focal cortical deficits. Similarly, some unusual CBD cases present with a frontal dementia and little motor dysfunction (Bergeron *et al.* 1996). There is therefore some clinical overlap between Pick's disease and CBD, as well as several pathological similarities. The precise relationship between these two disorders is unclear.

Investigations are usually unhelpful and the diagnosis of CBD remains clinical. CT or MR scans may show asymmetrical frontoparietal cerebral atrophy. PET studies show impaired nigrostriatal dopaminergic function and asymmetrical reductions in frontoparietal and thalamic blood flow and metabolic activity, corresponding to the areas of greatest neuronal degeneration (Sawle *et al.* 1991; Blin *et al.* 1992). Proton MRS may also detect cortical and subcortical involvement (Tedeschi *et al.* 1997).

The prognosis of CBD is poor, with most patients surviving between 5 and 10 years (Wenning *et al.* 1998). No effective treatment is available although clonazepam may help the myoclonus and tremor.

32.3.11 The problem of 'cerebrovascular parkinsonism'

The notion that cerebrovascular disease can cause 'parkinsonism' has caused much confusion and attracted much criticism.

Patients with multiple subcortical lacunar infarcts may develop a disturbance of gait, often with additional pseudobulbar and limb pyramidal signs, emotional lability, and dementia (subacute ateriosclerotic encephalopathy or Binswanger's disease). The legs show a curious inability to relax when examined, giving rise to an impression of rigidity referred to variously as paratonia or 'gegenhalten' (counterholding). There is usually a history of strokes, hypertension, or other vascular risk factors. The progression is stepwise with sudden deteriorations or recognizable acute lacunar strokes as well as periods of stabilization (Caplan 1995). This form of cerebrovascular disease has been recognized for many years and has been referred to as 'arteriosclerotic parkinsonism' (Critchley 1929). At first glance, the shuffling gait is superficially similar to that seen in Parkinson's disease with small steps, start hesitation, and freezing and has been described as 'lower half parkinsonism' (Thompson and Marsden 1987) but differs from Parkinson's disease because it is wide based and there is no festination or lack of arm swing. Mild rigidity and bradykinesia may be seen but this is symmetrical and there is no tremor or response to levodopa. Although Binswanger's disease has some similarities to Parkinson's disease, a distinction can usually be made on the basis of these clinical differences. Another helpful diagnostic point is that the gait disturbance in cerebrovascular disease is more severe than would be predicted from the physical signs detected on the examination couch. This has given rise to the notion of an apraxia of gait. Impaired function of the periventricular white matter of the frontal lobes is a feature of other disorders associated with this sort of gait, such as hydrocephalus, as well as cerebrovascular disease (etat lacunaire). CT scanning shows deep white matter periventricular low density changes and MRI reveals multiple lacunar subcortical infarcts. However, such neuroimaging abnormalities are common in the elderly, and must be interpreted with caution; the diagnosis of Binswanger's disease should be clinical and not radiological (Bennett *et al.* 1990). Although Critchley's description of Binswanger's disease as cerebrovascular parkinsonism has become unfashionable, it is not unreasonable providing that the clinical features (which were well described by Critchley) are borne in mind and not confused with those of idiopathic Parkinson's disease. A common dilemma in clinical practice is elderly patients with cerebrovascular risk factors and parkinsonism in whom the clinical features are not clear cut. In these individuals the possibility of both conditions occurring together cannot be excluded and a therapeutic trial of levodopa is the best policy.

Very occasionally, cerebrovascular disease produces an akinetic rigid syndrome similar to idiopathic Parkinson's disease (Hunter *et al.* 1978). Not only has levodopa responsive parkinsonism occurred (Mark *et al.* 1995) but the correct diagnosis is sometimes made only at post-mortem (Hughes *et al.* 1993*b*). It is difficult to be certain how often cerebrovascular disease produces true parkinsonism but such cases are probably rare.

32.3.12 Pallidal degenerations

These rare conditions are pathologically and clinically heterogeneous and there is no agreed classification. Onset may be in children or adults. They are often sporadic but autosomal recessive or dominant forms are well described (Jellinger 1968).

A progressive akinetic-rigid syndrome with or without additional dystonia is a characteristic phenotype. In some patients the dystonia is the dominant feature. Pathologically there may be a pure pallidal degeneration (Hunt 1917; Aizawa *et al.* 1991) or degeneration of the pallidum and other areas of the basal ganglia, especially the STN, substantia nigra, and striatum in various combinations. One striking disorder, pallido-ponto-nigral degeneration (rapid-onset dystonia parkinsonism) has a fast onset over hours or days of parkinsonism and dystonia, with additional features such as pyramidal signs, dysarthria, ophthalmoparesis, and dementia in some cases (Wszolek *et al.* 1992; Brashear *et al.* 1996). This condition is autosomal dominant, and is genetically heterogeneous. It has occurred with tau gene mutations on chromosome 17, Parkin gene mutations (see Section 32.3.3) and a gene locus on chromosome 19 (Wijker *et al.* 1996; Kramer *et al.* 1999). Occasionally, parkinsonism follows striatal necrosis (Miyoshi *et al.* 1969; Caparros-Lefebvre *et al.* 1997) inherited as a recessive or dominant trait and due to mitochondrial dysfunction (Thyagarajan *et al.* 1995). These patients usually have prominent dystonia but parkinsonism can occur.

Pallidopyramidal degeneration causes parkinsonism and pyramidal tract signs such as spasticity and extensor plantar responses (Davison 1954). There is sometimes a response to levodopa, even in pathologically confirmed cases. However, some other reports of levodopa responsive pallidopyramidal disease without pathological evidence of the diagnosis are difficult to evaluate as it is difficult to exclude dopa responsive dystonia (Section 32.4.5).

32.3.13 Other akinetic rigid states

Hereditary disorders

There are rare familial forms of parkinsonism without typical Lewy body pathology. Parkinsonism with depression and hypoventilation occurs in adult life with prominent apathy and mood change as well as respiratory irregularities which may be fatal (Perry *et al.* 1990). A good response to levodopa may be seen but the prognosis is poor. Inheritance is autosomal dominant. A dominantly inherited parkinsonism is seen with chromosome 17q21 linked fronto-temporal dementia due to tau gene mutation (Wilhelmsen *et al.* 1994). Hallervorden–Spatz disease is an autosomal recessive disorder causing degeneration principally of the pallidum and substantia nigra pars reticulata. The usual clinical features are severe dystonia, dementia, and spasticity in childhood, sometimes with retinal degeneration (Section 32.4.11) but an adult onset form has been described in which the presentation was familial adult onset parkinsonism (Jankovic *et al.* 1985). A hereditary X-linked dystonia–parkin-

sonism (Lubag) occurs in the Philippines and causes prominent dystonia with parkinsonism (Section 32.4.4). Parkinsonism may also occur in Huntington's disease, especially the juvenile Westphal variant (Section 32.5.2). Wilson's disease causes a large number of movement disorders including parkinsonism and must always be considered in patients with early onset (probably under 50 years) or atypical parkinsonism. Additional physical signs include corneal Kayser–Fleischer rings, unusual tremor, psychiatric abnormality, and liver dysfunction (Sternlieb *et al.* 1987). Patients in whom the condition is suspected should be screened by appropriate ophthalmological and biochemical testing (Section 32.8). Dopa responsive dystonia (DRD) may cause prominent parkinsonism, and may present as mild, easily treated parkinsonism in older patients. DRD may closely simulate young onset Parkinson's disease, with prominent lower limb dystonia (Section 32.4.5). However, there is an excellent and sustained response to levodopa without the development of fluctuation and dyskinesia which is so common in YOPD. This excellent response to small doses of levodopa may be the only way to establish the diagnosis in some cases. Parkinsonism is commonly seen in the adult onset

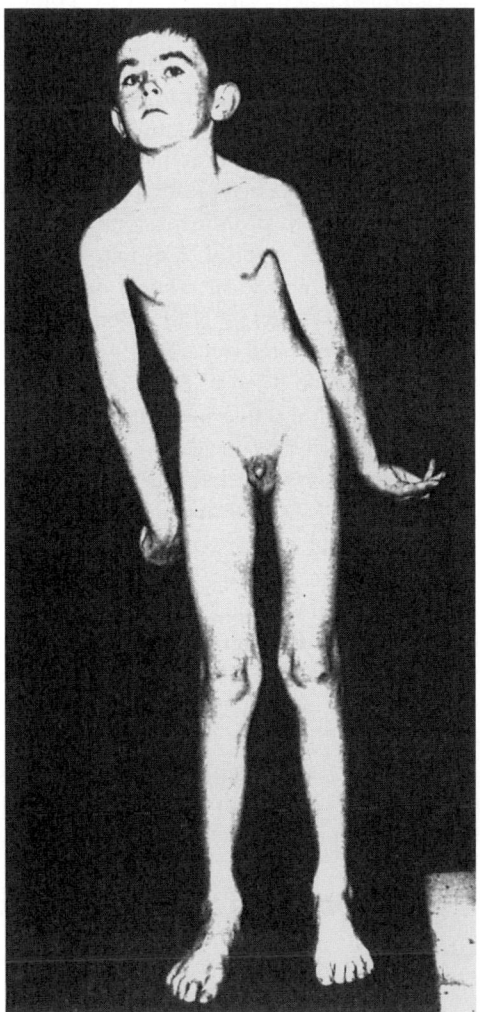

Fig. 32.13. A patient with generalized idiopathic torsion dystonia.

cerebellar degenerations, both sporadic and inherited. The akinetic rigid features are usually accompanied by other signs such as cerebellar ataxia, pyramidal signs, and peripheral neuropathy. Parkinsonism is especially typical of Machado–Joseph disease (*SCA3*) but may occur in other forms of degenerative cerebellar ataxia (Sections 31.9 and 31.10).

Degenerative disorders

The hemiparkinsonism–hemiatrophy syndrome is characterized by unilateral parkinsonism with a variable degree of atrophy of the same side of the body, sometimes just the hand or alternatively the face and limbs (Klawans 1981). The parkinsonism may become bilateral but is strikingly asymmetrical and there is sometimes contralateral cerebral atrophy detected on CT scans. Onset is typically in adult life and there may be slow progression. The response to levodopa is variable. Alzheimer's disease causes parkinsonism in addition to dementia in some patients. This is seen in advanced cases and is due to a number of factors including neuroleptic medication and coexistent Lewy body parkinsonism; some patients have a non-Lewy body degeneration of the substantia nigra (Morris *et al.* 1989). Some patients do not have any nigral abnormality when studied by PET or at post-mortem, indicating some other extranigral

process. Dopa responsive dystonia (see Section 32.4.4) can produce a similar phenotype (Greene *et al.* 2000).

Structural disease

Hydrocephalus typically presents with headache or with a combination of impaired gait, cognitive decline, and urinary incontinence. The gait disorder is similar to that seen in Binswanger's disease but some patients have had parkinsonism. This seems to be due to the effects of the hydrocephalus as well as coexistent Parkinson's disease or other forms of degenerative parkinsonism (Curran and Lang 1994). Some of these patients have responded to levodopa. Space occupying lesions such as tumours or subdural haematomas may very rarely cause parkinsonism, possibly due to compression of a cerebral peduncle or distortion of the basal ganglia. These cases have resembled Parkinson's disease initially and diagnosis can be delayed by the fact that brain scanning is not routine practice in otherwise typical parkinsonism.

Miscellaneous rare causes of parkinsonism

Cerebral anoxia may cause delayed parkinsonism and basal ganglia necrosis (Straussberg *et al.* 1993). Such patients are more likely to develop dystonia. Creutzfeldt–Jakob disease

Table 32.9. Hereditary dystonias

Type of dystonia	Subtypes	Genetics	Gene	Locus	Dystonia Gene
Primary torsion dystonia (PTD)		AD	Torsin A	9q34	DYT 1
		AD		8p21–q22	DYT 6
		AD		18p31	DYT 7
		AD	other loci		DYT 5
		Sporadic			
Dopa responsive dystonia (DRD)		AD	GTPCH1	14q22.3	DYT 5
		AR	Tyrosine	11p15.5	
		AR	hydroxylase 6-PTS		
Myoclonic dystonia		AD	Dopamine D2 receptor	7q21	DYT 11
Paroxysmal dystonias	Paroxysmal dystonic choreoathetosis (PDC)	AD	?	2q33–35	DYT 8
	Paroxysmal kinesiogenic choreoathetosis (PKC)	AD	?	16p11–12	DYT 10
	Intermediate PDC	AD	?		
Other hereditary dystonias	Rapidly progressive dystonia-parkinsonism	AD		19q13	DYT 12
	Deafness & dystonia	XL		Xq22	
	X-linked dystonia-parkinsonism	XL		Xq13	DYT 3
	Dystonia & mental retardation (Partington syndrome)	XL		Xp22	
	18q deletion syndrome	Sporadic mutation		18q22	

AD = autosomal dominant, AR = autosomal recessive, XL = X linked. For other abbreviations, see text. * existence of autosomal recessive PTD unlikely.

Table 32.10. Symptomatic dystonias

Category	Conditions
Rare metabolic disorders	**Wilson's disease***
	Caeruloplasmin deficiency
	Organic acidurias*
	GM1 gangliosidosis
	GM2 gangliosidosis
	Hexosaminidase A and B deficiency
	Lesch–Nyhan disease
	Neimann–Pick disease type C
	Metachromatic leucodystrophy
	Pelizaeus–Merzbacher disease
	Homocystinuria
	Neuronal ceroid lipofuscinosis (Kuf's)
	Triosephosphate isomerase deficiency
	Hartnup disease
Mitochondrial disorders	Leigh's disease*
	Leber's disease*
	Familial striatal necrosis*
Hereditary conditions	**Huntington's disease**
	Hereditary cerebellar degenerations
	Hallervorden–Spatz disease*
	Pallidal degenerations
	Neuroacanthocytosis
	Fahr syndrome
	Ataxia telangiectasia
Degenerative disorders	**Parkinson's disease**
	Multiple system atrophy
	Steele–Richardson–Olszewski disease
	Corticobasal degeneration
	Rett syndrome
Drug-induced dystonia	**Neuroleptics** (tardive dystonia)
	Levodopa (in Parkinson's disease)
	Others
Acquired disorders	**Athetoid cerebral palsy***
	Basal ganglia lesions, e.g. stroke, tumour, AVM
	Cerebral anoxia*
	Cerebral trauma
	Toxins,* e.g. manganese, CO, CS_2 methanol
	Osmotic myelinolysis
	Multiple sclerosis
	Hypoparathyroidism
	Encephalitis
	Haemolytic uraemic syndrome
	Wasp sting encephalopathy*
	Brainstem lesions
	Cervical cord lesions
	Peripheral trauma†

The principal causes of secondary dystonia are shown in bold type. Other causes are rare.
* Associated with low density basal ganglia lesions on CT/MRI.
† Probably exacerbates or precipitates PTD.

usually causes rapidly progressive dementia with myoclonus and ataxia but parkinsonism may occur occasionally (Sections 26.6.5, 34.12). Neuroacanthocytosis (Section 32.5.8) and Rett syndrome (Section 4.6.10) are distinctive disorders which can have akinetic rigid features. Parkinsonism also occurs in basal ganglia calcification. This may be secondary to hypoparathyroidism or it may be a hereditary disorder with normal calcium metabolism (Martinelli *et al.* 1993). Chronic liver failure, with repeated episodes of hepatic encephalopathy may be followed by the development of a chronic hepatocerebral degeneration, in which parkinsonism is a major feature.

32.4 The dystonias

32.4.1 Diagnosis and classification of dystonia

Dystonia has been defined as '*a syndrome of sustained muscle contractions, frequently causing twisting and repetitive movements or abnormal postures*' (Fahn *et al.* 1987). It is important to remember that dystonia is a type of involuntary movement and is no more a diagnosis than spasticity, ataxia, or any other physical sign although it is often used as a shorthand for its most common cause, primary torsion dystonia (PTD, see below). Dystonic movements are typically twisting and involve proximal more than distal muscles (Fig. 32.13). The eyes may close forcefully (blepharospasm), there may be jaw and tongue movements (oromandibular dystonia), or the neck may twist to one side, forward, or backwards (torticollis, antecollis, and retrocollis). If there is involvement of the bulbar muscles, there may be dysarthria, dysphagia, and impaired facial and tongue movements but no increased jaw jerk, the so-called 'striatal' pseudobulbar palsy. In the limbs, an arm will often twist and pronate and there may be spasm of the hand, especially with writing (writer's cramp) or other fine movements. Dystonia in a leg typically causes inversion and plantar flexion of the foot, often with extension of the big toe. This makes interpretation of the plantar response unreliable (the striatal pseudobabinski response or striatal foot). The trunk may be involved with scoliosis, extension, or flexion spasms (axial dystonia). Dystonic movements are often *action specific*, so that the hand may assume an abnormal posture only when writing and not during other actions such as shaving or typing. The gait may be abnormal with dystonic trunk and limb spasms and postures but the patient may be able to run or walk backwards normally. Action specificity may erroneously suggest a psychiatric disorder but is typical of dystonia. Sometimes there is *overflow dystonia* in which dystonic movements appear in other body parts which are not normally involved in the execution of a particular movement. Curiously, many patients display sensory tricks or *gestes antagonistiques* by which the movements may be suppressed, such as touching the face to correct torticollis, chewing to correct oromandibular dystonia, or holding a cane to correct a dystonic gait. There is considerable variation; the movements may be mobile and repetitive or fixed into abnormal postures. Sometimes, repetitive dystonic spasms lead to a tremulous appearance (myorhythmia) or jerking similar to myoclonus. The diagnosis of dystonia is clinical and may be difficult, requiring considerable experience.

Dystonia is often described clinically in terms of its anatomical extent. *Generalized dystonia* affects the legs, trunk, and often other body parts; *segmental dystonia* involves adjacent areas of a body region such as the cranial musculature or an arm and the neck; and *focal dystonia* affects only one site such as the neck, eyes, or a hand. *Hemidystonia* is usually due to a structural lesion of the contralateral basal ganglia.

The most important classification of dystonia is by aetiology (Tables 32.9 and 32.10). In clinical practice, the main distinction is between PTD and an alternative cause. A secondary dystonia is more likely in those with childhood or adolescent onset and with generalized dystonia. Hemidystonia is due to a contralateral cerebral structural lesion in 80 per cent of cases (Marsden and Quinn 1990).

32.4.2 **Primary torsion dystonia (dystonia musculorum deformans)**

Definition and prevalence

PTD causes a pure dystonic syndrome without any detectable underlying cause clinically or after investigation, and neuropathological abnormalities are absent. The concept of PTD was originally proposed to distinguish cases of dystonia without any obvious underlying cause from those due to Wilson's disease, lethargic encephalitis, or athetoid cerebral palsy (Herz 1944). The term is now rather confusing because although most patients with dystonia have PTD, a genetic aetiology has been established in many so that many cases of PTD are no longer 'idiopathic'.

The prevalence of PTD is approximately 330/million (Nutt *et al.* 1988) in the USA. The condition is more common in Ashkenazi Jews than would be expected by chance (Risch *et al.* 1995).

Diagnosis and clinical features

Although PTD may start in childhood, birth and early developmental milestones are normal and there should be no history of neonatal hypoxic-ischaemic encephalopathy or kernicterus. A detailed history is needed to distinguish PTD from dystonia caused by other neurological disorders or neuroleptic drugs (see Table 32.10). The symptoms and level of disability are obviously determined by the extent of the dystonia and the sites involved. PTD is highly variable, ranging from severe disabling generalized dystonia in childhood, to mild focal dystonia appearing in later life. Although some patients can have a mild postural tremor, no other neurological abnormalities occur. Dystonia is worse with emotion or stress and improved by relaxation; it disappears in sleep. There is a clear association between age and site of onset of PTD and the eventual severity of the dystonia. Generalized dystonia develops in the majority (80 per cent) of childhood onset

cases and about a third of adolescents; it is so rare (1–2 per cent) in adult onset cases (after age 20 years) that the diagnosis of PTD must be made with great caution. Most patients with PTD starting in adult life develop segmental or focal dystonia (Marsden and Harrison 1974; Fahn *et al.* 1987). The site of onset is also associated with age of onset and severity, so that early onset PTD usually starts in a leg, less commonly an arm. Later onset focal PTD usually starts in cranial or axial muscles or sometimes an arm. Consequently, most generalized cases start in childhood, focal cases appear mainly in adults (usually in the fourth to sixth decades), and segmental cases seem to commence over a wide age range (Fletcher *et al.* 1990).

Initially there are intermittent action-specific dystonic spasms but overflow dystonia (in other body areas during movement) and fixed dystonic postures may appear later. Affected children usually have a dystonic gait which may appear bizarre; a typical presentation at this age is inturning of a foot or a peculiar axial posture when walking or running. This may lead to a fall as the presenting feature. It is important to recognize the dystonic nature or action specificity of the movement to avoid the common misdiagnosis of psychiatric disease. Subsequent progression to generalized PTD is gradual over several years. Generalized PTD is severely incapacitating, leading to loss of walking and difficulty with upper limb function, speech, and swallowing. Such children may erroneously be thought to have athetoid cerebral palsy. Cognitive abilities, sphincter control, vision, hearing, sensory function, and the peripheral nerves are not affected and seizures do not occur. Eventually, speech and swallowing are affected but this is rare in the early stages. Once generalized dystonia has developed it is stable. Relentless and continuous deterioration throughout the life of the patient is not seen in PTD and suggests a secondary cause.

In adults the usual presentations are with writer's cramp, torticollis, or one of the other cranial focal dystonias. In most cases the dystonia remains localized and focal but in some there may be gradual progression over 5–10 years to contiguous body areas so that a segmental pattern evolves. Clinically, the various forms of focal PTD are fragments of generalized dystonia. In **torticollis**, there is intermittent or fixed turning of the head to one side. Sometimes the head moves backwards, forward, or laterally. In some patients this is a forceful slow movement, but in others it is tremulous. In such cases, the true nature of the tremor is indicated by an additional tilt or turn of the head due to the dystonia. Pain in the neck or shoulder is common and the torticollis may be more obvious when standing and walking than at rest. **Blepharospasm** causes forceful closure of the eyes with spasm of the orbicularis oculi muscles (Grandas *et al.* 1988). The eyes appear screwed up and the patient is unable to open them. This often occurs in bright sunlight or when watching television. In some patients the spasms are confined to the pretarsal section of the orbicularis oculi muscles so that the eyes lightly close (levator inhibition or apraxia of eyelid opening) (Elston 1992; Krack and Marion 1994). **Oromandibular dystonia** causes spasms of the jaw, tongue, and mouth. The jaw may open or forcefully close and the lip movements cause embarrassing facial movements. Chewing and eating are difficult along with speech. **Laryngeal dystonia** causes altered speech but with normal appearance of the larynx and cords at rest. Such patients are often thought to have a psychogenic disorder after a series of normal ENT examinations. The vocal cords may go into adductor spasm with a strained strangulated speech or forceful abduction which causes a quiet whispery voice. The problem may be permanent or intermittent and some patients are still able to sing or whisper normally. The most common upper limb dystonia is **writer's cramp**. During writing there are involuntary movements of the fingers or wrist; sometimes the whole arm adopts a dystonic posture. Writing may become impossible and some patients are forced to type or use the other hand which may subsequently become affected. This may affect writing only (simple writer's cramp) or other actions such as shaving (dystonic writer's cramp). Similar action-specific upper limb focal dystonia may be seen in typists, golfers, darts players, or musicians. **Axial dystonia** causes twisting, flexion, or extension of the spine, often worse when standing or walking but disappearing when lying supine. In some patients the trunk movement may be tremulous (Rivest and Marsden 1990). In all these forms of PTD remissions are uncommon and not usually sustained.

Genetics and aetiology

No consistent biochemical or pathological abnormality has been detected in PTD. In secondary dystonia altered dopaminergic function and basal ganglia lesions are frequently

Table 32.11. Investigations in suspected secondary dystonia

CT/MR scan

Nerve conduction studies

Evoked potentials (if clinically indicated)

Copper and caeruloplasmin levels
24-h urinary copper excretion
Slit lamp examination for KF rings

Biochemistry screen including calcium and liver function
Blood count and film for acanthocytes
CK level
α-Fetoprotein
Immunoglobulins
White cell enzymes
Blood and urinary amino acids
Urinary organic acids
Blood gases, lactate, pyruvate
CSF examination and lactate level
Skin and rectal biopsies (storage diseases)
Bone marrow examination (trephine for sea blue histiocytes)
Muscle biopsy (mitochondrial diseases)
DNA testing (mitochondrial diseases, Huntington's, cerebellar degenerations)

These investigations are intended as a guide only. The tests required in individual cases will be influenced by clinical probabilities and the age of the patient.

implicated but these have not been detected reliably in PTD. Some alterations of catecholamine levels have been reported (Hornykiewicz *et al.* 1988) but the significance of these is unclear and further studies are required. PET scanning has suggested mild alteration of nigrostriatal dopaminergic function but this is not marked (Playford *et al.* 1993). A basal ganglia mechanism underlying the dystonia is assumed on the basis of the frequent location of causative lesions in secondary dystonia but brainstem dysfunction may also be responsible (Zweig *et al.* 1988) and other areas of the CNS are sometimes implicated in secondary dystonia (Section 32.2.2). Clinical observations and an increased incidence among Ashkenazi Jews have long indicated a genetic basis for the disorder. About 50 per cent of patients with generalized or segmental PTD have affected relatives (Fletcher *et al.* 1990). It is now established that in the majority of generalized and segmental cases or those affected as children or young adults (which amounts to the same thing), PTD is caused by an autosomal dominant gene with 30–40 per cent penetrance and highly variable expression. A recessive form of PTD (DYT2) is unlikely. Similar inheritance has been demonstrated in Jewish and non-Jewish patients (Bressman *et al.* 1989; Fletcher *et al.* 1990). The higher incidence in the former is probably due to a genetic founder effect with a high gene frequency in Eastern Europe centuries ago (Fletcher *et al.* 1990). In families containing at least one case of early onset PTD, affected individuals may show only mild late onset focal dystonia or tremor and some obligate gene carriers are asymptomatic. There is also an increased family history of tremor and stuttering in such families suggesting that these may be minor manifestations of autosomal dominant PTD (Fletcher *et al.* 1991a). Sporadic cases are mainly due to new dominant mutations and inheritance of PTD from asymptomatic gene carrier parents; about 15 per cent may be non-genetic phenocopies. In the majority of Jewish and non-Jewish families with early onset limb dystonia, (Kramer *et al.* 1990; Warner *et al.* 1993) PTD is linked to a locus (DXT1) on chromosome 9q34. This gene has now been cloned and sequenced revealing a 3 base pair deletion in a gene encoding an ATP binding protein, torsinA (Ozelius *et al.* 1997).

In some non-Jewish families, autosomal dominant PTD is not linked to 9q34 (Bressman *et al.* 1994a,b, 1996; Holmgren *et al.* 1995; Bentivoglio *et al.* 1997). Clinically such families often contain affected individuals with prominent axial and cranial dystonia with later onset. In two American Mennonite families with early onset PTD, a gene on chromosome 8p21–8q22 (DYT6) appears to be responsible (Bressman *et al.* 1994a,b; Almasy *et al.* 1997). Among sporadic PTD cases, the DYT1 mutation is found in a few early onset generalized cases but is often absent (Valente *et al.* 1998; Brassat *et al.* 2000).

The genetic basis of the much more common adult onset focal PTD (in patients without more severely affected relatives) is less clear. In Germany, autosomal dominant torticollis is associated with a gene (DYT7) on chromosome 18p31 (Leube *et al.* 1996) and there is evidence that many patients with sporadic torticollis have inherited the same gene (Leube *et al.* 1997). The

9q34 PTD gene is not responsible for focal PTD in Jewish patients (Gasser *et al.* 1996). Two studies have shown that approximately 25 per cent of focal cases have affected relatives compared to 50 per cent of those with generalized or segmental disease (Waddy *et al.* 1991; Stojanovic *et al.* 1995). Accordingly, focal PTD may be more heterogeneous with a higher proportion of non-genetic cases possibly caused by environmental factors. These may also be involved in the highly varied expression of autosomal dominant PTD (Fletcher *et al.* 1991*b*). Overuse of a body part such as in musicians or manual workers has long been associated with the development of focal dystonia in the body part concerned. Such patients do not usually have the DYT1 mutation (Friedman *et al.* 2000). Moreover, there is a long recognized association between dystonia and preceding local trauma (Fletcher *et al.* 1991*c*). This cannot be due to trauma alone because a history of injury is no more common among PTD patients than controls (Fletcher *et al.* 1991). An interaction between trauma and a pre-existing (possibly genetic) predisposition seems possible. Examples of local injury or pain followed by dystonia include limb dystonia after fractures and lacerations, oromandibular dystonia after dental surgery, blepharospasm after eye disease, and torticollis after neck injuries. It should be noted that existing PTD may be exacerbated by surgical procedures and orthopaedic correction of dystonic deformity is therefore unwise (Fletcher *et al.* 1991*c*).

Investigations and diagnosis

The diagnosis of PTD is clinical but investigations are required to exclude other causes of dystonia, particularly Wilson's disease in some patients (Fahn *et al.* 1987). Athetoid cerebral palsy is excluded by enquiring about the perinatal history and subsequent motor developmental delay. Many other causes of secondary dystonia are also readily apparent from the patient's history which should not suggest any other cause, especially exposure to neuroleptic drugs. In PTD there are no other neurological abnormalities, intellect is preserved, and seizures do not occur. As has been mentioned, some patients do have a mild postural tremor. Some features of the dystonia might suggest a secondary cause rather than PTD such as lower limb onset or generalization in an adult, relentless deterioration without stabilization, early speech or swallowing involvement, hemidystonia, or the initial appearance of fixed dystonic postures. In patients with typical PTD, the degree of investigation will depend on age and severity. In younger patients (under 50) it is essential to exclude Wilson's disease by serum copper and caeruloplasmin estimations and a slit lamp examination for Kayser–Fleischer rings. If there is any doubt about the results a liver biopsy is indicated (Section 32.8). Most younger patients will also require MR brain scanning, routine blood count and film for acanthocytes, liver function tests, and calcium estimation. Older patients with typical late onset focal PTD probably do not require investigations. If there are atypical features to suggest a secondary dystonia, regardless of age, detailed investigation is required (Table 32.11) to exclude a secondary dystonia.

Treatment

It cannot be overemphasized that the diagnosis of PTD must not be made in younger patients without a therapeutic trial of levodopa to exclude dopa responsive dystonia (DRD) (Section 32.4.4). An adequate trial consists of 600 mg of levodopa per day (with a PDI) for at least 3 months. If there is no response, DRD is excluded and treatment for PTD can be initiated. High dose anticholinergic therapy, usually with benzhexol (trihexphenidyl), is the treatment of choice with over 50 per cent of patients obtaining significant improvement (Burke *et al.* 1986). The dose of benzhexol is initially very small with gradual slow increases over several months. Doses of up to 120 mg/day may be required and a useful response is unlikely below 30 mg daily. The drug is tolerated better in children than adults due to dose-related side effects including sedation, dry mouth, and blurred vision. Occasionally patients develop chorea (Nomoto *et al.* 1987). A better response is seen in patients treated soon after the onset of the dystonia (Greene *et al.* 1988). In patients with severe generalized dystonia, a combination of high dose benzhexol with tetrabenazine and a dopamine receptor blocker such as pimozide ('triple therapy') may be effective but at the expense of side effects such as parkinsonism and depression (Marsden *et al.* 1984*a*). Other drugs are of limited value. Baclofen may be helpful in some patients and there are occasional reports of improvement with benzodiazepines but these drugs have not been evaluated scientifically (Greene *et al.* 1988). Tetrabenazine alone may help in some cases (Jankovic and Orman 1988) but side effects are common. In some very severely affected patients with generalized dystonia, intrathecal baclofen has been effective (Albright *et al.* 1996; Paret *et al.* 1996) but in other patients the results were unimpressive (Ford *et al.* 1996).

Focal PTD is now frequently treated with local intramuscular type A botulinum toxin. The toxin binds to presynaptic cholinergic nerve terminals and cleaves proteins required for fusion of acetylcholine containing vesicles and the presynaptic membrane (Blasi *et al.* 1993). This leads to chemically induced denervation of the injected muscle. Weakness and atrophy appear after several days and the effect lasts for 3–6 months depending on the dose, the site treated, and the severity of the dystonia. This treatment has been used for over 10 years in a wide range of focal dystonias (Greene *et al.* 1994). In blepharospasm, over 90 per cent of patients improve for up to 4 months after periocular injections. Ptosis may occur in about 10 per cent of cases but is usually temporary; bruising and dryness of the eyes are occasionally troublesome. Some patients with pretarsal blepharospasm fail to respond unless the pretarsal orbicularis oculis muscle is specifically injected. In torticollis, 70–80 per cent of patients are improved in terms of reduced dystonia and relief of local muscular pain. The pattern of the head movement will determine the sites of injection. The effect lasts 3–4 months after which the treatment is repeated. The results with botulinum toxin are superior to anticholinergic therapy (Brans *et al.* 1996). Side effects include dysphagia in 10–20 per cent of cases but this is usually mild and resolves within

2 weeks. Occasionally patients develop severe dysphagia requiring nasogastric feeding in hospital and all patients must be warned of this possibility and offered prompt review if swallowing is badly affected. Some patients develop antibodies to the toxin which usually causes loss of effect. In these patients the type B toxin may be effective (Brin *et al.* 1999). This is more likely after larger doses and more frequent injections. Accordingly the minimum effective toxin dose should be used and patients should be treated as infrequently as their dystonia permits. Botulinum toxin injections may also improve writer's cramp (Cole *et al.* 1995; Wissel *et al.* 1996) and although most studies have used EMG guided injections, good results have been obtained without this (Rivest *et al.* 1991). Although the dystonia is reduced, weakness of the arm is inevitable if improvement is to be seen. EMG guided laryngeal injections have been effective in laryngeal dystonia (Greene *et al.* 1994) but adductor spasms respond better than whispering abductor dystonia. Other PTD patients with oromandibular dystonia, and dystonia of the lower limbs and axial muscles have been treated successfully with local botulinum toxin. Some patients who are not improved by drugs or botulinum toxin may respond to stereotactic thalamotomy (Andrew *et al.* 1983; Cardoso *et al.* 1995) but the results are unpredictable. Side effects including dysarthria may occur, especially after bilateral procedures. Those with peripheral and mainly unilateral dystonia tend to improve more. In patients with torticollis who do not respond to botulinum toxin, selective surgical denervation of the cervical muscles has been effective (Bertrand 1993). There is increasing interest in pallidotomy (Ondo *et al.* 1998) and pallidal stimulation (Kumar *et al.* 1999) in PTD and some secondary dystonias.

32.4.3 X-linked dystonia

A form of X-linked dystonia (DYT3) has been reported in the Philippines. Affected men usually develop focal dystonia at 30–45 years of age and this usually generalizes after a few years. There is prominent dystonia of the legs and often the axial and cranial areas with parkinsonism and tremor (Lee *et al.* 1976). Females are occasionally affected but not as severely. Pathologically there is gliosis and neuronal loss in the striatum and PET studies reveal impaired striatal metabolism but normal nigrostriatal dopaminergic function (Eidelberg *et al.* 1993*b*). The gene has been located on chromosome Xq13 (Haberhausen *et al.* 1995) but the molecular basis of the disorder is otherwise unclear. Treatment is ineffective.

32.4.4 Dopa responsive dystonia (DRD) (DYT5)

This is a rare disorder, probably accounting for 5–10 per cent of all childhood onset dystonia with a population frequency of about 0.5 per million (Nygaard *et al.* 1993). It is nevertheless, one of the most important clinical diagnoses in clinical neurology as it is effectively cured by small doses of levodopa, even

after many decades of severe neurological disability. DRD occurs in women three times more frequently and more severely than in men. Patients often have a family history suggesting autosomal dominant inheritance; penetrance of the DRD gene is approximately 45 per cent in women and 15 per cent in men. Typically the onset is in the first decade but some patients have a congenital onset with delayed motor milestones and others develop DRD in adolescence or adult life. In children dystonia of the legs and feet causes stiffness of the lower limbs, inturning of the feet, and toe walking (Nygaard 1995). The gait may appear dystonic or spastic and pyramidal signs including spasticity, ankle clonus, and extensor plantar responses are often present along with mild Parkinsonian cogwheel rigidity and bradykinesia of the upper limbs. Most patients gradually progress to generalized dystonia but other neurological features such as cognitive impairment or seizures do not occur. In some childhood onset cases the dystonia is mild and remains confined to the feet and others have focal dystonia such as torticollis. In older patients there is often mild parkinsonism, including rest tremor, showing an unusually good and sustained response to small doses of levodopa (Nygaard 1995). Diurnal fluctuation of symptoms with improvement in the morning or after sleep and increasing dystonia later in the day or after exercise is characteristic of DRD but may be absent.

Investigations are unhelpful in this condition; cerebral imaging is normal and correct diagnosis depends entirely on a high index of suspicion and readiness to deploy a therapeutic trial of levodopa in cases where DRD is even a remote clinical possibility. There is a particular danger of an erroneous diagnosis of athetoid or spastic diplegic cerebral palsy or hereditary spastic paraplegia from which DRD cannot always be reliably distinguished. This means that DRD must be considered in any child or young adult with dystonia or unexplained paraparesis or gait disorder. In DRD the response to levodopa is dramatic; dystonia is rapidly abolished even after decades without treatment. Although many patients require only 50–100 mg of levodopa per day (with a PDI) this is variable; accordingly it is advisable to try at least 600 mg (with a PDI) per day for 3 months before concluding that the patient does not have DRD.

A further diagnostic difficulty is the distinction between DRD and early onset Parkinson's disease in which prominent lower limb dystonia and parkinsonism may also occur (Section 32.3.3). In DRD, significant motor fluctuations and dyskinesias never develop whereas they appear at an early stage after starting levodopa in Parkinson's disease. Accordingly this distinction cannot always be made with confidence until the response to levodopa has been observed for a few years. It should be noted that a few patients with DRD do develop mild chorea on levodopa but this often disappears if the dose is reduced. An alternative but not widely available method is to examine the dopaminergic nigrostriatal system with PET; this is normal in DRD but abnormal in Parkinson's disease (Nygaard *et al.* 1992; Naumann *et al.* 1997).

Biochemically DRD is characterized by a striking reduction in CNS dopamine metabolism with reduced CSF dopamine metabolites and tetrahydrobiopterin (BH4, a co-factor for tyrosine hydroxylase) (Le Witt *et al.* 1986). Pathologically there are normal numbers of nigral neurons but these are hypopigmented (Rajput *et al.* 1994); striatal dopamine is reduced with normal levels of tyrosine hydroxylase immunoreactivity but reduced enzyme activity. The condition is caused by deletion (Furukawa *et al.* 2000) or point mutations of the GTP cyclohydrolase 1 (*GTPCH*) gene (Ichinose *et al.* 1994) which is located on chromosome 14q (Nygaard *et al.* 1993). *GTPCH* is required for tetrahydrobiopterin (BH4) synthesis, hence the reduced TH activity in the disorder. Some DRD families do not have a detectable GTPCH mutation (Bandmann *et al.* 1996) and the genetic basis of these cases is uncertain. There is a very rare autosomal recessive form of DRD caused by a missense point mutation of the TH gene (Bartholome and Ludecke 1998).

32.4.5 Paroxysmal dystonias

This is a heterogeneous group of disorders in which there are attacks of involuntary movements and complete recovery in between the episodes. The movements may be dystonic but are sometimes choreiform, ballistic, or mixed. For convenience they will be discussed with the dystonias. In some of the disorders the attacks are brief while others are more prolonged; some are triggered by movement while others are set off by other factors and paroxysmal dyskinesias may be familial or sporadic. In some cases, an underlying cause such as a focal brain lesion is apparent whereas others are idiopathic. Although other classifications have been proposed (Demirkiran and Jankovic 1995), the most clinically useful approach is to divide the paroxysmal dyskinesias as follows:

◆ brief attacks typically induced by movement (paroxysmal kinesigenic choreoathetosis);

◆ more prolonged, usually non-kinesigenic attacks;

◆ an intermediate form with longer attacks induced by prolonged exercise.

Paroxysmal kinesigenic choreoathetosis (PKC) (DYT10)

This condition usually develops in childhood or adolescence and is more common in females. The attacks are brief, lasting seconds or a few minutes and may occur many times a day. There is typically a prominent flurry of dystonic or choreiform movements which may be preceded by an altered sensation in the affected area such as stiffness or tingling. The movements may be unilateral or bilateral and although there may be falling, this is unusual. The majority of patients with PKC report that the episodes are triggered by sudden movement or a startle such as suddenly running or jumping up quickly from a seat but sometimes the initiating stimulus is absent or not related to movement such as hyperventilation or anxiety. There is no disturbance of consciousness or residual symptoms after the attack but there is a short refractory period during which another

attack cannot be induced. A good response to carbamazepine or other anticonvulsants is characteristic of PKC which is usually easily brought under control (Fahn 1994a; Wein *et al.* 1996). The majority of cases are idiopathic and these may be sporadic or familial with an autosomal dominant mode of inheritance. Investigations in such cases are all normal, including the EEG. Rarely PKC is secondary to some other underlying cerebral condition such as multiple sclerosis, head injury, stroke, or congenital cerebral malformations (Fahn 1994a). Most of the responsible lesions are in the thalamus, internal capsule, or basal ganglia but PKC may also follow brainstem or cervical cord lesions (Cosentino *et al.* 1996; Riley 1996). The attacks of PKC in multiple sclerosis often follow hyperventilation and are in many respects similar to the tonic spasms characteristic of that condition. There has been much debate as to whether PKC is a manifestation of epilepsy; this matter has never been entirely resolved. The preservation of consciousness and lack of post-ictal features do not exclude epilepsy although the nature of the movements suggests a subcortical basal ganglia origin and PKC is not currently regarded as a manifestation of epilepsy. This has obvious implications for employment and driving. The gene for PKC has been mapped to chromosome 16p11.2–12.1 (Bennett *et al.* 2000).

Paroxysmal (non-kinesigenic) dystonic choreoathetosis (PDC) (DYT8)

In PDC the attacks are also a mixture of dystonia and chorea but they are more prolonged, lasting minutes to hours. The frequency is much lower, with only two or three attacks per day at most and often less than this. Onset is more variable than with PKC, ranging from childhood up to middle age. The episodes are often precipitated by alcohol, caffeine, stress, or fatigue but not movement. Falling may be seen and a sensory aura is sometimes present. Most cases are idiopathic and these may be hereditary (autosomal dominant) or sporadic. In one family some affected relatives only had exercise-induced cramps while others had typical PDC attacks but only after prolonged exertion similar to that reported in the intermediate form (see below) (Schloesser *et al.* 1996). In familial or sporadic cases investigations are predictably normal and the diagnosis is clinical. Sporadic cases are often thought to be psychogenic and it may be difficult to exclude this possibility. Treatment is often unsuccessful but there may be a good response to clonazepam. Recently, autosomal dominant PDC has been assigned to a locus on chromosome 2q36–37 (Fink *et al.* 1996; Jarman *et al.* 1997) possibly involving the *SLC4A3* chloride/bicarbonate anion exchanger gene. Symptomatic PDC is less common than the hereditary form but has been reported with multiple sclerosis, a variety of other focal cerebral lesions, or hypoglycaemia.

Intermediate paroxysmal dystonic choreoathetosis (IDC)

The intermediate form is characterized by attacks which last 5–30 min, longer than in PKC but shorter than in PDC. They are induced by movement but this takes the form of prolonged exercise lasting several minutes (Lance 1977; Plant *et al.* 1984). There is no response to anticonvulsants or clonazepam. Most cases are familial with autosomal dominant inheritance, but a few sporadic cases have been reported.

32.4.6 Dyskinetic (athetoid) cerebral palsy

Cerebral palsy (CP) is a clinically and pathologically heterogeneous group of congenital disorders caused by damage to the immature brain, characterized by abnormalities of motor control (Section 4.2). Various motor abnormalities and other neurological impairments are seen and CP is divided into ataxic, spastic, and athetoid subtypes. In dyskinetic CP, the abnormal movements are principally dystonic and although the term athetosis was originally proposed to describe the movement disorder in these patients, there is no logical reason to use it other than as a historical diagnostic label for dyskinetic CP. Some clinicians differentiate dystonic and dyskinetic CP on the basis that the movements are slow or fixed in the former and more mobile in the latter but such variability has always been accommodated by the term dystonia. Nevertheless, the term dyskinetic CP is in common usage and will be used here. Dyskinetic CP mainly occurs in infants born at term; the birth histories are variable. In the past, severe neonatal jaundice, usually secondary to fetomaternal Rhesus or ABO blood group incompatibility, was a common cause of dyskinetic CP (*kernicterus*). Affected children had severe dystonia, deafness, dental abnormalities, abnormal eye movements, and mental retardation. Pathological changes affected the basal ganglia and brainstem (status dysmyelinatus). The other major group are those children with a history of significant perinatal asphyxia due to a clearly defined obstetric complication (Hagberg and Hagberg 1993). In these patients there will have been severe fetal distress and poor Apgar scores (<3) lasting 20 min with signs of significant neonatal hypoxic-ischaemic encephalopathy. These include hypotonia, impaired consciousness, irritability, and seizures. Pathologically there was damage attributed to ischaemic in the thalami and basal ganglia (status marmoratus) (Friede 1989). In many patients however, these features are absent and the birth history is normal. The aetiology of the dyskinetic CP in these patients is unknown. It seems unlikely that all cases of dyskinetic CP are due to perinatal asphyxia or kernicterus. Not all patients have ischaemic lesions in the basal ganglia on MRI and neuropathological studies have been limited. Not all patients have ischaemic lesions at autopsy and those who do may not be representative of the majority of dyskinetic CP patients who survive (Fletcher and Marsden 1996).

Clinically the patients may have signs of hypotonia in the neonatal period but this is variable. Some are normal initially but there is always abnormal motor development with delayed head control, sitting, and walking. Mild choreiform movements appear, often in the feet in the first few years and these gradually develop during childhood into generalized dystonia. Some patients are able to walk but others are severely disabled (Kyllerman *et al.* 1982). Additional signs are variably present and include spasticity, seizures, eye movement abnormalities, dysarthria, and deafness; cognitive function is often normal.

Some patients are stable for many years only to deteriorate markedly as adults. This may be due to additional cervical spondylotic myelopathy but others seem to have slowly progressive dystonia, spasticity, and dysarthria (Fletcher and Marsden 1996). The reasons for this are unknown. Some patients with dyskinetic CP have affected relatives and in single cases there is an increase in mean paternal age; this is indirect evidence that some of these cases may arise by fresh autosomal dominant genetic mutation (Fletcher and Foley 1993).

It is important not to diagnose dyskinetic CP without considering alternative diagnoses. A therapeutic trial of levodopa is essential to exclude dopa responsive dystonia (DRD) (Section 32.4.4) which may also cause motor delay and generalized dystonia. Some other patients with dyskinetic CP may improve partially with levodopa but not to the extent seen in DRD (Fletcher 1993). Other conditions which may cause marked dystonia in infancy are Lesch–Nyhan disease, Pelizaeus–Merzbacher disease, and the organic acidurias.

32.4.7 Delayed onset dystonia

It is well recognized that some brain lesions may be followed by the appearance of dystonia after an interval; the best-known example of this is the delayed leucoencephalopathy and pallidal necrosis following anoxic brain damage caused by carbon monoxide poisoning (Lee and Marsden 1994a). A similar delay in the appearance of dystonia may follow basal ganglia stroke, toxic brain damage, or head injury. In these situations, the dystonia appears after a variable delay ranging from a few days to several years and is often accompanied by spasticity and parkinsonism. A more difficult concept has been the suggestion that dystonia may appear many years after perinatal brain damage with normal intervening development (Burke *et al.* 1982a; Saint

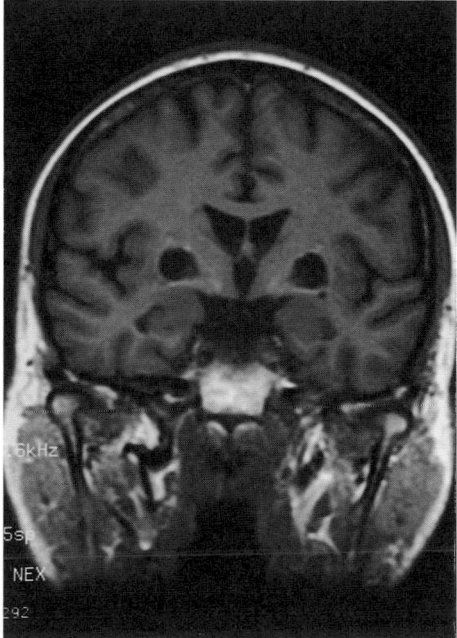

Fig. 32.14. MR scan appearance in striatal necrosis. The patient had dystonia and parkinsonism secondary to mitchondrial disease. (Courtesy of Dr A. Bowden, Consultant Neurologist, Walton Centre).

Hilaire *et al.* 1991). Such patients often have dystonia similar to ITD but were diagnosed as delayed onset dystonia following cerebral anoxia at birth purely on the basis of an abnormal perinatal history. It is difficult to be certain whether this interpretation is correct because a history of mild obstetric complications is common in normal individuals and such perinatal factors are poor predictors of neurological abnormalities unless very severe. Accordingly, it is unwise to assign much diagnostic relevance to mild abnormalities of parturition or transient indicators of perinatal hypoxia especially in those with subsequently normal motor milestones.

32.4.8 Post-encephalitic dystonia

Dystonia was often seen in patients who had survived an attack of lethargic encephalitis. Although parkinsonism was the most common complication (Section 32.3.6) some patients developed cranial or limb dystonia. In the early part of the twentieth century many cases of dystonia were attributed to encephalitis but the disorder is now very rare (Howard and Lees 1987).

32.4.9 Dystonia due to metabolic disorders

Many metabolic disorders may produce dystonia (see Table 32.10). Most of these are very rare and produce complex clinical disorders of which dystonia is only a part and often overshadowed by other features. The most important of these is *Wilson's disease* (Section 32.8). Other members of this group of dystonic disorders are rare and untreatable. There are several excellent reviews of these conditions to which the reader is directed for more detailed coverage (Barclay and Lang 1995; De Yebenes *et al.* 1996).

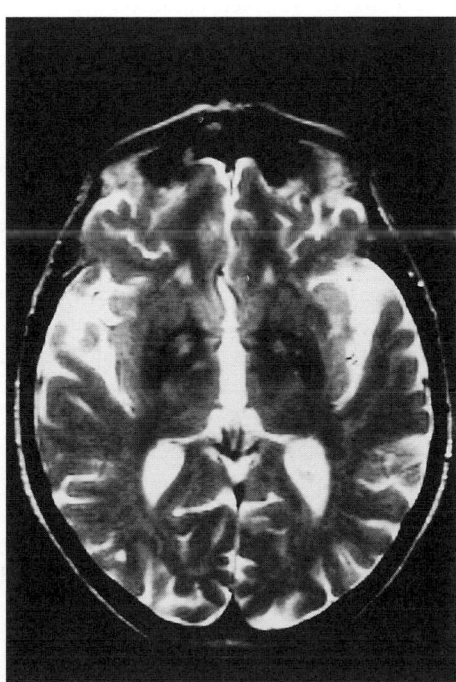

Fig. 32.15. MR brain scan of a patient with Hallervorden Spatz disease, showing the characteristic pallidal signal changes ('eye of the tiger sign')

Hereditary caeruloplasmin deficiency is very rare but is mentioned to distinguish it from Wilson's disease. Dementia, cranial dystonia, and diabetes are seen along with evidence of brain iron overload. There are abnormal MRI signals in the basal ganglia, brainstem, and dentate nuclei. Inheritance is autosomal recessive (Kawanami *et al.* 1996).

Organic acidurias (glutaric aciduria type 1 and methylmalonic aciduria) usually present in infancy with a severe encephalopathy and developmental delay; dystonia may be prominent and the diagnosis is established by urinary organic acid estimations (Section 4.10). Basal ganglia necrosis may be seen with CT or MRI. There is no effective treatment.

GM1 gangliosidosis (β-galactosidase deficiency) may present in adult life with dysarthria, dystonia, and parkinsonism. Dysmorphism and macular lesions are not seen unlike the infantile form. There may be putaminal lesions on CT or MRI and the diagnosis can be made by measuring β-galactosidase in leucocytes.

GM2 gangliosidosis (hexosaminidase deficiency) usually presents in infancy with a severe encephalopathy with myoclonus and seizures but later onset forms exist with dementia, psychiatric abnormalities, seizures, ataxia, and lower motor neuron findings. Dystonia may also occur but is not a prominent feature.

Lesch–Nyhan disease is an X-linked disorder caused by hypoxanthine-guanine phosphoribosyltransferase (HGPRT). Affected infants develop mental retardation, delayed motor development, self-mutilation, and dystonia. There is severe hyperuricaemia with renal stones and gouty arthritis. A partial HGPRT deficiency state occurs with similar but less severe clinical features.

Leucodystrophies may be associated with dystonia but this is rare and only a minor feature of metachromatic leucodystrophy (Section 29.6). Dystonia is much more typical of Pelizaeus–Merzbacher disease (X-linked sudanophilic leucodystrophy) which is characterized by nystagmus, ataxia, and dystonia in infancy. Leucocyte aryl-sulphatase A is reduced in metachromatic leucodystrophy, while Pelizaeus–Merzbacher disease can now be diagnosed by mutation screening of the proteolipid protein (PLP) gene on chromosome Xq22.

Neimann–Pick disease type C usually develops in infancy but a later onset form may occur. This causes a vertical supranuclear gaze palsy, ataxia, cataplexy and dystonia. There is an accumulation of sphingomyelin but sphingomyelinase levels are normal. Diagnosis is by bone marrow trephine to look for sea blue histiocytes or more reliably by filipin staining of cultured fibroblasts from a skin biopsy. The NPC1 gene is located on chromosome 18q11–12.

Homocystinuria is occasionally associated with dystonia but the cause is unclear. There may be vascular damage to the basal ganglia or alterations in striatal neurotransmission.

Kuf's disease is an adult onset form of neuronal ceroid lipofuscinosis. There is no visual failure and affected adults develop either a progressive myoclonic epilepsy or a dementia with cranial dystonia. Demonstration of osmiophilic fingerprint profiles or granular osmiophilic deposits by electron microscopy in rectal, skin, or liver biopsy is required for the diagnosis. Urinary sediment dolichol levels are also elevated but this test is not routinely available. There is no treatment.

Mitochondrial disorders are associated with a wide range of neurological features but dystonia is prominent in Leigh's disease, familial striatal necrosis, and in some cases of Leber's hereditary optic neuropathy (Hanna and Bhatia 1997). A diagnostic clue is the presence of striatal lesions on CT or MRI scans (Fig. 32.14). Leigh's disease may be caused by defects of oxidative phosphorylation (complex I, II, or IV deficiency) or pyruvate dehydrogenase deficiency and may be associated with mutations of nuclear or mitochondrial DNA. Dystonia may be prominent along with mental regression and brainstem signs especially respiratory irregularity, eye movement disorders, and ataxia. Familial striatal necrosis has also been linked to mitochondrial dysfunction and usually presents with dystonia and parkinsonism (Thyagarajan *et al.* 1995; Caparros-Lefebvre *et al.* 1997). Some patients with Leber's disease have also developed dystonia and striatal lesions (Marsden *et al.* 1986; Novotny *et al.* 1986). Clearly there is some overlap in the clinical features of these three forms of mitochondrial disease.

32.4.10 Dystonia in hereditary and degenerative disorders

Hallervorden–Spatz disease

This is a rare autosomal recessive disorder characterized by progressive dystonia, spasticity, and dementia (Dooling *et al.* 1974). The onset is usually before 20 years of age but adult onset cases have occurred (Jankovic *et al.* 1985). Rigidity of the legs is an early feature with dystonia and spasticity, brisk reflexes, and extensor plantar responses. Cognitive decline, retinitis pigmentosa, and sometimes seizures are additional features; relentless progression leads to generalized rigidity and dementia and survival is limited to a mean of 11 years. Later onset cases have presented with atypical parkinsonism (Section 32.3.13) dementia or chorea (Grimes *et al.* 2000). Investigations are often unhelpful but a characteristic appearance on T2 weighted MRI scans with pallidal hypointensity with a high signal centre 'eye of the tiger sign' may be seen (Fig. 32.15). Peripheral blood acanthocytes have been described as have sea blue histiocytes in the bone marrow. Pathologically there is increased iron deposition and axonal spheroid formation in the globus pallidus and substantia nigra pars reticulata. There is no effective treatment. A gene locus has been identified on chromosome 20 (Taylor *et al.* 1996).

There are several reports of probable variants of Hallervorden–Spatz disease. The HARP syndrome comprises hypoprebetalipoproteinaemia, acanthocytosis, retinitis pigmentosa, and pallidal degeneration (Orrell *et al.* 1995). The dystonia tends to affect cranial musculature and the characteristic brain MRI changes of Hallervorden–Spatz disease have been detected. Another case with parkinsonism, dementia, and suggestive MRI changes had pathological evidence of Hallervorden–Spatz disease and Lewy bodies in the substantia nigra (Tuite *et al.* 1996). There is an uncertain relationship between Hallervorden–Spatz disease and infantile neuroaxonal dystrophy based on similar pathological appearances.

Basal ganglia calcification (Fahr's syndrome)

This is a heterogeneous disorder in which there is idiopathic calcification of the basal ganglia and sometimes other brain areas together with neurological impairment. Calcification of the basal ganglia may be an incidental finding on CT scans and is usually mild and of no significance in this situation. Other specific neurological disorders such as cerebral anoxia, cerebral infections, disorders of calcium homeostasis, the Cockayne syndrome, Hallervorden–Spatz disease, and mitochondrial disorders may be associated with basal ganglia calcification and should be separated from the Fahr syndrome which refers to idiopathic cases which may be sporadic or autosomal dominant. Dystonia may be a prominent feature in these cases (Caraceni *et al.* 1974; Larsen *et al.* 1985) along with neuropsychological abnormalities consistent with basal ganglia dysfunction (Lopez-Villegas *et al.* 1996). The clinical phenotype may also include abnormal eye movements. In one multigenerational family, a gene locus was mapped to chromosome 14q (Geschwind *et al.* 2000).

Other hereditary and degenerative causes of dystonia

Other causes of dystonia in this group of conditions are shown in Table 32.10 and are dealt with separately. It should be noted that dystonia is often prominent in advanced Huntington's disease especially in the rigid Westphal variant in younger onset, paternally inherited cases (Section 32.5.2). Ataxia telangiectasia may present with a mainly dystonic syndrome (Bodensteiner *et al.* 1980) and skin changes may be absent or inconspicuous (Sections 19.5, 31.5.1). Diagnosis is facilitated by α-fetoprotein and immunoglobulin estimations. Dystonia may be prominent in the spinocerebellar degenerations, especially *SCA3*, and late onset degenerative cerebellar degenerations are one of the more common causes of secondary dystonia in clinical practice (see Chapter 31). Neuroacanthocytosis is associated with both chorea and dystonia and is discussed in Section 32.5.8. The Rett syndrome occurs only in girls and causes developmental regression, autism, stereotypic movements (especially of the hands), ataxia, bruxism, tremors, tics, and dystonia. Later there may be signs of parkinsonism (Fitzgerald *et al.* 1990).

32.4.11 Post-traumatic dystonia

There has been a frequently reported association between peripheral injuries or pain and the subsequent local development of dystonia. Although this has been noted for many years the mechanism is unclear and a causative link is speculative. Most cases have been in patients who develop various forms of focal adult onset PTD after local injuries (Section 32.4.2). Some of these patients may have a pre-existing genetic liability to dystonia, presumably PTD but this is unproven. Peripheral limb fractures, lacerations, and surgical procedures have figured prominently in these cases (Fletcher *et al.* 1991c) and patients with PTD should be warned of this possible risk prior to surgical operations. These should, as a consequence, be avoided whenever possible, especially misguided attempts at surgical correction of dystonic postures. In a survey of 104 cases of PTD, 17 gave a history of initiation or exacerbation of dystonia by trauma; recall bias is a possible explanation but patients with PTD do not in fact give a history of injury more often than matched controls (Fletcher *et al.* 1991*c*). Focal dystonias may follow repetitive use of a limb which may act as a form of soft tissue trauma (Section 34.4.2) sometimes in association with ulnar neuropathy (Ross *et al.* 1995). Such patients do not appear to carry the *DYT1* gene (Gasser *et al.* 1996). In another group of patients focal dystonic spasms develop in association with pain and reflex sympathetic dystrophy after local injury (Marsden *et al.* 1984*b*). The response to treatment in these patients is poor especially in those who have developed fixed abnormal postures and contractures although sympathetic blockade may provide some benefit. It can be difficult in some of these patients to exclude a psychogenic element and there have been spontaneous remissions. It is therefore probably unwise to recommend destructive peripheral surgical procedures or thalamotomy in these patients. Physiotherapy, anti-dystonia medications, and pain management form a reasonable policy.

32.4.12 Drug-induced dystonia

Acute transient and persistent tardive dystonia may follow the administration of neuroleptic drugs or other dopamine receptor blocking agents. These forms of dystonia are discussed in Section 32.9. Dystonia is also a common complication of levodopa or dopamine agonist therapy in Parkinson's disease and multiple system atrophy (Section 32.3). Although the effects of drugs affecting dopaminergic function are the best known and most important examples of drug-induced dystonia, many other agents have been implicated in small numbers of cases. These include tricyclic antidepressants and selective serotonin re-uptake inhibitors and buspirone. Some of these movement disorders have been persistent. Anticonvulsants have occasionally caused dystonia.

32.4.13 Dystonia caused by toxins

Various toxins may lead to dystonia, usually as part of a mixed extrapyramidal syndrome and with the characteristic features of a delay between the toxic exposure and the development of clinical signs and evidence from neuroimaging or neuropathological studies of damage to the globus pallidus. Toxic dystonia is reviewed in detail elsewhere (Chu *et al.* 1995). *Manganese* poisoning (Sections 5.7.4 and 32.3.5) usually causes parkinsonism with prominent dystonia especially involving gait. Dystonia

Table 32.12. Causes of chorea

Hereditary degenerative disorders	**Huntington's disease**
	Benign hereditary chorea
	DRPLA
	Hereditary spinocerebellar ataxias
	Fahr's syndrome
	Ataxia telangiectasia
Hereditary metabolic disorders	**Wilson's disease**
	Lesch–Nyhan disease
	Mitochondrial disease
Endocrine disorders	**Thyrotoxicosis**
	Pregnancy
	Addison's disease
Metabolic disorders	Hypo/hyperglycaemia
	Hypo/hypercalcaemia
	Non-Wilsonian hepatolenticular degeneration
Haematological disorders	**Neuroacanthocytosis**
	Antiphospholipid syndrome
	Polycythaemia rubra vera
	Sickle cell disease
Autoimmune conditions	**Systemic lupus erythematosus**
Infections	**Sydenham's chorea**
	Subacute sclerosing panencephalitis
	Creutzfeldt–Jakob disease
Vascular disorders	**Lacunar Infarction**
	Post-pump chorea
Drugs	Oral contraceptives
	Neuroleptics
	Levodopa
	Anticholinergics
	Other drugs
Other causes	Paroxysmal dyskinesias
	Focal lesions of the basal ganglia
	Senile chorea
	Athetoid cerebral palsy
	Toxin-related encephalopathies

DRPLA = dentatorubropallidoluysian atrophy. Bold type indicates the principal diagnostic considerations in cases of chorea.

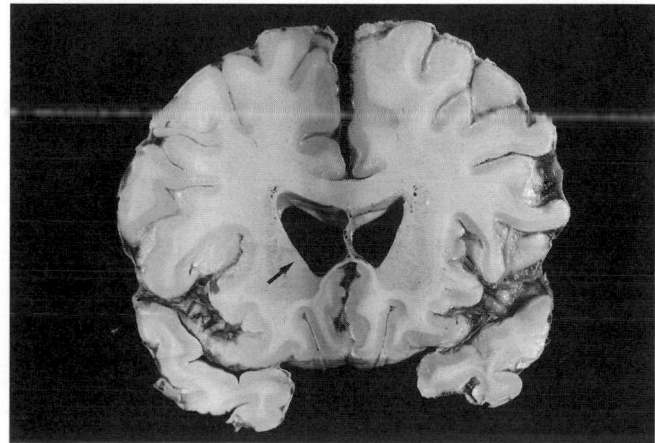

Fig. 32.16. Coronal brain section in Huntington's disease, showing almost total caudate atrophy (arrowed) and dilatation of the adjacent lateral ventricles (Vonsattel grade 5). (Courtesy of Dr J. Broome, Consultant Neuropathologist, Walton Centre).

has been reported after *carbon monoxide* exposure but this is rare. Most patients who survive the initial cerebral anoxia recover or are left with permanent neurological damage including mental changes, mutism, and rigidity due to spasticity and parkinsonism. Some develop a delayed post-anoxic encephalopathy in which parkinsonism and dystonia may occur but the former is usually much more prominent (Lee and Marsden 1994*b*). Many of these patients also recover spontaneously but the neurological damage to the basal ganglia and cerebral white matter is progressive in some. *Carbon disulphide* may produce an encephalopathy with delirium and parkinsonism as the main features but dystonia has occurred occasionally. *Cyanide* poisoning is usually fatal but parkinsonism and sometimes dementia and dystonia have occurred in a few survivors. This is associated with striatal and pallidal necrosis which is visible on CT or MRI scans. Dystonia has also followed poisoning with *disulphiram*.

32.4.14 Other secondary dystonias

As described in Section 32.2.2 dystonia may develop after focal brain lesions of various types, including tumours, arteriovenous malformations, and vascular lesions. These often involve the thalamus or putamen but not invariably. Dystonia has occasionally occurred in multiple sclerosis (Coleman *et al.* 1988) and has to be considered in the differential diagnosis of patients with paroxysmal dystonia. Parkinsonism and dystonia have also followed osmotic brain damage (Maraganore *et al.* 1992). Occasionally dystonia may occur in surprising clinical settings including brainstem haemorrhage and spinal cord lesions (Cammarota *et al.* 1995; Esteban Munoz *et al.* 1996).

32.5 Chorea and ballism

32.5.1 Diagnosis and classification of chorea

Chorea may be recognized clinically as irregular, low amplitude, rapid, movements of the extremities and the face. Mild chorea may be subtle and easy to dismiss as simple fidgetiness in an anxious patient. The movements are often disguised by the patient into apparently purposeful actions such as adjusting seating posture, clothing, or jewellery. More severe cases display obviously abnormal movements of the hands, feet, and face. Larger amplitude proximal choreiform movements may be violent and are referred to as ballism. Chorea may be partly suppressed by the patient but incompletely and not for long. Facial grimacing, eyebrow movements, and respiratory noises may be evident. In tardive dyskinesia, the movements of the face and tongue are choreiform but in this situation they are stereotyped and repetitive. Chorea may coexist with other movements, particularly dystonia which is usually more proximal, sustained, and twisting (Section 32.4.1) but the distinction is sometimes difficult. Chorea is simulated by the irregular sinuous movements of the fingers in pseudoathetosis due to severe proprioceptive loss of the upper limbs, commonly

caused by cervical myelopathy or large fibre peripheral neuropathy. The distinction is easily made by sensory testing during the neurological examination. The causes of chorea are shown in Table 32.12. This list is by no means exhaustive but many other causes of chorea are rare, based on very small numbers of reported cases or single reports and so are of limited clinical value. The conditions in bold type are the important considerations, either because they are regular causes of chorea in the clinic or because of the importance of the diagnosis, e.g. Wilson's disease. Some such as DRPLA and benign hereditary chorea are rare but very important in the differential diagnosis of Huntington's disease and therefore potential causes of diagnostic error in the clinic (see below).

32.5.2 Huntington's disease
Definition and prevalence

This is an autosomal dominant condition causing a movement disorder, usually chorea and mental changes. Huntington's disease (HD) is progressive and invariably fatal; there is no effective treatment. The prevalence is 4–10 per 100 000 in the UK with slightly lower rates in some parts of Europe and in North America (Harper 1991*b*). HD is caused by an unstable trinucleotide (CAG) repeat expansion in the *IT15* gene on chromosome 4p16.3 (Huntington's disease collaborative research group 1993) which encodes a 348 kDa protein, Huntingtin, widely expressed in neural and other tissues.

Pathology

In advanced cases the brain shows marked atrophy of the caudate and putamen with widening of the anterior horns of the lateral ventricles (Fig. 32.16). There is also atrophy of the cortex and subcortical white matter. Microscopically there is neuronal loss in the striatum and cerebral cortex and to a lesser extent in the thalami, other basal ganglia areas, brainstem, and sometimes cerebellum. The degree of striatal atrophy and neuronal loss is graded from 0 (absent) to 5 (severe) (Vonsattel *et al.* 1985). Although the degree of neuropathological change is related to age of onset, with older onset cases tending to have milder pathological changes, the relationship between clinical features and neuropathology is unreliable. Not only may clinically affected individuals, with the diagnosis confirmed by DNA analysis, have no detectable neuropathology but some asymptomatic individuals have had definite abnormalities. In the striatum, the main neuronal depletion affects medium spiny neurons with parallel reduction of striatal D_1 and D_2 receptors indicating simultaneous damage to the direct and indirect striatopallidal pathways. At present, the mechanism by which mutant Huntingtin, which is widely expressed throughout the brain, induces regionally selective neuronal loss is unknown. In animal models, similar neuropathological changes may be induced in the striatum by glutamate agonists, suggesting that the mechanism of cell death in HD is related to excessive excitatory neurotransmission but this is unproven in man. Studies of muscle energy metabolism in HD using $^{(31)}$P magnetic resonance spectroscopy indicate a possible role of mitochondrial dysfunction in HD as well as another polyglutamine (CAG repeat expansion) mediated disease dentatorubropallidoluysian atrophy (DRPLA) (Lodi *et al.* 2000).

Clinical features

HD may start at almost any age from early childhood to advanced old age and the clinical features are considerably influenced by the age of onset. The disorder usually starts between 30 and 50 with a mean of about 40 years although the mean age of onset in the general population rather than hospital-based series is approximately 5 years later (Harper 1991*b*). The juvenile HD variant with onset before 20 years accounts for about 5 per cent of the total and elderly onset disease (after age 60 years) occurs in up to 25 per cent of cases but less commonly in clinical series. The onset is gradual and most patients are diagnosed after several years of progressive motor and mental changes. About two-thirds of patients develop motor neurological symptoms at the onset, usually chorea, while the remainder present with personality or cognitive changes. Within this variable clinical picture, three broad phenotypes may be discerned: (a) 'classical' HD; (b) the juvenile onset variant; and (c) the elderly onset form.

The motor disorder of HD is much more complex and variable than is often realized. In classical HD, chorea is prominent and, along with the mental changes, becomes gradually more evident as the disease progresses. Even at this stage there is additional bradykinesia which contributes to abnormal movement (Thompson *et al.* 1988). As time passes, chorea often becomes overshadowed by increasing dystonia, rigidity, and bradykinesia which are associated with increasing immobility, postural instability, and eventual inability to walk. Spasticity with brisk tendon reflexes and extensor plantar responses may also appear but this is variable. The gait often becomes wide based and staggering with increasing falls, bradykinesia, and freezing. Eye movements are slowed at an early stage with difficulty initiating saccades, broken up pursuit movements, and impaired optokinetic responses. Dysarthria and dysphagia become increasingly apparent with a danger of aspiration pneumonia. Gradual weight loss is also common as HD progresses and many patients in the terminal stages of the disorder are in a cachectic state. This is probably not due to hyperkinetic movements which become less prominent in the later stages and is not related to nutritional intake. Many patients develop insomnia at night and somnolence by day which is disruptive for carers and other family members; incontinence occurs in 20 per cent of cases and epilepsy is slightly more common in HD than would be expected by chance. It should be noted that even within the phenotype of classical HD, the motor syndrome is variable. Not only is the severity of the chorea unpredictable but in some patients with the rigid form or Westphal variant of HD the clinical picture is dominated by rigidity from the outset. In these patients there is a combination of dystonia and parkinsonism and chorea may be absent. Most patients with the Westphal variant have juvenile onset HD but this is not always

the case (see below) and the two are not synonymous. Other patients have myoclonus (Thompson *et al.* 1994) or tics resembling Tourette's syndrome (Jankovic and Ashizawa 1995). The mental changes of classical HD usually evolve along with the movement disorder and are also variable. Early on there are changes in personality with altered mood, irritability, apathy, and anxiety. There may be a decline in work performance, deteriorating marital or family relationships, financial misjudgements, and altered sexual behaviour. Depression is often present in HD, sometimes appearing before any other symptoms, and often contributes significantly to impaired cognitive function (Morris 1991). Suicide and deliberate self-harm are also common in HD and are related to depression, the level of physical disability, and the extent of social support (Lipe *et al.* 1993). Dementia gradually becomes apparent in many patients and has been described as a subcortical dementia with slowing of thought processes, impaired long-term memory, and frontal lobe deficits (Marshall and Shoulson 1997). This probably reflects impaired subcortical basal ganglia function, involving the caudate to frontal lobe cortical loop (Section 32.2.1) as well as cortical pathology. Although it is often assumed that HD is invariably associated with dementia and several studies have reported a high incidence of this, vague and variable definitions of dementia and the confounding effects of depression make the true frequency difficult to establish. Some patients develop psychotic features, with hallucinations and delusions but this is uncommon. Others display obsessive compulsive features or altered sexual behaviour. It is common for there to be increasing apathy and social withdrawal (Marshall and Shoulson 1997) probably due to a combination of personality change, depression, and dementia. Survival in this form of HD is approximately 15 years from the onset but it is important to note that even within 'classical' HD (if such an entity can be defined) there is considerable variation. Some patients have a rapidly fatal illness lasting only a few years while others survive for up to 40 years (Harper 1991*b*). Sometimes the illness is remarkably benign with mild chorea, absent mental changes, minimal progression, and almost normal survival (MacMillan *et al.* 1993*a*).

The juvenile form of HD starts before the age of 20 years but sometimes in early childhood and usually takes the form of the rigid or Westphal variant. Such patients have almost always inherited the disease from an affected father. In these cases the onset is typically with progressive behavioural change and cognitive decline which evolves into severe mental impairment. This is accompanied by striking parkinsonism, dystonia, and rigidity. Eye movement abnormalities are prominent at an early stage along with brisk tendon reflexes, spasticity, and extensor plantar responses. Many of these patients develop seizures as well as dysarthria, dysphagia, and some have cerebellar signs or a postural tremor. Chorea can be present but is dominated by the severe rigidity and mental changes. Although juvenile HD is thought to have a more rapid course than classical disease, survival is actually similar (Roos *et al.* 1993). Moreover, a few early onset cases display a mild phenotype with chorea and prolonged survival (MacMillan *et al.* 1993*b*). In patients with onset after 60 years the disease is entirely different. Chorea is the main feature and mental changes may be inconspicuous or absent. Parkinsonism has been described but is rare. In these patients the disease runs a much more benign course but overall survival is similar due to other age-related causes of death. Although there is variation within the three age-related onset groups, the tendency for younger onset cases to have a more severe rigid form and older patients to have a milder illness with chorea and little rigidity is a useful clinical guide when considering the diagnosis of HD.

Genetics

HD is inherited as an autosomal dominant trait with full penetrance and 50 per cent risk to the offspring of affected individuals. This risk does not fall significantly until after the age of 40 years (Harper and Newcombe 1992). There is considerable variation in age of onset and severity even within families so that this is difficult to predict for relatives at risk. Anticipation, with a tendency for earlier age of onset in each generation has long been observed in HD. This is most noticeable with juvenile onset cases who usually have inherited the disorder from an affected father. Sporadic cases of HD without a family history certainly occur but an unreliable family history, premature death of a parent, or suspected non-paternity are often features of these cases and new mutations have been considered to be rare. Until recently, genetic testing was possible only with linked markers and this was difficult in many cases. With the discovery of the CAG repeat mutation in the Huntingtin gene, direct mutation testing on DNA samples is now possible for both affected and at risk individuals. Normal chromosomes contain 11–34 CAG repeats in 99 per cent of instances while 99 per cent of HD disease gene bearing chromosomes contain 36–121 repeats (Duayo et al. 1993; Kremer et al. 1994). Very occasional abnormal repeat numbers in control chromosomes have been attributed to HD homozygosity (individuals unexpectedly found to have two HD mutations), incidentally discovered HD gene carriers and laboratory errors (MacMillan et al. 1993b; Kremer et al. 1994). A few patients (probably about 1 per cent) diagnosed with HD have not had abnormal CAG repeat numbers; nearly all of these have been explained by inaccurate diagnosis or laboratory errors but occasional patients appear to have clinically and pathologically typical HD (Xuereb et al. 1996) presumably due to a different genetic mutation. An autosomal dominant Huntington-like disorder may be caused by a gene on chromosome 20p (Xiang et al. 1998) and an autosomal recessive disorder similar to HD is caused by a gene on chromosome 4p15.3 (Kambouris et al. 2000). Trinucleotide expansions in other genes are unlikely (Vuillaume et al. 2000). Unlike alleles with a normal CAG repeat number, HD CAG expansions are unstable and may lengthen or shorten during meiosis but with a preponderance of repeat number increases in affected offspring (Huntington's disease collaborative research group 1993). Most of the further increases are small but fathers sometimes transmit large increases suggesting that meiotic repeat length instability is greater in males. In sperm DNA there is therefore the combination of a stable normal repeat number

and a spread of different abnormal allele sizes (MacDonald et al. 1993). Longer CAG repeat lengths are associated with earlier disease onset with juvenile onset cases tending to have the greatest trinucleotide expansions. Accordingly, juvenile onset cases are usually of paternal origin because of the greater tendency for CAG repeat enlargement in spermatogenesis. A given CAG repeat length however, is associated with a range of ages of onset and so DNA analysis cannot reliably predict the onset of the disease in relatives at risk of HD (Craufurd and Dodge 1993). Among patients with a clinical diagnosis of HD and no family history, the HD mutation is frequently detected (MacMillan et al. 1993b; Davis et al. 1994) although some of these patients have unreliable family histories and may have had an affected parent. In other cases an allele of intermediate (30–38 repeats) size in an unaffected father has spontaneously enlarged into the HD range during spermatogenesis (Goldberg et al. 1993; Myers et al. 1993). Several examples of such new mutations arising in borderline paternal alleles have been described, usually in older fathers, indicating that there is a pool of premutations at the upper limit of the normal size range in the normal population from which new HD mutations arise. In some reports the relevant paternal allele has been just within the HD range suggesting that the father is in fact a HD gene carrier yet to develop elderly onset HD.

Diagnosis

As with most movement disorders, the exclusion of Wilson's disease is a priority in patients under the age of 50 years. A common difficulty is the combination of psychiatric illness and chorea in patients who have taken neuroleptic drugs. Some of these patients have tardive dyskinesia but others will have HD and the distinction may not be possible without DNA testing. Neuroacanthocytosis, DRPLA, benign hereditary chorea, late recurrences of rheumatic chorea, and new variant Creutzfeldt–Jakob disease (Zeidler et al. 1997) may resemble HD closely and confusion may arise in PTD and levodopa-induced chorea in Parkinson's disease. Areflexia does not occur in HD and suggests neuroacanthocytosis. HD must be considered in women presenting with chorea in pregnancy or taking oral contraceptives. In patients with a wide based ataxic gait, extrapyramidal features and abnormal eye movements it can be difficult to distinguish HD from a degenerative cerebellar ataxia. In these patients, the correct diagnosis may only become clear with follow-up observation or with DNA testing.

Investigations

In clinically affected patients neuroimaging often shows caudate atrophy although this may be absent and can occur in neuroacanthocytosis. Abnormal striatal function may be revealed by PET scans showing reduced basal ganglia metabolism and dopamine receptor levels but these tests are not specific or routinely available. Consequently, most investigations are useful only to exclude other diagnoses and include a full blood count, thyroid function tests, a blood film for acanthocytes, CK level, antinuclear factor, antiphospholipid antibodies, and calcium level. MR or CT scans may be helpful in cases of cerebrovascular chorea, Fahr syndrome, or focal lesions of the basal ganglia. Wilson's disease must be excluded in younger patients with serum copper and caeruloplasmin estimations and a slit lamp examination for Kayser–Fleischer rings. Many of the other causes of chorea in Table 32.12 are obvious from the history and so the need for additional tests varies. A definitive diagnosis of HD can be made by DNA analysis and may be particularly useful in diagnostically difficult cases, saving the patient from repeated negative investigations. Care should be taken to provide adequate counselling of the patient and, whenever possible, the family before confirmatory genetic testing and informed consent should be obtained. A genetic test is unwise without reasonable clinical grounds for the diagnosis, whatever the family history may suggest, as a positive test may not be diagnostically relevant in clinically dubious cases especially those presenting with behavioural or psychiatric problems.

Asymptomatic relatives

Relatives of those with HD often request medical advice because of concern over genetic risk or the significance of various symptoms. It is wise not to take a detailed history or examine such individuals unless they specifically request this and realize that a clinical evaluation is a form of diagnostic test as such people may be already affected with mild chorea or psychiatric abnormalities. Genetic counselling is the main requirement in these individuals who are usually at 50 per cent risk of developing HD. In sibs of apparently sporadic cases with definitely normal parents the risk is approximately 25 per cent as there may be a premutation in the father (Goldberg *et al.* 1993). In some presymptomatic gene carriers there are subtle physical signs or caudate atrophy on CT scans but it is usually impossible to predict an individual's genetic status and some relatives request genetic testing which must not be carried out without detailed counselling within the framework of nationally agreed guidelines (Craufurd and Tyler 1992). Genetic testing of minors is considered unethical and should be tactfully refused if requested by parents.

Management

There is no effective treatment for HD which usually progresses relentlessly. Psychological and social support together with genetic counselling are important. Chorea may be reduced by tetrabenazine or neuroleptic drugs such as sulpiride or haloperidol but is not indicated unless the movements are severe as suppression of chorea does not reduce disability (Shoulson 1981) and side effects may be troublesome. Depression sometimes responds to antidepressant medication or ECT. In rigid cases, parkinsonism may be improved with levodopa but this is modest. Psychotic features may be reduced with neuroleptic agents. Depending on the condition of the patient, referral for speech therapy, physiotherapy, and support from community social services may be indicated. Dysphagia may require a feeding gastrostomy but this always requires careful discussion with the patient and family. In some severely affected patients

community care may not be realistic and admission to a nursing home is appropriate. The complex medical, social, and legal aspects of management of HD are reviewed elsewhere (Morris and Tyler 1991).

32.5.3 Benign hereditary chorea

This is an autosomal dominant disorder causing non-progressive chorea without mental impairment (Pincus and Chutorian 1967). Penetrance of the gene is slightly reduced, especially in females. There is no progression and life expectancy is normal. The onset is in childhood whereas HD beginning at this age is usually severe with a rigid presentation (see above). Some reported cases have had ataxia, pyramidal signs, dysarthria, or tremor and in others there has been progression of the chorea and even cognitive decline. In patients with such additional signs the diagnosis should be regarded with suspicion as families thought to have benign hereditary chorea occasionally turn out to have the HD mutation (MacMillan *et al.* 1993*b*). A gene for benign hereditary chorea has been located on chromosome 14q (de Vries *et al.* 2000) but the condition is probably heterogeneous (Schrag *et al.* 2000).

32.5.4 Drug-induced chorea

Tardive dyskinesia caused by dopamine receptor blocking drugs is the most important example of drug-induced chorea (Section 32.9.2). Chorea is also caused by levodopa in patients with Parkinson's disease and is the main type of involuntary movement in dyskinetic patients (Section 32.3.1). Other causes of drug-induced chorea are rare and often based on one or a few reports only. The most commonly used drugs with this propensity are anticonvulsants, tricyclic antidepressants, SSRI antidepressants, and calcium channel blockers. Anticholinergics occasionally cause chorea which may cause confusion in patients receiving these drugs for dystonia (Nomoto *et al.* 1987).

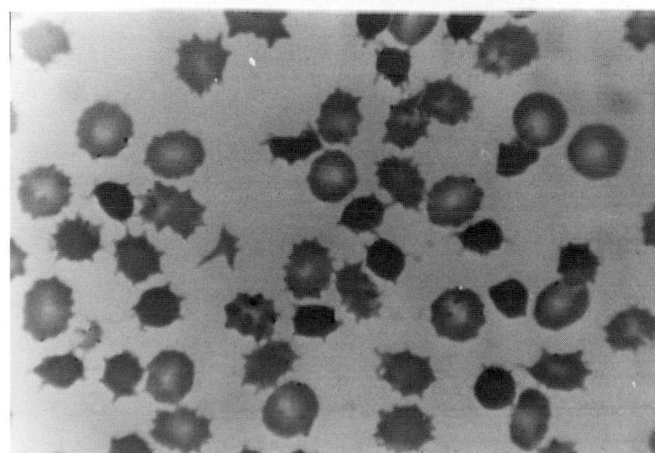

Fig. 32.17. Peripheral blood acanthocytes in neuroacanthocytosis.

32.5.5 **Sydenham's chorea**

This condition was described in the seventeenth century by Dr Thomas Sydenham and the association with rheumatic fever noted by Richard Bright in 1831. Previously a common condition and referred to as rheumatic chorea or St Vitus' dance, it is now rare in developed countries. Sydenham's chorea is triggered by a preceding infection with a group A streptococcus although there may be no clear history of this (Section 35.5). An immunological cross reaction between the streptococcal M protein and brain epitopes causes an autoimmune encephalitis. The condition occurs mainly in children and adolescents, more often in girls. There is a subacute onset of chorea, muscular weakness, hypotonia, and often prominent mental changes with emotional and behavioural abnormalities. The chorea may be unilateral and some patients develop frank hemiballismus (Vidakovic *et al.* 1994). The EEG shows slow wave changes and abnormal signal and swelling is noted in the basal ganglia on MRI scans (Heye *et al.* 1993; Giedd *et al.* 1995). PET scanning reveals increased striatal glucose metabolism (Weindl *et al.* 1993). The illness is usually at its worst for several weeks followed by gradual resolution over 3–6 months. In the acute stage the chorea may be reduced with neuroleptic medication such as haloperidol or sulpiride but sodium valproate is sometimes effective. In some cases there is a recurrence of chorea

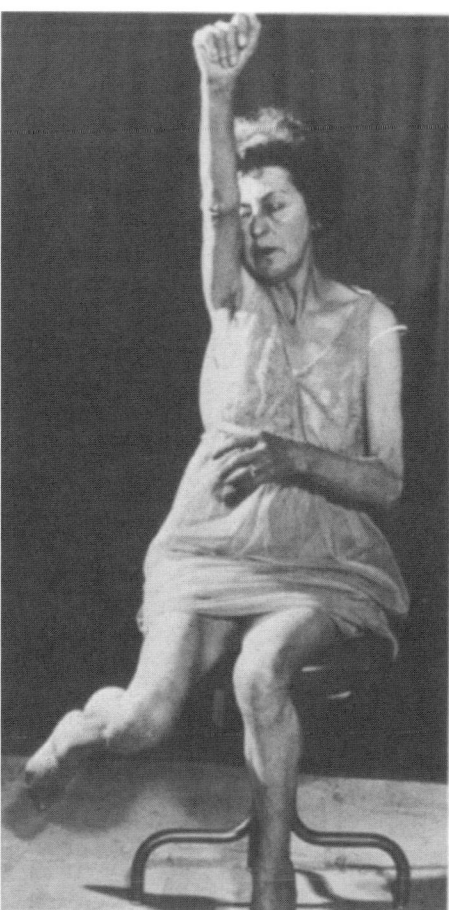

Fig. 32.18. A patient with right sided hemiballismus. Note the large amplitude of the involuntary movements.

many years later, even in old age, possibly due to residual striatal damage and age-related changes (Gibb and Lees 1989). This may cause diagnostic confusion with Huntington's disease.

32.5.6 **Chorea in systemic disease**

Chorea may be seen as a complication of the *antiphospholipid syndrome* associated with false positive syphilis serology, anticardiolipin antibodies, and the lupus anticoagulant (Section 28.2). Other features include thrombotic events such as stroke, deep venous thrombosis, migraine, recurrent abortion, and valvular heart disease. *Systemic lupus erythematosus* may also cause chorea, with or without the antiphospholipid syndrome. *Polycythemia rubra vera* is rarely associated with chorea, probably also due to basal ganglia ischaemia. Hyperthyroidism and other metabolic derangements including hypoglycaemia and hyperglycaemia may occasionally cause choreiform movements.

32.5.7 **Chorea associated with pregnancy and oral contraceptives**

Chorea occasionally occurs in pregnancy. This is much less common than it was, probably due to the decline in Sydenham's chorea. Typically, affected women had a history of previous Sydenham's chorea several years previously but this was not invariable. Other possible causes to consider are Huntington's disease, antiphospholipid syndrome, and SLE. Most cases resolve spontaneously after delivery. Chorea may occasionally develop in association with oestrogen containing oral contraceptives or topical creams (Nausieda *et al.* 1979) but the mechanism of this is unclear. The chorea resolves if the oestrogen is stopped.

32.5.8 **Neuroacanthocytosis (chorea-acanthocytosis)**

Acanthocytosis may occur in association with neurological disease in abetalipoproteinaemia, hypobetalipoproteinaemia (which mainly cause cerebellar ataxia), Hallervorden–Spatz disease and the HARP syndrome (Section 32.4.10), and neuroacanthocytosis. In neuroacanthocytosis there are peripheral

Table 32.13. Causes of tics

Primary tic disorders	Transient tic disorder
	Chronic motor tic disorder*
	Chronic vocal tic disorder*
	Tourette's syndrome
Secondary tic disorders	Huntington's disease
	Neuroacanthocytosis
	Drugs, mainly neuroleptics
	Encephalitis
	Focal basal ganglia lesions
	Rett syndrome

* May be variants of Tourette's syndrome.

blood acanthocytes but normal serum lipoproteins in association with neurological involvement. Typically there is chorea along with various additional features including orofacial dystonia, tics, parkinsonism, cognitive impairment, psychiatric abnormalities, and seizures (Hardie *et al.* 1991; Kartsounis and Hardie 1996). Patients typically have areflexia due to an axonal peripheral neuropathy (Section 12.7.5). Inheritance is unclear with a suggestion that some cases are X-linked. Pathologically there is atrophy of the striatum with neuronal loss and gliosis but the cerebral cortex is spared. Involvement of the substantia nigra and pallidum is variable. The diagnosis is suggested by the combination of chorea, with or without the other movement disorders, and areflexia. A fresh wet blood film shows excessive numbers of acanthocytes (Fig. 32.17), the blood CK is elevated, and lipoproteins are normal. CT scans may show caudate atrophy similar to that seen in Huntington's disease and PET scanning reveals reduced striatal glucose metabolism and dopaminergic function. Neurochemically there is striatal dopamine depletion (De Yebenes *et al.* 1988). There is no effective treatment for the condition which is progressive over 3–22 years (Rinne *et al.* 1994*b*).

Some patients with the McLeod syndrome have similar neurological features (Ho *et al.* 1996). In this X-linked condition there is acanthocytosis and abnormal expression of Kell blood group antigens with absent Kx antigen on erythrocytes. Several point mutations in the *XK* gene on the X chromosome. It is not known how many patients with neuroacanthocytosis have the McLeod syndrome.

32.5.9 Other causes of chorea and ballism

Chorea occurs as a feature of several other neurological disorders including DRPLA and other spinocerebellar degenerations, mitochondrial diseases (Nelson *et al.* 1995), various focal lesions of the basal ganglia (Lee and Marsden 1994*a*) including tumours and paroxysmal dystonias (Section 32.4.5). DRPLA is noteworthy because it may resemble Huntington's disease closely and is inherited as an autosomal dominant disorder (Section 31.9.6). Chorea has been reported as a complication of cerebrovascular disease in older patients with multiple lacunar cerebral infarcts, probably causing basal ganglia damage (Bhatia *et al.* 1994*b*). Some patients develop chorea after cardiopulmonary bypass usually for cardiac surgery in children. Recovery is variable and although the mechanism is unknown, basal ganglia ischaemia is possible. Senile chorea refers to the development of chorea in old age and is a heterogeneous condition. Many of these patients have Huntington's disease and some have cerebrovascular disease or late recurrence of Sydenham's chorea but others are unexplained.

Ballism is a clinically striking form of severe chorea which is commonly unilateral (Fig. 32.18) and associated with lesions of the subthalamic nucleus (Lee and Marsden 1994*a*). Vascular lesions account for most cases but imaging studies often fail to demonstrate subthalmic lesions and other causes including encephalitis, SLE, Sydenham's chorea, and metabolic disorders are sometimes responsible (Vidakovic *et al.* 1994).

32.6 Tics

32.6.1 Diagnosis and classification of tics

Tics are rapid brief jerks usually affecting the face, head, or upper body. They appear more semipurposeful and deliberate than dystonia, chorea, or myoclonus. They are repetitive and stereotyped and may be simple or complex. Simple motor tics are single brief movements such as blinking, head jerking, grimacing, or shrugging a shoulder and may be brief or more sustained ('dystonic tics'). Complex motor tics involve more elaborate stereotyped actions such as picking at the body or objects, rubbing or manipulative movements, mimicry or gestures. Vocal tics may be noises such as coughs, sniffs, or squeals while complex vocal tics consist of words and phrases. Tics are involuntary but can be suppressed more than other involuntary movements but with rising subjective tension followed by an exacerbation of tics as they are released. They are worse with anxiety or in certain social situations and relieved by distraction. Tics are preceded by an urge which is irresistible and relieved briefly by the movement. Some patients have more definite premonitory local sensations, 'sensory tics', and others describe an awareness of something in an external object 'phantom tics' which leads to a repetitive manipulation of the relevant object (Karp and Hallett 1996). The causes of tics are shown in Table 32.13.

32.6.2 Pathophysiology of tics

The mechanism of tics is unknown but is suspected to involve abnormal basal ganglia function. This is because some diseases in which tics occur have definite basal ganglia pathology such as Huntington's disease and neuroacanthocytosis. Some imaging studies in Tourette's syndrome have shown altered striatal anatomy (Singer *et al.* 1993; Hyde *et al.* 1995) and PET studies indicate reduced striatal metabolism (Stoetter *et al.* 1992). Altered brain dopaminergic function may be involved as tics may be both suppressed by dopamine blockers and caused by dopamine receptor hypersensitivity after neuroleptic therapy (Bharucha and Sethi 1995). PET studies however, indicate normal nigrostriatal dopamine function. There is no premovement potential prior to tics, consistent with their involuntary nature.

32.6.3 Gilles de la Tourette's syndrome

This condition was described in 1885 by Tourette in nine patients with motor and vocal tics. Tourette's syndrome (TS) starts before the age of 21, typically in childhood, causing multiple motor and subsequently vocal tics. The inheritance of TS is controversial but is likely to be autosomal dominant with reduced penetrance if psychological and physical manifestations are counted as expressions of the disorder, particularly in females (Pauls and Leckman 1986). To date, no gene locus has been identified. Motor tics include simple tics such as jerking, touching, or gesturing and complex tics in which there are more elaborate movements such as echopraxia (mimicking others) and copropraxia (obscene gestures). The movements may be mild and intermittent or continuous and severe enough to cause physical injury such as cervical myelopathy. Vocal tics similarly vary from simple noises to complex vocalizations such as echolalia (repeating others), palilalia (repeating the same syllable, word, or phrase repeatedly), and coprolalia (uttering obscene words). Some patients report internal mental palilalia or coprolalia. Although coprophenomena are a well-known feature of Tourette's syndrome, they are not required for the diagnosis and are seen in a minority of patients. An important

feature of the tics, especially vocalizations is that they are socially inappropriate and are distressing and embarrassing to the patient. In most patients the repertoire of tics changes at various times and the disorder shows intermittent exacerbations and periods of partial improvement. In addition to the tics, TS patients often have additional psychological disturbances (Robertson 1994). Obsessive compulsive disorder occurs in about 50 per cent of cases (Frankel *et al.* 1986; Jankovic 1987). The patients ruminate about recurring thoughts and have complex repetitive rituals which may seriously impede normal daily routines. Compulsions and tics are closely inter-

Table 32.14. Classifications of myoclonus

1. Clinical features	Anatomical extent	Generalized Multifocal Segmental Focal
	Exacerbating factors	Spontaneous Action Reflex
	Effect on muscle activity	Positive Negative
	Appearance	Rhythmic Irregular
2. Pathophysiological mechanism and site of origin	Cortical myoclonus Reticular reflex myoclonus Other subcortical myoclonus Spinal myoclonus Peripheral myoclonus	
3. Aetiology	Essential myoclonus	
	Primary epilepsy syndromes	
	Acquired metabolic disorders	Hepatic encephalopathy Uraemia Hyponatraemia Toxins
	Progressive cerebral disorders	Alzheimer's disease Corticobasal degeneration SSPE Creutzfeldt–Jakob disease Huntington's disease Diffuse Lewy body disease Spinocerebellar degenerations* Mitochondrial disease* Neuronal storage diseases* Lafora body disease* Coeliac disease* Whipple's disease* Biotin deficiency* Action myoclonus and renal failure* Other causes
	Posthypoxic myoclonus	
	Focal lesions of the cortex, brainstem, spinal cord, or peripheral nervous system	Tumour, AVM, encephalitis, ischaemia, trauma, demyelination, degeneration

SSPE = subacute, progressive panencephalitis: AVM = arteriovenous malformation.
* Aooount for most cases of 'progressive myoclonic encephalopathy' or the Ramsay Hunt syndrome (see text).

woven in many of these patients; compulsive touching and manipulating of objects or the body could be viewed as compulsions or as complex motor or phantom tics. Many patients also display evidence of attention deficit hyperactivity disorder (ADHD) with impulsiveness, inattention, and distractibility. This may cause serious educational, employment, and social difficulties. Self-mutilation of various forms also occurs in TS and is usually of a repetitive compulsive type (Robertson *et al.* 1989). Other psychological problems such as depression and anxiety are likely to be secondary to the handicaps experienced by these patients. Some patients have evidence of personality disorder with disruptive, aggressive, and antisocial behaviour. Intelligence is normal in TS but educational difficulties are common, mainly due to ADHD and may erroneously suggest a learning disability (Abwender *et al.* 1996). The overall prognosis is variable. TS tends to be worse during adolescence, especially in boys, but often improves thereafter. Remissions may occur in later adult life but only in 30–40 per cent of cases. Investigations in TS are unhelpful and the diagnosis is clinical, depending largely on the history. One of the most useful diagnostic points about TS is the early age of onset. A movement disorder appearing in adult life is unlikely to be TS. This is a key distinction from the secondary tic disorders in Table 32.13 which start later and usually have other clinical differences. TS is similarly differentiated from conditions such as hemifacial spasm or focal dystonias in which the onset will be much later, with different movements.

The management of TS is difficult. Mildly affected patients do not necessarily need drug treatment. Explanation, reassurance, and information are often adequate especially in children. Only if tics are severe enough to cause significant disability should medication be considered (Kurlan and Trinidad 1995) but, with the exception of neuroleptic drugs, few controlled trials have been reported. Clonidine, in doses up to 0.6 mg daily, is sometimes effective but this has been difficult to demonstrate in controlled studies especially at doses above 0.3 mg. More severe tics usually require a neuroleptic such as haloperidol or sulpiride. Several controlled studies have shown neuroleptics to be the most effective therapy for tics but they are not completely suppressed and side effects may occur including tardive dyskinesia (Bharucha and Sethi 1995). Other drugs are less well studied; tetrabenazine improves tics and is less likely to cause tardive dyskinesia, but may have other side effects. A reduction in tics has been reported with nicotine (Sanberg *et al.* 1997) and low dose dopamine agonists (Lipinski *et al.* 1997) but controlled studies are lacking. Some severe tics have been controlled with local injections of botulinum toxin (Jankovic 1994*a*). Clonazepam, calcium channel blockers, and tricyclic drugs have been used in TS but their effectiveness is doubtful. Obsessive–compulsive symptoms may be improved with SSRI drugs such as fluoxetine (20–40 mg daily) and ADHD has been improved with tricyclics, methyphenidate (Kurlan and Trinidad 1995), or selegiline (Jankovic 1993), although stimulant drugs may make tics worse. In patients with intolerable drug-resistant symptoms, anterior cingulotomy or limbic leucotomy has been employed.

32.6.4 Other tic disorders

Other causes of tics are shown in Table 32.13 and are discussed elsewhere in this chapter. Transient isolated tics are common in normal children and last less than a year before disappearing. They are of no significance. Only if they persist for longer than a year and are combined with other motor and vocal tics can a diagnosis of TS be made. The diagnosis in patients with chronic motor or vocal tics (but not both) is uncertain but such patients probably have TS (Kurlan *et al.* 1988). Tics also occur in adolescents with developmental disorders such as Rett's syndrome (Section 32.4.10). Some of the behavioural features of TS are seen in children with Asperger's syndrome (Section 4.4.2) and some of the latter have tics, indicating an overlap between these two disorders (Nass and Gutman 1997).

32.7 Myoclonus

32.7.1 Diagnosis and classification

Myoclonus refers to sudden and shock-like jerks due to bursts of muscle activity lasting 50–300 ms. There may also be brief pauses of muscle tone; these are referred to as negative myoclonus. In general, myoclonic jerks are involuntary, increased by movement, disrupt voluntary movements, and frequent. Negative myoclonus causes brief loss of muscle tone (asterixis) or postural lapses. The classifications of myoclonus are summarized in Table 32.14. These different classifications overlap; for example, cerebral anoxia or metabolic disturbances may cause cortical or reticular reflex myoclonus.

32.7.2 Cortical myoclonus

This is the most common type and produces generalized, multifocal, or focal myoclonus depending on the extent of the cortical pathological process. The jerks are often spontaneous but may be strikingly stimulus sensitive and exacerbated by movement. The EMG bursts during the jerks are short (10–50 ms) and associated with a preceding contralateral EEG cortical potential and, if there is stimulus sensitivity, abnormally large somatosensory evoked potentials (SSEPs) can be recorded over the corresponding area of sensorimotor cortex (Hallett *et al.* 1979). In patients with generalized as opposed to multifocal cortical myoclonus there is more rapid spread of the cortical discharge due to impaired cortico-cortical and transcallosal inhibition (Brown *et al.* 1996). Cranial nerve innervated musculature is activated in a strictly rostral–caudal sequence. Generalized or multifocal myoclonus may be spontaneous or triggered by tactile, visual, or auditory stimuli and may be seen with various forms of epilepsy or widespread cortical dysfunction due to anoxia, metabolic, toxic, or degenerative disorders (Section 32.7.10). Focal cortical myoclonus is a form of epilepsy and if spontaneous and repetitive it is the same as epilepsia partialis continua. It may be spontaneous or stimulus sensitive. Focal myoclonus is a symptom of localized cortical pathology such as a structural lesion, encephalitis, or an area of focal degeneration such as in corticobasal degeneration.

32.7.3 **Subcortical myoclonus**

In this form of myoclonus the jerks are generated between the cortex and the spinal cord, usually in the brainstem. There are two forms; reticular reflex myoclonus and so-called palatal myoclonus although the latter is more properly regarded as a form of tremor. In *reticular reflex myoclonus* the neuronal discharge arises in the brainstem reticular formation and spreads up the brainstem and then induces a generalized cortical discharge. Cranial nerve innervated muscles are activated in a caudal–rostral sequence and the body jerks are generalized, stimulus sensitive, and exacerbated by movement. This form of myoclonus is rare but can be seen in post-anoxic myoclonus, metabolic disorders, intoxications, and brainstem encephalitis (Kullmann *et al.* 1996). *Palatal myoclonus* is characterized by rhythmic movements of the palate at 0.5–3 Hz and there may be synchronous movements of the tongue, face, neck, or arms. In essential palatal myoclonus the movements are due to contraction of the tensor veli palatini and the patients report ear clicks; the condition disappears in sleep and there is no additional neurological impairment or evidence of an underlying cause. In symptomatic palatal myoclonus there are rhythmic contractions of the levator veli palatini which are not associated with ear clicking and persist in sleep. This form of palatal myoclonus is associated with lesions of the Guillain–Mollaret triangle (dentate–red nucleus–inferior olivary circuit) and hypertrophy of the inferior olivary nucleus (Deuschl *et al.* 1996). Various brainstem lesions have been associated with symptomatic palatal myoclonus including strokes, demyelination, and degenerative disorders (Howard *et al.* 1993).

Table 32.15. Causes of progressive myoclonic epilepsy and the Ramsay Hunt syndrome

Spinocerebellar degenerations	Unverricht–Lundborg disease
	DRPLA
	SCA14
Mitochondrial disorders	MERRF
	May–White syndrome
	Ekbom syndrome
Intestinal disease	Coeliac disease
	Whipple's disease
Other causes	Lafora body disease
	Creutzfeldt–Jakob disease
	Sialidosis
	Neuronal ceroid lipofuscinosis
	Gaucher's disease
	GM2 gangliosidosis
	Biotin deficiency
	Neuroaxonal dystrophy
	Action myoclonus-renal failure syndrome

DRPLA = dentatorubropallidoluysian atrophy; MERRF = myoclonic epilepsy with ragged red fibres.

32.7.4 **Spinal myoclonus**

Localized spinal lesions may produce segmental or focal myoclonic jerking in body areas supplied by the affected spinal segments. The jerks are rhythmic and spontaneous and persist in sleep. Spinal myoclonus is not usually stimulus sensitive or aggravated by movement. A variety of spinal lesions may be responsible including cervical spondylosis, tumours, demyelination, ischaemia, and arteriovenous malformations. In propriospinal myoclonus there are flexion or extension jerks of the neck, trunk, hips, and knees which are both spontaneous and stimulus sensitive. The myoclonus arises from a focal lesion and spreads up and down the cord to produce an extensive axial jerk (Brown *et al.* 1991a–d). Causes include trauma, myelitis, and tumour.

32.7.5 **Myoclonus of peripheral origin**

Spontaneous focal myoclonus in a limb or the trunk has occurred with nerve root, plexus, or peripheral nerve lesions (Marsden 1994). Causes have included peripheral nerve tumours, radiotherapy, electrocution, surgery, and spondylotic radiculopathy. Such lesions appear to induce repetitive discharges of groups of anterior horn cells by an unknown mechanism.

32.7.6 **Essential myoclonus and hereditary myoclonic dystonia**

In benign essential myoclonus there is the onset in childhood or adolescence of sudden myoclonic jerks affecting the face, arms, and trunk. The myoclonus is sometimes sensitive to sound and may be synchronous and bilateral or asymmetrical and multifocal. Severity is variable ranging from minimal twitching to severe myoclonus and there is autosomal dominant inheritance with variable penetrance. The disorder is benign and non-progressive and there are no additional neurological features. The EEG is normal and the myoclonus appears to be of subcortical origin (Quinn 1996). The jerks are characteristically sensitive to alcohol. Some of these patients also have signs of dystonia (Fahn and Sjaastad 1991) and families described as hereditary alcohol responsive myoclonic dystonia almost certainly have the same disorder (Quinn 1996). Occasionally there are sporadic cases of essential myoclonus without a family history. Treatment is difficult; clonazepam or anticholinergics may be partly effective. This condition is to be distinguished from patients with idiopathic torsion dystonia in whom jerky 'myoclonic' dystonic movements may be seen (Obeso *et al.* 1983). Various mutations of EPM2A have been identified but the function of the gene product, Laforin, is unknown (Minassian *et al.* 2000).

32.7.7 **Cerebral anoxic myoclonus (Lance Adams syndrome)**

Myoclonus may be a prominent feature in patients who have survived severe cerebral anoxia, typically following cardiorespiratory arrest due to asthma. There may be additional cognitive impairment, epilepsy, spasticity, and ataxia but this is variable. Most cases have stimulus sensitive, generalized or multifocal, cortical action myoclonus but reticular reflex myoclonus may occur occasionally (Brown *et al.* 1991*a–d*). Negative myoclonus with postural lapses also occurs and may be particularly disabling. Although some patients are severely affected due to action myoclonus, postural lapses, and other deficits, others may have a relatively pure myoclonic disorder and can improve gradually (Werhahn *et al.* 1997).

32.7.8 Spinocerebellar degenerations, progressive myoclonic epilepsies, and the Ramsay Hunt syndrome

This is a heterogeneous group of disorders which are grouped together because they share certain clinical features (Berkovic *et al.* 1986). Clinically there may be a combination of myoclonus and epilepsy with a variable degree of dementia or ataxia (progressive myoclonic epilepsy (Section 23.5.7)) or myoclonus and cerebellar ataxia with less prominent epilepsy and dementia (progressive myoclonic ataxia or the Ramsay Hunt syndrome). It is important to note that these are variations of the same clinical presentation which differ in emphasis but share a common differential diagnosis (Table 32.15). Several of these conditions are very rare causes and only the principal causes will be discussed here. In some patients, especially those with the Ramsay Hunt syndrome, a definite clinical or pathological diagnosis is elusive (Marsden *et al.* 1990).

- Unverricht–Lundborg disease is an autosomal recessive disorder caused by mutations of the Cystatin B gene on chromosome 21q22.3 (Pennacchio *et al.* 1996; Lalioti *et al.* 1997). The same disorder has been reported as Baltic, Finnish, and Mediterranean myoclonus. The onset is at 8–13 years with severe epilepsy and myoclonus; cerebellar ataxia, dysarthria, and mild intellectual impairment develop later and are less prominent. The prognosis is poor but some patients survive into adult life.

- DRPLA may also cause a Ramsay Hunt syndrome with ataxia and myoclonus (Section 31.8.6). Myoclonus may rarely occur in the olivopontocerebellar atrophy form of multiple system atrophy (Wenning *et al.* 1994*a*) but is usually inconspicuous. A combination of ataxia and myoclonus has been described in a family with autosomal dominant ataxia caused by the SCA14 gene on chromosome 19q (Yamashita *et al.* 2000).

- Whipple's disease may cause a variety of neurological syndromes including focal brain lesions, dementia, supranuclear gaze palsy, and myoclonus (Louis *et al.* 1996) (Section 34.13.7). This may occur independently of gastrointestinal malabsorption or other systemic features of the disorder. In some patients with neurological involvement, there is a rhythmic subcortical myoclonus affecting the extraocular and facial muscles (oculomasticatory myorhythmia) which may also affect the limbs. In most, but not all cases, the diagnosis is established by small bowel biopsy. It is possible to detect DNA from the causative organism *Tropheryma whippelii* in bowel or brain tissue (Lynch *et al.* 1997). Treatment is with antibiotics but the optimal regimen has not been determined.

- Coeliac disease is also associated with a range of neurological complications including peripheral neuropathy, encephalopathy, myelopathy, dementia, cerebellar ataxia, cerebral calcification, and seizures (Cooke and Smith 1966; Finelli *et al.* 1980). Some patients develop the Ramsay Hunt syndrome (Lu *et al.* 1993) in which there is stimulus sensitive cortical action myoclonus even without clear cortical pathology (Bhatia *et al.* 1995). Pathologically there may be degenerative changes or a CNS vasculitis (Rush *et al.* 1986; Mumford *et al.* 1996). The neurological features do not respond to a gluten free diet. Diagnosis is by small bowel biopsy and this should be considered in all cases of Ramsay Hunt syndrome even in the absence of gastrointestinal symptoms.

- Mitochondrial disease has many possible clinical presentations including progressive myoclonic epilepsy and is a cause of the Ramsay Hunt syndrome; when combined with the characteristic ragged red fibres on muscle biopsy (see Chapter 15) this is referred to as 'myoclonic epilepsy with ragged red fibres' (MERRF). The age of onset varies from childhood to adult life with myoclonus, epilepsy, ataxia, and sometimes deafness, muscle weakness, dementia, and short stature (Berkovic *et al.* 1989). The severity is variable within families and recurrence risks to relatives are low. MERRF is associated with various mutations of mitochondrial (mt) DNA. The most common is an A to G transition at position 8344 of the mtDNA genome in the tRNA lysine gene; other cases have a T to C mutation at position 8356 or the A to G 3243 mutation seen more commonly with MELAS (mitochondrial encephalomyopathy, lactic acidosis and stroke-like episodes) (Hanna and Bhatia 1997). Ekbom's syndrome and May–White syndrome are variants of MERRF, the former with additional subcutaneous lipomata and the latter with deafness. They are associated with the MERRF 8344 mutation and the latter also with a C insertion at position 7472 (Hanna and Bhatia 1997).

- Lafora body disease is an autosomal recessive disorder with onset in the second decade of myoclonus, seizures (frequently focal occipital attacks), and rapidly progressive dementia. A less rapidly progressive adult onset variant has been described (Footitt *et al.* 1997). The diagnosis is made by the presence of characteristic inclusions (Lafora bodies) in brain, liver, muscle, or skin biopsies. The biochemical defect is unclear and a gene (EPM2A) on chromosome 6q24 has been identified (Sainz *et al.* 1997). In one family with hereditary myoclonic dystonia, a missense point mutation of the D2 dopamine receptor gene (DRD2) was identified (Klein *et al.* 1999) but this has not been detected in other families (Klein *et al.* 2000). The prognosis is very poor with survival limited to a few years.

◆ Neuronal ceroid lipofuscinosis (see also Section 4) takes various forms and may present in childhood with progressive myoclonic epilepsy, visual failure, and dementia (Berkovic *et al.* 1986). There is also an adult onset form (Kuf's disease) which presents with progressive myoclonic epilepsy or a dementia with extrapyramidal signs (Section 32.4.9). There is no visual failure and the seizures may be photosensitive. Diagnosis is made by demonstrating characteristic finger-print bodies or granular osmiophilic deposits in muscle or rectal biopsies and can also be established by elevated urinary sediment dolichol levels (Berkovic *et al.* 1988).

◆ Sialidosis is caused by deficiency of α-N-neuraminidase (sialidase) and has two main clinical variants: late-onset, type I, with bilateral macular cherry-red spots and myoclonus, and infantile-onset, type II, with skeletal dysplasia, mental retardation, and hepatosplenomegaly but sometimes progressive myoclonic epilepsy. The sialidase gene on chromosome 6 (6p21.3) has different point mutations in sialidosis patients (Pshezhetsky *et al.* 1997). The diagnosis may be made by finding elevated urinary sialyloligosaccharides or deficiency of α-N-neuraminidase (Berkovic *et al.* 1986).

32.7.9 Prion diseases and other dementias

The combination of myoclonus with ataxia or dementia may be seen in several degenerative disorders. Cortical myoclonus is a prominent feature in Creutzfeldt–Jakob disease with ataxia and dementia (Section 34.12). A similar clinical picture is seen in subacute sclerosing panencephalitis (SSPE) (Section 34.9). In some patients with Alzheimer's disease there may also be myoclonus, especially some familial cases (Section 26.6.2). Other dementias may also cause myoclonus including Huntington's disease (Thompson *et al.* 1994), cortical Lewy body disease (Louis *et al.* 1997), and most strikingly in corticobasal degeneration (see above and Sections 32.3.10, 32.3.2, 32.5.2) (Rinne *et al.* 1994*b*). In these disorders the myoclonus is produced by widespread cortical pathology.

32.7.10 Metabolic, toxic, and other encephalopathies

Myoclonus is prominent in metabolic encephalopathy, especially negative myoclonus which produces the characteristic 'flapping tremor' seen in hypercapnia and liver failure. The most likely metabolic causes of myoclonic encephalopathy are uraemia, hepatic failure, and hyponatraemia. Bismuth ingestion causes a severe myoclonic encephalopathy (Gordon *et al.* 1995) and drugs are occasionally responsible such as antidepressants and anticonvulsants. Myoclonic encephalopathies may occur as a paraneoplastic syndrome (Anderson *et al.* 1988) or as a post-infectious phenomenon (Bhatia *et al.* 1992).

The *opsoclonus–myoclonus syndrome* is a rare disorder in which there is a gradual or abrupt onset of opsoclonus (Section 30.6.4), often with additional myoclonus. Some patients have ataxia, tremor, dysarthria, or altered consciousness. In children,

half of cases are paraneoplastic and usually improve after removal of the tumour, typically a neuroblastoma. The remainder are idiopathic and may improve with steroid therapy. In adults, half of cases are idiopathic and the remainder are post-infectious, paraneoplastic, toxic, or idiopathic (Caviness *et al.* 1995).

32.7.11 Treatment of myoclonus

This is determined by the site of origin of the myoclonus. In most cases of action myoclonus, which is the most disabling form, the jerks have a cortical origin. Cortical myoclonus responds to clonazepam, valproate, primidone, and piracetam (Brown *et al.* 1993). Better results are seen when these drugs are used in combination and when the underlying cause is not progressive. Severe focal cortical myoclonus may require surgical resection of a causative structural lesion while the myoclonus of corticobasal degeneration is resistant to treatment. Reticular reflex myoclonus responds less well to antimyoclonic drugs but may improve with clonazepam or fluoxetine (Obeso 1995). Palatal myoclonus has been treated with a wide range of drugs including clonazepam, anticholinergics, and local botulinum toxin (Varney *et al.* 1996). In spinal myoclonus the underlying cause should be treated where possible; clonazepam is sometimes helpful.

32.8 Wilson's disease

This is an autosomal recessive disorder in which an inability to excrete copper into bile leads to its accumulation in the liver and brain. Although rare it is one of the most important diagnoses in clinical neurology because early treatment may prevent or reverse otherwise permanent and fatal clinical manifestations. Unfortunately diagnosis is often delayed, with serious consequences.

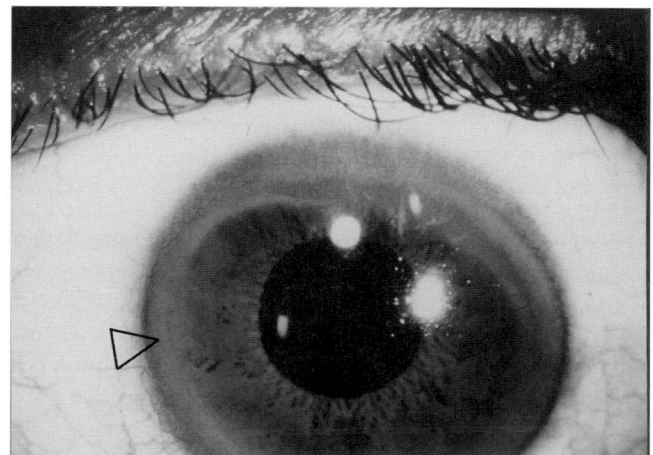

Fig. 32.19. A corneal Kayser Fleischer ring (arrowed) in Wilson's disease. The patient presented with writer's cramp, mild parkinsonism and a recent history of depression. See also Plate 25.

32.8.1 **Epidemiology, aetiology, and genetics**

The prevalence of Wilson's disease is thought to be 30 per million, with about 1 per cent of the population being heterozygotes (Scheinberg and Sternlieb 1984). Many cases are thought to be unrecognized although this is controversial and the frequency may be lower (Reilly *et al.* 1993). The cause of the disorder is mutation of a gene on chromosome 13q14.3 which encodes a copper transporting ATPase (Bull *et al.* 1993; Tanzi *et al.* 1993). There are several pathogenic mutations of the Wilson's disease gene (Thomas *et al.* 1995) but the effect of these is a failure to excrete copper into bile due to defective cellular transport. The inevitable accumulation of liver and subsequently brain copper causes tissue damage and the hepatic and neurological features of the disease.

Table 32.16. Movement disorders caused by neuroleptic drugs

Acute reactions	Acute dystonia
	Acute akathisia
	Neuroleptic malignant syndrome
Tardive syndromes	Tardive dyskinesia
	Tardive akathisia
	Tardive dystonia
	Tardive tremor
	Tardive Tourettism
	Tardive myoclonus
Parkinsonism	
Withdrawal reactions	Withdrawal emergent syndrome
	Covert/withdrawal dyskinesia
	Withdrawal akathisia

32.8.2 **Clinical features**

There is no correlation between the presence of liver or brain pathology and the clinical presentation. Even though liver damage is present in all symptomatic cases of Wilson's disease, the initial presentation is neurological in 40 per cent. The remainder present with liver disease, psychiatric manifestations, or occasionally renal, haematological, or skeletal problems. The disease usually starts between 5 and 40 years although a few patients have become unwell in their 50s (Marsden 1987).

Neurological Wilson's disease may develop very gradually, sometimes with intermittent acute deteriorations, or sometimes explosively and with rapid progression. Whatever the rate of onset, the end result is deterioration to severe neurological disability. There are three main types (Marsden 1987; Sternlieb *et al.* 1987). A dystonic form presents with dysarthria, dysphagia, and drooling of saliva due to dystonia of the face and bulbar musculature. In contrast to a pseudobulbar palsy, the jaw jerk is not increased. Eventually there may be a characteristic fixed facial dystonia and sometimes stridor. Dystonia of the limbs leads to rigidity, abnormal postures, and a dystonic gait. Inexorably the patient becomes severely dysarthric, unable to swallow, and immobile. In other cases there is an akinetic-rigid presentation with prominent resting or postural tremor and variable bradykinesia, rigidity, and facial immobility. The tremor of the arms may be very severe (wing beating tremor) causing injury. The third group of neurological cases are those with a cerebellar (pseudosclerotic) presentation in which there is gait ataxia, dysarthria, loss of limb co-ordination, and titubation of the head. There are usually additional extrapyramidal signs. Chorea is sometimes seen in Wilson's disease but tics and myoclonus are not characteristic. Other less common manifestations include brisk tendon reflexes, extensor plantar responses, seizures, and jerky pursuit eye movements. Restriction of eye movements is rare and sensory loss, visual impairment, or paralysis are not seen. It should be noted that the initial neurological symptoms of Wilson's disease are often mild, sometimes for years, with minimal or no physical signs and easily overlooked or misinterpreted as psychogenic, espe-

cially in the presence of psychiatric manifestations. Examples include a mild dysarthria, inco-ordination, subtle tremor, or dystonia and a slightly odd facial expression or gait. Late diagnosis is consequently common unless the condition is thought of in all patients under 50 with a movement disorder (Walshe and Yealland 1992). Some patients present with liver disease, either in the form of an acute hepatitis, fulminating liver failure, or advanced chronic cirrhosis. Others (about 20 per cent) initially develop insidious behavioural or psychiatric changes which may evolve into altered personality, depression, anxiety, or a psychosis with little to suggest the true diagnosis unless there is evidence of liver dysfunction or a neurological abnormality. Consequently, many patients are initially referred for psychiatric evaluation (Dening and Berrios 1989). Dementia may occur in Wilson's disease but is usually absent; it is difficult to assess the cognitive function of these severely disabled anarthric patients and a false impression of cognitive impairment is common. In many patients, severe psychiatric problems, and behavioural outbursts may be secondary to the physical and social consequences of the disease but this distinction is difficult to make (Sternlieb *et al.* 1987). Occasionally patients with Wilson's disease come to medical attention because of a haemolytic anaemia, bleeding disorder, renal dysfunction, osteomalacia, ricketts, or incidentally discovered laboratory tests.

In neurological Wilson's disease, patients almost always have corneal Kayser–Fleischer (KF) rings due to deposition of copper in Descemet's membrane (Fig. 32.19). The absence of KF rings in neurologically affected patients has occurred but is extremely rare (Demirkiran *et al.* 1996). The rings first appear in the superior cornea and may not be visible unless looked for specifically with a slit lamp by an experienced ophthalmologist who is familiar with their appearance. In patients with non-neurological presentations of Wilson's disease, KF rings are less reliable. Not only may they be absent in hepatic Wilson's disease but some other forms of liver disease such as primary biliary cirrhosis may be associated with them.

32.8.3 Laboratory diagnosis

Laboratory diagnosis of Wilson's disease should only be attempted in specialized laboratories. In 95 per cent of cases there is an associated deficiency of serum caeruloplasmin (Sternlieb *et al.* 1987) although the relevance of this to the pathophysiology of Wilson's disease is unknown. There is also an increase in urinary 24-h copper excretion but the total serum copper is misleading and of no value (Marsden 1987). It should be noted that these tests are occasionally difficult to interpret; caeruloplasmin is increased by oral contraceptives, pregnancy, and other forms of cholestatic liver disease and reduced in some Wilson's disease heterozygotes; in these situations a misleading result may occur. Urinary copper output is elevated in some renal disorders and in chronic liver disease. In most patients however, measurement of caeruloplasmin and examination of the eyes for KF rings will establish or exclude the diagnosis. If either test is abnormal or there is doubt about the interpretation of these tests, a liver biopsy will settle the matter. In Wilson's disease there is increased dry weight copper concentration and abnormal liver histology in all cases although histochemical staining for copper is notoriously unreliable. In suspected cases with a normal caeruloplasmin in whom a liver biopsy cannot be done, a radiocopper loading test may demonstrate a failure of incorporation of copper into caeruloplasmin (Sternlieb *et al.* 1987). A reasonable screening sequence in suspected cases or for siblings at risk is an ophthalmological assessment and measurement of caeruloplasmin and liver function tests; if there is any doubt after these investigations, a liver biopsy is required, especially to distinguish affected individuals from healthy heterozygotes.

Other tests are of limited value. Neuroimaging studies may show lesions in the basal ganglia, thalami, or brainstem (Roh *et al.* 1994) but these are not specific for Wilson's disease.

32.8.4 Treatment

In established Wilson's disease or presymptomatic patients the only hope of cure is to reduce the total body copper content. Penicillamine remains the principal copper chelating drug, leading to increased urinary copper excretion and a negative copper balance. About two-thirds of patients with neurological Wilson's disease improve but the remainder are severely disabled or die despite treatment (Walshe and Yealland 1993). Improvement may be seen within weeks but usually a few months of starting de-coppering therapy. A proportion of patients on penicillamine deteriorate neurologically in the early stages of treatment, possibly due to the mobilization of copper, even with gradual introduction of therapy. In addition, side effects from penicillamine are common, including acute sensitivity reactions, agranulocytosis, skin lesions, nephrotic syndrome, Goodpastures syndrome, SLE, and myaesthenia (Marsden 1987). Close clinical and laboratory monitoring of patients is therefore required. Alternative methods of reducing copper levels to be considered in patients unable to take penicillamine include trientene (Walshe 1982) and tetrathiomolybdate

(Brewer *et al.* 1994). Oral zinc reduces copper absorption and has been used in presymptomatic cases; its role in established Wilson's disease is less clear. It is important that treatment is continued for life if disastrous clinical deterioration is to be avoided. The extrapyramidal symptoms are difficult to treat but anticholinergics may improve dystonia (Walshe and Yealland 1993). In patients with severe liver damage, transplantation has been successful and may reverse some neurological features (Stracciari *et al.* 2000).

32.9 Drug-induced movement disorders

Numerous drugs may induce abnormal movements but the neuroleptic drugs and other dopamine receptor blocking agents are the most important. The effects of these drugs are summarized in Table 32.16. Drug-induced parkinsonism is discussed in Section 32.3.4.

32.9.1 Acute effects of neuroleptic drugs

Acute dystonic reactions

These are most commonly seen in young adults, usually males, given neuroleptics or other dopamine-receptor blocking drugs such as metoclopramide. There may be a family history of such reactions. The dystonia is often severe and dramatic with spasms affecting the eyes, face, mouth, and neck; oculogyric crises may occur. The attacks are often mistaken for a psychogenic reaction. The onset is within hours or a few days of starting treatment with the offending drug. The spasms persist for hours or days and are relieved by intravenous anticholinergics such as procyclidine, diazepam, or diphenhydramine (Miyasaki and Lang 1995). Such reactions occur in about 2.5 per cent of patients receiving dopamine receptor blockers (Rupniak *et al.* 1986) and other drugs are occasionally responsible.

Acute akathisia

Akathisia refers to an unpleasant subjective feeling of inner motor restlessness. Some relief is obtained by moving around and affected patients may walk up and down, continuously move their legs or repeatedly get up out of a chair. The onset is soon after exposure to neuroleptic drugs and is more common after higher doses. It is common, occurring in up to 50 per cent of patients receiving neuroleptics (Miyasaki and Lang 1995). The agitation caused by akathisia may be interpreted as worsening of the psychiatric disorder and may also threaten the patient's compliance with treatment. Some patients respond to a reduction in dosage or changing to a less potent neuroleptic. Others are relieved by anticholinergics and sometimes clonazepam or clonidine. β-Blockers have been reported to be highly effective but one recent study did not confirm this (Sachdev and Loneragan 1993).

Neuroleptic malignant syndrome

The neuroleptic malignant syndrome (NMS) is a potentially fatal idiosyncratic reaction to neuroleptic drugs (Section 5.5.2). It can occur after the initiation of treatment, following a change of drug or dose or at stable therapeutic doses. NMS is rare, occurring in less than 1 per cent of patients on neuroleptic medication; occasionally it has been associated with other drugs (Haddad 1994) or withdrawal of dopaminergic anti-Parkinsonian treatment. There is a rapid onset within 2–3 days of pyrexia, clouding of consciousness, rigidity, and autonomic disturbance (Buckley and Hutchinson 1995). There may be extrapyramidal signs, seizures, or delirium. Although the CK level is frequently elevated this is non-specific and there may be a leucocytosis or myoglobinuria. In some patients NMS develops more gradually and is less severe (Bristow and Kohen 1993). The differential diagnosis includes infection, encephalitis (which may have an initially psychiatric presentation), malignant hyperthermia (after anaesthesia), fulminating Wilson's disease, and lethal catatonia. The latter is clinically similar but rigidity occurs more gradually and it can occur without neuroleptic exposure. It has been suggested that NMS and lethal catatonia may be the same disorder (Buckley and Hutchinson 1995). Although a reduction in central dopaminergic transmission seems the likely cause of NMS, similar clinical features are seen with the 'serotonin syndrome' in which there is increased central 5HT activity caused by an interaction between monoamine oxidase inhibitors and SSRI antidepressant drugs (Sternbach 1991). NMS must be considered in any febrile patient on neuroleptic medication. Management consists of stopping the causative drug and correction of dehydration, fever, acidosis, or autonomic disturbances. Dantrolene, bromocriptine, or a combination of the two are reported to be beneficial and electroconvulsive therapy has been used successfully. Despite treatment, mortality remains high, up to 30 per cent. In those who recover, neuroleptics may be restarted after 2 weeks but with close supervision (Bristow and Kohen 1993; Miyasaki and Lang 1995).

32.9.2 Tardive effects of neuroleptic drugs

Tardive dyskinesia

Tardive dyskinesia (TD) is a notorious complication of chronic treatment with neuroleptic drugs. All dopamine receptor blocking drugs, including metoclopramide have the potential to cause TD but the newer atypical neuroleptics such as clozapine or olanzapine appear to be safer (Factor and Friedman 1997; Reus 1997). TD is often unmasked by a neuroleptic dose reduction or discontinuation of therapy but can develop on a stable dose. The likely cause is dopamine receptor supersensitivity as a result of chronic receptor blockade but other transmitters or a more complex imbalance of direct and indirect basal ganglia pathways may be involved (Feve et al. 1990). The reasons why only some patients are affected and for the delay in onset are unknown. The frequency of TD among neuroleptic treated patients is 15–20 per cent (Casey and Gerlach 1988) rising at about 5 per cent per year in the first 4 years of treatment (Gardos and Cole 1980). The elderly, females, and those with affective disorders or organic brain disease are more likely to be affected; although anticholinergics make established TD worse, they do not appear to confer increased risk. The significance of an association between TD and homozygosity for a particular allele (Ser9Gly) of the dopamine D3 receptor gene (Steen et al. 1997) is unclear. The movements are usually stereotypes or chorea involving the face and sometimes the trunk and limbs (Stacy et al. 1993). Typically there are repetitive tongue and lip smacking movements or grimacing. There may be additional trunk rocking or repetitive limb movement. In some patients TD is mild and may be unnoticed but in others it is disabling. Rarely, similar but spontaneous dyskinesias have been reported in untreated psychotic patients. Whether these movements were indeed similar to TD or were manifestations of an underlying condition such as Huntington's disease is unclear.

The treatment of TD depends on whether the patient's mental state requires continuing neuroleptic medication. If this is essential, increased blockade of supersensitive dopamine receptors by a higher neuroleptic dose or switching to a higher potency drug may be effective. In some patients, the use of an atypical neuroleptic such as clozapine, olanzapine, or quetiapine may allow remission of the TD while providing effective antipsychotic therapy (Factor and Friedman 1997; Simpson 2000). Dopamine depletion with tetrabenazine (Jankovic and Beach 1997) improves TD in 90 per cent of cases but side effects are often troublesome, especially sedation and depression. In contrast to acute drug-induced extrapyramidal effects, anticholinergics make TD worse and should be avoided or stopped. Alternatively, if the causative drug can safely be stopped, TD resolves in about a third of cases but this may take months or even years. While a remission is awaited, the dyskinesias may be worse but can be suppressed with tetrabenazine. Low doses of levodopa or dopamine agonists have been used to hasten dopamine receptor downregulation but were unsuccessful (Miyasaki and Lang 1995). In resistant cases improvement may be seen with other drugs including GABAergic agents such as baclofen, sodium valproate, and clonazepam. TD is a preventable disorder; neuroleptic drugs should be used sparingly and only when absolutely necessary. The use of limbic selective neuroleptics such as olanzapine offers the possibility of prevention (Reus 1997; Tran et al. 1997).

Tardive dystonia

In some patients, dystonic movements develop, with or without additional TD (Kang et al. 1988; Raja and Azzoni 1996). The dystonia is similar to that seen in PTD (Section 32.4.2) but tends to involve the neck and trunk more severely and rarely starts in a leg; like PTD the extent of the dystonia is determined by age with generalized cases tending to be younger. Tardive dystonia can develop at any stage after starting neuroleptic medication, often within a year, and is often disabling. It occurs at all ages but is more common in younger males. Remissions after stopping neuroleptic medication are uncommon and may take years to appear. Like TD, tardive dystonia responds to dopamine antagonists or tetrabenazine but by contrast it also improves with anticholinergics (Burke and Kang 1988; Miyasaki and Lang 1995). Cervical dystonia or blepharospasm may be treated with botulinum toxin while severe cases may require triple therapy (Section 32.4.2). Recently there have been reports of improvement with bilateral stereotactic pallidotomy (Weetman *et al.* 1997) and with clozapine (Friedman 1994; Trugman *et al.* 1994; Van Harten *et al.* 1996).

Tardive akathisia

Subjective motor restlessness similar to acute akathisia may also occur after chronic exposure to neuroleptics (Burke *et al.* 1982*b*). The patients are intensely restless and often unable to sit in a chair. There may be concomitant TD but more often any movements of the patient are clearly an attempt to obtain relief from the akathisia. Severe agitation may be mistaken for a worsening of the underlying psychiatric illness. Tardive akathisia, like other tardive phenomena, is often unmasked by a reduction of antipsychotic medication and is improved by restarting or increasing the neuroleptic while anticholinergics make the symptoms worse. This is the opposite pattern to that seen with acute akathisia. As with TD, tetrabenazine is often helpful. Some patients improve with propranolol or opiates such as codeine or dextropropoxyphene (Burke *et al.* 1989). Occasionally, patients develop delayed acute akathisia after an increase in neuroleptic dosage, a switch to a higher potency drug, or discontinuation of anticholinergic therapy; the precipitating changes in medication are helpful in making the distinction.

Other tardive phenomena

There have been rare reports of myoclonus, tics, and tremor as tardive effects (Stacy and Jankovic 1991; Bharucha and Sethi 1995). All have the hallmarks of tardive symptoms, namely appearance or exacerbation after neuroleptic reduction or discontinuation and improvement with tetrabenazine or increased dopamine receptor blockade. These reports are difficult to evaluate.

Withdrawal phenomena

In children, transient generalized chorea has been described after withdrawal of neuroleptic drugs. This 'withdrawal emergent syndrome (WES)' is analogous to TD but lasts only a few weeks (Polizos and Engelhardt 1978). A similar situation in adults exists with the appearance of TD for a few months after drug withdrawal (withdrawal dyskinesia) but this is simply TD which has resolved after stopping the causative drug. Covert dyskinesia refers to persistent TD which has been unmasked by stopping dopamine blockers. A similar phenomenon is seen with tardive akathisia which may appear after stopping a dopamine blocker (withdrawal akathisia) (Lang 1994).

32.9.3 **Other drug-induced dyskinesias**

Many different drugs cause dyskinesias or parkinsonism and a detailed review is beyond the scope of this chapter. Detailed reviews exist elsewhere (Miyasaki and Lang 1995). Most cases involve antidepressants, stimulants, anticonvulsants, and calcium channel blockers. Tricyclic antidepressants have been associated with action tremor, chorea, myoclonus, and dystonia (Vandel *et al.* 1997). These effects are rare and are often associated with overt toxicity. Selective serotonin re-uptake inhibitors such as fluoxetine may induce tardive dyskinesia, parkinsonism, and dystonia (Leo 1996). Lithium frequently causes tremor and in cases of toxicity may cause myoclonus and encephalopathy resembling Creutzfeldt–Jakob disease (Fear 1992). Stimulants such as amphetamines, methylphenidate, and cocaine are associated with tremors, chorea, tics, and stereotypes (Klawans and Weiner 1974). Phenytoin may cause myoclonus, asterixis, chorea, or dystonia; this is usually in association with toxicity and is more common with underlying striatal pathology (Miyasaki and Lang 1995). Sodium valproate is a cause of postural tremor and dystonia may be caused by gabapentin (Reeves *et al.* 1996). The main risk with calcium antagonists is parkinsonism (Section 32.3.4).

32.10 **Miscellaneous movement disorders**

A number of other disorders are conveniently considered along with the movement disorders. These often give rise to diagnostic problems unless their existence is remembered.

32.10.1 **Restless legs syndrome and periodic limb movements of sleep**

Restless legs syndrome (RLS) causes unpleasant sensations in the lower limbs with restlessness and sleep disturbance. Most cases are idiopathic but RLS can occur with uraemia, iron deficiency, lumbar radiculopathy, and some peripheral neuropathies. Onset is usually in older adults but this is not invariable and a family history of autosomal dominant inheritance is sometimes noted. The condition has been reviewed recently and diagnostic criteria suggested (Walters 1995). There should be a desire to move the legs with unpleasant sensory alterations (dysaesthesiae) in the legs, actual motor restlessness, worsening of symptoms at rest, in the evening, and at night, and partial relief with activity. The dysaesthesiae are often difficult for the patient to describe and may be referred to as aching, pulling, crawling, or tingling. The motor features include walking, stretching, or rubbing the legs and the patients often get up at night and pace the room to obtain some relief. Sleep is disrupted with resulting daytime sleepiness. Many patients develop frequent jerks of the legs and sometimes the arms while awaiting sleep at night. While asleep, there are characteristic slow, repetitive flexion movements of the legs, involving the ankle or the whole limb. These periodic limb movements of sleep (PLMS) occur in stage I or II sleep and last from 0.5 to 5 s. They also contribute to sleep fragmentation and daytime tiredness. The mechanism of RLS/PLMS is unclear but similar symptoms are seen in Parkinson's disease and neuroleptic-induced akathisia (see above) implicating abnormal central dopaminergic function. Improvement may be obtained with levodopa, dopamine agonists, clonazepam, or opiates such as codeine.

32.10.2 Other sleep-related movements

In normal individuals there may be generalized myoclonic jerks at the onset of sleep. Anxious individuals sometimes consult because of this but there is no pathological significance of these normal hypnic jerks. Some normal individuals also have brief multifocal myoclonic jerks of the limbs, referred to as physiological fragmentary myoclonus of sleep. This occurs in stages I, II, and REM sleep (Fish 1994) and rarely causes symptoms. In some individuals there is an excessive amount of fragmentary myoclonus of sleep which also occurs in stages III and IV and is associated with a variety of sleep disturbances including sleep apnoea and narcolepsy (Broughton et al. 1985).

Behavioural disturbances in non-REM sleep such as night terrors and sleepwalking and REM sleep-related behaviour disorder are discussed in Section 24.1.

Paroxysmal nocturnal dystonia (PND) is characterized by repetitive brief attacks of abnormal movements in sleep (Lugaresi et al. 1986). When PND was first described it was thought to be a sleep-related dyskinesia because the movements were thought to be dystonic and scalp EEG recordings were normal. However, it is now clear that this condition is actually a form of frontal lobe epilepsy in which attacks of bizarre motor activity from sleep are well recognized (Fish 1994).

32.10.3 Stiff man syndrome

In this condition there is a progressive rigidity of the trunk and proximal limbs with associated stimulus sensitive spasms. Many cases have now been described and diagnostic criteria proposed (Thompson 1994). Onset is usually between 30 and 60 years with slowly progressive rigidity of the trunk and later the proximal limbs over many years. There is a hyperlordotic posture with striking rigidity of the lumbar and abdominal muscles. The lumbar spasm and hyperlordosis persist when supine, in contrast to axial dystonia which is reduced at rest. Painful muscle spasms are superimposed upon the fixed rigidity. There are no other neurological signs and EMG recordings reveal continuous motor unit activity with normal motor units and no sign of denervation or peripheral neuropathy. There is an association with diabetes in about a third of cases and 10 per cent of patients also have epilepsy. Other autoimmune disorders sometimes coexist and a few cases are paraneoplastic (Levin 1997). Pathophysiologically, the continuous motor unit activity persists during attempted relaxation but is abolished by sleep, spinal, or general anaesthesia and by peripheral nerve block; this indicates a central origin of the abnormal motor activity. A number of exteroceptive polysynaptic spinal reflexes are exaggerated in stiff man syndrome (Meinck et al. 1984) suggesting abnormal inhibitory interneuronal function. There may also be

stimulus sensitive jerks of brainstem origin 'jerking stiff man syndrome' (Leigh et al. 1980). Antibodies to glutamic acid decarboxylase (GAD) are found in stiff man syndrome (Solimena et al. 1988) but are not present in all cases. These antibodies also cross react with pancreatic islet cells, gastric parietal cells, and thyroid antigens. The paraneoplastic stiff man syndrome is associated with different autoantibodies (De Camilli et al. 1993). In accord with the autoimmune inflammatory pathogenesis, oligoclonal bands and anti-GAD antibodies may be present in CSF and white matter lesions are occasionally seen on MR brain scans. No significant neuropathological abnormalities have been described but in one case there were minor abnormalities of inhibitory neurons in the cerebellum and spinal cord (Warich-Kirches et al. 1997). The spasms and stiffness are improved with high doses of diazepam, clonazepam, or baclofen but sedation is often troublesome and axial stiffness often persists; intrathecal baclofen has been successful in one patient (Seitz et al. 1995) but not in others (Silbert et al. 1995). There have been reports of improvement with steroids and plasma exchange (Vicari et al. 1989) but other patients have not responded (Harding et al. 1989). Intravenous immunoglobulin is also effective in some patients (Amato et al. 1994; Barker and Marsden 1997).

32.10.4 Progressive encephalomyelitis with rigidity and other forms of spinal rigidity

This condition is also associated with severe muscular rigidity and spasms but is more rapidly progressive and there is clinical and pathological evidence of an active encephalomyelitis, mainly affecting the brainstem and spinal cord. Some identical cases are paraneoplastic. Typically there is a subacute onset over weeks or months of rigidity of one or more limbs, usually the legs. Unlike the stiff man syndrome, there may be additional pain, sensory loss, dysaesthesiae, jerking, and weakness due to segmental spinal pathology; there may also be loss of tendon reflexes and extensor plantar responses. The rigidity becomes progressively worse with severe stimulus sensitive spasms of the trunk and limbs. Brainstem involvement is eventually seen with bulbar and oculomotor abnormalities. Progression is much quicker than stiff man syndrome with death occurring between 3 weeks and 3 years from onset. The spasms are abolished by sleep, anaesthesia, or nerve blocks consistent with a central origin and EMG may show additional denervation changes. Anti-GAD antibodies are usually absent but have been present in occasional atypical cases (Burn et al. 1991; Mitsumoto et al. 1991). The CSF contains a lymphocytic response and oligoclonal bands and areas of abnormal signal have been detected in the cerebral white matter and brainstem in some patients (Thompson 1994). Pathologically there are inflammatory changes in the brainstem and spinal cord, with long tact degeneration. There is no effective treatment although diazepam and baclofen may help the distressing spasms. One atypical case without pathological confirmation improved with steroids and plasma exchange (Fogan 1996). The relationship between progressive encephalomyelitis with rigidity and stiff man syndrome is unclear. Some patients have a less rapid course (Armon *et al.* 1996) while Brown has described patients with rigidity of the lower limbs, continuous motor unit activity, stimulus sensitive spasms, no axial involvement, or anti-GAD antibodies but a slowly progressive course over many years (Brown *et al.* 1997). This 'stiff leg syndrome' is probably a chronic spinal inter-neuronitis, clinically overlapping stiff man syndrome and pro-gressive encephalomyelitis with rigidity improvement may be seen with intravenous immunoglobulin (Souza-Lima *et al.* 2000). Occasionally, focal (usually cervical) spinal cord lesions such as neoplasms, syringomyelia, myelitis, trauma, and ischaemia may produce segmental rigidity with stimulus sensi-tive jerks (Thompson 1994).

32.10.5 Neuromyotonia and myokymia

Neuromyotonia refers to abnormal muscle stiffness caused by overactivity of peripheral nerve endings. There is rippling or twitching of the stiff muscles (clinical myokymia) and delayed relaxation but no percussion myotonia. This gives rise to gener-alized rigidity with sweating and rippling of muscles and abnormal postures of the limbs. EMG recordings show contin-uous motor unit activity which is abolished only by curare, indicating a peripheral nerve terminal origin. On EMG record-ings, there may be fasciculations, grouped motor unit dis-charges (also referred to as neurophysiological myokymia) and prolonged bursts of motor unit potentials. The presence of CSF oligoclonal bands and improvement after plasma exchange in many cases indicates an autoimmune mechanism (Sinha *et al.* 1991; Newsom-Davis and Mills 1993) and antibodies against peripheral nerve potassium channels have been detected (Shillito *et al.* 1995; Hart *et al.* 1997). Other cases are paraneo-plastic or associated with a peripheral neuropathy (Layzer 1995). Neuromyotonia also occurs in episodic ataxia type 2 caused by a mutation of the *KCNA1* potassium channel gene located at chromosome 12p13 (Comu *et al.* 1996).

32.10.6 Hemifacial spasm

This condition is included in this chapter as it is a common cause of involuntary facial movements and sometimes confused with tics and even dystonia of the face. There are irregular clonic and tonic contractions of one side of the face with simul-taneous eye closure, forehead contraction, and elevation of the angle of the mouth. There may be a mild facial weakness. The pattern of movement suggests an origin in the proximal part of the facial nerve in the posterior cranial fossa. Occasionally a tumour, arteriovenous malformation, or cyst is responsible but most cases are caused by microvascular compression of the facial nerve by a blood vessel which can be demonstrated by magnetic resonance tomographic angiography (Bernardi *et al.* 1993). The relative roles of local ephaptic transmission at the site of compression and abnormal facial nucleus hyper-excitability are unclear. Treatment is by microvascular surgical

decompression (Barker *et al.* 1995) or periocular botulinum toxin injections (Berardelli *et al.* 1993).

32.10.7 Painful feet and moving toes

In this rare condition there is pain in the lower limbs and con-tinuous writhing movements of the toes; occasionally the upper limbs are affected. The pain is the most prominent and early symptom and is severe, continuous, and similar to causalgia. Most cases are due to lesions of the spinal roots, lumbosacral plexus, or peripheral nerves; the latter may be traumatic or due to a diffuse neuropathy (Dressler *et al.* 1994). Some cases are idiopathic. The movements are occasionally seen without pain and are probably of central origin. Unless a surgically soluble lesion is identified, treatment is often ineffective although sym-pathetic blockade may be transiently helpful (Dressler *et al.* 1994).

32.10.8 Other movements originating in the peripheral nervous system

Various dyskinesias may appear after lesions of the peripheral nerves in addition to neuromyotonia, hemifacial spasm, and painful legs–moving toes syndrome. Dystonia after peripheral injury or overuse has been discussed in Section 32.4.11 and myoclonus of peripheral origin in Section 32.7.5. A curious phenomenon is the involuntary movements of limb stumps after amputation, often with phantom limb pain. The jerks may be transient or persistent and the mechanism by which they appear is unclear (Marion *et al.* 1989). Abnormal writhing movements of the abdominal wall are also reported after local surgery or trauma (Marsden 1994). These may be a form of post-traumatic dystonia.

32.10.9 Primary (pure) akinesia

Described mainly in Japan but also in the West, pure akinesia refers to the development of striking isolated slowness of gait, speech, and handwriting with no rigidity, tremor, dementia, or eye movement disorder (Matsuo *et al.* 1991; Riley *et al.* 1994). This appears to be a variant of Steele–Richardson–Olszewski disease, as some cases have had neuropathological confirmation of the diagnosis without the typical clinical signs in life. MRI and PET scanning also reveals similarities with Steele–Richardson–Olszewski disease (Taniwaki *et al.* 1992). A similar syndrome may occur with Lewy body disease (Quinn *et al.* 1989). There has been a report of improvement in gait using L-*threo*-3,4-dihydroxyphenylserine (3-0-DOPS) (Yamamoto *et al.* 1997).

32.10.10 Miscellaneous gait disorders

A disturbance of gait is a common effect of abnormal periph-eral motor or sensory function, as well as with pyramidal, cere-bellar, and extrapyramidal deficits. In some patients, the disorder of walking involves higher level dysfunction, particularly of the frontal lobes (Section 1.7.4). These disorders of gait often give rise to confusion, especially in the elderly in whom an erroneous diagnosis of Parkinson's disease is often made. The best known of these is the wide based shuffling *frontal gait disorder* associated with Binswanger's disease (Thompson and Marsden 1987); a similar gait is seen with other frontal lobe lesions such as atrophy, tumours, and hydrocephalus. There is a disproportionate degree of difficulty walking despite mild or absent neurological signs when the patient is examined at rest. There is shuffling (marche a petit pas), freezing, and start hesitation as well as a variable degree of dysequilibrium. The legs are often held stiff when examined due to an inability to relax them; this becomes more evident as the examiner passively moves the limbs (paratonia or gegenhalten). This gait is sometimes controversially referred to as *frontal lobe gait apraxia* due to the severe gait disturbance without corresponding motor or sensory deficit in the lower limbs (Nutt *et al.* 1993). In some patients with frontal pathology, the main deficit is a dysequilibrium of gait (*frontal ataxia of Bruns or frontal dysequilibrium*) in which the patient may be unable to sit or stand independently (Nutt *et al.* 1993). Postural reflexes are lost or inappropriate. In other patients there is a pure failure of gait initiation (*gait ignition failure or primary freezing of gait*) with start hesitation and freezing but no shuffling or falling (Atchison *et al.* 1993). These are probably all variations of a higher level gait disturbance caused by defective frontal lobe function and are common in the elderly. In some older patients, the gait is slow, laboured, and wide based but without falling, freezing, or shuffling; this probably reflects lack of confidence (Nutt *et al.* 1993).

32.10.11 Startle syndromes and hyperekplexia

The normal human auditory startle response is a polysynaptic reflex originating in the lower brainstem. The first activity is in the sternocleidomastoid, followed by the masseter and facial muscles and then by trunk and limb activation. There is conduction up the brainstem and caudally via slowly conducting reticulospinal pathways (Brown *et al.* 1991a–d). The auditory blink reflex precedes the startle response and is a separate phenomenon. Clinically there is eye closure, facial grimacing, flexion of the neck, trunk, and limbs, and autonomic changes with brief apnoea. Emotional and behavioural changes may follow.

Hereditary hyperekplexia

This is an autosomal dominant disorder characterized by abnormal excitability of the normal startle reflex. In the major form the onset is in infancy with stiffness and excessive startle reactions. There may be repeated cardiorespiratory arrests. In the older child, sudden noise or touch may cause two types of response; generalized tonic spasms with stiffening and falling and more frequent brief generalized startle responses (Brown *et al.* 1991a–d). The former may appear epileptic but there is no loss of consciousness. These attacks cause the child to adopt

a cautious gait and muscle stiffness also contributes to a curious hesitant walk and posture. There may be brisk reflexes and clonus in the legs. There is an increased incidence of epilepsy and learning disability in hyperekplexia, suggesting a widespread abnormality of cortical excitability. The EEG may show epileptiform activity. In the minor form, there is only an increased startle response, sometimes only with stress or intercurrent illness (Matsumoto and Hallett 1994). The major form of hereditary hyperekplexia is caused by mutations of the gene encoding the alpha 1 subunit of the glycine receptor on chromosome 5q (Shiang *et al.* 1993). Treatment is with clonazepam or valproate. The condition needs to be distinguished from startle-induced epilepsy which usually occurs in patients with congenital hemiparesis or severe generalized cerebral damage (Matsumoto and Hallett 1994).

Symptomatic hyperekplexia

Acquired hyperekplexia has been reported with brainstem lesions and sometimes ischaemic, traumatic, and inflammatory cerebral lesions (Matsumoto and Hallett 1994). Drugs are occasionally responsible but a number of sporadic adult onset cases are unexplained. None of these patients has the hereditary hyperekplexia mutation on chromosome 5 (Shiang *et al.* 1995).

Jumping, latah, and myriachit

In these conditions there is an excessive reaction to startle with a jump or start and then behavioural features such as automatic speech, echolalia, echopraxia, swearing, and aggression (Matsumoto and Hallett 1994). The cause of these conditions, which have similar core features, is unclear.

32.10.12 Mirror movements

Mirror movements are usually seen during voluntary finger movements which induce identical but involuntary movements on the contralateral side. They are usually seen in patients with a hemiparesis or a foramen magnum lesion and can occur in X-linked Kallmann's syndrome (Mayston *et al.* 1997). Such movements are normal during childhood and sometimes persist in healthy adults; they are more likely to be seen with increased effort, repetitive movement, and in the presence of pre-existing weakness. Some cases are familial. Mirror movements probably originate in the ipsilateral motor cortex, via the direct uncrossed corticospinal tract (Kanouchi *et al.* 1997).

32.10.13 Movement disorders in psychiatry

The majority of involuntary movements seen in psychiatric disease are tardive complications of neuroleptic treatment (Section 32.9). In addition, psychiatric features are prominent in some movement disorders and may be the presenting feature, such as Huntington's disease, Tourette's syndrome, dementia with Lewy bodies, and neuroacanthocytosis. Wilson's disease characteristically has a psychiatric presentation (Section 32.8.2). In some patients with conditions normally managed by psychiatrists, abnormal movements may also be a prominent feature and lead to diagnostic problems. Stereotypes are seen in autism and learning disability of various types. Rocking, rubbing, posturing, touching, bruxism, and self-injury are typical (Jankovic 1994b). Repetitive hand movements are seen in Rett's syndrome along with axial stereotypes and other dyskinesias such as dystonia and myoclonus (Fitzgerald *et al.* 1990). Some Rett's patients are Parkinsonian and others have ataxia, tremor, and respiratory irregularities. In schizophrenia there are spontaneous orofacial stereotypes similar to those seen in tardive dyskinesia (Fenton *et al.* 1994) as well as subtle abnormalities of fine motor control (Griffith *et al.* 1994). Mannerisms are normal actions performed in a bizarre or exaggerated way and are also a feature of schizophrenia. Catatonia is a confusing term first proposed by Kahlbaum in 1863 to describe what he believed was a distinct psychiatric disease but what is now known to be a heterogeneous syndrome. It is best considered as a behavioural disorder associated with abnormal motor behaviour but is sometimes used to refer to a subtype of schizophrenia in which catatonic features occur (Joseph 1992). Clinically, catatonic patients may have reduced or increased motor activity; some show mutism, akinesia, and a curious 'waxy flexibility' of the limbs whereby the examiner can put them into fixed positions for long periods (catalepsy). These patients may appear unco-operative or even stuporose. Others have abnormal psychomotor hyperactivity which is difficult to distinguish from mania. Either form can occur with autonomic instability and in some cases may lead to coma and death (lethal catatonia). In patients who have also received neuroleptic treatment, a diagnosis of neuroleptic malignant syndrome may be made (Buckley and Hutchinson 1995) unless the onset of similar symptoms prior to medication is noted. Whether catatonia, lethal catatonia, and the neuroleptic malignant syndrome can truly be distinguished is unclear. Catatonia may be caused by schizophrenia, depression, mania, or neurological disorders such as encephalitis, toxic encephalopathies, epilepsy, cerebral tumours, or neuroleptic drugs (Joseph 1992). Treatment will depend on the underlying cause but in psychiatric disease, a good response is often seen with intravenous diazepam or electroconvulsive treatment.

32.10.14 Psychogenic movement disorders

The great majority of movement disorders are organic and a diagnosis of a psychogenic condition should be made with caution. Commonly, patients with dystonia are incorrectly thought to have a psychiatric illness especially if the clinician is unfamiliar with the curious action specificity of the spasms. In those with Tourette's syndrome and tardive dyskinesia or akathisia, the movements are often assumed to be a behavioural manifestation of associated mental illness. Nevertheless, true psychogenic movement disorders do occur. These often take the form of dystonic spasms (Lang 1995), especially if there are features unlike PTD such as onset in a lower limb in an adult, with a fixed posture rather than a mobile action-specific spasm and associated pain. The distinction between post-traumatic focal dystonia and a psychogenic disorder can be very difficult and at

times impossible. Paroxysmal dyskinesias, resembling paroxysmal dystonic choreoathetosis are also sometimes psychogenic (Demirkiran and Jankovic 1995). Tremors which are intermittent and variable in frequency should also be viewed with suspicion although Wilson's disease (Section 32.8) is notorious for presenting with bizarre tremors and psychiatric manifestations. Other examples of non-organic movement disorders which often cause diagnostic problems include peculiar, unclassifiable gaits, excessive and unusual startle reactions, facial spasms, and even parkinsonism (Lang *et al.* 1995). Whenever possible, a diagnosis of a psychogenic disorder should be supported by other evidence such as non-organic weakness or sensory loss, the disappearance of movements with distraction or volitional movements, excessive and apparently deliberate slowness, unusual variability, and unexplained exacerbations or remissions. Such patients may have a past history of multiple medical symptoms of an uncertain nature, excessive fatigue, secondary gain in the form of family dynamics or social security benefits and involvement in litigation of some sort. None of these features is diagnostic as any may be present with organic illness; it is the overall picture which is suggestive (Fahn 1994b). At times, the matter may be impossible to resolve, in which case the diagnosis is best left open and the patient perhaps given the benefit of any doubt.

References

Aarsland, D., Andersen, K., Larsen, J. P. *et al.* (2001). Risk of dementia in Parkinson's disease. *Neurology*, **56**, 730–6.

Abwender, D. A., Como, P. G., Kurlan, R. *et al.* (1996). School problems in Tourette's syndrome. *Arch. Neurol.*, **53**, 509–11.

Adler, C. H., Sethi, K. D., Hauser, R. A. *et al.* (1997). Ropinirole for the treatment of early Parkinson's disease. The Ropinirole Study Group. *Neurology*, **49**, 393–9.

Aizawa, H., Kwak, S., Shimizu, T. *et al.* (1991). A case of adult onset pure pallidal degeneration. I. Clinical manifestations and neuropathological observations. *J. Neurol. Sci.*, **102**, 76–82.

Albright, A. L., Barry, M. J., Fasick, P. *et al.* (1996). Continuous intrathecal baclofen infusion for symptomatic generalized dystonia. *Neurosurgery*, **38**, 934–8; discussion 938–9.

Alexander, G. E. (1997). Anatomy of the basal ganglia and related motor structures. In: *Movement disorders: neurologic principles and practice* (ed. R. L. Watts and W. C. Koller), pp. 73–85. McGraw-Hill, New York.

Almasy, L., Bressman, S. B., Raymond, D. *et al.* (1997). Idiopathic torsion dystonia linked to chromosome 8 in two Mennonite families. *Ann. Neurol.*, **42**, 670–3.

Amato, A. A., Cornman, E. W., and Kissel, J. T. (1994). Treatment of stiff-man syndrome with intravenous immunoglobulin. *Neurology*, **44**, 1652–4.

Anderson, N. E., Budde-Steffen, C., Rosenblum, M. K. et al. (1988). Opsoclonus, myoclonus, ataxia, and encephalopathy in adults with cancer: a distinct paraneoplastic syndrome. Medicine (Baltimore), 67, 100–9.

Andrew, J., Fowler, C. J., and Harrison, M. J. G. (1983). Stereotaxic thalamotomy in 55 cases of dystonia. Brain, 106, 981–1000.

Arblaster, L. A., Lakie, M., Mutch, W. J. et al. (1993). A study of the early signs of drug induced parkinsonism. J. Neurol. Neurosurg. Psychiatry, 56, 301–3.

Armon, C., Swanson, J. W., McLean, J. M. et al. (1996). Subacute encephalomyelitis presenting as stiff-person syndrome: clinical, polygraphic, and pathologic correlations. Mov. Disord., 11, 701–9.

Atchison, P. R., Thompson, P. D., Frackowiak, R. S. et al. (1993). The syndrome of gait ignition failure: a report of six cases. Mov. Disord., 8, 285–92.

Averbuch-Heller, L., Paulson, G. W., Daroff, R. B. et al. (1999). Whipples disease mimicking progressive supranuclear palsy: the diagnostic value of eye movement recording. J. Neurol. Neurosurg. and Psychiat., 66, 532–5.

Bandmann, O., Nygaard, T. G., Surtees, R. et al. (1996). Dopa-responsive dystonia in British patients: new mutations of the GTP-cyclohydrolase I gene and evidence for genetic heterogeneity. Hum. Mol. Genet., 5, 403–6.

Barclay, C. L. and Lang, A. E. (1995). Other secondary dystonias. In: Handbook of dystonia (ed. J. K. C. Tsui and D. B. Calne), pp. 267–305. Marcel Dekker, New York.

Barclay, C. L. and Lang, A. E. (1997). Dystonia in progressive supranuclear palsy. J. Neurol. Neurosurg. Psychiatry, 62, 352–6.

Barker, F. G., 2nd, Jannetta, P. J., Bissonette, D. J. et al. (1995). Microvascular decompression for hemifacial spasm. J. Neurosurg., 82, 201–10.

Barker, R. A. and Marsden, C. D. (1997). Successful treatment of stiff man syndrome with intravenous immunoglobulin [letter]. J. Neurol. Neurosurg. Psychiatry, 62, 426–7.

Bartholome, K. and Ludecke, B. (1998). Mutations in the tyrosine hydroxylase gene cause various forms of L-dopa-responsive dystonia. Adv. Pharmacol., 42, 48–9.

Bennett, D. A., Wilson, R. S., Gilley, D. W. et al. (1990). Clinical diagnosis of Binswanger's disease. J. Neurol. Neurosurg. Psychiatry, 53, 961–5.

Bennett, L. B., Roach, E. S. and Bowcock, A. M. (2000). A locus for paroxysmal kinesigenic dyskinesia maps to human chromosome 16. Neurology, 54, 125–30.

Bentivoglio, A. R., Del Grosso, N., Albanese, A. et al. (1997). Non-DYT1 dystonia in a large Italian family. J. Neurol. Neurosurg. Psychiatry, 62, 357–60.

Berardelli, A., Formica, A., Mercuri, B. et al. (1993). Botulinum toxin treatment in patients with focal dystonia and hemifacial spasm. A multicenter study of the Italian Movement Disorder Group. Ital. J. Neurol. Sci., 14, 361–7.

Bergeron, C., Pollanen, M. S., Weyer, L. et al. (1996). Unusual clinical presentations of cortical-basal ganglionic degeneration. Ann. Neurol., 40, 893–900.

Berkovic, S. F., Andermann, F., Carpenter, S. et al. (1986). Progressive myoclonus epilepsies: specific causes and diagnosis. N. Engl. J. Med., 315, 296–305.

Berkovic, S. F., Carpenter, S., Andermann, F. et al. (1988). Kufs' disease: a critical reappraisal. Brain, 111, 27–62.

Berkovic, S. F., Carpenter, S., Evans, A. et al. (1989). Myoclonus epilepsy and ragged-red fibres (MERRF). 1. A clinical, pathological, biochemical, magnetic resonance spectrographic and positron emission tomographic study. Brain, 112, 1231–60.

Bernardi, B., Zimmerman, R. A., Savino, P. J. et al. (1993). Magnetic resonance tomographic angiography in the investigation of hemifacial spasm. Neuroradiology, 35, 606–11.

Bertoni, J. M., Brown, P., Goldfarb, L. G. et al. (1992). Familial Creutzfeldt–Jakob disease (codon 200 mutation) with supranuclear palsy. JAMA, 268, 2413–5.

Bertrand, C. M. (1993). Selective peripheral denervation for spasmodic torticollis: surgical technique, results, and observations in 260 cases. Surg. Neurol., 40, 96–103.

Bharucha, K. J. and Sethi, K. D. (1995). Tardive tourettism after exposure to neuroleptic therapy. Mov. Disord., 10, 791–3.

Bharucha, N. E., Bharucha, E. P., Bharucha, A. E. et al. (1988). Prevalence of Parkinson's disease in the Parsi community of Bombay, India. Arch. Neurol., 45, 1321–3.

Bhatia, K., Thompson, P. D., and Marsden, C. D. (1992). 'Isolated' postinfectious myoclonus. J. Neurol. Neurosurg. Psychiatry, 55, 1089–91.

Bhatia, K. P., Brown, P., Gregory, R. et al. (1995). Progressive myoclonic ataxia associated with coeliac disease. The myoclonus is of cortical origin, but the pathology is in the cerebellum. Brain, 118, 1087–93.

Bhatia, K. P., Lera, G., Luthert, P. J. et al. (1994). Vascular chorea: case report with pathology. Mov. Disord., 9, 447–50.

Bhatia, K. P. and Marsden, C. D. (1994). The behavioural and motor consequences of focal lesions of the basal ganglia in man. Brain, 117, 859–76.

Blasi, J., Chapman, E. R., Link, E. et al. (1993). Botulinum neurotoxin A selectively cleaves the synaptic protein SNAP-25. Nature, 365, 160–3.

Blin, J., Vidailhet, M. J., Pillon, B. et al. (1992). Corticobasal degeneration: decreased and asymmetrical glucose consumption as studied with PET. Mov. Disord., 7, 348–54.

Bodensteiner, J. B., Goldblum, R. M., and Golman, A. S. (1980). Progressive dystonia masking ataxia in ataxia telengiectasia. *Arch. Neurol.*, **37**, 464–5.

Boecker, H., Wills, A. J., Ceballos-Baumann, A. *et al.* (1997). Stereotactic thalamotomy in tremor-dominant Parkinson's disease: an H2$^{(15)}$O PET motor activation study. *Ann. Neurol.*, **41**, 108–11.

Boeve, B. F., Maraganore, D. M., Parisi, J. E. *et al.* (1999). Pathologic hetereneity in clinically diagnosed corticobasal degeneration. *Neurology*, **53**, 795–800.

Brans, J. W., Lindeboom, R., Snoek, J. W. *et al.* (1996). Botulinum toxin versus trihexyphenidyl in cervical dystonia: a prospective, randomized, double-blind controlled trial. *Neurology*, **46**, 1066–72.

Brashear, A., Farlow, M. R., Butler, I. J. *et al.* (1996). Variable phenotype of rapid-onset dystonia-parkinsonism. *Mov. Disord.*, **11**, 151–6.

Brassat, D., Camuzat, A., Vidailhet, M. *et al.* (2000). Frequency of the DYT1 mutation in primary torsion dystonia without family history. *Archives of Neurology*, **57**, 333–5.

Braune, S., Reinhardt, M., Schnitzer, R. *et al.* (1999). Cardiac uptake of [^{123}I]MIBG separates Pd from multiple system atrophy. *Neurology*, **54**, 1877–8.

Bressman, S. B., de Leon, D., Brin, M. F. *et al.* (1989). Idiopathic dystonia among Ashkenazi Jews: evidence for autosomal dominant inheritance. *Ann. Neurol.*, **26**, 612–20.

Bressman, S. B., Heiman, G. A., Nygaard, T. G. *et al.* (1994a). A study of idiopathic torsion dystonia in a non-Jewish family: evidence for genetic heterogeneity. *Neurology*, **44**, 283–7.

Bressman, S. B., Hunt, A. L., Heiman, G. A. *et al.* (1994b). Exclusion of the DYT1 locus in a non-Jewish family with early-onset dystonia. *Mov. Disord.*, **9**, 626–32.

Bressman, S. B., Warner, T. T., Almasy, L. *et al.* (1996). Exclusion of the DYT1 locus in familial torticollis. *Ann. Neurol.*, **40**, 681–4.

Brewer, G. J., Dick, R. D., Johnson, V. *et al.* (1994). Treatment of Wilson's disease with ammonium tetrathiomolybdate. I. Initial therapy in 17 neurologically affected patients. *Arch. Neurol.*, **51**, 545–54.

Brin, M. F., Lew, M. F., Adler, C. H. *et al.* (1999). Safety and efficacy of Neuro Bloc (botulinum toxin type B) in type A-resistant cervical dystonia. *Neurology*, **53**, 1431–38.

Bristow, M. F. and Kohen, D. (1993). How 'malignant' is the neuroleptic malignant syndrome? *BMJ*, **307**, 1223–4.

Brodal, A. (1981). *Neurological anatomy in relation to clinical medicine*. Oxford University Press, Oxford.

Brooks, D. J., Ibanez, V., Sawle, G. V. *et al.* (1992). Striatal D2 receptor status in patients with Parkinson's disease, striatonigral degeneration, and progressive supranuclear palsy, measured with ^{11}C-raclopride and positron emission tomography. *Ann. Neurol.*, **31**, 184–92.

Brooks, D. J., Salmon, E. P., Mathias, C. J. *et al.* (1990). The relationship between locomotor disability, autonomic dysfunction, and the integrity of the striatal dopaminergic system in patients with multiple system atrophy, pure autonomic failure, and Parkinson's disease, studied with PET. *Brain*, **113**, 1539–52.

Broughton, R., Tolentino, M. A., and Krelina, M. (1985). Excessive fragmentary myoclonus in non REM sleep: a report of 38 cases. *Electroenceph. Clin. Neurophysiol.*, **61**, 123–33.

Brown, P., Rothwell, J. C., Thompson, P. D. *et al.* (1991a). New observations on the normal auditory startle reflex in man. *Brain*, **114**, 1981–92.

Brown, P., Rothwell, J. C., Thompson, P. D. *et al.* (1991b). The hyperekplexias and their relationship to the normal startle reflex. *Brain*, **114**, 1903–28.

Brown, P., Thompson, P. D., Rothwell, J. C. *et al.* (1991c). Axial myoclonus of propriospinal origin. *Brain*, **114**, 197–214.

Brown, P., Thompson, P. D., Rothwell, J. C. *et al.* (1991d). A case of postanoxic encephalopathy with cortical action and brainstem reticular reflex myoclonus. *Mov. Disord.*, **6**, 139–44.

Brown, P., Steiger, M. J., Thompson, P. D. *et al.* (1993). Effectiveness of piracetam in cortical myoclonus. *Mov. Disord.*, **8**, 63–8.

Brown, P., Ridding, M. C., Werhahn, K. J. *et al.* (1996). Abnormalities of the balance between inhibition and excitation in the motor cortex of patients with cortical myoclonus. *Brain*, **119**, 309–17.

Brown, P., Rothwell, J. C., and Marsden, C. D. (1997). The stiff leg syndrome. *J. Neurol. Neurosurg. Psychiatry*, **62**, 31–7.

Buckley, P. F. and Hutchinson, M. (1995). Neuroleptic malignant syndrome [editorial]. *J. Neurol. Neurosurg. Psychiatry*, **58**, 271–3.

Bull, P. C., Thomas, G. R., Rommens, J. M. *et al.* (1993). The Wilson disease gene is a putative copper transporting P-type ATPase similar to the Menkes gene [published erratum appears in *Nat. Genet.*, **6** (2), 214, 1994]. *Nat. Genet.*, **5**, 327–37.

Burke, R. E., Fahn, S., and Gold, A. P. (1982a). Delayed onset dystonia in patients with static encephalopathy. *J. Neurol. Neurosurg. Psychiatry*, **43**, 787–97.

Burke, R. E., Fahn, S., Jankovic, J. *et al.* (1982b). Tardive dystonia: late onset and persistent dystonia caused by antipsychotic drugs. *Neurology*, **32**, 1335–46.

Burke, R. E., Fahn, S., and Marsden, C. D. (1986). Torsion dystonia: a double blind prospective trial of high dosage trihexphenidyl. *Neurology*, **36**, 160–4.

Burke, R. E. and Kang, U. J. (1988). Tardive dystonia: clinical aspects and treatment. *Adv. Neurol.*, **49**, 199–210.

Burke, R. E., Kang, U. J., Jankovic, J. et al. (1989). Tardive akathisia: an analysis of clinical features and response to open therapeutic trials. Mov. Disord., 4, 157–75.

Burn, D. J., Ball, J., Lees, A. J. et al. (1991). A case of progressive encephalomyelitis with rigidity and positive antiglutamic acid decarboxylase antibodies. J. Neurol. Neurosurg. Psychiatry, 54, 449–51.

Burn, D. J. and Brooks, D. J. (1993). Nigral dysfunction in drug-induced parkinsonism: an 18F-dopa PET study. Neurology, 43, 552–6.

Burn, D. J., Mark, M. H., Playford, E. D. et al. (1992). Parkinson's disease in twins studied with 18F-dopa and positron emission tomography. Neurology, 42, 1894–900.

Burn, D. J., Rinne, J. O., Quinn, N. P. et al. (1995). Striatal opioid receptor binding in Parkinson's disease, striatonigral degeneration and Steele–Richardson–Olszewski syndrome. A [11C]diprenorphine PET study. Brain, 118, 951–8.

Burn, D. J., Sawle, G. V., and Brooks, D. J. (1994). Differential diagnosis of Parkinson's disease, multiple system atrophy, and Steele–Richardson–Olszewski syndrome: discriminant analysis of striatal 18F-dopa PET data. J. Neurol. Neurosurg. Psychiatry, 57, 278–84.

Byrne, E. J., Lennox, G., Lowe, J. et al. (1989). Diffuse Lewy body disease: clinical features in 15 cases. J. Neurol. Neurosurg. Psychiatry, 52, 709–17.

Cammarota, A., Gershanik, O. S., Garcia, S. et al. (1995). Cervical dystonia due to spinal cord ependymoma: involvement of cervical cord segments in the pathogenesis of dystonia. Mov. Disord., 10, 500–3.

Caparros-Lefebvre, D., Destee, A., and Petit, H. (1997). Late onset familial dystonia: could mitochondrial deficits induce a diffuse lesioning process of the whole basal ganglia system? J. Neurol. Neurosurg. Psychiatry, 63, 196–203.

Caplan, L. R. (1995). Binswanger's disease—revisited. Neurology, 45, 626–33.

Caraceni, B., Broggi, G., and Avanzini, G. (1974). Familial idiopathic basal ganglia calcification exhibiting dystonia musculorum deformans features. Eur. Neurol., 12, 351–9.

Caraceni, T. (1994). A case for early levodopa treatment of Parkinson's disease. Clin. Neuropharmacol., 17, S38–42.

Cardoso, F., Jankovic, J., Grossman, R. G. et al. (1995). Outcome after stereotactic thalamotomy for dystonia and hemiballismus. Neurosurgery, 36, 501–7; discussion 507–8.

Carlson, J. H., Bergstrom, D. A., and Walters, J. R. (1987). Stimulation of both D1 and D2 receptors appears necessary for full expression of postsynaptic effects of dopamine agonists: a neurophysiological study. Brain Res., 400, 205–18.

Case records of the Massachusetts General Hospital (1993). A 75 year old man with right sided rigidity, dysarthria and abnormal gait. Case 46-1993. N. Engl. J. Med., 329, 1560–7.

Casey, D. E. and Gerlach, J. (1988). Tardive dyskinesia. Acta Psychiatr. Scand., 77, 369–78.

Caviness, J. N., Forsyth, P. A., Layton, D. D. et al. (1995). The movement disorder of adult opsoclonus. Mov. Disord., 10, 22–7.

Chu, N., Huang, C., Lu, C. et al. (1995). Dystonia caused by toxins. In: Handbook of dystonia (ed. J. K. C. Tsui and D. B. Calne), pp. 241–65. Marcel Dekker, New York.

Clarke, C. E., Speller, J. M. (2000). Pergolide versus bromocriptine for levodopa induced motor complications in Parkinson's disease. Cochrane Database Syst. Rev., pCD000236.

Cole, R., Hallett, M., and Cohen, L. G. (1995). Double-blind trial of botulinum toxin for treatment of focal hand dystonia. Mov. Disord., 10, 466–71.

Coleman, R. J., Quinn, N. P., and Marsden, C. D. (1988). Multiple sclerosis presenting as adult onset dystonia. Mov. Disord., 3, 329–32.

Collins, S. J., Ahlskog, J. E., Parisi, J. E. et al. (1995). Progressive supranuclear palsy: neuropathologically based diagnostic clinical criteria. J. Neurol. Neurosurg. Psychiatry, 58, 167–73.

Comu, S., Giuliani, M., and Narayanan, V. (1996). Episodic ataxia and myokymia syndrome: a new mutation of potassium channel gene Kv1.1. Ann. Neurol., 40, 684–7.

Conard, C., Andreadis, A., Trojanowski, J. Q. et al. (1997). Genetic evidence for the involvement of tau in progressive supranuclear palsy. Ann. Neurol., 41, 277–81.

Consensus Committee of the American Autonomic Society and the American Academy of Neurology (1996). Consensus statement on the definition of orthostatic hypotension, pure autonomic failure and multiple system atrophy. Neurology, 46, 1470.

Cooke, W. T. and Smith, W. T. (1966). Neurological disorders associated with adult coeliac disease. Brain, 89, 683–722.

Cosentino, C., Torres, L., Flores, M. et al. (1996). Paroxysmal kinesigenic dystonia and spinal cord lesion. Mov. Disord., 11, 453–5.

Counihan, T. J., Shinobu, L. A., Eskandar, E. N. et al. (2001). Outcomes following staged bilateral pallidotomy in advanced Parkinson's disease. Neurology, 56, 799–802.

Craufurd, D. and Dodge, A. (1993). Mutation size and age at onset of Huntington's disease. J. Med. Genet., 30, 1008–11.

Craufurd, D. and Tyler, A. (1992). Predictive testing for Huntington's disease: protocol of the UK Huntington's prediction consortium. J. Med. Genet., 29, 915–8.

Critchley, M. (1929). Arteriosclerotic parkinsonism. Brain, 52, 23 83.

Crossman, A. R., Mitchell, I. J., Sambrook, M. A. *et al.* (1988). Chorea and myoclonus in the monkey induced by gamma-aminobutyric acid antagonism in the lentiform complex. The site of drug action and a hypothesis for the neural mechanisms of chorea. *Brain*, 111, 1211–33.

Curran, T. and Lang, A. E. (1994). Parkinsonian syndromes associated with hydrocephalus: case reports, a review of the literature, and pathophysiological hypotheses. *Mov. Disord.*, 9, 508–20.

Daniel, S. E., de Bruin, V. M., and Lees, A. J. (1995). The clinical and pathological spectrum of Steele–Richardson–Olszewski syndrome (progressive supranuclear palsy): a reappraisal. *Brain*, 118, 759–70.

Davie, C. A., Wenning, G. K., Barker, G. J. *et al.* (1995). Differentiation of multiple system atrophy from idiopathic Parkinson's disease using proton magnetic resonance spectroscopy. *Ann. Neurol.*, 37, 204–10.

Davis, M. B., Bateman, D., Quinn, N. P. *et al.* (1994). Mutation analysis in patients with possible but apparently sporadic Huntington's disease. *Lancet*, 344, 714–7.

Davison, C. (1954). Pallidopyramidal disease. *J. Neuropathol. Exp. Neurol.*, 13, 50–9.

De Camilli, P., Thomas, A., and Cofiell, R. (1993). The synaptic vesicle associated protein amphiphysin is the 128 kD autoantigen of stiff man syndrome with breast cancer. *J. Exp. Med.*, 178, 2219–23.

De Rijk, M. C., Tzourio, C., Breteler, M. M. *et al.* (1997). Prevalence of parkinsonism and Parkinson's disease in Europe: the EUROPARKINSON Collaborative Study. European Community Concerted Action on the Epidemiology of Parkinson's disease. *J. Neurol. Neurosurg. Psychiatry*, 62, 10–5.

De Vries, B. B., Arts, W. F., Breedveld, G. J. *et al.* (2000). Benign hereditary chorea of early onset maps to chromosome 14q. *Am. J. Hum. Gen.*, 66, 136–42.

De Yebenes, J. G., Brin, M. F., Mena, M. A. *et al.* (1988). Neurochemical findings in neuroacanthocytosis. *Mov. Disord.*, 3, 300–12.

De Yebenes, J. G., Pernaute, R. S., and Tabernero, C. (1996). Symptomatic dystonias. In: *Movement disorders: neurologic principles and practice* (ed. R. L. Watts and W. C. Koller), pp. 455–75. McGraw-Hill, New York.

Defer, G. L., Geny, C., Ricolfi, F. *et al.* (1996). Long-term outcome of unilaterally transplanted parkinsonian patients. I. Clinical approach. *Brain*, 119, 41–50.

Deiber, M. P., Pollak, P., Passingham, R. *et al.* (1993). Thalamic stimulation and suppression of parkinsonian tremor. Evidence of a cerebellar deactivation using positron emission tomography. *Brain*, 116, 267–79.

Delisle, M. B., Murrell, J. R., Richardson, R. *et al.* (1999). A mutation at codon 279 (N279K) in exon 10 of the tau gene cause a taupathy with dementia and supranuclear palsy. *Acta Neuropathologica*, 98, 62–77.

DeLong, M. R. (1990). Primate models of movement disorders of basal ganglia origin. *Trends Neurosci.*, 13, 281–5.

Demirkiran, M. and Jankovic, J. (1995). Paroxysmal dyskinesias: clinical features and classification. *Ann. Neurol.*, 38, 571–9.

Demirkiran, M., Jankovic, J., Lewis, R. A. *et al.* (1996). Neurologic presentation of Wilson disease without Kayser–Fleischer rings. *Neurology*, 46, 1040–3.

Dening, T. R. and Berrios, G. E. (1989). Wilson's disease: psychiatric symptoms in 195 cases. *Arch. Gen. Psychiatry*, 46, 1126–34.

Deuschl, G., Toro, C., Matsumoto, J. *et al.* (1995). Movement-related cortical potentials in writer's cramp. *Ann. Neurol.*, 38, 862–8.

Deuschl, G., Toro, C., Valls-Sole, J. *et al.* (1996). Symptomatic and essential palatal tremor. 3. Abnormal motor learning. *J. Neurol. Neurosurg. Psychiatry*, 60, 520–5.

Dickson, D. W., Lin, W., Liu, W. K., Yen, S. H. (1999). Multiple system atrophy: a sporadic synucleinopathy. *Brain Pathology*, 9, 721–32.

Di Maria, E., Tabaton, M., Vigo, T. *et al.* (2000). Corticobasal degeneration shares a common genetic background with progressive supranuclear palsy. *Ann. of Neurol.*, 47, 374–7.

Dogali, M., Fazzini, E., Kolodny, E. *et al.* (1995). Stereotactic ventral pallidotomy for Parkinson's disease. *Neurology*, 45, 753–61.

Donnan, P. T., Steinke, D. T., Stubbings, C. *et al.* (2000). Selegicine and mortality in subjects with Parkinson's disease: A longitudinal community study. *Neurology*, 55, 1785–9.

Dooling, E. C., Schoene, W. C., and Richardson, E. P. (1974). Hallervorden–Spatz syndrome. *Arch. Neurol.*, 30, 70–83.

Dressler, D., Thompson, P. D., Gledhill, R. F. *et al.* (1994). The syndrome of painful legs and moving toes. *Mov. Disord.*, 9, 13–21.

Duayo, M., Ambrose, C., Myers, R. *et al.* (1993). Trinucleotide repeat length instability and age of onset in Huntington's disease. *Nat. Genet.*, 4, 387–92.

Dum, R. P. and Strick, P. L. (1991). The origin of corticospinal projections from premotor areas in the frontal lobe. *J. Neurosci.*, 11, 667–89.

Durif, F., Vidailhet, M., Assal, F. *et al.* (1997). Low-dose clozapine improves dyskinesias in Parkinson's disease. *Neurology*, 48, 658–62.

Durso, R., Evans, J. E., Josephs, E. *et al.* (1997). Central levodopa metabolism in Parkinson's disease after administration of stable isotope labelled levodopa. *Ann. Neurol.*, **42**, 300–4.

Eidelberg, D., Moeller, J. R., Ishikawa, T. *et al.* (1995). The metabolic topography of idiopathic torsion dystonia. *Brain*, **118**, 1473–84.

Eidelberg, D., Moeller, J. R., Ishikawa, T. *et al.* (1996). Regional metabolic correlates of surgical outcome following unilateral pallidotomy for Parkinson's disease. *Ann. Neurol.*, **39**, 450–9.

Eidelberg, D., Takikawa, S., Moeller, J. R. *et al.* (1993*a*). Striatal hypometabolism distinguishes striatonigral degeneration from Parkinson's disease. *Ann. Neurol.*, **33**, 518–27.

Eidelberg, D., Takikawa, S., Wilhelmsen, K. *et al.* (1993*b*). Positron emission tomographic findings in Filipino X-linked dystonia-parkinsonism. *Ann. Neurol.*, **34**, 185–91.

Elston, J. S. (1992). A new variant of blepharospasm. *J. Neurol. Neurosurg. Psychiatry*, **55**, 369–71.

Esteban Munoz, J., Tolosa, E., Saiz, A. *et al.* (1996). Upper-limb dystonia secondary to a midbrain hemorrhage [letter]. *Mov. Disord.*, **11**, 96–9.

Factor, S. A. and Friedman, J. H. (1997). The emerging role of clozapine in the treatment of movement disorders. *Mov. Disord.*, **12**, 483–96.

Fahn, S. (1994*a*). The paroxysmal dyskinesias. In: *Movement disorders*, Vol. 3 (ed. C. D. Marsden and S. Fahn), pp. 310–45. Butterworth-Heinemann, Oxford.

Fahn, S. (1994*b*). Psychogenic movement disorders. In: *Movement disorders*, Vol. 3 (ed. C. D. Marsden and S. Fahn), pp. 359–72. Butterworth-Heinemann, Oxford.

Fahn, S. (1996). Is levodopa toxic? *Neurology*, **47**, S184–95.

Fahn, S., Marsden, C. D., and Calne, D. B. (1987). Classification and investigation of dystonia. In: *Movement disorders*, Vol. 2 (ed. S. Fahn and C. D. Marsden), pp. 332–58. Butterworths, London.

Fahn, S. and Sjaastad, O. (1991). Hereditary essential myoclonus in a large Norwegian family. *Mov. Disord.*, **6**, 237–47.

Farrer, M., Guinn-Hardy, K., Muenter, M. *et al.* (1999). A chromosome 4p haplotype segregating with Parkinson's disease and postural tremor. *Hum. Mol. Genet.*, **8**, 81–5.

Fear, C. F. (1992). Drug induced Creutzfeldt Jacob like syndrome: a review. *Hum. Psychopharmacol.*, **7**, 89.

Fearnley, J. M. and Lees, A. J. (1991). Ageing and Parkinson's disease: substantia nigra regional selectivity. *Brain*, **114**, 2283–301.

Fearnley, J. M., Revesz, T., Brooks, D. J. *et al.* (1991). Diffuse Lewy body disease presenting with a supranuclear gaze palsy. *J. Neurol. Neurosurg. Psychiatry*, **54**, 159–61.

Federico, F., Simone, I. L., Lucivero, V. *et al.* (1997). Proton magnetic resonance spectroscopy in Parkinson's disease and progressive supranuclear palsy. *J. Neurol. Neurosurg. Psychiatry*, **62**, 239–42.

Fenton, W. S., Wyatt, R. J., and McGlashan, T. H. (1994). Risk factors for spontaneous dyskinesia in schizophrenia. *Arch. Gen. Psychiatry*, **51**, 643–50.

Feve, A., Angelard, B., Fenelon, G. *et al.* (1990). Neuroleptic induced tardive dyskinesia in the cebus monkey. *Mov. Disord.*, **7**, 32–7.

Finelli, P. F., McEntee, W. J., Ambler, M. *et al.* (1980). Adult celiac disease presenting as cerebellar syndrome. *Neurology*, **30**, 245–9.

Fink, J. K., Rainer, S., Wilkowski, J. *et al.* (1996). Paroxysmal dystonic choreoathetosis: tight linkage to chromosome 2q. *Am. J. Hum. Genet.*, **59**, 140–5.

Fish, D. R. (1994). Epilepsy masquerading as a movement disorder. In: *Movement disorders*, Vol. 3 (ed. C. D. Marsden and S. Fahn), pp. 346–58. Butterworth-Heinemann, Oxford.

Fitzgerald, P. M., Jankovic, J., Glaze, D. G. *et al.* (1990). Extrapyramidal involvement in Rett's syndrome. *Neurology*, **40**, 293–5.

Fletcher, N. A., Harding, A. E., and Marsden, C. D. (1990). A genetic study of idiopathic torsion dystonia in the United Kingdom. *Brain*, **113**, 379–95.

Fletcher, N. A., Harding, A. E., and Marsden, C. D. (1991*a*). A case–control study of idiopathic torsion dystonia. *Mov. Disord.*, **6**, 304–9.

Fletcher, N. A., Harding, A. E., and Marsden, C. D. (1991*b*). Intrafamilial correlation in idiopathic torsion dystonia. *Mov. Disord.*, **6**, 310–4.

Fletcher, N. A., Harding, A. E., and Marsden, C. D. (1991*c*). The relationship between trauma and idiopathic torsion dystonia. *J. Neurol. Neurosurg. Psychiatry*, **54**, 713–7.

Fletcher, N. A. and Foley, J. (1993). Parental age, genetic mutation and cerebral palsy. *J. Med. Genet.*, **30**, 44–6.

Fletcher, N. A., Thompson, P. D., Scadding, J. W. *et al.* (1993). Successful treatment of childhood onset symptomatic dystonia with levodopa. *J. Neurol. Neurosurg. Psychiatry*, **56**, 865–7.

Fletcher, N. A. and Marsden, C. D. (1996). Dyskinetic cerebral palsy: a clinical and genetic study. *Dev. Med. Child Neurol.*, **38**, 873–80.

Fogan, L. (1996). Progressive encephalomyelitis with rigidity responsive to plasmapheresis and immunosuppression. *Ann. Neurol.*, **40**, 451–3.

Footitt, D. R., Quinn, N., Kocen, R. S. *et al.* (1997). Familial Lafora body disease of late onset: report of four cases in one family and a review of the literature. *J. Neurol.*, **244**, 40–4.

Ford, B., Greene, P., Louis, E. D. *et al.* (1996). Use of intrathecal baclofen in the treatment of patients with dystonia. *Arch. Neurol.*, **53**, 1241–6.

Foster, N. L., Gilman, S., Berent, S. *et al.* (1992). Progressive subcortical gliosis and progressive supranuclear palsy can have similar clinical and PET abnormalities. *J. Neurol. Neurosurg. Psychiatry*, **55**, 707–13.

Frankel, J. P., Lees, A. J., Kempster, P. A. *et al.* (1990). Subcutaneous apomorphine in the treatment of Parkinson's disease. *J. Neurol. Neurosurg. Psychiatry*, **53**, 96–101.

Frankel, M., Cummings, J. L., Robertson, M. M. *et al.* (1986). Obsessions and compulsions in Gilles de la Tourette's syndrome. *Neurology*, **36**, 378–82.

Freed, C. R. Greene, P. E., Breeze, R. E. *et al.* (2001). Transplantation of embryonic neurons for severe Parkinson's disease. *New England Journal of Medicine*, **344**, 710–19.

Freeman, T. B., Olanow, C. W., Hauser, R. A. *et al.* (1995). Bilateral fetal nigral transplantation into the postcommissural putamen in Parkinson's disease. *Ann. Neurol.*, **38**, 379–88.

Friede, R. L. (1989). *Developmental neuropathology*, pp. 83–97. Springer, Berlin.

Friedman, J. H. (1994). Clozapine treatment of psychosis in patients with tardive dystonia: report of three cases. *Mov. Disord.*, **9**, 321–4.

Friedman, J. H., Factor, S. A. (2000). Atypical antipsychotics in the treatment of drug-induced psychosis in Parkinson's disease. *Movement Disorders*, **15**, 201–11.

Friedman, J. R. L., Klein, C., Leung, J. *et al.* (2000). The CAG deletion of the DYT1 gene is infrequent in musicians with focal dystonia. *Neurology*, **55**, 1417–18.

Frucht, S., Rogers, J. D., Greene, P. E. *et al.* (1999). Falling asleep at the wheel: motor vehicle mishaps in persons taking pramipexole and ropinirole. *Neurology*, **52**, 1908–10.

Furukawa, Y., Guttman, M., Sparagana, S. P. *et al.* (2000). Dopa responsive dystonia due to a large deletion in the GTP cyclohydrolose 1 gene. *Ann. Neurol.*, **47**, 517–20.

Gardos, G. and Cole, J. O. (1980). Overview: Public health issues in tardive dyskinesia. *Am. J. Psychiatry*, **137**, 776–81.

Gasser, T., Bove, C. M., Ozelius, L. J. *et al.* (1996). Haplotype analysis at the DYT1 locus in Ashkenazi Jewish patients with occupational hand dystonia. *Mov. Disord.*, **11**, 163–6.

Gasser, T., Muller-Myhsok, B., Wszolek, Z. K. *et al.* (1998). A susceptibility locus for Parkinson's disease maps to chromosome 2p13. *Nat. Genet.*, **18**, 262–5.

Geschwind, D. H., Loginov, M., Stern, J. M. (1999). Identification of a locus on chromosome 14q for idiopathic basal ganglia calcification (Fahr disease). *Am. J. Hum. Gen*, **65**, 764–72.

Gibb, W. R. and Lees, A. J. (1989). Tendency to late recurrence following rheumatic chorea. *Neurology*, **39**, 999.

Gibb, W. R., Lees, A. J., and Marsden, C. D. (1988). Pathological report of four patients presenting with cranial dystonias. *Mov. Disord.*, **3**, 211–21.

Giedd, J. N., Rapoport, J. L., Kruesi, M. J. *et al.* (1995). Sydenham's chorea: magnetic resonance imaging of the basal ganglia. *Neurology*, **45**, 2199–202.

Gilman, S. and Quinn, N. P. (1996). The relationship of multiple system atrophy to sporadic olivopontocerebellar atrophy and other forms of idiopathic late-onset cerebellar atrophy. *Neurology*, **46**, 1197–9.

Gilman, S., Sima, A. A., Junck, L. *et al.* (1996). Spinocerebellar ataxia type 1 with multiple system degeneration and glial cytoplasmic inclusions. *Ann. Neurol.*, **39**, 241–55.

Goetz, C. G. (1983). Drug induced parkinsonism and idiopathic Parkinson's disease. *Arch. Neurol.*, **40**, 325–6.

Goetz, C. G. and Stebbins, G. T. (1991). Effects of head trauma from motor vehicle accidents on Parkinson's disease. *Ann. Neurol.*, **29**, 191–3.

Golbe, L. (1991). Young onset Parkinson's disease: a clinical review. *Neurology*, **41**, 168–73.

Golbe, L. I. (1996). The epidemiology of progressive supranuclear palsy. *Adv. Neurol.*, **69**, 25–31.

Golbe, L. I., Di Iorio, G., Bonavita, V. *et al.* (1990). A large kindred with autosomal dominant Parkinson's disease. *Ann. Neurol.*, **27**, 276–82.

Goldberg, Y. P., Kremer, B., Andrew, S. E. *et al.* (1993). Molecular analysis of new mutations for Huntington's disease: intermediate alleles and sex of origin effects. *Nat. Genet.*, **5**, 174–9.

Gordon, M. F., Abrams, R. I., Rubin, D. B. *et al.* (1995). Bismuth subsalicylate toxicity as a cause of prolonged encephalopathy with myoclonus. *Mov. Disord.*, **10**, 220–2.

Grafman, J., Litvan, I., Gomez, C. *et al.* (1990). Frontal lobe function in progressive supranuclear palsy. *Arch. Neurol.*, **47**, 553–8.

Grafton, S. T., Waters, C., Sutton, J. *et al.* (1995). Pallidotomy increases activity of motor association cortex in Parkinson's disease: a positron emission tomographic study. *Ann. Neurol.*, **37**, 776–83.

Graham, J. G. and Oppenheimer, D. R. (1969). Orthostatic hypotension and nicotine sensitivity in a case of multiple system atrophy. *J. Neurol. Neurosurg. Psychiatry*, **32**, 28–34.

Grandas, F., Elston, J., Quinn, N. *et al.* (1988). Blepharospasm: a review of 264 patients. *J. Neurol. Neurosurg. Psychiatry*, **51**, 767–72.

Greene, P., Fahn, S., Brin, M. F. *et al.* (1994). Botulinum toxin therapy. In: *Movement disorders*, Vol. 3 (ed. C. D. Marsden and S. Fahn), pp. 477–502. Butterworth-Heinemann, Oxford.

Greene, P. E., Shale, H., and Fahn, S. (1988). Analysis of open label trials in torsion dystonia using high dosages of anticholinergics and other drugs. *Mov. Disord.*, **3**, 46–60.

Greene, P. E., Bressman, S. B., Ford, B., Hyland, K. (2000). Parkinsonism dystonia and hemiatrophy. *Movement Disorders*, **15**, 537–41.

Griffith, J. M., Adler, L. E., and Freedman, R. (1994). Fine motor performance in schizophrenia. *Neuropsychobiology*, **29**, 179–84.

Grimes, D. A., Lang, A. E., Bergeron, C. *et al.* (2000). Late adult onset chrorea with typical pathology of Hallervorden-Spatz syndrome. *Journal of Neurology, Neurosurgery and Psychiatry*, **69**, 392–5.

Guridi, J., Obeso, J. A. (2001). The subthalamic nucleus, hemiballismus and Parkinson's disease: reappraisal of a neurosurgical dogma. *Brain*, **124**, 5–19.

Haberhausen, G., Schmitt, I., Kohler, A. *et al.* (1995). Assignment of the dystonia-parkinsonism syndrome locus, DYT3, to a small region within a 1.8-Mb YAC contig of Xq13.1. *Am. J. Hum. Genet.*, **57**, 644–50.

Haddad, P. M. (1994). Neuroleptic malignant syndrome may be caused by other drugs. *BMJ*, **308**, 200.

Hagberg, B. and Hagberg, G. (1993). The origins of cerebral palsy. In: *Recent advances in paediatrics*, Vol. XI (ed. T. J. David), pp. 67–83. Churchill Livingstone, Edinburgh.

Hague, K., Lento, P., Morgello, S. *et al.* (1997). The distribution of Lewy bodies in pure autonomic failure: autopsy findings and review of the literature. *Acta Neuropathol. (Berlin)*, **94**, 192–6.

Hallett, M., Chadwick, D., and Marsden, C. D. (1979). Cortical reflex myoclonus. *Neurology*, **29**, 1107–25.

Hallett, M., Litvan, I. *et al.* (1999). Evaluation of surgery for Parkinson's disease. A report of the therapeutics and technology assessment subcommittee of the American Academy of Neurology. *Neurology*, **52**, 1910–21.

Hanna, M. G. and Bhatia, K. P. (1997). Movement disorders and mitochondrial dysfunction. *Cur. Opin. Neurol.*, **10**, 351–6.

Hardie, R. J. and Lees, A. J. (1988). Neuroleptic induced Parkinson's syndrome: clinical features and results of treatment with levodopa. *J. Neurol. Neurosurg. Psychiatry*, **8**, 850–4.

Hardie, R. J., Pullon, H. W. H., Harding, A. E. *et al.* (1991). Neuroacanthocytosis: a clinical, haematological and pathological study of 19 cases. *Brain*, **114**, 13–49.

Harding, A. E., Thompson, P. D., Kocen, R. S. *et al.* (1989). Plasma exchange and immunosuppression in the stiff man syndrome [letter]. *Lancet*, **2**, 915.

Harper, P. S. (1991a). The epidemiology of Huntington's disease. In: *Huntington's disease* (ed. P. S. Harper), pp. 251–80. W. B. Saunders, London.

Harper, P. S. (1991b). The natural history of Huntington's disease. In: *Huntington's disease* (ed. P. S. Harper), pp. 127–40. W. B. Saunders, London.

Harper, P. S. and Newcombe, R. G. (1992). Age at onset and life table risks in genetic counselling for Huntington's disease. *J. Med. Genet.*, **29**, 239–42.

Hart, I. K., Waters, C., Vincent, A. *et al.* (1997). Autoantibodies detected to expressed K$^+$ channels are implicated in neuromyotonia. *Ann. Neurol.*, **41**, 238–46.

Hauser, R. A., Freeman, T. B., and Olanow, C. W. (1995). Surgical therapies for Parkinson's disease. In: *Treatment of movement disorders* (ed. R. Kurlan), pp. 57–93. J. B. Lippincott, Philadelphia.

Hely, M. A., Morris, J. G., Reid, W. G. *et al.* (1994). The Sydney Multicentre Study of Parkinson's disease: a randomised, prospective five year study comparing low dose bromocriptine with low dose levodopa-carbidopa. *J. Neurol. Neurosurg. Psychiatry*, **57**, 903–10.

Herz, E. (1944). Dystonia. I. Historical review; analysis of dystonic symptoms and physiologic mechanisms involved. *Arch. Neurol. Psychiatry*, **51**, 305–18.

Heye, N., Jergas, M., Hotzinger, H. *et al.* (1993). Sydenham chorea: clinical, EEG, MRI and SPECT findings in the early staage of the disease. *J. Neurol.*, **240**, 121–3.

Ho, M. F., Chalmers, R. M., Davis, M. B. *et al.* (1996). A novel point mutation in the McLeod syndrome gene in neuroacanthocytosis. *Ann. Neurol.*, **39**, 672–5.

Hoenicka, J., Perez, M., Perez-Tur, J. *et al.* (1999). The tau gene AO allele and progressive supranuclear palsy. *Neurology*, **53**, 1219–25.

Holmgren, G., Ozelius, L., Forsgren, L. *et al.* (1995). Adult onset idiopathic torsion dystonia is excluded from the DYT 1 region (9q34) in a Swedish family. *J. Neurol. Neurosurg. Psychiatry*, **59**, 178–81.

Hornykiewicz, O., Kish, S. J., Becker, L. E. *et al.* (1988). Biochemical evidence for brain neurotransmitter changes in idiopathic torsion dystonia (dystonia musculorum deformans). *Adv. Neurol.*, **50**, 157–65.

Howard, R. S., Greenwood, R., Gawler, J. *et al.* (1993). A familial disorder associated with palatal myoclonus, other brainstem signs, tetraparesis, ataxia and Rosenthal fibre formation. *J. Neurol. Neurosurg. Psychiatry*, **56**, 977–81.

Howard, R. S. and Lees, A. J. (1987). Encephalitis lethargica. A report of four recent cases. *Brain*, **110**, 19–33.

Hughes, A. J., Bishop, S., Kleedorfer, B. *et al.* (1993a). Subcutaneous apomorphine in Parkinson's disease: response to chronic administration for up to five years. *Mov. Disord.*, **8**, 165–70.

Hughes, A. J., Daniel, S. E., Blankson, S. *et al.* (1993b). A clinicopathologic study of 100 cases of Parkinson's disease. *Arch. Neurol.*, **50**, 140–8.

Hughes, A. J., Daniel, S. E., Kilford, L. et al. (1992). Accuracy of clinical diagnosis of idiopathic Parkinson's disease: a clinico-pathological study of 100 cases. J. Neurol. Neurosurg. Psychiatry, 55, 181–4.

Hunt, J. R. (1917). Progressive atrophy of the globus pallidus (primary atrophy of the pallidal system): a system disease of the paralysis agitans type, characterised by atrophy of the motor cells of the corpus striatum. A contribution to the functions of the corpus striatum. Brain, 40, 58–148.

Hunter, R., Smith, J., Thomson, T. et al. (1978). Hemiparkinsonism with infarction of the ipsilateral substantia nigra. Neuropathol. Appl. Neurobiol., 4, 297–301.

Huntington's disease collaborative research group (1993). A novel gene that is unstable and expanded on Huntington's disease chromosomes. Cell, 72, 971–83.

Hyde, T. M., Stacey, M. E., Coppola, R. et al. (1995). Cerebral morphometric abnormalities in Tourette's syndrome: a quantitative MRI study of monozygotic twins. Neurology, 45, 1176–82.

Iacono, R. P., Kuniyoshi, S. M., Lonser, R. R. et al. (1996). Simultaneous bilateral pallidoansotomy for idiopathic dystonia musculorum deformans. Pediatr. Neurol., 14, 145–8.

Iacono, R. P., Shima, F., Lonser, R. R. et al. (1995). The results, indications, and physiology of posteroventral pallidotomy for patients with Parkinson's disease. Neurosurgery, 36, 1118–25; discussion 1125–7.

Ichinose, H., Ohye, T., Takahashi, E. et al. (1994). Hereditary progressive dystonia with marked diurnal fluctuations caused by mutations in the GTP cyclohydrolase I gene. Nat. Genet., 8, 236–42.

Ikoma, K., Samii, A., Mercuri, B. et al. (1996). Abnormal cortical motor excitability in dystonia. Neurology, 46, 1371–6.

Ito, M. (1984). The cerebellum and neural control. Raven Press, New York.

Jankovic, J. (1987). The neurology of tics. In: Movement disorders, Vol. 2 (ed. S. Fahn and C. D. Marsden), pp. 383–405. Butterworths, London.

Jankovic, J. (1993). Deprenyl in attention deficit associated with Tourette's syndrome. Arch. Neurol., 50, 286–8.

Jankovic, J. (1994a). Botulinum toxin in the treatment of dystonic tics. Mov. Disord., 9, 347–9.

Jankovic, J. (1994b). Stereotypies. In: Movement disorders, Vol. 3 (ed. S. Fahn and C. D. Marsden), pp. 503–17. Butterworth-Heinemann, Oxford.

Jankovic, J. and Ashizawa, T. (1995). Tourettism associated with Huntington's disease. Mov. Disord., 10, 103–5.

Jankovic, J. and Beach, J. (1997). Long-term effects of tetrabenazine in hyperkinetic movement disorders. Neurology, 48, 358–62.

Jankovic, J., Kirkpatrick, J. B., and Blomquist, K. A. (1985). Late onset Hallervorden–Spatz disease presenting as familial parkinsonism. Neurology, 35, 227–34.

Jankovic, J. and Orman, J. (1988). Tetrabenazine therapy of dystonia, chorea, tics, and other dyskinesias. Neurology, 38, 391–4.

Jarman, P. R., Davis, M. B., Hodgson, S. V. et al. (1997). Paroxysmal dystonic choreoathetosis. Genetic linkage studies in a British family. Brain, 120, 2125–30.

Jellinger, K. (1968). Progressive pallidumatrophie. J. Neurol. Sci., 6, 19–44.

Jenner, P. and Olanow, C. W. (1996). Oxidative stress and the pathogenesis of Parkinson's disease. Neurology, 47, S161–70.

Johnson, D. S. and Montgomery, E. B. (1997). Pathophysiology of cerebellar disorders. In: Movement disorders: neurologic principles and practice (ed. R. L. Watts and W. C. Koller), pp. 587–610. McGraw-Hill, New York.

Joseph, A. B. (1992). Catatonia. In: Movement disorders in neurology and psychiatry (ed. A. B. Joseph and R. R. Young), pp. 335–42. Blackwell, Boston.

Kaji, R., Ikeda, A., Ikeda, T. et al. (1995). Physiological study of cervical dystonia. Task-specific abnormality in contingent negative variation. Brain, 118, 511–22.

Kang, U. J., Burke, R. E., and Fahn, S. (1988). Tardive dystonia. Adv. Neurol., 50, 415–29.

Kambouris, M., Bohlega, S., Al-Tahan, A. et al. (2000). Localisation of the gene for a novel autosomal recessive neurodegenerative Huntington-like disorder to 4p15.3. Am. J. Hum. Gen., 66, 445–52.

Kanouchi, T., Yokota, T., Isa, F. et al. (1997). Role of the ipsilateral motor cortex in mirror movements. J. Neurol. Neurosurg. Psychiatry, 62, 629–32.

Karp, B. I. and Hallett, M. (1996). Extracorporeal phantom tics in Tourette's syndrome. Neurology, 46, 38–40.

Kartsounis, L. D. and Hardie, R. J. (1996). The pattern of cognitive impairments in neuroacanthocytosis. A frontosubcortical dementia. Arch. Neurol., 53, 77–80.

Kawanami, T., Kato, T., Daimon, M. et al. (1996). Hereditary caeruloplasmin deficiency: clinicopathological study of a patient. J. Neurol. Neurosurg. Psychiatry, 61, 506–9.

Kellett, M. W., Steiger, M. J. (1999). Deterioration in parkinsonism with low-dose pergolide. Journal of Neurology, 246, 309–11.

Kimber, J. R., Watson, L., and Mathias, C. J. (1997). Distinction of idiopathic Parkinson's disease from multiple system atrophy by stimulation of growth hormone release with clonidine. Lancet, 349, 1877–81.

Kitada, T., Asakawa, S., Hattori, N. et al. (1998). Mutations in the parkin gene cause autosomal recessive juvenile parkinsonism. Nature, 392, 605–8.

Klawans, H. L. (1981). Hemiparkinsonism as a late complication of hemiatrophy: a new syndrome. *Neurology*, **31**, 625–8.

Klawans, H. L. and Weiner, W. J. (1974). The effect of d amphetamine on choreiform movement disorders. *Neurology*, **24**, 314–8.

Klein, C., Brin, M. F., Kramer, P. *et al.* (1999). Association of a missense change in the D2 dopamine receptor with myoclonus dystonia. *Proc. Nat. Acad. Sci*, **96**, 5173–6.

Klein, C., Gurvich, N., Sena-Esteves, M. *et al.* (2000). Evaluation of the role of the D2 dopamine receptor receptor in myoclonus dystonia. *Ann. Neurol.*, **47**, 369–73.

Kordower, J. H., Freeman, T. B., and Snow, B. J. (1995). Neuropathological evidence of graft survival and striatal reinnervation after the transplantation of fetal mesencephalic tissue in a patient with Parkinson's disease. *N. Engl. J. Med.*, **332**, 1118–24.

Kosaka, K. (1993). Dementia and neuropathology in Lewy body disease. *Adv. Neurol.*, **60**, 456–63.

Kostic, V. S., Stojanovic-Svetel, M., and Kacar, A. (1996). Symptomatic dystonias associated with structural brain lesions: report of 16 cases. *Can. J. Neurol. Sci.*, **23**, 53–6.

Krack, P. and Marion, M. H. (1994). 'Apraxia of lid opening,' a focal eyelid dystonia: clinical study of 32 patients. *Mov. Disord.*, **9**, 610–5.

Kramer, P. L., de Leon, D., Ozelius, L. *et al.* (1990). Dystonia gene in Ashkenazi Jewish population is located on chromosome 9q32–34. *Ann. Neurol.*, **27**, 114–20.

Kramer, P. L., Mineta, M., Klein, C. *et al.* (1999). Rapid onset dystonia parkinsonism: linkage to chromosome 19q13. *Annals of Neurology*, **46**, 176–82.

Kremer, B., Goldberg, P., Andrew, S. E. *et al.* (1994). A worldwide study of the Huntington's disease mutation. The sensitivity and specificity of measuring CAG repeats. *N. Engl. J. Med.*, **330**, 1401–6.

Kruger, R., Kuhn, U., Muller, T. *et al.* (1998). Ala 30 Pro mutation in the gene encoding alpha-synuclein in Parkinson's disease. *Nat. Genet.*, **18**, 106–8.

Kulisevsky, J., Marti, M. J., Ferrer, I. *et al.* (1988). Meige syndrome: neuropathology of a case. *Mov. Disord.*, **3**, 170–5.

Kullmann, D. M., Howard, R. S., Miller, D. H. *et al.* (1996). Brainstem encephalopathy with stimulus-sensitive myoclonus leading to respiratory arrest, but with recovery: a description of two cases and review of the literature. *Mov. Disord.*, **11**, 715–8.

Kumar, R., Dagher, A., Hutchison, W. D. *et al.* (1999). Globus pallidus deep brain stimulation for generalised dystonia: clinical and PET investigation. *Neurology*, **53**, 871–4.

Kunig, G., Pogarell, O., Moller, J. C. *et al.* (1999). Pramipexole, a nonergot dopamine agonist, is effecive against rest tremor in intermediate to advanced Parkinson's disease. *Clinical Neuropharmacology*, **22**, 301–5.

Kurlan, R., Behr, J., Melved, L. *et al.* (1988). Transient tic disorder and the clinical spectrum of Tourette's syndrome. *Arch. Neurol.*, **45**, 1200–1.

Kurlan, R. and Trinidad, K. S. (1995). Treatment of tics. In: *Treatment of movement disorders* (ed. R. Kurlan), pp. 365–406. J. B. Lippincott, Philadelphia.

Kyllerman, M., Bager, B., Bensch, J. *et al.* (1982). Dyskinetic cerebral palsy I. Clinical categories, associated neurological abnormalities and incidences. *Acta Paediatr. Scand.*, **71**, 543–50.

Laitinen, L. V., Bergenheim, A. T., and Hariz, M. I. (1992). Leksell's posteroventral pallidotomy in the treatment of Parkinson's disease. *J. Neurosurg.*, **76**, 53–61.

Lalioti, M. D., Scott, H. S., Buresi, C. *et al.* (1997). Dodecamer repeat expansion in cystatin B gene in progressive myoclonus epilepsy. *Nature*, **386**, 847–51.

Lance, J. W. (1977). Familial paroxysmal dystonic choreoathetosis and its differentiation from related syndromes. *Ann. Neurol.*, **2**, 285–93.

Lang, A. E. (1994). Withdrawal akathisia: case reports and a proposed classification of chronic akathisia. *Mov. Disord.*, **9**, 188–92.

Lang, A. E. (1995). Psychogenic dystonia: a review of 18 cases. *Can. J. Neurol. Sci.*, **22**, 136–43.

Lang, A. E., Koller, W. C., and Fahn, S. (1995). Psychogenic parkinsonism. *Arch. Neurol.*, **52**, 802–10.

Langston, J., Ballard, P., Tetrud, J. *et al.* (1983). Chronic parkinsonism in humans due to a product of meperidine-analog synthesis. *Science*, **219**, 979–80.

Langston, J. W. (1996). The etiology of Parkinson's disease with emphasis on the MPTP story. *Neurology*, **47**, S153–60.

Larsen, J. P., Boas, J., Erdal, J. E. (2000). Does selegiline modify the progression of early Parkinson's disease? Results from a five-year study. The Norwegian-Danish study group. *European Journal of Neurology*, **6**, 539–47.

Larsen, T. A., Dunn, H. G., Jan, J. E. *et al.* (1985). Dystonia and calcification of the basal ganglia. *Neurology*, **35**, 533–7

Layzer, R. B. (1995). Neuromyotonia: a new autoimmune disease [editorial; comment]. *Ann. Neurol.*, **38**, 701–2.

Le Witt, P. A. *et al.* (1986). Terahydrobiopterin in dystonia: identification of abnormal metabolism and therapeutic trials. *Neurology*, **36**, 760–4.

Lee, L. V., Pascasio, F. M., Fuentes, F. D. *et al.* (1976). Torsion dystonia in Panay, Philippines. *Adv. Neurol.*, **14**, 137–51.

Lee, M. S. and Marsden, C. D. (1994a). Movement disorders following lesions of the thalamus or subthalamic region. *Mov. Disord.*, **9**, 493–507.

Lee, M. S. and Marsden, C. D. (1994b). Neurological sequelae following carbon monoxide poisoning: clinical course and outcome according to the clinical types and brain computed tomography scan findings. *Mov. Disord.*, **9**, 550–8.

Lees, A. J. (1987). The Steele–Richardson–Olszewski syndrome (Progressive supranuclear palsy). In: *Movement disorders*, Vol. 2 (ed. C. D. Marsden and S. Fahn), pp. 272–87. Butterworths, London.

Lees, A. J. (1995). Comparison of therapeutic effects and mortality data of levodopa and levodopa combined with selegiline in patients with early, mild Parkinson's disease. Parkinson's Disease Research Group of the United Kingdom. *BMJ*, **311**, 1602–7.

Lehericy, S., Vidailhet, M., Dormont, D. *et al.* (1996). Striatopallidal and thalamic dystonia. A magnetic resonance imaging anatomoclinical study. *Arch. Neurol.*, **53**, 241–50.

Leigh, P. N., Rothwell, J. C., Traub, M. *et al.* (1980). A patient with reflex myoclonus and muscle rigidity: 'jerking stiff man syndrome'. *J. Neurol. Neurosurg. Psychiatry*, **43**, 1125–31.

Lemon, R. N. (1988). The output map of the primate motor cortex. *Trends Neurosci.*, **11**, 501–6.

Leo, R. J. (1996). Movement disorders associated with the serotonin selective reuptake inhibitors. *J. Clin. Psychiatry*, **57**, 449–54.

Leroy, E., Boyer, R., Augburger, G. *et al.* (1998). The ubiquitin pathway in Parkinson's disease. *Nature*, **395**, 451–2.

Leube, B., Rudnicki, D., Ratzlaff, T. *et al.* (1996). Idiopathic torsion dystonia: assignment of a gene to chromosome 18p in a German family with adult onset, autosomal dominant inheritance and purely focal distribution. *Hum. Mol. Genet.*, **5**, 1673–7.

Leube, B., Hendgen, T., Kessler, K. R. *et al.* (1997). Sporadic focal dystonia in northwest Germany: molecular basis on chromosome 18p. *Ann. Neurol.*, **42**, 111–4.

Levin, K. H. (1997). Paraneoplastic neuromuscular syndromes. *Neurol. Clin.*, **15**, 597–614.

Limousin, P., Krack, P., Pollak, P. *et al.* (1998). Electrical stimulation of the subthalamic nucleus in advanced Parkinson's disease. *N. Engl. J. Med.*, **339**, 1105–11.

Lindvall, O., Sawle, G., Widner, H. *et al.* (1994). Evidence for long term survival and function of dopaminergic grafts in progressive Parkinson's disease. *Ann. Neurol.*, **35**, 172–80.

Lipe, H., Schultze, A., and Bird, T. D. (1993). Risk factors for suicide in Huntington's disease: a retrospective case controlled study. *Am. J. Med. Genet.*, **48**, 231–3.

Lipinski, J. F., Sallee, F. R., Jackson, C. *et al.* (1997). Dopamine agonist treatment of Tourette disorder in children: results of an open-label trial of pergolide. *Mov. Disord.*, **12**, 402–7.

Litvan, I., Agid, Y., Calne, D. *et al.* (1996a). Clinical research criteria for the diagnosis of progressive supranuclear palsy (Steele–Richardson–Olszewski syndrome): report of the NINDS-SPSP international workshop. *Neurology*, **47**, 1–9.

Litvan, I., Agid, Y., Jankovic, J. *et al.* (1996b). Accuracy of clinical criteria for the diagnosis of progressive supranuclear palsy (Steele–Richardson–Olszewski syndrome). *Neurology*, **46**, 922–30.

Litvan, I., Mangone, C. A., McKee, A. *et al.* (1996c). Natural history of progressive supranuclear palsy (Steele–Richardson–Olszewski syndrome) and clinical predictors of survival: a clinicopathological study. *J. Neurol. Neurosurg. Psychiatry*, **60**, 615–20.

Litvan, I., Mega, M. S., Cummings, J. L. *et al.* (1996d). Neuropsychiatric aspects of progressive supranuclear palsy. *Neurology*, **47**, 1184–9.

Litvan, I., Agid, Y., Goetz, C. *et al.* (1997a). Accuracy of the clinical diagnosis of corticobasal degeneration: a clinicopathologic study. *Neurology*, **48**, 119–25.

Litvan, I., Campbell, G., Mangone, C. A. *et al.* (1997b). Which clinical features differentiate progressive supranuclear palsy (Steele–Richardson–Olszewski syndrome) from related disorders? A clinicopathological study. *Brain*, **120**, 65–74.

Lodi, R., Schapira, A., Manners, D. *et al.* (2000). Abnormal in vivo skeletal muscle energy metabolism in Huntington's disease and dentatorubropallidoluysian atrophy. *Ann. Neurol.*, **48**, 72–6.

Logroscino, G., Marder, K., Cote, L. *et al.* (1996). Dietary lipids and antioxidants in Parkinson's disease: a population-based, case–control study. *Ann. Neurol.*, **39**, 89–94.

Lopez-Villegas, D., Kulisevsky, J., Deus, J. *et al.* (1996). Neuropsychological alterations in patients with computed tomography-detected basal ganglia calcification. *Arch. Neurol.*, **53**, 251–6.

Louis, E. D., Klatka, L. A., Liu, Y. *et al.* (1997). Comparison of extrapyramidal features in 31 pathologically confirmed cases of diffuse Lewy body disease and 34 pathologically confirmed cases of Parkinson's disease. *Neurology*, **48**, 376–80.

Louis, E. D., Lynch, T., Kaufmann, P. *et al.* (1996). Diagnostic guidelines in central nervous system Whipple's disease. *Ann. Neurol.*, **40**, 561–8.

Lozano, A. M., Lang, A. E., Galvez-Jimenez, N. *et al.* (1995). Effect of GPi pallidotomy on motor function in Parkinson's disease. *Lancet*, **346**, 1383–7.

Lu, C. S., Thompson, P. D., Quinn, N. P. *et al.* (1993). Ramsay Hunt syndrome and coeliac disease: a new association? *Mov. Disord.*, **1**, 209–19.

Lucking, C. B., Durr, A., Bonifati, B. *et al.* (2000). Association of early onset Parkinson's disease and Parkin gene mutations. *New Engl. J. Med.*, **342**, 1560–67.

Ludecke, B., Knappskog, P. M., Clayton, P. T. *et al.* (1996).

Recessively inherited L-DOPA-responsive parkinsonism in infancy caused by a point mutation (L205P) in the tyrosine hydroxylase gene. *Hum. Mol. Genet.*, **5**, 1023–8.

Lugaresi, E., Cirignotta, F., and Montagna, P. (1986). Nocturnal paroxysmal dystonia. *J. Neurol. Neurosurg. Psychiatry*, **49**, 375–80.

Lynch, T., Odel, J., Fredericks, D. N. *et al.* (1997). Polymerase chain reaction-based detection of *Tropheryma whippelii* in central nervous system Whipple's disease. *Ann. Neurol.*, **42**, 120–4.

MacDonald, M. E., Barnes, G., Srinidhi, J. *et al.* (1993). Gametic but not somatic instability of CAG repeat length in Huntington's disease. *J. Med. Genet.*, **30**, 982–86.

MacMillan, J. C., Morrison, P. J., Nevin, N. C. *et al.* (1993*a*). Identification of an expanded CAG repeat in the Huntington's disease gene (IT15) in a family reported to have benign hereditary chorea. *J. Med. Genet.*, **30**, 1012–3.

MacMillan, J. C., Snell, R. G., Tyler, A. *et al.* (1993*b*). Molecular analysis and clinical correlations of the Huntington's disease mutation. *Lancet*, **342**, 954–8.

Maher, E. R. and Lees, A. J. (1986). The clinical features and natural history of the Steele–Richardson–Olszewski syndrome (progressive supranuclear palsy). *Neurology*, **36**, 1005–8.

Maraganore, D. M., Folger, W. N., Swanson, J. W. *et al.* (1992). Movement disorders as sequelae of central pontine myelinolysis: report of three cases. *Mov. Disord.*, **7**, 142–8.

Maraganore, D. M., Harding, A. E., and Marsden, C. D. (1991). A clinical and genetic study of familial Parkinson's disease. *Mov. Disord.*, **6**, 205–11.

Marion, M. H., Gledhill, R. F., and Thompson, P. D. (1989). Spasms of amputation stumps: a report of 2 cases. *Mov. Disord.*, **4**, 1354–8.

Mark, M. H., Sage, J. I., Walters, A. S. *et al.* (1995). Binswanger's disease presenting as levodopa-responsive parkinsonism: clinicopathologic study of three cases. *Mov. Disord.*, **10**, 450–4.

Markopoulou, K., Wszolek, Z. K., and Pfeiffer, R. F. (1995). A Greek-American kindred with autosomal dominant, levodopa-responsive parkinsonism and anticipation. *Ann. Neurol.*, **38**, 373–8.

Marsden, C. D. and Harrison, M. G. J. (1974). Idiopathic torsion dystonia (dystonia musculorum deformans). A review of forty-two patients. *Brain*, **97**, 793–810.

Marsden, C. D., Marion, M.-H., and Sheehy, M. P. (1984*a*). The treatment of severe dystonia in children and adults. *J. Neurol. Neurosurg. Psychiatry*, **47**, 1166–73.

Marsden, C. D., Obeso, J. A., and Traub, M. M. (1984*b*). Muscle spasms associated with Sudeck's atrophy after injury. *BMJ*, **288**, 173–6.

Marsden, C. D., Lang, A. E., Quinn, N. P. *et al.* (1986). Familial dystonia and visual failure with striatal CT lucencies. *J. Neurol. Neurosurg. Psychiatry*, **49**, 500–19.

Marsden, C. D. (1987). Wilson's disease. *Q. J. Med.*, **65**, 959–66.

Marsden, C. D. and Rothwell, J. C. (1987). The physiology of idiopathic dystonia. *Can. J. Neurol. Sci.*, **14**, 521–7.

Marsden, C. D., Harding, A. E., Obeso, J. A. *et al.* (1990). Progressive myoclonic ataxia (the Ramsay Hunt syndrome). *Arch. Neurol.*, **47**, 1121–5.

Marsden, C. D. and Quinn, N. P. (1990). The dystonias. *BMJ*, **300**, 139–44.

Marsden, C. D. (1994). Peripheral movement disorders. In: *Movement disorders*, Vol. 3 (ed. C. D. Marsden and S. Fahn), pp. 406–17. Butterworth-Heinemann, Oxford.

Marsden, C. D. and Obeso, J. A. (1994). The functions of the basal ganglia and the paradox of stereotaxic surgery in Parkinson's disease. *Brain*, **117**, 877–97.

Marshall, F. J. and Shoulson, I. (1997). Clinical features and treatment of Huntington's disease. In: *Movement disorders: neurologic principles and practice* (ed. R. L. Watts and W. C. Koller), pp. 491–502. McGraw-Hill, New York.

Martinelli, P., Giuliani, S., Ippoliti, M. *et al.* (1993). Familial idiopathic strio-pallido-dentate calcifications with late onset extrapyramidal syndrome. *Mov. Disord.*, **8**, 220–2.

Masucci, E. F. and Kurtzke, J. F. (1989). Tremor in progressive supranuclear palsy. *Acta Neurol. Scand.*, **80**, 296–300.

Matsumine, H., Saito, M., Shimoda-Matsubayashi, S. *et al.* (1997). Localization of a gene for an autosomal recessive form of juvenile Parkinsonism to chromosome 6q25.2–27. *Am. J. Hum. Genet.*, **60**, 588–96.

Matsumoto, J. and Hallett, M. (1994). Startle syndromes. In: *Movement disorders*, Vol. 3 (ed. C. D. Marsden and S. Fahn), pp. 418–33. Butterworth-Heinemann, Oxford.

Matsuo, H., Takashima, H., Kishikawa, M. *et al.* (1991). Pure akinesia: an atypical manifestation of progressive supranuclear palsy. *J. Neurol. Neurosurg. Psychiatry*, **54**, 397–400.

Mayston, M. J., Harrison, L. M., Quinton, R. *et al.* (1997). Mirror movements in X-linked Kallmann's syndrome. I. A neurophysiological study. *Brain*, **120**, 1199–216.

McKeith, L. G., Galasko, D., Kosaka, K. *et al.* (1996). Consensus guidelines for the clinical and pathologic diagnosis of dementia with Lewy bodies (DLB): report of the consortium on DLB international workshop. *Neurology*, **47**, 1113–24.

McKeith, I., Del Ser, T., Spano, P. *et al.* (2000). Efficacy of rivastigmine in dementia with Lewy bodies: a randomised, double blind, placebo controlled international study. *Lancet*, **356**, 2031–6.

Meinck, H. M., Ricker, K., and Conrad, B. (1984). The stiff man syndrome: new pathophysiological aspects from abnormal exteroceptive reflexes and the response to clomipramine, clonidine and tizanidine. *J. Neurol. Neurosurg. Psychiatry*, **47**, 280–7.

Melamed, E., Achiron, A., Shapira, A. *et al.* (1991). Persistent and progressive parkinsonism after discontinuation of chronic neuroleptic therapy: an additional tardive syndrome? *Clin. Neuropharmacol.*, **14**, 273–8.

Menza, M. A., Cocchiola, J., and Golbe, L. I. (1995). Psychiatric symptoms in progressive supranuclear palsy. *Psychosomatics*, **36**, 550–4.

Merello, M. and Lees, A. J. (1992). Beginning-of-dose motor deterioration following the acute administration of levodopa and apomorphine in Parkinson's disease. *J. Neurol. Neurosurg. Psychiatry*, **55**, 1024–6.

Metzer, W. S., Newton, J. E., Steele, R. W. *et al.* (1989). HLA antigens in drug-induced parkinsonism. *Mov. Disord.*, **4**, 121–8.

Minassian, B. A., Ianzano, L., Meloche, M. *et al.* (2000). Mutation spectrum and predicted function of laforin in Lafora's progressive myoclonus epilepsy. *Neurology*, **55**, 341–6.

Mitsumoto, H., Schwartzman, M. J., Estes, M. L. *et al.* (1991). Sudden death and paroxysmal autonomic dysfunction in stiff-man syndrome. *J. Neurol.*, **238**, 91–6.

Miyasaki, J. M. and Lang, A. E. (1995). Treatment of drug induced movement disorders. In: *Treatment of movement disorders* (ed. R. Kurlan), pp. 429–76. J. B. Lippincott, Philadelphia.

Miyoshi, K., Matsuoka, T., and Mizushima, S. (1969). Familial holotopistic striatal necrosis. *Acta Neuropathol. (Berlin)*, **13**, 240–9.

Montastruc, J. L., Rascol, O., Senard, J. M. *et al.* (1994). A randomised controlled study comparing bromocriptine to which levodopa was later added, with levodopa alone in previously untreated patients with Parkinson's disease: a five year follow up. *J. Neurol. Neurosurg. Psychiatry*, **57**, 1034–8.

Morris, H. R., Janssen, J. C., Bandmann, O. *et al.* (1999). The tau gene AO polymorphism in progressive supranuclear palsy and related neurodegenerative disease. *J. Neurol. Neurosurg. Psychiat.*, **66**, 665–7.

Morris, J. C., Drazner, M., Fulling, K. *et al.* (1989). Clinical and pathological aspects of parkinsonism in Alzheimer's disease. A role for extranigral factors? *Arch. Neurol.*, **46**, 651–7.

Morris, M. (1991). Psychiatric aspects of Huntington's disease. In: *Huntington's disease* (ed. P. S. Harper), pp. 81–126. W. B. Saunders, London.

Morris, M. and Tyler, A. (1991). Management and therapy. In: *Huntington's disease* (ed. P. S. Harper), pp. 205–50. W. B. Saunders, London.

Mumford, C. J., Fletcher, N. A., Ironside, J. W. *et al.* (1996). Progressive ataxia, focal seizures, and malabsorption syndrome in a 41 year old woman [clinical conference]. *J. Neurol. Neurosurg. Psychiatry*, **60**, 225–30.

Muthane, U. B., Swamy, H. S., Satishchandra, P. *et al.* (1994). Early onset Parkinson's disease: are juvenile- and young-onset different? *Mov. Disord.*, **9**, 539–44.

Myers, R. H., MacDonald, M. E., Koroshetz, W. J. *et al.* (1993). De novo expansion of a (CAG)n repeat in sporadic Huntington's disease. *Nat. Genet.*, **5**, 168–73.

Nass, R. and Gutman, R. (1997). Boys with Asperger's disorder, exceptional verbal intelligence, tics, and clumsiness. *Dev. Med. Child Neurol.*, **39**, 691–5.

Naumann, M., Pirker, W., Reiners, K. *et al.* (1997). [^{123}I]beta-CIT single-photon emission tomography in DOPA-responsive dystonia. *Mov. Disord.*, **12**, 448–51.

Nausieda, P. A., Koller, W. C., Weiner, W. J. *et al.* (1979). Chorea induced by oral contraceptives. *Neurology*, **29**, 1605–9.

Neary, D., Snowdon, J. S., Shields, R. A. *et al.* (1987). Single photon emission tomography using ^{99m}Tc-HM-PAO in the investigation of dementia. *J. Neurol. Neurosurg. Psychiatry*, **50**, 1101–9.

Nelson, I., Hanna, M. G., Alsanjari, N. *et al.* (1995). A new mitochondrial DNA mutation associated with progressive dementia and chorea: a clinical, pathological, and molecular genetic study. *Ann. Neurol.*, **37**, 400–3.

Neshige, R., Luders, H., and Shibasaki, H. (1988). Recording of movement related potentials from scalp and cortex in man. *Brain*, **111**, 719–36.

Newman, G. C. (1985). Treatment of progressive supranuclear palsy with tricyclic antidepressants. *Neurology*, **35**, 1189–93.

Newsom-Davis, J. and Mills, K. R. (1993). Immunological associations of acquired neuromyotonia (Isaacs' syndrome). Report of five cases and literature review. *Brain*, **116**, 453–69.

Nomoto, M., Thompson, P. D., Sheehy, M. P. *et al.* (1987). Anticholinergic induced chorea in the treatment of focal dystonia. *Mov. Disord.*, **2**, 53–6.

Novotny, E. J., Singh, G., Wallace, D. C. *et al.* (1986). Lebers disease and dystonia: a mitochondrial disease. *Neurology*, **29**, 364–9.

Nutt, J. G., Muenter, M. D., Aronson, A. *et al.* (1988). Epidemiology of focal and generalised dystonia in Rochester, Minnesota. *Mov. Disord.*, **3**, 188–94.

Nutt, J. G., Marsden, C. D., and Thompson, P. D. (1993). Human walking and higher level gait disorders, particularly in the elderly. *Neurology*, **43**, 268–79.

Nutt, J. G. and Holford, N. H. (1996). The response to levodopa in Parkinson's disease: imposing pharmacological law and order. *Ann. Neurol.*, **39**, 561–73.

Nygaard, T. G. (1995). Dopa-responsive dystonia. *Curr. Opin. Neurol.*, **8**, 310–3.

Nygaard, T. G., Takahashi, H., Heiman, G. A. *et al.* (1992). Long-term treatment response and fluorodopa positron emission tomographic scanning of parkinsonism in a family with dopa-responsive dystonia. *Ann. Neurol.*, **32**, 603–8.

Nygaard, T. G., Wilhelmsen, K. C., Risch, N. J. *et al.* (1993). Linkage mapping of dopa-responsive dystonia (DRD) to chromosome 14q. *Nat. Genet.*, **5**, 386–91.

Obeso, J. A., Rothwell, J. C., Lang, A. E. *et al.* (1983). Myoclonic dystonia. *Neurology*, **33**, 825–30.

Obeso, J. A. and Martinez-Lage, J. M. (1992). Anticholinergics and amantadine. In: *Handbook of Parkinson's disease* (ed. W. C. Koller), pp. 383–90. Marcel Dekker, New York.

Obeso, J. A. (1995). Therapy of myoclonus. *Clin. Neurosci.*, **3**, 253–7.

Obeso, J. A., Linazasoro, G., Rothwell, J. C. *et al.* (1996). Assessing the effects of pallidotomy in Parkinson's disease [letter; comment]. *Lancet*, **347**, 1490.

Obeso, J. A., Guridi, J., and De Long, M. (1997). Surgery for Parkinson's disease [editorial]. *J. Neurol. Neurosurg. Psychiatry*, **62**, 2–8.

Oertel, W. H., Schwarz, J., Tatsch, K. *et al.* (1993). IBZM-SPECT as predictor for dopamimetic responsiveness of patients with de novo parkinsonian syndrome. *Adv. Neurol.*, **60**, 519–24.

Olanow, C. W. (1996). GPi pallidotomy—have we made a dent in Parkinson's disease? [editorial; comment]. *Ann. Neurol.*, **40**, 341–3.

Ondo, W. G., Desaloms, J. M., Janakovic, J. and Grossman, R. G. (1998). Pallidotomy for generalized dystonia. *Movement Disorder*, **13**, 693–8.

Orrell, R. W., Amrolia, P. J., Heald, A. *et al.* (1995). Acanthocytosis, retinitis pigmentosa, and pallidal degeneration: a report of three patients, including the second reported case with hypoprebetalipoproteinemia (HARP syndrome). *Neurology*, **45**, 487–92.

Otsuka, M., Ichiya, Y., Kuwabara, Y. *et al.* (1996). Differences in the reduced ^{18}F-Dopa uptakes of the caudate and the putamen in Parkinson's disease: correlations with the three main symptoms. *J. Neurol. Sci.*, **136**, 169–73.

Ozelius, L. J., Hewett, J. W., Page, C. E. *et al.* (1997). The early-onset torsion dystonia gene (DYT1) encodes an ATP-binding protein. *Nat. Genet.*, **17**, 40–8.

Pahwa, R. (1997). Toxin induced parkinsonian syndromes. In: *Movement disorders: neurologic principles and practice* (ed. R. L. Watts and W. C. Koller), pp. 315–23. McGraw-Hill, New York.

Pahwa, R., Wilkinson, S., Smith, D. *et al.* (1997). High-frequency stimulation of the globus pallidus for the treatment of Parkinson's disease. *Neurology*, **49**, 249–53.

Papp, M. I., Kahn, J. E., and Lantos, P. L. (1989). Glial cytoplasmic inclusions in the CNS of patients with multiple system atrophy (striatonigral degeneration, olivopontocerebellar atrophy and Shy–Drager syndrome). *J. Neurol. Sci.*, **94**, 79–100.

Papp, M. I. and Lantos, P. L. (1994). The distribution of oligodendroglial inclusions in multiple system atrophy and its relevance to clinical symptomatology. *Brain*, **117**, 235–43.

Paret, G., Tirosh, R., Ben Zeev, B. *et al.* (1996). Intrathecal baclofen for severe torsion dystonia in a child. *Acta Paediatr.*, **85**, 635–7.

Parkinson Study Group (1993). Effects of tocopherol and deprenyl on the progression of disability in early Parkinson's disease. *N. Engl. J. Med.*, **328**, 176–83.

Parkinson Study Group (1996). Impact of deprenyl and tocopherol treatment on Parkinson's disease in DATATOP patients requiring levodopa. *Ann. Neurol.*, **39**, 37–45.

Parkinson's Disease Research Group in the United Kingdom (1993). Comparisons of therapeutic effects of levodopa, levodopa and selegiline, and bromocriptine in patients with early, mild Parkinson's disease: three year interim report. *BMJ*, **307**, 469–72.

Passingham, R. E. (1987). Two cortical systems for directing movement. In: *Motor areas of the cerebral cortex*, pp. 151–64. John Wiley, Chichester.

Pauls, D. L. and Leckman, J. F. (1986). The inheritance of Gilles de la Tourette's syndrome and associated behaviours: evidence for autosomal dominant transmission. *N. Engl. J. Med.*, **315**, 993–7.

Pennacchio, L. A., Lehesjoki, A. E., Stone, N. E. *et al.* (1996). Mutations in the gene encoding cystatin B in progressive myoclonus epilepsy (EPM1). *Science*, **271**, 1731–4.

Perry, T. L., Wright, J. M., Berry, K. *et al.* (1990). Dominantly inherited apathy, central hypoventilation and Parkinson's syndrome: clinical, biochemical and neuropathological studies of 2 new cases. *Neurology*, **40**, 1882–7.

Peschanski, M., Defer, G., N. Guyen, J. P. *et al.* (1994). Bilateral motor improvement and alteration of L-dopa effect in two patients with Parkinson's disease following intrastriatal transplantation of foetal ventral mesencephalon. *Brain*, **117**, 487–99.

Piccini, P., Morrish, P. K., Turjanski, N. *et al.* (1997). Dopaminergic function in familial Parkinson's disease: a clinical and ^{18}F-dopa positron emission tomography study. *Ann. Neurol.*, **41**, 222–9.

Pillon, B., Blin, J., Vidailhet, M. *et al.* (1995). The neuropsychological pattern of corticobasal degeneration: comparison with progressive supranuclear palsy and Alzheimer's disease. *Neurology*, **45**, 1477–83.

Pincus, J. H. and Chutorian, A. (1967). Familial benign chorea with intention tremor: a clinical entity. *J. Paediatrics*, **70**, 724–9.

Plant, G. T., Williams, A. C., Earl, C. J. *et al.* (1984). Familial paroxysmal dystonia induced by exercise. *J. Neurol. Neurosurg. Psychiatry*, **47**, 275–9.

Plante-Bordeneuve, V., Davis, M. B., Maraganore, D. M. *et al.* (1994). Debrisoquine hydroxylase gene polymorphism in familial Parkinson's disease. *J. Neurol. Neurosurg. Psychiatry*, **57**, 911–3.

Plante-Bordeneuve, V., Taussig, D., Thomas, F. *et al.* (1995). A clinical and genetic study of familial cases of Parkinson's disease. *J. Neurol. Sci.*, **133**, 164–72.

Playford, E. D., Fletcher, N. A., Sawle, G. V. *et al.* (1993). Striatal [^{18}F]dopa uptake in familial idiopathic dystonia. *Brain*, **116**, 1191–9.

Plazzi, G., Cortelli, P., Montagna, P. *et al.* (1998) REM sleep behaviour disorder differentiates pure autonomic failure from multiple system atrophy with autonomic failure. *J. Neurol. Neurosurg. Psychiatry*, **64**, 683–5.

Poewe, W. H., Lees, A. J., and Stern, G. M. (1988). Dystonia in Parkinson's disease: clinical and pharmacological features. *Ann. Neurol.*, **23**, 73–8.

Polizos, P. and Engelhardt, D. M. (1978). Dyskinetic phenomena in children treated with psychotropic medications. *Psychpharmacol. Bull.*, **14**, 65–8.

Polymeropoulos, M. H., Lavedan, C., Leroy, E. *et al.* (1997). Mutation in the alpha-synuclein gene identified in families with Parkinson's disease [see comments]. *Science*, **276**, 2045–7.

Pramstaller, P. P., Wenning, G. K., Smith, S. J. *et al.* (1995). Nerve conduction studies, skeletal muscle EMG, and sphincter EMG in multiple system atrophy. *J. Neurol. Neurosurg. Psychiatry*, **58**, 618–21.

Pshezhetsky, A. V., Richard, C., Michaud, L. *et al.* (1997). Cloning, expression and chromosomal mapping of human lysosomal sialidase and characterization of mutations in sialidosis. *Nat. Genet.*, **15**, 316–20.

Quinn, N. P., Lang, A. E., Koller, W. C. *et al.* (1986). Painful Parkinson's disease. *Lancet*, **i**, 1366–9.

Quinn, N., Critchley, P., and Marsden, C. D. (1987). Young onset Parkinson's disease. *Mov. Disord.*, **2**, 73–91.

Quinn, N. P., Luthert, P., Honavar, M. *et al.* (1989). Pure akinesia due to Lewy body Parkinson's disease: a case with pathology. *Mov. Disord.*, **4**, 85–9.

Quinn, N. (1994). Multiple system atrophy. In: *Movement disorders*, Vol. 3 (ed. C. D. Marsden and S. Fahn), pp. 262–81. Butterworth-Heinemann, Oxford.

Quinn, N. P. (1996). Essential myoclonus and myoclonic dystonia. *Mov. Disord.*, **11**, 119–24.

Raja, M. and Azzoni, A. (1996). Tardive dystonia. Prevalence, risk factors and clinical features. *Ital. J. Neurol. Sci.*, **17**, 409–18.

Rajput, A. H., Rozdilsky, B., Hornykiewicz, O. *et al.* (1982). Reversible drug induced parkinsonism: clinicopathologic study of two cases. *Arch. Neurol.*, **39**, 644–6.

Rajput, A. H., Pahwa, R., Pahwa, P. *et al.* (1993). Prognostic significance of the onset mode in parkinsonism. *Neurology*, **43**, 829–30.

Rajput, A. H., Gibb, W. R., Zhong, X. H. *et al.* (1994). Dopa-responsive dystonia: pathological and biochemical observations in a case. *Ann. Neurol.*, **35**, 396–402.

Rajput, A. H., Rajput, A., Lang, A. E. *et al.* (1998). New use for an old drug: amantadine benefits levodopa induced dyskinesia. *Mov. Disord.*, **13**, 851.

Rascol, O., Brooks, D. J., Korczyn, A. D., *et al.* (2000). A five year study of the incidence of dyskinesia in patients with early parkinson's disease who were treated with ropinirole or levodopa. *New Engl. J. Med.*, **342**, 1484–91.

Reeves, A. L., So, E. L., Sharbrough, F. W. *et al.* (1996). Movement disorders associated with the use of gabapentin. *Epilepsia*, **37**, 988–90.

Reilly, M., Daly, L., and Hutchinson, M. (1993). An epidemiological study of Wilson's disease in the Republic of Ireland. *J. Neurol. Neurosurg. Psychiatry*, **56**, 298–300.

Remy, P., Zilbovicius, M., Leroy-Willig, A. *et al.* (1994). Movement- and task-related activations of motor cortical areas: a positron emission tomographic study. *Ann. Neurol.*, **36**, 19–26.

Reus, V. I. (1997). Olanzapine: a novel atypical neuroleptic agent. *Lancet*, **349**, 1264–5.

Revesz, T., Sangha, H., and Daniel, S. E. (1996). The nucleus raphe interpositus in the Steele–Richardson–Olszewski syndrome (progressive supranuclear palsy). *Brain*, **119**, 1137–43.

Ridding, M. C., Sheean, G., Rothwell, J. C. *et al.* (1995). Changes in the balance between motor cortical excitation and inhibition in focal, task specific dystonia. *J. Neurol. Neurosurg. Psychiatry*, **59**, 493–8.

Riley, D. E., Lang, A. E., Lewis, A. *et al.* (1990). Cortical-basal ganglionic degeneration. *Neurology*, **40**, 1203–12.

Riley, D. E. and Lang, A. E. (1993). The spectrum of levodopa related fluctuations in Parkinson's disease. *Neurology*, **43**, 1459–64.

Riley, D. E., Fogt, N., and Leigh, R. J. (1994). The syndrome of 'pure akinesia' and its relationship to progressive supranuclear palsy. *Neurology*, **44**, 1025–9.

Riley, D. E. (1996). Paroxysmal kinesigenic dystonia associated with a medullary lesion. *Mov. Disord.*, **11**, 738–40.

Rinne, U. K. (1985). Combined bromocriptine-levodopa therapy early in Parkinson's disease. *Neurology*, **35**, 1196–8.

Rinne, U. K. (1987). Early combination of bromocriptine and levodopa in the treatment of Parkinson's disease: a 5-year follow up. *Neurology*, **37**, 826–8.

Rinne, J. O., Lee, M. S., Thompson, P. D. *et al.* (1994). Corticobasal degeneration. A clinical study of 36 cases. *Brain*, **117**, 1183–96.

Rinne, J. O., Daniel, S. E., Scaravilli, F. *et al.* (1994). The neuropathological features of neuroacanthocytosis. *Mov. Disord.*, **9**, 297–304.

Rinne, J. O., Burn, D. J., Mathias, C. J. *et al.* (1995). Positron emission tomography studies on the dopaminergic system and striatal opioid binding in the olivopontocerebellar atrophy variant of multiple system atrophy. *Ann. Neurol.*, **37**, 568–73.

Rinne, U. K., Larsen, J. P., Siden, A. *et al.* (1998). Entacapone enhances the response to levodopa in parkinsonian patients with motor fluctuations. Nomecomt study group. *Neurology*, **51**, 1309–14.

Risch, N., de Leon, D., Ozelius, L. *et al.* (1995). Genetic analysis of idiopathic torsion dystonia in Ashkenazi Jews and their recent descent from a small founder population. *Nat. Genet.*, **9**, 152–9.

Rivest, J. and Marsden, C. D. (1990). Trunk and head tremor as isolated manifestations of dystonia. *Mov. Disord.*, **5**, 60–5.

Rivest, J., Lees, A. J., and Marsden, C. D. (1991). Writer's cramp: treatment with botulinum toxin injections. *Mov. Disord.*, **6**, 55–9.

Robertson, M. M., Trimble, M. R., and Lees, A. J. (1989). Self injurious behaviour and the Gilles de la Tourette syndrome: a clinical study and review of the literature. *Psychol. Med.*, **19**, 611–25.

Robertson, M. M. (1994). Gilles de la Tourette syndrome: an update. *J. Child Psychol. Psychiatry*, **35**, 597–611.

Roh, J. K., Lee, T. G., Wie, B. A. *et al.* (1994). Initial and follow-up brain MRI findings and correlation with the clinical course in Wilson's disease. *Neurology*, **44**, 1064–8.

Rojo, A., Pernaute, R. S., Fontan, A. *et al.* (1999). Clinical genetics of progressive supranuclear palsy. *Brain*, **122**, 1233–45.

Roos, R. A., Hermans, J., Vegter-van der Vlis, M. *et al.* (1993). Duration of illness in Huntington's disease is not related to age at onset. *J. Neurol. Neurosurg. Psychiatry*, **56**, 98–100.

Ross, M. H., Charness, M. E., Lee, D. *et al.* (1995). Does ulnar neuropathy predispose to focal dystonia? *Muscle Nerve*, **18**, 606–11.

Rothwell, J. (1994). *Control of human voluntary movement*. Chapman & Hall, London.

Rothwell, J. C., Vidailhet, M., Thompson, P. D. *et al.* (1994). The auditory startle response in progressive supranuclear palsy. *J. Neural Transm. Suppl.*, **42**, 43–50.

Rupniak, N. M., Jenner, P., and Marsden, C. D. (1986). Acute dystonia induced by neuroleptic drugs. *Psychopharmacology*, **88**, 403–19.

Rush, P. J., Inman, R., Bernstein, M. *et al.* (1986). Isolated vasculitis of the central nervous system in a patient with celiac disease. *Am. J. Med.*, **81**, 1092–4.

Sachdev, P. and Loneragan, C. (1993). Intravenous benztropine and propranolol challenges in acute neuroleptic-induced akathisia. *Clin. Neuropharmacol.*, **16**, 324–31.

Saint-Cry, J. A., Trepanier, L. L., Kumar, R. *et al.* (2000). Neuropsychological consequences of chronic bilateral stimulation of the subthalamic nucleus in Parkinson's disease. *Brain*, **123**, 2091–2117.

Saint Hilaire, M. H., Burke, R. E., Bressman, S. B. *et al.* (1991). Delayed-onset dystonia due to perinatal or early childhood asphyxia. *Neurology*, **41**, 216–22.

Sainz, J., Minassian, B. A., Serratosa, J. M. *et al.* (1997). Lafora progressive myoclonus epilepsy: narrowing the chromosome 6q24 locus by recombinations and homozygosities [letter]. *Am. J. Hum. Genet.*, **61**, 1205–9.

Salazar, G., Valls-Sole, J., Marti, M. J. *et al.* (2000). Postural and action myoclonus in patients with parkinsonian type multiple system atrophy. *Movement Disorders*, **15**, 77–83.

Sanberg, P. R., Silver, A. A., Shytle, R. D. *et al.* (1997). Nicotine for the treatment of Tourette's syndrome. *Pharmacol. Ther.*, **74**, 21–5.

Saver, J. L., Liu, G. T., and Charness, M. E. (1994). Idiopathic striopallidodentate calcification with prominent supranuclear abnormality of eye movement. *J. Neuroophthalmol.*, **14**, 29–33.

Sawle, G. V., Brooks, D. J., Marsden, C. D. *et al.* (1991). Corticobasal degeneration. A unique pattern of regional cortical oxygen hypometabolism and striatal fluorodopa uptake demonstrated by positron emission tomography. *Brain*, **114**, 541–56.

Schapira, A. H., Mann, V. M., Cooper, J. M. *et al.* (1990). Anatomic and disease specificity of NADH CoQ1 reductase (complex I) deficiency in Parkinson's disease. *J. Neurochem.*, **55**, 2142–5.

Schapira, A. H. (1994). Evidence for mitochondrial dysfunction in Parkinson's disease—a critical appraisal. *Mov. Disord.*, **9**, 125–38.

Scheinberg, I. H. and Sternlieb, I. (1984). *Wilson's disease*. W. B. Saunders, Philadelphia.

Schenck, C. H., Bundlie, S. R., and Mahowald, M. W. (1996). Delayed emergence of a parkinsonian disorder in 38% of 29 older men initially diagnosed with idiopathic rapid eye movement sleep behaviour disorder. *Neurology*, **46**, 388–93.

Schloesser, D. T., Ward, T. N., and Williamson, P. D. (1996). Familial paroxysmal dystonic choreoathetosis revisited. *Mov. Disord.*, 11, 317–20.

Schoenberg, B. S., Osuntokun, B. O., Adeuja, A. O. *et al.* (1988). Comparison of the prevalence of Parkinson's disease in black populations in the rural United States and in rural Nigeria: door-to-door community studies. *Neurology*, 38, 645–6.

Schwarz, J., Tatsch, K., Arnold, G. *et al.* (1993). ^{123}I-iodobenzamide-SPECT in 83 patients with de novo parkinsonism. *Neurology*, 43, S17–20.

Schwarz, J., Weis, S., Kraft, E. *et al.* (1996). Signal changes on MRI and increases in reactive microgliosis, astrogliosis, and iron in the putamen of two patients with multiple system atrophy. *J. Neurol. Neurosurg. Psychiatry*, 60, 98–101.

Scrag, A., Quinn, N. P., Bhatia, K. P. and Marsden, C. D. (2000). Benign hereditary chorea — entity or syndrome? *Movement Disorders*, 15, 280–8.

Seitz, R. J., Blank, B., Kiwit, J. C. *et al.* (1995). Stiff-person syndrome with anti-glutamic acid decarboxylase autoantibodies: complete remission of symptoms after intrathecal baclofen administration. *J. Neurol.*, 242, 618–22.

Sethi, K. D., Patel, B., and Meador, K. J. (1989). Metoclopramide-induced parkinsonism. *South Med. J.*, 82, 1581–2.

Shiang, R., Ryan, S. G., Zhu, Y. Z. *et al.* (1993). Mutations in the alpha 1 subunit of the inhibitory glycine receptor cause the dominant neurologic disorder, hyperekplexia. *Nat. Genet.*, 5, 351–8.

Shiang, R., Ryan, S. G., Zhu, Y. Z. *et al.* (1995). Mutational analysis of familial and sporadic hyperekplexia. *Ann. Neurol.*, 38, 85–91.

Shillito, P., Molenaar, P. C., Vincent, A. *et al.* (1995). Acquired neuromyotonia: evidence for autoantibodies directed against K$^+$ channels of peripheral nerves. *Ann. Neurol.*, 38, 714–22.

Shoulson, I. (1981). Huntington's disease: functional capacities in patients treated with neuroleptic and antidepressant drugs. *Neurology*, 31, 1333–5.

Shulman, L. M., Singer, C., Bean, J. A. *et al.* (1996). Internal tremor in patients with Parkinson's disease. *Mov. Disord.*, 11, 3–7.

Siegfried, J. and Lippitz, B. (1994). Bilateral chronic electrostimulation of ventroposterolateral pallidum: a new therapeutic approach for alleviating all parkinsonian symptoms. *Neurosurgery*, 35, 1126–9; discussion 1129–30.

Silbert, P. L., Gubbay, S. S., and Khangure, M. (1993). Multifocal astrocytoma masquerading as possible progressive supranuclear palsy [letter]. *J. Neurol. Neurosurg. Psychiatry*, 56, 220–1.

Silbert, P. L., Matsumoto, J. Y., McManis, P. G. *et al.* (1995). Intrathecal baclofen therapy in stiff-man syndrome: a double-blind, placebo-controlled trial. *Neurology*, 45, 1893–7.

Simpson, G. M. (2000). The treatment of tardive dyskinesia and tardive dystonia. *J. Clin. Psychiat.*, 61, 39–44.

Singer, H. S., Reiss, A. L., Brown, J. E. *et al.* (1993). Volumetric MRI changes in basal ganglia of children with Tourette's syndrome. *Neurology*, 43, 950–6.

Sinha, S., Newsom-Davis, J., Mills, K. *et al.* (1991). Autoimmune aetiology for acquired neuromyotonia (Isaacs' syndrome). *Lancet*, 338, 75–7.

Smith, C. A., Gough, A. C., Leigh, P. N. *et al.* (1992). Debrisoquine hydroxylase gene polymorphism and susceptibility to Parkinson's disease [published erratum appears in *Lancet*, 340 (8810), 64, 1992]. *Lancet*, 339, 1375–7.

Solimena, M., Folli, F., Denis-Donini, S. *et al.* (1988). Autoantibodies to glutamic acid decarboxylase in a patient with stiff man syndrome, epilepsy and type 1 diabetes mellitus. *N. Engl. J. Med.*, 318, 1012–20.

Souza-Lima, C. F., Ferraz, H. B., Braz, C. A. *et al.* (2000). Marked improvement in a stiff limb patient treated with intravenous immunoglobulin. *Movement Disorder*, 15, 358–9.

Stacy, M. and Jankovic, J. (1991). Tardive dyskinesia. *Curr. Opin. Neurol. Neurosurg.*, 4, 343–49.

Stacy, M., Cardoso, F., and Jankovic, J. (1993). Tardive stereotypy and other movement disorders in tardive dyskinesias. *Neurology*, 43, 937–41.

Stanford, P. M., Halliday, G. M., Brooks, W. S. *et al.* (2000). Progressive supranuclear palsy pathology caused by a novel silent mutation in exon 10 of the tau gene: expansion of the disease phenotype caused by tau gene mutations. *Brain*, 123, 880–93.

Steen, V. M., Lovlie, R., MacEwan, T. *et al.* (1997). Dopamine D3 receptor gene variant and susceptibility to tardive dyskinesia in schizophrenic patients. *Mol. Psychiat.*, 2, 139–45.

Sternbach, H. (1991). The serotonin syndrome. *Am. J. Psychiatry*, 148, 705–13.

Sternlieb, I., Giblin, D. R., and Scheinberg, I. H. (1987). Wilson's disease. In: *Movement disorders*, Vol. 2 (ed. C. D. Marsden and S. Fahn), pp. 288–302. Butterworths, London.

Stoetter, B., Braun, A. R., Randolph, C. *et al.* (1992). Functional neuroanatomy of Tourette's syndrome. Limbic–motor interactions studied with FDG PET. *Adv. Neurol.*, 58, 213–26.

Stojanovic, M., Cvetkovic, D., and Kostic, V. S. (1995). A genetic study of idiopathic focal dystonias. *J. Neurol.*, 242, 508–11.

Stracciari, A., Tempestini, A., Borghi, A *et al.* (2000). Effect of liver transplantation on neurological manifestations in Wilson's disease. *Arch. Neurol.*, 57, 384–6.

Straussberg, R., Shahar, E., Gat, R. *et al.* (1993). Delayed parkinsonism associated with hypotension in a child undergoing open-heart surgery. *Dev. Med. Child Neurol.*, 35, 1011–4.

Swerdlow, R. H., Parks, J. K., Miller, S. W. *et al.* (1996). Origin and functional consequences of the complex I defect in Parkinson's disease. *Ann. Neurol.*, 40, 663–71.

Tabaton, M., Rolleri, M., Masturzo, P. *et al.* (1995). Apolipoprotein E epsilon 4 allele frequency is not increased in progressive supranuclear palsy. *Neurology*, 45, 1764–5.

Tan, E. K., Khajavi, M., Thornb, J. I. *et al.* (2000). Variability and validity of polymorphism association studies in Parkinson's Disease. *Neurology*, 55, 533–8.

Taniwaki, T., Hosokawa, S., Goto, I. *et al.* (1992). Positron emission tomography (PET) in 'pure akinesia'. *J. Neurol. Sci.*, 107, 34–9.

Tanner, C. (1994). Epidemiological clues to the cause of Parkinson's disease. In: *Movement disorders*, Vol. 3 (ed. C. D. Marsden and S. Fahn), pp. 124–46. Butterworth-Heinemann, Oxford.

Tanner, C. M. and Goldman, S. M. (1996). Epidemiology of Parkinson's disease. *Neurol. Clin.*, 14, 317–35.

Tanzi, R. E., Petrukhin, K., Chernov, I. *et al.* (1993). The Wilson disease gene is a copper transporting ATPase with homology to the Menkes disease gene. *Nat. Genet.*, 5, 344–50.

Taylor, T. D., Litt, M., Kramer, P. *et al.* (1996). Homozygosity mapping of Hallervorden–Spatz syndrome to chromosome 20p12.3–p13. *Nat. Genet.*, 14, 479–81.

Tedeschi, G., Litvan, I., Bonavita, S. *et al.* (1997). Proton magnetic resonance spectroscopic imaging in progressive supranuclear palsy, Parkinson's disease and corticobasal degeneration. *Brain*, 120, 1541–52.

Thomas, G. R., Forbes, J. R., Roberts, E. A. *et al.* (1995). The Wilson disease gene: spectrum of mutations and their consequences [published erratum appears in *Nat. Genet.*, 9 (4), 451, 1995]. *Nat. Genet.*, 9, 210–7.

Thompson, P. D. and Marsden, C. D. (1987). Gait disoder of subacute arteriosclerotic encephalopathy: Binswanger's disease. *Mov. Disord.*, 2, 1–8.

Thompson, P. D., Berardelli, A., Rothwell, J. C. *et al.* (1988). The coexistence of bradykinesia and chorea in Huntington's disease and its implications for theories of basal ganglia control of movement. *Brain*, 111, 223–44.

Thompson, P. D. (1994). Stiff people. In: *Movement disorders*, Vol. 3 (ed. C. D. Marsden and S. Fahn), pp. 373–405. Butterworth-Heinemann, Oxford.

Thompson, P. D., Bhatia, K. P., Brown, P. *et al.* (1994). Cortical myoclonus in Huntington's disease. *Mov. Disord.*, 9, 633–41.

Thyagarajan, D., Shanske, S., Vazquez-Memije, M. *et al.* (1995). A novel mitochondrial ATPase 6 point mutation in familial bilateral striatal necrosis. *Ann. Neurol.*, 38, 468–72.

Tolosa, E., Montserrat, L., and Bayes, A. (1988). Blink reflex studies in focal dystonias: enhanced excitability of brainstem interneurons in cranial dystonia and spasmodic torticollis. *Mov. Disord.*, 3, 61–9.

Tran, P. V., Dellva, M. A., Tollefson, G. D. *et al.* (1997). Extrapyramidal symptoms and tolerability of olanzapine versus haloperidol in the acute treatment of schizophrenia. *J. Clin. Psychiatry*, 58, 205–11.

Trugman, J. M., Leadbetter, R., Zalis, M. E. *et al.* (1994). Treatment of severe axial tardive dystonia with clozapine: case report and hypothesis. *Mov. Disord.*, 9, 441–6.

Tuite, P. J., Provias, J. P., and Lang, A. E. (1996). Atypical dopa responsive parkinsonism in a patient with megalencephaly, midbrain Lewy body disease, and some pathological features of Hallervorden–Spatz disease. *J. Neurol. Neurosurg. Psychiatry*, 61, 523–7.

Uitti, R. J., Wharen, R. E., Jr., Turk, M. F. *et al.* (1997). Unilateral pallidotomy for Parkinson's disease: comparison of outcome in younger versus elderly patients. *Neurology*, 49, 1072–7.

Valente, E. M., Warner, T. T., Jarman, P. R. *et al.* (1998). The role of DYT1 in primary torsion dystonia in Europe. *Brain*, 121, 2335–40.

Valldeoriola, F., Valls-Sole, J., Tolosa, E. S. *et al.* (1995). Striated anal sphincter denervation in patients with progressive supranuclear palsy. *Mov. Disord.*, 10, 550–5.

Van der Kamp, W., Rothwell, J. C., Thompson, P. D. *et al.* (1995). The movement-related cortical potential is abnormal in patients with idiopathic torsion dystonia. *Mov. Disord.*, 10, 630–3.

Van Harten, P. N., Kampuis, D. J., and Matroos, G. E. (1996). Use of clozapine in tardive dystonia. *Prog. Neuropsychopharmacol. Biol. Psychiatry*, 20, 263–74.

Van Tol, H. H., Bunzow, J. R., Guan, H. C. *et al.* (1991). Cloning of the gene for a human dopamine D4 receptor with high affinity for the antipsychotic clozapine. *Nature*, 350, 610–4.

Vandel, P., Bonin, B., Leveque, E. *et al.* (1997). Tricyclic antidepressant-induced extrapyramidal side effects. *Eur. Neuropsychopharmacol.*, 7, 207–12.

Varney, S. M., Demetroulakos, J. L., Fletcher, M. H. *et al.* (1996). Palatal myoclonus: treatment with Clostridium botulinum toxin injection. *Otolaryngol. Head Neck Surg.*, 114, 317–20.

Verny, M., Duyckaerts, C., Agid, Y. *et al.* (1996). The significance of cortical pathology in progressive supranuclear palsy. Clinico-pathological data in 10 cases. *Brain*, 119, 1123–36.

Vicari, A. M., Folli, F., Pozza, G. *et al.* (1989). Plasmapheresis in the treatment of stiff-man syndrome [letter]. *N. Engl. J. Med.*, 320, 1499.

Vidakovic, A., Dragasevic, N., and Kostic, V. S. (1994). Hemiballism: report of 25 cases. *J. Neurol. Neurosurg. Psychiatry*, 57, 945–9.

Vonsattel, J.-P., Myers, R. H., Stevens, T. J. *et al.* (1985). Neuropathological classification of Huntington's disease. *J. Neuropathol. Exp. Neurol.*, 44, 559–77.

Vuillaume, I., Meynieu, P., Schraen-Maschke, S., Destee, A., Sablonierre, B. (2000). Absence of inidentified CAG expansion in patients with Huntington's disease like phenotype. *J. Neurol. Neurosurg. Psychiat.* 68, 672–5.

Waddy, H. M., Fletcher, N. A., Harding, A. E. *et al.* (1991). A genetic study of idiopathic focal dystonias. *Ann. Neurol.*, 29, 320–4.

Walshe, J. M. (1982). Treatment of Wilson's disease with trientene (triethylene tetramine) dihydrochloride. *Lancet*, i, 643–7.

Walshe, J. M. and Yealland, M. (1992). Wilson's disease: the problem of delayed diagnosis. *J. Neurol. Neurosurg. Psychiatry*, 55, 692 6.

Walshe, J. M. and Yealland, M. (1993). Chelation treatment of neurological Wilson's disease. *Q. J. Med.*, 86, 197–204.

Walters, A. S. (1995). Toward a better definition of the restless legs syndrome. The International Restless Legs Syndrome Study Group. *Mov. Disord.*, 10, 634–42.

Ward, C. D. (1994). Does selegiline delay progression of Parkinson's disease? A critical re-evaluation of the DATATOP study. *J. Neurol. Neurosurg. Psychiatry*, 57, 217–20.

Warich-Kirches, M., Von Bossanyi, P., Treuheit, T. *et al.* (1997). Stiff-man syndrome: possible autoimmune etiology targeted against GABA-ergic cells. *Clin. Neuropathol.*, 16, 214–9.

Warner, T. T., Fletcher, N. A., Davis, M. B. *et al.* (1993). Linkage analysis in British and French families with idiopathic torsion dystonia. *Brain*, 116, 739–44.

Watts, R. L., Mirra, S. S., and Richardson, E. P. (1997). Corticobasal ganglionic degeneration. In: *Movement disorders*, Vol. 3 (ed. C. D. Marsden and S. Fahn), pp. 282–99. Butterworth-Heinemann, Oxford.

Weetman, J., Anderson, I. M., Gregory, R. P. *et al.* (1997). Bilateral posteroventral pallidotomy for severe antipsychotic induced tardive dyskinesia and dystonia [letter]. *J. Neurol. Neurosurg. Psychiatry*, 63, 554–6.

Wein, T., Andermann, F., Silver, K. *et al.* (1996). Exquisite sensitivity of paroxysmal kinesigenic choreoathetosis to carbamazepine. *Neurology*, 47, 1104–6.

Weindl, A., Kuwert, T., Leenders, K. L. *et al.* (1993). Increased striatal glucose consumption in Sydenham's chorea. *Mov. Disord.*, 8, 437–44.

Wenning, G. K., Ben Shlomo, Y., Magalhaes, M. *et al.* (1994a). Clinical features and natural history of multiple system atrophy. An analysis of 100 cases. *Brain*, 117, 835–45.

Wenning, G. K., Jager, R., Kendall, B. *et al.* (1994b). Is cranial computerized tomography useful in the diagnosis of multiple system atrophy? *Mov. Disord.*, 9, 333–6.

Wenning, G. K., Quinn, N. P., Magalhaes, M. *et al.* (1994c). Minimal change multiple system atrophy. *Mov. Disord.*, 9, 161–6.

Wenning, G. K., Ben-Shlomo, Y., Magalhaes, M. *et al.* (1995). Clinicopathological study of 35 cases of multiple system atrophy. *J. Neurol. Neurosurg. Psychiatry*, 58, 160–6.

Wenning, G. K., Kraft, E., Beck, R. *et al.* (1997). Cerebellar presentation of multiple system atrophy. *Mov. Disord.*, 12, 115–7.

Wenning, G. K., Ben-Shlomo, Y., Hughes, A. *et al.* (2000). What clinical features are most useful to distinguish definite multiple system atrophy from Parkinson's disease? *J. Neurol. Neurosurg. Psychiat.*, 68, 434–40.

Wenning, G. K., Litvan, I., Jankovic, J. *et al.* (1998). Natural history and survival of 14 patients with corticobasal degeneration confirmed at postmortem examination. *J. Neurol. Neurosurg. Psychiatry*, 64, 184–9.

Werhahn, K. J., Brown, P., Thompson, P. D. *et al.* (1997). The clinical features and prognosis of chronic posthypoxic myoclonus. *Mov. Disord.*, 12, 216–20.

Wichmann, T. and DeLong, M. R. (1997). Physiology of the basal ganglia and pathophysiology of movement disorders of basal ganglia origin. In: *Movement disorders: neurologic principles and practice* (ed. R. L. Watts and W. C. Koller), pp. 87–97. McGraw-Hill, New York.

Wijker, M., Wszolek, Z. K., Wolters, E. C. *et al.* (1996). Localization of the gene for rapidly progressive autosomal dominant parkinsonism and dementia with pallido-ponto-nigral degeneration to chromosome 17q21. *Hum. Mol. Genet.*, 5, 151–4.

Wilhelmsen, K. C., Lynch, T., Pavlou, E. *et al.* (1994). Localisation of disinhibition-dementia-parkinsonism-amyotrophy complex to 17q21–22. *Am. J. Hum. Genet.*, 55, 1159–65.

Wilhelmsen, K. C., Mirel, D., Marder, K. *et al.* (1997). Is there a genetic susceptibility locus for Parkinson's disease on chromosome 22q13? *Ann. Neurol.*, 41, 813–7.

Will, R. G., Lees, A. J., Gibb, W. *et al.* (1988). A case of progressive subcortical gliosis presenting clinically as Steele–Richardson–Olszewski syndrome. *J. Neurol. Neurosurg. Psychiatry*, **51**, 1224–7.

Wissel, J., Kabus, C., Wenzel, R. *et al.* (1996). Botulinum toxin in writer's cramp: objective response evaluation in 31 patients. *J. Neurol. Neurosurg. Psychiatry*, **61**, 172–5.

Wszolek, Z. K., Pfeiffer, R. F., Bhatt, M. H. *et al.* (1992). Rapidly progressive autosomal dominant parkinsonism and dementia with pallido-ponto-nigral degeneration. *Ann. Neurol.*, **32**, 312–20.

Wszolek, Z. K., Pfeiffer, B., Fulgham, J. R. *et al.* (1995). Western Nebraska family (family D) with autosomal dominant parkinsonism. *Neurology*, **45**, 502–5.

Xiang, F., Almquist, E. W., Huq, M. *et al.* (1998). A Huntington disease-like neurodegenerative disorder maps to chromosome 20p. *Am. J. Hum. Gen.*, **63**, 1431–8.

Xuereb, J. H., MacMillan, J. C., Snell, R. *et al.* (1996). Neuropathological diagnosis and CAG repeat expansion in Huntington's disease. *J. Neurol. Neurosurg. Psychiatry*, **60**, 78–81.

Yamamoto, M., Fujii, S., Hatanaka, Y. (1997). Result of long-term administration of L-threo-3,4-dihydro-xyphenylserine in patients with pure akinesia as an early symptom of progressive supranuclear palsy. *Clin. Neuropharmacol.*, **20**, 371–3.

Yamashita, I., Sasaki, H., Yabe, I. *et al.* (2000). A novel locus for dominant cerebellar ataxia (SCA14) maps to a 10.2-cM interval flanked by D19S206 and D19S605 on chromosome 19q13.4-qter. *Ann. Neurol.*, **48**, 156–63.

Zeidler, M., Stewart, G. E., Barraclough, C. R. *et al.* (1997). New variant Creutzfeldt–Jakob disease: neurological features and diagnostic tests. *Lancet*, **350**, 903–7.

Zhang, Z. X. and Roman, G. C. (1993). Worldwide occurrence of Parkinson's disease: an updated review. *Neuroepidemiology*, **12**, 195–208.

Zweig, R. M., Hedreen, J. C., Jankel, W. R. *et al.* (1988). Pathology in brainstem regions of individuals with primary dystonia. *Neurology*, **38**, 702–6.

Neurological infection

Meningitis

Milne Anderson

33.1 Introduction

Infection of the central nervous system is usually described under three clinically descriptive headings: meningitis, encephalitis, and local suppuration. Most commonly, one of these syndromes dominates the clinical picture. However, two or rarely all three may co-exist in the same patient. The most frequent combination is meningitis with encephalitis. To some degree, the distinction is artificial because organisms do not recognize the anatomical boundary between meninx and brain parenchyma and most cases of meningitis suffer inflammation of underlying brain tissue, but this is not evident on examination. All three forms of infection share the signs of pyrexia, headache, drowsiness, and alteration of conscious level and focal neurology. Because the skull is effectively a rigid box, all three cause intracranial pressure (ICP) to rise as the soft structures inside become inflamed, and raised ICP is a major factor which contributes to neurological deterioration and morbidity in CNS infection. In cases of meningitis, signs of meningeal irritation predominate – neck stiffness, photophobia, vomiting, and irritability. Encephalitis results from infection of brain parenchyma and causes changes of mental state and deterioration of consciousness early in the evolution of the syndrome, to be followed by epileptic seizures and focal signs in a substantial proportion of cases. Local suppuration is the consequence of abscess or granuloma formation within brain substance or adjacent to the meninges. It is important to recognize that focal signs may also occur if infarction of brain tissue occurs from arteritis or phlebitis, or if encephalitis causes local necrosis. With any of these syndromes there may or may not be evidence of infection elsewhere in the body.

33.1.1 Definition of meningitis

In addition to infective causes, meningeal inflammation may result from irritation of the meninges by non-infectious causes such as blood from subarachnoid haemorrhage (Section 27.7), metastatic malignant cells (Section 18.10) and chemical irritants from ruptured brain cysts. The resulting clinical picture may be indistinguishable from infective meningitis without further investigation. For present purposes, the term 'meningitis' refers to the clinical syndrome in which signs of meningeal irritation predominate and that has been caused by an infectious agent. It has been customary to categorize meningitis as acute, subacute, or chronic in proportion to the speed of onset and clinical progression, and there is some diagnostic merit in so doing. Most cases are acute, presenting within hours or a day or so of onset of symptoms and most of these are caused by viruses or bacteria. Subacute cases evolve over days to a week or two and are caused by some bacteria and less commonly, fungi or parasites. Viruses are seldom implicated. Chronic meningitis evolves over weeks and may last for months or longer. Bacteria, fungi and parasites are likely causes.

Any infectious organism can cause meningitis if circumstances permit access to the neuraxis. Physical breach of the meninges following neurosurgery or skull fracture allows direct access of organisms to the CSF and brain. Immune suppression caused by diseases such as AIDS, or treatment regimes such as are given to transplant recipients or cancer sufferers, results in an increasing range of organisms reaching the brain so that each year there are more reports of exotic organisms and previously non-pathogenic agents causing meningitis and brain abscess. Once established within the neuraxis the organisms incite an inflammatory reaction in the CSF. Bacteria provoke an acute polymorphonuclear cellular response and this has led to the term 'pyogenic meningitis'. Rarely, fungi or parasites may cause a similar response. Viruses tend to induce a lymphocytic cellular response so causing the syndrome known as 'aseptic meningitis'. Approximately 80 per cent of cases of aseptic meningitis are caused by viruses. Most cases of acute meningitis are caused by viruses or bacteria. If conditions are favourable, any bacterium can cause meningitis, yet in practice most cases of bacterial meningitis are due to infection by a very small range of bacteria. The vast majority of cases are caused by meningococci, pneumococci, and *Haemophilus influenzae*. The age of the patient, geographical location, season of the year and presence of pre-existing disease may provide important clues to the nature of the pathogen.

Viral or aseptic meningitis is a benign, self-limiting condition in the main, although exceptions do occur. Bacterial meningitis was universally fatal prior to the antibiotics, and even now carries a substantial mortality and morbidity. Fungal and parasitic meningitides are often difficult to treat and also carry high mortality rates. In all forms of meningitis, the two major factors which lead to a poor outcome, are the state of consciousness of the patient on arrival in hospital and any delay in starting appropriate treatment. The former is beyond the control of the admitting doctor, but further deterioration can be obviated by ensuring that the patient is not left to languish in the Accident and Emergency Department while a bed is being identified to accommodate him. Inappropriate investigations are often ordered and carried out because a proper history has not been taken and this leads to further delay. There is little point in trying to take a history from a confused patient – much better to spend some time at the very beginning speaking to the relatives or friends or ambulance personnel, who can usually indicate what the main problem is. It is important to enquire if

there has been recent travel abroad and what the current state of immunization is. Bacterial meningitis can progress explosively, so if this diagnosis is suspected, antibiotics should immediately be administered parenterally on a 'best guess' basis while further investigation is undertaken. There have been theoretical objections to this course of action on the grounds that antibiotic administration will inhibit the culture and identification of causal organisms. This may be the case, but it is now becoming possible to diagnose infections by finding minute quantities of organism DNA in CSF by PCR and other techniques. Family practitioners should be encouraged to administer antibiotics on suspicion of meningitis when they first see the patient at home, and before they become embroiled in a prolonged telephone conversation to have the patient admitted.

33.1.2 Pathogenesis of meningitis

Pathogenic organisms which cause meningitis travel to the brain by one of three pathways:

1 by the bloodstream,

2 directly from suppurative infection in adjacent para-meningeal structures, and

3 by direct inoculation of organisms into the neuraxis by neurosurgery or trauma.

The first is the most common route. The blood-brain barrier (BBB) is a formidable obstacle to the entry of pathogenic organisms into the CNS, and such organisms must possess specific factors for virulence to broach those defences and invade neural structures. Once inside the CNS the organism is in an environment where the normal defence mechanisms which exist in the rest of the body, do not operate. Consequently, the potential for proliferation of organisms and disease production is greater.

Most of the common meningeal pathogens colonize the upper respiratory tract of humans. Data have been obtained from animal experiments which show that adherence to nasal mucosa is important for subsequent reactions which allow ingress of the organism to the neuraxis. Adherence is related to the presence of fimbriae in the cell wall. The character of the cell wall is also an important factor for virulence – those bacteria with a polysaccharide capsule are more invasive and virulent. The molecular basis of the polysaccharide varies between organisms and reflects their differing virulence. Natural antibodies including IgA are secreted by plasma cells in nasal epithelium and may interfere with adherence. The more successful pathogens secrete IgA protease which breaks down IgA and permits continuing adherence to nasal mucosa. By mechanisms that remain incompletely understood, bacteria cross the nasopharyngeal epithelium and enter the bloodstream. There they must combat host defence mechanisms, and the presence of a capsule is thought to protect against phagocytosis and complement activation. (Tunkel and Scheld 1993). The molecular status of the complement evading mechanism is unique for each major group of pathogenic organisms. The mechanisms by which bacteria penetrate the BBB remain unknown. The burden of bacteraemia may be relevant and organisms may be transported inside monocytes. Once inside the skull and within CSF there are few mechanisms to control the spread of bacteria. Complement levels are minimal, immunoglobulin levels are low and efficient opsonic attack on bacteria does not take place (Simberkoff *et al.*, 1980). Consequently, the effectiveness of CSF granulocytes is much reduced and bacterial replication increases. The host response to this bacterial invasion determines the clinical features of meningitis. Some complement does leak through inflamed meninges. Bacterial cell walls disintegrate releasing bacterial products that induce an inflammatory response in the CSF. Bacteria in CSF attract polymorphs chemotactically, particularly neutrophils. The mechanism by which they cross the BBB remains elusive. Granulocytes and lipopolysaccharide from several bacteria are potent inducers of inflammation. Cytokines, including interleukins 1 and 6, tumour necrosis factor and prostaglandins, are released into CSF. Adhesion molecules on vascular endothelial cells are activated, neutrophils bind to the epithelium and this assists their passage through vessel wall into the subarachnoid space or ventricles. Further disruption of the blood brain barrier ensues and inflammation spreads. Cerebral blood flow increases, inducing vasogenic cerebral oedema, and ICP rises. The inflammatory changes cause cytotoxic oedema and vasculitis which reduce cerebral blood flow and ICP rises further. The normal circulation of CSF from the subarachnoid space back into the blood of the venous sinuses is impaired and interstitial oedema puts ICP up further. The end result is derangement of cerebrovascular autoregulation and cerebral hyper- or hypo-perfusion further compromises the brain. (Tureen *et al.*, 1990). Many of these changes occur in the early stages of bacterial meningitis and efforts are now being made to devise adjunctive treatment regimes which will impede the inflammatory response and reduce ICP and maintain cerebral perfusion (Ashwal *et al.*, 1992).

33.1.3 Epidemiology of meningitis

Virtually any organism provided with direct access to the neauraxis, such as via a compound skull fracture, or by inoculation during a neurosurgical procedure, can cause meningitis. Immune suppression of severe degree, such as may occur with AIDS or other diseases which derange the immune system, or as a consequence of drug regimes in oncology or transplant medicine, for example, permits organisms which are normally nonpathogenic to overcome systemic defence mechanisms, and so gain access to the CSF and brain. The epidemiology of meningitis is complex and changes from year to year, and from place to place. Similar strains of the same organism can change their virulence characteristics, populations who may be susceptible to infection migrate, war and civil disruption produce reservoirs of pestilence in which many pathogens thrive, and the ease with which global travel is enjoyed by countless millions, some of whom may transport microbes to virgin regions, all contribute to changing patterns of disease. Also important are the seasonal breeding patterns of many insects and animals who act as reservoirs for infection.

The age of the patient is important – beyond the neonatal period approximately 70 per cent of cases of bacterial meningitis are caused by *Haemophilus influenzae*, *Neisseria meningitidis*, and *Streptococcus pneumoniae*. The success of immunization regimes in children and young adults against *Haemophilus* and more recently, the meningococcus, is altering the epidemiology of these infections in those areas of the globe where it has been possible to introduce immunization programmes. Nosocomially acquired forms of meningitis are increasing. Viral, fungal, and other forms have a different profile from the bacterial variety. Certain disease states predispose to infection by particular varieties of bacteria. Meningitis is found in all parts of the world, affects all races, and its occurrence is sporadic in the majority of cases. Epidemics do occur.

Viral meningitis

Viruses are the most common cause of the 'acute aseptic meningitis' syndrome, and account for more than 70 per cent of all cases world-wide. Viral meningitis follows systemic haematogenous infection. Certain viruses infect the meninges preferentially, others infect brain parenchyma and cause encephalitis. Many infect both and there is considerable overlap, which results in the clinical syndrome of meningo-encephalitis. The most common causes of viral meningitis are listed in Table 33.1. Many other viruses can rarely cause meningitis.

The majority of cases of viral meningitis occur in children and young adults and present throughout the year with peaks in summer and autumn in temperate regions. This probably relates to an increase in person to person transmission by faeco-oral contamination with enteroviruses at these times. The incidence of viral meningitis has been reported to be between 11 and 27 cases per 100 000 population per annum. This is a substantial underestimate because most cases of viral meningitis are benign and self limiting and determining the aetiology of the infection is not often the first priority – this tends to be the exclusion of potentially more serious bacterial meningitis. Now that more precise methods of identification are available, particularly PCR, it is possible to identify the cause of cases of aseptic meningitis in over 70 per cent of cases (Sawyer *et al.*, 1994).

Table 33.1. Viral causes of meningitis

Enteroviruses
Echo
Polio
Coxsackie
Arboviruses (varies with geography)
Herpes simplex type 2
Lymphocytic choriomeningitis
Varicella zoster
Mumps
HIV

Bacterial meningitis

The epidemiology of bacterial meningitis is complex and changing. It affects children under the age of 5 in the main – they account for over 70 per cent of cases, boys more than girls. Black and Hispanic populations are more at risk than Caucasians and this is thought to reflect poor socioeconomic conditions rather than any genetic predisposition. Most cases are sporadic. Neonates are affected by Gram negative enteric bacilli – *E coli* K1, *Klebsiella* species, and streptococci (usually group B) and *Listeria monocytogenes* which are picked up at birth, or nosocomially. *Haemophilus influenzae* and *Neisseria meningitidis* were the most common pathogens in children after the age of 1 month. This is still true of countries where immunization strategies against *H. influenzae* have not been instituted. Where they have, in USA and Europe, the incidence of this form of meningitis has fallen dramatically. The meningococcus is the only significant cause of epidemics. In sub Saharan Africa, epidemics occur annually due to strains of group A and C. Smaller epidemics have been reported from many countries throughout the world, and the causal strain has changed from country to country and from time to time. Transmission of meningococcal meningitis (and other forms) is enabled by close personal contact and the inhalation of airborne, infected droplets. This accounts for the tendency for outbreaks to occur within households, amongst school colleagues and friends, and in relatively closed populations, such as students in residence or recruits in military barracks.

In young adults the major pathogens are the meningococcus and the pneumococcus, the latter becoming more frequent with increasing age. In the elderly, Gram negative bacilli and *Listeria* assume major importance. All authorities agree that infection with *Listeria* appears to be on the increase as does infection acquired within hospitals (Durand *et al.*, 1993; Mylonakis *et al.*, 1998). Tuberculosis has never gone away and is a ubiquitous, continuing cause of meningitis, and not only in those with AIDS and other forms of immune compromise.

Underlying disease states

These may predispose the individual to infection by particular organisms. Fractures of the skull may result in direct inoculation of bacteria into CSF, particularly *Staphylococci*, Gram negative bacilli, and mixed infections with more than one organism. If a neurosurgical procedure becomes infected, it is almost always by a Gram negative bacillus. Compound fractures of the skull with CSF leaks to the exterior, invite infection by the pneumococcus in the main, and by Gram negative bacilli and by multiple organisms. Any case of recurrent meningitis should be investigated extensively for evidence of a previous skull fracture. In such cases it is important to recognize that there may not be a history of trauma, which may have been minor, or occurred so long before that it has been forgotten. The introduction of foreign material to the intracranial compartment, such as CSF shunts, is associated with infection by *Staphylococcus epidermidis*. Patients who have had the spleen removed and those with sickle cell disease, and alcoholics and liver cirrhotics are liable to pneumococcal meningitis. Diabetics may suffer from pneumococcal, staphylococcal, or Gram negative bacillary meningitis. Immune deficiency permits organisms easier access to the neuraxis, and different forms of immune defect favour specific bacteria. Cellular immune deficiency such as occurs with lymphomas and transplant recipients and AIDS render the patient liable to infection with intracellular organisms, most commonly *Listeria*. Neutropaenia renders the patient liable to meningitis from *Pseudomonas* and *Enterobacteriaciae*. Impairment of humoral immunity means that antibody production is deficient which favours infection by bacteria with capsules. Chronic lymphatic leukaemia, treated lymphomas and patients who have had radiotherapy and chemotherapy are at risk from infection by pneumococci, meningococci, *Haemophilus* and multiple organisms. Infection is often abrupt and overwhelming. During pregnancy and the peri-natal period, women are more susceptible to infection by *Listeria* and streptococci. These features are summarized in Table 33.2. It is often necessary to begin treatment of a suspected case of bacterial meningitis before the causal agent has been identified. Knowledge of any predisposing factors will enable antibiotic choices to be made appropriate to the most likely pathogen.

Tuberculous meningitis

This is found in communities throughout the world in proportion to the incidence of tuberculosis in the population. Perhaps 5–10 per cent of tuberculous (TB) infections manifest as TB meningitis which is invariably a complication of TB elsewhere

Table 33.2. Conditions which predispose to bacterial meningitis

Skull fracture	Staphylococci
	Gram negative bacilli
	Mixed infection
	Recurrent infection
Neurosurgery	Gram negative bacilli
CSF leak	Pneumococci
	Gram negative bacilli
	Mixed infection
CSF shunt	*Staphylococcus epidermidis*
Alcoholism	Pneumococcus
Liver cirrhosis	Pneumococcus
Sickle cell disease	Pneumococcus
Splenectomy	Pneumococcus
Diabetes	Pneumococcus
	Staphylococcus
	Gram negative bacilli
Peri-natal/pregnancy	Listeria
	Streptococci
Immune defect-lymphocytes -neutropaenia -humoral	Listeria
	Pseudomonas
	Pneumococci
	Haemophilus
	Meningococci
	Mixed infection

in the body, although that is not always clinically evident. Factors which are recognized to promote the spread of TB, are poor socio-economic conditions, overcrowding, malnutrition, poor hygiene, and lack of immunization programmes. Those most at risk of developing TB are children and young adults, ethnic minorities in industrialized nations and immigrants, and in the last decade and a half, people who have AIDS. HIV associated TB in urban areas has increased markedly in Britain and in the United States and in those countries with large AIDS populations, and is altering the epidemiology as an increasing number of cases are occurring in the adult age range, rather than in children. Most cases are still caused by *Mycobacterium tuberculosis*, but in the AIDS group, non-tuberculous mycobacteria, including the *M. avium* complex of organisms, are increasing as a cause of CNS infection, including meningitis. The epidemiology of the other more chronic forms of meningitis is briefly discussed under individual syndromes.

Fungal meningitis

There are more than 200,000 fungi known in the literature of which more than 100 are recognized to be pathogenic to man. Fungi in this group are saprophytes, widely distributed in nature, usually in humus enriched soils, and they are capable of infecting people with normal immune systems. They tend to be restricted in location – blastomycosis is found in North and Central America, coccidioidomycosis in south western USA, Central America and some northern regions of South America, paracoccidioidomycosis in Central and South America, histoplasmosis is endemic in central USA and may be found elsewhere. People working in these areas are most at risk of infection and rural occupations carry the highest risk. This explains why the vast majority of cases are found in males. It must not be forgotten that tourists to such areas can acquire infection that may not become evident until weeks or months later, which emphasizes how important it is to obtain a complete travel history from anyone suspected of suffering from meningitis. The cryptococcus is ubiquitous and meningitis may occur in those with normal immunity, but is seen most commonly in patients with immune deficit, particularly of cellular immunity such as AIDS, lymphoma and malignancy, and treatment with steroids. The route of infection is almost always by inhalation. Rarely, direct inoculation through a cut or graze takes place. The second group which can be classified 'opportunistic' does not normally affect those with intact immune systems. This is a disparate group and descriptions of novel infections are being added to, almost every day as the number of patients suffering immune suppression increases. *Candida* species are part of the normal flora of the human body and do not cause CNS disease unless there is some immune disturbance such as malignancy, steroid and broad spectrum antibiotic treatment, and AIDS. CNS infection occurs more readily if there is a conduit for organisms to invade the bloodstream and then the CSF, for example indwelling IV catheters or IV drug abuse. Cryptococcosis and candidiasis are the most common CNS mycoses. *Aspergillus* species can cause meningitis

in the immune suppressed, although in common with other opportunistic pathogens such as the *Zygomycetes*, local invasion, granuloma and abscess formation are more likely.

Parasitic meningitis

Parasites only very rarely cause meningitis. Much more commonly they cause encephalitis and the causes of parasitic encephalitis are described in Chapter 34. Amoebae, both *Naegleria* and *Acanthamoeba*, may cause forms of meningoencephalitis. *Naegleria* live in stagnant water and infect children and young adults, predominantly male, who play or swim in the water, to produce primary amoebic meningoencephalitis which can present exactly like acute bacterial meningitis. *Acanthamoebae* are more ubiquitous and can be found in dry soils and cause a granulomatous encephalitis which in some may resemble chronic meningitis. Males are affected much more frequently than females and there is often a predisposing condition with immuno-suppression such as AIDS. Infestation of humans by the rat lungworm, *Angiostrongylus*, causes eosinophilic meningitis. Cases have been reported from many parts of the world, particularly Thailand, India and the Far East, the Pacific Islands, and Africa.

33.1.4 The clinical features and differential diagnosis of meningitis

The clinical features of a classical case of meningitis are easy to recognize and are common to all types, no matter which organism has been the cause. Unfortunately, as many as 20 per cent of cases have atypical features. Acute meningitis presents within a few hours of the onset, or at the most, within a day or two. Viruses and bacteria are the cause. Fever, malaise, irritability, headache, photophobia, vomiting, neck stiffness, and confusion are the usual features. In the very young, the very old, the immune suppressed, and those with severe and overwhelming infection, these major clinical features may be absent, and this group may represent in excess of 20 per cent of all cases. Consequently, the threshold for considering a diagnosis of meningitis in these groups must be lowered. Children are most at risk, followed by young adults and the immune-suppressed, and the possibility of meningitis as a cause for their symptoms should be considered, particularly if there is lethargy, diminution in conscious level, drowsiness and pyrexia associated with neck stiffness. Fever is the sign most commonly present in more than 90 per cent of cases. The absence of pyrexia, and the presence of hypothermia in children, carries a very poor prognosis. Neck stiffness may not be evident in the early stages of meningitis, and its absence does not exclude a diagnosis of meningitis. Young children cannot complain of headache, and meningitis should be suspected if there is fever with behavioural change, increasing lethargy and diminution in mental status, and the declaration of epileptic seizures. The elderly may have no specific evidence of meningeal irritation and symptoms of confusion, lethargy and hallucinosis may be mistakenly attributed to concomitant illness or intercurrent infection. Conversely, neck stiffness in the elderly may be due to cervical spondylosis and confusion and hallucinations may result from intercurrent infection in chest or renal tract. It is not uncommon for cases of meningitis to have signs and symptoms of upper respiratory tract infection, or gastrointestinal disturbance, beforehand. Meningitis should therefore be considered as a diagnosis in those patients from the geriatric and paediatric age groups who are ill in a non-specific way, especially if they are pyrexial.

Epileptic seizures

These occur in up to 40 per cent of children with meningitis, and in a smaller proportion of older patients. The younger the brain, the more likely epilepsy is to be provoked by infection and pyrexia. If seizures are prolonged and continuous, CSF should be examined when it is judged safe to do so, and treatment with appropriate anticonvulsants and antibiotics must be given straight away to diminish the prospect of anoxic and metabolic brain damage. Convulsions may be the presenting feature of meningitis in any age group. Convulsions associated with pyrexia are a common problem in young children, and when they occur, raise the question 'is the convulsion due to the temperature or does the child have meningitis?'

CSF examination by lumbar puncture (LP) should be carried out as soon as possible if meningitis is suspected, and the place of LP in such children has long been debated. Evidence suggests that if the seizure is brief, if there is no associated neurological deficit or prolonged impairment of consciousness, and there are no signs of meningitis, it is reasonable to observe the child closely for a few hours and postpone LP.

Systemic infection

A search should be made for evidence of infection elsewhere in the body – is there a chest infection or pneumonia? Is there septic arthropathy or endocarditis? Different organisms have a propensity to cause particular infective complications, which may be useful in helping to reach a diagnosis, and these are discussed later under the particular organism. Skin rashes occur in a third of patients and should always be looked for, because they may be transient and localized. Meningococcal meningitis is accompanied by an early, diffuse maculopapular rash which may rapidly progress to petechiae and frank purpura in up to 60 per cent of cases. Viruses and other bacteria can also cause rashes, particularly Echo 9, staphylococci, pneumococci, *Haemophilus*, and *Listeria* species. Rashes may also be caused by reactions to antibiotics or other drugs, but this does not happen in the early stages of the disease. Shock and disseminated intravascular coagulation may complicate any severe bacterial meningitis and is most commonly seen in association with fulminant meningococcal septicaemia.

The time scale

The time scale and evolution of a case of meningitis may have diagnostic use. Viral meningitis is of acute onset, within hours or a day or so. Headache is a prominent feature and except in severe or complicated cases, consciousness is not impaired beyond drowsiness and the patient remains coherent and co-operative. Viral meningitis is usually benign and self-limiting. Acute bacterial meningitis comes on within hours or a day at the most. In some cases, particularly but not only of meningococcal infection, the onset may be fulminant with progression from the first symptoms to death compressed within a few hours. Bacterial meningitis is more likely to depress the level of consciousness and to produce raised intracranial pressure and focal neurological signs. Meningitis caused by TB and fungi is of more chronic evolution with symptoms and signs evolving over weeks or months.

Focal signs

Fifteen per cent of cases of bacterial meningitis develop focal neurological signs due to arteritis of intracranial arteries, often at the base of the brain, which gives rise to infarction of cerebral tissue and results in hemiparesis, hemisensory disturbance, hemianopia, or dysphasia. (Carpenter and Petersdorf 1962; Dodge and Swartz 1965; Swartz and Dodge 1965). Less commonly, cerebral venous thrombosis can cause focal signs with focal epileptic seizures. Rarely, the development of focal signs and seizures may indicate abscess formation. Cranial nerve palsies may develop from inflammation of the basal meninges. Raised intracranial pressure is present in every case of meningitis although it may not reach values which are clinically significant. Clinical indicators are impairment of conscious level from drowsiness to coma, increasing neck stiffness if there is cerebellar tonsillar herniation, sixth nerve palsies, and papilloedema. It is important to recognize that the absence of papilloedema does not mean that ICP is normal. A swollen optic disc associated with marked reduction of visual acuity may indicate septic optic neuritis. The level of consciousness is an important predictor of clinical outcome – the lower the Glasgow coma score, the higher the mortality which may reach 55 per cent in comatose adults. (Geiseler et al., 1980)

Electrolytes and serum osmolarity

These disturbances may occur, particularly in children. The syndrome of inappropriate secretion of antidiuretic hormone causes hyponatraemia. Overhydration of an unconscious patient is another cause of hyponatraemia in this group.

Differential diagnosis

The differential diagnosis of a case of meningitis is extensive (see Table 33.3).

Investigation

To distinguish the many infectious causes is often not possible at the bedside, and further tests are required including imaging of the intracranial contents and CSF examination when it is deemed safe. Brain abscess and subdural empyema may be clinically identical to severe meningitis, and brain imaging is necessary. Encephalitis is likely if there is significant impairment of consciousness or disturbance of intellect in the earlier stages.

Table 33.3. Meningitis – differential diagnosis

Infectious causes	Non-infectious causes
Encephalitis	Granulomatous angiitis
Brain abscess	Sarcoidosis
Subdural empyema	SLE
Septicaemia	Malignant meningitis
	Behçet's disease
	Whipple's disease
	Drug induced meningitis
	Brain tumour
	Subarachnoid haemorrhage
	Migraine
	Mollaret's syndrome
	Vogt–Koyanagi–Harada syndrome

Inflammation of the meninges may result from non-infectious causes such as intracranial granulomatous diseases and vasculitides including sarcoidosis, granulomatous angiitis of the CNS, systemic lupus erythematosis, Whipple's disease, Behçet's disease, and carcinomatous meningitis. The meningitic syndromes associated with these conditions are chronic rather than acute. There may be no other clinical evidence of the disease and meningitis can be the presenting feature. A further source for confusion is that pyrexia and neck stiffness may be prominent. Brain imaging with MR is often helpful because several of these diseases are associated with pathological changes of cerebral white matter. Lumbar puncture often reveals a cellular and monocytic CSF and it is important to have cytological and immunological examination of the cells undertaken. There have been individual cases reported of aseptic meningitis associated with the use of drugs, usually non-steroidal anti-intinflammatory drugs, trimethoprim, immunoglobulin, and some antibiotics. (Gordon *et al.*, 1990). Mollaret's syndrome of recurrent meningitis with predominantly lymphocytic and aseptic CSF is suspected by its recurrent nature. A recent association with Herpes simplex virus has been found. Brain tumours and raised intracranial pressure from hydrocephalus can cause marked neck stiffness and reduction in conscious level in association with cerebellar tonsillar herniation. Rarely, certain forms of brain tumour such as epidermoid cysts may leak their contents into the CSF and cause a chemical meningitis. Subarachnoid haemorrhage may not be classical with abrupt headache and may present with progressing headache over hours or days, neck stiffness, and pyrexia. CT scanning will demonstrate subarachnoid blood in the majority of patients and breakdown products of blood can be demonstrated in CSF for several days afterwards. Severe migraine may present in similar fashion, sometimes giving rise to a cellular response in the CSF. Diagnosis is by exclusion of subarachnoid blood. The Vogt-Koyanagi-Harada syndrome is a rare auto-immune syndrome with inflammatory changes in uvea, retina, meninges and skin, found in pigmented races. In the acute phase there may be lymphocytic meningitis.

33.2 Particular varieties of meningitis

Cases of meningitis share common features which are described above. Different pathogens produce clinical abnormalities peculiar to that particular organism, or which are common to organisms in the same group. This often has aetiological and diagnostic significance and the features of these forms of meningitis are described here.

33.2.1 Viral meningitis

Cases of viral meningitis occur throughout the year and affect children and young adults predominantly. In temperate climates, most cases occur in summer and autumn. The clinical picture is common to all infections and it is sometimes possible to find a sign or feature which indicates a specific pathogen such as parotitis with mumps. Characteristically, the onset is sudden with headache, pyrexia and neck stiffness, often preceded or accompanied by a non-specific upper respiratory infection or malaise. Nausea, irritability, lethargy, myalgia, and drowsiness are common. The appearance of focal neurological signs, seizures, or a deterioration of conscious level suggest that there has been progression to encephalitis. Symptoms resolve spontaneously in a few days and seldom persist beyond two weeks; and recovery is complete in most. In some, malaise, myalgia, and lassitude may continue for a few weeks. A rash may accompany enteroviral infections, myalgia and myocarditis may complicate coxsackie meningitis and HIV may have arthralgia and lymphadenopathy. In the early stages it may not be possible to differentiate viral meningitis from acute bacterial meningitis or, in some cases, subarachnoid haemorrhage and urgent CSF examination, with appropriate precautions, should be undertaken.

33.2.2 Bacterial meningitis

Many bacteria are capable of causing meningitis and this section deals with the clinical features of the most common infections.

Meningococcal meningitis

Meningococcal infection is found world-wide. The organism is an aerobic Gram negative diplococcus with a polysaccharide capsule. Variations in the structure of the capsule allow sub-classification into 13 serologically distinct sub-groups. Most disease is caused by organisms of groups A, B, C, and Y. Outbreaks caused by bacteria of these groups have occurred in many countries in past decades. Groups B and C have caused outbreaks in Britain, parts of Europe, and the United States. In industrialized nations, most cases occur in winter and spring. It is a disease of children and young adults and fewer than 10 per cent of cases occur in people over 45. The meningococcus infects humans only, and it colonizes the nasopharynx. Spread is by aerosol inhalation and close personal contact. The incidence of the carrier state varies greatly and is high in closed communities – from 30–60 per cent in military barracks and student halls of residence. Transmission of disease is carrier mediated. The characteristics which predispose to clinical infection remain ill-understood. The incubation period is short, less than 10 days and the clinical declaration of meningitis may be explosive. Features highly suggestive of meningococcal meningitis are the appearance of the typical rash on the trunk and legs. Beginning as petechiae which may be evident on palms and soles of feet, conjunctivae and mucous membranes, they coalesce to form purpura. This may extend, become bullous and lead to necrosis. If there is fulminant meningococcaemia, disseminated intravascular coagulation is triggered and ecchymoses appear which may progress to gangrene with resultant spontaneous amputation (Figure 33.1). Adrenal haemorrhage may result from severe meningococcal septicaemia and cause cardiovascular collapse, the Waterhouse–Friderichsen syndrome. In particularly fulminant cases, these findings may be evident before signs of meningitis are found. Myocarditis, pericarditis, and arthritis may be present and relate to circulating immune complexes.

Haemophilus influenzae meningitis

These bacteria are small, Gram negative cocco-bacilli and are either encapsulated or non-encapsulated. Encapsulated strains are divided into 6 types, a to f, which reflect antigenic properties of the capsule. Most severe infections are caused by the b type, Hib. This form of meningitis affects children under 5 years of age in more than 90 per cent of cases and is sporadic in the majority. It is found through out the world and asymptomatic nasopharyngeal colonization is common. Following the introduction of immunization programmes against Hib, particularly those using conjugate vaccines rather than older polysaccharide vaccines, the incidence of meningitis due to this organism has fallen dramatically in those countries where they have been adopted. Generally, the onset is less abrupt than the meningococcal form, although in some it may be abrupt and fulminant. Over 24 to 72 hours symptoms of upper respiratory infection develop, often accompanied by otitis media or sinusitis or epiglottitis. Signs of meningitis with neck stiffness and irritability follow. Epileptic seizures are common. Vascular complications may supervene (Figure 33.2). Some patients develop a rash which may have a petechial component. Response to antibiotics is rather slower than with other forms and fever often persists for some days. If it continues further, complications should be suspected – septic arthritis and osteomyelitis are well recognized. Subdural effusions are common and in the majority are not of continuing clinical significance and require no active treatment. Occasionally, surgical relief of pressure or eradication of infected effusion is necessary (Syrogiannopoulos *et al.*, 1986).

Pneumococcal meningitis

Streptococcus pneumoniae is a Gram positive non-motile encapsulated coccus. Virulence depends upon capsular polysaccharide characteristics and in the region of 84 capsular serotypes are recognized, of which 10 or so are responsible for the great majority of infections. They are part of the normal flora of the upper respiratory tract and as many as four serotypes have been recovered from the same patient. New strains colonize 25 per cent of the population each year. This form of meningitis is seen in adults and particular risk factors are sickle cell disease and haemoglobinopathies in young patients, splenectomy, alcoholism, drug abuse, head trauma and chronic otitis media, diabetes, and immune suppression. About half of all patients at the time of presentation with meningitis will have signs of pneumonia, otitis, or paranasal sinusitis. The clinical onset is usually abrupt and progression is rapid. Mental confusion, convulsions and focal signs from endarteritis and thrombophlebitis are common. In the immune suppressed, onset and progression are often explosive. Recurrent attacks of *Pneumococcal* meningitis should initiate a search for a CSF communication with the exterior.

Gram negative bacillary meningitis in adults

This form of meningitis is acquired in hospital and affects the immune suppressed, the elderly, and following neurosurgery. Most are caused by *E. coli. Klebsiella pneumoniae, Proteus* spp, and *Enterobacteriaeciae* spp; *Pseudomonas* and *Serratia* spp. cause most of the others. The clinical onset following trauma and neurosurgery tends to be insidious and relatively benign. If the infection is spontaneous the clinical course is fulminant with bacteraemia and shock.

Streptococcal meningitis

Most cases of meningitis are caused by Group B streptococci and affect neonates. There are six main serotypes and the

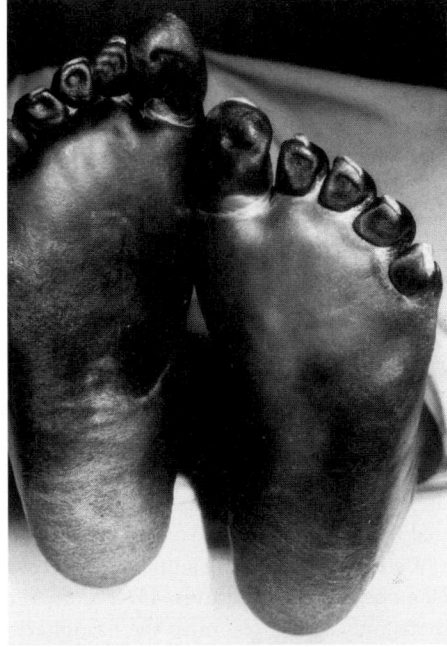

Fig. 33.1. Feet of a patient with meningococcal meningitis and septicaemia who has developed gangrene from peripheral vasculitis.

majority of cases are due to type 3. Adults are also infected. In half there is a predisposing cause such as senility, diabetes, childbirth, alcoholism, immune suppression, and AIDS (Dunne and Quagliarello 1993).

Listeria meningitis

Listeria monocytogenes is a Gram positive aerobic coccobacillus which is similar to diphtheroids on Gram stain. There are 11 serotypes and most infection is caused by three serotypes, 1a, 1b and 4b. Neonatal meningitis is acquired from the genital tract or from subclinical infection in the mother. Adult infection is sporadic and may affect normal people. Most have some form of immune disturbance such as diabetes, alcoholism, senility, or immune suppression associated with AIDS or cancer, haematological malignancy and renal tansplantation. The route of infection in non-puerperal cases is not known with certainty. Over 20 per cent seem to derive from contaminated foods – cheeses, vegetables, and undercooked meats. In neonates the onset of meningitis is usually more than 10 days after birth and symptoms may be quite non-specific such as failure to thrive. In adults the onset is seldom abrupt and progression may be rather indolent. In some, encephalitis with the brunt falling on the brainstem supervenes to cause ophthalmoparesis, cranial nerve palsies and upper motor neurone and cerebellar signs. Focal signs and epileptic seizures occur in a quarter of all cases (Mylonakis *et al.*, 1998).

33.2.3 Tuberculous meningitis

Tuberculosis continues to be a world-wide infection. Following improvements in sanitation and social circumstances, the availability of BCG immunization and the development of effective antibiotics, the incidence of all forms of TB infection decreased in the developed western world while in the developing world infection rates continued to rise and prevalence rates for exposure to TB by the age of 14 exceeded 80 per cent in some Asian countries. In some regions of the world where normal living standards have been disrupted by war and insurrection, TB has once more become a major health problem. Even in relatively stable social circumstances, TB infection has increased in vulnerable populations – racial and ethnic minorities, urban homeless and amongst those with AIDS. There has also been a change in the age range of persons affected. Formerly, CNS TB was a disease with a heavy childhood predominance, now the brunt of disease is falling on males aged from the third to the seventh decade. This represents both newly acquired and reactivated infection. The proportion of CNS infection has been difficult to determine because of the lack of notification in many countries – figures from Britain suggest that 10 per cent of all cases is a reasonable estimate (Wood and Anderson 1988). These figures are currently being skewed in the AIDS population where extrapulmonary TB occurs in 70 per cent of those with AIDS and TB (Slutsker *et al.*, 1993) and does not seem to be dependant on immune suppression – many cases have TB before immune compromise sets in. Most cases are caused by

the human strain of the organism. Bovine and avian mycobacterial infections in humans are rare. Atypical non-tuberculous mycobacterial infection may complicate AIDS.

Mycobacterium tuberculosis

This is a non-motile, aerobic bacillus with a thick cell wall containing a high lipid content that resists Gram staining and is rendered visible by the Ziehl-Neelson and other staining techniques. CNS infection is always secondary to TB infection elsewhere in the body. In most, the primary infection is pulmonary, mycobacteria having been inhaled which lodge in the alveoli and set up a peripheral Ghon focus. This is followed by central drainage to mediastinal lymph nodes. In the first few weeks, when there is an inadequate immune response, haematogenous spread of organisms takes place throughout the body. Within a month or so cell mediated immunity develops and T-lymphocytes stimulate mononuclear phagocytes. Both mycobacteria and phagocytes suffer many casualties and a tubercle forms with a caseous centre. Tissue hypersensitivity develops and the tuberculin skin test becomes positive. If host resistance is impaired, miliary TB with dissemination of small tubercles throughout the body occurs. If resistance is robust, the tubercles undergo fibrosis and resolve. Resolution may not be complete and viable organisms may be retained within the caseous centre and fibrous capsule. These organisms are capable of producing clinical infection if host resistance weakens and they are reactivated to proliferate and rupture from the caseous centre. TB meningitis occurs if a focus adjacent to CSF pathways ruptures and spreads mycobacteria throughout the subarachnoid space and cerebral ventricles. In rare cases, TB infection reaches the neuraxis by direct extension from contiguous structures such as spinal caries or tuberculous otitis.

Acute inflammatory TB meningitis covers the convexity of the cerebral hemispheres and the brunt falls on the basal meninges with green gelatinous exudation spreading outwards to block the interpeduncular cistern and the foramina of the fourth ventricle, and in severe cases the foramen magnum itself. Tuberculous nodules are frequent and mycobacteria are often plentiful. Meningeal arteries are always affected to some degree with inflammatory change in the vessel wall leading to thrombosis, predominantly of the internal carotid vessels at the base of the brain, the middle cerebral arteries, and the perforating vessels to the basal ganglia. The meningeal veins are also inflamed. There is always a component of associated encephalitis. CSF circulation is compromised because of obstruction to flow by adhesion of the basal meninges, aqueduct obstruction by debris or inflammation, and meningeal adhesions. Hydrocephalus is common. The clinical picture may therefore become confused with the development of focal signs and raised ICP. These may also result from the development of a tuberculoma or much more rarely, a tuberculous brain abscess

The clinical manifestations of TB meningitis are protean, to the degree that virtually any other neurological syndrome may be imitated. Since the time of Osler, it has been recognized that acute infectious diseases in children, particularly pertussis and measles and otitis media, commonly precipitate TB meningitis. Modern experience suggests that these observations may no longer be valid. Several attempts have been made to stage the disease but none has been satisfactory. In contrast to acute purulent bacterial meningitis, the onset and evolution of the disease is slow and insidious although in children it is sometimes of sudden onset and impossible to differentiate without CSF examination. Progression is slower in adults with some taking more than a month to see a doctor. At the onset, which may last 3 to 4 weeks, the signs and symptoms are quite nonspecific. Nausea, vomiting, malaise, apathy, irritability, anorexia and restlessness; depression, confusion and disturbed behaviour may occur in adults. The symptoms are so indefinite and at this stage, unaccompanied by signs, that a diagnosis of hysteria may be entertained, a possibility that Gowers warned of. Children may have nausea, vomiting, abdominal pain, and anorexia which may point to gastrointestinal pathology – continued unexplained vomiting in a child should always raise the spectrum of intracranial pathology. Headache is not commonly complained of, particularly in young children. Epileptic seizures may occur and if there is a focal component, parenchymal cerebral damage should be suspected, either from vascular complications or the development of a tuberculoma. By now, signs of meningeal irritation are usually to be found – neck stiffness, headache and photophobia together with a positive Kernig's sign. Most, but not all cases have pyrexia.

With disease progression the state of awareness and conscious level decline and signs of raised ICP including papilloedema become evident. This happens more frequently than in acute purulent meningitis. As the basal meninges become covered in exudate, cranial nerve palsies of the third, sixth and seventh nerve appear. Arteritis of the major cerebral vessels causes hemiparesis, dysphasia and movement disorders from basal ganglia infarction. Ophthalmologic examination of the fundi may reveal papilloedema or sometimes, optic atrophy consequent upon adhesive arachnoiditis. Choroidal tubercles may be evident in about 10 per cent of cases, and should be looked for. If there is hypothalamic disturbance, electrolytic and osmotic disturbances of the blood may be evident and should be strictly monitored. A predominantly spinal form of the disease may occur and can cause diagnostic confusion. In all cases, diligent search should be made for evidence of tuberculous infection elsewhere in the body, especially in the chest.

The differential diagnosis of TB meningitis is wide and includes other forms of sub-acute and chronic meningitis, also fungal varieties which often have pulmonary signs.

Systemic diseases which induce an inflammatory response in CSF, such as sarcoid and collagen/vascular disease can be difficult to distinguish. Brain tumours, metastases, and granulomas may produce focal signs and meningism.

33.2.4 Meningitis in the immune suppressed

Several forms of meningitis which affect the immune suppressed have already been described. Immune suppression renders the CNS and the whole human frame vulnerable to infection from organisms that would in normal circumstances be of no pathological consequence. The greater the degree of immune suppression, the wider the range of potential pathogens, and the greater ease by which they can spread throughout the body. Consequently, the onset and spread of such infection is often fulminating and devastating and CNS infection may only be part of a generalized reaction. Furthermore, because of the failure to mount an immune response, there may be no clinical evidence of meningitis – neck stiffness, pyrexia, photophobia and neurological signs are lacking. The only sign of deterioration may be the onset of circulatory collapse and sudden death. Particular forms of immune suppression predispose to infection with specific pathogens and some of these are detailed in Table 33.2. Enquiry must be made of potential exposure to pathogens including travel to foreign parts, exposure to animals and plants and insect vectors of disease, and to nosocomial sources. It must be emphasized that any organism, however unlikely, may be pathogenic in these circumstances. Neutropaenic patients are at risk of meningitis from *Pseudomonas* spp, *Enterobacteriaeciae* spp and Aspergillus. Those with a humoral defect are liable to meningitis from the pneumococcus, the meningococcus, *Haemophilus*, *Enterobacteriaeciae*, and multiple organisms. Cellular defects, including AIDS, render the patient vulnerable to *Listeria* and *Cryptococcus* meningitis (Aoun and Klatersky 1999, Rubin and Tolkoff-Rubin 1999). Once meningitis is suspected in such patients there should be no delay in instituting treatment which should be given as further investigations are carried out. Waiting for the results of tests before giving antibiotics or antifungals may turn out to be fatal for the patient.

33.2.5 Uncommon forms of meningitis

Many unusual pathogens have been reported as a cause of meningitis in patients suffering from AIDS, including meningitis caused by non-tuberculous mycobacteria. The features of these infections are discussed in Section 35.3.

Chronic meningitis may be caused by pathogens which are not native to the UK and may be imported. Rarely brucellosis may cause a meningoencephalitis (Section 35.6).

Meningitis due to fungi and parasites is rarely seen in patients who have no immune deficit and usually occurs in people who have travelled to foreign parts. They acquire the disease which remains asymptomatic during the incubation period, and weeks or months later, present with an illness which may be baffling to the unwary. It is necessary in every suspected case of meningitis to ensure that a full travel and recreational history is obtained and documented.

Cryptococcal meningitis

This affects those who suffer from immune suppression in the main, and can also infect those who have a normal immune system. The number of cases of cryptococcal meningitis is rising, primarily reflecting the spread of AIDS and immune suppression. Infection is acquired by inhaling spores and small yeast cells scattered in the environment. Most pulmonary infections are asymptomatic, some lead to infiltrates and granuloma formation. Cryptococcal infection, including meningitis, is clinically similar to TB. Acute meningitis is unusual, a chronic syndrome is usual. Headache, neck stiffness, vomiting, weight loss, and mild encephalitic features of disorientation, confusion, and memory loss are common and pressure signs, and cranial nerve palsies from basal meningeal adhesions follow. Focal signs may result from vascular compromise or granuloma formation. The syndrome evolves over months rather than weeks and there may be relapse and remission. There are no specific clinical diagnostic features. Diagnosis is by demonstration of yeast on India ink prepared fresh slide preparations in over 50 per cent of patients. Serum and CSF latex antigen tests are usually positive

Coccidioidomycosis

This is caused by *Coccidioides immitis*, a dimorphic fungus which inhabits dry, acid soils and is found in the south western United States, Central and South America. Arthrospores dislodged by man as he disturbs the soil, are inhaled and incite an inflammatory response in the lungs. In most, this is asymptomatic. In the others, a short lived 'flu like upper respiratory infection follows one week to one month after exposure. If this has been severe, cough, fever, chest pain, myalgia, headache, and a rash may be evident, sometimes erythema nodosum. The chest symptoms settle in two to three weeks but a few develop chronic pulmonary disease. Of the small minority who develop disseminated disease less than a half have chronic meningitis which comes on weeks or months, and sometimes more than a year later. Headache is often a prominent feature, raised ICP develops due to meningeal fibrosis, convulsions and focal signs appear. There are widespread intracranial microgranulomas which sometimes coalesce to form a space occupying granuloma. Untreated, it leads to death within a couple of years. Diagnosis can be made by CSF examination for complement fixing antibodies which are present in over 70 per cent of patients at the time of diagnosis, and become rapidly positive in the remainder.

Histoplasmosis

This is caused by *Histoplasma capsulatum*, is found world-wide and is endemic in the central United States. Fungal hyphae are inhaled and set up a self limiting pneumonitis. Both the immune competent and the immune suppressed are infected. Disseminated disease is rare, affects the normal and the immune compromised and carries a high mortality rate. Chronic meningitis and granuloma formation occur in about 20 per cent of these. Specific antibodies can be found in CSF by radioimmunassay and by complement fixation.

Paracoccidioidomycosis

This occurs in otherwise normal patients and is caused by inhalation of the spores of *Paracoccidioides brasiliensis*, found in the soil of Central and South America. This produces a granulomatous alveolitis and rarely, dissemination to the CNS takes place to cause chronic granulomatous meningitis.

Primary amoebic meningoencephalitis

This occurs when humans are infected by the parasites *Naegleria fowleri* or *Acanthamoeba*. The former causes acute purulent meningitis and the latter, a form of meningitis with focal granulomatous encephalitis. *Naegleria* are found in warm, stagnant water and soil and humans are infected when they swim in, or play near to still pools. Children and young adults are affected, boys much more than girls, and the immune system is intact. The onset is acute and is indistinguishable from acute bacterial meningitis. Progression is rapid with seizures and stupor supervening, followed by death in 3–4 days if the diagnosis is not made. This is difficult because CSF parameters are similar to bacterial meningitis but the Gram stain is negative. If the condition is suspected from the history of exposure to stagnant water, motile, amoeboid trophozoites may be seen in fresh, warm specimens on microscopy if the laboratory is alerted to look for them. Infection due to *Acanthamoeba* is less acute in onset and progression. Meningeal features accompanied by behavioural changes and focal signs progress over weeks and months, culminating in death. Trophozoites are not seen in CSF in this condition which is usually diagnosed after death. The only way to make the diagnosis in life is to identify parasites in biopsy tissue. Almost all cases die of the disease.

Eosinophilic meningitis

This occurs in Pacific regions and has spread to Africa, India, the Caribbean, Australia, and North America, carried there by rats on trading ships. *Angiostrongylus cantonensis* is a nematode which parasitizes the lungs of rats. Larvae infect a range of molluscs and humans are infected by eating uncooked vegetables which have been contaminated by snails. Once ingested, larvae migrate to the brain and set up meningitis – live worms have been recovered from brains. Within a month of ingestion of contaminated food, severe headache, vomiting, neck stiffness, paraesthesiae, and cranial nerve palsies appear. The eye may be involved with retinal haemorrhages and detachments. There may be blood eosinophilia and CSF examination reveals pleocytosis with the majority of cells being eosinophils. No specific treatment is available and steroids have been said to be useful (Pien and Pien 1999). Fortunately, most make a complete recovery within weeks. *Gnathostoma*, a nematode parasite of cats and dogs, can rarely cause a form of eosinophilic meningitis as can neurocysticercosis.

33.2.6 Recurrent meningitis

Meningeal disruption

The commonest cause for recurrent bacterial meningitis is a communication between the sub-arachnoid space containing CSF, and the exterior of the body. In adults, this is almost always due to previous head trauma resulting in a compound skull fracture with communication between the sub-arachnoid space and paranasal sinuses with fractures of the cribriform plate and the skull base, or between sub-arachnoid space and the middle ear. When CSF rhinorrhoea or otorhoea accompanies or precedes meningitis, diagnosis is not difficult although it may be difficult to determine the exact anatomical site of the communication. If there is no fluid leak, diagnosis may be delayed. Often, the head injury has happened so far in the past that its significance has been forgotten, or more rarely, was held to be insignificant. Even if no history of trauma is available, all cases of recurrent bacterial meningitis should be investigated fully to determine if there is a communication. The author recently found a communication from petrous bone to middle ear in a woman with recurrent meningitis who had suffered what was thought to be an insignificant head injury 40 years before and had a fracture which was found only after intricate CT scanning.

In children, head trauma remains a significant cause. The younger the child, the more likely it is that CSF pathways communicate with the outside as a consequence of a congenital abnormality, most often a fistulous connection from the middle ear. All such cases require an ENT review (Drummond *et al.*, 1999). Persisting fistulous tracts from meningocoeles are another potential source. In those patients in whom no physical communication with the exterior can be demonstrated, it is necessary to screen for congenital immunological defects.

The clinical features of meningitis in those cases are similar to those described above. The most common organism is *Strep. pneumoniae* which is present in about 75 per cent of all cases. *Haemophilus* and Gram negative bacilli have also been described and in practise almost any organism may be introduced to the neauraxis. There is some value in prescribing prophylactic penicillin whilst investigations are being undertaken to identify the communication. In those patients in whom an immune deficit is identified, correction of the deficit where possible, is the treatment of choice, and this may be accompanied by immunization against common pathogens.

Mollaret's meningitis

Recurrent episodes of an acute, aseptic, and predominantly lymphocytic, variety of meningitis were described by Mollaret. Lasting for up to a week at a time with spontaneous resolution, they would recur weeks or months later. For many years the aetiology has remained speculative and no infectious agent was identified. In the past decade an association with HSV type 2 and less commonly, type 1, infection has been established by demonstration of HSV DNA in CSF by PCR. There is often no history of herpetic infection elsewhere. It may be that treatment with acyclovir will prove to be useful.

Drugs

Recurrent aseptic meningitis has been described following exposure to a number of drugs including non-steroidal anti-inflammatory analgesics, antibiotics including penicillin, immune globulin, OKT3 monoclonal antibody, cytosine arabinose, and azathioprine. This list is not exhaustive and is being added to continually. Clinical features are similar to acute pyogenic meningitis and some may have a rash. CSF examination reveals a polymorphonuclear response with no organisms. Diagnosis is historical and it is essential to obtain a full and exhaustive drug history in all cases of recurrent meningitis. Demonstration that a particular drug is the cause can be confirmed by re-challenge, but this is not without hazard to the patient.

Recurring episodes of aseptic meningitis may occur in association with chronic systemic granulomatous and vasculitic diseases, such as sarcoidosis, systemic lupus erythematosis, Behçet's syndrome, cerebral vasculitides, meningeal metastatic disease, and sometimes brain tumours, usually cystic, that may disgorge their contents into the CSF of the ventricles or subarachnoid space and induce a chemical meningitis. Epidermoid cysts, craniopharyngiomas, and gliomas have been reported to cause this syndrome. Diagnosis is by identification of the underlying disease and it is necessary to exclude coincidental infection because many of these conditions may be associated with a degree of immune suppression.

33.2.7 Meningitis and neurosurgery

Infection rates following 'clean' neurosurgical procedures, that is elective procedures for non-infective conditions, are low, but not negligible. The average rate is in the order of 3–4 per cent and higher and lower rates are quoted, influenced by the type of procedure which is carried out and whether foreign material such as shunts or grafts have been introduced. Prophylactic antibiotics have been tried and opinion is divided over their routine use. All agree that the source of infection is in the operating theatre itself (Ingham *et al.*, 1991). It may be mundane – in the author's institution an outbreak of *Pseudomonas* meningitis was traced to a contaminated brush used to lather the scalp prior to shaving. Re-operations, deep craniotomies and prolonged procedures add to the risk. Traumatic cases and those penetrating paranasal sinuses carry the highest rates. Wound infections are caused by *Staph. aureus* spp. in the main and may progress to cause meningitis. Most cases of neurosurgical meningitis are due to Gram-negative bacilli – *Klebsiella pneumoniae*, *Acinetobacter* spp., and *E. coli*. It may be difficult to diagnose pyogenic meningitis at the onset because the evolution of the syndrome is insidious, post-operative patients often have headache and signs of meningeal irritation and pyrexia caused by blood in the subarachnoid space. Prolonged fever and reduced conscious level should suggest an infective cause and lead to CSF examination.

Shunt infection is common as is infection of subcutaneous reservoirs. Coagulase negative staphylococci are common pathogens, followed by *Staph. aureus* and gram-negative bacilli. Infection takes the form of non-specific malaise, pyrexia, lethargy, nausea, and vomiting and may be accompanied by septicaemia. Meningitis develops in a minority. Often it is necessary to remove the shunt or reservoir before eradication of the infection is achieved.

33.3 Investigation of meningitis

33.3.1 Prompt treatment

The diagnosis of meningitis must be immediately considered in any patient with fever, malaise, headache, neck stiffness, and irritability and it must be remembered that as many as 20 per cent of cases will not exhibit these classical signs. Together with the level of consciousness of the patient on admission, delay in starting antibiotic treatment is the most important adverse feature to affect the clinical outcome. In the past, it was considered of paramount importance to identify the infecting organism before administering antibiotics. Delay would occur when imaging of the cranial contents was undertaken in an effort to estimate whether ICP was raised and whether it was safe to carry out CSF examination by lumbar puncture. The best course of action now is to assume that all cases of suspected meningitis have raised ICP and to approach them accordingly. Antibiotics should be administered on a best guess basis while other tests and imaging are being carried out. Anxiety that prior antibiotic administration would increase the proportion of culture negative cases and lead to diagnostic and perhaps therapeutic confusion has not been justified, and the improvement in outcome confirms that the immediate treatment option is the best. Newer techniques such as PCR and immunoblotting permit detection of minute quantities of infecting material and confirmation of the organism even after antibiotics have been used – in many cases of established meningitis, abnormalities of the CSF and visible organisms in CSF will persist for more than 24 hours.

33.3.2 Blood cultures

In all cases, cultures should be taken from blood and any detected locus of infection. In more than half of cases of bacterial meningitis, the organism can be cultured from the blood. Abnormalities of the full blood count and a raised sedimentation rate are commonly found, indicate inflammation, and are seldom of diagnostic use. If the patient is shocked or purpuric, disseminated intravascular coagulation should be suspected and platelet count and coagulation studies should be performed. All patients should have their blood electrolytes monitored to detect the syndrome of inappropriate secretion of antidiuretic hormone.

33.3.3 Cerebrospinal fluid (CSF) examination

CSF by lumbar puncture remains the gold standard by which meningitis is diagnosed. However, to carry out a lumbar puncture in the presence of raised ICP is hazardous and potentially lethal and not a few deaths of meningitis patients have been caused by injudicious LP causing tonsillar herniation through foramen magnum and uncal herniation through the tentorial hiatus (Horwitz *et al.*, 1980). It can be difficult to decide when it is safe to carry out a lumbar puncture and experience and luck are necessary. Such a decision should not be left to the most junior member of the team – discussion with the consultant in charge is appropriate. If there are focal neurological signs, if the conscious level is depressed, if neck stiffness is marked (tonsillar herniation through foramen magnum makes the neck exceedingly stiff), if there is papilloedema or palsies of the sixth or third cranial nerve, it is best to defer lumbar puncture and continue treatment on a best guess basis. If there is a bleeding diathesis or coagulation defect these should be corrected. CSF should be sent to the laboratory to be examined immediately.

CSF is always abnormal in cases of meningitis. The pressure is almost always raised, even when the features listed above are absent. In bacterial meningitis and in the more chronic meningitides, the fluid is cloudy and may be discoloured. In viral meningitis it may be clear or slightly cloudy. The cell count of white blood cells, normally less than 5 per cu.mm, is increased in all forms of meningitis. In viral infections, in the first day or two, polymorphonuclear predominance may be seen, later lymphocytes take over. The cell count seldom rises over 100 per cu.mm. In most bacterial infections polymorphs predominate and the count can rise to the thousands. In more chronic bacterial infection such as TB, lymphocytes are the major cell type. Exceptions occur, and if organisms are not seen, treatment should be given according to the likely clinical diagnosis.

With bacterial meningitis it should be possible to identify the organism on microscopy after Gram staining in over 70 per cent of cases. This depends upon the amount of CSF examined, the burden of infection, how often the examination is carried and the experience of the observer. If no organisms are seen at first, there is value in carrying out a further examination 12 hours later. In 80 per cent of cases, it should be possible to culture bacteria from CSF. If fastidious or unusual pathogens are suspected, discussion of the clinical circumstances with the microbiologist will alert him to the need for special stains or culture techniques.

CSF glucose

At the same time as CSF is being obtained, venous blood should be drawn and sent for glucose level estimation. CSF glucose level is usually over 45 mg per dl. If the ratio of glucose in CSF: blood is less than 0.3 it is abnormal and is found in 75 per cent of patients with bacterial meningitis. Very low levels of CSF glucose are found with overwhelming infection, tuberculous, fungal and malignant meningitis. Values are usually normal with viral infections.

CSF protein

Levels are elevated in cases of meningitis and this reflects disruption of the blood brain barrier. Levels above 45 mg per dl in lumbar CSF are considered abnormal, and levels may be found one hundred fold or more, higher. This seldom has diagnostic significance.

Over the years, many tests have been devised with the purpose of providing a means to differentiate bacterial from viral and other forms of meningitis. Unfortunately, none has consistently been accurate and specific (Anderson 1984) and few laboratories employ them now. Recent advances in immunological techniques including western and southern blotting, and ELISA have greatly increased sensitivity to detect antibody and antigen in CSF and PCR has been applied to detect viral and bacterial nucleic acid fragments. These promise greater ease of diagnosis in future once the limits of sensitivity and specificity and cross contamination have been determined (DeBiasi and Tyler 1999). At present, the availability of such tests varies from laboratory to laboratory. The detection of cytokines such as tumour necrosis factors and interleukins as an indicator of the degree of the inflammatory response in CSF is under investigation. (Tauber and Moser 1999)

33.3.4 Imaging

Imaging of the cranial contents should be carried out in cases of meningitis if there are focal signs and if seriously raised intracranial pressure is suspected. It is also useful when there has been failure to respond to medical treatment or when complications are suspected. Expert neuroradiological interpretation should always be obtained if it is available because many of the changes are subtle and require experience to detect. Magnetic resonance imaging shows brain structure and white/grey matter differentiation better than CT and it is generally more sensitive. However, the time taken to acquire images is longer with MR, the patient must lie still within a claustrophobic metal tube and it is difficult to maintain an airway in an ill patient in a MR scanner. For these reasons, most patients with meningitis are scanned with CT (Fig. 33.2).

In the early stages of meningitis, no changes may be evident on the scans, which are normal. Meningeal enhancement over the cerebral cortex and at the base of the brain indicates

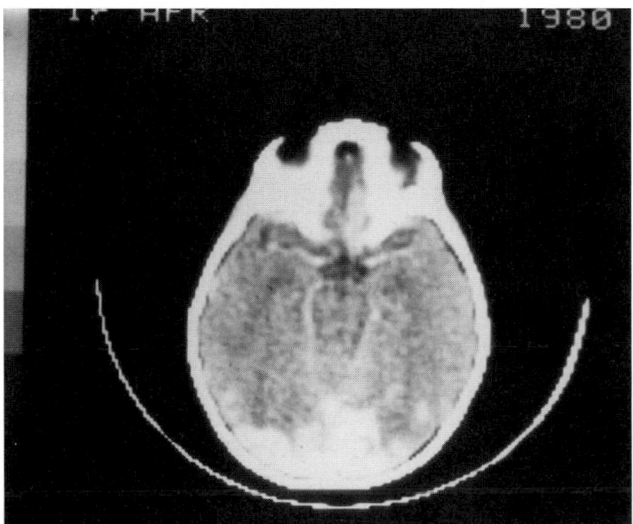

Fig. 33.2. Contrast-enhanced CT brain scan of a child with *Haemophilus* meningitis who has bilateral occipital venous infarcts.

inflammatory change. This is more evident following contrast injection. In severe cases, there may be enhancement of the ependymal lining of the ventricles. On MR scans, meningeal changes are more sensitive and enhancement may be more difficult to interpret. Small ventricles and effacement of sulci imply brain swelling and raised ICP. Hydrocephalus may result from CSF malabsorption caused by basal meningeal adhesions. Focal space occupation may point to abscess formation or cerebral infarction from arteritis or cerebral phlebitis. Subdural collections may complicate *Haemophilus* infection. Attention should be focused on the structures of the paranasal sinuses including the ethmoids and the sphenoidal sinus, mastoids and the integrity of the bone of the skull to detect any fractures or focus of infection. (Cabral *et al.*, 1987; Sze and Zimmermann 1988)

33.4 Treatment of meningitis

Once the diagnosis of meningitis has been considered, treatment regimes can be planned at the same time as diagnostic tests are taking place. In the case of viral and the more chronic forms of meningitis, there is not quite the same urgency required to choose antibiotics or chemotherapeutic agents. Their selection can often be made on a more precise basis as the results of investigations become available. When acute pyogenic meningitis is suspected, antibiotic choices must be made immediately and often on a best guess basis appropriate to the likely pathogen in the clinical circumstances, before bacteriological or serological confirmation is available. In all forms of meningitis, raised intracranial pressure consequent upon inflammatory changes inside the head, requires treatment. Attempts to modify the inflammatory process may aid reduction of ICP. Brain perfusion and nourishment must be maintained and regimes to achieve this are being developed.

33.4.1 Management of pressure and perfusion

The patient ill with meningitis is in a potentially volatile state when changes in circulation, ventilation and conscious level may occur at any time. Multi-system monitoring is necessary and this is best carried out in an intensive care unit. If there is a changing neurological deficit or deterioration in conscious level, intensive care is mandatory.

Several anti-inflammatory agents which act at different stages, including non-steroidal anti-inflammatories, pentoxifylline, naloxone, and monoclonal antibodies targeted against human β integrin, have been evaluated to determine if they will influence the changes induced by the breakdown of bacterial cell walls. To date, the only preparation which has provided a clinical effect has been dexamethasone (Townsend and Scheld 1993). Present evidence suggests that it is effective in diminishing morbidity in bacterial meningitis in children (McIntyre *et al.*, 1997) and results for adults are inconclusive (Thomas *et al.*, 1999). Anxieties have been expressed that steroid effects may be deleterious if the infecting organism is a pneumococcus with penicillin resistance. There does not seem to be any adverse effect on viral meningitis. Dexamethasone should be administered intravenously before antibiotics are given, and a dosage of 0.15 mg/kg body weight 6 hourly for no more than 4 days is suggested. Gastrointestinal bleeding is a real hazard and should be monitored for carefully. There is no place for prophylactic anticoagulation in the treatment of bacterial meningitis.

Intracranial pressure

This rises maximally in the first 48 hours and if there is clinical relapse. Deterioration in conscious level is a pointer to rising intracranial pressure. The aim in the management of raised ICP is to prevent secondary brain ischaemia by maintenance of cerebral perfusion. Autoregulation permits cerebral blood flow to stay fairly constant between a wide range of cerebral perfusion pressures. pO_2, pCO_2 and metabolic rate also have an effect on cerebral blood flow. As ICP rises, the perfusion pressure can be maintained by raising arterial pressure with vasopressor amines. Reduction of ICP achieves the same goal and is the preferred option. This can be done by instituting hyperventilation which causes cerebral blood flow to diminish by lessening vascular resistance. Raising the patient's head to at least an angle of 30 degrees improves venous drainage from the brain. Mannitol shrinks the brain temporarily by causing an osmotic flow from oedematous cerebral tissue into the blood. Dexamethasone is not usually effective in treating the cytotoxic form of oedema found with meningitis but is usually administered in a deteriorating situation. If ICP remains out of control despite these measures, barbiturate narcosis using a short acting preparation may be useful. ICP monitoring should be instituted before the neurological status and conscious level deteriorate sufficiently to cause a Glasgow coma score of 8 or less, or when focal signs appear. The preferred method is by the insertion of a ventricular catheter – hydrocephalus, which occurs in small proportion of cases, can be drained and intracranial pressure can be measured directly. Intracerebral haemorrhage and secondary infection are potential complications and it is prudent to give prophylactic antibiotics to cover Gram positive infection during the placement of the shunt. Measures to reduce ICP should be taken if recordings exceed 15 mmHg and certainly before they reach 20 mmHg. If pressure rises further, autoregulation will fail and brain damage will occur. (Pickard and Czosnyka 1993).

Epileptic seizures

These occur in about a third of all children with pyogenic meningitis and a smaller proportion of adults. These should be managed aggressively to prevent the development of status epilepticus. There have been no extensive comparisons of antiepileptic drugs in such circumstances. Custom, practice, and results favour phenytoin, reinforced by one of the shorter-acting intravenous preparations, if necessary. Drug management for the longer term can be reviewed once recovery from meningitis has taken place.

Fluid balance, electrolytes and osmolarity

These must be closely monitored, particularly in children who readily develop the syndrome of inappropriate secretion of antidiuretic hormone. Judicious restriction of fluid administration is appropriate to allow sodium levels to rise, and this must be done very carefully because hypovolaemia may exacerbate poor cerebral perfusion.

33.4.2 Antibiotics, antiviral agents, and specific treatments

In order to achieve bactericidal levels of antibiotics in CSF, concentrations of drugs must be in the order of 10–20 times higher than the minimal bactericidal concentration *in vitro* for the organism in question. Theoretically, the antibiotic should be lipid soluble to ease transfer across the blood brain barrier (BBB) but this does not pose practical problems because inflammation of the meninges breaks down the BBB and permits drugs to penetrate to CSF. It should be active within purulent and acidic CSF and the rate at which it is metabolized and cleared from CSF influences the dose and frequency of administration. There is no place for the administration of antibiotics intrathecally. In exceptional circumstances it may be necessary to instil antibiotics intraventricularly via a reservoir and shunt. For cases of bacterial meningitis, antibiotics should always be given intravenously. It is recommended that antibiotic choices are discussed with infectious disease consultants and bacteriologists who will have knowledge of local disease patterns, organism resistance, and nosocomial infection. The development of newer and more powerful antibiotics with a wider spectrum of activity has made the choice of antibiotics easier to make, but patterns of drug resistance change all the time. It is more and more necessary to initiate treatment immediately on an empirical basis, but this must not deter efforts to isolate the causal organism and determine antibiotic sensitivities. When these become available, the treatment regime can be altered as necessary.

Empirical antibiotic treatment for pyogenic meningitis is set out in Table 33.4.

Table 33.4. Empirical antibiotic treatment for pyogenic meningitis

Children and young adults	3rd generation cephalosporin
Adults	3rd generation cephalosporin
Elderly and immune compromised	3rd generation cephalosporin and ampicillin
Neurosurgery and trauma	3rd generation cephalosporin and nafcillin, flucloxacillin, or oxacillin
No history available	3rd generation cephalosporin, acyclovir, and metronidazole

Consider tuberculous meningitis in all cases

Penicillin

When organisms that are known to be sensitive to penicillin are present, penicillin remains the drug of choice. There is some evidence that prognosis can be improved if the practitioner who sees the child with meningitis at home gives an injection of penicillin before sending the patient to hospital (provided that there are no contraindications to penicillin). Because an increasing number of *Haemophilus* spp. are resistant to ampicillin and chloramphenicol, a third generation cephalosporin (ceftriaxone, cefotaxime or ceftizoxime) is preferred. Meningococci remain sensitive to penicillin in the vast majority of cases in Britain but resistant strains are being reported and some chloramphenicol resistant strains are being recognized. Increasingly, pneumococci are resistant to penicillin, approximately 6.5 per cent in Britain, and 25 per cent and higher in the United States and Europe. Resistance to cephalosporin is not yet a problem in Britain. If the patient has travelled from an area where drug resistance to any of these pathogens has been recorded, vancomycin or erythromycin may be used in addition to a third generation cephalosporin (Begg *et al.*, 1999).

The immune compromised and elderly

Listeria is a significant pathogen and ampicillin should be added to the regime. Following neurosurgery or head trauma, an antibiotic against Gram negative bacilli is necessary and it is prudent to cover *Staph. aureus*. The combination of a third generation cephalosporin with a flucloxacillin is usually adequate. Vancomycin is preferred if there is penicillin allergy and for MRSA. Cephalosporins are now considered to be more effective than aminoglycosides for the treatment of Gram negative bacillary meningitis and should be used. If *Psudomonas aeruginosa* is the cause, ceftazidime should be combined with an aminoglycoside.

    Shunt associated meningitis is treated with vancomycin to counter coagulase-negative *Staphylococci*. It is sometimes necessary to combine this with rifampicin. Removal of the shunt is usually needed to eradicate the infection. If meningitis is due to anaerobic organisms, metronidazole should be combined with penicillin. Dosage regimes, potential drug interactions and adverse effects are set out in several textbooks of pharmacology and in the British National Formulary, which is up-dated every 6 months and to which the reader is referred.

Newer antibiotics

Newer antibiotics have been developed with activity against organisms which cause meningitis. The reported number of cases in which they have been used to treat pyogenic meningitis is too small to date to permit recommendations about their use to be made. The length of time for which treatment should be given is variable, dependent upon the clinical response of the patient, and the nature of the infecting organism and the experience of the physician in charge. There are few objective scientific criteria on which to base the decision. On average, meningococcal infections require at least five days of parenteral antibiotics, *H. influenzae* 10 days and other forms, a minimum of 14 days. If the clinical response is not good, a review of the diagnosis and treatment is called for, together with repeat scanning to demonstrate complications such as abscess formation or sub-dural collection, and repeat CSF examination.

Tuberculous meningitis treatment

This is always started on an empirical basis because it takes several weeks to culture the organism and to determine antibiotic sensitivities. It is recommended that a specialist in tuberculosis is asked to advise about an appropriate drug regime because they will have knowledge of local sensitivity patterns and whether it is likely that drug resistant organisms have been imported. Multiple drug regimes are necessary to prevent the emergence of drug resistant strains. Prolonged follow up is needed to ensure compliance – failure to take the drugs is one of the commonest causes of treatment failure.. Contacts need to be traced and public health authorities notified – a statutory requirement in Britain. This is best done by a team familiar with the management of TB. Most regimes combine four or even five drugs in the beginning, and can be modified later if sensitivities become available. Usually rifampicin, pyrazinamide, isoniazid, and ethambutol are combined, with streptomycin added if the likelihood of drug resistance is high. Signs of clinical improvement are expected within a fortnight or so. Second line drugs are reserved for multi-drug resistant bacilli, or cases that have developed unacceptable toxic effects to one or more of the first line drugs. These drugs include capreomycin, cycloserine, para-aminosalicylic acid (PAS), ethionamide, kanamycin and amikacin and fluoroquinolones. All anti-TB drugs are potentially toxic and have a high incidence of side effects, which underscores the necessity for strict supervision by a team experienced in the management of TB. The length of time for which treatment should be given is determined by the clinical response. Short regimes of six months have been reported to be effective if sensitivities are known and include rifampicin and isoniazid. Longer treatment is usually necessary for a year or two years or longer if TB is associated with AIDS (Joint Tuberculosis Committee of the British Thoracic Society 1998). There is no good evidence that intrathecal steroids are of benefit in preventing adhesions and routine use of oral steroids has produced mixed results.

Viral meningitis

Viral meningitis does not require specific treatment because in the vast majority it is a benign self-limiting condition. This is fortuitous since none of the recognized anti-viral drugs is effective against the common causes of the aseptic meningitis syndrome. Meningitis caused by HSV might be expected to respond to acyclovir but this is seldom required because meningitis due to HSV is unusual, and is a benign self-limiting syndrome which does not need specific treatment. Symptomatic treatment to relieve headache should be given, by injection if needed and the patient and relatives should be reassured that the condition is benign and recovery will take place. It is increasingly difficult to allay public anxiety about meningitis as a consequence of hysterical reporting by the media. Relatives often put pressure on medical staff to administer antibiotics which are not necessary. Such requests can usually be deflected by discussion and explanation – if not, the author is prepared to give a short course of penicillin if there are no contraindications. It is prudent to review such patients once as an outpatient to allay anxieties about 'brain damage' from meningitis, if necessary by arranging a 'therapeutic' CT scan or EEG.

Fungal forms of meningitis

These can be treated now. Amphotercin B remains the standard therapy for most invasive mycoses but it is toxic. New lipid formulations have been developed which have fewer and less severe side effects, particularly nephrotoxicity. Amphotercin B can be used to treat meningitis due to candida, cryptococcosis, blastomycosis, histoplasmosis, coccidioidomycosis and para-coccidioidomycosis and aspergillosis. The pyrimidine drug, 5-fluorocytosine, has a limited spectrum and is toxic. Its use is limited to treatment of candida and cryptococcal meningitis in combination with amphotercin B. Of the azole antifungal drugs, miconazole and ketoconazole have been replaced by fluconazole and itraconazole. They are effective against the fungi listed above. One drawback is that they frequently interreact adversely with other drugs. Very extensive practice guidelines which include indications, dosage schedules, and adverse reactions have been issued by the Infectious Diseases Society of America in *Clinical Infectious Diseases* (2000) volume 30.

33.4.3 Management of family, contacts, and media

Public awareness of meningitis has increased exponentially, largely due to the media, much of it hysterical and ill-informed. A diagnosis of 'meningitis' induces alarm and it is important to establish sympathetic communication with the patient and relatives. Realistic reassurance about the likely course of the disease should be given and treatment regimes and the rationale for their use should be explained. Usually this is best done by a senior medical member of the team who should be prepared to make themselves available out of normal working hours. Relatives are often bewildered by the workings of an intensive care unit and they find it useful to have an explanation of what all the tubes and monitors are for. If surgical intervention such as a tracheostomy or burr holes is likely, then the procedures should be explained to the relations beforehand. Permission should be sought from the patient and relatives to discuss the illness with school, college, or work colleagues who will soon learn of the diagnosis and become alarmed that they may contract the disease. It should be anticipated that a diagnosis of meningitis will be communicated to the media, particularly if the patient is a child or college student and co-operation with media requests for information and interviews is advisable. This is best done by a senior member of the medical staff, not by an administrator or manager. In a unit that handles many such cases it is useful to have such a spokesperson

coached in media matters. A sympathetic interview can often allay public fears, a hostile one may compound them.

Once the organism has been identified, community and public health physicians can be notified. For certain infections, this is required by statute. If children or young adults in an institution are involved it is prudent to discuss the case with the local medical officer, no matter which organism is involved. If meningitis is caused by the meningococcus, 'kissing contacts', household contacts and school and college classmates need to be identified and offered prophylaxis with rifampicin. Infant and child contacts of *Haemophilus* infection may need to be contacted similarly and their immunization status ascertained – they can also be given prophylactic rifampicin. Such decisions and follow-up are best carried out by the MOH.

33.5 Outcome and sequelae

The vast majority of cases of viral meningitis make a complete recovery and have no further problem. Those cases caused by HIV infection adopt the prognosis of AIDS. The mortality rate for pyogenic meningitis varies according to organism, age, underlying predisposing factor, and clinical status when treatment began. Mortality is highest in infants and the elderly and may exceed 50 per cent. Rates of 5–10 per cent are found with meningococcal and *Haemophilus* meningitis. The infection rates for the latter have dropped so dramatically following immunization programmes that these figures may no longer apply. Pneumococcal meningitis has a higher mortality of between 10–30 per cent depending on any predisposing factors. *Listeria* varies from 9 per cent with no immune defect to 60 per cent or more with severe immune suppression. With TB meningitis, rates below 15 per cent are to be expected unless there is immune suppression. Fungal meningitis carries higher rates dependant upon the pathogen and underlying condition, and in some forms, treatment may have to be continued for life. With all forms of meningitis, if the patient is unconscious when treatment is started, 66 per cent mortality is to be expected.

Figures for the occurrence of complications during meningitis and the development of sequelae are difficult to interpret because reports have concentrated on a particular organism or a specific age group. Complications of pyogenic meningitis which are well recognized are epilepsy, brain infarction from basal arteritis or cerebral phlebitis, subdural collections, hydrocephalus due to basal adhesions, cranial nerve palsies, and less commonly, brain abscess. Systemic complications include septic shock, disseminated intravascular coagulation, and respiratory distress syndrome. Sequelae reflect complications and can be found in 10–20 per cent of survivors. Hearing loss, spasticity, blindness, behavioural disturbance, and epilepsy are the most common. Hydrocephalus occurs in less than 5 per cent and can become evident in later years as CSF absorption and circulation are disrupted as meningeal adhesions mature (Figure 33.3). Rare sequelae include the development of syringomyelia (Figure 33.4).

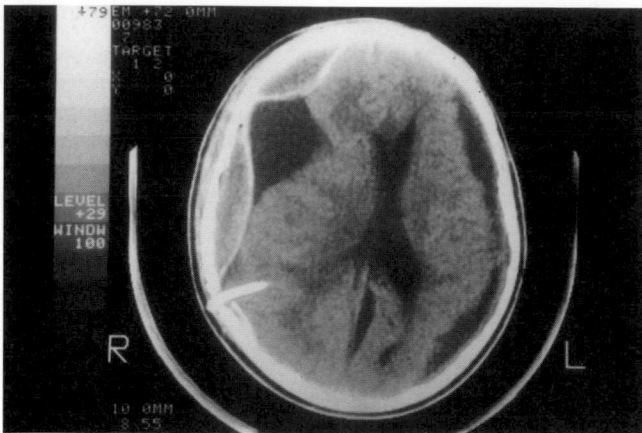

Fig. 33.3. Complications of sequelae. CT brain scan of a girl who suffered from pyogenic meningitis in early childhood and several years later became symptomatic from communicating hydrocephalus. Insertion of a ventricular shunt resulted in pressure reduction which led to the development of subdural and extradural haematomas.

33.6 Rehabilitation

Little has been written of the rehabilitation of patients who have had meningitis and suffered a neurological deficit. Often the deficit is subtle and may go unrecognized. Because deafness is such a common sequel it is important that all children who have had bacterial meningitis should have formal audiological assessment and if a deficit is noted, appropriate referral to paediatric, ENT, and educational services should be made. Behavioural and cognitive defects are common. If developmental milestones are delayed, or nursery and school performance lags behind that of peers or siblings, a full educational and neuropsychological appraisal should be carried out and an indi-

vidual development programme prepared. Epilepsy should be treated aggressively with appropriate AEDS with due attention to interaction with behavioural problems. Spasticity may be countered with antispastic medication including botulinus toxin, and physiotherapy. It is important to recognize that sequelae such as hydrocephalus or epilepsy may appear many years after apparently successful rehabilitation from meningitis.

33.7 Prevention

Immunization against the three main meningitic pathogens, *Haemophilus influenzae*, *Neisseria meningitidis*, and *Streptococcus pneumoniae*, is now possible. Where it has been introduced Hib vaccine has all but eliminated *Haemophilus* meningitis. Different vaccines have been developed. Current recommendations are to use a conjugate vaccine and offer it to all children and to adults with an increased risk of infection. Three doses are given at 2, 3 , and 4 months of age. A meningococcal polysaccharide vaccine is available against groups A and C and W135 and Y. Group B polysaccharide vaccines are poorly immunogenic and are not available for routine use. Conjugate vaccines are being developed and are under trial. A new group C conjugate vaccine has recently been introduced and it is intended that high risk populations will be targeted – children under 18 years of age and first year college and university students. Multivalent polysaccharide vaccine should be offered to asplenic patients and to those who are travelling to high risk areas such as northern regions of the Indian sub-continent, and sub-Saharan Africa. Vaccination is obligatory for Muslim pilgrims travelling to Saudi Arabia during Hajj. Advice should be obtained from infectious disease physicians on procedure for immunization against groups A and C during local outbreaks.

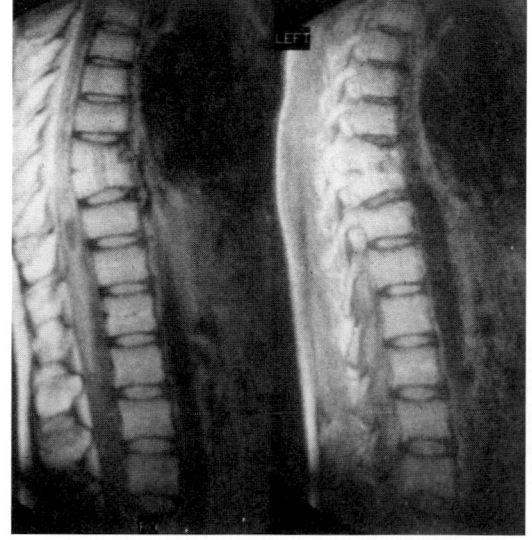

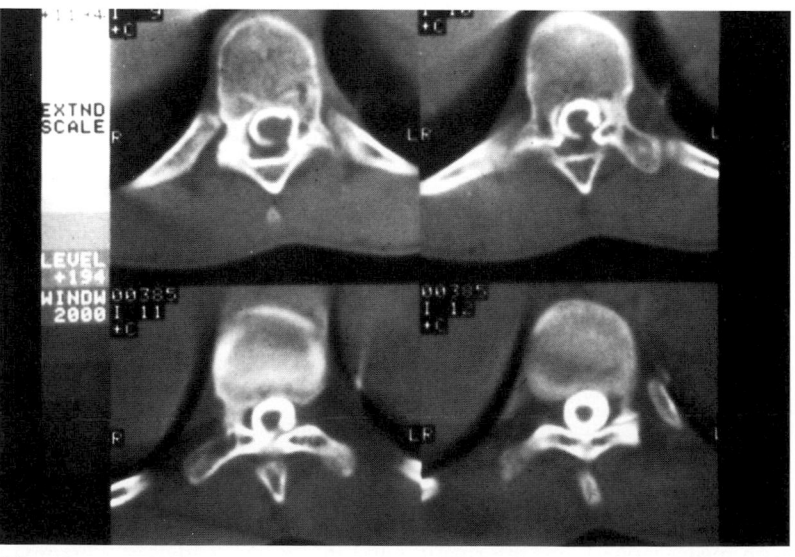

(A)   (B)

Fig. 33.4. Sagittal (a) and transverse (b) sections of a magnetic resonance scan of the thoracic spine showing a syrinx which has developed 10 years after recovery from TB meningitis. Bony involvement of adjacent vertebral bodies is evident. CSF dynamics were deranged at the foramen magnum due to meningeal adhesions.

A multivalent polysaccharide pneumococcal vaccine has been developed and should be offered to vulnerable populations. This includes those with chronic heart, lung, kidney or liver disease, asplenia, sickle cell disease, diabetes mellitus and immune deficiency. A conjugate vaccine will be available soon.

BCG should be given to infants as soon after birth as possible in areas with a high incidence of TB, otherwise to all individuals between the ages of 10 and 13.

References

Anderson, M. (1984). Bacterial meningitis. In: *Recent Advances in Clinical Neurology 4* (ed. G. H. Glaser and W. B. Matthews), pp. 87–121. Churchill Livingston, Edinburgh.

Aoun, M., and Klastersky, J. (1999). Infection in the immunodeficient patient. In *Clinical infectious diseases: a practical approach.* (eds. R. K. Root, F. Waldvogel, L. Corey, and W. E. Stamm), pp. 809–20. Oxford University Press, New York.

Ashwal, S., Tomasi, L., Schneider, S. *et al.* (1992). Bacterial meningitis in children: pathophysioogy and treatment. *Neurology* **42**, 739–48.

Begg, N., Cartwright, K. A., Cohen, J. *et al.* (1999). Consensus statement on diagnosis, investigation, treatment and prevention of acute bacterial meningitis in immunocompetent adults. British Infection Society Working Party. *J. Infect.*, **39**, 1–15.

Cabral, D. A., Flodmark, O., Farrell, K. *et al.* (1987). Prospective study of computed tomography in acute bacterial meningitis. *J. Pediatr.*, **111**, 201–5.

Carpenter, R. R., and Petersdorf R. G. (1962). The clinical spectrum of bacterial meningitis. *Am. J. Med.*, **33**, 262–75.

DeBiasi, R. L., and Tyler, K. L. (1999). Polymerase chain reaction in the diagnosis and management of central nervous system infections. *Arch. Neurol.*, **56**, 1215–19.

Dodge, P. R., and Swartz, M. N. (1965). Bacterial meningitis – A review of selected aspects II: special neurologic problems, post meningitic complications and clinicopathological correlations. *N. Engl. J. Med.*, **272**, 954–1010.

Drummond, D. S., de Jong, A. L., Giannoni, C. *et al.* (1999). Recurrent meningitis in the pediatric patient – the otolaryngologist's role. *Int. J. Pediatr Otorhinolaryngol.*, **48**, 199–208.

Dunne, D. W., and Quagliarello, V. (1993). Group B Streptococcal meningitis in adults. *Medicine* **27**, 1–10.

Durand, M. L., Calderwood, S. B., Weber, D. J. *et al.* (1993). Acute bacterial meningitis in adults. A review of 493 episodes. *N. Engl. J. Med.*, **328**, 21–8.

Geiseler, P. J., Nelson, K. E., Levin, S. *et al.* (1980). Community acquired purulent meningitis: a review of 1316 cases during the antibiotic era, 1954–1976. *Rev. Infect. Dis.*, **2**, 725–45.

Gordon, M. F., Allon, M., and Coyle, P. K. (1990). Drug induced meningitis. *Neurology* **40**, 163–4.

Ingham, H. R., Sisson, P. R., Mendelow, A. D. *et al.* (1991). Post operative and post traumatic infections. In: *Pyogenic Neurosurgical Infections*, pp. 177–94. Edward Arnold, London.

Joint Tuberculosis Committee of the British Thoracic Society (1998). Chemotherapy and management of tuberculosis in the United Kingdom: recommendations 1998. *Thorax* **53**, 536–48.

McIntyre, P. B., Berkey, C. S., King, S. M. *et al.* (1997). Dexamethasone as adjunctive therapy in bacterial meningitis. A meta-analysis of randomised clinical trials since 1988. *J.A.M.A.*, **278**, 925–31.

Mylonakis, E., Hohmann, E. L., and Calderwood, S. B. (1998). Central nervous system infection with *Listeria monocytogenes*. 33 years experience at a general hospital and review of 776 episodes from the literature. *Medicine (Baltimore)* **77**, 313–36.

Pickard, J. D., and Czosnyka, M. (1993). Management of raised intracranial pressure. *J. Neurol Neurosurg. Psychiat.*, **56**, 845–55.

Pien, F. D., and Pien, B. C. (1999). *Angiostrongylus cantonensis* eosinophilic meningitis. *Int. J. Infect. Dis.*, **3**, 161–3.

Rubin, R. H., and Tolkoff-Rubin, N. E. (1999). infection in the organ transplant recipient. In *Clinical infectious diseases: a practical approach*, pp. 821–28. (eds. R. K. Root, F. Waldvogel, L. Corey, W. E. Stamm). Oxford University Press, New York.

Sawyer, M. H., Holland, D., and Aintablian, N. (1994). Diagnosis of enteroviral central nervous system infection by polymerase chain reaction during a large community outbreak. *Pediatr. Inf. Dis.*, **13**, 177–82.

Simberkoff, M. S., Moldover, N. H., and Ranal, J. (1980). Absence of detectable bacterial and opsonic activities in normal and infected cerebrospinal fluids: a regional host defense deficiency. *J. Lab. Clin. Med.*, **95**, 362–72.

Slutsker, L., Castro, K. G., Ward, J. W. *et al.* (1993). Epidemiology of extra-pulmonary tuberculosis among persons with AIDS in the United States. *Clin. Inf. Dis.*, **16**, 513–18.

Swartz, M. N., and Dodge, P. R. (1965). Bacterial meningitis – a review of selected aspects. I. General clinical features, special problems and unusual meningeal reactions mimicking bacterial meningitis. *N. Engl. J. Med.*, **272**, 725–31.

Syrogiannopoulos, G. A., Nelson, J. D., and McCracken, G. H. (1986). Subdural collections of fluid in acute bacterial meningitis: A review of 136 cases. *Ped. Inf. Dis.*, **5**, 343–52.

Sze, G., and Zimmerman, R. D. (1988). The magnetic resonance imaging of infections and inflammatory diseases. *Radiol Clin North Amer* **26**, 839–59.

Tauber M. G., and Moser, B. (1999). Cytokines and chemokines in meningeal inflammation: biology and clinical implications. *Clin. Infect. Dis.* **28**, 1–11.

Thomas, R., Le Tulzo, Y., Bouget, J. *et al.* (1999). Trial of dexamethasone treatment for severe bacterial meningitis in adults. Adult Meningitis Steroid Group. *Intensive Care Med.*, **25**, 475–80.

Townsend, G. C., and Scheld, W. M. (1993). Adjunctive therapy for bacterial meningitis: Rationale for use, current status and prospects for the future. *Clin. Infect. Dis.*, **17**(**Suppl**), S537–49.

Tunkel, A. R, and Scheld, W. M. (1993). Pathogenesis and pathophysiology of bacterial meningitis. *Clin. Microbiol. Rev.*, **6**, 118–36.

Tureen, J. H., Dworkin, R. L., Kennedy, S. L. *et al.* (1990). Loss of cerebral autoregulation in experimental meningitis in rabbits. *J. Clin. Invest.*, **85**, 577–81.

Wood, M., and Anderson, M. (1988). Chronic meningitis. In *Neurological infections*, p. 174. (ed. J. Walton). W. B. Saunders, London.

CHAPTER 34

Encephalitis and other brain infections

Milne Anderson

34.1 Encephalitis. Introduction and definition

The term 'encephalitis' implies inflammatory change affecting brain parenchyma. By common usage the name refers to inflammation of the brain caused by infection. The anatomical distinction implied by the terms 'meningitis' and 'encephalitis' does not often exist in clinical practice for organisms do not usually recognize the borders between them, with the result that most cases of meningitis have a degree of underlying brain involvement, which may not be evident clinically or may be masked by the signs of meningitis. Likewise, primary encephalitis may have some meningitic features on examination, whence the term 'meningo-encephalitis'. The same organism may cause meningitis in one person and encephalitis in another, for reasons that we do not understand. Some organisms seem to cause only one clinical syndrome. Identical clinical syndromes may be caused by many different and varied pathogens—encephalitis may be caused by viruses, bacteria, fungi, and protozoa. The onset and evolution of the disease is most commonly acute, encephalitic features appearing within hours or at most a day or so, and usually following a non-specific prodrome which has evolved over a few days at the most. Chronic encephalitis has similar clinical features and the picture evolves over weeks or even months—it may reach a plateau or it may relapse and remit to a degree. Most cases of encephalitis are caused by viruses but protozoa such as malaria and toxoplasma and bacteria such as spirochaetes and rickettsiae can all cause acute encephalitis.

34.2 General considerations

Viral infections of the central nervous system (CNS) are usually complications of systemic viral infections, and it is understood that the distinction between neurotropic and non-neurotropic viruses is artificial when it is based on the CNS being primarily or secondarily infected. Commonly what happens is that virus enters the body through the skin as the result of an insect bite, or via the respiratory or gastrointestinal route, replicates at the site of entry and spills into the blood to cause a primary viraemia. Virus then concentrates in various locations such as lymph tissue, liver, and spleen following which secondary viraemia takes place. The mechanisms by which specific viruses target different organs are becoming understood and are beyond the scope of this discussion. Secondary viraemia produces a sufficiently large quantum of virus to force entry to the CNS via the vessels of the choroid plexus, the meninges, and the brain itself. The exact process by which virus broaches endothelium is not fully elucidated but it seems that virus associated with cells, and free virus, can cross. Other viruses such as HSV and rabies reach the brain by spreading from the periphery centripetally to the brain along peripheral or cranial nerve axons and across synapses. The mechanisms by which this takes place are being determined (Cassaday and

Whitley 1997). The physiology, genetic framework, and immunological competence of the host, are major factors in determining the location and the severity of viral disease of the CNS. By good fortune, encephalitis is a rare manifestation of common viral infections, and most patients who have systemic viral infections do not develop neurological signs.

In broad terms based on cause and pathogenesis, viral encephalitis can be grouped into three distinct categories:

◆ *Acute viral encephalitis* is due to direct invasion of the brain by virus, and the signs and symptoms result from this invasion and from the inflammatory change which it induces in the brain parenchyma.

◆ *Post-infectious encephalitis* is characterized pathologically by perivenous demyelination caused by allergic or immune mechanisms relating to viral infection.

◆ *Prion diseases.* The third group includes those encephalitides with a prolonged clinical evolution, known heretofore as the 'slow virus infections' and now as 'prion diseases'. The relationship of 'prions' (small *proteinaceous infective particles*— Prusiner 1982) to viruses is, at least, problematical and discussion of the clinical features of the diseases associated with 'prions' is included here by convention.

Viruses may be categorized in several different ways—according to nucleic acid content, size, sensitivity to lipid solvents, morphology and their method of development in cells, and their genetic relatedness. Viruses can be thought of as foreign entities with genomes of nucleic acid which parasitize a host cell to utilize that cell's synthetic apparatus to transfer the viral genome to other cells. The nucleic acid of each virus has a specific configuration and is either ribonucleic acid (RNA) or deoxoribonucleic acid (DNA) which is entwined in or is surrounded by proteins. This mature viral particle is called a 'virion'. Viruses multiply by adsorbing to a specific cell, penetrating the cell, and shedding the protein coat which surrounds the RNA or DNA: the viral genomic material is transcribed, replicated, and translated to produce proteins to assemble further viruses which are subsequently released as mature virions from the cell. This process varies according to the nature of the virus. A description of the complex interactions between virus and cell is beyond the scope of this text, and the reader is referred to virological treatises.

Each virus species contains only one form of nucleic acid, DNA or RNA. DNA viruses are usually double stranded, while RNA viruses tend to be single stranded, but the distinction is not absolute. DNA virus replication is like that of any cellular organism by transcription to messenger RNA and subsequent translation to polypeptides and protein. RNA virus replication may be direct by the formation of a complimentary RNA strand; or indirect by reverse transcription to a DNA provirus template from which identical RNA strands are then transcribed.

Viruses have been named in a haphazard fashion: some after the disease which they produce, such as rabies; others from the

Table 34.1. Viruses associated with neurological disease

DNA viruses	
Herpes virus	Herpes simplex 1 and 2
	Varicella–zoster
	Cytomegalovirus
	Epstein–Barr
Papovavirus	JC virus-progressive multifocal leucoencephalopathy
RNA viruses	
Retroviruses	HTLV-1—HAM-TSP
	HIV—AIDS
Picornovirus	
Enteroviruses	Poliomyelitis—polio
	Coxsakie
	Echovirus } — aseptic meningitis
Arenavirus	Lymphocytic choriomeningitis
Paramyxovirus	Influenza
	Mumps
Morbillivirus	Measles
Rhabdovirus	
Lyssavirus	Rabies
Bunyavirus	California and LaCrosse encephalitis
	Rift Valley fever
	Congo–Crimean haemorrhagic fever
Retrovirus	
Orbivirus	Colorado tick fever
Togavirus	
Alphavirus	Western, Eastern, and Venezuelan equine encephalitis
Flavivirus	Japanese, Murray Valley, and St Louis encephalitis
	Central European and Russian spring–summer encephalitis
	Louping ill
Rubivirus	Rubella

cytological appearance of infected tissue, hence cytomegalovirus; some from the anatomical site of their localization— enteroviruses; others from their ultrastructural appearance— arenaviruses; and others still from the geographical location where they were first isolated, as in Coxsakie virus. The main virus groups are listed in Table 34.1.

DNA viruses include *parvoviruses*. These are small viruses that do not cause neurological disease. *Papovaviruses* (*papilloma–polyoma–vacuolating* agent) include the *JC virus* of progressive multifocal leucoencephalopathy. *Adenoviruses* were originally isolated from lymphoid tissue, are associated with respiratory infection, and have been a rare cause of meningitis. The *herpes viruses* include the agents of herpes simplex, herpes zoster, cytomegalovirus, and Epstein–Barr virus (EBV). The *poxviruses* include the agent which caused smallpox, and are not of neurological importance.

RNA viruses include *picornoviruses* (*pico* (small)-*RNA-viruses*), which are divided into *enteroviruses* which normally replicate in the gastrointestinal tract, and *rhinoviruses* which cause the common cold and derive from the nose.

Togavirus (from *Toga* = a cloak) is the name thrown over a large group of viruses previously known as *arboviruses* (*ar*thropod-*bor*ne). The togaviruses include the *alphaviruses* which cause St Louis and Japanese encephalitis, and the *rubiviruses* which cause rubella. The *bunyaviruses* comprise the largest group of arboviruses and cause California and LaCrosse encephalitis. The name comes from Bumyamwera in Uganda, where the virus was first isolated. *Arenaviruses* are named after their morphology: on electron microscopy they show dense granules which resemble grains of sand (*arena* = sand), and include the *lymphocytic choriomeningitis virus*. *Coronaviruses* are named after the crown-like fringe that surrounds them, and are of no neurological significance. *Paramyxoviruses* include *mumps* and *measles viruses*. *Rhabdoviruses* are bullet shaped (*rhabdo* = rod) and include the *rabies* virus. *Retroviruses* are so-called because they contain the enzyme *reverse-transcriptase*, and provide the agents which cause AIDS and human T-cell leukaemia virus-I (HTLV-I) associated myelopathy.

The diagnosis of viral infection of the nervous system is seldom clinically difficult, by which is meant that meningitis, encephalitis, herpes zoster, and so on can usually be detected at the bedside. Careful attention to historical details, meticulous clinical examination, including search for current or past insect bites, appreciation of the significance of geographical and seasonal factors, including recent travel abroad to areas that are known to harbour insect vectors, and knowledge of the genetic background of the patient, will help to focus the differential diagnosis. Confirmation that a clinical syndrome is due to a particular virus requires demonstration of the presence of the virus or viral antigen in body tissue or fluids, or a specific antibody response to its presence. Even then there are difficulties: the presence of a virus may be due to a co-existing and unrelated infection, and serum antibody levels may be persistently raised from a previous infection, or the rise may represent an anamnestic generalized immune response to infection. There may also be difficulties with inadequate sensitivity of the tests employed, problems with cross-reactions that impair specificity, and timing the taking of specimens against the progression of the disease. Newer techniques have greatly increased the accuracy of serological diagnosis and now make it possible to detect viral nucleic acid in body fluid and tissue. In perhaps a third of all cases it is not possible to positively identify the pathogen.

Viral identification

Virus culture has not been greatly successful in the diagnosis of CNS infections, in large part due to the difficulty of obtaining specimens of neural tissue. It may be possible to cultivate virus from other sources but this is seldom fruitful. Traditionally, the demonstration of a fourfold rise in antibody titre between an acute phase and a convalescent serum sample to a specific virus has been sufficient to confirm the diagnosis. Numerous techniques that employ immunofluorescence and ELISA have greatly increased the sensitivity of diagnosis and the development of monoclonal antibodies has permitted the detection of viral antigen using these techniques. Rapid results can now be obtained by the use of IgM capture ELISA. Western blotting, in which electrophoretic gels use specific antibodies to trap antigen, is very sensitive. Viral nucleic acid can be detected and characterized by sensitive molecular techniques such as Southern blot hybridization and *in situ* hybridization. The polymerase chain reaction (PCR) is an exquisitely sensitive method to detect nucleic acid, capable of picking out a single viral genome in specimens that contain thousands of cells (Bell 1989; Jeffery and Bangham 1996; Jeffery *et al.* 1997; DeBiasi and Tyler 1999). Its application in Britain has been patchy, in some degree related to cost, but also due to problems of lack of specificity. With refinement, it is likely that the application of this technique may revolutionize diagnosis.

34.3 Clinical features and differential diagnosis of encephalitis

Viral encephalitis occurs throughout the world and is not rare. However, encephalitis is an unusual consequence of common viral infections, and only a small minority of patients with systemic viral infections develop clinical disease of the CNS. A list of the virus groups that cause encephalitis is found in Table 34.2. Encephalitis may be sporadic or epidemic. In the UK and Europe most cases are sporadic and are caused by herpes simplex and other herpes viruses. The success of immunization programmes with measles, mumps, and rubella vaccines (MMR) has seen a dramatic fall in the number of cases of encephalitis due to these viruses. In countries where these programmes are lacking, encephalitis due to these viruses still occurs to a significant degree. In the USA, sporadic and epidemic forms are caused by four main arboviruses, the agents that cause Eastern and Western encephalitis, St Louis and LaCrosse encephalitides. Elsewhere, Japanese B and other viruses are the cause of epidemics. The epidemiology of these different forms of encephalitis is varied and is discussed under the individual pathogens.

Table 34.2. Viral causes of encephalitis

Herpes simplex
Varicella–zoster
Cytomegalovirus
Epstein–Barr virus
Human herpes virus 6
B herpes virus
Mumps
Measles
Rabies
HIV
Arboviruses
JC virus

34.3.1 **Clinical features**

Most of the clinical features of encephalitis are common to all varieties. Some have specific features that are described later. There is often a prodrome of several days non-specific illness with fever, malaise, fatigue, and myalgia. With the onset of encephalitis the patient usually has signs of meningitis as well—headache, fever, and neck stiffness. Encephalitis is implied by signs of mental change: disorientation, behavioural and speech disturbance, and alteration of consciousness which may range from lethargy and drowsiness to deep coma. Epileptic seizures, generalized or focal, are common and focal neurological signs may appear: hemiparesis, cerebellar upset, sensory loss, spasticity, hallucinations, speech disturbance and other signs of parietal dysfunction, and memory upset. Signs may occur in other organ systems which may point to causal virus—for instance skin rashes which may be caused by measles or parotitis or orchitis from mumps.

34.3.2 **Differential diagnosis**

It will be readily acknowledged that such abnormalities occur in many other neurological conditions. Other non-viral forms of encephalitis have identical features. Meningitis of any severity, whether due to viral or other infectious agents, will affect mentation as it develops into meningo-encephalitis. Acute disseminated encephalomyelitis (Section 29.3.1) and even some of the more explosive varieties of multiple sclerosis and other varieties of CNS demyelination may have an encephalitic onset (Section 29.4). Intracranial suppuration, advanced primary or metastatic brain tumours, and raised intracranial pressure (ICP) from whatever cause may lead to coma and to neck stiffness from cerebellar tonsillar herniation. Intracranial haemorrhage can cause a similar picture, including pyrexia. Cerebral vasculitides either primary or secondary to collagen disease, not infrequently present as an encephalopathy and conditions which give rise to cerebral granulomas such as sarcoidosis, may be difficult to differentiate (Chapter 28). Encephalopathies that complicate metabolic disturbances such as kidney and liver failure often occur in the context of generalized infection and may be particularly difficult to diagnose (Chapter 25). Rare encephalopathies such as Wilson's disease (Section 32.8) must not be forgotten. The history may reveal a characteristic epidemiological pattern, the time of year and the disease known to occur in a particular community. Has there been a bite from or exposure to known insect vectors of disease? Enquiry must always be made about recent travel abroad and the activities which were undertaken during that time.

34.4 **Investigation**

34.4.1 **Virology**

When confronted by a possible case of viral encephalitis, investigation must be undertaken urgently to confirm the cause. At present, there is no specific treatment for most forms of viral encephalitis but this should not lessen the effort to establish a diagnosis that is necessary for prognostic and epidemiological reasons as well. As important, is the differentiation of those other conditions which can mimic encephalitis and may be amenable to other forms of treatment such as, for instance, bacterial meningitis and cerebral malaria. Haematological and biochemical tests are seldom of diagnostic help and are necessary to monitor satisfactory progress—electrolytic derangement may occur rapidly as a consequence of inappropriate secretion of antidiuretic hormone (ADH). Acute phase serum should be sent for antibody estimation, followed by a further specimen 10–14 days later. Specimens should be sent for viral culture and examination from obvious sites of infection or as required for specific infections such as rabies. Blood cultures should be taken and if it seems appropriate, blood films should be examined for malarial parasites.

34.4.2 **Cerebrospinal fluid**

Faced with a patient whose history and signs point to a diagnosis of encephalitis, it is imperative to examine the cerebrospinal fluid (CSF) by lumbar puncture, but this must not be done until it is considered safe to do so and after intracranial space occupation has been excluded by brain imaging. Even when no focal abnormality has been demonstrated, ICP may be dangerously high and cerebral oedema may develop with frightening rapidity. Judgement of the necessity for and safety of CSF examination in the individual patient requires clinical experience, and not a little luck, and such decisions should not be made by junior members of the team. CSF is usually under pressure and there is a pleocytosis that may vary from 10 cells/mm^3 to more than 2000 cells/mm^3. In the early stages these may be polymorphonuclear but in general they are lymphocytic unless there is a necrotizing component, in which case red cells are found. The protein content is raised and glucose is normal. By definition, bacteria are not found. Discussion with the virologist or microbiologist will indicate which tests are best to carry out on CSF, whether ELISA, DNA probes with hybridization, or nucleic acid amplification methods such as PCR, appropriate to the circumstances of the case (Tenover 1999). PCR is now accepted as the quickest and most accurate method by which to diagnose herpes simplex and other encephalitides—specific tests are discussed later under individual disease headings (Lakeman et al. 1995; Jeffery et al. 1997). The techniques of such investigations are being continually modified and newer commercial kits are available to laboratories almost by the month, which is one reason why timely discussion with laboratory experts is so important. Valuable advice may also be obtained from the Public Health Laboratory Service. An internet web site which I have found useful to access, and which can usually provide contemporary information or links, is that of the Center for Disease Control in Atlanta on www.cdc.gov.

34.4.3 **Electroencephalography**

The electroencephalogram is a useful non-invasive tool which can supply contributory, but seldom diagnostic, information. In cases of encephalitis it is usually abnormal and demonstrates diffuse slow wave activity that becomes slower with increasing severity. There may be focal abnormality reflecting greater structural change on one side of the brain and this seldom has diagnostic significance. In herpes simplex encephalitis abnormal EEG activity is commonly seen from one temporal lobe and this may spread to the other side as the disease progresses. This may be followed by spike and slow wave activity and periodic lateralized epileptiform discharges arising from a temporal lobe (Upton and Gumpert 1970; Smith *et al.* 1975). This is not pathognomonic. Characteristic appearances may be seen in certain stages of Creutzfeldt–Jakob disease (CJD) and in subacute sclerosing panencephalitis (Cobb 1966; Chiafolo *et al.* 1980). The EEG is useful in demonstrating and following up epileptic activity.

34.4.4 Imaging brain infection

As soon as is practicable, imaging of the intracranial contents should be undertaken. Neuroradiological help should be sought if it is easily available because some of the abnormalities are subtle, particularly in the early stages. Also a radiologist can advise about the best imaging sequence to be used appropriate to the clinical circumstances of the patient. With MR in particular, there is a wide range of pulse sequences and imaging planes that can be used. For encephalitis, MR is the modality of choice because it is superior to CT in demonstrating changes of cerebral oedema and white matter disturbance, infarction and derangement of the blood–brain barrier and contrast enhancement, structures in the posterior fossa, and it has virtually unlimited multiplanar imaging capability. CT is superior at interrogating bone. Unfortunately, there are some limitations to the use of MR with patients who are ill. It is necessary for them to lie still for about 30 min within a tube which some find claustrophobic. Any movement degrades the image and the acquisition time for some sequences can be quite long. This is not possible for patients who are ill or confused. If the patient has problems with his airway, is being ventilated or has ICP monitoring equipment *in situ*, the magnetic properties of the equipment prohibit its use with MR. Few units are equipped with non-metallic instruments. For these reasons CT is the more commonly used in emergency situations. Newer techniques to provide greater discrimination are continually being developed and when combined with contrast enhancement, produce images that are almost comparable to those obtained with MR. There is very little indication now for the use of conventional angiography in the investigation of brain infection— it is useful in the diagnosis of vasculitis and cerebral venous thrombosis.

In cases of viral encephalitis, no abnormality may be evident for the first few days of the illness. Changes which develop include diffuse brain swelling caused by oedema, white matter low density changes which may be diffuse or focal as in cases of herpes simplex encephalitis with predilection for the temporal lobes, sometimes associated with infarction. Later, atrophic changes may ensue. Imaging will identify areas of necrosis, granulomas, abscesses, neoplasm and venous thrombosis, and infarction. Certain changes are associated with particular conditions although these are not pathognomonic. They are described in the relevant sections.

34.5 Treatment

34.5.1 General measures

The general management of a patient with encephalitis is similar to the management of any unconscious or confused patient, care being taken to maintain adequate nutrition, hydration, and ventilation. Epileptic seizures need to be controlled and secondary infection must be prevented or treated vigorously if it occurs. In serious infection, raised ICP needs to be controlled (Barnett *et al.* 1988) to ensure adequate brain perfusion to prevent secondary ischaemia and infarction. ICP monitoring should be considered if the Glasgow Coma Scale falls to 8 or below, if there is radiological evidence of significant brain swelling or if there is mass effect. Hyperventilation and the administration of mannitol should be instituted (Pickard and Czosnyka 1993). There is no consensus on the use of dexamethasone or other steroids to reduce brain oedema. There is no clear evidence that steroids reduce the oedema found in intracranial infection and there are theoretical objections to their routine use. Most data relate to the use of dexamethasone in the treatment of herpes simplex encephalitis and childhood bacterial meningitis (Geiman and Smith 1992; McIntyre *et al.* 1997). In practice, dexamethasone is given to patients who have raised ICP and who continue to deteriorate. The availability of neuro-intensive care and a multidisciplinary approach to the care of such patients has produced undoubted improvement in their management.

34.5.2 Antiviral drugs

Specific treatment for viral encephalitis is available for only a minority of infections. Acyclovir has been shown to diminish the mortality rate blow 30 per cent in cases of herpes simplex encephalitis (Whitley *et al.* 1986). It is also useful for the treatment of varicella/zoster encephalitis. Related drugs, valacyclovir and famciclovir, are under investigation. Ganciclovir and foscarnet are of some use in cytomegalovirus infection (Diamond and Corey 1999). Treatment of AIDS and its neurological complication has improved and is now an extensive and complex field. Superadded and opportunistic infections should be treated immediately—toxoplasmosis responds to pyrimethamine and sulphadiazine, *Mycobacterium avium* complex disease can be treated with antibiotic combinations. Prolonged remission in AIDS can be brought about by suppressing the viral load in the blood with the use of antiretroviral combination therapy incorporating reverse transcriptase inhibitors (either nucleoside analogues or non-nucleoside drugs) and protease inhibitors (Corey 1999). Where appropriate, treatment regimes are discussed further under the headings of the individual infections.

Overall the prognosis for recovery from viral encephalitis is good but this depends greatly on the nature of the offending pathogen: rabies is universally fatal once established and herpes simplex encephalitis can be devastating.

34.6 The herpes viruses

Herpes viruses are widespread throughout the animal kingdom and, when a search has been made, a representative number has been found in most animal species examined. About 100 different herpes viruses are known and new ones are being added to the list. All share common structural features and many antigenic, biological, and chemical properties. All contain double stranded DNA enveloped in an icosahedral capsid with 262 capsomeres. The envelope contains lipid and glycoprotein, the latter providing unique antigenic properties to which the host responds. Any particular herpes virus is host-dependent and following primary infection, the virus becomes latent and is capable of reactivation many years later by an, as yet, unspecified stimulus. Viral DNA therefore remains in the host for the rest of its life. Man is the natural host to several of the herpes viruses and, very rarely, may be infected accidentally by a simian herpes virus. The nomenclature and classification of the herpes viruses remains contentious, and for the purposes of this chapter the popular names are used. Those viruses which cause disease in man are HSV-1 and -2, varicella–zoster, cytomegalovirus and EBV. Recently, human herpes virus 6 (HHV-6) has been found to produce encephalitis and B virus, a herpes virus found in Old World monkeys, has been transmitted to humans by animal bite, and person to person contact has been documented. One important factor that doubtless facilitates the property of latency is the ability of herpes viruses to pass from cell to adjacent cell by membrane fusion. In so doing, the virus avoids contact with extracellular antibodies and can also evade cells which do not have receptors for the virus on their surface.

34.6.1 Herpes simplex

The word 'herpes' has been in use since ancient times and may derive from Sanskrit. It has been used to describe a variety of skin lesions, and now refers to a vesicular exanthem, classically sited where skin and mucous membranes meet. It has long been recognized to be infectious and in the 1920s it was shown to be caused by a filterable virus. Smith *et al.* (1941) demonstrated intranuclear inclusions and subsequently isolated virus from the brain of a case of neonatal meningitis. Zarafonetis *et al.* (1944) demonstrated similar findings in an adult case with focal abnormalities. It has since become evident that herpes simplex encephalitis (HSE) has become the most common form of sporadic, and often fatal or disabling, encephalitis worldwide.

Two types of herpes simplex virus (HSV) are recognized to cause infection in humans: HSV-1 and HSV-2, which share some genomic characteristics and can be differentiated by antigenic, biological, and culture characteristics. Individual strains can be distinguished within the two types. HSV-1 is responsible for most of the non-genital 'above the belt' infections, while HSV-2 causes genital and neonatal infection, contracted 'below the belt'. Primary HSV infection occurs when a non-immune

person is infected with virus and this may or may not be clinically apparent. Antibodies and cell-mediated immunity are activated and persist for the life of the infected individual. In common with other herpes viruses, HSV shares the phenomenon of latency, by which the virus can lie dormant in cells in a non-productive state without causing cell death, and is capable of being reactivated at a later date and cause virus replication which may or may not result in disease.

The pathogenesis of latency remains poorly understood. As early as 1905, Cushing suspected that HSV could remain latent in sensory ganglia. It is now acknowledged that, following primary infection, virus is transmitted proximally along the axons of sensory nerves to reach the cell bodies in the craniospinal ganglia, where the viral genomes become repressed, being maintained in this state by the cell until the genome is reactivated to result in viral replication. This may lead to clinical disease, usually at the same site or within the same area of sensory supply as the primary infection. HSV has been found in the trigeminal ganglia of most people studied at routine necropsy. Many disparate stimuli may trigger reactivation of herpes—stress, infection, particularly pneumococcal and meningococcal, fever, irradiation, nerve root section, and dental manipulation.

Man is the reservoir and vector for HSV infection, which is universal and is transmitted by close personal contact. HSV-2 infections are acquired sexually or by inoculation of the neonate in the birth passage. HSV-1 is transmitted in saliva and other secretions from the eye and pharynx. Virus enters a mucous membrane, replicates and migrates up sensory axons and settles in the sensory ganglion. In most, the primary infection goes unnoticed and is inferred by the later demonstration of raised antibody titres to HSV. The prevalence of positive antibodies in an adult community reflects its socio-economic status: 30–50 per cent of higher socio-economic groups in the West have positive antibodies and this rises to 100 per cent for lower groups. HSV affects all races, both sexes, all nations, and occurs throughout the year. The mouth and lips are the most common sites of HSV-1 infection: the genitalia of HSV-2. The appearance of the characteristic ulcer may be accompanied by a mild systemic illness with pyrexia, malaise, and lymphadenopathy. The ulcers heal within 2 weeks. Recurrent disease from reactivation usually occurs at the site of the primary infection. In about 3 per cent of cases the eye is the site of primary attack. In those with eczema and other skin rashes, infection is liable to cause an extensive vesicular rash and in the immune suppressed, it may be catastrophic.

The most frequently devastating of herpetic infections occurs when the virus invades the brain and causes HSE. This is a rare complication of herpes infection with an estimated prevalence of 0.1–0.4 per 100 000 population per year. This is almost certainly an underestimate for it seems likely that milder forms of the disease go unreported and perhaps unrecognized. It is the most common form of sporadic encephalitis in Europe and North America and accounts for about 10–20 per cent of viral encephalitis cases (Corey and Spear 1986). It affects all age groups; one third of all cases occur under the age of 20, half over 50. It can result from primary infection in the young—perhaps as many as a third, but most cases are the result of reactivation of previous infection. In a few, it may be due to exogenous reinfection. It is not understood why HSE almost always occurs in previously fit, immunocompetent people who have circulating antibody to HSV. The vast majority of cases are caused by HSV-1.

Pathogenesis

The pathogenesis of HSE remains ill understood. Latent virus has been demonstrated in brain tissue but confirmation of reactivation within the brain has been elusive. It has been suggested that the virus may be reactivated in the olfactory bulb or trigeminal ganglion, thereafter travelling centrally along neurones. If this was the case it would be expected that reactivation of cutaneous infection in the same dermatome would follow, but this is not so: HSE is seldom associated with recurrent herpes labialis. It is possible that the virus may reach brain by spread from the olfactory mucosa along the olfactory bulb and tract to the infero-medial aspect of the temporal lobe, which is commonly infected in HSE. Such a hypothesis accords with necropsy findings and electron microscopic confirmation has been obtained (Ojeda *et al.* 1983). It may be, but has not been proved, that the strains of HSV which cause HSE have particular neurotropic qualities. HSE is no more common in immunocompromised patients than in those with normal immunity, and HSV is not isolated from the blood of patients with HSE, which makes it unlikely that infection is carried through the blood.

Pathologically, the changes of fatal HSE are those of a severe acute necrotizing encephalitis. The brain is swollen, congested with haemorrhagic damage of the temporal and frontal lobes to the degree of necrosis and liquefaction. Beyond these areas there is microscopic change—capillary congestion, perivascular infiltration, petechial haemorrhages on the surface of the brain, and inflammatory changes in the cortex and subcortical white matter. As virus spreads, neurones, oligodendrocytes, and astroglia all die. Eosinophilic intranuclear occlusions, Cowdry's type A inclusions, or Lipschutz bodies appear within glia and neurones, and are seen most often during the first week of infection. They are characteristic but not pathognomonic and may be found in other forms of herpes virus infection.

Clinical presentations

The clinical presentations of HSE are protean. The onset may be explosive but is more often insidious. Prodromal symptoms commonly last between 4 and 10 days and consist of malaise, fever, headache, and irritability. In more severe cases there is meningeal irritation, depression of conscious level, and epileptic seizures which may be generalized or focal. Signs of frontal and temporal lobe dysfunction follow, with personality change, memory loss, and psychiatric syndromes with hallucinations and—as the disease progresses—hemiparesis and parietal syndromes (Whitley *et al.* 1982). In as many as 87 per cent of cases, focal signs appear (Barza and Pauker 1980). As the infection spreads, signs of raised ICP supervene and dominate the

picture. Unless this can be reversed, it leads to decerebration and death. Mortality rates have varied according to the criteria used for diagnosis, and vary from 40 to 70 per cent in those who have developed focal signs, the prognosis being worse with increasing coma.

There are no clinical features of HSE which are diagnostic: even the presence of a cutaneous herpes is of no value since only a minority of patients with HSE will have them; furthermore, they appear with many other infections. The rapid onset of a pyrexial illness with confusion, obtundation, seizures, and focal signs is suggestive of HSE and demands instant further investigation. Blood investigations are of no value for immediate diagnosis, and HSE cannot be diagnosed by serum antibody tests alone. By the time that a diagnostic rise of fourfold or more of antibody levels has taken place, the opportunity for successful antiviral treatment has passed. Brain imaging should be undertaken, preferably with MR if the patient can tolerate the procedure. The appearances range from normal, through a tight brain to cerebral oedema. Focal abnormality is common with mass effect and infarctive changes in one or other or both temporal lobes (Fig. 34.1a) (Zimmermann *et al.* 1980; Demaerel *et al.* 1992). The EEG may show changes localizing to a temporal lobe with focal spike or slow wave activity, but these changes are not specific (Fig. 34.1b). If it is judged to be safe, CSF can be examined. Other infective conditions can be excluded and HSE can be positively diagnosed by detection of HSV DNA by PCR (Rowley *et al.* 1990; Lakeman *et al.* 1995). Non-specific changes of raised cell count, sometimes with red cells, protein content, and normal or reduced sugar level are commonly found.

Brain biopsy and the identification or culture of virus from biopsy specimens was the gold standard for the diagnosis of HSE. Unfortunately, this procedure carried a complication rate of at least 3 per cent of development of haemorrhage or brain swelling, and there was no guarantee that the appropriate area of the brain would be biopsied. There is now no place for brain biopsy to diagnose HSE. It is acknowledged that biopsy may be necessary in circumstances where the diagnosis is in doubt, and conditions such as granulomas or tumours require exclusion.

Treatment

Treatment of HSE in the past was with highly toxic antiviral drugs. Because of potential toxicity, accurate diagnosis was necessary before treatment could be instituted, and this usually meant that brain biopsy was required. The antiviral treatment of choice now for HSE is acyclovir (Whitley *et al.* 1986). Although not devoid of potential hazard, this is a considerable advance on what was available before and has revolutionized the treatment of suspected cases of HSE. When a case of suspected HSE is identified, it is my practice to begin treatment with acyclovir before the results of further investigations are known. Dosage schedules are subject to variation and the length of time for which treatment should be given is not well defined—at least 10 days is recommended. Treatment of epileptic seizures and cerebral oedema is usually necessary.

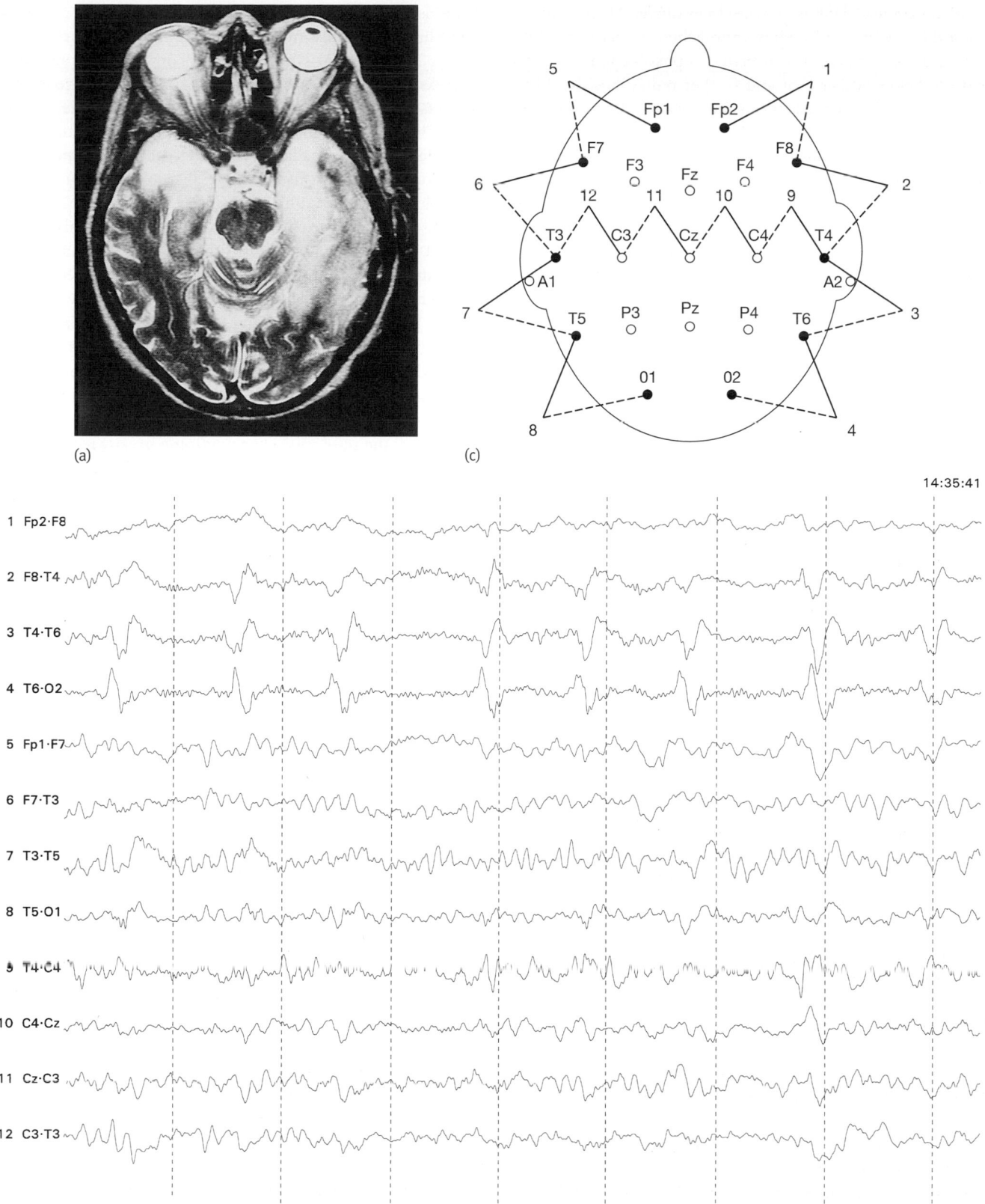

(a)

(c)

14:35:41

1 Fp2·F8

2 F8·T4

3 T4·T6

4 T6·O2

5 Fp1·F7

6 F7·T3

7 T3·T5

8 T5·O1

9 T4·C4

10 C4·Cz

11 Cz·C3

12 C3·T3

(b)

Fig. 34.1. Herpes simplex encephalitis. (a) MRI showing asymmetrical oedema and swelling of the temporal lobes, especially the medial portions (courtesy of Dr P. Anslow). (b) An EEG showing unilateral slow-wave complexes over the right temporal region, maximal at the T4 and T6 electrodes. These complexes are broader than in Creutzfeldt–Jakob disease, having a duration of up to 1 second, and they tend to repeat at longer intervals. The alpha rhythm is reduced over the affected right hemisphere. (Courtesy of Dr R. Kennett.) (c) The electrode montage used for the EEG. This was a bipolar montage, using 10–20 international electrode positions.

The outcome of HSE is not easy to evaluate. Before antiviral chemotherapy, mortality rates approached 70 per cent. With early diagnosis and rapid treatment it is possible to reduce this figure to below 30 per cent and further reductions should be possible if the diagnosis is considered earlier still. In those who survive, if there has been severe disease of the temporal lobes, epileptic seizures, personality disturbance, and memory defects, particularly for recent events, can be a considerable difficulty. Even in those who make good functional recoveries, formal neuropsychological tests may reveal subtle cognitive deficits (Gordon *et al.* 1990) and most have some form of persisting neurological sign or symptom (McGrath *et al.* 1997).

34.6.2 Varicella–zoster

Chicken-pox (varicella) and shingles (herpes zoster) are two commonplace diseases caused by the varicella–zoster virus (VZV). The association of 'chicken' with pox and varicella is obscure. 'Zoster' and 'shingles' derive from Greek and Latin and refer to the 'girdle' or 'belt' distribution of the rash in a typical attack of shingles. That the two conditions had a common origin was not appreciated until von Bokay (1909) noted that chicken-pox developed in children who had been exposed to adults with shingles. Proof of the hypothesis had to wait until the work of Weller and colleagues confirmed that the viruses causing the two conditions were identical (Weller 1953).

Chicken-pox results from primary VZV infection and is a disease of school-age children—about 95 per cent of the school-age population is infected. Shingles is due to reactivation of latent infection and affects adults. VZV is associated with several different neurological syndromes that may affect the central and peripheral nervous systems. The pathogenesis of these syndromes remains poorly understood and is influenced by the immune status and the age of the patient.

VZV is a DNA-containing herpes virus whose only natural host is man. It is the most infectious of the herpes viruses yet the most difficult to grow in culture. Chicken-pox is one of the childhood exanthems and is spread by droplets from the respiratory system and by direct contact. It tends to occur in epidemics each winter and spring. After an incubation period of 14 days a vesicular rash develops, accompanied by low grade fever and malaise. The rash appears in successive crops, so that lesions at different stages of development are present simultaneously, and it tends to affect the face and trunk rather than the limbs. Rarely, varicella pneumonia, hepatitis, secondary skin infections, and in the immune compromised, disseminated infection may ensue. Immunocompromised children are at particular risk of purpura fulminans and haemorrhagic varicella (Morgan and Smalley 1983).

Neurological complications of chicken-pox are rare and include encephalitis including cerebellar ataxia, aseptic meningitis, myelitis, and Guillain–Barré neuropathy. Formerly, Reye's syndrome was believed to be a complication of the infection. It is now held to be due to aspirin given to children to counter fever (Shope 1982). The incidence of neurological complications is about 1 : 1000 and 90 per cent of these will be encephalitis, in more than half taking the form of cerebellar ataxia. The cerebellar syndrome comes on a few days and up to 2 weeks after the onset of the rash. In a few, it may accompany the rash. It comes on gradually with dysarthria, ataxia, headache, and drowsiness. The generalized encephalitic form is of acute onset with headache, vomiting, drowsiness, and epileptic seizures which are usually generalized, with progression to hemiplegia, aphasia, cranial nerve palsies, and coma. Cerebellar ataxia, cerebral disturbance, and cranial nerve palsies may coexist in rare instances (Griffith *et al.* 1970; Johnson and Milbourn 1970; McKendall and Klawans 1978; Kennedy 1987). If the child is immunosuppressed, encephalitis may be devastating with dissemination of virus throughout the viscera and brain. The pathogenesis of encephalitis remains poorly understood: there has been necropsy evidence to support both direct invasion of the brain by virus, and an immune-mediated post-infectious encephalomyelitis.

Cases of the pure cerebellar syndrome usually recover completely and if there is confidence in the clinical diagnosis, no further investigation is needed. If there is doubt, or other pathology is suspected, brain imaging, CSF examination, and an EEG are called for. None of those shows diagnostic features. CT and MR changes range from a normal scan to cerebral oedema, white matter upset and subcortical plaque-like demyelinating lesions in cases of severe leucoencephalitis in the immune suppressed (Tenorio and Whitaker 1991; Lentz *et al.* 1993). CSF may show a lymphocytic pleocytosis and normal glucose. The EEG is abnormal in 25 per cent of the cerebellar ataxia cases with non-specific slow activity that soon reverts to normal. In the encephalitic form the EEG is more abnormal more frequently and for longer with diffuse slow activity and sometimes focal disturbance with seizure discharges. If necessary, antigen or antibody can be detected in CSF, but this is seldom necessary because the rash is quite characteristic.

Encephalitis is a rare complication of shingles (Section 12.14.5) in less than 1 per cent of cases. The old and immune compromised, and those with zoster affecting the cranial nerves, are most likely to be affected. It comes on a few days to a month or more following the development of the rash (Jemsek *et al.* 1983). The clinical features are those of encephalitis and the mortality rate is about 10 per cent. CSF, EEG, and cerebral imaging results are similar to those described above. Uncomplicated herpes zoster may have a pleocytic CSF so any abnormality found in encephalitic cases should be interpreted with caution. PCR for VZV DNA in CSF is positive (Puchhammer-Stockl *et al.* 1991).

Vascular syndromes accompany or succeed shingles by up to several months, as the result of a necrotizing granulomatous angiitis of small- and medium-sized cerebral vessels. Symptoms and signs are appropriate to the artery affected, and most frequently accompanies herpes zoster ophthalmicus (Verghese and Sugar 1986). Herpes virus particles have been found in artery walls associated with VZV antigen (Eidelberg *et al.* 1986; Fukumoto *et al.* 1986).

A syndrome has been described resembling progressive multifocal leucoencephalopathy—with white matter degeneration, type A intranuclear inclusions in oligodendrocytes, virus particles, and antigen to VZV virus—following a few months after zoster infection in patients who have been immune compromised by malignancy or AIDS (Horten *et al.* 1981).

About 10 per cent of cases of varicella encephalitis die and 25 per cent of the survivors have significant neurological sequelae—hemiparesis, epilepsy, developmental delay, and psychiatric disturbance (McKendall and Klawans 1978). Infantile hemiplegia from cerebral vasculopathy has been described (Caekbeke *et al.* 1990).

The complications of VZV infections which affect other parts of the nervous system are described elsewhere (Section 12.14.5).

Uncomplicated chicken-pox does not require specific treatment except in children who are immune compromised. They should be given specific varicella–zoster immune globulin (VZIG) as soon as possible after exposure to chicken-pox or shingles. A live attenuated varicella virus vaccine is available and is effective and may be offered to immune compromised children and others who may not have had chicken-pox in childhood if they are likely to come into contact with cases. Acyclovir is effective against VZV and it should be given as soon as the diagnosis is made. Whether it guards against the development of neurological complications has not yet been proved.

34.6.3 Cytomegalovirus

Cytomegalovirus (CMV) infections have been recognized since the turn of the previous century. The characteristic intranuclear inclusions found histologically in infected foetal tissue were misinterpreted as being the result of protozoan infection until the virus was isolated simultaneously in three laboratories in 1956, and it was named after the cytopathic effect which it produced in cell culture.

CMV is an atypical herpes virus with a double stranded DNA core, and shares the property of latency with the other herpes viruses. It can remain inactive within its human host, causing minimal disability. The host remains mobile and at intervals virus is produced and shed from various anatomical sites, particularly saliva, urine, and uterine cervical secretions. Consequently CMV is one of the most successful parasites of humans, and varying degrees of intimacy of contact can lead to infection so that almost 100 per cent of people from a poor socio-economic background, and 70 per cent with good hygienic conditions, have serological evidence of CMV infection, which in the vast majority is asymptomatic.

CMV is the most common pathogen to infect the foetus. This follows transplacental spread from maternal viraemia and affects up to 2.5 per cent of all live births. Fortunately, less than 5 per cent of those infected are symptomatic with evidence of cytomegalic inclusion disease (CID), although a proportion of those who are normal at birth develop problems later. CID affects many organs and the infant may have low birth weight, hepatosplenomegaly, jaundice, thrombocytopaenia, choroidoretinitis, and encephalitis with microcephaly, leading to mental retardation, seizures, spasticity, and deafness. Periventricular calcification is commonly seen on X-ray and on brain scanning, and ventricular dilatation. If asymptomatic infected infants are followed up neurological defects are found as they get older—up to 20 per cent have lower IQs and behavioural problems, minor inco-ordination and defects in perceptual skills and neural deafness (Griffiths 1987).

After the neonatal period, acquired primary or recurrent infection is usually symptomless. Occasionally there may be a mild non-specific illness like infectious mononucleosis. CMV may also be transmitted by infected blood and this results in a 'post-transfusion mononucleosis syndrome' in as many as 5 per cent of those infected.

Patients whose immune system is suppressed are particularly at risk of developing CMV infection, both primary and reactivated, and this often involves the CNS. In a retrospective survey of encephalitis associated with CMV, Arribas *et al.* (1996) found that only 3 per cent of cases were healthy before infection and 85 per cent had immune suppression from AIDS. The rest were immune suppressed for different reasons. Primary infection is usually symptomatic with persistent pyrexia which may last for a week, and is often fatal if bacterial or fungal infection supervenes. In some, disease may be limited to or accompanied by, severe choroidoretinitis. Transplant recipients are at risk of CMV infection. Most are primary from the allograft or blood products. Reactivation of latent infection may occur. Superinfection occurs when latent infection from a donor reactivates in the recipient. The organ that has been transplanted always fares worse than the rest of the body. The greater the degree of immune suppression, the higher the chance of developing CMV infection. Features are of persisting pyrexia from the second or third month post-transplant, much like septicaemia. Superadded infection, particularly *Pneumocystis pneumonitis*, carries a grave prognosis.

CMV is a common opportunistic pathogen which causes a form of encephalitis and affects other organs in patients with advanced AIDS (Drew 1988). Evidence of CMV infection has been found in brain at necropsy in up to a third of AIDS patients coming to necropsy (Snider *et al.* 1983; Vinters *et al.* 1989; Arribas *et al.* 1996). Unfortunately, it is impossible to determine in these patients, who have dementia, how much of their syndrome has been caused by HIV, or how much by CMV or other pathogens. It is also difficult to correlate pathological findings with clinical course. There is nothing specific about brain imaging (Clifford *et al.* 1996) and diagnosis requires the demonstration of CMV DNA in CSF (Cohen 1996; Wildemann *et al.* 1998). A distinct syndrome of ventriculoencephalitis caused by CMV in AIDS, characterized by simultaneous retinitis or other organ disease, mental change, large ventricles and periventricular enhancement on imaging, and CSF pleocytosis, has been described (Kalayjian *et al.* 1994). A form of brainstem encephalitis (Fuller *et al.* 1989), myelitis (Tucker *et al.* 1985), and a painful, progressive, ascending, lumbosacral radiculopathy (Miller *et al.* 1990) has also been described. Diagnosis is by demonstration of CMV DNA in CSF, usually by one of the PCR techniques. Treatment is with intravenous ganciclovir for 2 or 3 weeks and the clinical response is variable. It is used prophylactically in organ transplant recipients.

34.6.3 Epstein–Barr virus

Epstein–Barr virus (EBV) was discovered in 1964 in lymphoblasts from a case of Burkitt's lymphoma (Epstein *et al.* 1964). Burkitt anticipated that an infectious agent was the cause of the lymphocytic tumour which he described from a geographically limited area of Africa (Burkitt 1958). Consequent upon a serendipitous infection, further studies showed that EBV is the cause of infectious mononucleosis (IM) (Henle and Henle 1966). Association of EBV with several other conditions has been established—nasopharyngeal carcinoma, Hodgkin's disease, lethal midline granuloma, and hairy cell leukaemia— although a pathogenetic mechanism has not been established. IM has been associated with neurological complications since 1931 (Johansen 1931).

EBV is a member of the herpes group; it contains double stranded DNA and is structurally similar to other herpes viruses. Man is the only natural host. The only cells that have been shown to have receptors for EBV are B lymphocytes. EBV enters by infecting epithelial cells in the oropharynx whence infected B lymphocytes transport virus throughout the body via the blood. Many of these undergo transformation and stimulate a vigorous proliferation of T cells and natural killer cells many of which have 'suppressor' activity and appear as 'atypical lymphocytes' on peripheral blood films. As a consequence of this immune response, the symptoms of IM appear 30–60 days following infection. It is thought that EBV enters the brain via the B lymphocytes, and disease is brought about either by direct viral action or by local inflammatory response.

Epstein–Barr viral infection is ubiquitous and by the age of 30 the vast majority of adults show seropositivity. In areas of high population density and poor hygiene, almost everyone is infected by the age of three. Oral excretion of virus occurs and infection is spread by intimate oral contact and rarely, by blood transfusion (Gerber *et al.* 1969). In Western society IM is primarily a disease of adolescents. Symptoms develop abruptly with malaise, fever, headache, sore throat, cervical lymphadenopathy, and splenomegaly. There may be hepatomegaly, jaundice, myalgia, and the development of neurological syndromes. Sometimes there is an evanescent skin rash and periorbital oedema. In most, fever subsides within 2 weeks and there is complete recovery. In a few, lassitude persists and may develop into one of the chronic fatigue syndromes and depression. A causal link to EBV for these syndromes has not been proven (Amsterdam *et al.* 1986; Buchwald *et al.* 1987).

Characteristically, after the first week, there is a peripheral leucocytosis to 20 000/mm³ which includes 'atypical lymphocytes', T cells. In young adults with IM, 90 per cent develop heterophile antibodies that form the basis of the 'Paul–Bunnell' reaction, whose modern counterpart is the 'Monospot' test. For CNS disease, examination of CSF (or biopsy tissue from CNS lymphoma) for EBV DNA with PCR confirms the diagnosis.

Neurological complications occur in about 5 per cent of hospitalized cases (Gautier-Smith 1965) and probably fewer than 0.5 per cent of all cases. Aseptic meningitis is commonest and almost always resolves without sequelae. Encephalitis occurs in older children and young adults (Schnell *et al.* 1966) and very often affects the cerebellum (Bennett and Peters 1961). Some have been reported with personality change, some with extrapyramidal upset dependent upon the part of the brain most affected. Transverse myelitis has been recorded (Cotton and Webb-Poploe 1966) and Guillain–Barré polyneuropathy (Grose *et al.* 1975). Cranial nerve palsies, chiefly Bell's palsy, brachial plexopathies, and lumbosacral radiculopathy (Sharma *et al.* 1993) have been noted. EBV has been associated with CNS lymphomas in patients with normal immune systems and in those who have been immune suppressed from transplants, leukaemia, and AIDS (McMahon *et al.* 1991).

Most patients make a complete recovery. Treatment is symptomatic. Acyclovir and steroids have been tried for encephalitis and results have been conflicting. Lymphomas are treated with chemotherapy and/or radiation.

34.6.5 Human herpes virus 6

Human herpes virus 6 (HHV-6) has recently been discovered to have a role in human disease. In 1988 it was isolated from the blood of children who had suffered a roseola type of disease. CNS diseases with which it has since been linked are meningoencephalitis, retinitis, Guillain–Barré polyneuropathy, and epileptic seizures on the basis of serological studies and PCR studies of CSF and a causal relationship has not been definitely established (Kondo *et al.* 1993; Asano *et al* 1994; Caserta *et al.* 1994). Bassolasco *et al.* (1999) found HHV-6 DNA in CSF of 2.2 per cent of patients with neurological complications of AIDS. Other opportunistic infections, particularly CMV were present, and no definite relationship between HHV-6 and brain disease was found. Not enough is known to date to make any recommendations about treatment.

34.6.6 Herpes B virus

This is found in Old World monkeys and human disease has been described in persons bitten by a monkey and is therefore likely to occur only in laboratory workers. It has also been described following person to person contact. There have been very few cases and the clinical picture is of an ascending myelitis or encephalomyelitis. The onset is acute with neurological symptoms within 3–5 days and death has occurred within 2 weeks. A localized vesicular eruption occurs around the area of the bite, followed by regional lymphadenopathy then malaise, fever, myalgia, and neurological signs of myelitis and encephalitis (Sabin 1949; Holmes *et al.* 1990; Davenport *et al.* 1994).

34.7 Other viral encephalitides

34.7.1 Epidemic encephalitis

This form of encephalitis is caused by one of the arboviruses, the causal virus varying according to locality and season. *Arbovirus* derives from *arthropod-borne* virus, the term used to describe more than 450 strains of virus which are transmitted biologically by haematophagous arthropods such as mosquitoes, ticks, sandflies, and biting midges (*Phlebotomus* and *Culicoides*). Of these 450 strains, 60 are known to cause disease in man, such as dengue and yellow fever, where neurological involvement is of minor importance, or is caused by haemorrhagic or cardiovascular complications. There are in excess of 20 arboviruses that cause encephalitis in man (Table 34.3). All of them contain RNA and are classified in three families— Togaviridae, Bunyaviridae, and Reoviridae. Togaviridae are symmetrical spherical enveloped virions that range in size from 40 to 90 nm in diameter, and are subdivided by size into larger flaviviruses and smaller alphaviruses. Bunyaviridae are larger and the nucleocapsids have helical symmetry. The Reoviridae contain double stranded nucleic acid and have no envelope.

Vectors

All arboviral encephalitides are maintained by zoonoses with complex life cycles involving a non-human, vertebrate, primary host—usually birds and lower vertebrate—and a primary arthropod vector—usually a mosquito or tick. Many arboviruses have different vertebrate hosts and more than one vector. The mechanism of transmission is the same for all viruses. The mosquito or tick bites an infected rodent, primate, or bird, becomes infected, the virus replicates and spreads to the insect brain and salivary gland and within 2 weeks, the insect is infective. It bites a human, injecting virus in the process. This replicates in lymph nodes, spleen and vascular endothelium and viraemia develops. Most human infections are asymptomatic or lead to a mild flu-like illness of insidious onset with fever, headache, malaise, and myalgia. In the small number who develop encephalitis, virus enters the brain, probably by infecting vascular endothelial cells and diffusing through capillaries, spreads rapidly and infects neurones and glia which may die, and an inflammatory response ensues. Humans are infected by accident, and become 'dead end' hosts, because the viraemia which results is not of sufficient degree to infect a biting mosquito. The severity of the encephalitis varies with the strain of the infecting organism. The geographical distribution of the individual arbovirus is limited to particular regions of the world. Most cases of encephalitis occur in the summer, when arthropods are most active. Climatic factors are important—a late summer can prolong the period for potential infection. Worldwide, the most important cause of arbovirus encephalitis is Japanese B virus. In the USA there are four main agents, Eastern equine, Western equine, St Louis, and LaCrosse. Powessan virus causes a few cases in northern USA. Venezuelan equine encephalitis occurs in Central and South America. In Europe, arboviruses are transmitted by ticks and central European and Russian spring–summer encephalitis are the major forms. Other varieties exist in certain regions such as Murray Valley, West Nile, Semliki Forest encephalitis, and Colorado tick fever. Where merited, further descriptions are given under individual headings.

Clinical features

Signs and symptoms of arbovirus encephalitis are little different from other forms of viral encephalitis. Some forms have a more acute onset and progression and cause a more severe syndrome, others appear to have a predilection for certain areas of the brain. Features that are common to all, are drowsiness, headache, pyrexia, malaise, some neck stiffness, and sometimes epileptic seizures. Focal signs may develop less commonly than with other encephalitides. Routine blood tests are seldom helpful, EEG shows slow wave abnormality in proportion to the degree of impairment of awareness. Imaging with either CT or MR is often normal or may show a tight brain. In some cases of Japanese and St Louis encephalitis MR and CT have demonstrated abnormality in basal ganglia, brainstem, and substantia nigra (Misra *et al.* 1994; Cerna *et al.* 1999). The diagnosis of arbovirus encephalitis may be suspected if there is a history of exposure to insect bites in a geographical area known to harbour the virus. With ease of transcontinental travel, enquiry must be made of all suspected cases of encephalitis about recent movements, recreational and occupational activities—people who hike, camp, or work in forest and scrub exposed to mosquitoes and ticks have a higher exposure to insect bites. A high degree of suspicion is necessary—recently West Nile fever has occurred in New York (MMWR 1999) and in Romania in 1996 (Lundstrom 1999). With rare exceptions, an exact diagnosis cannot be made on medical grounds alone and laboratory evidence is required to confirm the diagnosis. Demonstrating a rise of antibody titre in paired serum samples has been the customary method now being overtaken by showing viral RNA in CSF by one of the PCR techniques or by demonstrating antigen or antibody by ELISA (Cuzzubbo *et al.* 1999).

Table 34.3. Major encephalitides caused by arboviruses

Reovirus	Colorado tick fever
Bunyavirus	California
	LaCrosse
	Jamestown Canyon
	Rift Valley
Togavirus	St Louis
	Japanese
	West Nile
	Murray Valley
	Far Eastern
	Kyasanur Forest
	Louping ill
	Powassan
	Eastern equine
	Western equine
	Venezuelan equine

34.7.2 Equine encephalitis

Eastern equine encephalitis

Eastern equine encephalitis is caused by an alphavirus and rarely afflicts humans. Wild birds of the Atlantic and Gulf coasts of the USA and Caribbean form the major reservoir. The principal vector is a mosquito, *Culiseta melanura*. Epidemics may occur in horses in summer and autumn and provide a warning that human cases may ensue. Human disease is sporadic. Some 4–10 days after the mosquito bite encephalitic symptoms appear. Seventy per cent of cases occur in children (Przelomski *et al.* 1988) and it is a particularly virulent infection with mortality rates varying from 30–70 per cent and survivors often have severe sequelae of mental retardation and epilepsy. There is no specific treatment or routine vaccine. Care should be taken to avoid mosquito bites.

Western equine encephalitis

Western equine encephalitis is caused by an alphavirus and causes more human diseases than the Eastern variety—mortality rate is 10 per cent. There are three different strains: the one from eastern USA is less severe than the two that occur in the west. The reservoir includes birds and small mammals in western USA, Canada, and eastern South America. The vectors are *C. melanura* in the east and *C. tarsalis* in the west. The disease is sporadic and peaks in early to mid-summer. Human disease occurs almost exclusively in the west of Canada and USA where the strains are more virulent. Infection is asymptomatic or very mild in the vast majority. Children are affected, males more than females, and may be left with permanent sequelae (Baker 1958). There is no specific treatment. A vaccine is available for those at high risk of infection.

Venezuelan equine encephalitis

Venezuelan equine encephalitis is caused by an alphavirus that causes disease in horses and man in Central and South America. Human disease follows epidemics in horses. It is less severe than the other equine encephalitides and fatalities are rare. The incubation period is a little longer, and CNS symptoms are usually confined to children and resolve within a week. Adults experience a mild flu-like illness. No specific treatment is available. A vaccine is available for people at occupational risk.

34.7.3 St Louis and Japanese encephalitis

St Louis encephalitis

St Louis encephalitis is caused by a flavivirus and is the most common mosquito-borne disease in USA. It exists in endemic and epidemic form throughout continental USA. The main reservoir is wild birds and the vectors are mosquitoes of the *Culex* species. In western states outbreaks occur after rainy periods, due to the habits of the mosquito vector, while in the mid-west and the east where the mosquito is different, epidemics appear after dry spells. Most cases are seen between July and October and clinical manifestations are more likely to affect the over 50s. Most have a mild flu-like illness, some have a mild meningitis, and only a few (less than 10 per cent) develop encephalitis (Brinker *et al.* 1979). There is no specific treatment.

Japanese encephalitis

Japanese encephalitis is the most common arbovirus encephalitis worldwide with in excess of 45 000 cases reported annually. The virus is a flavivirus. When first recognized, Japanese encephalitis carried a mortality rate approaching 50 per cent. This has fallen, but not to insignificant levels. Human disease occurs endemically in large areas of Southeast Asia, including Japan, Korea, China, Thailand, the Malaysian peninsula, Philippines, Borneo, Bangladesh, and large regions of India. The main reservoir is water birds and horses, pigs and goats function as an amplifying host reservoir. The vectors are varieties of *Culex* mosquitoes. The disease tends to follow annual patterns that relate to the geographical area and the vector. Most infections are mild or asymptomatic, when encephalitis occurs it can be devastating. Mortality rates average just over 10 per cent but in severe outbreaks, mortality of 50 per cent has been recorded. Encephalitis affects those less than 15 years and the old, in the main. The incubation period is 6–16 days and the signs can vary from flu, through aseptic meningitis, to rapidly progressive and fatal encephalitis (Dickerson *et al.* 1952; Kumar *et al.* 1994). If improvement is to occur, it begins within 4 days. Neurological sequelae are common in survivors. Diagnosis is by serological examination, CSF antibody estimation by IgM capture ELISA and most recently PCR of viral RNA in CSF. Brain imaging is not specific, and in common with other arbovirus encephalitides, lesions have been demonstrated in the extrapyramidal system (Misra *et al.* 1994). There is no specific treatment. A formalin inactivated vaccine is now available and has been used to good effect in Asia, and has been reported to be up to 90 per cent effective.

Other similar syndromes, transmitted by mosquitoes, have been described from localized areas and named accordingly. They are all variations on the same clinical theme and diagnosis and management are as described above. They include Murray Valley encephalitis from Victoria, Australia and Papua New Guinea. West Nile encephalitis is endemic in Egypt and Israel, Rocio encephalitis in the São Paolo region of Brazil, and Semliki Forest encephalitis in East Africa.

34.7.4 Tick-borne encephalitis

This group includes Russian spring–summer encephalitis, central European encephalitis, louping ill, Powessan virus encephalitis, and Colorado tick fever. The first four are caused by togaviruses, the last by an arbovirus of genus Reoviridae. They occur in wooded regions in northern latitudes and the disease may be endemic or sporadic. The vectors are species of Ixodid ticks and the hosts are small and not so small vertebrates—moles and rodents, and goat, sheep, and cattle. Virus may be transmitted in the milk of these last animals and this may be a source of infection. Man enters the woodlands and scrub for recreation or occupation and is bitten by a tick. In

Europe there are peaks of infection in early summer and autumn and this reflects tick activity. The neurological syndrome is acute and severe, more severe in children, and carries a mortality rate of approximately 20 per cent (Porterfield 1987). The Russian form is monophasic, the central European form is biphasic and less severe and occurs from Scandinavia to northern Greece. Diagnosis is serological and there is no specific treatment. An inactivated virus is available for people who are exposed in their occupation and it should be renewed annually.

Powessan virus is a flavivirus, found in *Ixodes* ticks in Canada and in mid and east USA. Human cases are rare and have been described in children. Louping ill has occurred in the UK for many years, causing a disease in sheep. Reported cases have been in laboratory workers as a benign biphasic illness with encephalitis in the second phases.

Colorado tick fever occurs in the western states of USA and Canada and is usually a benign infection. Few cases develop encephalitis. It occurs in early summer and affects those who go to forests for work or play. Chipmunks, squirrels, and deer mice are the reservoir and the wood tick, *Dermacentor andersonii*, is the vector. The incubation period is 3–6 days, then a sudden fever appears with myalgia, rigors, and headache. In about 10 per cent of cases a non-specific maculo-papular rash appears. The fever has a biphasic character with remission followed by reappearance (saddleback fever). In some cases full-blown encephalitis occurs. There may be haemorrhagic complications due to thrombocytopaenia and disseminated intravascular coagulation. Diagnosis is by serology and no specific treatment is possible (Goodpasture *et al.* 1978).

The California group of viruses are Bunyaviruses and include the agents which cause LaCrosse, California, and Jamestown Canyon virus. The clinical syndromes are similar, as are the viruses that are maintained by small rodents and the insect vector is the *Aedes* mosquito group. The diseases are endemic and there is usually a history of mosquito bite. Diagnosis is serological and now by PCR of CSF (Huang *et al.* 1999).

34.7.5 Rabies

Rabies has been recognized as a fearsome disease since Babylonian times. Hydrophobia, which results from pharyngeal spasm induced by attempts to drink, was described by Hippocrates and by Celsus who suggested that the causal noxious agent was transmitted in saliva from the bite of an infected animal. Pasteur also recognized this, and that the CNS was the region most infected. In 1885 he carried out his inoculation studies which demonstrated that people could be saved from this invariably fatal condition by inoculation, within a short time of the animal bite, of dried rabbit spinal cord which contained the agent in attenuated form (Pasteur 1885). In 1903 Negri noted the characteristic eosinophilic cytoplasmic inclusions in infected neurones, which were subsequently shown to be virus particles.

The *rabies virus* is a rhabdovirus, an RNA-containing bullet-shaped virus, in dimension 180 by 75 nm. It can be inactivated by ultraviolet and sunlight, desiccation, formalin, phenol, and importantly from a clinical standpoint, by detergents. It is distributed worldwide and is capable of infection of a large range of animal species, predominantly mammals, which provide a reservoir for the propagation of the disease. Mammals are the source of infection of man, the major species varying from continent to continent. Rabies is endemic in most parts of the world. Exceptions are the UK, Ireland, Australia and New Zealand, and most Pacific Islands including Hawaii, Antarctica, Japan, Taiwan, and some Caribbean and Mediterranean islands. Scandinavia, except for Denmark, is free. The insularity of these regions, strict quarantine regulations, and now mass immunization of populations of wild animals, has maintained the native fauna free of rabies. In other communities, such as the USA, measures such as muzzling of dogs and immunization regulations for domestic pets have reduced the risk of infection at the expense of shifting the main reservoir to skunks, foxes, racoons, and bats. Cats have now become a significant source. In Europe the main wild reservoir is the fox, followed by wolf, racoon, and dog. In Asia and Africa it is spread by wolves, jackals, and dogs, and small carnivores are also important; while in Central and South America vampire bats are the main source of the virus. Nevertheless, the vast majority of the 60 000 annual human deaths worldwide occur from canine contact (Haupt 1999). Rates of human rabies are highest in Asia, next in Africa. In USA the proportion of cases attributed to infection from bats has increased. Canine rabies was eradicated in Britain in 1922 and there have been no cases of rabies contracted in Britain since 1902, and the 21 recorded cases that have been treated here since, have been contracted abroad.

Transmission

Rabies is transmitted to man by inoculation of the virus in saliva from an infected animal through broken skin as the result of a bite. Non-bite transmission occurs very rarely—by aerosol inhalation in cavers visiting bat-infested caves, in laboratory workers, and by corneal transplantation from donors who had not been recognized to have the paralytic form of rabies. Human to human transmission of rabies has never been recognized, yet it remains a theoretical risk that a bite from a rabid patient could affect a medical attendant; so great care needs to be taken in nursing such people.

Following inoculation through the skin, the virus replicates locally, concentrates in the neuromuscular junction, enters the peripheral nerve axon via acetylcholine receptors and travels up the axon to the brain at a rate of approximately 3 mm/day. There it spreads to most areas of the brain and spinal cord and produces the clinical manifestations of the disease. It then disseminates throughout the body via the peripheral nerves, including those that go to the salivary glands, and is shed therefrom in saliva. Whether clinical infection follows a bite depends upon the severity of the bite (if shielded by clothing, penetration of the skin may be negligible), the viral load inoculated, the stage of the disease in the infecting animal and the location of the bite—bites nearer to the face and the brain produce symptoms quicker than bites to an extremity, and are more likely to result in clinical disease. About 15 per cent of bites from rabid dogs result in rabies in humans. Boys aged less than 15 years account for half of all cases and overall, about 80 per cent of cases are male.

After reaching the CNS virus replicates and spreads widely to produce a primary encephalomyelitis, with neuronal destruction, particularly affecting the brainstem, cerebral cortex, cerebellum, and Ammon's horn. The intraneural cytoplasmic eosinophilic inclusion body described by Negri is diagnostic and is found in 75 per cent of cases examined (Dupont and Earle 1965).

Incubation period

The incubation period of rabies in man varies enormously and cases have been described with onset of symptoms 1 week following exposure to several years later: up to six in a recent report (Smith et al. 1991). The average incubation period is between 3 weeks and 3 months in 90 per cent of cases when the time of the bite can be established accurately (Warrell 1976). It is shorter in children and in those with more severe bites to the head. In over 90 per cent of cases a history of a bite, usually from a dog, can be obtained (Lakhanpal and Sharma 1985). There is evidence that lack of a history of exposure is becoming more common, perhaps because the original bite seemed insignificant, took place too long before, was not recognized to be associated with rabies, or had been suppressed because of fear of treatment in children. The patient may be too ill to give a history and medical attendants may not suspect rabies (Smith et al. 1991). Consequent upon the massive increase in air travel, and international shifts of populations from war, pestilence, and political upheaval, it is necessary to consider rabies in the differential diagnosis of cases of encephalitis or of Guillain–Barré type polyneuropathy. Two cases of rabies presenting as encephalitis have been recognized in my practice in the UK in the past 20 years.

First symptoms

The first symptoms of rabies are entirely non-specific and may suggest flu—malaise, fever, chills, myalgia and headache, diarrhoea, nausea, and vomiting—and these may last for days. Discomfort, tingling, and pain at the site of the bite, now well-healed, are thought to indicate arrival of the virus at the spinal ganglion, to be followed within days by symptoms of cerebral involvement, hallucinations and nightmares, apprehension, depression, and agitation which progress to delirium, abnormal behaviour, and disruption of sleep pattern. Hallucinations, epileptic fits, and hyperventilation merge into the characteristic hydrophobic stage—the 'furious' form of the disease. It is important to recognize that in up to 20 per cent of cases the illness does not follow such a course, but results in spinal disturbance producing a clinical syndrome of the acute Guillain–Barré polyneuritic type—the 'dumb' form of the disease. It was from such cases which had not been recognized to be rabid, that corneas were removed for transplantation, with disastrous results.

Hydrophobia comes about from spasm of the pharyngeal and laryngeal muscles provoked by attempts to swallow, and in severe cases even by the sound of water or air wafting over the face. The spasms spread to other muscles and produce opisthotonos. The picture of hydrophobia, opisthotonos, convulsions, mania, and hyperexcitabilty is particularly distressing to relatives and attendants, more so because consciousness and awareness may be retained between times. Progression to coma and death within 10 days to a fortnight is inevitable. The average survival from onset is 18 days and this may be prolonged by a week with intensive care and ventilatory support. Raised ICP, autonomic dysfunction, and cardiac dysrythmia may require treatment. There have been reports of recovery from clinical rabies, but these have been questioned (Hattwick et al. 1972; Porras et al. 1976; Centers for Disease Control 1977). Each had received rabies vaccine.

Despite the current depressingly poor prognosis, earlier diagnosis and treatment may lead to a better outcome. All cases should be given the best available supportive treatment. They should be isolated. There is a theoretical risk that the disease may be transmitted to medical and nursing attendants so adequate protective clothing, including goggles, should be worn and all secretions should be regarded as potentially hazardous.

Diagnosis

The diagnosis of rabies on clinical grounds may be straightforward in a classical case when there is a history of an animal bite followed by the development of hydrophobia, but as often as not, and perhaps increasingly so, this is not immediately evident. The diagnosis should be considered in all cases of acute encephalitis, and of acute neuropathy especially if consciousness is clouded. Confirmation of the diagnosis requires demonstration of the virus in biopsy tissue, at necropsy, or on culture. Virus has been isolated from saliva, urine, and CSF. The preferred method of diagnosis at the time of writing is demonstration of rabies antigen by a fluorescent antibody technique on skin taken from a full thickness biopsy of the nape of the neck (Blenden et al. 1986). This is considered to be more sensitive and specific than fluorescent staining of cells obtained from corneal smears. Circulatory antibodies are seen within 10 days of clinical infection but interpretation may be difficult if postexposure immunization has been given. High levels of antibody in CSF probably reflect local production and are not seen following vaccination. The application of PCR to CSF promises to be useful in the diagnosis of rabies (DeBiasi and Tyler 1999).

Treatment

As soon as it is recognized that there has been exposure to a potentially rabid animal, by bite, scratch, or inhalation, postexposure treatment should be given. The wound should be thoroughly and vigorously cleansed with detergent and water to remove viral material before it reaches nerve endings. The wound should not be sutured provided it is not bleeding. Passive immunization should be induced by infiltrating the tissues surrounding the wound with human rabies immunoglobulin, and injecting the remainder into the buttock. Active immunity should be stimulated by injection of human diploid cell vaccine (HDVC) as soon as possible. Dosage schedules and precautions are to be found in Centers for Disease Control (1999) and can be downloaded from www.cdc.gov/ncidod/dvrd/rabies. Contacts, including nursing and medical staff treating patients with rabies should be given post-exposure prophylaxis (Mrak and Young 1994). Pre-exposure prophylaxis should be offered to those at risk such as veterinary workers, laboratory scientists, and animal handlers.

Once clinically evident, the treatment of rabies is supportive. There is no evidence that the use of corticosteroids, immune suppression, brain oedema reducing agents, interferon and other antiviral agents or antibiotics, has been of benefit in diagnosed cases. Antispastic agents, anticonvulsants, and muscle paralysing agents should be used as appropriate.

Prevention of rabies is a large and emotive topic tainted by politics and the activities of self-interested pressure groups. Fundamentally, it depends upon the control of animal reservoirs of infection. This may be achieved by immunizing domestic cats and dogs, by muzzling animals which may bite, and eliminating strays, and by subjecting animals introduced from abroad to a prolonged period of quarantine. Where such measures are not practicable the natives should be educated to avoid potentially dangerous animals, and measures should be instituted to maintain a barrier between sylvatic and enzootic rabies and the human population.

34.8 Encephalitis lethargica

This condition was first described by von Economo in 1917 and his name has been given to the disease—von Economo's encephalitis (see von Economo 1931). It probably first appeared in 1915 and during the following decade and a half, widespread epidemics occurred. The histological and epidemiological features of the disease have pointed to a viral, infectious aetiology but no virus has ever been isolated. It is probable that the disease has died out, certainly there has been no further epidemic. However, cases are still being described with similar clinical features (*Lancet* 1981; Rail *et al.* 1981; Blunt *et al.* 1997; Kun *et al.* 1999) and in the absence of an original, identified, causal agent, it cannot be denied that these may be cases of the same disease (Section 32.3.6). It seems likely that the clinical syndrome is defined more by the region of the brain which is affected, rather than the nature of the putative infecting organism, and that the aetiology of these cases is probably multifactorial.

The sexes were equally affected and no age group was exempt. Most cases occurred in early adult life, and during spring. The onset was acute, sometimes fulminant, with headache, malaise, myalgia, delirium, and convulsions. Less acute cases would develop a characteristic sleep disturbance with severe lethargy by day from which they could be roused, and insomnia by night. In a substantial and increasing proportion of cases the evolution of the condition would become chronic, and extrapyramidal manifestations would supervene, including frank parkinsonism with tremor, rigidity, and oculogyric crises. Some would have chorea or myoclonus. In the acute phase, pupillary abnormalities and disturbances of ocular movement were common. Epileptic seizures and signs of meningism were not common. CSF revealed no diagnostic features.

The pathological features were of diffuse congestion and oedema, occasionally with petechial haemorrhages, but these changes were seldom marked. Microscopy revealed neuronal degeneration with perivascular inflammatory change and infiltration with lymphocytes and plasma cells, most notably in substantia nigra, basal ganglia, and upper mid-brain grey matter, including the oculomotor nuclei.

Death rates varied, reaching 38.2 per cent in one large series, most patients died within the first month. Complete recovery occurred in only 25 per cent. Mental sequelae were common and included dementia in 25 per cent, depression, bradyphrenia and bradykinesis, and inability to concentrate. Varying degrees of parkinsonism were common, often associated with oculogyric crises, and lethargy. Relapses of the acute attack were recorded up to 20 years later. No treatment regime has been shown to be consistently beneficial—steroids have benefited two recent cases (Blunt *et al.* 1997).

34.9 Measles and subacute sclerosing panencephalitis

Measles is a highly infectious disease that affects children and young adults throughout the world. Before the development of an effective vaccine, 99 per cent of the population had been affected by the age of 20 and had antibodies to prove it, and this remains the case in Third World countries. Formerly a disease that affected the 5–9 years age group in the main, since the introduction of successful immunization, teenagers are more frequently infected. In the developing world, where there is little immunization, and where there is much malnutrition, measles devastates the under twos with a mortality of up to 10 per cent. Infection confers lifelong immunity.

Measles virus is an RNA virus and a member of the Paramyxoviridae, related to canine distemper virus and to rinderpest. It is possible for the virus of measles and canine distemper to persist in the CNS and produce chronic neurological disease. Measles appears to be an antigenically stable virus and the development of neurological complications was thought to be due variations in host susceptibility, age, and immune status, rather than to viral properties. However, there is now evidence that the virus found in cases of subacute sclerosing panencephalitis (SSPE) differs from wild virus because it has a deficient M protein, one of the virus-specific structural proteins. Antibody to M protein is low, while the antibody response to N and P proteins is particularly robust.

Measles is spread by aerosol droplets and respiratory inhalation and perhaps through the conjunctiva. Virus travels through the reticulo-endothelial system and the circulation. After an incubation period of 10 days, fever, malaise, conjunctival suffusion, and coryza appear. Koplik's spots, the pathognomonic sign of measles, appear as raised spots with white centres in the buccal and lower labial mucosa, fading as the rash develops at about 14 days on the face and behind the ears, and spreads centrifugally to involve the trunk and then the extremities. After 3 or 4 days the rash begins to fade, antibody is formed, and most patients make a good and complete recovery. Complications of measles are rare and include secondary infection of the rash, pneumonia, myocarditis, pericarditis, hepatitis, and neurological syndromes.

Neurological complications of measles which have been described are polyneuritis, transverse myelitis, acute hemiplegia, toxic encephalopathy and cerebellar ataxia, post-infectious encephalomyelitis, subacute inclusion body encephalitis (or measles inclusion body encephalitis), and SSPE (Ford 1928; Tyler 1957; Aarli 1974). Of these, post-infectious encephalitis accounts for 95 per cent. It occurs in patients with a normal immune system and who are over 2 years of age. The incidence approximates to 1 : 1000 of measles cases and rises with age. Subacute inclusion body encephalitis occurs in the immune compromised of any age and afflicts 1 in 10 of such patients who are affected by measles. SSPE occurs once in a million cases of measles and affects immunologically competent individuals, with a predilection for those less than 2 years.

Post-infectious measles encephalitis

Post-infectious measles encephalitis affects males and females equally. Signs begin to develop within 8 days of the onset, as the exanthem begins to subside. Fever recurs and encephalitis develops rapidly with convulsions, abnormal movements, focal paresis, ataxia, myoclonus, paraparesis and rarely, a pure myelitis (Johnson et al. 1984). Approximately 15 per cent die and more than 50 per cent have serious neurological sequelae. In contrast, uncomplicated measles carries a very good prognosis for complete recovery despite the observation that more than 50 per cent of children with measles have EEG abnormalities.

The pathological findings of post-infectious measles encephalitis share similar features with other viral post-infectious encephalitides—perivenous demyelination, gliosis, perivascular cuffing and in more severe cases, a frank haemorrhagic leucoencephalitis. The pathogenesis is thought to be similar to that of experimental allergic encephalomyelitis—an autoimmune demyelinating disease triggered by measles. Measles virus has only rarely been found in brain and it seems likely that the presence of virus triggers an abnormal immuno-regulatory response to myelin basic protein.

Subacute measles encephalitis occurs only in those who have been immune suppressed, most frequently children who have had leukaemia or lymphoma and have been irradiated. After an

attack of measles, some 2–6 months later, symptoms insidiously develop. Lethargy, mental confusion, epileptic seizures, myoclonus, and diffuse cerebral dysfunction, often affecting the parietal lobes, progress relentlessly to death in a few months (Hughes et al. 1993; Mustafa et al. 1993). Pathologically, inflammatory changes are seen throughout the brain and eosinophilic inclusions have been identified in the nuclei of neurones. Antibody titres are low or absent, which reflects immune suppression. Virus antigen has been found in brain tissue. EEG, CSF, and brain imaging show normal findings or non-specific changes only. With increased frequency of measles immunization in a population, this complication has markedly receded.

Subacute sclerosing panencephalitis

Subacute sclerosing panencephalitis (SSPE) has rejoiced in a plethora of names in the past including 'inclusion body encephalitis, nodular panencephalitis, subacute sclerosing leucoencephalitis' and finally 'subacute sclerosing panencephalitis'. A viral cause was postulated and Bouteille et al. (1965) demonstrated paramyxovirus structures in brain inclusion bodies. Two years later measles virus was cultivated from brain tissue and final confirmation of the relationship of measles to SSPE was obtained by the passage of the disease to animals (Katz et al. 1968). It is still not understood why SSPE, a progressive and fatal disease of the brain, should develop in a very small number of all the patients affected by measles every year. It is not known whether CNS infection occurs at the time of primary measles infection and simmers on for years before producing clinical signs, or whether it lies dormant in a site outside the CNS and spreads to the CNS not long before clinical signs become apparent. It seems likely that the former occurs, with virus entering the brain, probably by infection of cerebral capillary endothelium—measles virus containing immune complexes have been found in blood vessel wall (Kirk et al. 1991)—and mutates to a less invasive and more persistent form, which has defective coding for M protein. It seems likely that the persisting viral infection triggers an immune-mediated response which is responsible for the widespread demyelination.

The incidence of SSPE varies from country to country. It occurs 3–4 times more frequently in boys than girls, in younger children in a family, in rural rather than urban communities, and in lower socio-economic groups. All racial groups are affected and it seems that there is a higher incidence around the eastern Mediterranean littoral and in Arabs. Where effective immunization programmes have been introduced, SSPE is disappearing. Lack of measles immunization induces a significant risk factor (Miller et al. 1992). There does not seem to be a genetic predisposition.

The most important risk factor for the development of SSPE is suffering from measles at an early age, particularly within the first year of life. Almost all children with SSPE have a history of measles or measles immunization, and in those who do not, there is a history of household contact. The risk of contracting

SSPE after measles is of the order of 5–9 cases per million and drops to one-tenth following measles immunization.

SSPE is a disease of children who have been healthy. The average age of onset is 8–10 years and symptoms appear on average, 7 years after full recovery from measles. Ninety per cent of cases occur before the age of 16. The onset is insidious and may be recognized only in retrospect—emotional lability, behavioural alteration, impairment of scholastic performance, clumsiness, cognitive defects, ataxia, and epileptic seizures. The onset of myoclonic jerks that may be focal and soon become generalized, heralds the second stage of the disease. They become frequent and repetitive and correlate with the giant complexes seen on EEG (Fig. 2.12) (Yakub 1996). They may be provoked by sensory stimuli. Pyramidal and extrapyramidal signs with dystonia and dyskinesia appear. Akinetic seizures are common and there is inexorable progression to a vegetative state with dementia, decortication, and decerebration. Rarely, this may be interrupted by remission and exceptionally by stabilization of the disease. Progression is highly variable. Death may occur within weeks of onset, about half die within a year and most die within 2 years. Perhaps 4 per cent achieve remission (Risk and Haddad 1979).

Once myoclonus is evident the clinical diagnosis seldom presents difficulty and investigations provide confirmatory results. The EEG is genuinely useful with high voltage stereotyped slow wave complexes, often synchronous with clinical myoclonus, repeating every 8–10 s. CT and MR brain scans are not diagnostic and may show white matter change and atrophy. CSF examination is most useful and demonstrates great elevation of the gamma globulin fraction of the protein content due to the presence of measles antibody which is found in high concentration in unconcentrated fluid. PCR is reported to be useful (DeBiasi and Tyler 1999).

At necropsy, changes are evident in white and grey matter with neuronal degeneration, gliosis, proliferation of atrocytes, perivascular cuffing, lymphocytic and plasma cell infiltration and demyelination. Type A intranuclear inclusions are found in oligodendroglia and neurones. The changes are non-specific.

Treatment of the neurological complications of measles has not been effective in altering the natural history of the disease. All syndromes are treated symptomatically and general supportive treatment with anticonvulants, and haloperidol for behavioural upset, is given. Steroids, antiviral agents, and interferon have not been beneficial. SSPE is so infrequent that proper trials of the effects of treatment on its natural history have not been possible. Recent evidence suggests that alpha-interferon does not help (Fayad *et al.* 1997).

It is now well established that immunization against measles is effective and protects against neurological complications. Several vaccines are now available which are live attenuated strains, and now measles is combined with mumps and rubella in the 'MMR' vaccine. Both cellular and humoral responses are generated and seroconversion occurs in over 95 per cent of cases. The optimal age for immunization is after 15 months but in poorer communities, it may be necessary to immunize

within the first 12 months as maternal antibodies decline. There are few contra-indications to measles immunization. It may be given to HIV-positive children but probably should not be given to those who are severely immunocompromised.

34.10 Progressive multifocal leucoencephalopathy

Progressive multifocal leucoencephalopathy (PMLE) is the only neurological disease in humans caused by a papovavirus. It is an uncommon and almost always, fatal condition which affects hosts with defects of cellular immunity. It was first described by Astrom *et al.* (1958) as a complication of lymphoreticular disease.

Further reports recognized that other diseases associated with immune suppression such as sarcoidosis, carcinomatosis, organ transplantation, and immunosuppressive drug regimes, were associated with PMLE. It remained a rare condition until it was recognized that it was an increasingly frequent complication of AIDS, which reduces cell-mediated immunity, and is now recognized to be a major risk factor for PMLE. Cavenagh *et al.* (1959) suggested that PMLE may be caused by a virus, and Zu Rhein and Chou (1965), and Silverman and Rubinstein (1965), separately showed with the electron microscope that the oligodendrocytic inclusions were packed with virions which were morphologically similar to papovaviruses ('papova' derives from the first syllable of the names of the major sub-varieties of this type of DNA virus: the wart virus, *pa*pilloma; an oncogenic virus, *po*lyoma; and the *va*cuolating viruses). Padgett *et al.* (1971) grew and characterized a previously unknown polyoma virus from the brain of a patient with PMLE and named it the 'JC' virus after the initials of the patient's name. (This JC virus has nothing to do with Jakob–Creutzfeld disease.) Subsequent studies have confirmed that PMLE is caused by JC virus infection. Other patients with PMLE have been described where it was thought that Simian Virus 40 (SV40) was the cause, but it has since been shown that the SV40 isolates were contaminants from the monkey kidney cell lines employed.

On the basis of sero-epidemiological studies, exposure to JC virus is ubiquitous among adults of all races in the world. Seroconversion takes place during childhood and does not result in disease unless the subject becomes immune deficient. PMLE is the only disease known to be caused by the JC virus. The kidney is the site of latent JC virus infection and it is thought that when the immune system is suppressed, JC virus enters the circulation and travels to the brain, lung, and lymphoreticular system (Houff *et al.* 1988). In brain the oligodendrocytes become loaded with virus, with resultant cell destruction that leads to the breakdown of the myelin sheath and to the patchy demyelination which is so characteristic of the condition. It has been postulated that PMLE is due to reactivation of latent, previously, non-pathogenic JC virus infection. Mori *et al.* (1991) found evidence of JC virus DNA in oligodendroglia and astrocytes of elderly patients who had no evidence of PMLE. Others have found JC virus DNA in the brains of people, some of whom had AIDS and others did not, and who had no evidence of PMLE (Elsner and Dorries 1992; Quinlivan *et al.* 1992).

Pathology

The pathology of PMLE is characteristic. The JC virus produces a lysing infection of oligodendroglia which become large and spherical and have large inclusions. Astrocytes alter and show changes which are seen in malignancy. Inflammatory change is absent or minimal. There are multiple foci of white matter demyelination which coalesce as they enlarge. They are scattered throughout the cerebral hemispheres, cerebellum, and brainstem, and their location determines the clinical features. Initially they are most common at the junction of white and grey matter (which supports the notion that the virus reaches the brain by the bloodstream), and unlike multiple sclerosis the sub-pial and subependymal zones are relatively spared.

PMLE is found throughout the world and it may rarely occur in childhood. Prior to AIDS it was a very rare disease of the middle aged and elderly. Sufferers had conditions which reduced cellular immunity—carcinoma, lymphoreticular malignancy including Hodgkin's disease, lymphosarcoma and chronic lymphatic leukaemia, granulomatous conditions such as TB and sarcoidosis—or had been organ transplant recipients or patients treated with immunosuppressive drugs. In a few cases, no underlying condition was identified (Faris and Martinez 1972). With the evolution of AIDS, the picture changed. Now it is much more common and affects about 4 per cent of people with AIDS and is frequently the initial AIDS-defining illness (Berger *et al.* 1987).

Clinical features

The clinical features of PMLE are determined by the area of the brain which is involved in the pathological process. The onset is insidious and often difficult to recognize, even in retrospect, especially when it occurs in the evolution of an established predisposing disease. Much less commonly, PMLE may be the presenting manifestation of a previously undiagnosed illness which causes immune suppression, and rarely, the onset may be explosive and leads to the rapid demise of the patient. Such an explosive onset is seen more frequently in patients with AIDS. The progression of PMLE is relentless with a median survival reduced to 2–4 months. In 10 per cent the course is slightly more benign and exceptionally, survival may be for years. In patients who do not have AIDS, remissions have been reported (Price *et al.* 1983). The most common symptoms and signs are mental disturbance, and impairment of awareness and of consciousness. Multiple enlarging, but not space-occupying, lesions of white matter give rise to hamiparesis, parietal syndromes, visual pathway upset, pseudobulbar palsy, cortical blindness, dementia, and epileptic seizures; less commonly the white matter of the brainstem and cerebellum is affected with ataxia,

nystagmus, and bulbar palsies. Raised ICP is seldom a problem and headache is uncommon.

In the setting of established disease with immune suppression, such as lymphoma and AIDS, it will be readily understood that the clinical picture may also be caused by several other pathologies—metastatic carcinoma, or infection, other viral opportunistic infections or toxoplasmosis in AIDS. Further investigation is therefore necessary to confirm the diagnosis of PMLE.

Diagnosis

Brain imaging with CT, or preferably with more sensitive MRI (Fig. 34.2), reveals widespread, multiple, and often confluent, non-enhancing white matter lesions that do not occupy space (Berger *et al.* 1987; Whiteman *et al.* 1993). CSF examination is usually unremarkable or it may show a slight pleocytosis and some rise of the protein content. It is now possible to detect and crudely quantify JC virus in CSF and this may correlate with survival rates (Yiannoutsos *et al.* 1999). It is frequently necessary to resort to brain biopsy to diagnose PMLE, and also to exclude other pathologies such as lymphoma and other infection in AIDS patients. The characteristic pathological changes can usually be seen with light microscopy and virus particles can be seen with the electron microscope. A variety of immunocytological techniques and PCR can be used to demonstrate JC virus in tissue samples.

Treatment

Treatment of PMLE remains disappointing. Corticosteroids, cytosine arabinoside, transfer factor and other agents have not been effective. There is recent, unconfirmed evidence that survival time may be extended in AIDS patients with PMLE if they are given protease inhibitors (Dworkin *et al.* 1999).

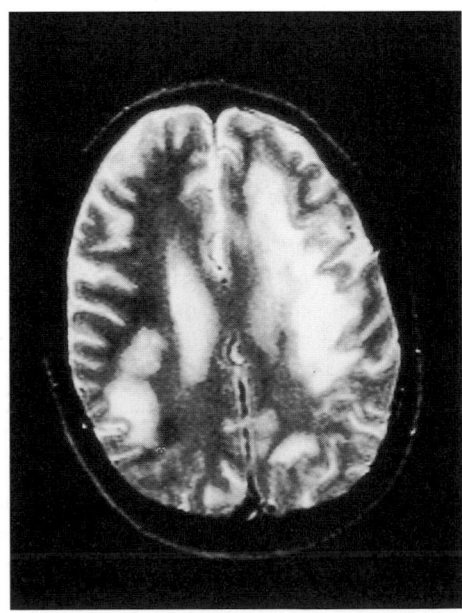

Fig. 34.2. Progressive multifocal leucoencephalopathy, showing widespread, multiple white matter lesions on MRI.

34.11 Retroviruses and HIV encephalopathy

Retroviruses are single stranded RNA viruses with reverse transcriptase activity which leads to DNA transcription of the virus and integration in the host genome where virus can lie dormant and escape immune attack. Two retroviruses cause neurological disease in humans, HTLV-I virus and HIV. Other retroviruses have been associated with human diseases but a causal relationship has not been confirmed. There are three sub-families of retroviruses—oncoviruses, spuma viruses, and lentiviruses. HTLV-I is an oncovirus and HIV is a lentivirus and they cause HTLV-I associated myelopathy (HAM) and AIDS, respectively. HAM and AIDS encephalopathy are discussed here, the neurological complications of AIDS are discussed in Section 35.3.

34.11.1 HTLV-I associated myelopathy (HAM)

HTLV-I associated myelopathy (HAM) is also known as tropical spastic paraparesis (TSP) (Section 20.6.4). The latter term was coined by Mani et al. (1969) to describe a spastic paraplegic syndrome in India which was similar to the spastic form of Jamaican neuropathy which had been described by Cruickshank (1956) and Montgomery et al. (1964). The syndrome has a far wider geographical distribution than was first suspected: cases have been described from the USA, Caribbean islands, Central and South America, Japan and the Far East, India, and Central and South Africa. In Europe it is found in immigrants from the Caribbean in Britain, France, and Italy (Bucher et al. 1990). In 1985 IgG antibodies to HTLV-I were found in the sera of 59 per cent of patients from Martinique with TSP and shortly after, antibodies to HTLV-I were found in the CSF and sera of Jamaican patients with TSP. At much the same time a myelopathy associated with HTLV-I infection was found in an endemic area in southern Japan, and was noted to be identical to TSP (Rodgers-Johnson et al. 1985). The clinical syndrome is now known as HAM (HTLV-I associated myelopathy).

HTLV-I is a type-C lymphotropic retrovirus which has a predilection for T4 lymphocytes. The virion is 110–140 nm in diameter, has a spherical core, and a Mg^{2+}-dependent reverse transcriptase of molecular weight >100 000. Lymphocytes which become infected are capable of indefinite growth and express specific surface viral antigens. The receptor has not yet been identified and transmission is from cell to cell. HTLV-I was first isolated from a patient with a cutaneous T-cell lymphoma and it soon became recognized that HTLV-I was associated with a unique form of adult T-cell leukaemia/lymphoma (ATL). Antibodies to HTLV-I were found to be prevalent in areas where ATL was endemic, particularly in Japan, and in the West Indies where the association between HTLV-I and TSP was made by Gessain et al. (1985). This association has been confirmed in many other areas of the world where HAM is found, and the geographical distribution of HAM is roughly co-terminous with that of ATL. ATL and HAM have been described in the same patient and the same strain of HTLV-I retrovirus has been isolated from separate patients with HAM and ATL.

It is now generally accepted that HTLV-I is the causal agent of HAM because there is intrathecal synthesis of antibody against HTLV-I and oligoclonal immunoglobulin bands in CSF react with viral antigen; virus has been isolated from cultured peripheral blood and CSF mononuclear cells; HTLV-I nucleic acid sequences have been identified in blood and CSF cells and viral antigen has been detected in CSF; and viral RNA has been detected in astrocytes in the CNS (Lehky et al. 1995). The epidemiology of HAM and HTLV-1 infection has been determined by using serological antibody detection. There is distinct geographical variation in the incidence of HTLV-I positivity and HAM. Southern Japan, the Caribbean, clusters in Panama, the Pacific coast of Colombia, and other areas of South America and equatorial regions of Africa, all have high rates. Studies of migrant populations demonstrate that infection is often acquired early in life and can travel with the individual to non-endemic areas to cause the disease decades later.

Seropositivity rates vary from up to 10 per cent in regions of Japan, 5 per cent in Jamaica, Barbados, and Haiti, 6 per cent in Venezuela, and 1–2 per cent of blacks in the southern USA. Among whites, only intravenous drug abusers show high levels of antibodies (Bucher et al. 1990). An age-dependent rise in seropositivity is a consistent finding in all groups studied, with a peak at 65. There is a low rate of myelopathy in relation to the frequency of seropositivity and it has been estimated that HTLV-I positive people have a less than 1 per cent chance of developing ATL or HAM. It has been suggested that these observations may be explained by cumulative exposure to an agent of low infectivity over the individual's lifetime. Disease expression is probably modified by genetic factors, environmental factors, or other acquired host factors.

The method of transmission is not evident in most cases. It can be passed on sexually from female to male, male to female most commonly, and male to male: from mother to child *in utero*, through breast milk, and via blood transfusion and intravenous drug abuse. (This last method is important for the transmission of HTLV-II.) Infected cells are transmitted in the blood, concentrate in regional lymph nodes, and disseminate through the body. How they infect the CNS is not known for sure: possibilities include direct infection of endothelial cells by virus in the blood, or by invasion of infected marrow derived lymphocytes. There is no evidence to implicate an insect vector in transmission. The length of time between infection and the declaration of diseases is not known in the naturally occurring form of the disease, and may be as short as 6 months if it is transmitted by blood (Kaplan et al. 1991).

How the neurological syndrome is produced is not known. It could be that the virus induces a host response which triggers mechanisms causing tissue injury, or an immune response from ongoing activation of immune cells, or there may be a direct toxic effect of the virus on oligodendroglia and astrocytes. The neuropathological changes seen in HAM are essentially those of chronic progressive inflammation. The changes predominate in, but are not confined to, the spinal cord and the brunt falls on the thoracic cord. The meninges surrounding the cord are thickened (Iwasaki 1990). Chronic meningo-encephalitis with perivascular cuffing and fibrosis, reactive astrocytic gliosis, and severe demyelination of pyramidal tracts and posterolateral columns leading to axonal loss, may all occur. Vasculitis and immune complex deposition in small vessels have also been described. Medulla, pons, and white matter of cerebrum and cerebellum may also have inflammatory changes.

Clinical manifestations

The clinical manifestations of HAM are of insidious onset and so may be difficult to interpret in the early stages. It may rarely be seen in childhood but usually occurs after the age of 30 with a peak age of clinical onset after 40 years. Females predominate with a 2 : 1 bias, and HAM is found in all socio-economic groups. There is difficulty with walking due to spasticity and weakness of the legs, usually symmetrical, with sensory symptoms of painful paraesthesiae in the legs, often with low back pain. Sphincter upset is common and is often an early feature. The course is slowly progressive over months and years and there are no remissions and no acute relapses. The physical signs are those of a spastic paraparesis with mild sensory loss, sphincter upset, and sometimes hyperreflexia of the upper limbs. Less commonly, cerebellar signs and evidence of cerebral and cranial nerve have been noted. The course is insidious over months and years in more than 75 per cent. The range is from 6 months to 26 years with an average of 8 years (Bucher *et al.* 1990). In addition to the features of myelopathy, some cases have been described with lower motor neurone features when the disease may mimic amyotrophic lateral sclerosis.

Diagnosis

The diagnosis of HAM is suggested by finding a chronic myelopathy in a person who lives in or who has migrated from an endemic area. MR imaging of the spine will exclude spinal compression and will demonstrate atrophy of the spinal cord and high intensity T2 weighted lesions in the cord. At least 50 per cent have lesions in brain white matter (Kira *et al.* 1988; Alcindor *et al.* 1992). Lesions have been found in the brain on MR scanning of people who have positive serology for HTLV-I and have no neurological signs. The EEG may show non-specific slow wave abnormalities and visual, somatosensory, and brainstem auditory evoked response estimates may be prolonged. Most patients are seropositive to HTLV-I. PCR may be necessary to distinguish positive results from HTLV-II in intravenous drug addicts. CSF examination may be normal but is more likely to demonstrate a raised mononuclear cell count and protein level. Over 70 per cent of cases have raised levels of intrathecal IgG antibody and HTLV-I specific antibodies are demonstrated in virtually all cases. CSF neopterin levels are raised in 55 per cent of cases in the CSF but only in 10 per cent of sera which suggests that there is a greater level of immune activation in the CNS than peripherally. A specific PCR test is available for CSF (DeBiasi and Tyler 1999).

Differential diagnosis

The differential diagnosis of HAM includes other myelopathies and causes of white matter lesions in the brain. Spinal compression is excluded by MR imaging, and if that is not available, by myelography. Weight is given to the suspected diagnosis if the patient lives in or has migrated from an endemic area, or if the patient has been exposed to blood transfusion, or if the patient abuses drugs.

Tropical ataxic neuropathies in Africa are usually associated with painful sensory loss and dermatitis, occur in relation to malnutrition, and are linked to ingestion of cassava and subsequent cyanide intoxication. Acute tropical spastic paraparesis may be linked to lathyrism in the Indian sub-continent or malnutrition or malabsorption in Africa. The spinal from of multiple sclerosis (MS) may be exactly like HAM—relapses and remissions and the occurrence of optic neuritis favour MS. Brain and spinal cord imaging can be very similar in the two conditions. AIDS may also cause a myelopathy and AIDS shares common epidemiological features with HTLV-I infection—sexual transmission, spread by blood transfusion and intravenous drug abuse, and mother to child infection. Dual infection with HTLV-I and HIV has been described in AIDS patients with myelopathy and the myelopathy has been of HAM type. It has been suggested that the presence of HIV increases the likelihood of the development of HAM in a person with both infections (Berger *et al.* 1991). The diagnosis of HAM requires the demonstration of specific antibody or virus or virus genes in spinal fluid or CSF cells.

Treatment

Treatment of HAM has been disappointing. Corticosteroids have not produced consistent improvement. There are recent reports of improvement following treatment with high dose alpha-interferon, but the numbers are small (Yamasaki *et al.* 1997). Immunomodulation, AZT, plasmaphoresis, and other treatments have not been consistently effective. The natural history of HAM is slow and progressive over many years, with increasing spasticity and eventually, a wheelchair existence. In several patients, the disease arrests.

34.11.2 HIV encephalopathy

Acquired immune deficiency syndrome (AIDS) was first recognized as a clinical syndrome in June 1981 when outbreaks of pneumonia caused by *Pneumocystis carinii*, and the occurrence of Kaposi's sarcoma, were described in previously healthy young homosexual men in the USA. It soon became evident that there was an epidemic of an immune-suppressive disease which was seen in homosexual males, intravenous drug abusers, haemophiliacs and others, and rendered the sufferers liable to life-threatening infection with opportunistic organisms, and to Kaposi's sarcoma and other forms of neoplasm. An infectious agent was suspected and in 1983, a retrovirus was isolated from a French patient with lymphadenopathy, found to be a retrovirus and was designated lymphadenopathy associated virus (LAV) (Barre-Sinoussi *et al.* 1983). The same group coined the term 'Human T-cell Lymphotropic Virus' to encompass a family of related viruses including leukaemia and AIDS retroviruses. The virus which they had isolated was confirmed as the cause of AIDS and was eventually designated Human Immunodeficiency Virus (HIV-1). A second retrovirus with some genomic differences has been isolated from AIDS patients from West Africa and termed HIV-2.

As more cases of AIDS were identified, it became evident that many patients with HIV infection had milder syndromes of prodromal immunodeficiency, persistent generalized lymphadenopathy (PGL) and AIDS-related complex (ARC), which would progress after a variable period to full-blown AIDS. The distinction between these syndromes has become blurred and their prognostic significance has diminished. It is now recognized that HIV infection impairs the response of the immune system and this results in a progression of disease from the initial stages with no symptoms through opportunistic infections of increasing severity and the development of malignancies and the full-blown clinical syndrome of AIDS. A description of the classification and clinical manifestation of AIDS is beyond the scope of this chapter and the reader is referred to specialist texts.

Following initial HIV infection, there is a phase of viraemia with a high plasma virus load. Virus attaches to T lymphocytes and macrophages via the CD 4 receptor. There is then a clinical lull that lasts for years, during which virus replicates at a slower rate and reduces the CD 4 lymphocyte count. As these cells become depleted to dangerous levels, virus replication increases, immunity becomes further deranged, and opportunistic infections and malignancies occur in the full-blown syndromes of AIDS. Arbitrarily, these phases may be correlated with the CD 4 cell count. The first, acute phase with seroconversion occurs within weeks of infection when the CD 4 count is normal. The lull phase, when the CD 4 count remains above 500/cmm, may last for years. When the count falls below 500/cmm, systemic complications begin to appear with increasing severity, until the count drops below 200/cmm, at which stage major opportunistic infection occurs. Factors which influence the severity and the rate of development of AIDS are not fully understood, and include the strain and virulence of the virus, the presence of concurrent viral infection such as with CMV, EBV, and herpes viruses which may facilitate entry of HIV to cells, and genetic factors—some individuals who have not developed HIV infection despite high risk and sustained exposure have been found to have a homozygous deletion of the CKR5 receptor which makes their cells less pervious to HIV. Modern treatment regimes have led to a reduction of viral load and prolongation of survival.

Following infection, most patients generate an immune response with antibody production to a wide range of viral structural proteins. Most of the standard serological assay techniques can be employed to detect HIV antibody. HIV RNA can be detected in a quantitative fashion by the application of PCR and has been further refined by incorporation of branched DNA amplification methods. It is possible now to monitor the viral load accurately, and this correlates well with disease activity and with the response to anti-retroviral treatment (Mellors *et al.* 1996).

Most cases of HIV infection have been contracted by virus inoculation from infected body fluids, or tissues, usually blood or semen, through sexual intercourse, intravenous drug administration, transfusion of contaminated blood products, and by transplacental transmission from mother to child. The epidemiology of AIDS is changing. Formerly a disease of male homosexuals and drug addicts, then of people who had received contaminated blood products, it is now spreading by heterosexual activity throughout the world, with the highest rates of increase in Africa and Asia.

HIV virus

The HIV virus is neurotropic and invasion of the nervous system occurs at an early stage. As many as 70 per cent of people with HIV infection will have clinical neurological disease, and this may occur at any stage (Levy *et al.* 1985). As many as 90 per cent of patients who die with AIDS will have neuropathological changes at necropsy (Kure *et al.* 1991). It may stem from direct infection of any part of the nervous system by the virus causing a primary meningitis, encephalitis, myelitis, peripheral neuritis, or myopathy. Secondary involvement of the nervous system occurs as a consequence of immune suppression permitting the development of primary or secondary brain neoplasia, or the development of CNS infection from a wide host of organisms, chief amongst which are toxoplasmosis, CMV infection, PMLE, and fungal meningitis. In this chapter, HIV encephalopathy is described. The other neurological complications of AIDS are dealt with in Section 35.3.

Primary HIV infection

Primary HIV infection is followed at about the time of seroconversion 2–6 weeks later by a flu-like syndrome. This resembles infectious mononucleosis, occurs in a variable, but high, proportion of patients, and is often associated with malaise, lymphadenopathy, and a rash. In about 10 per cent of these cases there is a self-limiting aseptic meningitis, or less commonly, mild encephalitis (Carne *et al.* 1985; Schacker *et al.* 1996). HIV RNA may be demonstrated in blood and CSF.

Dementia

Not long after AIDS was first described, it was recognized that patients would develop neurological dysfunction which could not be attributed to infection or to neoplasia. A progressive dementing illness was recognized and has been called HIV dementia, HIV encephalopathy, AIDS-dementia complex, and most recently, HIV-associated major cognitive/motor disorder (Janssen *et al.* 1991; Navia *et al.* 1986*a*). It is difficult to know the exact frequency of occurrence of the syndrome, not least because it is likely that some cases may go undiagnosed because the signs may be subtle and similar syndromes may be caused by concurrent encephalitides. A reasonable estimate would be that it affects at least 10–20 per cent of AIDS patients, the more advanced AIDS is, the higher the incidence of encephalopathy, and the more clinically severe. Rarely it can be the only and presenting feature of AIDS. It is one of the subcortical dementias and occurs most often in those whose CD 4 cell counts have fallen below 200/cmm and who already have AIDS. By the terminal stages of AIDS with CD 4 counts below 50/cmm almost all patients will have signs of AIDS encephalopathy.

With more subtle neuropsychological and neurophysiological assessment techniques it is possible to demonstrate mild cognitive defects in early HIV infection (Wilkie *et al.* 1990). Not all agree that such subtle abnormalities do herald decline into frank encephalopathy. In a recent study, a battery of investigations failed to demonstrate significant neurological deterioration in HIV patients until they developed AIDS and had a CD 4 count below 350/cmm (Harrison *et al.* 1998). In children, an encephalopathic presentation often appears before opportunistic infections, and is associated with developmental delay, microcephaly, and progressive motor disturbance with pseudobulbar palsy and sometimes with seizures (Scott 1991). In the beginning, the syndrome affects cognition then motor function becomes disturbed. The patient often has no complaints, attention has been drawn to apathy, lack of drive, mental slowing, difficulty with concentration, and poor memory, by family members and friends. This is followed by more obvious cognitive defects, decline in work performance, depression, and frustration. Often, the responses are slow and there is difficulty in formulating verbal replies and motor responses. Disruption of sleep rhythm, lack of sexual drive, and sometimes seizures occur. Subtle motor signs may be found on examination—mild dysdiadochokinesis, general hyper-reflexia, and the appearance of primitive reflexes, snout, pout, and grasp. Progression to a full-blown subcortical dementia ensues, paralleled by motor decline. Weakness may be spastic or extrapyramidal, some exhibit movement disorders, including myoclonus and marked ataxia of gait. Eye movement impairment is common. Deterioration is inexorable and leads to a vegetative state. Other manifestations of AIDS are often evident including wasting, lymphadenopathy, and alopecia.

Other neurological manifestations

Other neurological manifestations of AIDS commonly co-exist in patients with AIDS encephalopathy. These include myelopathy, opportunistic infection with toxoplasma, CMV, herpes, and PMLE which can cause a similar encephalitic picture, space occupying syndromes from abscess, granuloma, or tumour, metabolic encephalopathies, and cerebrovascular syndromes. Investigations are therefore directed to exclude or confirm the presence of these other syndromes, as much as they are to identify AIDS encephalopathy. MR brain scanning is obligatory to exclude these conditions. The findings in AIDS encephalopathy are not diagnostic and range from normal brain appearances through mild general atrophic changes with large ventricles and generous sulci, to gross cerebral atrophy and diffuse or focal white matter signal change (Levy *et al.* 1986; Olesen *et al.* 1988). Electroencephalography is no more specific than brain imaging.

CSF examination is not diagnostic and is necessary to determine if other infections co-exist. The cell count and protein content may be raised, HIV-specific antibody and oligoclonal bands are commonly present, and viral RNA can be demonstrated and quantified. Unfortunately, none of these findings confirms that the neurological syndrome is caused by HIV. Several surrogate markers in CSF for HIV encephalopathy have been assessed including neopterin, B2 microglobulin, tumour necrosis factor, and matrix metalloproteinases, and none has been shown to date to be useful in clinical practice.

Treatment

Treatment of HIV encephalopathy is now possible. Zidovudine, a nucleoside reverse transcriptase inhibitor, has been shown to produce improvement (Sidtis *et al.* 1993). Preliminary reports suggest that combinations of nucleoside reverse transcriptase inhibitors with protease inhibitors or with non-nucleoside reverse transcriptase inhibitors may be more effective.

34.12 Prion diseases

34.12.1 General considerations

The term 'prion' was coined by Prusiner in 1982 and referred to a *pro*teinaceous *in*fectious particle that he believed the agent which caused scrapie to be (Prusiner 1982). Scrapie is the name given in Scotland to a fatal disease of sheep which has been recognized for hundreds of years. Similar diseases have now been found in other animals—mink, deer, elk, kudu, puma, cheetah, domestic cats, and others, and in cattle, in the form of bovine spongiform encephalopathy. These diseases all share similar pathological features of brain histology—spongiform change in the cerebral hemispheres—and they have been found to be transmissible by inoculation into the same or other species. Since the 1920s spongiform change has been recognized in the brains of people dying from a form of rapidly progressive dementia described separately by Creutzfeldt and Jakob, now Creutzfeldt–Jakob disease (CJD), in a familial form of dementia with ataxia now known as the Gerstmann–Straussler–Scheinker syndrome (GSS), and in a curious form of progressive dementia associated with movement disorder, in a particular region of Papua New Guinea and known locally as 'Kuru'. In addition to their pathological similarities, these conditions have all shared the property of transmissibility to primates. The exact nature of the infectious agents has not yet been fully categorized, nor has the relationship of the human diseases to their animal counterparts. However, enough information now exists to suggest that this group of diseases is caused, or triggered by, a novel group of infectious agents, now called prions; and the changes which they induce in susceptible hosts to produce disease, are being unravelled. All of the spongiform encephalopathies have abnormal forms of prion protein (PrP) as constituents of the amyloid plaques which are found in the brain. One and possibly, two new diseases of humans have been added to this list recently, fatal familial insomnia (FFI) and new variant Creutzfeldt–Jakob disease (NVCJD). FFI is described elsewhere, descriptions of the other conditions follow.

34.12.2 Scrapie, kuru, and bovine spongiform encephalopathy

Scrapie

Scrapie is a disease of sheep that has been known to shepherds for centuries in Britain and on mainland Europe. It has many names which vary with locality, and the Scottish name, scrapie, is now the most widely used. It is found in sheep throughout the world with the exception of the Antipodes and Argentina. Scrapie refers to the scraping or scratching which the affected animal does against fence posts or trees, in order to obtain relief from the irritation which it experiences. The sheep becomes nervous and hypersensitive to sound and touch, develops pruritis, scrapes its fleece, and then becomes progressively inco-ordinate. Death occurs within weeks or months at the most. Within a flock, related animals tend to be affected, and recently, several genetic markers have been identified as risk factors for the disease. Histological examination of the brain reveals widespread spongiform change with vacuolation of the cytoplasm of neurones, neuronal cell loss, and amyloid deposition. In 1899, Besnoit succeeded in transmitting scrapie by inoculating infected tissue into a ewe, and Cuille and Chelle (1936) confirmed that it was transmissible by infecting sheep following intraocular inoculation, and they were able to demonstrate that the agent was filtrable. Despite the proximity of man to infected sheep over centuries, and man's habit of eating virtually all the body parts of sheep, no cases of 'naturally occurring' scrapie have been recorded in humans. Two cases have been recorded in laboratory workers who were accidently inoculated with infected material. In 1947, a similar disease was described in mink, transmissible mink encephalopathy.

Kuru

In the 1950s a disease, new to Western medicine, was being described from a remote area of Papua New Guinea by Gajdusek and Zigas (1957). Dating from the early part of the century, kuru affected a linguistic grouping of native peoples who used the Fore dialect. Women and children were predominantly affected and developed a progressive disease of swift evolution over a year on average, characterized by ataxia of gait, truncal ataxia, dysarthria, tremor, and titubation, usually with retention of intellect. Cerebellar deterioration became increasingly evident with disruption of eye movements and increasing disability, the appearance of pyramidal and extrapyramidal signs, and various forms of movement disorder, but apparently not myoclonus. Emotional lability, generalized muscle wasting and paralysis supervene and lead rapidly to death. Epidemiological studies linked the disease to the practice of cannibalism and it was felt that the higher incidence of the disease in women and children reflected their greater exposure to brain and offal of infected carcasses. Since cannibalism has reduced so has the occurrence of kuru, although new cases are still occurring which may be a function of a particularly long incubation period (Collinge and Palmer 1997).

Hadlow (1959) recognized that the spongiform nature of the pathological change in kuru brains had similarities to the changes seen with scrapie, and suggested that the disease may be transmissible. Kuru was transmitted to monkeys after intracerebral inoculation by Gajdusek et al. (1966) and 2 years later, the same group succeeded in transmitting CJD to monkeys using similar methods (Gibbs et al. 1968) and GSS followed in 1981 (Masters et al. 1981). The 'spongiform encephalopathies' now became the 'transmissible encephalopathies' although the nature of the infective agent remained elusive.

Bovine spongiform encephalopathy

In Britain in 1985 and 1986, isolated cases of cattle suffering from a progressive CNS degeneration were being reported. By 1988 this had become an epidemic. Examination of the brains of these animals revealed widespread spongiform change and the disease was called bovine spongiform encephalopathy (BSE). Both pathological and clinical similarities to scrapie were noted. BSE animals developed apprehension, hypersensitivity to stimuli, postural abnormalities, ataxia and this progressed rapidly to death. BSE has been shown to be transmissible to a range of animals including sheep, goats, mice, pigs, marmosets, monkeys, and mink. Following extensive epidemiological studies, it is now felt that the likely source of the disease in cattle is cross species transfer of scrapie infectious particles to cattle, in feed derived from sheep. In the 1970s a large number of surplus sheep were slaughtered and their carcasses were processed to animal protein feed and other by-products. There was no longer a market for tallow and like substances, so the process by which the carcasses were 'rendered' or dissolved was carried out at lower temperatures than before, and certain solvents were omitted. As a result, it is thought that scrapie particles remained viable, or reproducible, and were concentrated in the protein feed, and so infected the cattle. BSE has been found in Ireland, France, Switzerland, Portugal, Germany, Denmark, Italy, Canada, Oman, and the Falklands. In all of these countries, it seems likely that the source of infection has been meat or bone meal which originated from infected material in Britain. The British government has been obliged to institute measures to eradicate BSE from the national herd.

Parallel to, and a little later than, the evolution of the BSE saga, rare cases were appearing in Britain of a new variant of CJD (NVCJD) (Section 34.12.3) which had a different neuropathological profile, younger distribution and atypical clinical features (Will et al. 1996). Cases were also found in other countries that had BSE. It has been suggested that the appearance of this NVCJD is causally linked to the BSE epidemic by human ingestion of BSE contaminated meat, and may represent a further illustration of cross species infection.

34.12.3 Creutzfeldt–Jakob disease and allied encephalopathies

In 1920, Creutzfeldt described the case of a 22-year-old woman with progressive dementia and in 1921 Jakob described five

Table 34.4. Human prion diseases

Sporadic	Classical CJD
	?New variant CJD
Acquired	Iatrogenic CJD
	?New variant CJD
	Kuru
Inherited	Familial CJD
	GSS
	Fatal familial insomnia

cases of dementia with their pathological findings. Since then the name Creutzfelt–Jakob disease (CJD) has been ascribed to the syndrome (Section 26.6.5). The case which Creutzfeldt wrote has been shown not to have suffered from the disease which now bears his name, while at least two of the cases of Jakob did have the proper syndrome. The transmissibility of the condition has been well established, and its forms are human examples of prion diseases (Table 34.4).

CJD is a rare, rapidly progressive dementia which occurs worldwide with a frequency in the order of 0.5–1 case per million population. It affects both sexes and most racial groups. With the exception of infrequent familial clusters, its distribution appears to be random. About 15 per cent of cases are familial. The onset is insidious and the incubation period is unknown but certainly can run into many years. In iatrogenic cases, when the time of inoculation is known, the incubation period has been as short as 2 years. The average age of cases at onset is 60 years but some have been described with onset from 14 to 83 years.

Clinical features

In the beginning, symptoms are non-specific and variable, and no different from other forms of dementia—forgetfulness, fatigue, cognitive disturbance, depression and personality disorder, behavioural upset and derangement of sleep, weight loss, and malaise. CJD shares all of these symptoms with other dementias in the early stages, but CJD is much more quickly progressive—about 70 per cent of all cases are dead within 6 months. As other areas of the brain become affected, further signs appear and include sensory loss, visual upset, cortical blindness, ataxia, weakness, muscle wasting, spasticity, dysarthia, and epileptic seizures. Extrapyramidal signs of rigidity and bradykinesis and abnormal movements may appear. Myoclonus appears at any stage of the disease, and does, in most cases, at some stage. It may be asymmetrical at onset, asynchronous and susceptible to startle, appearing in one limb before spreading. The appearance of myoclonus is not diagnostic but it is highly suggestive of CJD. With progression, primitive reflexes appear together with autonomic disintegration, sometimes with central apnoea, wasting increases and the patient becomes vegetative and dies. Some rather atypical forms have been described. In the amyotrophic form, there is evidence of anterior horn cell degeneration. Doubt has been expressed that such cases may not be true CJD but ALS with dementia. Perhaps as many as 10 per cent of cases run a clinical course longer than 2 years, and some present with a cerebellar syn-

drome, the Brownell–Oppenheimer variant. When the brunt falls upon the parietal and occipital cortex, dyspraxia, agnosia, and cortical blindness indicate the Heidenheim form of the disease. There are no clinical features to distinguish the hereditary forms of CJD, which appear to be inherited as autosomal dominant, from the sporadic.

Iatrogenic CJD is clinically no different. Accidental inoculation of prions to humans has taken place by insertion of infected graft material such as dura mater or cornea, injection of growth hormone or gonadotropins harvested from human cadavers, and by the use of inadequately sterilized neurosurgical instruments. There is no conclusive evidence that blood transfusion has transmitted CJD. With inoculation near to the brain, the incubation period is shorter and the disease is similar to classical CJD, with peripheral injection such as growth hormone the incubation period is longer and the clinical syndrome is more of a progressive ataxic syndrome. There is some evidence that there may be a genetic susceptibility to iatrogenic CJD. There does not seem to be an increased risk of development of prion diseases by occupational exposure—there has not been a higher incidence of CJD in veterinary workers, shepherds, and herdsmen.

Gerstmann–Straussler–Scheinker disease (GSS) is a very rare form of autosomal dominant inherited progressive cerebellar ataxia with dementia. It begins between the ages of 20 and 50, with a mean age of onset of 42. Increasing clumsiness, ataxia, dysarthria, and dementia are followed by spasticity, weakness, rigidity, and tremor, sometimes myoclonic jerks and rapid progression to death within 1–5 years. Familial CJD and GSS share many clinical features, and it may not be possible to distinguish them on clinical or even on pathological grounds.

New variant CJD (NVCJD) has been described since the mid-1990s. Will et al. (1996) described 10 cases of CJD which differed from previous cases on clinical and specifically on neuropathological grounds. At the time of writing, some 48 such cases have now been reported to the CJD Surveillance Unit in Edinburgh (web site www.cjd.ed.ac.uk/index.htm and Department of Health web site www.doh.gov.uk/cjd/cjd1.htm) and increasingly, evidence suggests that its occurrence is linked to the ingestion of beef or beef products which have been contaminated by BSE. These cases differed from normal CJD by having a much younger age of onset at 27 years on average, by presenting with psychiatric problems with behavioural changes, and by developing ataxia and cerebellar dysfunction early in the course of the disease. Sensory upset with persistent limb and facial dysaesthesiae was prominent. Dementia, myoclonus, and movement disorder occurred late. None had the EEG features usually associated with CJD and pathological changes in the brain differed significantly from the classical appearances of CJD. The duration of disease is significantly longer than with classical CJD.

Neuropathology

The changes in CJD are widespread throughout the neuraxis, with neuronal loss in all layers of the cortex, astrocytic proliferation, and marked spongiform changes particularly in the deeper cortical layers. There is little demyelination, and spongiform change precedes neuronal loss and is due to the appearance of vacuoles within the cytoplasm of the neurophil. There is virtually no inflammatory change. Microglial proliferation with hyperplasia and hypertrophy, in relation to amyloid plaques, is seen. Amyloid plaques are found within the extracellular space, particularly in the cerebellar cortex (Masters and Richardson 1978). There is a wide spread of the distribution and severity of the pathological lesions and it has recently been recognized that spongiform change is not an exclusive feature of prion diseases (Bell and Ironside 1993). Amyloid plaques are seen in some cases of sporadic CJD, and with increasing concentration in kuru, inherited CJD, and GSS. The pathological changes seen in NVCJD are rather different. There is spongiform change in the cerebral cortex and in the basal ganglia and thalamus but the striking change is of widespread plaque formation in cerebrum and cerebellum, the plaques closely resembling those seen in kuru. The amyloid plaques which are seen in the transmissible encephalopathies contain abnormal forms of PrP.

Prion protein (PrP) is a normal protein found in most cell types and in the brain as a glycoprotein on the outer cell membrane. The coding gene for PrP is located on the short arm of chromosome 20, and the longer of its two exons contains the entire transcribed 253 codon region of the gene. Various different codon mutations have been described for familial CJD, GSS, and FFI, and it seems likely that variations in the genotype give rise to abnormal forms of PrP. Most cases of sporadic CJD are homozygous for a common PrP protein polymorphism. Cases of NVCJD have shown homozygosity for methionine at codon 129. These abnormal forms of PrP then accumulate in the brain in amyloid plaques, and are in some way responsible for the different phenotypes of CJD, so that one insertion or mutation may give rise to the extrapyramidal from of the disease, and a different mutation will produce another clinical form. It is likely that these abnormal forms of PrP represent the major component of the infectious agent (Collinge and Palmer 1997). How the pathological changes are induced is not yet understood, neither is the prevalence of infection known. Could it be that it is a ubiquitous infection, clinically inapparent in the population at large, and which manifests as disease only in those who are unfortunate enough to be genetically susceptible, or in whom mutation to a pathogenic form has taken place? Whatever the mechanism, it is now possible to define these forms of degenerative brain disease by identification of the associated pathogenic PrP gene mutation.

34.12.4 Diagnosis and management

Until the observation of myoclonus, or the obvious development of an extrapyramidal, anterior horn cell, cerebellar or parietal syndrome in association with dementia, or the demonstration of familial association, CJD does not differ from any of the other forms of progressive dementia, such as Alzheimer's disease and atherosclerosis, at least on clinical grounds (Section 26.6). Prion disease should be considered in the differential diagnosis of any atypical form of dementia or of progressive cerebellar degeneration. NVCJD must now be considered in the differential diagnosis of atypical psychiatric syndromes and encephalitides in young

people. The clinical spectrum of the prion diseases is now so wide that they must be considered in the differential diagnosis of many progressive neurological syndromes.

Investigations which are useful to diagnose CJD and other prion diseases are few. It is customary to carry out blood tests to exclude other forms of dementia such as neurosyphilis when the disease is in its early stages. Imaging of the brain should be carried out to exclude other pathology. There are no changes which are diagnostic of prion diseases and the appearances may be normal. Some authors have reported degenerative changes in various parts of the basal ganglia, white matter abnormalities, and cortical atrophy. The EEG becomes abnormal in all cases later in the evolution of the disease when diffuse slow wave activity is seen which is completely non-specific. In CJD, rhythmic and periodic bursts of high-amplitude bi- and triphasic sharp wave complexes may appear which may be synchronous with myoclonus (Fig. 34.3). These changes are characteristic, but not pathognomonic (Chiofalo *et al.* 1980).

CSF examination is not usually helpful as changes in the protein content are non-specific. In the past, histological examination of brain tissue obtained by surgical biopsy was sometimes helpful. This technique is no longer used because of the dangers of transmission of prions. The application of newer immunological and molecular genetic techniques to demonstrate various markers for prion disease has shown promise, but further experience has demonstrated that many of these techniques have not been sufficiently specific to be diagnostic (Hsich *et al.* 1996; Zerr *et al.* 1996; Otto *et al.* 1998). Most recently, demonstration of abnormal PrP in tonsil tissue obtained by biopsy during life (with appropriate precautions) appears to be the most accurate method available (Hill *et al.* 1997, 1999). In practice, in Britain, if a case of prion disease is suspected clinically, contact should be made with the CJD Surveillance Unit in Edinburgh, where advice is freely available on current diagnostic methodology.

No treatment has been demonstrated to be effective to limit the progression of prion diseases which are universally fatal. Symptomatic treatment is given for seizures, spasticity, and myoclonus, and is generally ineffective. Because of the infectious nature of prion diseases, staff treating such patients must take strict precautions, and all secretions from the patients must be treated as potentially infectious. Because of the resistance of prions to standard disinfecting agents special precautions are necessary. Surgical instrumentation should not be undertaken unless absolutely necessary and guidelines exist for the disposal of specimens, and surgical instruments, and for necropsy. People suspected of suffering from prion diseases should not donate blood and they are not suitable as donors for organ transplantation. If a hereditary form of prion disease is confirmed, genetic counselling should be offered along similar lines to that for Huntingdon's disease.

34.13 Non-viral encephalitis

Encephalitis which is clinically indistinguishable from the viral form of the disease, can be caused by other organisms, bacteria, and parasites. Commonly, the encephalitis is accompanied by

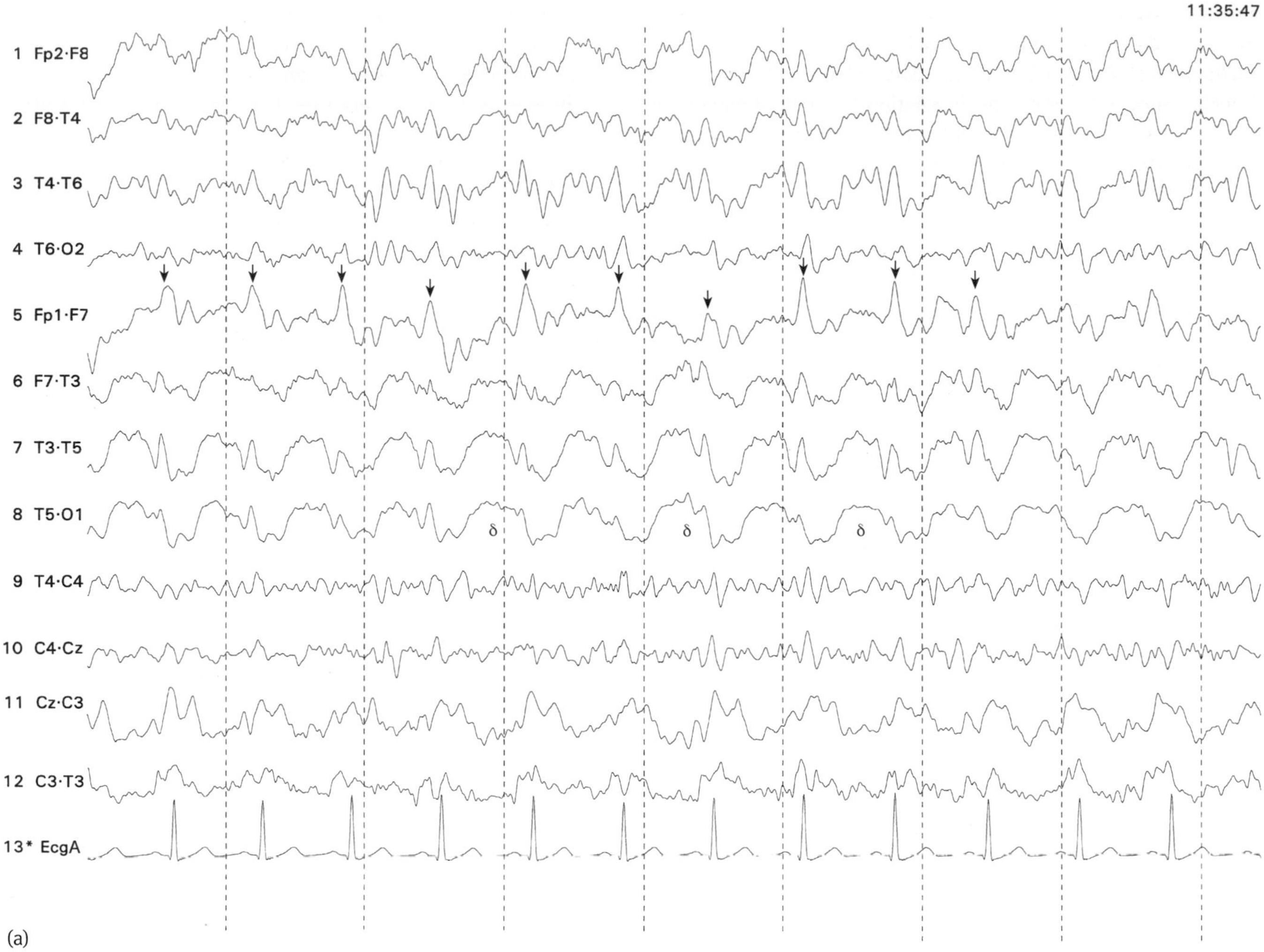

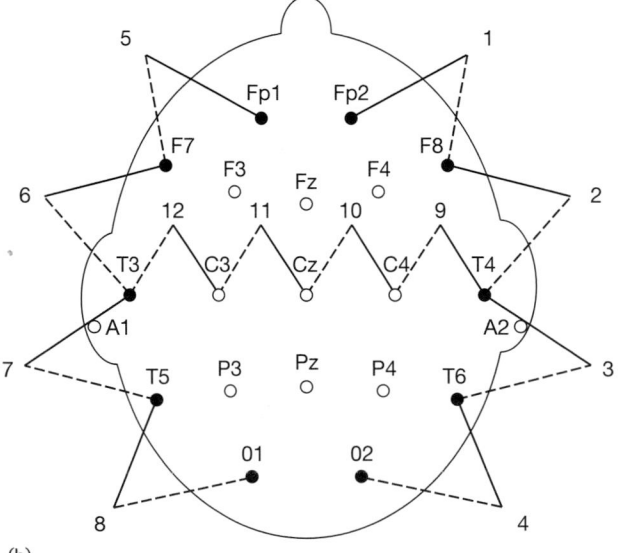

11:35:47
1 Fp2·F8
2 F8·T4
3 T4·T6
4 T6·O2
5 Fp1·F7
6 F7·T3
7 T3·T5
8 T5·O1
9 T4·C4
10 C4·Cz
11 Cz·C3
12 C3·T3
13* EcgA
δ
δ
δ

(a)

Fp1
Fp2
F7
F8
F3
Fz
F4
T3
C3
Cz
C4
T4
A1
A2
T5
P3
Pz
P4
T6
01
02
1
2
3
4
5
6
7
8
9
10
11
12

(b)

Fig. 34.3. Creutzfeldt–Jakob disease. (a) An EEG showing the characteristic finding of repetitive sharp waves or triphasic complexes. These are usually maximal anteriorly and may be asymmetrical (here maximal at FP1-F7, left frontal region). They repeat at 0.5–2-second intervals (see arrows) and have fairly short durations of up to 300 ms: The background EEG also contains an excess of delta slow-wave activity (δ), maximal on the left, and posterior dominant alpha rhythms, reduced on the left. (Courtesy of Dr R. Kennett). (b) The electrode montage used for the EEG. This was a bipolar montage, using 10–20 international electrode positions.

other clinical features which help to identify the aetiology—there are characteristic physical signs such as the eschar which occurs in Mediterranean spotted fever, or the rashes of other rickettsial diseases. The disease may be peculiar to a particular geographical area, such as the trypanosomiases, or it may occur in a specific season or in certain climatic conditions or in epidemic form such as typhus. Unfortunately, the ease with which continents can be hurdled with modern air travel, makes it necessary for the doctor who attends a patient with encephalitis, to pay particular and focused attention to the history of recent travel, and potential exposure to insect vectors of disease and other pathogens to which the patient may have been exposed in the course of recreation or occupation. Once the possibility has been entertained that the cause of the syndrome may be exotic by comparison to local epidemiology, it is not usually too difficult to narrow the field when a travel history is known. Fortunately, advances in molecular biology have made it possible to provide quick and reliable tests which will confirm the pathogen within a short time. For many of these encephalitides, curative treatment is possible provided the diagnosis is made expeditiously. Few neurologists will have had exposure to all of these varieties of infectious encephalitis and a quick phone call, e-mail, or fax to a colleague in the Infectious and Tropical Diseases department, locally or abroad, will usually provide reassuring advice. I have found that Government Departments and WHO have often been helpful in this way.

34.13.1 Chlamydial diseases

Three species of chlamydiae can cause human disease; *Chlamydia trachomatis*, *Chlamydia pneumoniae*, and *Chlamydia psittaci*. The first causes trachoma in dry areas of the Third World, and it is a major cause of sexually transmitted diseases throughout the world. Man is the only host and neurological complications are rare. *Chlamydia pneumoniae* has been recognized as an organism separate from *C. psittaci* since the 1980s and it produces clinical syndromes similar to that produced by *C. psittaci*. Man is the only host, unlike *C. psittaci*, which occurs in a wide range of birds and mammals. Humans are infected accidentally following exposure to infected birds.

Chlamydiae are coccoid, obligate, intracellular pathogens which contain DNA and RNA. *Chlamydia psittaci* causes infection in a large variety of birds—not just the psittacine family of parrots, budgerigars, and cockatoos—but also finches, pigeons, pheasants, seabirds, and poultry. The disease produced is more correctly termed 'ornithosis'. In birds, infection is commonly asymptomatic and the organism is shed in faeces, from the beak and contaminates the feathers. Human infection results from inhalation of the organism or by ingestion after handling contaminated plumage. Those occupationally exposed to birds such as pet shop owners and poultry workers are at particular risk, as are pigeon fanciers. However, even a short period of exposure may be sufficient to result in infection. Person to person transmission is rare. Laboratory personnel are at risk of potentially serious infection and should be warned of the suspected diagnosis when specimens are dispatched. The organism is pathogenic to the lung and infection can range from asymptomatic, to severe and potentially fatal, atypical pneumonia. Liver, spleen, meninges, brain, and heart may also be involved.

Pathologically, there are lymphocytic exudates in the pulmonary alveoli and interstitial spaces. The lungs become heavily congested and macrophages containing inclusion bodies are characteristic. When the brain is infected, there is oedema and congestion and with evidence of direct neuronal invasion, chromatolysis and intracytoplasmic inclusions in neurones and meningeal cells.

The incubation period varies from 4 to 15 days and in some, may be as long as a month. Clinical features may vary widely. Many merely have a mild upper respiratory tract infection which may not be recognized as anything more than a common cold. In others, there is abrupt onset of fever, rigors, and chills, with severe headache, myalgia, and a persistent dry cough. There is a relative bradycardia and few signs to be found on examination of the chest, which is at variance with the abnormalities often seen on chest X-ray. The white cell count is often normal and in as many as 25 per cent of cases there may be leucopenia. In most, infection subsides within 2 weeks. In severe cases, endocarditis, hepatitis, and more severe respiratory involvement may supervene. A minority develop meningo-encephalitis which may progress to coma. Rarely, meningo-encephalitis may predominate from the outset (Crosse 1990). Other neurological syndromes have been described including transverse myelitis, cranial nerve palsies, and cerebellar disturbance (Carr-Lake and Narr 1976). There are no specific features and diagnosis depends on the recognition of the atypical pneumonia, or that the patient has been exposed to potentially infected birds. Provided diagnosis and treatment are timely, mortality rates should not be above 5 per cent, although there is a greater risk in pregnant women.

Diagnosis is confirmed by isolation of the organism from respiratory secretions (which is hazardous to laboratory staff) or by the demonstration of antibody rise in acute and convalescent sera. PCR examination of tissue or fluid, and enzyme immunoassays are being developed, but there have been some problems with cross reactions.

Treatment of chlamydial infection is with tetracycline, erythromycin, or clarythromycin. Some of the newer quinolones are also effective. For neurological disease, parenteral administration is preferred, and a prolonged course is often necessary because of the risk of relapse. Steps should be taken to identify the source of infection with the co-operation of local public health authorities.

Aseptic meningitis and meningo-encephalitis have been described as rare accompaniments of the second or lymphatic stage of *lymphogranuloma venereum*, caused by certain strains of *C. trachomatis*. Recent reports have suggested that infection with *C. pneumoniae*, on the basis of serological testing, may play some part in the development of cerebral and coronary artery atherosclerosis. It should be observed that several other organisms have been similarly implicated on fairly specious grounds, and at present, there is no firm evidence to substantiate these claims.

34.13.2 Rickettsial infections

Rickettsiae are Gram-negative, cocco-bacillary, obligate intracellular bacteria that cause a range of diseases, including acute meningo-encephalitis. Their definitive hosts are rodents and other mammals such as dogs, and the vectors which transmit them to man are ticks, lice, fleas, or mites. On the basis of the clinical syndromes which they produce in humans, and on their antigenicity and growth characteristics, they are divided into three main groups, the spotted fever group, the typhus group, and the scrub typhus group (Table 34.5). Q fever, due to infection with *Coxiella burnetii*, is contained in a fourth group that includes infections caused by *Erlichia* species, which can rarely cause an acute meningo-encephalitis. Rickettsiae are inoculated into the human body by the bite of the vector insect, or by scratching of contaminated insect material though skin or mucous membrane. They penetrate host cells where they multiply then spread throughout the body via the bloodstream and lymphatics. Characteristically, they produce a widespread vasculitis which increases vascular permeability, produces oedema and endothelial cell injury, activates inflammatory and coagulation mechanisms, and may result in widespread organ damage due to thrombosis, haemorrhage, and shock. When this occurs in the brain, meningo-encephalitis results. Q fever is probably acquired through inhalation of the organism from infected animal products. The incubation period, progression, and clinical features of the different syndromes varies, but all generally share the features of high pyrexia, skin rash, headache, and myalgia, and if neurological features develop, meningo-encephalitis is evident by the second week. Other similar diseases with a localized geographical distribution and caused by related rickettsial organisms are being continually described with slight variations on the same clinical theme.

Rocky Mountain Spotted fever

This condition was first described from the Rocky Mountain region of the USA and it soon became evident that the same disease occurred throughout the western hemisphere. The natural cycle of infection is maintained by small mammals and ixoxid ticks which bite and infect humans. The wood tick and the dog tick (*Dermacentor andersoni* and *variabilis*, respectively) are the principal vectors. There is a higher incidence of disease in children and males, probably reflecting proximity to dogs and occupational exposure. However, with increased foreign travel and exposure to insect vectors when following outdoor tourist activities, the rickettsial diseases may be encountered anywhere in the world and in any ethnic and social group. There is variation between the virulence of infection and the old, infirm, diabetic, or alcoholic are said to suffer more severe disease. Blacks with glucose-6-phosphate dehydrogenase deficiency develop particularly virulent disease.

The incubation period is about 1 week and varies in proportion to the bite inoculum. Most patients can remember and report the insect bite. Fever with rigors, chills, malaise, headache, myalgia, conjunctival injection, and photophobia and diffuse oedema come on suddenly, to be followed by a distinctive rash by the third to the fifth day of the illness—it is maculopapular, erythematous on the wrists and ankles and spreads centrally to the trunk and it often becomes petechial and sometimes purpuric with haemorrhagic necrosis and gangrene in severe cases, which may mimic meningococcal septicaemia. Headache is invariable, and a variable proportion, perhaps as many as 25 per cent, of patients progress to develop encephalitis with drowsiness, confusion, convulsions, followed by stupor and coma if they are not treated appropriately. Most forms of focal, neurological disturbance have been described but these are uncommon (Helmick *et al.* 1984; Kirk *et al.* 1990). The overall mortality varies up to 10 per cent and is worsened by any delay in the institution of antibiotic treatment. Because of this, treatment should be instituted immediately on clinical suspicion—it may turn out to be fatal to await laboratory diagnosis.

Blood tests are seldom helpful in the acute stage—rise in serum antibody titre is useful but takes time. CSF examination reveals non-specific changes with a rise in the cell count and protein content and may be normal. EEG will show non-specific slowing. Cerebral imaging with CT or MR is usually normal and may show non-specific white matter abnormality. Immunofluorescence of skin biopsy is said to be specific but not very sensitive and is not widely available. PCR of CSF, blood, and skin biopsy specimens is undergoing evaluation.

The treatments of choice are tetracycline or doxycycline for 10 days to a fortnight, for adults, and chloramphenicol to be considered for young children to avoid the teeth stains which may complicate treatment with tetracycline (Shaked 1991). Appropriate supportive treatment is given and steroids have been used although the evidence that they are routinely efficacious is lacking.

Table 34.5. Human rickettsial diseases

Group	Organism	Vector	Geography	Disease
Spotted fever	*R. rickettsii*	Tick	North, Central, South America	Rocky Mountain spotted fever
	R. conorii	Tick	Mediterranean, Asia, Africa	Bouttoneuse fever
	R. australis	Tick	Northern Australia	Queensland tick typhus
	R. siberica	Tick	Asia	North Asian tick typhus
	R. akari	Mite	USA, Russian Federation, Asia	Rickettsialpox
Typhus	*R. prowazekii*	Louse	Ubiquitous	Epidemic typhus
	R. typhi	Flea	Ubiquitous	Murine typhus
Scrub typhus	*R. tsutsugamushi*	Mites	Asia, Pacific Australia	Scrub typhus
Other	*C. burnettii*	None	Ubiquitous	Q fever

Mediterranean Spotted fever (Boutonneuse fever)

This condition is caused by *R. conori* which is usually inoculated into humans by the brown dog tick *Rhipicephalus sanguineus*. Different vectors and hosts are found in central Europe and in Russia, Ukraine, and around the Black and Caspian seas, and all cause different forms of spotted fevers. In the Mediterranean variety, at the site of inoculation the organisms reproduce and produce local inflammation with endothelial vasculitis which raises an erythematous papule. The centre of the papule becomes necrotic and dark coloured, the 'tache noire', which is characteristic. From there, spread takes place to local lymph nodes then to the general circulation. In 7 days or thereby, symptoms similar to those of Rocky Mountain Spotted fever appear—fever, headache, myalgia, arthralgia, lymphadenopathy, and rash. Meningism and encephalopathic features occur in up to 20 per cent of cases. Laboratory investigations, EEG, and brain imaging produce similar appearances to those of RMSF. Diagnosis is clinical, based on the findings of fever, rash, and eschar, and can be confirmed by antibody studies. PCR is being evaluated. Treatment with tetracycline or chloramphenicol is given as described above. The outcome is usually excellent and mortality rates of about 1 per cent should be expected (Raoult *et al.* 1986). An excellent account of similar Rickettsial diseases and their epidemiology is to be found in Beati and Raoult (1998).

Epidemic and murine typhus

Epidemic and murine typhus are clinically similar. Epidemic typhus occurs in conditions of overcrowding and poor sanitation such as accompany war, natural disasters, and civil insurrection. It is caused by *R. prowazekii* and transmitted by the louse. Murine typhus is linked to the distribution of rats, is transmitted by the rat flea and is caused by *R. typhi*. The incubation period is about 2 weeks. The clinical syndrome of the two diseases resembles a severe form of RMSF with the abrupt onset of fever, headache, myalgia, and a spreading macular and petechial rash, delirium, and encephalopathy. White spots (typhus nodules) may be evident in the retina on fundoscopy. Investigations and treatment are similar to those described above. The outcome from murine typhus is usually excellent For epidemic typhus, mortality rates may be high, in proportion to the degree of debilitation of the population at the time of onset of the epidemic. Brill–Zinsser disease is a form of recrudescent typhus which may occur in people who have recovered from typhus years before. It may represent a diminution in host immunity. The clinical features are those of a mild form of epidemic typhus but the rash may be lacking, in which case diagnosis depends on eliciting a history of previous typhus infection. The response to tetracycline is usually good.

Scrub typhus

Scrub typhus is found in the Far East, particularly in southeastern Asia. It is caused by *R. tsutsugamuchi* and is transmitted to man by the bite of 'chiggers', mite larvae. The clinical features are of fever, general lymphadenopathy, and an eschar at the site of the bite. Headache and myalgia are invariable and as many as 10 per cent develop features of encephalitis. A rash on the trunk, spreading to the limbs, is common. Confirmation of the diagnosis is serological and PCR has been developed and is accurate. Treatment is with tetracycline.

Q fever

Q fever is caused by *Coxiella burnetii*, a cocco-bacillus. It infects a large number of animal species, usually asymptomatically, where it localizes to the uterus and mammary glands. Direct or indirect exposure to infected animals may result in clinical disease in humans. Infection usually results from aerosol inhalation of infected material. This may take several forms which include an acute self-limiting febrile illness, pneumonia, endocarditis, hepatitis, aseptic meningitis, and encephalitis. Neurological complications are in fact quite rare, although one group reported transient neurological features such as hallucinations, speech disturbance, and facial pain in 23 per cent of patients in one outbreak (Smith *et al.* 1993). Patients who are immune compromised may be more at risk of developing disease. Investigations and treatment are similar to those described above.

34.13.3 Mycoplasma infection

The two major mycoplasma organisms which are associated with neurological disease are *Mycoplasma pneumoniae* and *Mycoplasma hominis*. The latter is found in the genitourinary tract and may be a cause of neonatal meningitis. It has been isolated from rare cases of brain abscess. *Mycoplasma pneumoniae* has been associated with several neurological syndromes. It is one of the smallest bacteria, about 200 nm in diameter, and it does not have a rigid cell wall. It causes an atypical form of pneumonia in a minority of patients. In the majority who become symptomatic, an influenza-like illness creeps on after 2–3 weeks incubation with severe coughing, headache, and myalgia. Young adults, children, and adolescents are affected most frequently. The infection is transmitted by inhalation.

Neurological complications have been reported in up to 7 per cent of hospitalized cases and occur from 3 to 30 days after the upper respiratory infection (Sterner and Biberfeld 1969). Aseptic meningitis, encephalitis, cerebellar syndrome, Guillain–Barré polyneuropathy, transverse myelitis, and cranial nerve palsies have all been described. The pathogenic mechanisms are not always clear—in some it seems that direct CNS invasion occurs and in others there may be an immune mediated form of post-infectious encephalitis perhaps with immune complex vasculopathy (Behan *et al.* 1986; Nishimura *et al.* 1996). Diagnosis can be made by the detection of cold haemagglutins in the serum of a patient with neurological complications after an upper respiratory infection. Their absence does not exclude the diagnosis as their presence is fairly non-specific. Increase in serum antibody titres can be confirmatory. PCR of CSF is likely to prove useful (DeBiasi and Tyler 1999). Erythromycin, doxycycline, or tetracycline for 2 weeks is effective treatment for the acute respiratory infection and the response of neurological disease is variable and probably depends on the pathogenic mechanism. Perhaps one-third of patients have persisting neurological signs and severe meningo-encephalitis carries a poor prognosis.

34.13.2 Malaria

Malaria is the most important parasitic disease which affects humans in the world. In the region of two billion people live in malarial endemic zones, 300 million or more are affected each year, the majority in Africa, and as many as three million die each year. The increase in global travel means that malaria can be seen in any country in the world, having been contracted abroad in the tropics. In Britain, 2500 cases were recorded by the Malaria Reference Laboratory in 1996, 1283 of which caused by falciparum malaria (Jones 1998), and these numbers are rising. Involvement of the brain occurs only in those affected by *Plasmodium falciparum* and cerebral malaria results. For practical purposes, *P. vivax*, *P. ovale*, and *P. malariae* do not cause cerebral malaria—those cases which have been reported have probably been of dual infection with *P. falciparum* and another plasmodium. The death rate from cerebral malaria varies from 10 to 50 per cent. Cerebral malaria is an acute diffuse encephalopathy with fever, which can kill within 72 h if not recognized and treated. It is well to consider that a patient with *P. falciparum* infection and any disturbance of CNS function, has cerebral malaria, and treat accordingly. Delay in making the diagnosis contributes significantly to the high mortality rate. For the purposes of research and uniformity of definition, Warrell *et al.* (1982) proposed that cerebral malaria be defined as unrousable coma in patients with acute falciparum malaria and asexual parasites seen on blood smears, and who have no other cause for the coma. People who live in endemic areas may acquire a degree of immunity which diminishes with time. Those most at risk of developing severe malaria are the traveller who has no immunity and visits an endemic area to be exposed for the first time, the emigrant returning from a long stay abroad, whose immunity has lapsed, pregnant women, children in malarious areas between the ages of 6 months and 3 years who have lost maternally acquired immunity, and those who have become immune suppressed. The presence of haemoglobin S offers some protection against falciparum infection. However, it is not necessary to have travelled to an endemic area to contract malaria. Cases have been reported of cerebral malaria developing in people who have not been out of Britain and are thought to have acquired the disease by being bitten by infected mosquitoes that have been imported to the country by aircraft flying from endemic areas—some may have been bitten while sitting in aircraft during stopovers in the tropics, so-called 'runway malaria' (Conlon *et al.* 1990).

Transmission

Malaria occurs in countries lying between the latitudes 60 °N and 40 °S which includes most of Africa, Central and South America, regions in the Middle East, Iran, the Indian sub-continent, Southeast Asia, the Philippines, Borneo, and southern China. Infrequently, malaria may be contracted from infected blood transfused in endemic areas, or from needle sharing amongst drug addicts. The vast majority of cases of cerebral malaria result from humans being bitten by the female *Anopheles* mosquito which harbours the falciparum parasite. When they feed they inject sporozoites into the blood. They circulate and are rapidly cleared by the liver where they enter the hepatocytes and reproduce asexually, forming schizonts. One to three weeks later they rupture into the circulation as motile merozoites and quickly invade red blood cells and they can be seen on blood films under the microscope. They feed on haemoglobin and further asexual reproduction takes place. The progeny mature through the stages of merozoite and trophozoite, multiplying approximately tenfold, following which they rupture out of the erythrocyte and parasitize other unaffected red cells. Cells of any age are affected so there is no limit on the potential degree of parasitaemia. If the parasite load is high severe haemolysis may ensue. This rupture and dispersal takes place approximately every 48 h, and causes fever. Some of the merozoites develop into the sexual gametocyte stage and they are ingested by the female mosquito during her blood meal, undergo sexual replication within the mosquito to form infective sporozoites which are inoculated into another human when the mosquito next bites.

Pathophysiology

The manifestations of cerebral malaria result from a series of complex and not fully understood, interactions within the cerebral vasculature which are mediated by vascular, humoral, and haematological factors. The rheology of parasitized erythrocytes is disturbed in cerebral malaria and they adhere to the endothelium of brain capillaries and 'sludge' the circulation by mechanical occlusion. Changes take place in the erythrocyte wall which develops cone-shaped knobs which adhere to endothelial cell membranes (MacPherson *et al.* 1985) and the cells are sequestrated. The molecular basis for these changes is not yet understood and several red cell surface molecules and receptor molecules are currently under study and further description is beyond the scope of this chapter. Cytokines released by macrophages, tumour necrosis factor, interleukins, and other vasoactive substances have been found to be raised in cases of cerebral malaria. Whether increased vascular permeability is important is the subject of dispute (Patnaik *et al.* 1994). The blood–brain barrier is disrupted (Brown *et al.* 1999). However the changes are brought about, they result in a fall in cerebral perfusion and hypoxia, shift to anaerobic metabolism and increased production of CSF lactate. Hypoglycaemia from hepatic glycogen depletion, malabsoprtion of glucose from the gut, and increased metabolism of glucose by a large biomass of parasites, and metabolic acidosis may compound these changes, as may acute tubular necrosis and the adult respiratory distress syndrome. A proportion of patients with cerebral malaria have coexisting infections including pneumonia, urinary tract infections, septicaemia, and bacterial meningitis, each of which can exacerbate decline. Disseminated intravascular coagulation is another potential complication. Whether cerebral oedema occurs and ICP is significantly raised, has been the subject of debate. Cerebral oedema has been observed in necropsy specimens and it has been claimed that this has been an agonal manifestation. The CSF pressure has been found to be high at the time of lumbar puncture in a group of African children (Newton *et al.* 1991) yet Looareesuwan *et al.* (1983) found in a CT study that there was no evidence of cerebral oedema and Warrell *et al.* (1982) found that administration of dexamethazone did not improve prognosis. However, Looareesuwan *et al.* (1995) found evidence of gross cerebral oedema and tonsillar herniation in a study using brain MR imaging. It would be rather surprising if a disease which caused intracranial vascular changes and microthrombosis did not raise ICP, and appropriate precautions should be taken if CSF examination by lumbar puncture is necessary.

Clinical features

The clinical features of cerebral malaria are protean. In non-endemic areas the diagnosis is not infrequently delayed or missed altogether, with fatal consequences. Any person from an endemic area or who has visited an endemic area, or even who may be exposed to aircraft from such a region, and who falls ill with a pyrexia and cerebral symptoms, should be considered to be a possible case of cerebral malaria and investigated and treated accordingly. It is also important to remember that falciparum malaria may affect organ systems other than the brain and the presentation may reflect this. In adults the symptoms and signs of cerebral involvement usually follow a few days of pyrexia and non-specific malaise which may be mistaken for influenza. Characteristically, there are paroxysms of chills, rigors, and fever, with headache and myalgia, which may recur. The temperature usually remains elevated. In some, the onset may be abrupt and patients who are very ill may be hypothermic rather than pyrexial. Cerebral malaria may occur at any time during falciparum infection, even after effective treatment has been started. Evidence of cerebral involvement manifests by a decrease in the conscious level gradually to coma. This may be punctuated by epileptic seizures, commonly non-focal, in 45 per cent of patients. Before coma supervenes, there may be signs of an organic brain syndrome with confusion, disorientation, agitation, and psychosis. Some develop focal weakness and movement disorders. Meningism and opisthotonus may occur and as cerebral involvement increases decerebrate and decorticate posturing may be seen. Retinal haemorrhages may be found, and bruxism is common. Anaemia and jaundice are frequent accompaniments and hepatosplenomegaly is common. Disseminated intravascular coagulation, pulmonary oedema, and blackwater fever from haemolysis are serious complications. Prolonged coma and frequent convulsions should prompt a search for hypogylcaemia or other metabolic disturbance, and for pyogenic meningitis. Severely ill patients are liable to Gram-negative septicaemia.

In children, disease evolution is often much more rapid and they are even more likely to have epileptic seizures. Cough, diarrhoea, anorexia, and vomiting are common. Retinal haemorrhages are found and similar neurological signs to adults. Differentiation from bacterial meningitis can be difficult (Berkley *et al.* 1999). Recovery from coma with treatment is quicker in children—children improve within 24 h while adults may take 3 days.

Diagnosis

Confirmation of the diagnosis of malaria must be obtained immediately. If it is not possible to access a suitable laboratory, treatment should be started straight away. Thick and thin blood films should be examined by an experienced parasitologist after appropriate staining. If the blood smears are negative, treatment should be given anyway, and smears repeated every 8 or 12 h. A full blood count, urea, electrolytes, blood gases, and sugar, should be monitored. It is not necessary to examine the CSF unless bacterial meningitis is suspected, in which cases, precautions for raised ICP should be taken. It may be safer to treat empirically with antibiotics and forego CSF examination. Electroencephalography shows non-specific changes of encephalopathy and may be useful to detect subclinical epileptic activity. Brain imaging with CT or MR may reveal normal appearances or a tight oedematous brain and is useful to exclude other pathology. Newer tests based on the detection of histidine-rich protein which is produced in the knobs which are seen on the walls of parasitized red cells have been developed and are being evaluated—these include the ParaSight-FTM and the Malaria PfTM tests which are rapid dipstick type tests, said to be sensitive, specific, and easy to use (Shiff *et al.* 1993; Durrheim *et al.* 1998).

Treatment

Chloroquine used to be the drug of choice for the treatment of cerebral malaria, but the emergence of resistant parasites in many regions has reduced its usefulness and quinine is now the drug of choice. Quinine is not available in the USA where quinidine gluconate is used instead. Quinine is given by slow intravenous infusion in a dose of 10 mg/kg over 2–4 h. For patients who have acquired disease in Southeast Asia it is advisable to double the loading dose. Quinine should never be given by bolus injection. Check should be made that the patient has not received quinine, quinidine, or mefloquine within 24 h before giving treatment, and since these drugs are cardiotoxic, close monitoring of cardiac status is required. Drug levels should be monitored to achieve therapeutic concentrations. Quinine can reduce blood sugar levels quite significantly and this requires careful attention. When the patient regains consciousness, oral treatment with quinine 600 mg/12 h can be given. Treatment with quinine should be followed by either pyrimethamine-sulphdoxine (Fansidar) or doxycycline.

Newer drugs derived from sweet wormwood (*Artemeia annua*), artemisinin, artemether, and artesunate, suggest that they clear parisitaemia quicker than quinine and they seem to be safe and effective. The results of further trials are awaited.

Supportive treatment on an intensive care unit should be given paying particular attention to the control of epileptic seizures, monitoring anaemia, hypoglycaemia, renal function, and lung function. Antibiotics may be needed for Gram-negative septicaemia or meningitis. It may be necessary to treat cerebral oedema. If the parasite load is particularly high, exchange transfusion may be needed.

Outcome

Neurological sequelae occur in 5–10 per cent of cases and take the form of epilepsy, mental retardation, spasticity, behavioural upset, focal signs if there has been brain infarction, and a cerebellar syndrome. Mortality rates vary according to the state of the patient at diagnosis and are worse if there has been any delay. Intensive care can reduce the overall mortality rate of up to 25 per cent.

Prophylaxis against malaria is possible by avoiding mosquito bites by the use of appropriate clothing and mosquito nets, and by taking prophylactic drugs before and during the time of visits to endemic areas. Patterns of drug resistance vary in different parts of the world and advice should be sought from an expert in tropical diseases on the regime best suited to the geography.

34.13.5 Trypanosomiasis

Trypanosomes affect man and his livestock. There are two quite distinct forms of trypanosomiasis which affect humans, predominantly in rural areas, are caused by different organisms, occur in separate continents, and cause diseases with quite characteristic features. African trypanosomiasis or sleeping sickness is caused by trypanosomes of the group *brucei* and affects the CNS in humans. American trypanosomiasis or Chaga's disease is caused by *Trypanosoma cruzi* and affects the heart and bowel predominantly, and CNS features are relatively rare.

African trypanosomiasis

There are two forms of this disease which correspond roughly to the epidemiological regions in which they occur between the latitudes of 15 °N and 15 °S in Africa. The Gambian or West African form occurs in the western and central parts, the Rhodesian or East African form of trypanosomiaisis occurs in the east and there is overlap in the middle where they meet. Both forms are fatal if not treated. Gambian sleeping sickness has a slower and more protracted course than Rhodesian. The former is caused by *Trypanosoma brucei gambiense*, the latter by *Trypanosoma brucei rhodesiense*, but the two strains of protozoa may be morphologically indistinguishable. Trypanosomes are elongated motile protozoa, 10–30 μm long with a central nucleus and they are propelled by an undulating membrane and flagellum.

The sleeping sicknesses are transmitted by male and female tsetse flies of the species *Glossina*. The trypanosomes undergo a developmental cycle in the fly which remains infective for its life span of several months. Once injected into the human host, the trypanosomes multiply locally, cause inflammatory change which may result in a chancre, and spread via the lymphatics and bloodstream throughout the body, including the CNS, invading the intercellular and extracellular fluids of many organs, causing febrile attacks which relate to waves of parasitaemia, as they go. In the CNS the meninges become congested and infiltrated by lymphocytes and large plasma cells which are full of immunoglobulin, known as Mott cells. There is a complex and incompletely understood relationship between the trypanosome and the body's immune system which allows the organism to alter its antigenic disposition when challenged by the host defences. This results in recurring production of immunoglobulin to each wave of parasitaemia, and may lead to a build up of large levels of gammaglobulinaemia. They can remain latent in the CNS, in the choroid plexus and elsewhere, and can re-invade the CNS from time to time. There they cause a meningo-encephalitis.

The clinical features of Rhodesian sleeping sickness are more severe and acute than those of the Gambian variety, which tends to be more indolent. A chancre may form at the site of the bite, and lasts for 2 or 3 weeks. This is associated with the manifestations of haematological and lymphatic disease—weakness, myalgia, arthralgia, lymphadenopathy and splenomegaly, pruritis and skin rashes, recurrent fever, and malaise. These features may persist for months or years. CNS involvement is indicated by personality change, memory failure, persistent headache, and disturbance of the sleep rhythm with insomnia at night and somnolence during the day. Psychotic episodes and organic brain syndromes develop as the disease progresses, and pyramidal, extrapyramidal, cerebellar signs, together with convulsions, become evident. Mycardial and pericardial disease is often evident in Rhodesian sleeping sickness. Untreated, patients become increasingly obtunded and lapse into coma in months with the Rhodesian form, and a longer period for the Gambian form.

Diagnosis is not difficult when the disease occurs in endemic areas. Few cases occur in Britain, and the history of travel from an endemic area is important. Demonstration of the parasite is necessary before commencing treatment, which can be quite toxic. Samples of the initial skin lesion, lymph nodes, blood, or centrifuged CSF are concentrated and examined. The use of PCR to demonstrate trypanosome DNA in blood (Kabiri *et al.* 1999) and CSF (Truc *et al.* 1999) promises much. The CSF should be examined in all cases and any increase of cell count or elevation of protein level should be taken as evidence of CNS disease. Detection of antigen in serum and CSF by ELISA has shown high levels of accuracy (Nantulya *et al.* 1992).

Treatment of cerebral trypanosomiasis is difficult and toxic. Three drugs are useful for the treatment of the blood and lymph node stage of the disease, suramin, pentamidine, and melarsoprol, and only the last is effective against CNS disease. These drugs are all potentially highly toxic and it is best to consult a tropical diseases expert on their use. An encephalopathy may follow treatment with melarsoprol and this may be prevented by the simultaneous administration of steroids. Drug combinations are being studied to determine if they are more effective than single regimes.

American trypanosomiasis (Chaga's disease)

This from of trypanosomiasis occurs in South and Central America and as far north as southern Texas. It is caused by *Trypanosoma cruzi* which is transmitted by bugs of the *Triatoma* genus. Many different mammals function as hosts and there are some strain differences in the organism which lead to variations in virulence and disease syndromes. Humans are bitten by the bug and develop the acute stage of infection with local lymphatic invasion followed by secondary haematogenous dissemination and the organisms lodge in other tissue sites. Haematogenous spread is recurrent and during this phase, which lasts for 2 or 3 months, there are symptoms and signs of generalized infection. Immune defences build up and the disease becomes quiescent for years, sometimes for the rest of the patient's life. Years later the chronic stage becomes evident, usually with cardiomyopathy or with gastro-intestinal disease which leads to mega-oesophagus or mega-colon. Rarely, in the acute phase, there may be a sudden meningo-encephalitis when the brain becomes invaded by trypanosomes. Sometimes this can take the form of localized necrotizing encephalitis. These acute meningo-encephalitides carry a high mortality, sometimes approaching 50 per cent, and are seen more frequently in young children. In immune suppressed patients, and in those with AIDS, full-blown encephalitis may occur at any time, in relation to variation of immune status. In chronic Chaga's disease, frank encephalitis is rare, but CNS involvement may be evident as minor cerebral dysfunction, epilepsy, behaviour, and cognitive disorders in children, polyneuropathy and stroke as a consequence of cardiomyopathy (Kirchhoff 1993; Pitella 1993).

Diagnosis is by demonstration of the parasite in the bloodstream and detection of antibody or antigen in the blood. Drugs which are effective are niphotimox and benzonidazole, but treatment of CNS disease is often disappointing.

34.13.6 Other parasites

Isolated case reports have appeared in the literature over the years of cases of meningo-encephalitis from which various parasites have been identified. Most of these are medical curiosities, and usually, the offending pathogen has been discovered after the death of the patient. *Micronema, Angiostrongylus cantonensis, Lagochilascaris, Baylisascaris, Gnathostoma*, and other nematode parasites have all been implicated in such cases (Lowichik and Siegel 1995). Other parasites cause encephalitis rarely, but often enough to produce a recognizable clinical syndrome.

Primary amoebic encephalitis results from infection by free living amoebae of the species *Naegleria fowleri*. This is a ubiquitous organism that lives in moist soils and most cases have been reported in children who have been swimming in infected water. Amoebae enter the nasal cavity, and ascend to the brain along the olfactory nerves and blood vessels to the meninges and spread thereafter to cause florid necrotizing inflammation. The clinical syndrome comes on suddenly with a severe meningo-encephalitis which has no distinguishing features, and the clue to diagnosis is exposure to stagnant water (Carter 1968). Special examination of fresh, warm specimens of CSF are necessary to demonstrate motile trophozoites. Prognosis is poor and most die rapidly. Survival has been described in patients treated with high doses of parenteral amphotercin. Rifampicin, miconazole, and tetracycline may enhance the effect of amphotercin. *Acanthamoeba* and *Balamuthia* species can cause a subacute or chronic, granulomatous, meningo-encephalitis, and tends to affect immunocompromised people and can cause disease in those whose immune response is intact. Amoebae are not found in the CSF and the diagnosis is not usually made during life unless there has been some reason to biopsy the brain or meninges. Prognosis is almost hopeless, which provides some justification for aggressive treatment with amphotercin.

34.13.7 Whipple's disease

In 1907, George Whipple published a case report of a man of 36 who developed weight loss, steatorrhoea, and arthropathy and soon died. Necropsy revealed infiltration of the intestinal lymph glands by deposits of fats, fatty acids, mononuclear and polynuclear giant cells, and 'foamy' mononuclear cells in the intestinal mucosa. He named it an intestinal lypodystrophy and noted the presence of peculiar rod-shaped organisms in gland tissue, and he mused that they might be of aetiological significance (Whipple 1907). In succeeding years, electron microscopic observations have confirmed the presence of a rod-shaped bacillus, weakly Gram-positive, 1–2 μm long with a thick outer wall which stains with PAS dyes. It is exceptionally difficult to culture and its presence in body tissues can be inferred by the identification of a 16S rRNA gene sequence using PCR. This gene sequence has a phylogenetic association with *Actinomycetes* and the bacillus is thought to be a novel actinomycete which has been named *Tropheryma whippelii*. The method of infection and pathogenesis are not known. Because of the gastrointestinal location of the disease, it is thought to be contracted by ingestion following which it disseminates through the body via lymph and blood. In addition to the gut, the CNS, eyes, heart, lungs, and skin and joints may be involved and the disease may present in any of these systems. As many as 15 per cent of cases do not have gastrointestinal symptoms and jejunal biopsy may be normal (Durand *et al.* 1997).

Clinical features

Whipple's disease is rare. It affects men more than women, and occurs at any age, most commonly with onset in the 40s. Usually there is diarrhoea with malabsorption, weight loss, wasting, pyrexia, sometimes of unknown origin, and lymphadenopathy. Onset is insidious and progress is often atypical. Between 5 and 40 per cent have neurological manifestations and in as many as 5 per cent the disease may be confined to the CNS (Keinath *et al.* 1985; Fleming *et al.* 1988). The most frequent CNS manifestations are dementia, ocular movement disturbance, movement disorders, particularly myoclonus, hypothalamic upset, epilepsy, ataxia, meningitis, and focal cerebral signs. Headache is common. Ophthalmoplegia is of supranuclear type and affects vertical rather than horizontal movement. Internuclear ophthalmoplegia has been described. Movement disorders may affect the eyes—oculomasticatory myorhythmia and oculo-facial-skeletal myorhythmia are said to be diagnostic. Certainly, the triad of dementia, ophthalmoplegia, and myoclonus is highly suggestive of Whipple's disease. Diagnostic guidelines for neurological Whipple's disease have been proposed (Louis *et al.* 1996).

Diagnosis

Diagnosis is by demonstration of a positive PCR against *T. whippelii* in material from affected tissue, including CSF. CT and MR imaging of the brain may show atrophy, mass lesions and contrast enhancement, white matter high signal areas, ring enhancing lesions, and hydrocephalus. Differential diagnosis is wide and includes the dementias, encephalopathies, CNS vasculitides, demyelination, granulomatous disease, and chronic CNS infection. If movement disorder is present with dementia Creutzfeldt–Jakob disease merits exclusion.

Treatment

Treatment is with antibiotics. The regime currently in favour is a combination of parenteral penicillin and streptomycin for a minimum of 14 days, followed by cotrimoxazole orally for up to 2 years; or parenteral ceftriaxone for a month followed by 2 years of oral cefixime. This length of treatment is necessary because of the high incidence of relapse. PCR is now recognized to be the best test to monitor progress and it is necessary to check CSF as well as bowel for negative results before discontinuing treatment (Ramzan *et al.* 1997).

34.14 Intracranial suppuration

34.14.1 General considerations

Brain abscess, subdural empyema, and extradural abscess are all forms of intracranial suppuration. They share common clinical features—they occur relatively infrequently, they present as emergencies, diagnosis is commonly delayed because of lack of familiarity with the clinical picture, morbidity and mortality from each of these conditions remains high, and the incidence of sequelae is considerable. They also share common aetiological factors although there is some evidence that patterns of infection are changing. It might be expected that any form of suppuration would be accompanied by obvious clinical signs of infection such as pyrexia, tachycardia, and malaise. While this does happen, systemic manifestations of infection and inflammation are not always present when the site of suppura-

tion is intracranial, and this may obscure the true diagnosis. If there are overt foci of infection, this considerably aids diagnosis, and specimens from them should be obtained forthwith. It is imperative that such foci be eradicated at the same time as the intracranial problem is being treated. The clinical profiles of brain abscess, subdural empyema, and extradural abscess are sufficiently distinct to warrant separate descriptions.

34.14.2 Brain abscess: clinical features and differential diagnosis

The incidence of brain abscess is generally held to be about 1 in 10 000 of all general hospital admissions in the Western world, approximating to five cases per million population per annum. All agree that this is an underestimate of the true incidence because a proportion are first diagnosed at necropsy, and the spread of HIV infection and other diseases which cause immune suppression has produced a large population vulnerable to opportunistic infection by an ever increasing range of pathogens. It is probable that the number of patients who develop brain abscess is rising, and more cases are being diagnosed as imaging techniques have become more discriminating. Males are affected about twice as often as females although the sex difference is diminishing. The median age is 30–45 years with 25 per cent occurring under the age of 15 and it is unusual for brain abscess to occur under the age of 2 years (deLouvois *et al.* 1977; McLelland *et al.* 1978; Seydoux and Francioli 1992). However, it may be that in the very young age groups abscesses are misdiagnosed as meningitis.

Source of infection

Bacteria reach the brain by three main routes; by the bloodstream, by extension from a contiguous focus of infection, or by being directly inoculated into the brain substance by trauma or by neurosurgery which is not aseptic (Table 34.6). It seems unlikely that spread through CSF plays a part. The route of infection cannot be identified with certainty in about 20 per cent of cases. Formerly spread from an adjacent infection such as otitis or paranasal sinusitis was the most common mechanism but this is now being overtaken by blood-borne infection. Brain abscess is rare in bacterial endocarditis and experimental work has shown that if the blood–brain barrier remains intact, bacteraemia does not lead to brain abscess formation; bacteria cannot set up a nidus of infection in undamaged brain (Molinari *et al.* 1973). It is necessary for there to be a microscopic area of necrosis, either microinfarction from embolism or from hypoxaemia, or from adjacent infection causing thrombophlebitis, for an abscess to take root. Once started, an abscess develops through a series of stages which are well documented and are reproducible under experimental conditions. Furthermore, the pathological changes of these stages of evolution correlate very well with clinical progression and CT brain scan appearances, and it is necessary to bear in mind the timing of imaging in relation to the onset of symptoms when interpreting the scans. Other factors which influence the rate of develop-

Table 34.6. Brain abscess—predisposition and bacteriology

Primary infection	Site of abscess	Organism
Ear	Temporal lobe/cerebellum	Streptococci Enterobateriaceae Bacillus fragilis
Paranasal sinuses	Frontal/deep temporal lobe. Subdural empyema Staphylococci	Streptococci Bacteroides Enterobacteriaceae
Dental sepsis/instrumentation	Multiple	Mixed includes: Fusobacteria Bacteroides Streptococci
Chest, AV malformation, endocarditis	Multiple	Streptococci Staphylococci Bacteroides Fusobacterium
Immune suppression	Multiple	Fungi Toxoplasma Enterobacteriaceae Nocardia Mycobacteria Any organism

ment of an abscess are the quantum and duration of bacteraemia, the virulence of the infecting organism and the host resistance, and the magnitude of preceding embolism.

The first stage is of early cerebritis with perivascular inflammatory change and oedema surrounding the area of brain necrosis. Late cerebritis is characterized by necrosis of the centre, fibroblasts and neovascularity appear at the periphery and begin to form a capsule. Astrocytic reaction is induced and white matter oedema spreads. Early capsule formation continues with the development of further fibroblasts, peripheral vascularity, oedema, and reactive astrocytosis. Late capsule formation proceeds after about a fortnight as it thickens and puts down collagen (Britt *et al.* 1981; Britt and Enzmann 1983).

The sources of primary infection which seed brain abscesses are many. There is a degree of correlation between the source of infection, the part of the brain in which the abscess grows, and the pathogenic organism (Table 34.6). Otogenic infection,

which is diminishing in frequency in the Western world, but not in the Third World, spreads to the temporal lobe (Fig. 34.4) or cerebellum and is likely to be caused by a mixed flora which may include aerobic or anaerobic streptococci, enterobacteriaceae, and *Bacillus fragilis*. Paranasal sinusitis predisposes to frontal lobe and deep temporal lobe abscesses and to subdural empyema. The offending organisms include streptococci, including *Strep millerii*, staphylococci, bacteroides, and enterobacteriaceae. Blood-borne infection may settle anywhere in the brain and may give rise to multiple and multiloculated abscesses. The distribution of the middle cerebral artery is favoured and they occur near the grey–white matter junction where the blood flow is not so rich. The source is often in the chest, and may be a lung abscess or bronchiectasis, congenital heart disease, particularly with right to left shunt, or pulmonary arteriovenous fistula. The organisms are varied and include streptococci, anaerobic, microaerophilic and *viridans*, bacteroides, fusobacterium, and staphylococci. Another cause of bacteraemia is peridontal infection, either spontaneous or caused to flare up by dental manipulation. This gives rise to mixed infections with fusobacteria, bacteroides, and streptococci. Other procedures which may give rise to bacteraemia are instrumentation of the oesophagus, gastrointestinal and urinary tract, and to pelvic structures. Abscesses which result from implantation of organisms by trauma or neurosurgery occur in relation to the wound or tract of the injury and the organisms are staphylococci, streptococci, clostridia, or enterobacteriaceae. It very seldom happens that bacterial meningitis gives rise to a brain abscess—it may be that this happens more commonly in infants in which case the organism is likely to be a Gram-negative bacillus. In patients who suffer immune sup-

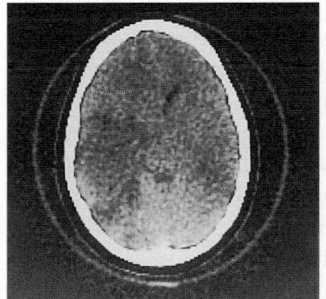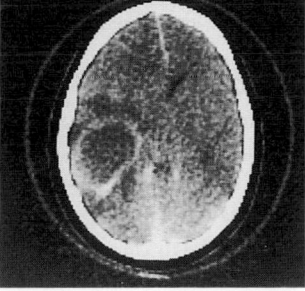

Fig. 34.4. Otogenic cerebral abscess in the temporal lobe shown by CT scan unenhanced (left) and contrast enhanced (right).

pression by virtue of disease or its treatment, the CNS is vulnerable to attack by a very wide range of organisms, most of which would not be virulent enough to cause infection in normal circumstances. Because of the lack of an immune reaction to infection, such patients may not exhibit the clinical signs that would normally be found, and, by the time of presentation, the infection may be overwhelming. In such circumstances, the lesions are often multiple. Fungi, toxoplasma, enterobacteriaceae, nocardia, and mycobacterial infection have all to be considered in addition to the usual pathogens.

The ability to isolate an organism from abscess pus depends very much on close liaison with the microbiology laboratory and it is prudent to involve the microbiologist from the very beginning of the patient's work up. The microbiologist will need to know of any obvious foci of infection, whether antibiotics have been administered, are there any underlying predisposing factors? Care should be taken that there is no delay in transport of the specimens to the laboratory and that proper culture media are set up for fastidious organisms and for anaerobes and fungi. The yield of positive cultures can be increased significantly when such measures are taken (deLouvois *et al.* 1977).

Clinical features

The presentation of brain abscesses is variable and depends on the virulence of the organism, the host defences, the age of the patient, the severity of the primary infection, and the site and number of brain abscesses. The onset may be fulminant, leading to death within days or even hours, particularly if an abscess ruptures into the cerebral ventricles. In others, the evolution may be over months, and in one case which I have seen, following a head injury, some years passed between the injury which caused a compound frontal skull fracture and the later

development of a frontal brain abscess. In most, the duration of symptoms by the time of presentation is 2 weeks. Headache occurs in most patients and there are no specific features. It may be generalized or localized, continuous or intermittent. Pyrexia occurs in only about 50 per cent. Focal signs appropriate to the site of the lesion commonly develop, in as many as half of all cases, and may include epileptic seizures which occur commonly and are more likely to be generalized. Brain abscesses occupy space and together with the surrounding oedema, lead to raised ICP. Some disturbance of the conscious level and sensorium is usual—from lethargy to coma in severe cases. Prognosis is closely related to the level of consciousness at the time of admission. Neck stiffness may be evident and may suggest a degree of meningitis. If fever is present or if signs of infection elsewhere in the body are evident then the diagnosis is not usually too difficult to reach. Since these signs are absent as often as not, it is not uncommon to initially misdiagnose brain abscesses as intracranial tumours, infarction, haemorrhage with clot formation, necrotizing encephalitis, severe migraine, stroke, or meningitis. CT brain scan typically shows a contrast-enhancing ring surrounded by oedema (Fig. 34.4). Intracranial vasculitis and non-infective granulomas as well as malignant tumours and multiple sclerosis (Fig. 34.5) may all present clinically like an abscess, complete with raised temperature and scan appearances of ring-enhancing lesions (Nielsen *et al.* 1982; Chun *et al.* 1986; Mampalan and Rosenblum 1988). In young children and infants the clinical picture may be quite atypical. The head may enlarge from increasing ICP and may be associated with vomiting and epileptic seizures so mimicking a brain tumour or hydrocephalus from congenital abnormality.

34.14.3 Subdural empyema

Subdural empyema refers to the accumulation of pus in the potential space between the dura and arachnoid mater. It is more likely to collect over the convexities of the cerebral hemispheres, in the parafalcine region and above the tentorium cerebelli because brain is not as closely applied to the dura in these areas as it is in the region of the venous sinuses. Fewer than 10 per cent occur in the posterior fossa. Subdural empyema shares similar pathogenetic mechanisms with brain abscess and they not infrequently occur together. Subdural pus results from extension of infection from the ear or from paranasal sinusitis, or less frequently from osteomyelitis of the skull. Rarely, it may be caused by haematogenous spread or by direct implantation of organisms following cranial trauma. In young children the subdural effusions which accompany meningitis may become infected. The causal organisms reflect the underlying predisposition—in adults aerobic and anaerobic streptococci, staphylococci, and Gram-negative organisms predominate—in children and infants *Haemophilus influenzae*, pneumococci, and Gram-negative bacteria are the most frequent. It is important to remember that in circumstances favourable to the organism, any one may become pathogenic, including fungi.

More than half of all patients are less than 20 years old and there is a male : female ratio of 2 : 1. The clinical presentation is

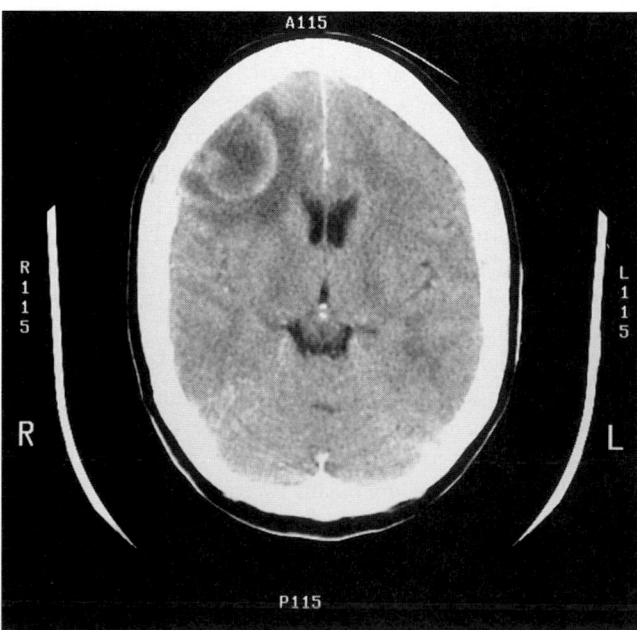

Fig. 34.5. CT brain scan of a patient with multiple sclerosis, showing a ring enhancing right frontal lesion, thought to be an abscess, which showed signs of acute multiple sclerosis on biopsy.

acute, within 2 weeks, sometimes explosive, and usually includes overt signs of infection such as pyrexia, tachycardia, and rigors, perhaps with evidence of local infection; a painful tender face, pain over the mastoid process, or tenderness on palpation over the paranasal sinuses. There may have been non-specific malaise for a few days. There are signs of raised ICP—drowsiness, decreased conscious level which may progress to coma, neck stiffness, papilloedema, and sixth or third cranial nerve palsies. Focal signs of hemiparesis, dysphasia, nystagmus, and ataxia may point to the region of the brain that is primarily affected, either by direct pressure and inflammation from the pus, or by vascular damage from superficial thrombophlebitis. Epilepsy is common, much more so than with intracerebral abscess, and is often focal. As many as two-thirds of all patients may be so afflicted. If subdural empyema is suspected, anticonvulsants should be given straight away. A collection of pus in the parafalcine area of the brain may cause a monoparesis of the leg, paraparesis and sphincter upset, mimicking a spinal cord lesion. The diagnosis should be considered in any patient with focal signs or symptoms accompanied by pyrexia and epileptic seizures (Bannister *et al.* 1981; Miller *et al.* 1987; Dill *et al.* 1995; Nathoo *et al.* 1999).

34.14.4 Extradural brain abscess

Also known as epidural brain abscess, this condition refers to the collection of pus in the extradural, or epidural space, i.e. the potential space which exists between the outside of the dura mater and the inside of the skull. Normally there is no separation of the two. If sepsis occurs in adjacent structures such as the skull bones in mastoiditis or osteomyelitis, following trauma or paranasal infection, pus can spread to this space and strip the dura from the underlying bone, and in the process cause hyperaemia of the meninges and fibrin deposition and thrombophlebitis. Unfortunately, one of the increasingly frequent causes of introducing sepsis is neurosurgery (Hlavin *et al.* 1994). The organisms which cause extradural abscesses are those of the underlying cause of sepsis—chief amongst which are streptococci, anaerobes, and staphylococci, but a variegation of organisms has been described including fungi.

Cranial extradural infection is rare and is less common than spinal extradural infection. It may occur in any age group and in either sex. Unlike the other forms of intracranial suppuration, the signs of local infection tend to over-ride those of neurological dysfunction. Focal and neurological signs and raised ICP are uncommon. It is more likely that local pain, tenderness, and oedema will be found on examination of the skull. Localized headache is common as are signs of systemic infection. In fungal infections and in some of the more chronic bacterial infections, including TB, the evolution of the disease to hospital presentation may take months.

34.14.5 Investigation

A high index of suspicion is required in order to make an expeditious diagnosis of intracranial suppuration. In brain abscess signs of infection are often lacking, in subdural and extradural infection they are commonly present. All patients should have a full blood count and ESR examination carried out, together with electrolyte estimation and CRP level. Other blood tests should be carried out according to clinical indications. If there is an obvious site of infection, specimens should be obtained for culture, if necessary by needle aspiration, and X-rays obtained according to clinical need. Lumbar puncture to examine CSF should never be undertaken if these pathologies are suspected, because each may be associated with a rise of ICP to potentially lethal levels. X-rays of the skull may reveal changes of sinusitis, mastoiditis, osteomyelitis, and shift of the pineal to indicate midline shift from cerebral space occupation. Such changes are seen more readily and in better detail by scanning. Consequently, skull X-rays are seldom carried out nowadays. Electroencephalography may be asked for, particularly if the patient presents with epileptic seizures. Localized discharges may be found in relation to an abscess causing brain irritation but these are in no way specific for infection; neither are the changes of focal slow wave activity which are also commonly seen.

The best way to diagnose suspected intracranial suppuration is to image it with CT or MR. MR is in general more sensitive than CT but it does have limitations when the patient is acutely ill (Section 34.4.4). The changes seen on scans must be interpreted with critical attention to the time at which they were undertaken in relation to the clinical evolution of the disease. It is always best to obtain the help of a neuroradiologist if at all possible, because the changes may be subtle and similar to those produced by several other disease states. There should be no inhibition in asking for repeat scans to determine if there has been change in the radiological appearances for these can occur rapidly and when this happens, it may serve to distinguish an abscess from an area of infarction or a tumour. It is also necessary to use contrast enhancement with CT, otherwise lesions may be missed (Fitzpatrick and Gan 1999). On CT scan the earliest stages of the evolution of a cerebral abscess, cerebritis, appears as a low-density abnormality which may have some surrounding oedema and a little space occupation. Later, surrounding oedema and space occupation increase and the centre of the abscess develops a much lower density, and as the capsule of the abscess matures, ring enhancement following the injection of contrast media, takes place (Fig. 34.3). It is possible to identify the location and number of lesions, and the presence of hydrocephalus and mass effect.

Unfortunately, such imaging changes, although characteristic, are not specific for they may be seen with high-grade gliomas and metastases and with some forms of granuloma. Haemorrhagic infarction and bleeding from arteriovenous anomalies has also caused confusion, as has relapsing multiple sclerosis. The condition of the paranasal sinuses, including the sphenoidal sinus, and mastoid air cells should be noted, and search made for skull fractures and cranial defects. MR imaging is superior to CT in the early detection of cerebritis and in determining the extent of white matter change. The application of newer techniques such as diffusion weighting MR imaging promises greater discrimination between abscesses and other pathology in the future (Weisberg 1984; Davidson and Steiner 1985; Schroth *et al.* 1987; Kim *et al.* 1998; Miller *et al.* 1988; Desprechins *et al.* 1999). The appearances of subdural empyema are of an extracerebral collection of density lower than brain with a rim of enhancement following contrast injection. Extradural collections show as low-density areas inside the skull with a thick densely enhancing ring at the periphery. Changes of infection may be evident in the adjacent bone (Weingarten *et al.* 1987; Tsuchiya *et al.* 1992; Nathoo *et al.* 1999).

34.14.6 Treatment

The sooner that treatment with appropriate antibiotics is given, the better is the prognosis for all forms of intracranial suppuration. If there is likely to be a delay before imaging or surgery or even transfer to a specialist unit (as happens more frequently in the NHS of today), empirical antibiotic treatment should be given immediately. The regime can be altered later if necessary. Diligent search must be made for the source of infection, specimens taken, and the source eradicated. Supportive treatment aimed at the maintenance of circulation and the correction of hypoxaemia should be given. Electrolytic upset and derangement of serum osmolality are not uncommon and need to be monitored and corrected. Raised ICP is often a problem. There are no clear data on the effects of steroid treatment, beneficial or otherwise, when used to reduce ICP in these conditions—most practitioners use them if the clinical situation is deteriorating. More acutely, pressure monitoring is advisable if it is available, and hyperventilation and mannitol can be given in the short term. We do not know if such measures are consistently beneficial in the long term. Epileptic seizures are treated with anticonvulsants. The incidence of epileptic attacks is very high in subdural empyema and I believe that prophylaptic anticonvulsants should be given as soon as the diagnosis is suspected. Whether they are needed in the longer term can be reviewed.

In all forms of intracranial suppuration, samples of pus and infected tissue should be obtained as soon as possible. There is no agreement on the form of surgery which is best, or when it should be timed, in the treatment of brain abscess. If accessible and not in too risky an area, an abscess should be aspirated surgically. Stereotactic techniques have improved precision and biopsy yield and have reduced surgical morbidity (Apuzzo *et al.* 1987; Mamelak *et al.* 1995; Barlas *et al.* 1999). The appearances should be monitored by repeat scanning and if the lesion or lesions do not show reduction in size, they should be re-aspirated, and the treatment regime re-assessed. In this respect, MR probably does have some advantage over CT in that the detail seen on scan is rather more precise and there is no known radiation hazard of repeat MR scanning. Multiple abscesses should be treated in this way too. There is some evidence that adequate reduction in abscess size and eventual resolution can be obtained by medical treatment alone without the need for aspiration (Boom and Tuazon 1985). While this is possible, it is undoubtedly better to have a specimen of infected tissue to determine the nature and the antibiotic sensitivity of the infect-

ing organism. If the patient is immune suppressed, the threshold for surgical aspiration is lowered because the spectrum of organisms which may be causing the abscess is so much wider. In patients with AIDS, toxoplasmosis is the likely cause of lesions which look like abscesses. However, the appearances are not specific. A reasonable course of action would be to treat for toxoplasmosis with pyrimethamine and sulphadiazine and folinic acid (to counter pyrimethamine effects on haematogenesis), and monitor progress closely. If the appearances are atypical, if blood serology for toxoplasmosis is negative, if there is clinical progression, or if there is no evidence of clinical and radiological improvement within a fortnight on treatment, aspiration should take place.

Surgical treatment is necessary for subdural empyema. I have some doubts about the adequacy of burr-hole aspiration alone because it is possible to miss small loci of pus and craniotomy with wide exploration of the exposed brain is recommended (Bannister *et al.* 1981; Morgan and Williams 1985; Feuerman *et al.* 1989). Widespread exploration, excision of infected material and bone, and later cranioplasty, are used for extradural infection.

The choice of antibiotic used will be determined by several factors which will include the likely causal organism, the ability of the drug to penetrate into CSF and into the pus in the abscess cavity, and it must be active in the presence of pus. Our knowledge of penetration and activity of the newer antibiotics is not good. At present the favoured empirical regime combines penicillin intravenously in a dose of 24 mega units each day for an average sized adult, with chloramphenicol 1 g intravenously every 6 h and metronidazole 500 mg intravenously every 8 h. Some prefer to give a third generation cephalosporin, usually cefotaxime or ceftriaxone, in preference to penicillin and chloramphenicol. Other antibiotics will be given according to the results of cultures and it is prudent to discuss the best treatment regime with one or all of bacteriologist, pharmacologist, and infectious diseases physician. In order to prevent confusion, the neurologist should retain overall responsibility for the prescription of drugs. The length of time for which drugs should be given and the frequency that blood levels should be checked, depend upon the circumstances of the individual patient and improvement of scan appearances. In this respect, it is important to recognize that abscesses which appear to be cured clinically may show changes, including contrast enhancement, for months afterwards. Parenteral treatment is usually given for 1–2 months, followed by a variable regime of oral treatment, if appropriate. Unfortunately, we do not have trial data on which to base decisions about antibiotic regimes.

34.14.7 Outcome and sequelae

The introduction of CT brought about a dramatic reduction in the mortality rate for brain abscess and for subdural empyema, and to a lesser degree, for extradural haematoma. There had been a reduction with the introduction of antibiotics, but the ability to localize the lesions accurately, and to monitor their progress, has been the major factor in reducing death rates from

80 per cent or thereby, in the pre-antibiotic era, to contemporary levels of less than 5 per cent. Doubtless many other factors have contributed to this improvement, including the introduction of stereotactic surgical techniques, the development of newer antibiotics, and improvement in intensive care. Nevertheless, it remains true that delay in diagnosis and the administration of antibiotics, has an adverse effect on the outcome. Harrison (1982) found that in a proportion of cases, clinical and historical evidence of fever and infection had been disregarded, and I fear that the same may happen in some cases even today. Increasing impairment of conscious level also carries a poor prognosis. Inappropriate use of antibiotics may be another factor (Yang 1981). The mortality rate for the treatment of subdural empyema has been variably reported and approximates to 20–25 per cent.

The major sequelae suffered by survivors of brain abscess are epilepsy, focal neurological deficit, and mental changes. Epilepsy has occurred in more than 50 per cent of survivors and is more frequent if the patient is young, if the abscess has been in the frontal, temporal, or parietal region, and if seizures have occurred in the acute phase. The longer the follow up, the greater is the number of survivors who will develop seizures. Generalized seizures are more common than focal and usually begin within 5 years. In the UK, for an ordinary driving licence at the time of writing, the regulations require the patient to be banned from driving for a minimum period of 1 year from treatment of a cerebral abscess, and 2 years for a subdural empyema, provided they remain seizure free. For a professional driving licence, the prospective risk for the development of epilepsy is so high, that revocation of the licence is required, and restoration will not be contemplated until the applicant has been seizure free for 10 years. Focal deficits occur in between 25 and 50 per cent of survivors. Mental changes are almost certainly under-reported and affect at least 20 per cent.

After subdural empyema, improvement from focal disturbance is much better. Epilepsy is a considerable problem. Cowie and Williams (1983) found that in their series, 63 per cent of cases had seizures during the acute phase of the illness. Of these, only 29 per cent continued to have seizures. However, of those who had no seizures in the acute phase, 42 per cent went on to have fits. There is a case to recommend prophylactic treatment with anti-epileptic drugs to all patients with intracranial and subdural abscess, but there is no evidence that this protects against the development of epilepsy.

34.15 Intracranial granulomas and cysts

Granulomas and cysts of the brain can be caused by infections. In some cases, the same agents which cause meningitis and, sometimes encephalitis, can also induce foci of inflammation within brain parenchyma, which enlarge to cause solid granulomas or fluid filled cysts which do not suppurate. The factors that lead the same infectious agent to give rise to meningitis in one patient, and a granuloma in another, or both in the same patient, are not fully understood. In such cases, it will be readily recognized that the clinical picture may be complicated. Granulomas and cysts often present with focal signs, features of space occupation, and with epilepsy, and may be complicated by the clinical features of meningitis. The same clinical picture is caused by a wide variety of pathogens. It is usually not possible to differentiate these syndromes without cranial imaging, which has revolutionized management and greatly improved the prognosis for most of these conditions. Signs of infection elsewhere in the body, perhaps peculiar to a particular organism, the geographical location or the seasonal timing of an outbreak, or the association with an occupation or leisure pastimes which may provoke exposure to a specific disease, can all provide clues to the cause. In a significant number of cases, even after these factors have been determined, there may still be a choice of diagnoses and it is necessary to revert to surgical biopsy of the lesion. As with other infections, delay in making a diagnosis leads to a poorer prognosis.

34.15.1 Tuberculoma

The aetiology and pathogenesis of intracranial tuberculomas is similar to that of tuberculous meningitis (Section 33.2.3). Mycobacteria reach the brain via the bloodstream and form tubercles which grow and become surrounded by a fibrous capsule which surrounds a caseous core with Langhans cells, epitheliod cells and lymphocytes, and organisms may be evident. The lesions may be single or multiple, and may vary in size from small nodules to large, well circumscribed tumours several centimetres in diameter which may be macroscopically indistinguishable from meningiomas—to the degree of inducing its own blood supply from the meninges. The consistency and degree of fibrous encapsulation can vary too, so that a tuberculoma may be mistaken for a glial tumour. Not all tumours are discreet and nodular and it is possible to have an extensive multilocular tuberculoma, or a thin film of tuberculoma tissue over the surface of the brain adherent to the meninges, much like an *en plaque* meningioma. Rarely, but less so now than formerly, the centre of the tuberculoma may liquefy to become an abscess. It has been reported that such abscesses caused a more florid and toxic clinical presentation. This has not been our experience. We have been able to distinguish tuberculous abscess from tuberculous granuloma only after imaging, and because of the relative rarity of the former, stereotactic biopsy has always been carried out to obtain information about the organism.

Before the advent of chemotherapy, tuberculomas were common, accounting for 34 per cent of space occupying lesions found in a necropsy series in Leeds (Garland and Armitage 1933). In the developing world where TB remains endemic, tuberculomas still account for a similar proportion of brain tumours, to the degree that it is often appropriate to treat for TB as soon as a space occupying lesion is found, and monitor the clinical status. Biopsy or surgical removal is carried out if there is no improvement or the patient deteriorates. Formerly, tuberculomas affected children in the main, but now the

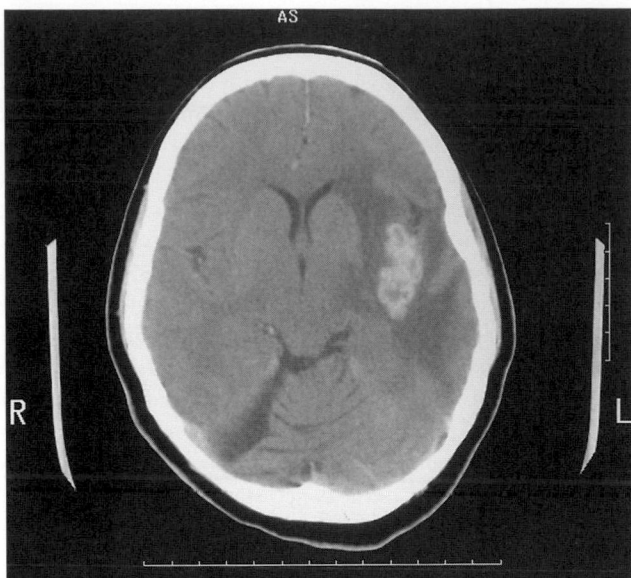

Fig. 34.6. CT brain scan showing a developing tuberculoma in the left Sylvian fissure. The Indian lady had been treated with sensitivity-proven anti-TB drugs throughout.

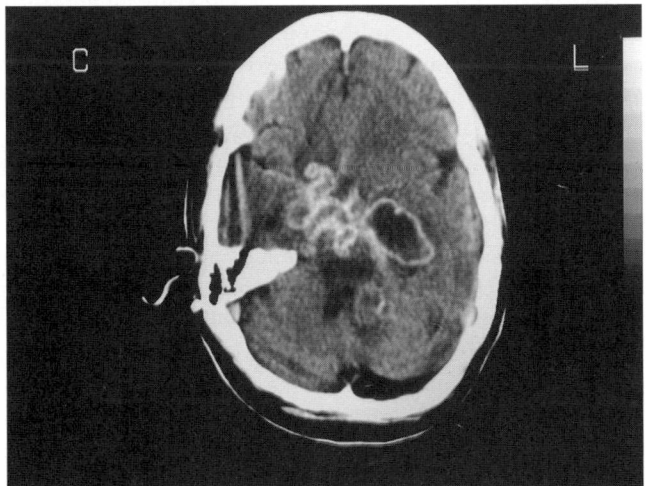

Fig. 34.7. TB abscess and tuberculomas which developed in an Indian lady who did not take prescribed anti-TB chemotherapy in her homeland.

emphasis is shifting to adults and any age group may be affected. Approximately 10–15 per cent of cases of tuberculous meningitis are complicated by the development of tuberculomas, and this may happen even with adequate and appropriate chemotherapy (Fig. 34.6). Similarly, further tuberculomas may develop as the index one resolves (Fig. 34.7). In the majority of cases, tuberculomas develop as the sole neurological syndrome, and there is commonly no clinical evidence of TB elsewhere in the body. In such cases the diagnosis may be inferred by the racial origin of the patient or by travel from a known tuberculous region. In England, we have seen intracranial tuberculomas in all racial groups, and there is a higher frequency in immigrants from India, Pakistan, Southeast Asia, the Carib-

bean, Africa, and Ireland, and more so if immigration has been recent.

Tuberculomas and abscesses may occur in any area of the brain and the symptoms and signs are appropriate to the area of the brain affected. Multiple tuberculomas may produce a confusing clinical picture in the same vein as multiple metastases. Presentation may be as a space occupying lesion with symptoms and signs of raised ICP, with focal neurological signs, or with epilepsy, either generalized or focal. The presentation of the syndrome is seldom acute, tending to evolve over weeks or months although exceptions do occur. There is usually no evidence of TB elsewhere in the body—if there is the diagnosis becomes easier. Similarly, clinical and laboratory indices of infection or inflammation are lacking, more often than not. The patients often appear very well clinically. Brain imaging with CT or MRI has revolutionized the management of this condition. The appearances are not diagnostic and may mimic virtually any other from of intracranial space occupying lesion (Selvapandian *et al.* 1994). The common appearance of a tuberculoma is of a low or equi-dense lesion surrounded by oedema, often with microscopic calcification, and a surrounding rim of enhancement following contrast. Lobulated rings and discs may also be seen (Mishra and Goyal 1999). If a tuberculoma is suspected, the CSF should not be examined.

A search must be made for evidence of TB elsewhere in the body and a chest X-ray should be done. Mantoux testing is positive in about two-thirds of cases but this is not diagnostic. In those cases that do not show evidence of other TB infection, a definitive diagnosis can be made only by examination of tissue obtained by biopsy. In patients who present with single or multiple lesions and in whom space occupation is not a problem, and who are of a recognized at-risk racial grouping, our practice is to look for evidence of TB elsewhere and to treat with anti-TB chemotherapy, closely monitoring the appearance of the lesions with serial scans, and with frequent clinical assessments. If there is evidence of scan or clinical deterioration, surgical biopsy is undertaken. Unfortunately, tuberculomas can enlarge or develop *de novo* despite anti-TB chemotherapy, and this may be a source of confusion. The threshold for biopsy is much lower in patients with immune suppression and AIDS and who have lesions which look like abscesses. There does not seem to be a great risk of causing TB meningitis or dissemination of TB to other parts of the body from these procedures, provided the patient is already on chemotherapy.

Once the diagnosis of tuberculoma has been reached an antituberculous drug regime is decided upon, appropriate to the circumstances of the patient, in the same way as treatment for TB meningitis. Discussion with a physician experienced in the treatment of TB who will have knowledge of local patterns of drug resistance, is always recommended (Section 33.2.3). The same physician will be able to organize tracing family and work place contacts and appropriate notification of disease. The length of time for which treatment should be given approximates to that for TB meningitis and is influenced by improvement in scan appearances. Raised ICP can be treated with dexamathasone and other agents if needed, apparently without causing increased hazard of disease dissemination. Epilepsy is controlled with anticonvulsant drugs.

Provided the diagnosis is made expeditiously, and a full course of anti-TB treatment is given, the outcome is usually excellent, and complete recovery is possible. The prognosis is not good for drug resistant strains, or for those with AIDS. For reasons that this author does not understand, some cases are seen who do not respond to chemotherapy at all, despite the bacillus having been shown to be sensitive in the laboratory, and blood and CSF drug levels having been within the recognized therapeutic ranges.

34.15.2 Other bacterial causes

Other bacterial infections which may cause granulomas inside the head include *Nocardia* (Section 34.15.3), rarely *Brucella*, and syphilis which may cause a gumma. It is likely that more and varied infections, usually starting as meningitis and leading to the formation of granulomas will be described in those who are immune suppressed. The clue to granuloma formation is the appearance of focal signs in the context of meningo-encephalitis and the diagnosis can be confirmed by brain imaging. Those syndromes associated with specific organisms are described under the organism title.

34.15.3 Nocardiosis

Nocardiosis is an opportunistic infection of man which occurs in patients who are immune suppressed by reason of treatment or disease—lymphoreticular neoplasia, organ transplantation, connective tissue disease, malignancy, pulmonary alveolar proteinosis, chronic high dose glucocorticoid treatment, and HIV. Six species of *Nocardia* cause disease in man, *Nocardia asteroides* predominates and infection takes the form of invasive pulmonary disease acquired by inhalation, with multiple abscess formation which may disseminate via the bloodstream and seed in the brain to cause abscesses there in as many as 20 per cent of cases. Much less commonly cutaneous infection by the other species produces cellulitis and mycetoma. *Nocardia* are aerobic Gram-positive bacteria which grow in tissue as a widely spreading mycelium. They differ from fungi.

The neurological manifestations of nocardial disease are those of brain abscess with signs of space occupation and raised ICP, focal deficit, and epilepsy. There is usually evidence of pulmonary infection ranging from localized pneumonitis to fulminating pneumonia and lung abscess. There is nothing characteristic of nocardial brain abscess, and the clue to diagnosis comes from the underlying associated condition. Rarely, there may be meningitis or invasion of adjacent skull bone with osteomyelitis. Brain imaging with CT or MR shows characteristics of brain abscess with cystic space occupation, rim enhancement and surrounding oedema and the lesions may be multiple. Diagnosis is by demonstration of the organism in pus obtained from a lesion by stereotactic biopsy. Some advocate surgical excision of the abscesses. Treatment is with sulphonamides and trimethoprim for at least a year. Minocycline or

amikacin together with a third generation cephalosporin is an alternative combination (Mamelak *et al.* 1994). Mortality rates are high and vary from 30 to 60 per cent.

34.15.4 Actinomycosis

Actinomyces which cause actinomycosis are Gram-positive anaerobic microbes and are normal commensals of the mouth and pharynx of humans. Virtually all human infection is caused by *Actinomyces israeli*. The organisms invade the tissue when trauma, usually minor, occurs to skin or mucous membrane. Risk factors include dental extraction and caries, trauma to the head, chronic middle ear disease, and osteomyelitis. Once in the tissues, they cause suppuration and inflammatory change and induce small granuloma formation which coalesces to form abscesses. These spread by invasion of adjacent tissue and pus is discharged through the sinuses which are formed. Neurological disease is rare, complicates no more than 3 per cent of all cases, and results from direct spread of craniofacial disease, or haematogenous dissemination from lung disease. The most common lesion is a brain abscess. Subdural and epidural abscesses are less common. Meningo-encephalitis and actino-mycotic granulomas have also been described. Brain scan appearances are not diagnostic and mimic other kinds of abscess and skull osteomyelitis. Diagnosis is not difficult if there is evidence of suppurating, discharging sinuses, and is confirmed by demonstration of the characteristic sulphur granules and demonstration of the organism in pus or biopsy tissue. Treatment is by surgical extirpation of diseased tissue as far as is possible, and drainage of pus. Penicillin is the drug of choice, and prolonged treatment for up to 1 year may be required. Tetracycline and erythromycin are alternatives. Secondary infection is common and requires treatment according to culture results. The overall mortality is about a quarter and a substantial proportion of survivors have neurological abnormalities (Smego 1987).

34.15.5 Aspergillosis

Aspergillus species are saprophytic fungal moulds which are found throughout the world in soil and water and vegetable matter. Transmission to humans occurs through inhalation of the fungus, consequently the brunt of infection falls upon the lungs and the upper respiratory passages. In people with an intact immune system, infection is usually limited to the lungs and nasopharynx, where abscesses, granulomas, pneumonia, and chronic granulomatous disease develop. There is seldom spread elsewhere: sometimes there is invasion of adjacent structures from nasopharyngeal disease. In the immune compromised, invasive aspergillosis results and the disease spreads by the bloodstream to other organs including brain. Those conditions which predispose to invasive disease include neutropaenia, and haematological malignancy, organ transplantation, chronic corticosteroid treatment, i.v. drug abuse, and other chronic debilitating states. Several varieties of *Aspergillus* can cause human disease, and the vast majority of cases are caused by *A. fumigatus* and *A. flavus*. Aspergillosis is found worldwide, in all races, both sexes, and in any age group from neonate to senility. CNS disease usually results from haematogenous dissemination but it may also occur by direct extension from paranasal or orbital granulomas or via emmisary veins. The pattern of CNS involvement varies; direct extension results in abscess formation in the frontal and temporal lobes and this may be single or multiple and can develop over weeks or months and is often associated with granuloma formation; haematogenous dissemination causes acute disease with multiple necrotizing abscesses. Because hyphae of the fungus invade blood vessels, such infection gives rise to thrombosis and infarction, and in some cases, true 'mycotic' aneurysms are formed. Stroke syndromes are therefore commonly found with *Aspergillus* infection.

The clinical syndromes of aspergillosis are many and reflect the area of brain affected and the underlying lesion. Abscesses and granulomas present as space occupying lesions with raised ICP and focal signs and epilepsy, basal granulomas cause multiple cranial nerve palsies and ophthalmoplegia, arterial invasion results in abrupt stroke syndromes. Rarely, meningitis may occur.

There are no specific features which point to a diagnosis of aspergillosis—it should be suspected in the immune suppressed who develop a brain abscess, granuloma, or stroke. Brain imaging will show abscess formation and infarction or haemorrhage, perhaps with paranasal granulomas (Ashdown *et al.* 1994; DeLone *et al.* 1999). Diagnosis is by demonstration of fungal elements in biopsy tissue. Serological tests have not been helpful. Recent reports suggest that PCR for *Aspergillus* DNA in CSF is useful (Kami *et al.* 1999) but this may not always be appropriate when there is space occupation. Once the diagnosis has been established, treatment is with amphotercin and surgical extirpation of the lesion or lesions whenever possible (Denning and Stevens 1990). Concomitant therapy with rifampicin, ketoconazole, and itraconazole has been tried and individual reports have noted success. The outcome is often poor and the mortality rate exceeds 50 per cent for the immune compromised.

34.15.6 Blastomycosis

Blastomyces dermatidis is a dimorphic yeast which was formerly thought to be peculiar to the south and central USA and the Great Lakes region. Most cases have been recorded from these areas but reports from Africa and South America and rarer reports from other regions have confirmed that the organism is ubiquitous and probably resides in the soil. Infection is acquired by inhalation, occurs almost always in males who have worked outdoors or who have engaged in outdoor pursuits, and produces an acute chest infection which is usually self-limiting and has similarities to coccidioidomycosis and histoplasmosis. More cases are being seen in AIDS patients. In a few, dissemination to other organs takes place by the bloodstream. If the CNS is involved a chronic meningitic syndrome occurs and rarely, an abscess or granuloma may develop in the brain. Invariably,

there is evidence of pulmonary or cutaneous disease. The clinical and imaging features are similar to other CNS granulomas and abscesses and diagnosis depends upon the demonstration of fungal material on biopsy specimens (Roos *et al.* 1987). Serodiagnostic and skin tests are suggestive but not conclusive. Treatment of CNS disease is with amphotercin, ketoconazole, and itraconazole.

34.15.7 Coccidioidomycosis

Coccidioidomycosis is caused by the dimorphic fungus *Coccidioides immitis* which exists in soil in southern USA, Mexico, and parts of South America. The spores are inhaled by people who work in or visit these areas and give rise to pulmonary infection which is asymptomatic in the majority. Others develop a self-limiting flu-like illness with fever, cough, often accompanied by erythema nodosum, 1 week to 1 month after infection. In less than 1 per cent, spread beyond the respiratory system occurs and one-third of these develop CNS involvement, almost always a form of chronic meningitis which comes on weeks or months later. Blacks, pregnant women, people on steroids, diabetics, and now people with AIDS, are at greater risk of development of CNS complications (Bronnimann *et al.* 1987).

The clinical features of coccidioidomycotic meningitis are no different from any other form of meningitis. It produces a chronic mononuclear response with a high eosinophil count in the CSF. There is a granulomatous response in the meninges. Focal signs may be caused by granuloma formation, abscess, or from infarction consequent upon obliterative arteritis (Bouza *et al.* 1981). Brain imaging is necessary to demonstrate these features and to determine whether there is hydrocephalus prior to CSF examination. Diagnosis is by demonstration of raised complement fixing antibodies in CSF from the beginning and the titres tend to reflect activity of disease and can be used to monitor the progress of therapy. It is possible to culture the fungus from CSF in up to one-third of cases, but this takes time.

Treatment is with fluconazole and amphotercin which may need to be installed intrathecally. It is usually necessary to continue treatment for a prolonged time and relapse is common. The mortality rate is high.

34.15.8 Mucormycosis

Mucormycosis refers to infection with fungi of the Mucoraceae family. It is used interchangeably, although semantically inaccurately, with phycomycosis and zygomycosis (the class of fungi named Phycomycetes or Zygomycetes includes the family Mucoraceae). The major pathogens in this group are of the genera *Rhizopus*, *Absidia*, *Mucor*, and *Cunninghamella*. They are found throughout the world and they grow in soil and decaying vegetable matter. Less than 5 per cent of cases occur in normal hosts. Seventy per cent occur in diabetics who become acidotic, and acidosis from other conditions can predispose to development of rhinocerebral mucormycosis. Other groups at risk are the severely malnourished, the immune suppressed, particularly those who have lymphoma and blood malignancy and those who have suffered extensive trauma (Lehrer *et al.* 1980). Recently, there have been reports of association with treatment by deferoxamine (Vlasveld and Sweder von Asbeck 1991). The spores are inhaled or inoculated through damaged skin or mucosa. An acute suppurative pyogenic necrosis is produced with granuloma formation if the process is more chronic. These fungi have an affinity for arteries which they penetrate, inducing thrombosis and infarction and causing distal embolization and the formation of true mycotic aneurysms. CNS disease occurs in about one-third of cases and the portal of entry is by the bloodstream or by contiguous spread from palate or paranasal sinuses and orbit.

The classical presentation is of painful proptosis associated with visual loss in a diabetic. The fungus then extends by the venous system into adjacent brain. Nasal ulcers and cutaneous necrosis are not uncommon. The patient is ill and there is usually pyrexia. As contiguous cranial nerves are picked off, multiple palsies occur and infarction of blood vessels leads to focal neurological signs. Abscesses distant from the site of local infection may be set up and cause confusing localizing signs. Progression of disease is rapid and secondary infection may occur.

Brain imaging with CT or MR will show invasion of paranasal and orbital spaces and brain, by granuloma, together with destructive bony erosion and areas of infarction. Confirmation of the diagnosis is by demonstration and subsequent culture of the fungus from scrapings or biopsy specimens. CSF examination is not helpful, nor is blood serology. Treatment is by surgical extirpation of the fungal material in so far as is possible, and this may require the combined efforts of neurosurgeon, ENT surgeon, maxillo-facial surgeon, and ophthalmic surgeon. At the same time antifungal agents should be administered, the best of which in this circumstance, is amphotercin B. Ketoconazole has been reported to be effective. Equally important is prompt and aggressive treatment of the underlying predisposing condition such as diabetic ketoacidosis. A few survivors have been reported but rhinocerebral mucormycosis remains the most rapidly fatal of CNS fungal diseases.

34.15.9 **Toxoplasmosis**

Toxoplasmosis is caused by infection by the coccidian protozoan *Toxoplasma gondii.* (The gondi is a north African rodent.) Infection is found in man and other animals throughout the world and almost any warm-blooded animal, including birds, can act as an intermediate host but the cat is the definitive host in which the parasitic life cycle is completed. They excrete oocysts in their faeces which are resistant to most insults, and they can remain infective for months. Humans become infected by ingesting foodstuffs or water contaminated by cat droppings, or by eating infected meat which has not been fully cooked, or by picking up infection in the uterus. Most infections in normal immunocompetent hosts are of no clinical significance. Several

factors influence human susceptibility including proximity to cats, dietary habits, climate, and sanitary provision. There is a wide variation in seropositivity throughout the world with highest rates being recorded in France, UK, and USA. The incidence of infection increases with age. The clinical manifestations of toxoplasma infection are influenced by the immunological competence of the host. In most people who are immunologically competent, infection is asymptomatic. In a minority there is a benign, transient flu-like illness with malaise, lymphadenopathy, maculopapular rash, and myalgia. This may be complicated by hepatitis, meningo-encephalitis, or myocarditis. If the immune system is compromised as it is with AIDS, infection can be devastating, either by dissemination of primary infection, or more frequently, by re-activation of latent infection. Toxoplasma encephalitis is almost always caused by reactivation. Up to 40 per cent of AIDS patients are so infected and as many as 30 per cent die of toxoplasmosis in Europe. Cerebral toxoplasmosis usually occurs in patients whose CD4 cell counts are less than $200/\mu l$ and in as many as half, it is the AIDS defining event. There may be racial and geographic susceptibility.

Toxoplasma in the brain can cause a localized, relatively indolent granuloma, multiple miliary granulomas, focal encephalitic change with necrosis and abscess formation with poorly defined capsules, or a diffuse necrotizing encephalitis and combinations of all of these. Lesions are commonly multiple. Any part of the CNS can be affected and there is some predilection for deeper structures in the region of the basal ganglia and midline. In AIDS patients there are multiple areas of focal necrotizing encephalitis which contain tissue cysts and extracellular tachyzoites (Luft *et al.* 1984).

The clinical syndromes approximate to a diffuse encephalitis or an enlarging intracranial mass lesion or a combination of these. The onset is variable, from insidious to explosive with non-focal or focal symptoms and signs according to the location and nature of the process. Headache, confusion, fever, epileptic seizures, behavioural changes, and altered mental status are common. Focal neurological signs develop and with involvement of deep brain structures, extrapyramidal signs and movement disorders have been described (Porter and Sande 1992; Luft *et al.* 1993).

Patients who are suspected of having cerebral toxoplasmosis should have the diagnosis confirmed by a combination of brain imaging and serological testing. A PCR for toxoplasma DNA in CSF is under evaluation. MR is more sensitive than CT and will show lesions which CT has missed, thus it is the imaging modality of choice. Single or more usually, multiple solid or cystic spherical lesions with ring enhancement, surrounding oedema, and space occupation, are common and occur in up to 90 per cent of patients. The appearances are not pathognomonic (Farkash *et al.* 1986; Navia *et al.* 1986b). Multiple lesions favour toxoplasmosis, a single lesion favours lymphoma but there is overlap. In patients who are immunocompetent, a single positive IgG blood titre is a sensitive indicator of infection. In AIDS and other immunocompromised patients, raised or rising titres do not necessarily indicate active infection.

However, absence of an IgG response implies that the syndrome may not be due to toxoplasmosis and another cause should be sought. Definitive diagnosis rests with demonstration of the parasite in biopsy material from an affected area of brain. A presumptive diagnosis of cerebral toxoplasmosis may be made by monitoring clinical and radiological improvement following a trial of treatment. This course of action would be appropriate for a patient with positive serology and who had multiple lesions on scanning and there was no other obvious diagnosis. Those with a single cerebral lesion, particularly if serology is negative, would best have biopsy undertaken and this is imperative for those who have not shown a satisfactory response to treatment.

The primary therapy for cerebral toxoplasmosis is pyrimethamine combined with sulphadiazine. This is given together with folinic acid for 6 weeks, following which lifelong treatment with smaller doses for chronic disease suppression is necessary in AIDS patients. In patients who may react adversely to sulphadiazine, clindamycin may be used. Other drugs including azithromycin and clarithromycin are under evaluation. Space occupying lesions may require surgical decompression or aspiration. Prevention of disease is difficult and avoidance of close contact with cats and ensuring that meat for human consumption is well cooked, may diminish the risk of infection in the vulnerable.

34.15.10 Cysticercosis

Cysticercosis refers to infestation of humans by the larval form of the pork tapeworm, *Taenia solium*. Laennec invented the term 'cysticercus' from the Greek words 'kystis', meaning bladder, and 'kerkos', meaning tail. A bladder with a tail describes the appearance of the larva. *Taenia solium* is a cestode and a common tapeworm which infests the intestine of man. It occurs worldwide and particularly high rates of infestation have been reported from Central and South America, Africa, India, and the Far East. Pockets of infestation occur in areas of Europe such as Poland and there may be some relationship to the culinary habits of the populace who eat uncooked or undercooked pork. Improvements in veterinary hygiene practices have led to a marked reduction in cases in developed countries where cases may be found in immigrants and in people who have travelled to endemic areas. The adult tapeworm parasitizes the small intestine of man (the definitive host) and can grow to a length of some metres. Segments of the worm containing ova are deposited in faeces which may contaminate the environment to be ingested by pigs, the intermediate host. In the pig the eggs hatch and the embryos migrate through intestinal wall, into the bloodstream and are distributed to various tissues, particularly muscle, where the embryos develop into cysticerci. When infested pork is eaten by man, cysticerci, stimulated by gastric acid, penetrate the wall of the small bowel, attach themselves to the mucosa and become adult *Taenia*. Man can also become the intermediate host by ingesting food contaminated by his own faecal material if personal hygiene is poor. The clinical manifestations of cysticercosis are determined by the severity of the

Table 34.7. Forms of CNS cysticercosis

Brain parenchymal cysts
Intraventricular cysts
Spinal cord cysts
Meningeal syndromes
Vascular syndromes

infestation and the immunological reaction provoked, and by the site where the cysticerci lodge. The incubation period is variable and may be as short as a few months or as long as several years. Most clinical cases occur between the ages of 20 and 50 but any age or race and either sex may be affected. There have been various classifications of the clinical features of CNS disease; that in Table 34.7 is favoured. These syndromes are not mutually exclusive and two or more forms of the disease may co-exist.

Clinical features

Brain parenchymal cysts commonly declare themselves with epileptic seizures which may be generalized or focal, in over 50 per cent of cases. Focal neurological syndromes appropriate to the area of the brain involved may occur. In a minority dementia and bilateral signs may reflect multiplicity of lesions throughout the hemispheres. Intraventricular cysts usually cause obstruction to CSF flow and result in acute hydrocephalus with signs of raised ICP. If the lesion is pedunculated, acute attacks of hydrocephalus may result in the manner of colloid cysts. Spinal cysticercosis occurs in less than 5 per cent of cases and produces signs of spinal cord compression, often in the high cervical region. Meningeal cysticercosis results from a basal arachnoiditis and manifests as hydrocephalus complicated by cranial nerve palsies. In some, chronic meningitis is produced. It is only in recent years that it has been recognized that vascular occlusion may occur from obliteration of the vessels at the base of the brain or more peripherally, which have been affected by arachnoiditis so causing stroke syndromes in the distribution of these vessels. This is a frequent cause of stroke amongst the young in endemic areas (Del Brutto 1992).

Neurological syndromes

The neurological syndromes of cysticercosis may mimic stroke, meningitis, tumour, abscess, raised ICP, and dementia, and diagnosis is greatly aided by a history of exposure through travel in endemic areas. However, there is adequate documentation of acquisition of the disease by societies who do not eat pork, by infection from immigrants from endemic areas (Schantz *et al.* 1992). Consequently, neurocysticercosis must be considered in the differential diagnosis of the above syndromes worldwide. Signs of cysticercosis elsewhere in the body aid diagnosis and subcutaneous intramuscular nodules should be sought—they may be found in between 5 and 50 per cent of cases dependent upon geographical location. Serological tests have not provided a good index of activity of neurological disease and various tests to demonstrate antibody to or antigen from cysticerci have been developed. At the time of writing the most specific and sensitive test is the enzyme linked immuno-electrotransfer blotting antibody detection (EITB) estimation which can be carried out on serum and CSF. Brain imaging with CT or MR is essential for diagnosis of neurocysticercosis. The appearances depend upon the degree of maturity of the cyst activity—active lesions show as round hypodense or iso-dense masses with surrounding oedema. As the cysts cause less inflammatory reaction they begin to calcify. Extensive infestation with multiple cysts at different stages of development may be seen. Ventricular enlargement from obstruction either from cysts or basal arachnoiditis may be evident. Diagnosis can be confirmed by stereotactic biopsy and demonstration of larval components.

Treatment

Treatment is symptomatic with relief of intracranial hypertension by shunting, surgical removal of lesions which are space occupying, and the prescription of anti-epileptic drugs for seizures. Specific anti-cysticercal treatment with praziquantel and albendazole has been reported to have been effective in reducing the number and the size of cysts, and in cutting down the number of seizures. Doubt has been cast on the efficacy of such treatment (Carpio *et al.* 1995; Salinas *et al.* 1999).

34.15.11 Schistosomiasis

Schistosomiasis is endemic in the tropics and subtropics and affects more than 200 million people in more than 70 countries. Travellers to these countries are at risk of infection if they come into contact with the cercariae by swimming in, or drinking, contaminated water. Three species of schistosome infect man, *S. haematobium*, *S. mansoni*, and *S. japonicum*. Other species may cause human disease but only rarely. Schistosomes are digenetic trematodes which reproduce sexually in definitive hosts, man, and asexually in intermediate hosts, snails. The adult worms live in the portal or mesenteric veins of man (*S. mansoni* and *japonicum*) or the vesical plexus (*S. haematobium*). Eggs are produced which develop into miracidia which penetrate bowel or bladder and are excreted. In regions of poor sanitation they contaminate fresh water, infect susceptible snails, and develop in the tissues to become cercariae. These mature, leave the snail, and swim in the water. Humans are infected by swimming in, or drinking, contaminated water. Cercariae penetrate skin or gut mucosa, become shistosomula, and travel via the bloodstream and lymphatics to the lungs whence they are dispersed throughout the body in the circulation. They then settle in the mesenteric or vesical venous plexuses where they mature into adult worms. Chronic schistosomal infection results from the immunological reaction and granuloma formation incited by eggs trapped in the venous plexuses and this gives rise to hepatosplenic and urinary obstructive disease.

CNS disease occurs in less than 5 per cent of cases and comes about when eggs travel through the pelvic venous plexuses to the venous plexuses surrounding the spinal cord and causes spinal schistosomiasis. Cerebral schistosomiasis probably results from transport of the eggs to the brain via the veinous plexuses and not by arterial embolization. Each species of schistosome can affect the brain or the spinal cord. *S. japonicum* favours brain almost exclusively, *S. haematobium* the spinal cord, and *S. mansoni* both (Ariizumi 1963; Pitella and Lana-Peixoto 1981). Schistosomal infestation is endemic in Africa, the Middle East, Egypt, Sudan, South America, Southeast Asia, China, the Philippines, and Japan.

Acute cerebral schistosomiasis presents as a fulminating encephalitis or encephalomyelitis with pyrexia and skin rashes, seizures, pyramidal signs, confusion, and neck stiffness. Some may progress to coma. Examination of peripheral blood reveals an eosinophilic pleocytosis and CSF also shows a pleocytosis. It probably is a form of allergic encephalopathy and most patients recover.

Chronic cerebral schistosomiasis results from granuloma formation in the brain and may declare itself many years after the original infestation. Presentation is of a focal cerebral lesion which may occupy space. Epilepsy is common. Brain imaging with CT or MR reveals enhancing mass lesions often with surrounding oedema—appearances which are seen with other granulomas or tumours. Diagnosis depends upon the recognition of schistosomiasis elsewhere and the finding of eggs in stool or urine. Biopsy of the granuloma may show diagnostic changes and eggs. Serological tests using schistosomal antigen and ELISA are useful.

Spinal schistosomiasis presents as a transverse myelitis, intrathecal granuloma, or conus syndrome with radiculopathy (Haribhai *et al.* 1991).

Treatment of schistosomiasis is effective. Praziquantel is the drug of choice and is effective against all three species. Metrifonate is effective against *S. haematobium* only. If space occupation is a problem, surgical removal of the lesions may be necessary otherwise if the diagnosis has been made with confidence, it may be sufficient to treat with praziquantel and monitor the resolution of granulomas with serial brain imaging (Watt *et al.* 1986). Steroids may be used to reduce oedema and modify any inflammatory reactions.

34.15.12 Paragonimiasis

Paragonimiasis is caused by infestation with the lung fluke trematode of the genus *Paragonimus*. Seven species cause disease in man. *P. westermani* is the predominant species to cause disease in man. China, Japan, the Philippines, Korea and Thailand, regions of Africa, and South America and Central America are endemic areas. Man is infected accidentally by ingesting infested raw or undercooked crayfish or crabs. They have derived the infestation from freshwater snails that have picked up miracidia in the water, shed by man from infected pulmonary cysts and the cycle is complete. After ingestion by man, the organisms penetrate the gut wall into the peritoneum and penetrate the diaphragm into lung where they mature into flukes and lay eggs. These rupture into a bronchiole and eggs, blood, and debris are expectorated. The route by which the CNS becomes infected is by migration of the organism via the veins or vascular fascial sheaths through the jugular foramen. Dissemination may also take place by the bloodstream. The fluke or the eggs incite an inflammatory response which becomes granulomatous and fibrotic with time and may later calcify. The CNS is involved in less than 1 per cent of all cases and the clinical syndromes include meningo-encephalitis (Oh 1968), basal arachnoiditis, and multiple granuloma formation. Meningitis presents acutely, granulomas are usually insidious in evolution producing focal signs, seizures, and space occupation. Optic atrophy caused by adhesive arachnoiditis is not uncommon. Brain imaging with CT or MR will demonstrate space occupying multiple granulomas with a tendency to coalesce. Ring-like enhancing lesions occurring in clusters are seen in the active stages (Cha *et al.* 1994). In more chronic lesions ring calcification may be seen. There may be an eosinophilic response in the blood. Chest X-ray is abnormal in most cases and eggs may be found in sputum and faeces. Complement fixation and immunoblot antibody tests are useful and may be done on blood and CSF. Treatment with praziquantel, with steroids to cover any inflammatory reaction, is effective. In chronic cases residual signs and seizures are common.

34.15.13 Echinococcosis

Echinococcosis or hydatid disease is caused by the larval cysts or hydatids (water droplet) of the tapeworm *Echinococcus granulosus*. Other species of *Echinococcus* have been known to cause disease in man, including *E. multilocularis*, but such infestation is rare and produces alveolar hydatid disease in which the cerebral cysts are multiple and multiloculated and filled with rather denser material. *Echinococcus granulosus* is a common parasite of dogs which is the definitive host for the adult worm which lives in the small intestine. Eggs are discharged in faeces, and are ingested by farm animals, usually sheep. Inside the intermediate host, the organism penetrates gut wall and travels in the veins or lymphatics to other tissues where it forms an enlarging cyst. Dogs are infected by eating infected flesh or offal. Man is accidentally infected by coming into contact with the eggs in the faeces of dogs, commonly in the coats of dogs where the larvae lodge. The disease is widespread in those parts of the world where sheep are kept and where dogs are used to tend them—South America, Europe, Australia, New Zealand, Mediterranean countries, Britain, and Central Asia.

Children are particularly liable to infection, perhaps because of their affinity to dogs and their poor hygiene habit. Once ingested, the eggs penetrate duodenal wall and travel in the veins of the portal system to the liver where most are trapped. Some manage to squeeze through and travel via the heart to the lungs where most of the surviving eggs are trapped. A few of these manage to get through to the general circulation and are distributed throughout the body with very few lodging in brain. This filtering mechanism accounts for the frequency with which different organs develop hydatids—liver 65 per cent, lung 20 per cent, brain 2 per cent. Once in the brain the larvae

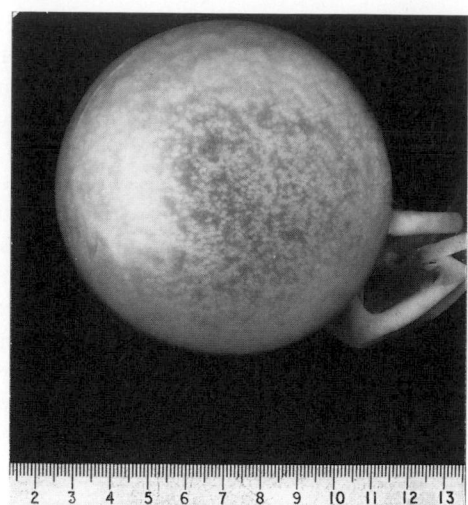

Fig. 34.8. Hydatid cyst, 9 cm in diameter, removed from the brain of an English boy of farming stock.

form a double layered cyst which slowly enlarges and may grow to a prodigious size (Fig. 34.8). Symptoms are of increasing ICP with focal signs appearing late if at all. Schroeder's diagnostic tetrad is useful—a child from a rural sheep rearing area, in good general health, with signs of raised ICP, and with ill defined focal signs (Schroeder 1941). In some cases the larvae lodge in bone of the skull or vertebrae and cysts form there to cause pressure on adjacent structures with resulting multiple cranial nerve palsies or paraparesis.

The diagnosis of cerebral hydatid disease is suggested by the finding of raised ICP in a person from a sheep rearing zone. The diagnosis is confirmed by brain imaging with CT or MR which will demonstrate one or sometimes multiple, large, spherical, space occupying cysts filled with fluid of the same radiological density as CSF (Ersahin *et al.* 1993). Immunological tests may be useful, but are not infrequently negative with brain cysts. CSF should not be examined because of raised ICP. Signs of hydatids elsewhere such as in liver or lung, lend support to the diagnosis. It is important that a hydatid cyst should be differentiated from other cystic brain lesions because the surgical technique for removal is specific. Great care should be taken not to puncture the cysts because to do so allows fluid containing daughter cysts to spread to form further hydatids. An ingenious method of removal was devised by Arana-Iniguez in which saline is injected between the outer layer of the hydatid and the brain, forcing the cyst to the surface where it can be delivered intact and removed (Arana-Iniguez and San-Julian 1955). If cysts are removed intact the prognosis is excellent. Albendizole has been used for treatment of bony disease and for inoperable cysts but the results have not been encouraging.

34.15.14 Amoebal infestation

Cerebral amoebiasis occurs as a rare complication of amoebic dysentery and is to be distinguished from the meningo-encephalitis caused by *Naegleria*. Amoebic dysentery is caused by *Entamoeba histolytica* which colonizes the large bowel and is found in many countries throughout the world including Central and South America, Africa, Southeast Asia, and other areas. It may penetrate bowel and lead to hepatic abscesses in 10 per cent, or less commonly, lung abscesses. Rarely, it will lead to the formation of brain abscesses which are often multiple and invasive and destructive. Clinical features are of a focal expanding cerebral lesion in a patient who is ill and has hepatic involvement and a history of dysentery. Brain imaging shows changes of developing abscesses as described above. Diagnosis is usually made by demonstration of amoebic trophozoites in biopsy material and by demonstration of trophozoites or cysts in faecal samples. The prognosis is almost uniformly poor. Recommended treatment is with aspiration of abscess contents and systemic metronidazole.

34.15.15 Other parasitic infestations

In certain regions of the world and in exceptional circumstances, several other parasites may cause infection in the CNS. The exceptional circumstances often include immune suppression of the host, or trauma which permits access to the neuraxis which would otherwise be denied. Sometimes travel to an inaccessible area invites exposure to exotic organisms. The clinical syndromes which result usually do not have pathognomonic features and the clue to the diagnosis of meningo-encephalitis or brain abscess or granuloma in these cases depends upon recognition of the abnormal circumstances in which infection has been acquired. Commonly the correct diagnosis is not reached until after death.

Tapeworms

Infection by the larval form of the cestode tapeworm, *Spirometra*, causes sparganosis. Dogs and cats are parasitized and man is infected by drinking water contaminated by the larvae or by eating raw meat of infected snakes or frogs—Asia and South America are the main reservoirs. The larvae penetrate gut and migrate to other tissue, usually muscle, where they produce subcutaneous cysts. Only rarely is the CNS involved by a cerebral granuloma which functions as a space occupying mass (Tsai *et al.* 1993). Diagnosis is by stereotactic biopsy. Treatment is by excision if possible. There is little information concerning the efficacy of treatment with albendazole or praziquantel. Spinal granulomas have also been described.

Coenurosis is caused by infestation with the larval form of some species of dog tapeworm, most commonly *Taenia multiceps* in Europe, Africa, and South America, and *T. serialis* in Europe and North America. Other species do not cause significant CNS infection. Sheep are intermediate hosts and man is infected in the same way as with cysticercosis. Cysts, usually solitary, develop in brain and cause a space occupying syndrome. Basal arachnoiditis may contribute to this. Imaging demonstrates a cystic mass in or about the ventricles (Pau *et al.* 1987). Treatment is by surgical excision.

Filariasis

Meningo-encephalitis has been described in filariasis (van Bogaert *et al.* 1955) and an eosinophilic meningitis from infection by the larvae of *Angiostrongylus* (Fuller *et al.* 1993). It is to be anticipated that with the spread of immune suppression and improved diagnostic techniques, reports of even more exotic infestations will appear in the literature.

34.16 Miscellaneous bacterial infections

The CNS may be involved by infections which are not primarily neurotrophic. For instance, the common cold may induce severe and prolonged headache and headache is a common accompaniment of many generalized infections. Some infections which focus on other systems may involve the CNS almost incidentally—the viral haemorrhagic fevers Lassa fever, Yellow fever, Ebola disease, and others, which may disrupt coagulation mechanisms, lead to widespread bleeding which may affect any organ including the brain. Recently recognized bacteria have, in a similar way, been associated with CNS syndromes although the burden of their infection usually falls on other systems. Some of these infections occur in geographic areas limited by the distribution of the vectors responsible for transmission of the disease such as ehrlichiosis. Others, such as bartonellosis, may cause neurological syndromes in the immune suppressed. Individual case reports are to be found of CNS infection in the immune suppressed by an increasing range of bacteria which are not normally pathogenic to the CNS. This spectrum will expand in future.

34.16.1 Ehrlichiosis

Three species of *Ehrlichia* have been implicated in causing human disease. Most commonly, *E. chaffeensis* has been the agent. These are small coccobacilli like *Rickettsiae* and they are thought to transmit disease via tick vectors. In some regions, the vectors are the same ticks which carry the agents of Lyme disease and Babesiosis; co-infection may occur. Most cases have been described from the USA but cases have been reported from Europe, Africa, and Asia. In the summer months, patients are bitten by a tick and develop a non-specific flu-like illness 2 weeks later associated with a rash. In severe cases, disseminated intravascular coagulation and encephalopathy or meningitis may ensue. Diagnosis is by finding positive serology in the blood of those with an appropriate clinical syndrome and exposure to ticks. PCR is both sensitive and specific (Dumler and Bakken 1995). Treatment is with doxycycline or rifampicin.

34.16.2 Bartonella

Bartonella bacilliformis is the aetiological agent of Oroya fever, a bacteraemic infection limited to the Andes region and characterized by fever, headache, encephalopathy, lymphadenopathy, and anaemia. It carries a high mortality rate if untreated.

Cat scratch disease is caused by infection with *Bartonella hense-lae* and is ubiquitous. Fleas carried by cats are the vectors and infection occurs in normal humans and in those who are immune suppressed, particularly with AIDS. In this group, the onset is commonly insidious with malaise, myalgia, fatigue, and recurring headache and fever. Progression to encephalopathy or meningo-encephalitis may follow; this may be impossible to distinguish from HIV-associated encephalopathy. In the immunocompetent by contrast, the onset may be quite acute. Bacillary angiomatosis may occur in both normals and the immunosuppressed. A form of retinitis leading to sudden loss of visual acuity is a common feature. Diagnosis is serological and treatment is with doxycycline (Adal *et al.* 1994). Treatment for 3 months or more may be needed in those with AIDS and relapse may require long-term treatment.

34.17 Spirochaetal diseases

34.17.1 Syphilis: primary and secondary

Syphilis derives from the name of a shepherd in a poem by Fracastorius in 1521, who was crippled (*Syphilos Gr.* maimed) by the disease, having offended the Gods. It is not known where the disease originated. Reports of infection of almost epidemic proportions began to appear in Europe at the end of the fifteenth and the beginning of the sixteenth centuries, and it was thought to originate from the New World. Dementia para-lytica was described by the end of the eighteenth century and during the nineteenth century descriptions of general paresis of the insane (GPI), tabes dorsalis, and syphilitic arteritis appeared. In the early days of the twentieth century, the causal organism *Treponema pallidum* had been identified and linked to GPI. The Wasserman complement fixation diagnostic test was devised in the first decade and treatment with Salvarsan and malaria was described. Penicillin was first used in 1943 and remains the mainstay of treatment to this day.

The organism which causes syphilis is a spirochaete, *Treponema pallidum*. It is a flexible, spiral organism with a corkscrew motion which can be observed by dark ground illumination through the microscope and is 5–15 μm in length. It is fastidious and requires heat, light, and moisture for survival, which are provided by contact with warm living tissue. It does not survive long without animal contact. Infection in humans occurs as a result of warm and moist contact, venereal in the vast majority. Congenital disease is caused by transplacental transfer. Treponemes spiral through mucous membranes which have been abraded, multiply locally, and pass rapidly to regional lymph nodes, thence via lymph and blood throughout the body. Invaded tissues react with lymphocytic and plasma cell infiltration causing endarteritis and giving rise eventually to fibrosis and scarification. This reaction may remain quiescent for years to be resurrected years later, pro-ducing new clinical manifestations. By convention, congenital syphilis is separated from acquired syphilis, and of the latter, three phases of infection are recognized, primary, secondary, and terti-ary. Neurological disease does not usually accompany primary infection although treponemes may be isolated from CSF at this stage. The CNS may be implicated in secondary syphilis and is a common site for tertiary syphilis.

Syphilis affects every race throughout the world, both sexes and any age group. The true incidence is almost certainly under-reported because of reluctance to admit to the disease and also because the clinical manifestations may be minimal at the onset or masked by another co-existing sexually acquired infection. Following the introduction of effective treatment with penicillin, the incidence diminished, and tertiary syphilis declined dramatically. However, this position has not been maintained, and syphilis continues to present a health hazard, particularly in HIV-positive males. The natural history of syphilitic infection is greatly modified by antibiotic treatment and it is impossible to predict who will develop late manifesta-tions of the disease. The primary disease occurs within weeks, or at the most, 3 months of infection. Secondary syphilis follows after 1–6 months and tertiary syphilis can appear within 2–3 years or as long as 20 years or more, after the first infection.

Primary syphilis usually takes the form of a chancre, or genital ulcer, 3–6 weeks after infection. This is associated with inguinal adenopathy. There may be other, co-existing sexually transmitted infection and this may obscure the clinical picture. Treated or untreated, the chancre and adenopathy resolve after some weeks. Secondary syphilis comes on 2–4 months later and is manifest by the development of skin lesions—papular, macular, or vesicular rashes, condylomata lata around the genitals, and patchy alopecia. In this stage, rare CNS manifestations include acute meningitis. Following recovery from this phase, without treatment, patients may be asymptomatic for many years, as the disease lies latent, the only evidence of syphilitic infection being found in serological tests. In perhaps as many as 35 per cent of such cases, tertiary syphilis develops. This affects skin, locomotor system, cardiovas-cular system, viscera, and the CNS. When the CNS is involved, the term 'neurosyphilis' applies—clearly this may encompass the meningitis of secondary infection. Common usage infers that neurosyphilis means tertiary involvement of the CNS.

34.17.2 Neurosyphilis

Approximately 10 per cent of cases of tertiary syphilis affect the CNS. The clinical syndromes of neurosyphilis are several and more than one may occur in the same patient. Consequently, none of the clinical classifications is entirely satisfactory, but this is not of too great moment since the treatment for each is basically the same—penicillin with symptomatic management as necessary. The account of the clinical syndromes by Wilson (1940) remains unsurpassed. The following classification is based on that (Table 34.8).

By definition, asymptomatic neurosyphilis has no clinical manifestations and the diagnosis is based on the finding of abnormalities on CSF examination—sometimes a raised cell count and always positive immunological tests. The significance of this form of the disease is that, without adequate treatment, and sometimes despite apparently adequate treatment, parenchymal neurosyphilis may develop later.

Table 34.8. Classification of neurosyphilis

1. Asymptomatic
2. Meningeal
3. Meningovascular
4. General paresis of the insane (GPI)
5. Tabes dorsalis
6. Optic atrophy
7. Spinal parenchymal
8. Gumma
9. Osteitis of skull and spine
10. Neurosyphilis with HIV

Meningeal syphilis

Meningeal syphilis may develop at any time following primary infection. Most commonly this takes the form of acute or subacute meningitis about 2 years after the initial infection. A more chronic form with meningeal granulomatous change may lead to multiple cranial nerve palsies, hydrocephalus, Argyll Robertson pupils, seizures, and focal signs (Merritt and Moore 1935). CSF examination reveals meningitic change with raised cell count, protein, and reduced glucose content. Immunological tests for syphilis are positive.

Meningovascular syphilis

Meningovascular syphilis follows initial infection by 5 years or more on average, and is brought about by endarteritis of large and medium cerebral vessels, giving rise to stroke syndromes from infarction. The meninges are also affected with granulomas and adhesions and spinal cord disease is not infrequent. Strokes in the young may be manifestations of meningovascular syphilis. Blood and CSF tests for syphilis are positive.

General paresis of the insane

General paresis of the insane (GPI) or dementia paralytica, used to affect about 5 per cent of untreated syphilitics. Symptoms appear 10–15 years after primary infection and result from structural degeneration of the cerebrum with neuronal loss, cerebral atrophy, and glial proliferation. Onset is insidious with psychiatric symptoms predominating—memory loss, delusions, often of grandeur, disinhibition, emotional outbursts, and erratic behaviour, deterioration of personal habits and hygiene, and disintegration of symbolic thought lead to professional disaster and social catastrophe. Further parenchymal damage results in clumsiness, inco-ordination, epilepsy, cranial nerve palsies, Argyll Robertson pupils, long tract signs, frank dementia, and sphincter incontinence. Blood and CSF tests are abnormal.

Tabes dorsalis

Tabes dorsalis or locomotor ataxia is more common in men, comes on later than GPI—on average 10–20 years from first infection, and is often associated with other varieties of paren-

chymal disease. The initial symptoms are sensory. Lancinating, sudden, lightning pains affect the legs and less frequently, trunk and arms. They are repeated, exquisitely painful, and have a tendency to occur in clusters over several days or longer, at a time. Similar painful crises may disturb the abdominal viscera to cause severe abdominal pain, vomiting, paralytic ileus, and rarely may cause similar crises of bowel and bladder. Paraesthesiae and sensory diminution affect the feet and legs and sometimes the trunk in a cape or girdle distribution. Loss of posterior column function causes postural ataxia and unsteadiness of gait, more evident in the dark when visual clues are lost. Tendon reflexes are reduced and later lost, associated with hypotonia. Hypotonia leads to hypermobility of joints, which combined with sensory loss results in repeated and increasing trauma to joints. These become disorganized and grossly arthritic and swollen as first described by Charcot. Trophic ulceration occurs over areas of skin lacking sensation and which are subjected to pressure, usually in the feet. Argyll Robertson pupils (eccentric, irregular, with depigmentation of the iris and failure of reaction to light with retention of the reaction of accommodation) are seen in more than half of cases of tabes. Optic atrophy is common as are oculomotor palsies and result in a characteristic facial appearance with bilateral ptosis leading to compensatory frontalis over-reaction. Other forms of neurosyphilis commonly co-exist. CSF and blood usually show positive changes of syphilis, but may be normal in advanced, 'burnt out' cases.

Syphilitic optic atrophy

Syphilitic optic atrophy is the result of damage to the optic nerve fibres from chronic inflammatory changes and progresses insidiously to complete blindness on average 8 years after first infection and commonly accompanies tabes dorsalis.

Spinal parenchymal neurosyphilis

Spinal parenchymal neurosyphilis is caused by meningomyelitis, hypertrophic pachymengitis, and spinal cord infarction. Spinal cord syndromes incorporating radiculopathy appropriate to the level of disease are found. All spinal syndromes carry a high risk of vascular complication from physical intervention, and neurosurgery is almost always best avoided.

Gummas

Gummas are rubbery nodules of inflammatory tissue and produce signs by virtue of their space occupying characteristics. They are exceptionally rare and are likely to be misdiagnosed as neoplasms or granulomas unless specific serological tests are undertaken (Punt 1983).

Syphilitic osteitis

Syphilitic osteitis of the skull and vertebrae is really no more than a historical oddity nowadays. Signs are caused by secondary pressure on adjacent spinal cord or brain.

Associated HIV infection

It may be argued that neurosyphilis associated with HIV infection should not be categorized separately because the clinical manifestations incorporate each and several of the syndromes described above. However, it has been reported that HIV patients who have syphilis have a greater likelihood of developing secondary syphilis, are likely to have atypical manifestations of neurosyphilis, and atypical serological tests, including false positive tests for syphilis. It may not be possible to differentiate the neurological damage caused by HIV from that caused by syphilis and both syphilis and HIV may produce CSF abnormalities. It was thought that the response of such patients to treatment with penicillin was suboptimal (Gordon *et al.* 1994). Recent studies indicate that the problem may not be as serious as once feared (Simon 1994). Nevertheless, the combination of the two pathologies in the same patient can be confusing, and produces a diagnostic scenario distinct from straightforward neurosyphilis (Johns *et al.* 1987; Katz *et al.* 1993).

Congenital syphilis

Congenital syphilis is always contracted by transplacental passage of the treponeme. Abortion or stillbirth may ensue, or the infant may have syphilis at birth. Transplacental infection is more likely if the mother has primary or secondary disease. In most infants with early congenital syphilis (before 2 years) signs become evident between 2 weeks and 2 months and may appear later, manifesting as secondary syphilis in several organs. Nasal discharge or snuffles, is common, hepatosplenomegaly, osteochondritis, choroidoretinitis, skin eruptions, and failure to thrive are amongst the features. In late congenital syphilis there may be no signs, infection being indicated by positive blood tests. Signs of infection include interstitial keratitis, choroidoretinitis, optic atrophy, perforation of the nasal septum and palate, anterior bowing of the tibia, painless arthropathy resulting in Clutton's joints, deafness, and peg-like deformities of the teeth—Hutchinson's teeth.

34.17.3 Diagnosis and treatment of syphilis

Dark field microscopy of specimens from chancres and the identification of *Treponema pallidum* is the quickest and best test for the diagnosis of primary syphilis. Direct fluorescent antibody staining of the organism has about the same sensitivity. In later forms of syphilis the diagnosis is made by serological tests which broadly fall into two groups—non-treponemal tests which rely on reagin antibodies which are non-specific globulin complexes, and treponemal tests which utilize specific antibodies. Very recently, PCR has been used to detect treponemal genetic material in tissues and CSF and promises to be a highly specific and sensitive tool for the diagnosis of neurosyphilis. The Venereal Disease Reference Laboratory test (VDRL) and the Wassermann tests are examples of non-treponemal tests and they become positive within 4–6 weeks of infection and are positive in virtually all patients with neurological syphilis. Unfortunately, reagin antibody is not specific

for syphilis, therefore a specific treponemal antibody test such as the fluorescent treponemal antibody-absorbed (FTA-ABS) or *Treponema pallidum* haemagglutination assay (TPHA) is necessary to confirm that the cause is treponemal infection. The FTA-ABS and TPHA when applied to CSF are highly specific for neurosyphilis. The non-treponemal tests are easily quantitated and higher titres indicate disease activity. Following successful treatment of primary and secondary disease these tests may revert to normal. In neurological syphilis, they usually remain positive. Anxieties have been expressed that the sensitivity and accuracy of both treponemal and non-treponemal tests in patients with impairment of cellular immunity such as AIDS, may be disturbed. It is probable that such occurrences are rare and the tests can be interpreted normally in HIV patients. In neurosyphilis, other changes which are found in the CSF are raised cell counts with lymphocytic pleocytosis, particularly with GPI, increased protein content, and increased immunoglobulin content. These are less marked in tabes and in long standing cases, there may be no significant changes other than positive serology.

There are no diagnostic radiological features of neurosyphilis. Plain X-rays may reveal disorganization of joints in tabes dorsalis—similar changes may be seen in cases of syringomyelia and severe diabetic neuropathy. Brain imaging with MR or CT may reveal infarcts in meningovascular syphilis, general atrophic changes in GPI, and atrophic or pachymeningitic features on spinal imaging in cases of tabes. Conventional or MR angiography of the cerebral arteries in young stroke syndromes may show occlusion or variation in calibre of vessels, indicating arteritis.

The treatment of all forms of neurosyphilis is briefly stated—penicillin. If allergy to penicillin is a problem, erythromycin or a cephalosporin, are suitable alternatives. There is no good evidence that *T. pallidum* has developed resistance to penicillin. Many different dosage regimes have been advocated. Most agree that oral treatment is not appropriate and it is better to err on the side of too much than too little. My current practice is to give 24 million units of benzyl penicillin IV in divided dose for a minimum of 2 weeks. If no improvement in CSF parameters occurs after 3 or 4 months, the course is repeated. Erythromycin 500 mg every 6 h for 30 days is an alternative regime. Penicillin is treponemicidal and lyses the organisms whereby large quantities of antigenic material are released into the bloodstream. This may result in a Jarisch–Herxheimer type of reaction with confusion, delirium, convulsions, and pyrexia. Steroids reduce the severity of such reactions and should be administered routinely before the first dose of antibiotic is given and for 48 h thereafter. Symptomatic treatment is given for other manifestations—antiepileptic drugs for seizures, orthopaedic treatment for unstable joints. Lightning pains and crises in tabes may respond to treatment with carbamazepine, reinforced with amitryptiline at night. Recent experience with gabapentin suggests that it may be helpful.

The prognosis following treatment of neurological syphilis is related to how early treatment has been given in the course of the disease, and whether irreversible parenchymal change has taken place in brain or spinal cord. It should be possible to arrest the progress of disease in three-quarters of the cases of meningovascular disease and in a lesser proportion of cases of GPI and tabes.

34.17.4 Lyme disease

Lyme disease is a form of borreliosis, characterized by cutaneous, arthritic, cardiological, and neurological manifestations, and takes its name from the Lyme district of Connecticut, USA. In the early 1970s a cluster of juvenile cases were thought to have juvenile rheumatoid arthritis, and provided the stimulus for the description of the disease by Steere *et al.* (1977). It became evident that many of the cases had suffered an insect bite and developed an unusual skin lesion thereafter, (erythema chronicum migrans, ECM), before going on to develop arthritis, and in some cases, cardiac and neurological complications. It became evident that it was an arthropod-borne infection, and that the skin lesions had been described in Sweden and associated with tick bites in the early twentieth century. Furthermore, the connection between ECM and arthritic and neurological disease had been documented from several places in Europe in the first half of the twentieth century and it has since been demonstrated that the American and European diseases are caused by very similar spirochaetes.

As more information accumulates, it is becoming evident that the manifestations of Lyme disease may occur worldwide. Endemic areas are found in USA, Europe, Central Asia, China and the Far East, and in Australia. It is anticipated that other continents will be found to harbour the disease. The causal organism is *Borrelia burgdorferi* in the USA and in Europe and almost identical borrelia, *B. garinii* and *B. afzellii* from Europe and Asia. The species difference probably accounts for geographical variations of clinical manifestations—arthritis is more common in USA, cutaneous and neurological disease in Europe. The vectors for the disease are hard-bodied ticks of the genus *Ixodes* and different species carry the infecting organism in different countries. What is common to them all is they are found in forest and scrub and are most active in late spring and early summer, which accounts for the seasonal variation of disease. Deer, mice, and many other small mammals and birds are the hosts. Infection in humans is contracted when a tick bites man when he visits woodlands for work or recreation, and spirochaetes are inoculated. Clinical symptoms appear after an incubation period of 3–31 days and accord with tissue invasion—*Borreliae* have been isolated from skin, blood, CSF, and joint fluid. More chronic manifestations appear months to years later and are almost certainly due to autoimmune mechanisms.

The clinical features of Lyme disease are now described as developing in three stages. Stage 1 is of early, localized infection. Stage 2 is of early, disseminated infection and stage 3 is of late or persisting infection. Not all patients pass through all of the stages and presentation varies. It is a multisystem disease which, if not recognized, can become chronic and disabling.

The early, localized stage is preceded by a tick bite, but this may be remembered by only about a third of all patients. After a week to a month, ECM appears at the site of the bite, and may cause considerable itching. There may be mild flu-like reaction and regional lymphadenopathy and the skin lesion subsides.

Following haematogenous spread of the spirochaetes weeks to months after the bite, early, disseminated disease manifests with further cutaneous manifestations, adenopathy and fatigue, myalgia, and mild meningo-encephalitis. With progression, the organisms localize to the nervous system in between 15 and 50 per cent, higher figures being found in Europe. Cardiac disturbance, usually with dysrhythmias, myocarditis, or pericarditis, occurs in a minority. In North America, recurrent arthropathies ensue in up to 40 per cent, much less in Europe.

Late, persisting disease most commonly involves the musculoskeletal system with polyarthralgia followed by erosive bone disease. There is often a characteristic skin lesion, acrodermatitis chronica atrophicans, particularly in European cases. Neurological disturbance in the form of encephalomyelopathy, polyneuritis, optic neuritis, cerebral vasculitis, and mental and cognitive dysfunction have all been recognized as late manifestations. Neurological manifestations which occur in the early disseminated phase include polyneuritis and radiculitis, cranial neuropathies, and meningo-encephalitis. Polyneuritis is commonly asymmetrical, painful, and predominantly motor (Section 12.14.3). Guillain–Barré syndrome like features may be seen (Garcia-Monco and Benach 1995; Halperin 1998). Electrophysiology commonly shows signs of axonal disturbance, often in a radicular distribution and CSF examination may reveal a pleocytosis. Cranial neuropathies most frequently affect the seventh nerve and other nerves are involved less often, including the second. There is nothing specific about the meningo-encephalitis which is associated with CSF pleocytosis. The protein content may be raised and serological tests and PCR are positive.

If there is a history of tick bite and if it is followed by ECM, the diagnosis of Lyme disease is not difficult. However, this is available in a minority of cases only. Therefore, any patient with meningo-encephalitis, chronic lymphocytic meningitis, cranial neuritis including Bell's palsy, polyradiculitis, or polyneuritis may harbour the disease. If arthropathy co-exists, the chances of Lyme disease are higher. EEG, peripheral electrophysiology and brain scans, CT and MR, may be abnormal, but the abnormalities are not specific. Diagnosis depends on the demonstration of raised antibody titres in blood and CSF, and now PCR against borrelia DNA is specific and sensitive.

In order to reduce the chance of sequelae, treatment should be given as soon as possible after diagnosis. There have been no large-scale trials of antibiotics so optimal regimes have not been determined. Doxycycline or tetracycline for 14 days is recommended for early disease. Amoxicillin, penicillin, and erythromycin are also effective. For those with neurological disease, especially if chronic, i.v. penicillin, ceftriaxone, or cefutaxime is recommended. A mild form of Jarisch–Herxheimer reaction may occur, but this seldom requires steroid treatment.

The outlook is good. In more chronic cases, more than 1-month-long course of antibiotics may be necessary.

34.17.5 Relapsing fever

The relapsing fevers are caused by infection of humans by various species of *Borreliae*, which are Gram-negative, helical bacteria. Before 1980, the term Borreliosis was used synonymously with relapsing fever, but the recognition that Lyme disease, which is not a relapsing fever, was caused by *Borrelia burgdorferi* has led to the name 'relapsing fever' being resurrected to describe the syndromes caused by non-Lyme *Borreliae*.

Relapsing fever is transmitted to man by ticks of the soft-shelled *Ornithodoros* species which harbour many species of *Borreliae*, and live in remote, forested areas at elevation, or by lice which transmit infection due to *B. recurrentis*. The louse-borne variety is now limited to the horn of Africa and the Sudan, while tick-borne disease is found in Africa, Asia, and the Americas. Ticks form an arthropod reservoir for the disease and become infectious when they feed on infected rodents. When they subsequently bite man they transmit *Borreliae* in their saliva. The clinical syndrome which is produced is the same, no matter which species of *Borrelia* is implicated.

The incubation period varies from 3 to 15 days with an average of a week. Onset is sudden with pyrexia, headache, rigors, myalgia, disturbance of sleep rhythm, confusion, delirium, and meningism. A petechial rash occurs in some and the conjunctivae are injected. In severe cases, thrombocytopaenia and consumptive coagulopathy may complicate the picture (Southern and Sanford 1969). Without treatment, the febrile episode resolves after a few days, only to recur a week later and this cycle may be repeated several times. There are clinical similarities to malaria and arboviral and rickettsial encephalitides. Diagnosis is by demonstration of the organism in blood smears, best taken during febrile attacks. Serum antibodies can be detected by ELISA and immunoblotting techniques. Treatment is effective with antibiotics, and penicillin, erythromycin, and chloramphenicol have all been given successfully. A Jarisch–Hexheimer reaction may occur.

34.17.6 Leptospirosis

Leptospirosis is a zoonotic disease which affects many species of mammals throughout the world. It is caused by several species of *Leptospira*, Gram-negative, motile, helical, thin bacteria. They persist in the renal and genital tracts of carrier animals and are excreted in their fluids. They survive in water for a long time and in damp soils and animal tissues. Man becomes infected by contact with infected tissues, urine, or water and transmission takes place through the skin, conjunctivae, or mucous membranes. Infection is more common in those who arc cxposed to rats, other rodents, and livestock: sewer workers, veterinary attendants, and abattoir workers, or those who by recreation are infected by contaminated water: swimmers, water skiers, windsurfers. The disease is found throughout the world and in the USA and elsewhere dogs are the most important carriers in the urban setting.

The manifestations of leptospirosis vary according to the age and health of the patient, and with the character and type of the infecting organism. Subclinical infections are common and symptomatic disease is usually mild. Only about 10 per cent develop Weil's disease involving the liver and kidneys. The incubation period ranges from 3 to 30 days and the clinical onset is abrupt with pyrexia, headache, myalgia and malaise, cough, chest pain, conjunctival suffusion, and photophobia. A maculopapular rash appears in 30 per cent of cases and there may be lymphadenopathy. This corresponds to the period of leptospiraemia. After a week, there is clinical improvement and the patient becomes afebrile for a day or two, following which the second phase of the illness occurs, corresponding to the development of specific antibodies. Lymphocytic meningitis with CSF cell counts in the hundreds occurs and resolves within a few days. CSF abnormalities may persist for several weeks. A minority go on to develop more severe manifestations of a generalized vasculitis which results in renal failure, jaundice, myocarditis, skin, and mucosal haemorrhages, and culminates in hepato-renal failure and death, if there is no response to treatment (Edwards and Domm 1960; Lecour *et al.* 1989). Mortality rates up to 40 per cent have been recorded in outbreaks associated with *L. icterohaemorrhagiae* and *copenhageni* infection.

The diagnosis of leptospirosis is usually made with serological tests. The organism may be cultured from blood and urine if samples are taken within the first fortnight. PCR for leptospiral DNA in blood, urine, and CSF is under evaluation. ELISA for antibodies in blood samples taken a fortnight apart, or in a single sample of CSF, will demonstrate positive titres.

Most cases of leptospirosis do not require specific treatment and management is symptomatic. If the disease is thought to be severe, antibiotic treatment with penicillin should be given (Watt *et al.* 1988), doxycycline if there is penicillin allergy. Steroids should be given to cover the first few doses because a Jarisch–Herxheimer type of reaction may occur. In severe cases, dialysis and intensive care may be needed.

References

Aarli, J. A. (1974). Nervous complications of measles: clinical manifestations and prognosis. *Eur. Neurol.*, **12**, 79–93.

Adal, K. A., Cockerell, C. J., and Petri, W. A. (1994). Cat scratch disease, bacillary angiomastosis and other infections due to Rochalimaea. *N. Engl. J. Med.*, **330**, 1509–15.

Alcindor, F., Valderrama, R., Canaveggio, M. *et al.* (1992). Imaging of human T-lymphotropic virus type 1-associated chronic progressive myeloneuropathies. *Neuroradiology*, **35**, 69–74.

Amsterdam, J. D., Henle, W., Winokur, A. *et al.* (1986). Serum antibodies to Epstein–Barr virus in patients with major depressive disorder. *Am. J. Psychiatry*, **143**, 1593–6.

Appuzzo, M. L., Chandrasoma, P. R., Cohen, D. *et al.* (1987). Computed imaging stereotaxy: experience and perspective related to 500 procedures applied to brain masses. *Neurosurgery*, **20**, 930–7.

Arana-Iniguez, R. and San-Julian, J. (1955). Hydatid cysts of the brain. *J. Neurosurg.*, **12**, 323–35.

Ariizumi, M. (1963). Cerebral schistosomiasis japonica: report of one operated case and fifty clinical cases. *Am. J. Trop. Med. Hyg.*, **12**, 40–5.

Arribas, J. R., Storch, G. A., Clifford, D. B. *et al.* (1996). Cytomegalovirus encephalitis. *Ann. Intern. Med.*, **125**, 577–87.

Asano, Y., Yoshikawa, T., Suga, S. *et al.* (1994). Clinical features of infants with primary human herpes virus 6 infection (exanthem subitum, roseola infantum). *Pediatrics*, **93**, 104–8.

Ashdown, B. C., Tien, R. D., and Felsberg, G. J. (1994). Aspergillosis of the brain and paranasal sinuses in immunocompromised patients: CT and MR imaging findings. *Am. J. Roentgenol.*, **162**, 155–9.

Astrom, K. E., Mancall, E. L., and Richardson, E. P. (1958). Progressive multifocal leukoencephalopathy. *Brain*, **81**, 93–111.

Baker, A. B. (1958). Western equine encephalitis. Clinical features. *Neurology*, **8**, 880–1.

Bannister, G., Williams, B., and Smith, S. (1981). Treatment of subdural empyema. *J. Neurosurg.*, **55**, 82–8.

Barlas, O., Sencer, A., Erkan, K. *et al.* (1999). Stereotactic surgery in the management of brain abscess. *Surg. Neurol.*, **52**, 404–10.

Barnett, G. H., Ropper, A. H., and Romeo, J. (1988). Intracranial pressure and outcome in adult encephalitis. *J. Neurosurg.*, **68**, 585–8.

Barre-Sinoussi, F., Chermann, J. C., Rey, F. *et al.* (1983). Isolation of a T-lymphotropic retrovirus from a patient at risk from acquired immune deficiency syndrome (AIDS). *Science*, **220**, 868–71.

Barza, M. and Pauker, S. G. (1980). The decision to biopsy, treat or wait in suspected herpes simplex encephalitis. *Ann. Intern. Med.*, **92**, 641–9.

Bassolasco, S., Marenzi, M., Dahl, H. *et al.* (1999). Human herpesvirus 6 in cerebrospinal fluid of patients infected with HIV: frequency and clinical significance. *J. Neurol. Neurosurg. Psychiatry*, **67**, 789–92.

Beati, L. and Raoult, D. (1998). Mediterranean spotted fever and other spotted fever group rickettsiae. In: *Zoonoses*, Chap. 21 (ed. S. R. Palmer, L. Soulsby, and D. I. H. Simpson), pp. 217–40. Oxford University Press, Oxford.

Behan, P. O., Feldman, R. G., Segerra, J. M. *et al.* (1986). Neurological aspects of mycoplasmal infection. *Acta Neurol. Scand.*, **74**, 314–22.

Bell, J. (1989). The polymerase chain reaction. *Immunol. Today*, **10**, 351–5.

Bell, J. E. and Ironside, J. W. (1993). Neuropathology of spongiform encephalopathies in humans. *Br. Med. Bull.*, **49**, 738–77.

Bennett, D. R. and Peters, H. A. (1961). Acute cerebellar syndrome secondary to infectious mononucleosis in a 52-year old man. *Ann. Intern. Med.*, **55**, 147–9.

Berger, J. R., Kaszovitz, B., Post, J. D. *et al.* (1987). Progressive multifocal leukoencephalopathy associated with human immune deficiency virus infection. *Ann. Intern. Med.*, **107**, 78–87.

Berger, J. R., Raffanti, S., Svenningsson, A. *et al.* (1991). The role of HTLV in HIV-1 neurologic disease. *Neurology*, **41**, 197–202.

Berkley, J. A., Mwangi, I., Mellington, F. *et al.* (1999). Cerebral malaria versus bacterial meningitis in children with impaired consciousness. *Q. J. Med.*, **92**, 151–7.

Blenden, D. C., Creech, W., and Torres-Anjel, M. J. (1986). Use of immunofluorescence examination to detect rabies virus antigen in skin of humans with clinical encephalitis. *J. Infect. Dis.*, **154**, 698–701.

Blunt, S. B., Lane, R. J., Turjanski, N. *et al.* (1997). Clinical features and management of two cases of encephalitis lethargica. *Mov. Disord.*, **12**, 354–9.

Boom, W. H. and Tuazon, C. V. (1985). Successful treatment of multiple brain abscesses with antibiotics alone. *Rev. Infect. Dis.*, **7**, 189–99.

Bouteille, M., Fontaine, C., Vedrenne, C. *et al.* (1965). Sur un cas d'encephalite subaigue a inclusions. Etude anotomo-clinique et ultrastructurale. *Rev. Neurol.*, **113**, 454–8.

Bouza, E., Dryer, J. A., Hewitt, W. L., and Meyer, R. D. (1981). Coccidioidal meningitis: an analysis of 31 cases and revue of the literature. *Medicine*, **60**, 139–72.

Brinker, K. R., Paulson, G., and Monath, T. P. (1979). St Louis encephalitis in Ohio, September 1975: clinical and EEG studies in 16 cases. *Arch. Intern. Med.*, **139**, 561–6.

Britt, R. H., Enzmann, D. R., and Yeager, A. S. (1981). Neuropathological and computerised tomographic findings in experimental brain abscess. *J. Neurosurg.*, **55**, 590–603.

Britt, R. H. and Enzmann, D. R. (1983). Clinical stages of human brain abscesses on serial CT scans after contrast infusion: computerised tomographic, neuropathological and clinical considerations. *J. Neurosurg.*, **59**, 972–89.

Bronnimann, D. A., Adam, R. G., and Galgiani, J. N. (1987). Coccidioidomycosis in the acquired immunodeficiency syndrome. *Ann. Intern. Med.*, **106**, 372–9.

Brown, H., Hien, T. T., Day, N. *et al.* (1999). Evidence of blood–brain dysfunction in cerebral malaria. *Neuropath. Appl. Neurobiol.*, 25, 331–40.

Bucher, B., Poupard, J. A., Vernant, J.-C. *et al.* (1990). Tropical neuromyelopathies and retroviruses: a review. *Rev. Infect. Dis.*, 12, 890–9.

Buchwald, D., Sullivan, J. L., and Komaroff, A. L. (1987). Frequency of 'Chronic active Epstein–Barr virus infection' in a general practice. *JAMA*, 257, 2303–7.

Burkitt, D. (1958). A sarcoma involving the jaws in African children. *Br. J. Surg.*, 46, 218.

Caekbeke, J. F. V., Peters, A. C. B., Vandvik, B. *et al.* (1990). Cerebral vasculopathy associated with primary varicella infection. *Arch. Neurol.*, 47, 1033–5.

Carne, C. A., Tedder, R. S., Smith, A. *et al.* (1985). Acute encephalopathy coincident with seroconversion for HTLV-III antibody. *Lancet*, ii, 1206–8.

Carpio, A., Santillan, F., Leon, P. *et al.* (1995). Is the course of neurocysticercosis modified by treatment with antihelminthic agents? *Arch. Intern. Med.*, 155, 1982–8.

Carr-Locke, D. L. and Nair, H. J. (1976). Neurological presentation of psittacosis during a small outbreak in Leicestershire. *Br. Med. J.*, ii, 853–4.

Carter, R. F. (1968). Primary amoebic meningoencephalitis: clinical, pathological and epidemiological features of six cases. *J. Pathol. Bacteriol.*, 96, 1–25.

Caserta, M. T., Hall, C. B., Scnabel, K. *et al.* (1994). Neuroinvasion and persistence of human herpes virus 6 in children. *J. Infect. Dis.*, 170, 1586–9.

Cassady, K. A. and Whitley, R. J. (1997). Pathogenesis and pathophysiology of viral infections of the central nervous system. In: *Infections of the central system*, 2nd edn (ed. W. M. Scheld, R. J. Whitley, and D. T. Durack), pp. 7–22. Lippincott-Raven, Philadelphia.

Cavenagh, J. B., Greenbaum, D., Marshall, A. H. E. *et al.* (1959). Cerebral demyelination associated with disorders of the reticulo-endothelial system. *Lancet*, ii, 525–9.

Centers for Disease Control (1977). Rabies in a laboratory worker—New York. *MMWR*, 26, 183–4.

Centers for Disease Control (1999). Human rabies prevention—United States, 1999. Recommendations of the advisory committee on immunisation practices (ACIP). *MMWR*, 48, 1–22.

Cerna, F., Mehard, B., Luby, J. P. *et al.* (1999). St Louis encephalitis and the substantia nigra: MR imaging evaluation. *Am. J. Neuroradiol.*, 20, 1281–3.

Cha, S. H., Chang, K. H., Cho, S. Y. *et al.* (1994). Cerebral paragonimiasis in early active stage: CT and MR features. *Am. J. Roentgenol.*, 162, 141–5.

Chiofalo, N., Fuentes, A., and Galves, S. (1980). Serial EEG findings in 27 cases of Creutzfeldt–Jacob disease. *Arch. Neurol.*, 37, 143–5.

Chun, C. H., Johnson, J. D., Hofstetter, M. *et al.* (1986). Brain abscess. A study of 45 consecutive cases. *Medicine*, 65, 415–31.

Clifford, D. B., Arribas, J. R., Storch, G. A. *et al.* (1996). Magnetic resonance brain imaging lacks sensitivity for AIDS associated cytomegalovirus encephalitis. *J. Neurovirol.*, 2, 397–403.

Cobb, W. (1966). The periodic events of subacute sclerosing panencephalitis. *Electroenceph. Clin. Neurophysiol.*, 21, 278–94.

Cohen, B. A. (1996). Prognosis and response to therapy of cytomegalovirus encephalitis and meningomyelitis in AIDS. *Neurology*, 46, 444–50.

Collinge, J. and Palmer, M. S. (1997). Human prion diseases. In: *Prion diseases* (ed. J. Collinge and M. S. Palmer), pp. 18–56. Oxford University Press, Oxford.

Conlon, C. P., Berendt, A. R., Dawson, K. *et al.* (1990). 'Runway malaria'. *Lancet*, 335, 472–3.

Corey, L. and Spear, P. (1986). Infections with herpes simplex viruses. *N. Engl. J. Med.*, 314, 749–57.

Corey, L. (1999). Antiretroviral therapy. In: *Clinical infectious diseases* (ed. R. H. Root, F. Waldvogel, L. Corey, and W. E. Stamm), pp. 959–64. Oxford University Press, Oxford.

Cotton, P. B. and Webb-Poploe, M. M. (1966). Acute transverse myelitis as a complication of glandular fever. *Br. Med. J.*, 1, 654–5.

Cowie, R. and Williams, B. (1983). Late seizures and morbidity after subdural empyema. *J. Neurosurg.*, 58, 569–73.

Crosse, B. A. (1990). Psittacosis: a clinical review. *J. Infect.*, 21, 251–9.

Cruickshank, E. K. (1956). A neurological syndrome of uncertain origin—review of 100 cases. *West Indian Med. J.*, 5, 147–58.

Cuille, J. and Chelle, P. L. (1936). La maladie dite tremblante du mouton, est-elle inoculable? *C. R. Acad. Sci.*, 203, 1552–4.

Cuzzubbo, A. J., Endy, T. P., Vaughn, D. W. *et al.* (1999). Evaluation of a new commercially available immunoglobulin M capture enzyme-linked immunosorbent assay for diagnosis of Japanese encephalitis infections. *J. Clin. Microbiol.*, 37, 3738–41.

Davenport, D. S., Johnson, D. R., Holmes, G. P. *et al.* (1994). Diagnosis and management of human B virus (Herpesvirus simiae) infections in Michigan. *Clin. Infect. Dis.*, 19, 33–41.

Davidson, H. D. and Steiner, R. E. (1985). Magnetic resonance imaging in infections of the central nervous system. *Am. J. Neuroradiol.*, 6, 499–504.

DeBiasi, R. L. and Tyler, K. L. (1999). Polymerase chain reaction in the diagnosis and management of central nervous system infections. *Arch. Neurol.*, **56**, 1215–9.

Del Brutto, O. H. (1992). Cysticercosis and cerebrovascular disease: a review. *J. Neurol. Neurosurg. Psychiatry*, **55**, 252–4.

DeLone, D. R., Goldstein, R. A., Petermann, G. *et al.* (1999). Disseminated aspergillosis involving the brain: distribution and imaging characteristics. *Am. J. Neuroradiol.*, **20**, 1597–604.

DeLouvois, J., Gortvai, P., and Hurley, R. (1977). Bacteriology of abscesses of the central nervous system: a multicentre prospective study. *Br. Med. J.*, **ii**, 981–4.

Demaerel, P., Wilms, G., Robberecht, W. *et al.* (1992). MRI of herpes simplex encephalitis. *Neuroradiology*, **34**, 490–3.

Denning, D. W. and Stevens, D. A. (1990). Antifungal and surgical treatment of invasive aspergillosis: a review of 2,121 published cases. *Rev. Infect. Dis.*, **12**, 1147–201.

Desprechins, B., Stadnik, T., Koerts, G. *et al.* (1999). Use of diffusion-weighted MR imaging in differential diagnosis between intracerebral necrotic tumors and cerebral abscesses. *Am. J. Neuroradiol.*, **20**, 1252–7.

Diamond, C. and Corey, L. (1999). Antiviral drugs and therapy. In: *Clinical infectious diseases* (ed. R. H. Root, F. Waldvogel, L. Corey, and W. E. Stamm), pp. 349–64. Oxford University Press, Oxford.

Dickerson, R. B., Newton, R. J., and Hansen, J. E. (1952). Diagnosis and immediate prognosis of Japanese B encephalitis. *Am. J. Med.*, **12**, 277–90.

Dill, S. R., Cobbs, C. G., and McDonald, C. K. (1995). Subdural empyema: analysis of 32 cases and review. *Clin. Infect. Dis.*, **20**, 372–86.

Drew, W. L. (1988). Cytomegalovirus infection in patients with AIDS. *J. Infect. Dis.*, **158**, 449–56.

Dumler, J. S. and Bakken, J. S. (1995). Ehrlichial diseases of humans: emerging tick-borne infections. *Clin. Infect. Dis.*, **20**, 1102–10.

Dupont, J. R. and Earle, K. M. (1965). Human rabies encephalitis: a study of 49 fatal cases, with a review of the literature. *Neurology, Minneapolis*, **15**, 1023–34.

Durand, D. V., Lecomte, C., Cathbras, P. *et al.* (1997). Whipple disease. Clinical review of 52 cases. *Medicine (Baltimore)*, **76**, 170–84.

Durrheim, D. N., LaGrange, J. J. P., Govere, J. *et al.* (1998). Accuracy of a rapid immunochromatographic card test for *Plasmodium falciparum* in a malaria control programme in South Africa. *Trans. R. Soc. Trop. Med. Hyg.*, **92**, 32–3.

Dworkin, M. S., Wan, P. C., Hanson, D. L. *et al.* (1999). Progressive multifocal leukoencephalopathy: improved survival of human immunodeficiency virus-infected patients in the proteases inhibitor era. *J. Infect. Dis.*, **180**, 621–5.

Edwards, G. A. and Domm, B. M. (1960). Human leptospirosis. *Medicine*, **39**, 117–56.

Eidelberg, C., Sotrel, A., Horoupian, D. S. *et al.* (1986). Thrombotic cerebral vasculopathy associated with herpes zoster. *Ann. Neurol.*, **19**, 7–14.

Elsner, C. and Dorries, K. (1992). Evidence of human polyoma virus BK and JC infection in normal brain tissue. *Virology*, **191**, 72–80.

Epstein, M. A., Barr, Y. M., and Achomg, B. G. (1964). Virus particles in cultured lymphoblasts from Burkitt's lymphoma. *Lancet*, **1**, 702–3.

Ersahin, Y., Mutluer, S., and Guzelbag, E. (1993). Intracranial hydatid cysts in children. *Neurosurgery*, **33**, 219–25.

Farkash, A. E., Maccabee, P. J., Sher, J. H. *et al.* (1986). CNS toxoplasmosis in acquired immune deficiency syndrome: a clinical–pathological–radiological review of 12 cases. *J. Neurol.*, **49**, 744–8.

Fayad, M. N., Yamount, B. I., and Mroueh, S. (1997). Alpha interferon in the treatment of subacute sclerosing panencephalitis. *J. Child Neurol.*, **12**, 486–8.

Feuerman, T., Wackym, P. A., Gade, G. F. *et al.* (1989). Craniotomy improves outcome in subdural empyema. *Surg. Neurol.*, **32**, 105–10.

Fitzpatrick, M. O. and Gan, P. (1999). Contrast enhanced computed tomography in the early diagnosis of cerebral abscess. *Br. Med. J.*, **319**, 239–40.

Fleming, J. L., Wiesner, R. H., and Shorter, R. G. (1988). Whipple's disease: clinical, biochemical and histolopathological features and assessment of treatment in 29 patients. *Mayo Clin. Proc.*, **63**, 539–51.

Ford, F. R. (1928). The nervous complications of measles. *Bull. Johns Hopkins Hosp.*, **43**, 140–55.

Fukumoto, S., Kinjo, M., Hokamura, K. *et al.* (1986). Subarachnoid haemorrhage and granulomatous angiitis of the basilar artery: demonstration of the varicella-zoster-virus in the basilar artery lesions. *Stroke*, **17**, 1024–8.

Fuller, A. Q., Munckhoff, W., Kiers, L. *et al.* (1993). Eosinophilic meningitis due to *Angiostrongylus cantonensis*. *West. J. Med.*, **159**, 78–80.

Fuller, G. N., Guiloff, R. J., Scaravalli, F. *et al.* (1989). Combined HIV–CMV encephalitis presenting with brainstem signs (review). *J. Neurol. Neurosurg. Psychiatry*, **52**, 975–9.

Gajdusek, D. C., Gibbs, C. J. J., and Alpers, M. P. (1966). Experimental transmission of a kuru-like syndrome to chimpanzees. *Nature*, **209**, 794–6.

Gajdusek, D. C. and Zigas, V. (1957). Degenerative disease of the central nervous system in New Guinea: the endemic occurrence of 'Kuru' in the native population. *N. Engl. J. Med.*, **257**, 974–8.

Garcia-Monco, J. L. and Benach, J. L. (1995). Lyme neuroborreliosis. *Ann. Neurol.*, **37**, 691–702.

Garland, H. G. and Armitage, G. (1933). Intracranial tuberculoma. *J. Pathol. Bacteriol.*, **37**, 461–71.

Gautier-Smith, P. C. (1965). Neurological complications of glandular fever. *Brain*, **88**, 232–4.

Geiman, B. J. and Smith, A. L. (1992). Dexamethasone and bacterial meningitis. A meta-analysis of randomized controlled trials. *West. J. Med.*, **157**, 27–31.

Gerber, P., Walsh, J. H., and Rosenblum, E. N. (1969). Association of E–B virus with the post perfusion syndrome. *Lancet*, **1**, 593–5.

Gessain, A., Vernant, J. C., Barin, A. *et al.* (1985). Antibodies to human-lymphotropic virus type 1 in patients with tropical spastic paraparesis. *Lancet*, **ii**, 407–410.

Gibbs, C. J. J., Gajdusek, D. C., Asher, D. M. *et al.* (1968). Creutzfeldt–Jakob disease (spongiform encephalopathy): transmission to the chimpanzee. *Science*, **161**, 388–9.

Goodpasture, H. C., Poland, J. D., and Francy, D. B. (1978). Colorado tick fever: clinical epidemiology and laboratory aspects of 228 cases in Colorado in 1973–1974. *Ann. Intern. Med.*, **88**, 303–10.

Gordon, B., Selnes, O. A., and Hart, J. (1990). Long term cognitive sequelae of acyclovir-treated herpes simplex encephalitis. *Arch. Neurol.*, **47**, 646–7.

Gordon, S. M., Eaton, M. E., George, R. *et al.* (1994). The response of symptomatic neurosyphilis to high dose intravenous penicillin G in patients with human immunodeficiency virus infection. *New Engl. J. Med.*, **331**, 1469–73.

Griffith, J. F., Salam, M. V., and Adams, R. D. (1970). The nervous system diseases associated with varicella. *Acta Neurol. Scand.*, **46**, 279–300.

Griffiths, P. D. (1987). Cytomegalovirus. In: *Principles and practice of clinical virology* (ed. A. J. Zuckerman, J. E. Banatlava, and J. R. Pattison), pp. 75–109. Wiley, Chichester.

Grose, C., Henle, W., Henle, G. *et al.* (1975). Primary Epstein–Barr virus infections in acute neurological diseases. *N. Engl. J. Med.*, **292**, 392–5.

Hadlow, W. J. (1959). Scrapie and kuru. *Lancet*, **ii**, 289–90.

Halperin, J. J. (1998). Nervous system Lyme disease. *J. Neurol. Sci.*, **153**, 182–91.

Haribhai, H. C., Bhigjee, A. I., Bill, P. L. A. *et al.* (1991). Spinal cord schistosomiasis. *Brain*, **114**, 709–26.

Harrison, M. J. G. (1982). The clinical presentation abscess. *Q. J. Med.*, **51**, 461–8.

Harrison, M. J. G., Newman, S. P., Hall-Craggs, M. A. *et al.* (1998). Evidence of CNS impairment in HIV infection: clinical, neuropsychological, EEG, and MRI/MRS study. *J. Neurol. Neurosurg. Psychiatry*, **65**, 301–7.

Hattwick, M. A. W., Weiss, T. T., Stechschulte, C. J. *et al.* (1972). Recovery from rabies. A case report. *Ann. Intern. Med.*, **76**, 931–42.

Haupt, W. (1999). Rabies—risk of exposure and current trends in prevention of human cases. *Vaccine*, **17**, 1742–9.

Helmick, C. G., Bernard, K. W., and D'Angelo, L. J. (1984). Rocky Mountain Spotted Fever: clinical, laboratory and epidemiological features of 262 cases. *J. Infect. Dis.*, **150**, 480–8.

Henle, G. and Henle, W. (1966). Immunofluorescence in cells derived from Burkitt's lymphoma. *J. Bacteriol.*, **91**, 1248–56.

Hill, A. F., Zeidler, M., Ironside, J. *et al.* (1997). Diagnosis of new variant Creutzfeldt–Jakob disease by tonsil biopsy. *Lancet*, **349**, 99–100.

Hill, A. F., Butterworth, R. J., Jioner, S. *et al.* (1999). Investigation of variant Creutzfeldt–Jakob disease and other human prion diseases with tonsil biopsy samples. *Lancet*, **353**, 183–9.

Hlavin, M. L., Kaminski, H. J., Fenstemaker, R. A. *et al.* (1994). Intracranial suppuration: a modern decade of post operative subdural empyema and epidural abscess. *Neurosurgery*, **34**, 974–80.

Holmes, G. P., Hilliard, J. K., and Klontz, K. C. (1990). B virus (herpes virus simiae) infection in humans: epidemiological investigation of a cluster. *Ann. Intern. Med.*, **112**, 833–9.

Horten, B., Price, R. W., and Jiminez, D. (1981). Multifocal varicella-zoster virus leukoencephalitis temporarily remote from herpes zoster. *Ann. Neurol.*, **9**, 251–66.

Houff, S. A., Major, E. O., Katz, D. A. *et al.* (1988). Involvement of JC virus-infected mononuclear cells from the bone marrow and spleen in the pathogenesis of progressive multifocal leukoencephalopathy. *New Engl. J. Med.*, **318**, 301–5.

Hsich, G., Kenney, K., Gibbs, C. J. *et al.* (1996). The 14-3-3-brain protein in cerebrospinal fluid as a marker for transmissible spongiform encephalopathies. *N. Engl. J. Med.*, **335**, 924–30.

Huang, C., Campbell, W., Grady, L. *et al.* (1999). Diagnosis of Jamestown Canyon encephalitis by polymerase chain reaction. *Clin. Infect. Dis.*, **28**, 1294–7.

Hughes, I., Jenney, M. E. M., Newton, R. W. *et al.* (1993). Measles encephalitis during immunosuppressive treatment for acute lymphoblastic leukaemia. *Arch. Dis. Child.*, **68**, 775–8.

Iwasaki, Y. (1990). Pathology of chronic myelopathy associated with HTLV-1 infection (HAM/TSP). *J. Neurol. Sci.*, **96**, 103–23.

Janssen, R. J., Cornblath, D. R., Epstein, L. G. *et al.* (1991). Nomenclature and research case definitions for neurologic manifestations of human immunodeficiency virus-type 1 (HIV-1) infection. *Neurology*, **41**, 778–85.

Jeffery, K. J. M. and Bangham, C. R. M. (1996). Recent advances in the laboratory diagnosis of central nervous system infections. *Curr. Opin. Infect. Dis.*, **9**, 132–7.

Jeffery, K. J. M., Read, S. J., Peto, T. E. O. *et al.* (1997). Diagnosis of viral infections of the central nervous system: clinical interpretation of PCR results. *Lancet*, **349**, 313–7.

Jemsek, J., Greenberg, S. B., Taber, L. *et al.* (1983). Herpes zoster-associated encephalitis: clinicopathologic report of 12 cases and review of the literature. *Medicine (Baltimore)*, **62**, 81–97.

Johansen, A. H. (1931). Serous meningitis and infectious mononucleosis. *Acta Med. Scand.*, **76**, 269–72.

Johns, D. R., Tierney, M., and Fenelstein, D. (1987). Alteration in the natural history of neurosyphilis by concurrent infection with the human immunodeficiency virus. *N. Engl. J. Med.*, **316**, 1569–72.

Johnson, R. T. and Milbourn, P. E. (1970). Central nervous system manifestations of chicken pox. *Can. Med. Assoc. J.*, **102**, 831–4.

Johnson, R. T., Griffen, D. E., Hirsch, R. L. *et al.* (1984). Measles encephalomyelitis—clinical and immunologic studies. *N. Engl. J. Med.*, **310**, 137–41.

Jones, M. E. (1998). Modern malaria. *Proc. R. Coll. Physicians Edinb.*, **28**, 370–82.

Kabiri, M., Franco, J. R., Simarro, P. P. *et al.* (1999). Detection of *Trypanosoma brucei gambiense* in sleeping sickness suspects by PCR amplification of expression-site-associated genes 6 and 7. *Trop. Med. Int. Health*, **4**, 658–61.

Kalayjian, R. C., Cohen, M. L., Bonomo, R. A. *et al.* (1994). Cytomegalovirus ventriculoencephalitis in AIDS. A syndrome with distinct clinical and pathologic features. *Medicine*, **72**, 67–77.

Kami, M., Ogawa, S., Kanda, Y. *et al.* (1999). Early diagnosis of central nervous system aspergillosis using polymerase chain reaction, latex agglutination test, and enzyme-linked immunosorbent assay. *Br. J. Haematol.*, **106**, 536–7.

Kaplan, J. E., Litchfield, B., Roualt, C. *et al.* (1991). HTLV-1 associated myelopathy associated with blood transfusion in the United States. *Neurology*, **41**, 192–7.

Katz, D. A., Berger, J. R., and Duncan, R. C. (1993). Neurosyphilis. A comparative study of the effects of infection with human immunodeficiency virus. *Arch. Neurol.*, **50**, 243–9.

Katz, M., Rorke, L. B., Masland, W. S. *et al.* (1968). Transmission of an encephalitogenic agent from brains of patients with subacute sclerosing panencephalitis to ferrets. *N. Engl. J. Med.*, **279**, 793–8.

Keinath, R. D., Merrell, D. E., Vlietstra, R. *et al.* (1985). Antibiotic treatment and relapse in Whipple's disease. Long term follow up of 88 patients. *Gastroenterology*, **88**, 1867–73.

Kennedy, P. G. E. (1987). Neurological complications of varicella-zoster virus. In: *Infections of the nervous system* (ed. P. G. E. Kennedy and R. T. Johnson), pp. 177–208. Butterworth, London.

Kim, Y. J., Chang, K. H., Song, I. C. *et al.* (1998). Brain abscess and necrotic or cystic brain tumor: discrimination with signal intensity on diffusion-weighted MR imaging. *Am. J. Roentgenol.*, **171**, 1487–90.

Kira, J.-I., Minato, S.-I., Itoyama, Y. *et al.* (1988). Leukoencephalopathy in HTLV-1 associated myelopathy: MRI and EEG data. *J. Neurol. Sci.*, **87**, 221–32.

Kirchhoff, L. V. (1993). American trypanosomiasis (Chaga's disease): a tropical disease now in the United States. *New Engl. J. Med.*, **329**, 639–44.

Kirk, J., Zhou, A. L., McQuaid, S. *et al.* (1991). Cerebral endothelial cell infection by measles virus in subacute sclerosing panencephalitis: ultrastructural and *in situ* hybridization evidence. *Neuropathol. Appl. Neurobiol.*, **17**, 289–97.

Kirk, L. J., Fine, P. D., Sexton, J. D. *et al.* (1990). Rocky Mountain Spotted Fever: a clinical review based on 48 confirmed cases 1943–1986. *Medicine*, **69**, 35–45.

Kondo, K., Nagafuji, H., Hata, A. *et al.* (1993). Association of human herpes virus 6 infection of the central nervous system with recurrence of febrile convulsions. *J. Infect. Dis.*, **167**, 1197–200.

Kumar, R., Selvan, A. S., and Sharma, S. (1994). Clinical predictors of Japanese encephalitis. *Neuroepidemiology*, **13**, 97–102.

Kun, L. N., Yian, S. Y., Haur, L. S. *et al.* (1999). Bilateral substantia nigra changes on MRI in a patient with encephalitis lethargica. *Neurology*, **53**, 1860–2.

Kure, K., Llena, J. F., Lyman, W. D. *et al.* (1991). Human immunodeficiency virus-1 infection of the nervous system: an autopsy study of 268 adult, pediatric and fetal brains. *Hum. Pathol.*, **22**, 700–10.

Lakeman, F. D., Whitley, R. J., the NIAID Collaborative Antiviral Study Group (1965). Diagnosis of herpes simplex encephalitis: application of polymerase chain reaction to cerebrospinal fluid from brain-biopsied patients and correlation with disease. *J. Infect. Dis.*, **171**, 857–63.

Lakhanpal, U. and Sharma, R. C. (1985). An epidemiological study of 177 cases of human rabies. *Int. J. Epidemiol.*, **14**, 614–7.

Lancet (1981). Encephalitis lethargica. *Lancet*, **ii**, 1396–7.

Lecour, H., Miranda, M., Magro, C. *et al.* (1989). Human leptospirosis—a review of 50 cases. *Infection*, **17**, 8–12.

Lehky, T. J., Fox, C. H., Koenig, S. et al. (1995). Detection of human T-lymphotropic virus type 1 (HTLV-1) Tax RNA in the central nervous system of HTLV-1 associated myeloparthy/tropical spastic paraparesis patients by in situ hybridisation. Ann. Neurol., 37, 167–75.

Lehrer, R. I., Howard, D. H., Syperd, P. S. et al. (1980). Mucormycosis. Ann. Intern. Med., 93, 93–108.

Lentz, D., Jordan, J. E., Pike, G. B. et al. (1993). MRI in varicella-zoster virus leukoencephalitis in the immunocompromised host. J. Comput. Assist. Tomogr., 17, 313–6.

Levy, R. M., Bredesen, D. E., and Rosenblum, M. L. (1985). Neurological manifestations of the acquired immunodeficiency syndrome: analysis of 50 patients. J. Neurosurg., 62, 475–95.

Levy, R. M., Rosenbloom, S., and Perrett, L. V. (1986). Neuroradiologic findings in AIDS: a review of 200 cases. Am. J. Roentgenol., 147, 977–83.

Looareesuwan, S., Warrell, D. A., White, D. A. et al. (1983). Do patients with cerebral malaria have cerebral oedema? A computed tomography study. Lancet, 1, 434–7.

Looareesuwan, S., Wilairatana, P., Krishna, S. et al. (1995). Magnetic resonance imaging of the brain in patients with cerebral oedema. Clin. Infect. Dis., 21, 300–9.

Louis, E. D., Lynch, T., Kaufmann, P. et al. (1996). Diagnostic guidelines in central nervous system Whipple's disease. Ann. Neurol., 40, 561–8.

Lowichik, A. and Siegel, J. D. (1995). Parasitic infections of the central nervous system in children. Part 1: Congenital infections and meningoencephalitis. J. Child Neurol., 10, 4–17.

Luft, B. J., Brooks, R. G., Conley, F. K. et al. (1984). Toxoplasmic encephalitis in patients with acquired immune deficiency syndrome. JAMA, 252, 913–7.

Luft, B. J., Hafner, R., Korzun, A. H. et al. (1993). Toxoplasmic encephalitis in patients with the acquired immunodeficiency syndrome. N. Engl. J. Med., 329, 995–1000.

Lundstrom, J. O. (1999). Mosquito-borne viruses in western Europe: a review. J. Vector Ecol., 24, 1–39.

MacPherson, G. G., Warrell, M. J., White, N. J. et al. (1985). Human cerebral malaria: a quantitative ultrastructural analysis of parasitised erythrocyte sequestration. Am. J. Pathol., 119, 385–401.

Mamelak, A. N., Obana, W. G., Flaherty, J. F. et al. (1994). Nocardia brain abscess: treatment strategies and factors influencing outcome. Neurosurgery, 35, 622–31.

Mamclak, A. N., Mampelan, T. J., Obana, W. G. et al. (1995). Improved management of multiple brain abscesses: a combined medical and surgical approach. Neurosurgery, 36, 76–85.

Mampalam, T. J. and Rosenblum, M. L. (1988). Trends in the management of bacterial brain abscesses; a review of 102 cases over 17 years. Neurosurgery, 23, 451–8.

Mani, K. S., Mani, A. J., and Montgomery, R. D. (1969). A spastic paraplegic syndrome in south India. J. Neurol. Sci., 9, 179–99.

Masters, C. L., Gajdusek, D. C., and Gibbs, C. J. J. (1981). Creutzfeldt–Jakob disease virus isolations from the Gerstmann–Straussler syndrome with an analysis of the various forms of amyloid plaque deposition in the virus-induced spongiform encephalopathies. Brain, 104, 559–88.

Masters, C. L. and Richardson, E. P. (1978). Subacute spongiform encephalopathy (Creutzfeldt–Jakob disease). The nature and progression of spongiform change. Brain, 101, 333–44.

McGrath, N., Anderson, N. E., Croxson, M. C. et al. (1997). Herpes simplex encephalitis treated with acyclovir: diagnosis and long term outcome. J. Neurol. Neurosurg. Psychiatry, 63, 321–6.

McIntyre, P. B., Berkey, C. S., King, S. M. et al. (1997). Dexamethasone as adjunctive therapy in bacterial meningitis. A meta-analysis of randomized clinical trials since 1988. JAMA, 278, 925–31.

McKendall, R. R. and Klawans, H. L. (1978). Nervous system complications of varicella-zoster. In: Handbook of clinical neurology, Vol. 34 (ed. P. J. Vinken and G. W. Bruyn), pp. 161–83. North-Holland, Amsterdam.

McLelland, C. J., Craig, B. F., and Crockaed, H. A. (1978). Brain abscesses in Northern Ireland: a thirty year community review. J. Neurol. Neurosurg. Psychiatry, 41, 451–8.

McMahon, E. M. E., Glass, J. D., Hayward, S. D. et al. (1991). Epstein–Barr virus in AIDS related primary central nervous system lymphoma. Lancet, 338, 969–73.

Mellors, J. W., Kingsley, L. A., Rinaldo, C. R. et al. (1996). Prognosis in HIV-1 infection predicted by the quantity of virus in plasma. Science, 272, 1167–70.

Merritt, H. H. and Moore, M. (1935). Acute syphilitic meningitis. Medicine, 14, 119–83.

Miller, C., Farrington, C. P., and Harbert, K. (1992). The epidemiology of subacute sclerosing panencephalitis in England and Wales 1970–1989. Int. J. Epidemiol., 21, 998–1006.

Miller, E. S., Dias, P. S., and Uttley, D. (1987). Management of subdural empyema: a series of 24 cases. J. Neurol. Neurosurg. Psychiatry, 50, 1415–8.

Miller, E. S., Psrilal, S. D., and Uttley, D. (1988). Scanning in the management of intracranial abscess: a review of 100 cases. Br. J. Neurosurg., 2, 439–46.

Miller, R. G., Storey, J. R., and Greco, C. M. (1990) Ganciclovir in the treatment of progressive AIDS-related polyradiculaopathy. *Neurology*, **40**, 569–74.

Mishra, N. K. and Goyal, M. (1999). Imaging of CNS tuberculosis. In: *Neurology in tropics* (ed. J. S. Chopra and I. M. S. Sawnhney), pp. 370–90. Churchill Livingstone, New Delhi.

Misra, U. K., Kalita, J., Jain, S. K. *et al.* (1994). Radiological and neurophysiological changes in Japanese encephalitis. *J. Neurol. Neurosurg. Psychiatry*, **57**, 1484–7.

MMWR (1999). Outbreak of West Nile-like viral encephalitis—New York, 1999. *MMWR*, **48**, 845–9.

Molinari, G. F., Smith, L., Goldstein, M. N. *et al.* (1973). Brain abscess from septic embolism: an experimental model. *Neurology*, **23**, 1205–10.

Montgomery, R. D., Cruickshank, E. K., Robertson, W. B. *et al.* (1964). Clinical and pathological observations on Jamaican neuropathy: a report of 206 cases. *Brain*, **87**, 425–62.

Morgan, D. W. and Williams, B. (1985). Posterior fossa subdural empyema. *Brain*, **108**, 983–93.

Morgan, E. R. and Smalley, L. A. (1983). Varicella in immunocompromised children. *Am. J. Dis. Child.*, **137**, 883–5.

Mori, M., Kurata, H., Tajima, M. *et al.* (1991). J C Virus detection by in situ hybridization in brain tissue from elderly patients. *Ann. Neurol.*, **29**, 428–432.

Mrak, R. E. and Young, L. (1994). Rabies encephalitis in humans: pathology, pathogenesis and pathophysiology. *J. Neuropathol. Exp. Neurol.*, **53**, 1–10.

Mustafa, M. M., Weitman, S. D., Winick, N. J. *et al.* (1993). Subacute measles encephalitis in the young immunocompromised host: report of two cases diagnosed by polymerase chain reaction and treated with ribavirin and review of the literature. *Clin. Infect. Dis.*, **16**, 654–60.

Nantulya, V. M., Doua, F., and Molisha, S. (1992). Diagnosis of *Trypanosoma brucei gambiense* sleeping sickness using an antigen detection enzyme-linked immunosorbent assay. *Trans. R. Soc. Trop. Med. Hyg.*, **86**, 42–5.

Nathoo, N., Nadvi, S. S., van Dellen, J. R. *et al.* (1999). Intracranial subdural empyemas in the era of computed tomography: a review of 699 cases. *Neurosurgery*, **44**, 529–35.

Navia, B. A., Jordan, B. D., and Price, R. W. (1986*a*). The AIDS–dementia complex. 1 Clinical features. *Ann. Neurol.*, **19**, 517–24.

Navia, B. A., Petito, C. K., Gold, J. W. M. *et al.* (1986*b*). Cerebral toxoplasmosis complicating the acquired immune deficiency syndrome: clinical and neuropathological findings in 27 patients. *Ann. Neurol.*, **19**, 224–38.

Newton, C. R. J. C., Kirkham, F. J., Winstanley, P. A. *et al.* (1991). Intracranial pressure in African children with cerebral malaria. *Lancet*, **337**, 573–6.

Nielsen, H., Gyldensted, C., and Harmsen, A. (1982). Cerebral abscess: etiology and pathogenesis, symptoms, diagnosis and treatment. *Acta Neurol. Scand.*, **65**, 609–22.

Nishimura, M., Saida, T., Kuroki, S. *et al.* (1996). Post infectious encephalitis with anti-galactocerebroside antibody subsequent to *Mycoplasma pneumoniae* infection. *J. Neurol. Sci.*, **140**, 91–5.

Oh, S. J. (1968). Paragonimus meningitis. *J. Neurol. Sci.*, **6**, 419–33.

Ojeda, V. J., Archer, M., Robetson, T. A., and Bucens, M. R. (1983). Necropsy study of the olfactory portal of entry in herpes simplex encephalitis. *Med. J. Aust.*, **1**, 79–81.

Olesen, W. L., Longo, F. M., Mills, C. M. *et al.* (1988). White matter disease in AIDS: findings at MR imaging. *Radiology*, **169**, 445–8.

Otto, M., Wiltfrang, J., Schutz, E. *et al.* (1998). Diagnosis of Creutzfeldt–Jakob disease by measurement of S100 protein in serum: prospective case–control study. *Br. Med. J.*, **316**, 577–82.

Padgett, B. L., Walker, D. L., Zu Rhein, G. M. *et al.* (1971). Cultivation of papova like virus from human brain with progressive multifocal leukoencephalopathy. *Lancet*, **I**, 1257–60.

Pasteur, L. (1885). Methode pour prevenir la rage apres morsure. *C. R. Acad. Sci. (Paris)*, **101**, 765–74.

Patnaik, J. K., Das, B. S., and Mishra, S. K. (1994). Vascular clogging, mononuclear cell margination and enhanced vascular permeability in the pathogenesis of human cerebral malaria. *Am. J. Trop. Med. Hyg.*, **51**, 642–7.

Pau, A., Turtas, S., Brambilla, M. *et al.* (1987). Computed tomography and magnetic resonance imaging of cerebral coenurosis. *Surg. Neurol.*, **27**, 548–52.

Pickard, J. D. and Czosnyka, M. (1993). Management of raised intracranial pressure. *J. Neurol. Neurosurg. Psychiatry*, **56**, 845–55.

Pitella, J. E. (1993). Central nervous sytem involvement in Chaga's disease: an updating. *Rev. Inst. Med. Trop. Sao Paulo*, **35**, 111–6.

Pitella, J. E. H. and Lana-Peixoto, M. A. (1981). Brain involvement in hepatosplenic schistosomiasis mansoni. *Brain*, **104**, 621–32.

Porras, C., Barboza, J. J., Fuenzalida, E. *et al.* (1976). Recovery from rabies in man. *Ann. Intern. Med.*, **85**, 44–8.

Porter, S. B. and Sande, M. A. (1992). Toxoplasmosis of the central nervous system in the acquired immunodeficiency syndrome. *N. Engl. J. Med.*, **327**, 1643–8.

Porterfield, J. S. (1987). Alphaviruses, flaviviruses, and bunyaviridae. In: *Principles and practice of clinical virology* (ed. A. J. Zuckerman, J. E. Banatlava, and J. R. Pattison), pp. 419–31. Wiley, Chichester.

Price, R. W., Nielsen, S., Horten, B. *et al.* (1983). Progressive multifocal leukoencephalopathy: a burnt out case. *Ann. Neurol.*, **13**, 484–90.

Prusiner, S. B. (1982). Novel proteinaceous infectious particles cause scrapie. *Science*, **216**, 136–44.

Przelomski, M. M., O'Rourke, E., and Grady, G. F. (1988). Eastern equine encephalitis in Massachusetts: a report of 16 cases: 1970–1984. *Neurology*, **38**, 736–9.

Puchhammer-Stockl, E., Popow-Kraupp, T., Heinz, F. X. *et al.* (1991). Detection of varicella-zoster virus DNA by polymerase chain reaction in the cerebrospinal fluid of patients suffering from neurological complications associated with chickenpox or herpes zoster. *J. Clin. Microbiol.*, **29**, 1513–6.

Punt, J. (1983). Multiple cerebral gummata. *J. Neurosurg.*, **59**, 959–61.

Quinlivan, E. B., Norris, M., Bouldin, T. W. *et al.* (1992). Subclinical central nervous system infection with JC virus in patients with AIDS. *J. Infect. Dis.*, **166**, 80–5.

Rail, D., Scholtz, C., and Swash, M. (1981). Post-encephalitic parkinsonism in current experience. *J. Neurol. Neurosurg. Psychiatry*, **44**, 670–6.

Ramzan, N. N., Loftus, E., and Burgart, L. J. (1997). Diagnosis and monitoring of Whipple disease by polymerase chain reaction. *Ann. Intern. Med.*, **126**, 520–7.

Raoult, D., Zuchelli, P., Weiller, P. J. *et al.* (1986). Incidence, clinical observations and risk factors in the severe form of Mediterranean spotted fever among patients admitted to hospital in Marseilles 1983–1984. *J. Infect.*, **12**, 111–6.

Risk, W. S. and Haddad, F. S. (1979). The variable natural history of subacute sclerosing panencephalitis. *Arch. Neurol.*, **36**, 610–4.

Rodgers-Johnson, P. E. B., Gajdusek, D. C., Morgan, OstC. *et al.* (1985). HTLV-1 and HTLV-III antibodies and tropical spastic paraparesis. *Lancet*, **ii**, 1247–8.

Roos, K. L., Bryan, J. P., Maggio, W. M. *et al.* (1987). Intracranial blastomycoma. *Medicine*, **66**, 224–35.

Rowley, A., Lakeman, F. D., Whitley, R. J. *et al.* (1990). Rapid detection of herpes simplex virus DNA in cerebrospinal fluid of patients with herpes simplex encephalitis. *Lancet*, **1**, 440–1.

Sabin, A. B. (1949). Fatal B virus encephalomyelitis in a physician working with monkeys. *J. Clin. Invest.*, **28**, 808.

Salinas, R., Counsell, C., Prasad, K. *et al.* (1999). Treating neurocysticercosis medically: a systematic review of randomised controlled trials. *Trop. Med. Int. Health*, **4**, 713–8.

Schacker, T., Collier, A. C., Hughes, J. *et al.* (1996). Clinical and epidemiologic features of primary HIV infection. *Ann. Intern. Med.*, **125**, 257–64.

Schantz, P. M., Moore, A. C., Munoz, J. L. *et al.* (1992). Neurocysticercosis in an orthodox Jewish community in New York city. *N. Engl. J. Med.*, **327**, 692–5.

Schnell, R. G., Dyck, P. J., Bowie, E. J. W. *et al.* (1966). Infectious mononucleosis: neurologic and EEG findings. *Medicine*, **45**, 51–63.

Schroeder, A. H. (1941). Diagnostico del quiste hidatico cerebral y su tratamiento. *Anales Inst. Neurologia (Montevideo)*, **3**, 11–38.

Schroth, G., Kretzschmar, K., Gawaehn, J. *et al.* (1987). Advantage of magnetic resonance imaging in the diagnosis of cerebral infections. *Neuroradiology*, **29**, 120–6.

Scott, G. B. (1991). HIV infection in children: clinical features and management. *J. Acquir. Immune Defic. Syndr.*, **4**, 109–15.

Selvapandian, S., Rajshekhar, V., Chandy, M. J. *et al.* (1994). Predictive value of computed tomography-based diagnosis of intracranial tuberculomas. *Neurosurgery*, **35**, 845–50.

Seydoux, C. and Francioli, P. (1992). Bacterial brain abscess: factors influencing mortality and sequelae. *Clin. Infect. Dis.*, **15**, 394–401.

Shaked, Y. (1991). Rickettsial infections of the central nervous system: the role of prompt antimicrobial therapy. *Q. J. Med.*, **79**, 301–6.

Sharma, K. R., Sriram, S., Fries, T. *et al.* (1993). Lumbosacral radiculoplexopathy as a manifestation of Epstein–Barr virus infection. *Neurology*, **43**, 2250–4.

Shiff, C. J., Premji, Z., and Minjas, J. N. (1993). The rapid manual ParaSight-FO test. A new diagnostic tool for *Plasmodium falciparum* infection. *Trans. R. Soc. Trop. Med. Hyg.*, **87**, 646–8.

Shope, T. C. (1982). Chickenpox encephalitis and encephalopathy: evidence for differing pathogenesis. *Yale J. Biol. Med.*, **55**, 321–7.

Sidtis, J. J., Gatsonis, C., Price, R. W. *et al.* (1993). Zidovudine treatment of AIDS dementia complex: results of a placebo-controlled trial. *Ann. Neurol.*, **33**, 343–9.

Silverman, L. and Rubenstein, L. J. (1965). Electron microscope observations in a case of progressive multifocal leukoencephalopathy. *Acta Neuropath.*, **5**, 215–44.

Simon, R. P. (1994). Neurosyphilis. *Neurology*, **44**, 2228–30.

Smego, R. A. (1987). Actinomycosis of the central nervous system. *Rev. Infect. Dis.*, **9**, 855–65.

Smith, D. L., Ayres, J. G., Blair, I. *et al.* (1993). A large Q fever outbreak in the West Midlands: clinical aspects. *Respir. Med.*, **87**, 509–16.

Smith, J. B., Westmorland, B. F., Reagan, T. J. *et al.* (1975). A distinctive clinical EEG profile in herpes simplex encephalitis. *Mayo Clin. Proc.*, **50**, 469–74.

Smith, J. S., Fishbein, D. B., Rupprecht, C. E. *et al.* (1991). Unexplained rabies in three immigrants in the United States. A virologic investigation. *N. Engl. J. Med.*, **324**, 205–11.

Smith, M. G., Lennette, E. H., and Reames, H. R. (1941). Isolation of virus of herpes simplex and demonstration of intranuclear inclusions in a case of acute encephalitis. *Am. J. Path.*, **17**, 55–68.

Snider, W. D., Simpson, D. M., Nielson, S. *et al.* (1983). Neurological complications of acquired immune deficiency syndrome: analysis of 50 patients. *Ann. Neurol.*, **14**, 403–18.

Southern, P. M. and Sanford, J. P. (1969). Relapsing fever: a clinical and microbiological review. *Medicine*, **48**, 129–49.

Steere, A. C., Malawista, S. E., and Snydman, D. R. (1977). Lyme arthritis: an epidemic of oligoarticular arthritis in children and adults in three Connecticut communities. *Arthritis Rheum.*, **20**, 7–17.

Sterner, G. and Biberfeld, G. (1969). Central nervous system complications of *Mycoplasma pneumonia* infection. *Scand. J. Infect. Dis.*, **1**, 203–8.

Tenorio, G. and Whitaker, J. N. (1991). Steroid dependant post varicella encephalomyelitis. *J. Child Neurol.*, **6**, 45–8.

Tenover, F. C. (1999). Specimen management and rapid detection of infectious agents. In: *Clinical infectious diseases* (ed. R. K. Root, F. Waldvogel, L. Corey, and W. E. Stamm), pp. 137–44. Oxford University Press, Oxford.

Truc, P., Jamonneau, V., Cuny, G. *et al.* (1999). Use of polymerase chain reaction in human African trypanosomiasis stage determination and follow-up. *Bull. World Health Organ.*, **77**, 745–8.

Tsai, M. D., Chang, C. N., Ho, Y. S., *et al.* (1993). Cerebral sparganosis diagnosed and treated with stereotactic techniques. *J. Neurosurg.*, **78**, 129–32.

Tsuchiya, K., Makita, K., Furui, S. *et al.* (1992). Contrast-enhanced magnetic resonance imaging of sub- and epidural empyemas. *Neuroradiology*, **34**, 494–6.

Tucker, T., Dix, R. D., Katzen, C. *et al.* (1985). Cytomegalovirus and herpes simplex virus ascending myelitis in a patient with acquired immune deficiency syndrome. *Ann. Neurol.*, **18**, 74–9.

Tyler, H. R. (1957). Neurological complications of rubella (measles). *Medicine*, **36**, 147–58.

Upton, A. and Gumpert, J. (1970). Electroencephalography in the diagnosis of herpes-simplex encephalitis. *Lancet*, **I**, 650–2.

Verghese, A. and Sugar, A. M. (1986). Herpes zoster ophthalmicus and granulomatous angiitis. *J. Am. Geriatr. Soc.*, **34**, 309–12.

Vinters, H. V., Kwok, M. K., Ho, H. W. *et al.* (1989). Cytomegalovirus in the nervous system of patients with the acquired immune deficiency syndrome. *Brain*, **112**, 245–68.

Vlasveld, L. T., Sweder von Asbeck, B. (1991). Treatment with deferoxamine: a real risk factor for mucormycosis? *Nephron*, **57**, 487–9.

Von Bokay, J. (1909). Uber den atiologischen Zusammenhang der varizellen mit gewissen Fallen von Herpes Zoster. *Wien Klin. Wochenschr.*, **22**, 1323–42.

Von Economo, C. (1931) *Encephalitis lethargica: its sequelae and treatment* (trans. K. O. Newman). Oxford University Press, London.

Warrell, D. A. (1976). The clinical picture of rabies in man. *Trans. R. Soc. Trop. Med. Hyg.*, **70**, 188–95.

Warrell, D. A., Looareesuwan, S., Warrell, M. J. *et al.* (1982). Dexamethasone proves deleterious in cerebral malaria. A double blind trial in 100 consecutive patients. *N. Engl. J. Med.*, **306**, 313–9.

Watt, G., Adopon, B., Long, G. W. *et al.* (1986). Praziquantel in treatment of cerebral schistosomiasis. *Lancet*, **ii**, 529–32.

Watt, G., Padre, L. P., Tuazon, M. L., Calubaquib, C. *et al.* (1988). Placebo-controlled trial of intravenous penicillin for severe and late leptospirosis. *Lancet*, **I**, 433–5.

Weingarten, K., Zimmerman, R. D., and Becker, R. D. (1987). Subdural and epidural empyemas: MR imaging. *Am. J. Neuroradiol.*, **10**, 81–7.

Weisberg, L. (1984). Clinical–CT correlations in intracranial suppurative (bacterial) disease. *Neurology*, **34**, 509–10.

Weller, T. H. (1953). Serial propagation *in vitro* of agents producing inclusion bodies derived from varicella and herpes zoster. *Proc. Soc. Exp. Biol. Med.*, **83**, 340–6.

Whipple, G. H. (1907). A hitherto undescribed disease characterized anatomically by deposits of fat and fatty acids in the intestinal and mesenteric lymphatic tissues. *Johns Hopkins Hosp. Bull.*, **18**, 382–91.

Whiteman, M. L., Post, M. J. D., Berger, J. R. *et al.* (1993). PML in 47 HIV seropositive patients: neuroimaging with clinical and pathological correlation. *Radiology*, **187**, 233–40.

Whitley, R. J., Lakeman, A. D., Linneman, C. *et al.* (1982). Herpes simplex encephalitis: clinical assessment. *JAMA*, **247**, 317–20.

Whitley, R. J., Alford, C. A., Hirsch, M. S. *et al.* (1986). Vidarabine versus acyclovir therapy of herpes simplex encephalitis. *N. Engl. J. Med.*, **314**, 144–9.

Wildemann, B., Haas, J., Lynen, N. *et al.* (1998). Diagnosis of cytomegalovirus encephalitis in patients with AIDS by quantitation of cytomegalovirus genomes in cells of cerebrospinal fluid. *Neurology*, **50**, 693–7.

Wilkie, F. L., Eisdorfer, C., Morgan, R. *et al.* (1990). Cognition in early Human Immunodeficiency Virus infection. *Arch. Neurol.*, **47**, 433–40.

Will, R. G., Ironside, J. W., Zeidler, M. *et al.* (1996). A new variant of Creutzfeldt–Jakob disease in the UK. *Lancet*, **347**, 921–5.

Wilson, S. A. K. (1940). Neurosyphilis. In: *Neurology*, Vol. 1 (ed. A. N. Bruce), pp. 455–69. Edward Arnold, London.

Yakub, B. A. (1996). Subacute sclerosing panencephalitis (SSPE): early diagnosis, prognostic factors and natural history. *J. Neurol. Sci.*, **139**, 227–34.

Yamasaki, K., Kira, J., Koyanagi, Y. *et al.* (1997). Long term, high dose interferon-alpha treatment in HTLV-1 associated myelopathy/tropical spastic paraparesis: a combined clinical, virological and immunological study. *J. Neurol. Sci.*, **147**, 135–44.

Yang, S. Y. (1981). Brain abscess: a review of 400 cases. *J. Neurosurg.*, **55**, 794–9.

Yiannoutsos, C. T., Major, E. O., Curfman, B. *et al.* (1999). Relation of JC virus DNA in the cerebrospinal fluid to survival in acquired immunodeficiency syndrome patients with biopsy-proven progressive multifocal leukoencephalopathy. *Ann. Neurol.*, **45**, 816–21.

Zarafonetis, C. J. D., Smadel, J. E., Abams, J. W. *et al.* (1944). Fatal herpes simplex encephalitis in man. *Am. J. Path.*, **20**, 429–45.

Zerr, I., Bodemer, M., Otto, M. *et al.* (1996). Diagnosis of Creutzfeldt–Jakob disease by two-dimensional gel electrophoresis of cerebrospinal fluid. *Lancet*, **348**, 846–9.

Zimmermann, R. D., Russell, E. J., Leeds, N. *et al.* (1980). CT in the early diagnosis of herpes simplex encephalitis. *Am. J. Roentgen*, **134**, 61–6.

Zu Rhein, G. M. and Chou, S. M. (1965). Particles resembling papova viruses in human cerebral demyelinating disease. *Science*, **148**, 1477–9.

CHAPTER 35

Complications of systemic infections and immunizations

Milne Anderson

35.1 Introduction and general considerations

This chapter discusses neurological conditions which are associated with infection by particular organisms, but in which the neurological disorder is brought about not by the direct pathogenic effects of the organisms themselves, but by the immunological reactions which they induce in the host, or as a result of the toxins which they produce. In rheumatic fever, infective endocarditis, and vaccine related encephalopathies, the immunological reaction induces a response which incites antigen:antibody reactions that result in pathological tissue responses. In AIDS, by contrast, the immunological response is essentially negative with breakdown of mechanisms, predominantly cellular, which normally counter infection. Consequently, both pathogenic and opportunistic organisms can gain access to the neuraxis and produce a wide range of infectious syndromes. Furthermore, more than one infective agent may be involved and the clinical syndrome may be caused by the HIV virus itself, modified by additional pathogens to produce a confusing mixture of signs. Tetanus and pertussis produce toxins which act at sites distant from the focus of infection. In all of these circumstances, measures must be taken to counter the secondary pathogenic mechanisms in addition to those which have a direct effect on the organism, in order to provide significant clinical improvement.

35.2 **Septic encephalopathy**

Septic encephalopathy is an ill defined yet well recognized state of disordered cerebral function which occurs in patients in the clinical setting of severe generalized infection. The incidence of sepsis and septic shock are not known because the entities are so ill defined but they are on the increase and sepsis of various forms is the most common cause of death on intensive care units. Factors which have contributed to this are the widespread use of antibiotics effective against Gram negative and Gram positive infection, an explosion in the population of patients who are immune suppressed from disease, immunotherapy and chemotherapy, increased use of invasive procedures, and aggressive surgical interventions. Approximately 50 per cent of patients with septic shock have a bacteraemia, Gram negative in the majority, Gram positive and mixed in the remainder with some due to fungi and viruses. Most cases have an underlying cause which predisposes to the dissemination of infection such as tissue damage from trauma or burns, diabetes, drug abuse, AIDS, organ failure, and chemotherapy. In some there is no underlying cause and sepsis is the consequence of infection by a particularly virulent organism.

35.2.1 **Pathophysiology**

The pathophysiology is poorly understood and is certainly multifactorial. Mechanisms which have been postulated, and for which there is some evidence, are brain microabscesses, diffuse microemboli, metabolic derangement, damage from bacteria and bacterial breakdown products, hypoxia and poor cerebral perfusion, and in some, the toxic effects of drugs. Bacterial components are released into the circulation, endotoxin in Gram negative infection, exotoxins in the case of other organisms such as *Staphylococci* and *Streptococci*. These activate the complement system and the coagulation/fibrinolysis mechanisms and trigger the breakdown of kallikreins to bradykinin which causes hypotension and increases vascular permeability. Cellular stimulation, phagocytic, neutrophil and endothelial, releases cytokines which in turn stimulate or over-stimulate, the inflammatory cascade. The complex interaction of these and other mechanisms produces the clinical manifestations of sepsis which manifest in several organ systems, including the brain, to cause septic encephalopathy (Glauser *et al.* 1991, Parillo 1993).

35.2.2 **Clinical signs**

The clinical signs of septic encephalopathy often appear early and are non-specific. Alteration of mental status is always present and is usually the first sign of brain disturbance. Drowsiness, confusion, disorientation, inattention, restlessness, and hallucinations, which progress to coma are usual. Spasticity or rigidity often accompanies coma. Epileptic seizures may occur but their presence and the declaration of focal signs should prompt a search for underlying structural brain pathology – septic encephalopathy is seldom accompanied by focal neurology (Young *et al.*, 1990). Signs of generalized sepsis, hypothermia, hypotension, thrombocytopaenia, and involvement of other organ systems, hepatic, renal, respiratory, or cardiac, are usual. Often, there is multiple organ failure. Search must be made for a focus of infection if it has not already been identified.

35.2.3 **Diagnosis**

Diagnosis of septic encephalopathy requires the exclusion of other causes of diffuse cerebral dysfunction. Anoxia and hypotension must be identified and corrected because their persistence will result in irreversible brain damage. Septic encephalopathy is usually reversible provided the underlying cause of sepsis can be treated, and treatment is given quickly. Mortality increases markedly with reduction of the Glasgow Coma Scale count (Eidelman *et al.*, 1996). Meningitis can be excluded by CSF examination – in most cases of septic encephalopathy the CSF findings are unremarkable. Brain imaging is usually normal (Bolton *et al.*, 1993). If it is clinically possible, MR brain imaging is preferred because of its ability to identify small areas of infarction, white matter abnormality, and microabscesses better than CT. In this circumstance the most sensitive indicator of brain dysfunction is the EEG. It can exclude significant encephalopathy and roughly quantify the degree of cerebral dysfunction – changes vary from excessive theta activity in mild encephalopathy, through delta then triphasic waves to suppression or burst suppression in the most severe encephalopathies (Young *et al.*, 1992). The EEG is particularly useful in monitoring the progress of septic encephalopathy. Blood cultures should be done, together with a full blood count and coagulation screen, blood gas measurement and appropriate tests for organ dysfunction.

33.2.4 **Treatment**

Treatment of septic encephalopathy is essentially that of the underlying condition. Antibiotics are given in high dose intravenously appropriate to the causal organism. Pus should be evacuated surgically. Cardiovascular and ventilatory support and the management of coagulopathy are imperative. It is important to review all drugs being used to determine if any may be contributing to the syndrome. Therapeutic attempts to manipulate the inflammatory response have not produced much success to date. The prognosis for septic encephalopathy is very much the prognosis of the underlying cause and if this can be treated expeditiously and hypoxia and hypoperfusion of brain tissue can be avoided, prospects for complete recovery are good.

35.3 **Neurological complications of AIDS**

Disease of the nervous system is common in HIV infection and occurs in as many as 70 per cent of all cases. It usually occurs in those who are already immune suppressed from AIDS and in

Table 35.1. Neurological complications of HIV infection

Primary	Secondary
Meningitis (seroconversion)	Opportunistic infection
Encephalopathy	Primary and secondary neoplasia
Myelopathy	Side-effects of drugs
Neuropathy	Metabolic derangement
Myopathy	Vascular
Combinations	Combinations

about 20 per cent of those who are HIV positive, neurological disease defines the onset of clinical AIDS. Asymptomatic disease occurs in a further proportion because necropsy series have shown neuropathological changes in more than 90 per cent of the brains of people who die of AIDS (Gray *et al.*, 1988). The spectrum of neurological syndromes is large and encompasses all parts of the nervous system from the deepest reaches of the brain to the most peripheral outpost in muscle. There are numerous ways in which such disease may be classified. One classification is into those conditions which result from direct infection by the HIV virus, primary complications, and those which arise as a consequence of the functional derangement which the virus has produced elsewhere and then secondarily infects the nervous system, secondary infection (Table 35.1).

35.3.1 **Primary neurological complications**

These stem from infection of the nervous system by the virus and include encephalopathy, myelopathy, neuropathy, and myopathy. Secondary complications are brought about by immune suppression permitting infection or neoplasia to disrupt neurological function directly or by causing other pathology which will disrupt it, such as the side-effects of drug treatment, metabolic derangement, or vascular impairment. A further and perhaps more practical clinical differentiation is between non-focal and focal syndromes. A strategy for management of the neurological complications of AIDS is offered, following a description of the complications.

Meningitis at the time of seroconversion and the encephalopathy associated with HIV infection are described in Section 34.11. Myelopathy complicating AIDS is caused by several different pathologies. Most common is a vacuolar myelopathy caused by the HIV virus, neuropathological signs of which may be identified in as many of 30 per cent of patients dying of AIDS – not all have clinical evidence of the condition. Characteristically, there is progressive (over weeks to months) spastic paraparesis which may be asymmetrical, sensory disturbance, sphincter upset, and proprioceptive impairment (Petito *et al.*, 1985). This is akin to the clinical features of sub-acute combined degeneration of the cord. The neuropathological changes are most marked in the thoracic area with vacuolation within the myelin of the dorsal and lateral columns, relative preservation of axons, microglial nodules, and multinucleate giant cells full of virus. Polyneuropathy and encephalopathy often co-exist.

The most common neuropathy seen in AIDS is a distal, symmetrical, sensorimotor polyneuropathy in which painful dysaesthesiae are often predominant (Section 12.14.2). Neurophysiological studies suggest axonal disturbance and this has been confirmed by biopsy. Although direct infection by HIV virus has been suspected, it has not been proven and it may be cytokine mediated. Autonomic neuropathy with postural hypotension, bowel disturbance and cardiac dysrythmia often co-exists. Similar clinical findings occur secondary to nutritional deficiencies and drugs. Inflammatory, demyelinating polyneuropathies of both the acute and the chronic relapsing type, are described associated with HIV infection (Leger *et al.*, 1989; Simpson and Wolfe 1991).

A primary myopathy, HIV-associated myopathy, occurs when the CD4 cell counts are below 500/ml. The clinical features are of limb girdle weakness, muscle tenderness, wasting and increase in creatine phosphokinase, exactly like idiopathic polymyositis (Section 15.7) (Simpson and Bender 1988). Electromyographic and biopsy features are also similar.

35.3.2 **Secondary complications**

Opportunistic infection is the most common. The risk of development of infection is in direct proportion to the degree of immune suppression which is indicated by the CD4 cell count. Agents which are common pathogens are listed in Table 35.2.

Cytomegalovirus infections

Cytomegalovirus infection is the most frequent viral opportunistic infection in AIDS and evidence of infection is found in 30 per cent of brains at necropsy. Correlation with clinical infection is not always evident. For details of the encephalitic features of CMV infection see Section 34.6.3. The presentation and evolution of encephalitis are measured in weeks (Holland *et al.*, 1994). Rarely CMV encephalitis may cause a mass cerebral lesion. CMV has been associated with a painful, asymmetrical polyradiculoneuropathy, usually with sphincter disturbance

Table 35.2. Opportunistic CNS pathogens in AIDS

Viruses	Cytomegalovirus
	JC virus (PML)
	HSV
	VZV
	EB virus (lymphoma)
Bacteria	TB
	Syphilis
	Mycobacterium avium
	Nocardia
	Brain abscess – mixed
Fungi	Cryptococcus
	Candida
	Histoplasma
	Aspergillus
Protozoa	Toxoplasma
	Pneumocystis carinii

(Section 12.14.2). CSF examination reveals polymorphonuclear leucocytosis and CMV can be cultured from CSF in about half of all cases. PCR is reported to be confirmatory.

Progressive multifocal leucoencephalopathy

Progressive multifocal leucoencephalopathy caused by the JC virus complicates AIDS in up to 5 per cent of cases and is often the AIDS defining event (Section 34.10). Infections by Herpes simplex and varicella zoster virus are described in Sections 34.6.1 and 34.6.2.

Epstein-Barr virus

Epstein-Barr virus (see Chapter 34.6.4) is associated with the development of primary CNS lymphoma in AIDS. Primary lymphoma develops in up to 4 per cent of AIDS patients and is the second most common cause of intracranial space occupation. It usually develops in those with CD4 cell counts less than 100/ml. The clinical features are of mental disturbance with confusion, hallucinations, memory disturbance, focal signs and epileptic seizures, obtundation and features of raised ICP. There is often fever and meningeal involvement with neck stiffness. Lesions are often multiple and signs may be confusing. (Baumgartner *et al.*, 1990; MacMahon *et al.*, 1991).

Tuberculosis

Tuberculous pulmonary infection is common in AIDS patients, particularly in drug addicts. Extrapulmonary TB occurs in some 70 per cent and in a small minority this affects the CNS to cause meningitis which has the same features as TB in non-AIDS patients (Berenguer *et al.*, 1992) (Section 33.2.3). Tuberculomas and TB abscesses have been recorded. Atypical mycobacteria, including *M. avium-intracellulare* have a tendency to cause granulomas which may be multiple.

Syphilis and neurosyphilis

Syphilis and neurosyphilis are common in AIDS patients and AIDS seems to increase the risk of earlier development of neurosyphilis (Section 34.17.2). The condition may be asymptomatic and found at CSF examination (Berger 1991). If the definition is taken as a positive CSF-VDRL test then the incidence of neurosyphilis, asymptomatic or symptomatic, approximates to 5 per cent in high risk populations. The clinical features are the same as those in the non-HIV population, although some unusual manifestations have been recorded. It is unclear if the co-existence of HIV infection alters the natural history of neurosyphilis – response to medication may be impaired (Marra *et al.*, 1996). There is evidence that higher dose drug regimes are needed to obtain control of the infection – relapse following treatment with previously accepted dosages is not infrequent (Malone *et al.*, 1995).

Cryptococcal meningitis

Cryptococcal meningitis is one of the most common CNS infections in AIDS. *Cryptococcus neoformans* is an encapsulated yeast which is found throughout the world in soil and animal and bird droppings. Most infections follow inhalation of the small yeast form of the fungus which sets up pulmonary infection, usually without signs, and infection is limited to lung and lymph node. In the immune compromised, an interstitial pneumonitis may occur. Reactivation of the primary pulmonary infection occurs when cellular immune defences fail and dissemination takes place via the bloodstream to other organs, most commonly the CNS. There a chronic form of meningitis occurs. A small number may develop cerebral granulomas.

Cryptococcal meningitis occurs in approximately 7 per cent of AIDS patients and this figure can be reduced if prophylactic antifungals are given. The clinical features are non-specific debility and fatigue and the development over 3 or 4 weeks of neck stiffness, headache, fever, irritability, confusion, and neurological signs. Cranial nerve palsies may ensue. Symptoms and signs may persist for months. In severe immune depression, onset may be acute or even explosive. The differential diagnosis includes other causes of meningitis. Diagnosis is by CSF examination which reveals a mononuclear pleocytosis, raised protein content and positive cryptococcal antigen, presence of yeast forms under the microscope after staining with India ink, and a positive PCR. *Cryptococci* can often be cultured. Treatment is with a combination of Amphotercin B combined with fluconazole for two weeks, followed by fluconazole for 3 months and in reduced dose for the rest of the patient's life. If maintenance therapy is not given as many as 80 per cent will relapse.

Candida spp., part of the normal human flora can pass into the bloodstream of AIDS patients and cause a chronic form of meningitis. *Aspergillus* and *Histoplasma* can also cause similar syndromes. The diagnosis is by direct observation of the fungus in CSF, demonstration of fungal antigen or a positive PCR in CSF. *Aspergillus* and *Mucorales* are more likely to produce a cerebral granuloma than meningitis in AIDS patients.

Toxoplasmosis

The clinical details of toxoplasmosis are enumerated in Section 34.15.9 (Luft and Remington 1992; and Porter and Sande 1992). 20–30 per cent of AIDS patients will develop toxoplasmic encephalitis and this will be due to reactivation of latent infection in 95 per cent. *Toxoplasma* encephalitis is the most common cause of focal masses inside the heads of AIDS patients. Definitive diagnosis can only be made by brain biopsy but a presumptive diagnosis may be made if there is a response to treatment with pyrimethamine and sulphadiazine.

Metastatic disease

Metastatic malignant disease may affect the CNS in AIDS. Non-CNS lymphoma may spread to involve brain or spinal cord, with malignant meningitis and multiple cranial nerve palsies the most common manifestations. Exceptionally, Kaposi's sarcoma has spread to CNS.

Drug side-effects

Drug treatment in AIDS commonly cause side-effects and complications in the nervous system. Neuropathies are recognized complications of nucleoside analogue antiretroviral drugs, isoniazid and vincristine (Section 12.18.9). In some cases of HIV-associated neuropathies, the addition of one of these drugs has been sufficient to cause deterioration in the neuropathy. Zidovudine has caused a myopathy similar to HIV-associated myopathy after prolonged high dose treatment. Zidovudine has been reported to have a toxic effect on muscle mitochondria (Peters *et al.*, 1993). Improvement has been noted after zidovudine has been withdrawn.

Cerebrovascular complications

Cerebrovascular complications occur in AIDS due to several causes. Emboli may result from endocarditis. Infarction may follow thrombosis caused by cerebral vasculitis and infection with VZV, syphilis, *Aspergillus*, or *Mucorales*. Haemorrhage may be the end result of drug-induced thrombocytopaenia or DIC.

35.3.3 Management

Management of a patient who is known to be HIV positive and develops neurological complications must be undertaken urgently. Often the neurological syndrome defines that the patient has developed AIDS. Conversely, it may not be known that the subject is HIV positive when neurological signs appear. It follows that a high index of suspicion that there may be underlying HIV infection, is necessary when these infectious syndromes declare themselves *de novo*. Enquiry must be made of occupational, recreational, geographical or travel exposure to potential pathogens, no matter how exotic. Search is made on physical examination for any locus of infection and specimens taken if one is found. The CD4 status should be assessed – the greater the degree of immune suppression the wider the range of possible pathogens, and the greater chance of multiple infection (and the poorer the prognosis). Blood cultures should be set up. Whether there are focal neurological signs or not, brain imaging should be undertaken. By choice this would be MR with and without gadolinium injection. White matter abnormalities are better delineated and early changes of meningitis and abscess are more evident than with CT. If the patient cannot tolerate MR then CT with contrast enhancement is adequate. If there is no mass lesion on the scan a decision should be made to examine the CSF provided there is no cerebral oedema. Microscopy, culture, serological tests, and PCR against the diseases listed above should be carried out. Non-space occupying white matter abnormalities, diffuse or patchy, seen on scan may be caused by viral encephalitides including AIDS encephalopathy and PMLE.

If a mass lesion or lesions are seen on the scan, the most likely causes in descending order are toxoplasmic encephalitis, lymphoma, pyogenic abscess, or parasitic or fungal granuloma. Infarction and haemorrhage are usually easy to distinguish from these. Metastatic neoplasia may cause confusion. If the mass or masses are causing significantly raised ICP, surgical decompression should be undertaken when possible, and representative tissue removed for histology and culture. If raised ICP is not a problem the results of toxoplasma serology will influence management. If negative, stereotactic biopsy of a lesion should be undertaken. If serology is positive and the patient's condition is stable, it is reasonable to treat for toxoplasmosis, keep the patient under close observation, and rescan within two weeks. If clinical progress and scan appearances continue to show improvement, it is reasonable to continue with pyrimethamine and sulphadiazine and have follow up scans. If there is no clinical or radiological improvement after 2 weeks, or if there is obvious deterioration, stereotactic biopsy should be undertaken forthwith and the treatment regime adjusted according to results. If dexamethasone or other agents have been used to reduce brain oedema, appropriate allowance must be made when assessing clinical and radiological improvement.

There have been some reports suggesting that ancillary radiological techniques such as SPECT, PET, and manipulation of MR data can allow discrimination between white matter abnormalities caused by AIDS encephalopathy, PMLE, and lymphoma (Ernst *et al.*, 1999; Hoffman *et al.*, 1993; Ruiz *et al.*, 1994). Experience is not yet sufficient to provide a definitive answer.

35.4 Infective endocarditis

Infective endocarditis is an infection of the heart, especially the endothelial lining. Heart valve leaflets are predominantly involved and in certain circumstances, chordae tendinae, mural endocardium or intracardiac foreign bodies such as prosthetic valves or pacing electrodes may be subject to infection. Because cardiac endothelium is resistant to infection, there needs to be some pre-existing abnormality or anomaly to which sterile platelet and fibrin containing thrombi can adhere and form, such as abnormal valves. If bacteraemia occurs, however transient, organisms adhere to these previously sterile thrombi and multiply there. The clinical manifestations of infective endocarditis are caused by local cardiac damage which these organisms induce, and by the damage caused peripherally by embolization producing local infarction and often setting up one or multiple loci of infection. Sometimes, particularly virulent organisms such as *Staphylococcus aureus* will cause infection on normal cardiac endothelial structures. A large spectrum of organisms has been recognized to cause infective endocarditis and in practice most cases are caused by a small spectrum which share the ability to survive in the circulation, to adhere to endothelium, and to propagate in vegetations. The central nervous system is the site where many of these emboli lodge. Persisting bacteraemia is a constant feature of infective endocarditis and induces immunological changes that contribute to the development of vasculitis and other clinical manifestations.

There are two forms of endocarditis, acute and subacute, the distinction between the two being based on the speed of evolution of the clinical picture which has usually been related to the virulence of the infecting organism. Acute endocarditis is associated with rapid progression over days, obvious toxicity and constitutional symptoms, rapid development of cardiac disease, and metastatic infection. There is often no evidence of pre-existing cardiac disease and the causal organisms have been virulent – *Staph. aureus*, *Streptococci*, gonococci, and *Haemophilus*. Subacute endocarditis is a more indolent condition which affects an already diseased heart, has less evidence of toxicity and evolves over weeks or months. Peripheral manifestations are fewer and the organisms are less virulent – *Strep. viridans* is the most common and a wide range of organisms have been identified including enterococci and Gram negative coccobacilli from the mouth and throat – transient bacteraemia is commonplace after teeth brushing and following iatrogenic instrumentation. Fungi and parasites may rarely cause endocarditis.

35.4.1 Incidence

The incidence of infective endocarditis has remained surprisingly constant over the years at approximately 2–4 cases per 100 000 per annum in developed countries. However, the pattern of infection keeps changing, and the distinction between acute and sub-acute disease has blurred. Underlying conditions which predispose to infective endocarditis are rheumatic heart disease, particularly in developing countries, congenital heart disease – bicuspid aortic valve is important in older patients, degenerative disease with atheroma in the elderly, cardiac surgery with prosthetic valves, pacemakers, and systemic arterial shunts. Mitral valve prolapse has been described as a significant predisposing factor but this may have been exaggerated. To cause endocarditis, it is necessary for organisms to access the bloodstream and conditions which predispose to this include iatrogenic instrumentation, haemodialysis, dental manipulation, tissue trauma and burns, and intravenous drug addiction. IV drug addiction carries a very high risk of septicaemia and is increasing as a cause of infective endocarditis. Immune suppression from AIDs and other causes permits cardiac colonization by a wide range of organisms including fungi. In approximately 5 per cent of patients, no organism can be detected, usually because of prior antibiotic administration. In such cases, diagnosis can be confirmed by serological tests or PCR.

35.4.2 Clinical manifestations

The clinical manifestations of infective endocarditis derive from a combination of four main mechanisms – cardiac tissue destruction from valve and other vegetations, distal embolization and infarction, metastatic infection from bacteraemia, and tissue damage due to immune complex deposition and local complement activation. Constitutional symptoms derive from bacteraemia. The signs and symptoms vary enormously. Fever is the most common sign and it may not be evident in the ill or elderly. Cardiac murmurs are the next most common manifestation and are heard in 80 per cent of patients. They may change or be evanescent. Malaise, night sweats, weight loss, and arthralgia are common, as is splenomegaly. Anaemia is invariable. Osler's nodes (tender nodules found on the pulp of the fingers), splinter haemorrhages and petechiae, finger clubbing,

and retinal haemorrhages were formerly commonplace and are seen less frequently now because the diagnosis is usually made earlier before these lesions have had time to develop. Congestive cardiac failure develops in up to half of all patients. Peripheral embolism causes signs appropriate to the organ involved. Renal dysfunction from immune mediated glomerulonephritis may occur in 15 per cent of patients. Neurological complications occur in 19 to 40 per cent with an average of 30 per cent—which has remained constant over the years. The presentation of endocarditis may be entirely neurological and any stroke in a young person should prompt a search for underlying endocarditis (Lerner and Weinstein 1966; Osler 1885; Pruitt *et al.*, 1978).

35.4.3 Neurological complications

Neurological complications of endocarditis occur equally in the sexes and increase with age. They are usually associated with abnormalities of the valves on the left side of the heart, the most common being embolic stroke. If the organism is virulent, stroke occurs earlier. Embolism takes place to the distribution of the middle cerebral artery in the vast majority of cases; consequently signs are of hemiparesis, hemisensory deficit, and dysphasia. It is rare for brain stem to be affected and rarer still for spinal cord. Emboli are often multiple so that signs may be complex. If the embolus is small and disintegrates, TIAs occur (Figure 35.1). Intracranial haemorrhage occurs in about 5 per cent of cases and may be intracerebral or subarachnoid. It is caused by rupture of mycotic aneurysms in most, in some by transformation of infarction to haemorrhage by the use of anticoagulant drugs. Mycotic aneurysms are

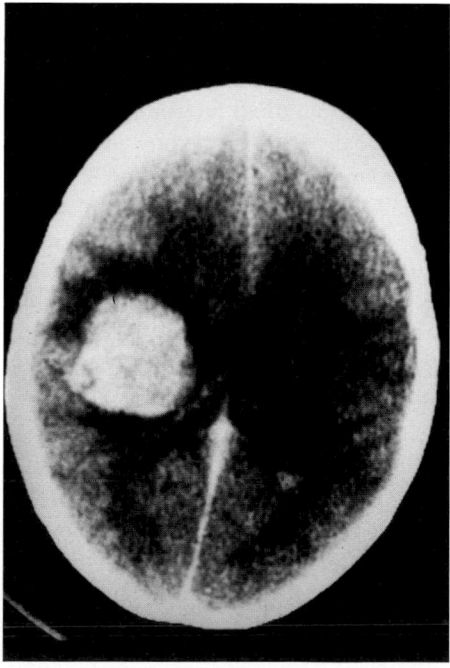

Fig. 35.1. Subacute bacterial endocarditis: contrast-enhanced CT brain scan showing right frontoparietal haematoma.

caused by infected emboli lodging in vasa vasorum causing local infection and arteritis which leads to weakening of the vessel wall and subsequent aneurysm formation. This is most frequent in middle cerebral artery territory, and they tend to be distal rather than proximal and they grow rapidly. They may rupture into brain or into the subarachnoid space.

Brain abscesses occur in up to 4 per cent of cases and are caused by emboli to the brain which set up a nidus of infection. They are often multiple. Meningitis, both septic and aseptic, is recognized in 10 per cent of cases who have neurological complications. Epileptic seizures occur in about 10 per cent, and may be generalized or focal. Focal seizures imply underlying structural brain damage and this is usually caused by brain infarction.

20 per cent of neurological cases are accompanied by a miscellany of symptoms and signs which have been loosely grouped under the term 'toxic encephalopathy' or 'septic encephalopathy'. These include confusion, confabulation, disorientation, personality change, and decrease of conscious level, and coma. Many factors contribute to this, including anoxia, metabolic disturbance, and immune arteritis. Immune complex deposition has been postulated as a cause but remains unproven.

35.4.4 Diagnosis

Diagnosis is suggested by the clinical findings of changing cardiac murmurs and evidence of peripheral embolism in a toxic, ill patient, and is confirmed by the demonstration of infecting organisms in blood cultures and vegetations on cardiac valves by echocardiography. In more indolent infection, cardiac murmurs may not be so evident. Blood cultures are positive in more than 90 per cent of patients who have not received antibiotics. The more frequently cultures are taken, the higher the positive yield is likely to be. Search should be made for fastidious and exotic organisms and serological tests and PCR for organisms such as *Legionella*, *Brucella*, *Coxiella*, and others should be set up. Anaemia of normochromic, normocytic type is common, there is peripheral leucocytosis and the ESR is invariably raised, often to values over 100 mm per hour. CRP is also elevated. Cardiac investigations including ECG and echocardiography are necessary. A cardiologist should be invited to supervise these and advise about the most appropriate echo technique. Urinalysis reveals proteinuria and haematuria in half of all patients. Brain imaging is indicated when there are neurological complications, and if the patient can tolerate it, MRI is to be preferred. Abscess formation, infarction, haemorrhage, cerebral oedema, and mycotic aneurysms may be identified by angiographic sequences. If this is not available, conventional arteriography will yield sufficient information to decide surgical strategy (Figure 35.2). CSF examination seldom provides sufficient information to alter clinical management and is contraindicated if there are focal lesions or signs of raised ICP. It may be necessary if there is neck stiffness and clinical suspicion of meningitis. Criteria for the diagnosis of infective endocarditis may be found in Durack *et al.*, (1994), the Duke criteria.

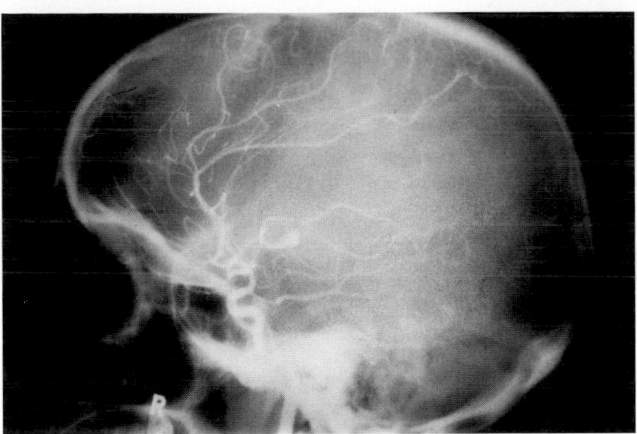

Fig. 35.2. Subacute bacterial endocarditis: right middle cerebral artery mycotic aneurysm (demonstrated by conventional angiography) which had ruptured to cause the intracerebral haematoma illustrated in Fig. 35.1.

35.4.5 Treatment

Treatment requires the eradication of the infecting organism and management of complications. Antibiotics (or antifungal drugs if indicated) are administered according to the causal organism and the antibiotic sensitivities obtained. In theory, bactericidal drugs are to be preferred and high blood concentrations are necessary for the drugs to penetrate relatively avascular cardiac vegetations. Therefore, it is necessary to administer these parenterally and for a prolonged period. Advice for the most appropriate antibiotic regimes should be sought from a bacteriologist and a consultant in infectious diseases. Cardiological input will be required to monitor heart status and treat failure and advise on surgery for heart valve damage. Cardiac surgical intervention is often necessary.

The treatment of neurological complications is usually straightforward. Meningitis is treated with antibiotics; similarly multiple brain abscesses unless they occupy space or fail to respond to antibiotics, in which case they should be drained surgically using stereotactic techniques. There is no general consensus regarding the treatment of cerebral emboli – should a heart valve with a vegetation source of emboli be replaced? And if so, after how many episodes? Each case must be assessed individually. Anticoagulant treatment for recurrent emboli complicating infective endocarditis should not be given in the author's view, because of the danger of haemorrhage into the affected brain. The place of adjunctive treatment with aspirin has not yet been defined. Intracerebral haemorrhage does not require active surgical treatment unless the haematoma functions as an expanding space occupying lesion. A search should be made for an underlying mycotic aneurysm with angiography, and conventional angiography retains the advantage over MR as it allows better delineation of the neck and surgical anatomy. These are uncommon lesions and complicate infective endocarditis in less than 5 per cent of cases (Pruitt *et al.*, 1978; Salgado *et al.*, 1989). The indications for surgical treatment remain controversial largely because a proportion of unruptured aneurysms will resolve given antibiotic treatment over a prolonged period (Brust *et al.*, 1990). Most agree that a mycotic aneurysm associated with intracerebral or subarchnoid haemorrhage should be treated surgically. For others it would seem reasonable to repeat angiography to determine if there is an increase in size of the aneurysm and, if there is, proceed to surgical treatment provided the position of the aneurysm and the clinical state of the patient allow. In this circumstance, MR angiography has the advantage. The size of the aneurysm is not a good indicator of subsequent rupture.

35.4.6 Outcome

Treatment outcomes for infective endocarditis depend upon the virulence of the infecting organism, the nature of any underlying cardiac lesion, any delay in diagnosis, and the presence of complications. Mycotic aneurysms carry a high mortality whether they rupture or not – on average 45 per cent. Meningitis and multiple cerebral abscesses have mortality rates approaching 80 per cent. Recurrent endocarditis occurs in up to 4 per cent of cases with a higher incidence in drug addicts. Chemoprophylaxis has been recommended for patient groups with cardiac lesions which are thought to predispose to the development of endocarditis, and surgical or dental procedures have been identified which may cause bacteraemia and lead to infection. However, the efficacy of chemoprophylaxis has not been proved.

35.5 Rheumatic fever

Rheumatic fever is the name given to the disease entity which follows upper respiratory infection by some types of Group A streptococci. Formerly a common infection of childhood, its incidence diminished dramatically in Europe and North America in the 1950s and 1960s concurrently with improvements in social conditions and the increased availability of antibiotics, particularly penicillin. In these countries the disease is seldom seen and, as a consequence, is more difficult to diagnose. The annual incidence is believed to be about 0.5 affected per 100,000 children of school age. The need to be constantly alert to its occurrence was demonstrated by outbreaks in the United States in the 1980s, which affected military institutions and reasonably affluent communities in five cities. In developing countries the incidence is increasing and is about 100–200 per 100,000 of school age children. Current understanding is that rheumatic fever is caused by a disturbed host autoimmune response to infection by particular serotypes of Group A β-hacmolytic streptococci (M types 3, 5, 18, 19, 24 and others). A surface protein of the bacterial wall, protein M, carries specific epitopes and is instrumental in the disease process but the exact mechanisms are not yet understood. Bacterial breakdown products are released from the pharynx and induce an immunological cross reaction with other tissues, particularly heart muscle and valves (Olivier 2000). This reaction with other body tissues

accounts for the various manifestations in other systems which are characteristic of rheumatic fever (Bisno 1991). It may be that a degree of genetic susceptibility predisposes to these reactions. The risk of developing rheumatic fever following tonsillitis or pharyngitis which has not been treated with antibiotics, is less than 1 per cent.

Any age group and either sex can be afflicted by rheumatic fever and the commonest age group at presentation is 5 to 15 years. It occurs more commonly in populations of lower socio-economic status (because of overcrowding). Typically between two and six weeks following an attack of tonsillitis or pharyngitis symptoms of rheumatic fever appear. There is fever which may be irregular, malaise, and generalized toxicity.

35.5.1 General features

Carditis, polyarthritis, chorea, subcutaneous nodules, and erythema marginatum occur in frequencies which vary from population to population and with age. Young children tend to have carditis (40 per cent and includes myocarditis, pericarditis, and valvular disease), while older patients tend to have arthritis. The arthritis is typically fleeting, polyarticular, and involves the large joints and afflicts about 70 per cent of patients.

Ten per cent have subcutaneous nodules which appear on the extensor surfaces of the wrists, elbows, and knees. Five per cent have erythema marginatum. About 10 per cent develop chorea and this figure is higher in reports from some areas, particularly South America. Criteria for the diagnosis of rheumatic fever have been devised based on criteria proposed by Jones in the 1940s (Table 35.3).

35.5.2 Rheumatic chorea

Rheumatic chorea (also known as Sydenham's chorea or St Vitus dance) is one of the common manifestations of rheumatic fever (Section 32.5.5). It affects children much more commonly than adults and females more than males. There is often no obvious history of rheumatic fever and for the onset to be insidious. Consequently, Sydenham's chorea should be considered in the differential diagnosis of any movement disorder in a young person. At first, abnormal movements may be intermittent and

Table 35.3. Criteria for the diagnosis of rheumatic fever

Diagnosis requires evidence of previous streptococcal infection plus	
1. two major criteria, or	
2. one major plus two minor criteria	
Major criteria	Carditis
	Arthritis
	Subcutaneous nodules
	Erythema marginatum
	Chorea
Minor criteria	Clinical findings including arthralgia and pyrexia
	Laboratory findings (raised ESR, CRP, ASO titre)

tic-like and they are often misinterpreted as being of hysterical origin. Onset can also be explosive with generalized and often violent, choreic movements which involve limbs and trunk and face. It has been said to subside during sleep but this has not been the author's experience. In 20 per cent of cases only one side is affected. Commonly, the patient is more emotional than usual. The average duration of chorea is only two to three months but some persist for much longer, in some for years (Cardoso *et al.*, 1999). It has been said that chorea is less likely to be followed by long-term cardiac problems but the incidence of accompanying carditis has been recorded at up to 30 per cent. There is a slight chance of recurrence and females who have had Sydenham's chorea may develop chorea later when they become pregnant or if they take the contraceptive pill.

Diagnosis

Investigations to confirm a diagnosis of Sydenham's chorea include demonstration of previous streptococcal infection by serological means and application of the above diagnostic criteria for rheumatic fever. Cerebral imaging with CT or MR is usually normal. Sedation may be necessary for these procedures if movements are particularly violent. It has been assumed that some functional derangement of basal ganglial structures, perhaps of an immunological or vasculitic basis underpins the mechanism of chorea in these cases. Anti-neuronal antibodies have been found in some and in others there has been an increase in CSF IgG but these findings are not consistent. CSF examination is not diagnostically useful. Few scan abnormalities have been documented. High signal on T2 weighted MR images have been reported in caudate and putamen (Castillo *et al.*, 1999) and vasculitic changes in major cerebral vessels (Ryan and Antony 1999).

The diagnosis of Sydenham's chorea is not difficult if it occurs in the setting of rheumatic fever. If not, other conditions which should be excluded are Huntington's disease in older patients, Wilson's disease in teenagers and young adults and the syndrome of Gilles de la Torette. In younger patients white matter degenerations and metabolic encephalopathies may produce movement disorders, but intellect and mentation are usually disturbed with these conditions. Cerebral neoplasia must be excluded if the chorea is one sided. Pregnancy and exposure to oral contraceptives may cause chorea in young women.

Treatment

Treatment of Sydenham's chorea is that of rheumatic fever firstly, followed by treatment of the movement disorder if it persists. A cardiac assessment should be carried out. β-haemolytic streptococci remain exquisitely sensitive to penicillin which should be administered. Other manifestations of rheumatic fever are treated with aspirin reinforced with steroids if necessary. There is no good evidence that the administration of steroids influences chorea significantly. Haloperidol and tetrabenazine have been used to try to influence chorea.

35.6 Brucellosis

In humans, brucellosis is caused by infection by species that belong to the genus Brucella. It was first described by Marston in 1861 and Bruce, who was working for the Army Medical Service in Malta, cultured a micrococcus from the spleen of a fatal case and named it *Micrococcus melitensis* after the old name for Malta. The name was changed to *Brucella melitensis* in his honour in 1920. Zammit, a Maltese colleague of Bruce found antibodies against the organism in the serum of goats and Horrocks isolated the organism from the milk of an infected goat in 1905. Concurrently, Bang isolated *B. abortus* from cattle in Denmark and slightly later in 1914, Traum isolated *B. suis* from sows. Evans recognized the relationship between these organisms and their diseases in 1918 and she established that milk was the source of the infection.

Brucellosis is a disease of animals which spreads to humans who ingest infected, unpasteurized milk, milk products such as cheese, or undercooked meat, or come in contact with the organism by occupational contact with animals. The bacterium enters through abrasions or by inhalation. There are six species of *Brucella* – *melitensis, abortus, suis, canis, neotomae,* and *ovis*. The last two do not cause human disease and *B. canis* very seldom does. *B. melitensis* infects sheep, goats, and camels; *B. abortus* infects cattle and *B. suis*, pigs and other species such as reindeer and hare. Brucellosis is found throughout the world and the incidence is probably increasing but this is difficult to prove. It is endemic in Asia, Africa, Central and South America, and in several Mediterranean countries. In Britain most cases are caused by *B. abortus* and *B. melintensis* is imported. In the United States *B. suis* is the major pathogen, *B. melitensis* in the Mediterranean.

Once the organism has entered the bloodstream it travels to regional lymph nodes, thence to the reticulo-endothelial system, particularly spleen, liver, bone marrow and lymph nodes, where granulomas with epithelioid and giant cells similar to sarcoidosis, and other chronic granulomatous conditions, are formed. These are full of bacteria and may progress to abscess formation. Endocarditis, osteomyelitis, and genitourinary tract granulomas occur rarely. Neurological involvement includes acute and chronic vascular inflammation, diffuse meningeal inflammation and adhesions occasionally associated with non-caseating granulomas and encephalitic changes, brain oedema, and white matter degeneration. Perineural infiltration of nerve roots may take place (Larbrisseau *et al.*, 1978). Bone of the vertebral column, discs and joints may be invaded by granuloma.

Brucella organisms are non-motile, unencapsulated Gram negative coccobacilli which are faculatatively intracellular. This last property makes it difficult to eradicate the infection with antibiotics and prolonged courses are often necessary. Pasteurization kills the organism.

35.6.1 Common manifestations

Brucellosis most commonly manifests as the acute form. Both sexes and any age are affected. The incubation period may be as

Table 35.4. Neurological syndromes of Brucellosis

Acute	meningo-encephalitis
Chronic	meningitis
	encephalitis
	focal granuloma
	vasculitis and infarction
	cranial and peripheral multiple mononeuropathy
	myelopathy
	radiculopathy
	central demyelination
	psychiatric?

short as one to three weeks, and may be as long as six months. Headache, weakness, malaise, back pain, and arthralgia are accompanied by fever, sweating, and shivering with a tendency to be more marked towards evenings. Progression may be insidious and evidence of disease spreading to other systems, particularly osteo-articular, ensues (Young 1983). Classically, intermittent and irregular fever (undulant) with backache and sciatica is associated with lymphadenopathy and splenomegaly. The nervous system is affected in about 5 per cent of all cases (Al-Deeb *et al.*, 1989; Bahemuka *et al.*, 1988; Shakir *et al.*, 1987). The clinical syndromes of neurobrucellosis are several and diverse and may affect any part of the central and peripheral nervous system. More than one syndrome may be present to further confuse the picture (Table 35.4).

The clinical features of meningitis and encephalitis are similar to those of other chronic forms such as TB or fungal meningitis, from which brucella can be distinguished only with further tests. The course is often chronic and relapsing. Focal granulomas can occur anywhere throughout the neuraxis and the signs reflect their location. Epileptic seizures are not uncommon and raised intracranial pressure may cause papilloedema. Vasculitis of the major cerebral vessels gives rise to focal signs as a result of infarction. Sub-arachnoid haemorrhage from rupture of mycotic aneurysms has been described (McLean *et al.*, 1992) and embolization from endocarditis is a rare complication. Multiple mononeuropathy affecting the cranial nerves, particularly VIII, VII, V and the oculomotor nerves, occurs due to perineural inflammation. Peripheral nerves may be similarly affected and usually involves the legs. Myelopathy and radiculopathy, often combined, have a tendency to occur in the lower thoracic and lumbosacral regions and have been caused by transverse myelitis, infarction, arachnoiditis, epidural abscess or spondylitis, and compression of cord and nerve roots. Central demyelination has been described, and papillitis and optic neuritis and may represent an immunologically mediated reaction. Whether there is a specific psychiatric syndrome associated with brucellosis has been the subject of considerable argument. There is no doubt that many of the neurological syndromes are misdiagnosed or diagnosed late, and more than one patient has been accused of malingering. Depression is common and organic brain damage may lead to psychiatric syndromes including psychoses.

35.6.2 Differential diagnosis

The differential diagnosis of neurobrucellosis includes many syndromes. In the acute phase, bacterial and viral meningo-encephalitides, including herpes encephalitis, must be excluded. Chronic disease is similar to TB and fungal meningitis and granulomas, TB spondylitis and pyogenic infections, Lyme disease, syphilis, sarcoidosis and Behçet's disease. The tendency of neurobrucellosis to exhibit a relapsing course can be very like multiple sclerosis and the scan appearances and CSF abnormalities may be similar.

35.6.3 Diagnosis

In an endemic area, diagnosis is usually not too difficult once it has been considered. Confirmation can be obtained by culture of the organism from blood, CSF, bone marrow, or lymph node. This is positive in about 25 per cent of cases. A presumptive diagnosis can be made by demonstrating rising titres of specific antibody in serum. Both IgM and IgG rise, the latter more slowly. Discussion with the laboratory is appropriate to determine the most appropriate technique – CIE, IF, and ELISA have all been applied. Raised titres of IgG are found in CSF in cases of meningitis, there is lymphocytic pleocytosis and raised protein content. The application of PCR to both blood and CSF promises to increase specificity and diagnostic accuracy (Matar *et al.*, 1996). The radiological abnormalities of neurobrucellosis are not specific. Plain X-rays of the spine may indicate sacroileitis and erosion of vertebrae. CT scanning of the brain may indicate granuloma formation or infarction, of the spine, bony erosion. MR imaging of the brain will show white matter abnormalities to better advantage and of the spine, soft tissue granulomatous change and spinal block. Isotope bone scanning can highlight inflammatory changes in bone and joint before they become evident on CT or MR. None of these changes is specific – similar appearances are seen with chronic pyogenic, tuberculous and fungal infections.

35.6.4 Treatment

Treatment of brucellosis is with antibiotics. In the more chronic forms this can be difficult because of the ability of *Brucella* to remain protected within the monocyte–phagocyte environment. As a consequence, relapses are frequent. Commonly used regimes combine doxycycline with streptomycin or rifampicin for 6 weeks to 2 months with appropriate precautions for the use of streptomycin. For acute cases, a combination of tetracycline and rifampicin for two weeks would appear to be adequate. In more chronic cases, particularly those with polyradiculopathy and granulomas, antibiotic treatment may have to be given for 6 months or more. Repeat courses may be needed. It is prudent to cover the first few days of antibiotic treatment with steroids to diminish the risk of a Jarisch–Herxheimer reaction. Some reports suggest that concurrent prednisolone treatment is useful in those with arachnoiditis and cranial nerve palsies (Al-Deeb *et al.*, 1988). With adequate and timely antibiotic treatment most cases make a complete recovery and the relapse rate should be less than 10 per cent. It is prudent to keep all cases under surveillance for a year after the cessation of treatment. Antibody levels fall but the clinical correlation between complete recovery and the levels is not absolute. Results with PCR are encouraging (Morata *et al.*, 1999).

35.6.5 Prevention

Prevention of brucellosis in humans depends on eradication of the infection in animals and the pasteurization of milk for human consumption. Immunization of those at risk, such as vets and those involved in animal husbandry, has been used, but has not been completely effective.

35.7 Tetanus

Tetanus (literally 'muscular spasm') is the name given to a condition known since ancient times, caused by infection due to *Claustridium tetani*, which causes muscle spasms. It was recognized by Hippocrates, and Aretaeus of Cappodoccia gave a graphic account of the clinical manifestations. The organism was identified from soil by Nicolaier in 1884 who recognized that it produced a toxin with similarities to strychnine. Two years later Rosenbach found the bacillus in man. Four years later, Behring and Kitasato were able to demonstrate that the disease could be prevented by immunization and in the same year Faber found a heat-labile toxin. Small amounts of toxin injected into animals would induce immunity which could be passively transferred to humans and the use of antitoxic serum prevented the development of tetanus in the wounded during the First World War. In countries where tetanus immunization has been introduced, the incidence of clinical tetanus has declined dramatically. There are probably in excess of one million cases of tetanus in the world each year. Neonatal tetanus accounts for about 50 per cent of all cases.

Clostridium tetani is an anaerobic Gram-positive bacillus which is slowly motile and produces a terminal spore as it matures, looking like a tennis racket or distaff under the microscope (hence the name *Clostridium*). These spores are highly resistant to heat, disinfectants, and antibiotics and may lie dormant in soil for many years. They are ubiquitous and are found in soils of all kinds, particularly in ones which have been enriched with moisture and manure (either human or animal). Human infection occurs with contamination of cuts, burns, animal bites, or even insect bites. Any age group is at risk, but particularly neonates in undeveloped countries who are born in unhygienic conditions where the umbilicus becomes contaminated by spores. Infection is more likely if the wound is particularly traumatic and associated with tissue damage. However, inoculation can take place via apparently innocuous pricks which penetrate the skin, e.g. rose thorns. Forgetting such incidents may account for the observation that no history of trauma is obtained in a small proportion of cases. Tetanus

may follow childbirth or abortion, intravenous drug abuse, surgical operations, and body piercing. Otitis media and mastoiditis may be sources of infection.

When the spores are introduced to damaged tissues they are activated to the vegetative form in anaerobic conditions and produce the tetanus toxin, tetanospasmin, which is neurotoxic, disseminates throughout the body, and causes clinical tetanus. Another toxin, tetanolysin, is also produced which has the ability to disrupt cell membranes and damage tissue adjacent to the wound. Its part in the pathogenesis of tetanus is not understood.

Tetanospasmin is produced by pathogenic strains of *C. tetani* – strains which do not produce tetenospasmin do not cause tetanus. Tetanospamin is a single polypeptide chain which is broken by endogenous proteases to produce a light and a heavy sub-chain which are linked co-valently by a disulphide bridge. The heavy sub-chain can be cleaved by papain treatment to produce a smaller fragment known as the C fragment, leaving the disulphide joined A-B fragment. The exact mechanisms by which these produce the manifestations of tetanus have not been fully elucidated. It is thought that fragment C binds to neural ganglioside receptors at presynaptic end plate junctions, and the light chain inhibits transmitter release. Fragment C may facilitate trans-synaptic transport of toxin. However it functions, once tetanospasmin has entered the presynaptic vesicle it can inhibit transmitter release for as long as several weeks. It can also be translocated by retrograde axonal transport and transynaptic migration to neurones in spinal cord and brain. Tetanospasmin also circulates in the blood and spreads to endplates throughout the body. Circulating toxin can be neutralized by antitoxin but once it has crossed the neural membrane it cannot be inactivated. Within the CNS it migrates to inhibitory cells where GABA release is prevented and this increases the activity of α-motoneurones resulting in muscular hypertonicity. Inhibitory reflexes are also disrupted which means that stimulation of the motor system produces intense contraction of all muscle groups, both agonist and antagonist, to cause tetanic muscle spasm. The sympathetic nervous system is also affected, leading to signs of sympathetic over-activity.

Four clinical varieties of tetanus are recognized and reflect the host reaction to infection, the quantum of tetanospasmin production, and the site of action of the toxin (Table 35.5).

35.7.1 Incubation

The incubation period for the development of tetanus reflects the time from spore inoculation to toxin production and symptom onset, and this may be as short as 24 hours or as long

Table 35.5. Clinical varieties of tetanus

Local
Cephalic
Generalized
Neonatal

as several months but usually falls within one to three weeks. The shorter the incubation period, the more severe the infection and the poorer the prognosis. Distal wounds have a longer period than those proximate to the CNS and large wounds with a greater inoculum produce symptoms sooner.

35.7.2 Localized tetanus

Localized tetanus refers to rigidity and spasm of muscle in proximity to the site of inoculation. It may be associated with local weakness and muscle pain, and it may persist for weeks. Such patients have some degree of immunity with sufficient circulating antibody to bind to toxin to prevent it reaching the CNS, but not enough to prevent local disturbance. If treated it has a very low mortality. The danger is that it may progress to generalized tetanus if not recognized and the toxin is not neutralized with antitoxin.

35.7.3 Cephalic tetanus

Cephalic tetanus is a localized form in which signs are limited to the lower cranial nerves. There is facial weakness, and trismus (from the Greek 'to grate' alluding to the grinding of teeth from spasm of the masseter muscles), dysphagia and, rarely, involvement of the extraocular muscles. It occurs in less than 1 per cent of cases and tends to be associated with head wounds and otitis media (Dastur *et al.*, 1977; DeSouza *et al.*, 1992; Vakil *et al.*, 1973).

35.7.4 Generalized tetanus

Generalized tetanus is the most frequently recognized form of the disease in adults. There is often ill-defined malaise for a day or so, followed by muscle spasms and trismus. The jaw muscles become tight on chewing and progresses to inability to open the mouth fully because of muscle rigidity leading to 'lockjaw'. As the facial and jaw muscles become more rigid, facial expression becomes fixed in a grimace, 'risus sardonicus'. Rigidity of abdominal and paraspinal muscles accompanies these changes and spasm spreads with neck retraction and opisthotonus. Recurrent spasms of muscles occur, either spontaneously or reflexly, in response to stimuli. Respiratory muscle involvement leads to periods of apnoea and cyanosis, paraspinal muscle contraction may be of such severity that vertebral or other fractures are caused. Spasm of laryngeal and pharyngeal muscle may cause choking. Without treatment, the patient's sensorium and consciousness remain intact (Weinstein 1973). Autonomic dysfunction, with sympathetic hyperactivity may follow with tachycardia, hypertension, and cardiac dysrhythmia (Kerr *et al.*, 1968; Wright *et al.*, 1989) and sudden death (Trujillo *et al.*, 1987). Provided supportive intensive care treatment is provided, improvement occurs in most patients within 4 weeks. If antitoxin is not given the disease persists for as long as tetanospasmin is produced. Patients who develop tetanus should be actively immunized against it because an adequate immune response is not always triggered by the disease as the amount of toxin produced may not be sufficient.

35.7.5 Neonatal tetanus

Neonatal tetanus follows contamination of the umbilical stump in new-borns. It occurs in populations who have not been immunized (antibodies from the mother will transfer to the baby and confer protection in early life). After 5–7 days the baby becomes weak and irritable and fails to feed. Muscle rigidity, spasms, apnoea, and cyanosis follow and the infant rapidly becomes dehydrated and hypotensive. Autonomic disturbance ensues and is often fatal. Mortality rates often exceed 50 per cent.

35.7.6 Diagnosis

The diagnosis of tetanus must rely on clinical factors because there is no specific diagnostic test which will be positive in the early stages. Unfortunately, blood tests and electromyography do not help. Strychnine poisoning is the only condition which produces similar clinical features. Adverse reactions to psychotropic drugs may produce muscular rigidity and dystonia, sometimes to the severity of opisthotonus. Meningitis will feature neck stiffness, and the stiff man syndrome is decidedly more chronic.

35.7.7 Treatment

Treatment is essentially supportive. Intensive care has greatly improved prognosis by preventing death from respiratory and cardiovascular failure (Trujillo *et al.*, 1987). The wound which has provided the portal of entry should be thoroughly cleansed and damaged tissue removed. Muscular spasms should be controlled with antispastic agents. Benzodiazepines have been used most commonly and successful results have been reported with midazolam. Baclofen has been used, both systemically and intrathecally, and dantrolene may have a place. If these measure fail to control spasms, neuromuscular blockade becomes necessary. Concurrently, the immune status of the patient should be established by estimation of serum anti-tetanus antibodies. Human tetanus immunoglobulin should be given to neutralize circulating tetanospasmin which has not yet entered the CNS. Intrathecal use of immunoglobulin has been advocated but does not seem to be more useful than systemic treatment. Active immunization should be given. Autonomic overactivity is controlled with a combination of α – and β – adrenergic blockade.

35.7.8 Complications

Complications of tetanus include hypoxia, respiratory failure, and pneumonia. Isolated neuropathies of the lower cranial nerves and of peripheral nerves may occur, and may be part of a more generalized 'critical care polyneuropathy'. Fractures of vertebrae and long bones may follow violent muscle spasm as may rhabdomyolysis in severe cases.

35.7.9 Prevention

Tetanus can be prevented if active immunization of populations at risk is undertaken. In Britain tetanus immunization is combined with diphtheria and pertussis in DTP, and dosage schedules can be found in the British National Formulary. A series of three intramuscular injections at monthly intervals during the first months of life confers immunity for some years. Booster doses are given before 5 years and on leaving school. Any person suffering a wound which may have become contaminated with spores should have a booster dose if 10 years or more have elapsed since the last immunization.

35.8 Pertussis (whooping cough)

Despite wide ranging immunization programmes, pertussis or whooping cough remains a significant infectious disease in all continents of the world, and a major cause of child mortality in the developing world where it has not been possible to mount or to maintain effective rates of immunization. In those regions of the world where immunization has been carried out for years, mortality and morbidity from pertussis dropped to very low levels, but it has not been possible to maintain this improvement. The main reason is that popular anxieties about potential side-effects of the vaccine, particularly encephalopathy, led to a drop in the take-up rate and lessening of herd immunity with a consequent rise in the number of cases. There has been a resurgence of the disease in countries such as Russia and Iraq, where war and civil insurrection have made it impossible to continue with immunization programmes. There is some evidence that immunity in adults diminishes with age and that if re-immunization is not undertaken, they can become infected and develop whooping cough. Formerly a disease of children of kindergarten or primary school age, it is being seen with greater frequency in infants who have not yet been immunized, and in young adults. Some 5 to 6,000 cases are reported annually in the United States.

Pertussis is caused by *Bordetella pertussis*. This is a small Gram–negative coccobacillus related to Haemophilus. Pertussis is transmitted by person-to-person contact and inhalation of aerosol droplets from an infected person. The respiratory tract becomes colonized and after an incubation period which can vary from one to three weeks, signs of the first stage of infection appear. There is non-specific malaise, catarrh, and a dry cough that increases in severity, associated with lacrimation, sneezing, coryza, and low fever. This is the time when patients are most infectious. After one to two weeks the distinctive paroxysmal stage follows in which the patient has severe spells of violent coughing, gagging and vomiting, severe enough to interfere with breathing and cause apnoea and cyanosis. As the spasm ends, the violent intake of air gives rise to the characteristic 'whoop' which gives the disease its name. The paroxysms of coughing are frequently repeated throughout the day and are extremely exhausting for the patient. If the patient has some immunity, the duration of this stage may only be a few days, if there is no immunity it may last for weeks. Most make a complete recovery. Complications, if they occur, do so during the paroxysmal stage and include pneumonia, subconjunctival haemorrhage, pneumothorax, and neurological problems in between one and five per cent of cases.

35.8.1 Pathophysiology

The pathophysiology of pertussis infection is complex and not yet fully understood. The organisms do not invade tissues but produce a series of powerful biologically active substances or toxins which are thought to control the virulence of the organisms and to influence the symptomatology of the illness. Included in these are pertussis toxin (lymphocytosis promoting factor), agglutinogens, filamentous haemaglutinin, pertactin and tracheal cytotoxin and endotoxin. These are variously implicated in attaching to target cells, damaging ciliated respiratory cells and tracheal cells, suppressing immune effector cells, and modification of macrophages, and promotion of lymphocytosis. They are immunologically important and recognition that they may function as protective antigens has led to their incorporation in acellular vaccines (Kerr and Matthews 2000; Hewlett 1997).

35.8.2 Diagnosis

The diagnosis of pertussis is made by culture of the organism from throat swabs, but this can be difficult and takes time. Serological tests are useful and PCR has now been used, and is both sensitive and specific (Meade and Bollen 1994). One notable feature of pertussis is the occurrence of an absolute lymphocytosis during the late catarrhal and early paroxysmal phase of the illness.

35.8.3 Complications

The neurological complications of pertussis include epileptic seizures and encephalopathy. These are found most commonly in children under the age of ten but can occur in adults (Halperin and Marrie 1991). There are no characteristic features – epileptic seizures may be generalized or focal, there may be focal neurological signs, and conscious level is depressed. The pathophysiology is multifactorial. Hypoxia may occur during paroxysms of coughing, and intracranial pressure may be forced up during the paroxysms to cause intracranial haemorrhages. Pertussis toxin and accompanying inflammatory changes may have a direct toxic effect on the CNS and this may be exacerbated by concomitant hypoglycaemia and metabolic disturbance.

35.8.4 Treatment

Treatment of pertussis with antibiotics should be carried out as soon as the diagnosis is suspected. Erythromycin is the antibiotic of choice and should be given for 14 days. An alternative is trimethoprim-sulfamethoxazole. Newer antibiotics are undergoing assessment.

35.8.5 Prevention

Immunization against pertussis is available and is effective. It is usually administered along with diphtheria and tetanus as DTP or triple vaccine. Details of immunization schedules and dosages are to be found in the British National formulary. Triple vaccine incorporates a whole cell pertussis component and adverse reactions include local pain and swelling at the injection site, pyrexia and irritability, and rarely convulsions and encephalopathy. Acellular pertussis vaccines are being developed.

In the 1970s reports appeared of presumed pertussis vaccine-associated encephalopathies and the resultant publicity led to a drastic fall off in the rate of immunization of the general population. Subsequent studies both in Britain and the United States showed that no significant statistical link could be made between whole cell pertussis vaccine and encephalopathy, neurological damage, and death. The risk of permanent brain damage in previously normal children who have been given pertussis vaccine is estimated at 1 per 310,000 immunizations which is substantially less than the incidence of encephalopathy from pertussis itself (Ad Hoc Committee 1991; Miller *et al.*, 1993; Therapeutics and Technology Assessment Subcommittee 1992).

35.9 Vaccine related encephalopathies

Certain individuals have developed neurological disorders, usually of an encephalitic or myelopathic nature, following apparent recovery from acute infections, mainly viral. Studies demonstrated that there was an immunological basis for the syndrome and the term 'post infectious encephalomyelitis' was applied. Clinically and pathologically identical syndromes were seen following immunization or vaccination and the terms 'post-vaccinial or post-immunization encephalomyelitis' were given to them. The pathological substrate common to all is acute disseminated encephalomyelitis (ADEM) in some degree and there is overlap in particularly acute cases with acute haemorrhagic leukoencephalopathy. Excellent clinical accounts are to be found in Miller and Stanton (1954) and Spillane and Wells (1964). For the purposes of this discussion, the term 'vaccine associated encephalopathy' (VAE) is used.

The original descriptions related to cases which developed following vaccination against smallpox with vaccinia virus. With the demise of smallpox in 1977 and subsequent discontinuation of vaccinia immunization, the incidence of VAE has fallen from reported figures of between 1:63 to 1:300,00 to nil. Other immunizations which have been associated with VAE and ADEM are measles, rabies, diphtheria/ tetanus toxoid, pertussis, influenza, and Japanese B encephalitis. One feature common to all of these has been the presence of brain tissue containing myelin or myelin- derived proteins. As vaccines have become modified and purified to be free of such immunogens, the incidence of VAE has diminished. It is felt that VAE resulting in ADEM is a T-cell mediated autoimmune response against myelin basic protein (Hemachudha *et al.*, 1987; Johnson *et al.*, 1984). It is not clear why some people develop VAE while the majority exposed to the same agents do not. This may relate to genetic control of the immune response.

Pathologically, the changes in the brain are of acute swelling and venous engorgement of white matter. There is perivascular oedema and mononuclear cell infiltration. Demyelination with relative axonal sparing occurs and lipid-laden macrophages are evident. Clinical features are variable, presumably in proportion to the vigour of the immune response. Days, or more usually, within two to three weeks following immunization, an encephalitic illness ensues, characterized by headache, fever, confusion, obtundation, epileptic seizures, sometimes focal neurological signs, hemiparesis, hemisensory disturbance, movement disorder, ataxia, optic neuritis, and progression to coma. There may be evidence of myelopathy. Mortality rates as high as 40 per cent have been reported; nearer 10 per cent is the norm. Significant neurological sequelae are common.

Routine blood investigations are seldom helpful. The EEG is abnormal showing diffuse slow wave activity, sometimes with localization and seizure activity, but this is quite non-specific. Brain imaging with CT, or preferably MR, demonstrate white matter changes, which may enhance, ranging from circumscribed lumps invading grey matter and sometimes occupying space, to coalescing, infiltrative regions of white matter disturbance with oedema. These lesions are often widespread and multiple (Kepes 1993; Kesselring *et al.*, 1990). CSF is usually abnormal with a rise in protein, mononuclear pleocytosis, and an increase in immunoglobulin content and myelin basic protein levels.

35.9.1 Treatment

No specific therapy is available. Supportive treatment with maintenance of vital functions, administration of anti-epileptic drugs as necessary, reduction of brain oedema with dexamethasone, osmotic agents and hyperventilation, and the management of intercurrent infection, should be given. Corticosteroids are usually given as anti-inflammatory agents but there is no good evidence that they are efficacious. It is as well to persist with aggressive therapy in apparently hopeless circumstances because, despite the high mortality and morbidity, in some the outcome may be surprisingly good. With modern acellular vaccines and vaccines free of neural proteins the risk of development of encephalopathy following immunization is in most cases virtually nil, and in all cases less than the risk of neurological complications developing from the native infection itself.

References

Ad Hoc Committee for the Child Neurology Society Consensus Statement on Pertussis Immunization and the Central Nervous System. (1991). Pertussis immunization and the Central Nervous System. *Ann. Neurol.*, **29**, 458–60.

Al-Deeb, S. M., Yaqub, B. A., Sharif, H. S. *et al.* (1989). Neurobrucellosis: clinical characteristics, diagnosis and outcome. *Neurology* **39**, 498–501.

Bahemuka, M., Shemena, A. R., and Panayiotopoulos, C. P. (1988). Neurological syndromes of brucellosis. *J. Neurol. Neurosurg. Psychiatry.*, **51**, 1017–21.

Baumgartner, J. E., Rachlin, J. R., Beckstead, J. H. *et al.* (1990). Primary central nervous system lymphomas: natural history and response to radiation therapy in 55 patients with acquired immunodeficiency syndrome. *J. Neurosurg.*, **73**, 206–11.

Berenguer, J,. Moreno, S., Laguna, F. *et al.* (1992). Tuberculous meningitis in patients infected with the human immunodeficiency virus. *N. Engl. J. Med.*, **326**, 668–72.

Berger, J. R. (1991). Neurosyphilis in human immunodeficiency virus type-1 seropositive individuals. *Arch. Neurol.*, **48**, 700–2.

Bisno, A. L. (1991). Group A streptococcal infections and acute rheumatic fever. *N. Engl. J. Med.*, **325**, 783–93.

Bolton, C. F., Young, G. B., and Zochodne, D. W. (1993). The neurological complications of sepsis. *Ann. Neurol.*, **33**, 94–100.

Brust, J. C. M., Dickenson, P. C. T., and Hughes, J. E. O. (1990). The diagnosis and treatment of cerebral mycotic aneurysm. *Ann. Neurol.*, **27**, 238–46.

Cardoso, F., Vargas, A..P, Oliveira, L. D. *et al.* (1999). Persistent Sydenham's chorea. *Mov. Disord.*, **14**, 805–7.

Castillo, M., Kwock, L., and Arbelaez, A. (1999). Sydenham's chorea: MRI and proton spectroscopy. *Neuroradiology* **41**, 943–5.

Dastur, F. D., Shahani, M. T., Dastoor, D. H. *et al.* (1977). Cephalic tetanus: demonstration of a dual lesion. *J. Neurol. Neurosurg. Psychiatry* **40**, 782–6.

DeSouza, C. E., Karnad, D. R., and Tilve, G. H. (1992). Clinical and bacteriological profile of the ear in otogenic tetanus: a case control study. *J. Laryngol. Otol.*, **106**, 1051–4.

Durack, D. T., Lukes, A. S., Bright, D. K. *et al.* (1994). New criteria for diagnosis of infective endocarditis: utilisation of specific echocardiographic findings. *Am. J. Med.*, **96**, 200–9.

Eidelman, L. A., Putterman, D., Putterman, C. *et al.* (1996). The spectrum of septic encephalopathy. Definitions, etiologies and mortalities. *J.A.M.A.*, **275**, 470–3.

Ernst, T., Chang, L., Witt, M. *et al.* (1999). Progressive multifocal leukoencephalopathy and human immunodeficiency virus-associated white matter lesions in AIDS: magnetization transfer MR imaging. *Radiology* **210**, 539–43.

Glauser, M. P., Zanetti, G., Baumgartner, J. D. *et al.* (1991). Septic shock: pathogenesis *Lancet* **338**, 732–6.

Gray, F., Gherardi, R., and Scaravilli, F. (1988). The neuropathology of the acquired immune deficiency syndrome (AIDS). *Brain* **111**, 245–66.

Halperin, S. A. and Marrie, T. J. (1991). Pertussis encephalopathy in an adult: case report and review. *Rev. Infect. Dis.*, **13**, 1043–7.

Hemachudha, T., Griffen, D. E., Giffels, J. J. *et al.* (1987). Myelin basic protein as an encephalitogen in encephalomyelitis and polyneuritis following rabies vaccination. *N. Engl. J. Med.*, **316**, 369–74.

Hewlett, E. L. (1997). Pertussis: current concepts of pathogenesis and prevention. *Pediatr. Inf. Dis. J.*, **16**, S78–84.

Hoffman, J. M. and Waskin, H. A. (1993). FDG–PET in differentiating lymphoma from nonmalignant central nervous system lesions in patients with AIDS. *J. Nucl. Med.*, **34**, 5676–5.

Holland, N. R., Power, C., Matthews, V. P. *et al.* (1994). Cytomegalovirus encephalitis in acquired immunodeficiency syndrome (AIDS). *Neurology* **44**, 507–14.

Johnson, R. T., Griffen, D. E., Hirsch, R. L. *et al.* (1984). Measles encephalitis: clinical and immunological studies. *N. Engl. J. Med.*, **310**, 137–41.

Kepes, J. J. (1993). Large focal tumor-like demyelinating lesions of the brain: intermediate entity between multiple sclerosis and acute disseminated encephalomyelitis? A study of 31 patients. *Ann. Neurol.*, **33**, 18–27.

Kerr, J. H., Corbett, J. L., Prys–Roberts, C. *et al.* (1968). Involvement of the sympathetic nervous system in tetanus. Studies in 82 cases. *Lancet* **II**, 236–41.

Kerr, J. R. and Matthews, R. C. (2000). Bordetella pertussis infection: pathogenesis, diagnosis, management and the role of protective immunity. *Eur. J. Clin. Microbiol. Infect. Dis.*, **19**, 77–88.

Kesselring, J., Miller, D. H., Robb, S. A. *et al.* (1990). Acute disseminated encephalomyelitis. MRI findings and the distinction from multiple sclerosis. *Brain* **113**, 291–302.

Larbrisseau, A., Maravi, E., and Agulera, F. (1978). The neurological complications of brucellosis. *Can. J. Neurol. Sci.*, **5**, 369–76.

Leger, J. M., Bouche, P., Bogert, F. *et al.* (1989). The spectrum of polyneuropathies in patients infected with HIV. *J. Neurol., Neurosurg., Psychiatry* **52**, 1369–74.

Lerner, P. I., and Weinstein, L. (1966). Infective endocarditis in the antibiotic era. *N. Engl. J. Med.*, **274**, 199–206, 259–66, 323–31, 388–93.

Luft, B. J., and Remington, J. S. (1992). Toxoplasmic encephalitis in AIDS. *Clin. Inf. Dis.*, **15**, 211–22.

MacMahon, E. M., Glass, J. D., and Hayward, S. D. (1991). Epstein-Barr virus in AIDS-related primary central nervous system lymphoma. *Lancet* **338**, 969–73.

Malone, J. L., Wallace, M. R., Hendrick, B. B. *et al.* (1995). Syphilis and neurosyphilis in a human immunodeficiency virus type-1 seropositive population: evidence for frequent serological relapse after therapy. *Am. J. Med.*, **99**, 55–63.

Marra, C. M., Longstreth, W. T., Maxwell, C. L. *et al.* (1996). Resolution of serum and cerebrospinal fluid abnormalities after treatment of neurosyphilis: influence of concomitant human immunodeficiency virus infection. *Sex Transm. Dis.*, **23**, 184–9.

Matar, G. M., Khnisser, I. A., Abdelnoor, A. M. (1996) Rapid laboratory confirmation of human brucellosis by PCR analysis of a target sequence on the 31-kilodalton Brucella antigen DNA. *J. Clin. Microbiol.*, **34**, 477–8.

McLean, D. R., Russell, N., Khan, M. Y. (1992). Neurobrucellosis: clinical and therapeutic features. *Clin. Infect. Dis.*, **15**, 582–90.

Meade, B. D., and Bollen, A. (1994). Recommendations for the use of the polymerase chain reaction in the diagnosis of *Bordetella pertussis* infections. *J. Med. Microbiol.*, **41**, 51–5.

Miller, D., Madge, N., Diamond, J. *et al.* (1993). Pertussis immunisation and acute serious neurological illnesses in children. *Brit. Med. J.*, **307**, 1171–6.

Miller, H. G., and Stanton, J. B. (1954). Neurological sequelae of prophylactic inoculation. *Q. J. Med.*, **23**, 1–27.

Morata, P., Queipo-Ortuna, M. I., and Reguera, J. M. (1999). Post treatment follow up of brucellosis by PCR assay. *J. Clin. Microbiol.*, **37**, 4163–6.

Olivier, C. (2000). Rheumatic fever – is it still a problem? *J. Antimicrob. Chemother.*, **45**, 13–21.

Osler, W. (1885). Gulstonian lectures on malignant endocarditis. *Lancet* **I**, 415–18, 459–64, 505–8.

Parillo, J. E. (1993). Pathogenetic mechanisms of septic shock *N. Engl. J. Med.*, **328**, 1471–7.

Peters, B. S., Winer, J., Landon, D. N. *et al.* (1993). Mitochondrial myopathy associated with chronic zidovudine therapy in AIDS. *Q. J. Med.*, **86**, 5–15.

Petito, C. K., Navia, B. A., Cgo, E. S. *et al.* (1985). Vacuolar myelopathy pathologically resembling subacute combined degeneration in patients with the acquired immunodeficiency syndrome. *N. Engl. J. Med.*, **312**, 874–9.

Porter, S. B., and Sande, M. A. (1992). Toxoplasmosis of the central nervous system in the acquired immunodeficiency syndrome. *N. Engl. J. Med.*, **327**, 1643–8.

Pruitt, A. A., Rubin, R. H., and Karchmer, A. W. (1978). Neurologic complications of bacterial endocarditis. *Medicine* **57**, 329–47.

Ruiz, A., Ganz, W. I., Post, M. J, *et al.* (1994). Use of thallium-201 brain SPECT to differentiate cerebral lymphoma from toxplasma encephalitis in AIDS patients. *Am. J. Neuroradiol.*, **15**, 1885–94.

Ryan, M. M., and Antony, J. H. (1999). Cerebral vasculitis in a case of Sydenham's chorea. *J. Child. Neurol.*, **14**, 815–18.

Salgado, A. V., Furlan, A .J., Keys, T. F. *et al.* (1989). Neurologic complications of endocarditis: A 12–year experience. *Neurology* **39**, 173–8.

Shakir, R. A., Al-Din, A. S. N., and Araj, G. F. (1987). Clinical categories of neurobrucellosis: a report of 19 cases. *Brain* **110**, 213–223.

Simpson, D. E., and Wolfe, D. E. (1991). Neuromuscular complications of HIV infection and its treatment. *AIDS* **5**, 917–26.

Simpson, D. M., and Bender, A. N. (1988). Human immunodeficiency virus-associated myopathy: analysis of eleven patients. *Ann. Neurol.*, **24**, 79–84.

Spillane, J. D., and Wells, C. E. C. (1964). The neurology of Jennerian vaccination. A clinical account of the neurological complications which occurred during the smallpox epidemic in South Wales in 1962. *Brain* **87**, 1–44.

Therapeutics and Technology Assessment Subcommittee of the American Academy of Neurology (1992). Assessment : DTP vaccination. *Neurology* **42**, 471–2.

Trujillo, M. H., Castillo, A., Espana, J. *et al.* (1987). Impact of intensive care management on the prognosis of tetanus. *Chest* **92**, 63–5.

Trujillo, M. H., Castillo, A., Espana, J. *et al.* (1987). Impact of intensive care management on the prognosis of tetanus: Analysis of 641 cases. *Chest* **92**, 63–5.

Vakil, B. J., Singhal, B. S., Pandya, S. S. *et al.* (1973). Cephalic tetanus. *Neurology* **23**, 1091–5.

Weinstein, L. (1973). Current concepts: tetanus. *N. Engl. J. Med.*, **289**, 1293–6.

Wright, D. K., Lalloo, U. G., Nayiager, S. *et al.* (1989). Autonomic nervous system dysfunction in severe tetanus: current perspectives. *Crit. Care Med.*, **17**, 370–5.

Young, E. J. (1983). Human brucellosis. *Rev. Infect. Dis.*, **5**, 821–42.

Young, G. B., Bolton, C. F., Archibald, Y. M. *et al.* (1992). The electroencephalogram in sepsis-associated encephalopathy. *J. Clin. Neurophysiol.*, **9**, 145–52.

Young, G. B., Bolton, C. F., Austin, T. W. *et al.* (1990). The encephalopathy associated with septic illness. *Clin. Invest. Med.*, **13**: 297–304.

Index

Note: The alphabetical order is letter-by-letter. Page numbers in *italic* refer to figures and/or tables separate from the main text.

mens may be needed to obtain positive findings because of the focal nature of deposits. Normal skin sites of more than 3 mm from a lesion or sites in areas not commonly involved may test negative for such IgA deposits.

IgA ANTIENDOMYSIAL (IgA-EmA), IgA ANTI-TISSUE TRANSGLUTAMINASE (IgA ANTI-tTG), IgA-RETICULIN, AND IgA-GLIADIN AUTOANTIBODIES.

Gluten sensitivity presents as celiac disease or dermatitis herpetiformis. Tissue transglutaminase has been implicated as the major autoantigen of gluten sensitive disease. Sera from patients with either form of gluten sensitive disease react with tissue transglutaminase and epidermal (type 3) transglutaminase. Antibodies in dermatitis herpetiformis patients show a markedly higher avidity for epidermal transglutaminase and these patients have an antibody population specific for this enzyme. Epidermal transglutaminase, rather than tissue transglutaminase, is the dominant autoantigen in dermatitis herpetiformis.[17]

Circulating antibodies to endomysium, tissue transglutaminase, reticulin, and gliadin occur in patients with gluten-sensitive enteropathy (i.e., dermatitis herpetiformis and celiac disease). IgA antiendomysial antibodies to the endomysium (an intermyofibrial substance) on esophageal smooth muscle are found in the serum of patients with dermatitis herpetiformis. Tissue transglutaminase (an enzyme that metabolizes gliadin) has been identified as the target antigen of anti-endomysium antibodies.[18,19] (IgA-EmA) antibodies disappear with strict adherence to a gluten-free diet and reappear when gluten is consumed. Serologic studies for the presence of IgA-EmA are highly specific and are found in approximately 70% of all patients with dermatitis herpetiformis who are not on a gluten-free diet, in almost 100% of patients with dermatitis herpetiformis and a grade 3 or 4 flattening of the intestinal mucosa, and in all untreated patients with celiac disease. The antibodies are absent in linear IgA bullous dermatosis. The titers of IgA-EmA parallel the degree of jejunal involvement. The incidence of antibody decreases to 0% when gluten is strictly avoided for 3 months. The test is especially useful for patients in whom the histologic and direct immunofluorescence studies are negative or equivocal. Reticulin antibodies occur in 36% of patients. Antigliadin antibodies are detected in two thirds of dermatitis herpetiformis patients and are not disease-specific because increased frequencies of these antibodies are also detected in patients with pemphigus and pemphigoid. Measurement of tissue transglutaminase autoantibodies may evolve as a new screening and follow-up method. Circulating IgA autoantibodies to tTG are not detectable in linear IgA disease or other subepidermal autoimmune bullous diseases. The levels of IgA anti-tTG antibodies reflect the extent of histopathologic changes of the jejunal mucosa in dermatitis herpetiformis.

TRIAL OF SULFONES.

Patients with a classic history and vesicular eruption may be given a trial of sulfone therapy if they are very uncomfortable. The dramatic relief of symptoms within hours or a few days supports the diagnosis of dermatitis herpetiformis.

Treatment

DAPSONE OR SULFAPYRIDINE. These drugs control but do not cure the disease. Dapsone is more effective than sulfapyridine. The mechanism of action is unknown but possibly is explained by lysosomal enzyme stabilization. For adults, the initial dosage of dapsone is 100 to 150 mg given orally once a day. Itching and burning are controlled in 12 to 48 hours, and new lesions gradually stop appearing. The dosage is adjusted to the lowest level that provides acceptable relief; this is usually in the range of 50 to 200 mg/day. Some patients' symptoms are controlled with 25 mg/day, whereas others may require up to 400 mg/day. Probenecid blocks the renal excretion of dapsone, and rifampin increases the rate of plasma clearance. Dapsone produces dose-related hemolysis, anemia, and methemoglobinemia somewhat in all patients. A leukocyte count and hemoglobin determination should be done weekly when possible for the first month, monthly for 6 months, and semiannually thereafter. Methemoglobinemia, although not usually a significant problem, may cause a blue-gray cyanosis. The coadministration of cimetidine is reported to reduce dapsone-dependent methemoglobinemia in dermatitis herpetiformis patients.[20] Patients with glucose-6-phosphate dehydrogenase (G6PD) deficiency may have a profound hemolysis during sulfone or sulfapyridine therapy, and those at risk of having the deficiency (African Americans, Asians, and those of Mediterranean descent) should have a G6PD level measurement before starting therapy.

Sulfapyridine, a short-acting sulfonamide (starting dosage, 500 to 1500 mg/day), can be substituted for dapsone and does not cause neuropathy. Consider sulfapyridine for patients who can not tolerate dapsone.

Sulfapyridine is difficult to obtain. Sulfasalazine (Azulfidine) is metabolized to 5-ASA (mesalamine) and sulfapyridine and may be considered if sulfapyridine can not be obtained.

Adverse reactions. Peripheral motor neuropathy may develop during the first few months of dapsone therapy. Generally, high dosages from 200 to 500 mg/day or high cumulative doses in the range of 25 to 600 gm have been implicated.[21] Typically, the distal upper and lower extremities, particularly the hand muscles, are involved. Paresthesia and weakness are the most common complaints, and atrophy of interosseus muscles is often found. Patients complain of difficulty with manual tasks and gait disturbance. Foot-drop is a common manifestation. Rarely, sensory involvement manifested by paresthesia, diminished pain, and numbness accompanies the motor disorder.[22] Symptoms slowly but invariably improve over months to years when the medication is stopped. Agranulocytosis and aplastic anemia rarely occur but have resulted in death.

Dapsone hypersensitivity syndrome. The dapsone hypersensitivity syndrome usually appears 4 weeks or longer after starting the drug. It consists of a mononucleosis like illness with fever, malaise, and lymphadenopathy. Exanthematous skin eruptions usually resolve within 2 weeks of stopping dapsone.[23] Hypersensitivity hepatitis has been reported as a component of the syndrome. Hypothyroidism may develop 3 months after the onset of DHS. Blood and liver function study results usually become normal within a few months after the patient stops taking dapsone. Prednisone is the preferred treatment. Prednisone is slowly tapered for more than 1 month while the function of affected organs is monitored to minimize recurrences. Dapsone appears to be safe during pregnancy.[24]

GLUTEN-FREE DIET. Strict adherence to a gluten-free diet (avoid foods containing wheat, rye, and barley) for at least 6 months allows most patients to begin a decrease in or possibly a discontinuation of sulfone therapy. The diet has to be followed for many months (often 2 years) before medications can be discontinued.[25] Although intestinal villous architecture improves, symptoms and lesions recur in 1 to 3 weeks if a normal diet is resumed. Current evidence indicates that a gluten-free diet needs to be continued indefinitely. Patients found to have a linear IgA immunofluorescence pattern do not have villous atrophy and do not respond to a gluten-free diet. Oats can be included in a gluten-free diet without deleterious effects to the skin or intestine.[26,27] Wheat starch–based gluten-free flour products were not harmful in the treatment of celiac disease and dermatitis herpetiformis.[28]

Products must be chosen carefully, because some so-called gluten-free foods contain high levels of gliadin, the enterotoxic agent in gluten.[29] Gluten is in all grains except rice and corn. There are many online sources of gluten-free foods such as ENER-G Foods, Inc. (www.ener-g.com), 1-800-331-5222. The Gluten Intolerance Group of North America (www.gluten.net) publishes a newsletter and offers other services.

ELEMENTAL DIET. Dietary factors other than gluten may be important in the pathogenesis of dermatitis herpetiformis. Various substances can act as antigens; if the antigens can be eliminated, no new harmful immune complexes are formed. Most antigens that lead to humoral immune responses are proteins; therefore a diet without full proteins (elemental diet) is not likely to contain major antigens. In one study, a diet of amino acids, fat, and carbohydrates produced a rapid benefit and allowed a significant reduction in the dosage of dapsone within 2 weeks.[30] A significant improvement in clinical disease activity, independent of gluten administration, and in small bowel morphology are also seen with an elemental diet.[31]

TETRACYCLINE AND NICOTINAMIDE. Successful treatment of dermatitis herpetiformis and linear IgA bullous dermatosis[32] with tetracycline (500 mg one to three times daily) or minocycline (100 mg twice daily) and nicotinamide (500 mg two or three times daily) is reported. Stopping either nicotinamide or minocycline resulted in a flare-up of the dermatitis herpetiformis. A combination of heparin, tetracycline and nicotinamide is also reported to be effective.[33]

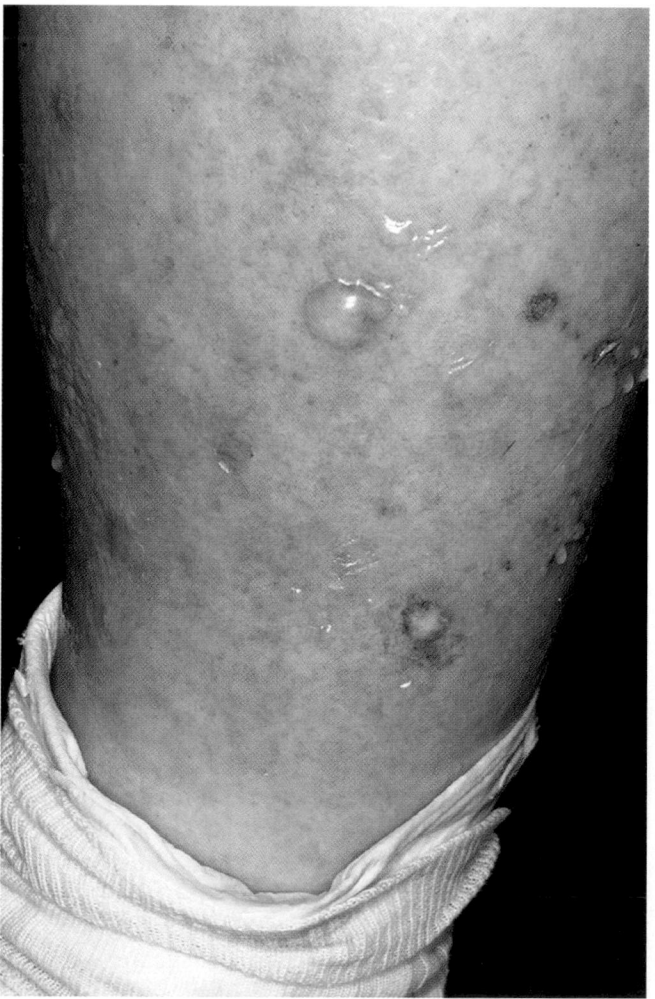

A

Bullae in Diabetic Persons

Crops of bullae may appear abruptly in diabetic persons, usually on the feet and lower legs. They usually develop overnight without preceding trauma. There is little pain or discomfort. Different epidermal split levels and subepidermal separation have been reported.[34] The bullae arise from a noninflamed base, are usually multiple, and vary in size from 1 to several cm.[35] Occasionally they are huge, involving the entire dorsum of the foot or a major portion of the lower leg (Figure 16-7). The bullae are tense and rupture in approximately 1 week, leaving a deep, painless ulcer that forms a firmly adherent crust. Even if not infected, these large ulcers take many weeks to heal. Many patients never have another episode, whereas others have recurrences.

No immunopathologic features are found. The cause is unknown, but is possibly ischemic.[36]

TREATMENT. Ulcers may be compressed several times a day with tepid Burrow's solution. The treatment of deeper erosions and ulcers is described in Chapter 3.

Pemphigus

Pemphigus (from the Greek *pemphix,* meaning bubble or blister) is a rare, group of autoimmune, intraepidermal blistering diseases involving the skin and mucous membranes.[37] The group includes pemphigus vulgaris and pemphigus foliaceus. Both were usually fatal before glucocorticoid therapy. The difference between the two disorders is the level of the epidermis at which acantholysis (loss of cohesion of epithelium) occurs: the suprabasilar level in pemphigus vulgaris and the subcorneal level in pemphigus foliaceus. Other members of the pemphigus group are paraneoplastic pemphigus, which generally occurs in patients with lymphoma, and drug-induced pemphigus, which usually develops after taking penicillamine.[38]

There are 0.1 to 0.5 cases of pemphigus per 100,000 per year. The disease is associated with HLA-DR4, DQ8 haplotypes dominantly distributed among Jewish patients and these plus DR6, DQ5 haplotypes in non-Jewish patients.[39] The mean age of onset is in the sixth decade. Lever classifies pemphigus into two categories: pemphigus vulgaris, with pemphigus vegetans considered to be a variant; and pemphigus foliaceus, with pemphigus erythematosus designating the localized disease.[40] Pemphigus is a disease that is more heard of than seen. Autoantibodies in pemphigus vulgaris attack normal proteins within the desmosomal structure that causes cell-to-cell separation.

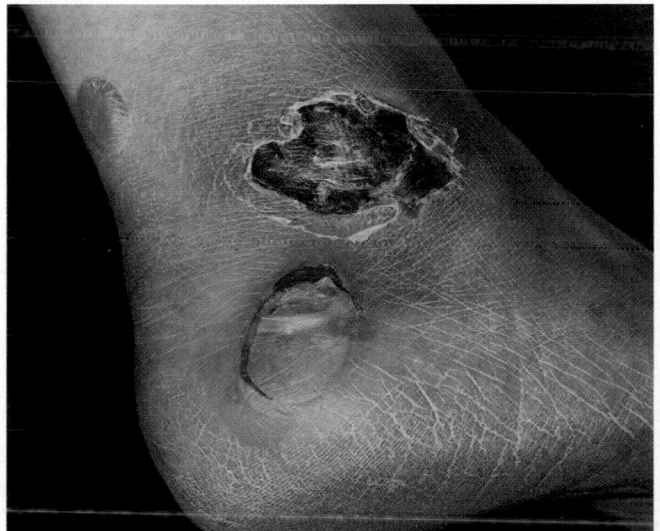

B

Figure 16-7 Bullosis diabeticorum. Blisters appear spontaneously without any trauma on nonerythematous skin. Blisters usually occur on the lower legs and feet but may occur on the arms. Blisters may be very large. There is little discomfort. Lesions heal spontaneously.

PEMPHIGUS VULGARIS

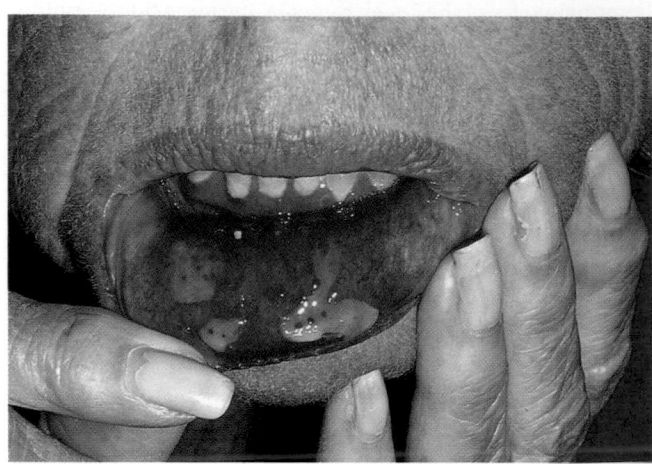

Figure 16-8 Pemphigus vulgaris presents with oral lesions in over 50% of patients. Most patients have oral lesions. Oral lesions may be the only manifestation of the disease or they may precede the onset of skin lesions by several months.

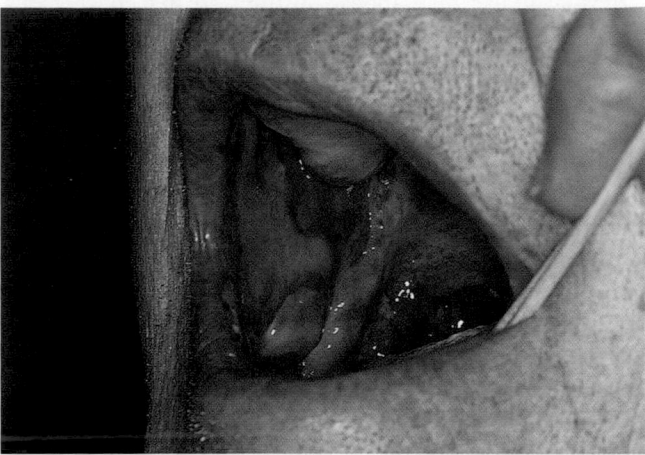

Figure 16-9 Intact bullae are rarely found in the mouth. Painful erosions are the typical finding, and they are slow to heal. Erosions are found in all areas of the oral cavity and may involve the larynx. Pain interferes with eating.

Figure 16-10 Flaccid blisters rupture easily because the roof, which consists only of a thin portion of the upper epidermis, is very fragile. Healing is with brown hyperpigmentation, but without scarring.

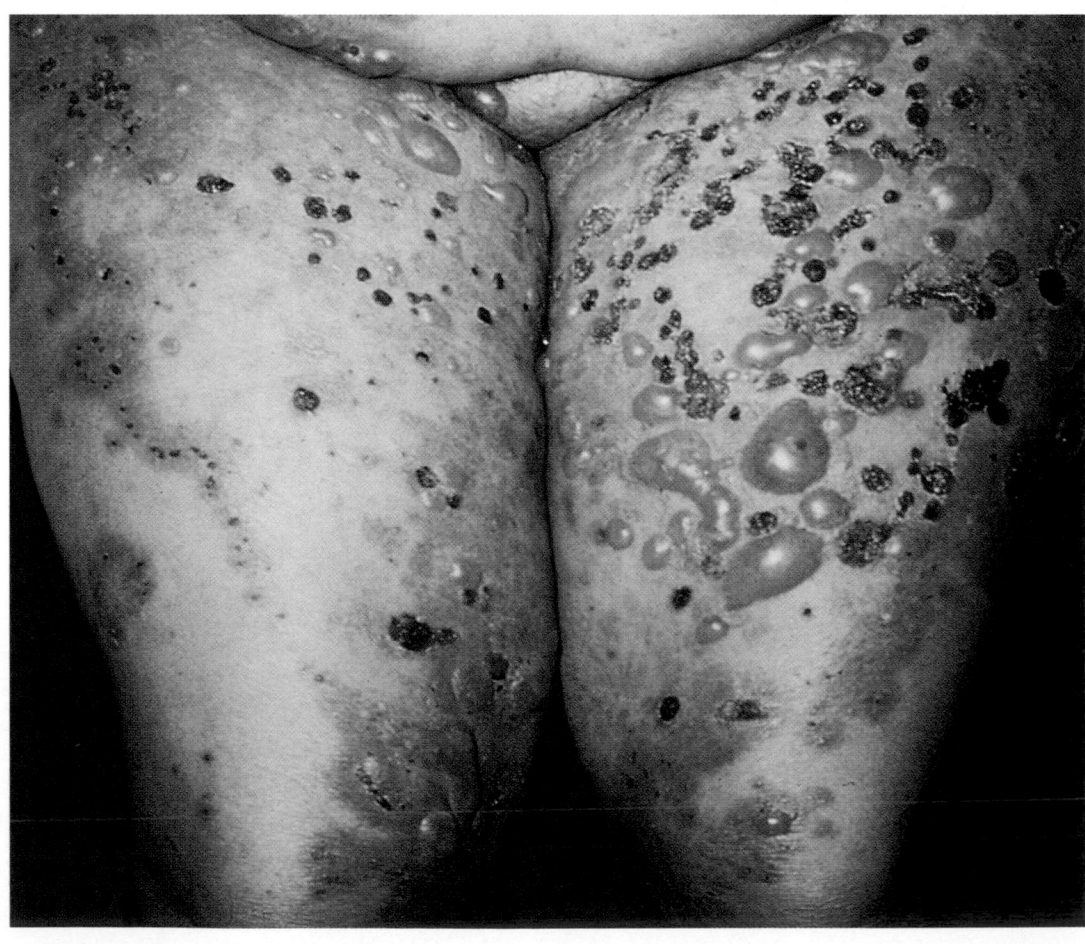

Pathophysiology

Pemphigus is the result of the interaction between genetically predisposed individuals and possibly some exogenous factor. The presence of foci of pemphigus foliaceus (fogo selvagem) in rural South America suggests that the disorder can be triggered in susceptible persons by an environmental agent (probably an unidentified infectious agent), whose antigens mimic those of desmoglein 1, and that clinical disease evolves in the persons who have the most vigorous immune response to desmoglein 1. Both idiopathic and induced pemphigus have the same human leukocyte antigen (HLA) pattern.

Desmoglein

The structural integrity of the epidermis depends on the sharing of desmosomes by neighboring keratinocytes. Desmosomal connections are broken and reform as keratinocytes migrates from the basal layer toward the skin surface. Desmoglein is a cell-to-cell adhesion molecule contained in desmosomes that contributes to the strength of the intercellular desmosomal bridge. There are three isotypes of desmoglein, Dsg1, Dsg2, and Dsg3. Dsg2 is expressed in all desmosome-possessing tissues, Dsg1 and Dsg3 are restricted to stratified squamous epithelia, where blister formation is found in patients with pemphigus.

DSG1 AND DSG3 AUTOANTIBODIES. Circulating IgG autoantibodies are directed against the normal desmoglein proteins within the desmosomal structure on the cell surface of keratinocyte. The autoantibodies destroy the adhesion between epidermal cells allowing fluid to accumulates in the gaps in the epidermis to form blisters. The target molecule of pemphigus autoantibodies is a transmembrane desmosomal component, desmoglein 3 (Dsg3) in pemphigus vulgaris (PV) and Dsg1 in pemphigus foliaceus (PF).

Patients with mucosal dominant PV are negative for anti-Dsg1 antibodies but positive for Dsg3 antibodies. Patients with mucocutaneous PV have both anti-Dsg3 and anti-Dsg1 IgG antibodies. Patients with PF have only anti-Dsg1 IgG.[41, 42]

Pemphigus vulgaris

Pemphigus vulgaris is the most common form of pemphigus.[43] Painful oral erosions usually precede the onset of skin blisters by weeks or months (Figures 16-8 and 16-9). Involvement of other mucosal surfaces occurs in patients with widespread disease. The soft palate was involved in 80% of cases at initial presentation.[44] Nonpruritic flaccid blisters varying in size from 1 to several cm appear gradually on normal or erythematous skin and may be localized for a considerable time. The most common sites are the scalp, face, axilla, and oral cavity. Blisters invariably become generalized if left untreated (Figure 16-10). The blisters rupture easily because the vesicle roof, which consists of only a thin portion of the upper epidermis, is fragile (Figure 16-11). Application of pressure to small intact bullae causes the fluid to dissect laterally into the midepidermal areas altered by bound IgG (Nikolsky's sign).

Exposed erosions last for weeks before healing with brown hyperpigmentation but without scarring. Blisters, erosions, and lines of erythema may appear in the esophageal mucosa.[45] Death formerly occurred in all cases, usually from cutaneous infection, but now occurs in only 10% of cases, usually from complications of steroid therapy. Sunlight exposure is harmful.[46]

Pemphigus vegetans is a variant of pemphigus vulgaris that presents with large verrucous confluent plaques and pustules localized to flexural areas in the axilla and groin.

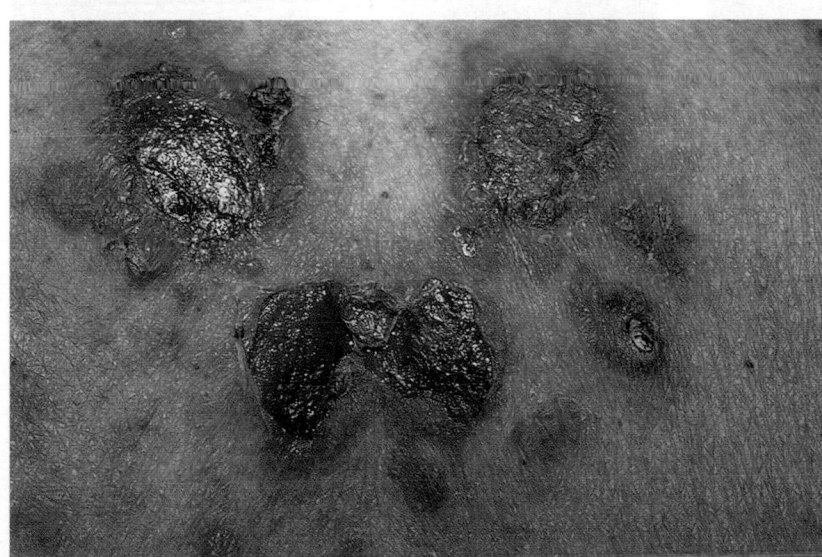

Figure 16-11 Fragile blisters rupture easily to form painful erosions. Finger pressure separates normal-appearing epidermis, producing an erosion (Nikolsky's sign). Pressure on the edge of a blister spreads the blister into unaffected skin.

Pemphigus foliaceus, IgA pemphigus, and pemphigus erythematosus

The age of onset varies more widely in pemphigus foliaceus and pemphigus erythematosus than in pemphigus vulgaris, and there is no racial prevalence. Oral lesions are rarely present. Pemphigus foliaceus begins gradually on the face (Figures 16-12 and 16-13) in a "butterfly" distribution or first appears on the scalp, chest, or upper back in a seborrheic distribution.

Pemphigus foliaceus

Pemphigus foliaceus (superficial pemphigus) presents with recurrent shallow erosions, erythema, scaling, and crusting. Small flaccid blisters may occur but they are superficial, very fragile, and rupture easily. Serum leaks out and desiccates, forming the localized or broad areas of crust (Figures 16-14 and 16-15). Intact thin-walled blisters are sometimes seen near the edge of the erosions. The site of blister formation in the horizontal plane of the stratum corneum can be demonstrated in skin biopsy specimens after the upper portion of the epidermis has been dislodged with lateral finger pressure (Nikolsky's sign). IgA pemphigus has clinical and histologic similarity to subcorneal pustular dermatosis and pemphigus foliaceus. IgA antibodies are bound to the epidermal cell surface, and half of the patients have circulating IgA anti–cell surface antibodies.[47,48]

Skin lesions of pemphigus foliaceus are generally well demarcated and do not extend into large eroded areas as those of pemphigus vulgaris. Mucous membrane involvement is uncommon. Pemphigus foliaceus may remain localized for years and it has a better prognosis than pemphigus vulgaris.

Pemphigus erythematosus

Pemphigus erythematosus, also known as Senear-Usher syndrome, may actually be a combination of localized pemphigus foliaceus and systemic lupus erythematosus (see Figure 16-12), because many of these patients have a positive antinuclear antibody. If the eruption becomes more diffuse or generalized, the term pemphigus foliaceus is used. The disease may last for years and may be fatal if not treated.

Fogo selvagem

Fogo selvagem (Portuguese for "wild fire") is an endemic form of pemphigus foliaceus found in certain rural areas of South America, including Brazil, Colombia, Bolivia, Peru, and Venezuela, as well as in Tunisia. It occurs in jungle areas but the disease disappears when the jungle is cleared. Environmental triggers such as an infectious agent have been proposed to induce Fogo selvagem. Fogo selvagem occurs in children and young adults and may affect several family members. This endemic variant is clinically indistinguishable from nonendemic pemphigus foliaceus.

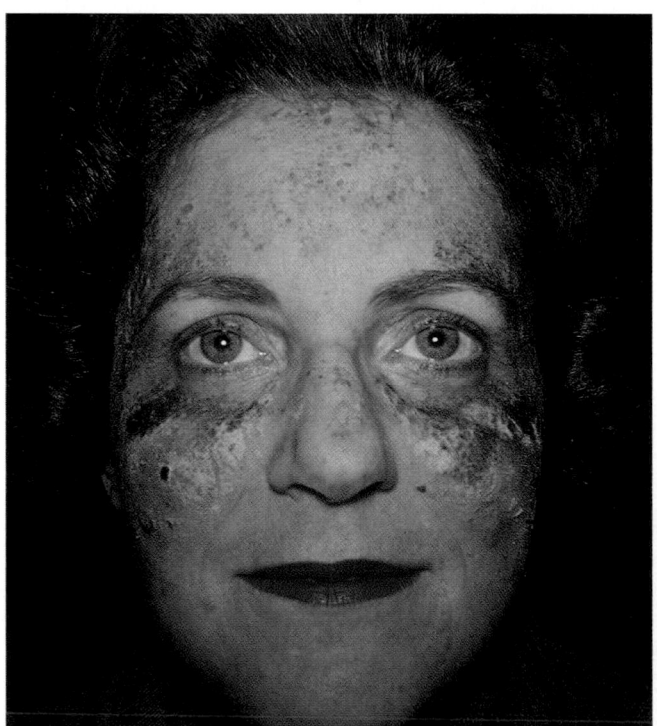

Figure 16-12 Pemphigus erythematosus. Serum and crust with occasional vesicles are present on the face in a butterfly distribution.

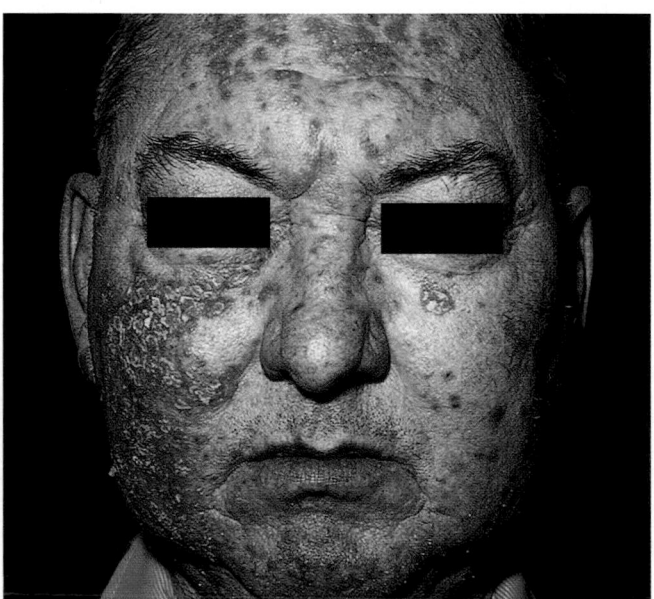

Figure 16-13 Pemphigus foliaceous. Scaly, crusted erosions appear on an erythematosus base. They may be confined to seborrheic areas on the face and trunk. The mucous membranes are usually not involved.

PEMPHIGUS FOLIACEUS

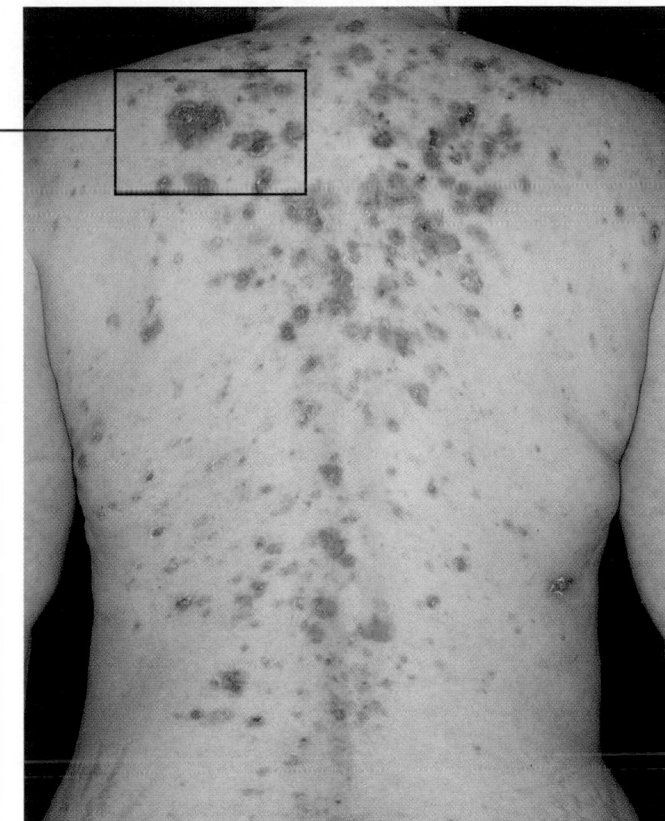

Figure 16-14 The symmetrical distribution of red, eroded, crusted lesions. Occasionally vesicles are seen at the edge of a lesion.

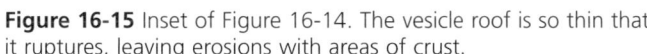

Figure 16-15 Inset of Figure 16-14. The vesicle roof is so thin that it ruptures, leaving erosions with areas of crust.

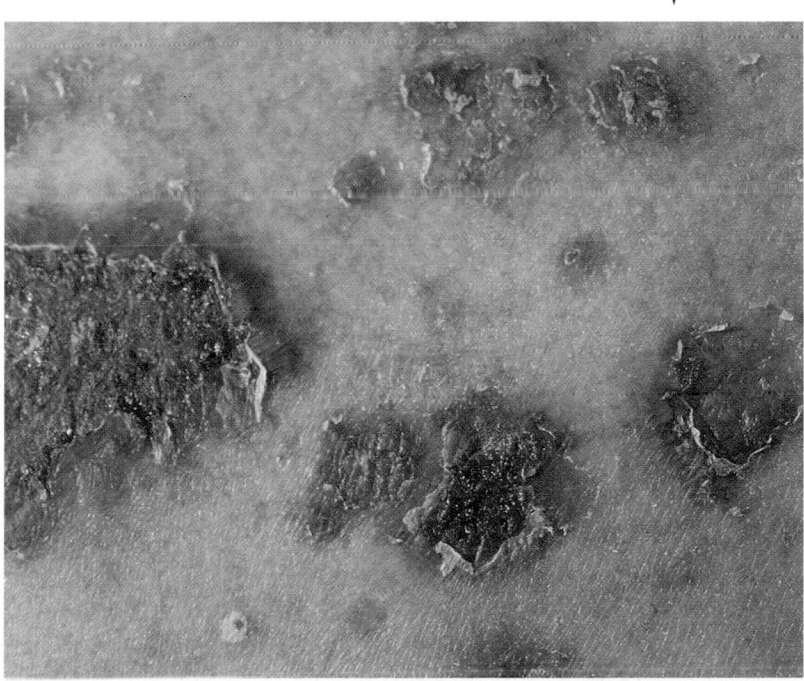

Diagnosis of pemphigus

SKIN BIOPSY FOR LIGHT MICROSCOPY. Histologic studies may yield key findings in cases that are negative by direct immunofluorescence. A small, early vesicle or skin adjacent to a blister biopsied with a 3- or 4-mm punch shows an intraepidermal bulla and acantholysis (separation of epidermal cells near the blister following dissolution of the intercellular cement substance). The basal epidermal cells become detached from each other but remain attached to the basement membrane. There is a mild-to-moderate infiltrate of eosinophils (Figures 16-16 and 16-17).

DIRECT IMMUNOFLUORESCENCE OF SKIN. Two biopsies are recommended. One biopsy specimen should be taken from the edge of a fresh lesion and the second from an adjacent normal area. Two biopsies are especially helpful in evaluation of oral lesions because lesional sites are frequently denuded. Mucosal biopsies should be taken 0.5 cm from a lesion because closer sites may be negative. Specimens are deposited in Michel's transport media available from specialized laboratories around the country. These are transported unrefrigerated. Perilesional biopsies of skin or mucous membranes usually reveal IgG, strong IgG4 and frequently C3 in the intercellular areas in patients with all clinical variants of pemphigus.

INDIRECT IMMUNOFLUORESCENCE. Serum IgG antibodies directed against the keratinocyte cell surface can be demonstrated by indirect immunofluorescent staining and are present in all forms of true pemphigus in approximately 75% of patients with active disease. Take blood in a red top tube. A combination of indirect immunofluorescence on two substrates (monkey and guinea pig esophagus) and ELISA tests for Dsg1 and Dsg3 affords the greatest sensitivity and highest level of confidence in the diagnosis of pemphigus. ELISA for Dsg1 and Dsg3 distinguishes between pemphigus vulgaris and foliaceus. Cases that have both skin and mucosal lesions have both Dsg3 and Dsg1 antibodies (Table 16-1).

In some cases, the level of circulating intercellular substance IgG antibody reflects the activity of disease, rising during periods of activity and falling or disappearing during times of remission.[49] Many patients show a poor correlation between the titer of circulating antibody and disease activity. Therefore management of pemphigus should be guided by clinical disease activity rather than by the pemphigus antibody titer. In some cases periodic serum tests to detect changes in titers are helpful in evaluating the clinical course.[50] Serum should be tested every 2 to 3 weeks until remission and every 1 to 6 months thereafter.

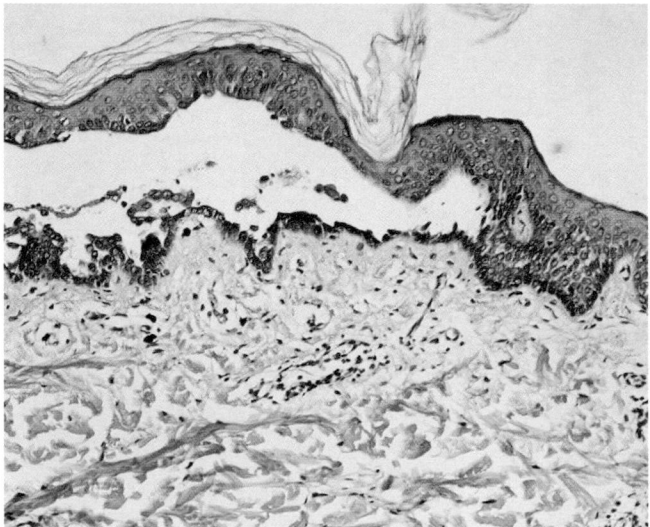

Figure 16-16 Pemphigus vulgaris. The epidermal separation occurs low in the epidermis.

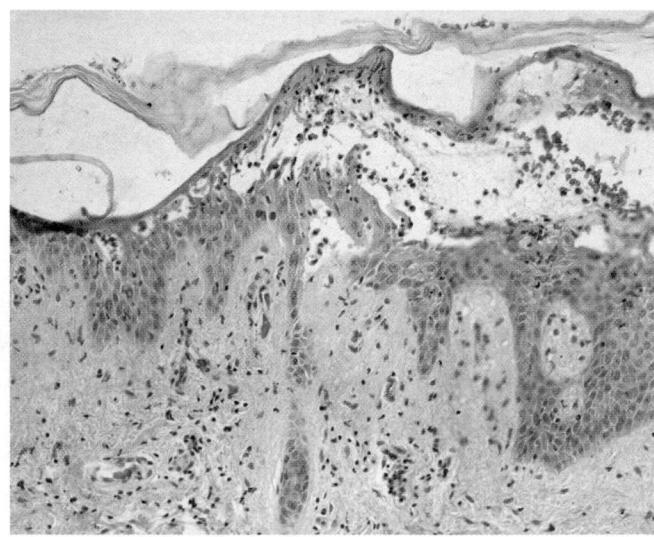

Figure 16-17 Pemphigus foliaceus. The intraepidermal spearation appears high in the epidermis.

Treatment

CORTICOSTEROIDS AND IMMUNOSUPPRESSIVE AGENTS.
Systemic glucocorticosteroids are still the mainstay of therapy. Very high-dose regimens (more than 120 mg/day)[40,51] provide no benefit over the low-dose regimens with respect to the frequency of relapse or the incidence of complications.[52]

TOPICAL STEROIDS.
Patients with mild pemphigus vulgaris or pemphigus foliaceus responded to clobetasol propionate 0.05% cream applied to mucosal lesions and involved skin twice a day for at least 15 days, then progressively tapered.[53]

ADJUVANTS.
Because of the potential toxicity of systemic corticosteroids, another drug may be initiated long term. The adjuvant therapy (corticosteroid-sparing medication) is initiated with or after starting corticosteroids. Although there are no controlled studies most experts believe that immunosuppressive agents have a steroid sparing effect. They may decrease the side effects of steroid therapy by allowing the use of lower steroid dosages and lead to increased remission rates. Others disagree and feel that the improved prognosis of pemphigus in recent years is due to the use of lower dosages of corticosteroids, and the improved treatment of corticosteroid complications. The most commonly used agents are cyclophosphamide (1.5 to 2.5 mg/kg/day),[54] and azathioprine (1.5 to 2.5 mg/kg/day).[55] Methotrexate is rarely used because of the reported high incidence of severe infections.

CYCLOPHOSPHAMIDE.
Cyclophosphamide may be the most effective drug but it is toxic. Side effects include bone marrow suppression, hemorrhagic cystitis, bladder fibrosis, reversible alopecia, and an increased risk of bladder carcinoma and lymphoma. Monitor urinalysis and blood cell counts. Encourage oral fluid intake to decrease the risk of bladder fibrosis and hemorrhagic cystitis.

AZATHIOPRINE.
Azathioprine causes bone marrow suppression, hepatotoxicity, and an increased risk of malignancy that is lower than that of cyclophosphamide. Monitoring blood cell counts and liver function tests. Detailed prescribing information for azathioprine is found on page 570.

INTRAVENOUS IMMUNOGLOBULIN.
In patients who do not respond to conventional immunosuppressants, intravenous immunoglobulin (IVIG) appears to be an effective treatment alternative. Its early use is of significant benefit in patients who may experience life-threatening complications from immunosuppression. IVIG is effective as monotherapy. Several courses of treatment may be required to obtain a durable remission.[56,57]

Many other agents have been tried alone or as adjuvants. These include chlorambucil, mycophenolate mofetil,[58,59] dapsone,[60] cyclosporine,[61,62] gold,[63] plasma exchange,[64] extracorporeal photopheresis,[65] IVIG,[66] and tetracycline 2 gm/day.[67] A large series demonstrated that combination treatment with corticosteroids and cyclosporine, 5 mg/kg, offers no advantage over treatment with corticosteroids alone in patients with pemphigus.[68]

Approach to treatment
Therapeutic choices are determined by the patient's age, degree of involvement, the rate of disease progression, and the subtype of pemphigus.[37]

PREDNISONE.
Elderly patients with mild to moderate disease can be treated with prednisone, at 40 mg/day, along with cyclophosphamide or azathioprine. Patients with more severe disease may require 60 to 80 mg/day of prednisone. The dosage of prednisone is tapered to a level that controls most disease activity. Attempts are made to use an alternate-day regimen to minimize side effects. During the prednisone taper, the immunosuppressive agent is continued at full dosage. The speed of the prednisone taper is determined by the level of disease activity. It is not necessary to have the disease totally suppressed before lowering the prednisone.

Patients who cannot take steroids may be treated with cyclophosphamide or azathioprine alone. Patients who fail to respond to corticosteroids and immunosuppressive agents can be treated with plasmapheresis, extracorporeal photophoresis or IVIG.

Many patients with pemphigus foliaceus can be treated with potent topical steroids[53] or low doses of corticosteroids. Hydroxychloroquine 200 mg twice a day was reported to be an effective adjuvant in patients with persistent and widespread pemphigus foliaceus. This was especially true when photosensitivity was present.[69] The combination of nicotinamide (1.5 gm/day) and tetracycline (2 gm/day) or minocycline (100 mg twice a day) was found to be an effective alternative to steroids in pemphigus foliaceus and a steroid-sparing adjuvant, rather than a steroid alternative for pemphigus vulgaris.[70] Dapsone may also be effective.

Sunlight exposure is harmful. Protection from sunlight should be part of the treatment.[46]

Course and remission
It is possible to eventually induce complete and durable remissions in most patients with pemphigus that permit systemic therapy to be safely discontinued without a flare in disease activity. The proportion of patients in whom this can be achieved increases steadily with time, and therapy can be discontinued in approximately 75% of patients after 10 years.[71]

DETERMINING REMISSION AND WHEN TO STOP TREATMENT.
Treatment is stopped when patients are clinically free of disease and when they have a negative finding on direct immunofluorescence. The titers of circulating antibody have a rough correlation with disease activity, but they are not accurate enough to determine when to stop therapy. A skin biopsy for direct immunofluorescence can predict when a patient is in remission and be used to predict relapse. A negative direct immunofluorescence finding suggests that there is immunologic remission and 80% of patients with a negative direct immunofluorescence study remained disease free for the next 5 years.[72]

Pemphigus in association with other diseases

Myasthenia gravis and thymoma have been reported on many occasions in association with pemphigus (usually erythematosus and vulgaris).[73] The clinical course is variable, but myasthenia gravis develops in most patients, followed by the detection of thymus disease, and finally by the appearance of pemphigus. Malignancy, usually of the lymphoid or reticuloendothelial system, occurs more frequently in patients with pemphigus than in normal persons. Paraneoplastic pemphigus is described in the following sections.

Drug-induced versus drug-triggered pemphigus

Drugs implicated in pemphigus can be divided into two main groups according to their chemical structure: those containing a sulfhydryl radical (thiol drugs or SH drugs) and nonthiol drugs. Penicillamine (a thiol drug) was the first drug re-ported to induce pemphigus (Figure 16-18). Pemphigus foliaceus has been reported in approximately 5% of patients taking 500 to 2000 mg of D-penicillamine or captopril[74] for 2 months to 4 years.[75] Most cases were mild. Patients with pemphigus induced by SH drugs (drugs containing a sulfhydryl radical, e.g., penicillamine or captopril) show spontaneous recovery in 39.4% and 52.6% of cases, respectively, once the drug is discontinued.[76,77]

Pemphigus induced by other drugs shows spontaneous recovery in only 15% of cases. This suggests that penicillamine (SH drugs) induces pemphigus, whereas other drugs only trigger the disease in patients with a predisposition.[78,79]

The pemphigus-like eruption is not always limited, and the mortality approaches 10%.[80]

The autoantibody response is similar in both spontaneous and drug-related disease. Therefore a similar molecular mechanism in the two types of pemphigus is suggested.[81,82]

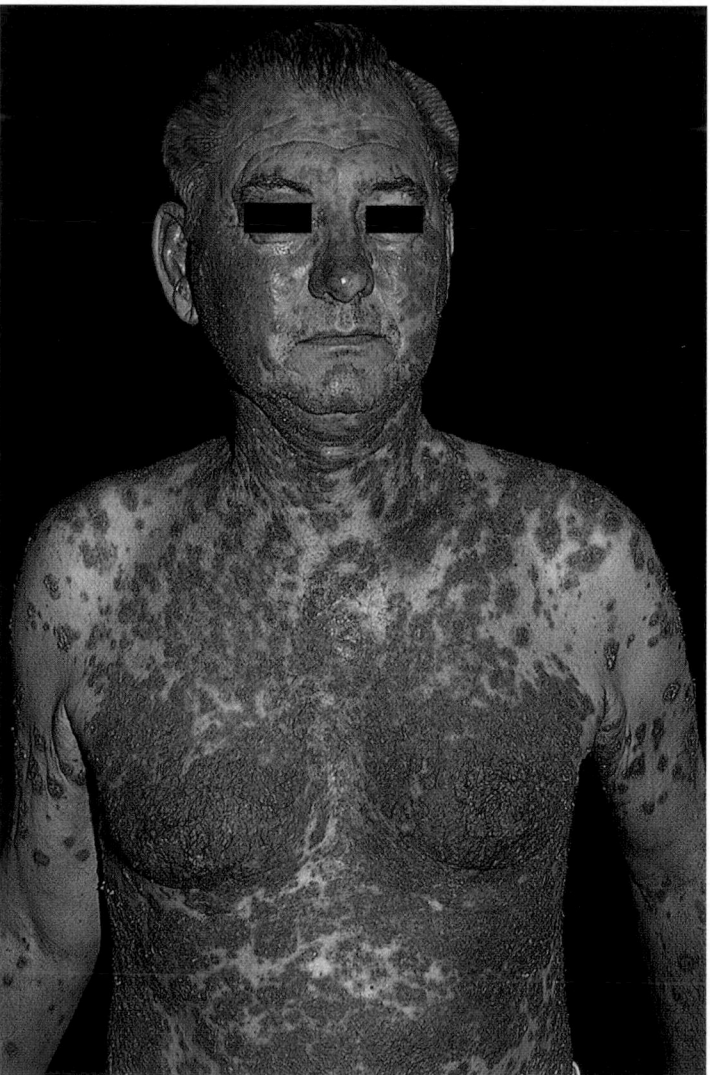

Figure 16-18 Drug-induced pemphigus (penicillamine). The eruption may not develop until months after starting the drug. Lesions produced by the thiol drugs (penicillamine) usually present as pemphigus foliaceous with scaling and crusts concentrated on the trunk. Oral lesions do not occur. Non–thiol drugs present with a pemphigus vulgaris pattern with flaccid blisters and oral erosions.

Paraneoplastic pemphigus (neoplasia-associated pemphigus)

Paraneoplastic pemphigus is an autoimmune disease that accompanies an overt or occult neoplasm and causes blisters. It has clinical and histologic features of both Stevens-Johnson syndrome and pemphigus vulgaris.[83] There are painful mucosal ulcerations, conjunctival reactions, and polymorphous skin lesions on the trunk and extremities that usually progress to blisters (Box 16-1). Antibodies against epithelial proteins are present in desmosomes and hemidesmosomes in the epidermis and respiratory epithelium. The prognosis is poor except for some patients who undergo total resection of their neoplasm. Progressive respiratory failure with clinical features of bronchiolitis obliterans is frequently the cause of death.

Neoplasia-associated pemphigus may be a more precise term for this disorder because the course of the blistering eruption does not always parallel the course of the underlying cancer.

Laboratory diagnosis of paraneoplastic pemphigus

HISTOLOGIC STUDIES. The histologic findings show features of pemphigus and erythema multiforme. There are intraepithelial clefts with epidermal acantholysis. In addition, there are dyskeratotic keratinocytes, vacuolar change of the basilar epidermis, and epidermal exocytosis of inflammatory cells.[84,85]

DIRECT IMMUNOFLUORESCENCE. Testing of mucous membrane and skin biopsies shows cell surface deposits of IgG and C3 along with granular basement membrane deposits of C3.

INDIRECT IMMUNOFLUORESCENCE. Indirect immunofluorescence with rat bladder substrate is used to differentiate PNP from classic pemphigus. Circulating IgG anti–cell-surface and anti-cytoplasmic antibodies occur in a pattern and intensity unique to these patients[86] (Table 16-4).

The Pemphigoid Group of Diseases

Bullous pemphigoid, herpes gestationis, and cicatricial pemphigoid are autoimmune subepidermal blistering diseases with circulating IgG and basement membrane zone–bound IgG antibodies and C3.[87]

Bullous pemphigoid

Bullous pemphigoid (BP) is a rare, relatively benign, autoimmune subepidermal bullous disease of the elderly. Like patients with other autoimmune diseases, they have an immune response to constituents of normal tissue. There is no racial or gender prevalence. Pemphigoid is a disease of the elderly, with most cases occurring after age 60, although cases have been reported in children. There have been many reports of the coexistence of bullous pemphigoid with other disorders, but their association is probably coincidental.[88] There is little evidence of an association of bullous pemphigoid with internal malignancy.[89-91] Drugs are often suspected of causing pemphigoid[92]; stopping medication or changing to a different oral medication may help.

Pathophysiology

BP is mediated by autoantibodies that bind to the bullous pemphigoid antigens 230 (BP230) a cytoplasmic component and 180 (BP180), a transmembrane glycoprotein component of hemidesmosomes of epidermal basal cells.[93,94] Skin-fixed and circulating IgG autoantibodies target one or both BP antigens. These IgG autoantibodies are found both circulating and bound in the lamina lucida region of the basement membrane zone (BMZ) of the epidermis. The BMZ-bound autoantibodies result in activation of complement and chemotaxis and degranulation of leukocytes. The leukocytes release proteolytic enzymes that cause basement membrane destruction, resulting in dermal-epidermal separation. The final result is a subepidermal blister.

Box 16-1 Criteria for the Diagnosis of Neoplasia-Induced Pemphigus

(A patient is considered to have neoplasia-induced pemphigus if all three major or two major and two or more minor criteria are met.)

Major criteria	Minor criteria
Polymorphous mucocutaneous eruption	Positive cytoplasmic staining of rat bladder epithelium by indirect immunofluorescence
Concurrent internal neoplasia	Intercellular and basement membrane zone immunoreactants on direct immunofluorescence of perilesional tissue
Characteristic serum immunoprecipitation findings	Acantholysis in biopsy specimen from at least one anatomic site of involvement

From Camisa C: Arch Dermatol 1993; 129:883.

CLINICAL MANIFESTATIONS. Oral blisters (24%), if present, are mild and transient. Pemphigoid begins with a localized area of erythema or with pruritic urticarial plaques that gradually become more edematous and extensive. A diagnosis of hives is frequently made in this preblistering stage. The amount of itching varies but is usually moderate to severe. A group of elderly patients had itching for a mean period of 10 months before the diagnosis was made.[95] In most cases the plaques turn dark red or cyanotic in 1 to 3 weeks, resembling erythema multiforme, as vesicles and bullae rapidly appear on their surface.

The eruption is usually generalized. The most common sites are the lower part of the abdomen, the groin, and the flexor surfaces of the arms and legs. The palms and soles are affected (Figures 16-19 and 16-20). Involvement of genital mucous membranes occurs in 7% of patients. The 1- to 7-cm bullae appear isolated or in clusters and are tense with good structural integrity, in contrast to the large, flaccid, easily ruptured bullae of pemphigus. Firm pressure on the blister will not result in extension into normal skin as occurs in pemphigus; therefore Nikolsky's sign is negative. Most bullae rupture within a week, leaving an eroded base that, unlike the situation with pemphigus, does not spread and heals rapidly.

Many localized clinical variants of bullous pemphigoid have been reported (vesicular, vegetating, hyperkeratotic, erythrodermic) that have the same histologic and immunologic characteristics as generalized bullous pemphigoid. Bullous pemphigoid may occur at sites of trauma and with little spread of the condition outside such areas.[96,97] The diagnosis is confirmed with histologic studies and direct and/or indirect immunofluorescence. See the next section on localized bullous pemphigoid.

DIFFERENTIAL DIAGNOSIS. The differential diagnosis includes epidermolysis bullosa acquisita, dermatitis herpetiformis, pemphigus, bullous systemic lupus erythematosus, and bullous drug eruptions.

COURSE AND PROGNOSIS. The course is variable. Untreated pemphigoid may remain localized and undergo spontaneous remission, or it may become generalized. Generalized BP has a poor prognosis especially in older patients and those in poor general condition. The prognosis was documented in 82 bullous pemphigoid patients treated with a variety of medications. The mortality rate at 1 year was 19%, and treatment was believed to be contributory in seven deaths.[98] The duration varied from 9 weeks to 17 years. The remission rate was 30% at 2 years and 50% at 3 years. Late re-

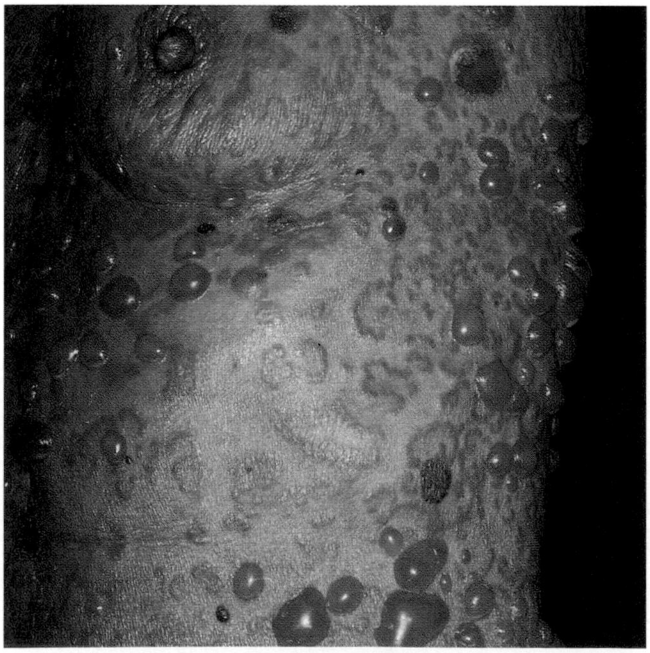

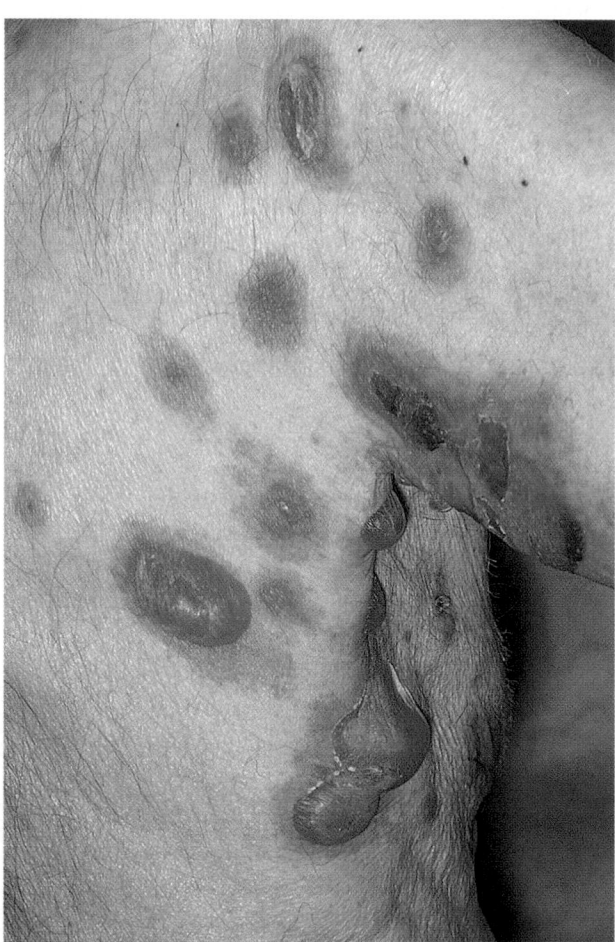

Figure 16-19 Bullous pemphigoid. Generalized eruption with tense blisters arising from an edematous, erythematous annular base.

Figure 16-20 Bullous pemphigoid. Urticarial lesions may appear weeks or months before the appearance of blisters. Bullae occur on normal-appearing and erythematous skin. They heal without scarring or milia formation.

lapse was observed after disease-free intervals of more than 5 years. Throughout this impressive disease, patients remain afebrile, relatively comfortable, and ambulatory. No clinical, immunologic, or immunogenetic factors are predictive of disease duration.[98]

Of the factors related to bullous pemphigoid activity (duration; pruritus; and number and extent of blisters, eosinophilia, and serum antibodies), only generalized pemphigoid was predictive of death in comparison with localized forms.[99] The presence of circulating autoantibodies against BP180 autoantigen but not autoantibodies against BP230 was found to be significantly more frequent (60% vs. 25%) in BP patients who died within the first year of treatment.[100] Older patients who required a higher dosage of oral glucocorticosteroids at hospital discharge and who had low serum albumin levels were at higher risk of death within the first year after hospitalization.[101]

LABORATORY. Peripheral blood eosinophilia occurs in 50% of patients, and elevated serum IgE in 85%. Remission of BP is paralleled by a decrease of serum levels of IgE and the different IgG subclasses reactive with BP180.[102]

Skin biopsy for light microscopy. There are two important features to demonstrate in biopsy specimens of bullous diseases: the level of cleft formation (i.e., intraepidermal or subepidermal) and the presence or absence of an inflammatory infiltrate, as well as the type of cell present (eosinophils or neutrophils, etc.). Bullae in pemphigoid may arise from inflamed (infiltrate-rich) or noninflamed (infiltrate-poor) skin; the most information is provided through a biopsy on an early bulla on inflamed skin. Histologically, there are subepidermal bullae with eosinophils in the dermis and bullae cavities (Figure 16-21).

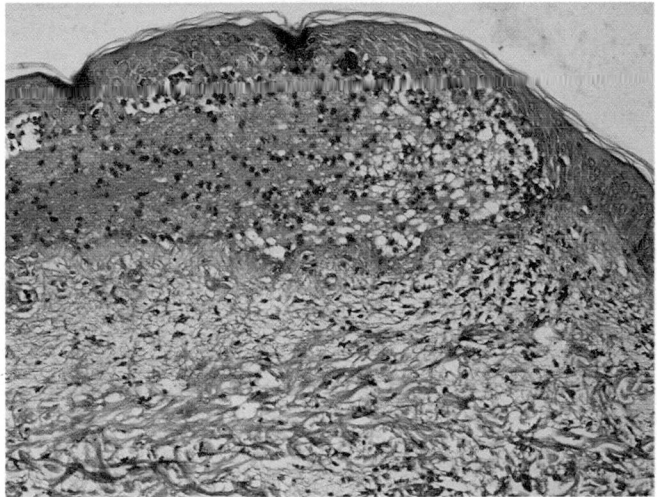

Figure 16-21 Bullous pemphigoid. A subepidermal blister contains numerous eosinophils.

Direct immunofluorescence of skin. Another 3- or 4-mm punch biopsy specimen is taken and submitted in special transport media. The highest diagnostic yield for direct immunofluorescence (DIF) comes from biopsy specimens of inflamed skin next to a blister. DIF results are positive in a high percentage of patients even after treatment is initiated. The yield is 62% from oral mucosal biopsy specimens.[103]

DIF shows IgG and/or C3 and, sometimes, IgA, IgM, and fibrin in a linear band at the BMZ. Similar findings can be observed in epidermolysis bullosa acquisita, cicatricial pemphigoid, herpes gestationis and bullous eruption of systemic lupus erythematosus. Therefore indirect immunofluorescence studies are necessary to complete the evaluation. Bullous pemphigoid and epidermolysis bullosa acquisita (EBA) are characterized by linear IgG deposits along the BMZ. Patients with EBA are more likely to have IgG staining without concomitant C3 deposition than are patients with bullous pemphigoid.[104] Biopsy specimens treated with 1 M sodium chloride separate through the lamina lucida. The IgG appears in the dermal side of the split specimens in EBA and predominantly or exclusively in the epidermal side in bullous pemphigoid. DIF studies relate to treatment responses. As the disease subsides, complement C3 deposits disappear. Normal skin of the forearm can be used for such studies.

Indirect immunofluorescence. Most cases of BP can be diagnosed with serologic studies.[105] By indirect immunofluorescence microscopy using NaCl-separated human skin, 87% of cases reveal circulating serum IgG antibodies.[94]

These antibodies detect the 230-kd major or the 160- to 180-kd minor bullous pemphigoid antigens synthesized by keratinocytes. Some BP sera recognize both antigen proteins, while others detect only BP230 or BP180 or none. Their level does not correlate with disease activity as it does in pemphigus. In sera analyzed for reactivity with BP180, autoantibodies are detected in 90% by immunoblot analysis or by ELISA. In contrast to indirect immunofluorescence reactivity that reflects reactivity to both BP180 and BP230, serum levels of autoantibodies to BP180 correlate with disease activity in BP. Therefore assaying reactivity to BP180 may be a helpful guide for disease management.[100,106,107]

Approximately 10% to 15% of patients may not have detectable circulating autoantibodies using salt-split skin indirect immunofluorescence studies; these patients should be evaluated using the salt-split skin direct immunofluorescence assay.

TREATMENT. The degree of involvement and the rate of disease progression dictate treatment.

Itching is controlled with hydroxyzine (Atarax) 10 to 50 mg every 4 hours as needed. Systemic steroids combined with immunosuppressive agents such as azathioprine, cyclophosphamide, methotrexate, or chlorambucil have been the mainstay of therapy. Antibiotics, dapsone, and topical steroids may be a safe and effective alternative for some patients. For more information, see the treatment section for cicatricial pemphigoid.

Topical steroids. A study showed that topical corticosteroid therapy is effective for limited,[108] moderate, and severe bullous pemphigoid and is superior to oral corticosteroid therapy for extensive disease. Patients received either topical clobetasol propionate cream (40 gm per day) or oral prednisone (0.5 mg per kilogram of body weight per day) for those with moderate disease, and 1 mg per kilogram per day for those with extensive disease. Disease was controlled at 3 weeks in the entire topical corticosteroid group. Severe complications occurred in 29% of the topical-corticosteroid group and in 54% in the oral-prednisone group.[109]

Antibiotics. Studies have reported an excellent clinical response when localized or generalized bullous pemphigoid was treated with tetracycline, minocycline, or erythromycin, with or without niacinamide.[99] The recommended schedules are tetracycline or erythromycin 1.0 to 2.5 gm/day, or minocycline 200 mg/day and niacinamide 1.5 to 2.5 gm/day. Patients with generalized bullous pemphigoid were treated with tetracycline (2 gm daily) without niacinamide.[110] Bulla formation was significantly reduced within 1 week and stopped within 1 to 3 weeks. The 2-gm dosage was maintained for 1 to 2 months, decreased by 500-mg decrements every month, and then stopped. These drugs may suppress the inflammatory response at the BMZ, inhibit neutrophil chemotaxis, and increase cohesion of the dermoepidermal junction. The effect may be enhanced by a synergetic effect of niacinamide.

Sulfones. The efficacy of dapsone is limited.[111] Patients who have a neutrophil-predominant infiltrate may be the best candidates for this drug. The response occurs within 2 weeks; the dosage is usually 100 mg/day of dapsone. The dosage is regulated according to the patient's response. Dapsone therapy is described in detail in the dermatitis herpetiformis treatment section earlier in this chapter.

Prednisone and immunosuppressive drugs (adjuvant therapy). The mainstay of therapy in past years has been systemic corticosteroids. Noncontrolled trials have reported the use of adjuvant therapies with steroid-sparing effects. These have included azathioprine,[112] cyclophosphamide, chlorambucil, and methotrexate. A large, randomized, multicenter, unblinded study was designed to assess the efficacy of azathioprine or plasma exchange when added to conventional dosages of prednisolone. The study demonstrated that neither azathioprine nor plasma exchange is effective enough to be used routinely as an adjuvant to corticosteroids in the management of bullous pemphigoid.[113]

Patients who do not respond to attempts to control their conditions with topical steroids, antibiotics and dapsone and require suppression may be treated with prednisone or prednisolone. Most authorities recommend an initial dosage of 0.75 to 1 mg/kg per day in two daily doses. Most patients are controlled in 28 days and the dosage can be gradually tapered. The schedule used in one study was to taper to a daily dose of 0.5 mg/kg at 3 months and 0.2 mg/kg at 6 months.[113]

The time required for resolution with prednisone depends on the number of blisters on day 1.[114] The addition of dapsone to the existing regimen of corticosteroids may help to produce a clinical remission, to lower the dosage of prednisone, and to taper off prednisone more easily.[115]

Consider adjuvant immunosuppressive therapy with azathioprine if dapsone and prednisone fail. As the disease comes under control the prednisone therapy is tapered to every other day and then stopped. Azathioprine is continued for another 3 to 6 months and stopped when the disease has cleared. Cyclophosphamide is also used as a steroid sparring drug. It is more toxic than azathioprine and is reserved for elderly patients who have extensive disease who do not tolerate azathioprine

Ultraviolet light and scratching may induce bullae and should be avoided.[116] One should consider stopping or changing oral medications that are sometimes suspected of causing pemphigoid.

Azathioprine. Azathioprine as a single agent may be considered for older patients with more significant disease who do not respond to dapsone or antibiotics and who do not tolerate prednisone. Younger patients are usually not treated with azathioprine because of the increase risk of malignant neoplasms. Patients respond within 3 to 6 months of treatment. Treatment may then be stopped and restarted with disease flares.

The risk of azathioprine-induced myelosuppression can be predicted by detecting patients with intermediate or low thiopurine methyltransferase (TPMT) activity.

TPMT levels are evaluated to ensure the patient receives adequate levels of azathioprine. Korman recommends the following guidelines for azathioprine regimens.[117] Patients who are homozygous for the low TPMT allele (TPMT level, <5.0 U/mL of red blood cells; 0.3% of whites) should not receive azathioprine because they have a high likelihood of developing pancytopenia. Patients with intermediate TPMT activity (11% of whites) with levels of 5.0 to 13.7 U/mL should receive approximately 0.5 mg/kg of azathioprine and patients with TPMT levels of 13.7 to 19.0 U/mL should receive approximately 1.5 mg/kg of azathioprine. Patients with TPMT levels of 19.0 (89% of whites) should receive 2.5 mg/kg of azathioprine.[118]

Methotrexate. Low-dose oral pulse methotrexate may be an effective alternative in patients with generalized bullous pemphigoid. Oral methotrexate, at an initial dosage of 5 mg/wk and increased by 2.5 mg/wk to a maximum of 12.5 mg/wk was given to elderly patients with generalized bullous pemphigoid who were not responding to potent topical steroids. The disease was controlled in the majority of patients with 5 to 7.5 mg of methotrexate per week.[119]

OTHER TREATMENTS. Cyclosporine, chlorambucil, mycophenolate mofetil,[120] plasmapheresis, intravenous immunoglobulins[121] have all been used in patients with severe progressive disease.

Localized pemphigoid

Cicatricial pemphigoid (mucosal surfaces), localized childhood vulvar pemphigoid, pretibial pemphigoid[122] (nonscarring bullous lesions predominantly on the legs of women), localized chronic pemphigoid of Brunsting-Perry[123] (crops of grouped blisters on the head and neck that heal with atrophic scars), dyshidrosiform pemphigoid[124] (vesiculobullous hemorrhagic lesions of the palms and soles), and pemphigoid vegetans (erosive and vegetating plaques)[125] are variants of localized pemphigoid. These patients possess the same circulating IgG autoantibodies as patients with generalized bullous pemphigoid.[126] Direct immunofluorescence is, however, a less useful diagnostic test in localized bullous pemphigoid; the intensity of the reaction correlates roughly with extent of disease.[127]

MUCOUS MEMBRANE PEMPHIGOID. Cicatricial pemphigoid, or mucous membrane pemphigoid (MMP), is a rare, chronic, subepidermal blistering and scarring disease.[128,129] It is characterized by the production of autoantibodies against basement membrane zone antigens (lamina lucida proteins involved in human keratinocyte adhesion to extracellular matrix). MMP affects persons older than 40 years of age and has a 2:1 predilection for women.

The oral cavity and the eye are most frequently involved.[130] Unlike bullous pemphigoid, there are few remissions.

Oral disease. The mouth is involved in 85% of cases. Desquamative gingivitis is the most frequent manifestation. The gingiva appears red with diffuse or patchy involvement (Figure 16-22). Oral vesiculobullous lesions form, then rupture, leaving clean, noninflamed erosions that are relatively painless and do not interfere with eating. The vermilion border of the lips is spared, in contrast to the situation with pemphigus. Hoarseness is a sign of laryngeal involvement (8% of cases). A subset of patients have only oral disease which has a relatively benign course compared with patients with oral cavity and other mucosae and skin involvement.[131]

Ocular disease. The eye is involved in 65% of cases. Unilateral conjunctivitis is often the initial presentation; within 2 years the disease is usually bilateral. Fibrosis beneath the conjunctival epithelium is the primary destructive process. Gradual shrinkage of the conjunctiva leads to obliteration of the conjunctival sac (Figure 16-23). Reduced tearing with erosion and neovascularization of the cornea leads to corneal opacification and perforation. Fibrous conjunctival adhesions become more numerous; the disease leads to blindness in approximately 20% of cases. Prolonged periods of remission after stopping therapy occur in one third of patients. Follow-up must be continued for life, because relapse occurs in 22% of those who were in remission and not undergoing therapy.[132]

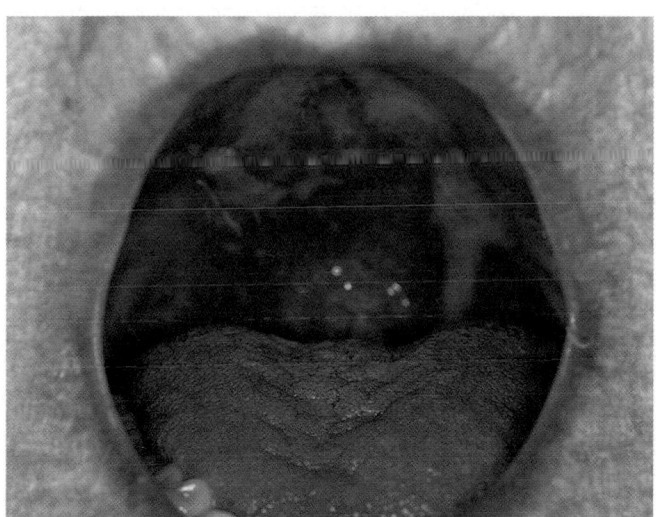

Figure 16-22 Cicatricial pemphigoid. Recurrent, painful erosions occur in the mouth. Scarring may lead to esophageal stenosis.

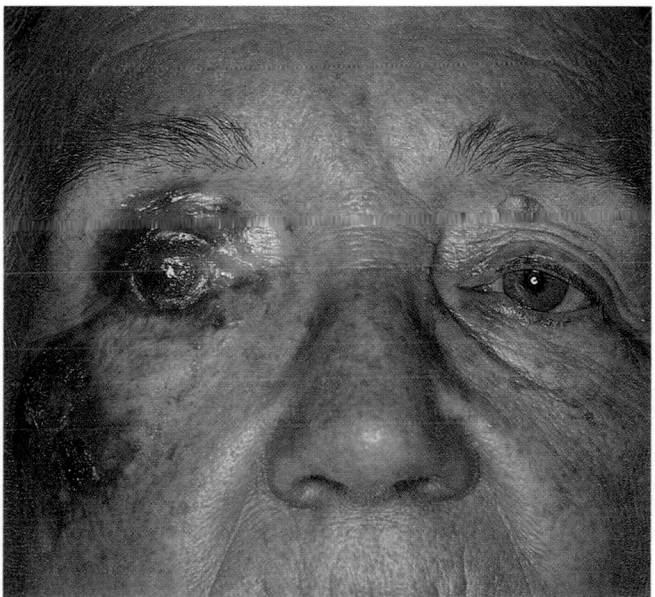

Figure 16-23 Cicatricial pemphigoid. Patients with ocular involvement present with pain, conjunctivitis, and conjunctival erosions, which leads to development of entropion and many other ocular changes, including opacification and blindness.

Skin disease. Cutaneous lesions develop in approximately 25% of patients that consist of scattered tense vesicles or bullae that arise from a red base, usually on the face, neck, and scalp. Vesicles rupture and leave an erosion that eventually heals with or without atrophic scars. Fibrous adhesions and atrophy can occur on the penis, vulva, vagina (17% of cases), and anus. When there is involvement of the head and neck but not the mucous membrane, the disease is known as the Brunsting-Perry type of cicatricial pemphigoid.

DIAGNOSIS. The biopsy shows a subepidermal bulla with little inflammation. Direct immunofluorescence of lesional, perilesional, and normal mucous membrane biopsy specimens shows linear deposition of complement and IgG and, less often, IgA. Circulating IgG and IgA antibodies are found in 10% of cases with routine techniques and up to 82% when salt-split human skin is used as a substrate. The autoantibodies bind to the epidermal roof in most cases.[133]

TREATMENT. Patients with MMP are treated like those with bullous pemphigoid (see the treatment section for bullous pemphigoid). Treatment is guided by the extent of disease and the site of involvement. Ocular, laryngeal, esophageal, and genital involvement are treated aggressively.

Plan of therapy. Treat localized disease with topical therapy and use intralesional steroids if that fails. Start dapsone if topical therapy is ineffective. Patients not responsive to dapsone after 12 weeks are treated with prednisone with or without dapsone. Immunosuppressive agents and prednisone are used if dapsone fails.[134] Cyclophosphamide is tried first; azathioprine is the alternate choice. The response is slow. The skin and oral lesions respond more quickly and predictably than the eye lesions. Most patients require long-term suppression. Taper and withdraw drugs when a remission is achieved.

Topical therapy

ORAL CAVITY. Debride dead tissue from the oral mucosa. Hydrogen peroxide, elixir of dexamethasone, and elixir of diphenhydramine are each diluted with tap water to a concentration of 1:4 or 1:6, as tolerated.[135] They are not swallowed. Before meals patients rinse with hydrogen peroxide and diphenhydramine (reduces pain, does not suppress taste completely as does viscous lidocaine). After meals patients rinse with hydrogen peroxide to remove food particles and debris, then with dexamethasone for its antiinflammatory effect. Between meals and before bedtime, patients rinse with hydrogen peroxide, then with dexamethasone. This schedule is demanding but effective. Treat oral lesions with fluocinonide gel, which is more adherent and results in better patient compliance than triamcinolone acetonide in Orabase. Food can be puréed in a blender if eating is painful.

EYES. Lubricate frequently with artificial tears and ointments. Infection of the lids is treated with topical or systemic antibiotics. Topical steroids are not effective.

Intralesional therapy. Lesions of the skin, oral cavity, nose, genitalia, and anus respond to intralesional steroids. Inject high in the dermis to avoid atrophy. Use triamcinolone acetonide (dilution of 5 to 10 mg/mL); repeat every 2 to 4 weeks.

Systemic therapy

DAPSONE. Dapsone (75 to 200 mg/day) is the drug of first choice; it controls the inflammation[136] in most patients and achieves a remission in others.[137]

CORTICOSTEROIDS. Prednisone (0.75 to 1 mg/kg per day) is used. The initial dose depends on the severity of the disease. A twice-daily dosage is used during the acute stage and changed to single daily morning dose after new blister formation stops. Taper dosage slowly to avoid a relapse.

IMMUNOSUPPRESSIVE AGENTS (ADJUVANT THERAPY). Immunosuppressive agents have a corticosteroid-sparing effect. They are started when corticosteroids are initiated or shortly afterward. Cyclophosphamide (1.5 to 2.5 mg/kg/day) is superior to azathioprine but is more toxic. Azathioprine is the alternate choice. A significant response requires 8 to 12 weeks.

ANTIBIOTICS. Infections of the mucous membranes and skin are treated with systemic antibiotics (e.g., doxycycline 200 mg/day).

Surgical therapy. Surgery to deal with scarring and to prevent blindness, upper airway stenosis, or esophageal stricture is performed after disease activity has stopped.

LOCALIZED VULVAR PEMPHIGOID. Childhood localized vulvar pemphigoid is a morphologic variant of bullous pemphigoid.[138,139] Patients present with recurrent vulvar vesicles and ulcers. Scarring may or may not occur. As with generalized pemphigoid, direct immunofluorescence shows linear IgG and C3 at the basement membrane, and indirect immunofluorescence is positive in some cases. Lesions may be treated with a group III through V topical steroid. Oral erythromycin may be effective, as is reported for generalized pemphigoid. Periodic outbreaks have been reported to occur for 3 years. Cases have been misdiagnosed as child abuse.[140,141]

Benign chronic bullous dermatosis of childhood

Chronic bullous dermatosis of childhood is a rare, nonhereditary, subepidermal blistering disease with clinical features similar to those of bullous pemphigoid and dermatitis herpetiformis except that there is only moderate itching.[142] Large, tense subepidermal bullae appear in clusters on the face (particularly around the mouth), lower trunk, inner thighs, and genitalia. A significant number of patients have linear IgA deposits at the BMZ, circulating IgA anti-BMZ antibodies,[143] and normal jejunal biopsy results.[144,145] The prognosis is good: the disease eventually clears after remissions and exacerbations, and always before puberty. Corticosteroids are used only if dapsone fails.

Herpes gestationis (pemphigoid gestationis)

Herpes gestationis (HG), an intensely pruritic, blistering disease of pregnancy, occurs in fewer than 1 in 50,000 pregnancies.[146] There is a genetic predisposition; 90% of patients express class II antigens (HLA-DR3 and HLA-DR4) and a class III antigen (C4).[147] HG appears to be mediated by an Ig-G1 specific for a 180-kd component of hemidesmosomes. The disease may appear for the first time during any pregnancy, but once it has occurred, it tends to reappear earlier and be more severe during any subsequent pregnancy. The disorder usually appears during the second or third trimester but may occur from the second week to the early postpartum period. It disappears 1 or 2 months after delivery and recurs with subsequent pregnancies. The newborn fetus has cutaneous involvement 10% of the time. HG is associated with an increase in prematurity.[148]

CLINICAL PRESENTATION. The intensity of disease varies. HG may be subclinical or mild and nonvesicular during one pregnancy, and explosive and vesiculobullous during another.[149] Edematous plaques occur in crops on the abdomen and extremities and coalesce into bizarre polycyclic rings covering wide areas of the skin (Figure 16-24). As with pemphigoid, within days to weeks the tense blisters evolve from the edematous plaques, rupture to leave slowly healing denuded areas, and heal without scarring; they do cause postinflammatory hyperpigmentation. Spontaneous clearing may be seen during the latter period of the pregnancy, but flares are seen at the time of delivery in 75% to 80% of cases. Mild recurrences may occur with menstruation and the use of oral contraceptives. Mucous membrane involvement is rare.

DIAGNOSIS. Biopsy specimens taken from inflamed skin adjacent to a blister exhibit histologic features similar to those of pemphigoid. A bandlike deposit of C3 in most cases and IgG in 10% of cases can be demonstrated at the BMZ by direct immunofluorescence. Circulating IgG (the so-called herpes gestationis factor) is difficult to find with conventional indirect immunofluorescence techniques. The herpes gestationis factor avidly fixes complement. Therefore a special technique, complement immunofluorescence, which requires a fresh source of complement, is most successful. The herpes gestationis factor can pass through the placenta and may be responsible for the transient pemphigoid-like skin lesions present in some newborns of affected mothers.[150] Peripheral eosinophilia is the only other common laboratory abnormality.

TREATMENT. Mild cases of pemphigoid gestationis may respond to topical corticosteroid therapy with or without orally administered antihistamines Most patients require prednisone (0.5 to 1.0 mg/kg per day) in divided doses.[151] There appears to be no difference in the frequency of uncomplicated live births in patients with pemphigoid gestationis treated with systemic glucocorticoids versus those treated with topical agents. If systemic glucocorticoids are administered during pregnancy, newborns are at risk for development of reversible adrenal insufficiency. As with pemphigoid, the dosage is adjusted to disease response.

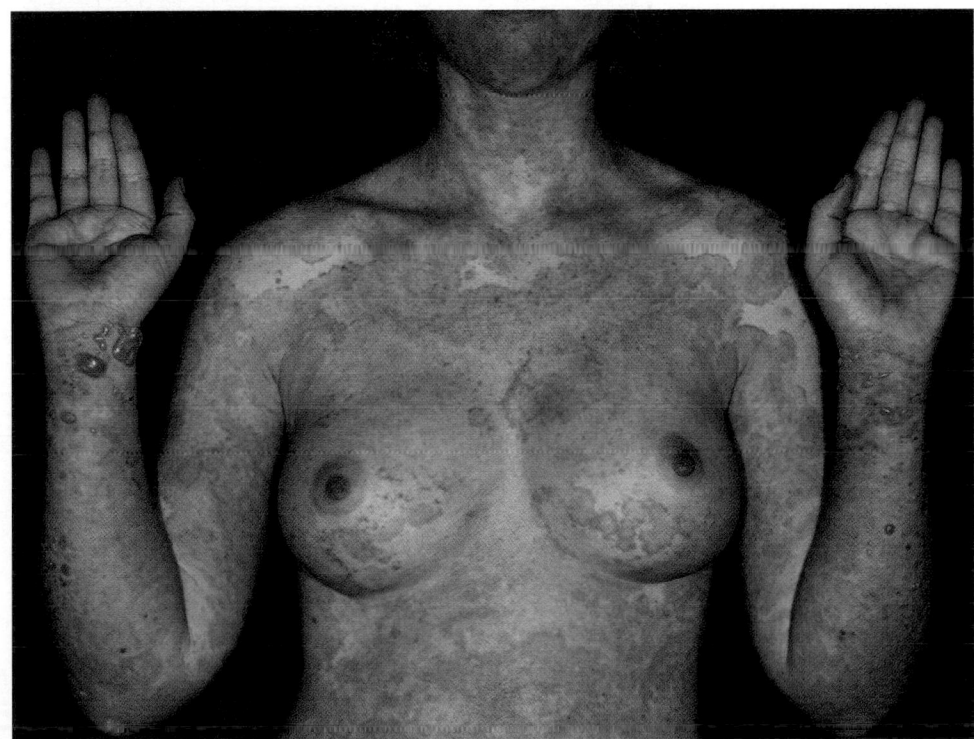

Figure 16-24 Herpes gestationis. Blisters arise from erythematous, edematous polycyclic rings.

Pemphigoid-like Disease

Epidermolysis bullosa acquisita

Epidermolysis bullosa acquisita (EBA) is a rare, chronic, subepidermal, mucocutaneous blistering disease characterized by skin fragility and spontaneous, as well as trauma-induced, blisters that heal with scar formation and milia.

The clinical and histologic picture may mimic bullous or cicatricial pemphigoid and bullous systemic lupus erythematosus. It is characterized by a chronic course, poor response to therapy, and occasional remissions. It is seen in children[152] and adults. There are two distinctive clinical presentations that are not mutually exclusive.[153] Diagnosis requires immunofluorescence studies of serum and biopsy specimens.

TYPE VII COLLAGEN. EBA is associated with autoimmunity to type VII collagen. Type VII collagen (the protein component of anchoring fibrils that fortify the attachment of the epidermis to the dermis) is the target molecule in EBA. Autoantibodies interfere with type VII collagen function and are believed to play an important role in the pathogenesis of sub-lamina densa blister formation in this disease.

CLASSIC EPIDERMOLYSIS BULLOSA ACQUISITA. The classical or mechanobullous form of EBA is characterized by skin fragility, trauma-induced blisters and erosions with mild mucous membrane involvement and healing with dense scars. It resembles the dystrophic forms of inherited epidermolysis bullosa. Classic EBA presents with tense blisters on a noninflammatory base. They appear in trauma-prone areas of the palms, soles, elbows, and knees. The lesions heal with scarring and milia formation that resembles porphyria cutanea tarda (Figure 16-25). Some of these patients may have a scarring alopecia and nail dystrophy.

EBA may extensively (or predominantly) affect mucosal epithelia in a manner resembling cicatricial pemphigoid.[154] Ocular involvement is common, but visual loss is rare.

BULLOUS PEMPHIGOID-LIKE EPIDERMOLYSIS BULLOSA ACQUISITA. Approximately 50% of patients with EBA present this type of clinical picture early in the course of their disease. Tense blisters on an inflammatory base are widely distributed on the trunk and flexural surfaces. There is pruritus, minimal skin fragility, and healing of some of the lesions without scarring and milia.

DIAGNOSIS. Special immunofluorescence tests are required to differentiate EBA from bullous pemphigoid (see Table 16-5). Direct immunofluorescence of perilesional skin shows linear and homogeneous deposits of IgG and C3[155] in the BMZ, bullous pemphigoid shows the same picture. These two diseases can be distinguished by studies of serum tested by indirect immunofluorescence on salt-split normal skin or by obtaining a fresh perilesional skin biopsy, inducing a split at the lamina lucida, and testing for the site of IgG deposition by direct immunofluorescence. Deposition of IgG on the dermal side of the separation differentiates EBA from bullous pemphigoid, which shows IgG on the epidermal side of the separation.[156,157] Indirect immunofluorescence studies of serum with 1 mol/L NaCl-separated human skin shows IgG anti-BMZ autoantibody (antitype VII collagen antibodies) bound to the dermal side of the separation.

TREATMENT. Most patients respond poorly to topical and systemic therapy. Some patients respond to high-dose prednisone therapy. Colchicine (0.6 to 1.5 mg a day for up to 4 years),[158] cyclosporine (6 mg/kg/day),[159] and high-dose[160] or low-dose intravenous immunoglobulins[161] may be effective.[162,163]

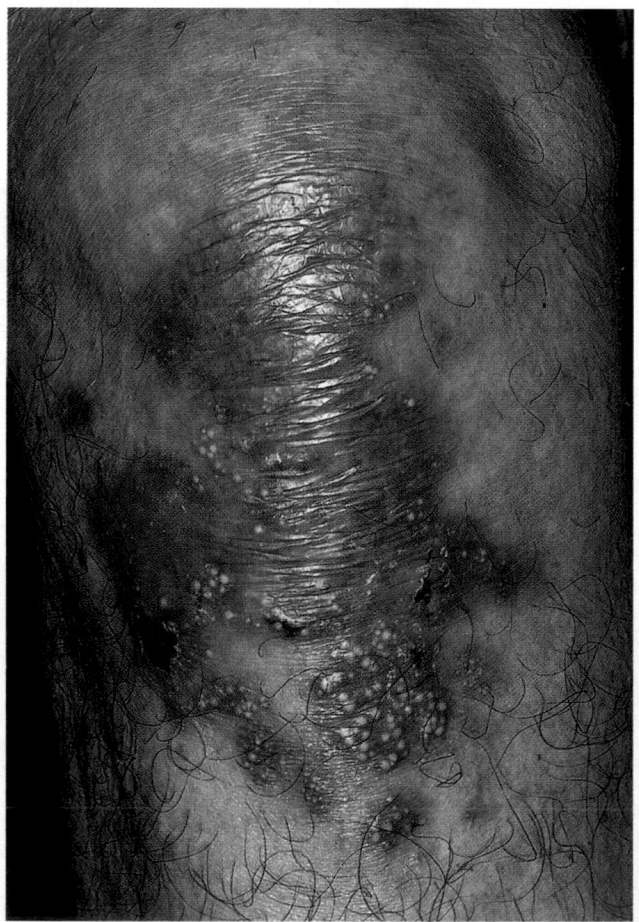

Figure 16-25 Epidermolysis bullosa acquisita. There are several forms of the disease. The mildly inflammatory form is the most common and presents with vesicles and bullae on the extensor surfaces of the hands, elbows, and knees. This form resembles the dominantly inherited form of epidermolysis bullosa dystrophica and heals with scar and milia formation.

Benign Familial Chronic Pemphigus

Benign familial chronic pemphigus (Hailey-Hailey disease) is a rare, autosomal dominant, intraepidermal, nonscarring bullous disease characterized by erosions, blisters, and warty papules.[164] The disease first appears in adolescence or early adult life, usually during the summer; it is characterized by remissions and exacerbations. Lesions develop on areas exposed to ultraviolet light (nape of the neck and back) and on areas subjected to friction and maceration (axillae and groin) (Figure 16-26). Friction, heat, and sweating exacerbate the lesions, and pain may limit physical activities. Infection with staphylococci, herpes simplex virus,[165] or *Candida* may also precipitate the disease. Longitudinal white bands are present in the fingernails in 71% of patients.[166] Suction tests on clinically normal skin demonstrated a widespread subclinical abnormality in keratinocyte adhesion.[167] An ultraviolet provocation test has been used to identify genetic carriers of Hailey-Hailey disease.[168]

NONINTERTRIGINOUS LESIONS. The eruption begins with a group of pruritic vesicles arising from a red or noninflamed base; they are grouped in an annular or serpiginous pattern. The vesicles rupture quickly and are replaced by an advancing rim of scale and crust similar to that seen in impetigo and tinea. The active border extends peripherally, leaving a pale, hypopigmented center. New crops of vesicles appear on the border but rupture so quickly that they may not be appreciated. These moist, indurated plaques ooze serum. Lesions may heal spontaneously in colder weather.

INTERTRIGINOUS LESIONS. Vesicles sometimes appear in intertriginous lesions, but most often the patient has broad, moist, red, fissured areas or vegetating warty papules and plaques that do not extend beyond the opposing skin surfaces of the groin or axillae.[169] Intertriginous lesions are chronic and respond slowly to therapy, especially in obese patients.

TREATMENT

Nonintertriginous lesions. Oral antibiotic therapy (e.g., erythromycin, dicloxacillin, or a cephalosporin) should be started, followed in 3 or 4 days by administration of a group III through V topical steroid. Most lesions of the back and neck respond quickly to this simple program, and treatment is stopped when the lesions have healed. Sunscreens should be worn on exposed surfaces in the summer.

Intertriginous lesions. Groin and axillary lesions may be infected with bacteria and yeast. Therapy with one of the above oral antibiotics is started, and antiyeast creams (e.g., ketoconazole) are applied. Cream is applied to moist lesions and compressed with cool Burow's or silver nitrate solution. Compressing is discontinued once the surfaces are dry, and group V topical steroid creams are applied twice a day until lesions have healed.[166] Chronic and unresponsive lesions have been treated successfully by excision, topical cyclosporine,[170] carbon dioxide laser,[171,172] split-thickness skin grafting,[173] and dermabrasion.[174]

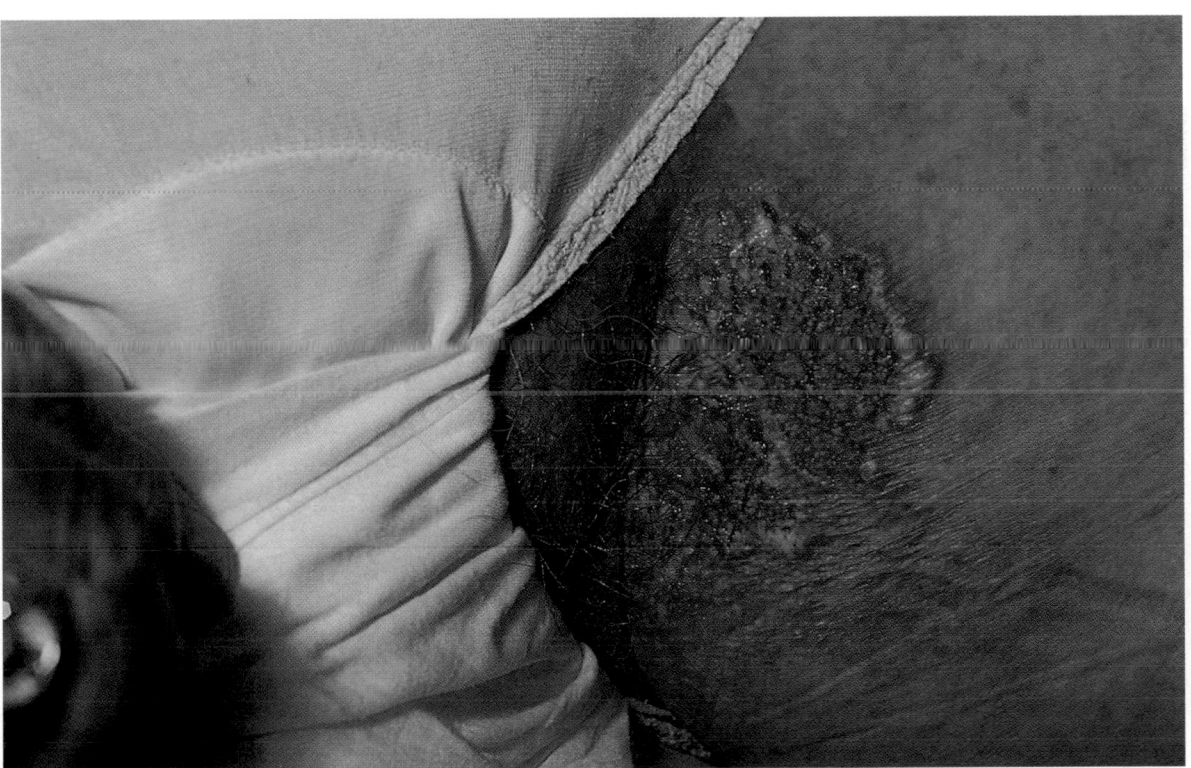

Figure 16-26 Benign familial chronic pemphigus. Erythematous annular plaques with vesicles and scale near the advancing border.

Epidermolysis Bullosa

Epidermolysis bullosa is a term given to three major groups and approximately 16 variants of rare dominant and recessive genetic diseases in which minor trauma causes noninflammatory blistering (mechanobullous diseases).[175] These diseases are classified as scarring or nonscarring and histologically by the level of blister formation.

The National Epidermolysis Bullosa Registry assists patients and physicians in determining what form of epidermolysis they have and advises them on treatment, medical management, and genetic counseling. Approximately 50 epidermolysis cases occur per 1 million live births in the United States. Of these cases, approximately 92% are epidermolysis bullosa simplex, 5% are dystrophic epidermolysis bullosa, and 1% are junctional epidermolysis bullosa.

CLINICAL CLASSIFICATION (SCARRING VS. NONSCARRING). The clinical classification is based on the presence or absence of dystrophic changes and scarring. The intraepidermal forms (epidermolysis bullosa simplex) do not scar. Junctional forms (junctional epidermolysis bullosa) manifest as atrophy. Dermal forms (dystrophic epidermolysis) result in atrophy and scarring.

HISTOLOGIC CLASSIFICATION (LEVEL OF BLISTER FORMATION). Classification is based on light and electron microscopic levels of separation:

Split-through epidermal basal cells—intraepidermal types
Split-through basement membrane area—junctional types
Split-through upper dermis—dermal forms

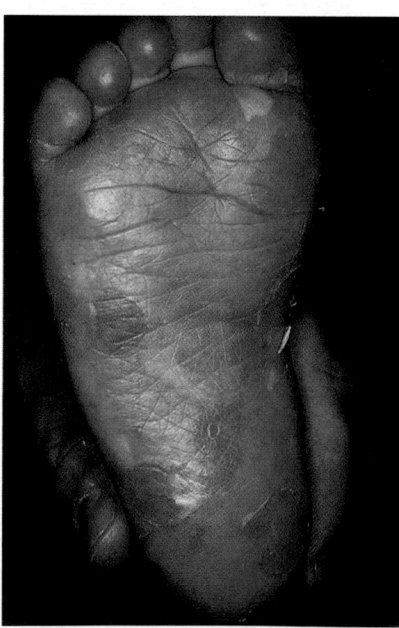

Figure 16-27 Epidermolysis bullosa simplex. Fragility of the skin results in non-scarring blisters caused by little or no trauma. There are several subtypes. Mild blistering of the hands and feet is called Weber-Cockayne disease. The inheritance is autosomal dominant.

Epidermolysis bullosa simplex. The disease is autosomal dominant. Sporadic cases may arise by new mutation. Blistering begins in infancy or childhood, especially on the hands and feet or any other point of trauma, and heals without scarring (Figure 16-27). The major complication is infection.

Junctional epidermolysis bullosa. The disease is autosomal recessive. In most cases severe generalized blistering of the skin with the exception of the palms and soles begins in infancy. There is no scarring. Extensive involvement of the mouth, larynx, eyes, and esophagus is often present. The dentition may become defective. Most patients die in early childhood.

Dystrophic epidermolysis bullosa. The disease may be either autosomal dominant or autosomal recessive. There is great variation in the severity of the several forms of dystrophic epidermolysis bullosa. The severe, recessive form exhibits repeated cycles of blistering and scarring that lead to fusion of the digits, producing the so-called mitten deformity (Figure 16-28).

DIAGNOSIS. Electron microscopic examination of the skin is the standard for diagnosis. Monoclonal antibodies have recently been used for diagnosis. Immunofluorescence tests for localization of type IV collagen, laminin, and pemphigoid antibodies in the roof or floor of bullae help differentiate the forms of epidermolysis bullosa.

MANAGEMENT. Patients must avoid trauma. Dilantin, a known collagenase inhibitor, is not an effective treatment for recessive dystrophic epidermolysis bullosa. Genetic counseling is essential, and fetal skin biopsy techniques have been developed for prenatal diagnosis. Additional information can be obtained from the Dystrophic Epidermolysis Bullosa Research Foundation, 141 Fifth Avenue, Suite 7-S, New York, NY 10010; 1-212-693-6610.

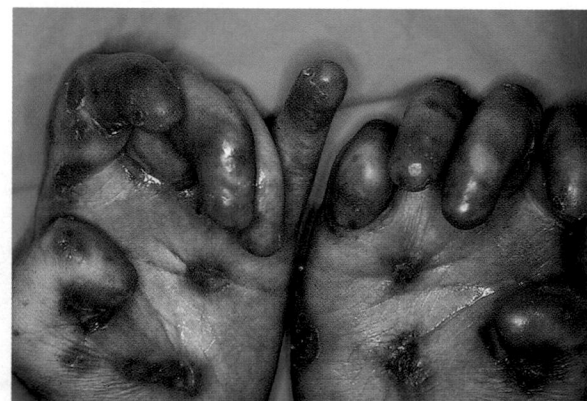

Figure 16-28 Dystrophic epidermolysis bullosa is characterized by blistering in response to the slightest trauma. Repetitive trauma leads to a mitten-like deformity with digits encased in an epidermal "cocoon."

The Newborn with Blisters, Pustules, Erosions, and Ulcerations

There are more than 30 diseases in the newborn that can present with blisters, pustules, erosions, and ulcerations (Boxes 16-2 to 16-4). For diagnostic purposes they are divided into infectious causes, common transient skin lesions, and uncommon and rare causes (Table 16-6). The most common transient diseases are described below. A complete list is presented in the boxes below. The following laboratory tests may be helpful: bacterial, viral, or fungal cultures; Gram stain; Wright's stain; Tzanck smears; potassium hydroxide (KOH) preparations; and skin biopsies.

DIAGNOSIS. The diagnosis is usually based on clinical findings. The Tzanck smear should be the first test performed. It detects herpes infection (multinucleated giant cells) and noninfectious pustular eruptions (eosinophils, neutrophils).[176,177] Gram stain and potassium hydroxide preparation detect bacterial and fungal infections.

The main benign transient neonatal types of pustulosis are erythema toxicum neonatorum, transient neonatal pustular melanosis, and neonatal acne.

Text continued on p. 582.

Box 16-2 Conditions Where Pustules or Vesicles Predominate

Common causes

Erythema toxicum neonatorum

Miliaria

Neonatal acne

Neonatal candidiasis

Neonatal pustular melanosis

Staphylococcal pyoderma

Uncommon causes

Acropustulosis of infancy

Congenital candidiasis

Herpes simplex

Incontinentia pigmenti

Scabies

Rare causes

Acrodermatitis enteropathica

Congenital self-healing histiocytosis

Cytomegalovirus

Eosinophilic pustular folliculitis

Hyperimmunoglobulin E syndrome

Listeria monocytogenes

Neonatal Behçet's disease

Varicella

From Frieden IJ: Curr Probl Dermatol 1992; 4:123.

Box 16-3 Conditions Where Bullae May Predominate

Common causes

Bullous impetigo

Sucking blisters

Uncommon causes

Epidermolysis bullosa

Staphylococcal scalded skin syndrome

Rare causes

Acrodermatitis enteropathica

Aplasia cutis congenita

Chronic bullous dermatosis of childhood

Congenital protein C or S deficiency

Congenital syphilis

Diffuse cutaneous mastocytosis

Ectodermal dysplasias

Epidermolytic hyperkeratosis

Erythropoietic porphyria

Maternal bullous disease

Neonatal varicella

Perinatal gangrene of the buttock

Pseudomonal infection

Toxic epidermal necrolysis

From Frieden IJ: Curr Probl Dermatol 1992; 4:123.

Box 16-4 Conditions Where Erosions or Ulcerations May Predominate

Common causes

Skin changes due to perinatal or neonatal trauma

Sucking blisters

Uncommon causes

Aplasia cutis congenita

Epidermolysis bullosa

Herpes simplex, especially congenital

Staphylococcal scalded skin syndrome

Rare causes

Aspergillus infection

Congenital erosive and vesicular dermatosis

Congenital protein C deficiency

Ectodermal dysplasias

Group B streptococcal infection

Hemangiomas and vascular malformations

Intrauterine varicella infection

Neonatal Behçet's disease

Neonatal lupus erythematosus

Pseudomonas aeruginosa (ecthyma gangrenosum)

Perinatal gangrene of the buttock

Toxic epidermal necrolysis

From Frieden IJ: Curr Probl Dermatol 1992; 4:123.

Table 16-6 Differential Diagnosis: Blisters and Pustules in the Newborn

Disease	Usual age	Skin: morphology
Infectious causes		
Staphylococcal pyoderma	Few days to weeks	Pustules, bullae, occasional vesicles
Staphylococcal scalded skin syndrome	3-7 d; occasionally older	Erythema, cutaneous tenderness, superficial blisters, erosions
Group A streptococcal disease	Few days to weeks	Isolated pustules, honey-crusted areas
Group B streptococcal disease	At birth or first few days	Vesicles, bullae, erosions, honey-crusted lesions
Listeria monocytogenes	Usually at birth	Hemorrhagic pustules and petechiae
Haemophilus influenzae	Birth or first few days	Vesicles and crusted areas
Pseudomonas aeruginosa	Days to weeks	Erythema, pustules, hemorrhagic bullae, necrotic ulcerations
Congenital syphilis	Usually at birth	Blisters or erosions on dusky or hemorrhagic base
Congenital candidiasis	At birth or first week	Erythema and fine papules evolve into vesicles and pustules
Neonatal candidiasis	Weeks to months	Scaly red patches with satellite papules and pustules
Aspergillus	5 d +	Morphology: pustules rapidly evolve to other ulcers
Neonatal herpes simplex	Usual: 5-14 d	Vesicles, crusts, erosions may be grouped or not. May follow dermatome
Intrauterine herpes simplex	At birth	Vesicles, widespread bullae, erosions, scars, missing skin
Fetal varicella infection	At birth	Usually scarring, limb hypoplasia, erosions
Neonatal Varicella	0-14 d	Vesicles on an erythematous base; may be very numerous
Scabies	3-4 weeks or later	Papules, nodules, crusted area
Transient skin lesions		
Erythema toxicum neonatorum	Usually 24-48 h	Erythematous macules, papules, and pustules
Neonatal pustular melanosis	At birth	Pustules without erythema; hyperpigmented macules; some have collarette of scale
Miliaria crystallina	Usually first week of life	Dewdrop-like vesicles, very superficial, no erythema
Miliaria rubra	Days to weeks	Erythematous papules with superimposed pustules
Sucking blisters	At birth	Flaccid bulla or bullae on nonerythematous base
Neonatal acne	3-4 weeks	Comedones, papules, pustules
Skin changes of perinatal/neonatal trauma	Birth to few days	Erosions on scalp, perineal or scalp gangrene (rare)
Uncommon and rare causes		
Perinatal gangrene of the buttock	First few hours to days of life	Erythema or blanching, then localized gangrene, hemorrhagic bulla
Acropustulosis of infancy	Birth or first days or weeks	Vesicles and pustules

From Frieden IJ: Curr Probl Dermatol 1992; 4:123.

CNS, Central nervous system.

Skin: usual distribution	Clinical: other	Diagnosis/findings
Mainly diaper area, periumbilical	Boys more than girls; may be in epidemic setting	Gram stain: polymorphonuclear neutrophilic leukocytes, gram + cocci in clusters. Bacterial culture
Generalized, begins on the face; blistering and erosions in areas of mechanical stress	Irritability, fever	Skin biopsy: separation upper epidermis. Bacterial cultures: blood, urine, etc.
No specific area predisposed	Moist umbilical stump; occasional cellulitis, meningitis, pneumonia	Gram stain: gram + cocci in chains. Bacterial l cuture
No specific area predisposed	Pneumonia, bacteremia	Gram stain: gram + cocci chains. Bacterial culture
Generalized, especially trunk and extremities	Septic; respiratory distress; maternal	Gram stain: gram + rods. Bacterial culture
No specific area predisposed	Bacteremia, meningitis may be present	Gram stain: small gram-bacilli. Bacterial culture
Any area; may concentrate in diaper area	Prematurity, history of surgery, GI or pulmonary anomalies are risk factors	Skin or tissue Gram stain: gram-negative rods. Cultures of skin, blood, etc.
Palms, soles, knees, abdomen	Low birth weight, hepatosplenomegaly, metaphyseal dystrophy	Dark field of involved skin. Incompletely treated maternal syphilis
Any part of body; palms and soles often involved	Prematurity, foreign body in cervix or uterus are risk factors	KOH: hyphae, budding yeast
Diaper area or intertriginous areas	Usually none; previous antibiotic prescribed	KOH: hyphae, budding yeast
Any area	Extreme prematurity/ immunocompromised host	Skin biopsy: septate hyphae. Tissue fungal culture
Anywhere; scalp monitor site, torso, oral lesions are most frequent sites	Signs of sepsis; irritability and lethargy; eye, CNS are frequent sites of disease	Tzanck, viral culture
Anywhere on body	Low birth weight; microcephaly, chorioretinitis	Tzanck, viral culture
Anywhere; usually extremities	Maternal varicella first trimester	Tzanck, viral culture
Generalized distribution	Maternal varicella 7 d before to 2 d after delivery	Tzanck, viral culture
Generalized, palms, soles	Others in family with itching or rash	Scabies prep: mites (eggs, feces)
Buttocks, torso, proximal extremities. No palms, soles	Usually term infants over 2500 gm	Wright's stain: eosinophils
Anywhere; most common on forehead, behind ears, neck, back, fingers, toes	Term infants; more common in black infants	Wright's stain: PMNs, occasional eosinophils
Forehead, upper trunk, volar forearms most common sites	May be history of warm incubator, occlusive clothing, dressings	Usually clinical; Wright's Gram stain negative
Same as miliaria crystalline	Same as miliaria crystalline	Usually clinical; skin biopsy if doubt
Radial forearm, wrist, hand, dorsal, thumb, index finger	Infants sucks vigorously on affected areas	Clinical diagnosis
Mainly cheeks, forehead	Comedones clue to diagnosis	Clinical diagnosis
Scalp, perineum, heels	History fetal monitoring, vacuum extraction, neonatal intensive care	Usually clinical diagnosis
Buttock, perineal area; unilateral	Variable history, umbilical artery catheterization	Clinical diagnosis
Hands and feet, especially medial	Severe pruritus; lesions come in crops on palms and soles	Clinical. Skin biopsy: intraepidermal pustule

Continued

Table 16-6 Differential Diagnosis: Blisters and Pustules in the Newborn—cont'd

Disease	Usual age	Skin: morphology
Congenital self-healing histiocytosis	Usually at birth	Erythematous papules, pustules, vesicles, crusting
Diffuse cutaneous mastocytosis	Birth, first weeks of life	Bullae, infiltrated skin, hives, dermographism
Maternal bullous disease	At birth	Tense or flaccid bullae or erosions
Neonatal lupus erythematosus	Birth, first few days	Erosions, other scaly or atrophic plaques
Neonatal Behçet's disease	Congenital or first few days	Mucous membrane erosions, pustules, and necrotic ulcers
Chronic bullous dermatosis of childhood	One congenital case	Tense blisters, often grouped with rosettes, sausage-shaped
Toxic epidermal necrolysis	Birth to few weeks of age	Diffuse skin erythema, tenderness, erosions
Erosive and vesicular dermatosis	Birth	Vesicles and erosions
Hemangiomas and vascular malformations	Birth or first few weeks	Ulcerations overlie macular erythema or obvious vascular anomaly
Eosinophilic pustular folliculitis	Birth or later	Multiple pustules, crusted area
Acrodermatitis enteropathica	Weeks to months	Sharply demarcated psoriasiform plaques, sometimes vesicles and bullae
Epidermolysis bullosa	Birth, rarely later	Bullae or erosions, milla nail dystrophy in dystrophic EB, occasional aplasia cutis
Epidermolytic hyperkeratosis	Birth	Bullae, erosions, ichthyotic areas of skin
Incontinentia pigmenti	Birth or first weeks	Linear streaks of erythematous papules and vesicles
Hyperimmunoglobulin E syndrome	Days to weeks	Multiple vesicles, grouped and individual
Aplasia cutis congenital	Birth	One or multiple membrane-covered, depressed areas of skin or raw, ulcerated areas
Ectodermal dysplasias (ED)	Congenital or early infancy	Vesicles or bullae
Erythropoietic porphyria	Early infancy	Vesicles or bullae
Protein C or S deficiency	Birth or first days of life	Hemorrhagic bullae and cutaneous infarctions

From Frieden IJ: Curr Probl Dermatol 1992; 4:123.

CNS, Central nervous system.

Skin: Usual distribution	Clinical: other	Diagnosis/findings
Generalized distribution	Check lymph nodes, liver, spleen, blood, bones	Skin biopsy: large histiocytes
Generalized distribution, bleeding, diatheses	Wheezing, diarrhea	Skin biopsy: infiltrate of mast cells
Generalized distribution	Maternal history of blistering disease	Maternal history, direct immunofluorescence
Face, upper torso	Occasional pancytopenia; heart block	Skin biopsy: epidermal atrophy and vascular interface dermatitis; positive maternal neonatal serology (anti-SSA, SSB)
Oral, genital mucosa; extremities, especially periungual	Maternal history of Behçet's disease	Circulating immune complexes; elevated IgG, decreased total hemolytic complement
Generalized; may concentrate in perineum	Neonatal case: severe eye involvement, milia	Skin biopsy: subepidermal bulla direct immunofluorescence: linear IgA
Generalized distribution	Graft-vs.-host disease Klebsiella sepsis, etc	Skin biopsy: full-thickness necrosis
Generalized, over 75% of body	? infection or placental infarctions	? Clinical
Ear, lip, perineum, extremities	Contiguous vascular anomaly usually evident	Clinical
Scalp, hands, feet	Frequent eosinophilia	Skin biopsy: folliculitis with eosinophils
Periorificial and acral	Diarrhea, irritability, alopecia, history of hyperalimentation	Serum zinc level less than 50
Anywhere, especially extremities, mucosa	Other epithelial tissues, that is, GI, genitourinary, cornea, trachea, may be affected	Skin biopsy for electron microscopy or immunofluorescence mapping
Generalized; blisters more on hands and feet	Family history may be positive	Skin biopsy: big keratohyaline granules
Generalized following Blaschko's lines	Family history may be positive; eye, CNS, and other abnormalities	Skin biopsy: eosinophilic spongiosis and dyskeratosis
Generalized distribution	Recurrent S. aureus infection, eosinophilia	? Clinical (IgE not high in newborn period)
Usually scalp, may be elsewhere	May be associated with epidermal nevus, placental infarctions, etc.	Clinical or skin biopsy
Depends on specific kind; acral in some; Blaschko's lines in Goltz syndrome	Sweating, limb, oral abnormalities, vary with specific kind of ED	Usually clinical diagnosis
Photodistribution	Hemolytic anemia, pink urine	High porphyrins in blood, urine
May be focal or generalized	Blood picture consistent with disseminated intravascular coagulation	Absent protein C or S in blood

COMMON TRANSIENT SKIN LESIONS

Erythema toxicum neonatorum. Lesions are not present at birth. Erythema toxicum neonatorum (ETN) (toxic erythema of the newborn) occurs in 20% to 50% of term infants—usually second and later deliveries—who are otherwise healthy. It is rare in premature infants and in those weighing less than 2500 gm. Most cases occur between 24 and 48 hours of age.

The rash often begins on the face; the trunk, proximal extremities, and buttocks are commonly involved. Palms and soles are not affected. Lesions may localize at pressure sites. Four types of lesions occur: macules, wheals, papules, and pustules. Tiny papules and pustules are superimposed on macules or wheals. New lesions appear as older lesions resolve. Wright's stain of a pustule shows numerous eosinophils. Peripheral eosinophilia is unusual.

Transient neonatal pustular melanosis. Lesions are present at birth but may be overlooked for 1 or 2 days. Transient neonatal pustular melanosis (TNPM) occurs in 2% to 5% of term blacks and 0.6% of whites who are otherwise healthy. Vesiculopustules, with no underlying erythema, rupture and form a hyperpigmented macule with a collarette of scale. Lesions may be solitary or grouped; most are 2 to 3 mm. They are located on the forehead, behind the ears, under the chin, on the neck and back, and on the hands and feet. The palms and soles may be affected. Lesions are very superficial, located within or just beneath the stratum corneum. Wright's stain shows polymorphonuclear neutrophilic leukocytes (PMNs); eosinophils may predominate. No treatment is necessary. Pustules resolve in a few days; pigmented macules may last for several weeks to months.

A clear-cut differentiation between TNPM and ETN is not always possible. The name sterile transient neonatal pustulosis has been proposed to unify these conditions.

Neonatal acne. Lesions occur 1 to 2 weeks after birth in approximately 20% of newborns. Comedones, papules, and pustules occur in the same distribution as in adolescent acne. Lesions resolve spontaneously.

Miliaria. Lesions occur approximately 1 week after birth. Miliaria or heat rash occurs in warm climates, while warming in an incubator, during a fever, or from wearing occlusive dressings or warm clothing. Eccrine sweat-duct occlusion is the initial event. The duct ruptures, leaks sweat into the surrounding tissues, and induces an inflammatory response. Occlusion occurs at two different levels to produce two distinct forms of miliaria. In miliaria crystallina, occlusion of the eccrine duct at the skin surface results in accumulation of sweat under the stratum corneum. The lesion appears as a clear dewdrop. There is little or no erythema. The vesicles appear individually or in clusters. Miliaria rubra results from occlusion of the intraepidermal section of the eccrine sweat duct. Papules and vesicles surrounded by a red halo or diffuse erythema develop as the inflammatory response develops. A cool water compress and proper ventilation are all that is necessary to treat this self-limited process.

References

1. Yancey K, Egan C: Pemphigoid: clinical, histologic, immunopathologic, and therapeutic considerations [clinical conference], JAMA 2000; 284(3):350.

2. Mutasim D, Adams B: Immunofluorescence in dermatology, J Am Acad Dermatol 2001; 45:803; quiz 822.

3. Egan C, et al: Dermatitis herpetiformis: a review of fifty-four patients, Ir J Med Sci 1997; 166:241.

4. Cuartero BG, et al: Dermatitis herpetiformis vs. celiac disease, Ann Esp Pediatr 1992; 37:307.

5. Hall RP, Otley C: Immunogenetics of dermatitis herpetiformis, Semin Dermatol 1991; 10:240.

6. Ermacora E, et al: Long-term follow-up of dermatitis herpetiformis in children, J Am Acad Dermatol 1986; 15:24.

7. Cunningham MJ, Zone JJ: Thyroid abnormalities in dermatitis herpetiformis: prevalence of clinical thyroid disease and thyroid autoantibodies, Ann Intern Med 1985; 102:194.

8. Aine L, et al: Coeliac-type dental enamel defects in patients with dermatitis herpetiformis, Acta Derm Venereol 1992; 72:25.

9. Lahteenoja H, et al: Oral mucosa is frequently affected in patients with dermatitis herpetiformis [letter], Arch Dermatol 1998; 134(6):756.

10. Klein P, Callen J: Drug-induced linear IgA bullous dermatosis after vancomycin discontinuance in a patient with renal insufficiency, J Am Acad Dermatol 2000; 42(2 Pt 2):316.

11. Dieterich W, et al: Antibodies to tissue transglutaminase as serologic markers in patients with dermatitis herpetiformis, J Invest Dermatol 1999; 113:133.

12. Volta U, et al: Correlation between IgA antiendomysial antibodies and subtotal villous atrophy in dermatitis herpetiformis, J Clin Gastroenterol 1992; 14:298.

13. Lewis H, et al: Protective effect of gluten-free diet against development of lymphoma in dermatitis herpetiformis, Br J Dermatol 1996;135(3):363.

14. Collin P, Pukkala E, Reunala T: Malignancy and survival in dermatitis herpetiformis: a comparison with coeliac disease, Gut 1996; 38(4):528.

15. Smith SB, et al: Linear IgA bullous dermatosis v dermatitis herpetiformis: quantitative measurements of dermoepidermal alterations, Arch Dermatol 1984; 120:324.

16. Husz S, et al: Development of a system for detection of circulating antibodies against hemidesmosomal proteins in patients with bullous pemphigoid [In Process Citation], Arch Dermatol Res 2000; 292:217.

17. Sardy M, et al: Epidermal transglutaminase (TGase 3) is the autoantigen of dermatitis herpetiformis, J Exp Med 2002; 195:747.

18. Dieterich W, et al: Antibodies to tissue transglutaminase as serologic markers in patients with dermatitis herpetiformis, J Invest Dermatol 1999; 113:133.

19. Koop I, et al: Detection of autoantibodies against tissue transglutaminase in patients with celiac disease and dermatitis herpetiformis [In Process Citation], Am J Gastroenterol 2000; 95:2009.

20. Coleman MD, et al: The use of cimetidine to reduce dapsone-dependent methaemoglobinaemia in dermatitis herpetiformis patients, Br J Clin Pharmacol 1992; 34:244.

21. Waldinger TP, et al: Dapsone induced peripheral neuropathy, Arch Dermatol 1984; 120:356.

22. Ahrens EM, Meckler RJ, Callen JP: Dapsone-induced peripheral neuropathy, Int J Dermatol 1986; 25:314.

23. Kumar RH, et al: Dapsone syndrome—a five year retrospective analysis, Indian J Lepr 1998; 70:271.

24. Kahn G. Dapsone is safe during pregnancy, J Am Acad Dermatol 1985; 13:838.

25. Garioch JJ, et al: 25 years' experience of a gluten-free diet in the treatment of dermatitis herpetiformis, Br J Dermatol 1994; 131:541.

26. Reunala T, et al: Tolerance to oats in dermatitis herpetiformis, Gut 1998; 43:490.

27. Hardman C, et al: Absence of toxicity of oats in patients with dermatitis herpetiformis [see comments], N Engl J Med 1997; 337:1884.

28. Kaukinen K, et al: Wheat starch-containing gluten-free flour products in the treatment of coeliac disease and dermatitis herpetiformis: A long-term follow-up study, Scand J Gastroenterol 1999; 34:163.

29. Ciclitira PJ, et al: Evaluation of a gluten free product containing wheat gliadin in patients with coeliac disease, BMJ 1984; 289:83.

30. van de Meer JB: Gluten-free diet and elemental diet in dermatitis herpetiformis, Int J Dermatol 1990; 29:679.

31. Kadunce DP, et al: The effect of an elemental diet with and without gluten on disease activity in dermatitis herpetiformis, J Invest Dermatol 1991; 97:175.

32. Peoples D, Fivenson DP: Linear IgA bullous dermatosis: successful treatment with tetracycline and nicotinamide, J Am Acad Dermatol 1992; 26:498.

33. Shah S, Ormerod A: Dermatitis herpetiformis effectively treated with heparin, tetracycline and nicotinamide, Clin Exp Dermatol 2000; 25:204.

34. Toonstra J: Bullosis diabeticorum: report of a case with a review of the literature, J Am Acad Dermatol 1985; 13:799.

35. Bernstein JE, et al: Bullous eruption of diabetes mellitus, Arch Dermatol 1979; 115:324.

36. Goodfield MJD, et al: Bullosis diabeticorum, J Am Acad Dermatol 1986; 15:1292.

37. Korman N: New and emerging therapies in the treatment of blistering diseases, Dermatol Clin 2000; 18:127, ix.

38. Edelson R: Pemphigus—decoding the cellular language of cutaneous autoimmunity, N Engl J Med 2000; 343:60.

39. Ahmed AR, et al: Linkage of pemphigus vulgaris antibody to the major histocompatibility complex in healthy relatives of patients, J Exp Med 1993; 177:419.

40. Lever WF: Pemphigus and pemphigoid, a review of the advances made since 1964, J Am Acad Dermatol 1979; 1:1.

41. Amagai M, et al: The clinical phenotype of pemphigus is defined by the anti-desmoglein autoantibody profile, J Am Acad Dermatol 1999; 40:167.

42. Amagai M: Autoimmunity against desmosomal cadherins in pemphigus, J Dermatol Sci 1999; 20(2):92.

43. Becker BA, Gaspari AA. Pemphigus vulgaris and vegetans, Dermatol Clin 1993; 11:429.

44. Lamey PJ, et al: Oral presentation of pemphigus vulgaris and its response to systemic steroid therapy, Oral Surg Oral Med Oral Pathol 1992; 74:54.

45. Trattner A, et al: Esophageal involvement in pemphigus vulgaris: A clinical, histologic, and immunopathologic study, J Am Acad Dermatol 1991; 24:223.

46. Reis V, et al: UVB-induced acantholysis in endemic pemphigus foliaceus (fogo selvagem) and pemphigus vulgaris, J Am Acad Dermatol 2000; 42:571.

47. Supapannachart N, Mutasim DF: The distribution of IgA pemphigus antigen in human skin and the role of IgA anti-cell surface antibodies in the induction of intraepidermal acantholysis, Arch Dermatol 1993; 129:605.

48. Beutner EH, et al: IgA pemphigus foliaceus. Report of two cases and a review of the literature, J Am Acad Dermatol 1989; 20:89.

49. Sams WM, Gammon WR: Mechanism of lesion production in pemphigus and pemphigoid, J Am Acad Dermatol 1982; 6:431.

50. David M, et al: The usefulness of immunofluorescent tests in pemphigus patients in clinical remission, Br J Derm 1989; 120:391.

51. Lever WF, Schaumburg-Lever G: Treatment of pemphigus vulgaris, Arch Dermatol 1984; 120:44.

52. Ratnam KV, et al: Pemphigus therapy with oral prednisolone regimens: A 5-year study, Int J Dermatol 1990; 29:363.

53. Dumas V, et al: The treatment of mild pemphigus vulgaris and pemphigus foliaceus with a topical corticosteroid, Br J Dermatol 1999; 140:1127.

54. Ahmed AR, Hombal S: Use of cyclophosphamide in azathioprine failures in pemphigus, J Am Acad Dermatol 1987; 17:437.

55. Aberer W, et al: Azathioprine in the treatment of pemphigus vulgaris, J Am Acad Dermatol 1987; 16:527.

56. Bystryn J-C, et al: Treatment of pemphigus with intravenous immunoglobulin, J Am Acad Dermatol 2002; 47:358.

57. Ahmed A, Sami N: Intravenous immunoglobulin therapy for patients with pemphigus foliaceus unresponsive to conventional therapy, J Am Acad Dermatol 2002; 46:42.

58. Enk A, Knop J: Mycophenolate is effective in the treatment of pemphigus vulgaris [see comments], Arch Dermatol 1999; 135(1):54.

59. Nousari H, et al: Mycophenolate mofetil in autoimmune and inflammatory skin disorders, J Am Acad Dermatol 1999; 40:265.

60. Basset N, et al: Dapsone as initial treatment in superficial pemphigus, Arch Dermatol 1987; 123:783.

61. Mobini N, Padilla TJ, Ahmed A: Long-term remission in selected patients with pemphigus vulgaris treated with cyclosporine, J Am Acad Dermatol 1997; 36:264.

62. Lapidoth M, et al: The efficacy of combined treatment with prednisone and cyclosporine in patients with pemphigus: preliminary study, J Am Acad Dermatol 1994; 30:752.

63. Pandya A, Dyke C: Treatment of pemphigus with gold, Arch Dermatol 1998; 134:1104.

64. Bystryn JC: Plasmapheresis therapy of pemphigus, Arch Dermatol 1988; 124:1702.

65. Wollina U, Lange D, Looks A: Short-time extracorporeal photochemotherapy in the treatment of drug-resistant autoimmune bullous diseases, Dermatology 1999; 198:140.

66. Ahmed A: Intravenous immunoglobulin therapy in the treatment of patients with pemphigus vulgaris unresponsive to conventional immunosuppressive treatment, J Am Acad Dermatol 1987; 16:527.

67. Calebotta A, et al: Pemphigus vulgaris: benefits of tetracycline as adjuvant therapy in a series of thirteen patients, Int J Dermatol 1999; 38:217.

68. Ioannides D, Chrysomallis F, Bystryn J: Ineffectiveness of cyclosporine as an adjuvant to corticosteroids in the treatment of pemphigus, Arch Dermatol 2000; 136:868.

69. Hymes SR, Jordon RE: Pemphigus foliaceus. Use of antimalarial agents as adjuvant therapy, Arch Dermatol 1992; 128:1462.

70. Chaffins ML, et al: Treatment of pemphigus and linear IgA dermatosis with nicotinamide and tetracycline: a review of 13 cases, J Am Acad Dermatol 1993; 28:998.

71. Herbst A, Bystryn J: Patterns of remission in pemphigus vulgaris, J Am Acad Dermatol 2000; 42:422.

72. Ratnam KV, Pang BK: Pemphigus in remission: value of negative direct immunofluorescence in management, J Am Acad Dermatol 1994; 30:547.

73. Cruz PD, Coldiron BM, Sontheimer RD: Concurrent features of cutaneous lupus erythematosus and pemphigus erythematosus following myasthenia gravis and thymoma, J Am Acad Dermatol 1987; 16:472.

74. Kuechle MK, et al: Angiotensin-converting enzyme inhibitor-induced pemphigus: three cases and literature review, Mayo Clin Proc 1994; 69:1166.

75. Ahmed R: Pemphigus associated with D-penicillamine. In Ahmed AR, moderator: Pemphigus: current concepts, Ann Intern Med 1980; 92:396.

76. Levy RS, Fisher M, Alter JN: Penicillamine: review and cutaneous manifestations, J Am Acad Dermatol 1983; 8:548.

77. Mutasim DF, et al: Drug-induced pemphigus, Dermatol Clin 1993; 11:463.

78. Wolf R, et al: Drug-induced versus drug-triggered pemphigus, Dermatologica 1991; 182:207.

79. Goldberg I, Kashman Y, Brenner S: The induction of pemphigus by phenol drugs, Int J Dermatol 1999; 38:888.

80. Kohn SR: Fatal penicillamine-induced pemphigus foliaceus-like dermatosis, Arch Dermatol 1986; 122:17.

81. Brenner S, Bialy-Golan A, Crost N: Dipyrone in the induction of pemphigus, J Am Acad Dermatol 1997; 36:488.

82. Brenner S, Bialy-Golan A, Anhalt G: Recognition of pemphigus antigens in drug-induced pemphigus vulgaris and pemphigus foliaceus, J Am Acad Dermatol 1997; 36:919.

83. Robinson N, et al: The new pemphigus variants [see comments], J Am Acad Dermatol 1999; 40:649; quiz 672.

84. Mehregan DR, et al: Paraneoplastic pemphigus: a subset of patients with pemphigus and neoplasia, J Cutan Pathol 1993; 20:203.

85. Horn TD, Anhalt GJ: Histologic features of paraneoplastic pemphigus, Arch Dermatol 1992; 128:1091.

86. Helou J, et al: Accuracy of indirect immunofluorescence testing in the diagnosis of paraneoplastic pemphigus, J Am Acad Dermatol 1995; 32:441.

87. Yancey K, Egan C: Pemphigoid: clinical, histologic, immunopathologic, and therapeutic considerations [clinical conference], JAMA 2000; 284:350.

88. Taylor G, et al: Bullous pemphigoid and autoimmunity, J Am Acad Dermatol 1993; 29:181.

89. Venning VA, Wojnarowska F: The association of bullous pemphigoid and malignant disease: a case control study, Br J Dermatol 1990; 123:439.

90. Ortiz LJ, et al: Bullous pemphigoid and malignancy, Bol Asoc Med P R 1990; 82:458.

91. Lindelof B, et al: Pemphigoid and cancer, Arch Dermatol 1990; 126:66.

92. Smith EP, et al: Antigen identification in drug-induced bullous pemphigoid, J Am Acad Dermatol 1993; 29:879.

93. Kippes W, et al: [Immunopathologic changes in 115 patients with bullous pemphigoid], Hautarzt 1999; 50:866.

94. Nakatani C, Muramatsu T, Shirai T: Immunoreactivity of bullous pemphigoid (BP) autoantibodies against the NC16A and C-terminal domains of the 180 kDa BP antigen (BP180): immunoblot analysis and enzyme-linked immunosorbent assay using BP180 recombinant proteins, Br J Dermatol 1998; 139:365.

95. Bingham EA, et al: Prolonged pruritus and bullous pemphigoid, Clin Exp Dermatol 1984; 9:564.

96. Macfarlane AW, Verbov JL: Trauma-induced bullous pemphigoid, Clin Exp Dermatol 1989; 14:245.

97. Liu HH, et al: Clinical variants of pemphigoid, Int J Dermatol 1986; 25:17.

98. Venning VA, Wojnarowska F: Lack of predictive factors for the clinical course of bullous pemphigoid, J Am Acad Dermatol 1992; 26:585.

99. Hornschuh B, et al: Treatment of 16 patients with bullous pemphigoid with oral tetracycline and niacinamide and topical clobetasol, J Am Acad Dermatol 1997; 36:101.

100. Schmidt E, et al: Serum levels of autoantibodies to BP180 correlate with disease activity in patients with bullous pemphigoid [see comments], Arch Dermatol 2000; 136:174.

101. Razany B, et al: Risk factors for lethal outcome in patients with bullous pemphigoid, Arch Dermatol 2002; 138:903.

102. Dopp R, et al: IgG4 and IgE are the major immunoglobulins targeting the NC16A domain of BP180 in Bullous pemphigoid: serum levels of these immunoglobulins reflect disease activity, J Am Acad Dermatol 2000; 42(4):577.

103. Anstey A, et al: Determination of the optimum site for diagnostic biopsy for direct immunofluorescence in bullous pemphigoid, Clin Exp Dermatol 1990; 15:438.

104. Smoller BR, Woodley DT: Differences in direct immunofluorescence staining patterns in epidermolysis bullosa acquisita and bullous pemphigoid, J Am Acad Dermatol 1992; 27:674.

105. Chimanovitch I, et al: Bullous pemphigoid of childhood: autoantibodies target the same epitopes within the NC16A domain of BP180 as autoantibodies in bullous pemphigoid of adulthood, Arch Dermatol 2000; 136(4):527.

106. Schmidt E, et al: Autoantibodies to BP180 associated with bullous pemphigoid release interleukin-6 and interleukin-8 from cultured human keratinocytes, J Invest Dermatol 2000; 115:842.

107. Schmidt E, Brocker E, Zillikens D: [New aspects on the pathogenesis of bullous pemphigoid], Hautarzt 2000; 51:637.

108. Zimmermann R, Faure M, Claudy A: [Prospective study of treatment of bullous pemphigoid by a class I topical corticosteroid (see comments)]. Ann Dermatol Venereol 1999; 126:13.

109. Joly P, et al: A comparison of oral and topical corticosteroids in patients with bullous pemphigoid, N Engl J Med 2002; 346:321.

110. Thomas I, et al: Treatment of generalized bullous pemphigoid with oral tetracycline, J Am Acad Dermatol 1993; 28:74.

111. Bouscarat F, et al: Treatment of bullous pemphigoid with dapsone: retrospective study of thirty-six cases, J Am Acad Dermatol 1996; 34:683.

112. Ahmed AR, Maize JC, Provost TT: Bullous pemphigoid: clinical and immunologic follow-up after successful therapy, Arch Dermatol 1977; 113:1043.

113. Guillaume JC, et al: Controlled trial of azathioprine and plasma exchange in addition to prednisolone in the treatment of bullous pemphigoid, Arch Dermatol 1993; 129:49.

114. Chosidow O, et al: Pharmacokinetics of prednisone and prednisolone in bullous pemphigoid patients, Int J Clin Pharmacol Ther Toxicol 1991; 29:376.

115. Jeffes E, Ahmed AR: Adjuvant therapy of bullous pemphigoid with dapsone, Clin Exp Dermatol 1989; 14:132.

116. Dahl MC, Cook LJ: Lesions induced by trauma in pemphigoid, Br J Dermatol 1979; 101:469.

117. Korman N: Bullous pemphigoid. The latest in diagnosis, prognosis, and therapy [editorial; comment], Arch Dermatol 1998; 134:1137.

118. Tavadia S, et al: Screening for azathioprine toxicity: a pharmacoeconomic analysis based on a target case, J Am Acad Dermatol 2000; 42:628.

119. Heilborn J, et al: Low-dose oral pulse methotrexate as monotherapy in elderly patients with bullous pemphigoid, J Am Acad Dermatol 1999; 40:741.

120. Grundmann-Kollmann M, et al: Mycophenolate mofetil: a new therapeutic option in the treatment of blistering autoimmune diseases, J Am Acad Dermatol 1999; 40:957.

121. Harman K, Black M: High-dose intravenous immune globulin for the treatment of autoimmune blistering diseases: an evaluation of its use in 14 cases, Br J Dermatol 1999; 140:865.

122. Borradori L, et al: Localized pretibial pemphigoid and pemphigoid nodularis, J Am Acad Dermatol 1992; 27:863.

123. Leenutaphong V, et al: Localized cicatricial pemphigoid (Brunsting-Perry): electron microscopic study, J Am Acad Dermatol 1989; 21:1089.

124. Descamps V, et al: Dyshidrosiform pemphigoid: report of three cases, J Am Acad Dermatol 1992; 26:651.

125. Chan LS, et al: Pemphigoid vegetans represents a bullous pemphigoid variant. Patient's IgG autoantibodies identify the major bullous pemphigoid antigen, J Am Acad Dermatol 1993; 28:331.

126. Domloge-Hultsch N, et al: Autoantibodies from patients with localized and generalized bullous pemphigoid immunoprecipitate the same 230-kd keratinocyte antigen, Arch Dermatol 1990; 126:1337.

127. Weigand DA, Clements MK: Direct immunofluorescence in bullous pemphigoid: effects of extent and location of lesions, J Am Acad Dermatol 1989; 20:437.

128. Ahmed AR, et al: Cicatricial pemphigoid, J Am Acad Dermatol 1991; 24:987.

129. Mutasim DF, et al: Cicatricial pemphigoid, Dermatol Clin 1993; 11:499.

130. Ahmed AR, Hombal SM: Cicatricial pemphigoid, Int J Dermatol 1986; 25:90.

131. Mobini N, Nagarwalla N, Ahmed A: Oral pemphigoid. Subset of cicatricial pemphigoid? Oral Surg Oral Med Oral Pathol Oral Radiol Endocrinol 1998; 85:37.

132. Neumann R, et al: Remission and recurrence after withdrawal of therapy for ocular cicatricial pemphigoid, Ophthalmology 1991; 98:858.

133. Sarret Y, et al: Salt-split human skin substrate for the immunofluorescent screening of serum from patients with cicatricial pemphigoid and a new method of immunoprecipitation with IgA antibodies, J Am Acad Dermatol 1991; 24:952.

134. Tauber J, et al: Systemic chemotherapy for ocular cicatricial pemphigoid, Cornea 1991; 10:185.

135. Fleming T, Korman N: Cicatricial pemphigoid, J Am Acad Dermatol 2000; 43:571; quiz 591.

136. Fern AI, et al: Dapsone therapy for the acute inflammatory phase of ocular pemphigoid, Br J Ophthalmol 1992; 76:1332.

137. Rogers RS III, Seehafer JR, Perry HO: Treatment of cicatricial (benign mucous membrane) pemphigoid with dapsone, J Am Acad Dermatol 1982; 6:215.

138. Saad RW, et al: Childhood localized vulvar pemphigoid is a true variant of bullous pemphigoid, Arch Dermatol 1992; 128:807.

139. Guenther LC, Shum D: Localized childhood vulvar pemphigoid, J Am Acad Dermatol 1990; 22:762.

140. Levine V, et al: Localized vulvar pemphigoid in a child misdiagnosed as sexual abuse, Arch Dermatol 1992; 128:804.

141. Marren P, et al: Vulvar involvement in autoimmune bullous diseases, J Reprod Med 1993; 38:101.

142. Marsden RA, et al: A study of benign chronic bullous dermatosis of childhood and comparison with dermatitis herpetiformis and bullous pemphigoid occurring in childhood, Clin Exp Dermatol 1980; 5:159.

143. Roberts LJ, Sontheimer RD: Chronic bullous dermatosis of childhood: immunopathologic studies, Pediatr Dermatol 1987, 4.6.

144. Sweren RJ, Burnett JW: Benign chronic bullous dermatosis of childhood: a review, Cutis 1982; 29:350.

145. Wojnarowska F, et al: Chronic bullous disease of childhood, childhood cicatricial pemphigoid, and linear IgA disease of adults, J Am Acad Dermatol 1988; 19:792.

146. Shornick JK: Herpes gestationis, J Am Acad Dermatol 1987; 17:539.

147. Shornick JK, et al: Complement polymorphism in herpes gestationis: association with C4 null allele, J Am Acad Dermatol 1993; 29:545.

148. Shornick JK, Black MM: Fetal risks in herpes gestationis, J Am Acad Dermatol 1992; 26:63.

149. Shornick JK: Herpes gestationis, Dermatol Clin 1993; 11:527.

150. Shornick JK, et al: Herpes gestationis: clinical and histologic features of twenty-eight cases, J Am Acad Dermatol 1983; 8:214.

151. Engineer L, Bhol K, Ahmed A: Pemphigoid gestationis: a review, Am J Obstet Gynecol 2000; 183:483.

152. Arpey CJ, et al: Childhood epidermolysis bullosa acquisita. Report of three cases and review of literature, J Am Acad Dermatol 1991; 24:706.

153. Woodley DT: Epidermolysis bullosa acquisita, Progr Dermatol 1988; 22:1.

154. Luke M, et al: Mucosal morbidity in patients with epidermolysis bullosa acquisita, Arch Dermatol 1999; 135:954.

155. Mooney E, et al: Studies on complement deposits in epidermolysis bullosa acquisita and bullous pemphigoid, Arch Dermatol 1992; 128:58.

156. Gammon WR, et al: Direct immunofluorescence studies of sodium chloride-separated skin in the differential diagnosis of bullous pemphigoid and epidermolysis bullosa acquisita, J Am Acad Dermatol 1990; 22:664.

157. Domloge-Hultsch N, et al: Direct immunofluorescence microscopy of 1 mol/L sodium chloride-treated patient skin, J Am Acad Dermatol 1991; 24:946.

158. Cunningham B, Kirchmann T, Woodley D: Colchicine for epidermolysis bullosa acquisita, J Am Acad Dermatol 1996; 34:781.

159. Mallett RB, Holden CA: Clearing of epidermolysis bullosa acquisita with cyclosporine, J Am Acad Dermatol 1991; 24:1034.

160. Jolles S, Hughes J, Whittaker S: Dermatological uses of high-dose intravenous immunoglobulin, Arch Dermatol 1998; 134:80.

161. Kofler H, et al: Intravenous immunoglobulin treatment in therapy-resistant epidermolysis bullosa acquisita, J Am Acad Dermatol 1997; 36:331.

162. Engineer L, Ahmed A: Emerging treatment for epidermolysis bullosa acquisita, J Am Acad Dermatol 2001; 44:818.

163. Engineer L, Ahmed A: Role of intravenous immunoglobulin in the treatment of bullous pemphigoid: analysis of current data, J Am Acad Dermatol 2001; 44:83.

164. Richard G, et al: Genetics of Hailey-Hailey familial chronic benign pemphigus, Dermatol Monatsschr 1990; 176:673.

586 Clinical Dermatology

165. Peppiatt T, et al: Hailey-Hailey disease-exacerbation by herpes simplex virus and patch tests, Clin Exp Dermatol 1992; 17:201.

166. Burge SM: Hailey-Hailey disease: the clinical features, response to treatment and prognosis, Br J Dermatol 1992; 126:275.

167. Burge SM, et al: Hailey-Hailey disease: a widespread abnormality of cell adhesion, Br J Dermatol 1991; 124:329.

168. Richard G, et al: Hailey-Hailey disease. Early detection of heterozygotes by an ultraviolet provocation tests-clinical relevance of the method, Hautarzt 1993; 44:376.

169. Langenberg A, et al: Genital benign chronic pemphigus (Hailey-Hailey disease) presenting as condylomas, J Am Acad Dermatol 1992; 26:951.

170. Jitsukawa K, et al: Topical cyclosporine in chronic benign familial pemphigus (Hailey-Hailey disease), J Am Acad Dermatol 1992; 27:625.

171. Kartamaa M, Reitamo S: Familial benign chronic pemphigus (Hailey-Hailey disease). Treatment with carbon dioxide laser vaporization, Arch Dermatol 1992; 128:646.

172. McElroy JA, et al: Carbon dioxide laser vaporization of recalcitrant symptomatic plaques of Hailey-Hailey disease and Darier's disease, J Am Acad Dermatol 1990; 23:893.

173. Menz P, Jackson IT, Connolly S: Surgical control of Hailey-Hailey disease, Br J Plast Surg 1987; 40:557.

174. Kirtschig G, et al: Treatment of Hailey-Hailey disease by dermabrasion, J Am Acad Dermatol 1993; 28:784.

175. Uitto J, Christiano AM: Inherited epidermolysis bullosa: Clinical features, molecular genetics, and pathoetiologic mechanisms, Dermatol Clin 1993; 11:549.

176. Van Praag M, et al: Diagnosis and treatment of pustular disorders in the neonate, Pediatr Dermatol 1997; 14:131.

177. Nanda S, et al: Analytical study of pustular eruptions in neonates [In Process Citation], Pediatr Dermatol 2002; 19:210.

Connective tissue diseases (lupus, dermatomyositis, scleroderma, overlap syndromes) are a group of multisystem illnesses of unknown etiology. They have no typical pattern of onset, duration, or organ involvement. This variability makes classification and diagnosis difficult; therefore a list of clinical diagnostic criteria has been established for each entity and is tabulated in the text.

Connective tissue diseases can be more accurately described as autoimmune diseases. Many serum antibodies directed at cellular components (autoantibodies) have been found in each disease and are probably responsible for the clinical manifestations.

Diagnosis

The diagnosis of connective tissue disease is made by the clinical picture. Antibodies to cell components (typically nuclear antigens) are present in these multisystem disorders. Detecting and defining them helps support the clinical diagnosis and provides information about subsets of disease and prognosis. A large number of antibodies are reported in the literature. Each systemic autoimmune disease has a characteristic antinuclear antibody (ANA) spectrum. Patients often produce multiple autoantibodies. The problem is knowing which tests to order and how to interpret them. An approach to the diagnosis of connective tissue diseases is shown in the diagram on pp. 588 and 589.

Antinuclear antibody testing

ANAs are detected by the indirect immunofluorescence tests. They are performed by applying test serum to a tissue section (human laryngeal epithelioma cancer cell line [Hep-2 cells]). Antibodies to nuclear antigens attach to the various components of the nucleus. Fluorescein-labeled antihuman immunoglobulins are applied to the preparation and react with ANAs that have attached to the nucleus. The preparation is visualized with a fluorescent microscope. Diverse patterns of nuclear fluorescence (homogeneous, peripheral, speckled, or nucleolar) reflect the binding of antibodies to different nuclear components. Nuclear staining patterns were once used as criteria for subsetting,[1] but, with the availability of direct measurements for specific autoantibodies, pattern identification has become less important. The test requires interpretation by visual inspection and consequently lacks a high degree of specificity.

APPROACH TO THE DIAGNOSIS OF CONNECTIVE TISSUE DISEASES*

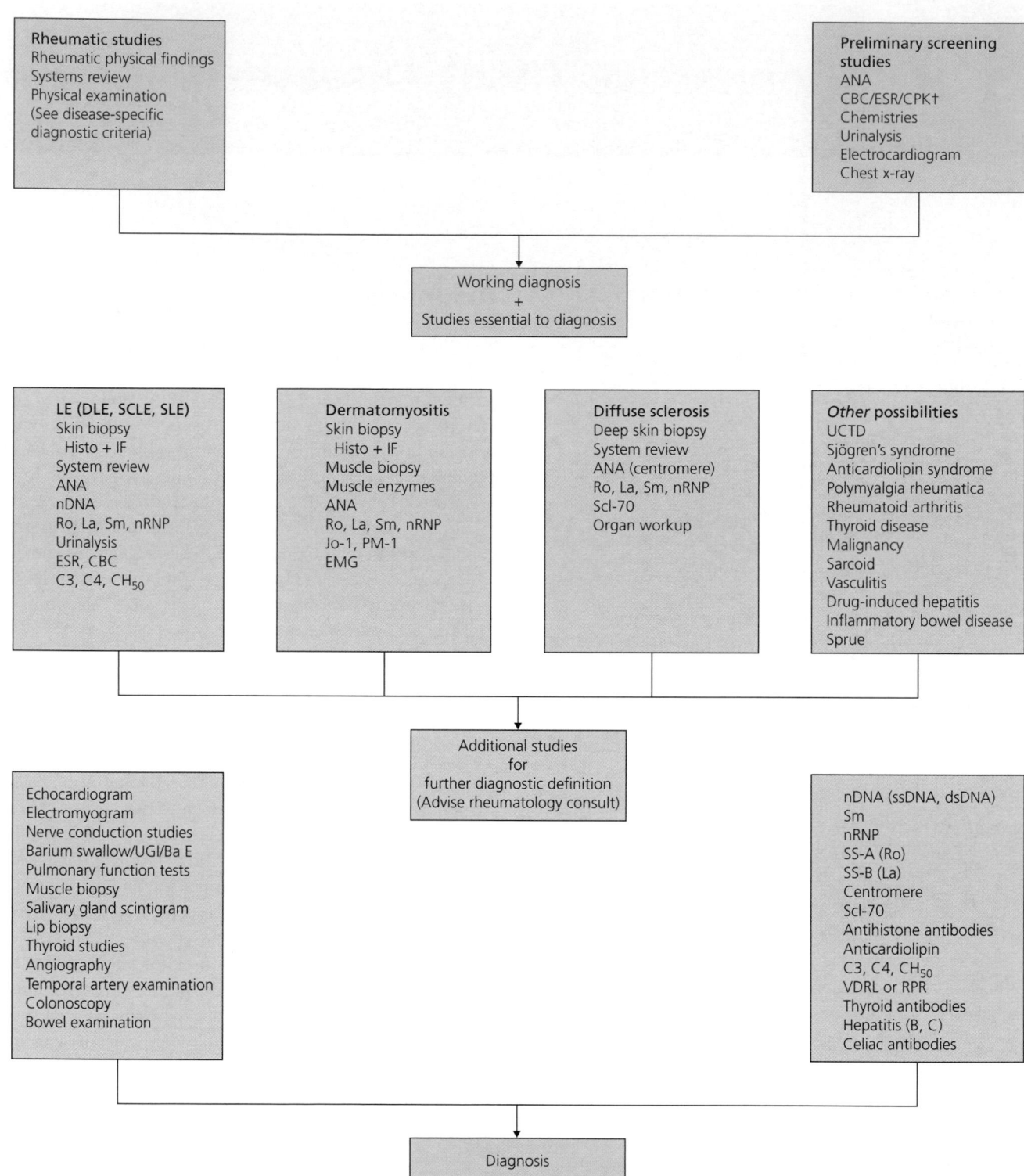

Rheumatic studies
Rheumatic physical findings
Systems review
Physical examination
(See disease-specific
diagnostic criteria)

**Preliminary screening
studies**
ANA
CBC/ESR/CPK†
Chemistries
Urinalysis
Electrocardiogram
Chest x-ray

Working diagnosis
+
Studies essential to diagnosis

LE (DLE, SCLE, SLE)
Skin biopsy
  Histo + IF
System review
ANA
nDNA
Ro, La, Sm, nRNP
Urinalysis
ESR, CBC
C3, C4, CH$_{50}$

Dermatomyositis
Skin biopsy
  Histo + IF
Muscle biopsy
Muscle enzymes
ANA
Ro, La, Sm, nRNP
Jo-1, PM-1
EMG

Diffuse sclerosis
Deep skin biopsy
System review
ANA (centromere)
Ro, La, Sm, nRNP
Scl-70
Organ workup

Other possibilities
UCTD
Sjögren's syndrome
Anticardiolipin syndrome
Polymyalgia rheumatica
Rheumatoid arthritis
Thyroid disease
Malignancy
Sarcoid
Vasculitis
Drug-induced hepatitis
Inflammatory bowel disease
Sprue

Additional studies
for
further diagnostic definition
(Advise rheumatology consult)

Echocardiogram
Electromyogram
Nerve conduction studies
Barium swallow/UGI/Ba E
Pulmonary function tests
Muscle biopsy
Salivary gland scintigram
Lip biopsy
Thyroid studies
Angiography
Temporal artery examination
Colonoscopy
Bowel examination

nDNA (ssDNA, dsDNA)
Sm
nRNP
SS-A (Ro)
SS-B (La)
Centromere
Scl-70
Antihistone antibodies
Anticardiolipin
C3, C4, CH$_{50}$
VDRL or RPR
Thyroid antibodies
Hepatitis (B, C)
Celiac antibodies

Diagnosis

*Flow sheet designed by Constance Passas, M.D. (rheumatologist).
†*CBC,* Complete blood count; *ESR,* erythrocyte sedimentation rate; *CPK,* creatine phosphokinase; *IF,* immunofluorescence; *UCTD,* undifferentiated
connective tissue disease (formerly mixed CTD); *EMG,* electromyogram; *ENA,* extractable nuclear antigens; *SLE,* systemic lupus erythematosus;
PSS, progressive systemic sclerosis; *SCLE,* subacute cutaneous lupus erythematosus; *DLE,* discoid lupus erythematosus.

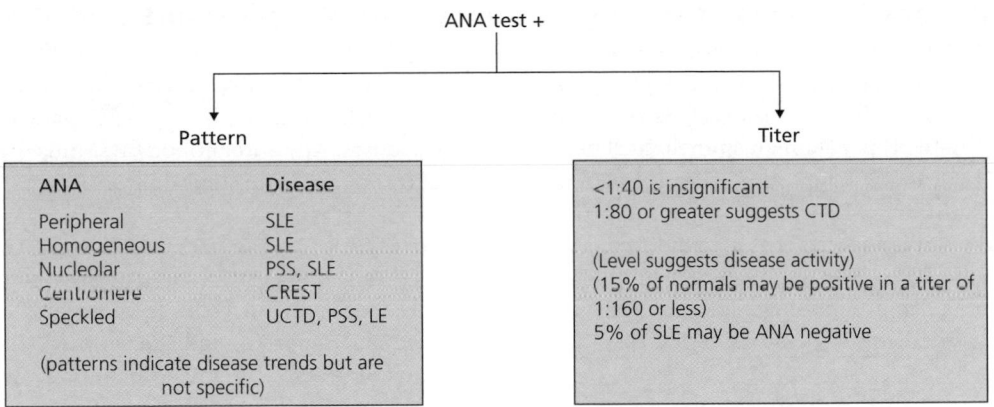

SEROLOGIC PROFILES IN CONNECTIVE TISSUE DISEASES

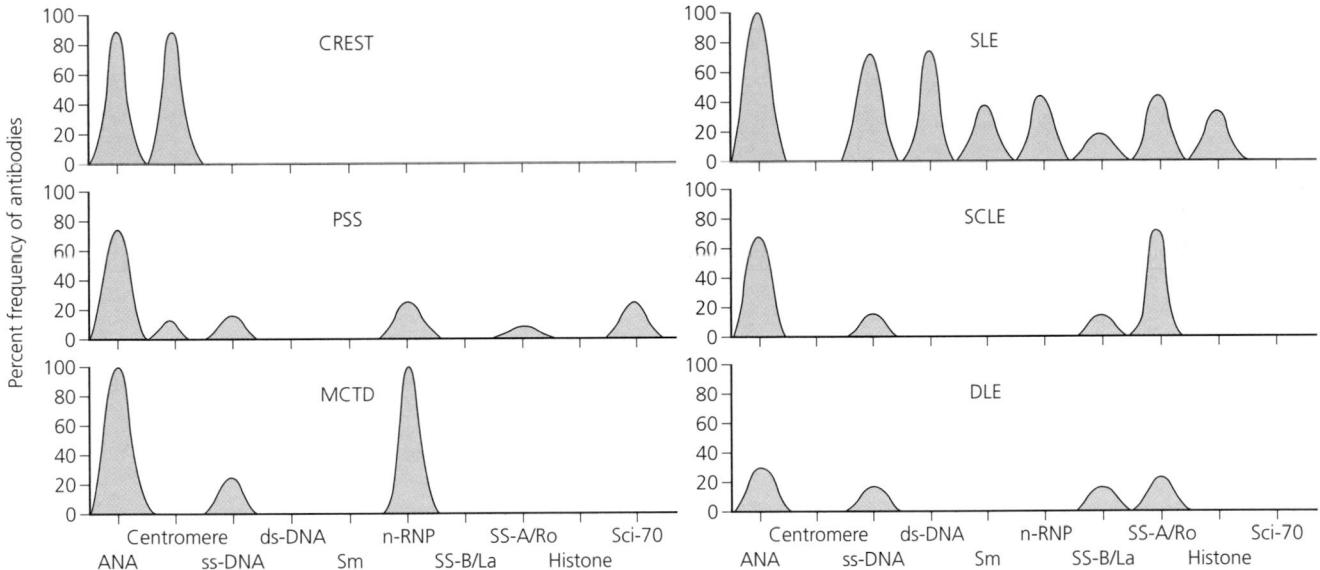

ANTINUCLEAR ANTIBODY SCREENING. ANA is the first test to order when collagen vascular disease is suspected (Table 17-1). The routine test method used is indirect immunofluorescence on mouse liver substrate. If results of this test are negative, ANA on HEp-2 (human epithelial cell tissue substrate) should be ordered; many ANA-negative patients react with HEp-2 substrate. Many laboratories use HEp-2 routinely. A negative result suggests that a connective tissue disease is unlikely; a positive result, especially a high titer in a patient with appropriate clinical findings, supports a diagnosis of a connective tissue disease.

FALSE-POSITIVE TEST RESULTS. Positive results occur in normal blood donors and in patients with chronic liver disease, neoplasms, or active chronic infections. These patients usually have lower titers than those in patients with autoimmune diseases. Any autoantibody test must be interpreted in the context of available clinical information.

ANTINUCLEAR ANTIBODY PATTERNS AND TITERS. If ANA is positive, one of the six patterns (homogeneous, peripheral, speckled, nucleolar, centromere, cytoplasmic) is identified and reported, and the serum is titered. The patterns are not specific for any autoantibody or disease entity, and a positive result must be confirmed by using more specific tests. A number of specific antibodies can cause each pattern. The ANA test determines that ANAs of a certain group are present, but it does not identify them.

SPECIFIC DIAGNOSTIC ANTIBODY TESTS. Specific antibody tests should be ordered. The clinical presentation and ANA pattern help to determine which test to order (Tables 17-2 and 17-3). Some laboratories offer tests for groups of antigens (i.e., ANA profiles).

Table 17-1 ANA-Screening Test

ANA (on HEp-2 cells)	Frequency of ANA positivity (%)
Systemic lupus erythematosus	95-100
Drug-induced lupus erythematosus	100
Scleroderma	60-95
Sjögren's syndrome	80
Polymyositis-dermatomyositis	49-74
Rheumatoid arthritis	40-60
Mixed connective tissue disease	100
Normal	<4

Modified from Harmon CE: Med Clin North Am 1985; 69:547.

Table 17-2 Autoantibody Tests for Connective Tissue Diseases

Antibody	Clinical significance
Antinuclear antibodies	Screening for SLE and PSS
Centromere antibodies	Marker for CREST
nDNA antibodies	Marker for SLE
DNP antibodies	Marker for SLE
Histone antibodies	To exclude drug-induced LE
ENA: Sm antibodies	Marker for SLE
RNP antibodies	SLE, MCTD, scleroderma
SS-A (Ro)/SS-B (La)	SLE, Sjögren's syndrome,
Antibodies	SCLE, and others
Scl-70 antibodies	Marker for scleroderma
Jo-1 antibodies	Marker for polymyositis
PCNA	SLE with high incidence of proliferative glomerulonephritis
Ku (Ki) antibodies	Polymyositis/scleroderma overlap, SLE
Phospholipid antibodies (lupus anticoagulant)	Marker for SLE subset with thrombosis: frequent aborters

Modified from Handbook: clinical relevance of tests, Buffalo, NY: IMMCO Diagnostics, 1993.
SLE, Systemic lupus erythematosus; *PSS,* progressive systemic sclerosis; *DNP,* deoxyribonuclear protein; *LE,* lupus erythematosus; *ENA,* extractable nuclear antigens; *MCTD,* mixed connective tissue disease; *SCLE,* subacute cutaneous lupus erythematosus; *PCNA,* proliferating cell nuclear antigen.

Table 17-3 Diagnostic Significance of Immunologic Findings in Serum and Skin Biopsies in Connective Tissue Diseases

Disease	Biopsy findings: direct immunofluorescence	Serum findings	Relevance
Systemic LE	LE band (granular immune deposits, IgG, and/or IgM) IgA, C3 at DEJ in lesional and/or normal skin: (over 90% in sun-exposed skin)	ANA elevated titers (about 95%-99%); nDNA antibodies about 50%-75%; DNP antibodies <50%; Sm antibodies in about 20%; RNP antibodies in about 5%-30%; SS-A antibodies in about 30%-40%; SS-B antibodies in about 1%-15%; phospholipids antibodies in about 30%-50%: PCNA antibodies in about 2%-10%: Ku(Ki) antibodies in about 10%	DIF, ANA, and ENA usually diagnostic; nDNA and Sm antibodies diagnostic markers
Discoid LE	LE band, mostly IgG and C in lesion ONLY	Essentially negative; ANA titers usually in normal range	LE band highly characteristic
Subacute cutaneous LE	LE band in lesion	ANA positive in 70%; SS-A (Ro) antibodies positive in more than 60%	DIF and anti-SS-A (Ro) highly characteristic
Neonatal LE	LE band in lesion (about 50%)	ANA positive in 30%; antibodies to SS-A (Ro) in 100%; antibodies to SS-B (La) in about 60%	DIF and anti-SS-A (Ro) highly characteristic
Drug-induced LE	LE band in lesion (rare)	ANA positive in more than 90%; histone positive about 90%; other antibodies to nDNA and ENA negative	DIF and histone antibodies in absence of other nuclear antibodies highly characteristic
Mixed connective tissue disease	Nuclear IgG or LE band in normal and/or lesional epidermis	Speckled ANA antibodies in more than 95% and RNP antibodies in more than 90%	Serology and/or DIF of nuclei diagnostic for MCTD, SLE, or PSS
Sjögren's syndrome	Negative	ANA positive in about 55%; antibodies to SS-A (Ro) in 43%–88%; SS-B (La) in 14%-60%; RF positive	Positive serum results support diagnosis
Progressive systemic sclerosis (scleroderma)	Nucleolar IgG in epidermis in few cases; most negative	ANA (about 85%) speckled or nucleolar; centromere antibody in CREST (70% to 90%); Scl-70 antibodies in diffuse sclerosis (45%) and in acrosclerosis (15% to 20%)	DIF limited value; centromere antibodies diagnostic marker in CREST; Scl-70 antibodies diagnostic marker in scleroderma
Polymyositis/ dermatomyositis	Negative	ANA usually positive (more than 80%); Jo-1 antibodies in 30% PM, 10% DM; SS-A (Ro) antibodies in 55% PM/Scleroderma overlap; Ku (Ki) antibodies in 10% PM/scleroderma overlap	Limited value, but positive serum results support diagnosis
Rheumatoid arthritis	Negative	ANA usually negative or low titer; RF positive in about 90%; RNA positive in about 70% to 90% and 95% of RF-negative cases	Positive serum results support diagnosis

Modified from Handbook: clinical relevance of tests, Buffalo, NY: IMMCO Diagnostics, 1993.

LE, Lupus erythematosus; *DEJ*, dermal-epidermal junction; *DNP*, deoxyribonuclear protein; *PCNA*, proliferating cell nuclear antigen; *DIF*, direct immunofluorescence; *ENA*, extractable nuclear antigen; *MCTD*, mixed connective tissue disease; *SLE*, systemic lupus erythematosus; *PSS*, progressive systemic sclerosis; *RF*, rheumatoid factor; *PM*, polymyositis; *DM*, dermatomyositis; *RANA*, antibodies to rheumatoid arthritis associated nuclear antigen.

Lupus Erythematosus

Clinical classification

Systemic lupus erythematosus (SLE) is a multisystem disease of unknown origin characterized by the production of numerous diverse types of autoantibodies that, through immune mechanisms in various tissues, cause several combinations of clinical signs, symptoms (Table 17-4), and laboratory abnormalities (Table 17-5). The natural history of SLE is characterized by episodes of relapses, flares, and remissions. The outcome is highly variable, ranging from remission to death.

The prevalence of LE in North America and northern Europe is about 40 per 100,000 population. There appears to be a higher incidence in African Americans and Hispanics. More than 80% of cases occur in women during childbearing years.

The American College of Rheumatology classification criteria for systemic lupus erythematosus (SLE) were updated in 1997 (www.rheumatology.org) (see Table 17-4). The presence of four or more of the 11 parameters, serially or simultaneously, is believed to be compatible with the diagnosis of LE. Those criteria in a modified form are illustrated in Figure 17-1.

Table 17-4 American College of Rheumatology: The 1997 Revised Criteria for Classification of Systemic Lupus Erythematosus*

Definition	Criterion
1. Malar rash	Fixed erythema, flat or raised, over the malar eminences, tending to spare the nasolabial folds
2. Discoid rash	Erythematous raised patches with adherent keratotic scaling and follicular plugging; atrophic scarring may occur in older lesions
3. Photosensitivity	Skin rash as a result of unusual reaction to sunlight, by patient history or physician observation
4. Oral ulcers	Oral or nasopharyngeal ulceration, usually painless, observed by physician
5. Arthritis	Nonerosive arthritis involving 2 or more peripheral joints, characterized by tenderness, swelling, or effusion
6. Serositis	a) Pleuritis—convincing history of pleuritic pain or rubbing heard by a physician or evidence of pleural effusion *OR* b) Pericarditis—documented by ECG or rub or evidence of pericardial effusion
7. Renal disorder	a) Persistent proteinuria greater than 0.5 gm per day or greater than 3+ if quantitation not performed *OR* b) Cellular casts—may be red cell, hemoglobin, granular, tubular, or mixed
8. Neurologic disorder	a) Seizures—in the absence of offending drugs or known metabolic derangements; e.g., uremia, ketoacidosis, or electrolyte imbalance *OR* b) Psychosis—in the absence of offending drugs or known metabolic derangements, e.g., uremia, ketoacidosis, or electrolyte imbalance
9. Hematologic disorder	a) Hemolytic anemia—with reticulocytosis *OR* b) Leukopenia—less than 4,000/mm³ total on 2 or more occasions *OR* c) Lymphopenia—less than 1,500/mm³ on 2 or more occasions *OR* d) Thrombocytopenia—less than 100,000/mm³ in the absence of offending drugs
10. Immunologic disorder	a) Anti-DNA: antibody to native DNA in abnormal titer *OR* b) Anti-Sm: presence of antibody to Sm nuclear antigen *OR* c) Positive finding of antiphospholipid antibodies based on 1) an abnormal serum level of IgG or IgM anticardiolipin antibodies, 2) a positive test result for lupus anticoagulant using a standard method, or 3) a false-positive serologic test for syphilis known to be positive for at least 6 months and confirmed by *Treponema pallidum* immobilization or fluorescent treponemal antibody absorption test. Standard methods should be used in testing for the presence of antiphospholipid
11. Antinuclear antibody	An abnormal titer of antinuclear antibody by immunofluorescence or an equivalent assay at any point in time and in the absence of drugs known to be associated with "drug-induced lupus" syndrome

Hochberg MC: Arthritis Rheum 1997; 40:1725.

* The proposed classification is based on 11 criteria. For the purpose of identifying patients in clinical studies, a person shall be said to have systemic lupus erythematosus if any four or more of the 11 criteria are present, serially or simultaneously, during any interval of observation.

Subsets of cutaneous lupus erythematosus

Attempts have been made to group patients into subsets to define more homogeneous groups with a predictable course or response to treatment. Subsets of LE have been defined by cutaneous manifestations present in some form in most patients with lupus.[2] The classification in Table 17-5 divides cutaneous LE into three types on the basis of the clinical appearance of the skin lesion: chronic cutaneous LE (scarring, discoid LE [DLE]), subacute cutaneous LE (SCLE), and acute cutaneous LE (ALE). A comparison of laboratory findings in these subsets is shown in Table 17-6.

An overview of the lupus syndromes appears in the diagram on p. 595.

Table 17-5 Classification of Cutaneous Lupus Erythematosus

Type	Clinical forms	Clinical and laboratory features	Histologic features
DLE, 15%-20%*	Localized Generalized (lesions above and below the neck) Hypertrophic	Usually localized, chronic, scarring lesions of head or neck region or both lasting months to years Usually no extracutaneous disease (5% of patients develop SLE) Antinuclear antibodies occasionally present in low titer; anticytoplasmic antibodies not present Anti-dsDNA antibodies rarely present Subepidermal immunoglobulin deposits commonly found in lesions (75%) but rarely present in uninvolved skin Simultaneous occurrence of severe systemic lupus erythematosus with nephritis is rare	Hydropic degeneration of the epidermal basal cell layer with focal epidermal atrophy Heavy mononuclear cell infiltrate in upper dermis, periappendiceal and perivascular regions, extending into the deep dermis
SCLE, 10%-15%*	Papulosquamous (psoriasiform), 8% Annular-polycyclic, 5%*	Usually widespread, nonscarring lesions with associated scaling, depigmentation, and telangiectasias on face, neck, upper and extensor arms (photosensitive distribution) lasting weeks to months; lesions often exacerbated by exposure to sun Usually associated with extracutaneous disease, but severe renal or central nervous system disease uncommon Antinuclear and anticytoplasmic antibodies frequently present (60% of patients) Anti-dsDNA antibodies present in low serum concentrations in 30% of patients; hypocomplementemia rare HLA-A1, B8, and DR3 significantly increased Subepidermal immunoglobulin deposits present in only 50% of lesions and 30% of uninvolved skin	Marked hydropic changes along epidermal basal cell layer Moderate mononuclear cell infiltrate in superficial dermis only Pilosebaceous atrophy, hyperkeratosis; direct IF staining reveals discrete, speckled IgG deposits in the basal cell cytoplasm associated with Ro/SSA antibodies
Acute cutaneous LE, 30%-50%*	Localized, indurated erythematous lesions (malar areas of face—butterfly rash) Widespread indurated erythema (face, scalp, neck, upper chest, shoulders, extensor arms, backs of hands)	Transient (hours to days) Multisystem disease usually present; renal disease common Antinuclear antibodies usually present Anti-dsDNA antibodies present in 60%–80% of patients, often in high concentration; hypocomplementemia common Subepidermal immunoglobulin deposits commonly found in lesional (>95%) and exposed nonlesional (75%) skin	Hydropic changes along epidermal basal layer Sparse mononuclear cell infiltrate and upper dermal edema

Modified from Gilliam JN, Sontheimer RD: J Am Acad Dermatol 1981; 4:471; and Valesk JE, et al: J Am Acad Dermatol 1992; 27:194.

dsDNA, Double-stranded DNA.

*Estimated percentage incidence in systemic lupus erythematosus.

Table 17-6 Comparison of Laboratory Findings in the Cutaneous Subsets of Lupus Erythematosus

Finding	DLE (%)	SCLE (%)	ALE (%)
ANA titer (≥1:160)	4	63	98
Anti-dsDNA	Rare	30	60–80
ESR greater than 30	Few	59	90
LE cell preparation	2	55	80
Low C3 or CH_{50}	Rare	Rare	90
WBC count less than 4000	7	19	17
Rheumatoid factor latex test positive	15	19	37
Low hemoglobin level	Few	15	50
VDRL biologic false-positive	Few	7	22
Direct immunofluorescence and the lupus band test			
Lesion	90	60	95
Normal sun-exposed	0	46	75
Normal nonexposed	0	26	50

ANA, Antinuclear antibody; *ESR,* erythrocyte sedimentation rate; *LE,* lupus erythematosus; *WBC,* white blood cell; *VDRL,* Venereal Diseases Research Laboratories (test).

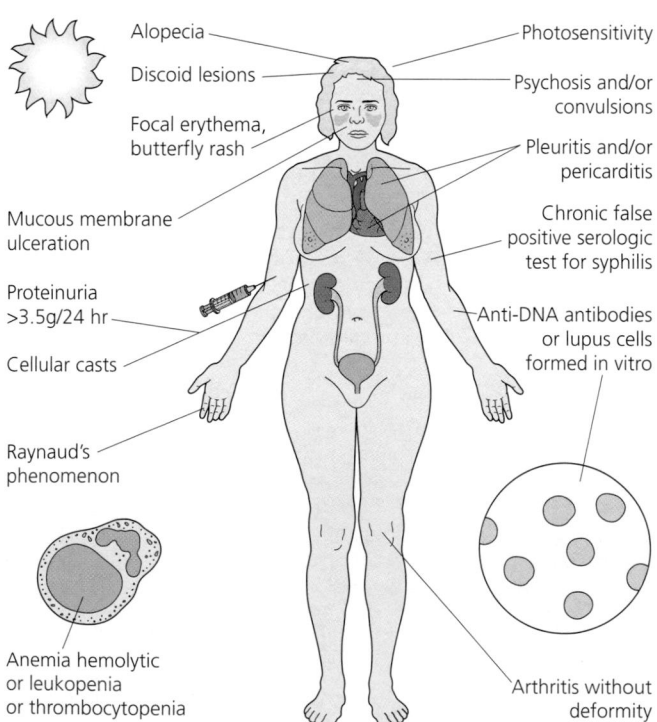

Figure 17-1 Clinical and laboratory characteristics of systemic lupus erythematosus (SLE). *(Modified from American Rheumatism Association [ARA] criteria.)*

OVERVIEW OF LUPUS SYNDROMES:
AUTOANTIBODY PROFILES AND CUTANEOUS MANIFESTATIONS

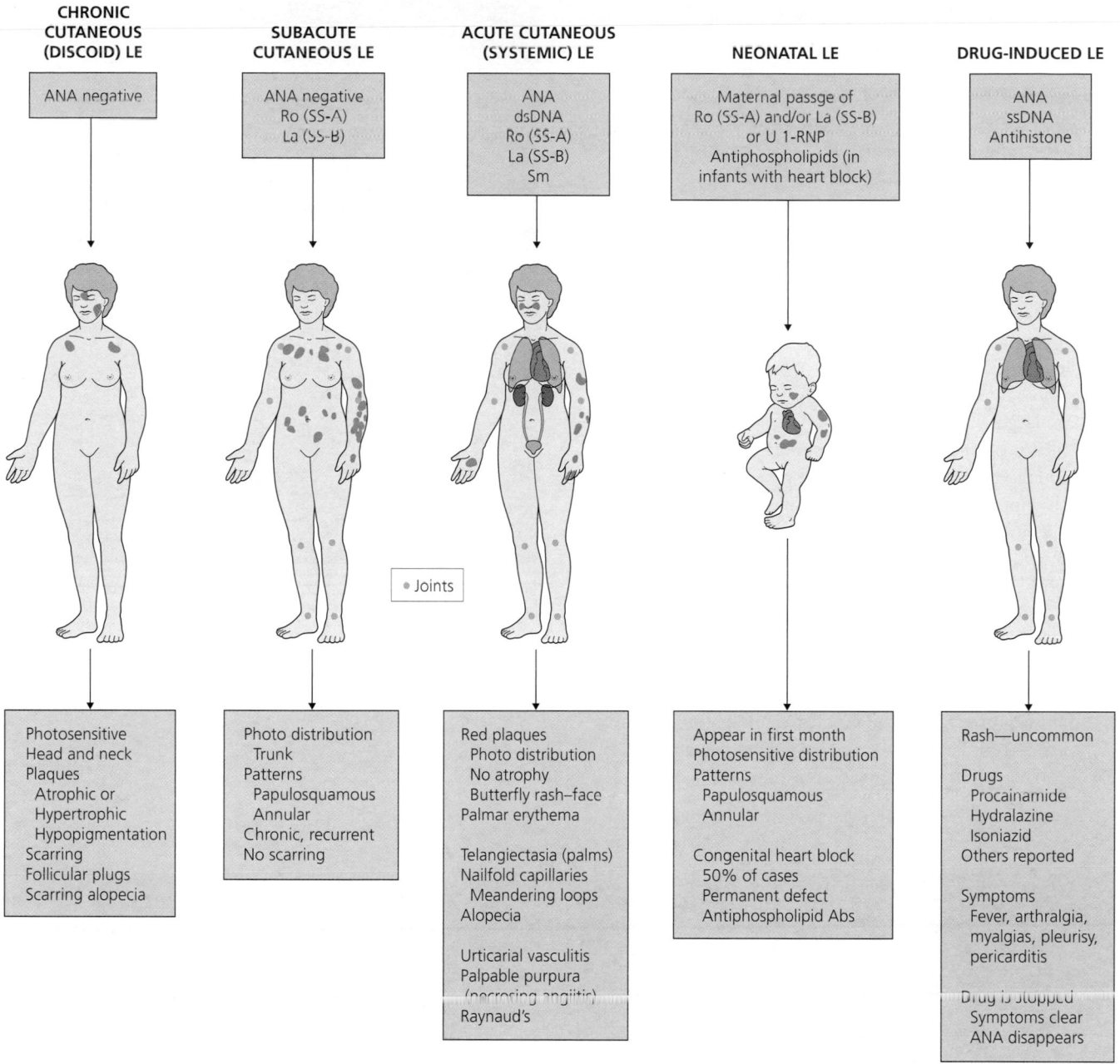

CHRONIC CUTANEOUS (DISCOID) LE

ANA negative

Photosensitive
Head and neck
Plaques
  Atrophic or
  Hypertrophic
  Hypopigmentation
Scarring
Follicular plugs
Scarring alopecia

SUBACUTE CUTANEOUS LE

ANA negative
Ro (SS-A)
La (SS-B)

Photo distribution
  Trunk
Patterns
  Papulosquamous
  Annular
Chronic, recurrent
No scarring

ACUTE CUTANEOUS (SYSTEMIC) LE

ANA
dsDNA
Ro (SS-A)
La (SS-B)
Sm

• Joints

Red plaques
  Photo distribution
  No atrophy
  Butterfly rash–face
Palmar erythema

Telangiectasia (palms)
Nailfold capillaries
  Meandering loops
Alopecia

Urticarial vasculitis
Palpable purpura
(necrosing angiitis)
Raynaud's

NEONATAL LE

Maternal passge of
Ro (SS-A) and/or La (SS-B)
or U 1-RNP
Antiphospholipids (in
infants with heart block)

Appear in first month
Photosensitive distribution
Patterns
  Papulosquamous
  Annular

Congenital heart block
  50% of cases
  Permanent defect
  Antiphospholipid Abs

DRUG-INDUCED LE

ANA
ssDNA
Antihistone

Rash—uncommon

Drugs
  Procainamide
  Hydralazine
  Isoniazid
  Others reported

Symptoms
  Fever, arthralgia,
  myalgias, pleurisy,
  pericarditis

Drug is stopped
  Symptoms clear
  ANA disappears

Chronic cutaneous lupus erythematosus

Patients with DLE have a low incidence of systemic disease. The disease is more common in females, and it has a peak incidence in the fourth decade. Less than 2% of patients with DLE develop the disease before 10 years of age. Trauma and ultraviolet light exposure (UVB) may initiate and exacerbate lesions. There are several clinical variations (Table 17-5).

The most common manifestation is the discoid LE lesion. Lesions are sharply demarcated and can be round, thus giving rise to the term *discoid* (or disclike). The face and scalp are the most commonly affected areas, but lesions may occur on any body surface. Lesions are usually asymmetrically distributed and begin as asymptomatic, well-defined, elevated, red-to-violaceous, 1- to 2-cm, flat-topped plaques with firmly adherent scale (Figure 17-2). The scale penetrates into the orifices of the hair follicle. Peeling the scale reveals an undersurface that has the appearance of a carpet penetrated by several carpet tacks; it is called carpet tack scale (Figure 17-3). Carpet tack scale is most apparent on the face and scalp where the follicular orifices are larger.

Atrophy occurs in both the epidermis and the dermis. Epidermal atrophy occurs early and gives the surface either a smooth white or a wrinkled appearance. Hypopigmentation is particularly disfiguring for blacks (Figure 17-4). Follicular plugs may be prominent (Figure 17-5). These lesions endure for months and either resolve spontaneously or progress with further atrophy, ultimately forming smooth white or hyperpigmented depressed scars with telangiectasia and scarring alopecia.[3,4] Occasionally plaques become thick (hypertrophic DLE). DLE can cover wide areas of the face, causing disfigurement (Figure 17-5). The laboratory and histologic features are outlined in Tables 17-5 and 17-6. The presence of anti-ssDNA occurs with widespread active disease.[5]

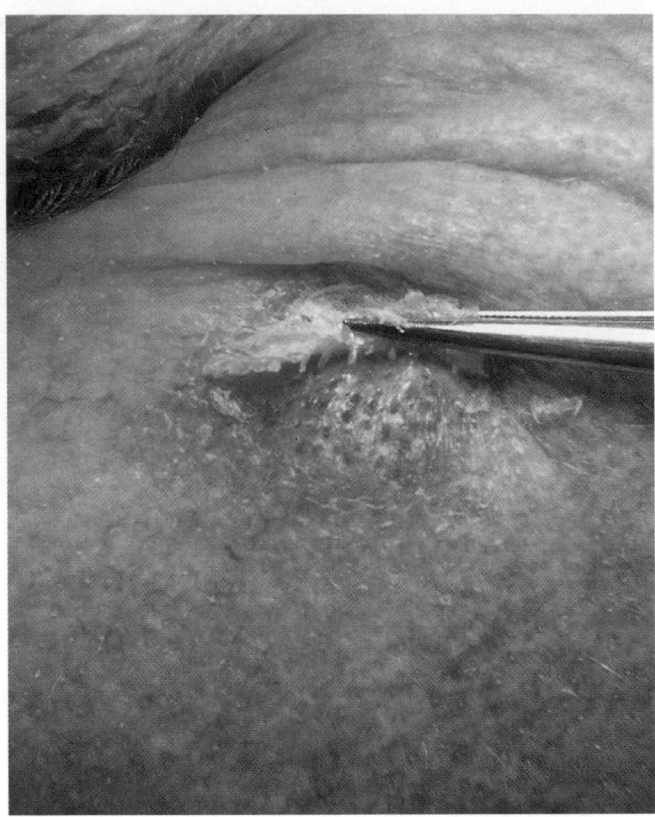

Figure 17-3 Chronic cutaneous LE (discoid LE). Carpet tack scale created by keratin plugs that penetrate deep into the hair follicle.

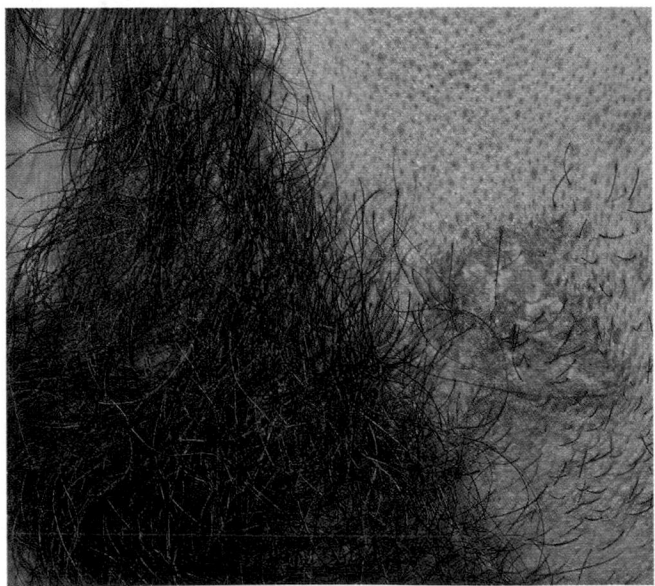

Figure 17-2 Chronic cutaneous LE (discoid LE). An early lesion. Well-defined, elevated, flat-topped plaques with adherent scale.

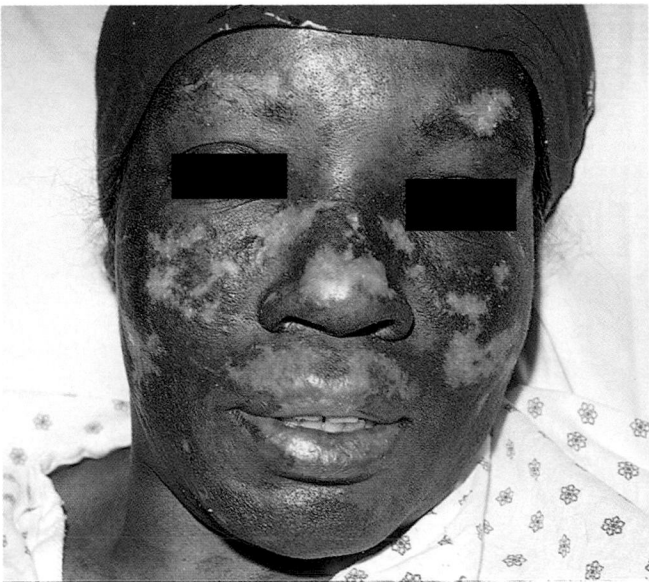

Figure 17-4 Discoid LE is more common in blacks. The typical hypopigmented lesions are disfiguring.

CHRONIC CUTANEOUS LE (DISCOID LE)

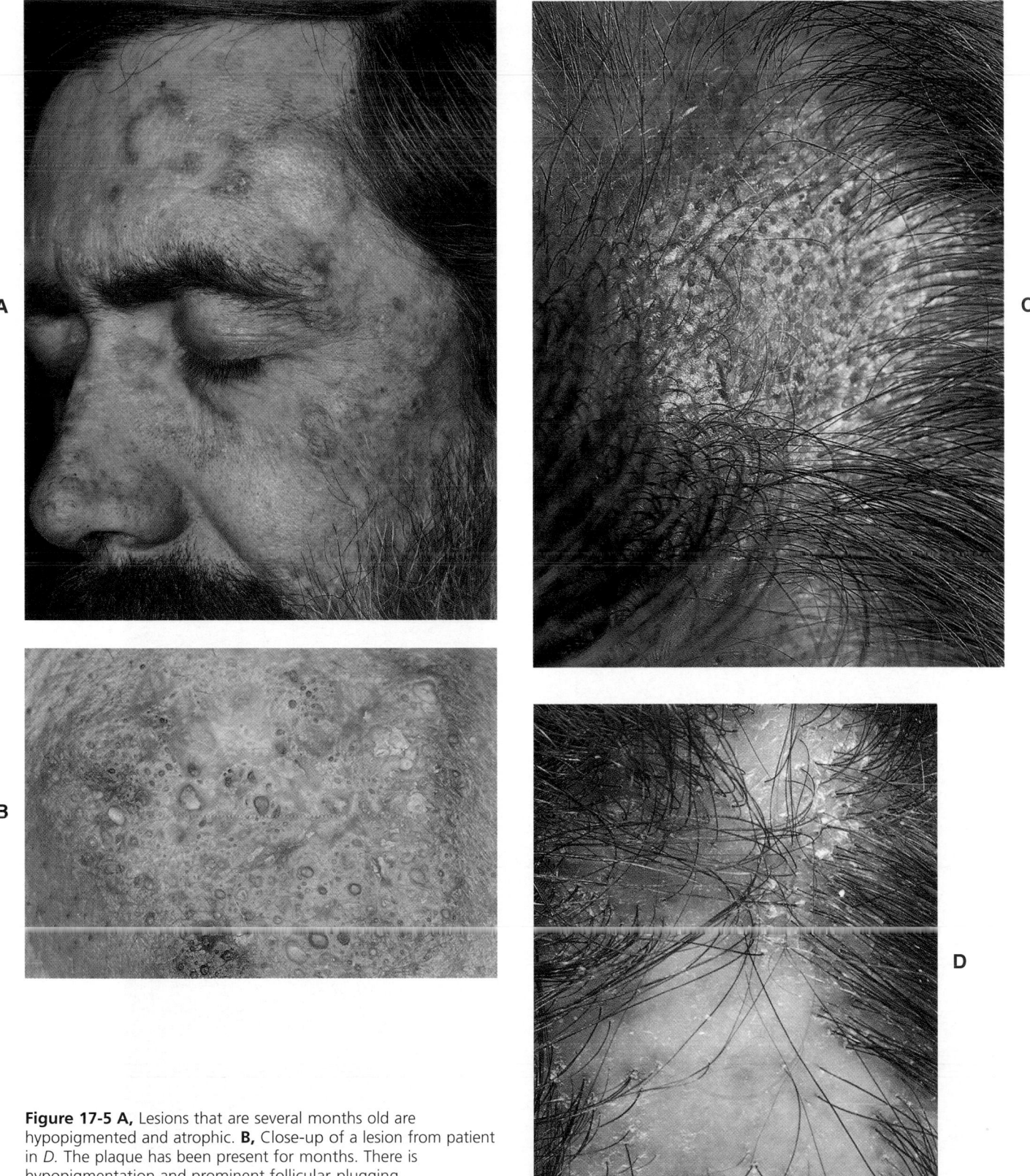

Figure 17-5 A, Lesions that are several months old are hypopigmented and atrophic. **B,** Close-up of a lesion from patient in *D*. The plaque has been present for months. There is hypopigmentation and prominent follicular plugging.
C, Prominent follicular plugging in a plaque of discoid LE located in the scalp. **D,** Scarring alopecia of the scalp; end-stage disease.

Subacute cutaneous lupus erythematosus

Subacute cutaneous lupus erythematosus (SCLE) encompasses the clinical spectrum of cutaneous LE between the chronic, destructive DLE and the erythema of acute cutaneous LE. However, SCLE can be associated with the full spectrum of LE-associated phenomena (Table 17-5). Like DLE, the individual lesions of SCLE may last for months; in contrast to DLE, they heal without scarring. Most patients with SCLE are white females. SCLE may be induced by a variety of drugs, most notably hydrochlorothiazide and calcium channel blockers.

Two morphologic varieties are a papulosquamous pattern (Figure 17-6) and an annular-polycyclic pattern (Figure 17-7). Both occur most often on the trunk; one predominates. The lesions spare the knuckles, the inner aspects of the arms, the axillae, and the lateral part of the trunk.[6] They are rarely seen below the waist. A subtle gray hypopigmentation and telangiectasia are frequently seen in the center of annular lesions, bordered by erythema and a superficial scale. Follicular plugging, adherent hyperkeratosis, scarring, and dermal atrophy that are characteristic of DLE are not prominent features of SCLE. Hypopigmentation and telangiectasia become more evident as individual lesions resolve. The hypopigmentation fades after several months, but the telangiectasia may persist. The disease tends to be chronic and recurrent, lasting for years. SCLE and antibodies to Ro/SSA have been associated with hydrochlorothiazide therapy.[7]

Figure 17-6 Subacute cutaneous LE (papulosquamous pattern). Lesions are confined to exposed areas on the upper half of the body.

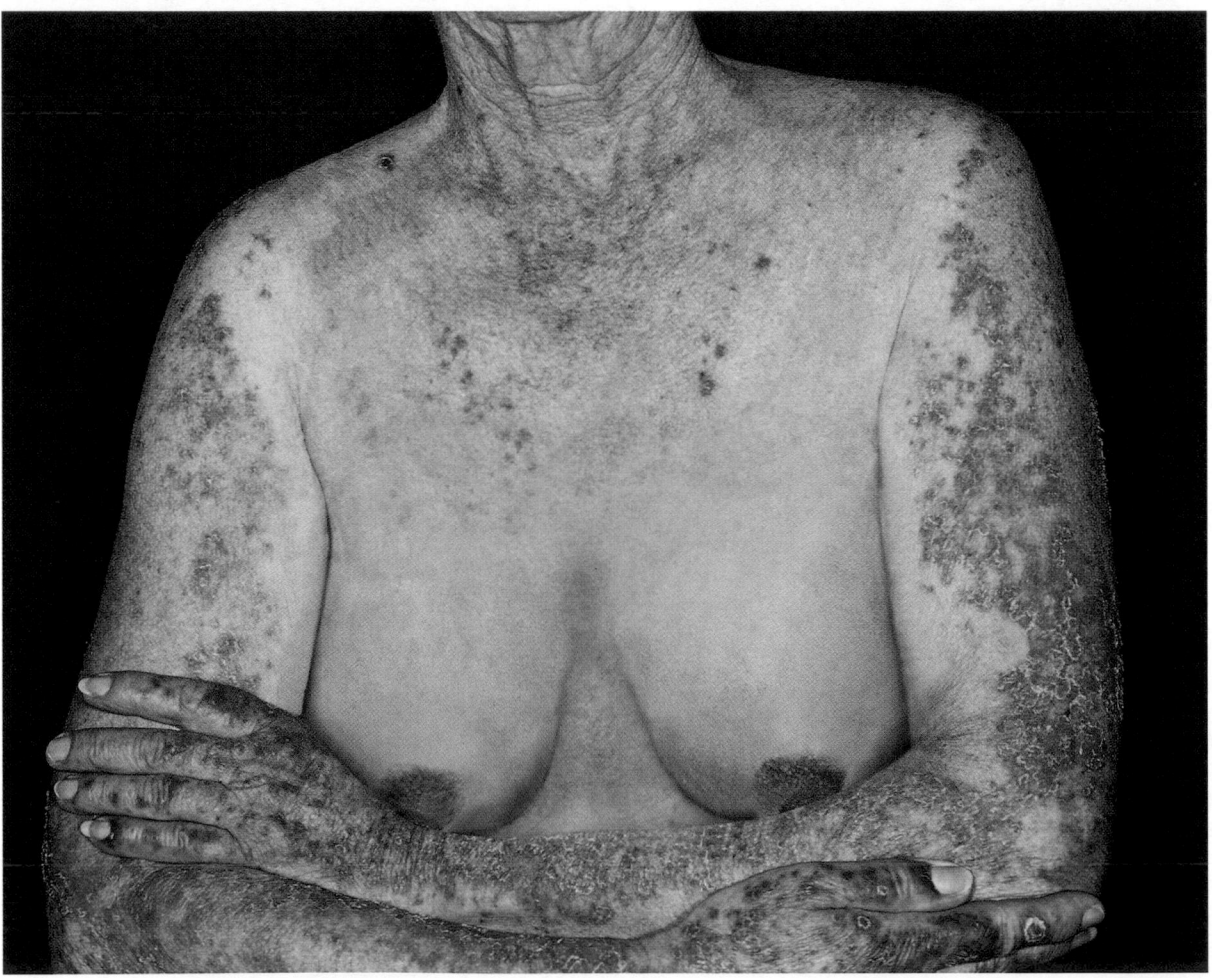

Other dermatologic manifestations are photosensitivity (85% to 52%), periungual telangiectasia (51% to 22%), discoid LE (35% to 19%), and vasculitis (12%).[6,8] Systemic manifestations (arthritis/arthralgia [74% to 43%], renal disease [19% to 11%], serositis [12%], and central nervous system [CNS] symptoms [19% to 6%]) are not severe and follow a benign course.[8]

The laboratory and histologic features of SCLE are outlined in Tables 17-5 and 17-6. Antibodies to Ro/SSA are present in 29% of patients.[8]

Figure 17-7 Subacute cutaneous LE (annular-polycyclic pattern). The annular plaques have an erythematous scaly border, the central area is hypopigmented, and the eruption is confined to the back and hands.

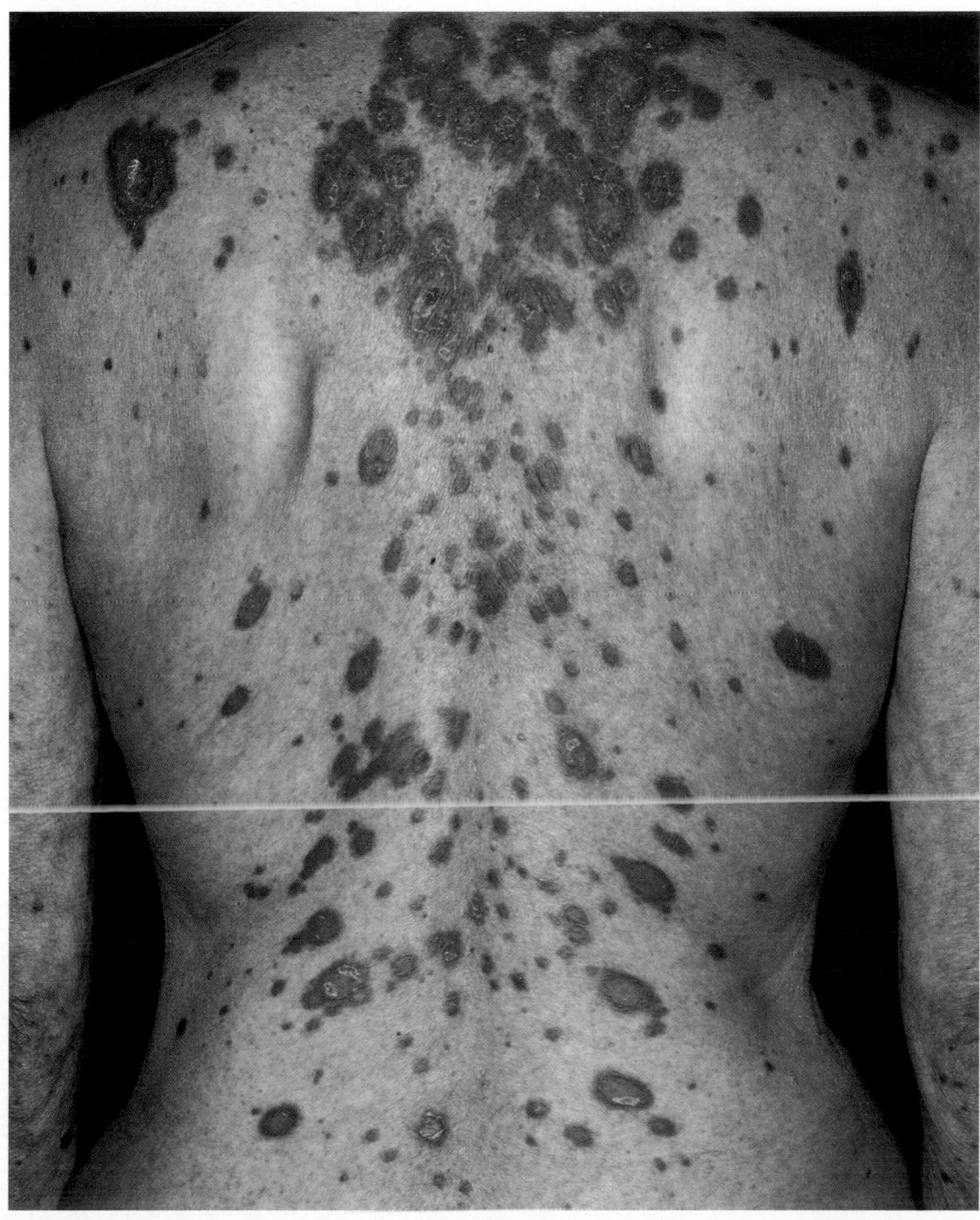

Systemic lupus erythematosus

The rash of systemic lupus erythematosus SLE consists of superficial-to-indurated, nonpruritic, erythematous-to-violaceous plaques; these occur primarily on sun-exposed areas of the face, chest, shoulders, extensor arms, and backs of the hands (see Figure 17-8). There may be fine scaling on the surface, but atrophy does not occur. Superficial erythematous plaques may last for a few days, becoming more intense as disease activity increases and fading with improvement in systemic symptoms. The most indurated hivelike plaques remain relatively fixed in shape and may persist for months. The classic butterfly rash (Figure 17-9) over the malar and nasal area occurs in 10% to 50% of patients with ALE, but it is not the most common cutaneous presentation.

The main causes of morbidity and mortality and the main immunologic parameters in SLE were analyzed for 1,000 patients (female to male ratio, 10:1) in a 5-year multicenter study. Table 17-7 shows the frequencies of the main SLE clinical manifestations during the 5-year study. Table 17-8 shows the frequencies of the clinical manifestations according to the immunologic parameters at the beginning of the study. Table 17-9 shows autoantibodies commonly present in sera of patients with systemic lupus erythematosus.

Oral steroids were used in 65.2%, antimalarial agents in 40.2%, nonsteroidal anti-inflammatory drugs in 28.4%, antiaggregants (mainly aspirin) in 13.6%, azathioprine in 13.1%, pulse cyclophosphamide in 8.5%, oral cyclophosphamide in 7.4%, and anticoagulants (heparin, warfarin, or coumadin) in 6.9%.

The most frequent causes of death were active SLE (28.9%), infections (28.9%), and thromboses (26.7%). Most patients who died of active SLE had progressive frequently multisystemic disease. The most frequent infections were bacterial sepsis of pulmonary (8.9%), abdominal (8.9%), and urinary (6.7%) origin. A survival probability of 95% at 5 years was found.[10]

Table 17-7 Clinical Manifestations Related to SLE

SLE manifestation	Percent
Arthritis	41.3
Malar rash	26.4
Nephropathy	22.2
Photosensitivity	18.7
Fever	13.9
Neurologic involvement	13.6
Raynaud's phenomenon	13.2
Serositis	12.9
Thrombocytopenia	9.5
Oral ulcers	8.9
Thrombosis	7.2
Livedo reticularis	5.5
Discoid lesions	5.4
Subacute cutaneous lesions	4.6
Myositis	4
Hemolytic anemia	3.3

Adapted from Cervera R: Medicine 1999; 78.

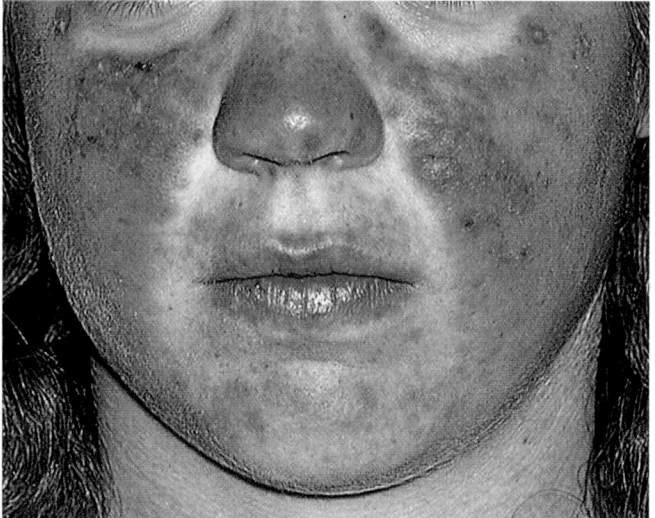

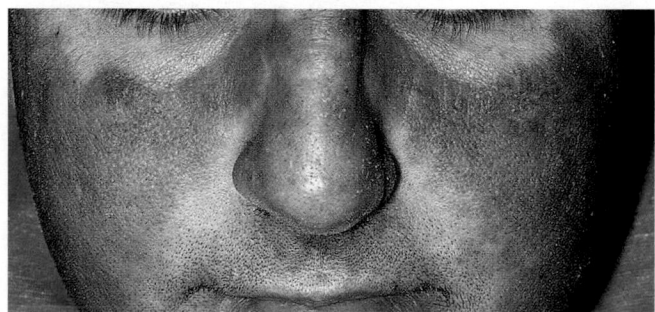

Figure 17-9 Acute cutaneous LE (systemic LE). The classic butterfly rash occurs in 10% to 50% of patients with acute LE.

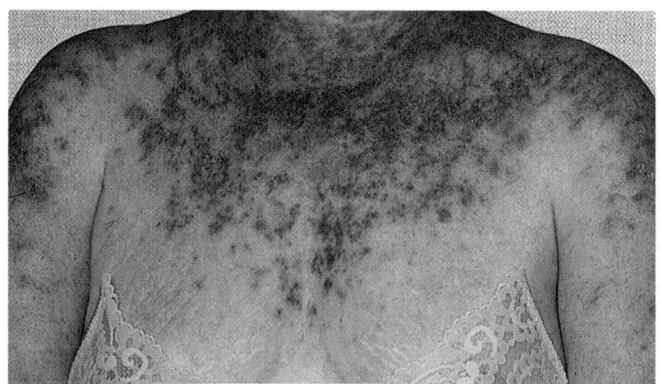

Figure 17-8 Exposure to sun produces a nonpruritic, scaling eruption that does not become atrophic.

Table 17-8 Clinical Manifestations Related to SLE by Autoantibody Pattern

SLE manifestation	High DNA (n = 779)	Ro(SS-A) (n = 254)	La(SS-B) (n = 192)	RNP (n = 131)	RF (n = 180)	IgG aCL (n = 204)	IgM aCL (n = 108)	LA (n = 94)
Arthritis	51	51	38	51	44	34	40	45
Nephropathy	32	24	23	26	15	26	25	26
Malar rash	30	30	25	34	27	21	23	26
Photosensitivity	23	21	19	25	19	20	17	17
Serositis	17	13	15	14	13	11	9	18
Fever	17	16	18	17	12	18	19	19
Raynaud's phenomenon	14	16	13	33	19	11	11	12
Neurologic involvement	12	13	13	10	14	17	14	
Oral ulcers	11	7	8	15	13	10	15	9
Thrombocytopenia	11	7	9	11	6	14	12	25
Thrombosis	7	7	5	8	3	11	8	13
Livedo reticularis	6	5	3	6	10	5	6	3
Hemolytic anemia	5	5	2	6	2	5	8	5
Myositis	5	3	3	8	6	3	4	1
Discoid lesions	4	8	96	12	4	4	6	11
Subacute lesions	4	8	7	10	5	3	5	8

Adapted from Cervera R: Medicine 1999; 78.

Values are percentages. A multicenter prospective study of 1000 patients.

n = Number of patients.

DNA, Deoxyribonucleic acid; *RF,* rheumatoid factor; *RNP,* ribonucleoprotein.

Table 17-9 Autoantibodies Commonly Present in Sera of Patients with Systemic Lupus Erythematosus

Autoantibody	Frequency of occurrence	FANA pattern in Hep-2 cells	Clinical associations
SLE-specific dsDNA	30% to 70% SLE	Nucleoplasmic, homogeneous	Virtually diagnostic of SLE, common in lupus nephritis, in some patients parallels disease activity
Sm	15% to 30% SLE	Nucleoplasmic, coarse speckled	Associated with U1-RNP antibodies
SLE-nonspecific Histones	>95% drug-induced SLE	Nucleoplasmic, homogeneous	Associated with anti-DNA antibodies
Ro/SSA	24% to 60% SLE	Nucleoplasmic, fine speckled	Subacute cutaneous SLE, neonatal lupus syndrome, SLE with C2 and C4 deficiencies
	88% to 96% Sjogren's syndrome		In patients with Sjögren's associated with vasculitis, hypergamma-globulinemia, +RF
	18% PM-DM, 5% PSS, 5% RA		
LA/SSB	9% to 34% SLE	Nucleoplasmic, fine speckled	Present in 90% mothers with infants born with neonatal lupus syndrome
	71% to 87% Sjögren's syndrome		
U1RNP	30% to 40% SLE	Nucleoplasmic, coarse speckled	Often present in association with anti-Sm antibodies
	Almost all patients with MCTD		Features of SLE, scleroderma, or DM-PM

Adapted from Evans J: Clin Chest Med 1998; 19.

FANA, Fluorescent antinuclear antibody; *SLE,* systemic lupus erythematosus; *MCTD,* mixed connective tissue disease; *DM-PM,* dermatomyositis-polymyositis; *RF,* rheumatoid factor; *RA,* rheumatoid arthritis; *PSS,* progressive systemic sclerosis.

Other cutaneous signs of lupus erythematosus

TELANGIECTASIA. Telangiectasia is a prominent feature of connective tissue disease. Telangiectasia occurs on the palms and fingers in association with palmar erythema; it resembles that observed in liver disease and pregnancy (Figures 17-10 and 17-11). Short, linear telangiectasias are a frequent finding in SLE. Using the ophthalmoscope technique described later in this chapter, nailfold capillary microscopy reveals tortuous, "meandering" capillary loops in 53% of patients with SLE.[11] Usually some disorganization of the capillary pattern is present, but avascular areas are rare, and the capillaries are not widened (see Figure 17-22).

ALOPECIA. Alopecia is one of the major features of SLE and occurs in more than 20% of cases. Both scarring and non-scarring alopecia occur. Nonscarring hair loss occurs more frequently in SLE, and scarring alopecia is more common in DLE. In nonscarring alopecia the scalp may show focal or diffuse areas of erythema and scale similar to that seen with seborrheic dermatitis. The hair, especially in the frontal areas, becomes coarse and dry. The fragile, poorly formed shafts break, leaving patches of short, unmanageable hair, called lupus hair. The scalp and hair eventually become normal as disease activity wanes.

URTICARIA. The reported incidence of urticaria or urticaria-like lesions with LE varies between 7% and 28%.[12] Urticaria is the presenting sign in approximately 5% of cases.[13] Clinically, lesions may be indistinguishable from typical hives; but unlike hives, they are usually nonpruritic, persist for days, and remain relatively fixed in position. This clinical presentation is typical of urticarial vasculitis. In most cases a biopsy reveals necrotizing vasculitis, and the lupus band test is generally positive. Therefore the hivelike lesions are probably a result of immune complex deposition rather than a manifestation of allergy.

RAYNAUD'S PHENOMENON. Raynaud's phenomenon is another major diagnostic criterion for SLE. It occurs in 20% or more of SLE patients and may precede other signs and symptoms of SLE by months or years.[15] Progression to digital ulceration is more common in scleroderma.

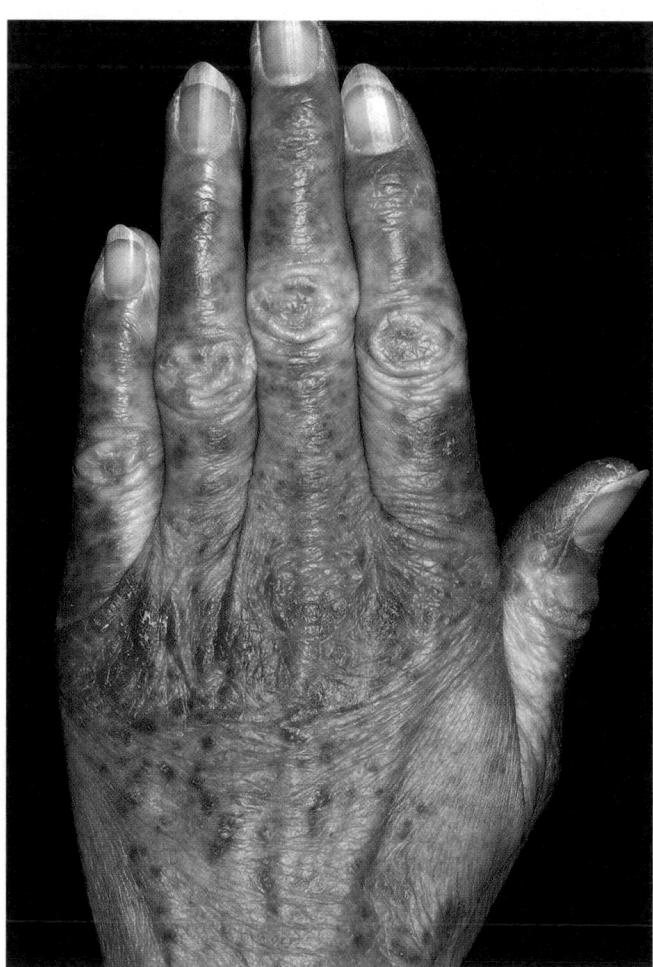

Figure 17-10 Cutaneous LE. In contrast to dermatomyositis, erythema and telangiectasia spare the knuckles.

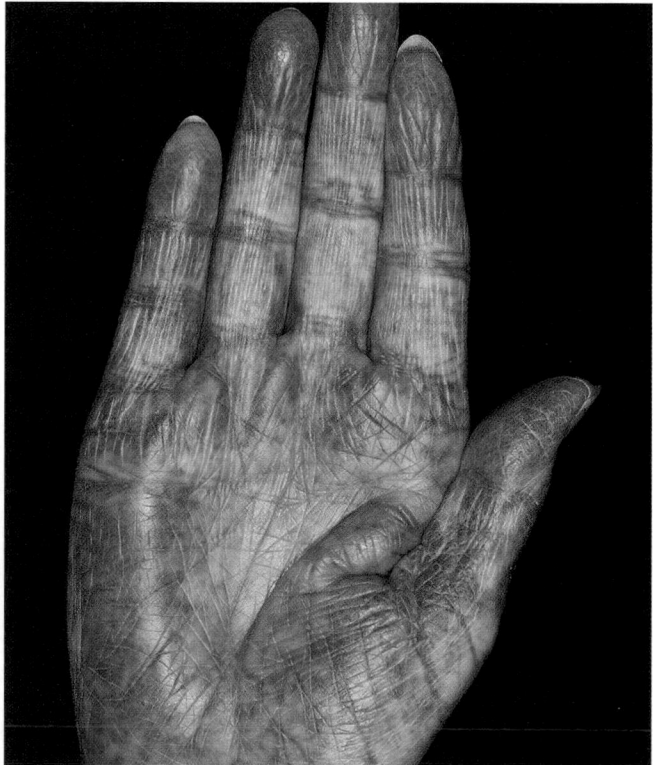

Figure 17-11 Cutaneous LE. Erythema and telangiectasia may appear on the palms.

Drug-induced lupus erythematosus

Many drugs have been reported to cause a syndrome similar to systemic lupus erythematosus. Many patients with probable drug-induced lupus erythematosus (DILE) have the clinical picture and serologic findings typical for lupus.[16,17]

Diagnostic criteria for DILE include:

1. Exposure (3 weeks to 2 years) to a drug suspected to induce DILE
2. No history for SLE prior to the use of the drug therapy
3. Detection of positive ANA with at least one clinical sign of SLE
4. Rapid improvement and gradual fall in the ANA and other serologic findings upon withdrawal of the drug

More than 80 drugs have been associated with DILE. Drugs responsible for the development of DILE can be divided into four groups.

1. Drugs for which there are well-controlled studies and their role for inducing DILE has been documented (hydralazine, procainamide, isoniazid, methyldopa, chlorpromazine, and quinidine).
2. Drugs possibly related to DILE (anticonvulsant agents, antithyroid drugs, penicillamine, sulfasalazine, beta-blockers, and lithium).
3. Drugs suggested as causes for DILE but lacking well-controlled studies (gold salts, penicillin, tetracycline, phenylbutazone, estrogens and oral contraceptives, griseofulvin).
4. Drugs recently reported to induce DILE (minocycline, valproate, calcium-channel blockers, interferon, interleukin-2 [IL-2]).

DRUGS. Procainamide is the most common cause of drug-related lupus in the United States. Up to 80% of patients taking procainamide have a positive ANA test result. Approximately 30% of that group have clinical symptoms. Patients treated with the usual doses of hydralazine have a relatively low incidence of positivity for ANAs and a very low rate of occurrence of the clinical syndrome.[18]

CLINICAL PRESENTATION. Most commonly the onset of symptoms occurs many months after the drug has been initiated. DILE resembles mild SLE. It usually occurs in older age groups; SLE commonly occurs in young women. DILE is characterized by arthralgia and/or arthritis (80% to 90%), myalgia (up to 50%), serositis (pleurisy and pericarditis), fever, hepatomegaly, splenomegaly, and skin manifestation. Arthralgia or arthritis is sometimes the only clinical symptom. The small joints are usually affected. There is no central nervous system involvement.

SKIN MANIFESTATIONS. Skin manifestations appear in 25% to 53% of patients and include lesions compatible with the typical lesions of SLE. Butterfly rash, alopecia, discoid lesions, and mucosal ulcers, are usually absent. Some drugs (e.g., hydrochlorothiazide, captopril, calcium channel blockers, terbinafine) induce skin and clinical symptoms compatible with the diagnosis of subacute cutaneous LE. These include photosensitivity, annular or squamous lesions, and Ro/SS A antibodies.

LABORATORY FINDINGS. ANA is an important marker for DILE. The incidence ranges up to 90% in hydralazine-related DILE, but ANA may be absent. The pattern of ANA is homogeneous or speckled. ANA may persist in falling titers for a long period after halting the implicated drug. Antinuclear antibodies in DILE are fairly specific and mainly directed against histones or single-stranded DNA (ssDNA). The histone antibodies are specific for DILE, but they might be detected in 20% of the patients with SLE. Anemia, leukocytopenia, thrombocytopenia are rarely reported. Involvement of the kidney has been reported in cases treated with D-penicillamine, hydralazine, griseofulvin, procainamide, and anticonvulsants. Acute hepatitis accompanies DILE associated with minocycline. Anti-dsDNA antibodies are absent and serum complement levels are normal. The histologic picture is not specific.

GENETIC FACTORS. A liver acetyltransferase enzyme inactivates some of these drugs. Patients can be categorized as either slow or fast acetylators. The rate of drug acetylation is genetically determined. Rapid acetylators have a much lower incidence of hydralazine-induced DILE. Slow acetylators are at high risk for developing DILE. Acetylation patterns are important for patients treated with hydralazine, procainamide, isoniazid, and sulfonamides.[19] HLA-DR4 and DILE are closely related. Seventy-three percent of patients with hydralazine-related DILE have HLA-DR4.

PROGNOSIS. DILE is a mild form of SLE. DILE resolves in weeks and rarely in years after drug withdrawal. The ANA level typically remains elevated after symptoms have resolved on an average of 4 months. Acute severe hepatitis sometimes occurs in patients with DILE secondary to minocycline.

TREATMENT. DILE does not usually require treatment. Patients with pericarditis, pleural effusions, or pulmonary infiltrates often require prednisone. They respond quickly, and prednisone can be tapered and then discontinued over a few months.[20] Symptomatic patients may also respond to antimalarial agents.

Neonatal lupus erythematosus

Neonatal LE (NLE) is a rare disorder caused by transplacental autoantibodies from the mother to the fetus. This syndrome is characterized by one or more of the following findings: subacute cutaneous lupus-like annular and polycyclic lesions, congenital heart block, cardiomyopathy, cholestatic hepatitis, and thrombocytopenia.[21] Connective tissue disease may develop in adulthood. NLE is caused by the transplacental passage of maternal IgG anti-Ro/SSA and/or anti-La/SSB or anti-U1RNP.[22] Most babies of mothers with anti-Ro/SSA, anti-La/SSB, or anti-U1RNP autoantibodies do not develop NLE. There is no way to determine which fetus or infant will be affected. Anti-Ro/SSA are the predominant autoantibodies, and are found in approximately 95% of cases.[22]

The skin lesions (present in approximately 50% of affected infants) usually appear within the first month of life and may be initiated by sun exposure. Lesions present with plaques of erythema with central atrophy. A periorbital "owl-eye" or "eye mask" facial rash is common. Lesions appear on the, scalp (Figure 17-12), arms and legs, trunk, and groin. Crusted lesions predominated in male infants.[23] The lesions heal without scarring or atrophy within 6 months.[24] The autoantibodies disappear with the rash. The congenital heart block (present in approximately 50% of affected infants) is a permanent defect that develops in utero during the late second and the third trimesters of pregnancy. Many babies require pacemakers, and approximately 10% die of complications related to cardiac disease. The proposed cause is that the anti-Ro/SSA antibody binds with an autoantigen in the heart and produces an inflammatory process, resulting in fibrotic replacement and destruction of one or more of the following: the sinoatrial bundle, the atrioventricular bundle, or the bundle of His.[25]

Approximately 50% of mothers have clinical features of either Sjögren's syndrome or LE at the time of birth, but more than 85%, with time, demonstrate the onset of sicca symptoms (dry eyes, dry mouth) and/or joint stiffness, arthralgias, or swelling.[26] Of anti-Ro/SSA-positive patients, 90% to 95% possess either the HLA-DR2 or -DR3 phenotype.[27] Of lupus patients with abnormal fetal heart rate, 100% have antibodies to phospholipids (lupus anticoagulant).

MANAGEMENT. Two lesional skin biopsies are taken: one for hematoxylin and eosin and the other for immunofluorescence. The finding of anti-Ro/SSA antibody in the infant and mother confirms the diagnosis. Mothers are advised that the risk of a similarly affected infant in subsequent pregnancies is approximately 25%.[26] Patients with heart block may be asymptomatic or require pacemakers.

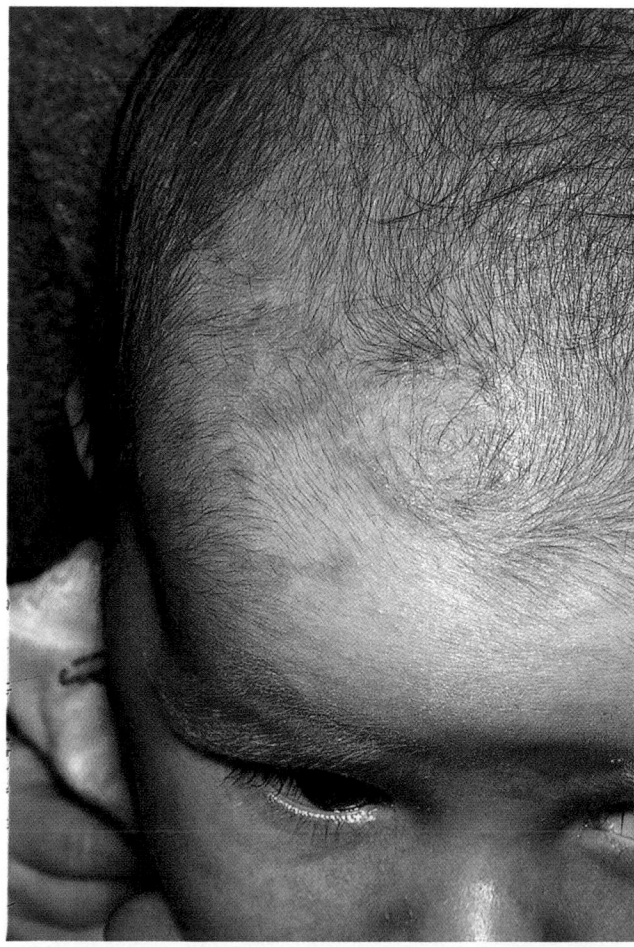

Figure 17-12 Neonatal lupus. Annular erythematous plaques with a slight scale usually appear on the head slightly after birth. Sun exposed areas of the arms and trunk may also be involved. Telangiectasia is often prominent. Skin lesions resolve with time.

Diagnosis and management of cutaneous lupus erythematosus

Lupus is an uncommon disease that has been described extensively in the medical literature and in the lay press. Some patients are familiar with the term and fear the worst when informed of their diagnosis. They should be assured that the disease in the majority of patients can be controlled with existing therapy, but that periodic clinical and laboratory evaluations are necessary to monitor disease activity.

Management consists of defining the type of cutaneous subset, performing a physical examination to document systemic symptoms, obtaining a battery of relevant blood studies as a baseline for diagnosis and later comparison as disease activity changes (Box 17-1), obtaining a biopsy specimen of lesional skin for routine histologic studies and immunofluorescence, and, if appropriate, obtaining a biopsy specimen of nonlesional skin for immunofluorescence and topical and/or systemic treatment. A discussion of systemic symptom management is beyond the scope of this book.

LABORATORY STUDIES. A compilation of some of the studies used for the evaluation of LE is listed in the Box 17-1. Patients with chronic cutaneous LE but without evidence of systemic disease should have a similar evaluation for documentation, because a few of these patients may later develop SLE. A comparison of the laboratory findings in the cutaneous subsets of LE is found in Table 17-6. Changes in values of some of these tests may reflect changes in disease activity.

Box 17-1 Workup for Suspected Cutaneous Lupus Erythematosus (DLE, SCLE, SLE)

History and physical examination
Skin lesion biopsy for histologic studies
CBC, ESR, platelet count
ANA
Anti-nDNA
Anti-RNP (U1RNP)
Anti-Ro (SS-A), Anti-La (SS-B), SM
Serologic tests
Urinalysis

Optional tests

Serum protein electrophoresis
Circulating immune complexes
Immunofluorescence skin biopsy
Antiphospholipid antibodies
Total hemolytic complement (if abnormal, C3, C2, C4 levels)
Creatinine clearance

ANTINUCLEAR AND ANTICYTOPLASMIC ANTIBODIES. The production of antinuclear and anticytoplasmic antibodies is a fundamental characteristic of LE. Numerous diverse antibodies are produced, and most laboratories have access to facilities that can measure the antibodies listed in Table 17-2. Measurement of these antibodies provides valuable information for diagnosis and prognosis. Quantitative measurement of some of these antibodies, such as anti–double-stranded DNA, can be made, and changes in levels assist in determining disease activity.

Measurement of ANA was the first test available for directly measuring antinuclear antibodies in a qualitative and quantitative manner. The test is positive in the vast majority of patients with LE (see Tables 17-1, 17-3, and 17-5) and is an important screening test.

The ANA test is a nonspecific test that detects many types of antinuclear antibodies. The significance of titers varies with different laboratories, but generally titers below 1:16 are believed to be negative, whereas titers above 1:64 indicate possible SLE. Extremely high titers such as 1:32,000 may be found. Unfortunately the titer level or change of titer has not been a reliable indicator of disease activity.

ANTINUCLEAR ANTIBODY PATTERNS. The pattern of the ANA may correlate with specific antibodies, but interpretation of patterns should be attempted only by experts.

SKIN BIOPSY. A biopsy of skin lesions provides important diagnostic information. The histologic characteristics are listed in Table 17-5.

Lupus band test. The term lupus band test (LBT) refers to direct immunofluorescence examination of normal sun-protected, normal sun-exposed, or lesional skin. Deposits of one or more immunoglobulins are found at the dermoepidermal junction and in the walls of dermal vessels in patients with DLE, SCLE, and SLE. Immunofluorescence may be helpful when the diagnosis is in question. Antibody testing has reduced the need for immunofluorescence testing.

Treatment

SUNSCREENS. Photosensitivity is a major factor in all types of cutaneous LE. Sunlight in the ultraviolet-B (UVB) and ultraviolet-A (UVA) regions can induce and exacerbate all forms of lupus erythematosus. Patients should avoid direct exposure to sunlight, particularly during the summer and between the hours of 10 AM and 3 PM and exposure through window glass.[28] Broad-spectrum sunscreens with a sun protection factor of maximum value (greater than 15) that block UVB and UVA light should be applied if sun exposure is anticipated. Zinc oxide and titanium dioxide containing sunscreen block UVA and UVB light. Patients should be encouraged to apply sunscreens as a routine procedure after morning washing during the summer months.

TOPICAL CORTICOSTEROIDS. Topical corticosteroids are the agents of first choice for all forms of cutaneous LE. Groups I through V topical steroids are required to control DLE. They may be applied three times a day to all active lesions, including those on the face. Patients should be encouraged to restrict application to the active lesion and to avoid normal surrounding skin. Lesions of SCLE and ALE may be treated with groups III through V topical steroid applied three times a day. Those who do not respond should be advanced to group II topical steroids. Discontinue treatment when lesions have cleared.

INTRALESIONAL CORTICOSTEROIDS. DLE lesions that are resistant to topical steroids may be managed well with periodic intralesional injections of steroids (e.g., equal parts of 1% Xylocaine or saline and triamcinolone acetonide [Kenalog] 10 mg/mL). Lesions frequently become inactive after a single injection and may remain in remission for months. The steroid should be injected with a 27- or 30-gauge needle with sufficient solution to blanch the lesion—approximately 0.1 mL/1.0 cm lesion.

ANTIMALARIAL AGENTS. The antimalarial agents remain the cornerstone of treatment because of their effectiveness and safety. They are effective in the treatment of all forms of cutaneous LE. The recommended safe and effective dosage for an individual weighing 150 pounds is 200 mg of hydroxychloroquine (Plaquenil) twice a day.[29] Patients can be maintained on this dosage as long as needed, but they should have periodic eye evaluations. Antimalarial agents are maintained at the recommended dosages until the lesions resolve. They are then reduced to the lowest possible dosage to maintain control. Patients with quiescent SLE who are taking hydroxychloroquine are less likely to have a clinical flare-up if they are maintained on the drug. The discontinuation of treatment in patients with quiescent disease is associated with a 2.5-fold increase in the risk of new clinical manifestations or, in the case of previous manifestations, a recurrence or an increase in severity.[30]

Patients with cutaneous LE who smoke are significantly less likely to respond to antimalarial therapy.[31]

Antimalarial ocular toxicity. Fear of retinal toxicity resulted in a substantial reduction in the use of antimalarial drugs, but it was later discovered that excessive daily dosages influenced retinal damage. No cases of retinopathy have been reported when the dose of hydroxychloroquine did not exceed 6.5 mg/kg/day and with therapy that did not extend longer than 10 years.[32] By performing serial testing of the foveal reflex and of the reaction of visual fields to red targets,[33] the ophthalmologist can detect a state of "premaculopathy." While the patient is on therapy, premaculopathy is defined as the loss of foveal reflex or the development of paracentral scotomata to red test objects. It is a state of functional loss that is reversible by discontinuation of the drug. Testing is done before treatment and every 12 to 18 months during therapy. The package insert recommends baseline screening and follow-up eye examinations every 3 months. Screening at such intervals is unlikely to be cost-effective at the recommended dosage when a patient has had less than 10 years of therapy. Patients taking high doses of antimalarial agents or with decreased renal function need more frequent examinations. Visual field testing can be performed by Amsler grid. It is simple, inexpensive, and easily administered at home by the patient and can screen for shallow relative paracentral scotomas.[32]

DAPSONE. Antimalarial agents are the drugs of first choice for cutaneous LE when topical steroids have failed. Dapsone (initial dosage 100 mg/day) is an effective alternative for all forms of cutaneous LE.[34–39] The dosage is adjusted after evaluation of clinical response and side effects. Dapsone therapy is described on p. 557.

ORAL CORTICOSTEROIDS. Occasionally patients with cutaneous LE do not respond to topical steroids, antimalarial agents, or dapsone. Such patients should discontinue other forms of therapy and begin prednisone at dosages high enough to control the disease (e.g., 20 mg twice a day), until control is obtained. Oral steroids are then tapered and discontinued; the patient is once more given a trial of conventional therapy.

OTHER TREATMENTS. Azathioprine (100 to 150 mg/day),[40–42] methotrexate,[43] thalidomide (50 to 300 mg/day),[44] and acitretin (50 mg/day)[45] are effective for severe, chloroquine-resistant DLE. Isotretinoin (1 mg/kg/day) is reported to be effective for patients with DLE and SCLE.[46]

Dermatomyositis and Polymyositis

Dermatomyositis (DM) and polymyositis (PM) are rare inflammatory muscle diseases.[47,48] The term *polymyositis* is reserved for cases in which skin inflammation is absent. Although patients of any age may be affected, most patients are either children or adults older than 40 years of age. Adult DM can be associated with malignancy and collagen vascular diseases. The clinical picture varies considerably, and the following classification and diagnostic criteria (Box 17-2) of the idiopathic inflammatory myopathies have been suggested.[49,50]

Classification of idiopathic inflammatory myopathies

Group I	PM
Group II	DM
Group III	PM or DM with malignancy
Group IV	Childhood PM or DM
Group V	PM or DM associated with collagen-vascular disease

Polymyositis

Symmetric proximal muscular weakness, especially of the hips and thighs, is characteristic of PM. The onset is insidious; patients first note difficulty rising from a chair. Neck muscles are commonly involved, leading to weakness in raising the head ("drooped head"). Dysfunction of the pharyngeal muscles may lead to dysphagia and aspiration pneumonia. Respiratory muscles of the chest wall can be involved. Distal strength is usually preserved. Myalgias can occur, and tenderness is uncommon. Arthralgias are a presenting sign in 41% of patients.[51] Weakness progresses over weeks to months;

spontaneous remission may occur. Deep tendon reflexes remain normal, and atrophy occurs late in the course of the disease. The muscle changes are indistinguishable from those seen in DM.

Dermatomyositis

The associated features of PM may precede by months, accompany, or follow the skin signs. Proximal muscle weakness is the most common presenting manifestation; the rash is present in 40% of patients when they are first evaluated.[52,53] The cutaneous changes sometimes precede the onset of muscle weakness by more than a year.[54] The course of adult DM may be acute, chronic, recurrent, or cyclic. DM tends to be a more severe disease than PM,[54] with a more severe myopathy. DM occurs in all age groups and equally in males and females. Malignancy seems to be associated with skin disease. Malignancy occurs in patients with dermatomyositis who do not have muscle disease, but the incidence of malignancy is not increased in patients with the muscle disease alone (i.e., polymyositis).

AMYOPATHIC DERMATOMYOSITIS. The term *amyopathic dermatomyositis* has been applied to three groups of patients: those with cutaneous changes only, those with cutaneous changes only at baseline with subsequent development of myositis, and those with cutaneous changes with normal muscle enzyme serum levels at baseline but with myositis demonstrated by electromyography and/or muscle biopsy specimens.[55,56,57]

DERMATOLOGIC MANIFESTATIONS. There are six dermatologic features of DM: the pathognomonic heliotrope, Gottron's papules, a photosensitive violaceous eruption, periungual telangiectasia, poikiloderma, and scaly red scalp.

Heliotrope erythema of eyelids. Heliotrope erythema of the eyelids (heliotrope: violet color) is a term used to describe the violaceous discoloration around the eyes (Figure 17-13). It is a pathognomonic sign of DM. Periorbital edema and violet discoloration may be either the earliest cutaneous sign or a residual finding as diffuse erythema fades.

Box 17-2 Diagnostic Criteria for Dermatomyositis and Polymyositis

Major criteria

Proximal symmetric muscle weakness

Compatible muscle biopsy

Myopathy or inflammatory myositis

Elevated skeletal muscle enzymes (e.g., CPK, aldolase, SGOT)

Compatible dermatologic features

Exclusion of other disorders causing myopathy

Neurologic disease

Muscular dystrophies

Infections

Toxins

Endocrinopathies

Confidence limits

Definite PM: three or four criteria (DM + rash)

Probable PM: two criteria (DM + rash)

Possible PM: one criterion (DM + rash)

Modified from Bohan A, et al: Medicine 1977; 56:255; and Callen JP: Dis Mon 1987; 33:237.

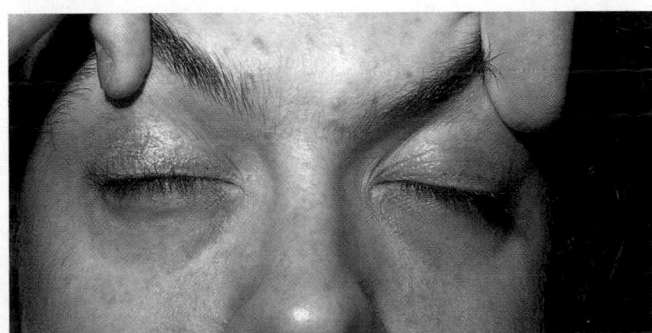

Figure 17-13 Dermatomyositis. Heliotrope (violaceous) discoloration around the eyes and periorbital edema.

DERMATOMYOSITIS

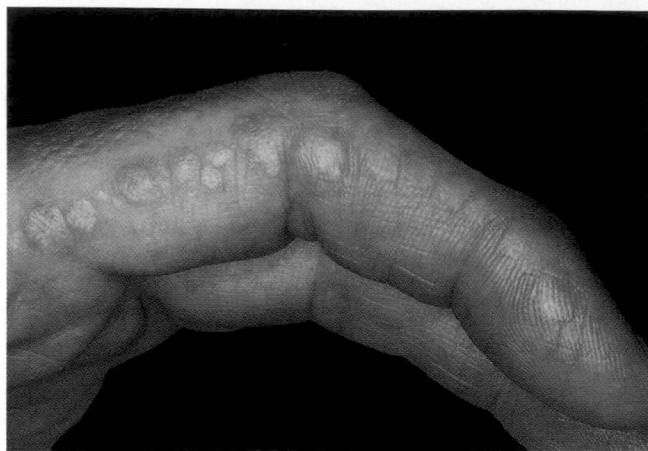

Figure 17-14 Gottron's papules, a pathognomonic sign of dermatomyositis, are round, smooth, violaceous-to-red, flat-topped papules that occur over the knuckles and along the sides of the fingers.

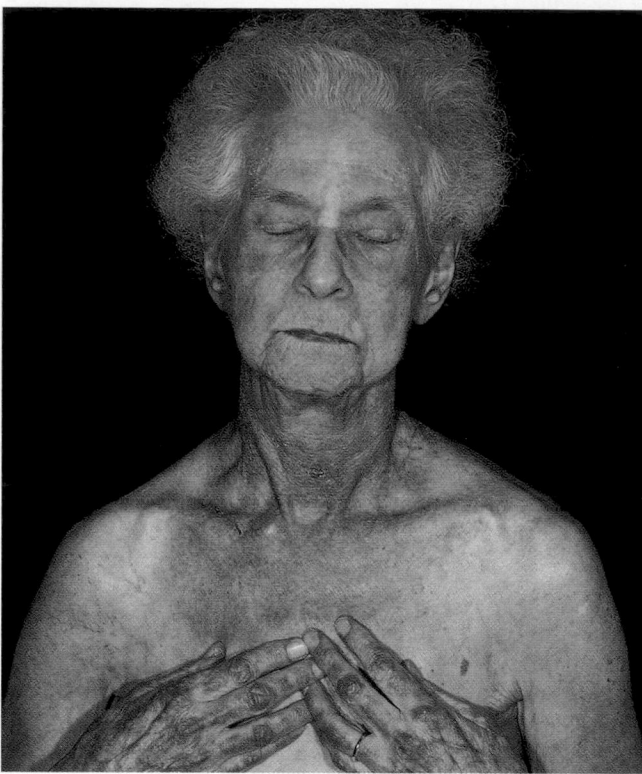

Figure 17-15 Violaceous scaling patches on the face and dorsal interphalangeal joints. The knuckles are involved; they are spared in SLE.

Figure 17-16 Violaceous erythema and Gottron's papules may occur over the knuckles and spare the skin over the phalanges.

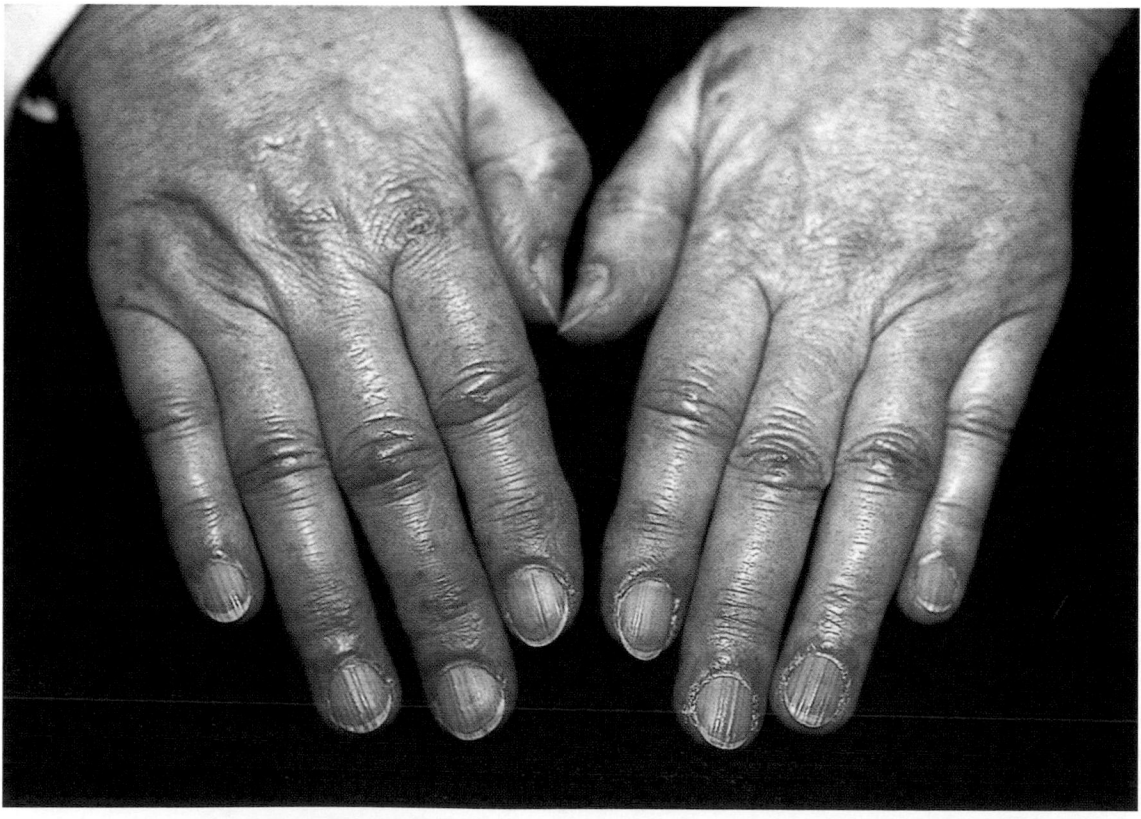

Gottron's papules. Gottron's papules, a pathognomonic sign of DM, are round, 0.2- to 1-cm, smooth, violaceous-to-red, flat-topped papules that occur over the knuckles, along the sides of the fingers (Figure 17-14), and sometimes over the knees and elbows. Lupus of the back of the hand usually spares the knuckles (see Figure 17-10). Several lesions appear simultaneously any time during the course of the disease; they tend to remain fixed in position. Approximately 60% to 80% of DM patients have Gottron's papules sometime during the course of the disease.

Violaceous scaling patches. A characteristic violet erythema with or without scaling occurs in a localized or diffuse distribution. The localized eruption appears symmetrically over bony prominences such as the knees, elbows, and interphalangeal joints (Figures 17-15 and 17-16). DM typically involves the knuckles and spares the skin over the phalanges (see Figure 17-16). The distribution is reversed in SLE when the skin over the phalanges is involved and the knuckles are spared (see Figure 17-10). The diffuse form begins as a patchy, diffuse, dusky-red or violet erythema of the sun-exposed areas of the face, neck, back, and arms and later may involve the buttocks and legs. Over time the rash becomes confluent, and involved areas become minimally raised and slightly scaly. A diffuse, deep red erythema (malignant erythema) may appear superimposed on the existing eruption in patients with an evolving malignancy. Photosensitivity is common. The rash tends to be confined to sun-exposed areas and is worse after sun exposure.

Periungual erythema and telangiectasia. Clinically these are similar to those seen in other connective tissue diseases. The telangiectasia is most prominent on the proximal nailfold and appears as irregular, red, linear streaks (Figure 17-17). Nailfold capillary microscopy using the ophthalmoscope (see Figure 17-23) reveals a pattern identical to that seen in scleroderma but quite different from that seen in SLE. Therefore this technique may help to distinguish DM from SLE. The cuticles are thick, rough, hyperkeratotic, and irregular (moth-eaten appearance).

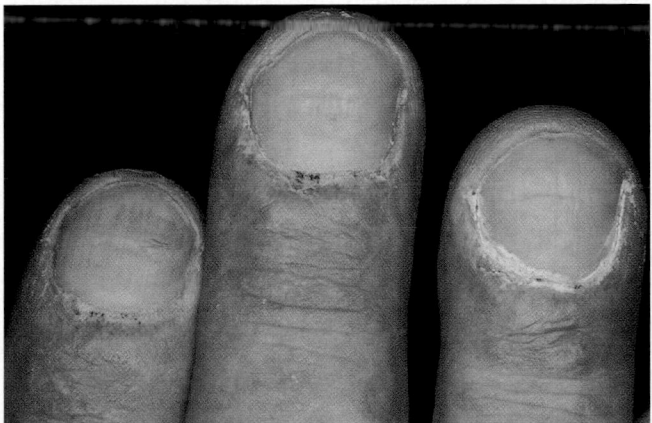

Figure 17-17 Dermatomyositis. Periungual erythema and telangiectasia similar to that seen in other connective tissue diseases.

Poikiloderma. Late in the course of the disease, as the erythema fades, a highly characteristic pattern may occur in the same sun-exposed areas occupied by the diffuse erythema. Poikiloderma is a descriptive term for the pattern that consists of finely mottled white areas and brown pigmentation, telangiectasia, and atrophy. Poikiloderma also occurs as an isolated phenomenon with mycosis fungoides and other rare dermatologic conditions.

Scaly red scalp. Scalp scaling may be a sign of DM. Erythematous, scaly, atrophic scalp lesions initially diagnosed as psoriasis, seborrheic dermatitis, or lupus erythematosus were reported in a series of patients with DM.[58]

DIFFERENTIAL DIAGNOSIS. A diagnosis of psoriasis might be made if scale forms on poikilodermatous patches especially if there is no photodistribution. T-cell lymphoma or lupus might be confused with poikiloderma. Differential diagnoses of early skin lesions include polymorphic light eruption, contact dermatitis, and atopic dermatitis.

DERMATOMYOSITIS WITH MALIGNANCY. There is an increased incidence of malignancy in adult DM and PM.[59,60] Therefore PM/DM may occur as a paraneoplastic syndrome. This association appears to correspond most closely with the dermatologic manifestations, as it occurs in patients with dermatomyositis who do not have muscle disease, but the incidence of malignancy is lower in patients with the muscle disease alone (i.e., polymyositis). The incidence of malignancy in patients with dermatomyositis without myositis corresponds to that seen in patients with fully developed dermatomyositis. The association is largely with malignant neoplasms diagnosed at or before the time of diagnosis of PM and DM.[61] Therefore steps aimed at early cancer detection and treatment must be taken. Patients older than 50 years of age are at greatest risk. The cancer incidence declines steadily with increasing years since initial diagnosis of PM/DM. The cancer risk is increased approximately sixfold during the first year, but is lower during the second year, with no significant excesses in subsequent years of follow-up.[62] Therefore among long-term survivors of PM/DM, there is little evidence to warrant extensive preventive and screening measures after 2 years. Tumors may appear at any site, but significant excesses are observed for cancers of lung, ovary, lymphatic and hematopoietic systems, and nasopharyngeal areas. In 30% of patients the tumor appeared first, and symptoms of DM subsequently appeared, with a mean interval of 16 months. The rash and symptoms of DM may clear following resection of the tumor. Recurrence of dermatomyositis may indicate the occurrence of a second primary malignancy or recurrent cancer.

CHILDHOOD DERMATOMYOSITIS. Juvenile dermatomyositis is characterized by a nonsuppurative myositis that causes symmetric weakness, rash, and vasculitis affecting the gastrointestinal tract and the myocardium.[63] Skin lesions are similar to those in adult dermatomyositis. The female-to-male ratio is 2:1. The average of onset is 7.8 years.

Calcinosis of subcutaneous tissue (occurs in approximately two thirds of patients and is complicated by recurrent infections),[64] muscle atrophy, residual proximal weakness, contractures, Raynaud's phenomenon, and arthritis are possible late sequelae.[65] Approximately 50% of children have a very acute, rapidly progressive disease, whereas the remainder present subacutely with rash and a gradually progressive weakness of muscles, joint contractures, and, very infrequently, calcinosis.[66] The course of treated patients is variable: 25% are well in 2 years, 31% experience recurrences when steroids are stopped after remission, and 44% have continuous disease for more than 2 years despite continual corticosteroid therapy.[67]

Elevations in erythrocyte sedimentation rate, lactate dehydrogenase, and aspartate aminotransferase (AST) occur commonly. Elevations in creatine kinase (CK) and aldolase may be delayed, especially in patients who demonstrate gradual onset of disease. Therefore serial laboratory values are recommended.[68] The creatine phosphokinase concentration is elevated when there is acute muscle damage; antinuclear antibodies are usually present. The clinical course, incidence of calcinosis, and survival improve significantly with intensive early therapy with corticosteroids and physical therapy; as many as 92% survive and as many as 85% are functionally normal after 5 years.[69] The incidence of cancer is low. Death can occur in the acute phase due to myocarditis, progressive unresponsive myositis, perforation of the bowel as a sequel to vasculitis ulceration, or, occasionally, lung involvement. Muscle biopsy specimens studied by electron microscopy show tuboreticular inclusions.[68]

OVERLAP SYNDROMES. Myositis may occur during the course of other connective tissue diseases such as scleroderma, rheumatoid arthritis, and LE. The most common association is with scleroderma and is termed *sclerodermatomyositis.* Sclerodermatomyositis is a distinct overlap syndrome, with features of SLE, scleroderma, and PM; it is called mixed connective tissue disease. Of these patients, 80% are females, and the peak age of onset is 35 to 40 years of age. Clinically, females come to the physician with swollen hands and tapered fingers, Raynaud's phenomenon, abnormal esophageal motility, myositis, and lymphadenopathy. High titers of antibody (anti-RNP) to an extractable nuclear antigen called ribonucleoprotein (RNP) occur in all such patients but are not unique to mixed connective tissue disease. ANA is present, but Sm is absent.

DIAGNOSIS. Diagnostic measures include muscle biopsy from weak muscles, skin biopsy of involved skin, and electromyography and measurement of muscle enzymes (Box 17-3). One or more of these parameters may be normal at the time of diagnosis or during the course of the disease; therefore a complete evaluation is needed in all cases.[70]

Muscle enzymes. Muscle enzymes are released when muscle cell damage occurs. The following serum muscle enzymes may be elevated: creatine kinase (CK), serum glutamic oxaloacetic transaminase (SGOT), alanine aminotransferase (ALT), lactic dehydrogenase (LDH), AST, or aldolase. Measure all muscle enzymes (CK, aldolase, LDH, ALT, AST) because elevation of only one enzyme can occur. Serum muscle enzymes are measured for diagnostic purposes and to monitor disease activity. Although some patients with myositis have normal CKs, most experts use the CK as a guide to clinical response or reactivation of the myositis. These changes can occur months before or after a change in clinical course, predicting improvement or therapy failure. Measuring urinary creatine (not creatinine) in a 24-hour collection is an early and sensitive indicator of muscle injury and a better indicator of activity than the serum creatine kinase. The test is especially useful when serum creatine is normal.

Histology of skin lesions. Histopathologic findings are similar to cutaneous lupus erythematosus with hyperkeratosis, vacuolization of the basal keratinocytes, melanin incontinence, perivascular lymphocytic infiltrate, and epidermal atrophy.

Muscle biopsy. Muscle biopsies from the same patient may vary. Several specimens may have to be taken to demonstrate an abnormality.[71] A weak muscle should be sampled, usually from a proximal muscle group such as the biceps or quadriceps. Magnetic resonance imaging (MRI) can be used to accurately localize an affected area for biopsy. Avoid muscles where electromyography had already been done or where injectable anesthetics have been used. Dermatomyositis is a complement-mediated microvasculopathy and will show muscle fiber and capillary damage. Lymphocytes and macrophages partially invade non-necrotic fibers.[72]

Electromyographic studies. These studies are indicated to diagnose the disease but not to follow disease activity.

Magnetic resonance imaging. MRI may help to establish the diagnosis, to find an appropriate muscle biopsy site, and to monitor the progress of the disease.[73] MRI findings include subcutaneous edema, increased water content of the muscle, intramuscular calcium deposits, and fatty infiltration or atrophy of the muscle.

Phosphorus 31 magnetic resonance spectroscopy. MRS is a noninvasive test that can be used when decisions are made about changes in therapy. It provides the most reliable data to document flare-ups of disease activity and periods of relative inactivity.[74]

Box 17-3 Workup for Suspected Dermatomyositis

- Skin biopsy for histology and immunofluorescence
- Muscle biopsy
- Muscle enzymes
- Electromyography
- ANA
- Antibodies-SSA (Ro), SSB (La), Sm, nRNP, Jo-1, PM-1

Antibody tests. Specific autoantibody tests (ANA, Jo-1, SSA [Ro], Ku [Ki]) should be ordered (see Tables 17-1 to 17-3, 17-10). These tests are of limited value in making the diagnosis, but positive serum results help to support it. Serologic studies such as rheumatoid factor, ANA, anti-Ro/SSA, anti-La/SSB, and anti-RNP are performed to rule out associated collagen vascular diseases. Positive low-titer ANA occurs in most cases, even in the absence of connective tissue disease. Anti-Ku antibodies are associated with myositis overlap with scleroderma or systemic lupus erythematosus.

EVALUATION FOR POSSIBLE MALIGNANCY. Patients with DM should be evaluated for internal malignancy.[75] Complete history and physical examination in a search for malignancy should be repeated at certain intervals (e.g., every 6 months, particularly in the older age group of patients). All unusual signs, symptoms, and laboratory values should be pursued. The cancer risk is increased about sixfold during the first year, but is lower during the second year, with no significant excesses in subsequent years of follow-up.[62] Therefore among long-term survivors of PM/DM, there is little evi-

Box 17-4 Initial Evaluation for Malignancy
History and physical examination
Complete blood count
Comprehensive metabolic panel
Tests for blood in stool
CT scans of chest and abdomen
Ultrasound pelvis (women)
Mammography
Endoscopic studies of upper and lower GI tract (according to patient's age)
ENT evaluation (especially for Southeast Asia patients)
Adapted from Sparsa A, et al: Arch Dermatol 2002; 138:885.

Table 17-10 Autoantibodies Commonly Present in Sera of Patients with Idiopathic Inflammatory Myopathies

Autoantibody	Frequency of occurrence	FANA pattern in Hep-2 cells	Clinical associations
Myositis specific Anti-synthetase antibodies		35% to 40%	Found exclusively or most commonly in PM-DM or PM-DM overlap
Jo-1	20% PM-DM	Speckled cytoplasmic	Interstitial lung disease, arthritis, Raynaud's phenomenon, and mechanic's hands = "antisynthetase syndrome"
PL-7	3% to 5% PM-DM	Speckled cytoplasmic	Antisynthetase syndrome
PL-12	3% PM-DM	Speckled cytoplasmic	Antisynthetase syndrome
EJ	<3% PM	Cytoplasmic	Antisynthetase syndrome
OJ	<3% PM/DM	Undescribed	Antisynthetase syndrome
SRP	4% to 5% PM-DM	Nucleolar and speckled cytoplasmic	Severe disease, poor prognosis
KJ	<1% PM	Dense speckled cytoplasmic	ILD, PM, Raynaud's
Mas	<1% PM	Not described	? History of alcohol abuse
Fer	<1% PM	Not described	Localized myositis
Mi-2	5% to 35% PM-DM	Fine speckled nuclear	V-sign rash, nailfold changes
Other autoantibodies Ku	5% to 12% PM-DM	Homogenous nuclear and nucleolar	Overlap syndrome
PM-Scl	8% to 25% PM/ overlap	Homogenous nuclear and nucleolar	Overlap syndrome
Ro/SSA	5% to 10% PM-DM	Fine speckled nuclear	Sicca symptoms, overlap syndrome
U1-RNP	12% PM-DM	Coarse speckled	Overlap syndrome

Adapted from Evans J: Clin Chest Med 1998; 19.
PM, Polymyositis; *DM,* dermatomyositis; *SRP,* signal recognition particle; *ILD,* interstitial lung disease; *RP,* Raynaud's phenomenon; *RNP,* ribonucleoprotein.

dence to warrant extensive preventive and screening measures after 2 years. Tumors may appear at any site but significant excesses are observed for cancers of lung, ovary, lymphatic and hematopoietic systems, and nasopharyngeal areas. The signs and symptoms of DM often clear shortly after the removal of a malignancy.

TREATMENT. Untreated patients die, are crippled, or survive without sequelae. Oral corticosteroids are the treatment of first choice for most adults who have skin and muscle symptoms. Adjuvant immunosuppressive drugs are used if muscle symptoms do not respond to oral steroids. Physical therapy is essential to prevent joint contractures and muscle atrophy. Skin disease is treated with group I or II topical steroids and sunscreen.

Corticosteroids. Patients respond better if treatment is started as soon as possible after diagnosis.[76] Oral prednisone (0.5 to 1.5 mg/kg) is given in a single daily dose (not every-other-day dosing) until serum CK is normal. Most patients begin to improve after the first month. Muscle strength improvement usually lags behind decreasing CK values. The dosage is lowered over a 12- to 24-month period as disease activity improves, as indicated by improving clinical signs and decreasing levels of muscle enzymes. Another regimen involves (1) oral prednisone in a divided daily dose of 40 to 60 mg/day (1-2 mg/kg in children) until the CK has normalized; (2) consolidation of the prednisone into a single daily dose, which is then reduced by one fourth every 3 to 4 weeks only if the CK value is still normal; and (3) continuation of the prednisone until a maintenance dose of 5 to 10 mg/day is reached, at which time this dosage is continued for 1 year.[77] Progressive weakness with normal or no increase in CK values suggests steroid myopathy. Reduction of neck flexor strength is seen with dermatomyositis. Neck flexor strength is unchanged if steroid myopathy is developing.

Consider adjunctive therapy if there is no improvement in muscle strength after 3 months of therapy.

Methotrexate. Methotrexate is first-line adjuvant therapy in patients unresponsive to steroids. Start oral methotrexate at 7.5 to 10 mg per week, increased by 2.5 mg per week to total of 25 mg per week.[78] Intravenous dosage is 10 mg per week, increased by 2.5 mg per week to total of 0.5 to 0.8 mg per kg. Taper steroid dose as dosage increases. Side effects occur frequently and include stomatitis, gastrointestinal symptoms, pneumonitis, pruritus, fever, neutropenia, hepatic fibrosis, and cirrhosis. One to 3 mg of folic acid daily minimizes side effects. A pretreatment liver biopsy is performed for patients with liver disease.

Azathioprine (Imuran). Start oral medication with 2 to 3 mg/kg per day (usually 100 to 200 mg/day) tapered to 1 mg/kg per day once steroid is tapered to 15 mg per day. Reduce dosage monthly by 25-mg intervals. Maintenance dosage is 50 mg per day. Screen patients for thiopurine methyltransferase deficiency before treatment (see p. 570). Adverse effects include gastrointestinal symptoms, leukopenia from bone marrow suppression and increased risk of lymphoma, and hepatotoxicity.

Cyclophosphamide (Cytoxan). The drug is less effective than azathioprine. Start oral medication at 1 to 3 mg/kg per day or intravenous dose at 2 to 4 mg/kg per day, with prednisone. There is an increased risk of malignancy.

Cyclosporine and intravenous immunoglobulin are effective alternative treatments. Cyclosporine is very effective but nephrotoxic. Intravenous immunoglobulin is very expensive.

Treating cutaneous disease. The cutaneous eruption often resists systemic therapy. Group IV and V topical steroids reduce the erythema but do not clear the eruption. Exposure to sunlight should be minimized; broad-spectrum sunscreens are important. Antimalarials are sometimes effective in treating the cutaneous lesions of DM. Hydroxychloroquine sulfate (200 to 400 mg/day) is prescribed.[52] Antimalarial drugs have no effect on muscle disease. Non-life threatening cutaneous reactions (79% generalized morbilliform eruptions) may occur in one third of patients.[79]

Physical therapy. Bed rest is essential for patients with active muscle disease. Physical therapy is very important in the management of DM to prevent atrophy and contractures. Prednisone and immunosuppressive agents treat inflammation, but they do not make muscles strong. An aggressive-passive physical therapy program should be started, and, as muscle pain decreases, an active exercise program should begin.

PROGNOSIS. There is a poor prognosis when muscle weakness has existed for more than 4 months before diagnosis,[70] with dysphagia, pulmonary disease and malignancy,[50] and for DM patients with a lack of creatine kinase elevation.[80] The cumulative survival rate is as high as 73% after 8 years.[53]

Scleroderma

Scleroderma is a disease characterized by sclerosis of the skin and visceral organs, vasculopathy (Raynaud's phenomenon), and autoantibodies. The spectrum of disease is wide, with systemic and localized forms (Box 17-5).

Systemic sclerosis

Systemic sclerosis has a reported incidence of 2 to 12 cases per million people per year. There are two major subsets of the systemic forms: diffuse scleroderma and CREST syndrome. The criteria for the diagnosis of scleroderma are listed in Box 17-6. CREST (calcinosis cutis, Raynaud's phenomenon, esophageal involvement, sclerodactyly, telangiectasia) syndrome is slowly progressive. Diffuse scleroderma can be rapidly progressive and potentially fatal; there is symmetric fibrous thickening and hardening (sclerosis) of the skin and fibrous and degenerative changes in synovium, digital arteries, and certain internal organs, most notably the esophagus, intestinal tract, heart, lungs, and kidneys (Tables 17-11 and 17-12).[81]

Overlap syndromes exist in which typical scleroderma skin changes accompany a variety of other skin and internal diseases.

Localized scleroderma is restricted to the skin in an asymmetric manner. The other forms are rare and are not discussed here. Raynaud's phenomenon precedes or is an early manifestation in the majority of cases. All forms of scleroderma are more common in females.

Chemically induced scleroderma

Scleroderma-like diseases can be induced by a number of chemical compounds, such as plastics, solvents, and drugs. Contaminated rapeseed oil is the cause of toxic oil syndrome, and l-tryptophan induces eosinophilia-myalgia syndrome. Paraffin and silicon can trigger so-called adjuvant disease. Long-term exposure to silica can lead to idiopathic scleroderma.[82,83] This supports the hypothesis that collagen disease may be attributable to the occupations of hypersusceptible persons.

Diffuse scleroderma

INITIAL SIGNS AND SYMPTOMS. Presenting signs are skin thickening of the hands and/or Raynaud's phenomenon (64%)[84]; rheumatic complaints, including arthralgias and stiffness of the knees (30%); or weakness, weight loss, easy fatigability, stiffness, edema, and diffuse musculoskeletal aching.

Box 17-5 Classification of Scleroderma and Scleroderma-Like Disorders

Systemic sclerosis

Diffuse scleroderma (10% of cases of systemic sclerosis)

    Skin—bilateral symmetric fibrosis of skin, face, proximal and distal portions of the extremities

    Visceral disease—relatively early appearance

CREST syndrome (90% of cases of systemic sclerosis)

    Skin—relatively limited involvement, often confined to fingers and face

    Visceral disease—delayed appearance

Overlap syndromes

    Sclerodermatomyositis

    Mixed connective tissue diseases

Localized scleroderma

Morphea

    Plaquelike

    Guttate

    Generalized

    Subcutaneous and keloid morphea

Linear scleroderma

En coup de sabre (with or without facial hemiatrophy)

Chemical-induced scleroderma-like conditions

Vinyl chloride disease

    Pentazocine-induced fibrosis

    Bleomycin-induced

Eosinophilic fasciitis pseudoscleroderma

Edematous (scleredema, scleromyxedema)

Indurative (amyloidosis, porphyria cutanea tarda, carcinoid syndrome, phenylketonuria)

Atrophic (progeria, Werner's syndrome, lichen sclerosis et atrophicus)

Adapted from Masi AT, et al: Bull Rheum Dis 1981; 3:1.

Box 17-6 Scleroderma Criteria

Major criteria

Proximal sclerosis—single major criterion (91% sensitivity and greater than 99% specificity)*

Minor criteria

Sclerodactyly

Digital pitting scars of fingertips or loss of substance of the finger pad

Pulmonary fibrosis-bibasilar

One major criterion or two or more minor criteria were found in 97% of patients with definite systemic sclerosis, but in only 2% of the comparison patients with SLE, PM/DM, or Raynaud's phenomenon†

* From American Rheumatism Association: Arthritis Rheum 1980; 23:581.

† Excludes localized scleroderma and pseudoscleroderma.

Table 17-11 Organ Involvement in Progressive Systemic Sclerosis

Organ	Involvement (%)
Skin	98
Esophageal atrophy or fibrosis	74
Small intestinal atrophy or fibrosis	48
Large intestinal atrophy or fibrosis	39
Myocardial fibrosis	81
Pericardium*	53
Pericardial effusion	35
Pulmonary interstitial fibrosis	74
Pleural disease	81
Kidneys†	58
Skeletal muscle atrophy	41
Skeletal muscle round cell infiltration	8
Thyroid (fibrosis)	24
Adrenal atrophy	26
Cancer	2

Adapted from D'Angelo WA, et al: Am J Med 1969; 46:428.

* Pericarditis (fibrous or fibrinous) or pericardial adhesions.

† Any of the following: 1) fibrinoid necrosis of afferent arterioles or glomeruli; 2) hyperplasia of interlobular artery; or 3) thickening of basement membrane or wire-loop.

SKIN. The disease typically remains confined to the fingers, hands, and face for months or years but may progress to involve the forearms, legs, and eventually the entire body (Figures 17-18 and 17-19). In both systemic sclerosis and CREST syndrome there are three stages of skin disease: (1) edematous, (2) indurative or sclerotic, and (3) atrophic.[85]

In the edematous phase the skin is thickened and swollen and appears tense, with nonpitting edema producing the classic early signs of a masklike facies and "sausaging" of the fingers (Figure 17-19). Hand motion is restricted. The disease progresses to the indurative phase, and skin becomes hard, stiff, and bound down. Hand motion is further restricted. Hair loss and anhidrosis reflect fibrosis and degeneration of appendages. Mottled brown pigmented and hypopigmented areas occur on the forearms, upper thorax, chest, and scalp. Ulcerations, telangiectasia, and atrophy gradually appear. The skin of the fingers and hands becomes thin, shiny, smooth, and tightly bound down with the fingers contracted (sclerodactyly: "claw deformity") (Figure 17-20, A). The fingers narrow or taper distally, and the terminal phalanges become shortened as a result of distal bone resorption.

Repeated and increasingly severe attacks of Raynaud's phenomenon lead to fingertip ulcerations that leave pitted or star-shaped scars (Figure 17-20, B). Facial skin contracts and appears fixed to bone. The nose becomes beak shaped, and the skin about the mouth is drawn into furrows that radiate from the mouth (Figure 17-21). The curvature of the mouth becomes smaller, and the lips are thinned. Telangiectatic mats appear on the hands, face, and trunk, and dilated capillary loops are found at the proximal nailfold. Atrophy and softening of the dermis eventually make the skin more pliable.

Table 17-12 Signs of Visceral Involvement in Systemic Sclerosis

	Mild	Severe
Raynaud's	Less than 5 times a day	More than 15 times/day, or digital ulcerations, or both
Esophagus	Dysphagia to solid foods; normal barium swallow	Dysphagia to solid and soft foods and weight loss (>10%); abnormal barium swallow with dilation of the lower two thirds of the esophagus
Lung	No symptoms: vital capacity >70% predicted and CO_2-diffusing capacity between 50% and 75% of predicted, PO_2	Dyspnea + vital capacity <50% of predicted or Co_2-diffusing capacity <33% of predicted, Po_2 <69 mm Hg
Heart	Nonspecific ST	T changes; angina; definite ischemic changes by ECG; hypokinesis by MUGA scan or an ejection fraction <30%
Muscle	Mild EMG or CK abnormalities	Definite myositis clinically, biochemically, by EMG, or by muscle biopsy
Kidney	Mild hypertension or a serum creatine 1.5 times normal, or a creatine clearance <80%, or a 24-hour protein of <500 mg	Refractory hypertension, or a serum creatine 4 times normal, or a creatine clearance <20%, or a 24-hour protein <3 gm

ECG, electrocardiogram; *EMG*, electromyogram; *CK*, creatine kinase; *MUGA*, multiunit gated acquisition.

RAYNAUD'S PHENOMENON. Raynaud's syndrome is a vasospastic disorder precipitated by temperature changes. The term *Raynaud's phenomenon* is used when the changes occur in scleroderma or other connective tissue diseases, and the term *Raynaud's disease* is used when the syndrome occurs in the absence of other conditions. Raynaud's phenomenon is the first symptom of systemic sclerosis in 47% of patients, preceding the onset of sclerodermatous skin changes by several months or years. It occurs during the course of the disease in 90% to 95% of patients.[86] One study showed that 18% of patients with Raynaud's syndrome had systemic sclerosis.[87] The phenomenon does not commonly occur with morphea or other localized forms of scleroderma.

Raynaud's phenomenon represents an episodic vasoconstriction of the digital arteries and arterioles that is precipitated by cold or stress. It is much more common in women. There are three stages during a single episode: pallor (white), in which vasospasm causes the fingers to turn white, cold, numb, and painful; cyanosis (blue), in which relaxation of vasospasm occurs; and hyperemia (red), in which relaxation results in reactive hyperemia and the fingers turn red.

Nailfold capillary patterns as detected by nailfold capillary microscopy may help distinguish Raynaud's disease (no scleroderma) from Raynaud's phenomenon (associated with scleroderma). A decrease in capillary loops[88,89] occurs in Raynaud's phenomenon. This fact may help to predict which cases of Raynaud's syndrome will evolve into systemic sclerosis.

TELANGIECTASIAS. The telangiectasias of CREST syndrome and scleroderma have a unique morphology. They occur as flat (macular), 0.5-cm, rectangular collections of uniform, tiny vessels; these are the so-called telangiectatic mats (Figure 17-20, A). These mats are most commonly found on the face, lips, palms, and backs of the hands. Telangiectasias may be present around the lips, tongue, and mucous membranes. Involvement of the oral mucosa also suggests Rendu-Osler-Weber disease (hereditary hemorrhagic telangiectasia).

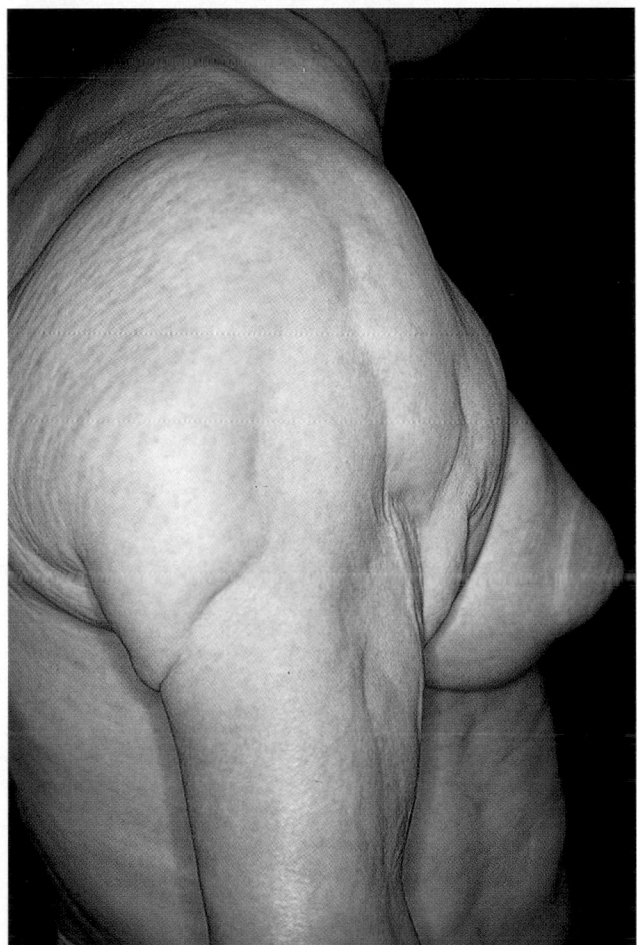

Figure 17-18 Scleroderma. Diffuse systemic sclerosis. Diffuse sclerosis of the limbs.

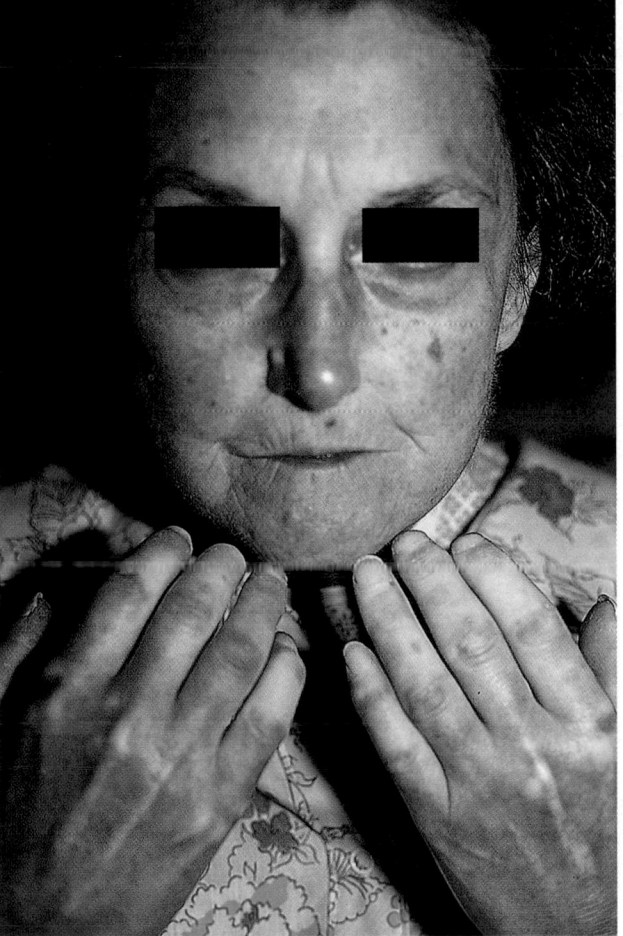

Figure 17-19 Scleroderma. The hands may be edematous and swollen early in the disease. These changes progress to other areas including the face. This edematous stage precedes the sclerotic stage.

SCLERODERMA

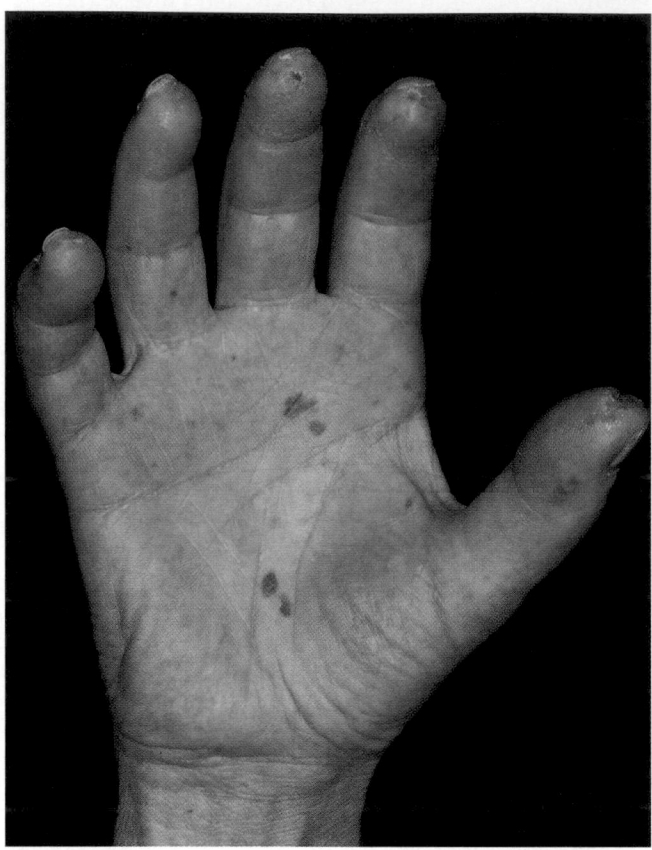

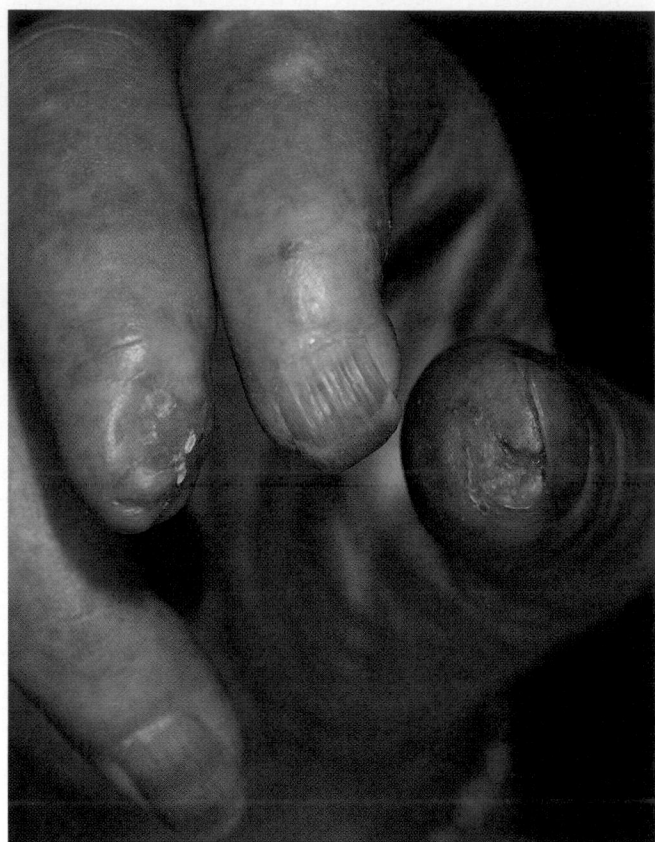

A, The skin is tightly bound down. The fingers are contracted. Telangiectatic mats are evident on the palms. There are fingertip ulcerations.

B, Fingertips are narrowed, and the fingers are shortened as a result of distal bone resorption.

Figure 17-20

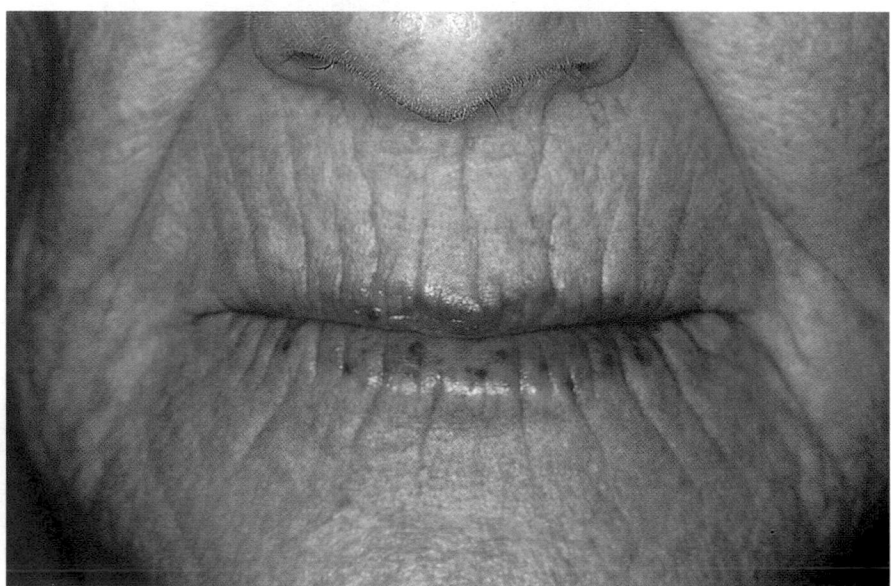

Figure 17-21 Telangiectasias are most obvious in the perioral area and neck. The skin about the mouth is drawn into furrows that radiate from the mouth.

GASTROINTESTINAL TRACT. Fibrosis and atrophy of smooth muscle can occur in any part of the gastrointestinal (GI) tract. Approximately 10% of patients may have GI symptoms before the appearance of skin changes.[90] Dysphagia is the most common sign of GI involvement.

Esophageal dysfunction with hypomotility, dysphagia, reflux esophagitis, and fibrotic strictures occurs in approximately 90% of patients. Gastroesophageal reflux rather than impaired motility is the major cause of esophageal symptoms.[91] Cinefluoroscopic and manometric studies reveal reduced or absent peristalsis of the lower third of the esophagus. Extremely sensitive, noninvasive scintigraphic procedures are available for quantitative assessment of esophageal function.[92,93] There is no increased frequency of esophageal carcinoma.[94]

Intestinal dilation and hypoperistalsis are the most common small bowel abnormalities. They lead to a "stagnant loop" syndrome with bacterial overgrowth, malabsorption, and steatorrhea. A characteristic mucosal fold pattern is called the hide-bound small bowel of scleroderma.[95] Bleeding gastric telangiectasias located primarily in the upper part of the GI tract can result in severe blood loss.[96] Wide-mouthed sacculations, loss of colonic haustration, and constipation occur with colonic involvement.

LUNGS. Lung disease is a frequent cause of death. Abnormal pulmonary function studies with reduced vital and total lung capacity are usually the first signs of lung disease. Dyspnea is the most common symptom; moist basilar rales are the most frequent sign. Interstitial fibrosis and thickening of the alveolar septa are the most common histologic changes. Fibrotic changes typically involve the lower lung fields, and pleural effusions are unusual. A diffuse reticulonodular interstitial pattern in a basilar distribution may be seen in the chest radiograph. Pulmonary hypertension occurs in 33% of patients.[97]

KIDNEYS. Renal disease and hypertension are the major causes of death in patients with systemic scleroderma. The appearance of proteinuria, hypertension, or azotemia are poor prognostic signs, and death usually occurs in less than 1 year.[98]

OTHER ORGANS. Myocardial fibrosis results in arrhythmias, and pulmonary fibrosis leads to pulmonary hypertension and right-sided heart failure. Polyarthralgia or arthritis was among the initial symptoms in 41% of patients.[99,100] Sclerosis of the frenulum may immobilize the tongue. Fibrosis of the minor salivary glands may cause the clinical features of Sjögren's syndrome.

PROGNOSIS. Baseline factors that are most predictive of a poor outcome (rapidly progressive disease and early death) included the presence of abnormal cardiopulmonary signs and abnormal urine sediment (pyuria, hematuria).[101] A subset of patients with scleroderma with antibodies to centromere and histone have severe pulmonary or vascular disease.[102]

CREST syndrome

A more benign, chronic, and localized variant of scleroderma is called CREST syndrome (formerly known as acrosclerosis). The five clinical features of this disease (calcinosis cutis, Raynaud's phenomenon, esophageal involvement, sclerodactyly, and telangiectasia) are discussed in the section on systemic sclerosis. Calcinosis is a unique feature of CREST.

CALCINOSIS. Subcutaneous calcinosis occurs most commonly on the palmar aspects of the tips of the fingers. Calcinosis also occurs over the bony prominences of the knees, elbows, spine, and iliac crests. The deposits appear as firm, subcutaneous nodules that may eventually rupture at the surface, discharging fragments of calcium. In response to this foreign material, the skin surrounding the calcium becomes painful, red, and sometimes chronically infected, requiring courses of oral antibiotics.

Although patients with CREST syndrome can progress to more involved systemic disease, those with the clinical and serologic markers of the syndrome have a more benign course than patients with diffuse scleroderma.

The clinical differentiation between CREST syndrome and Osler's disease (telangiectasia hereditaria hemorrhagica) is difficult because telangiectasia may be the most prominent clinical feature in both disorders. However, patients with CREST syndrome usually have anticentromere antibodies in the serum.

Diagnosis of diffuse scleroderma

Specific circulating antibodies are useful in establishing the diagnosis. Most other laboratory studies are nonspecific (Box 17-7).

AUTOANTIBODIES. Antinuclear antibodies can be detected in more than 85% to 95% of patients with systemic sclerosis. Centromere antibody is found most frequently in patients with limited disease; they are found in as many as 96% of patients with CREST or acroscleroderma and sclerosis limited to the digits,[103] and in only 21% of patients with diffuse sclerosis[104] (Table 17-13).

Box 17-7 Workup for Diffuse Sclerosis
• Deep skin biopsy
• System review
• Office nailfold capillary microscopy
• ANA (centromere)
• Antibodies-SSA (Ro), SSB (La), Sm, nRNP Scl-70
• Organ workup

Table 17-13 Autoantibodies Commonly Present in Sera of Patients with Scleroderma

Autoantibody	Frequency of occurrence	FANA pattern in Hep-2 cells	Clinical associations
ACA	20% to 59% scleroderma	Diffuse punctate speckled nuclear metaphase plate in dividing cells	Limited scleroderma, Raynaud's, less pulmonary fibrosis and renal crisis
Scl-70	20% to 30% scleroderma	Homogeneous nuclear and speckled nucleolar	Diffuse skin involvement, pulmonary interstitial fibrosis, peripheral vascular disease,? association with cancer
Th/To	4% to 10% scleroderma	Homogeneous nucleolar	? Association with puffy fingers, small-bowel involvement, low thyroid, less arthritis
Fibrillarin (U3-RNP)	6% to 8% scleroderma	Clumpy nucleolar	More common in patients of African descent and with diffuse disease, more severe disease
RNA polymerase I	4% to 20% scleroderma	Speckled nucleolar	Diffuse disease
RNA polymerase II	4% scleroderma	Speckled nucleolar	Diffuse disease, also found in patients with SLE and overlap
RNA polymerase III	23% scleroderma	Nuclear speckled	Diffuse disease
PM-Scl	2% to 5% scleroderma	Homogeneous nucleolar	Overlap with PM-DM

Adapted from Evans J: Clin Chest Med 1998; 19.

ACA, Anticentromere antibody; *PM-DM,* polymyositis-dermatomyositis; *SLE,* systemic lupus erythematosus.

The frequency of antibodies in patients with systemic sclerosis is as follows: centromere (21% to 32%), Scl-70 (45%), and nucleolar (15%). More than one of the three antibodies is rarely demonstrated in any one serum. One of them is found in two thirds of sera from patients with SSc. Scl-70 antibody is found almost exclusively in sera from patients with extensive SSc (involving the skin of the trunk).[105]

A subset of patients with antibodies to centromere and histone have severe pulmonary or vascular disease.[102]

OTHER STUDIES. Hypergammaglobulinemia (most often IgG) occurs in approximately 50% of patients. The ESR is elevated (20 to 80) in 60% of cases.[86] There are many other nonspecific findings.

Office nailfold capillary microscopy

A technique has been described for characterizing the telangiectasias seen in the proximal nailfold of the various connective tissue diseases. The scleroderma pattern is distinctive and is also seen in dermatomyositis. Familiarity with this technique may help to differentiate patients with lupus and dermatomyositis from patients who have cutaneous eruptions that appear to be similar. The technique used by Minkin and Rabhan[11] is as follows:

A drop of mineral oil is placed on each nailfold. The ophthalmoscope is set at 40×, resulting in a 10× magnification. The instrument is placed close to, but not in touch with, the oil. Generally the capillaries are best seen in the nailfold of the fourth finger. Because the field of observation is smaller than in wide-field microscopy, the ophthalmoscope must be moved over the entire nailfold. A technique for using a television camera to record nailfold capillary characteristics has been described.[106]

NORMAL. In normal people the capillaries are seen as fine, regular loops with a small, even space between the afferent and efferent limbs, in a row perpendicular to the nail (Figure 17-22).

OVERLAP SYNDROMES (SCLERODERMA, DERMATOMYOSITIS). The scleroderma pattern (megacapillaries and/or avascularity) (Figure 17-23) seen in 74% of patients with scleroderma consists of enlarged and deformed capillaries with dilation of both limbs of the loop, which is often engorged with blood ("sausage loop"). There is marked disorganization of the loop arrangement. Loss of capillaries produces many avascular areas and disruption of the orderly appearance of the capillary bed. Patients with Raynaud's phenomenon who present with avascularity and/or a mean of more than two megacapillaries per digit are likely to progress to a scleroderma spectrum disorder.[107-109] The same pattern is seen in 82% of patients with dermatomyositis.

MIXED CONNECTIVE TISSUE DISEASE. The scleroderma pattern is present in 63%, the lupus pattern in 22%; 73% have bushy capillary formation. The presence of bushy capillaries suggests mixed connective tissue disease (Figure 17-24).[109]

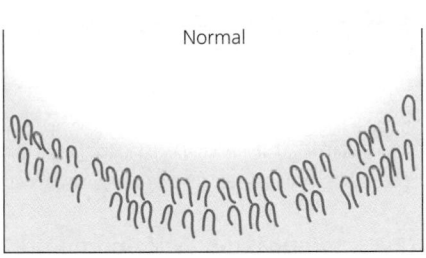

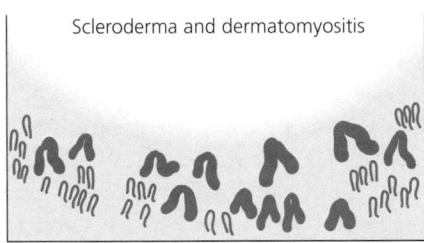

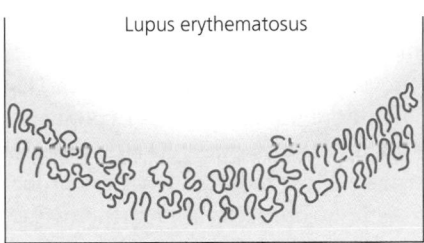

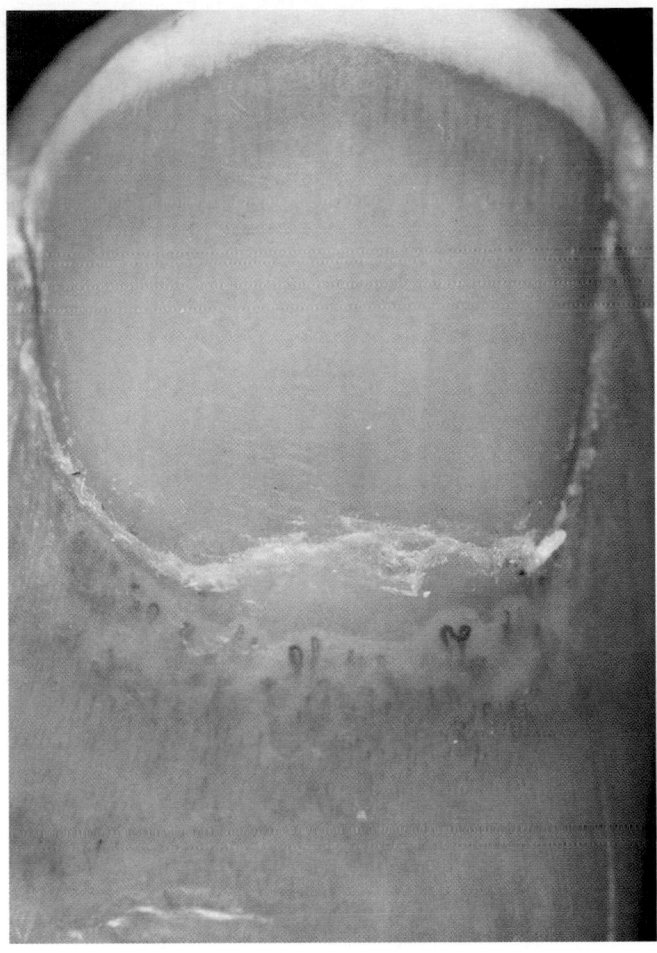

Figure 17-22 Office nailfold capillary microscopy. In normal people the capillaries are seen as fine regular loops. In scleroderma and dermatomyositis the capillary loops are enlarged, deformed, and dilated. Many capillary loops have been lost. In lupus the capillaries are tortuous but there is little dilation of capillary loops. (*From Minkin W, Rabhan NB: J Am Acad Dermatol 7:190, 1982.*)

Figure 17-23 Nailfold capillary microscopy, scleroderma, dermatomyositis. The dilated, tortuous capillary loops and avascular areas are obvious. There are enlarged and deformed, dilated capillaries. Loss of capillaries has produced many avascular areas. Normal capillary loops are seen near the bottom of the picture.

LUPUS. In lupus there are tortuous, "meandering" capillary loops, but there is relatively little dilation of the capillary limbs. At times the loop length is increased and may resemble a renal glomerulus. There is usually some disorganization of the capillary pattern, but only rarely are avascular areas seen.

The changes are distinctive enough that a relatively inexperienced observer can accurately distinguish between patients with scleroderma and those with systemic LE or rheumatoid arthritis.[110] There is a close association between the degree of visible capillary abnormalities and organ involvement.[111]

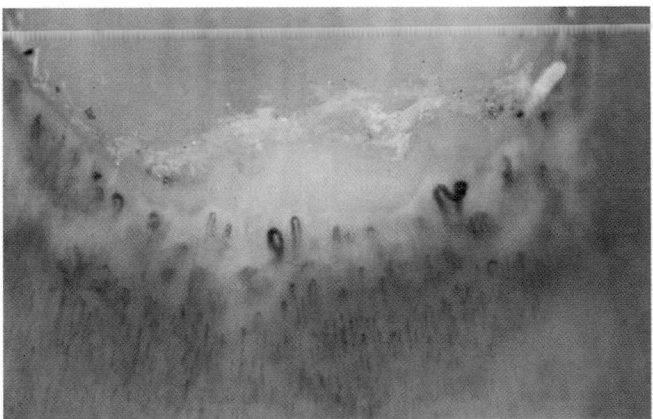

Figure 17-24 Nailfold capillary microscopy. Mixed connective tissue disease. Presence of bushy capillaries is suggestive of mixed connective tissue disease.

Treatment

SYSTEMIC THERAPY. Penicillamine, methotrexate, photopheresis, relaxin, interferons, and cyclosporine have all been studied in controlled trials with variable outcomes. Many other case reports for other drugs exist. There is no overall effective therapy.

Penicillamine (500 to 1500 mg/day) is often the treatment of choice for progressive systemic sclerosis. The clinical response to this agent is variable. There is no advantage to using penicillamine in doses higher than 125 mg every other day.[112]

MANAGEMENT OF CUTANEOUS DISEASE. Cutaneous ulcers are protected with an occlusive dressing such as DuoDerm. Ischemic digital-tip ulcers may be protected with a small plastic "cage." Infection is signaled by abrupt erythema, swelling, and increased pain and is usually due to *Staphylococcus.* Adequate skin lubrication is difficult to maintain. Patients should bathe less and use moisturizers. Pruritus tends to occur early in the course of diffuse disease, especially over the forearms, and disappears after months or several years. Antipruritic moisturizers such as Sarna lotion may help.

No satisfactory medical approaches to calcinosis have yet been developed. Simple surgical excision may be performed if the overlying skin is intact and is not infiltrated with calcium, which may interfere with wound healing. When skin breakdown and draining fistulous tracts occur from deeper deposits in deeper levels, primary wound closure is not possible. Intense, sterile, inflammatory reactions surrounding hydroxyapatite deposits, along with constitutional symptoms such as low-grade fever, may be dramatically improved by a course of oral colchicine 0.5 mg once or twice daily for 7 to 10 days.

A daily physical therapy program emphasizing full range of motion of all large joints is important.

Localized scleroderma

Raynaud's phenomenon, acrosclerosis, or involvement of internal organs does not occur in localized scleroderma. There are three variants: morphea, linear scleroderma, and en coup de sabre.

Morphea

Morphea is more common in females; it can occur at any age but is more common after age 30. Like scleroderma, morphea begins spontaneously and involves thickening or sclerosis of the skin. The two diseases differ in appearance, in the extent of the lesions, and in evolution. Scleroderma appears as a bound-down skin thickening with minor skin color change, progresses to involve large contiguous areas of skin, and does not improve with time. The lesions of morphea begin as one-to-several circumscribed areas of purplish induration (Figure 17-25).

After weeks or months, the major portion of the central region of discoloration becomes thickened, firm, hairless, and ivory-colored. The smooth, dull, white, waxy surface is elevated, in contrast to the diffusely bound-down skin of scleroderma. The violaceous or lilac-colored active inflammatory border is a highly characteristic feature of morphea. During the active stage, the round-to-oval plaques slowly extend peripherally but do not increase very much in size. Active lesions persist for 1 to 25 years. Inactive lesions leave their mark. Although much of the induration and skin thickening disappear, previously involved sites may exhibit atrophy and a mottled brown hyperpigmentation at the border and in the previously thickened plaque area (Figure 17-26). The remainder of the lesion becomes hypopigmented.

Multiple small, white plaques (guttate morphea) are a rare form of morphea. Most reported cases are probably cases of lichen sclerosis et atrophicus; in fact, the two diseases may appear simultaneously in the same patient.[113]

LABORATORY DIAGNOSIS. Anti-DNA antibodies have been reported in some children. The presence of antihistone antibodies (AHAs) has been demonstrated in localized scleroderma. AHAs were detected in 42% of patients with localized scleroderma and in 87% of patients with generalized morphea.[114,115] The presence of AHAs strongly correlated with the number of morphea lesions, the total number of lesions, and the number of involved areas of the body. ANAs did not correlate with the presence or number of linear lesions. The relationship of morphea to *Borrelia* infection remains undetermined.

BIOPSY. The histopathologic features vary with the course of the disease. Early active lesions reveal inflammatory cells in the dermis and subcutaneous tissue. Inflammation is most marked at the violaceous border. The collagen becomes eosinophilic and increases to occupy portions of the subcutaneous fat. Inflammation and sclerosis diminish with time.

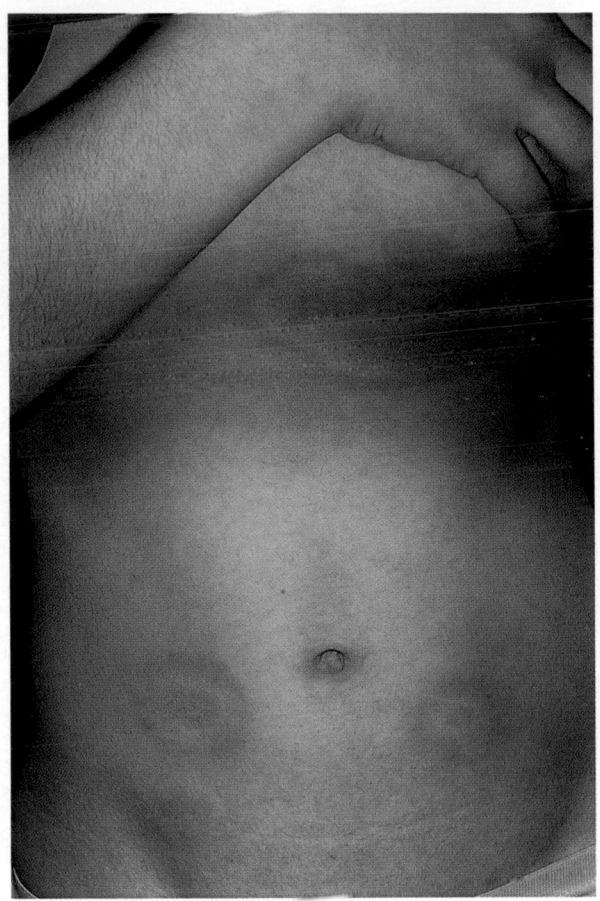

Figure 17-25 Morphea. A single or few oval areas of nonpitting erythema and edema typically appears on the trunk. A violaceous border (lilac ring) surrounds the indurated area. The center of the lesion then develops smooth, ivory-colored hairless plaques, and the ability to sweat is lost.

TREATMENT. Asymptomatic plaques should probably be left alone to resolve spontaneously. Topical steroids and occlusion may induce slight improvement.

Inducing atrophy by infiltrating with triamcinolone acetonide (10 mg/mL) may be useful in areas where skin thickening has resulted in discomfort or limitation of motion. Thickened tissue offers great resistance to infiltration, and scattered pitted areas of atrophy rather than a uniform decrease in plaque thickness may result.

Hydroxychloroquine sulfate (200 mg) may be considered for patients who have multiple lesions that on skin biopsy are shown to be in an active inflammatory stage.[116] The adult dosage is 200 mg of hydroxychloroquine twice a day. Induration may be markedly reduced or disappear in 2 to 4 months. The medication should be discontinued after lesions improve. The fundi should be examined by an ophthalmologist before antimalarials are started and should be monitored periodically. Oral calcitriol (1,25 dihydroxy vitamin D3) 0.50 to 0.75 mg for 3 to 7 months showed a beneficial effect in generalized morphea during an open study.[117] Rapidly deteriorating, generalized morphea has been helped with sulfasalazine (Azulfidine) 1 to 4 gm/day.[118]

Calcipotriene ointment (Dovonex) 0.005% may be an effective treatment for localized scleroderma. Calcipotriene ointment 0.005% was applied without occlusion in the morning but with occlusion at night. The effects of the application are evident by 1 month.[119]

Figure 17-26
Morphea. Lesions persist for months or years. They eventually become soft, atrophic, and hypopigmented or hyperpigmented.

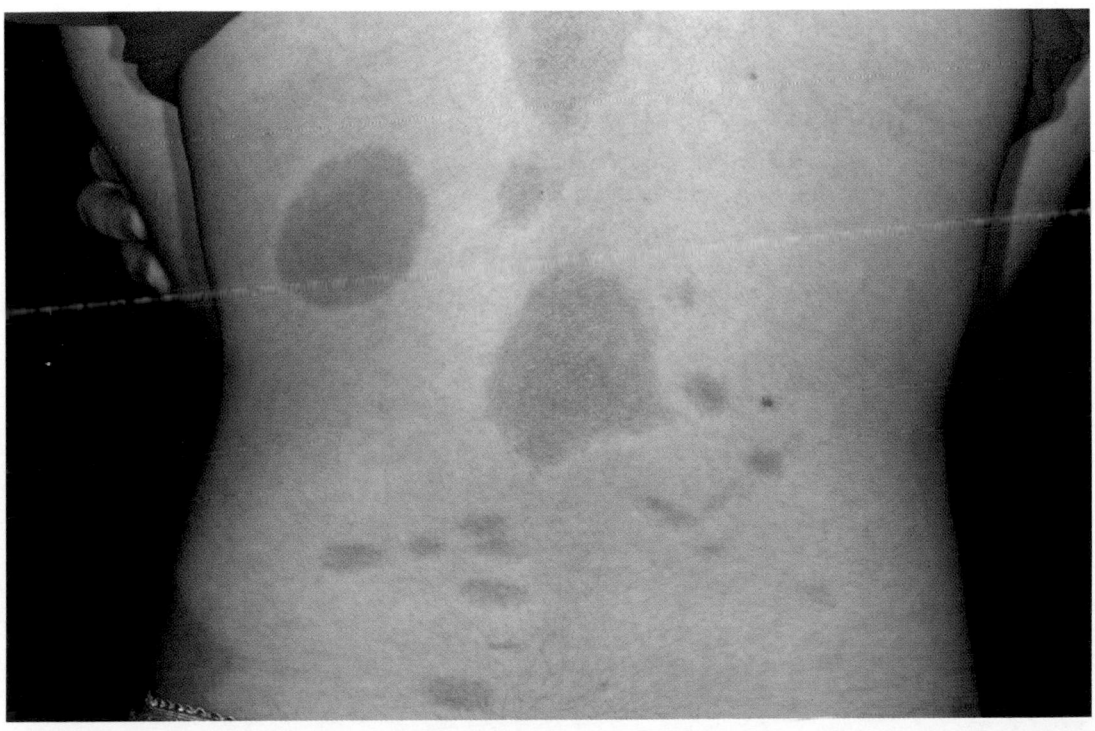

Linear scleroderma

Lesions of linear scleroderma have bands of sclerotic skin that often cross joint lines and lead to mild, but occasionally severe and disabling, joint contractures. Unlike oval plaque morphea, the inflammatory and fibrotic process may involve the underlying subcutaneous tissue and muscle, causing the fibrotic band to be more firmly anchored (Figure 17-27). One large study provides the following data.[120] The female-to-male ratio is 4:1, and 83% of patients are younger than 25 years old when the disease begins. Trauma to the involved site precedes the lesions in 23% of cases. The onset is usually slow and insidious. Most lesions occur on the extremities, and two or more lesions appear simultaneously (61%), often bilaterally (46%). Joint contractures occur in 56% of patients. The typical patient has active disease for 2 to 3 years. It remains controversial whether linear scleroderma follows Blaschko's lines.

LABORATORY. In one study, peripheral blood eosinophilia (200 to 2500 cells/mm³) occurred in 50% of patients with early active disease and declined with time.[121] The frequency of antinuclear antibodies (HEp-2 cells) was 46%. Antibodies to single-stranded DNA were present in 50% of patients and were more common in those with joint contractures and disease duration of greater than 2 years, but the level of antibody does not correlate with extent of disease.[122] Morphea occurred in 50% of patients.

TREATMENT. Early and continued physical therapy is crucial to maintain adequate joint motion. Methotrexate (MTX), 0.3 to 0.6 mg/kg per week and pulse intravenous methylprednisolone, 30 mg/kg for 3 days monthly for 3 months was effective after 3 months of treatment.[123] Low-dose UVA1 phototherapy can be highly effective for sclerotic plaques, even in patients with advanced localized scleroderma and with lesions rapidly evolving.[124] PUVA-cream therapy may be effective.[125]

En coup de sabre

The most distinct form of localized scleroderma is morphea of the frontoparietal face and scalp regions, called en coup de sabre, so named because it appears that the blade of a sabre has struck a sharp, deep, vertical line on the face (Figure 17-28). The involved site may show all of the features of morphea. In time, atrophy of one side of the face may occur, giving the impression that a blade was turned to the side to remove a thickness of skin after landing vertically. Frontoparietal scleroderma may occur along the lines of Blaschko.[126]

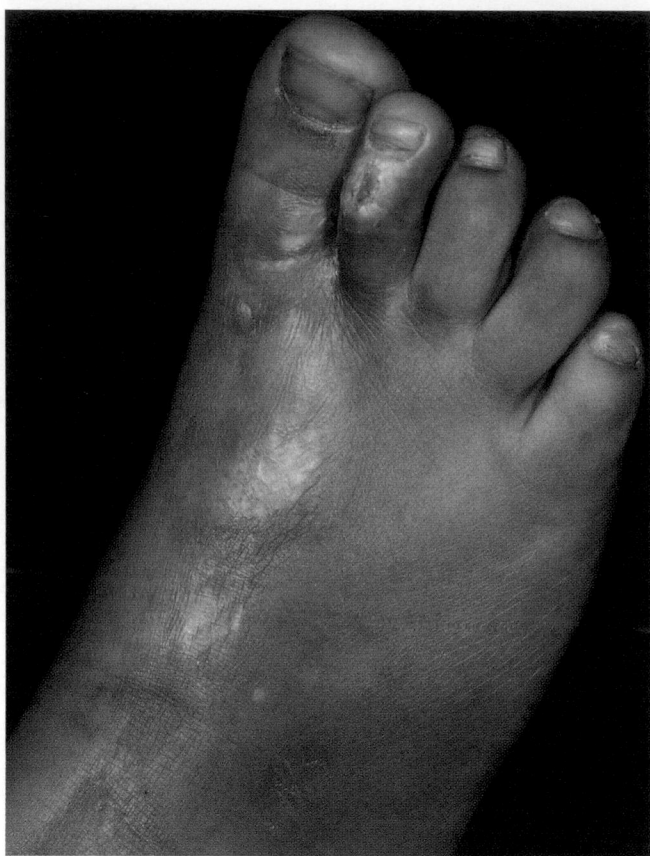

Figure 17-27 Linear morphea occurs as a single linear band, usually along the length of a limb. The deep fascia is closer to the dermis than on the trunk. This may explain why lesions may be fixed to underlying structures and extend to muscle or bone.

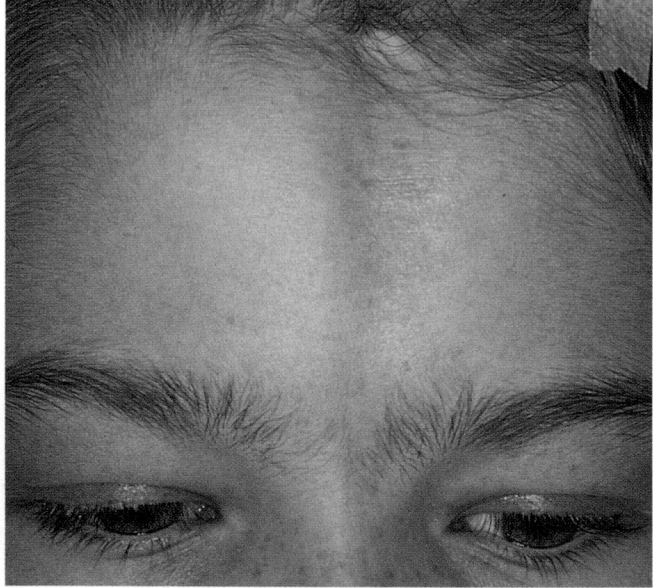

Figure 17-28 Frontoparietal linear morphea (en coup de sabre) is a depression suggestive of a stroke from a sword. Extensive lesions may cause hemifacial atrophy.

References

1. Provost TT: Subsets in systemic lupus erythematosus: Review article, J Invest Dermatol 1979; 72:110.

2. Gilliam JN, Sontheimer RD: Distinctive cutaneous subsets in the spectrum of lupus erythematosus, J Am Acad Dermatol 1981; 4:471.

3. de B, D., et al: The sequelae of chronic cutaneous lupus erythematosus, Lupus 1992; 1:181.

4. Wilson CL, et al: Scarring alopecia in discoid lupus erythematosus, Br J Dermatol 1992; 126:307.

5. Callen JP, Fowler JF, Kulick KB: Serologic and clinical features of patients with discoid lupus erythematosus: Relationship of antibodies to single-stranded deoxyribonucleic acid and of other antinuclear antibody subsets to clinical manifestations, J Am Acad Dermatol 1985; 13:748.

6. Sontheimer RD, Thomas JR, Gilliam JN: Subacute cutaneous lupus erythematosus: A cutaneous marker for a distinctive lupus erythematosus subset, Arch Dermatol 1979; 115:1409.

7. Reed BR, et al: Subacute cutaneous lupus erythematosus associated with hydrochlorothiazide therapy., Ann Intern Med 1985; 103:49.

8. Callen JP, et al: Subacute cutaneous lupus erythematosus: Clinical, serologic, and immunogenetic studies of forty-nine patients seen in a nonreferral setting, J Am Acad Dermatol 1986; 15:1227.

9. Reference deleted in proofs.

10. Cervera R, et al: Morbidity and mortality in systemic lupus erythematosus during a 5-year period. A multicenter prospective study of 1,000 patients, European Working Party on Systemic Lupus Erythematosus, Medicine (Baltimore) 1999; 78(3):167.

11. Minkin W, Rabhan NB: Office nail fold capillary microscopy using ophthalmoscope, J Am Acad Dermatol 1982; 7:190.

12. O'Loughlin, Schroeter AL, Jordan RE: Chronic urticaria-like lesions in systemic lupus erythematosus, Arch Dermatol 1978; 114:879.

13. Sanchez NP, et al: The clinical and histopathologic spectrums of urticarial vasculitis: Study of forty cases, J Am Acad Dermatol 1982; 7:599.

14. Reference deleted in proofs.

15. Kallenberg CGM, Wouda AA: The systemic involvement and immunologic findings in patients presenting with Raynaud's phenomenon, Am J Med 1980; 69:675.

16. Pramatarov K: Drug-induced lupus erythematosus, Clin Dermatol 1998; 16(3):367.

17. Callen J: Drug-induced cutaneous lupus erythematosus, a distinct syndrome that is frequently unrecognized, J Am Acad Dermatol 2001; 45(2):315.

18. Litwin A, et al: Immunologic effects of hydralazine in hypertensive patients, Arthritis Rheum 1981; 24:1074.

19. Reidenberg MM, et al: Acetylator phenotype in idiopathic systemic lupus erythematosus, Arthritis Rheum 1980; 23:569.

20. Rothfield N: Current approach to SLE and its subsets, Dis Mon 1982; October.

21. Lee L: Neonatal lupus: Clinical features, therapy, and pathogenesis, Curr Rheumatol Rep 2001; 3(5):391.

22. Lee LA: Neonatal lupus erythematosus, J Invest Dermatol 1993; 100:9S.

23. Weston W, Morelli J, Lee L: The clinical spectrum of anti-Ro-positive cutaneous neonatal lupus erythematosus, J Am Acad Dermatol 1999; 40(5 Pt 1):675.

24. Lee LA: Maternal autoantibodies and pregnancy-II: The neonatal lupus syndrome, Baillieres Clin Rheumatol 1990; 4:69.

25. Alexander E, et al: Anti-Ro/SS-A antibodies in the pathophysiology of congenital heart block in neonatal lupus syndrome, an experimental model. In vitro electrophysiologic and immunocytochemical studies, Arthritis Rheum 1992; 35:176.

26. McCune AB, Weston WL, Lee LA: Maternal and fetal outcome in neonatal lupus erythematosus, Ann Intern Med 1987; 106:518.

27. Ivarellos A, et al: Relationship of HLA-DR and MT antigens to autoantibody expression in systemic lupus erythematosus, Arthritis Rheum 1983; 26:1533.

28. Kuhn A, et al: Phototesting in lupus erythematosus: A 15-year experience, J Am Acad Dermatol 2001; 45(1):86.

29. Potter B: Hydroxychloroquine, Cutis 1993; 52:229.

30. The Hydroxychloroquine Study Group: A randomized study of the effect of withdrawing hydroxychloroquine sulfate in systemic lupus erythematosus, N Engl J Med 1991; 324:150.

31. Jewell M, McCauliffe D: Patients with cutaneous lupus erythematosus who smoke are less responsive to antimalarial treatment, J Am Acad Dermatol 2000; 42(6):983.

32. Van BM, Piette W: Antimalarials, Dermatol Clin 2001; 19(1): 147, ix.

33. Weiner A, et al: Hydroxychloroquine retinopathy, Am J Ophthalmol 1991; 112:528.

34. Coburn PR, Shuster D: Dapsone and discoid lupus erythematosus, Br J Dermatol 1982; 106:105.

35. Ruzicka T, Goerz G: Dapsone in the treatment of lupus erythematosus, Br J Dermatol 1981; 104:53.

36. Hall RP, et al: Bullous eruption of systemic lupus erythematosus-dramatic response to dapsone therapy, Ann Intern Med 1982; 97:167.

37. Matthews CNA, Saihan EM, Warin RP: Urticarial-like lesions associated with systemic lupus erythematosus: Response to dapsone, Br J Dermatol 1978; 99:455.

38. Holtman JH, et al: Dapsone is an effective therapy for the skin lesions of subacute cutaneous lupus erythematosus and urticarial vasculitis in a patient with C2 deficiency, J Rheumatol 1990; 17:1222.

39. Lindskov R, Reymann F: Dapsone in the treatment of cutaneous lupus erythematosus, Dermatologica 1986; 172:214.

40. Tsokos GC, Caughman SW, Klippel JH: Successful treatment of generalized discoid skin lesions with azathioprine, Arch Dermatol 1985; 121:1323.

41. Shehade S: Successful treatment of generalized discoid skin lesions with azathioprine, Arch Dermatol 1986; 122:376.

42. Callen JP, et al: Safety and efficacy of a broad-spectrum sunscreen in patients with discoid or subacute cutaneous lupus erythematosus, Cutis 1991; 47:130.

43. Kuhn A, et al: Methotrexate treatment for refractory subacute cutaneous lupus erythematosus, J Am Acad Dermatol 2002; 46(4):600.

44. Duong D, et al: American experience with low-dose thalidomide therapy for severe cutaneous lupus erythematosus, Arch Dermatol 1999; 135(9):1079.

45. Ruzicka T, et al: Treatment of cutaneous lupus erythematosus with acitretin and hydroxychloroquine, Br J Dermatol 1992; 127:513.

46. Newton RC, et al: Mechanism-oriented assessment of isotretinoin in chronic or subacute cutaneous lupus erythematosus, Arch Dermatol 1986; 122:170.

47. Caro I: Dermatomyositis, Semin Cutan Med Surg 2001; 20(1):38.

48. Kovacs S, Kovacs S: Dermatomyositis, J Am Acad Dermatol 1998; 39(6):899; quiz 921.

49. Pearson CM, Bohan A: The spectrum of dermatomyositis. Symposium on rheumatic diseases, Med Clin North Am 1977; 61:439.

50. Bohan A, et al: A computer-assisted analysis of 153 patients with polymyositis and dermatomyositis, Medicine 1977; 56:255.

51. Hoffman GS, et al: Presentation, treatment and prognosis of idiopathic inflammatory muscle disease in a rural hospital, Am J Med 1983; 75:433.

52. Callen JP: Dermatomyositis, Dis Mon 1987; 33:305.

53. Hochberg MC, Feldman D, Stevens MB: Adult onset polymyositis/dermatomyositis: An analysis of clinical and laboratory features and survival in 76 patients with a review of the literature, Semin Arthritis Rheu 1986; 15:168.

54. Rockerbie NR, et al: Cutaneous changes of dermatomyositis precede muscle weakness, J Am Acad Dermatol 1989; 20:629.

55. Jorizzo J: Dermatomyositis: practical aspects, Arch Dermatol 2002; 138(1):114.

56. el-Azhary R, Pakzad S: Amyopathic dermatomyositis: Retrospective review of 37 cases, J Am Acad Dermatol 2002; 46(4):560.

57. Sontheimer R: Would a new name hasten the acceptance of amyopathic dermatomyositis (dermatomyositis sine myositis) as a distinctive subset within the idiopathic inflammatory dermatomyopathies spectrum of clinical illness? J Am Acad Dermatol 2002; 46(4):626.

58. Kasteler JS, Callen JP: Scalp involvement in dermatomyositis: Often overlooked or misdiagnosed, JAMA 1994; 272:1939.

59. Sigurgeirsson B, et al: Risk of cancer in patients with dermatomyositis or polymyositis. A population-based study, N Engl J Med 1992; 326:363.

60. Bonnetblanc JM, et al: Dermatomyositis and malignancy. A multicenter cooperative study, Dermatologica 1990; 180:212.

61. Manchul LE, et al: The frequency of malignant neoplasms in patients with polymyositis-dermatomyositis: A controlled study, Arch Intern Med 1985; 145:1835.

62. Chow W, et al: Cancer risk following polymyositis and dermatomyositis: A nationwide cohort study in Denmark, Cancer Causes Control 1995; 6(1):9.

63. Pachman LM: Juvenile dermatomyositis: A clinical overview, Pediatr Rev 1990; 12:117.

64. Moore EC, et al: Staphylococcal infections in childhood dermatomyositis-association with the development of calcinosis, raised IgE concentrations and granulocyte chemotactic defect, Ann Rheum Dis 1992; 51:378.

65. Hiketa T, et al: Juvenile dermatomyositis: A statistical study of 114 patients with dermatomyositis, J Dermatol 1992; 19:470.

66. Ansell BM: Juvenile dermatomyositis, J Rheumatol Suppl 1992; 33:60.

67. Spencer CH, et al: Course of treated juvenile dermatomyositis, J Pediatr 1984; 105:399.

68. Peloro T, et al: Juvenile dermatomyositis: A retrospective review of a 30-year experience, J Am Acad Dermatol 2001; 45(1):28.

69. Fisler RE, et al: Aggressive management of juvenile dermatomyositis results in improved outcome and decreased incidence of calcinosis, J Am Acad Dermatol 2002; 47:505.

70. Tymms KE, Webb J: Dermatopolymyositis and other connective tissue diseases: A review of 105 cases, J Rheumatol 1985; 12:1140.

71. Bohan A, Peter JB: Polymyositis and dermatomyositis, N Engl J Med 1975; 292:344.

72. Carpenter S, Karpati G: The pathological diagnosis of specific inflammatory myopathies, Brain Pathol 1992; 2:13.

73. Fraser DD, Frank JA, Dalakas M: Magnetic resonance imaging in the idiopathic inflammatory myopathies, J Rheumatol 1991; 18:1693.

74. Park JH, et al: MRI and P-31 magnetic resonance spectroscopy provide unique quantitative data useful in the longitudinal management of patients with dermatomyositis, Arthritis Rheum 1994; 37:736.

75. Sparsa , et al: Routine vs. extensive malignancy search for adult dermatomyositis and polymyositis, Arch Dermatol 2002; 138:885.

76. Joffe M, et al: Drug therapy of the idiopathic inflammatory myopathies: Predictors of response to prednisone, azathioprine, and methotrexate and a comparison of their efficacy, Am J Med 1993; 94(4):379.

77. Drake L, et al: Guidelines of care for dermatomyositis. American Academy of Dermatology, J Am Acad Dermatol 1996; 34 (5 Pt 1):824.

78. Miller LC, et al: Methotrexate treatment of recalcitrant childhood dermatomyositis, Arthritis Rheum 1992; 35:1143.

79. Pelle MT, Callen JP: Adverse cutaneous reactions to hydroxychloroquin are more common in patients with dermatomyositis than in patients with cutaneous lupus erythematosus, Arch Dermatol 2002; 138:1231.

80. Fudman EJ, Schnitzer TJ: Dermatomyositis without creatine kinase elevation: A poor prognostic sign, Am J Med 1986; 80:329.

81. Rodman GP: When is scleroderma not scleroderma? The differential diagnosis of progressive systemic sclerosis, Bull Rheum Dis 1981; 31:7.

82. Haustein UF, et al: Chemically-induced scleroderma, Hautarzt 1992; 43:469.

83. Pelmear PL, et al: Occupationally induced scleroderma, J Occup Med 1992; 34:20.

84. Rodman GP: The natural history of progressive systemic sclerosis (diffuse scleroderma), Bull Rheum Dis 1963; 13:301.

85. Rocco VK, Hurd ER: Scleroderma and scleroderma-like disorders, Semin Arthritis Rheum 1986; 16:22.

86. Tuffanelli DL, Winkelmann RK: Systemic scleroderma: A clinical study of 727 cases, Arch Dermatol 1961; 84:359.

87. Blunt RJ, Porter JM: Raynaud syndrome, Semin Arthritis Rheum 1981; 10:281.

88. Houtman PM, et al: Diagnostic significance of nailfold capillary patterns in patients with Raynaud's phenomenon, J Rheumatol 1986; 13:556.

89. Lee P, et al: Digital blood flow and nailfold capillary microscopy in Raynaud's phenomenon, J Rheumatol 1986; 13:564.

90. Kinder RR, Fleischman R: Systemic scleroderma: A review of organ systems, Int J Dermatol 1974; 13:362.

91 Orringer MB, et al: Gastroesophageal reflux in esophageal scleroderma: Diagnosis and implications, Ann Thorac Surg 1976; 21:601.

92. Davidson A, Russell C, Littlejohn GO: Assessment of esophageal abnormalities in progressive systemic sclerosis using radionuclide transit, J Rheumatol 1985; 12:472.

93. Carette S, et al: Radionuclide esophageal transit in progressive systemic sclerosis, J Rheumatol 1985; 12:478.

94. Segel MC, et al: Systemic sclerosis (scleroderma) and esophageal adenocarcinoma: Is increased patient screening necessary? Gastroenterology 1985; 89:485.

95. Horowitz AL, Meyers MA: The "hide-bound" small bowel of scleroderma: Characteristic mucosal fold pattern, Am J Roentgen Rad Ther Nucl Med 1973; 119:332.

96. Allende HD, Ona FV, Noronha AI: Bleeding gastric telangiectasia. Complication of Raynaud's phenomenon, esophageal motor dysfunction, sclerodactyly, and telangiectasia (REST) syndrome, Am J Gastroenterol 1981; 75:354.

97. Ungerer RG, et al: Prevalence and clinical correlates of pulmonary arterial hypertension in progressive systemic sclerosis, Am J Med 1983; 75:65.

98. Cannon PJ, et al: The relationship of hypertension and renal failure in scleroderma (progressive systemic sclerosis) to structural and functional abnormalities of the renal cortical circulation, Medicine 1974; 53:1.

99. Rodman GP, Medsger TA, Jr: The rheumatic manifestations of progressive systemic sclerosis (scleroderma), Clin Orthop 1968; 57:81.

100. Rodman GP, Medsger TA, Jr: Musculoskeletal involvement in progressive systemic sclerosis (scleroderma), Bull Rheum Dis 1966; 17:419.

101. Bulpitt KJ, et al: Early undifferentiated connective tissue disease: III. Outcome and prognostic indicators in early scleroderma (systemic sclerosis), Ann Intern Med 1993; 118:602.

102. Martin L, et al: Identification of a subset of patients with scleroderma with severe pulmonary and vascular disease by the presence of autoantibodies to centromere and histone, Ann Rheum Dis 1993; 52:780.

103. Tuffanelli DL, et al: Anticentromere and anticentriole antibodies in the scleroderma spectrum, Arch Dermatol 1983; 119:560.

104. Giordano M, et al: Different antibody patterns and different prognosis in patients with scleroderma with various extent of skin sclerosis, J Rheumatol 1986; 13:911.

105. Ullman S, et al: Serology in patients with scleroderma, Ugeskr Laeger 1993; 155:472.

106. Studer A, et al: Quantitative nailfold capillary microscopy in cutaneous and systemic lupus erythematosus and localized and systemic scleroderma, J Am Acad Dermatol 1991; 24:941.

107. Zufferey P, et al: Prognostic significance of nailfold capillary microscopy in patients with Raynaud's phenomenon and scleroderma-pattern abnormalities. A six-year follow-up study, Clin Rheumatol 1992; 11:536.

108. Marlcy HR. Capillary abnormalities. Raynaud's phenomenon, and systemic sclerosis in patients with localized scleroderma, Arch Dermatol 1992; 128:630.

109. Granier F, et al: Nailfold capillary microscopy in mixed connective tissue disease, Arthritis Rheum 1986; 29:189.

110. McGill NW, Gow PJ: Nailfold capillaroscopy: A blinded study of its discriminatory value in scleroderma, systemic lupus erythematosus, and rheumatoid arthritis, Aust NZ J Med 1986; 16:457.

111. Schmidt K-U, Mensing H: Are nailfold capillary changes indicators of organ involvement in progressive systemic sclerosis? Dermatologica 1988; 176:18.

112. Clements P: Penicillamine in the treatment of systemic sclerosis, Curr Rheumatol Rep 1999; 1(1):38.

113. Uitto J, Santa C, Bauer EA: Morphea and lichen sclerosus et atrophicus, J Am Acad Dermatol 1980; 3:271.

114. Sato S, et al: Clinical characteristics associated with antihistone antibodies in patients with localized scleroderma, J Am Acad Dermatol 1994; 31:567.

115. Sato S, et al: Antigen specificity of antihistone antibodies in localized scleroderma, Arch Dermatol 1994; 130:1273.

116. Winkelmann RK: Localized cutaneous scleroderma, Semin Dermatol 1985; 4:90.

117. Hulshof MM, et al: Oral calcitriol as a new therapeutic modality for generalized morphea, Arch Dermatol 1994; 130:1290.

118. Czarnecki DB, Taft EH: Generalized morphea successfully treated with salazopyrin, Acta Derm Venereol (Stockh) 1982; 62:81.

119. Cunningham B, et al: Topical calcipotriene for morphea/linear scleroderma, J Am Acad Dermatol 1998; 39(2 Pt 1):211.

120. Falanga V, et al: Linear scleroderma. Clinical spectrum, prognosis, and laboratory abnormalities, Ann Intern Med 1986; 104:849.

121. Falanga V, Medsger TA, Jr: Frequency, levels, and significance of blood eosinophilia in systemic sclerosis, localized scleroderma, and eosinophilic fasciitis, J Am Acad Dermatol 1987; 17:648.

122. Falanga V, Medsger TA, Reichlin M: High titers of antibodies to single-stranded DNA in linear scleroderma, Arch Dermatol 1985; 121:345.

123. Uziel Y, et al: Methotrexate and corticosteroid therapy for pediatric localized scleroderma, J Pediatr 2000; 136(1):91.

124. Kerscher M, et al: Low-dose UVA phototherapy for treatment of localized scleroderma, J Am Acad Dermatol 1998; 38(1):21.

125. Grundmann-Kollmann M, et al: PUVA-cream photochemotherapy for the treatment of localized scleroderma, J Am Acad Dermatol 2000; 43(4):675.

126. Soma Y, Fujimoto M: Frontoparietal scleroderma (en coup de sabre) following Blaschko's lines, J Am Acad Dermatol 1998; 38(2 Pt 2):366.

Hypersensitivity Syndromes

Hypersensitivity syndromes are displayed in the diagram on p. 627.

Erythema Multiforme

Erythema multiforme (EM) is a relatively common, acute, often recurrent inflammatory disease. Many factors have been implicated in the etiology of EM, including numerous infectious agents, drugs, physical agents, x-ray therapy, pregnancy, and internal malignancies. In approximately 50% of cases no cause can be found. EM is commonly associated with a preceding acute upper respiratory tract infection, herpes simplex infection (HSV), or mycoplasma pneumoniae infection such as primary atypical pneumonia.[1]

CLASSIFICATION. A new classification, based on the pattern and distribution of cutaneous lesions, separates erythema multiforme major from Stevens-Johnson syndrome (SJS) and toxic epidermal necrolysis[2–4] (see the section on Stevens-Johnson syndrome). Erythema multiforme differs from Stevens-Johnson syndrome and toxic epidermal necrolysis by occurrence in younger males, frequent recurrences, less fever, milder mucosal lesions, and lack of association with collagen vascular diseases, human immunodeficiency virus infection, or cancer. Recent or recurrent herpes is the principal risk factor for EM. Drugs have higher etiologic fractions for Stevens-Johnson syndrome and toxic epidermal necrolysis.[4]

HERPES ASSOCIATED WITH RECURRENT EM. Herpes-associated EM develops in only a few of the many individuals who experience recurrent herpes simplex virus infection. EM develops in some adults and children[5] after each episode of herpes simplex.[6] Skin biopsy specimens of EM lesions from patients with recurrent disease showed HSV-specific DNA in most cases.[7]

Pathogenesis

Studies suggest that immune complex formation and subsequent deposition in the cutaneous microvasculature may play a role in the pathogenesis of EM. Circulating complexes and deposition of C_3, IgM, and fibrin around the upper dermal blood vessels have been found in the majority of patients with EM.[8] Histologically, a mononuclear cell infiltrate is present about these same upper dermal blood vessels; in the other immune complex–mediated cutaneous vasculitis (leukocytoclastic vasculitis), polymorphonuclear leukocytes are present.

EM shows lichenoid inflammatory infiltrate and epidermal necrosis that mainly affected the basal layer.[2] Necrotic keratinocytes range from individual cells to confluent epidermal necrosis. The epidermo-dermal junction shows changes ranging from vacuolar alteration up to subepidermal blisters. The dermal infiltrate is mostly perivascular.[9] SJS has a predominantly necrotic pattern in which major epidermal

HYPERSENSITIVITY SYNDROMES

ERYTHEMA MULTIFORME	STEVENS-JOHNSON SYNDROME	TOXIC EPIDERMAL NECROLYSIS	ERYTHEMA NODOSUM	SWEET'S SYNDROME (ACUTE FEBRILE NEUTROPHILIC DERMATOSIS)

Herpes simplex
Mycoplasm pneumoniae
Other infections
Drugs
Malignancies
Others
	Drugs
	  Phenytoin
	  Phenobarbital
	  Sulfonamides
	  Penicillins
	  Others
	Infections
		Drugs
		  Phenytoin
		  Phenobarbital
		  Sulfonamides
		  Ampicillin
		  Allopurinol
		  Thiacetazone
		  Isoniazid
		  NSAIDs
		Others
			Infections
			  Streptococci
			  Tuberculosis
			  Coccidioidomycosis
			  Others
			Drugs
			  Sulfonamides
			  Oral contraceptives
			Systemic illness
			  Sarcoidosis
			  Ulcerative colitis
			  Crohn's disease
			  Lymphoma
			  Leukemia
			Pregnancy
				Infections
				Autoimmune
				  disorders
				Lymphoma
				Solid tumors

• Joints (arthritis or arthralgias)

ERYTHEMA MULTIFORME	STEVENS-JOHNSON SYNDROME	TOXIC EPIDERMAL NECROLYSIS	ERYTHEMA NODOSUM	SWEET'S SYNDROME

Age 20-40
Prodrome
Few symptoms
 	
Urticarial papules
Target lesions or
  vesicles and bullae
  Backs of hands
  Palms
  Soles
  Extensor limbs
  Generalized
Mucous membranes
  Minimal lesions
Recur in crops for
  2 to 3 weeks
Oral lesions (few)
	Children, young
	  adults
	Prodrome
	  URI symptoms
	  Fever (high)
	  Sore throat
	  Cough
	
	Bullae
	Crops of lesions
	  Skin
	  Conjunctivae
	  Mouth
	  Genitalia
	Ulcerative stomatitis
	Corneal ulcerations
	Hacking cough
	  Pneumonitis
		Prodrome
		  Fever
		  Headache
		  Sore throat
		
		SJS-like mucous
		  membrane disease
		Stomatitis
		Conjuctivitis
		Hot erythema
		Painful skin
		Blisters and bullae
		Detachment of the
		  epidermis—diffuse
		Bronchopneumonia
		Septicemia
			Female:male 3:1
			Age 20-40
			Prodrome
			  Fever
			  Malaise
			
			Skin
			  Red swellings
			  Shins
			  Forearms (lateral
			    surfaces)
			Arthralgias
			Arthritis
			Hilar adenopathy
				Female:male 3:1
				Middle-aged
				Influenza-like illness or intestinal infection
				
				Skin lesions
				  1-3 weeks later
				Nonspecific infection
				  Respiratory tract
				  GI tract
				Painful red, round
				  plaques
				Fever or
				Low temperature
				Malaise
				Arthralgias
				Arthritis
				Conjunctivitis
				
				Polys >70%
				Leukocytosis >8000

necrosis and minimal inflammatory infiltration are found. Acrosyringeal concentration of keratinocyte necrosis in EM occurs in drug-related cases and is more likely to be accompanied by a dermal inflammatory infiltrate containing eosinophils. Drug concentration in sweat may explain this pattern with subsequent toxic and immunologic mechanisms leading to the fully evolved lesion.[10] Erythema multiforme has a high density cell infiltrate rich in T-lymphocytes. In contrast, toxic epidermal necrolysis is characterized by a cell-poor infiltrate in which macrophages and dendrocytes predominate. Such differences indicate a distinct pathogenesis for these diseases.[11]

Clinical manifestations

The prodromal symptoms, morphologic configuration of the lesions, and intensity of systemic symptoms vary. Milder forms of the disease may be preceded by malaise, fever, or itching and burning at the site where the eruption will occur. The cutaneous eruptions are most distinctive, and classification is based on their form. Mucosal lesions may occur in up to 70% of cases. The most common sites are the lips and buccal mucosa.

TARGET LESIONS AND PAPULES. Target lesions and papules are the most characteristic eruptions. Dusky red, round maculopapules appear suddenly in a symmetric pattern on the backs of the hands and feet and the extensor aspect of the forearms and legs. The trunk may be involved in more severe cases. Early lesions itch, burn, or are asymptomatic. The diagnosis may not be suspected until the nonspecific early lesions evolve into target lesions during a 24- to 48-hour period (Figures 18-1 and 18-3). The classic "iris" or target lesion results from centrifugal spread of the red maculopapule to a circumference of 1 to 3 cm as the center becomes cyanotic, purpuric, or vesicular. The mature target lesion consists of two distinct zones: an inner zone of acute epidermal injury with necrosis or blisters and an outer zone of erythema. There may be a middle zone of pale edema. Partially formed targets with annular borders or target lesions on the palms and soles are less distinctive and clinically resemble urticaria. Individual lesions heal in 1 or 2 weeks without scarring but with hypopigmentation or hyperpigmentation, while new lesions appear in crops.

Bullae and erosions may be present in the oral cavity. The entire episode lasts for approximately 1 month.

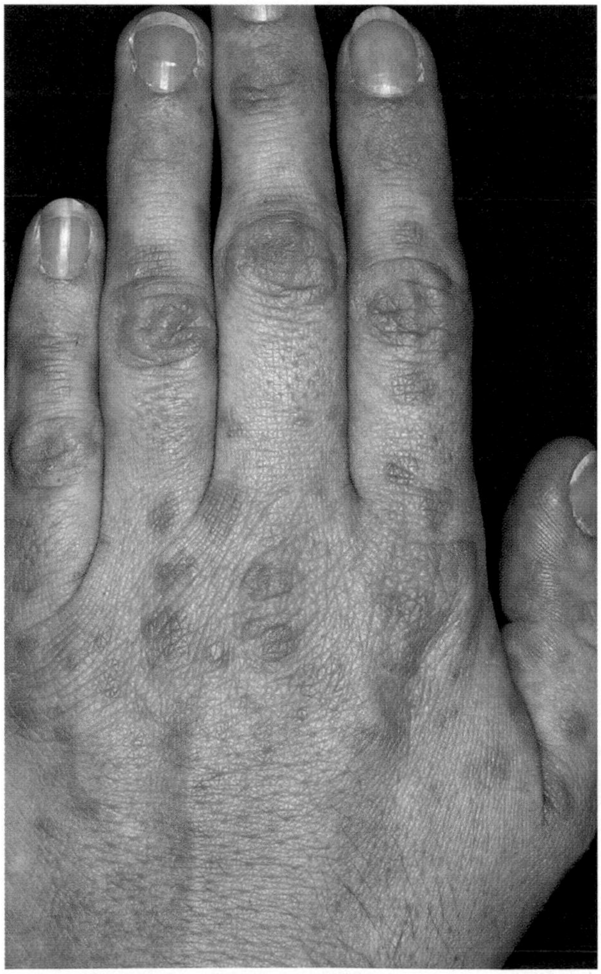

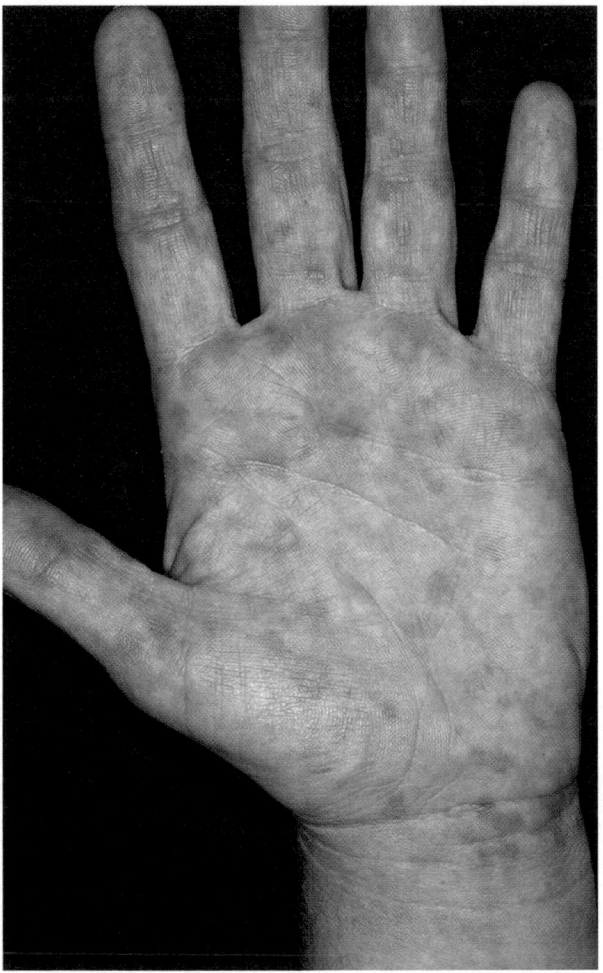

Figure 18-1 Erythema multiforme. Target lesions begin as dull red macules that develop a vesicle in the center. The periphery becomes cyanotic.

Figure 18-2 Erythema multiforme. Target lesions on the palms and soles are highly characteristic of erythema multiforme.

LABORATORY INVESTIGATIONS. Elevated erythrocyte sedimentation rate and moderate leukocytosis are found in the more severe cases. Biopsy is performed for atypical cases. Direct immunofluorescence may be needed to exclude other bullous diseases.

TREATMENT. Mild cases are not treated. Patients with many target lesions respond rapidly to a 1- to 3-week course of prednisone. Prednisone (40 to 80 mg/day) is continued until control is achieved and is then tapered rapidly in 1 week. Treatment with prednisone can successfully abort a recurrence. Oral acyclovir (400 mg twice a day) used continually prevents herpes-associated recurrent EM in many cases[12] (Figure 18-4). Herpes-associated EM is not prevented if oral acyclovir is administered after a herpes simplex recurrence is evident, and it is of no value after EM has occurred.[13] Acyclovir has been used by some patients continually for years without any apparent ill effects. Recurrent erythema multiforme patients should receive oral acyclovir (where

HSV is not an obvious precipitating factor) for 6 months. Valacyclovir and famciclovir are absorbed better than acyclovir and may be used for patients who do not respond to acyclovir.[14] If these treatments fail, dapsone or antimalarial drugs may be tried. Partial or complete suppression was evident in patients treated with dapsone (100 to 150 mg daily). Azathioprine was used successfully in patients with severe disease for whom all other treatments had failed. The response to treatment was dose-dependent (100 to 150 mg daily).[15] The condition recurred on discontinuation of therapy.

Patients with chronic recurrent EM were given thalidomide 100 mg/day after other treatments had failed, particularly acyclovir and prednisone. Thalidomide was given at the beginning of an episode. The duration of the episodes was reduced by 11 days on the average. Patients with frequent recurrent EM were given continuous treatment. Lesions disappeared within 5 to 8 days, and remission was maintained with low-dose treatment.[16]

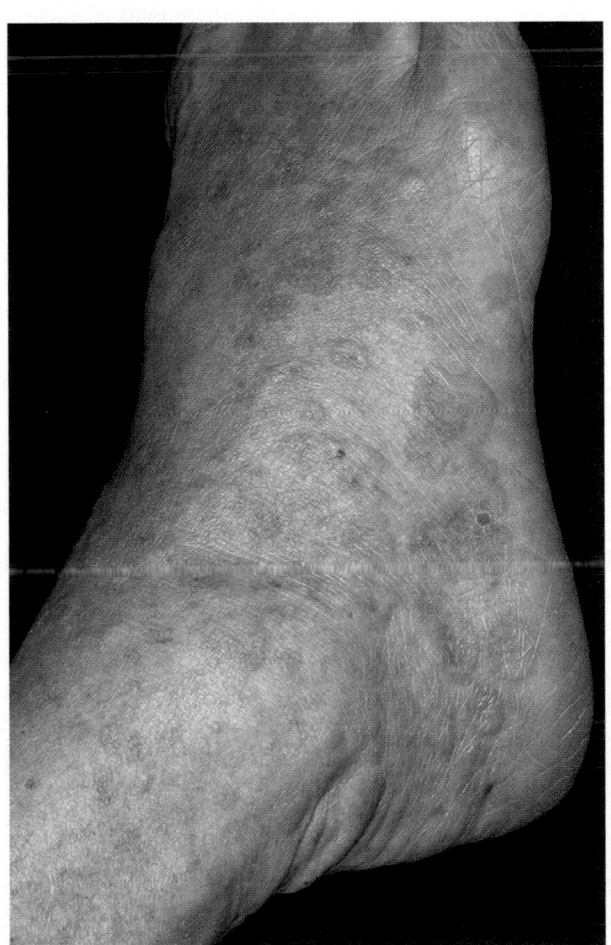

Figure 18-3 Erythema multiforme. Lesions are concentrated on the distal extremities.

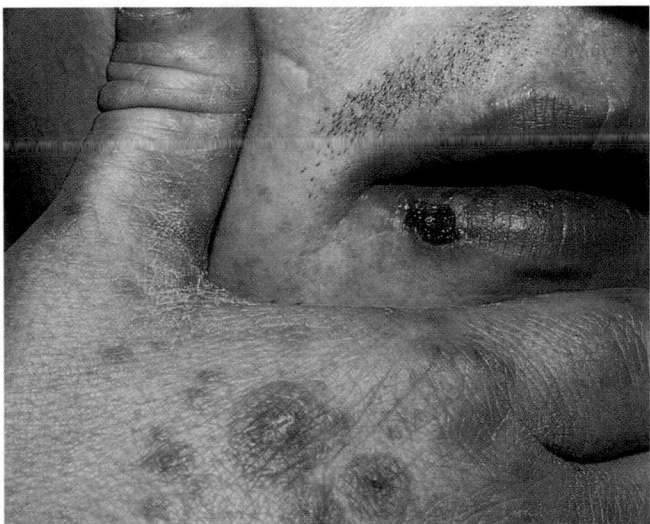

Figure 18-4 Erythema multiforme. An episode may be precipitated by herpes simplex infection.

The Stevens-Johnson Syndrome/Toxic Epidermal Necrolysis Spectrum of Disease

Stevens-Johnson syndrome (SJS) and toxic epidermal necrolysis (TEN) have traditionally been considered the most severe forms of erythema multiforme (EM). It was recently proposed that EM major is distinct from SJS and TEN on the basis of clinical criteria. The proposed concept is to separate an EM spectrum from an SJS/TEN spectrum. EM, characterized by typical target lesions, is a postinfectious disorder, often recurrent but with low morbidity. The second, characterized by widespread blisters and purpuric macules, is usually a severe drug-induced reaction with high morbidity and a poor prognosis. In this concept, SJS and TEN might be only types of the same drug-induced process that vary in severity.[4, 17] A three-grade classification has been proposed:

Grade 1: SJS mucosal erosions and epidermal detachment below 10%

Grade 2: Overlap SJS/TEN epidermal detachment between 10% and 30%

Grade 3: TEN epidermal detachment more than 30%

Stevens-Johnson syndrome

Vesiculobullous disease of the skin, mouth, eyes, and genitals is called Stevens-Johnson syndrome. The disease occurs most often in children and young adults. The cutaneous eruption is preceded by symptoms of an upper respiratory infection. A harsh, hacking cough and patchy changes on chest radiograph examination indicate pulmonary involvement. Patients with limited disease may be weak and lethargic, but the prognosis is good with conservative treatment. Mortality approaches 10% for patients with extensive disease. Fever is high during the active stages. Oral lesions may continue for months.

SKIN LESIONS. Skin lesions in SJS are flat atypical targets or purpuric maculae that are widespread or distributed on the trunk, palms, and soles (Figures 18-5 and 18-6). This is in contrast to the lesions in erythema multiforme, which consist of typical or raised atypical targets or raised edematous papules that are located on the extremities and/or the face.[18] New crops of lesions appear, but the disease is self-limited and resolves in approximately 1 month if there are no complications.

MUCOSAL LESIONS. Bullae occur suddenly 1 to 14 days after the prodromal symptoms, appearing on the conjunctivae, mucous membranes of the nares, mouth (Figure 18-7), anorectal junction, vulvovaginal region, and urethral meatus. Ulcerative stomatitis leading to hemorrhagic crusting is the most characteristic feature.

OCULAR SYMPTOMS. Corneal ulcerations may lead to blindness. Severe ocular mucosal injury that occurs in Stevens-Johnson syndrome may be a precipitating factor in the development of ocular cicatricial pemphigoid, a chronic, scarring inflammation of the ocular mucosae that can lead to blindness. The time between the onset of Stevens-Johnson syndrome and cicatricial pemphigoid ranges from a few months to 31 years.[19]

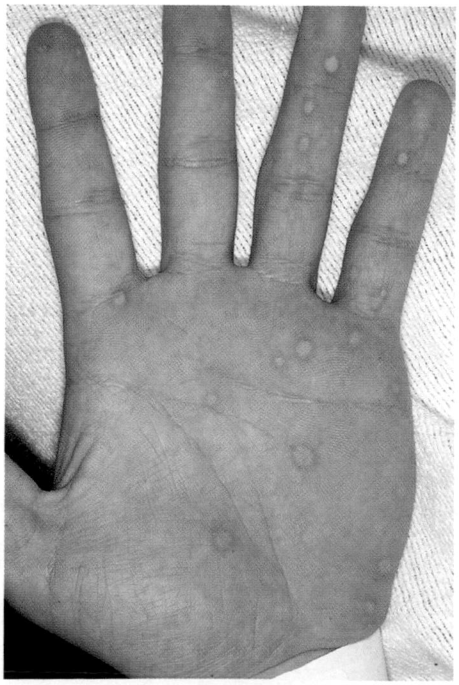

Figure 18-5 Stevens-Johnson syndrome. Vesicles that do not form the typical target of erythema multiforme may appear on the palms and soles.

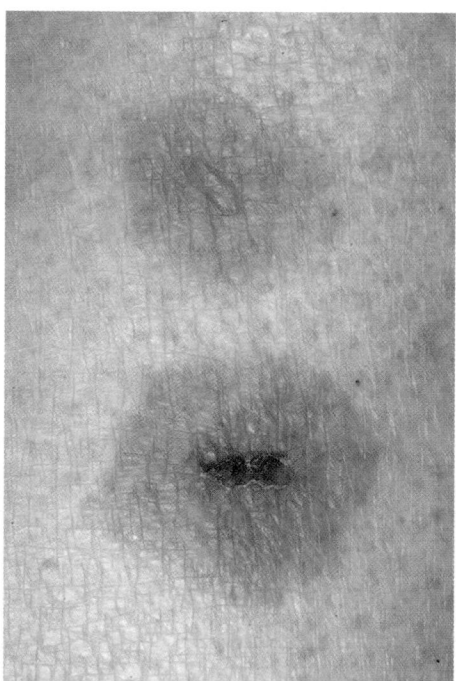

Figure 18-6 Stevens-Johnson syndrome. Atypical target lesions consist of round red macules, some of which have a central vesicle. There may be just a few lesions on the trunk.

ETIOLOGY. Drugs are the most common cause (phenytoin, phenobarbital, sulfonamides, penicillins). The disease occurs most often in patients treated for seizure disorders. Upper respiratory tract infection, gastrointestinal (GI) disorders, Mycoplasma pneumoniae infection,[20] and herpes simplex virus infection are all implicated. Possible causes should be sought diligently so that recurrences can be avoided.

DIAGNOSIS. A skin biopsy should be performed if the classic lesions are not present. Direct immunofluorescence may be helpful in nontypical cases[21] (see Table 16-4).

TREATMENT. The use of corticosteroids remains controversial. A study of children suggests that treatment with systemic corticosteroids may be associated with delayed recovery and significant side effects.[22] Other studies conclude that corticosteroids are beneficial and may be life-saving.[23,24] Many physicians presented with a sick child who has extensive cutaneous, ocular, and oral lesions elect to treat with oral steroids; most often prednisone (20 to 30 mg twice a day) is given until new lesions no longer appear; it is then tapered rapidly.

Itching can be controlled with antihistamines. Cutaneous blisters are treated with cool, wet Burrow's compresses. Topical steroids should not be applied to eroded areas. Papules and plaques may respond to group II to V topical steroids. Frequent rinsing with lidocaine hydrochloride (Xylocaine Viscous) may relieve oral symptoms. Patients may tolerate only a liquid or soft diet. Ocular involvement is monitored by an ophthalmologist to minimize conjunctival scarring. Antiseptic eye drops and separation on synechiae are required. Vitamin A administered topically and systemically was reported to be effective for lacrimal hyposecretion.[25] Secondary infection is treated with oral antibiotics. Stevens-Johnson syndrome associated with herpes simplex virus may be prevented by early use of acyclovir and prednisone.[26]

STEVENS-JOHNSON SYNDROME

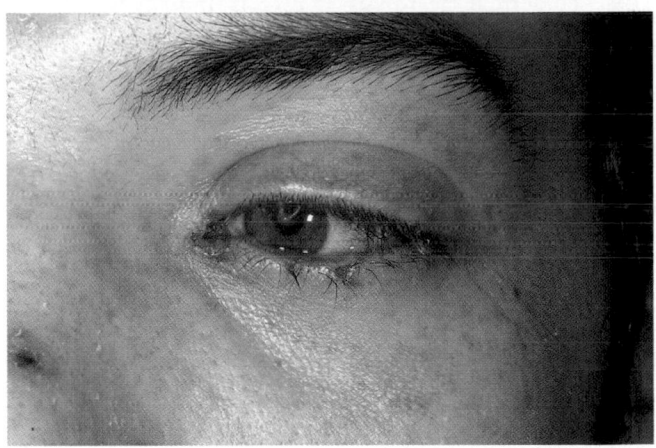

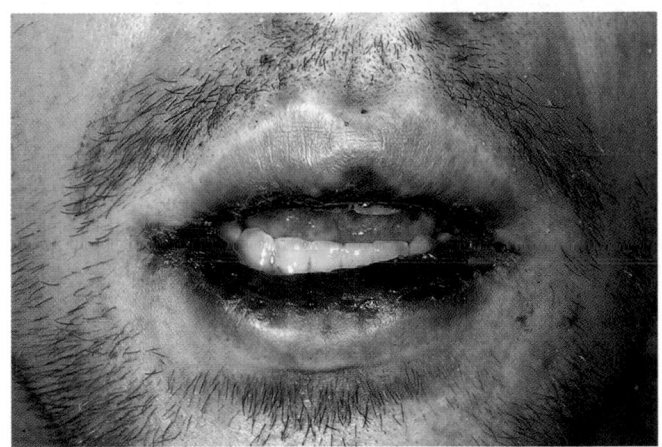

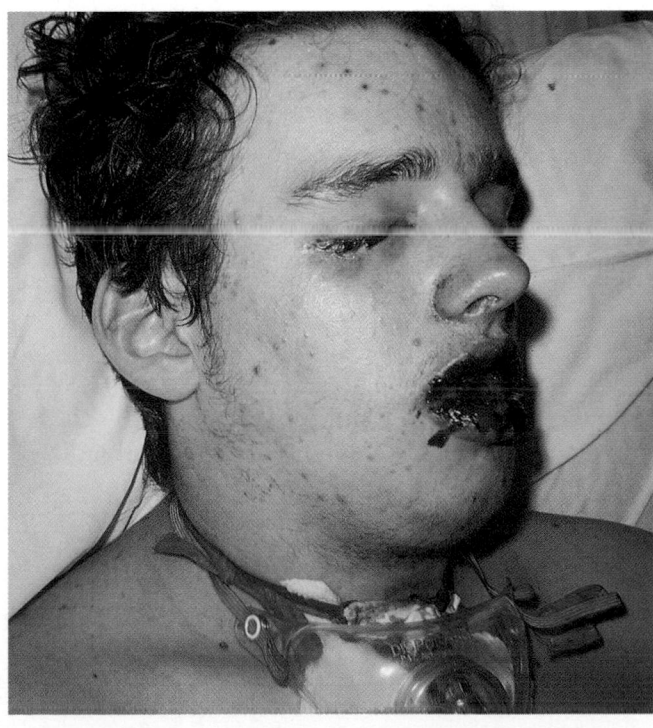

Figure 18-7 Bullae are present on the conjunctivae and in the mouth. Sloughing, ulceration, and necrosis in the oral cavity interfere with eating. Genital lesions cause dysuria and interfere with voiding.

Toxic epidermal necrolysis

Toxic epidermal necrolysis (TEN) is initially seen with Stevens-Johnson–like mucous membrane disease and progresses to diffuse, generalized detachment of the epidermis through the dermoepidermal junction.[27, 28] This full-thickness loss of the epidermis results in a high mortality rate. Fluid loss is not a major problem; death is usually caused by overwhelming sepsis originating in denuded skin or lungs. TEN is rare, occurring in 1.3 cases per million per year.[29]

The mortality rate is 1% to 5% for Stevens-Johnson syndrome, and 34% to 40% for TEN. Mortality is not affected by the type of drug responsible. In contrast to previous series, today there is a high prevalence of human immunodeficiency virus infection among patients with TEN. This high rate of HIV infection is linked to an increased use of sulfonamides—mainly sulfadiazine—in these patients.[30-32] TEN may occur after bone marrow transplantation.[33] It seems to be related to a drug reaction to sulfonamides as often as to acute graft-vs.-host disease.

TOXIC EPIDERMAL NECROLYSIS VS. STAPHYLOCOCCAL SCALDED SKIN SYNDROME. This life-threatening disease is similar in appearance to the staphylococcal scalded skin syndrome (SSSS), which is induced by a staphylococcal toxin. The split in SSSS, however, is high in the epidermis, just below the stratum corneum, permitting rapid healing of the epidermis without danger of infection. The diagnosis of either TEN or SSSS can be made rapidly by examination of a skin biopsy by frozen section technique.

PATHOLOGY AND PATHOGENESIS. Histologically there is an early mild interface dermatitis that evolves into full-thickness necrosis of the epidermis. Keratinocytes from patients with TEN were found to undergo extensive apoptosis.[34] There is subepidermal blister formation, keratinocyte necrosis, and a sparse lymphohistiocytic infiltrate around superficial dermal blood vessels. Lymphopenia is frequently documented. Cytotoxic T cells (CD8+ lymphocytes) may contribute to the pathogenesis of blister formation by causing degeneration and necrosis of drug-altered keratinocytes.[35-38]

ETIOLOGY. The causes of TEN are the same as those of Stevens-Johnson syndrome, but drugs are most frequently implicated in TEN. The reaction is independent of dosage. In two large series, the culprit drugs included antibiotics (40%), anticonvulsants (11%), and analgesics (5% to 23%). Developing countries have a higher incidence of reactions to antituberculous drugs.[39] The most frequent underlying diseases justifying drug treatment are infections (52.7%) and pain (36%). Challenge tests are absolutely contraindicated in Stevens-Johnson syndrome and toxic epidermal necrolysis.[40] TEN and other severe cutaneous adverse drug reactions may be linked to an inherited defect in the detoxification of drug metabolites. In a few predisposed patients, a drug metabolite may bind to proteins in the epidermis and trigger an immune response, leading to immunoallergic cutaneous adverse drug reaction.[41]

MEDICATIONS. The use of antibacterial sulfonamides, anticonvulsant agents, oxicam NSAIDs, allopurinol, chlormezanone, and corticosteroids is associated with large increases in the risk of Stevens-Johnson syndrome or toxic epidermal necrolysis. The excess risk of these drugs does not exceed five cases per million users per week.[42] The risk of developing TEN from antiepileptic drugs is highest in the first 8 weeks after onset of treatment.[43]

The following drugs are most commonly implicated:
Sulfonamides
Trimethoprim-sulfamethoxazole
Chlormezanone
Aminopenicillins
Quinolones
Cephalosporins
Acetaminophen
Carbamazepine
Phenobarbital
Phenytoin
Valproic acid
NSAIDs
Allopurinol
Corticosteroids

PRODROMAL SYMPTOMS. Fever is the most frequent prodromal symptom. Symptoms suggestive of an upper respiratory tract infection, such as headache and sore throat, usually precede the appearance of skin lesions by 1 or 2 weeks. Stomatitis, conjunctivitis, and pruritus occur 1 to 2 days before the onset of the rash.

SKIN. TEN begins with diffuse, hot erythema covering wide areas. In hours the skin becomes painful, and with slight thumb pressure the skin wrinkles, slides laterally, and separates from the dermis (Figure 18-8, A). This ominous sign (Nikolsky's sign) (Figure 18-8, B) heralds the onset of a life-threatening event. Small blisters and large bullae may appear. Nonerythematous skin usually remains intact, and the scalp is spared.

MUCOUS MEMBRANES. Inflammation, blistering, and erosion of the mucosal surfaces, especially the oropharynx, are early and characteristic findings. The vaginal tract epithelium frequently blisters and erodes. Pain and erosion of oral mucous membranes interfere with oral intake, and nasogastric or duodenal tube feeding is often required. The rest of the gastrointestinal tract functions normally if sepsis does not occur.

EYES. Severe eye involvement is a constant feature. Purulent conjunctivitis leads to swelling, crusting, and ulceration with pain and photophobia. Complications include conjunctival erosions with subsequent revascularization, fibrous adhesions, and corneal ulceration and blindness. Photophobia, mucinous discharge, and decreased visual acuity may last for years.

TOXIC EPIDERMAL NECROLYSIS

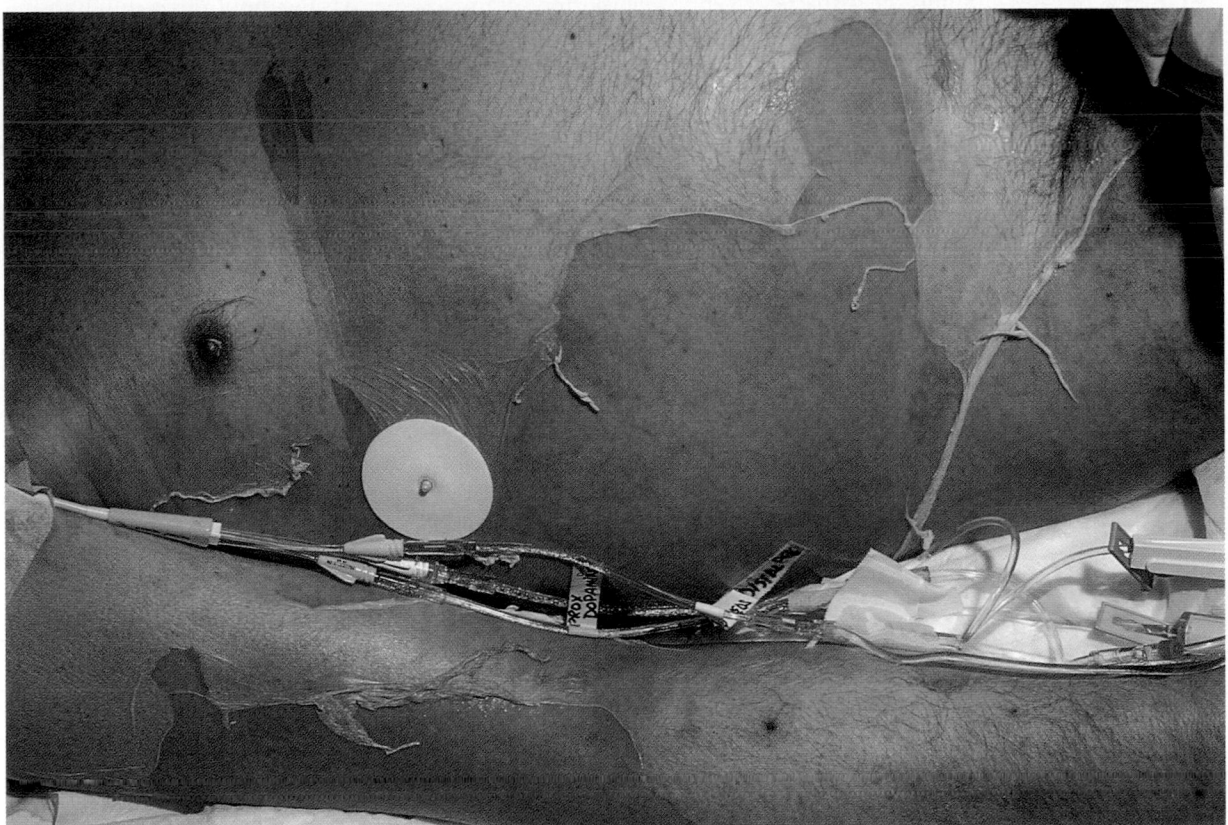

A, Large sheets of full-thickness epidermis are shed.

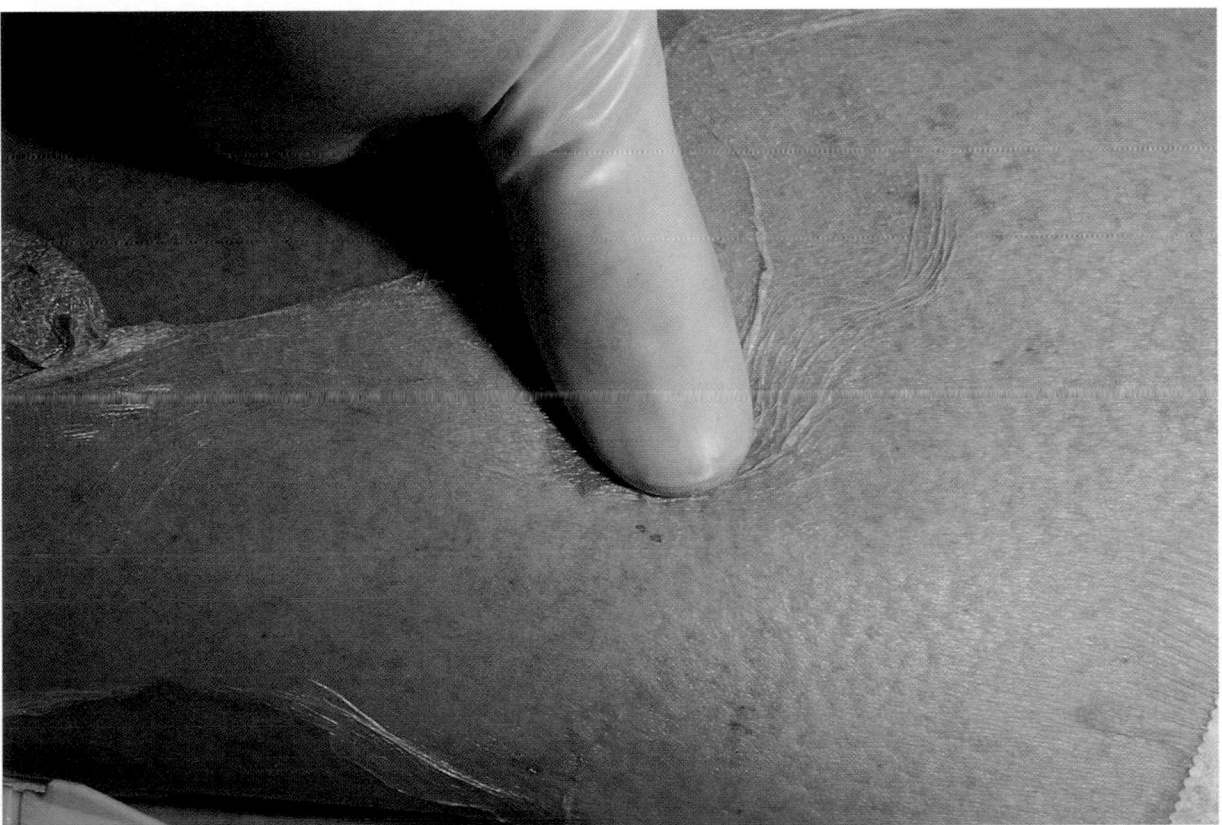

B, Toxic epidermal necrolysis begins with diffuse, hot erythema. In hours the skin becomes painful, and with slight thumb pressure the skin wrinkles, slides laterally, and separates from the dermis (Nikolsky's sign).

Figure 18-8

RESPIRATORY TRACT. Involvement of bronchial epithelium was noted in 27% of cases and must be suspected when dyspnea, bronchial hypersecretion, normal chest radiograph, and marked hypoxemia are present during the early stages of toxic epidermal necrosis. Bronchial injury indicates a poor prognosis.[44] Life-threatening acute respiratory decompensation requiring ventilatory support and long-term pulmonary function abnormalities may occur. Patients should be closely monitored for pulmonary complications.[45] Bronchopneumonia occurs in 30% of reported cases and is the cause of death in many cases. Many patients require intubation or ventilatory support. Respiratory failure can occur, with mucus retention and sloughing of the tracheobronchial mucosa.

INFECTION. Septicemia and gram-negative pneumonia are the most common causes of death. The lungs and denuded skin are the common portals of entry. The incidence of positive blood culture results is very high when central venous lines are used. Intravenous lines are changed or discontinued if it is probable that they are the source of positive blood culture findings. The urethra is often involved, but the use of Foley catheters can be avoided in many cases.

FLUID AND ELECTROLYTE LOSS. Fluid loss in TEN is not as severe as it is in burn patients, but significant losses can occur if grafts are not applied. Apparently, the acute-phase reactants that create massive edema after thermal injury are not released in TEN.

OTHER COMPLICATIONS. Leukopenia of uncertain cause may occur. Toxins (e.g., from absorbed silver sulfadiazine) or immune complexes may be the cause.[46-49] In one series, renal involvement consisting of hematuria, proteinuria, and elevated serum creatine occurred in 50% of patients with Stevens-Johnson syndrome.[50]

TREATMENT

Systemic steroids. The use of systemic steroids is still controversial,[51,52] but most authors recommend that steroids not be used.[53]

Steroids cannot prevent the occurrence of TEN, even in high dosages.[54] Patients treated for other diseases with glucocorticosteroids for at least 1 week before the first dermatologic sign of TEN showed no difference in mortality compared with untreated patients.[55] This suggests that steroids do not protect the epidermis from drug-induced keratolysis. Improved survival rates have been reported when patients with TEN have been treated without steroids.[56]

Cyclosporine. Patients with TEN treated with cyclosporine A (3 mg/kg per day) without other immunosuppressive agents experienced rapid reepithelialization and a low mortality rate. This regimen was more effective than a series of patients previously treated with cyclophosphamide and corticosteroids.[57,58]

Cyclophosphamide. In one study, cyclophosphamide (100 to 300 mg/day intravenously for 5 days) stopped the blistering, pain, and erythema in a few days. Reepithelialization rapidly occurred in 4 to 5 days.[35] Cyclophosphamide inhibits cell-mediated cytotoxicity.

Plasma exchange and immunoglobulins. Plasma exchange resulted in complete remission in two series.[59,60] Plasmapheresis is a safe intervention in extremely ill patients and may reduce the mortality rate.[61] IVIG is a safe and effective treatment for TEN adults and children. Early treatment with IVIG at a total dose of 3g/kg over 3 consecutive days (1g/kg per day for 3 days) is recommended.[62]

Burn center treatment. TEN has pathophysiologic similarities to partial-thickness burn injury. The management of major fluid and electrolyte derangements, the intensive nutritional support, and the management of extensive cutaneous injuries with ready access to biologic and semisynthetic wound dressings are best accomplished in a multidisciplinary burn center.[63]

The current trend toward prolonged treatment in outside facilities before referral to a burn center is detrimental to the care of patients with TEN. The overall rate of bacteremia, septicemia, and mortality is significantly reduced with early (< or = 7 days) referral to a regional burn center.[64,65]

Separation at the junction of the dermis and epidermis leaves totally viable dermis and intact skin appendages. If the dermis can be protected from toxic detergents, salves, or desiccation, rapid resurfacing by proliferation of epithelium from the skin appendages will occur in approximately 14 days without scarring.[66] Silver sulfadiazine and mafenide acetate (Sulfamylon) delay epithelialization. A new dressing designed for patients with burns (Soft-Dorb, DeRoyal Industries Inc, Powell, TN) can be impregnated with 0.5% silver nitrate solution and allows for a moist wound-healing. It can be left in place for 2 to 3 days, which prevents further damage to the skin. Extensive early debridement of necrotic skin areas followed by wound coverage with Biobrane,[67] (Dow B. Hickam, Inc, Sugarland, TX), a temporary semisynthetic skin substitute, decreased pain and fluid loss, and possibly facilitated epithelialization.

Erythema Nodosum

Erythema nodosum (EN) is a nodular erythematous eruption that is usually limited to the extensor aspects of the extremities. EN represents a hypersensitivity reaction to a variety of antigenic stimuli and may be observed in association with several diseases (infections, immunopathies, malignancies) and during drug therapy (with halides, sulfonamides, oral contraceptives). Approximately 55% of cases are idiopathic. Laboratory tests show no specific abnormalities except those related to an underlying disease. Familial EN is reported, with affected family members showing a common haplotype.[68] The incidence has decreased in the antibiotic era. EN is seen more frequently in females. The peak incidence occurs between the ages of 18 and 34 years. The female:male ratio is 5:1.[69]

CLINICAL MANIFESTATIONS AND COURSE. Prodromal symptoms of fatigue and malaise or symptoms of an upper respiratory infection precede the eruption by 1 to 3 weeks. The clinical picture is that of a nonspecific systemic illness, with low-grade fever (60%), malaise (67%), arthralgias (64%), and arthritis (31%). Pulmonary hilar adenopathy may develop as part of the hypersensitivity reaction of EN and is seen in cases with diverse causes.

JOINT SYMPTOMS. Arthralgia occurs in more than 50% of patients and begins during the eruptive phase or precedes the eruption by 2 to 8 weeks. Symptoms may disappear in a few weeks or persist for 2 years, but they always resolve without destructive joint changes. The rheumatoid factor is negative. Joint symptoms consist of erythema, swelling, and tenderness over the joint, sometimes with effusions; arthralgia and morning stiffness, most commonly in the knee, but any joint may be affected; and polyarthralgia lasting for days.

SKIN ERUPTION. The eruptive phase begins with flulike symptoms of fever and generalized aching. The characteristic lesions begin as red, nodelike swellings over the shins; as a rule, both legs are affected. Similar lesions may appear on the extensor aspects of the forearms, thighs, and trunk (Figure 18-9). The border is poorly defined, with size varying from 2 to 6 cm. Lesions are oval, and their long axis corresponds to that of the limb. During the first week the lesions become tense, hard, and painful; during the second week they become fluctuant, as in an abscess, but never suppurate. The color changes in the second week from bright red to bluish or livid; as absorption progresses, it gradually fades to a yellowish hue, resembling a bruise; this disappears in 1 or 2 weeks as the overlying skin desquamates. The individual lesions last approximately 2 weeks, but new lesions sometimes continue to appear for 3 to 6 weeks. Aching of the legs and swelling of the ankles may persist for weeks. The condition may recur for months or years.

PATHOGENESIS AND ETIOLOGY. Erythema nodosum is probably a delayed hypersensitivity reaction to a variety of antigens; circulating immune complexes have not been found in idiopathic or uncomplicated cases.[70] EN is a reaction pattern elicited by many different diseases (Box 18-1). In one large series, 32.5% of cases were idiopathic.[71] The most common cause today is streptococcal infection[72] and noninfectious inflammatory diseases in children[73] and streptococcal infection and sarcoidosis in adults. Dental treatment and the possible presence of infectious dental foci should be considered in the differential diagnosis. EN is reported following dental treatment associated with gingival bleeding or due to infectious dental foci.[74] Many other causes of EN have been reported; most consist of single histories. New etiologies continue to be described.

FUNGAL INFECTIONS. Coccidioidomycosis (San Joaquin Valley fever) is the most common cause of EN in the west and southwest United States. In approximately 4% of males and 10% of females, the primary fungal infection, which may be

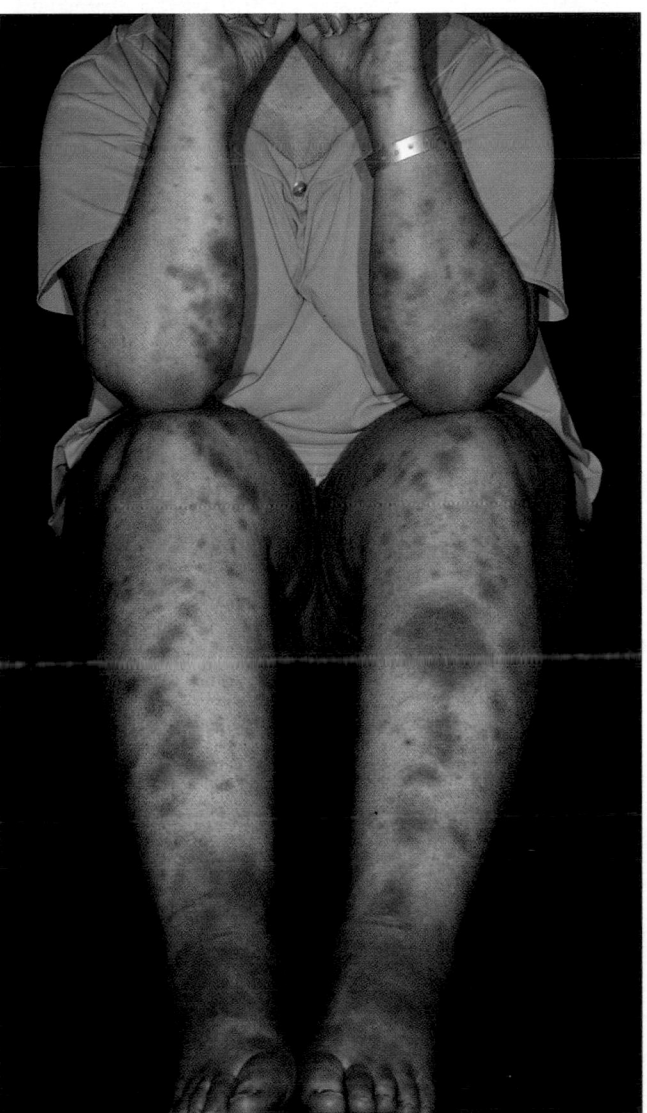

Figure 18-9 Erythema nodosum. Red node-like swelling in the characteristic distribution.

asymptomatic or involve symptoms of an upper respiratory infection, is followed by the development of EN. The lesions appear when the skin-test result becomes positive, 3 days to 3 weeks after the end of the fever caused by the fungal infection. Dissemination and serious disease develop more often in pregnant patients with coccidioidomycosis than in the general population. Erythema nodosum appears to be a salient marker of a positive outcome for pregnant patients, more so than for the general population.

Histoplasmosis, blastomycosis, and lymphogranuloma venereum may cause EN. Leprosy is another possible inciting factor. Clinically, erythema nodosum leprosum resembles EN, but the histologic picture is that of leukocytoclastic vasculitis.

INFLAMMATORY BOWEL DISEASE. Inflammatory bowel diseases such as ulcerative colitis and regional ileitis may trigger EN, usually during active disease with symptoms of abdominal complaints and diarrhea. The mean duration of chronic ulcerative colitis before the onset of EN is 5 years, and the EN is controlled with adequate therapy of the colitis.[75] *Yersinia enterocolitica*, a gram-negative bacillus that causes acute diarrhea and abdominal pain, is a reported cause.

DRUGS. Sulfonamides, bromides, and oral contraceptives have been reported to cause EN. Several other drugs, such as antibiotics, barbiturates, and salicylates, are often suspected but seldom proved causes.

SARCOIDOSIS. EN occurs in up to 39% of cases of sarcoidosis and has also been observed in pregnant women.[76] Seasonal clustering of sarcoidosis presenting with EN has been reported. This suggests a common environmental trigger in the etiology of sarcoidosis.[76]

Box 18-1 Erythema Nodosum—The Most Common Causes

Infections
Streptococci
Tuberculosis
Psittacosis
Yersiniosis
Lymphogranuloma venereum
Cat-scratch disease
Coccidioidomycosis
Upper respiratory infection

Drugs
Sulphonamides
Bromides
Oral contraceptives

Systemic Illnesses
Sarcoidosis
Inflammatory bowel disease
Hodgkin's disease

Pregnancy

LYMPHOMA. EN should be considered as a warning signal of impending relapse in a patient with a history of Hodgkin's disease.[77] Patients in whom erythema nodosum was associated with non-Hodgkin's lymphoma have an extremely protracted course. Erythema nodosum associated with non-Hodgkin's lymphoma may precede the diagnosis of lymphoma by months.[78]

DIAGNOSIS. Initial evaluation should include throat culture, antistreptolysin titer, chest radiograph, purified protein derivative skin test, and ESR. The ESR is elevated in all patients with EN.

Patients with GI symptoms should have a stool culture for *Y. enterocolitica, Salmonella,* and *Campylobacter.* Bilateral hilar adenopathy on chest radiograph examination does not establish the diagnosis of sarcoidosis, because hilar adenopathy occurs in EN produced by coccidioidomycosis, histoplasmosis, tuberculosis, streptococcal infections, lymphoma, and as a nonspecific reaction in many cases.[79]

BIOPSY. The clinical picture is characteristic in most cases, and a biopsy is not required. Histologic confirmation is desirable in atypical cases.[80] An excisional rather than a punch biopsy is necessary to sample the subcutaneous fat adequately. Tissue sections show lymphohistiocytic infiltrate, granulomatous inflammation, and fibrosis in the septa of the subcutaneous fat; these are all features of a septal panniculitis.

DIFFERENTIAL DIAGNOSIS. In Weber-Christian panniculitis, localized areas of subcutaneous inflammation tend to occur on the thighs and trunk rather than on the lower legs. Lesions may suppurate and heal with atrophy and localized depressions. Superficial and deep thrombophlebitis and erysipelas must also be differentiated from EN.

TREATMENT. EN in most instances is a self-limited disease and requires only symptomatic relief with salicylates and bed rest. Indomethacin (250 mg three times daily) or naproxen (250 mg twice daily) may be more effective than aspirin. Cases that are recurrent, unusually painful, or long lasting require a more vigorous approach.

A supersaturated solution of potassium iodide[83] (5 drops three times daily) in orange juice is started. Increase the dose by 1 drop per dose per day until the patient responds. Relief of lesional tenderness, arthralgia, and fever may occur in 24 hours. Most lesions completely subside within 10 to 14 days. However, potassium iodide is not effective for all patients with EN. Patients who receive medication shortly after the initial onset of EN respond more satisfactorily than those with chronic EN. Side effects include nasal catarrh and headache. Hyperthyroidism may occur with long-term use.

Corticosteroids are effective but seldom necessary in self-limited diseases. Recurrence following discontinuation of treatment is common, and underlying infectious disease may be worsened.[84]

There is limited experience with colchicine, hydroxychloroquine, and dapsone.

Vasculitis

Cutaneous vasculitis encompasses a highly heterogeneous group of disorders of diverse etiology, pathogenesis, and clinical features (Boxes 18-2 to 18-4 and Table 18-1).[85,86]

CLASSIFICATION. Vasculitis, or angiitis, defined as inflammation of the vessel wall, is probably initiated by immune complex deposition. The cutaneous vasculitic diseases are classified according to the type of inflammatory cell within the vessel walls (neutrophil, lymphocyte, or histiocyte) and the size and type of blood vessel involved (venule, arteriole, artery, or vein). Some vasculitic diseases are limited to the skin; others involve vessels in many different organs.

CLINICAL PRESENTATION. The clinical presentation varies with the size of the blood vessel involved and the intensity of the inflammation (Table 18-1; see the comparison of vasculitic syndromes on p. 640). Small-vessel vasculitis—arteriole, capillary, venule—most commonly affects the skin and rarely causes serious internal organ dysfunction, except when the kidney is involved.

There are numerous cutaneous diseases that histologically show some degree of vessel inflammation. Only those diseases that have inflammation severe enough to cause necrosis of vessel walls are discussed here. Necrotizing angiitis is the term given to this group of diseases. These diseases have clinical features that allow one to predict that vessel inflammation and necrosis are taking place and to identify the size of vessel involved[87,88] (see Table 18-1).

Box 18-2 Major Categories of Noninfectious Vasculitis*

Large-vessel vasculitis

Giant-cell arteritis

Takayasu's arteritis

Medium-sized vessel vasculitis

Polyarteritis nodosa

Kawasaki's disease

Primary granulomatous central nervous system vasculitis

Small-vessel vasculitis

ANCA-associated small-vessel vasculitis

   Microscopic polyangitis

   Wegener's granulomatosis

   Churg-Strauss syndrome

   Drug-induced ANCA-associated vasculitis

Immune-complex small-vessel vasculitis

   Henoch-Schönlein purpura

   Cryoglobulinemic vasculitis

   Lupus vasculitis

   Rheumatoid vasculitis

   Sjögren's syndrome vasculitis

   Hypocomplementemic urticarial vasculitis

   Behcet's disease

   Goodpasture's syndrome

   Serum-sickness vasculitis

   Drug-induced immune-complex vasculitis

   Infection-induced immune-complex vasculitis

Paraneoplastic small-vessel vasculitis

   Lymphorproliferative neoplasm-induced vasculitis

   Myeloproliferative neoplasm-induced vasculitis

   Carcinoma-induced vasculitis

Inflammatory bowel disease vasculitis

From Jennette JC, Falk RJ: N Engl J Med 1997; 1512.

*Vascular inflammation is categorized as either infectious vasculitis, which is caused by the direct invasion of vessel walls by pathogens (e.g., rickettsial organisms in Rocky Mountain spotted fever), or noninfectious vasculitis, which is not caused by the direct invasion of vessel walls by pathogens (although infections can indirectly induce noninfectious vasculitis, for example, by generating pathogenic immune complexes). ANCA denotes antineutrophil cytoplasmic autoantibodies.

Box 18-3 Names and Definitions of Vasculitis Adopted by the Chapel Hill Consensus Conference on the Nomenclature of Systemic Vasculitis

Large-vessel vasculitis

Giant cell (temporal) arteritis	Granulomatous arteritis of the aorta and its major branches, with a predilection for the extracranial branches of the carotid artery; *often involves the temporal artery; usually occurs in patients older than 50 y and is often associated with polymyalgia rheumatica*
Takayasu arteritis	Granulomatous inflammation of the aorta and its major branches; *usually occurs in patients younger than 50 y*

Medium-sized vessel vasculitis

Polyarteritis nodosa (classic PAN)	Necrotizing inflammation of medium-sized or small arteries without glomerulonephritis or vasculitis in arterioles, capillaries, or venules
Kawasaki disease	Arteritis involving the large, medium-sized, or small arteries and associated with mucocutaneous lymph node syndrome; *coronary arteries are often involved; aorta and veins may be involved; usually occurs in children*

Small-vessel vasculitis

Wegener's granulomatosis	Granulomatous inflammation involving the respiratory tract and necrotizing vasculitis affecting small- to medium-sized vessels (e.g., capillaries, venules, arterioles, and arteries); *necrotizing glomerulonephritis is common*
Churg-Strauss syndrome	Eosinophil-rich and granulomatous inflammation involving the respiratory tract, necrotizing vasculitis affecting small- to medium-sized vessels, and associated with asthma and eosinophilia
Microscopic polyangiitis	Necrotizing vasculitis, with few or no immune deposits, affecting small vessels (e.g., capillaries, venules, or arterioles); *necrotizing arteritis involving small and medium-sized arteries may be present; necrotizing glomerulonephritis is very common; pulmonary capillaritis often occurs*
Henoch-Schönlein purpura	Vasculitis, with IgA-dominant immune deposits, affecting small vessels (e.g., capillaries, venules, or arterioles); *typically involves skin, gut, and glomeruli and is associated with arthralgias or arthritis*
Essential cryoglobulinemic vasculitis	Vasculitis, with cryoglobulin immune deposits, affecting small vessels (e.g., capillaries, venules, or arterioles), and associated with cryoglobulins in serum; *skin and glomeruli are often involved*
Cutaneous leukocytoclastic angiitis	Isolated cutaneous leukocytoclastic angiitis without systemic vasculitis or glomerulonephritis

From Jennette JC, Falk RJ: N Engl J Med 1997; 1512.

Table 18-1 Comparison of Organ Involvement in Various Vasculitides

Organ System	PAN	WG	MPA	CSS	CV	UV	HSP
Cutaneous	50	40	50	55	90	100	90
Pulmonary	30	90	35	60	<5	10	<5
Renal	30	80	90	35	25	<5	50
Ear, nose, throat	7	90	25	50	<5	<5	<5
Musculoskeletal	70	60	60	50	70	40	75
Neurologic	60	50	35	70	40	<5	10
Gastrointestinal	30	50	40	45	30	15	60

From Fiorentino DF: J Am Acad Dermatol 2003; 48:311.
PAN, Polyarteritis nodosa; *WG,* Wegener's granulomatosis; *MPA,* microscopic polyangiitis; *CSS,* Churg-Strauss syndrome; *CV,* cryoglobulinemic vasculitis; *UV,* urticarial vasculitis; *HSP,* Henoch-Schönlein purpura.

Box 18-4 The American College of Rheumatology Classification Criteria for Vasculitis

Giant-cell (temporal) arteritis (GCA)

1. Age >50 y at onset
2. New type of headache
3. Abnormal temporal artery on clinical examination (tenderness to palpation or decreased pulsation)
4. Elevated erythrocyte sedimentation rate
5. Temporal artery biopsy showing vasculitis

Three criteria classify GCA with sensitivity of 93.5% and specificity of 91.2%

Takayasu's arteritis (TA)

1. Age less than 40 yr at onset
2. Limb claudication
3. Decreased brachial artery pulses
4. BP >10 mm Hg difference between two arms
5. Bruits
6. Arteriogram normal

Three criteria classify TA with sensitivity of 90.5% and specificity of 97.8%

Polyarteritis nodosa (PAN)

1. Weight loss >4 kg
2. Livedo reticularis
3. Testicular pain or tenderness
4. Myalgias, myopathy, or tenderness
5. Neuropathy
6. Hypertension (diastolic BP >90 mm Hg)
7. Renal impairment (elevated BUN or creatine)
8. Hepatitis B virus
9. Abnormal arteriography
10. Biopsy of artery showing PAN

Three criteria classify PAN with sensitivity of 82.2% and specificity of 86.6%

Wegener's granulomatosis (WG)

1. Nasal or oral inflammation
2. Chest x-ray showing nodules, infiltrates (fixed), or cavities
3. Microscopic hematuria or red cell casts in urine
4. Granulomatous inflammation on biopsy (within vessel wall or perivascular)

Two criteria classify WG with sensitivity of 88.2% and specificity of 92.0%

Churg-Strauss syndrome (CSS)

1. Asthma
2. Eosinophilia (>10%)
3. Neuropathy
4. Pulmonary infiltrates (nonfixed)
5. Sinusitis
6. Extravascular eosinophils on biopsy

Four criteria classify CSS with sensitivity of 85% and specificity of 99.7%

Hypersensitivity vasculitis

1. Age >16 yr at onset
2. Medications that may have precipitated event
3. Palpable purpura
4. Cutaneous eruption
5. Positive biopsy results

Three criteria classify HSV with sensitivity of 71.0% and specificity of 83.9%

Henoch-Schönlein purpura (HSP)

1. Palpable purpura
2. Age at onset <20y
3. Bowel angina
4. Vessel wall granulocytes on biopsy

Two criteria classify HSP with sensitivity of 87% and specificity of 88%

BP, Blood pressure; *BUN,* blood urea nitrogen; *PMN,* polymorphonuclear cells.

Table 18-2 Clinical Signs of Necrotizing Vasculitis with Respect to Vessel Size Involved

Signs	Diseases
Small vessels (arteriole, capillary, venule)	
Urticaria reflects minimal vessel inflammation and necrosis.	Hypersensitivity vasculitis
Palpable purpura: exudation and hemorrhage from damaged vessels produce the most characteristic lesion of small-vessel necrotizing vasculitis. The lesion is a red, slightly elevated papule that does not blanch on application of external pressure.	Henoch-Schönlein purpura Essential mixed cryoglobulinemia Vasculitis associated with connective tissue disease Vasculitis associated with malignancies Serum sickness and serum sickness-like reactions
Nodules, bullae, or ulcers may be present if vessel wall inflammation and necrosis are intense.	Chronic urticaria (urticarial vasculitis) Urticarial prodrome of acute hepatitis type B infection
Large vessels (small- and medium-sized muscular arteries)	
Subcutaneous nodules, ulceration, and ecchymoses result from necrosis and thrombosis of larger vessels, which lead to infarction.	Polyarteritis nodosa Churg-Strauss syndrome Wegener's granulomatosis Giant cell (temporal) arteritis

VASCULITIC SYNDROMES

Large- to medium-sized artery	Small artery	Arteriole	Capillary	Venule	Vein
Branches directed to extremities, head, neck Main visceral arteries (renal, hepatic, coronary, mesenteric)	Skin nodules	Purpura			
	Distal arterial radicals (subcutaneous and deep dermal arteries)				

Chronic infection
Acute strep infection
Drug
Hepatitis B
ANCA

ANCA

ANCA

Streptococcal or viral URI
IgA, IC

Drugs
Infections
CTD
Neoplasms
IC

Polyarteritis Nodosa

Wegener's Granulomatosis

Churg-Strauss Syndrome

Henoch-Schönlein Purpura

Hypersensitivity Vasculitis

• Joints (arthritis or arthralgias)

---

* Weight loss
* Testicular pain
* Myalgias, weakness, or leg tenderness
* Mono- or poly-neuropathy
* Diastolic BP >90

Skin
  Livedo reticularis
  Nodules
  Ulcers

* Elevated BUN or creatine
* Hepatitis B surface antigen or antibody
* Arteriographic abnormality
* Granulocytes in artery wall

p-ANCA

---

* Oral ulcers or nasal discharge (purulent or bloody)
* Hemoptysis

Skin
  Palpable purpura

* Chest x-ray
  Nodules
  Infiltrates (fixed) or cavities
* Microhematuria or red cell casts
* Granulomatous inflammation Peri- or extra-vascular area (artery or arteriole)

c-ANCA

---

* Asthma
* History of allergy
* Mono- or poly-neuropathy
Fever

Skin
  Palpable purpura
  Nodules
  Ulcers

* Eosinophilia >10%
* Paranasal sinus abnormality
* Extravascular eosinophils

Elevated IgE
Pulmonary infiltrates (nonfixed)

p-ANCA

---

* Age <20
* GI bleeding
Abdominal pain
Arthralgia
Scrotal swelling

Skin
  Palpable purpura

* Skin
  Extravascular or perivascular granulocytes
Hematuria
Proteinuria
IgA-glomeruli
IgA-arterioles (skin)

---

* Age >16
* Medication at onset
Neuropathy
Abdominal pain
Arthralgia
GI bleeding

Skin
  * Palpable purpura
  * Maculopapular rash

* Skin—peri- or extravascular granulocytes
ESR elevated
Hematuria
Proteinuria

---

*1990 American College of Rheumatology criteria of diagnosis.
ANCA, Antineutrophil cytoplasmic autoantibodies.
IC, Immune complex mediate.

ANTINEUTROPHIL CYTOPLASMIC ANTIBODIES. The diagnosis and classification of vasculitis has been revolutionized by the discovery of serum antineutrophil cytoplasmic autoantibodies (ANCAs) (Table 18-3). ANCAs are a serologic marker for many forms of necrotizing vasculitis. Use of ANCA testing provides a significant diagnostic advantage over reliance on biopsy findings alone in patients whose differential diagnosis includes any of the vasculitic diseases. Two staining patterns may be identified using immunofluorescence (IFA) on ethanol fixed neutrophils: either a diffuse granular staining of the cytoplasm (cytoplasmic, or C-ANCA) or concentration of fluorescence around the nucleus (perinuclear, or P-ANCA).

Antineutrophil cytoplasmic autoantibody–associated vasculitis. ANCA-associated small-vessel vasculitis is the most common primary systemic small-vessel vasculitis in adults and includes three major categories: Wegener's granulomatosis, microscopic polyangiitis, and Churg-Strauss syndrome. Most patients with Wegener's granulomatosis have PR3-ANCA (cytoplasmic ANCA or C-ANCA); most patients with microscopic polyangiitis or Churg-Strauss syndrome have MPO-ANCA (perinuclear ANCA or P-ANCA). Approximately 10% of patients with typical Wegener's granulomatosis or microscopic polyangiitis have negative assays for ANCA; therefore ANCA negativity does not rule out these diseases. The specificity of ANCA positivity is not absolute; a positive result is not diagnostic for an ANCA-associated vasculitis, especially if the result of an indirect immunofluorescence assay has not been confirmed by the more specific enzyme immunoassay (EIA) technique. Patients are usually screened with the indirect immunofluorescence (IFA) test. The EIA is performed when the IFA test result is positive to identify the antigen. A more comprehensive strategy would be to order the IFA and EIA.

A positive test result for C- or P-ANCA predicts a 96% probability that necrotizing vasculitis or crescentic glomerulonephritis will develop; a negative test result portends a 93% probability that the patient does not have these diseases. ANCAs are reliable monitors of disease activity because antibody titers decline when patients go into remission with effective immunosuppressive therapy and increase with relapse.

Table 18-3 Frequency and Type of ANCA Found in Various Vasculitic and Nonvasculitic Disorders

Disease	ANCA (frequency)
Wegener's granulomatosis	C-ANCA (75%-80%)
	P-ANCA (10%-15%)
	Negative (5%-15%)
Microscopic polyangiitis/idiopathic crescentic GN	C-ANCA (25%-35%)
	P-ANCA (50%-60%)
	Negative (5%-10%)
Churg-Strauss syndrome	C-ANCA (10%-15%)
	P-ANCA (55%-6%)
	Negative (30%)
Drug-induced vasculitis	P-ANCA (?)
Rheumatoid arthritis/ Felty's syndrome	P-ANCA (30%-70%) A-ANCA
SLE	P-ANCA (20%-30%) A-ANCA
Ulcerative colitis	P-ANCA (50%-70%)
Crohn's disease	(20%-40%)
Sclerosing cholangiitis	P-ANCA (60%-70%)
Primary biliary cirrhosis	P-ANCA (30%-40%)
Autoimmune hepatitis	C-ANCA (45%)
	P-ANCA (33%-90%)
Chronic infections	C-ANCA
	P-ANCA (?)
	A-ANCA

Fiorentino DF: J Am Acad Dermatol 2003; 48:311.

Vasculitis of Small Vessels

Most diseases characterized by necrotizing inflammation of small blood vessels have a number of features in common. Skin lesions reflect various degrees of small-vessel necrotizing inflammation; the most common is palpable purpura (see Table 18-2).

ETIOLOGY. There is hypersensitivity to various antigens (drugs, chemicals, microorganisms, and endogenous antigens) with formation of circulating immune complexes that are deposited in walls of vessels. Some of the diseases reported to be associated with hypersensitivity vasculitis and the incidence of these diseases are listed in Table 18-4.

In many cases, the cause is not determined.

PATHOGENESIS. The vessel-bound immune complexes activate complement that is chemotactic for neutrophils. Neutrophils adhere to endothelial cells and migrate into the surrounding connective tissue. Activated endothelial cells release inflammatory mediators (cytokines) that attract inflammatory cells. There is an inflammatory response in the walls of small vessels in which leukocytes, by release of lysosomal enzymes, damage vessel walls, causing extravasation of erythrocytes. The term leukocytoclastic vasculitis describes the histologic pattern produced when leukocytes fragment (i.e., undergo leukocytoclasis during the inflammatory process, leaving nuclear debris or "dust").

Table 18-4 Causal Agents, Associated Conditions, and Vasculitis Syndromes Identified

	% of Patients
Cause/association	
Hepatitis C virus	19.0
Hepatitis B virus	5.0
Other infections	4.0
Drug intake	9.6
Underlying malignant neoplasm	10.0
Connective-tissue diseases	8.4
Behçet disease	2.0
Rheumatological disease	2.4
Essential mixed cryoglobulinemia	1.3
Inflammatory bowel disease	2.5
Miscellaneous	3.0
Vasculitic syndrome	
Hypersensitivity vasculitis	64.0
Polyarteritis nodosa	6.0
Pustular vasculitis	6.0
Henoch-Schönlein purpura	5.2
Livedo vasculitis	4.5
Urticarial vasculitis	3.2
Rheumatoid vasculitis	3.2
Erythema elevatum diutinum	2.6
Churg-Strauss vasculitis	2.0

From Sais G: Arch Dematol 1998; 34:309.

Hypersensitivity vasculitis

Cutaneous small-vessel vasculitis (leukocytoclastic vasculitis, hypersensitivity vasculitis) is the most commonly seen form of small-vessel necrotizing vasculitis. The disease may be limited to the skin or may involve many different organs and be coexistent with many other diseases. Histologically there is fibrinoid necrosis of small dermal blood vessels, leukocytoclasis, endothelial cell swelling, and extravasation of red blood cells (RBCs).

SKIN LESIONS. Prodromal symptoms include fever, malaise, myalgia, and joint pain. The characteristic lesions are referred to as palpable purpura. The lesions begin as asymptomatic, localized areas of cutaneous hemorrhage that acquire substance and become palpable as blood leaks out of damaged vessels (Figure 18-10). Lesions may coalesce, producing large areas of purpura (Figure 18-11). Nodules and urticarial lesions may appear. Hemorrhagic blisters and ulcers may arise from these purpuric areas and indicate more severe vessel inflammation and necrosis (Figure 18-12). A few-to-numerous discrete, purpuric lesions are most commonly seen on the lower extremities but may occur on any dependent area, including the back if the patient is bedridden, or the arms. Ankle and lower leg edema may occur with lower leg lesions.

Small lesions itch and are painful; nodules, ulcers, and bullae may be very painful.

Lesions appear in crops, last for 1 to 4 weeks, and heal with residual scarring and hyperpigmentation. Patients may experience one episode if a drug or viral infection is the cause or multiple episodes when the lesions are associated with a systemic disease, such as rheumatoid arthritis or systemic lupus erythematosus. Recurrent crops of new lesions may appear for weeks, months, or years. The disease is usually self-limited and confined to the skin.

DURATION. In one study the disease resolved in less than 6 months in 46.9% of the patients and persisted in 43.8%. The duration of the cutaneous vasculitis ranged from 1 week to 318 months. The average duration of cutaneous lesions was 27.9 months.

SYSTEMIC DISEASE. Hypersensitivity vasculitis has many systemic manifestations; the numbers in parentheses in the following discussion indicate the approximate percentage of involvement.[89-91]

An analysis of cutaneous hypersensitivity vasculitis in patients seen by two practicing dermatologists showed that the disease has a better prognosis with less systemic involvement than in those patients seen at medical center clinics.[92, 93]

SMALL VESSEL VASCULITIS

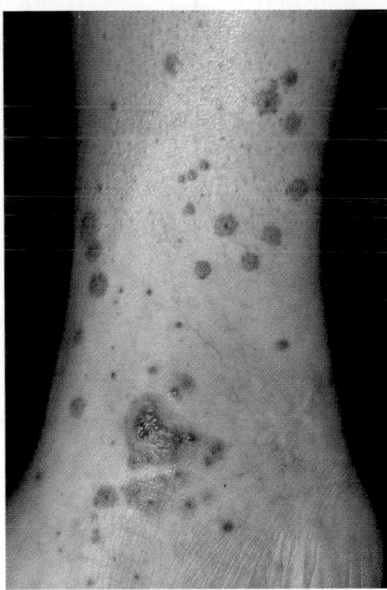

Figure 18-10 Palpable purpura are most often found on the lower legs.

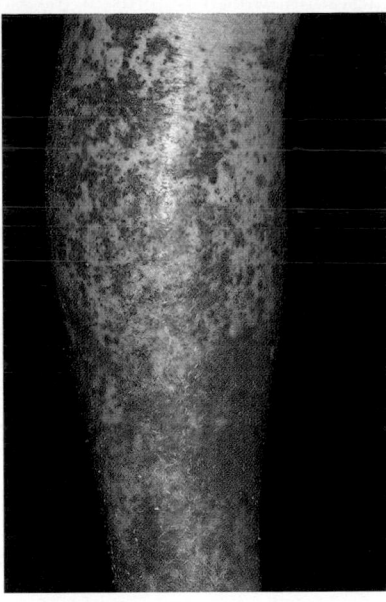

Figure 18-11 Lesions may be barely palpable and coalesce into broad hemorrhagic areas.

Figure 18-12 An intense eruption with lesions that have coalesced and ulcerated.

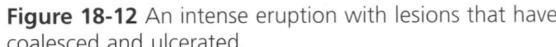

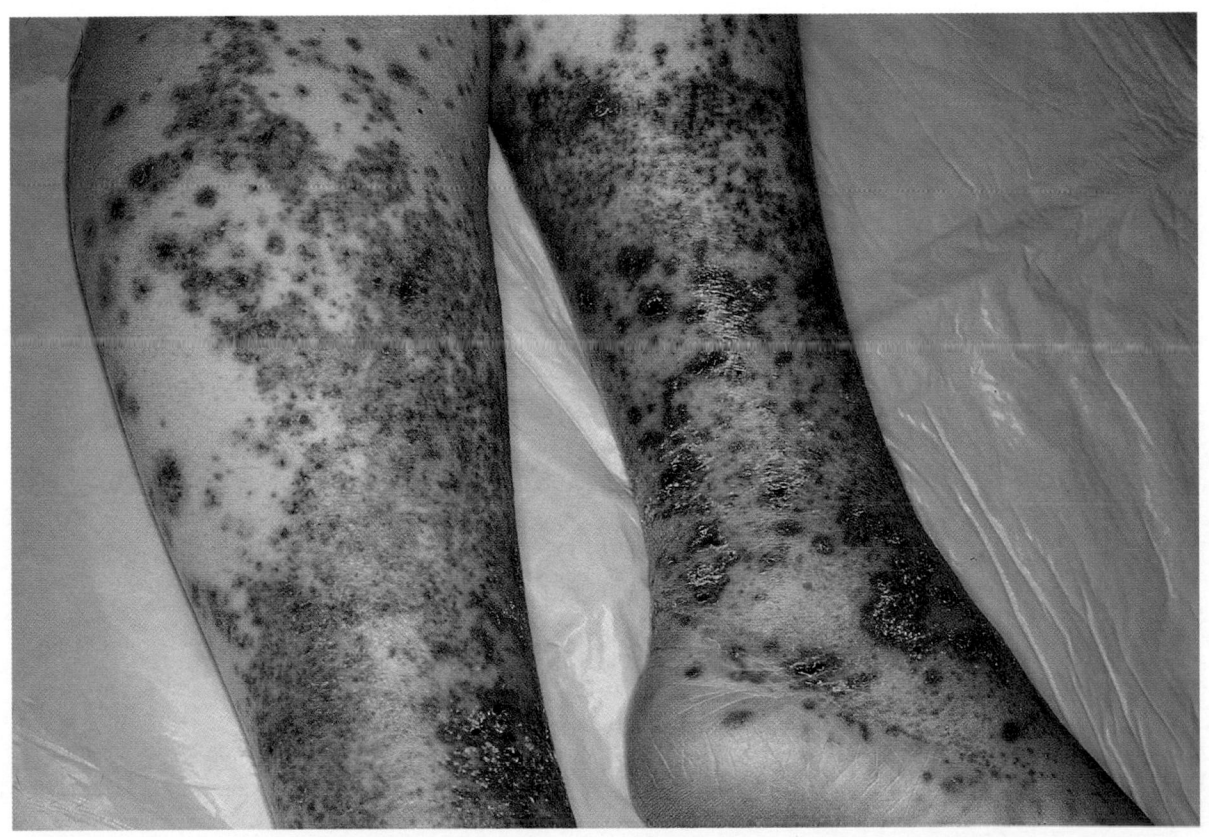

- Kidneys (50%): Kidney disease is the most common systemic manifestation. Mild vasculitis of the kidneys causes microscopic hematuria and proteinuria. Necrotizing glomerulitis or diffuse glomerulonephritis may lead to chronic renal insufficiency and death.
- Nervous system (40%): Peripheral neuropathy with hypoesthesia or paresthesia is more common than central nervous system involvement.
- Gastrointestinal tract (36%): Vasculitis of the bowel causes abdominal pain, nausea, vomiting, diarrhea, and melena.
- Lung (30%): Pulmonary vasculitis may be asymptomatic, detected only as nodular or diffuse infiltrates on chest film; it also may be symptomatic, with cough, shortness of breath, and hemoptysis.
- Joints (30%): Symptoms vary from pain to erythema and swelling.
- Heart (50%): Myocardial angiitis produces arrhythmias and congestive heart failure.

Indicators of systemic disease are listed in Box 18-5.

PHYSICAL EXAMINATION. Look for systemic disease with a complete history and physical examination. Examine ear, nose, and throat for signs of Wegener's granulomatosis.

LABORATORY STUDIES. Studies to consider are listed in Box 18-6. Decreased levels of complement components are more often present in vasculitis associated with rheumatoid arthritis, systemic lupus erythematosus, cryoglobulinemia, Sjögren's syndrome, or urticarial vasculitis. Every patient should be screened for renal involvement.

Order ANCA tests when systemic vasculitis is suspected. The ESR is almost always increased during active vasculitis. A normal ESR in a patient with purpura suggests that immune complex disease is absent. Low complement levels are associated with other features such as renal disease, arthritis, and the presence of immunoreactants deposited along the basement membrane zone of the epidermis.[94]

The frequency of abnormal tests is listed in Table 18-5.

SKIN BIOPSY. The clinical presentation is so characteristic that a biopsy is generally not necessary. In doubtful cases, a punch biopsy should be taken from an early active lesion. The characteristic mixed infiltrate of mononuclear cells and neutrophils, fibrinoid necrosis of blood vessel walls, and nuclear dust from neutrophil fragmentation (leukocytoclasis) will be obscured if ulcerated lesions are sampled. Patients with deeper levels of vasculitis (down to the lower half of the reticular dermis) have evidence of a more severe clinical disease with systemic involvement.

IMMUNOFLUORESCENT STUDIES. Immunofluorescent studies may be done if the diagnosis cannot be determined from the clinical presentation and skin biopsy. Immune complexes are phagocytized rapidly after deposition in the vessels. Therefore the best time for biopsy of a vessel for immunofluorescence is within the first 24 hours after the lesion forms.

Box 18-5 Indicators of Systemic Vasculitis in 160 Patients with Leukocytoclastic Vasculitis*

Extracutaneous involvement histologically confirmed
Persistent hematuria and abnormal proteinuria
Renal biopsy showing vasculitis
Electromyogram evidence of mixed (motor and sensory) abnormalities
Peripheral nerve biopsy showing vasculitis
Intestinal biopsy showing vasculitis
Vasculitic changes shown on abdominal angiography

From Sais G: Arch Dermatol 1998; 34:309.
*Systemic involvement was documented in 20% of the patients.

Box 18-6 Tests to Consider for Evaluation of Cutaneous Small-Vessel Vasculitis

Initial laboratory evaluation
Complete blood cell count
Erythrocyte sedimentation rate
Urinalysis
Stool guaiac tests
Serum chemistry profile
Antinuclear antibodies
Antineutrophil cytoplasmic autoantibodies
Chest radiography
Rheumatoid factor
Cryoglobulins
Complement (total)
Hepatitis B virus
Hepatitis C virus

Adults with persistent fever, abnormal blood smears, risk for HIV infection, severe vasculitis
Anticardiolipin
Antistreptolysin O titer
Anti-DNA, anti-Ro, anti-LA antibodies
Electrocardiography
HIV serology
Platelet counts
Prothrombin and partial thromboplastin times
Serum creatine
Serum immunoglobulin determination
Serum protein electrophoresis
Throat culture
Urinary protein determination (24-hour)

Adapted from Blanco R, et al: Medicine 1998; 77:403.

The most common immunoreactants present in and around blood vessels are IgM, C3, and fibrin. The presence of IgA in blood vessels of a child with vasculitis suggests the diagnosis of Henoch-Schönlein purpura.

TREATMENT. Identify and remove the offending antigen (i.e., drug, chemical, or infection). No other treatment may be necessary, and the disease may clear spontaneously. In other instances the disease persists or becomes recurrent.

Topical corticosteroids and topical antibiotic creams may be helpful. Prednisone, 60 to 80 mg per day, controls systemic symptoms and cutaneous ulceration. Taper slowly (3 to 6 weeks) to prevent rebound. Nonsteroidal anti-inflammatory drugs (acetylsalicylic acid, indomethacin) may be used for persistent or necrotic lesions, myalgias, fever, and arthralgia.

Colchicine, which inhibits neutrophil chemotaxis, in doses of 0.6 mg twice to three times daily, might be helpful in chronic forms of the disease.[93,95-97] Effects are seen in 7 to 10 days, and colchicine is tapered and discontinued when lesions resolve. Treatment can be continued for months if necessary, and side effects are minimal.

Dapsone 100 to 150 mg per day controlled three patients in whom disease was confined to the skin.[98] Potassium iodide (0.3-1.5 g four times daily) is useful in nodular vasculitis. H1 antihistamines alone or with H2 antihistamines alleviate pruritus and block histamine-induced endothelial gap formation with resultant trapping of immune complexes. Azathioprine 150 mg/day was used in patients with recalcitrant disease or steroid-induced side effects and produced a good clinical response in 4 to 8 weeks.[93] Cyclophosphamide 2 mg/kg per day induced remissions in patients with multiple-organ involvement who were not controlled with prednisone.[99] Methotrexate (10-25 mg/wk) or cyclosporine (3-5 mg/kg per day) are alternatives for patients with a rapidly progressing course and systemic involvement. Hydroxychloroquine is not effective.

Henoch-Schönlein purpura

Henoch-Schönlein purpura (HSP), or anaphylactoid purpura, is an acute leukocytoclastic vasculitis that occurs mainly in children between the ages of 2 and 10, although adult cases are reported. It is the most common systemic vasculitis in children and is characterized by vascular deposition of IgA-dominant immune complexes, and preferentially involves venules, capillaries, and arterioles. There are palpable purpura over the legs and buttocks, abdominal pain (63%), GI bleeding (33%), arthralgia (82%), nephritis (40%), hematuria (see Table 18-6), and, histologically, by leukocytoclastic vasculitis.[100] It is a self-limited illness, but one third of patients will have one or more recurrences of symptoms.

PROGNOSIS. HSP is usually benign and self-limiting; the degree of renal involvement determines the prognosis. The long-term prognosis is excellent for both adults and children.[101] In 50% of cases, there are recurrences, typically in the first 3 months; these are milder and more common in patients with nephritis.

ADULTS VS. CHILDREN. The frequency of previous drug treatment, primarily antibiotics or analgesics, is similar in both groups, but previous upper respiratory tract infection is more frequent among the children. No precipitating event is found in 72% of the adults and 66% of the children.[101] Adults have a lower frequency of abdominal pain and fever and a higher frequency of joint symptoms. Adults have more frequent and severe renal involvement. An increased erythrocyte sedimentation rate is more frequent in the adults. Complete recovery occurs in 93.9% of children and in 89.2% of adults. Adults required more aggressive therapy, consisting of steroids and/or cytotoxic agents. However, the final outcome of HSP is equally good in adults and children.[101]

Table 18-5 Routine Laboratory Studies in 160 Patients with Leukocytoclastic Vasculitis

ESR > 20 mm/h	52.4%
Anemia	37%
Pathologic urine sediment	21.7%
Hypergammaglobulinemia (>24 gm/L)	20%
24-hour proteinuria > 0.3 gm	19%
Leukocytosis	18%
Elevated transaminase levels	18%
Urea level > 9.7 mmol/L	16%
Creatine > 130 µmol/L	13%
Thrombocytosis	10%
Eosinophilia	2.5%
From Sais G: Arch Dermatol 1998; 34:309.	

Table 18-6 Clinical Features in 25 Patients with Henoch-Schönlein Purpura

Purpura	100%
Arthralgia	84%
Abdominal pain	76%
Nephritis	44%
Gastrointestinal bleeding	40%
Miscellaneous	
Encephalopathy	8%
Orchitis	4%
From Saulsbury FT: Pediatr Dermatol 1984; 1:195.	

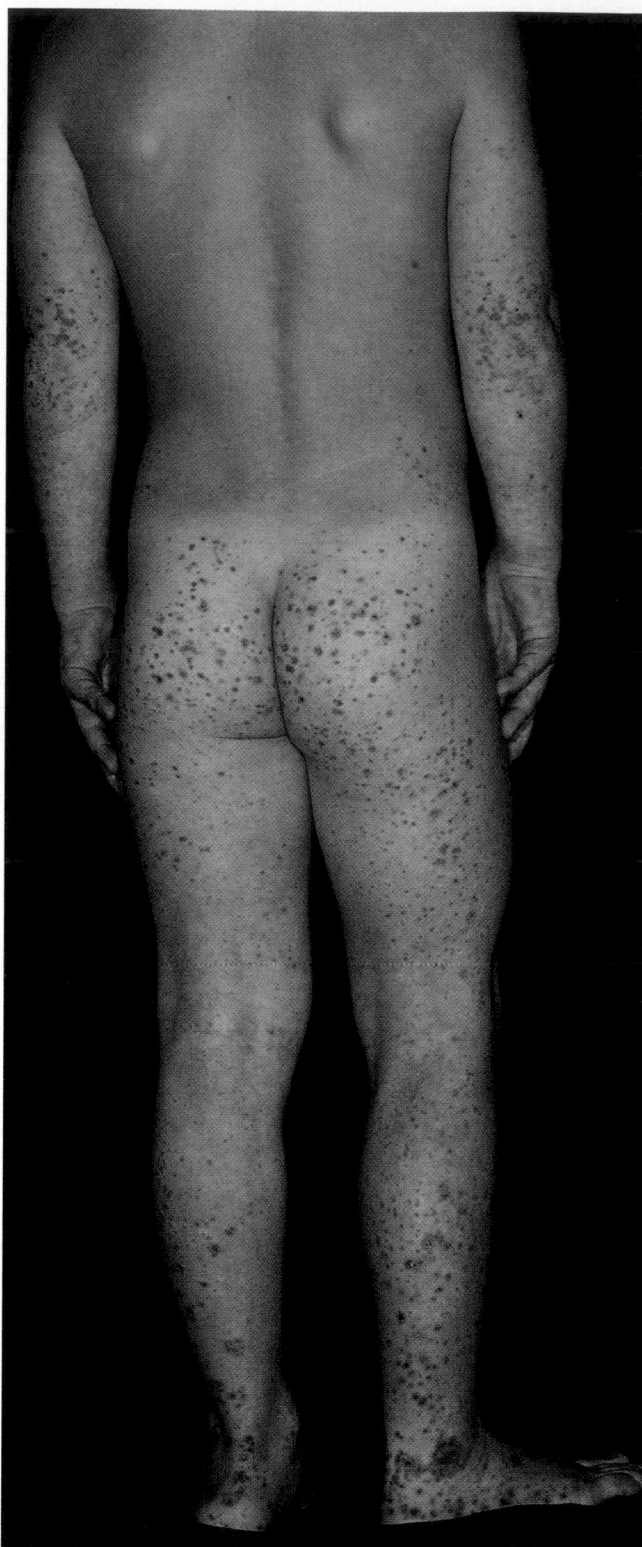

Figure 18-13 Henoch-Schönlein purpura. Palpable purpuric lesions are most common on the lower extremities and buttocks but can appear on the arms, face, and ears; the trunk is usually spared.

ETIOLOGY. HSP tends to occur in the springtime; a streptococcal or viral upper respiratory infection may precede the disease by 1 to 3 weeks. A cluster of cases was reported, suggesting that HSP is caused by person-to-person spread of an infectious agent of the respiratory tract to susceptible hosts.[102]

A number of infectious agents and drugs have been implicated, but the etiology of HSP remains unknown.

Immunoglobulin A. IgA plays a critical role in the immunopathogenesis of HSP. There are increased serum IgA concentrations, IgA-containing circulating immune complexes, and IgA deposition in vessel walls and renal mesangium. There are 2 subclasses of IgA, but HSP is associated with abnormalities involving IgA1 exclusively and not IgA2. All of its features are attributable to the widespread vasculitis believed to be initiated by entrapment of circulating IgA-containing immune complexes in blood vessel walls in the skin, kidneys, and GI tract.

CLINICAL FEATURES. Prodromal symptoms include anorexia and fever. The clinical features of HSP are as follows.[103]

Skin. Nonthrombocytopenic palpable purpura is most common on the lower extremities and buttocks but can appear on the arms, face, and ears; the trunk is usually spared (Figure 18-13). The lesions evolve from urticarial papules into the classic leukocytoclastic vasculitic lesions within 48 hours. The lesions are 2 to 10 mm in diameter and appear in crops among coalescent ecchymoses and pinpoint petechiae. Lesions fade in several days, more rapidly with bed rest, leaving brown macules. New lesions appear with ambulation. Seventy-seven percent present with cutaneous signs; 10% have no leg involvement; 4.5% have edema of the hands, feet, or face.[104]

Abdominal symptoms. GI symptoms occur in 40% to 60% of patients; these include colicky pain, nausea, vomiting, upper GI bleeding, diarrhea, and bloody stool and are potentially the most serious manifestations. Although GI bleeding occurs in 52% of patients, it is self-limiting, and blood transfusions have not been required.[105] Symptoms precede the skin disease by up to 2 weeks and simulate a number of inflammatory or surgically treated bowel diseases. Major complications of abdominal involvement develop in 4.6%, of which intussusception is by far the most common. The intussusceptum is confined to the small bowel in 58% and it is frequently inaccessible to demonstration by contrast enema.

Ultrasound is the imaging modality of choice. It provides an easy, noninvasive, objective method of monitoring patient progress. It allows direct visualization of bowel involvement and detection of complications such as intussusception. It also demonstrates edematous hemorrhagic infiltration of the intestinal wall, which can occur in the duodenal, jejunal, and ileal segments.[106] Ultrasonography complements serial clinical assessment, clarifies the nature of the gastrointestinal involvement, and reduces the likelihood of unnecessary surgery.

Routine abdominal radiographs are not recommended, unless perforation is clinically suspected.[107]

Upper GI endoscopy can be useful. Inflammation of the duodenum, especially of the second part, is characteristic of HSP. Upper GI endoscopy shows redness, swelling, petechiae or hemorrhage, or erosions and ulceration of the mucosa. Histology of mucosal biopsy specimens shows nonspecific inflammation with positive staining for IgA in the capillaries.[108]

Joint symptoms. Arthralgia, probably resulting from painful periarticular edema rather than from inflammatory joint disease, involves the ankles, knees, and dorsum of the hands and feet in more than 80% of patients. It is often incapacitating, but it is self-limiting and nondeforming.

Nephritis. The long-term prognosis of HSP is directly dependent on the severity of renal involvement. Nephritis occurs in 20% to 50% of children. The renal disease is usually milder in children and almost always heals. The onset may be acute or delayed. Acute nephritis occurs from 1 to 12 days after the onset of other signs and symptoms. The onset of renal involvement may be delayed for weeks or months in a substantial proportion of patients. Microscopic hematuria is a constant feature, but episodes of gross hematuria occur in 40% of patients with nephritis. Proteinuria and hematuria are found in about 40% of cases. Urinary abnormalities can persist for 2 to 5 years in patients who develop nephritis in the acute phase of HSP. Progression to nephrotic syndrome and acute and chronic renal failure is possible.[109]

When HSP presents with more than just microhematuria, only 72% of cases proceed to complete recovery.[110] Heavy proteinuria at onset, focal sclerotic and tubulointerstitial changes, and crescents and capsular adhesions are poor prognostic indicators. After a follow-up of at least 8 years, 53% of patients are clinically in remission. Evidence of renal disease may reappear after apparent complete recovery. Childhood HS nephritis requires long-term follow-up, especially during pregnancy. A study of 78 subjects who had HS nephritis during childhood (at a mean of 23.4 years after onset) showed that severity of clinical presentation and initial findings on renal biopsy correlate well with outcome but have poor predictive value in individuals. Forty-four percent of patients who had nephritic or nephrotic syndromes at onset have hypertension or impaired renal function; 82% of those who presented with hematuria (with or without proteinuria) are normal. Sixteen of 44 full-term pregnancies were complicated by proteinuria and/or hypertension, even in the absence of active renal disease.[111]

The renal pathologic findings present a spectrum, from mild focal glomerulitis to necrotizing or proliferative glomerulonephritis with diffuse mesangial proliferation. Diffuse mesangial deposits of IgA are seen on immunofluorescent studies. HS nephritis may be the single most common form of crescentic glomerulonephritis, accounting for 30% of cases.[110]

Adults. A multicenter collaborative study of 152 patients compared the progression of renal disease in children and adults with HPS nephritis. Crescents were found in 36% of adults and 34.6% of children, nephrotic-range proteinuria in 29.5% of adults and 28.1% of children and functional impairment in 24.1% of adults and 36.9% of children. The outcome was similar for both age groups (remission, 32.5% of adults and 31.6% of children; renal function impairment, 31.6% of adults and 24.5% of children). End-stage renal disease was observed in 15.8% of adults and in 7% of children. None of the children died, and adult survival was 97% at 5 years. In adults at presentation, renal function impairment, as well as proteinuria higher than 1.5 gm per day and hypertension, were negative prognostic factors. In children no definite level of proteinuria, hypertension, or other data were found to be associated with poor prognosis.[112]

A recent infectious history, pyrexia, the spread of purpura to the trunk, and biologic markers of inflammation are predictive factors for renal involvement.[113]

Acute scrotal swelling. Acute scrotal swelling may be the presenting manifestation and occur in up to 15% of boys with HSP. The vasculitis of HSP may involve the scrotum and clinically mimic diseases requiring surgical intervention, such as testicular torsion or an incarcerated inguinal hernia. Sonographic findings include an enlarged, rounded epididymis, thickened scrotal skin, and a hydrocele with intact vascular flow in the testicles. Nuclear imaging may be used to assess testicular perfusion.[114] The sonographic findings in the scrotum are sufficiently characteristic to allow distinction from torsion in most cases. These findings help prevent unnecessary surgical exploration.[115]

PATHOLOGY. The pathology of HSP is that of an acute vasculitis of arterioles and venules in the superficial dermis and the bowel. Immunofluorescence staining of tissues usually reveals the presence of IgA in the walls of the arterioles and in the renal glomeruli. The serum IgA level is frequently higher than normal.

DIAGNOSIS. There are no diagnostic laboratory tests. CBC, ANA, platelet counts, and coagulation studies are normal. The ESR may be elevated, and the serum complement level may be depressed. In one study, serum IgA concentrations were increased in 44% of children.[116] Direct immunofluorescent studies show IgA deposition in blood vessels (75% in affected skin and 67% in uninvolved skin) of the superficial dermis.[117] IgA1 is the dominant IgA subclass.[118]

IgA in vessel walls is a sensitive and specific marker that helps to solidify the diagnosis of HSP. This finding should not be used as the sole criterion for making the diagnosis because it is seen in many other disorders, such as venous stasis and erythema nodosum. One study revealed a significant correlation between plasma levels of anaphylatoxins C3a and C4a and plasma creatine in patients with nephritis.[119] The role of IgA ANCA has not been defined.[120]

MANAGEMENT. The offending antigen must be identified and removed. The possibilities include infections, malignancies, foods, and drugs. Patients with ANCA-associated small-vessel vasculitis who present with purpura, abdominal pain, and nephritis but do not have IgA immune deposits do not have Henoch-Schönlein purpura and do not have a good prognosis and should be treated quickly with immunosuppressive therapy.

Corticosteroids. The joint pain, inflammation, and painful cutaneous edema are treated with analgesics, nonsteroidal antiinflammatory agents, and corticosteroids. Corticosteroid therapy may hasten the resolution of arthritis and abdominal pain but does not prevent recurrences. Corticosteroids in usual doses have no effect on established nephritis. The optimal management of HSP-associated gastrointestinal and renal involvement has not yet been determined. Reports favor a short course of oral corticosteroids for severe abdominal pain and immunosuppressive therapy for patients with progressive nephritis.[121]

Treatment with corticosteroids may be useful in early disease before infarction has taken place.[122] In a short-term, double-blind, crossover trial, prednisone had no effect on IgA nephropathy.[110] One study showed that early corticosteroid therapy does not prevent delayed nephritis in children.[123] Another study claims that prednisone given for 2 weeks may prevent nephritis in children who do not already have it when first seen.[110]

Cyclophosphamide. An intensive immunosuppressive regimen that combines prednisone and cyclophosphamide at high doses was shown to be effective in healing Henoch-Schönlein renal disease.[124,125]

Azathioprine. Early treatment for severe nephritis with prednisone and azathioprine prevented progression of chronic changes and improved outcome.[126,127]

Immunoglobulin. An open prospective trial using intravenous immunoglobulin (2 gm/kg per month) followed by 6 months of intramuscular immunoglobulins (IMIG, 0.35 mL/kg every 15 days) was able to slow or to stop the decline in the glomerular filtration rate, to reduce proteinuria, hematuria, leukocyturia and the histologic index of activity on renal biopsy in patients with severe forms of IgA nephropathy (IGAN) and HSP.[128] An adult with HSP nephritis with massive proteinuria who failed to respond to oral prednisolone had a partial improvement with steroid pulse therapy. High-dose intravenous immunoglobulin treatment was introduced, and a dramatic improvement of proteinuria was noted.[129]

Antinuclear Cytoplasmic Antibody–Associated Small-Vessel Vasculitis

ANCA-associated small-vessel vasculitis is the most common primary systemic small-vessel vasculitis in adults and includes Wegener's granulomatosis, microscopic polyangiitis, and Churg-Strauss syndrome. Wegener's granulomatosis has necrotizing granulomatous inflammation and no asthma; Churg-Strauss syndrome presents with asthma, eosinophilia, and necrotizing granulomatous inflammation; and microscopic polyangiitis has no granulomatous inflammation or asthma. An identical pauci-immune necrotizing and crescentic glomerulonephritis occurs in all three diseases. Rapid diagnosis and treatment is critical because life-threatening injury to organs often develops quickly. A small number of patients with typical clinical and pathological features of these diseases are ANCA-negative.

Wegener's granulomatosis

Wegener's granulomatosis is a rare, fatal, necrotizing, granulomatous vasculitis that occurs in children and adults (Boxes 18-3 to 18-5). More than 90% of patients with Wegener's granulomatosis have upper or lower respiratory tract disease or both.

CLINICAL MANIFESTATIONS. Manifestations of upper respiratory tract disease are sinus pain and purulent drainage, nasal mucosal ulceration with epistaxis, and otitis media. Necrosis of the nasal septum with perforation or saddle-nose deformation and injury to the facial nerve by otitis media resulting in facial paralysis may occur. Tracheal inflammation and sclerosis cause stridor and may lead to dangerous airway stenosis. Necrotizing granulomatous pulmonary inflammation produces nodular radiographic densities, whereas alveolar capillaritis causes pulmonary hemorrhage with less fixed and more irregular infiltrates. Approximately 80% of patients will develop glomerulonephritis.

Cutaneous signs. Fourteen percent to 47% have skin disease with histopathologic findings of necrotizing vasculitis,[130] granulomatous vasculitis, or palisading granuloma.[131] In one study there were palpable purpura (35%), oral ulcers (20%), skin nodules (8%), skin ulcers (7%), and necrotic papules (7%). Dermatologic manifestations were associated with a higher frequency of articular and renal involvement (68% vs. 25% and 80% vs. 47%, respectively).[132]

Churg-Strauss syndrome

Churg-Strauss syndrome (see Boxes 18-3 to 18-5) has three phases: allergic rhinitis and asthma; eosinophilic infiltrative disease, such as eosinophilic pneumonia or gastroenteritis; and systemic small-vessel vasculitis with granulomatous inflammation. All patients have eosinophilia (more than 10% eosinophils in the blood).

Vessels are grossly affected, as in polyarteritis nodosa, but histologically these vessels show granulomatous inflammation in addition to leukocyte invasion. Multisystem visceral and cutaneous disease similar to polyarteritis nodosa follows the initial triad of signs and symptoms with hypertension, abdominal pain, neurologic involvement, and pneumonia. The skin is involved in approximately 50% of cases showing palpable purpura, ulcers, infarcts, and deep cutaneous or subcutaneous nodules.[133] Cutaneous involvement generally parallels the systemic course. Antineutrophil cytoplasmic antibodies (p-ANCA) are found in about 60% of cases. Renal involvement is infrequent. Coronary arteritis and myocarditis account for 50% of deaths.

Microscopic polyangiitis

Microscopic polyangiitis is a systemic necrotizing small-vessel vasculitis without granulomatous inflammation. It is primarily associated with necrotizing and crescentic glomerulonephritis and pulmonary capillaritis. Cutaneous manifestations are frequent; palpable purpura occurs in 40% of cases. There is a prodromal phase of constitutional upset, fever arthralgia, and myalgia and elevated inflammatory indexes, such as C-reactive protein level and ESR. Glomerulonephritis occurs in 96% of cases, and pulmonary involvement occurs in 50% of cases. Most patients have p-ANCA. Positive ANCA and negative serologic test results for hepatitis B help differentiate microscopic polyangiitis from polyarteritis nodosa. The distinction between microscopic polyangiitis and polyarteritis nodosa is sometimes difficult.[134,135] Treat with methylprednisolone, cyclophosphamide, and possibly plasmapheresis.

TREATMENT OF ANCA-ASSOCIATED VASCULITIS. The standard therapy for generalized ANCA-associated vasculitis is at least one year of corticosteroid and oral cyclophospamide therapy. Cyclophosphamide causes hemorrhagic cystitis and increases the risk if bladder cancer and lymphoproliferative disease, myelodysplasia, and infertility. The vasculitis returns in 50% of patients, often after the reduction or discontinuation of therapy. Azathioprine is less toxic than cyclophosphamide. Early substitution of azathioprine for cyclophosphamide after remission (usually at three months) can reduce the rate of toxic effects associated with long-term cyclophosphamide treatment.[136]

Antinuclear Cytoplasmic Antibody–Negative Small-Vessel Vasculitis

ESSENTIAL MIXED CRYOGLOBULINEMIA

Cryoglobulins. Three types of cryoglobulinemia are distinguished based on the composition of the proteins:

Type I is composed of monoclonal immunoglobulin and is associated with multiple myeloma. There are large amounts of cryoprecipitate that can produce thrombosis, necrosis, and ulceration.

Type II (mixed): monoclonal IgM and polyclonal IgG antibodies.

Type III (mixed): polyclonal IgM and polyclonal IgG antibodies.

Both mixed types of cryoglobulinemia possess anti-IgG or rheumatoid factor activity. Mixed types have smaller amounts of cryoprecipitate that can be deposited in tissue and lead to vasculitis.

CRYOGLOBULINEMIA. Cryoglobulinemia may be found in a number of disorders. Mixed cryoglobulins are immune complexes that cause systemic vasculitis with a variety of symptoms. The features are recurrent palpable purpura of the lower extremities (100%), polyarthralgias without arthritis (72%), and renal disease (55%). The average age is 50 years. The arthralgias are a common presenting symptom and recur throughout the course of the disease. Patients describe a "gelling" of joints on exposure to cold. Clinical signs of renal disease are proteinuria, diastolic hypertension, edema, and renal failure. The prognosis is poor for patients with renal disease.

The serum cryoglobulin concentration does not correlate with disease activity (vasculitis or glomerulonephritis). Serum protein electrophoresis shows diffuse polyclonal hypergammaglobulinemia without any homogeneous bands in 60% of patients. Most patients have infection with hepatitis C virus, which is thought to be etiologic. A distinctive and diagnostically useful complement abnormality is the presence of very low levels of early components (especially C_4) with normal or slightly low C_3 levels.

The ESR is elevated. The main cause of morbidity is progressive glomerulonephritis (50% of patients), which most often has a type I membranoproliferative phenotype.

Cutaneous vasculitis and arthralgias require no therapy or are treated with aspirin or other nonsteroidal antiinflammatory agents.

Serious visceral involvement, such as in glomerulonephritis, usually requires treatment with corticosteroids combined with a cytotoxic drug.

Neutrophilic Dermatoses

Neutrophilic dermatosis represents a continuous spectrum encompassing five entities: subcorneal pustular dermatosis, Sweet's syndrome, erythema elevatum diutinum, pyoderma gangrenosum, and neutrophilic eccrine hidradenitis. The different neutrophilic dermatoses are manifestations of a potentially multisystemic neutrophilic disease. All may present with pustules, plaques, nodules, and ulcerations. Histologically, a neutrophilic infiltrate appears at variable levels in the epidermis, dermis, and subcutaneous tissue. Systemic manifestations include generalized symptoms and joint, renal, ocular, and lung involvement. There is an overlap in the clinical manifestations of the four entities.[137] Subcorneal pustular dermatosis and neutrophilic eccrine hidradenitis are very rare and not described here.

Sweet's syndrome (acute febrile neutrophilic dermatosis)

Sweet, in 1964, described a disease with four features: fever; leukocytosis; acute, tender, red plaques; and a papillary dermal infiltrate of neutrophils. This led to the name acute febrile neutrophilic dermatosis. Larger series of patients showed that fever and neutrophilia are not consistently present. The diagnosis is based on the two constant features, a typical eruption and the characteristic histologic features; thus the eponym Sweet's syndrome (SS) is used. The criteria of the diagnosis of SS are listed in Box 18-7.

Box 18-7 Diagnostic Criteria for Sweet's Syndrome*

Major criteria

1. Abrupt onset of tender or painful erythematous plaques or nodules occasionally with vesicles, pustules, or bullae
2. Predominantly neutrophilic infiltration in the dermis without leukocytoclastic vasculitis

Minor criteria

1. Preceded by a nonspecific respiratory or gastrointestinal tract infection or vaccination or associated with:
   - Inflammatory diseases such as chronic autoimmune disorders and infections
   - Hemoproliferative disorders or solid malignant tumors
   - Pregnancy
2. Accompanied by periods of general malaise and fever (>38°C)
3. Laboratory values during onset: ESR >20 mm; C-reactive protein positive; segmented-nuclear neutrophils and stabs >70% in peripheral blood smear; leukocytosis >8000 (three of four of these values necessary)
4. Excellent response to treatment with systemic corticosteroids or potassium iodide

Modified from von den Driesch P: J Am Acad Dermatol 1994; 31:535.

*Both major and two minor criteria are needed for diagnosis.

Eighty-six percent of patients are women with a preceding upper respiratory infection. The mean age at presentation is 56 years (range, 22 to 82 years). SS is common in Japan. A genetic predisposition is possible; HLA-Bw54 was found to be a risk factor in a series of Japanese patients with SS.

ETIOLOGY. Sweet's syndrome can be classified based upon the clinical setting in which it occurs: classical or idiopathic Sweet's syndrome, malignancy-associated Sweet's syndrome, and drug-induced Sweet's syndrome.[138]

SYSTEMIC DISEASES. SS is a reactive phenomenon and should be considered a cutaneous marker of systemic disease.[139] Careful systemic evaluation is indicated, especially when cutaneous lesions are severe or hematologic values are abnormal. Approximately 20% of cases are associated with malignancy, predominantly hematological, especially acute myelogenous leukemia. An underlying condition (streptococcal infection, inflammatory bowel disease, nonlymphocytic leukemia and other hematologic malignancies, solid tumors, pregnancy) is found in up to 50% of cases. Attacks of SS may precede the hematologic diagnosis by 3 months to 6 years, so that close evaluation of patients in the "idiopathic" group is required.

There is now good evidence that treatment with hematopoietic growth factors, including granulocyte colony-stimulating factor, which is used to treat acute myelogenous leukemia[140,141], and granulocyte-macrophage colony-stimulating factor, can cause Sweet's syndrome.[142] Lesions typically occur when the patient has leukocytosis and neutrophilia but not when the patient is neutropenic. However, G-CSF may cause SS in neutropenic patients because of the induction of stem cell proliferation, the differentiation of neutrophils, and the prolongation of neutrophil survival.[143]

CLINICAL MANIFESTATIONS. Acute, tender, erythematous plaques, nodes, pseudovesicles and, occasionally, blisters with an annular or arciform (Figures 18-14 and 18-15) pattern occur on the head, neck, legs, and arms, particularly the back of the hands and fingers (Figure 18-16). The trunk is rarely involved. Fever (50%); arthralgia or arthritis (62%); eye involvement, most frequently conjunctivitis or iridocyclitis (38%); and oral aphthae (13%) are associated features. Differential diagnosis includes erythema multiforme, erythema nodosum, adverse drug reaction, and urticaria.[144-146] Recurrences are common and affect up to one third of patients.[147]

LABORATORY STUDIES. Studies show a moderate neutrophilia (less than 50%), elevated ESR (greater than 30 mm/hr) (90%), and a slight increase in alkaline phosphatase (83%). Skin biopsy shows a papillary and mid-dermal mixed infiltrate of polymorphonuclear leukocytes with nuclear fragmentation and histiocytic cells. The infiltrate is predominantly perivascular with endothelial-cell swelling in some vessels, but vasculitic changes (thrombosis; deposition of fibrin, complement, or immunoglobulins within the vessel walls; red blood cell extravasation; inflammatory infiltration of vascular walls) are absent in early lesions.[148,149]

Vasculitis occurs secondary to noxious products released from neutrophils. Blood vessels in lesions of longer duration are more likely to develop vasculitis than those of shorter duration because of prolonged exposure to noxious metabolites. Therefore, vasculitis does not exclude a diagnosis of Sweet's syndrome.[150]

TREATMENT. Systemic corticosteroids (prednisone 0.5 to 1.5 mg/kg of body weight per day) produce rapid improvement and are the "gold standard" for treatment. The temperature, WBC count, and eruption improve within 72 hours. The skin lesions clear within 3 to 9 days. Abnormal laboratory values rapidly return to normal. There are, however, frequent recurrences. Corticosteroids are tapered within 2 to 6 weeks to zero. Resolution of the eruption is occasionally followed by milia and scarring. The disease clears spontaneously in some

patients. Topical and/or intralesional corticosteroids may be effective as either monotherapy or adjuvant therapy.

Oral potassium iodide[138,151] or colchicine[152] may induce rapid resolution. Patients who have a potential systemic infection or in whom corticosteroids are contraindicated can use these agents as a first-line therapy.

In one study, indomethacin, 150 mg per day, was given for the first week, and 100 mg per day was given for 2 additional weeks. Seventeen of 18 patients had a good initial response; fever and arthralgias were markedly attenuated within 48 hours, and eruptions cleared between 7 and 14 days. Patients whose cutaneous lesions continued to develop were successfully treated with prednisone (1 mg/kg per day). No patient had a relapse after discontinuation of indomethacin.[153]

Other alternatives to corticosteroid treatment include dapsone, doxycycline, clofazimine, and cyclosporine.[154] All of these drugs influence migration and other functions of neutrophils.

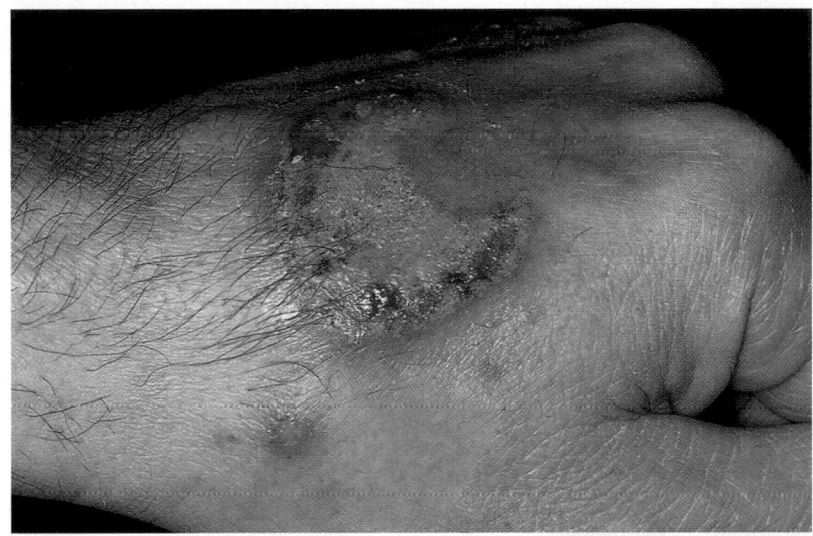

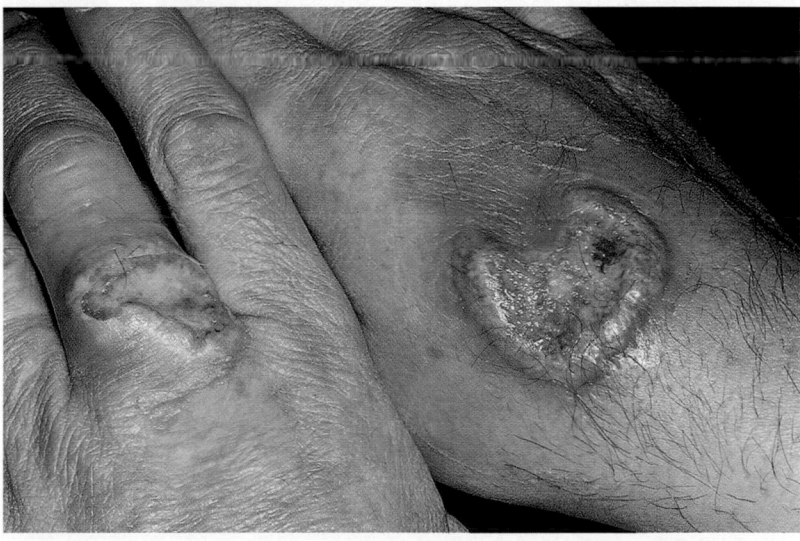

Figure 18-14 Sweet's syndrome. Red-blue papules may coalesce into round plaques. The edges are sometimes studded with pustules. Edema at the border of the lesion can produce a vesicular appearance.

Figure 18-15 Sweet's syndrome and pyoderma gangrenosum occur at sites of minor trauma (pathergy).

SWEET'S SYNDROME

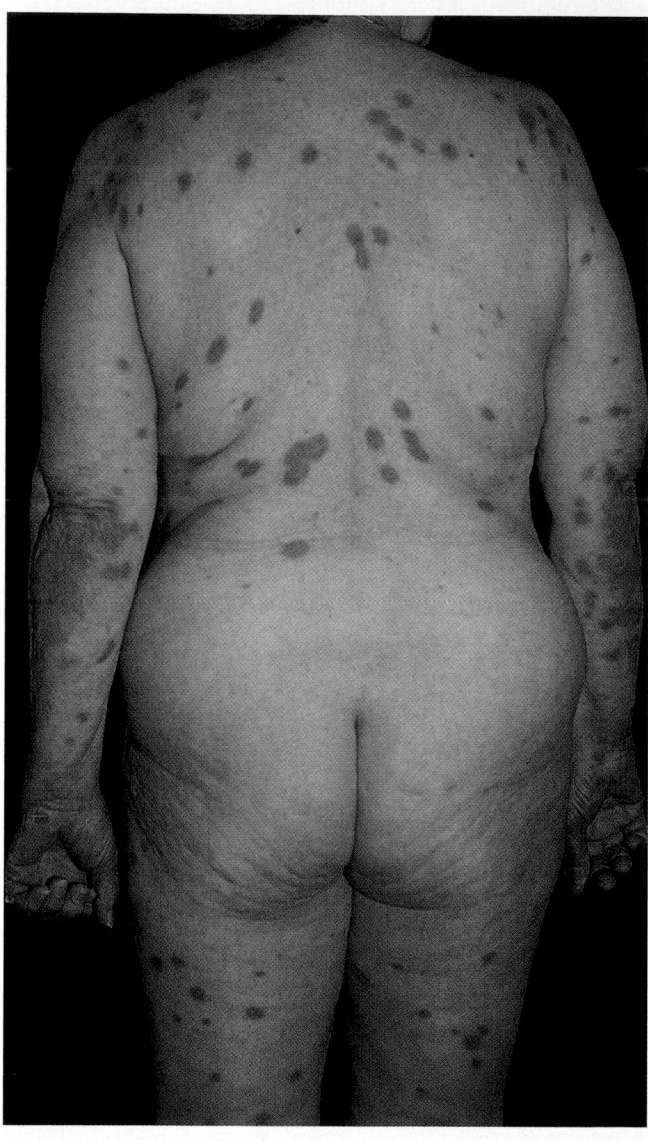

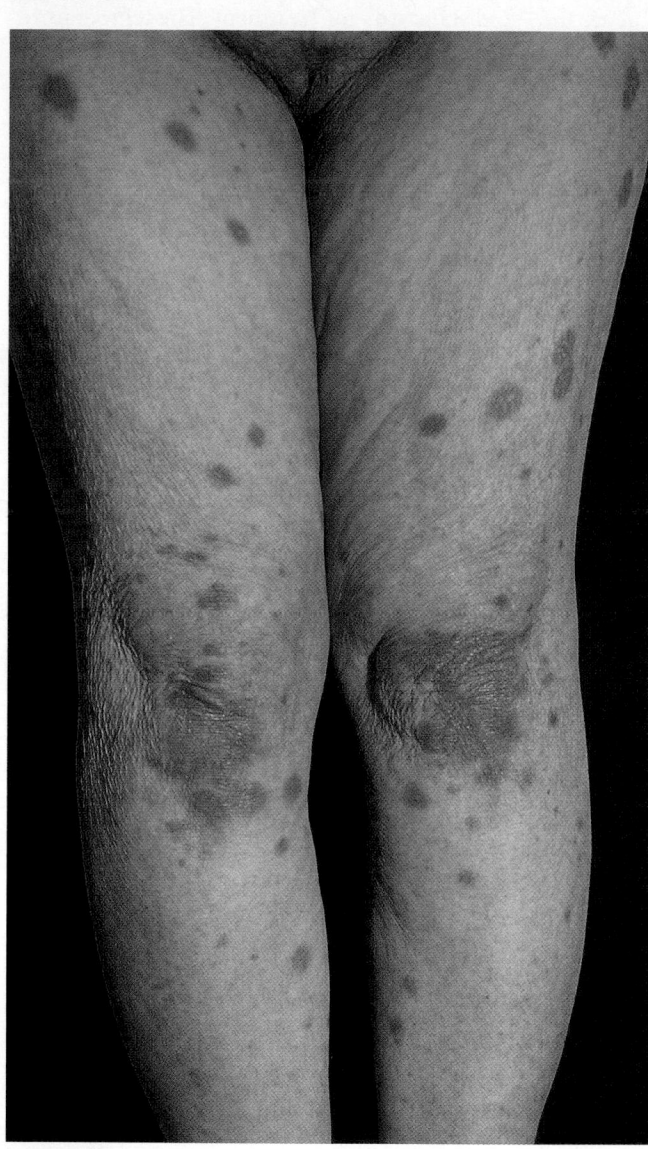

A, Multiple, painful, sharply demarcated, erythematous plaques occur on the neck, upper chest, back, and extremities.

B, Plaques are painful and burning but not itching. The surface is mamillated (papular) or may contain pustules.

Figure 18-16

Erythema elevatum diutinum

Erythema elevatum diutinum (EED) is a rare skin disease (average age, 53 years; range, 32 to 65 years). There are persistent, non-purpuric, deep, brown-red–to–purple papules, nodules, and plaques. Blisters and ulcers can develop. Lesions are symmetrically distributed on extensor surfaces on the extremities with a preference for joint regions. Occasionally lesions are found on the buttocks, face, and torso. EED may be a complication of HIV infection.[155] Cutaneous lesions may closely resemble Kaposi's sarcoma and other malignant neoplasms.[156] The lesions are often accompanied by arthralgias (in approximately 40% of patients) and drug intolerance.

ETIOLOGY. EED is most likely caused by immune complex deposition (Arthus reaction) in the dermal vessels. Excess exposure to antigens (recurrent infections) or situations in which high levels of antibody occur (e.g., paraproteinemias) are likely to result in immune complexes. The cause of this disorder might be an allergic reaction to streptococcal superantigens. Associated medical problems include hypergammaglobulinemia, both monoclonal (IgA clonal gammopathies)[157] and polyclonal[158]; multiple myeloma; and myelodysplasia. EED may precede the myeloproliferative disorders by up to 7.8 years. Chronic infection or recurrent infections (both streptococcal and non-streptococcal) are also reported.

HISTOLOGY. Early lesions show leukocytoclastic vasculitis and a massive dermal infiltrate composed mainly of neutrophils, histiocytes/macrophages, and Langerhans' cells. Later lesions contain patterned (storiform or concentric) fibrosis and a dermal infiltrate of lymphocytes and histiocytes/macrophages and Langerhans' cells.[159] Lipid material forms in some older lesions. The term extracellular cholesterosis is used to describe this process.

LABORATORY STUDIES. Laboratory studies to consider for patients with EED include skin biopsy, serum protein electrophoresis, quantitative immunoglobulins, immunoelectrophoresis, cryoglobulins, and complement studies (C3, C4, and CH50). Direct immunofluorescence studies are generally nondiagnostic.

TREATMENT. Dapsone (e.g., 100 mg per day) is the treatment of choice.[160] One case of EED that was unresponsive to dapsone was successfully treated with colchicine.[161]

Pyoderma gangrenosum

Pyoderma gangrenosum (PG) is a rare, poorly understood, noninfectious neutrophilic ulcerating skin disease.[162] It often occurs in patients with chronic underlying inflammatory or malignant disease such as ulcerative colitis, rheumatoid arthritis,[163] chronic active hepatitis, Crohn's disease, IgA monoclonal gammopathy,[164] and hematologic and lymphoreticular malignancies, but in 40% to 50% of patients, no associated disease is found. Trauma (pathergy) may precede PG in a few

patients.[165] The disease is recurrent in approximately 30% of patients. In rare instances, PG occurs in children; thus it should be considered in the differential diagnosis of pustular disorders in children with underlying conditions such as ulcerative colitis.[166] A seronegative arthritis affecting large joints is present in approximately 40% of cases.

CUTANEOUS MANIFESTATIONS. Lesions are most commonly found on the lower legs (Figure 18-17), but they may occur on the thighs, buttocks, chest, head, neck, and anywhere on the skin.[167] One study showed that lesions were multiple in 71%, and more than 50% were situated below the knees. The lesion begins as a tender, red macule or papule, pustule, nodule, or bulla. Pustules or vesicles appear on the surface, and the surrounding skin becomes dusky red and indurated. A necrotizing inflammatory process extends peripherally from the primary lesion, resulting in a necrotic ulcer or ulcers with a purulent base with an undetermined purple-to-red margin and a halo of surrounding erythema (Figures 18-18 and 18-19). The fully evolved lesion is generally less than 10 cm, but it may be enormous. The lesions tend to endure, lasting months to years, and heal with cribriform scarring.

BOWEL DISEASE. PG occurs in both ulcerative colitis and in Crohn's disease. Approximately 50% of PG cases occur in association with ulcerative colitis.[75] Approximately 2% of patients with active and extensive ulcerative colitis have PG[168], and another 4% of patients with active ulcerative colitis have erythema nodosum, which in its early stages can be confused with PG. Males and females are affected equally. The mean duration of chronic ulcerative colitis before the appearance of erythema nodosum and PG is 5 and 10 years, respectively.[75,169] The lesions generally appear during the course of active bowel disease, but they also occur in inactive colitis or less severe disease and may not appear until after colectomy. Pyoderma resolved without intestinal resection in two thirds of patients. Healing after intestinal resection is unpredictable regarding both timing and extent of resection.[170]

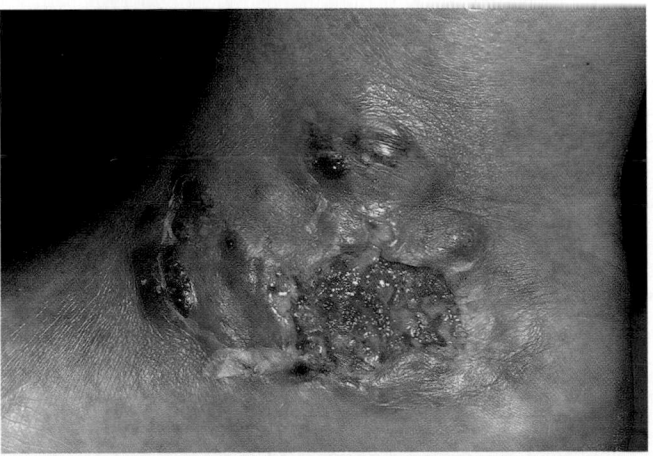

Figure 18-17 Pyoderma gangrenosum. Lesions are most often found on the legs.

DIAGNOSIS. The diagnosis is based on clinical and pathologic features and requires exclusion of conditions that produce ulcerations (Boxes 18-8 and 18-9). The diagnosis is difficult to make because of the condition's ability to mimic other ulcerative lesions and its lack of specific laboratory and pathologic findings. Histopathologically, PG evolves from folliculitis and abscess formation; it may also show leukocytoclastic vasculitis. The lesions then evolve to suppurative granulomatous dermatitis and finally regress with prominent fibroplasia.[171] These changes are nonspecific; therefore biopsy is of little diagnostic value. No specific abnormal laboratory determination has been found that is useful to diagnosis. Serum protein immunoelectrophoresis may be ordered to test for monoclonal gammopathy.

TREATMENT. Systemic corticosteroids and cyclosporine are the most common treatment for extensive disease. Combinations of corticosteroids with cytotoxic drugs such as azathioprine, cyclophosphamide, or chlorambucil are used in patients with disease that is resistant to corticosteroids.[172] Many other treatments are reported. Trauma must be avoided.

Steroids. The small early lesion may be aborted with an intralesional injection of triamcinolone acetonide (Kenalog 10 mg/mL or 40 mg/mL).[173] Group II to V topical steroids with or without occlusion may be effective.

Systemic corticosteroids are the most consistently reported effective treatment for larger active or fully evolved lesions. Steroids probably do little to alter the natural course of the disease, and in many cases lesions recur after treatment is stopped. Prednisone 40 to 80 mg daily is required for initial control, and the dosage is then tapered and stopped.

Topical tacrolimus. Tacrolimus ointment 0.1 (Protopic)[174] may be effective for mild or early cutaneous lesions.

Oral immunosuppressive agents. Immunosuppressive agents may be the most effective treatment. Mycophenolate mofetil, an immunosuppressive agent used almost exclusively in transplantation medicine, may be effective in combination with cyclosporine A.[175] There are many case reports of cyclosporine used as monotherapy. Intravenous bolus cyclophosphamide is reported to be effective in inducing a remission.[176] Oral chlorambucil 2 to 4 mg/day in combination with prednisone or used alone is an effective corticosteroid-sparing agent.[177]

IVIG. Dramatic improvement was reported with high-dose intravenous immunoglobulin (IVIG) (400 mg/kg per day for 5 consecutive days). After 1 week, there was an arrest in the progression of the ulcers and a marked reduction in pain. Two weeks later clinical improvement of the ulcers was observed. Subsequently, IVIG was given at a dose of 1 g/kg per day for 2 consecutive days.[178] The progression of disease was stopped within a few days with short-term combination therapy consisting of high-dose intravenous immunoglobulins and systemic corticosteroids.[165]

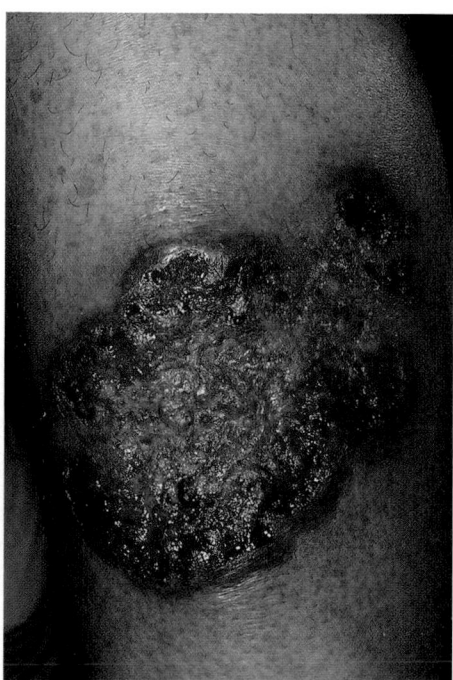

Figure 18-18 Pyoderma gangrenosum. The classic presentation of rapidly progressive, painful, suppurative cutaneous ulcers with edematous, boggy, blue, undermined, and necrotic borders.

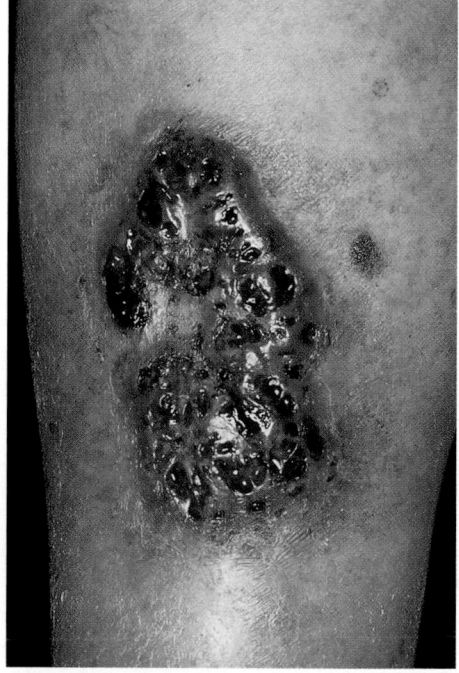

Figure 18-19 Pyoderma gangrenosum. Neutrophilic dermatoses inflammatory disorders have in common a tendency for pathergy (induction of the inflammatory process after skin trauma).

Box 18-8 Approach to the Patient With Suspected Pyoderma Gangrenosum

Important historical data

Markedly painful ulcer

Rapid progression of ulceration

Type of skin lesion preceding the ulcer (papule, pustule, or vesicle)

Minor trauma (pathergy) preceding development of the ulcer

Symptoms of an associated disease (e.g., inflammatory bowel disease or arthritis)

Drug history (e.g., bromides, iodide, hydroxyurea, or granulocyte-macrophage colony-stimulating factor)

Characteristic features of ulcer on physical examination

Tenderness

Necrosis

Irregular violaceous border

Undermined, rolled edges

Skin biopsy

Aim: to rule out diagnoses that mimic pyoderma gangrenosum

Protocol:

Elliptical incisional biopsy preferable to punch biopsy; include inflamed border and ulcer edge at a depth that includes subcutaneous fat

Specimen from inflamed border—routine histology (hematoxylin-and-eosin staining) and special staining Gram's (methenamine silver and Fite) to detect microorganisms

Specimen from edge of ulcer—culture in appropriate culture media (to detect bacteria, fungi, and atypical myobacteria)

Laboratory investigations

Aims: to identify associated diseases and to rule out diagnoses that mimic pyoderma gangrenosum

Investigations to consider:

Complete blood count

Erythrocyte sedimentation rate

Blood chemistry (liver- and kidney-function tests)

Protein electrophoresis

Chest radiography

Colonoscopy

Coagulation panel (including antiphospholipid-antibody screening)

Antineutrophilic cytoplasmic antibodies

Cryoglobulins

Venous- and arterial-function studies

Close, continuous follow-up

Monitor response to and side effects of therapy

If no response to treatment, reconsider diagnosis and repeat biopsy

From Weenig RH, et al: N Engl J Med 2002; 347:1412.

Box 18-9 Ulcers Resembling Pyoderma Gangrenosum

Cause of cutaneous ulceration

Vascular occlusive or venous disease

Antiphospholipid-antibody syndrome

Livedoid vasculopathy

Venous stasis ulceration

Small-vessel occlusive artery disease

Type I cryoglobulinemia

Klippel-Trénaunay-Weber syndrome

Vasculitis

Wegener's granulomatosis

Polyarteritis nodosa

Cryoglobulinemic (mixed) vasculitis

Takayasu's arteritis

Leukocytoclastic vasculitis plus secondary infection

Cutaneous involvement of malignant process

Lymphoma

Angiocentric T-cell lymphoma

Anaplastic large-cell T-cell lymphoma

Mycosis fungoides bullosa

Unspecified lymphomas

Leukemia cutis

Langerhans'-cell histiocytosis

Primary cutaneous infection

Deep fungal infection

Sporotrichosis

Aspergillosis

Cryptococcosis

Zygomycosis

Penicillium marneffei infection

Herpes simplex virus type 2

Cutaneous tuberculosis

Mycobacterium ulcerans (Buruli ulcer)

Amebiasis cutis

Drug-induced or exogenous tissue injury

Munchausen's syndrome or factitial disorder

Hydroxyurea-induced ulceration

Contact vulvitis

Injection-drug abuse with secondary infection

Bromoderma

Loxoscelism (bite of a brown recluse spider)

Drug-induced lupus

Other inflammatory disorders

Cutaneous Crohn's disease

Ulcerative necrobiosis lipoidica

From Weenig RH, et al: N Engl J Med 2002; 347:1412.

Schamberg's disease

Schamberg's disease (progressive pigmented purpuric dermatosis, purpura simplex) is an uncommon eruption characterized by petechiae and patches of brownish pigmentation (hemosiderin deposits), particularly on the lower extremities. Patients are frightened by this vasculitic-appearing eruption, but there is no hematologic disease, venous insufficiency, or associated internal disease. Males are affected more often than females. Children are also affected.[179] Lesions remain for months or years and present only a cosmetic problem. Histologically, there is inflammation and hemorrhage without fibrinoid necrosis of vessels. The cause is unknown, but a cellular immune reaction may play a role.[180] In some patients, the eruption was related to medications.[181]

CLINICAL MANIFESTATIONS. Asymptomatic, irregular, orange-brown patches of varying shapes and sizes appear (Figure 18-20). The most characteristic feature is orange-brown, pinhead-sized "cayenne pepper" spots. Mild erythema and scaling sometimes cause slight itching. Lesions are most common on the lower legs, but they can appear on the upper body. New spots can appear and older ones can fade. In contrast to hypersensitivity vasculitis (palpable purpura), the lesions are macular.

MANAGEMENT. The patient should be assured that there is no systemic disease. Three patients were treated with pentoxifylline, 100 mg tid for 8 weeks. A significant response was observed within 2 to 3 weeks. One patient had recurrence after discontinuation of this treatment but promptly responded to resumption of therapy. No adverse effects were noted in any patients.[182] Another report of four patients treated with pentoxifylline (Trental), 400 mg daily, showed that the drug had no benefit.[183] Inform patients that the pigmentation lasts for years and can be covered with cosmetics, such as Dermablend, if desired. Mild itching and erythema respond quickly to group V topical steroids. Lesions persist, but 67% eventually clear.[184]

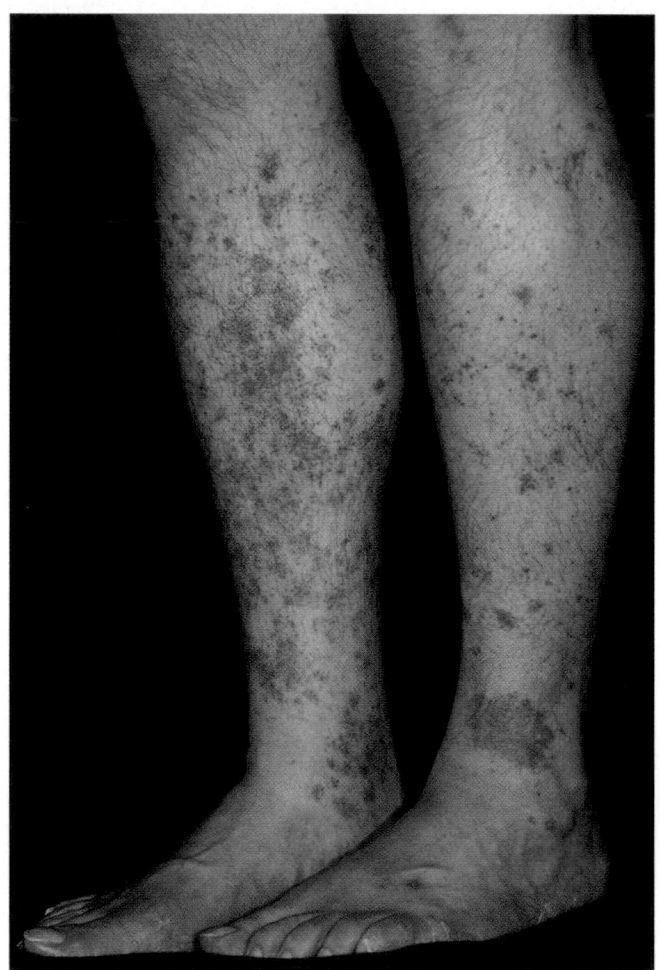

A, Asymptomatic, irregular, orange-brown patches of varying shapes and sizes occur most often on the lower extremities.

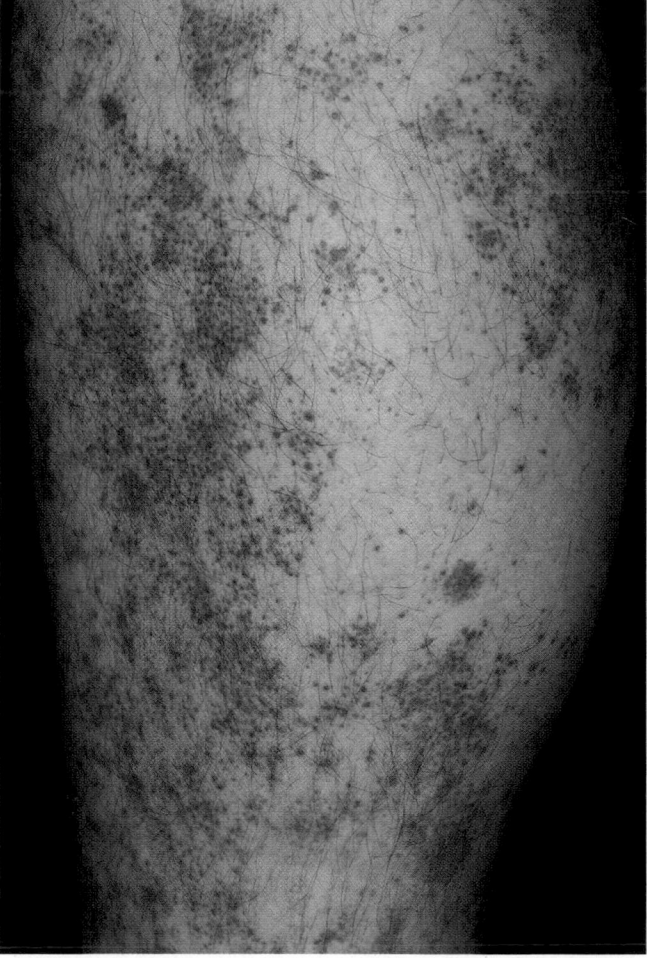

B, The most characteristic feature is the orange-brown, pinhead-sized "cayenne pepper" spots.

Figure 18-20 Schamberg's disease.

References

1. Villiger R, et al: Precipitants in 42 cases of erythema multiforme, Eur J Pediatr 1999; 158(11):929.

2. Cote B, et al: Clinicopathologic correlation in erythema multiforme and Stevens-Johnson syndrome, Arch Dermatol 1995; 131(11):1268.

3. Assier H, et al: Erythema multiforme with mucous membrane involvement and Stevens-Johnson syndrome are clinically different disorders with distinct causes [see comments], Arch Dermatol 1995; 131(5):539.

4. Auquier-Dunant A, et al: Correlations between clinical patterns and causes of erythema multiforme majus, Stevens-Johnson syndrome, and toxic epidermal necrolysis, Arch Dermatol 2002; 138:1019.

5. Weston WL, et al: Herpes simplex virus in childhood erythema multiforme, Pediatrics 1992; 89:32.

6. Nesbit SP, Gobetti JP: Multiple recurrence of oral erythema multiforme after secondary herpes simplex: report of case and review of literature, JAMA 1986; 112:348.

7. Imafuku S, et al: Expression of herpes simplex virus DNA fragments located in epidermal keratinocytes and germinative cells is associated with the development of erythema multiforme lesions, J Invest Dermatol 1997; 109(4):550.

8. Finan MC, Schroeter AL: Cutaneous immunofluorescence study of erythema multiforme: correlation with light microscopic patterns and etiologic agents, J Am Acad Dermatol 1984; 10:497.

9. Rzany B, et al: Histopathological and epidemiological characteristics of patients with erythema exudativum multiforme major, Stevens-Johnson syndrome and toxic epidermal necrolysis, Br J Dermatol 1996; 135(1):6.

10. Zohdi-Mofid M, Horn T: Acrosyringeal concentration of necrotic keratinocytes in erythema multiforme: a clue to drug etiology. Clinicopathologic review of 29 cases, J Cutan Pathol 1997; 24(4):235.

11. Paquet P, Pierard G: Erythema multiforme and toxic epidermal necrolysis: a comparative study, Am J Dermatopathol 1997; 19(2):127.

12. Tatnall F, Schofield J, Leigh I: A double-blind, placebo-controlled trial of continuous acyclovir therapy in recurrent erythema multiforme, Br J Dermatol 1995; 132(2):267.

13. Huff JC: Acyclovir for recurrent erythema multiforme caused by herpes simplex, J Am Acad Dermatol 1988; 18:197.

14. Kerob D, et al: Recurrent erythema multiforme unresponsive to acyclovir prophylaxis and responsive to valacyclovir continuous therapy [letter], Arch Dermatol 1998; 134(7):876.

15. Schofield JK, et al: Recurrent erythema multiforme: clinical features and treatment in a large series of patients, Br J Dermatol 1993; 128:542.

16. Cherouati K, et al: [Treatment by thalidomide of chronic multiforme erythema: its recurrent and continuous variants. A retrospective study of 26 patients], Ann Dermatol Venereol 1996; 123(6-7):375.

17. Bastuji-Garin S, et al: A clinical classification of cases of toxic epidermal necrolysis Stevens-Johnson syndrome and erythema multiforme, Arch Dermatol 1993; 129:92.

18. Haudrey MD, et al: Erythema multiforme with mucous membrane involvement and Stevens-Johnson syndrome are clinically different disorders with distinct causes, Arch Dermatol 1995; 131:539.

19. Chan LS, et al: Ocular cicatricial pemphigoid occurring as a sequela of Stevens-Johnson syndrome, JAMA 1991; 266:1543.

20. Levy M, Shear NH: Mycoplasma pneumoniae infections and Stevens-Johnson syndrome. Report of eight cases and review of the literature, Clin Pediatr 1991; 30:42.

21. Buchkell LL, Mackel SE, Jordan RE: Erythema multiforme: direct immunofluorescence studies and detection of circulating immune complexes, J Invest Dermatol 1980; 74:372.

22. Rasmussen JE: Erythema multiforme in children: response to treatment with systemic corticosteroids, Br J Dermatol 1976; 95:181.

23. Patterson R, et al: Stevens-Johnson syndrome (SJS): effectiveness of corticosteroids in management and recurrent SJS, Allergy Proc 1992; 13:89.

24. Tripathi A, et al: Corticosteroid therapy in an additional 13 cases of Stevens-Johnson syndrome: a total series of 67 cases, Allergy Asthma Proc 2000; 21(2):101.

25. Singer L, et al: Vitamin A in Stevens-Johnson syndrome, Ann Ophthalmol 1989; 21:209.

26. Detjen PF, et al: Herpes simplex virus associated with recurrent Stevens-Johnson syndrome. A management strategy, Arch Intern Med 1992; 152:1513.

27. Avakian R, et al: Toxic epidermal necrolysis: a review, J Am Acad Dermatol 1991; 25:69.

28. Roujeau JC, et al: Toxic epidermal necrolysis (Lyell syndrome), J Am Acad Dermatol 1990; 23:1063.

29. Roujeau JC, et al: Toxic epidermal necrolysis (Lyell syndrome). Incidence and drug etiology in France, 1981-1985, Arch Dermatol 1990; 126:37.

30. Correia O, et al: Evolving pattern of drug-induced toxic epidermal necrolysis, Dermatology 1993; 186:32.

31. Saiag P, et al: Drug-induced toxic epidermal necrolysis (Lyell syndrome) in patients infected with the human immunodeficiency virus, J Am Acad Dermatol 1992; 26:567.

32. Kimura S, et al: Three cases of acquired immunodeficiency syndrome complicated with toxic epidermal necrolysis, Jpn J Med 1991; 30:553.

33. Villada G, et al: Toxic epidermal necrolysis after bone marrow transplantation: study of nine cases, J Am Acad Dermatol 1990; 23:870.

34. Paul C, et al: Apoptosis as a mechanism of keratinocyte death in toxic epidermal necrolysis, Br J Dermatol 1996; 134(4):710.

35. Heng MC, Allen SG: Efficacy of cyclophosphamide in toxic epidermal necrolysis. Clinical and pathophysiologic aspects, J Am Acad Dermatol 1991; 25:778.

36. Correia O, et al: Cutaneous T-cell recruitment in toxic epidermal necrolysis. Further evidence of CD8+ lymphocyte involvement, Arch Dermatol 1993; 129:466.

37. Villada G, et al: Immunopathology of toxic epidermal necrolysis. Keratinocytes HLA-DR expression, Langerhans cells, and mononuclear cells: an immunopathologic study of five cases, Arch Dermatol 1992; 128:50.

38. Miyauchi H, et al: T-cell subsets in drug-induced toxic epidermal necrolysis. Possible pathogenic mechanism induced by CD8-positive T cells, Arch Dermatol 1991; 127:851.

39. Leenutaphong V, et al: Stevens-Johnson syndrome and toxic epidermal necrolysis in Thailand, Int J Dermatol 1993; 32:428.

40. Breathnach S: Management of drug eruptions: Part II. Diagnosis and treatment, Australas J Dermatol 1995; 36(4):187.

41. Wolkenstein P, et al: Metabolic predisposition to cutaneous adverse drug reactions, Arch Dermatol 1995; 131:544.

42. Roujeau J, et al: Medication use and the risk of Stevens-Johnson syndrome or toxic epidermal necrolysis [see comments], N Engl J Med 1995; 333(24):1600.

43. Rzany B, et al: Risk of Stevens-Johnson syndrome and toxic epidermal necrolysis during first weeks of antiepileptic therapy: a case-control study. Study Group of the International Case Control Study on Severe Cutaneous Adverse Reactions, Lancet 1999; 353(9171):2190.

44. Lebargy F, et al: Pulmonary complications in toxic epidermal necrolysis: a prospective clinical study, Intensive Care Med 1997; 23(12):1237.

45. McIvor R, et al: Acute and chronic respiratory complications of toxic epidermal necrolysis, J Burn Care Rehabil 1996; 17(3):237.

46. Kim PS, et al: Stevens-Johnson syndrome and toxic epidermal necrolysis: a pathophysiologic review with recommendations for a treatment protocol, J Burn Care Rehabil 1983; 4:91.

47. Goens J, et al: Haematological disturbances and immune mechanisms in toxic epidermal necrolysis, Br J Dermatol 1986; 114:255.

48. Vermeer BJ, Claas FJH: Toxic epidermal necrolysis (letter), Arch Dermatol 1985; 121:715.

49. Roujeau JC, et al: Granulocytes, lymphocytes, and toxic epidermal necrolysis, Arch Dermatol 1985; 121:305.

50. Ting HC, Adam BA: Stevens-Johnson syndrome: a review of 34 cases, Int J Dermatol 1985; 24:587.

51. Tegelberg-Stassen MJ, et al: Management of nonstaphylococcal toxic epidermal necrolysis: follow-up study of 16 case histories, Dermatologica 1990; 180:124.

52. Patterson R, et al: Erythema multiforme and Stevens-Johnson syndrome. Descriptive and therapeutic controversy, Chest 1990; 98:331.

53. Peters W, et al: Toxic epidermal necrolysis: a burn-centre challenge, Can Med Assoc J 1991; 144:1477.

54. Guibal F, et al: Characteristics of toxic epidermal necrolysis in patients undergoing long-term glucocorticoid therapy [see comments], Arch Dermatol 1995; 131(6):669.

55. Rzany B, et al: Toxic epidermal necrolysis in patients receiving glucocorticosteroids, Acta Derm Venereol 1991; 71:171.

56. Halebian PH, et al: Improved burn center survival of patients with toxic epidermal necrolysis managed without corticosteroids, Ann Surg 1986; 204:503.

57. Arevalo J, et al: Treatment of toxic epidermal necrolysis with cyclosporin A, J Trauma 2000; 48(3):473.

58. Paquet P, Pierard G: Would cyclosporin A be beneficial to mitigate drug-induced toxic epidermal necrolysis? Dermatology 1999; 198(2):198.

59. Sakellariou G, et al: Plasma exchange (PE) treatment in drug-induced toxic epidermal necrolysis (TEN), Int J Artif Organs 1991; 14:634.

60. Chaidemenos G, et al: Plasmapheresis in toxic epidermal necrolysis, Int J Dermatol 1997; 36(3):218.

61. Egan C, et al: Plasmapheresis as an adjunct treatment in toxic epidermal necrolysis, J Am Acad Dermatol 1999; 40(3):458.

62. Prins C, et al: Treatment of toxic epidermal necrolysis with high-dose intravenous immunoglobulins, Arch Dermatol 2003; 139:26.

63. Yarbrough DR: Treatment of toxic epidermal necrolysis in a burn center, J S C Med Assoc 1997; 93(9):347.

64. McGee T, Munster A: Toxic epidermal necrolysis syndrome: mortality rate reduced with early referral to regional burn center, Plast Reconstr Surg 1998; 102(4):1018.

65. Murphy J, Purdue G, Hunt J: Toxic epidermal necrolysis, J Burn Care Rehabil 1997; 18(5):417.

66. Smoot ER: Treatment issues in the care of patients with toxic epidermal necrolysis, Burns 1999; 25(5):439.

67. Arevalo J, Lorente J: Skin coverage with Biobrane biomaterial for the treatment of patients with toxic epidermal necrolysis, J Burn Care Rehabil 1999; 20(5):406.

68. Elkayam O, et al: Familial erythema nodosum, Arthritis Rheum 1991; 34:1177.

69. Cribier B, et al: Erythema nodosum and associated diseases. A study of 129 cases, Int J Dermatol 1998; 37(9):667.

70. Fox MD, Schwartz RA: Erythema nodosum, Am Fam Physician 1992; 46:818.

71. Atanes A, et al: Erythema nodosum: a study of 160 cases, Med Clin (Barc) 1991; 96:169.

72. Labbe L, et al: Erythema nodosum in children: a study of 27 patients, Pediatr Dermatol 1996; 13(6):447.

73. Hassink R, et al: Conditions currently associated with erythema nodosum in Swiss children, Eur J Pediatr 1997; 156(11):851.

74. Kirch W, Duhrsen U: Erythema nodosum of dental origin, Clin Invest Med 1992; 70:1073.

75. Mir-Madjlessi SH, Taylor JS, Farmer RG: Clinical course and evolution of erythema nodosum and pyoderma gangrenosum in chronic ulcerative colitis: a study of 42 patients, Am J Gastroenterol 1985; 80:615.

76. Wilsher M: Seasonal clustering of sarcoidosis presenting with erythema nodosum, Eur Respir J 1998; 12(5):1197.

77. Taillan B, et al: Erythema nodosum and Hodgkin's disease, Clin Rheumatol 1990; 9:397.

78. Bohn S, Buchner S, Itin P: [Erythema nodosum: 112 cases. Epidemiology, clinical aspects and histopathology (see comments)], Schweiz Med Wochenschr 1997; 127(27-28):1168.

79. Lofgren S: Erythema nodosum: studies on etiology and pathogenesis in 185 adult cases, Acta Med Scand 1946; 174 [suppl]:1.

80. Sanz V, et al: Erythema nodosum versus nodular vasculitis, Int J Dermatol 1993; 32:108.

81. Reference deleted in proofs.

82. Reference deleted in proofs.

83. Sterling J, Heymann W: Potassium iodide in dermatology: a 19th century drug for the 21st century-uses, pharmacology, adverse effects, and contraindications, J Am Acad Dermatol 2000; 43(4):691.

84. Soderstron RM, Krull EA: Erythema nodosum: a review, Cutis 1978; 21:806.

85. Jennette J, Falk R: Small-vessel vasculitis. N Engl J Med 1997; 337(21):1512.

86. Lotti T, et al: Cutaneous small-vessel vasculitis, J Am Acad Dermatol 1998; 39(5 Pt 1):667; quiz 688.

87. Bacon PA: Systemic vasculitic syndromes, Curr Opin Rheumatol 1993; 5:5.

88. Soter NA: Clinical presentations and mechanisms of necrotizing angiitis of the skin, J Invest Dermatol 1976; 67:354.

89. Ramsay C, Fry L: Allergic vasculitis: clinical and histological features and incidence of renal involvement, Br J Dermatol 1969; 81:96.

90. Winkelman RK, Ditto WB: Cutaneous and visceral syndromes of necrotizing or "allergic" angiitis: a study of thirty-eight cases, Medicine 1964; 43:59.

91. Lopez LR, et al: Gastrointestinal involvement in leukocytoclastic vasculitis and polyarteritis nodosa, J Rheumatol 1980; 7:677.

92. Ekenstram EA, Callen JP: Cutaneous leukocytoclastic vasculitis, Arch Dermatol 1984; 120:484.

93. Callen JP, Ekenstam EA: Cutaneous leukocytoclastic vasculitis: clinical experience in 44 patients, South Med J 1987; 80:848.

94. Sanchez NP, Van H, Daniel SWP: Clinical and histopathologic spectrum of necrotizing vasculitis: report of findings in 101 cases, Arch Dermatol 1985; 121:220.

95. Sais G, et al: Colchicine in the treatment of cutaneous leukocytoclastic vasculitis. Results of a prospective, randomized controlled trial, Arch Dermatol 1995; 131(12):1399.

96. Sullivan T, King L, Boyd A: Colchicine in dermatology, J Am Acad Dermatol 1998; 39(6):993.

97. Callen JP: Colchicine is effective in controlling chronic cutaneous leukocytoclastic vasculitis, J Am Acad Dermatol 1985; 13:193.

98. Fredenberg MF, Malkinson FD: Sulfone therapy in the treatment of leukocytoclastic vasculitis: report of three cases, J Am Acad Dermatol 1987; 16:772.

99. Fauci AS: Cyclophosphamide, N Engl J Med 1979; 301:235.

100. Saulsbury F: Henoch-Schonlein purpura in children. Report of 100 patients and review of the literature, Medicine 1999; 78(6):395.

101. Blanco R, et al: Henoch-Schonlein purpura in adulthood and childhood: two different expressions of the same syndrome [see comments], Arthritis Rheum 1997; 40(5):859.

102. Farley TA, et al: Epidemiology of a cluster of Henoch-Schönlein purpura, Am J Dis Child 1989; 143:798.

103. Saulsbury FT: Henoch-Schönlein purpura, Pediatr Dermatol 1984; 1:195.

104. Nussinovitch M, et al: Cutaneous manifestations of Henoch-Schonlein purpura in young children, Pediatr Dermatol 1998; 15(6):426.

105. Cull DL, et al: Surgical implications of Henoch-Schönlein purpura, Pediatr Surg 1990; 25:741.

106. Couture A, et al: Evaluation of abdominal pain in Henoch-Schönlein syndrome by high frequency ultrasound, Pediatr Radiol 1992; 22:12.

107. Connolly B, O'Halpin D: Sonographic evaluation of the abdomen in Henoch-Schonlein purpura, Clin Radiol 1994; 49(5):320.

108. Kato S, et al: Gastrointestinal endoscopy in Henoch-Schönlein purpura, Eur J Pediatr 1992; 151:482.

109. Linne T, et al: Renal function and biopsy changes during the course of Henoch-Schönlein glomerulonephritis, Acta Paediatr Scand 1983; 72:97.

110. Gauthier B: Schönlein-Henoch nephritis and IgA nephropathy in children, Curr Opin Pediatr 1993; 5:180.

111. Goldstein AR, et al: Long-term follow-up of childhood Henoch-Schönlein nephritis, Lancet 1992; 339:280.

112. Coppo R, et al: Long-term prognosis of Henoch-Schonlein nephritis in adults and children. Italian Group of Renal Immunopathology Collaborative Study on Henoch-Schonlein purpura, Nephrol Dial Transplant 1997; 12(11):2277.

113. Tancrede-Bohin E, et al: Schonlein-Henoch purpura in adult patients. Predictive factors for IgA glomerulonephritis in a retrospective study of 57 cases [see comments], Arch Dermatol 1997; 133(4):438.

114. Ben-Sira L: Severe scrotal pain in boys with Henoch-Schonlein purpura: incidence and sonography [Record Supplied By Publisher], Pediatr Radiol 2000; 30(2):125.

115. O'Brien WM, et al: Acute scrotal swelling in Henoch-Schönlein syndrome: evaluation with testicular scanning, Urology 1993; 41:366.

116. Petersen S, et al: Immunoglobulin and complement studies in children with Schönlein-Henoch syndrome and other vasculitic diseases, Acta Paediatr Scand 1991; 80:1037.

117. Van H, Gibson LE, Schroeter AL: Henoch-Schönlein vasculitis: direct immunofluorescence study of uninvolved skin, J Am Acad Dermatol 1986; 15:665.

118. Egan C: IgA1 is the major IgA subclass in cutaneous blood vessels in henoch-Schonlein purpura. [In Process Citation], Br J Dermatol 1999; 141(5):859.

119. Abou-Ragheb HH, et al: Plasma levels of the anaphylatoxins C3a and C4a in patients with IgA nephropathy/Henoch-Schönlein nephritis, Nephron 1992; 62:22.

120. Helander SD, et al: Henoch-Schönlein purpura: clinicopathologic correlation of cutaneous vascular IgA deposits and the relationship to leukocytoclastic vasculitis, Acta Derm Venereol 1995; 75:125.

121. Szer I: Gastrointestinal and renal involvement in vasculitis: management strategies in Henoch-Schönlein purpura, Cleve Clin J Med 1999; 66(5):312.

122. Wang YJ, et al: Clinical studies of Henoch-Schönlein purpura in Chinese children, Chung Hua I Hsueh Tsa Chih 1993; 51:345.

123. Saulsbury FT: Corticosteroid therapy does not prevent nephritis in Henoch-Schönlein purpura, Pediatr Nephrol 1993; 7:69.

124. Faedda R, et al: Regression of Henoch-Schonlein disease with intensive immunosuppressive treatment, Clin Pharmacol Ther 1996; 60(5):576.

125. Iijima K, et al: Multiple combined therapy for severe Henoch-Schonlein nephritis in children, Pediatr Nephrol 1998; 12(3):244.

126. Foster B: Effective therapy for severe Henoch-Schonlein purpura nephritis with prednisone and azathioprine: a clinical and histopathologic study [Record Supplied By Publisher], J Pediatr 2000; 136(3):370.

127. Bergstein J, Leiser J, Andreoli S: Response of crescentic Henoch-Schoenlein purpura nephritis to corticosteroid and azathioprine therapy, Clin Nephrol 1998; 49(1):9.

128. Rostoker G, et al: Immunomodulation with low-dose immunoglobulins for moderate IgA nephropathy and Henoch-Schonlein purpura. Preliminary results of a prospective uncontrolled trial [see comments], Nephron 1995; 69(3):327.

129. Kusuda A, et al: Successful treatment of adult-onset Henoch-Schonlein purpura nephritis with high-dose immunoglobulins, Intern Med 1999; 38(4):376.

130. Mangold MC, Callen JP: Cutaneous leukocytoclastic vasculitis associated with active Wegener's granulomatosis, J Am Acad Dermatol 1992; 26:579.

131. Patten SF, Tomecki KJ: Wegener's granulomatosis: cutaneous and oral mucosal disease, J Am Acad Dermatol 1993; 28:710.

132. Francès C, et al: Wegener's granulomatosis: dermatologic manifestation in 75 cases with clinicopathologic correlation, Arch Dermatol 1994; 130:861.

133. Davis M, et al: Cutaneous manifestations of Churg-Strauss syndrome: a clinicopathologic correlation, J Am Acad Dermatol 1997; 37(2 Pt 1):199.

134. Matteson E: Small-vessel vasculitis, N Engl J Med 1998; 338(14):994.

135. Kirkland G, et al: Classical polyarteritis nodosa and microscopic polyarteritis with medium vessel involvement—a comparison of the clinical and laboratory features, Clin Nephrol 1997; 47(3):176.

136. Jayne D, et al: A randomized trial of maintenance therapy for vasculitis associated with antineutrophil cytoplasmic autoantibodies, NEJM 2003; 349:36.

137. Vignon-Pennamen MD, Wallach D: Cutaneous manifestations of neutrophilic disease. A study of seven cases, Dermatologica 1991; 183:255.

138. Cohen P, Kurzrock R: Sweet's syndrome: a review of current treatment options, Am J Clin Dermatol 2002; 3(2):117.

139. Fett D, Gibson L, Su W: Sweet's syndrome: systemic signs and symptoms and associated disorders [see comments], Mayo Clin Proc 1995; 70(3):234.

140. Paydas S, Sahin B, Zorludemir S: Sweet's syndrome accompanying leukaemia: seven cases and review of the literature, Leuk Res 2000; 24(1):83.

141. Jain K: Sweet's syndrome associated with granulocyte colony-stimulating factor, Cutis 1996; 57(2):107.

142. Merkel P: Drugs associated with vasculitis, Curr Opin Rheumatol 1998; 10(1):45.

143. Prevost-Blank P, Shwayder T: Sweet's syndrome secondary to granulocyte colony-stimulating factor, J Am Acad Dermatol 1996; 35(6):995.

144. Sitjas D, et al: Acute febrile neutrophilic dermatosis (Sweet's syndrome), Int J Dermatol 1993; 32:261.

145. Smolle J, Kresbach H: Acute febrile neutrophilic dermatosis (Sweet syndrome). A retrospective clinical and histological analysis, Hautarzt 1990; 41:549.

146. Kemmett D, Hunter JA: Sweet's syndrome: a clinicopathologic review of twenty-nine cases, J Am Acad Dermatol 1990; 23:503.

147. Ginarte M, Garcia DI, Toribio J: [Sweet's syndrome: a study of 16 cases], Med Clin 1997; 109(15):588.

148. Going JJ, et al: Sweet's syndrome: histological and immunohistochemical study of 15 cases, J Clin Pathol 1987; 40:175.

149. Jordaan HF: Acute febrile neutrophilic dermatosis. A histopathological study of 37 patients and a review of the literature, Am J Dermatopathol 1989; 11:99.

150. Malone J, et al: Vascular inflammation (vasculitis) in sweet syndrome: a clinicopathologic study of 28 biopsy specimens from 21 patients, Arch Dermatol 2002; 138(3):345.

151. Honma K, et al: Potassium iodide inhibits neutrophil chemotaxis, Acta Derm Venereol 1990; 70:247.

152. Ritter S, et al: Long-term suppression of chronic Sweet's syndrome with colchicine, J Am Acad Dermatol 2002; 47(2):323.

153. Jeanfils S, et al: Indomethacin treatment of eighteen patients with Sweet's syndrome, J Am Acad Dermatol 1997; 36(3 Pt 1): 436.

154. von d, Driesch P: Sweet's syndrome (acute febrile neutrophilic dermatosis), J Am Acad Dermatol 1994; 31:535.

155. Muratori S: Erythema elevatum diutinum and HIV infection: a report of five cases [In Process Citation], Br J Dermatol 1999; 141(2):335.

156. Shanks J, et al: Nodular erythema elevatum diutinum mimicking cutaneous neoplasms, Histopathology 1997; 31(1):91.

157. Yiannias JA, et al: Erythema elevatum diutinum: a clinical and histopathologic study of 13 patients, J Am Acad Dermatol 1992; 26:38.

158. Wilkinson SM, et al: Erythema elevatum diutinum: a clinico-pathological study, Clin Exp Dermatol 1992; 17:87.

159. Carlson J, Le BP: Localized chronic fibrosing vasculitis of the skin: an inflammatory reaction that occurs in settings other than erythema elevatum diutinum and granuloma faciale, Am J Surg Pathol 1997; 21(6):698.

160. Grabbe J, et al: Erythema elevatum diutinum—evidence for disease-dependent leucocyte alterations and response to dapsone, Br J Dermatol 2000; 143(2):415.

161. Henriksson R, et al: Erythema elevatum diutinum-a case successfully treated with colchicine, Clin Exp Dermatol 1989; 14:451.

162. Bennett M, et al: Pyoderma gangrenosum. A comparison of typical and atypical forms with an emphasis on time to remission. Case review of 86 patients from 2 institutions, Medicine 2000; 79(1):37.

163. Ko CB, et al: Pyoderma gangrenosum: associations revisited, Int J Dermatol 1992; 31:574.

164. Powell FC, et al: Pyoderma gangrenosum and monoclonal gammopathy, Arch Dermatol 1983; 119:468.

165. Gleichmann U, et al: [Post-traumatic pyoderma gangrenosum: combination therapy with intravenous immunoglobulins and systemic corticosteroids], Hautarzt 1999; 50(12):879.

166. Barnes L, et al: Pustular pyoderma gangrenosum associated with ulcerative colitis in childhood: report of two cases and review of the literature, J Am Acad Dermatol 1986; 15:608.

167. von dDP. Pyoderma gangrenosum: a report of 44 cases with follow-up, Br J Dermatol 1997; 137(6):1000.

168. Basler RSW: Ulcerative colitis and the skin, Med Clin North Am 1980; 64:941.

169. Thornton JR, et al: Pyoderma gangrenosum and ulcerative colitis, Gut 1980; 21:247.

170. Levitt MD, et al: Pyoderma gangrenosum in inflammatory bowel disease, Br J Surg 1991; 78:676.

171. Hurwitz RM, Haseman JH: The evolution of pyoderma gangrenosum: a clinicopathologic correlation, Am J Dermatopathol 1993; 15:28.

172. Wollina U: Clinical management of pyoderma gangrenosum, Am J Clin Dermatol 2002; 3(3):149.

173. Goldstein F, Krain R, Thornton JL: Intralesional steroid therapy of pyoderma gangrenosum, J Clin Gastroenterol 1985; 7:499.

174. Nasr I: Topical tacrolimus in dermatology, Clin Exp Dermatol 2000; 25(3):250.

175. Michel S, et al: [Therapy-resistant pyoderma gangrenosum—treatment with mycophenolate mofetil and cyclosporine A], Hautarzt 1999; 50(6):428.

176. Reynoso-von DC, et al: Intravenous cyclophosphamide pulses in pyoderma gangrenosum: an open trial, J Rheumatol 1997; 24(4):689.

177. Burruss J, Farmer E, Callen J: Chlorambucil is an effective corticosteroid-sparing agent for recalcitrant pyoderma gangrenosum, J Am Acad Dermatol 1996; 35(5 Pt 1):720.

178. Hagman J, et al: The use of high-dose immunoglobulin in the treatment of pyoderma gangrenosum [In Process Citation], J Dermatolog Treat 2001; 12(1):19.

179. Draelos ZK, Hansen RC: Schamberg's purpura in children: case study and literature review, Clin Pediatr 1987; 26:659.

180. Ghersetich I, et al: Cell infiltrate in progressive pigmented purpura (Schamberg's disease): immunophenotype, adhesion receptors, and intercellular relationships, Int J Dermatol 1995; 34(12):846.

181. Abeck D, et al: Acetaminophen-induced progressive pigmentary purpura (Schamberg's disease), J Am Acad Dermatol 1992; 27:123.

182. Kano Y, et al: Successful treatment of Schamberg's disease with pentoxifylline [see comments], J Am Acad Dermatol 1997; 36(5 Pt 2):827.

183. Burkhart C, Burkhart K: Pentoxifylline for Schamberg's disease [letter; comment], J Am Acad Dermatol 1998; 39(2 Pt 1):298.

184. Ratnam KV, et al: Purpura simplex (inflammatory purpura without vasculitis): a clinicopathologic study of 174 cases, J Am Acad Dermatol 1991; 25:642.

Light-Related Diseases and Disorders of Pigmentation

Photobiology

Sunlight has profound effects on the skin and is associated with a variety of diseases (see Boxes 19-1 and 19-2). Ultraviolet (UV) light causes most photobiologic skin reactions and diseases.[1] The accepted unit for measurement of the wavelength of light is the *nanometer* (nm). The solar radiation that reaches the earth is a continuous spectrum consisting of wavelengths of electromagnetic energy above 290 nm. By convention, UV light is divided into UVA (320 to 400 nm; long wave, black light), UVB (290 to 320 nm; middle wave, sunburn), and UVC (100 to 290 nm; short wave, germicidal). UVA is further subdivided into two regions: short-wave UVA, or UVA II (320 to 340 nm), and long-wave UVA, or UVA I (340 to 400 nm). The ratio of UVA to UVB is 20:1, and two thirds of this UVA is UVA I. Eighty percent of UVB and 70% of UVA radiation occur between the hours of 10 AM and 2 PM. More than 90% of UV may penetrate clouds. UV radiation generates reactive oxygen species that damage skin.

UVA. UVA causes immediate and delayed tanning and contributes little to erythema and burning. It is constant throughout the day and throughout the year. The longer wavelengths of UVA can penetrate more deeply, reaching the dermis and subcutaneous fat. Chronic exposure to UVA radiation causes the connective tissue degeneration seen in photoaging, photocarcinogenesis, and immunosuppression. Photocarcinogenesis is augmented in patients who are immunosuppressed for organ transplantation. UVA augments the carcinogenic effects of UVB. UVA penetrates window glass and interacts with topical and systemic chemicals and medication. It produces photoallergic and phototoxic reactions.

UVB. UVB produces the most harmful effects and is greatest during the summer. Snow and ice reflect UVB radiation. UVB delivers a high amount of energy to the stratum corneum and superficial layers of the epidermis and is primarily responsible for sunburn, suntan, inflammation, delayed erythema, and pigmentation changes. It produces tanning more efficiently than does UVA. Chronic effects include photoaging, immunosuppression, and photocarcinogenesis. It is most intense when the sun is directly overhead between 10 AM and 2 PM. UVB is absorbed by window glass. Prior exposure to UVA enhances the sunburn reaction from UVB.

UVC. UVC is almost completely absorbed by the ozone layer and is transmitted only by artificial sources such as germicidal lamps and mercury arc lamps.

Box 19-1 Photosensitivity Diseases: Diseases Characterized by the Development of a Cutaneous Eruption After Exposure to Light

Idiopathic
Polymorphous light eruption
Actinic prurigo
Hydroa vacciniforme
Hydroa aestivale
Chronic actinic dermatitis
Solar urticaria
Degenerative and neoplastic
Actinic damage
Actinic keratosis
Basal cell carcinoma
Squamous cell carcinoma
Malignant melanoma
Secondary to exogenous agents
Phototoxicity: Contact and systemic
Photoallergy: Contact and systemic
Drug eruptions
Metabolic
Erythropoietic porphyria
Erythropoietic protoporphyria
Porphyria cutanea tarda
Variegate porphyria
Photoexacerbated dermatoses
Autoimmune diseases
  Lupus erythematosus
  Dermatomyositis
  Pemphigus
  Pemphigus foliaceus
  Bullous pemphigoid

Genodermatoses
Familial benign chronic pemphigus
Keratosis follicularis (Darier's disease)
Bloom's syndrome
Rothmund-Thompson syndrome
Kindler syndrome
Cockayne's syndrome
Xeroderma pigmentosum
Trichothiodystrophy
Hartnup disease
Infectious disease
Herpes simplex labialis
Nutritional deficiencies
Pellagra
Pyridoxine deficiency
Primary dermatologic diseases
Atopic dermatitis
Transient acantholytic dermatosis
Disseminated superficial actinic porokeratosis
Lichen planus actinicus
Psoriasis
Reticular erythematous mucinosis
Acne rosacea
Acne
Darier's disease
Hailey-Hailey disease

Adapted from Lim HW, Epstein J: J Am Acad Dermatol 1997; 36:84.

Sun-Damaged Skin

SUNLIGHT-SKIN INTERACTION. DNA is mutated by UVB. Absorption of UVA leads to the release of reactive oxygen species that cause oxidation of lipids and proteins that affect DNA repair, produce dyspigmentation, and cause photoaging and carcinogenesis.

AGING VERSUS SUN DAMAGE. Sun exposure is the major cause of the undesirable skin changes often inaccurately perceived as aging. These changes, known as *photoaging*, are caused primarily by repeated sun exposure and not by the passage of time. Many of the clinical signs attributed to aging are actually manifestations of solar damage. The two processes are biologically different. The difference can best be demonstrated to patients by comparing the appearance of the skin under the arm near the axillae with the sun-exposed surface of the lower arm.

NORMAL AGING. The skin begins to show signs of aging by ages 30 to 35. Aged skin is thin, fragile, and inelastic. The epidermis becomes thin. There is a gradual loss of blood vessels, dermal collagen, fat, and the number of elastic fibers. There is a reduction in the density of hair follicles, sweat ducts, and sebaceous glands, resulting in a reduction in perspiration and sebum production. Potent steroids should not be used on aged skin with few blood vessels because the steroids are not cleared from the skin as easily as in younger persons.

The skin becomes atrophic and fragile when subcutaneous tissue is lost. Elastic fibers are responsible for the elasticity and resilience of the skin. In normal aging, there is loss and fragmentation of elastic fibers, which result in fine wrinkles that resemble crumpled cigarette paper. These shallow wrinkles disappear by stretching. The skin is easily distorted, but it recoils slowly.

Box 19-2 Most Common Photodermatoses According to Age the Symptoms First Occur

Childhood

Juvenile spring eruption
(lesions on ears in spring)

Polymorphous light eruption
(itchy lesion in V area of neck and elsewhere)

Erythropoietic protoporphyria
(burning pain, increased protoporphyrin levels in red blood cells)

Actinic prurigo
(lesions on bridge of nose, HLA-DR4)

Hydroa vacciniforme
(very rare, scar formation)

Adulthood

Polymorphous light eruption
(females with itchy lesion in V of neck and elsewhere)

Drug-induced photosensitivity
(all sun-exposed areas, positive phototest results)

Solar urticaria
(lesions appear within 5-10 mi and disappear in 1-2 h)
(Urticaria on phototesting)

Lupus erythematosus
(anti-Ro/SS-A antibodies, skin immunofluorescence)

Porphyria cutanea tarda
(porphyrin determinations)

Old age

Chronic actinic dermatitis
(persistent redness of face in elderly man)

Drug-induced photosensitivity
(all sun-exposed areas, positive phototest results)

Cutaneous T-cell lymphoma
(CD4+ cells on histological examination)

Dermatomyositis
(creatine level in 24-hour urine)

Adapted from Roelandts R: Arch Dermatol 2000; 136:1152.

Box 19-3 Sun-Induced Skin Changes

Texture changes

Solar elastosis
  Thickened, wrinkled, yellowish skin

Atrophy
  Thinning of the skin; fine wrinkling, prominent blood vessels, easy bruising and tearing of the skin, often with many linear scars

Wrinkles
  Deep—do not disappear by stretching
    Posterior neck sun damage (cutis rhomboidalis nuchae)
    Thickened skin is crisscrossed by deep lines creating rhomboidal patterns

Vascular Changes

Diffuse erythema
  Most apparent in fair-skinned people

Ecchymoses and stellate pseudoscars
  Bleeding into the skin follows minor trauma—only on exposed surfaces of the back of the hands and arms; associated with atrophy, ease of skin tearing, and linear scars

Telangiectasias
  Cheeks, nose, and ears

Venous lake
  Round purple ectatic vessels—lower lips and ears

Pigmentation Changes

Freckles
  Small, oval, brown macules—primarily on the face

Lentigo
  Large brown macules—face, back of the hands, arms, chest, upper back

Guttate hypomelanosis
  Discrete, round, white macules—lower legs and arms

Brown and white pigmentation (irregular)
  Deep brown with areas of hypopigmentation

Poikiloderma of civatte
  Reddish-brown reticulated pigmentation with telangiectasias, atrophy, and prominent hair follicles—chest and neck

Papular changes

Nevi
  More numerous on sun-exposed surfaces in predisposed individuals

Yellow papules (solar elastosis)
  Dull-to-bright yellow papules that may coalesce to form plaques

Seborrheic keratosis
  Discrete superficial (stuck-on) lesions—more numerous in sun-exposed areas; flat on extremities, elevated on the trunk

Comedones and cysts around the eyes (Favre-Racouchot syndrome)

PHOTOAGING. Photoaging refers to those skin changes superimposed on intrinsic aging by chronic sun exposure[2] (Box 19-3). Unprotected, chronically exposed children can acquire significant actinic damage by the time they reach age 15. The effects of this damage may become apparent after age 20. Sun-damaged skin is characterized by *elastosis* (a coarsening and yellow discoloration of the skin), irregular pigmentation, roughness or dryness, telangiectasia, atrophy, deep wrinkling, follicular plugging, and a variety of benign and malignant neoplasms.[3] The epidermis thickens. Although many different cells are affected, it is the elastotic material that accounts for the most striking effects of sun damage.

Solar elastosis is a sign highly characteristic of severe sun damage (Figure 19-1). There is massive deposition in the upper dermis of an abnormal, yellow, amorphous elastotic material that does not form functional elastic fibers. This altered connective tissue does not have the resilient properties of elastic tissue.

Wrinkling becomes coarse and deep rather than fine, and the skin is thickened (Figure 19-2). These wrinkles do not disappear by stretching.[4] Sun-induced wrinkling on the back of the neck shows a series of crisscrossed lines (Figure 19-3) that form a rhomboidal pattern *(cutis rhomboidalis nuchae)*.

Reactive hyperplasia of melanocytes causes persistent pigmentation in the form of freckles, lentigines, and irregular hyperpigmentation and hypopigmentation on the hands, forearms, legs, chest, and back (Figure 19-3).

Chronic sun exposure disrupts the maturation of keratinocytes, causing scaling, roughness, seborrheic keratosis (Figures 19-4 to 19-6), actinic keratosis, actinic cheilitis, and squamous cell carcinoma.

Blood vessels diminish in number, and the walls of the remaining vessels become thin. Blood vessels need connective tissue for support. Bleeding occurs with the slightest trauma to the sun-damaged surfaces of the forearms and hands but not to the unexposed surfaces. Haphazard scarring may follow (Figure 19-7). Making patients aware of this difference convinces them that they do not have a platelet abnormality.

Comedones form about the eyes (Figures 19-8 and 19-9).

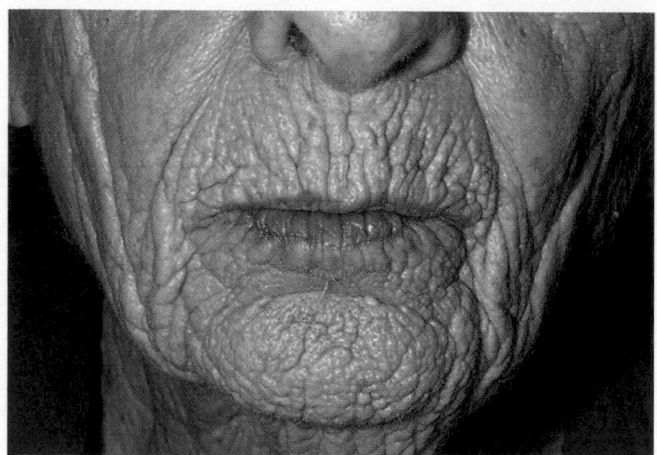

Figure 19-2 Leathered wrinkling is a sign of severe sun damage.

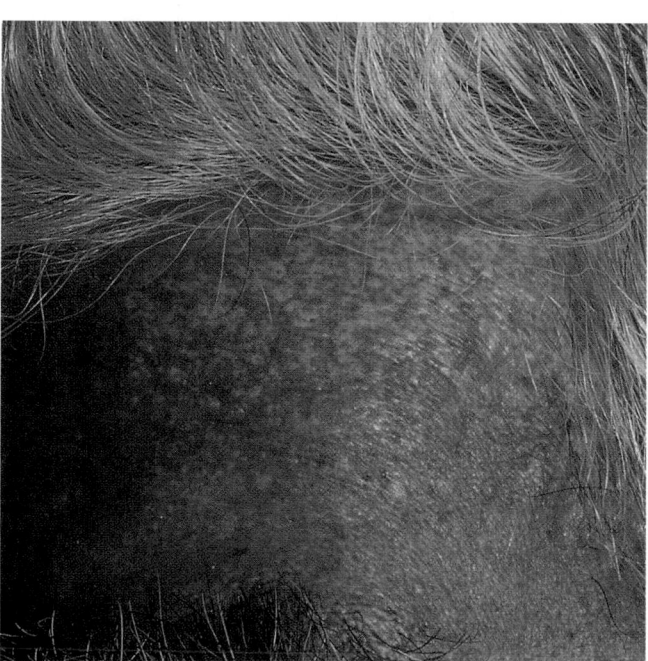

Figure 19-1 Solar elastosis. Numerous yellowish globules in the dermis can be seen through the thin, atrophic epidermis.

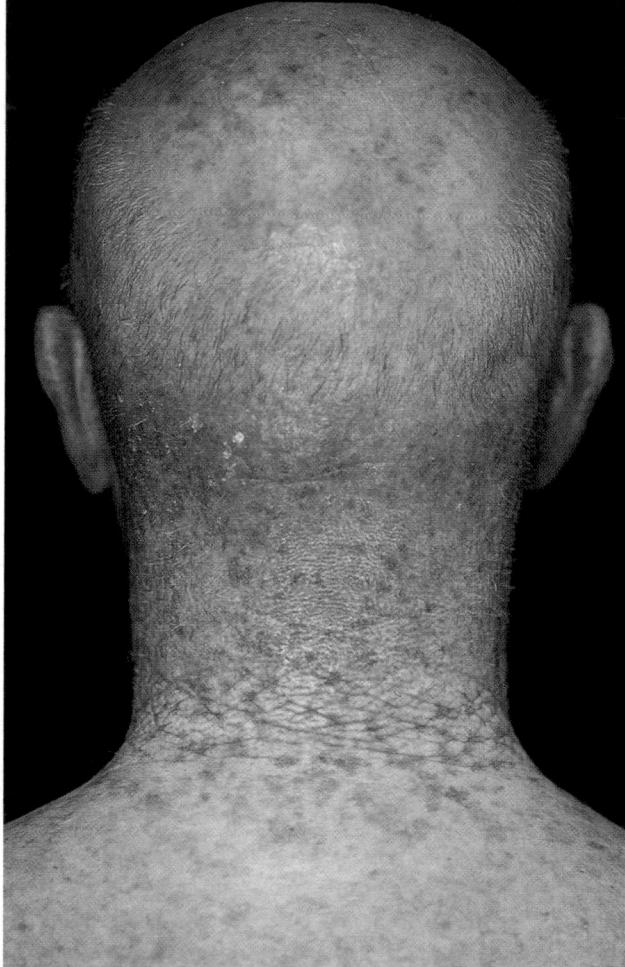

Figure 19-3 Reactive hyperplasia of melanocytes causes lentigines on the upper back. Diffuse persistent erythema is most prominent in fair-skinned people. Sun-induced wrinkling on the back of the neck shows a series of crisscrossed lines.

PHOTOAGING

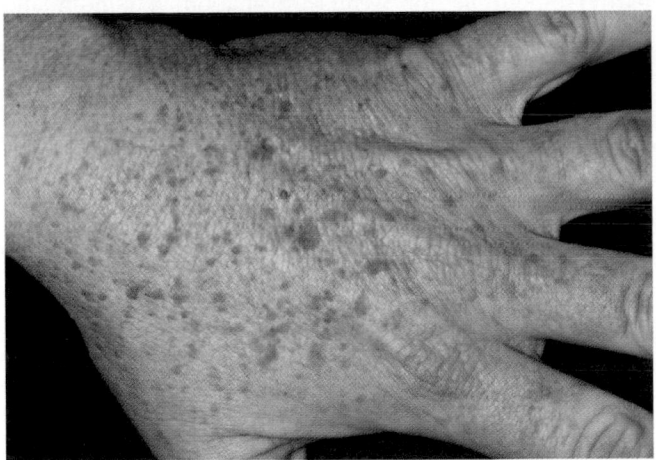

Figure 19-4 Slightly elevated seborrheic keratoses occur on the back of the hands and may be misdiagnosed as solar lentigines.

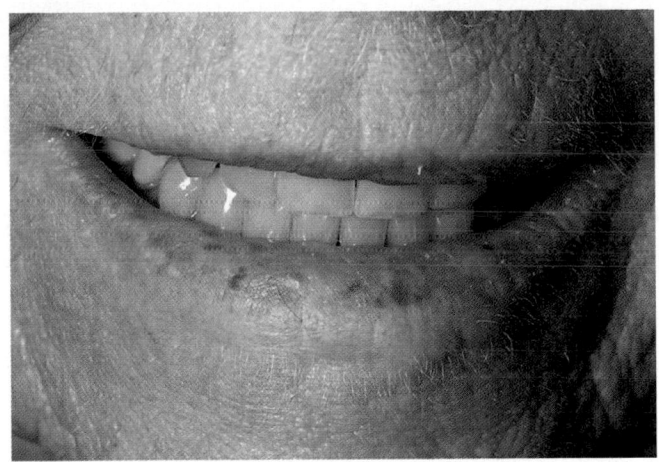

Figure 19-5 Sun damage causes lower lip atrophy with loss of normal skin lines.

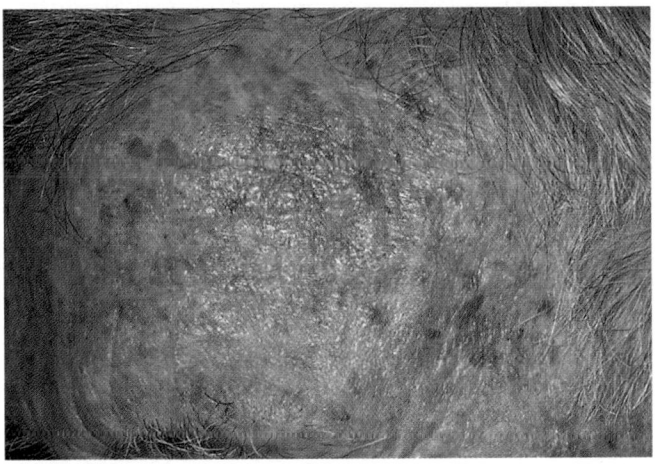

Figure 19-6 Variations in pigmentation and diffuse actinic keratosis may occur after years of sun exposure.

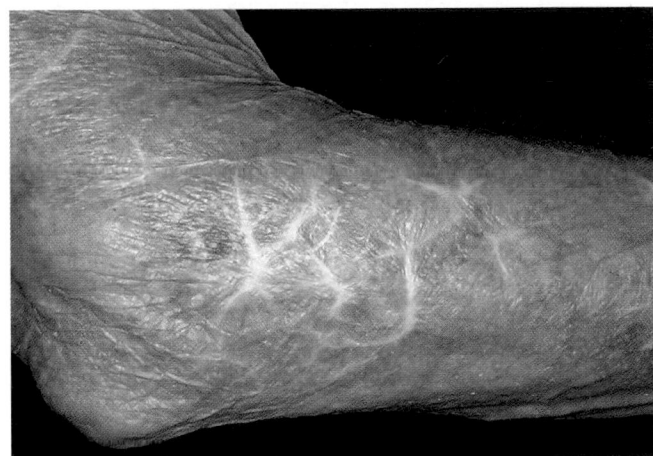

Figure 19-7 Fragile sun-damaged skin is easily torn and heals with haphazard scars called stellate pseudoscars.

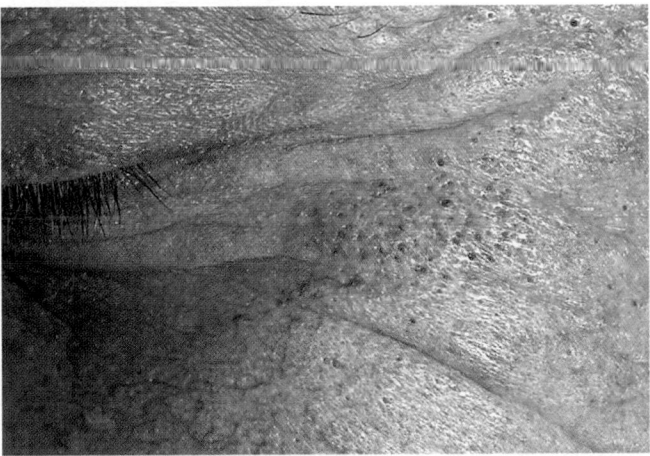

Figure 19-8 Actinic comedones. Open and closed comedones are present in the periorbital areas. Acne-like inflammation does not occur.

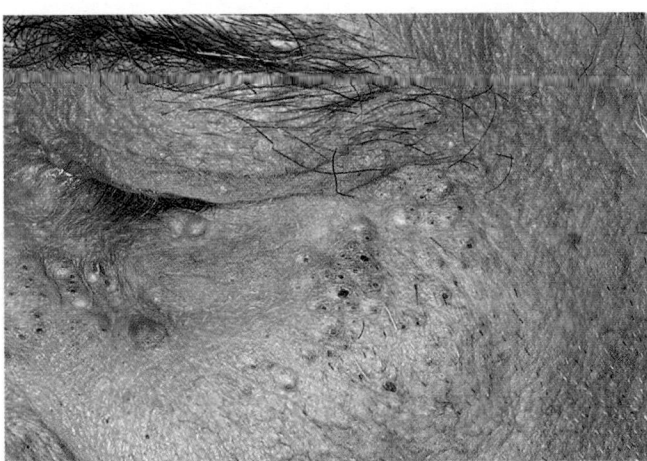

Figure 19-9 Actinic comedones may become very large and can easily be expressed with a comedone extractor.

Treatment of photoaging

Photoaging is treated with either topical treatments or resurfacing through chemical peels, dermabrasion, or lasers.

TOPICAL TREATMENT. Topical treatments have the following characteristics.

1. Noninvasive
2. Slow to produce changes (latency period is 3 to 6 months)
3. Maintenance of improvements requires continued use
4. Medication is expensive

Photoaging responds to treatment with topical retinoids such as tretinoin and tazarotene. The improvement is retinoid specific and not secondary to irritation. Improvement can be achieved without excessive use of medication, thereby minimizing the occurrence of irritation. Some skin peeling is unavoidable.

TOPICAL TRETINOIN AND TAZAROTENE. Topical retinoids provide some reversal of photodamaged skin (Box 19-4). Objective improvements in wrinkling are seen after 3 to 6 months. *Dyspigmentation* (brown spots and mottled hyperpigmentation), surface roughness, and fine wrinkles respond best. The greatest response to therapy occurs during the initial 6 to 9 months.

Repeated applications of retinoids produce a skin reaction resembling irritation. This reaction is characterized by redness and desquamation, signs that correspond histologically to alterations in the stratum corneum and epidermal hyperplasia. Initially patients experience skin tightening and a pink glow. This smoothening occurs within 1 to 2 weeks of treatment. It is the first sign of improvement, and it occurs because the stratum corneum is thinner and more compact, and the epidermal layer is thicker and spongiotic. Increased proliferation of basal keratinocytes eventually doubles the epidermal thickness.

Box 19-4 Topical Tretinoin and Tazarotene— Effects of Treatment

Fine wrinkling—improved
Coarse wrinkling—improved
Tactile roughness—improved
Lentigines—reduction in number
Freckles—reduction in color
Actinic keratoses—decrease in number
Telangiectasia—did not improve
Cutaneous reaction
Dermatitis—(1 to 10 weeks) xerosis, mild scaling, irritation
Increased pinkness, "rosy glow"
Inflammation—(3+ months) of presumed subclinical actinic keratoses

Collagen formation is reduced in photoaged skin and is partly responsible for wrinkle formation. Tretinoin and tazarotene increase collagen levels in photoaged skin; the end result is wrinkle effacement. Effacement of fine wrinkles occurs after 3 to 4 months of tretinoin therapy. The deepest coarse facial wrinkles are still evident. Despite continued improvement in wrinkle effacement, the epidermal histology reverts to the pretherapy state.

Hyperpigmented lesions are a predominant component of photoaging in Chinese and Japanese persons; tretinoin cream lightens the hyperpigmentation of photoaging in these patients.[5] Tretinoin therapy for individuals with darker skin pigmentation is safe. Postinflammatory dyspigmentation at sites of retinoid dermatitis does not occur in black and Asian patients.

RETINOID APPLICATION PROCEDURES. The response to retinoid may be dose dependent; higher concentrations in one study were more effective.[6] Many patients experience a "retinoid dermatitis" with erythema and peeling. It is unnecessary to push retinoid use to the point that brisk retinoid dermatitis develops to achieve maximum clinical improvement of photoaged skin. A 48-week regimen of once-daily treatment with medication, followed by treatment 3 times weekly for an additional 24 weeks, maintains and, in some cases, even enhances the improvements in photoaged skin. Treatment on a once-a-week basis with retinoids is less effective in sustaining the clinical improvement achieved by the initial treatment regimen of tretinoin on a once-daily basis. Some reversal of the beneficial effects of tretinoin treatment is observed after discontinuation of therapy for 24 weeks, which indicates the need to continue tretinoin therapy to maintain clinical improvement.[7]

Begin with nighttime application. Start treatment with cream-based tretinoin (0.025%), emollient-based tretinoin (Renova 0.05% or 0.02%) or cream-based tazarotene (Avage 0.1). A gradual introduction to treatment using every-other-day application is appropriate for patients with sensitive skin (usually type I; Table 19-1), followed by more frequent applications when patients accommodate. Apply moisturizing cosmetics or lubricating lotions if dryness occurs. Maximum response occurs after 8 to 12 months of treatment; thereafter application frequency should be reduced to 3 or 4 times a week to maintain improvement.

SUN PROTECTION DURING USE. Encourage the daily use of sunscreens. Increased "photosensitivity" during tretinoin use is not an accelerated sunburn response. No increased risk of photocarcinogenesis has been detected in humans.

TRETINOIN USE AND PREGNANCY. The data on routine clinical use of topical tretinoin indicate that there is no increased risk for pregnant women. However, spontaneous malformation of the fetus occasionally occurs in "normal" pregnancies. It may therefore be prudent to postpone tretinoin therapy for patients who are actively trying to conceive, to avoid wrongful blame for congenital defects that may occur by chance.[8]

ALPHA-HYDROXY ACIDS CREAMS. Alpha-hydroxy acids (AHAs) have been promoted as improving the appearance of photodamaged skin. The Food and Drug Administration has mandated that the concentration of AHAs in cosmetics cannot exceed 10%. Cosmetologists can use a concentration of glycolic or lactic acid of up to 30%. Physicians can use glycolic acid peels of higher concentration and provide lotions with acid concentrations of greater than 10%. The low concentration in cosmetics has only a modest effect on photoaging.

ESTROGEN REPLACEMENT. Statistically significant reductions in dry skin and skin wrinkling occur with estrogen replacement.[9]

Resurfacing procedures

Resurfacing procedures have the following characteristics.
1. Results occur quickly.
2. Perioperative morbidity ranges from mild to significant.
3. Complications occur such as scarring and hypopigmentation.
4. Improvements may have to be maintained with topical treatments.
5. Treatment is expensive.

Resurfacing occurs at three levels.
1. Superficial–wounds from the stratum corneum through the papillary dermis (0.06 mm)
2. Medium depth–wounds of the upper reticular dermis (0.45 to 0.6 mm)
3. Deep–midreticular dermal wounds (0.6 to 0.8 mm)

Epidermal healing comes from the adnexal epithelium. A high density of adnexa (hair follicles, eccrine sweat ducts) occurs on the face. Nonfacial epithelium has a low density of adnexa and can tolerate only superficial resurfacing. The deeper the wound, the greater the amount of collagen regeneration. Light peels, light laser resurfacing, or microdermabrasion does not achieve the deep resurfacing results needed for deeper lines.

GLYCOLIC ACID PEELS. Controversy exists whether glycolic acid peels have clinical benefits beyond the controlled skin wounding seen with any peel. One study showed that application of 50% glycolic acid peels spaced 1 week apart for 4 weeks to photodamaged skin produced improvement in texture, a reduced number of solar keratoses, and a decrease in fine wrinkling. However, other studies showed no improvement.[9]

DEEPER CHEMICAL PEELS. Chemical peels can produce destruction at all three levels. Upper-dermal (medium-depth) and mid-dermal (deep) peels cause histologic changes that can reverse some aspects of photoaging. Phenol and trichloroacetic acid peels can produce very gratifying results; their use requires special training.

MICRODERMABRASION. The microdermabrasion machine shoots micronized aluminum oxide crystals at the skin with vacuum removal. This "lunch time peel" is advertised as involving "no pain, no anesthesia, no recuperation, no acids, no side effects." The machine is capable of wounding from superficial to light-medium depths. Nonphysicians use this machine. They do not wound the skin deep enough to produce significant results.

DERMABRASION. Dermabrasion produced with high-speed abraders can produce gratifying results. After treatment, the epidermal thickness returns to normal, and there are increased collagen and elastic fibers. Dermabrasion is especially effective when used with trichloroacetic acid peels. Dermabrasion is a technically difficult procedure that is performed by dermatologic and plastic surgeons.

LASER RESURFACING. Resurfacing treats photodamaged skin by wounding. The injury removes the photodamaged area of the epidermis and stimulates collagen production in the dermis. There are many different lasers that produce wounding at all levels. The Ultrapulsed CO_2 laser can achieve varying depths of destruction by changing the power setting and number of passes. Persistent improvement similar to that seen with dermabrasion occurs. The ablation of other lasers such as Er:YAG is less aggressive than CO_2 laser ablation.

Table 19-1 Skin Types		
Skin type*	Sensitivity to UV light†	Sunburn and tanning history
I	Very sensitive	Always burns easily; never tans
II	Very sensitive	Always burns easily; tans minimally
III	Sensitive	Burns moderately; tans gradually and uniformly (light brown)
IV	Moderately sensitive	Burns minimally; always tans well (moderate brown)
V	Minimally sensitive	Rarely burns; tans profusely (dark brown)
VI	Insensitive	Never burns; deeply pigmented (black)

Adapted from Pathak MA: J Dermatol Surg Oncol 1987; 13:739.

*Constitutive color of unexposed buttock skin of individuals of skin types I to III is white and of skin type IV, white or faintly brown.

Individuals with skin type V have brown buttock skin, and those with skin type VI have dark brown or black buttock skin.

†Based on first 30 to 45 minutes of sun exposure after winter season or no sun exposure.

Suntan and Sunburn

Light-induced skin changes depend on the intensity and duration of exposure and genetic factors.

SUNTAN. A tan protects the body from photoinjury, but UV-induced injury must occur to produce a tan. Therefore intentional suntanning is unwise. Repeated brief exposures sufficient to induce tanning add to long-term damage. In general for a given individual, the deeper the tan, the more skin damage is sustained in achieving the tan.

Tanning follows moderate and intense sun exposure and occurs in two stages. The first stage, immediate pigment darkening (IPD), is caused primarily by UVA. The skin becomes brown while exposed but fades rapidly after exposure. IPD is caused by a photochemical change in existing melanin, not by an increase in melanin. A lasting tan requires the synthesis of new melanin; a more lasting tan becomes visible within 72 hours.

TANNING PARLORS. Evidence shows that tans of comparable degrees acquired from different UV sources are similar in the amount of photodamage and skin cancer risk that accompany a tan. Large amounts of radiation are delivered in a short time in commercial tanning parlors. This accelerates photoaging and increases the risk of skin cancer.

SUNBURN. Forty-three percent of white US children experienced one or more sunburns during the year.[10] The sunburn reaction occurs in stages. With sufficient exposure, erythema appears within minutes (immediate erythema), fades, and then reappears and persists for days (delayed erythema). Vascular permeability of varying degrees results in edema and blisters. Desquamation occurs within a week. Systemic and topical corticosteroids have little or no clinically important effect on the sunburn reaction. Systemic and topical nonsteroidal antiinflammatory drugs, when used at dosages to achieve optimal serum levels for anti-inflammatory effect, only result in an early and mild reduction of UVB-induced erythema.[11] Sunburn is best treated with cool, wet compresses. Topical anesthetic preparations that contain lidocaine provide some relief. Benzocaine, incorporated into some sunburn preparations, is a sensitizer and should be avoided. Protection with sunscreens can, if used properly, prevent burning in even fair-skinned individuals.

Sun Protection

UV-induced damage to collagen and elastic fibers and a number of skin cancers[12] can be greatly reduced by high *sun protection factor* (SPF; see later) sunscreens and other methods to reduce sun exposure (Box 19-5). Sun protection may allow for repair of damaged skin. New collagen and elastin may form, and precancerous changes may regress. Substantial lifetime sun exposure occurs with brief incidental exposures such as working outdoors, participating in recreational activities, and walking outside for lunch; therefore, many people need daily protection.

METHODS OF SUN PROTECTION. Natural protection is provided by the stratum corneum and the skin pigment, melanin. People vary widely in their natural ability to tan or burn. A sun-reactive skin typing system has been devised to classify individuals as to their ability to tan or burn. These categories (see Table 19-1) are useful guides for devising programs for sun protection.

Recommendations for minimizing sun exposure are listed (see Box 19-5). Sunburns are particularly harmful, and great emphasis should be placed on preventing burns. Patients frequently relate that permanent freckling occurred on the upper back after one severe burn. People who take short winter vacations in the south are particularly apt to burn. Total sun exposure during a lifetime is greatest on the face, back of the neck, bald head, upper chest, forearms, backs of the hands, and exposed lower legs. The effects of sunlight can readily be appreciated by comparing the lateral (sun-exposed) surfaces with the medial (sun-protected) surfaces of the forearms of older individuals.

CLOTHING. Clothing is the best protection. Weave tightness and fabric type determine the potential for photoprotection. Stretched or wet fabric is less effective. Darker colors provide greater protection than lighter colors. Some manufacturers market special clothing with SPF ratings, including Solumbra (Sun Precautions, Everett, WA, 1-800-882-7860, 1-888-Solumbra, www.solumbra.com). See the formulary for a complete list of clothing manufacturers.

Box 19-5 Protection Against UV Damage
Use a sunscreen SPF of at least 12 to 30 daily.
Apply sunscreen 15 to 30 minutes before going outdoors.
Reapply sunscreen every 2 hours or after exposure to water.
Avoid peak sunlight hours (10 AM and 3 PM).
Wear dark, loose, dry clothing with a tight weave, wide-brim hat, long-sleeved shirt, pants.
Consider taking oral antioxidant supplements daily:
1 to 2 gm/d of L-ascorbic acid (vitamin C)
500 to 1000 IU of alpha-tocopherol (vitamin E)
25,000 IU of vitamin A

PROTECTING THE YOUNG. Significant sun exposure occurs during the early years of life when children spend hours playing outside. A study showed that regular use of a sunscreen with an SPF of 15 during the first 18 years of life reduces the lifetime incidence of basal and squamous cell carcinoma by 78%.[13] All children should be protected with high-number SPF sunscreens. One-piece bathing suits that cover the trunk, upper arms, and legs are ideal for children.

SUNSCREENS. Sunscreens are topical agents that protect the skin from UV light. Guidelines for their application are listed in Box 19-5. Sunscreens should not be used as a means of allowing more time in the sun; this negates their beneficial effects.

Sunscreens are topical agents that absorb, scatter, or reflect ultraviolet radiation (UVR) and visible light.[14] UVA agents absorb radiation in the spectral range of 320 to 400 nm. UVB agents absorb radiation in the range of 290 to 320 nm.

The Food and Drug Administration (FDA) has issued the final monograph for sunscreen drug products for over-the-counter human use. This establishes conditions for safety, efficacy, and labeling. The regulations reduce the number of allowable sunscreen ingredients (Box 19-6). The monograph specifies an upper limit of SPF 30; any product with an SPF greater than 30 can be labeled only as SPF 30 plus or SPF 30+.

The absorption spectra of some of these sunscreens are shown in Figure 19-10.

PHYSICAL SUNSCREENS. Physical sunscreens (referred to as *inorganic* or *nonchemical sunscreens*) are composed of particles that scatter and reflect light. They contain titanium dioxide or zinc oxide and block a wide spectrum of light. Titanium dioxide protects against UVB and UVA II. Zinc oxide protects against UVB, UVA II, and UVA I. No irritant or sensitization reactions have been reported with either ingredient. These opaque formulations block UVA and therefore are effective for photosensitizing diseases such as polymorphous light eruption, the porphyrias, and lupus erythematosus. Physical sunscreens can be especially useful in areas that burn easily, such as the nose and lips.

CHEMICAL SUNSCREENS. Chemical sunscreens absorb radiation. Newer broad-spectrum chemical sunscreens include a combination of chemicals that absorb both UVB and UVA radiation. Para-aminobenzoic acid (PABA) was the first chemical sunscreen agent, but its potential to cause allergic reactions has limited its use. Chemical sunscreens include PABA esters, salicylates, cinnamates, and benzophenones.

WATER-RESISTANT SUNSCREENS. Many new preparations resist removal by bathing. The vehicle is the most important factor in determining water resistance. A water-resistant product maintains the SPF level after 40 minutes of water immersion. A waterproof product is tested after 80 minutes of water immersion.

Box 19-6 Food and Drug Administration Sunscreen Final Monograph Ingredients

Drug name	Concentration (%)	Absorbance
Aminobenzoic acid	15	UVB
Avobenzone	2-3	UVA I
Cinoxate	3	UVB
Dioxybenzone	3	UVB, UVA II
Homosalate	15	UVB
Meradimate	5	UVA II
Octocrylene	10	UVB
Octinoxate	7.5	UVB
Octisalate	5	UVB
Oxybenzone	6	UVB, UVA II
Padimate-O	8	UVB
Ensilozole	4	UVB
Sulisobenzone	10	UVB, UVA II
Titanium dioxide	2-25	Physical
Trolamine salicylate	12	UVB
Zinc oxide	2-20	Physical

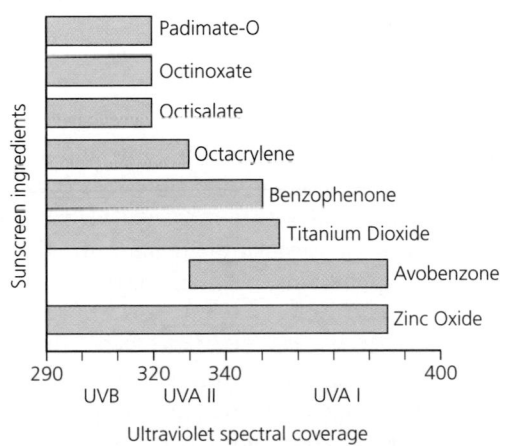

Figure 19-10 Absorption spectra of sunscreen components

SUN PROTECTION FACTOR. The effectiveness of sunscreens is expressed as the SPF. The SPF is defined as the ratio of the least amount of UVB energy (minimum erythema dose) required to produce a minimum erythema reaction through a sunscreen product film to the amount of energy required to produce the same erythema without any sunscreen application. For an individual who wears a sunscreen with an SPF of 8, 8 times longer than usual is required to develop erythema. The SPF for commercially available products is derived from tests with application of a uniform amount of sunscreen that is thicker than most individuals routinely use. A substantial amount of sunscreen must be applied to obtain a full SPF rating.

CHOICE OF SUNSCREEN STRENGTH. A sunscreen with an SPF of 15 or greater is recommended under most conditions. Sun protection does not increase proportionally with the designated SPF. In the higher range of SPFs, the differences become less meaningful. An SPF of 15 indicates 93% protection; an SPF of 34 indicates 97% protection.

FREQUENCY OF USE. The majority of lifetime sun exposure occurs during multiple brief exposures that are not intended to produce tanning; therefore daily sun protection should be encouraged. People who sunburn easily or those who have light complexions or sun-sensitivity disorders should use a high SPF sunscreen every day, all year round, particularly if they live in more equatorial latitudes. Sunscreens should be applied once in the morning and reapplied every two hours or after swimming and heavy exercise. Encourage people to have sunscreens available in the bathroom and to make morning application part of their daily ritual. Sunscreen may fail to prevent sunburn if it is washed off during swimming or if it is not applied to all exposed skin.[15] The protection against sunburn afforded by a reapplication of sunscreen relative to a single application is significant. Compared with the first application, the second sunscreen application affords 3.1 times more protection against minimal UVR-induced erythema. The combined effect of two sunscreen applications gives 2.5 times better protection from UVR than does a single sunscreen application.[16]

GLASS FILTERS. Glass filters out UVB but transmits UVA. Protective coatings applied to glass can block UVA radiation. Llumar window film (1-800-2-llumar, www.llumar.com) is a microthin film that is installed onto home and automobile glass surfaces to provide solar protection. It screens out 99% of the UV rays. Glass filters are indicated for patients with multiple skin cancers, transplant patients with skin cancers, and patients with photosensitive dermatoses.

ADVERSE REACTIONS TO SUNSCREENS. Allergic reactions occur more frequently to preservatives or fragrances than to the active ingredients. Irritation to creams is much more common than allergy to a component. Burning or stinging may be experienced in the eye area. Sunscreen active ingredients may cause photocontact allergic reactions. Most patients who develop photocontact dermatitis to sunscreens are patients with photodermatides.

VITAMINS C AND E AND CAROTENOIDS. The daily use of 2 gm of ascorbic acid (vitamin C) combined with 1000 IU of D-alphatocopherol (vitamin E) reduces the sunburn reaction, which might indicate a consequent reduced risk for later sequelae of UV-induced skin damage.[17] Another study showed that a combination of carotenoids (25 mg total carotenoids/d) and vitamin E (500 IU) provided protection against erythema.[18]

VITAMIN D LEVELS. Regular use of sunscreens does not result in vitamin D levels outside the normal range.[19]

SUNLESS OR SELF-TANNING LOTIONS. Sunless or self-tanning lotions contain dihydroxyacetone (DHA), which darkens the skin by staining. The preparations are nontoxic. The site of action of DHA is the stratum corneum. Staining of skin occurs when DHA combines with free amino groups in skin proteins (keratin) in the stratum corneum to form brown products called *melanoidins*. Little to no sunscreen protection is provided by their use. Some products are formulated with standard sunscreens.

The newer preparations are cosmetically acceptable, as opposed to the orange color that was produced by older formulations.

APPLICATION TECHNIQUE OF SELF-TANNING LOTIONS. Care, skill, and experience are necessary with using these products. The most even color is obtained when the skin is lightly buffed or abraded before application to enhance its smoothness.[20] Tinted products may assist the inexperienced user in uniformly applying the product.

The depth of color directly correlates with thickness and compactness of the stratum corneum. Rougher, hyperkeratotic skin takes up the color more unevenly, as does older skin or mottled or freckled skin. Scars color poorly. Even application is required, with lighter application around elbows, knees, and ankles to avoid excessive darkening in these areas. Care also needs to be taken around the hairline, where lighter hair may darken. Hands need to be washed immediately after use to avoid darkening of the palms, fingers, and nails. A color change may be observed within 1 hour after application. Maximal darkening may take 8 to 24 hours to develop. Individuals can make several successive applications every few hours to achieve their desired color. Color may last 5 to 7 days with a single application. Depending on anatomic application, the same color can be maintained with repeat applications every 1 to 4 days.[21] The face requires fewer applications to maintain the color than the extremities.

INDICATIONS. The color achieved is dependent on skin type. People with skin type II or III (medium complexion) obtain the best results. Results are not as good in older individuals with roughened, hyperkeratotic skin or those with mottled pigmentation with freckling. These products camouflage leg spider veins and vitiligo.

Polymorphous Light Eruption

Polymorphous light (PML) eruption is the most common light-induced skin disease seen by the practitioner. It is a long-standing, slowly ameliorating disease; the risk for lupus erythematosus is not increased.[22] Not only does the clinical picture vary, but symptoms may vary over the years. There are several morphologic subtypes,[23] but individual patients tend to develop the same type each year. Lesions usually heal without scarring. The eruption appears first on limited areas but becomes more extensive during subsequent summers. Most people with PML eruption have exacerbations each summer for many years; a few have temporary remissions. The disease may begin at any age. The amount of light exposure needed to elicit an eruption varies greatly from one patient to another. Patients can tolerate a certain minimum exposure time, such as 30 minutes, after which the eruption appears. Light sensitivity decreases with repeated sun exposure; this phenomenon is referred to as *hardening*. The eruption may cease to appear after days or weeks of repeated sun exposure. Those exposed to sunlight year round rarely acquire PML eruption. Most patients have symptoms 2 hours after exposure. In a 7-year follow-up study, 57% of patients reported a decreased sun sensitivity, including 11% in whom the PML eruption totally cleared; none of the patients developed systemic lupus erythematosus.[24]

HEREDITARY PML ERUPTION (ACTINIC PRURIGO). Hereditary PML eruption occurs in the Inuit of North America and in native Americans of North, Central, and South America. Its transmission appears to be autosomal dominant with incomplete penetrance and variable expressivity. In northern latitudes, the eruption appears on sun-exposed areas of the body as early as March and persists through October.[25] The face is the most commonly involved area. The majority of patients are sensitive to UVA light. The younger ages of onset (up to 20 years of age) are associated with cheilitis and more acute eruptions and are more likely to improve over 5 years. Those who develop actinic prurigo as adults (21 years of age and older) tend to have a milder and more persistent dermatosis.[26]

CLINICAL PRESENTATION. Women are affected more often than are men. The mean age at onset is 34 years (5 to 82 years). For men the mean age is 46 years and for women, 28 years. The most common initial symptoms are burning, itching, and erythema.[27] The eruption usually lasts for 2 or 3 days, but in some cases it does not clear until the end of summer.

Many patients experience malaise, chills, headache, and nausea starting approximately 4 hours after exposure but lasting only 1 or 2 hours. The most commonly involved areas are the V of the chest (the area exposed by open-necked shirts), the backs of the hands, extensor aspects of the forearms, and the lower legs of women. Reports vary as to the wavelength of light responsible for inducing lesions. The wavelength of light necessary to elicit the eruption varies with each patient. Many react to UVB, others to UVA,[28] or some to both.[29]

CLINICAL SUBTYPES. There are a number of clinical types of PML eruption.[23]

Papular type. The papular type is the most common form (Figure 19-11). Small papules are disseminated or densely aggregated on a patchy erythema.

Plaque type. The plaque type is the second most common pattern. Plaques may be superficial or urticarial. They may coalesce to form larger plaques and at times are eczematous (Figures 19-12 and 19-13).

Papulovesicular type. The papulovesicular type is less common. It occurs primarily on the arms, lower limbs, and V area of the chest and usually begins with urticarial plaques from which groups of vesicles arise (Figure 19-14). Itching is common and is usually moderate or marked.[30] This form occurs almost exclusively in women.

Eczematous type. Erythema, papules, scale, and sometimes vesicles occur. Eczematous lesions occur almost exclusively in men.

Erythema multiforme type. Erythema multiforme–type lesions and distribution are similar to those of classic erythema multiforme, with lesions most frequent on the backs of the hands and extensor forearms.

Hemorrhagic type. The hemorrhagic type may first appear as hemorrhagic papules or purpura. This form is rare.

Differential diagnosis. The papular form resembles atopic dermatitis. PML eruption is less pruritic and occurs in a sun-exposed distribution, not in crease areas, as does atopic dermatitis.

Systemic and discoid lupus erythematosus plaque–like lesions and histology may be identical to PML eruptions. The characteristic direct and indirect immunofluorescence patterns of lupus erythematosus clarify the diagnosis.

DIAGNOSIS. The histologic features are not diagnostic. Immunofluorescence is negative. Phototesting is not essential but, when performed, must include both UVB and UVA testing.

POLYMORPHOUS LIGHT ERUPTION

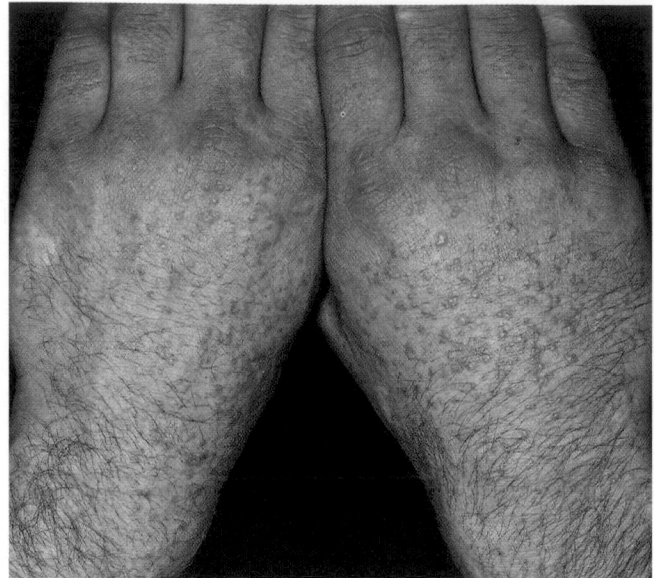

Figure 19-11 Papular type.

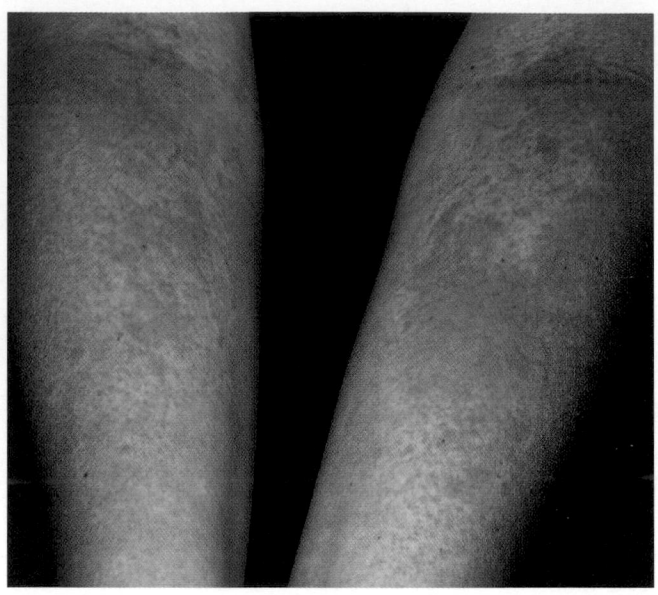

Figure 19-12 Plaque type.

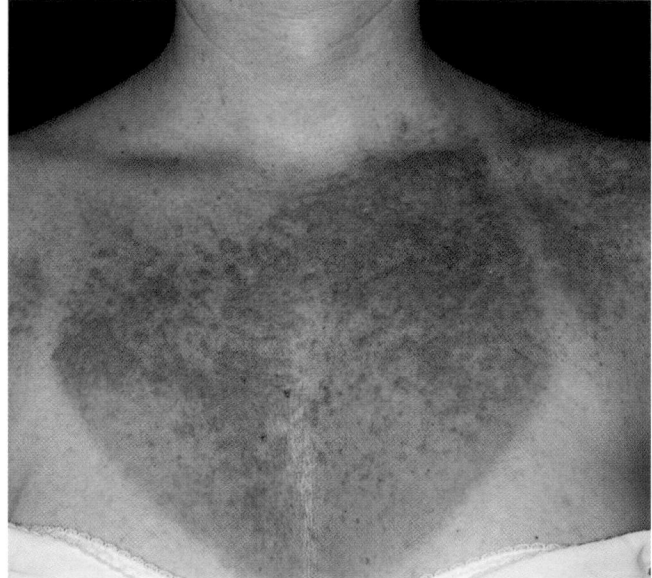

Figure 19-13 Plaque type.

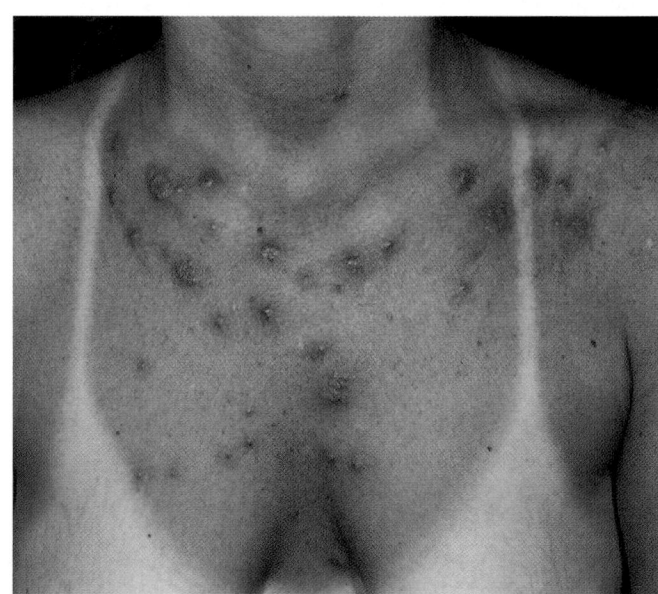

Figure 19-14 Papulovesicular type.

Treatment

Topical steroids, antimalarial agents, and beta-carotene are often disappointing. Prophylactic therapy with sunscreens is partially effective. In the case of minor complaints, patients can become disease free by using sunscreens and gradually increasing sun exposure in the spring. Phototherapy and photochemotherapy are most effective.

TOPICAL AND ORAL STEROIDS. Short, intermittent 3- to 14-day courses of groups I to V topical steroids are effective.[31] Groups II through V topical steroids reduce pruritus and hasten resolution. Short courses of oral steroids are useful for very itchy, widespread eruptions or for patients who flare during a course of phototherapy or photochemotherapy.

PROTECTION. Sun exposure during times of maximum intensity (between 11 AM and 3 PM) should be avoided. Sunscreens with maximum sun-protecting factors should be used. Those containing parsol 1789 (avobenzone), zinc oxide, and titanium dioxide are the most effective[32,33] (total block SPF 60, 1-800-332-5536, www.totalblock.com). Protective clothing should be worn over involved areas. The most sensitive patients are advised about filters for car windows (llumar UV shield, 1-888-2-Uvshield, www.llumar.com) and fluorescent lighting at home.

DESENSITIZATION WITH PHOTOTHERAPY. The sensitivity of human skin to UV radiation decreases after exposure to UV radiation. Adaptation occurs by exposing patients to small and controlled doses of light. Doses small enough not to cause any abnormal reaction but large enough to increase the tolerance of the skin to light are used. A regular series of such exposures, with small increments in exposure time, can result in an appreciable tolerance. Increments of 10% per exposure are given as long as there are no adverse reactions.[27] This is the so-called *phenomenon of hardening*. This practice is safe; therefore controlled exposure to sunlight or artificial UV light sources should be the first type of treatment. Patients treated with UVB in the dermatologist's office receive five exposures per week for 3 weeks in the spring, with gradually increasing exposure doses.[34,35,36] Hardening may also be accomplished with either UVA (340 to 400 nm)[37] or UVA and UVB (300 to 400 nm) (10 exposures to UV light).[38]

PSORALEN UVA (PUVA). Trioxsalen and natural sunlight[38] treatment is simple and effective for patients who do not improve with the above routine measures and for those who have significant eruptions each summer. A 5-mg dose of trioxsalen should be given for every 20 to 25 pounds of body weight (average dose, 5 to 6 tablets), followed by sunlight in 2 hours or more. In the early spring the patient should be exposed to 15 minutes of sunlight the first day, and the exposure should be increased by several minutes each day. Topical steroids should be applied if the disease is activated by treatment. Maximum protection is reached 3 weeks after a 1-week course of treatment, and a single course offers a minimum of 6 weeks of protection. The course is repeated each month during the spring and summer months. Protective glasses such as NoIR should be worn for the remainder of the day after taking psoralens.

The same treatment can be acquired in the dermatologist's office using artificial UVA light and 8-methoxypsoralen. A remission can be obtained for most patients by treatment two or three times each week for 4 to 12 weeks in the early spring.[29,35,36,39] (See the section on treatment of psoriasis for details.)

ANTIMALARIAL DRUGS. Antimalarial drugs may be effective and should be considered for patients who are not protected by sunscreens and do not respond to UVB or PUVA phototherapy.[40] Antimalarials need to be used only during the summer months; therefore the total necessary dose is small. A 3-month trial (hydroxychloroquine 400 mg/day for the first month and 200 mg/day thereafter) has been effective in reducing rash and irritation.[41] Although the risk of eye damage is slight, ophthalmologic examinations should be obtained periodically to monitor for antimalarial toxicity.

Beta-carotene is somewhat effective for prophylactic treatment of PML eruption, but the skin turns yellow-orange. In one study, only 30% of patients responded satisfactorily to a dosage of 3 mg/kg body weight continued throughout the summer.[39]

Hydroa Aestivale and Hydroa Vacciniforme

Hydroa aestivale (summer prurigo of Hutchinson) and hydroa vacciniforme are rare but very distinctive light-induced eruptions. They may represent a type of PML eruption that is peculiar to children. The onset is before puberty (average age at onset is about 6 years), and males are affected more frequently than females. It begins with moderate erythema and itching within 1 to 2 hours of sun exposure. The lesions of hydroa aestivale consist of papules with weeping and crusting. The symmetric photodistributed eruption is most prominent on the face, ears, and backs of the hands (Figure 19-15). Involvement of non–sun-exposed areas, especially the buttocks, is not uncommon. The rash fades but may persist through the winter months. There is evidence of genetic transmission. In many cases, UVB light reproduces the lesions.

Hydroa vacciniforme (Figure 19-16) is similar to hydroa aestivale, except that tense, umbilicated vesicles resembling smallpox appear on the face, ears, chest, and backs of the hands; after they break and form a crust, they may heal with scarring.

Broad-band UVB therapy may be effective for hydroa vacciniforme. UVA light reproduced the eruption in one case.[42] Both diseases usually clear after puberty. Avoidance of the sun and use of sunscreens, group V topical steroids, and wet compresses and antimalarials can control these diseases.

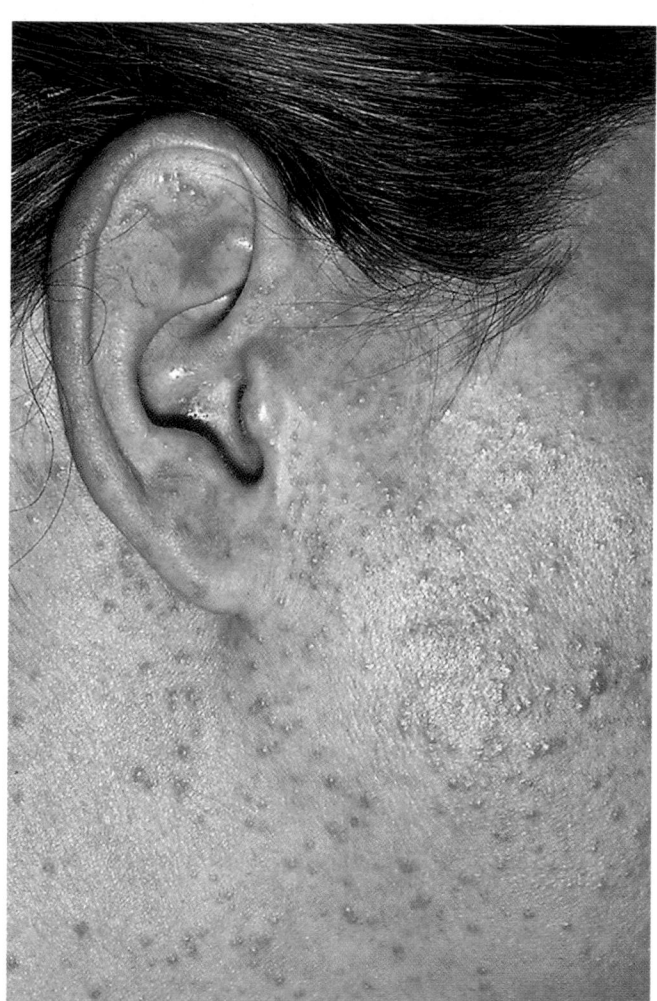

Figure 19-15 Hydroa aestivale. Papules appear on sun-exposed skin and may progress to weeping and crusting.

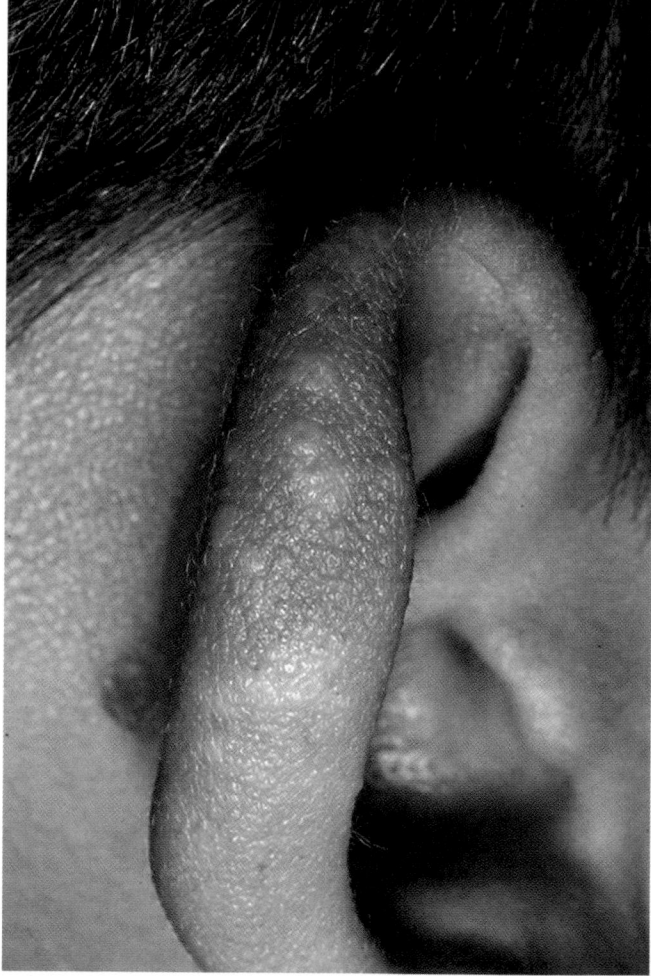

Figure 19-16 Hydroa vacciniforme. Papules and pustules appear on exposed areas of the face and ears. Lesions become umbilicated and sometimes necrotic. They may heal with hypopigmented depressed scars.

Porphyrias

The porphyrias are a group of diseases caused by inborn enzymatic defects in the heme biosynthetic pathway (Table 19-2). Each type of porphyria is associated with a specific enzymatic defect that results in an excess of a specific porphyrin (Table 19-3). The porphyrias are classified into two groups, erythropoietic and hepatic, on the basis of the principal site of the specific enzymatic defect. They are differentiated by measuring heme precursors in urine, feces, erythrocytes, and plasma. Most forms are inherited as Mendelian autosomal dominants.

Two main types of clinical manifestation occur: life-threatening attacks of acute porphyria and skin photosensitization. Attacks of the acute porphyrias (acute intermittent porphyria, variegate porphyria, and hereditary coproporphyria) are important because they may be life threatening. The nonacute porphyrias (porphyria cutanea tarda and erythropoietic porphyria) present as skin photosensitization.

The skin lesions in porphyria cutanea tarda (the most common cutaneous porphyria), variegate porphyria, hereditary coproporphyria, and congenital erythropoietic porphyria are similar: mechanical fragility, subepidermal bullae, hypertrichosis, and pigmentation. Erythropoietic protoporphyria (EPP) is characterized by acute photosensitivity without these lesions.

All types show excess porphyrin metabolites in blood, urine, or feces and in various tissues such as skin and liver. Porphyrins are red-brown pigments. Certain porphyrin metabolites (porphyrinogens) accumulate in the skin and are auto-oxidized to become porphyrins. Porphyrins absorb UVA light in the 400- to 410-nm range (Soret band). These excited porphyrins generate peroxides that cause the blisters seen in porphyria cutanea tarda and variegate porphyria.

Porphyria cutanea tarda

Porphyria cutanea tarda (PCT) is the most common type of porphyria. PCT results from a deficiency of hepatic uroporphyrinogen decarboxylase activity. Both acquired and familial forms exist and are commonly associated in adults with liver disease and hepatic iron overload. The acquired ("sporadic") form is most often precipitated by alcohol.[43] Estrogens, oral contraceptives, certain environmental pollutants, and iron overloading may precipitate PCT. There is also a dominantly inherited form. Most people who consume alcohol or take estrogens do not develop porphyria; therefore it is likely that genetic factors are important in the pathogenesis of nonfamilial cases. This genetic predisposition may explain why some patients on chronic hemodialysis develop PCT.[44] Some of these patients with chronic renal failure have highly increased uroporphyrin concentrations.

HEPATITIS C AND PCT. There is a strong association between hepatitis C virus (HCV) infection and PCT. PCT has also been associated with mutations in the hemochromatosis gene (*HFE*) that are associated with HLA-linked hereditary hemochromatosis. The prevalence of HCV infection (56%) and mutations in *HFE* (73%) are high among North American patients with PCT. Thirty-two of 39 PCT patients with HCV were men, all of whom used alcohol. In contrast, 22 of 31 PCT patients without HCV infection were women, 12 of whom had taken estrogens. The HCV-positive group was more likely to have used illicit intravenous drugs and to have had several (more than four) sex partners.[45] All PCT patients should be tested for HCV infection and for *HFE* mutations. Although HCV infection is a trigger for PCT, preclinical PCT is rare in chronic HCV infection in the United States.

CLINICAL MANIFESTATIONS. The clinical features in order of frequency are blistering in sun-exposed areas (Figures 19-17 and 19-18), increased skin fragility, facial hypertrichosis, hyperpigmentation, sclerodermoid changes, and dystrophic calcification with ulceration.[46] The milia occur in previously blistered sites on the hand (Figure 19-19). The classic form of epidermolysis bullosa acquisita has similar features (see Chapter 16).

DIAGNOSIS. The patient's urine may have a red-brown discoloration ("port-wine urine") from high levels of porphyrin pigments, and it may show a bright pink fluorescence under a Wood's light (Wood's light is a blue light with an emission peak of 360 nm). PCT may be confused with other forms of porphyria and other bullous diseases. Assays of fecal, plasma, urinary, and red blood cell porphyrins should be ordered, especially if other forms of porphyria are in the differential diagnosis. The diagnosis is confirmed by demonstrating an elevated urine uroporphyrin level. A 24-hour collection of urine contains different amounts of the various porphyrins in ratios that can be diagnostic. The proportion reported as uroporphyrin dominates the urinary assay in PCT, usually being present in a ratio of 4:1 or more to the coproporphyrin proportion. Quantitative assays of the various porphyrins must be performed to obtain a reliable diagnosis. Biopsy specimens for direct immunofluorescence are taken from the edge of lesions.

Treatment

PHLEBOTOMY. Iron overload is one of the factors that trigger the disease; iron removal by phlebotomy is the treatment of choice.[47] It reduces hepatic iron stores and produces remissions of several years' duration. One unit of blood should be removed every 2 to 4 weeks until the hemoglobin drops to 10 gm/dl or until the serum iron drops to 50 mg/dl. The average number of units required for remission varies between 8 and 14.[48] Measurement of plasma uroporphyrin is an effective way to monitor the progress of patients with PCT. Treatment should continue until plasma uroporphyrin levels drop under 10 mmol/L.[49] Plasma ferritin levels can also be used as a guide to treatment by venisection. Phlebotomy can be terminated when iron stores, as reflected by plasma ferritin concentration, have fallen to low normal limits.[50]

Table 19-2 Clinical Features of the Porphyrias

Type of porphyria	Heredity	Age of onset	Cutaneous manifestations	Extra-cutaneous manifestations	Laboratory findings			
					Urine	Feces	Erythrocytes	Plasma fluorescence emission peak (nm)
Erythropoietic								
Erythropoietic porphyria	AR*	Infancy	Blisters Severe scarring	Red teeth Hemolytic anemia	Uro I Copro I	Copro I	Uro I Stable fluorescence	615
Erythropoietic proto-porphyria	AD	Childhood	Burning Edema Thickening Rarely blisters	Rarely occurs Fatal liver disease Gallstones	Negative	Protopor-phyrin contin-uously	Protopor-phyrin Transient fluorescence	632
Hepatic, Erythropoietic								
Hepatoerythro-poietic porphyria	AR	Infancy	Blisters Severe scarring Thickening	Decreased liver function	Uro I Uro III	Copro I Copro III Isocoproporphyrin	Protopor-phyrin	
Hepatic								
Acute inter-mittent porphyria	AD	Adolescence	Negative	Abdominal pain Neuropathy Psychosis	ALA and PBG contin-uously	Negative	Negative	615
Variegate porphyria	AD	Young adult-hood	Same as porphyria cutanea tarda	Same as acute inter-mittent porphyria	ALA and PBG during attacks Copro > Uro	Protopor-phyrin contin-uously Some Copro X-por-phyrin	Negative	624–626
Porphyria cutanea tarda	AD	Middle age	Blisters Scarring Thickening Scleroderma-like features	Decreased liver function Siderosis	Uro I > Uro III contin-uously Continuous fluores-cence	Isocoproporphyrin > Copro	Negative	615
Hereditary copropor-phyria	AD	Young adult-hood	Same as porphyria cutanea tarda	Same as acute inter-mittent porphyria	Copro, ALA, and PBG during attacks	Copro III contin-uously	Negative	615

Modified from Sekula SA, Tschen JA, Rosen T: Am Fam Physician 1986; 33:219.

Uro, Uroporphyrin; *Copro*, coproporphyrin; *ALA*, aminolevulinic acid; *PBG*, porphobilinogen; *AR*, autosomal recessive; *AD*, autosomal dominant.

Table 19-3 Classification of the Porphyrias

Type of porphyria	Enzyme defect	Recommended tests
Erythropoietic		
Erythropoietic porphyria	Uroporphyrinogen III cosynthetase	Urine porphyrins, erythrocyte porphyrins
Erythropoietic protoporphyria	Ferrochelatase (heme synthetase)	Urine, fecal, erythrocyte porphyrins
Hepatic, Erythropoietic		
Hepatoerythropoietic porphyria	Ferrochelatase, uroporphyrinogen decarboxylase	Urine, fecal, erythrocyte porphyrins
Hepatic		
Acute intermittent porphyria	Uroporphyrinogen 1 synthetase	Urine PBG, porphyrins; erythrocyte uroporphyrinogen I synthetase; erythrocyte δ-aminolevulinate dehydratase
Variegate porphyria	Protoporphyrinogen oxidase	Urine PBG, porphyrins; fecal porphyrins (erythrocyte uroporphyrinogen I synthetase and δ-aminolevulinate dehydratase may be necessary)
Porphyria cutanea tarda	Uroporphyrinogen decarboxylase	Urine porphyrins
Hereditary coproporphyria	Coproporphyrinogen oxidase	Urine PBG, porphyrins; fecal porphyrins (erythrocyte uroporphyrinogen I synthase and δ-aminolevulinate dehydratase may be necessary)
Intoxication porphyria (chemicals)		
	Variable	Erythrocyte porphyrins; urine δ-ALA, PBG, porphyrins; fecal porphyrins*

PBG, Porphobilinogen; *ALA*, δ-aminolevulinate.

In some cases the quantitation of erythrocyte zinc protoporphyrin is necessary to distinguish intoxication porphyria from protoporphyrin.

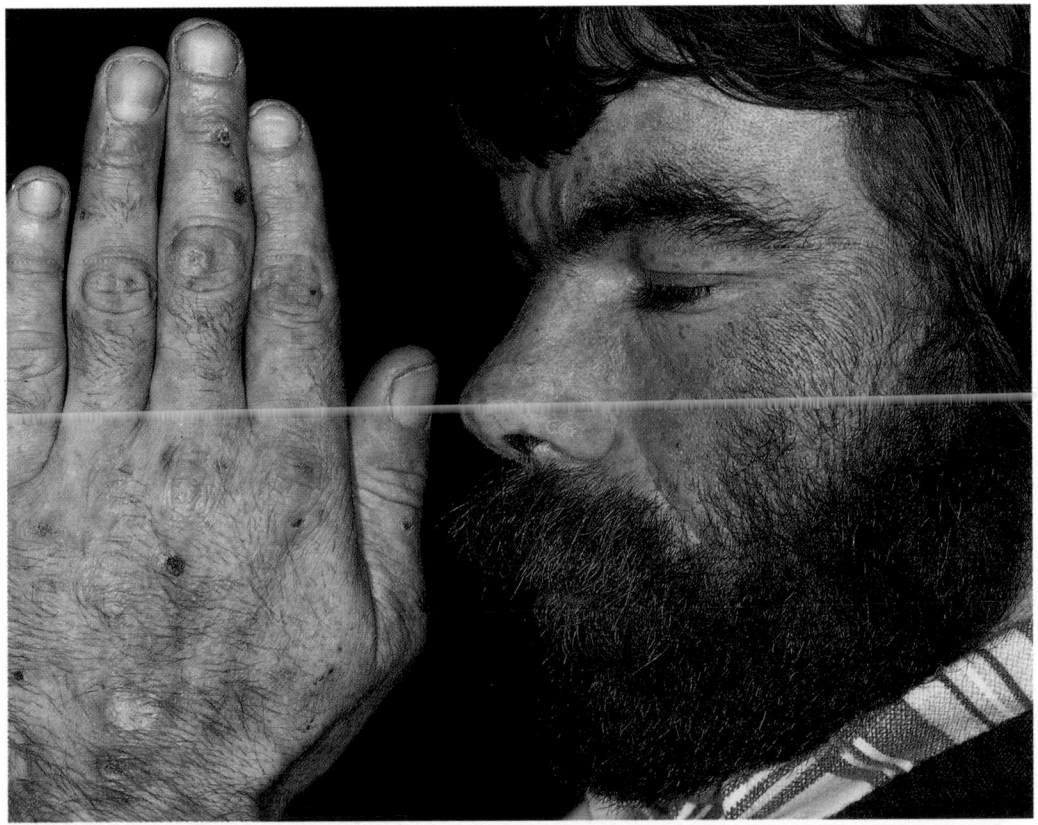

Figure 19-17 Porphyria cutanea tarda. There is increased facial hair around the eyes. Chronic sun exposure has resulted in blistering, erosions, and atrophic scars on the backs of the hands.

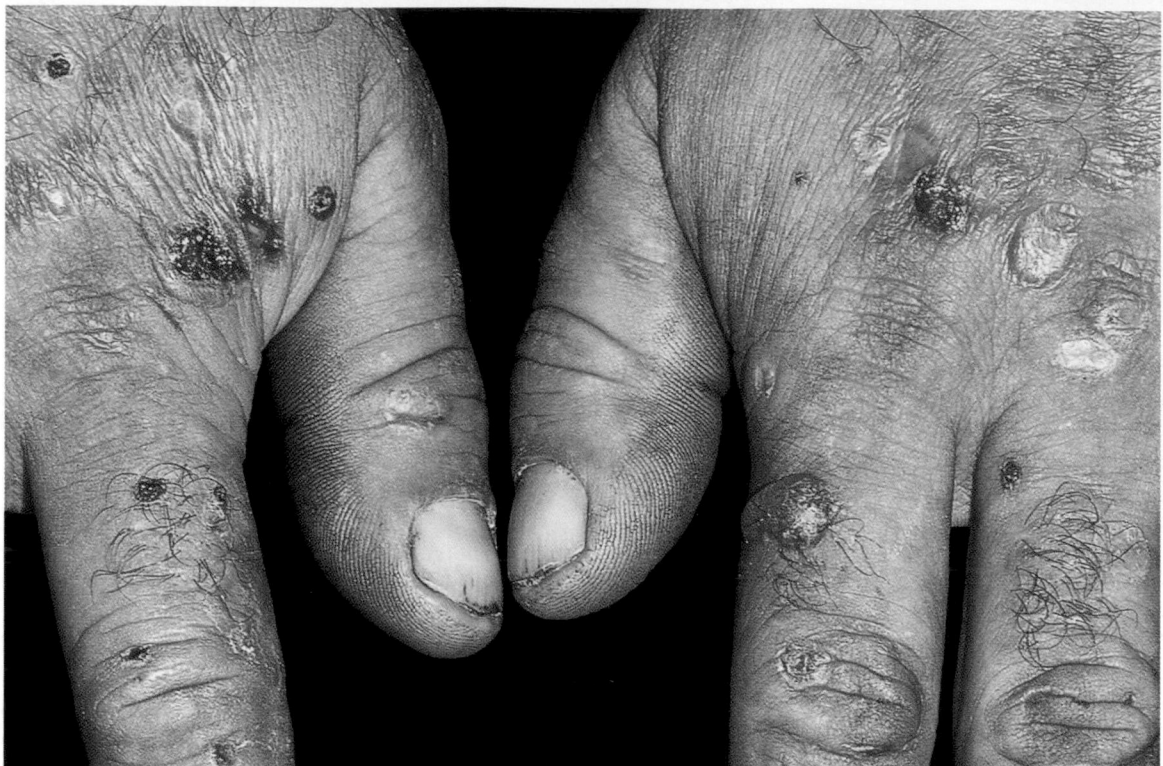

Figure 19-18 Fragile sun-exposed skin develops erosions and bullae after mechanical trauma. This is most commonly seen on the dorsal aspects of the hands and forearms. Healing results in scars, milia, and hyperpigmented and hypopigmented atrophic patches.

CHLOROQUINE. Chloroquine in very low dosages may also be used.[51] Chloroquine causes the release of hepatic tissue-bound uroporphyrin, and subsequently it is rapidly eliminated by the plasma and excreted by the urine. A too-rapid release of porphyrins might severely affect liver function. Complete clinical and biochemical response has occurred with the use of chloroquine 125 to 250 mg twice weekly for 8 to 18 months. Remission in most patients has been for more than 4 years.[52]

Combined treatment with repeated bleeding and chloroquine results in remission in an average of 3.5 months. The time necessary for remission with chloroquine alone is 10.2 months; the time for remission with phlebotomy alone is 12.5 months.[53]

Complete elimination of alcohol and exposure to other hepatotoxins resulted in complete clinical clearing of bullae and skin fragility in 2 months to 2 years in one series of patients.[54]

Sunscreens that block UVA light should be used. Physical sunblockers that contain titanium dioxide are moderately effective.[55]

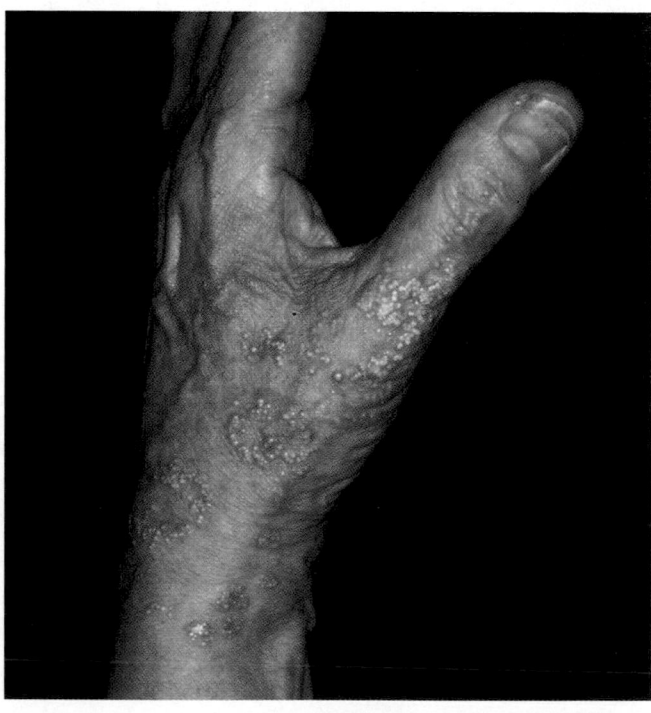

Figure 19-19 Porphyria cutanea tarda. White milia form during the healing process.

Pseudoporphyria

Pseudoporphyria is a therapy-induced bullous photosensitivity disorder. It is a condition that mimics PCT in almost every aspect, except that porphyrin levels in the urine, plasma, and stools are normal. It has been attributed to drugs, UVA irradiation (tanning beds)[56], excessive sun exposure, and chronic renal failure/dialysis.[57]

CLINICAL MANIFESTATIONS. There is increased skin fragility, easy bruising, and light-provoked bullae on the dorsum of the hand followed by healing with scarring and milia (Figure 19-20). The onset of bullae may occur 1 week after the drug has been initiated or may not occur for months. An important clue to the diagnosis is that few patients with pseudoporphyria have hypertrichosis, hyperpigmentation, or the sclerodermoid changes found in PCT.[58]

DRUGS. Naproxen, a propionic acid derivative, is the nonsteroidal anti-inflammatory drug (NSAID) most frequently linked to pseudoporphyria. Most cases of naproxen-induced pseudoporphyria occur in children. Pseudoporphyria was reported in up to 12% of patients with juvenile rheumatoid arthritis[59] who were treated with naproxen. Naproxen-induced pseudoporphyria in adults occurs primarily in women. Patients who require NSAIDs and develop pseudoporphyria should be switched to agents that are less photosensitizing, such as diclofenac, indomethacin, and sulindac. Other drugs, including tetracyclines, furosemide, nalidixic acid, dapsone, oxaprozin, and nabumetone, are implicated.[60]

TANNING BEDS. Most patients are young women with fair skin. Vesicles and bullae occur on the dorsal hands, but other areas may be involved. Skin fragility, scarring, and milia occur. Some patients had been taking medications (NSAIDs, furosemide, tetracycline, oral contraceptives).[57]

CHRONIC RENAL FAILURE/DIALYSIS. Pseudoporphyria has been reported in patients undergoing hemodialysis or peritoneal dialysis and in cases of chronic renal failure without accompanying dialysis.[61]

LABORATORY FINDINGS. The histologic (subepidermal bullae with no inflammation, thickened dermal capillary walls with deposition of periodic acid/Schiff—positive material) and immunofluorescent (granular deposits of IgG and C3 at the dermoepidermal junction and in the upper dermal vasculature) findings are identical to those found in PCT. Porphyrin levels in the urine, plasma, and stools are normal. Because of difficulties in interpreting urinary testing in the setting of dialysis, plasma porphyrins and fecal porphyrins should also be assayed in the evaluation of patients with chronic renal failure who have bullous dermatoses.

TREATMENT. Stopping the drug is curative in most cases, but remission may not occur for months.

Figure 19-20 Pseudoporphyria. Light-provoked bullae on the back of the hands, followed by healing with scarring, is precipitated by certain drugs such as naproxen.

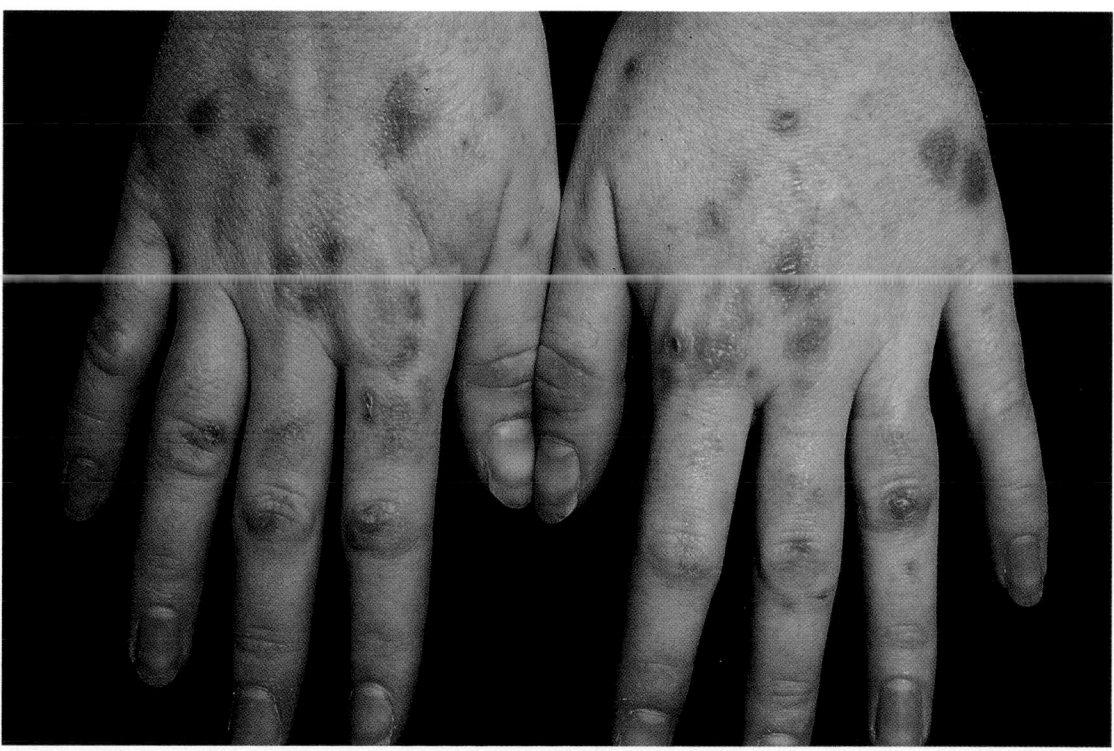

Erythropoietic protoporphyria

EPP differs clinically from PCT.[62] This disease begins in childhood. There are few or no blisters; rather, children complain of burning and redness when exposed to sun or UV light. There are no porphyrins in the urine. EPP is an autosomal dominant hereditary disorder with irregular penetrance. It is characterized by a deficiency of ferrochelatase, the terminal enzyme in the heme biosynthetic pathway that catalyzes the insertion of ferrous iron into protoporphyrin to form heme. The enzyme deficiency causes the accumulation of the photoreactive molecule protoporphyrin in various tissues. Protoporphyrin overproduction occurs mainly in erythroid tissue. Circulating erythrocytes leak protoporphyrin, which accumulates in skin cells. The release of protoporphyrin from erythrocytes is greatly increased if the erythrocytes are exposed to small amounts of light. The cutaneous symptoms are elicited by protoporphyrin-sensitized photodamage of endothelial cells.[63]

CLINICAL MANIFESTATIONS. The disease is often suspected in infancy or childhood when patients cry or complain of burning of the skin on the face and hands within minutes of sun exposure. Exposure through window glass also elicits symptoms. Hours later, diffuse swelling or erythema appears, and burning persists (Figure 19-21). Purpura may occur, but vesiculation is uncommon. Often, acute changes are not seen. The period of sun exposure required to elicit burning varies from day to day. Several hours of exposure may be tolerated. A "priming phenomenon" has been reported.[64] A certain duration of exposure "primes" the skin so that a short period of additional sun exposure in the same area, even the next day, produces symptoms. It may then take several days after symptoms have developed to regain the usual degree of tolerance. Patients may present with a waxy, cobblestone-like induration of the involved skin. When this

change occurs over the knuckles and fingers, the hands look old ("old knuckles"). This is a pathognomonic change in children. Depressed scars form on the nose, cheeks, and dorsum of the hands. Large second-degree phototoxic burns of the abdominal wall have occurred after prolonged exposure to light during surgery.[65]

Most treated patients function well and have a normal life span. Protoporphyrins may accumulate in hepatocytes and cause liver disease.

LIVER DISEASE. Excess protoporphyrin affects hepatobiliary structures, and a spectrum of changes, which range from ultrastructural bile canalicular damage to cirrhosis or acute hepatic failure, may occur. The course is unpredictable. Patients may be stable for several years after evidence of liver function abnormalities. Then, within weeks, hepatic failure may develop, requiring urgent orthotopic liver transplantation.[65,66] Gallstones may occur in young children.

LABORATORY. Erythrocyte and plasma protoporphyrin and fecal protoporphyrin levels are elevated (see Table 19-2). Fluorescence microscopy is a highly reliable screening test for the detection of increased red cell porphyrins.[67] The urine is normal. Red blood cell protoporphyrins are also increased in iron deficiency anemia and lead poisoning, but photosensitivity is absent. Liver biopsy may show periportal fibrosis.

TREATMENT. Oral beta-carotene (Solatene 30 mg) is helpful in treating the skin photosensitivity.[68,69] Improvement occurs within 1 month of initiating treatment. The children's dosage is 30 mg once, twice, or three times a day. The adult dosage is 60 to 180 mg/day. The skin becomes yellow in 4 to 6 weeks; stools are orange. Therapy is used from early spring through the fall. Pyridoxine was associated with a marked reduction in photosensitivity without evidence of adverse effects in two patients who were only moderately responsive to beta-carotene and sunscreens. The reported effective dosage is 25 to 100 mg/hour for 6 to 10 doses during the day; protection was maintained when the dosage was lowered to 100 mg three times a day.[70] Iron therapy may be considered for prophylaxis of hepatic failure.[71,72] Red blood cell exchange transfusions have been reported to be effective. Cholestyramine 4 gm three times a day is reported to decrease photosensitivity and porphyrin levels.[73] Photoprotection against UVA by chemical sunscreens and physical sunscreens that contain microfine titanium dioxide is helpful. Products containing microfine titanium dioxide offer superior photoprotection for patients who are abnormally sensitive to long-wavelength UV radiation.[55]

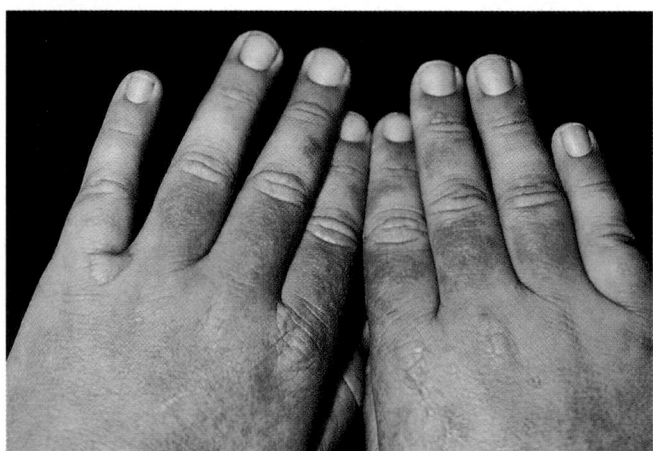

Figure 19-21 Erythropoietic protoporphyria. There are few or no blisters. Burning and redness occur with sun exposure. *(Courtesy Maureen Poh-Fitzpatrick, M.D.)*

Phototoxic Reactions

Phototoxic reactions are nonallergic cutaneous responses induced by a variety of topical and systemic agents. The frequency of these eruptions has decreased as informed physicians, aware of the photosensitive potential of certain drugs, have chosen alternatives. Phototoxicity occurs when a photosensitizer is absorbed into the skin either topically or systemically in appropriate concentrations and is exposed to adequate amounts of specific wavelengths of light, usually UVA. Theoretically, if sufficient quantities of chemical and light are delivered, the reaction should occur in all exposed individuals. In fact, the response varies.

TOPICAL EXPOSURE. Exposure to plants or chemicals that contain light-sensitizing compounds followed by exposure to certain activating wavelengths of UV light produces a highly characteristic eruption. A minimum response consists of an almost imperceptible erythema, followed by prolonged hyperpigmentation. A maximum response consists of tingling of the exposed skin and erythema that occur shortly after exposure, followed within hours by burning edema and vesiculation at the end of 24 hours. This is followed by a bullous reaction that lasts for days (Figure 19-22). Linear streaks (similar to poison ivy) of erythema and vesicles produced by drawing the offending agent across the skin surface are particularly characteristic of topical exposure (Figure 19-23). Desquamation occurs, and residual hyperpigmentation may persist for 1 year or longer.

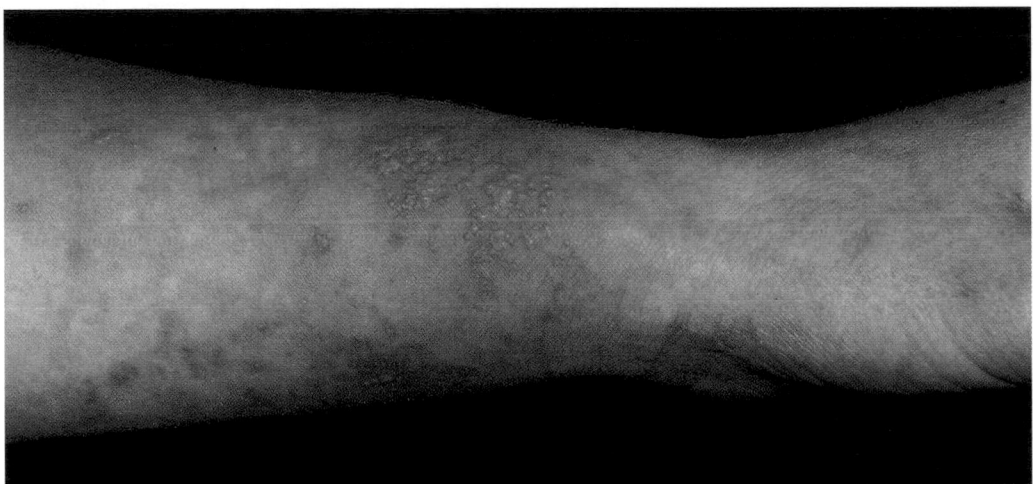

A, Diffuse erythema and vesiculation occurred 24 hours after preparing celery in a commercial processing plant.

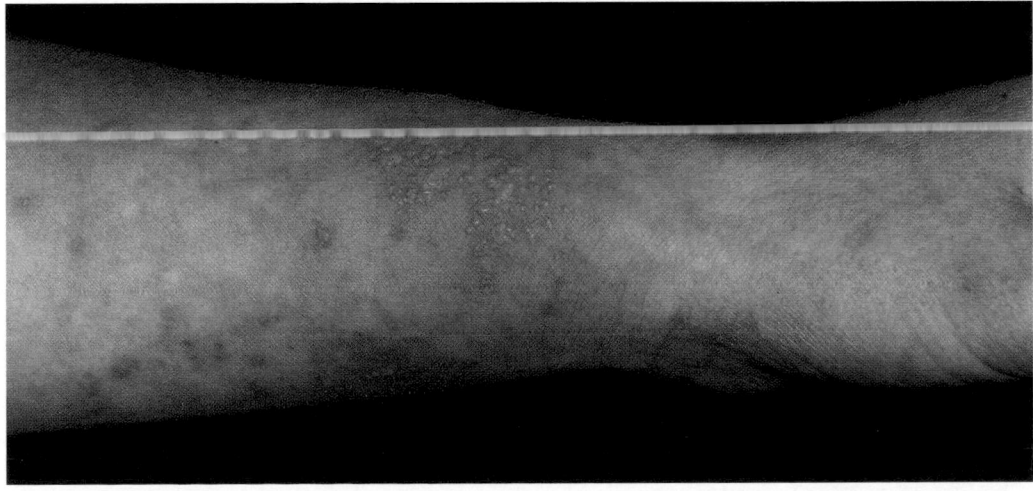

B, The patient pictured in *A* developed diffuse hyperpigmentation in the previously inflamed areas 2 weeks after the acute episode.

Figure 19-22 Phototoxic eruption.

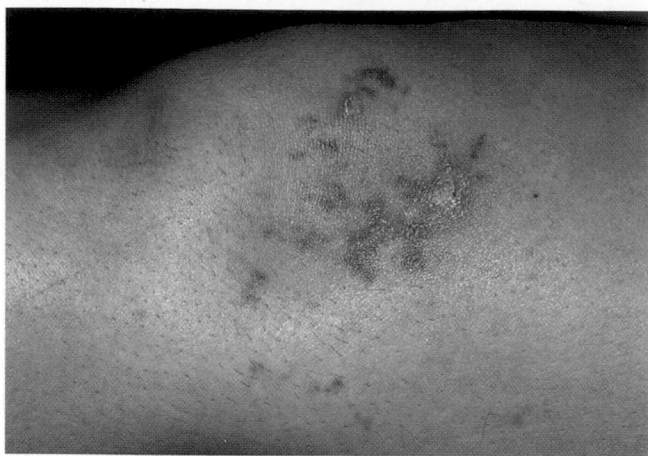

Figure 19-23 Phytophotodermatitis. Exposure to substances that contain psoralen compounds such as lime juice followed by sun exposure can cause erythema and vesicles that heal with brown hyperpigmentation.

Box 19-7 Agents Causing Phototoxic Reactions
Internal drugs
Chlorpromazine
Chlorothiazides
Tetracyclines
Demeclocycline (Declomycin)
8-Methoxypsoralens
Trimethylpsoralen
Nalidixic acid
Amiodarone
Piroxicam (Feldene)
Sulfonamides
Furosemide
Topical agents
Coal tar derivatives
Perfumes
Plants containing psoralen compounds (phytophotodermatitis)
Celery
Gas plant (burning bush, dittany)
Meadow grass (agrimony)
Parsnip (wild parsnip)
Persian limes
Wild angelica
Angelica
Cow parsley
Carrot (wild)
Fig (wild)
Sweet orange
False bishop's weed
Hogweed
Rue
Many others reported, but rare

PHYTOPHOTODERMATITIS. Exposure to plants[74] that contain light-sensitizing compounds[75] such as furanocoumarins (psoralens) can cause intense reactions. Examples are exposure to celery by salad makers and grocery workers,[76] wild parsnip in meadows, the rind and pulp of limes,[77-79] berlock dermatitis caused by the psoralen compounds in oil of bergamot (used in some perfumes) (Figure 19-24), and the leaves and young fruits of figs.[80]

The distribution of phototoxic reactions is sharply limited to areas of sun exposure. Topical exposure to solutions or plants produces bizarre patterns of inflammation, such as streaks from brushing against a plant or haphazard lines from celery juice.

DRUGS. Exposure to certain drugs[81,82] may result in a generalized intense erythema in sun-exposed skin (Box 19-7). Long lists of drugs reported to cause photosensitivity have been compiled; these are misleading because many are from single case reports. Thiazide diuretics are common offenders.[83] The characteristic areas are the forehead, nose, malar eminences, cheeks, upper ears, lateral and posterior neck, V of the chest, extensor surfaces of the forearms, backs of the hands, and prominences of the pretibial and calf areas. The upper eyelids, nasolabial folds, and submental areas are typically spared. *Photo-onycholysis,* which is the separation of the nails from the nailbeds, may occur with drugs such as demeclocycline hydrochloride (Declomycin) and tetracycline.

MANAGEMENT. In most instances, withdrawal of the drug results in clearance of the clinical reaction. The patient should never take the offending drug again. In rare instances, photosensitivity persists for months or years. These patients may benefit from treatment with PUVA.[84] Topical steroids provide some relief, but oral steroids are often necessary. When simple elimination fails to establish the offending agent, phototesting by physicians experienced with such procedures should be performed.[85]

Photoallergy

Photoallergic reactions are uncommon. UV light initiates a reaction between skin protein and a chemical or drug to form an antigen. A delayed hypersensitivity reaction follows, and the clinical presentation is, like poison ivy, eczematous inflammation. Plant and pesticide allergens should be included in the patch and photo-patch test series used for the evaluation of patients with suspected photoallergy.[86] Photoallergic contact dermatitis to PABA and structurally related PABA sunscreen has been documented.[87] Some patients without additional drug exposure continue to have flares for years when exposed to sunlight; this is termed a *persistent light reaction*.

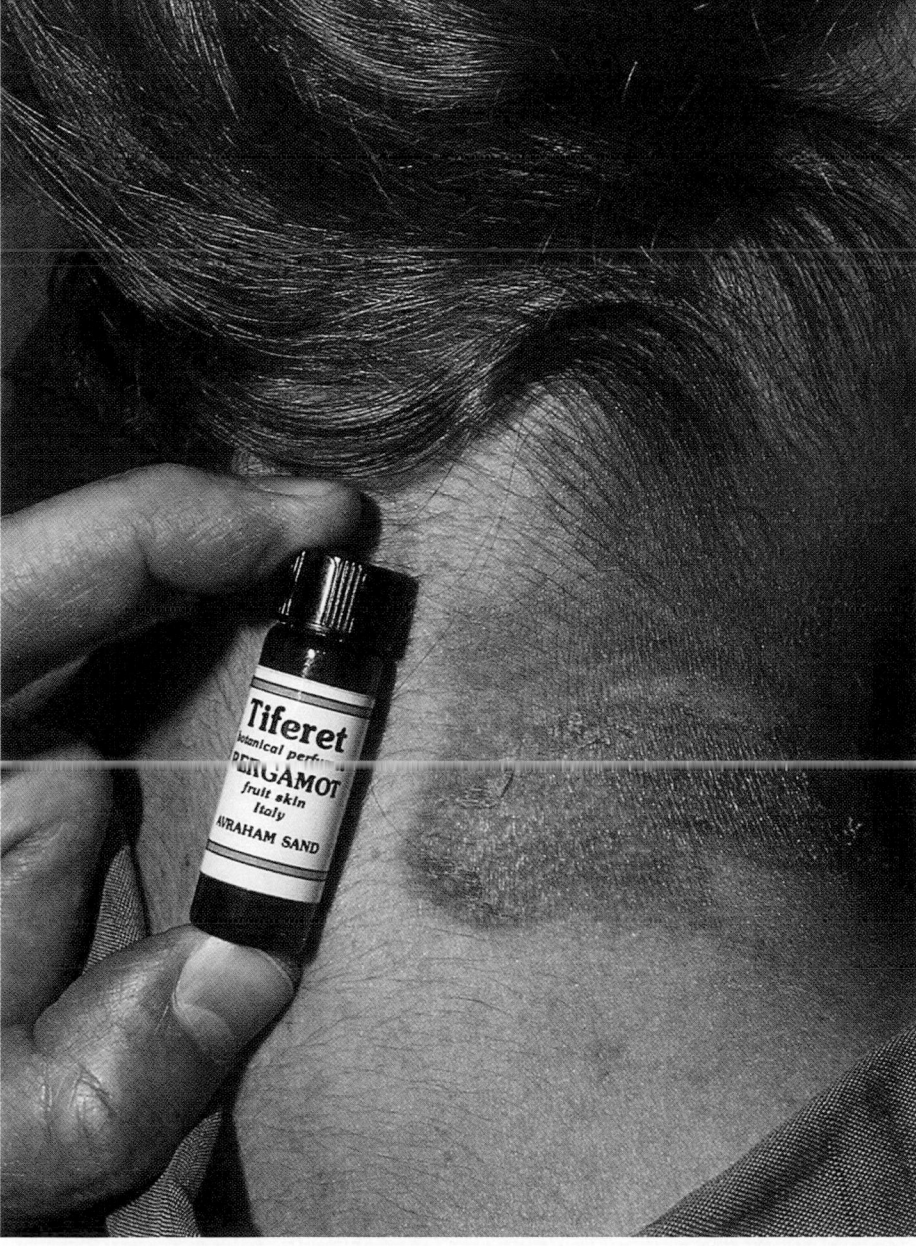

Figure 19-24 Phototoxic reaction (berlock dermatitis). Oil of bergamot (used in some perfumes) contains psoralens, which can cause erythema followed by prolonged hyperpigmentation after exposure to light.

Table 19-4 Disorders of Pigmentation

Hypopigmentation	Hyperpigmentation
Acquired	Circumscribed brown
Chemical-induced	Café-au-lait spots
Halo nevus	Diabetic dermopathy
Idiopathic guttate	Erythema ab igne
hypomelanosis	Fixed drug eruption
Leprosy	Freckles
Leukoderma associated	Lentigo in children
with melanoma	Peutz-Jeghers syndrome
Pityriasis alba	Lentigo in adults
Postinflammatory	Melasma
hypopigmentation	Phytophotodermatitis
Tinea versicolor	Diffuse brown
Vitiligo	Addison's disease
Congenital	Biliary cirrhosis
Albinism, partial	Hemochromatosis
(piebaldism)	Malignant melanoma
Albinism, total	(metastatic)
Nevus anemicus	
Nevus depigmentosus	
Piebaldism	
Tuberous sclerosis	

Disorders of Hypopigmentation

Diseases that present with hypopigmentation or hyperpigmentation are listed in Table 19-4. The most common and distinctive are described in the following paragraphs.

Vitiligo

The word *vitiligo* may be derived from the Greek *vitelius*, signifying a "calf's white patches." Vitiligo is an acquired loss of pigmentation characterized histologically by absence of epidermal melanocytes. It may be an autoimmune disease associated with antibodies (vitiligo antibodies) to melanocytes,[88] but the pathogenesis is still not understood. Studies suggest there is some genetic mechanism involved in the etiology of vitiligo and that it is polygenic in nature.[89] There is a positive family history in at least 30% of cases. Both sexes are affected equally. Approximately 1% of the population is affected; 50% of cases begin before age 20. The pigment loss may be localized or generalized.[90] Many patients are embarrassed. Physicians should be especially alert to the effects of disfigurement.[91]

CLINICAL MANIFESTATIONS. There are two types (A and B) (Table 19-5). In the more common type A (generalized), there is a fairly symmetric pattern of white macules with well-defined borders. The borders may have a red halo (inflammatory vitiligo) or a rim of hyperpigmentation. The loss of pigmentation may not be apparent in fair-skinned individuals, but it may be disfiguring in blacks. Initially the disease is limited; it then progresses slowly over years. Commonly involved sites include the backs of the hands, the face, and body folds, including axillae and genitalia (Figures 19-25 to 19-28). White areas are common around body openings such as the eyes, nostrils, mouth, nipples, umbilicus, and anus. The palms, soles, scalp, lips, and mucous membranes may be affected. Vitiligo occurs at sites of trauma (Köebner's phenomenon), such as around the elbows and in previously sunburned skin. Many patients with vitiligo develop halo nevi. An acrofacial or lip-tip type (involving lips and digits) also occurs.

Table 19-5 Vitiligo (Types A and B) Clinical Manifestations

	Type A	Type B
Distribution	Nondermatomal	Dermatomal (zosteriform)
Ratio	3	1
Onset	Any age (50% before age 20)	Young
Activity	Lifelong	Rapid spread 1 year
Associated with halo nevus	Yes	No
Köebner's phenomenon	Yes	No
Associated with immunologic diseases	Yes	No

Modified from Koga M, Tango T: Br J Dermatol 1988; 118:223.

VITILIGO

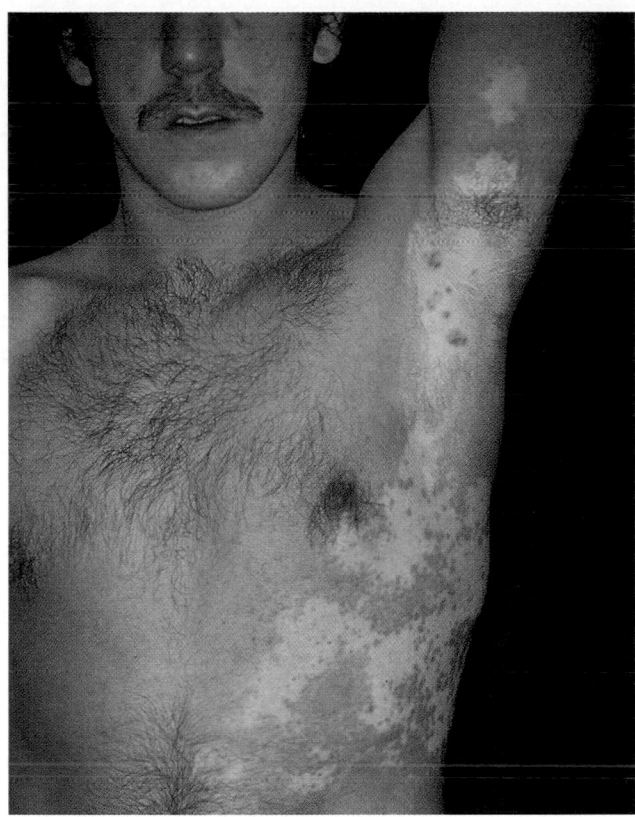

Figure 19-25 Body folds, including the axillae, are commonly involved. Wood's light examination may be necessary to demonstrate this in patients with light skin.

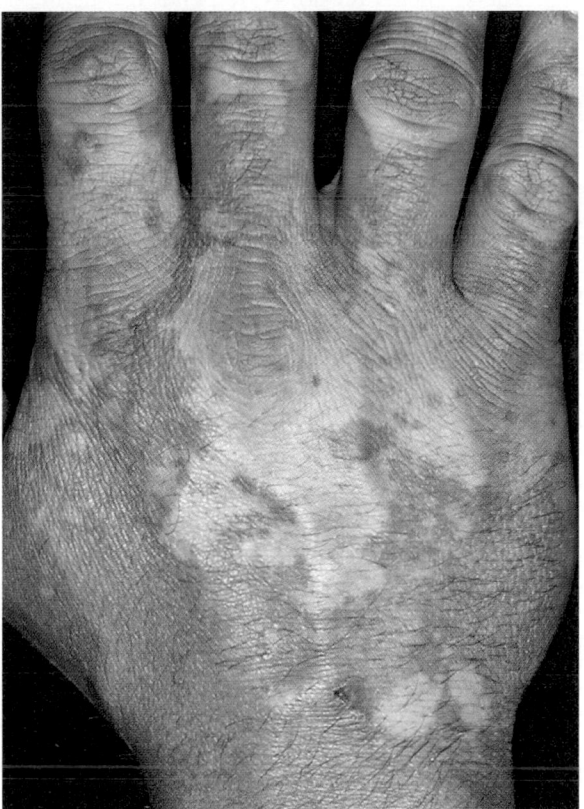

Figure 19-26 The back of the hand is a commonly involved site.

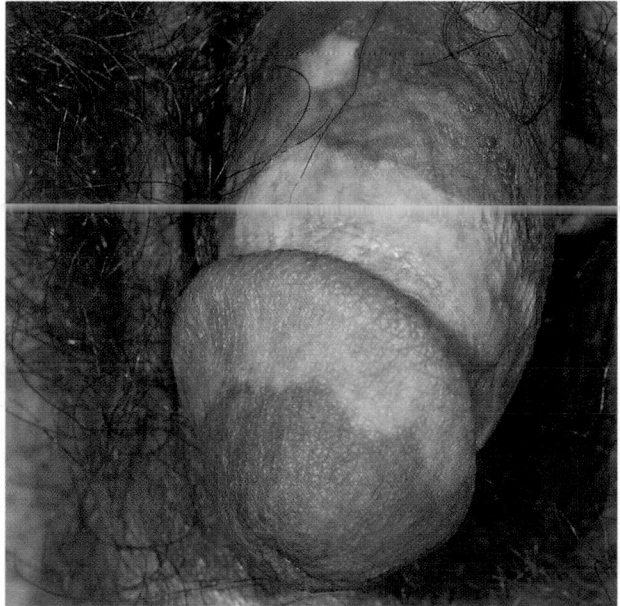

Figure 19-27 The penis is a commonly involved site.

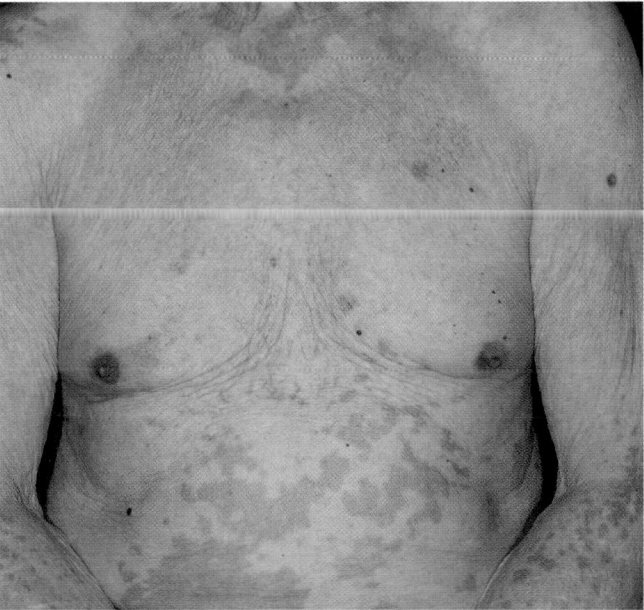

Figure 19-28 There is almost total loss of pigment. Monobenzone (Benoquin), a potent depigmenting agent, could be used for cosmetic purposes to remove the remaining pigment.

Segmental vitiligo (type B) occurs in an asymmetric distribution. The segments do not correspond to a dermatomal distribution. It is common in segmental forms for the hair follicles to be depigmented, indicating an absence of follicular melanocytes. The onset is earlier than the generalized form. There is a decreased association with autoimmune disease.

CHILDHOOD VITILIGO. Childhood vitiligo is a distinct subset of vitiligo. There is an increased incidence of segmental vitiligo (type B vitiligo), of autoimmune and/or endocrine disease, of premature graying in immediate and extended family members, and of organ-specific antibodies, in addition to a poor response to topical PUVA therapy.[92]

PSYCHOLOGIC IMPACT. Vitiligo can have a major impact on personality. Feelings of stress, embarrassment, self-consciousness, and low self esteem can occur. Patients claim the disease interferes with sexual relationships. The psychologic impact can be profound in deeply pigmented races. The disease can have serious social stigma in some cultures.

EYE, EAR, AND MENINGEAL FINDINGS. Vitiligo affects all melanocytes. Depigmented areas in the pigment epithelium of the retina and choroid occur in up to 40% of vitiligo patients. The incidence of uveitis is elevated. The membranous labyrinth of the inner ear contains melanocytes. Minor hearing problems can occur. The Vogt-Koyanagi-Harada syndrome consists of vitiligo with many other associated findings; the most common are meningismus, hearing loss, alopecia, tinnitus, and poliosis. The aseptic meningitis may be due to destruction of leptomeningeal melanocytes. The disease appears in the fourth to fifth decade and is more common in women and in persons with dark pigmentation.

ASSOCIATED DISEASES. Most patients with vitiligo have no other associated findings; however, vitiligo has been reported to be associated with alopecia areata, hypothyroidism, Graves' disease, Addison's disease, pernicious anemia, insulin-dependent diabetes mellitus, uveitis, chronic mucocutaneous candidiasis, the polyglandular autoimmune syndromes, and melanoma.[93] Thyroid disorders have been reported in as many as 30% of vitiligo patients.[94] Circulating autoantibodies such as antithyroglobulin and antimicrosomal and antiparietal cell antibodies have been found in more than 50% of patients.[95]

WOOD'S LIGHT EXAMINATION. Examination with the Wood's light in a dark room accentuates the hypopigmented areas and is useful for examining patients with light complexions. The axillae, anus, and genitalia should be carefully examined. These areas are frequently involved but often clinically nonapparent without the Wood's light. Vitiligo may be a predictor of metastases in melanoma patients, and a Wood's light examination may show early subtle changes in these patients.

STUDIES. Obtain a thyroid-stimulating hormone level and complete blood count with indices and blood sugar level to rule out thyroid disease, pernicious anemia, and diabetes mellitus.

RESOURCES. The National Vitiligo Foundation provides information and support for patients (611 South Fleishel Avenue, Tyler, TX 75701; telephone: (903) 531-0074; Fax: (903) 525-1234; e-mail: www.nvfi.org/menu.htm).

INDICATIONS FOR TREATMENT. Treatment is necessary for patients in whom the disease causes emotional and social distress. Vitiligo in individuals with fair complexions is usually not a significant cosmetic problem. The condition becomes more apparent in the summer months when tanning accentuates normal skin. Tanning may be prevented with sunscreens that have an SPF of 15 or higher. Vitiligo is a significant cosmetic problem in people with dark complexions, and repigmentation with psoralens may be worthwhile.

MECHANISM OF REPIGMENTATION. The goal of treatment is to restore melanocytes to the skin. Therapy involves stimulating melanocytes within the hair follicle to proliferate and migrate back into depigmented skin. Depigmented skin is devoid of melanocytes in the epidermis. Melanotic melanocytes in the bulb and infundibulum of the hair follicle are absent in vitiliginous skin. Repigmentation is caused by activation and migration of melanocytes from a melanocytic reservoir located in the hair follicles. Therefore skin with little or no hair (hands and feet) or with white hair responds poorly to treatment. Inactive amelanotic melanocytes in the middle and lower parts of the follicle and the outer root sheath are still present. These cells can be activated by treatment to acquire enzymes for melanogenesis. They proliferate and mature as they migrate up the hair follicle into the epidermis and spread centrifugally. When a vitiliginous spot repigments, it repigments from the follicle and spreads outward. This process is slow and requires at least 6 to 12 months of treatment. The face, arms, trunk, and legs respond best.

Melanocytes divide rapidly after any inflammatory process or after UV irradiation. PUVA produces inflammation in the skin at the depth of the hair follicle. Cytokines released by the inflammatory process may stimulate melanocytes to proliferate and migrate out.

GUIDELINES FOR THE TREATMENT OF VITILIGO. Evidence-based guidelines for the treatment of vitiligo in children and in adults have been established.[96] A treatment scheme is found in Table 19-6.

Table 19-6 Treatment Scheme for Vitiligo

	Clinical type of vitiligo	First-choice therapy*	Alternative therapies*
Children <12 y	All	Class 3 corticosteroids (and UVA); course, 6-9 mo (aged <6 y, no UVA)	Local UVB (311 nm); course, 6-12 mo Topical psoralen—UVA; course, 6-12 mo
Adults	Localized (≤2% depigmentation)	Class 3 corticosteroids (and UVA); course, 6-9 mo	Local UVB (311 nm); course, 6-12 mo Topical psoralen—UVA; course, 6-12 mo
	Generalized (>2% depigmentation)	UVB (311 nm); course, 6-24 mo	Oral psoralen—UVA; course, 6-24 mo
	Segmental or stable	Autologous transplantation (until 100% repigmentation)	Class 3 corticosteroids (and UVA); course, 6-9 mo UVB (311 nm); course, 6-24 mo
	Lip-tip	Autologous transplantation (until 100% repigmentation)	Micropigmentation (until 100% repigmentation)
	Therapy-resistant and/or generalized (>80% depigmentation)	Depigmentation with bleaching cream and/or laser (until 100% depigmentation)	None

From Njoo M, et al: Arch Dermatol 1999; 135:1514.

*The course is expressed as a range from minimum to maximum.

CHILDREN. Vitiligo can be associated with significant psychologic trauma; early treatment is more effective. Early lesions may respond better to therapy. Repigmentation therapies stimulate the melanocytic reserves in the hair follicles. Follicular melanocytes are mostly destroyed in older lesions and response to repigmentation therapy is poor.

For children younger than 12 years, treatment with class 3 topical corticosteroids (e.g., fluticasone propionate [Cutivate] or betamethasone valerate) is recommended as the first-choice therapy. This choice is made regardless of the clinical type. When no repigmentation is observed after 6 months, localized UVB therapy or topical PUVA therapy could be prescribed and the "skin-saving principle" applied (i.e., parts of the body where no lesions are present [especially the face] should be shielded during treatments). Parts of the body that have repigmented satisfactorily during the course of the therapy should, if possible, be shielded during subsequent treatments (e.g., trousers should be worn). In children, genital areas should be protected during UV exposures. Treatment with topical corticosteroid may be combined with UVA radiation. Comparative studies have shown that the combined treatment with fluticasone and UVA led to a greater repigmentation than did treatment with either fluticasone or UVA alone.[97] A facial tanner or a sun bed may be used as the UVA source.[96]

ADULTS. Treatment choice is guided by clinical type. Patients with localized vitiligo can be treated with class 3 corticosteroids combined with UVA therapy. If there is no response after 6 months, localized UVB or topical PUVA therapy can be given as an alternative. Narrowband UVB therapy is recommended as the most effective and safest therapy for generalized vitiligo. A minimum treatment duration of 6 months is recommended. Responsive patients can be given

this treatment for a maximum of 24 months. After the first course of 1 year, a resting period of 3 months is recommended to minimize the annual cumulative dose of UVB.

Segmental and lip-tip vitiligo (lips and digits) is best treated with autologous transplantation.

In patients with extensive areas of depigmentation (80%) and/or disfiguring lesions on the face who do not respond to repigmentation therapies, depigmentation of the residual melanin should be considered. During and on completion of the therapy, patients should minimize sun exposure and apply broad-spectrum sunscreens. The use of a potent bleaching cream and/or laser therapy (e.g., the Q-switched ruby laser) is considered to be the cornerstone of depigmentation therapy for these patients.

In all cases, advice regarding the use of camouflage and sun-blocking agents should always be given. If necessary, psychologic counseling may be recommended.[96]

NARROW-BAND UVB. Narrow-band (311 nm) UVB radiation provides a new alternative to conventional PUVA therapy without many of the adverse effects associated with PUVA therapy. UVB therapy may stimulate release of cytokines and inflammatory mediators in the skin that stimulate melanocyte migration and proliferation. Narrow-band UVB lamps produce less erythema, and hyperkeratosis is not observed after long-term irradiation. Treatments are given two or three times weekly, and exposure times are usually no longer than 5 minutes.[98] Narrow-band UVB therapy is effective and safe in childhood vitiligo.[99] As with other forms of phototherapy, the face and trunk had better repigmentation than distal extremities.

Some patients spontaneously repigment, sometimes after moderate sun exposure. UVB or PUVA can then be used to encourage further repigmentation. Reevaluate patients every 2 or 3 months. Therapy should be stopped if no color returns after this period. Patients who respond usually keep their pigment. Patients who have actively spreading vitiligo should not be treated; treatment does not halt the spread of the disease.

PUVASOL (PSORALENS AND SUNLIGHT). The following program is to be used with natural sunlight. Start with trioxsalen, which is less phototoxic than methoxsalen. The dose (see p. 673) should be taken 2 to 4 hours before measured periods of sun exposure. Maximum solar radiation is received between 11 AM and 3 PM. The patient should be treated only twice each week during the first 2 weeks to determine the degree of sun sensitivity. Treatments may be more frequent after this initial period. A persistent, faint erythema is the desired result. The schedule in Table 19-7 is suitable for most patients.

RESPONSE TO TREATMENT. Improvement begins with perifollicular pigmentation, which then enlarges. Repigmentation occurs at the borders but at a slower rate. Best results are obtained on the face and neck. The face begins to respond after 25 treatments; other areas, after 50. Results are poor on the hands and feet and over bony prominences. Focal vitiligo responds better than generalized vitiligo (i.e., it responds to 100 treatments or less, whereas generalized vitiligo requires as many as 200 treatments).[100] Most patients who respond do not develop new areas of pigment loss. The appearance of new or enlarged macules indicates the possible beginning of treatment failure. Maintenance therapy is not required. Totally repigmented macules should remain filled with 85% certainty; those incompletely filled in are likely to reverse and depigment.

TOPICAL THERAPY. Topical psoralens and topical steroids have been used with some success in patients with limited areas of pigmentation (see Box 19-6). Some dermatologists who have years of experience with phototherapy will not use topical psoralens. They believe that the potential for phototoxicity to produce severe burns is too great. The edges where there is residual pigmentation always hyperpigment; this disappears with time.

IMMUNOMODULATORS. Tacrolimus ointment (Protopic) and pimecrolimus (Elidel) have been used to treat vitiligo. These medications are well tolerated and can be used for prolonged periods without steroid-like side effects. Varying degrees of pigmentation have been experienced.

GRAFTING AND TRANSPLANTATION. Several surgical procedures have been developed for treating depigmented skin; these include grafting suction-blistered epidermis, minigrafts, and transplantation of in vitro–cultured epidermis-bearing melanocytes.

SYSTEMIC STEROIDS. Systemic corticosteroids can arrest the progression of vitiligo and lead to repigmentation in a significant proportion of patients, but they may also produce unacceptable side effects. Oral minipulse therapy with 5 mg betamethasone/dexamethasone was reported to arrest the progression and induce spontaneous repigmentation in some vitiligo patients. To minimize the side effects, betamethasone as a single oral dose was taken after breakfast on 2 consecutive days per week. The progression of the disease was arrested in 89% with active disease, whereas some patients needed an increase in the dosage to 7.5 mg/day to achieve a complete arrest of lesions. Within 2 to 4 months, 80% of the patients started having spontaneous repigmentation of the existing lesions that progressed with continued treatment.[102]

COSMETICS. For cosmetic purposes, lesions may be temporarily dyed brown with Dy-O-Derm or Vita-Dye. Cosmetics that camouflage (i.e., Dermablend and Covermark; see the Formulary) effectively hide the white patches. Each product is available in several shades.

The sunless or self-tanning lotions that contain dihydroxyacetone (DHA) darken the skin by staining. These preparations work best in vitiligo patients with skin phototypes II and III and are particularly useful if their normal skin is already tanned. The major problem is color blending and matching at the border of vitiliginous and normal skin.[20]

DEPIGMENTATION OF REMAINING NORMAL SKIN. Patients with more than 40% involvement of the skin surface may choose to remove the remaining normal skin pigment with 20% monobenzone (Benoquin cream). It is not always successful in achieving complete depigmentation. Monobenzone destroys melanocytes and can cause contact dermatitis. Therefore, as a test before starting generalized therapy, monobenzone should be applied to a single pigmented spot daily for 1 week. Thereafter larger pigmented areas are treated twice daily for 1 year or longer, not 4 months as is stated in *The Physicians' Desk Reference*. Application for 3 to 4 years may be necessary. Resistant areas such as the hands are treated with monobenzone under Saran Wrap occlusion. Patients may note an inflammatory response within the pigmented skin but not in the white skin. The monobenzone can be diluted to a 10%, 5%, or lower concentration for these patients. A group VI topical steroid may also be used to control inflammation.

Table 19-7 Treatment of Vitiligo with Psoralens: Suggested Sun Exposure Guide		
	Basic skin color	
Treatment	**Light**	**Medium**
Initial exposure	15 min	20 min
Second exposure	20 min	25 min
Third exposure	25 min	30 min
Fourth exposure	30 min	35 min
Subsequent exposures	Gradually increase exposure on the basis of erythema and tenderness	

Depigmentation is usually done in regions to limit drug absorption. Start with the face and upper extremity areas and then treat lower extremity sites. Truncal areas are last, and many patients choose to leave their trunk its normal color. The rate of depigmentation can vary from weeks to 4 years.

People assisting others with application of monobenzone must wear gloves and use applicators to prevent depigmenting their own skin.

Patients must understand that this is a permanent procedure. They will be sun sensitive for the rest of their lives and must use sunscreen during sun exposure. The results of treatment are usually very gratifying.

Patients who would like some skin color after treatment can use beta-carotene (Solatene) 60 mg 3 times a day for 10 weeks, followed by 30 mg 3 times a day for maintenance (Tishcon Corporation, [800] 866-0978).

Idiopathic guttate hypomelanosis

Idiopathic guttate hypomelanosis (white spots on the arms and legs) is characterized by 2- to 5-mm white spots with sharply demarcated borders. They are located on the exposed areas of hands, forearms, and lower legs of middle-aged and older people (Figure 19-29). Patients have signs of early aging and sun exposure, including seborrheic keratoses, lentigines, and xerosis in the same areas. A subset of these patients has lesions unrelated to sun exposure.[101] The condition is asymptomatic. Lesions show a decrease in the number of melanocytes.[103] Melanin is absent in basal keratinocytes. Treatment with tretinoin for 4 months restores the elasticity, with a partial restoration of pigmentation.[104]

Pityriasis alba

Pityriasis alba is a common finding (5% of children) that is probably more usual in patients with the atopic diathesis (see p. 119). The condition appears in most instances before puberty. The face, neck, and arms are the most common sites. The lesions begin as a nonspecific erythema and gradually become scaly and hypopigmented. The hypopigmentation is transient and caused by mild dermal inflammation and the UV screening effect of the scaly skin. The condition gradually improves after puberty. Treatment consists of lubrication. Mild inflammation responds to group V topical steroids, but the degree of pigmentation is not affected by any treatment.

The condition is often confused with vitiligo and tinea versicolor. Vitiligo does not scale. The potassium hydroxide preparation is positive in tinea versicolor.

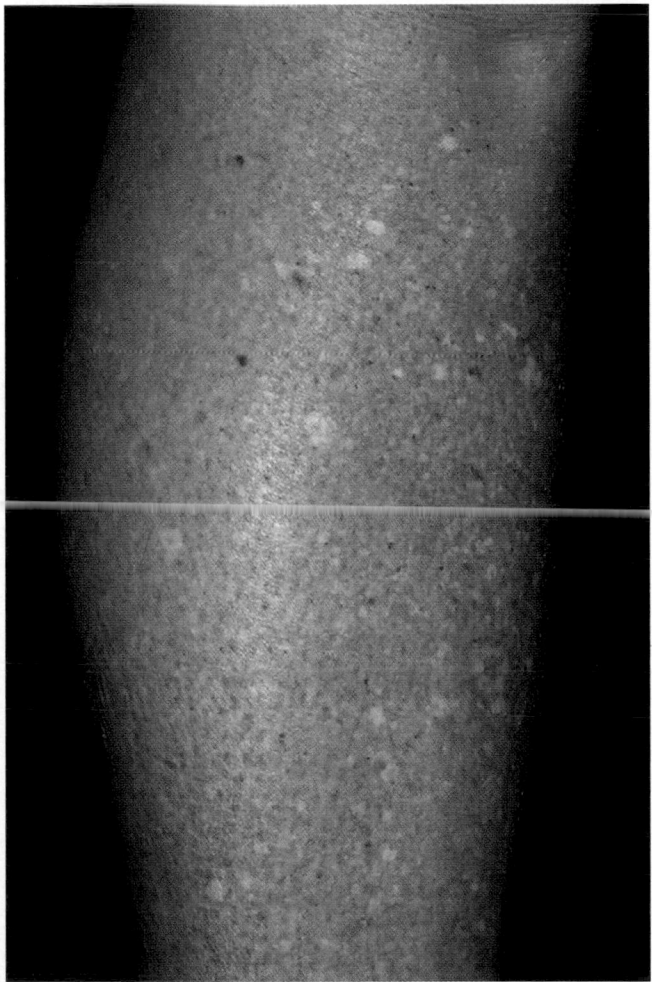

Figure 19-29 Idiopathic guttate hypomelanosis. White spots on the arms and lower legs occur in the middle-aged and the elderly.

Nevus anemicus

Nevus anemicus is a congenital localized pharmacologic cutaneous anomaly most often seen on the trunk.[105] It may be linked with certain genodermatoses, including neurofibromatosis. The lesion usually consists of a well-defined white macule with an irregular border, often surrounded by smaller white macules beyond the border of the major lesion (Figure 19-30). Histologically the skin appears normal; the pale color has been attributed to local blood vessel sensitivity to catecholamines. Hence, it has been called a *pharmacologic nevus*. Special stains confirm the presence of melanin and melanocytes. There is a lack of dermatitis within the margins of nevus anemicus in generalized contact dermatitis.[106] The lesion is most often confused with tinea versicolor or vitiligo. The white macule lacks the scale of tinea and, during Wood's light examination, does not become as prominent as vitiligo. Friction or cold or heat application fails to induce erythema in the involved areas. Treatment is not required. Camouflage make-up hides the lesion.

Tuberous sclerosis

Hypopigmented macules (oval, ash leaf-shaped, or stippled) that are concentrated on the arms, legs, and trunk are the earliest signs of tuberous sclerosis[107,108] (Figure 19-31; see also Chapter 26). They are present in 40% to 90% of patients with the disease, and they number from 1 to 32 in affected individuals. Minimally visible hypopigmented spots are more easily visualized with the Wood's lamp. As noted, Wood's light is a blue light with an emission peak of 360 nm. The blue end of visible light is absorbed by epidermal pigmentation. If there is no epidermal pigmentation in a site, the area will appear nonpigmented compared with the surrounding skin.[109]

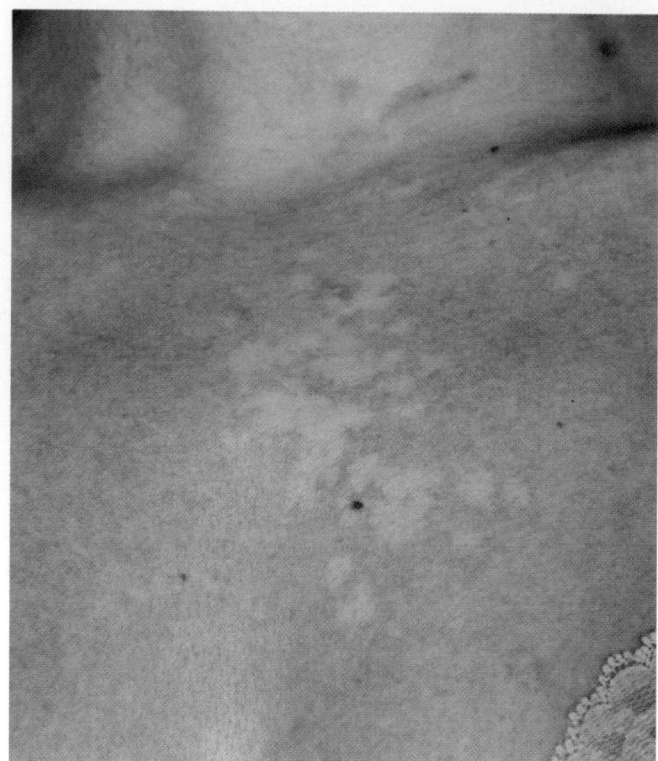

Figure 19-30 Nevus anemicus.

Figure 19-31 Tuberous sclerosis. Ash leaf-shaped hypopigmented macules.

Disorders of Hyperpigmentation

FRECKLES (EPHELIDES) VS. LENTIGO. Ephelides and solar lentigines are different types of pigmented lesions.[110] Solar lentigines are more prevalent than ephelides, increase in prevalence and number with higher age, are most prevalent on the trunk, and occur more frequently in males. Ephelides loose their prevalence with age, become equally distributed on the face, arms, and trunk, and occur more frequently in females. An intimate association of ephelides, but not solar lentigines, has been found with hair color and skin type.

Freckles

Freckles, or ephelides, are small, red or light brown macules that are promoted by sun exposure and fade during the winter months. They are usually confined to the face, arms, and back. The number varies from a few spots on the face to hundreds of confluent macules on the face and arms. They occur as an autosomal dominant trait and are most often found in individuals with fair complexions. The use of sunscreens prevents the appearance of new freckles and helps prevent the darkening of existing freckles that typically accompanies sun exposure.

Lentigo in children

A lentigo is a small (0.5- to 2-cm) tan, brown, or black oval-to-round macule that is darker than a freckle and is not affected by sunlight. Freckles darken with sun exposure. Lentigines may increase in number during childhood and adult life or fade at any time. The Peutz-Jeghers syndrome refers to mucocutaneous pigmentation consisting of many blue-brown lentigines, less than 0.5 cm in diameter, on the buccal mucosa and other areas of the glabrous skin, accompanied by generalized intestinal polyposis.[111,112]

Lentigo in adults

Lentigo, or liver spots, occurs in sun-exposed areas of the face, arms, and hands (Figure 19-32). The lesions vary in size from 0.2 to 2 cm and become more numerous with advancing age. Facial solar lentigines frequently lack the rete ridge hyperplasia classically associated with lentigines from other anatomic sites.[113]

A biopsy should be taken from any lentigo that develops a highly irregular border, localized increase in pigmentation, or localized thickening to rule out lentigo maligna melanoma. Cryotherapy is an effective treatment, but hypopigmentation is a possible side effect. Topical 0.1% tretinoin cream or 0.1% tazarotene cream (Avage) significantly improves both clinical and microscopic manifestations of liver spots. After 10 months, 83% of patients with facial lesions who were treated with tretinoin had lightening of these lesions. The lesions do not return for at least 6 months after therapy is discontinued.[114]

A single course of Q-switched ruby laser exposure completely clears lesions on the arms and hands. Peeling solution with glycolic acid is ineffective.[115]

Hyperpigmented lesions are a predominant component of photoaging in Chinese and Japanese persons; 0.1% tretinoin cream significantly lightens the hyperpigmentation of photoaging in these patients.[5] Hydroquinone preparations are occasionally useful for bleaching these lesions.

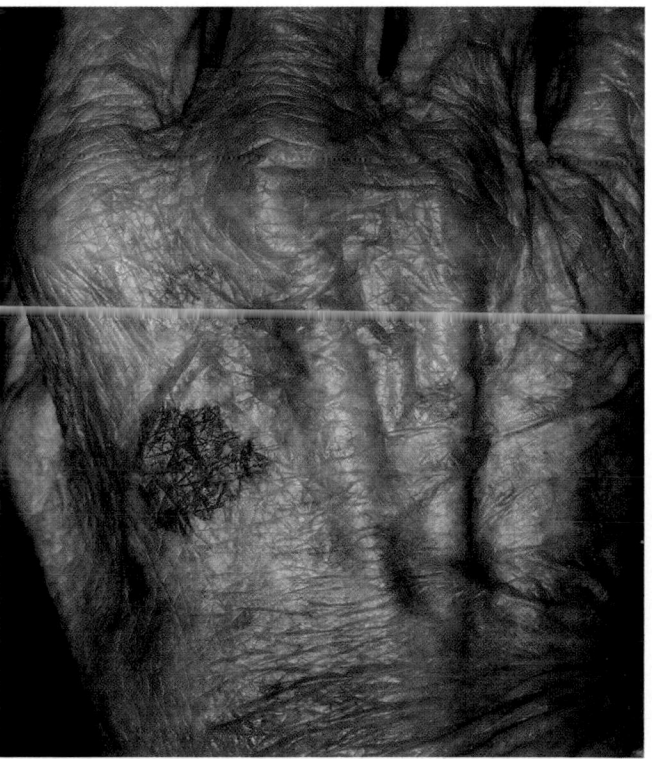

Figure 19-32 Lentigo (liver spots). Brown macules that appear in chronically sun exposed areas.

Melasma

Melasma (chloasma, or mask of pregnancy) is a common acquired symmetric brown hyperpigmentation involving the face and neck in genetically predisposed women.[116] The psychosocial impact can be devastating. The pigmentation develops slowly without signs of inflammation and may be faint or dark.

ETIOLOGY. Genetic factors and UV radiation are the most important causes. Other causes include pregnancy, oral contraceptives, estrogen-progesterone therapies, thyroid dysfunction, cosmetics, and phototoxic and antiseizure drugs. Melasma may not resolve after delivery or withdrawal of oral contraceptives. Mild subclinical ovarian dysfunction may be present in some patients.[117]

CLINICAL AND HISTOLOGIC PATTERNS. There are three clinical patterns: centrofacial, malar, and mandibular. There are four types based on Wood's light examination: (1) the epidermal type has increased melanin in the basal, suprabasal, and stratum corneum layers. The pigmentation is intensified by Wood's light examination. (2) The dermal type does not show enhancement with the Wood's light. Melanophages are found in the superficial dermis and in the deep dermis, (3) a mixed-type epidermal and dermal pigment type that shows no or slight enhancement with the Wood's light, and (4) Wood's lamp inapparent, which is seen in dark individuals. The epidermal type responds to depigmenting agents; the dermal pigmentation resists the action of bleaching agents. Three histologic patterns of pigmentation have been described: epidermal, dermal, and mixed.

There is an increased number and activity of melanocytes in the epidermis and an increased number of melanophages in the dermis. The forehead, malar eminences, upper lip, and chin are most frequently affected (Figure 19-33). Melasma occurs during the second or third trimester of pregnancy, gradually fades after delivery, and darkens with subsequent pregnancies. Melasma occurs in some women taking oral contraceptives.[118]

TREATMENT. Melasma is difficult to treat. Treatments include hypopigmenting agents, chemical peels, and lasers. Cosmetics (such as Dermablend) may be used to camouflage the pigmentation. Cosmetics are heavy and objectionable to some patients.

SUN PROTECTION. UV radiation has a significant effect on the pathogenesis of melasma. Sun exposure must be minimized. Sunscreens that block both UVA and UVB light should be used. Titanium dioxide– and zinc oxide–containing sunscreens reflect UVA and UVB. There are several brands.

HYPOPIGMENTING AGENTS. Hydroquinone is the most effective topically applied bleaching agent. This agent is available in 2% concentrations without prescription (Porcelana) and by prescription in 3% (Melanex) and 4% (Claripel, Eldoquin-Forte, Eldopaque-Forte, Solaquin Forte, Lustra, Lustra-AF) concentrations (see the Formulary). Higher extemporaneously compounded concentrations of hydroquinone (as high as 10%) can be prescribed for difficult cases. The medication should be applied twice daily—once in the morning and before bedtime. Hydroquinone is an irritant and a sensitizer, and skin should be tested for sensitivity before use by applying a small amount to the cheek or arm once each day for 2 days (open patch testing). The development of erythema or vesiculation indicates an allergic reaction and precludes further use. These preparations must be used for months and in many cases result in gradual depigmentation. Skin must be protected with broad-spectrum sunscreens both during and after treatment. Tretinoin (Retin-A) enhances the epidermal penetration of hydroquinone and is often prescribed to be used at a different time of day. Start with a low concentration of tretinoin. Increase the concentration until slight irritation occurs. Hydroquinones also bleach freckles and lentigines but not café-au-lait spots or pigmented nevi.

TRI-LUMA CREAM. Tri-Luma Cream is a combination product containing 4.0% hydroquinone, 0.05% tretinoin, and 0.01% fluocinolone acetonide. The recommended course of therapy is qd for 8 weeks. Significant results have been seen after the first 4 weeks of treatment. After 8 weeks of treatment, 13% to 38% of the patients achieved clearing of melasma. It is more effective than any of the single agent treatments.

TRETINOIN. Topical tretinoin used alone produces significant clinical improvement of melasma, mainly due to reduction in epidermal pigment. Improvement occurs slowly and may require up to a year of treatment.[119,120]

AZELAIC ACID. Azelaic acid (Azelex) is used to treat acne and melasma. It has selective effects on hyperactive and abnormal melanocytes and minimal effects on normally pigmented human skin, freckles, and senile lentigines. It is reported to be as effective as 4% hydroquinone. Azelaic acid with tretinoin caused more skin lightening after 3 months than did azelaic acid alone.[121]

CHEMICAL PEELS. Superficial, medium, and deep chemical peels are used to treat melasma in lighter-complexioned whites. Trichloroacetic acid and alpha-hydroxy acids have been used; they are somewhat effective.[122] Darker complexioned individuals are poor candidates for chemical peels because postinflammatory hyperpigmentation frequently occurs.

LASERS. Several types of lasers have been used with mixed results. Pulsed CO_2 laser followed by Q-switched alexandrite laser in the treatment of dermal-type melasma is reported effective. The combination is proposed to be effective by first destroying the abnormal melanocytes with the pulsed CO_2 laser and then selectively eliminating the dermal melanin with the alexandrite laser.[123]

MELASMA

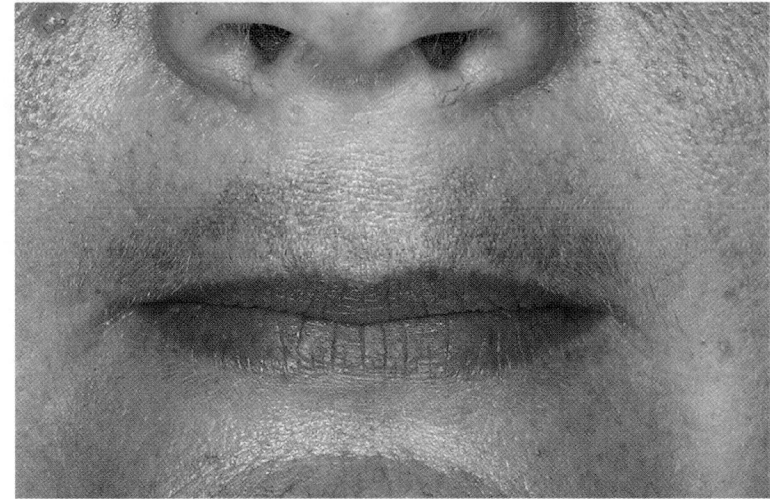

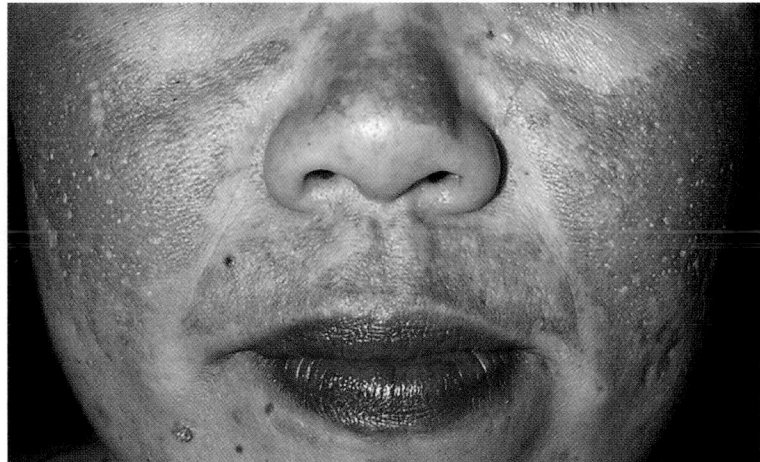

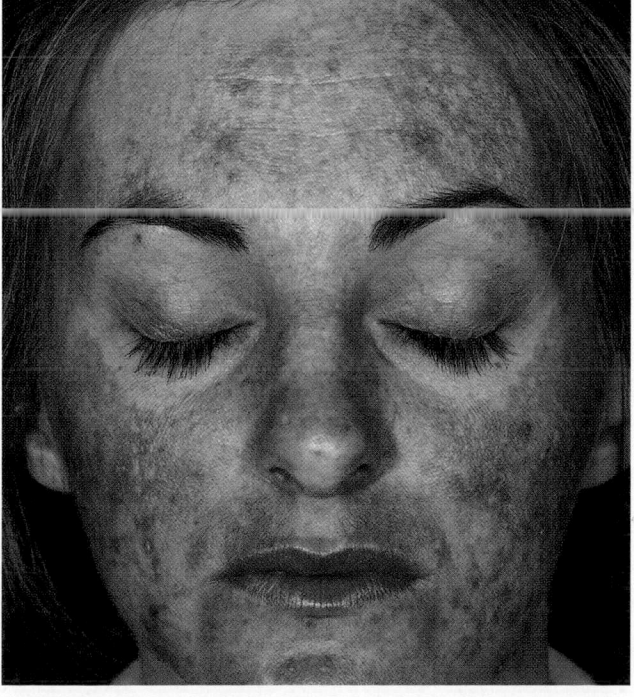

Figure 19-33 Diffuse brown hyperpigmentation may occur during pregnancy or while taking oral contraceptives. The upper lip, malar eminences, and forehead are the most frequently affected.

Café-au-lait spots

Café-au-lait spots are uniformly pale brown macules that vary in size from 0.5 to 20 cm and can be found on any cutaneous surface (Figure 19-34) (see also Chapter 26, p. 905.). They may be present at birth, are estimated to be present in 10% to 20% of normal children, and increase in number and size with age. Six or more spots greater than 1.5 cm in diameter are presumptive evidence of neurofibromatosis (von Recklinghausen's disease) in young children over 5 years of age. In children under 5 years of age, five or more café-au-lait spots greater than 0.5 cm in diameter suggest the diagnosis of neurofibromatosis. Café-au-lait spots are present in 90% to 100% of patients with von Recklinghausen's disease. Smaller spots 1 to 4 cm in diameter in the axillae (axillary freckling or Crowe's sign) are a rare but diagnostic sign of neurofibromatosis. There is no increased incidence of café-au-lait spots in tuberous sclerosis.[124] Lesions that are similar but that have a more irregular border (shaped like "the coast of Maine") are seen in polyostotic fibrous dysplasia (Albright's syndrome). The smooth, regular border of the café-au-lait macules of neurofibromatosis has been compared with "the coast of California."

Macromelanosomes, or larger-than-normal pigment granules, have been detected with the electron microscope in the café-au-lait spots of some patients with neurofibromatosis, but their absence does not rule out the diagnosis. Café-au-lait spots cannot be lightened by hydroquinone bleaching agents. Q-switched laser and erbium:YAG laser treatments have been reported to be effective.[125]

Diabetic dermopathy

Diabetic dermopathy is the most common cutaneous marker of diabetes mellitus and is present in 40% of diabetic patients. Diabetic dermopathy is a clinical sign of an increased likelihood of internal complications in diabetic patients.[126]

Lesions are asymptomatic, round, atrophic hyperpigmented areas on the shins (shin spots). They begin as round-to-oval, flat-topped, red, scaly papules that may become eroded. The lesions eventually clear or heal with epidermal atrophy or hyperpigmentation. They may also appear on the forearms, the anterior surface of the lower thighs, and the sides of the feet. Men are affected twice as often as women. They may be initiated by trauma.

Erythema ab igne

Chronic exposure to heat from a wood stove, fireplace, electric blanket, electric heater, hot water bottle, or hot compress may cause a distinctive cutaneous eruption with a reticular pattern. The eruption initially appears as bands of erythema, but brown hyperpigmentation develops with repeated exposure (Figure 19-35).

Erythema ab igne may develop in patients who apply local heat or hot water bottles to painful metastatic and primary tumors.[127]

The pigmentation, caused by melanin,[128] may fade in time or may be permanent. The eruption must be differentiated from livido reticularis, which occurs with diseases such as leukocytoclastic vasculitis. Livido reticularis is a reddish-purple reticular pigmentation, probably caused by restricted blood flow through the horizontal venous plexus. The color persists, but brown hyperpigmentation does not occur.

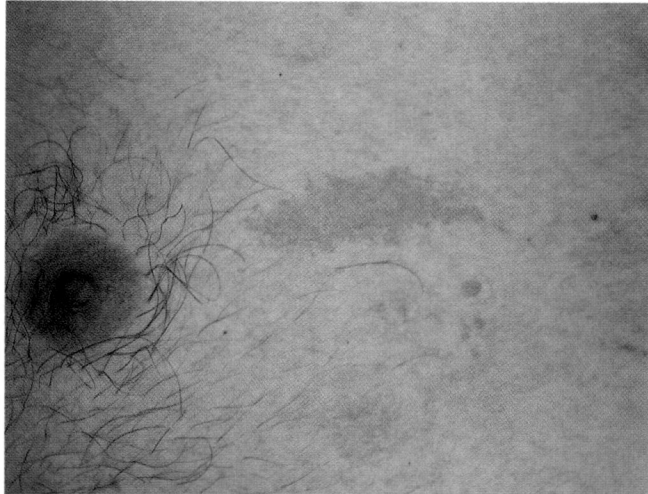

Figure 19-34 Café-au-lait spots. Irregular brown macules that are found in 10% to 20% of normal children. Number and size are increased in neurofibromatosis. (See Figure 26-11.)

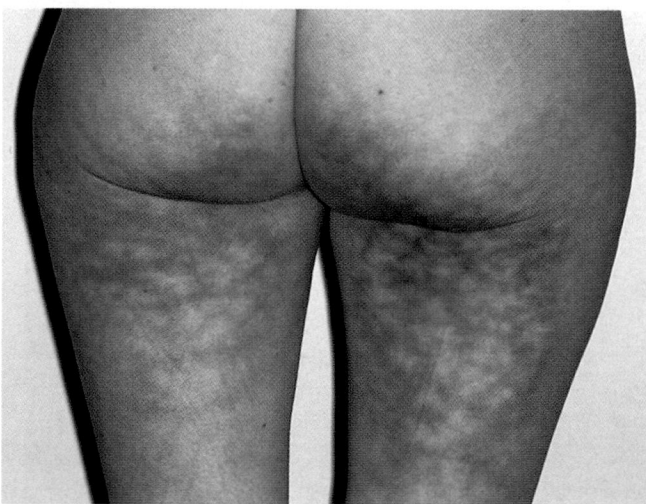

Figure 19-35 Erythema ab igne. Reticular brown hyperpigmentation that develops in areas chronically exposed to heat. A heating pad used for several months produced the eruption depicted here.

References

1. De BH, et al: Modern approaches to photoprotection, Dermatol Clin 2000; 18(4):577.

2. Taylor, et al: Photoaging/photodamage and photoprotection, J Am Acad Dermatol 1990; 22:1.

3. Gilchrest BA: Overview of skin aging, J Cutaneous Aging Cosmetic Dermatol 1988; 1:1.

4. Tsuji T, et al: Two types of wrinkles in aged persons (letter), Arch Dermatol 1986; 122:22.

5. Griffiths CE, et al: Topical tretinoin (retinoic acid) treatment of hyperpigmented lesions associated with photoaging in Chinese and Japanese patients: a vehicle-controlled trial, J Am Acad Dermatol 1994; 30:76.

6. Kang S, et al: Tazarotene cream for the treatment of facial photodamage: a multicenter, investigator-masked, randomized, vehicle-controlled, parallel comparison of 0.01%, 0.025%, 0.05%, and 0.1% tazarotene creams with 0.05% tretinoin emollient cream applied once daily for 24 weeks, Arch Dermatol 2001; 137(12):1597.

7. Olsen E, et al: Sustained improvement in photodamaged skin with reduced tretinoin emollient cream treatment regimen: effect of once-weekly and three-times-weekly applications, J Am Acad Dermatol 1997; 37(2 Pt 1):227.

8. Kang S, Voorhees J: Photoaging therapy with topical tretinoin: an evidence-based analysis, J Am Acad Dermatol 1998; 39 (2 Pt 3):S55.

9. Lawrence N: New and emerging treatments for photoaging, Dermatol Clin 2000; 18(1):99.

10. Hall H, et al: Factors associated with sunburn in white children aged 6 months to 11 years, Am J Prev Med 2001; 20(1):9.

11. Driscoll M, Wagner R: Clinical management of the acute sunburn reaction, Cutis 2000; 66(1):53.

12. Wulf HC, et al: Sunscreens for delay of ultraviolet induction of skin tumors, J Am Acad Dermatol 1982; 7:194.

13. Stern RS, Weinstein MC, Baker SG: Risk reduction for non-melanoma skin cancer with childhood sunscreen use, Arch Dermatol 1986; 122:537.

14. Patel NP, Highton A, Moy RL: Properties of topical sunscreen formulations, J Dermatol Surg Oncol 1992; 18:316.

15. Wright M, Wright S, Wagner R: Mechanisms of sunscreen failure [In Process Citation], J Am Acad Dermatol 2001; 44(5):781.

16. Pruim B, Green A: Photobiological aspects of sunscreen re-application, Australas J Dermatol 1999; 40(1):14.

17. Eberlein-Konig B, Placzek M, Przybilla B: Protective effect against sunburn of combined systemic ascorbic acid (vitamin C) and d-alpha-tocopherol (vitamin E), J Am Acad Dermatol 1998; 38(1):45.

18. Stahl W, et al: Carotenoids and carotenoids plus vitamin E protect against ultraviolet-induced erythema in humans, Am J Clin Nutr 2000; 71(3):795.

19. Marks R, et al: The effect of regular sunscreen use on vitamin D levels in an Australian population, Arch Dermatol 1995; 131:415.

20. Levy SB: Dihydroxyacetone-containing sunless or self-tanning lotions, J Am Acad Dermatol 1992; 27:989.

21. Levy S: Tanning preparations, Dermatol Clin 2000; 18(4):591.

22. Hasan T, et al: Disease associations in polymorphous light eruption. A long-term follow-up study of 94 patients, Arch Dermatol 1998; 134(9):1081.

23. Holzle E, et al: Polymorphous light eruption, J Invest Dermatol 1987; 88(suppl):32.

24. Jansen CT, Karvonen J: Polymorphous light eruption, Arch Dermatol 1984; 120:862.

25. Fusaro RM, Johnson JA: Topical photoprotection for hereditary polymorphic light eruption of American Indians, J Am Acad Dermatol 1991; 24:744.

26. Lane PR, et al: Actinic prurigo: clinical features and prognosis, J Am Acad Dermatol 1992; 26:683.

27. Boonstra H, et al: Polymorphous light eruption: A clinical, photobiologic, and follow-up study of 110 patients, J Am Acad Dermatol 2000; 42(2 Pt 1):199.

28. Holzle E, et al: Polymorphous light eruption: experimental reproduction of skin lesions, J Am Acad Dermatol 1982; 7:111.

29. Ortel B, et al: Polymorphous light eruption: action spectrum and photoprotection, J Am Acad Dermatol 1986; 14:748.

30. Elpern DJ, Morison WL: Papulovesicular light eruption, Arch Dermatol 1985; 121:1286.

31. Lane PR, et al: Treatment of actinic prurigo with intermittent short-course topical 0.05% clobetasol 17-propionate. A preliminary report, Arch Dermatol 1985; 121:1286.

32. Allas S, et al: Comparison of the ability of 2 sunscreens to protect against polymorphous light eruption induced by a UV-A/UV-B metal halide lamp [letter], Arch Dermatol 1999; 135(11):1421.

33. Bissonnette R, et al: Comparison of UVA protection afforded by high sun protection factor sunscreens, J Am Acad Dermatol 2000; 43(6):1036.

34. Morison WL, et al: UVB phototherapy and prophylaxis of polymorphous light eruption, Br J Dermatol 1982; 106:231.

35. Murphy GM, et al: Prophylactic PUVA and UVB therapy in polymorphic light eruption: a controlled trial, Br J Dermatol 1987; 116:531.

36. Addo HA, Sharma SC: UVB phototherapy and photochemotherapy (PUVA) in the treatment of polymorphic light eruption and solar urticaria, Br J Dermatol 1987; 116:539.

37. Berg N, et al: Ultraviolet A phototherapy and trimethylpsoralen UVA photochemotherapy in polymorphous light eruption: a controlled study, Photodermatol Photoimmunol Photomed 1994; 10:139.

38. Rucker BU, et al: Ultraviolet light hardening in polymorphous light eruption: a controlled study comparing different emission spectra, Photodermatol Photoimmunol Photomed 1991; 8:73.

39. Parrish JA, et al: Comparison of PUVA and beta-carotene in the treatment of polymorphous light eruption, Br J Dermatol 1979; 100:187.

40. Epstein JH: Polymorphous light eruption, J Am Acad Dermatol 1980; 3:329.

41. Murphy GM, Hawk JLM, Magnus IA: Hydroxychloroquine in polymorphic light eruption: a controlled trial with drug and visual sensitivity monitoring, Br J Dermatol 1987; 116:379.

42. Eramo LR, Garden JM, Esterly NB: Hydroa vacciniforme, Arch Dermatol 1986; 122:1310.

43. Thiers BH: The porphyrias, J Am Acad Dermatol 1981; 5:621.

44. Poh-Fitzpatrick M, et al: Porphyria cutanea tarda in two patients treated with hemodialysis for chronic renal failure, N Engl J Med 1978; 299:292.

45. Bonkovsky H, et al: Porphyria cutanea tarda, hepatitis C, and HFE gene mutations in North America, Hepatology 1998; 27(6):1661,

46. Grossman M, et al: Porphyria cutanea tarda: clinical features and laboratory findings in 40 patients, Am J Med 1979; 67:277.

47. Sampietro M, Fiorelli G, Fargion S: Iron overload in porphyria cutanea tarda, Haematologica 1999; 84(3):248.

48. Cripps DJ: Hospital management of the dermatologic patient: the porphyrias, Semin Dermatol 1986; 5:55.

49. Adjarov D, Kerimova M: Effective control of patients with porphyria cutanea tarda by measuring plasma uroporphyrin, Clin Exp Dermatol 1991; 16:254.

50. Ratnaike S, et al: Plasma ferritin levels as a guide to the treatment of porphyria cutanea tarda by venesection, Australas J Dermatol 1988; 29(1):3.

51. Adjarov D, et al: Choice of therapy in porphyria cutanea tarda, Clin Exp Dermatol 1996; 21(6):461.

52. Kordac V, et al: Chloroquine in the treatment of porphyria cutanea tarda, N Engl J Med 1977; 296.

53. Seubert S, et al: Results of treament of porphyria cutanea tarda with bloodletting and chloroquine, Z Hautkr 1990; 65:223.

54. Topi GC, Amantea A, Griso D: Recovery from porphyria cutanea tarda with no specific therapy other than avoidance of hepatic toxins, Br J Dermatol 1984; 111:75.

55. Diffey BL, Farr PM: Sunscreen protection against UVB, UVA and blue light: an in vivo and in vitro comparison, Br J Dermatol 1991; 124:258.

56. Stenberg A: Pseudoporphyria and sunbeds, Acta Derm Venereol 1990; 70:354.

57. Green J, Manders S: Pseudoporphyria, J Am Acad Dermatol 2000; 17(6):480.

58. Poh-Fitzpatrick MB: Porphyria, pseudoporphyria, pseudo-pseudoporphyria, Arch Dermatol 1986; 122:403.

59. De SB, et al: Pseudoporphyria and nonsteroidal antiinflammatory agents in children with juvenile idiopathic arthritis, Pediatr Dermatol 2000; 17(6):480.

60. La Duca J, Bouman P, Gaspari A: Nonsteroidal antiinflammatory drug-induced pseudoporphyria: A case series [epub ahead of print] [record supplied by publisher], J Cutan Med Surg 2002.

61. Poh-Fitzpatrick MB, Sosin AE, Bemis J: Porphyrin levels in plasma and erythrocytes of chronic hemodialysis patients, J Am Acad Dermatol 1982; 7:100.

62. Todd D: Erythropoietic protoporphyria, Br J Dermatol 1994; 131(6):751.

63. Brun A, Sandberg S: Mechanisms of photosensitivity in porphyric patients with special emphasis on erythropoietic protoporphyria, J Photochem Photobiol B 1991; 10:285.

64. Poh-Fitzpatrick MB: The "priming phenomenon" in the acute phototoxicity of erythropoietic protoporphyria, J Am Acad Dermatol 1989; 21:311.

65. Shehade SA, et al: Predictable and unpredictable hazards of erythropoietic protoporphyria, Clin Exp Dermatol 1991; 16:185.

66. Mercurio MG, et al: Terminal hepatic failure in erythropoietic protoporphyria, J Am Acad Dermatol 1993; 29:829.

67. Todd DJ, et al: Erythropoietic protoporphyria. The problem of a suitable screening test, Acta Derm Venereol 1990; 70:347.

68. Mathews-Roth MM, et al: Beta-carotene as a photoprotective agent in erythropoietic protoporphyria, N Engl J Med 1970; 282:1231.

69. Mathews-Roth MM: Erythropoietic protoporphyria: diagnosis and treatment, N Engl J Med 1977; 297:98.

70. Ross JB, Moss MA: Relief of the photosensitivity of erythropoietic protoporphyria by pyridoxine, J Am Acad Dermatol 1990; 22:340.

71. Gordeuk VR, et al: Iron therapy for hepatic dysfunction in erythropoietic photoporphyria, Ann Intern Med 1986; 105:27.

72. Mercurio M, et al: Terminal hepatic failure in erythropoietic protoporphyria, J Am Acad Dermatol 1993; 29(5 Pt 2):829.

73. McCullough A, et al: Fecal protoporphyrin excretion in erythropoietic protoporphyria: effect of cholestyramine and bile acid feeding, Gastroenterology 1988; 94(1):177.

74. Kavli G, Volden G: Phytophotodermatitis, Photodermatology 1984; 1:65.

75. Benezra C, Ducombs G: Molecular aspects of allergic contact dermatitis to plants: recent progress in phytodermatochemistry, Dermatosen 1987; 35:4.

76. Berkley SF, et al: Dermatitis in grocery workers associated with high natural concentrations of furanocoumarins in celery, Ann Intern Med 1986; 105:351.

77. Gross TP, et al: An outbreak of phototoxic dermatitis due to limes, Am J Epidemiol 1987; 125:509.

78. White W: Club Med dermatitis, N Engl J Med 1986; 314:319.

79. Nigg HN, et al: Phototoxic coumarins in limes, Food Chem Toxicol 1993; 31:331.

80. Watemberg N, et al: Phytophotodermatitis due to figs, Cutis 1991; 48:151.

81. Ljunggren B, Bjellerup M: Systemic drug photosensitivity, Photodermatology 1986; 3:26.

82. Epstein JH, Wintroub BU: Photosensitivity due to drugs, Drugs 1985; 30:42.

83. Addo HA, Ferguson J, Frain-Bell W: Thiazide-induced photosensitivity: a study of 33 subjects, Br J Dermatol 1987; 116:749.

84. Robinson HN, Morison WL, Hood AF: Thiazide diuretic therapy and chronic photosensitivity, Arch Dermatol 1985; 121: 522.

85. Holzle E, et al: Photopatch testing: the 5-year experience of the German, Austrian and Swiss Photopatch Test Group, J Am Acad Dermatol 1991; 25:59.

86. Mark K, et al: Allergic contact and photoallergic contact dermatitis to plant and pesticide allergens, Arch Dermatol 1999; 135(1):67.

87. Thune C: Contact and photocontact allergy to sunscreens, Photodermatology 1984; 1:5.

88. Naughton GK, Reggiardo D, Bystryn J-C: Correlation between vitiligo antibodies and extent of depigmentation in vitiligo, J Am Acad Dermatol 1986; 15:978.

89. Bhatia PS, et al: Genetic nature of vitiligo, J Dermatol Sci 1992; 4:180.

90. Lerner AB, Norland JJ: Vitiligo: the loss of pigment in skin, hair, and eyes: J Dermatol 1978; 5:1.

91. Porter JR, et al: The effect of vitiligo on sexual relationships, J Am Acad Dermatol 1990; 22:221.

92. Halder RM, et al: Childhood vitiligo, J Am Acad Dermatol 1987; 16:948.

93. Bolognia JL, Pawelek JM: Biology of hypopigmentation, J Am Acad Dermatol 1988; 19:217.

94. Cunliffe WJ, et al: Vitiligo, thyroid disease, and autoimmunity, Br J Dermatol 1968; 80:135.

95. Korkij W, et al: Tissue-specific autoantibodies and autoimmune disorders in vitiligo and alopecia areata: a retrospective study, J Cutan Pathol 1984; 11:522.

96. Njoo M, et al: The development of guidelines for the treatment of vitiligo, Clinical Epidemiology Unit of the Istituto Dermopatico dell'Immacolata-Istituto di Recovero e Cura a Carattere Scientifico (IDI-IRCCS) and the Archives of Dermatology, Arch Dermatol 1999; 135(12):1514.

97. Westerhof W, et al: Left-right comparison study of the combination of fluticasone propionate and UV-A vs. either fluticasone propionate or UV-A alone for the long-term treatment of vitiligo, Arch Dermatol 1999; 135(9):1061.

98. Scherschun L, Kim J, Lim H: Narrow-band ultraviolet B is a useful and well-tolerated treatment for vitiligo, J Am Acad Dermatol 2001; 44(6):999.

99. Njoo M, Bos J, Westerhof W: Treatment of generalized vitiligo in children with narrow-band (TL-01) UVB radiation therapy, J Am Acad Dermatol 2000; 42(2 Pt 1):245.

100. Lassus A, et al: Treament of vitiligo with oral methoxsalen and UVA, Photodermatology 1984; 1:170.

101. Falabella R, et al: On the pathogenesis of idiopathic guttate hypomelanosis, J Am Acad Dermatol 1987; 16:35.

102. Pasricha JS, Khaitan BK: Oral mini-pulse therapy with betamethasone in vitiligo patients having extensive or fast-spreading disease, Int J Dermatol 1993; 32:753.

103. Wallace M, et al: Numbers and differentiation status of melanocytes in idiopathic guttate hypomelanosis, J Cutan Pathol 1998; 25(7):375.

104. Pagnoni A, et al: Hypopigmented macules of photodamaged skin and their treatment with topical tretinoin, Acta Derm Venereol 1999; 79(4):305.

105. Ahkami R, Schwartz R: Nevus anemicus, Dermatology 1999; 198(4):327.

106. Mizutani H, et al: Loss of cutaneous delayed hypersensitivity reactions in nevus anemicus. Evidence for close concordance of cutaneous delayed hypersensitivity and endothelial E-selectin expression, Arch Dermatol 1997; 133(5):617.

107. Hurwitz S, Braverman IM: White spots in tuberous sclerosis, J Pediatr 1970; 77:587.

108. Fitzpatrick TB, et al: White leaf-shaped macules, earliest visible sign of tuberous sclerosis, Arch Dermatol 1968; 98:1.

109. Kurlemann G, Schuierer G: Images in clinical medicine. Ash-leaf spots in tuberous sclerosis, N Engl J Med 1998; 338(26):1887.

110. Bastiaens M, et al: Ephelides are more related to pigmentary constitutional host factors than solar lentigines, Pigment Cell Res 1999; 12(5):316.

111. Reid JD: Intestinal carcinoma in the Peutz-Jeghers syndrome, JAMA 1974; 229:833.

112. Papaioannon A, Critselis A: Malignant changes in the Peutz-Jeghers syndrome, N Engl J Med 1973; 289:694.

113. Andersen W, Labadie R, Bhawan J: Histopathology of solar lentigines of the face: a quantitative study, J Am Acad Dermatol 1997; 36(3 Pt 1):444.

114. Rafal ES, et al: Topical tretinoin (retinoic acid) treatment for liver spots associated with photodamage, N Engl J Med 1992; 326:368.

115. Kopera D, Hohenleutner U, Landthaler M: Q-switched ruby laser application is safe and effective for the management of actinic lentigo (topical glycolic acid is not), Acta Derm Venereol 1996; 76(6):461.

116. Grimes P: Melasma. Etiologic and therapeutic considerations, Arch Dermatol 1995; 131(12):1453.

117. Hassan I, et al: Hormonal milieu in the maintenance of melasma in fertile women, J Dermatol 1998; 25(8):510.

118. Sanchez NP, et al: Melasma: a clinical, light microscopic, ultrastructural, immunofluorescence study, J Am Acad Dermatol 1981; 4:698.

119. Griffiths CE, et al: Topical tretinoin (retinoic acid) improves melasma. A vehicle-controlled, clinical trial, Br J Dermatol 1993; 129:415.

120. Kimbrough-Green C, et al: Topical retinoic acid (tretinoin) for melasma in black patients. A vehicle-controlled clinical trial, Arch Dermatol 1994; 130(6):727.

121. Breathnach A: Melanin hyperpigmentation of skin: melasma, topical treatment with azelaic acid, and other therapies, Cutis 1996; 57(1 Suppl):36.

122. Cotellessa C, et al: The use of chemical peelings in the treatment of different cutaneous hyperpigmentations, Dermatol Surg 1999; 25(6):450.

123. Nouri K, et al: Combination treatment of melasma with pulsed CO_2 laser followed by Q-switched alexandrite laser: a pilot study, Dermatol Surg 1999; 25(6):494.

124. Bell SD, MacDonald DM: The prevalence of café-au-lait patches in tuberous sclerosis, Clin Exp Dermatol 1985; 10:562.

125. Alora M, Arndt K: Treatment of a café-au-lait macule with the erbium:YAG laser, J Am Acad Dermatol 2001; 45(4):566.

126. Shemer A, et al: Diabetic dermopathy and internal complications in diabetes mellitus, Int J Dermatol 1998; 37(2):113.

127. Dellavalle R, Gillum P: Erythema ab igne following heating/cooling blanket use in the intensive care unit, Cutis 2000; 66(2):136.

128. Hurwitz RM, Tisserand ME: Erythema ab igne, Arch Dermatol 1987; 123:21.

Benign Skin Tumors

Seborrheic Keratoses

Seborrheic keratoses (SKs) and nevi are the most common benign cutaneous neoplasms. SKs are of unknown origin and have no malignant potential. One must be familiar with all of the characteristics and variants of these lesions to differentiate them from other lesions and to prevent unnecessary destructive procedures.[1] SKs can be easily and quickly removed and, if the procedure is correctly executed, heal with little or no scarring. Most people develop at least one SK at some point in their lives. SKs appear in a substantial proportion of people younger than 30 years.[2] The term *senile keratosis* is no longer appropriate for these lesions. The number varies from less than 20 in most individuals to numerous lesions on the face or trunk. Patients refer to them as warts, but SKs do not contain human papilloma viruses.[3]

SURFACE CHARACTERISTICS. The surface of SKs is either smooth with tiny, round, embedded pearls or rough, dry, and cracked. They are sharply circumscribed and vary from 0.2 cm to more than 3 cm in diameter. They appear to be stuck to the skin surface and, in fact, occur totally within the epidermis. The surface characteristics vary with the age of the lesion and its location. Those on the extremities are often subtle, flat, or minimally raised and are slightly scaly with accentuated skin lines. Lesions on the face and trunk vary considerably in appearance, but the characteristics common to all lesions are the well-circumscribed border, the stuck-on appearance, and the variable tan-brown-black color (Figures 20-1 to 20-6). When the border is irregular and notched, the SK resembles a malignant melanoma.

Smooth or rough surfaced. The surface characteristics show considerable variation (see diagram on p. 700). Smooth-surfaced, dome-shaped tumors have white or black pearls of keratin, are 1 mm in diameter, and are embedded in the surface. These horn pearls are easily seen with a hand lens. The presence of horn cysts on the surface helps to confirm the diagnosis of an SK. Horn cysts are also found on the surface of some dermal nevi. The rough-surfaced SKs are the most common. They are oval-to-round, flattened domes with a granular or irregular surface that crumbles when picked.

SEBORRHEIC KERATOSIS

Irregular or smooth surface; marked papillomatosis causes an irregular surface that retains keratin

Epidermis thickens; immature keratinocytes accumulate

Horn cysts (horn pearls)

Focal keratination occurs to produce horn cysts

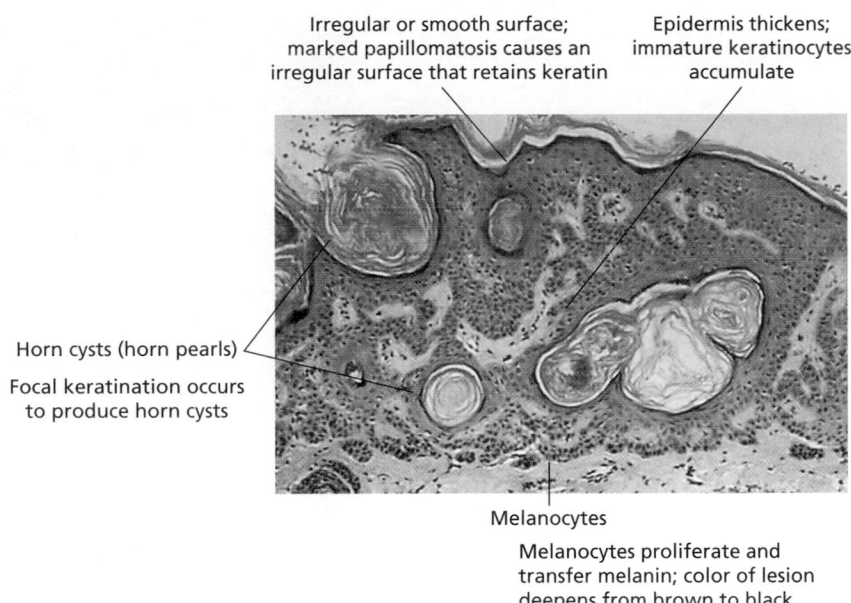

Melanocytes

Melanocytes proliferate and transfer melanin; color of lesion deepens from brown to black

Figure 20-1 Cross-section shows embedded horn cysts.

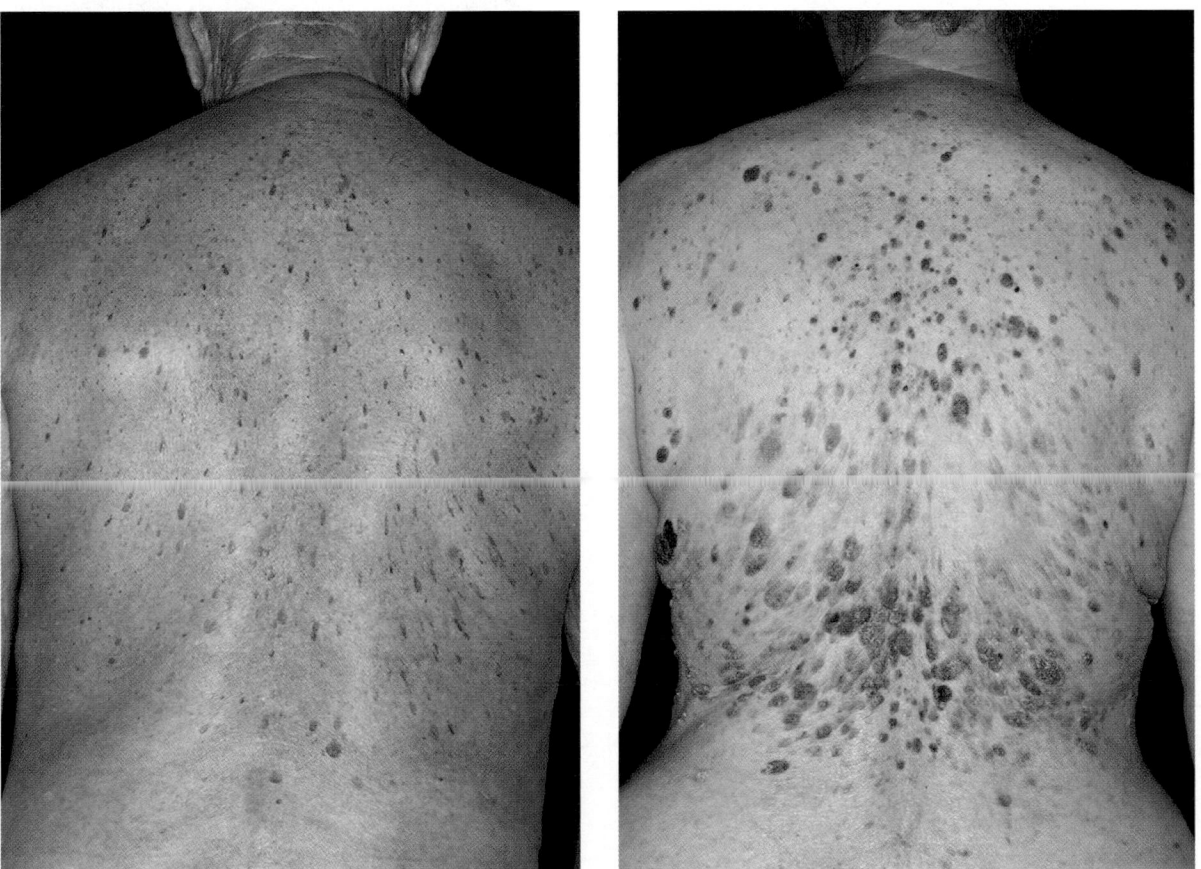

Figure 20-2 Lesions are very common on the back; an individual may have numerous lesions on the sun-exposed back and none on the buttocks.

SEBORRHEIC KERATOSIS

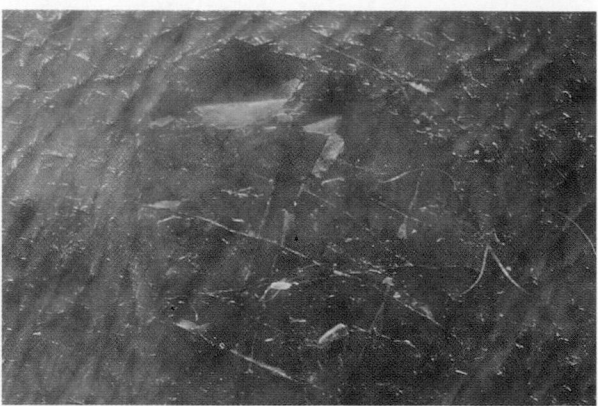

ROUGH-SURFACE LESIONS

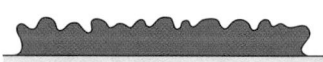

Flat; some scale; light color

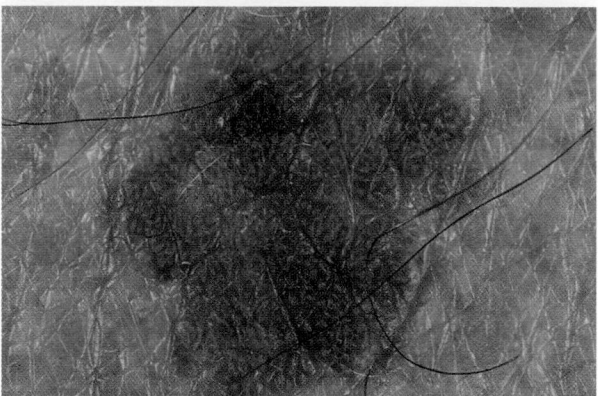

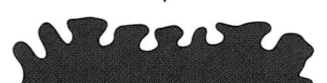

Height increase; lesion appears "stuck on" to surface; color darkens

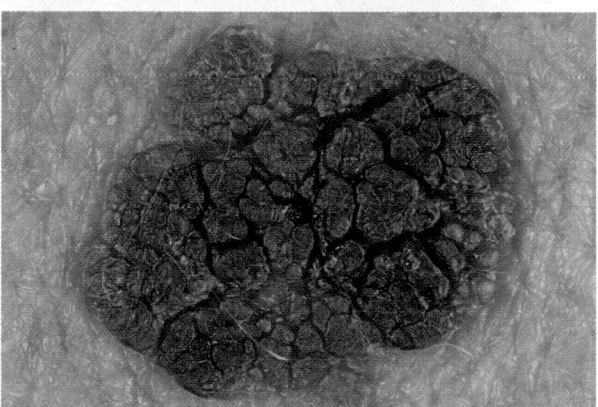

Deep surface cracks appear; keratin can be peeled off; brown or black

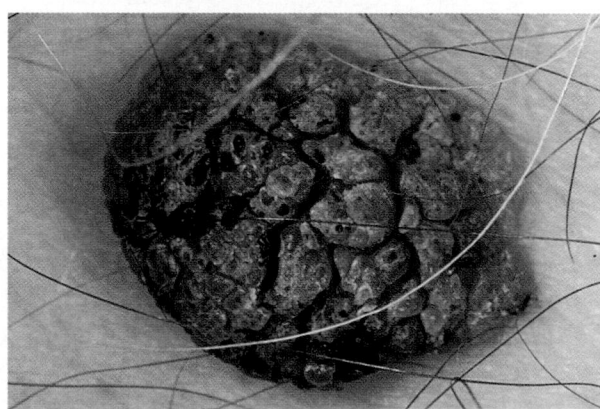

SEBORRHEIC KERATOSIS

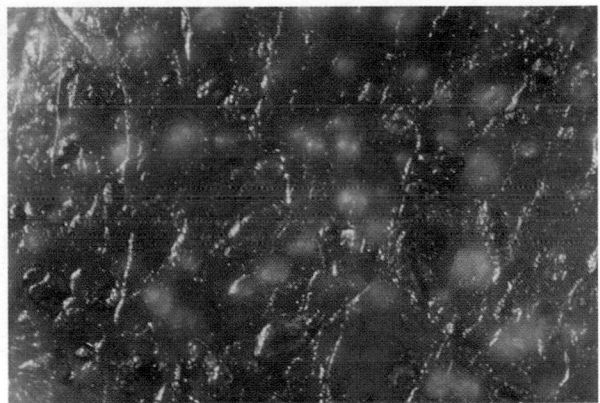

SMOOTH-SURFACE LESIONS

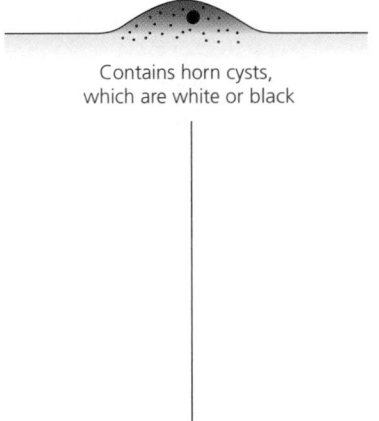

Contains horn cysts,
which are white or black

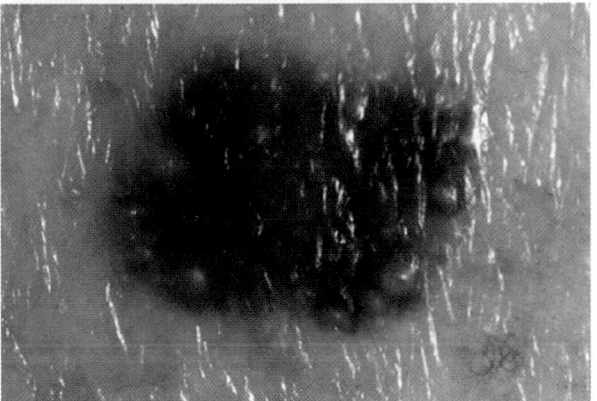

Height increases; horn cysts become
more numerous

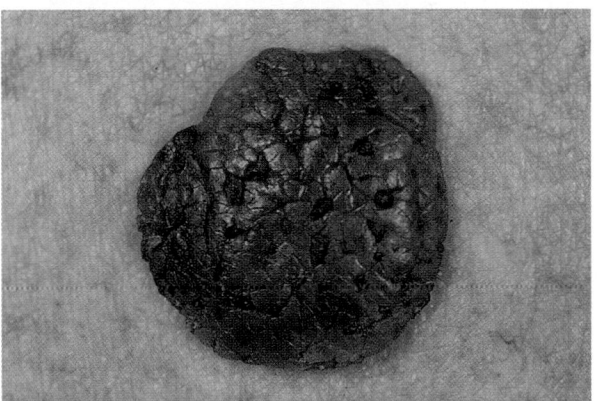

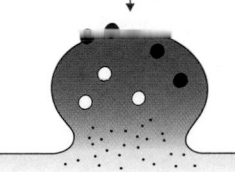

Smooth, dome-shaped papule;
horn cysts project from surface

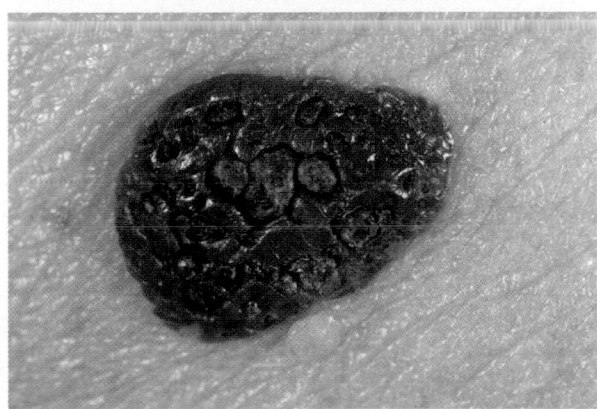

SEBORRHEIC KERATOSIS

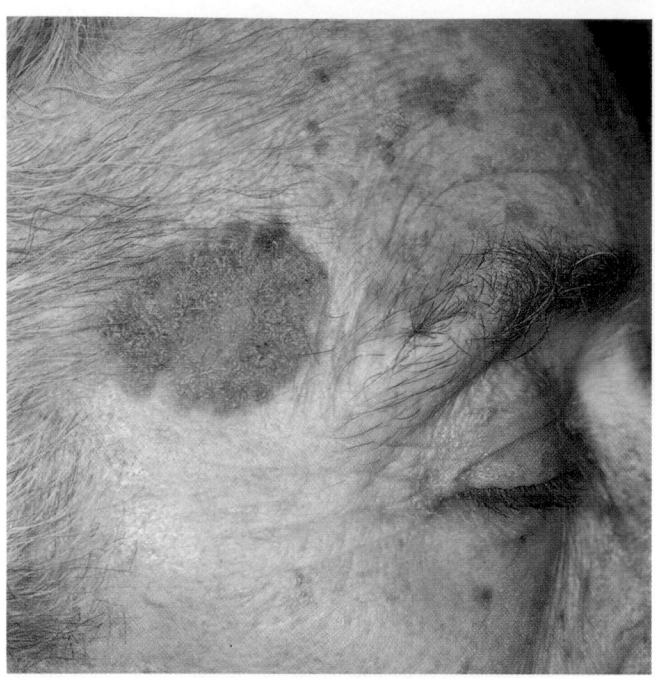

Figure 20-3 Very large lesions may form along the hairline and temple. Flat lesions are usually brown.

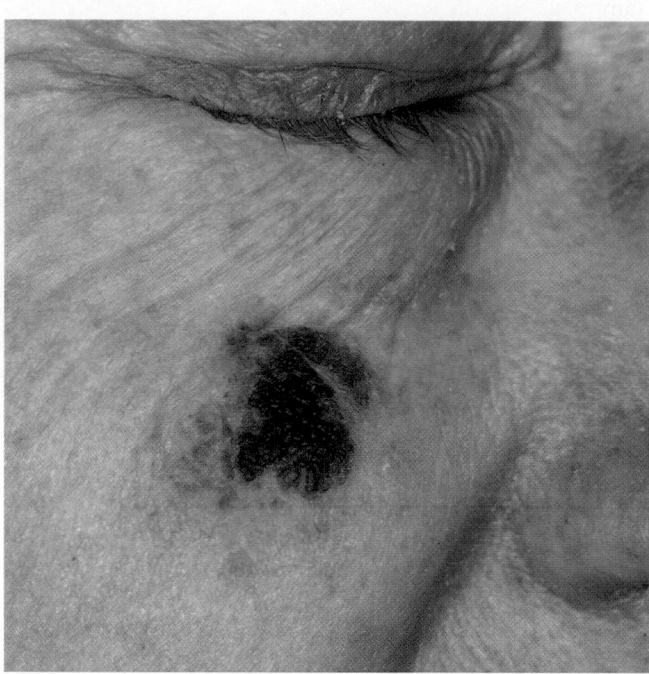

Figure 20-4 Thicker lesions may become dark brown or black.

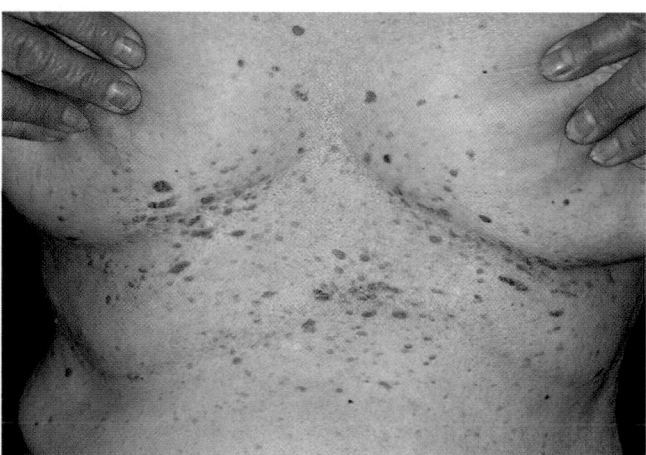

Figure 20-5 Lesions are commonly found under the breasts. Maceration may cause keratosis to become red and irritated.

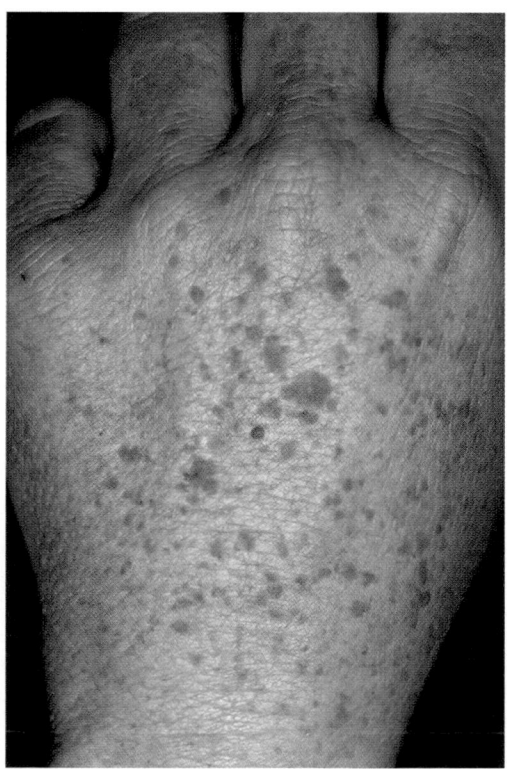

Figure 20-6 Sun exposure causes keratosis on the back of the hand in predisposed individuals.

SEBORRHEIC KERATOSIS VS. MALIGNANT MELANOMA. Many patients present with dark, irregular, sometimes irritated SKs and worry that they are melanomas. SKs can show many of the features of a malignant melanoma, including an irregular border and variable pigmentation (Figures 20-7 to 20-10). The key differential diagnostic features are the surface characteristics. Melanomas have a smooth surface that varies in elevation and in color, density, and shade. SKs preserve a uniform appearance over their entire surface. Examination with a hand lens is very helpful. Many SKs occur in sun-exposed areas.

ACCURACY OF DIAGNOSIS. When a clinical diagnosis of SK is made with confidence, the lesion is often left untreated or a destructive method of removal is used. The diagnostic accuracy must be high to justify such practices, which do not yield material for histopathologic confirmation. A diagnostic accuracy of greater than 99% was established by dermatologists in a study. The extremely high diagnostic accuracy of greater than 99% justifies common clinical practice. A biopsy should be performed in cases of diagnostic doubt.[4] Submit for histological examination all specimens that have been removed.[5]

MELANOMA MIMICS

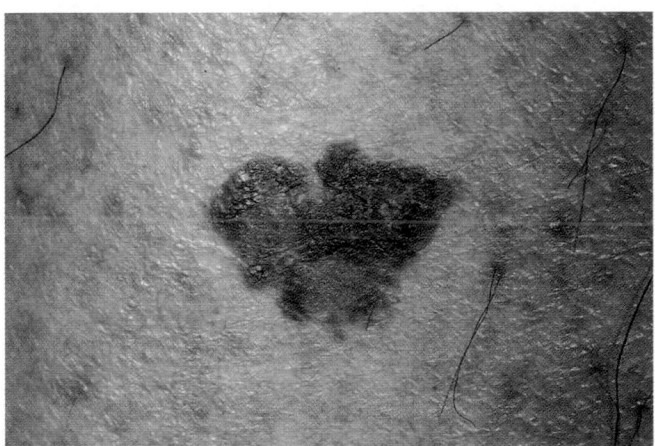

Figure 20-7 There is variation in pigmentation, and the border is irregular and notched, but the surface is regular with dense keratin.

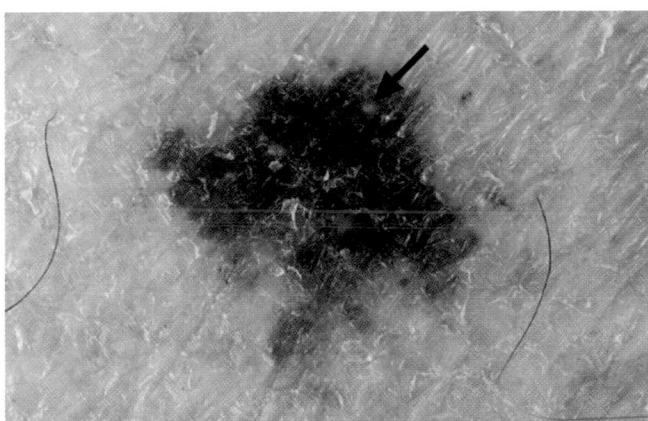

Figure 20-8 This black irregular lesion resembles a melanoma. The white horn pearl imbedded in the surface *(arrow)* supports the diagnosis of seborrheic keratosis.

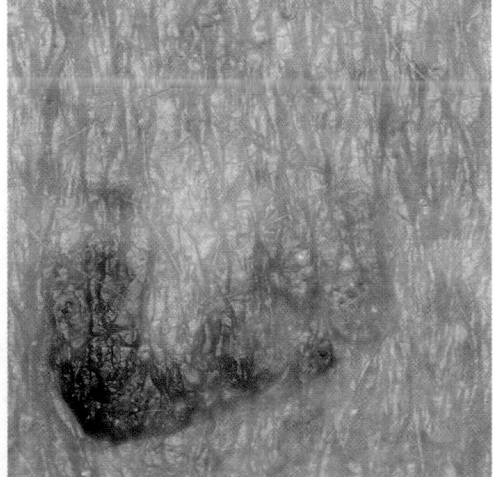

Figure 20-9 This flat lesion has many features of a superficial spreading melanoma. The colors are variable and the white area looks like an area of tumor regression.

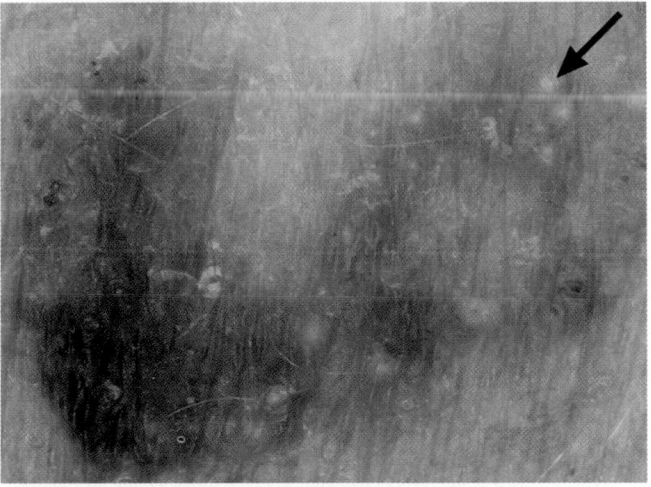

Figure 20-10 A magnified view shows several horn cysts *(arrow)* that are typically found in seborrheic keratoses and rarely present in melanoma

IRRITATED SEBORRHEIC KERATOSIS. Although generally asymptomatic, SKs can be a source of itching, especially in the elderly, who have a tendency to unconsciously manipulate these protruding growths. Irritation can be aggravated by chafing from clothing or from maceration in intertriginous areas, such as under the breasts and in the groin. When inflamed, SKs become slightly swollen and develop an irregular, red flare in the surrounding skin. Itching and erythema can then appear spontaneously in other SKs that have not been manipulated (Figure 20-11) and in areas without SKs. A halo of eczema can appear around SKs; the inflamed border is red, scaly, and may represent a localized form of nummular (coin-shaped) dermatitis.[6] The only treatment is to apply topical steroids or to remove all inflamed lesions. With continued inflammation, the SK loses most of its normal characteristics and becomes a bright red, oozing mass with a friable surface that itches intensely and resembles an advanced melanoma or a pyogenic granuloma.

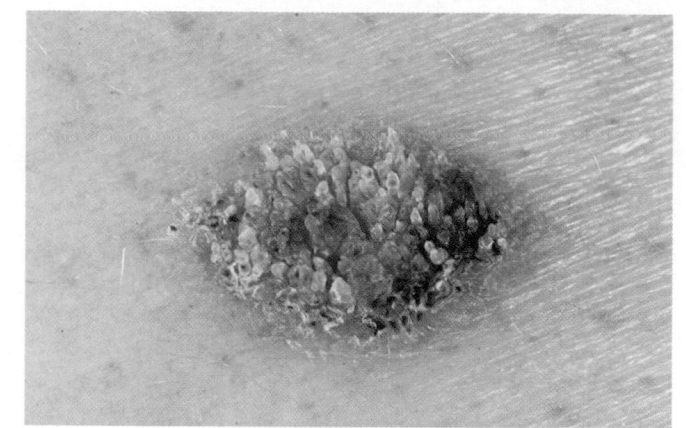

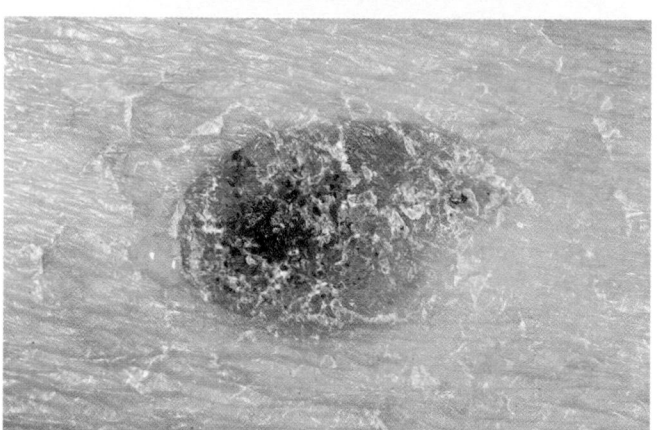

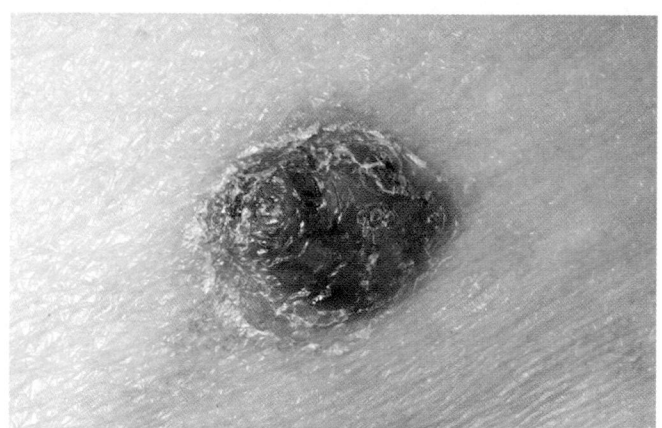

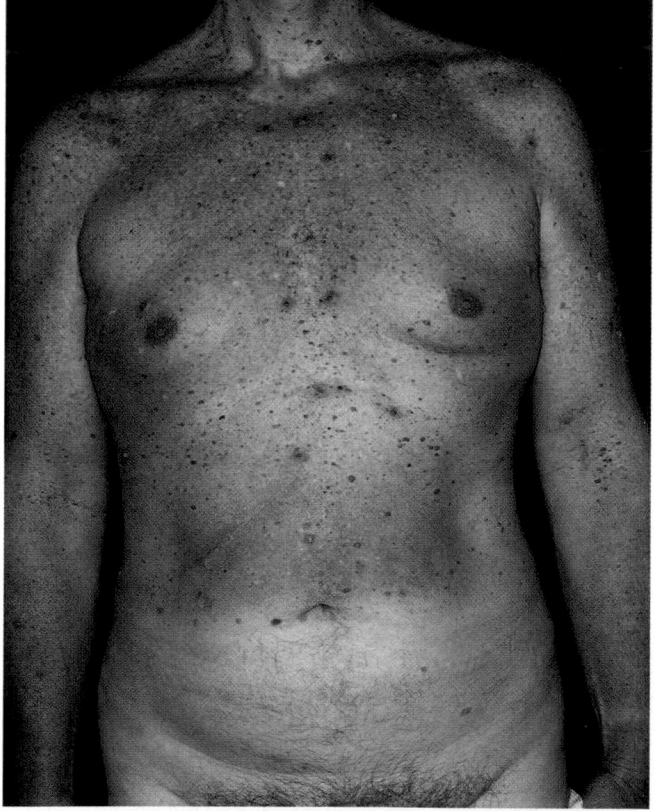

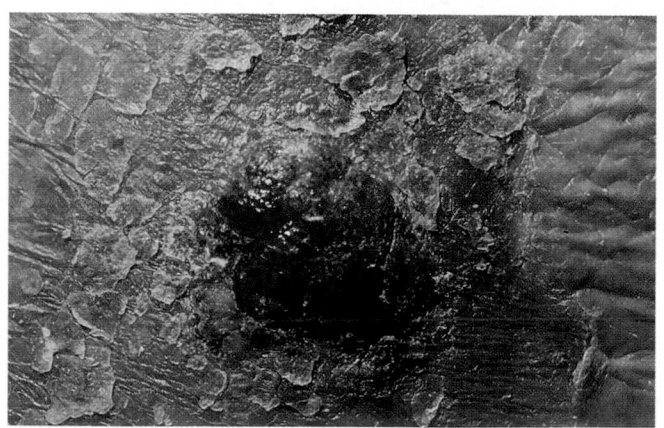

Figure 20-11 Irritated seborrheic keratosis. **A,** Most lesions are solitary but many keratoses may become inflamed at once. **B,** Minimal inflammation at the base. **C,** Surface characteristics are less distinct as inflammation intensifies. **D,** Dense scale and crust obliterate diagnostic features. **E,** This red, oozing mass has lost all diagnostic characteristics and resembles a pyogenic granuloma or melanoma.

SIGN OF LESER-TRÉLAT (ERUPTIVE SK AS A SIGN OF INTERNAL MALIGNANCY). The sudden appearance of or sudden increase in the number and size of SKs on noninflamed skin has been reported to be a sign of internal malignancy (see Figure 26-1). There is a controversy over the sign's validity. Several papers refute its existence,[7,8] but single case reports are regularly published.[9] The average age at the time of onset is 61 years. The most common type of associated malignancy is adenocarcinoma (69%); the stomach (40%) is most often involved. In one study, 70% of patients had paraneoplastic disorders such as acanthosis nigricans, acquired ichthyosis, and lanugo hair.[10] Paraneoplastic disorders are cutaneous changes that signal the presence of various internal malignancies. A tumor-produced humoral factor (e.g., transforming growth factor-alpha) could be responsible for the acute eruption of the seborrheic keratoses.

Most patients have metastatic disease when the keratoses appear.[11] The SKs often parallel the course of the malignancy, decreasing in number and size following surgical or chemotherapeutic intervention and returning with recurrence of the cancer, but this is not always the case. Patients with numerous SKs need not be evaluated for malignancy unless the lesions erupt abruptly. Erythrodermatous or eczematous skin[12] can promote the appearance of keratoses, and association with internal malignancy would not be considered in this instance.[13] Keratoses that appear during the course of widespread inflammatory skin disease may regress after the inflammation resolves.[14]

TREATMENT. Lesions are removed for cosmetic purposes or to eliminate a source of irritation. Since these growths appear entirely within the epidermis, scalpel excision is unnecessary. They are easily removed with cryosurgery or curettage. Lesions to be curetted are first anesthetized with Xylocaine introduced with a needle. With multiple strokes, a small curette is smoothly drawn through the lesion (see Chapter 27). SKs on the face or on other areas with inappreciable underlying support can be softened before curettage with the electric needle. Monsel's solution controls bleeding, and the site remains exposed to heal. Some lesions are tenaciously fixed to the skin and resist curettage; others are on sites that are difficult to curette, such as the eyelid. These can be dissected with curved, blunt-tipped scissors. Cryosurgery is effective for thin SKs but post-treatment hyperpigmentation or hypopigmentation is a possible side effect.

Stucco Keratoses

Stucco keratoses, sometimes referred to as barnacles, are common, nearly inconspicuous, papular, warty lesions[15] occurring on the lower legs (Figure 20-12), especially around the Achilles tendon area, the dorsum of the foot, and the forearms of the elderly. The 1- to 10-mm, round, very dry, stuck-on lesions are considered by most patients to be simply manifestations of dry skin. The dry surface scale is easily picked intact from the skin without bleeding, but it recurs shortly thereafter. The lesions can be removed with curettage or cryosurgery.

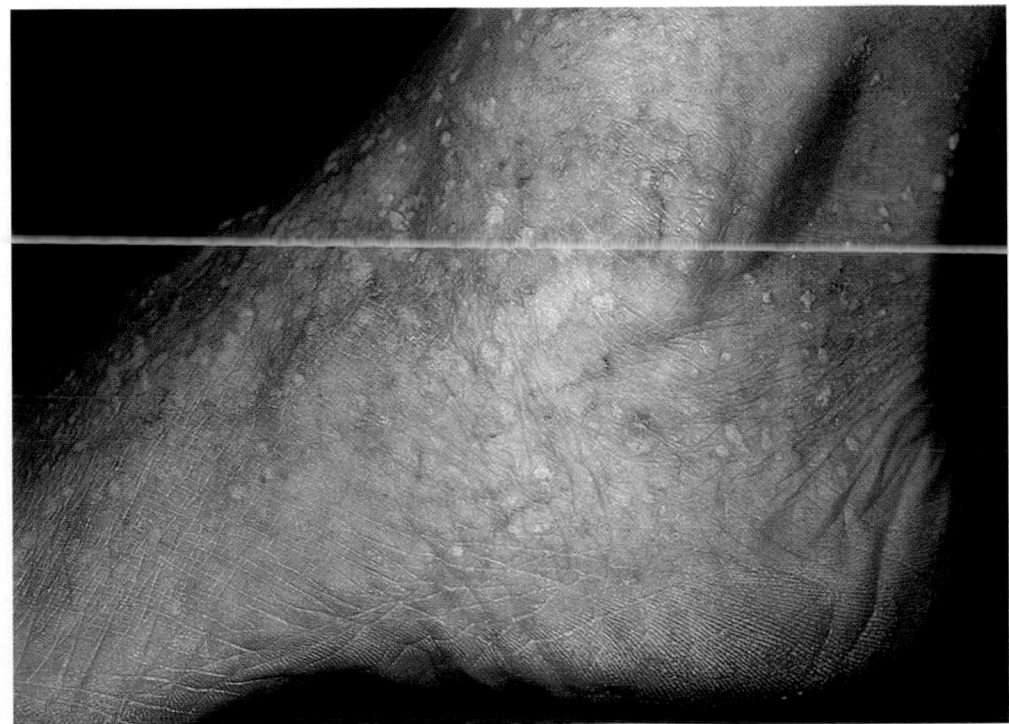

Figure 20-12 Stucco keratosis. Multiple small, scaling lesions in a typical location.

Dermatosis Papulosa Nigra

Young and middle-aged blacks may develop multiple brown-black, 2- to 3-mm, smooth, dome-shaped papules on the face (Figure 20-13).[16] They probably represent a type of SK. Patients who desire removal should be informed that white, hypopigmented scarring may result. The patient's response should be determined by curetting or freezing one or two lesions and permitting them to heal completely.

Cutaneous Horn

Cutaneous horn refers to a hard, conical projection composed of keratin and resembling an animal horn. It occurs on the face, ears, and hands (Figure 20-14) and may become very long. Warts, SKs, actinic keratosis, and squamous cell carcinoma may all retain keratin and produce horns. Cryosurgery, local scissor excision, or surgical excision performs treatment.

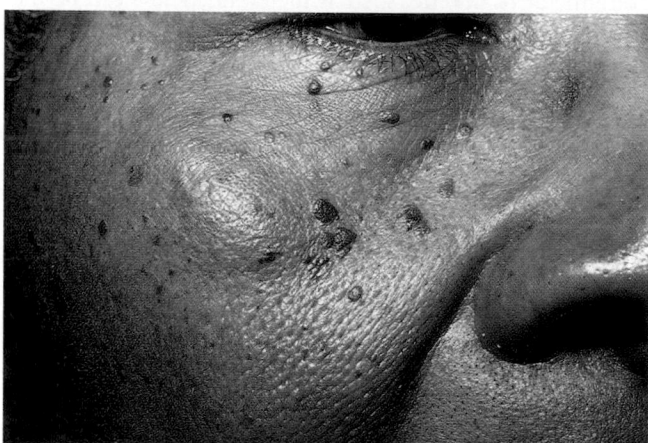

Figure 20-13 Dermatosis papulosa nigra. Lesions begin after puberty in blacks and slowly increase in number. They are smooth, brown-black papules that occur on the malar area of the face and forehead.

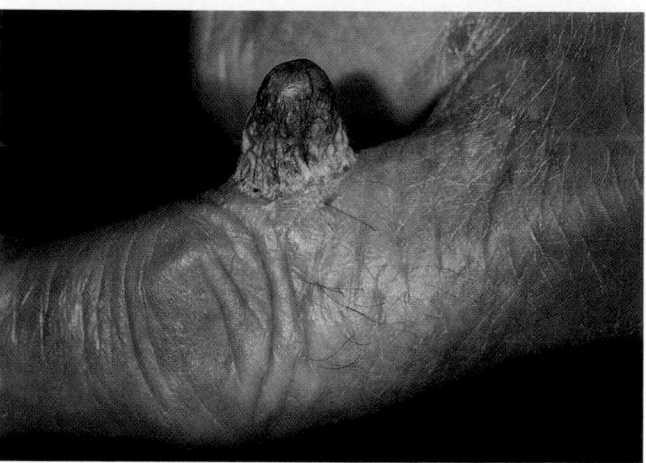

Figure 20-14 Cutaneous horn. A biopsy showed this lesion to be an actinic keratosis.

Skin Tags (Acrochordon) and Polyps

SKIN TAGS. Skin tags are common tumors found in approximately 25% of males and females. They occur more often and in greater number in obese patients. The most frequent affected area is the axilla (48%), followed by the neck (35%) and inguinal region. The majority of carriers (71%) have no more than three skin tags per location. They can begin in the second decade, with a steady increase in frequency up to the fifth decade; above this age there is no further growth.[19] The skin tags begin as a tiny, brown or skin-colored, oval excrescence attached by a short, broad-to-narrow stalk (Figures 20-15 to 20-18). With time, the tumor can increase to 1 cm as the stalk becomes long and narrow. Patients complain that when they wear clothing or jewelry, these tumors are annoying. The stalks are easily removed by scissor excision or with a light touch of the electrocautery. Local anesthesia is usually not necessary.

POLYPS. Skin polyps have a long, narrow stalk and a broad tip (Figures 20-19 to 20-21). Sometimes they become twisted and compromise the blood supply. Lesions then turn dark brown or black. This sudden change is alarming to patients (see Figure 20-21). Polypoid growths may be skin tags, nevi, or melanomas. Polyps occur on the eyelids (see Figure 20-16), groin, axilla, or any skin surface except the palms and soles.

SKIN TAGS AND COLONIC POLYPS. A series of articles claimed that there is an association between skin tags and adenomatous polyps. A study of 150 consecutive patients who underwent colonoscopy concluded that skin tags as markers of colon neoplasms are insufficient to warrant endoscopic examination.

SKIN TAGS AND POLYPS

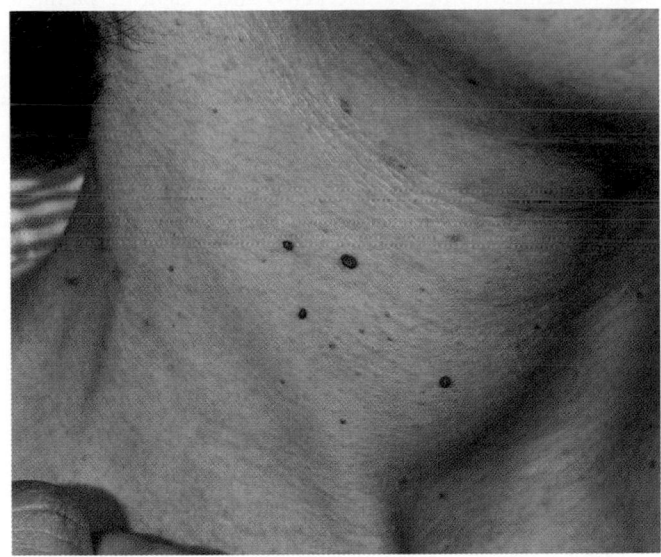

Figure 20-15 Multiple round, black, oval excrescences attached by a short broad-to-narrow stalk.

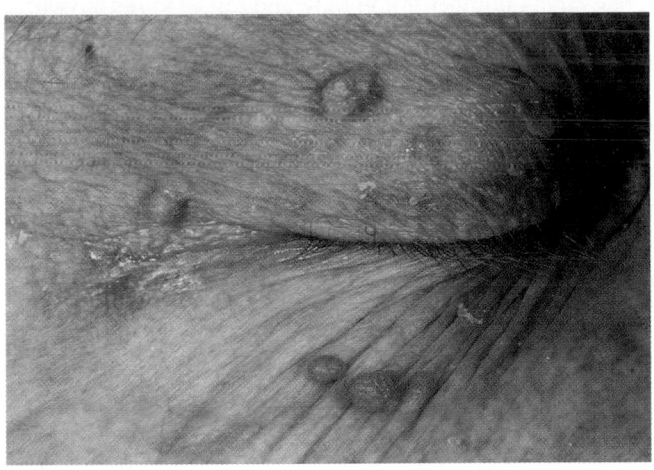

Figure 20-16 Skin tags and polyps are frequently present on the lids.

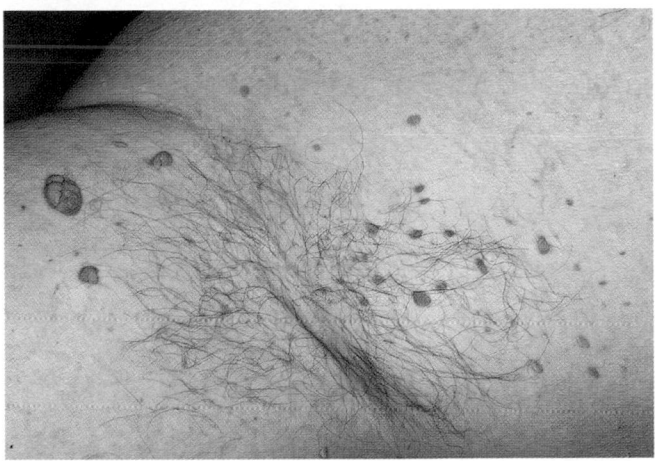

Figure 20-17 Skin tags are commonly found in the axilla. There is great variation in the number of lesions.

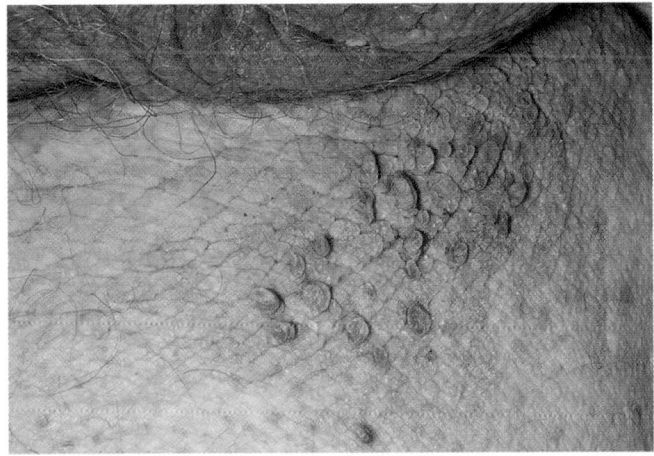

Figure 20-18 Skin tags may be numerous in the groin. Obesity predisposes to this dense clustered pattern.

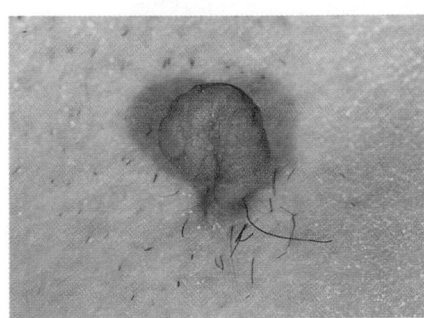

Figure 20-19 A polypoid mass on a long, narrow stalk. Some nevi have an identical appearance.

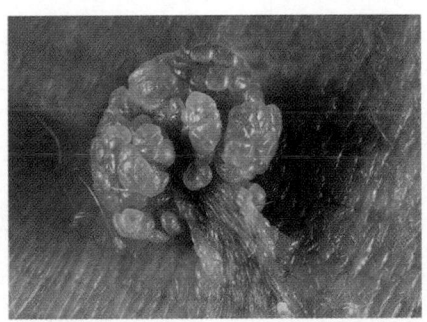

Figure 20-20 Polyp. Polyps contain a long stalk and a broad tip. A biopsy showed this lesion to be a dermal nevus.

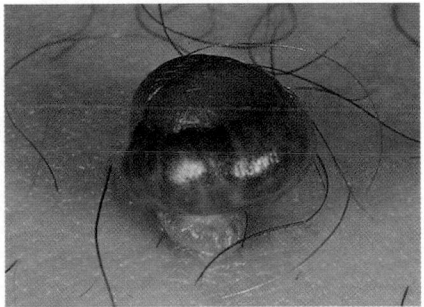

Figure 20-21 Infarcted polyp. Torsion on the stalk can compromise the blood supply. Lesions turn blue-black in hours to days.

Dermatofibroma

Dermatofibromas are common, benign, asymptomatic-to-slightly itchy lesions occurring more frequently in females. They vary in number from 1 to 10 and can be found anywhere on the extremities and trunk, but they are most likely to occur on the anterior surface of the lower legs. Dermatofibromas may not be tumors; rather, they may represent a fibrous reaction to trauma, a viral infection, or an insect bite. They appear as 3- to 10-mm, slightly raised, pink-brown, sometimes scaly, hard growths that retract beneath the skin surface during attempts to compress and elevate them with the thumb and index finger (Figures 20-22 to 20-25). Multiple dermatofibromas (i.e., more than 15) are very rare but have been reported with systemic lupus erythematosus,[20,21] with and without immunosuppressive therapy. Dermatoscopic examination shows a central white scarlike patch and a delicate pigment network at the periphery (see Figure 20-40).[22]

TREATMENT. Some patients object to the color of the lesion and therefore request excision. These lesions are most commonly found on the lower legs, where elliptic excisions closed with sutures may result in wide, unsightly scars. An alternative is to shave the brown surface with a #15 surgical blade and allow the wound to granulate and reepithelialize. The healed area remains hard because a portion of the fibrous tissue has remained. The brown color may reappear in some lesions. Conservative cryosurgery may also eliminate the color and part of the tumor.[23]

DERMATOFIBROMA

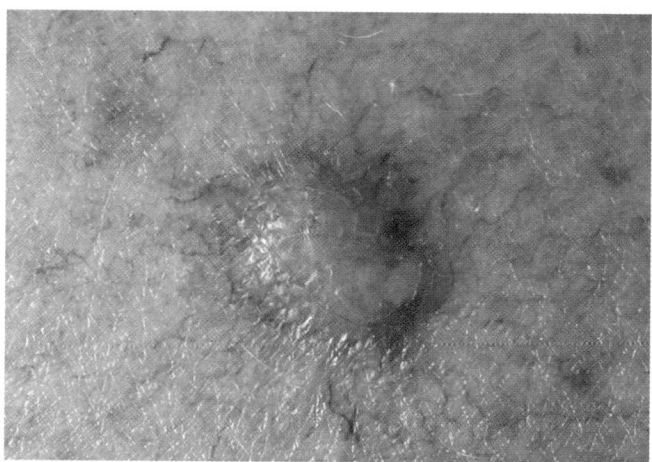

Figure 20-22 Early lesions have a well defined border with an irregular red surface. Brown pigmentation may occur at the periphery after months or years. Pigmentation may extend onto the lesion but almost never reaches the center. Patients often suspect melanoma at this stage.

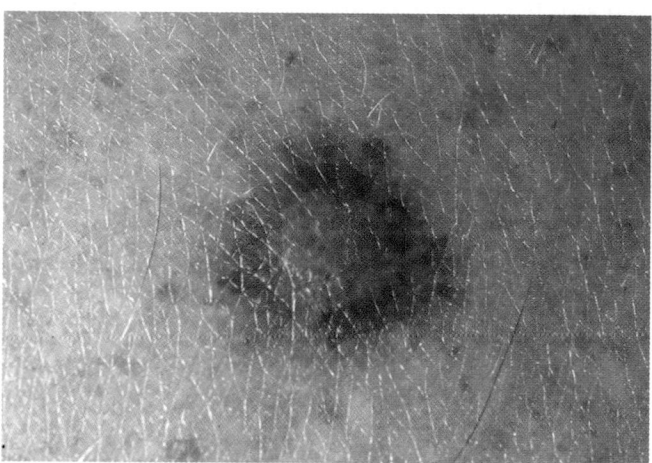

Figure 20-23 A typical lesion on the lower leg that is slightly elevated, round, and hyperpigmented, with a scaling surface.

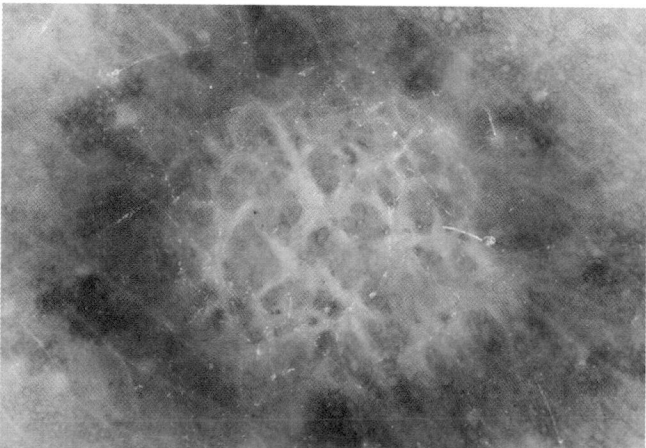

Figure 20-24 Dermoscopy (see p. 798) reveals a white lacy center surrounded by a uniform network.

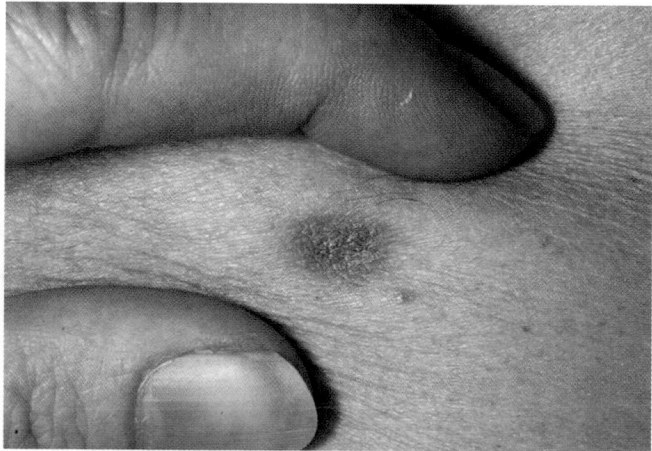

Figure 20-25 Retraction sign. Dermatofibromas retract beneath the skin during attempts to compress and elevate them.

Hypertrophic Scars and Keloids

Injury or surgery in a predisposed individual can result in an abnormally large scar. A hypertrophic scar is inappropriately large but remains confined to the wound site and in time regrooooo; a keloid extends beyond the margins of injury (Figures 20-26 to 20-29) and usually is constant and stable without any tendency to subside.[24] Hypertrophic scars may regress with time and occur earlier after injury (usually within 4 weeks); keloidal scars may begin later, even years after the event. There are histologic differences between hypertrophic scars and keloids. Large collagen bundles occur in keloidal scars but not in hypertrophic scars. Keloids are often symptomatic, and complaints arise because of tenderness, pain, and hyperesthesia, particularly in the early stages of development. Keloids are most common on the shoulders and chest, but they may occur on any skin surface. Blacks are more susceptible and sometimes are victims of facial keloids. Some patients with cystic acne of the back and chest form numerous keloidal scars.

TREATMENT. There is no routinely effective therapy for all keloids, but a variety of treatment methods exists,[25,26,27] including intralesional steroid injection, surgical correction, cryotherapy, compression therapy, and irradiation.

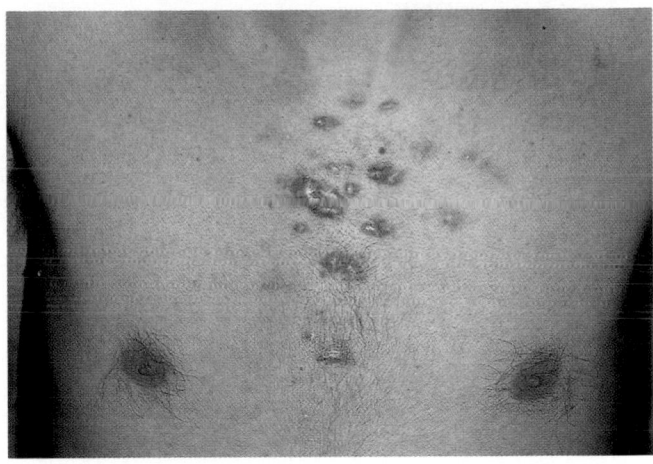

Figure 20-27 Keloids form in predisposed individuals following cystic acne.

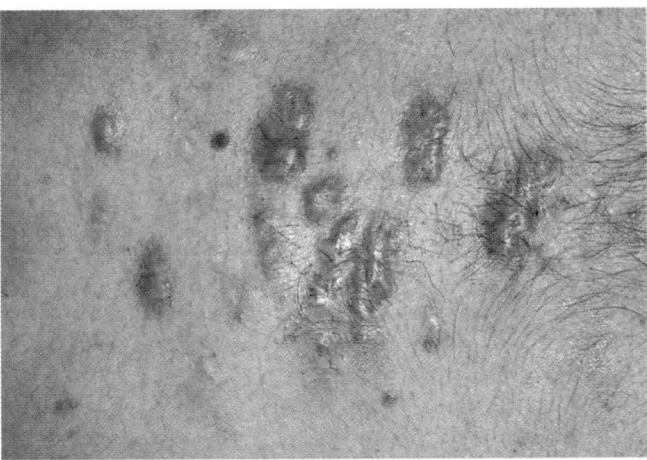

Figure 20-28 Keloids on the chest and extremities are raised with a flat surface. The base is wider than the top.

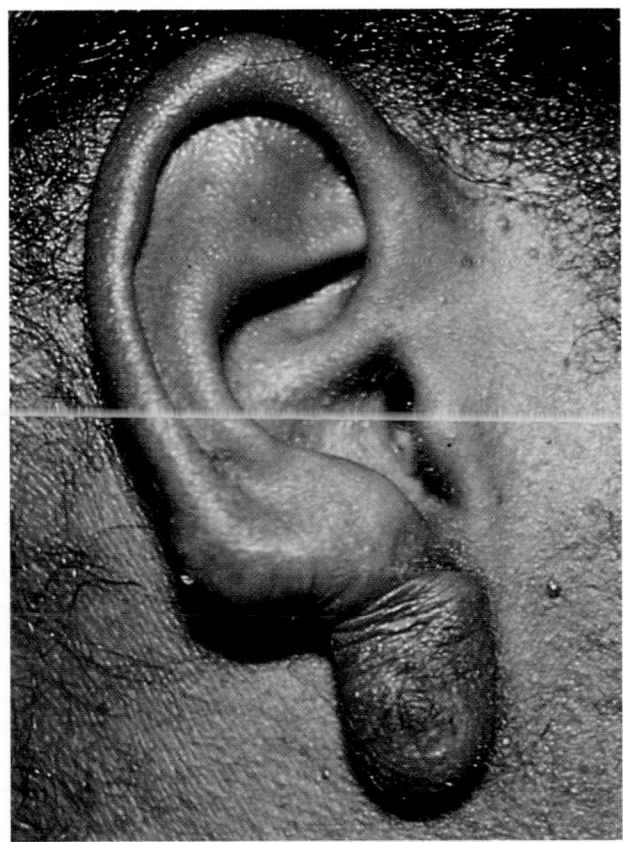

Figure 20-26 Keloid. Huge keloids may form on the ear lobes after any surgical procedure.

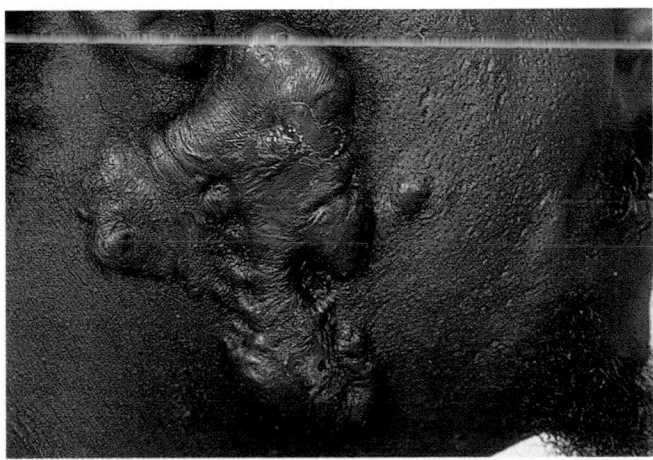

Figure 20-29 Blacks develop keloids most commonly on the earlobes and face.

INTRALESIONAL STEROID INJECTIONS. Fresh, small, and narrow lesions are treated with intralesional injections of corticosteroids every 2 to 4 weeks. Early keloids have softer proliferating connective tissue and are more inclined to improve with intralesional injections than are older, inactive lesions. When the lesion shrinks to near the skin surface, the frequency and concentration of injections should be decreased to avoid overcompensation and telangiectasia. Inducing atrophy with an intralesional injection of triamcinolone acetonide (Kenalog) 10 to 40 mg/ml is adequate for most small lesions; a 27- or 30-gauge needle is used. The 40 mg/ml concentration is preferred for most patients. To distribute the suspension evenly, the triamcinolone should be injected while continuously advancing the needle. Particles of steroid that have not been properly dispersed remain visible as white flecks in the scar tissue. The pressure of the injection should be firm until the lesion blanches. Light cryosurgery before the injection facilitates the process. Nitrogen is applied briefly for 2 to 4 seconds until the skin frosts. The keloid is injected 10 to 15 minutes later. This allows better dispersal of the steroid and minimizes deposition into surrounding normal tissue.[28]

SURGERY AND INTRALESIONAL STEROID INJECTIONS. Surgical excision removes the bulk of the scar and has the potential to replace a broad-based scar with a thin scar. Surgical removal alone is associated with a 55% to 100% recurrence rate,[25] but better results are realized when intralesional steroids are used following surgery. A typical treatment program involves injecting triamcinolone acetonide 10 to 40 mg/ml into the wound edges after excision. Treatment of the healed site is repeated at 2- to 4-week intervals for 6 months.

CRYOTHERAPY. Cryotherapy can produce flattening in some patients. In one study, cryotherapy with a hand-held liquid nitrogen spray unit resulted in complete flattening in 73% of keloids, most of which were less than 2 years old. At each treatment session, the entire lesion was treated with two or three freeze-thaw cycles. Lesions required 2 to 10 treatment sessions. A topical antibiotic cream and dressing were applied each day during the 1-month healing process. Side effects were limited to hypopigmentation and atrophy.[28] Cryotherapy has been used with corticosteroid injections. Darker skinned patients are at greater risk for hypopigmentation.[29]

SILICONE GEL SHEETING. The effectiveness of silicone gel sheeting (e.g., Epi-Derm, Sil-K, Cica-Care, ReJuveness, DuraSil, Silastic Gel Sheeting) and other occlusive dressings in treating keloidal and hypertrophic scars is uncertain. It is claimed that these dressings can prevent keloids from recurring after surgery. In a controlled analysis of fresh surgical incisions, silicone gel sheeting significantly inhibited the formation of hypertrophic scars. Sheeting is used for at least 12 hours daily for 2 months.[30] Beneficial effects are not related to pressure.[31]

RADIATION THERAPY WITH SURGERY. Radiation after surgical excision can prevent recurrence of keloidal scars in approximately 75% of cases at 1-year follow-up. This is higher than the rate controls treated with surgical excision alone, which appear to be approximately 40%. The most frequently used treatment was superficial x rays of 900 cGy or greater in fractions given within 10 days of surgery. Radiation is usually given within 24 hours after surgery to subdue the second-generation fibroblasts. It should be performed within 10 days of the surgery and is of no additional benefit when performed before surgery.[24]

5-FLUOROURACIL. 5-fluorouracil (50 mg/cc) intralesionally is used in the treatment of inflamed hypertrophic scars, both as an individual agent and with low-dose intralesional corticosteroids plus pulsed dye laser therapy. Frequent initial injections (once to thrice weekly) were found to be more efficacious with decreasing frequency (weekly to monthly) during a period of stabilization and resolution of the scars. The combination of 5-FU and Kenalog was more effective and less painful. The addition of the pulsed dye laser treatments simultaneous with injection therapy was found to be most effective.[32]

BLEOMYCIN. Bleomycin may be effective. In one study bleomycin (1.5 IU/ml) was dripped onto the scars, after infiltration with local anesthetic, and then the skin was punctured repeatedly with a 25-gauge needle to allow penetration into the dermis. Between 2 to 5 treatments were required at 1- to 4-month intervals. Complete flattening was obtained in 3 of the 7 keloidal scars, with highly significant flattening (90%) in the others.[33]

PULSED DYE LASER. The 585-nm pulsed dye laser is effective in reducing symptoms, color, and height in keloidal scars.[34] Multiple treatment sessions are suggested for achieving greater response.[35]

Keratoacanthoma

Keratoacanthoma (KA) is a relatively common, benign, epithelial tumor that was previously considered to be a variant of squamous cell carcinoma. The etiology is unknown. No human papillomavirus-DNA sequences were detected in lesions by polymerase chain reaction.[36] It is a disease of the elderly (mean age, 64 years) with an annual incidence rate of 104 per 100,000.[37] It is not associated with internal malignancy. There may be a seasonal presentation of keratoacanthoma that suggests that ultraviolet radiation has an acute effect on the development of KA.[38] KAs may develop in sites of previous trauma.

Most cases are the "crateriform" type, which grow rapidly then undergo spontaneous regression. Less than 2% belong to the rare destructive variants with no regression and persistent invasive growth. These are referred to as keratoacanthoma marginatum centrifugum and mutilating keratoacanthomas and can lead to severe defects.

Muir-Torre syndrome is a rare autosomal dominant genodermatosis that is characterized by the presence of at least one sebaceous gland tumor and a minimum of one internal malignancy. Keratoacanthomas have been noted in 23% of patients. The most commonly associated neoplasms are colorectal (61%) and genitourinary (22%).[39]

KA begins as a smooth, dome-shaped, red papule that resembles molluscum contagiosum. In a few weeks the tumor may rapidly expand to 1 or 2 cm and develop a central keratin-filled crater that is frequently filled with crust (Figure 20-30). The growth retains its smooth surface, unlike a squamous cell carcinoma. Untreated, growth stops in approximately 6 weeks, and the tumor remains unchanged for an indefinite period. In the majority of cases it then regresses slowly over 2 to 12 months and frequently heals with scarring. The limbs, particularly the sun-exposed hands and arms, are the most common site; the trunk is the second most common site, but KA may occur on any skin surface, including the anal area.[40] On occasion, multiple KAs appear, or a single lesion extends over several centimeters. These variants resist treatment and are unlikely to undergo spontaneous remission.

DIFFERENTIATING SQUAMOUS CELL CARCINOMA FROM KERATOACANTHOMA. Squamous cell carcinoma (SCC) and KA are sometimes difficult to distinguish by histopathological examination, since cytological features are similar in both tumors. Many of the criteria commonly used for the differential diagnosis of SCC and KA are not reliable. Atypical or difficult cases should therefore be considered and treated as SCC.[41]

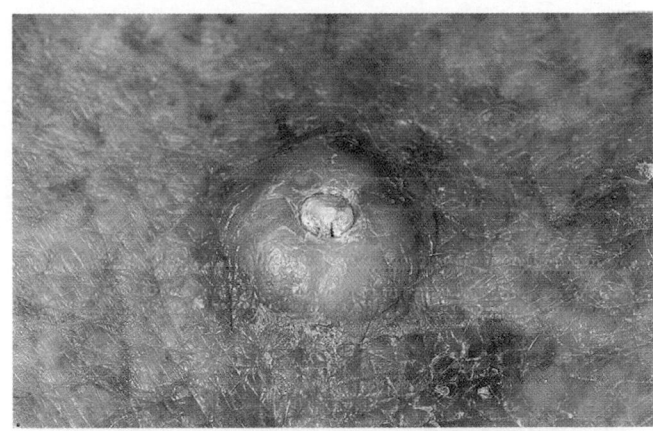

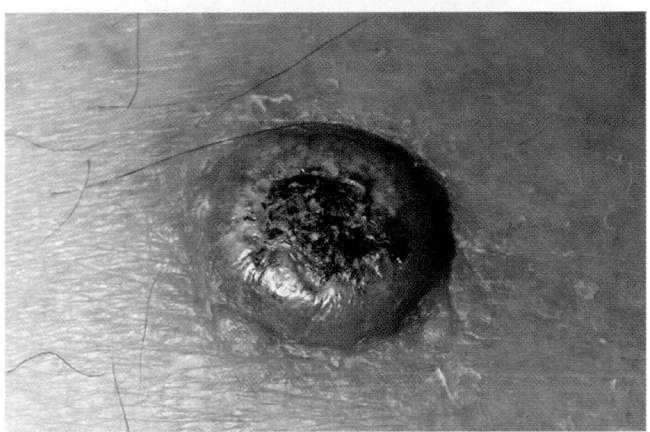

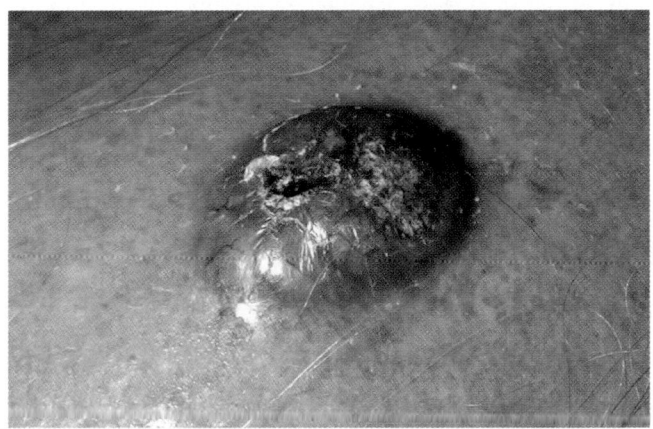

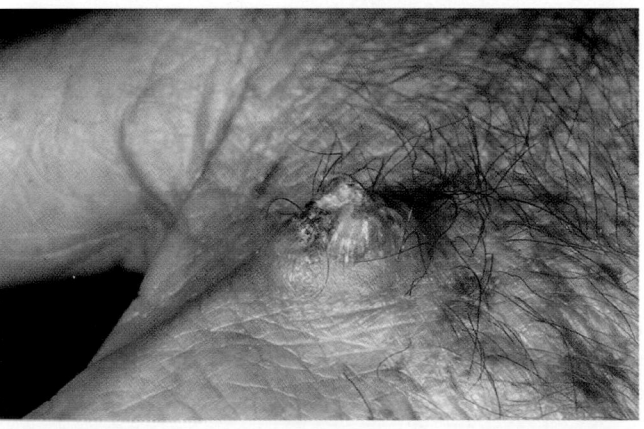

Figure 20-30 Keratoacanthoma. Lesions are solitary, smooth, dome-shaped red papules or nodules. They have a central keratin plug. Most occur on sun-exposed surfaces of the face and dorsum of the upper extremities.

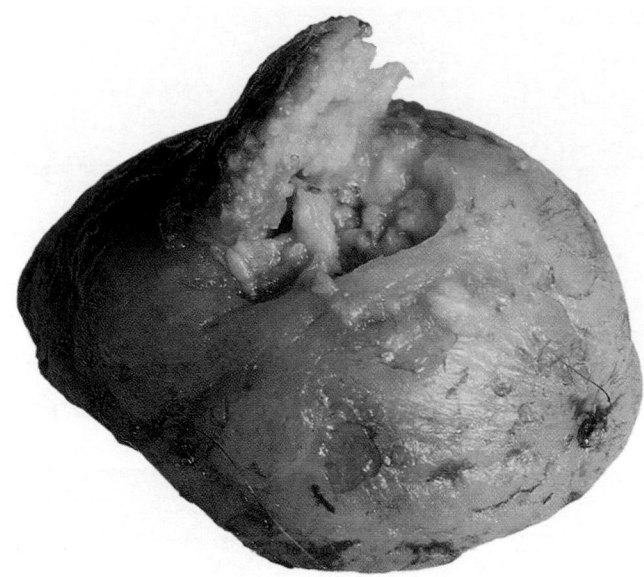

Figure 20-31 The central crust has been elevated from this blunt dissected lesion.

TREATMENT. There is no advantage to waiting for spontaneous regression to occur, since most KAs ultimately heal with scarring. KAs are treated surgically or medically. KAs may recur.

SURGERY. Electrodesiccation and curettage[42] or blunt dissection (Figure 20-31)[43] (see Chapter 27) are efficient and effective for smaller lesions. Excision is effective for large tumors.

5-FLUOROURACIL (TOPICAL). Topical 5% fluorouracil cream (Efudex) applied three times a day in the rapid growth phase cured most lesions in 1 to 6 weeks.[44,45] If possible the central crust should be removed to enhance penetration of medicine. The cream is applied to the lesion and its immediate vicinity, preferably under tape occlusion. Pretreatment with 6% salicylic acid gel (Keralyt) or 40% urea cream (Vanamide) for lesions on the forearms, hands, or legs enhances penetration of the 5-fluorouracil cream. Lesions on the face and lips may clear in 1 or 2 weeks, but as long as 6 weeks is required for lesions in other areas to respond.

5-FLUOROURACIL (INTRALESIONAL INJECTION). Excellent results have been reported with 5-fluorouracil injections.[44,46] The tumor is injected with the undiluted solution of 5-fluorouracil 50 mg/ml (available as fluorouracil injection in 500 mg/10 ml ampules). The usual amount is 0.1 to 2 ml, depending on the size of the tumor, injected tangentially into the slopes and then under the tumor. Extravasation of 5-fluorouracil from the central crater causes the amounts absorbed to be less than the amounts injected. Injections are given at 1- to 4-week intervals, depending on the response to treatment. Repeat injections are postponed if a lesion is undergoing necrosis. Patients should be evaluated at weekly intervals. This technique is especially useful for large KAs in difficult locations.[47] Intralesional 5-fluorouracil may be ineffective for older KAs that are not rapidly proliferating. Reported time for healing varies from 1 to 9 weeks.

IMIQUIMOD. Topical treatment with imiquimod cream (Aldara) every other day for 4 to 12 weeks caused complete regression in 4 patients. No recurrence occurred.[48]

PODOPHYLLUM RESIN. Podophyllum (20%) in compound tincture of benzoin or alcohol may cure KAs. Remove the central crust and apply podophyllum with a cotton swab. Repeat the treatment every 2 weeks until the lesion disappears.

METHOTREXATE (INTRALESIONAL INJECTION). Nine patients with solitary KAs were treated with intralesional methotrexate (MTX). MTX is injected superficially and directly into the lesion at a dose of 12.5 mg/ml. Injections are given at 2-week intervals. Necrosis of the lesion usually begins 5 to 8 days after injection. If complete response is not obtained after two injections, excision is indicated. The mean time to clearing was 3 weeks, with a range of 2 to 4 weeks. All lesions cleared completely; none recurred. Total cumulative dose ranged from 5 to 50 mg. The average amount of MTX per injection was 15 mg. No side effects were noted, and cosmetic results were very good.[49] Pancytopenia after treatment of keratoacanthoma by single lesional methotrexate infiltration is reported.[50]

INTERFERON ALFA-2a (INTRALESIONAL INJECTION). Six large KAs were treated with intralesional interferon alfa-2a. Regression occurred in five cases in 3 to 7 weeks, with excellent cosmetic results. The main side effect was pain during injection.[51]

RADIOTHERAPY. KAs that are recurrent after surgical excision or those in which resection would result in cosmetic deformity may benefit from radiotherapy (total doses from 3500 cGy in 15 fractions to 5600 cGy in 28 fractions).[52-54]

ISOTRETINOIN. Patients with multiple KAs have been treated with oral isotretinoin[55] and oral etretinate.[56] Patients with a solitary KA may respond to a short course of isotretinoin.[57] Nine of twelve patients achieved complete resolution of the KA. The average duration of isotretinoin therapy was 6.3 weeks (range, 10 days to 12 weeks) in dosages of 0.5 to 1.0 mg/kg/day.[58]

An initial trial of oral isotretinoin is an alternative to immediate surgical excision for the treatment of large keratoacanthomas in instances when tumor removal would cause considerable cosmetic deformity.[59]

Epidermal Nevus

The term *epidermal nevus* is commonly used to describe a group of cutaneous hamartomas linked by common clinical and histologic features. Linear epidermal nevus or nevus unius lateris (a linear, unilateral, wartlike nevus), nevus verrucosus (a localized, wartlike nevus), and ichthyosis hystrix (an irregular, bilateral, truncal nevus) are some of the names given to variants of epidermal nevus. Inflammatory linear verrucous epidermal nevus (ILVEN) is characterized by intensely erythematous, pruritic, inflammatory papules that occur as linear bands along the lines of Blaschko. The term *nevus* means a congenital defect of the skin characterized by the localized excess of one or more types of cells. Histologically the cells are identical to or closely resemble normal cells. Epidermal nevus should be used as a general term to designate an excess of one type of epidermally derived cells (e.g., squamous cell or sebocyte). However, the term is commonly reserved for congenital growths in which the predominant cell is the keratinocyte. These nevi arise from the pluripotential germinative cells in the basal layer of the embryonic epidermis. These cells give rise to keratinocytes and skin appendages (hair follicles, sweat glands).

CLINICAL CHARACTERISTICS. These well-circumscribed growths are present at birth or appear in infancy or childhood. They are round, oval, or oblong; elevated; flat-topped; yellow-tan to dark brown; and have a uniformly warty or velvety surface with sharp borders (Figures 20-32 and 20-33). They appear more commonly on the head and neck; 13% of patients have widespread lesions. Blaschko described a system of lines on the skin that linear nevi follow.[60] These lines represent a developmental growth pattern of the skin (Figure 20-34). Epidermal nevi may spread beyond their original distribution; further progression is unlikely after late adolescence. Nevi present at birth and those on the head are less likely to spread. In spite of their unusual appearance and occasional itching, they are generally inconsequential. Occasionally the growths are very large and disfiguring. Patients with epidermal nevi are at significant risk of having other anomalies in other organ systems.[61] Abnormalities are more likely in patients with widespread nevi. The most common systems involved are skeletal, neurologic, and ocular.

Figure 20-32 Epidermal nevus. A congenital lesion, which is often linear, and has a dark brown, warty, or velvety surface.

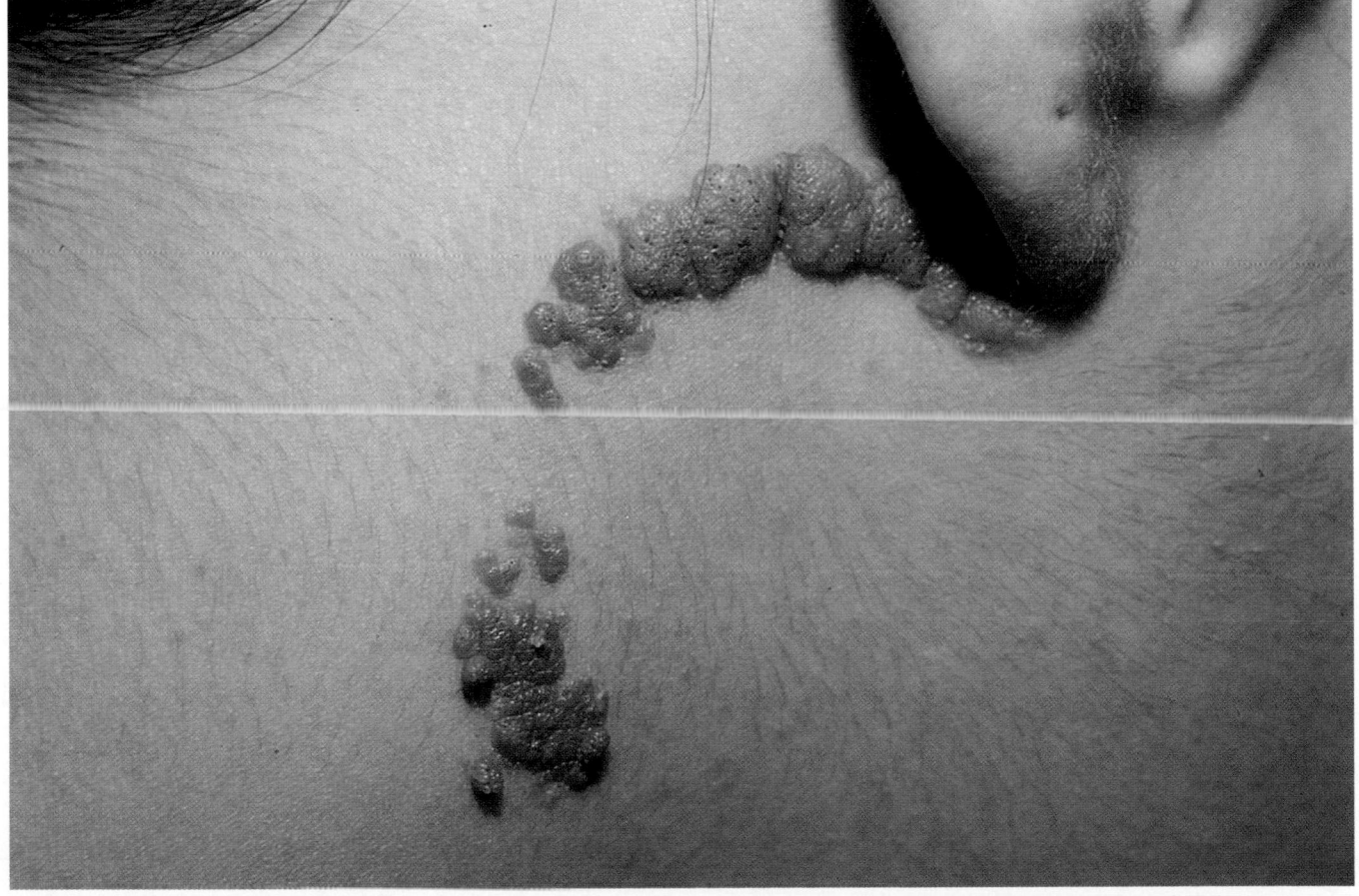

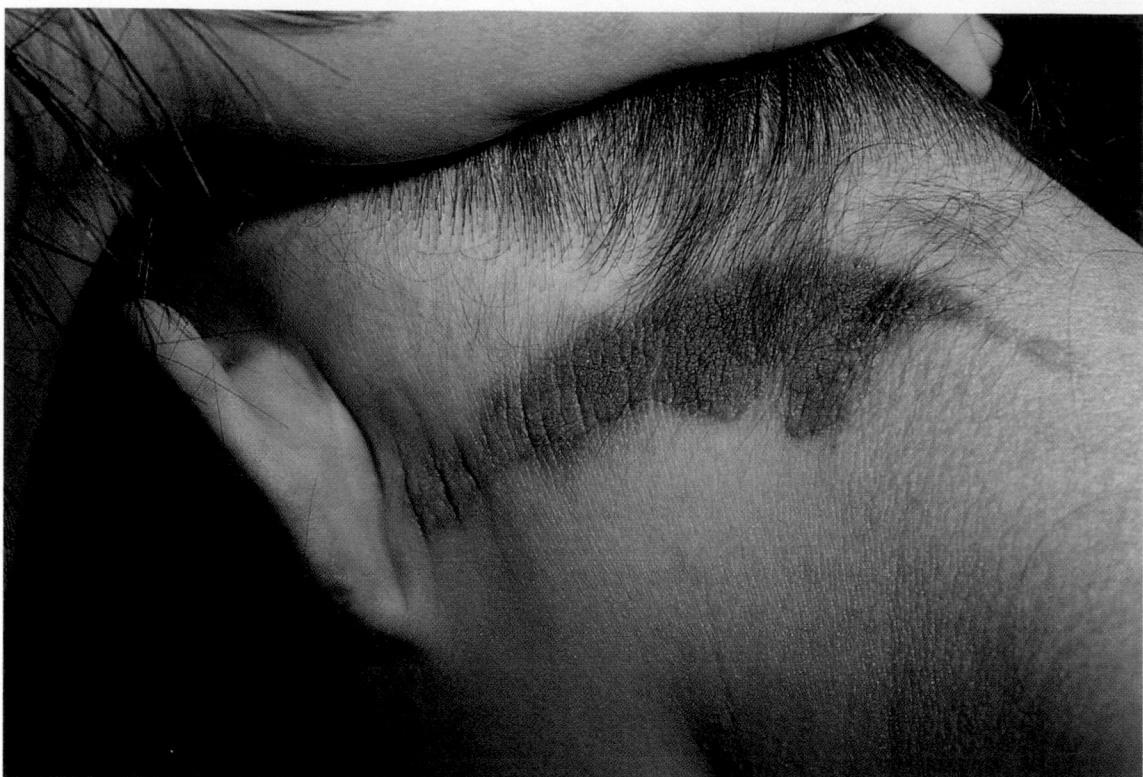

Figure 20-33 Epidermal nevus. A flat, broad lesion that follows Blaschko's lines.

GENETIC COUNSELING. The very rare epidermal nevus syndrome consists of extensive epidermal nevi associated with skeletal, ocular, and central nervous system disorders.[62-65] Small lesions are sporadic. Patients do not have a family history of epidermal nevi. Most cases of epidermal nevus syndrome occur sporadically, but there is some suspicion that an autosomal dominant transmission may be present. Inform patients that genetic transmission is possible with large epidermal nevi but that the data is inadequate to make an accurate determination.

The cause of epidermal nevus syndrome is unknown. Possible explanations are faulty migration and development of embryonic tissue or a developmental error in separation of the ectoderm from the neural tube. Treatment may be attempted with cryosurgery[66] or dermabrasion, but the growths may recur; plastic surgery excision produces the most predictable results.

TREATMENT. Inflammatory linear verrucous epidermal nevus (ILVEN) is treated to relieve discomfort and improve cosmetic appearance. Reported therapeutic approaches include dermabrasion, cryotherapy, laser therapy, and partial-thickness excision. Full-thickness surgical excision is effective definitive treatment.[67] Inflamed and noninflamed linear verrucous epidermal nevus improved using topical 0.1% tretinoin cream and 5% 5-fluorouracil. The creams were applied separately and rubbed into the skin sequentially using equal amounts and occluded with a gauze bandage. Dramatic clearing occurred in 10 weeks.[68]

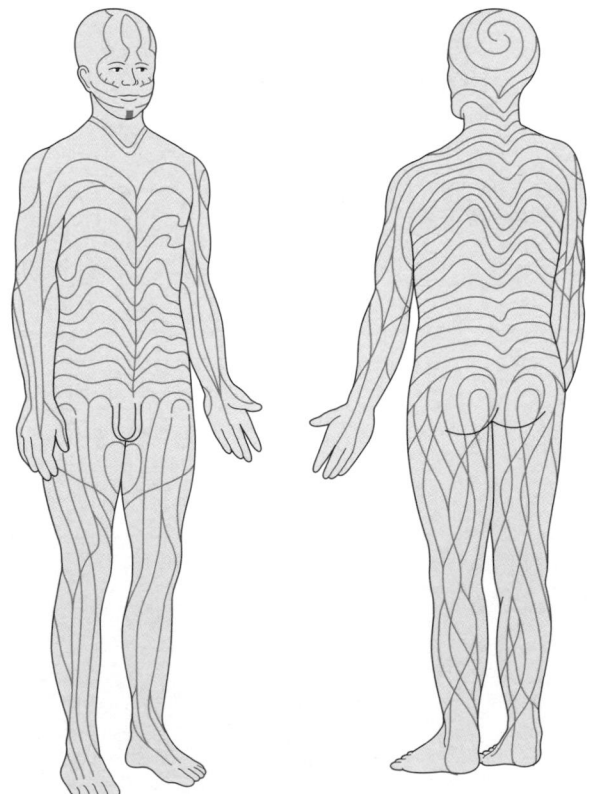

Figure 20-34 Blaschko's lines.

Nevus Sebaceous

Nevus sebaceous is a distinctive growth most commonly found on the scalp, followed by the forehead and retroauricular region.[69,70] Involvement of the neck and trunk is exceptional. A nevus of epithelial and nonepithelial skin components, nevus sebaceous sustains age-related modifications in morphology. The nevus occurs singly and is asymptomatic. Two thirds of cases are present at birth; the others develop in infancy or early childhood. Males and females are equally affected. The very rare nevus sebaceous of Jadassohn syndrome consists of the triad of a linear sebaceous nevus, convulsions, and mental retardation. A variety of congenital malformations of the ocular, skeletal, vascular, and urogenital systems have been described in association with nevus sebaceous.[71,72] Neurological abnormalities have been reported in patients with sebaceous nevi, but the incidence is low. It is recommended that patients with sebaceous nevi have a neurological assessment and that imaging be performed on all those in whom clinical abnormalities are demonstrated, as well as on those patients with large nevi involving the centrofacial area.[73]

Most lesions are sporadic, but cases of inherited nevus sebaceous have been reported.[74]

EVOLUTION OF LESIONS. Lesions are oval to linear, varying from 0.5 × 1 cm to 7 × 9 cm. The three-stage evolution of the nevoid condition (newborn, puberty, adult) parallels the natural histologic differentiation of normal sebaceous glands. The lesions in infants and younger children are smooth to gently papillated, waxy, hairless thickenings (Figure 20-35). During puberty there is a massive development of sebaceous glands with epidermal hyperplasia within the lesions (Figure 20-36). At this stage they change clinically by developing a verrucous mulberry irregularity of the surface covered with numerous, closely aggregated, yellow-to-dark brown papules. When this transformation becomes noticeable, parents become worried and seek medical attention. In approximately 20% of the cases, a third phase of evolution involves the development of secondary neoplasia in the mass of the nevus.

TUMORS ARISING IN NEVUS SEBACEUS. A number of benign and malignant "nevoid tumors" may occur. Prophylactic surgical excision during childhood is often recommended. The rate of malignant tumors is very low. Benign neoplasms are common. Trichoblastoma and not basal cell carcinoma is the most frequent follicular tumor, showing a striking female predominance. Most tumors occur in adults older than 40 years; therefore prophylactic surgery in young children is of uncertain benefit. Clinical follow-up is probably sufficient, and even those cases with clinical changes often prove to be benign tumors. The malignant degenerations are relatively low grade; only a few cases of metastasis are reported.[75]

TREATMENT. Most tumors occur in adults older than 40 years. Therefore prophylactic surgery in young children is of uncertain benefit. Clinical follow-up is probably sufficient. Most cases with clinical changes most often prove to be benign tumors. Plastic surgical excision is the most effective treatment. Attempts at local destruction with electrocautery or cryosurgery may lead to recurrence.

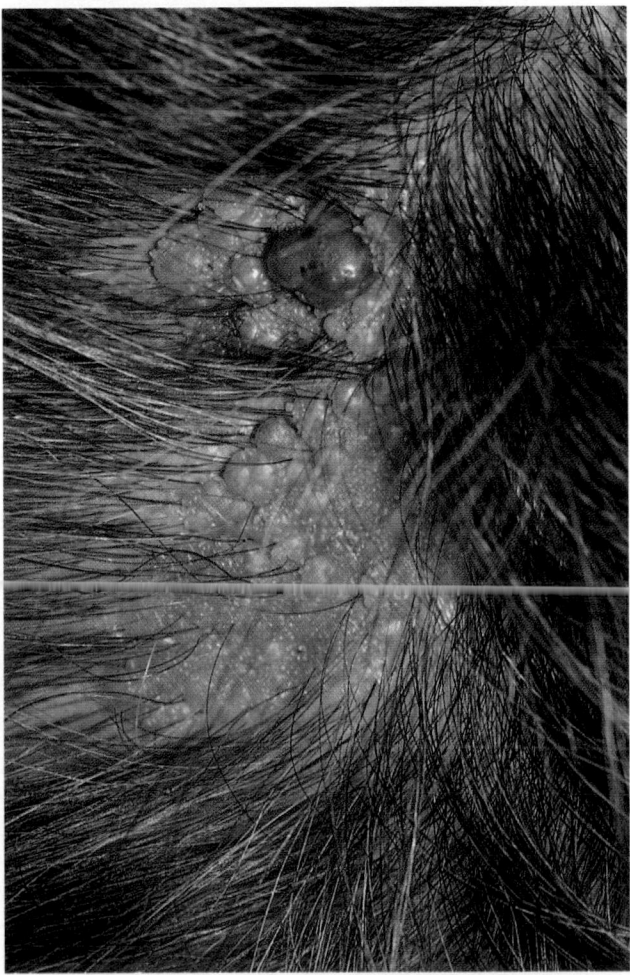

Figure 20-36 Nevus sebaceous. A white globular surface indicative of sebaceous gland hyperplasia that occurs after puberty.

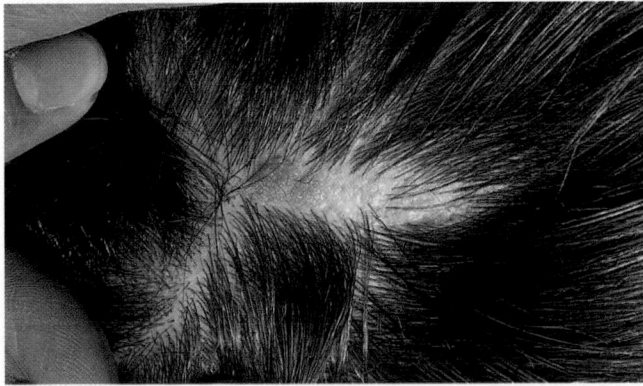

Figure 20-35 Nevus sebaceous. A typical lesion on the scalp of a prepubertal male.

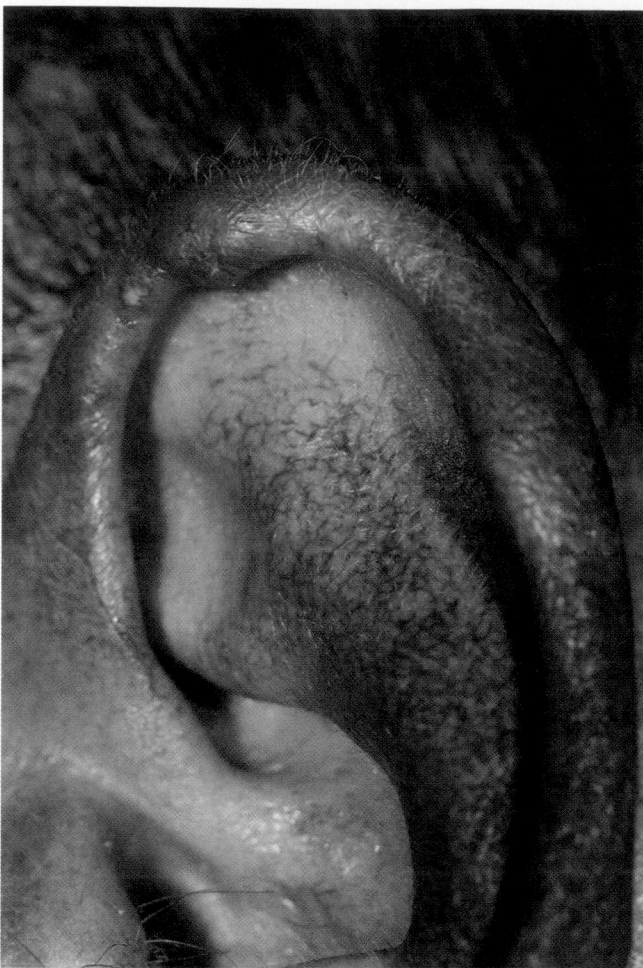

Figure 20-37 Chondrodermatitis nodularis chronica helicis. A painful, firm nodule with scaling in the center, occupying a commonly observed site on the lateral surface of the helix.

Chondrodermatitis Nodularis Chronica Helicis

This uncommon disorder occurs on the lateral surface of the helix (Figure 20-37) and occasionally on the antihelix, a site rarely occupied by other growths. One (occasionally more) firm, 2- to 6-mm nodule appears spontaneously. It subsequently develops a central scale that lacks the keratinous plug of a keratoacanthoma (Figure 20-38). Removal of the scale reveals a small central erosion. Unlike the full distended margins of a squamous or basal cell carcinoma, the sides of this mass slope down from the center (Figure 20-39). The small mass is dull red to white and is painful. During the active stage, the base may become red and swollen; pain is constant. Pressure of any type becomes intolerable. As the mass attains its maximum size, it becomes lighter in color but remains symptomatic. The cause of this disorder is unknown, but chronic sun exposure may be a factor. Men over the age of 40 account for 90% of the patients.

Histologically the dermis shows collagen degeneration with granulation tissue, edema, and inflammation.

TREATMENT

Medical management. Medical management is often unsatisfactory. A special pillow relieves pressure. Contact: CNH Pillow, PO Box 1247, Abilene, TX 79604, (915) 672-2162. Intralesional triamcinolone acetonide (10 to 40 mg/ml) once every 2 to 3 weeks until clear may be sufficient.[76] There is some degree of persistent pain throughout treatment. The CO_2 laser may be used to vaporize the cutaneous nodules and involved cartilage.[77] Cryotherapy also has been used.

Surgical management. A simple and effective treatment is to excise the nodule with scissors, curet the base, and gently electrodesiccate to eradicate all foci of inflammation. Bleeding is controlled with Monsel's solution. The wound granulates and heals with a defect (see Chapter 27). Recurrences are common if all sites of inflammation have not been eradicated. Several other techniques have been described.[78,79]

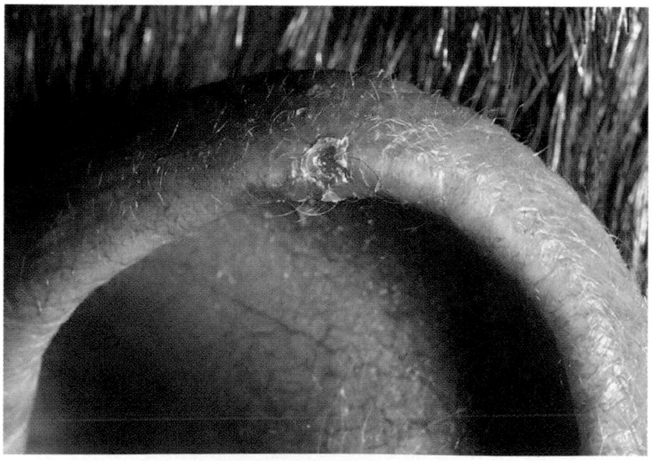

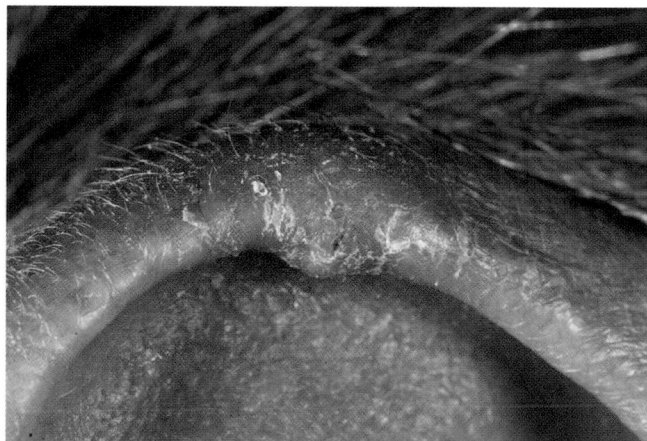

Figure 20-38 Chondrodermatitis nodularis. Shown is an early lesion with a central crust on the most common site, the apex of the helix.

Figure 20-39 Chondrodermatitis nodularis. A long-standing lesion with a dense rolled edge and a central crust.

Epidermal Cyst

The common epidermal or sebaceous cyst occurs primarily on the face, back or base of the ears, chest, and back or on almost any skin surface (Figures 20-40 to 20-43). Children who are brought to the physician with epidermal cysts or patients with epidermal cysts in unusual areas such as the legs should be suspected of having Gardner's syndrome (see Chapter 26). The cyst wall is lined with stratified squamous epithelium, which produces keratin. The round, protruding, smooth-surfaced mass is movable and varies in size from a few millimeters to several centimeters. The cyst communicates with the surface through a narrow channel, and the surface opening appears as a small, round, sometimes imperceptible, keratin-filled orifice (i.e., a blackhead) (see Figure 20-41). Epidermal cysts may originate from comedones; such lesions are superficial, with a large, black, keratinous plug on the surface. They are referred to as giant comedones and are commonly found on the back. Cysts may remain small for years or may progressively develop. Spontaneous rupture of the wall results in discharge of the soft, yellow keratin into the dermis. A tremendous inflammatory response ensues, and the sterile purulent material either points and drains through the surface or is slowly reabsorbed (Figure 20-44). If the wall is destroyed during the inflammatory process, the cyst will not recur.

TREATMENT. Like boils, fluctuant, inflamed cysts must be drained and evacuated. Small cysts are removed by making a linear incision with a #11 blade over the surface and, if possible, through the orifice. The soft keratinous material is expressed through the incision, and the remaining material is dislodged with a #1 curette. After total evacuation, firm pressure generally forces the cyst wall through the incision, where it can be grasped with the forceps and separated from connective tissue with scissors (this technique is illustrated in Chapter 27). To absorb blood and serum, the wound is compressed for several minutes. If necessary, the wound edges may be supported with Steri-Strips. Excision is the procedure of choice for large cysts. Cysts may also be excised and sutured or dissected (Figure 20-45).

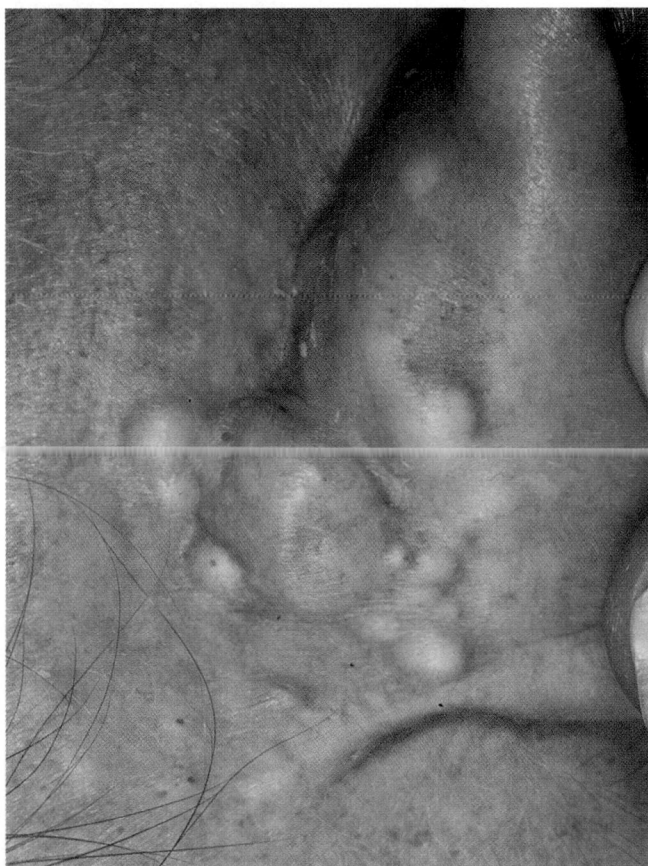

Figure 20-40 The posterior auricular fold is a common place to find one or many epidermal cysts.

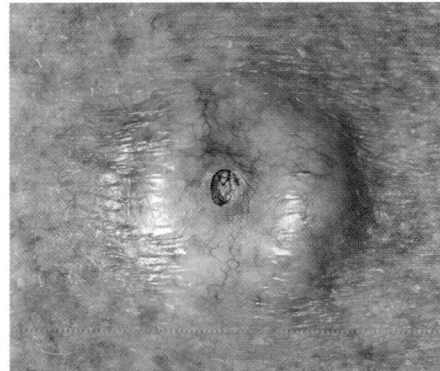

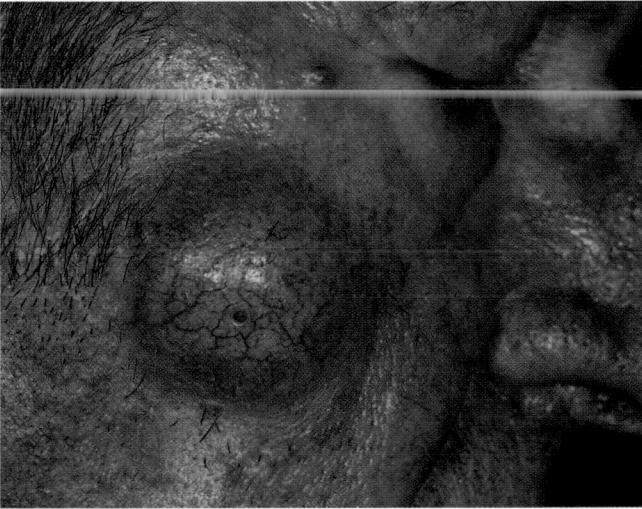

Figure 20-41 The keratin-filled orifice (blackhead) communicating with the surface is not usually as prominent as illustrated here.

EPIDERMAL CYSTS

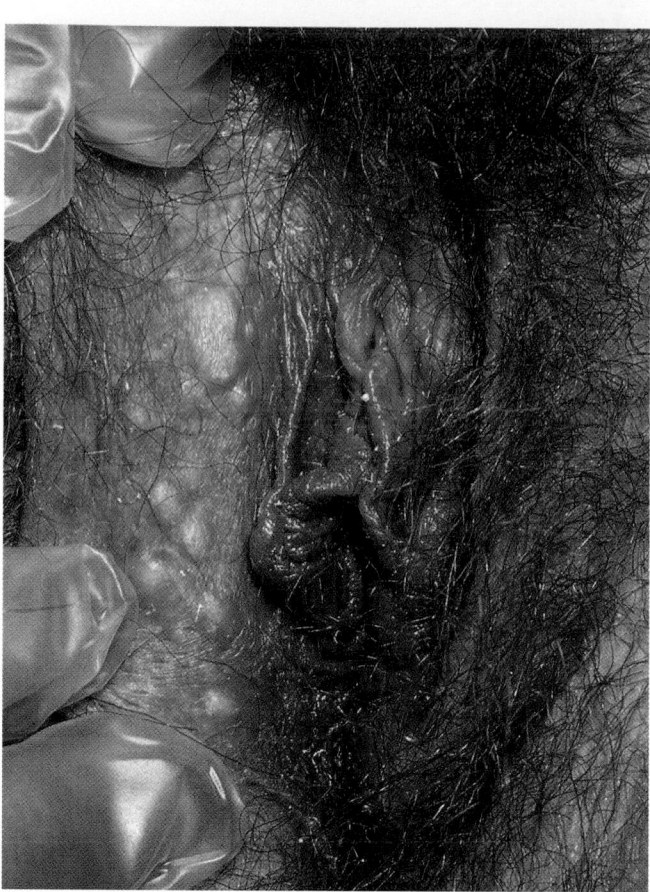

Figure 20-42 Epidermal cysts occur in areas where sebaceous glands are large and numerous, such as on the labia.

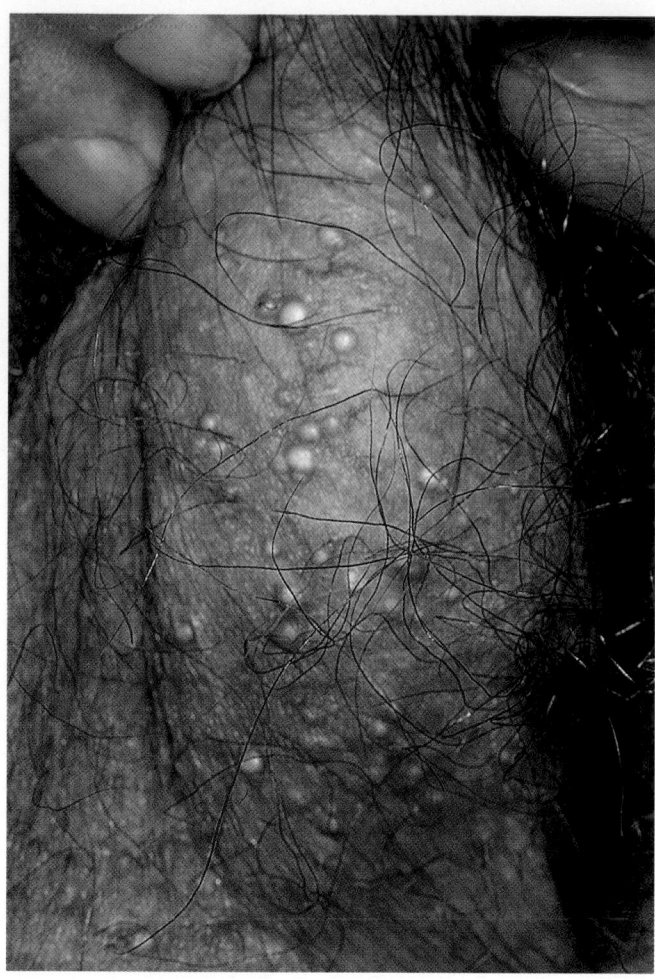

Figure 20-43 Epidermal cysts are common on the scrotum. Lesions may be few or numerous and vary in size. Some are larger than a centimeter.

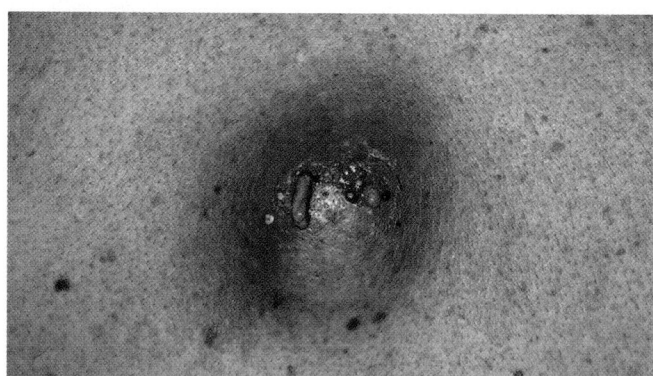

Figure 20-44 A ruptured epidermal cyst results in intense inflammation and resembles a furuncle.

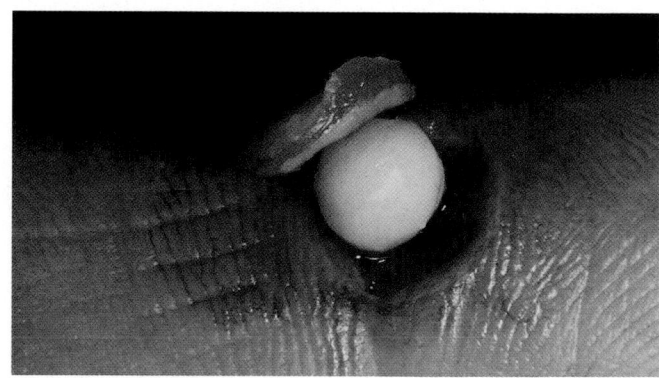

Figure 20-45 Epidermal cyst. The lesion has been dissected intact.

Pilar Cyst (Wen)

Pilar cysts occur in the scalp and, like epidermal cysts, are freely movable. They are frequently multiple and may become large masses (Figures 20-46 and 20-47). The epithelial-lined wall produces keratin of a different quality than that of the epidermal cyst, but rupture of the wall creates the same intense reaction. The cyst contains concentric layers of dry keratin, which over time may become macerated, soft, and cheesy (Figure 20-48).

TREATMENT. Except for the largest structures, pilar cysts can be satisfactorily removed through a linear excision, avoiding suture closure. The following procedure should be used (this procedure is illustrated in Chapter 27):

1. Cut the hair over the cyst and make a 3- to 10-mm linear incision.
2. With firm pressure, express the contents and dislodge remaining fragments with a #1 curette.
3. Firmly press the curette against the inner wall of the cyst and move it back and forth to dislodge the cyst from its surroundings. The wall is firm and has a smooth, glazed surface that is easily separated from connective tissue.
4. Hold the cut edge of the cyst with forceps and, while applying continuous pressure to the sides of the wound, separate the cyst from the supporting connective tissue with a blunt dissecting instrument such as a Schamberg or blunt-tipped scissors. The cyst will literally pop out of the wound.
5. To control bleeding, apply firm pressure for 5 minutes. Dressings or bandages are unnecessary.

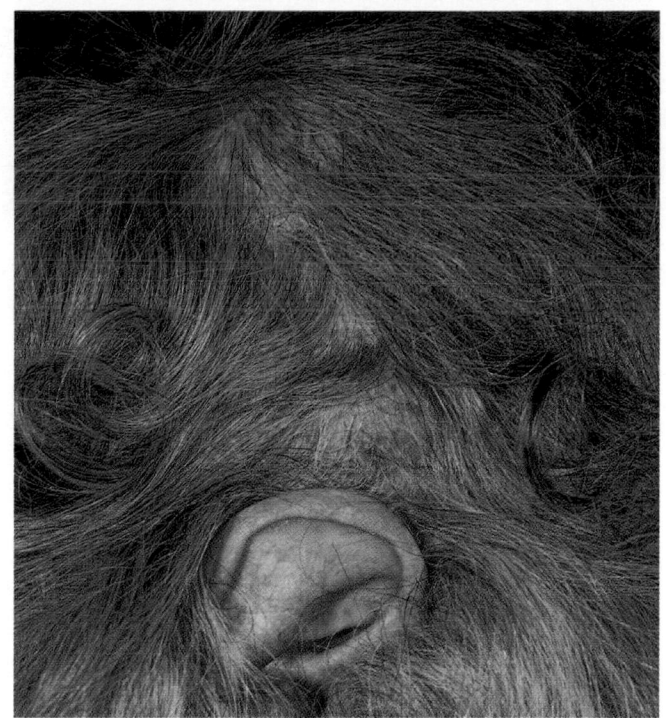

Figure 20-46 Pilar cyst. A freely movable cystic mass found on the scalp. Communication with the surface is rarely observed.

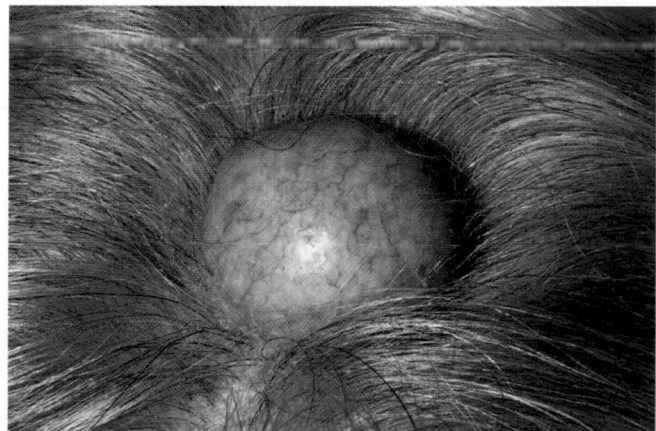

Figure 20-47 Pilar cyst. This very large cyst is more prominent than most lesions. Expansion of the cyst has destroyed hair follicles.

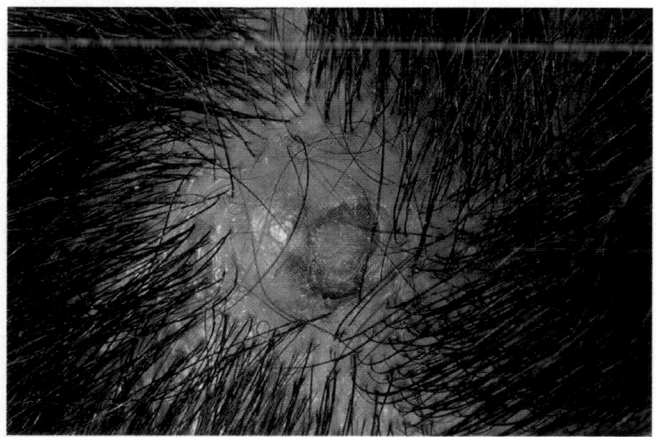

Figure 20-48 Pilar cyst. The cyst has spontaneously ruptured and is discharging amorphous cyst contents onto the skin surface.

Senile Sebaceous Hyperplasia

Senile sebaceous hyperplasia consists of small tumors composed of enlarged sebaceous glands. They begin as pale yellow, slightly elevated papules; with time they become yellow, dome-shaped, and umbilicated (Figures 20-49 to 20-51). Senile sebaceous hyperplasia with telangiectasia may be mistaken for a basal cell carcinoma (see Figures 20-51 and 20-52). However, close examination of the surface with a hand lens shows a haphazard distribution of vessels on the surface of basal cell carcinoma, whereas the vessels in sebaceous hyperplasia occur only in the valleys between the small yellow lobules. The lesions occur after age 30 in 25% of the population and gradually become more numerous. There is no relationship between the skin type and the occurrence of these lesions. They are commonly found on the forehead, cheeks (see Figure 20-49), lower lid, and nose. The etiology remains unclear; chronic solar exposure is not a likely cause.[80]

TREATMENT. Treatment consists of removal of the elevated portion of the papule. A pitted scar results if the entire structure is removed with a curette. The superficial portion of the lesion may be removed by shave excision or destroyed with conservative surface or intralesional electrosurgery.[81] Bichloracetic acid can be used for treatment. A tiny amount of acid is carefully applied to the surface with a wooden applicator stick. A stinging sensation occurs and lasts for 24 hours. Polysporin ointment is applied twice a day for 1 week. The treated area forms a crust, heals with residual erythema, and fades over time.[82] Patients with numerous lesions have been reported. Most lesions regress after one treatment with 3 stacked pulses of the 585-nm pulsed-dye laser.[83]

Oral isotretinoin in very low dosages (10 to 20 mg qd) is dramatically effective for patients with numerous lesions. All lesions clear within 2 weeks but recur after the medication is stopped.[84] Patients can often maintain control with low dosages of isotretinoin (e.g., 10 mg once or twice each week). It has been speculated that longer treatment (more than 12 weeks) may result in perifollicular fibrosis in the region formerly occupied by the sebaceous gland and may offer a long-term remission. Optimum treatment and dosage schedules have not been established. Intermittent low-dose isotretinoin may be the best approach. Long-term isotretinoin therapy may be associated with many side effects.

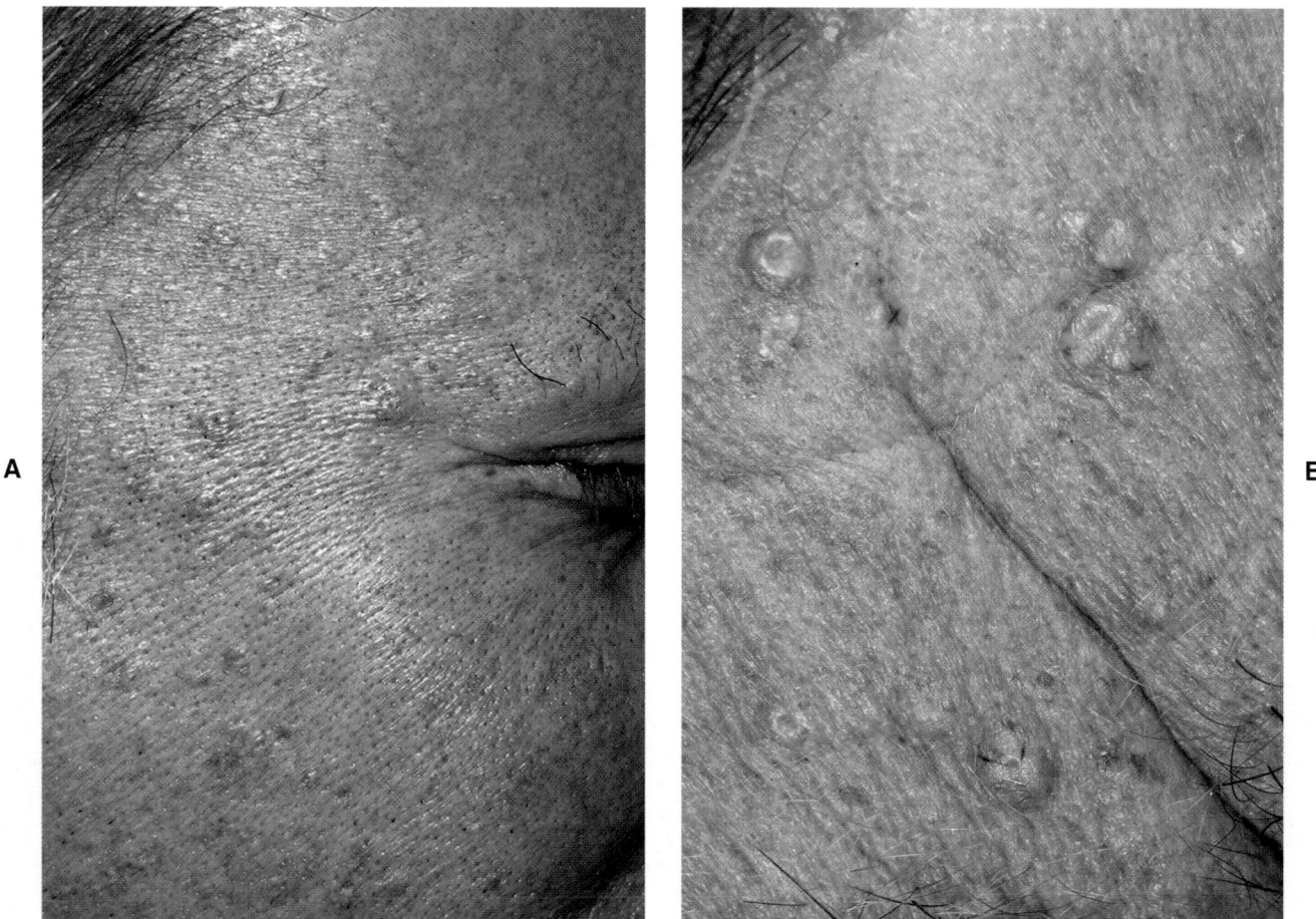

Figure 20-49 A, Senile sebaceous hyperplasia (cheek). Note central umbilication. **B,** Central umbilication can be seen in this close view.

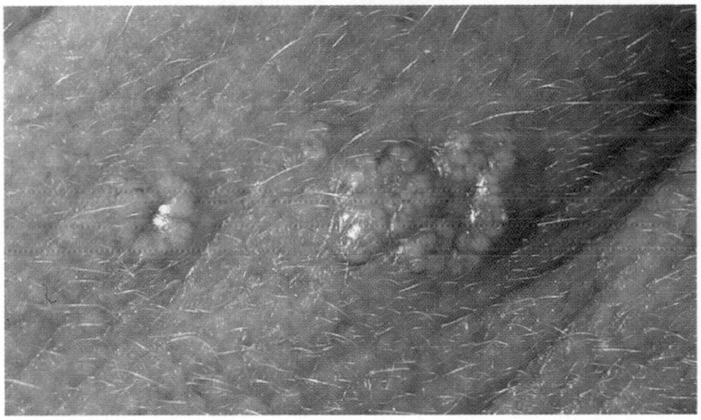

Syringoma

Syringomas are sweat duct tumors composed of small, firm, flesh-colored dermal papules that occur on the lower lids (Figures 20-53 and 20-54) and, less commonly, on the forehead, chest, and abdomen. Lesions may develop at any age, but they initially appear most frequently during the third and fourth decades; they then slowly become more numerous. The tumors have no malignant potential. They may be removed for cosmetic purposes by electrodesiccation and curettage[85] or excised by gently elevating the small mass with forceps or the curved bevel of a 25-gauge needle and cut out with curved scissors or shaved with a #11 scalpel blade. The oval wound is left to heal by secondary intention.[86,87]

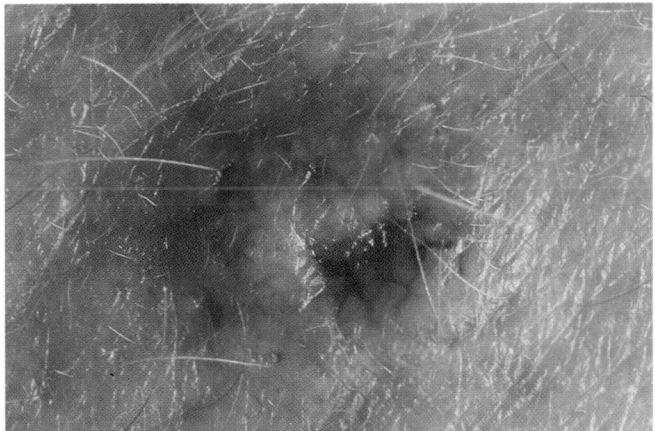

Figure 20-50 Sebaceous hyperplasia. A single lesion shows a collection of white-yellow globules. This lesion does not have central umbilication.

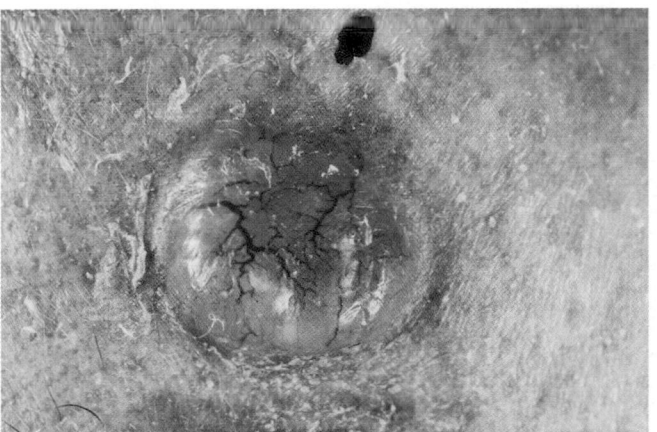

Figure 20-51 Sebaceous hyperplasia. A magnified lesion shows well-defined yellow lobules. Small blood vessels occur between the lobules. Compare this with the position of the blood vessels in a basal cell epithelioma.

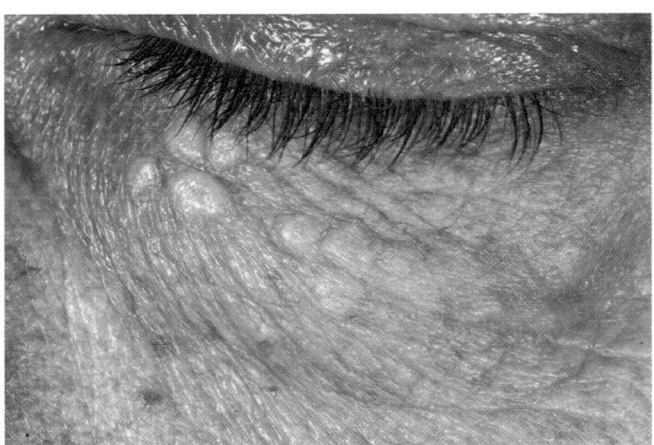

Figure 20-53 Syringoma. Yellow-white round and flat-topped papules most commonly found on the lower lids.

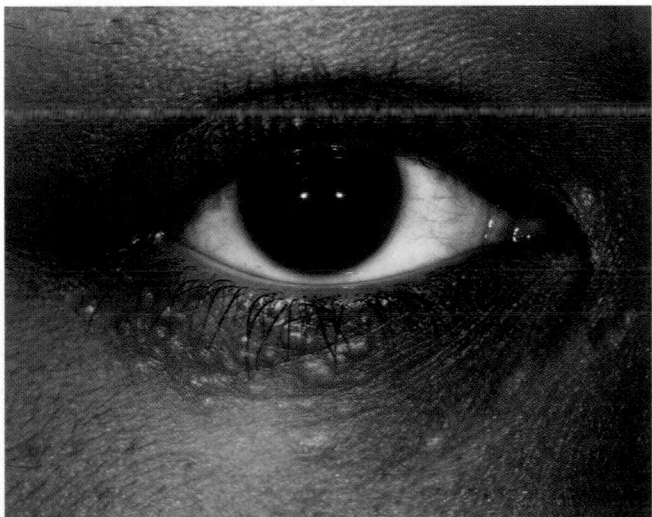

Figure 20-52 Basal cell carcinoma. The blood vessels are haphazardly distributed over the entire surface.

Figure 20-54 Syringoma on the lower lid of a young woman.

References

1. Stern RE, Boudreaux C, Arndt KA: Diagnostic accuracy and appropriateness of care for seborrheic keratoses. A pilot study of an approach to quality assurance for cutaneous surgery, JAMA 1991; 265:74.

2. Gill D, Dorevitch A, Marks R: The prevalence of seborrheic keratoses in people aged 15 to 30 years: is the term senile keratosis redundant? Arch Dermatol 2000; 136(6):759.

3. Zhu WY, et al: Detection of human papillomavirus DNA in seborrheic keratosis by polymerase chain reaction, J Dermatol Sci 1992; 4:166.

4. Murphy M, et al: Accuracy of diagnosis of seborrheic keratoses in a dermatology clinic, Arch Dermatol 2000; 136(6):800.

5. Izikson L, et al: Prevalence of melanoma clinically resembling seborrheic keratosis: analysis of 9204 cases, Arch Dermatol 2002; 138(12):1562.

6. Tegner E, et al: Halo dermatitis around tumours, Acta Derm Venereol 1990; 70:31.

7. Grob JJ, et al: The relation between seborrheic keratoses and malignant solid tumours: a case-control study, Acta Derm Venereol 1991; 71:166.

8. Lindelof B, et al: Seborrheic keratoses and cancer, J Am Acad Dermatol 1992; 26:947.

9. Heaphy MR, Millns JL, Schroeter AL: The sign of Leser-Trelat in a case of adenocarcinoma of the lung, J Am Acad Dermtol 2000; 43(2 pt2):386.

10. Holdiness MR: The sign of Leser-Trelat: a review, Int J Dermatol 1986; 25:564.

11. Czarnecki DB, et al: The sign of Leser-Trelat, Australas J Dermatol 1983; 24:93.

12. Flugman SL, et al: Transient eruptive seborrheic keratosis associated with erythrodermic psoriasis and erythrodermic drug eruptions : report of two cases, J Am Acad Dermatol 2001 ; (6 suppl) : S212.

13. Brown FC: Sign of Leser-Trelat, Arch Dermatol 1974; 110:129.

14. Berman A, Winkelmann RK: Seborrheic keratoses: appearance in course of exfoliative erythroderma and regression associated with histologic mononuclear cell inflammation, Arch Dermatol 1982; 118:615.

15. Shall L, Marks R: Stucco keratoses. A clinico-pathological study, Acta Derm Venereol 1991; 71:258.

16. Graham R: What is dermatosis papularis nigra? Practitioner 1989; 233:635.

17. Spitalny AD, Lavery LA: Acquired fibrokeratoma of the heel, J Foot Surg 1992; 31:509.

18. Reference deleted in proofs.

19. Reference deleted in proofs.

20. Lu I, Cohen RR, Grossman ME: Multiple dermatofibromas in women with HIV infection and systemic lupus erythematosus, J Am Acad Dermatol 1995; 32:901.

21. Niiyama S, Happle R, Hoffmann R: Guess what! Multiple disseminated dermatofibromas in a woman with systemic lupus erythematosus, Eur J Dermatol 2001; 11(5):475.

22. Ferrari A, et al: Central white scarlike patch: a dermatoscopic clue for the diagnosis of dermatofibroma, J Am Acad Dermatol 2000; 43(6):1123.

23. Lanigan SW, Robinson TWE: Cryotherapy for dermatofibromas, Clin Exp Dermatol 1987; 12:121.

24. Shaffer JJ, Taylor SC, Cook-Bolden F: Keloidal scars: a review with a critical look at therapeutic options, J Am Acad Dermatol 2002; 46(2 Suppl Understanding):S63.

25. Lawrence WT: In search of the optimal treatment of keloids: report of a series and a review of the literature, Ann Plast Surg 1991; 27:164.

26. Nemeth AJ: Keloids and hypertrophic scars, J Dermatol Surg Oncol 1993; 19:738.

27. Datubo-Brown DD: Keloids: a review of the literature, Br J Plast Surg 1990; 43:70.

28. Rusciani L, et al: Use of cryotherapy in the treatment of keloids, J Dermatol Surg Oncol 1993; 19:529.

29. Ceilley RI, Babin RW: The combined use of cryosurgery and intralesional injections of suspensions of fluorinated adrenocorticosteroids for reducing keloids and hypertrophic scars, J Dermatol Surg Oncol 1979; 5:54.

30. Ahn ST, Monafo WW, Mustoe TA: Topical silicone gel for the prevention and treatment of hypertrophic scar, Arch Surg 1991; 126:499.

31. Sawada Y, Sone K: Hydration and occlusion treatment for hypertrophic scars and keloids, Br J Plast Surg 1992; 45:599.

32. Manuskiatti W, Fitzpatrick RE: Treatment response of keloidal and hypertrophic sternotomy scars: comparison among intralesional corticosteroid, 5-fluorouracil, and 585-nm flashlamp-pumped pulsed-dye laser treatments, Arch Dermatol 2002; 138(9):1149.

33. Espana A, Solano T, Quintanilla E, Bleomycin in the treatment of keloids and hypertrophic scars by multiple needle punctures, Dermatol Surg 2001; 27(1):23.

34. Alster T, Williams C: Treatment of keloid sternotomy scars with 585 nm flashlamp-pumped pulsed-dye laser, Lancet 1995; 345(8959):1198.

35. Manuskiatti W, Fitzpatrick R, Goldman M: Energy density and numbers of treatment affect response of keloidal and hypertrophic sternotomy scars to the 585-nm flashlamp-pumped pulsed-dye laser, J Am Acad Dermatol 2001; 45(4):557.

36. Viviano E, Sorce M, Mantegna M: Solitary keratoacanthomas in immunocompetent patients: no detection of papillomavirus DNA by polymerase chain reaction, New Microbiol 2001; 24(3):295.

37. Chuang TY, et al: Keratoacanthoma in Kauai, Hawaii: the first documented incidence in a defined population, Arch Dermatol 1993; 129:317.

38. Dufresne R, Marrero G, Robinson-Bostom L: Seasonal presentation of keratoacanthomas in Rhode Island, Br J Dermatol 1997; 136(2):227.

39. Akhtar S, et al: Muir-Torre syndrome: case report of a patient with concurrent jejunal and ureteral cancer and a review of the literature [see comments], J Am Acad Dermatol 1999; 41(5 Pt 1):681.

40. Kuppers F, et al: Keratoacanthoma in the differential diagnosis of anal carcinoma: difficult diagnosis, easy therapy. Report of three cases. [In Process Citation], Dis Colon Rectum 2000; 43(3):427.

41. Cribier B, Asch P, Grosshans E: Differentiating squamous cell carcinoma from keratoacanthoma using histopathological criteria. Is it possible? A study of 296 cases, Dermatology 1999; 199(3):208.

42. Nedwich JA: Evaluation of curettage and electrodesiccation in treatment of keratoacanthoma, Australas J Dermatol 1991; 32:137.

43. Habif TP: Extirpation of keratoacanthomas by blunt dissection, J Dermatol Surg Oncol 1980; 6:652.

44. Goette DK, Odom RB: Successful treatment of keratoacanthoma with intralesional fluorouracil, J Am Acad Dermatol 1980; 2:212.

45. Gray R, Meland N: Topical 5-fluorouracil as primary therapy for keratoacanthoma, Ann Plast Surg 2000; 44(1):82.

46. Eubanks SW, et al: Treatment of multiple keratoacanthomas with intralesional fluorouracil, J Am Acad Dermatol 1982; 7:126.

47. Parker CM, Hanke W: Large keratoacanthomas in difficult locations treated with intralesional 5-fluorouracil, J Am Acad Dermatol 1986; 14:770.

48. Dendorf M, et al: Topical treatment with imiquimod may induce regression of facial keratoacanthoma, Eur J Dermatol (France) 2003; 13(1):80.

49. Spieth K, Gille J, Kaufmann R: Intralesional methotrexate as effective treatment in solitary giant keratoacanthoma of the lower lip, Dermatology 2000; 200(4):317.

50. Goebeler M, et al: Pancytopenia after treatment of keratoacanthoma by single lesional methotrexate infiltration, Arch Dermatol 2001; 137(8):1104.

51. Grob JJ, et al: Large keratoacanthomas treated with intralesional interferon alfa-2a, J Am Acad Dermatol 1993; 29:237.

52. Caccialanza M, Sopelana N: Radiation therapy of keratoacanthomas: results in 55 patients, Int J Radiat Oncol Biol Phys 1989; 16:475.

53. Farina AT, et al: Radiotherapy for aggressive and destructive keratoacanthomas, J Dermatol Surg Oncol 1977; 3:177.

54. Donahue B, et al: Treatment of aggressive keratoacanthomas by radiotherapy, J Am Acad Dermatol 1990; 23:489.

55. Schaller M, et al: Multiple keratoacanthomas, giant keratoacanthoma and keratoacanthoma centrifugum marginatum: development in a single patient and treatment with oral isotretinoin, Acta Derm Venereol 1996. 76(1):40.

56. Lo SA, et al: [Keratoacanthoma centrifugum marginatum. Possible etiological role of papillomavirus and therapeutic response to etretinate], Ann Dermatol Venereol 1996; 123(10):660.

57. Canas G, Robson K, Arpey C: Persistent keratoacanthoma: challenges in management, Dermatol Surg 1998; 24(12):1364.

58. Goldberg LH, et al: Treatment of solitary keratoacanthomas with oral isotretinoin, J Am Acad Dermatol 1990; 23:934.

59. Wong W, et al: Treatment of a recurrent keratoacanthoma with oral isotretinoin, Int J Dermatol 1994; 33(8):579.

60. Taieb A, et al: Lichen striatus: a Blaschko linear acquired inflammatory skin eruption, J Am Acad Dermatol 1991; 25:637.

61. Rogers M, McCrossin I, Commens C: Epidermal nevi and the epidermal nevus syndrome: a review of 131 cases, J Am Acad Dermatol 1989; 20:476.

62. Solomon LM, Esterly NB: Epidermal and other congenital organoid nevi, Curr Probl Pediatr, 1975; 6:1.

63. Goldberg LH, Collins SAB, Siegel DM: The epidermal nevus syndrome: case report and review, Pediatr Dermatol 1987; 4:27.

64. Happle R: How many epidermal nevus syndromes exist?: a clinico-genetic classification, J Am Acad Dermatol 1991. 25:557.

65. Hodge JA, Ray MC, Flynn KJ: The epidermal nevus syndrome, Int J Dermatol 1991; 30:91.

66. Fox BJ, Lapins NA: Comparison of treatment modalities for epidermal nevus: a case report and review, J Dermatol Surg Oncol 1983; 11:879.

67. Lee B, et al: Full-thickness surgical excision for the treatment of inflammatory linear verrucous epidermal nevus, Ann Plast Surg 2001; 47(3):285.

68. Kim J, Chang M, Shwayder T: Topical tretinoin and 5-fluorouracil in the treatment of linear verrucous epidermal nevus, J Am Acad Dermatol 2000; 43(1 Pt 1):129.

69. Alessi E, Sala F: Nevus sebaceous: a clinicopathologic study of its evolution, Am J Dermatopathol 1986; 8:27.

70. Weng CJ, et al: Jadassohn's nevus sebaceous of the head and face, Ann Plast Surg 1990; 25:100.

71. Kang WH, Koh YJ, Chun SI: Nevus sebaceous syndrome associated with intracranial arteriovenous malformation, Int J Dermatol 1987; 26:382.

72. Diven DG, et al: Nevus sebaceous associated with major ophthalmologic abnormalities, Arch Dermatol 1987; 123:383.

73. Davies D, Rogers M: Review of neurological manifestations in 196 patients with sebaceous naevi, Australas J Dermatol 2002; 43(1):20.

74. Sahl W, Jr: Familial nevus sebaceous of Jadassohn: occurrence in three generations, J Am Acad Dermatol 1990; 22:853.

75. Cribier B, et al: Tumors arising in nevus sebaceus: a study of 596 cases, J Am Acad Dermatol 2000; 42 (2 Pt 1): 263.

76. Cox N, Denham P: Intralesional triamcinolone for chondrodermatitis nodularis: a follow-up study of 60 patients, Br J Dermatol 2002; 146(4):712.

77. Taylor MB: Chondrodermatitis nodularis chronica helicis. Successful treatment with the carbon dioxide laser, J Dermatol Surg Oncol 1991; 17:862.

78. Coldiron BM: The surgical management of chondrodermatitis nodularis chronica helicis, J Dermatol Surg Oncol 1991; 17:902.

79. Lawrence CM: The treatment of chondrodermatitis nodularis with cartilage removal alone, Arch Dermatol, 1991; 127:530.

80. Kumar P, Marks R: Sebaceous gland hyperplasia and senile comedones: a prevalence study in elderly hospitalized patients, Br J Dermatol 1987; 117:231.

81. Bader R, Scarborough D: Surgical pearl: intralesional electrodesiccation of sebaceous hyperplasia, J Am Acad Dermatol 2000; 42(1 Pt 1):127.

82. Rosian R, et al: The treatment of benign sebaceous hyperplasia with the topical application of bichloracetic acid, J Dermatol Surg Oncol 1991; 17:876.

83. Aghassi D, et al: Elucidating the pulsed-dye laser treatment of sebaceous hyperplasia in vivo with real-time confocal scanning laser microscopy, J Am Acad Dermatol 2000; 43(1 Pt 1):49.

84. Burton CS, Sawchuk WS: Premature sebaceous gland hyperplasia: successful treatment with isotretinoin, J Am Acad Dermatol 1985; 12:182.

85. Stevenson TR, Swanson NA: Syringoma: removal by electrodesiccation and curettage, Ann Plast Surg 1985; 15:151.

86. Moreno-Gonzalez J, Rios-Arizpe S: A modified technique for excision of syringomas, J Dermatol Surg Oncol 1989; 15:796.

87. Maloney ME: An easy method for removal of syringoma, J Dermatol Surg Oncol 1982; 8:973.

Premalignant and Malignant Nonmelanoma Skin Tumors

Basal Cell Carcinoma

Basal cell carcinoma (BCC) is the most common invasive malignant cutaneous neoplasm found in humans.[1] The most common presenting complaint is a bleeding or scabbing sore that heals and recurs. Unfortunately, there is a tendency to regard BCC as nonmalignant because the tumor rarely metastasizes. BCC advances by direct extension and destroys normal tissue. Left untreated or inadequately treated, the cancer can destroy the whole side of the face or penetrate subcutaneous tissue into the bone and brain.

BASAL CELL CARCINOMA VS. SQUAMOUS CELL CARCINOMA. BCC and squamous cell carcinoma (SCC) are referred to as nonmelanoma skin cancers. A number of differences between these two tumors exist (Table 21-1). The relationship with ultraviolet (UV) radiation is stronger for SCC. SCCs of the head and neck occur on areas receiving maximal irradiation. The distribution of BCC on the face does not correspond well with areas of maximal sun exposure. Many occur on sun-protected sites, such as the inner canthus and behind the ears. Approximately one third of all BCCs occur on areas of the skin that receive little or no UV radiation and, unlike SCCs, they are uncommon on the back of the hands and on the forearms.[2] Increasing grade of wrinkling is associated with a progressive reduction in risk of a BCC.[3]

LOCATION. Eighty-five percent of all BCCs appear on the head and neck region; 25% to 30% occur on the nose alone, the most common site. BCC is rarely found on the backs of the hands, although this site receives a significant amount of solar radiation. Tumors also occur in sites protected from the sun, such as the genitals and breasts. BCC in blacks is rare.

INCIDENCE. The tumor may occur at any age, but the incidence of BCC increases markedly after age 40. The incidence in younger people is increasing, possibly as a result of increased sun exposure.[4]

Pathophysiology

BCCs arise from basal keratinocytes of the epidermis and adnexal structures (hair follicles, eccrine sweat ducts). UVB radiation damages deoxyribonucleic acid (DNA) and its repair system and alters the immune system. BCC grows by direct extension and appears to require the surrounding stroma to support its growth. This may explain why the cells are not capable of metastasizing through blood vessels or lymphatics.

The course of BCC is unpredictable. BCC can remain small for years with little tendency to grow, particularly in the elderly, or it may grow rapidly or proceed by successive spurts of extension of tumor and partial regression. BCC occurs at the site of previous trauma, such as scars, thermal burns, and injury. BCC occurs years later at sites treated with ionizing radiation. The tumor appears 3 months to 7 or more years later at the site of a previous injury.[5]

Table 21-1 Basal Cell Carcinoma vs. Squamous Cell Carcinoma

Incidence	Basal cell carcinoma	Squamous cell carcinoma
Males	175 per 100,000 Minnesota 849 per 100,000 Australia	106 per 100,000 Pacific Northwest 166 per 100,000 Australia
Females	124 per 100,000 Minnesota 605 per 100,000 Australia	30 per 100,000 Pacific Northwest
United States 1999	800,000	200,000
United States 1978 Number per 100,000 person-years	247 (males) 150 (females)	65 (males) 24 (females)
Distribution	Face, head, neck: distribution does not correspond well with areas of maximal sun exposure Occurs on relatively sun-protected sites, such as the inner canthus and behind the ears One third occur on areas that receive little or no UV radiation Uncommon on back of the hands and on forearms	Head, neck: areas of maximal irradiation
Age	20% occur in patients younger than 50 yr of age	Uncommon in the young
Celtic ancestry: fair skin, blue eyes, red or fair hair, inability to tan	Risk low: patients do not have phenotypic markers of high risk	High risk
Most important risk factor	Inability to tan	Cumulative sun exposure. Increasing age more important than tanning ability
UV exposure patterns	Intermittent sun exposure Childhood and adolescent sun exposure	Cumulative exposure. Childhood and adolescent sun exposure
Other environmental exposures		Chronic ulceration and inflammation, scarring dermatosis, immunosuppressed states, human papillomavirus infection, chemical carcinogens (coal-tar products), psoralens and UVA, arsenic, cigarette smoking
Risk of developing a subsequent nonmelanoma skin cancer of the same type	3-year cumulative risk of a subsequent BCC after an index BCC is 44% BCC patients are 8 times more likely to develop another BCC than a first SCC 3-year cumulative risk of developing a BCC for patients with a history of an SCC is 43%	3-year cumulative risk of a subsequent SCC after an index SCC is 18% Risk of developing an SCC in patients with a prior BCC is 6%
Genodermatoses	Xeroderma pigmentosum Nevoid BCC syndrome	Xeroderma pigmentosum Epidermodysplasia verruciformis

Adapted from Leman JA, et al: Arch Dermatol 2001; 137:1239; and Marcil I, Stern RS: Arch Dermatol 2000; 136:1524.

Histologic characteristics

The cells of a BCC resemble those of the basal layer of the epidermis. They are basophilic, have a large nucleus, and appear to form a basal layer by forming an orderly line around the periphery of tumor nests in the dermis, a feature referred to as palisading (Figure 21-1).

There are five major histologic patterns.[6]

1. Nodular (21%): a rounded mass of neoplastic cells with well-defined peripheral contours. Peripheral palisading is well developed (Figure 21-1).
2. Superficial (17%): contains buds of atypical basal cells extending from the basal layer of the epidermis (Figure 21-2).
3. Micronodular (15%): small, rounded nodules of tumor about the size of hair bulbs. Tumor islands are rounded, well demarcated, and demonstrate peripheral palisading.
4. Infiltrative (7%): tumor islands vary in size and show a jagged configuration.
5. Morpheaform (1%): numerous small, elongated islands containing a few cells that appear as strands or cords in a fibrous stroma.

A mixed pattern (two or more major histologic patterns) is present in 38.5% of cases.

Clinical types

BCC occurs in many different clinical forms, which vary in appearance and malignant potential.

NODULAR BASAL CELL CARCINOMA. Nodular BCC is the most common form of BCC. The lesion begins as a pearly white or pink, dome-shaped papule resembling a molluscum contagiosum or dermal nevus (Figures 21-3 and 21-4). The mass extends peripherally. The lesion may remain flat. Traction on the surrounding skin accentuates the pearly border. Telangiectatic vessels become prominent and easily recognizable through the thin epidermis as the lesion enlarges. The growth pattern is irregular, forming an oval mass whereby the surface may become multilobular. The center frequently ulcerates and bleeds and subsequently accumulates crust and scale (see Figure 21-4). Ulcerated BCCs were formerly designated rodent ulcers.

Ulcerated areas heal with scarring, and patients often assume their conditions are improving. This cycle of growth, ulceration, and healing continues as the mass extends peripherally and deeper; masses of enormous size may be attained. BCCs may present as nonhealing leg ulcers. Biopsy specimens should be taken of leg ulcers that do not respond to treatment.[7] The tissue mass of a nodular BCC has a distinctive consistency that can be appreciated during curettage or biopsy. It has poor cohesive forces and collapses or breaks down when manipulated with a curette. This is an important diagnostic feature that supports the clinical impression during the biopsy procedure.

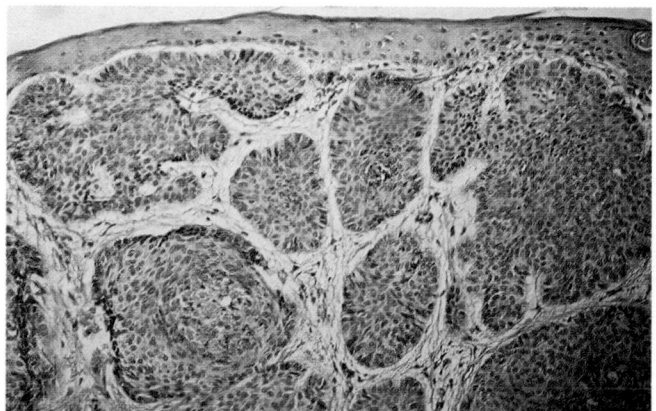

Figure 21-1 Nodular basal cell carcinoma. Nests of atypical basal cells are found in the dermis.

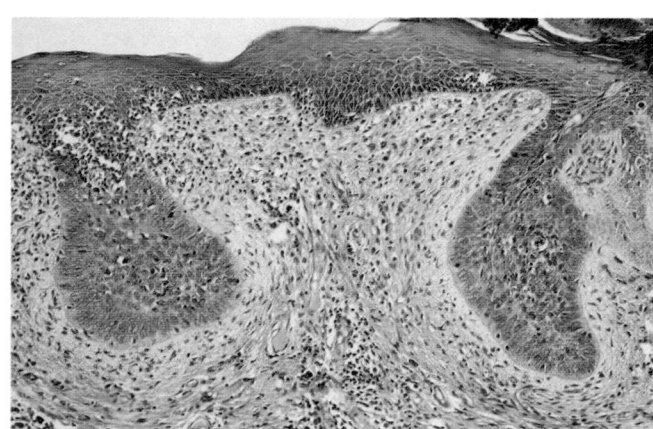

Figure 21-2 Superficial basal cell carcinoma. Buds of atypical basal cells extending from the basal layer of the epidermis.

NODULAR BASAL CELL CARCINOMA

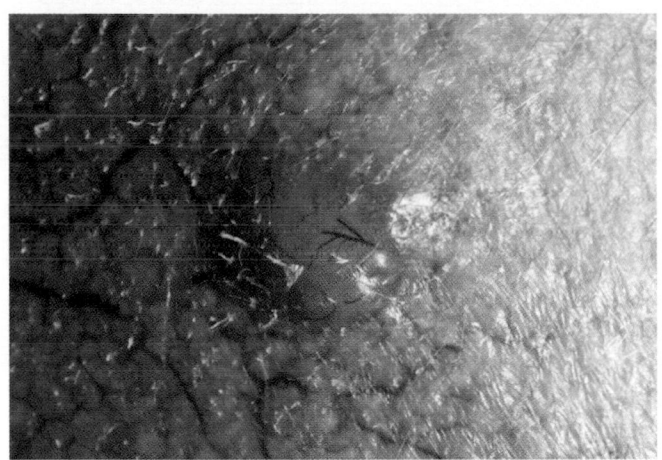

A, Classic presentation. A pink pearly white papule with prominent telangiectatic vessels.

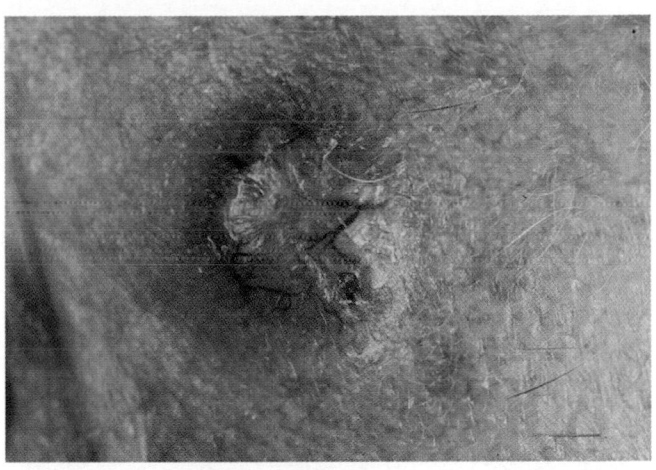

B, Lesion is not pearly white and resembles a dermal nevus.

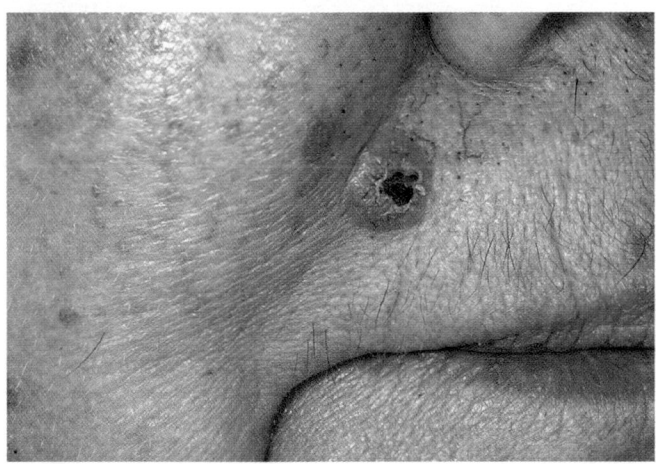

C, Central crusting occurs as the lesion enlarges.

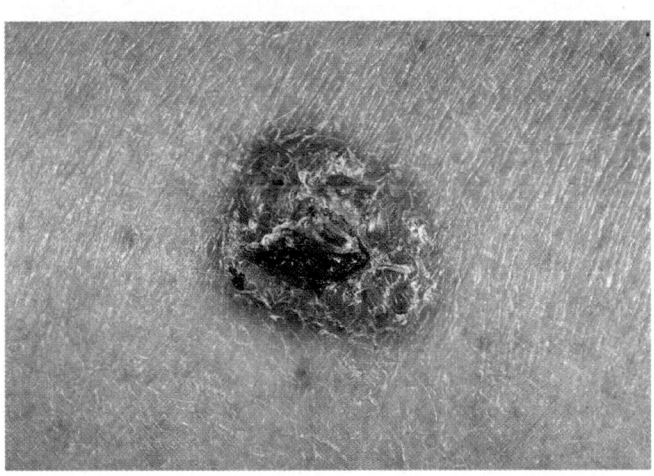

D, A dome-shaped papule covered with scale resembles an irritated seborrheic keratosis.

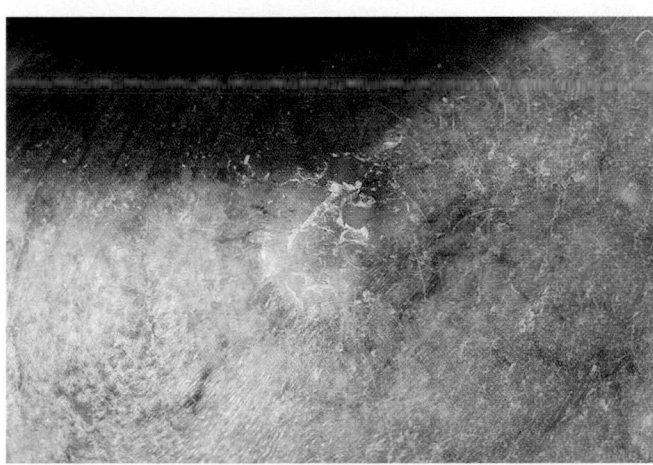

E, Tension on the surrounding skin accentuated this tiny translucent lesion with surface telangiectasia.

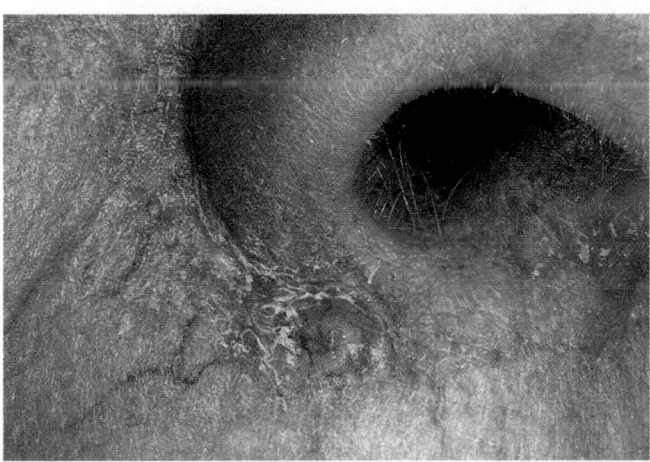

F, Small lesions can be missed on physical examination.

Figure 21-3

NODULAR BASAL CELL CARCINOMA

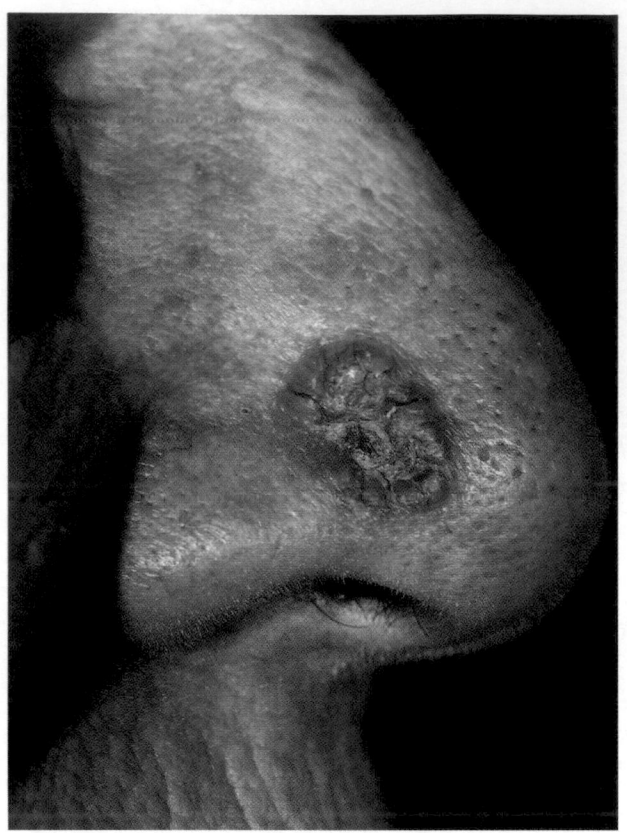

A, The center is ulcerated and is covered with a crust.

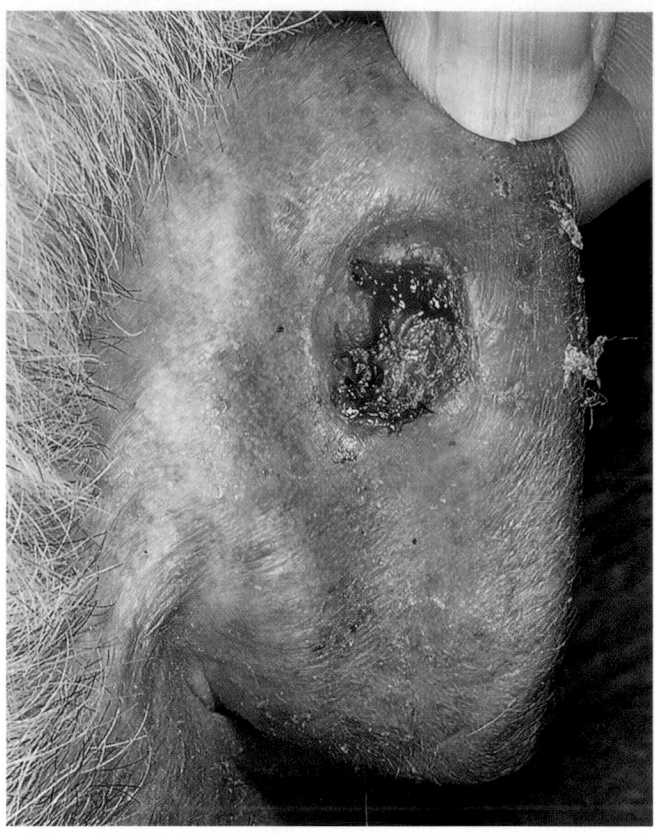

B, This lesion appeared to be inflammatory and was treated with topical steroids. After repeated cycles of healing and ulceration, a biopsy proved the diagnosis.

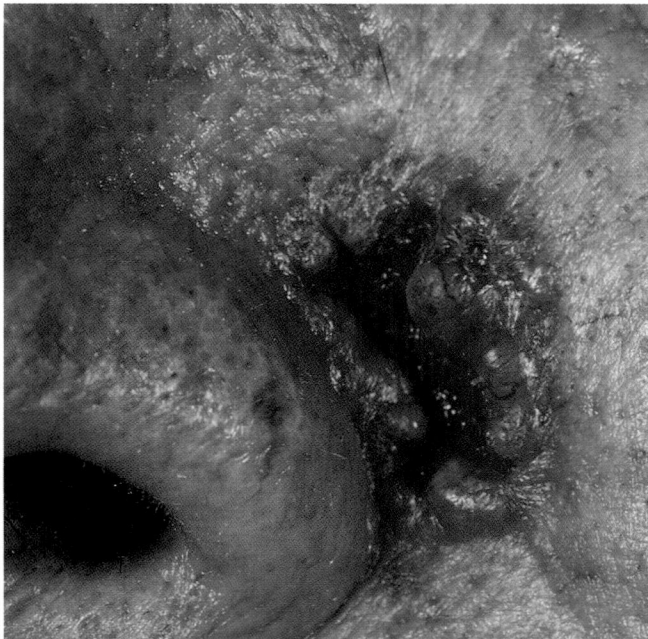

C, A deep ulcer is surrounded by a nodular tumor. In the past this type of lesion was referred to as a *rodent ulcer.*

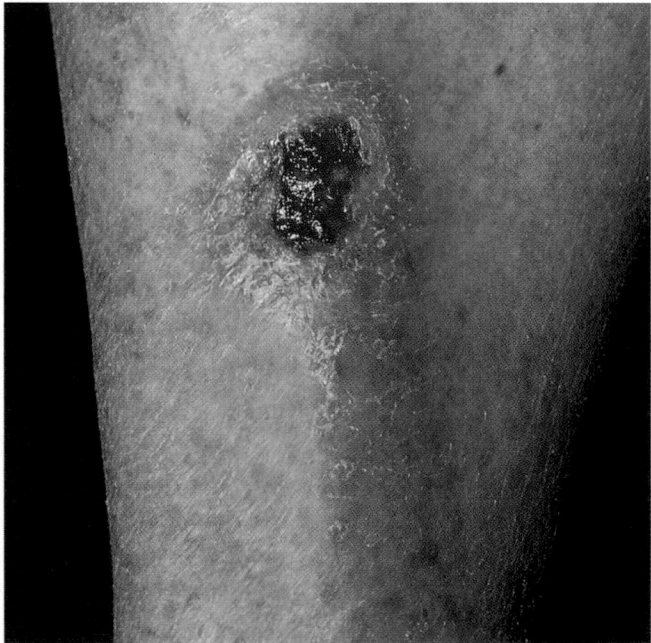

D, Lesions can appear anywhere on the body. Suspect basal cell carcinoma when a small leg ulcer fails to heal after conventional therapy. Close examination reveals a nodular border.

Figure 21-4

PIGMENTED BASAL CELL CARCINOMA. BCCs may contain melanin that imparts a brown, black, or blue color through all or part of the lesion. Clinically, the lesion resembles a melanoma or pigmented seborrheic keratosis, but close inspection reveals the characteristically elevated, pearly white, translucent border (Figure 21-5). Surface microscopy (dermoscopy, p. 798) may be used for more accurate diagnosis. Pigmented BCC must not have a pigment network and must have 1 or more of the following 6 positive features: large gray-blue ovoid nests, multiple gray-blue globules, maple leaflike areas, spoke wheel areas, ulceration, and arborizing "treelike" telangiectasia.[8] A biopsy confirms the diagnosis. The histologic pattern most frequently associated with pigment is the nodular pattern.[9]

CYSTIC BASAL CELL CARCINOMA. This variant of nodular BCC appears as a smooth, round, cystic mass. Cystic BCC behaves like nodular BCC.

SCLEROSING OR MORPHEAFORM BASAL CELL CARCINOMA. Morpheaform BCC is an insidious tumor possessing innocuous surface characteristics that can mask its potential for deep, wide extension. The tumor is waxy, firm, flat-to-slightly raised, either pale white or yellowish, and resembles localized scleroderma, thus the designation morpheaform (Figure 21-6). The borders are indistinct and blend with normal skin. Lesions may become depressed and firm, resembling a scar. The tissue is rigid and difficult or impossible to remove with a curette. Localization of this tumor by inspection or biopsy is impossible. The average subclinical extension beyond clinically delineated borders was 7.2 mm in one study.[10] Treatment consists of wide excision or, preferably, Mohs' micrographic surgery.

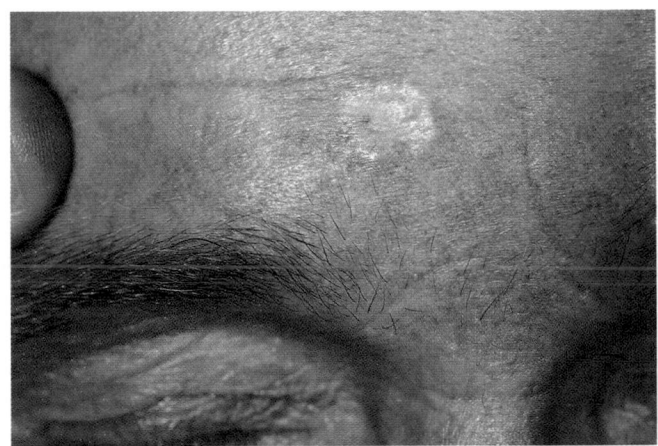

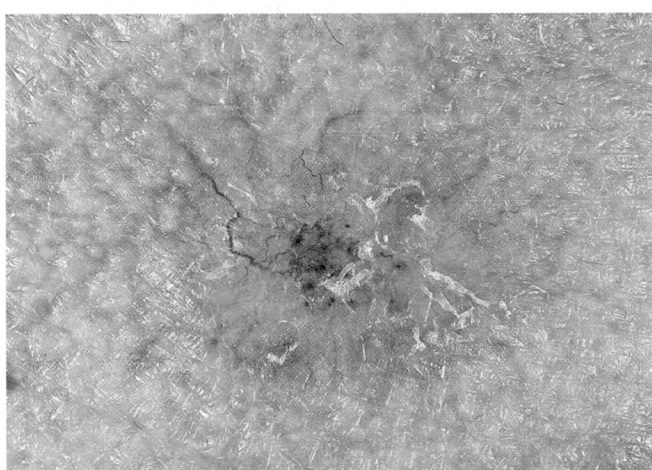

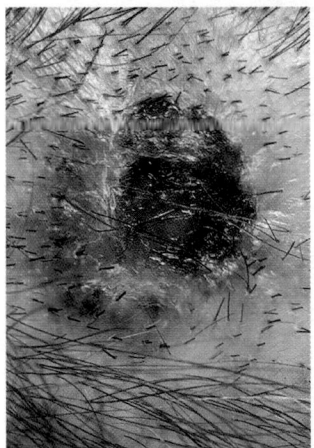 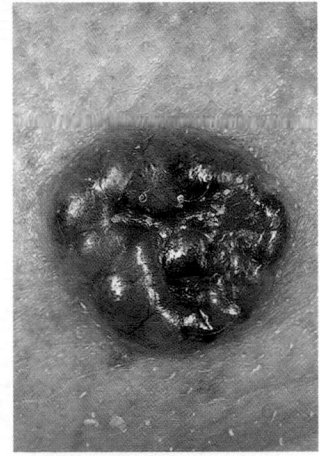

Figure 21-5 Pigmented basal cell carcinoma. Variable amounts of melanin are seen in these special types of nodular basal cell carcinomas.

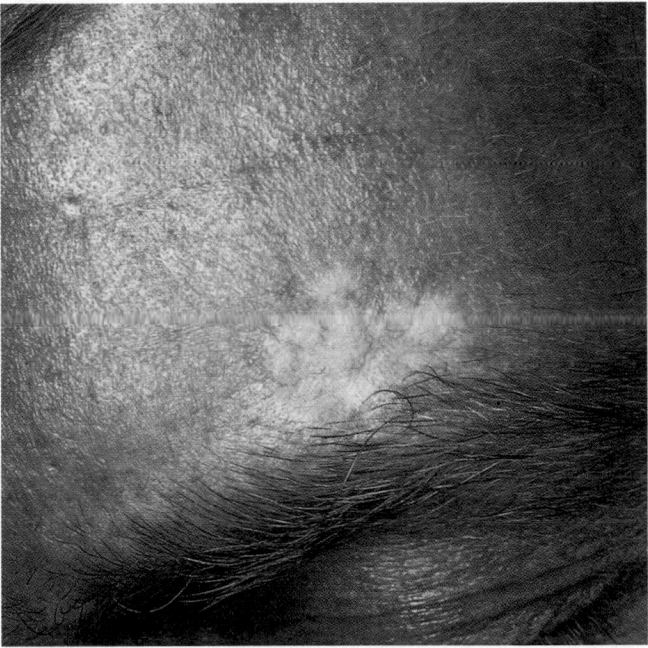

Figure 21-6 Sclerosing basal cell carcinoma. These hard yellow masses may have ill-defined borders.

SUPERFICIAL BASAL CELL CARCINOMA. The least aggressive BCC is the superficial BCC. This tumor occurs most frequently on the trunk and extremities but may occur on the face. There may be one or more lesions. The tumor spreads peripherally, sometimes for several centimeters, and invades after considerable time. Slowly growing lesions may be present for years before patients seek help. The circumscribed, round-to-oval, red, scaling plaque resembles a plaque of eczema, psoriasis, extramammary Paget's disease, or Bowen's disease (Figure 21-7, A to E). However, careful inspection of the border reveals its thin, raised, pearly white nature (Figure 21-7, E). The characteristic features can also be appreciated by eliminating the redness with lateral finger pressure.

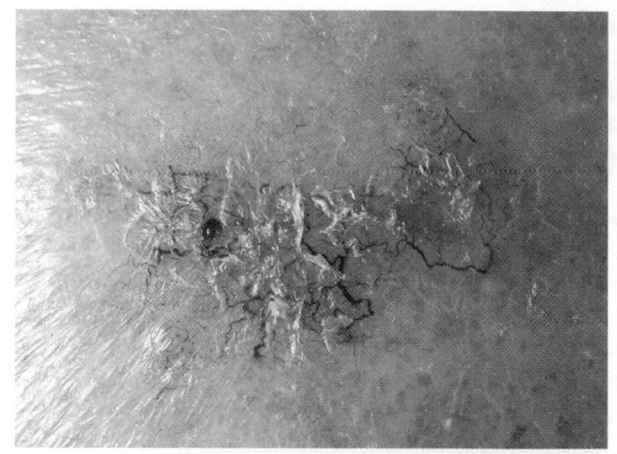
B

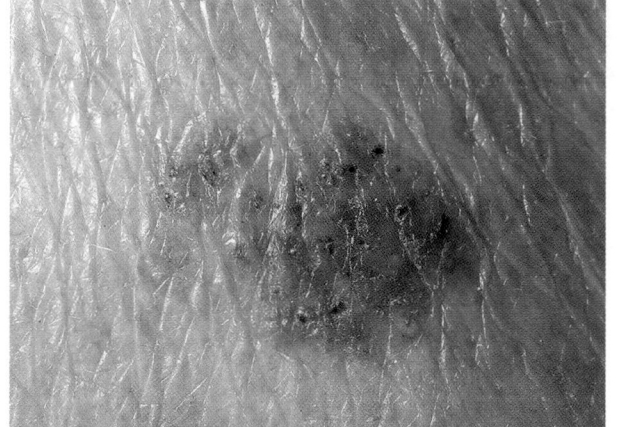
C

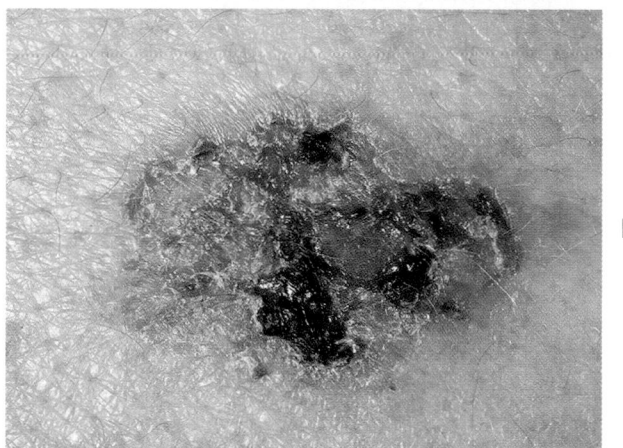
D

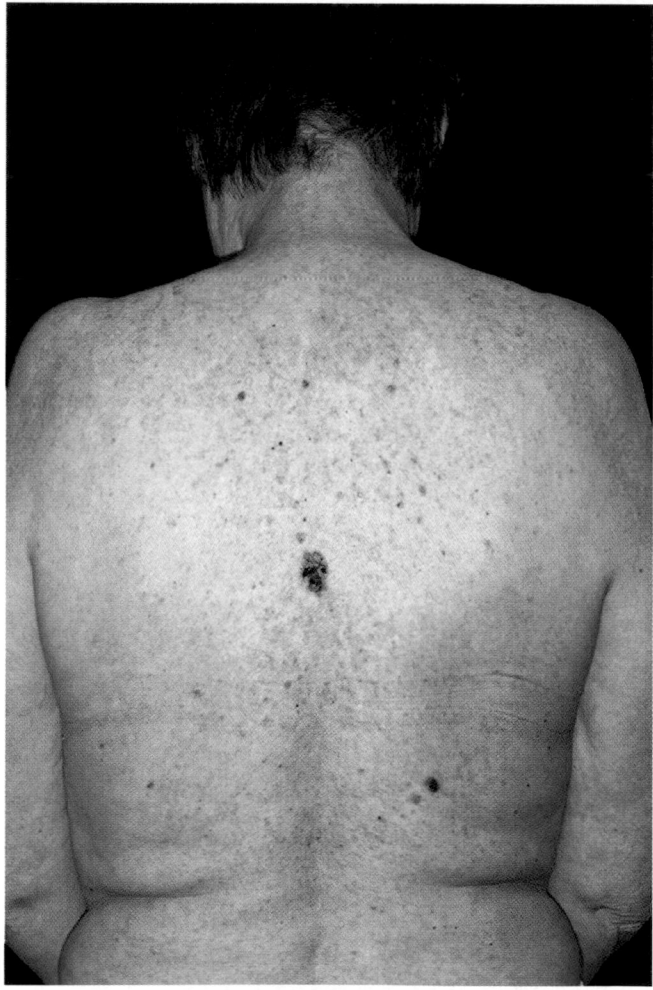
A

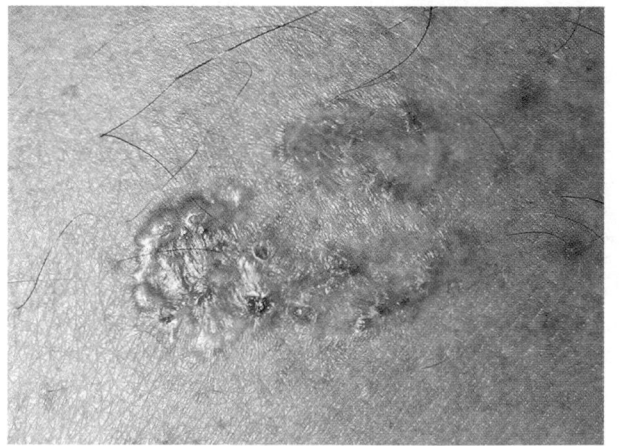
E

Figure 21-7 Superficial basal cell carcinoma. **A,** The trunk is the most common site. **B,** Telangiectasia may be prominent. **C,** Lesions resemble eczema or psoriasis. **D,** Crust and scale occur as the lesion enlarges. **E,** Tension on surrounding skin accentuates the raised border.

NEVOID BASAL CELL CARCINOMA SYNDROME (GORLIN-GOLTZ SYNDROME).

This rare disease is inherited as an autosomal dominant trait with high penetrance and variable expressivity. The gene is located on chromosome 9q22.3-q31.[11, 12] It has the following major features: multiple BCCs appear at birth or in early childhood; numerous small pits on the palms and soles (Figure 21-8) (50% to 87%); epithelium-lined jaw cysts, which commonly cause symptoms (65% to 90%); ectopic calcification with lamellar calcification of falx cerebri (80%); and a variety of skeletal abnormalities, especially of the ribs, skull, and spine (70% to 75%).[13] A characteristic facies is present in approximately 70% of patients. Physical findings include "coarse face" (54%), relative macrocephaly (50%), hypertelorism (42%) and frontal bossing (27%).[14]

Numerous associated anomalies may be present (see Box 21-1).[15, 16] There is great variation in the number and behavior of the nevoid BCC. The median number is eight. Although many patients have no BCCs or just a few, more than 1000 BCCs can be present.[17] The first tumor occurs at 23 years of age (mean).[14] Locally destructive tumors are not seen before puberty. Aggressive tumor behavior can occur after puberty, and all patients must be observed closely. Most of the highly invasive tumors involve embryonic cleft areas of the face. Development of multiple BCCs is enhanced by exposure to light and x-ray irradiation,[18] but they also occur on unexposed surfaces.[19] Multiple bilateral jaw cysts are the presenting complaint in approximately 50% of patients; a dentist, R.J. Gorlin, discovered the syndrome. The cysts appear during the first decade of life and displace the child's teeth, often in the premolar area.[20] The first cyst occurs in 80% by the age of 20 years. The number of cysts ranges from one to 28 (median, three). They cause pain, drainage, and jaw swelling. The occurrence of multiple skeletal anomalies is highly suggestive

and may be the earliest clue to the diagnosis of nevoid BCC syndrome in children. Complete or partial bridging of the sella turcica is present in 75% of patients. Splayed and bifurcated ribs occur in 40% of patients. Ovarian fibromas were diagnosed by ultrasound in (17%) at 30 years of age (mean).

The initial evaluation of patients suspected of having BCC syndrome should include the following: (1) family history; (2) dental consultations; and (3) radiographs of jaws, skull, chest, spinal column, and hands. Radiographs show calcification of the falx cerebri (65%) or tentorium cerebelli (20%); bridged sella (68%), bifid ribs (26%), and flame-shaped lucencies of the phalanges; and metacarpal and carpal bones of the hands (30%).[14]

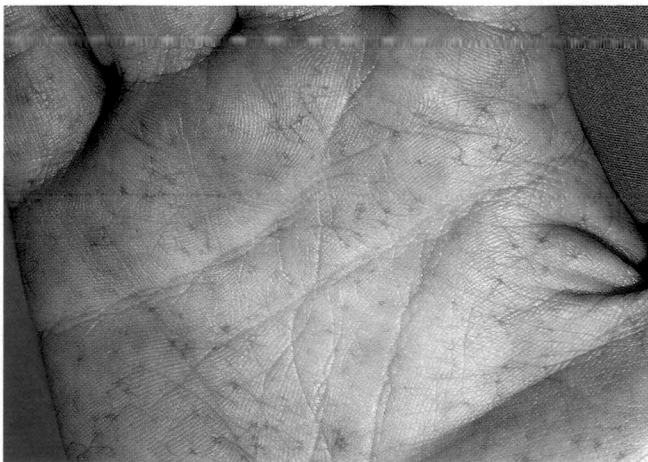

Figure 21-8 Nevoid BCC syndrome. Numerous small pits occur in the palms and soles.

Box 21-1 Nevoid Basal Cell Carcinoma Syndrome
Skin
Multiple nevoid basal cell carcinomas
Pits—palms and soles (50% to 65%)
Milia, cysts (epithelial and sebaceous)
Face and mouth
Multiple jaw cysts (65% to 90%)
Presenting complaint in 50%
Characteristic facies (70%)
Mandibular prognathism
Broadening of the nasal root (25%)
Frontal/temporoparietal bossing
Ocular hypertelorism
Central nervous system
Lamellar calcification of falx cerebri (90%)
Bridging of the sella turcica (75%)
Mental retardation
Electroencephalographic abnormalities
Skeletal system anomalies (70% to 75%)
Rib anomalies (55%): bifurcation and splaying (40%), synostotic or partial agenesis, or rudimentary cervical ribs
Vertebrae (65%): kyphoscoliosis (50%), spina bifida occulta (40%)
Shortened metacarpals (usually 4th, 5th, or both) (28%)
Bone cysts—phalanges and other bones (46%)
Many others
Others
Lymphomesenteric cysts
Ovarian fibromas or cysts
Kimonis VE et al: Am J Med Genet 1997; 69:299.

Management and risk of recurrence

There are several factors to consider before choosing the best treatment modality.[21] The most important are clinical presentation, cell type, tumor size, and location. The diagram below presents a treatment algorithm for BCE.

CLINICAL TYPE. Nodular and superficial BCCs are the least aggressive and can be completely removed by electrodesiccation and curettage or by simple surgical excision.

HISTOLOGIC TYPE. The micronodular, infiltrative, and morpheaform BCCs have a higher incidence of positive tumor margins (18.6%, 26.5%, and 33.3%, respectively) after excision and have the greatest recurrence rate.[6] Clinically, BCCs with these patterns have poorly defined borders and are not apparent during physical examination.[22] They subtly extend into surrounding tissue and are easily missed by blind treatment techniques such as surgical excision. An average of 7.2 mm of subclinical tumor extension was found in morpheaform BCCs in one study, compared with 2.1 mm of extension in well-circumscribed nodular lesions.[10] Routine pathologic examination of surgically excised BCCs may not detect a small nodule or strand of BCC on the other side of the excision margin. These tumors need more aggressive treatment with wide excision or microscopically controlled surgery.

TUMOR SIZE. In general, electrodesiccation and curettage afford excellent results for small (less than 1 cm) nodular BCCs located on the forehead and cheeks. Nodular BCCs on the forehead and cheek that are larger and have well-defined margins should be excised and closed; electrosurgery for large tumors may result in large, unsightly scars. The margins of sclerosing BCCs cannot be determined by inspection, and either excision or, preferably, Mohs' micrographic surgery should be performed. Superficial BCCs of any size can be adequately removed by electrosurgery or treated medically with imiquimod cream (Aldara).

LOCATION. Tumors around the nose, eye, and ear require special consideration. Lesions of the nose greater than 1 cm, lesions of the margin of the eyelid and the vermilion border of the lip, lesions involving cartilage, and sclerosing epitheliomas respond poorly to electrodesiccation and curettage.[23] BCCs of the medial canthus are particularly dangerous. The skin rests close to bone and cartilage, and tumor cells initially invade and proceed to migrate undetected along periosteum or perichondrium. Healing occurs over inadequately treated tumors, and deep invasion and lateral extension can remain undetected, resulting in a tumor of massive proportions. Extension to the eye and brain is possible.

RISK OF RECURRENCE WITH ELECTRODESICCATION AND CURETTAGE (ED&C). Low-, intermediate-, and high-risk sites for recurrence following ED&C of primary BCC have been defined. The neck, trunk, and extremities are considered low-risk sites with a 5-year recurrence rate of 8.6%. The scalp, forehead, and temples are of intermediate risk with a 12.9% recurrence rate. High-risk sites, such as the nose, eyelids, chin, jaw, and ear, have a recurrence rate of 17.5%.[24] To achieve a 95% cure rate for ED&C at middle-risk sites, lesions should measure less than 1 cm in diameter, and in high-risk areas a 95% cure rate for ED&C may be achieved by selecting lesions less than 6 mm in diameter.

RELATIVE RISK AND FOLLOW-UP. Patients treated for BCC should be observed periodically for 5 years or longer.[25] Of patients with one BCC, a second BCC develops in 36% to 50% during the 5 years after treatment.[26, 27] In another series, another BCC developed in 41% of patients who had two or more previous skin cancers.[28]

BASAL CELL CARCINOMA

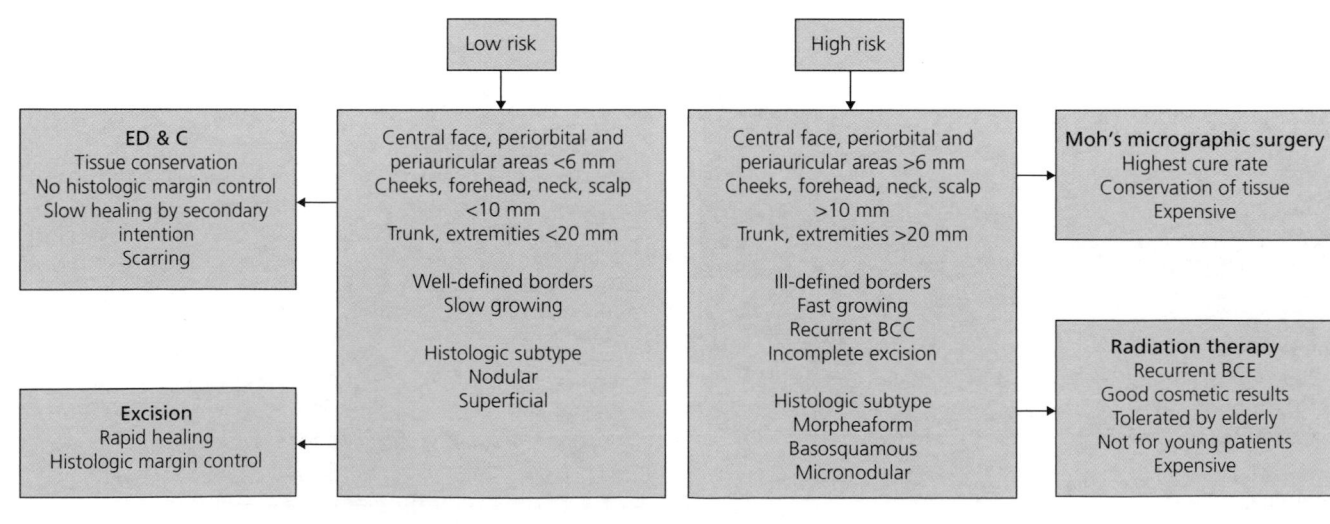

Adapted from Martinez JC, Otley CC: MayoClin Proc 2001;76:1253.

Recurrent basal cell carcinoma

CLINICAL PRESENTATION. Inadequately treated BCC may recur. The tumor may be superficial in the scar tissue, on the border, or deep in the dermis or subcutaneous fat (Figure 21-19). The clinical presentation of recurrent BCC sometimes differs from the original tumor. A tumor that infiltrates scar tissue produces a subtle change in color and consistency that is easily missed. Erosions that appear spontaneously at the border or in the scar are suspicious. The characteristic pearly white border is often absent, but biopsy of the erosion with the curette can reveal the soft, amorphous, gelatinous tissue of BCC extending deep and laterally well beyond the border of the erosion. Deep recurrences show a normal or a brownish erythematous surface and can be confused with epidermal cysts.[29]

Histologic picture, anatomic location, and size are factors in predicting recurrence.

Histologic type. Tumors of the morpheaform and basosquamous varieties have the greatest recurrence rate. BCCs that histologically show poor palisading or have a micronodular (islands of tumor) and/or infiltrating strand pattern without sclerotic stroma clinically have poorly defined borders and are not apparent during physical examination.[22]

They subtly extend into surrounding tissue and are easily missed by blind treatment techniques such as surgical excision. An average of 7.2 mm of subclinical tumor extension was found in morpheaform BCCs in one study, compared with 2.1 mm of extension in well-circumscribed nodular lesions.[10] As mentioned previously, routine pathologic examination of surgically excised BCCs may not detect a small nodule or strand of BCC on the other side of the excision margin. These tumors need more aggressive treatment with wide excision or microscopically controlled surgery.

Location. Increasing diameter of the lesion and location of the lesion on various sites of the head, especially the nose and ear, are associated with an increased risk of recurrence, whereas location on the neck, trunk, limbs, or genitalia is associated with a decreased risk of recurrence with curettage-electrodesiccation, radiation therapy, and surgical excision.[30] BCCs on the nose or perinasal area may infiltrate along the perichondrium or penetrate into the embryonic fusion plane of the nasolabial fold, resulting in subclinical extension.

Size. The larger the tumor, the greater the chance of recurrence; increased subclinical extension is seen with larger tumors.

Figure 21-9 Recurrent basal cell carcinoma. A haphazard nodular tumor with telangiectasia surrounds and infiltrates under scar tissue.

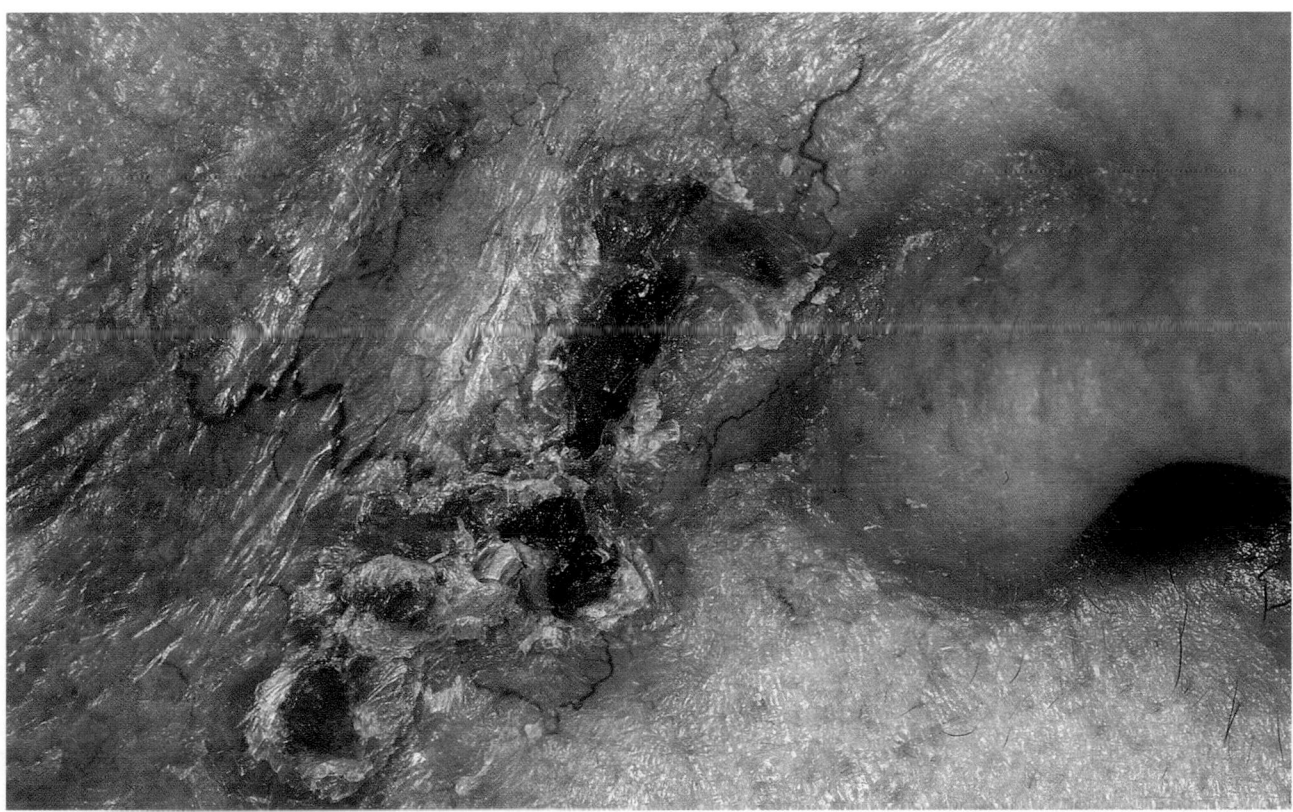

Treatment

The following section outlines various treatment modalities.[31] Specific techniques are described in Chapter 27.

RECOMMENDED FOLLOW-UP EVALUATION. Patients with BCC may benefit from a once-yearly complete skin examination. Because the risk of a subsequent BCC decreases 3 years after an index tumor, the need for continued surveillance of patients with a BCC who have remained tumor-free after 3 years is probably limited.[32]

BIOPSY. Biopsy alone of a small BCC often appears curative with no clinical evidence of residual tumor. Two thirds of clinically disease-free biopsy sites were shown to contain microscopic foci of BCC.[33]

ELECTRODESICCATION AND CURETTAGE. ED&C is most beneficial for nodular BCCs less than 6 mm in diameter, regardless of anatomic site; selected larger BCCs, depending on their anatomic site; and superficial BCCs.[24,34-37] It is not appropriate for morpheaform BCCs because margins cannot be clinically defined. Lesions on the nose and nasolabial folds may be treated if they are well defined and very small; otherwise, these high-risk areas should be treated by Mohs' micrographic surgery. ED&C is particularly useful for ear lesions, where mobilization of skin for closure after excision is difficult.

Curettage requires firm dermis on all sides and below the tumor to enable the curette to distinguish between dermis and soft tumor (Figure 21-10). If the tumor encroaches on the fat, the curette cannot distinguish between fat and soft tumor, and an alternate procedure must be used. Curettage should be avoided for lesions on the back and shoulders, where the dermis is thick, unless the BCCs are superficial and small. Proper technique requires vigorous curettage, usually two to three times; therefore lesions on the eyelid or lip area are treated by other methods. It is especially useful for lower extremity tumors, where tissue mobilization for excision may be difficult.

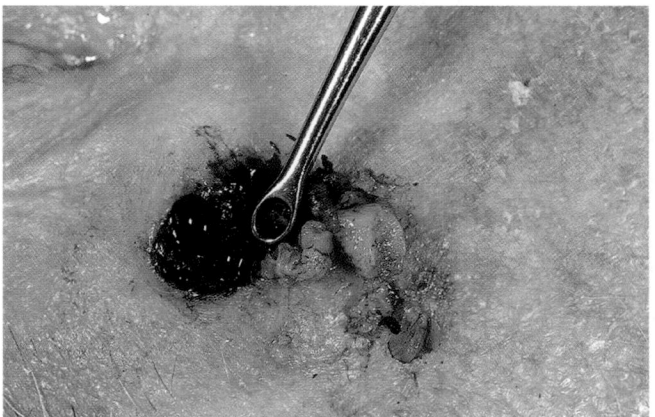

Figure 21-10 Nodular basal cell carcinoma. Curettage easily disrupts the poorly cohesive tumor.

Wounds created by electrosurgery ooze serum and accumulate crust during a 2- to 6-week healing period. The recurrence rate for ED&C performed by a fully trained dermatologist is 5.7%. The overall recurrence rate for surgical excision is 5.3%.[38] The technique is explained in Chapter 27.

EXCISION SURGERY. Excision surgery is preferred for large tumors with well-defined borders on the cheeks, forehead, trunk, and legs. The cosmetic result is good and healing time is less than that required for electrosurgery. Excision with primary closure is technically difficult on the ears and nose. The advantage of feeling the tumor with a curette is lost and adequate margins must be taken. A 98% cure rate was achieved in one study when BCCs less than 2 cm were excised with excisional margins of 4 mm around the tumor.[39] One large series revealed 5-year recurrence rates of BCCs excised from various anatomic sites: 0.7% on the neck, trunk, and extremities; 3.2% on the head if lesions were less than 6 mm in diameter; 5.2% on the head if lesions were 6 to 9 mm in diameter; and 9.0% on the head if lesions were 10 mm or more in diameter.[40]

Preoperative curettage. Preoperative curettage may assist the surgeon in better defining the tumor border and decreases the frequency of positive margins in the management of BCC. It offers a 24% reduction in surgical failure rates in the treatment of BCC. Curettage showed no benefit in the treatment of SCC. It is postulated that SCC differs from noninvasive BCC in that SCC invades as small nests in the absence of mucinous stroma and therefore does not loosen as readily from its surrounding matrix as would BCC. Thus, although preexcisional curettage of SCC does no harm, it may not improve surgical cure rates.[41]

Incompletely resected basal cell carcinoma. Adequate excision, peripherally and in depth, is the key to surgical control, and the demonstration of tumor cells at the margins of excision is associated with recurrence rates of more than 30%. Data support the policy of immediate re-excision or Mohs' micrographic surgery for all patients with incompletely excised basal cell carcinomas rather than a "wait-and-see" policy after incomplete excision.[42-44] Re-excision may not be necessary if the patient's life span is limited or if treatment of a possible recurrence would not be difficult.

CRYOSURGERY. Cryosurgery with liquid nitrogen delivered with a spray apparatus or a cryoprobe is appropriate for small-to-large BCCs of the nodular and superficial types with clearly definable margins (laterally and in depth).[45] It is not indicated for tumors deeper than 3 mm unless thermocouples are used to measure depth of freeze. A biopsy is performed as a separate operation before the cryosurgical procedure to determine cell type and extent of the tumor or just before the cryosurgery if there is no doubt about the diagnosis. Postoperative pain is moderate to severe. The appearance of a wound a few days after treatment is sometimes alarming to patients. Cryosurgery techniques are explained in Chapter 27.

MOHS' MICROGRAPHIC SURGERY. Mohs' surgery is a microscopically controlled technique that may be used for all types and sizes of BCCs. The procedure is unnecessarily destructive for smaller lesions or for lesions with well-defined clinical margins, such as nodular or superficial multicentric BCCs.

Mohs' surgery is the treatment of choice for most sclerosing BCCs and other BCCs with poorly defined clinical margins; for tumors in areas of potentially high recurrence (Box 21-2), such as the nose or eyelid; for very large primary tumors; and for large, recurrent BCCs.[46] The technique is explained in Chapter 27.

RADIATION. Radiation is useful for elderly patients who cannot tolerate minor surgical procedures. For areas in which preservation of normal surrounding tissue is of prime consideration (e.g., around the eyelids and lips), radiation therapy may produce the best cosmetic result.

The overall 5-year recurrence rate is 7.4%. BCCs less than 10 mm in diameter on the head have a 5-year recurrence rate of 4.4%,[47] whereas those 10 mm or greater in diameter have a rate of 9.5%. The proportion of recurrence-free treatment sites with a good or excellent long-term cosmetic outcome after radiation therapy (63%) is lower than that of curettage-electrodesiccation (91%) and of surgical excision (84%).[48]

Radiation therapy is an effective method of treating recurrent BCCs that are smaller than 1 cm.[49] Therefore, if the long-term cosmetic outcome after treatment is not an overriding concern, x-ray therapy is an effective modality for many primary and recurrent BCCs. The treatment requires a number of outpatient visits that may be difficult for debilitated patients.

IMIQUIMOD 5% CREAM (ALDARA). Imiquimod is an immune response modifier that induces cytokines related to cell-mediated immune responses including interferon-alfa, interferon-gamma, and interleukin 12. Patient-administered imiquimod 5% cream administered daily for a period of 6 weeks effectively treated superficial BCE. Local skin reactions are common but well tolerated.[50, 51]

5-FLUOROURACIL. 5-fluorouracil (5-FU) should not be used for the treatment of any BCCs, with the exception of some that occur in the rare basal cell nevus syndrome.[52] 5-FU can destroy the surface tumor without affecting deeper cells.

INTRALESIONAL INTERFERON-ALFA AND PHOTODYNAMIC THERAPY. These are new experimental methods of therapy and are not likely to become important therapeutic modalities.[53]

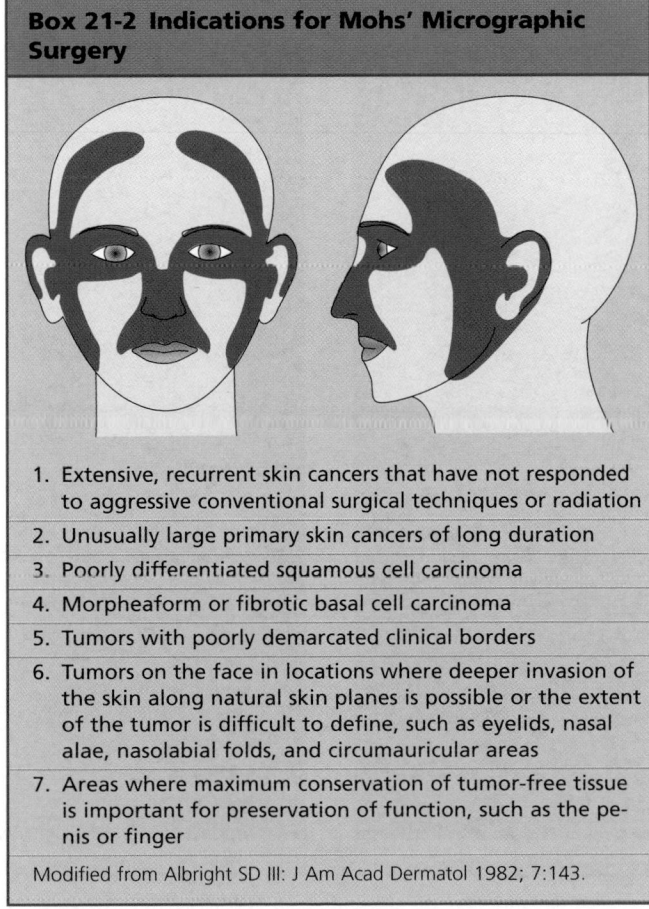

Box 21-2 Indications for Mohs' Micrographic Surgery

1. Extensive, recurrent skin cancers that have not responded to aggressive conventional surgical techniques or radiation
2. Unusually large primary skin cancers of long duration
3. Poorly differentiated squamous cell carcinoma
4. Morpheaform or fibrotic basal cell carcinoma
5. Tumors with poorly demarcated clinical borders
6. Tumors on the face in locations where deeper invasion of the skin along natural skin planes is possible or the extent of the tumor is difficult to define, such as eyelids, nasal alae, nasolabial folds, and circumauricular areas
7. Areas where maximum conservation of tumor-free tissue is important for preservation of function, such as the penis or finger

Modified from Albright SD III: J Am Acad Dermatol 1982; 7:143.

Actinic Keratosis

Actinic keratosis (AK) (solar keratosis) is a squamous cell carcinoma confined to the epidermis. The lesions are common, sun-induced, and increase in number with age. Most lesions remain superficial. Lesions that extend more deeply to involve the papillary and/or reticular dermis are termed *squamous cell carcinoma* (SCC).[54]

The potential for change cannot be predicted by clinical signs or histologic characteristics. Thick lesions are worrisome. Patients with AKs need periodic evaluation and usually repetitive treatments to prevent the development of aggressive cancers. Individuals with light complexions are more susceptible than those with dark complexions. Years of sun exposure are required to induce sufficient damage to cause lesions. Actinic keratoses may undergo spontaneous remission if sunlight exposure is reduced, but new lesions may appear.[55] Patients often present with lesions that were first noticed during the summer, suggesting that the lesions may become more active after sunlight exposure. Immunosuppression is a risk factor. SCC is up to 65 times as likely to develop in transplant patients as controls. Lesions appear 2 to 4 years after transplantation and increase in frequency.[56]

Perspective for the patient

An AK is an intraepidermal SCC. This definition is useful for the clinician and pathologist, but it confuses and worries the patient. The term actinic keratosis without the word cancer is appropriate for patients. Patients need to understand that these lesions can become thicker and change into invasive cancers but the chance of that happening is small. Periodic examinations, treatment, and preventive measures (sunscreens, clothing) are necessary.

CLINICAL PRESENTATION. Actinic keratoses begin as an area of increased vascularity, with the skin surface becoming slightly rough. Texture is the key to diagnosing early lesions. They are better recognized by palpation than by inspection. Very gradually an adherent, yellow, sharp scale forms. Removal of the scale may cause bleeding (Figures 21-11 to 21-13). Most lesions vary in size from 3 to 6 mm. The extent of disease varies from a single lesion to involvement of the entire forehead, balding scalp, or temples. AK can progress into thickened or hypertrophic lesions. Thickened lesions can progress to squamous cell carcinoma and be clinically indistinguishable from squamous cell carcinoma. Induration, inflammation, and oozing suggest degeneration into malignancy.

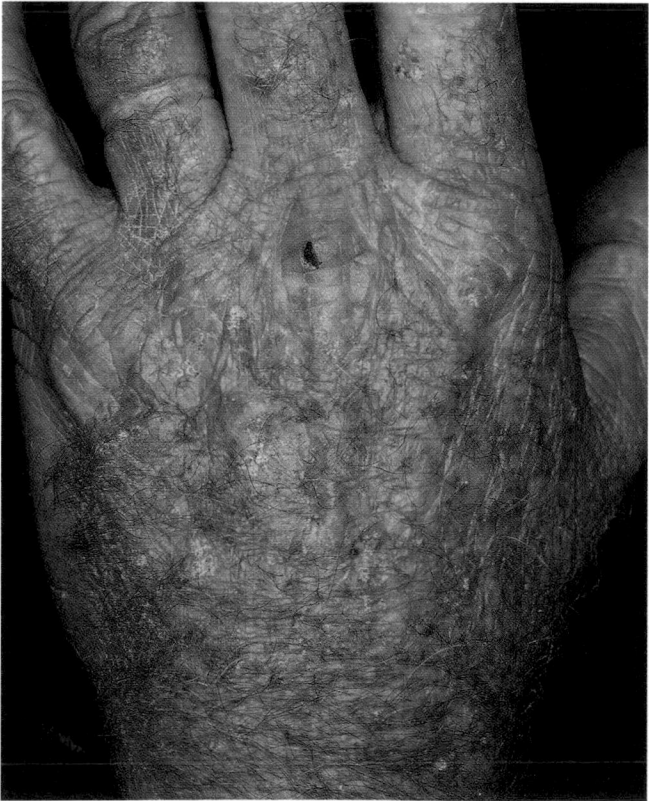

Figure 21-11 Actinic keratosis. Several oval-to-round, red, indurated lesions with adherent scale.

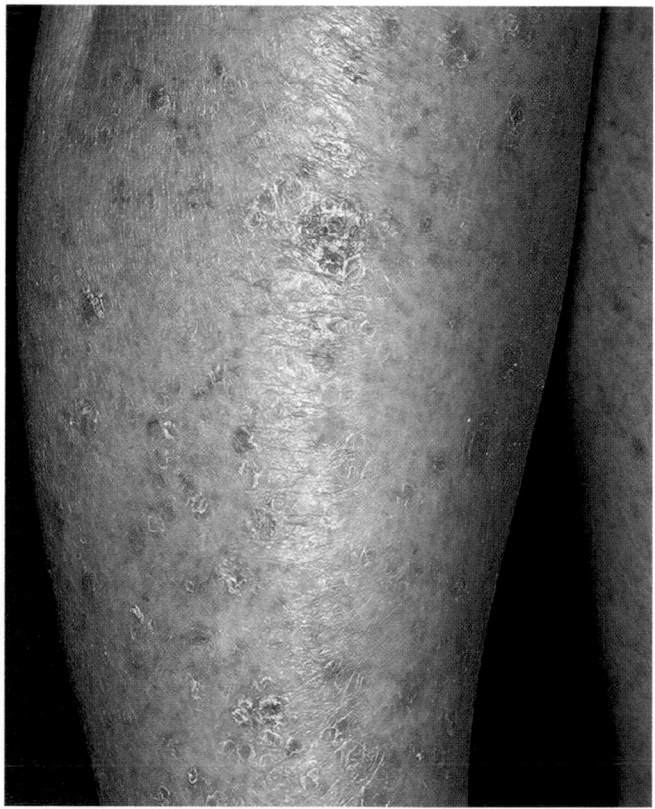

Figure 21-12 Actinic keratoses may appear in large numbers on unexposed arms and legs.

ACTINIC KERATOSIS

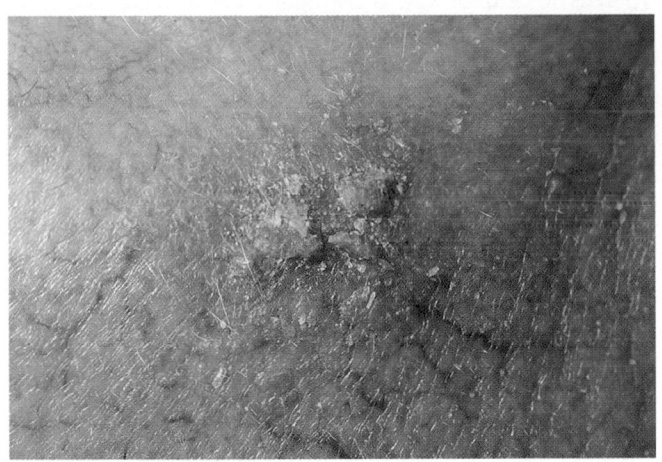

A, Classic lesion with sharp, adherent scale on a red base.

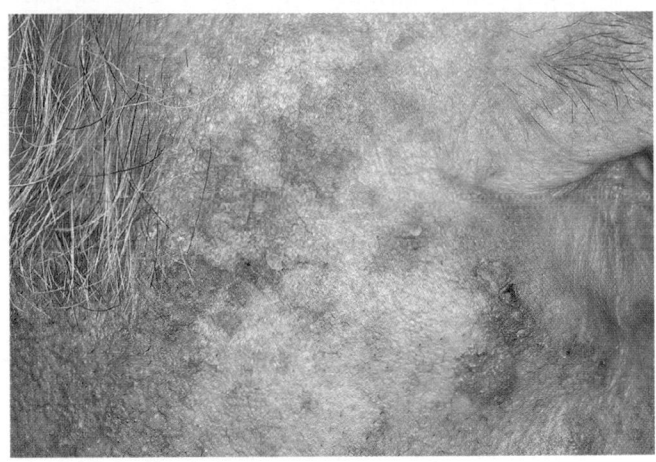

B, Many lesions may appear on the face. The surrounding skin is irregularly pigmented with dilated blood vessels.

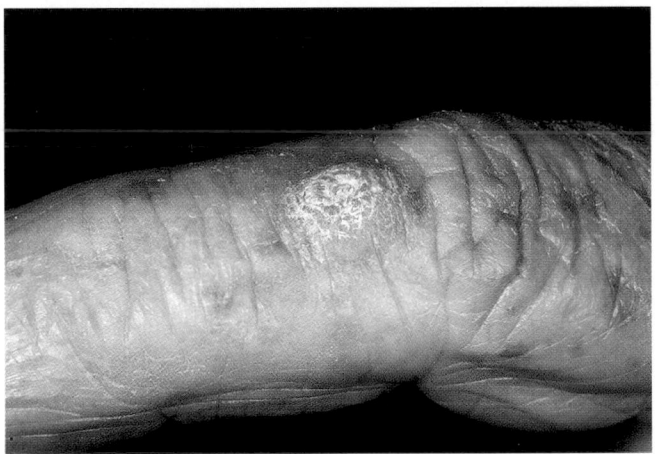

C, Thicker lesions may degenerate into squamous cell carcinomas.

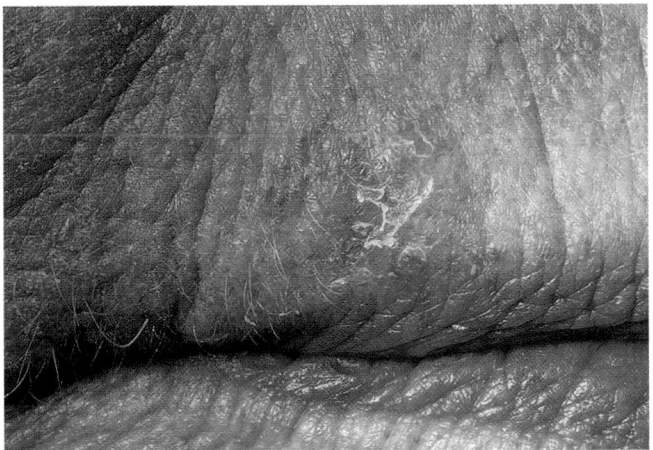

D, Keratoses on the lips may be deeper than they appear.

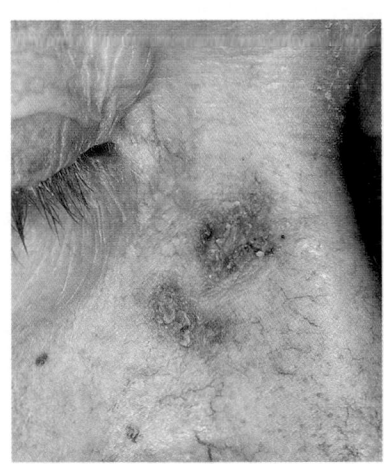

E, Large keratoses may have considerable depth.

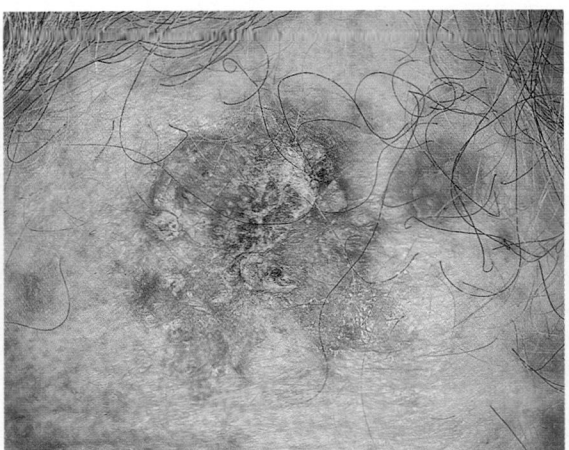

F, Very large lesions take months or years to form.

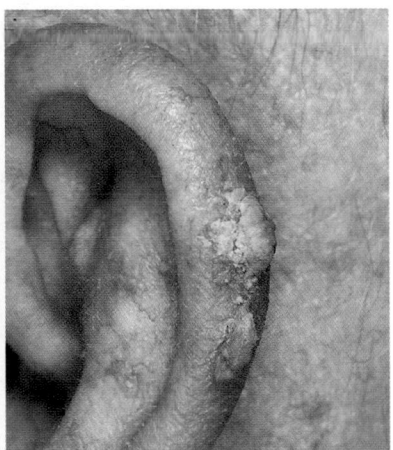

G, Squamous cell carcinoma has an identical appearance.

Figure 21-13

CLINICAL VARIANTS. Clinical variants include cutaneous horn, spreading pigmented AK, and actinic cheilitis. Cutaneous horn is a hypertrophic AK that accumulates keratin to become a conical hyperkeratotic protuberance (see Figure 20-14). Pigmented AKs resemble a scaling lentigo, seborrheic keratosis, or melanoma (Figures 21-14 and 21-15). Actinic cheilitis is AK occurring on the lower lips. The lips are rough, scaly, red, and may show fissuring, scaliness, and ulcerations (Figures 21-16 and 21-17). These findings can be seen in SCC of the lip. SCCs of the lip have approximately an 11% metastatic rate, which is higher than other cutaneous squamous cell carcinomas.[57]

TRANSFORMATION INTO SQUAMOUS CELL CARCINOMA.
After several years, a small percentage of lesions may increase in size and thickness, extend into the dermis, and be a risk for metastatic disease. A very low yearly transformation rate for single lesions can translate into a substantial lifetime risk of transformation for patients with several actinic keratoses. The average number of AK per person is 7.7. The likelihood of an AK developing into a SCC is estimated to be 0.085% per lesion per year. Therefore, SCC would develop at a rate of at least 10.2% over 10 years.[54,58] Up to 60% of SCCs develop from actinic keratosis.[59] Squamous cell carcinomas that evolve from actinic keratosis are not aggressive but may eventually metastasize.[60]

ACTINIC KERATOSIS VS. SQUAMOUS CELL CARCINOMA.
There is no definite way to distinguish between an AK and an SCC without a biopsy. There is a continuum of clinical signs that makes distinction difficult. An increase in the thickness, redness, pain, ulceration, and size only suggests progression to SCC, but it is impossible to predict the point at which an individual AK will evolve into an invasive SCC. Lesions thought to be actinic keratoses or those not responding to treatment may actually be SCCs. Therefore treatment should be aggressive and patients monitored closely to prevent progression.[57]

PATHOPHYSIOLOGY AND HISTOLOGY. Ultraviolet radiation initiates the process by inducing mutations in DNA usually in the p53 tumor-suppressor gene in keratinocytes. Cells with dysfunctional p53 may, with additional exposure to UV radiation, be promoted to undergo an uncontrolled clonal cellular proliferation in the epidermis to produce an AK. Additional exposure to radiation may convert the AK into a SCC. Histologically, an AK consists of abnormal epithelial cells confined to the epidermis. The features of the cells are identical to those found in invasive squamous cell carcinoma, including those that have metastasized.[54] The cells have large pleomorphic nuclei and acidophilic cytoplasm (Figure 21-18). Some are in mitosis. They show signs of faulty cornification with dyskeratotic cells and parakeratosis.[61] The term "squamous cell carcinoma in situ" is frequently used to describe a lesion with abnormal cells confined to the epidermis. The follicles are not involved, so there is no follicular plugging. Penetration through the dermoepidermal junction and into the dermis indicates the development of an invasive SCC.

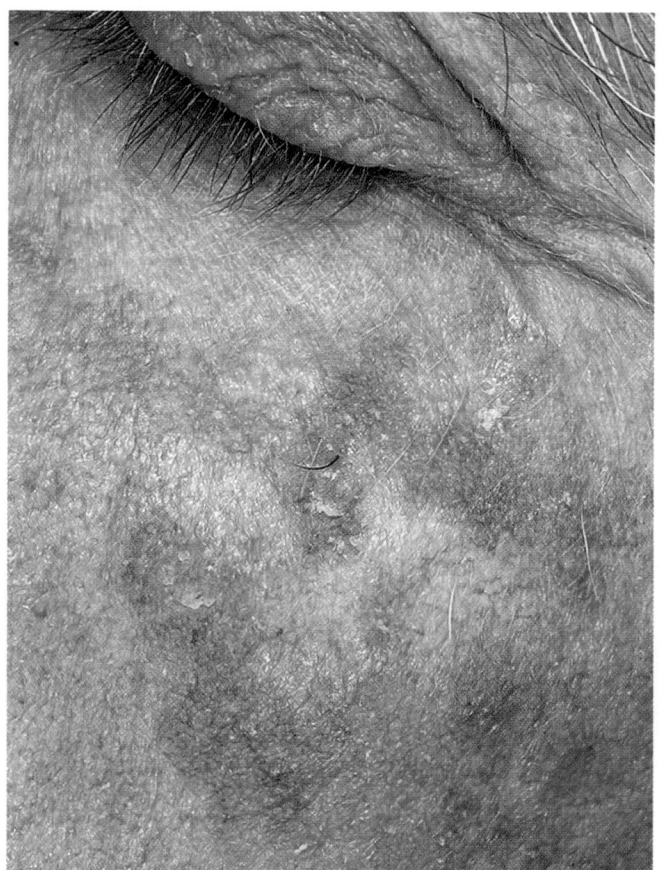

Figure 21-14 Pigmented actinic keratosis.

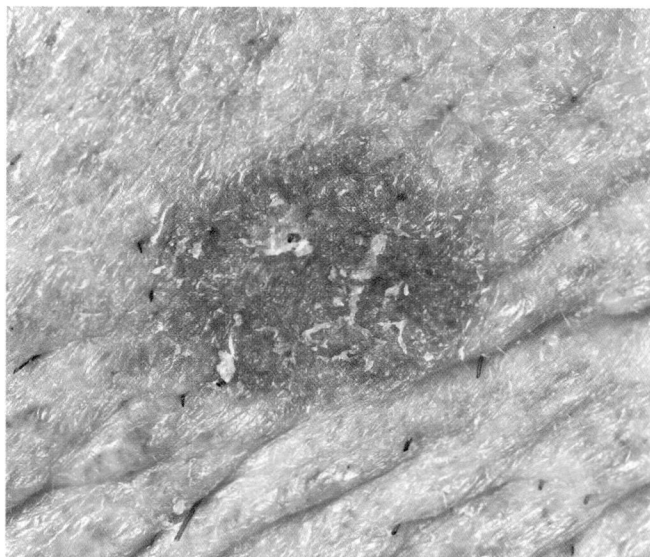

Figure 21-15 Pigmented actinic keratosis.

ACTINIC KERATOSIS

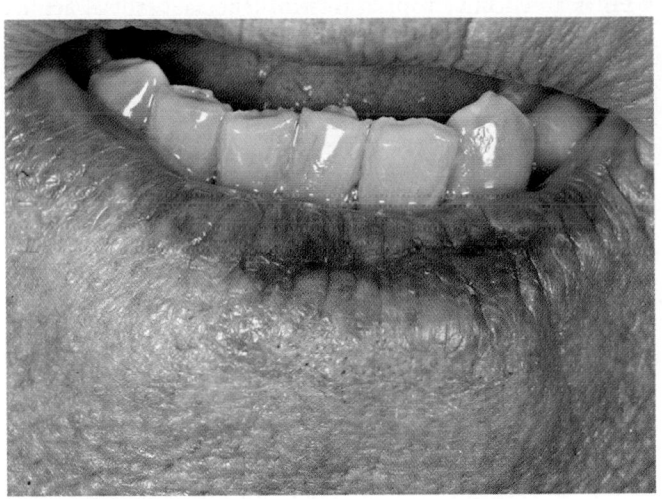

Figure 21-16 Broad superficial lesions may be present for months to years with little progression. These respond to topical 5-fluorouacil.

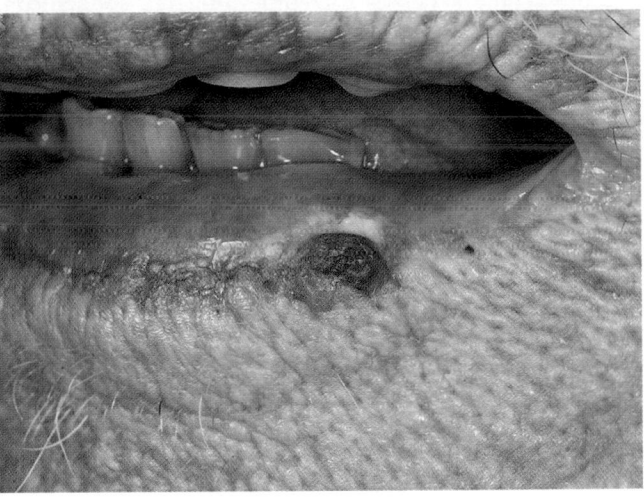

Figure 21-17 The depth of this lesion is difficult to judge by physical examination. Surgery is the most reliable treatment.

Figure 21-18 Keratin and crust are present on the surface. Atypical epithelial cells are confined to the epidermis and do not involve the follicular structure.

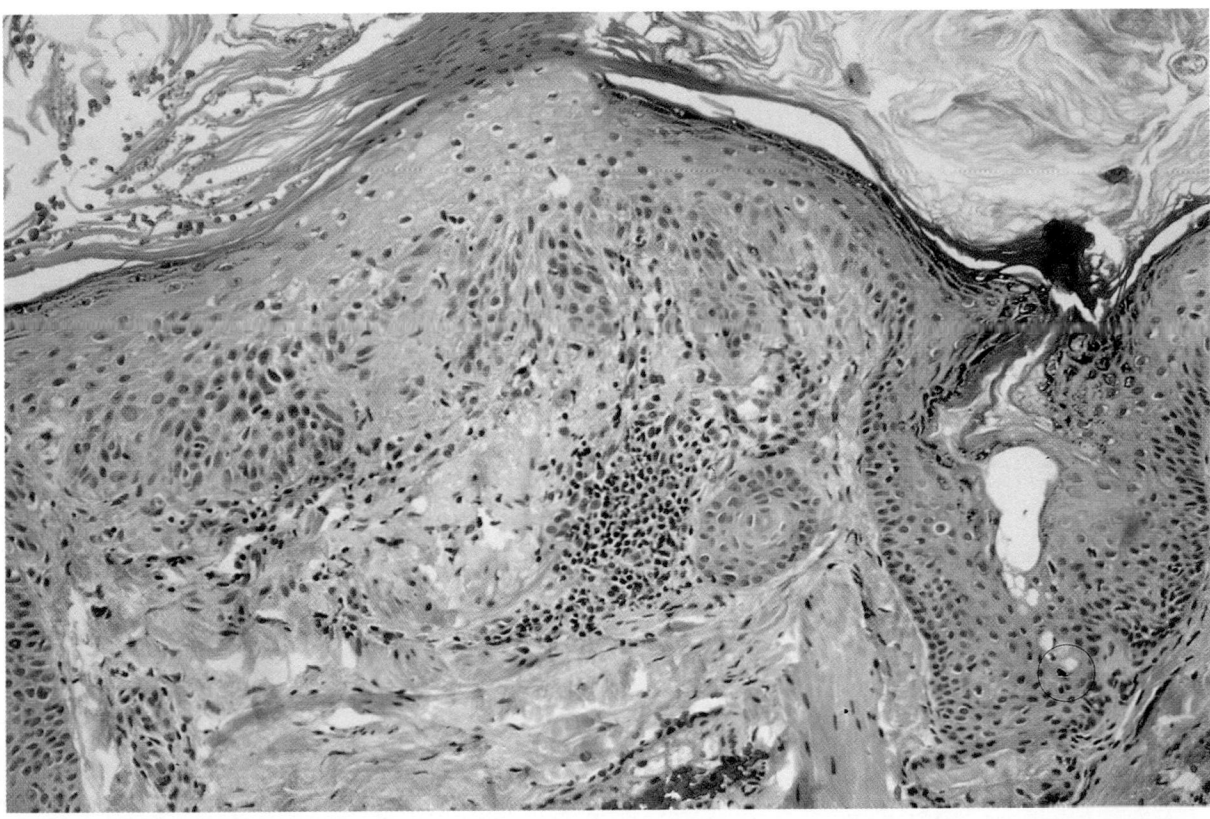

Management

Because actinic keratoses sometimes undergo spontaneous remission, definitive treatment may be delayed for patients with a few superficial lesions. Small lesions should be reexamined at a later date for spontaneous remission. Patients should make every effort to prevent further sun damage. This does not mean that patients must hibernate for a lifetime, but they should understand techniques to reduce sunlight exposure. There is a continuum and a progression from actinic keratoses to squamous cell carcinoma so that there is no way to reliably distinguish clinically between the two diagnoses. Because it can be impossible to distinguish between an actinic keratosis and squamous cell carcinoma, treatment of actinic keratoses should be aggressive to stop the progression to squamous cell carcinoma.[57] All patients with actinic keratosis should be examined carefully for basal cell carcinomas.

CRYOTHERAPY. Cryotherapy is the treatment of choice for most isolated, superficial, actinic keratoses.[62] Actinic keratosis resides in the epithelium. Cryotherapy with liquid nitrogen causes the separation of the epidermis and dermis, resulting in a highly specific, nonscarring method of therapy for superficial lesions. Patients with darker complexions may develop hypopigmented areas after freezing, and treating multiple lesions on the faces of such patients may result in white-spotted faces. Topical 5-FU is the best alternative.

SURGICAL REMOVAL. Individual indurated lesions or those with thick crusts should be removed with minor surgical procedures. It is unnecessary to biopsy lesions less than 0.5 cm. Larger lesions or those occurring about or on the vermilion border of the lips should be examined. Electrodesiccation and curettage easily remove small, thicker lesions. The CO_2 laser may be superior to vermilionectomy for actinic cheilitis too extensive to be treated with topical 5-FU.[63,64]

SUNSCREENS. Regular use of sunscreens prevents the development of solar keratoses.[65] Sunscreens that contain a combination of ingredients to block both the UVA and UVB spectrum of ultraviolet light are most effective. Sunscreens are best applied in the morning on days when sun exposure is anticipated. Sunscreens should be applied to the face, lower lip, ears, back of the neck, and backs of the hands and forearms. Hats should cover bald heads. The physician should explain that although sunscreens are used, additional lesions might occur, but that many superficial areas of involvement may actually improve.[55]

TOPICAL CHEMOTHERAPY WITH 5-FLUOROURACIL. 5-FU is an effective topical treatment for superficial actinic keratosis. Thicker lesions, especially those on the scalp, may evolve into squamous cell carcinomas and should be treated with more aggressive techniques.[66] The agent is incorporated into rapidly dividing cells, resulting in cell death. Normal cells are less affected and clinically appear to be unaffected. Inflammation is induced during this process. Thick, indurated lesions become most inflamed and may best be managed by surgically removing them before instituting topical chemotherapy. The available preparations of 5-FU are listed in Table 21-2 and in the Formulary.

Patients should be cautioned about the various stages of inflammation encountered during treatment. Considerable discomfort may be experienced for 1 week or more during periods of intense inflammation. Pain can be minimized if only small areas are treated at one time; however, many patients wish to treat the full face instead of prolonging the unsightly erythema and crusting for weeks. Lesions on the back of the hands, arms, and lower legs require longer periods of treatment than those on the face (Table 21-3). Patients with a small number of lesions may be treated during the summer or winter. Patients with a large number of lesions who work outdoors are best treated in the winter. Pharmaceutical companies that manufacture 5-FU supply patient information sheets and videos with color photographs of the various stages of inflammation.

Table 21-2 Preparations for Treatment of Actinic Keratosis

Product	Active ingredient	Packaging
Carac	0.5% Fluorouracil	30 gm cream
Efudex	2% Fluorouracil 5% Fluorouracil 5% Fluorouracil	10 ml liquid 10 ml liquid 25 gm cream
Fluoroplex	1% Fluorouracil 1% Fluorouracil	30 ml solution 30 gm cream
Aldara	5% Imiquimod	Cream—box of 12 packets
Solaraze gel	3% Diclofenac sodium	25 gm, 50 gm cream

Table 21-3 Guidelines for Duration of 5-FU Therapy According to Site

Site	Early signs of inflammation (days)	Duration of treatment (weeks)
Face, lips	3-5	2-4
Scalp	4-7	3-5
Neck	4-7	2-4
Arms, hands, legs	10-14	4-8
Back	10-14	4-6
Chest	10-14	4-6

Adapted from Goette KD: J Am Acad Dermatol 1981; 4:633.

Treatment technique (5-FU) and expected results

5-FU is available as a 0.5%, 1%, and 5% cream and a 1% and 2% solution. The 1% solution is helpful for the scalp, and the 2% solution is used for individual lesions. Carac (5-fluorouracil 0.5% cream), a new formulation, is applied once daily for up to 4 weeks as tolerated.[71] Irritation resolves with 2 weeks of cessation of treatment. Efudex or Fluoroplex is applied twice a day for 2 to 4 weeks. Applying 5-FU preparations two or three times a week is less effective.[72] Significant irritation and discomfort is frequently encountered. Petrolatum may be applied between 5-FU applications to soothe raw, dry, and cracked areas. Oral pain medication (e.g., acetaminophen with codeine) controls pain at the peak of inflammation. Instruction handouts and videos supplied by 5-FU manufacturers are very helpful.

TOPICAL CHEMOTHERAPY WITH IMIQUIMOD.

Imiquimod (Aldara) 5% cream is an immune response modifier approved for the treatment of genital warts. Imiquimod applied three times a week for 6 to 8 weeks successfully cleared all actinic keratosis. In the event of a local skin reaction, treatment was modified to two times per week.[67] Imiquimod is also effective for treatment of superficial basal cell cancers.

DICLOFENAC SODIUM.

Topical gel containing 3% diclofenac in 2.5% hyaluronic acid produced a cure (all lesions fully resolved) in 47% of patients compared with 19% of patients using placebo after 3 months of treatment. Mild-to-moderate skin irritation has been reported in up to 72% of patients.[68]

INFLAMMATORY RESPONSE AND PHYSICIAN SUPERVISION.

In the early inflammatory phase, erythema first appears in treated areas at predictable intervals (see Table 21-3). In the severe inflammatory phase (Figures 21-19 to 21-21), erythema, edema, burning, stinging, and oozing reach maximum intensity at different intervals, depending on the site treated and the thickness of the lesions. In the lesion disintegration phase (Figures 21-19, B, 21-20, and 21-21), erosion or ulceration, intense inflammation, discomfort, pain, crusting, eschar formation, and evidence of reepithelialization occur. When this phase is reached, treatment stops. Table 21-3 lists the approximate duration of treatment. Patients should be evaluated every 1 or 2 weeks during the treatment period. This irritating treatment is a major event for the patient. They are physically and mentally traumatized, and they will have many questions. Patients need close supervision, encouragement, and reassurance. They frequently call the office during treatment. The

ACTINIC KERATOSIS—TREATMENT WITH TOPICAL 5-FU

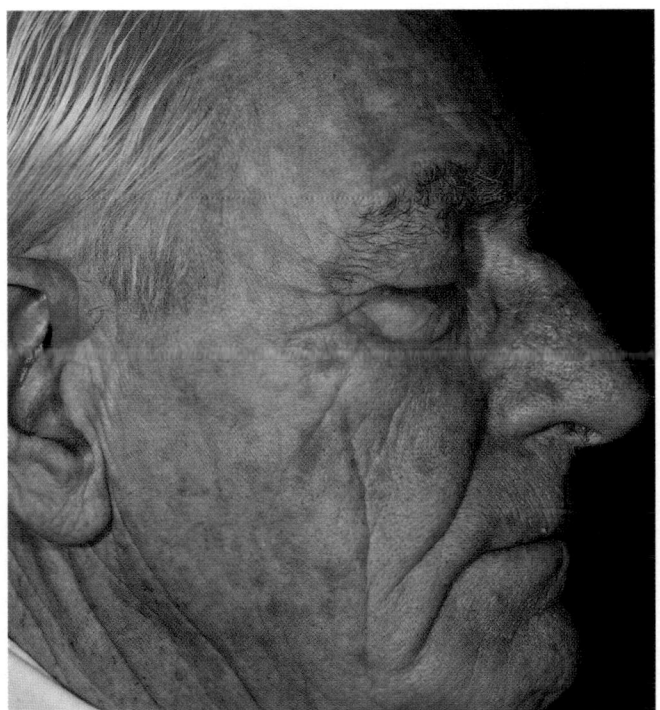

A, Diffuse involvement of the forehead. Lesions are superficial. Lesions on the cheek were not clinically apparent.

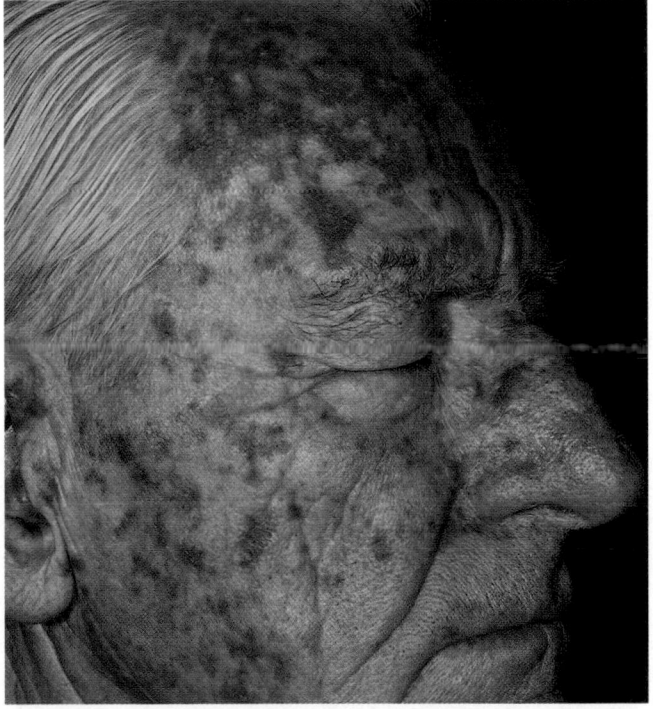

B, Maximum intensity of inflammation was reached 3 weeks after starting treatment. The medication has inflamed the cheek lesions that were not clinically apparent before treatment.

Figure 21-19

clinician must determine the endpoint of treatment and be prepared to manage excessive inflammation with wet compresses and group V to VI topical steroids. Infection responds to Bactroban ointment or oral antibiotics. Sunscreens can be irritating and not used during treatment. Sun exposure is avoided by using hats and clothing. Women may tolerate bland liquid makeup.

TOPICAL STEROIDS. Some authors suggest using topical steroids during the entire treatment period to suppress inflammation and decrease patient discomfort. This technique, however, may make it difficult to determine when therapy should be stopped.

ACTINIC KERATOSIS OF THE FACE. Patients with mild damage consisting of erythema and scaling can be treated with tretinoin cream 0.05% alone for several months. Small, superficial lesions that do not respond can then be treated with 5-FU or cryosurgery. Patients with many lesions can be pretreated with tretinoin cream applied once each day for 1 to 3 months. Pretreatment with tretinoin may improve the quality of the dermis and reduce subsequent treatment time with 5-FU. Tretinoin 0.025% cream should be prescribed for patients with sensitive skin. 5-FU may then be applied alone or in combination with tretinoin to complete the treatment program. Combination therapy may shorten the treatment period, but it produces more intense inflammation.

ACTINIC KERATOSES OF THE UPPER AND LOWER EXTREMITIES. These lesions are frequently multiple, hyperkeratotic, and distributed over a large area. Hyperkeratosis tends to limit penetration of topical 5-FU. Lesions on the extremities require longer treatment than those on the face. Lesions may be pretreated for a week or two or longer with bid applications of tretinoin 0.025% gel or 12% ammonium lactate to reduce hyperkeratosis, which interferes with 5-FU penetration. Plastic (Saran Wrap) occlusion is sometimes used to facilitate 5-FU penetration of thicker lesions.

ACTINIC CHEILITIS. Actinic cheilitis is treated effectively with 5-FU cream (Figure 21-22); however, pain and excessive crusting can make this a very unpleasant experience. Some authors suggest using 5% 5-FU cream three times a day for 14 to 18 days to obtain the optimal reaction in the shortest time.[73] The objective is to reduce the morbidity to 2 weeks. Application of 5% lidocaine ointment relieves pain.

Cool compresses are applied several times each day if inflammation is intense. Group V topical steroids may be applied to red areas to suppress inflammation and pruritus. Appearance of a purulent exudate suggests infection; when this occurs, oral antistaphylococcal antibiotics or Bactroban ointment should be prescribed. In the healing phase, residual erythema and hyperpigmentation persist for several weeks.

CONTACT ALLERGY TO 5-FU. Contact allergy to 5-FU should be suspected if intense erythema and vesiculation occur (Figure 21-23). Patch testing is not reliable because many patients who are allergic to 5-FU do not show a positive patch test reaction.

PROGNOSIS. Patients should remain free of lesions for months and possibly years, but recurrences can be anticipated. Frequently, unsupervised patients inadequately treat their own newly evolving lesions, resulting in surface healing but untreated deeper abnormal cells. For this reason, no refills should be indicated on the initial prescription, and patients should be instructed to discard medication when treatment is finished.

ACID PEELS. Glycolic acid is an alpha hydroxy acid that is useful as a chemical peeling agent. Actinic keratoses involve epidermal hyperplasia and retention of stratum corneum. Alpha hydroxy acids applied topically in high concentrations (30% to 70% glycolic acid) cause epidermolysis and elimination of keratosis.[74] Fluorouracil cream may be used for 5 to 7 days prior to the peel to "light up" and identify the lesions. Glycolic acid is applied with a cotton swab to the keratoses, is left on for 5 to 10 minutes, and is then removed with alcohol. Trichloroacetic acid (35%) and Jessner's solution (14 gm of resorcinol, 14 gm of lactic acid, and 14 gm of salicylic acid dissolved in ethanol to make a final solution of 100 ml) induce a medium-depth peel and equal fluorouracil in efficacy.[75]

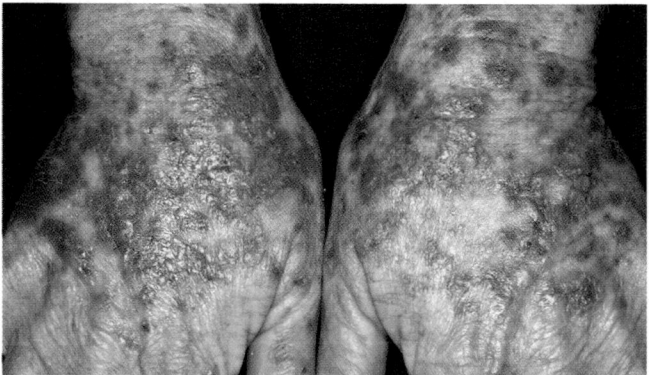

Figure 21-20 Actinic keratosis 4 weeks after starting 5-fluorouracil.

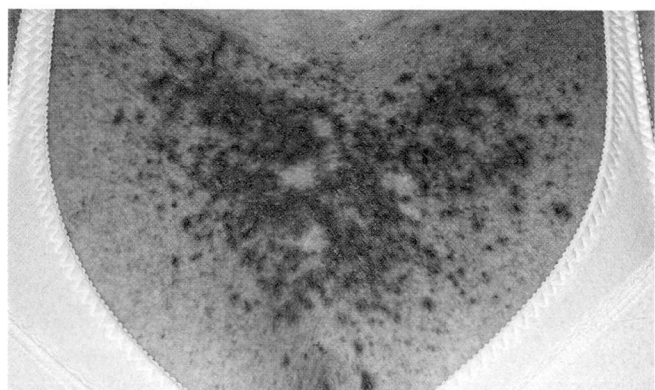

Figure 21-21 Actinic keratosis 3 weeks after starting 5-fluorouracil.

TREATMENT WITH TOPICAL 5-FU

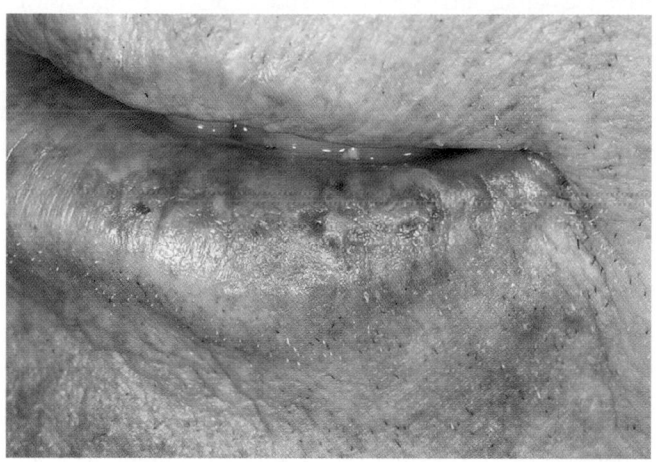

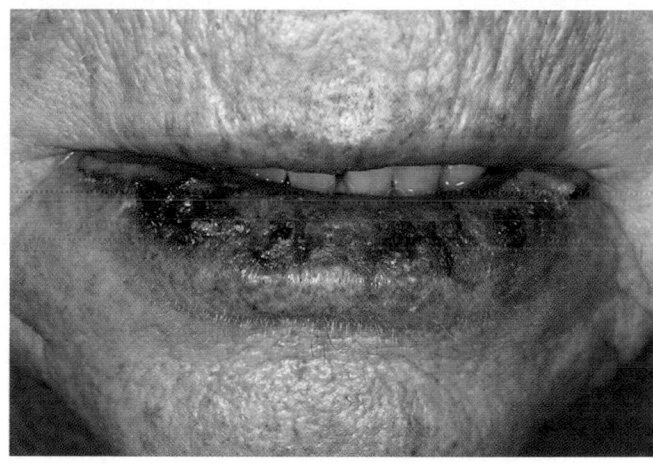

A, Before treatment. The lower lip is pink-white and smooth. The non-exposed upper lip is normal.

B, Two weeks after starting topical 5-FU. The entire lower lip is ulcerated.

Figure 21-22 Actinic cheilitis.

Figure 21-23 Contact dermatitis to 5-fluorouracil. Inflammation intensified more rapidly than expected. The patient continued to apply 5-fluorouracil because he understood that intense inflammation was to be expected. Examination showed vesiculation characteristic of contact dermatitis. Patch testing to the 5-FU cream proved the diagnosis.

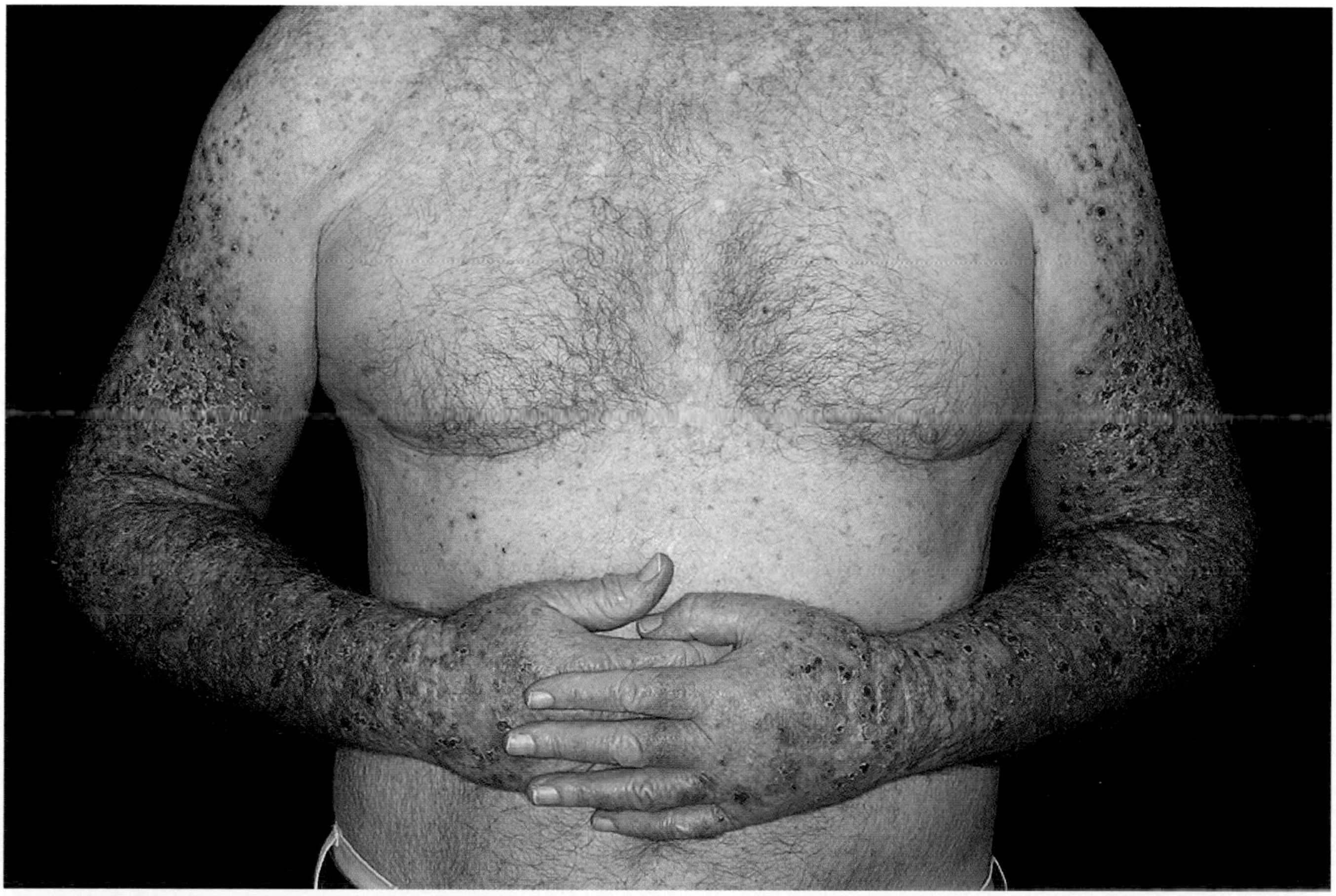

Squamous Cell Carcinoma

Nonmelanoma skin cancer is the most common cancer in the United States—1.3 million cases are expected in 2001. Approximately 80% of nonmelanoma skin cancers are BCC, and 20% are SCC. SCC is the second most common cancer among whites. Unlike BCCs, cutaneous SCCs are associated with a substantial risk of metastasis.[76]

Squamous cell carcinoma arises in the epithelium and is common in the middle-aged and elderly population. SCCs are often separated into two major groups based on their malignant potential. Those arising in areas of prior radiation or thermal injury, in chronic draining sinuses, and in chronic ulcers are typically aggressive and have a high frequency of metastasis. SCCs originating in actinically damaged skin are less aggressive and less likely to metastasize.

ETIOLOGY AND RISK FACTORS. UVB radiation is important for the induction of SCC. Risk factors include exposure to sunlight during childhood, sunburns, ionizing radiation, light skin, hazel or blue eyes, blonde or red hair, outdoor occupations, freckling, or facial telangiectasia, living in the South, and psoriasis treatment with oral psoralen and ultraviolet A radiation (PUVA). Arsenic, used in medications in the past, and in drinking water produces tumors and carcinoma in situ. Human papillomavirus types 6 and 11 are found in tumors of the genitalia and type 16 in periungual tumors. UVB radiation damages DNA (by inducing the formation of pyrimidine dimers) and its repair system and alters the immune system. UVB radiation induces mutation of p53 tumor-suppressor genes. These mutations are found in SCC. Keratinocytes undergo clonal expansion and form actinic keratosis. Uncontrolled proliferation of abnormal cells leads to squamous-cell carcinoma in situ and invasive squamous-cell carcinoma.

Cell-mediated immunity and immune function may be modulated by UVB radiation. Immunosuppression leads to a great increase in the risk of SCC. Renal-transplant recipients have a 253-fold increase in the risk of SCC.[77] Longer wavelength UVA radiation damages DNA and is also carcinogenic. SCC arises in skin that has been damaged by thermal burns or chronic inflammation. It also occurs from epidermal diseases of unknown origin, such as Bowen's disease (Box 21-3).

LOCATION. Like basal cell carcinoma, SCCs are most common in sun-exposed areas; however, the distribution is different.[78] SCCs are common on the scalp, backs of the hands, and the superior surface of the pinna; BCC is rarely found on these sites.

INCIDENCE. In 1994 in the United States, the lifetime risk of squamous-cell carcinoma was 9% to 14% among men and 4% to 9% among women. The incidence is highest in lower latitudes such as the southern United States and Australia. The incidence increases rapidly with age and sun exposure and is approximately twice as high in men as in women. A sharp increase in incidence during the past two decades has been documented.

COMMON PRECURSOR LESIONS. Actinic keratosis is the most common precursor of SCC. They begin on sun-exposed skin as isolated or multiple 2- to 6-mm flat pink, brown, rough lesions that are more easily felt than seen. Early lesions may involute. Lesion may persist for long periods without changing. A small number become thicker, accumulate scale, and evolve into SCC. Another form of SCC in situ is Bowen's disease, which presents as a sharply demarcated, erythematous, velvety, or scaly plaques on sun-exposed areas. The red smooth plaques of Bowen's disease on the glans penis of uncircumcised men are called erythroplasia of Queyrat.

PATHOPHYSIOLOGY. Atypical squamous cells originate in the epidermis from keratinocytes and proliferate indefinitely. A flat, scaly lesion becomes an indurated SCC when cells penetrate the epidermal basement membrane and proliferate into the dermis.

CLINICAL MANIFESTATIONS. SCCs arising from actinic keratosis may have a thick, adherent scale. The tumor is soft and freely movable and may have a red, inflamed base. These lesions are most frequently observed on the bald scalp, forehead, ears, and backs of the hands (Figures 21-24 and 21-25). Cutaneous horns may begin as actinic keratosis and degenerate into SCC. SCCs originating on the lip (Figures 21-26 and 21-27) or from apparently normal skin are aggressive and metastasize to the regional lymph nodes and beyond.

Those SCCs beginning in actinically damaged skin, but not from actinic keratosis, appear as firm, movable, elevated masses with a sharply defined border and little surface scale. SCCs that arise in actinically damaged skin were previously thought to have a minimal potential for metastasis; however, such lesions may be aggressive.

Box 21-3 Lesions from Which Squamous Cell Carcinoma Originates
Actinic keratosis
Cutaneous horn
Bowen's disease   Erythroplasia of Queyrat

Chemical exposure
    Arsenic (internal)
    Tar (external), except therapeutic tars

Leukoplakia
Lichen sclerosis et atrophicus (vulva)

Sites of chronic infection
    Chronic sinus tracts
    Osteomyelitis

Thermal burn scars (Marjolin's ulcer)   Radiation-damaged skin

SQUAMOUS CELL CARCINOMA

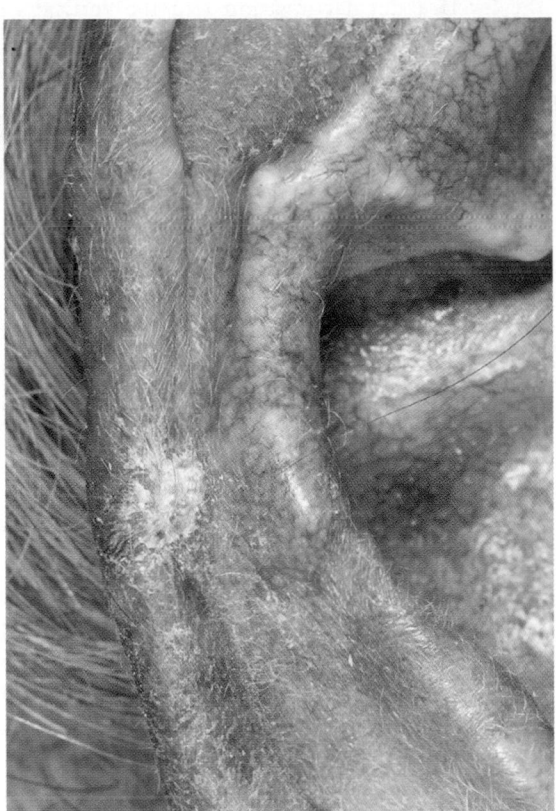

Figure 21-24 A red, keratotic papule with dense surface scale. Lesions may be misinterpreted as actinic keratosis. Cryotherapy may destroy the surface but leave deeper malignant cells untreated. Check draining lymph nodes.

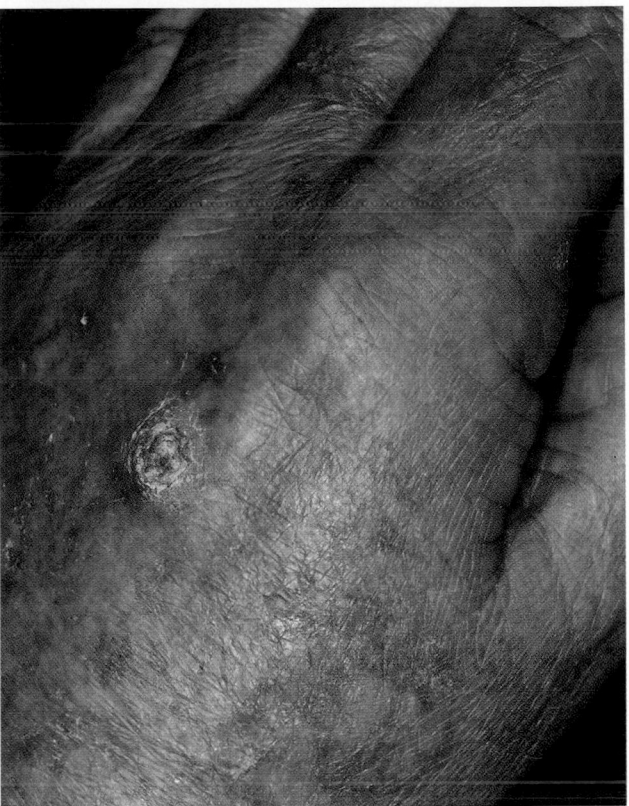

Figure 21-25 Nodular lesions may be painful. The lesion had been treated several times in the past with cryotherapy. It has been present for 2 years and demonstrated little progression in depth.

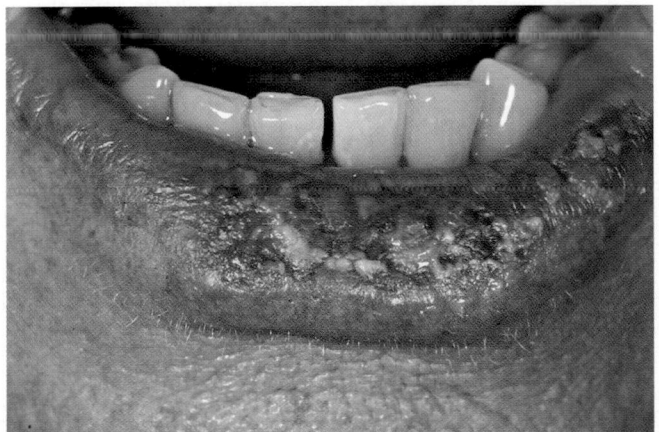

Figure 21-26 Several ulcerated lesions are present on the lower lip of this patient who has spent years working outdoors.

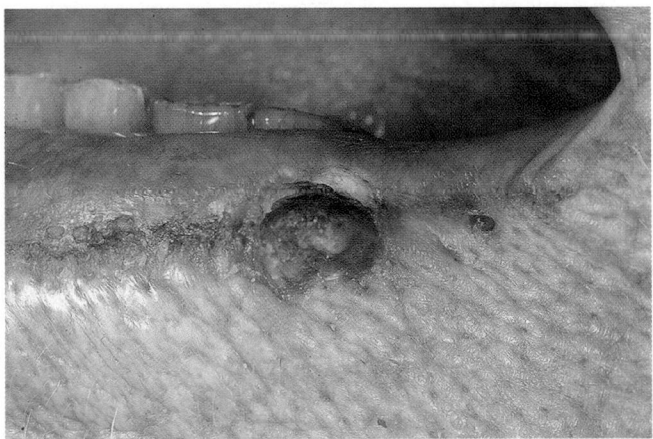

Figure 21-27 The sun-exposed lower lip is a common site. Palpation reveals a deep nodular mass.

KERATOACANTHOMAS VS. SQUAMOUS CELL CARCINOMA. Keratoacanthomas are sometimes difficult to differentiate from SCC. Keratoacanthomas appear suddenly and grow rapidly (see p. 711). They reach a certain size, usually 0.5 cm to 2.0 cm, stop growing, and then regress weeks to months later. They begin as red- to flesh-colored, dome-shaped papules with a smooth surface and a central crater filled with a keratinous plug. The pathologist sometimes has difficulty differentiating the benign keratoacanthoma from SCC. Tumors that cannot be classified are treated as SCCs.

METASTATIC POTENTIAL. The potential for SCCs to metastasize is related to the size, location, degree of differentiation, histologic evidence of perineural involvement, immunologic status and depth of invasion (Table 21-4).[79,80] SCC first metastasizes to regional lymph nodes in the majority of cases.

TUMOR SIZE AND DEPTH. In one study, no carcinoma less than 2 mm thick metastasized. Tumors between 2 and 6 mm thick with moderate differentiation and a depth of invasion that does not extend beyond the subcutis can be classified as low-risk carcinomas. The risk of metastasis is high for undifferentiated carcinomas greater than 6 mm thick that have infiltrated the musculature, the perichondrium, or the periosteum.[81] Another study of SCCs on the trunk and extremities showed that, like melanoma, tumor behavior correlated best with the level of dermal invasion and the vertical tumor thickness. Tumors that recurred were at least 4 mm thick and involved the deep half of the dermis or deeper structures. All tumors that proved fatal were at least 10 mm thick.[82] Investigators concluded that patients whose tumors penetrate through the dermis or exceed 8 mm in thickness are at high risk of recurrence or death.

LOCATION. Tumors on the scalp, forehead, ears, nose, and lips are at higher risk for metastases.[83] Tumors developing at sites of chronic inflammation, such as ulcers, scar tissue, and previous radiation sites also have higher rates of metastasis.

IMMUNOLOGIC STATUS. Host immune surveillance plays a role in determining the metastatic potential of SCC.[84] Patients with lymphoproliferative disorders, renal transplants, and those undergoing chronic oral corticosteroid therapy are at high risk. Renal-transplant recipients are at increased risk for skin cancer, most frequently SCC.[85] SCCs are also more aggressive in renal transplant patients, in whom they are associated with a higher risk of metastasis than in the general population. HLA-B mismatching is significantly associated with the risk of SCC in renal-transplant recipients, as is HLA-DR homozygosity.[86]

MODE OF SPREAD. Cutaneous SCC may spread by (1) expansion and infiltration, (2) shelving or skating, (3) conduit spread, or (4) metastasis.[87,88] SCC grows locally by expansion and infiltration. When the tumor reaches a hard surface (muscle, cartilage, bone), it may spread laterally (shelves or skates) under normal skin along facial or capsular planes, muscle, perichondrium, and periosteum. Shelving and skating occur in areas with little subcutaneous tissue, such as the scalp, ears, eyelids, nose, and upper lips. The spreading of a tumor along the nerve or vessel in the perineural or perivascular space is called conduit spread. This occurs in areas with major nerve trunks on the head and neck. Failure to recognize these three local modes of spread may result in an inadequate surgical procedure. Most SCCs are located on the head and neck. These metastasize, primarily by way of the lymphatics, initially to the superficial (first echelon) draining lymph nodes, then spread to deeper (second echelon) nodes. Distant metastasis occurs by hematogenous dissemination most commonly to the lungs, liver, brain, skin, or bone. SCCs originating on the lip[89,90] (see Figures 21-26 and 21-27) and pinna metastasize in 10% to 20% of cases.

TREATMENT. Guidelines of care for cutaneous SCC have been established by the American Academy of Dermatology.[91] See the diagram for treatment on p. 747. Small SCCs evolving from actinic keratosis are treated by electrodesiccation and curettage. Larger tumors or those on or near the vermilion border of the lips are best excised and should include the subcutaneous fat.[78] Histologic microstaging may help to direct therapy. Tumors thinner than 4 mm can be managed by sim-

Table 21-4 Influence of Tumor Variables on Local Recurrence and Metastasis of Squamous Cell Carcinoma

Factor	Local recurrence	Metastasis
Size		
<2 cm	7.4%	9.1%
≥2 cm	15.2%	30.3%
Depth		
<4 mm/Clark I to II	5.3%	6.7%
≥4 mm/Clark IV, V	17.2%	45.7%
Differentiation		
Well differentiated	13.6%	9.2%
Poorly differentiated	28.6%	32.8%
Site		
Sun-exposed	7.9%	5.2%
Ear	18.7%	11.0%
Lip	10.5%	13.7%
Scar carcinoma (non-sun-exposed)	N/A	37.9%
Previous treatment	23.3%	30.3%
Perineural involvement	47.2%	47.3%
Immunosuppression	N/A	12.9%

From Rowe DE, Carroll RJ, Day CL: J Am Acad Dermatol 1992; 26:976.
N/A, Not available

SQUAMOUS CELL CARCINOMA

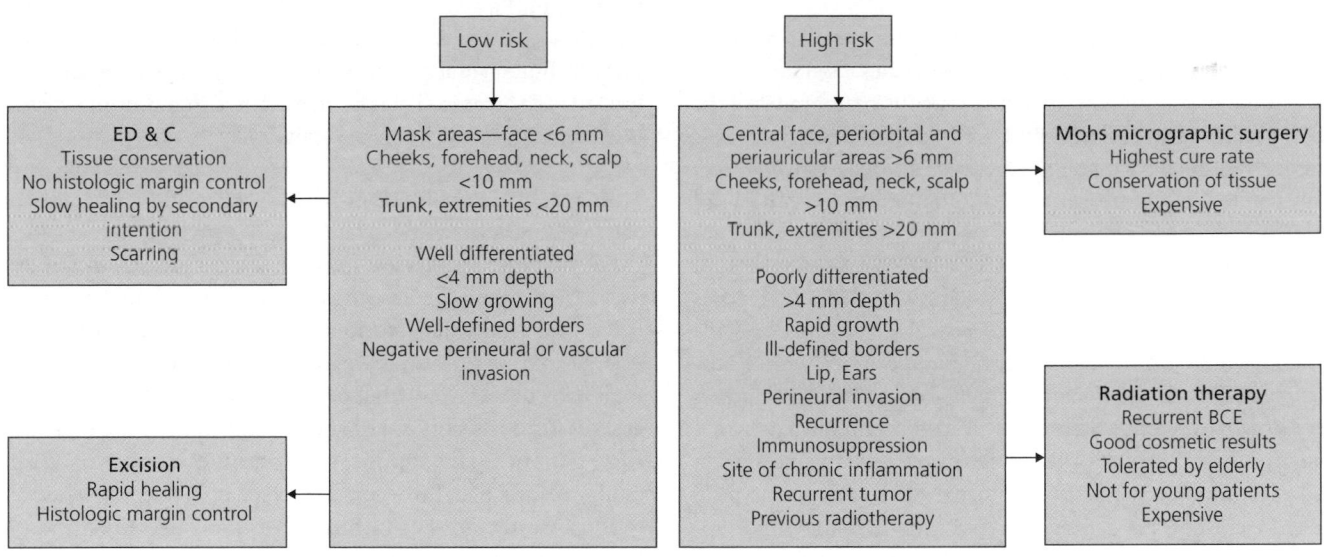

Adapted from Martinez JC, Otley CC: MayoClin Proc 2001;76:1253.
MillerSJ: Dermatol Surg 2000;26:289. Johnson Tm, et. al: J AM Acad Dermatol 1992;26:467.

ple local removal. Patients with lesions that are between 4 and 8 mm thick or that exhibit deep dermal invasion should undergo excision. Tumors that penetrate through the dermis are staged by the surgeon and treated with several modalities including excisional and Mohs' surgery,[79] neck dissection, radiation therapy, and chemotherapy.[79,92] Larger tumors or those about the nose and eyes require special consideration (see p. 735). Surgical margins for excision of primary cutaneous SCCs have been proposed (Table 21-5).[83]

When SCC metastasizes, it spreads first to local nodal groups. The combination of Mohs' micrographic surgery and sentinel lymphadenectomy may be an option for management of SCCs at high risk for metastasis.[93]

RECOMMENDED FOLLOW-UP EVALUATION. SCC patients may benefit from a once-yearly complete skin examination. Since the risk of subsequent SCC increases with number of previous SCCs, patients with multiple previous SCCs might merit more frequent examination.[91]

Squamous Cell Carcinoma of the Extremities (Marjolin's Ulcer)

Marjolin's ulcer is a term that refers to malignant changes occurring in chronic ulcers and wounds of the skin,[94] sinuses, and previous burns.[95] Most lesions are reported in burns. The majority of these lesions are found on the extremities. Development times for burn scar carcinomas of more than 30 years have been noted. Different cultures appear to have markedly different susceptibilities to Marjolin's ulcer. Japan, Northern India, and China report high incidences of burn-scar carcinoma. SCCs that occur at sites of chronic inflammation are more aggressive than those that develop from actinic keratosis or Bowen's disease. Their appearance is masked by inflamed hypertrophic tissue.

The overall metastatic rate is greater than 40%. The incidence of regional lymph node involvement from burn-scar carcinoma is approximately 35%. The 5-year survival rate for lower extremity lesions is approximately 30%.[96] Because of the focal nature of malignant change in burn scars, excisional biopsy should be performed. Punch biopsies may be negative.[97]

Wide local excision has proven unreliable for grade II and grade III disease; amputation and prophylactic node irradiation is recommended.[98] Wide local excision is reserved only for very small lesions that can be radically excised or for grade I lesions.

Table 21-5 Surgical Guidelines for Primary Squamous Cell Carcinoma

Size	Histologic grade	Anatomic location	Depth of invasion	Surgical margin
<2 cm	1	Low risk*	Dermis	4 mm
≥2 cm	2,3,4	High risk†	Subcutaneous tissue	6 mm

From Brodland DG, Zitelli JA: 1992; 27:241.
*Includes tumors less than 1 cm located in "high-risk" areas.
†Scalp, ears, eyelids, nose, and lips.

Bowen's Disease

Bowen's disease, also referred to as squamous cell carcinoma in situ, appears mainly on sun-exposed sites. Squamous cell carcinoma in situ presenting on the mucous membranes of the glans penis, vulva, and oral mucosa is known as erythroplasia of Queyrat. Bowen's disease presents as a slowly growing, red, scaly patch. Lesions are found most often on the lower limbs of women and on the scalp and ears of men.[99] Typical lesions are slightly elevated, red, scaly plaques with surface fissures and foci of pigmentation. The borders are well defined (Figures 21-28 to 21-31), and lesions closely resemble psoriasis, chronic eczema, actinic keratosis, superficial basal cell carcinoma, seborrheic keratosis, and malignant melanoma. The plaque grows very slowly by lateral extension and may eventually, after several months or years, invade the dermis, producing induration and ulceration. When confined to the epidermis the atypical cells, in contrast to actinic keratosis, involve epidermal appendages, particularly the hair follicle (see Figure 21-32). In contrast to actinic keratosis, the basal cells in Bowen's disease are normal.[100] Atypical cells are also found at the periphery of lesions in clinically uninvolved skin. Atypical cells in the epidermal lining of the hair follicle, although still confined to the epidermis, are deeper and more difficult to reach by treatment modalities such as topical 5-FU or electrosurgery, which only permit access to superficial areas.

Immunohistochemistry may sometimes be valuable in differentiating Paget's disease, superficial spreading melanoma, and Bowen's disease.[101] The cause of Bowen's disease is unknown, but several patients with this disease were formerly treated with arsenic. There is no evidence that Bowen's disease is a skin marker for internal malignancy.[102-104]

TREATMENT. Small lesions may be successfully treated with electrodesiccation and curettage, cryosurgery, or excisional surgery. Larger lesions are treated with excisional surgery[105,106] or 5-FU cream applied twice a day for 4 to 8 weeks. Treatment is discontinued when erosion and superficial necrosis occur. A large area surrounding the lesion should be treated in order to destroy the clinically inapparent disease. Some authors suggest plastic occlusion to enhance penetration to the hair follicle.[107] A once-daily application of imiquimod 5% cream (Aldara) for up to 16 weeks was very effective; 93% had no residual tumor present in their 6-week posttreatment biopsy specimens. Imiquimod is a topical immune response modifier that stimulates the production of interferon alfa and other cytokines. It is inconveniently packaged in small foil envelopes. Express medication through a hole created with a pin to conserve medication. Bowen's disease has been successfully treated in renal transplant patients with 5% imiquimod and 5% 5-fluorouracil therapy.[108]

Close follow-up of patients after treatment is required because recurrences are relatively common. Recurrence is related to follicular involvement and ill-defined lateral margins. If left untreated, development of invasive carcinoma is possible but uncommon.

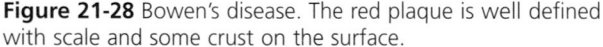

Figure 21-28 Bowen's disease. The red plaque is well defined with scale and some crust on the surface.

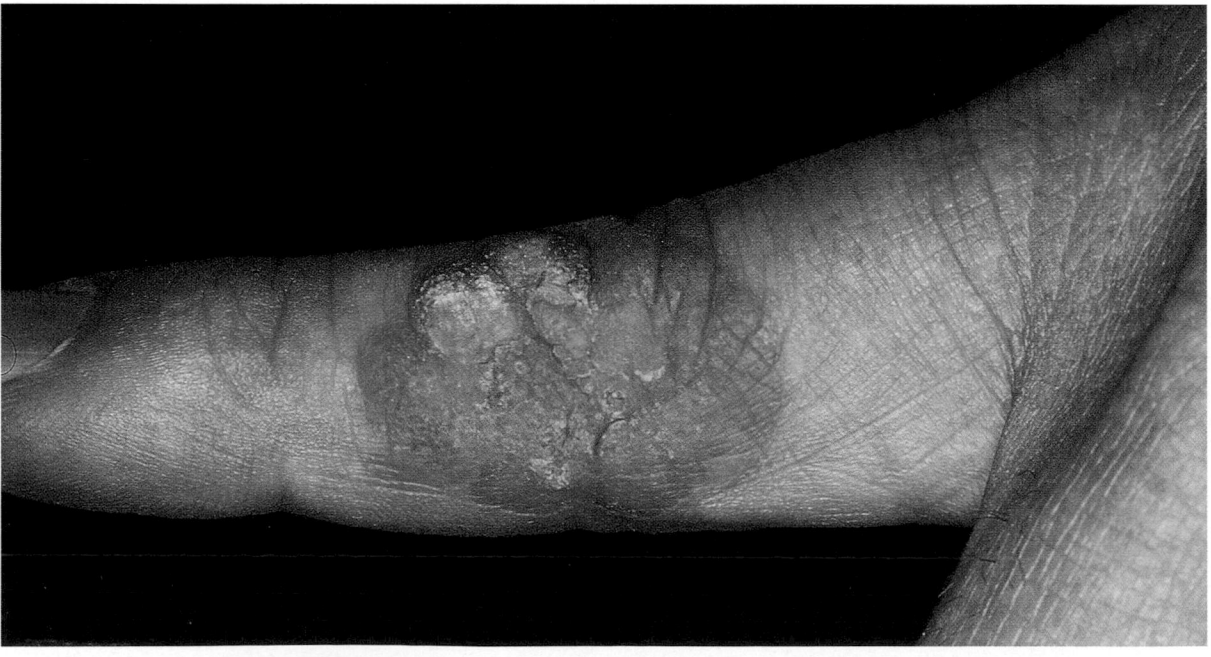

BOWEN'S DISEASE

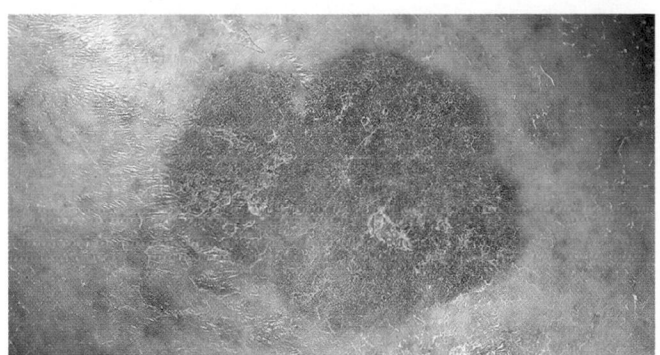

Figure 21-29 This thin lesion is pigmented and sharply demarcated.

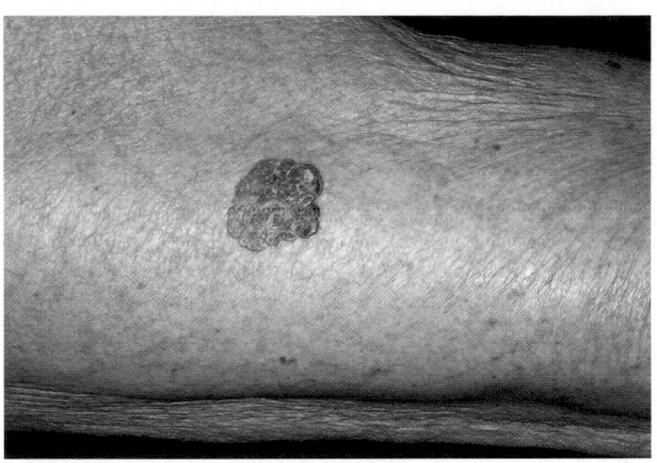

A

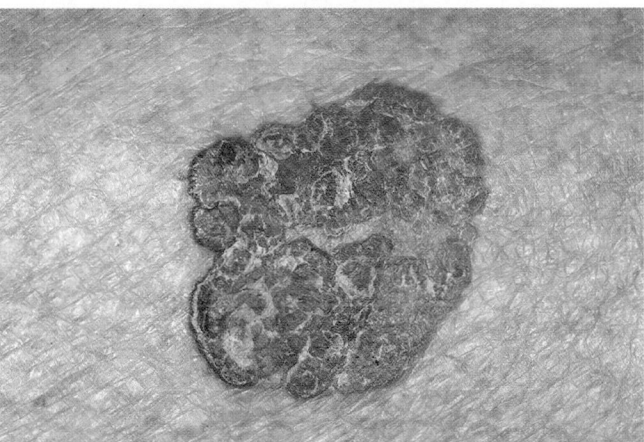

B

Figure 21-30 A, This sharply demarcated, erythematous plaque with an irregular border had been present for months. The surface was hyperkeratotic and crusted. **B,** Scale and crust are prominent. Lesions can become fissured and ulcerated.

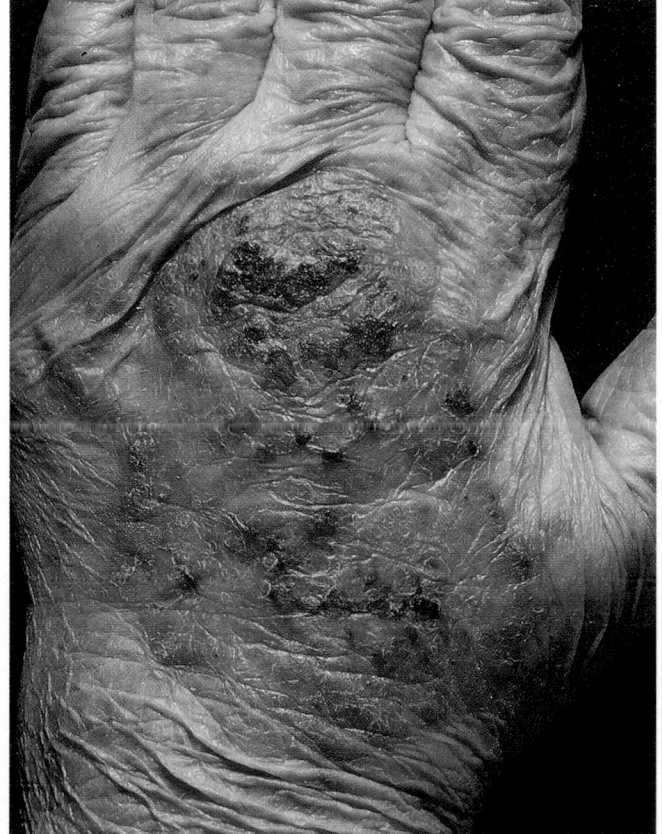

Figure 21-31 A large plaque that was misdiagnosed as tinea and psoriasis. Scale and crust form on a surface that intermittently oozes serum.

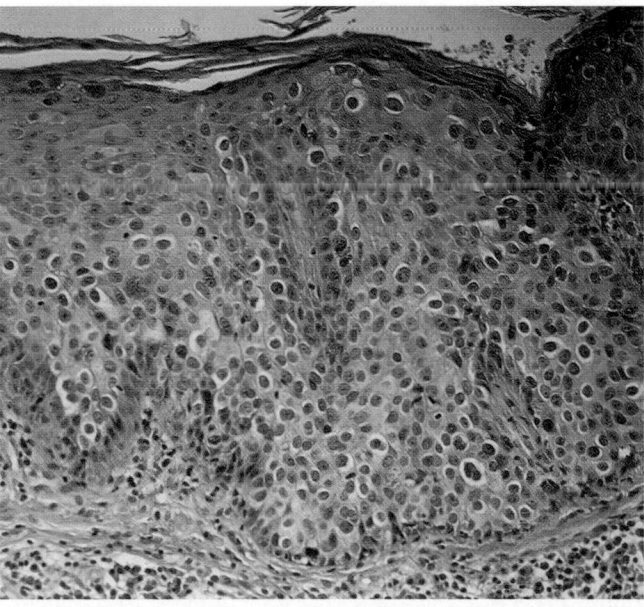

Figure 21-32 Atypical cells are present throughout the entire thickness of the epidermis. The dermoepidermal junction remains distinct and intact.

Erythroplasia of Queyrat

Clinically and histologically, erythroplasia of Queyrat of the penis resembles Bowen's disease and is probably the same entity. It is a carcinoma in situ that mainly occurs on the glans penis, the prepuce, or the urethral meatus of elderly males. It appears exclusively under the foreskin of the uncircumcised penis and is a moist, slightly raised, well-defined, red, smooth or velvety plaque (Figure 21-33). A coinfection with human papillomavirus type 8 and carcinogenic genital human papillomavirus types has been demonstrated.[109] Analogous to Bowen's disease of the skin, erythroplasia of Queyrat grows very slowly and has the potential for degeneration into squamous cell carcinoma. Similar lesions may occur on the vulva. 5-FU cream or imiquimod cream (Aldara) are treatment options. Recurrences are unlikely because the hair follicles that serve as foci for recurrence are absent on the penile mucosa.[110] A 3- to 4-week course is usually required. Use of 5% lidocaine ointment is recommended for pain. Neodymium:YAG or carbon dioxide laser therapy provides excellent cosmetic and functional results. However, the high incidence of recurrence indicates the need for careful followup and patient self-examination.[111] Erythroplasia involving the distal glans penis around the urethra and extending into the urethral meatus may require Mohs' microscopically controlled surgery.

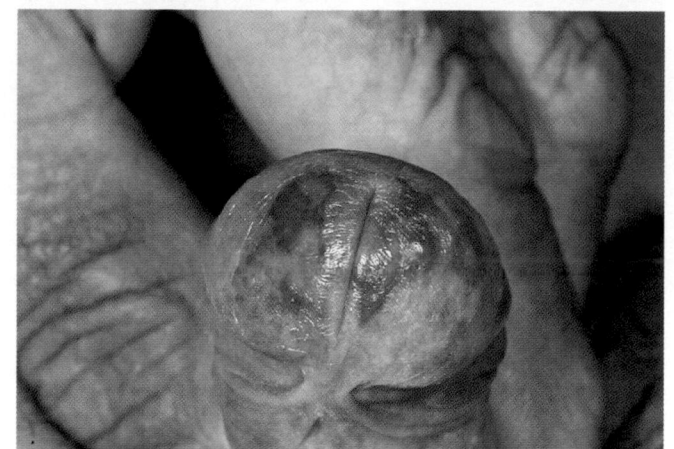

B

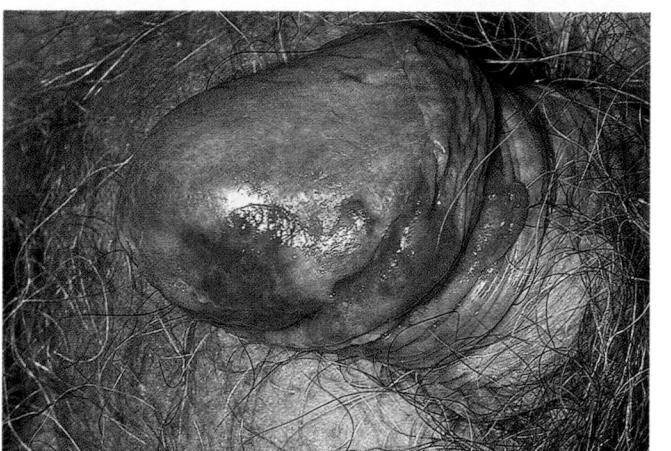

C

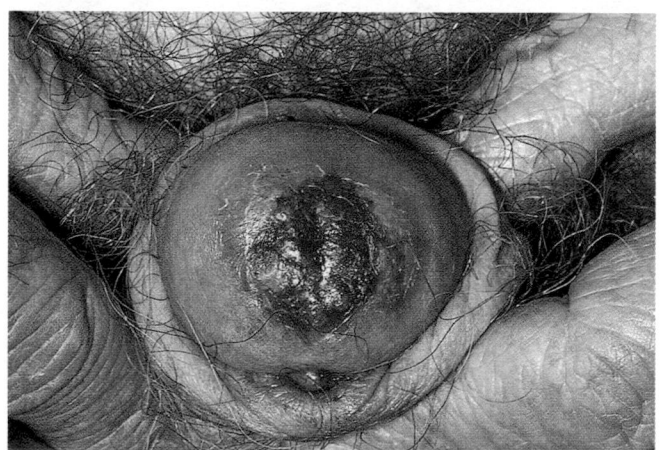

D

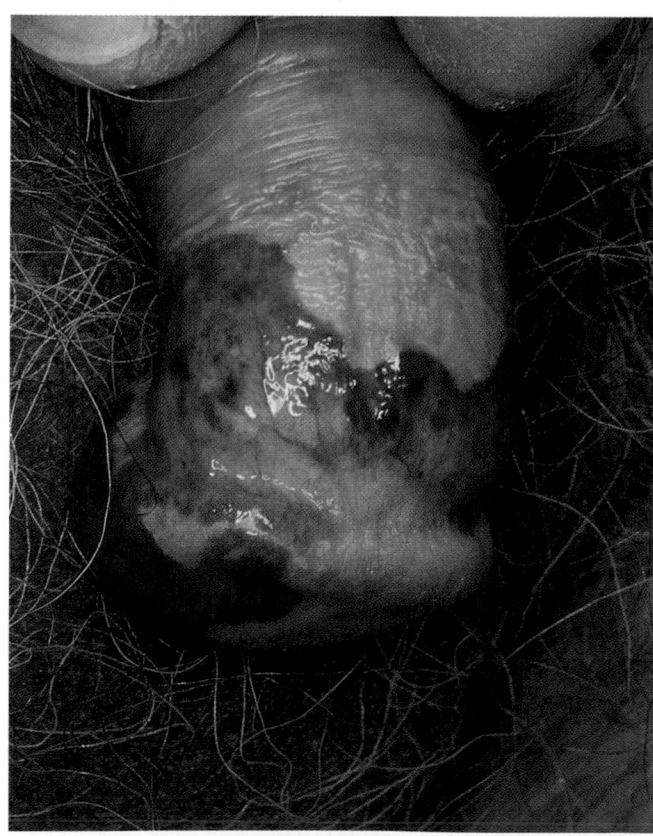

A

Figure 21-33 A, Erythroplasia of Queyrat. A moist, glistening, slightly raised plaque. **B,** A minimally raised plaque with variable texture. **C,** A broad lesion involving the glans and shaft. It occurs most often in uncircumcised men. **D,** An early lesion surrounding the urethral meatus.

Leukoplakia

Leukoplakia is the most common premalignant lesion of the oral mucosa. Leukoplakia is a clinical term used to describe a range of nonspecific white lesions, from slightly raised, white, translucent areas to dense, white, opaque lesions, with or without ulceration on the vermilion border of the lips (Figure 21-34), oral mucosa, or vulva. When a biopsy is taken, the term leukoplakia should be replaced by the diagnosis obtained histologically. Smoking is the most common cause of oral lesions,[112] but chronic irritation from carious teeth or malaligned dentures and betel nut chewing[113] (Taiwan) are also causes.

CLINICAL PRESENTATION. The most common sites of oral leukoplakia are the commissures and the buccal mucosa. Leukoplakias in the floor of mouth more often present in smokers than in non-smokers. Leukoplakias on the borders of the tongue are more common among non-smokers than smokers.[114] A particularly aggressive form of oral leukoplakia that begins with hyperkeratosis, spreads to become multifocal and verruciform in appearance, and later becomes malignant has been termed proliferative verrucous leukoplakia. Lesions are often bilateral and affect mandibular, alveolar, and buccal mucosa.[115]

MALIGNANT DEGENERATION. SCC develops in 17% of all patients with leukoplakia.[116,117] In one study of 500 patients with oral leukoplakia, there was SCC in 9.6% of cases and dysplasia in an additional 24%. One study found a 2.9% annual malignant transformation rate for patients with leukoplakia.[118] Almost 50% of oral SCCs are associated with or preceded by leukoplakia.[119] Leukoplakia on the floor of the mouth and the ventral surface of the tongue is associated with the highest risk of cancer.[120]

Degeneration to carcinoma takes 1 to 20 years. Clinically, the patches are white, slightly elevated, usually well-defined plaques that show little tendency to extend peripherally.

DIFFERENTIAL DIAGNOSIS. The differential diagnosis includes candidiasis, lichen planus, habitual cheek biting, white sponge nevus, and secondary syphilis. A lesion unique to acquired immunodeficiency syndrome (AIDS), termed *hairy leukoplakia*, presents as an asymptomatic, slightly raised, poorly demarcated lesion with a corrugated or "hairy" surface composed of white papillary projections. It occurs principally on the lateral borders of the tongue (Figure 11-26). Candida organisms are frequently observed on the lesion surface. Human papilloma virus and Epstein-Barr virus have been identified in the lesions. Dyskeratosis congenita is a congenital multisystem disorder, characterized by skin pigmentation, dystrophic nails, and leukoplakia.

HISTOLOGIC CHARACTERISTICS. Histologic changes occur, varying from mild scaling and epidermal thickening with minimal inflammation to varying degrees of dysplasia or carcinoma in situ.[121] The clinical appearance of leukoplakia does not generally correlate well with the histopathologic change; therefore biopsy should be performed for all cases to determine which are precancerous.[122] Small lesions may be biopsied and simply followed if the histology is benign. Plaques that histologically exhibit atypical features should be excised, electrodesiccated, destroyed with the laser,[123] or frozen with liquid nitrogen.[124]

PROGNOSIS. There are no reliable predictors of which leukoplakia lesions will develop into SCC. The increasing incidence of head and neck cancers emphasizes the importance of early identification of which oral white patches will develop into carcinomas. The DNA content (ploidy) in cells of oral leukoplakia can be used to predict the risk of oral carcinoma. Cells in lesions are classified as diploid (normal), tetraploid (intermediate), or aneuploid (abnormal). A carcinoma developed in 3% with diploid lesions, in 60% with tetraploid lesions, and in 84% with aneuploid lesions. The cumulative disease-free survival rate was 97% among the group with diploid lesions, 40% among the group with tetraploid lesions, and 16% among the group with aneuploid lesions.[125] Ploidy is determined with a multistep procedure performed on paraffin-embedded tissue samples.

TREATMENT. Many lesions clear spontaneously or regress when cigarette or pipe smoking is stopped. If a young man with leukoplakic lesions stops using tobacco for six weeks, most of his leukoplakic lesions will resolve clinically.[126] Long-term follow-up is desirable to check for recurrences.

Leukoplakia of the vulva and the lip can be successfully treated with 5-FU. Lip lesions are treated twice daily with applications of 1% 5-FU solution until erythema and erosions become marked in approximately 10 to 21 days. Discomfort is intense and can be relieved with cool compresses or topical lidocaine gel. Localized dysplastic oral leukoplakia is treated with surgical excision, electrosurgery, cryosurgery or CO_2 laser evaporation.[127,128] Tretinoin (Retin-A) gel shows only a limited effect in controlling oral leukoplakia.[129]

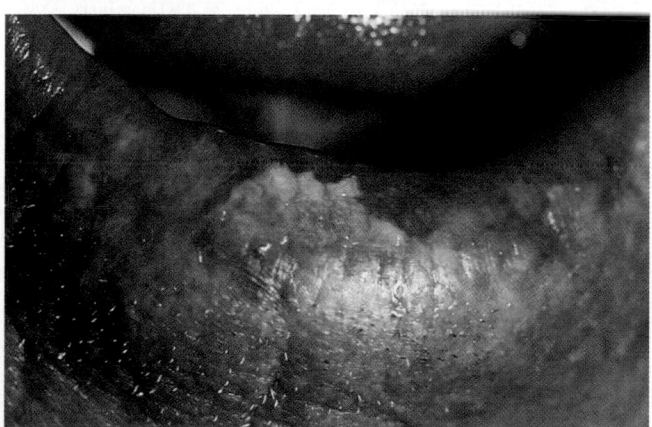

Figure 21-34 Leukoplakia. A thin white plaque had been present on the lip for over 2 years. The patient smoked.

VERRUCOUS CARCINOMA

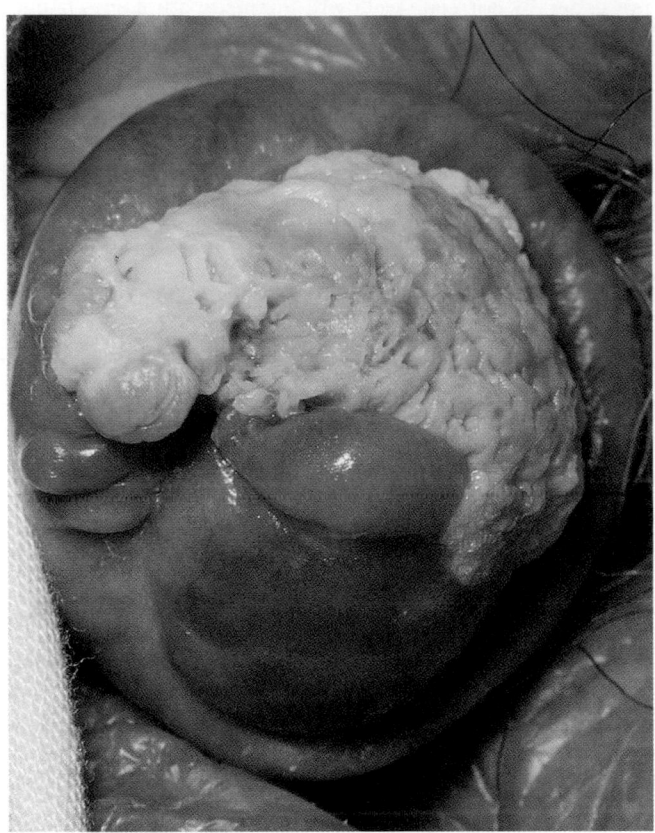

Figure 21-35 The giant condylomata of Buschke-Löwenstein occurs on the male and female genitalia. They initially appear as warts, but grow relentlessly despite multiple attempts at conservative topical and surgical treatment.

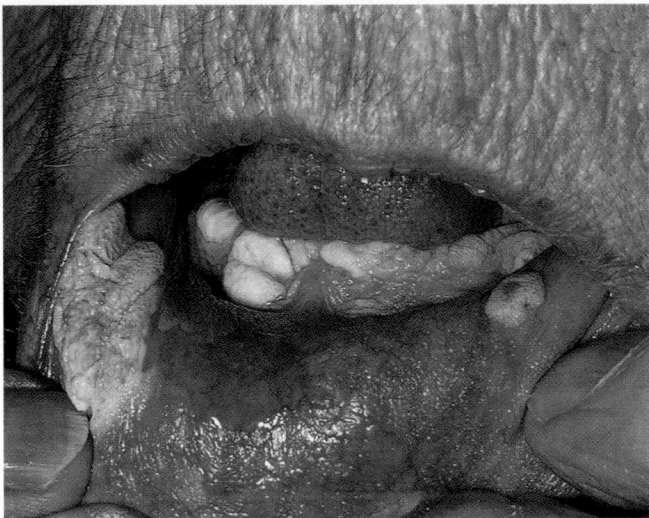

Figure 21-36 Oral florid papillomatosis. A white verrucous growth that may extend widely over the oral mucosa.

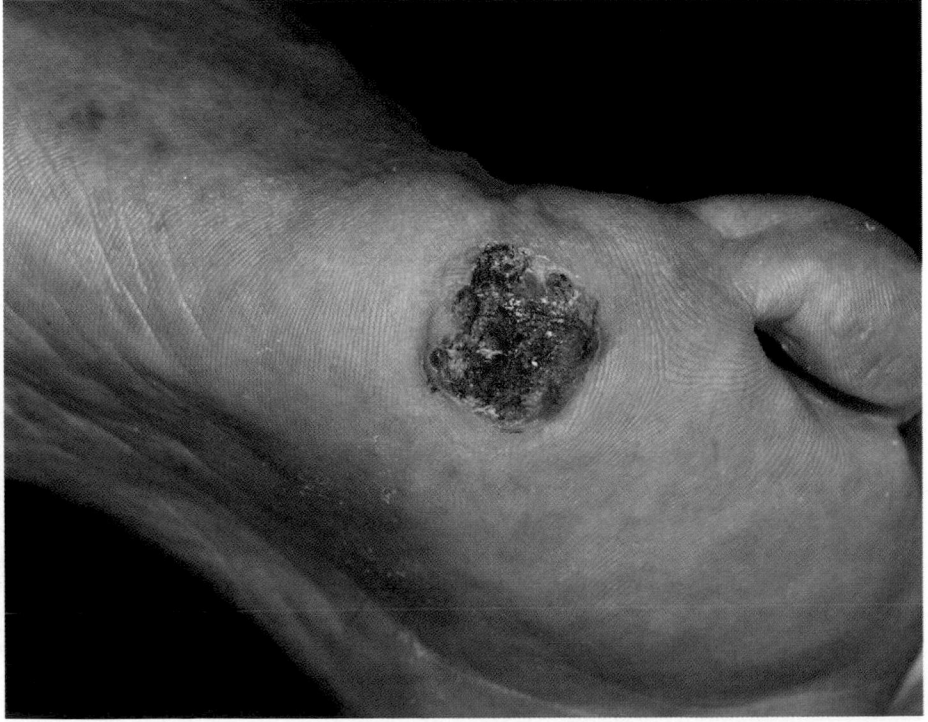

Figure 21-37 Epithelioma cuniculatum. A lesion was present for months and was suspected of being a plantar wart.

Verrucous Carcinoma

Verrucous carcinoma (VC) is a term encompassing three rare entities: epithelioma cuniculatum (plantar surface of the foot), giant condylomata of Buschke-Löwenstein (perineum) (Figure 21-35), and oral florid papillomatosis (Figure 21-36).[130] Verrucous carcinoma can occur at other sites. They typically develop at sites of chronic irritation and inflammation. The term *verrucous carcinoma* was coined to denote a locally aggressive, exophytic, low-grade squamous cell carcinoma with little metastatic potential. Verrucous carcinomas have been reported on many other skin surfaces.[131] Verrucous carcinomas are probably caused by human papilloma viruses (HPV) and are most often associated with HPV-6 and -11.[132,133] They are thought to represent an intermediate lesion in a pathologic continuum from condyloma to squamous cell carcinoma. All three entities have similar biologic potential and show bulky, exophytic, fungating growth, with a high degree of cellular differentiation histologically. A slowly growing tumor extends in surface area and locally compresses and displaces rather than infiltrating contiguous structures and rarely metastasizes. Histologically, the tumor displays massive epidermal thickening with local invasion minus cellular atypia. In their early stages, all tumors may be mistaken for warts (Figure 21-37). However, tumors are unresponsive to locally destructive procedures and slowly, over months or years, increase in size, become indurated, and deeply penetrate the dermis. Conservative local excision,[134] Mohs' microscopically controlled surgery,[135] radiation therapy,[136] CO_2 laser[137] and systemic chemotherapy,[138] acitretin,[139] and intralesional interferon[140] have all been advocated.

BUSCHKE-LÖWENSTEIN TUMOR. This tumor, a carcinoma-like condylomata acuminata, is verrucous carcinoma of the anogenital mucosal surface. The incidence varies from 5% to 24% of all penile cancers. These tumors occur most commonly in uncircumcised men on the glans and prepuce and have the same clinical appearance on the vulva, vagina, cervix,[141] and anorectum. Transformation into invasive carcinoma has been described.[142]

ORAL FLORID PAPILLOMATOSIS. The incidence of VC among oral carcinomas is 2% to 12%. These very rare tumors are most often reported in white men between 55 and 65 years of age. Tobacco chewing is a risk factor. Many patients have poor oral hygiene or dentures. Early lesions appear as white patches on a red base. Lesions develop into extensive grey-white, warty tumors with a deeply cleaved surface on the gingival mucosa and may extend to the entire oral mucosa and into the larynx and trachea.[143] Local aggression with bone, muscle, and salivary gland invasion occurred in 53% of cases in one study.[144] White sponge nevus is autosomal dominant and is characterized by white lesions that appear from birth to adolescence.

VERRUCOUS CARCINOMA (EPITHELIOMA CUNICULATUM) PLANTARE. This tumor occurs in older men with a mean age of 60. Exophytic tumors with ulceration and sinuses draining foul-smelling discharge cause pain and bleeding. This tumor mimics a variety of other skin lesions with its insidious onset.[145,146] Plantar warts, ischemic ulcers, melanoma, and SCC must be considered.

Arsenical Keratoses and Other Arsenic-Related Skin Diseases

Pentavalent, inorganic arsenic, dispensed years ago as Fowler's solution (potassium arsenite solution) for psoriasis and other diseases, may cause a number of problems. Arsenical keratoses are discrete, round, wartlike, or pointed keratotic lesions that appear 20 or more years after chronic arsenic ingestion (Figure 21-38). Arsenical keratoses may degenerate into squamous cell carcinoma. Lesions are most common on the palms and soles but may occur elsewhere. Bowen's disease, multiple basal cell carcinomas, and changes in pigmentation characterized by small, round, white macules ("raindrops on a hyperpigmented background") are additional findings in patients with chronic arsenic ingestion. A significant excess of bladder cancer mortality occurred in patients treated with Fowler's solution.[147] Exposure to Chinese proprietary medicines containing inorganic arsenic poses a risk for the development of cutaneous and systemic malignancies.[148]

Chronic arsenic toxicity from drinking well water polluted with arsenic has been reported.[149] No treatment is necessary for arsenical keratosis unless signs of degeneration occur.

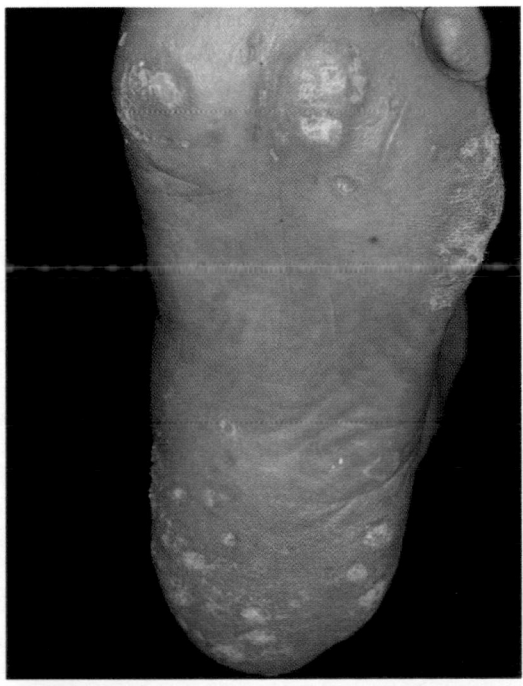

Figure 21-38 Arsenical keratoses. Discrete, wartlike, keratotic lesions occur on the palms and soles.

Cutaneous T-Cell Lymphoma

The term *cutaneous T-cell lymphoma* (CTCL) encompasses a group of distinct lymphomatous neoplasms of helper T cells that present in the skin but later may involve lymph nodes, peripheral blood cells, and the viscera. Mycosis fungoides, Sézary syndrome, and lymphoma cutis are all examples of CTCL. The malignant cells have a marked affinity for the skin, particularly the epidermis, often leading to formation of Pautrier's intraepidermal abscesses. The disease progresses to systemic involvement as the cells lose their affinity for the epidermis. Greater awareness and earlier detection have suggested that CTCL has replaced Hodgkin's disease as the most common adult lymphoma. Unlike other closely related diseases (e.g., adult T-cell leukemic lymphoma), CTCL does not appear to be communicable. Patients with CTCL are heterogeneous with respect to immunocompetence, and this heterogeneity affects their clinical course and response to therapy. The disease was thought to be confined to the elderly, but newer diagnostic techniques show that it starts insidiously in younger adults. A persistent eruption, even in youths and young adults, should be thoroughly evaluated for possible CTCL. Early detection is essential because the disease has an excellent prognosis in the initial stage when it is confined to the skin. The disease is fatal once systemic spread has occurred. The most common forms of CTCL are mycosis fungoides (MF) and Sézary syndrome (SS), the leukemic phase of MF.

MOLECULAR THEORY OF ORIGIN. CTCL is a malignancy of a single clone of CD4-positive T cells. Each patient develops a unique clone of malignant cells with unique surface receptors. The disease advances with the development of progressively more aggressive subclones. Initially, Langerhans' cells carry antigens from the skin to peripheral lymph nodes, where they present the antigens to CD4-positive T cells and convert them to cutaneous T-cell lymphoma cells (CTCL cells). The T cells acquire cutaneous lymphoid antigen (CLA) on their surfaces, which acts as a skin-selective homing receptor.[150] CLA permits adherence of the T cell to dermal blood vessels, giving the cells the ability to infiltrate the skin.[151] A unique feature of early stage CTCL is epidermotropism, in which malignant cells are found in the proximity of the epidermis, where the cellular growth environment is conducive to their proliferation. A second set of antigenic peptides permits immunologic attack against the malignant cells through the use of photopheresis.

REFERRAL. Establishing a diagnosis of cutaneous lymphoma is complicated. Patients suspected of having this disease are referred to a tertiary care center.

DIAGNOSIS. The diagnosis is made by recognizing the clinical characteristics of the various stages of the disease and is supported by histopathology. Multiple biopsies at different sites are useful. It is important to biopsy suspected lesions early enough so that potentially curative treatment can be initiated. Immunophenotypic and gene rearrangement studies can confirm clinical suspicion when histology is equivocal. Evaluation for systemic involvement includes examination of peripheral blood for Sézary cells and biopsy of palpable lymph nodes.

Mycosis fungoides

The name mycosis fungoides is misleading because the disease is not fungal in origin. MF is a T-cell lymphoma that appears to originate in the skin. MF is twice as common in men as in women. Most cases are diagnosed in the fifth and sixth decades, but individuals can develop this disease in childhood and adolescence. African Americans are twice as likely to be affected as whites. The incidence has increased threefold (from 0.19 cases to 0.42 cases per 100,000 population) in the past 20 years. The course is unpredictable, sometimes lasting less than 1 year or lingering for decades.

DISEASE PROGRESSION. There are four phases in the evolution of the disease: pre-MF, patch (flat, scaly, red, sometimes pruritic), plaque, and tumor. Most patients with patches or plaques do not have disease progression. Lesions from the last three phases may be present simultaneously. Erythroderma may occur at any time. There are many clinical variants. Lymphadenopathy may develop at any stage. Survival time is less than 3 years once the tumor phase begins. Despite the new laboratory diagnostic methods, recognition of the physical signs of the disease by the clinician and routine histology are still the most sensitive methods of detection.

INITIAL BIOPSY. An initial punch biopsy will confirm the lymphoid nature of a lesion. Then early MF must be distinguished from inflammatory disorders. Obtaining a 1 cm shave biopsy specimen and section it longitudinally. The tissue can be placed flat onto a piece of paper to prevent curling during formalin fixation. Obtaining fresh-frozen tissue for early MF is routinely performed at some academic centers.

Most neoplasms can be classified as lymphoid or nonlymphoid and benign or malignant based on the growth pattern and cytologic features. Patch- or plaque-stage lesions are usually diagnosed on the basis of light microscopic features and clinical correlation. Early MF resembles inflammatory dermatoses, and pathologists often cannot make a diagnosis with confidence. Immunohistochemistry is frequently inconclusive.

HISTOLOGIC CHARACTERISTICS. CTCL presents a difficult diagnostic challenge for the pathologist. Histologic scores do not always correlate with the stages of disease and are not an accurate predictor of clinical outcome. The histologic diagnosis of MF is difficult because many subtle changes, most of which may be present to some degree in many inflammatory and neoplastic cutaneous conditions may be present. A combination of histologic parameters can be used to establish a microscopic diagnosis of MF without the necessity of confirmatory immunophenotyping in the vast majority of cases. The most specific features to discriminate between MF and benign inflammatory diseases are Pautrier's microabscesses (atypical lymphocytes in collections within the epidermis), haloed lymphocytes (caused by retraction artifact surrounding intraepidermal lymphocytes), exocytosis (presence of lymphocytes in the epidermis), hyperconvoluted intraepidermal lymphocytes, and lymphocytes aligned within the basal layer. Few cases demonstrate all histologic features. Haloed lymphocytes are the most accurate discriminator of MF from non-MF.[152] Stop topical therapy (steroids, light therapy) for at least 2 weeks before performing a skin biopsy.

IMMUNOPHENOTYPING. Immunohistochemical studies for B and T cell markers are performed on all suspected cutaneous lymphomas. Antibody studies on paraffin and fresh tissue specimens can confirm that the process is lymphocytic and identifies the type of lymphocyte (T cell vs. B cell vs. natural killer cell) and subsets of these cells based on their immunophenotype (eg, CD3$^+$/CD4$^+$ T-helper cells [TH] or CD3+/CD8+ T cytotoxic/suppressor [TC] cells). The hallmark is the T helper/inducer subset marker, CD4.

GENE REARRANGEMENT ANALYSIS. Clonal rearrangement of T-cell receptor (TCR) genes can be demonstrated in lesional tissue in most cases. Gene rearrangement analysis (GRA) is used to identify and quantitate cell clones. Clonal proliferation from a single lymphocyte is a feature of malignancy. Populations of neoplastic lymphocytes contain the same gene rearrangement. Populations of reactive lymphocytes contain a mixture of gene rearrangements. The Southern blot technique requires DNA extracted from fresh-frozen tissue. Polymerase chain reaction (PCR) can use DNA extracted from unstained sections of archived, formalin-fixed tissue. PCR-GRA can be used to monitor the response to therapy by detecting the presence or absence of the malignant clone in the skin or blood.

STAGING PROCEDURES. A baseline workup includes physical examination. Document the presence of lymphadenopathy and hepatosplenomegaly. Obtain a complete blood cell count (review the buffy coat smear for Sézary cells), biopsy with gene rearrangement analysis, flow cytometric studies of the blood to detect a circulating malignant clone, and computed tomographic scanning of the chest, abdomen, and pelvis.

STAGING. Cancer staging systems stratify cases according to prognosis so that therapy can be given to homogeneous subsets. Most cancers are staged by the TNM system. The T stage describes the tumor, N the nodal status, and M the presence or absence of metastasis. A modified staging classification describes new prognostic subsets (Box 21-4 and Table 21-6).

PROGNOSIS. The prognosis for patch-stage or (<10%) limited plaques is similar to that for normal age-matched controls. Patients with T3 and T4 disease who are older than 60 years at diagnosis or with elevated serum lactate dehydrogenase levels have a median survival of approximately 3 years. Five-year survival for tumor and erythrodermic stages decreases to approximately 40% (Table 21-6).[153]

Box 21-4 Modified TNM and Staging Classification for Cutaneous T-Cell Lymphoma	
T:	Skin
T1:	Patches and/or plaques covering <10% of the skin surface
T2a*:	Patches (>10% of the skin surface)
T2b*:	Plaques (>10% of the skin surface)
T3:	Tumor stage
T4:	Generalized erythroderma (80% or more of skin surface)
N:	Lymph nodes
N0:	No clinically abnormal peripheral lymph nodes, pathology negative
N1:	Clinically abnormal peripheral lymph nodes, pathology negative
N2:	No clinically abnormal peripheral lymph nodes, pathology positive
N3:	Clinically abnormal peripheral lymph nodes, pathology positive
B:	Peripheral blood
B0:	Atypical circulating cells not present (<5%)
B1:	Atypical circulating cells present (5%)
M:	Visceral organs
M0:	No visceral organ involvement
M1:	Visceral organ involvement (confirmed by pathology)

*The T2 stage is divided into two subgroups on the basis of the depth of the infiltrate (determined histologically) and cytology.

Table 21-6 Modified Overall Staging System for Mycosis Fungoides and Survival*

Clinical stage	TNM classification			Survival 5 yr	Survival 10 yr	Survival 5 yr	Survival 10 yr	Survival 15 yr
IA	T1	N0	M0	95.1	84.6	91.7	82.5	79.0
IB	T2a	N0	M0	83.5	—			
IIA	T1,2a	N1	M0	90.2	—	78.3	52.6	44.7
IIB	T2b	N0,1	M0	75.0	50.0			
IIIA	T3	N0,1	M0	44.9	31.1	47.2	32.9	19.9
IIIB	T4	N0,1	M0	49.3	34.5			
IVA	T1-4	N2,3	M0					
IVB	T1-4	N0-3	M1					

Adapted from Kashani-Sabet M, McMillan A, Zackheim: J Am Acad Dermatol 2001; 45:700.

CLINICAL PRESENTATIONS

Pre-MF. The pre-MF phase is the first phase in which the diagnosis is suspected, but it cannot be made by clinical or histologic criteria. This premycotic phase persists for months or years and is suspected when inflammation persists and recurs after repeated courses of topical steroids. Spontaneous remissions do occur. Nonspecific pruritic eruptions or pruritus alone may be the only manifestation. A red, scaly, eczematous-like or psoriasis-like eruption and an atrophic, mottled, telangiectatic eruption referred to as large-patch parapsoriasis or poikiloderma vasculare atrophicans may occur. These two latter dermatoses possess characteristic features that allow one to predict with a greater degree of certainty that the evolution of typical MF may occur. These dermatoses can be present for as long as 35 years before the plaques and tumors of MF develop.

Eczematous form. The eczematous form presents with persistent, nonspecific, flat, red, itchy, eczematous areas that resemble asteatotic eczema or atopic dermatitis, except that the lesions tend to remain fixed in location and size, and the margins are sharply delineated (Figures 21-39 and 21-40).

The poikilodermatous-parapsoriasis lesion. Lesions of parapsoriasis en plaques are sharply circumscribed and have a faint erythema and sometimes a yellowish cast, a fine scale, and a slightly wrinkled surface. On the trunk and limbs, the lesions are usually 1 to 5 cm and round, oval, or fingerlike (digitate dermatosis). On the buttocks and thighs, where they occur more commonly, lesions present as patches as large as 15 cm. Patients with long-standing parapsoriasis-like lesions that are resistant to conventional treatment require careful monitoring for the possible development of cutaneous lymphoma.[154]

Poikiloderma vasculare atrophicans is a term used to describe lesions that have telangiectasia; "cigarette-paper" skin with fine, wrinkly atrophy; and mottled pigmentation (Figure 21-41). The appearance of poikilodermatous changes is an ominous sign. The terms *parapsoriasis variegata* or *parapsoriasis lichenoides* are used to describe variants of these lesions that present with a netlike or reticulated pattern.

Histologic examination shows chronic, nonspecific inflammation in the dermis. The infiltrate may be present as a band in the upper dermis. The inflammatory cells may be polymorphic, and the epidermis may be thickened. A scant number of lymphocytes may be found in the epidermis.

Patch stage. The disease enters the patch stage when histologic changes are characteristic of MF. The morphology of the lesion does not necessarily change.

Plaque stage. The plaque stage is entered gradually when dusky red-to-brown, sometimes scaly areas become elevated above the surrounding uninvolved skin because of acanthosis (thickening of the epidermis). Plaques can arise from uninvolved skin. Itching becomes more persistent and intense and may be intolerable. The plaques vary in shape with round, oval, arciform, or serpiginous patterns, occasionally with central clearing. The extent of involvement varies from a few isolated areas to a major portion of the skin (Figures 21-42 to 21-44). Infiltration of the entire skin produces a thickened red hide with scale (exfoliative dermatitis) or without scale (erythroderma). MF may begin as exfoliative erythroderma. Infiltration and plaques in hairy areas may produce alopecia. Histologically, the plaques exhibit a superficial, deep, perivascular lymphocytic infiltrate with collections of lymphocytes (Pautrier's microabscesses) within a thickened epidermis. The infiltrate becomes mixed (lymphocytes, eosinophils, and plasma cells) as the plaque stage progresses. Some of the lymphocytes are atypical, having a large, hyperconvoluted or cerebriform nucleus ("mycosis cell") (see Figure 21-49). The plaque stage persists for an indefinite period. Plaques regress, remain stationary, or evolve into nodules and tumors.

Tumor stage. Tumors develop from preexisting plaques or erythroderma, or they may originate from red or normal skin (Figures 21-45 to 21-47). Itching may decrease in intensity. Tumors vary in size, some becoming huge or mushroom-shaped (thus the term *mycosis fungoides*, which has been in use for 150 years). Necrosis and ulceration of plaques and tumors are common.

In the early stages, the disease remains confined to the skin. Superficial lymphadenopathy may be detected in the plaque stage, and deep lymphadenopathy with visceral metastasis, such as to the spleen, lungs, or gastrointestinal tract, may occur during the tumor stage.[28]

PRE-MYCOSIS FUNGOIDES AND PATCH STAGE

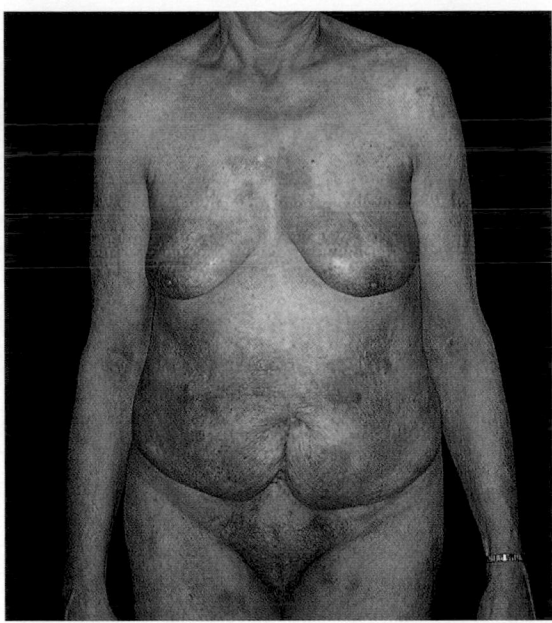

Figure 21-39 The eczematous or patch phase presents with red macules that have a fine scale. Lesions may be multiple. Itching is variable. Lesions are hypopigmented or hyperpigmented in dark-skinned individuals. Patches slowly evolve into plaques.

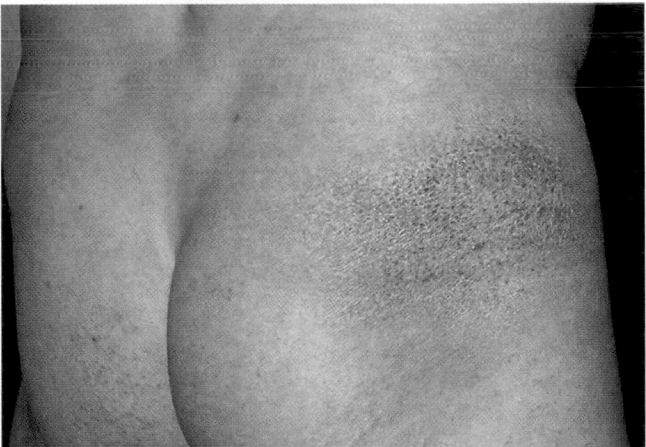

Figure 21-40 Patches may affect any area but they are found most often in sun-protected locations such as the buttock and lower trunk. Early lesions look like nummular eczema. They tend to remain fixed in location for months.

Figure 21-41 Mycosis fungoides (poikiloderma vasculare atrophicans). Red-brown hyperpigmented plaques with an atrophic, wrinkled surface tend to remain fixed in location.

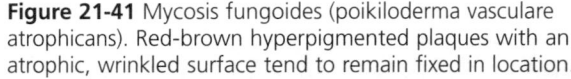

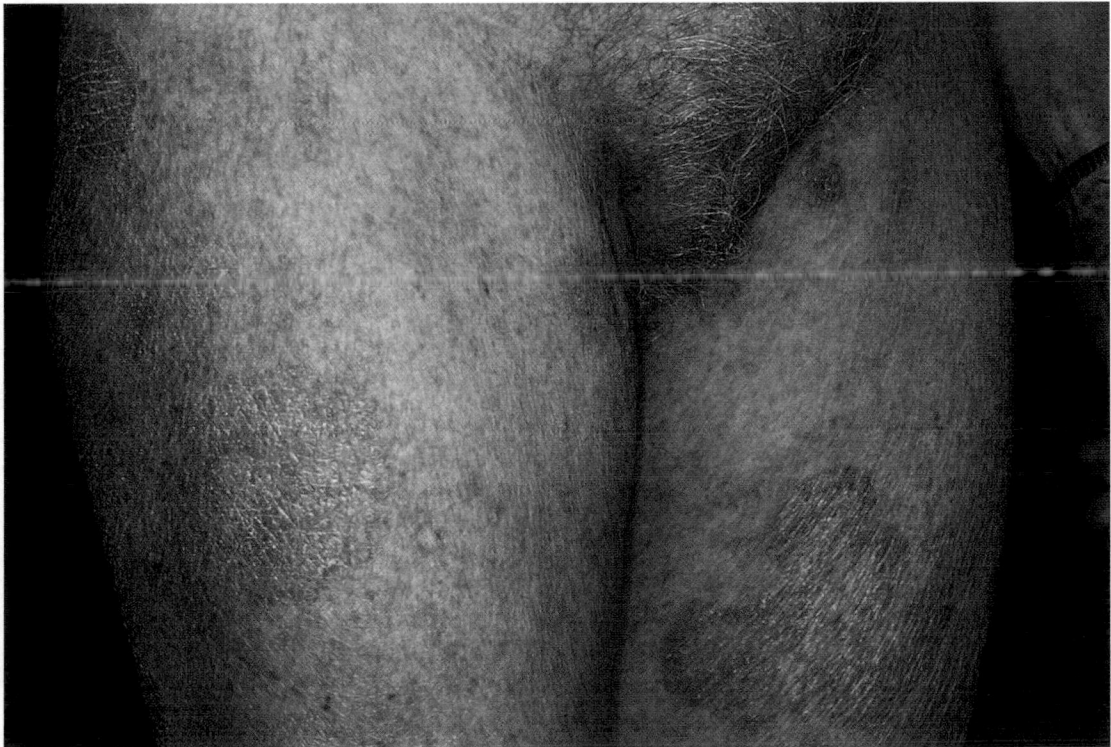

MYCOSIS FUNGOIDES—PLAQUE STAGE

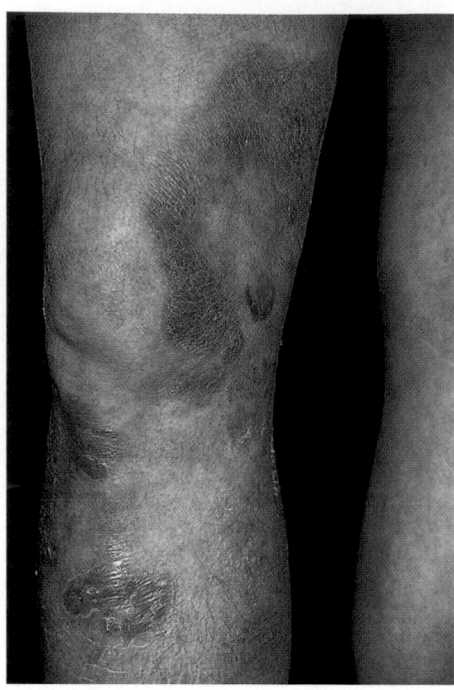

Figure 21-42 Early plaques have a fine scaling surface. The well-demarcated, erythematous lesions slowly evolve into tumors.

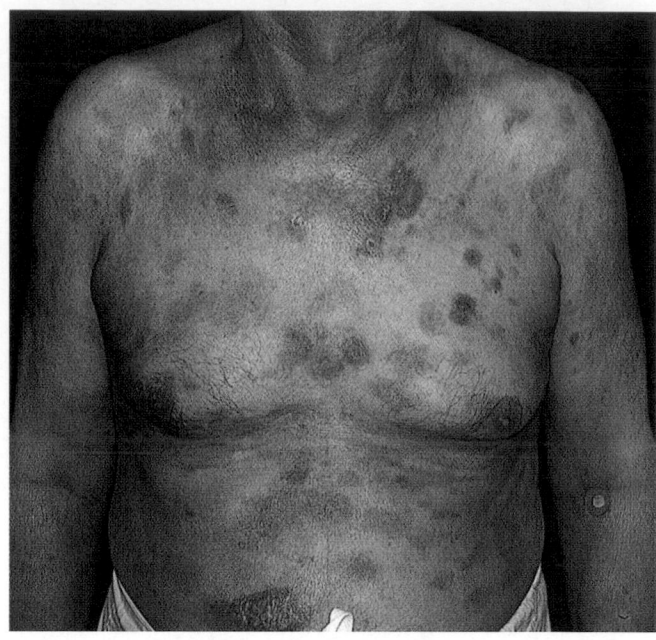

Figure 21-43 Annular or serpiginous plaques may be numerous. Central clearing may occur. Itching may be intense at this stage.

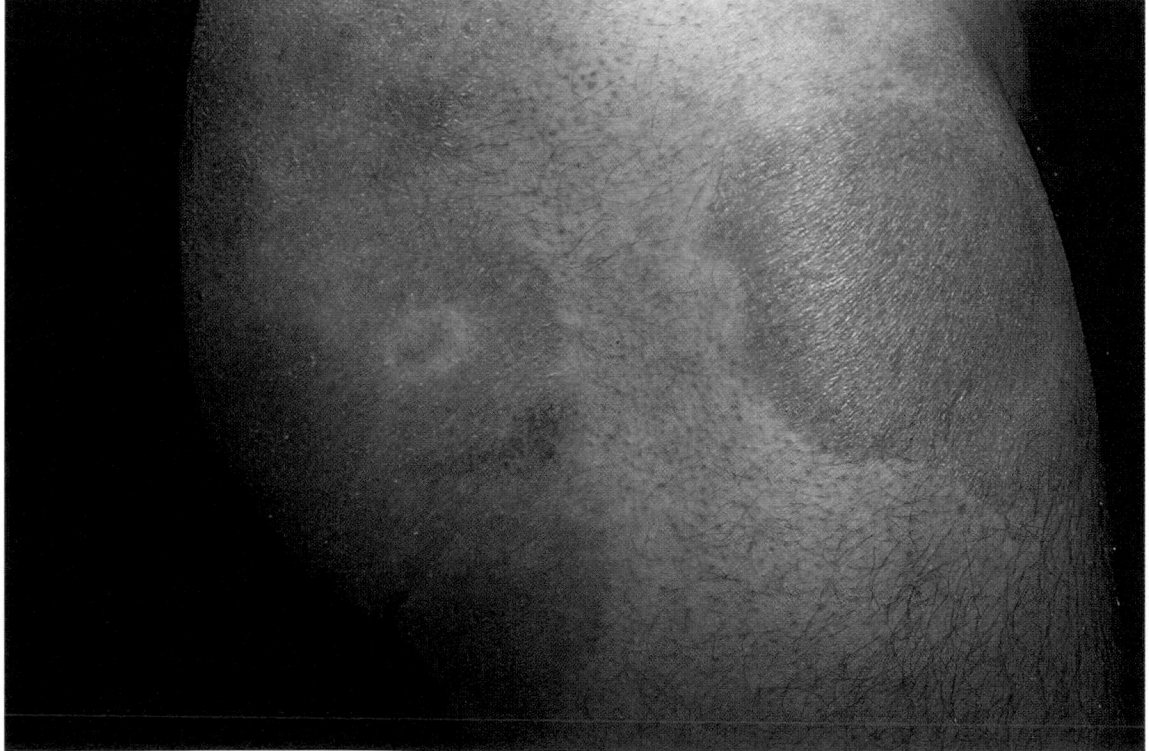

Figure 21-44 Large plaques have slowly evolved from stable macular, scaling, eczematous-appearing lesions.

MYCOSIS FUNGOIDES—TUMOR STAGE

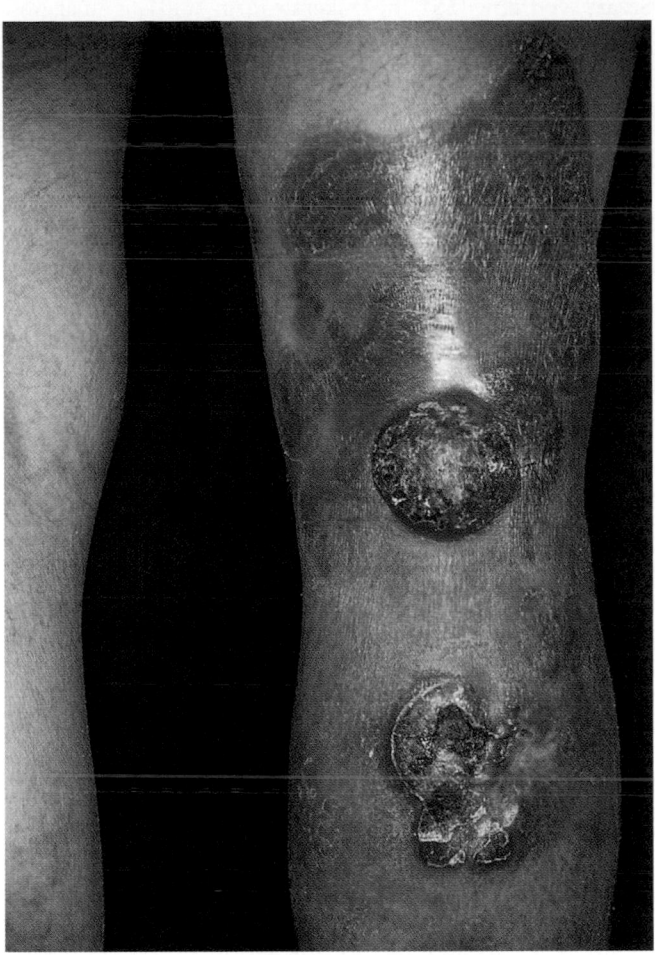

Figure 21-45 Red-violet, dome-shaped tumors may be exophytic or ulcerated.

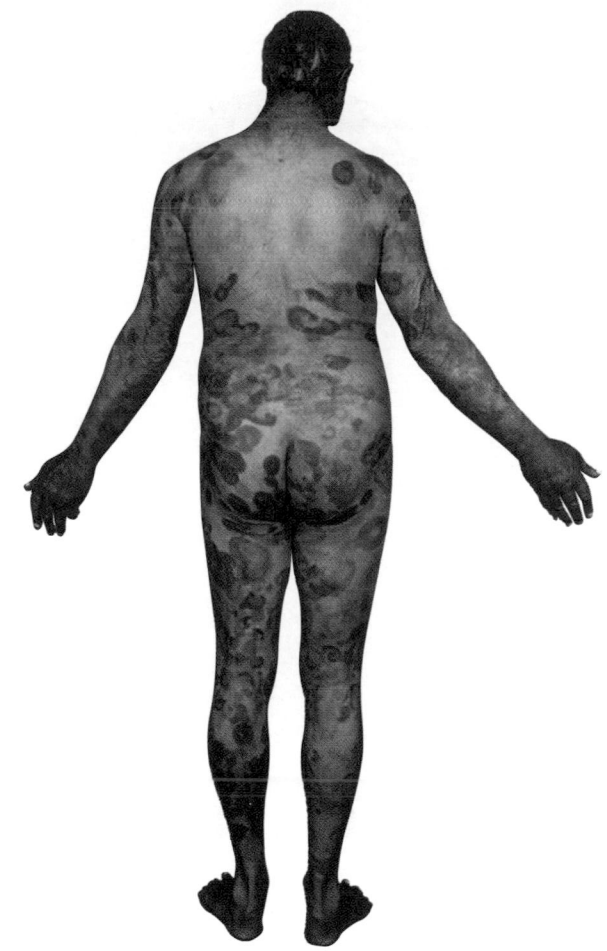

Figure 21-46 Widespread tumors have an annular and serpiginous pattern with central clearing.

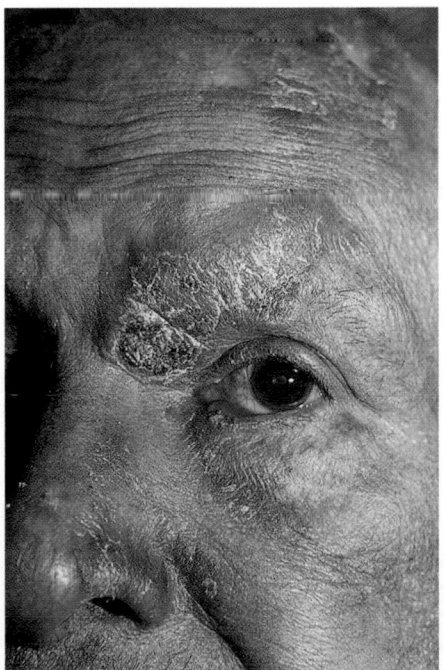

Figure 21-47 Tumors are ulcerated and exophytic. They resemble a mycotic infection; thus the archaic term *mycosis fungoides.*

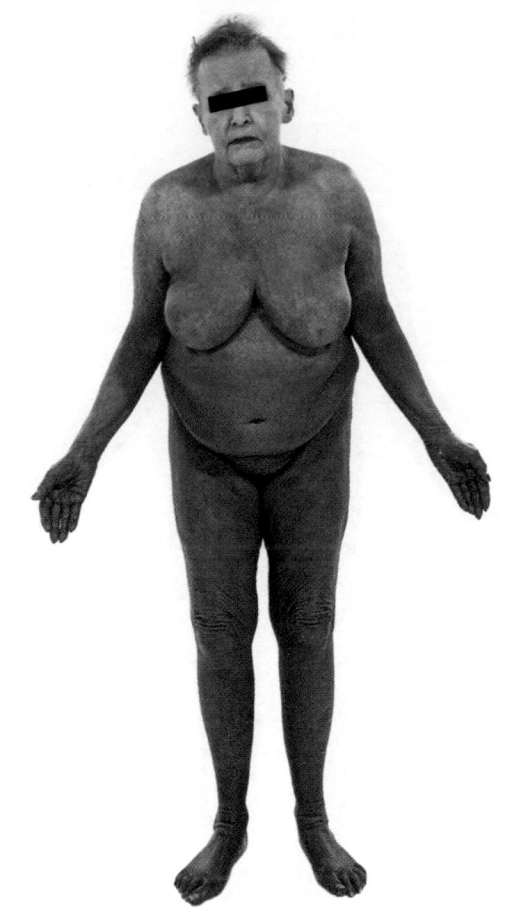

Figure 21-48 Sézary syndrome. Generalized erythroderma with scaling and thickening of the palms and soles.

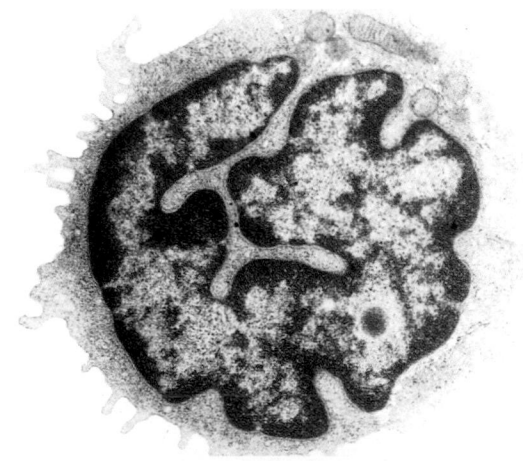

Figure 21-49 Sézary cells. Nuclei are hyperconvoluted.

Sézary syndrome

Sézary syndrome (SS), the leukemic form of MF, is an aggressive lymphoma (Figure 21-48). The estimated 5-year survival rate is 11%. SS consists of the triad of erythroderma, lymphadenopathy, and cerebriform lymphocytes (Sézary cells) in the peripheral blood, lymph nodes, and skin. Patients may have generalized pruritus, exfoliative dermatitis and thickening of the skin, ectropion, alopecia, and thickening of the palms and soles. The erythema may wax and wane during the day, or it may disappear and be replaced by plaques and tumors. Evidence supporting the diagnosis includes Sézary cells comprising more than 5% to 20% of circulating lymphocytes or more than 1,000/mm³, an expanded population of $CD4^+/CD7^-$ circulating lymphocytes by flow cytometry, an elevated CD4/CD8 ratio, or a clonal TCR gene rearrangement. Skin biopsy may reveal features resembling those found in the early stages of classic MF. Circulating cells with hyperconvoluted nuclei (Sézary cells) appear to be identical to those found in the skin infiltrates of MF (Figure 21-49).

TREATMENT. (See the diagram on p. 761.) Some experts think that the disease can be cured with aggressive treatment when disease is confined to the skin. Stable, localized, nonplaque disease may last for years. Because of the efficacy of topical nitrogen mustard, PUVA, and electron beam therapy in inducing and maintaining remissions, we now rarely see rapid evolution of the disease in patients whose CTCL is diagnosed early. Patients with clinical stage IA mycosis fungoides who are treated do not have an altered life expectancy. Less than 10% progress to more advanced stages and few die of disease.[155] Therapy for CTCL is dependent on the clinical stage. The goal of therapy is to achieve and maintain a remission or obtain palliation in advanced cases. Clinically visible disease should be treated. Patients in remission should be observed indefinitely. Maintenance therapy is routine at some centers.

Topical nitrogen mustard. Topical mechlorethamine is a cost-effective and convenient therapy for patients with limited patch and plaque mycosis fungoides.[155] Topical nitrogen mustard (10 mg vial) has been used for more than 20 years and is useful in controlling early stage disease. There is no systemic absorption (laboratory monitoring not required). An aqueous solution (10 to 20 mg/dL) is prepared by the patient or an ointment (10 to 20 mg HM2/100 gm Aquaphor) is prepared by the pharmacist. Solution is applied once daily with a cloth or brush to the entire body surface except the groin. Areas of disease activity may become inflamed. After several weeks, treatment is limited to affected area. Slow responders are treated bid or with higher concentrations (30 to 40 mg/dl). Application is continued until complete clearance. A 2- to 6-month trial of daily application of solution (either lesional or total body surface) or a 6- to 12-month trial is suggested. This is followed by maintenance therapy (average 6 months).[156] Acute or delayed hypersensitivity reactions (5% with ointment, >30 % with aqueous) occur. Desensitization is then accomplished, and treatment is

CUTANEOUS T-CELL LYMPHOMA

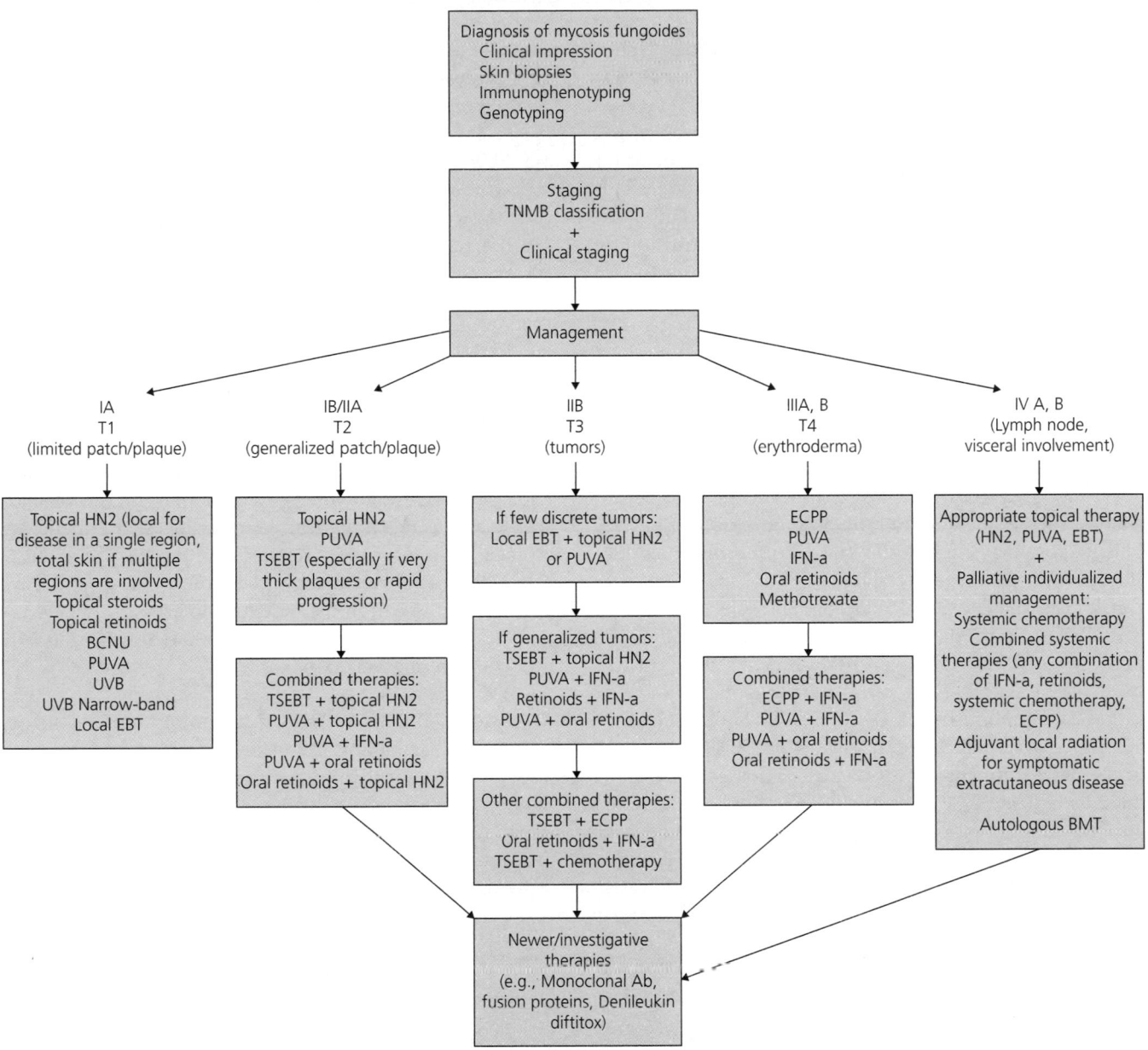

HN2, Mechlorethamine; BCNU, carmustine; UVA, ultraviolet B; PUVA, psoralen + ultraviolet A; EBT, electron beam therapy; TSEBT, total skin electron beam therapy; ECPP, extracorporeal photopheresis; IFN-a, interferon alfa; Denileukin diftitox, fusion proteins DAB389-interleukin-2 (IL-2) (Ontak); Targretin (Bexarotene) pills gel; Panretin; Tazarotene.

Adapted from Kim YH, Hoppe RT: Semin Oncol 1999; 26:276.

resumed. Complete responses were achieved in 80%, 68%, and 61% of patients in stages IA, IB, and IIA of the disease, respectively.[157] Topical carmustine (BCNU) is also effective, but systemic absorption occurs. Telangiectasias may develop where the drug is applied.[158] Although the response rate to total skin electron beam therapy was superior to that of topical mechlorethamine, the long-term survival results were similar. Keep medication refrigerated. Medication is available from several pharmacists, including Crown Drugs (Philadelphia, Pa.) or the Yale Medical Center Pharmacy (New Haven, Conn.).

Topical corticosteroids. Topical corticosteroids, especially class I compounds, are an effective treatment for patch-stage mycosis fungoides. Corticosteroids produced total response rates of 94% (complete response, 63%) in T1 disease, which is comparable to the results seen with topical chemotherapy. The complete response rate decreased to 25% in T2 disease. Most patients were treated with clobetasol propionate emollient cream.[159]

Bexarotene. Bexarotene 1% retinoid gel (Targretin) has an overall response rate of 44% to 63% (complete response, 8% to 21%) in patients with refractory stage IA-IIA CTCL. The predominant side effect is mild to moderate local irritation or rash.[160] The medication is very expensive.

PUVA and UVB. CTCL often begins in sun-shielded regions, such as the buttocks and inferior surface of breasts. This suggests that sun exposure to the trunk and extremities alters the environment of certain regions of the skin so that CTCL cells find those sites inhospitable. This may explain why UVB or PUVA therapy can maintain a patient in remission. PUVA is very effective in the limited, "thin," plaque stage of CTCL.[161,162] High rates of remission are induced within 2 to 6 months with a regimen of two or three treatments per week, increasing the dosage of UVA by 0.5 J/cm2 in alternate treatments, as tolerated. The dosage is held constant, then slowly tapered to once per week, once per 2 weeks, once per month, once every other month for 6 months, and then once every 3 months for an indefinite period. Total response rates of 95% (complete response in 79% of T1 cases, 59% of T2 cases) is reported. Duration of remission averaged 3.6 years with maintenance PUVA at least once per month.[163] Complete remission occurs faster compared with topical therapy.

Traditional broadband UVB phototherapy (280-320 nm) has been associated with an 83% total and complete response rate in T1 disease.[164] However, long-wave UVA penetrates deeper into the dermal infiltrates than UVB. "Shadowed" areas (scalp, perineum, axillae, skinfolds, soles) may not receive adequate exposure. The combination of interferon and PUVA showed high complete remissions in preliminary studies.[165]

Total skin electron beam therapy. Management of stage IB/IIA (generalized patch/plaque, T2) disease is with HN2, PUVA, TSEBT and UVB. TSEBT should be considered as initial therapy for patients with aggressive disease, extensive thick plaques, or who fail HN2 or PUVA. TSEB therapy is the most reliable method for inducing complete remission in generalized patches, plaques, and tumors. Complete response rates of up to 98% for limited plaques and 36% for tumors is reported.[166] The majority of patients have a relapse within 5 years. After attaining complete remission with TSEB, some physicians initiate adjuvant therapy, most commonly topical nitrogen mustard. Adjuvant HN2 or oral PUVA should be administered for at least 6 months after a complete response to TSEBT.[167] A total of ~36 Gy is given over ~10 wks with a 1 wk split after 18 to 20 Gy. "Shadowed" areas need supplemental treatment.[156] Adverse effects are erythema, desquamation, alopecia, loss of nails, and inability to sweat.

Extracorporeal photopheresis. Extracorporeal photopheresis is useful for treating Sézary syndrome and the erythrodermic phase of MF. It is also effective alone or in combination with adjunctive therapy[168] for extensive patch or plaque disease and some tumor-stage disease. Remissions longer than 3 years have been achieved in some patients. Photopheresis involves long-wave radiation (UVA) of leukocytes taken from the patient who has ingested 8-methoxypsoralen, with subsequent reinfusion of the leukocytes to the patient.[169-171] The treatment is given on 2 consecutive days every month for 6 months. Patients who have a CD4:CD8 ratio of less than or equal to 5 do better than those with few or no CD8+ cells in their skin.[172]

ADVANCED DISEASE. Individual tumors respond to orthovoltage x-irradiation. All of the treatments for advanced disease may be initially successful in inducing remissions, but none appears to prolong survival. Many new agents are being tested. Anti–T-monoclonal antibodies and recombinant fusion proteins (denileukin diftitox; trade name Ontak) may prove useful for extracutaneous disease.

LYMPHOMATOID PAPULOSIS. Lymphomatoid papulosis is a rare disease in which the skin lesions have a neoplastic-like histology, but the clinical course is benign and chronic.[173] Five percent to 20% of cases evolve into a lymphoma (MF, T-immunoblastic lymphoma, and Hodgkin's disease). Crops of reddish-brown papules undergo central necrosis and spontaneous healing with scar formation. Lesions persist for 2 to 4 weeks before resolving. Papules arise in crops over the trunk and extremities for months to years. The new lesions itch or are painful.

Paget's Disease of the Breast

Paget's disease of the breast results from invasion of the epidermis of the nipple, areola, and surrounding skin by malignant cells originating from an underlying ductal carcinoma.[174] An underlying carcinoma of the breast may be palpated, but in approximately 40% of cases, the cancer is clinically impalpable and radiologically undetectable.[175, 176]

CLINICAL PRESENTATION. The disease begins insidiously in one breast with a small area of erythema on the nipple that drains serous fluid and forms a crust (Figures 21-50 and 21-51). The inflammation is usually attributed to trauma, and partial healing comforts the patient. Patients equate lumps rather than inflammatory changes with cancer and, consequently, the disease continues. Malignant cells migrate through the epidermis, and the disease becomes initially apparent on the areola and, at a much later date (a year or more), on the surrounding skin (Figure 21-50). The process appears eczematous, but the plaque is indurated and has sharp margins, which remain relatively fixed for weeks. Ulceration is a late finding. Paget's disease of the male nipple is very rare and is more aggressive than in females.

DIAGNOSIS. Clinically and histologically, the process is very similar to Bowen's disease; however, Bowen's disease of the nipple is very rare. A crucial point to note is that Paget's disease of the breast is a rare, unilateral disease, whereas eczematous inflammation of the nipples is common and almost invariably bilateral. Cytologic diagnosis can be made from nipple scrape smears.[177] A biopsy may be studied with conventional stains and immunohistochemistry. Immunocytochemical techniques are more reliable for distinguishing

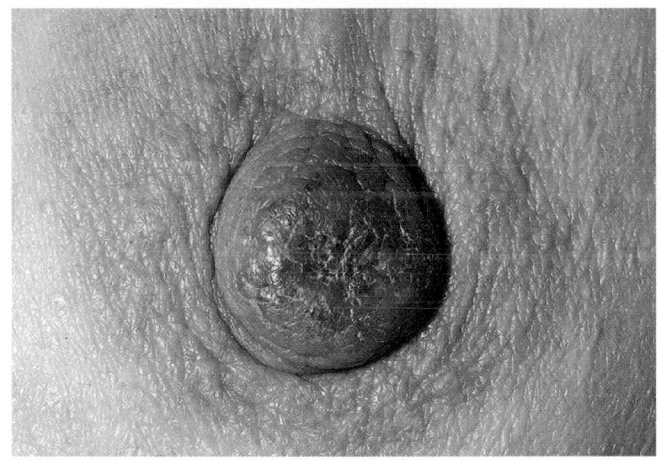

Figure 21-50 Paget's disease. Early lesions are subtle and present with erythema, scale, and crust. They may ooze serum. A diagnosis of irritation or eczema may be suspected. The infiltrating process spreads to the areola and beyond.

Paget's disease from superficial spreading malignant melanoma and from primary intraepidermal carcinoma than conventional mucin histochemistry using diastase periodic-acid-Schiff (d-AS) with and without Alcian blue. Positive immunoreactivity occurs with cytokeratin (CAM 5.2), c-erb B-2 oncoprotein (21N), and carcinoembryonic antigen (CEA). CEA is seen in virtually all cases of mammary Paget's disease, with consistent negative immunoreactivity in melanoma and other tumor types.[178,179]

TREATMENT. After biopsy, treatment is surgical. Cone excision of the nipple-areola complex was described as inadequate in one study.[180] Another study reported success with local radiotherapy when disease was confined to the nipple.[181]

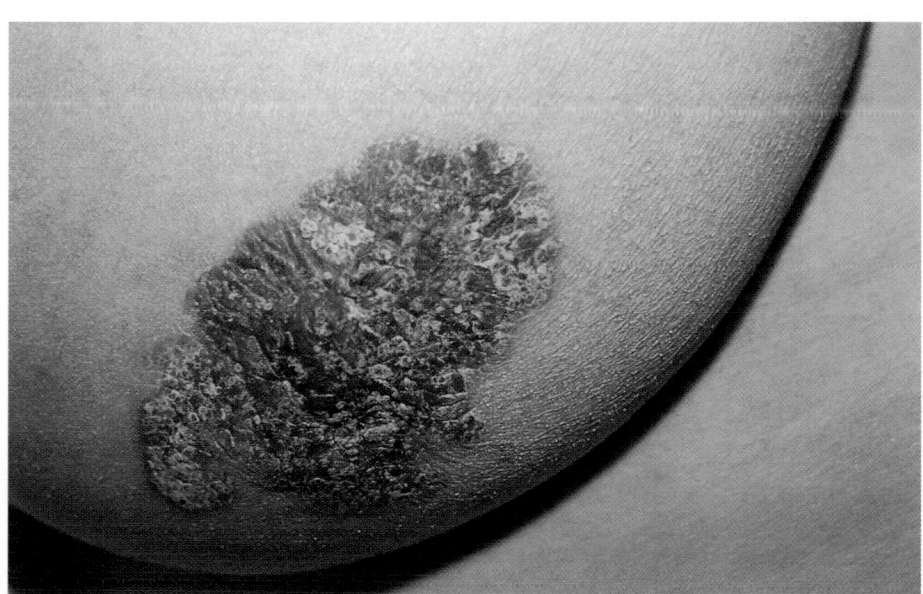

Figure 21-51 A red, scaling plaque drains serous fluid and forms a crust. The lesion appears eczematous but, unlike eczema, is unilateral.

Extramammary Paget's Disease

Extramammary Paget's disease is a rare cutaneous adenocarcinoma that occurs in elderly women more often than in men and is located in the vulva, scrotum, axilla, or the perianal area. Various histochemical studies suggest evidence of sweat gland derivation of the disease.[182,183]

ASSOCIATION WITH UNDERLYING MALIGNANCY. The disease may be associated with an underlying adenocarcinoma or carcinoma of the rectum, and 26% of affected patients ultimately die either from the disease itself or from an associated internal malignancy. Twenty-four percent have an associated underlying cutaneous adnexal adenocarcinoma. These patients have a higher mortality rate (46%) than patients with extramammary Paget's disease without underlying cutaneous adnexal adenocarcinoma. Twelve percent of patients with extramammary Paget's disease have an associated concurrent underlying internal malignancy.[184] The location of the underlying internal malignancy is closely related to the location of the cutaneous disease; that is, a perianal location is associated with adenocarcinoma of the digestive system, a penile location is associated with genitourinary malignancy, etc. As with Paget's disease of the breast, the epidermis is infiltrated with malignant cells that migrate laterally. Biopsy often reveals cells that are exterior to the clinically apparent areas, a fact that explains the high rate of recurrence after excision.

CLINICAL PRESENTATION. The disease in males and females appears as a white-to-red, scaling or macerated, infiltrated, eroded, or ulcerated plaque, most frequently observed on the labia majora (Figure 21-52) and scrotum[185] (Figure 21-53). Persistent itching and burning is common. The clinical presentation closely resembles lichen sclerosus et atrophicus, lichen simplex chronicus, leukoplakia, Bowen's disease, or chronic yeast infection.

HISTOLOGIC CHARACTERISTICS. Histologically, Paget's disease resembles Bowen's disease and superficial spreading melanoma. Paget's cells are mucin positive, as determined by Hale's colloidal iron stain. The cytoplasm is often PAS-positive and stains with Alcian blue at pH 2.5. Immunoperoxidase stains are helpful in establishing the diagnosis and in excluding conditions that resemble Paget's disease. Most cases are CEA positive.[186] CEA is a sweat gland marker. Antikeratin stains Bowen's disease and anti-S-100 protein stain is positive in melanoma.

MANAGEMENT. Conventional surgical excision or Mohs' micrographic surgery,[187] followed optionally by radiation therapy,[188,189] is the treatment for regionally confined disease. A nonradical conservative surgical approach has been advocated. In one study, skinning vulvectomy with split-thickness skin graft, hemivulvectomy, and simple vulvectomy produced excellent results for patients with limited disease without an underlying adenocarcinoma.[190] Fluorescein given intravenously helps to visualize disease margins with the use of an ultraviolet light.[191] Recurrent Paget's disease of the vulva has been treated successfully with topical bleomycin.[192] All patients with extramammary Paget's disease should have a careful physical examination to search for internal malignancy.

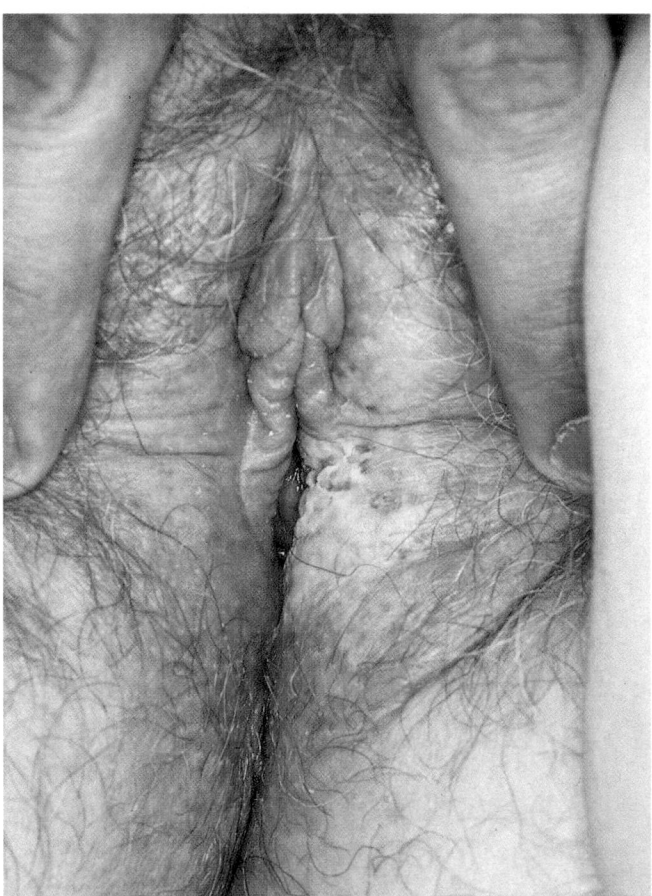

Figure 21-52 Extramammary Paget's disease. A white, eroded plaque with ill-defined borders on the labia.

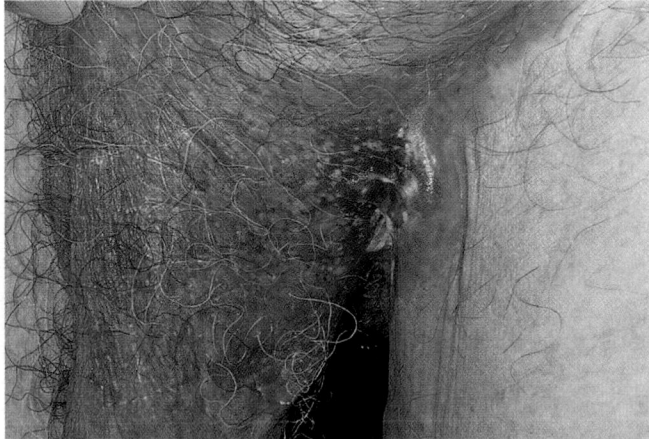

Figure 21-53 Extramammary Paget's disease. Three biopsies were taken before malignant cells were demonstrated at the periphery of this chronic ulcer at the base of the scrotum.

Cutaneous Metastasis

The incidence of cutaneous metastasis in patients with malignancy is approximately 2% to 10%.[193-197] Cutaneous metastases may be the first sign of extranodal metastatic disease, particularly in patients with melanoma, breast cancer, or mucosal cancers of the head and neck.[198] In a series of papers, Brownstein and Helwig[195-197] stated several aspects of cutaneous metastasis. They determined the incidence and relative importance of the gender of the patient, the location of the metastatic growth, the morphology of the metastatic lesion, and the histologic features of the metastatic lesion in identifying the site of the primary tumor. The incidence of some of these features is summarized in Tables 21-7 and 21-8 and is illustrated in Figure 21-54. The most helpful information for localizing the primary tumor is the sex of the patient and the location of the skin tumor.

MORPHOLOGIC CHARACTERISTICS. The most common representation of cutaneous metastasis is an aggregate of discrete, firm, nontender, skin-colored nodules that appear suddenly, grow rapidly, attain a certain size (often 2 cm), and remain stationary (Figure 21-55). Accurate clinical diagnosis is rare; the lesions are most frequently diagnosed as cysts or benign fibrous tumors. In several instances, the clinical picture is that of a vascular tumor such as a pyogenic granuloma, hemangioma, or Kaposi's sarcoma (Figure 21-56). The periumbilical Sister Mary Joseph's nodule heralds an underlying gastric tumor.

Table 21-7 Origins of Skin Metastases

Men			Women		
Primary site	Cases with skin metastases	%	Primary site	Cases with skin metastases	%
Lung	132	22.4	Breast	380	71.0
Melanoma	103	17.5	Melanoma	49	9.1
Colon and rectum	104	17.7	Colon and rectum	26	4.8
Oral cavity	68	11.6	Ovary	20	3.7
Kidney	35	6.0	Lung	15	2.8
Upper digestive tract	35	6.0	Unknown	9	1.6
Breast	12	2.0	Oral cavity	9	1.6
Stomach	29	4.9	Endometrium	4	0.7
Esophagus	18	3.1	Urinary bladder	6	1.1
Urinary bladder	11	1.9	Uterine cervix	6	1.1
Unknown	11	1.9	Stomach	3	0.6
Pancreas	13	2.2	Bile ducts	3	0.6
Larynx	7	1.2	Pancreas	4	0.6
Liver	4	0.7	Nasal sinuses	3	0.5
TOTAL	**587**			**535**	

Adapted from Lookingbill DP, Spangler N, et al: J Am Acad Dermatol 1993; 29:228-236; and Brownstein MH, Helwig EB: Cancer 1972; 29:1298.

Table 21-8 Sites of Distant Skin Metastases

Primary site	Scalp	Face	Neck	Shoulders	Chest	Back	Abdomen	Upper extremities	Lower extremities
Breast	18	2	12	11	4	37	15	16	9
Melanoma	10	7	21	7	28	8	10	21	25
Unknown	4	3	5	0	1	2	5	2	6
Lung	2	1	2	0	9	2	7	1	1
Oral cavity	2	2	4	0	1	1	0	1	0
Colon and rectum	1	1	0	0	2	2	2	0	0

Modified from Lookingbill DP, Spangler N, et al: J Am Acad Dermatol 1993; 29:228.

CUTANEOUS METASTASIS

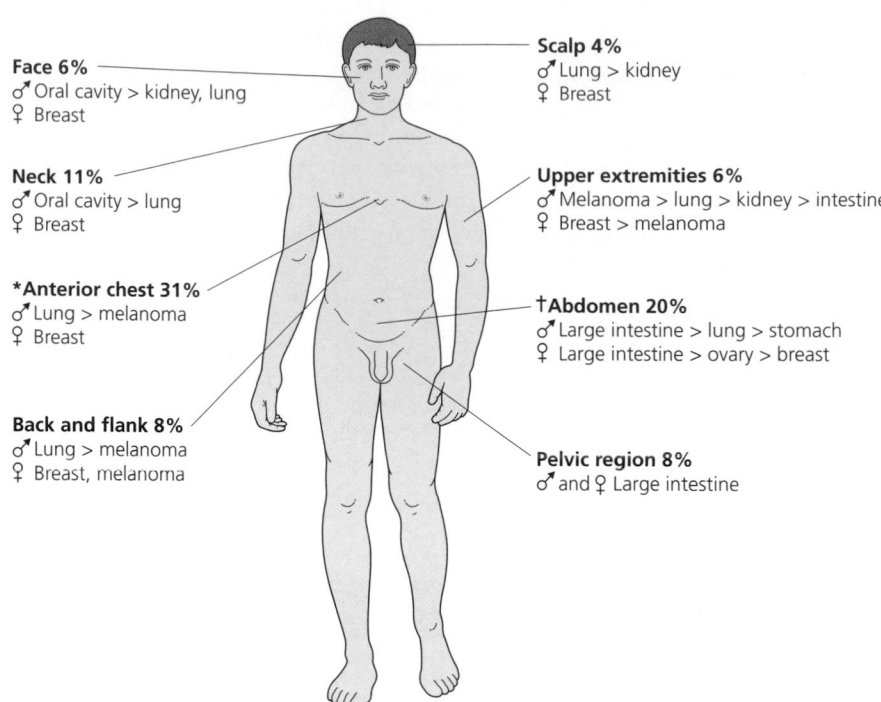

Scalp 4%
♂ Lung > kidney
♀ Breast

Face 6%
♂ Oral cavity > kidney, lung
♀ Breast

Neck 11%
♂ Oral cavity > lung
♀ Breast

Upper extremities 6%
♂ Melanoma > lung > kidney > intestine
♀ Breast > melanoma

*Anterior chest 31%
♂ Lung > melanoma
♀ Breast

†Abdomen 20%
♂ Large intestine > lung > stomach
♀ Large intestine > ovary > breast

Back and flank 8%
♂ Lung > melanoma
♀ Breast, melanoma

Pelvic region 8%
♂ and ♀ Large intestine

Figure 21-54 Patterns of cutaneous metastasis. 724 patients. Percentages are of the total number of cases. *(Modified from Brownstein MN, Helwig EB: Arch Dermatol 105:862, 1972.)*

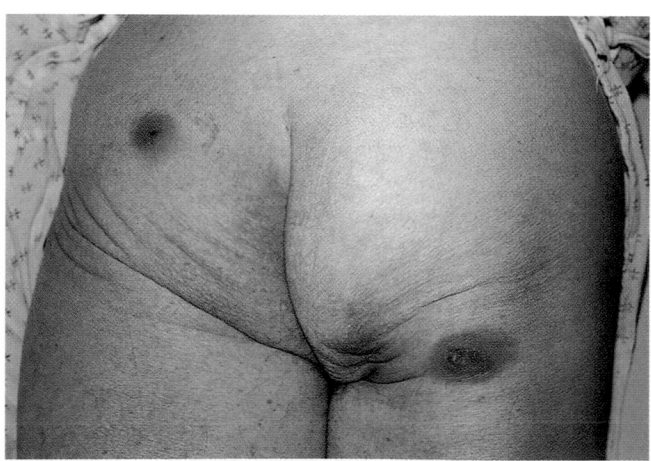

Figure 21-55 Metastatic carcinoma. The nodules had remained fixed in size after an initial rapid growth.

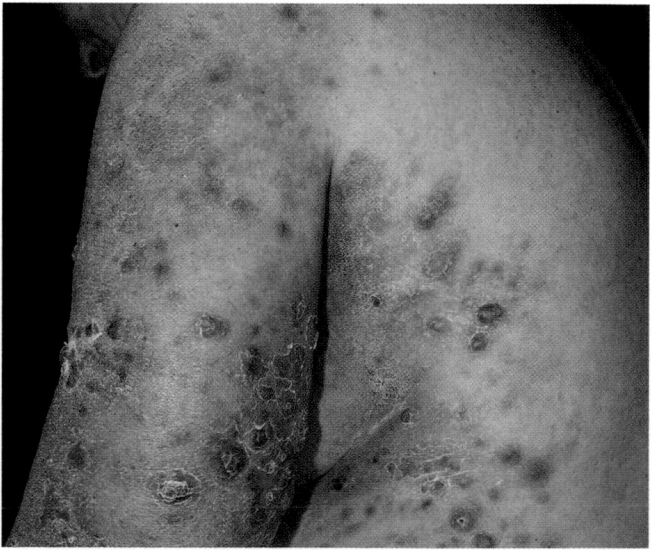

Figure 21-56 Metastatic carcinoma of the breast. Nodules appear vascular and resemble Kaposi's sarcoma.

The second most common pattern of cutaneous metastasis is inflammation with erythema, edema, warmth (Figures 21-57 and 21-58), and tenderness. The primary tumor is usually in the breast, and malignant cells spread to the subepidermal lymphatic vessels, where they create obstruction. The initial diagnosis is frequently a bacterial infection, such as erysipelas or cellulitis. The patient is, however, afebrile and appears to be healthy.

The third and least common pattern simulates a cicatricial condition and resembles discoid lupus erythematosus or morphea. Asymptomatic sclerodermoid plaques, sometimes associated with hair loss (alopecia neoplastica), are most frequently located on the scalp and are caused by metastasis from breast cancer in women and lung or kidney tumors in men. Carcinoma en cuirasse is seen with breast cancer and appears as a hard, infiltrated plaque with a leathery appearance that results from fibrosis and lymph stasis.

HISTOLOGIC CHARACTERISTICS. In general, the histologic features of primary and metastatic tumors are similar, but metastatic tumors are often less differentiated. Frequently, biopsy specimens are not interpreted as originating from a distant site. Adenocarcinoma metastatic to the skin is most often secondary to cancer of the large intestine, lung, or breast. Squamous cell carcinoma metastatic to the skin customarily originates from the oral cavity, lung, or esophagus. Undifferentiated lesions usually originate from the breast or lungs.

MODE OF SPREAD. Tumors that invade veins, such as carcinoma of the kidney and lung, frequently present as cutaneous metastasis occurring in diverse skin sites distant from the primary tumor. Cancers that invade lymphatics, such as carcinoma of the breast and squamous cell carcinoma of the oral cavity, appear late in the course of the disease and may invade skin overlying the primary tumor.[88]

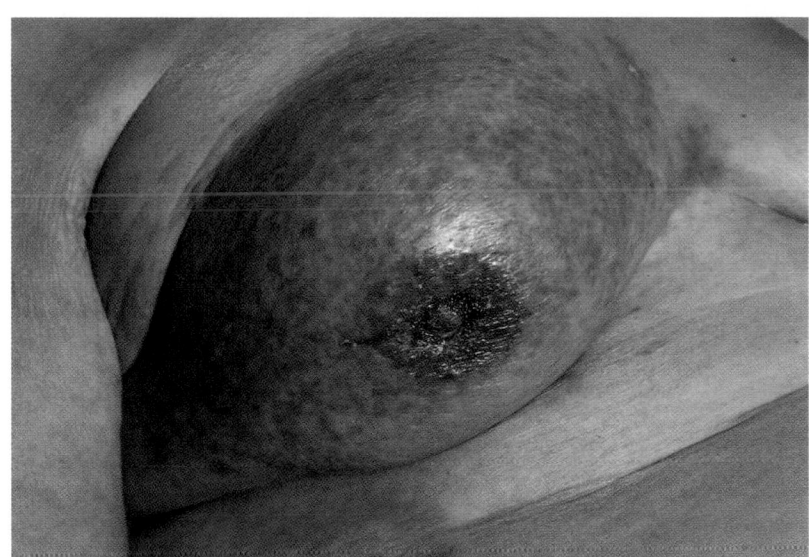

Figure 21-57 Inflammatory cutaneous metastasis with erythema, edema, and crusting.

Figure 21-58 Inflammatory cutaneous metastasis. Erosion and crusting resemble infected eczema.

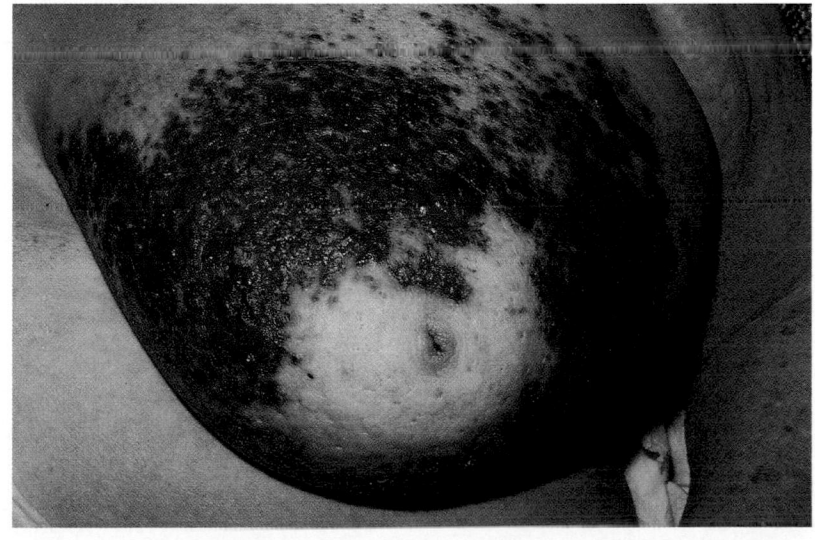

References

1. Preston DS, Stern RS: Nonmelanoma cancers of the skin, N Engl J Med 1992; 327:1649.

2. Leman J, McHenry P: Basal cell carcinoma: still an enigma, Arch Dermatol 2001; 137(9):1239.

3. Brooke R, et al: Discordance between facial wrinkling and the presence of basal cell carcinoma, Arch Dermatol 2001; 137(6):751.

4. Cox NH: Basal cell carcinoma in young adults, Br J Dermatol 1992; 127:26.

5. Rustin MHA., Chambers TJ, Munro DD: Post-traumatic basal cell carcinomas, Clin Exp Dermatol 1984; 9:379.

6. Sexton M, et al: Histologic pattern analysis of basal cell carcinoma. Study of a series of 1039 consecutive neoplasms, J Am Acad Dermatol 1990; 23:1118.

7. Phillips TJ, et al: Nonhealing leg ulcers: a manifestation of basal cell carcinoma, J Am Acad Dermatol 1991; 25:47.

8. Menzies S, et al: Surface microscopy of pigmented basal cell carcinoma, Arch Dermatol 2000; 136(8):1012.

9. Maloney ME, et al: Pigmented basal cell carcinoma: investigation of 70 cases, J Am Acad Dermatol 1992; 27:74.

10. Salasche SJ, Amonette RA: Morpheaform basal cell epitheliomas: a study of subclinical extensions in a series of 51 cases, J Dermatol Surg Oncol 1981; 7:387.

11. Farndon PA, et al: Location of gene for Gorlin syndrome, Lancet 1992; 339:581.

12. Chenevix-Trench G, et al: Further localization of the gene for nevoid basal cell carcinoma syndrome (NBCCS) in 15 Australasian families: linkage and loss of heterozygosity, Am J Hum Genet 1993; 53:760.

13. Gorlin RJ: Nevoid basal-cell carcinoma syndrome, Medicine 1987; 66:98.

14. Kimonis V, et al: Clinical manifestations in 105 persons with nevoid basal cell carcinoma syndrome, Am J Med Genet 1997; 69(3):299.

15. Gutierrez MM, Mora RG: Nevoid basal carcinoma syndrome. A review and case report of a patient with unilateral basal cell nevus syndrome, J Am Acad Dermatol 1986; 15:1023.

16. Evans DG, et al: Complications of the nevoid basal cell carcinoma syndrome: results of a population based study, J Med Genet 1993; 30:460.

17. Pratt MD, Jackson R: Nevoid basal cell carcinoma syndrome. A 15-year follow-up of cases in Ottawa and the Ottawa valley, J Am Acad Dermatol 1987; 16:964.

18. Howell JB: Nevoid basal cell carcinoma syndrome, J Am Acad Dermatol 1984; 11:98.

19. Goldstein AM, et al: Sun exposure and basal cell carcinomas in the nevoid basal cell carcinoma syndrome, J Am Acad Dermatol 1993; 29:34.

20. Correl RW: Bilateral cysts of the jaw occurring with multiple skin lesions, J Am Dent Assoc 1980; 101:978.

21. Drake LA, et al: Guidelines of care for basal cell carcinoma. The American Academy of Dermatology Committee on Guidelines of Care, J Am Acad Dermatol 1992; 26:117.

22. Lang PG, Maize JC: Histologic evolution of recurrent basal cell carcinoma and treatment implications, J Am Acad Dermatol 1986; 14:186.

23. Crissey J: Curettage and electrodesiccation as a method of treatment for epitheliomas of the skin, J Surg Oncol 1971; 3(3):287.

24. Silverman MK, et al: Recurrence rates of treated basal cell carcinomas. Part 2: Curettage-electrodesiccation, J Dermatol Surg Oncol 1991; 17:720.

25. McDaniel WE: Adequate follow up for treated basal cell carcinoma, Arch Dermatol 1986; 122:243.

26. Marghoob A, et al: Risk of another basal cell carcinoma developing after treatment of a basal cell carcinoma, J Am Acad Dermatol 1993; 28:22.

27. Karagas MR, et al: Risk of subsequent basal cell carcinoma and squamous cell carcinoma of the skin among patients with prior skin cancer. Skin Cancer Prevention Study Group, JAMA 1992; 267:3305.

28. Epstein E.H., et al: Mycosis fungoides: survival, prognostic features, response to therapy, and autopsy findings, Medicine 1972; 15:61.

29. Leonforte JF: Deep recurrent basal cell epithelioma, J Am Acad Dermatol 1987; 16:1257.

30. Dubin N, Kopf AW: Multivariate risk score for recurrence of cutaneous basal cell carcinomas.,Arch Dermatol 1983; 119:373.

31. Thissen M, Neumann M, Schouten L: A systematic review of treatment modalities for primary basal cell carcinomas, Arch Dermatol 1999; 135(10):1177.

32. Marcil I, Stern R: Risk of developing a subsequent nonmelanoma skin cancer in patients with a history of non-melanoma skin cancer: a critical review of the literature and meta-analysis, Arch Dermatol 2000; 136(12):1524.

33. Holmkvist K, Rogers G, Dahl P: Incidence of residual basal cell carcinoma in patients who appear tumor free after biopsy, J Am Acad Dermatol 1999; 41(4):600.

34. McDaniel WE: Therapy for basal cell epitheliomas by curettage only, Arch Dermatol 1983; 119:901.

35. Spiller WF, Spiller RF: Treatment of basal cell epithelioma by curettage and electrodesiccation, J Am Acad Dermatol 1984; 11:808.

36. Kopf AW, et al: Curettage-electrodesiccation treatment of basal cell carcinomas, Arch Dermatol 1977; 113:439.

37. Salasche SJ: Curettage and electrodesiccation in the treatment of midfacial basal cell epithelioma, J Am Acad Dermatol 1983; 8:496.

38. Alexiades-Armena Kas M, et al: The appropriateness of curettage and electrodesiccation for the treatment of basal cell carcinomas, Arch Derm 2000; 136(6):800.

39. Wolf DJ, Zitelli JA: Surgical margins for basal cell carcinoma, Arch Dermatol 1987; 123:340.

40. Silverman MK, et al: Recurrence rates of treated basal cell carcinomas. Part 3: Surgical excision, J Dermatol Surg Oncol 1992; 18:471.

41. Chiller K, et al: Efficacy of curettage before excision in clearing surgical margins of nonmelanoma skin cancer, Arch Dermatol 2000; 136(11):1327.

42. Richmond JD, Davie RM: The significance of incomplete excision in patients with basal cell carcinoma, Br J Plast Surg 1987; 40:63.

43. Robinson J, Fisher S: Recurrent basal cell carcinoma after incomplete resection, Arch Dermatol 2000; 136(11):1318.

44. Berlin J, et al: The significance of tumor persistence after incomplete excision of basal cell carcinoma, J Am Acad Dermatol 2002; 46(4):549.

45. Torre D: Cryosurgery of basal cell carcinoma, J Am Acad Dermatol1986; 15:917.

46. Buker JL, Amonette RA: Micrographic surgery, Clin Dermatol 1992; 10:309.

47. Wilder RB, et al: Basal cell carcinoma treated with radiation therapy, Cancer 1991; 68:2134.

48. Silverman MK, et al: Recurrence rates of treated basal cell carcinomas. Part 4: X-ray therapy. J Dermatol Surg Oncol 1992; 18:549.

49. Wilder RB, et al: Recurrent basal cell carcinoma treated with radiation therapy, Arch Dermatol 1991; 127:1668.

50. Marks R, et al: Imiquimod 5% cream in the treatment of superficial basal cell carcinoma: results of a multicenter 6-week dose-response trial, J Am Acad Dermatol 2001; 44(5):807.

51. Beutner K, et al: Therapeutic response of basal cell carcinoma to the immune response modifier imiquimod 5% cream, J Am Acad Dermatol 1999; 41(6):1002.

52. Labandter HP, Ryan RF: 5-fluorouracil in management of Gorlin's syndrome, N Engl J Med 1978; 298:913.

53. Stenquist B, et al: Treatment of aggressive basal cell carcinoma with intralesional interferon: evaluation of efficacy by Mohs' surgery, J Am Acad Dermatol 1992; 27:65.

54. Cockerell C: Histopathology of incipient intraepidermal squamous cell carcinoma ("actinic keratosis"), J Am Acad Dermatol 2000; 42(1 Pt 2):11.

55. Marks R, et al: Spontaneous remission of solar keratoses: the case for conservative management, Br J Dermatol 1986; 115:649.

56. Jensen P, Moller B, Hansen S: Skin cancer in kidney and heart transplant recipients and different long-term immunosuppressive therapy regimens, J Am Acad Dermatol 2000; 42(2 Pt 1):307.

57. Moy R: Clinical presentation of actinic keratoses and squamous cell carcinoma, J Am Acad Dermatol 2000; 42(1 Pt 2):8.

58. Dodson JM, et al: Malignant potential of actinic keratoses and the controversy over treatment. A patient-oriented perspective, Arch Dermatol 1991; 127:1029.

59. Marks R, Rennie G, Selwood TS: Malignant transformation of solar keratoses to squamous cell carcinoma, Lancet 1988; 1:795.

60. Moller R, Reymann F, Hou-Jensen K: Metastases in dermatological patients with squamous cell carcinoma, Arch Dermatol 1979; 115:703.

61. Heaphy M, Ackerman A: The nature of solar keratosis: a critical review in historical perspective, J Am Acad Dermatol 2000; 43(1 Pt 1):138.

62. Feldman S, et al: Destructive procedures are the standard of care for treatment of actinic keratoses, J Am Acad Dermatol 1999; 40(1):43.

63. Alamillos-Granados FJ, et al: Carbon dioxide laser vermilionectomy for actinic cheilitis, J Oral Maxillofac Surg 1993; 51:118.

64. Johnson TM, et al: Carbon dioxide laser treatment of actinic cheilitis. Clinicohistopathologic correlation to determine the optimal depth of destruction, J Am Acad Dermatol 1992; 27:737.

65. Thompson SC, et al: Reduction of solar keratoses by regular sunscreen use, N Engl J Med 1993; 329:1147.

66. Goette DK: Topical chemotherapy with 5-fluorouracil. A review, J Am Acad Dermatol 1981; 4:633.

67. Stockfleth E, et al: Successful treatment of actinic keratosis with imiquimod cream 5%: a report of six cases, Br J Dermatol 2001; 144(5):1050.

68. Wolf J., et al:Topical 3.0% diclofenac in 2.5% hyaluronan gel in the treatment of actinic keratoses, Int J Dermatol 2001; 40(11):709.

69. Reference deleted in proofs.

70. Reference deleted in proofs.

71. Loven K, et al: Evaluation of the efficacy and tolerability of 0.5% fluorouracil cream and 5% fluorouracil cream applied to each side of the face in patients with actinic keratosis [In Process Citation], Clin Ther 2002; 24(6):990.

72. Pearlman DL: Weekly pulse dosing: effective and comfortable topical 5-fluorouracil treatment of multiple facial actinic keratoses, J Am Acad Dermatol 1991; 25:665.

73. Bennett R, et al: Current management using 5-fluorouracil: 1985, Cutis 1985; 218.

74. Moy LS, et al: Glycolic acid peels for the treatment of wrinkles and photoaging, J Dermatol Surg Oncol 1993; 19:243.

75. Lawrence N, et al: A comparison of the efficacy and safety of Jessner's solution and 35% trichloroacetic acid vs. 5% fluorouracil in the treatment of widespread facial actinic keratosis, Arch Dermatol 1995; 131:176.

76. Alam M, Ratner D: Cutaneous squamous-cell carcinoma, N Engl J Med 2001; 344(13):975.

77. Hartevelt MM, et al: Incidence of skin cancer after renal transplantation in the Netherlands, Transplantation 1990; 49:506.

78. Kwa RE, Campana K, Moy RL: Biology of cutaneous squamous cell carcinoma, J Am Acad Dermatol 1992; 26:1.

79. Rowe DE, et al: Prognostic factors for local recurrence, metastasis, and survival rates in squamous cell carcinoma of the skin, ear, and lip. Implications for treatment modality selection, J Am Acad Dermatol 1992; 26:976.

80. Dinehart SM, Pollack SV: Metastases from squamous cell carcinoma of the skin and lip, J Am Acad Dermatol 1989; 21:241.

81. Breuninger H, et al: Microstaging of squamous cell carcinomas, Am J Clin Pathol 1990;94:624.

82. Friedman HI, Cooper PH, Wanebo HJ: Prognostic and therapeutic use of microstaging of cutaneous squamous cell carcinoma of the trunk and extremities, Cancer 1985; 56:1099.

83. Brodland DG, Zitelli JA: Surgical margins for excision of primary cutaneous squamous cell carcinoma, J Am Acad Dermatol 1992; 27:241.

84. Dinehart SM, et al: Immunosuppression in patients with metastatic squamous cell carcinoma from the skin, J Dermatol Surg Oncol 1990; 16:271.

85. Boyle J, et al: Cancer, warts, and sunshine in renal transplant patients: a case-control study, Lancet 1984; 1:702.

86. Bavinck JN, et al: Relation between skin cancer and HLA antigens in renal-transplant recipients, N Engl J Med 1991; 325:843.

87. Johnson TM, et al: Squamous cell carcinoma of the skin (excluding lip and oral mucosa), J Am Acad Dermatol 1992; 26:467.

88. Brodland DG, Zitelli JA: Mechanisms of metastasis, J Am Acad Dermatol 1992; 27:1.

89. Hosal IN, et al: Squamous cell carcinoma of the lower lip, Am J Otolaryngol 1992; 13:363.

90. McGregor GI, et al: Impact of cervical lymph node metastases from squamous cell cancer of the lip, Am J Surg 1992; 163:469.

91. Task F: Cutaneous, Squamous, Cell, Carcinoma, Guidelines of care for cutaneous squamous cell carcinoma. Committee on Guidelines of Care, J Am Acad Dermatol 1993. 28:628.

92. Sadek H, et al: Treatment of advanced squamous cell carcinoma of the skin with cisplatin, 5-fluorouracil, and bleomycin, Cancer 1990; 66:1692.

93. Weisberg N, Bertagnolli M, Becker D: Combined sentinel lymphadenectomy and Mohs' micrographic surgery for high-risk cutaneous squamous cell carcinoma, J Am Acad Dermatol 2000; 43(3):483.

94. Stankard CE, et al: Chronic pressure ulcer carcinomas, Ann Plast Surg 1993; 30:274.

95. Fleming MD, et al: Marjolin's ulcer: a review and reevaluation of a difficult problem, J Burn Care Rehabil 1990; 11:460.

96. Novick M, et al: Burn scar carcinoma: a review and analysis of 46 cases, J Trauma 1977; 17:808.

97. Phillips T, et al: Burn scar carcinoma. Diagnosis and management, Dermatol Surg 1998; 24(5):561.

98. Lifeso RM, Bull CA: Squamous cell carcinoma of the extremities, Cancer 1985; 55:2862.

99. Kossard S, Rosen R: Cutaneous Bowen's disease. An analysis of 1001 cases according to age, sex, and site, J Am Acad Dermatol 1992; 27:406.

100. Ishida H, et al: Comparative histochemical study of Bowen's disease and actinic keratosis: preserved normal basal cells in Bowen's disease [In Process Citation], Eur J Histochem 2001; 45(2):177.

101. Reed W, et al: Immunohistology is valuable in distinguishing between Paget's disease, Bowen's disease, and superficial spreading malignant melanoma, Histopathology 1990; 16:583.

102. Chuang TY, et al: Bowen's disease (squamous cell carcinoma in situ) as a skin marker for internal malignancy: a case-control study, Am J Prev Med 1990; 6:238.

103. Chute CG, et al: The subsequent risk of internal cancer with Bowen's disease, JAMA 1991; 266:816.

104. Lycka BA: Bowen's disease and internal malignancy. A meta-analysis, Int J Dermatol 1989; 28:531.

105. Rasmussen OO, Christiansen J: Conservative management of Bowen's disease of the anus, Int J Colorectal Dis 1989; 4:164.

106. Beck DE, Fazio VW: Premalignant lesions of the anal margin, South Med J 1989; 82:470.

107. Sturm HM: Bowen's disease and 5-fluorouracil, J Am Acad Dermatol 1979; 1:513.

108. Smith K, Germain M, Skelton H: Squamous cell carcinoma in situ (Bowen's disease) in renal transplant patients treated with 5% imiquimod and 5% 5-fluorouracil therapy, Dermatol Surg 2001; 27(6):561.

109. Wieland U, et al: Erythroplasia of queyrat: coinfection with cutaneous carcinogenic human papillomavirus type 8 and genital papillomaviruses in a carcinoma in situ, J Invest Dermatol 2000; 115(3):396.

110. Goette DK, et al: Erythroplasia of Queyrat: treatment with topically applied 5-fluorouracil, JAMA 1975; 232: 934.

111. van BB, et al: Laser therapy for carcinoma in situ of the penis, J Urol 2001; 166(5):1670.

112. Banoczy J, Gintner Z, Dombi C: Tobacco use and oral leukoplakia, J Dent Educ 2001; 65(4):322.

113. Shiu M, et al: Risk factors for leukoplakia and malignant transformation to oral carcinoma: a leukoplakia cohort in Taiwan, Br J Cancer 2000;82(11):1871.

114. Schepman K, et al: Tobacco usage in relation to the anatomical site of oral leukoplakia, Oral Dis 2001; 7(1):25.

115. Zakrzewska J, et al: Proliferative verrucous leukoplakia: a report of ten cases, Oral Surg Oral Med Oral Pathol Oral Radiol Endod 1996; 82(4):396.

116. Silverman S, Jr., Gorsky M, Lozada F: Oral leukoplakia and malignant transformation: a follow-up study of 257 patients, Cancer 1984; 53:563.

117. Dorey JL, et al: Oral leukoplakia: current concepts in diagnosis, management, and malignant potential, Int J Dermatol 1984; 23:638.

118. Schepman K, et al: Malignant transformation of oral leukoplakia: a follow-up study of a hospital-based population of 166 patients with oral leukoplakia from The Netherlands, Oral Oncol 1998; 34(4):270.

119. Schepman K, et al: Concomitant leukoplakia in patients with oral squamous cell carcinoma, Oral Dis 1999; 5(3):206.

120. Kramer IRH: Oral leukoplakia, J R Soc Med 1980; 73:765.

121. Crissman JD, et al: Premalignant lesions of the upper aerodigestive tract: pathologic classification, J Cell Biochem Suppl 1993; 1:49.

122. Shklar G: Oral leukoplakia, N Engl J Med 1986; 315:1544.

123. Horch HH, Gerlach KL: CO2 laser treatment of oral dysplastic precancerous lesions: a preliminary report, Lasers Surg Med 1982; 2:179.

124. Al-Drouby HAL: Oral leukoplakia and cryotherapy, Br Dent J 1983; 155:124.

125. Sudbo J, et al: DNA content as a prognostic marker in patients with oral leukoplakia, N Engl J Med 2001; 344(17):1270.

126. Martin G, et al: Oral leukoplakia status six weeks after cessation of smokeless tobacco use, J Am Dent Assoc 1999; 130(7):945.

127. Gooris P, et al: Carbon dioxide laser evaporation of leukoplakia of the lower lip: a retrospective evaluation, Oral Oncol 1999; 35(5):490.

128. Schoelch M, et al: Laser management of oral leukoplakias: a follow-up study of 70 patients, Laryngoscope 1999; 109(6):949.

129. Epstein J, Gorsky M: Topical application of vitamin A to oral leukoplakia: a clinical case series, Cancer 1999; 86(6):921.

130. S RA: Verrucous carcinoma of the skin and mucosa, J Am Acad Dermatol 1995; 32:1.

131. Kao GF, Graham JH, Helwig HB: Carcinoma cuniculatum (verrucous carcinoma of the skin): a clinicopathologic study of 46 cases with ultrastructural observations, Cancer 1982; 49:2395.

132. Rubben A., et al: Rearrangements of the upstream regulatory region of human papillomavirus type 6 can be found in both Buschke-Lowenstein tumours and in condylomata acuminata, J Gen Virol 1992; 73:3147.

133. Noel JC, et al: Verrucous carcinoma of the penis: importance of human papillomavirus typing for diagnosis and therapeutic decision, Eur Urol 1992; 22:83.

134. Koch B, et al: National survey of head and neck verrucous carcinoma: patterns of presentation, care, and outcome, Cancer 2001; 92(1):110.

135. Mora RG: Microscopically controlled surgery (Mohs' chemosurgery) for treatment of verrucous squamous cell carcinoma of the foot (epithelioma cuniculatum), J Am Acad Dermatol 1983; 8:354.

136. Reinecke L, Thornley AL: Case report: radiotherapy-an effective treatment for vaginal verrucous carcinoma, Br J Radiol 1993; 66:375.

137. Persky M: Carbon dioxide laser treatment of oral florid papillomatosis, J Dermatol Surg Oncol 1984; 10:64.

138. Ilkay AK, et al: Buschke-Lowenstein tumor: therapeutic options including systemic chemotherapy, Urology 1993; 42:599.

139. Mehta R, Rytina E, Sterling J: Treatment of verrucous carcinoma of vulva with acitretin, Br J Dermatol 2000; 142(6):1195.

140. Geusau A, et al: Regression of deeply infiltrating giant condyloma (Buschke-Lowenstein tumor) following long-term intralesional interferon alfa therapy, Arch Dermatol 2000; 136(6):707.

141. Schwartz RA: Buschke-Lowenstein tumor: verrucous carcinoma of the penis, J Am Acad Dermatol 1990; 23:723.

142. Creasman C, et al: Malignant transformation of anorectal giant condyloma acuminatum (Buschke-Loewenstein tumor), Dis Colon Rectum 1989; 32:481.

143. Cannon CR, Hayne ST: Concurrent verrucous carcinomas of the lip and buccal mucosa, South Med J 1993; 86:691.

144. Rajendran R, et al: Ackerman's tumour (verrucous carcinoma) of the oral cavity: a histopathologic study of 426 cases, Singapore Dent J 1989; 14:48.

145. Smith P, Jr, et al: Verrucous carcinoma: epithelioma cuniculatum plantare, J Foot Surg 1992; 31:324.

146. Fugate DS, Romash MM: Carcinoma cuniculatum (verrucous carcinoma) of the foot, Foot Ankle 1989; 9:257.

147. Cuzick J, et al: Ingested arsenic, keratoses, and bladder cancer, Am J Epidemiol 1992; 136:417.

148. Wong S, Tan K, Goh C: Cutaneous manifestations of chronic arsenicism: review of seventeen cases, J Am Acad Dermatol 1998; 38(2 Pt 1):179.

149. Guha MD, et al: Arsenic levels in drinking water and the prevalence of skin lesions in West Bengal, India, Int J Epidemiol 1998; 27(5):871.

150. Borowitz MJ, et al: Abnormalities of circulating T-cell subpopulations in patients with cutaneous T-cell lymphoma: cutaneous lymphocyte-associated antigen expression on T cells correlates with extent of disease, Leukemia 1993; 7:859.

151. Berg EL, et al:The cutaneous lymphocyte antigen is a skin lymphocyte homing receptor for the vascular lectin endothelial cell-leukocyte adhesion molecule-1, J Exp Med 1991; 174:1461.

152. Smoller B., et al: Reassessment of histologic parameters in the diagnosis of mycosis fungoides, Am J Surg Pathol 1995; 19(12):1423.

153. Fung M, et al: Practical evaluation and management of cutaneous lymphoma, J Am Acad Dermatol 2002; 46(3):325; quiz:358.

154. Kikuchi A., et al: Parapsoriasis en plaques: its potential for progression to malignant lymphoma, J Am Acad Dermatol 1993; 29:419.

155. Kim Y, et al: Clinical stage IA (limited patch and plaque) mycosis fungoides. A long-term outcome analysis, Arch Dermatol 1996; 132(11):1309.

156. Kim Y, Hoppe R: Mycosis fungoides and the Sezary syndrome, Semin Oncol 1999; 26(3):276.

157. Vonderheid EC, et al: Long-term efficacy, curative potential, and carcinogenicity of topical mechlorethamine chemotherapy in cutaneous T cell lymphoma, J Am Acad Dermatol 1989; 20:416.

158. Zackheim HS, et al: Topical carmustine (BCNU) for mycosis fungoides and related disorders: a 10-year experience, J Am Acad Dermatol 1983; 9:363.

159. Zackheim H, Kashani-Sabet M, Amin S: Topical corticosteroids for mycosis fungoides. Experience in 79 patients, Arch Dermatol 1998; 134(8):949.

160. Breneman D, et al: Phase 1 and 2 trial of bexarotene gel for skin-directed treatment of patients with cutaneous T-cell lymphoma, Arch Dermatol 2002; 138(3):325.

161. Rosenbaum MM, et al: Photochemotherapy in cutaneous T cell lymphoma and parapsoriasis en plaques: long-term follow-up in forty-three patients, J Am Acad Dermatol 1985; 13:613.

162. Honigsmann H, et al: Photochemotherapy for cutaneous T cell lymphoma: a follow-up study, J Am Acad Dermatol 1984; 10:238.

163. Herrmann J, et al: Treatment of mycosis fungoides with photochemotherapy (PUVA): long-term follow-up, J Am Acad Dermatol 1995; 33(2 Pt 1):234.

164. Ramsey DL, et al: Ultraviolet-B phototherapy for early-stage cutaneous T-cell lymphoma, Arch Dermatol 1992; 128:931.

165. M EN, et al: Complete remission in psoralen and UV-A (PUVA)-refractory mycosis fungoides-type cutaneous T-cell lymphoma with combined interferon alfa and PUVA, Arch Dermatol 1993; 129:747.

166. Hoppe R: Total skin electron beam therapy in the management of mycosis fungoides, Front Radiat Ther Oncol 1991; 25:80; discussion: 132.

167. Chinn D, et al: Total skin electron beam therapy with or without adjuvant topical nitrogen mustard or nitrogen mustard alone as initial treatment of T2 and T3 mycosis fungoides, Int J Radiat Oncol Biol Phys 1999; 43(5):951.

168. Bunn PA, Jr, et al: Systemic therapy of cutaneous T-cell lymphomas (mycosis fungoides and Sézary syndrome), Ann Intern Med 1994; 121:592.

169. Edelson R, et al: Treatment of cutaneous T-cell lymphoma by extracorporeal photochemotherapy. Preliminary results, N Engl J Med 1987; 316:297.

170. Zic J, et al: Extracorporeal photopheresis for treatment of cutaneous T-cell lymphoma, J Am Acad Dermatol 1992; 27:729.

171. Heald P, et al: Treatment of erythrodermic cutaneous T-cell lymphoma with extracorporeal photochemotherapy, J Am Acad Dermatol 1992; 27:427.

172. Armus S, et al: Photopheresis for the treatment of cutaneous T cell lymphoma, J Am Acad Dermatol 1990; 23:898.

173. Karp DL, Horn TD: Lymphomatoid papulosis, J Am Acad Dermatol 1994; 30:379.

174. Paone JF, Baker RR: Pathogenesis and treatment of Paget's disease of the breast, Cancer 1981; 48:825.

175. Vielh P, et al: Paget's disease of the nipple without clinically and radiologically detectable breast tumor. Histochemical and immunohistochemical study of 44 cases, Pathol Res Pract 1993; 189:150.

176. Ikeda DM, et al: Paget disease of the nipple: radiologic-pathologic correlation, Radiology 1993; 189:89.

177. Samarasinghe D, et al: Cytological diagnosis of Paget's disease of the nipple by scrape smears: a report of five cases, Diagn Cytopathol 1993; 9:291.

178. Hitchcock A: Routine diagnosis of mammary Paget's disease. A modern approach, Am J Surg Pathol 1992; 16:58.

179. Haerslev T, Krag J: Expression of cytokeratin and erbB-2 oncoprotein in Paget's disease of the nipple. An immunohistochemical study, APMIS 1992; 100:1041.

180. Dixon AR, et al: Paget's disease of the nipple, Br J Surg 1991; 78:722.

181. el-Sharkawi A., Waters JS: The place for conservative treatment in the management of Paget's disease of the nipple, Eur J Surg Oncol 1992; 18:301.

182. Merot Y, et al: Extramammary Paget's disease of the perianal and perineal regions, Arch Dermatol 1985; 121:750.

183. Hamm H, Vroom TM, Czarnetzki BM: Extramammary Paget's cells: further evidence of sweat gland derivation, J Am Acad Dermatol 1986; 15:1275.

184. Chanda JJ: Extramammary Paget's disease: prognosis and relationship to internal malignancy, J Am Acad Dermatol 1985; 13:1009.

185. Reedy MB, et al: Paget's disease of the scrotum: a case report and review of current literature, Tex Med 1991; 87:77.

186. Helm KF, et al: Immunohistochemical stains in extramammary Paget's disease, Am J Dermatopathol 1992; 14:402.

187. Coldiron BM, et al: Surgical treatment of extramammary Paget's disease. A report of six cases and a reexamination of Mohs' micrographic surgery compared with conventional surgical excision, Cancer 1991; 67:933.

188. Besa P, et al: Extramammary Paget's disease of the perineal skin: role of radiotherapy, Int J Radiat Oncol Biol Phys 1992; 24:73.

189. Brierley JD, Stockdale AD: Radiotherapy: an effective treatment for extramammary Paget's disease, Clin Oncol 1991; 3:3.

190. Bergen S, et al: Conservative management of extramammary Paget's disease of the vulva, Gynecol Oncol 1989; 33:151.

191. Misas JE, et al: Vulvar Paget disease: fluorescein-aided visualization of margins, Obstet Gynecol 1991; 77:156.

192. Watring WG, et al: Treatment of recurrent Paget's disease of the vulva with topical bleomycin, Cancer 1978; 41:10.

193. Lookingbill DP, et al: Cutaneous metastases in patients with metastatic carcinoma: a retrospective study of 4020 patients, J Am Acad Dermatol 1993; 29:228.

194. Lookingbill DP, et al: Skin involvement as the presenting sign of internal carcinoma. A retrospective study of 7316 cancer patients, J Am Acad Dermatol 1990; 22:19.

195. Brownstein MH, Helwig EB: Metastatic tumors of the skin, Cancer 1972; 29:1298.

196. Brownstein MH, Helwig EB: Patterns of cutaneous metastasis, Arch Dermatol 1972; 105:862.

197. Brownstein MH, Helwig EB: Spread of tumors to the skin, Arch Dermatol 1973; 107:80.

198. Poole S, Fenske NA: Cutaneous markers of internal malignancy. I. Malignant involvement of the skin and the genodermatoses, J Am Acad Dermatol 1993; 28:1.

Nevi and Malignant Melanoma

Melanocytic Nevi

Nevi, or moles, are benign tumors composed of nevus cells that are derived from melanocytes. Many myths surround moles; for example, that hairs should not be plucked from moles or that moles should not be removed or disturbed. These myths should be clarified.

NEVUS CELLS. The nevus cell differs from melanocytes. The nevus cell is larger, lacks dendrites, has more abundant cytoplasm, and contains coarse granules. Nevus cells aggregate in groups (nests) or proliferate in a non-nested pattern in the basal region at the dermoepidermal junction. Nevus cells in the dermis are classified into types A (epithelioid), B (lymphocytoid), and C (neuroid). Through a process of maturation and downward migration, type A epidermal nevus cells develop into type B cells and then into type C dermal nevus cells.

INCIDENCE AND EVOLUTION. Moles are so common that they appear on virtually every person. They are present in 1% of newborns and increase in incidence throughout infancy and childhood. The incidence peaks in the forth to fifth decades. Nevi then diminish in number with advancing age.

Size and pigmentation may increase at puberty and during pregnancy. Nevi may occur anywhere on the cutaneous surface. There is a strong correlation between sun exposure and the number of nevi. Acquired nevi on the buttock or female breast are unusual.

NEVI VS. MELANOMA. Nevi exist in a variety of characteristic forms that must be readily recognized to distinguish them from malignant melanoma. Except for certain types, such as large congenital nevi and atypical moles, most nevi have a very low malignant potential.

Nevi vary in size, shape, surface characteristics, and color. The important fact to remember is that each individual nevus tends to remain uniform in color and shape. Although various shades of brown and black may be present in a single lesion, the colors are distributed over the surface in a uniform pattern.

Melanomas consist of malignant pigment cells that grow and extend with little constraint through the epidermis and into the dermis. Such unrestricted growth produces a lesion with a haphazard or disorganized appearance, which varies in shape, color, and surface characteristics. Nevertheless, the characteristics of uniformity cannot always be relied on to differentiate benign from malignant lesions because very early melanomas may appear quite uniform, having a round or oval shape with a uniform brown color.

EXAMINATION WITH A HAND LENS AND DERMOSCOPE. Careful inspection of suspicious lesions with a powerful hand lens and dermoscope will reveal a number of features that can not be appreciated with the naked eye. Dermoscopy is discussed on page 798.

Common moles

Nevi may be classified as acquired or congenital, but a clinical classification based on appearance and conventional nomenclature is used here.[1] Common acquired nevi appear after 6 months of age. They enlarge and increase in number through the third and fourth decades and then slowly disappear. Most are less than 5 mm in diameter. Fifty-five percent of adults have between 10 and 45 nevi greater than 2 mm in diameter.[2] Nevi tend to be concentrated on sun-exposed sites.

CLASSIFICATION. Common moles are subdivided into three types—junction, compound, and dermal—based on the location of the nevus cells in the skin (see diagram below). The three types represent sequential developmental stages in the life history of a mole. During childhood, nevi begin as flat junction nevi in which the nevus cells are located at the dermoepidermal junction. They evolve into compound nevi when some of the cells migrate into the dermis. Migration of all of the nevus cells into the dermis results in a dermal nevus. Dermal nevi usually form only in adults, but this evolution does not consistently occur.[1] Nevi with cells confined to the dermoepidermal junction area tend to be flat, whereas those with cells confined to the dermis are usually elevated.

JUNCTION NEVI. Junction nevi are flat (macular) or slightly elevated, and they are light brown to brown-black with uniform pigmentation that may be slightly irregular (Figure 22-1). The surface is smooth and flat to slightly elevated, and the border is round or oval and symmetric. Most lesions are hairless. Junction nevi vary in size from 0.1 to 0.6 cm; some are larger. Junction nevi may change into compound nevi after childhood, but they remain as junction nevi on palms, soles, and genitalia. Junction nevi are rare at birth and generally develop after the age of 2 years. Degeneration into melanoma is very rare.

COMPOUND NEVI. Compound nevi are slightly elevated and flesh colored or brown. They are elevated and smooth or warty and become more elevated with increasing age (Figure 22-2). They are uniformly round, oval, and symmetric. Hair may be present. If a white halo appears at the periphery of the lesion, it is referred to as a halo nevus.

DEVELOPMENTAL STAGES IN THE LIFE HISTORY OF COMMON MOLES

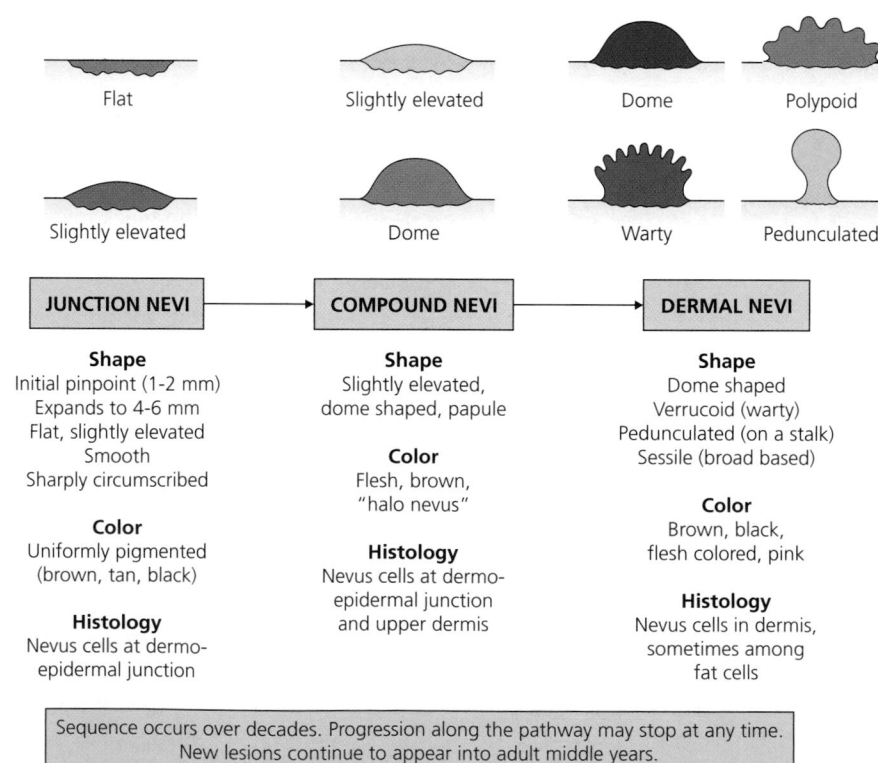

| Flat | Slightly elevated | Dome | Polypoid |
| Slightly elevated | Dome | Warty | Pedunculated |

JUNCTION NEVI → **COMPOUND NEVI** → **DERMAL NEVI**

JUNCTION NEVI	**COMPOUND NEVI**	**DERMAL NEVI**
Shape Initial pinpoint (1-2 mm) Expands to 4-6 mm Flat, slightly elevated Smooth Sharply circumscribed	**Shape** Slightly elevated, dome shaped, papule	**Shape** Dome shaped Verrucoid (warty) Pedunculated (on a stalk) Sessile (broad based)
Color Uniformly pigmented (brown, tan, black)	**Color** Flesh, brown, "halo nevus"	**Color** Brown, black, flesh colored, pink
Histology Nevus cells at dermo- epidermal junction	**Histology** Nevus cells at dermo- epidermal junction and upper dermis	**Histology** Nevus cells in dermis, sometimes among fat cells

Sequence occurs over decades. Progression along the pathway may stop at any time.
New lesions continue to appear into adult middle years.

MELANOCYTIC NEVI

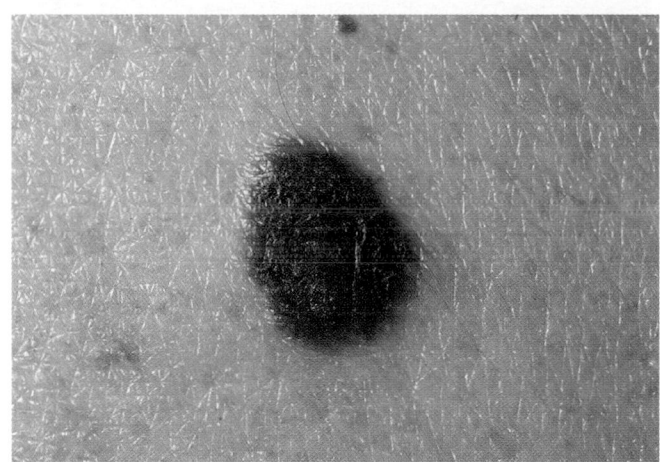

Figure 22-1 Junction nevus. The lesion is slightly raised, dark, and uniform.

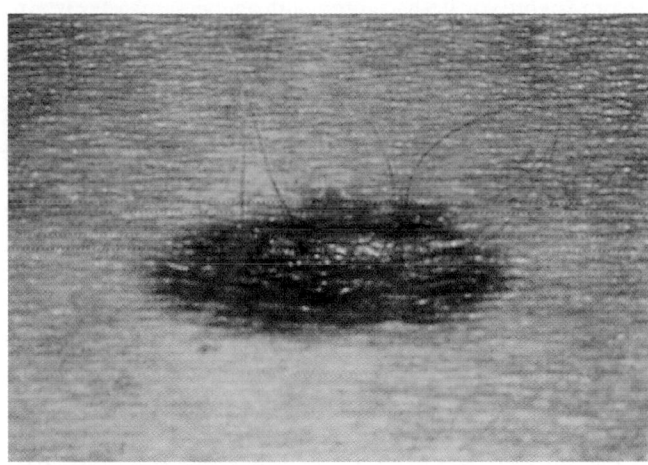

Figure 22-2 Compound nevus. The surface is covered with uniform brown-black dots.

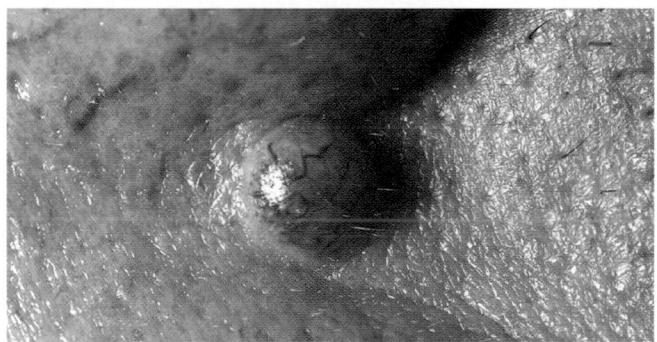

Figure 22-3 Dermal nevus. Flesh colored with surface vessels; resembles basal cell carcinoma.

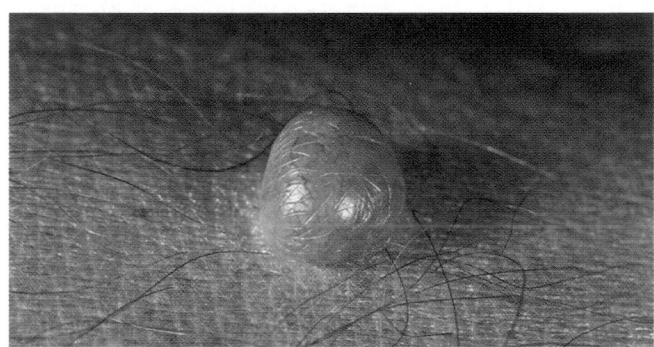

Figure 22-4 Dermal nevus. Dome shaped.

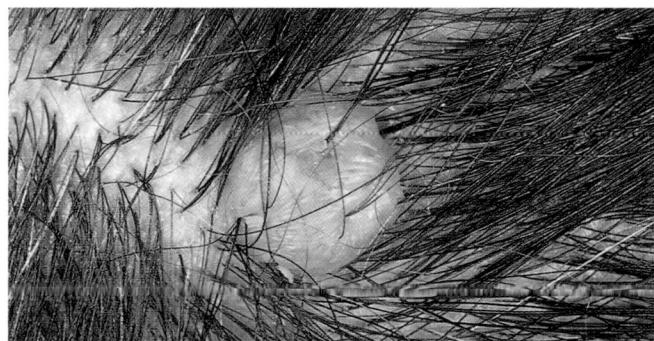

Figure 22-5 Dermal nevus. Flesh colored and dome shaped.

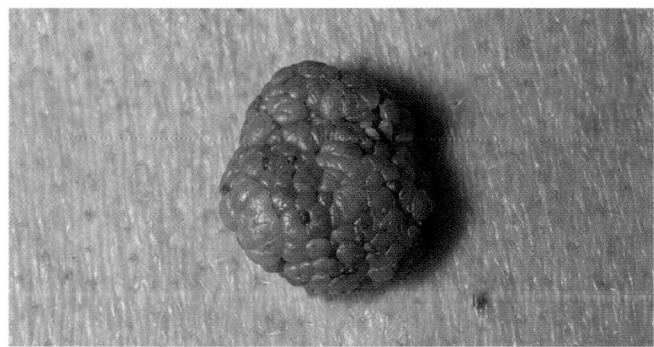

Figure 22-6 Dermal nevus. Warty (verrucous) surface.

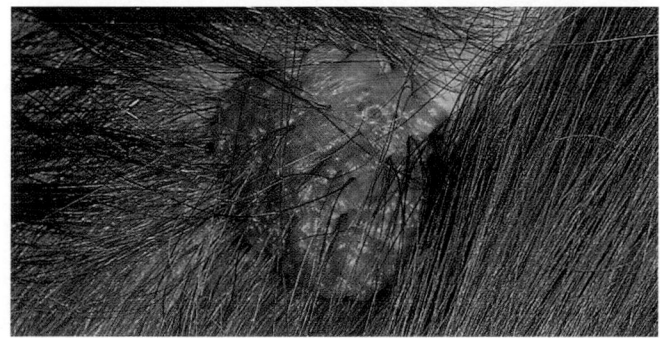

Figure 22-7 Dermal nevus. Polypoid.

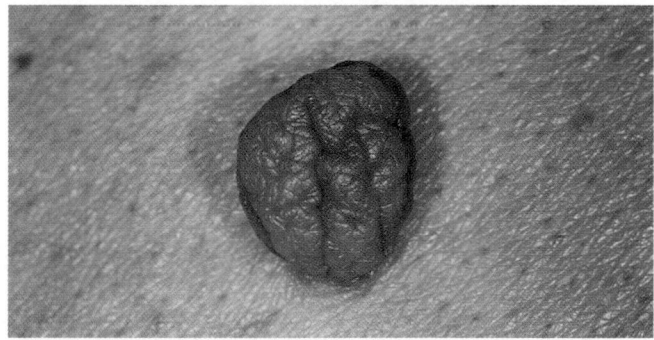

Figure 22-8 Dermal nevus. Pedunculated with a soft, flabby, wrinkled surface.

DERMAL NEVI. Dermal nevi are brown or black, but may become lighter or flesh-colored with age. Lesions vary in size from a few millimeters to a centimeter. The variety of shapes reflects the evolutionary process in which moles extend downward with age and nevus cells degenerate and become replaced by fat and fibrous tissue.

Dome-shaped lesions are the most common (Figures 22-3 through 22-5). They generally appear on the face and are symmetric, with a smooth surface. They may be white or translucent, with telangiectatic vessels on the surface mimicking basal cell carcinoma. The structure may be warty (Figure 22-6) or polypoid (Figure 22-7). Pedunculated lesions with a narrow stalk are located on the trunk, neck, axilla, and groin. They may appear as a soft, flabby, wrinkled sack (Figure 22-8).

Elevated nevi are exposed and are prone to trauma from clothing and other stimuli, often causing them to bleed and inflame, influencing some patients to suspect malignancy. White borders may appear, creating a halo nevus. Degeneration to melanoma is very rare, but dermal nevi may resemble nodular melanoma; therefore knowledge of duration is important.

Management
SUSPICIOUS LESIONS. Any pigmented lesion suspected of being malignant should be biopsied or referred for a second opinion. Suspicious lesions should be completely removed by excisional biopsy down to and including subcutaneous tissue.

NEVI. Patients frequently request removal of nevi for cosmetic purposes. It is good practice to biopsy all pigmented lesions; therefore total removal by electrocautery should be avoided. Nevi are removed either by shave excision or by simple excision and closure with sutures. Most common nevi are small and consequently, shave excision is adequate.

RECURRENT PREVIOUSLY EXCISED NEVI (PSEUDO-MELANOMA). Weeks to months after incomplete removal of a nevus, brown macular pigmentation may appear in the scar (Figure 22-9). Some nevus cells remain with shave excision and partial repigmentation is possible. Residual pigmentation may be removed with electrocautery or cryosurgery. An unusual histologic picture resembling melanoma (pseudomelanoma) may follow partial removal of nevi.[3-5] If the repigmented area is excised, the pathologist should always be notified that the submitted tissue was acquired from a previously treated area. Histologically, the melanocytes appear atypical but are confined to the epidermis, and there is no lateral spread of individual melanocytes.

NEVI WITH SMALL DARK SPOTS. A small percentage of small dark dots within melanocytic nevi are due to melanoma. These roundish areas of brown or black hyperpigmentation measure 3 mm or less in diameter and are located peripherally.[6] Biopsy specimens of nevi with small dark dots should be sectioned to ensure histologic examination of this focus of hyperpigmentation.

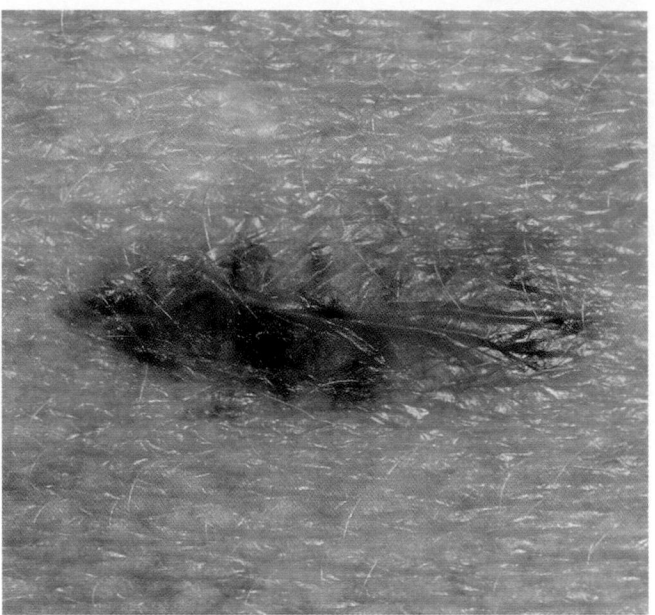

Figure 22-9 Recurrent, previously excised nevi (pseudomelanoma). Brown, macular pigmentation may appear in the scar of an incompletely removed nevus.

Special forms
Special forms of pigmented lesions include congenital nevus, halo nevus, speckled lentiginous nevus, Becker's nevus, benign juvenile melanoma (Spitz nevus), blue nevus, and labial melanotic macules.

CONGENITAL NEVI. Congenital nevi (birthmarks) are present at birth and vary in size from a few millimeters to several centimeters, covering wide areas of the trunk, extremity, or the face. Some lesions first become apparent during infancy. Not all pigmented lesions present at birth are congenital nevi; café-au-lait spots may also be present at birth. The largest lesions are referred to as giant hairy nevi. Giant congenital nevi on the trunk are referred to as bathing trunk nevi. Congenital nevi may contain hair; if present, it is usually coarse. Such nevi are uniformly pigmented, with various shades of brown or black predominating, but red or pink may be a minor or sometimes predominant color. Most are flat at birth but become thicker during childhood, and the surface becomes verrucous and sometimes nodular.

Size. Congenital nevi are arbitrarily divided into groups according to their size in infancy: small (<1.5 cm in diameter), medium (1.5 to 20 cm in diameter), and large (>20 cm in diameter).

Histologic characteristics. Nevus cells occur: (1) in the lower two thirds of the dermis, occasionally extending into the subcutis; (2) between collagen bundles distributed as single cells or cells in single file or both; and (3) in the lower two thirds of the reticular dermis or subcutis associated with appendages, nerves, and vessels. Some congenital nevi do not have these microscopic features. Large congenital nevi usually do have the classic microscopic findings of congenital nevi, whereas small congenital nevi most often do not show these classic features. Medium-sized congenital nevi may or may not show these classic microscopic features.

Malignant potential. The malignant potential of congenital nevi may be dependent on the histologic pattern of the lesion rather than the clinical size. Small congenital nevi frequently lack melanocytes in the deeper dermis. The increased risk of melanoma formation in large congenital nevi may be a result of transformation of cells residing deep in the dermis.[7]

SMALL CONGENITAL NEVI. The incidence of malignant degeneration in small congenital nevi (<1.5 cm in diameter) is extremely low and prophylactic removal is not essential (Figure 22-10). Almost all melanomas arising in small congenital nevi are of the epidermal variety. Therefore clinical observation will detect malignant changes in small congenital nevi. If small congenital nevi are to be excised, delaying this procedure until just before puberty would be appropriate because small congenital nevi do not unergo malignant transformation in prepubertal age groups.

MEDIUM-SIZED CONGENITAL NEVI. The risk of the occurrence of malignant melanoma in medium-sized (1.5 to 19.9 cm in diameter) congenital melanocytic nevi is the subject of controversy (Figures 22-11 and 22-12). Universally accepted recommendations regarding the management of such lesions have not been made. A short-term follow-up study showed no increased risk for malignant melanoma arising in banal-appearing medium-sized lesions or that prophylactic excision of all such lesions is mandatory. Lifelong medical observation seems a reasonable alternative for many medium-sized congenital melanocytic nevi.[8]

Another approach would be to perform a punch or small incisional biopsy. If the histologic pattern is that of an acquired nevus (superficial variant of congenital nevi), then the malignant potential is extremely low, and any malignant transformation would most likely be of the epidermal variety, which would be detectable by clinical observation. If the histologic pattern is that of the deeper dermal tumor, then a significant risk may be present; prophylactic excision at the earliest stage possible would be indicated.[9]

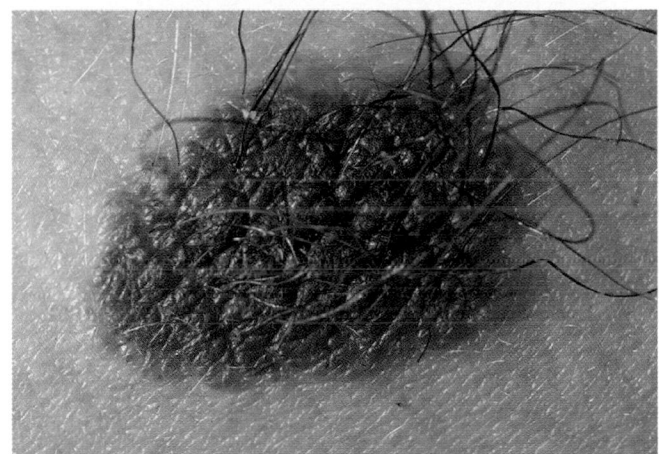

Figure 22-10 A small congenital nevus has a uniform cobblestone surface and is covered with hair.

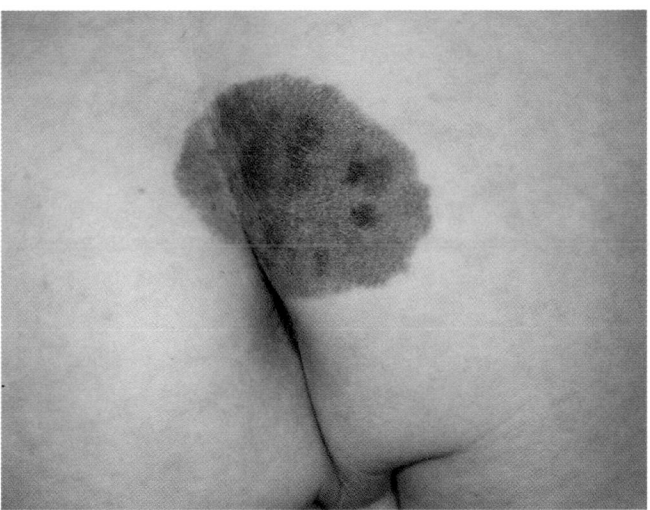

Figure 22-11 Medium-sized congenital nevus. Pigmentation is variable and nonuniform, but a biopsy showed all such areas were benign.

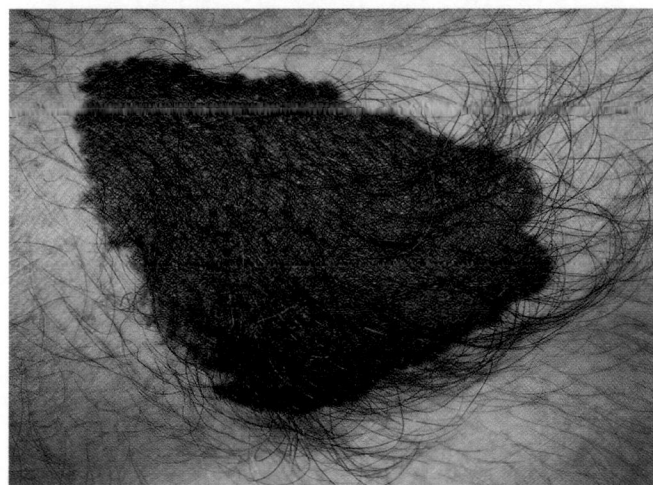

Figure 22-12 Medium-sized congenital nevus. The border is irregular and appears notched, but that characteristic is maintained in a uniform manner around the entire border.

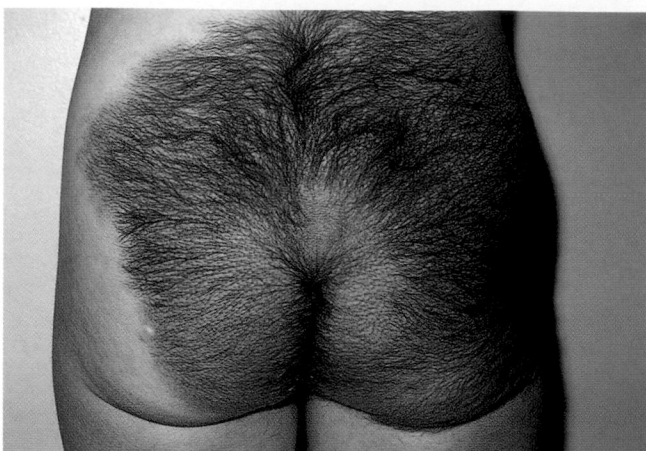

Figure 22-13 Large congenital hairy nevus.

LARGE CONGENITAL NEVI. Large congenital melanocytic nevi (comprising 5% body surface area or greater in preadolescents and more than 20 cm in adolescents and adults) may undergo malignant transformation (Figures 22-13 and 22-14).[10] The incidence ranges from 1.8% to 7.1%. Approximately half of the melanomas occur by 3 to 5 years of age. Therefore large, thick lesions should be removed as soon as possible. Large congenital nevi lighten with time and most nodules occur before the age of 2 years. There is an initial darkening with a subsequent significant lightening with age accompanied by increased surface irregularities, nodules, and hair growth. The most common anatomic site is the trunk. Most are associated with satellite congenital nevi, which can be extensive and involve a variety of sites. As many as two thirds of melanomas developing in giant congenital melanocytic nevi have nonepidermal origins. Therefore clinical observation will fail to detect most malignant transformations in these patients. Currettage offers an adequate alternative to surgical excision when performed during the first 2 weeks of life.[10a]

SPECKLED LENTIGINOUS NEVUS. Speckled lentiginous nevus (nevus spilus) is a common hairless, oval or irregularly shaped brown lesion that is dotted with darker brown-to-black spots. They may appear at any age. Lesions can appear at birth or in early infancy as lightly colored café-au-lait macules. Pigmented macules and papules then develop over a period of months to years. Lesions may be very large. It has been suggested that speckled lentiginous nevus is a subtype of congenital melanocytic nevus.[11] The brown area is usually flat, and the black dots may be slightly elevated and contain typical nevus cells (Figure 22-15). The spots range from 1 to 3 mm in diameter and may be lentigines, junctional, compound, or intradermal nevi. The background hyperpigmentation histologically has the features of a lentigo or café-au-lait macule. There is considerable variation in size, ranging from 1 to 20 cm. The anatomic position or time of onset is not related to sun exposure. Transformation into melanoma is rare. The risk of transformation may be similar to classic congenital nevi of similar size. Examine lesions periodically and educate the patient regarding the clinical signs of melanoma. Routine excision is not necessary. Biopsy suspicious areas. Speckled lentiginous nevus is flat and necessitates excision and closure if the patient desires removal.

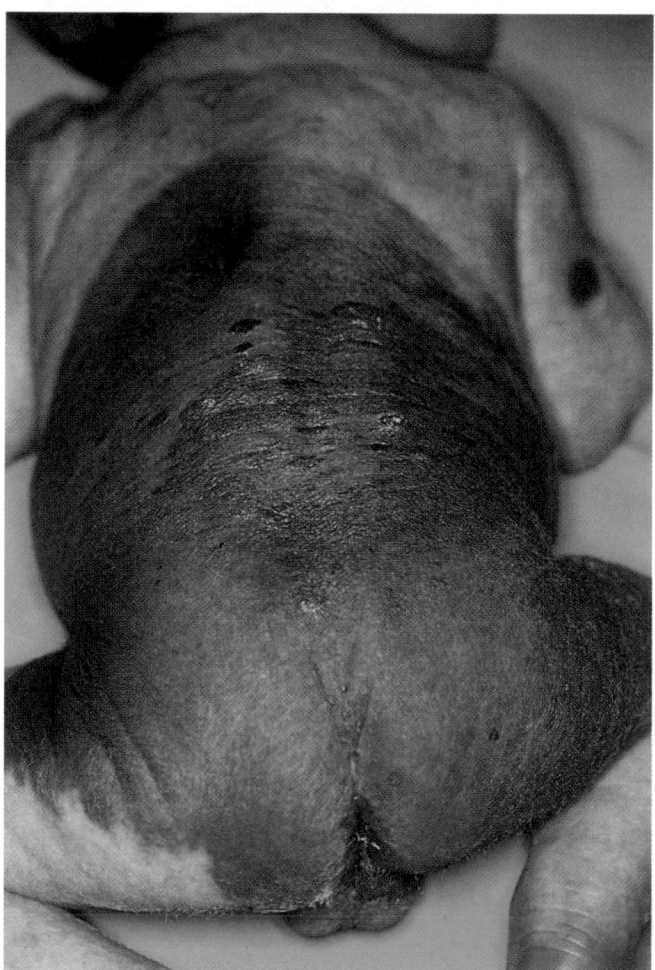

Figure 22-14 Giant congenital nevus (bathing trunk nevus).

SPECKLED LENTIGINOUS NEVUS

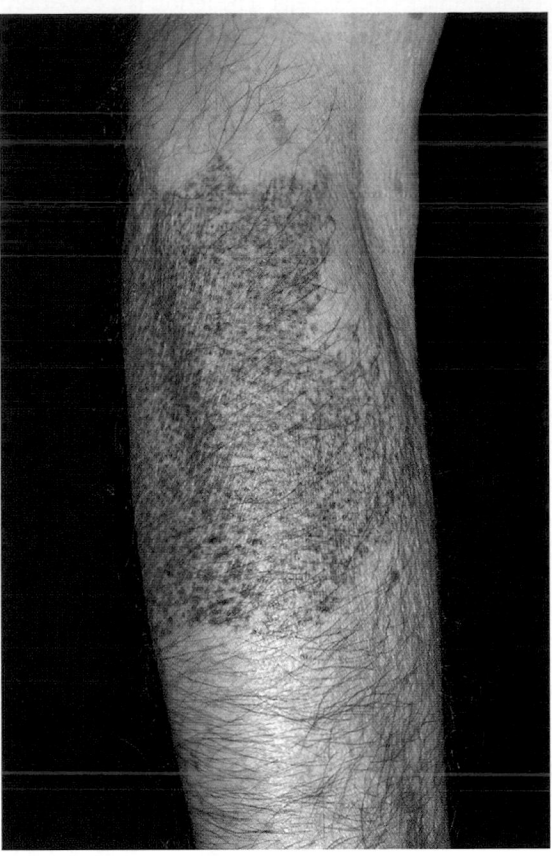

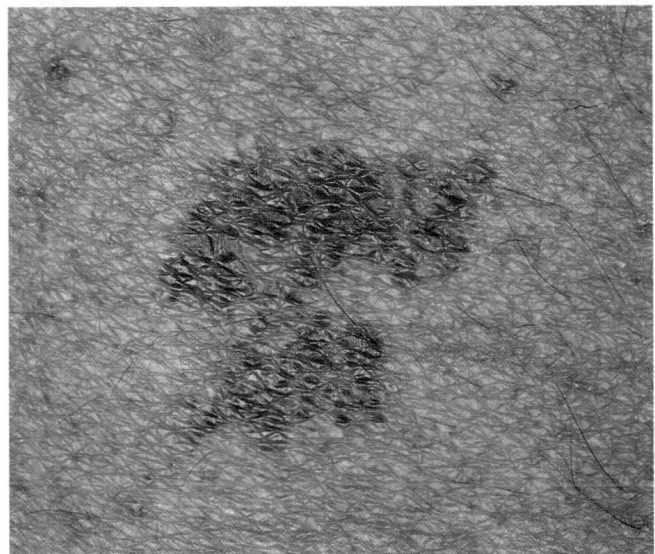

A, A large, brown, macular lesion resembling a café-au-lait spot. Tiny black papules are uniformly distributed over the surface.

B, The macular pigmentation is less prominent than in the lesion illustrated in *A*.

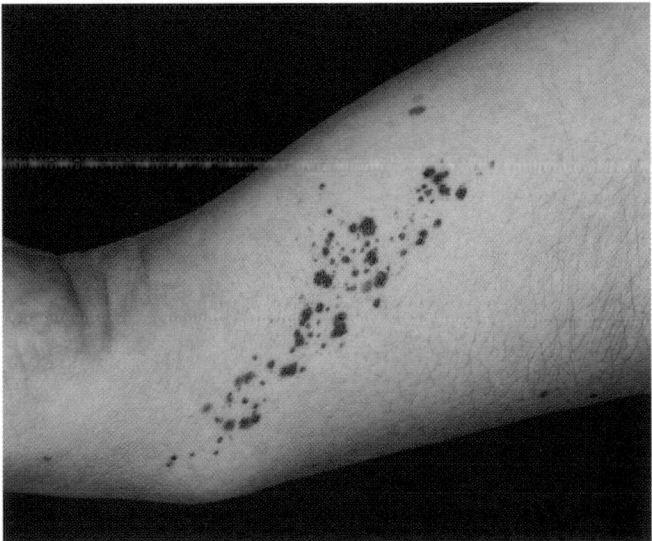

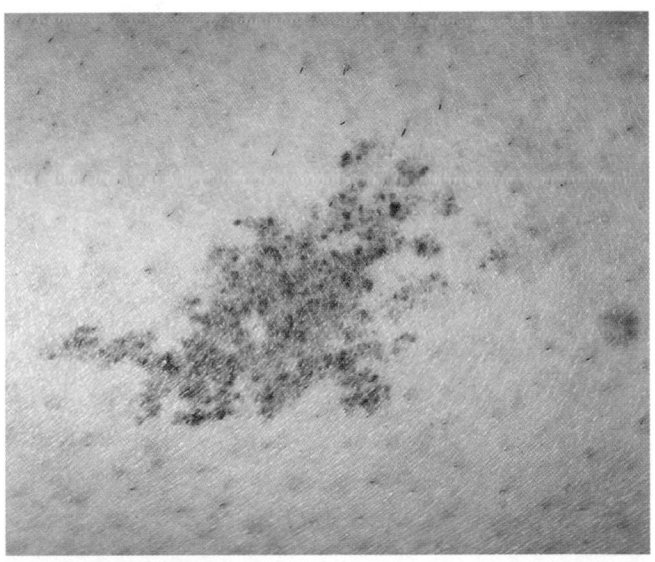

C, The macular pigmentation is almost entirely absent. The multiple papules containing nevus cells predominate.

D, Macular pigmentation is variable.

Figure 22-15

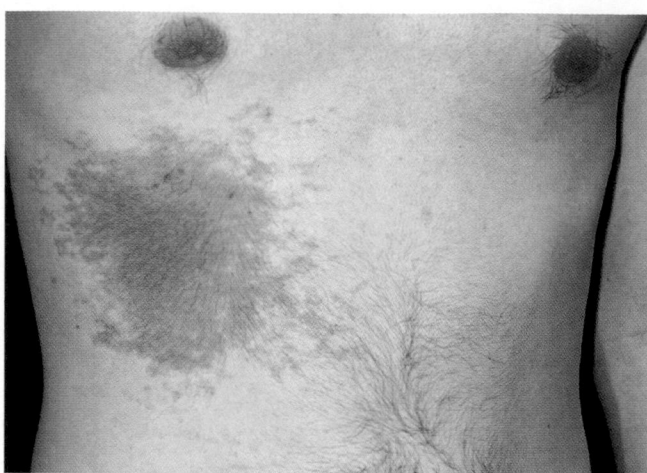

Figure 22-16 Becker's nevus. This irregular lesion contains no hair. It has been stable in size for years.

BECKER'S NEVUS. Becker's nevus is not a nevocellular nevus because it lacks nevus cells. The lesion is a developmental anomaly consisting of either a brown macule (Figure 22-16), a patch of hair (Figure 22-17), or both (Figure 22-18). Nonhairy lesions may later develop hair. The lesions appear in adolescent men on the shoulder, submammary area, and upper and lower back.[12] Becker's nevus varies in size and may enlarge to cover the entire upper arm or shoulder. The border is irregular and sharply demarcated. Malignancy has never been reported.

Becker's nevus syndrome is the presence of an epithelial nevus showing hyperpigmentation, increased hairiness and hamartomatous augmentation of smooth muscle fibers, and other developmental defects such as ipsilateral hypoplasia of the breast and skeletal anomalies including scoliosis, spina bifida occulta, or ipsilateral hypoplasia of a limb.[13] The Becker's nevus syndrome usually occurs sporadically.

Becker's nevus is usually too large to remove by excision. The hair may be shaved or permanently removed. Laser removal of hair and pigmentation is reported.

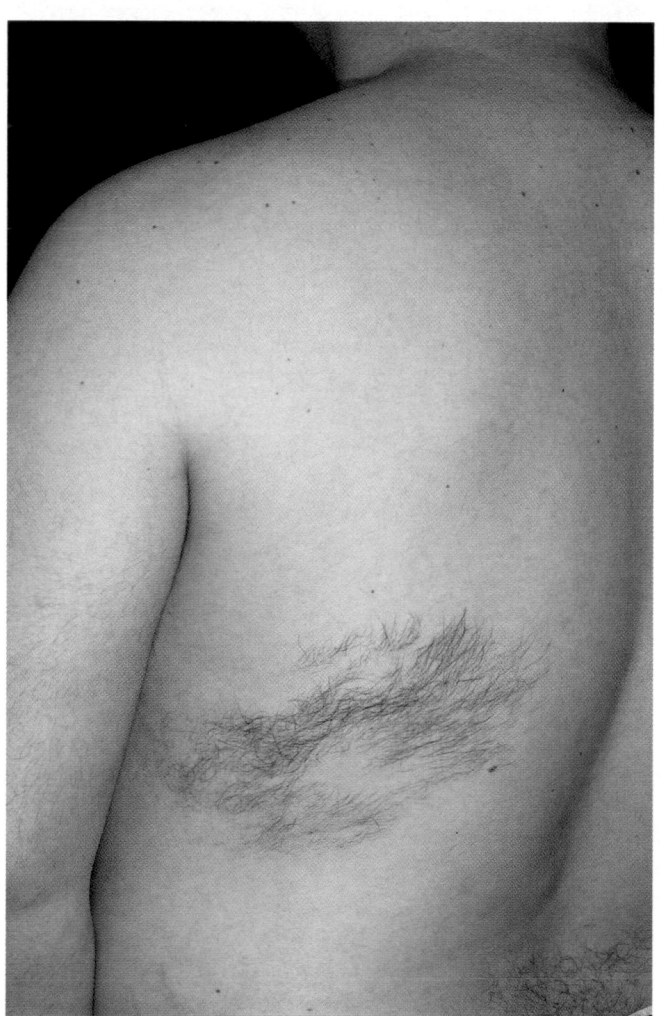

Figure 22-17 Becker's nevus. This lesion contains no pigmentation.

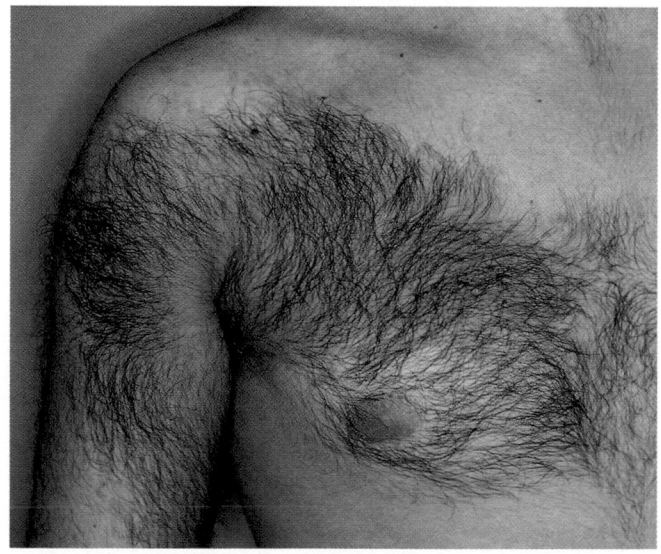

Figure 22-18 Becker's nevus. A typical lesion with macular pigmentation and hair.

HALO NEVI. A compound or dermal nevus that develops a white border is called a halo nevus. The incidence in the population is estimated to be 1%. Halo nevi are found most commonly in children. The average age of onset is 15 years. The depigmented halo is symmetric and round or oval with a sharply demarcated border (Figure 22-19). There are no melanocytes in the halo area.

HISTOLOGIC CHARACTERISTICS. T lymphocytes at the site of depigmentation suggest that these cells participate in the halo phenomenon.[14] Most halo nevi are located on the trunk; they never occur on palms and soles. They may occur as an isolated phenomenon, or several nevi may spontaneously develop halos. Halos may repigment with time, or the nevus may disappear. Repigmentation often takes place over months or years; however, it does not always occur. Repigmentation does not follow removal of the nevus. The incidence of vitiligo may be increased in patients with halo nevi. A halo may rarely develop around malignant melanoma, but in such instances it is usually not symmetric.

Removal of a halo nevus is unnecessary unless the nevus has atypical features. Parental concern over this impressive change is often reason for a conservative excision. In such cases, the mole part of a halo nevus may be removed by shave or excision.

SPITZ NEVUS. Spitz nevus, or benign juvenile melanoma, is most common in children but does appear in adults. The term *melanoma* is used because the clinical and histologic appearance is similar to melanoma. They are hairless, red or reddish-brown, dome-shaped papules or nodules with a smooth (Figure 22-20) or warty surface; they vary in size from 0.3 to 1.5 cm.[15] The color is caused by increased vascularity, and bleeding sometimes follows trauma. Spitz nevi are usually solitary but may be multiple. They appear suddenly and, contrary to slowly evolving common moles, patients can sometimes date their onset. The Spitz nevus should be removed for microscopic examination. Histologic differentiation from melanoma is sometimes difficult.

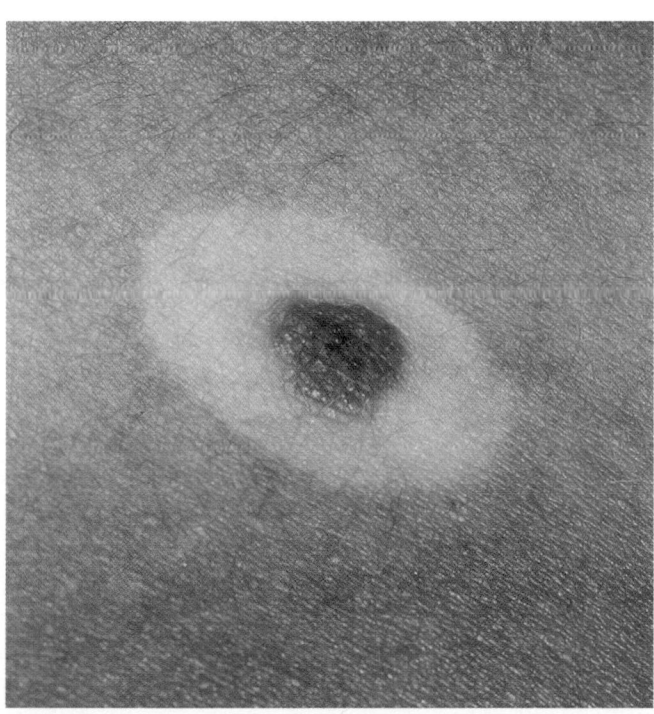

Figure 22-19 Halo nevus. A sharply defined, white halo surrounds this compound nevus.

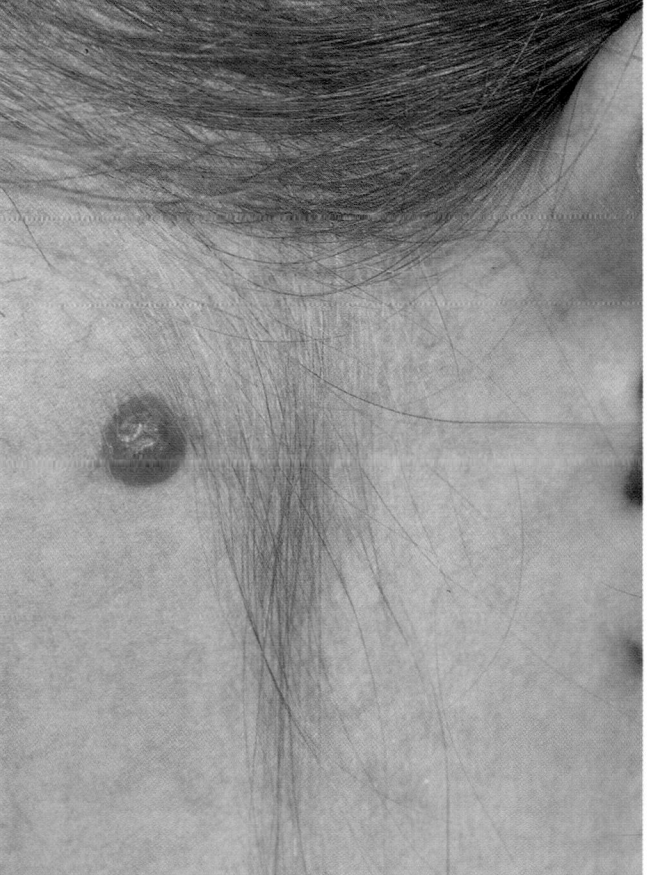

Figure 22-20 Benign juvenile melanoma (Spitz nevus). A reddish, dome-shaped nodule that generally appears in children.

BLUE NEVUS. The blue nevus is a slightly elevated, round, regular nevus, usually less than 0.5 cm, and contains large amounts of pigment located in the dermis (Figure 22-21). The brown pigment absorbs the longer wavelengths of light and scatters blue light (Tyndall effect). The blue nevus appears in childhood and is most common on the extremities and dorsum of the hands. A rare variant, the cellular blue nevus, is larger (usually greater than 1 cm) and nodular and is frequently located on the buttock.

Melanomas are reported arising in association with a common or cellular blue nevus and arising de novo and resembling cellular blue nevi.[16] Blue nevi may be removed for cosmetic purposes.

LABIAL MELANOTIC MACULE. Brown macules on the lower lip are relatively common, especially in young adult women (Figure 22-22). Histologically, they resemble freckles and not lentigo, but unlike freckles, they do not darken with sun exposure. They are benign.[17] Cryotherapy or laser surgery is used for patients who request treatment.

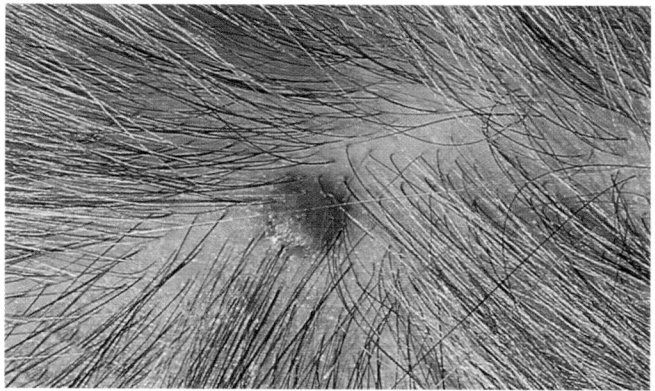

Figure 22-21 Blue nevus. Most lesions are small and round.

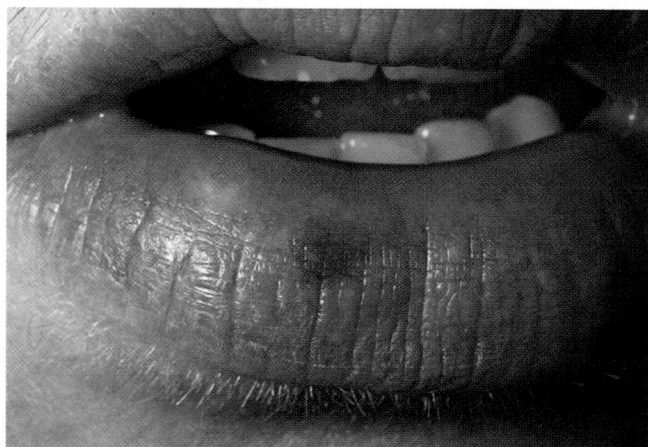

Figure 22-22 Labial melanotic macule. These common lesions worry the patient who suspects melanoma. They are benign.

Atypical nevi

Atypical nevi, also referred to as dysplastic nevi, may be inherited in a familial pattern or occur sporadically. They are usually larger than 5 mm in diameter and are either flat or flat with a raised center ("fried egg") (Table 22-1). They are darkly or irregularly pigmented with shades of brown and pink and usually have irregular or indistinct borders.[18] Dysplastic nevi are common, with a prevalence rate of about 5%. Dysplastic nevi differ from common acquired nevi by (1) beginning to appear near puberty instead of in childhood; (2) continuing to develop past the fourth decade. Atypical nevi are a "marker" for patients at an increased risk for development of melanoma and a precursor lesion to melanoma. No data are available to assess what effect prophylactic removal has on decreasing the risk for future development of melanoma.

FAMILIAL MELANOMA AND MELANOMA PRECURSORS. Cutaneous melanoma may occur as isolated, so-called sporadic cases; in association with multiple atypical nevi; or in familial clusters, in which case it is referred to as the atypical mole syndrome (AMS), formerly known as dysplastic nevus syndrome. In the late 1970s, the dysplastic nevus (DN) or atypical mole (AM) was identified in melanoma-prone families. It was then determined that AMs are cutaneous markers that identify specific family members who are at increased risk for melanoma. The AM may also be the single most important precursor lesion of melanoma. These nevi may occur in persons from melanoma-prone families and in persons who lack both a family history and a personal history of melanoma.[19]

ATYPICAL MOLE SYNDROME AND FAMILIAL MELANOMA. Numerous families with multiple melanoma patients have been reported. These patients usually develop melanoma at a young age, have a predisposition to multiple primary melanomas, and have the tendency to develop thin, superficial-spreading melanomas. Large, unusual-looking moles were initially recognized as a precursor to melanoma in patients with familial cutaneous melanoma. This syndrome was named B-K mole syndrome from two of the probands, and the precursor nevi were designated as B-K moles and later referred to as dysplastic nevi.[20] The syndrome is now called the atypical-mole syndrome. Recent estimates suggest that approximately 32,000 persons in the United States have familial atypical mole syndrome with familial melanoma, accounting for approximately 5.5% of all melanomas diagnosed in this country.[21] Hereditary malignant melanoma and atypical moles represent pleiotropic effects of a Mendelian autosomal dominant gene with high penetrance.[22]

One study showed that the hereditary cutaneous malignant melanoma/atypical mole syndrome does not predispose to other cancers.[23]

DEFINITION. The National Institutes of Health (NIH) Consensus Conference on Diagnosis and Treatment of Early Melanoma has defined the familial atypical mole and melanoma syndrome as (1) the occurrence of malignant melanoma in one or more first- or second-degree relatives; (2) a large number of melanocytic nevi (MN), often more than 50, some of which are atypical and often variable in size; and (3) melanocytic nevi that demonstrate certain histologic features. AMS probably represents a spectrum. At one end all members of a kindred have AMs and some have malignant melanoma (MM). At the other end are persons with one AM without a personal or family history of MM.

ASSOCIATION WITH MELANOMA. Patients with AMS, familial or sporadic, are at significant risk for developing melanoma.[24,25] Atypical moles have been observed in 8% of patients with nonfamilial (sporadic) melanoma, and the transformation into superficial-spreading melanoma has been photographically documented. Family members without atypical moles do not show any apparent increase in melanoma risk. The frequency of sporadic AMs in the general population is unknown.

Atypical moles are found on the skin of 90% of patients with hereditary melanomas, and more than 50% of melanomas in this group are associated histologically with and probably evolve from atypical moles.[26-29] The lifetime risk of developing cutaneous melanoma among the white population in the United States is approximately 0.8%, or one in 125. Persons who have AMs and no family members with the disease have a 6% risk of developing melanoma.[30] Persons who have AMs and a history of melanoma have a 10% risk of getting a second melanoma; persons who have AMs and have a family member with melanoma have a 15% risk. The lifetime risk of melanoma approaches 100% for those people with AMs from families with two or more first-degree relatives who have cutaneous melanoma.[31,32]

Among atypical mole–bearing family members, those patients with melanoma have very large numbers of nevi more frequently than patients with AMs without melanoma. Family members with AMs have more nevi than do patients who have only common acquired nevi.

Table 22-1 Differences Between Atypical Moles and Common Nevi

Characteristics	Atypical moles	Common nevi
Distribution	Back most common, upper and lower limbs, sun-protected areas, female breasts, scalp, buttock, groin	Usually sun-exposed areas; most above the waist
Number	Less than 10 to greater than 100	10 to 40
Age at onset	Appear as normal nevi at age 2 to 6; increase in number and size at puberty; new nevi appear throughout life	Absent at birth; appear at age 2 to 6; grow vertically in uniform manner throughout life; several may appear at puberty
Size	Usually greater than 5 mm and commonly greater than 10 mm	Usually less than 6 mm
Shape and contour	Irregular border; flat (macular) areas; margin fades into surrounding skin, always has a macular component	Round, symmetric, uniformly macular or papular smooth border
Color	Variable within a single lesion; brown, black, red, pink	Uniform tan, brown, black; darken during pregnancy or at adolescence; become lighter with age
Histologic characteristics	Persistent lentiginous melanocytic hyperplasia Melanocytic nuclear atypia* Lamellar fibroplasias Concentric eosinophilic fibroplasias Sparse, patchy lymphocytic infiltration	Nevus cells at the dermoepidermal junction and/or in the dermis

Modified from Greene MH, et al: N Engl J Med 1985; 312:91.
*May not be essential to make diagnosis.

Clinical features of atypical moles

MORPHOLOGY. These unusual nevi differ in a number of important ways from typical acquired pigmented nevi or moles[33] (Table 22-1). Atypical moles are larger than common moles. They have a mixture of colors, including tan, brown, pink, and black. The border is irregular and indistinct and often fades into the surrounding skin. The surface is complex and variable, with both macular and papular components. A characteristic presentation is a pigmented papule surrounded by a macular collar of pigmentation ("fried-egg lesion") (Figures 22-23 and 22-24). In one study, the total number of nevi and macular components were the only useful features to predict histologic melanocytic dysplasia. However, "fried-egg lesions" often do not display histologic melanocytic dysplasia. In contrast, the absence of a macular component in melanocytic nevi in a person with fewer than 13 total body nevi accurately predicts the absence of melanocytic dysplasia on histologic examination.[34]

SURFACE CHARACTERISTICS. The surface characteristics of atypical nevi are distinctive and can be appreciated with a hand lens and dermascope (see page 799).

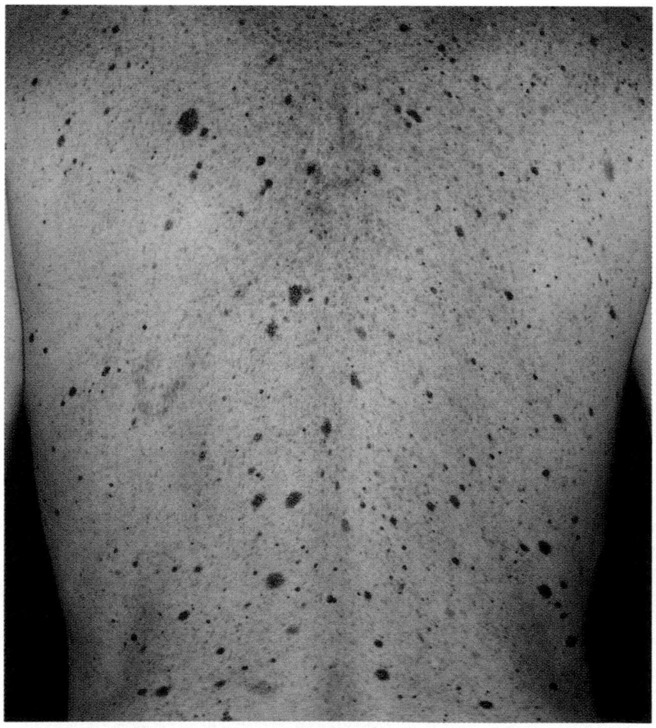

DEVELOPMENT AND DISTRIBUTION. Atypical moles are not present at birth, but begin to appear in the mid-childhood years as typical common moles. The appearance changes at puberty, and newer lesions continue to appear well after the age of 40.[35] Common moles occur most often on sun-exposed areas. AMs occur in those locations and at unusual sites such as the scalp, buttocks, and breast. The predilection sites for melanoma in familial AMS patients of both sexes correspond with the distribution of nevi; in males nevi and melanoma counts are higher on the back; in females both the back and the lower extremities are affected. These findings strongly suggest an association between nevus distribution and melanoma occurrence and site in familial AMS.[36]

HISTOLOGIC CHARACTERISTICS. The NIH Consensus Conference listed the histologic criteria as follows: architectural disorder with asymmetry, subepidermal (concentric eosinophilic and/or lamellar) fibroplasia, and lentiginous melanocytic hyperplasia with spindle or epithelioid melanocytes aggregating in nests of variable size and forming bridges between adjacent rete ridges. Melanocytic atypia may be present to a variable degree. In addition, there may be dermal infiltration with lymphocytes, as well as the "shoulder" phenomenon (intraepidermal melanocytes extending singly or in nests beyond the main dermal component).[37]

MANAGEMENT. Recommendations for treatment of patients with AMs have been given in the National Institutes of Health Consensus Development Conference statement, October 24 to 26, 1983.[33] These, along with other recommendations, are given in Box 22-1.

Figure 22-23 Atypical nevi. There are numerous large nevi present. Superficial spreading melanomas have been removed from the upper back and the midline on the left side (note scars). Nevi are larger than 1 cm and irregularly pigmented.

Box 22-1 Recommendations for the Management of AMS

- Examine total cutaneous surface every 3 to 12 mo, beginning around puberty
- Use hair-blower for scalp examination
- Consider total cutaneous photographs as baseline
- Excise lesions suspected to be melanoma
- Educate patient on self-examination of skin
- Recommend sun avoidance and/or protection
- Suggest screening of blood relatives for AM and MM
- Suggest regular ophthalmologic examinations for ocular nevi and ocular melanoma

ATYPICAL MOLES

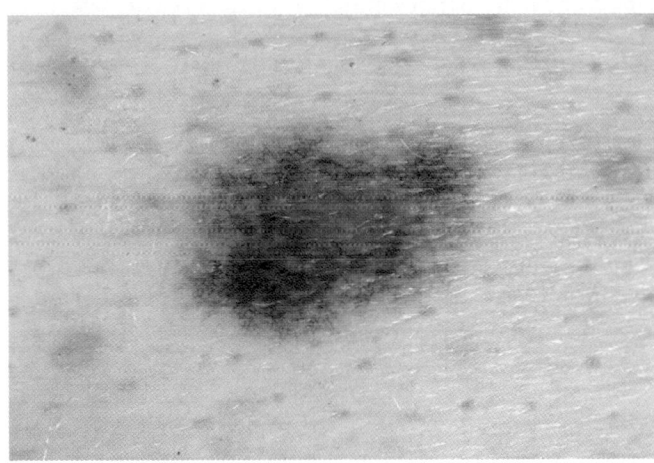

A, Macular, variable pigmentation, ill-defined borders.

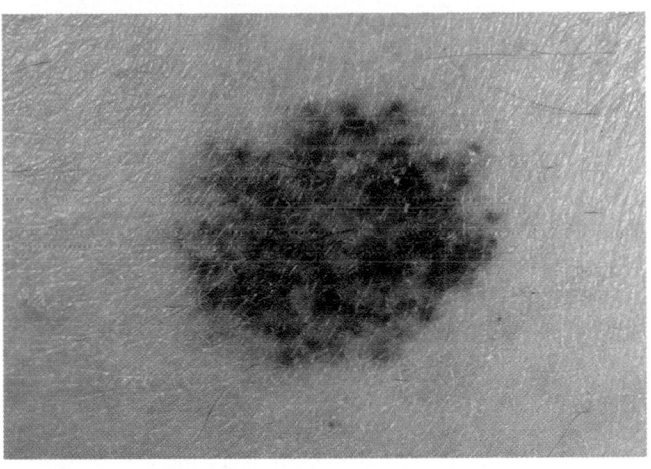

B, Macular, complex pigmentation, notched border.

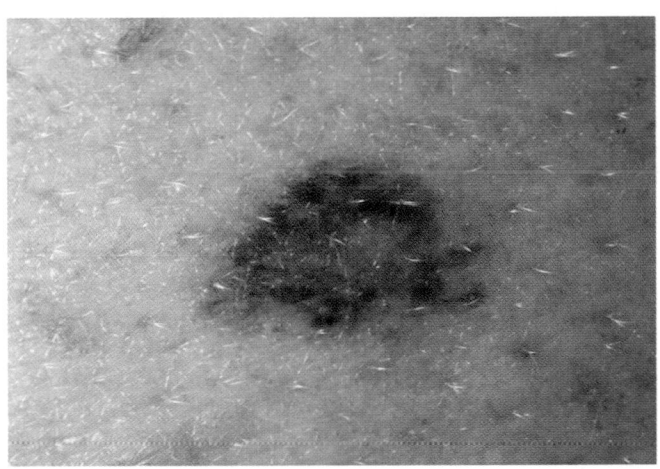

C, Macular, variable pigmentation, fades at border.

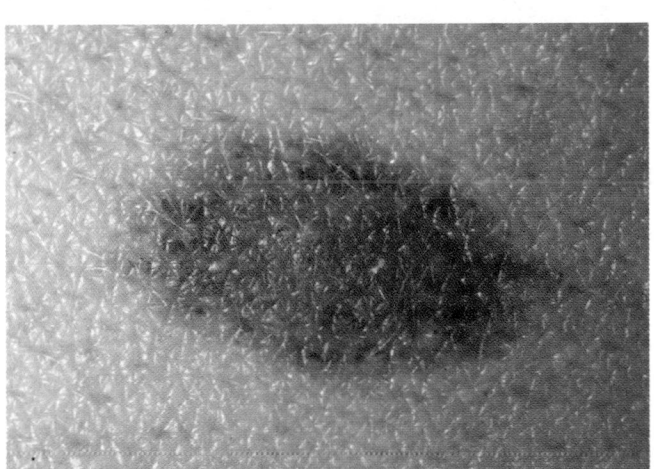

D, Papular, large lesion.

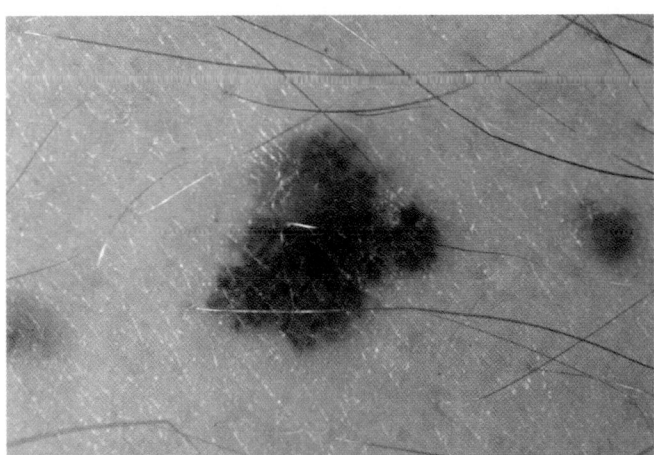

E, Macular, papular, variable pigmentation, irregular border.

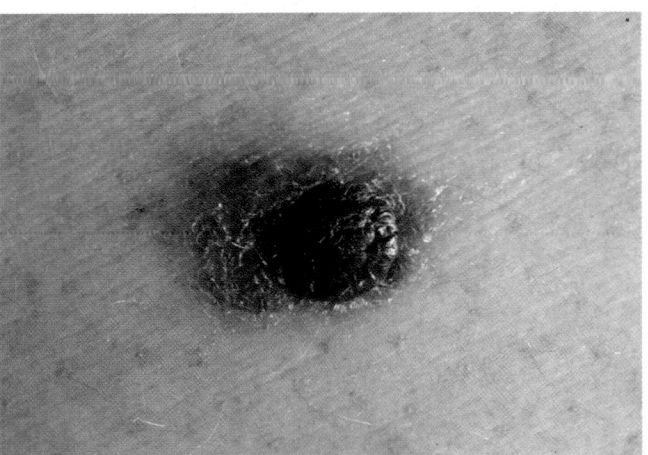

F, "Fried egg pattern," raised with dark center, macular periphery, pigmentation fades at border.

Figure 22-24

Malignant Melanoma

Malignant melanoma is a malignancy of melanocytes that occurs in the skin, eyes, ears, gastrointestinal tract, leptomeninges, and oral and genital mucous membranes. One of the most dangerous tumors, melanoma has the ability to metastasize to any organ, including the brain and heart.

RISK FOR MELANOMA. The risk factors for melanoma are listed in Table 22-2. The incidence of melanoma has tripled in Caucasians during the last 40 years. Their lifetime risk of cutaneous melanoma in 1987 was 1 in 123. The lifetime risk is estimated to increase to one in 50 by 2010. The highest incidence is in Australia and New Zealand. Melanoma is responsible for 75% of skin cancer deaths in the United States. Melanoma develops one twentieth as frequently in African

Americans as in whites, and the incidence in Hispanic persons is one sixth that in whites. The median age of melanoma diagnosis is 53 years. It is the most common cancer in women aged 25 to 29 years.

ULTRAVIOLET RADIATION EXPOSURE. Increased exposure to ultraviolet (UV) radiation is considered to be a factor for the increased incidence of melanoma. Sunburns are a risk factor for melanoma.[39] Sunburns are primarily due to UVB (280 to 320 nm) radiation. Melanomas are also increased in people exposed to ultraviolet A (UVA) radiation. High doses of UVA radiation are received in sun beds and with exposure to psoralen and UVA (PUVA) therapy.

PUVA and risk of melanoma. Oral methoxsalen (psoralen) and ultraviolet A radiation (PUVA) is effective therapy for psoriasis and other skin conditions. It is carcinogenic. An increased risk of melanoma is observed beginning 15 years after first exposure to oral methoxsalen (psoralen) and ultraviolet A radiation (PUVA). This risk is greater in patients exposed to high doses of PUVA, appears to be increasing with the passage of time, and should be considered in determining the risks and benefits of this therapy.[40]

RISK AND SUN EXPOSURE. Increased recreational sun exposure and alterations of the upper atmosphere by pollutants resulting in increased radiation may be the two most important factors in the disproportionate rise in the incidence of melanoma. People who suntan poorly or sunburn easily or who have had multiple or severe sunburns have a twofold to threefold increased risk for developing cutaneous melanoma. Individuals with recreational and vacation sun exposure who experience acute episodic exposures to sunlight may be at greater risk than those with constant occupational sun exposure. Continuous UV radiation exposure, either in adult life or during adolescence, seems to play a protective role in melanoma risk. Those with outdoor occupations have been found to have a lower risk of acquiring melanoma. Intermittent exposure is associated with significant risk increases of melanoma.[41] It is postulated that sunlight causes cutaneous immunosuppression.

SUNSCREEN EFFECTIVENESS. Chemical sunscreens block UVB but are less effective at blocking UVA, which makes up 90% to 95% of ultraviolet energy in the solar spectrum. Sunscreens prevent erythema and sunburn, but inhibit accommodation of the skin to sunlight; therefore their use may permit excessive exposure of the skin to UVA. Laboratory data suggest that melanoma is promoted by UVA; therefore UVB sunscreens might not be effective in preventing melanoma. Sunscreen use may give people a false sense of security and encourage excessive exposure. Hats, protective clothing, and avoiding sunbathing are more protective than chemical sunscreens. For white, freckled children, the use of a broad-spectrum sunscreen with a high sun protection factor attenuates the development of nevi and, by deduction, decreases the risk of developing a melanoma.[42] Sunscreens

Table 22-2 Risk Factors for Developing Cutaneous Melanoma	
Risk status	**Relative risk***
Greatly increased risk	
Personal history of atypical moles, family history melanoma, and greater than 75-100 moles	35
Previous nonmelanoma skin cancer	17
Congenital nevus (giant, >20 cm)	15-5
History of melanoma	9-10
Family history of melanoma in parent, sibling, or children	8
Immunosuppression	8-6
Moderately increased risk	
Clinically atypical nevi (2-9)	7.3-4.9 No family history of melanoma/ sporadic atypical nevi
Large number of nevi	
(51-100)	5.0-3.0
(26-50)	4.4-1.8
Chronic tanning with UVA (PUVA treatments [>250] for psoriasis)	5.4
Modestly increased risk	
Repeated blistering sunburns	
(3)	3.8
(2)	1.7
Freckling	3.0
Fair skin, inability to tan	2.6
Red or blond hair	2.2
Clinically atypical nevus (1)	2.3

Adapted from Robinson JK: Dermatol Nurs 2000; 12:397.

*The relative risk is the degree of increased risk for persons with the risk factor(s) as compared with persons without the risk factor. If the relative risk is 1, there is no increased risk.

that contain zinc oxide or titanium dioxide reflect light and are referred to as physical rather than chemical sunscreens. These compounds effectively block UVA light.

ABCDs OF MALIGNANT MELANOMA RECOGNITION. The goal is to recognize melanomas at the earliest stage. Compared to common acquired melanocytic nevi, malignant melanomas tend to have Asymmetry, Border irregularity, Color variation, and Diameter enlargement. Changes in shape and color are important early signs and should always arouse suspicion. Ulceration and bleeding are late signs; hope of cure diminishes greatly if the diagnosis has not been made before such changes occur. The specific signs that appear during the evolution of each type of melanoma are listed and illustrated on the following pages. A list of all possible changes at all stages of development is given in Table 22-3.

CHARACTERISTICS OF BENIGN MOLES. Moles evolve and change during life. All of the changes occur over long periods of time and are nearly imperceptible. Circumferential enlargement occurs in common nevi of children. Benign ac-

quired nevi progress from lentigo simplex, to flat pigmented junctional nevi, to elevated pigmented compound nevi, to more elevated skin-colored intradermal nevi over decades. Intradermal nevi continue to elevate as collagen is laid down over nests of nevus cells in the upper dermis. Therefore the distance between the dermoepidermal junction and the top of the underlying intradermal nevus increases with age.[43]

Benign moles have a more uniform tan, brown, or black color. The border is regular and the lesion is roughly symmetric; if the lesion could be folded in half, the two halves would superimpose. Most acquired benign moles are 6 mm or less in diameter and appear early in life.

RECENT CHANGE IN A MOLE. The patient's description of a change in a mole may be the earliest sign of melanoma. Changing color, developing erythematous or hyperpigmented halos, increase in diameter, height, or asymmetry of borders or changing surface characteristics, pruritus, pain, bleeding, ulceration, or tenderness all suggest evolution into melanoma.

Table 22-3 Signs Suggesting Malignancy in Pigmented Lesions

Sign	Implication
Change in color	
Sudden darkening; brown, black	Increased number of tumor cells, the density of which varies within the lesion, creating irregular pigmentation
Spread of color into previously normal skin	Tumor cells migrating through epidermis at various speeds and in different directions (horizontal growth phase)
Red	Vasodilation and inflammation
White	Areas of regression or inflammation
Blue	Pigment deep in dermis, sign of increasing depth of tumor
Change in characteristics of border	
Irregular outline	Malignant cells migrating horizontally at different rates
Satellite pigmentation	Cells migrating beyond confines of primary tumor
Development of depigmented halo	Destruction of melanocytes by possible immunologic reaction and inflammation
Changes in surface characteristics	
Scaliness	
Erosion	
Oozing	
Crusting	
Bleeding	
Ulceration	
Elevation	
Loss of normal skin lines	
Development of symptoms	
Pruritus	
Tenderness	
Pain	

PRECURSOR LESIONS

Acquired melanocytic nevi. People with an increased number of benign melanocytic nevi have an increased risk for the development of melanoma. The number at which point the risk becomes significant varies from person to person, depending on factors such as family history and sun exposure. Because 80% of all patients have up to 50 benign nevi, a practical "cut-off" number of nevi over which patients might be at an increased risk for the development of melanoma would be 50. The relative risk for these patients has ranged from 3 to 15 when compared with the relative risk for patients with either no nevi or fewer than five nevi.[2]

Atypical nevi. Atypical nevi may be observed in persons with or without melanoma and may be inherited in a familial pattern or occur sporadically. They are usually larger than 5 mm in diameter and are either flat or flat with a raised center ("fried egg"). They are darkly or irregularly pigmented with shades of brown and pink and usually have irregular or indistinct borders. Patients with atypical nevi outside of the familial melanoma setting have an increased risk for the development of melanoma but the rate is much lower. One clinically atypical nevus was associated with a twofold risk for the development of melanoma, whereas 10 or more atypical nevi conferred a 12-fold increased risk over patients without atypical nevi.[44,45]

Congenital nevi. The malignant potential of congenital nevi is dependent on size and histologic pattern. See page 776.

Four major clinical-histopathologic subtypes

Melanoma either begins de novo or develops from a preexisting lesion, such as a congenital or atypical mole. A classification into several different types was devised after observing that the microscopic anatomy of the tumor at the periphery of the elevated tumor mass was variable and possessed characteristic patterns that could be correlated with distinctive clinical presentations. The proposed types are superficial spreading melanoma (SSM), lentigo maligna melanoma (LMM), nodular melanoma (NM), and acral-lentiginous melanoma (ALM).

Many, but not all,[46] pathologists recognize these various clinicopathologic types of melanoma. Some melanomas do not conform to this clinicopathologic classification and may be labeled exclusively malignant melanoma. Malignant melanoma may be a single entity that has various clinical and histologic forms varying with the degree of differentiation of the tumor cell. The potential for a melanocyte to degenerate and become neoplastic is probably influenced by a number of factors, including degree of skin pigmentation, heredity, immunologic status, quantity of solar radiation, gender of the individual, and anatomic position on the body.

GROWTH CHARACTERISTICS. Once a melanocyte becomes neoplastic, constraints on its localization are removed, and it may leave its assigned position at the basal layer of the epidermis. A well-differentiated malignant melanocyte retains its affinity for the epidermis and may grow slowly horizontally, only to be restrained or eliminated in some areas by a still-competent immunologic system. Years of slow growth and regression by a number of such cells on the face produces the LMM.

A more immature group of cells would be more aggressive and extend and regress at a faster rate, stimulating new vessel formation and inflammation. Such biologic behavior could be expected to produce the SSM. Melanomas in which the cells are extending laterally are considered to be in the horizontal (radial) growth phase. This phase may endure for months or years.

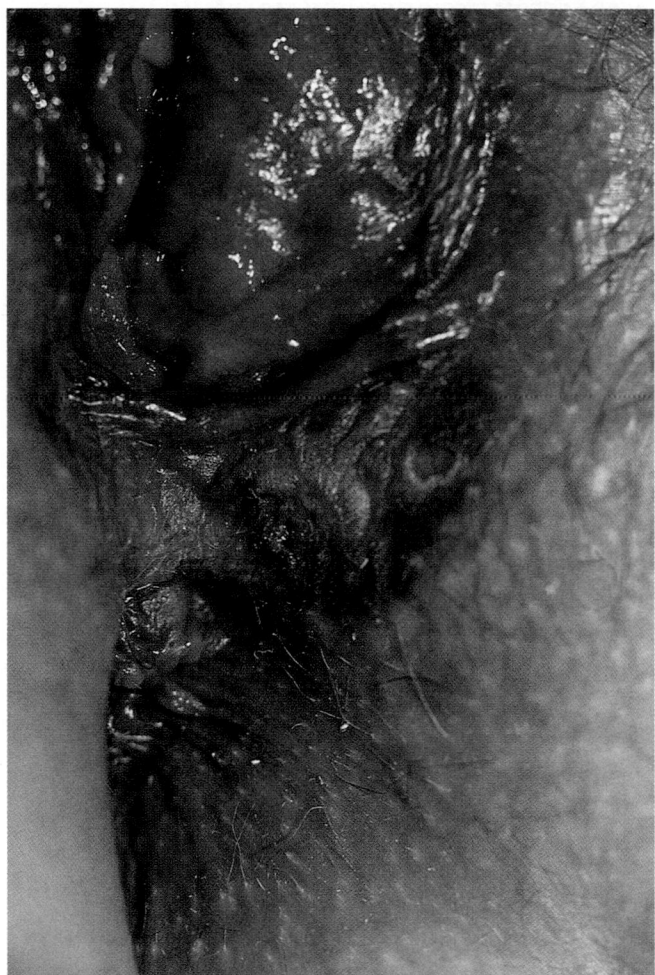

Figure 22-25 Superficial spreading melanoma. Modesty prevented the patient from asking the physician about this lesion on the vulva, which had been present for 2 years. Fortunately, it was discovered during a complete examination of the skin.

A poorly differentiated cell knows no bounds, has no affinity for the epidermis, and grows both horizontally and vertically, producing a mass or NM. Melanomas in which cells have begun to grow vertically into the dermis and form a mass are considered to be in the vertical growth phase. The validity of the type classification has yet to be settled; however, it does enable one to understand the growth and evolution of malignant melanoma; and therefore is an aid to making an early diagnosis. The various types of melanomas have specific characteristics.

Superficial spreading melanoma

SSM (Box 22-2) is most common in middle age, from the fourth to fifth decade. It develops anywhere on the body (Figure 22-25), but most frequently on the upper back of both sexes and on the legs of women (Figure 22-26). SSM begins in a nonspecific manner and then changes shape by radial spread and regression (Figure 22-27). The random migration of cells, along with the process of regression, results in lesions with an endless variety of shapes and sizes. The shape is bizarre if left untreated for years. The hallmark of SSM is the haphazard combination of many colors, but it may be uniformly brown or black. Colors may become more diverse as time proceeds. A dull red color is frequently observed, which may occupy a small area or may dominate the lesion. The precursor radial growth phase may last for months or for more than 10 years. Nodules appear when the lesion is approximately 2.5 cm in diameter.

Box 22-2 Superficial Spreading Melanoma
70% of melanomas
Diameter >6 mm
Trunk in men and women and the legs in women
Irregular asymmetric borders
Begins as flat or elevated brown lesion
Evolves into black, blue, red, white colors

Figure 22-26 Distribution of superficial spreading melanoma of the skin in men and women. (*From* Causes and effects of changes in stratospheric ozone: *Washington, DC, National Academy Press. Courtesy New York University Melanoma Cooperative Group and the National Academy Press.*)

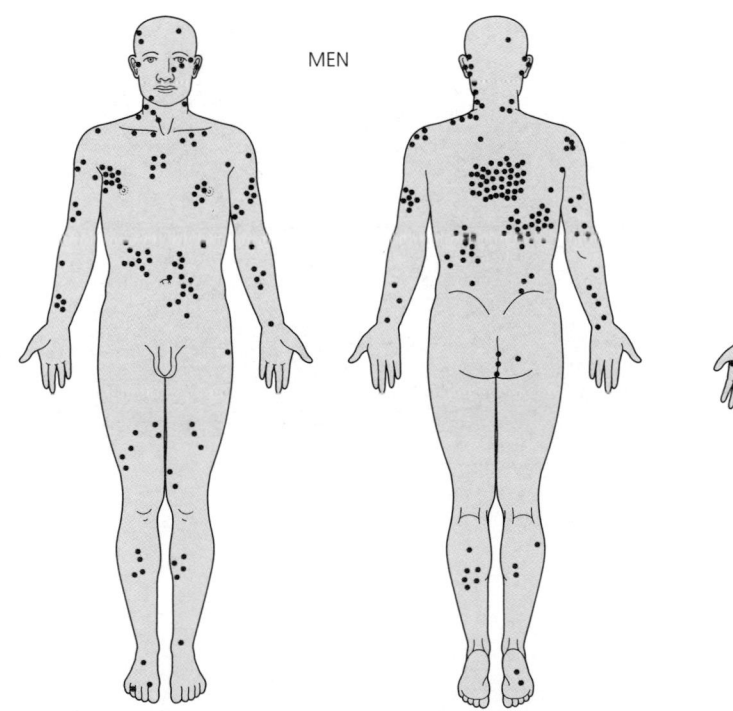
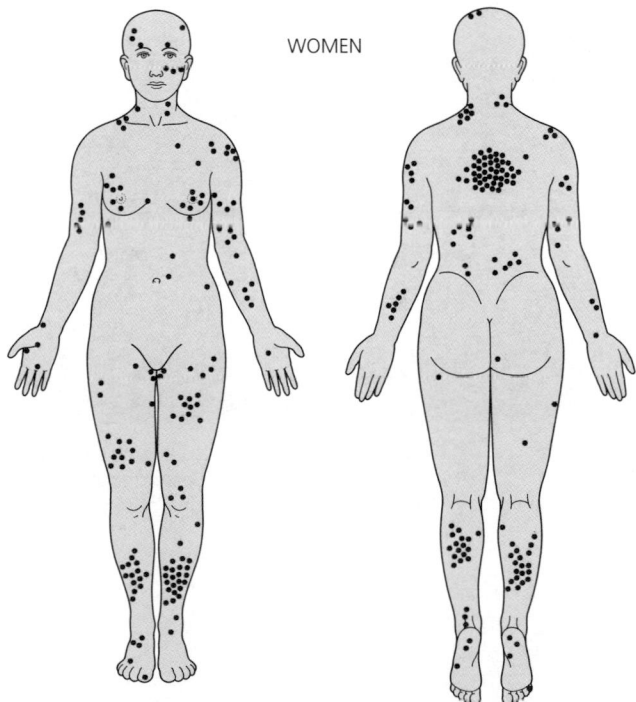

MEN

WOMEN

SUPERFICIAL SPREADING MELANOMA

Initial phase (months to years)
1. Flat, not palpable
2. Color variation slight
3. Indistinguishable from other early melanomas

Brown, brown-black
Slight focal blue
Faint red and white

0 to 0.6 cm

Radial growth phase (months to 10 years)
1. Border irregular
2. Areas of regression appear with angular notching
3. Thick areas appear at about 2.5 cm—herald onset of vertical phase

Colors become
more pronounced

Angular notching

0.6 to 2.5 cm

Vertical growth phase (months to years)
1. Numerous patterns, depending on degree of growth and regression
2. Tumors palpable
   Plaquelike elevation at border
   Nodules in center
3. Areas of ulceration and scaling

Highly regressed
area

or

Striking contrast
in colors

Blue-gray
Blue-black
Red and white

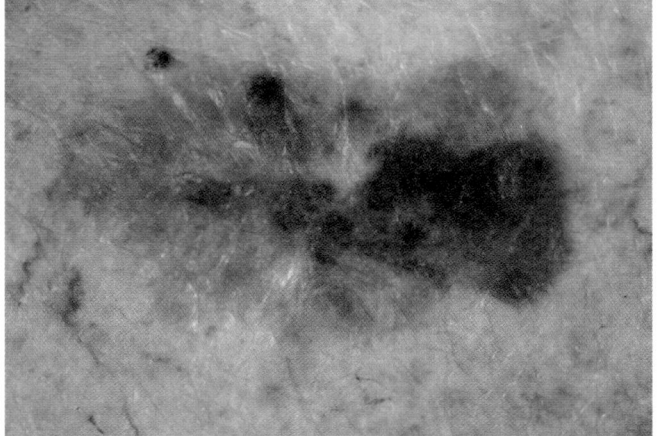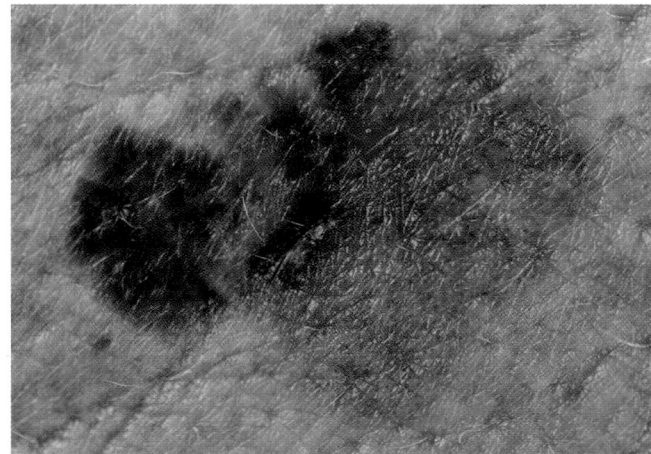

Figure 22-27 Superficial spreading melanomas in all stages of development. The small early lesions have irregular borders, irregular pigmentation, and small white areas indicating regression. The largest tumors show an accentuation of all of these features.

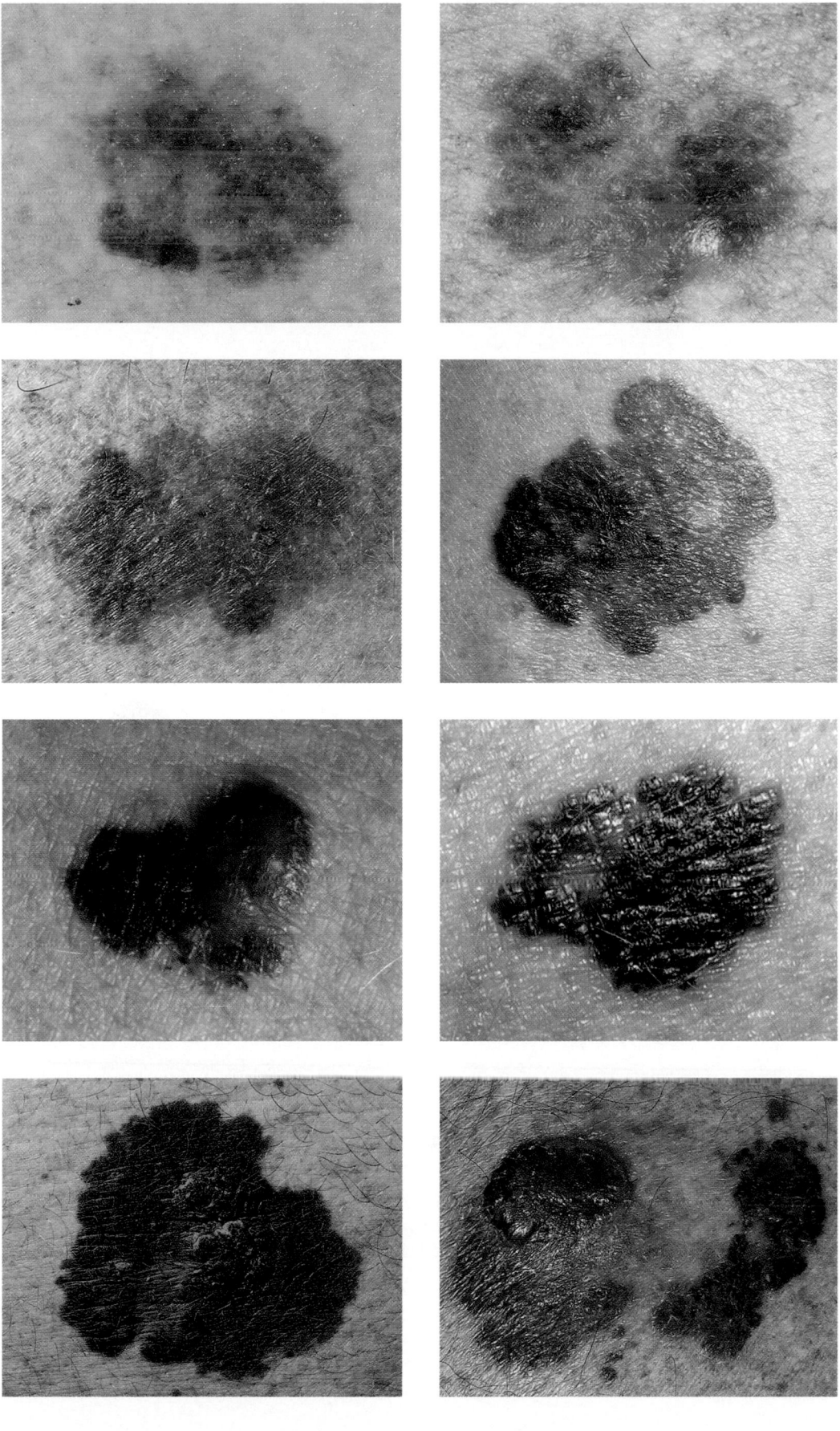

Nodular melanoma

NM (Figure 22-28, Box 22-3) occurs most often in the fifth or sixth decade. It is more frequent in males than females, with a ratio of 2:1. It is found anywhere on the body. NM is most commonly dark brown, red-brown, or red-black and is dome-shaped, polypoid, or pedunculated. It is occasionally amelanotic (flesh-colored) and resembles flesh-colored dermal nevi or basal cell carcinoma. These amelanotic melanomas represent 1.8% to 8.1% of all melanomas.[47] NM is the type of melanoma most frequently misdiagnosed because it resembles a blood blister, hemangioma, dermal nevus, seborrheic keratosis, or dermatofibroma (see p. 797).

Box 22-3 Nodular Melanoma
15%-20% of melanomas
Trunk and legs
Rapid growth: weeks, months
Brown-to-black papule or nodule
Ulcerates and bleeds

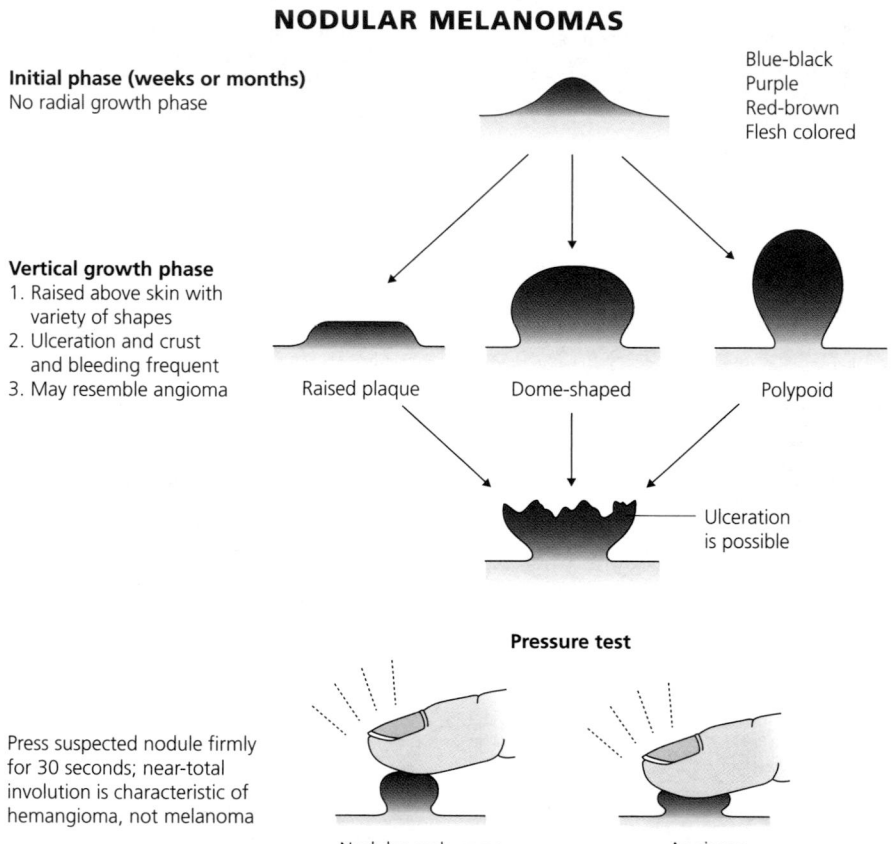

NODULAR MELANOMAS

Initial phase (weeks or months)
No radial growth phase

Blue-black
Purple
Red-brown
Flesh colored

Vertical growth phase
1. Raised above skin with variety of shapes
2. Ulceration and crust and bleeding frequent
3. May resemble angioma

Raised plaque   Dome-shaped   Polypoid

Ulceration is possible

Pressure test

Press suspected nodule firmly for 30 seconds; near-total involution is characteristic of hemangioma, not melanoma

Nodular melanoma   Angioma

Figure 22-28 There are raised plaque, dome-shaped, and polypoid lesions. Some appear to be originating from nevi. A halo has developed around one of the plaque-shaped melanomas.

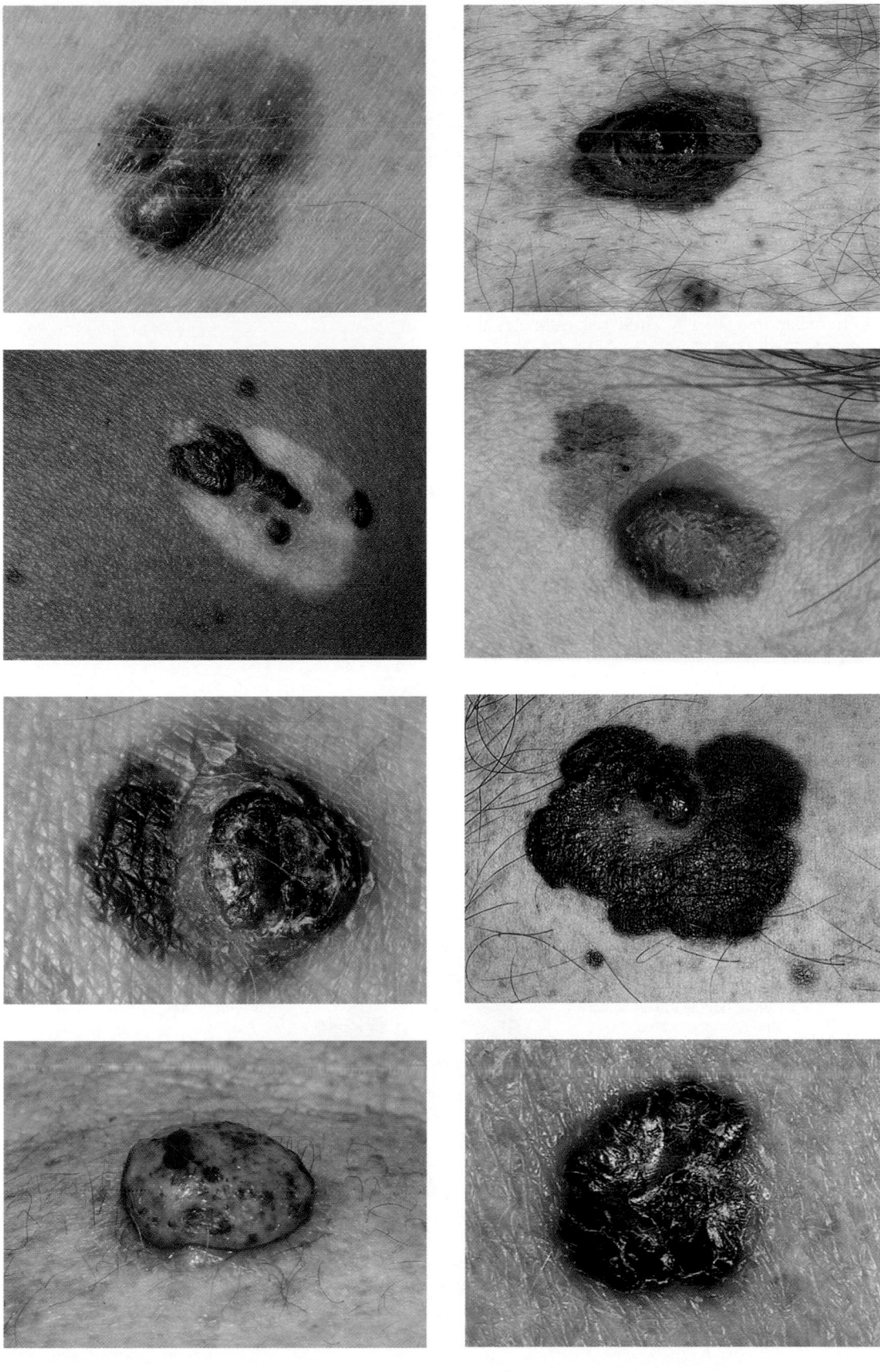

Lentigo maligna melanoma

LMM (Figure 22-29, Box 22-4) usually presents in the sixth or seventh decade. Most are located on the face, but 10% are on other exposed sites, such as arms and legs. The radial growth phase is called lentigo maligna (LM) or Hutchinson's freckle. The radial growth phase may last for years and never develop a vertical growth phase. The risk of progression of LM to LMM varies with age, but is lower than commonly believed. For a patient aged 45 years with LM, the estimated risk of developing LMM by age 75 is 3.3%. Estimated lifetime risk of transformation to melanoma is 4.7%. For a patient aged 65 years with LM, the risk of developing LMM is 1.2%, and the lifetime risk of transformation to melanoma is 2.2%. These risk estimates apply to patients in whom LM is discovered incidentally.[48]

LMM may have a complex patten. Years of migration and regression can produce lesions with a shape more varied and bizarre than that of SSM. The color is more uniform than SSM, but red and white may later occur. Tumors are generally in the center of the lesion, away from the border. LMM may ulcerate or undergo changes similar to other lesions when they enter the tumor stage. Nodules are usually single and generally appear when the lesion has assumed a size of 5 to 7 cm but may occur in much smaller lesions. LMM does not have a better prognosis than other forms of melanoma; as with other types of melanoma, the prognosis depends on tumor thickness.[49]

LENTIGO MALIGNA-MELANOMA

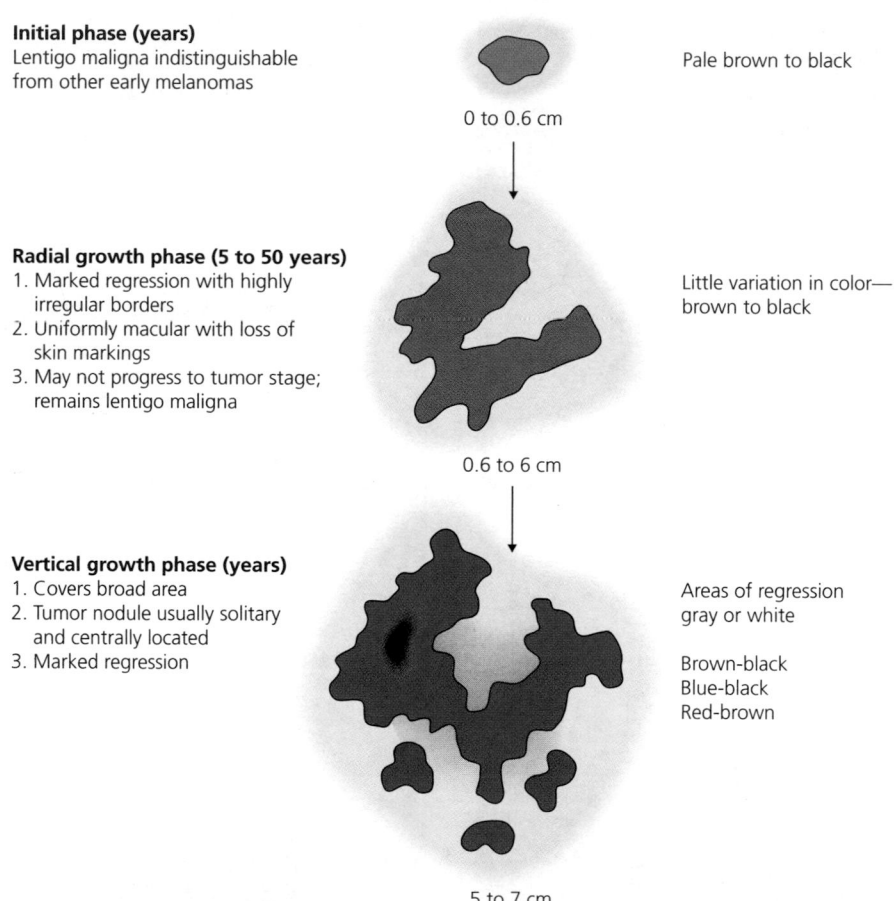

Initial phase (years)
Lentigo maligna indistinguishable from other early melanomas

0 to 0.6 cm

Pale brown to black

Radial growth phase (5 to 50 years)
1. Marked regression with highly irregular borders
2. Uniformly macular with loss of skin markings
3. May not progress to tumor stage; remains lentigo maligna

0.6 to 6 cm

Little variation in color— brown to black

Vertical growth phase (years)
1. Covers broad area
2. Tumor nodule usually solitary and centrally located
3. Marked regression

5 to 7 cm

Areas of regression gray or white

Brown-black
Blue-black
Red-brown

Figure 22-29 The lesions grow slowly and regress for several years, forming highly irregular borders. The color remains brown or black until the tumor stage is reached.

Box 22-4 Lentigo Maligna Melanoma

- 4%-15% of melanomas
- Head, neck, and arms (sun-damaged skin)
- Average age 65
- Slow growth 5-20 years
- Arises in <10% of intraepithelial precursor lesions (lentigo maligna)
- Precursor lesion usually large (3-6 cm diameter)
- Precursor lesion exists for 10-15 years
- Brown-to-black macular pigmentation
- Raised blue-black nodules

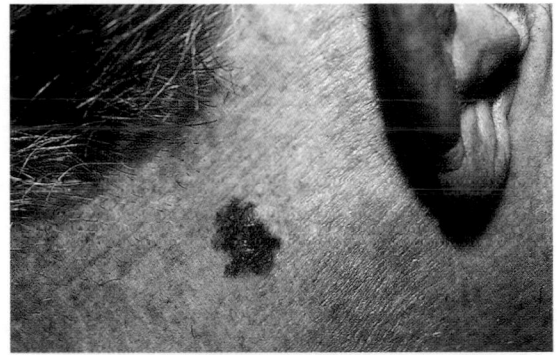

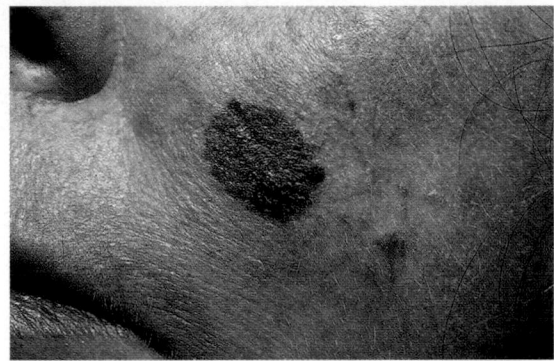

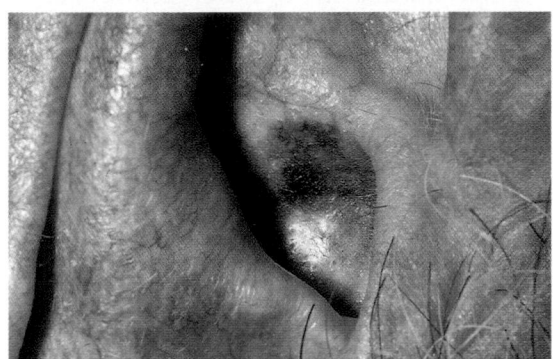

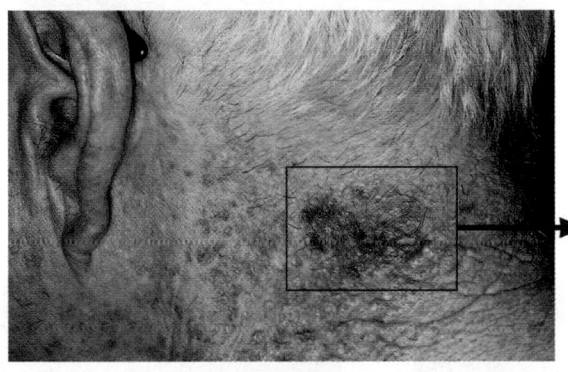

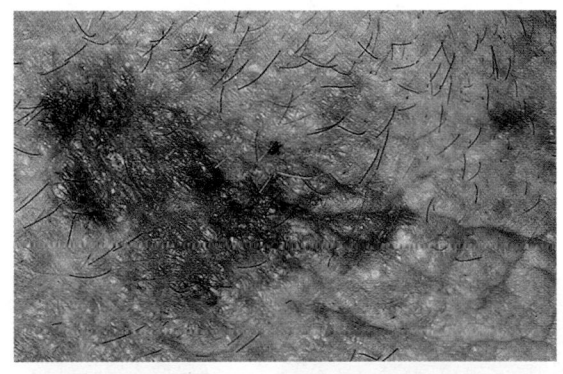

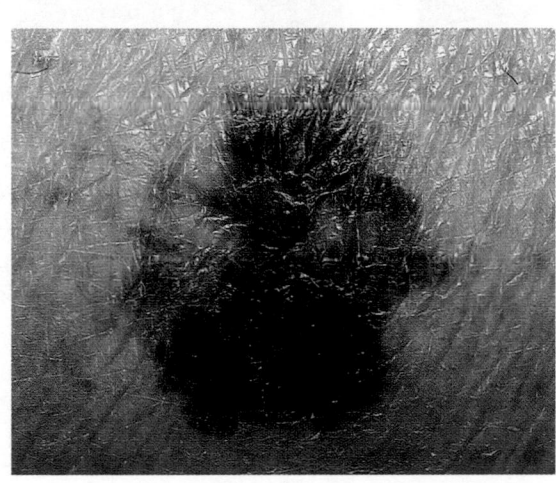

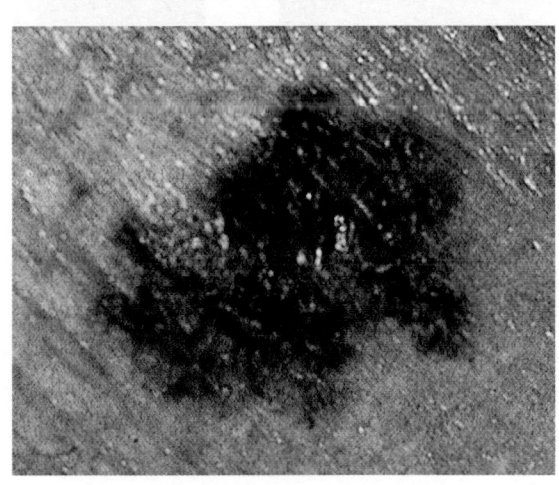

Acral lentiginous melanoma

ALM (Figures 22-30 to 22-33, Box 22-5) appears on the palms,[50] soles, terminal phalanges, and mucous membranes.[51] Similar in clinical presentation to LM and LMM, ALM has the same colors and tendency to remain flat. Like LM, plantar melanomas may remain latent for a number of years, making patients with these lesions good candidates for therapeutic cures if detected early.[52] ALM is most frequent in African Americans and Asians. The sole of the foot is the most prevalent site of malignant melanoma in non-whites. Small areas of elevation may be associated with deep invasion; the tumor is very aggressive and metastasizes early. The sudden appearance of a pigmented band originating at the proximal nail fold (Hutchinson's sign) is suggestive of acral-lentiginous melanoma (Figure 22-31). Acquired melanocytic lesions on the sole larger than 7 mm in maximum diameter should be examined histologically.

RARE TYPES. The following melanoma variants account for less than 2% of melanomas: Melanoma arising from congenital nevus, mucosal (lentiginous) melanoma, ocular melanoma, malignant blue nevus, amelanotic melanoma (no pigment), and desmoplastic/neurotropic melanoma (markedly fibrotic stroma).

Box 22-5 Acral Lentiginous Melanoma
2%-8% of melanomas in whites
30%-75% of melanomas in African Americans, Asians, and Hispanics
Palms, soles
Under nail plate: Hutchinson sign (pigment spreads to proximal and lateral nailfolds)

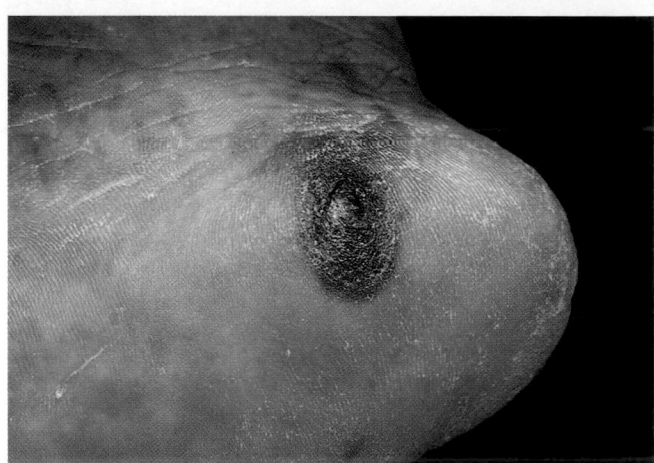

Figure 22-30 Acral lentiginous melanoma. A large, dark, flat lesion.

ACRAL LENTIGINOUS MELANOMA

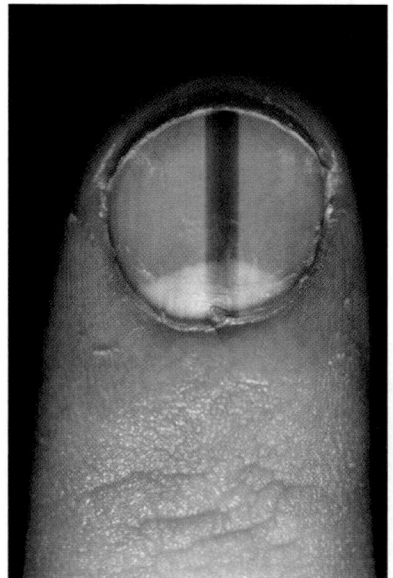

Figure 22-31 The sudden appearance of a pigmented band at the proximal nail fold is suggestive of melanoma.

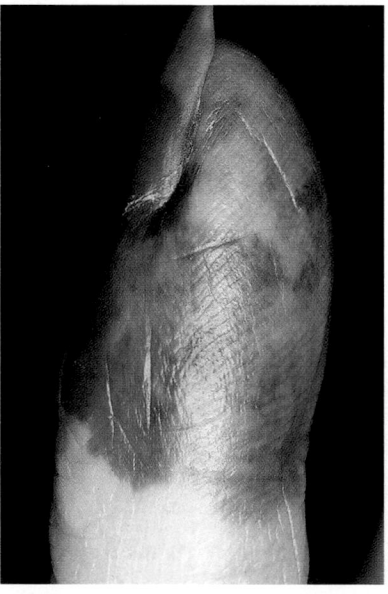

Figure 22-32 Periungual spread of pigmentation from a melanoma to the proximal and lateral nail folds is called Hutchinson's sign.

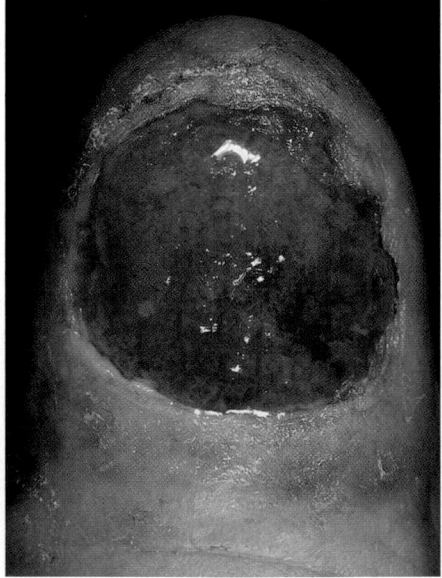

Figure 22-33 Melanoma involving the entire nail bed.

Benign lesions that resemble melanoma

Typical nevi or other lesions, such as those of seborrheic keratosis, angiomas, and dermatofibromas may have features that suggest melanoma. Biopsy specimens of these lesions should be obtained (Figures 22-34 to 22-37).

Lesion examination

OBSERVATION PLUS MAGNIFICATION PLUS DERMOS-COPY. Several different lesions can be recognized by observation or magnification with a 10× ocular. The 10× ocular is a superior instrument for studying the surface characteristics of seborrheic keratosis, basal cell carcinoma, dermatofibroma, compound nevi, dermal nevi, halo nevi, and hemangiomas. Many lesions can be scanned quickly. The dermoscope is an invaluable instrument for examination of flat to slightly raised pigmented lesions such as atypical nevi and lesions suspected of being melanoma. Examining numerous seborrheic keratoses with a dermoscope is inefficient. The horn pearls and keratin structure are clearly appreciated with 10× ocular magnification.

SCREENING FOR MELANOMA. Most pigmented lesions can be diagnosed on the basis of clinical criteria. Examination of the surface with 10× magnification is highly recommended for the initial evaluation of all skin growths. However, there are many small lesions in which the distinction between a benign and malignant process cannot be made by observation and magnification. Dermoscopy is useful for the diagnosis of these doubtful skin lesions.

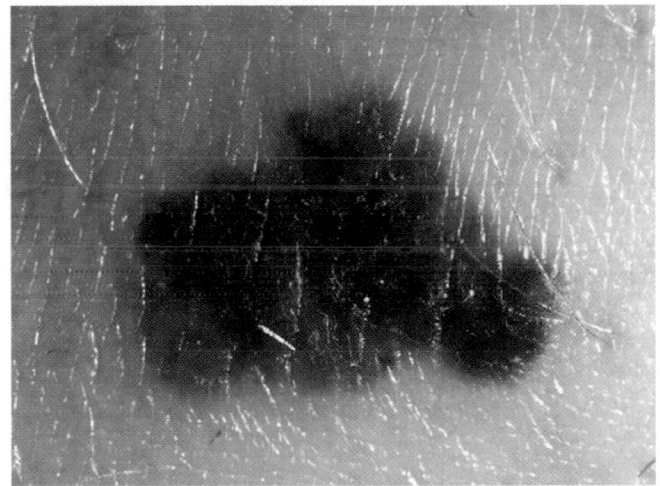

Figure 22-35 Melanoma mimic. Compound nevus with an irregular border.

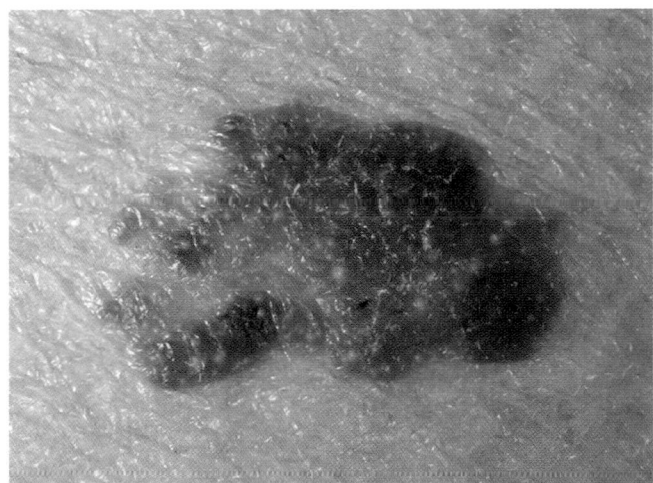

Figure 22-36 Melanoma mimic. Seborrheic keratosis with variable pigmentation and an irregular border. The horn peals (typical of a seborrheic keratosis) suggest that the lesion is benign.

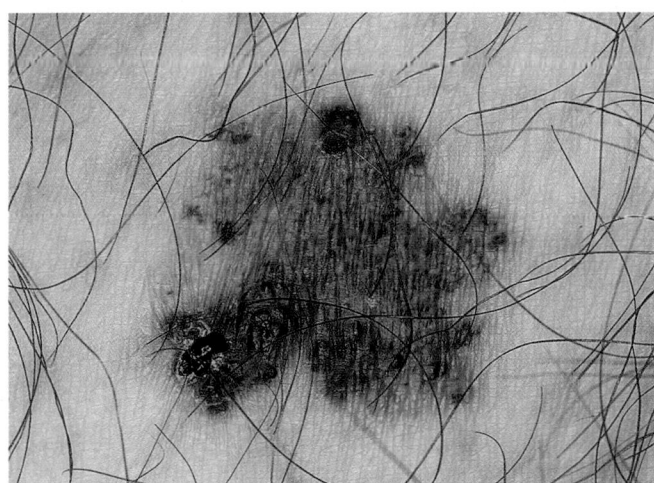

Figure 22-34 Melanoma mimic. Hemangioma with an irregular border and variable pigmentation.

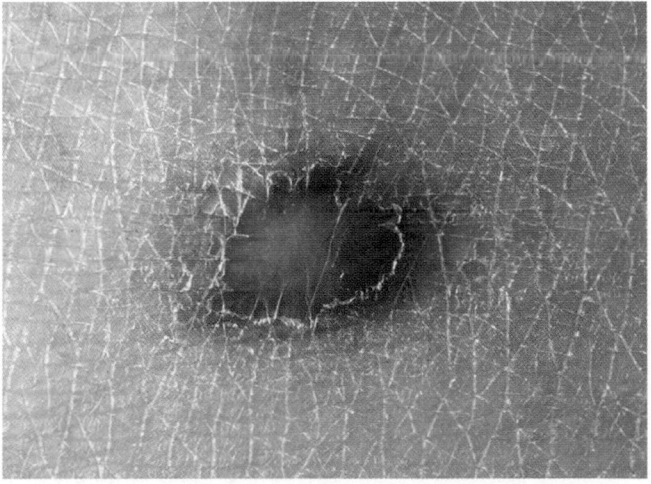

Figure 22-37 Melanoma mimic. Dermatofibroma with dark pigmentation at the border.

Dermoscopy

Dermoscopy (epiluminescent microscopy, dermoscopy, magnified oil immersion diascopy) is a technique used to see a variety of patterns (Table 22-4) and structures in lesions that are not discernible to the naked eye (www.dermoscopy.org). Lotion or mineral oil may be applied to the surface of the lesion to make the epidermis more transparent. Then examination with a 10× ocular, a microscope ocular eyepiece (held upside down) or a dermoscope (Figure 22-38) (available from surgical supply houses) reveals several features that are helpful in differentiating between benign and malignant pigmented lesions. The DermLite™ and DermoGenius are highly accurate oil-free pocket epiluminescent microscopes. A clear and deep view into pigmented lesions can be made in seconds with these instruments. Many lesions can be examined in a short time. Dermoscopy provides additional criteria for the diagnosis of melanoma (see p. 803).

Dermoscopy tables

- Patterns, p. 798
- Benign pigmented lesions, p. 800
- Atypical nevi, pp. 802-803
- 7-pt checklist for the diagnosis of melanoma, pp. 804-805

Table 22-4 Patterns Seen with Dermoscopy

Pattern	Diagnostic significance	Histology
Reticulated pattern or brown pigment "network"	A network of brownish lines over a tan background	Pigment in the epidermal basal cells. It is regular or irregular, narrow or wide
Diffuse pigmentation or blotches	Irregularly shaped, dark brown or black areas of pigmentation of various sizes. Some resemble "ink spots"	Areas where there is melanin in all levels of the epidermis and/or upper dermis
Brown globules	Circular to oval pigmented structures	Nests of melanocytes or melanophages at the dermoepidermal junction or in the upper dermis
Black dots	Sharply circumscribed and round. Various sizes but often very small	Focal collection of melanin in the stratum corneum
Depigmented or hypopigmented areas	Zones of relatively lighter pigmentation	Patchy areas of the epidermis that contain less melanin or a relatively thinned epidermis where telangiectasias are often noticeable
White areas	These areas have no pigment. Areas of "regression" in melanomas	Zones with no melanin in the epidermis and dermis. Areas of fibroplasia and telangiectasias
Grey blue areas	Irregular, confluent, gray-blue to whitish blue diffuse pigmentation	Fibrosis and melanophages or melanocytes of midreticular dermis location. Melanin in the deeper dermis causes the blue hue
Radial streaming pseudopods	Linear brown to black streaks radiate from the border of a pigmented lesion into surrounding skin. Also seen in the central areas of lightly pigmented melanomas. Pseudopods are curved extensions	Radially arranged nests. Confluent pigmented junctional nests at the periphery
Milia-like cysts (pseudocysts)	White or black round structures imbedded in a seborrheic keratosis or papillomatous dermal nevus	Intraepidermal horn globules underneath the surface
Comedo-like openings	White or black round structures protruding from the surface of a seborrheic keratosis or papillomatous dermal nevus	Intraepidermal horn globules reaching the surface. Keratin plugs in adnexal ostia
Telangiectasia	Short red hairlike strands	Dilated vessels in the papillary dermis
Red-blue areas	Red round globules	Dilated vascular spaces in the papillary dermis in hemangiomas or angiokeratoma
Leaf-like areas	Flecks of pigment in a pearly white papule	Pigmented clusters in a basal cell carcinoma
Central white scarlike patch + delicate pigment network at the periphery	Dermatofibroma	Epidermal hyperplasia and pigment in the basal layer

Adapted from Bahmer F, et al: J Am Acad Dermatol 1990; 23:1159.

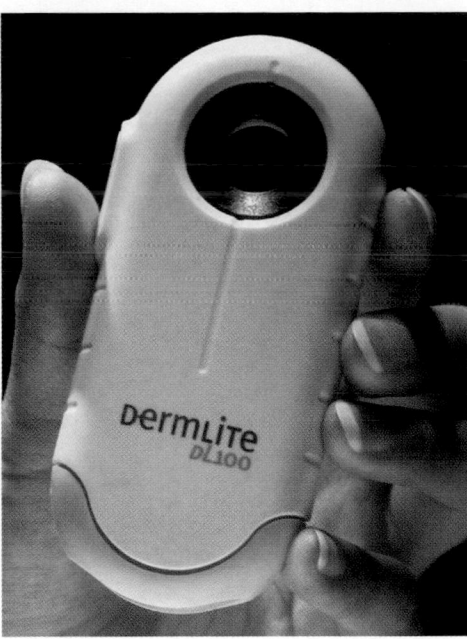

Figure 22-38 Dermoscope.

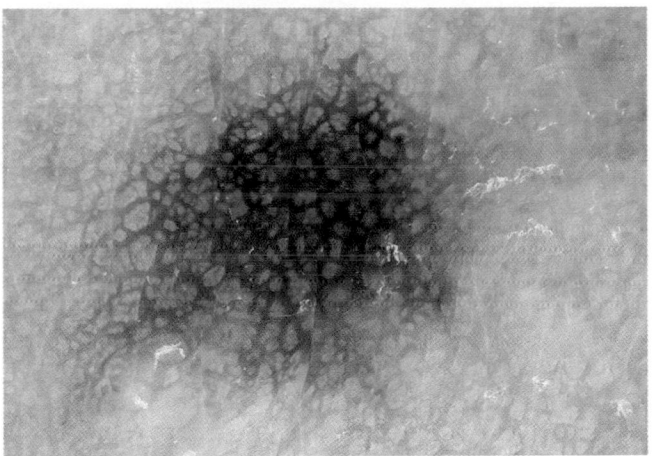

Figure 22-39 Dermoscopy (junction nevus). The uniform pigment network is more prominent in the center.

The pigment network

The presence of a pigment network usually implies that the lesion is melanocytic (Figure 22-39). The pattern may be subtle or present only in a small area. The network of common lesions such as lentigo and junctional nevi fades and thins at the periphery. The typical honeycomb-like pattern of the pigment network on the trunk and proximal extremities results from pigmentation along the rete ridges. The pseudonetwork patterns on the face, palms, and soles result from junctional pigment outlining hair follicles, sebaceous glands, and eccrine ducts. Pigment on the palms and soles outlines linear skin markings along or across the skin furrows resulting in a parallel, lattice, or fibrillar pattern. Growing melanomas distort the normal skin anatomy and cause variation in pigmentation patterns and structures. Networks in melanomas are variable. Thin melanomas and melanomas in situ may have only very subtle pigmentation changes. Subtle thickening and darkening of pigment network lines may be seen near the periphery in early lesions. As Breslow thickness increases, the pigment network tends to become more variable in thickness and color density. The lines become thick and dark. They also become darker near the periphery. These result from wide and shallow pigmented rete ridges. Pseudopods and radial streaming occur at the edge of a region of thickened, darkened network at the periphery.

Approach to diagnosis of pigmented lesions by dermoscopy[53]:

1. Determine if a pigment network is present and determine its characteristics and make an initial diagnosis.
2. Group lesions by their relative degrees of heterogeneity and eccentricity of the pigment network.
3. If a network is not seen, look for typical patterns of benign lesions and melanoma mimickers.
4. Use the information to guide management.

Many lesions will lack classic dermoscopy features of melanoma. This ill-defined group of possible early melanomas will include many atypical nevi. Clinical judgment using all available information must be used to make the decision to excise or observe. Total number of lesions, history of melanoma, family history, body site, and surgical morbidity such as scarring are factors to consider before making the final management decision.

DERMATOSCOPIC CHARACTERISTICS OF BENIGN PIGMENTED LESIONS. The dermatoscopic characteristics of benign melanocytic nevi are described[54] in Table 22-5, and an example is shown in Figure 22-40.

Classification of atypical melanocytic nevi

Clinical classification

The clinical diagnosis of atypical melanocytic nevi is established when at least three of the following characteristics are present:

Diameter greater than 5 mm
Ill-defined borders
Irregular margin
Varying shades in the lesion
Presence of papular and macular components

Dermoscopic classification

STRUCTURAL FEATURES PLUS DISTRIBUTION OF PIGMENTATION. The following dermatoscopic classification allows characterization of the different dermatoscopic types of atypical nevi. Knowledge of these dermatoscopic types should reduce unnecessary surgery for benign melanocytic lesions.[55]

Atypical nevi are classified according to structural features, that is, reticular, globular, or homogeneous patterns or combinations of these types. The nevi are also characterized by distribution of pigmentation (Tables 22-7 and 22-8).

Table 22-5 Dermoscopic Characteristics of Benign Pigmented Lesions

Lesion	History	Clinical presentation	Dermoscopy
Congenital melanocytic nevi	Present at birth or shortly after. Change over time; may enlarge and develop more hairs and new nodules	Brown or black, smooth or pebbly texture, tan and dark, speckled background, increased terminal hairs	Globular or homogenous pattern. Globules of varying shapes, sizes, and numbers. Globules may have a dense "cobble-stone" arrangement. There may be no pigment network. Milia-like cysts may be seen
Melanocytic nevi (junctional nevi, compound nevi, dermal nevi)	Acquired in early child-hood. Increase in number and size. Regress after third decade	Begin as brown macules and can progress to dome-shaped, cerebriform, or pedunculated papules	Most have one or more of the following features: a network, globules, dots, streaks, and structureless areas. The structures usually are regular in shape and size and have a uniform distribution
Junctional nevi	Become thicker during adolescence. Usually change color and sometimes develop hair	Macular, light to dark brown, symmetrical, and smoothly textured. Center darker than periphery	Honeycomb-like network pattern—uniform and homogeneous distribution. Network often prominent in the center and fades toward the edges. Network in center often obscured by heavy pigmentation. Small black dots and globules may be present
Compound nevi	Become thicker during adolescence. Change color and sometimes develop hair	Slightly raised or papillomatous. Uniform light to dark brown	Network pattern is less prominent. Central pigmentation is less intense. Globules (distributed uniformly) may be present. Large globules may form a cobblestone pattern
Dermal nevi		Smooth or papillomatous surface. elevated, dome-shaped, sessile or pedunculated papules or nodules that are light brown	No network or black dots. Red dots and lines correspond to dilated blood vessels. A few globules may be present. Globules may be angulated
Spitz Nevi	Most seen in children. Firm, round, 2- to 8-mm papule. Face most common location	Smooth dome-shaped, variable telangiectases, and uniform color, (usually pink or tan to dark brown)	1. Starburst pattern (50% of cases)- A black-blue-whitish structureless center surrounded by a thickened network that ends abruptly at the periphery. Pigmented streaks radiate from the periphery. This resembles a bursting star 2. Globular pattern (25% of cases)- uniform distribution of globules and dots throughout or globules at the periphery surrounding a brown to blue-gray center
Blue nevi		Dome-shaped papules. Diffuse slate-gray to blue	Blue pigmentation distributed throughout. No globules, dots, or network (because the pigment is located in the dermis)
Halo nevi	Several may be present. The central nevus may disappear. Eventually the halo may disappear	Zone of hypopigmentation around a melanocytic neoplasm	Central nevus is light-brown and structureless. Occasional dots and globules
Lentigines and ephelides			Pigment networks, usually with relatively thin and lightly pigmented network lines
"Ink spot" lentigines			Have a dark (nearly black) network that is irregular, with marked variation in line thickness
Dermatofibromas			Usually have a flat ring of lightly pigmented network around a central hypopigmented papule

Adapted from Rao BK, Wang SQ, Murphy FP: Derm Clin 2001; 19:269.

NEVI

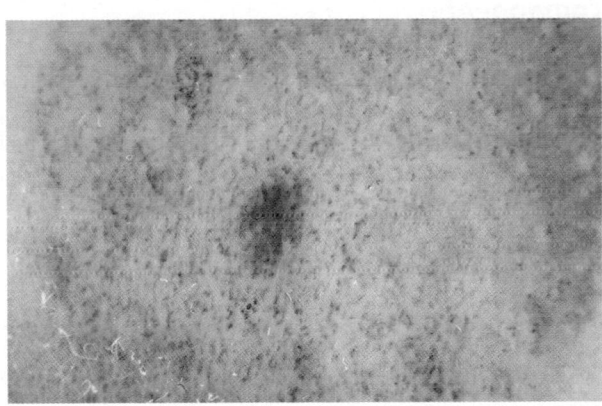

Congenital nevus

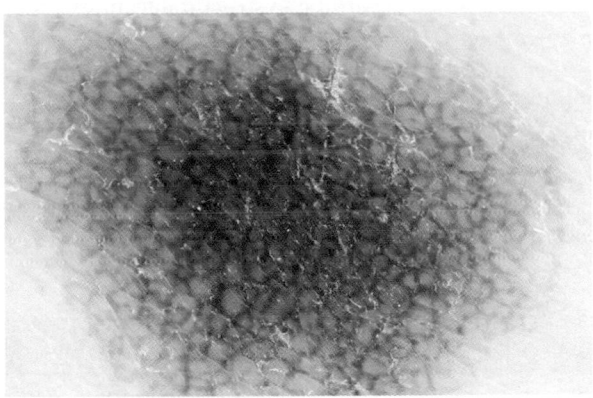

Junctional nevus

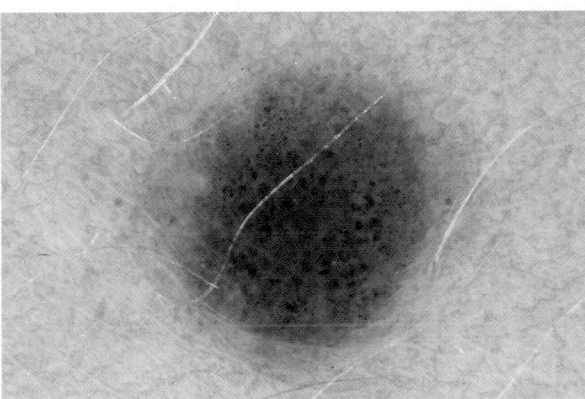

Compound nevus

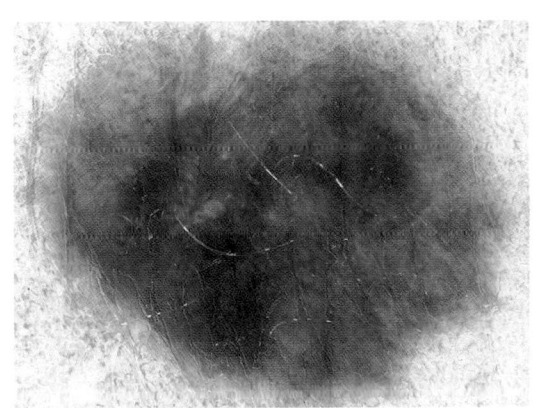

Blue nevus

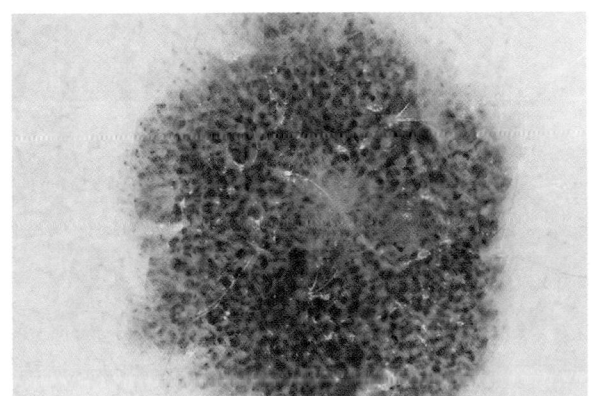

Halo nevus

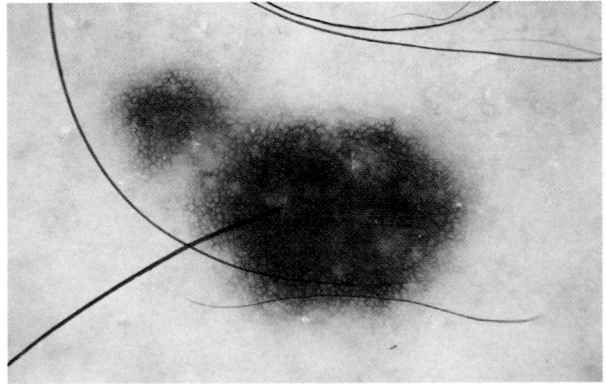

Lentigo

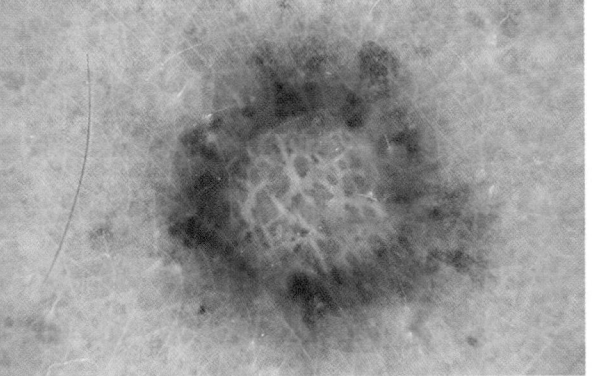

Dermatofibroma

Figure 22-40

Classification by main structural components

Nevi are first classified according to structural features: reticular pigment network, pigmented globules, and homogeneous pigmentation (Table 22-6). When a clear predominance of one of these structural components is seen, the nevus is classified as reticular, globular, or homogeneous.

Classification by combinations of structural components

In the case of the dominant presence of two structural components, the nevus is classified as reticular-globular, reticular-homogeneous, or globular-homogeneous (Table 22-6). No single nevus shows all three structural components. The most common are the reticular type, followed by the reticular-homogeneous and globular-homogeneous types.

Table 22-6 Dermoscopic Types of Atypical Melanocytic Nevi—Structural Features

Type	Definition and predominant features
Clear predominance of one structural component	
Reticular	Pigment network
Globular	Numerous globules or dots
Homogeneous	Homogeneous brown pigmentation
Dominant presence of two structural components	
Reticular-globular	>3 meshes of pigment network with >3 globules of dots
Reticular-homogeneous	>3 meshes of pigment network with homogeneous brown pigmentation in at least one quarter of the lesion
Globular-homogeneous	>3 globules or dots with homogeneous brown pigmentation in at least one quarter of the lesion
Unclassified	No specific pattern

DERMOSCOPIC TYPES OF ATYPICAL MELANOCYTIC NEVI

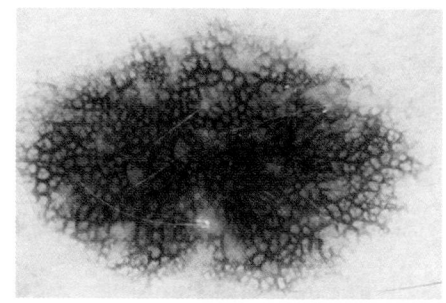

Reticular

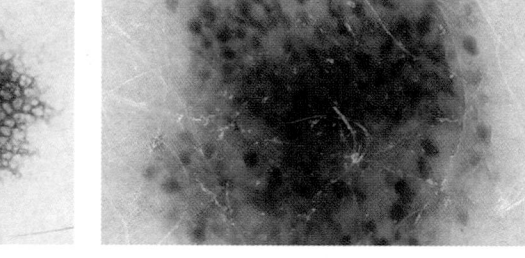

Globular

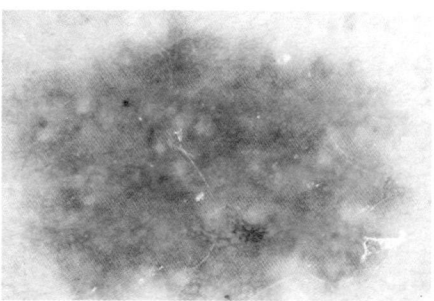

Homogeneous

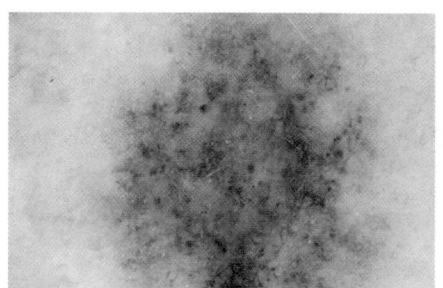

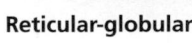

Reticular-globular

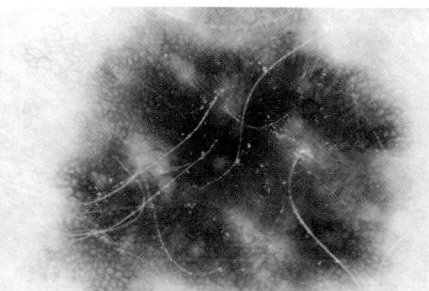

Reticular-homogeneous

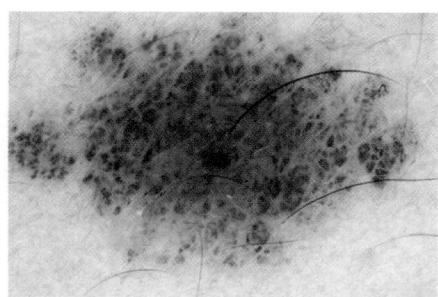

Globular-homogeneous

Classification by distribution of pigmentation

The distribution of the pigmentation is then classified as central hyperpigmented or hypopigmented, eccentric peripheral hyperpigmented or hypopigmented, and multifocal hyperpigmented or hypopigmented (Table 22-7). In cases where hyperpigmentation and hypopigmentation are present, classification is based on the predominant distribution of color.

Interpretation and management

Most individuals have one predominant type of nevus. A lesion that does not belong to the predominant type of nevus in a given patient should be considered an atypical lesion and therefore deserving of special attention.

Table 22-7 Dermoscopic Types of Atypical Melanocytic Nevi—Distribution of Pigmentation	
Pigmentation	**Definition**
Central hyperpigmented	Hyperpigmented area (significantly darker than the entire lesion) surrounded by fainter parts of the lesion
Eccentric peripheral hyperpigmented	Hyperpigmented area (significantly darker than the entire lesion) reaching 1 part of the border of the lesion
Central hypopigmented	Hypopigmented area (significantly fainter than the entire lesion) surrounded by darker parts of the lesion
Eccentric peripheral hypopigmented	Hypopigmented area (significantly fainter than the entire lesion) reaching 1 part of the border of the lesion
Multifocal hyperpigmented and hypopigmented	Patchy distribution of hyperpigmented and hypopigmented areas
Adapted from Hofmann-Wellenhof R, Blum A, Wolf IH, et al: Arch Dermatol 2001; 137:1575.	

DERMOSCOPIC TYPES OF ATYPICAL MELANOCYTIC NEVI

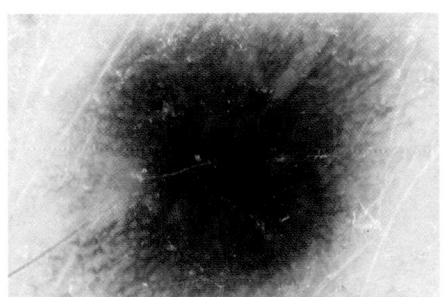

Central hyperpigmented

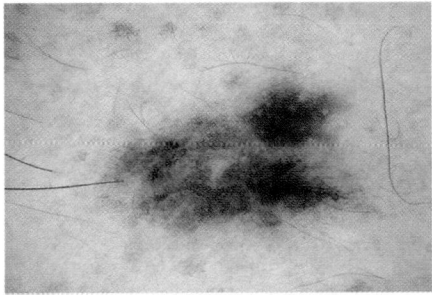

Eccentric peripheral hyperpigmented

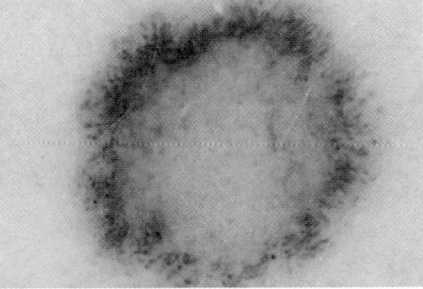

Central hypopigmented

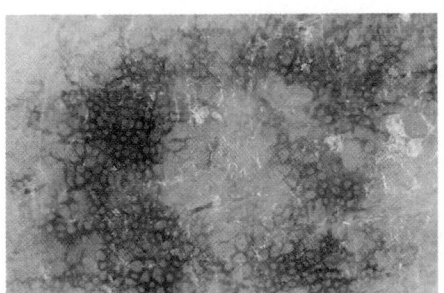

Central hypopigmented

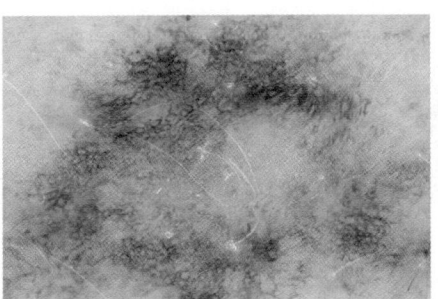

Eccentric peripheral hypopigmented

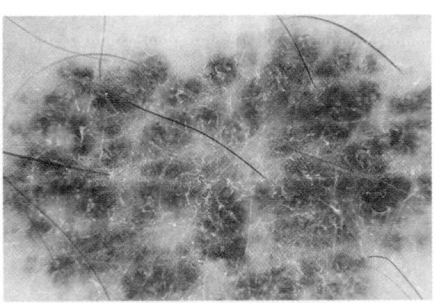

Multifocal hyperpigmented and hypopigmented

Table 22-8 7-Point Checklist: Definition and Histopathologic Correlates of the Seven Melanoma-Specific Dermoscopic Criteria (See text on p. 806)

ELM criterion	Definition	Histopathologic correlates	7-point score* (A minimum score of 3 is required for the diagnosis of melanoma)
1. Atypical pigment network	Black, brown, or gray network with irregular meshes and thick lines	Irregular and broadened rete ridges	2
2. Blue-whitish veil	Irregular, confluent, gray-blue to whitish-blue diffuse pigmentation	Acanthotic epidermis with focal hypergranulosis above sheets of heavily pigmented melanocytes in the dermis	2
3. Atypical vascular pattern	Linear-irregular or dotted vessels not clearly combined with regression structures	Neovascularization	2
4. Irregular streaks	Irregular, more or less confluent, linear structures not clearly combined with pigment network lines	Confluent junctional nests of melanocytes	1

Table 22-8 7-Point Checklist: Definition and Histopathologic Correlates of the Seven Melanoma-Specific Dermoscopic Criteria (See text on p. 806)

ELM criterion	Definition	Histopathologic correlates	7-point score* (A minimum score of 3 is required for the diagnosis of melanoma)
5. Irregular pigmentation	Black, brown, and/or gray pigmented areas with irregular shape and/or distribution	Hyperpigmentation throughout the epidermis and/or upper dermis	1
6. Irregular dots/globules	Black, brown, and/or gray round to oval, variously sized structures irregularly distributed within the lesion	Pigment aggregates within stratum corneum, epidermis, dermoepidermal junction, or papillary dermis	1
7. Regression structures	White areas (white scarlike areas) and blue areas (gray-blue areas, peppering, multiple blue-gray dots) may be associated, thus featuring so-called blue-whitish areas virtually indistinguishable from blue whitish veil	Thickened papillary dermis with fibrosis and/or variable amounts of melanophages	1

Adapted from Argenziano G, et al: Arch Dermatol 1998; 134:1563; and the Consensus Net Meeting on Dermoscopy (CNMD) 2000 (under the auspices of the European Society of Dermato-Oncology).

*By addition of the individual scores a minimum total score of 3 is required for the diagnosis of melanoma.

Atypical nevi with the reticular pattern and uneven pigmentation are especially prone to over-diagnosis as melanoma. The most common heterogeneous distribution of pigmentation is multifocal hyperpigmentation or hypopigmentation, followed by central hypopigmentation and central hyperpigmentation. Eccentric peripheral hyperpigmentation is often found in malignant melanoma. Atypical nevi with eccentric peripheral hyperpigmentation should be regarded as the most relevant simulators of melanoma within the morphologic spectrum of atypical nevi. Therefore this type of nevus should be excised or monitored using digital dermoscopy at 3-month intervals. When the eccentric peripheral hyperpigmentation increases, excision of the lesion is necessary.

Dermoscopic characteristics of melanoma

A standardized terminology for dermoscopy patterns was established in 1989.[56] A number of diagnostic methods using these criteria have been devised. Pattern analysis is based on the assessment of numerous individual criteria. It is accurate but complicated. The ABCD rule of dermoscopy was established in 1994. It is based on analysis of the lesion's Asymmetry, Border, Color, and different Dermoscopic structures. The ABCD rule was easier to learn but less accurate. A new 7-point checklist system (Table 22-8) using simplified pattern analysis is accurate and easy to learn.[57] The 7-point checklist, compared with the ABCD rule, allows better diagnostic accuracy because of the tendency of the ABCD rule to overclassify atypical nevi as melanomas.

THE 7-POINT CHECKLIST. A dermoscopic score is determined for each lesion based on the presence of three major criteria and four minor criteria. The major criteria are an atypical network, a blue-gray veil, and an atypical vascular pattern. The minor criteria are irregular streaks, irregular pigmentation, irregular dots or globules, and regression. A score of 2 is given to each of three major criteria, and a score of 1 is given to each of four minor criteria. A total score of 3 or more suggests melanoma. For a melanoma to be diagnosed, identification of at least 1 major and 1 minor criterion (or 3 minor criteria) is required. Melanocytic nevi usually have a score less than 3, and a score of 3 suggests the lesion may be an atypical nevus.

These criteria serve only as guidelines. Lesions with a suspicious score should be excised.

Limitations of dermoscopy

Dermoscopy may enhance the clinician's ability to diagnose melanoma. Knowledge and experience are required. Even experienced users may obtain a false sense of security in 20% or more cases of melanoma that lack classic dermoscopy features of melanoma. The dermoscopy feature most common in thin melanomas (Breslow thickness of <0.75 mm) is an irregular pigment network. Atypical nevi often have hyperpigmentation and bridging of the rete ridges, which give them a similar appearance by dermoscopy. Dermoscopy criteria for melanoma variants such as amelanotic melanomas, desmo-

plastic melanomas, lentigo maligna melanoma, or nevoid melanoms are lacking. A patient's report of change in a lesion is an important risk factor for melanoma. Approximately 10% of melanomas have no characteristic dermoscopy findings. The decision to perform a biopsy of a lesion of moderate to high clinical suspicion for melanoma before dermoscopy observation should not be changed by the lack of dermoscopy criteria for melanoma.[9]

Pregnancy, oral contraceptives, prognosis, and risk

On the basis of a limited number of controlled studies, it does not appear that pregnancy before, after, or at the time of diagnosis of stage I MM influences the 5-year survival rate.[58, 59]

Oral contraceptive use does not seem to increase the risk of malignant melanoma,[60] except possibly for women aged 30 to 40 years who used oral contraception for 10 years or more or who started to use oral contraception 15 years or more before the diagnosis.[61]

Management

Biopsy

Whenever possible, excise the lesion for diagnostic purposes using narrow margins (2 to 3 mm of normal skin). Wider margins (>1 cm) may disrupt cutaneous lymphatic flow and affect the ability to identify the sentinel node(s).[62] Incisional biopsy does not adversely affect survival. A punch biopsy technique is appropriate when the suspicion for melanoma is low, when the lesion is large, or when it is impractical to perform an excision. Punch through the thickest part of the lesion. Perform a repeat biopsy if the initial biopsy specimen is inadequate for accurate histologic diagnosis or staging. Shave biopsies are discouraged because partial removal of the primary melanoma may not provide accurate Breslow-depth measurement.

Histologic findings

Superficial spreading melanoma, lentigo maligna melanoma, and acral lentiginous melanoma initially have an in situ (radial growth phase) and in time may enter a vertical growth phase.[63] Lateral intraepidermal extension of melanoma cells occurs in all subtypes except nodular melanoma.

RADIAL GROWTH PHASE TUMORS. Large and atypical melanocytes first proliferate in the epidermis above the epidermal basement membrane. They are arranged haphazardly at the dermal-epidermal junction, show upward (pagetoid) migration, and lack the biologic potential to metastasize. They then invade the papillary dermis (Clark level 2). Malignant cells confined above the epidermal basement membrane (in situ) or in the papillary dermis (microinvasive) are called radial growth phase melanomas. These are almost always less than 0.76 mm thick.

VERTICAL GROWTH PHASE TUMORS. Tumors that have invaded the reticular dermis have entered the vertical growth phase. They have metastatic potential. There are mitoses and nuclear pleomorphism. Cells fail to mature as the tumor extends downward into the dermis. Clark levels 3 and 4 tumors are usually in the vertical growth phase.

TUMOR THICKNESS (BRESLOW MICROSTAGE). Tumor thickness, as defined by the Breslow depth, is the most important histologic determinant of prognosis. The tumor is step sectioned (Figure 22-41). The section with the deepest level of penetration of tumor is used to measure thickness. An ocular micrometer is placed on the microscope. The pathologist measures the thickness of the tumor in millimeters from the top of the granular cell layer (or base of superficial ulceration) to the deepest part of the tumor. The report is given as Breslow level, followed by the depth reported in millimeters.

ULCERATION. The presence of ulceration microscopically, defined as the loss of epidermis overlying the melanoma, is the next most important histologic determinant of patient prognosis and should be used to upstage patients with melanoma when present.

TUMOR THICKNESS (CLARK LEVEL). Clark levels measure tumor invasion anatomically. The tumor depth is reported by anatomic site (e.g., epidermis, depth in dermis, etc.) and assigned a Clark level of invasion (see Figure 22-41). Clark levels appear to affect prognosis only in thinner (<1 mm depth) melanomas.

PATHOLOGY REPORT. The pathologist determines the following: Tumor thickness in millimeters (Breslow's level) and presence of ulceration.

Reporting of other histologic features is encouraged, but may not be related to prognosis: Clark's level, growth phase, tumor infiltrating lymphocytes, mitotic rate, regression, angiolymphatic invasion, microsatellitosis, neurotropism, and histologic subtype are reported by many pathologists.

MITOTIC RATE. The mitotic rate per square millimeter is reported.

TUMOR-INFILTRATING LYMPHOCYTES. The degree to which lymphocytes infiltrate and disrupt the tumor cell.

HISTOLOGIC REGRESSION. Areas of epidermis that have no recognizable tumor and are flanked by areas of melanoma indicate regression.

Special stains. The pathologist may use immunohistochemical staining for lineage (S-100, homatropine methylbromide 45) or proliferation markers (proliferating cell nuclear antigen, Ki67) in difficult cases.

Biopsy specimen
Sections cut by pathologist

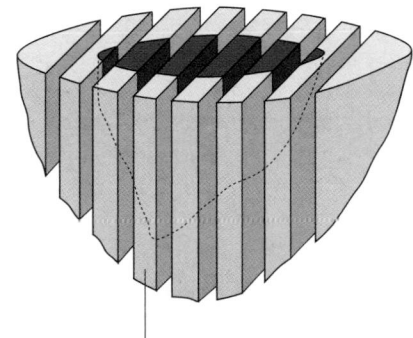

Section with deepest penetration of tumor; this section used to report Breslow microstage and Clark level

Figure 22-41 To obtain the Breslow microstage, an ocular micrometer mounted on the microscope is used. Measurement is made from the granular cell layer to the section with the deepest penetration of tumor. When ulceration is present at the surface, measurement starts at the ulcer base.

Breslow microstage

Clark levels 1–5

Depth of invasion in millimeters

0
1.0
2.0
3.0
4.0

Granular cell layer

Epidermis

Papillary dermis

Reticular dermis

Subcutaneous fat

1. Intraepidermal

2. In papillary dermis

3. Fills papillary dermis

4. Reticular dermis

5. Enters fat

Tumor pictured—reported by pathologist as:
1. Depth of invasion 3.3 mm
2. Clark level 4

Excision after biopsy (resection margins)

Complete surgical removal of the entire neoplasm must be accomplished with histologic verification of removal. Recommended surgical margins based on depth of the tumor (Breslow measurement) and diameter of the melanoma[9] are listed in Table 22-9.

Compromises are necessary for lesions on the digits and face. Excising to fascia may not be necessary for melanoma tumors confined to the upper levels of the skin, while wider cutaneous margins may be appropriate for large in situ tumors.[64]

Metastatic staging and prognosis

The presence or absence of micrometastasis in the sentinel lymph node (SLN) is the most important prognostic factor for recurrence and the most powerful predictor of survival.

SENTINEL LYMPH NODE BIOPSY. The SLN is defined as the first node in the lymphatic basin that drains the lesion and is at the greatest risk for the development of metastasis. Although no survival benefit has been proven for the procedure, the staging information is useful in identifying patients who may benefit from further surgery or adjuvant therapy.[65]

Indication. SLN biopsy is appropriate for melanomas deeper than 1.0 mm and for tumors 1 mm or less when histologic ulceration is present and/or classified as Clark level 4 or higher. The SLN biopsy is inappropriate for nonulcerated Clark level 2 or 3 melanomas 0.75 mm or less in depth and uncertain in tumors 0.76 to 1.0 mm deep unless they are ulcerated or Clark level 4 or higher.[66]

Procedure. Preoperative radiographic mapping (lymphoscintigraphy) and vital blue dye injection around the primary melanoma or biopsy scar (at the time of wide local excision or reexcision) is performed to identify and remove the initial draining regional node(s). Some centers use technetium 99m–labeled radioisotope and a hand-held gamma probe. The sentinel node is examined for micrometastasis with histology and immunohistochemistry. A therapeutic lymph node dissection is performed if micrometastasis is present. Preceding diagnostic excisions of malignant melanoma with a maximum margin of 10 mm do not alter the lymphatic flow or interfere with accurately obtaining the SLN of the primary tumor.[62]

There are several reasons to perform sentinel lymph node biopsy.[67] It improves the accuracy of staging and provides valuable prognostic information to guide treatment decisions. It facilitates early therapeutic lymph node dissection for those patients with nodal metastases. SLN biopsy identifies patients who are candidates for adjuvant therapy with interferon alfa-2b and identifies homogeneous patient populations for entry onto clinical trials of adjuvant therapy agents.

ELECTIVE LYMPH NODE DISSECTION. Patients with clinically enlarged lymph nodes and no evidence of distant disease should undergo a complete regional lymph node dissection. The value of elective lymph node dissection for other patients has not been defined.

Initial diagnostic workup

Routine imaging studies including chest radiography and blood work have limited, if any, value in the initial workup of asymptomatic patients with primary cutaneous melanoma 4 mm or less in thickness. On the other hand, negative results may alleviate patient anxiety. Indications for initial imaging studies and blood work are most appropriately directed based on findings from a thorough medical history and thorough physical examination.

Follow-up examinations

Follow patients to detect asymptomatic metastases and additional primary melanomas.[68] Demonstrate self-examination of skin and lymph nodes. Routine physician examinations are performed at least annually. History and physical examination directs the need for laboratory tests and imaging studies.

An overview of the management of melanoma is shown in the diagram on p. 809.

Table 22-9 Surgical Margins for Excision of Melanoma		
Melanoma—diameter of lesion	**Surgical margins based on histologic depth (Breslow) of lesion**	
	Breslow depth <2.0 mm	Breslow depth 2.0-4.0 mm
Trunk, proximal extremities, <2.0 cm	1.0 cm	2.0 cm
Trunk, proximal extremities, >2.0 cm	1.5 cm	2.0 cm
Head, neck, hands, feet, <3.0 cm	1.5 cm	2.0 cm
Head, neck, hands, feet, >3.0 cm	2.5 cm	2.5 cm
Adapted from Kanzler MH, Mraz-Gernhard S: J Am Acad Dermatol 2001; 45:260.		

Follow-up intervals

Patients with thicker tumors have elevated risk of recurrence in the early years after diagnosis and need to be followed more frequently. Follow-up interval of 1 to 4 times per year, depending on the thickness of the lesion and other risk factors, for 2 years after diagnosis and one to two times per year thereafter is reasonable. Table 22-10 and the diagram below provide a guide for follow-up intervals.

Recurrence may develop after 10 years or more of a patient being disease free. Late recurrence may be local, and survival subsequent to treatment of these metastases is often protracted. Therefore patients with cutaneous melanoma should be observed for life.

Table 22-10 Follow-up Guidelines

Breslow depth (mm)	History and physical examination	Chest radiography (CXR)/laboratory studies*
Stage IA	6 months × 2 years 12 months thereafter	No
Stage I/II 1.0-4.0 mm	4-6 months × 3 years 12 months thereafter	Initial: CXR, optional CBC, LFT Follow-up: Yearly CXR, optional CBC, LDH
Stage I/II >4.0 mm	4-6 months × 3 years 12 months thereafter	Initial: CXR, optional CBC, LFT Follow-up: Yearly CXR, optional CBC, LDH
Stage III/IV	3-4 months × 5 years 12 months thereafter	Initial: CXR and CT scans† Initial: CBC, LFTs Follow-up: q 6-12 mo CXR, LFT

Adapted from Robinson JK: Dermatol Nurs 2000; 12:397.

*LFT are LDH, AST, ALT, and Alk Phos.

†CT scans and blood studies based on physical examination findings.

MANAGEMENT OF MELANOMA

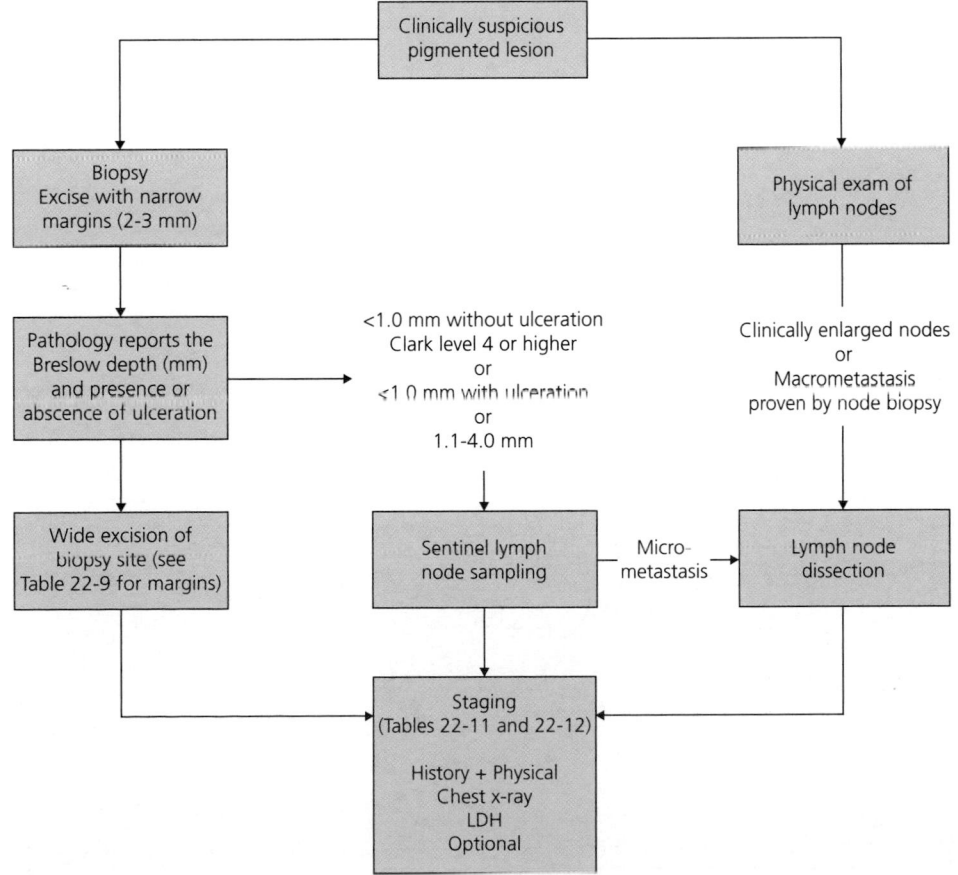

Staging and Prognosis

Melanoma staging system

The staging system for cutaneous melanoma under the auspices of the American Joint Committee on Cancer was revised in 2002.[69,70] Tumor/node/metastasis criteria and stage grouping and prognosis for melanoma were established (Tables 22-11 to 22-13).

Major revisions in the tumor-node-metastasis criteria

1. Melanoma thickness and ulceration, but not level of invasion, is used in the T category (except for T1 melanomas). Clark level is included only in thin primary tumors (<1 mm depth, stages IA and IB) because its prognostic value is minimal in thicker primary melanoma.
2. The number of metastatic lymph nodes rather than their gross dimensions and the delineation of clinically occult (i.e., microscopic) versus clinically apparent (i.e., macroscopic) nodal metastases is used in the N category. Microscopic regional lymph node metastasis is detected by sentinel lymph node biopsy and differentiated from macroscopic nodal metastasis determined by physical examination and surgery.

3. The site of distant metastases and the presence of elevated serum lactic dehydrogenase are used in the M category.
4. An upstaging of all patients with stage I, II, and III disease occurs when a primary melanoma is ulcerated.
5. A merging of satellite metastases around a primary melanoma and in-transit metastases into a single staging entity that is grouped into stage III disease.
6. A new convention for defining clinical and pathologic staging to take into account the staging information gained from intraoperative lymphatic mapping and sentinel node biopsy.

Medical Treatment

Adjuvant high-dose interferon IFN alfa produces increases in relapse-free survival rates and overall survival rates in selected patients. Interferon alfa-2b therapy is used for patients with regional nodal and/or in-transit metastasis and for node-negative patients with primary melanomas deeper than 4 mm. The use of interferon alfa-2b therapy is uncertain in patients with ulcerated intermediate primary tumors (2.01 to 4.0 mm in depth) and inappropriate for node-negative patients with nonulcerated tumors less than 4.0 mm deep.[66] Vaccines and biologic response modifiers show promise in prolonging survival.

Table 22-11 Tumor/Node/Metastasis Classification for Melanoma

T classification		
T1	<1.0 mm	a: without ulceration
T1		b: with ulceration or Clark's level IV or V
T2	1.01-2.0 mm	a: without ulceration
T2		b: with ulceration
T3	2.01-4.0 mm	a: without ulceration
T3		b: with ulceration
T4	>4.0	a: without ulceration
T4		b: with ulceration
N classification		
N1	One lymph node	a: micrometastasis b: macrometastasis
N2	2-3 lymph nodes	a: micrometastasis b: macrometastasis c: in-transit Met(s)/satellites(s) without metastatic lymph nodes
N3	4 or more metastatic lymph nodes, matted lymph nodes, or combinations of in-transit met(s)/satellite(s), or ulcerated melanoma and metastatic nodes(s)	
M classification		
M1a	Distant skin, sub-Q, or lymph node mets	Normal LDH
M1b	Lung mets	Normal LDH
M1c	All other visceral mets Any distant mets	Normal LDH Elevated LDH with any M

From Balch CM: J Clin Oncol 2001; 19:3635.

Table 22-12 Pathologic Stage Grouping

0	Tis	NO	MO
IA	T1a	NO	MO
IB	T1b	NO	MO
	T2a	NO	MO
IIA	T2b	NO	MO
	T3a	NO	MO
IIB	T3b	NO	MO
	T4a	NO	MO
IIC	T4b	NO	MO
IIIA	T1-4a	N1a	MO
	T1-4a	N2a	MO
IIIB	T1-4b	N1a	MO
	T1-4b	N2a	MO
	T1-4a	N1b	MO
	T1-4a	N2b	MO
	T1-4a/b	N2c	MO
IIIC	T1-4b	N1b	MO
	T1-4b	N2b	MO
	Any T	N3	MO
IV	Any T	Any N	Any M

From Balch CM: J Clin Oncol 2001; 19:3635.
Tis, in situ.

Treatment of Lentigo Maligna

Lentigo maligna is found predominantly in areas of actinic damage where cosmetically unsatisfactory scars may result from conventional surgery. Cryosurgery is an efficient alternative to conventional surgery provided that patients are selected properly and extension of cryonecrosis is monitored.[71] Several case reports suggest that lentigo maligna responds to 5% imiquimod cream (Aldara).

Table 22-13 Survival Rates for Melanoma TNM and Staging Categories

Pathologic stage	TNM	Thickness (mm)	Ulceration	No. + nodes	Nodal size	Distant metastasis	1-Year	2-Year	5-Year	10-Year
IA	T1a	1	No	0	—	—	99.7	99.0	95.3	87.9
IB	T1b	1	Yes or level IV, V	0	—	—	99.8	98.7	90.9	83.1
	T2a	1.01-2.0	No	0	—	—	99.5	97.3	89.0	79.2
IIA	T2b	1.01-2.0	Yes	0	—	—	98.2	92.9	77.4	64.4
	T3a	2.01-4.0	No	0	—	—	98.7	94.3	78.7	63.8
IIB	T3b	2.01-4.0	Yes	0	—	—	95.1	84.8	63.0	50.8
	T4a	>4.0	No	0	—	—	94.8	88.6	67.4	53.9
IIC	T4b	>4.0	Yes	0		—	89.9	70.7	45.1	32.3
IIIA	N1a	Any	No	1	Micro	—	95.9	88.0	69.5	63.0
	N2a	Any	No	2-3	Micro	—	93.0	82.7	63.3	56.9
IIIB	N1a	Any	Yes	1	Micro	—	93.3	75.0	52.8	37.8
	N2a	Any	Yes	2-3	Micro	—	92.0	81.0	49.6	35.9
	N1b	Any	No	1	Macro	—	88.5	78.5	59.0	47.7
	N2b	Any	No	2-3	Macro	—	76.8	65.6	46.3	39.2
IIIC	N1b	Any	Yes	1	Macro	—	77.9	54.2	29.0	24.4
	N2b	Any	Yes	2-3	Macro	—	74.3	44.1	24.0	15.0
	N3	Any	Any	4	Micro/macro	—	71.0	49.8	26.7	18.4
IV	M1a	Any	Any	Any	Any	Skin, SQ	59.3	36.7	18.8	15.7
	M1b	Any	Any	Any	Any	Lung	57.0	23.1	6.7	2.5
	M1c	Any	Any	Any	Any	Other visceral	40.6	23.6	9.5	6.0

From Balch CM: J Clin Oncol 2001; 19:3635.

References

1. Cochran AJ, et al: Nevi, other than dysplastic and Spitz nevi, Semin Diagn Pathol 1993; 10:3.

2. Kanzler M, Mraz-Gernhard S: Treatment of primary cutaneous melanoma, JAMA 2001; 285:1819.

3. Connors RC, Ackerman AB: Histologic pseudomalignancies of the skin, Arch Dermatol 1976; 112:1767.

4. Ronnen M, et al: Pseudomelanoma following treatment with surgical excision and intralesional triamcinolone acetonide to prevent keloid formation, Int J Dermatol 1987; 25:533.

5. Park HK, et al: Recurrent melanocytic nevi: clinical and histologic review of 175 cases, J Am Acad Dermatol 1987; 17:285.

6. Bolognia JL, et al: The significance of eccentric foci of hyperpigmentation ("small dark dots") within melanocytic nevi, Arch Dermatol 1994; 130:1013.

7. Jerdan M, et al: Neuroectodermal neoplasms arising in congenital nevi, Am J Dermatopathol 1985; 7:41.

8. Sahin S, et al: Risk of melanoma in medium-sized congenital melanocytic nevi: a follow-up study, J Am Acad Dermatol 1998; 39:428.

9. Kanzler M, Mraz-Gernhard S: Primary cutaneous malignant melanoma and its precursor lesions: diagnostic and therapeutic overview, J Am Acad Dermatol 2001; 45:260.

10. Egan C, et al: Cutaneous melanoma risk and phenotypic changes in large congenital nevi: a follow-up study of 46 patients, J Am Acad Dermatol 1998; 39:923.

10a. De Raeve LE, Roseeuw DI: Curettage of giant congenital melanocytic nevi in neonates: a decade later, Arch Dermatol 2002 138: 943.

11. Schaffer J, et al: Speckled lentiginous nevus: within the spectrum of congenital melanocytic nevi, Arch Dermatol 2001; 137:172.

12. Bart RS, Kopf A: Extensive melanosis and hypertrichosis (Becker's nevus), J Dermatol Surg Oncol 1977; 3:379.

13. Happle R, Koopman R: Becker nevus syndrome, Am J Med Genet 1997; 68:357.

14. Zeff R, et al: The immune response in halo nevi, J Am Acad Dermatol 1997; 37:620.

15. Rapini R: Spitz nevus or melanoma? Semin Cutan Med Surg 1999; 18:56.

16. Granter S, et al: Melanoma associated with blue nevus and melanoma mimicking cellular blue nevus: a clinicopathologic study of 10 cases on the spectrum of so-called 'malignant blue nevus,' Am J Surg Pathol 2001; 25:316.

17. Gupta G, Williams R, Mackie R: The labial melanotic macule: a review of 79 cases. Br J Dermatol 1997; 136:772.

18. Rhodes AR, et al: Risk factors for cutaneous melanoma, JAMA 1987; 258:3146.

19. Newton JA: Familial melanoma, Clin Exp Dermatol 1993; 18:5.

20. Pellegrini AE: The dysplastic nevus syndrome: What is it? Am J Dermatopathol 1982; 4:453.

21. Kraemer KH, et al: Dysplastic nevi and cutaneous melanoma risk (letter), Lancet 1983; 2:1076.

22. Goldstein AM, et al: The inheritance pattern of dysplastic naevi in families of dysplastic naevus patients, Melanoma Res 1993; 3:15.

23. Greene MH, et al: Hereditary melanoma and the dysplastic nevus syndrome: the risk of cancers other than melanoma, J Am Acad Dermatol 1987; 16:792.

24. Marghoob AA, et al: Risk of cutaneous malignant melanoma in patients with "classic" atypical mole syndrome, Arch Dermatol 1994; 130:993.

25. Kang S, et al: Melanoma risk in individuals with clinically atypical nevi, Arch Dermatol 1994; 130:999.

26. Reimer RR, et al: Precursor lesions in familial melanoma, a new genetic preneoplastic syndrome, JAMA 1978; 239:744.

27. Elder DE, et al: Dysplastic nevus syndrome: a phenotypic association of sporadic cutaneous melanoma, Cancer 1980; 46:1787.

28. Happle R, et al: Arguments in favor of a polygenic inheritance of precursor nevi, J Am Acad Dermatol 1982; 6:540.

29. Greene MH, et al: Precursor naevi in cutaneous malignant melanoma: a proposed nomenclature, Lancet 1980; 2:1024.

30. Kousseff BG: The genetics of malignant melanomas, Ann Plast Surg 1992; 28:11.

31. Kraemer KN, et al: Risk of cutaneous melanoma in dysplastic nevus syndrome types A and B, N Engl J Med 1986; 315:1615.

32. Greene MH, et al: Melanoma risk in familial dysplastic nevus syndrome (abstract), J Invest Dermatol 1984; 82:424.

33. Precursors to malignant melanoma, National Institutes of Health Consensus Development Conference Statement, Oct 24-26, 1983, J Am Acad Dermatol 1984; 10:83.

34. Roush GC, et al: Prediction of histologic melanocytic dysplasia from clinical observation, J Am Acad Dermatol 1993; 29:555.

35. Halpern AC, et al: Natural history of dysplastic nevi, J Am Acad Dermatol 1993; 29:51.

36. Crijns MB, et al: On naevi and melanomas in dysplastic naevus syndrome patients, Clin Exp Dermatol 1993; 18:248.

37. NIH Consensus conference: Diagnosis and treatment of early melanoma, JAMA 1992; 268:1314.

38. Hall H, et al: Update on the incidence and mortality from melanoma in the United States, J Am Acad Dermatol 1999; 40:35.

39. Wang S, et al: Ultraviolet A and melanoma: a review, J Am Acad Dermatol 2001;44:837.

40. Stern R: The risk of melanoma in association with long-term exposure to PUVA, J Am Acad Dermatol 2001; 44:755.

41. Cattaruzza M: The relationship between melanoma and continuous or intermittent exposure to uv radiation [record supplied by publisher], Arch Dermatol 2000; 136:773.

42. Bigby M: Sunscreens, nevi, and melanoma revisited, Arch Dermatol 2000; 136:1549.

43. Kittler H, et al: Frequency and characteristics of enlarging common melanocytic nevi, Arch Dermatol 2000; 136:316.

44. Greene M, et al: High risk of malignant melanoma in melanoma-prone families with dysplastic nevi, Ann Intern Med 1985; 102:458.

45. Tucker M, et al: Clinically recognized dysplastic nevi. A central risk factor for cutaneous melanoma, JAMA 1997; 277:1439.

46. Ackerman AB, David KM: A unifying concept of malignant melanoma: biologic aspects, Hum Pathol 1986; 17:438.

47. Koch S, Lange J: Amelanotic melanoma: the great masquerader, J Am Acad Dermatol 2000; 42:731.

48. Weinstock MA, Sober AJ: The risk of progression of lentigo maligna to lentigo maligna melanoma, Br J Dermatol, 1987; 116:303.

49. Koh HK, et al: Lentigo maligna melanoma has no better prognosis than other types of melanoma, J Clin Oncol 1984; 2:994.

50. Dwyer PK, et al: Plantar malignant melanoma in a white caucasian population, Br J Dermatol 1993; 128:115.

51. Sutherland CM, et al: Acral lentiginous melanoma, Am J Surg 1993; 166:64.

52. Scrivner D, et al: Plantar lentiginous melanoma, Cancer 1987; 60:2502.

53. Kenet R, Kenet B: Risk stratification. A practical approach to using epiluminescence microscopy/dermoscopy in melanoma screening, Dermatol Clin 2001; 19:327.

54. Rao B, Wang S, Murphy F: Typical dermoscopic patterns of benign melanocytic nevi, Dermatol Clin 2001; 19:269.

55. Hofmann-Wellenhof R, et al: Dermoscopic classification of atypical melanocytic nevi (Clark nevi), Arch Dermatol 2001; 137:1575.

56. Bahmer F, et al: Terminology in surface microscopy. Consensus meeting of the Committee on Analytical Morphology of the Arbeitsgemeinschaft Dermatologische Forschung, Hamburg, Federal Republic of Germany, Nov. 17, 1989, J Am Acad Dermatol 1990; 23:1159.

57. Argenziano G, et al: Epiluminescence microscopy for the diagnosis of doubtful melanocytic skin lesions. Comparison of the ABCD rule of dermoscopy and a new 7-point checklist based on pattern analysis, Arch Dermatol 1998; 134:1563.

58. Driscoll MS, et al: Does pregnancy influence the prognosis of malignant melanoma? J Am Acad Dermatol 1993; 29:619.

59. Kjems E, Krag C: Melanoma and pregnancy. A review, Acta Oncol 1993; 32:371.

60. Palmer JR, et al: Oral contraceptive use and risk of cutaneous malignant melanoma, Cancer Causes Control 1992; 3:547.

61. Le MG, et al: Oral contraceptive use and risk of cutaneous malignant melanoma in a case-control study of French women, Cancer Causes Control, 1992; 3:199.

62. Koller J, Rettenbacher L: The influence of diagnostic biopsies on the sentinel lymph node detection in cutaneous melanoma, Arch Dermatol 2000; 136:1176.

63. Ming M: The histopathologic misdiagnosis of melanoma: sources and consequences of "false positives" and "false negatives," J Am Acad Dermatol 2000; 43:704.

64. Macht S: Depth of excision of melanomas, JAMA 2001; 286:167.

65. Connelly T: Sentinel lymph node mapping and biopsy in the evaluation of primary melanoma, J Am Acad Dermatol 2001; 44.876.

66. Dubois R, et al: Developing indications for the use of sentinel lymph node biopsy and adjuvant high-dose interferon alfa-2b in melanoma, Arch Dermatol 2001; 137:1217.

67. McMasters K, et al: Sentinel lymph node biopsy for melanoma: controversy despite widespread agreement, J Clin Oncol 2001;19:2851.

68. Chartier T, Bigby M: Rational follow-up recommendations for patients with melanoma, Arch Dermatol 2000; 136:1145.

69. Balch C, et al: Final version of the American Joint Committee on Cancer staging system for cutaneous melanoma, J Clin Oncol 2001; 19:3635.

70. Balch C, et al: Prognostic factors analysis of 17,600 melanoma patients: validation of the American Joint Committee on Cancer melanoma staging system, J Clin Oncol 2001; 19:3622.

71. Bohler-Sommeregger K, et al: Cryosurgery of lentigo maligna, Plast Reconstr Surg 1992; 90:436:

Vascular Tumors and Malformations

❑ **Congenital vascular lesions**
  Hemangiomas of infancy
  Malformations

❑ **Acquired vascular lesions**
  Cherry angioma
  Angiokeratomas
  Venous lake
  Lymphangioma circumscriptum
  Pyogenic granuloma (lobular capillary
    hemangioma)
  Kaposi's sarcoma

❑ **Telangiectasias**
  Spider angioma
  Hereditary hemorrhagic telangiectasia
  Unilateral nevoid telangiectasia syndrome
  Scleroderma
  Generalized essential telangiectasia

Congenital Vascular Lesions

A number of different congenital vascular lesions occur in the skin. Most represent developmental malformations and do not appear to be genetically determined. Vascular structures may be abnormal in size, abnormal in numbers, or both. These varied lesions have been referred to by many terms that have since been abandoned in favor of a simple classification, consisting of two groups, that is based on history and physical examination. The two major categories are hemangiomas and vascular malformations (Table 23-1 and Box 23-1).[1]

Table 23-1 Congenital Vascular Lesions

	Hemangiomas of infancy	Malformations
Occurrence	40% present at birth Most occur in first year of life	99% present at birth
Location	Common on face, any area	Common on limbs, any area

Appearance	Well delineated
	  Red (superficial)
	  Blue (deep)
		Poorly circumscribed

Course	Rapid neonatal growth Slow involution	No change in size Grows in proportion to child No involution
Vessel type	Predominantly arterial	Predominately venous, but any combination of capillary, venous, arterial, and lymphatic components can occur

Histology	Proliferative phase
	  Proliferation of plump endothelial cells
	Involuting phase
	  Fibrosis, fatty infiltration
	  Diminished cellularity, increased number
	    of mast cells
		Normal endothelial turnover
		Normal number of mast cells
		Flattened endothelium

Hemangiomas of infancy

Hemangiomas of infancy are benign neoplasms that result from rapid proliferation of endothelial cells. After an initial proliferating phase, many undergo complete regression with fibrosis. The color depends on its location. Hemangiomas involving the papillary dermis (superficial strawberry hemangiomas) are red; those in the reticular dermis and subcutaneous fat are blue or colorless (deep, cavernous hemangiomas). All have the same vascular components and histopathology. Early hemangiomas are highly cellular, and numerous mast cells are present in the stroma. Lumina are more obvious and larger as the lesion matures. Vascular spaces may have features of capillaries, venules, and arterioles. Progressive interstitial fibrosis occurs during regression. Thrombocytopenic purpura and chronic consumption coagulopathy complicating very large hemangiomas is named Kasabach-Merritt syndrome.

Box 23-1 Congenital Vascular Lesions

Hemangiomas of infancy
    Superficial (strawberry)
    Deep (cavernous)
    Mixed (involves dermis and subcutis)

Malformations
    Salmon patch
    Nevus flammeus
    Syndromes
        Sturge-Weber
        Cobb
        Klippel-Trenaunay-Weber
    Maffucci's

Other arteriovenous malformations

Superficial hemangiomas

Superficial (strawberry) hemangioma may be present at birth but more often appears within the first 2 weeks of life in 1% to 3% of infants; the female-to-male ratio is 3:1. Many children have one, but 15% to 20% have several. Most are small, harmless birthmarks that proliferate for 8 to 18 months and then slowly regress over the next 5 to 8 years, leaving normal or slightly blemished skin. They consist of a collection of dilated vessels in the dermis surrounded by masses of proliferating endothelial cells. These cells are responsible for the unique growth characteristics. The lesions begin as nodular masses or as flat, ill-defined, telangiectatic macules that are mistaken for bruises. Superficial hemangiomas grow rapidly for weeks or months, forming nodular, protuberant, compressible masses of a few millimeters to several centimeters. In rare instances the lesions may almost cover an entire limb. They are bright red with well-defined borders (Figure 23-1).

Figure 23-1 Strawberry hemangioma. A nodular, protuberant mass consisting of dilated vessels in the dermis that undergoes spontaneous involution in more than 90% of the cases.

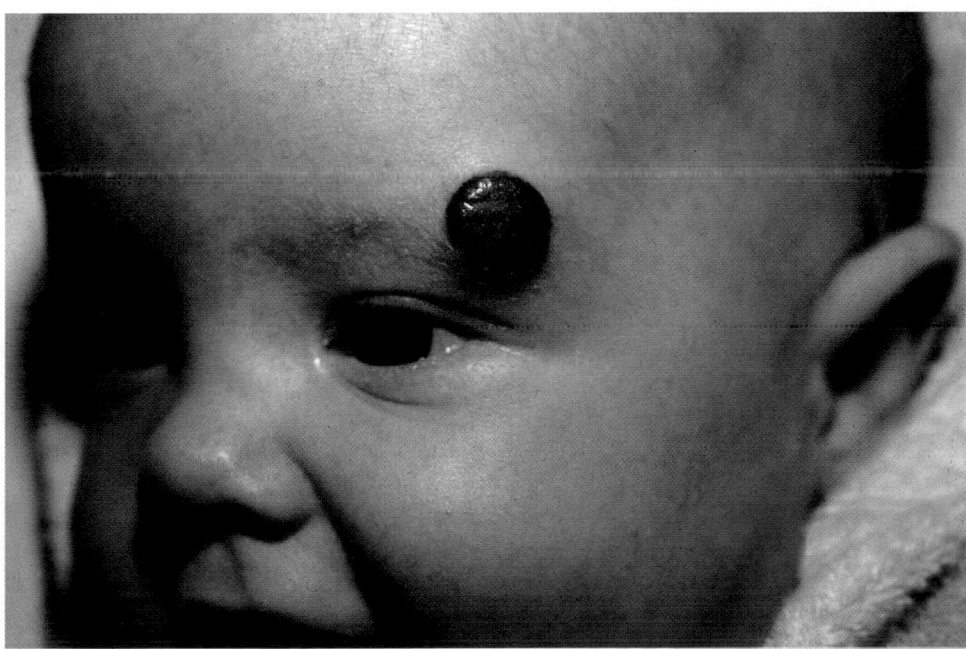

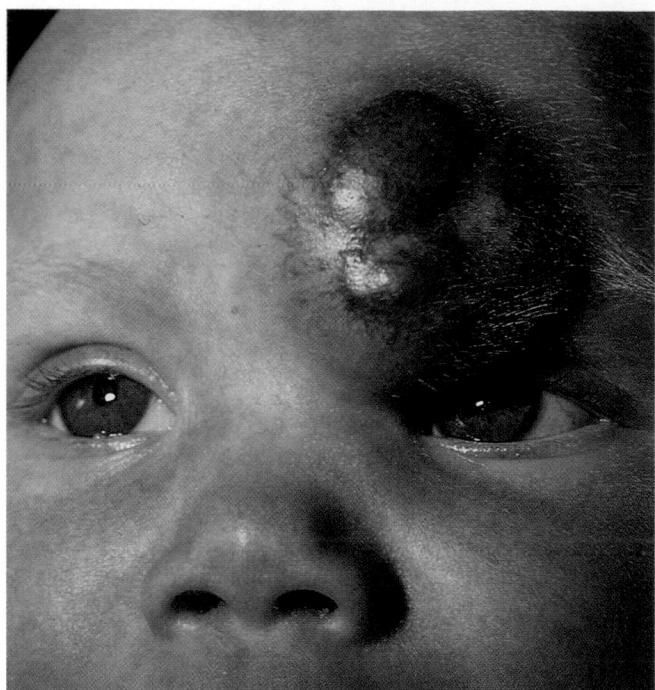

Figure 23-2 Strawberry hemangioma. A rapidly growing mass that is encroaching on the orbit.

Vital structures can be compressed (Figure 23-2), and rapidly growing areas may ulcerate. Larger lesions (>6 cm) ulcerate more frequently.[2]

Hemangiomas may block vision, interfere with feeding or respiration, or obstruct the external auditory canal. Recurrent bleeding may complicate ulceration. Most have a benign course. An inactive phase lasting several months is followed by fibrosis and involution. About 30% resolve by the third birthday, 50% by the fifth, and 70% by the seventh.[3] The mass shrinks and fades in color during the scarring process. Involution begins in most cases by age 3; those present after ages 7 to 9 infrequently undergo further regression. Regression is characterized by normal-appearing skin (approximately 70% of cases) or by atrophy, scarring, telangiectasia, pigmentation changes, and deformity.

MANAGEMENT

Nonintervention. Lesions that are relatively small and indolent should remain untouched if they are to involute spontaneously. In most cases, the result is very satisfactory. Patients should be seen regularly to reassure their parents and to monitor growth (measurements, photographs). Small areas of bleeding and ulceration are treated with cool, wet compresses. Lesions with functional impairment, deep ulceration, or infection need treatment. Facial lesions that pose a cosmetic problem are also considered for treatment. Ultrasound, roentgenography, or magnetic resonance imaging are performed in infants with multiple cutaneous hemangiomas to rule out visceral involvement.

Treating ulcers and rapidly proliferating lesions. Ulceration is the most frequent complication. It usually occurs during the proliferation phase. It is more common in areas of trauma. Ulcerations are painful, may become infected, and heal with scarring. Ulceration is managed with local wound care, topical and systemic antibiotics, systemic and intralesional corticosteroids, flashlamp pulsed-dye laser, interferon alfa-2a, and pain medication.[2,4]

Local wound care. Compresses (saline, Burrow's solution) reduce and absorb exudate and debride. Metronidazole gel or mupirocin ointment treats infection.

Petroleum jelly (Vaseline)-impregnated gauze and barrier creams are used for ulceration around the anus and female genitalia. Occlusive dressings (e.g., polyurethane film dressing) act as a barrier, control pain, and encourage healing.

Infection. Systemic antibiotics (first-generation cephalosporines) are used frequently.

Corticosteroids. Rapidly growing lesions or those that have the potential to interfere with vital structures such as the eyes, auditory canals, and airways or those that threaten permanent disfigurement should be treated initially with prednisone given in divided doses twice a day. The proliferative phase is inhibited and the hemangioma shrinks. Treatment should be maintained until cessation of growth or shrinkage of the hemangioma is accomplished. Most lesions stabilize and markedly regress in 2 to 4 weeks. Prednisone may then be given in a single, early-morning dose tapered on an alternate-day schedule for a few weeks and then discontinued. The pace of tapering depends on several factors (i.e., the age of the infant, the indication for treatment, any toxic effects, and any rebound growth). Administration of oral prednisone or prednisolone (2 to 3 mg/kg per day) given over a mean of 1.8 months before tapering had a response of 84% in stabilizing or shrinking most growing cutaneous hemangiomas.[5]

Because nearly 40% of patients reported rebound with tapering, brief courses of 2 to 3 weeks' duration are probably inadequate. Occasionally, higher doses and longer treatment may be required. A second course of treatment is given for recurrences. Lesions that do not regress by late childhood may be evaluated for surgical excision.

Intralesional steroids. Intralesional steroids (triamcinolone, 10 to 20 mg/mL, with a maximum injection of 3 to 5 mg/kg per procedure) are used for rapidly expanding and ulcerated lesions. Multiple injections into the tumor are used and the procedure may be repeated a few times at 4- to 8-week intervals.[6] Periorbital hemangiomas have been associated with ophthalmic complications in 40% to 80% of cases.[7] Strabismus and amblyopia are the most common. Intralesional steroids are frequently used by the ophthalmologist to treat lesions that do not respond to oral steroids (Box 23-2).[8,9] In most cases, clinical response is noticed within 1 to 3 days. The first change is a blanching of the vascular pattern, followed by a rapid regression in the size of the mass. Involution is most rapid in the first or second week after treatment. Retinal occlusion is a potential risk. Surgery is used for lesions that do not respond to corticosteroids.

Interferon alfa-2b. Interferon alfa-2b (an antiangiogenic protein) is an option for steroid-resistant, organ-interfering and/or life-threatening giant hemangiomas. It slowly halts the growth of hemangiomas and may result in a higher rate of shrinkage than seen with corticosteroids. Subcutaneous injections of 1 to 3 million U/m^2 per day of interferon alfa-2b during the first month and subsequently every 48 to 72 hours, depending on the evolution in each case, were used. Treatment lasts from 3 to 12 months. Volume reduction and remission of their complications occurs. Therapy is generally well tolerated in children. Side effects include fever, neutropenia, and an increase in serum aminotransferase levels and neurotoxicity. Fever and malaise are treated with acetaminophen. The occurrence of spastic diplegia was reported in 5 of 26 children treated with interferon alfa-2a. The neurologic changes improved in two patients but in the remaining 3, paralysis was permanent.[10] Therefore most experts limit the use of interferon alfa to those infants with life-threatening or severely function-threatening hemangiomas that have failed to respond to steroid therapy. Decreased urinary basic fibroblast growth factor (bFGF) levels correlated with hemangioma involution. Patients who receive interferon alfa-2b and prednisone seem to improve faster. Imaging studies and urinary (bFGF) levels are used to monitor treatment response.[11]

Lasers. The vascular specific pulsed dye laser (flashlamp-pumped) is the treatment of choice for superficial cutaneous hemangiomas at sites of potential functional impairment and on the face. The yellow laser light is absorbed by oxyhemoglobin. Short pulses are used so that only targeted vessels are heated without affecting surrounding tissue. Hemangiomas with a deep component do not respond because the effect of the pulsed dye laser (PDL) is limited by its depth of vascular injury (1.2 mm). Even totally superficial capillary hemangiomas that were greater than 3 to 4 mm in thickness respond slowly and incompletely after several treatments.[12]

Early therapeutic intervention may not prevent proliferative growth of the deeper or subcutaneous component of the hemangioma.[13] Guidelines for the recommendation of laser therapy include periorificial location and the potential for functional impairment, ulceration or location over an area of increased risk of ulceration, such as the diaper region, and anatomic areas where there is a concern for cosmetic disfigurement. Consider treatment of facial hemangiomas that do not regress by the school-age years to relieve the social burden on young patients. Pulsed dye lasers are also effective for removing residual telangiectasias associated with regression. At least 75% of patients can achieve 50% lesional lightening. Infants may be more responsive than adults. Generally six treatment sessions are required; further treatments are often beneficial. Lesional reduction can be significant.

Pain is intolerable for infants and young children. Topical or general anesthesia is required. Immediate skin darkening is secondary to an intravascular coagulum. The blackening resolves in a week or two. The safety record is excellent. Scarring, fibrosis atrophy, cutaneous depression, and pigmentary changes develop in about 1% of patients.

There are no age restrictions for pulsed dye laser treatment; even premature infants have safely undergone therapy.[14,15] Superficial coagulation with argon lasers and deeper coagulation with Nd:YAG lasers are associated with significant scarring and generally are not used.

Topical imiquimod. Imiquimod cream was used to treat infantile hemangiomas in the proliferative phase. The cream was applied three times per week for 4 weeks. Because of inflammation with erythema and crusting, a rest period of 2 weeks was given. A marked reduction of inflammation and size was observed. Treatment was restarted and continued for 2 more weeks. Complete regression was noted 4 weeks later.

Surgery. Most hemangiomas are managed medically. Esthetic correction may be delayed until after involution at the age of 8 to 10 years. Some experts recommend early surgery, especially in children with very large or mixed (subcutaneous and cutaneous) head and neck cutaneous or mucosal hemangiomas where irreversible and unaesthetic scars are predictable. Excisional surgery is indicated for small pedunculated hemangiomas and nasal and eyelid lesions that do not respond to other treatments.

Box 23-2 Guidelines for the Use of Intralesional Steroids in Periorbital Hemangiomas

Evaluation

History and physical examination

Computed tomography scan

Avoidance of immunization with live virus vaccines

Short-acting, light, general anesthetics

Pharmacologic agent

Triamcinolone, 10 to 20 mg/mL, with a maximum injection of 3 to 5 mg/kg per procedure

Procedure

Anterior approach to the eyelid is preferred

Multiple injection sites: 0.1 cc aliquot

Aspirate before injecting (27- or 30-gauge needle)

Digital pressure is then applied to avoid hematomas

Repeat up to three times at 8-week intervals or until regression has ceased

Deep hemangiomas

Deep (cavernous) hemangiomas are collections of dilated vessels deep in the dermis and subcutaneous tissue that are present at birth. Apparently localized and superficial venous lesions may coexist with venous ectasias and deep vein anomalies. Clinically they appear as pale, skin-colored, red, or blue masses that are ill defined and rounded (Figure 23-3). Most are asymptomatic. Hyperhidrosis over the lesion is common, and often there are recurrent episodes of thrombophlebitis in or near the lesions. Like superficial hemangiomas, the lesions enlarge for several months, become stationary for an indefinite period, and undergo spontaneous resolution. They are managed like superficial hemangiomas.

KASABACH-MERRITT SYNDROME. Kasabach-Merritt syndrome is a variant of disseminated intravascular coagulation (DIC) in which platelets and clotting factors are locally consumed within a giant hemangioma. This disorder is suspected when children with large hemangiomas present with pallor, petechiae ecchymoses, easy bruising, prolonged bleeding from superficial abrasions, or rapid changes in the size or appearance of the hemangioma. There is thrombocytopenia, microangiopathic hemolytic anemia, and an acute or chronic consumption coagulopathy in association with a rapidly enlarging hemangioma (Figure 23-4).[16] The cause of DIC is not known, but blood is static in the venous sinusoids, and both platelets and contact factors may be activated by the abnormal endothelium. Kasabach-Merritt syndrome occurs most often in young infants during the first few weeks of life, but it may occur in adults.

The majority of hemangiomas are very large and occur on the limbs or trunk. Prednisone 2 to 4 mg/kg/day is indicated when the hemangioma rapidly enlarges and the platelet count drops precipitously. The initial response is often inadequate, and combined steroid/radiation treatment is then indicated. Interferon (IFN)-alpha therapy is added and steroids are tapered if the addition of radiation failed.[17,18]

HEMANGIOMAS ASSOCIATED WITH CONGENITAL ABNORMALITIES. The association of hemangiomas with congenital abnormalities is rare. Most of the vascular lesions associated with congenital malformations and syndromes are malformations, such as the port-wine stain, or other true vascular malformations and are not hemangiomas. A few malformation syndromes have an association with cutaneous hemangiomas. These include PHACE syndrome (posterior fossa brain malformation, multiple hemangiomas, arterial anomalies, coarctation of the aorta, cardiac defects, eye abnormalities); midline abdominal and sternal defects in conjunction with facial hemangiomas; and spinal cord and vertebral abnormalities with sacral hemangiomas. Large facial hemangiomas (occupying at least one quarter to one half of the facial surface) may be linked to the Dandy-Walker malformation (cystic expansion of the fourth ventricle into the posterior cranial fossa) or other posterior fossa brain abnormalities (e.g., hypoplastic cerebellum, posterior fossa arachnoid cyst).[19] Ophthalmologic disorders (choroidal hemangioma, microphthalmos, and strabismus) may also be present. Brain-imaging studies should be performed on all asymptomatic infants with extensive facial hemangiomas to assess for hydrocephalus and fourth-ventricle anomalies.

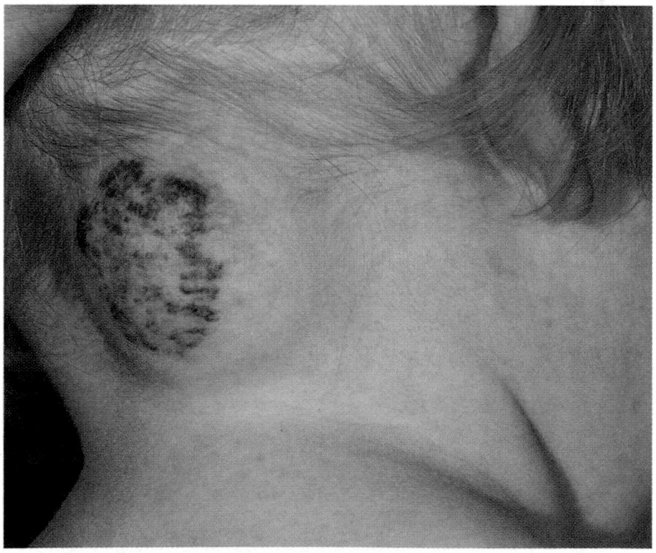

Figure 23-3 Cavernous hemangioma. Cavernous hemangioma is a collection of dilated vessels deep in the dermis and subcutaneous tissue that presents as a pale, skin-colored, red, or blue mass.

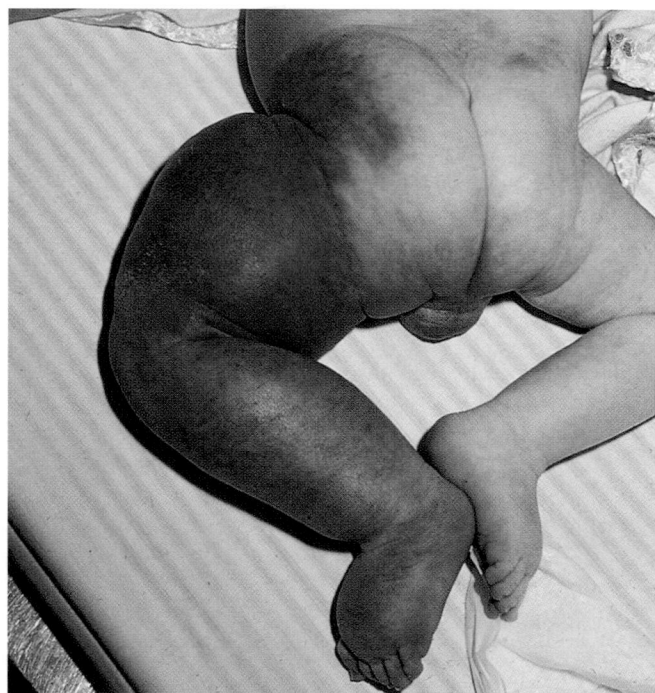

Figure 23-4 Kasabach-Meritt syndrome. Thrombocytopenia, microangiopathic hemolytic anemia, and an acute or chronic consumption coagulopathy occur in association with a rapidly enlarging hemangioma. *(Courtesy Nancy B. Esterly, M.D.)*

Malformations

Vascular malformations are anomalies that result from in-born errors of vascular morphogenesis. They are congenital (present at birth). There is no cellular proliferation in enlarging vascular malformations. They expand with the child's growth because of progressive ectasia resulting from changes in blood or lymphatic flow and pressure.

Nevus flammeus (port-wine stains)

Nevus flammeus are congenital vascular malformations that commonly involve the face and neck of newborns, although lesions have been described in nearly all sites, including mucous membranes. The lesion is a vascular ectasia rather than a proliferative process. It results from progressive vascular dilatation of preexisting blood vessels. There is a decrease in nerve fibers associated with the ectatic blood vessels, and it is postulated that the lesion results from a neural deficiency of sympathetic innervation of the blood vessels.

In most cases these distinctive lesions are developmental anomalies that are not genetically transmitted. They are present at birth in 0.1% to 0.3% of infants. Nevus flammeus are a significant cosmetic problem that does not fade with age. These nevi are usually unilateral; they frequently occur on the face, but they also appear elsewhere (Figure 23-5). They may be a few millimeters in diameter or may cover an entire limb

(Figure 23-6). Size remains stable throughout life. Nevus flammeus appears at birth as flat, irregular, red-to-purple patches. Initially the lesions are smooth, but later they may become papular, simulating a cobblestone surface. Two thirds of all patients develop nodularity or hypertrophy by the fifth decade of life. Unlike the salmon patch, nevus flammeus tends to darken with age. The entire depth of the dermis contains numerous dilated capillaries. Approximately 10% of all patients with facial port-wine stains have glaucoma without leptomeningeal involvement. Ipsilateral glaucoma is frequent when nevus flammeus involves both the ophthalmologic and maxillary divisions of the trigeminal nerve, but it is unlikely when the face is affected in either one of the upper divisions of the fifth cranial nerve or solely below the eye. Dilated conjunctival vessels are common when the lids are involved, but this finding is not correlated with the presence or absence of glaucoma.

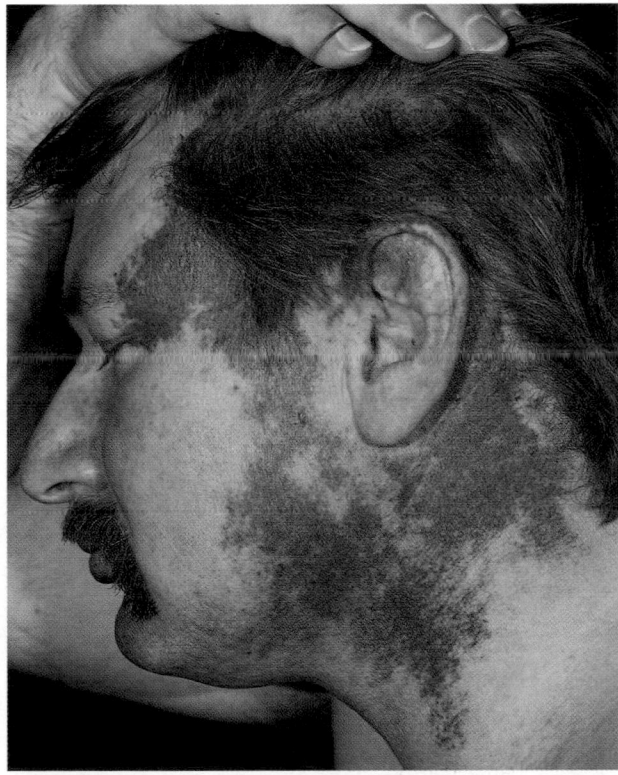

Figure 23-5 Nevus flammeus. An extensive lesion with a relatively smooth surface.

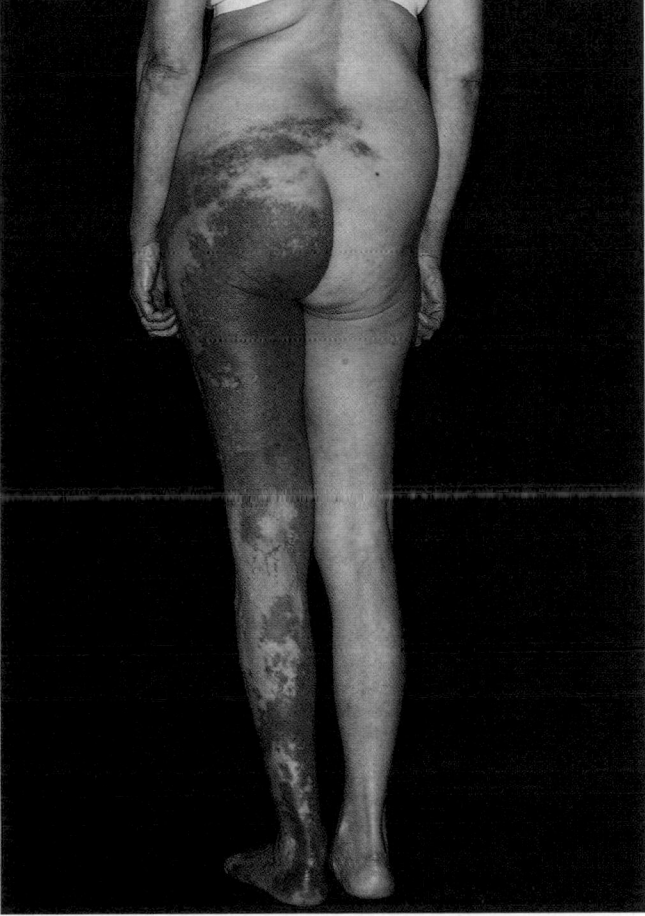

Figure 23-6 Nevus flammeus covering the entire lower limb. The affected limb is 2 inches longer than the normal side.

Table 23-2 Neurocutaneous Syndromes with Vascular Abnormalities

	Cobb syndrome	Sturge-Weber syndrome	Rendu-Osler-Weber syndrome
Synonym	Cutaneomeningo-spinal angiomatosis	Encephalotrigeminal angiomatosis	Hereditary hemorrhagic telangiectasia
Inheritance	Not familial	Dominant partial trisomy or not familial	Autosomal-dominant
Sex distribution	More in males	Equal	Equal
Age of onset	Childhood or adolescence	Two thirds with hemangioma at birth	Childhood
Skin lesion	Port-wine stain or angiokeratomas in dermatomal distribution corresponding within segment or two of area of spinal cord involvement*	Ipsilateral capillary angioma or port-wine stain in distribution of superior and middle branches of the trigeminal nerve*; associated cavernous changes may occur. No consistent relationship between extent of skin lesion and degree of meningeal involvement	Telangiectasia (skin and mucous membranes)*
CNS findings	Arteriovenous or venous angioma of the spinal cord* Neurologic signs of cord compression or anoxia	Angioma of meninges* Intracranial gyriform calcifications Mental retardation (60%)* Epilepsy (usually focal)* Hemiparesis contralateral to skin lesions* Visual impairment (50% have one or more of various eye abnormalities)*	Angiomas in the brain or spinal cord with signs of localized tumor
Associated findings	Angioma of vertebrae Renal angioma Kyphoscoliosis	Renal angioma Coarctation of aorta High, arched palate Abnormally developed ears	Pulmonary arteriovenous anastomoses Hemorrhage from lesions in mouth, GI tract, and GU tract and associated anemia
Diagnostic aids	Lateral spine x-ray film Computed tomography Magnetic resonance imaging	EEG Computed tomography Magnetic resonance imaging	Computed tomography Magnetic resonance imaging
Treatment	Surgical removal of spinal cord angioma if possible	Anticonvulsants Surgical removal of intracranial lesion if possible Cosmetic procedures for skin lesions	Cautery of bleeding lesions

From Jessen T, Thompson S, Smith EB: Arch Dermatol 1977; 113:1582.

CNS, Central nervous system; *GI,* gastrointestinal; *GU,* genitourinary; *EEG,* electroencephalogram.

* Major component of this syndrome.

Fabry-Anderson syndrome	Ataxia telangiectasia	von Hippel-Lindau disease
Angiokeratoma corporis diffusum	Cephalo-oculocutaneous telangiectasia	Angiomatosis retinae et cerebelli syndrome
Recessive trait (X chromosome)	Autosomal recessive	Autosomal dominant
Males tend to full syndrome: Angiokeratomas Extremity pain High blood pressure Cardiomegaly Albuminuria Hypohidrosis	Equal	Equal
Childhood	Childhood	Adult
Small, clustered angiokeratomas (symmetric, mucosal, increased over bony prominences) Palmar mottling	Telangiectasia (increased in sun-exposed areas)* Inelasticity	Port-wine stains in some; most with no cutaneous lesions Café-au-lait spots
Cerebral vascular accidents Neuronal glycolipid deposition (peripheral neuritis)	Progressive cerebellar ataxia (voluntary movements)* Ocular telangiectasia (spread from canthal fold)* Peculiar eye movements (nystagmus, poor control)* Retarded Slow dysarthric speech Decreased tendon reflexes	Cerebellar hemangioblastoma and cyst* Spinal hemangioblastoma (rarely) Retinal hemangiomas (tangle of vessels away from disc)*
Stooped posture Slender limbs; thin, weak muscles Dilated, tortuous conjunctival and retinal vessels Varicose veins and stasis edema Scant facial hair Hypogonadism	Sinopulmonary infections* Hypoplastic or absent thymus Small spleen Retarded growth Malignancies (reticulum cell sarcoma, Hodgkin's disease, lymphosarcoma, gastric carcinoma)	Pheochromocytoma Pancreatic cysts Hepatic angiomas Renal hypernephromas (20%) Polycythema (erythropoietic substance from tumor)
Urinary glycolipids (ceramide trihexoside) Slit lamp Biopsy—renal or marrow (lipid deposits)	Diminished or absent IgA Increased serum alpha-fetoprotein	Hemogram (polycythemia) Urinalysis, excretory urograms Computed tomography Magnetic resonance imaging
Symptomatic	Control infections Plasma infusions (IgA) Thymus transplant Transfer factor	Supportive

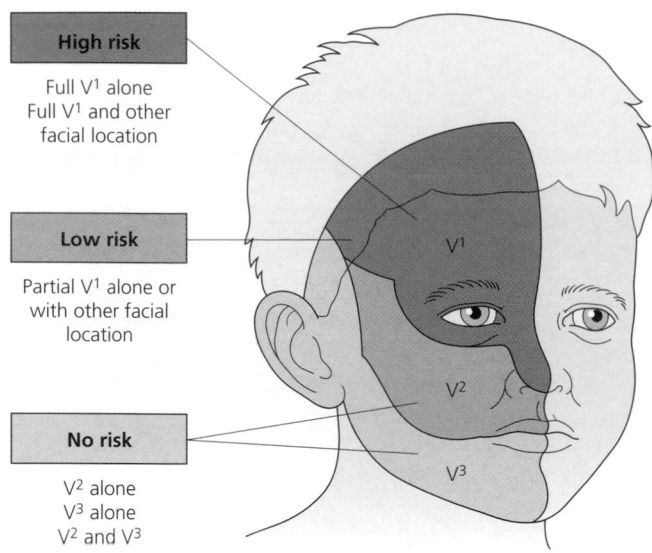

High risk

Full V¹ alone
Full V¹ and other
facial location

Low risk

Partial V¹ alone or
with other facial
location

No risk

V² alone
V³ alone
V² and V³

V¹

V²

V³

Figure 23-7 Facial port-wine stains and risk of Sturge-Weber syndrome. *(Adapted from Enjolvas O, Riche MC, Merland JJ: Pediatrics 76:48, 1985.)*

Box 23-3 Sturge-Weber Syndrome (encephalotrigeminal angiomatosis)

Vascular malformations of the central nervous system and the face (port-wine stain or nevus flammeus) in a V1 trigeminal nerve distribution

Port-wine stain (capillary malformation)

- Involves the ophthalmic branch of the trigeminal nerve, in particular the upper eyelid and supraorbital region
- May extend into the maxillary (V2) and mandibular (V3) regions
- May have associated soft tissue and bony overgrowth
- May be hidden in scalp or mouth
- May be absent in the forme fruste of Sturge-Weber

Leptomeningeal malformation

- Usually ipsilateral to port-wine stain
- Capillary and venous anomalies
- No correlation between the size of facial and CNS malformations
- Characteristic computed tomography/magnetic resonance imaging findings may allow diagnosis in patients before onset of CNS manifestations

CNS manifestations

- Seizures
- Mental retardation
- Contralateral hemiplegia or hemisensory deficits
- Contralateral homonymous hemianopsia (impaired vision in half of the visual field)

Ocular involvement

- Ipsilateral to the port-wine stain
- Can be seen with V1 or V2 involvement
- Glaucoma
- Buphthalmos (enlargement of the ocular globe)
- Vascular malformations of the conjunctiva, episclera, choroid, and retina

From Mirowski GW, et al: J Am Acad Dermatol 1999 41: 772.

SYSTEMIC SYNDROMES. Nevus flammeus may be a component of neurocutaneous syndromes (Table 23-2), such as Sturge-Weber syndrome (nevus flammeus of the trigeminal area) (Figure 23-7) or Klippel-Trenaunay-Weber syndrome. When it occurs over the midline of the back, nevus flammeus may be associated with an underlying spinal cord arteriovenous malformation.

Sturge-Weber syndrome. Sturge-Weber syndrome (Box 23-3) consists of a large facial nevus flammeus in the distribution of the ophthalmologic division of the trigeminal nerve (forehead, eye, and maxillary area) and ipsilateral leptomeningeal angiomatosis (Figures 23-8 and 23-9). Bilateral nevus flammeus occurs in 40% of patients. Epilepsy and mental retardation occur in many patients. Glaucoma, buphthalmos, and blindness are present in 30% to 60% of cases. Patients who do not have nevus flammeus on the areas served by branches V1 and V2 of the trigeminal nerve have no signs or symptoms of eye and/or central nervous system (CNS) involvement (see Figure 23-7). Nevus flammeus of the eyelids, bilateral distribution of the birthmark, and unilateral nevus flammeus involving all three branches of the trigeminal nerve are associated with a significantly higher likelihood of having eye and/or CNS complications. Twenty-four percent of those with bilateral trigeminal nerve nevus flammeus have eye and/or CNS involvement, compared with 6% of those with unilateral lesions. All those who have eye and/or CNS complications have port-wine stain involvement of the eyelids; in 91% both upper and lower eyelids are involved, whereas in 9% only the lower eyelid is involved. None of those with upper eyelid nevus flammeus alone have eye and/or CNS complications.[20] In summary, patients with nevus flammeus of the eyelids, bilateral lesions, and unilateral lesions involving all three divisions of the trigeminal nerve should be studied for glaucoma or for CNS lesions.[20]

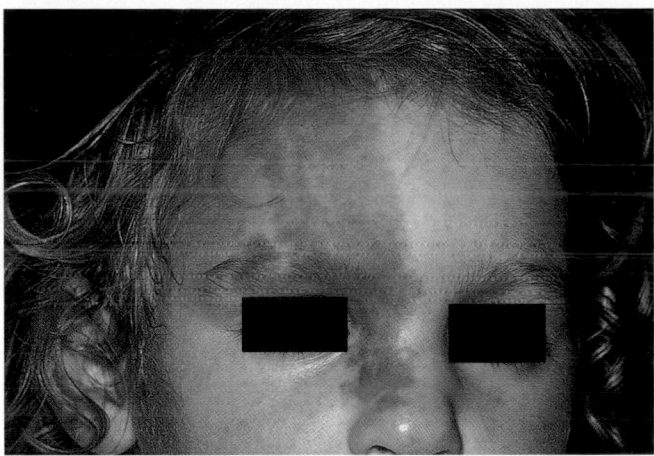

Figure 23-8 Sturge-Weber syndrome. Involvement of the entire V1 area puts the patient at a high risk of having Sturge-Weber syndrome.

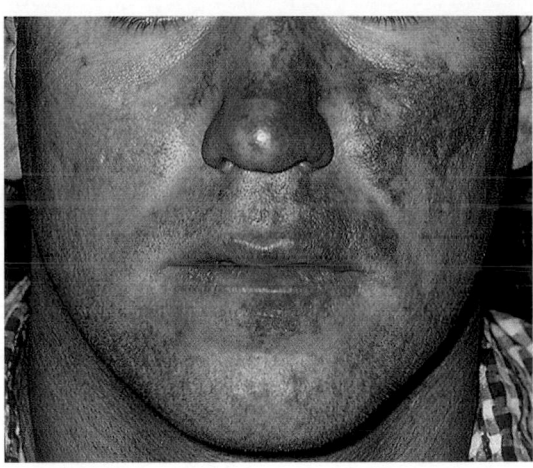

Figure 23-9 Port-wine stain involving V2. There were no CNS or ocular findings of Sturge-Weber syndrome.

Klippel-Trenaunay syndrome. The syndrome is characterized by the triad of capillary and venous malformations, venous varicosity, and hyperplasia of soft tissue—and possibly bone—in the affected area. If in addition there is an arteriovenous fistula, the term *Parkes-Weber syndrome* is used. The lower limb is the most commonly involved area.

TREATMENT. Nevus flammeus have the potential to cause lasting detrimental psychologic effects.

Lasers. Laser therapy is effective for midline lesions in adults and children. Centrofacial lesions and lesions involving maxillary areas in adults and children respond less favorably than lesions located elsewhere on the head and neck.

Individuals are treated as outpatients; patients under 12 years of age usually require some form of sedation or anesthesia, since the procedure is painful and cooperation during the procedure is necessary.

Cosmetics. The cosmetic appearance of some patients with nevus flammeus can be significantly improved by using the tinted waterproof makeup Covermark. Covermark is sold on the Internet (www.covermark.com). Dermablend is a similar product that is generally available in department stores or at www.dermablend.com.

Salmon patches

Salmon patches (stork bite, angel's kiss) are actually variants of nevus flammeus; they are present in approximately 40% to 70% of newborns. They are red, irregular, macular patches resulting from dilation of dermal capillaries. The most common site is on the nape of the neck (Figure 23-10), where the lesion is referred to as a stork bite. They are often inconspicuous and covered by hair. Patches that occur on the glabella and upper eyelids are sometimes mistaken for pressure or forceps clamp marks. Salmon patches on the face fade within a year, but those on the nape may persist for life. Medial nevus flammeus involving sacral skin are also frequent and often persist into adult life.

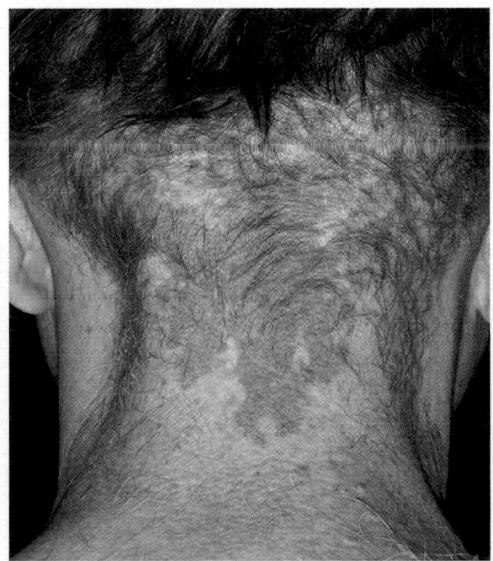

Figure 23-10 Salmon patch (stork bite). A variant of nevus flammeus found in many individuals on the nape of the neck.

Acquired Vascular Lesions

Cherry angioma

The most common vascular malformation is the benign cherry or senile angioma. These 0.5- to 5-mm, smooth, firm, deep red papules (Figure 23-11) occur in virtually everyone after age 30 and numerically increase with age. Patients recognize them as new growths, prompting concerns about malignancy. They are most common on the trunk and vary in number from a few to hundreds. Some pregnant women show an increased number of cherry angiomas during pregnancy that involute in the postpartum period.

Trauma produces slight bleeding. The papules are easily removed by scissor excision or electrodesiccation and curettage.

Angiokeratomas

Angiokeratomas are lesions characterized by dilation of the superficial dermal blood vessels and hyperkeratosis of the overlying epidermis. The term is applied to four different vascular malformations. The most common are angiokeratomas of the scrotum (Fordyce) (Figure 23-12, A) or vulva,[21] characterized by multiple 2- to 3-mm, red-to-purple papules that occasionally bleed with trauma (Fig. 23-12, B). The onset is between the ages of 20 and 50 years. Increased venous pressure may be implicated, such as occurs with pregnancy and hemorrhoids. If desired, removal is performed by simple scissor excision or electrodesiccation and curettage. The other forms of angiokeratomas are rare. They consist of red-brown-black, hyperkeratotic plaques varying in size and distribution. Numerous cutaneous angiokeratomas (angiokeratoma corporis diffusum) are part of Fabry's disease (see Table 23-2).

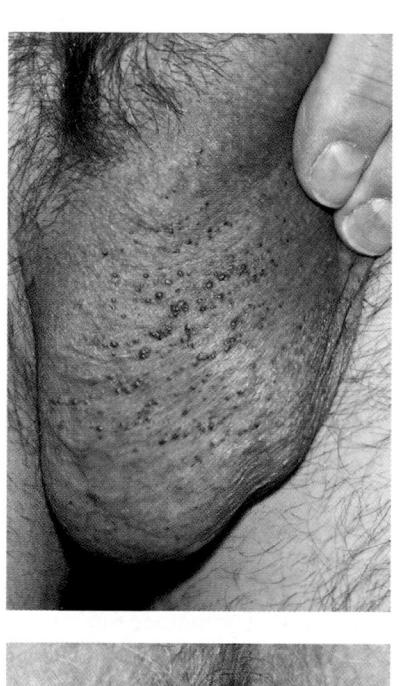

A

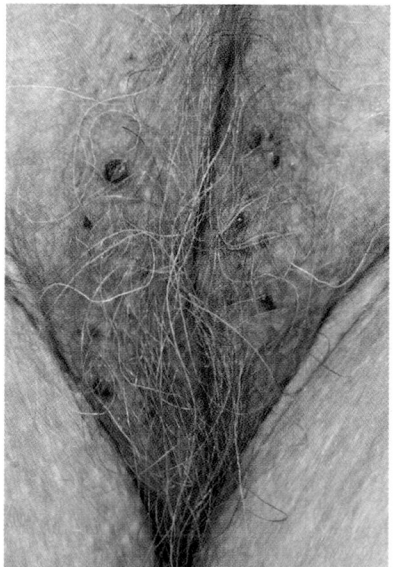

B

Figure 23-11 Cherry angioma. Multiple small, red papules commonly occur on the trunk.

Figure 23-12 Angiokeratomas (Fordyce). Multiple red-to-purple papules consisting of multiple small blood vessels.

Venous lake

Venous lakes are dark blue, slightly elevated, 0.2- to 1-cm, dome-shaped lesions composed of a dilated, blood-filled vascular channel. They are common on sun-exposed surfaces of the vermilion border of the lip (Figure 23-13, A), face and the ears (Figure 23-13, B).[22] Lesions resemble melanoma, but firm compression forces the blood out and proves they are vascular. They occasionally bleed following trauma and can be removed by electrodesiccation or with lasers.

Lymphangioma circumscriptum

These uncommon but distinctive hamartomatous malformations consist of dilated lymph channels, which may be filled with serosanguineous fluid, that communicate with deeper lymph channels. The appearance of the lesions has been compared to a mass of frog's eggs ("frog spawn"). They consist of tiny to 5-mm, grouped, translucent or hemorrhagic vesicles on a dull red or brown base (Figure 23-14). Some lesions contain a mixture of vascular and lymph channels. Lesions may appear in the setting of postmastectomy lymphedema as a result of lymphatic damage following surgery and radiation.[23] This is referred to as secondary lymphangioma (lymphangiectasis).

The malformations consist of a collection of subcutaneous lymphatic cisterns with a thick muscle coat that communicates through dilated channels lined with lymphatic endothelium with the superficial vesicles. There is no communication between the cysts and the adjacent normal lymphatics.[24] The contraction of the muscle coat may force fluid to the surface and create the vesicles. The depth and extent of involvement cannot be adequately estimated from the cutaneous examination. Magnetic resonance imaging has been used to demonstrate accurately the true extent of involvement.[25]

TREATMENT. Treatment is indicated for cosmetic reasons and to prevent leakage of fluid and recurrent infection. The lesions recur unless the deep communicating cisterns are removed or destroyed. Small groups of surface vessels can be destroyed by electrosurgery. Surgical removal of the subcutaneous cisterns, leaving sufficient skin for primary closure, results in acceptable cure rates. Residual skin vesicles separated from their underlying cysts regress.[26] Surface lymphatic vessels are vaporized, and communicating channels to deeper cisterns are sealed with the CO_2 laser,[27] which, unlike the argon laser, is not color dependent for vaporization.

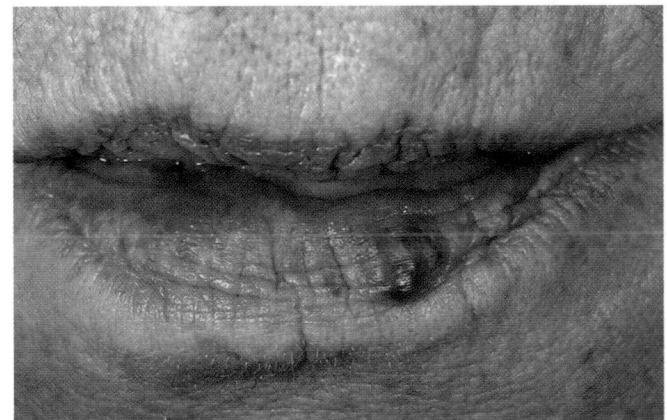

A

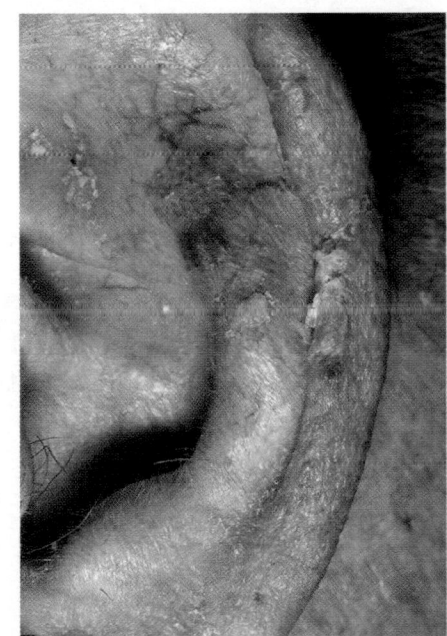

B

Figure 23-13 Venous lake. Dark blue papules caused by dilation of venules found on the vermillion border of the lower lips, ears, neck and face. Several lesions may be present. Compression forces the blood out and flattens the lesion, proving that it is not a melanoma. Actinic damage is probably the cause.

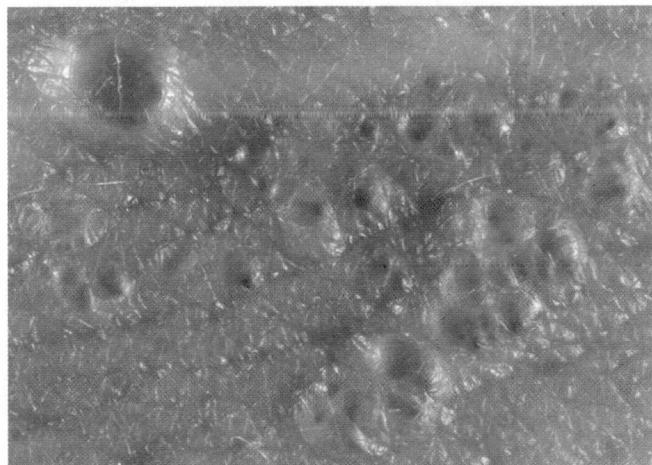

Figure 23-14 Lymphangioma circumscriptum. Dilated lymph channels. Appearance has been compared to a mass of frog's eggs ("frog spawn"). Lesions are filled with clear or blood-tinged fluid.

Pyogenic granuloma (lobular capillary hemangioma)

Pyogenic granuloma is a benign acquired vascular lesion of the skin and mucous membranes that is common in children and young adults.[28] It often appears as a response to a injury or hormonal factors. Pyogenic granuloma may develop in cysts of acne patients treated with isotretinoin. Lesions are small (less than 1 cm), rapidly growing, yellow-to-bright red, dome-shaped (Figures 23-15 and 23-16), fragile protrusions that have a glistening, moist-to-scaly surface.[29] The base of the lesion is often surrounded by a collarette of scale (Figure 23-17). They are most commonly seen on the head and neck region and on the extremities, especially the fingers. Pyogenic granuloma occurs in pregnant women (pregnancy epulis) and is found primarily in the gingiva.[30] The word epulis is used to describe a localized growth on the gingiva.

The slightest trauma causes bleeding that is difficult to control. The dermis is composed of a mass of capillaries. Pyogenic suggests an infectious origin, but the lesion is neither a hemangioma nor a neoplasm. It is an inflammatory and hyperplastic condition, better interpreted as a florid expression of granulation tissue proliferation. Pyogenic granuloma-like lesions occur in patients with acquired immunodeficiency syndrome (AIDS) who develop cat-scratch disease (bacillary angiomatosis).

TREATMENT. Treatment consists of firm and thorough curettage of the base and border. Electrodesiccation is often necessary to eradicate the lesions completely and to control bleeding. Pyogenic granuloma recurs if the smallest piece of abnormal tissue remains.[31] Multiple recurrent lesions are more common in adolescents or young adults, and they occur after attempts of electrodesiccation or surgical removal of the primary single lesion.[31a] Spontaneous resolution usually occurs within 6 months. Pregnancy epulis usually regresses following childbirth.

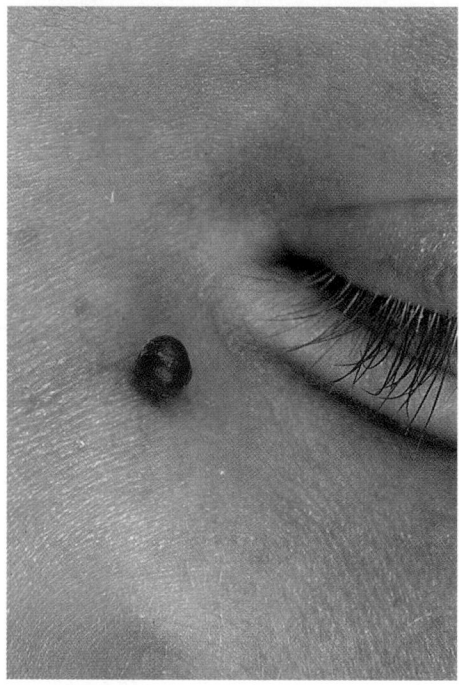

Figure 23-16 Pyogenic granuloma. Most lesions are small. The major complaint is profuse and prolonged bleeding.

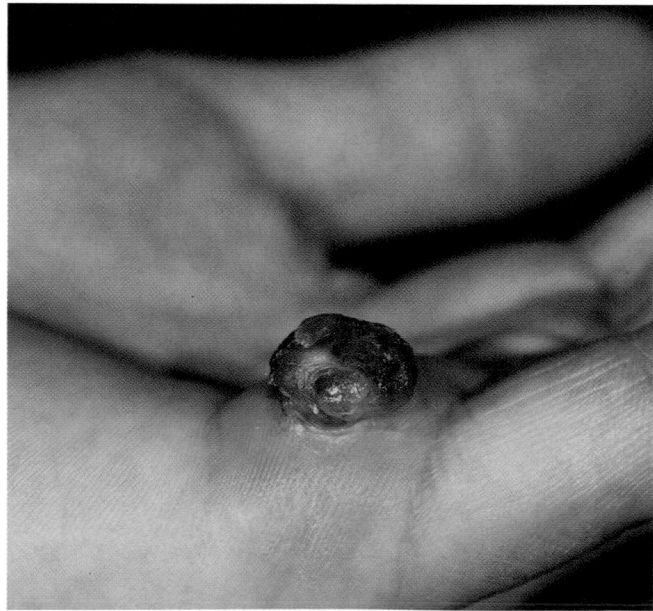

Figure 23-15 Pyogenic granuloma. A dome-shaped tumor with a moist, fragile surface. The lesion may bleed profusely with the slightest trauma.

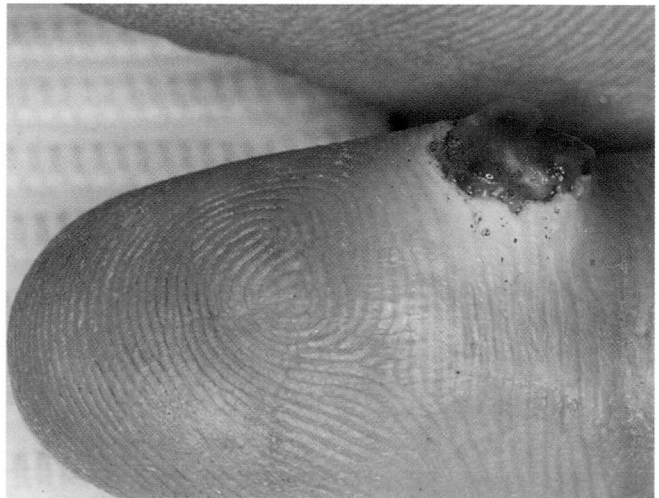

Figure 23-17 Side view of a pyogenic granuloma demonstrating the white collarette of scale often observed at the base.

Bacillary angiomatosis

Bacillary angiomatosis is an infectious disease caused by two species of Bartonella: *B. quintana* and *B. henselae*. Cats may serve as a reservoir of the disease in some patients. A cat scratch or bite may transmit the bacteria. The disease affects 1 to 2 per 1000 AIDS patients, but a few cases are reported in immunocompetent patients.[32]

Bacillary angiomatosis may involve skin, internal organs, or both and may be accompanied by systemic symptoms.

Skin lesions may be solitary or multiple, and some patients have a widespread eruption with innumerable lesions. The lesions begin as red to purple pinpoint-size papules that increase in size to form nodules and tumors. Superficial lesions resemble pyogenic granuloma; deeper lesions appear as red subcutaneous nodules that may enlarge to several centimeters in diameter. Involvement of the oral and genital mucous membranes is also frequent.

Blood, skin, or visceral cultures confirm the infection. Organisms are demonstrated in tissue with the Warthin-Starry stain. Most patients have advanced AIDS with CD4+ lymphocytic counts of less than 200 cells/mm³. Histologically there is a capillary proliferation. The presence of neutrophils and leukocytoclastic debris supports the diagnosis. Masses of bacteria appear as aggregates of granular, purple material with hematoxylin-eosin stain. The aggregates are also demonstrated with the Warthin-Starry stain. Bacillary angiomatosis responds to oral erythromycin or tetracycline, although repeat courses may be necessary because the disease has a tendency to relapse.

Kaposi's sarcoma

Kaposi's sarcoma (KS), or multiple idiopathic hemorrhagic sarcomas, are vascular neoplasms that were rarely seen before the AIDS era. Kaposi's sarcoma can be divided into four subsets on the basis of clinical and epidemiologic criteria (Table 23-3).[33] The incidence of second malignancies (especially lymphoreticular neoplasms) is increased in classic Kaposi's sarcoma and in Kaposi's sarcoma patients with AIDS. Classic and AIDS-associated Kaposi's sarcoma may be caused by a new herpes virus.[34]

PATHOGENESIS. Human herpes virus 8 in the presence of host immunosuppression is the primary factor in the development of all forms of Kaposi's sarcoma. The pathogenesis of AIDS-related KS involves human herpes virus type 8, altered expression and response to cytokines, and stimulation of KS growth by the HIV-1 transactivating protein Tat. Tat promotes the growth of spindle cells of endothelial origin only in the presence of inflammatory cytokines. Serologic studies show that, unlike other human herpes viruses, Kaposi's sarcoma associated herpes virus is not ubiquitous. Like other human herpes viruses, most primary infections appear to be asymptomatic. The virus can be transmitted sexually and by other means. The virus has been found in saliva and semen of infected persons. The highest rates of infection are in Central Africa. Homosexual men, regardless of their HIV serostatus, have an asymptomatic infection rate of almost 40%.

Table 23-3 Clinical Features of Kaposi's Sarcoma

	Classic	African cutaneous	African lymphadenopathic	AIDS	Immunosuppressive
Epidemiology	Sporadic (endemic)	Endemic	Endemic	Endemic	Sporadic
Age (years)	50-70	<10, >20	<10	25-42	20-80
Mean age	68	35	<10	35	—
M:F ratio	3:1	10-15:1	1-2:1	Male, homosexual	10-1.7:1
Incidence	0.02	—	0.1-0.85*†	40%-70%, up to 90%	—
% Cancers diagnosed	0.06	—	9%	—	—
Sites	Legs, feet	Extremities	Nodes	Head, neck, upper aspect of trunk	Variable
Lesion type	Nodular	Nodular, florid, infiltrating	Lymphadenopathic	Macules, plaques, nodules	Nodules
Node involvement	Rare	Uncommon, indolent	Expected	Common	Variable
Course	Indolent	Locally aggressive	Aggressive	Fulminant	Fulminant
Treatment response	Good	Good	Good initially	Poor	Variable

From Piette WW: J Am Acad Dermatol 1987; 16:855.
* Cases/100,000 population
† Representative incidence figures from Tanzania.

CLASSIC KAPOSI'S SARCOMA. The rare classic form generally appears on the hands, feet, or lower legs and progresses up the arms and legs. It begins as violaceous macules and papules and very slowly progresses to form plaques with multiple red-purple nodules (Figure 23-18). It occurs almost exclusively in elderly males of Jewish, Greek, or Italian descent. The male to female ratio is 15 to 1. Progression of this disease in the elderly is slow (years or decades) and, although lymph node and visceral involvement can occur, most of these patients die of unrelated causes. Immunocompetent asymptomatic patients with little progression can simply be observed. Excision or intralesional injection interferon alfa-2b (1 million to 3 million U) is effective for single lesions. Single dose radiation is effective for patients with a few lesions. A course of wide area radiotherapy is effective for extensive disease. Patients with extensive or recurrent disease can also be treated with chemotherapy or a combination of surgery, chemotherapy, and radiation.

ENDEMIC AFRICAN KAPOSI'S SARCOMA. Kaposi's sarcoma in HIV-negative and HIV-positive patients is the most frequently occurring tumor in central Africa. It accounts for up to 50% of tumors reported in men in some countries. There are two forms: the cutaneous and the lymphatic. Both are rare in patients between 10 and 20 years of age. The cutaneous form typically occurs in men (median age, 41 years) with indolent disease and nodules or plaques on edematous limbs. Lymph node or systemic involvement is uncommon. The aggressive lymphadenopathic form is seen in children younger than 10 years of age. In eastern and southern Africa, Kaposi's sarcoma makes up 25% to 50% of soft-tissue sarcomas in children and 2% to 10% of all cancers in children. Cutaneous lesions may surface; the prognosis is poor.[35] Endemic Kaposi's sarcoma responds to local radiation therapy or chemotherapy.[36] Complete (32%) and partial (54%) regression of cutaneous lesions was achieved with radiation therapy, which is the treatment of choice for this disease.[37]

KAPOSI'S SARCOMA ASSOCIATED WITH IMMUNO-SUPPRESSION. Kaposi's sarcoma develops in 0.1% to 5.3% of transplant recipients (especially in certain ethnic groups), 67% to 80% are men. The median interval from organ transplantation to the diagnosis of Kaposi's sarcoma is 30 months. A primary herpes 8 infection transmitted by the transplanted organs is a possible source. This type of Kaposi's sarcoma is aggressive, involving lymph nodes, mucosa, and visceral organs in about half of patients, sometimes in the absence of skin lesions. Some tumors regressed after therapy was withdrawn,[38] and others responded to radiation and chemotherapy.

EPIDEMIC OR AIDS-RELATED KAPOSI'S SYNDROME. The incidence of Kaposi's sarcoma in American men with AIDS decreased from 40% in 1981 to less than 20% in 1992. It is the most common tumor that occurs in patients infected with the human immunodeficiency virus. KS occurs in roughly 20% of HIV-infected homosexual men, 3% of heterosexual intravenous drug users, 3% of transfusion recipients, 3% of women or children, and 1% of hemophiliacs.

Kaposi's syndrome probably occurs as a multicentric rather than a metastatic disease in AIDS. Unlike the classic form, lesions are often multifocal and widespread when first detected. They are most commonly found on the trunk and the head and neck areas. Mucous membranes are involved.[39] They initially form slightly raised, oval or elongated, poorly demarcated, rust-colored infiltrates. Rapid progression to red or purple nodules and plaques may follow (Figure 23-19 and see Figures 11-33 to 11-36). They may look like granulation tissue, stasis dermatitis, pyogenic granuloma, or capil-

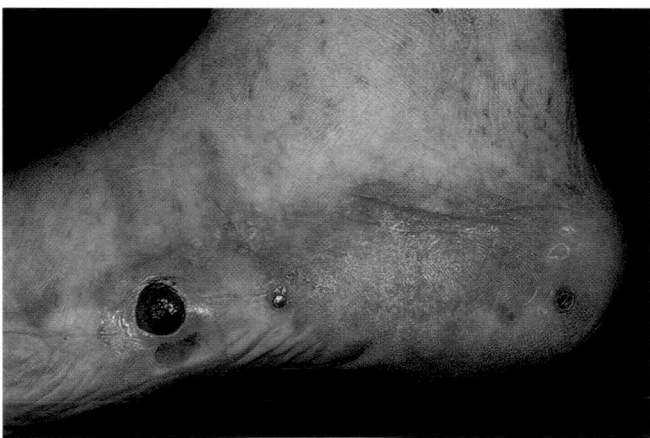

Figure 23-18 Kaposi's sarcoma. Most lesions are on the lower extremities. Here there are plaques and tumors.

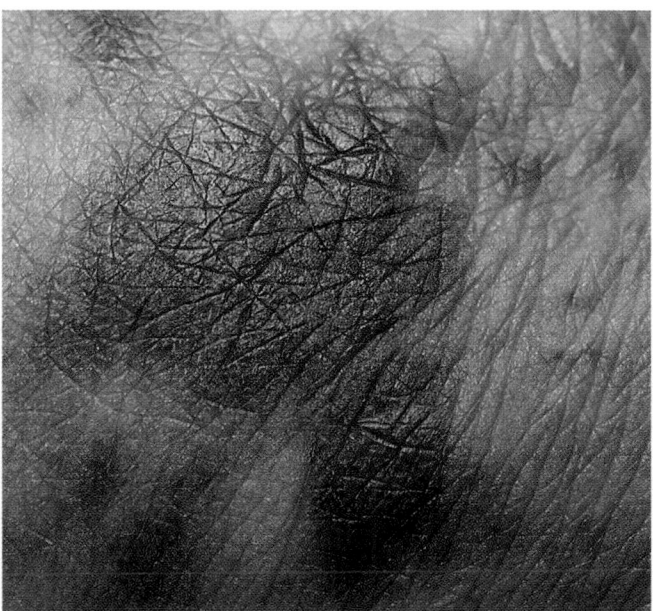

Figure 23-19 Kaposi's sarcoma. Early lesion consisting of violaceous macules and plaques.

lary hemangiomas.[40] More than half of the patients have generalized lymphadenopathy at the time of first examination. Eventually most patients develop extracutaneous disease (oral cavity, gastrointestinal [GI] tract, lungs, and lymph nodes) (see Chapter 11). It is important to treat cutaneous lesions for cosmetic purposes, because their presence is a constant reminder of a fatal disease. Limited cutaneous disease is treated with alitretinoin gel (Panretin),[41] intralesional vinblastine, radiation therapy,[42] laser therapy, or cryotherapy. Antiretroviral therapy helps resolve immunosuppression and slows progression or shrinks Kaposi's sarcoma. The response is unpredictable and other treatments are required. The response to radiation therapy and chemotherapy is less than in classic Kaposi's sarcoma.

TREATMENT. The goals are palliation of symptoms; shrinkage of tumors to alleviate edema, organ compromise, or psychological stress; and prevention of disease progression. Local and systemic therapies are used. Observation is appropriate for immunocompetent asymptomatic patients with little progression of disease over a long period. In some cases the disease regresses spontaneously.[34,43]

HAART. Highly active anti-HIV therapy or HAART can be used as first-line of therapy for KS. Anti-retrovirals are associated with a decreased proportion of new AIDS-KS cases and regression in the size of existing KS lesions. Regression and resolution of cutaneous and visceral lesions have been reported. HAART prolongs the time to treatment failure of anti-KS therapies.

Surgery. Excision is appropriate for single lesions and resectable recurrences.

Liquid nitrogen cryotherapy. Liquid nitrogen cryotherapy is easily applied as a primary therapy. A complete response is observed in 80% of treated Kaposi's sarcoma lesions. There is often persistent Kaposi's sarcoma in the deeper dermis under the treated site, but the cosmetic effect is excellent. Patients receive an average of three treatments per lesion. Treatment is repeated at 3-week intervals, allowing adequate healing time. One treatment consisted of two freeze-thaw cycles, with thaw times ranging from 11 to 60 seconds per cycle (range, 10 to 20 seconds for macular lesions and 30 to 60 seconds for papular lesions).[44] Treatment is well tolerated. Blistering occurs frequently, but pain is limited. Secondary infection does not occur. Keep treated lesions covered until they heal, because blister fluid may contain HIV.

Intralesional chemotherapy. Intralesional chemotherapy is more effective than cryotherapy for nodular lesions greater than 1 cm in diameter. It is also useful for the treatment of symptomatic oral lesions. Postinflammatory hyperpigmentation may respond to cryotherapy or may be camouflaged with cosmetics. Vinblastine is prepared from stock solutions to the desired concentration. Vinblastine-containing syringes can be stored under refrigeration after preparation. Vinblastine 0.1 mg (0.5 ml of a 0.2 mg/ml solution) is injected per square centimeter of lesion. Oral lesions and larger cutaneous lesions respond best to 0.2 mg/cm². In this setting, increasing the concentration of vinblastine to 0.4 to 0.6 mg/ml is recommended to reduce the volume injected per square centimeter of lesion to 0.5 ml. A maximum total dose of 2 mg during clinic visits is recommended. After a healing interval of 3 weeks, each treated lesion may require an additional 1 to 2 injections for maximal response.[45] Pain lasts for 1 to 2 days. Local anesthesia does not reduce the efficacy of treatment or the pain experienced by the patient.

Topical retinoids. Alitretinoin (Panretin) used for 12 to 16 weeks produced a response rate of 36%. Alitretinoin gel may be used for KS, which is not severe enough to use systemic chemotherapy and for patients who have received systemic chemotherapy and want to treat lesions that remain.[41]

Alitretinoin is not indicated when systemic anti-KS therapy is required (e.g., in patients with more than 10 cutaneous lesions in the prior month, symptomatic lymphedema, symptomatic pulmonary KS, or symptomatic visceral involvement).

Radiation therapy. Radiation therapy was the primary form of local therapy for Kaposi's sarcoma before the AIDS epidemic. Response rates of greater than 80% were achieved.[46] Radiation therapy is indicated for large tumor masses, especially those that interfere with normal function. Patients with a few lesions in a limited area respond well to single doses of radiation (8 to 12 Gy). Megavoltage electrons, supervoltage photons, and whole-body-surface electron-beam therapy have all produced excellent responses.[47,48]

Cytotoxic therapy. Immunosuppressive medications favor proliferation of KS. Therefore systemic chemotherapy should be reserved for patients with extensive disease that has already failed to respond to antiretroviral therapy.[49] Cytotoxic therapy is considered for rapidly progressive disease (10 or more new cutaneous lesions/month), lymphedema, pulmonary KS, and widespread symptomatic visceral disease. The Klein regimen of weekly outpatient intravenous vinblastine (4 to 6 mg) is one of the first lines of treatment. Doxorubicin, bleomycin, vincristine, and other drugs have been used.[50]

Interferon. Subcutaneous, intravenous, or intralesional interferon alfa all resulted in remissions, but the high doses required lead to an impaired quality of life.[51]

Telangiectasias

Telangiectasias are permanently dilated, small blood vessels consisting of venules, capillaries, or arterioles. The maximum diameter is 1 mm. Vessels appear as single strands, in groups as small macules, or with a central punctum. They accompany a variety of diseases and sometimes are clues to the underlying diagnosis (Box 23-4). Telangiectasias are usually only a cosmetic problem; they rarely bleed.

Spider angioma

Spider angiomas (nevus araneus) form as arterioles (spider bodies), become more prominent near the surface of the skin, and radiate capillaries (spider legs) (Figures 23-20 and 23-21). They are present in 10% to 15% of normal adults and young children. Once formed, they tend to be permanent. Bleeding rarely occurs. The face, neck, upper part of the trunk, and arm are involved in adults. In children they are most often seen on the hands and fingers. They increase in number with liver disease and during pregnancy and are probably stimulated by higher-than-normal estrogen concentrations. Lesions usually disappear at the end of the pregnancy. Spider angiomas should be distinguished from the flat patches of tiny vessels of uniform size (telangiectatic mats) seen in scleroderma.

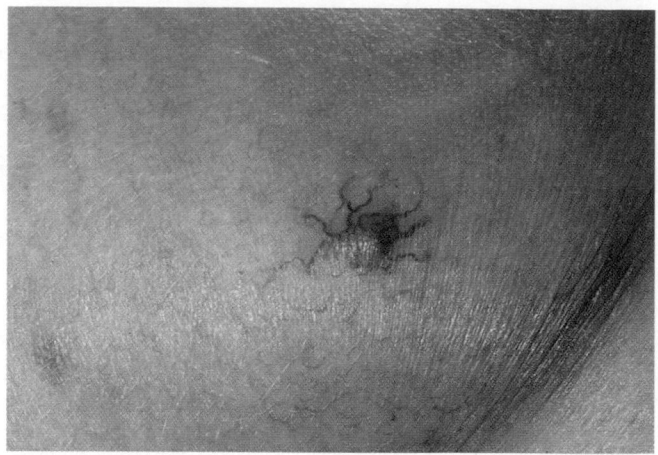

Figure 23-20 Spider angioma. Lesions appear in 10% to 15% of children and adults. Most patients have one or two lesions. They are found most commonly on the face, upper part of the trunk, and backs of the hands. Lesions may occur during pregnancy and resolve months after delivery. Suspect liver disease in patients with many lesions.

Box 23-4 Classification of Telangiectasia

Primary (cause unkown)

Ataxia telangiectasia
Generalized essential telangiectasia
Hemorrhagic hereditary telangiectasia (Rendu-Osler-Weber syndrome)
Spider angiomas
Unilateral nevoid telangiectasia syndrome

Secondary (part of known entity)

Actinically damaged skin
After laser or electrosurgery
After cryosurgery
Basal cell carcinoma
Collagen vascular disease
    Dermatomyositis
    Lupus erythematosus
    Scleroderma
Cushing's syndrome
Estrogen excess
    Cirrhosis
    Oral contraceptives
    Pregnancy
Metastatic carcinoma
Necrobiosis lipoidica diabeticorum
Poikilodermas
Pseudoxanthoma elasticum
Radiation therapy injury
Rosacea
Telangiectasia macularis eruptiva perstans (generalized cutaneous mastocytosis)
Topical steroid induced
Xeroderma pigmentosa

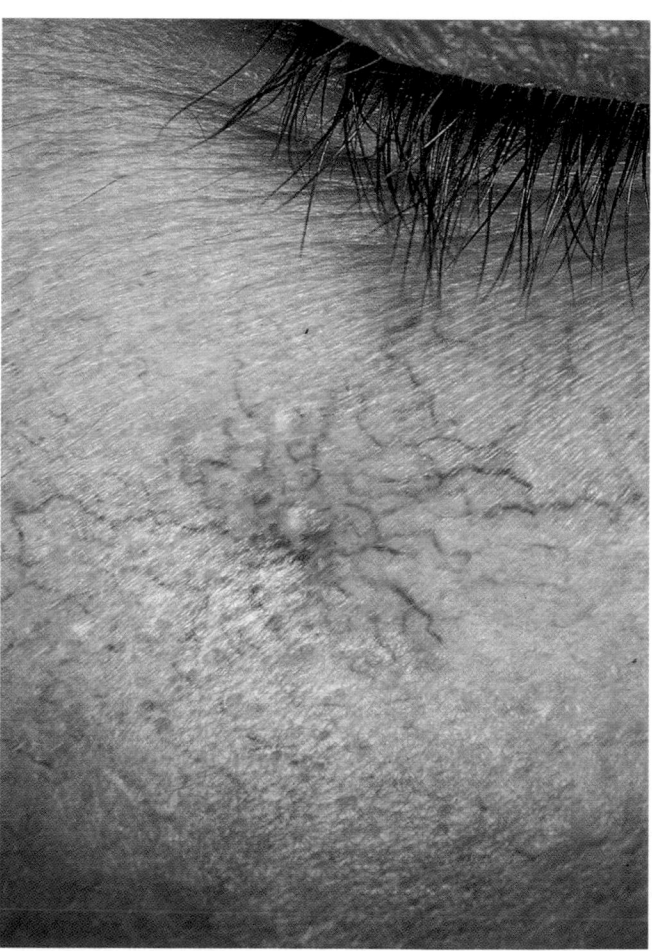

Figure 23-21 Spider angioma. Well-defined, dilated vessels radiate from a central point.

TREATMENT. Local anesthesia is optional in the following procedure for treatment. The blood is forced out of the spider by pressing firmly on the lesion; with continuous pressure, the finger is moved slightly to one side to expose the central arteriole, and the central arteriole is gently electrodesiccated. If the arteriole has been destroyed, the radiating capillaries may not fill. Incompletely destroyed lesions may recur. Vigorous desiccation may cause a pitted scar. Recurrences are uncommon. Lasers are also effective.

Hereditary hemorrhagic telangiectasia

Hereditary hemorrhagic telangiectasia (HHT) (Osler-Weber-Rendu disease) is an autosomal dominant disease[52] characterized by epistaxis, cutaneous telangiectases, and visceral arteriovenous malformations that affect many organs.[53,54] The characteristic lesions begin as tiny, flat telangiectasias, with a few vessels radiating from a single point. Arterioles in the dermis become dilated and communicate directly with the venules without intervening capillaries. Engorged lesions are fragile and bleed easily with the slightest trauma. Few to numerous lesions occur primarily on the lips, tongue (Figure 23-22), nasal mucosa, forearms, hands, fingers, palms and soles, under the nails, and throughout the gastrointestinal tract, but any skin area or internal organ may be involved. Epistaxis is the most common manifestation. It may require multiple transfusions and oral iron. Recurrent epistaxis begins by the age of 10 years and becomes more severe in later decades. Although lesions may be prominent during childhood, they are most often so small and subtle that stretching the lip is required to accentuate them. By the third or fourth decade, telangiectasias become more apparent, and the diagnosis is easily made. HHT is the most common cause of pulmonary arteriovenous fistula; 5% to 15% of persons with HHT have pulmonary arteriovenous malformations. High-resolution helical computed tomographic scanning without the use of contrast material demonstrates the vessels. Chest radiography, arterial-blood gas measurements, and finger oximetry are screening test for suspected pulmonary arteriovenous malformations. Most lesions occur near the bases of the lungs.

The distribution and clinical appearance of the telangiectasia in the CREST syndrome (calcinosis, Raynaud's phenomenon, esophageal involvement, sclerodactyly, telangiectasia) and HHT are very similar.[55]

Recurrent bleeding from nasal or gastrointestinal telangiectasia is fatal in a small number of cases. GI bleeding usually starts in the fifth or sixth decade.

TREATMENT. Bleeding points are treated by electrocautery. Local hyperfibrinolysis has been demonstrated in lesions mediated by an increase in tissue plasminogen activator. This finding provides a basis for the use of antifibrinolytic drugs. Epistaxis improved and hemoglobin levels increased with tranexamic acid (1 g four times daily), an antifibrinolytic drug that is 10 times as potent as aminocaproic acid and has a longer half-life.[56] Intranasal tranexamic acid is also effective.[57]

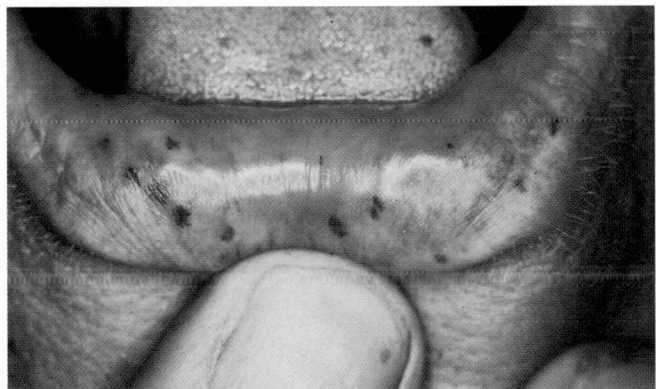

Figure 23-22 Hereditary hemorrhagic telangiectasia. Telangiectases are found on the lips, oral mucosa, nasal mucosa, skin, and conjunctiva. Epistaxis is the most common manifestation of the disease. Blood transfusions may be required.

Unilateral nevoid telangiectasia syndrome

Numerous threadlike telangiectasias that appear in a unilateral dermatomal distribution are called unilateral superficial telangiectasias. There are acquired and congenital forms. The congenital form is more common in males. The acquired form begins with states of increasing estrogen blood levels: (1) at puberty in females, (2) during pregnancy (Figure 23-23), or (3) with alcoholic cirrhosis. In subsequent pregnancies the syndrome recurs once it has appeared, although it may appear for the first time during a second pregnancy.[58,59] Most cases involve the trigeminal, C3, C4, or adjacent dermatomes. The distribution suggests an estrogen-sensitive nevoid anomaly.[60] Telangiectases may involve the oral and gastric mucosa. Lesions may clear as levels of estrogen decrease.

Pulsed dye laser, 585 nm, is effective treatment, but the response is short-lived, with a 100% recurrence.

Scleroderma

The telangiectasias of CREST syndrome and scleroderma have a unique morphology. They occur as flat (macular), 0.5-cm, rectangular collections of uniform tiny vessels; these are the so-called telangiectatic mats (see Figure 17-18). These mats are most commonly found on the face, lips, palms, and backs of the hands. Telangiectasias may be present around the lips, tongue, and mucous membranes. Involvement of the oral mucosa also suggests Rendu-Osler-Weber disease.

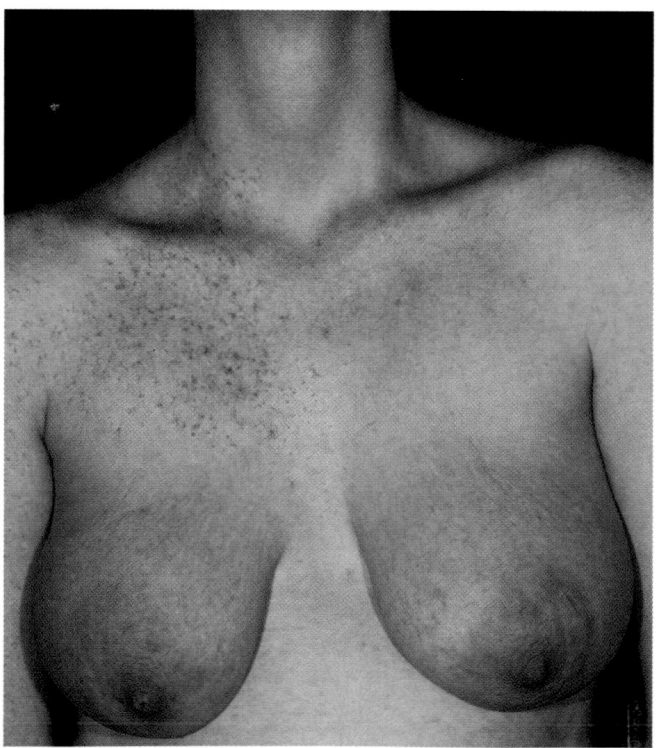

Figure 23-23 Unilateral nevoid telangiectasia syndrome. Telangiectasia appeared on the right chest and arm during pregnancy.

Generalized essential telangiectasia

Widespread idiopathic telangiectasia (generalized essential telangiectasia) is a rare disorder characterized by the development and gradual spreading of telangiectases. It is seen primarily in women and is sometimes familial. The average age at onset is 38 years. For no apparent reason telangiectases start to appear in the lower extremities and progress steadily to involve the skin of the trunk, the arms, and the face. General health is not affected, and standard laboratory tests are normal. Conjunctival telangiectases are rarely reported.

The telangiectasias slowly progress over years or decades and are not accompanied by associated systemic problems. Autosomal dominant transmission has been suggested. Lesions have been reported to resolve with tetracycline.[61] Successful treatment with the 585-nm flashlamp-pumped pulsed dye laser is reported.

References

1. Mulliken JB, Glowacki J: Hemangiomas and vascular malformations in infants and children: a classification based on endothelial characteristics, Plast Reconstr Surg 1982; 69:412.

2. Kim H, Colombo M, Frieden I: Ulcerated hemangiomas: clinical characteristics and response to therapy, J Am Acad Dermatol 2001; 44:962.

3. Illingworth RS: Thoughts on the treatment of vascular nevi, Arch Dis Child 1976; 51:138.

4. Dinehart S, Kincannon J, Geronemus R: Hemangiomas: evaluation and treatment, Dermatol Surg 2001; 27:475.

5. Bennett M, et al: Oral corticosteroid use is effective for cutaneous hemangiomas: an evidence-based evaluation, Arch Dermatol 2001; 137(9):1208.

6. Brockner AL, Frieden IJ: Hemangiomas of infancy, J Am Acad Dermatol 2003; 48:477.

7. Stigmar G, et al: Ophthalmic sequelae of infantile hemangiomas of the eyelids and orbit, Am J Ophthalmol 1978; 85:806.

8. Kushner BJ: The treatment of periorbital infantile hemangioma with intralesional corticosteroid [and discussion by Edgerton MT: 525-526.], Plast Reconst Surg 1985; 76:517.

9. Reyes BA: Intralesional steroids in cutaneous hemangioma, J Dermatol Surg Oncol 1989; 15:828.

10. Barlow CF, et al: Spastic diplegia as complication of interferon alfa-2a treatment of hemangiomas of infancy, J Pediatr 1998; 132:527.

11. Chang E, et al: Successful treatment of infantile hemangiomas with interferon-alpha-2b, J Pediatr Hematol Oncol, 1997; 19:237.

12. Garden J, Bakus A: Laser treatment of port-wine stains and hemangiomas, Dermatol Clin, 1997; 15:373.

13. Poetke M, Philipp C, Berlien H: Flashlamp-pumped pulsed dye laser for hemangiomas in infancy: treatment of superficial vs mixed hemangiomas, Arch Dermatol 2000; 136:628.

14. Garden JM, et al: Treatment of cutaneous hemangiomas by the flashlamp-pumped pulsed dye laser: prospective analysis, J Pediatr 1992; 120:555.

15. Garden JM, Bakus AD: Clinical efficacy of the pulsed dye laser in the treatment of vascular lesions, J Dermatol Surg Oncol 1993; 19:321.

16. Esterly NB: Kasabach-Merritt syndrome in infants, J Am Acad Dermatol 1983; 8:504.

17. Hesselmann S, et al: Case report: Kasabach-Merritt syndrome: a review of the therapeutic options and a case report of successful treatment with radiotherapy and interferon alpha, Br J Radiol 2002; 75(890):180.

18. Shin H, Ryu K, Ahn H: Stepwise multimodal approach in the treatment of Kasabach-Merritt syndrome, Pediatr Int 2000; 42(6):620.

19. Burns AJ, Kaplan LC, Mulliken JB: Is there an association between hemangioma and syndromes with dysmorphic features? Pediatrics 1991; 88:1257.

20. Tallman B, et al: Location of port-wine stains and the likelihood of ophthalmic and/or central nervous system complications, Pediatrics 1991; 87:323.

21. Novick NL: Angiokeratoma vulvae, J Am Acad Dermatol, 1985; 12:561.

22. Goldberg LH, Altman AR: Venous lakes of the ears, Cutis 1985; Dec:472.

23. Leshin B, Whitaker DC, Foucar E: Lymphangioma circumscriptum following mastectomy and radiation therapy, J Am Acad Dermatol 1986; 15:1117.

24. Whimster IW: The pathology of lymphangioma circumscriptum, Br J Dermatol 1976; 94:473.

25. McAlvany JP, et al: Magnetic resonance imaging in the evaluation of lymphangioma circumscriptum, Arch Dermatol 1993; 129:194.

26. Browse NL, et al: Surgical management of lymphangioma circumscriptum, Br J Surg 1986; 73:585.

27. Bailin PL, Kantor GR, Wheeland RG: Carbon dioxide laser vaporization of lymphangioma circumscriptum, J Am Acad Dermatol 1986; 14:257.

28. Harris M, et al: Lobular capillary hemangiomas: An epidemiologic report, with emphasis on cutaneous lesions, J Am Acad Dermatol 2000; 42(6):1012.

29. Ro BI: Granuloma pyogenicum, Int J Dermatol 1986; 25:634.

30. Daley TD, et al: Pregnancy tumor: an analysis, Oral Surg Oral Med Oral Pathol 1991; 72:196.

31. Patrice SJ, et al: Pyogenic granuloma (lobular capillary hemangioma): a clinicopathologic study of 178 cases, Pediatr Dermatol 1991; 8:267.

31a. Taira JW, et al: Lobular capillary hemangioma (pyogenic granuloma) with satellitosis, J Am Acad Dermatol 1992; 27:297.

32. Plettenberg A, et al: Bacillary angiomatosis in HIV-infected patients—an epidemiological and clinical study, Dermatology 2000; 201(4):326.

33. Tappero JW, et al: Kaposi's sarcoma. Epidemiology, pathogenesis, histology, clinical spectrum, staging criteria and therapy, J Am Acad Dermatol 1993; 28:371.

34. Mitsuyasu R: Update on the pathogenesis and treatment of Kaposi sarcoma, Curr Opin Oncol 2000; 12:174.

35. Ziegler JL: Endemic Kaposi's sarcoma in Africa and local volcanic soils, Lancet 1993; 342:1348.

36. Stein ME, et al: Endemic African Kaposi's sarcoma: clinical and therapeutic implications. 10-year experience in the Johannesburg Hospital (1980-1990), Oncology 1994; 51:63.

37. Stein ME, et al: Radiation therapy in endemic (African) Kaposi's sarcoma, Int J Radiat Oncol Biol Phys 1993; 27:1181.

38. Trattner A, et al: The appearance of Kaposi sarcoma during corticosteroid therapy, Cancer 1993; 72:1779.

39. Mitsuyasu RT: Clinical aspects of AIDS-related Kaposi's sarcoma, Curr Opin Oncol 1993; 5:835.

40. Safai B, et al: The natural history of Kaposi's sarcoma in the acquired immunodeficiency syndrome, Ann Intern Med 1985; 103:747.

41. Duvic M, et al: Topical treatment of cutaneous lesions of acquired immunodeficiency syndrome-related Kaposi sarcoma using a litretinoin gel, Arch Dermatol 2000; 136(12):1544.

42. Kirova Y, et al: Radiotherapy in the management of epidemic Kaposi's sarcoma: a retrospective study of 643 cases, Radiother Oncol 1998; 46:19.

43. Mitsuyasu R: AIDS-related Kaposi's sarcoma: current treatment options, future trends, Oncology 2000; 14:867; discussion 878, 881, 887.

44. Tappero JW, et al: Cryotherapy for cutaneous Kaposi's sarcoma (KS) associated with acquired immune deficiency syndrome (AIDS): a phase II trial, J Acquir Immune Defic Syndr 1991; 4:839.

45. Boudreaux AA, et al: Intralesional vinblastine for cutaneous Kaposi's sarcoma associated with acquired immunodeficiency syndrome. A clinical trial to evaluate efficacy and discomfort associated with infection, J Am Acad Dermatol 1993; 28:61.

46. Harrison M, et al: Response and cosmetic outcome of two fractionation regimens for AIDS-related Kaposi's sarcoma, Radiother Oncol 1998; 46:23.

47. Berson AM, et al: Radiation therapy for AIDS-related Kaposi's sarcoma, Int J Radiat Oncol Biol Phys 1990; 19:569.

48. Stelzer KJ, Griffin TW: A randomized prospective trial of radiation therapy for AIDS-associated Kaposi's sarcoma, Int J Radiat Oncol Biol Phys 1993; 27:1057.

49. Gascon P, Schwartz R: Kaposi's sarcoma. New treatment modalities, Dermatol Clin 2000; 18(1):169.

50. Dezube B: Acquired immunodeficiency syndrome-related Kaposi's sarcoma: clinical features, staging, and treatment, Semin Oncol 2000; 27(4):424.

51. Krown S: Management of Kaposi sarcoma: the role of interferon and thalidomide, Curr Opin Oncol 2001; 13:374.

52. Trembath R, et al: Clinical and molecular genetic features of pulmonary hypertension in patients with hereditary hemorrhagic telangiectasia, N Engl J Med 2001; 345:325.

53. Shovlin C, et al: Diagnostic criteria for hereditary hemorrhagic telangiectasia (Rendu-Osler-Weber syndrome), Am J Med Genet 2000; 91:66.

54. Garcia-Tsao G, et al: Liver disease in patients with hereditary hemorrhagic telangiectasia, N Engl J Med 2000; 343:931.

55. Lee J, Ben-Aviv D, Covello S: The diagnostic quandary of hereditary haemorrhagic telangiectasia vs. CREST syndrome, Br J Dermatol 2001; 145(4):646.

56. Sabba C, Gallitelli M, Palasciano G: Efficacy of unusually high doses of tranexamic acid for the treatment of epistaxis in hereditary hemorrhagic telangiectasia, N Engl J Med 2001; 345:926.

57. Klepfish A, Berrebi A, Schattner A: Intranasal tranexamic acid treatment for severe epistaxis in hereditary hemorrhagic telangiectasia, Arch Intern Med 2001; 161:767.

58. Wilkin JK, et al: Unilateral dermatomal superficial telangiectasia, J Am Acad Dermatol 1983; 8:468.

59. Tok J, et al: Unilateral nevoid telangiectasia syndrome, Cutis 1994; 53:53.

60. Uhlin SR, McCarty KS Jr: Unilateral nevoid telangiectatic syndrome: the role of estrogen and progesterone receptors, Arch Dermatol 1983; 119:226.

61. Shelley WB: Essential progressive telangiectasia, JAMA 1971; 210:1343.

Physicians are frequently confronted with hair-related problems. Most complaints are from patients with early onset pattern baldness. The physician must be able to recognize this normal, inherited hair loss pattern so that detailed and expensive evaluations can be avoided. Other patients have complaints about abnormal hair growth; these diseases must be recognized and not dismissed as balding. The signs of hair loss or excess growth are at times subtle. The signs usually seen with cutaneous disease, such as inflammation, may be absent. A systematic approach to evaluation is essential.

Anatomy

HAIR FOLLICLE. Humans have about 5 million hair follicles at birth. No follicles are formed after birth, but their size changes under the influence of androgens. The hair follicle is formed in the embryo by a club-shaped epidermal, down growth, the primary epithelial germ that is invaginated from below by a flame-shaped, capillary-containing dermal structure called the papilla of the hair follicle. The central cells of the down growth form the hair matrix, the cells of which form the hair shaft and its surrounding structures. The ma-

trix lies deep within the subcutaneous fat. The mature follicle contains a hair shaft, two surrounding sheaths, and a germinative bulb (Figure 24-1). The follicle is divided into three sections. The infundibulum extends from the surface to the sebaceous gland duct. The isthmus extends from the duct down to the insertion of the erector muscle. The inferior segment, which exists only during the growing (anagen) phase, extends from the muscle insertion to the base of the matrix. The matrix contains the cells that proliferate to form the hair shaft (Figure 24-2). The mitotic rate of the hair matrix is greater than that of any other organ. The cells begin to differentiate at the top of the bulb. The inner and outer root sheaths protect and mold the growing hair. The inner root sheath disintegrates at the duct of the sebaceous gland. Hair growth is greatly influenced by any stress or disease process that can alter mitotic activity.

HAIR STRUCTURE. The hair shaft is dead protein. It is formed by compact cells that are covered by a delicate cuticle composed of platelike scales. The living cells in the matrix multiply more rapidly than those in any other normal human tissue. They push up into the follicular canal, undergo dehydration, and form the hair shaft, which consists of a dense, hard mass of keratinized cells. Normal hairs have a pointed tip. The hair in the follicular canal forms a cylinder of uniform diameter. Short hairs with tapered tips have either short growth cycles or have experienced the recent onset of anagen.

The growing shaft is surrounded by several concentric layers (see Figure 24-2). The outermost glycogen-rich layer is called the outer root sheath. It is static and continuous with the epidermis. The inner root sheath (Henle's layer, Huxley's layer, and cuticle) is visible as a gelatinous mass when the hair is plucked. It protects and molds the growing hair but disintegrates before reaching the surface at the infundibulum.

The hair shaft that emerges has three layers—an outer cuticle, a cortex, and sometimes an inner medulla—all of which are composed of dead protein. The cuticle protects and holds the cortex cells together. Split ends result if the cuticle is damaged by brushing or chemical cosmetic treatments. The cortex cells in the growing hair shaft rapidly synthesize and accumulate proteins while in the lower regions of the hair follicle. Systemic diseases and drugs may interfere with the metabolism of these cells and reduce the hair shaft diameter.

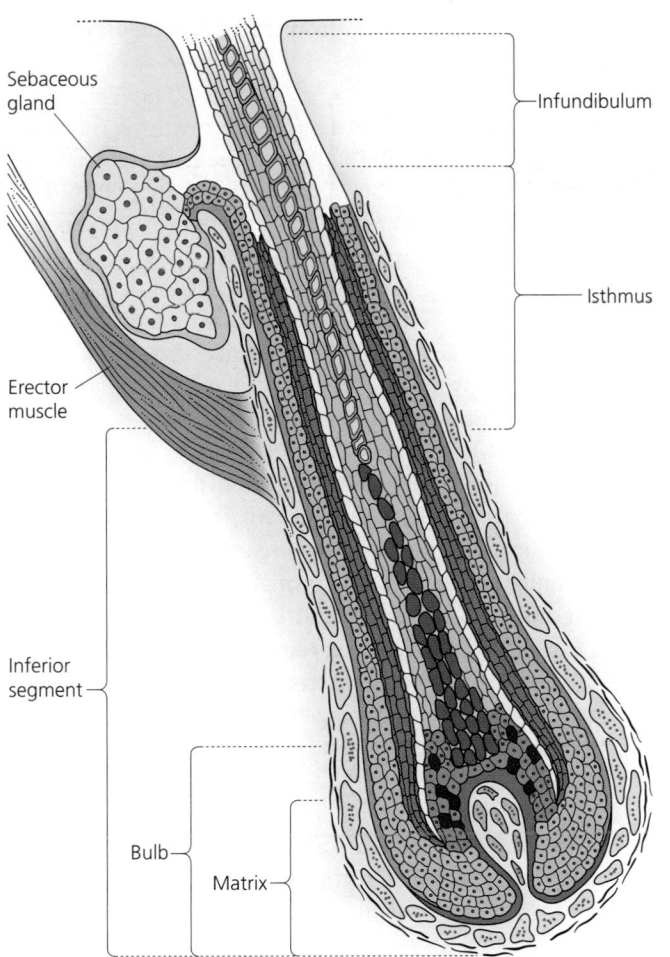

Sebaceous gland

Erector muscle

Inferior segment

Bulb

Matrix

Infundibulum

Isthmus

Figure 24-1 Hair follicle. Longitudinal section showing the three sections: the infundibulum, the isthmus, and the inferior segment.

Figure 24-2 Hair bulb. The outer and inner root sheaths mold and protect the growing hair shaft. The hair shaft consists of the medulla, hair cortex, and cuticle.

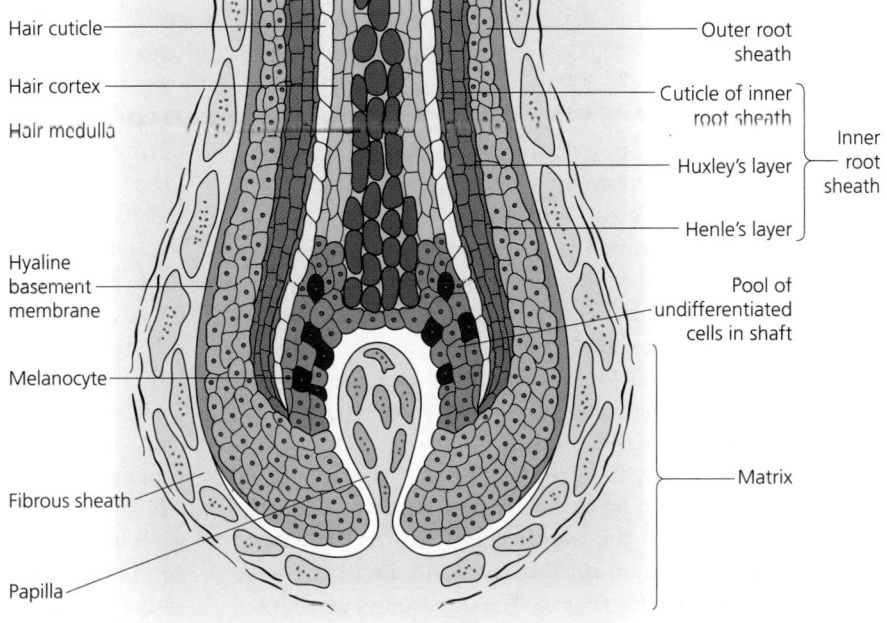

Hair cuticle

Hair cortex

Hair medulla

Hyaline basement membrane

Melanocyte

Fibrous sheath

Papilla

Outer root sheath

Cuticle of inner root sheath

Huxley's layer

Henle's layer

Inner root sheath

Pool of undifferentiated cells in shaft

Matrix

Pigment-containing melanosomes are acquired deep in the bulb matrix and are deposited in the cortical and medullary cells.

TYPES OF HAIR. There are three types of hair.[1] Thick, pigmented hairs are called terminal hairs. Terminal hairs on the top of the head and in the beard, axillary, and pubic areas are influenced by androgens. Androgens are important in regulating hair growth. At puberty, androgens increase the size of follicles in the beard, chest, and limbs and decrease the size of follicles in the bitemporal region, which reshapes the hairline in men and many women.

Lanugo hairs are the fine hairs found on the fetus; similar fine hairs (peach fuzz) found on the adult are called vellus hairs. Vellus hair is short, fine, relatively nonpigmented and covers much of the body. Hair on the rest of the body is independent of androgens.

Physiology

Cycling of hair follicles depends on the interaction of the follicular epithelium with the dermal papilla. The dermal papilla induces hair-follicle formation from the overlying epithelium at the onset of each new follicular cycle. The bulge consists of cells in the outer-root sheath, which is located near the insertion of the arrector pili muscle (Figure 24-3). The dermal papilla interacts with germ cells in the hair-follicle bulge to regenerate the lower follicle. Stem cells in the bulge portion of the outer-root migrate out of the follicle and regenerate the epidermis after injury.

Rapidly proliferating matrix cells in the hair bulb produce the hair shaft. The matrix cells differentiate, move upward and are compressed and funneled into their final shape by the rigid inner-root sheath. The shape (curvature) of the inner root sheath determines the shape of the hair. The bulk of the hair shaft is called the cortex. Pigment in the hair shaft is produced by melanocytes interspersed among the matrix cells. The volume of the dermal papilla determines the diameter of the hair shaft.

Hair growth cycle

The average scalp has more than 100,000 hairs. The growth phase of scalp hair is approximately 1000 days (range, 2 to 6 years). Hair in other areas, such as the eyebrows and eyelashes, has a shorter growth phase (1 to 6 months). Scalp hair grows 0.3 to 0.4 mm/day, or approximately 6 inches a year.

Humans have a mosaic growth pattern; hair growth and loss are not cyclic or seasonal, as in some mammals, but occur at random, so that hair loss is continuous (see Figure 24-3). Each hair follicle perpetually goes through three stages in the hair growth cycle: catagen (transitional phase), telogen (resting phase), and anagen (growing phase) (Figure 24-4). Approximately 90% to 95% of hairs are in the anagen phase, and 5% to 10% are in the telogen phase. Up to 100 telogen hairs are lost each day from the head, and about the same number of follicles enter anagen. The duration of anagen determines the length of hair, and the volume of the hair bulb determines the diameter.

Anagen and telogen hairs from hair-plucked preparation are shown in Figure 24-5.

ANAGEN (GROWTH). The anagen or growth phase begins with resumption of mitotic activity in the hair bulb and dermal papilla. Interactions between the dermal papilla and the overlying follicular epithelium are required for the onset of anagen. The follicle grows down and meets the dermal papilla, recapitulating the embryonic events of development of the hair follicle. A new hair shaft forms and forces the tightly held club hair out. During anagen, hair grows at an average rate of 0.35 mm/day, or 1 cm in 28 days[2]; this rate diminishes with age.

Hair follicles in different areas of the body produce hairs of different lengths. The length is proportional to the duration of the anagen cycle. Scalp hair remains in an active growing phase for an average of 2 to 6 years. The active growing phase is much shorter and the resting stage is longer for hair on the arms, legs, eyelashes, and eyebrows (30 to 45 days), which explains why these hairs remain short. Approximately 90% to 95% of scalp hairs are in an active growing phase at any one time. Continuous anagen occurs in some dogs (e.g., poodles) and in merino sheep; these animals do not lose or shed hair.

CATAGEN (INVOLUTION). Catagen is a process of involution that occurs with cell death in follicular keratinocytes. It is the phase of acute follicular regression that signals the end of anagen. Less than 1% of scalp hairs are in this 2- to 3-week transitional phase at any one time. Cell division in the hair matrix stops, and the resting, or catagen, stage begins. The outer root sheath degenerates and retracts around the widened lower portion of the hair shaft to become a club hair. The lower follicle shrinks away from the connective tissue papilla and ascends to the level of the insertion of the erector muscle. The dermal papilla condenses and moves upward, coming to rest underneath the hair-follicle bulge. The completion of catagen is marked by formation of the normal club hair.

TELOGEN (REST). All activity ceases and the structure rests during the telogen phase. The telogen phase in the scalp lasts for 2 to 3 months before the scalp follicles reenter the anagen stage and the cycle is repeated. The percentage of follicles in the telogen stage varies according to the body region. Approximately 5% to 10% of scalp hairs are in the telogen phase at any one time, and these follicles are randomly distributed. The telogen phase is much longer in eyebrow, eyelash, trunk, arm, and leg hair. Approximately 40% to 50% of follicles on the trunk are in telogen phase. The inactive dead hair, or club hair, has a solid, hard, dry, white node at its proximal end; the white color is due to a lack of pigment. The club hair is firmly held in place and then ejected. A new anagen hair grows and replaces the shed telogen hair. Approximately 25 to 100 telogen hairs are shed each day; possibly twice this number are lost on the days the hair is shampooed. Seasonal shedding occurs in other animals but is random in humans.

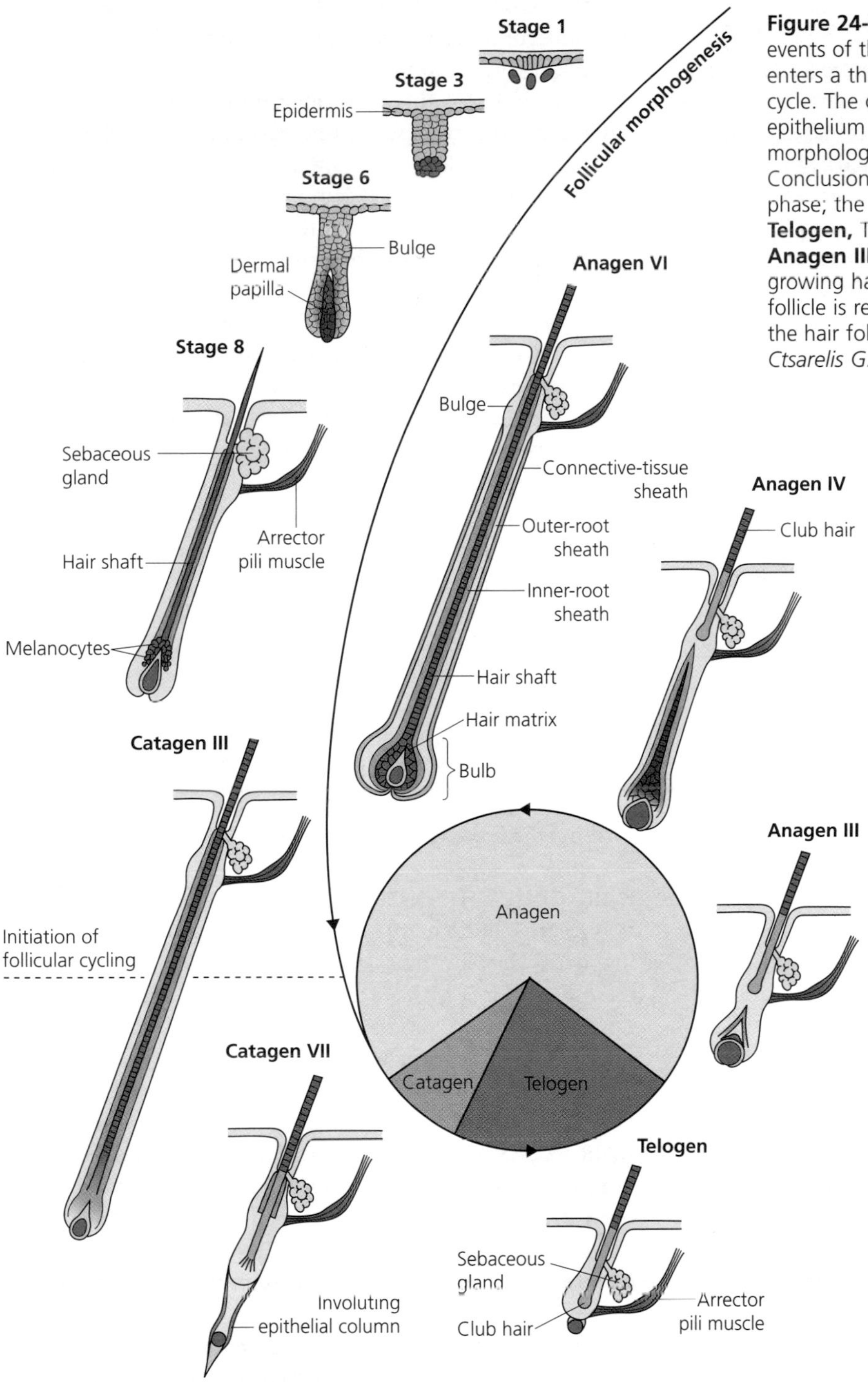

Stage 1

Stage 3

Epidermis

Stage 6

Follicular morphogenesis

Dermal papilla

Bulge

Anagen VI

Bulge

Connective-tissue sheath

Outer-root sheath

Inner-root sheath

Hair shaft

Hair matrix

Bulb

Stage 8

Sebaceous gland

Hair shaft

Arrector pili muscle

Melanocytes

Catagen III

Initiation of follicular cycling

Catagen VII

Involuting epithelial column

Anagen

Catagen

Telogen

Anagen IV

Club hair

Anagen III

Telogen

Sebaceous gland

Club hair

Arrector pili muscle

Figure 24-3 Stages 1, 3, 6, and 8 represent the embryonic events of the development of the hair follicle. The follicle then enters a three-stage (anagen, catagen, and telogen) growth cycle. The cycle depends on the interaction of the follicular epithelium and the dermal papilla. The roman numerals indicate morphologic substages of anagen and catagen. **Catagen III,** Conclusion of the growth phase. **Catagen VII,** Transition phase; the inferior segment separates from the papilla. **Telogen,** The hair ascends to the level of the erector muscle. **Anagen III,** The growing cycle resumes. **Anagen IV,** The growing hair forces the club hair out. **Anagen VI,** The mature follicle is restored. The pie chart shows the proportion of time the hair follicle spends in each stage. *(Adapted from Paus R, Ctsarelis G: NEJM 1999; 341:491.)*

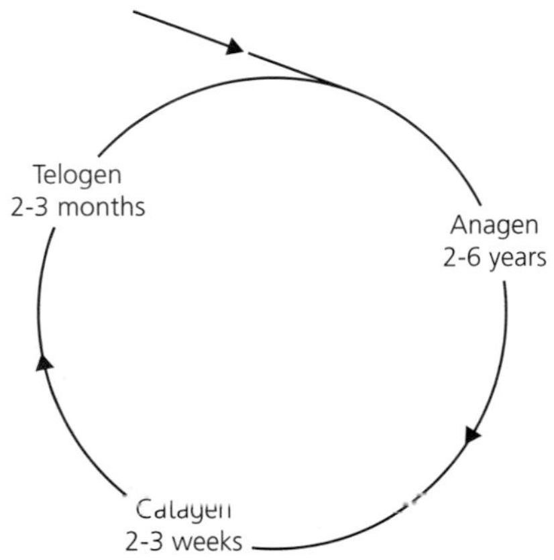

Telogen 2-3 months

Anagen 2-6 years

Catagen 2-3 weeks

Figure 24-4 Hair growth cycle—scalp.

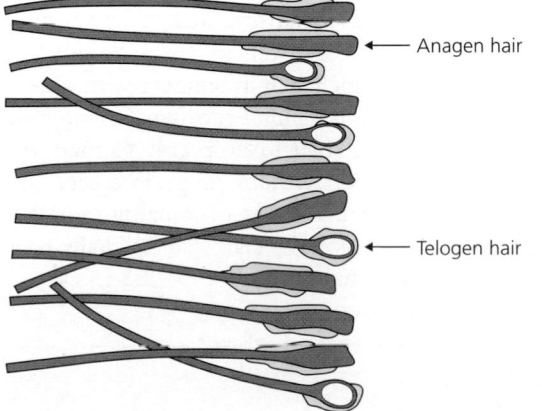

Anagen hair

Telogen hair

Figure 24-5 Hair pluck preparation showing anagen and telogen hairs.

Evaluation of Hair Loss

The causes of hair loss (alopecia) are numerous. Most hair problems seen by the practitioner are due to changes in hair-follicle cycling. Scarring alopecias are due to other causes. A classification is used here that is based primarily on distribution and scarring (i.e., localized [patchy] vs. generalized and scarring vs. nonscarring). A systematic approach for evaluation of hair loss is outlined in Box 24-1 and Table 24-1. The evaluation of the woman who complains that "My hair is falling out in large amounts" is presented in the diagram on p. 840.

Diagnosis of hair disease

HISTORY. Inquire about drugs, severe diet restriction, vitamin A supplementation, and thyroid symptoms. Determine the time of onset and the duration of hair loss. Abrupt-onset telogen effluvium is most often related to a specific event. Gradual or imperceptible onsets are more complicated and involve possible shortened anagen, as well as a differential diagnosis that includes alopecia areata, androgenetic alopecia, and diffuse primary scarring alopecias.

PHYSICAL EXAMINATION. Examine the scalp surface and hair shafts. Microscopically examine hair ends and hair shaft diameters. Hair density may be reduced by 50% before hair thinning becomes clinically apparent; therefore observation is an inaccurate method of evaluating density and loss.

HAIR PULL TEST. For the hair pull test, obtain a sample 3 cm above the auricle. Tightly grasp 20 to 40 hairs firmly between the thumb and forefinger. Exert a slow, constant traction to slightly tent the scalp, and slide the fingers up the hair shafts. There should be fewer than six club hairs extracted. Repeat the count on the opposite side of the head and in two other areas. Examine the hair bulbs.

Box 24-1 Systematic Approach to Evaluation of Hair Loss	
History	**Diagnostic procedures**
Sudden vs. gradual loss	Hair pull test
Presence of systemic disease or high fever	Daily counts Part width
Recent psychologic or physical stress	Possible trichotillomania
Medication or chemical exposure	Potassium hydroxide examination for fungi
Examination	**Scalp biopsy**
Localized vs. generalized	
Scarring vs. nonscarring	
Inflammatory vs. noninflammatory	**Hormone studies**
Density: normal or decreased	
Presence of follicular plugging	
Skin disease in other areas	

DAILY COUNTS. The patient collects hair lost in the first morning combing and includes those lost during washing for 14 days, saving them in clear plastic bags. The patient counts the hairs and records the number on the bags. Examine the hairs under the microscope to determine if the bulbs are anagen or telogen. Daily hair shed counts are not necessary if the pull test is positive. It is normal to lose up to 100 hairs daily and 200 to 250 hairs on the day of shampooing. If the hair is shampooed daily, the counts should be less than 100.

PART WIDTH. Make a coronal part with a comb over the vertex. Note the part width. Make a series of parallel parts over the vertex and visually compare the part diameter. Do the same over the occipital and temporal scalp. Visually compare the part diameters in the different anatomic scalp areas. Hair density is greatest in childhood and decreases progressively with age. The hair is less dense in the vertex in both sexes, and thinning increases with age.

HAIR SHAFT EXAMINATION (CLIP TESTS). Grasp 25 to 30 hairs between the thumb and forefinger just at the scalp surface. Cut the hair between the fingers and the scalp. Hair just above the fingers is cut and discarded. Float the hairs onto a wet microscope slide and cover with another slide. Evaluate hair shaft diameter and structure. There are many rare diseases that produce shaft structural abnormalities such as pili torti in which the hair is twisted on its axis.

HAIR GROWTH WINDOW. Select an area where the hair fails to grow and an area that can be covered by the remaining hair. Cut the hair short, then shave a 2.0-cm² area. Occlude the area with an occlusive dressing and remove it in 1 week if trichotillomania is suspected. Normal growth is 2.5 mm in 1 week and 1 cm in 1 month. This test proves to the patient that the hair is growing.

HAIR PLUCK—TRICHOGRAM. This is a painful technique but is still used by some clinicians. Abruptly extract hairs from the scalp with a rubber-tipped needle holder. Cut the excess hair 1 cm from the roots, float the hairs onto a wet microscope slide or Petri dish, and examine with a hand lens (see Figure 24-5).

Telogen hairs have small, unpigmented, ovoid bulbs and do not contain an internal root sheath. Anagen hairs have larger, elongated, pigmented (if hair is pigmented) bulbs shaped like the end of a broom, surrounded by a gelatinous internal root sheath.

There are diseases in which hair fragments with absent bulbs are obtained during a hair pull. Processes that interfere with cell division cause the shaft to be poorly formed and therefore apt to break under tension. Alopecia areata, antimetabolite therapy, and small doses of ionizing radiation interrupt the mitotic activity in the cells that normally contribute cells to the growing hair.

Table 24-1 A Simplified Tool for the Diagnosis of Alopecia (This scheme will diagnose 97% of cases of alopecia)

Disease	Scalp	Pattern	Pull test	Laboratory	Treatment
Diffuse loss (non-scarring)					
Telogen effluvium	Normal	Diffuse	Increased telogen	Disease specific	Disease specific
Diffuse alopecia areata	Normal	Irregularly diffuse	Increased telogen	—	Topical immunotherapy
Androgenic alopecia (men)	Normal	Hamilton (Figure 24-6)	Negative	—	Minoxidil Finasteride 1 mg Surgery
Androgenetic alopecia (women)	Normal	Ludwig (Figure 24-7)	Negative	Testosterone DHEAs	Minoxidil Oral contraceptives Spironolactone
Systemic disease (thyroid, iron deficiency, systemic lupus erythematosus, dermatomyositis)	Normal in most	Diffuse	Normal or increased telogen	Thyroid function Iron/IBC ANA	Disease specific
Patchy loss (scarring)					
Lichen planopilaris	Hairs trapped in "islands"	Patchy	Negative	Biopsy Immuno-fluorescence	Hydroxychloroquine Cyclosporine
Discoid lupus erythematosus	Atrophy, dys-pigmentation, follicular plugging	Patchy	Negative	Biopsy	Intralesionalsteroids Hydroxychloroquine
Folliculitis decalvans	Pustules at periphery Bogginess	Patchy	Negative	Bacterial Culture Biopsy	Rifampicin Clindamycin Other antibiotics
Pseudopelade	Scarring, non-inflammatory	Moth-eaten pattern	Negative	Biopsy Immuno-fluorescence	Topical steroids Hydroxychloroquine
Follicular degen-eration syndrome	Scarring in localized pattern	Patchy over crown	Negative	Biopsy	Avoid hair traction
Patchy loss (non-scarring)					
Alopecia localized	Normal	Patchy + exclamation mark hairs	May be + at margins	KOH children	Intralesional Steroids Minoxidil Anthralin
Tinea capitis	Scale or papules or pustules	Patchy	Hair breakage	KOH Fungal culture	Oral antifungal antibiotics
Traction alopecia	± Scarring	Patchy, marginal	Hair breakage	—	Avoid
Trichotillomania	± Scarring, normal	Patchy with stubble	Usually negative	—	Fluoxetine, others Psychotherapy
Syphilis	Normal	Moth-eaten	Increased telogen	RPR	Penicillin
Hair breakage	Normal	Patchy or marginal	Broken hairs	—	—

Adapted from Robert RL: Dermatol Clin 1996; 14.

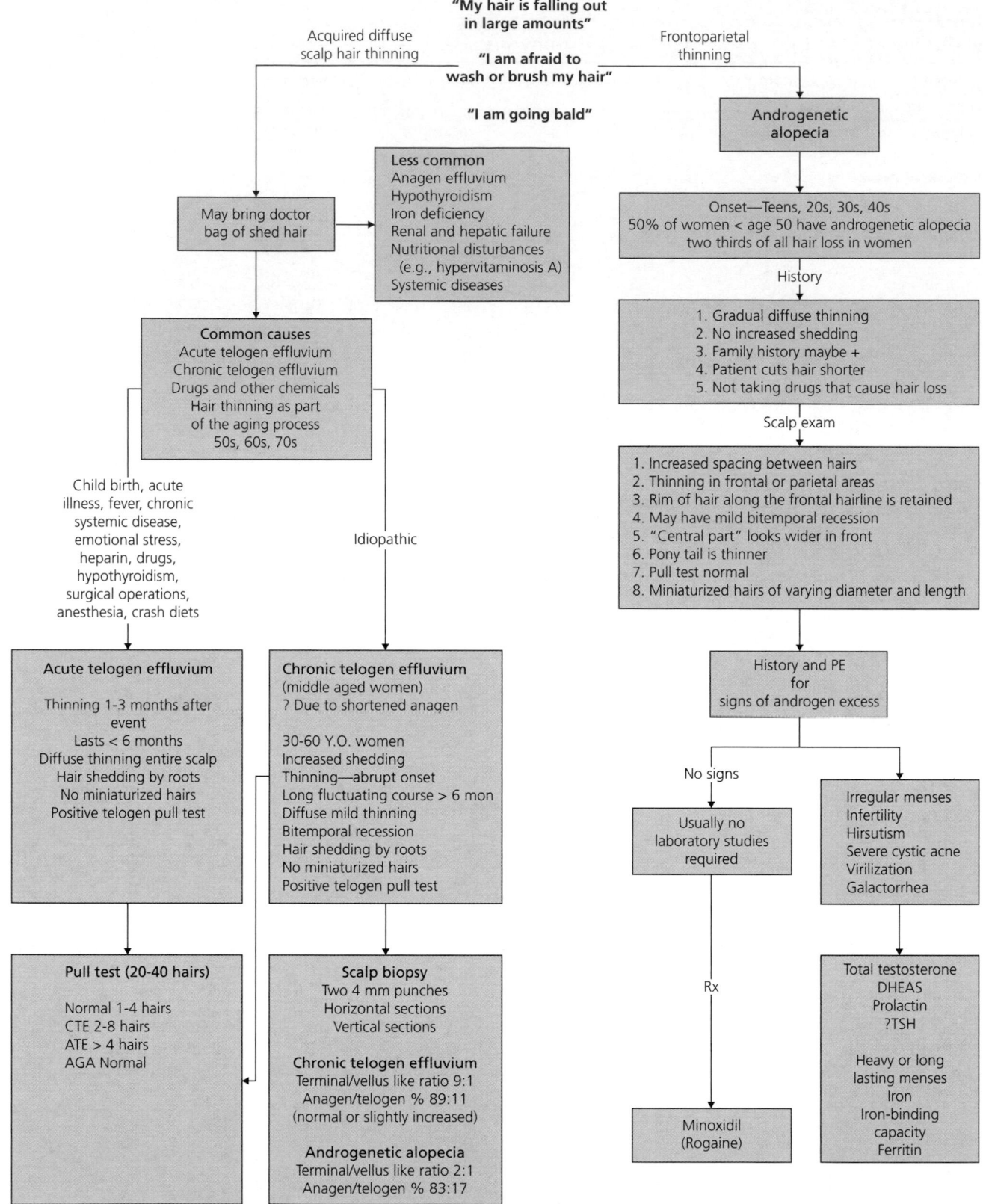

"My hair is falling out in large amounts"

Acquired diffuse scalp hair thinning

"I am afraid to wash or brush my hair"

Frontoparietal thinning

"I am going bald"

May bring doctor bag of shed hair

Less common
Anagen effluvium
Hypothyroidism
Iron deficiency
Renal and hepatic failure
Nutritional disturbances
(e.g., hypervitaminosis A)
Systemic diseases

Androgenetic alopecia

Onset—Teens, 20s, 30s, 40s
50% of women < age 50 have androgenetic alopecia
two thirds of all hair loss in women

Common causes
Acute telogen effluvium
Chronic telogen effluvium
Drugs and other chemicals
Hair thinning as part
of the aging process
50s, 60s, 70s

History
1. Gradual diffuse thinning
2. No increased shedding
3. Family history maybe +
4. Patient cuts hair shorter
5. Not taking drugs that cause hair loss

Scalp exam
1. Increased spacing between hairs
2. Thinning in frontal or parietal areas
3. Rim of hair along the frontal hairline is retained
4. May have mild bitemporal recession
5. "Central part" looks wider in front
6. Pony tail is thinner
7. Pull test normal
8. Miniaturized hairs of varying diameter and length

Child birth, acute illness, fever, chronic systemic disease, emotional stress, heparin, drugs, hypothyroidism, surgical operations, anesthesia, crash diets

Idiopathic

History and PE
for
signs of androgen excess

Acute telogen effluvium

Thinning 1-3 months after event
Lasts < 6 months
Diffuse thinning entire scalp
Hair shedding by roots
No miniaturized hairs
Positive telogen pull test

Chronic telogen effluvium
(middle aged women)
? Due to shortened anagen

30-60 Y.O. women
Increased shedding
Thinning—abrupt onset
Long fluctuating course > 6 mon
Diffuse mild thinning
Bitemporal recession
Hair shedding by roots
No miniaturized hairs
Positive telogen pull test

No signs

Usually no
laboratory studies
required

Irregular menses
Infertility
Hirsutism
Severe cystic acne
Virilization
Galactorrhea

Pull test (20-40 hairs)

Normal 1-4 hairs
CTE 2-8 hairs
ATE > 4 hairs
AGA Normal

Scalp biopsy
Two 4 mm punches
Horizontal sections
Vertical sections

Chronic telogen effluvium
Terminal/vellus like ratio 9:1
Anagen/telogen % 89:11
(normal or slightly increased)

Androgenetic alopecia
Terminal/vellus like ratio 2:1
Anagen/telogen % 83:17

Rx

Minoxidil
(Rogaine)

Total testosterone
DHEAS
Prolactin
?TSH

Heavy or long
lasting menses
Iron
Iron-binding
capacity
Ferritin

CTE Chronic telogen effluvium
ATE Acute telogen effluvium
AGA Androgenetic alopecia

Generalized Hair Loss

Diffuse hair loss (Box 24-2 and Table 24-2) usually occurs without inflammation or scarring. The loss affects hairs throughout the scalp in a more or less uniform pattern. The hair pull test is important for differential diagnosis.

TELOGEN EFFLUVIUM. A number of events have been documented that prematurely terminate anagen and cause an abnormally high number of normal hairs to enter the resting, or telogen, phase (see Box 24-2).[3] The follicle is not diseased but has had its biologic clock reset and undergoes a normal involutional process. Usually no more than 50% of the patient's hair is affected. Scarring and inflammation are absent. Resting hairs on the scalp are retained for approximately 100 days before they are lost; therefore telogen hair loss should occur approximately 3 months after the event that terminated normal hair growth.

Kligman[4] explained this process and identified the various precipitating events (see Box 24-2). The most common causes are briefly discussed here. High fever from any cause may result in a sudden diffuse loss of club hairs 2 to 3 months later. Hair loss begins abruptly and lasts for approximately 4 weeks. Hair pluck tests show telogen counts that vary from 30% to 60%. Full recovery can be expected.

Severe emotional and physical traumas have been documented to cause diffuse hair loss. Hair loss has been reported to occur 2 weeks after severe psychologic or physical trauma, but because that is too short a time for the induction of the telogen phase, the loss must have occurred by another mechanism. Some individuals may experience increased shedding due to idiopathic shortening of anagen (a short anagen syndrome). They have increased shedding and decreased hair length. For every 50% reduction in the duration of anagen, there is a corresponding doubling of follicles in telogen.

POSTPARTUM HAIR LOSS. The percentage of follicles in telogen progressively decreases during pregnancy, particularly during the last trimester. Diffuse but primarily frontotemporal hair loss occurs in a significant number of women 1 to 4 months after childbirth. The loss can be quite significant, but recovery occurs in less than 1 year. Hair growth usually returns to the prepregnancy state.

DRUGS. Cytotoxic drugs that directly affect hair matrix cell proliferation cause profound hair loss, inducing an anagen effluvium. A large number of drugs probably cause telogen effluvia. These are listed in Box 24-3.

Box 24-2 Hair Loss

Generalized*	Localized†
Telogen effluvium	Androgenic alopecia
Acute blood loss	Male pattern
Childbirth	Female pattern
Crash diets	Hirsutism
(inadequate protein)	Alopecia areata
Drugs	Trichotillomania
Coumarins	Traction alopecia
Heparin	Scarring alopecia
Propanolol	Developmental defects:
Vitamin A	aplasia cutis
High fever	Physical injury: burns,
Hypothyroidism and	pressure
hyperthyroidism	Infection
Physical stress (e.g., surgery)	Fungal: kerion
Physiologic (e.g., neonate)	Bacterial: folliculitis,
Psychologic stress	furuncle
Severe illness (e.g.,	Viral: herpes zoster
systemic lupus	Neoplasms
erythematosus)	Metastatic carcinoma
Anagen effluvium	Sclerosing basal cell
Cancer chemotherapeutic	carcinoma
agents	Others
Poisoning	Lupus erythematosus
Thallium (rat poison)	Lichen planus
Arsenic	Cicatricial pemphigoid
Radiation therapy	**Scleroderma**
Generalized patchy	
Secondary syphilis:	
"moth eaten"	
alopecia	

*Diffuse, uniform loss, but many hairs left randomly distributed in area of loss.

†Most or all hair missing from involved area.

Table 24-2 Features Differentiating Telogen Effluvium and Anagen Effluvium

Clinical presentation	Telogen	Anagen
Onset of shedding after insult	2–4 months	1–4 weeks
Percent hair lost	20–50	80–90
Type of hair lost	Normal club (white bulb)	Anagen hair (pigmented bulb)
Hair shaft	Normal	Narrowed or fractured

Box 24-3 Drugs Probably Associated With Telogen Effluvium

Aminosalicylic acid	Enalapril
Amphetamines	Etretinate
Bromocriptine	Levodopa
Captopril	Lithium
Carbamazepine	Metoprolol
Cimetidine	Propanolol
Coumadin	Pyridostigmine
Danazol	Trimethadione

ANAGEN EFFLUVIUM. Anagen effluvium (see Box 24-2 and Table 24-2) is the abrupt loss of hair from follicles that are in their growing phase. An abrupt insult to the metabolic and follicular reproductive apparatus must be delivered to create such an event. Cancer chemotherapeutic agents and radiation therapy are capable of such an insult. The rapidly dividing cells of the matrix and cortex are affected. The insult causes a change in the rate of hair growth but does not convert the follicle to a different growth phase, as occurs in telogen effluvium. High concentrations of antimetabolites or radiation bring the entire metabolic process to an abrupt halt, and the entire hair and hair root are shed intact. The only hairs left are those in the telogen phase. These are dead, wedged into the hair canal, and unaffected by any acute event. The stem cells of the hair follicles are spared because of their slow cycling, and they generate a new hair bulb. Insults of less intensity slow the mitotic rate of the bulb and cortex cells, causing bulb deformity and narrowing of the lower hair shaft. Narrow, weakened hair shafts are easily broken and shed without bulbs. Since 90% of scalp hairs are in the anagen phase, a large number of hairs can be affected. Patients with 10% to 20% of their hair remaining after an insult almost certainly have had an anagen effluvium. Minoxidil 2% topical has no benefit in the prevention of chemotherapy-induced alopecia.[5]

Localized Hair Loss

Androgenic alopecia in men (male-pattern baldness)

Baldness in men is not a disease, but rather a physiologic reaction induced by androgens in genetically predisposed men. The pattern of inheritance is probably polygenic. Thinning of the hair begins between the ages of 12 and 40 years, and about half the population expresses this trait before the age of 50.

HAMILTON PATTERNS. The progression and various patterns of hair loss are classified by Hamilton (Figure 24-6). Triangular frontotemporal recession occurs normally in most young men (type I) and women after puberty. The first signs of balding are increased frontotemporal recession accompanied by midfrontal recession (type II). Hair loss in a round area on the vertex follows, and the density of hair decreases, sometimes rapidly, over the top of the scalp (types III through VII).

PATHOPHYSIOLOGY. Androgenic alopecia is due to the progressive shortening of successive anagen cycles. There are two populations of scalp follicles: androgen-sensitive follicles on the top and androgen-independent follicles on the sides and back of the scalp. In genetically predisposed individuals, and under the influence of androgens, predisposed follicles are gradually miniaturized, and large, pigmented hairs (terminal hairs) are replaced by thin, depigmented hairs (vellus hairs).

Inflammation surrounds the bulge area of the outer-root sheath. The inflammation may damage the follicle stem cells, which results in a decrease in hair-follicle density. Hair follicles are still present, but removing androgens or treatment with minoxidil or finasteride does not result in the conversion of miniaturized follicles back to terminal ones.

Figure 24-6 Norwood/Hamilton classification of male-pattern baldness.

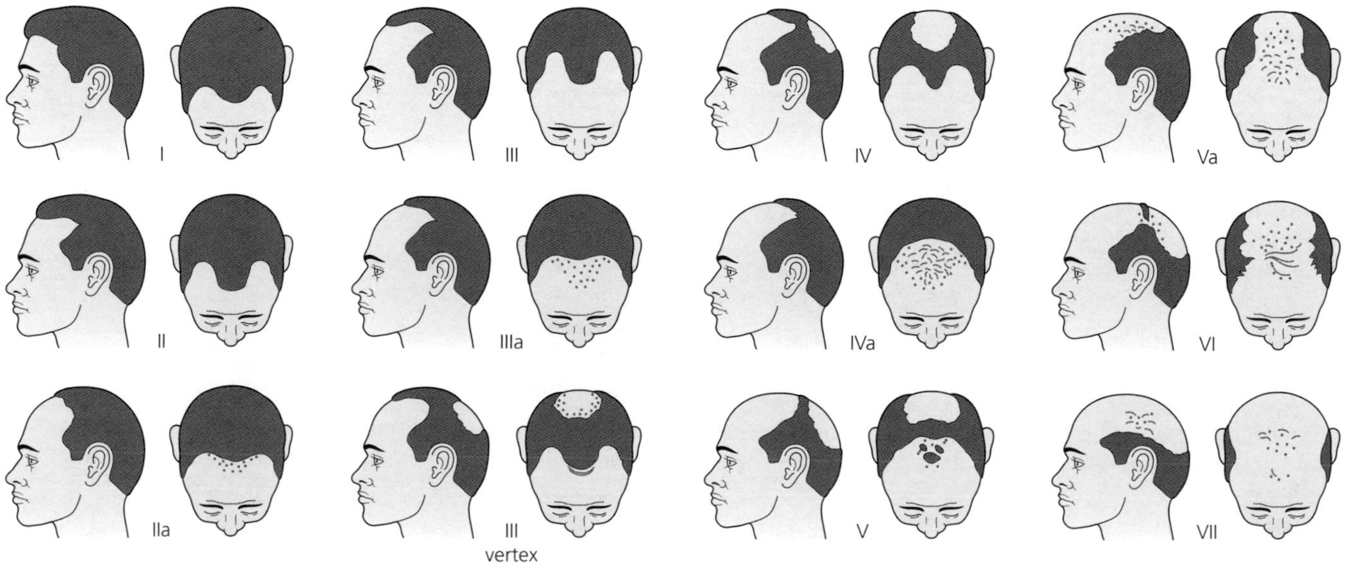

Skin androgen metabolism. Testosterone is converted to the more potent dihydrotestosterone by 5α-reductase. Skin cells contain 5α-reductase (types I and II). The type I enzyme is found in sebaceous glands, and the type II enzyme is found in hair follicles and the prostate gland. Testosterone and dihydrotestosterone act on androgen receptors in the dermal papilla. They increase the size of hair follicles in androgen-dependent areas such as the beard area during adolescence, but later in life dihydrotestosterone binds to the follicle androgen receptor and activates transformation of large, terminal follicles to miniaturized follicles. The duration of anagen shortens with successive hair cycles, and the follicles become smaller, producing shorter, finer hairs. Androgenetic alopecia does not develop in men with a congenital absence of 5α-reductase type II. Finasteride, which inhibits 5α-reductase type II, slows or reverses the progression of androgenetic alopecia.

TREATMENT. The desire for treatment varies. Some men accept the inevitable; others find baldness intolerable. Topical treatment (minoxidil), oral (finasteride) treatment, and several surgical procedures are available. The drugs can enlarge existing hairs and retard thinning in the vertex and the frontal regions. They have no benefit for men who are bald or those with bitemporal recession without hair. Benefits are seen in 6 to 12 months. Treatment must be continued indefinitely. If treatment is stopped, benefits are lost within 6 to 12 months, and hair density will be the same as before treatment. Patients who begin balding at an early age are most distressed and are tempted to consult nonphysician "experts" at hair clinics. These clinics offer a variety of topical preparations, none of which has any value. Selected patients may be referred for hair transplants, plastic surgical rotation flaps, or wigs.

Minoxidil. Minoxidil was developed to treat hypertension. It increases the duration of anagen, causes follicles at rest to grow, and enlarges miniaturized follicles. These effects occur in only a minority of patients. Minoxidil 2% (Rogaine) and 5% (Extra Strength Rogaine) are available over the counter. Generic brands of the 2% solution are available. One milliliter of solution is applied twice daily and spread lightly with a finger. A new applicator conveniently and effectively applies the medication. Minoxidil increases nonvellus hairs. Spontaneous reversal to the pretreatment state occurs in 1 to 3 months after stopping treatment.[6] Ideal candidates are men younger than 30 years of age who have been losing hair for less than 5 years. The solutions produce a modest increase in hair on scalps of young men and women with mild to moderate hair loss, with continuous bid application for years to maintain the effect.[7] Unpublished studies in women did not find differences between 2% and 5% minoxidil, but many clinicians recommend that women use the 5% solution. A 48-week study in men found a mean increase in hairs per square centimeter of 12.7 with 2% minoxidil, and 18.5 with 5% minoxidil. One study found that topical use of 2% minoxidil caused small but statistically significant increases in left ventricular end-diastolic volume, cardiac output, and left ventricular mass.[8] Dizziness and tachycardia have been reported with 2% solution. Local irritation, itching, dryness, and erythema may occur and are likely due to the vehicle of alcohol and propylene glycol. The medication is applied to a dry scalp twice a day. The hair should not be wet for at least an hour afterward. About one third of these patients grow hair that is long enough to be cut or combed. Hair growth is evident in 8 to 12 months. Minoxidil may stop or retard the progression of male-pattern baldness.

Finasteride. Finasteride (Propecia 1 mg) taken daily is an effective oral therapy for androgenetic alopecia in men. Some physicians prescribe finasteride (Proscar 5 mg) and instruct patients to split the 5-mg tablet with a pill splitter into four equal parts. The cost savings is considerable.

Androgenetic alopecia (male pattern hair loss) is caused by androgen-dependent miniaturization of scalp hair follicles, with scalp dihydrotestosterone (DHT) implicated as a contributing cause. Finasteride blocks 5α-reductase type II which inhibits the conversion of testosterone to dihydrotestosterone and decreases serum and cutaneous dihydrotestosterone concentrations. This slows further hair loss, inhibits androgen-dependent miniaturization of hair follicles and improves hair growth and hair weight[9] in men with androgenetic alopecia.

In men with male pattern hair loss, finasteride 1 mg/day slowed the progression of hair loss and increased hair growth in clinical trials over 2 years.[10] Efficacy is evident within 3 months of therapy. The drug produces progressive increases in hair counts at 6 and 12 months. The improvement is maintained through the second year. Therapy leads to slowing of further hair loss.

Finasteride is effective in men with vertex male pattern hair loss and hair loss in the anterior/mid area of the scalp.[11] It may not be effective for men who are older than 60 years of age because type 2 5α-reductase activity in the scalp may not be as high as in younger men.

In postmenopausal women with androgenetic alopecia, finasteride 1 mg/day taken for 12 months did not increase hair growth or slow the progression of hair thinning.[12] Finasteride is contraindicated in women who are or may potentially be pregnant because of the risk that inhibition of conversion of fetal testosterone to DHT could impair virilization of a male fetus. Approximately 20% to 30% of men do not respond. Treatment must be continued indefinitely.

SIDE EFFECTS. In the first year, 4.2% of men report side effects related to sexual dysfunction, which resolved both after discontinuation and spontaneously in many men who chose to remain on drug treatment. No other significant adverse effects related to finasteride treatment are observed. In men 18 to 41 years old who were taking 1 mg of finasteride daily, serum prostate-specific antigen levels decreased by 0.2 ng/ml, which is insignificant.[13] Finasteride decreases serum prostate-specific antigen levels by about 50% in older men.

Finasteride is beneficial in women with hirsutism, but the drug should be used cautiously in women because of its potential feminizing effects on male fetuses.

HAIR TRANSPLANTS. Hair transplants have been used successfully for years to permanently restore hair. Age is not a determining factor. Androgen-independent hairs from the lateral and posterior areas of the scalp are used. The surgeon must have a sense of aesthetics to properly design the anterior hairline. There are many techniques used for harvesting and implanting the graphs. The techniques are constantly changing and improving.

SCALP REDUCTION AND FLAPS. An anterior-posterior elliptic excision of bald vertex scalp with primary closure can provide an instant hair effect. The procedure can be repeated every 4 weeks until hair margins converge or scalp tissue becomes too thin. Grafts or flaps may be used later to fill any remaining void. Alternately, several types of flaps can be designed by the creative surgeon to fill voids.

HAIR WEAVES. Hair weaves have been refined by the HAIR CLUB FOR MEN (1-800-677-7700) in the United States. They create a matrix of crisscrossing, transparent fibers, fitted and shaped to the client's thinning area. The matrix is porous, allowing the scalp to "breathe." New hair is added to the matrix strand by strand to re-create the pattern and hair flow of the client's own hair. The matrix is then fused to the client's remaining growing hair using a medical adhesive called Polyfuse. The client returns to HAIR CLUB FOR MEN for haircuts and to replace the Polyfuse every 5 weeks. Clients are generally very satisfied with the process and prefer it to a wig.

Adrenal androgenic female-pattern alopecia

Chronic, progressive, diffuse hair loss in women in their 20s and 30s is a frequently encountered complaint. These women, who usually have a normal menstrual cycle and lack any abnormalities on physical examination, have been classified as having "male-pattern baldness," a genetic trait, and have been dismissed without further evaluation. Recent studies have shown that some of these women have increased levels of the serum adrenal androgen dehydroepiandrosterone sulfate (DHEA-S) and a distinct pattern of central scalp alopecia, which has been called adrenal androgenic female-pattern alopecia.

Male-pattern baldness results in a gradual regression of the hair on the central scalp and gradual frontotemporal recession, as well as a gradual decrease in hair shaft diameter in the areas of hair loss. In contrast, most women with diffuse alopecia experience a gradual loss of hair on the central scalp, with retention of the normal hairline without frontotemporal recession. There is a variety of anagen hair diameters. With advancing age, the central thinning becomes more pronounced; in contrast to male-pattern baldness, a fringe of hair along the frontal hairline persists (Figure 24-7).[14] In exceptional cases, a course similar to that in men is seen, with deep frontotemporal recession.

LABORATORY FINDINGS. The laboratory investigation of female patients with diffuse alopecia with both female and male patterns is outlined in Table 24-3. Laboratory evaluation for some androgenic alopecia patients should initially include determination of the serum DHEA-S and total serum testosterone (T) levels, testosterone-estradiol–binding globulin (TeBG) for the T/TeBG ratio, and serum prolactin levels.[15]

TREATMENT. A 2% topical minoxidil solution (Rogaine/Regaine) was significantly more effective than placebo in the treatment of female androgenic alopecia.[16, 17] A 5% solution is available.

See treatment for androgenic alopecia in men and hirsutism.

Table 24-3 Laboratory Values for Evaluation of Diffuse Female Alopecia

Laboratory parameter	Female-pattern alopecia	Female-pattern alopecia with hirsutism	Male-pattern alopecia (frontotemporal recession)
DHEA-S*	Normal or elevated	Normal or elevated	Elevated
T	Normal	Normal or elevated	Elevated
TeBG	Normal	Decreased or normal	Decreased or normal
T/TeBG Prolactin†	Normal	Elevated	Elevated

*DHEA-S, dehydroepiandrosterone sulphate; T, total serum testosterone; TeBG, testosterone-estradiol–binding globulin; T/TeBG, androgenic index.
†If elevated, suspect pituitary disease (e.g., pituitary prolactin secreting adenoma).

FEMALE PATTERN—ALOPECIA

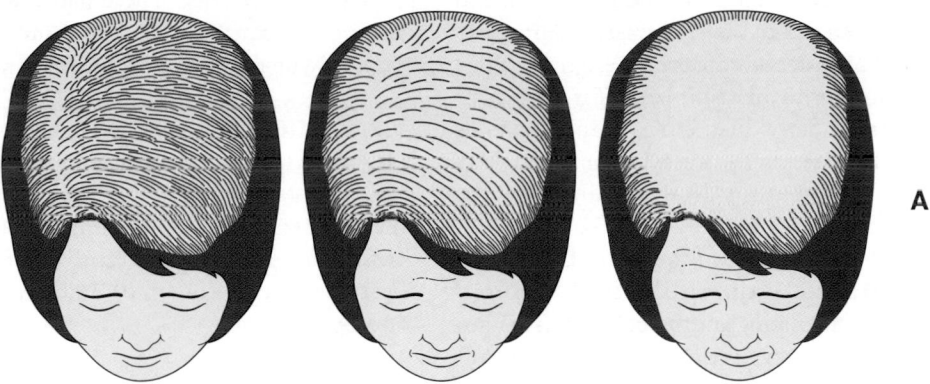

A

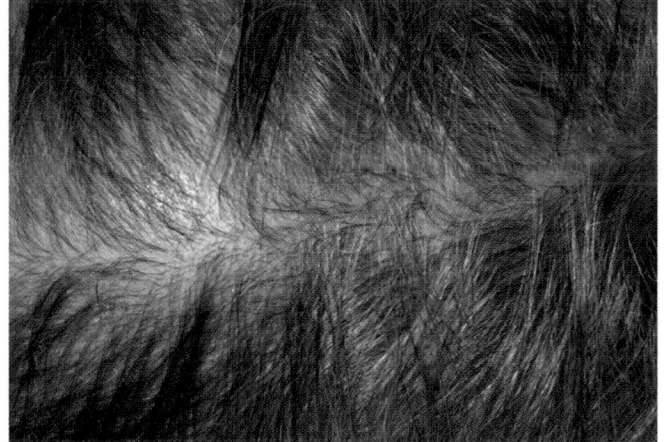

B

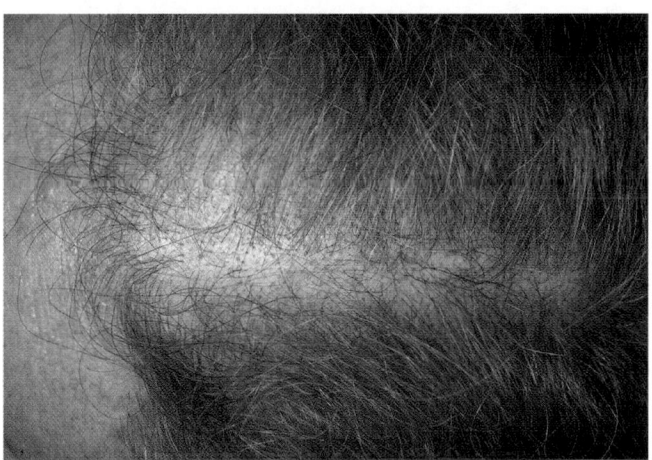

C

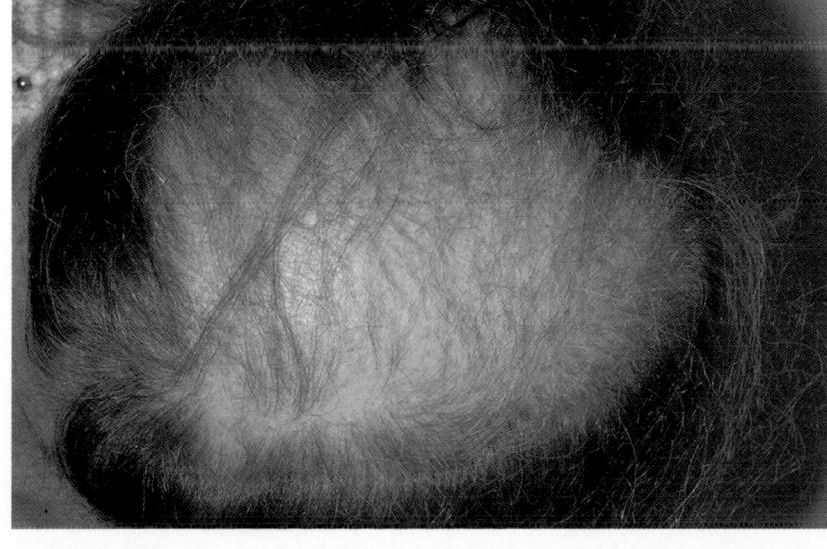

D

Figure 24-7 A, Ludwig pattern. Evolution of the female type of androgenic alopecia. **B,** Widening of the hair part is an initial change. **C,** More extensive widening of the hair part. **D,** Diffuse hair loss over the crown. The frontal hair line is preserved.

Hirsutism

Hirsutism is the presence of terminal (thick, dark) hairs in females in a male-like pattern such as on the face, chest, and areolae. It affects between 5% and 10% of women. Hirsutism is usually benign and of cosmetic concern.

Hirsutism in women with masculinizing signs, particularly if they arise after puberty, may indicate an ovarian or adrenal neoplasm. There are many causes of hirsutism (Box 24-4). The degree of hirsutism is determined by the Ferriman-Gallwey score (Table 24-4).

IDIOPATHIC HIRSUTISM. Hirsute patients with normal ovulatory function and circulating androgen levels have idiopathic hirsutism (IH). A history of regular menses is not sufficient to exclude ovulatory dysfunction, since up to 40% of hirsute women with menses are anovulatory. The excessive body hair is due to increased sensitivity of the pilosebaceous unit to normal plasma levels of androgen. These women may have increased numbers of androgen receptors and increased 5α-reductase activity. These patients respond to antiandrogen or 5α-reductase inhibitor therapy (finasteride).[18] Less than 20% of all hirsute women have IH.

VIRILIZATION. Virilization is the combination of hirsutism plus other signs of masculinization, such as deepening of the voice and temporal balding (Box 24-5). Virilization may be the sign of an ovarian or adrenal tumor. Virilization is associated with markedly increased androgen production by the ovary or adrenal (or both) and markedly increased plasma androgens.

OVARIAN VIRILIZATION. Rare androgen-secreting ovarian tumors can cause virilization. The onset of hirsutism and virilization is more abrupt than in women with polycystic ovary syndrome. Ovarian tumors may secrete a variety of hormones including thyroxine.

ADRENAL VIRILIZATION. Adrenal virilization is most commonly caused by congenital adrenal hyperplasia (21-hydroxylase deficiency). The diagnosis is usually made at birth because of sexual ambiguity. Less severe forms are termed late-onset adrenal hyperplasia, and hirsutism begins at puberty. Adrenal tumors are a rare cause of androgen excess in women.

Box 24-4 Causes of Hirsutism

Hirsutism without virilization	Hirsutism with virilization
Genetic	Ovarian
Polycystic ovary syndrome	Polycystic ovary syndrome
Racial	Hyperthecosis
Familial	HAIR-AN syndrome (hyperandrogenism, insulin resistance, acanthosis nigricans)
Physiologic	
Puberty	
Pregnancy	Tumors
Menopause	Adrenal
Endocrine	Congenital adrenal hyperplasias (classic and attenuated forms)
Hypothyroidism	
Acromegaly	
Congenital lesions	21-hydroxylase deficiency
Hurler's syndrome	11-hydroxylase deficiency (rare)
Trisomy E	
De Lange's syndrome	3β-hydroxysteroid dehydrogenase deficiency (rare)
Porphyria	
Hamartomas	Tumors
Drugs	ACTH-dependent Cushing's syndrome
Androgens	
Diazoxide	
Glucocorticoids	
Minoxidil	
Oral contraceptives (progestational components)	
Phenytoin	
CNS lesions	
Multiple sclerosis	
Encephalitis	
Hyperostosis frontalis interna	
Achard-Thiers syndrome	

Box 24-5 Hirsutism and Virilization—Clinical Findings in Women

Hirsutism: Excessive hair growth in women in 9 key androgen-sensitive anatomic sites.
Face
Chest
Areola
Linea alba
Lower back
Upper back
Buttock
Inner thigh
External genitalia
Virilization: The combination of hirsutism plus:
Acne and increased sebum production
Clitoral hypertrophy
Decrease in breast size
Deepening of the voice
Frontotemporal balding
Increased muscle mass
Infrequent or absent menses
Heightened libido
Hirsutism
Malodorous perspiration

Table 24-4 The Ferriman-Gallwey Hirsute Score for Women

Site	Definition	Grade
Upper lip	A few hairs at the outer margin	1
	A small moustache at outer margin	2
	A moustache extending halfway from outer margin	3
	A moustache extending to the midline	4
Chin	A few scattered hairs	1
	Scattered hairs with small concentrations	2
	Complete cover light	3
	Complete cover heavy	4
Chest	Circumareolar hairs	1
	Circumareolar hairs with mid-line hair	2
	Fusion of circumareolar hairs with mid-line hair giving three-fourths cover	3
	Complete cover	4
Upper back	A few scattered hairs	1
	More than a few scattered hairs but still scattered	2
	Complete cover light	3
	Complete cover heavy	4
Lower back	A sacral tuft of hair	1
	A sacral tuft of hair with some lateral extension	2
	Three-quarter cover	3
	Complete cover	4
Upper abdomen	A few midline hairs	1
	Rather more but still mid-line	2
	Half cover	3
	Complete cover	4
Lower abdomen	A few mid-line hairs	1
	A mid-line streak of hair	2
	A mid-line band of hair	3
	An inverted V-shaped growth	4
Upper arm	Sparse growth affecting not more than a quarter of the limb surface	1
	More than a quarter coverage but still incomplete	2
	Complete cover light	3
	Complete cover heavy	4
Thigh	Sparse growth affecting not more than one fourth of the limb surface	1
	More than one-fourth coverage but still incomplete	2
	Complete cover light	3
	Complete cover heavy	4

Where:

• Grade 0 indicates the absence of terminal hair

Ferriman-Gallwey hormonal hair score =

= (grade for upper lip) + (grade for chin) + (grade for chest) + (grade for upper back) + (grade for lower back) + (grade for upper abdomen) + (grade for lower abdomen) + (grade for upper arm) + (grade for thigh)

Interpretation:

• Minimum hormonal hair score: 0
• Maximum hormonal hair score: 36
• The higher the score, the more hirsute the woman.
• A score more than 6 in a white woman indicates an abnormal hair distribution.
• Each ethnic group may have a different upper limit of normal.

*Hirsutism in women is measured by the degree of hair growth in nine body regions.

BODY HAIR. The number of hairs per unit area is determined by genetic factors. Mediterranean men and women have more body hairs per unit area than Asians. Hair follicles cover the entire body except for the lips, palms, and soles. There are two types of hair follicles: vellus and terminal. Most women have some terminal hair in the so-called male sexual pattern around the areolae and extending from the pubis in the midline of the abdomen. In women, excess androgen production stimulates vellus hairs to develop into long, coarse, pigmented terminal hairs in most areas of the body except the scalp, where terminal hairs are converted to vellus hairs, resulting in balding. Women in whom hirsutism develops after puberty, especially if accompanied by signs of virilization such as infrequent or absent menses, have an abnormal condition and require further evaluation.

Pathophysiology

Hirsutism is caused by high androgen levels (from ovaries or adrenal glands) or by hair follicles that are more sensitive to normal androgen levels. Free testosterone is the androgen that causes hair growth.

Androgens are produced by the adrenals and ovaries. They are transported in the blood by sex hormone–binding globulin (SHBG) to the hair follicle where they are converted and bind to androgen receptors. Overproduction of androgens, increased conversion of androgen at the follicle, decreased metabolism, and enhanced receptor binding are potential causes of hirsutism.

Testosterone stimulates the growth of thick, dark hair. Estrogens slow growth and produce finer, lighter hairs. Progesterone has a minimal effect. Serum levels of testosterone are regulated by SHBG. SHBG levels increase with higher estrogen levels, such with oral contraceptive therapy. Increased SHBG levels lower the activity of circulating testosterone. Lower levels of SHBG increase the availability of free testosterone. SHBG levels decrease in response to the following:
- Adrenal hyperplasia (congenital or delayed-onset)
- Cushing syndrome
- Excess growth hormone
- Exogenous androgens
- Hyperinsulinemia
- Hyperprolactinemia
- Obesity
- Polycystic ovary syndrome

CIRCULATING ANDROGENS. The primary mechanism leading to the development of hirsutism and virilization is increased secretion of testosterone and other androgens by the ovaries or adrenal glands. The principal sources of circulating androgens in normal women are summarized in Figure 24-8. The higher the production of androgens, the greater the degree of virilization. The four primary circulating androgenic steroids in women are dehydroepiandrosterone (DHEA) and its sulfate (DHEA-S), androstenedione, and testosterone.

Approximately 50% of the testosterone is secreted from the ovaries and adrenal glands. The remainder is produced from metabolism in the liver, fat, and skin of the prehormones androstenedione, DHEA, and DHEA-S. Androstenedione is produced by both the ovaries and the adrenal glands. DHEA-S originates from the adrenal glands. The liver is the major site of testosterone metabolism. Testosterone overproduction overwhelms the liver's clearance capabilities, and excessive testosterone appears in the circulation. The hair follicle then becomes a site to metabolize the excess testosterone.

Metabolism of excess testosterone by the hair follicle leads to excessive coarse hair production.

ANDROGENS AND FOLLICLES. Testosterone binds to androgen receptors in the hair follicle. The follicular enzyme 5α-reductase is activated and transforms receptor-bound testosterone to 5α-dihydrotestosterone (DHT). The activated hormones stimulate follicular proliferation, resulting in the growth of thick (terminal) hair. Androgen-dependent follicles are located in the beard area, upper back, shoulders, sternum, axillae, and pubis (Figures 24-9 and 24-10). Axillary and pubic follicles are very sensitive to low levels of androgens, whereas follicles on the face and trunk respond only to high levels of androgens. Excess androgens can transform vellus hair in these regions to terminal hair (thick, pigmented hair) and produce hirsutism. Frontotemporal scalp hair recession often is seen with hirsutism.

ANDROGEN PRODUCTION IN HIRSUTISM. Mean plasma androgen levels are elevated in women with hirsutism, but there is considerable overlap in values among normal women and women with idiopathic hirsutism and polycystic ovary syndrome. Between 25% and 60% of hirsute women have a normal total plasma testosterone level. A normal plasma testosterone level is found in 80% of women with normal menses. Testosterone production rates are almost always elevated in hirsute women. A normal random plasma testosterone level in a hirsute woman frequently does not accurately reflect the testosterone production rate. The free plasma testosterone level is a more sensitive index of increased testosterone production in women with hirsutism than is the total testosterone level.[19]

DIAGNOSIS OF HIRSUTISM. Determine age of onset, severity, and rate of progression. Hirsutism that begins at puberty may be caused by polycystic ovary syndrome or hyperthecosis, idiopathic hirsutism, or late-onset adrenal hyperplasia. Sudden onset of hirsutism suggests an iatrogenic cause (drugs, etc.) or, if associated with virilization, a tumor of the ovary or adrenal gland. The presence of acanthosis nigricans suggests the diagnosis of the HAIR-AN syndrome in association with PCOS or hyperthecosis. Clitorimegaly, male-pattern baldness, and other virilizing signs suggest an ovarian or adrenal tumor.

HIRSUTISM

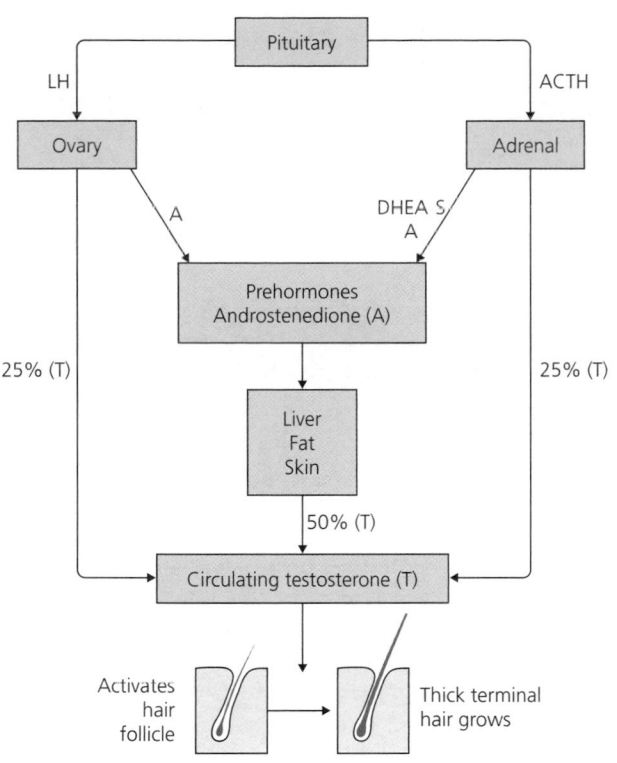

Figure 24-8 Androgen-dependent hirsutism.
T = testosterone; DHEA = dehydroepiandrosterone;
DHEA-S = dehydroepiandrosterone sulfate;
A = androstenedione.

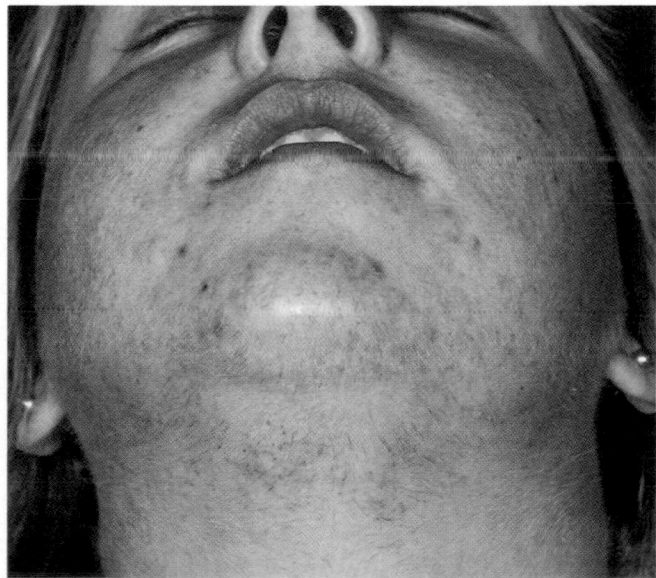

Figure 24-9 Hirsutism (grades II and III). Growth of terminal hair on the chin and neck of a young woman.

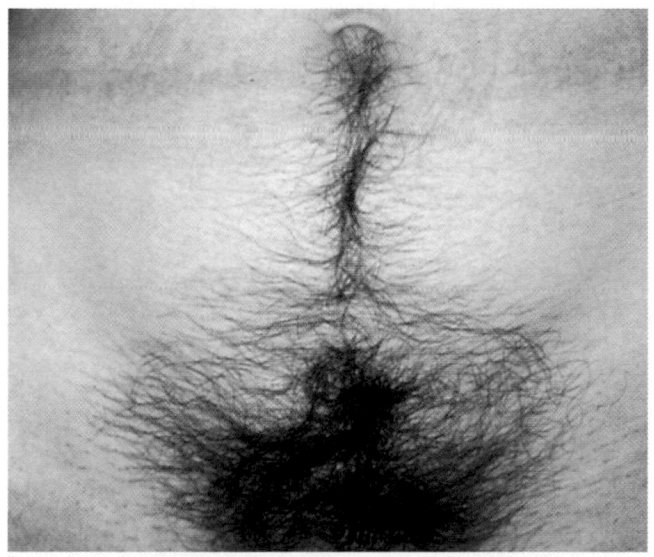

Figure 24-10 Hirsutism. A prominent escutcheon in a woman.

EXAMINATION AND TESTS. A systematic approach for the evaluation of hirsutism is outlined in Boxes 24-6 and 24-7 and in the diagram on p. 851. Measure serum testosterone and DHEA-S levels. If mild hirsutism and normal or near-normal levels of testosterone and DHEA-S are present, more extensive testing is usually not indicated if the history sug-

gests polycystic ovary syndrome. Serum testosterone is markedly elevated in ovarian causes of virilization, and DHEA-S is elevated in cases of virilization of adrenal origin. If there is a family history of adrenal hyperplasia or if the symptoms of hirsutism are more severe, basal 17-OHP should be measured.

Box 24-6 Evaluation of Hirsutism

Determine that hirsutism actually exists

Document degree and distribution. Drug-induced hirsutism (other than androgens) consists of increase in fine hairs (lanugo-like) that is not restricted to androgen-dependent areas

Classify degree of hirsutism

(based on distribution and number of terminal hairs) See Ferriman-Gallwey model (page 847)

History

Serious disease is suggested by onset of hirsutism well after puberty, rapid progression of hair growth, balding, deepening of the voice, and increased libido

Idiopathic hirsutism, polycystic ovary disease, and late-onset attenuated congenital adrenal hyperplasia (21-hydroxylase deficiency) usually start at puberty with slowly progressive hair growth. Weight gain and menstrual irregularity are often seen

Polycystic ovary disease is the most common cause of hyperandrogenism in women. These women show no signs of virilization and minor degrees of hirsutism

Physical examination

Look for signs of virilization

Determine "clitoral index": the product of the vertical and horizontal dimensions of the glans clitoris—normal range, 9-35 mm². Unequivocal clitoral enlargement (>100 mm²) suggests severe hyperandrogenicity and is not usually seen in polycystic ovary disease, idiopathic hirsutism, or congenital adrenal hyperplasia

Pelvic examination: 50% of ovarian tumors are palpable

Palpate abdomen for adrenal masses

Acanthosis nigricans suggests insulin resistance

Examine for signs of Cushing's disease

Perform initial laboratory studies

Serum dehydroepiandrosterone sulfate (DHEA-S)

Total or free testosterone

Consider more detailed initial workup for patients with virilization or other complications (see Box 24-7)

Perform follow-up studies or refer to endocrinologist

Adapted from Rittmaster RS, Loriaux DL: Ann Intern Med 1987; 106:95.

Data from Birnbaum MD, Rose LI: Fertil Steril 1979; 32:536; Rittmaster RS, Loriaux DL: Ann Intern Med 1987; 106:95; and Braunstein GD: Female reproductive disorders. In Hershman JM, ed: Management of endocrine disorders. Philadelphia, Lea & Febiger, 1980.

Box 24-7 Laboratory Evaluation for Complicated Cases of Hirsutism

Initial visit

Virilization (determine degree of severity)

Serum testosterone* and free testosterone (Determine level of circulating testosterone, whatever its origin)

Testosterone-estradiol–binding globulin (To assess the influence of any excess androgenic hormone, whatever its origin. Androgens depress liver synthesis of this binding protein)

Serum 17-hydroxyprogesterone (between 7:00 and 9:00 AM) (if history suggestive of congenital adrenal hyperplasia)

Serum dehydroepiandrosterone sulfate (DHEA-S)[†]

Serum androstenedione[‡]

Serum LH and FSH

Serum thyroxine

Ovarian sonography (ultrasound)

With these tests, the diagnosis can be established in more than 95% of patients at the first visit

Subsequent visits

Testosterone: normal or slightly elevated

No further investigation

Testosterone: markedly elevated

Repeat testosterone test

Computed tomography (adrenal glands)

ACTH stimulation test for confirmation—if 17-hydroxyprogesterone elevated

Surgical exploration

Urinary free cortisol + overnight dexamethasone suppression test (if Cushing's syndrome suspected)

Ovarian/adrenal vein catheterization

Prolactin levels rule out prolactin-secreting tumor

Data from Morris DV: Clin Obstet Gynecol 1985; 12:649; Hammond MG, Talbert LM, Groff TR: Postgrad Med 1986; 79:107.

*Serum testosterone levels fluctuate with the menstrual cycle, peaking at midcycle.

†Serum DHEA-S is used as a marker of adrenal androgen production because serum concentrations do not vary with the menstrual cycle and there is little diurnal fluctuation.

‡Serum A concentrations vary as much as 50% over a 24-hour period. There is an increase in mean plasma A levels during midcycle.

SCREENING TESTS
TOTAL OR FREE TESTOSTERONE + DHEA-S

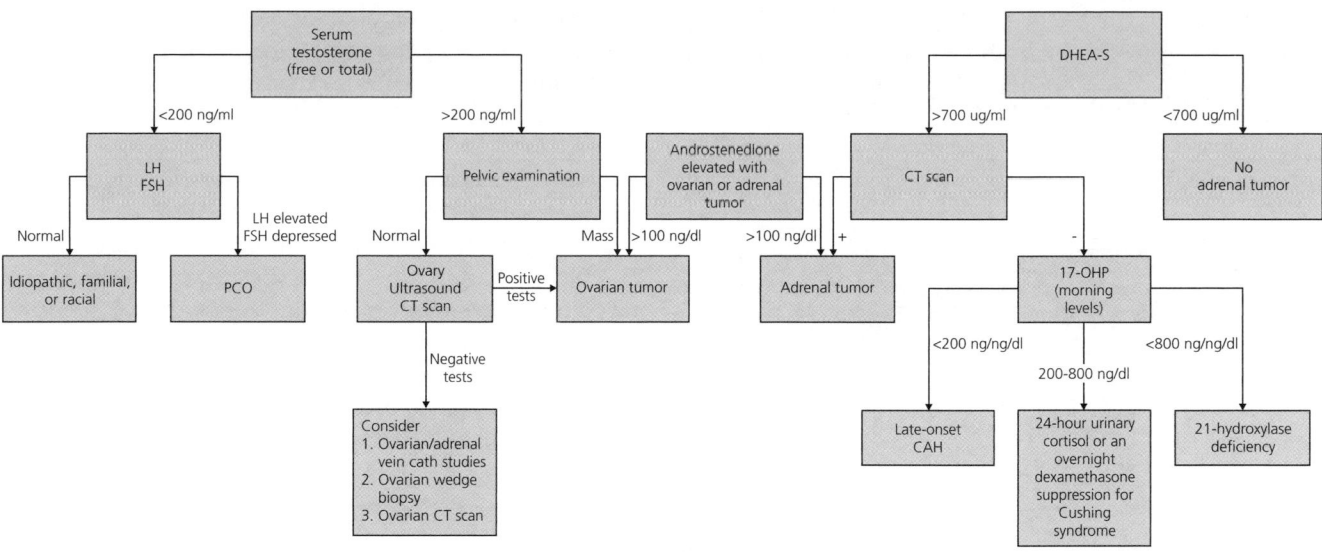

DHEA-S, Dehydroepiandrosterone sulfate; PCOD, polycystic ovary disease; LH, lutinizing hormone; FSH, follicle-stimulating hormone; 17 OHP, 17-hydroxyprogesterone; CAH, congenital adrenal hyperplasia

POLYCYSTIC OVARY SYNDROME. Polycystic ovary syndrome (PCOS) is the most frequent cause of anovulatory infertility and hirsutism. It is a heterogeneous syndrome that affects 6% of women of reproductive age. The etiology is unknown. The onset is in the peripubertal years. There is insulin resistance, androgen excess, and abnormal gonadotropin secretion. There are signs and symptoms of elevated androgen levels, menstrual irregularity, and amenorrhea.

A genetic defect may cause an increase in intraovarian androgens and stop ovulation. The polycystic ovary forms when an anovulatory state exists. Bilaterally enlarged polycystic ovaries develop, defined by the presence of more than eight follicles per ovary, with the follicles less than 10 mm in diameter. These findings are seen on ultrasound examinations in more than 90% of women with PCOS, but they are also present in up to 25% of normal women. Serum testosterone and LH are elevated in most affected women. Women present with menstrual irregularities, infertility, and androgen excess symptoms of hirsutism and acne. Some women have normal cycles. Virilizing signs such as clitorimegaly, deepening of the voice, temporal balding, or masculinization of body habitus are almost always absent. Obesity is present in up to 70% of patients.

PCOS is associated with hyperinsulinemia, insulin resistance, an increased risk for type 2 diabetes mellitus, acanthosis nigricans, lipid abnormalities, and hypertension. Hyperinsulinemia may be the cause of the overproduction of ovarian androgens. The risk of endometrial cancer is three times higher than in normal women.

Diagnosis. In the absence of pregnancy and when amenorrhea or oligomenorrhea has persisted for 6 months or longer without a diagnosis, a careful history and physical examination should be undertaken, with particular attention to patterns of hair distribution and a search for acanthosis nigricans.

The diagnosis of PCOS is primarily clinical (Boxes 24-8 and 24-9). Many women have elevated testosterone, LH, and fasting insulin and reduced levels of sex hormone-binding globulin. Many consider an LH-to-FSH ratio of 3:1 diagnostic. Ultrasound shows more than eight ovarian follicles (less than 10 mm in diameter).

Treatment. Weight reduction, diet, and exercise are essential. Monthly progestin therapy such as medroxyprogesterone (Provera) controls endometrial proliferation but does not suppress ovarian androgen production.

Low-dose oral contraceptive pills prevent endometrial hyperplasia and cancer and treat hirsutism and acne. Antiandrogens may be combined with oral contraceptive pills for the treatment of hirsutism. Spironolactone (25 to 100 mg twice daily) or flutamide (250 mg twice daily) are effective. Clomiphene citrate (Clomid) is used for patients who desire pregnancy. Metformin (Glucophage) improves insulin sensitivity, decreases serum LH and free testosterone levels, and may restore menstrual cycles.

Box 24-8 Diagnostic Criteria for Polycystic Ovary Syndrome*

Clinical features

Amenorrhea, oligomenorrhea or dysfunctional uterine bleeding

Anovulatory infertility

Hirsutism and/or acne

Central obesity

Endocrine abnormalities on laboratory tests

Elevated androgen (i.e., testosterone) levels

Elevated luteinizing hormone concentration with normal to mildly elevated follicle-stimulating hormone level

Insulin resistance with hyperinsulinemia

Radiologic abnormalities on ultrasound examination

Multiple (nine or more) subcortical follicular cysts

Increased ovarian stromal density and/or volume

Exclusion of other etiologies

Prolactinoma

Virilizing tumors of adrenal or ovarian tumors

Congenital adrenal hyperplasia

Cushing's syndrome

Adapted from Hunter MH, Sterrett JJ: Am Fam Physician 2000; 62.
*The diagnosis is based on the presence of some or all of the common clinical features and is confirmed by the presence of biochemical or radiologic evidence of endocrine abnormality and the exclusion of other etiologies.

Box 24-9 Polycystic Ovary Syndrome Workup (Evaluation of chronic hyperandrogenic anovulatory women)

Urine human chorionic gonadotropin (exclude pregnancy)

Prolactin (rule out prolactinoma)

Testosterone (mildly elevated, rule out virilizing tumors)

Luteinizing hormone (usually high)

Follicle-stimulating hormone (low or normal)

Fasting glucose (elevated)

Lipid profile, including total, low-density lipoprotein and high-density lipoprotein cholesterol levels (rule out cardiovascular disease)

Order in selected patients

Pelvic ultrasound examination

Dehydroepiandrosterone sulfate level* (screen for adrenal tumor)

17-hydroxyprogesterone level (screen for adult-onset congenital adrenal hyperplasia)

Dexamethasone suppression test (for cortisol excess—hypertension, central obesity, etc.)

Adapted from Hunter MH: Am Fam Physician 2000; 62.

TREATMENT OF HIRSUTISM. Hirsutism cannot be cured, only suppressed. The problem is cosmetic, and the decision to treat must be made after consideration of the potential side effects of medication. Many women find excess hair intolerable and choose to tolerate side effects.

Treatment begins after ovarian and adrenal disease has been investigated and, if present, is dealt with appropriately (Box 24-10).

Oral contraceptives reduce free testosterone. Low-dose glucocorticoids (dexamethasone, prednisone) suppress adrenal gland production and lower DHEA-S levels. Spironolactone and cyproterone acetate are androgen receptor competitive inhibitors. Spironolactone is used extensively in the United States to treat hirsutism. Cyproterone acetate is available in other countries. Patients are treated and observed during a 3-month suppression period. Hair growth neither lessens nor worsens during this period. Improvement is observed within 6 to 12 months.

Finasteride is beneficial in women with hirsutism, but the drug should be used cautiously because of its potential feminizing effects on male fetuses.

Initiating treatment. Standard treatment is combination oral contraceptives (COCs) and androgen receptor blockers. Norgestimate (Ortho Tri-Cyclen) is a low androgenic progestin and is a good first choice. Spironolactone is usually the first choice for an androgen receptor blocker. Start with 25 mg twice daily and increase to 50 mg twice daily. If there is no improvement after 3 to 6 months, the dose can be increased to a maximum of 100 mg twice daily. In cases of intolerance or lack of improvement, flutamide at a starting dose of 125 to 250 mg/day can be considered. Liver function studies every 2 weeks for the first month, then monthly thereafter, are required in patients receiving flutamide. Finasteride, 1 or 5 mg/day can be considered for women who

Box 24-10 Treatment Options for Hirsutism

Androgen receptor blockers
    Spironolactone
    Flutamide
    Cyproterone acetate

Ovarian suppression
    Combination oral contraceptives

Adrenal suppression
    Low-dose corticosteroids

5α-reductase inhibition
    Finasteride

do not tolerate androgen receptor blockers. Finasteride is contraindicated in pregnancy. The drugs take from 6 to 9 months to improve hirsutism. In responsive patients, dexamethasone may be used at low doses (associated with an antiandrogen) to prolong the length of the remission. Finasteride may be used as an alternative to low-dose antiandrogen therapy, but the results are often less satisfactory.[20] Cessation of antiandrogen therapy is followed by recurrence.[21]

Combination oral contraceptives. Combination oral contraceptives (COCs) reduce the cutaneous androgen effect by suppressing gonadotropin release (luteinizing hormone), which results in suppression of ovarian androgen production. COCs regulate the menstrual cycle in oligomenorrheic women and reduce side effects of androgen receptor blockers. COCs reduce hair growth in women with idiopathic hirsutism and polycystic ovary disease and in oligomenorrhea with hyperandrogenism.

The estrogen component of COCs decreases the ovarian and adrenal androgen production and stimulates the liver to produce increased quantities of sex hormone-binding globulin (SHBG). The circulating globulin binds and decreases the concentration of active serum androgens. The criteria for choosing COCs are the same as for hirsutism and acne. A decrease in SHBG may occur with some COCs due to low estrogenic activities. This decrease allows increased circulating amounts of free androgen of adrenal or ovarian origin. COCs with progestins that have low androgenic-to-progestin activity ratios (e.g., desogestrel, ethynodiol diacetate, gestodene, norethindrone) and COCs with moderate-to-high estrogen contents are most effective (see list of COCs in formulary). Ortho Tri-Cyclen, Ortho-Cyclen, and Ovcon 35 meet these criteria.

COCs containing new progestogens have very restricted effectiveness in the short term (6 cycles), but their long-term use (greater than 12 cycles) cures mild-to-moderate hirsutism and improves severe hirsutism. In women being treated with antiandrogens, COCs are important to provide control of the menstrual cycle and contraception.

Spironolactone. Spironolactone is an aldosterone antagonist that is used as a diuretic and an antihypertensive agent. Spironolactone has antiandrogen properties. It acts at the hair follicle as an androgen receptor competitive inhibitor, resulting in decreased production of dihydrotestosterone, and suppresses androgen production by the gonad and adrenal glands. Antiandrogens do not induce hair loss, but the hair shaft diameter decreases in size, and color lightens. The drug is best suited to women with idiopathic hirsutism with normal menses. Pregnancy is contraindicated during spironolactone use. Spironolactone is not useful for women with a slight degree of hirsutism. Various studies have used spironolactone in the range of 25 to 100 mg given twice daily. Spironolactone's effectiveness is dosage-dependent: low dosages are less active than other antiandrogens, whereas high dosages (200 mg/day) are very effective at the cost of several adverse effects (particularly dysfunctional uterine bleeding), but the concomitant use of combination oral contraceptives may prevent these adverse effects.

The most common side effects are increased menstrual frequency, nausea, and fatigue. The menstrual irregularity can be treated with oral contraceptives. The drug is contraindicated in women with renal insufficiency because of the risk of hyperkalemia.

Flutamide. Flutamide (Eulexin) is a pure antiandrogen approved for prostate carcinoma that blocks androgen receptors and inhibits hair growth. It is very effective in treating hirsutism within 6 to 12 months. A low dose regimen with an initial treatment period using 250 mg/day to achieve satisfactory results, followed by a long maintenance treatment period using 125 mg/day is effective.[22] Dry skin is very frequent during treatment, and hepatotoxicity is possible at high dosages.

Finasteride. Finasteride, a 5α-reductase type 2 inhibitor, blocks the formation of DHT from testosterone. It is approved for use in the 5 mg dosage (Proscar) for benign prostate enlargement and in the 1 mg dose (Propecia) for androgenetic alopecia in men. It is the least effective antiandrogen, but a dosage of 5 mg/day decreases hirsutism without adverse effects. The drug could potentially feminize a male fetus; therefore pregnancy must be avoided. Oral contraceptives may be taken with finasteride.

Cyproterone acetate. Cyproterone acetate (available outside the United States) is a moderately potent antiandrogen. It is a progestogen that suppresses gonadotropin secretion and acts by blocking androgen receptors. It is used in Europe and in other countries to treat hirsutism. It is often used in women who have elevated testosterone with polycystic ovary syndrome. Dosages ranging from 2 to 200 mg/day, generally in combination with ethynyl estradiol, are used. Cyproterone acetate is taken up in adipose tissue and then slowly released, thus rendering the patient susceptible to menstrual irregularity. A reversed sequential regimen was developed to avoid this side effect. It consists of giving cyproterone acetate on days 5 through 15 of the cycle in dosages initially of 50 to 100 mg/day. Ethynyl estradiol is given in a dosage of 50 mg daily from days 5 through 26 of the cycle. Dosage reduction is possible once effective remission of hirsutism occurs. A combination oral contraceptive (Diane) containing cyproterone acetate (2 mg) and estrogen ethinyl estradiol (50 mg) is sometimes used for maintenance. Side effects include nausea, weight gain, breast tenderness, breakthrough bleeding, headache, decreased libido, and depression.

Glucocorticoids. Glucocorticoids are most effective for patients whose hirsutism is of short duration. Glucocorticoids suppress adrenocorticotropic hormone (ACTH) and thereby diminish adrenal androgen production. They are used to treat women with congenital adrenal hyperplasia (classic and attenuated forms) and other conditions with increased levels of DHEA-S. Low dosages of glucocorticoids suppress androgen but not adrenal glucocorticoid production. Dexamethasone (0.25 to 1 mg) or prednisone (5 to 7.5 mg) is administered at bedtime. Nighttime administration reduces the early-morning peak of ACTH secretion and generally does not cause the typical side effects of glucocorticoid excess or prolonged adrenal suppression. Dosage adjustments must be made because the dosage required for adrenal suppression, particularly with dexamethasone, varies widely among patients. DHEA-S and morning cortisol levels should be monitored. DHEA-S levels should fall to near-normal range, and cortisol levels should be maintained at normal levels. Treatment is stopped after 1 year, and the patient is observed. Decreased hair growth occurs in approximately 30% to 50% of patients.

COSMETIC APPROACH. Excess facial hair may be plucked, shaved, bleached, wax stripped, or removed by chemical depilatories. These treatments only temporarily alleviate the problem because irritation or plucking rapidly induces the anagen stage and hair-follicle growth.[23] Electrolysis and selective photothermolysis with the use of lasers destroy the hair shaft, outer root sheath, bulge, and dermal papilla of the hair follicles. The extent of the destruction determines whether the follicle regenerates.

Shaving. Shaving is effective. Shaving does not increase the thickness or rate of growth, but women are reluctant to use this technique. Stubble may be noticeable with thicker hair. Shave with the grain to avoid folliculitis.

Waxing and plucking. Waxing and plucking remove hair at the root. Waxing is painful. The results can last up to 6 weeks. Folliculitis and hyperpigmentation can occur.

Bleaching. Pigment in hair can be removed with over-the-counter peroxide bleaching agents (Jolen Crème Bleach, etc.). This is effective for women with light skin that is close to the color of bleached hair. Dark skin makes bleached hair look more prominent. Irritation can occur.

Depilatories. Thioglycolates (Nair, Better Off hair remover cream, etc.) are available over the counter. They break down the hair shaft and penetrate into the hair follicle to remove some of the hair below skin level. Therefore this treatment lasts longer than shaving. Some women do not tolerate the irritation.

Electrolysis. Permanent follicular destruction with an electrical probe that is passed into the follicle is a good option for women with small areas of facial hair. There are three techniques. Galvanic electrolysis uses direct current to generate sodium hydroxide, which destroys follicular epithelium. Thermolysis damages follicles with heat generated with high-frequency alternating current. The blend method is a combination of galvanic and thermolysis electrolysis. Cost, pain, and time are considerations. Hypertrophic scars are possible; therefore, test a small area first. This procedure requires experience and good technique.

Lasers. Laser and flashlamp technology are the most efficient methods of long-term hair removal currently available. Lasers selectively destroy the hair follicle without damage to adjacent tissues. All these lasers work on the principle of selective photothermolysis, with the melanin in the hair follicles as the chromophobe. Selective photothermolysis relies on the absorption of a brief radiation pulse by specific pigmented targets, which generates and confines the heat to that selected target. Hair removal is most successful in patients with lighter skin colors and dark-colored hairs. Hair removal systems include: ruby laser (694 nm), alexandrite laser (755 nm), diode laser (800 nm), intense pulsed light source (590 to 1200 nm) and the neodymium:yttrium-aluminium-garnet (Nd:YAG) laser (1064 nm), with or without the application of carbon suspension. The Nd:YAG laser is less efficacious, but more suited to patients with darker colored skin. Multiple treatments are necessary. Hair clearance, after repeated treatments, of 30% to 50% is generally reported 6 months after the last treatment. Temporary adverse effects include erythema and perifollicular edema, which are common. Crusting, vesiculation, hypopigmentation, and hyperpigmentation (depending on skin color and other factors) may also occur.[24]

Vaniqa. Eflornithine HCl topical cream (Vaniqa) slows facial hair growth by blocking ornithine decarboxylase, an enzyme found in the hair follicle of the skin needed for hair growth. This results in slower hair growth and improved appearance where Vaniqa is applied. Vaniqa does not permanently remove hair. It is applied twice daily. The patient continues to use hair removal techniques as needed in conjunction with Vaniqa. Improvement may be seen as early as 4 to 8 weeks. Stop treatment if no improvement is seen after 6 months of use. In about 8 weeks after stopping treatment with Vaniqa, the hair will return to the same condition as before beginning treatment.

Alopecia areata

Alopecia areata (AA) is a common asymptomatic disease characterized by the rapid onset of total hair loss in a sharply defined, usually round, area.[25] The diagnosis is made by observation. Any hair-bearing surface may be affected. The cause is unknown. An interaction between genetic and environmental factors may trigger the disease. Alopecia areata is a partial loss of scalp hair; alopecia totalis is 100% loss of scalp hair, and alopecia universalis is 100% loss of hair on the scalp and body.

Prevalence

The prevalence of AA in the United States is 0.1% to 0.2% of the population. Sixty percent of patients present with their first patch before 20 years of age. Familial incidence is 37% in patients who had their first patch by 30 years of age and 7.1% with the first patch after 30 years of age.[25]

CLINICAL PRESENTATION. A wide spectrum of involvement is seen. Most patients report the sudden occurrence of one or several 1- to 4-cm areas of hair loss on the scalp that can be easily concealed by covering with adjacent hair. The skin is smooth and white or may have short stubs of hair. The hair shaft in AA is poorly formed and breaks on reaching the surface (Figure 24-11, A). Some patients complain of itching, tenderness, or a burning sensation before the patches appear.

AA appears to progress as a wave of follicles prematurely enters telogen.[26] The event weakens or narrows the hair shaft, which continues to grow before the telogen phase is complete. Most weakened hairs fracture when they reach the surface. The affected hairs that are often found retained at the periphery of a lesion have a normal upper shaft and a narrowed base—"exclamation point" hair.

Regrowth begins in 1 to 3 months and may be followed by loss in the same or other areas. The new hair is usually of the same color and texture, but it may be fine and white (Figure 24-11, B). Occasionally the white color remains. The eyelashes, beard, and, rarely, other parts of the body may be involved. Total hair loss of the scalp (alopecia totalis) (Figure 24-11, D), seen most frequently in young people, may be accompanied by cycles of growth and loss, but the prognosis for long-term regrowth is poor. Total body hair loss (alopecia universalis) is very rare.

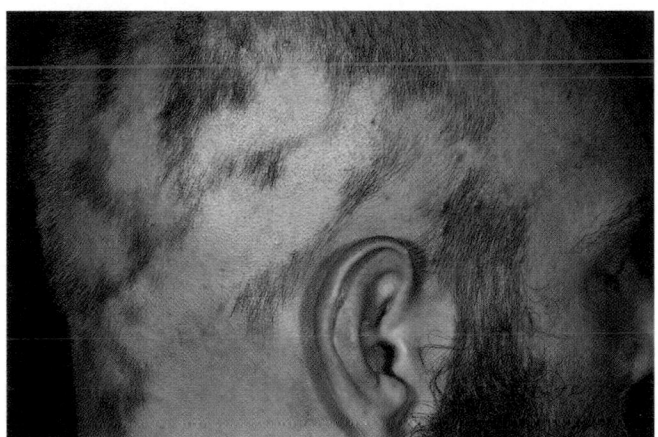

A, Multiple round and oval patches of hair loss.

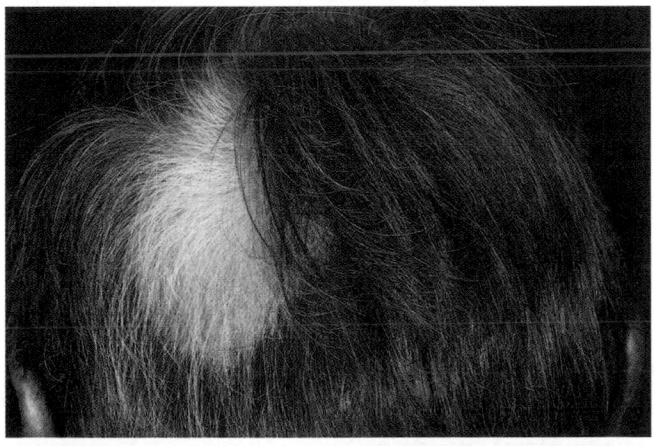

B, The regrown hair is white.

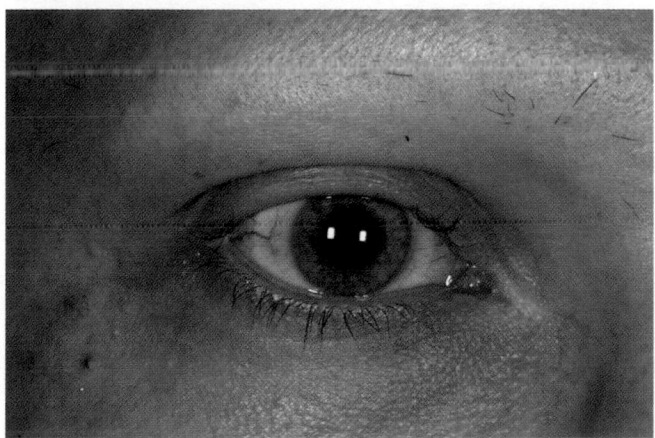

C, Loss of eyelashes and eyebrows is a common finding.

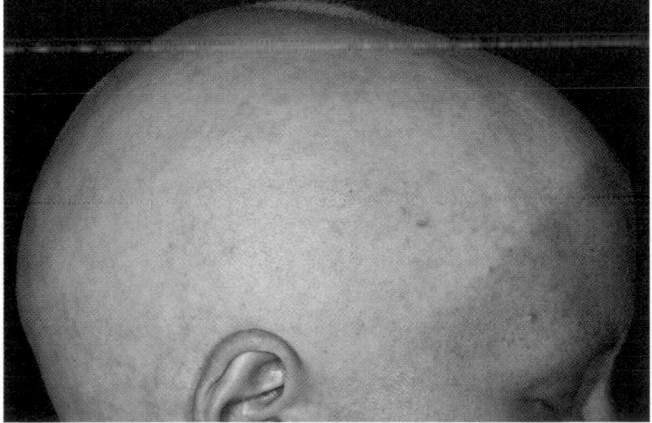

D, Alopecia totalis. The hair has regrown for short periods. The prognosis for normal regrowth is poor.

Figure 24-11 Alopecia areata.

PSYCHOLOGICAL IMPLICATIONS. Hair plays an important role in one's appearance and self-image, and sudden hair loss in a bizarre pattern is psychologically painful.[27] It affects the quality of life and limits social freedom. Those affected equate partial hair loss with balding and fear total hair loss. The appearance is striking, and people stare. AA is devastating for image-conscious teenagers. Patients make attempts to hide bald spots by covering them with adjacent long hairs. Those with extensive loss who cannot adequately camouflage the spots may go into hiding or obtain a wig. A network of support groups across the country is available to help people cope with fears, loneliness, and concerns. The National Alopecia Areata Foundation, 710 C St., Ste. 11, San Rafael, CA 94901-3853 (415-456-4644; *www.alopeciaareata.com*), provides informational brochures, newsletters, research, updates, sources of scalp prostheses, videotapes for schoolchildren, and locations of support groups and holds an annual conference to help patients cope with the condition. The physician can provide continuing support for this difficult problem.

NAIL CHANGES. Nail dystrophy may be associated with AA. The incidence is 10% to 66%. Pitting with an irregular pattern or in organized transverse or longitudinal rows and longitudinal striations resulting in sandpaper appearance may be seen in one to all of the nails of some patients with AA (Figure 24-12).[28] Dystrophy precedes, coincides with, or occurs after resolution of AA.

PROGNOSIS. The course is unpredictable; recovery may be complete or partial. Several episodes of loss and regrowth are typical. The prognosis for total permanent regrowth in cases with limited involvement is excellent. Most patients entirely regrow hair within 1 year without treatment; 10% develop chronic disease and may never regrow hair. Patients with a family history of AA, young age at onset, immune diseases, nail dystrophy, atopy, and extensive hair loss have a poor prognosis.[29]

DIFFERENTIAL DIAGNOSIS. The differential diagnosis includes trichotillomania and telogen effluvium. In trichotillomania there are short and broken hairs. A 4-mm punch biopsy may be required. Hair loss occurs over the entire scalp with telogen effluvium. The "moth-eaten" or diffuse alopecia of secondary syphilis may be confused with AA.[30]

ETIOLOGY. The etiology is unknown. Genetic factors are important. There is a higher incidence of a family history in patients with AA. Stress is frequently cited. One study concludes that there is little evidence that emotional stress plays a significant role in the pathogenesis of AA.[31]

IMMUNOLOGIC FACTORS. AA may be an autoimmune disease mediated by T lymphocytes directed to hair follicles. There are associations between AA and autoimmune disorders. An incidence of 8% to 11.8% in the frequency of thyroid disease is reported. AA patients have an increased prevalence of antithyroid and thyroid microsomal antibodies. AA patients have a fourfold greater incidence of vitiligo. The significance of these findings is unknown.

PATHOLOGY. A peribulbar lymphocytic infiltrate ("swarm of bees") with no scarring is characteristic. The acute follicular inflammation attacks the hair bulb in the subcutaneous fat. This inflammation terminates the anagen stage, forcing the follicle into catagen. Since the bulge area is spared, a new hair bulb and shaft grow at the start of the anagen stage, once the inflammation has subsided or has been controlled with glucocorticoids.

TREATMENT. Treatments control, do not cure, and do not prevent spread. Treatment according to age and severity is listed in Boxes 24-11 and 24-12.

Box 24-11 Treatment for Patients With Alopecia Areata According to Age and Severity of Condition
Patients < 10 years of age
5% topical minoxidil solution, topical glucocorticoid, or both
Anthralin (short contact)*
Patients >10 years of age
<50% of scalp affected
Intralesional glucocorticoid, 5% topical minoxidil solution, or both, with or without topical glucocorticoid
Anthralin (short contact)*
>50% of scalp affected
5% Topical minoxidil solution, with or without topical glucocorticoid
Topical immunotherapy
Anthralin (short contact)*
Oral glucocorticoid
Scalp prosthesis
Eyebrows and beard affected
Intralesional glucocorticoid, 5% topical minoxidil solution, or both
From Price VH: N Engl J Med 1999; 341.
*Anthralin is left on the scalp for 20 to 60 minutes.

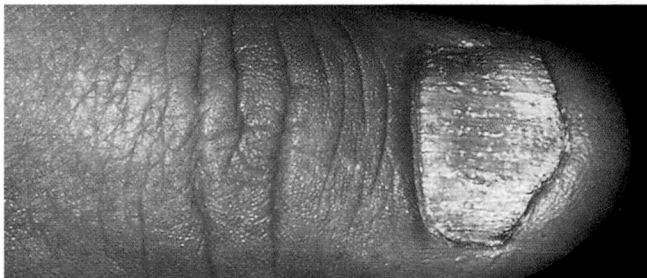

Figure 24-12 Shallow pitting occurs in some patients with alopecia areata.

Box 24-12 Suggested Methods of Treatment for Alopecia Areata

Intralesional glucocorticoid

All sites

The preferred compound is triamcinolone acetonide (10 mg/ml), administered with a 3-ml syringe with a 30-gauge 1½-inch long needle. Concentrations of 2.5 to 8 mg/ml may also be used, 2.5 mg/ml is used for the beard area and eyebrows. Inject 0.1 ml or less into the mid-dermis at multiple sites 1 cm apart; do not raise wheal or inject into subcutaneous tissue. Repeat every 4 to 6 weeks; if atrophy of the skin occurs, do not reinject affected site until atrophy resolves. Optional topical anesthesia may be used: apply a mixture of 2.5% lidocaine and 2.5% prilocaine (EMLA cream) in a thick layer to intact skin and cover with occlusive dressing for 1 hour before injections are given; remove cream immediately before injections.

Scalp

The maximal dose is 20 mg per visit. When more than 50% of scalp is affected, inject only selected sites.

Eyebrows

The maximal dose is 1.25 mg per visit injected into the mid-dermis of each brow at five or six sites (for a total of 2.5 mg to both brows).

Beard

The maximal dose is 7.5 mg per visit.

5% Topical minoxidil solution

Scalp and beard

The maximal dose is 1 ml per application. Apply twice daily to affected sites. Spread solution with fingers. Wash hands afterward. This treatment is not effective for patients with total (100%) loss of scalp hair.

Eyebrows

Apply two applications to each eyebrow with a finger twice daily using a mirror to ensure precise placement. Hold a cotton ball over the eye for protection. Wash hands afterward.

Anthralin (short contact)*

Apply 0.5 to 1% anthralin cream to affected scalp once daily; leave on 20 to 30 minutes daily for 2 wk, then 45 minutes daily for 2 wk, up to a maximum of 1 hour daily. Wash hands afterward, and avoid getting anthralin in the eyes.

Remove from scalp with mineral oil, then wash off with soap and water. Do not use on brows or beard. Some patients tolerate overnight application.

Topical glucocorticoid

Apply twice daily.

Topical immunotherapy

Use diphencyprone or squaric acid dibutyl ester to induce contact sensitization. For initial sensitization, apply 2% solution of selected contact allergen in acetone to a 4-cm² area on one side of the scalp. After initial sensitization, apply diluted solution of contact allergen weekly to same half of scalp in two coats. The patient washes off the allergen after 48 hr after both the sensitizing application and subsequent weekly applications. Adjust concentration of allergen according to the response to the previous week's treatment. Desired responses include mild itching, erythema, and scaling.

Concentrations of allergen that elicit responses range from 0.0001%, 0.001%, 0.01%, 0.025%, 0.05%, 0.1%, 0.25%, 0.5%, and 1.0% to 2.0%. After hair growth is established on the treated side (in 3 to 12 months), then both sides of the scalp are treated. Apply contact sensitizer with wooden applicator tipped with generous amount of cotton (the physician or nurse applying weekly treatment must wear gloves). To minimize side effects it is recommended that the allergen be applied in a physician's office and not be given to the patient for use at home.

Oral glucocorticoids

Active, extensive, or rapidly spreading alopecia areata

For patients weighing >60 kg the recommended treatment is 40 mg of oral prednisone daily for 1 wk; then 35 mg daily for 1 wk; 30 mg daily for 1 wk; 25 mg daily for 1 wk; 20 mg daily for 3 days; 15 mg daily for 3 days; 10 mg daily for 3 days; and 5 mg daily for 3 days. Prednisone may be used with 5% topical minoxidil solution twice daily and intralesional triamcinolone acetonide injections given as above, every 4 to 6 weeks. Topical therapy should be continued twice daily with or without intralesional injections every 4 to 6 weeks after prednisone is tapered.

Active, less extensive alopecia areata

Twenty mg of oral prednisone should be given daily or every other day; dose should be tapered slowly by increments of 1 mg after the condition is stable.

Adapted from Price VH: N Engl J Med 1999; 341.

*Anthralin is left on the scalp for 20 to 60 minutes.

Observation. The majority of patients with a few small areas of hair loss can be assured that the prognosis for regrowth is excellent. If there is great anxiety or if bald areas cannot be concealed, then intralesional injections should be considered.

Topical steroids. Topical steroids are of little value.

Intralesional injections. Intralesional corticosteroid injections are first-line therapy for patients with less than 50% of scalp involvement. Regrowth is seen in 4 to 8 weeks. Repeat injections every 4 to 6 weeks. Atrophy occurs with larger volumes and concentrations of triamcinolone and with injections that are too superficial. Children younger than 10 years may not tolerate the pain. Stop treatment if there is no response after 6 months of treatment. Intralesional steroid injections do not alter the course of the disease, and the hair may once again be shed.

Minoxidil (topical solution). Minoxidil (Rogaine 5% solution) must be applied twice daily. The 5% concentration is more effective. The response is variable. Hair regrowth occurs in 20% to 45% in patients with 20% to 99% scalp involvement.[32] The response is slow and requires months of treatment. Initial hair regrowth is usually seen after 12 weeks. Minoxidil does not change the course of the disease, and continual use is required to sustain growth.[32] Anthralin or betamethasone dipropionate enhances the efficacy of minoxidil solution. Anthralin is applied 2 hours after the second minoxidil application. Betamethasone dipropionate cream is applied twice daily, 30 minutes after each use of minoxidil. These treatments are not effective for alopecia totalis/universalis.

Anthralin. Anthralin results in regrowth in 20% to 25% of patients. Irritation is not necessary, and short-contact therapy is effective. Side effects include irritation, scaling, folliculitis, and regional lymphadenopathy. Protect treated skin from sun exposure. Anthralin temporarily stains the skin. It may have a nonspecific immunomodulating effect. The treatment is safe and may be considered for refractory cases. Combination therapy with 5% minoxidil plus 0.5% anthralin is more effective than when either drug is used as a single agent.[33] New hair growth is seen within 3 months. Anthralin is a good choice for children.

Topical immunotherapy. Topical immunotherapy with contact sensitizers is the most effective treatment for chronic, severe AA.[34] The mechanism is not clear, but it probably has an immunomodulating effect. Squaric acid dibutyl ester (SADBE), and diphenylcyclopropenone (DPCP) are used.[35,36] The success rate in the most experienced hands is approximately 60% in patients with 25% to 99% scalp involvement. This is not routine therapy and is not available in some teaching centers.

Systemic corticosteroids. Systemic corticosteroids are effective but rarely used. The side effects, high relapse rate, long treatment periods, and inability to change prognosis limit their use.[37] Young adult patients with active disease affecting more than 50% of the scalp are the best candidates. A 6-week taper of prednisone resulted in 25% regrowth in 30% to 47% of patients with mild to extensive AA, alopecia totalis, or alopecia universalis, with predictable and transient side effects. Patients with recent-onset AA (1 year) and a bald surface of greater than 30% of the scalp were given 250 mg intravenously of methylprednisolone twice a day on 3 successive days. The course of the ongoing episode of AA was stopped in eight patients. At the 6-month follow-up, a regrowth on 80% to 100% of the bald surfaces was observed in six patients.[38]

Cyclosporine. Oral cyclosporine is effective for treatment of AA.[39] However, the side effects, high recurrence rate, and long treatment periods limit the use of this drug.

Hair weaves and wigs. See treatment section under androgenic alopecia in men. High-quality wigs are available.

Trichotillomania

Trichotillomania is defined as recurrent pulling out of hair, resulting in noticeable hair loss, with increased tension immediately before pulling or when attempting to resist the behavior. Pleasure, gratification, or relief when pulling out the hair is characteristic.[40]

PREVALENCE. Prevalence rates range from 0.6% to 13%. This conscious or subconscious habit or tic is most commonly performed by young children, adolescents, and women. Many children have a benign, self-limited form of hair pulling. The average age of onset is 11 to 13 years. The female-male ratio is 2.5:1. Increased prevalence has been documented in adults with anxiety and with affective disorders.

DERMATOLOGIC MANIFESTATIONS. Hair is twisted around the finger and pulled or rubbed until extracted or broken. The favorite site is the easily reached frontoparietal region of the scalp, but any scalp area or the eyebrows and eyelashes may be attacked. The affected area has an irregular angulated border, and the density of hair is greatly reduced; but the site is never bald, as in alopecia areata. Several short, broken hairs of varying lengths are randomly distributed in the involved site. Hair that grows beyond 0.5 to 1 cm can be grasped by small fingers and extracted (Figures 24-13 and 24-14).

PSYCHIATRIC MANIFESTATIONS. The symptom may first manifest during inactive periods in the classroom, while watching television, or in bed while waiting to fall asleep. Parents seldom notice the behavior. In many children trichotillomania is triggered by hospitalizations or medical interventions, problems at home, or difficulties at school. Cases also occur with severe sibling rivalry, a disturbed parent-child relationship, and mental retardation.[41] Comorbidity with mood and anxiety disorders and in patients with a primary depressive illness increases in incidence, with trichotillomania arising in adolescence and adulthood.[42] Some psychiatrists classify it as an obsessive-compulsive disorder in adults.[43]

The course is chronic, with remissions and exacerbations. Patients can spend 1 to 3 hours per day pulling hair that results in severe hair loss, suffering, and loss of productive social and work relationships. Shame is a prominent component. Hair pullers fear discovery and avoid health care visits and worry about being critically judged. Psychological suffering is intense.

DIAGNOSIS. First, the patient should be asked if he or she manipulates the hair. Parents or teachers may be aware of the habit. A potassium hydroxide and Wood's light examination rules out noninflammatory tinea capitis. Areas of alopecia areata are completely devoid of hair. In questionable cases, a hair pluck can be performed from the diseased areas; in trichotillomania, it shows no telogen hair roots. Nearly 100% of the hairs are in the active-growing, anagen phase. The absence of telogen hairs is the reason no hair is released on gentle hair traction. Skin biopsy specimens (4- or 5-mm punch extending into the subcutaneous tissue) show normal hairs, absence of hairs in follicles, and no infiltration of leukocytes. Catagen hairs are present in 74%, pigment casts in 61%, and traumatized hair bulbs in 21%; these findings are most evident in areas affected for less than 8 weeks.[44]

TREATMENT. A summary of treatment strategies is listed in Box 24-13. Many patients are psychologically stable[45] and require only a discussion of the problem with an understanding physician or parent. Many of these cases resolve spontaneously. Advise parents to divert the child's attention when hair is being pulled and to be accepting and supportive rather than judgmental or punitive. Patients with extensive involvement or those who persist in the habit should undergo psychiatric evaluation. The relative effectiveness and long-term benefits of behavioral and drug treatments are not established. For more information contact the Trichotillomania Learning Center (TLC), 1215 Mission Street, Santa Cruz, CA 95060 (831-457-1004; www.trich.org).

Box 24-13 Guidelines for the Treatment of Trichotillomania

- Adequate physician-patient relationship to improve insight, acknowledgment of disease, and compliance with treatment
- Evaluate all sites of pulling
- Assess motivation for treatment
- Inquire about trichophagia
- Consider psychiatric referral
- Evaluate and treat comorbid conditions (e.g., skin picking, mood disorders, anxiety disorders)
- Guide patient to educational and support groups
- Institute modified habit reversal
- Evaluate pharmacotherapy:
  Clomipramine (evaluating the adverse effects of clomipramine) or SSRIs
  Add low doses of neuroleptics (haloperidol, pimozide, or risperidone) in cases of partial or unsustained response to antidepressants (clomipramine or SSRIs)
  Lithium carbonate
  Naltrexone
- Consider introducing posthypnotic suggestions
- Institute relapse-prevention strategies

Modified from Koran LM: Trichotillomania. In: Obsessive-compulsive and related disorders in adults. A comprehensive clinical guide. Cambridge (UK): University Press; 1999:185.

Traction (cosmetic) alopecia

Prolonged tension created by certain hairstyles, such as braids or pony tails, hair rollers, and hot hair-straightening combs, may result in temporary or, rarely, permanent hair loss in an area corresponding exactly to the stressed hair. The scalp may appear normal or may show evidence of inflammation or scarring.

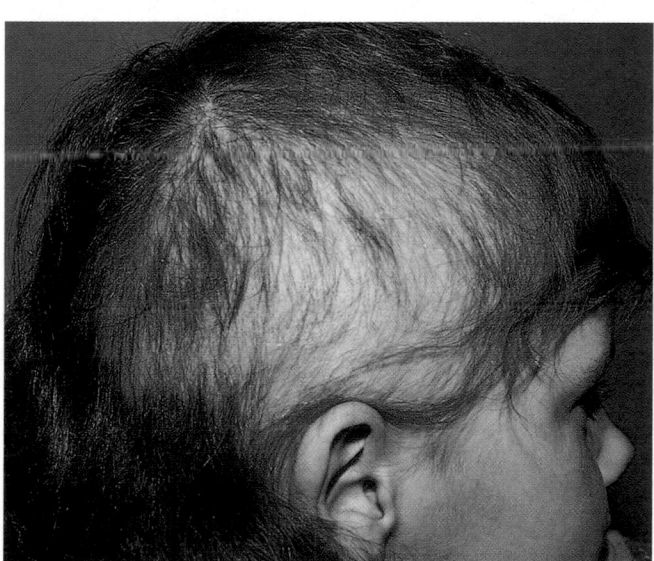

Figure 24-13 Hair has been manually extracted from a wide area of the scalp. There is no inflammation or scarring.

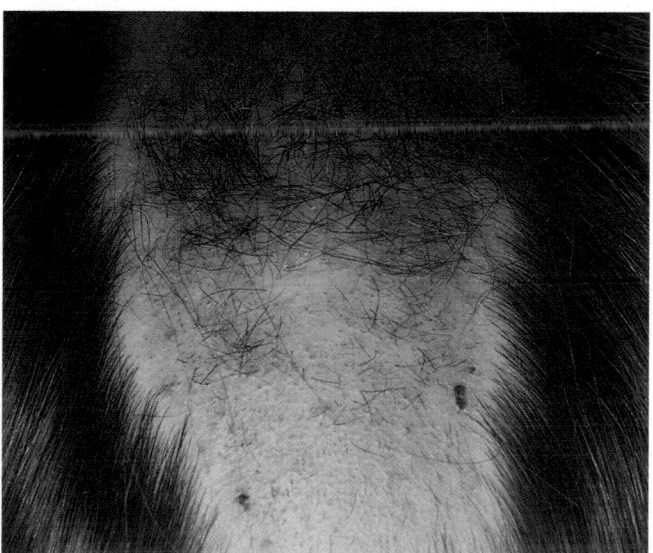

Figure 24-14 Several short hairs are randomly distributed in the involved site.

Scarring alopecia

The classification of scarring alopecia is confusing. The cicatricial or scarring alopecias result in irreversible hair loss.[46] They occur with either destruction of the follicle or scarring of the reticular dermis. The most commonly recognized entities are described here (see Table 24-1).

Central centrifugal scarring alopecia

The term *central centrifugal scarring alopecia* has been used to describe four diseases (follicular degeneration syndrome, pseudopelade, folliculitis decalvans, tufted folliculitis) that some think are clinical subsets of the same process. They have the following features[47]:

- Hair loss on the crown or vertex
- Progressive disease with eventual "burnout"
- Symmetrical expansion
- Most active disease at the periphery

FOLLICULAR DEGENERATION SYNDROME. This disease is common and occurs most often in African Americans. Scarring alopecia is most prominent on the crown. There is premature desquamation of the inner root sheath and migration of the hair shafts through the outer root sheath. The inner root sheath disappears very low in the follicle below the isthmus. Premature desquamation of the inner root sheath is found in inflamed and noninflamed follicles and in the "normal" scalp. There is a spectrum of severity from slowly progressive (over decades) and relatively noninflammatory disease to rapidly progressive (over years) and highly inflammatory disease. Patients with highly inflammatory disease would have been described as having folliculitis decalvans. The end stage may be described as pseudopelade.

PSEUDOPELADE. Pseudopelade is an archaic term that designates a slowly progressive cicatricial alopecia without clinically evident folliculitis. It does not describe any one disease entity but represents the end stage of various forms of scarring alopecia. Pseudopelade of Brocq was a term originally used to describe white adult males with asymptomatic, irregularly shaped, widely distributed clusters of hairless patches that are at times atrophic. Periods of disease progression are followed by dormant periods.

FOLLICULITIS DECALVANS. Folliculitis decalvans is a chronic pustular eruption of the scalp resulting in patchy permanent alopecia. Late-stage lesions show wide areas of scarring with active pustular lesions at the margins (Figure 24-15). The etiology is unknown. Chronic bacterial folliculitis or altered host immune responses are proposed mechanisms. *Staphylococcus aureus* may be cultured from pustular lesions. Biopsy specimens of early lesions show follicular neutrophilic abscesses in the infundibula or upper or mid levels of the follicle. Late lesions show dermal lymphocytes, destruction of follicles, and dermal scarring. Systemic and topical antibiotics (mupirocin) and daily bactericidal antibiotic treatment of the nasal vestibules to eliminate the carrier state of *Staphylococcus* may help. One, two, or three 10-week courses of a combination of 300 mg of rifampicin and 300 mg of clindamycin twice daily for 10 weeks arrested the disease. Dapsone 100 mg per day was effective.[48] Some patients have areas of tufted folliculitis. Tufted hair folliculitis (a possible variant of folliculitis decalvans) is characterized by follicular fusion in which multiple hair tufts emerge from a single dilated follicular orifice. These two entities may form part of a spectrum of a single disease.

TUFTED FOLLICULITIS. Tufted folliculitis (TF) may not be a specific disease but an end stage of other diseases such as folliculitis decalvans or acne keloidalis. Patients present with an inflamed scalp with pustules from which *S. aureus* can be cultured.[49] It leads to patches of scarring alopecia within which multiple hair tufts emerge from dilated follicular orifices (Figure 24-16). Tufted folliculitis can be differentiated from folliculitis decalvans only by finding several hair tufts scattered within patches of scarring alopecia.

Tufting of hair is caused by clustering of adjacent follicular units due to a fibrosing process and to retention of telogen hairs within the involved follicular units.

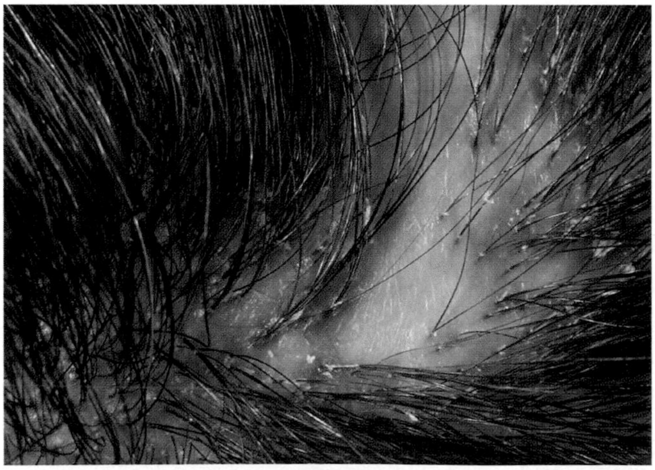

Figure 24-15 Folliculitis decalvans. End stage with a few pustules.

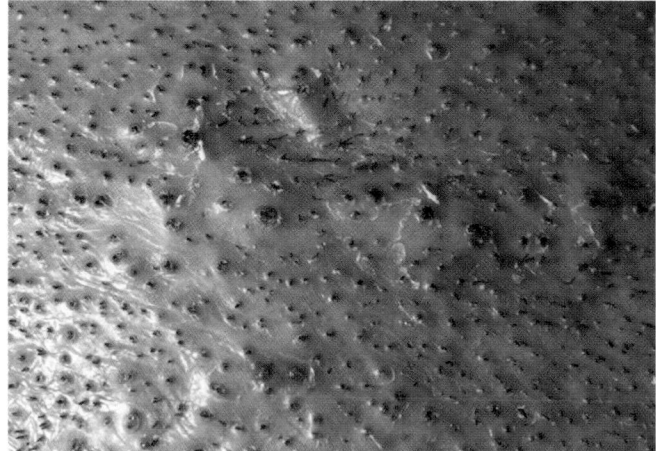

Figure 24-16 Tufted folliculitis. Multiple hairs in a single orifice.

Acne keloidalis

Acne keloidalis (AK) usually affects young black men. Small, follicular papules with occasional pustules occur on the occipital scalp and posterior neck. They coalesce into firm papules and become thick and elevated (Figure 24-17). Abscesses and sinuses with pus may develop. There are no symptoms or mild burning or itching. Histologically there is inflammation, fibroplasia, and disappearance of sebaceous glands.[47] Treatment is discussed on page 283.

Dissecting cellulitis

This uncommon disease most often affects young adult African-American men. Multiple inflammatory nodules are concentrated on the crown, vertex, and occiput. They evolve into coalescing, boggy, fluctuant, oval, and linear ridges that eventually discharge purulent material (Figure 24-18). There may be little or no pain.[47] The presence of hair follicles appears to be essential for disease progression. Eventually, dense dermal fibrosis, sinus tract formation, hypertrophic scarring, and permanent hair loss occur. This condition, along with hidradenitis suppurativa and acne conglobata, form the "follicular occlusion triad." Isotretinoin is effective.[50]

Lichen planopilaris

Lichen planus presents with erythema and perifollicular scaling or as scattered foci of partial hair loss. It may be insidious or fulminate. Large areas of the scalp may be involved. Other skin and mucosal lesions of lichen planus may be present. Histologic verification is required for diagnosis. Biopsy of early lesions shows lichenoid interface inflammation involving only the follicles and the perifollicular dermis.[51] Immunofluorescence in active stages shows cytoid body staining by anti-IgM and anti-IgA. Intralesional steroids are not very effective. Hydroxychloroquine may be effective with long-term use (months to years). Cyclosporine may be considered.

Chronic cutaneous lupus erythematosus

Chronic cutaneous lupus erythematosus (discoid lupus erythematosus) is a common cause of scarring alopecia (see page 596). Women are more often affected. Early discrete bald patches look like pseudopelade or lichen planopilaris. Late lesions are more pronounced and clinically diagnostic. The combination of diffuse scaling, erythema, telangiectases, and mottled hyperpigmentation within areas of scarring is highly characteristic. Follicular plugging and epidermal atrophy occur (Figure 24-19). With time, plugged follicles disappear, and the skin becomes smooth, atrophic, and scarred. Biopsy of early lesions shows follicular inflammatory changes; late lesions show scarring in the reticular dermis. Immunofluorescent studies are not useful. Treatment includes intralesional steroids and antimalarials (hydroxychloroquine).

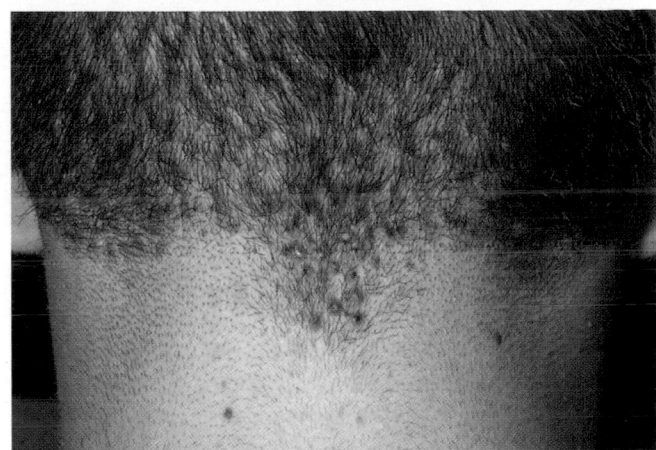

Figure 24-17 Acne keloidalis.

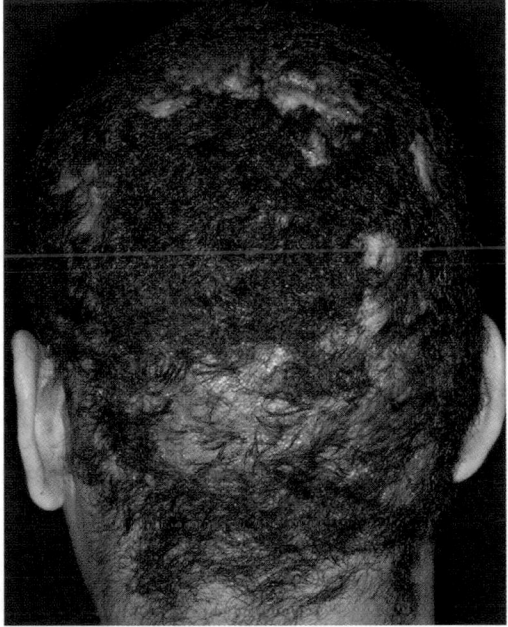

Figure 24-18 Dissecting cellulitis.

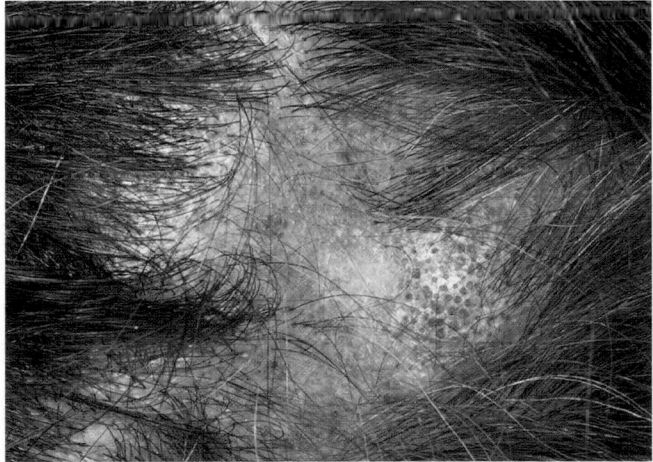

Figure 24-19 Discoid lupus.

Trichomycosis

Trichomycosis is an asymptomatic infection of axillary or pubic hair caused by a corynebacterium. The hair shaft becomes coated with adherent yellow (occasionally red or black), firm concretions[52] (Figure 24-20). Hyperhidrosis is often present. The hair is shaved, and hyperhidrosis is controlled with antiperspirants. Naftifine hydrochloride 1% cream (Naftin) is effective for superficial fungal infections and also has antibacterial properties. It is reportedly effective for trichomycosis.[53]

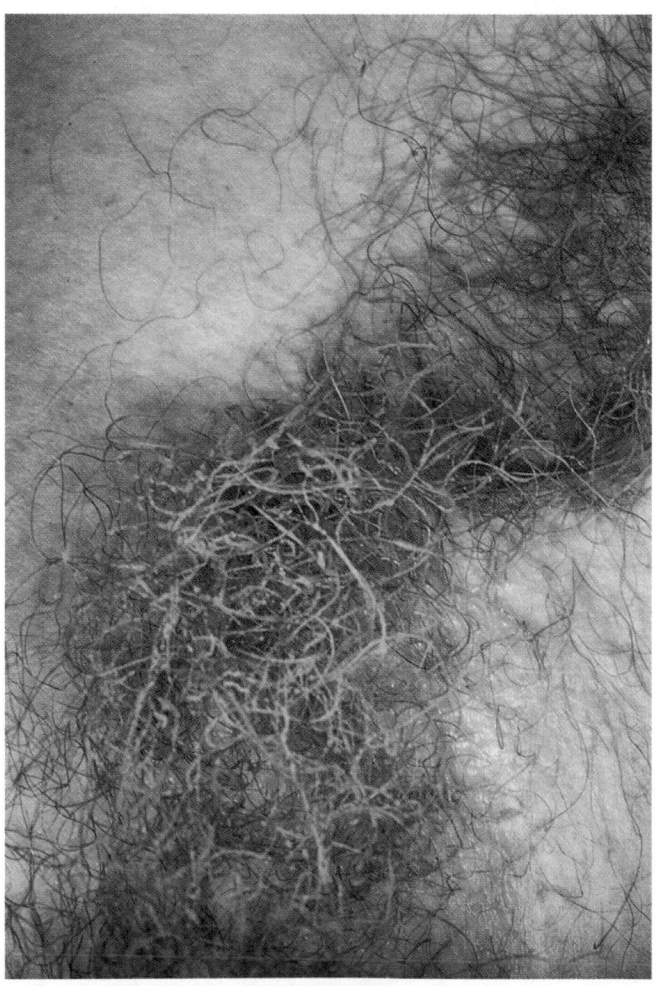

Figure 24-20 Trichomycosis axillaris. Yellow concretions are adherent to the axillary hair. These concretions are composed of a mass of diphtheroid organisms and not fungi.

References

1. Paus R, Cotsarelis G: The biology of hair follicles, N Engl J Med 1999; 341491-7.
2. Munro DD: Hair growth measurement using intradermal sulphur 35 L-cystine, Arch Dermatol 1966; 93:119.
3. Headington JT. Telogen effluvium, Arch Dermatol 1993; 129:356.
4. Kligman AM: Pathologic dynamics of human hair loss. I. Telogen effluvium, Arch Dermatol 1961; 83:175.
5. Granai CO, et al: The use of minoxidil to attempt to prevent alopecia during chemotherapy for gynecologic malignancies, Eur J Gynaecol Oncol 1991; 12:129.
6. Olsen EA, Weiner MS: Topical minoxidil in male pattern baldness: effects of discontinuation of treatment, J Am Acad Dermatol 1987; 17:97.
7. Rietschel RL, Duncan SH: Safety and efficacy of topical minoxidil in the management of androgenetic alopecia, J Am Acad Dermatol 1987; 16:677.
8. Sawaya M, Shapiro J: Androgenetic alopecia. New approved and unapproved treatments, Dermatol Clin 2000; 18:47, viii.
9. Price V, et al: Changes in hair weight and hair count in men with androgenetic alopecia after treatment with finasteride, 1 mg, daily, J Am Acad Dermatol 2002; 46(4):517.
10. Kaufman K, et al: Finasteride in the treatment of men with androgenetic alopecia. Finasteride Male Pattern Hair Loss Study Group, J Am Acad Dermatol 1998; 39:578.
11. Leyden J, et al: Finasteride in the treatment of men with frontal male pattern hair loss, J Am Acad Dermatol 1999; 40:930.
12. Price V, et al: Lack of efficacy of finasteride in postmenopausal women with androgenetic alopecia, J Am Acad Dermatol 2000; 43:768.
13. Walsh P: Treatment with finasteride preserves usefulness of prostate-specific antigen in the detection of prostate cancer: results of a randomized, double-blind, placebo-controlled clinical trial, J Urol 1999; 161:350.
14. Ludwig E: Classification of the types of androgenic alopecia (common baldness) occurring in the female sex, Br J Dermatol 1977; 97:247.
15. Pitts RL: Serum elevation of dehydroepiandrosterone sulfate associated with male pattern baldness in young men, J Am Acad Dermatol 1987; 16:571.
16. De V, et al: Androgenetic alopecia in the female. Treatment with 2% topical minoxidil solution, Arch Dermatol 1994; 130:303.
17. Jacobs JP, et al: Use of topical minoxidil therapy for androgenetic alopecia in women, Int J Dermatol 1993; 32:758.
18. Azziz R, Carmina E, Sawaya M: Idiopathic hirsutism, Endocr Rev 2000; 21(4):347.
19. Leshin M: Southwestern internal medicine conference: hirsutism, Am J Med Sci 1987; 294:369.
20. Carmina E: A risk-benefit assessment of pharmacological therapies for hirsutism, Drug Saf 2001; 24(4):267.
21. Yucelten D, et al: Recurrence rate of hirsutism after 3 different antiandrogen therapies, J Am Acad Dermatol 1999; 41(1):64.
22. Venturoli S, et al: Low-dose flutamide (125 mg/day) as maintenance therapy in the treatment of hirsutism, Horm Res 2001; 56(1-2):25.
23. Richards RN, McKenzie MA, Meharg GE: Electroepilation (electrolysis) in hirsutism, J Am Acad Dermatol 1986; 15:693.
24. Liew S: Laser hair removal: guidelines for management, Am J Clin Dermatol 2002; 3(2):107.
25. Madani S, Shapiro J: Alopecia areata update, J Am Acad Dermatol 2000; 42:549; quiz 567.

26. Messenger AG, Slater DN, Bleehen SS: Alopecia areata: alterations in the hair growth cycle and correlation with the follicular pathology, Br J Dermatol 1986; 114:337.

27. Beard HO: Social and psychological implications of alopecia areata, J Am Acad Dermatol 1986; 14:697.

28. Dotz WI, Lieber CD, Vogt PJ: Leukonychia punctata and pitted nails in alopecia areata, Arch Dermatol 1985; 121:1452.

29. Mitchell A, Krull E: Alopecia areata: pathogenesis and treatment, J Am Acad Dermatol 1984; 111:763.

30. Lee JY, Hsu ML: Alopecia syphilitica, a simulator of alopecia areata: histopathology and differential diagnosis, J Cutan Pathol 1991; 18:87.

31. van D, et al: Can alopecia areata be triggered by emotional stress? An uncontrolled evaluation of 178 patients with extensive hair loss, Acta Derm Venereol 1992; 72:279.

32. Price VH: Double-blind, placebo-controlled evaluation of topical minoxidil in extensive alopecia areata, J Am Acad Dermatol 1987; 16:730.

33. Fiedler VC, et al: Treatment-resistant alopecia areata. Response to combination therapy with minoxidil plus anthralin, Arch Dermatol 1990; 126:756.

34. Rokhsar C, et al: Efficacy of topical sensitizers in the treatment of alopecia areata, J Am Acad Dermatol 1998; 39:751.

35. Pericin M, Trueb R: Topical immunotherapy of severe alopecia areata with diphenylcyclopropenone: evaluation of 68 cases, Dermatology 1998; 196:418.

36. Cotellessa C, et al: The use of topical diphenylcyclopropenone for the treatment of extensive alopecia areata, J Am Acad Dermatol 2001; 44:73.

37. Alabdulkareem A, Abahussein A, Okoro A: Severe alopecia areata treated with systemic corticosteroids, Int J Dermatol 1998; 37:622.

38. Perriard-Wolfensberger J, et al: Pulse of methylprednisolone in alopecia areata, Dermatology 1993; 187:282.

39. Gupta AK, et al: Oral cyclosporine for the treatment of alopecia areata. A clinical and immunohistochemical analysis, J Am Acad Dermatol 1990; 22:242.

40. Hautmann G, Hercogova J, Lotti T: Trichotillomania, J Am Acad Dermatol 2002; 46(6):807.

41. Oranje AP, Peereboom-Wynia JDR, De R: Trichotillomania in childhood, J Am Acad Dermatol 1986; 15:614.

42. Swedo SE, Rapoport JL: Annotation: trichotillomania, J Child Psychol Psychiatry 1991; 32:401.

43. Christenson GA, et al: Characteristics of 60 adult chronic hair pullers, Am J Psychiatry 1991; 148:365.

44. Muller SA: Trichotillomania: a histopathologic study in sixty-six patients, J Am Acad Dermatol 1990; 23:56.

45. Christenson GA, et al: Personality and clinical characteristics in patients with trichotillomania, J Clin Psychiatry 1992; 53:407.

46. Headington J: Cicatricial alopecia, Dermatol Clin 1996; 14:773.

47. Sperling L, Solomon A, Whiting D: A new look at scarring alopecia, Arch Dermatol 2000; 136(2):235.

48. Powell J, Dawber R, Gatter K: Folliculitis decalvans including tufted folliculitis: clinical, histological and therapeutic findings, Br J Dermatol 1999; 140:328.

49. Kunte C, Loeser C, Wolff H: Folliculitis spinulosa decalvans: successful therapy with dapsone, J Am Acad Dermatol 1998; 39:891.

50. Scerri L, Williams H, Allen B: Dissecting cellulitis of the scalp: response to isotretinoin, Br J Dermatol 1996; 134(6):1105.

51. Annessi G, et al: A clinicopathologic study of scarring alopecia due to lichen planus: comparison with scarring alopecia in discoid lupus erythematosus and pseudopelade, Am J Dermatopathol 1999; 21:324.

52. Levit F: Trichomycosis axillaris: a different view, J Am Acad Dermatol 1988; 18:778.

53. Rosen T, et al: Naftifine treatment of trichomycosis pubis, Int J Dermatol 1991; 30:667.

See pages 866 to 867 for 24 photos of the most common nail disorders.

Anatomy and Physiology

ANATOMY. The nail unit consists of several components (Figure 25-1). The nail plate is hard, translucent, dead keratin. The nailfold includes the skin surrounding the lateral and proximal aspects of the nail plate. The proximal nailfold overlies the matrix. Its keratin layer extends onto the proximal nail plate to form the cuticle. Capillary loops at the tip of the proximal nailfold are normally small and inapparent, but they become distinct in diseases such as systemic lupus erythematosus and scleroderma. The proximal nailfold epithelium covers the proximal nail plate for a few millimeters and then makes a 180-degree turn and curves back into direct contact with the nail plate. It makes another 180-degree turn and becomes continuous with the nail matrix.

The matrix epithelium synthesizes 90% of the nail plate. The lunula (white half-moon), which is visible through the nail plate, is the distal aspect of the nail matrix. It is continuous with the nail bed. The nail bed extends from the distal nail matrix to the hyponychium. As the nail streams distally, material is added to the undersurface of the nail, thickening it and making it densely adherent to the nail bed.[1] The nail bed consists of parallel longitudinal ridges with small blood vessels at their base (Figure 25-2). Bleeding induced by trauma or vessel disease, such as lupus, occurs in the depths of these grooves, producing the splinter hemorrhage pattern viewed through the nail plate. The hyponychium is a short segment of skin lacking nail cover; it begins at the distal nail bed and terminates at the distal groove.

NAIL BIOPSY. Ungual biopsies are used to diagnose tumors, inflammatory disease, and infections. The ideal ungual biopsy is performed after avulsion of the plate. This allows clear visualization of the matrix and bed. A punch or excisional biopsy technique is chosen, which provides a sufficient amount of tissue and produces a minimal amount of scarring.

NAIL PLATE AVULSION. One or two percent lidocaine without epinephrine is injected with a 30-gauge needle into the lateral and proximal nailfolds, or a digital block may be used. Carbocaine may be used and is longer acting. Wait at least 3 to 5 minutes after injection until the nail apparatus is fully anesthetized. A wide Penrose drain is used as a tourniquet for no more than 10 minutes. The nailfolds are loosened from the nail plate with a 2- to 3-mm nail elevator, 2- to 3-mm dental spatula, or mosquito forceps. The same instrument is then placed under the distal edge of the nail plate and gently pushed distally to proximally to separate the nail plate from the underlying nail bed. Rock the instrument back and forth to ensure full nail-plate/nail-bed separation. Grasp the nail plate with a Kelly hemostat or nail-grasping forceps and gently remove it. After the procedure, the wound is dressed with Polysporin ointment, Telfa, tube gauze, and then tape.[2]

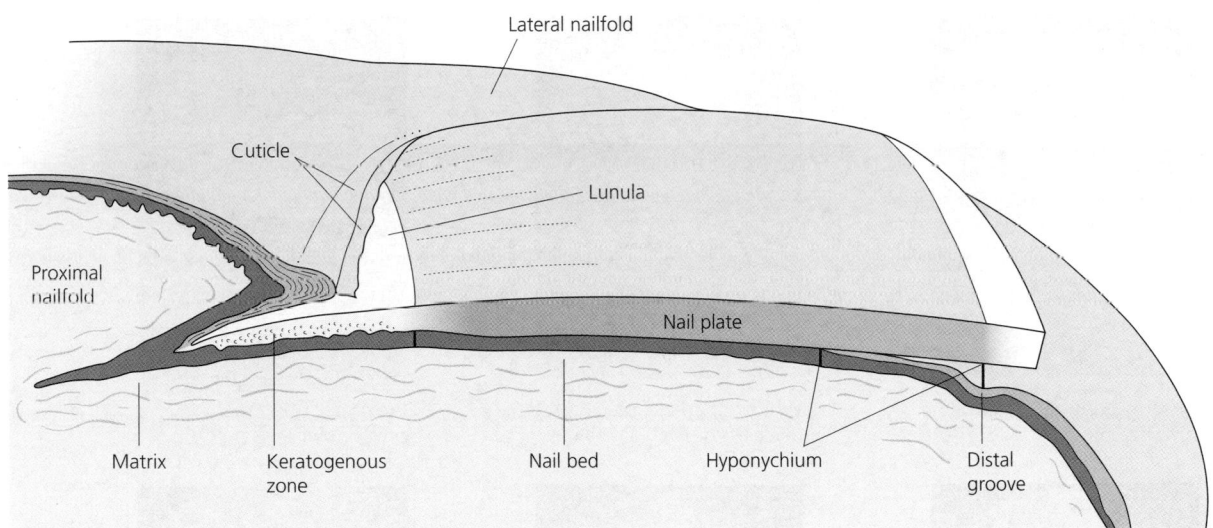

Figure 25-1 Diagrammatic drawing of an adult fingertip, showing nail structures through a longitudinal midline plane.

PARONYCHIAL BIOPSY. Paronychial (proximal and lateral nailfold) lesions can be biopsied by a shave biopsy or a punch biopsy or removed en bloc by blunt dissection. Elliptic excisional biopsies of the proximal nailfold are performed with the long axis oriented horizontally. Be aware of the insertion of the extensor tendon. Elliptic excisions of the lateral nailfold are oriented longitudinally.

NAIL-MATRIX BIOPSY. Nail-matrix biopsy may cause permanent nail dystrophy. The most common reason to biopsy the nail matrix is to exclude the diagnosis of melanoma in a patient with a longitudinal, pigmented band. Care must be taken in nail matrix biopsy to minimize the risk of permanent nail dystrophy.[3] For longitudinal bands that are 3 mm or narrower, a simple punch biopsy to excise the focus of pigmentation in the matrix is sufficient. More complicated excisional techniques to sample wider lesions are best performed by dermatologic surgeons.[4]

GROWTH RATES. Nails grow continuously, but their growth rate decreases both with age and poor circulation. Fingernails, which grow faster than toenails, grow at a rate of 0.5 to 2 mm per week. It takes approximately 5.5 months for a fingernail to grow from the matrix to the free edge and approximately 12 to 18 months for a toenail to be replaced. A reduction in the rate of matrix-cell division occurs during systemic diseases such as scarlet fever, causing thinning of the nail plate (Beau's lines).

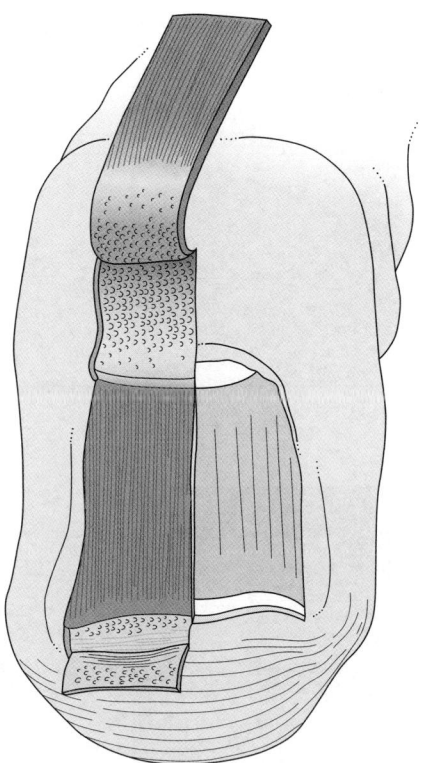

Figure 25-2 Dermal topography underlying nail unit. The nail bed consists of parallel longitudinal ridges with small blood vessels at their base. Anatomic pathology of splinter hemorrhages is obvious.

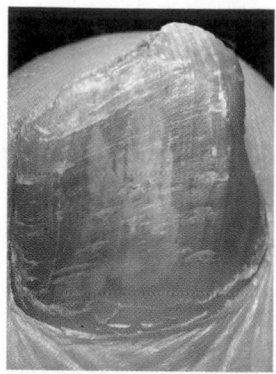

Distal subungual onycho-
mycosis, pp. 875, 876

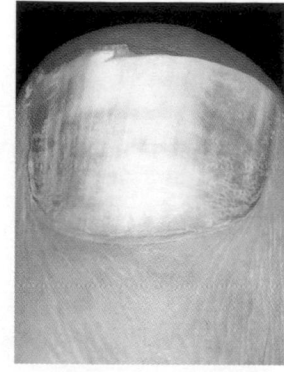

White superficial onycho-
mycosis, p. 876

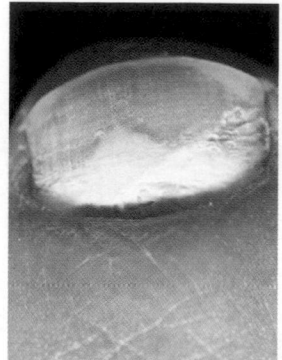

Proximal subungual
onychomycosis, p. 876

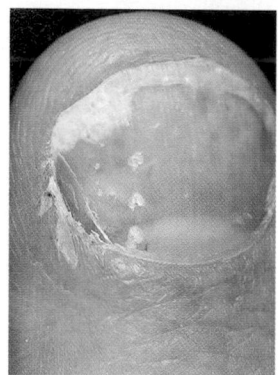

Psoriasis—pitting,
pp. 219, 869

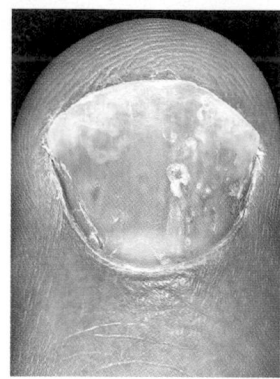

Psoriasis—onycholysis,
p. 869

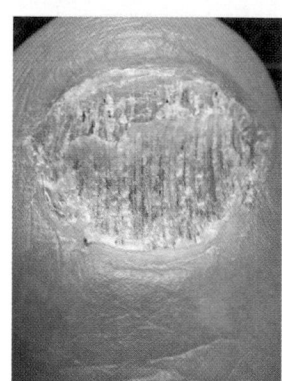

Psoriasis-plate alteration,
pp. 219, 869, 872

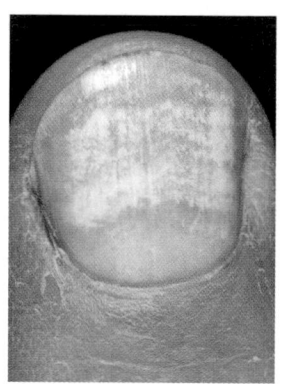

Leukonychia, p. 882

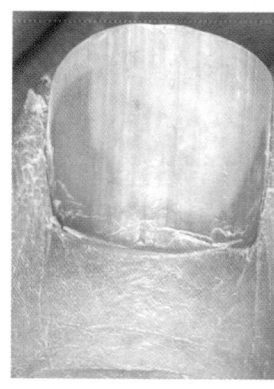

Onycholysis—secondary
infection, p. 881

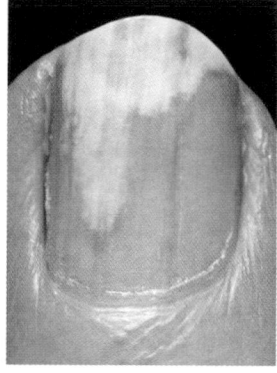

Onycholysis—trauma,
p. 880

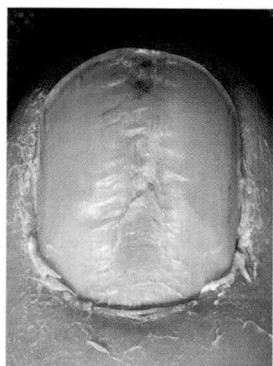

Habit-tic deformity, p. 883

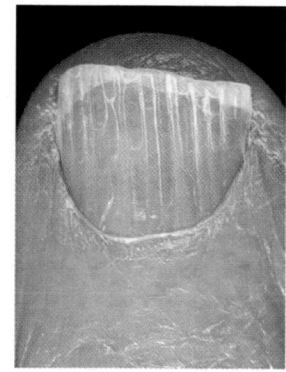

Ridging, p. 868

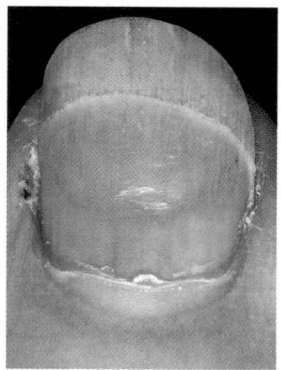

Beau's lines, p. 884

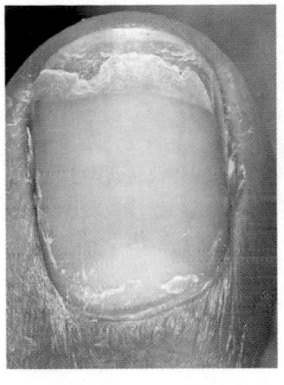

Distal splitting, p. 883

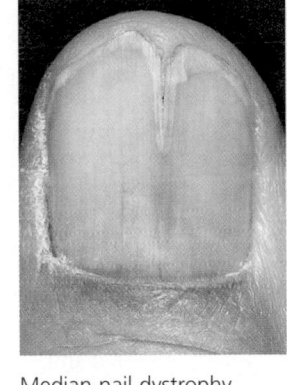

Median nail dystrophy,
p. 884

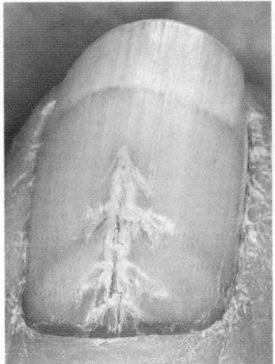

Median nail dystrophy,
p. 884

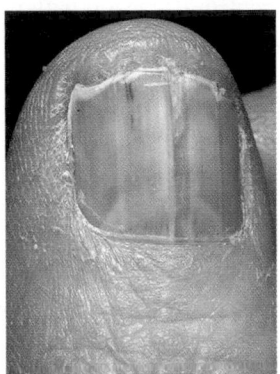

Darier's disease, p. 871

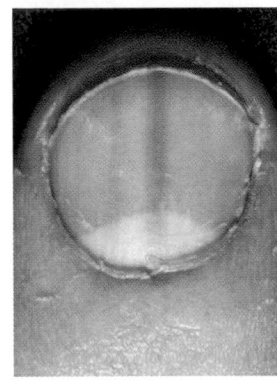

Pigmented band,
pp. 796, 868

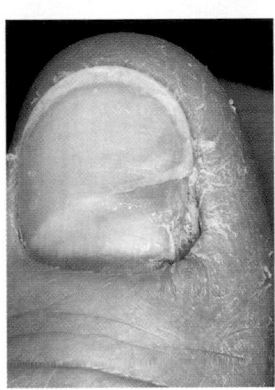

Chronic paronychia, p. 872

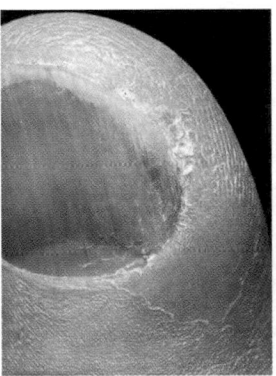

Acute paronychia, p. 871

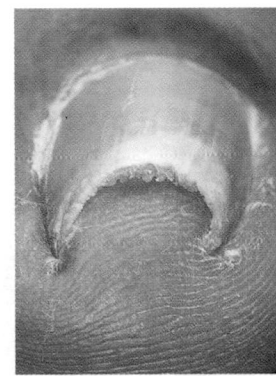

Pincer nail, p. 884

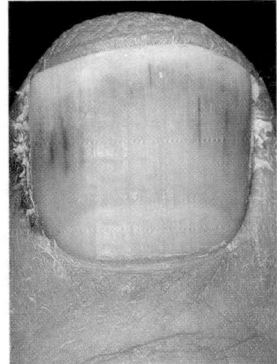

Splinter hemorrhages,
p. 865

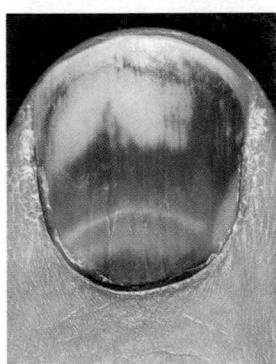

Trauma, p. 882

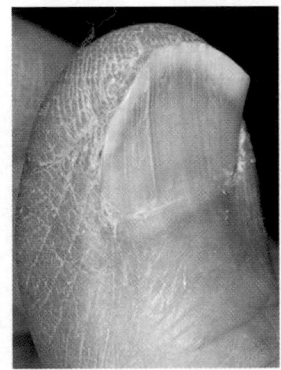

Spoon nails, p. 885

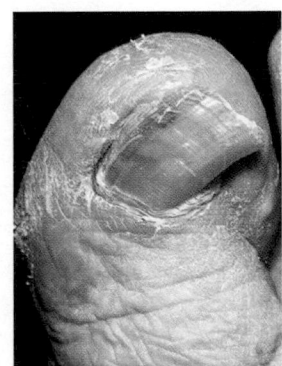

Plate hypertrophy, p. 883

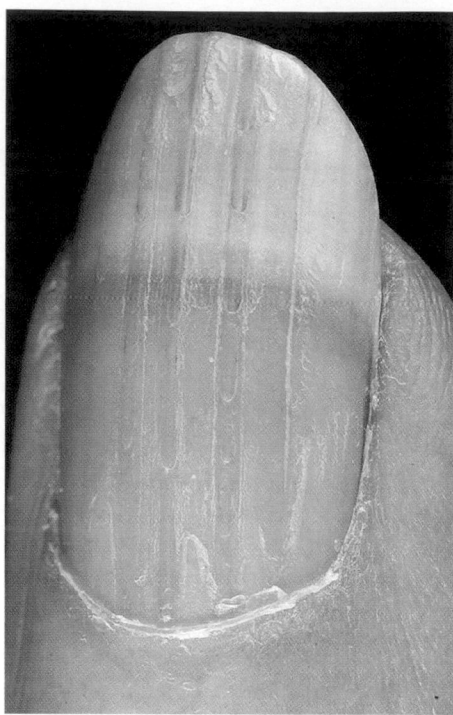

Figure 25-3 Longitudinal ridging. Parallel elevated nail ridges are a common aging change. This change does not indicate any deficiency.

Normal Variations

The shape and opacity of the nail varies considerably among individuals. Aging may increase or decrease nail thickness. Longitudinal ridging (Figure 25-3) is common in aging, but this variant is occasionally observed among the young. Beading occurs at all ages but is more common in the elderly (Figure 25-4). The beads cover part or most of the plate surface and are arranged longitudinally. A pigmented band or bands occur in more than 90% of blacks (Figure 25-5). The sudden appearance of such a band in whites necessitates further investigation.

Nail structure can be altered by primary skin diseases, infections, trauma, internal diseases, congenital syndromes, and tumors. A more detailed discussion with illustrations of the most commonly encountered entities is presented in the following sections.

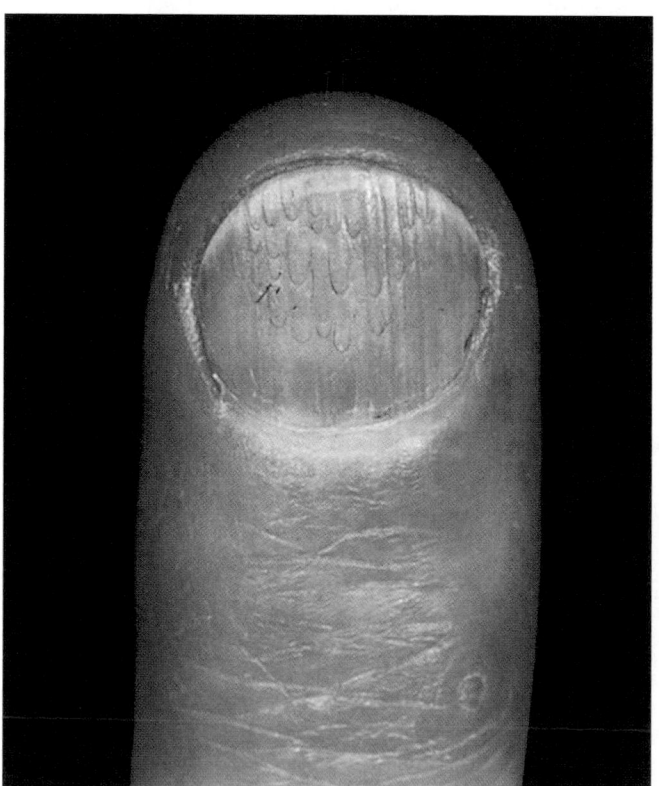

Figure 25-4 Longitudinal ridging and beading. A variant of normal, most commonly seen in the elderly.

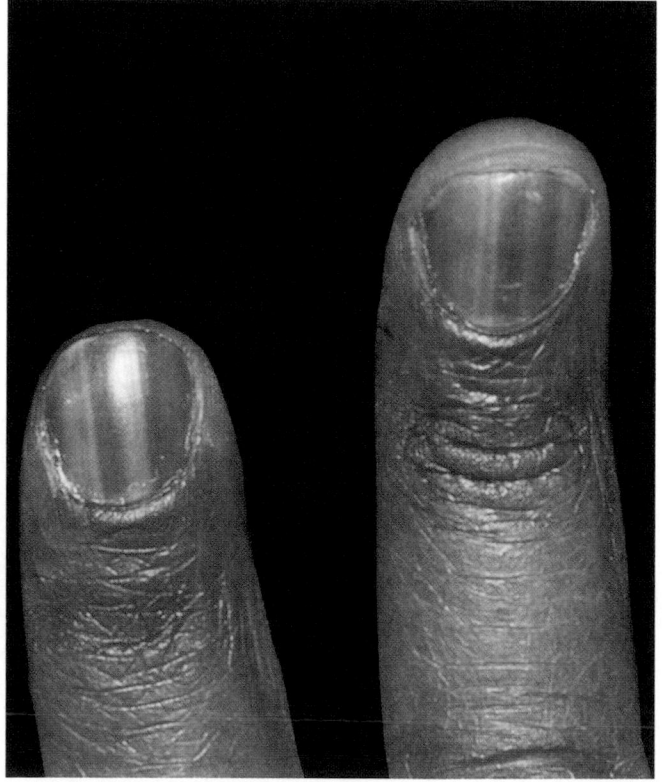

Figure 25-5 Pigmented bands occur as a normal finding in more than 90% of blacks.

Nail Disorders Associated with Skin Disease

PSORIASIS. Nail changes are characteristic of psoriasis, and the nails of patients should be examined. These changes offer supporting evidence for the diagnosis of psoriasis when skin changes are equivocal or absent.

The incidence of nail involvement in psoriasis varies from 10% to 50%. Nail involvement usually occurs simultaneously with skin disease but may occur as an isolated finding. Over 50% of patients suffer from pain, and many are restricted in their daily activities.

PITTING. Pitting, or sharply defined ice pick–like depressions in the nail plate, is the most common finding (Figure 25-6). The number, distribution, patterns, and depth vary. Nail plate cells are shed in much the same way as psoriatic scale is shed, leaving a variable number of tiny, punched-out depressions on the nail plate surface. They emerge from under the cuticle and grow out with the nail. Many other cutaneous diseases may cause pitting (e.g., eczema, fungal infections, and alopecia areata), or it may occur as an isolated finding in a normal variation.

ONYCHOLYSIS. Psoriasis of the hyponychium results in the accumulation of yellow, scaly debris that elevates the nail plate. The debris is commonly mistaken for nail fungus infection. Psoriasis of the nail bed causes separation of the nail from the nail bed. Unlike the uniform separation caused by pressure on the tips of long nails, the nail detaches in an irregular manner (Figure 25-7). The nail plate turns yellow, simulating a fungal infection. Separation begins at the distal groove or under the nail plate and may involve several nails.

NAIL DEFORMITY. Extensive involvement of the nail matrix results in a nail losing its structural integrity, resulting in fragmentation and crumbling. Gross alteration of the nail plate surface and nail-bed splinter hemorrhages are common (Figure 25-8).

OIL SPOT LESION. Psoriasis of the nail bed may cause localized separation of the nail plate. Cellular debris and serum accumulates in this space. The brown, yellow color (Figure 25-9) observed through the nail plate looks like a spot of oil.

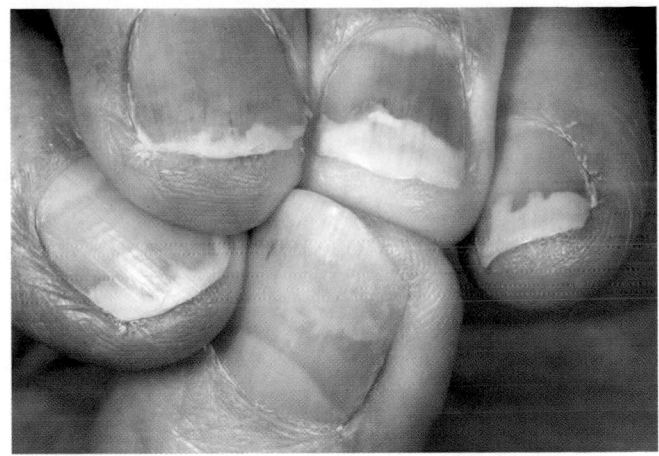

Figure 25-7 Psoriasis. Separation of the nail plate from the nail bed (onycholysis) may be present on several nails. Fungal infections have a similar appearance.

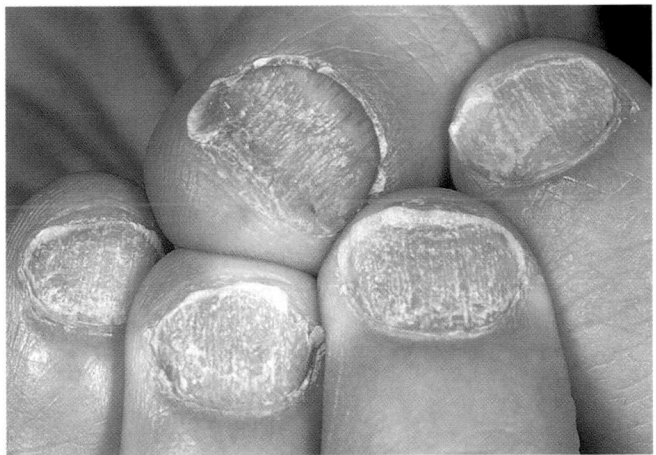

Figure 25-8 Psoriasis of the entire nail matrix causes grossly deformed nails.

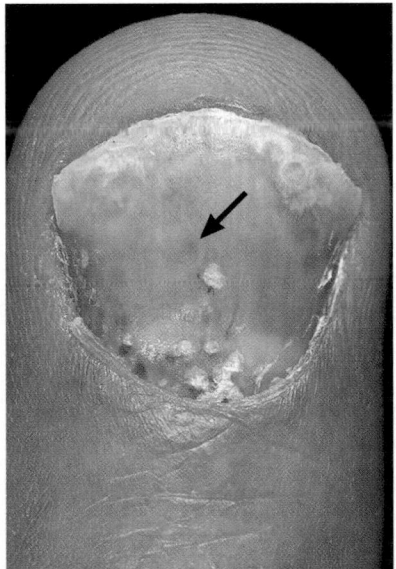

Figure 25-9 Psoriasis of the nail bed causes serum to leak under the nail plate and make an "oil spot" *(arrow)*.

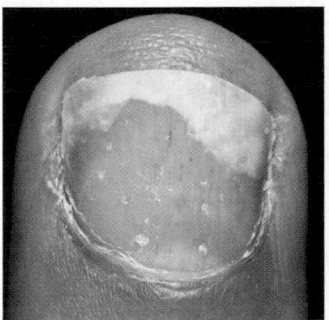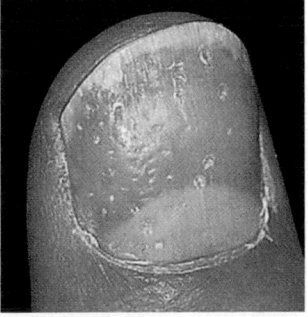

Figure 25-6 Psoriasis. Pitting is the most common nail change found in psoriasis.

TREATMENT. Nail psoriasis is difficult to treat, but may respond to different approaches used alone or together.[5,6] Relapse is common. Nail may improve when patients are treated with systemic agents such as cyclosporine, methotrexate, or acitretin.

Triamcinolone acetonide. Intralesional injections at monthly intervals into the matrix with triamcinolone acetonide (Kenalog) (2.5 to 10 mg/ml) delivered with a 30-gauge needle is the standard treatment for psoriatic nail disease used by most dermatologists. A simplified protocol has been proposed. Triamcinolone acetonide (0.4 mL, 10 mg/mL) is injected, following ring block, at each of four periungual sites: two at the nail matrix and one in each lateral nail fold, directed medially towards the nail bed. This method is utilized to achieve delivery of the agent to both the nail matrix and nail bed. If needed, a second set of injections is administered after 2 months. Subungual hyperkeratosis, ridging, and thickening respond well. Benefits are sustained for at least 9 months. Onycholysis and pitting are less responsive.[7]

Calcipotriol. Calcipotriol ointment or a combination of betamethasone dipropionate (64 mg/g) and salicylic acid (0.03 g/g) ointment are reported to reduce subungual hyperkeratosis in nail bed psoriasis by about 40% after the medication is applied bid to affected nails for 5 months.[8]

Tazarotene. Tazarotene 0.1% gel (Tazorac) is applied each evening for up to 24 weeks to fingernails. Medication can be used under occlusion or unoccluded. Tazarotene gel reduced onycholysis (in occluded and nonoccluded nails) and pitting (in occluded nails).[9]

Anthralin. Topical anthralin resulted in moderate improvement in 60% of patients after 5 months. Onycholysis and pachyonychia both responded, and the number of pits was markedly decreased in some cases. An ointment of 0.4% to 2.0% anthralin in petrolatum was applied to the affected nail bed once a day and washed away with water after 30 minutes. Then 10% triethanolamine cream was applied to prevent pigmentation. The main side effect was reversible pigmentation of the nail plate.[10]

There is little merit in treating psoriatic nails with photochemotherapy (PUVA) or topical 5-fluorouracil (5-FU).

PUSTULAR PSORIASIS OF THE NAIL APPARATUS.
Pustular psoriasis of the nail bed, matrix, or surrounding skin is common and may be painful. It has a chronic course and poor response to treatment. Severe cases are treated with systemic retinoids. Topical calcipotriol is effective in about 50% of patients with localized disorder and is also useful as maintenance therapy after retinoid treatment.[11]

LICHEN PLANUS. Approximately 25% of patients with nail lichen planus (LP) have LP in other sites before or after the onset of nail lesions. Nail LP usually appears during the fifth or sixth decade of life. The matrix, nail bed, and nailfolds may be involved in producing a variety of changes, few of which are characteristic. Minimal inflammation of the matrix induces longitudinal grooving and ridging, which are the most common findings of LP of the nail. The development of severe and early destruction of the nail matrix with scarring characterizes a small subset of patients with nail LP.[12] A pterygium, caused by adhesion of a depressed proximal nailfold to the scarred matrix, may occur after intense matrix inflammation (Figure 25-10). The nail plate distal to this focus is either absent or thinned out. In most cases, nail LP is self-limiting or promptly regresses with treatment. Permanent damage to the nail is uncommon, even in patients with diffuse involvement of the matrix. Matrix lesions may respond to intralesional triamcinolone acetonide (2.5 to 5 mg/ml) delivered with a 30-gauge needle every 3 or 4 weeks. Severe cases respond to prednisone (20 to 40 mg/day). This may require a long course of treatment in which the possible risks may outnumber the advantages. Onychomycosis may be confused clinically with lichen planus.

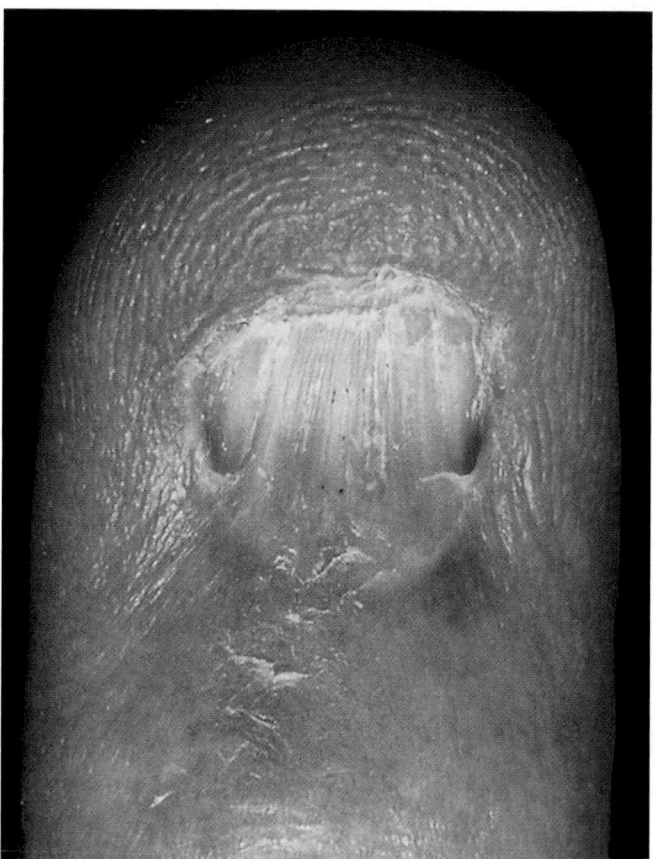

Figure 25-10 Lichen planus. Inflammation of the matrix results in adhesion of the proximal nailfold to the scarred matrix, a pterygium.

ALOPECIA AREATA. A few patients with alopecia areata have shallow pitting or surface stippling in a uniform or grid-like pattern (Figure 25-11).

DARIER'S DISEASE. A number of nail changes are reported with Darier's disease, but white, longitudinal streaks are the most common and the most characteristic (p. 867).

Acquired Disorders

Bacterial and viral infections

ACUTE PARONYCHIA. The rapid onset of painful, bright red swelling of the proximal and lateral nailfold may occur spontaneously or may follow trauma or manipulation (Figures 25-12 and 25-13). Superficial infections present with an accumulation of purulent material behind the cuticle (Figure 25-12). The small abscess is drained by inserting the pointed end of a comedone extractor or similar instrument between the proximal nailfold and the nail plate (Figure 25-14). Pain is abruptly relieved. A diffuse, painful swelling suggests deeper infection, and cases that do not respond to anti-staphylococcal antibiotics may require deep incision. Acute paronychia rarely evolves into chronic paronychia.

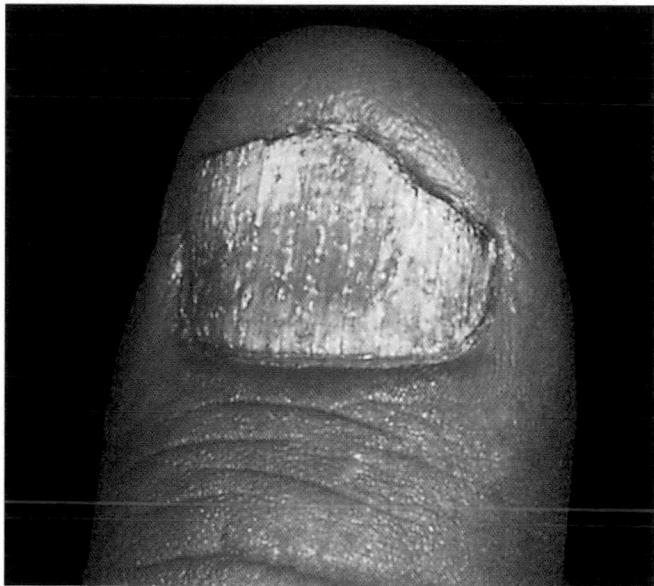

Figure 25-11 Alopecia areata. Shallow pitting occurs in some patients with alopecia areata.

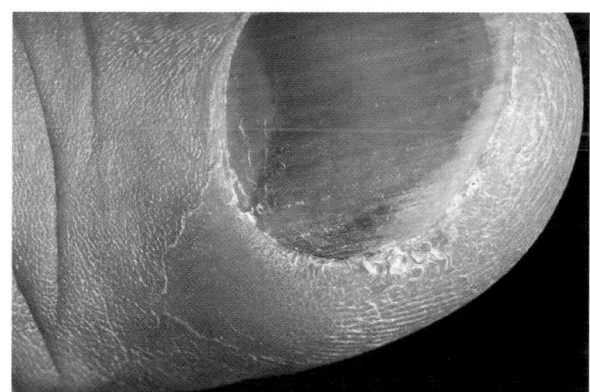

Figure 25-13 Acute paronychia. Acute pain and swelling of the lateral nailfold may follow any form of trauma (biting, sucking, chemical irritants).

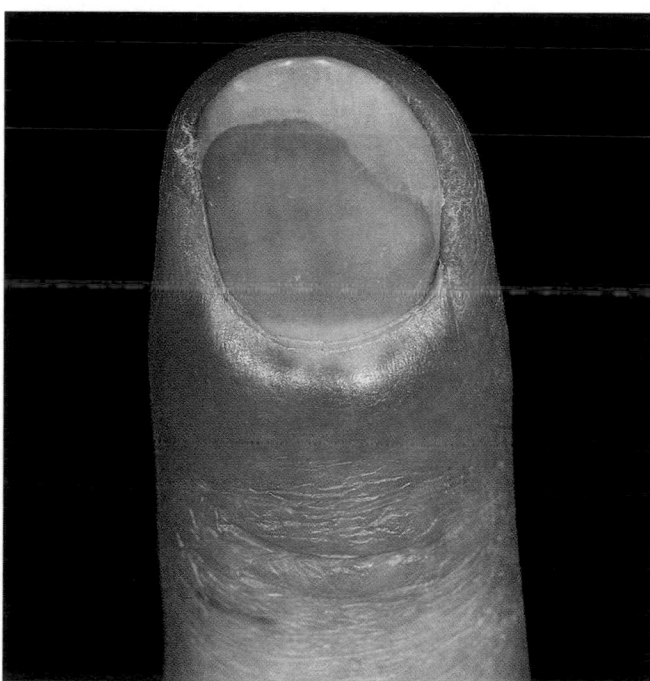

Figure 25-12 Acute paronychia. Erythema and purulent material occur at the proximal nailfold.

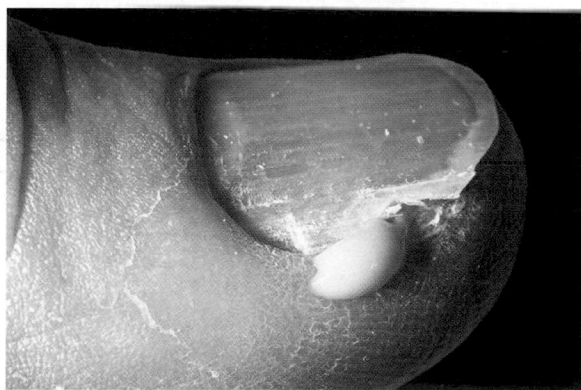

Figure 25-14 Acute paronychia. Elevation of the lateral nailfold releases a large amount of purulent material. Pain is relieved immediately. Flush the cavity with normal saline.

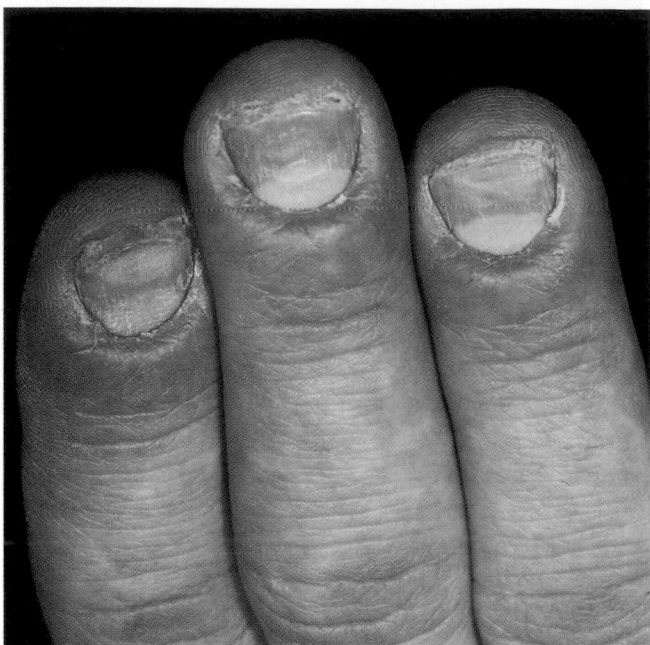

Figure 25-15 Chronic paronychia. Erythema and swelling of the nailfolds. The cuticle is absent. Chronic inflammation has caused horizontal ridging of the nails.

CHRONIC PARONYCHIA. Chronic paronychia is not a yeast infection, but rather an inflammation of the proximal nailfold.[13] Chronic paronychia evolves slowly and presents initially with tenderness and mild swelling about the proximal and lateral nailfolds (Figure 25-15). Significant contact irritant exposure is a major cause. Individuals whose hands are repeatedly exposed to moisture (e.g., bakers, dishwashers, and dentists) are at greatest risk. Manipulation of the cuticle accelerates the process. Typically, many or all fingers are involved simultaneously. The cuticle separates from the nail plate, leaving the space between the proximal nailfold and the nail plate exposed to infection. Many organisms, both pathogens and contaminants, thrive in this warm, moist intertriginous space. The skin about the nail becomes pale red, tender or painful, and swollen. Occasionally a small quantity of pus can be expressed from under the proximal nailfold. A culture of this material may grow *Candida* or gram-positive and gram-negative organisms. *Candida* is probably just a colonizer of the proximal nail fold rather than a direct cause of the disease. It disappears when the physiologic barrier is restored.[13] The nail plate is not infected and maintains its integrity, although its surface becomes brown and rippled. There is no subungual thickening such as that present in some fungal infections. The process is chronic and responds very slowly to treatment. Psoriasis of the fingers may present in a similar form (Figure 25-16).

Figure 25-16 Psoriasis of the proximal and lateral nailfolds and nail matrix produces erythema, swelling and nail plate distortion. Differentiation from chronic paronychia may be difficult. Nail pits suggest psoriasis.

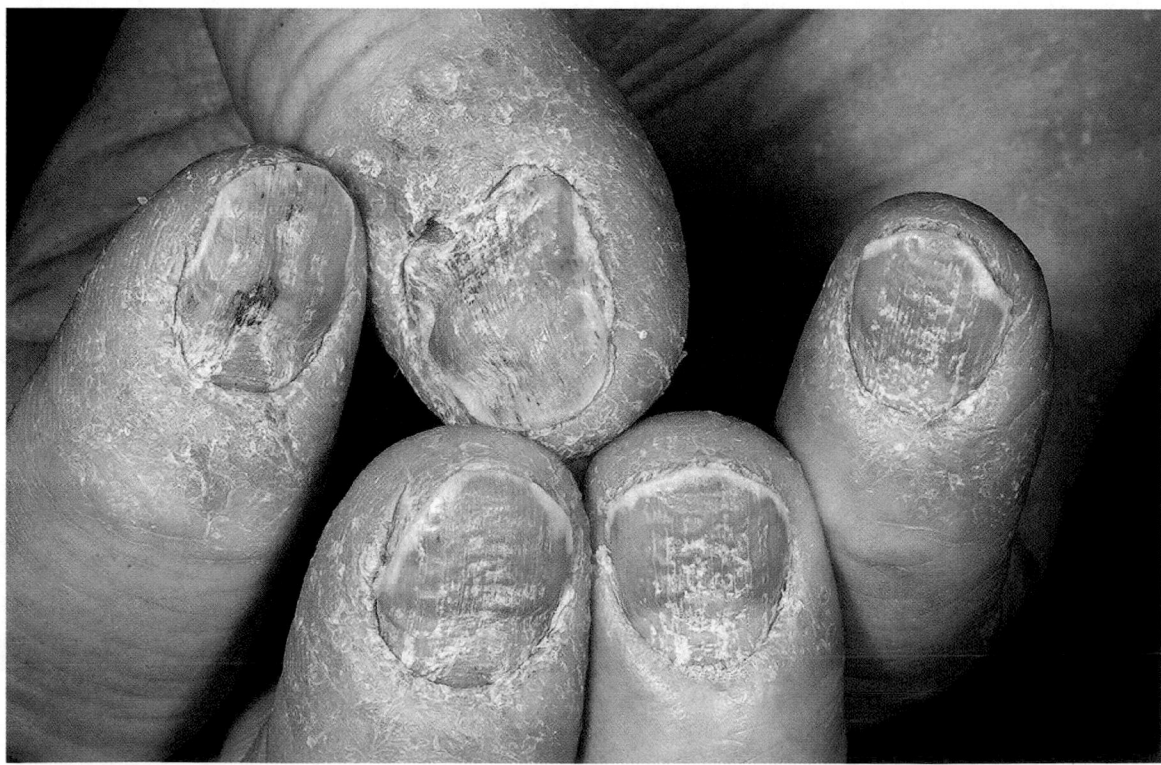

Treatment. Resolution of chronic paronychia depends on avoiding exposure to contact irritants and on treatment of underlying inflammation and infection.[14] Every attempt must be made to keep the proximal nailfold dry. Patients should refrain from washing dishes and from washing their own hair. Rubber or plastic gloves are of some value, but moisture accumulates in them with prolonged use. The hands stay dry if a cotton glove is worn under the rubber glove. Controlling inflammation is the primary goal. Topical steroid creams (group 5) applied bid for up to 3 weeks are more effective than systemic antifungals.[13] Oral antibiotics do not penetrate this distal site in sufficient concentration, and the variety of organisms is too numerous to respond to a single oral agent. Treatments to keep the space between the nail plate and proximal nailfold may help. Place fungoid tincture (miconazole) or one or two drops of 3% thymol in 70% ethanol (compounded by a pharmacist) at the proximal nailfold and wait for this liquid to flow by capillary action into the space created by the absent cuticle. Slight elevation of the proximal nailfold with a flat toothpick facilitates penetration. This should be repeated two or three times a day for weeks, until the cuticle is re-formed. The cuticle may never re-form in patients with long-standing inflammation. Fluconazole (200 mg/day) for 1 to 4 weeks may control chronic inflammation. Short courses of fluconazole may have to be repeated as the infection recurs.

DRUG-INDUCED PARONYCHIA. The protease inhibitors lamivudine and indinavir, used to treat human immunodeficiency virus, have been reported to cause paronychia and ingrown toenails in about 4% of patients receiving these drugs. Pyogenic granuloma-like lesions, staphylococcal superinfection, onycholysis, and severe skin dryness may also be present. The nails of the great toes are usually affected.[15] The lesions appear 2 to 12 months after starting treatment.[16] Complete regression of skin manifestations occurs within 9 to 12 weeks after the drugs are withdrawn. Inhibition of endogenous proteases may explain the initial hypertrophy of the nail fold and the subsequent development of pyogenic granuloma-like lesions.[17]

***PSEUDOMONAS* INFECTION.** Repeated exposure to soap and water causes maceration of the hyponychium and softening of the nail plate. Separation of the nail plate (onycholysis) exposes a damp, macerated space between the nail plate and the nail bed, which is a fertile site for the growth of *Pseudomonas.* The nail plate assumes a green-black color (Figure 25-17). There is little discomfort or inflammation. This presentation may be confused with subungual hematoma (see Figure 25-36), but the absence of pain with *Pseudomonas* infection establishes the diagnosis. Apply a few drops of a mixture of one part chlorine bleach/four parts water under the nail three times a day. Vinegar (acetic acid) may also be used.

HERPETIC WHITLOW. Dentists and nurses used to be at risk of acquiring herpes simplex infection of the fingertip. The risk has greatly diminished with the use of gloves. The appearance and course of the disease resembles that at other body sites, except that there is extreme pain from the swollen fingertips (see Figure 25-18). Herpes simplex virus infection in AIDS patients is characterized by atypical presentations and unusual locations. Herpetic fingers infections in these patients may rapidly progress to the complete destruction of nail structures.[18]

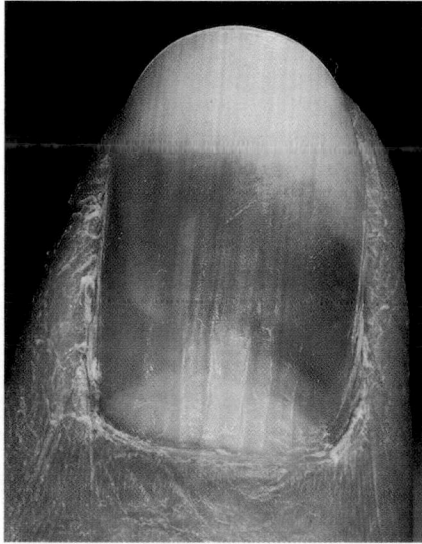

Figure 25-17 *Pseudomonas* colonized the space between the nail and the nail plate after onycholysis occurred, imparting a green color to the nail plate.

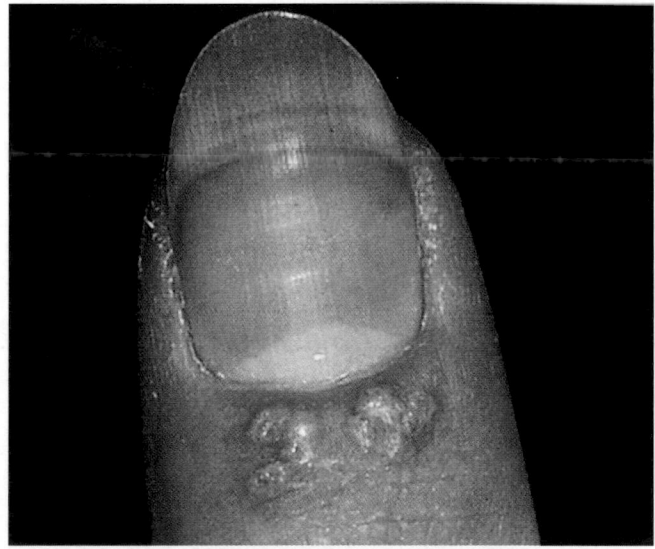

Figure 25-18 Herpes simplex of the finger (herpetic whitlow). Innoculation followed examination of a patient's mouth.

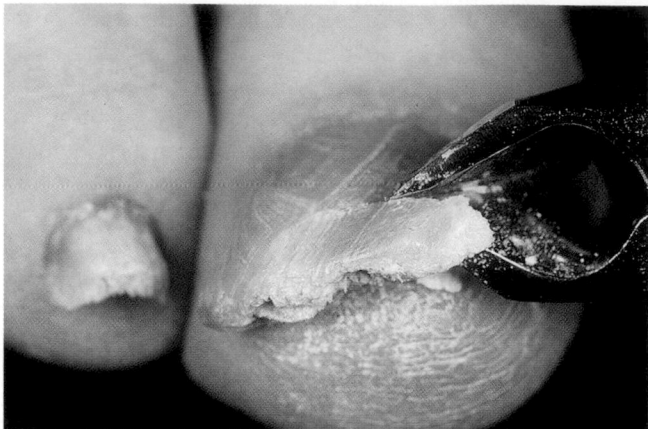

Figure 25-19 Clip the nail plate to relieve pain and expose subungual material for KOH examination and to obtain a nail sample for histology for evaluation of onychomycosis.

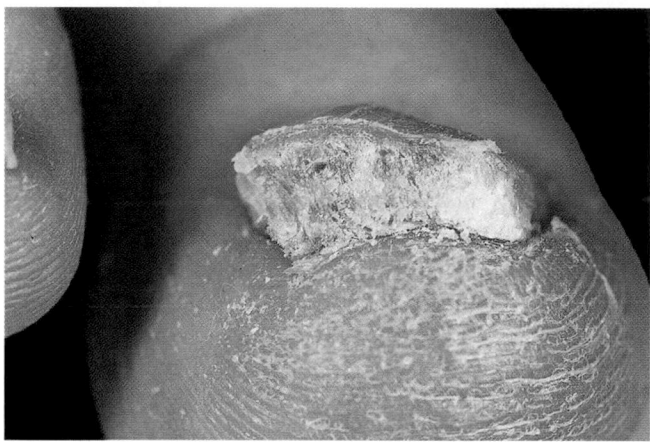

Figure 25-20 Subungual debris has been exposed for sampling. Reduce thick nails with an anvil cutter to relieve shoe pressure.

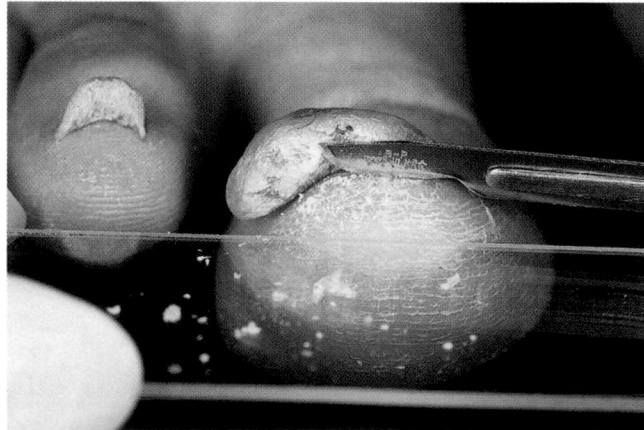

Figure 25-21 Remove subungual debris for KOH fungal examination.

Fungal nail infections

Tinea of the nails is also called tinea unguium. Dermatophytes *T. rubrum* and *T. mentagrophytes* are responsible for most fingernail and toenail infections, but the so-called nonpathogenic fungi (contaminants), and *Candida* can also infect the nail plate.[19] Multiple pathogens may be present in a single nail. Nail infection may occur simultaneously with hand or foot tinea or may occur as an isolated phenomenon. Toenail infections occur in 15% to 20% of the population between 40 and 60 years of age. The disease may also occur in children.

Trauma predisposes to infection. There is a tendency to label any process involving the nail plate as a fungal infection, but many other cutaneous diseases can change the structure of the nail. Fifty percent of thick nails are not infected with fungus. Many patients with nail disease have psoriasis and are not infected with fungus. Differential diagnosis is discussed at the end of this section.

TINEA VS. PSORIASIS. Differentiation of fungal infection from dystrophic changes resulting from psoriasis or other causes is difficult. Potassium hydroxide (KOH) preparations, culture and, occasionally, nail unit biopsy specimens are used. These tests are time-consuming and may yield false-negative results. Histologic examination of distal nail clipping specimens by routine histology and periodic acid-Schiff (PAS) staining is an accurate and simple method for differentiating onychomycosis from nail psoriasis (Figure 25-19). It is equal to culture and superior to KOH preparation in leading to the correct diagnosis of dermatophyte infection.[20]

LABORATORY DIAGNOSIS. The diagnosis of fungal nail infection may be established with both a potassium hydroxide (KOH) examination and a culture. Physicians without the facilities to perform a KOH or culture may obtain these services from local or specialty laboratories, such as the University Center for Medical Mycology, Department of Dermatology, 11100 Euclid Avenue, Cleveland, OH, 44106-5028; 1-800-4MYC-LAB, www.medicalmycology.org. They provide convenient containers for specimen collection. Confirm the species of fungus before starting oral antifungal treatment. When performing cultures, obtain crumbling debris from under several nails and at different parts (proximal and distal areas of infection) of the infected nail (Figure 25-20). Collect subungual debris from under the distal edge of the nail with a curet. Sample the nail surface with a curet or scrape it with a #15 scalpel blade (Figure 25-21). Fungi are found in the nail plate and in the cornified cells of the nail bed. Hyphae that are present in the nail plate may not be viable; therefore sample the cornified cells of the nail bed if possible.

Nail collection techniques for culture. First swab the nail plate with alcohol to remove bacteria. Fragments of nail-plate and nail bed scrapings are inoculated onto Sabouraud's medium with and without antibiotics to identify the fungal species. Use fresh Sabouraud's with antibiotics. Antibiotics degrade in old media and do not effec-

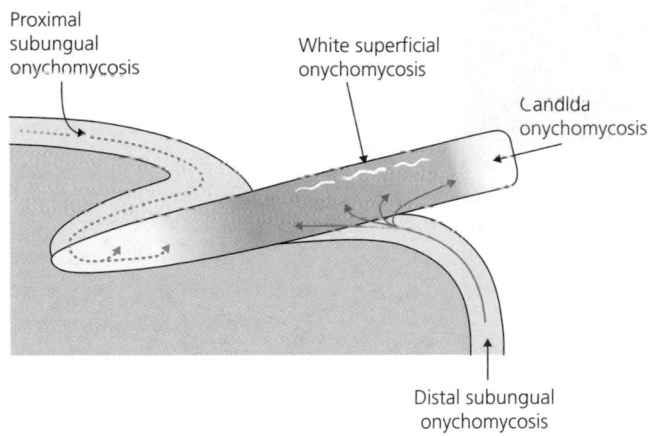

Figure 25-22 Four types of onychomycosis showing different entry points by infecting organisms.

tively suppress bacterial contaminants. The dermatophyte test medium contains the antibiotic cycloheximide and phenol red as a pH indicator. Dermatophytes release alkaline metabolites that turn the medium from yellow to red in 7 to 14 days. Some nondermatophytes, such as Scopulariopsis, Aspergillus, Penicillium, black molds, and yeast, may cause a color change and give a false-positive reaction.[21] The nail plate and hard debris can be adequately softened for direct examination by leaving the fragments, along with several drops of potassium hydroxide, in a watch glass covered with a Petri dish for 24 hours. (See Chapter 13 on fungal infections for details of the KOH examination.)

PATTERNS OF INFECTION. There are four distinct patterns of nail infection.[22] Several patterns of infection may occur simultaneously in the nail plate. Trichophyton rubrum and *T. mentagrophytes* invade the nail plate more frequently than *T. violaceum* or *T. tonsurans*. Aspergillus, Cephalosporium, Fusarium, and Scopulariopsis, generally considered contaminants or nonpathogens, have been isolated from infected nails. They may be found in any pattern of nail infection, especially distal subungual onychomycosis and white superficial onychomycosis. The contaminants do not respond to griseofulvin or the newer oral antifungal agents. The four patterns of nail infection are illustrated in Figure 25-22.

Distal subungual onychomycosis. Distal subungual onychomycosis (Figures 25-23 and 25-24) is the most common pattern of nail invasion. Fungi invade the hyponychium, the distal area of the nail bed. The distal nail plate turns yellow or white as an accumulation of hyperkeratotic debris causes the nail to rise and separate from the underlying bed. Fungus grows in the substance of the plate, causing it to crumble and fragment. A large mass composed of thick nail plate and underlying debris may cause discomfort with footwear.

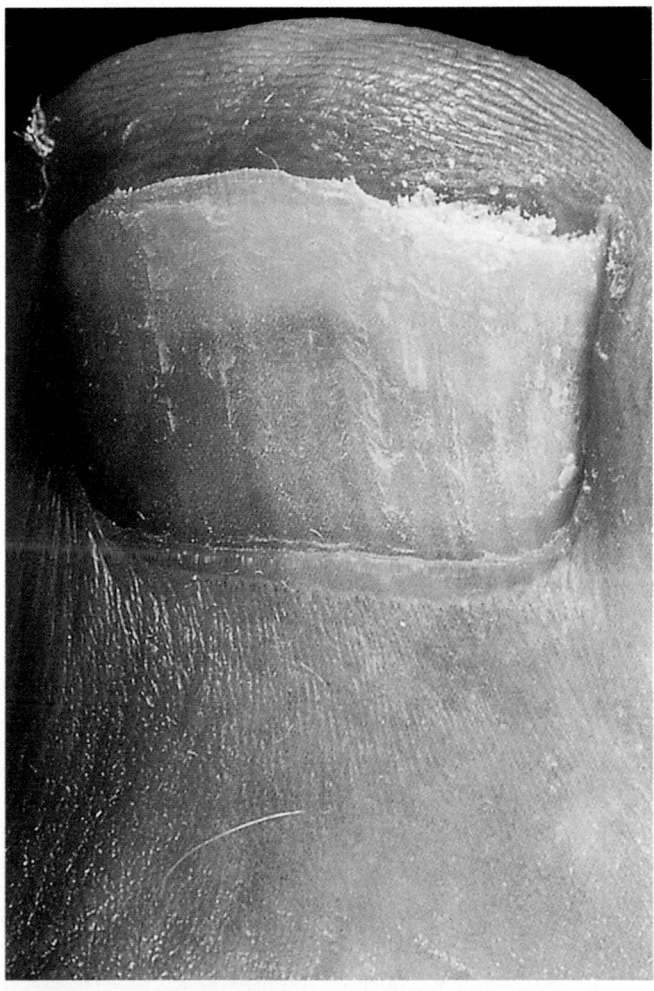

Figure 25-23 Distal subungual onychomycosis. Early changes showing subungual debris at the distal end of the nail plate.

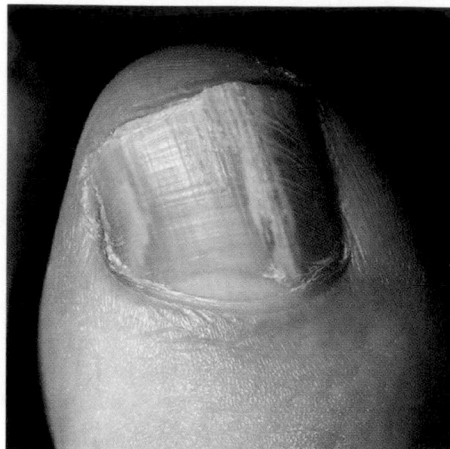

Figure 25-24 Distal subungual onychomycosis. The infection has progressed proximally to form a linear channel. Channeling is a highly characteristic feature of a fungal infection.

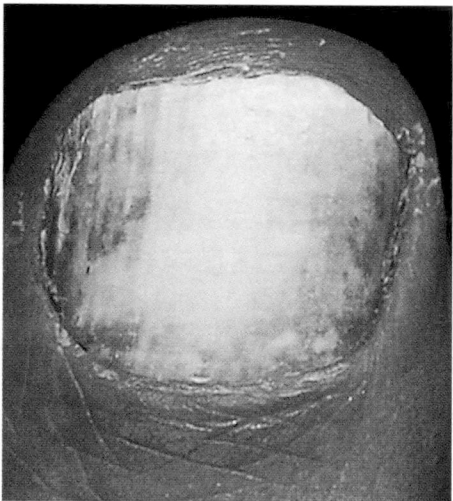

Figure 25-25 White superficial onychomycosis. The surface is soft, dry, and powdery and can easily be scraped away. The nail plate is not thickened and does not separate from the nailbed.

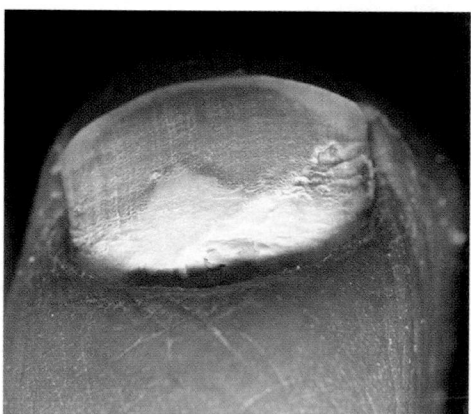

Figure 25-26 Proximal subungual onychomycosis. Fungal invasion of the proximal plate produces leukonychia. Infection may involve the entire thickness of the proximal plate.

White superficial onychomycosis. This is caused by surface invasion of the nail plate, most often by *T. mentagrophytes*. The surface of the nail is soft, dry, and powdery and can easily be scraped away (Figure 25-25). The nail plate is not thickened and remains adherent to the nail bed.

Proximal subungual onychomycosis. Microorganisms enter the posterior nailfold-cuticle area, migrate to the underlying matrix, and finally invade the nail plate from below. Infection occurs within the substance of the nail plate, but the surface remains intact. Hyperkeratotic debris accumulates and causes the nail to separate (Figure 25-26). Transverse white bands begin at the proximal nail plate and are carried distally with outward growth of the nail plate. *T. rubrum* is the most common cause. This is the most common pattern seen in patients with AIDS.

Candida onychomycosis. Nail-plate infection caused by *C. albicans* is seen almost exclusively in chronic mucocutaneous candidiasis. It generally involves all of the fingernails (Figure 25-16). The nail plate thickens and turns yellow-brown.

There are many other patterns of infection. Linear, yellow, or dark brown streaks appear at the distal end and grow proximally in some patterns. In others, some or all of the nail plate may appear yellow; in these areas, the nail can be separated from the underlying bed.

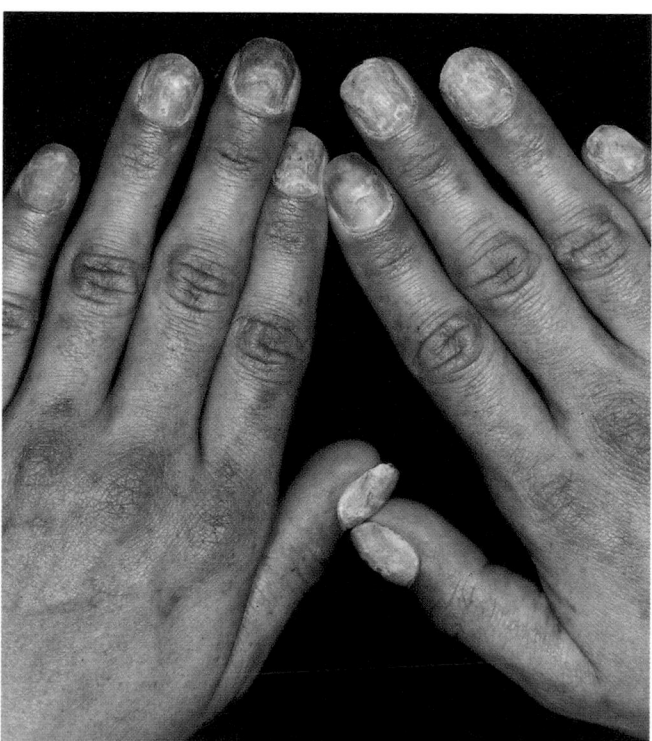

Figure 25-27 *Candida* onychomycosis in a patient with chronic mucocutaneous candidiasis. All of the fingernails are infected.

DIFFERENTIAL DIAGNOSIS. Psoriasis is most commonly confused with onychomycosis, and the two diseases may co-exist. More confusion exists, since psoriatic nail disease may present as an isolated phenomenon without other cutaneous signs. The single distinguishing feature of psoriasis, pitting of the nail-plate surface, is not a feature of fungal infection. Leukonychia, the occurrence of white spots or bands that appear proximally and proceed out with the nail, is probably caused by minor trauma and may be confused with proximal subungual onychomycosis. Eczema or habitual picking of the proximal nailfold induces the nail plate to be wavy and ridged, but its substance remains intact and hard. Numerous, less common nail diseases may be confused with tinea unguium.

GENETIC PREDISPOSITION. Trichophyton rubrum onychomycosis frequently occurs in several members of the same family in different generations. The infection is rare in persons marrying into infected families. Predisposed individuals may acquire *Trichophyton rubrum* infection in childhood from their infected parents. The infection remains asymptomatic and localized to the plantar region. Nail invasion begins in adult life, possibly from nail trauma.

QUALITY OF LIFE ISSUES. Onychomycosis physically and psychologically affects patients' lives. It is capable of having a negative effect on quality of life via social stigma and disrupting daily activities. The problems are embarrassment, functional problems at work, reduction in social activities, fear of spreading the infection to others, and a significant incidence of pain.[23] Onychomycosis can interfere with standing, walking, and exercising. Associated physical impairments can result in paresthesia, pain, discomfort, and loss of manual dexterity. Patients may also suffer from loss of self-esteem and social interaction. Insurance companies consider this disease a *cosmetic nuisance* and are reluctant to pay for treatment unless the patient is physically impaired by the disease.

TREATMENT

*Oral agents—**Terbinafine, itraconazole, fluconazole.*** These drugs penetrate keratinizing tissue. The levels reached in nail plate exceed those in plasma. Therapeutic levels persist in nails for at least one month after discontinuation of therapy. Terbinafine has higher cure rates and a slower relapse rate. Itraconazole can influence the level of many drugs. Terbinafine is relatively free of interactions. Table 25-1 discusses recommended dosages.

CONTINUOUS TERBINAFINE. Continuous terbinafine (250 mg/day for 12 weeks) is significantly more effective than intermittent itraconazole (400 mg/day for 1 week in every 4 weeks for 12 weeks) in the treatment of toenail onychomycosis.[24] A large comparative study produced the following data. At week 72 the mycological cure rates were 75.5% for terbinafine and 38.3% in the itraconazole group.[25] The high rates of cure achieved by terbinafine are maintained more than 2 years. The failure and relapse rates seen with itracona-

zole are much higher.[26] Terbinafine 250 mg daily for 12 weeks is significantly more effective in the treatment of onychomycosis than fluconazole 150 mg once weekly for either 12 or 24 weeks. Mycological cure rates at 60 weeks were: terbinafine group (89%) and fluconazole groups (51% and 49%). Complete clinical cure of the target nail at week 60 was 67% in the terbinafine group, compared with 21% and 32% in the fluconazole groups, respectively.[27]

Itraconazole should be taken with a full meal to ensure maximal absorption.

Griseofulvin is less effective than the newer antifungal agents. Periodic debridement of infected nail during the course of treatment may increase the cure rate.

INTERMITTENT TERBINAFINE. The tested regimens for the use of current antifungals are not optimal. Zaias treated patients with onychomycosis with 250 mg of oral terbinafine daily for 1 week of every month for 11 or more months, until the mycotic nail bed had been completely replaced by new, nonmycotic nail bed.

Patients were examined monthly for evidence of proximal extension of the nail bed lesion beneath a reference notch that had been cut into the overlying nail plate of the target nail to mark the proximal limit of the nail bed lesion at the beginning of treatment. Any proximal extension of the lesion below the reference notch during treatment was a treatment failure, and treatment was stopped. The cure rate was 90%.

Itraconazole was less effective.[28]

DIFFICULT CASES. Patients with lateral nail edge infection, yellow streaks, and total dystrophic onychomycosis are often resistant to treatment and may require longer courses of treatment. Some physicians use PENLAC (Ciclopirox nail laquer) with oral antifungal drugs to enhance effectiveness.

Table 25-1 Oral Antifungal Agents for Treating Tinea of the Nails

Drug	Dosage
Fluconazole (Diflucan)	One 150-mg dose each week for 9 months
Itraconazole (Sporanox)	200 mg/day for 12 weeks for toenails, 6 weeks for fingernails "Pulse dosing": 400 mg/day for first week of each month Fingernails 2-3 pulses Toenails 3-4 pulses
Terbinafine	250 mg/day (12 weeks for toenails, 6 weeks for fingernails)

PREVENTING RECURRENCE. PENLAC applied to the nail and nailfold two to three times each week may prevent recurrence after a course of oral antifungal medication. Preventing recurrence of tinea pedis may prevent recurrence of onychomycosis. There is evidence that prolonged use of a topical antifungal agent applied around the toes, after clinical response of onychomycosis to an oral agent, may prevent nail reinfection.[29] Use of a topical antifungal cream for 1 year after clinical cure of onychomycosis has prevented reinfection in the 12-month follow-up period.[30] A weekly application of terbinafine cream in the nail area, between the toes and on the soles would be a reasonable prevention program. Trauma to the tip of nails from tight-fitting shoes may be the single most important event for encouraging hyphae invasion in the region of the hyponychium that leads to distal subungual onychomycosis. Shoes or boots that create a confined, damp, and warm atmosphere facilitate the development of fungal infection. Protect feet in communal showers. Medicated powders applied directly to the toe webs and soles (not poured into shoes) will help maintain a dry environment.

DRUG INTERACTIONS. Itraconazole has an affinity for cytochrome P-450 enzymes and therefore has the potential for interactions. Terbinafine is not metabolized through this system and has little potential for drug-drug interactions. Drug interactions are usually less severe with fluconazole than with itraconazole.[28,29]

LABORATORY MONITORING. Many physicians check liver function and complete blood counts prior to and at six weeks during treatment with terbinafine. Laboratory tests are not required during pulse dosing of itraconazole.

SAFETY OF ORAL AGENTS. Terbinafine and itraconazole are promoted in the media. Patients are given the impression that they cause many side effects, especially liver disease. These drugs have been used in Europe and the United States for several years. They have a very low incidence of serious side effects.[31]

Assessing drug effectiveness. The method described here is used to assess patients with distal subungual onychomycosis[29] (Figure 25-28). When an effective dosage of an oral antifungal agent is given, it acts as a barrier to further proximal nail invasion by the fungus (Figure 25-29). A superficial horizontal cut is made with a scalpel in the midline on the normal nail plate, adjacent to the onychomycotic border. The groove is filled with ink or dye, and a measurement is

Figure 25-28 Determination of drug effectiveness in onychomycosis. Diagrammatic drawing of the objective method for determining drug effectiveness with antifungal agents in onychomycosis. Chronologic sequence of events in a patient cured with the minimum effective daily dose. *PNF,* proximal nailfold. The brown areas are clinical onychomycosis. *X* is a superficial cut made on the normal nail plate adjacent to the onychomycotic border. *Y* is the distance from the proximal nailfold to the onychomycotic border (*X*) and reflects normal nail present. An effective dosage acts as a barrier as in nails 2 through 5. The initial drug dosage became ineffective (nail 8) and required an increase in the drug dose to achieve a cure (nails 9 and 10). (*From Zaias N, Drachman D: J Am Acad Dermatol 1983; 9:912.*)

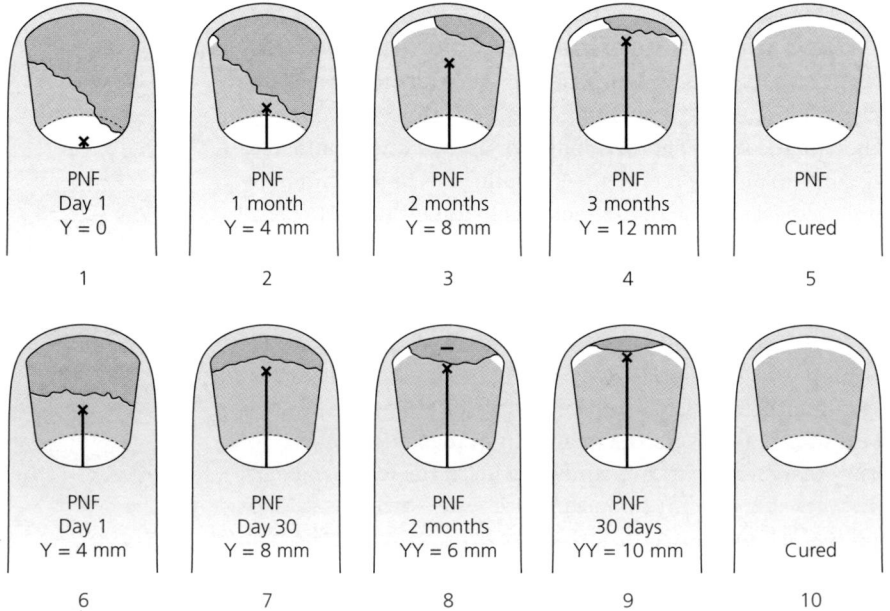

taken from this point to the proximal nailfold's edge. If an effective dosage is given, the onychomycotic area does not invade proximal to the mark; then the amount of new plate should reflect the normal nail-plate production. The patient returns in 1 month. In most normal, healthy subjects, 1.5 to 2 mm of nail plate grows per month from the large toenails and 3 to 4 mm of nail plate grows per month from the fingernails. If the fungus invades proximal to the horizontal scalpel groove, then the dosage of medication is increased and the measuring process starts anew.

TOPICAL AGENTS (PENLAC). Ciclopirox nail lacquer 8% (PENLAC) is approved for mild to moderate onychomycosis of the fingers and toes resulting from Trichophyton rubrum without lunula involvement. The nail lacquer is applied once daily to the affected nail, 5 mm of the surrounding skin and, if possible, to the nail bed, hyponychium, and undersurface of the nail plate. Each new application should be placed over the old one and all coats removed with alcohol once a week. After evaporation of volatile solvents in the lacquer, the concentration of ciclopirox in the remaining lacquer film reaches approximately 35%, providing a high concentration gradient for penetration into the nail.[32] The management program includes removal of the unattached, infected nails as frequently as once per month. At the end of the 48-week treatment period, the mycologic cure rate (negative culture and negative light microscopy) was 29%.[32]

Mechanical reduction of infected nail plate. A nail clipper with plier handles may be used to remove substantial amounts of hard, thick debris. One should insert the pointed tip of the instrument as far down as possible between the diseased nail and the nail bed. Adherent thick nail plate can be reduced by sanding or cutting the surface layers with the clippers. Removal of the infected nail may accelerate resolution of the infection.

Surgical removal. Painful or extremely infected nails (usually the nail of the first toe) can be removed by a simple surgical procedure (see p. 864).

Nonsurgical avulsion of nail dystrophies. Symptomatic dystrophic nails may be painlessly removed with a urea compound (Figure 25-30). The technique has its greatest application in removing hypertrophic mycotic nails and can be used to treat other hypertrophic nail conditions of the nail plate, such as psoriatic nails.[33] The procedure also facilitates subsequent treatment with topical antifungal agents. The technique removes only grossly diseased or dystrophic nails, not normal nails. Forty percent urea gel (Carmol-40 gel, Vanamide cream) is commercially available or by prescription.

Cloth adhesive tape is used to cover the normal skin surrounding the affected nail plate, which has been pretreated with tincture of benzoin. The urea cream is generously applied directly to the nail surface and covered with a piece of plastic wrap. This in turn is covered with a finger that is cut from a plastic glove and held in place with adhesive tape. Patients are instructed to keep the area completely dry with the aid of plastic gloves or booties.

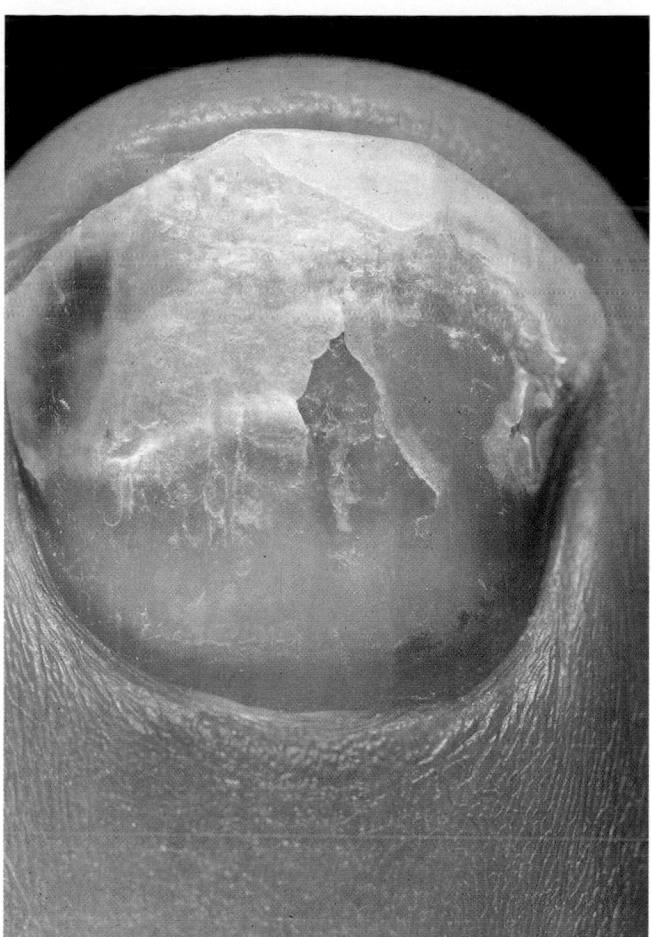

Figure 25-29 Distal subungual onychomycosis treated for 8 weeks. A distinct border separates the normal nail from the infected distal nail plate.

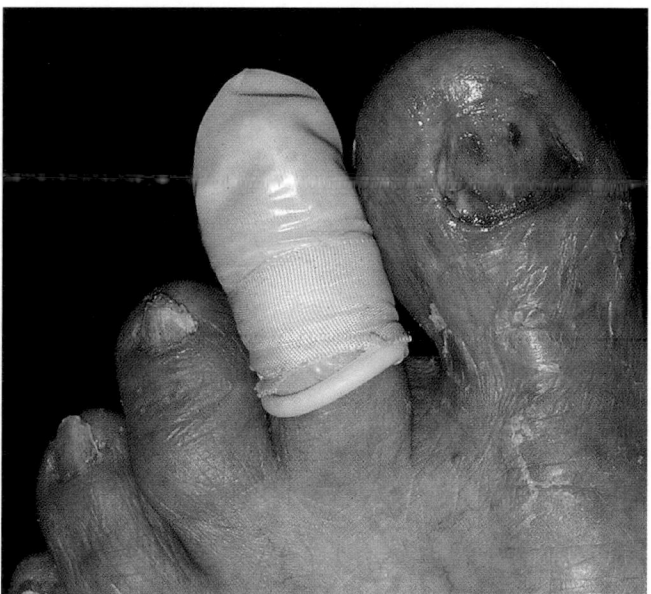

Figure 25-30 Nonsurgical avulsion of nail dystrophies. A 40% urea medication is occluded to remove infected nail plate.

An alternate technique uses adhesive felt (mole skin) and waterproof, stretchable tape (Blenderm). A nail-shaped hole is cut in a piece of moleskin, and the moleskin is applied, sticky surface down, on the dorsal aspect of the toe so that just the nail is exposed through the hole. The well is filled with the urea cream and covered with Blenderm tape.[34] The patient returns to the physician in 7 to 10 days. At that time the treated nails are removed, when possible, by either lifting the entire nail plate from the nail bed or by cutting the abnormal portions with a nail cutter. This is followed by light curettage until a clinically normal nail is reached at all margins.

Trauma

ONYCHOLYSIS. Onycholysis, the painless separation of the nail from the nail bed, is common. Separation usually begins at the distal groove and progresses irregularly and proximally, causing part or most of the plate to become separated. The nonadherent portion of the nail is opaque with a white (Figure 25-31), yellow (Figures 25-32 and 25-33), or green tinge. The causes of onycholysis include psoriasis, trauma, *Candida* or *Pseudomonas* infections, internal drugs, PUVA photochemotherapy,[35] contact with chemicals, maceration from prolonged immersion, and allergic contact dermatitis (e.g., to nail hardener and adhesives).[36] Onycholysis is known to be associated with thyroid disease (especially hyperthyroidism). Consider screening patients with unexplained onycholysis for asymptomatic thyroid disease.[37]

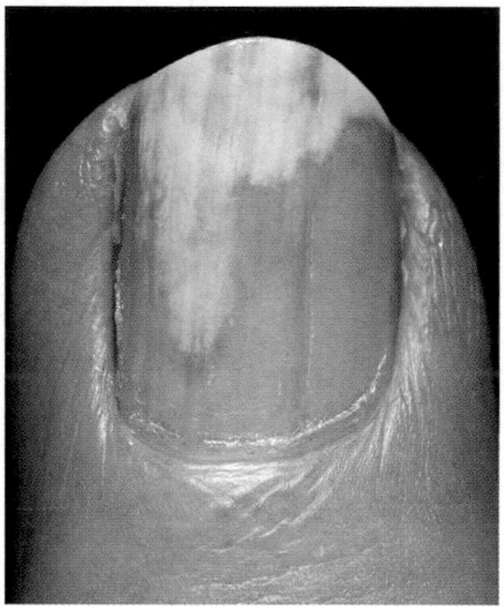

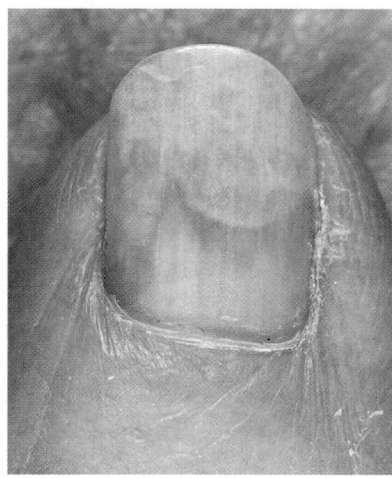

Figure 25-31 Onycholysis. Separation of the nail plate starts at the distal groove. Minor trauma to long fingernails is the most common cause.

Figure 25-32 Onycholysis. The yellow color may indicate a secondary *Candida* infection. Psoriasis and tinea have a similar appearance.

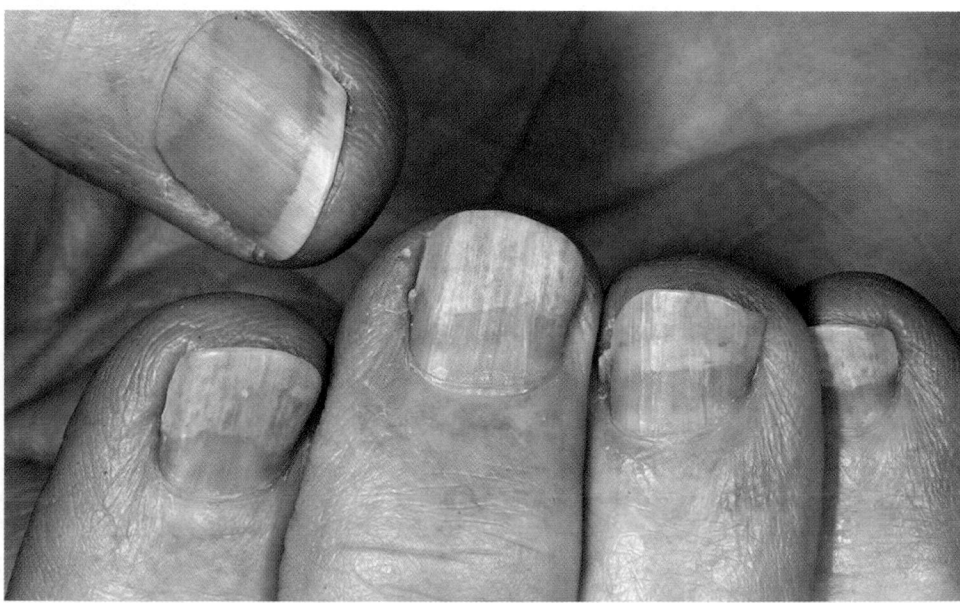

Figure 25-33 Onycholysis. Involvement of many nails simultaneously is the typical presentation.

When other signs of skin disease are absent, onycholysis is most frequently seen in women with long fingernails. With normal activity, the extended nail inadvertently strikes objects and acts as a lever to pry the nail from the nail bed. Forcing a stylus between the nail plate and bed while manicuring can cause separation.

TREATMENT. All of the separated nail is removed, and the fingers are kept dry. Removing the separated nail eliminates the lever, and dryness discourages infection. One should not cover the cut nails; occlusion promotes maceration. Any form of manipulation should be discouraged. Avoid exposure to contact irritants. Yeast commonly grows in the space between nail and nailbed. Use liquid topical agents that can flow under the nail such as fungoid tincture that contains miconazole. Use oral fluconazole (Diflucan) for resistant cases. A short course of fluconazole (e.g., 150 mg qd for 5 to 7 days) may have to be repeated as the nail grows out.

PHOTOONYCHOLYSIS. Onycholysis may be precipitated by exposure to ultraviolet radiation. Photoonycholysis may occur with the use of tetracycline antibiotics and cytotoxic drugs. Nail changes with the taxanes, primarily docetaxel, are reported in up to 30% to 40% of patients. Prolonged weekly paclitaxel, other taxanes, and anthracyclines cause onycholysis in some patients, which may be precipitated by exposure to sunlight. Patients receiving these drugs should protect their nails from sunlight.[38] The reaction does not warrant discontinuation of therapy.

NAIL AND CUTICLE BITING. Nail biting is a nervous habit that usually begins in childhood and lasts for years. One or all nails may be chewed as far as the lunula. The nail plate is chiseled and bitten from the nail bed by the teeth. Nail growth occurs during periods of physical activity, but periods of physical inactivity seem to promote zealous nail biting. Thin strips of skin on the lateral and proximal nailfold may also be stripped (Figure 25-34).

Patients are aware of their habit but seem powerless to control it. In one study mild aversion such as painting the nail plate with a distasteful preparation such as Nail Cure (Purepac) or Sally Hansen Nail Biter resulted in significant improvements in nail length. A second effective method of habit reversal is to have the person perform a competing response whenever they have the urge to nail bite or found themselves biting their nails.[39]

NAIL PLATE EXCORIATION. Digging or excoriating the nail plate is much less common than biting. This destructive practice may result in gross deformity of the nail plate.

HANGNAIL. Triangular strips of skin may separate from the lateral nailfolds, particularly during the winter months. Attempts at removal may cause pain and extension of the tear into the dermis. Separated skin should be cut before extension occurs. Constant lubrication of the fingertips with skin creams (e.g., Aquaphor ointment) and avoidance of repeated hand immersion in water is beneficial.

INGROWN TOENAIL. Ingrown fingernails and toenails are common; the large toe is most frequently affected. The nail pierces the lateral nailfold and enters the dermis, where it acts as a foreign body. The first signs are pain and swelling. The area of penetration becomes purulent and edematous as exuberant granulation tissue grows alongside the penetrating nail (Figure 25-35). Ingrown nails are caused by lateral pressure of poorly fitting shoes, improper or excessive trimming of the lateral nail plate, or trauma.

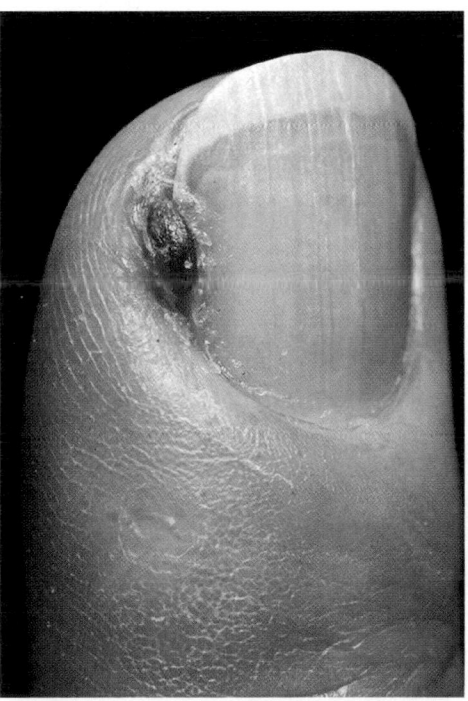

Figure 25-35 An ingrown nail has stimulated the formation of granulation tissue.

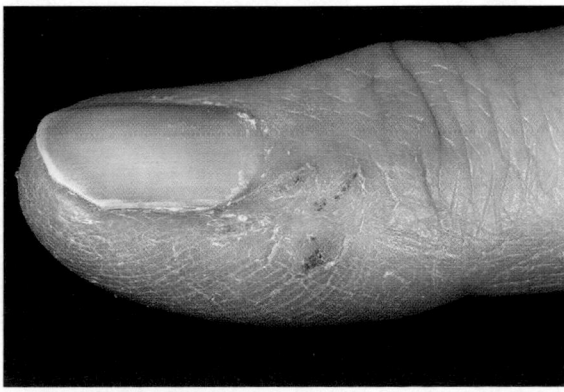

Figure 25-34 Nail and cuticle biting.

TREATMENT

Ingrown nail without inflammation. Separate the distal anterior tip and lateral edges of an ingrown toenail from the adjacent soft tissue with a wisp of absorbent cotton coated with collodion. This gives immediate relief of pain and provides a firm runway for further growth of the nail. The collodion fixes the cotton in place, waterproofs the area, and permits bathing. The cotton insert may need reinsertion in 3 to 6 weeks. Cotton without collodion may be used, but it may have to be replaced frequently. This method is not applicable to patients with infected acute inflammation of the lateral nailfold.[40]

Ingrown nail with inflammation. The lateral nailfold is infiltrated with 1% or 2% lidocaine (Xylocaine). Nail-splitting scissors are inserted under the ingrown nail parallel to the lateral nailfold. The tip is inserted toward the matrix until resistance is met, and the wedge-shaped nail is then cut and removed. Granulation tissue is reduced with a silver nitrate application or removed with a curet. For a few days, the inflamed site is treated with a Burrow's cool, wet compress until the swelling and inflammation have subsided. Shoes should be worn that allow the toes to fall naturally, without compression. The new nail is forced up and over the lateral nailfold by inserting cotton under the lateral nail margin and allowing it to remain in place for days or weeks.

Recurrent ingrown nail. Patients with recurrent ingrown nails may require the use of liquid phenol for permanent destruction of the lateral portions of the nail matrix.[41-44] The use of oral antibiotics as an adjunctive therapy in treating ingrown toenails does not play a role in decreasing the healing time or postprocedure morbidity.[45]

SUBUNGUAL HEMATOMA. Subungual hematoma (Figure 25-36) may be caused by trauma to the nail plate, which causes immediate bleeding and pain. The quantity of blood may be sufficient to cause separation and loss of the nail plate. The traditional method of puncturing the nail with a red-hot paperclip tip remains the quickest and most effective method of draining the blood. Alternatively, a carbon dioxide laser can be used to melt the nail at the center of the discolored area and decompress the hematoma.[46] No anesthesia is required with this procedure. Trephining the nail with a hand drill, dental drill, or a fine-point scalpel blade can be painful because of the pressure required to puncture the nail. Often digital nerve block is necessary when drilling methods are used. Trauma to the proximal nailfold causes hemorrhage that may not be apparent for days. The nail plate may emerge from the nailfold with bloodstains that remain until the nail grows out. Young children with subungual hematoma may be victims of child abuse.[47]

NAIL HYPERTROPHY. Gross thickening of the nail plate may occur with tight-fitting shoes or other forms of chronic trauma. The nail plate is brown, very thick, and points to one side (Figure 25-37). Shoes compress the nail plate against the toe and cause pain. The substance of the nail plate may be reduced with sandpaper or a file, or the nail can be removed and the nail matrix permanently destroyed with phenol so that the nail will not regrow.[41]

WHITE SPOTS OR BANDS. White spots (leukonychia punctata) in the nail plate, a very common finding, possibly result from cuticle manipulation or other mild forms of trauma (Figure 25-38). The spots or bands may appear at the lunula or may appear spontaneously in the nail plate and subsequently disappear or grow with the nail.[48] Psoriasis of the mid nail matrix can also produce this change.

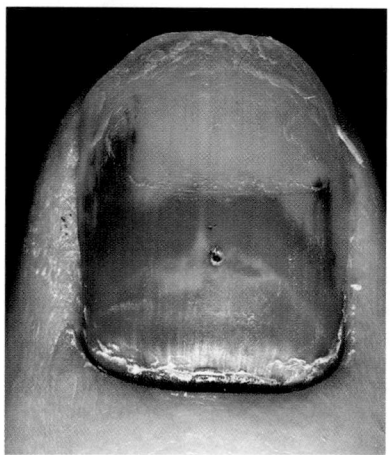

Figure 25-36 Subungual hematoma. A *Proteus* or *Pseudomonas* infection might be suspected if there were no history of trauma.

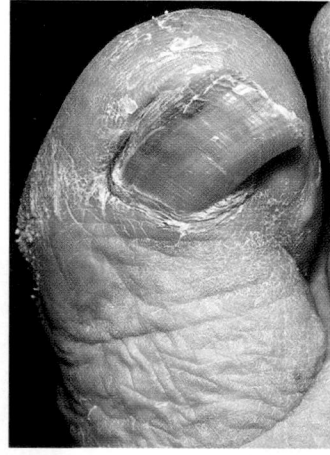

Figure 25-37 Nail hypertrophy. The nail plate becomes thick and distorted, often causing discomfort when shoes are worn.

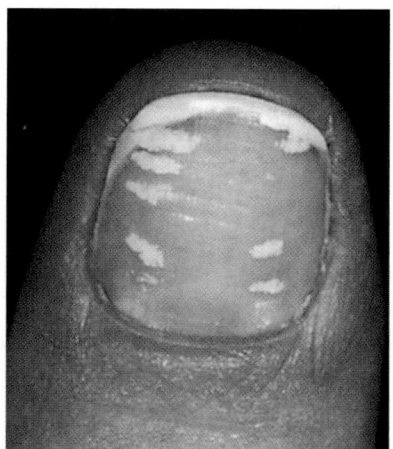

Figure 25-38 White spots (leukonychia punctata). A common finding often mistaken for a fungal infection.

DISTAL PLATE SPLITTING (BRITTLE NAILS). The splitting into layers or peeling of the distal nail plate may resemble or be analogous to the scaling of dry skin (Figure 25-39). This nail change is found in approximately 20% of the adult population.[49] Repeated water immersion and the frequent use of nail polish removers increases the incidence of brittle nails, particularly in women.[50] Local measures to rehydrate the nail plate should be initiated. A moisturizer may be applied after the nails have been soaked in water. Protection with rubber over-cotton gloves and application of heavy lubricants (e.g., Aquaphor ointment) directly to the nail plate provide improvement. The moisturizing agent may be applied under occlusion with a white cotton glove or sock.[51] Nail enamel may slow the evaporation of water from the nail plate. It should be removed and reapplied no more than once a week. A number of nail conditioning products (e.g., Elon nail products) are available from Dartmouth pharmaceuticals online (www.ilovemynails.com) and in pharmacies.

Patients with brittle nails who receive the B-complex vitamin biotin (2.5 mg/day) may improve and have up to a 25% increase in nail-plate thickness.[52,53]

HABIT-TIC DEFORMITY. Habit-tic deformity is a common finding and is caused by biting or picking a section of the proximal nailfold of the thumb with the index fingernail. Although the condition is most common to the thumbnails, all nails can be affected. The lesion is often noted as an inci-

dental finding in a patient seeking treatment for another cutaneous disease. The resulting defect consists of a longitudinal band of horizontal grooves that often have a yellow discoloration. The band extends from the proximal nailfold to the tip of the nail (Figure 25-40). This should not be confused with the nail rippling that occurs with chronic paronychia or chronic eczematous inflammation of the proximal nailfold. The ripples of chronic inflammation appear as rounded waves (Figure 25-41), in contrast to the closely spaced, sharp grooves produced by continual manipulation.

The method of formation is demonstrated for the patient. Some patients are not aware of their habit, and others who admit to nail picking may not realize that they have created the defect. Patients who discontinue manipulation are able to grow relatively normal nails; there are those, however, who find it impossible to stop.

From a psychiatric perspective, it is often unclear how to classify habit-tic disorders. The heterogeneity of behaviors complicates the diagnostic process. In some cases it might be classified as obsessive-compulsive disorder. In other cases, the behavior is automatic, bearing similarities to the impulse control disorder trichotillomania, which may be related to obsessive-compulsive disorders. Obsessive-compulsive disorder sometimes responds to the serotonin reuptake inhibitor fluoxetine (Prozac), and patients with habit-tic deformity may respond to this medication.[54]

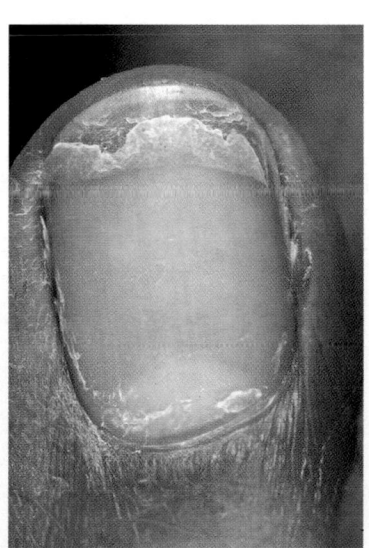

Figure 25-39 Distal nail splitting. The nail splits into layers or the distal nail plate peels, a change analogous to the scaling of dry skin.

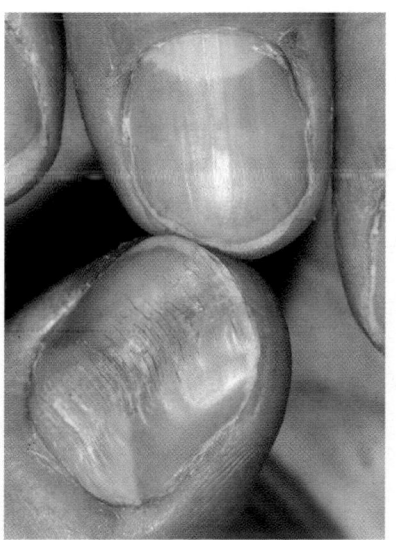

Figure 25-40 Habit-tic derformity. A common finding on the thumbs caused by picking the proximal nailfold with the index finger.

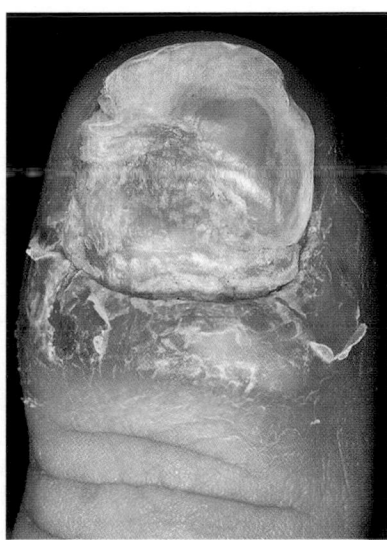

Figure 25-41 Nail rippling caused by chronic inflammation of the proximal nailfold. A normal nail grows once the eczema has been controlled.

MEDIAN NAIL DYSTROPHY. Median nail dystrophy is a distinctive nail-plate change of unknown origin. A longitudinal split appears in the center of the nail plate. Several fine cracks project from the line laterally, giving the appearance of a fir tree. The thumb is most often affected (Figure 25-42). There is no treatment, and after a few months or years the nail can be expected to return to normal. Recurrences are possible.

PINCER NAILS (CURVATURE). Inward folding of the lateral edges of the nail results in a tube- or pincer-shaped nail (Figure 25-43). The nail bed is drawn up into the tube and may become painful. The toenails are more commonly involved than the fingernails. Shoe compression is thought to cause pincer nails, but the etiology is uncertain. If pain is significant, surgical removal of the nail or reconstruction of the nail unit is required.

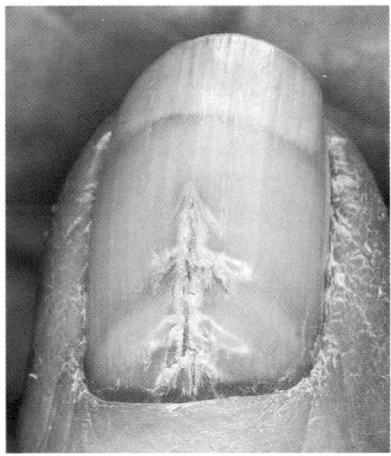

Figure 25-42 Median nail dystrophy.

The Nail and Internal Disease

BEAU'S LINES. Beau's lines are transverse depressions of all of the nails that appear at the base of the lunula weeks after a stressful event has temporarily interrupted nail formation (Figure 25-44). The lines progress distally with normal nail growth and eventually disappear at the free edge. They develop in response to many diseases, such as syphilis, uncontrolled diabetes mellitus, myocarditis, peripheral vascular disease, and zinc deficiency, and to illnesses accompanied by high fevers, such as scarlet fever, measles, mumps, hand-foot-mouth disease,[55] and pneumonia,[56] and to chemotherapeutic agents.[57]

YELLOW NAIL SYNDROME. The spontaneous appearance of yellow nails occurs before, during, or after certain respiratory diseases and in diseases associated with lymphedema. Patients note that nail growth slows and appears to stop. The nail plate may become excessively curved, and it turns dark yellow (Figure 25-45). The surface remains smooth or acquires transverse ridges, indicating variations in the growth rate; nails grow at less than half the normal rate. Partial or total separation of the nail plate may occur. The nails show an increased curvature about the long axis, the cuticles and lunulae are lost, and usually all the nails are involved. The nails grow very slowly, at a rate of 0.1 to 0.25 mm/week, compared with 0.5 to 2 mm/week for normal adult fingernails. Nails that grow slowly often become thicker.[58] The diseases reported to be associated with yellow nail syndrome are edema of the lower extremities, facial edema, pleural effusion, bronchiectasis, sinusitis,[59] bronchitis, and chronic respiratory infections.[60] The lymphatic impairment associated with yellow nail syndrome appears to be secondary, and predominantly functional in nature, rather than as a result of structural changes.[61] Yellowish nail pigmentation has been

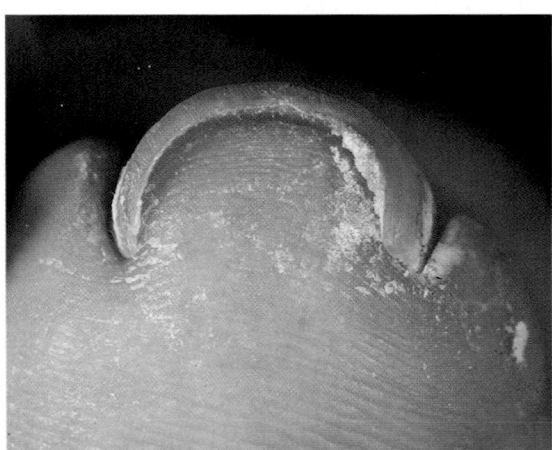

Figure 25-43 Pincer nails (overcurvature). Inward folding of the lateral edges of the nail results in a tube- or pincer-shaped nail.

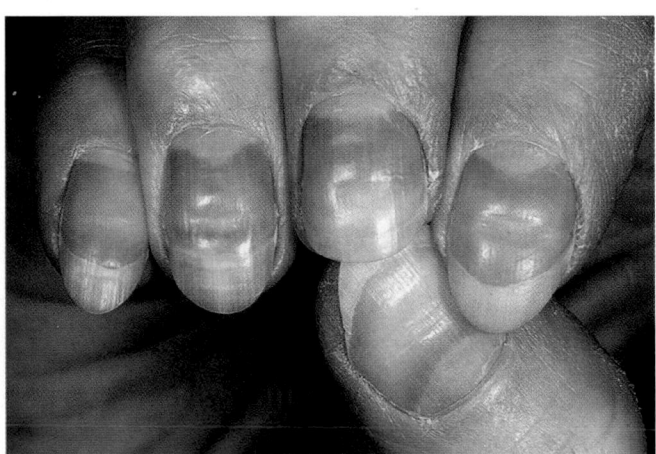

Figure 25-44 Beau's lines. A transverse depression of the nail plate that occurs several weeks after certain illnesses.

reported in patients with AIDS. The nails may spontaneously improve, even when the associated disease does not improve.[62,63] Oral vitamin E in dosages of up to 800 IU/day for up to 18 months may help. Yellow nails that were treated with a 5% vitamin E solution (containing DL-alpha-tocopherol in dimethyl sulfoxide), two drops twice a day to the nail plate, showed marked clinical improvement and an increase in nail-growth rate.[64]

SPOON NAILS. Lateral elevation and central depression of the nail plate cause the nail to be spoon shaped; this is called koilonychia (Figure 25-46). Spoon nails are seen in normal children and may persist a lifetime without any associated abnormalities. The spontaneous onset of spoon nails has been reported to occur with iron-deficiency anemia and in 50% of patients with idiopathic hemochromatosis.[65] The nail reverts to normal when the anemia is corrected.

FINGER CLUBBING. Finger clubbing (Hippocratic nails) is a distinct feature associated with a number of diseases, but it may occur as a normal variant. The distal phalanges of the fingers and toes are enlarged to a rounded, bulbous shape. The nail enlarges and becomes curved, hard, and thickened (Figure 25-47). The angle made by the proximal nailfold and nail plate (Lovibond's angle) increases and approaches or exceeds 180 degrees. The proximal nailfold feels as though it is floating on the underlying tissue. Clubbing is associated with a variety of lung diseases, cardiovascular disease, cirrhosis, colitis, and thyroid disease. In one study, one third of patients with lung cancer had evidence of clubbing as defined by a new digital index of clubbing.[66] The changes are permanent.

TERRY'S NAILS. Terry's nails are white or light pink but retain a 0.5- to 3-mm normal, pink, distal band (Figure 25-48). The findings are associated with cirrhosis, chronic congestive heart failure, adult-onset diabetes mellitus, and age.[67] It has been speculated that Terry's nails are a part of aging and that associated diseases "age" the nail. These changes are not associated with hypoalbuminemia or anemia.

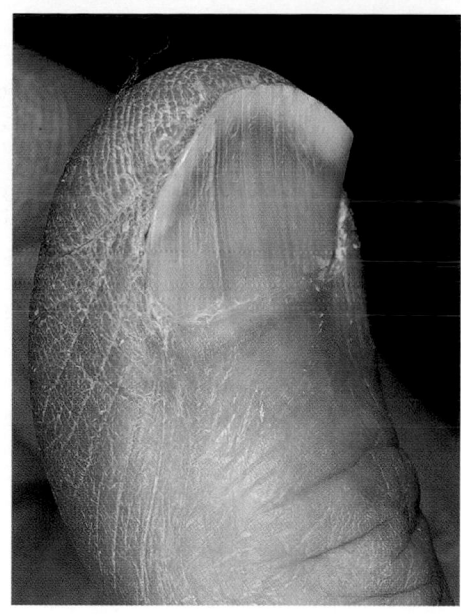

Figure 25-46 Spoon nails (koilonychia). Most cases are a variant of normal.

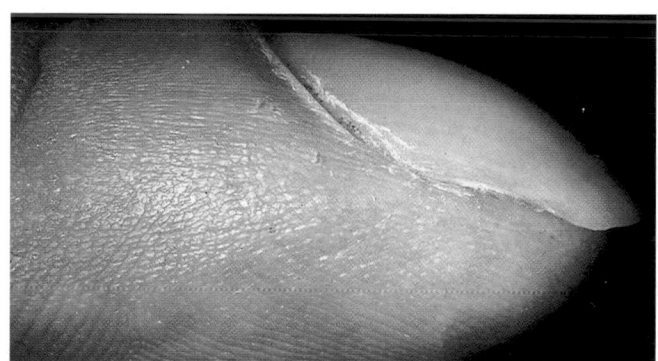

Figure 25-47 Finger clubbing. The distal phalanges are enlarged to a rounded, bulbous shape. The nail enlarges and becomes curved, hard, and thickened.

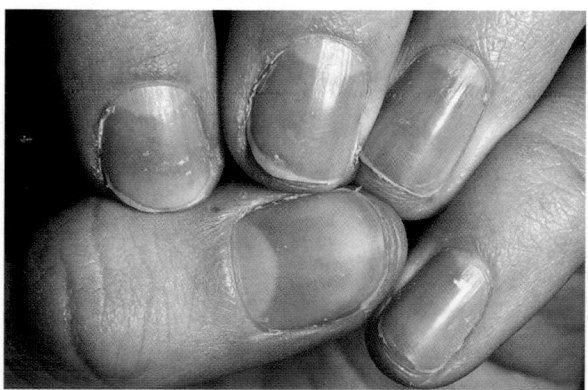

Figure 25-45 Yellow nail syndrome.

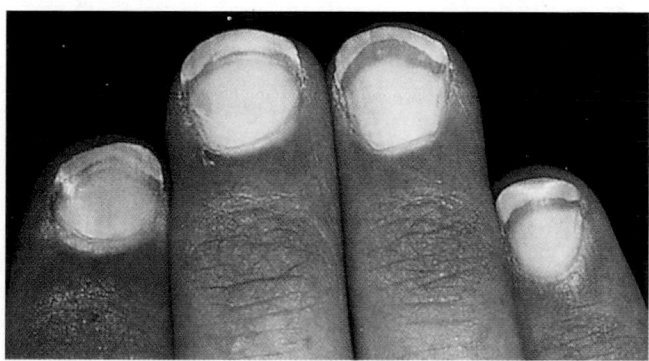

Figure 25-48 Terry's nails. The nail bed is white with only a narrow zone of pink at the distal end.

Congenital Anomalies

Numerous congenital syndromes involve nail changes. The most widely understood syndromes all have autosomal dominant inheritance patterns.

Among other signs of pachyonychia congenita, there are yellow, very thick nail beds with elevated nails, palmar and plantar hyperkeratosis, and white keratotic thickening of the tongue. Some patients have erupted teeth at birth. In nail-patella syndrome, there are defective short nails and small or absent patella, in addition to other signs.

Color and Drug-Induced Changes

Changes in nail color may result from a color change in the nail plate or in the nail bed. Several articles[68,69,70] list changes associated with nail pigmentation. Some of these changes are listed in Tables 25-2 and 25-3. Cancer chemotherapeutic drugs have been associated with a variety of changes in the nail unit (Table 25-4).

Table 25-2 Color Changes of Nails

Etiology	Pattern of color change
Brown nails	
Antimalarial drugs	Diffuse blue, brown
Cancer chemotherapeutic agents (Table 25-4)	Transverse black bands
Hyperbilirubinemia	Diffuse brown
Junctional nevi	Longitudinal brown bands
Malnutrition	Diffuse brown or black bands
Melanocyte stimulating hormone oversecretion	Longitudinal brown bands
Addison's disease	
Cushing's disease (after adrenalectomy)	
Pituitary tumor	
Melanoma	Longitudinal bands, may increase with width (Hutchinson's sign)
Normal finding in more than 90% of blacks	Longitudinal brown bands
Photographic developer	Diffuse brown
Green nails	
Pseudomonas	Green streaks and patches
Yellow nails	
Yellow-nail syndrome	Diffuse yellow
Onycholysis	Distal nail separation
Blue nails (blacks)	
Zidovudine treatment for AIDS	Diffuse blue
Antimalarial drugs	Diffuse blue
Minocycline	Diffuse blue
Wilson's disease	Diffuse blue
Hemorrhage	Irregular

Table 25-3 White Nail or Nail-Bed Changes

Disease	Clinical appearance
Anemia	Diffuse white
Arsenic	Mee's lines: transverse white lines
Cirrhosis	Terry's nails: most of nail, zone of pink at distal end (Figure 25-48)
Congenital leukonychia (autosomal dominant; variety of patterns)	Syndrome of leukonychia, knuckle pads, deafness; isolated finding; partial white
Darier's disease	Longitudinal white streaks
Half-and-half nail	Proximal white, distal pink; azotemia
High fevers (some diseases)	Transverse white lines
Hypoalbuminemia	Muehrcke's lines: stationary paired transverse bands
Hypocalcemia	Variable white
Malnutrition	Diffuse white
Pellagra	Diffuse milky white
Punctate leukonychia	Common white spots
Tinea and yeast	Variable patterns
Thallium toxicity (rat poison)	Variable white
Trauma	Repeated manicure: transverse striations
Zinc deficiency	Diffuse white

Table 25-4 Nail Changes Induced by Cancer Chemotherapeutic Drugs

Drug	Apparent change	Site of action/mechanism/comments
Adriamycin (doxorubicin)	Onycholysis; hyperpigmentation; transverse pigmented bands; longitudinal gray, brown, and black pigmented bands; bluish nails	Nail-bed and matrix toxicity
Bleomycin (patient also taking vinblastine)	Onycholysis; "dystrophy"; longitudinal pigmented bands; shedding; thickening of nail bed; darkening of nail cuticle	Nail-bed or matrix toxicity
Cancer chemotherapeutic drugs in general	Slow growth; sometimes Beau's lines	Matrix toxicity
	White transverse lines (Mee's lines)	Combination chemotherapy (doxorubicin, cyclophosphamide, vincristine)—nail plate
Cyclophosphamide (Cytoxan)	Hyperpigmentation; transverse pigmented bands; longitudinal pigmented band	Nail-bed and nail-plate color change matrix and bed toxicity
Dacarbazine (DTIC)	Hyperpigmentation	Matrix toxicity
Daunorubicin	Transverse brown-black bands	Probable matrix toxicity
5-fluorouracil (topical and systemic)	Diffuse blue superficial pigment; hyperpigmentation; onycholysis "Dystrophy"; paronychial inflammation; pain and thickening of nail bed; transverse striations, half and half–like nail changes	Superficial blue pigment may be scraped off
Genetic tendency for nail pigmentation postchemotherapy	Brownish	Probable matrix toxicity
Hydroxyurea	Atrophic, brittle nails	Nail-matrix toxicity
Melphalan (Alkeran)	Longitudinal pigmented bands	Nail bed—increase in melanin in basal melanocytes, matrix toxicity
Mercaptopurine	Nail shedding	Probable cytotoxic and photosensitivity effect on bed and matrix
Methotrexate	Hyperpigmentation, acute paronychia	Probable matrix toxicity
Nitrogen mustard	Hyperpigmentation	Probable matrix toxicity
Nitrosoureas	Hyperpigmentation	Probable matrix toxicity

From Daniell CR III, Scher RK: J Am Acad Dermatol 1984; 10:250.

Tumors

A limited number of tumors have been reported to occur about and under the nails (Table 25-5).

WARTS. The most common periungual growth is the periungual wart. It is discussed in Chapter 12. Warts are most common in children who bite their nails. Warts on the lateral nailfold and on the fingertip may extend deeply under the nail (Figure 25-49). A longitudinal nail groove may result from warts situated over the nail matrix. Warts are epidermal growths, but, if massive, they can erode the underlying bony matrix by displacement.

DIGITAL MUCOUS CYSTS. Digital mucous cysts (focal mucinosis) are not true cysts but rather a focal collection of mucin lacking a cystic lining. These soft, dome-shaped, translucent, pink-white structures occur on the dorsal surface of the distal phalanx of the middle-aged and the elderly (Figure 25-50). These structures contain a clear, viscous, jellylike substance that exudes if the cyst is incised. There are two types. The cysts on the proximal nailfold are not connected to the joint space or tendon sheath. They result from localized fibroblast proliferation. Compression of the nail-matrix cells induces a longitudinal nail groove. The cysts located on the dorsal-lateral finger at the distal interphalangeal (DIP) joint are probably caused by herniation of tendon sheaths or joint linings and are related to ganglion and synovial cysts.[71]

Simple surgical excision, intralesional steroid injections, and unroofing of the cyst followed by electrodesiccation and curettage have a high recurrence rate.[72]

Excision of the lesion with its pedicle and associated portions of the joint capsule affords a high cure rate but may result in subsequent partial loss of motion.[73]

Cryosurgery. Cryosurgery using either the open-spray or the cryoprobe technique yields a cure rate of up to 75%.[74] A local anesthetic is injected before treatment. The roof of the cyst is removed with scissors and the gelatinous material is expelled to facilitate freezing of the base of the lesion. Either a flat cryoprobe of approximately the same size as the cyst or a direct intermittent open spray to the center of the lesion is applied. The freeze time is 30 to 40 seconds when the

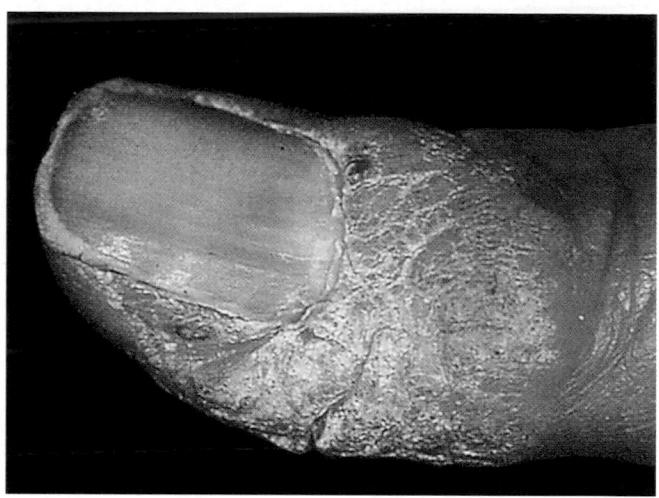

Figure 25-49 Periungual wart.

Table 25-5 Nail-Unit Tumors	
Diagnosis	**Clinical findings**
Malignant	
Squamous cell	Verrucous lesion, onycholysis, or subungual carcinoma growth; nail-plate destruction
Bowen's disease	Hyperkeratosis and onycholysis
Melanoma	Longitudinal brown subungual band; pigmented macule extending onto the periungual skin (Hutchinson's sign); mass below the nail, loss of nail plate, ulceration
Benign	
Myxoid cyst	Dome-shaped, translucent, proximal nailfold
Acquired digital fibrokeratoma	Looks like a garlic clove with the outer skin stripped off; usually projects from proximal nail groove
Glomas tumor	Red or blue suffusion beneath the nail plate; pressure blanches capillaries and causes pain
Giant cell tumor of tendon sheath	Arises from synovial lining cells associated with the distal interphalangeal joint synovia and tendons; firm and deeply fixed to the underlying fibrous tissue; does not arise on the nail unit
Exostosis	A painful, bony growth; x-ray film confirms diagnosis
Warts	May occur on any surface about the nail; spread by nail biting
Keratoacanthoma	Rapidly growing mass, central crust
Pyogenic granuloma	Red, vascular excrescence often devoid of an epithelial cover; profuse bleeding with slight trauma

cryoprobe technique is used and 20 to 30 seconds when the open-spray technique is used. The treated site becomes edematous and exudative, and a bulla develops in most cases. Healing is complete in 4 to 6 weeks. Lesions can be re-treated if necessary.

Multiple punctures. A high cure rate may be achieved with the simple technique of repeated punctures and expression of the cyst contents (Figure 25-50, B). Cysts that resisted multiple needlings are usually reduced to small, asymptomatic nodules. Without anesthesia, the cyst is punctured with a medium-sized hypodermic needle (26 gauge) to a depth of 3 to 5 mm. The clear contents, sometimes tinged with blood, are squeezed out by fingertip pressure. The patient is given a supply of needles to repeat the procedure at home if the cyst recurs. From 1 to 10 or more needlings result in a cure or in an asymptomatic lesion.

Carbon dioxide laser. Carbon dioxide laser vaporization performed under local anesthesia resulted in complete remission in four out of six patients. No side effects of therapy occurred.[75]

PYOGENIC GRANULOMA. Pyogenic granuloma occasionally occurs in the lateral nailfold. This benign mass of vascular tissue is removed with thorough desiccation and curettage (Figure 25-51). Recurrences are common if any residual tissue is left. Periungual malignant melanoma can mimic pyogenic granuloma.

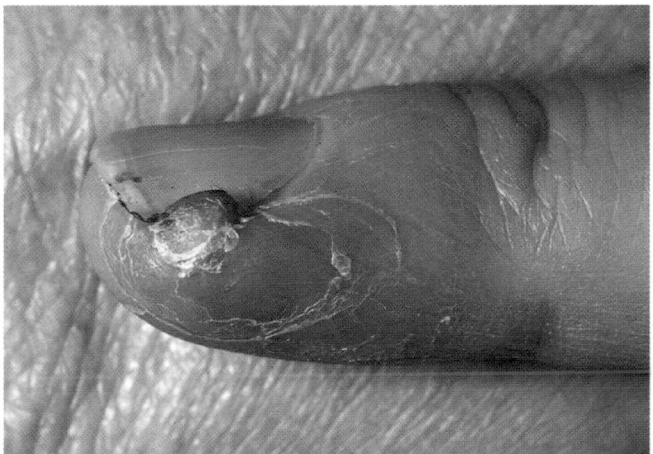

A, Lesions may form at the lateral nailfold and be caused by an ingrown nail.

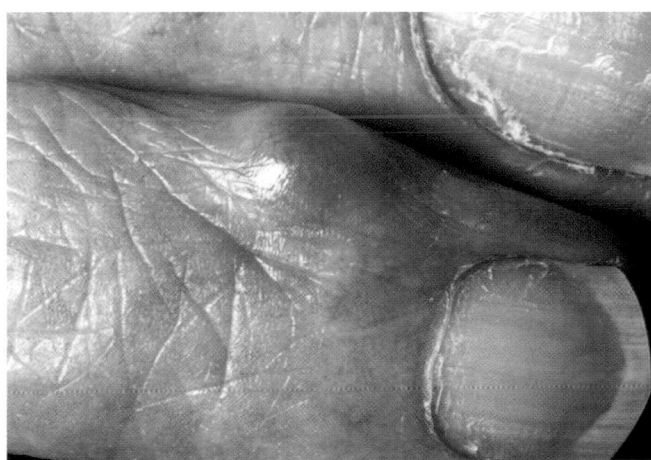

A, Digital mucous cyst. Intact cyst.

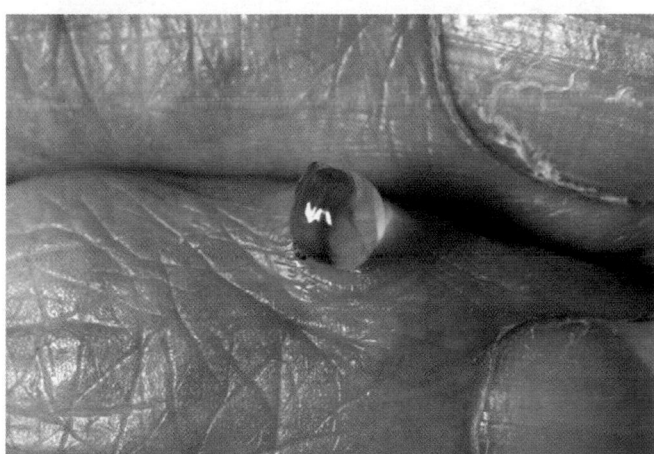

B, Incision with a #11 surgical blade. A clear, sometimes blood-tinged, viscous, jellylike substance exudes when the cyst is incised.

Figure 25-50

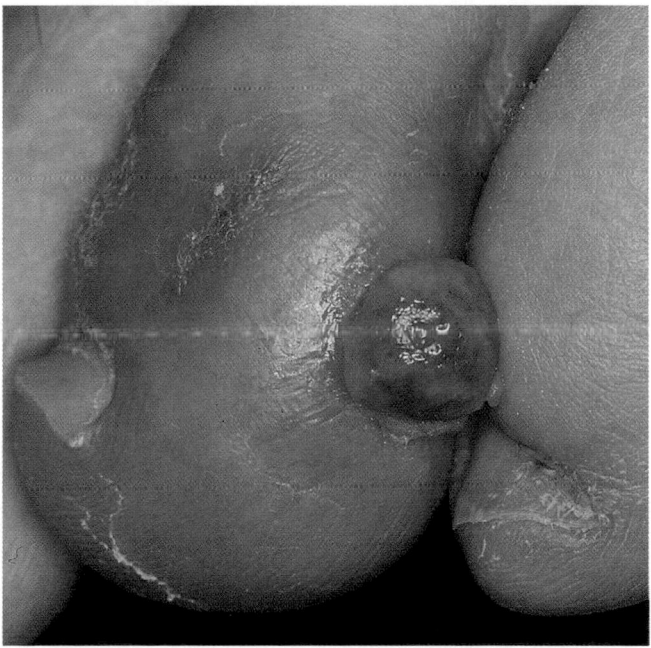

B, Pyogenic granuloma. A pedunculated nodule with a smooth, glistening surface. The surface frequently becomes crusted, eroded, or ulcerated. Minor trauma may produce considerable bleeding.

Figure 25-51 Pyogenic granuloma.

NEVI AND MELANOMA. Junctional nevi can appear in the nail matrix and produce a brown pigmented band. Brown longitudinal bands are common in blacks (see Figure 25-5) but rare in whites. Melanoma of the nail region, or melanotic whitlow, although rare, is a distinctive lesion (see Figure 22-52). Most are classified as acral lentiginous melanomas. The growth is usually painless and slow, and it can occur anywhere around or under the nail.[76] The lesion may present as a pigmented band that increases in width. There has not been enough experience to make specific recommendations concerning the management of pigmented bands in whites. The spontaneous appearance of such a band is noteworthy to most physicians, who promptly require a biopsy. Benign subungual nevi are rare in whites, so subungual nevoid lesions should be regarded as malignant until proved otherwise.[77]

Melanocytes in normal nail matrices are distributed in the basal layer and in the lower half of the epithelium. Therefore malignant melanoma of the nail matrix can arise from melanocytes situated in the squamous epithelium above the basal layer.

ABCDEF CRITERIA. The most salient features of subungual melanoma can be summarized according to the newly devised criteria that may be categorized under the first letters of the alphabet, namely ABCDEF of subungual melanoma. In this system A stands for age (peak incidence being in the 5th to 7th decades of life) and African Americans, Asians, and Native Americans in whom subungual melanoma accounts for up to one third of all melanoma cases. B stands for brown to black and with breadth of 3 mm or more and variegated borders. C stands for change in the nail band or lack of change in the nail morphology despite, presumably, adequate treatment. D stands for the digit most commonly involved, E stands for extension of the pigment onto the proximal and/or lateral nailfold (i.e., Hutchinson's sign), and F stands for family or personal history of dysplastic nevus or melanoma.[78]

Hutchinson's sign. Hutchinson's sign, periungual extension of brown-black pigmentation from longitudinal melanonychia onto the proximal and lateral nailfolds, is an important indicator of subungual melanoma. Periungual hyperpigmentation also occurs in Bowen's disease of the nail unit. Hyperpigmentation of the nail bed and matrix may reflect through the "transparent" nailfolds simulating Hutchinson's sign.[79]

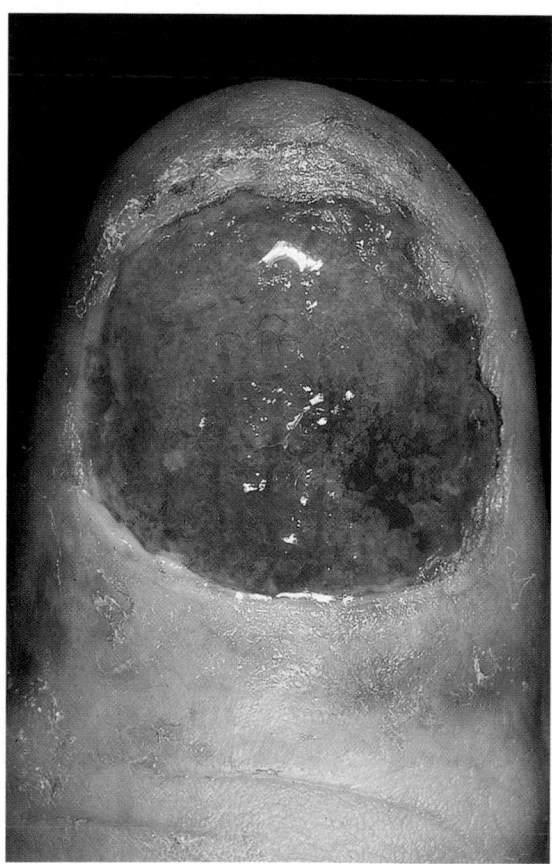

Figure 25-52 Melanoma involving the entire nail bed. This is a rare presentation.

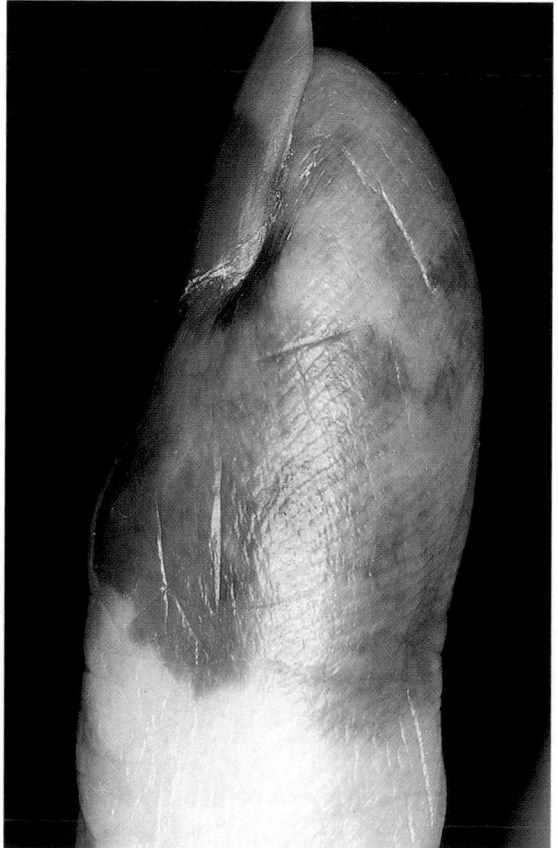

Figure 25-53 Hutchinson's sign. Extension of pigmentation onto the nail folds is a classic sign of subungual melanoma.

References

1. Johnson M, Comaish JS, Shuster S: Nail is produced by the normal nail bed: a controversy resolved, Br J Dermatol 1991; 125:27.

2. Daniel CR: Basic nail plate avulsion, J Dermatol Surg Oncol 1992; 18:685.

3. Fleegler EJ: A surgical approach to melanonychia striata, J Dermatol Surg Oncol 1992; 18:708.

4. Rich P: Nail biopsy. Indications and methods, J Dermatol Surg Oncol 1992; 18:673.

5. De BD: Management of nail psoriasis [In Process Citation], Clin Exp Dermatol 2000; 25(5):357.

6. Van LS, Scher R. Developments in the treatment of nail psoriasis, melanonychia striata, and onychomycosis. A review of the literature, Dermatol Clin 2000; 18(1):37.

7. de BD, Lawrence C: A simplified protocol of steroid injection for psoriatic nail dystrophy, Br J Dermatol 1998; 138(1):90.

8. Tosti A, et al: Calcipotriol ointment in nail psoriasis: a controlled double-blind comparison with betamethasone dipropionate and salicylic acid, Br J Dermatol 1998; 139(4):655.

9. Scher R, Stiller M, Zhu Y, Tazarotene 0.1% gel in the treatment of fingernail psoriasis: a double-blind, randomized, vehicle-controlled study, Cutis 2001; 68(5):355.

10. Yamamoto T, Katayama I, Nishioka K: Topical anthralin therapy for refractory nail psoriasis, J Dermatol 1998; 25(4):231.

11. Piraccini B, et al: Pustular psoriasis of the nails: treatment and long-term follow-up of 46 patients, Br J Dermatol 2001; 144(5):1000.

12. Tosti A, et al: Nail lichen planus: clinical and pathologic study of twenty-four patients, J Am Acad Dermatol 1993; 28:724.

13. Tosti A, et al: Topical steroids versus systemic antifungals in the treatment of chronic paronychia: an open, randomized double blind study and double dummy study, J Am Acad Dermatol 2002; 47:73.

14. Daniel CR, et al: Chronic paronychia and onycholysis: a thirteen-year experience, Cutis 1996; 58(6):397.

15. Alam M, Scher R: Indinavir-related recurrent paronychia and ingrown toenails, Cutis 1999; 64(4):277.

16. Tosti A, et al: Paronychia associated with antiretroviral therapy, Br J Dermatol 1999; 140(6):1165.

17. Bouscarat F, Bouchard C, Bouhour D: Paronychia and pyogenic granuloma of the great toes in patients treated with indinavir [letter], N Engl J Med 1998; 338(24):1776.

18. Robayna M, et al: Destructive herpetic whitlow in AIDS: report of three cases, Br J Dermatol 1997; 137(5):812.

19. Haneke E: Fungal infections of the nail, Semin Dermatol 1991; 10:41.

20. Machler B, Kirsner R, Elgart G: Routine histologic examination for the diagnosis of onychomycosis: an evaluation of sensitivity and specificity, Cutis 1998; 61(4):217.

21. Cooper A: The diagnosis of nail fungal infections, Arch Dermatol 1991; 127:1566.

22. Zaias N: Onychomycosis, Arch Dermatol 1972; 105:273.

23. Drake L, et al: The impact of onychomycosis on quality of life: development of an international onychomycosis-specific questionnaire to measure patient quality of life, J Am Acad Dermatol 1999; 41(2 Pt 1):189.

24. Crawford F, et al: Oral treatments for toenail onychomycosis, Arch Dermatol 2002; 138:811.

25. Evans E, Sigurgeirsson B: Double blind, randomised study of continuous terbinafine compared with intermittent itraconazole in treatment of toenail onychomycosis. The LION Study Group, BMJ 1999; 318(7190):1031.

26. De CC, Hindryckx P: Long-term outcomes in the treatment of toenail onychomycosis, Br J Dermatol 1999; 141(Suppl 56):15.

27. Havu V, et al: A double-blind, randomized study to compare the efficacy and safety of terbinafine (Lamisil) with fluconazole (Diflucan) in the treatment of onychomycosis, Br J Dermatol 2000; 142(1):97.

28. Zaias N, et al: Onychomycosis treated until the nail is replaced by normal growth or there is failure, Arch Dermatol 2000; 136(7):940.

29. Zaias N, Drachman D: A method for the determination of drug effectiveness in onychomycosis: trials with ketoconazole and griseofulvin ultramicrosize, J Am Acad Dermatol 1983; 9:912.

30. Ciclopirox (Penlac) nail lacquer for onychomycosis, Med Lett Drugs Ther 2000; 42(1080):51.

31. Hall M, et al: Safety of oral terbinafine: results of a postmarketing surveillance study in 25,884 patients, Arch Dermatol 1997; 133(10):1213.

32. Bohn M, Kraemer K: Dermatopharmacology of ciclopirox nail lacquer topical solution 8% in the treatment of onychomycosis [Record Supplied By Publisher], J Am Acad Dermatol 2000; 43 Pt 2(4):S57.

33. South DA, Farber EM: Urea ointment in the nonsurgical avulsion of nail dystrophies: a reappraisal, Cutis 1982; 25:609.

34. Averill RW, Scher RK: Simplified nail taping with urea ointment for nonsurgical nail avulsion, Cutis 1986; Oct:231.

35. Morgan JM, et al: Onycholysis in a case of atopic eczema treated with PUVA photochemotherapy, Clin Exp Dermatol 1992; 17:65.

36. Guin J, Baas K, Nelson-Adesokan P: Contact sensitization to cyanoacrylate adhesive as a cause of severe onychodystrophy, Int J Dermatol 1998; 37(1):31.

37. Nakatsui T, Lin A: Onycholysis and thyroid disease: report of three cases, J Cutan Med Surg 1998; 3(1):40.

38. Hussain S, et al: Onycholysis as a complication of systemic chemotherapy: report of five cases associated with prolonged weekly paclitaxel therapy and review of the literature, Cancer 2000; 88(10):2367.

39. Allen K: Chronic nailbiting: a controlled comparison of competing response and mild aversion treatments, Behav Res Ther 1996; 34(3):269.

40. Ilfeld FW: Ingrown toenail treated with cotton collodion insert, Foot Ankle 1991; 11:312.

41. Siegle RJ, Harkness J, Swanson NA: Phenol alcohol technique for permanent matricectomy, Arch Dermatol 1984; 120:348.

42. Siegle RJ, Stewart R: Recalcitrant ingrowing nails. Surgical approaches, J Dermatol Surg Oncol 1992; 18:744.

43. Ceilley RI, Collison DW: Matricectomy, J Dermatol Surg Oncol 1992; 18:728.

44. Felton P, Weaver T: Phenol and alcohol chemical matrixectomy in diabetic versus nondiabetic patients. A retrospective study, J Am Podiatr Med Assoc 1999; 89(8):410.

45. Reyzelman A, et al: Are antibiotics necessary in the treatment of locally infected ingrown toenails? [In Process Citation], Arch Fam Med 2000; 9(9):930.

46. Helms A, Brodell R: Surgical pearl: prompt treatment of subungual hematoma by decompression, J Am Acad Dermatol 2000; 42(3):508.

47. Gavin L, et al: Chronic subungual hematomas: a presumed immunologic puzzle resolved with a diagnosis of child abuse, Arch Pediatr Adolesc Med 1997; 151(1):103.

48. Zaun H. Leukonychias, Semin Dermatol 1991; 10:17.

49. Lubach D, et al: Incidence of brittle nails, Dermatologica 1986; 172:144.

50. Lubach D, Beckers P: Wet working conditions increase brittleness of nails, but do not cause it, Dermatology 1992; 185:120.

51. Cohen PR, Scher RK: Geriatric nail disorders: diagnosis and treatment, J Am Acad Dermatol 1992; 26:521.

52. Hochman LG, et al: Brittle nails: response to daily biotin supplementation, Cutis 1993; 51:303.

53. Colombo VE, et al: Treatment of brittle fingernails and onychoschizia with biotin: scanning electron microscopy, J Am Acad Dermatol 1990; 23:1127.

54. Vittorio C, Phillips K: Treatment of habit-tic deformity with fluoxetine, Arch Dermatol 1997; 133(10):1203.

55. Clementz G, Mancini A: Nail matrix arrest following hand-foot-mouth disease: a report of five children, Pediatr Dermatol 2000; 17(1):7.

56. Sweren RJ, Burnett JW: Multiple Beau's lines, Cutis 1982; 29:41.

57. Ben-Dayan D, et al: Transverse nail ridgings (Beau's lines) induced by chemotherapy [see comments], Acta Haematol 1994; 91(2):89.

58. Moffitt D, de BD: Yellow nail syndrome: the nail that grows half as fast grows twice as thick, Clin Exp Dermatol 2000; 25(1):21.

59. Varney V, et al: Rhinitis, sinusitis and the yellow nail syndrome: a review of symptoms and response to treatment in 17 patients, Clin Otolaryngol 1994; 19(3):237.

60. Venincie PY, Dicken CH: Yellow nail syndrome: report of five cases, J Am Acad Dermatol 1984; 10:187.

61. Bull R, Fenton D, Mortimer P: Lymphatic function in the yellow nail syndrome, Br J Dermatol 1996; 134(2):307.

62. De CSD, et al: Yellow nail syndrome, J Am Acad Dermatol 1990; 22:608.

63. Pavlidakey GP, Hashimoto K, Blum D: Yellow nail syndrome, J Am Acad Dermatol 1984; 11:509.

64. Williams HC, et al: Successful use of topical vitamin E solution in the treatment of nail changes in yellow nail syndrome, Arch Dermatol 1991; 127:1023.

65. Chevrant-Breton J, et al: Cutaneous manifestations of idiopathic hemochromatosis, Arch Dermatol 1977; 113:161.

66. Baughman R, et al: Prevalence of digital clubbing in bronchogenic carcinoma by a new digital index, Clin Exp Rheumatol 1998; 16(1):21.

67. Holzberg M, Walker HK: Terry's nails: revised definition and new correlations, Lancet 1984, April.896.

68. Daniel CR III, Scher RK: Nail changes secondary to systemic drugs or ingestants, J Am Acad Dermatol 1984; 10:250.

69. Daniel CR III, Osment LS: Nail pigmentation abnormalities: their importance and proper examination, Cutis 1982; 30:348.

70. Unamuno P, et al: Leukonychia due to cytostatic agents, Clin Exp Dermatol 1992; 17:273.

71. Newmeyer et al: Mucous cysts: the dorsal digital interphalangeal joint ganglion, Plast Reconstr Surg 1974; 53:313.

72. Sonnex TS: Digital myxoid cysts: a review, Cutis 1986; Feb:89.

73. Miller PK, et al: Focal mucinosis (myxoid cyst). Surgical therapy, J Dermatol Surg Oncol 1992; 18:716.

74. Kuflik EG: Specific indications for cryosurgery of the nail unit. Myxoid cysts and periungual verrucae, J Dermatol Surg Oncol 1992; 18:702.

75. Karrer S, et al: Treatment of digital mucous cysts with a carbon dioxide laser, Acta Dermatol Venereol 1999; 79(3):224.

76. Mikhail GR: Subungual epidermoid carcinoma, J Am Acad Dermatol 1984; 11:291.

77. Shukla VK, Hughes LE: How common are benign subungual naevi? Eur J Surg Oncol 1992; 18:249.

78. Levit E, et al: The ABC rule for clinical detection of subungual melanoma, J Am Acad Dermatol 2000; 42(2 Pt 1):269.

79. Baran R, Kechijian P: Hutchinson's sign: a reappraisal, J Am Acad Dermatol 1996; 34(1):87.

❑ **Internal cancer and skin disease**
  Cutaneous paraneoplastic syndromes

❑ **Cutaneous manifestations of diabetes mellitus**
  Necrobiosis lipoidica
  Granuloma annulare

❑ **Acanthosis nigricans**

❑ **Xanthomas and dyslipoproteinemia**

❑ **Neurofibromatosis**

❑ **Tuberous sclerosis**

❑ **Cancer-associated genodermatoses**
  Cowden's disease (multiple hamartoma
    syndrome)
  Muir-Torre syndrome
  Gardner's syndrome

❑ **Pseudoxanthoma elasticum**

❑ **Guide to information for families with
  inherited skin disorders**

Certain cutaneous diseases are frequently associated with internal disease. The skin disease itself may be inconsequential, but its presence should prompt investigation of possible related internal disorders. A selected group of such diseases is discussed in this chapter. Pigmentary skin changes associated with internal diseases are also discussed in Chapter 19.

Internal Cancer and Skin Disease

The skin can be associated with internal malignancy in a variety of ways. The skin lesions may be a marker for an inherited syndrome (i.e., the genodermatoses), may represent a reaction to the tumor (the paraneoplastic syndromes) (Figure 26-1), may be caused by a carcinogen, may occur as a result of treatment, or may represent direct tumor extension or metastasis to the skin.[1-4] These disease associations are listed in Table 26-1 and in Boxes 26-1 and 26-2. Syndromes in which genodermatosis is associated with cancer are discussed later in this chapter.

Cutaneous paraneoplastic syndromes

Paraneoplastic syndromes (PNSs) are diseases that appear before or concurrently with an internal malignancy. They represent a remote or systemic effect of a neoplasm (see Box 26-1). There is a wide range of categories of PNSs, including endocrine, neurologic, hematologic, rheumatic, renal, and cutaneous.[5] They may be the initial clue to the presence of an underlying neoplasm.[5] The activity of a PNS can parallel the

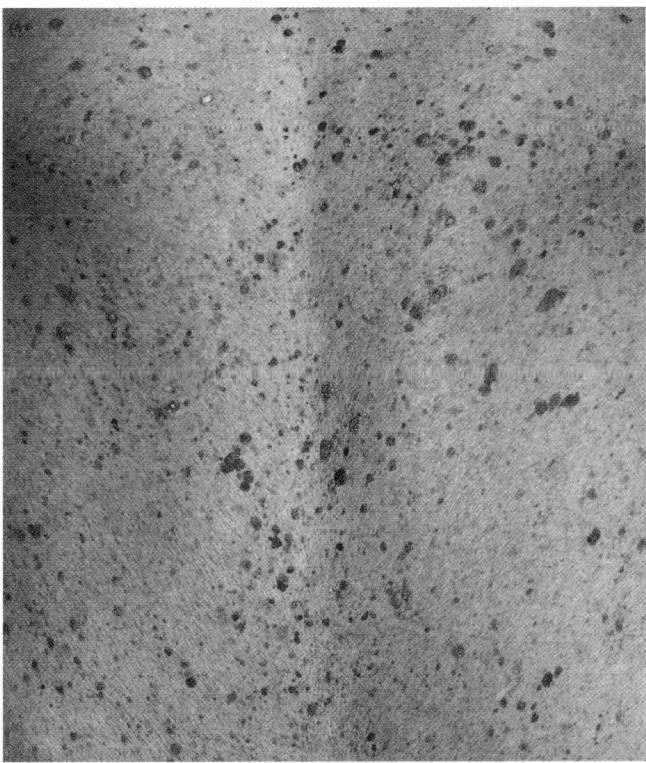

Figure 26-1 A paraneoplastic syndrome; the Leser-Trélat sign. The rapid onset of numerous seborrheic keratoses can be associated with an internal malignancy.

Table 26-1 Cutaneous Lesions and Internal Malignancy

Syndrome	Clinical presentation	Malignancy
Ataxia telangiectasia	Cerebellar ataxia, telangiectasia (e.g., pinna, bulbar conjunctiva)	Reticulum cell sarcoma, Hodgkin's, gastric
Alopecia mucinosa	Patch of follicular papules and boggy infiltrate, face, trunk, scalp	Mycosis fungoides
Amyloidosis	Macroglossia; smooth tongue; shiny, translucent, waxy papules on eyelids, nasolabial folds, lips, and intertriginous areas; "pinch purpura"—skin bleeds with trauma	Multiple myeloma
Acanthosis nigricans	Adult onset in absence of obesity, endocrinopathy, and family history; hyperkeratotic, hyperpigmented skin folds in flexural areas (neck, axillae, antecubital fossa, breast, groin)	Abdominal cancer, other adenocarcinomas
Bazex's syndrome (acrokeratosis paraneoplastica)	Three stages: (1) psoriasiform lesions, tips of fingers and toes; (2) keratoderma, hands and feet; (3) lesions extend locally and new lesions appear on knees, legs, thighs, arms	Carcinoma of esophagus, tongue, lower lip, upper lobes of the lungs
Bloom's syndrome	Erythema face ("butterfly area"), stunted growth	Acute leukemia
Carcinoid syndrome	Episodes of flushing (face, neck, chest), dyspnea, asthma, diarrhea, murmur of pulmonary stenosis and insufficiency	Serotonin-containing tumor of body parts such as appendix, small intestine, bronchus
Cowden's syndrome (multiple hamartoma syndrome)	Warty papules on face, hands, mouth	Breast, thyroid
Dermatomyositis (adult)	Heliotrope erythema eyelids, bluish-red plaques on knuckles	Breast, gastrointestinal, genitourinary, lung, ovary
Erythema gyratum repens	Rapidly moving waxy bands of erythema with serpiginous outline and "wood grain" pattern	Breast, lung, stomach, bladder, prostate
Gardner's syndrome	Epidermal cysts, cutaneous osteomas and fibromas, polyps in small and large intestine	Adenocarcinoma of colon
Glucagonoma syndrome	Migratory necrolytic erythema in intertriginous and dependent areas, elevated serum glucagon levels	Glucagon-secreting alpha cell tumor of the pancreas
Hypertrichosis lanuginosa (acquired)	Long hair on face and trunk	Bronchus, gallbladder, rectum
Ichthyosis (acquired)	Generalized scaling, prominent on extremities, spares the flexural area	Hodgkin's disease; other lymphoproliferative malignancies; cancer of lung, breast, cervix
Kaposi's sarcoma	Red papular and nodular neoplasms most common on lower legs	Internal organ Kaposi's sarcoma, high incidence of other cancers
Leser-Trélat sign	Sudden appearance (3–6 months) and rapid increase in size and number of seborrheic keratoses	Colon, breast
Melanosis (generalized)	Generalized cutaneous melanosis	Metastatic melanoma
Metastases to the skin	Metastasis to any cutaneous site	Variety of tumors
Muir-Torre syndrome	Multiple sebaceous adenomas	Visceral carcinomas
Paget's disease (breast)	Eczematous crusted lesion of nipple, areola	Breast
Paget's disease (extramammary)	Eroded scaling plaques of vulva, scrotum, axilla, perianal, groin	Cervical cancer and adenocarcinoma of anus and rectum
Palmoplantar keratoderma (tylosis)	Skin thickening of palms and soles	Gastrointestinal carcinomas
Paraneoplastic pemphigus	Blisters, erosive stomatitis	Lymphoid malignancies, thymomas, sarcomas

Table 26-1 Cutaneous Lesions and Internal Malignancy—cont'd

Syndrome	Clinical presentation	Malignancy
Peutz-Jeghers syndrome	Pigmented macules on lips and oral mucosa, polyposis of small intestine	Adenocarcinoma of stomach, duodenum, colon
Sipple's syndrome	Multiple mucosal neuromas	Medullary carcinoma of thyroid, C cell neoplasia, pheochromocytoma
Sweet's syndrome	Fever, painful cutaneous plaques	Hematologic malignancies
Urticaria pigmentosa (disseminated maculopapular form)	Brown-red macules and papules that contain mast cells and urticate when traumatized	Hematologic malignancies
von Hippel-Lindau disease	Angiomas of skin, angiomatosis of cerebellum or medulla	Hypernephroma, pheochromocytoma
Von Recklinghausen's neurofibromatosis	Café-au-lait spots, white macules, multiple cutaneous neuromas, internal neuromas	Malignant neurilemoma, astrocytoma, pheochromocytoma
Wiskott-Aldrich syndrome	Eczematous lesions in atopic dermatitis distribution	Reticuloendothelial malignancy

Box 26-1 Cancer Syndromes Associated with Cutaneous Disease

Inherited syndromes with cutaneous signs—the genodermatoses (those associated with internal malignancies)

Howel-Evans syndrome (palmo-plantar keratoderma) (Dermatosis associated with, but not caused by, the tumor)
Ataxia telangiectasia
Basal cell nevus syndrome (Gorlin's syndrome)
Cowden's disease (multiple hamartoma syndrome)
Cronkhite-Canada syndrome
Gardner's syndrome
Immunodeficiency syndromes
Multiple mucosal neuroma syndrome
Peutz-Jeghers syndrome
Torre-Muir syndrome
von Hippel-Lindau syndrome
von Recklinghausen's syndrome
Werner's syndrome
Wiskott-Aldrich syndrome

Paraneoplastic syndromes (cutaneous reactions to internal malignancies)

Acanthosis nigricans
Acquired hypertrichosis lanuginosa
Acquired ichthyosis
Bazek's syndrome
Carcinoid-flushing
Dermatomyositis
Erythema gyratum repens
Erythroderma
Glucagonoma syndrome
Herpes zoster
Keratoacanthomas
Leser-Trélat sign
Migratory thrombophlebitis
Multiple eruptive angiomas
Pruritus
Pyoderma gangrenosum
Raynaud's syndrome—atypical
Urticaria

Hormone-secreting tumors

APUDoma
Ectopic ACTH syndrome
Carcinoid syndrome
Glucagonoma syndrome

Carcinogen-induced skin cancers

Arsenical keratosis
Bowen's disease of covered skin

Diseases with rapid onset of cutaneous disease

Acanthosis nigricans
Acquired ichthyosis
Eczematous reactions
Eruptive seborrheic keratosis—Leser-Trélat sign
Eruptive lanugo hair—hypertrichosis lanuginose (acquisita)
Erythema gyratum repens
Figurate erythemas
Multiple eruptive angiomata

course of the tumor and thus be used as a marker of remission or recurrence. PNSs are estimated to occur in 7% to 15% of patients with cancer.

The cutaneous changes are thought to result from the production of biologically active hormones, growth factors, or antigen-antibody interactions induced by or produced by the tumor.[6,7] Many of these syndromes, such as acanthosis nigricans, are proliferative skin disorders. Products secreted by the tumor, such as transforming growth factor alpha, may stimulate keratinocytes to proliferate.[8]

Cutaneous Manifestations of Diabetes Mellitus

Approximately 30% of patients with diabetes mellitus develop a skin disorder sometime during the course of disease.[9] A list of these disorders follows:[10]

Candida infections (mouth, genital)
Carotenodermia (yellow skin)
Diabetic bullae
Diabetic dermopathy (shin spots)
Diabetic thick skin
Erythema (face, lower legs, feet)
External otitis
Finger pebbles
Foot ulcers
Acanthosis nigricans (insulin resistance syndromes)
Gas gangrene (nonclostridial)
Granuloma annulare (localized or generalized)
Insulin lipodystrophy
Necrobiosis lipoidica
Yellow nails
Perforating disorders
Eruptive xanthomas

Necrobiosis lipoidica

Necrobiosis lipoidica (NL) is a disease of unknown origin, but more than 50% of the patients with NL are generally insulin dependent. The previous term *necrobiosis lipoidica diabeticorum* was changed because a significant minority of patients do not have diabetes. The skin lesions may appear years before the onset of diabetes, and most patients with diabetes do not develop NL. The disease may occur at any age, but it most commonly appears in the third and fourth decades. Most of the patients are females, and in most cases the lesions are confined to the anterior surfaces of the lower legs[11] (Figure 26-2).

The eruption begins as an oval, violaceous patch and expands slowly. The advancing border is red, and the central area turns yellow-brown. The central area atrophies and has a waxy surface; telangiectasias become prominent (Figure 26-2, B and C). Ulceration occurs, particularly following trauma, in 13% of cases (Figure 26-2, D).[12] In many instances the clinical presentation is so characteristic that biopsy is not required.[13]

TREATMENT

Topical and intralesional steroids. Topical and intralesional steroids arrest inflammation but promote further atrophy. One large plaque completely involuted after 6 weeks of clobetasol propionate under occlusion.[14] Intralesional injections effectively control small areas of NL, but the concentration of triamcinolone acetonide (10 mg/ml) should be diluted with saline or Xylocaine to 2.5 mg/ml to avoid atrophy.

Systemic corticosteroids. A 5-week course of systemic corticosteroids resulted in complete cessation of disease activity and no recurrence in a mean follow-up period of 7 months in 6 patients; however, restitution of atrophic skin lesions was not achieved.[15] Ulceration of NL was successfully treated with oral prednisolone.[12]

Pentoxifylline. Pentoxifylline (Trental) 400 mg three times a day resulted in significant improvement after 1 month of treatment in one patient. Ulcerating NL, resistant to acetylsalicylic acid, healed completely within 8 weeks of administration of 400 mg pentoxifylline twice a day.[16] Pentoxifylline is thought to decrease blood viscosity by increasing fibrinolysis and red blood cell deformability and also to inhibit platelet aggregation.

Aspirin and dipyridamole. A number of changes in the microvasculature occur in the dermis of plaques of NL. The proposed cause is either an immune complex–mediated vasculitis with vascular occlusion in the small vessels or a delayed hypersensitivity reaction. The increased tendency to show spontaneous platelet aggregation may also play a role in vascular occlusion. Treatment has been used to inhibit these changes. Low-dose aspirin and dipyridamole are thought to inhibit platelet aggregation, but reports concerning their efficacy in healing ulcers in plaques of NL are conflicting.[17-19] The recommended treatment is aspirin (3.5 mg/kg every 48 hours),[20] which for the average patient is 325 gm (one tablet), or dipyridamole (Persantine) (25-, 50-, or 75-mg tablets) (2 to 3 mg/kg/day), which for the average patient is 150 to 200 mg daily in divided doses.[21] For effective control of ulceration, platelet-inhibition therapy must be used for a minimum of 3 to 7 months. Recommended treatment schedules should be followed because there is evidence that higher dosages can decrease treatment effectiveness.

Other treatments. Cyclosporine, mycophenolate mofetil, photochemotherapy with topical PUVA, and chloroquine[22] are reported to be effective.[23]

Skin grafting. Skin grafting is effective for extensive disease.[24]

NECROBIOSIS LIPOIDICA

A, Erythematous violaceous plaques on the anterior surfaces of the lower legs.

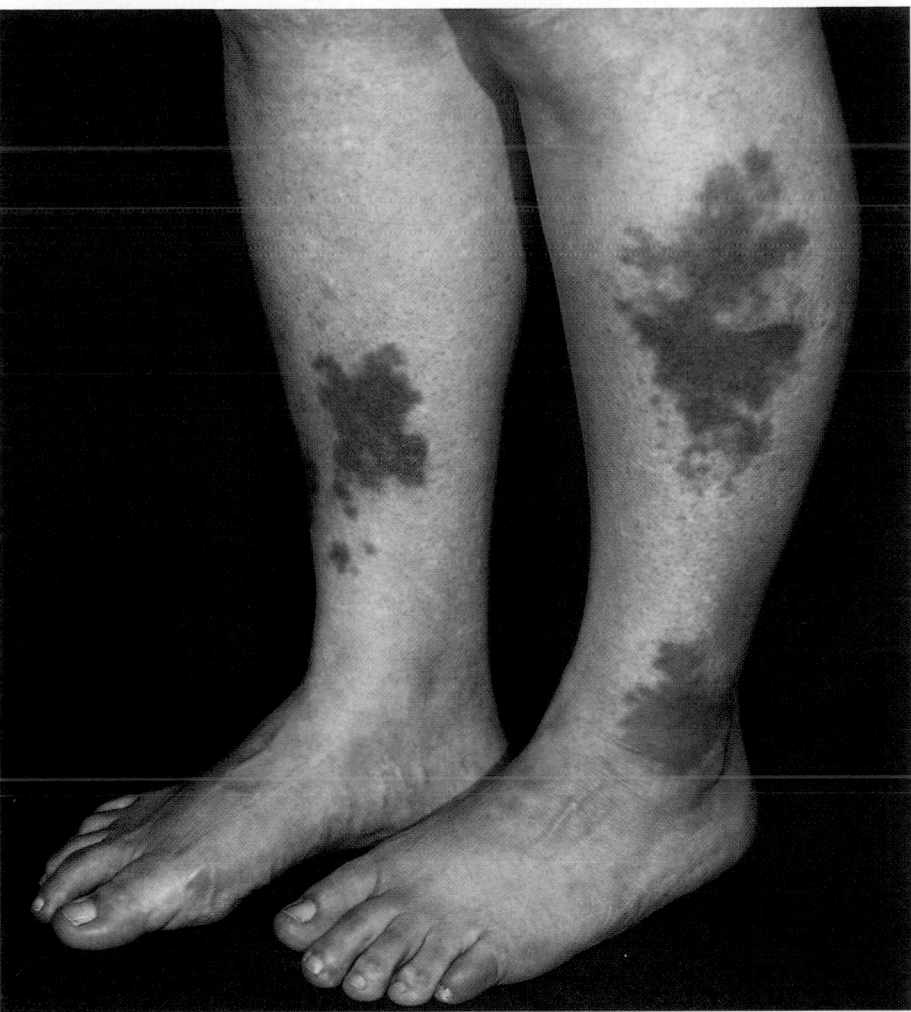

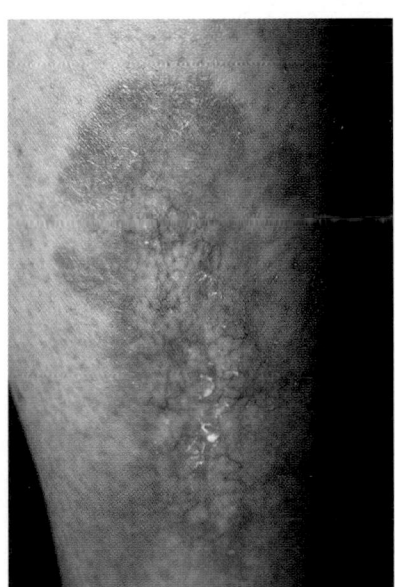

B, The central area is waxy yellow with prominent telangiectasia.

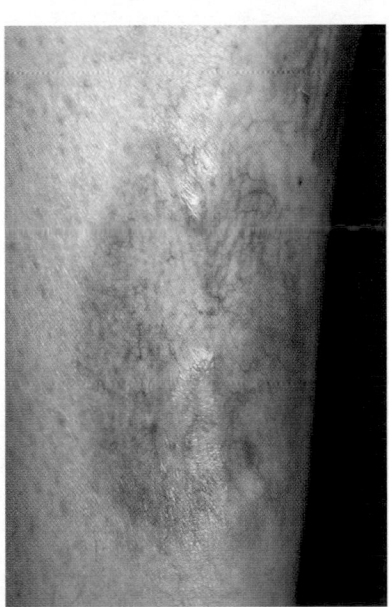

C, End-stage disease with atrophy and telangiectasia.

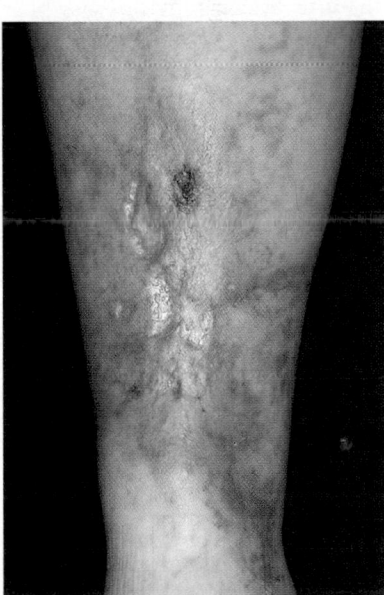

D, Severe disease with dense fibrosis and ulceration.

Figure 26-2

Granuloma annulare

There are conflicting reports about the association of granuloma annulare (GA) with diabetes mellitus. A case-control study failed to reveal any statistically significant correlation between GA and type 2 diabetes mellitus.[25] Most patients with the localized form of granuloma annulare do not have clinical or laboratory evidence of diabetes. The association between disseminated granuloma annulare and diabetes has been established, but the frequency is unknown.[26] In a retrospective study 12% of patients with GA had diabetes mellitus. Those patients suffered significantly more often from chronic relapsing GA than nondiabetic patients.[27] Granuloma annulare can be associated with HIV and can present at all stages of HIV infection. Generalized GA is the most common clinical pattern in HIV infection.[28]

CLINICAL PRESENTATION. Granuloma annulare is characterized by a ring of small, firm, flesh-colored or red papules. The localized form, most common in young adult females, is most frequently found on the lateral or dorsal surfaces of the hands and feet (Figure 26-3). The disease begins with an asymptomatic, flesh-colored papule that undergoes central involution. Over months, a ring of papules slowly increases in diameter to 0.5 to 5 cm (Figure 26-4). The duration of the disease is highly variable. Many lesions undergo spontaneous involution without scarring, whereas others last for years. The familial occurrence of granuloma annulare is uncommon but has been noted in siblings, twins, and successive generations.[29]

Disseminated granuloma annulare occurs in adults and appears with numerous flesh-colored or erythematous papules, some of which form annular rings. The papules may be accentuated in sun-exposed areas. The course is variable; many lesions persist for years.

Figure 26-3 Granuloma annulare. The dorsal surfaces of the hands and feet and the extensor aspects of the arms and legs are the most common sites. Lesions are either papular or broad superficial plaques.

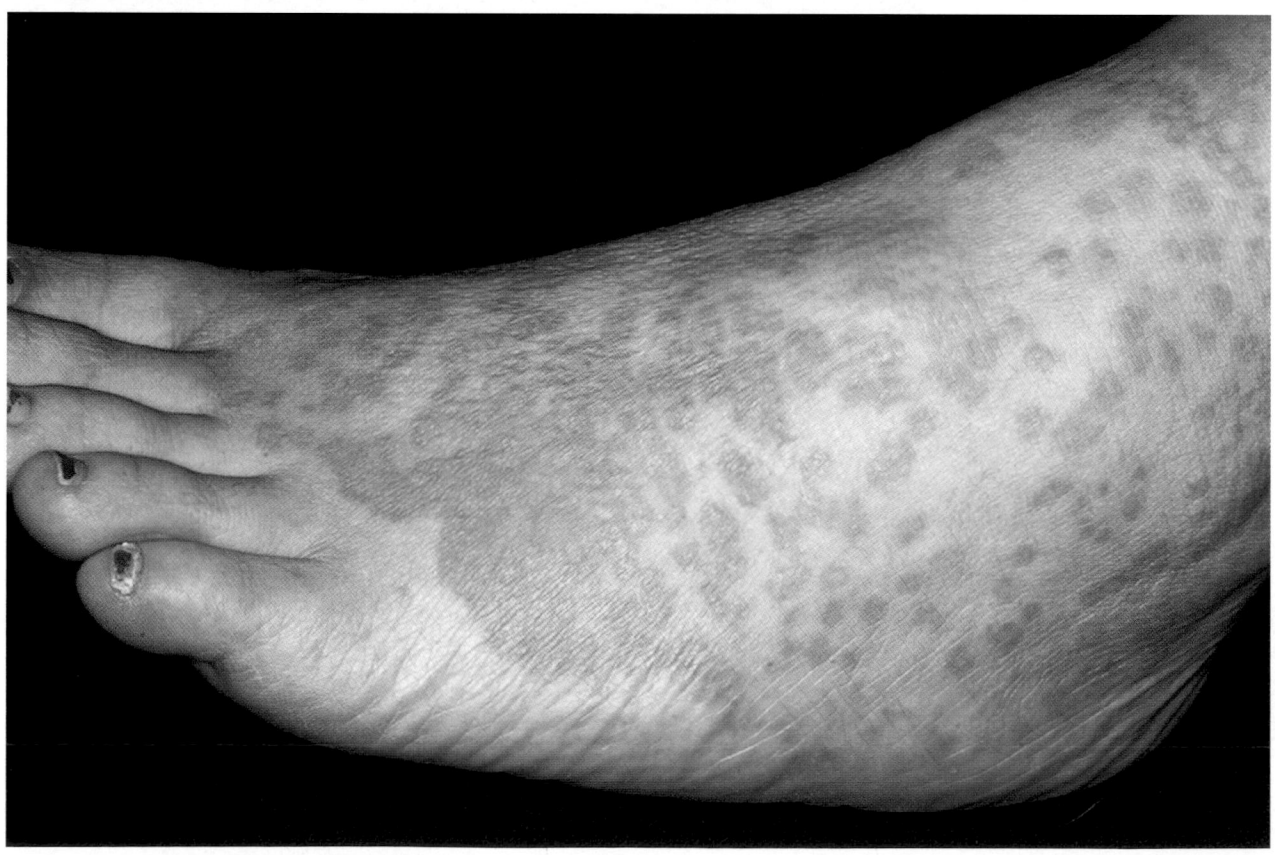

Generalized perforating granuloma annulare is characterized by 1- to 4-mm umbilicated papules on the extremities and is most commonly seen in children and young adults. Biopsy shows transepithelial elimination of degenerating collagen fibers. A high incidence of perforating granuloma annulare has been reported in the Hawaiian Islands.[30]

Subcutaneous granuloma annulare occurs in children. A painless subcutaneous nodule(s) in the lower anterior tibial region or foot and the scalp, typically in the occiput, are the most common presenting features.[31] The mean age at presentation is 3.9 years. Diagnosis requires an excisional biopsy. Lesions may recur after excision. Lesions may resolve spontaneously and recur after excision. No record of progression to systemic illness is reported.[32,33]

DIAGNOSIS. The clinical presentation is characteristic, and biopsy may not be required. The histology shows collagen degeneration, a feature similar to that seen in necrobiosis lipoidica.

TREATMENT. Localized lesions are asymptomatic and are best left untreated. Those patients troubled by appearance may be treated with intralesional injections of triamcinolone acetonide (2.5 to 5 mg/ml). The solution should be injected only into the elevated border. Topical steroids have little effect. Clobetasol propionate lotion left under the completely occlusive patch DuoDerm was effective after 4 weeks. Occlusion may be used for 8 to 12 hours each day. Atrophy is a possible side effect.[34] A single 10 to 60 second freeze-thaw cycle using nitrous oxide or liquid nitrogen applied with closed probes produced resolution in 80.6% of patients.[35] Disseminated granuloma annulare has been reported to respond to dapsone,[36,37] isotretinoin,[38,39] etretinate,[40] hydroxychloroquine,[41,42] cyclosporine (3 mg/kg),[43] niacinamide (1.5 gm/day), and PUVA.[44]

Three women who had had disseminated GA for more than 1 year were treated with vitamin E 400 IU daily and Zileuton 2400 mg daily. All responded within 3 months with complete clinical clearing.[45]

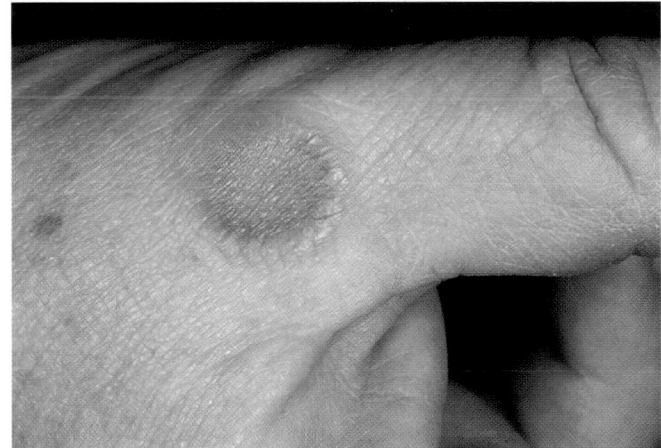

A

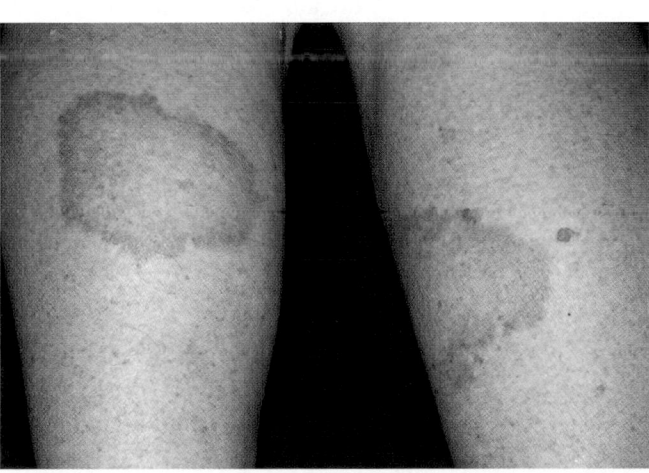

C

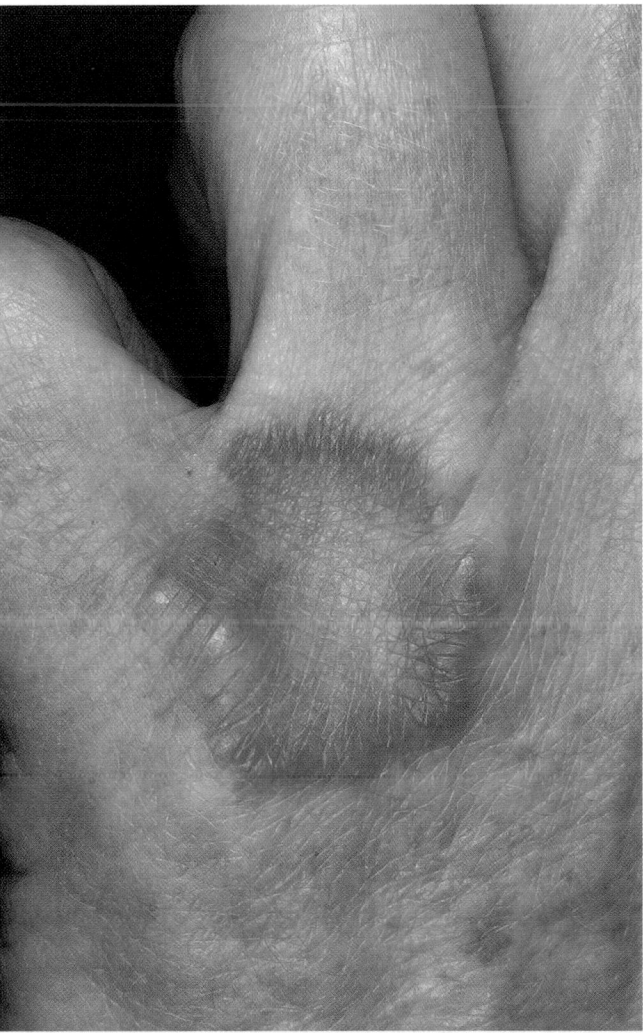

B

Figure 26-4 Granuloma annulare. **A,** A ring of flesh-colored to red papules slowly expands. **B,** The border is either papular or smooth, and the center is depressed. **C,** Round and annular lesion can extend over wide areas.

Acanthosis Nigricans

Acanthosis nigricans (AN) is a nonspecific reaction pattern that may accompany obesity; diabetes; excess corticosteroids; pineal tumors; other endocrine disorders (Box 26-2); multiple genetic variants; drugs such as nicotinic acid, estrogens, and corticosteroids; and adenocarcinoma. AN is classified into malignant and benign forms (Box 26-3).

CLINICAL CHARACTERISTICS. In all cases the disease presents with symmetric, brown thickening of the skin. In time the skin may become quite thickened as the lesion develops a leathery, warty, or papillomatous surface (Figure 26-5). The lesions range in severity from slight discoloration of a small area to extensive involvement of wide areas. The most common site of involvement is the axillae, but the changes may be observed in the flexural areas of the posterior neck (Figure 26-6) and groin, the belt line, over the dorsal surfaces of the fingers, in the mouth, and around the areolae of the breasts and umbilicus. During the process there is papillary hypertrophy, hyperkeratosis, and an increased number of melanocytes in the epidermis.

BENIGN ACANTHOSIS NIGRICANS. The majority of cases are idiopathic and are associated with obesity; this process is referred to as pseudoacanthosis nigricans. There is a high prevalence of AN in obese adults. There is a positive correlation between the development of AN and the severity of the obesity. It is postulated that heat, friction, and maceration in the flexural folds are the cause, but in one study of obese patients, those with acanthosis nigricans had fasting plasma insulin levels that were markedly higher than those without acanthosis nigricans. Therefore acanthosis nigricans may be a cutaneous marker of hyperinsulinemia in obese individuals.[46,47] Young children have low prevalences of obesity and acanthosis nigricans, but the prevalences of both increases with increasing age. Nearly 40% of Native American teenagers, 13% of African American, 6% of Hispanic, and less than 1% of white, non-Hispanic children between the ages of 10 and 19 have AN. AN identifies a subgroup within an ethnic group that has the highest insulin concentration, the most severe insulin resistance, and the highest risk for the development of type 2 diabetes.[48]

The interaction between excessive amounts of circulating insulin with insulin-like growth factor receptors on keratinocytes may lead to the development of acanthosis nigricans.[49]

In rare instances acanthosis nigricans may occur as an autosomal dominant trait with no obesity, associated endocrinopathies, or congenital abnormalities; it may appear at birth or during childhood and is accentuated at puberty.[50]

DRUG-INDUCED AN. Drug-induced acanthosis nigricans has occurred with the use of nicotinic acid[51] and, rarely, with other agents.[52]

ENDOCRINE SYNDROMES WITH AN. In a large and heterogeneous group of conditions, insulin action at the cellular level is markedly reduced[53] (see Box 26-2). Acanthosis nigricans appears to represent a cutaneous marker of tissue insulin resistance, irrespective of its cause (antibodies to the insulin receptor or congenital or acquired defects of receptor or postreceptor function).[54-58] These patients may not require insulin therapy, and many do not have diabetes. For patients without diabetes, insulin resistance is established by the documentation of high levels of circulating insulin or by the observation of an impaired response to exogenous insulin. Prolonged hypersecretion of insulin may lead to pancreatic exhaustion, glucose intolerance, and type II diabetes.

Box 26-2 Endocrine Syndromes with Acanthosis Nigricans (Most Have Insulin Resistance + Hyperinsulinemia + AN)

Insulin-resistant states
    Type A syndrome
    Type B syndrome
    Lipoatrophic diabetes
    Leprechaunism
    Acral hypertrophy syndrome
    Pinealoma
    Pineal hyperplasia syndrome
Hyperandrogenic states
    Type A and B syndromes
    Polycystic ovary disease
    Ovarian hyperthecosis
    Stromal luteoma
    Ovarian dermoid cysts
Acromegaly
Cushing's disease
Pituitary basophilism
Obesity
Hypothyroidism
Addison's disease
Hypogonadal syndrome with insulin resistance
Prader-Willi syndrome
Alstrom syndrome

Adapted from: Lowella EE, Fenske NA: JAAD 1996; 34:892.

Box 26-3 Classification of Acanthosis Nigricans

Benign
    Obesity related
    Hereditary (many syndromes)
    Endocrine syndromes
Malignant

Two syndromes of insulin resistance and acanthosis nigricans are of special interest and discussed in the following.

Type A syndrome. Type A syndrome is also called the HAIR-AN syndrome, is characterized by hyperandrogenemia (HA), extreme insulin resistance (IR), and acanthosis nigricans occurring in the absence of obesity or lipoatrophy. It is distinguished from type B insulin resistance by a lack of antibodies to the insulin receptor or other evidence of autoimmune disease. It is familial and affects mainly black women who have the onset of acanthosis nigricans in infancy or childhood. There are signs of virilization or accelerated growth. These include acne, hirsutism, androgenetic alopecia, amenorrhea, increased libido, increased muscle mass, loss of breast tissue, clitoromegaly, and infertility. The causes include ovarian or adrenal gland tumors, polycystic ovaries, congenital or acquired adrenal hyperplasia, Cushing's disease, drugs, and gonadal dysgenesis. The AN is usually generalized, with rapid progression during the prepubertal period and early reproductive years. The cause of HA is thought to be related to extreme insulinemia. Patients have high plasma levels of testosterone, normal DHEA-S, 24-hour urinary 17-ketosteroids and 17-hydroxyprogesterone, and normal basal gonadotropins (LH, FSH).

Type B syndrome. Type B syndrome occurs in older women with signs of autoimmune disease, including circulating antibodies to the insulin receptor. The average age at onset is 39 years. These patients have AN of varying severity and most have only laboratory evidence of autoimmunity such as leukopenia and high titers of anti-DNA antibodies. Patients have uncontrolled diabetes mellitus, acanthosis nigricans, and, in premenopausal women, ovarian hyperandrogenism.

The vulva is a common place to find acanthosis nigricans in obese, hirsute, hyperandrogenic, insulin-resistant women.[59]

TREATMENT. Lesions are usually asymptomatic and do not require treatment. Reducing thicker lesions in areas of maceration may decrease odor and promote comfort. Lac-Hydrin, a 12% lactic acid cream, applied as needed may soften lesions. Retinoic acid (Retin-A cream or gel) applied each day, or less often if irritation occurs, is effective.[60] Oral isotretinoin (Accutane) is useful, but acanthosis nigricans recurs when the drug is discontinued.[61]

MALIGNANT ACANTHOSIS NIGRICANS. The cases of greatest concern are those originating in nonobese adult patients. These cases may result from secretion of tumor products with insulin-like activity or transforming growth factor alpha, which stimulates keratinocytes to proliferate.[8] These patients must be evaluated for internal malignancy. The stomach is the most common site,[62] but cancer in several other areas has been reported.[63] Malignant AN has a different clinical appearance. Lesions develop rapidly and tend to be more severe and extensive. Hyperpigmentation is prominent and is not limited to the hyperkeratotic areas. Mucous membrane involvement and thickening of the palms and soles occur more frequently. Itching is common.

In approximately one third of patients, the skin lesions precede the clinical manifestations of cancer, and in several cases they have disappeared with successful removal of the tumor.[64] A recurrence of acanthosis nigricans may mark the recurrence or metastasis of the previously treated cancer. In patients with malignant acanthosis, chemotherapy may relieve many of the distressing cutaneous symptoms.[65]

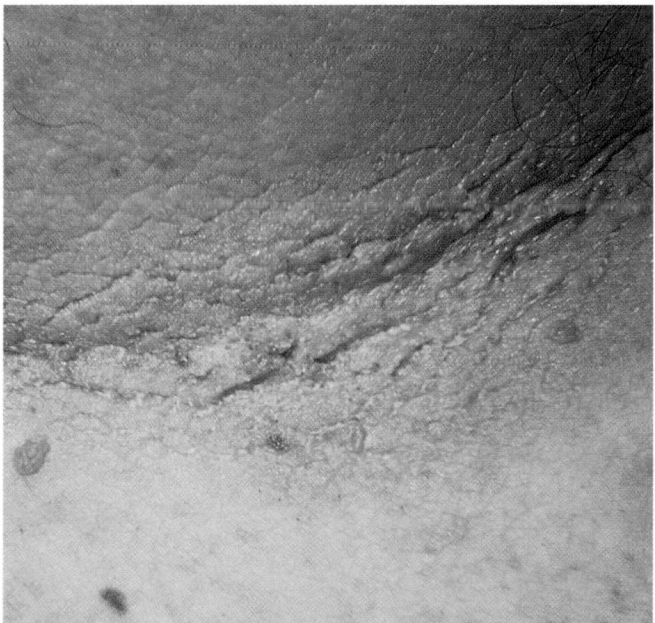

Figure 26-5 Acanthosis nigricans. The skin is brown and thickened and has a papillomatous surface.

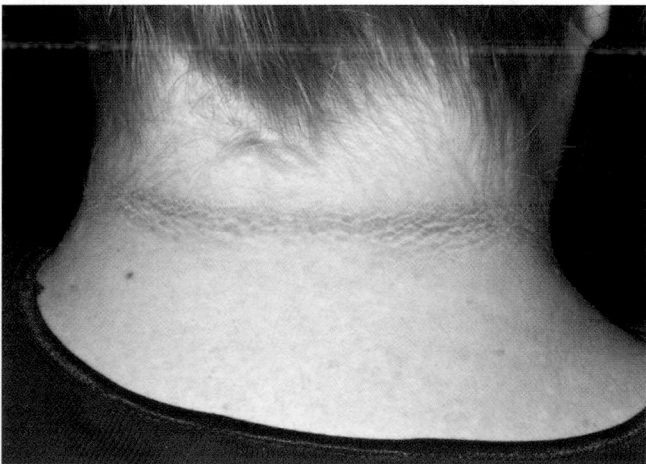

Figure 26-6 Acanthosis nigricans of the neck. The patient was obese.

Xanthomas and Dyslipoproteinemia

The plasma lipids and lipoprotein levels are under the control of a number of genetic and environmental influences. Abnormalities in a number of these lipids or subfractions result in dyslipoproteinemias and xanthomas. Xanthomas are lipid deposits in the skin and tendons that occur secondary to a lipid abnormality. These localized deposits are yellow and are frequently very firm. Although certain types of xanthomas are characteristic of certain lipid abnormalities, none is absolutely specific because the same form of xanthomas occurs in many different diseases[66]; further investigation is always required. The molecular defect of various lipid disorders is now known; however, the classification and diagnosis are still based on history and clinical presentation (Table 26-2).

PATHOPHYSIOLOGY. The liver secretes lipoproteins, which are particles composed of various combinations of cholesterol and triglycerides. These particles are made water soluble to facilitate transport to peripheral tissues by polar phospho-lipids and 12 different specific proteins termed apolipoproteins. The apolipoproteins also serve as cofactors for plasma enzymes and interact with cell surface receptors. Lipoproteins are divided into five major classes: chylomicrons, very low-density lipoproteins (VLDL), intermediate-density lipoproteins (IDL), low-density lipoproteins (LDL), and high-density lipoproteins (HDL). LDL and HDL have each been divided into two subfractions.

CLASSIFICATION: PRIMARY VS. SECONDARY HYPER-LIPOPROTEINEMIA. Dyslipoproteinemias are categorized as primary or secondary. Primary conditions (Table 26-3) are genetically determined and were grouped by Fredrickson into five or six types on the basis of specific lipoprotein elevations.[67] This classification recognizes elevations of chylomicrons (type I), VLDL or pre-beta lipoproteins (type IV), "broad beta" disease (or type III hyperlipoprotcinemia), beta lipoproteins (LDL) (type II), and elevations of both chylomicrons and VLDL (type V). In addition, the combined elevations in pre-beta (VLDL) and beta (LDL) lipoproteins were

Table 26-2 Xanthomas

Type	Clinical characteristics	Associated lipid abnormality
Xanthelasma	Inner or outer canthus; plane or papular	No lipid abnormality; increased frequency of apo E-ND phenotype and hyperapobetalipoproteinemia; type II*
Eruptive	Crops of discrete yellow papules on an erythematous base on buttocks, extensor aspects of elbows and knees; lesions clear when triglycerides return to normal	Indicative of hypertriglyceridemia and seen with types I, II, IV, and rarely III and diabetes mellitus
Plane	Palms and palmar creases, eyelids, face, neck, chest	Biliary cirrhosis; type III; reported in types II, IV
Tuberous	Lipid deposits in dermis and subcutaneous tissue; plaquelike or nodular; frequently found on the elbows or knees	Hypertriglyceridemia (familial or acquired); types II and III; biliary cirrhosis
Tendinous	Nodules involving the elbows, knees, Achilles tendon, and dorsum of hands and feet	Indicates hypercholesterolemia; type II, occasionally III

* There are five types of familial hyperlipidemia.

Table 26-3 Primary Dyslipidemia (the Genetic Dyslipidemias)

Phenotype	Lipoprotein at increased concentration	Cholesterol concentration	Triglyceride concentration	Dermatologic lesion(s)
I	Chylomicrons	+	+ + + +	Eruptive xanthomas
IIa	LDL	+ + + +	+	Tendon, tuberous, and intertriginous xanthomas; xanthelasma
IIb	VLDL and LDL	+ + + +	+ +	Tendon, tuberous, and intertriginous xanthomas; xanthelasma
III	IDL	+ + +	+ + +	Palmar xanthomas
IV	VLDL	+	+ + +	Eruptive xanthomas
V	Chylomicrons and VLDL	+ +	+ + + +	Eruptive xanthomas

recognized as type IIb hyperlipoproteinemia. This older classification still provides a useful conceptual framework. It, however, does not include HDL cholesterol nor does it differentiate severe monogenic lipoprotein disorders from the more common polygenic disorders. The World Health Organization has classified lipoprotein disorders on the basis of arbitrary cut-points, but the traditional classification will be used in this text.

Secondary hyperlipoproteinemias occur as a result of another disease process that can induce symptoms (Box 26-4), lipoprotein changes, and xanthomas that mimic the primary syndromes. Diagnosis should be made as follows:

1. Determine the type of xanthoma.
2. Measure fasting blood levels of cholesterol, triglycerides, and HDL, VLDL and LDL.
3. Rule out secondary diseases (Box 26-4). The diagnosis of primary hyperlipoproteinemia is one of exclusion.
   a. Thyroid, liver, renal function tests
   b. Glucose tolerance tests
   c. Complete blood count (CBC), serum, and urine immunoelectrophoresis
   d. Chest x-ray film, bone marrow
   e. Antinuclear antibodies (ANA)

XANTHELASMA AND PLANE XANTHOMAS. Plane xanthomas occur in several areas of the body and are flat or slightly elevated (Figures 26-7 and 26-8). Xanthelasma is the most common form (see Figure 26-7). Xanthelasma can be associated with familial hypercholesterolemia, phenotype IIa or IIb, but 50% of the patients have normal cholesterol levels. Longevity studies have shown that xanthelasma, with or without hypercholesterolemia, is one of the main risk factors for death from atherosclerotic disease. Further study of these patients with normal cholesterol and triglycerides often reveals an elevated LDL and VLDL and decreased HDL.[68] This profile is found for patients who have a high risk of atherosclerotic

Box 26-4 Acquired Disorders of Lipoprotein Metabolism
Hypercholesterolemia
Nephrotic syndrome
Hypothyroidism
Dysgammaglobulinemia
Acute intermittent porphyria
Obstructive liver disease
Combined hyperlipidemia
Nephrotic syndrome
Hypothyroidism
Glucocorticoid excess/Cushing's disease
Diuretics
Uncontrolled diabetes
Hypertriglyceridemia
Diabetes mellitus
Uremia
Sepsis
Obesity
Systemic lupus erythematosus
Dysgammaglobulinemia
Glycogen storage disease, type I
Lipodystrophy
Drugs
Alcohol
Estrogens
β-adrenergic blocking agents
Isotretinoin (13-*cis*-retinoic acid)

cardiovascular disease. Studies show that numerous people with xanthelasma have an elevated apolipoprotein B[69] and other fractions that are known to be atherogenic. It may be that all patients with xanthelasma have an increased risk for atherosclerosis.

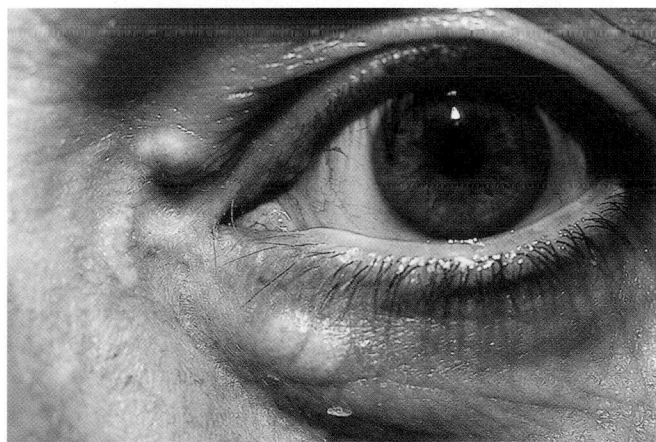

Figure 26-7 Xanthelasma. Lesions are usually located on the medial side of the lids.

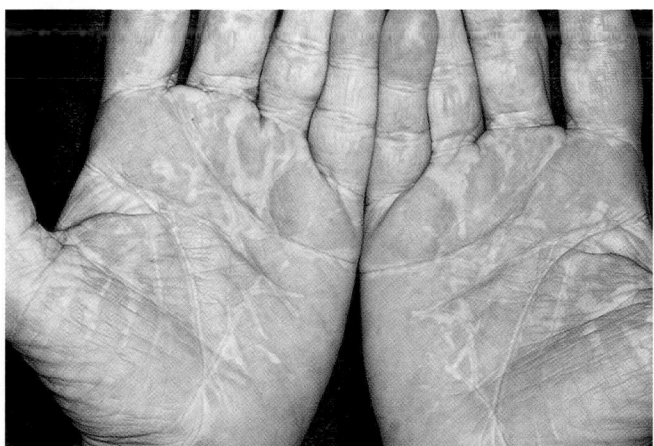

Figure 26-8 Plane xanthomas (macular) of the palms are characteristic of type III dysbetalipoproteinemia.

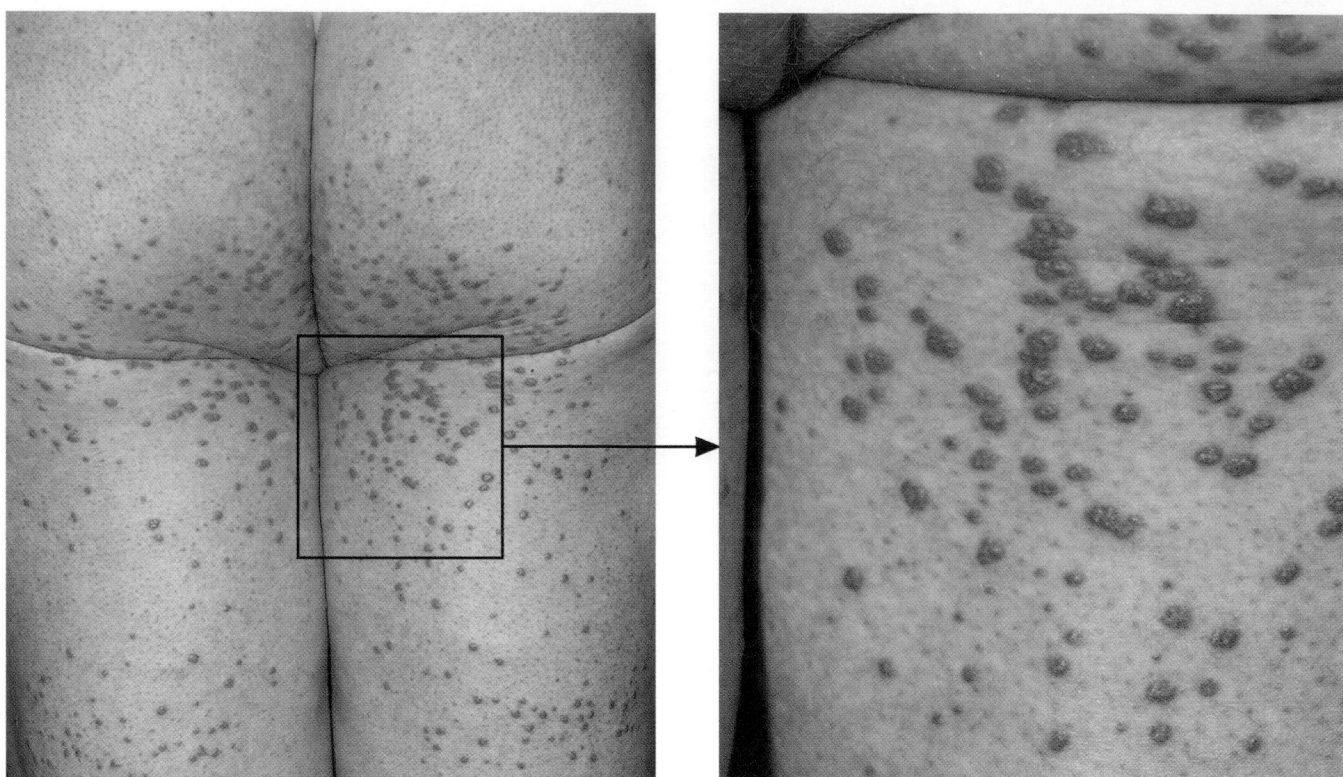

Figure 26-9 Eruptive xanthomas are found on the buttocks, shoulders, and the extensor surfaces of the extremities. The red-yellow papules erupt abruptly and may resolve in a few weeks. Pruritus is common. They are a sign of hypertriglyceridemia and appear in secondary hyperlipidemias (e.g., diabetes).

ERUPTIVE XANTHOMAS. These are yellow, 1- to 4-mm papules with a red halo around the base. They appear suddenly in crops on extensor surfaces of the arms, legs, and buttocks and over pressure points (Figure 26-9). Lesions clear rapidly when serum lipid levels are lowered.

TUBEROUS XANTHOMAS. These are slowly evolving yellow papules, nodules, or tumors that occur on the knees, elbows, and extensor surfaces of the body and the palms (Figure 26-10).

TENDINOUS XANTHOMAS. These smooth, deeply situated nodules are attached to tendons, ligaments, and fascia. They are most often found on the Achilles tendons and the dorsal aspects of the fingers.

REGRESSION OF XANTHOMAS. Certain xanthomas disappear with treatment.[70] The eruptive and palmar xanthomas can regress rapidly. The eruptive type of tuberous xanthomas can disappear. Tendinous xanthomatous lesions tend to persist.

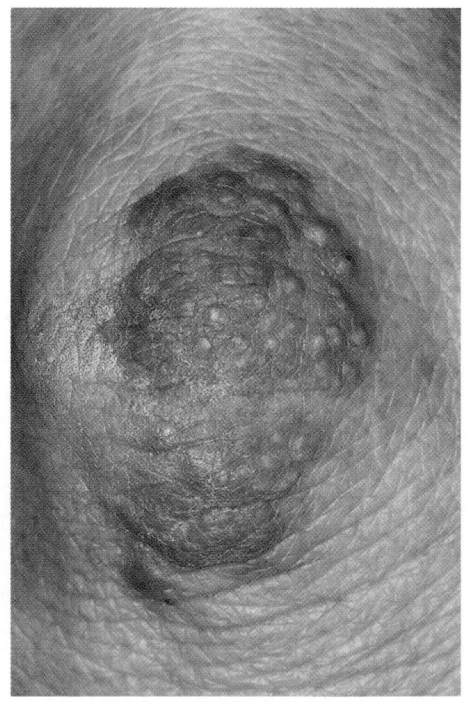

Figure 26-10 Tuberous xanthomas are painless, red-yellow nodules that develop in pressure areas.

Neurofibromatosis

The neurofibromatoses comprise at least two autosomal dominant disorders with an incidence of approximately 1 in 3000. These diseases have tumors surrounding nerves. Neurofibromatosis 1 (NF1) is the most common and is characterized by congenital lesions of the skin, central nervous system, bone, and endocrine glands. The cardinal features of the disorder are café-au-lait spots, axillary freckling, cutaneous neurofibromas, and iris hamartomas (Lisch nodules). Common complications include learning disability, scoliosis, and optic gliomas. Neurofibromatosis 2 (NF2) is characterized by bilateral acoustic neuromas and other nerve tumors. Skin and other systemic manifestations are minimal or absent.[71] Café-au-lait macules, freckling, and neurofibromas localized to a segment of the body are called segmental neurofibromatosis (NF5).[72] The NF1 gene is located on chromosome 17 and the NF2 gene is found on chromosome 22.

NEUROFIBROMATOSIS 1. NF1 is a disorder of neural crest–derived cells characterized by the presence of café-au-lait spots, multiple neurofibromas, and Lisch nodules (pigmented iris hamartomas); there are several other less common features. There is considerable variation of manifestations within the same family. It occurs in approximately one of every 3500 births and affects both sexes with equal frequency and severity. Neurofibromatosis is one of the most common mutations in humans; at least half of the cases represent new mutations.

CLINICAL MANIFESTATIONS

Café-au-lait spots. Café-au-lait spots are light-colored-to-brown macules (see Chapter 19). The criteria for establishing the diagnosis with reference to the number and size of café-au-lait spots[73] are listed in Box 26-5. The spots are present in virtually every patient with neurofibromatosis, usually at birth, but they may not appear for months. Their size and number increase with age (Figure 26-11, A). Intertriginous freckling, a pathognomonic sign, may occur in the axillae, inframammary region, and groin (Figure 26-11, B). Café-au-lait macules alone are not absolutely diagnostic of NF1, regardless of their size and number.

Box 26-5 Diagnostic Criteria for Neurofibromatosis 1 (NF1)
Six or more café-au-lait macules
1.5 cm in postpubertal individuals
0.5 cm in prepubertal individuals
Two or more neurofibromas of any type *or*
One or more plexiform neurofibromas
Freckling of axillae or inguinal area
Bilateral optic gliomas
Two or more Lisch nodules
Sphenoid wing dysplasia *or*
Congenital bowing *or*
Thinning of the long bone cortex (with or without pseudoarthrosis)
First-degree relative with NF1 by these criteria
NF1 diagnosis: Two or more features
Adapted from National Institutes of Health Consensus Development Conference. Neurofibromatosis. Conference statement. Arch Neurol 1988; 45:576.

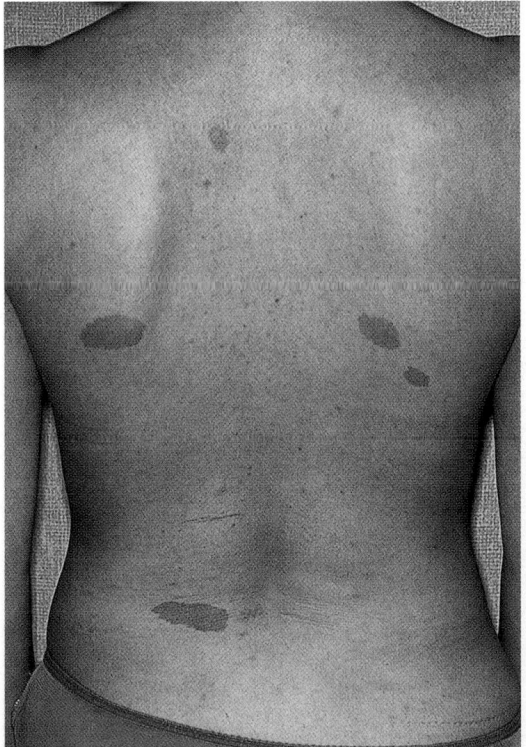

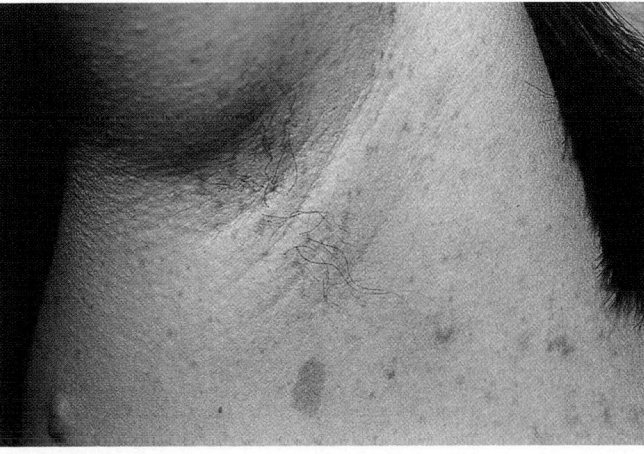

Figure 26-11 von Recklinghausen's neurofibromatosis. **A,** Café-au-lait spots vary in size and have a smooth border. **B,** Axillary freckling (Crowe sign) is a pathognomonic sign.

A

B

PRESUMPTIVE EVIDENCE OF NEUROFIBROMATOSIS

- Six or more café-au-lait macules over 5 mm in greatest diameter if prepubertal
- Six or more café-au-lait macules over 15 mm in greatest diameter if postpubertal

NEUROFIBROMAS. Tumors are usually not present in childhood, but they begin to appear at puberty. Tumors increase in both number and size as the patient ages. Some patients have only a few small tumors, whereas others develop hundreds over the entire body surface, including the palms and soles (Figure 26-12).

There are three different types of cutaneous tumors. The most common is sessile or pedunculated. Early tumors are soft, dome-shaped papules or nodules that have a distinctive violaceous hue. Digital pressure on the soft tumor causes invagination or "button-holing." When the soft tumors attain a certain size, they bend and hang or become pendulous. The plexiform neuroma is an elongated tumor that occurs along the course of peripheral nerves. Elephantiasis neuromatosa is a term used to describe a diffuse tumor of nerve trunks that extends into surrounding tissues, causing gross deformity. This form of neuroma produced the facial deformity in Joseph Merrick of London, England, the man who was described in the play and movie, *The Elephant Man.* Most tumors are benign, but malignant degeneration to a neurofibrosarcoma or malignant schwannoma has been reported in approximately 2% of cases[74]; it rarely occurs before age 40.

LISCH NODULES. Lisch nodules (LNs) are pigmented, melanocytic,[75] iris hamartomas (Figure 26-13).[76] They increase in number with age and are asymptomatic. The prevalence of LNs and neurofibromas according to age is shown in Figure 26-14. All adults with neurofibromatosis who are 21 years of age or older have LNs. LNs have never been seen in the absence of neurofibromatosis. They are never the only clinical sign of NF1. They are more likely to be present in younger patients than are neurofibromas (see Figure 26-14) and therefore help to make the diagnosis in younger patients.[77] No association has been found between LNs and overall clinical severity. They are markers for the von Recklinghausen's neurofibromatosis gene; they may be present in immediate relatives who have no cutaneous or other specific signs of the disease.[78] LNs may be seen without the aid of instruments, but slit-lamp examination is essential for differentiation from iris freckles or nevi. Iris freckles are flat and have a lacework structure, whereas LNs are raised, round, dome-shaped, brown papules that are present in both eyes.

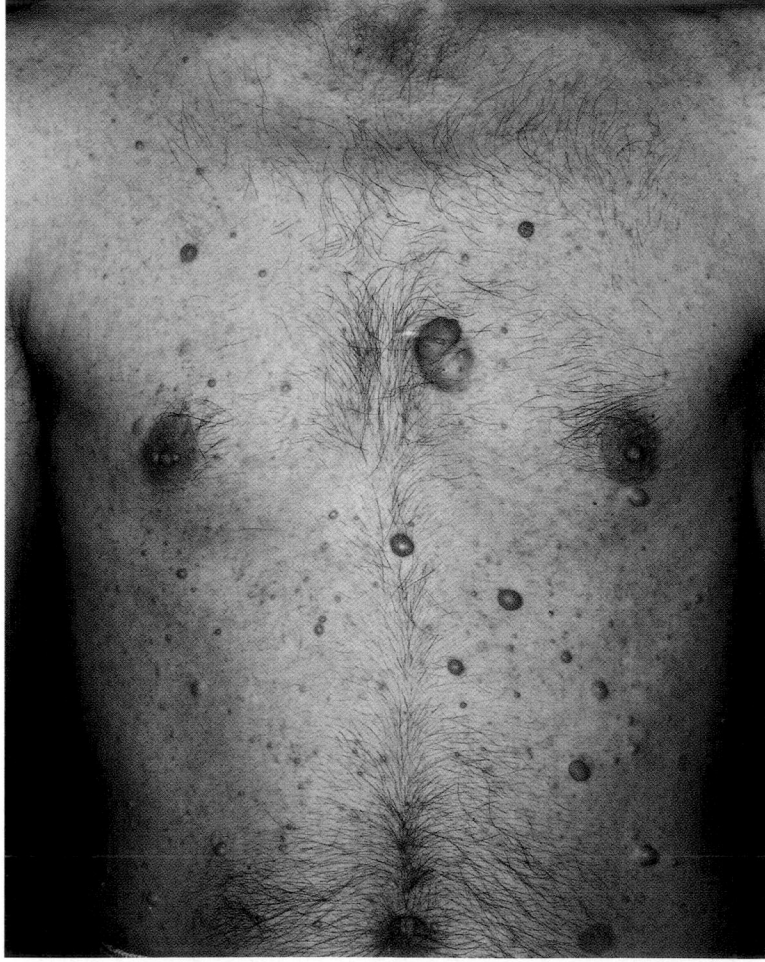

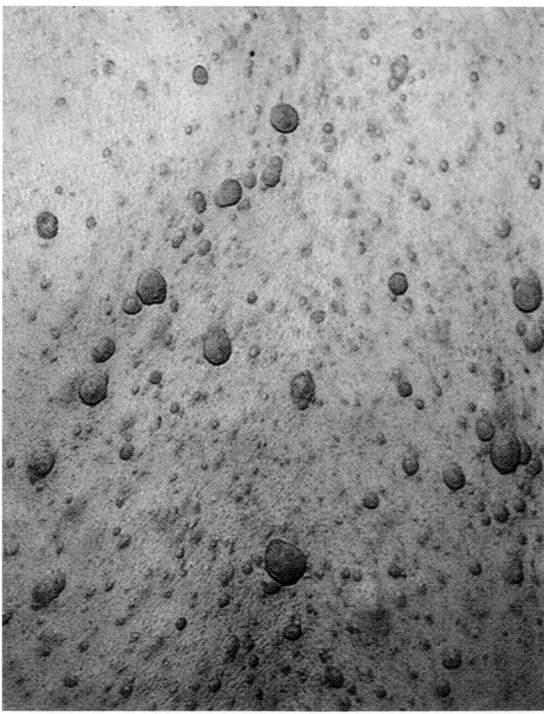

Figure 26-12 von Recklinghausen's neurofibromatosis. Adult patient with hundreds of neurofibromas.

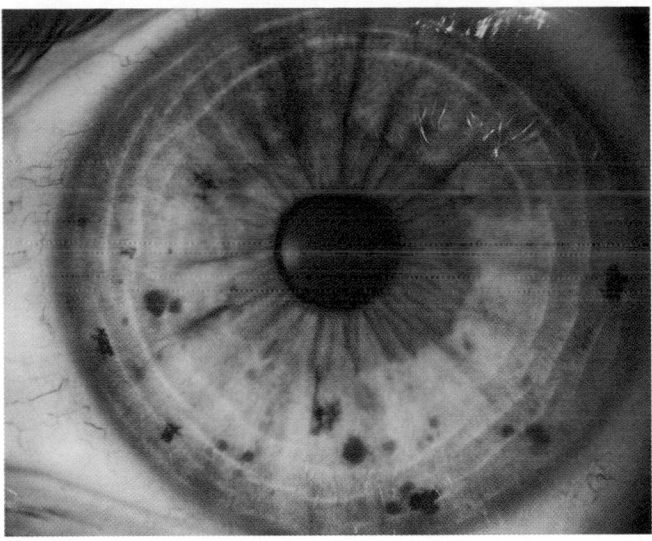

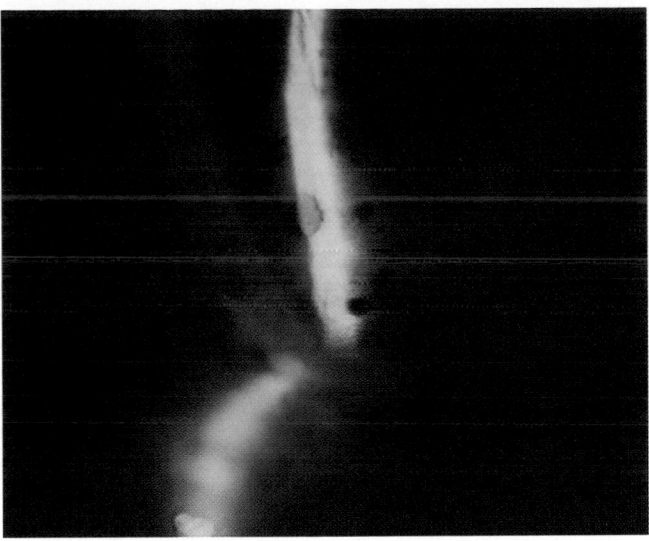

A, Lisch nodules—pigmented iris hamartomas are present in more than 60% of patients with neurofibromatosis who are 7 years of age or older.

B, Slit-lamp examination is essential for differentiation from iris freckles. Iris freckles are flat and have a lace-work structure; Lisch nodules are raised, round, fluffy, and light brown. (*Courtesy Lucian Szmyd, M.D.*)

Figure 26-13 von Recklinghausen's neurofibromatosis—Lisch nodules.

SYSTEMIC MANIFESTATIONS. Neurofibromatosis has a broad spectrum of systemic manifestations; the most important are listed in Box 26-6.

NATURAL HISTORY. Survival rates are significantly impaired for relatives with neurofibromatosis, are worse in probands, and are worst in female probands. Malignant neoplasms or benign central nervous system tumors occur in 45% of probands. Compared with the general population, male relatives with neurofibromatosis have the same rate of neoplasms, whereas female relatives have a nearly twofold higher rate. Nervous system tumors are disproportionately represented.[79]

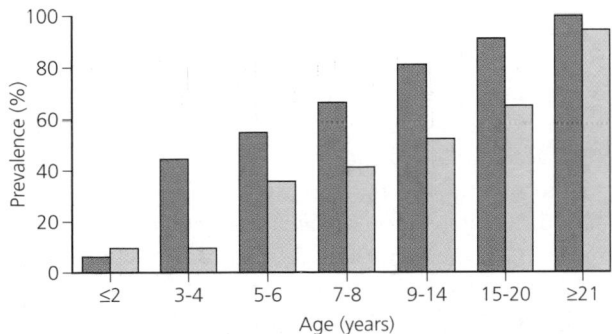

Figure 26-14 Prevalence of Lisch nodules (dark blue bars) and neurofibromas (light blue bars) in 167 patients with neurofibromatosis 1, according to age. (*Modified from Lubs ML et al: N Engl J Med 324:1264, 1991.*)

Box 26-6 Systemic Manifestations of Neurofibromatosis
Central nervous system tumors
Optic gliomas
Astrocytomas, acoustic neuromas, meningiomas, neurilemomas
Constipation
Headache
Intellectual handicap
Kyphoscoliosis
Macrocephaly
Malignant disease
Neurofibrosarcoma
Malignant schwannoma
Neuroblastoma
Wilm's tumors
Rhabdomyosarcoma
Leukemia
Pheochromocytomas
Premature or delayed puberty
Pseudarthrosis (tibia, radius)
Seizures
Speech impediment
Short stature
From Riccardi VM: N Engl J Med 1981; 305:1617.

DIAGNOSIS. NF1 is considered to be present in an individual with two of the criteria listed in Box 26-5, provided no other disease accounts for the findings.[80]

NF1 should be suspected in children with a large head circumference (above the 97th percentile for age) and one of the following: a mild cognitive impairment, a learning disability, or a selective visual-spatial impairment.

SEGMENTAL NEUROFIBROMATOSIS (NF5).

Segmental neurofibromatosis (neurofibromatosis type V) is a rare disorder characterized by café-a-lait macules and neurofibromas, or only neurofibromas, limited to one region of the body (Figure 26-15). Segmental neurofibromatosis has only

been described in about 100 patients. The median age at onset is 28 years. The neurofibromas most commonly occupied either a cervical or thoracic dermatome and were unilateral. Café-au-lait macules were present in 26% of patients. Axillary freckling occurs in only 10% of patients. Most patients with segmental neurofibromatosis (93%) do not have a family history of neurofibromatosis.[72] A postzygotic somatic mutation in a primitive neural crest cell is the most likely causative mechanism for this cutaneous hamartoma.[81, 82] The lesions are strictly unilateral and noninherited in most cases; however, in a few patients, the disease becomes generalized.[83] These patients should be examined for LNs and other signs of neurofibromatosis.

GENETIC COUNSELING. The patient's offspring, both male and female, have a 50% chance of inheriting this autosomal dominant disease. The penetrance is virtually 100%, but the expressivity is extremely variable. The severity of the disease is highest in those born to an affected mother.[84] Fifty percent of cases are new mutations in which the parents are unaffected. All family members and relatives should be examined for the triad of Lisch iris nodules, solitary neurofibromas, and café-au-lait spots.[78]

The LN is a reliable indicator of NF1; slit-lamp examination is important to establish the diagnosis. All people above the age of 20 who have NF1 also have LNs.[77] Therefore minimally affected and unaffected parents and adult siblings can be identified. If the diagnosis is in doubt and a child has no LNs, the examination should be repeated periodically. LNs often appear before neurofibromas. Adult siblings and adult children of affected persons can be counseled that their risk of having affected children is the same (approximately 1 in 3500) as that of the parents of patients with sporadic cases if all three elements of the triad are absent.[85] Patients who have a segmental pattern of neurofibromatosis should be counseled that genetic transmission of their trait, though rare, is possible.[86]

MANAGEMENT. There are more than 60 neurofibromatosis clinics in the United States. These clinics are usually based at teaching centers where a group of specialists provides a team approach to management. The National Neurofibromatosis Foundation has a list of clinics and can be reached by calling (800) 323-7938. A genetic counselor is available to speak to the physician or the patient. Neurofibromatosis, Inc. provides support and services to NF families (1-800-942-6825) or on the web at www.nfinc.org.

Cutaneous tumors may be excised. The patient must be followed closely to detect malignant degeneration of neurofibromas. Genetic counseling is of utmost importance. Periodic complete evaluations are required to detect the numerous possible internal manifestations. Magnetic resonance imaging with gadolinium enhancement is the primary neuroimaging modality used for diagnosis, management, and screening of family members.[87,88]

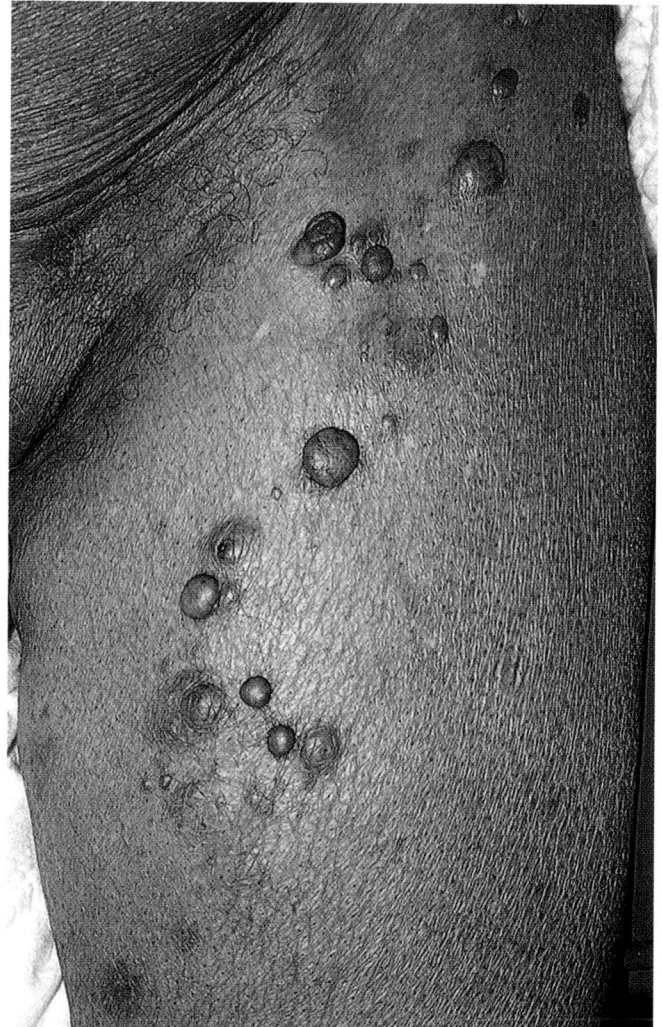

Figure 26-15 Segmental neurofibromatosis (NF5). Tumors are restricted to a segment of skin.

Tuberous Sclerosis

Tuberous sclerosis (epiloia) is an autosomal dominant disease of variable penetrance that is characterized by multiple hamartomas of the skin, central nervous system, kidneys, heart, retina, and other organs. The skin lesions (adenoma sebaceum, shagreen patch, white macules, or periungual fibromas) are reliable markers of the disease. Tuberous sclerosis affects at least 1 in 6000 people; two thirds of cases occur sporadically; one third are familial. Mildly affected individuals may be undiagnosed. The triad of epilepsy, angiofibromas (adenoma sebaceum), and mental retardation (the Vogt triad) that is typically associated with tuberous sclerosis is present in only 25% of patients. Mental retardation may be present in less than 50%.

Box 26-7 Revised Diagnostic Criteria for Tuberous Sclerosis Complex (TSC)*

Major features

1. Facial angiofibromas or forehead plaque
2. Non-traumatic ungual or periungual fibroma
3. Hypomelanotic macules (more than three)
4. Shagreen patch (connective tissue nevus)
5. Multiple retinal nodular hamartomas
6. Cortical tuber (a)
7. Subependymal nodule
8. Subependymal giant cell astrocytoma
9. Cardiac rhabdomyoma, single or multiple
10. Lymphangiomyomatosis (b)
11. Renal angiomyolipoma (b)

Minor features

1. Multiple randomly distributed pits in dental enamel
2. Hamartomatous rectal polyps (c)
3. Bone cysts (d)
4. Cerebral white matter migration lines (a, d, e)
5. Gingival fibromas
6. Non-renal hamartoma (c)
7. Retinal achromic patch
8. "Confetti" skin lesions
9. Multiple renal cysts (c)

Definite TSC: Either 2 major features or 1 major feature with 2 minor features

Probable TSC: One major feature and one minor feature

Possible TSC: Either 1 major feature or 2 or more minor features

(a) When cerebral cortical dysplasia and cerebral white matter migration tracts occur together, they should be counted as one rather than two features of TSC.

(b) When both lymphangiomyomatosis and renal angiomyolipomas are present, other features of TSC should be present before a definitive diagnosis is assigned.

(c) Histologic confirmation is suggested.

(d) Radiographic confirmation is sufficient.

(e) One panel member recommended that three or more radial migration lines consitute a major feature.

*From the 1998 Tuberous Sclerosis Alliance, consensus conference[89] and National Institutes of Health consensus conference: tuberous sclerosis complex.[90]

DIAGNOSTIC CRITERIA. In July 1998 the Tuberous Sclerosis Alliance (www.tsalliance.org) (800-225-NTSA), then known as the National Tuberous Sclerosis Association, convened a consensus conference and developed a revised scheme for TS diagnostic criteria (Box 26-7).

The new diagnostic criteria eliminated any single finding as specifically distinctive or characteristic of the disease. Originally, cortical tubers were believed to be pathognomonic. Evidence now suggests that radiographic brain imaging and histologic studies are unable to distinguish these tubers from isolated cortical dysplasia. Two other types of brain lesions—subependymal giant cell astrocytomas and subependymal nodules—can be distinguished from cortical tubers and from each other. The two subependymal lesions have a histologic and radiographic appearance that differs from the cortical tuber, whereas the giant cell astrocytoma is the only one that tends to enlarge. It is important to distinguish between the three different brain lesions for identification and monitoring purposes. Dermatologic manifestations are especially important in diagnosing TS.

CLINICAL MANIFESTATIONS. The time course of tuberous sclerosis lesions is illustrated in the diagram below.

Adenoma sebaceum. Adenoma sebaceum is the most common cutaneous manifestation of tuberous sclerosis.[91] The lesions consist of smooth, firm, 1- to 5-mm, yellow-pink papules with fine telangiectasia (Figure 26-16). Their color and location suggest an origin from sebaceous glands, but these growths are benign hamartomas composed of fibrous and vascular tissue (angiofibromas). The angiofibromas are located on the nasolabial folds, cheeks, chin and, occasionally, on the forehead, scalp, and ears. The number varies from a few inconspicuous lesions to dense clusters of papules. They are rare at birth but may begin to appear by ages 2 to 3 and proliferate during puberty. They may be mistaken for multiple trichoepitheliomas, an autosomal dominant condition that appears on the central face. A secondary feature, the "forehead plaque," is a large angiofibroma. Patients with the autosomal dominant disorder multiple endocrine neoplasia type 1 (MEN1) can develop multiple angiofibromas and several other types of cutaneous tumors in addition to tumors of pituitary, parathyroid, and entero-pancreatic endocrine tissues.[92]

Time Course of TS lesions

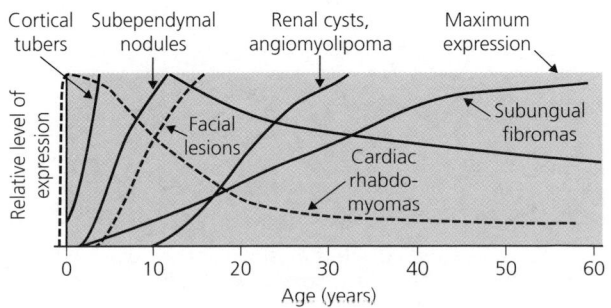

TUBEROUS SCLEROSIS

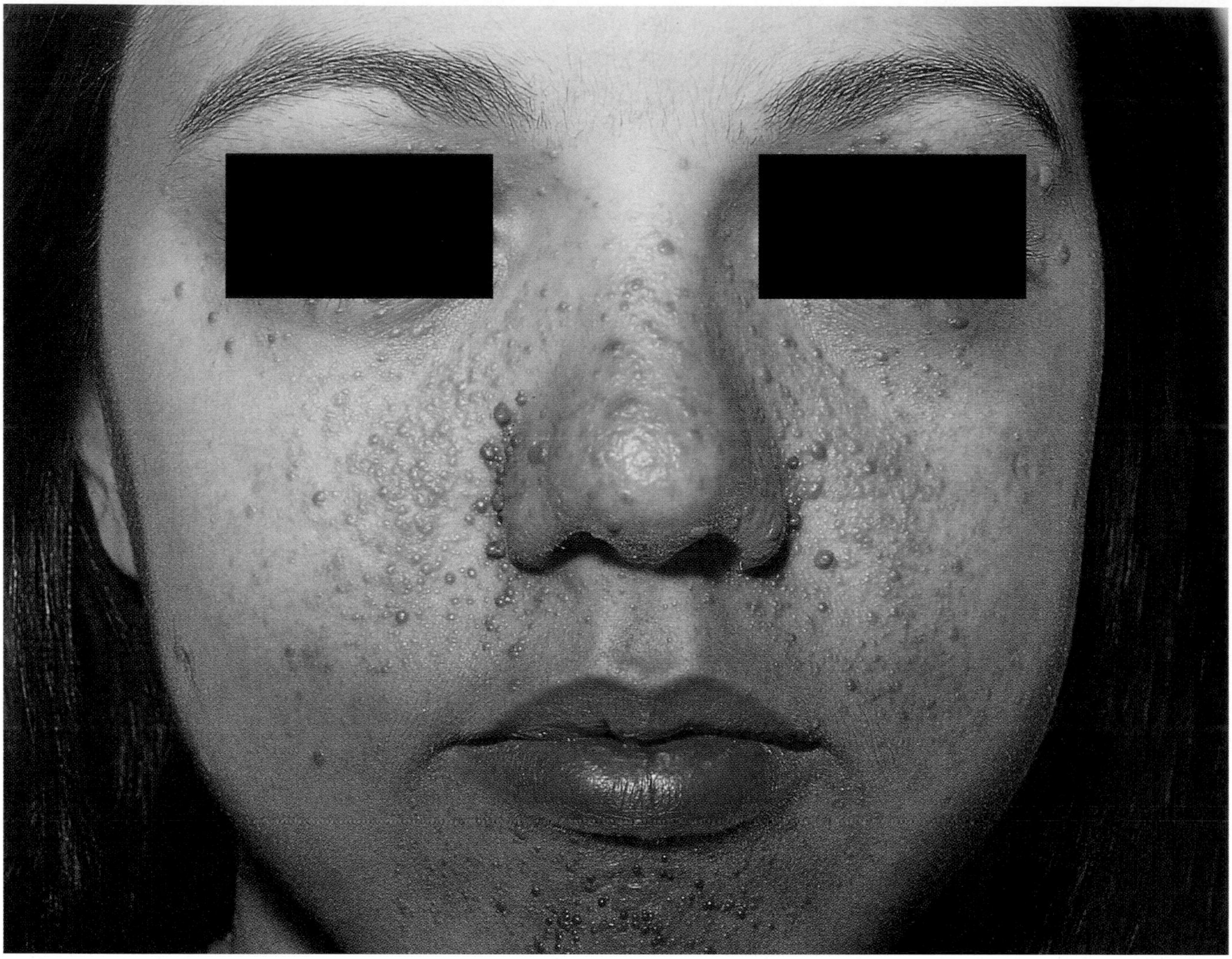

Figure 26-16 Adenoma sebaceum appears during childhood or early adolescence. These angiofibromas first appear as flat, pink macules and later become papular. Lesions may bleed easily.

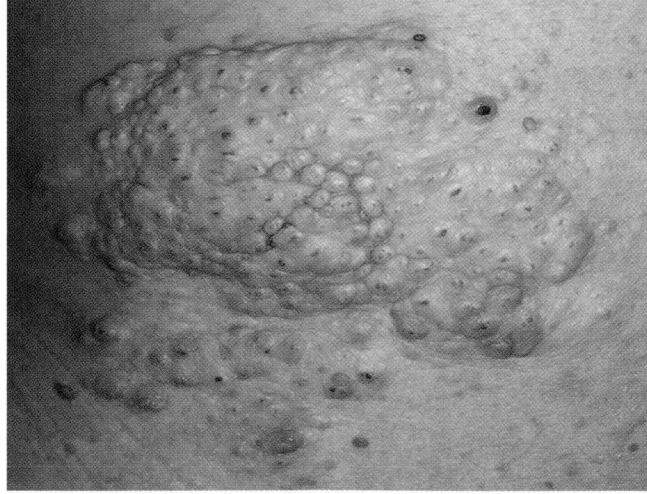

Figure 26-17 Shagreen patch is most commonly found in the lumbosacral region. The patch appears in childhood or early adolescence.

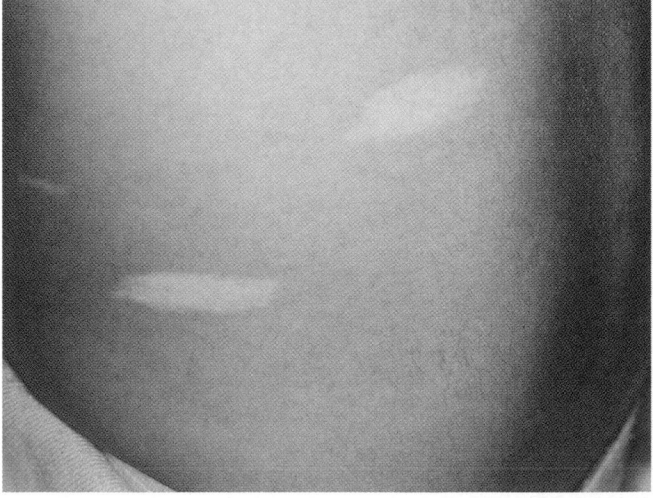

Figure 26-18 Ash leaf macules (hypomelanotic macules) are often present at birth.

Shagreen patch. The shagreen patch is highly characteristic of tuberous sclerosis and occurs in as many as 80% of patients; it occurs in early childhood and may be the first sign of disease. The lesion varies in size from 1 to 10 cm. There is usually one lesion, but several may be present. They are soft, flesh-colored-to-yellow plaques with an irregular surface that has been likened to pigskin (Figure 26-17). The lesion consists of dermal connective tissue and appears most commonly in the lumbosacral region.

Whitish macules and white tufts of hair. Hypomelanotic macules (oval, ash-leaf shaped, stippled, or "confetti shaped") are randomly distributed with a concentration on the arms, legs, and trunk. They are the earliest sign of tuberous sclerosis (Figure 26-18).[93] They are present in 40% to 90% of patients with the disease and number from 1 to 32 in affected individuals.[94-96] The white macules are present at birth and increase in number and size throughout life. They vary from 0.5 to 12 cm in diameter. The "confetti" macules are the rarest of the three types and consist of numerous 1- to 3-mm macules. The Wood's light can be used to accentuate the white macules and is particularly useful for examining patients with light skin. A biopsy shows melanocytes, thus excluding the diagnosis of vitiligo. Hypopigmented macules, present at birth, are not invariably associated with tuberous sclerosis, but their presence is an indication for further study. It is essential that the diagnosis be established as soon as possible so that parents can obtain genetic counseling. A tuft of white hair with no depigmentation of the scalp skin underlying the white tuft has been reported as an early sign of tuberous sclerosis.[97]

Periungual fibromas. Periungual fibromas appear at or after puberty in approximately 50% of cases. They are smooth, flesh-colored, conical projections that emerge from the nailfolds of the toenail and fingernail (Figure 26-19).

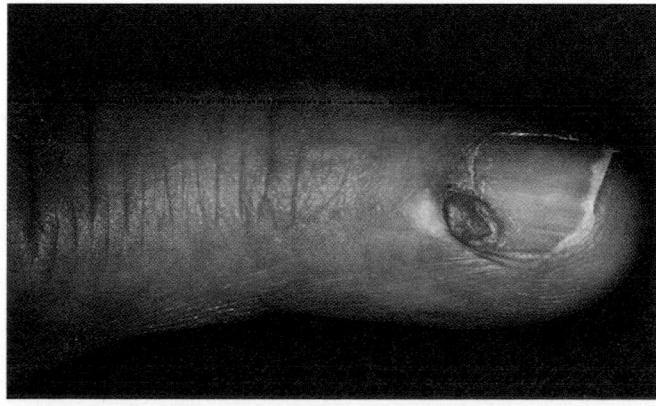

Figure 26-19 Tuberous sclerosis. Periungual fibromas.

SYSTEMIC MANIFESTATIONS. Mental retardation occurs in less than 50% of cases. Subependymal nodules and cortical and white matter tubers are characteristic of tuberous sclerosis. Sclerotic patches (tubers) consisting of astrocytes and giant cells are scattered throughout the cortical gray matter. Calcium is deposited in tubers and may be detected shortly after birth by computed tomography (CT) scan, magnetic resonance imaging (MRI), or x-ray films and is found in 90% of affected children.[98,99] Brain lesions cause seizures in more than 90% of patients. Benign tumors consisting of vascular fibrous tissue and fat and smooth muscle are found in numerous organs, including the kidneys, liver, and gastrointestinal tract. Gray or yellow retinal plaques occur in 25% of cases. The incidence of enamel pitting in the adult is 100%. A dental disclosing solution swabbed on dry teeth exposes the pits.[100]

GENETIC COUNSELING. TS belongs to the family of tumor-suppressor-gene syndromes. These genes normally function as cellular "brakes." When they lose their function (as a result of mutations), uncontrolled proliferation and tumor formation occur. Affected patients typically have one inactivating mutation in either the TSC1 or TSC2 gene in all germ-line and somatic cells.[101] The patient's offspring, both male and female, have a 50% chance of inheriting this autosomal dominant disease. The penetrance is high, but expressivity is variable. Patients with normal parents acquire the disease from a new mutation.

Approximately 50% of TSC families show genetic linkage to TSC1 and 50% to TSC2. Among sporadic TSC cases, mutations in TSC2 are more frequent and often accompanied by more severe neurologic deficits. Intellectual disability is significantly more frequent in TSC2 sporadic cases than in TSC1 sporadic cases.[102] The TSC1 (chromosome 9) and TSC2 (chromosome 16) genes encode distinct proteins, hamartin, and tuberin, respectively, which are widely expressed in the brain. Mosaicism is the phenomenon in which a fraction of, rather than all, germ-line and somatic cells contain a mutation of chromosomal abnormality. It occurs in all genetic disorders in which spontaneous mutations occur. Because of this phenomenon, some patients' mutation may not be detected in present methods of testing. The failure to detect mosaicism has important implications for genetic counseling.[103]

The Tuberous Sclerosis Alliance provides information and support for physicians, patients, and families. The headquarters is at 8000 Corporate Drive, Suite 120, Landover, MD 20785; (800) 225-NTSA.

DIAGNOSIS AND MANAGEMENT. The diagnosis of tuberous sclerosis must be sought in infants with white macules, white hair tufts, or other cutaneous signs. The diagnosis may be established by demonstrating brain calcifications that may occur in early infancy. Brain lesions in tuberous sclerosis are of three kinds; cortical tubers, white matter abnormalities, and subependymal nodules. CT demonstrates calcified subependymal nodules. MR imaging demonstrates more

Table 26-4 Summary of Testing Recommendations of the Tuberous Sclerosis Consensus Conference

Assessment	Initial testing	Repeat testing
Neurodevelopmental testing	At diagnosis and at school entry	As indicated
Ophthalmic examination	At diagnosis	As indicated
Electroencephalography	If seizures occur	As indicated for seizure management
Electrocardiography	At diagnosis	As indicated
Echocardiography	If cardiac symptoms occur	If cardiac dysfunction occurs
Renal ultrasonography	At diagnosis	Every 1 to 3 years
Chest computed tomography	At adulthood (women only)	If pulmonary dysfunction occurs
Cranial computed tomography*	At diagnosis	Children/adolescents: every 1 to 3 years
Cranial magnetic resonance imaging*	At diagnosis	Children/adolescents: every 1 to 3 years

Roach ES, et al: J Child Neurol 1999; 14:401.

*Either cranial computed tomography or magnetic resonance imaging, but usually not both.

clearly cortical, and white matter lesions than CT.[104,105] A positive scan result is often obtainable before the calcifications are present on skull x-ray films and even before the pathognomonic cutaneous findings appear.

Facial angiofibromas may be surgically removed for cosmetic purposes by electrosurgery, cryosurgery, dermabrasion, or lasers.

DIAGNOSTIC STUDIES. In newly diagnosed patients, testing (Table 26-4) helps confirm the diagnosis and to identify complications. For patients with an established diagnosis, studies can identify treatable complications. Tests sometimes provide evidence of disease in asymptomatic relatives of children with tuberous sclerosis complex. Affected relatives who have abnormal tests usually have at least subtle findings.

Cancer-Associated Genodermatoses

An overview of the familial multiple cancer syndromes with cutaneous findings appears in the diagram on p. 913.

Cowden's disease (multiple hamartoma syndrome)

Cowden's disease (multiple hamartoma syndrome) is a multisystem disease inherited as an autosomal dominant trait with incomplete penetrance and variable expression. It is characterized by multiple hamartomas of ectodermal, endodermal, and mesodermal origin; a high incidence of malignant tumors of the breast and/or thyroid gland. The mucocutaneous manifestations are the most characteristic feature and are the key to diagnosis. The diagnostic criteria for Cowden's disease are listed in Box 26-8.

Box 26-8 Cowden's Syndrome Diagnostic Criteria

Pathognomonic criteria

    Mucocutaneous lesions
        Multiple facial trichilemmomas
        Papillomatous papules
        Mucosal lesions
        Acral keratoses

Major criteria

    Breast cancer
    Thyroid cancer, especially follicular thyroid carcinoma
    Macroencephaly
    Hamartomatous outgrowths of cerebellum (Lhermitte-Duclos disease)

Minor criteria

    Thyroid lesions (e.g., adenoma or goiter)
    Mental retardation (IQ 75)
    Hamartomatous intestinal polyps
    Fibrocystic disease of the breast
    Lipomas
    Fibromas
    Genitourinary tumors or malformations

Operational diagnosis for individual

(1) Mucocutaneous lesions alone if

    a. Six facial papules with 3 trichilemmomas
    b. Cutaneous facial papules and oral mucosal papillomatosis
    c. Oral mucosal papillomatosis and acral keratoses
    d. Six or more palmar/plantar keratoses

or

(2) Two major criteria, but one must include macrocephaly or Lhermitte-Duclos disease

or

(3) One major and 3 minor criteria

or

(4) Four minor criteria

Adapted from Lindor NM, Greene MH: J Natl Cancer Inst 1998; 90:1059, and from Hensin Tsao: J Am Acad Dermatol 2000; 42:939.

FAMILIAL MULTIPLE CANCER SYNDROMES
AUTOSOMAL DOMINANT "CANCER FAMILY SYNDROMES"

Cowden's disease
(Multiple hamartoma syndrome)

Muir-Torre syndrome

Gardner's syndrome
(Familial adenomatous polyposis
with extraintestinal manifestations)

Females

Mucocutaneous lesions
  Facial papules
  Oral papules
  Hand keratosis

Breast lesions
  Cancer
  Fibrocystic

Thyroid
  Goiter
  Carcinoma

Males = females

Skin tumors
  Sebaceous gland
  (at least 1)

Keratoacanthomas

Internal tumors
  Colorectal
  Genitourinary
  Breast

• Solid tumors

Males = females

Skin signs
  Epidermal cysts

Osteomas (palpable)
  Skull
  Jaw

Pigmented ocular
  fundus lesions

Colon
  Polyps > 100
  Adenocarcinoma

Thyroid carcinoma

MUCOCUTANEOUS LESIONS. Facial papules and oral mucosal papillomatosis are the most sensitive indicators of the disease. The asymptomatic cutaneous lesions are usually noticed at age 20, and no further progression of lesions is seen after the age of 30. The principal cutaneous lesion is a papule that may be smooth or keratotic. Cutaneous facial papules are of two types: Lichenoid, flesh-colored, flat-topped papules are found in the centrofacial and periorificial areas; and flesh-colored, elongated, verrucoid, papillomatous lesions are found clustered around the mouth, nose, eyes, and on the ears. The majority of these lesions are trichilemmomas.[106] The differential diagnosis of these facial papules includes Darier's disease and adenoma sebaceum found in tuberous sclerosis. Acral keratoses are located primarily on

the dorsum of the hands and feet. They resemble flat warts (i.e., they are flesh-colored, flat-topped papules 1 to 4 mm in diameter). Palmoplantar keratoses are isolated, pinpoint-to-pea-sized, translucent, hard papules that may show a central depression.[107]

The oral lesions are white, smooth-surfaced papules, 1 to 3 mm in diameter, that often coalesce, giving a cobblestone appearance. They are located primarily on the gingival, labial, and palatal surfaces.

BREAST LESIONS. Breast lesions are the most important and potentially serious abnormality of Cowden's disease.[108,109] Ductal adenocarcinoma occurs in more than 30% of patients, and fibrocystic disease occurs in 60% of patients. The median age of diagnosis of breast cancer is 41 years. All women with Cowden's disease should be considered for prophylactic bilateral total mastectomy by their third decade of life.[110,111]

THYROID GLAND LESIONS. Palpable enlargement (goiter and adenoma) is the most frequently reported internal abnormality of Cowden's disease. Carcinoma is reported in several cases.

A wide variety of other abnormalities and malignancies have been reported, but the incidence is low.

Muir-Torre syndrome

Muir-Torre syndrome (MTS) is a rare autosomal dominant genodermatosis characterized by at least one sebaceous gland tumor[112a] and a minimum of one internal malignancy. The common presentation is the presence of sebaceous tumors along with a low-grade visceral malignancy. The presence of sebaceous tumors warrants a search for an internal malignancy. This syndrome is now considered a subtype of the more common hereditary nonpolyposis colorectal cancer syndrome (HNPCC). The MTS and HNPCC syndrome are associated with hMSH2 gene mutations.

SKIN TUMORS. Sebaceous tumors appear before the internal malignancy in 22%, concurrently in 6%, and after the internal malignancy in 56%.[112a] The sebaceous gland tumors (adenoma, sebaceoma, epithelioma, or carcinoma) usually occur on the trunk, face, and scalp (Figure 26-20). They vary from small, asymptomatic papules or nodules that resemble cysts or benign tumors to waxy papules. The syndrome may occur in individuals with a single sebaceous gland tumor.[112] Some benign sebaceous neoplasms in MTS might have a high potential for malignant transformation or may be well-differentiated sebaceous carcinomas with low-grade malignancy, mimicking sebaceous adenoma/sebaceoma.[113]

Single or multiple keratoacanthomas occur in approximately 20% of patients. The median age for the appearance of the skin lesions is 53 years (range, 23 to 89 years).[114] Sebaceous gland tumors in the general population are rare. A tumor diagnosed as a sebaceous adenoma, sebaceous epithelioma, or sebaceous carcinoma should alert the clinician to the possibility of visceral cancer in both the patient and in family members. Sebaceous hyperplasia commonly seen on the face is not associated with malignancy.

INTERNAL TUMORS. The most commonly associated neoplasms are colorectal (47%); 58% of these tumors occur proximal to or at the splenic flexure.

MTS patients have a genetic predilection to hereditary nonpolyposis colorectal cancer (HNPCC). There are at least eight other major cancer susceptibility syndromes that infer an increased risk for colorectal cancer and/or colorectal polyposis. Therefore the differential diagnosis of hereditary colorectal cancer can be complex.[114a] Genitourinary tumors

(21%), breast carcinomas (12%), and hematologic disorders (9%) are also common.[115] Fifty-three percent of patients develop one cancer, 37% develop two to three cancers, and 10% develop four to nine cancers. Cutaneous lesions occur before or concurrent with the diagnosis of the initial cancer in 63% of patients. The median age for the detection of the initial visceral neoplasm is 53 years (range, 23 to 89 years).[114] A few cases have been associated with polyps in the colon, but widespread gastrointestinal polyposis is rare. There is a relatively low potential for malignancy in both cutaneous and internal tumors, but metastasis from internal malignancies does occur, particularly from colon cancer.[116]

EPIDEMIOLOGY. Muir-Torre syndrome may appear de novo,[117] but there is often a variable family history of cutaneous and/or internal tumors. Males and females are equally affected. This may be one of the four subtypes of cancer family syndrome characterized by a genetically determined (autosomal dominant) predisposition to multiple visceral malignancies that arise at an early age and pursue a relatively benign course. As in cancer family syndrome, colon cancers in Muir-Torre syndrome are often more proximal to the splenic flexure than in the general populace.[118]

MANAGEMENT. Regular follow-up and search for new malignancy and evaluation and monitoring of family members is necessary. Patients and their families should be counseled about genetic predisposition.

TREATMENT. The combination of interferon with retinoids may prevent tumor development. A patient with multiple sebaceous tumors, keratoacanthomas, and internal cancers was treated with interferon (IFN-alpha2a) s.c. 3 × 10(6) U three times a week along with 50 mg isotretinoin daily and topical isotretinoin gel. During a follow-up of 29 months, only 1 sebaceous skin tumor developed. No evidence of internal tumor development or recurrence was found.

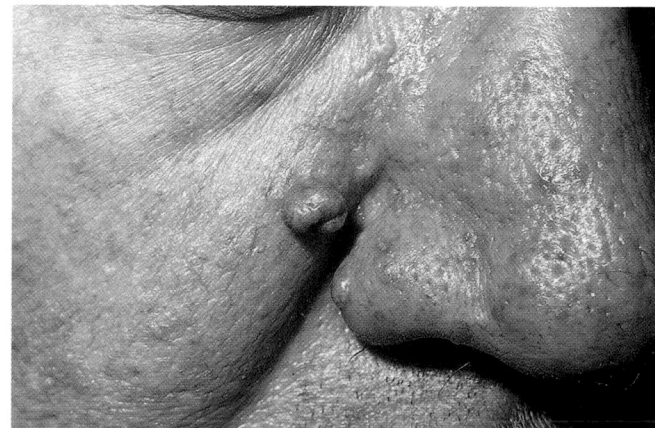

Figure 26-20 Muir-Torre syndrome. A sebaceous adenoma is the most characteristic marker of the disease.

Gardner's syndrome

Gardner's syndrome (familial adenomatous polyposis with extraintestinal manifestations) is an autosomal dominantly transmitted disease with a similar penetrance in both sexes of nearly 100%. It consists of intestinal polyposis, epidermal cysts, multiple osteomas, mesenteric fibromas,[119] desmoid tumors,[120] pigmented ocular fundus lesions, unerupted teeth, and odontomas.[121] The incidence is approximately 1 of 8300 to 1 of 16,000 births.[122] The adenomatous polyposis coli (APC) gene on chromosome 5q21 is altered by point mutations in the germ line of Gardner's syndrome patients. The identification of these genes should aid in the counseling of patients with genetic predispositions to colorectal cancer.[123-125]

CUTANEOUS SIGNS. Polyposis is a nearly constant feature, but epidermal cysts occur in approximately 35%. Epidermal cysts are frequently the presenting complaint and appear most often on the head and neck, but they frequently also occur in areas such as the legs, where epidermal cysts are rarely found. Gardner's syndrome should be considered in patients with epidermal cysts in unusual areas. The cysts can occur in childhood, but the average age at onset is 13 years.[126] They range from a few to many lesions and can be small or large enough to distort normal structures. Osteomas can be recognized clinically and radiographically in childhood. They most commonly appear on the head and neck and can be seen and felt.

Osteomas. Multiple osteomas, especially of the skull and jaws, are found in a number of affected and at-risk relatives. In some, these "markers" are found early in life, before the appearance of colonic polyps. Radiography of the jaws may serve as a valuable tool for the early detection of carriers of Gardner's syndrome.[127]

Pigmented ocular fundus lesions. Pigmented ocular fundus lesions are a reliable clinical marker for the disease and are found in 90% of patients and 47% of relatives who are at a 50% risk for Gardner's syndrome.[128,129] The presence of bilateral lesions, multiple lesions (more than four), or both is a specific and sensitive clinical marker for the syndrome. The lesions are discrete, darkly pigmented, and round, oval, or kidney shaped[128]; they range in size from 0.1 to 1 (or more) optic-disc diameters. One to 30 lesions may be present.

Thyroid carcinoma. Carcinoma of the thyroid gland is frequently reported in these patients. It has the following characteristics: female predominance (89%), youth (average 23.6; range, 16 to 40 years), papillary form (88%), and multicentricity (70%).[130] Most (55.5%) thyroid carcinomas were discovered 1 to 17 years after familial adenomatous polyposis was identified, although some have been found before (29.6%) or at the same time (14.8%) it was diagnosed.[131] The high frequency of multicentric papillary thyroid carcinoma warrants aggressive diagnostic screening at regular intervals with neck palpation and ultrasonography.

Colonic polyps and cancer. Colonic polyps can be detected before the patient reaches puberty. They are usually asymptomatic, number greater than 100, and invariably progress to adenocarcinoma. Sulindac reduces the number and size of colorectal adenomas in patients with familial adenomatous polyposis, but its effect is incomplete, and it is unlikely to replace colectomy as primary therapy.[132] Gardner's syndrome patients who undergo aggressive bowel surgery when polyps are detected can have a normal life span. All family members should be examined. Genetic counseling is essential for this autosomal dominantly inherited disease.

Pseudoxanthoma Elasticum

Pseudoxanthoma elasticum (PXE) is an inherited defect of elastic tissue with many systemic manifestations. The diagnosis relies on clinical features and the histologic demonstration of abnormal, calcified elastic fibers.[133] The disease varies widely in its degree of expression. The estimated prevalence is 1:160,000. The name *pseudoxanthoma elasticum* refers only to the cutaneous aspect of the disease, although the skin is the least severely involved organ. The syndrome is characterized by flexurally distributed, yellowish papules; vascular complications, such as accelerated atherosclerosis; hypertension; intermittent claudication; gastrointestinal bleeding; angioid streaks in the ocular fundus; blindness; and many other disorders. Calcification and fragmentation of elastic fibers of the dermis, in the media and intima of the blood vessels, and in other organs cause the complications. Patients with PXE are usually diagnosed in the third to fourth decades of life.

GENETICS. PXE is a genetic disease with different modes of inheritance and much variance in clinical expression. There is both autosomal dominant and autosomal recessive inheritance. Ninety percent of patients appear to have a sporadic or autosomal recessive inheritance pattern with early onset (average age of 13 years) and a female to male ratio of 2:1.

SKIN LESIONS. The most common presentation consists of numerous tiny, yellowish grouped papules arranged in lines in flexural areas. The most commonly affected sites are the neck and axillae (Figure 26-21). The antecubital and popliteal fossae, inguinal region, and periumbilical area may also be involved. Mucous membrane involvement can occur, most commonly on the inner aspect of the lower lip. The appearance has been compared to the skin of a plucked chicken. In severe cases the skin may be lax and hang in folds. The lesions have a xanthomatous quality; thus the designation pseudoxanthoma. The condition may be difficult to recognize if the skin is mildly affected. Degenerated and calcified elastic fibers are found internally and histologically in the skin. The onset of symptoms usually occurs in the second decade of life, although there is marked variability, and the disease is rarely diagnosed in childhood.

OCULAR CHANGES. Angioid streaks (AS) are present in over 80% of patients with PXE (Figure 26-22). Angioid streaks are seen as red-to-brown bands that vary in pigmentation. They look like irregular blood vessels and are almost always bilateral. Bruch membrane is a collagen- and elastin-containing membrane between the retina and the choroid. Degeneration of the elastic portion of Bruchs' membrane results in breaks in the thickened and calcified membrane. Formation of these rents is followed by a proliferation of the pigment epithelium over the rents. Deep brown streaks simulating blood vessels radiate in a spokelike pattern directly beyond the optic disc. Retinal changes may first be observed after the age of 20. These ocular findings may be the only sign of disease for many years. There may be a loss of central vision. Decreased visual acuity usually occurs, but complete blindness is rare.

Fluorescein angiography may show increased fluorescence in the early phase resulting from atrophy of the retinal pig-

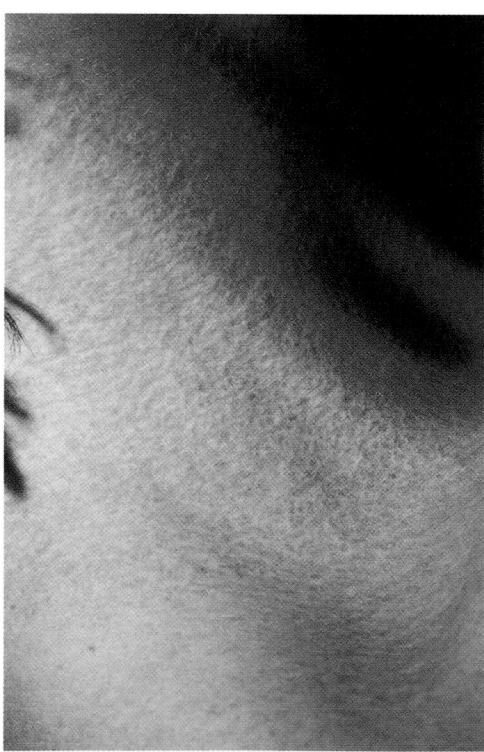

Figure 26-21 Pseudoxanthoma elasticum. Yellowish papules are found in flexural areas such as the neck and axillae.

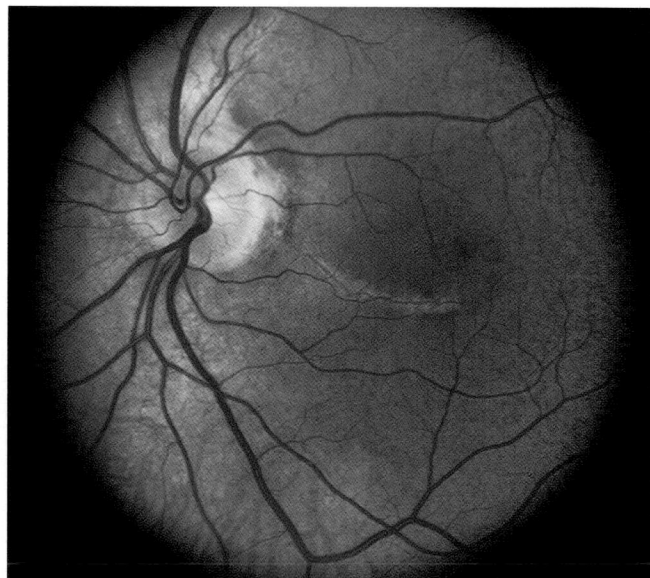

Figure 26-22 Pseudoxanthoma elasticum. Angioid streaks (cracking and fissuring of the retina) result from calcification of the elastic fibers in Bruch's membrane of the retina.

ment epithelium overlying an intact choriocapillaris. Defects in the Bruch membrane may predispose to choroidal neovascular ingrowth, which can result in subretinal hemorrhage and ultimately disciform degeneration. Macular involvement with loss of vision usually appears after age 40 years and may be a result of retinal pigment epithelium atrophy or choroidal neovascular membrane. Choroidal neovascular membranes may be treated with treatment laser photocoagulation.

Mottled hyperpigmentation is an early finding, consisting of a speckled, yellowish mottling of the posterior pole temporal to the macula. This appearance, called *peau d'orange,* is believed to be caused by changes in the retinal pigmented epithelium overlying a calcified and degenerating Bruchs' membrane. This finding is virtually pathognomonic of PXE and may be present in the first decade of the disease, before the appearance of the angioid streaks.[134] Although PXE is commonly diagnosed in patients with angioid streaks, these findings can also occur in Paget's disease of bone and sickle cell anemia.

CARDIOVASCULAR DISEASE. Calcification of the internal elastic laminae of the coronary arteries leads to narrowing of vessel lumina of mostly medium-sized arteries, resulting in symptoms similar to those of accelerated atherosclerosis.[135] Cardiovascular complications are common. Hypertension, premature atherosclerosis, angina pectoris, myocardial infarction, diminished arterial pulses, and intermittent claudication can occur. In the absence of cardiac risk factors, patients with myocardial infarction or other signs of atherosclerotic vascular disease at an early age should be investigated for PXE.

HEMORRHAGIC DIATHESIS. Gastrointestinal bleeding has resulted in fatalities. Superficial erosive lesions can be found in the gastrointestinal tract, but bleeding can occur without a source. Yellowish papular lesions have been found on the gastric mucosa. Other reported sites include subarachnoid, retinal, renal, uterine, bladder, nasal, and joint bleeding.

DIAGNOSIS. The absence of skin lesions should not be used to exclude the disorder. Nonlesional flexural skin biopsy can be used to establish the diagnosis. Histologic criteria are essential for the diagnosis of PXE. A skin biopsy demonstrating calcification and fragmentation and clumping of elastic fibers in the deep dermis or of scars in randomly chosen sites or in normal-appearing flexural skin is the gold standard for diagnosis.[136,137] Verhoeff-van Gieson staining reveals the elastic tissue changes. Von Kossa stain shows calcified elastic tissue in the middle and deep dermis.

Skin examination and fundus examination should be performed in all first-degree relatives of PXE patients, and scar or flexural biopsies should be considered if there is any suggestion of the disease. Perform a funduscopic examination on patients with early onset of cardiovascular symptoms without significant risk factors. If eye changes are found, biopsy scars and/or axillary skin.

Guide to Information for Families with Inherited Skin Disorders

National Center for Education in Maternal and Child Health (NCEMCH)
2000 15th Street, North, Suite 701
Arlington, VA 22201-2617
(703) 524-7802
www.ncemch.org

Genetic Alliance (formerly The Alliance of Genetic Support Groups, Inc.)
4301 Connecticut Avenue, NW, #404
Washington, DC 20008-2304
(202) 966-5557
(800) 336-GENE
www.geneticalliance.org/

National Organization for Rare Disorders (NORD)
P.O. Box 8923
New Fairfield, CT 06812-8923
(203) 746-6518
www.rarediseases.org/

National Neurofibromatosis Foundation, Inc.
95 Pine Street, 16th Floor
New York, NY 10005
(212) 344-NNFF(6633)
(800) 323-7938
www.nf.org

Tuberous Sclerosis Alliance
801 Roeder Road, Suite 750
Silver Spring, MD 20910
(301) 562-9890
(800) 225-6872
www.tsalliance.org/

In addition to these organizations, most medical genetics centers are happy to provide information about such groups. The address and telephone number of the nearest center can be obtained by contacting the American Board of Medical Genetics, 9650 Rockville Pike, Bethesda, MD 20814; (301) 571-1825, www.abmg.org.

References

1. McLean DI: Cutaneous paraneoplastic syndromes, Arch Dermatol 1986; 122:765.

2. Thiers BH: Dermatologic manifestations of internal cancer, CA-A CA, J Clinicians 1986; 36:130.

3. Callen JP: Skin signs of internal malignancy: fact, fancy, and fiction, Semin Dermatol 1984; 3:340.

4. Elewski BE, Gilgor RS: Eruptive lesions and malignancy, Int J Dermatol 1985; 24:617.

5. Kurzrock R, Cohen P: Cutaneous paraneoplastic syndromes in solid tumors, Am J Med 1995; 99(6):662.

6. Ellis DL, et al: Melanoma, growth factors, acanthosis nigricans, the sign of Leser-Trélat, and multiple acrochordons: a possible role for alpha-transforming growth factor in cutaneous paraneoplastic syndromes, N Engl J Med 1987; 317: 1582.

7. Abeloff MD: Paraneoplastic syndromes: a window on the biology of cancer, N Engl J Med 1986; 317:1598.

8. Wilgenbus K, et al: Further evidence that acanthosis nigricans maligna is linked to enhanced secretion by the tumour of transforming growth factor alpha, Arch Dermatol Res 1992; 284:266.

9. Sibbald R, Landolt S, Toth D: Skin and diabetes, Endocrinol Metab Clin North Am 1996; 25(2):463.

10. Perez MI, Kohn SR: Cutaneous manifestations of diabetes mellitus, J Am Acad Dermatol 1994; 30:519.

11. Lowitt MH, Dover JS: Necrobiosis lipoidica, J Am Acad Dermatol 1991; 25: 735.

12. Dwyer CM, Dick D: Ulceration in necrobiosis lipoidica: a case report and study, Clin Exp Dermatol 1993; 18:366.

13. Ferringer T, Miller F: Cutaneous manifestations of diabetes mellitus [In Process Citation], Dermatol Clin 2002; 20(3):483.

14. Goette DK: Resolution of necrobiosis lipoidica with exclusive clobetasol propionate treatment, J Am Acad Dermatol 1990; 22:855.

15. Petzelbauer P, et al: Necrobiosis lipoidica: treatment with systemic corticosteroids, Br J Dermatol 1992; 126:542.

16. Noz KC, et al: Ulcerating necrobiosis lipoidica effectively treated with pentoxifylline, Clin Exp Dermatol 1993; 18:78.

17. Statham B, Finlay AY, Marks R: A randomized double-blind comparison of an aspirin dipyridamole combination versus a placebo in the treatment of necrobiosis lipoidica, Acta Derm Venereol 1981; 61:270.

18. Eldor A, Diaz EG, Naparstek E: Treatment of diabetic necrobiosis with aspirin and dipyridamole, N Engl J Med 1977; 297:1033.

19. Beck H, et al: Treatment of necrobiosis lipoidica with low- dose acetylsalicylic acid: a randomized double-blind trial, Acta Derm Venereol 1985; 65:230.

20. Karkavitsas K, et al: Aspirin in the management of necrobiosis lipoidica, Acta Derm Venereol 1982; 62:183.

21. Unge G, Tornling G: Treatment of diabetic necrobiosis with aspirin or pipyridamole, N Engl J Med 1978; 299:1366.

22. Nguyen K, Washenik K, Shupack J: Necrobiosis lipoidica diabeticorum treated with chloroquine, J Am Acad Dermatol 2002; 46(2 Suppl Case Reports): S34.

23. Tidman M: Management of necrobiosis lipoidica [In Process Citation], Clin Exp Dermatol 2002; 27(4):328.

24. Youshock E, Beninson J: Necrobiosis lipoidica: treatment with porcine dressings, split-thickness skin grafts and pressure garments: a case report and review of treatment modalities, Angiology 1985; 36:821.

25. Nebesio C, Lewis C, Chuang T: Lack of an association between granuloma annulare and type 2 diabetes mellitus, Br J Dermatol 2002; 146(1):122.

26. Haim S, Friedman-Birnbaum R, Shafrir A: Generalized granuloma annulare: relationship to diabetes mellitus as revealed in 8 cases, Br J Dermatol 1970; 83:302.

27. Studer E, Calza A, Saurat J: Precipitating factors and associated diseases in 84 patients with granuloma annulare: a retrospective study, Dermatology 1996; 193(4):364.

28. Toro J, et al: Granuloma annulare and human immunodeficiency virus infection [see comments], Arch Dermatol 1999; 135(11):1341.

29. Friedman SJ, Winkelmann RK: Familial granuloma annulare: report of two cases and review of the literature, J Am Acad Dermatol 1987; 16:600.

30. Samlaska CP, et al: Generalized perforating granuloma annulare, J Am Acad Dermatol 1992; 27:319.

31. McDermott M, et al: Deep granuloma annulare (pseudorheumatoid nodule) in children: clinicopathologic study of 35 cases, Pediatr Dev Pathol 1998; 1(4): 300.

32. Davids JR, et al: Subcutaneous granuloma annulare: recognition and treatment, J Pediatr Orthop 1993; 13:582.

33. Felner E, Steinberg J, Weinberg A: Subcutaneous granuloma annulare: a review of 47 cases, Pediatrics 1997; 100(6):965.

34. Volden G:Successful treatment of chronic skin diseases with clobetasol propionate and a hydrocolloid occlusive dressing, Acta Derm Venereol 1992; 2(1):69.

35. Blume-Peytavi U, et al: Successful outcome of cryosurgery in patients with granuloma annulare, Br J Dermatol 1994; 130(4):494.

36. Saied N, Schwartz RA, Estes SA: Treatment of generalized annulare with dapsone, Arch Dermatol 1980; 116:1345.

37. Steiner A, Pehamberger H, Wolff K: Sulfone treatment of granuloma annulare, J Am Acad Dermatol 1985; 13:1004.

38. Schleicher SM, Milstein HJ: Resolution of disseminated granuloma annulare following isotretinoin therapy, Cutis 1985; Aug:147.

39. Czarnecki D, Gin D: The response of generalized granuloma annulare to dapsone, Acta Derm Venereol 1986; 66(1):82.

40. Botella-Estrada R, et al: Disseminated granuloma annulare: resolution with etretinate therapy, J Am Acad Dermatol 1992; 26:777.

41. Simon M, von den Driesch P: Antimalarials for control of disseminated granuloma annulare in children, J Am Acad Dermatol 1994; 31(6):1064.

42. Carlin MC, Ratz JL: A case of generalized granuloma annulare responding to hydroxychloroquine, Cleve Clin J Med 1987; 54:229.

43. Fiallo P: Cyclosporin for the treatment of granuloma annulare, Br J Dermatol 1998; 138(2):369.

44. Setterfield J, Huilgol S, Black M: Generalised granuloma annulare successfully treated with PUVA, Clin Exp Dermatol 1999; 24(6):458.

45. Smith K, Norwood C, Skelton H: Treatment of disseminated granuloma annulare with a 5-lipoxygenase inhibitor and vitamin E, Br J Dermatol 2002; 146(4):667.

46. Stone OJ: Acanthosis nigricans-decreased extracellular matrix viscosity: cancer, obesity, diabetes, corticosteroids, somatotrophin, Med Hypotheses 1993; 40:154.

47. Hud J, Jr., et al: Prevalence and significance of acanthosis nigricans in an adult obese population, Arch Dermatol 1992; 128:941.

48. Stuart C, et al: Acanthosis nigricans, J Basic Clin Physiol Pharmacol 1998; 9(2-4):407.

49. Cruz P, Jr.; Hud J, Jr: Excess insulin binding to insulin-like growth factor receptors: proposed mechanism for acanthosis nigrican, J Invest Dermatol 1992; 98:82S.

50. Tasjian D, Jarratt M: Familial acanthosis nigricans, Arch Dermatol 1984; 120:1351.

51. Coates P, et al: Resolution of nicotinic acid-induced acanthosis nigricans by substitution of an analogue (acipimox) in a patient with type V hyperlipidaemia, Br J Dermatol 1992; 126.412.

52. Pedro S: Drug-induced acanthosis nigricans, N Engl J Med 1974; 291:422.

53. Moller DE, Flier JS: Insulin resistance-mechanisms, syndromes, and implications, N Eng J Med 1991; 325:938.

54. Stuart CA, et al: Insulin resistance with acanthosis nigricans: the roles of obesity and androgen excess, Metabolism 1986; 35:197.

55. Stuart CA, et al: Prevalence of acanthosis nigricans in an unselected population, Am J Med 1989; 87:269.

56. Plourde PV, Marks JG, Jr, Hammond JM: Acanthosis nigricans and insulin resistance, J Am Acad Dermatol 1984; 10:887.

57. Cohen P, et al: Insulin resistance and acanthosis nigricans: evidence for a postbinding defect in vivo, Metabolism 1990; 39:1006.

58. Rendon MI, et al: Acanthosis nigricans: a cutaneous marker of tissue resistance to insulin, J Am Acad Dermatol 1989; 21:461.

59. Grasinger CC, et al: Vulvar acanthosis nigricans: a marker for insulin resistance in hirsute women, Fertil Steril 1993; 59:583.

60. Darmstadt GL, Yokel BK, Horn TD: Treatment of acanthosis nigricans with tretinoin, Arch Dermatol 1991; 127:1139.

61. Katz RA: Treatment of acanthosis nigricans with oral isotretinoin, Arch Dermatol 1980; 116:110.

62. Rigel DS, Jacobs MI: Malignant acanthosis nigricans: a review, J Dermatol Surg Oncol 1980; 6:923.

63. Curth HO, et al: The site and histology of the cancer associated with acanthosis nigricans, Cancer 1962; 15:433.

64. Brown J, Winkelmann RK: Acanthosis nigricans: study of 90 cases, Medicine 1968. 47:33.

65. Anderson S, Hudson-Peacock M, Muller A: Malignant acanthosis nigricans: potential role of chemotherapy, Br J Dermatol 1999; 141(4):714.

66. Cruz PD, Jr., East C, Bergstresser PR: Dermal, subcutaneous, and tendon xanthomas: diagnostic markers for specific lipoprotein disorders, J Am Acad Dermatol 1988; 19:95.

67. Fredrickson DS, Lees RS: A system for phenotyping hyperlipoproteinemia, Circulation 1965; 31:321.

68. Bergman R: The pathogenesis and clinical significance of xanthelasma palpebrarum, J Am Acad Dermatol 1994; 30:236.

69. Douste-Blazy P, et al: Increased frequency of Apo E-ND phenotype and hyperapobeta-lipoproteinemia in normolipidemic subjects with xanthelasmas of the eyelids; Ann Intern Med 1982; 96:164.

70. Illingworth D: Management of hypercholesterolemia, Med Clin North Am 2000; 84(1):23.

71. Mulvihill JJ, et al: NIH conference. Neurofibromatosis 1 (Recklinghausen disease) and neurofibromatosis 2 (bilateral acoustic neurofibromatosis). An update, Ann Intern Med 1990; 113:39.

72. Hager C, Cohen P, Tschen J: Segmental neurofibromatosis: case reports and review, J Am Acad Dermatol 1997; 37(5 Pt 2):864.

73. Crowe FW, Schull WJ, Neel JV: A clinical, pathologic, and genetic study of multiple neurofibromatosis, Adv Neurol 1981; 29:33.

74. Hope DG, Mulvihill JJ: Malignancy in neurofibromatosis, Adv Neurol 1981; 29:33.

75. Williamson TH, et al: Structure of Lisch nodules in neurofibromatosis type 1, Ophthalmic Paediatr Genet 1991; 12:11.

76. Lewis RA, Riccardi VM: von Recklinghausen neurofibromatosis: incidence of iris hamartomata, Ophthalmology 1981; 88:348.

77. Lubs ML, et al: Lisch nodules in neurofibromatosis type 1, N Engl J Med 1991; 324:1264.

78. Toonstra J, et al: Are Lisch nodules an ocular marker of the neurofibromatosis gene in otherwise unaffected family members? Dermatologica 1987; 174:232.

79. Sorensen SA, Mulvihill JJ, Nielsen A: Long-term follow-up of von Recklinghausen neurofibromatosis, N Engl J Med 1986; 314:1010.

80. Neurofibromatosis, C., Statement, National Institutes of Health Consensus Development Conference, Arch Neurol 1988; 45:575.

81. Trattner A, et al: Segmental neurofibromatosis, J Am Acad Dermatol 1990; 23:866.

82. Riccardi VM: Neurofibromatosis: the importance of localized or otherwise atypical forms, Arch Dermatol 1987; 123:882.

83. Roth RR, Martines R, James WD: Segmental neurofibromatosis, Arch Dermatol 1987; 123:917.

84. Miller M, Hall JG: Possible maternal effect on severity of neurofibromatosis, Lancet 1978; 11:1071.

85. Riccardi VM: Neurofibromatosis: past, present, and future, N Engl J Med 1991; 324:1283.

86. Sloan JB, et al: Genetic counseling in segmental neurofibromatosis, J Am Acad Dermatol 1990; 22:461.

87. Truhan AP, Filipek PA: Magnetic resonance imaging: Its role in the neuroradiologic evaluation of neurofibromatosis, tuberous sclerosis, and Sturge-Weber syndrome, Arch Dermatol 1993; 129:219.

88. Shu HH, et al: Neurofibromatosis: MR imaging findings involving the head and spine, AJR 1993; 160:159.

89. Roach E, et al: Tuberous Sclerosis Consensus Conference: recommendations for diagnostic evaluation. National Tuberous Sclerosis Association, J Child Neurol 1999; 14(6):401.

90. Hyman M, Whittemore V: National Institutes of Health consensus conference: tuberous sclerosis complex, Arch Neurol 2000; 57(5):662.

91. Nickel WR, Reed WB: Tuberous sclerosis, Arch Dermatol 962; 85:209.

92. Pack S, et al: Cutaneous tumors in patients with multiple endocrine neoplasia type 1 show allelic deletion of the MEN1 gene, J Invest Dermatol 1998; 110(4):438.

93. Hurwitz S, Braverman IM: White spots in tuberous sclerosis, J Pediatr 1970; 77:587.

94. Roth JC, Epstein CJ: Infantile spasms and hypopigmented macules: early manifestations of tuberous sclerosis, Arch Neurol 1971; 20:547.

95. Fois A, et al: Early signs of tuberous sclerosis in infancy and childhood, Helv Paediatr Acta 1973; 28:313.

96. Jozwiak S: Diagnostic value of clinical features and supplementary investigations in tuberous sclerosis in children, Acta Paediatr Hung 1992; 32:71.

97. McWilliam RC, Stephenson JBP: Depigmented hair: the earliest sign of tuberous sclerosis, Arch Dis Child 1978; 53:961.

98. Burkhart CG, El-Shaar A: Computerized axial tomography in the early diagnosis of tuberous sclerosis, J Am Acad Dermatol 1981; 4:59.

99. Menor F, et al: Neuroimaging in tuberous sclerosis: a clinicoradiological evaluation in pediatric patients, Pediatr Radiol 1992; 22:485.

100. Mlynarczyk G: Enamel pitting. A common sign of tuberous sclerosis, Ann N Y Acad Sci 1991; 615:367.

101. Crino P, Henske E: New developments in the neurobiology of the tuberous sclerosis complex, Neurology 1999; 53(7):1384.

102. Jones A, et al: Comprehensive mutation analysis of TSC1 and TSC2: and phenotypic correlations in 150 families with tuberous sclerosis, Am J Hum Genet 1999; 64(5):1305.

103. Kwiatkowska J, et al: Mosaicism in tuberous sclerosis as a potential cause of the failure of molecular diagnosis, N Engl J Med 1999; 340(9):703.

104. Inoue Y, et al: CT and MR imaging of cerebral tuberous sclerosis, Brain Dev 1998; 20(4):209.

105. Evans J, Curtis J: The radiological appearances of tuberous sclerosis, Br J Radiol 2000; 73(865):91.

106. Brownstein MH, et al: The dermatopathology of Cowden's syndrome, Br J Dermatol 1979; 100:667.

107. Salem OS, Steck WD: Cowden's disease (multiple hamartoma and neoplasia syndrome): a case report and review of the English literature, J Am Acad Dermatol 1983; 8:686.

108. Schrager C, et al: Clinical and pathological features of breast disease in Cowden's syndrome: an underrecognized syndrome with an increased risk of breast cancer, Hum Pathol 1998; 29(1):47.

109. Schrager C, et al: Similarities of cutaneous and breast pathology in Cowden's Syndrome, Exp Dermatol 1998; 7(6):380.

110. Williard W, et al: Cowden's disease. A case report with analyses at the molecular level, Cancer 1992; 69:2969.

111. Walton BJ, et al: Cowden's disease: a further indication for prophylactic mastectomy, Surgery 1986; 90:82.

112. Rothenberg J, et al: The Muir-Torre (Torre's) syndrome: the significance of a solitary sebaceous tumor, J Am Acad Dermatol 1990; 23:638.

112a. Akhtar S, et al: Muir-Torre syndrome: case report of a patient with concurrent jejunal and ureteral cancer and a review of the literature [see comments], J Am Acad Dermatol 1999; 41:681.

113. Misago N, Narisawa Y: Sebaceous neoplasms in Muir-Torre syndrome, Am J Dermatopathol 2000; 22:155.

114. Cohen PR, et al: Association of sebaceous gland tumors and internal malignancy: the Muir-Torre syndrome, Am J Med 1991; 90:606.

114a. Hampel H, Peltomaki P: Hereditary colorectal cancer: risk assessment and management, Clin Genet 2000; 58:89.

115. Cohen PR: Muir-Torre syndrome in patients with hematologic malignancies, Am J Hematol 1992; 40:64.

116. Finan MC, Connolly SM: Sebaceous gland tumors and systemic disease: a clinicopathologic analysis, Medicine 1984; 63:232.

117. Bisceglia M, Zenarola P: Muir-Torre syndrome: a case report, Tumori 1991; 77:277.

118. Lynch HT, et al: The cancer family syndrome: rare cutaneous phenotypic linkage of Torre's syndrome, Ann Intern Med 1981; 141:607.

119. Burke AP, et al: Mesenteric fibromatosis. A follow-up study, Arch Pathol Lab Med 1990; 114:832.

120. Zissiadis A, et al: Desmoid tumor in Gardner's syndrome, Am Surg 1990; 56:305.

121. Jones K, Korzcak P: The diagnostic significance and management of Gardner's syndrome, Br J Oral Maxillofac Surg 1990; 28:80.

122. Sanchez MA, et al: Be aware of Gardner's syndrome: a review of the literature, Am J Gastroenterol 1979; 71:68.

123. Paraskeva C, Williams AC: Cell and molecular biology of gastrointestinal tract cancer, Curr Opin Oncol 1992; 4:707.

124. Pathak S, et al: Identification of colon cancer-predisposed individuals: a cytogenetic analysis, Am J Gastroenterol 1991; 86:679.

125. Powell SM, et al: Molecular diagnosis of familial adenomatous polyposis, N Engl J Med 1993; 329:1982.

126. Leppard B, Bussey HJR: Epidermoid cysts, polyposis coli and Gardner's syndrome, Br J Surg 1975; 62:387.

127. Halling F, et al: Clinical and radiological findings in Gardner's syndrome: a case report and follow-up study, Dentomaxillofac Radiol 1992; 21:93.

128. Traboulsi EI, et al: A clinicopathologic study of the eyes in familial adenomatous polyposis with extracolonic manifestations (Gardner's syndrome), Am J Ophthalmol 1990; 110:550.

129. Iwama T, et al: Association of congenital hypertrophy of the retinal pigment epithelium with familial adenomatous polyposis, Br J Surg 1990; 77:273.

130. Kelly MD, et al: Carcinoma of the thyroid gland and Gardner's syndrome, Aust N Z J Surg 1993; 63:505.

131. Bell B, Mazzaferri EL: Familial adenomatous polyposis (Gardner's syndrome) and thyroid carcinoma. A case report and review of the literature, Dig Dis Sci 1993; 38:185.

132. Giardiello FM, et al: Treatment of colonic and rectal adenomas with sulindac in familial adenomatous polyposis, N Engl J Med 1993; 328:1313.

133. Sherer D, Sapadin A, Lebwohl M: Pseudoxanthoma elasticum: an update, Dermatology 1999; 199(1):3.

134. Pisani M, et al: Mottled hyperpigmentation of the fundus oculi associated with angioid streaks in pseudoxanthoma elasticum, G Ital Dermatol Venereol 1990; 125:569.

135. Lebwohl M, et al: Brief report: occult pseudoxanthoma elasticum in patients with premature cardiovascular disease, N Engl J Med 1993; 329:1237.

136. Lebwohl M, et al: Diagnosis of pseudoxanthoma elasticum by scar biopsy in patients without characteristic skin lesions. N Engl J Med 1987; 317:347.

137. Hausser I, Anton-Lamprecht I: Early preclinical diagnosis of dominant pseudoxanthoma elasticum by specific ultrastructural changes of dermal elastic and collagen tissue in a family at risk, Hum Genet 1991; 87:693.

- ❑ **Local anesthesia**

- ❑ **Hemostasis**

- ❑ **Wound healing**
  Postoperative wound care

- ❑ **Skin biopsy**
  Punch biopsy
  Shave biopsy and shave excision
  Simple scissor excision

- ❑ **Electrodesiccation and curettage**

- ❑ **Curettage**

- ❑ **Blunt dissection**

- ❑ **Cryosurgery**

- ❑ **Extraction of cysts**

- ❑ **Mohs' micrographic surgery**

- ❑ **Chemical peels**

- ❑ **Filling materials**

- ❑ **Liposuction**

- ❑ **Lasers**

- ❑ **Botulinum toxin**

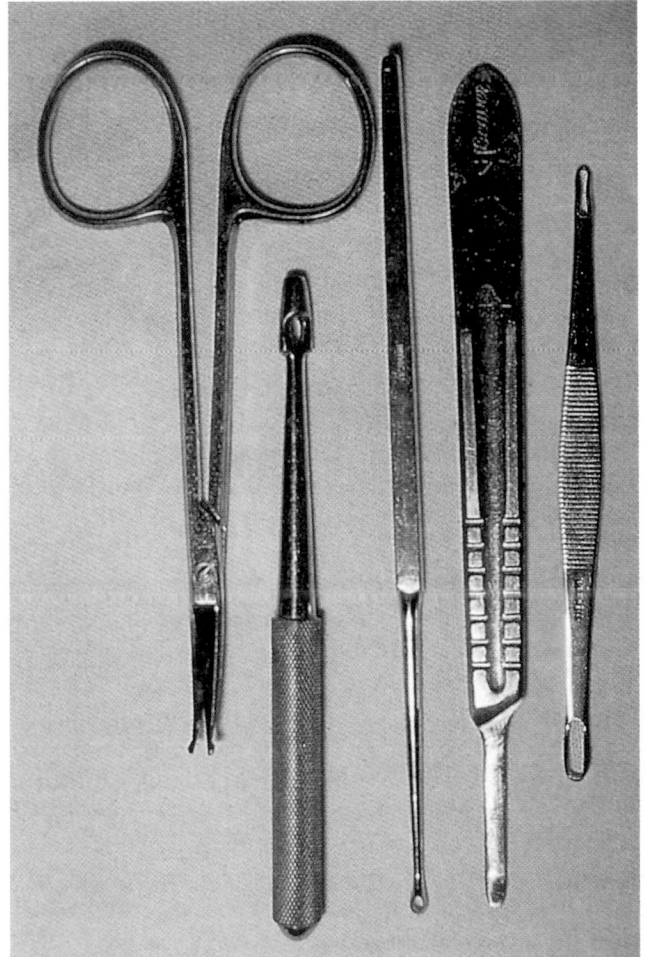

Figure 27-1 Instruments used for basic dermatologic surgical procedures. From left to right: curved probe-tipped scissors, 3-mm dermal punch, #1 curet, blunt dissector, Schamberg comedo expressor.

Punch biopsy, shave biopsy, electrodesiccation and curettage, blunt dissection, and simple excision and suture closure are the basic techniques that physicians who treat skin disease should learn. One should be familiar with the more sophisticated techniques, such as Mohs' micrographic surgery, so that referral to physicians who perform these techniques can be made at the proper time. The instruments used for most basic dermatologic surgical procedures are shown in Figure 27-1.

Local Anesthesia

Lidocaine (Xylocaine) 1% or 2%, with or without epinephrine, is used for most surgical procedures.[1] The onset of anesthesia is almost instantaneous, and the duration is adequate for most minor procedures. A 27- or, preferably, a 30-gauge needle is used.

EPINEPHRINE. The vasoconstriction induced by epinephrine prevents absorption of lidocaine, prolongs anesthesia, and controls bleeding. Xylocaine with epinephrine is generally not used on fingertips. Very small quantities are usually tolerated on the nose and pinna.

LIDOCAINE ALLERGY. Allergy to lidocaine is very rare.[2,3] Most patients who claim to be allergic have had a vasovagal response. Bacteriostatic saline is an alternative for patients who are allergic to lidocaine (see the following discussion).

PAIN REDUCTION. Anesthetics produce a sharp pain during skin infiltration. Pain is greater with rapid injections and can be minimized with slow injections through a 30-gauge needle. The needle should be inserted slowly but firmly into the dermis. A needlestick at 90 degrees to the skin surface causes less pain because fewer nerves are transversed by the needle.[4] The skin is rapidly pinched between the thumb and forefinger and shaken just before and during the injection.[5] Pinching the skin in the area to be injected either distracts the patient or blocks the transmission of pain impulses caused by the injections. Placing the needle distal to the area of pinched skin is more effective. Anesthesia is initiated by injecting a tiny amount of fluid; after a few seconds, infiltration is continued slowly until the skin surrounding the lesion blanches. A wheal can be raised by inserting the needle almost vertically. Penetration of the thick palm and sole skin is very painful. The area about the nostrils is very sensitive. Intrafollicular injection into the large follicles of the nose and cheeks minimizes pain. Superficial injections into the penis and vulva are well tolerated.

PAINLESS ANESTHESIA. Icing the lesion for 1 minute numbs the skin and minimizes needle-penetration pain. Adequate anesthesia with little or no infiltration pain can be induced with the following preparations. Bacteriostatic saline and lidocaine diluted with bacteriostatic saline solution are less painful than 1% lidocaine with sodium bicarbonate. It is unlikely that the pain of infiltration is a simple function of the pH of the anesthetic solution.[6]

Bacteriostatic saline. Commercially available bacteriostatic saline contains benzyl alcohol, which acts as a painless anesthetic. The anesthetic effect dissipates rapidly when injected subcutaneously. The volume of saline required to achieve anesthesia is at least 2 to 3 times that required when using 1% lidocaine and is of brief duration.

Saline and epinephrine. The addition of epinephrine 3 ml of 1 mg/ml (1:100,000 dil.) to 30 ml of bacteriostatic saline extends the duration of anesthesia from 4 minutes to 120 minutes. Bacteriostatic saline should not be used as an anesthetic for newborns.

Saline diluted with lidocaine. A mixture of saline (27 ml) and lidocaine 1% with or without epinephrine (3 ml) is also effective.

Buffered lidocaine. The addition of sodium bicarbonate reduces the pain produced by infiltration of lidocaine with or without epinephrine.[7] One milliliter of Neutra-Caine, a 7.5% sodium bicarbonate buffer solution, is added to 5 ml of lidocaine or bupivacaine. Buffered lidocaine and epinephrine maintain greater than a 90% concentration 2 weeks after buffering when stored at 0° to 4° C. This permits batch buffering and storage for up to 2 weeks when properly refrigerated.[8] $NaHCO_3$ enhances the killing effect that has been described for lidocaine alone. The inability to recover common pathogenic bacteria from biopsy specimens could be the result of exposure to lidocaine buffered with $NaHCO_3$. Warming the local mixture to 40° C reduces the discomfort of injection even further.[9]

The ice-saline–lidocaine technique. This is a simple method of minimizing pain when obtaining local anesthesia. Cryogel packs are applied before the local anesthetic injection to minimize the pain of piercing the skin with the injection needle. The surgical field is then infiltrated with benzyl alcohol–containing normal saline. Subsequently, lidocaine with epinephrine can be infiltrated without discomfort.[10]

EMLA, ELA-Max. EMLA is a mixture of 2.5% lidocaine and 2.5% prilocaine in an oil and water emulsion. ELA-Max is a topical anesthetic cream with 4% lidocaine at pH 7.4. These agents should be applied to the desired area for approximately 1 hour under an occlusive dressing. They provide effective analgesia, making them useful for superficial surgery, split-thickness skin grafts, venipuncture, argon laser treatment, epilation, and debridement of infected ulcers. Other indications have included use in postherpetic neuralgia, hyperhidrosis, painful ulcers, and inhibition of itching and burning.[11] A single application of ELA-Max in a child weighing less than 10 kg and between 10 and 20 kg should not be applied over an area larger than 100 cm².

Hemostasis

Monsel's solution (ferric subsulfate) is a valuable agent for providing rapid hemostasis. It is particularly effective in controlling bleeding after curettage of seborrheic keratosis and basal cell carcinoma. Immediate hemostasis is most efficiently achieved if the solution is applied when the wound is not bleeding. To exert tension and stop bleeding, the thumb and index finger are placed at the opposite edges of the wound, and the skin is stretched. The blood is then wiped with gauze, the Monsel's solution is applied with a cotton-tipped applicator, and the tension is maintained for approximately 15 seconds. The lack of blood flow apparently allows more complete coagulation.

MONSEL'S ARTIFACT. When a biopsy is repeated, an area of skin that has been treated with Monsel's solution has a pigmented artifact that can interfere with histologic interpretation. The use of Monsel's solution should be avoided after biopsies of pigmented lesions or tumors that may prove to be diagnostic problems. The pathologist should be informed if Monsel's solution had been used.[12]

Wound Healing

Types of cutaneous wounds

FULL-THICKNESS WOUNDS. The epidermis and the full thickness of the dermis are lost. The defect is deeper than the adnexa (hair follicles, eccrine sweat ducts). These wounds heal by contraction (associated with myofibroblast development), granulation tissue formation (with fibroplasia and neovascularization), and reepithelialization. Contraction causes a 40% decrease in the size of the wound. Epithelialization occurs from the wound edges.

PARTIAL-THICKNESS WOUNDS. The epidermis and some portion of the dermis with parts of the adnexa remain in the wound bed. Such wounds are produced by shave excisions, curettage and electrodesiccation, dermabrasion, chemical peels, and carbon dioxide (CO_2) laser surgery. These wounds heal quickly through reepithelialization from the wound edges and adnexal structures in the base of the wound. Wound contraction is minimal when only the most superficial portion of the dermis has been lost.

Physiology of wound healing

WOUND CONTRACTION AND SCAR FORMATION. Wound contraction begins at 1 week after the wound occurs. Light colonization with pathogenic bacteria may not interfere, but infection inhibits healing. Tensile strength in a wound increases progressively up to 1 year after the wound occurs. Tensile strength in a healed wound is always less than 80% of normal. Healing time is related to the logarithm of the area. The width of the wound is a better predictor of healing time than is the area in which the wound occurred. Wounds created by destructive techniques (e.g., cryosurgery, electrosurgery, laser surgery, and chemical cautery) heal more slowly than clean wounds created by scalpel or curet surgery.

CELLULAR CHANGES. Neutrophils appear in a wound 6 hours after the event, reach their greatest number after 24 to 48 hours, and start to disappear after 72 hours. Neutrophils are not crucial to wound healing; neutropenia does not interfere with healing. Fibroblasts populate the wound after 48 to 72 hours. Their growth is enhanced by low oxygen and high lactate levels. Fibroblasts synthesize collagen and elastin. Myofibroblasts are modified fibroblasts that resemble smooth muscle cells in morphology and function. They contain large amounts of contractile proteins and are responsible for wound contraction.[13]

REEPITHELIALIZATION. Epidermal healing first depends on epidermal cell migration (first 24 hours) and later on epidermal cell mitosis, which peaks after 48 hours. Keratinocytes initially migrate over a matrix of fibronectin, fibrin, collagen, and elastin. This matrix acts as a structural support for cell migration. Epidermal migration and proliferation occur from the epithelial cells at the edge of the wound and from appendageal structures remaining in the wound bed. The rate of reepithelialization is directly related to the moistness of the wound. Open, dry wounds reepithelialize slower than occluded, moist wounds. The migration of keratinocytes beneath a dry crust is slower than migration over an occluded, moist wound, where the plane of epithelial cell migration lies near the wound surface (Figure 27-2).

Figure 27-2 Occlusive dressing. The effects of tissue humidity on reepithelialization are shown. Occlusive dressings allow epithelialization to occur at the wound surface. In open wounds the epithelium migrates beneath a desiccated crust and devitalized dermis.

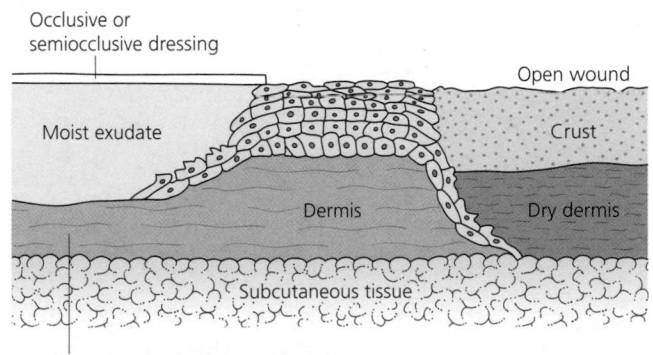

Impairment of wound healing

TOPICAL THERAPY. Topical steroids may interfere with healing because of their antiinflammatory action (Table 27-1).

ANTISEPTIC SOLUTIONS. One percent povidone-iodine, 3% hydrogen peroxide, and 0.5% chlorhexidine solutions are toxic for fibroblasts and keratinocytes and may delay the formation of granulation tissue.

HEMOSTATIC SOLUTIONS. Monsel's solution (ferric subsulfate), 30% aluminum chloride, and silver nitrate produce tissue necrosis and delay reepithelialization. The effect on small wounds is minimal.

Contact dermatitis

Contact allergic reactions may occur with tapes and antibiotic ointments. Neomycin is a common sensitizer and should be avoided. Polysporin and Bacitracin are not common sensitizers.

SYSTEMIC FACTORS. Malnutrition interferes with healing. Vitamin C and zinc deficiencies lead to poor healing. Systemic steroids in a dosage greater than 10 mg a day interfere with healing. Clinical experience suggests no impairment of wound healing for patients taking chemotherapeutic drugs.

Wound dressings

WOUND DRESSINGS—MECHANISM OF ACTION. Occlusion of wounds leads to faster healing.[14] The process of neovascularization within granulation tissue is stimulated by hypoxic conditions such as those that occur beneath occlusive, oxygen-impermeable dressings. Occlusive dressings prevent crust formation and drying of the wound bed. The rate of epithelialization is faster under occlusive dressings.

Wound fluid under occlusive dressings is favorable to fibroblast proliferation. Adhesive occlusive dressings may remove newly formed epithelium. Hydrocolloid adhesive occlusive dressings prevent entry of bacteria into the wound. The use of occlusive dressings in chronic wounds leads to less pain, better granulation tissue, and painless wound debridement. In acute wounds, occlusive dressings promote bacterial growth but result in faster reepithelialization.

FUNCTION. Protection with dressings exerts pressure and maintains a moist wound environment. They reduce pain when applied to partial-thickness wounds. Topical antimicrobial agents that may enhance reepithelialization include neomycin, polymyxin B, Neosporin ointment, silver sulfadiazine, and 20% benzoyl peroxide lotion. Hexachlorophene, chlorhexidine, and alcohol may retard reepithelialization.[15]

OCCLUSIVE DRESSINGS. Crust formation is suppressed if the surface of the wound is kept moist by an occlusive film or by gauze applied over Polysporin. The level of adequate tissue humidity is then very close to the skin surface, and the epidermis migrates rapidly over the moist bed. Patients treated with occlusive dressings tend to have softer, smoother, smaller, and more superficial scars. There does not seem to be an increased incidence of infection with occlusive dressings. Occlusive dressings reduce wound pain. So-called oxygen-permeable membranes do not seem to transmit oxygen to the wound.[16] Many synthetic occlusive dressings are available for a variety of wounds (see Chapter 3); examples of clinical uses include the following:
   • Arterial and venous catheter sites
   • Burns
   • Decubitus ulcers
   • Dermabrasion site after tattoo removal
   • Leg ulcers following pinch grafts
   • Mohs' micrographic wounds
   • Skin graft donor sites
   • Stasis ulcers
   • Surgical incisions
   • Traumatic wounds

APPLICATION TECHNIQUES

Occlusive dressings. Occlusive dressings (e.g., Duoderm) are best suited to chronic wounds, such as venous ulcers. Good preparation of surrounding skin by cleansing with hydrogen peroxide and drying with gauze ensures secure adhesion. Excess skin oil is removed with alcohol. At least 2.5 cm of margin around the wound should be allowed to prevent leakage. The length of time occlusive dressings should stay on a wound varies; dressings should be left in place until they start leaking fluid from their sides. Early removal of dressings can lead to stripping of delicate new epithelium. Initially, dressings usually need to be changed every other day. Thereafter, they may be left in place for many days if excess fluid does not accumulate. Dressings applied over fresh wounds accumulate large amounts of fluid that can be removed by needle aspiration.

Table 27-1 Topical Agents that Affect Epidermal Migration	
Agents	Relative rate of healing (%)*
Triamcinolone acetonide ointment (0.1%)	−34
Furacin	−30
USP Petrolatum	−8
Eucerin	+5
Benoxyl lotion base (benzoyl peroxide preparation)	+14
Silvadene cream	+28
Neosporin ointment	+28
Telfa dressing	+14
*Compared with untreated.	

Patients who disrupt new epithelium by careless removal of adherent dressings should use a nonadherent dressing such as Vigilon.[17] Dressings should not be applied to inflamed eczematous skin at the borders of stasis ulcers.

Semipermeable dressings. Semipermeable dressings (Opsite, Tegaderm) are an option for partial-thickness open wounds. These are changed when the amount of wound exudate becomes excessive. Vigilon is an oxygen-permeable dressing that consists of 4% polyethylene oxide and 96% water. It absorbs its own weight of exudate and, with the exterior polyethylene film removed, excess exudate can be absorbed by overlying absorbent dressings. Vigilon is nonadherent and maintains a moist wound environment. Vigilon is removed and a new dressing is applied every 24 to 48 hours.

Postoperative wound care (Box 27-1)

Partial and full-thickness open wounds
1. Avoid alcohol and aspirin in the immediate postoperative period.
2. Keep wounds covered and moist (e.g., with Polysporin or Bacitracin) to prevent crusts.
3. Bathing of granulating wounds is allowed. Avoid cleansing with hydrogen peroxide or povidone-iodine.
4. Undressed sutured wounds can be washed with soap and water twice a day starting the morning after surgery.

Sutured wounds
OFFICE
1. Semipermeable tape strips (e.g., Steristrips, Clearon skin closures) reduce tension across the suture line. Spaces left between the strips allow wound exudate to escape and to be absorbed by the overlying dressing.
2. A nonadherent primary dressing may then be applied, taped in place, and covered with a pressure dressing applied (bulky gauze) and secured by adhesive tape.
3. Tissue adhesives (tincture of benzoin, Mastisol) are applied to the skin to increase the adherence of tape to the skin.
4. Pressure dressings (applied for 24 to 36 hours) reduce the risk of hematoma formation following the excision of cysts.

HOME. Small wounds do not require dressing for more than 24 to 48 hours.
1. Change dressing once or twice daily. The dressing may be left in place for uncomplicated dry wounds until the sutures are removed.
2. Cleanse with a mild liquid soap, sterile saline, or hydrogen peroxide solution.
3. An antibiotic ointment (e.g., Bacitracin) is applied and the wound is covered with a nonadherent dressing. The antibiotic ointment reduces the risk of the contact layer of the dressing adhering to the wound bed.
4. A pressure dressing is applied if required.

EXCESS GRANULATION TISSUE. Granulation tissue is a loose collection of fibroblasts, inflammatory cells, and new vessels in an edematous matrix that forms at the base of open wounds. It provides a foundation for reepithelialization. Excessive granulation tissue rises above the wound surface, imposing a barrier to the inward-migrating epidermis. Certain areas, such as the scalp, temples, and lower legs, are prone to form exuberant granulation tissue in open surgical wounds or ulcers. Excess granulation tissue must be removed or suppressed. One technique is to curet the tissue and rub the base with a silver nitrate stick.

Scarlet red gauze. Recurrent granulation tissue can be very effectively suppressed with scarlet red gauze, which is available in prepackaged wrappers. The deep purple-colored gauze is applied over the tissue, covered with white gauze, and secured with tape. The dressing is changed daily until reepithelialization is complete. The results can be amazing.

SCAR FORMATION. The evolution of a scar takes several months. New scars are thick and vascular, but gradually, over months, they become less vascular, nonbulky, and flat. Scars that remain thick (hypertrophic scars) or become inappropriately large (keloids) can be treated with intralesional steroids (see Chapter 20).

Box 27-1 Wound Management Guidelines

1. Use antiseptics for disinfection of intact skin only.
2. Select a method of wounding that minimizes tissue necrosis.
3. Use pinpoint electrocoagulation, pressure, topical thrombin, collagen, or gelatin rather than caustic agents to establish hemostasis.
4. Apply topical antibiotics to the wound instead of antiseptics to prevent wound infection and to accelerate healing.
5. Substitute tap water for hydrogen peroxide to cleanse wounds.
6. Use nonadherent occlusive dressing on wounds to accelerate healing.

From Brown CD, Zitelli JA: J Dermatol Surg Oncol 1993; 19:732.

Skin Biopsy

A skin biopsy can be performed simply in the office. Several techniques are practiced, and each has specific advantages (Table 27-2).

CHOICE OF SITE. Generally, biopsies should not be taken from lesions below the knee if other sites are available. Specimens from this area are sometimes difficult for the pathologist to interpret, particularly specimens taken from older patients, in whom mild inflammation and pigmentation produced by stasis may be present. On the face, particularly in the elderly, the arteries are superficial at the following three locations: the temple lateral to the eyebrow (the temporal artery), the nasolabial fold as it intersects the alae (angular artery), and the supraorbital notch at the medial end of the brow (the supraorbital artery). Arteries may be injured by a deep punch biopsy at these sites.

SELECTION OF LESION FOR BIOPSY. As a general rule, biopsies should be taken from lesions that are fresh but well developed. Very early lesions may not have developed diagnostic histologic features, and older lesions may be excoriated or crusted. However, it is important to perform biopsies of very early lesions for diagnosis of vesiculobullous diseases, such as pemphigus and dermatitis herpetiformis. Chronic diseases such as discoid lupus erythematosus may not develop diagnostic features for weeks; biopsies of older lesions should be performed in these cases.

Punch biopsy

A full thickness of skin can easily be obtained with a cylindric dermal punch biopsy tool. Disposable punches are very convenient (e.g., the Baker-Cummins punch). They are available in 2-mm, 3-mm, 3.5-mm, 4-mm, and 6-mm widths. The 3-mm punch is adequate for most lesions. Biopsies of the face may be performed with a 2-mm punch to minimize scarring. The resulting wound has smooth, round edges and heals with a slightly depressed scar.

Table 27-2 Dermatologic Biopsy Techniques

Type of biopsy	Indications
Punch	Most superficial inflammatory and bullous diseases; benign and malignant tumors except malignant melanoma
Shave	Superficial benign and malignant tumors (e.g., seborrheic keratoses, warts, dome-shaped nevi, and non-melanoma malignancies)
Excision	Deep inflammatory diseases (e.g., erythema nodosum); malignant melanoma

The procedure is adequate for the diagnosis of most tumors. If possible, lesions suspected of being malignant melanoma should be removed completely intact with an excisional biopsy. The quantity of tissue may be inadequate for diagnosis of inflammatory diseases and diseases of adipose tissue, such as erythema nodosum.

Suturing round or oval defects produced by the punch may decrease healing time. Healing by secondary intention is slow but cosmetically acceptable.

PUNCH BIOPSY TECHNIQUE. The site is prepared for biopsy with an alcohol pad; a sterile technique is not required. Local anesthesia is induced with 1% lidocaine with epinephrine. Epinephrine is avoided for biopsy near the fingertips. The injection is positioned around and under but not directly into the lesion.

The surrounding tissue is supported by stretching the skin with the thumb and index finger of the free hand. The punch is rotated back and forth between the thumb and forefinger while it is simultaneously pushed vertically into the tissue. Resistance is felt while the instrument penetrates through the dermis but ceases as the punch sinks quickly on entry into the subcutaneous tissue (Figure 27-3, A and B).

The punch is withdrawn and the cylindric piece of tissue is gently supported with smooth-tipped forceps; the specimen is cut deep with scissors to include subcutaneous tissue. Forceps with teeth may crush the specimen (Figure 27-3, C).

The tissue is immediately transferred to a preservative, and bleeding is controlled with gauze pressure or Monsel's solution (Figure 27-3, D). Some surgeons prefer to apply a single suture to punch defects larger than 3 mm.

Shave biopsy and shave excision

Shave biopsy and shave excision are useful for elevated lesions and when a full thickness of tissue is unimportant. The technique, therefore, is not useful for most inflammatory skin diseases. Shave excision of nevi produces excellent cosmetic results. Any pigmented lesion suspected of being a melanoma should be totally removed by excisional biopsy.

SHAVE TECHNIQUE. The lesion is elevated from the surrounding skin by infiltration with lidocaine. The surrounding skin is supported with the thumb and forefinger of the free hand. The flat surface of a #15 surgical blade is laid against the skin next to the lesion. With long strokes, the blade is smoothly drawn through the lesion; back-and-forth sawing motions produce a jagged surface (Figure 27-4). Several strokes may be required around the periphery of larger lesions. The last attachment of skin may be severed more easily with scissors than with a scalpel blade. Rough edges and contours can be smoothed with electrocautery, and bleeding can be controlled with Monsel's solution.

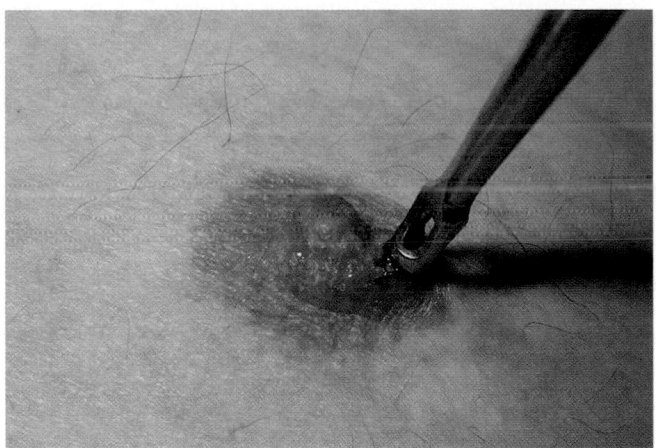

A, The dermal punch is rotated back and forth while gently advancing it through the dermis into the subcutaneous tissue.

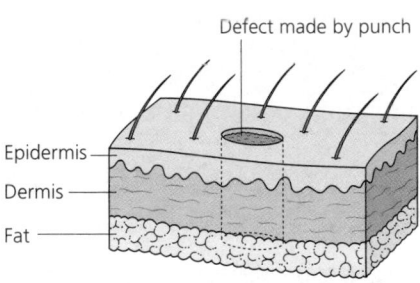

B, The punch should be introduced through the dermis and into the fat.

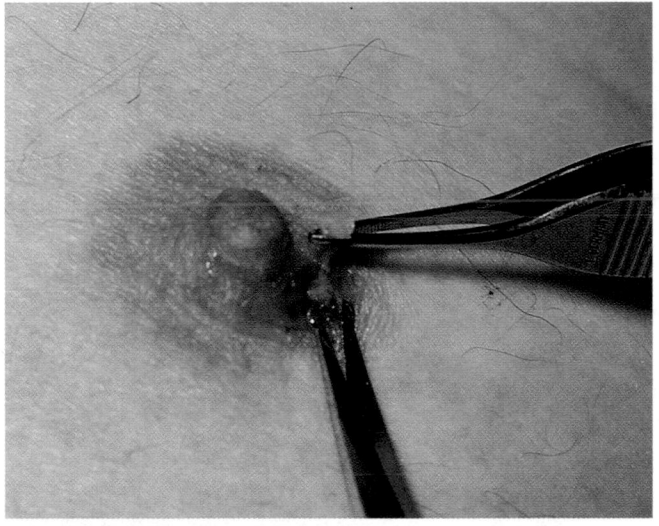

C, The cylindric piece of tissue is gently supported with forceps and cut deep to include subcutaneous tissue.

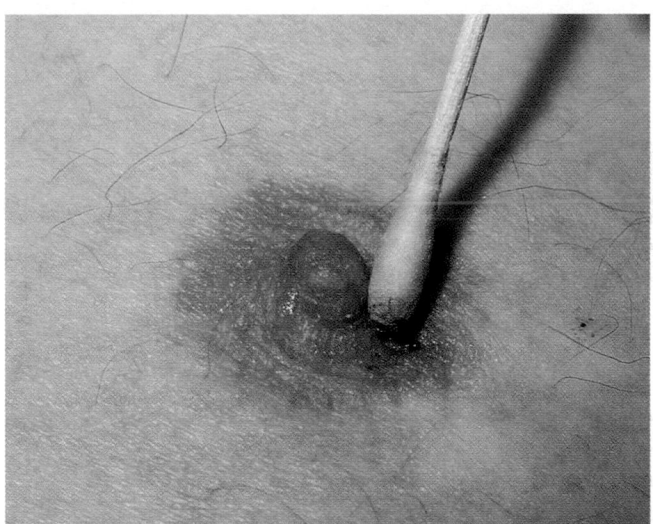

D, Bleeding is controlled with Monsel's solution.

Figure 27-3 Punch biopsy.

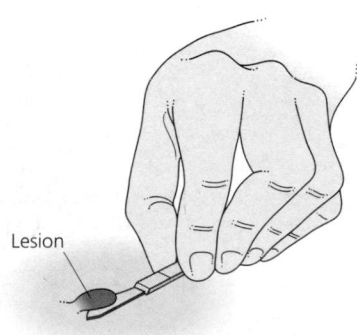

Figure 27-4 Shave excision. The curved surgical blade is laid flat on the skin surface and smoothly drawn through the base of the lesion.

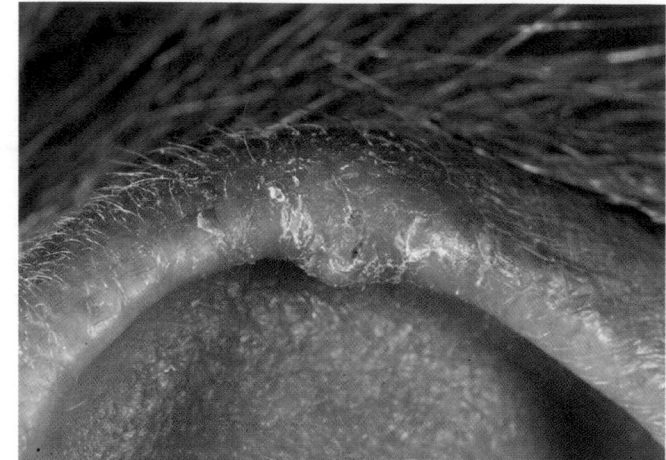

A

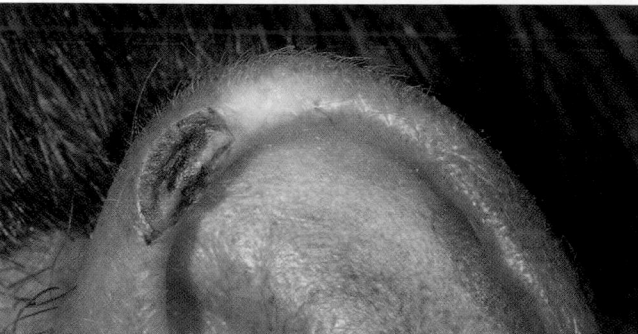

B

Figure 27-6 Simple scissor excision.

Simple scissor excision

Firm lesions that resist curettage may be removed by simple scissor excision. Polypoid and dome-shaped nevi, firm seborrheic keratoses, warts, and corns are removed by resting the curved section of curved, probe-pointed scissors on the skin surface and cutting about the border while slowly advancing the tip of the scissors toward the center of the lesion. The curet is used to remove any remaining tissue fragments. The resulting defect is usually smooth and remains on the same plane as the skin surface (Figures 27-5 and 27-6). Rough edges and contours can be smoothed with electrocautery.

A, Chondrodermatitis nodularis chronica helicis before scissor excision.
B, The lesion was excised, and the surface healed with a white, smooth scar. Another lesion appeared anterior to the first and was excised by scissor excision. Note the exposed cartilage.

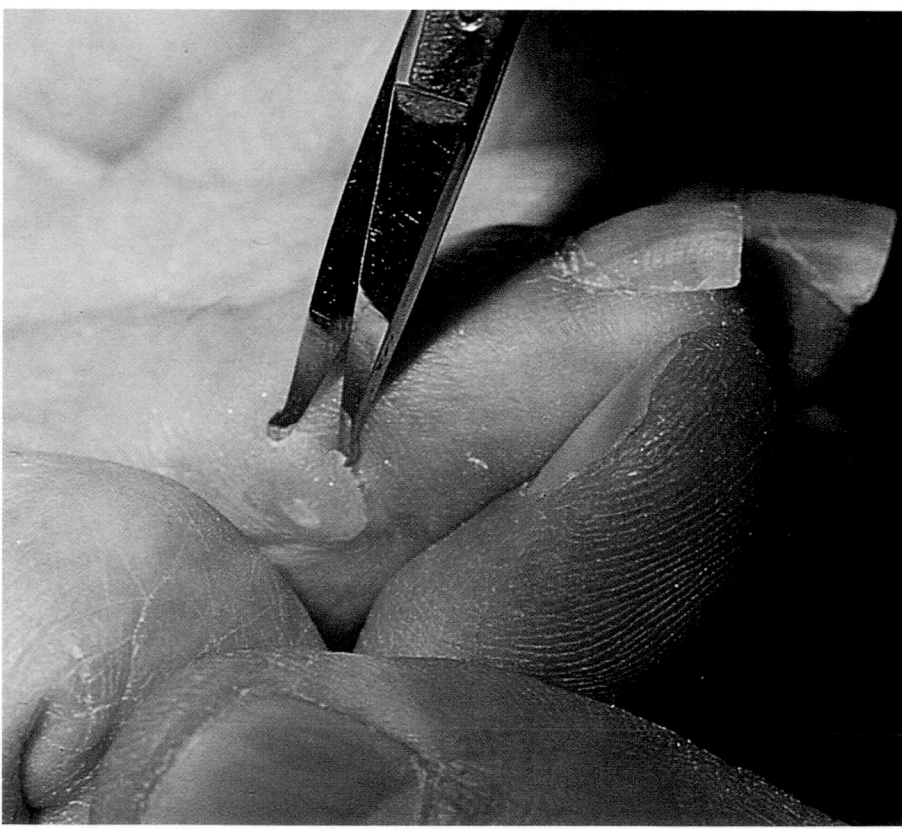

Figure 27-5 Scissor excision of a corn.

Electrodesiccation and Curettage

INDICATIONS. Electrodesiccation and curettage (ED&C) is an invaluable technique for removing a variety of superficial skin lesions, such as seborrheic keratoses, basal cell epitheliomas, squamous cell carcinomas, pyogenic granulomas, granulation tissue, and genital warts. Electrodesiccation without curettage is sufficient for spider angiomas; small digitate, filiform, and genital warts; and small skin tags about the neck and axillae. The curet may be used without electrodesiccation to remove soft seborrheic and actinic keratoses and filiform warts.

EQUIPMENT. The required instruments are an electrodesiccation unit and a set of sharp dermal curets. Many inexpensive electrosurgical office units are capable of executing electrodesiccation, fulguration, and coagulation. Examples of commonly used electrosurgical office units are the Electricator, Hyfrecator, Bantam Bovie, and Ritter coagulator.

PACEMAKER PATIENTS. Modern pacemakers are very resistant to electrical interference. Simple electrosurgery of small lesions on relatively healthy patients who have pacemakers poses negligible risks. Both cardiac pacemakers and defibrillators can, however, be affected by electrosurgery.[18] The cardiologist can assist in defining the patient's risks and dependency on the device, preoperatively preparing the patient, and assisting in selecting the appropriate precautionary measures once the input of the appropriate electrosurgical technique is known.

Techniques

Electrodesiccation and fulguration are accomplished without the use of an indifferent electrode. The effects are superficial; electrodesiccation and fulguration are the techniques of choice for most dermatologic applications.[19,20] Coagulation produces greater tissue destruction and requires the use of an indifferent electrode.[21]

FULGURATION. The surface to be treated should be dry and relatively free of blood. The pointed electrode is held slightly away from the tissue surface; a "sparking" occurs, resulting in superficial dehydration (Figure 27-7, A). The tissues in the immediate surrounding area are charred. Hemostasis can be accomplished only if the field is dry.

DESICCATION. The pointed electrode contacts the skin surface or is inserted slightly into the tissue (Figure 27-7, B). The resulting char of the tissue is essentially produced by fulguration. As with fulguration, hemostasis is possible only if the field is wiped dry.

ELECTROCOAGULATION. The bipolar setting is required. The active electrode (needle, small ball) is placed in contact with the tissue. Because of increased amperage, tissue necrosis tends to be more extensive than that produced by fulguration or desiccation. The greater production of heat and the conduction of current along vessels makes hemostasis possible in a bloody field.

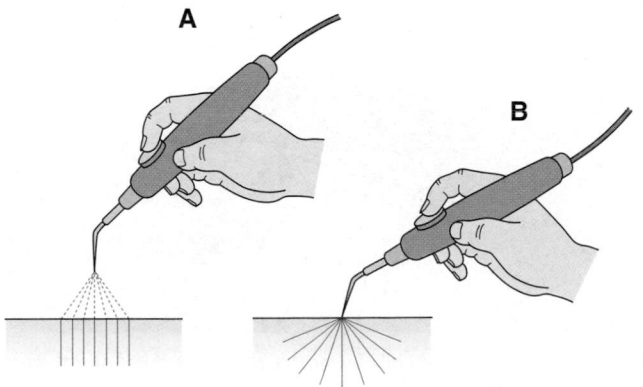

Figure 27-7 A, Electrofulguration—the needle is held above the skin surface. **B,** Electrodesiccation—the needle touches the skin surface. (*From Boughton RS, Spencer SK: J Am Acad Dermatol 862-867, 1987.*)

Curettage

Curettage is a scraping or scooping technique used to remove soft tumors, such as seborrheic keratoses, or tissues that have been softened by electrosurgery. Superficial growths are removed with minimal destruction of normal tissue. In many instances curettage is followed by electrodesiccation to control bleeding and destroy remaining fragments of tissue. Electrodesiccation, however, results in more hypopigmentation and scarring.

INDICATIONS. Seborrheic keratoses, warts, molluscum contagiosum, actinic keratoses, Bowen's disease, basal cell carcinoma, and squamous cell carcinoma may all be treated by curettage with or without electrosurgery.

INSTRUMENTS. A dermal curet has a round or oval, sharp ring. Curets are available in diameters ranging from 1 to 7 mm. Instruments with smaller diameters are most useful for minor procedures.

Techniques—curettage

Local anesthesia is induced with 1% lidocaine with epinephrine injected with a 27- or 30-gauge needle.

PENCIL TECHNIQUE. The pencil technique is best for most soft lesions. Fine, precise movements are possible. The handle of the curet is grasped like a pencil between the thumb and the index and middle fingers. The base of the palm rests on the skin for stability. The skin around the lesion is stretched and held taut by the fingers of the surgeon's free hand. With several smooth, firm strokes (Figure 27-8, A and B), the curet is drawn through the tissue. The curet may be pulled toward the surgeon with the index finger[22,23] or pushed away with the thumb. The surgeon may actually feel the consistency of the tumor with the curet. This is very helpful when curetting nodular basal cell epithelioma, which has a firm, gelatin-like consistency. The dermis at the base of the tumor is very firm and resists curettage. The interface between the tumor and the dermis is not as distinct in elderly patients with actinically damaged dermal connective tissue. Bleeding is controlled with Monsel's solution.

Techniques—electrodesiccation and curettage of basal cell carcinoma[24,25]

The technique for electrodesiccation and curettage of nodular and superficial basal cell carcinoma (BCC) is as follows: Local anesthesia is induced with 1% lidocaine and epinephrine. The surrounding tissue is supported with the finger, and the soft, friable tumor, which has a less cohesive texture, is curetted until firm dermis is reached. The underlying dermal fibrous tissue is hard, unyielding, and almost impossible to dislodge. The soft-textured tumor offers little resistance to the curet, and more than 90% of the tumor mass can be quickly removed (Figure 27-8, B). The entire surface and border is electrodesiccated or coagulated by slowly drawing the probe back and forth until a uniform char has been created at the base. The charred tissue is removed with the curet, and the desiccation and curettage is repeated two more times or until a normal tissue plane is observed and developed throughout. Desiccating and curetting is continued approximately 0.5 cm beyond the visible borders of the lesion to ensure that microscopic extensions of the tumor are destroyed. Active bleeding from the base may indicate residual tumor. Tumor-free dermis oozes blood in a uniform manner. Bleeding is controlled with Monsel's solution.

POSTOPERATIVE CARE. The wound may be left exposed to the air or may be covered with a bandage or light dressing. Daily washing with soap and water is encouraged. For large surgical defects that are allowed to heal by secondary intention, infection is prevented and crust formation is discouraged by applying Vaseline or an ointment-based topical antibiotic such as Bacitracin. The wound may be washed and intermittently covered with an adhesive bandage or gauze if desired.

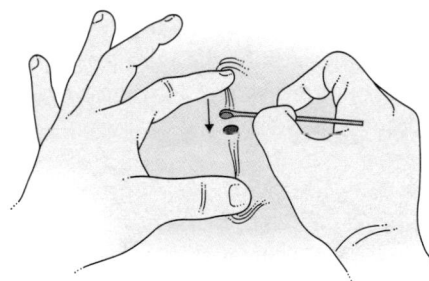

A, Pencil technique demonstrating method of holding curet and two-way tension planes for stabilizing the lesion.

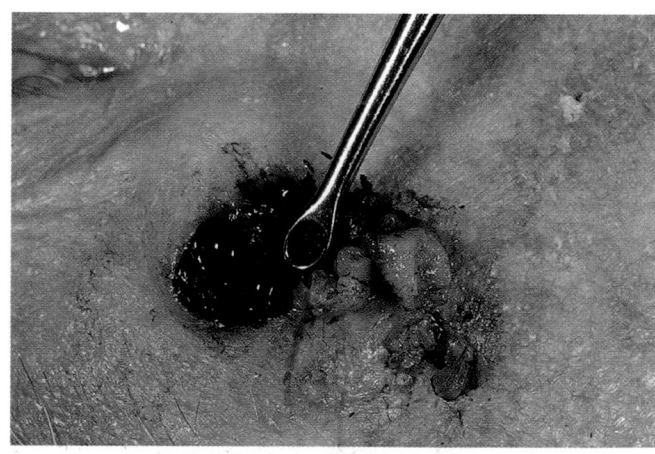

B, Curettage of a basal cell carcinoma with a #1 curet and the pencil technique.

Figure 27-8 Curettage technique.

Blunt Dissection

Blunt dissection is a simple surgical procedure for removing epidermal tumors, such as warts[26,27] and keratoacanthoma[28]; the technique is fast, effective, and usually nonscarring. In many instances it is superior both to electrodesiccation and curettage and to excision because normal tissue is not disturbed.

Blunt dissectors are available commercially or may be homemade by altering the blade end of a Bard-Parker handle by flattening it with a grinding wheel and bending the tip approximately 30 degrees. A Schamberg acne expressor may also be used as a blunt dissecting instrument.

Technique

The patient may be premedicated with analgesics for lesions in which postoperative pain is anticipated, such as with large plantar or periungual warts. The procedure is relatively painless when performed on areas other than the palms and soles.

Local anesthesia is induced with 2% lidocaine with epinephrine.

A plane of dissection is established by inserting the tip of blunt-tipped scissors between the lesion and normal skin and cutting the skin circumferentially (Figure 27-9, A).

The blunt dissector is inserted in the plane of cleavage; the intact lesion can be separated easily with short, firm strokes from the surrounding and underlying normal tissue (Figure 27-9, B). At the conclusion of this gross dissection, the blunt dissector is drawn firmly back and forth over the exposed surface of the bed to ensure that no tissue fragments remain (Figure 27-9, C).

Bleeding is controlled with Monsel's solution. A bandage is placed on the wound, and the patient is advised to change it daily for 3 to 4 days. Thereafter, the wound is left exposed. The patient should be cautioned that moderate to intense pain may occur for 15 minutes to 2 hours after blunt dissection of periungual and plantar warts.

Cryosurgery

Small, superficial, nonmalignant lesions may be quickly and effectively treated by freezing with liquid nitrogen (boiling point −196° C). Cryosurgery for malignant lesions requires experience and sophisticated equipment with thermocouples that measure the depth of freeze.[29,30] Severe pain may result from freezing thick areas, such as the palms and soles, or areas that are anatomically confined, such as the area about the nails.[31] Lesions located on these areas are best treated with other methods. Epithelial cells, melanocytes, and nerve tissue are more susceptible to cold injury than is the connective tissue of the dermis and vessels.

INDICATIONS. Cryosurgery is very effective for common and genital warts, actinic keratoses, thin seborrheic keratoses, lentigines, and molluscum contagiosum.[32] The superficial

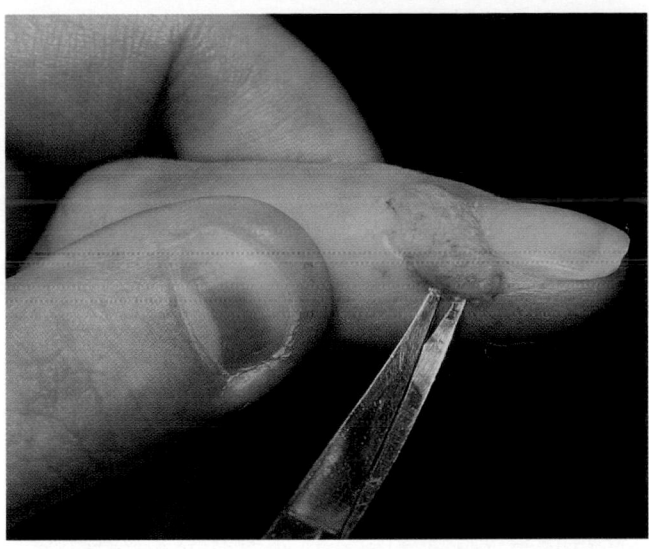

A, A plane of dissection is established by cutting circumferentially around the lesion with probe-tipped curved scissors.

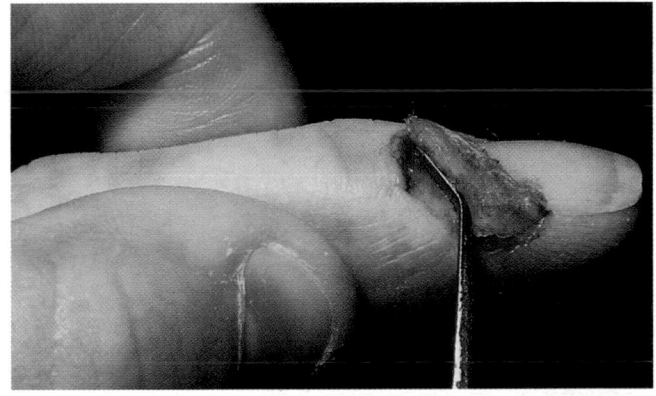

B, The blunt dissector is inserted in the plane of cleavage and firmly pressed against the lesion with several short, firm strokes.

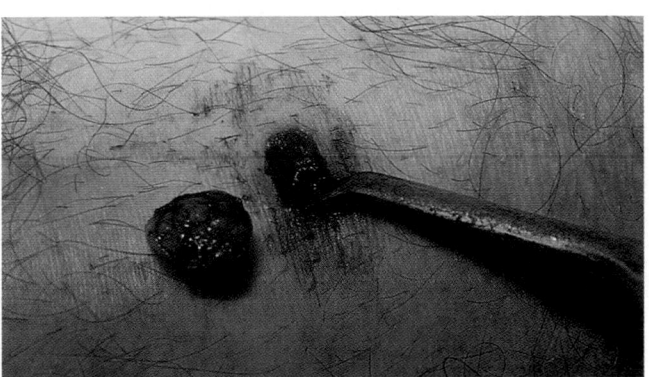

C, The blunt dissector is drawn firmly back and forth over the exposed surface to remove remaining fragments of tissue.

Figure 27-9 Blunt dissection of a wart.

portions of dermatofibromas and sebaceous hyperplasia can be destroyed by freezing. Thick seborrheic keratoses are best removed with the curet.

EQUIPMENT. Liquid nitrogen is available in most cities and may be stored in the office in 1- to 2-gallon tanks for approximately 10 days. Cotton swabs have been used to administer the nitrogen, but they are capable of transmitting virus particles. It is now recommended that nitrogen be administered with a direct spray or contact probe with an autoclavable tip.[33] A number of relatively inexpensive cryospray instruments are available, such as the Cry-Ac (Owen Instruments).

Technique

Maximum tissue destruction occurs with rapid freezing and slow thawing. Repeated freeze-thaw cycles increase cell damage.[34] Pain is moderate to intense during freezing. The depth of freeze is approximately 1.5 the lateral spread.[35] The end point of a 1- to 3-mm rim of freeze around the lesions corresponds to a thaw time of approximately 20 to 40 seconds and is adequate for epidermal lesions such as warts and actinic keratoses. Longer freeze-thaw times destroy portions of the dermis. The technique should be used conservatively; it is better to undertreat a lesion and re-treat it at a later date than to freeze it too vigorously, destroy excessive amounts of normal tissue, and create hypopigmentation. Repetitive pinching of the skin during cryosurgery lessens perceived pain.[4]

Thin lesions. Seborrheic keratoses, flat warts, and actinic keratoses form a crust in 7 to 10 days and fall off. Broad, flat seborrheic keratoses may be frozen in sections (Figure 27-10, A); freezing from the center of a large lesion results in a freeze that is too deep.

Thick lesions. A hemorrhagic bulla must be created to treat warts effectively. Warts require more prolonged freezing than do thin seborrheic and actinic keratoses and heal in 2 to 3 weeks.

C&C (cryoanesthesia and cutting or curetting). For raised lesions such as thick seborrheic keratoses and small dermal nevi (less than 5 mm), cryospray may be used to achieve quick cryoanesthesia. The raised portion is then removed with a curet or is cut flush to the skin surface with scissors or a scalpel. Treatment of nevi with the C&C method has an added advantage: any pigment that remains at the base of the lesion can be destroyed by short freezing the base.

"Dip-stick" method. A large cotton-tipped swab is prepared by winding the tip to a point. The applicator is dipped into the nitrogen tank, and the tip is immediately applied to the center of the lesion. A white, hard area of freeze rapidly propagates in all directions. The swab is removed after a 1- to 3-mm rim of freeze surrounding the lesion has been established. The swab is then discarded.

Cryospray. Benign, superficial lesions are usually treated for 5 to 15 seconds to establish a 1- to 3-mm rim of freeze extending beyond the lesion.

POSTCRYOSURGERY. Erythema and edema occur within minutes of thawing. Superficial freezing causes separation at the dermoepidermal junction and can produce a vesicle or bulla. Bullae are likely to occur on the arms and hands (Figure 27-10, B), and they can be large and hemorrhagic. They resolve within a few days but sometimes require drainage if discomfort occurs. Cryosurgery wounds are slower to epithelialize than are laser or scalpel wounds.

COMPLICATIONS. Scarring is minimal with superficial freezing; the cosmetic results are equal to or better than those obtained with desiccation and curettage. If hypertrophic scarring; significant hypopigmentation or hyperpigmentation; or oozing, weeping wounds occur after treatment of warts or keratoses, freezing was too aggressive. Hyperpigmentation occurs in people with darker complexions. The trunk and legs are the areas most likely to form round, hyperpigmented macules after cryosurgery.

The nerves are superficial on the lateral aspects of the digits,[36] the angle of the jaw, and the ulnar fossa of the elbow. Cryosurgery should be avoided in these areas to prevent nerve damage.

Melanocytes are very sensitive to cold injury, and healing with hypopigmentation is common. Cryosurgery should be used with caution for dark-complected individuals.

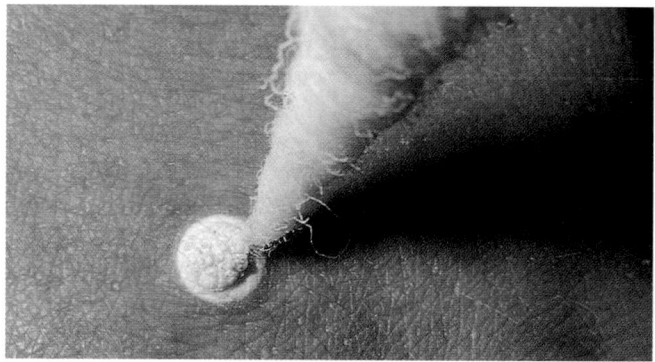

A, The nitrogen-soaked, cotton-tipped applicator is applied to the surface until a 1-mm rim of frozen tissue has been established.

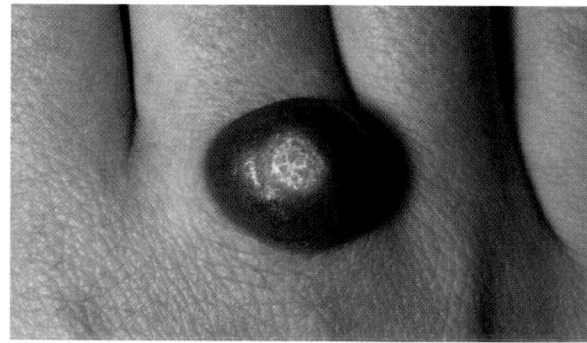

B, Hemorrhagic bullae can occur 24 to 48 hours after cryosurgery. This is most likely to occur on the arms and hands.

Figure 27-10 Cryosurgery.

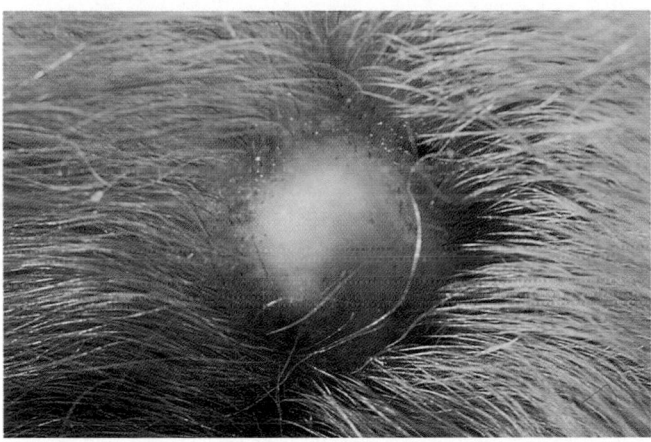

A, Make a linear incision (3 to 10 mm) through the skin and into the cyst with a pointed-tipped #11 surgical blade.

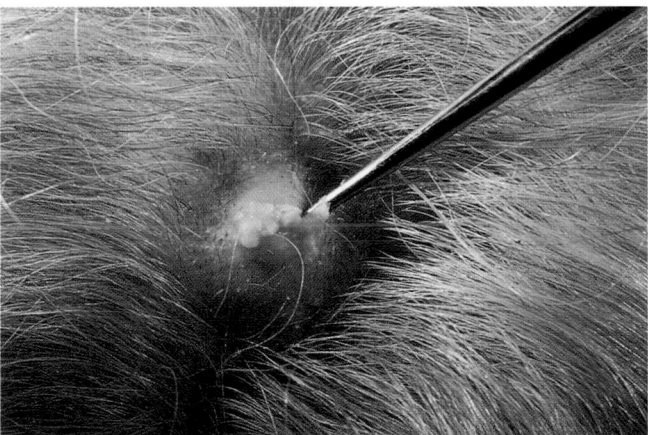

B, Insert a 1- to 3-mm curet through the incision and dislodge and remove as much of the cyst contents as possible. Compress the surrounding skin to force the cyst contents through the small incision.

Extraction of Cysts

A quick, simple technique is available for the removal of small epidermal (sebaceous) and pilar (scalp wens) cysts. Normal tissue is not removed, sutures are unnecessary, and there is little scarring.

Technique

After induction of local anesthesia, a linear incision (3 to 10 mm) is made through the skin and into the cyst with a pointed-tipped #11 surgical blade (Figure 27-11, A). The surrounding skin is compressed to force the cyst contents through the small incision. A 1- to 3-mm curet is inserted through the incision, and any remaining fragments of material are dislodged and removed (Figure 27-11, B). After total evacuation, firm pressure forces a part or all of the cyst wall through the incision, where it can be grasped with the forceps (Figure 27-11, C) and separated with scissors from connective tissue (Figure 27-11, D). To absorb blood and serum, the wound is compressed for several minutes, then covered with a small dressing. The area can be washed the next day.

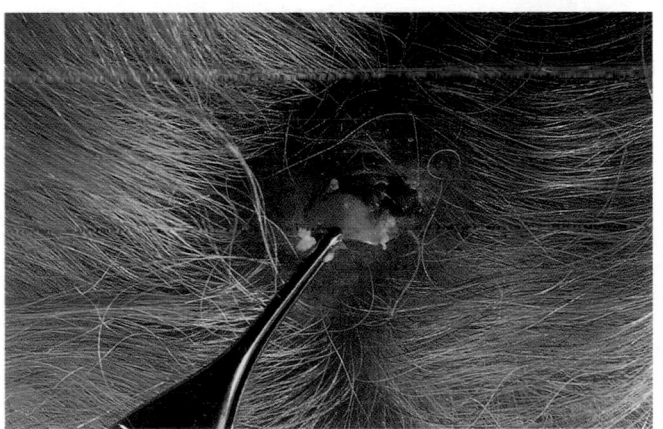

C, After total evacuation, firm pressure forces a part or all of the cyst wall through the incision. The cyst wall is grasped with forceps.

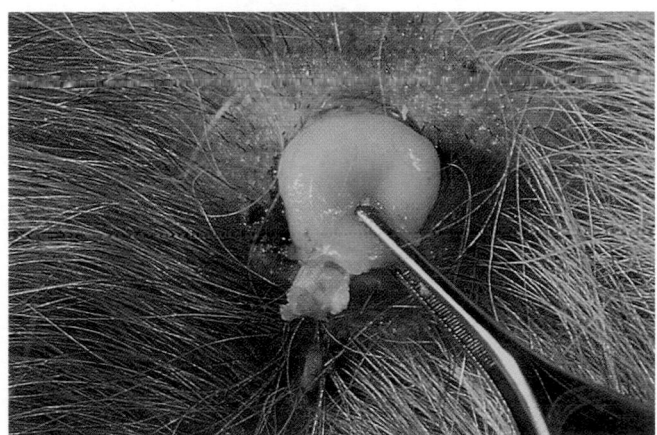

D, The cyst is separated with scissors from connective tissue and removed.

Figure 27-11 Extraction of cysts.

Mohs' Micrographic Surgery

Rather than increase in a sphere-shaped mass, certain skin tumors, such as basal cell epithelioma, transmit random, fingerlike projections into the surrounding connective tissue. These tumor strands may go undetected with standard desiccation and curettage or excision techniques, resulting in recurrence. In the past, multiple procedures were performed on unfortunate patients who, after a series of unsuccessful procedures, acquired a diffuse, poorly defined mass of substantial proportions.

In 1941 Frederick Mohs described a microscopically guided method of tracing and removing basal cell carcinomas.[37] Since then the technique has been used to treat many contiguously spreading skin cancers.[38] The procedure has been modified and is usually performed on fresh tissue in 1 day on an outpatient basis. Tissue is removed in thin layers, and all margins of the specimen are mapped to determine whether tumor remains. Cure rates are very high. The technique is tissue sparing: the tumor is precisely identified, and maximum amounts of normal skin can be retained.[39]

Technique

The clinically apparent area is removed with a curet (Figure 27-12). In the past, a chemical fixative—zinc chloride paste—was applied and allowed to penetrate the tissue. Paste application resulted in the use of the now outdated term, *Mohs' chemosurgery*. Currently, the fixation step is omitted, thus the designation *fresh tissue technique*.[40-42]

A thin, horizontal layer of tissue is removed with a scalpel and divided into more convenient smaller specimens for frozen section. Two adjacent edges of tissue are dyed red and blue to provide spatial orientation. A diagram of the section is prepared, and the number and color coding is indicated on the map. Specimens are mounted in a cryostat and then sectioned. Cut sections are stained and microscopically examined.

The location of the tumor cells is indicated on a map, and the above steps are repeated only in areas with tumors until a cancer-free plane is reached.

Figure 27-12 Microscopically guided excision of cutaneous tumors—Mohs' microscopic surgery.

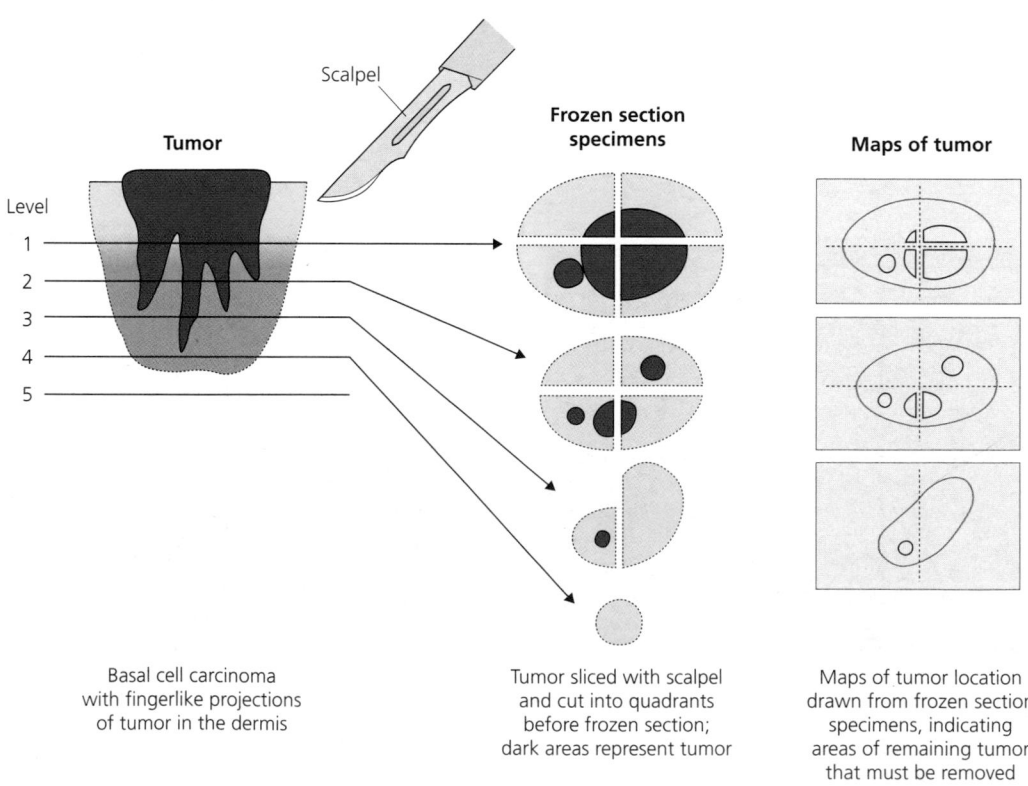

Basal cell carcinoma with fingerlike projections of tumor in the dermis

Tumor sliced with scalpel and cut into quadrants before frozen section; dark areas represent tumor

Maps of tumor location drawn from frozen section specimens, indicating areas of remaining tumor that must be removed

The defect created by the fresh tissue technique can heal by secondary intention or can be closed primarily. Flaps were found to be preferable to skin grafts for facial repair, with forehead and nasolabial flaps particularly useful for the nose.[41] Cure rates of 94% to 99%[44] have been achieved (Figure 27-13).

The advantages of the microscopically controlled technique are that it preserves maximum amounts of normal tissue around the cancer, and it provides great reliability in determining adequate margins of excision. The disadvantage is that it is time-consuming, requiring hours or days to perform.

The indications for Mohs' micrographic surgery[42] are listed in Box 27-2.

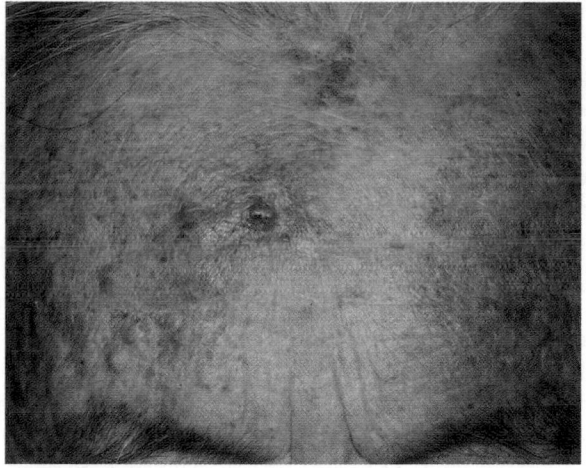

A, Sclerosing basal cell carcinoma. A small nodule is surrounded by an ill-defined erythematous area of induration.

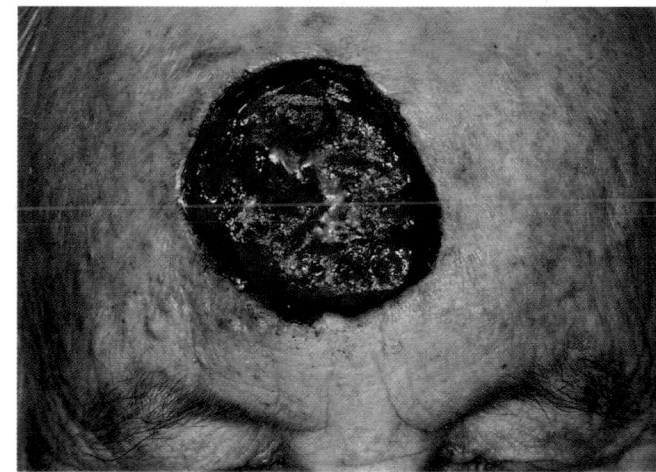

B, Mohs' micrographic surgery reveals the extent of the tumor shown, which clinically appeared to be rather small.

Box 27-2 Indications for Mohs' Micrographic Surgery

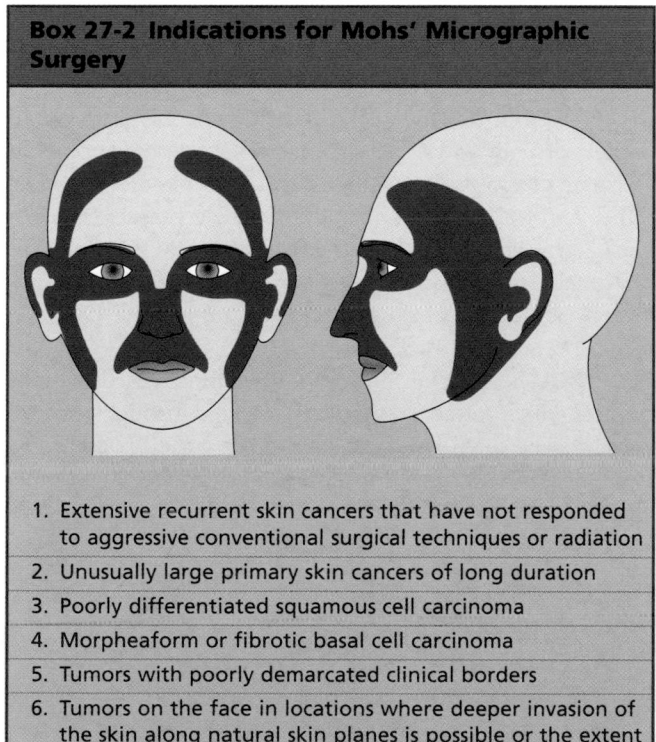

1. Extensive recurrent skin cancers that have not responded to aggressive conventional surgical techniques or radiation
2. Unusually large primary skin cancers of long duration
3. Poorly differentiated squamous cell carcinoma
4. Morpheaform or fibrotic basal cell carcinoma
5. Tumors with poorly demarcated clinical borders
6. Tumors on the face in locations where deeper invasion of the skin along natural skin planes is possible or the extent of the tumor is difficult to define, such as eyelids, nasal alae, nasolabial folds, and circumauricular areas
7. Areas where maximum conservation of tumor-free tissue is important for preservation of function, such as the penis or finger

Modified from Albright SD III: J Am Acad Dermatol 1982; 7:143.

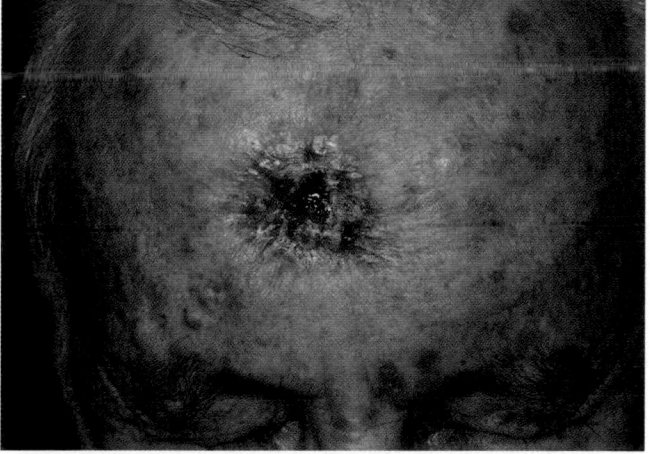

C, Six weeks after Mohs' micrographic surgery. The defect is healing by secondary intention.

Figure 27-13 Mohs' micrographic surgery technique.

Chemical Peels

Chemical peeling of facial skin is commonly performed by aesthetic surgeons. Peeling produces a controlled, partial-thickness chemical burn of the epidermis and the outer dermis. Several techniques are available to fine-tune the depth of the peel. Regeneration of peeled skin from follicular and eccrine duct epithelium results in a fresh, orderly, organized epidermis. In the dermis, a new 2- to 3-mm band of dense, compact, orderly collagen is formed between the epidermis and the underlying damaged dermis, which results in effective ablation of the fine wrinkles in the skin and a reduction of pigmentation. These clinical and histologic changes are long-lasting (15 to 20 years) and may be permanent for some patients. The local complications of peeling include pigmentation changes, scarring, milia, ectropion, infection, activation of herpes simplex, and toxic shock syndrome.[43] Chemical facial exfoliation can be deep, medium, or superficial, depending on the depth of penetration of the caustic agent used.

DEEP PEELS TO THE DEEP RETICULAR DERMIS. Phenol (carbolic acid), when used in the Baker's formula (3 ml phenol, 2 ml water, 8 drops 0.25% septisol [hexachlorophene soap], 3 drops croton oil), provides dramatic results but has the potential for systemic complications. Phenol is a protein precipitant that causes rapid denaturation of the surface keratin and other proteins in the epidermis and outer dermis. This burn injury extends to a depth of approximately 2 to 3 mm. Phenol is rapidly absorbed into the circulation and may cause cardiac arrhythmias. Full epithelialization occurs in 6 to 7 days. Phenol peels are best suited to fair-skinned women and can provide substantial improvement in rhytidosis and actinic damage.

MEDIUM-DEPTH PEELS TO THE OUTER PAPILLARY DERMIS. The results of medium-depth peels with trichloroacetic acid (TCA) are not as profound. TCA (35% to 50%) peels lighten pigmentary problems and improve rhytides with minimal potential for systemic toxicity, but local complications, including scarring and pigmentary changes, are still possible.

SUPERFICIAL PEELS TO THE OUTER PAPILLARY DERMIS. Superficial peels with TCA (10% to 25%) and many other agents, when performed repeatedly, improve pigmentary irregularities and may improve some minor surface changes and impart a fresher appearance to facial skin.[44] Glycolic acid is an alpha hydroxy acid that is also used as a chemical peeling agent. Glycolic acid (50% to 70%) produces superficial peels that remove actinic keratoses, fine wrinkles, lentigines, melasma, and seborrheic keratoses. As with other peels, the depth of penetration can be titrated by the timed duration of the application of the acid. Peels are left on the skin for 3 to 7 minutes and can be repeated 3 to 4 times. Glycolic acid can be used to peel skin of all skin types with minimal risk.[45]

Filling Materials

Soft tissue implants are now available for the treatment of facial wrinkles, acne scars, and surgical defects. Bovine collagen (Zyderm I and II) is placed in the superficial dermis for correction of superficial wrinkle lines. Zyplast, a cross-linked bovine collagen product, is placed deeper and can raise depressed areas, such as those of acne scars, deep nasolabial folds, and surgical defects. Some patients are allergic to this material. Dermalogen is an injectable human tissue matrix implant procured from donor tissue. No allergy testing is needed. Cosmoderm and CosmoPlast contain collagen derived from cultures of human fibroblast cells grown in the laboratory. No skin testing is required.

Autologous fatty tissue injection is a surgical technique and does not require FDA approval. Adipocytes are harvested with a needle, washed, and reinjected. The poor viability of harvested cells has limited the effectiveness of this technique.

Liposuction

Liposuction surgery is a safe technique when performed by a fully trained, experienced physician. Patients under 40 years of age with good skin elasticity are the best candidates, but patients ranging in age from 16 to over 70 can be successfully treated. Previously, body contouring by surgical excision of fat produced large scars. Fat is removed through half-inch incisions during liposuction.

INDICATIONS. With a variety of new instruments and techniques, virtually any area can be treated—the small pot belly, the spare tire, hips, lateral thighs, and "love handles" on men. Other appropriate areas include the male breasts (gynecomastia), the chin, the neck, anterior axillary fat folds, and the proximal arms. Lipomas are easily extracted. Liposuction is used by some surgeons during face-lift surgery.[46]

TECHNIQUE. A radial tunneling procedure is used. A small cannula with a rounded aperture is inserted through a ½-inch incision. The cannula is pushed into the fat to break it loose from the fibrous stroma. Multiple to-and-fro movements mechanically disrupt the fat and create tunnels. The loosened fat is removed with a very powerful suction.

Lasers

There are several types of lasers used to treat cutaneous disease[47] (Table 27-3).

PHOTOTHERMOLYSIS. Laser light is absorbed by chromophores, light-absorbing components of skin (melanin, hemoglobin, water, tattoo ink). The absorbed energy is converted to thermal energy with heating of the chromophore. If a targeted tissue (chromophore) strongly absorbs a selected wavelength, and the pulse duration is shorter than the thermal relaxation time (cooling time) of the tissue, then only selective thermal injury will occur. By limiting thermal damage to the target chromophore, less injury occurs to the surrounding tissue, with a reduced risk for scarring.

HOW LASERS WORK. Lasers apply an electric charge that activates a medium, usually a gas-like carbon dioxide or a crystal such as a ruby rod. The activated medium releases light, which is focused by mirrors and released in a beam. The laser apparatus consists of three elements. The pumping system is the power supply. The flashlamp is one type of pumping system. The lasing medium supplies the electrons needed for stimulated emission of radiation. It can be gaseous (argon, carbon dioxide, He-Ne, copper vapor, excimer, kryton), liquid (tunable dye), solid (alexandrite, ruby, Nd:YAG, Er:YAG, Ga:As) or comprised of free electrons. The optical cavity consists of two parallel mirrors (one partially reflective) enclosing the lasing medium that is excited by the pumping system.

The wavelength of light is determined by the laser medium present in the optical cavity.

Table 27-3 Lasers in Dermatology

Wavelength (NM)	Laser	Indications
488-514 (blue-green)	Argon (continuous)	Telangiectases, thick PWS in adults; epidermal pigmented lesions
504-690 (green-yellow-red)	Argon-pumped tunable dye (continuous)	Telangiectases, thick PWS in adults; epidermal pigmented lesions; photodynamic therapy
510 (green)	Flashlamp-pumped dye (short-pulsed)	Epidermal pigmented lesions; red tattoos
511 (green)	Copper vapor/bromide (pseudo-continuous)	Epidermal pigmented lesions
521; 531 (green)	Krypton (continuous)	Epidermal pigmented lesions
532 (green)	KTP (pseudo-continuous)	Telangiectases, thick PWS in adults; epidermal pigmented lesions
532 (green)	KTP (long-pulsed)	Telangiectases, PWS in adults; epidermal pigmented lesions
532 (green)	Frequency-doubled Q-switched Nd:YAG (pulsed)	Epidermal pigmented lesions; red tattoos
568 (yellow)	Krypton (continuous)	Telangiectases, thick PWS in adults
578 (yellow)	Copper vapor/bromide (pseudo-continuous)	Telangiectases, thick PWS in adults
585-600 (yellow)	Flashlamp-pumped dye (long-pulsed)	PWS, PWS in children, telangiectases, warts, hypertrophic scars, striae
694 (red)	Q-switched ruby (pulsed)	Epidermal and dermal pigmented lesions; blue, black, and green tattoos
694 (red)	Ruby (long-pulsed)	Hair removal; dermal pigmented lesions
755 (infrared)	Q-switched alexandrite (pulsed)	Epidermal and dermal pigmented lesions; blue, black and green tattoos
755 (infrared)	Alexandrite (long-pulsed)	Hair removal
810 (infrared)	Diode (long-pulsed)	Hair removal
1064 (infrared)	Q-switched Nd:YAG (pulsed)	Dermal pigmented lesions; blue, and black tattoos
1064 (infrared)	Nd:YAG (long-pulsed)	Hair removal
1064 (infrared)	Nd:YAG (continuous)	Deep coagulation of tissue
1320 (infrared)	Nd:YAG (pulsed)	Nonablative skin resurfacing
2940 (infrared)	Er:YAG (pulsed)	Skin resurfacing
10600 (infrared)	Carbon dioxide (continuous; pulsed)	Coagulation, vaporization, and cutting of tissue; skin resurfacing

Adapted from: Hruza GJ: Skin & Aging, Jan 2000.
PWS, Port-wine stain.

LASER TYPES. Continuous wave lasers (argon, argon-pumped tunable dye, krypton) produce a laser beam that is emitted continually. Most of the skin is heated by conduction during the long exposure, regardless of the wavelength. Pulsed lasers produce a beam that is emitted in individual short pulses with a long period (0.1 to 1 sec) between pulses.

Q-switching refers to a switch that allows the release of all of the laser energy in one powerful pulse. The target is heated at such a rapid rate that it shatters. Short-pulse (Q-switched ruby, alexandrite Nd:YAG) lasers are used for smaller structures (melanosomes, tattoo ink particles).

Carbon dioxide lasers have different lasing modes. In the continuous wave mode, the laser beam coagulates, vaporizes, or cuts tissue. The "ultra-pulse" and scanned modes achieve complete tissue vaporization with little collateral damage; they are used for skin resurfacing to remove wrinkles and scars.

VASCULAR LESIONS. Lasers are used to treat congenital and acquired vascular lesions, including port-wine stains, hemangiomas, facial telangiectasias, poikiloderma, cherry angiomas, venous lakes, and spider leg veins. The chromophore targeted is hemoglobin. Energy absorption by hemoglobin results in local thermal damage.

The flashlamp-pumped pulsed dye laser revolutionized the treatment of port-wine stains in infants and in adults, where resolution of the port-wine stain is excellent, with a scarring rate of approximately 1% and only occasional temporary hyperpigmentation. The following lasers are used to treat vascular lesions: the argon at 488 to 514 nm; the frequency-doubled Nd:YAG at 532 nm; the krypton at 568 nm; the argon dye at 577 to 600 nm; the copper vapor at 578 nm; and the pulsed dye at 585, 595, and 600 nm. No one laser is ideal for all types of vascular lesions. Lasers with longer wavelengths penetrate more deeply.

Tattoos and pigmented lesions. Treatment of benign pigmented lesions with a predominant epidermal component (solar lentigines, ephelides, melasma, nevus of Ota), and red, blue, black, and green tattoos are effectively treated with Q-switched lasers. Café-au-lait macules, Becker's nevi, and melasma have a variable response to lasers. "Q-switching" lasers produce very high power and extremely short pulses of light. Q-switched lasers are the ruby at 695-nm, the Nd:YAG at 1064 nm in the near-infrared spectrum and 532 nm in the green light spectrum, and the alexandrite at 755 nm. The chromophores for these lasers are melanin and tattoo pigment. The wavelengths of these lasers are long enough to penetrate into the dermis where there is tattoo ink or dermal pigment.[47]

The ultrashort pulse duration of these lasers produce photoacoustic waves that breaks tattoo particles into smaller pieces. Tattoo fragments are phagocytosed and removed. Blue-black tattoos respond best to the Q-switched ruby and 1064-nm Nd:YAG lasers; green tattoos respond to the alexandrite laser; and red tattoos are treated by the 532-nm Nd:YAG laser. Professional tattoos do not respond as quickly as amateur tattoos.

Non-Q-switched lasers are also used to treat pigmented lesions with the flash lamp-pumped pulsed dye with a green light at 510 nm and the krypton, which simultaneously produces a green light at 521 nm and 530 nm and a yellow light at 568 nm.

Skin resurfacing. Skin resurfacing is used for the treatment of facial wrinkles and acne scarring. The lasers used for skin resurfacing are the CO_2 at 10,600 nm and the Er:YAG at 2940 nm. Water is the chromophore targeted. The heat results in vaporization of the tissue. Peripheral thermal damage and scarring are minimized with the new superpulsed lasers and computerized scanning. Darker skin patients may have unacceptable alterations in pigmentation.

Hair removal. Lasers provide effective and possibly permanent hair removal, with minimal discomfort and low risk for scarring. The Nd:YAG laser at 1064 nm; the ruby, long-pulse alexandrite, and diode lasers; and nonlaser pulsed-light source are used for hair removal. The laser light penetrates into the dermis, where it is absorbed by melanin in the follicle. The pulse width must be long enough to allow thermal damage to occur to the hair follicle. The normal-mode ruby laser has a pulse duration that is between the thermal relaxation time for the hair follicle and allows for greater thermal conduction and destruction of the follicle. A cooling hand piece is placed at the skin surface to conduct heat away from the epidermis and minimize thermal damage. Hair removal with the ruby laser is more effective in the fair-skinned, dark-haired patient. Nonlaser pulsed-light sources are also used.

Botulinum Toxin

This is the most popular nonsurgical cosmetic procedure performed in the United States. Botulinum toxin is available in Europe and the United States. Products from different companies vary in their effectiveness. Botulinum toxin type A is an unstable protein. It should be used shortly after it is reconstituted with saline. Each patient must be evaluated individually. The dosage and number of injections is tailored to the patient's muscles. Injections are delivered into the belly of the muscle. Botox injections take 3 to 7 days to work and last 3 to 5 months. Men tend to require more Botox. Avoid aspirin and other blood thinners a week before injection.

INDICATIONS AND SIDE EFFECTS. Botulinum toxin A is approved for the treatment of glabellar lines. About 20 units of Botox is injected into the procerus and corrugator supercilii muscles. The maximum response rate occurs 30 days after treatment. Headache occurs in 13% of patients; eyelid ptosis occurs in 3% of treated patients.

The glabellar complex, forehead, and crow's feet are the most commonly treated areas. Botox is not a substitute for blepharoplasty, nor will it take care of redundant skin. Complications include bruising, headache, ptosis, diplopia, and under- or over-correction. Ecchymosis is common after injecting crow's feet and can be minimized by injecting superficially and by icing. Treatment around the mouth and neck (for horizontal lines and for softening hypertrophied platysmal cords) is technically more difficult, and side effects include dysphagias, dysphonias, and weak, "floppy" necks. Diffusion into other muscles is minimized by keeping injections small, precise, and well away from potential trouble areas. Avoid overdilution of the product. Some physicians dilute a vial of botulinum toxin with up to 10 cc of sterile saline. Others use 2 cc to get a concentration of 5 U per 0.1 mL. The more concentrated toxin results in less diffusion.

References

1. Huang W, Vidimos A: Topical anesthetics in dermatology, J Am Acad Dermatol 2000; 43(2 Pt 1):286.

2. Ruzicka T, et al: Allergy to local anesthetics: comparison of patch test with prick and intradermal test results, J Am Acad Dermatol 1987; 16:1202.

3. Glinert RJ, Zachary CB: Local anesthetic allergy. Its recognition and avoidance, J Dermatol Surg Oncol 1991; 17:491.

4. Fosko S: Reply [Record Supplied By Publisher], J Am Acad Dermatol 1999; 41(6):1048.

5. Fosko S, Gibney M, Harrison B: Repetitive pinching of the skin during lidocaine infiltration reduces patient discomfort, J Am Acad Dermatol 1998; 39(1):74.

6. Lugo-Janer G, et al: Less painful alternatives for local anesthesia, J Dermatol Surg Oncol 1993; 19:237.

7. McKay W, Morris R, Mushlin P: Sodium bicarbonate attenuates pain on skin infiltration with lidocaine, with or without epinephrine, Anesth Analg 1987; 66:572.

8. Larson PO, et al: Stability of buffered lidocaine and epinephrine used for local anesthesia, J Dermatol Surg Oncol 1991; 17:411.

9. Mader TJ, et al: Reducing pain of local anesthetic infiltration: warming and buffering have a synergistic effect, Ann Emerg Med 1994; 23:550.

10. Swinehart JM: The ice-saline-Xylocaine technique. A simple method for minimizing pain in obtaining local anesthesia, J Dermatol Surg Oncol 1992; 18:28.

11. Lycka BA: BMLA. A new and effective topical anesthetic, J Dermatol Surg Oncol 1992; 18:859.

12. Olmstead PM, Lund HZ, Leonard DD: Monsel's solution: a histologic nuisance, J Dermatol Surg Oncol 1980; 3:492.

13. Telfer NR, Moy RL: Wound care after office procedures, J Dermatol Surg Oncol 1993; 19:722.

14. Eaglstein WH: Occlusive dressings, J Dermatol Surg Oncol 1993; 19:716.

15. Brown CD, Zitelli JA: A review of topical agents for wounds and methods of wounding. Guidelines for wound management, J Dermatol Surg Oncol 1993; 19:732.

16. Varghese MC, et al: Local environment of chronic wounds under synthetic dressings, Arch Dermatol 1986; 122:52.

17. Falanga V: Occlusive wound dressings: why, when, which? Arch Dermatol 1988; 124:872.

18. Riordan A, Gamache C, Fosko S: Electrosurgery and cardiac devices, J Am Acad Dermatol 1997; 37(2 Pt 1):250.

19. Sheridan A, Dawber R: Curettage, electrosurgery and skin cancer, Australas J Dermatol 2000; 41(1):19.

20. Goldman G: The current status of curettage and electrodesiccation [In Process Citation], Dermatol Clin 2002; 20(3):569, ix .

21. Boughton RS, Spencer SK: Electrosurgical fundamentals, J Am Acad Dermatol 1987; 16:862.

22. Adam JE: The technic of curettage surgery, J Am Acad Dermatol 1986; 15:697.

23. Mohs FE: The technic of curettage surgery, J Am Acad Dermatol 1987 (letter); 16:886.

24. Whelan CS, Deckers PJ: Electrocoagulation for skin cancer: an old oncologic tool revisited, Cancer 1981; 47:2280.

25. Salasche SJ: Curettage and electrodesiccation in the treatment of midfacial basal cell epithelioma, J Am Acad Dermatol 1983; 8:496.

26. Pringle WM, Helms BC: Treatment of plantar warts by blunt dissection, Arch Dermatol 1973; 108:79.

27. Habif TP, Graf FA: Extirpation of subungual and periungual warts by blunt dissection, J Dermatol Surg Oncol 1981; 7:553.

28. Habif TP: Extirpation of keratoacanthomas by blunt dissection, J Dermatol Surg Oncol 1980; 6:652.

29. Kuflik EG, Gage AA: The five-year cure rate achieved by cryosurgery for skin cancer, J Am Acad Dermatol 1991; 24:1002.

30. Torre D: Cryosurgery of basal cell carcinoma, J Am Acad Dermatol 1986; 15:929.

31. Kuflik EG: Specific indications for cryosurgery of the nail unit. Myxoid cysts and periungual verrucae, J Dermatol Surg Oncol 1992; 18:702.

32. Kuflik EG: Cryosurgery updated, J Am Acad Dermatol 1994; 31:925.

33. Boulier IC, et al: Disposable attachments in cryosurgery: a useful adjunct in the treatment of HIV-associated neoplasms, J Dermatol Surg Oncol 1991; 17:277.

34. Farrant J, Walter CA: The cryobiological basis for cryosurgery, J Dermatol Surg Oncol 1977; 3:403.

35. Torre D: Understanding the relationship between lateral spread of freeze and depth of freeze, J Dermatol Surg Oncol 1979; 5:51.

36. Elton RF: Complications of cutaneous cryosurgery, J Am Acad Dermatol 1983; 8:513.

37. Mohs FE: Chemosurgery, a microscopically controlled method of cancer excision, Arch Surg 1941; 42:279.

38. Bennett RG: Current concepts in Mohs micrographic surgery, Dermatol Clin 1991; 9:777.

39. Roenigk RK: Mohs' micrographic surgery, Mayo Clin Proc 1988; 63:175.

40. Tromovitch TA, Stegman SJ: Microscopic-controlled excision of cutaneous tumors: chemosurgery, fresh tissue technique, Cancer 1978; 41:653.

41. Rudolph R, Miller SH: Reconstruction after Mohs cancer excision, Clin Plast Surg 1993; 20:157.

42. Albright SD: Treatment of skin cancer using multiple modalities, J Am Acad Dermatol 1982; 7:143.

43. Peters W: The chemical peel, Ann Plast Surg 1991; 26:564.

44. Matarasso SL, Glogau RG: Chemical face peels, Dermatol Clin 1991; 9:131.

45. Moy LS, et al: Glycolic acid peels for the treatment of wrinkles and photoaging, J Dermatol Surg Oncol 1993; 19:243.

46. Field LM: Lipo-suction surgery: a review, J Dermatol Surg Oncol 1984; 10:530.

47. Massey R, et al: Lasers in dermatology: a review, Cutis 2001; 67(6):47.

Appendix Dermatology and the Recently Returned Traveler

Table 1 Causes of Dermatologic Nodules and Cysts

Disease	Etiologic agent	Comments
Bacterial		
Bartonellosis	*Bartonella bacilliformis*	Multiple, may be verrucous
	B. quintana	Variety of skin lesions described
Cat-scratch disease	Usually *B. henselae*	
Glanders	*Pseudomonas mallei*	
Granuloma inguinale	*Calymmatobacterium granulomatis*	
Leprosy	*Mycobacterium leprae*	
Leptospirosis	Multiple serovars of *Leptospira interrogans*	
Lyme disease	*Borrelia burgdorferi*	Rare
Lymphogranuloma venereum	*Chlamydia trachomatis* immunotypes L1, L2, L3	
Mycetoma	Multiple species of bacteria and fungi	Begins as subcutaneous nodule
Mycobacteriosis	*Mycobacterium marinum*	Often multiple nodules
	M. ulcerans	Begins as nodule
	M. tuberculosis	
Rhinoscleroma	*Klebsiella rhinoscleromatis*	Usually infects nose
Syphilis	*Treponema pallidum* ssp. *pallidum*	Endemic and venereal
Yaws	*T. pallidum* ssp. *pertenue*	
Fungal		
Blastomycosis	*Blastomyces dermatitidis*	
Chromomycosis	Several different fungi	
Coccidioidomycosis	*Coccidioides immitis*	
Cryptococcus	*Cryptococcus neoformans*	
Histoplasmosis	*Histoplasma capsulatum* var. *capsulatum*	
	H. capsulatum var. *duboisii*	Found in Africa
Lobomycosis	*Loboa loboi*	
Mycetoma	Multiple species of bacteria and fungi	
Penicilliosis	*Penicillium marneffei*	
Sporotrichosis	*Sporothrix schenckii*	
Helminthic		
Coenurosis	Several species of tapeworms	
Cutaneous larva migrans	Primarily *Ancylostoma braziliense* and *A. caninum*	Larvae of dog and cat hookworms
Cysticercosis	*Taenia solium*	May be multiple
Dirofilariasis	*Dirofilaria immitis* and other *Dirofilaria* species	
Dracunculiasis	*Dracunculus medinensis*	

Table 1 Causes of Dermatologic Nodules and Cysts—cont'd

Disease	Etiologic agent	Comments
Echinococcus	Primarily *Echinococcus granulosus* and *E. multilocularis*	
Filariasis	*Wuchereria bancrofti, Brugia malayi*	Mass in scrotum
Gnathostomiasis	*Gnathostoma spinigerum*	
Loiasis	*Loa loa*	Inflammatory swellings
Onchocerciasis	*Onchocerca volvulus*	Painless, mobile, dermal nodules
Paragonimiasis	Primarily *Paragonimus westermani*	
Schistomiasis	Primarily *Schistosoma haematobium, S. japonicum,* and *S. mansoni*	Verrucous, vegetating
Sparganosis	Tapeworm larvae of genus *Spirometra*	
Visceral larva migrans	Primarily *Toxocara canis* and other roundworms	
Protozoan		
Amebiasis, cutaneous	*Entamoeba histolytica*	
Leishmaniasis, cutaneous and mucocutaneous	Multiple species of *Leishmania*	Single or multiple ulceration
Leishmaniasis, visceral post kala-azar	Primarily *L. donovani*	Widespread nodules
Trypanosomiasis, African	*Trypanosoma brucei gambiense*	Chancre at bite site
	T. Brucei rhodesiense	
Trypanosomiasis, American	*T. cruzi*	Chagoma
Viral		
Orf	Orf virus	Becomes ulcerated, crusted
Pseudocowpox	Milker's node virus	Milker's nodule
Arthropod bites and infestations		
Myiasis	Larvae of flies of the order *Diptera*	
Scabies	*Sarcoptes scabiei* var. *hominis*	Penile nodule and other lesions
Tick granuloma	Several species of ticks	Retained portion of tick, small nodule; may be pruritic; may persist for months or longer
Tungiasis	*Tunga penetrans*	

From Wilson ME: A world guide to infections: diseases, distribution, diagnosis, New York, 1991, Oxford University Press.

Table 2 Causes of Ulcerative Dermatologic Lesions

Disease	Etiologic agent	Comments
Bacterial		
Anthrax*	*Bacillus anthracis*	Hemorrhagic; surrounding oedema
Chancroid*	*Haemophilus ducreyi*	Painful, shallow ulcer, ragged edge; single or multiple
Diphtheria, cutaneous*	*Corynebacterium diphtheriae*	Shallow ulcer
Glanders*	*Pseudomonas mallei*	Ulceration of nodules
Granuloma inguinale*	*Calymmatobacterium granulomatis*	Painless ulcer
Leprosy	*Mycobacterium leprae*	Neuropathic ulcer
Lymphogranuloma venereum*	*Chlamydia trachomatis* immunotypes L1, L2, L3	Late ulceration
Melioidosis*	*Burkholderia pseudomallei*	Necrotic ulcer with local cellulitis lymphangitis
Mycetoma*	Multiple species of bacteria and fungi	Ulcer, sinus tracts
Mycobacteriosis*	*Mycobacterium marinum*	Nodules may ulcerate
	M. ulcerans	Deep ulcer
	M. tuberculosis	Papule that ulcerates at primary inoculation site
Plague	*Yersinia pestis*	Near primary inoculation site; breakdown of bubo
Rickettsial infections*	Multiple rickettsial species	Eschars at site of arthropod bite for some spotted fevers and typhus fevers
Syphilis, venereal*	*Treponema pallidum* ssp. *pallidum*	Painless ulcer with indurated edge
Tropical ulcer*	Multiple species of bacteria	Painful necrotic ulcer
Tularemia*	*Francisella tularensis*	Ulcerated nodule
Yaws*	*T. pallidum* ssp. *pertenue*	Papule ulcerates, papillomatous surface
Fungal		
All invasive fungal infections (e.g., histoplasmosis, coccidioidomycosis, cryptococcosis) may cause ulcerative skin lesions. Deep abscesses and sinus tracts may form.		
Helminthic		
Dracunculiasis	*Dracunculus medinenis*	Ulcer at site of eruption of worm
Protozoan		
Amebiasis, cutaneous	*Entamoeba histolytica*	Painful, rapidly growing ulcers; necrotic
Leishmaniasis	Multiple *Leishmania* species	Cutaneous and mucocutaneous
Viral		
Orf*	Orf virus	
Herpes simplex*	Herpes simplex virus	
Arthropod bites and infestations		
Spider bites*	Brown recluse and other spiders	Gangrenous slough at bite site
Myiasis*	Larvae of flies of the order *Diptera*	
Tungiasis*	*Tunga penetrans*	

From Wilson ME: A world guide to infections: diseases, distribution, diagnosis, New York, 1991, Oxford University Press.
*Primary inoculation site.

Table 3 Causes of Migratory Dermatologic Lesions

Disease	Etiologic agent	Comments
Cutaneous larva migrans	Primarily *Ancylostoma braziliense* and *A. caninum*	Larvae of dog and cat hookworms
Dracunculiasis	*Dracunculus medinensis*	Movement of worm just below dermis before eruption
Fascioliasis	*Fasciola hepatica* *F. gigantica*	Migratory areas of inflammation, especially with *F. gigantica*
Gnathostomiasis	*Gnathostoma spinigerum*	Migratory inflammatory lesions, 1 cm/h or faster when subcutaneous
Hookworm	Primarily *Ancylostoma duodenale* and *Necator americanus*	
Loiasis	*Loa loa*	Migratory inflammatory swellings; worm may be visible crossing conjunctivae
Myiasis	Larvae of flies of the order *Diptera*	Visible movement of maggot(s) within the lesion may be noted
		Larvae of some *Diptera* (e.g., *Hypoderma*) migrate in soft tissues
Paragonimiasis	Primarily *Paragonimus szechuanesis* and *P. westermani*	Subcutaneous migratory swelling or subcutaneous nodules
Sparganosis	Tapeworm larvae of the genus *Spirometra*	
Strongyloidiasis	*Strongyloides stercoralis*	Migratory, serpiginous lesions (larva currens), 5-10 cm/h

From Wilson ME: A world guide to infections: diseases, distribution, diagnosis, New York, 1991, Oxford University Press.

Table 4 Causes of Pruritic Lesions

Disease	Etiologic agent	Diagnostic test
Helminthic*		
Cercarial dermatitis	Species of avian and small mammal schistosomes	
Cutaneous larva migrans	Primarily *Ancylostoma braziliense* and *A. caninum*	
Dracunculiasis	*Dracunculus medinensis*	Identification of discharged motile larvae
Enterobiasis (pinworms)	*Enterobius vermicularis*	Identification of eggs and adult worms with perianal tape test
Gnathostomiasis	*Gnathostoma spinigerum*	Identification of larva in surgical specimen
Hookworm	*A. duodenale* *Necator americanus*	Identification of eggs in stool
Loiasis	*Loa loa*	Extraction and identification of adult worm, e.g., from conjunctivae; serologic tests are also available by special arrangement
Onchocerciasis	*Onchocerca volvulus*	Identification of microfilariae in skin snip or of adult worm in excised nodule
Schistosomiasis (early)	Primarily *Schistosoma haematobium, S. japonicum,* and *S. mansoni*	
Strongyloidiasis	*Strongyloides stercoralis*	Identification of larvae in stool, small bowel contents; rarely in sputum, peritoneal fluid, urine, CSF or pleural fluid
Trypanosomiasis, African	*Trypanosoma brucei gambiense* *Trypanosoma brucei rhodesiense*	Pruritus and chancre during or shortly after penetration. Usual diagnostic methods are not useful at this point in infection
Arthropod bites and infestations		
Myiasis	Larvae of flies of order *Diptera*	Identification of larvae
Fleas	*Pulex irritans,* human flea, and animal fleas	Identification of flea
Lice (body and crab)	*Pediculus humanus capitis,* head louse	Identification of louse
	P. humanus humanus, body/clothing louse	
	Pthirus pubis, pubic/crab louse	
Mosquitoes	Many species of mosquitoes	
Scabies	*S. scabiei* var. *hominis*	Identification of mite, or its eggs or feces on skin scraping of burrows or in tissue sections of skin biopsy
Coelenterata		
Seabather's eruption	*Edwardsiella lineata,* larvae of adult sea anemone *Linuche unguiculata,* larvae of jellyfish	

From Wilson ME: A world guide to infections: diseases, distribution, diagnosis, New York, 1991, Oxford University Press.

*In the helminthic infections, parasites and eggs are not often in stool when skin lesions appear. Also, pruritus may be transient or intermittent. All helminthic infections may cause urticaria.

Dermatologic Formulary

ACNE MEDICATIONS

Retinoids

	Base	Concentration	Packaging
Retin-A (Tretinoin)	Cream	0.025%	20 gm
			45 gm
		0.05%	20 gm
			45 gm
		0.1%	20 gm
			45 gm

Retinoids

	Base	Concentration	Packaging
	Gel	0.01%	15 gm 45 gm
		0.025%	15 gm 45 gm
	Liquid	0.05%	28 ml
Retin-A Micro (Tretinoin)	Gel	0.1%	20 gm 45 gm
		0.04%	20 gm 45 gm
Tazorac (Tazarotene)	Gel	0.1%	30 gm 100 gm
		0.05%	30 gm 100 gm
	Cream	0.1%	15 gm 30 gm 60 gm
		0.5%	15 gm 30 gm 60 gm
Differin (Adapalene)	Gel	0.1%	45 gm
	Cream	0.1%	45 gm
	Pledgets	0.1%	1 box
	Solution	0.1%	30 ml
Azelex (Azelaic acid)	20% cream	20% acid	30 gm, 50 gm

Benzoyl Peroxide Cleansers

Product	Formulation	Packaging
Benzac AC wash 2.5%	Liquid 2.5%	8 oz
Benzac AC wash 5%	Liquid 5%	8 oz
Benzac AC wash 10%	Liquid 10%	8 oz
Benzac W wash (Rx)	Liquid 5%	4 oz, 8 oz
Benzac W wash (Rx)	Liquid 10%	8 oz
Brevoxyl Cleansing Lotion (Rx)	Liquid 4%	10.5 oz
Brevoxyl Cleansing Lotion (Rx)	Liquid 8%	10.5 oz
Brevoxyl Creamy Wash	Liquid 4%	6 oz tube
Brevoxyl Creamy Wash	Liquid 8%	6 oz tube
Desquam-X 5% wash (Rx)	Liquid 5%	150 ml
Desquam-X 10% wash (Rx)	Liquid 10%	150 ml
Desquam-X 10% bar (Rx)	Bar 10%	4 oz bar
Panoxyl 5 bar (otc)	Bar 5%	4 oz bar
Panoxyl 10 bar (otc)	Bar 10%	4 oz bar
Triaz 3%	Liquid 3%	6 oz, 12 oz
Triaz 6%	Liquid 6%	6 oz, 12 oz
Triaz 9 %	Liquid 9%	6 oz, 12 oz

Benzoyl Peroxide Gels (2.5% to 3.0%)

Product	Base	Packaging
Benzac W 2.5	Water	60 gm, 90 gm
Benzac AC 2.5%	Water	60 gm, 90 gm
Clear By Design (otc)	Water	45 gm, 90 gm
Desquam-X 2.5%	Water	1.5 oz
Desquam-E 2.5	Water	1.5 oz
Panoxyl AQ 2.5	Water	60 gm, 120 gm
Triaz 3%	Water	42.5 gm

Benzoyl Peroxide Gels (4% to 8%)

Product	Base	Packaging
Benoxyl 5 (otc)	Water	1 oz, 2 oz
Benzac 5	12% alcohol	60 gm
Benzac AC 5%	Water	60 gm, 90 gm
Benzac W 5	Water	60 gm, 90 gm
Brevoxyl 4% (Rx)	Water	42.5 gm, 90 gm
Brevoxyl 8% (Rx)	Water	42.5 gm, 90 gm
5-Benzagel	14% alcohol	42.5 gm, 85 gm
Clinac BPO	7%	45 gm
Desquam-X 5	Water	45 gm, 90 gm
Desquam-E 5	Water	1.5 oz
Neutrogena Acne Mask 5%		2 oz tube
Panoxyl 5	20% alcohol	60 gm, 120 gm
Panoxyl AQ 5	Water	60 gm, 120 gm
Sulfoxyl Regular 5 (contains 2.5% sulfur)	Water	30 ml
Triaz 6%	Water	42.5 gm

Benzoyl Peroxide Gels (10%)

Product	Base	Packaging
Acne-Aid (otc)	Flesh-tinted	1.8 oz
Benoxyl 10 (otc)	Water	1 oz, 2 oz
Benzac 10	12% alcohol	60 gm
Benzac AC 10%	Water	60 gm, 90 gm
Benzac W 10	Water	60 gm, 90 gm
10-Benzagel	14% alcohol	42.5 gm, 85 gm
Desquam-X 10	Water	42.5 gm, 85 gm
Desquam-E 10	Water	1.5 oz
Panoxyl 10	20% alcohol	60 gm, 120 gm
Panoxyl AQ 10	Water	60 gm, 120 gm
Sulfoxyl Strong 10 (contains 5% sulfur)	Water	2 oz

Topical Antibiotics for Acne

Product	Antibiotics	Packaging
Akne-Mycin	2% erythromycin	25 gm ointment
A/T/S	2% erythromycin	60 ml liquid
A/T/S gel	2% erythromycin	60 ml liquid
Azelex	20% azelaic acid	30 gm, 50 gm cream
Benzaclin	1% clindamycin 5% benzoyl peroxide	25 gm, 50 gm gel
Benzamycin	3% erythromycin 5% benzoyl peroxide	23.3, 46.6 gm gel
Benzamycin Pak	3% erythromycin 5% benzoyl peroxide	60 packets
Cleocin T	1% clindamycin	30 gm, 60 ml liquid 30 gm, 60 ml gel 60 ml lotion #60 pledgets
Clindagel	1% clindamycin	42 gm, 77 gm gel
Clindets	1% clindamycin	#60 pledgets
Duac gel	1% clindamycin 5% benzoyl peroxide	45 gm gel
Emgel	2% erythromycin	27 gm, 50 gm gel
Erycette	2% erythromycin	#60 swabs
EryDerm	2% erythromycin	60 ml liquid
Erygel	2% erythromycin	30 gm, 60 gm gel

Continued

Topical Antibiotics for Acne (cont'd)

Product	Antibiotics	Packaging
Erymax	2% erythromycin	2 oz, 4 oz liquid
Finacea	15% azelaic acid	30 gm gel
Klaron 10%	10% sodium sulfacetamide	4 oz bottle
Plexion TS (topical suspension)	5% sulfur, 10% sodium sulfacetamide	30 gm tube
Plexion Cleanser	5% sulfur, 10% sodium sulfacetamide	6 oz tube, 12 oz
Staticin	1.5% erythromycin	60 ml liquid
Theramycin Z	2% erythromycin	60 ml liquid

Drying-Keratolytic Antibiotic Preparations

Product	Sulfur	Other	Packaging
Avar	5%	10% sodium sulfacetamide	45 gm Aqueous Gel
Avar Green	5%	10% sodium sulfacetamide	45 gm Aqueous Gel with green pigment to mask redness
Clenia	5%	10% sodium sulfacetamide	1 oz emollient cream
Plexion TS (topical suspension)	5%	10% sodium sulfacetamide	30 gm tube
Plexion SCT	5%	10% sodium sulfacetamide	4 oz
Rosula	5%	10% sodium sulfacetamide	45 ml Aqueous Gel with 10% urea
Sulfacet-R lotion (Rx)	5%	10% sodium sulfacetamide	25 ml
Sulfacet-R lotion TF (tint-free)	5%	10% sodium sulfacetamide	25 ml
Sulfoxyl lotion regular (Rx)	2%	5% benzoyl peroxide	59 ml
Sulfoxyl lotion strong (Rx)	5%	10% benzoyl peroxide	59 ml

Medicated Bar Cleansers for Acne

Product	Active ingredient	Packaging
Acne-Aid Cleansing Bar	6.3% surfactant	4 oz, 5.8 oz bars
Panoxyl Bar 5%, 10%	Benzoyl peroxide	4 oz bar
Salicylic acid soap	2% salicylic acid	4 oz bar
Sulfur soap	10% sulfur	116 gm bar

Medicated Cleansers for Acne

Product	Active ingredient	Packaging
AVAR cleanser	5% sulfur, 10% sodium sulfacetamide	8 oz pump
Brasivol	Aluminum oxide scrub particles	Base, fine, medium, rough
Clenia	5% sulfur, 10% sodium sulfacetamide	6 oz, 12 oz foaming wash
Neutrogena Oil-Free Acne Wash	2% salicylic acid	6 oz pump
Ovace wash	10% sodium sulfacetamide	6 oz, 12 oz
Plexion Cleanser	5% sulfur, 10% sodium sulfacetamide	6 oz, 12 oz
Rosanil	5% sulfur, 10% sodium sulfacetamide	6 oz
SalAc Foam	2% salicylic acid	100 gm canister
SalAc	2% salicylic acid	6 oz bottle

Isotretinoin (Accutane, Amnesteen, Sotret)

Capsules	10 mg
	20 mg
	40 mg

Dosing Isotretinoin by Body Weight

Body weight		Total mg/day		
Kilograms	Pounds	0.5 mg/kg	1 mg/kg	2 mg/kg
40	88	20	40	80
50	110	25	50	100
60	132	30	60	120
70	154	35	70	140
80	176	40	80	160
90	198	45	90	180
100	220	50	100	200

Antiwrinkle Cream

Product	Active ingredient	Packaging
Renova 0.02% emollient	Tretinoin	40 gm
Renova 0.05% emollient	Tretinoin	40 gm
Avage 0.1 cream	Tazarotene	30 gm

Vitamins for Acne

Nicomide tablet contains: nicotinamide 750 mg, zinc 25 mg, folic acid 500 mg
Usual dose is one tablet bid

ANTIBIOTICS (ORAL)

Generic	Brand name	Preparation*	Adult dosage (mg unless noted)
Cephalosporins			
Cephradine	Velosef	250, 500 mg	1-2 gm/24h (bid, qid)
Cephalexin	Keflex	250, 500 mg	250-1000 qid
Cefdinir	Omnicef	300 mg tablet, oral suspension	300 mg bid
Cefadroxil	Duricef	500, 1000 mg	1 gm-24h (qd-bid)
Second-generation			
Cefaclor	Ceclor	250, 500 mg	250-500 tid
Cefuroxime	Ceftin	125, 250, 500 mg	250-500 bid
Cefprozil	Cefzil	250, 500 mg 125 mg/5 ml 250 mg/5 ml	250 bid-500 qd
Cefixime	Suprax	200, 400 mg	200 bid, 400 qd
Fluoroquinolones			
Ofloxacin	Floxin	200, 300, 400 mg	200-400 mg q12h
Ciprofloxacin	Cipro	500, 750 mg	500-750 bid
Macrolides			
Erythromycin (ethylstearate)	E.E.S., E-Mycin, Pediamycin	250, 400 mg	250-800 qid*
Erythromycin (enteric coated)	ERYC, Ery-Tab, E-Mycin	125, 250, 330, 500 mg	250-500 q6h*
Clarithromycin	Biaxin	250, 500 mg	250-500 mg bid
Azithromycin	Zithromax	250 mg 200 mg oral suspension	500 mg first day 250 qd 3 4 days
Penicillins			
Ampicillin	Amcill	250, 500 mg	250-500 qid
Penicillin V	Pen-Vee K, etc.	250, 500 mg	250-500 qid
Dicloxacillin	Dynapen	125, 250, 500 mg	125-500 q6h
Cloxacillin	Generic	250, 500 mg	500 mg qid
Amoxicillin	Generic	250, 500 mg	250-500 tid
Amoxicillin clavulanate	Augmentin	250, 500 mg	250-500 q8h
Sulfonamides, sulfones			
Sulfamethoxazole-trimethoprim	Bactrim DS, Septra DS	800 mg/160 mg	1 tablet bid
Dapsone	Generic	25, 100 mg	50-300 mg qid
Tetracyclines			
Clindamycin	Cleocin	75, 150, 300 mg	150-300 q6h
Demeclocycline	Declomycin	150 mg	150 mg qid, or 300 mg bid
Doxycycline	Monodox, Vibramycin, Doryx, Adoxa	50, 75, 100 mg	100-200/24h (qid-bid)
Minocycline	Dynacin tablets	50, 75, 100 mg	100-200/24h (qid-bid)

*Many preparations available in liquid form.

ANTIBIOTICS (TOPICAL)*

Generic name	Brand name	Preparation*
Bacitracin	Baciguent ointment	15, 30, 120 gm
Chloramphenicol	Chloromycetin cream	30 gm
Clioquinol and 1% HC	Vioform cream	20 gm
Gentamycin	Garamycin cream, ointment, solution	15 gm, 5 ml solution
Iodoquinol and 0.5% or 1% HC	Vytone	1 oz tube
Mafenide acetate	Sulfamylon cream	60, 120, 480 gm
Metronidazole	MetroGel cream, lotion	45 gm, 1 oz lotion
	Noritate	30 gm
Mupirocin 2%	Bactroban cream, ointment	15, 30 gm
Neomycin	Many brands	7.5-60 gm
Nitrofurazone	Furacin cream	28 gm
Polymyxin and bacitracin	Polysporin ointment (many brands)	15, 30 gm (ointment)
	Neosporin powder	10 gm (powder)
Polymyxin, neomycin, and bacitracin	Neosporin (many brands)	15, 30 gm
Povidone-iodine	Betadine ointment	30 gm
Silver sulfadiazine	Silvadene cream	20, 50, 85, 400 gm

*Topical antibiotics for acne are listed in the acne medication section.

ANTIFUNGAL AGENTS (ORAL)

Brand name	Generic name	Packaging
Diflucan	Fluconazole	50, 100, 150, 200 mg
Fulvicin P/G	Griseofulvin ultramicrosize	125, 165, 250, 330 mg
Fulvicin U/F	Griseofulvin microsize	250, 500 mg; 125 mg/ml suspension
Grifulvin V	Griseofulvin microsize	250, 500 mg; 125 mg/5 ml in 4 oz bottle
Gris-PEG	Griseofulvin ultramicrosize	125, 250 mg
Mycosatin	Mystatin	500,000, 1 million U capsules 100,000 U/ml suspension
Nizoral	Ketoconazole	200 mg
Lamisil	Terbinafine	250 mg
Sporanox	Itraconazole	100 mg
Mycelex troches for oral Candida		10 mg troche; bottle of 70 or 140 Dissolve 5/day in mouth for 14 days

ANTIFUNGAL AGENTS (TOPICAL)

Topical Agents Active Against Dermatophytes and Candida

Brand name	Generic name	Packaging
Exelderm	Sulconazole	15, 30, 60 gm cream 30 ml solution
Lamisil (not for Candida)	Terbinafine hydrochloride cream	12, 24 gm cream 30 ml dropper or spray
Loprox	Ciclopirox olamine	15, 30, 90 gm cream 30, 100 gel 30, 60 ml topical suspension
Lotrimin	Clotrimazole	Several creams and solutions 15, 30, 45, 90 gm cream 10, 30 ml solution
Lotrisone*	Clotrimazole and betamethasone Dipropionate	15, 45 gm cream 30 ml lotion
Micatin	Miconazole	0.5 oz cream 3.5 oz spray liquid 3.5 oz spray powder
Naftin	Naftifine	15, 30, 60 gm cream 20, 40, 60 gm gel
Nizoral	Ketoconazole	15, 30, 60 gm
Oxistat	Oxiconazole	15, 30, 60 gm cream 30 ml lotion
Penlac	Ciclopirox	6.6 ml nail lacquer solution
Spectazole	Econazole	15, 30, 85 gm cream

*A preparation containing an antifungal agent and potent topical steroid; it is useful for inflamed fungal infections. Potent topical steroids should be used only for short durations in intertriginous areas such as the groin. Change to an antifungal agent once inflammation is controlled.

Topical Agents Active Against Candida

Brand name	Generic name	Packaging
Fungizone	Amphotericin B	20 gm cream 30 ml lotion
Fungoid tincture	Miconazole	2 oz bottle liquid
Mycostatin	Nystatin	30 gm cream
Mycolog II*	Nystatin and triamcinolone	15, 30, 60 gm cream or ointment
Mycelex troches†	Clotrimazole	10 mg troche Bottle of 70

*A preparation containing an anti-Candida agent and topical steroid; it is useful for inflamed yeast infections. Topical steroids should be used only for short durations in intertriginous areas such as the groin. Change to an anti-Candida agent once inflammation is controlled.
†Dissolve in mouth 5/day for 14 days.

Agents Effective for Treating Tinea Versicolor

Brand name	Generic name	Packaging*	Directions
DHS Zinc (or any other zinc shampoo)	2% pyrithione zinc	6 oz, 12 oz	Apply to trunk, arms, and thighs for 10 min; shower off; repeat for 14 days
Exelderm	Sulconazole	15, 30, 60 gm 30 ml bottle	qd for 14 days
Lamisil	Terbinafine hydrochloride	24 gm pump	qd for 14 days
Loprox	Ciclopirox olamine	15, 30, 60 gm cream	qd for 14 days
Lotrimin	Clotrimazole	15, 30, 45, 90 gm cream	qd for 14 days
Micatin	Miconazole	0.5 oz cream	bid 3 weeks
Sebulex	2% sulfur, 2% salicylic acid	240 ml lotion	Apply qhs, wash off in morning, for 7 days
Selsun lotion	2.5% selenium sulfide	generic lotion	Apply daily for 10 min for 7 consecutive days
Spectazole	Econazole	15, 30, 85 gm cream	qd for 14 days
Nizoral	Ketaconazole	200 mg tablet 15, 30, 60 cream gm	Single 400 mg dose each month or 200 mg qd 5 days
		120 ml shampoo	Apply once and rinse off
Diflucan	Fluconazole	50, 100, 150, 200 mg	Single 300-mg dose
Sporanox	Itraconazole	100 mg	200 mg for 7 days

*Many sizes of these preparations are available. Generally it is most economical to prescribe the largest-size container because a large area must be treated.

ANTIHISTAMINES

Medications for Urticaria

Drug	Initial dose (adult)	Maximal dose* (adult)	Liquid formulation	Tablet formulation
H1-receptor antagonists				
Nonsedating *				
Fexofenadine (Allegra)	180 mg qd	180 mg bid	—	30 mg, 60 mg, 180 mg
Desloratadine (Clarinex)	5 mg	10 mg	—	5 mg
Loratadine (Claritin)	10 mg qd	20 mg bid	5 mg/5 ml	10 mg
Cetirizine (Zyrtec)	10 mg qd	10 mg bid	5 mg/5 ml	5 mg, 10 mg
Sedating				
Hydroxyzine (Atarax)	10 mg qid	50 mg qid	10 mg/5 ml Susp. 25 mg/5 ml	10 mg, 25 mg, 50 mg, 100 mg
Diphenhydramine (Benadryl)	25 mg bid	50 mg qid	Elixir 12.5 mg/5 ml Syrup 6.25 mg/5 ml	25, 50 mg 12.5 mg chew tab
Cyproheptadine (Periactin)	4 mg qid	8 mg qid	2 mg/5 ml	8 mg
H2-receptor antagonists				
Cimetidine (Tagamet)	400 mg bid	800 mg bid	300 mg/5 cc	200 mg, 300 mg, 400 mg, 800 mg
Ranitidine (Zantac)	150 mg bid	300 mg bid	75 mg/5 cc	150 mg, 300 mg
Famotidine Pepcid)	20 mg bid	40 mg bid	40 mg/5 cc	20 mg, 40 mg
H1- and H2-receptor antagonist				
Doxepin (Sinequan)	10 mg qid	50 mg qid	10 mg/ml	10 mg, 25 mg, 50 mg, 75 mg, 100 mg, 150 mg
Corticosteroids				
Prednisone	20 mg qod with gradual taper	Many other dose schedules	5 mg/5 ml	2.5 mg, 5 mg, 10 mg, 20 mg, 50 mg
Methylprednisolone (Medrol)	16 mg qod with gradual tapering	Many other dose schedules	—	2 mg, 4 mg, 8 mg, 16 mg, 24 mg, 32 mg
Leukotriene antagonists				
Zafirlukast (Accolate)	20 mg bid	—	—	10 mg, 20 mg
Montelukast (Singulair)	10 mg qd	—	—	4 mg chewable, 5 mg chewable, 10 mg
Epinephrine	**Injection**			
• Ana-Guard (1:1000)	0.3 mL/dose SC			
• EpiPen (1:1000)	0.3 mg/dose			
• EpiPen Jr (1:2000)	Children<12 yr: 0.15 mg/dose			
Immunotherapy				
Cyclosporin	2-3 mg/kg daily	4-6 mg/kg daily	100 mg/ml	25 mg, 50 mg, 100 mg
Methotrexate	2.5 mg PO bid for 3 days of the week	5 mg PO bid for 3 days of the week	25 mg/ml	2.5 mg

*Higher dosages than recommended by the manufacturer may be required for maximum therapeutic effect.

ANTINEOPLASTIC AGENTS (TOPICAL)

	Product	Packaging
Aldara	5% imiquimod	Box of 12 packets
Carac	0.5% fluorouracil	30 gm tube
Fluoroplex	1% fluorouracil 1% fluorouracil	30 ml solution 30 gm cream
Efudex	2% fluorouracil 5% fluorouracil 5% fluorouracil	10 ml liquid 10 ml liquid 25 gm cream

ANTIPERSPIRANTS

Brand name	Active ingredient	Packaging
Certain-Dri (otc)	Aluminum chloride (hexahydrate)	1, 2 oz roll-on Pump spray (nonaerosol)
Drysol (Rx)	20% aluminum chloride (hexahydrate) in 93% anhydrous ethyl alcohol	35 ml bottle with Dab-O-Matic applicator 37.5 ml bottle
Hypercare	20% aluminum chloride (hexahydrate) in 93% anhydrous ethyl alcohol	37.5 ml bottle and 35 cc and 60 cc bottle with Dab-O-Matic applicator
Lazerformalyde solution (Rx)	10% formaldehyde	3 oz roll-on
Formaldehyde-10 spray	10% formaldehyde	2 oz spray bottle
Xerac AC (Rx)	6.25% aluminum chloride (hexahydrate) in 96% anhydrous ethyl alcohol	35, 60 ml bottles with Dab-O-Matic applicator

Drionic Therapy for Hyperhidrosis (Iontophoresis)

Iontophoresis (the application of low-level electric current to the surface of the skin) results in reduced production of sweat at that site. A battery-operated device conforming to the shape of the treated area, using tap water–wetted pads in contact with the skin of the palms, soles, or axillae, is available for patient self-use. Four to 15 treatments 20 minutes long inhibit sweat for up to 6 weeks; 95% of patients showed improvement in 2 weeks, and 86% remained improved at 6 weeks. Minor retreatment every 6 weeks is needed to sustain inhibition. Biopsies reveal hyperkeratotic plugs within sweat ducts following treatment.

Three devices (Drionic Hands, Drionic Axillae, Drionic Feet) are available at $125.00 per pair. They may be ordered by the patient from General Medical Co, Dept DM-8, 1935 Armacost Ave., Los Angeles, CA 90025. (www.drionic.com)

More complicated devices are available from other manufacturers.

ANTIPRURITIC CREAMS AND LOTIONS

Brand name	Active ingredient	Packaging
Eucerin itch relief	menthol 0.15%	6.8 oz spray
Neutrogena antiitch moisturizer	camphor 0.1%, dimethacone 0.1%	10.1 oz
PrameGel	1% pramoxine, 0.5% menthol	
Pramosone cream 1%, 2.5%	Hydrocortisone & Pramoxine HCL	1oz, 2 oz
Pramosone lotion 1%	Hydrocortisone & Pramoxine HCL	2 oz, 4 oz, 8 oz
Pramosone lotion 2.5%	Hydrocortisone & Pramoxine HCL	2 oz, 4 oz
Pramosone ointment 1%, 2.5%	Hydrocortisone & Pramoxine HCL	1 oz
Sarna	0.5% each of camphor, menthol	7.5 oz bottle
Zonalon	5% doxepin	45 gm

ANTIVIRAL AGENTS

Abreva (docosanol) 2 gm (otc)
Denavir (penciclovir), 1.5 gm ointment
Famvir (famciclovir), 125, 250, 500 mg tablets
Valtrex (valacyclovir), 500 mg, 1 gm capsules
Zovirax (acyclovir), 200, 400, 800 mg capsules
Zovirax ointment 5%, 3 and 15 gm tubes

Topical Therapy for Postherpetic Neuralgia
Zostrix (capsaicin, 0.075% cream), 1 oz tube (otc)

CONTRACEPTIVES (ORAL)

Drug	Progestin (mg)	Estrogen (ethinyl estradiol mg)
Desogen	Desogestrel 0.15	30
Ortho-Cept	Desogestrel 0.15	30
Ortho-Cyclen	Norgestimate 0.25	35
Ortho Tri-Cyclen	Norgestimate 0.25	35
Ovcon-35	Norethindrone 0.4	
Brevicon 21, 28	Norethindrone 0.5	35
Modicon 21, 28	Norethindrone 0.5	35
Ortho-Novum 7/7/7*	Norethindrone 0.5, 0.75, 1.0	35
Ortho-Novum 10-11*	Norethindrone 0.5, 1.0	35
N.E.E. 10/11 21, 28	Norethindrone 0.5, 1.0	35
Tri-Norinyl*	Norethindrone 0.5, 1.0, 0.5	35
Norinyl 1 1 35 21, 28	Norethindrone 1.0	35
Ortho 1/35 21	Norethindrone 1.0	35
Demulen 1/50 21, 28	Ethynodiol diacetate 1.0	50
Demulen 1/35 21, 28	Ethynodiol diacetate 1.0	35
Triphasil 21, 28	Levonorgestrel 0.05, 0.075, 0.125	30, 40, 30
Tri-Levlen 21, 28	Levonorgestrel 0.05, 0.075, 0.125	30, 40, 30
Levlen 21, 28	Levonorgestrol 0.15	30
Nordette 21, 28	Levonorgestrol 0.15	30
Lo/Ovral 21, 28	Norgestrel 0.3	30
Ovral	Norgestrel 0.5	50
Loestrin 1/20	Norethindrone 1.0	20
Loestrin 1.5/30	Norethindrone 1.5	30

Modified from The Medical Letter 1992; 34 (885), Dec 11; and Dickey RP: Managing contraceptive pill patients, ed 4, Durant, OK, 1986, Creative Informatics.

*Many oral contraceptives are available in both 21- and 28-day regimens. Total androgenic effect of a pill depends on the balance between the estrogen and progestin agent. Pills with low androgenicity are better for acne, alopecia, and hirsutism. Individual response to pills varies. Some women with acne improve with pills with high androgenicity.

CORTICOSTEROIDS (TOPICAL)*

Group	Brand name	%	Generic name	Tube size (gm unless noted)
I	Condran tape		Flurandrenolide	small roll, large roll, patches
	Cormax cream	0.05	Clobetasol propionate	15, 30, 45
	Cormax ointment	0.05		15, 30, 45
	Cormax scalp solution	0.05		25 ml, 50 ml
	Ultravate cream	0.05	Halobetasol propionate	15, 50
	Ultravate ointment	0.05		15, 50
	Diprolene lotion	0.05	Augmented betamethasone dipropionate	30 ml, 60 ml
	Diprolene ointment	0.05		15, 50
	Diprolene gel	0.05		15, 50
	Olux foam	0.05	Clobetasol propionate	50 gm, 100 gm can
	Psorcon ointment	0.05	Diflorasone diacetate	15, 30, 60
	Temovate-E cream	0.05	Clobetasol propionate	15, 30, 45, 60
	Temovate ointment	0.05	Clobetasol propionate	15, 30, 45, 60
	Temovate gel	0.05	Clobetasol propionate	15, 30, 60
II	Cyclocort ointment	0.1	Amcinonide	15, 30, 60
	Diprolene AF cream	0.05	Augmented betamethasone dipropionate	15, 50
	Diprosone ointment	0.05	Betamethasone dipropionate	15, 45
	Diprosone aerosol	0.1	Betamethasone dipropionate	85 gm can
	Elocon ointment	0.1	Mometasone furoate	
	Halog cream	0.1	Halcinonide	15, 30, 60
	Halog ointment	0.1		15, 30, 60
	Halog solution	0.1		20, 60 ml
	Halog-E cream	0.1		30, 60
	Lidex cream	0.05	Fluocinonide	15, 30, 60, 120
	Lidex -E	0.05	Fluocinonide	15, 30, 60
	Lidex gel	0.05		15, 30, 60
	Lidex ointment	0.05		30, 60
	Lidex solution	0.05		20, 60 ml
	Psorcon-E cream	0.05	Diflorasone diacetate	15, 30, 60
	Psorcon-E ointment	0.05		15, 30, 60
	Topicort cream	0.25	Desoximetasone	15, 60
	Topicort gel	0.05		15, 60
	Topicort ointment	0.25		15, 60
III	Alphatrex cream	0.05	Betamethasone dipropionate	45
	Alphatrex ointment	0.05		45
	Aristocort A cream	0.5	Triamcinolone acetonide	15
	Betatrex ointment	0.1	Betamethasone valerate	45
	Cutivate ointment	0.005	Fluticasone propionate	15, 30, 60
	Cyclocort lotion	0.1	Amcinonide	20, 60 ml
	Cyclocort cream	0.1	Amcinonide	15, 30, 60
	Diprosone cream	0.05	Betamethasone dipropionate	15, 45
	Diprosone lotion	0.05	Betamethasone dipropionate	20, 60 ml
	Elocon ointment	0.1	Mometasone furoate	15, 45
	Kenalog cream	0.5	Triamcinolone acetonide	20
IV	Aristocort A ointment	0.1	Triamcinolone acetonide	15, 60
	Cordran ointment	0.05	Flurandrenolide	15, 30, 60
	Cyclocort cream	0.1	Amcinonide	15, 30, 60
	Dermatop-E ointment	0.1	Prednicarbate	15, 60

Group	Brand name	%	Generic name	Tube size (gm; unless noted)
	Elocon cream	0.1	Mometasone furoate	15, 45
	Elocon lotion	0.1		30, 60 ml
	Kenalog ointment	0.1	Triamcinolone acetonide	15, 60
	Luxig foam	0.12	Betamethasone valerate	50 gm, 100 gm can
	Synalar ointment	0.025	Fluocinolone acetonide	15, 60
	Westcort ointment	0.2	Hydrocortisone	15, 45, 60
V	Aristocort cream	0.1	Triamcinolone acetonide	15
	Betatrex cream	0.1	Betamethasone valerate	45
	Cloderm cream	0.1	Clocortolone pivalate	15, 45
	Cordran SP cream	0.05	Flurandrenolide	15, 30, 60
	Cordran lotion	0.5		15, 60 ml
	Cordran ointment	0.025		15, 30, 60
	Cutivate cream	0.05	Fluticasone propionate	15, 30, 60
	Dermatop-E cream	0.1	Prednicarbate	15, 60
	DesOwen ointment	0.05	Desonide	15, 60
	Kenalog cream	0.1	Triamcinolone acetonide	15, 60, 80
	Kenalog lotion	0.1		60 ml
	Locoid lipocream	0.1	Hydrocortisone butyrate	15, 45
	Locoid cream	0.1	Hydrocortisone butyrate	15, 45
	Locoid ointment	0.1		15, 45
	Locoid solution			20, 60 cc
	Synalar cream	0.025	Fluocinolone acetonide	15, 60
	Synemol cream	0.025	Fluocinolone acetonide	60
	Tridesilon ointment	0.05	Desonide	15, 60
	Westcort cream	0.2	Hydrocortisone valerate	15, 45, 60
VI	Aclovate cream	0.05	Prednicarbate	15, 45, 60
	Aclovate ointment	0.05	Prednicarbate	15, 45, 60
	Aristocort A cream	0.025	Triamcinolone acetonide	15, 60
	Capex shampoo	0.01	Fluocinolone acetonide	120 ml
	Dermasmooth	0.01	Fluocinolone acetonide	4 oz
	Cordran SP cream	0.025	Flurandrenolide	30, 60
	DesOwen cream	0.05	Desonide	15, 60, 90
	DesOwen lotion	0.05		2, 4 oz
	Kenalog lotion	0.025	Triamcinalone acetonide	60 ml
	Synalar solution	0.01		20, 60 ml
VII	Epifoam	1.0	Hydrocortisone acetate	10 gm can
	Hytone cream	2.5	Hydrocortisone	1, 2 oz
	Hytone lotion	2.5		2 oz
	Hytone ointment	2.5		1 oz
	Lacticare HC lotion	1.0	Hydrocortisone	4 oz
		2.5		2 oz
	Pramosone	1.0	Hydrocortisone acetate 1 pramoxine	2, 4, 8 oz lotion
				1, 2 oz cream
				1 oz ointment
		2.5		2, 4, oz lotion
				1, 2 oz cream
				1 oz ointment
		1.0	Hydrocortisone	Many brands

Listed by potency group: group I is the most potent.

CORTICOSTEROIDS (ORAL)

Generic name	Brand name	Preparation	Equivalent dose (mg)
Betamethasone	Celestone	0.6 mg, 0.6 mg/5 ml	0.6
Cortisol (hydrocortisone)	Cortef	5, 10, 20 mg	20
	Hydrocortone	10, 20 mg	20
Cortisone	Cortone	25 mg	25
Dexamethasone	Decadron	0.25, 0.5, 0.75, 1.5, 4, 6 mg	0.75
Dexamethasone	Hexadrol	0.5, 0.75, 1.5, 4 mg, 5 mg/5ml	0.75
Methylprednisolone	Medrol	2, 4, 8, 16, 24, 32 mg	4
Prednisolone	Delta-Cortef	5 mg	5
	Prelone	15 mg/5 ml	5
Prednisone	Deltasone	1, 2.5, 5, 10, 20, 50 mg	5
	Liquid Pred	5 mg/5 ml	5
	Metricorten	1, 5 mg	5
	Orasone	1, 5, 10, 20, 50 mg	5
Triamcinolone	Aristocort	1, 2, 4, 8, 16 mg, 2 mg/5 ml	4
	Kenacort	1, 2, 4, 8 mg, 4 mg/5ml	4

DEPIGMENTING AND COSMETIC COVERING AGENTS

Skin Bleaches and Depigmenting Agents

Brand name	Active ingredient	Sun protectant	Packaging
Benoquin cream (Rx)*	20% monobenzone	None	1¼ oz tube
Claripel	4% hydroquinone	Sunscreen	28 gm, 45 gm tube
Eldopaque Forte 4% cream (Rx)†	4% hydroquinone	Sunblock	1 oz tube
Eldoquin Forte 4% cream (Rx)	4% hydroquinone	None	1 oz tube
Glyquin	4% hydroquinone	Sunscreen	1 oz jar
Glyquin XM	4% hydroquinone Vitamins C & E Hyaluronic acid	Sunscreen	1 oz jar
Lustra	4% hydroquinone	None	1 oz, 2 oz jar
Lustra AF	4% hydroquinone	Sunscreen	1 oz, 2 oz jar
Alustra	4% hydroquinone Retinol	None	1 oz jar
Melanex topical solution‡	3% hydroquinone	None	1 oz bottle
Solaquin Forte 4% cream (Rx)	4% hydroquinone	Sunscreen	1 oz tube
Solaquin Forte 4% gel (Rx)	4% hydroquinone	Sunscreen	1 oz tube
Solage	2% mequinol 0.01% tretinoin	none	30 ml
TriLuma	4% hydroquinone 0.01% fluocinolone acetonide 0.05% tretinoin	none	30 gm
Ultraquin	Hydroquinone crystals for compounding		

*Indicated for extensive vitiligo to depigment entire body.
†Flesh-tinted cream base.
‡Packaged with a narrow plastic and broad tip sponge applicator.

Masking Agents (Cosmetic Covering Agents)			
Brand name	**Base**	**Packaging**	**Shades**
Covermark*	Cream	Many products	9-10
Dermablend cover cream*	Cream	Many products	21
Dy-O-Derm†	Liquid	4 oz	
Vitady†	Liquid	15 ml	

*Waterproof concealing makeup.
†A solution to mask vitiligo; transmits most UVA radiation, so it can be used concurrently with psoralens in vitiligo therapy.

HAIR RESTORATION PRODUCTS

Propecia	Finasteride	1 mg
Rogaine	Minoxidil solution 2% for women, 5% for men	60 ml bottle

IMMUNOMODULATORS (TOPICAL)

Steroid Free Topical Antiinflammatory Agents		
Elidel cream 1%	Pimecrolimus	15g, 30 gm, 100 gm
Protopic ointment 0.1 %	Tacrolimus	30 gm, 60 gm, 100 gm
Protopic ointment 0.03 %	Tacrolimus	30 gm, 60 gm, 100 gm

LUBRICATING AGENTS

Emollients

Emollients are complex mixtures containing many ingredients. They are listed under their primary ingredient.

Emollients Containing Urea		
Urea promotes hydration and removal of excess keratin.		
Product	**Active ingredients**	**Packaging**
Carmol 10 lotion	10% urea	6 oz
Carmol 20 cream	20% urea	3 oz
Carmol 40 lotion (Rx)	40% urea	8 oz
Carmol 40 gel (Rx)	40% urea	10 m
Carmol 40 cream (Rx)	40% urea	1oz, 3 oz, 7 oz
Ultra Mide lotion	25% urea	8 oz
Vanamide urea cream	40% urea	85 gm, 199 gm

Emollients Containing Lactic Acid

Lactic acid promotes hydration and removal of excess keratin.

Product	Active ingredients	Packaging
Amlactin cream	12%	4.9 oz
Amlactin AP cream	12%	4.9 oz anti-itch cream + 1% pramoxine
Amlactin lotion	12%	8 oz, 14 oz
Epilyt lotion	5%	4 oz
Lac-Hydrin cream (Rx)	12%	385 gm bottles
Lac-Hydrin lotion (Rx)	12%	400 gm
Lacticare lotion	5%	8, 12 oz bottles
Lactinol lotion	10%	8 oz
U-Lactin lotion	—	8 oz

Ointments

Ointments containing petrolatum
Aquaphor
DML Forté
Elta
Eucerin
Moisturel
Greaseless ointments
Acid Mantle
Unibase

Gel That Removes Excess Keratin

Keralyt gel, 6% salicylic acid and propylene glycol, 1 oz

PROTECTING BARRIER CREAMS

Brand/generic name	Size	Use
Dermaguard	2, 12 oz	Industrial (protects against acids)
Desitin ointment	30, 60, 120, 240, 480 gm	Protective ointment
Ivy Shield	1.25, 4, 16 oz	Helps prevent poison ivy and oak dermatitis
Kerodex 51	120, 480 gm	Protective cream for dry, oily work
Kerodex 71	120, 480 gm	Protective cream (water repellent)
pH-Stabil	60, 240 gm	Protective cream
SBR-Lipocream	30, 100 gm	Protective cream
TheraSeal	6 oz	Protective cream
Zinc oxide		
20% ointment	60 gm	Protective ointment
25% paste	30, 60, 480 gm	Protective paste

PSORIASIS AND SEBORRHEIC DERMATITIS (SHAMPOOS)

Antimicrobial Antiseborrheic Shampoos (Pyrithione Zinc and Others)

Brand name	Active ingredient	Packaging
Capitrol (Rx)	2% chloroxine	85 gm
DHS Zinc	2% pyrithione zinc	8, 12 oz
Head & Shoulders	2% pyrithione zinc	400 ml
Nizoral	2% ketoconazole	4 oz
ZNP Bar	2% pyrithione zinc	4.2 oz bar

Selenium Sulfide Shampoos

Brand name	Concentration	Packaging
Selsun	2.5%	120 ml
Selsun Blue	1%	120, 210, 330 ml
Head & Shoulders Intensive Treatment	1%	400 ml

Tar and Tar-Combination Shampoos

Brand name	Concentration	Packaging
Ala Seb T	5% coal tar solution 2% colloidal sulfur 2% salicylic acid	4 oz, 12 oz
Denorex	2% coal tar gel 2% coal tar lotion	60, 120 ml 120, 240 ml
DHS Tar	0.5% coal tar USP	4, 8, 16 oz
DHS Tar gel	0.5% coal tar USP	8 oz
Ionil T	1.0 % coal tar USP	16 oz
Liquor carbonis detergens	10-15% coal tar	Any amount in Green soap*
Neutrogena T/gel	2% Newtar	4.4, 8.5, 16 oz
Neutrogena T/gel extra strength	4% Newtar (1% coal tar)	6 oz
Neutrogena T/sal	3% salicylic acid	4.5 oz
Packer's pine tar	0.82% pine tar	180 ml
Pentrax tar	5% crude coal tar	8 oz
Pentrax Gold	2% crude coal tar	5.7 oz
Polytar	1% mixture of tars	6 oz, 12 oz
Sebutone	0.5% coal tar, 2% salicylic acid, 2% sulfur	120, 240 gm lotion
Tarsum	2% coal tar	4, 8 oz
Tegrin Medicated	5% coal tar extract	60, 132 ml cream 112.5, 198 ml lotion
Theraplex T shampoo	1% coal tar	8 oz
Tiseb-T	0.5% coal tar	
Vanseb-T	5% coal tar	120 ml lotion
Xseb-T plus	10% crude coal tar	4, 8 oz
Zetar	1% whole coal tar	180 ml

*Pharmacist compounded.

Sulfur and Salicylic Acid Shampoos

Product	Sulfur	Salicylic acid	Packaging
Ala-Seb	2%	2%	4oz, 12 oz
Ionil Plus		2%	240 ml
DHS Sal		3%	4 oz
Meted	5%	3%	120 ml
Salicylic Acid & Sulfur Soap	5%	3%	4.1 oz
Sebulex	2%	2%	120 ml 120, 240 ml
Sulfoam	2%		4, 8, 16 oz
Tiseb	—	2%	8 oz
Vanseb	2%	1%	90 gm cream 120 ml lotion
Xseb	—	4%	4, 8 oz
P & S	—	2%	4, 8 oz

Antiseborrheic Preparations

Brand name	Active ingredient	Packaging
DermaZinc Therapy spray/drops	(0.25%) zinc pyrithione	4 oz
Loprox gel	Ciclopirox	45 gm
Nizoral cream	Ketoconazole	15, 30, 60 gm
Ovace wash	10% sulfacetamide sodium	6 oz, 12 oz
Ovace foam	10% sulfacetamide sodium	50 gm, 100 gm can
Carmol scalp treatment lotion	10% sulfacetamide sodium	90 gm

Corticosteroid, Tar, and Other Medicated Scalp Preparations and Shampoos

Brand name	Active ingredient	Base	Packaging
Derma-smoothe/FS (Rx)	Fluocinolone acetonide 0.01%	Peanut oil	120 ml
P & S liquid	Less than 1% phenol, NaCl	Paraffin oil	120, 240 ml
Estar Therapeutic Tar Gel	5% coal tar	Water	3 oz
10% liquor carbonis detergens in Nivea oil*	Liquor carbonis detergens, 8, 16 oz	Nivea oil	Prescribe
Capex shampoo (Rx)	0.01% fluocinolone acetonide		120 ml
Overnight scalp treatment	2% salicylic acid	Spray	6 oz

*Pharmacist compounded.

PSORIASIS MEDICATIONS (ORAL)

Psoralens

Brand name	Active ingredient	Packaging
Oxsoralen lotion	Methoxsalen 1% lotion	1 oz bottle
Oxsoralen-Ultra	Methoxsalen (liquid form)	10 mg capsules, bottle of 50 (green capsules)
8-MOP	Methoxsalen (crystalline form)	10 mg capsules, bottle of 30 (pink capsules)
Trisoralen tablets	Trioxsalen	5 mg tablets, bottles of 28, 100

Recommended Oxsoralen-Ultra Dosage According to Weight

Patient's weight		Dose	
(kg)	(lbs)	Low	High
<30	<65	10	10
30-50	65-100	10	20
51-65	101-145	20	30
66-80	146-175	20	40
81-90	176-200	30	50
91-115	200-250	30	60
>115	>250	40	70

Acitretin (Soriatane)

Capsules	10, 25 mg

Methotrexate

Tablets	2.5, 5, 7.5, 10, 15 mg	
Preservative-free injection	25 mg/ml	2, 4, 8 ml vials
Powder for injection	20 mg, 1 gm	20 ml vials or single-use vials

PSORIASIS MEDICATIONS (TOPICAL)

Anthralin (Dithranol)

Brand name	Concentration (%)	Base	Packaging
Drithocreme	0.1	Cream	50 gm tube
Drithocreme HP 1%	1	Cream	50 gm tube
Dritho-Scalp	0.5	Cream	50 gm tube*
Psoriatec	1.0	Cream	50 gm tube
*With special applicator.			

Anthralin Stain-Prevention Treatment

Brand name	Active ingredient	Packaging	Use
CuraStain	Triethanolamine	4 oz cream or spray	Dermatologic stain remover; apply to surrounding skin and lesions before wash-off. Apply to lesions after wash-off.

Topical Retinoids

Tazorac (tazarotene)

Gel	0.05%, 0.1%	30 gm 100 gm
Cream	0.05%, 0.1%	15 gm 30 gm 60 gm

Topical Vitamin D$_3$ Analog

Brand name	Active ingredient	Packaging
Dovonex ointment	Calcipotriene .05	30, 60, 100 gm tubes
Dovonex cream	Calcipotriene .05	30, 60, 100 gm tubes

Tar-Containing Bath Oil

Brand name	Size	Packaging
Balnetar	2.5% coal tar	240 ml
Doak Oil	2% tar distillate	240 ml
Doak Oil Forte	5% tar distillate	120 ml
Lavatar	33.3% tar distillate	120, 480 ml
Polytar Bath	25% polytar	240 ml
Zetar emulsion (Rx)	30% whole coal tar	177 ml (6 oz)

Tar Creams and Solutions

Brand name	Concentration	Other ingredient(s)	Base	Packaging
Aqua Tar	2.5% coal tar extract	—	Gel (water base)	90 gm
Cutar	7.5% LCD		Emulsion	6 oz, 1 gal
Doak Tar Lotion	5% tar distillate	—	Lotion	4 oz
Elta lite tar	10% LCD		Lotion	8 oz
Elta tar	10% coal tar		Cream	3.8, 16 oz
Estar	5% coal tar	13.8% alcohol	Gel	90 gm
Fototar	2% coal tar, USP	—	Cream	85 gm, 1 lb jar
Fototar Stik	5% coal tar, USP	—	Wax	15 gm
Ichthyol	10% ichthammol	—	Ointment	30 gm
Liquor carbonis detergens*	20% coal tar solution	—	Solution	4 oz, pt, gal
Mazon cream	0.18% coal tar	1% salicylic acid, 1% resorcinol, 0.5% benzoic acid	Cream	
Oxipor VHC	48.5% coal tar solution	1% salicylic acid	Lotion	2 oz, 4 oz
P & S Plus	8% coal tar solution	2% salicylic acid	Gel	105 gm
Packer's	5.87% pine tar		Soap	
PolyTar Soap	Blend of tars		Soap	Bar
Pragmatar	4% coal tar distillate	3% salicylic acid, 3% sulfur	Ointment	
PsoriGel	7.5% coal tar solution	1% alcohol	Gel	4 oz
T/Derm	5% coal tar extract	Alcohol free	Oil	4 oz
Tegrin Medicated	5% crude coal tar extract		Lotion Cream	6 oz 60, 132 gm
Unguentum Bossi	5% tar distillate	5% ammoniated Hg	Ointment	60, 480 gm

*Used by the pharmacist for compounding in Unibase and other ointment bases.

Gel That Removes Excess Keratin

Keralyt Gel, 6% salicylic acid and propylene glycol, 1 oz

ROSACEA MEDICATIONS (TOPICAL)

Brand name	Generic name	Packaging
Avar	5% sulfur, 10% sodium sulfacetamide	45 gm Aqueous Gel
Avar Green	5% sulfur, 10% sodium sulfacetamide	45 gm Aqueous Gel with green pigment to mask redness
Clenia	5% sulfur, 10% sodium sulfacetamide	1 oz emollient cream (alcohol free) 6 oz, 12 oz foaming wash
Finacea 15%	Azelaic acid	30 gm gel
Klaron 10%	10% sodium sulfacetamide	2 oz bottle
Metro Gel 0.75%	Metronidazole	45 gm tube
Metro Cream 0.75%	Metronidazole	45 gm tube
Metro Lotion 0.75%	Metronidazole	2 oz bottle
Noritate Cream 1%	Metronidazole	30 gm tube
Sulfacet-R lotion	5% sulfur, 10% sodium sulfacetamide	25 gm bottle
Sulfacet-R lotion (tint free)	5% sulfur, 10% sodium sulfacetamide	25 gm bottle
Plexion TS (topical suspension)	5% sulfur, 10% sodium sulfacetamide	30 gm tube
Plexion Cleanser	5% sulfur, 10% sodium sulfacetamide	6 oz tube
Rosula	5% sulfur, 10% sodium sulfacetamide	45 ml Aqueous Gel with 10% urea

Vitamins for Rosacea
Nicomide tablet contains nicotinamide 750 mg, zinc 25 mg, folic acid 500 mg
Usual dose is one tablet bid

SCABICIDES AND PEDICULOCIDES

Scabicides

Brand name	Generic name	Packaging
Acticin	Permethrin	5% cream: 60 gm
Elimite	Permethrin	5% cream: 60 gm
Eurax*	Crotamiton	10% cream: 60 gm 10% lotion: 2 oz, 1 pt
Kwell	Lindane	1% cream: 2 oz, 16 oz 1% lotion: 2 oz, 16 oz
Kwell shampoo	Lindane	1% lotion: 2 oz, 16 oz
5%-10% precipitated	Sulfur	Sulfur in petrolatum†
Stromectol	Ivermectin‡	6 mg tablets‡

*Eurax has been reported to be less effective than lindane.
†Pharmacist compounded.
‡See p. 504.

Pediculocides

Brand name	Generic name	Packaging
A-200 (otc)	0.33% pyrethrins	30 gm gel
A-200 Pyrinate Gel shampoo (otc)	0.17% pyrethrins	2, 4 oz shampoo
NIX cream rinse	Permethrin	2 oz
Ovide	0.5% malathion	2 oz lotion
R & C shampoo (otc)	0.3% pyrethrins	2, 4 oz shampoo
RID (otc)	0.3% pyrethrins	2 oz, 4 oz, 1 gal liquid

*For removal of lice eggs (nits); does not kill lice.

SHAMPOO—FRAGRANCE FREE, DYE FREE

DHS Clear, 8, 16 oz

SOAP-FREE CLEANSERS

Often used in the management of atopic dermatitis.	
Aquanil lotion	8, 16 oz
Cetaphil lotion	4, 8, 16 oz
Cetaphil Daily Facial Cleanser	8 oz
Moisturel sensitive skin cleanser	8.75 oz
Neutrogena—nondrying	5.5 oz
SFC lotion	8, 16 oz

SOAPS—BAR (MILD, NONIRRITATING)

Alpha-Keri	Dove	Oilatum
Basis glycerin	Neutrogena dry skin	Purpose
Basis superfatted	Nivea Creme	Shepard's moisturizing
Cetaphil	Cetaphil anti-bacterial	

SUNPROTECTIVE CLOTHING

Coolibar 952-922-1445 www.coolibar.com
A full line of sunprotective clothing and glasses

Radicool Australia 714-220-4900 ext. 224 www.radicoolaustralia.com
A full line of 100 SPF+ swimwear

Sunday Afternoons 888-874-2642 www.sundayafternoons.com
Sunprotective hats and clothing

SunPrecautions 800-882-7860 www.sunprecautions.com
A full line of sunprotective clothing

Tilley Endurables 800-338-2797 www.tilley.com
Sunprotective clothing and hats

Tuga Sun Protective sunwear 800-428-TUGA www.plangea.com
UPF 50+ Children's swimwear

Wallaroo Hat Company 888-925-2766 www.wallaroohats.com
UPF 50+ hats

VAGINAL ANTI-*CANDIDA* AGENTS

Topical Therapy for Acute *Candida* Vaginitis

Drug	Formulation	Dosage
Butoconazole	Cream	5 gm at bedtime for 3 days
Clotrimazole	Cream, 1%	5 gm at bedtime for 7 to 14 days
	Cream, 10%	5 gm single application
	Vaginal tablet, 100 mg	1 tablet at bedtime for 7 days or 2 tablets at bedtime for 7 days
	Vaginal tablet, 500 mg	1 tablet once
Miconazole	Cream, 2%	5 gm at bedtime for 7 days
	Vaginal suppository, 100 mg	1 suppository at bedtime for 7 days
	Vaginal suppository, 200 mg	1 suppository at bedtime for 3 days
	Vaginal suppository, 1200 mg	1 suppository once
Econazole	Vaginal tablet, 150 mg	1 tablet at bedtime for 3 days
Fenticonazole	Cream, 2%	5 gm at bedtime for 7 days
Tioconazole	Cream, 2% Cream, 6.5%	5 gm at bedtime for 3 days 5 gm at bedtime in a single dose
Terconazole	Cream, 0.4% Cream, 0.8% Vaginal suppository	5 gm at bedtime for 7 days 5 gm at bedtime for 3 days 80 mg at bedtime for 3 days
Nystatin	Vaginal tablet, 100,000 U	1 tablet at bedtime for 14 days

Preparation for Restoration and Maintenance of Vaginal Acidity

Aci-Jel therapeutic vaginal jelly, 0.921% acetic acid, 85 gm tube, 1 full applicator morning and evening

WART MEDICATIONS

Cantharidin

Brand name	Contents	Packaging
Cantharone	0.7% cantharidin	7.5 ml
Cantharone Plus	30% sal acid, 5% podophyllin, 1% cantharidin	7.5 ml

Order these products from KRONOS Pharmacy, 800-723-7455; Dormer Laboratories Inc., www.dormer.com, 416-242-6167; Pharmascience Inc., www.pharmascience.com

Silver Nitrate

Product	Silver nitrate	Packaging
Silver nitrate	10%	30 ml solution
Silver nitrate	10%	30 gm ointment
Silver nitrate sticks		Packages of 12

Salicylic Acid Preparations for Treating Warts, Calluses, and Hyperkeratotic Skin (all otc)

Brand name	Salicylic acid (%)	Packaging
Compound W		
Liquid	17	9.3 ml liquid
Gel	17	7.5 gm gel
Duofilm	17	15 gm gel
Duofilm patch	40	18 in box
Keralyt	6	30 gm gel
Mediplast	40	Plaster
Trans-Plantar	21	Cartons of 20 mm 25 patches, securing tapes, and cleaning file
Trans-Ver-Sal	15	Cartons of 6, 12, or 20 mm (15 or 40 pads), securing tapes, and emery file
Many other brands available		

Podophyllin/Podofilox

Brand name	Podophyllin	Packaging
Condylox gel	0.5% podofilox (podophyllotoxin)	3.5 gm
Condylox solution	0.5% podofilox (podophyllotoxin)	3.5 ml
Podocon-25	25% in benzoin tincture	15 ml
Pododerm	25% in benzoin tincture	5 ml

Interferon
Intron-A (interferon alfa-2b), 10 million IU vial
Alferon N injection (interferon alfa-N3) 1 ml

Dichloracetic Acid—Keratolytic and Cauterizing	
Dichloroacetic acid	1 oz, 2 oz
Order from Delasco 800-831-6273, www.delasco.com	

WET DRESSINGS

Generic/brand name	Active ingredient
Acetic acid	Vinegar is 5% acetic acid
AluWets crystals	Aluminum chloride hexahydrate
Buro-Sol powder	Aluminum acetate
Burrow's solution (Domeboro, Bluboro, Pedi-Boro, Buro-Sol)	Aluminum acetate
Domeboro otic solution	2% acetic acid (60 ml)
Domeboro powder, Bluboro, Pedi-Boro	Aluminum sulfate, calcium acetate (boxes of 12, 100 packets)
Domeboro tablets, Bluboro, Pedi-Boro	Aluminum sulfate, calcium acetate (boxes of 2, 100 tablets)
Potassium permanganate	0.025%-0.1%, stains skin purple
Silver nitrate	0.1%-0.5%, stains skin black (prepared by pharmacist)

PHARMACISTS THAT WILL COMPOUND MEDICATIONS

Custom Scripts
800-226-7094
www.custom-rx.com

Index

Page references followed by *t* or *b* indicate tables or boxes, respectively. References in *italics* indicate illustrations and figures.

Regional Differential Diagnoses

Anus
Candidiasis 445
Condyloma lata (secondary syphilis) 318
Extramammary Paget's disease 764
Gonorrhea 332
Herpes simplex/zoster 381
Hidradenitis suppurativa 202
Lichen sclerosis et atrophicus 257
Lichen simplex chronicus 54
Psoriasis (gluteal pinking) 211
Streptococcal cellulitis 277
Syphilis (primary—chancre) 317
Vitiligo 684
Warts 364

Areolae (breast)
Eczema 45
Fox-Fordyce spots 169
Paget's disease 763
Seborrheic keratosis 702

Arms and forearms
Acne 192
Atopic dermatitis 111
Cat-scratch disease 528
Dermatitis herpetiformis (elbows) 554
Dermatomyositis 607
Eruptive xanthoma 904
Erythema multiforme 626
Granuloma annulare 898
Herpes zoster 394
Insect bite 533
Keratoacanthoma 711
Keratosis pilaris 116
Leukocytoclastic vasculitis 642
Lichen planus 250
Lupus erythematosus 600
Neurotic excoriations 68
Nummular eczema 54
Pigmentary demarcation lines
Pityriasis alba (white spots) 118
Polymorphic light eruption 671

Prurigo nodularis 68
Purpura (in sun-damaged skin) 662
Scabies 497
Scleroderma 613
Seborrheic keratosis (flat) 664
Sporotrichoid spread
Squamous cell carcinoma 744
Stellate pseudo scars 665
Sweet's syndrome 650
Swimming pool granuloma (mycobacteria) 304
Tinea 420

Axillae
Acanthosis nigricans 900
Acrochordons 706
Candidiasis 447
Contact dermatitis 85
Erythrasma 419
Fox-Fordyce spots 169
Freckling-Crowe's Sign (von Recklinghausen's disease) 906
Furunculosis 286
Hailey-Hailey disease 551
Hidradenitis suppurativa 202
Impetigo 267
Lice 506
Pseudoxanthoma elasticum 916
Scabies 497
Striae distensae 37
Tinea 420
Trichomycosis axillaris 862

Back
Acne 174
Amyloidosis 894
Atrophoderma
Becker's nevus 780
Cutaneous T cell lymphoma 754
Dermatographism 142
Erythema ab igne 694
Keloids—acne scars 709
Lichen spinulosis
Melanoma 790
Nevus anemicus 690
Notalgia paresthetica

Pityriasis lichenoides et varioliformis acuta (PLEVA) 261
Seborrheic keratosis 698
Striae distensae 37
Tinea versicolor 451
Transient acantholytic dermatosis (Grover's disease)

Buttocks
Cutaneous T cell lymphoma 754
Erythema ab igne 694
Furunculosis 286
Herpes simplex (females) 386
Hidradenitis suppurativa 202
Psoriasis 212
Scabies 497
Striae distensae 37
Tinea 421

Chest
Acne 174
Actinic keratosis 736
Darier's disease
Eruptive syringoma 4
Eruptive vellus hair cyst
Keloids 16
Nevus anemicus 3
Seborrheic dermatitis 242
Steatocystoma multiplex 451
Tinea versicolor 451
Transient acantholytic dermatitis (Grover's disease)

Chin
Acne 172
Atopic dermatitis 108
Basal cell carcinoma 720
Dental sinus
Epidermal cyst 717
Impetigo 267
Perioral dermatitis 30
Warts (flat) 373

Ear
Actinic keratosis 736
Atypical fibroxanthoma
Basal cell carcinoma 720

Bowen's disease 748
Cellulitis 294
Chondrodermatitis nodularis chronica helicis 716
Eczema (infected) 296
Epidermal cyst 717
Hydroa vacciniforme 674
Keloid (lobe) 709
Lupus erythematosus (discoid) 596
Lymphangitis 294
Melanoma 795
Ochronosis 3
Pseudocyst
Psoriasis 218
Ramsey-Hunt syndrome (herpes zoster) 399
Relapsing polychondritis
Seborrheic dermatitis 242
Squamous cell carcinoma 744
Tophi (gout)
Venous lake 825

Elbows and knees
Calcinosis cutis/CREST 617
Dermatitis herpetiformis 554
Erythema multiforme 491
Gout
Granuloma annulare 898
Lichen simplex chronicus 54
Psoriasis 210
Rheumatoid nodule
Scabies 497
Xanthoma 902

Face
Actinic keratosis 742
Adenoma sebaceum 4
Alopecia mucinosa 894
Angioedema 129
Atopic dermatitis 108
Basal cell carcinoma 720
Cowden's disease 912
CREST 617
Dermatosis papulosa nigra 706
Eczema 85
Erysipelas 273

Face—cont'd

Favre Racouchot (senile comedones) 194
Granuloma faciale
Herpes simplex 381
Herpes zoster 394
Impetigo 267
Keratoacanthoma 711
Lentigo maligna 794
Lupus erythematosus (discoid) 596
Lupus erythematosus (systemic) 600
Lymphocytoma cutis
Melasma 3
Molluscum contagiosum 344
Nevus sebaceous 715
Pemphigus erythematosus 559
Perioral dermatitis 30
Pilomatrixoma
Pityriasis alba (white spots) 118
Psoriasis 214
Rosacea 198
Scleroderma 613
Sebaceous hyperplasia 720
Seborrheic dermatitis 242
Seborrheic keratosis 698
Secondary syphilis 318
Spitz's nevus 781
Squamous cell carcinoma 744
Steroid rosacea 30
Sweet's syndrome 627
Sycosis barbae (folliculitis-beard) 282
Tinea 434
Trichoepitheliomas 909
Warts (flat) 373
Wegener's granulomatosis 640

Foot (dorsum and sides)

Calcaneal petechiae (black heel) 374
Contact dermatitis 85
Cutaneous larva migrans 537
Erythema multiforme 491
Granuloma annulare 898

Hand, foot, and mouth disease 462
Keratoderma blennorrhagica (Reiter's disease) 216
Lichen planus 250
Lichen simplex chronicus 54
Painful fat herniation (piezogenic papules)
Pernio
Pyogenic granuloma 826
Scabies 497
Stucco keratosis 705
Tinea 413

Foot (sole)

Arsenical keratosis 753
Corn (clavus) 374
Cutaneous larva migrans 537
Dyshidrotic eczema
Epidermolysis bullosum 576
Erythema multiforme 491
Hand, foot, and mouth disease 462
Hyperkeratosis 580
Immersion foot
Juvenile plantar dermatosis
Keratoderma
Keratoderma blennorrhagica (Reiter's disease) 216
Lichen planus 252
Melanoma 796
Nevi 774
Pitted keratolysis 416
Pityriasis rubra pilaris 240
Psoriasis (pustular) 214
Pyogenic granuloma 826
Rocky Mountain spotted fever 524
Scabies (infants) 502
Syphilis (secondary) 318
Tinea 413
Tinea (bullous) 414
Verrucous carcinoma 753
Wart

Forehead

Actinic keratosis 736
Basal cell carcinoma 720
Flat warts 373

Herpes zoster 394
Psoriasis 214
Scleroderma (en coup de sabre) 622
Sebaceous hyperplasia 720
Seborrheic dermatitis 242
Seborrheic keratosis 698
Sweet's syndrome 627

Groin

Acrochordons (skin tags) 706
Candidiasis 440
Condyloma 338
Erythrasma 419
Extramammary Paget's disease 764
Hailey-Hailey disease 551
Hidradenitis suppurativa 202
Histiocytosis X 580
Intertrigo 15
Lichen simplex chronicus 54
Molluscum contagiosum 344
Pemphigus vegetans 561
Psoriasis (without scale) 211
Seborrheic keratosis 698
Striae (topical steroids) 15
Tinea 417

Hand (dorsa)

Acquired digital fibrokeratoma 888
Acrosclerosis 617
Actinic keratosis 736
Atopic dermatitis 105
Atypical mycobacteria 304
Blue nevus 782
Calcinosis cutis/CREST 617
Cat-scratch disease 528
Contact dermatitis 85
Cowden's disease 912
Dermatomyositis 607
Erysipeloid 287
Erythema multiforme 491
Gonorrhea 330
Granuloma annulare 898
Herpes simplex/zoster 381
Impetigo 267
Keratoacanthoma 711
Lentigo 691

Lichen planus 250
Lupus erythematosus (systemic) 600
Mucous cyst (finger) 888
Orf (finger)
Paronychia (acute, chronic) 871, 872
Pityriasis rubra pilaris 240
Polymorphic light eruption 671
Porphyria cutanea tarda 675
Pseudo PCT (porphyria cutanea tarda) 675
Psoriasis 215
Pyogenic granuloma 826
Scabies 497
Scleroderma 613
Seborrheic keratosis 664
Sporotrichosis 8
Squamous cell carcinoma 745
Stucco keratosis 705
Sweet's syndrome 651
Swimming pool granuloma 744
Tinea 425
Tularemia (ulcer)
Vesicular "id reaction" 59
Xanthoma 902

Hands (palms)

Basal-cell nevus syndrome (pits) 731
Calluses/corns 374
Contact dermatitis 85
Cowden's disease 912
Dyshidrotic eczema 58
Eczema 50
Erythema multiforme 491
Hand, foot, and mouth disease 462
Keratoderma 894
Keratolysis exfoliativa 55
Lichen planus (vesicles) 250
Lupus erythematosus 592
Melanoma
Pityriasis rubra pilaris 240
Pompholyx 59
Psoriasis 214
Pyogenic granuloma 826
Rocky Mountain spotted fever 524

Continued

Scabies (infants) 502
Syphilis (secondary) 318
Tinea 425
Vesicular "id reaction" 59
Wart 371

Inframammary
Acrochordon (skin tags)
  707
Candidiasis 440
Contact dermatitis 85
Intertrigo 418
Psoriasis (without scale)
Seborrheic keratoses 702
Tinea versicolor 451

Leg
Basal cell carcinoma 728
Bites 533
Bowen's disease 748
Dermatofibroma 708
Disseminated superficial ac-
  tinic porokeratosis
Ecthyma 272
Ecthyma gangrenosum 298
Eruptive xanthomas 904
Kaposi's sarcoma 827
Livedo reticularis
Lupus panniculus
Majocchi's granuloma
  (tinea) 422
Melanoma 791
Nummular eczema 54
Panniculitis 75
Pityriasis lichenoides et
  varioliformis acuta
  (PLEVA) 261
Porokeratosis of Mibelli
Prurigo nodularis 68
Pyoderma gangrenosum 653
Squamous cell carcinoma
  744
Urticarial vasculitis 154
Vasculitis (nodular lesions)
  637
Wegener's granulomatosis
  640
Churg-Strauss syndrome
  640
Polyarteritis nodosa 640
Weber-Christian disease

Legs—lower
Bites 533
Cellulitis 273
Dermatofibroma 708
Diabetic bullae 559
Diabetic dermopathy (shin
  spots) 694
Erysipelas 273
Erythema induratum
Erythema nodosum 635
Flat warts 373
Folliculitis 279
Granuloma annulare 898
Henoch-Schönlein purpura
  640
Ichthyosis vulgaris 115
Idiopathic guttate hypome-
  lanosis 689
Leukocytoclastic vasculitis
  642
Lichen planus 250
Lichen simplex chronicus
  54
Majocchi's granuloma
  (tinea) 422
Myxedema (pretibial)
Necrobiosis lipoidica 14
Purpura 17
Schamberg's purpura 656
Stasis dermatitis 72
Subcutaneous fat necrosis
  (associated with
  pancreatitis)
Sweet's syndrome 652
Vasculitis (nodular lesions)
  637
Weber-Christian disease
Xerosis 60

Lips
Actinic cheilitis 738
Allergic contact dermatitis
  84
Angioedema 129
Aphthous ulcer
Fordyce spots (upper lips)
  169
Herpes simplex 381
Labial melanotic macule 782
Leukoplakia 751
Mucous cyst
Perlèche 450
Pyogenic granuloma 826

Squamous cell carcinoma
  744
Venous lake 825
Wart

Neck (side and front)
Acanthosis nigricans 900
Acne 171
Acrochordon (skin tags)
  706
Atopic dermatitis 112
Berloque dermatitis 683
Contact dermatitis 85
Dental sinus
Elastosis perforans
  serpiginosa
Epidermal cyst 717
Folliculitis 279
Impetigo 267
Pityriasis rosea 246
Poikiloderma of Civatte
  663
Pseudofolliculitis 280
Pseudoxanthoma elasticum
  916
Sycosis barbae (fungal,
  bacterial) 282
Tinea 421
Wart 372

Neck (back)
Acne 171
Acne keloidalis 283
Actinic keratosis 736
Cutis rhomboidalis nuchae
  664
Epidermal cyst 717
Folliculitis 279
Furunculosis
Herpes zoster 394
Lichen simplex chronicus
  54
Neurotic excoriations 68
Salmon patch 823
Tinea 421

Nose
Acne 171
Actinic keratosis 736
Adenoma sebaceum 910
Basal cell carcinoma 720
Discoid lupus
  erythematosus 861

Fissure (nostril) 15
Granulosa rubra nasi
Herpes simplex 381
Herpes zoster 394
Impetigo 267
Lupus erythematosus 600
Nasal crease
Nevus 775
Rhinophyma 200
Rosacea 198
Seborrheic dermatitis 242
Squamous cell carcinoma
  744
Telangiectasias 199
Trichofolliculoma
Wegener's granulomatosis
  640

Penis
Aphthae (Behcet's
  syndrome) 14
Balanitis circinata (Reiter's
  syndrome) 216
Bite (human) 529
Bowenoid papulosis 343
Candidiasis (under fore-
  skin) 445
Chancroid 327
Condyloma (warts) 337
Contact dermatitis
  (condoms) 85
Erythroplasia of Queyrat
  (Bowen's disease) 750
Factitious
Fixed drug eruption 492
Giant condyloma
  (Buschke-Lowenstein)
  749
Granuloma inguinale 329
Herpes simplex/zoster 381
Lichen nitidus 4
Lichen planus 255
Lichen sclerosis et atrophi-
  cus (balanitis xerotica
  obliterans) 258
Lymphogranuloma
  venereum 325
Molluscum contagiosum
  344
Nevus
Pearly penile papules 339
Pediculosis (lice) 506
Penile melanosis